Oxford Textbook of
Palliative Medicine

Oxford Textbook of
Palliative
Medicine

FOURTH EDITION

Edited by

Geoffrey Hanks

Nathan I. Cherny

Nicholas A. Christakis

Marie Fallon

Stein Kaasa

Russell K. Portenoy

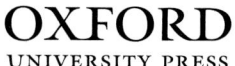

OXFORD

UNIVERSITY PRESS

OXFORD

UNIVERSITY PRESS

Great Clarendon Street, Oxford OX2 6DP

Oxford University Press is a department of the University of Oxford.
It furthers the University's objective of excellence in research, scholarship,
and education by publishing worldwide in

Oxford New York

Auckland Cape Town Dar es Salaam Hong Kong Karachi
Kuala Lumpur Madrid Melbourne Mexico City Nairobi
New Delhi Shanghai Taipei Toronto

With offices in

Argentina Austria Brazil Chile Czech Republic France Greece
Guatemala Hungary Italy Japan Poland Portugal Singapore
South Korea Switzerland Thailand Turkey Ukraine Vietnam

Oxford is a registered trade mark of Oxford University Press
in the UK and in certain other countries

Published in the United States
by Oxford University Press Inc., New York

First edition published 1993
First published in paperback 1995
Second edition published 1998
Reprinted 1998
Second edition published in paperback 1999
Reprinted 2001, 2003
Third edition published 2004
Fourth edition published 2010

British Library Cataloguing in Publication Data is available

Library of Congress Cataloging in Publication Data is available

Typeset in Minion
by Cepha Imaging Private Ltd., Bangalore, India
Printed in Italy
on acid-free paper by Rotolito Lombarda SpA

ISBN 978-0-19-857029-5

10 9 8 7 6 5 4 3 2 1

Summary of contents

Contents

Section 10 The management of common symptoms and disorders

Preface to the fourth edition

This fourth edition of the *Oxford Textbook of Palliative Medicine* is the first without Derek Doyle as one of the editors. Derek has been the driving force behind this book from the beginning and an inspiration to the now hundreds of contributors and editors who have been involved and who have made the book so successful. Derek has always been first to meet the deadlines, indefatigable in dealing with problems, always ready to take on extra work and fill the gaps, a prodigious writer and editor, and a real pioneer of palliative medicine around the world. We have missed his involvement with this new edition and hope that we have maintained the standard.

Kenneth Calman also steps down as an editor this time. The original idea for the textbook was Ken's and he recruited Derek Doyle and Geoffrey Hanks some 20 years ago to start work on the project. Ken had to withdraw shortly afterwards when he became Chief Medical Officer in Scotland, the first of a succession of appointments to some of the most senior positions in health care and academia in the UK. Sir Kenneth was able to join us in editing the third edition of the textbook but has retired as an editor and is now Chancellor of Glasgow University.

Four new editors have joined Geoffrey Hanks and Nathan Cherny in this new edition. The editors are eminent physicians who are widely recognized as leading authorities in what continues to be a rapidly expanding field. In recent years, there has been major progress in the United States, with recognition of palliative medicine as a subspeciality and the development of formal mechanisms for board certification. This is an important step forward for palliative medicine and will have an impact much further afield. With the participation of Russell K. Portenoy and Nicholas A. Christakis as editors of this volume, there is greater balance between European and North American authors.

Also joining the editorial team is Marie Fallon from Edinburgh and Stein Kaasa from Trondheim in Norway. They further broaden the geographical representation of this edition, and like the other editors, bring the perspective of established researchers in different fields relevant to palliative care. Editors with a practical appreciation of research imperatives are particularly important now, with strides being made in palliative medicine research, particularly in recent years with regard to funding, research capacity, and the creation of infrastructure to support research through new academic departments of palliative medicine.

From the outset, the *Oxford Textbook of Palliative Medicine* was designed to present practical clinical advice backed up by the most up-to-date scientific data. The emerging discipline of palliative medicine is a cross cutting-speciality, which overlaps many areas of medicine and depends on a multi-disciplinary approach to ensure the optimal care of patients with serious or life-threatening illnesses. What has become evident in the progress from one edition of the textbook to the next is that the evidence base for palliative care is growing, and the need to provide practice guidance in the translation of research into clinical care must be a primary goal of enterprises such as this book.

This edition of the *Oxford Textbook of Palliative Medicine* includes new authors for many chapters and many completely new chapters. There are some changes to the structure of the book, which are outlined in the *Introduction*. As in previous editions, the overarching aim has been to maintain both a high standard of excellence for all the content and a freshness of approach and emphasis reflective of the evolving discipline. To all of our authors, both those who have contributed to the current edition and those who have stood down, we record our most grateful thanks. We appreciate the contribution of your knowledge and experience to this textbook.

As always we thank our publishers and in particular Georgia Pinteau and her colleagues for their continuing support and enthusiasm for this textbook. Our particular thanks also to our secretaries who have made an enormous and vital contribution to the textbook: to Debbie Ashby in Bristol, Harriet Harris in Edinburgh, Nancy Smith in Boston, Gunn-Heidi Tobekk in Trondheim, Marilyn Herleth in New York, and Rama Sapir in Jerusalem.

And finally, we dedicate this textbook to the colleagues with whom we work, those who have taught and inspired us, and most of all to those we serve, our patients and their families.

Geoffrey Hanks
Nathan I. Cherny
Nicholas A. Christakis
Marie Fallon
Stein Kaasa
Russell K. Portenoy
April 2009

Preface to the third edition

We continue to be delighted with the success of this textbook and grateful for the many comments and suggestions sent to us by colleagues round the world. In the few years since the last edition was published many new palliative care services have been established, Palliative Medicine has been recognized as a specialty in more countries, and everywhere this textbook has come to be recognized as the definitive text on a fast-developing subject.

Our editorial team has changed. Our sense of loss when Neil MacDonald had to retire from the team was, to some extent, eased when he agreed to write several chapters and when we found not one, but two distinguished colleagues to replace him. Neither needs much introduction. Nathan Cherny, an Australian–trained physician works in Jerusalem, but is equally well known and respected in the United States where he pursued his studies in Memorial Sloan Kettering Cancer Center in New York. Sir Kenneth Calman, now Vice Chancellor of Durham University, England was previously the first professor of oncology in the University of Glasgow and instrumental in establishing palliative care services in that city before becoming, in turn, the Chief Medical Officer, Scotland and Chief Medical Officer, England.

We introduced many changes and innovations into the second edition and in this, the third edition, we have made even more changes—many of them suggested by readers. In many respects this is a new book; so comprehensive are the changes. There are new chapters devoted to palliative medicine in the context of care of the elderly and intensive care. A chapter is devoted to complementary and alternative medicine in relation to patients receiving palliative care, and a whole section to the contributions to palliative medicine of allied health professionals as they are now termed.

Increasingly it is being recognized that the principles of palliative medicine are applicable in the care of people with non-malignant conditions.

Reflecting that we have introduced chapters on non-malignant respiratory disease, non-malignant neurological disease, cardiac disease, dietary and nutritional problems, while many other sections from previous editions have been totally rewritten, often by new authors whom we have been delighted to welcome to this work.

So important do we regard education and training in our subject that this section has also been rewritten and the opportunity taken to introduce new ideas and new technologies such as internet learning and video conferencing. Readers will not be surprised to see lists of recommended websites, and references to websites.

We feel privileged to have worked with contributors from so many countries including Australia, Canada, China, Germany, India, Israel, Italy, Norway, Sweden, and the United States. All exceedingly busy, they have willingly written for our textbook and shared their wealth of knowledge and clinical experience. Our especial thanks, however, must go to our secretaries, Debbie Ashby in Bristol and Judith Sunter in Durham, to our professional colleagues, to Catherine Barnes and all at Oxford University Press, and to Mukesh of Newgen Imaging.

As with previous editions we dedicate this textbook to suffering patients around the world and to our colleagues who care for them.

Derek Doyle
Geoffrey Hanks
Nathan I. Cherny
Kenneth Calman
September 2003

Preface to the second edition

When the first edition of this textbook was published in 1993 we were honoured to receive many appreciative reviews: several of them raised points to consider in a second edition and offered most constructive suggestions. We have been able to add comments from colleagues all over the world, to all of whom we express our appreciation. Our publishers have persuaded us to produce a new edition into which we can incorporate the many points raised.

Several people commented that the textbook appeared to be exclusively for doctors, yet palliative care, as is so frequently stated in the text, is team caring, interprofessional in fact rather than multiprofessional. We make no apology for it being a *medical textbook* for that is exactly what we intended and explained in the Preface to the first edition. We continue to see a need for a medical reference book whilst fully respecting and appreciating the roles of colleagues in other professions. In the same way we feel the title is right in referring to *palliative medicine* rather than palliative care or hospice care but readers will notice that throughout the text, wherever team collaboration is mentioned, the word used is *care* rather than *medicine*, and the much-loved word *hospice* is used when that is the title of a particular unit or service.

Another important comment was that the first edition appeared to focus on malignant disease although the principles of palliative medicine are said to apply to all diseases. In particular, some colleagues asked why a section had not been devoted exclusively to palliation in the geriatric population. The first comment has been addressed in this new edition by requesting all our contributors to demonstrate the relevance of palliative medicine across the clinical spectrum, where necessary highlighting special areas and issues for attention. We sought the opinion of specialist geriatricians and in the light of their comments have decided not to devote a special chapter to their patients.

What we *have* done is to introduce completely new chapters and make the book bigger and even more comprehensive. The increasingly important contribution of interventional radiology has been recognized with a full chapter, as have the subjects of audit and the economics of palliative medicine, and AIDS in children. A new chapter is devoted to pruritus and sweating, another to pain assessment, and yet another to pharmacological aspects of palliative medicine.

The section on cultural issues was appreciated by many readers and in this new edition it has been expanded with the additions of chapters on the cultures of sub-Saharan Africa, China and Japan, and Australian indigenous peoples, reflecting the worldwide spread and appropriateness of palliative medicine. A new team of authors has written the ethics section and, in recognition of the ethical issues in caring for children, a new chapter has been introduced on ethical issues in paediatric palliative medicine. Even when chapter titles have not been changed readers will find that many alterations have been made in the text, much new material added, and many new references cited, reflecting the considerable advances in this specialty in a very few years.

We pay tribute to those contributors to the first edition who so graciously agreed to stand down and hand over the baton to other authorities, and welcome our many new colleagues. To them all we express very sincere thanks for all the time, work, and endless patience they have so generously shared with us.

We have enjoyed working with our friends in Oxford University Press and make no apology for singling out Dr Irene Butcher whose skills, patience, and wisdom seem to us to be limitless. Finally, but with great sincerity, we acknowledge our immeasureable debt to our assistants, secretaries, and colleagues who in diverse ways made this new edition possible.

Derek Doyle
Geoffrey W.C. Hanks
Neil MacDonald
October 1997

Preface to the first edition

We offer this new textbook as our contribution to modern palliative medicine. Our readers deserve some explanation about its contents and our fellow contributors our *unqualified* appreciation and respect.

Until quite recently terminal care, as it used to be called, consisted of little more than 'tender loving care' married to pain and symptom control using basic drugs skilfully prescribed. Some argued that there was little else to it and certainly not sufficient to merit a major textbook. We felt differently as, clearly, do many others who have made the subject their life's work. We were conscious of how much can be done, how much there is to learn, and how little we ourselves knew. Equally we were aware of how much our colleagues in related disciplines and specialties could share with us, how much valuable research had been done and how much remains to be done. Hence this textbook. Our aim has been to produce as comprehensive a book as possible, with a body of knowledge based on sound research as well as extensive clinical experience. To some extent we believe we have succeeded. Readers will note differing opinions, each firmly held by those with that level of experience and authority. We have made no attempt to reconcile all such differences for they are important. They demonstrate where dogmatism may be inappropriate and where further studies are still needed. Having said that, we have been impressed with the unanimity demonstrated in most areas and the professional open-mindedness and humility displayed by our contributors.

On many more occasions than might have been expected, we have been reminded what a strong scientific base palliative medicine is built on. Little of what has been written is merely anecdotal, valuable as that can be. Much has been studied and researched, forming the basis of this textbook.

Inevitably some will criticize the book as too much related to, and reflecting, 'Westernized' medical practice without due attention to the needs of the 'palliative care Third World'. Throughout, we have never ignored the needs of those having to work with limited resources but have tried to demonstrate not only what can be done in the medically-sophisticated world but also by colleagues less fortunate than ourselves. Treatment regimens include basic principles as well as sophisticated techniques, always emphasizing the totality of care, and the roles and needs not only of other professionals but also the relatives. We are deeply conscious that, while for a few, palliative medicine is the final stage of years of sophisticated therapeutic management, for millions of others all they can ever hope for is that its benefits will eventually become available to them and their families.

Clearly it would be impossible to detail each drug, each with as many different proprietary names, for every country where this book may be read. Rather we have chosen to use generic names.

Palliative medicine impinges on and frequently overlaps with many other medical specialties. Gone are the days when a patient receiving palliative care never again had further investigations or benefited from the advice of surgeons and oncologists. We have tried to demonstrate the contributions of other specialists by inviting them to share their knowledge and their contributions with us and have been honoured by their unstinting willingness to do so. Technical details of their work would have been out of place in such a textbook but readers will appreciate how they too can contribute to the complex kaleidoscope which confronts us and challenges us in palliative medicine.

In the same way in which we have encouraged these coauthors to share their wisdom in their own way, so too have we not attempted to impose a consistency of style on their writing but left them to express their thoughts and share their deeply-held feelings in their own inimitable way. We believe that this has enriched the book.

To our contributors we offer our profound thanks and respect. Few have worked alone; most have been assisted by many others, perhaps unnamed in this book, and by clinician colleagues who have acted for them when their writing took up days and weeks of precious time. To them all, named and unnamed, we extend our appreciation. They have all borne with our demands and our criticisms with unfailing patience making us appreciate what sensitive, understanding clinicians they must be.

Traditionally all authors and editors close with a grateful tribute to their publishers. In our case we would go further. We could never have dared to expect such patience with our shortcomings, such guidance when we so often called for it, and such genuine interest in, and enthusiasm for, our subject and this book. We are deeply grateful. We feel particularly privileged to have worked with Dr Irene Butcher who was an unfailing source of encouragement, support, and advice. No editors could have been better served.

Our secretaries deserve a special mention. Irene Turnbull (Edinburgh), Felicity Fleetwood (London), and Sheila Parr and Patricia McDonald (Edmonton) have given unstintingly of their skills, time, and loyalty, and to each we offer our unqualified thanks.

We dedicate this textbook to the colleagues with whom we work, those who have taught and inspired us and, most of all, to those we serve, our patients and their families.

Derek Doyle
Geoffrey W.C. Hanks
Neil MacDonald

Foreword

When the first edition of *the Oxford Textbook of Palliative Medicine* was published in 1993, St. Christopher's Hospice in London had recently celebrated its first quarter century, palliative medicine had been recognized as a sub-specialty of internal medicine 5 years before in the United Kingdom, and palliative care, as it was more usually called when speaking of team-caring, was still in its infancy in most other countries. It was appropriate and helpful to readers for Dame Cicely Saunders to focus on the history of the 'Hospice Movement' as she did in its Foreword. The launch of this new edition, the fourth in only 16 years, says much about the remarkable growth of palliative medicine, its acceptance, and its standing worldwide. It challenges us to take a critical look at what is happening in our burgeoning subject and ask where palliative medicine is going in our rapidly changing world. There are some important questions.

Is the knowledge base of palliative medicine growing?

One of the many questions put to those negotiating for specialty status for palliative medicine in the United Kingdom in 1987 was, 'Is there a sufficient knowledge base to justify such status and, if so, do you expect it to grow?' Subsequent history and each edition of this textbook are proof that the positive and very enthusiastic response they gave was fully justified. Much of this is due to the steadily increasing research being done within palliative medicine itself. Some is because palliative medicine is at last being recognized as relevant in non-malignant conditions. Much is because of the newfound interest in palliative medicine and its scientific basis on the part of colleagues in other related disciplines. Today, most of palliative medicine is based on sound research but we must all recognize the importance of those core aspects of it which, up to now, have not lent themselves to existing research models. That fact does not make them any less valid or important. In subsequent editions of this book, scientific evaluation of them may be a feature. Whilst in no way detracting from the exciting accumulation of knowledge referred to, it has to be noted (as will be mentioned later in this Foreword) that some of the advances involve sophisticated diagnostic technology and therapeutics, the understandable absence of which in resource-limited countries must not deter doctors there from practising palliative medicine.

Do people today understand what palliative medicine is?

This question may surprise some readers, but as recently as the launch of the first edition of this book, there was much confusion.

Even today, the answer is not a simple one. The fact that palliative medicine is increasingly being adopted worldwide does not mean it is understood. Ask some nurses, some members of professions allied to medicine, health-care planners, the public, local and national politicians and, most crucially, our patients, and widespread confusion will be evident. Much of the blame for that lies with palliative medicine/care workers themselves. Feeling that all existing definitions are inadequate we have kept devising new ones—usually longer, more wordy, more complex, and convoluted—leading not to clarity but to confusion. We have chosen to discard some of the original names for what we do—terminal care, care of the dying, continuing care—in favour of something regarded as more euphemistic by speaking of continuing care, palliative care, or supportive care, wrongly assuming that they are easier to understand and to describe to all who need to know. We have emphasized that palliative care embodies the essential features of all good care—whatever the pathology, the stage of the illness, the place of care, or the prognosis, whatever the age, gender, race, social status, or religious faith of the patient. Having implied that the principles of palliative care might, indeed should, have been employed from the time of diagnosis and be the hallmark of all good care from then on, we have now reverted to calling it 'end-of-life care'. In so doing, we are telling all who are interested what they had long suspected—palliative care is care for those at the end of life and embraces terminal and supportive care. It is the 'principles', which have universal relevance.

Perhaps there would have been less confusion if the principles had been listed or explained. They include the centrality of the patient and family, the need for attention to detail, the necessity for excellent communications, the consummate skill of listening without speaking, the relief of suffering whatever its cause, heightened sensitivity to unspoken fears and unmentioned suffering and last, but not least, empathy (but not sympathy) in abundance. Surely no one would deny that these are the cardinal features of all good care!

Does any of this matter? Yes it does. Because its 'principles are those of all good care' many professional colleagues in other branches of medicine regard themselves as already providing it (which is probably true) and see little reason formally to introduce these principles into their care regimens at earlier stages, or to develop their knowledge and skill bases through further training.

The result is unrelieved unnecessary suffering of patients and families, greater demands on specialist palliative care services when predictable crises develop, and missed opportunities to inculcate the principles of palliative medicine in all our young successors. Those working in specialist palliative medicine cannot rest until every patient has access to their expertise and every doctor has had formal instruction (and examination) in its principles.

Because these principles are appropriate, indeed are essential, in the management of all chronic, life-threatening, or at any rate life-shortening, conditions, some have chosen to regard it as synonymous with care of the elderly, care of the chronic sick, care of the many neurological patients for whom there is no cure, and an alternative to advice from pain specialists. If we are honest, much as we can often offer such patients, we do not have the expertise or the resources to become 'all things to all men' nor should we try to.

Clarification of what we do might hopefully stop people equating palliative care with euthanasia or physician-assisted suicide (PAS) and might improve care in general and specialist hospitals and care homes where most patients end their days, rather than at home where they would prefer to be. This textbook is a salutary reminder that none of us can rest until the skilled recognition, measurement, and relief of suffering in all its forms becomes the norm in every care programme in hospital or home. We are a long way from that!

Is palliative medicine research-based?

Reference has already been made to the historic negotiations leading to specialty status for palliative medicine. Another important question asked of the negotiators was whether or not palliative medicine was researched-based and how important its practitioners regarded research. Those who asked such questions had good reasons for doing so. With the notable exception of pain management, almost all other therapeutic regimens in use were based on considerable clinical experience but not robust studies. Indeed much that was recommended in the first edition of this book was anecdotal. The questioners may also have heard of reluctance on the part of many palliative medicine physicians to engage in research for fear of adding to patient distress, invading privacy, being accused of experimentation and, being very honest, not having the necessary training and experience in research methodology. It has also to be remembered that many of the pioneer palliative care units in the United Kingdom as in other countries were operated by the voluntary sector. Their generous donors feared that engaging in research would reduce patient-dignity, make patients feel like numbers rather than people, and raise fears that they were used as 'guinea pigs' and might lessen charitable giving on which they depended.

Even since the first edition of this book, the scene has changed dramatically. Most of what is recommended in the pages that follow has been scientifically evaluated. The reference lists are longer than ever. Worthwhile research is being carried out in every academic palliative medicine service and all major clinical units. Leading scientists are setting the pace, training young recruits (though there are certainly not enough of them) eager to engage in research. Two of the highlights of recent years have been the establishment of regional, national, and international research bodies bringing together research workers to enable better collaboration (though still grossly under-funded) and the development of excellent scientific journals in this field, each of the editors of this book

having contributed to this progress. There is no longer any reason for sceptics to regard palliative medicine as 'soft'.

Palliative care (for once again we are speaking of the coordinated work of many team members) is right to be proud and grateful for the vast sums of money donated for patient care, all being put to excellent use as the public clearly recognizes. Palliative medicine research and education, on the other hand, do not have, and probably never will have, the high profile and appeal of research and professional training which characterize cancer, chest and heart disease, strokes, and chronic neurological conditions. Philanthropists will never become famous by funding palliative medicine research. Centuries may pass before a Nobel Prize is won by one of our discipline.

Are we teaching and training appropriately? One of the toughest challenges facing palliative medicine is bringing the needs of research and professional training to the attention of major funding bodies. Perhaps this calls for an international initiative, for the problem is certainly an international one, bigger than any of the existing national or international groups or bodies speaking for palliative medicine.

We have good reason to be delighted, if a little surprised, that so many excellent young physicians are now opting for careers in palliative medicine, particularly in the increasing number of countries where it has specialty status. As governments respond to consumer demands for more specialist palliative care services, the need for more such young specialists will continue to grow. We must resist the temptation to lower requirements and reduce training times to meet such demands. At the same time, we must recognize that the luxury of continuity of care by one physician may have gone for ever as more and more new recruits to our specialty are women working part-time.

More importantly, we must recognize that few patients need specialist palliative medicine, which should be available primarily for those with complex problems, rare conditions, or for those needing the input of many members of the specialist interdisciplinary palliative care team. The vast majority of people (some have suggested 90 per cent) can be, should be, cared for by their general practitioner (GP)/family physician in their own homes, but herein lies the problem. They need to be trained, and there is evidence that few get such comprehensive training beyond the relief of pain. Increasingly, their palliative medicine tutors have themselves had little experience in community care/general practice. All too easily, palliative medicine comes to be seen by GPs and consultants as an exercise in clinical pharmacology, the juggling of opioids, when what most GPs say they want is more guidance on aspects of nursing care, psychosocial, and spiritual care, but not if they are too time-consuming for today's general practice. This issue of how much time must be spent with terminally ill patients is important and one that palliative medicine workers seldom address. It is a myth that more time must be spent with them than with most others because they want to unburden their hearts and delve deep into existentialism. That myth discourages some from offering real palliative care and creates around us— palliative medicine specialists—an aura of mystery we do not deserve.

Some will retort that expecting the modern GP to offer better, more comprehensive palliative care is wishful thinking. Excellent as their care may be during office hours, they may not be on call in the evenings and at weekends; they may no longer do house calls; they may feel they know all they need to about the pharmaco-therapeutics of palliative medicine and need only the additional, skilled input of community nurses for their dying patients. Only the voice of patients and relatives—the consumers—will change this situation and the inspired charismatic teaching of palliative medicine specialists and GP tutors who hopefully have had appropriate training in education methodology.

One of the great advances in the 16 years' lifetime of this book has been the development of hospital palliative care services, reducing the need for transfers to free-standing hospices by making palliative care available in every specialist unit of secondary and tertiary hospitals. They continue to remind us that palliative medicine was never established exclusively for cancer patients or those with motor neuron disease. Some have even suggested that such services deskill other staff. It certainly remains to be demonstrated that they develop palliative medicine skills throughout the hospital and from there into the community. Proof of what they can achieve, and what they cannot do, is urgently needed, if we are to improve both care provision and professional training.

In short, there is a heavy burden of responsibility on already over-worked palliative medicine doctors to focus the training and teaching they give to others where it will have maximum impact. The notion that the principal, the most important, providers of such care are those working in specialist units must be dispelled. If the highest quality palliative medicine is to be made available to the 90 per cent of patients under the care of their family doctors, in their homes or care homes, and the most appropriate use be made of specialist services, then we cannot rest until in-depth courses on community palliative medicine are available for every doctor working in the community.

Is palliative medicine adapting to our fast-changing society or being changed by it?

Change is not always synonymous with progress or improvement. Few would say our society is changing faster than it has done for a very long time. This Foreword is being written near the end of 2008 with the world financial markets in turmoil, an international credit crisis, millions worldwide facing unemployment or loss of homes and/or pensions, companies and institutions previously synonymous with stability and probity now facing liquidation, and many now joining in the blame-game. Charities, great and small, report reduced donations and fewer people volunteering their time and skills. What few would deny is that there has been much evidence of greed and its consequences. For many people, the new god had become money and the driving force of life, the accumulation of wealth and possessions. Deny is as most politicians will predictably do, the state is regarded as more important than the individual, the accumulation of wealth and its trappings more relevant goals than the dignity of the individual. What most strikes the worried, bemused onlooker is how small the world now seems. Within hours of bad news in one country, another on the other side of the world feels the financial or economic tsunami.

We are a small planet with more in common than we choose to admit. One day we can be feeling safe, the next, fragile, and not a little frightened. Wherever we are, whatever our race, our culture, our beliefs, our colour, our health-care system, our fundamental needs are the same. What should excite us in palliative medicine is the realization that what the world, and each individual in it, needs are the tenets we hold dear in palliative medicine, those cornerstones on which we are built—human kindness and empathy, respect for dignity, and humankind's profound need to feel wanted,

valued, and trusted, all married to appreciative, non-judgemental mutual respect. These features seem in short supply in societies more familiar with today's cynicism, scepticism, mutual suspicion, self-preservation, and strident religious and political fundamentalism.

However, a small world has a positive side. It makes it easier for the best features of palliative medicine and its clinical advances to spread more quickly and to be adopted. Many of us have been defensive when palliative medicine has been described as yet another feature of the privileged medicine of the affluent West—sometimes described as the cherry on the cream on the top of an already rich cake! The taunt has some justification however! Do we in the advantaged West always remember those providing palliative medicine in less-privileged countries when we publish our papers, produce new guidelines, or promote new technology? Are we interested in the lone doctor serving a scattered population of thousands far from any teaching hospital or specialist palliative medicine service or the colleague working in a country with a dose ceiling on opioids (if they are even available) and the persistent fear of opiophobia? How often do we remind ourselves that for more than three-quarters of the world population, cure, or even worthwhile life-prolongation, is unrealistic and unattainable? Worldwide, the most valuable skills that any doctor can possess are those of palliative medicine (though the term may be unknown to them).

Even in the few years since the first edition, the world of medicine, including palliative medicine, has become more complicated, more sophisticated, largely evident in its use of diagnostic technology. If there are funds to pay for it, and staff to operate and interpret it, well and good. What is not right is implying that such sophistication is essential for good palliative care when we all know that in vast areas of the world no such sophistication is possible. If appropriate analgesia was ever to be withheld because there was no scanner, it would be as unforgivable as what happened when some of us were junior doctors—no analgesia was given, no pain was relieved until a diagnosis had been made. Sophistication is a luxury, not a pre-requisite for good palliative medicine wherever the patient is being cared for. It is time for us to re-examine our therapeutic regimens and ask if they have become over-complicated, perhaps reflecting our 'persona' rather than therapeutic necessity.

Changes in hospitals and in doctoring

Two critically important features of our times are the changed, and still changing, role of hospitals and, secondly, the changed perception of what doctors aim for. Once places where patients might receive good nursing care for weeks, or longer if they needed it, today, hospitals are diagnostic or day-surgery centres, their efficiency measured in the shortest length of stay achieved or the highest 'through-put' figures. Questions are asked when beds are 'blocked' by the chronic sick or, worse still, by the dying. Better to send such patients home under the care of GPs/family physicians whether or not the practicalities of that have been assessed, or in the case of the elderly, to care homes where, all too often, only lip service is given to palliative care.

There is the tacit assumption—and one that is unfounded and wrong—that the primary goal of a doctor should be to cure, or if that is impossible, to maintain life for as long as possible, sometimes without any thought being given to what we mean by life and whether it has any residual quality. Palliative medicine is most certainly not about abbreviating life. Neither is it about prolonging it without due thought to its quality, though it is worth recalling that many people receiving palliative care, their suffering skilfully relieved, live much longer than was ever thought possible.

The paradox is that much as terminally ill patients say they want to stay at home as long as possible they seldom get that 'privilege' and most die where they have least wanted to be—in a general hospital, possibly in a unit unfamiliar to them. The reasons are obvious. In their own homes, if they need out-of-hours medical attention, they are more likely to be seen by a doctor unfamiliar with them or their problems and medications than by a doctor from their practice. As every palliative medicine physician knows, the success or failure of home care largely depends on the relatives. If they feel supported and appreciated, and not under societal pressure to have their loved one admitted somewhere, care at home is possible, If not, as much for their sake as that of the patient, transfer to hospital will be requested.

Can hospitals measure palliative medicine efficiency?

Behind this question lies the groundswell of frustration and dismay, increasingly being expressed by doctors and nurses in Western countries, about the time they must spend (and, as most would say, waste) in data collection designed to measure 'clinical efficiency'. They resent their work being evaluated and checked on by what they describe as 'tick-box mentality'.

Nobody denies that targets are essential. They are valid scientific tools and useful when they are appropriate to the work being done, the activity being measured and, putting it another way, when the questions being asked are legitimate questions. Inappropriate questions are those which bear no relation whatsoever to the care of people receiving palliative medicine. They are often based on wrong assumptions—something is valid if it can be measured/counted and conversely, if something cannot be counted it is not important; if a box can be ticked showing that some question was asked or procedure carried out it can be assumed it helped the patient; the shorter the time a patient occupies a hospital bed the more efficient that ward is, and conversely, the longer the length of stay the less efficient the ward/unit is. The list of illustrations is endless. The frustration experienced by clinicians, including palliative medicine physicians, is distressing and needless; the effect on our patients something we should be deeply concerned about. The inappropriate targets being set in palliative care (for once again this affects all team members) and the 'tick-box completions' to support them is the work of those who know little or nothing about palliative medicine. They are people who do not realize how seldom our patients 'waste' our time, who do not know how many of our patients already feel a burden without being made to feel just

another statistic, and, in short, do not know what we do, why we do it, how we do it, and how committed we are to superb—effective and efficient—patient care.

The question is whether palliative care clinicians need to follow the herd 'because management says we must' or are confident enough to demonstrate more appropriate targets and better means of achieving them. Can we not set about demonstrating to management what palliative medicine is all about, telling them what our patients are always telling us about their needs, explaining how we can and will measure relief of pain and every other form of suffering, and how we can demonstrate that what they have been expecting us to do does not measure what is at the heart of palliative medicine and nobody knows that better than we do! Arrogant? Not the way we have traditionally behaved in palliative medicine? Possibly, but palliative medicine is at risk of losing some of its unique identity.

Are we changing with the times?

We all recognize that we are an ageing society. Living longer means more degenerative conditions, more dementia, more dependency extending over much longer, three or four generations of one family alive and interdependent, greater mobility, speedier communications, ever-more expensive medications, a more demanding (and possibly a more litigious) public—these are but a few of tomorrow's challenges. The question is not 'are we changing' but 'are we flexible enough to change without dropping standards' or so blending into our various health-care system that we lose some identity, some of that rich, creative 'uniqueness' that has characterized palliative medicine and palliative care for the past 50 years. Are we producing the leaders, the teachers, the researchers, the writers we shall need even before the fifth edition appears. This new edition shows that our leaders are very conscious of these challenges.

Palliative medicine does more than offer superb comfort care to those on their final journey of life, protracted as that last stage may be as a result of the ministrations of so many of our professional colleagues. It says to the lonely 'you are not alone'. It says to the fearful 'we are near you and understand'. It says to those who wonder if they have achieved anything, if they will ever be missed, 'thank you for teaching us what we so needed to know'. It says what everyone in the world at some time or other wants to hear 'you matter because you are you!'.

Palliative medicine must be one of the few branches of medicine which prompts the patient to tell us what we find so difficult to understand, 'I feel safe now!'.

Derek Doyle
Edinburgh, 2009.

Contributor affiliations

Andy Adam, Professor of Interventional Radiology, Department of Radiology, Guy's and St Thomas' Hospital, NHS Foundation Trust, London, UK

Linda Armstrong, Consultant Speech and Language Therapist, Perth, UK

Greg G. Bailly, Assistant Professor, Department of Urology, Dalhousie University, Halifax, Canada

Jane Ellen Barr, Director of Wound Healing, NSLIJHS Long Island University Medical Center New Hyde Park, New York

Vickie Baracos, Division of Palliative Care Medicine, Department of Oncology, University of Alberta, Edmonton, Canada

Claudia Bausewein, The Cicely Saunders Foundation Research Training Fellow, King's College London, UK

Stephen Bayles, Assistant Professor, Vanderbilt-Bill Wilkerson Center for Otolaryngology and Communication Sciences, Nashville, USA

Michaela Bercovitch, Sheba Medical Center, Tel Aviv, Israel

Cheryl R. Billante, Vanderbilt Voice Center, Nashville, USA

Stewart Bond, Research Associate, John A. Hartford Foundation Claire M. Fagin Fellow, Vanderbilt University School of Nursing, Nashville, USA

Gian Domenico Borasio, Professor of Palliative Medicine, Interdisciplinary Center for Palliative Medicine and Department of Neurology, Munich University Hospital, Munich, Germany

Georg Bosshard, Researcher, Institute of Legal Medicine University of Zürich, Switzerland

Mark Bower, Professor of Oncology, Consultant Medical Oncologist, Chelsea & Westminster Hospital, London, UK

William Breitbart, Chief, Psychiatry Service, Memorial Sloan Kettering Cancer Centre New York, USA

Stephen C. Brown, Academic Professor, Department of Anesthesia, Hospital for Sick Children, Toronto, Canada

Eduardo Bruera, Department of Palliative Care and Rehabilitation Medicine, The University of Texas M. D. Anderson Cancer Center, Houston, Texas

Gary Buckholz, San Diego Hospice, USA

Ira R. Byock, Professor and Director of Palliative Medicine, Dartmouth-Hitchcock Medical Center, New Hampshire, USA

Kenneth Calman, Chancellor, University of Glasgow, UK

David Cameron, Associate Professor, Department of Family Medicine, University of Pretoria, South Africa

Augusto Caraceni, Director, Pain Therapy, Palliative Care and Rehabilitation, National Cancer Institute, Milan, Italy

David Casarett, Center for Health Equity Research and Promotion at the Philadelphia VA Medical Center, and the Division of Geriatrics, Institute on Aging, Leonard Davis Institute of Health Economics and the Center for Bioethics at the University of Pennsylvania, USA

David J. Casper, Memorial Sloan–Kettering Cancer Center, and Cornell University Weill College of Medicine, New York, USA

J. Brian Cassel, Senior Analyst, VCU Massey Cancer Center, Richmond Virginia, USA

Barrie Cassileth, Chief, Integrative Medicine Service, Memorial Sloan–Kettering Cancer Center, New York, USA

Raphael Catane, Professor and Chief of Medical Oncology, Department of Medical Oncology, Sheba Medical Center, Tel Aviv, Israel

Fiona Cathcart, (Retired) Consultant Clinical Psychologist, St Columba's Hospice, Edinburgh, UK

E Joanna Chambers, Consultant in Clinical Oncology and Palliative Medicine, North Bristol NHS Trust, Southmead Hospital, Bristol, UK

Kin-Sang Chan, Chief of Service and Consultant, Pulmonary and Palliative Care Unit, Haven of Hope Hospital, Kowloon, Hong Kong

Nathan I. Cherny, Norman Levan Chair of Humanistic Medicine, Director Cancer Pain and Palliative Medicine, Department of Oncology, Shaare Zedek Medical Center, Jerusalem, Israel

Andrea Cheville, Associate Professor, Physical Medicine, Mayo Clinic, Minnesota, USA

Harvey Max Chochinov, Professor and Canada Research Chair in Palliative Care, University of Manitoba; Director, Manitoba Palliative Care Research Unit, CancerCare Manitoba, Canada

Nicholas A. Christakis, Professor of Medicine and Professor of Medical Sociology, Harvard Medical School, and Attending Physician, Mt. Auburn Hospital, Cambridge, MA

David Clark, Chair of Medical Sociology and Director of the International Observatory on End of Life Care, Institute for Health Research, Lancaster University, UK

Anthony Cmelak, Assistant Professor, Department of Radiation Oncology, Vanderbilt-Ingram Cancer Center, Nashville, USA

S. L. Cohen, Bloomsbury Institute of Intensive Care Medicine, University College London Division of Medicine, UK

John J. Collins, Head, Pain and Palliative Care Service, The Children's Hospital at Westmead, Sydney, Australia

Lesley A. Colvin, Consultant/ Senior Lecturer in Anaesthesia & Pain Medicine, University of Edinburgh, UK

Franco De Conno, Director, Rehabilitation and Palliative Care Unit, National Cancer Institute (Foundation), Milan, Italy

Stephen R. Connor, Vice President, for Research, & International Development at the National Hospice & Palliative Care Organization (NHPCO) in Alexandria, Virginia, USA

Jill Cooper, Senior Occupational Therapist, Royal Marsden Hospital, London, UK

Michael J. Cousins, Professor and Head, Department of Anaesthesia and Pain Management, Royal North Shore Hospital, University of Sydney, Australia

Sarah Cox, Consultant in Palliative Care, Chelsea & Westminster Hospital, London, UK

Nessa Coyle, International Association Hospice and Palliative Care, Houston, USA

David Currow, Professor of Palliative Medicine, Department of Palliative and Supportive Services, Division of Medicine, Flinders University, Bedford Park, Australia

LaVera Crawley, Assistant Professor (Research), Department of Paediatrics, Stanford University Center for Biomedical Ethics, California, USA

Carolyn L. Datta, Specialist Registrar in Palliative Medicine, The Ayrshire Hospice, Ayr, UK

Isobel Davidson, Department of Dietetics, Greater Glasgow and Clyde Acute Services Division and Reader Dietetics, Nutrition and Biological Sciences, School of Health Sciences, Queen Margaret University, Edinburgh, UK

Betty Davies, Professor and Chair, Family Health Care Nursing Department, University of California San Francisco, USA

Gary Deng, Integrative Medicine Service, Memorial Sloan–Kettering Cancer Center, New York, USA

A. H. Dickenson, Department of Pharmacology, *University College London*, UK

Ellie Dowling, Vanderbilt-Bill Wilkerson Center for Otolaryngology and Communication Sciences, Nashville, USA

Michael Downing, Medical Director of Victoria Hospice Society, Victoria, Canada

Derek Doyle, National Council for Palliative Care, England, Wales and North Ireland and Scottish Partnership for Palliative Care, Edinburgh, UK

Francis G. Dunn, Consultant Cardiologist/Clinical Director, Cardio-Thoracic Directorate, Stobhill NHS Trust, Glasgow, UK

Frank Elsner, Chair, Physician Education Taskforce, European Association for Palliative Care, Germany

Anne English, Physiotherapy Clinical Specialist, Dove House Hospice, Hull, UK

Mary Ersek, Associate Professor, University of Pennsylvania, School of Nursing, Philadelphia, PA, USA

Marie Fallon, St Columba's Hospice Chair of Palliative Medicine, University of Edinburgh, UK

Lesley Fallowfield, Professor of Psycho-Oncology, Director, Psychosocial Oncology Group Cancer Research UK, Brighton and Sussex Medical School, University of Sussex, Brighton, UK

John T. Farrar, Assistant Professor of Epidemiology, University of Pennsylvania, USA

Kenneth C. H. Fearon, Professor of Surgical Oncology, Edinburgh University and Consultant in Colorectal Surgery, Western General Hospital, Edinburgh, UK

Betty R. Ferrell, Research Scientist, City of Hope National Medical Center, Duarte, CA USA

Frank D. Ferris, San Diego Hospice, USA

Jacqueline Filshie, Consultant Anaesthetist, Royal Marsden Hospital, London, UK

Perry G. Fine, Professor of Anesthesiology, University of Utah, Salt Lake City; Attending Physician, Pain Management Center, University of Utah, Salt Lake City, USA

Nanna Brix Finnerup, Danish Pain Research Center and Department of Neurology, Aarhus University Hospital, Aarhus, Denmark

Joseph J. Fins, Chief, Division of Medical Ethics; Professor of Medicine, Public Health, and Medicine in Psychiatry, Weill Cornell Medical College, New York, USA

Anne Marie Flores, Assistant Professor of Orthopaedics and Rehabilitation, Vanderbilt University Medical Center, Nashville, USA

Kathleen Foley, Pain and Palliative, Care Service, Memorial Sloan Kettering Cancer Centre New York, USA

Karen Forbes, Consultant Physician and Macmillan Professorial Teaching Fellow in Palliative Medicine, University Hospitals Bristol and University of Bristol, UK

Nicos I. Fotiadis, Consultant Interventional Radiologist, Barts and The London NHS Trust, London, UK

Deborah Franklin, Assistant Professor, Department of Rehabilitation Medicine; Director, Comprehensive Acute Rehabilitation Unit; Director, Cancer Rehabilitation, Thomas Jefferson University, Philadelphia, USA

Paul Glare, Chief, Palliative Pain Service, Department of Medicine, Memorial Sloan-Kettering Cancer Centre, New York, USA

Margaret Gibbs, senior pharmacist, St Christopher's Hospice, London, UK

Nathan E. Goldstein, Director, Integrated Fellowship in Palliative Medicine; Assistant Professor, Brookdale Department of Geriatrics, Mount Sinai School of Medicine, New York; James J. Peters Veterans Affairs Medical Center, New York, USA

Fiona Graham, Senior Lecturer in General Practice at the University of Central Lancashire, Preston, UK

Patricia Grocott, Reader, King's College London, UK

Kirsten Haman, Research Assistant Professor, Department of Psychiatry, Vanderbilt University Medical Center, Nashville, USA

Geoffrey Hanks, Professor of Palliative Medicine, University of Bristol, UK

Mike Harlos, Professor, Faculty of Medicine, University of Manitoba; Medical Director, Palliative Care Program, Winnipeg Regional Health Authority, Canada

Rev. James M. Harper, III, The Midwest CPE Program c/o Research Medical Center Pastoral Care Dept., Kansas City, USA

Dagny Faksvåg Haugen, Helse Bergen Haukeland University Hospital, Bergen, Norway

John H. Healey, Orthopaedic Surgery Service, Department of Surgery, Memorial Sloan-Kettering Cancer Center, Affiliated with Weill Medical College of Cornell University, New York. USA

Meg Hegarty, Repatriation General Hospital, Daw Park, Australia

Keela Herr, Professor & Chair, Adult & Gerontology Nursing, College of Nursing, University of Iowa, USA

Irene J. Higginson, Professor of Palliative Care and Policy, Head of Department, Consultant in Palliative Medicine, School of Medicine of Guy's, King's and St Thomas', King's College London, UK

Peter J. Hoskin, Consultant in Clinical Oncology, Mount Vernon Cancer Centre, Middlesex, and Professor in Clinical Oncology, University College London, UK

Jane M. Ingham, Professor, Palliative Medicine, St Vincents Clinical School, The University of New South Wales; and Director, The Cunningham Centre for Palliative Care, Sacred Heart Hospice, NSW, Australia

Liz Jamieson, Cancer Research UK London Psychosocial Group, UK

David Jeffrey, Honorary Senior Lecturer in Palliative Medicine, University of Edinburgh, UK

Troels Staehelin Jensen, Danish Pain Research Center and Department of Neurology, Aarhus University Hospital, Aarhus, Denmark

Stein Kaasa, Professor in Palliative medicine and Head of the Palliative Medicine Unit, Department of Cancer Research and Molecular Medicine Faculty of medicine, NTNU and St. Olavs University Hospital; National Cancer Director, Directorate for Health and Social Affairs, Trondheim, Norway

Menelaos Karanikolas, Assistant Professor of Anesthesiology, Washington University School of Medicine, St. Louis, USA; and Assistant Professor, Dept. of Anaesthesiology and Critical Care Medicine, University of Patras Medical School; Rion, Greece

Vaughan Keeley, Consultant in Palliative Medicine, Derby, UK

Jeremy Keen, Consultant Physician in Palliative Care and Lead Clinician in Palliative Care, Highland Hospice, Inverness, UK

Deborah Kirklin, Honorary Senior Lecturer, Medical Ethics and Humanities, University College London, UK

David W. Kissane, Chair, Department of Psychiatry & Behavioral Sciences, Memorial Sloan-Kettering Cancer Center, New York, USA

Jonathan Koffman, Lecturer in Palliative Care, Department of Palliative Care, Policy and Rehabilitation, King's College School of Medicine, Weston Education Centre, London, UK

Eric L. Krakauer, Centre for Palliative Care, Harvard Medical School; and Palliative Care Service, Massachusetts General Hospital, Boston, USA

Linda J. Kristjanson, Deputy Vice-Chancellor, Research and Development, Curtin University of Technology, Australia

Robert S. Krouse, Department of Surgery, Southern Arizona Veterans Affairs Health Care System and the University of Arizona, Tucson, USA

Suresh Kumar, Neighbourhood Network in Palliative Care Contact Point, Institute of Palliative Medicine, Medical College, Calicut, Kerala, India

Vic Larcher, Consultant in Paediatric Palliative Medicine, Great Ormond Street Hospital, London, UK

Richard M. Leach, Consultant Physician and Honorary Senior Lecturer, Guy's and St Thomas' Hospital Trust and GKT School of Medicine, St Thomas' Campus, London, UK

S. Lawrence Librach, Head, Division of Palliative Care, University of Toronto, Canada

Liliana De Lima, Executive Director, International Association for Hospice and Palliative Care, Houston, USA

John Håvard Loge, Professor, Department of Behavioural Sciences in Medicine, University of Oslo, Oslo, Norway

Charles L. Loprinzi, Professor of Oncology, Mayo Clinic, Minnesota, USA

Karl Lorenz, Veterans Administration, Greater Los Angeles Healthcare System; Veterans Integrated Palliative Program; David Geffen School of Medicine at University of California at Los Angeles and RAND Health, Santa Monica, California, USA

Stefan Lorenzl, Grosshadern Hospital Neurology Clinic, Munich University Hospital, Munich, Germany

Michal Lotem, Sharett Institute of Oncology, Hadassah Hebrew University Hospital, Jerusalem, Israel

David Lussier, Director, Geriatric Pain Clinic, McGill University Health Center, Montreal, Canada

Alison MacDonald, Lecturer and specialist Speech and Language Therapist, Speech and Hearing Sciences, Queen Margaret University, Edinburgh, UK

Neil MacDonald, McGill Cancer Nutrition and Rehabilitation Program, Department of Oncology, McGill University, Montreal, Canada

Kathryn A. Mannix, Consultant in Palliative Medicine, Newcastle upon Tyne Hospitals Foundation NHS Trust; Marie Curie Hospice, Newcastle upon Tyne, UK

Cinzia Martini, Rehabilitation and Palliative Care Unit, National Cancer Institute (Foundation), Milan, Italy

Lars Johan Materstvedt, Department of Philosophy, Norwegian University of Science and Technology, Trondheim, Norway

Susan E. McClement, Associate Professor, Faculty of Nursing, University of Manitoba; Research Associate, Manitoba Palliative Care Research Unit, CancerCare Manitoba, Canada

Andrew D. McGavigan, Clinical Research Fellow, Cardio-Respiratory Directorate, Stobhill Hospital, Glasgow, UK

Patricia A. McGrath. Scientific Director, Divisional Center of Pain Management and Pain Research, Anesthesia, Hospital for Sick Children, Toronto, Canada

Malcolm McIllmurray, Professor of medical oncology, Royal Lancaster Infirmary, Lancaster, UK

Henry J. McQuay, Nuffield Professor of Clinical Anaesthetics, Nuffield Department of Anaesthetics, University of Oxford, UK

Diane E. Meier, Director, Lilian and Benjamin Hertzberg Palliative Care Institute; Professor, Brookdale Department of Geriatrics and Adult Development; Catherine Gaisman Professor of Medical Ethics; Director, Center to Advance Palliative Care, Mount Sinai School of Medicine, New York, USA

Sebastiano Mercadante, Consultant in Pain and Palliative Care, Pain Relief and Palliative Care Unit, La Maddelena Cancer Center, Palermo, Italy

Jennifer Miller, Acting Chair, HIV/AIDs, Oncology & Palliative Care, The College of Occupational Therapists, London, UK

Anthoulla Mohamudally, Clinical Fellow, Cunningham Centre for Palliative Care, Sacred Heart Hospice, St. Vincent's Hospital, NSW, Australia

Barbara Monroe, Chief Executive, St Christopher's Hospice, London, UK

Andrew Moore, Pain Research, Nuffield Department of Anaesthetics, University of Oxford, UK

Anna C. Muriel, Assistant Professor of Psychiatry Harvard Medical School. Chief, Division of Pediatric Psychosocial Oncology Dana-Farber Cancer Institute, Boston, MA

Barbara A. Murphy, Associate Professor, Department of Medicine, Vanderbilt-Ingram Cancer Center, Nashville, USA

Friedemann Nauck, Professor of Palliative Medicine, Department of Palliative Medicine, University of Göttingen, Germany

Elizabeth G. Nilson, Assistant Professor of Public Health, Assistant Professor of Medicine, Weill Cornell Medical College, New York, USA

Richard W. Norman, Professor, Department of Urology, Dalhousie University, Halifax, Canada

Clare O'Callaghan, University of Melbourne, Sessional Music Therapist, Oncology, Hematology and Palliative Care, Austin and Repatriation Medical Center, Parkville, Australia

Norma O'Leary, Consultant in Palliative Medicine, Our Lady of Lourdes Hospital, Drogheda, Co.Louth and Co.Meath

Stacy Orloff, Vice President of Palliative Care and Community Programs, *The Hospice,* Florida Suncoast, Florida, USA

Diane Palac, Dartmouth-Hitchcock Medical Center, General Internal Medicine, One Medical Center Drive, Lebanon, USA

Joan T. Panke, Executive director of the DC Partnership to Improve End-of-Life Care in Washington, USA

Sophie Pautex, Pain and Palliative Care Consultant, Department of Rehabilitation and Geriatrics, University Hospital Geneva, Switzerland

Nicholas Park, North Bristol NHS Trust, UK

Steven D. Passik, Associate Attending Psychologist, Department of Psychiatry and Behavioral Sciences, Memorial Sloan-Kettering Cancer center, New York, USA

Nik K. Patel, North Bristol NHS Trust, UK

Jose Pereira, Leenaards Foundation Chair and Professor of Palliative Care, University of Lausanne and University of Geneva, Switzerland; Adjunct Professor, Divisions of Palliative Medicine, University of Calgary and University of Alberta, Canada

Mark R. Pittelkow, Professor of Dermatology, Mayo Clinic, Minnesota, USA

Michael Piza, Project Officer, The Cunningham Centre for Palliative Care, Sacred Heart Hospice; and Conjoint Associate Lecturer, St Vincents Clinical School, University of New South Wales, Sydney, Australia

David Praill, Help the Hospices and Worldwide Palliative Care Alliance, London, UK

Russell K. Portenoy, Chairman and Gerald J. and Dorothy R. Friedman Chair in Pain Medicine and Palliative Care, Department of Pain Medicine and Palliative Care, Beth Israel Medical Center, New York, NY, USA, and Professor of Neurology and Anesthesiology, Albert Einstein College of Medicine, Bronx, New York, USA

TJ. Prendergast, Associate Professor of Medicine and Anesthesiology at Dartmouth Hitchcock Medical Center, New York, USA

Thomas E. Quinn, Patient Care Services, Massachusetts General Hospital, Boston, USA

M.R. Rajagopal, Professor of Pain and Palliative Medicine, SUT Academy of Medical Sciences, Trivandrum, Kerala, India

Dilini Rajapakse, Consultant in Paediatric Palliative Medicine, Great Ormond Street Hospital, London, UK

Amanda Ramirez, Cancer Research UK London Psychosocial Group, UK

Paula K. Rauch, Child Psychiatrist, Harvard Medical School; Massachusetts General Hospital, Boston, USA

Claud Regnard, Consultant in Palliative Medicine, St Oswald's Hospice, Newcastle upon Tyne, UK

Alison Richardson, Cancer Research UK London Psychosocial Group, UK

Rosemary Richardson, Department of Dietetics, Greater Glasgow and Clyde Acute Services Division and Dietetics, Nutrition and Biological Sciences, School of Health Sciences, Queen Margaret University, Edinburgh, UK

Sheila Ridner, Assistant Professor, Vanderbilt University School of Nursing, Nashville, USA

Carla Ripamonti, Consultant in Medical Oncology and Clinical Pharmacology, Rehabilitation and Palliative Care, Istituto Nazionale dei Tumori, Milan, Italy

Clive J.C. Roberts, Consultant Senior Lecturer in Clinical Pharmacology and Therapeutics, Department of Medicine, University Hospitals Bristol and University of Bristol, UK

Diane Robinson, Physiotherapy Clinical Specialist, St Catherine's Hospice, Scarborough, UK

Vicky Robinson, Consultant Nurse, St Christopher's Hospice, London, UK

Angela Rogers, Senior Research Fellow, University of Southampton, UK

Gordon D. Rubenfeld, Chief, Program in Trauma, Emergency, and Critical Care, Sunnybrook Health Sciences Centre, University of Toronto

Rabbi Jonathan E. Rudnick, Vice-President, Community Chaplain, Rabbinical Association of Greater Kansas City, USA

Tarun Sabharwal, Consultant Interventional Radiologist, Department of Radiology, St Thomas's Hospital, London, UK

Megan B. Sands, Staff Specialist Palliative Medicine, Department of Palliative Care, Prince of Wales Hospital; and Conjoint Lecturer, Prince of Wales Clinical School, University of New South Wales, Sydney, Australia

Michael J. Sateia, Professor of Psychiatry, Chief, Section of Sleep Medicine, Dartmouth Medical School, Lebanon, USA

Alberto Sbanotto, Physician, Department of Neurology, Istituto Nazionale dei Tumori, Milan, Italy

Erin Schweers Cornelius, Department of Education and Psychological Studies, University of Miami, Coral Gables, Florida

Michael M.K. Sham, Consultant in Palliative Care and Chest Medicine, Nam Long Hospital, Hong Kong

Harold Siden, Department of Pediatrics, University of British Columbia; Canuck Place Children's Hospice, Vancouver, Canada

Fabio Simonetti, Physician, Neurology Unit, Rehabilitation and Palliative Care, Istituto Nazionale dei Tumori, Milan, Italy

Christian Sinclair, Kansas City Hospice and Palliative Care, Kansas City, USA

Per Sjøgren, Danish Society of Palliative Medicine, Copenhagen, Denmark

Thomas J. Smith, Chair, Hematology-Oncology and Palliative Care, VCU Massey Cancer Center, Virginia, USA

Karen E. Steinhauser, Health Scientist, VA Medical Center; Associate Professor, Duke University Medical Center

Michael M. Stevens, Senior Staff Specialist and Head, Oncology Unit, The Children's Hospital at Westmead, Sydney, Australia

Patrick Stone, Division of Mental Health, St George's University of London, London

Florian Strasser, Oncology and Palliative Medicine, Section Oncology/Hematology, Department Internal Medicine, Kantonsspital, St.Gallen, Switzerland

Annette F. Street, Professor, Cancer and Palliative Care Studies, La Trobe University/Director, Austin Health Clinical School of Nursing, La Trobe University - Bundoora, Melbourne, Australia

Robert A. Swarm, Chief, Division of Pain Management, Associate Professor of Anesthesiology, Washington University School of Medicine, St. Louis, USA

Nigel Sykes, Head of Medicine, Consultant in Palliative Medicine, St. Christopher's Hospice, London, UK

Martin H. N. Tattersall, Professor of Cancer Medicine, Medical Psychology Research Unit, Department of Medicine, University of Sydney; and Department of Medical Oncology, Royal Prince Alfred Hospital, Camperdown, NSW 2040, Australia

Emma Teasdale, Cancer Research UK London Psychosocial Group, UK

John W. Thompson, Hon. Physician and Honorary Consultant in Medical Studies, St Oswald's Hospice, Newcastle upon Tyne, UK

Anne Berit Thorsen, Associate Consultant in Palliative Care, Palliative Care Unit, Haven of Hope Hospital, Hong Kong

James A. Tulsky, Professor of Medicine and Nursing, Director, Center for Palliative Care, VA and Duke Medical Centers

A. Robert Turner, Professor of Medicine, Clinical Haematology and Medical Oncology, University of Alberta, Canada

Doris M.W. Tse, Chief of Service, Department of Medicine and Geriatrics, Caritas Medical Centre, Hong Kong

Robert Twycross, Emeritus Clinical Reader in Palliative Medicine, Oxford University, UK

Wakenda K. Tyler, Orthopaedic Surgery Service, Department of Surgery, Memorial Sloan-Kettering Cancer Center, Affiliated with Weill Medical College of Cornell University, New York, USA

Mary L.S. Vachon, Departments of Psychiatry and Public Health Sciences, University of Toronto, Canada

Vittorio Ventafriddas (Late) Scientific Director, Fondazione Floriani, Milan, Italy

Raymond Voltz, Chair, Department of Palliative Medicine, Centre for Integrated Oncology, University Hospital Cologne, Germany

Ladislav Volicer, School of Aging Studies, University of South Florida, Tampa, USA

Charles F. von Gunten, Associate Clinical Professor of Medicine, Cancer Symptom Control Program, University of California San Diego; Provost of The Institute for Palliative Medicine at San Diego Hospice, USA

Sharon Watanabe, Department of Symptom Control and Palliative Care, Cross Cancer Institute, Edmonton, Alberta, Canada

Philip Wiffen, Pain Research, Nuffield Department of Anaesthetics, University of Oxford, UK

R. M. Gordon-Williams, Department of Pharmacology, University College London, UK

Panarut Wisawatapnimit, Doctoral Student, School of Nursing, Vanderbilt University, Nashville, USA

Deborah Witt Sherman, Division of Nursing, New York University, USA

Roger Woodruff, Director of Palliative Care, Austin Health, Melbourne, Australia

Michèle J. M. Wood, Senior Lecturer in Art Therapy at University of Hertfordshire, UK

Sriram Yennurajalingam, Palliative Care & Rehabilitation Medicine, MD Anderson Cancer Center

Talia Zaider, Memorial Sloan-Kettering Cancer Center, New York, USA

Giovambattista Zeppetella, Medical Director, St Clare Hospice, Honorary Consultant Princess Alexandra NHS Trust, Harlow, UK

SECTION 1

Introduction to the fourth edition: facing the challenges of continuity and change

Geoffrey Hanks, Nathan I. Cherny, Russell K. Portenoy, Stein Kaasa, Marie Fallon, and Nicholas Christakis

The fourth edition of the *Oxford Textbook of Palliative Medicine* reflects the continuity, development, and evolution of the art and science of caring for the incurably ill and dying. The editorial board of the textbook reflects this same theme of continuity and evolution. Professor Geoffrey Hanks, a stalwart of all three previous editions has led the editorial team. He has been supported by Nathan I. Cherny (an editor from the previous edition) and by an international team of new editors including Marie Fallon (Scotland), Russell K. Portenoy (USA), Stein Kaasa (Norway), and Nicholas Christakis (USA).

The *Oxford Textbook of Palliative Medicine* has evolved to increasing become a truly international text. We now have 193 contributors from 16 countries and 6 continents. This new edition is a major reworking of the textbook with multiple new chapters and new authors. The book has been substantially restructured with new sections on the interdisciplinary team, geriatric palliative medicine, disease modification in advanced cancer, and a section devoted to specific neoplastic diseases. Additionally, some of the pre-existing sections have been restructured. This is particularly true for the subsection on pain in which there are now new chapters on bone pain, neuropathic pain, and breakthrough pain.

As much as we would like to call our contributor list the best and the brightest, we are well aware of the depth of talent and thoughtfulness that exist in the world of palliative medicine. It is in this sense of humility that we invite you to be reviewers and contributors to help make this textbook a very real and living endeavour by taking time to write back to the editors with your feedback about the book or its individual chapters. This information will be used for the development of subsequent editions. To this end we invite you to send feedback to editors@OTPM4.org

As editors, we are well aware of the tensions in the palliative care world regarding the evolution of palliative medicine. We embrace this tension as a challenge to address issues of continuity, development, and change as a theme of this edition.

Continuity: cardinal concepts underlying the philosophy of palliative medicine

Palliative medicine asserts boldly and optimistically that even in the face of overwhelming illness suffering can and must be relieved. This assertion is derived from a rights ethos. There may be pragmatic, economic, geopolitical, or social reasons that make it difficult to provide palliative care, but these do not diminish from duty of care to seek the adequate relief of suffering of persons with incurable illness.

The factors that motivate palliative medicine practitioners to do what they do in the face of great challenges are the underlying axioms of our endeavours. Beyond intuition we believe that it is important to articulate why we make the personal and professional investment in attempting to address intense human suffering in the context of incurable illness and impeding death.

Care, compassion, and empathy and justice

Care is the recognition that the well-being of others is a matter of consequence. As an integral part of the human experience, it is a motivating force that influences the nature and dynamic of interpersonal behaviours. Compassion is that aspect of care that recognizes the emotional dimension of the human experience.

Empathy, the ability to perceive and to understand the emotional experience of others and to relate to it a meaningful and appropriate manner, predicates care and compassion. In the clinical context, an empathic connection occurs when the carer understands what their patient is experiencing, and when this is communicated (verbally or non-verbally) such that the patient feels that they are understood. The empathic connection is often therapeutic in itself. Beyond that, it is a motivating bond which also facilitates the trust necessary to forge an effective therapeutic relationship.

There is a linear relationship between empathy, care, and perception of justice. The rights claim to adequate relief of suffering is derived from the empathic experience; i.e. that unnecessary suffering is a profound matter of consequence and that it demands a constructive response. Empathy, care, and compassion motivate sensitivity, respect, compassion, concern, charity, generosity, altruism and, sometimes, self sacrifice. The absence of care implies that the well-being of the other is inconsequential and, in its absence, human interaction is often characterized by insensitivity, neglect, or negligence.

Resilience

In taking on the task of palliative care, we, as health-care providers willingly expose ourselves to physical, emotional, and existential distress on a daily basis. Caring for patients and their families in this context day after day (and, in many cases, for years on end), challenges us. We are challenged as professionals and as individuals; each with our own families, needs, and outside stressors. We are challenged as health-care teams; the differential stressors borne by members of the care team can strain and challenge even the best of collaborative relationships.

As caregivers, resilience is the quality that enables us to withstand and to develop despite the tidal surge of suffering that we dare to confront with skills, dedication, and good intentions. As teams, resilience is the flexible, binding matrix that keeps us working constructively together despite forces of team stress, conflict, interpersonal frictions, and grievances that would potentially fragment or undermine our ability to deliver care.

By virtue of self-selection, clinicians choosing to enter into a career of palliative care often have a strong perception of personal resilience. In most cases, palliative care clinicians have chosen their career paths and are thus self-interested partners in developing and preserving their ability to function, to contribute, and to rise above the suffering we help relieve. Not all, however, who work in palliative care, do so by choice. Interns, resident staff, nursing students, administrative and support staffs are often find themselves in palliative care by consignment rather than by choice. For those without innate resilience or good supports, this can be a high-stress challenge that can only be endured if given support understanding and an environment that helps foster coping and resilience.

The patients and families we seek to help have not chosen their fate. How they cope, or are helped to cope, hinges on both meticulous care and on the fostering of resilience in the patient, the individual family members, and of the family as a unit. Some patients come with rich sources of personal and family resilience; many, however come to us overwhelmed and bereft. Beyond the relief of physical symptoms, the processes of adaptive coping and of psychological and spiritual healing all demand the nurturing of coping and courage.

Courage

For the incurably ill, fear is a part of life. There is just so much to fear; death, physical distress, and debilitation, dependency, and so many losses. Loss of potency, of beauty, of control over biologic function, of mental faculties, of future hopes, of separation, of and of life itself.

Courage takes many forms in the lives of our patients. Finding the courage to seek meaning in a life to be foreshortened and to be able to savour the available life whilst, at the same time, grieving the hopes and dreams, that cannot and will not be fulfiled. Courage to confront difficult decisions about treatment options that have both the potential to either improve quality of life or possibly to undermine it. No one wants to live with a gastrostomy, to wear a diaper, to have an intercostal catheter, to have limb amputated, or to undergo endoscopic stent insertion. In making such benevolent recommendations, we ask a lot of the patients' resources. Yet, for many of our patients, the courage to submit to such procedures will ultimately allow them to live better than they did without.

We often ask of our patients to make the switch from seeking more and better life to accepting the inevitability of impending death. Not only is their courage in choosing the activist or interventionalist option 'to do'; there is courage, sometimes even greater courage, in making decisions to desist from, to forgo, or to withdraw treatments or interventions.

Humility and audacity

The magnitude of the issues that our patients confront challenge the limits of the art and science of palliative medicine. Understanding the limits of what can be reasonably expected from our care, treatments, and interventions emphasize the need to present treatment plans with both hope and humility. Often, there will be no one best management option, and, in presenting therapeutic options, we need to explain not only what we know, but also the uncertainties involved.

An excess of optimistic and overconfident hubris regarding the anticipated outcome of treatments risks undermining credibility. This affects the way in which we present anticipated outcomes from treatment recommendations. Desisting from saying some intervention or treatment 'will help', rather, invoking the contingency 'may help', a commitment to vigilant monitoring of outcomes with a readiness to readdress the treatment plan project an honesty and a commitment to care that encourages and fosters trust.

Honest and humble evaluation of what we can reasonably expect from our care outcomes make us aware of the limits of resources, therapeutic efficacy, and of knowledge that limit our ability to provide optimal outcomes for all. It is this critical element of humility that provides the impetus to programme development, political activism to improve resource allocation and, importantly, research to improve the knowledge base of palliative medicine.

For all of its inherent wisdom, there is a tension between palliative medicine and the humility of the Serenity Prayer. The Serenity Prayer asks us to 'Accept the things we cannot change, to change the things we can and to have the wisdom to know the difference'. The importance of the issues that we confront in palliative medicine impels us to seek ways to shift the boundaries between the 'things that cannot be changed' and those that are amenable to intervention and change. This is the dimension of audacity and the imperative of research.

Sensitivity to differences

There is no one best way to deal with life-threatening illness and indeed cultural, religious, and interpersonal factors strongly affect individual approaches. Individualized care needs to recognize and address a range of potential responses to the issues and decisions faced by our patients and their families.

While cultural sensitivity is important, it is equally important to recognize the heterogeneity with different cultural and religious communities. Indeed, reductionist anthropological approaches with cultural stereotyping are best avoided in favour of a more individualized approach that explores the values and goals of the individual patient and their family.

Trust

Through empathy, compassion, honesty, humility, sensitivity, and diligence, we aim to develop a bond of trust. We aim to build a trust that is sufficiently robust such that patients and their families feel secure in their care to facilitate effective care planning and delivery, courage, and resilience despite the profound difficulties of their circumstances.

Development: education, sevice delivery, availability, and theraputics

Education

The maturing of palliative medicine as a profession has been accompanied by the ongoing development of palliative medicine education and educational resources all over the world.

Increasingly, medical schools around the world are recognizing the importance of undergraduate training in the principles of palliative care. It is widely recognized that palliative care is an excellent format for modelling the principles of the bio-psycho-social model of health care that is now widely accepted as the standard of care. Curricula have been developed and published by multiple countries, universities, and individual faculties and there are a plethora of teaching models and aids that have been published and disseminated.

Advanced training in palliative medicine has taken multiple strides forward since the publication of the last edition of the Textbook. The outstanding development has been the recognition, in 2007, of Hospice and Palliative Medicine as a sub-specialty by the American Boards of Medical Specialties. After years of intense effort by a dedicated core of clinicians and researchers, this is a landmark achievement that is likely to impact on similar licencing authorities around the globe. Indeed, palliative medicine is now a recognized medical specialty or sub-specialty in 16 countries, and in others application for specialty or sub-specialty accreditation are underway or pending.

There is no consensus as to how to best train palliative medicine specialists. The content and duration of advanced training programmes varies greatly around the globe; 1 year in the United States, 3 years in the United Kingdom and Australia. Some programmes insist on a research component and others make no such demand. Given that the level of training not only affects competence and service delivery, but also impacts on the function and well-being of specialist clinicians working in the field, the issues of the adequacy of training are salient. How best to adequately equip specialist palliative care clinicians remains an open question worthy of further evaluation and research.

Worldwide, there is an increasing recognition that almost all physicians need some degree of proficiency in palliative medicine. This is specifically true for specialists working in high-mortality fields such as oncology, intensive care, geriatrics, neurology, nephrology, cardiology, and internal medicine. In all of these named specialties there have been important developments over the past 10 years. These are reflected in curricula development, training initiatives, publications, and research. Despite this, actual changes in training in practice have been, at best, inconsistent and at worst, disappointing. Overall, progress is evidenced but, in most of these specialties, the development of a high level of skill and understanding of palliative medicine remains a goal that has yet to be achieved.

Research in palliative care

Basic, clinical, sociological, and psychological research are all critical to expand the boundaries of knowledge in order to optimize patient care. This truism is valid for the medical endeavour in general, and is particularly relevant for palliative medicine in which the evidence base of practice is still relatively underdeveloped. The proliferation of research relevant to the care of the incurably ill has been a critical part of the maturation of palliative medicine. Research findings have sharpened out understanding of the mechanisms of symptoms we seek to relieve, helped define the limits of old approaches, and have uncovered new approaches to challenging and difficult problems that have previously been refractory to older approaches. Indeed, this edition of the Textbook is replete with multiple new approaches and insights that have been derived from these research endeavours.

By its nature, research in palliative medicine is very broad in its scope. Social science and psychical research are as important in our field as are basic science and therapeutic studies. The care of the incurably ill and their families is a 'complex system' challenge requiring multiple inputs, resource allocation, pharmacotherapeutic and psychological skills, and social understanding. All of these factors are increasingly represented in the growing research culture that we seek to encourage and cultivate.

Funding for palliative care research remains a challenge. Because many of the agents used for palliative care are not under patent, industry sponsorship is not widely available. In recent years, we have witnessed the development of research consortiums in palliative care that have been able to (successfully) submit grant proposals for complex interdisciplinary research endeavours. There is ongoing need to advocate for better funding for palliative care research.

Service delivery

The past decade has seen a flourishing of palliative medicine services in different settings worldwide. This has been well documented and monitored by the International Observatory of End of Life Care Project. There is not a region in the world that has not observed growth in palliative medicine services in the past 10 years. While there are areas where penetration and integration are tremendous, there are others in which programme development is still evolving and, sadly, many in which services are scarce and rudimentary. Programmes promoting education and service development, such as those championed by the Open Society Institute, the National Cancer Institute of the United States, and the European Society of Medical Oncology have made a substantial contribution in many countries with less developed services.

There are now a great many models of palliative medicine service delivery: inpatient and home-based hospices, hospital consultation services, acute palliative care wards and day hospitals, ambulatory clinics, and mobile clinics. Although the underlying principles and philosophy are consistent, the spectrum of observed problems may be profoundly different in different care settings.

This is particularly true with the increasing movement towards 'upstream palliative medicine' in which palliative medicine is being delivered at an earlier stage of the trajectory of illness. The issues confronted by clinicians working in early stage palliative medicine units, such as those in acute palliative medicine units, are often quite different from those confronted by clinicians who are providing immediate end-of-life care. The goals of care are different with a greater emphasis on function and, often, life prolongation (even in the face of incurable disease). In such cases, the duration of care will be prolonged and the fluctuating status of illness (with treatment-induced remissions and relapses) may involve rapidly changing care needs with changing problems lists and priorities.

Journals

There are now more than 10 peer-reviewed journals dedicated to issues of palliative care (Table 1.1). Additionally, the major journals of many other sub-specialties have increasingly embraced the palliative care issues which now feature ever more prominently. Dedicated palliative care sections in general journals, such as have appeared in the *British Medical Journal* and *JAMA*, bring palliative care to a wider audience and are particularly commended.

Table 1.1 Palliative care journals

American Journal of Hospice and Palliative Care
BMC Palliative Care
Death Studies
European Journal of Palliative Care
International Journal of Palliative Nursing
Journal of Psychosocial Oncology
Journal of Pain and Palliative Care Pharmacotherapy
Journal of Pain and Symptom Management
Journal of Palliative Care
Journal of Palliative Medicine
Omega
Palliative and Support Care
Palliative Medicine
Progress in Palliative Care
Psychooncology
Supportive Care in Cancer
Journal of Supportive Oncology

Evolution: change and challenges in palliative medicine

One of the early axioms of palliative care is that it sought to provide an alternative to 'aggressive' or 'highly technical' medical care. Indeed palliative care was often presented as 'strong' on care and 'low' on technology. In the sixties and early seventies, when these concepts were initially articulated, low-technology options were often indeed the very best that could be offered to help relieve patient distress. At that time there were very few truly effective palliative anti-tumour options beyond radiotherapy, and endoscopy and interventional radiology were in their absolute infancy.

The extraordinary development of non-curative, but potentially beneficial, interventions to address so many of the conditions, symptoms, and complications confronted by patients has created new opportunities, new tensions, and new dilemmas for palliative medicine clinicians.

New therapeutic opportunities

The last 20 years have seen dramatic changes in the non-curative treatment options for many of the conditions we encounter, particularly in cancer and HIV. With the introduction of a widening repertoire of treatment approaches, the natural history of advanced cancer and HIV infection have seen radical changes. While many, if not most of these, interventions are not curative, they have created new opportunities to control the ravages of disease, thus reducing symptoms and also by changing the natural history of the disease. Some interventions may add months, others, possibly years to survival.

Whereas previously it was often the role of the palliative medicine clinician to present a counterpoint to the high morbidity and low likely benefit of chemotherapy, the recent developments in the field of palliative anti-tumour therapies have added a whole new outlook for many patients. These developments have necessitated a change in the relationship between palliative medicine and medical oncology.

Furthermore, in order for palliative medicine clinicians to maintain credibility, they now need a far greater sophistication in the understanding of palliative approaches that change the course of the underlying disease: be it in cancer care, retroviral care, or in the management of other degenerative conditions where disease modification is available.

New palliative interventions exist not only for specific disease states but for also for specific disease complications and symptoms. Endoscopic interventions and interventional radiology have radically broadened the range of options in the cases of obstruction of luminal structures (GI, GU, vascular, and respiratory). These approaches have altered the management of intestinal, biliary, ureteric, and bronchial obstruction, venous compression syndromes, and in select cases pain management. Surgical approaches have made major changes to the management of complications of cancer such as spinal cord compression, brain metastases, and impending fractures (see sections 10 and 11).

Palliative medicine clinicians are challenged to take an increasing role in the development and evaluation of these sorts of interventions.

New tensions

Concern is often expressed that the increased availability of technical interventions to relieve distress somehow diminishes from the ability to care, or from the heart of palliative care. It is sometime asserted that palliative care is being excessively 'medicalized'.

However, just as there is a romantic image of the 19th-century physician at the bedside of his patient dying of TB offering possibly a tincture of opium but predominantly as a source of comfort, there is also a tendency of romanticizing the days of palliative care when many of these new palliative interventions were not yet available.

Interventional palliative care needs to be used judiciously. When it is considered among the possibly appropriate treatment options, it needs to be discussed with patients in an appropriate perspective: presenting likelihood of benefit, risks, and alternative approaches. Given the choice, many patients are interested approaches that offer the possibility of life prolongation or symptom relief through these interventions. However, compassionate patient-based care or interventional palliative care should never be presented as 'either or' options.

Many dying patients are not in a rush to die and their desire for life-prolonging treatments is often appropriate. Although the WHO definition of palliative care includes the statement that palliative 'intends neither to hasten nor postpone death', one must recognize that there is a difference between prolonging dying and prolonging a life in the face of incurable illness. Unfortunately, this is often confused, leading people to believe that non-curative disease-modifying drugs or other high-tech palliative interventions are not part of the palliative care. The consequence of this confusion is substantial: and indeed some patients are denied palliative care services because there are interested in these interventions or treatments, and others are denied access to treatments that would otherwise serve their goals of care because they are in a palliative care clinical pathway.

New challenges

Many of the service delivery models for palliative care were developed with the aim of offering a more cost-effective way of managing patients with incurable illness. Indeed, this was not only the advertised advantage, but programmes were budgeted based on assumptions of great savings for the health-care funders.

How are palliative care services, whose budgets are based on the assumption that palliative care is cheaper, going to manage with these new technologies? This is a major challenge that is not well answered. Many hospices are forced to limit or even preclude the accessibility to palliative interventions, many restrict access to patients who are no longer receiving disease-modifying treatments, some are financially compromised in their valiant attempts to provide all of the potentially helpful options for patients who are needing palliative care services over a longer time frame (by virtue of disease modification).

How different health-care systems cope with the changing face of palliative care is going to have to be part of the next edition. We don't yet have the answers.

In conclusion

Although we may now be professional carers, at some times in our lives our loved ones or we ourselves will be the people needing the care that we espouse and deliver. Professor Balfour Mount would express this in his widely quoted aphorism that 'we are all in the same boat'. As palliative carers too, we are all in the same boat: despite our varying settings and circumstances, we are challenged by the same spectrum of problems, challenges, and questions.

In this text you will find some of the answers to many of the questions. Humility demands that we recognize that, with what we know, not all of the questions can yet be answered. Indeed, often the best that can be offered is a range of suboptimal options to be considered and possibly tried on a sequential basis. This underlies the imperative to work together to push the boundaries of what we know, and how we apply it to the care of the incurably ill.

We hope that this Fourth Edition of the *Oxford Textbook of Palliative Medicine* will help in that endeavour.

SECTION 2

The worldwide status of palliative care

2.1

International progress in creating palliative medicine as a specialized discipline

David Clark

The mid-20th century saw some important changes occurring in Western medicine and health care. New specialties were advancing rapidly, innovative treatments were proliferating, and there was an increasing emphasis on the cure and rehabilitation of those with serious illness. Around the same time, death in the hospital, rather than at home, became more common in many societies, and in this setting, the dying patient or 'hopeless case' was often viewed as a failure of medical practice[1]. The focus of modern medicine moved farther away from the care of those at the end of life and appeared to be preoccupied with new interventions focused on cure rather than palliation.

These changes in medicine were accompanied, in many countries, by intense regulation of opioids in medical practice. Public policies contributed to the reality that many patients with cancer could not obtain adequate pain relief. Both doctors and patients were concerned about the possibility of addiction to opioids, and in some settings, the endurance of pain without resorting to powerful drugs was portrayed as a test of moral fortitude and an 'inevitable' aspect of advanced malignancy[2]. The development of pain management as a medical sub-specialty may have helped encourage a focus on procedures and de-emphasize the routine use of opioids, such as morphine. In many clinical settings around the world, the use of oral opioids for pain-related to advanced illness was impossible or considered a 'last resort'[3].

Although many of these concerns about the structures of care and the availability of opioid therapy for pain remain today, a small number of European and North American clinicians and researchers in the 1940s and 1950s did begin to show interest in the social and medical aspects of care for dying patients and in the different ways of understanding and relieving cancer pain. As a result, progress in 'whole person' care, specifically focused on populations with suffering related to serious and advanced illnesses, and improvements in the specific modalities of pain and symptom management, have been made.

In 1953, John Bonica published the first textbook of pain medicine, in which the role of morphine was reappraised. He wrote, '... in spite of what has been and will be said, it is my opinion that narcotic drugs, particularly morphine, when *properly used* have no pharmacological rivals in the management of intractable pain associated with inoperable disease'[4]. His groundbreaking work was followed by numerous studies of the problems experienced by patients and families affected by advanced disease, particularly cancer, and the insights that emerged from this work strongly influenced later activists in palliative care[5,6].

This momentum continued in the early 1960s, with studies on bereavement[7] and on terminal cancer at home[8,9], as well as in some key editorials that appeared in the *Lancet* [10] and the *British Medical Journal*[11]. Although these did much to raise interest in the problems of care for the dying, it was still the case, as the psychiatrist John Hinton noted, 'the large number of articles in which remembered experience is distilled into advice on the management of dying awesomely overshadows the few papers attempting to measure the degree of success or failure of treatment'[12]. Over time, however, there was a shift from 'anecdote to evidence' in publications about the care of the dying, and a research-based approach to improving care at the end of life began to be more visible[13]. Within a few years, there was also sociological interest in these issues, found in ethnographic studies of the care of the dying in American hospitals[14] and also in surveys of bereaved relatives who were asked about the experiences of the deceased person in the last year of life[15].

The rise of hospice and palliative care in a distinctly modern guise took place against this backdrop of modest, but growing, clinical, educational, and research interest[16]. It was in the late 1950s that the nurse, social worker, and physician, Dr Cicely Saunders, first began to play an instrumental role in establishing the modern science and art of caring for patients with advanced malignant disease. She founded the world's first modern hospice at St Christopher's in South London, which opened in 1967. Cicely Saunders focused her attention on patients in the final stages of cancer, especially those with the most complex problems, and she was key to defining a new knowledge base of care for those dying from malignancies.

The writings of Cicely Saunders relied heavily on individual patient experiences, and she was assiduous in collecting these. A report on a series of 340 cases in 1960[17] was followed by a report on 1100 by 1967[18]. A striking feature of her papers was their articulation of the relationship between physical and mental suffering.

This reached full expression in the concept of 'total pain'[19], which included physical distress, mental distress, social problems, and emotional difficulties, and captured so comprehensively by the patient who told her, 'All of me is wrong'[20]. Such ideas were also linked to a hard-headed approach to pain management. Her message was simple, 'constant pain needs constant control', and she argued for analgesics to be employed in a fixed scheduled dosing regimen, which would ensure that pain was prevented, rather than alleviated, once it had become established. She also advocated that analgesics be used progressively to address poorly controlled pain, culminating in the regular use of so-called strong opioids such as morphine. Against accepted wisdom, Saunders argued that the concern about the problem of addiction was misguided in this setting, and patients receiving such medications could live out their lives in comfort and quality. She also showed that opioids given orally were effective and they worked by relieving pain, not just by masking it. A lifelong opponent of euthanasia, she also pressed tirelessly for the proper relief of suffering without the hastening of death[21].

During this period in the late 1960s and early 1970s, parallel developments were taking place elsewhere. From the outset, ideas developed at St. Christopher's were applied differently in other places and contexts. Cicely Saunders was part of an international network of like-minded people in North America, India and Sri Lanka (then Ceylon), Australia, France, Switzerland, the Netherlands, and communist Poland, as revealed in her remarkable and extensive correspondence at the time[22]. It came to be accepted in several countries that the principles of hospice care for cancer patients could be practised in many settings, including specialist inpatient units and in home-care and day-care services. Likewise, hospital units and support teams, which brought the new thinking about the care of those with advanced malignant disease into the very heartlands of acute cancer medicine, were established.

In 1973, John Bonica hosted the first international pain meeting, providing a forum for debate, discussion, and the development of systems to improve pain relief in oncology and other fields[23]. Interaction between pain and 'terminal care' experts began to increase. In 1982, a meeting, which tackled the problem of cancer pain at the population level, was convened by Jan Stjernsward, Head of the World Health Organization (WHO) Cancer Unit[24]. Four years later, the WHO published its guide to cancer pain relief[25] with a view to relieving cancer pain worldwide by the early 21st century. In this guide, the clinical approach to cancer pain relief was conceptualized as a 'ladder,' with the regular administration of oral morphine as a linchpin of clinical practice. The WHO first endorsed a definition of palliative care created by a group of world leaders during an expert committee meeting in 1989[26]. The most recent definition[27] of palliative care to appear from the WHO is:

Palliative care is an approach that improves the quality of life of patients and their families facing the problems associated with life-threatening illness, through the prevention and relief of suffering by means of early identification and impeccable assessment and treatment of pain and other problems, physical, psychosocial, and spiritual.

Palliative care is generally defined as follows:

◆ Provides relief from pain and other distressing symptoms.

◆ Affirms life and regards dying as a normal process.

◆ Intends neither to hasten or postpone death.

◆ Integrates the psychological and spiritual aspects of patient care.

◆ Offers a support system to help patients live as actively as possible until death.

◆ Offers a support system to help the family cope during the patient's illness and in their own bereavement.

◆ Uses a team approach to address the needs of patients and their families, including bereavement counselling, if indicated.

◆ Enhances quality of life, and may also positively influence the course of illness.

◆ Is applicable early in the course of illness, in conjunction with other therapies that are intended to prolong life, such as chemotherapy or radiation therapy, and includes those investigations needed to better understand and manage distressing clinical complications.

These are large and complex claims, and there are concerns about the extent to which palliative care services are achieving them, either due to a lack of coverage or because the services do not have the capacity to deliver interdisciplinary care at this level of sophistication. There is growing evidence of increased palliative care development around the world, but progress is uneven and many regions are still underserved.

Around the world

In the wake of developments at the local level, and as hospice and palliative care services became established in individual countries, there quickly emerged a range of international associations created to promote and develop the work of hospice and palliative care, as well as the cognate field of pain medicine. These focused on professional development, education, and training; on clinical innovation and research; and on lobbying and advocacy. Table 2.1.1 contains a timeline of these international organizations and initiatives[28,29].

A comprehensive review of palliative care developments in some of the English-speaking countries (the United Kingdom, United States, Canada, Australia, and New Zealand), where progress has been most significant, acknowledges that each had different starting points for palliative care development, but 'in the longer run, most countries tend to develop a mix of independent, hospital-based, and community-based services'[30].

Hospice services in the United States grew dramatically from the first organization, which was opened in New Haven, Connecticut in 1974, to more than 3000 providers by the end of the 20th century. In 1982, a major milestone was achieved with the designation of hospice as an entitlement funded under the Federal Medicare programme. During the 1990s, two private foundations developed extensive programmes concerned with improving the culture of end-of-life care in American society. The Robert Wood Johnson Foundation created the Last Acts initiative and the Open Society Institute established the Project on Death in America. An influential report by the Institute of Medicine (IOM), published in 1997, sought to strengthen popular and professional understanding of the need for good care at the end of life and acknowledged the value of specialist recognition for palliative medicine[31]. In 2004, the National Institutes of Health held a 'State-of-the-Science' meeting

Table 2.1.1 Pan-national associations and initiatives in hospice and palliative care.

1973	International Association for the Study of Pain, founded Issaquah, Washington, USA
1976	1st International Congress on the Care of the Terminally Ill, Montreal, Canada
1977	Hospice Information Service, founded at St Christopher's Hospice, London, UK
1980	International Hospice Institute, became International Hospice Institute and College (1995) and International Association for Hospice and Palliative Care (1999)
1982	World Health Organization Cancer Pain Programme initiated
1988	European Association of Palliative Care founded in Milan, Italy
1998	Poznan Declaration leads to the foundation of the Eastern and Central European Palliative Task Force (1999)
1999	Foundation for Hospices in Sub-Saharan Africa founded in USA
2000	Latin American Association of Palliative care founded
2001	Asia Pacific Hospice Palliative Care Network founded
2002	UK Forum for Hospice and Palliative Care Worldwide founded by Help the Hospices
	Hospice Information Service re-launched as Hospice Information a joint venture between Help the Hospices and St Christopher's Hospice
2004	African Palliative Care Association founded
2005	First World Hospice and Palliative Care Day

on Improving End-of-Life Care, which brought together prominent clinicians and researchers to focus on defining and understanding major considerations related to end-of-life care, and developing interventions for symptom management, social and spiritual care, and caregiver support[32].

In neighbouring Canada, where Balfour Mount first coined the term 'palliative care' in 1974[33], a Senate report in 2000 stated that no extension of palliative care provision had occurred in the previous 5 years, and fewer than 5 per cent of people received such care. In response, the government set out recommendations for further development among the country's 600 services[34].

In Latin America, there was evidence of faltering progress. Palliative care services existed in seven countries, with the greatest development in Argentina[35]. A major problem there, as in other developing regions, was one of poor opioid availability, an issue highlighted in the 1994 Declaration of Florianopolis[36].

The first evidence of hospice developments in the Asia Pacific region came with a service for dying patients in Korea, at the Calvary Hospice of Kangung. This sole service was established by the Catholic Sisters of the Little Company of Mary in 1965, and had increased to 60 such services by 1999[37]. In Japan, the first hospice was also Christian, established in the Yodogwa Christian Hospital in 1973; by the end of the century, the country had 80 inpatient units[38]. In Australia, the country that established the world's first chair in palliative care, commonwealth and state funds increased steadily from 1980 onward, and by 2002, there were 250 designated palliative care services[39]. Although protocols for the WHO three-step analgesic ladder were first introduced into China in 1991, and there were said to be hundreds of palliative care services

in urban areas by 2002, little is actually known about the state of palliative care in the world's most populous country[40].

An extensive review of hospice and palliative care developments in India has mapped the existence of services state by state and explored the perspectives and experiences of those involved, with a view to stimulating development[41]. The study found that 135 hospice and palliative care services existed in 16 states. These were usually concentrated in large cities, with the exception of the state of Kerala, where services were much more widespread. Non-government organizations, and public and private hospitals and hospices, were the predominant sources of palliative care. Nevertheless, successful models exist in Kerala for the development of affordable, sustainable community-based hospice and palliative care services[42], and these may have potential for replication elsewhere.

A review of hospice and palliative care developments in Africa mapped the existence of services country by country and explored the perspectives and experiences of those involved[43]. No identified hospice or palliative care activity could be found in 21 countries; capacity-building activity was underway to promote hospice and palliative care delivery in 11 countries; localized provision of hospice and palliative care was in place in a further 11; and services were achieving some measure of integration with mainstream health care and gaining wider policy recognition in four countries. The authors concluded that models exist in Uganda, Kenya, South Africa, and Zimbabwe for the development of affordable, sustainable, community-based hospice and palliative care services, and the newly formed African Palliative Care Association has huge potential to promote innovation in a context where interest in the development of hospice and palliative care in Africa has never been greater.

In the former communist countries of Eastern Europe and Central Asia, there were few palliative care developments during the years of Soviet domination. Most initiatives can be traced to the early 1990s, after which many projects got underway. These have been documented in detail[44], and there is evidence of some service provision in 23 out of 28 countries in the region. Poland and Russia have the most advanced programmes of palliative care, with considerable achievements in Romania and Hungary as well. Nevertheless, in a region of over 400 million people, there were just 467 palliative care services in 2002, more than half of which were found in a single country, Poland.

Palliative care in Western Europe made rapid progress from the early 1980s, but even by the late 1990s, there were still striking variations in provision across countries[45]. After the founding of St Christopher's in England, in 1967, it was only a few years before the first services began to appear elsewhere: in Norway (1973), Sweden (1977), Italy (1980), Germany (1983), Spain (1984), Belgium (1985), France (1986), and the Netherlands (1991). In all of these countries, the provision of palliative care has moved beyond isolated examples of pioneering services run by enthusiastic founders and is being delivered in a variety of settings (domiciliary, quasi-domiciliary, and institutional), though these are not given uniform priority everywhere.

The Council of Europe published a set of guidelines on palliative care in 2003 and described it as an essential and basic service for the whole population[46]. Its recommendations appear to have been used quite actively in some countries with less-developed palliative care systems, particularly in Eastern Europe, where they have served as a tool for advocacy and lobbying. Policy issues relating

Table 2.1.2 Categorization of palliative care development (countries by group).

Group 4 Approaching integration N=35/234 (15%)	Argentina, Australia, Austria, Belgium, Canada, Chile, Costa Rica, Denmark, Finland, France, Germany, Hong Kong, Hungary, Iceland, Ireland, Israel, Italy, Japan, Kenya, Malaysia, Mongolia, New Zealand, Netherlands, Norway, Poland, Romania, Singapore, Slovenia, South Africa, Spain, Sweden, Switzerland, Uganda, United Kingdom, United States of America
Group 3 Localized provision N=80 (34%)	Aland Islands, Albania, Armenia, Azerbaijan, Bangladesh, Barbados, Belarus, Bermuda, Bosnia and Herzegovina, Botswana, Brazil, Bulgaria, Cameroon, Cayman Islands, China, Colombia, Congo, Croatia, Cuba, Cyprus, Czech Republic, Dominican Republic, Ecuador, Egypt, El Salvador, Estonia, Georgia, Gibraltar, Greece, Guadeloupe, Guatemala, Guernsey, Guyana, Honduras, India, Indonesia, Iraq, Isle of Man, Jamaica, Jersey, Jordan, Kazakhstan, Korea (South), Kyrgyzstan, Latvia, Lithuania, Luxembourg, Macao, Macedonia, Malawi, Malta, Mexico, Moldova, Morocco, Myanmar, Nepal, Nigeria, Pakistan, Panama, Peru, Philippines, Portugal, Russia, Saudi Arabia, Serbia, Sierra Leone, Slovakia, Sri Lanka, Swaziland, Tanzania, Thailand, The Gambia, Trinidad and Tobago, Ukraine, Uruguay, United Arab Emirates, Venezuela, Viet Nam, Zambia Zimbabwe
Group 2 Capacity building N=41 (18%)	Algeria, Bahrain, Belize, Bolivia, British Virgin Islands, Brunei, Cambodia, Democratic Republic of Congo, Cote d'Ivoire, Dominica, Ethiopia, Fiji, Ghana, Haiti, Holy See (Vatican), Iran, Kuwait, Lebanon, Lesotho, Madagascar, Mauritius, Mozambique, Namibia, Nicaragua, Oman, Palestinian Authority, Papua New Guinea, Paraguay, Qatar, Reunion, Rwanda, Saint Lucia, Seychelles, Sudan, Suriname, Tajikistan, The Bahamas, Tunisia, Turkey, Uzbekistan, Puerto Rico
Group 1 No known activity N=78 (33%)	Afghanistan, American Samoa, Andorra, Angola, Anguilla, Antigua and Barbuda, Aruba, Benin, Bhutan, Burkina Faso, Burundi, Cape Verdi, Central African Republic, Chad, Comoros, Cook Islands, Djibouti, Equatorial Guinea, Eritrea, Falkland Islands, Faroe Islands, French Guiana, French Polynesia, Gabon, Greenland, Grenada, Guam, Guinea, Guinea-Bissau, Kiribati, Korea (DPR), Laos, Liberia, Libya, Liechtenstein, Maldives, Mali, Marshall Islands, Martinique, Mauritania, Mayotte, Micronesia, Monaco, Montenegro, Montserrat, Nauru, Netherlands Antilles, New Caledonia, Niger, Niue, Norfolk Island, Northern Mariana Islands, Palau, Pitcairn, Saint Helena, Saint Kits and Nevis, Saint Pierre and Miquelon, Saint Vincent and the Grenadines, Samoa, San Marino, Sao Tome and Principe, Senegal, Solomon Islands, Somalia, Svalbard, Syria, Timor-Leste, Togo, Tokelau, Tonga, Turkmenistan, Turks and Caicos Islands, Tuvalu, U.S. Virgin Islands, Vanuatu, Wallis and Fortuna, Western Sahara, Yemen

Source: Wright *et al.*, (2008).

to end-of-life care in Europe also have been raised by other non-governmental and inter-governmental organizations. At palliative care conferences in 1995 (Barcelona)[47] and 1998 (Poznan)[48], exhortatory declarations were made, calling for government action on palliative care at the national level and drawing attention to key problems and issues facing palliative care as it developed internationally. By 2003, the European Society for Medical Oncology[49] was giving greater recognition to palliative care. In 2004, the European Federation of Older Persons launched a campaign to make palliative care a priority topic on the European health agenda[50]. The same year, WHO Europe produced an important document on *Better Palliative Care for Older People*. Its aim was 'to incorporate palliative care for serious chronic progressive illnesses within ageing policies, and to promote better care toward the end of life'[51]. Its companion volume, *Palliative Care: The Solid Facts* is a resource for policy makers in a context where 'the evidence available on palliative care is not complete and ... there are differences in what can be offered across the European region'[52]. In 2007, a set of 'commitments' for palliative care improvement was entered into by palliative care associations at the Budapest Congress of the European Association for Palliative Care[53]. Despite the powerful symbolic language of these and other documents, however, evidence of their impact remains unclear[54].

A study conducted in 2006 by the International Observatory on End of Life Care[55] categorized hospice–palliative care development in every country of the world, using the United Nations listing of 234 countries. The study used a four-part typology to describe the level of hospice–palliative care in each country: (1) no known hospice–palliative care activity, (2) capacity-building activity but no services yet operational, (3) countries with localized hospice–palliative care provision, and (4) countries where hospice

and palliative care activities are approaching integration with mainstream health-care providers. In total, 115 of the world's 234 countries have established one or more hospice–palliative care service. Yet only 35 (15 per cent) countries have achieved a measure of integration with other mainstream service providers together with wider policy recognition. In 78 (33 per cent) countries, no palliative care activity can be identified. Table 2.1.2 lists all countries by group.

Specialty recognition

The published literature contains a small, but growing, comparative perspective on hospice and palliative care developments in different regions of the world[56,57]. It appears that the global categorization of palliative care development is closely correlated with the state of palliative medicine as a field of specialization at the country level. The 35 countries with the highest level of palliative care development are also those in which the most substantial strides have been made towards specialty recognition for palliative medicine. The International Observatory on End of Life Care archives contain evidence of just 17 countries worldwide that have established palliative medicine as a specialty or sub-specialty (see Table 2.1.3). Within this group, there is considerable variation in the procedures that govern specialty status.

The designation of palliative medicine as a specialty or sub-specialty in a country does not mean that there is a uniform 'currency' of specialization for the field. Health-care systems differ considerably in how they accredit medical practitioners, and especially in their accreditation of specialist training, and this is reflected in the recognition of palliative medicine in different places. There are also resource implications, which affect how training is supported,

Table 2.1.3 Countries with palliative medicine as a specialty or sub-specialty.

UK	1987
Ireland	1995
Hong Kong	1998
Poland	1999
Romania	2000
New Zealand	2001
Germany	2006
Latvia	2005
Australia	2005
Czech Republic	2005
Malaysia	2005
Slovakia	2005
Argentina	2006
USA	2006
Georgia	2007
France	2007
Philippines	NK

although these do not explain the wide variations in length of training that can be observed.

Centeno et al.[58] reported on a survey of palliative medicine specialization in the WHO European region, covering 52 countries. They found that palliative medicine has official certification in just seven European countries. Full specialty status exists in the United Kingdom (1987) and Ireland (1995). In other countries, palliative medicine is regarded as a sub-specialty, which consists of a second specialization following certification in a full specialty; this is the case in Poland (1999), Romania (2000), Slovakia (2005), Germany (2006), and France (2007). In nine other countries, there was evidence of discussion and actions in process relating to certification in palliative medicine. In the Czech Republic, Norway, and Sweden, the certification process is at an advanced stage of development; in the Czech Republic, the plans are for a specialty in palliative medicine and pain management. The process of certification has also started in Finland, Iceland, and Spain. In Latvia, palliative medicine is certified as a specific area, but work is being carried out to achieve sub-specialty certification. In Spain, the relevant qualification will follow certification in another specialty and is referred to as a 'specific area of competency'.

Elsewhere in Europe, progress toward specialization is less clear but there is information to show that there are at least postgraduate courses or university diplomas in Italy, Lithuania, Portugal, Belgium, Bosnia and Herzegovina, Estonia, Georgia, Hungary, and Luxembourg. The Nordic Specialist Course in Palliative Medicine, begun in 2001, brings together five countries, is a particularly sophisticated example of its type, and is a likely precursor to specialty recognition[59].

The status of palliative medicine and its development at the country level remains rather under-documented in the published literature. Problems in understanding this history are also compounded by the fact that some authors have restricted their focus to *palliative medicine* (as is the purpose here), whereas others have attended more generally to the development of palliative care. The development of palliative medicine has been described in more detail for a small number of countries and is reviewed here.

In the United Kingdom, three factors conjoined in the 1980s to build a platform for the broad consolidation of the new field of activity: a medical association was formed to support its practitioners; a scientific journal was established; and recognition was given to palliative medicine as an area of specialization—the first country in the world to do so[60]. In 1987, palliative medicine was established as a sub-specialty of general medicine, initially on a 7-year 'novitiate,' which when successfully concluded, led to the creation of a specialty in its own right. Indeed, the specialty broke new ground in accepting as an appropriate qualification for entry, membership of the Royal Colleges of Physicians, Radiology, and Anaesthetics. Initially, membership of the Royal College of General Practitioners was not recognized as a mode of entry, though considerable protest and further campaigning led to its recognition within a few years. In 1987, all doctors working full time in hospices were granted specialist registration. Thereafter, entrants into higher medical training for the new specialty were required to be Members of the Royal Colleges of Physicians, General Practitioners or Psychiatrists, or Fellows of the Royal College of Surgeons. This was modified in 2002 to include Members of the Irish College of General Practitioners and Fellows of the Royal Colleges of Radiologists and Anaesthetists. The 4-year training programme in the United Kingdom was designed to equip trainees with skills to practice palliative medicine in any setting. The training generally includes at least 2 years within specialist palliative care teams—hospice- or hospital-based—combined with a range of relevant training in chronic pain management, oncology, community services, or paediatric palliative care. Importantly, United Kingdom programmes also require competence in a range of essential management skills, including recruiting and managing staff, and service development. In 2005, it was noted that 'In practice, most recruits into the specialty today have had several years' experience in general medicine, oncology, or radiotherapy, after gaining their higher qualification, but only a few have had experience of specialist palliative medicine as a senior house officer (SHO)[61]. In 2007, Professor John Tooke's inquiry into medical careers recommended that medical training should consist of: (1) one foundation year (similar to house officer year), (2) 3 years of general training in a broad mix of specialties, and (3) followed by 4 to 5 years in higher specialist training. Progression through the three stages will require achievement of competencies and will involve selection—and this will become the new framework for those training in palliative medicine.

Developments in Ireland took a similar path when, in 1989, the first post of consultant physician in palliative medicine was created in Dublin. Then, in the mid-1990s, the Irish Medical Council considered the inclusion of palliative medicine in its list of recognized specialties. Such recognition required evidence of a significant corpus of knowledge specific to palliative medicine, over and above that which would be within the competence of any registered medical practitioner, as well as the existence of a recognized body to oversee developments in the new specialty, including training and education. The Minister for Health and Children approved the inclusion of palliative medicine amongst the list of recognized Irish medical specialties in June 1995[62].

Hong Kong recognized palliative medicine as a specialty in 1998, under the Hong Kong College of Physicians of the Academy of Medicine. The training consists of a 4-year dual-accreditation programme in conjunction with internal medicine[63]. Palliative medicine as a medical sub-specialty was introduced in Poland in 1999; it takes 2 years to complete the training at one of the 14 centres with specialist accreditation[64]. In the following year, full specialty recognition was given to palliative medicine in Romania. Here, the training requires completion of a 12-week course (8 weeks' theory and 4 weeks' clinical practice)[65].

The Royal Australasian College of Physicians (RACP) established a pathway for sub-specialty training in palliative medicine in 1991, with a 3-year training programme. But as palliative medicine was not on the federal government's list of medical specialties, the fellows emerging from the programme were classified as specialists in General Medicine. In 1999, a Chapter of Palliative Medicine was created within the Adult Medical Division of the RACP, again with its own training pathway and in order to create a second entry point to specialist training, this one with a 2-year training programme. The result was that all doctors, whether new graduates or specialist practitioners, had a defined pathway into specialized training in palliative medicine. This quickly led to specialty recognition in New Zealand, which was achieved in 2001. In Australia, the process proved longer and more complex, culminating in recognition of the new specialty by the Minister for Health in 2005[66].

Palliative medicine was recognized in Slovakia as a sub-specialty beginning in January 2005. At the beginning of 2006, The Federal Medical Chamber in Germany passed a new regulation for sub-specialization in palliative medicine under the control of the Board of Palliative Medicine, which requires 6 months of practice in a palliative medicine unit[67].

The development of palliative medicine in the United States has been seen in three phases[68]: (1) the period until the work of Elizabeth Kubler Ross and Cicely Saunders became known, (2) the development of hospice programmes across the country, and (3) the development of a distinct and officially recognized sub-specialty of medicine. Within this scheme, the path to sub-specialty recognition for palliative medicine in the United States began in 1988 with the creation of the Academy of Hospice Physicians, later the American Academy of Hospice and Palliative Medicine. Further progress was made in the 1990s when the Institute of Medicine, the American College of Physicians, and the American Board of Internal Medicine all highlighted the need for greater physician competency in the care of persons with terminal illness. In 2006, the Accreditation Council for Graduate Medical Education (ACGME) and the American Board of Medical Specialties (ABMS) approved and recognized a new specialty in hospice and palliative medicine. This has led to a transition in the physician certification process from the independent American Board of Hospice and Palliative Medicine to the ABMS, and a transition in the accreditation of training programmes from another independent organization to the ACGME[69]. In this process, hospice and palliative medicine has become a sub-specialty of no fewer than 11 primary specialties, a first in the history of the ABMS. Formal certification of physicians and accreditation of training programmes begin in 2008.

There are some major anomalies in how palliative medicine is recognized and accredited. Canada is a country that has played a major role in the development of modern palliative care, but yet has not attained specialty status for palliative medicine, to serious detrimental effect, in the eyes of at least one senior commentator[70]. Another senior figure in the field maintains that the question of whether to seek specialty or sub-specialty status can only be decided at the country level, but notes that the only countries where palliative medicine has made much impact on professional education and clinical practice are those where physicians are working full time in the field, whether or not specialty recognition exists[71].

At the same time, specialty recognition can be seen as a turning point in hospice and palliative care history[72]. It has been noted that 'the original heated debate that accompanied the development of palliative medicine as a medical specialty in the United Kingdom in 1987 has continued in all other countries where the effort has been made to develop the specialty'[73]. For some, specialization is seen as the key to integration of palliative care into the mainstream health system and a major platform from which to develop an evidence-based model of practice that is crucial to long-term viability. Others appear concerned that specialization will bring about an overemphasis on physical symptoms at the expense of psychosocial and spiritual concerns. There have been claims that forces of medicalization and routinization[74] are at work, or even that the 'holism' of palliative care philosophy masks a new, more subtle form of surveillance of the dying and bereaved in modern society[75]. Even in the early 1990s, a palliative medicine physician could raise concerns about a specialty narrowly bounded by the practice of 'symptomatology' and thereby failing to create the conditions for deeper, personal 'healing'[76].

As the specialty develops, its medical attention tends to focus on pain and symptom management as a set of problems within the relief of suffering—giving weight to the charge of creeping medicalization. At the same time, it is precisely in this biomedical area of palliative care that measurable and striking successes are to be found in the use of pain-relieving and symptom-controlling technologies, some of which seem to have not yet percolated into the wider health-care system.

One theme that can be identified across all of these developments is the recognition that palliative care is an area of medicine for which the health-care system as a whole should take responsibility. This finds its most articulate expression in the concept that palliative care should be seen as a *public health issue*[77] and the knowledge and skills of palliative care must be translated into evidence-based, cost-effective interventions, which can reach everyone in the population. To be effective, this requires governments to adopt policies in support of palliative care at all appropriate levels of the health-care system and for these policies to have community support and endorsement. The WHO has been the most powerful advocate of this approach, though it now finds favour with palliative care experts in many contexts.

It has been suggested that palliative medicine has the advantage of being a new and emerging specialty, relatively unencumbered by vested interests, and capable of avoiding the mistakes sometimes made in other areas of medicine, in particular, the risk of achieving a lot for a few; however, the needs of the majority remain unmet[78]. For such an approach, it is important that we have a worldwide perspective, accompanied by specific knowledge of local problems and issues and how they might be overcome. Careful thought also needs to be given to the contribution that specialization in palliative medicine can make to the global need for appropriate care of those with advanced disease and those facing death. The fate of palliative medicine is only one of the factors that will determine how dying people are cared for, both now and in the future.

References

1. Gavey, C.J. (1952). *The management of the "hopeless" case*. H.K. Lewis, London.

2. Seymour, J. and Clark, D. (2005). The modern history of morphine use in cancer pain. *European Journal of Palliative Care*, 12(4), 152–5.

3. Baszanger, I. (1998). Inventing pain medicine. *From the laboratory to the clinic*. Rutgers University Press, New Brunswick.

4. Bonica, J.J. (1953). *The management of pain: with special emphasis on the use of analgesic block in diagnosis, prognosis and therapy*. Henry Kimpton, London.

5. Bailey, M. (1959). A survey of the social needs of patients with incurable lung cancer. *The Almoner*, 11(10), 379–97.

6. Aitken-Swan, J. and Paterson, R. (1955). The cancer patient: delay in help seeking. *British Medical Journal*, March 12, 623–31.

7. Murray Parkes, C. (1964). Recent bereavement as a cause of mental illness. *British Journal of Psychiatry*, 110, 198–204.

8. Wilkes, E. (1964). Cancer outside hospital. *The Lancet*, June 20, 1379–81.

9. Wilkes, E. (1965). Terminal cancer at home. *The Lancet*, April 10, 799–801.

10. Leading article. (1961). Euthanasia. *The Lancet*, August 12, 351–2.

11. Leading article. (1963). Distress in dying. *British Medical Journal*, August 17, 400–1.

12. Hinton, J. (1965). Problems in the care of the dying. *Journal of Chronic Diseases*, 17, 201–5.

13. Clark, D. (1999). Cradled to the grave? Pre-conditions for the hospice movement in the UK, 1948–67. *Mortality*, 4(3), 225–47.

14. Glaser, B. and Strauss, A. (1965). *Awareness of dying*, Aldine, Chicago, Il.

15. Cartwright, A., Hockey, J., and Anderson, J.L. (1973). *Life before death*. Routledge, London.

16. Clark, D. (2002). Between hope and acceptance: the medicalisation of dying. *British Medical Journal*, 324, 905–7.

17. Saunders, C. (1960). Drug treatment of patients in the terminal stages of cancer. *Current Medicine and Drugs*, 1(1) July, 16–28.

18. Saunders, C. (1967). The care of the terminal stages of cancer. *Annals of the Royal College of Surgeons*, 41 (Supplementary issue Summer), 162–9.

19. Clark, D. (1999). 'Total pain', disciplinary power and the body in the work of Cicely Saunders 1958–67. *Social Science and Medicine*, 49(6), 727–36.

20. Saunders, C. (1964). The symptomatic treatment of incurable malignant disease. *Prescriber's Journal*, 4(4), 68–73.

21. Saunders, C. (1975). (Member of Church of England Board of Social Responsibility Working Party) *On dying well: An Anglican contribution to the debate on euthanasia*. Church Information Office, London.

22. Clark, D. (2002). *Cicely Saunders Founder of the hospice movement, selected letters 1959–999*, Oxford University Press, Oxford.

23. Seymour, J., Clark, D., and Winslow, M. (2005). Pain and palliative care: the emergence of new specialties. *Journal of Pain and Symptom Management*, 29(1), 2–13.

24. Meldrum, M. (2005). The ladder and the clock: cancer pain and public policy at the end of the twentieth century. *Journal of Pain and Symptom Management*, 29(1), 41–54.

25. World Health Organization. (1986). *Cancer pain relief*. World Health Organization, Geneva.

26. World Health Organization. (1990). *Cancer pain relief and palliative care*. WHO Technical Report Series 804. World Health Organization, Geneva.

27. Sepúlveda, C., Marlin, A., Yoshida, T. *et al.* (2002). Palliative care: The World Health Organization's global perspective. *Journal of Pain and Symptom Management*, 24(2), 91–6.

28. http://www.library.ucla.edu/libraries/biomed/his/painexhibit/panel10.htm, accessed 6 November 2007.

29. Richardson, H., Praill, D., and Jackson, A. (2002). The UK Forum for Hospice and Palliative Care Overseas. *European Journal of Palliative Care*, 9(2), 72–3.

30. Lewis, M. (2007). *Medicine and the care of the dying. A modern history* p.157, Oxford University Press, New York.

31. Field, M.J. and Cassel, C.K. (eds.) (1997). *Approaching death. Improving care at the end of life*. National Academy Press, Washington.

32. Grady, P.A. (2005). Introduction: Papers from the National Institutes of Health State-of- the Science Conference on Improving End of Life Care. *Journal of Palliative Medicine*, 8 (Suppl 1), s-1–s-3.

33. Mount, B. (1997). The Royal Victoria Hospital Palliative Care Service: a Canadian experience. In *Hospice Care on the International Scene* (eds. C. Saunders and R. Kastenbaum), Springer, New York.

34. Carstairs, S. and Chochinov, H. (2001). Politics, palliation and Canadian progress in end-of-life care. *Journal of Palliative Medicine*, 4(3), 396–69.

35. De Lima, L. (2001). Advances in palliative care in Latin America and the Caribbean: ongoing projects of the Pan American Health Association (PAHO). *Journal of Palliative Medicine*, 4(2), 228–31.

36. Stjernswärd, J., Bruera, E., Joranson, D. *et al.* (1995). Opioid availability in Latin America: The Declaration of Florianopolis. *Journal of Pain and Symptom Management*, 10(3), 233–6.

37. Chung, Y. (1999). Palliative care in Korea: a nursing point of view. *Progress in Palliative Care*, 8(1), 12–16.

38. Maruyama, T.C. (1999). *Hospice care and culture*. Ashgate, Aldershot.

39. Hunt, R., Fazekas, B.S., Luke, C.G. *et al.* (2002). The coverage of cancer patients by designated palliative services: a population-based study, South Australia, 1999. *Palliative Medicine*, 16, 403–9.

40. Wang, X.S., Yu, S., Gu, W. *et al.* (2002). China: status of pain and palliative care. *Journal of Pain and Symptom Management*, 24(2), 177–9.

41. McDermott, E., Selman, L., Wright, M. *et al.* (2006). Hospice and palliative care development in India. Poster presented at the 4th Research Congress of the European Association for Palliative Care, Venice.

42. Shabeer, C. and Kumar, S. (2005). Palliative care in the developing world: a social experiment in India. *European Journal of Palliative Care*, 13(2), 76–79.

43. Wright, M. and Clark, D. (2006). *Hospice and palliative care development in Africa. A review of developments and challenges*. Oxford University Press, Oxford.

44. Clark, D. and Wright, M. (2003). *Transitions in end of life care. Hospice and related developments in Eastern Europe and Central Asia*. Open University Press, Buckingham.

45. Have, H. and Clark, D. (eds.) (2002). *The ethics of palliative care. European perspectives*. Open University Press, Buckingham.

46. Recommendation Rec. (2003). 24 of the Committee of Ministers to member states on the Organization of palliative care and explanatory memorandum (adopted by the Committee of Ministers on 12 November 2003 at the 860th meeting of the Ministers' Deputies).

47. Barcelona Declaration on Palliative Care. (1995). *European Journal of Palliative Care*, 3(1), 15.

48. Poznan Declaration. (1998). *European Journal of Palliative Care*, 6(2), 61–65.

49. Cherny, N.I., Catane, R., and Kosmidis, P. (2003). ESMO takes a stand on supportive and palliative care. *Annals of Oncology*, 14(9), 1335–7.

50. See: http://www.eurag-europe.org/palliativ-en.htm, accessed 6 November 2007.

51. Davies, E. and Higginson, I.J. (eds.) (2004). *Better palliative care for older people*. World Health Organization, Copenhagen.

52. Davies, E. and Higginson, I.J. (eds.) (2004). *Palliative care: The solid facts*. World Health Organization, Copenhagen.

53. Radbruch, Foley, L., De Lima *et al.* (2007). The Budapest Commitments: setting the goals. A joint initiative by the European Association for Palliative Care, the International Association for Hospice and Palliative Care and Help the Hospices. *Palliative Medicine*, 21(4), 269–71.

54. Clark, D. and Centeno, C. (2006). Palliative care in Europe: an emerging approach to comparative analysis. *Clinical Medicine*, 6(2), 197–201.

55. Wright, M., Wood, J., Lynch, T. *et al.* (2008). Mapping levels of palliative care development: A global view. *Journal of Pain and Symptom Management*, 35(5), 469–85.

56. Saunders, C. and Kastenbaum, R., (eds.) (1997). *Hospice care on the international scene*. Springer, New York.

57. Bingley, A.F. and Clark, D. (forthcoming). *Palliative Care Developments in the region represented by the Middle East Cancer Consortium: A review and comparative analysis*. National Cancer Institute: Bethesda, MD.

58. Centeno, C., Noguera, A., Lynch, T. *et al.* (2008). Official certification of doctors working in palliative medicine in Europe: data from an EAPC study in 52 European countries. *Palliative Medicine*, **21**, 683–7.

59. http://www.dspam.suite.dk/nordicprogram2007–09.pdf, accessed 6 November 2007.

60. Clark, D. (2006). The development of palliative medicine in the UK and Ireland. In *Textbook of palliative medicine* (eds. E. Bruera, I. Higginson, C. Ripamonti, *et al.*), pp. 3–9. Hodder Arnold, London.

61. Doyle, D. (2005). Palliative medicine: the first 18 years of a new sub-specialty of General Medicine. *Journal of the Royal College of Physicians of Edinburgh*, **35**, 199–205.

62. O'Brien, T. and Clark, D. (2005). A national plan for palliative care – the Irish experience. In *Palliative care in Ireland* (eds. J. Ling and L. O'Siorain), pp. 3–18. Open University Press, Maidenhead.

63. Hoy, A.M. (2004). Training specialists in palliative medicine. In *Oxford textbook of palliative medicine* (eds. D. Doyle, G. Hanks, N. Cherny, *et al.*), pp. 1167–8. Oxford University Press, Oxford.

64. Centeno, C., Noguera, A., Lynch, T. *et al.* (2008). Official certification of doctors working in palliative medicine in Europe: data from an EAPC study in 52 European countries. *Palliative Medicine*, **21**, 683–7.

65. Centeno, C., Noguera, A., Lynch T. *et al.* (2008). Official certification of doctors working in palliative medicine in Europe: data from an EAPC study in 52 European countries. *Palliative Medicine*, **21**, 683–7.

66. Cairns, W. (2007). A short history of palliative medicine in Australia. *Cancer Forum*, **31**(1), 6–9.

67. Centeno, C., Noguera, A., Lynch, T. *et al.* (2008). Official certification of doctors working in palliative medicine in Europe: data from an EAPC study in 52 European countries. *Palliative Medicine*, **21**, 683–7.

68. Ryndes, T. and von Gunten, C.F. The development of palliative medicine in the USA. In *Textbook of palliative medicine* (eds. E. Bruera, I. Higginson, C. Ripamonti, *et al.*), pp. 29–35. Hodder Arnold, London.

69. Schonwetter, R. (2006). Hospice and palliative medicine goes mainstream. *Journal of Palliative Medicine*, **9**(6), 1240–2.

70. Macdonald, N. (2006). The development of palliative care in Canada. In *Textbook of palliative medicine* (eds. E. Bruera, I. Higginson, C. Ripamonti, *et al.*), pp. 22–8. Hodder Arnold, London.

71. Doyle, D. (1997). Palliative medicine training for physicians. *Journal of Neurology*, **24** (Suppl 4), S26–S29.

72. Fordham, S., Dowrick, C., and May, C. (1998). Palliative medicine: is it really specialist territory? *Journal of the Royal Society of Medicine*, **91**, 568–72.

73. Bruera, E. and Pace, E.A. (2006). Palliative care versus palliative medicine. In *Textbook of palliative medicine* (eds. E. Bruera, I. Higginson, C. Ripamonti, *et al.*), pp. 64–7. Hodder Arnold, London.

74. Hoy, A. (1999). Routinisation and medicalisation. *European Journal of Palliative Care*, **6**, 178.

75. Clark, D. (1999). 'Total pain', disciplinary power and the body in the work of Cicely Saunders, 1958–1967. *Social Science and Medicine*, **49**, 727–36.

76. Kearney, M. (1992). Palliative medicine – just another specialty? *Palliative Medicine*, **6**, 39–46.

77. Stjernsward, J., Foley, K.M., Ferris, F.D. *et al.* (2007). The public health strategy for palliative care. *Journal of Pain and Symptom Management*, **33**(5), 486–93.

78. Stjernsward, J. and Clark, D. (2003). Palliative medicine – a global perspective. In *Oxford textbook of palliative medicine* (eds. D. Doyle, G.W.C. Hanks, N. Cherny, *et al.*), (2003), 3rd edition. pp. 1199–224. Oxford University Press, Oxford.

2.2

Lessons learned from hospice in the United States of America

Stephen R. Connor and Perry G. Fine

Introduction

Hospice care in the USA is both envied and criticized. It is an experiment that continues to evolve. What began as a version of inpatient hospice care transplanted from the St Christopher's Hospice model in the United Kingdom is now a large health-care system that greatly emphasizes home care rather than inpatient care. Although the establishment of the federal Medicare Hospice Benefit in 1982 was followed by enormous growth, the benefit has been a two-edged sword for hospice. It is an economic engine, and at the same time, a self-limiting mechanism.

This chapter explores the history of hospice in the USA within the broader context of palliative care. It describes the growth and development of hospice as a health-care system, provides details about its regulation and economics, and presents its major challenges, both present and future.

History of hospice care in the USA

The seeds of hospice care in the USA were planted through a series of lectures given by Dame Cicely Saunders at the invitation of Florence Wald, then Dean of the School of Nursing at Yale University. These visits led to the founding of the first hospice in the USA in 1971. This first hospice, located in New Haven, Connecticut, began by providing home care services in 1973 and later built a large inpatient facility in Branford[1]. For the next several years, the idea of hospice care spread throughout the USA, and by 1980 there were 138 hospice programmes providing care across the country. All of these early programmes were small not-for-profit groups that mainly delivered home care to small numbers of patients and families, primarily in suburbs and generally well-resourced communities.

This critical mass began to be large enough to call itself a movement, which led to the formation of the National Hospice Organization in 1978. In 1979, the first hospice standards were published and the first large meeting of hospice leaders in Washington, DC occurred. The newly formed association saw its major task as growing hospice care throughout the USA. They recognized that for hospice programmes to continue to grow, a reliable source of funding would be necessary. There was considerable support from both legislators and government agencies to find a way for hospice to succeed, but little was known about how hospice care should be organized, delivered, and funded.

The Health Care Finance Administration (subsequently renamed the Centers for Medicare and Medicaid Services), a branch of the United States Department of Health, Education and Welfare (subsequently renamed the Department of Health and Human Services), agreed to allow a national hospice demonstration project to capture essential information on costs and services. Twenty-six hospices were selected to participate in the project and were reimbursed for their services. At the conclusion of the demonstration project, government and hospice representatives believed that they had a model for how hospice care could be organized and funded, and a bill was introduced to Congress to create a new Medicare entitlement for hospice care.

While developing this legislation, there was much negotiation and compromise. To gain reimbursement for care, hospices were forced to accept a number of provisions that had not been a part of how hospice in the USA had operated up to that point. Following this legislation, patients had to be certified by two physicians as having a life expectancy of 6 months or less, they could not receive both palliative and curative care simultaneously, they had to sign a consent indicating that they understood that they were receiving palliative and not curative care, and the benefit was limited to a total of 7 months. A sunset provision required that the Congressional Budget Office report on the impact of hospice care in 7 years and that Congress would have to pass a new law to make the benefit permanent based on the outcomes of the report.

In an interesting footnote to this history, the restriction on curative treatment was a demand of then President Ronald Reagan's budget director David Stockman who was concerned that providing both palliative and curative care would be too expensive. Contrasting with this administrative regulation, the original US hospice standards described hospice care as providing 'appropriate therapy', which is 'always a mixture of palliative and curative therapies'.

The Medicare Hospice Benefit became law in 1982 and the first hospices were certified by Medicare in 1983. It was slow going at first. Most hospices in the USA were ambivalent about receiving government reimbursement for care. Many opposed the benefit, fearing that government payment and regulations would ruin the spirit of hospice care that had been so carefully nurtured in the early formative years. Ten years would pass before hospice would embrace the benefit as a mechanism for growth. Many programmes were content to remain small and selective in delivering hospice care.

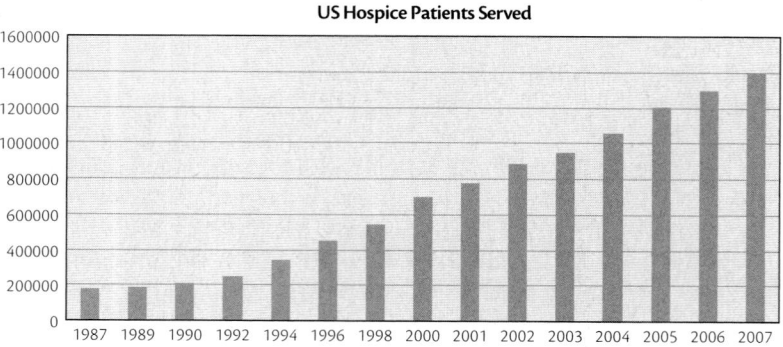

Figure 2.2.1 Hospice patients served in the USA, 1987–2007. *Source:* National Hospice and Palliative Care Organization, used with permission.

Hospice care has grown in the last 26 years from a small and insignificant part of the US health-care system to the fastest growing sector of the Medicare budget. The National Hospice and Palliative Care Organization (NHPCO), formerly the National Hospice Organization, estimates that there were 177 000 patients served in 1987 and 20 years later, in 2007, there were more than 1.4 million hospice patients served (Fig. 2.2.1)[2].

Medicare, which is the federally funded health-care programme for individuals who are 65 years and older or who are disabled, is the largest payer of hospice care in the USA. In 2007, total payments for hospice care under Medicare exceeded $10 billion. Approximately 84 per cent of hospice patients have Medicare as their primary insurance and Medicare pays for 87 per cent of hospice days of care. Medicare, however, is not the only payer of hospice care. The remaining payment sources include Medicaid (a state-run health-care programme for the poor who are not yet eligible for Medicare), which accounts for about 5 per cent of payments, and a variety of private insurance programmes, which also account for about 5 per cent of payments[2].

Hospice care under the Medicare model, which is emulated by Medicaid and many private payers, is a capitated system in which programmes are paid one of four per diem payments for each day of patient enrolment, depending on the care provided to the patient. The levels of care, their definitions, and national averages of utilization are summarized in Table 2.2.1. Payment rates for these levels of care are indexed annually and are adjusted for urban areas with higher salary costs. There are additional payment rules

including a requirement that no more than 20 per cent of days can be at the inpatient level of care and a cap that limits total payments to a hospice provider based on an annually adjusted amount.

Challenges for hospice and palliative care in the USA

Determining prognosis

According to Medicare regulations, eligibility for initial hospice admission requires that two physicians attest that the terminal illness has a prognosis of 6 months or less if the disease runs its normal course. After admission to the programme, recertification of prognosis is required by one physician at defined intervals (after each of two initial 90-day benefit periods, and then after each of an unlimited number of subsequent 60-day periods). Given the biases and limitations of the art of physician prognostication[4], determining this 6-month eligibility for hospice care is a significant medical and emotional challenge.

This challenge may relate to the perception that acknowledging a limited prognosis will have adverse outcomes. This perception, which may be expressed by patients and families, and by health professionals as well, is not supported by empirical data. Studies on the impact of truth telling have never found evidence that it hastens death. On the contrary, appropriate candor often helps patients overcome a growing sense of lonely apprehension[5]. More recent evidence[6] shows that hospice enrolment may increase survival for

Table 2.2.1 Hospice care under the Medicare model.

Level of care	Definition	National averages of utilization	Payment rate*
Routine Home Care	Patients in personal residence, nursing home, or assisted living facility receiving routine home care	96 per cent of patient days	$139.97 per diem
Continuous Home Care	Patients during periods of crisis in lieu of hospitalization, from 8 to 24 h of (nursing) care provided in the home setting for brief periods	<1 per cent of patient days	$34.4/h
General Inpatient Care	Short-term inpatient care when symptom management or other medical care cannot be accomplished in another setting, or when there is a breakdown of home-based caregiving	3 per cent of patient days	$622.66 per diem
Inpatient Respite Care	Up to 5 days' inpatient care solely to provide a break to caregivers	<1 per cent of patient days	$144.79 per diem

*For the 2008/2009 Federal fiscal year. National averages adjusted by CBSA.

some patients, perhaps due to more consistent monitoring or less exposure to the hazards of over treatment.

From the medical perspective, the ability to accurately prognosticate survival is limited, particularly for diseases other than cancer and for periods beyond a few weeks[4]. In the mid-1990s, the National Hospice Organization published guidelines for determining life expectancy for cancer and several non-cancer disease states as a way of providing hospices and referring physicians a rudimentary means of screening patients. The goal was to tap clinical experience and provide a response to the question, 'Is this patient more or less likely to die from their disease in less than 6 months if it runs its usual course?' In so doing, access to hospice might improve. The Hospice Fiscal Intermediaries (i.e. payers) for hospice services provided to patients receiving the Medicare benefit converted these 'guidelines' into 'policies' that are used to review hospice claims. If the policy criteria are met, the hospice can expect payment. If not, the hospice can still be paid but must provide a rationale as to why the patient is terminally ill.

The creation of these policies (also called 'local medical review policies' or 'local coverage determinations') spurred great controversy within the hospice community, with some believing that, as policies, they would serve as a barrier to hospice admission. Others have used these to educate referral sources on how to identify 'hospice eligible patients' and to reassure referring physicians that their patients meet eligibility requirements for this benefit. From a purely empirical perspective, the coverage policies have never been validated.

Notwithstanding ongoing concerns regarding the validity and utility of these policies, hospice enrolment in the USA has grown at a double-digit pace over the last decade. Length of stay, however, has remained lower than ideal, except for some patients with non-malignant conditions. Linking eligibility for the Medicare benefit to a 6-month prognosis may have had the unintended consequence of encouraging very late referrals, both because of the connection between hospice and death, which rendered the programme unattractive to the many patients, families, and physicians who are not comfortable with a direct approach to end-of-life issues, and because physicians may be concerned that earlier referral is against regulations. Most patients admitted to hospice die within weeks and are unable to make optimal use of the services provided by these programmes.

Although prognostication for cancer patients is generally more predictable than for patients with non-malignant conditions, cancer is becoming more of a chronic illness for many patients, for whom prognostic uncertainty is increasing as well[7]. Some progress is being made in improving the accuracy of determining prognosis through the use of tools such as the Palliative Performance Scale[8], the Minimum Data Set[9], and more definitive clinical determinants of end-stage disease in specific chronic conditions such as amyotrophic lateral sclerosis[10] and chronic renal failure[11]. This is of great importance and hopefully will accelerate with more detailed observational studies and the wider use of validated instruments. At present, however, lack of prognostic confidence reinforces avoidance of the subject of life expectancy and impedes appropriate care planning, and for Medicare beneficiaries (accounting for over 75 per cent of deaths in the USA), also imposes significant potential financial consequences for hospice programmes. Prognostic uncertainty therefore also contributes to a tension in the current reimbursement structure of the health-care system for patients with chronic

progressive illnesses, and this influences the dynamics of hospice practice in the USA.

Length of service

During the original hospice demonstration project, the average length of service for hospice patients was about 70 days. Currently, average hospice length of service is 67 days, which has rebounded from a low of 48 days. This average is skewed by a minority of patients with relatively long lengths of stay and a more meaningful measure is the median length of service, which continued to stay near 20 days. Hospice length of service has a bimodal distribution with more than 30 per cent of patients dying in 7 days or fewer after admission. Conversely, the rate of patients on service more than 180 days has risen to 13 per cent.

The optimal length of hospice service is unknown and is likely to vary with the specific concerns of the patient and family. One estimate suggests that a duration of 60–90 days would be likely to benefit most of those admitted to these programmes[12]. This amount of time may be needed to effectively manage symptoms, understand the medical issues sufficiently to prevent unnecessary hospitalizations and anticipate symptoms and other needs, and establish the type of therapeutic relationship with the patient and family that may facilitate self-determination at the end of life.

The observation that most patients admitted to hospice programmes have eschewed further disease-modifying therapy and subsequently receive aggressive symptomatic treatments, including opioids, may raise concern that hospice admission hastens death. This concern may further link hospice with death in the minds of both professional and lay audiences, and in this way increase the reluctance of physicians to refer, or patients to accept referral, to these programmes. Empirical studies have not confirmed the concern that hospice admission hastens death. Among other observations, a recent survey demonstrated that aggressive use of opioid analgesics by hospice programmes has no appreciable influence on timing of death[13]. This should help reduce concern among patients, families and health-care professionals, and encourage referrals early enough so that the benefits from admission have a chance to materialize.

Economics of hospice: tax-exempt and non-tax-exempt status

While in the USA the majority of hospices are still not-for-profit, there has been considerable growth in the proportion of non-tax-exempt ('for-profit') hospices in the USA during the last 10 years. The chief differences between these two financial structures are that tax-exempt programmes are allowed to use charitable financial gifts to support operations and any surplus funds are not subject to state or federal business taxes. However, non-tax-exempt programmes can provide incentives for staff through profit-sharing and stimulate outside investment by offering potential profits, especially through the mechanism of publicly traded stocks. Given the profit motive, these hospice programmes have a strong incentive to grow.

Before 1985, there was only one non-tax-exempt hospice in the USA. At present, nearly half of the more than 4700 hospice locations are for-profit. These programmes now serve a majority of the total hospice population.

While some have suggested that the advent of for-profit hospices is not a positive development in the USA, risking an erosion of the hospice philosophy of care, several factors should be considered.

For-profit hospices have achieved substantial growth because of their relative willingness to increase outreach to the underserved, including inner city residents, patients with non-cancer diagnoses, and nursing home residents. The non-tax-exempt sector tends to devote more resources to outreach to referral sources in order to grow. To meet the needs of referrers, these programmes also have developed and implemented innovative processes to be quickly responsive to referrals. Whereas there may be less sense of community ownership, especially in hospice chains (multi-site programmes with a central corporate structure), there is more access to capital for growth, there is an ability to benefit from economies of scale (e.g. purchasing power for pharmaceuticals), and there are incentives for increased efficiencies such as leading-edge information management systems.

Not-for-profit hospices are usually more mission-driven, locally owned and more broadly responsive to diverse community needs. Volunteers are more plentiful, and more community grief and bereavement services are offered. In general, the total amount of care delivered by non-tax-exempt and tax-exempt hospices is similar, although there may be a somewhat different mix of services. All Medicare Certified Hospices must adhere to the same federally mandated conditions of participation.

Access and quality

The biggest challenges facing hospice in the USA are to ensure minimal variability in the consistency and quality of services (including the training and credentialling, and the knowledge, skills and experience, of management and clinical staff) and to achieve unfettered access to care in a timely manner. Achieving access for vulnerable and disenfranchised populations including the homeless, prisoners, ethnic minorities, paediatric patients, those with uncertain or indeterminate prognoses, veterans, the poor and uneducated, and those in very rural areas continues to be a challenge. Likewise, measuring and improving the quality of palliative care is a major challenge.

Some improvement has been seen in moving hospice from a mostly white suburban population to a more mainstream population. In 2007, the proportion of hospice patients who are Caucasian dropped to 81 per cent[2], moving closer to parity with general population demographics. This required more effective outreach to Hispanic/Latino, African American, and Asian populations. However access to hospice for minority populations continues to be a concern and African American patients have been found to have less access in most parts of the United States[13]. In cooperation with the Veterans Administration, NHPCO has developed a Veterans Hospice Partnership Programme that is improving access for veterans, and a 'rural toolkit' has been constructed to promote hospice care in the very large and sparsely populated areas that exist throughout the USA. Similarly, the Institute of Medicine (a branch of the United States National Academy of Science) had described a lack of paediatric palliative care services. Consequently, programmes initiated by NHPCO's Children's Project on Palliative/Hospice Services, Children's Hospice International, the Initiative for Paediatric Palliative Care, and others have made access to care for dying children a high priority.

Progress has been made in measuring the quality of hospice and palliative care. NHPCO launched a national Quality Initiative and, in partnership with Brown University in Providence, Rhode Island, has developed a national quality benchmarking service for hospices (www.nhpco.org/research). Currently, this service has been adopted by more than 1000 hospices and permits the comparison of family evaluations of hospice care[14] and family evaluations of palliative care. The NHPCO system also provides comparative results from standardized patient evaluations of care, staff evaluations of the work environment, and family evaluations of the quality of bereavement services. Data also are being collected from more than 3700 hospice sites on quantities of care[15] and a research agenda has been published[16].

Evolution of hospice care: the palliative care movement in the USA

A broader palliative care movement in the USA, largely based in hospitals, emerged in the 1990s out of the hospice movement. The melding of palliative care with traditional hospice care in the USA is best exemplified by the name adaptations made by the respective membership and professional societies. The National Hospice Organization was renamed NHPCO, and now includes both hospice and palliative care members. This organization is avidly working to develop a supportive infrastructure for palliative care programmes. In a similar way, the original Academy of Hospice Physicians changed into the American Academy of Hospice and Palliative Medicine, a professional organization of approximately 3000 physicians that is committed to supporting and advancing the field. In parallel, the Hospice and Palliative Nurses Association has evolved and now has a large membership and a credentialling process. In the interdisciplinary spirit, these two professional associations have held their annual meetings together over the last few years.

The palliative care movement in the USA has been driven largely by the recognition of the serious and highly prevalent unmet needs of patients with chronic progressive illnesses and their families in acute care facilities. These needs overlap those experienced by patients with advanced illness, who are eligible for hospice services. Thus, specialist-level palliative care may address the concerns of patients with life-threatening disease, and their families, at a time when hospice referral is not possible, or when hospice referral is possible but not accessible or desired by the patient. Given the link between hospice and death, palliative care may offer a more acceptable path for patients and families who are hospice-eligible but do not want to acknowledge the imminence of death or whose circumstances warrant a level of medical care that cannot be medically or financially supported by hospice programmes. Access to specialist-level palliative care and hospice care ideally can provide for comprehensive, coordinated, and integrated care throughout the continuum of various sites of care and diagnoses/conditions[17]. This is something to strive for, and can be represented by the model shown in Figure 2.2.2.

In the USA, the number and quality of palliative care services have been growing rapidly, most notably in hospital settings. The Centre to Advance Palliative Care, initially supported by the Robert Wood Johnson Foundation and led by Dr Diane Meier at Mount Sinai Medical Centre in New York City, has provided organizational support and training to assist in the development of these programmes (www.capc.org). Community-based and freestanding palliative care programmes have been slower to develop, though currently 64 per cent of NHPCO's hospice members are working to integrate and coordinate pre-hospice palliative care and hospice at end of life.

In the latter half of the 1990s and early 2000s, another philanthropy, the Soros Open Society Institute, funded the Project on

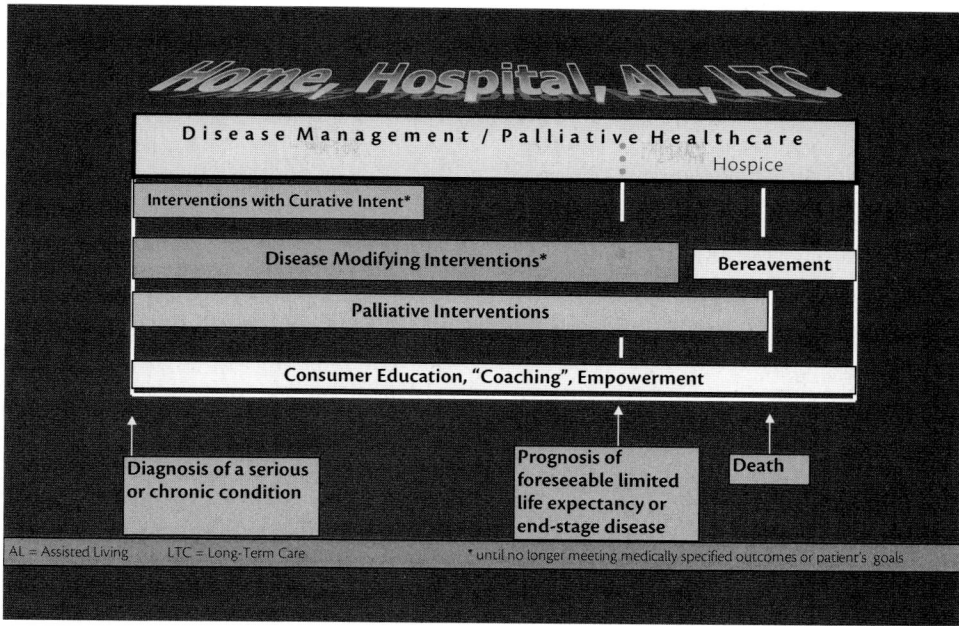

Figure 2.2.2 Conceptual model of a fully integrated and coordinated health-care system for patients with chronic progressive illness. Adapted from: Fine, P.G., and Davis, M. (2005). Hospice: comprehensive care at the end of life. *Anesthesiology Clinics of North America*, **24**, 181–204, used with permission.

Death in America, under the leadership of Dr Kathleen Foley of Memorial Sloan Kettering Cancer Center in New York City. This initiative, which has now ended, supported a Scholar's Programme (led by Dr Susan Block of Harvard Medical School), which created a corps of academically-based palliative care professionals to sustain, promote, and develop the discipline of palliative medicine.

This era also saw the founding of the first department at a major medical centre devoted to palliative care. Although medical schools have not yet developed departments of this type, the creation of a department-level entity at a university-affiliated hospital by Dr Russell Portenoy reflected progress in the academic acceptance of this new discipline.

In 2004, a National Consensus Project for Quality Palliative Care was created and published a consensus-based Guideline for Quality Palliative Care[18]. This document was subsequently endorsed by many health organizations, furthering a major cultural shift in American medicine, and giving credence and impetus to this burgeoning area of health care.

Notwithstanding these very positive changes, there remain great obstacles to the mainstreaming or 'normalizing' of palliative care throughout the US health-care continuum. Palliative care providers may have initially avoided the negative connotations that hospice has with death, but recognition is growing that the health-care community and public also associates palliative care with impending mortality. With this, the field faces the same challenges as hospice in gaining consumer and physician acceptance.

Equally important, there is no payment stream established for most of the professional services provided by palliative care programmes. Only physicians and Nurse Practitioners can bill, and the time and effort of other nurses, social workers, chaplains, consulting pharmacists, and others must be covered by revenue generated in other ways. The lack of a payment stream impedes the development of new services and the expansion of those that have been created.

Although there is a case to be made to institutions that these services are cost-minimizing through their ability to shorten hospital length of stay and reduce resource use of those patients referred, the supporting data are meagre and each hospital has individual exigencies that may preclude the simple generalization of positive economic analyses. Until a clear revenue stream is established to support interdisciplinary palliative care, the further development of programmes will depend on insecure sources, including competitive hospital budgets and philanthropy. Moreover, other than the approximately 1299 hospital-based palliative care programmes currently reported by the Centre to Advance Palliative Care, it is difficult to determine the growth and utilization of community-based palliative care services without a distinct payment stream (insurance benefit) to serve as a data resource.

In the USA, it is likely that some combination of economic pressures brought on by the demographics of a longer-living population with multiple chronic conditions; the potential for significant cost savings through crisis prevention, early intervention and advance care planning; and increasing consumer demand for supportive (palliative) services will ultimately create changes in the various systems supporting both non-hospice-based palliative care and traditional hospice venues. The path that these changes will follow has not been defined yet.

The most recent change of great import in the USA with regard to hospice and palliative care is the approval of Palliative Medicine as a bona fide sub-specialty by the American Board of Medical Specialties. This approval translates into a certification process for specialists in hospice and palliative medicine that mirrors the processes developed for other medical subspecialties. This development has been coupled with the acceptance of Hospice and Palliative Medicine Fellowships (post-residency training programmes) by the Accreditation Council for Graduate Medical Education. As of 2008, physicians may seek advanced training in an accredited programme, and through this experience or other paths, obtain formal board certification in Hospice and Palliative Medicine. This change establishes credibility and authority to the physician component of both hospice and palliative care programmes. With both formal recognition and postgraduate training programmes for physicians, palliative care and hospice programmes will have better and stronger ties to 'mainstream' health-care systems and mechanism for developing a well-trained, dedicated and expert-level physicians workforce. This mechanism will of course require many years to realize an adequate supply of specialists and the rather large gap between the growing need for highly skilled hospice/palliative medicine physicians and their availability will concurrently drive efforts to develop mid-career education and mentoring programmes.

Although there are many challenges ahead, the progress made in a relatively brief amount of time is great cause for optimism. If there is a single lesson to be gained from a retelling of 'the hospice story' in the USA, it is that a small group of dedicated people with a powerful vision, a strong sense of purpose and unwavering tenacity can create great positive change.

Further reading

Byock, I. (1997). *Dying well*. The Berkeley Publishing Group, New York.

Connor, S. (2009). *The essential guide to hospice and palliative care*, 2nd Edition. Routledge, Philadelphia, PA.

Fine, P.G. *The Hospice Companion* (2008). Oxford University Press, New York.

Lattanzi-Licht, M., Mahoney, J.J., and Miller, G.W. (1998). *The hospice choice: in pursuit of a peaceful death*. Simon & Schuster, New York.

Stoddard, S. (1992). *The hospice movement: a better way of caring for the dying*, Revised edition.Vintage Books, New York.

References

1. Connor, S.R. (1998). *Hospice: practice, pitfalls, and promise*, p. 5. Taylor & Francis, Washington, DC.
2. National Hospice and Palliative Care Organization. (2008). *NHPCO facts and figures: Hospice care in America*. Retrieved from http://www.nhpco.org/files/public/Statistics_Research/NHPCO_facts-and-figures_2008.pdf on 22 October 2008.
3. Christakis, N.A. (1999). *Death foretold: prophecy and prognosis in medical care*. University of Chicago Press, Chicago, IL.
4. Weisman, A.D., and Hackett, T.P. (1967). Denial as a social act. In *Psychodynamic studies on aging: creativity, reminiscing and dying* (eds. S. Levin, and R.J. Kahana), pp. 79–110. International Universities Press, New York.
5. Connor, S., Pyenson, B., Fitch, K. *et al.* (2007). Comparing hospice and non-hospice patient survival among patients who die within a 3-year window. *Journal of the Pain and Symptom Management*, **33** (3), 238–46.
6. Lamont, E.B. and Christakis, N.A. (2003). Complexities in prognostication in advanced cancer: "to help them live their lives the way they want to". *Journal of the American Medical Association*, **290**, 98–104.
7. Harrold, J., Rickerson, E., Carroll, J.T. *et al.* (2005). Is the palliative performance scale a useful predictor of mortality in a heterogeneous hospice population? *Journal of Palliative Medicine*, **8**, 503–9.
8. Morris, J.N., Hawes, C., Fries, B.E. *et al.* (1990). Designing the national resident assessment inventory for nursing homes. *Gerontologist*, **3**, 293–307.
9. McCluskey, L. and Houseman, G. (2004). Medicare hospice referral criteria for patients with amyotrophic lateral sclerosis: a need for improvement. *Journal of Palliative Medicine*, **7**, 47–53.
10. Murray, A.M., Arko, C., Chen, S.C. *et al.* (2006). Use of hospice in the United States dialysis population. *Clinical Journal of the American Society Nephrology*, **1**, 1248–55.
11. Iwashyna, T.J. and Christakis, N.A. (1998). Attitude and selfreported practice regarding hospice referral in a national sample of internists. *Palliative Medicine*, **1**, 241–8.
12. Portenoy, R., Sibirceva, U., Smout, R. *et al.* (2006). Opioid use and survival at the end of life: A survey of a hospice population. *Journal of Pain and Symptom Management*, **32**(6), 532–40.
13. Connor, S., Elwert, F., Spence, C. *et al.* (2008). Racial disparity in hospice use in the United States in 2002. *Palliative Medicine*, **22**, 2005–13.
14. Connor, S.R., Teno, J., Spence, C. *et al.* (2005). Family evaluation of hospice care: results from voluntary submission of data via website. *Journal of Pain and Symptom Management*, **30**, 9–17.
15. Connor, S.R., Tecca, M., Lund Person, J. *et al.* (2004). Measuring hospice care: the National Hospice and Palliative Care Organization National Hospice Data Set. *Journal of Pain and Symptom Management*, **28**, 316–28.
16. National Hospice and Palliative Care Organization. (2004). Development of the NHPCO research agenda. *Journal of Pain and Symptom Management*, **28**, 488–96.
17. Fine, P.G. and Davis, M. (2006). Hospice: comprehensive care at the end of life. *Anesthesiology Clinics of North America*, **24**, 181–204.
18. National Consensus Project for Quality Palliative Care. (2004). Clinical practice guidelines for quality palliative care. Retrieved from http://www.nationalconsensusproject.org

Providing palliative care in resource-poor countries

M.R. Rajagopal and Robert Twycross

Introduction

Palliative care is a prominent feature of the programmes of the World Health Organization (WHO), particularly cancer and AIDS. Given the fact that the total annual number of deaths in developing countries will soon reach 50 million, and that about two-third of dying patients would probably benefit from palliative care, the only way for universal access to be achieved in resource-poor countries will be by adopting a public health approach. The patterns which have evolved, for example, in the UK and the USA are far too expensive and, if transplanted into resource-poor countries, would not reach more than a small percentage of those in need.

Present reality

Not just a question of resources

China and India, each with populations in excess of 1 billion, are the two countries with the greatest number of poor people[1]. Palliative care in China is still in the early stages of development. In India, where palliative care services have been slowly developing for over 20 years, <1 per cent of the needy have access to it[2]. The Continent of Africa has a total population of >800 million divided between 47 individual countries. The poverty in most of these countries is widespread and often extreme. In only four African countries is there anything approaching a country-wide network of palliative care services, namely Kenya, Uganda, Zimbabwe, and South Africa[3,4].

Yet, in China and India (and in many other resource-poor countries), for those who can afford it, the latest medical technology is available in well-equipped expensive hospitals; what is not available is the relatively inexpensive option of palliative care. Reasons for this include the allure of hi-tech medicine for the medical profession and political short-sightedness.

India has a national system in which, theoretically, primary health care is available free for all citizens, together with secondary and tertiary referral centres. However, in practice, the cost of treatment is shifted to the patient. A private health insurance system exists but is affordable only by the rich; the average person cannot afford it. Paradoxically, even for the rich, palliative care is generally not available. Thus, universal access to palliative care is more than a question of resources; the public, health-care professionals, policy makers, and administrators all need to be educated about the scope and benefits of palliative care.

Complementary and alternative medicine

More than 200 different treatments come under the broad heading of complementary and alternative medicine[5]. It is estimated that, worldwide, about two-thirds of cancer patients resort to some form of complementary or alternative therapy[6]. However, objective evidence of effectiveness for most of these treatments is not available. A review of research into 19 complementary treatments published in 2000–2005 concluded that 'further research is warranted'[7].

Resorting to alternative systems of medicine may deprive a patient of the chance of a cure in a potentially curable condition. Further, most are expensive compared to the cost of palliative care. Many practitioners of alternative medicine encourage belief in cure even when this is not realistic. This leads to false hope, and the patient and family are prevented from preparing for the fatal outcome and/or accessing palliative care.

In a survey of 440 patients with advanced cancer seen in a palliative care clinic in India, 147 (33 per cent) were using some form of alternative medicine as the definitive therapy for their cancer[8]. Of these, 84 were receiving Ayurvedic remedies (traditional Indian medicine); 46 were taking homeopathic remedies; and 17 were receiving one of several others. None was cured.

All systems of medicine need to be evaluated, and used to the patient's advantage[9]. This is not an easy task because different systems of medicine are based on different sets of principles which often create major methodological difficulties in research. However, in South Africa, active steps have been taken to enlist the positive support of traditional healers, particularly in the care of patients with AIDS, by educating them about palliative care.

Poverty and disease

Even if not already poor, people with disabling diseases are particularly vulnerable to poverty. The disease often deprives the person and their family of income, and the treatment necessitates considerable expenditure. In a study in rural Kerala, South India, of those below the poverty line, the main reason for the poverty in nearly 30 per cent was the cost of medical treatment[10].

A survey of people with disabilities in India found that the cost of medical treatment, purchase and maintenance of special devices, and travel costs to medical and rehabilitation centres varied from 3 days to 2 years' income, with a mean of 2 months[11]. In relation to cancer, given the high cost of treatment, the financial implications are even worse, and often include the cost of repeated travel to and from a distant medical centre.

Beliefs and attitudes

Societal attitudes can either help or hinder. In some societies it is considered a person's duty to respect and care for elders, and thus a culture of care is likely to be ingrained. On the other hand, a fatalistic attitude towards suffering and death may limit care. Further, religious objections to opioids can be a major barrier to pain relief. In some cultures, it is considered a bad omen to talk of death. This creates a major barrier to communication, and the 'wall of silence' (or the 'conspiracy of words') is likely to increase anxiety and suffering for the patient.

Social structures

One of the positive points in many developing countries is a strong family structure. Relatives rally round when a family member is unwell, though they seldom know what to do except by intuition. A patient left alone in a hospital or other institution is the exception rather than the rule. This offers the potential of a strong workforce for palliative care delivery. Thus, empowering the family to care for the patient is well worth the time and efforts of the caring team. Removing misconceptions like the fear of contagion and teaching basic nursing skills (including changing wound dressings) and simple lymphoedema massage can make a dramatic difference.

On the negative side, a large number of relatives could deprive the patient and spouse of privacy. When a person is ill, the responsibility for taking decisions is often assumed by the family who, with good intentions, may deny the person their right to take decisions for themself. Controversy within the family regarding choice of treatment can cause confusion and increase distress, and may even result in the patient being denied the most appropriate treatment. The family may block all efforts by the caring team to communicate the diagnosis and the details of management to the patient. The family may also demand the continuation of futile curative or life-sustaining treatment, unmindful of the wishes of the patient. In societies in which the family can override the autonomy of the patient, the caring team has the difficult task of convincing all the family members of the most appropriate course of action, before they are allowed to talk directly to the patient.

Implications of the disease and treatment on the family

The need to care for the ill person creates enormous physical and psychosocial stresses for the family. In most of the developing world with very limited or no access to free medical care, available finance within the family is frequently all spent on the patient, with nothing left for the rest of the family. Even in an affluent country, it has been documented that, in >10 per cent of cases, family members become ill or unable to function normally because of the associated stresses[12]. The situation is likely to be significantly worse in resource-poor countries.

Major psychological problems among family members go undetected. Family members lose jobs because they have to care for the patient and, in countries with high unemployment, often the loss of a job is for life. Children drop out of school, either because the family can no longer afford the fees or because they are recruited to the family's workforce. The psychological problems of children are often the most neglected; most palliative care teams cannot extend the scope of their service to address these.

Social changes

An increasing cause of suffering in developing countries is the radical impact on the social system caused by industrialization. This is resulting in a steady migration of young adults from villages to cities. By 2050, two-thirds of the world's population will live in cities. Existing support systems are being disrupted without an adequate replacement within the emerging new order. Because of the population shift, it is increasingly impossible for young adults to look after the old and ailing left behind in the villages. Further, in the past, family gatherings and rituals helped to blunt the grief of loss after the death of a loved one but, increasingly, there is now nothing left in place to support the bereaved.

Social support

Palliative care includes psychological and social support as well as physical care. Palliative care teams can educate family members and friends about the illness, the patient's needs and about how they can help. In some societies, cancer is feared partly because it is believed to be contagious. In such circumstances, removing the fear of contagion can make a dramatic improvement in the family's quality of life.

However, the over-riding social problem in resource-poor countries is financial. Many palliative care teams try to socially rehabilitate patients and families, e.g. by endeavouring to find employment for their fitter patients, and for families when the breadwinner is afflicted. This is not easy considering the background of high levels of unemployment. Many also try to support schooling for patients' children.

There is often pressure on palliative care teams to find resources for curative treatment. This is clearly beyond the remit of a palliative care service. Even so, it is not easy to tell a person with a potentially curable condition, 'We have no money for chemotherapy. You must wait until you get pain; then we can help you'.

The AIDS pandemic

In sub-Saharan Africa, HIV/AIDS has overtaken cancer in terms of numbers and social impact. In some African countries, more than 30 per cent of the adult population are HIV-positive. Often it is the main breadwinner who is affected. Hundreds of thousands of children are 'AIDS orphans'. Thus, from a public health and planning point of view, it is necessary to include the ongoing cost of caring for the orphans (Figs. 2.3.1 and 2.3.2). This will further restrict the financial resources available for the care of patients.

Further, financial support from the international donor community may well be conditional, e.g. limited to people who are HIV-positive. Unfortunately this disadvantages many dying patients, including most of those with cancer—whose symptomatic end-stage may well be longer in countries with poor or non-existent oncology services.

The disease spectrum

In resource-poor countries, there is often confusion about which diseases fall within the remit of palliative care. Thus, those with

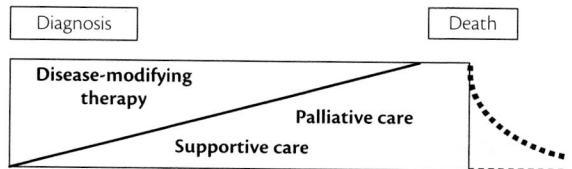

Figure 2.3.1 Diagram illustrating the relationship of palliative care of early days to disease-modifying/curative treatment.

advanced cancer get quality care but those with advanced chronic obstructive pulmonary disease do not, even though their suffering may be no less. Further, the original WHO description of palliative care as applicable when 'the disease is no longer amenable to curative treatment' caused suffering by effectively denying symptom relief and psychosocial support when anticancer treatment was still in progress.

Home, hospital, or hospice?

Many resource-poor countries start to introduce palliative care by building an inpatient hospice. However, although a Western-style hospice may be relevant as a training centre for health-care professionals, such a facility in a resource-poor country cannot reach large numbers. In any case, most people would prefer to stay in their home, however humble that may be, provided they receive adequate support.

The marginalized in affluent countries

A lot of suffering also exists in the midst of affluence, e.g. in the Middle East[13]. Many countries there have state-of-the-art technology for diagnostic and curative management but no palliative care. Even where there are palliative care facilities, patients still have to be hospitalized when strong opioids are needed because it is illegal for patients to have such drugs at home. The fatwa which stated that 'there is no objection against using these analgesics (opium and other analgesics) in advanced cancer patients because this is a necessity' seemed to be a major positive step[14]. However, 7 years later, it has had little impact on the person in pain. Hopefully, in the Middle East, things will soon show definite improvement as more countries there establish palliative care services.

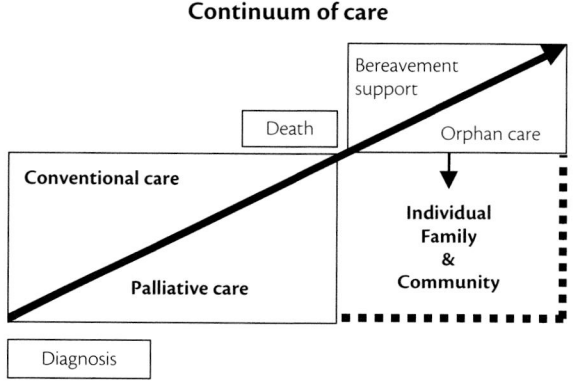

Continuum of care

Figure 2.3.2 Modified diagram illustrating the extension of palliative programmes in sub-Saharan Africa (Defilippi K, South Coast Hospice, KWaZulu Natal, South Africa).

Creative solutions

The problems are daunting but, fortunately, creative and affordable solutions are being identified which make use of relatively simple methods, applicable and sustainable at the community level. However, for these to succeed, both political and public commitment are essential. To achieve this amid all the other claims on very limited health resources (e.g. US $12 per capita per annum in Uganda) there needs to be strong well-reasoned advocacy from community groups, the health professions, and the wider public, such as has been the case in relation to AIDS. We include two examples of successful development.

Uganda

Uganda is the only country in Africa which has made palliative care for people with AIDS and cancer a priority in its National Health Plan, where it is classed as 'essential clinical care'[15–18]. Uganda has established all the foundation measures as recommended by WHO[19]:

- a clear national policy has been agreed;
- education in palliative care is incorporated into the undergraduate curricula of doctors and nurses;
- courses and workshops in pain relief and palliative care are available to health-care professionals at all levels;
- affordable morphine is produced generically within the country;
- the Ministry of Health has published guidelines for handling morphine and other strong opioids[20];
- nurses qualified in palliative care are able to prescribe morphine.

Hospice Africa Uganda is the major resource for education and training in palliative care at all levels and has developed models for community and home-based care[21,22]. The AIDS Support Organization provides counselling and support services[23], and the Mildmay Center for HIV/AIDS Care in Entebbe is extending its activities from a referral centre to rural home-based care. Church hospitals complement the government health services. Three home-care services have been established in the country by faith-based organizations. All these services are linked together through the Palliative Care Association of Uganda, set up as an Non-Governmental Organization (NGO) in 2000.

Uganda was a key demonstration country in WHO's community health approach to palliative care for HIV/AIDS and cancer patients in Africa, a joint project between Botswana, Ethiopia, Tanzania, Uganda, and Zimbabwe[24]. Hospice Africa Uganda also holds workshops in other African countries, sensitizing them to the need for establishing foundation measures for palliative care in education, drug availability, and policy as well as running training courses for health-care professionals[25].

Uganda has demonstrated the importance and success of a harmoniously integrated governmental approach with clear policies and a decentralized community-based approach, linked to its HIV/AIDS programme[4]. Uganda and Zambia are the only two African countries where the prevalence of HIV/AIDS in the population has declined[26]. It currently stands at 6–7 per cent (down from 30 per cent in Uganda), and is a strong evidence of the value of strategic policy-making. Through advocacy from Hospice Africa Uganda, funded initially by the Royal Air Force (advocacy and training in Tanzania) and later by the Diana, Princess of Wales Memorial

Fund, affordable oral morphine has been introduced to Tanzania, Malawi, Nigeria, and Cameroon.

In 2005, the African Palliative Care Association was established with its headquarters in Kampala. The Association works closely with existing palliative care services throughout Africa. So far, links have been established with 17/47 countries in Africa.

India

With about 2.4 million people with cancer and with a similiar number HIV-positive[27], India has a vast reservoir of suffering. In the 1980s, there were only a few pain clinics in various parts of India. Modern palliative care was first introduced in 1986 in the form of Shanti Avedna Ashram, a Western-style hospice in Mumbai. However, the more widespread development of palliative care was minimal until 1993 when the Indian Association of Palliative Care was launched and the Pain and Palliative Care Society (PPCS) in Calicut, Kerala was founded[27].

In 1995, the PPCS was designated a WHO Demonstration Project for a community-based ('bottom-up') approach. It succeeded in developing an effective low-cost home-care system based on an outpatient clinic functioning 6 days a week, supported by home visits when possible, and inpatient facility when essential[28]. By its example, the PPCS motivated an increasing number of doctors and members of the public. By working with lay volunteers, a network of 33 palliative care clinics developed in the surrounding part of Kerala over the next 7 years[28,29].

These clinics are housed almost anywhere—in an empty shop space in the market, a public library, or a small rented building. Typically, the clinics are NGOs and function 1–2 days per week. They provide outpatient care through a volunteer doctor, often working on their weekly day off. Some offer home visits to those too unwell to come to the clinic; a few have inpatient facilities. Generally, the NGOs raise the necessary financial resources locally, often by regular modest donations from hundreds (sometimes thousands) of members of the general public.

Because there are no support systems for the chronically ill, palliative care services are not restricted to people with cancer and AIDS, but extend to:

◆ stable chronic disorders, such as post-traumatic paraplegia;

◆ fluctuating chronic disorders, such as filarial lymphoedema and sickle-cell disease;

◆ slowly progressive diseases, such as peripheral vascular disease;

◆ all end-stage progressive diseases, such as renal failure and chronic obstructive pulmonary disease with respiratory failure.

Trained volunteers take on much of the psychosocial support and, like some relatives, often undertake nursing tasks (including changing wound dressings) and simple lymphoedema massage. In the absence of a state social security system, palliative care teams have provided financial assistance to enable some patients to travel to the outpatient clinic, and for rehabilitation of families.

Since the turn of the century, Neighbourhood Networks in Palliative Care have been established[30]. These are mainly volunteer-driven and community-owned. Most financial needs are provided by local fund-raising. The strong roots in the community ensure that coverage is good in the locality and that continuity of care is better than with the earlier doctor-led clinics. Trained lay volunteers identify people in their locality who would benefit from palliative care, make home visits and offer psychosocial support, in addition to acting as a link between the patient and the health-care professional.

Questions have been raised about the quality of care that such teams can give[31]. There are concerns about the feasibility of volunteers attempting to provide psychological support. Clearly, there is need for the Neighbourhood Networks to be evaluated systematically[32]. Even so, there is little doubt that community involvement has increased community awareness and extended support to many more patients and families.

The Kerala experience also emphasizes that, if palliative care is developed before the establishment of wide-ranging chronic care facilities, it is likely to incorporate a wide spectrum of patient categories. In Kerala, the definition of palliative care has effectively become *the active total care in the community of patients with a chronic disorder or an advanced disease, and their families.* Palliative care is seen more in terms of helping patients (and their families) make a transition from being passive victims to empowered persons rather than in helping them adjust to the imminent inevitably of death—which may be decades away (Table 2.3.1).

Hospital-based Pain and Palliative Care Clinics, already established in several major hospitals, are still necessary for patients with end-stage disease and intractable pain or other refractory symptoms, and for patients with chronic non-malignant pain. Such centers are also necessary for teaching and training purposes, and for hosting diploma and other postgraduate courses.

The Indian Association of Palliative Care has been a major force in bringing together palliative care workers in a large country and in sharing ideas. With support from the USA (National Cancer Institute and the WHO Collaborating Center in Madison, Wisconsin), Pallium India, an NGO, has catalysed the development of three palliative care centers in North and North-East India. With support from the International Network for Cancer Treatment and Research and the American Cancer Society, it has also facilitated

Table 2.3.1 Disease spectrum of patients seen at a rural palliative care clinic in Kerala[a].

Diagnosis	Number of patients
Malignant disease	83
Cerebrovascular accidents with residual paralysis and sequelae	25
Bedfast in advanced age	16
Paraplegia/tetraplegia	10
Advanced chronic obstructive pulmonary disease	2
Dementia	2
Cerebral palsy	1
Muscular dystrophy	1
Intervertebral disc prolapse with intractable pain	1
Pyonephrosis (symptom management in conjunction with definitive treatment)	1
Chronic liver disease	1

[a] Alpha Pain Clinic, Edamuttam, Trissur District; 42 per cent did not have cancer.

the initiation of a palliative care training center in the MNJ Institute of Oncology, Hyderabad, Andhra Pradesh.

Although most palliative care delivery in India has been driven by NGOs, government involvement has also been important. The Indian Association of Palliative Care and other NGOs, working with Pain and Policy Studies Group of Madison-Wisconsin, have had several major successes in relation to Government. For example:

◆ palliative care centres have been exempted from the need for a 'drug licence', thereby enabling them to dispense drugs without an obligation to employ a qualified pharmacist, something which most centres could not afford[33];

◆ narcotic regulations have been simplified in 13 of 28 states[34];

◆ an uninterrupted supply of morphine sulphate powder has been guaranteed from Government Opium and Alkaloid factories[35];

◆ palliative care is now part of the National Cancer Control Programme (with effect from 2007).

It is hoped that this last achievement will result in the formation of a palliative care department in every Regional Cancer Center in India, and at least one palliative care service in every state before the end of the next 5-year plan in 2012.

Foundation measures for a public health approach

The Ugandan and Indian experiences demonstrate that a certain pattern of activities will bring success. Palliative care should be integrated with, and not separated from, the mainstream of health care. A public health approach means that the methods adopted must be scientifically valid as well as acceptable, sustainable, and affordable at the community level[36,37]. Ideally, there should be a comprehensive generic plan for the development of a palliative care programme for cancer, AIDS, other end-stage disease, and the care of older people with chronic illnesses which can be implemented worldwide. Inevitably, there will be some disease-specific measures; for example, antiretroviral drugs for those infected with HIV.

According to the WHO, there are three foundation measures which are essential in order to achieve a successful public health approach to the development of palliative care (Fig. 2.3.3)[38,39].

Policy

Hitherto, the development of palliative care has come about mostly as a result of the efforts of local and national palliative care 'champions' and associated NGOs. However, to achieve population-wide coverage, palliative care needs to be integrated into mainstream health care. This is unlikely to occur unless it becomes Government policy for palliative care to be an essential or core element of the national health services, coupled with an action plan for implementation.

For example, since 1991, in line with the three-pronged Cancer Control Programme of the WHO, it has been the policy of successive Indian governments that palliative care should be an integral component of cancer care. However, it was only in 2005 that palliative care experts were included in the task force for formulating the future strategy for the ongoing National Cancer Control Programme.

Institutional policy

It is likely that a palliative care service in a resource-poor country will sooner or later become swamped with patients, and that the service will have to expand indefinitely and/or reduce the quality of the care. So, given the likelihood of an increasing demand for care, it is essential for new services to have a policy which deals with this eventuality. If possible, such a policy should be based on a properly conducted needs assessment and consideration should be given to establishing new more local services, thereby improving access to palliative care. In all this, it is important to keep the following points in mind:

◆ *Patients' needs should come first.* This is not automatically the case; the success of the organization or department may effectively become the team's main concern. If commitment to the organization exceeds commitment to the patients, there is a likelihood that we end up building monuments and that patients, though essential, become a nuisance.

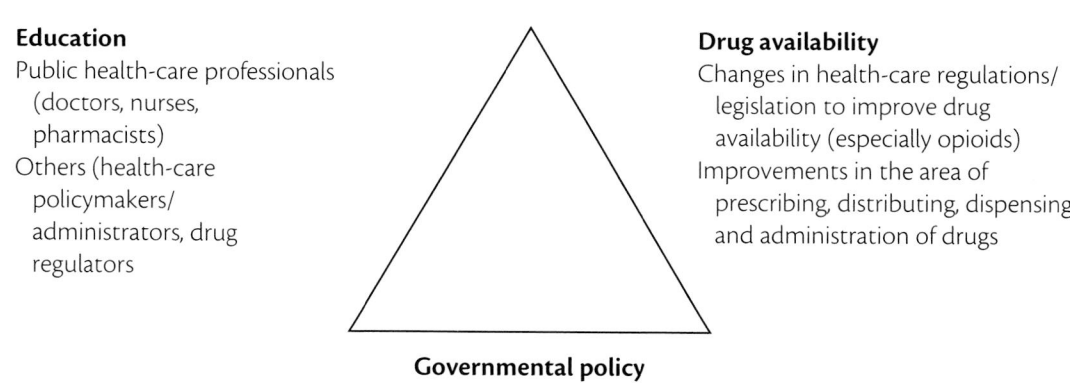

Education
Public health-care professionals
   (doctors, nurses,
   pharmacists)
Others (health-care
   policymakers/
   administrators, drug
   regulators

Drug availability
Changes in health-care regulations/
   legislation to improve drug
   availability (especially opioids)
Improvements in the area of
   prescribing, distributing, dispensing,
   and administration of drugs

Governmental policy
National or state policy declaring that palliative care
   should be an integral part of basic health care, and
   including a plan of action to achieve this target

Figure 2.3.3 Foundation measures necessary for an effective national programme.

◆ *The palliative care delivery system should be realistic and sustainable.* The delivery system has to be adapted to the local cultural and economic situation. It is clearly unjust to give superlative care at great cost to 250 inpatients per annum if 2500 others (or more) are denied any help. The Western inpatient hospice system cannot be translated in its entirety to developing countries. Further, experience in Uganda and India have shown that care at home, supported by an outpatient clinic and occasional home visits, is cost-effective in terms of achieving population-wide coverage, with a 'back-up' inpatient facility for those with overwhelming problems, or no family and home.

◆ *A partnership in care needs to be established with the family.* The strength in many resource-poor countries lies in their strong family structure. Enough trained nurses will never be affordable to care for literally millions of patients. However, success is still possible by empowering the relatives to care for the patient, establishing a partnership in care.

◆ *A partnership in care also needs to be established with the patient.* The average villager is capable of making brave and intelligent decisions regarding treatment options. Formal education and intelligence are not synonymous. Doctors have no right to force decisions on the patient.

◆ *The family's finances need to be considered before recommending treatment.*

◆ *Make use of existing resources.* Constructing new palliative care centres is likely to exhaust available resources, and should be discouraged. Wherever possible, existing facilities should be made use of, i.e. hospitals and primary health centres.

◆ *Deficiencies in existing facilities need to be supplemented by NGOs.* Ways must be found to complement existing services, thereby 'plugging gaps' and evolving a seamless integrated service. Experience has shown that, with determination and diplomacy, it is generally possible for NGOs to work successfully alongside national health services.

◆ *Volunteers can be the backbone of the palliative care service.* There are numerous individuals who are kind-hearted and willing to help. However, this potential work force needs to be trained and properly managed[40].

◆ *Advocacy is essential.* A strategy is necessary to influence policy and to improve funding and drug availability. There is need both to approach Health Department decision-makers directly and to influence them indirectly through the public. The mass media— press, television, radio—have an important role to play in this.

Education

The carers, whether professional, volunteer, or family, all need training to enable them to acquire the necessary attitude, knowledge, and skills. Indeed, education about palliative care must be extended to the public at large, policy-makers and health service administrators.

Generally, there is always resistance to change. In relation to palliative care, those most resistant or indifferent to the need for change have often been other doctors, notably leaders within other specialties—including oncology. Palliative care is often seen as an admission of failure (something which many doctors find very hard). The fact that most major cancer centres around the world still do not have a fully fledged and fully integrated palliative care service must be regarded as a black mark on the medical profession.

Public education

Unfortunately, scientific proof of benefit does not automatically mean enhanced clinical practice. It needs persistent effort to effect change. Experience has repeatedly shown that the general public is often more open to new ideas than health-care professionals or administrators. Even when a specialist is reluctant to refer patients to a palliative care service, repeated demands by patients eventually force a change in attitude. Public demand can also lead to administrative reforms. Advocacy programmes have an important role to play, as shown by tobacco control programmes.

Education of the public is also needed because palliative care should be a partnership between patient, family, health-care professionals, and volunteers. Without sufficient understanding of its full scope, palliative care may end up being only 'terminal care', with the patient being denied help until the last few days of life. Further, if patients (and families) believe that morphine is addictive, a reluctance to take it may result in avoidable suffering.

Public understanding is also necessary to overcome the current problem of over-medicalization of death. It is a disturbing paradox that, in cities in resource-poor countries, the dying are often subjected to futile high-tech interventions. People with irreversible end-stage disease frequently die while still on ventilators, the family ruined by the high cost of futile treatment, and with children forced to discontinue their education. There is often public discussion about euthanasia but rarely about the possibilities of palliative care. It is up to the palliative care fraternity to bring these issues to public attention. Possible educational activities include:

◆ using the mass media to assist in changing public opinion and attitudes, and in influencing public action;

◆ public awareness programmes as part of community activities;

◆ incorporating palliative care and related matters in school and college curricula[41,42].

Professional education

Medical training needs to address not only knowledge acquisition (*head*) but also attitudes (*heart*), and skills (*hands*). All three are essential, particularly in palliative care. Although it is effective in conveying book knowledge, didactic training seldom changes practice because it seldom changes attitudes and does not improve skills. The best way to learn any aspect of medicine is by the bedside, including 'hands-on' training. Unfortunately, this cannot always be arranged. When a short didactic course is all that can be offered, it helps if:

◆ 1–2 sessions include a clinical presentation with the patient in the classroom;

◆ course participants spend 1–2 h observing a palliative clinic in action;

◆ course participants join in a home visit.

Drug availability

It is generally agreed that analgesics are the mainstay of cancer pain management[43]. Policies and recommendations for rational public health implementation are available[44–46], and essential drug policies have been established[25,47–49].

Despite this, limited drug availability, specifically of morphine, continues to be a major obstacle to the development of palliative care[44]. The ability of drug regulatory authorities to block or hinder the ready availability of cheap generic oral preparations of morphine is amazing. David Joranson, Distinguished Scientist at the Pain & Policy Studies Group, University of Wisconsin Comprehensive Cancer Center, a WHO Collaborating Center for Policy and Communications in Cancer Care, has helped local palliative care activists in many countries over the last 15–20 years[50]. But it seems that one has to be Houdini to escape from the ensnarement of bureaucratic (and indifferent) red tape[33]. This is a black mark, but more for the civil service than the medical profession.

However, widespread poverty in resource-poor countries dictates that, unless drugs are inexpensive, overcoming regulatory barriers alone does not translate into pain relief. Paradoxically, expensive drugs are frequently available in such countries, but not cheap formulations like ordinary (normal release) morphine (Table 2.3.2). The power of drug companies to buy influence over every key group in health care—doctors, NGOs, charities, patient groups, journalists, politicians—is deeply disturbing[51,52]. In the absence of close monitoring, questionable practices go undocumented in developing countries.

Put at its simplest, the pharmaceutical industry tends to promote expensive new analgesics. As this is not balanced by education in the use of less expensive drugs, this shifts the balance in favour of expensive drugs. It is shameful that many institutions have expensive sustained-release morphine, but not inexpensive ordinary morphine preparations. Many centres use transdermal fentanyl as the first-line strong opioid. Limited resources are thus spent unnecessarily, and thousands of other people are denied pain relief in consequence. Pharmaco-economics are an important aspect of the development of palliative care services, to prevent limited resources being unnecessarily frittered away.

Essential steps in creating a strategy

An action plan with short-term, medium-term, and long-term goals should be created. This should take account of both the positives and the negatives:

◆ What is already available and what is not?

◆ Do we have a trained doctor and nurse?

Table 2.3.2 Relative cost of opioids in India.

Name of drug	Dose	Cost (US $/24 h)
Dextropropoxyphene	130 mg q6h	0.25
Codeine	60 mg q4h	1.00
Tramadol	100 mg q6h	1.50
Morphine (normal release)	10 mg q4h	0.16
Morphine (sustained release)	30 mg q12h	0.40
Fentanyl (transdermal)	25 mcg/h[a]	8.00

[a] some institutions have transdermal fentanyl but not morphine, even though the use of both is controlled by the same regulations.

◆ Are our colleagues sufficiently educated to refer appropriate patients to the new service?

◆ Is the public aware of the positive implications of a palliative care service?

◆ Do we know how to procure strong opioids, particularly inexpensive preparations of morphine?

◆ Do we have enough money for an uninterrupted supply of essential drugs?[53]

◆ How much free treatment will we be able to provide?

◆ Can we train and use volunteers to act as the link between the patients and the health-care professionals?

◆ Can any part of the work be undertaken by existing organizations?

◆ Is it possible to combine palliative care advocacy with tobacco control activities and cancer awareness programmes, and vice versa?

The action plan should include a timetable, with stated deadlines, for educational activities and drug availability. Periodic reviews are crucial.

Both pioneering and palliative care are emotionally demanding. It is easy for those simultaneously setting up services and campaigning for governmental support to become exhausted. There is a need to interact with others, both within the palliative care team of professionals and volunteers, and with an evolving group of committed supporters. Many times, a problem shared becomes a problem halved.

Conclusion

It has been said that history alternates between charisma and routinization. In this context, charisma refers to the ability of exceptional individuals to act as a catalyst for social change, and acknowledges the impact of personality in bringing about radical innovation in institutions and established beliefs. In relation to the evolution of palliative care in the UK, USA, and other English-speaking Western countries, Cicely Saunders was the initial charismatic influence. Now, in countries where palliative care is well established and fully integrated into the national health service, a major challenge is to prevent palliative care moving from the creative and disruptive influence of charisma to the cosy ambience of routinization. It is crucial to the continuing development of palliative care worldwide that palliative care remains *a movement with momentum*, manifesting an ongoing creative tension between charisma and routinization. Fortunately, so far, this often seems to be the case.

Thus, it is heartening that in many countries palliative care is breaking out of its original cocoon, and is imaginatively and compassionately responding to neglected and unsupported suffering of many kinds in the community. There is a continuing need for inspired leadership—and an ongoing positive partnership between community, NGOs, health-care professionals, and government. In practice, we should anticipate that much of the 'active total care' will be provided by trained family members in the patients' homes and by trained volunteers, with the dedicated support of the professionals.

The 20th century was a time of unparalleled, and at times incredible, advances in medical science and the treatment of disease. Let us hope that the 21st century will be the time when medicine generally becomes holistic, with attention being paid to the whole person, rather than just to the disease process. Although much still needs to be done, much has been achieved. Thankfully, the light at the end of the tunnel is growing both in size and in intensity.

References

1. Tully, M. (1991). *No full stops in India*. Peguin Books India, New Delhi.
2. Rajagopal, M.R. and Joranson, D. (2007) Opioid availability—an update. *Journal of Pain and Symptom Management*, **33**, 615–22.
3. Harding, R. and Higginson, I.J. (2005). Palliative care in sub-Saharan Africa. *Lancet*, **365**, 1971–7.
4. Wright, M. and Clark, D. (2006). *Hospice and palliative care in Africa—a review of developements and challenges*. Oxford University Press, Oxford.
5. Hemming, L. and Maher, D. (2005). Complementary therapies in palliative care: a summary of current evidence. *British Journal of Community Nursing*, **10**, 448–52.
6. Ott, M.J. (2002). Complementary and alternative therapies in cancer symptom management. *Cancer Practice*, **10**, 162–6.
7. Ernst, E. *et al.* (2006) Complementary/alternative medicine for supportive cancer care: development of the evidence-base. *Supportive Care in Cancer*, **15**, 565–8.
8. Sureshkumar, K. and Rajagopal, M.R. (1996). Palliative care in Kerala. Problems at presentation in 440 patients with advanced cancer in a south Indian state. *Palliative Medicine*, **10**, 293–8.
9. Ramesh, P. *et al.* (1998). Managing morphine-induced constipation: a controlled comparison of an ayurvedic formulation and senna. *Journal of Pain and Symptom Management*, **16**, 240–4.
10. George, A.T. Catastrophic health care expenditure and impoverishment in Kerala: an analysis based on NSSO 55th round. [Dissertation]: Jawaharlal Nehru University; 2005.
11. National Human Rights Commission. (2006). *Disability: definitions, estimates and causes*. Retrieved from: http://nhrc.nic.in/Publications/Disability/chapter01.html
12. Emanuel, E.J. *et al.* (2000). Understanding economic and other burdens of terminal illness: the experience of patients and their caregivers. *Annals of Internal Medicine*, **132**, 451–9.
13. Bedikian, A.Y. and Thompson, S.E. (1995). Saudi community attitudes towards cancer. *Annals of Saudi Medicine*, **15**, 161–7.
14. Isbister, W.H. (2002). A "good" fatwa. *British Medical Journal*, **325**, 1227.
15. Jagwe, J.G. and Barnard, D. (2002). The introduction of palliative care in Uganda. *Journal of Palliative Medicine*, **5**, 160–3.
16.. Merriman, A. (2002). Uganda: current status of palliative care. *Journal of Pain and Symptom Management*, **24**, 252–6.
17. Republic of Uganda (1999) *National health policy*. Ministry of Health, Kampala.
18. Republic of Uganda (2000). *National sector strategic plan* 2000/01–2004/05. Ministry of Health, Kampala.
19. Stjernsward, J. *et al.* (1996). The World Health Organization Cancer Pain and Palliative Care Program. Past, present, and future. *Journal of Pain and Symptom Management*, **12**, 65–72.
20. Republic of Uganda (2001). *Guidelines for handling class A drugs—Uganda*. Ministry of Health, Kampala.
21. Hospice Africa Uganda (2006). *HAU strategic plan 2006–2011*. HAU, Kampala.
22. Merriman, A. and Heller, K. (2002). *Hospice Uganda—a model palliative care initiative in Africa: an interview with Anne Merriman*. In Innovations in end of life care. Retrieved from:http://www.edc.org/lastacts
23. Anonymous (1995). *TASO Uganda: the inside story. Participatory evaluation of HIV/AIDS counselling, medical and social services 1993–1994*. WHO, Kampala: TASO and Geneva.
24. World Health Organization. (2004). *A community health approach to palliative care for HIV/AIDS and cancer patients in sub-Saharan Africa*. WHO, Geneva.
25. Hospice Africa Uganda. (2006). *Palliative medicine—pain and symptom control in the cancer and/or AIDS patient in Uganda and other African countries* (4e). Hospice Africa Uganda, Kampala.
26. Hunter, S. (2000). *Reshaping societies. HIV/AIDS and social changes: a resource book for planning, programs and policy making*. Hudson Run Press, Glen Falls, New York.
27. AIDS and HIV information from Avert.org. India: HIV and AIDS statistics. http://www.avert.org/indiaaids.htm accessed 15 October 2008.
28. Rajagopal, M.R. and Kumar, S. (1999). A model for delivery of palliative care in India—the Calicut experiment. *Journal of Palliative Care*, **15**, 44–9.
29. Rajagopal, M.R. and Venkateswaran, C. (2003). Palliative care in India: successes and limitations. *Journal of Pain and Palliative Care Pharmacotherapy*, **17**, 121–8; discussion 129–30.
30. Kumar, S. (2004). Learning from low income countries: what are the lessons?: Palliative care can be delivered through neighbourhood networks. *British Medical Journal*, **329**, 1184.
31. Gupta, H. (2004). How basic is palliative care? *International Journal of Palliative Nursing*, **10**, 600–1.
32. Downing, J. *et al.* (2005). How basic is palliative care? Responses to Harmala Gupta. *International Journal of Palliative Nursing*, **11**, 34–9.
33. Joranson, D.E. *et al.* (2002). Improving access to opioid analgesics for palliative care in India. *Journal of Pain and Symptom Management*, **24**, 152–9.
34. Palat, G. and Rajagopal, M. (2006). Pain relief on a shoe-string budget: Experience from Kerala, India. *Proceedings of the 11th World Congress on Pain* (eds. H. Flor. *et al.*). IASP Press, Seattle.
35. Rajagopal, M.R. *et al.* (2001). Medical use, misuse, and diversion of opioids in India. *Lancet*, **358**, 139–43.
36. Gómez-Batiste, X. (1994). Catalonia's five-year plan: basic principles. *European Journal of Palliative Care*, **1**, 45–9.
37. Nair, M. (1988). *Ten year action Plan for cancer control in Kerala*. Trivandrum, Kerala.
38. World Health Organization (1990). *Cancer pain relief and palliative care. Technical Report Series 804*. WHO, Geneva.
39. World Health Organization. (2002). *National Cancer Control Programmes. Policies and managerial guidelines* (2e), p. 84. WHO, Geneva.
40. Livingstone, H. (2002). Pain relief in the developing world: the experience of hospice Africa-Uganda. In *Pain and palliative care in the developing World and marginalized populations* (eds. M.R. Rajagopal, *et al.*), pp. 107–18. Haworth Medical Press, New York.
41. Department of Education and Skills. (1999). *A teacher's guide to personal, social and health education*. The Stationery Office, London.
42. Abras, M.A. (2002). Teaching children to understand death and grieving. *European Journal of Palliative Care*, **6**, 256–7.
43. World Health Organization. (1986). *Cancer pain relief*. WHO, Geneva.
44. World Health Organization. (1996). *Cancer pain relief: with a guide to opioid availability* (2e). WHO, Geneva.
45. Stjernsward, J. (2002). Uganda: initiating a government public health approach to pain relief and palliative care. *Journal of Pain and Symptom Management*, **24**, 257–64.
46. Foley, K. *et al.* (2002). Palliative care in resource-poor settings. In *A guide to supportive and palliative care of people with HIV/AIDS* (eds. J. O'Neil and P. Selwyn). HRSA, HIV/AIDS Bureau, Rockville, MD.
47. Pretoria Primary Health Care. (1998). *Standard treatment guidelines and essential drugs list*. Directorate Pharmaceutical Programmes and Planning, Pretoria.

48. Harare Ministry of Health and Child Welfare. (1989). *Essential Drug List for Zimbabwe (EDLIZ), including guidelines for treatment of medical conditions common in Zimbabwe.*

49. Ministry of Health and Social Affairs. (2002). *Lag (2002:160) om Lakemedelsformaner m.m.* Socialdepartementet, Stockholm. Available from: http://www.lagrummet.gov.se and http://www.mpa.se

50. Mosoiu, D. *et al.* (2006). Reform of drug control policy for palliative care in Romania. *Lancet,* **367,** 2110–7.

51. Angell, M. (2004). *The truth about the drug companies: how they deceive us and what to do about it.* Random House, New York.

52. Ferner, R.E. (2005). The influence of big pharma. *British Medical Journal,* **330,** 855–6.

53. De Lima, L. (2006). The international association for hospice and palliative care list of essential medicines for palliative care. *Palliative Medicine,* **20,** 647–51.

Ensuring palliative medicine availability: the development of the IAHPC list of essential medicines for palliative care

Liliana De Lima, Derek Doyle,
Neil MacDonald, Eric L. Krakauer,
Karl Lorenz, David Praill, and Kathleen Foley

Introduction

The essential medicines concept

According to the World Health Organization (WHO), *essential medicines* are those that satisfy the primary health-care needs of the population[1]. The concept was laid down by WHO in 1977 with the recommendation that essential medicines be selected with due regard to disease prevalence, evidence on efficacy and safety, and comparative cost-effectiveness. Essential medicines are intended to be available at all times in adequate amounts, in the appropriate dosage forms, with assured quality, and at a price the individual and the community can afford.

The essential drugs concept can be applied in all countries and at various levels (national, provincial, municipality, hospital) and is especially valuable in resource-poor settings, as it seeks to prioritize medications and thereby improve access to treatment. Focusing formularies on essential drugs may lower costs due to economies of scale.

In addition to the concept, the WHO also developed a Model List of Essential Medicines which is updated every 2 years. The concept and the WHO Model List are presented to countries so that governments can construct their own essential medicines policies and lists.

Over a period of more than 30 years, the Essential Medicines concept provided a basis for numerous national essential medicines programmes whereby countries developed their own essential medicines lists based on local needs. Use of this concept by countries around the world has had a considerable impact: The number of people with access to essential drugs has grown from roughly 2.1 billion in 1977 to an estimated 3.8 billion in 1999, and the number of countries that have formulated or updated a national drug policy grew from 14 in 1989 to 66 in 1999. By the end of 1999, more than 150 WHO Member States had a national essential medications list; and 127 of the lists had been revised within the previous 5 years[2].

Inadequate access to medications: a persistent problem

According to data from the WHO, in spite of recent progress, a large part of the world's population still has little or no access to essential and often life-saving medicines. This results in enormous unnecessary suffering and loss of life, particularly among the poor, and massive damage to national economies. It has been estimated that one-third of the world's population lacks access to the most basic essential medications. The problem is particularly severe in the poorest parts of Africa and Asia[3].

In 1986, the WHO and its Expert Committee on Cancer Pain Relief developed an effective analgesic method for the relief of cancer pain. The method relies on the availability of opioid analgesics, including morphine, codeine, and others. Known as the *Three-Step Analgesic Ladder*[4], it has been widely disseminated and is based on the use of the oral route for its convenience and effectiveness. Both morphine and codeine are included in the WHO Model List in the Analgesics section. However, several reports from the WHO, the United Nations (UN), the International Narcotics Control Board (INCB), and other organizations indicate that opioid analgesics are insufficiently available, particularly in developing countries[5–9]. Prescription of morphine and other potent opioids may be restricted to a small percentage of physicians by requiring a special registration procedure. In many countries opioid use is prohibited or limited due to high prices and national laws or by limiting the dosages, the concentrations, or the duration of therapy, regardless of the patients' needs[10–13].

The INCB and WHO have jointly identified the following obstacles to availability of opioid analgesics[7,8]:

- misinterpretation of the International treaties by national drug regulatory authorities;

- legislative, regulatory, and administrative impediments that exist in various countries and that lead to the under-utilization of opioids;

- sub-optimal medical, nursing, and pharmacy practices;

- misperceptions and lack of knowledge of health-care workers about the role and safety of opioid analgesics and about the availability and use of alternative treatments;

- shortage of health-care workers and facilities (including the infrastructure for opioid distribution);

- financial constraints of drug markets, resulting in higher costs, both to the country and to the individual patient;

- structural constraints such as difficulties encountered by pharmaceutical companies to introduce opioids into a market; and

- constraints on availability stemming from governmental action to combat drug abuse.

Many organizations, individuals, academic centres, advocacy groups, and pain and palliative-care organizations are working to improve access to analgesic medications. Recently, palliative-care groups also have been advocating for the availability of other medications needed to treat the most common symptoms in palliative care.

Essential medicines for palliative care

The 14th edition of the WHO Essential Medicines Model List included a section called 'Medicines Used in Palliative Care' (Section 8.4), which did not include a list of medications for palliative care but the following paragraph:

> The WHO Expert Committee on the Selection and Use of Essential Medicines recommended that all the drugs mentioned in the WHO publication Cancer Pain Relief: With a Guide to Opioid Availability, second edition, be considered essential. The drugs are included in the relevant sections of the Model List, according to their therapeutic use, e.g. analgesics[14].

Appendix 2.4.1 includes the list of medications mentioned in the WHO publication *Cancer Pain Relief with a Guide to Opioid Availability*[7] and referenced in the above paragraph.

To remedy this deficit, the WHO Cancer Control Programme requested help from the International Association for Hospice and Palliative Care (IAHPC) to develop a list of essential medicines for palliative care. This chapter describes the process used by IAHPC to develop the list which was proposed as the Essential Medicines List for Palliative Care for the WHO.

Process

The Cancer Control Programme of the WHO requested that a list be prepared based on recommendations from an international palliative care expert committee using two criteria: **efficacy** and **safety**. Once it received the list the WHO planned to carry out **cost-effectiveness** analysis and evidence-based reviews of the recommended medications. In response, the IAHPC formed a Task Force which included board members of the IAHPC and external advisors.

Table 2.4.1 Symptoms rated as most common in palliative care by international experts.

Pain:	
Mild to moderate	
Moderate to severe	
Bone	
Neuropathic	
Visceral	
Dyspnoea	Fatigue
Terminal respiratory congestion	Anxiety
Dry mouth	Depression
Hiccups	Delirium
Anorexia–cachexia	Insomnia
Constipation	Terminal restlessness
Diarrhoea	Sweating
Nausea	
Vomiting	

Appendix 2.4.3 includes the names of the members of the Task Force as well as the names of individuals who collaborated and the roles they played in the project.

The Task Force developed a plan of action with the following steps.

First step—developing a set of guiding principles:

The Task Force requested help from Derek Doyle to prepare a set of guiding principles and an ethical framework for the discussion and for future use and application of the list. The set of Guiding Principles are included in Appendix 2.4.2. The Guiding Principles state that the primary goal of developing the list should be to benefit patients and provide a method for developing the list that is transparent and honest.

Second step—identification of the most prevalent symptoms in palliative care

Members of the Task Force agreed that the best approach to build a list of essential medicines in palliative care was to start with a list of the most common symptoms in palliative care[15–17]. It was also agreed that the group would not address disease-modifying medications for underlying conditions, including cancer, HIV, and other infections or diseases.

An initial list of 21 symptoms prevalent in palliative-care patients was developed by the committee (Table 2.4.1).

Third step—first list: identification of the appropriate medications to treat these symptoms:

IAHPC board members and other palliative-care leaders from around the world were asked to propose appropriate medications for the symptoms identified in the second step.

Of a total of 40, 34 physicians responded (85 per cent), 15 were from developing countries. In total, they recommended 147 products. This initial list was decreased to 120 by removing non-medications (i.e. oxygen) and duplicates.

Fourth step—second list: online survey using a modified Delphi process

The modified Delphi survey process has been described elsewhere[18,19]. An online survey consisting of 19 rating panels (one for each symptom and four for pain: mild to moderate, moderate to severe, visceral pain, and bone pain) was sent by email to 112 physicians, pharmacists, and pharmacologists (77 from developing countries). The names and contact information for these professionals were provided by the members of the Task Force, the IAHPC board members, and from the membership database of IAHPC.

Using a scale of 1–9, participants were asked to rate the effectiveness and safety of each medication using the following definitions from the Institute of Medicine in the USA[20]:

a. Effectiveness: a drug class or medication is defined as effective for treating a specific symptom in a palliative-care population based on consideration of:

Evidence of treatment effectiveness: the strongest evidence is derived from randomized controlled trials (RCTs), but other experimental designs, observational studies, and expert opinion are also useful in rating this issue in the absence of RCTs. With respect to drug class, the evidence should be consistent across drugs within a group. Ratings of 1–3 mean that the drug class or medication is not effective for treating that specific symptom in palliative-care populations; ratings of 4–6 mean that there will be considerable variability in the effectiveness of that drug class or medication for treating that specific symptom in palliative-care populations; and ratings of 7–9 mean that drug class or medication is very effective for treating that specific symptom.

b. Safety: the safety profile of an agent, when used in a clinically appropriate manner, is sufficiently known (and/or described) in the target and/or general population so that adverse events can be anticipated and, if possible, prevented; or, when they occur, can be duly recognized and mitigated. In addition, the safety profile of one agent should be viewed in context of its pertinent comparators.

Ratings of 1–3 mean that drug class or medication is not safe for use in palliative-care populations; ratings of 4–6 mean that there will be considerable variability in the safety of using a drug class or medication in palliative-care populations; and ratings of 7–9 mean that the drug class or medication is very safe to use in this population.

Seventy-one participants (63 per cent) responded to the modified Delphi survey. Following the guidelines from the request by WHO which required that the list should be based on the consensus of pain and palliative-care individuals, the working group determined that only those medications for which at least 50 per cent of the respondents rated 7 or above for both safety and efficacy, would be included in the final discussion and selection process.

There was consensus among the respondents about the effectiveness and safety of 48 medications for 18 of the 23 symptoms.

Fifth step—final list of essential medicines in palliative care

Twenty-eight global, regional, and professional organizations working in pain and palliative care were invited to a meeting in Salzburg, Austria, from April 30th to May 2nd, 2006. Thirty-one representatives from 26 of these organizations attended. Appendix 2.4.3 includes the list of participants and organizations represented in the meeting. This meeting was co-funded and hosted by the International Palliative Care Initiative of the Open Society Institute (OSI). Participants received a copy of the then current version of the *WHO Model List of Essential Medicines* (14th edition), as well as the results of the modified Delphi survey which also showed the ratings that each medication received.

Participants were divided into three working groups. Each group considered medications for a specific set of symptoms:

(1) medications used to treat mental health symptoms,

(2) medications to treat pain, and

(3) medications to treat gastrointestinal symptoms.

A few additional symptoms (e.g. hiccups) were randomly assigned to each group.

Led by a moderator, each group held a structured discussion addressing agreement and disagreement about medications under consideration as 'essential medications' for each symptom. Groups were instructed to base the discussions especially on those medications which at least 50 per cent of the respondents rated as both safe and effective (score of 7 or above). For several groups of medications, in which the Delphi survey did not result in the 50 per cent consensus as described, the group was asked to review the comprehensive list and make recommendations based on their expertise.

Using the results from the modified Delphi survey and by a process of reaching consensus, each group identified the medications they considered essential for each symptom. The Chairs of each group then shared the results with all participants and a general discussion ensued. When there were differences of opinion, alternatives were discussed and the best option was decided by consensus. Thus, each of the medications included in the IAHPC List was reviewed and approved by the conference participants as a whole.

Results

The conference participants agreed with the respondents to the modified Delphi survey in that there is not enough evidence to recommend any medications as both safe and effective for five of the symptoms—bone pain, dry mouth, fatigue, hiccups, and sweating—and asserted that additional research is needed to identify safe and effective medications for these symptoms.

The IAHPC List includes 33 medications and is presented in Table 2.4.2. Fourteen were included in the WHO Model List for the treatment of conditions common in palliative care. A medication listed in one section of the WHO Model List does not preclude its inclusion in another section if the medication is determined by WHO to be essential for the treatment of more than one condition.

In Table 2.4.2, the third column describes the IAHPC indication(s) for palliative care. The fourth column identifies those medications on the IAHPC List which were at the time, included in the *WHO Model List of Essential Medicines* (14th edition) as well as the indications for these medicines specified by WHO.

IAHPC copyrighted the IAHPC List with the purpose of ensuring that it could be freely accessed, copied, disseminated, duplicated, and distributed.

The IAHPC, WWPCA, and other organizations have disseminated the IAHPC List of Medications through press releases, newsletters, and pain and palliative care journals. A special request was sent to the editors of pain and palliative care journals asking them to assist in dissemination. Several journals accepted this invitation and have published reports, editorials, and papers since then[21–26].

Table 2.4.2 IAHPC List of essential medicines for palliative care©.

Medication	Formulation	Indication for palliative care	WHO Essential Medicines Model List Section, subsection and indication
Amitriptyline*	50–150 mg tablets	Depression Neuropathic pain	24.2.1—Depressive disorders
Bisacodyl	10 mg tablets 10 mg rectal suppositories	Constipation	Not included
Carbamazepine**	100–200 mg tablet	Neuropathic pain	5—Anticonvulsants/antiepileptics 24.2.2—Bipolar disorders
Citalopram (*or any other equivalent generic SSRI except paroxetine and fluvoxamine*)	20 mg tablets 10 mg/5 ml oral solution 20–40 mg injectable	Depression	Not included
Codeine	30 mg tablets	Diarrhoea Pain—mild to moderate	2.2—Opioid analgesics 17.5.3—Antidiarrhoeal
Dexamethasone	0.5–4 mg tablets 4 mg/ml injectable	Anorexia Nausea Neuropathic pain Vomiting	3—Antiallergics and anaphylaxis 8.3—Hormones and antihormones
Diazepam	2.5 –10 mg tablets 5 mg/ml injectable 10 mg rectal suppository	Anxiety	1.3—Preoperative sedation short term procedures 5—Anticonvulsants/antiepileptics 24.3—Generalized anxiety, sleep disorders
Diclofenac	25–50 mg tablets 50 and 75 mg/3 ml injectable	Pain—mild to moderate	Not included
Diphenhydramine	25 mg tablets 50 mg/ml injectable	Nausea Vomiting	Not included
Fentanyl (transdermal patch)	25 µg/h 50 µg/h	Pain—moderate to severe	Not included
Gabapentin	tablets 300 mg or 400 mg	Neuropathic pain	Not included
Haloperidol	0.5–5 mg tablets 0.5–5 mg drops 0.5–5 mg/ml injectable	Delirium Nausea Vomiting Terminal restlessness	24.1—Psychotic disorders
Hyoscine butylbromide	20 mg/ml oral solution 10 mg tablets 10 mg/ml injectable	Nausea Terminal respiratory congestion Visceral pain Vomiting	Not included
Ibuprofen	200 mg tablets 400 mg tablets	Pain—mild to moderate	2.1—Non-opioids and NSAIMs
Levomepromazine	5–50 mg tablets 25 mg/ml injectable	Delirium Terminal restlessness	Not included
Loperamide	2 mg tablets	Diarrhoea	Not included
Lorazepam***	0.5–2 mg tablets 2 mg/ml liquid/drops 2–4mg/ml injectable	Anxiety Insomnia	Not included
Megestrol acetate	160 mg tablets 40 mg/ml solution	Anorexia	Not included

(continued)

Table 2.4.2 (Continued) IAHPC List of essential medicines for palliative care©.

Medication	Formulation	Indication for palliative care	WHO Essential Medicines Model List Section, subsection and indication
Methadone (immediate release)	5mg tablets 1 mg/ml oral solution	Pain—moderate to severe	24.5—Substance dependence
Metoclopramide	10 mg tablets 5 mg/ml injectable	Nausea Vomiting	17.2—Antiemetics
Midazolam	1–5 mg/ml injectable	Anxiety Terminal restlessness	Not included
Mineral oil enema			Not included
Mirtazapine *(or any other generic dual action NassA or SNRI)*	15–30 mg tablets 7.5–15 mg injectable	Depression	Not included
Morphine	Immediate release: 10–60 mg tablets Immediate release: 10 mg/5 ml oral solution Immediate release: 10 mg/ml injectable Sustained release: 10 mg tablets Sustained release: 30 mg tablets	Dyspnoea Pain—moderate to severe	2.2—Opioid analgesics (Only immediate release is included in the WHO Model List (14th edition). Sustained release morphine is not) **Note**: this statement is no longer true. The 15th edition of the WHO Model List includes sustained release morphine
Octreotide	100 mcg/ml injectable	Diarrhoea Vomiting	Not included
Oral rehydration salts		Diarrhoea	17.5.1—Oral rehydration
Oxycodone	5 mg tablet	Pain—moderate to severe	Not included
Paracetamol (acetaminophen)	100–500 mg tablets 500 mg rectal suppositories	Pain—mild to moderate	2.1—Non-opioids and NSAIMs
Prednisolone (as an alternative to dexamethasone)	5 mg tablet	Anorexia	3—Antiallergics and anaphylaxis 8.3—Hormones and antihormones 21.2—Anti-inflammatory agents
Senna	8.6 mg tablets	Constipation	17.4—Laxatives
Tramadol	50 mg immediate release tablets/capsules 100 mg/ml oral solution 50 mg/ml injectable	Pain—mild to moderate	Not included
Trazodone	25–75 mg tablets 50 mg injectable	Insomnia	Not included
Zolpidem (still patented)	5–10 mg tablets	Insomnia	Not included

Complementary: *Require special training and/or delivery method.*

* Side-effects limit dose.

** Alternatives to amitriptyline and tricyclic antidepressants (should have at least one drug other than dexamethasone).

*** For short term use in insomnia.

Notes:

Non-benzodiazepines should be used in the elderly.

Non-steroidal anti-inflammatory medicines (NSAIMs) should be used for brief periods of time.

NO GOVERNMENT SHOULD APPROVE MODIFIED RELEASE MORPHINE, FENTANYL OR OXYCODONE WITHOUT ALSO GUARANTEEING WIDELY AVAILABLE NORMAL RELEASE ORAL MORPHINE.

This list is copyrighted by IAHPC. The organization provides permission for free reproduction, printing, and publication of this list with appropriate credit and reference to copyright.

Limitations of the list

This project focused on medications to treat the most common symptoms in a limited number of diseases recognizing that it will need to be expanded to address other conditions and symptoms in the future. Some of these concerns are particularly important in resource-poor settings and may be only partially addressed within the scope of the project.

Additionally, the list was developed for adult patients and it does not address the needs and formulations of other patient groups both in terms of specific drugs and formulations. A list of Essential Medicines in Palliative Care for children is currently being developed by WHO. In the same way, a list of Essential Medicines for the elderly needs to be developed, with special medications and formulations for this special patient population.

The project did not address cost issues as they were addressed in the Critical Reviews commissioned later by the WHO.

Advocacy

As the holder of the copyrights to the IAHPC List of Essential Medicines for Palliative Care, the IAHPC has granted permission to all those interested to reproduce and use the list as an advocacy tool to promote access to palliative care. It especially encourages use of the list as a model for countries in which there currently is limited availability and problems of accessing opioid analgesics and other medications for palliative care and for development of national lists tailored to local needs and resources.

Recent developments

During the second half of 2006, the IAHPC submitted the IAHPC List to the WHO for review and possible addition of the medications to the WHO Model List. In March 2007, WHO convened the Expert Committee on Essential Medicines in Geneva during which the IAHPC was represented by the coordinator of the project (LDL). In addition to presenting the complete list for consideration by the WHO and the Expert Committee, the IAHPC also presented two individual applications: modified-release morphine as an additional formulation to the existing list of morphine formulations in the opioid analgesic section (Section 2.2), and fluoxetine for depressive disorders (Section 24.2.1) in the WHO Model List.

After analyzing the IAHPC List, the WHO Expert Committee members decided that it was necessary to present applications for individual medications and not a collective list. The applications for modified-release morphine and fluoxetine were included in the sections mentioned above in the 15th edition of the WHO Model List[27]. In the same way, the paragraph under the palliative care section was modified for the following:

Medicines used in palliative care

The WHO Expert Committee recognizes the importance of listing specific medicines in the Palliative Care Section. Some medicines currently used in palliative care are included in the relevant sections of the Model List, according to their therapeutic use, e.g. analgesics. The Guidelines for Palliative Care that were referenced in the previous list are in need of update. The Committee expects applications for medicines needed for palliative care to be submitted for the next meeting.

The WPCA, in collaboration with the IAHPC and the European Association for Palliative Care (EAPC), has recently put in place a strategy to encourage and support hospice and palliative care national associations to work in different areas including medications. This strategy was launched as the Budapest Commitments during the 10th Congress of the EAPC in June 2007. Among the several recommendations, the Budapest Commitment calls associations to help ensure the availability and access to the IAHPC List of Essential Medicines in Palliative Care for patients in need[28]. The WPCA will provide guidance to the national associations in this process to support national associations, and a follow up meeting is planned for the 11th Congress of the EAPC in 2009.

Future

The IAHPC, WPCA, and pan-national associations, aim to ensure that global health institutions, non-governmental organizations (NGOs), and other multi-lateral organizations such as the World Bank are aware of the issue of access to medicines for pain relief and palliative care; and that national associations are aware of the key issues relating to the IAHPC List of Essential Medicines for Palliative Care.

The IAHPC and all the organizations involved in this process welcome suggestions on ways to continue to improve the List of Essential Medicines for Palliative Care and to improve access to medications for patients in need.

Conclusion

The majority of the medications included in the IAHPC List are simple and inexpensive while a few require special training or delivery methods. The process of compiling the list demonstrated how often simple, inexpensive medications can be as effective in the management of symptoms as expensive ones. Treatment protocols and drug formulations newly developed in affluent countries and aggressively marketed are not necessarily more efficacious and safe than existing ones. In the process of selecting the medications, the group was careful to recommend only those for which sufficient experience and information is available to ensure both their efficacy and safety.

It is hoped that the concept of Essential Medicines and, more specifically, the IAHPC List of Essential Medicines in Palliative Care, will result in increased access to adequate treatment for patients who have uncontrolled symptoms. Governments, policy makers, and health-care providers should take the necessary steps to ensure that all patients in need have access to the medications in the List of Essential Medicines in Palliative Care.

Acknowledgements

The costs of travel for representatives from developing countries and room and board for all the participants to the meeting in Salzburg were covered by IAHPC and the Palliative Care Initiative of the Open Society Institute (OSI). The cost of travel for representatives from organizations in developed countries was funded by their respective organizations. Karl Lorenz was supported by an Advanced Career Development Award from the Department of Veterans Affairs HSR&D.

References

1. World Health Organization (2006). *Essential medicines: definition and concept*. Retrieved from http://www.who.int/medicines/services/essmedicines_def/en/index.html on 6 December 2006

2. World Health Organization. (2003). *Framework for action in essential drugs and medicines policy*. WHO, Geneva.

3. World Health Organization. (2000). *Essential drugs and medicines policy. the essential drug strategy*. WHO, Geneva.

4. World Health Organization. (1990). *Cancer pain relief and palliative care*. Report of a WHO Expert Committee, World Health Organization Technical Report Series No 804; Geneva: WHO.

5. UN Economic and Social Council. (2005). *Resolution 2025/25; Treatment of Pain using opioid analgesics*. Adopted at the 36th Plenary Meeting, July 22, 2005. NY, UN ECOSOC.

6. United Nations. (1996). *Availability of opiates for medical needs*. Special report prepared pursuant to Economic and Social Council resolutions 1990/31 and 1991/43. New York: UN.

7. World Health Organization. (1996). *Cancer pain relief with a guide to opioid availability*, 2nd edition. WHO, Geneva.

8. International Narcotics Board. (2000). UN Drug Control Body concerned over inadequate medical supply of narcotic drugs to relieve pain and suffering. Press Release, Vienna: INCB, February 23.

9. Pain & Policy Studies Group. (2007). Improving Availability of essential pain medicine for cancer and HIV/AIDS pain relief: Report for 2006. Madison, WI: University of Wisconsin Pain & Policy Studies Group/WHO Collaborating Centre for Policy and Communicationsin Cancer Care.

10. De Lima, L., Sweeney, C., Palmer, J.L. *et al.* (2004). Potent analgesics are more expensive for patients in developing countries: a comparative study. *Journal of Pain and Palliative Care Pharmacotherapy*; 18(1).

11. Blengini, C., Joranson, D.E., and Ryan, K.M. (2003). Italy reforms national policy for cancer pain relief and opioids. *European Journal of Cancer*, 12(1), 28–34.

12. Mosoiu, D., Ryan, K.M., Joranson, D.E. *et al.* (2006). Reforming drug control policy for palliative care in Romania. *The Lancet*, 367, 2110–7.

13. Joranson, D. (1999). Availability of opioids for cancer pain: recent trends, assessment of system barriers, new World Health Organization Guidelines and the Risk of Diversion. *Journal of Pain and Symptom Management*, 18, 358–68.

14. World Health Organization. (2005). *Essential Medicines: WHO Model List*, 14th edition, WHO, Geneva. Retrieved from http://whqlibdoc.who.int/hq/2005/a87017_eng.pdf on 6 December 2006

15. Solano, J.P., Gomes, B., and Higginson, I. (2006). A comparison of symptom prevalence in far advanced cancer, AIDS, heart disease, chronic obstructive pulmonary disease and renal disease. *Journal of Pain and Symptom Management*, 13(1), 58–69.

16. Carr, D., Goudas, L., Lawrence, D. *et al.* (2002). Management of cancer symptoms: pain, depression, and fatigue. Evidence Report / Technology Assessment Number 61. Agency for Healthcare Research and Quality U.S. Department of Health and Human Services.

17. Plan, W.M., and Arnold, R.M. (2005). Terminal care: the last weeks of life. *Journal of Palliative Medicine*, 8(5), 1042–54.

18. Custer, R.L., Scarcella, J.A., and Stewart, B.R. (1999). The modified Delphi technique: a rotational modification. *Journal of Vocational and Technical Education*, 15(2), 1–10.

19. Linstone, H.A., and Turoff, M. (eds.) (1975). *The Delphi method: Techniques and applications*. New Jersey Institute of Technology. Retrieved from http://www.is.njit.edu/pubs/delphibook/ on 28 January 2006.

20. Institute of Medicine. (2001). *Crossing the quality chasm: a new health system for the 21st century*. The National Academies Press, Washington, DC.

21. Observations (2006). IAHPC issues List of Essential Palliative Care Drugs. *Supportive Oncology*, 4(8).

22. Doyle, D. (2006). The International Association for Hospice and Palliative Care List of Essential Medicines for Palliative Care. *Palliative Medicine*, 20, 645–6.

23. De Lima, L. (2006). The International Association for Hospice and Palliative Care List of Essential Medicines for Palliative Care. *Palliative Medicine*, 20, 647–51.

24. De Lima, L., MacDonald, N., and Doyle, D. (2006). IAHPC List of Essential Medicines for Palliative Care: summary of process for editors of pain and palliative care journals. *Journal of Palliative Care*, 22(4), 300–4.

25. De Lima, L. (2007). International Association for Hospice and Palliative Care List of Essential Medicines for Palliative Care. *Annals of Oncology*, 18(2), 395–9.

26. De Lima, L., Krakauer, E.L., Lorenz, K. *et al.* (2007). Ensuring palliative medicines availability: the development of the IAHPC List of Essential Medicines for Palliative Care. *Journal of Pain and Symptom Management*, 33(5), 521–6.

27. World Health Organization. (2007). *WHO Model List of Essential Medicines*, 15th edition. WHO, Geneva.

28. Radbruch, L., De Lima, L., Praill, D. *et al.* (2007). The Budapest Commitments – a framework for palliative care development. A joint initiative by the European Association for Palliative Care (EAPC), the International Association for Hospice and Palliative Care (IAHPC) and the Worldwide Palliative Care Alliance (WPCA). *European Journal of Palliative Care*, 2007: *Book of Abstracts, 10th Congress of the EAPC*, Budapest. EAPC.

Appendix 2.4.1 Medicines included in the WHO publication *Cancer Pain Relief with a Guide to Opioid Availability (2nd edition)*[7]

ASA, alcohol, amitriptyline, betamethasone, bisacodyl, bupivacaine, buprenorphine, carbamazepine, choline magnesium, codeine, chlorocresol, chlorpromazine, cyclizine, desipramine, dexamethasone, dextropropoxyphene, diazepam, diclofenac, diflunisal, dihydrocodeine, dimenhydrinate, docusate, haloperidol, hydromorphone, hyoscine butylbromide, ibuprofen, indometacin, imipramine, levorphanol, lidocaine, methadone, morphine, naloxone, naproxen, oxycodone, paracetamol, pethidine, phenol, prednisone, prednisolone, prochlorperazine, senna, standardized opium, tramadol, trisalicylate, valproic acid.

Appendix 2.4.2 Guiding Principles for the development, use and application of the *IAHPC List of Essential Medicines for Palliative Care*

a) The *IAHPC List of Essential Medicines for Palliative Care* will be produced by a representative group of palliative care specialists, each with very considerable experience in this discipline. Some work in countries where palliative care is well established and developing rapidly, others in countries at earlier stages of development. They come from countries differing in resources and the technical capabilities of their health-care systems; in culture; and in their ethnic, linguistic, and religious traditions. These specialists are each affiliated to, and represent, national and international associations and societies for the study and provision of palliative care.

These palliative medicine specialists share a commitment to the provision of palliative care to all who need it irrespective of race, color, creed, class, or financial means. They believe that:

◆ Every person with a life threatening illness has the right to receive appropriate palliative care.

◆ It is the responsibility of every clinician to provide appropriate palliative care to those who need it.

◆ Persons receiving palliative care should be enabled to receive it in the place of their choice.

b) The *IAHPC List of Essential Medicines for Palliative Care* is not a directive but is offered for guidance. Important as the cost of medicines is in every country, the list does not use low cost as a primary criterion, but rather efficacy and safety. The cost is a political issue which needs to be addressed by governments, advocacy and professional groups, and by multi-lateral organizations such as WHO.

c) The *IAHPC List of Essential Medicines for Palliative Care* has been produced with only one aim—to facilitate provision of the best possible care for all those with advanced life-threatening illness, uninfluenced by commercial or political considerations.

d) The *IAHPC List of Essential Medicines for Palliative Care* will be of little or no use if:

◆ clinicians and students in health-care disciplines are not taught how to use these medicines in the palliative care setting;

◆ the medicines are not made available and accessible, if needs be by appropriate legislation;

◆ the list is not brought to the attention of physicians, nurses and pharmacists by relevant government, professional and academic bodies, professional journals and charities involved in promotion and supporting the provision of palliative care; and

◆ countries do not have in place, or are not prepared to produce, National Palliative Care Policies/Guidelines.

e) The *IAHPC List of Essential Medicines for Palliative Care* is not an endorsement of any product, does not assume similar pharmacological action or adverse effects among medications within the same class, and should not be read as promoting a proprietary preparation.

f) The *IAHPC List of Essential Medicines for Palliative Care* will need to be reviewed and revised on a regular basis, taking into account research findings, changes in practice, and constructive comments from palliative care workers worldwide.

The following recommendations flow from the principles listed above:

i) Every effort should be made to ensure ready availability and accessibility of all essential medicines before approving more expensive but equally efficacious formulations.

ii) Every effort should be made to ensure that prescribing physicians and pharmacists are made aware of comparative costs of drugs on the essential medicines list and their more expensive competitors with equivalent therapeutic benefit.

iii) Every encouragement should be given to editors of scientific and in particular palliative care journals to encourage the publication of the essential medicines list for palliative care.

iv) Every effort should be made to get charities supporting palliative care providers and educators to encourage recipients of their funds to use and promote the drugs on the essential medicine list in preference to more expensive ones with equivalent therapeutic benefit.

v) All trainees in palliative care—whether medical, nursing, pharmacy, clinical psychology—should be made aware of the *IAHPC Essential Medicines List for Palliative Care*, should be prepared to be examined on it, and should understand why drugs were selected for the list.

vi) The *IAHPC List of Essential Medicines for Palliative Care* should be brought to the attention of the groups being set up in many countries to keep politicians informed about palliative care so that policy and law makers may learn of the benefits of such a list and of the pressing need for legislation to establish availability and accessibility of the medicines. They should know what is being done in other countries to promote and provide palliative care to all who need it, irrespective of race, creed, or financial means.

vii) The *IAHPC List of Essential Medicines for Palliative Care* should be studied by all the national and international professional associations and societies represented by the specialists who have drawn it up, and their considered opinions and suggestions on it should be taken into account when the list is finalized and subsequently updated.

Appendix 2.4.3 Pain and palliative care organizations represented in the Salzburg meeting.

Name	Representing	Country
Adams, Vanessa	Velindre NHS Trust and Hospice Africa Uganda	UK and Uganda
Alexander, Carla	National Association for Palliative Care (NHPCO)	USA
Aapro, Matti	Multi-national Ass. For Supportive Care in Cancer (MASCC)	Switzerland
Callaway, Mary	International Palliative Care Initiative—Open Society Institute	USA
Cleary, James	American Academy of Hospice and Palliative Medicine (AAHPM)	USA
Daeninck, Paul	Canadian Society of Palliative Care Physicians	Canada
De Conno, Franco	European Association for Palliative Care (EAPC)	Italy
Doyle, Derek	National Council for Palliative Care	UK
Filbert, Marilene	European Association for Palliative Care (EAPC)	France
Foley, Kathleen	International Palliative Care Initiative—Open Society Institute	USA
Goh, Cynthia	Asia Pacific Hospice Palliative Care Association (APHN)	Singapore

(continued)

Appendix 2.4.3 (Continued) Pain and palliative care organizations represented in the Salzburg meeting.

Grassi, Luigi	International Psycho Oncology Society (IPOS) and World Psychiatric Association (WPA)	Italy
Gwyther, Elizabeth	Hospice and Palliative Care Association of South Africa (HPCA)	South Africa
Hanks, Geoffrey	International Assoc. for the Study of Pain (IASP)	UK
Krakauer, Eric	Centre for Palliative Care, Harvard Medical School	USA
Law, Freida	Li Ka Shing Foundation	China
Luczak, Jacek	Eastern and Central Europe Palliative Care Task Force (ECEPT)	Poland
Merriman, Anne	African Palliative Care Association (APCA)	Uganda
Praill, David	Help the Hospices	UK
Rowett, Debra	Palliative Care Australia (PCA)	Australia
Rubach, Maryna	European Society of Medical Oncology (ESMO)	Poland
Serdar, Erdine	European Federation of IASP Chapters (EAFIC)	Turkey
Wenk, Roberto	Latin America Association for Palliative Care (ALCP)	Argentina
IAHPC		
De Lima, Liliana	International Association for Hospice & Palliative Care (IAHPC)	USA
MacDonald, Neil	International Association for Hospice & Palliative Care (IAHPC)	Canada
Ripamonti, Carla	International Association for Hospice & Palliative Care (IAHPC)	Italy
WHO		
Hill, Suzanne	WHO—Dept of Medicines Policy and Standards	Switzerland
Scholten, Willem	WHO—Dept of Medicines Policy and Standards	Switzerland
Sepulveda, Cecilia	WHO—Cancer Control Programme	Switzerland

SECTION 3

The challenge of palliative medicine

The problem of suffering and the principles of assessment in palliative medicine

Nathan I. Cherny

Despite the advances of modern medicine, many illnesses continue to evade cure. Chronic progressive incurable illness is a major cause of disability, distress, suffering, and, ultimately, death. This is true for many causes of cancer, progressive neurologic disorders, AIDS, and other disorders of vital organs. Progressive chronic diseases of this ilk are most common in late adulthood and old age, but they occur in all ages.

When cure is not possible, as often it is not, the relief of suffering is the cardinal goal of medicine. Recognition of this axiom is at the heart of the philosophy, science, and practice of palliative medicine.

Understanding suffering

For the patient with incurable illnesses such as cancer, the goals of care may be stated as the alleviation of suffering, the optimization of quality of life until death ensues, and the provision of comfort in death[1,2]. Persistent suffering that is inadequately relieved (or the anticipation of this situation) undermines, for the sufferer, the value of life. Without hope that this situation will be relieved, patients, their families, and professional health-care providers may see elective death by suicide, euthanasia, or assisted suicide as their only alternatives. The truth of the perception that patients need to be killed or assisted to kill themselves to be adequately relieved of suffering depends upon the adequacy of the available measures to relieve suffering. The essence of the controversy is the problem of suffering.

The alleviation of suffering is universally acknowledged as a cardinal goal of medical care[1,3–9]. The ability to formulate a response to the challenge of suffering requires a clinically relevant understanding of the nature of the problem. Paradoxically, however, the medical literature on the nature of suffering is sparse. Cassell described suffering as arising from a threat to the integrity of the person, and elucidated multiple factors that may contribute to that threat[10,11]. He asserts, however, that the nature of suffering precludes the development of a clinical taxonomy, and that the ability to recognize suffering is an acquired skill[11]. Cicely Saunders has described a model of suffering as 'Total Pain'. Although this model does not define the nature of the problem, it does outline some of the various physical, psychological, emotional, existential, and social factors that contribute to the experience[12].

Defining suffering

In the cancer setting, clinical and psychosocial research has helped define the scope and prevalence of distresses experienced by patients, their families, and their attending health-care professionals, and has highlighted the complex interrelations between these groups. Based on a review of this research, a new definition of suffering and a taxonomy of factors that may contribute to the experience was proposed[13]. According to this model, suffering is defined as an aversive experience characterized by the perception of personal distress that is generated by adverse factors that undermine quality of life[13]. The defining characteristics of suffering include: (1) the presence of perceptual capacity (sentience), (2) that the factors undermining quality of life are appraised as distressing, and (3) that the experience is aversive. According to this definition, suffering is a phenomenon of conscious human existence, the intensity of which is determined by the number and severity of the factors diminishing from quality of life, the processes of appraisal, and perception. Each of these variables is amenable to therapeutic interventions.

The triangular model of suffering

The encounter with terminal illness is a potential cause of great distress to patients, their families, and the professional caregivers attending them. Among patients with advanced cancer, for instance, at least two-thirds of patients with advanced cancer have significant pain and numerous other physical symptoms can equally diminish the patient's quality of life. Furthermore, many patients endure enormous psychological distress, and in some cases, from an existential perspective that, even without pain or other physical symptoms, continued life is without meaning. For the families and loved ones of patients there is, likewise, great distress in this process: anticipated loss, standing witness to the physical and emotional distress of the patient, and bearing the burdens of care. Finally, professional caregivers may potentially be stressed by the suffering, which they witness, and which challenges their clinical and emotional resources.

According to this model[13], the suffering of each of these three groups is inextricably interrelated such that the perceived distress

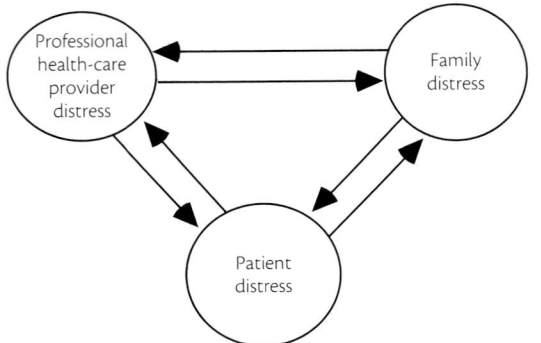

Figure 3.1.1 The interrelationship between the distress of the patient, the family, and the health-care providers.

of any one of these three groups may amplify the distress of the others (Fig. 3.1.1).

Suffering, personal growth, and resilience

The potential for personal development and net positive gain in overcoming situations of adversity and suffering is widely recognized. This potential, however, is predicated on the ability to cope with the prevailing problems and challenges. It is the phenomenon of coping that generates the potential for growth and reward[14,15]. Coping does not occur if the demands of the situation are overwhelming (as distinct from merely being appraised as overwhelming). For example, the patient with inadequately relieved pain, shortness of breath, or vomiting, may be absolutely unable to address issues related to their offspring and spouse. The spouse and offspring who are overwhelmed by problems of daily-care requirements may be absolutely unable to appreciate time with the patient. Suffering in chronic debilitating illness cannot be eliminated, but if adequate relief is achieved, then coping and growth can occur. By understanding and addressing the factors that may potentially overwhelm the patient, family, and health-care providers, the necessary pre-conditions for coping and growth are established.

The potential for growth and adaptation are related to the quality and process of resilience. Resilience is the capacity of an individual person or a social system to grow and to develop in the face of very difficult circumstances[16]. Often, the problems to be overcome may open up access to some hitherto hidden inner resources in a person, and trigger off a growth process. If certain problems turn out to be positive challenges stimulating growth, others will be destructive. So, in a difficult situation, growth will sometimes happen in spite of problems, sometimes thanks to them, and in many situations, it will be a mixture of both. Resilience is not limited to victims and patients, but also to their families and friends, and to the staff providing care. Resilience has several important attributes: resilience is not an absolute; rather, it is a relative personal attribute, which may vary over time. It consists of dimensions of resistance to adversity and the ability to make constructive adaptation. This latter characteristic implies the capacity to transform a negative event into an element of growth. It is important to emphasize that resilience does not ignore the need to dealing with problems and negative situations; it involves processes of grieving and negative emotions, such as sadness and fear, but also involves looking for positive elements to rebuild life. Reliance does not invoke denial, but, rather,

a realistic view of the situation that is not exclusively determined by problems, and which recognizes that identification of positives is necessary for coping and growth.

Relieving suffering: a right

It is widely held that terminally ill patients have a right to adequate relief of uncontrolled suffering. Indeed, the World Health Organization asserts that the relief of pain and other symptoms is a right of the patient with advanced and incurable cancer[17] and the right to the adequate provision of palliative care for the terminally ill has been ratified by the American Medical Association, Academy of Psychosomatic Medicine, American Academy of Hospice and Palliative Medicine, American Board of Hospice and Palliative Medicine, American College of Chest Physicians, American Pain Society, and the National Kidney Foundation[18]. The right has legal status recognized by the supreme court of the United States[19] and in Israeli statute law defining the rights of the dying[20].

The corollary of this right is the responsibility of caregivers to ensure that adequate provisions are made for relief. The formulation of a therapeutic response requires an understanding of the phenomenon of suffering and of the factors that contribute to it. Failure to appreciate, or to effectively address, the full diversity of contributing factors may confound effective therapeutic strategies.

Cancer as a model of suffering and terminal illness

The interrelated elements of suffering in terminal illness are well illustrated by an evaluation of the distress among cancer patients, their families, and the caring health-care providers.

Patient distress

Physical symptoms (see Section 10)

Prevalence data suggest that 70–90 per cent of patients with advanced cancer will have significant pain that requires the use of opioid drugs[21]. Persistent pain interferes with the ability to eat[22], sleep[23], think, interact with others[24], and is correlated with fatigue in cancer patients[25] and depression and anxiety[26].

The prevalence of symptoms other than pain in the advanced cancer patient have been well documented in the hospice and palliative care literature[27]: multiple concurrent physical symptoms are common during the last weeks of life with a particularly high prevalence of fatigue and generalized weakness[28], and in the last few days of life, dyspnoea, delirium, nausea, and vomiting are most common[29–35].

The data on the prevalence of physical symptoms among children with advanced and incurable cancer are similarly dramatic. In a Swedish survey of the parents of dying children, the symptoms that had a moderate or high impact of the child's well-being were: physical fatigue (86 per cent), reduced mobility (76 per cent), pain (73 per cent), and decreased appetite (71 per cent)[36]. Findings from an English survey were similar; pain was observed in 71–92 per cent of children and the other major symptoms were anorexia, weight loss, and weakness[37].

Interestingly and importantly, the prevalence of symptoms in disease other than cancer has recently been reviewed in a study that evaluated the relative prevalence of 11 common symptoms (pain, depression, anxiety, confusion, fatigue, dyspnoea, insomnia, nausea, constipation, diarrhoea, anorexia) among end-stage patients suffering from five common, chronic, and progressive diseases (cancer, AIDS, heart disease, chronic obstructive pulmonary disease, and renal disease). Three symptoms—pain, breathlessness, and fatigue—were found among more than 50 per cent of patients, for all five diseases. The great similarity in the spectrum of symptoms seen across all illness groups suggests that there are a number of common symptoms found as patients approach death in both malignant and non-malignant chronic illnesses[38].

Psychological symptoms (see Chapters 15.2 and 15.5)

The prevalence of psychiatric distress in cancer patients is a subject of dispute, and the prevalence of the problem has been variably estimated from 12 per cent[39], 40 per cent[40], to upward of 60 per cent of patients with far advanced cancer[41,42]. Whatever the prevalence, there is agreement that the most common problems are adjustment disorders, depression, anxiety, and delirium[40,41,43]. All four of these symptoms may contribute to the development of suicidal thoughts, and indeed, psychiatric disorders are present in the vast majority cancer patients who are suicidal[44]. Assessment of suicidal cancer patients at the Memorial Sloan-Kettering Cancer Center by the Psychiatry Service diagnosed one-third with major depression, 20 per cent with a delirium, and 50 per cent with an adjustment disorder with anxious and depressed features at the time of evaluation[44].

Factors that adversely influence the prevalence and severity of psychological distress are: the presence of advanced disease; distressing physical symptoms (especially pain)[26,45]; disability; unresolved previous experiences of loss or separation[46]; feelings of frustration and hopelessness[46]; a lack of perceived support from at least one loved person[47]; strained interpersonal relationships[47]; controlling personality trait[48]; difficulties in adapting to the illness and its implications[49]; economic concerns; impaired cognitive abilities[46]; and unsatisfactory communication regarding illness or treatment (particularly, where there has been the precipitous disclosure of poor prognosis without allowance for a process of adjustment and assimilation of information)[50]. Uncontrolled pain is an important precipitant of psychological distress and is a suicide risk factor. In a large prospective study of psychological symptoms in cancer patients[45], the prevalence of cancer-related pain was 39 per cent in those who had a psychiatric diagnosis and only 19 per cent in those without such a diagnosis. Indeed, it has been observed that psychiatric symptoms commonly resolve with adequate pain relief[26].

Spiritual and existential distress (see Chapter 15.1)

The importance of spirituality in care of the dying is increasingly acknowledged by clinicians, researchers, and educators in end-of-life care. The Institute of Medicine[51] lists spiritual well-being as one of six domains of quality supportive care of the dying. Consequentially, exploring this dimension of well-being is an important part of routine physician inquiry, especially among patients with advanced and incurable illness[52].

Defining existential issues such as spirituality is challenging and definitions abound. One comprehensive review of the health literature documented 92 definitions of the term 'spirituality'[53]. This review identified seven definitional themes: relationship to God, a spiritual being, a higher power, or a reality greater than the self; not of the self; transcendence or connectedness to a bigger picture but unrelated to a belief in a higher being; a conviction that there is more to life than what we can observe materially; meaning and purpose in life; life force of the person, integrating aspect of the person; and summative definitions that combined multiple themes. In another interesting study that evaluated Buddhist and Christian terminally ill patients in Taiwan[54], 10 themes in four broad categories emerged: communion with self (self-identity, wholeness, inner peace); communion with others (love, reconciliation); communion with nature (inspiration, creativity); and communion with a higher being (faithfulness, hope, gratitude).

Positive connections to life around us inspire a conscious or unconscious perception that life has significance, purpose, and meaning. This is of practical consequence; particularly in the context of discovering or building connections. These connection may be with God, relations, projects, responsibilities, special objects, rituals, non-sectarian religion or philosophy, or even the shared appreciation of beauty, poetry, or music[55]. While the source or inspiration for such significance will vary from person to person, what they hold in common is their ability to imbue life with an overarching sense of purpose and meaning, including a sustained investment in life itself.

Within the religious worldview, spirituality is usually associated with a sense of connectedness to a God, whereas within the secular realm, it often invokes a search for significance and meaning. According to Viktor Frankl, having a sense that one's life has meaning involves the conviction that one is fulfilling a unique role and purpose in a life. He suggests that life is a gift that comes with a responsibility to live to one's full potential as a human being, and that through this process, one can achieve a sense of peace, contentment, or even transcendence through connectedness with something greater than oneself. He describes central paths to fulfil one's potential as a human being through: (1) involvement in creative or productive actions, (2) life experience, and (3) connectedness and love. Of these three paths he ascribes greatest importance to connectedness and love[56].

A study of 248 cancer outpatients found that spiritual or existential needs were commonly unmet. The most common of these were help in overcoming fears (51 per cent), finding hope (42 per cent) and meaning in life (40 per cent), finding spiritual resources (39 per cent), and having someone to talk about the meaning of life and death (25 per cent)[57].

Common existential issues for patients with advanced cancer include hopelessness, futility, meaninglessness, disappointment, remorse, death anxiety, and disruption of personal identity. Existential distresses may be related to past, present, or future concerns. Current personal integrity, the sense of who one is as a person, can be disrupted by changes in body image; somatic, intellectual, social, and professional function; and in perceived attractiveness as a person and as a sexual partner[10,58]. For some patients, retrospection can trigger profound disappointment (from unfulfilled aspirations or a deprecation of the value of previous achievements), or remorse from unresolved guilt[10,58,59].

If life is perceived to offer, at best, comfort in the setting of fading potency or, at worst, ongoing physical and emotional distress as days pass slowly until death, anticipation of the future may be associated with feelings of hopelessness, futility, or meaninglessness, such that the patient sees no value in continuing to live. Death anxiety is common among cancer patients; surveys have shown that 50–80 per cent of terminally ill patients have concerns or troubling thoughts about death, and that only a minority achieve an untroubled acceptance of death[58]. Together, these symptoms have been labelled a 'demoralization syndrome'[60].

Although these existential issues are sometimes referred to as 'spiritual', they appear to be universal, and independent of religion and religious practice[59,61].

Family/social distress

The perception by the patient of the distress of family, friends, and health-care providers, can further amplify the patient's distress, and thus contribute to the nihilistic conclusion that ongoing existence only constitutes a perpetuation of the burden to self and to others.

Family distress (see Chapter 15.3)

The development of advanced cancer in a family member impacts upon the entire family. The challenges confronting the family: to acknowledge the ending of life as they have known it, and to define a new way of constructively living out their final days together as best possible, engender great stresses[62]. Among the contributing factors to the ensuing distress are empathic suffering with the distress of the patient; grief and bereavement; role changes; and the physical, financial, and psychological sequelae of the burdens of care[63]. Furthermore, the family carers of cancer patients have been shown to constitute a vulnerable population. In one study, almost a quarter of the family caregivers for the terminally ill had chronic health problems themselves[64], and others have highlighted the further detriment to health incurred by family carers[65]. A very high prevalence of anxiety and adjustment difficulties have also been identified among family members, the severity of which is often as great as that of the patients themselves[66,67].

Psychosocial factors

A review of the data on the impact of cancer on the family members identified 11 major issues for family members: emotional strain, physical demands, uncertainty, fear that the patient will die, alteration in roles and lifestyles, financial concerns, ways to comfort the patient, perceived inadequacy of care services, existential concerns, sexuality, and non-convergent needs among family members[68]. These issues can be profoundly influenced by the trajectory of the illness. For example, a long illness characterized by a remitting and relapsing course may produce persistent anxiety and uncertainty, which can produce severe emotional fatigue[69,70]. To resolve those feelings, family members may, in some circumstances, hope for the patient's rapid demise. In contrast, when the time from diagnosis to impending death has been short, there may be little opportunity for family members to come to terms with the presence of life-threatening illness, let alone impending death.

Psychological problems of anxiety, depression, and adjustment disorder are common among family members of patients with advanced cancer. Studies of family cohesiveness indicate that these problems are more prevalent in families with low levels of cohesiveness and high levels of conflict[71]. Good communication within the family mitigates against psychological distress in general[71] and anxiety in particular[72].

Grief

In most cases, the pre-terminal phase of the cancer experience is associated with a period of anticipatory grieving[73] in which the family undergoes a transition associated with the patient's 'fading away'[62]. In one study[62], the onset of this transition was generally heralded by a deterioration in the patient's condition that challenged ongoing denial. The most heralding events were unrecoverable weakness; loss of independence in ambulation and personal care; and loss of mental clarity. These events are distressing in that they constitute losses, diminish hope for recovery, and focus attention on the inevitability of the patient's demise.

Caregiver burden

Although most patients die in the hospital setting, most of the care prior to dying is carried out at home by the family members with the support of health-care professionals. The care of a terminally ill family member greatly strains the physical, emotional, and psychological resources of the family unit and its individual members.

Home care often involves participation in personal hygiene needs, administration of medication by non-invasive or invasive routes, attention to nutritional needs, psychological support, and emergency management of such problems as pain, dyspnoea, or bleeding. The heavy physical work of transferring a weak or immobile patient, and attending to other needs (such as laundering or cleaning), is often further compounded by exhaustion due to sleep deprivation due to anxious thoughts or patient-care needs. For many, this is a new experience, and the uncertainties about the dying process and the ability to cope with the problems that lie ahead may become a focus for anxiety or ruminative thoughts. Family caregivers may be ill-prepared to assume these tasks, requiring information on the disease and treatment, as well as instruction in technical and care skills. Moreover, caregiving must be balanced against already established roles and role responsibilities.

Financial distress

Financial distress has been under-appreciated and is often neglected in routine care[74]. Studies comparing the relative costs of home and hospital-based terminal care[75,76] have generally neglected the financial and social costs to the family. In the National Hospice Study, 26 per cent of primary caretakers either left their work or lost their jobs, and 60 per cent reported a significant reduction in income due to either absenteeism or a change in work arrangements[77]. Permanent loss of employment occurred most frequently among those who could least afford it: older women and low-income families[77]. The costs of caring for a family member can leave the surviving family with severely compromised resources[78]. This distress is often exacerbated by inadequate insurance coverage.

Caregiver conflicts

The caregiver may experience profound conflict in this situation: conflict between the desire to provide adequate relief of distressing symptoms while, at the same time, wanting to preserve their loved one's alertness, and to avoid hastening death; and conflict between the duty to care for a loved one and to care for oneself, and one's other responsibilities. Additionally, there is often conflict between caregiving family members regarding goals of care, limits of care, and aggressiveness of care[79]. Guilt, anger, denial, and other emotional influences sometimes compel family members into conflicted opinions whether to treat a devastating illness aggressively or discontinue life-sustaining measures[80]. These conflicts may reflect low levels of pre-existing cohesiveness, or, they may threaten family closeness and collaboration in previously cohesive families.

Family needs

The needs of the families of patients with advanced cancer have been surveyed by several researchers[81–88]. The prompt and effective relief of patient symptoms is a major priority for family members, as are the needs for education in the comfort care of the patient, and for physician and nursing availability[83,89]. Families often express the need for communication from health-care providers that is honest, direct, and compassionate, in which family concerns and opinions are heard and valued, and that conveys information that can help in patient care. Material supports such as a hospital bed, and professional supports in the framework of family meetings are similarly valued. Commonly unmet needs include the need to receive assurance of the patient's comfort; to be informed of the patient's condition; to ventilate emotions; to receive comfort and support from family members; and to receive acceptance, support, and comfort from health-care professionals.

Risk identification

The endurability of the burdens of care is an important consideration in long-term care planning; the family members' current and future welfare is an important consideration when care demands are great and supportive resources for home care are limited[90]. In a large retrospective survey, 22 per cent of families of terminally ill patients were unable or unwilling to provide personal or medical care[91].

The identification of populations at particularly high risk for early intervention is facilitated by an assessment of stressors, particular family needs, and the resources available to the family. In a survey of bereavement, counsellors highlighted several different risk factors: perceived lack of caregiver social support (70 per cent), caregiver history of drug/alcohol abuse (68 per cent), poor caregiver coping skills (68 per cent), caregiver history of mental illness (67 per cent), and patient is a child (63 per cent)[92].

Another approach has been to look at global family functioning as a predictor of coping. In a large longitudinal study, Kissane and colleagues identified characteristics of families with high prevalence of distress and poor coping[93]. Families classified as 'hostile' were characterized by low cohesiveness, low expressiveness, and high conflict. Family members typically described family life as fraught with frequent arguing, little teamwork, or felt closeness among members, and minimal communication. Families classified as 'sullen' were also characterized by reduced cohesiveness and expressiveness, but only mild-to-moderate conflict. Reports of overt hostility were low in this group, suggesting that anger is muted, with depression gaining more prominence as the anger is directed inwards.

In contrast, the attributes identified to facilitate effective function include: the ability to work cohesively, prior successful experience in handling stress, a substantial and flexible repertoire of coping strategies, family stability, financial security, the availability of outside supports to which the family is receptive, and a readiness to view this difficult period as potentially growth-producing[94]. Kissane identified two positive patterns of family function predictive of good coping. 'Supportive families' described family life as intimate and mutually supportive, with open and honest communication among its members, tolerance of emotional expression, and little to no escalation in conflict. Similarly, 'conflict-resolving' families, which had cohesiveness and above-average expressiveness, but also the presence of conflict but with good conflict management (characterized by the ability to both voice and resolve differences between family members)[93].

Health-care professional distress (see Section 15)
Stressors

Health-care professionals may experience distress due to the constant exposure to suffering, loss, and grief that they are expected to be able to ease or relieve. Among the stressors experienced by professionals working in this field are: patients who experience high morbidity and mortality; high work pressure; frequent life and death decisions (which sometimes occur in ambiguous circumstances); high consumer expectations; inter-staff conflict; severe patient dependency, debilitation or disfigurement; severe emotional distress among patients and their families; and issues relating to suffering and distress caused by the treatments themselves[95]. It's not unusual for clinicians to bond strongly with patients who remind them of someone special in their lives or identify with patients who are similar to themselves in age, appearance, or background[96]. Identification with patients can revive personal pain and heighten feelings of guilt or a lack of control, resulting in burnout[97].

Physician distress

Stress and burnout are common phenomenon among clinicians managing patients with incurable cancer. Among oncologists, various studies have demonstrated prevalence rates of 25–56 per cent[98-101]. Multiple factors contribute to stress in oncology clinicians. There is an increasing awareness of the major contribution of workload and life balance issues[101,102]: volume overload, difficulty balancing personal and professional lives, inadequate staffing to do the job properly, the challenge of keeping current with medical literature, and pressures to obtain grants and to publish. Mounting administrative issues add to this. These include a mounting bureaucratic burden of dealing with governmental and insurance reimbursement issues, administrative duties/office management, applying for/maintaining grant support, and being responsible for the quality of the work of other staff. Interpersonal conflict and difficulties in relationships with colleagues, junior staff, nurses, administrative staff, and administration are common. To all of these, are added the challenges of end-of-life care: dealing and being involved with the physical and emotional suffering of patients, delivering bad news, and having to deal with distressed, angry, or blaming relatives.

Oncologists must deal daily with stressed patients and families, disproportionate hopes and expectations, emotionally laden dialogues with patients and families, and the limitations of treatments that are unable to deliver cures. Burnout results from overwhelming stress that creates an imbalance between the professional's needs and the rewards derived from the job itself.

Regarding the contribution of end-of-life on oncologist burnout, an ESMO survey of almost 900 medical oncologists, regarding their attitudes to and involvement with the management of advanced cancer[103], found that just over a third of respondents reported that they feel emotionally burned out by having to deal with too many deaths. This predilection to burnout was associated closely with negative attitudes to involvement in supportive and palliative care and low levels of actual involvement or referral to palliative care colleagues. This study suggest that burnout from end-of-life care, was not so much associated to over-exposure but rather to poor attitudinal preparedness and aberrant role definition. These findings suggest that positive attitudes and involvement in palliative care are all resilience factors that helps prevent burnout caused by exposure to advanced cancer.

In a survey of 81 French general practitioners[104], 86 per cent endorsed the assertion that encounters with death were a cause of physician suffering. The major causes of physician suffering were the end of the doctor–patient relationship (58 per cent); feelings of uselessness (55 per cent) and failure (38 per cent); increased awareness of their own mortality (49 per cent); and the presence of 'questions without answers' (31 per cent). The most commonly reported feelings that were experienced by these physicians at the bedside of the dying patient were sadness (94 per cent), helplessness (89 per cent), failure (61 per cent), disappointment (59 per cent), and loneliness (51 per cent).

Nursing distress

Studies of nurses working in palliative care have yielded mixed results; an international study evaluating stress levels and coping mechanisms among professionals who work with illness and death found that palliative care and hospice workers had less stress and better coping than those in other fields[105]. Despite that, the potential for exhaustion and burnout is well described[105,106]. Major sources of stress include perceived deficiencies in symptom control, deep emotional involvement in work, dealing with young patients, dealing with the emotional needs of distressed relatives, and conflict with the participating physicians over the goals of care[107–109].

Research among nurses have demonstrated both vulnerability and resilience factors. Personality characteristics such as perfectionism and over-involvement with patients may contribute to compassion fatigue or burnout. Self-esteem, sense of mastery and purpose, in life and a clear philosophy of life are protective factors.

Younger nurses with fewer years of experience report higher levels of distress[110]. A qualitative study of palliative care professionals found that less-experienced clinicians focused on the technical aspects of care. Clinicians with more than 10 years' experience focused on their commitment to patient and family and developing trusting and open therapeutic relationships. They were also likely to recognize the stressful nature of end-of-life care and to understand the experience from the perspective of the patient and family, as well as the meaning of the experience to themselves, both personally and professionally[111].

Assessment and planning

An effective approach to the alleviation of suffering for patients with incurable or terminal illness is predicated upon careful case assessment, identification of care needs, formulation of a multidisciplinary therapeutic intervention to address those needs, and the provision of ongoing monitoring with readiness to reevaluate the care plan as problems arise or needs change.

Assessment

An appreciation of the full diversity of factors that may contribute to suffering underscores the need for a methodical approach to the assessment of each individual case. The objectives of the assessment are to identify current problems that are a source of distress to each of the parties, to assess their care needs, and to evaluate the adequacy of the available resources. This evaluation must incorporate: medical variables in the patient, family, and available community medical system; psychological variables in the patient, family, and psychosocial community supports; and social and financial variables in the patient and family. Since both the patient and the family are part of the unit of care, assessment requires discussion with both. The clinician must maintain a clinical posture that affirms relief of suffering as the central goal of therapy, and which encourages open and effective communication about perceived problems.

Patient assessment

The prevalence of poorly controlled pain and other physical symptoms, and the impact of these factors on the lives of all involved, emphasize the importance of addressing these issues at the earliest opportunity. The early establishment of good symptom control conveys concern, builds the trust of patients and their families, and facilitates the ability to address other important issues.

Patient variables that must be assessed include the disease status, expected disease progression, present functional level, symptoms, current therapies, and anticipated future problems. Of particular importance is the patient's level of function, reflecting his or her mobility (e.g. fully bedbound or fully mobile without aids), ability to communicate (from severe as with brain tumours to minimal impairment), ability to perform activities of daily living, bowel and bladder function (from incontinence to full self-care), and level of alertness (from coma to full alertness). The use of validated pain and symptom assessment instruments can provide a format for communication between the patient and health-care professionals and can also be used to monitor the adequacy of therapy.

It is important to ascertain the patient and the family's understanding of the nature and extent of the illness and their expectations of treatment and outcome. As part of this process, the clinician must develop an understanding of the patient's prioritization of the sometimes conflicting goals of care: optimization of comfort, function (interactional function in particular), and duration of survival.

Family assessment

Family assessment should encompass medical variables, psychosocial concerns, and the adequacy and availability of supports. Evaluation of the willingness and ability of home carers to provide home care and the availability of supports are essential. Concurrent medical problems in a family member, particularly a primary caregiver, need to be evaluated, since the viability of the home-care plan may depend upon the family member's ability to participate in care. Since the ability of families to cope with homecare is largely determined by the nature of the available home-care supports[112–114], the family assessment must include an assessment of available health-care professional and community supports.

It is important to ascertain the family's understanding of the nature and extent of the patient's cancer and their expectations of treatment and outcome. Discrepancies between what is known and understood by the patient and the family should be identified, and the reasons for these discrepancies should be tactfully explored. Knowledge deficits may have been deliberately maintained; the family or patient not wanting information overload, the patient protecting the family from knowledge of poor prognosis, or the family protecting the patient from the impact of such information[115,116]. This part of the assessment requires a non-judgemental posture, and sensitivity to psychological and cultural factors that may influence the transmission of information.

Health-care professional assessment

Evaluation of the professional caregiver supports usually requires greater detail than that which can be provided by the patient and family alone. To effectively plan for ongoing care, the clinical coordinator must understand the limitations of the involved health-care professionals (knowledge, experience, and availability for home care), their difficulties in coping with the situation, and their perceived needs to improve the care outcome. As previously described, the coping of professional caregivers may be severely strained by issues pertaining to communication; conflict with the patient, family, or colleagues, perceived therapeutic failure; excessive workload or emotional strain; and difficult therapeutic or ethical decisions.

Awareness of this interrelated construct enables the clinician to construct a series of critical questions regarding each of these domains, the answers to which constitute the basis of a patient assessment.

The patient

Who is the patient and what is their social context? It is critically important to be aware of who is this person who now needs care. This includes collection of information about basic demographics, family structure, other significant relationships, professional and education history, and place of dwelling. This phase should also incorporate past medical history and significant elements of family health and social history.

What is the patient's illness, and where is the patient in the natural history of the condition? More often than not, this information will be available from the referring clinician and the patient's medical record. Specific information is required regarding the diagnosis, sites of disease, active medical problems, and anticipated prognosis. Anticipated prognosis relates not only to life expectancy, rather a broader concept that incorporates the projected course of illness and anticipated complications or problems.

Is the patient clear-headed, if not why not? Cognitive impairment is very common among patients with advanced cancer and among other patients needing palliative care[117–119]. The presence of delirium impairs the ability to obtain direct information from the patient and will impair the ability to directly address many of the subsequent assessment issues without involvement of family and healthcare providers. When cognitive impairment is identified, efforts should be made to identify reversible contributing factors. The chronology of the problem must be assessed, including pre-morbid level of function, the time course of the deterioration in cognitive function, precipitating or alleviating factors, and other features of co-morbidity that may help identify the underlying problem. In this setting, the clinician will need to obtain the greater part of the clinical information from the family members or other involved observers. Since iatrogenic cognitive impairment caused by centrally acting drugs is common, it is important to review the patient's drug chart and to ask about the ingestion of any other substances (such as 'medicinal' mushrooms) which may be implicated.

What does the patient understand of the illness? Care planning and further evaluations require that the clinician is aware of the extent of the patient's familiarity with his/her condition and what the patient's communication preferences are. Although there is extensive data indicating that most patients want accurate information regarding their medical status, this is not universal[120]. Some patients want only limited information and a few want no information[120]. Excessive candor in the setting of impaired coping, or in a patient who expresses a desire not to receive information may constitute a maleficent assault[120–122].

What are the current goals of care? The goals of care are often complex, but can generally be grouped into three broad categories: (1) prolonging survival, (2) optimizing comfort, and (3) optimizing function[123]. The relative priority of these goals provides an essential context for therapeutic decision-making[124]. The prioritization of these goals is a dynamic phenomenon which changes with the evolution of the disease. For some patients requiring palliative care, the optimization of comfort, function, and survival may share equal priority, whereas the provision of comfort usually assumes overriding priority as death approaches.

Awareness of goals has major implications for care and therapeutic decision-making and it influences the evaluation process. When patients equally prioritize optimal comfort and function, the therapeutic intent is to achieve an adequate degree of relief without compromising cognitive and physical function. In this setting, impairments to physical, psychological, or social function require careful evaluation in order to guide care needs. When, however, comfort is the overriding goal of care, and the overriding intent is to achieve relief of discomfort, there may be areas of function or of disease status that are no longer an essential part of the assessment.

What are the physical consequences of the illness? Is the patient coping? Are there physical problems that are not well controlled? Patients needing palliative care are typically polysymptomatic and often have severe limitations in activities of daily living. Data from a number of studies have demonstrated that patients commonly have 6–10 active distressing symptoms[27]. Symptom assessment aims to identify the active symptoms, their severity, and the degree of distress that they are engendering for the patient. Several well-validated tools have been developed to help screen patients for physical and psychological symptoms and to monitor their severity. Pain in particular needs detailed evaluation; this is addressed in greater detail in Chapter 10.1.

Symptom evaluation must be accompanied an evaluation of function. This should incorporate activities of daily living such as ambulation, toileting, dressing, eating, sleeping, and sexual function (if clinically appropriate).

The extent of the physical examination will be determined, in part, by the patient's prevailing condition and the goals of care. The physical examination often helps refine the differential diagnosis of problems indicated by the clinical history. Details of physical examination are beyond the scope of this introduction: suffice it to say that special attention must be paid to common problems associated with advanced illness including mouth care and skin integrity, as well as to sites incriminated by the patient's symptoms or which may be commonly involved in the disease from which the patient suffers. When the patient suffers from pain or from neurologic symptoms, the valuation should incorporate a neurologic examination.

All relevant pre-existing diagnostic investigations should be reviewed. These often reveal important information that may explain current symptoms or help focus the need for any future diagnostic interventions.

Psychologically, how is the patient coping? What is he/she thinking? What are his/her active fears or concerns? Fear, anxiety, sadness, depression, and sleep disturbance are among the most common symptoms of advanced cancer. They are a substantial cause of distress, undermine coping, and are a major contributing factor for suicidal ideation and the desire for death. Patients should be asked how they are coping. This serves as a useful opening to explore more specific psychological and social issues. Inquiry about coping conveys concern. This, in turn contributes to the development of trust and facilitates development of the therapeutic relationship.

Specific inquiry should be made regarding feelings of sadness, anxiety, or persistent fears. If acknowledged, these symptoms should be further evaluated to identify the contributing factors, severity of the symptoms, and the impact of the psychological distress on patient function.

When patients express fears or anxiety, it is important to clarify the specific fears. Often, fears are based either on misinformation or on anticipated problems that are very unlikely to occur. In other situations, patient fears are appropriate but are magnified either by poor communication or by a lack of communication. Patients with advanced cancer often harbour fears of uncontrolled pain, dyspnoea, or some other form of uncontrolled suffering at the end of life. These fears can be addressed through counselling, a commitment to continuity of care, and to adequate palliation, and meticulous clinical follow-up with implementation of those commitments.

On a day-to-day basis, how is the patient coping and do they have adequate supports? Effective day-to-day coping requires an integration between physical, psychological, and disease-related factors in coordination with environmental factors related to family, friend, and health-care supports. This complex interaction must be evaluated. Asking patients about their day-to-day coping is a technique to open a dialogue regarding this complex interaction. Similarly, one can ask the patient if they have adequate supports. Support and coping are deliberately general queries that may evoke responses, relating very diverse issues and concerns. Commonly expressed concerns include financial concerns, fears of family burnout, lack of availability of medical and nursing staff, difficulties in obtaining parking at the hospital, communication concerns with clinical staff, and inadequately controlled symptoms.

What are the deeper thoughts that the patient harbours? What sort of life have they had? Do they have unfulfilled dreams or aspirations? What have been the things that have made them sad or happy? How do they see the future? Existential and spiritual issues may relate to the past, present, or future. As people approach the end of life, they commonly have many thoughts relating to the life that they have lived, issues of legacy, the life that they are currently living and concerns the time that remains ahead of them. Additionally, many patients harbour transcendental thoughts relating to their place in the world, their relationship to God, and thoughts related to afterlife. These concerns are universal, cross-cultural, and are probably intrinsic to mortal life. The relative weight of these issues is influenced by culture, past, cognitive function, and the place in the life cycle at which the patient is confronting their mortality.

Evaluating these deeply personal issues requires the prior development of a trusting relationship. Exploration and disclosure of these issues is usually undertaken over time. In many instances, the patient may chose to disclose and discuss different issues with different staff members. This may reflect interpersonal dynamics, specific clinical skills, or perceived roles. Information sharing, with the patient's permission, with other members of the interdisciplinary team helps sensitize other participating caregivers to the specific cares, concerns, and sensitivities of the patient. When patients feel understood, they are more likely to feel trust in the care team and environment.

Life review techniques can help identify points of meaning, important issues of legacy, as well as unresolved issues related to the past such as remorse, unfulfilled ambitions, or guilt. Direct questioning can be used to evaluate the patient coping in the family, at work, and in significant relationships.

Fear of death is commonplace. Specific death-related fears may include fears of pain, dyspnoea, loss of control, medical abandonment or overtreatment, oblivion, and concern for surviving family members. Frequently, specific goals or uncompleted tasks will be identified. This information may be critical for life planning in the time that remains for the patient.

What future problems are anticipated? What provisional steps can be taken to cover contingencies? Careful contingency planning can help avoid crises. Contingency planning should relate to specific anticipated physical problems (such as pain, dyspnoea, immobility, wound breakdown, or bleeding), psychological problems (such as anxiety, sleep disturbance, or delirium), and home-care problems (such as failing supports, family burnout, or access problems). By identifying probable contingencies, one can implement and prepare a backup plan. Examples of this sort of planning include: provision of opioids and antipsychotics, if pain or delirium are anticipated, oxygen—if hypoxaemia is anticipated, and bathroom railing—if immobility is anticipated. When home death is anticipated, it is helpful to have a prepared programme for the family of who needs to be called with all phone numbers prepared and any paperwork ready and available.

In some circumstances, the nature of the anticipated contingency may be such that it may impact on the immediate care plan. This is especially true when catastrophic bleeding from a carotid or femoral blowout is anticipated. If the patient lives alone or with a companion, who may be significantly traumatized by this sort of horrid event, anticipatory admission to a hospital or palliative care unit may be appropriate. This is true for patients who may suffer asphyxiation from upper airway tumour.

Family

Who is the family and what is there social context? This is well achieved using a family map. Critical issues for assessment of each family member include: age, place of residence, health status, occupation, nuclear family relationships, geographic and emotional proximity to the patient. Some family members may have unresolved past issues with the patient and, as far as is possible, it is helpful to identify these.

How is the physical and psychological well-being of the family member? Since advanced and incurable illnesses are most commonly a problem of the elderly, often the caring family member may be in poor physical health. Similarly, significant illness in a family is a major emotional stress and indeed, family members often suffer from anxiety, depression, and adjustment disorders or difficulty. It is important that the members of the care team be aware of these factors as they will impact on the ability of the family member to participate in care and they indicate specific care needs of their own.

What do the family members understand of the patient's condition and the goals of care? Discrepancies between the patient's and the family members' understanding of the patients' diagnosis, treatments, anticipated outcomes of treatment, prognosis, and goals of care are commonplace[125]. It is only by asking family members what they understand of the illness that these discrepancies can be identified. When discrepancies are identified, the clinician must evaluate if there is a specific reason that they exist. Occasionally, the patient may have specifically requested that information not be disclosed to family members or to a specific family member. When this has been the case, the reasons for concealment of this sort should be explored with the patient.

Emotionally, how are they coping with the prevailing situation? Are they adequately supported? Are they coping? Life-threatening disease in a family member is a major life stress. Coping with this sort of stress is very variable and it has both psychological and physical dimensions. When emotional coping is difficult or when failure of coping occurs, this impacts on everyone else involved in the care dynamic including the patient, other family members, and the professional health-care team[126]. Coping with physical care needs can be severely compromised when there is a failure of emotional coping. It is, therefore important to explore issues of emotional coping of the family members. Common issues include anticipatory grief, anxiety, and depression. Changes in the patient's condition commonly precipitate transient adjustment disorders that may manifest as anxiety, panic, depression, psychomotor retardation, or acting-out.

Physically, how are they coping with the prevailing situation? Are they adequately supported? It is important to evaluate the family members' ability to cope with the patient's care needs, to identify the role of pre-emptive or remedial assistance when available, and to identify impending breakdown in coping (which may require urgent intervention such as respite admission)[127–129]. This process aims to evaluate the limits of the family's coping resources for home care. If the patient's care needs exceed these limits, other care plans will need to be activated. Coping with physical care needs can be supported by the provision of appropriate physical supports (such as a wheelchair, hospital bed, toileting equipment), education in care provision, and professional or volunteer assistance.

What are the deeper thoughts that the family members harbour? What sort of life have they had? Do they have unfulfilled dreams or aspirations? What have been the things that have made them sad or happy? How do they see the future? Life-threatening illness in a spouse, sibling, or parent threatens a significant relationship, and it impacts on the way family members relate to their past, present, and future. Family members may suffer the same spectrum of existential issues as the patients themselves[130]. As with the patient, life review techniques may identify unfilled ambitions, regrets, and remorse related to relationship issues with the patient, as well as help highlight positive aspects of their shared experiences. The patient's illness may have altered the structure of the family relationships. Often, evaluation of future goals can identify specific targets that may not be achievable with the involvement of the patient unless they are brought forward. In many instances, discussion of these issues has facilitated the bringing forward of major life events such as weddings, long-distance travel, or family reunions.

What are their concerns for the future? Family members often have specific fears regarding anticipated future events in relation to the patient. Common fears include fears of: uncontrolled pain, confusion, incontinence, loss of ambulatory function, bleeding, addiction, abandonment, and lack of supports. Once identified, these fears are often amenable to intervention either through counselling, information transfer, family meetings, or the development of clear contingency plans and lines of communication.

Have they suffered other losses in the past? In what circumstances? How did they deal with them? How are these losses impacting on what is happening now? Previous grief experiences impact on the distress of impending bereavement[131,132]. Knowing about the experiences of previous losses can help the professional caregiver address issues related to the current situation. Family members who have experienced multiple grief experiences may be suffering from cumulative losses. In other situations, family members have fears based on the previous death experiences. Consequently, it is important to ask family members about previous death experiences: What happened? How did they cope? Did the experience leave them with any specific fears or hopes regarding death and end-of-life care?

Health-care providers

Who is involved in the patient's care? Patients commonly have multiple professionals involved in their care. It is critical to identify them, their roles, the limits of their availability, the cost of their services, and the extent of their communication. Contact details should be made available and clear lines of communication and responsibility established. A clinician should be nominated as the coordinating clinician who is ultimately responsible for the coordination of professional caregiver activities.

What is the experience and expertise of the professional health-care providers with the prevailing problems? Health-care professionals constitute a heterogeneous group. Professionals vary greatly in their experience and training and attitudes regarding palliative care and end-of-life care. Since knowledge deficits are endemic, it is important to understand the specific professional background of each of the participating clinicians. Where lack of experience or lack of knowledge in palliative care is identified in the care team, special provision for expert backup or remedial education may be required.

What do the professional health-care providers understand of the illness and of the goals of care? It is important to clarify the understanding of all participating caregivers regarding the goals of care and of their specific care goals. Miscommunication of the goals of care, or lack of concordance between professional caregivers on this issue can contribute to conflict and confusion.

What are the limits of care that they can reasonably provide? Do they have adequate human resources to deal with the prevailing problems? Are they coping? Usually, there are limits to the professional services and personnel resources available for the care of patients. These limits need to be determined. Once determined, it is important to assess the likelihood that they will be adequate to meet the patients and family's care needs. When the care needs are great and the professional caregiver resources are limited, it is important to assess professional caregiver coping. When there is mismatch between care needs and available services, particularly in the setting of home care, alternative care arrangements in hospital or a palliative care department or hospice may need to be considered.

How are they coping with the emotional impact of the situation? Caring for incurable patients and their families places a great stress on the emotional coping resources of health-care professionals and sometimes professionals feel inadequately prepared for the emotion-laden nature of this work. Consequently, it is important to assess the coping of the members of the care team with the emotional issues to which they are being exposed. As part of this assessment, it is important to check that the emotional care burden is being distributed between the professional carers and that there is provision for debriefing.

Do they have adequate physical resources? Home care of patients needing palliative care often requires equipment such as a hospital bed, ambulating assist devices (such as a walking frame or wheel chair), toileting equipment, oxygen, suction device, or

Table 3.1.1 The dimensions of patient distress, management approaches, and potential therapeutic resources.

Dimension	Distress	Intervention(s)	Therapists
Physical	Pain Other physical symptoms Physical disability	Comprehensive pain management Comprehensive therapy Physiatric review and therapy	MD, Nur, Anesth, PCS, Physiat, OT, PT.
Psychological	Anxiety Depression Adjustment difficulties Cognitive impairment Unresolved previous loss or separation Control	Careful assessment for reversible factors Psychotherapy ± pharmacotherapy Cognitive or behavioural interventions	Onc, Nur, SW, Psych, Neur, PCS
Social	Strained family relationships Unsatisfactory communication regarding illness or treatment Economic	Family assessment, supportive intervention Assessment and facilitation Assessment and support	MD, Nur, SW, Psych, PCS
	Family related Feeling an excessive care burden Feeling an excessive emotional burden Feeling an excessive economic burden	Address issues of family distress	See Table 3.1.2
	Doctor related Lack of MD attention to current problems Lack of empathic support from MD MD excessively hopeful or pessimistic	Evaluate limits of available medical supports Expert consultation	PCS, Psych, SW, Nurs
Existential	Current personal integrity Changes in body image and function Changes in intellectual function Changes in social and professional function Changes in attractiveness as a sexual partner	Attention to reversible factors Use of prosthetic, cosmetic, orthotic, or functional supports Cognitive, behavioural and supportive psychotherapies to enhance coping	MD, Nur, SW, Phys, Psych, Chap, PCS, Physiat, OT, PT, ST, Cosmet
	Retrospective distress Disappointment Remorse	Cognitive restructuring Life-review techniques	SW, Psych, Chap, MD, Nurs, PCS, MT, RecT
	Anticipation Hopelessness Futility Meaninglessness Death concerns	Cognitive restructuring and goal reprioritization Identification of short-term achievable goals Abandonment of unachievable goals Addressing fears associated with death	Psych, SW, MD, Nur, Chap, PCS, ClinEth

Note:

Chap	Chaplain	PCS	Palliative Care Specialist
ClinEth	Clinical Ethicist	Physiat	Physiatrist
Cosmet	Cosmetician	Psych	Psychiatrist
MD	Doctor	PT	Physical Therapist
MT	Music Therapist	RecT	Recreation Therapist
Nurs	Nurse	SW	Social Worker
OT	Occupational Therapist		

Source: reproduced with permission from Cherny, N.I., Coyle, N., Foley, K.M. (1994). Suffering in the advanced cancer patient: a definition and taxonomy. *Journal of Palliative Care*, **10**(2), 57–70.

specific medications. It is incumbent to evaluate what resources are needed and the evaluate availability and cost (if any).

What future problems are anticipated? What provisional steps can be taken to cover contingencies? The issue of contingency planning was addressed as part of the patient assessment. The evaluation of the care services must include an evaluation of the implementation of the contingency arrangements. Lines of communications should be clarified, and the extent of available cover for emergencies checked. If the need for admission is foreseen, communication including a letter of introduction should be prepared in advance. When it is anticipated that the patient will die in the near future,

there should be clear instructions for the family indicating who to contact including the details of funeral company contacts.

Formulating a care plan

Based on this assessment, one can formulate a care plan that addresses all aspects of the care trilogy: patient, family, and caregivers. The formulation can be summarized in a document or report that describes:

1   The medical condition of the patient and the goals of care

2   Description of the involved family and professional carers

3   Patient issues: physical, psychological, existential, social, communication, understanding

4   Family issues: physical, psychological, existential, social, communication, understanding

5   Professional carer issues: staffing, training, resources, resource/need match, emotional coping

6   Coping assessment: patient, family, and professional staff

7   Contingency planning: anticipated contingencies, planned interventions

Tables 3.1.1 and 3.1.2 illustrate interdisciplinary care plans to address patient and family needs in each of the dimensions of care.

Implementation of ongoing assessment

Advanced incurable illness leading towards death is characterized by the potential for rapid and dramatic change and the overall tendency for change, increasing dependency, and an increasingly complex confluence of physical, psychological, existential, ethical, and social concerns. Just as care for the palliative care patient is a longitudinal commitment, so is assessment. Consequently, this assessment must be repeated at appropriate intervals, which will be determined by the rate of change in the patient's clinical condition or at points of major change in goals, care plan, or the patient's condition.

Family meetings

A common source of distress for patient, family, and professional carers occurs when there is a lack of coordination in the desired goals of patient care. The goals of care are often complex, but can generally be grouped into three broad categories: (1) prolonging survival, (2) optimizing comfort, and (3) optimizing function. The relative priority of these goals provides an essential context for therapeutic decision-making. The prioritization of these goals is a dynamic phenomenon, which changes with the evolution of the disease: whereas the optimization of comfort, function, and survival may share equal priority during the phase of ambulatory palliation, the provision of comfort usually assumes overriding priority as death approaches. When patients equally prioritize optimal comfort and function, the therapeutic intent is to achieve an adequate degree of relief without compromising cognitive and physical function. When comfort is the overriding goal of care, the overriding intent is to achieve relief. In the latter circumstance, there is a willingness to continue therapies that may impair function, or even foreshorten life expectancy.

Family meetings, with relevant members of the professional health-care team, provide a useful format for discussing the needs

Table 3.1.2 The dimensions of family member distress, management approaches, and potential therapeutic resources.

Dimension	Distress	Intervention	Therapist(s)
Patient related	Patient in physical distress Patient in psychological distress Patient in existential distress	Treat patient and support family Treat patient and support family Treat patient and support family	MD, Nurs, Psych, Chap, ClinEth
Physical	Illness Physical disability	Comprehensive therapy Physiatric review and therapy	MD, Nur,
Psychological	Anxiety Depression Adjustment difficulties Unresolved previous loss or separation Uncertainty	Psychotherapy ± pharmacotherapy Cognitive or behavioural interventions	MD, Nur, SW, Psych, Neur, PCS Chap
Social	Alteration in roles and lifestyles Unsatisfactory communication regarding illness or treatment Lack of comfort and support from family members Lack of support and comfort from health-care professionals Non-convergent needs among family members Economic/ employment	Acknowledge difficulties Explore specific problems of family and supports Assess information needs and address them Provide sensitive information and express readiness to provide appropriate supports Express readiness to deal with whatever difficulties may arise Identify family members in need of psychological or psychiatric support.	MD, Nur, SW, Psych, PCS
Personal resources	Excessive physical demands Excessive complexity of care Exhaustion	Optimize home supports Provide effective backup Consider alternative care arrangements Consider respite care	SW, Nurs, MD

Chap	Chaplain	PCS	Palliative Care Specialist	
ClinEth	Clinical Ethicist	Physiat	Physiatrist	
Cosmet	Cosmetician	Psych	Psychiatrist	
MD	Doctor	PT	Physical Therapist	
MT	Music Therapist	RecT	Recreation Therapist	
Nurs	Nurse	SW	Social Worker	
OT	Occupational Therapist			

Source: reproduced with permission from Cherny, N.I., Coyle, N., Foley, K.M. (1994). Suffering in the advanced cancer patient: a definition and taxonomy. *Journal of Palliative Care,* **10**(2), 57–70.

of all parties involved, clarifying care goals, sharing and exploring concerns, and developing a therapeutic plan that adequately addresses those needs. The participants should be determined on an individual case basis. Since the family is an appropriate unit of care, and its members have a right to confidentiality, it may be appropriate, on occasion, to meet without the participation of the patient, to address their concerns and needs. Meetings with the participation of all persons who are involved can open communication, improve coordination in the formulation of a care plan, and facilitate better personal coping for each of the individuals involved.

Formulation and implementation of a care plan

Coordination of the many participants in this sort of multi-disciplinary care requires an identified leader for each case. This role is usually filled by either a physician or nurse, and the specific person may change in the course of an illness as the predominant care needs change. For example, with the progression of the cancer from a diagnostic stage to a palliative stage, the responsibility may shift sequentially from a surgeon, to a medical oncologist, and finally, to a palliative care care nurse. The coordinator, or case manager, is responsible for monitoring the degree to which care needs are being met, and for facilitating change when necessary. Similarly, the well-being and function of the health-care professionals must be monitored, ensuring the availability of appropriate manpower and expertise to effectively manage the prevailing problems. For security and safety in the event of a clinical crisis, it is essential that the patient and family have access to a contact person with 24-h availability. This model represents a family-centred, multi-disciplinary, collaborative approach between physicians, nurses, social workers, other therapists, and community supports.

Conclusion

An understanding of the nature of suffering and of the factors that contribute to it are essential to the task of palliative medicine. Suffering is a complex human experience, which requires evaluation in order to construct an effective therapeutic response that is appropriate to presenting problems. An effective approach incorporates careful case assessment, identification of care needs, formulation of a multi-disciplinary therapeutic intervention to address those needs, and the provision of ongoing monitoring with readiness to re-evaluate the care plan as problems arise or needs change.

References

1. Wanzer, S.H., Federman, D.D., Adelstein, S.J. et al. (1989). The physician's responsibility toward hopelessly ill patients. A second look. *New England Journal of Medicine*, **320**(13), 844–9.
2. Duggleby, W. and Berry, P. (2005). Transitions and shifting goals of care for palliative patients and their families. *Clinical Journal of Oncology Nursing*, **9**(4), 425–8.
3. Roy, D.J. (1991). Relief of suffering: the doctor's mandate [editorial]. *Journal of Palliative Care*, **7**(4), 3–4.
4. Angell, M. (1982). The quality of mercy [editorial]. *New England Journal of Medicine*, **306**(2), 98–9.
5. American Medical Association. (1996). Good care of the dying patient. Council on Scientific Affairs, American Medical Association. *Journal of the American Medical Association*, **275**(6), 474–8.
6. American Nurses Association Center for Ethics and Human Rights Task Force on the nurse's role in end-of-life decisions. (1992). Compendium of position statements on the nurse's role in end-of-life decisions. American Nurses Association Center for Ethics and Human Rights Task Force on the nurse's role in end-of-life decisions. ANA Publ (PR-9.65M), 1–13.
7. President's Commission for the Study of Ethical Problems in Medical and Biomedical and Behavioral Research. (1983). *Deciding to Forgo Life Sustaining Treatment: Ethical and Legal Issues in Treatment Decisions*. Washington: U.S. Government Printing Office.
8. Rich, B.A. (2001). Physicians' legal duty to relieve suffering. *Western Journal of Medicine*, **175**(3), 151–2.
9. Roy, D.J. (1993). Biology and meaning in suffering. *Journal of Palliative Care*, **9**(2), 3–4.
10. Cassell, E.J. (1982). The nature of suffering and the goals of medicine. *New England Journal of Medicine*, **306**(11), 639–45.
11. Cassell, E.J. (1991). Recognizing suffering. *Hastings Center Reports*, **21**(3), 24–31.
12. Saunders, C. (1984). The philosophy of terminal care. In *The management of terminal malignant disease* (ed. C. Saunders), pp. 232–41. Baltimore: Arnold Publishers.
13. Cherny, N.I., Coyle, N., and Foley, K.M. (1994). Suffering in the advanced cancer patient: a definition and taxonomy. *Journal of Palliative Care*, **10**(2), 57–70.
14. Lazarus, R.S. (1985). The psychology of stress and coping. *Issues in Mental Health Nursing*, **7**(1-4), 399–418.
15. Folkman, S., Lazarus, R.S., Gruen, R.J. et al. (1986). Appraisal, coping, health status, and psychological symptoms. *Journal of Personal and Social Psychology*, **50**(3), 571–9.
16. Vanistendael, S. (1996). *Growth in the Muddle of Life: Resilience: Building on People's Strengths*. International Catholic Child Bureau.
17. World Health Organization (1996). *Cancer Pain Relief*, 2nd edition. Geneva: World Health Organization.
18. Cassel, C.K. and Foley, K.M. (1999). *Principles for Care of Patients at the End of Life: An Emerging Consensus among the Specialties of Medicine*. MY: Milbank Memorial Fund.
19. Burt, R.A. (1997). The Supreme Court speaks—not assisted suicide but a constitutional right to palliative care. *New England Journal of Medicine*, **337**(17), 1234–6.
20. Steinberg, A. and Sprung, C.L. (2006). The dying patient: new Israeli legislation. *Intensive Care Medicine*, **32**(8), 1234–7.
21. van den Beuken-van Everdingen, M., de Rijke, J., Kessels, A. et al. (2007). Prevalence of pain in patients with cancer: a systematic review of the past 40 years. *Annals of Oncology*, **18**, 1437–49.
22. Feuz, A. and Rapin, C.H. (1994). An observational study of the role of pain control and food adaptation of elderly patients with terminal cancer. *Journal of the American Dietetic Association*, **94**(7), 767–70.
23. Hugel, H., Ellershaw, J.E., Cook, L. et al. (2004). The prevalence, key causes and management of insomnia in palliative care patients. *Journal of Pain and Symptom Management*, **27**(4), 316–21.
24. Ferrell, B.R. (1995). The impact of pain on quality of life. A decade of research. *Nursing Clinics of North America*, **30**(4), 609–24.
25. Burrows, M., Dibble, S.L., and Miaskowski, C. (1998). Differences in outcomes among patients experiencing different types of cancer-related pain. *Oncology Nursing Forum*, **25**(4), 735–41.
26. Mystakidou, K., Tsilika, E., Parpa, E. et al. (2006). Psychological distress of patients with advanced cancer: influence and contribution of pain severity and pain interference. *Cancer Nursing*, **29**(5), 400–5.
27. Teunissen, S.C., Wesker, W., Kruitwagen, C. et al. (2007). Symptom Prevalence in Patients with Incurable Cancer: A Systematic Review. *Journal of Pain and Symptom Management*, **34**(1), 94–104.
28. Chang, V.T., Hwang, S.S., Feuerman, M. et al. (2000). Symptom and quality of life survey of medical oncology patients at a veterans affairs medical center: A role for symptom assessment. *Cancer*, **88**(5), 1175–83.
29. Coyle, N. (1990). The last four weeks of life. *American Journal of Nursing*, **90**(12), 75–6, 78.

30. Ventafridda, V., Ripamonti, C., De Conno, F. *et al.* (1990). Symptom prevalence and control during cancer patients' last days of life. *Journal of Palliative Care*, **6**(3), 7–11.

31. Henteleff, P.D. (1991). Symptom prevalence and control during cancer patients' last days of life. *Journal of Palliative Care*, **7**(2), 50–1.

32. Johanson, G.A. Symptom character and prevalence during cancer patients' last days of life. *American Journal of Hospital Palliative Care*, **8**(2), 6–8, 18.

33. Reuben, D.B., Mor, V., and Hiris, J. (1988). Clinical symptoms and length of survival in patients with terminal cancer. *Archives of Internal Medicine*, **148**(7), 1586–91.

34. Fainsinger, R., Miller, M.J., Bruera, E. *et al.* (1991). Symptom control during the last week of life on a palliative care unit. *Journal of Palliative Care*, **7**(1), 5–11.

35. Lichter, I. and Hunt, E. (1990). The last 48 hours of life. *Journal of Palliative Care*, **6**(4), 7–15.

36. Jalmsell, L., Kreicbergs, U., Onelov, E. *et al.* (2006). Symptoms affecting children with malignancies during the last month of life: a nationwide follow-up. *Pediatrics*, **117**(4), 1314–20.

37. Goldman, A., Hewitt, M., Collins, G.S. *et al.* (2006). Symptoms in children/young people with progressive malignant disease: United Kingdom Children's Cancer Study Group/Paediatric Oncology Nurses Forum survey. *Pediatrics*, **117**(6), e1179–86.

38. Solano, J.P., Gomes, B., and Higginson, I.J. (2006). A Comparison of Symptom Prevalence in Far Advanced Cancer, AIDS, Heart Disease, Chronic Obstructive Pulmonary Disease and Renal Disease. *Journal of Pain and Symptom Management*, **31**(1), 58–69.

39. Kadan-Lottick, N.S., Vanderwerker, L.C., Block, S.D. *et al.* (2005). Psychiatric disorders and mental health service use in patients with advanced cancer: a report from the coping with cancer study. *Cancer*, **104**(12), 2872–81.

40. Grabsch, B., Clarke, D.M., Love, A. *et al.* (2006). Psychological morbidity and quality of life in women with advanced breast cancer: a cross-sectional survey. *Palliative Support Care*, **4**(1), 47–56.

41. Breitbart, W. and Jacobsen, P.B. (1996). Psychiatric symptom management in terminal care. *Clinical Geriatric Medicine*, **12**(2), 329–47.

42. Breitbart, W., Bruera, E., Chochinov, H. *et al.* (1995). Neuropsychiatric syndromes and psychological symptoms in patients with advanced cancer. *Journal of Pain and Symptom Management*, **10**(2), 131–41.

43. Portenoy, R.K., Thaler, H.T., Kornblith, A.B. *et al.* (1994). Symptom prevalence, characteristics and distress in a cancer population. *Quality of Life Research*, **3**(3), 183–9.

44. Breitbart, W. (1988). Suicide in cancer patients. *Scandinavian Journal of Social Medicine*, **16**(3), 149–53.

45. Derogatis, L.R., Morrow, G.R., Fetting, J. *et al.* (1983). The prevalence of psychiatric disorders among cancer patients. *Journal of the American Medical Association*, **249**(6), 751–7.

46. Nordin, K., Berglund, G., Glimelius, B. *et al.* (2001). Predicting anxiety and depression among cancer patients: a clinical model. *European Journal of Cancer*, **37**(3), 376–84.

47. Stedeford, A. (1984). Psychological aspects of the management of terminal cancer. *Comprehensive Therapy*, **10**(1), 35–40.

48. Watson, M., Pruyn, J., Greer, S. *et al.* (1990). Locus of control and adjustment to cancer. *Psychological Reports*, **66**(1), 39–48.

49. Farberow, N.L., Schneiderman, E.S., and Leonard, C.V. (1963). *Suicide among general medical and surgical hospital patients with malignant neoplasms*. Washington: US Veterans Administration.

50. Mager, W.M. and Andrykowski, M.A. (2002). Communication in the cancer 'bad news' consultation: patient perceptions and psychological adjustment. *Psychooncology*, **11**(1), 35–46.

51. Field, M.J., Cassel, E.K., (eds.) (1997). *Approaching Death: Improving Care at the End of Life*. Washington, DC: National Academy Press.

52. Ambuel, B. (2003). Taking a spiritual history #19. *Journal of Palliative Medicine*, **6**(6), 932–3.

53. Unruh, A.M., Versnel, J., and Kerr, N. (2002). Spirituality unplugged: a review of commonalities and contentions, and a resolution. *Canadian Journal of Occupation Therapy*, **69**(1), 5–19.

54. Chao, C.S., Chen, C.H., and Yen, M. (2002). The essence of spirituality of terminally ill patients. *Journal of Nursing Research*, **10**(4), 237–45.

55. Vanistendael, S. (2007). Resilience and spirituality. In *Resilience and Palliative Care*, (eds. Monroe, B. and Oliviere, D.). Oxford: Oxford University Press.

56. Frankl, V. (1992). *Man's Search for Meaning: An Introduction to Logotherapy*, Beacon Press.

57. Moadel, A., Morgan, C., Fatone, A. *et al.* (1999). Seeking meaning and hope: self-reported spiritual and existential needs among an ethnically-diverse cancer patient population. *Psychooncology*, **8**(5), 378–85.

58. Bolmsjo, I. (2000). Existential issues in palliative care—interviews with cancer patients. *Journal of Palliative Care*, **16**(2), 20–4.

59. Yalom, I.D. (1980). *Existential Psychotherapy*. New York: Basic Books.

60. Kissane, D.W., Clarke, D.M., and Street, A.F. (2001). Demoralization syndrome—a relevant psychiatric diagnosis for palliative care. *Journal of Palliative Care*, **17**(1), 12–21.

61. Kissane, D.W. (2000). Psychospiritual and existential distress. The challenge for palliative care. *Australian Family Physician*, **29**(11), 1022–5.

62. Davies, B., Reimer, J.C., and Martens, N. (1990).Families in supportive care—Part I: The transition of fading away: the nature of the transition. *Journal of Palliative Care*, **6**(3), 12–20.

63. McPherson, G. (2003). Patients with cancer often felt a need to conceal their distress to protect family, friends, and doctors. *Evidence Based Nursing*, **6**(3), 95.

64. West, S.R., Harris, B.J., Warren, A. *et al.* (1986). A retrospective study of patients with cancer in their terminal year. *New Zealand Medical Journal*, **99**(798), 197–200.

65. Schachter, S. (1992). Quality of life for families in the management of home care patients with advanced cancer. *Journal of Palliative Care*, **8**(3), 61–6.

66. Grov, E.K., Dahl, A.A., Moum, T. *et al.* (2005). Anxiety, depression, and quality of life in caregivers of patients with cancer in late palliative phase. *Annals of Oncology*, **16**, 1185–91.

67. Grov, E.K., Fossa, S.D., Sorebo, O. *et al.* (2006). Primary caregivers of cancer patients in the palliative phase: A path analysis of variables influencing their burden. *Social Science Medicine*, **63**, 2429–39.

68. Lewis, F. (1986). The impact of cancer on the family: a critical analysis of the research literature. *Patient Education and Counseling*, **8**, 269–89.

69. Steele, R.G. (2000). Trajectory of certain death at an unknown time: children with neurodegenerative life-threatening illnesses. *Cancer Journal of Nursing Research*, **32**(3), 49–67.

70. Blood, G.W., Simpson, K.C., Dineen, M. *et al.* (1994). Spouses of individuals with laryngeal cancer: caregiver strain and burden. *Journal of Communication Disorders*, **27**(1), 19–35.

71. Ozono, S., Saeki, T., Inoue, S. *et al.* (2005). Family functioning and psychological distress among Japanese breast cancer patients and families. *Support Care Cancer*, **13**(12), 1044–50.

72. Edwards, B. and Clarke, V. (2004). The psychological impact of a cancer diagnosis on families: the influence of family functioning and patients' illness characteristics on depression and anxiety. *Psychooncology*, **13**(8), 562–76.

73. Kissane, D.W., McKenzie, D.P., and Bloch, S. (1997). Family coping and bereavement outcome. *Palliative Medicine*, **11**(3), 191–201.

74. Rabow, M.W., Hauser, J.M., and Adams, J. (2004). Supporting family caregivers at the end of life: "they don't know what they don't know". *Journal of the American Medical Association*, **291**(4), 483–91.

75. Ventafridda, V., De Conno, F., Vigano, A. *et al.* (1989). Comparison of home and hospital care of advanced cancer patients. *Tumori*, **75**(6), 619–25.

76. Beck-Friis, B., Norberg, H., and Strang, P. (1991). Cost analysis and ethical aspects of hospital-based home-care for

terminal cancer patients. *Scandinavian Journal of Primary Health Care*, **9**(4), 259–64.

77. Muurinen, J.M. (1986).The economics of informal care. Labor market effects in the National Hospice Study. *Medical Care*, 24(11), 1007–17.

78. Grunfeld, E., Coyle, D., Whelan, T. *et al.* (2004). Family caregiver burden: results of a longitudinal study of breast cancer patients and their principal caregivers. *Canadian Medical Association Journal*, **170**(12), 1795–801.

79. Kramer, B.J., Boelk, A.Z., and Auer, C. (2006). Family conflict at the end of life: lessons learned in a model program for vulnerable older adults. *Journal of Palliative Medicine*, 9(3), 791–801.

80. Bloche, M.G. (2005). Managing conflict at the end of life. *New England Journal of Medicine*, 352(23), 2371–3.

81. Kristjanson, L.J. (1989). Quality of terminal care: salient indicators identified by families. *Journal of Palliative Care*, 5(1), 21–30.

82. Kristjanson, L.J., Atwood, J., and Degner, L.F. (1995). Validity and reliability of the family inventory of needs (FIN): measuring the care needs of families of advanced cancer patients. *Journal of Nursing Measurement*, 3(2),109–26.

83. Kristjanson, L.J., Leis, A., Koop, P.M. *et al.* (1997). Family members' care expectations, care perceptions, and satisfaction with advanced cancer care: results of a multi-site pilot study. *Journal of Palliative Care*, **13**(4), 5–13.

84. Ferrell, B.R., Cohen, M.Z., Rhiner, M. *et al.* (1991). Pain as a metaphor for illness. Part II: Family caregivers' management of pain. *Oncology Nursing Forum*, **18**(8), 1315–21.

85. Ferrell, B.R., Rhiner, M., Cohen, M.Z. *et al.* (1991). Pain as a metaphor for illness. Part I: Impact of cancer pain on family caregivers. *Oncology Nursing Forum*, **18**(8), 1303–9.

86. Milberg, A. and Strang, P. (2000). Met and unmet needs in hospital-based home care: qualitative evaluation through open-ended questions. *Palliative Medicine*, 14(6), 533–4.

87. Soothill, K., Morris, S.M., Harman, J. *et al.* (2001). The significant unmet needs of cancer patients: probing psychosocial concerns. *Support Care Cancer*, 9(8), 597–605.

88. Scott, G., Whyler, N., and Grant, G. (2001). A study of family carers of people with a life-threatening illness 1: the carers' needs analysis. *International Journal of Palliative Nursing*, 7(6), 290–1.

89. Fridriksdottir, N., Sigurdardottir, V., and Gunnarsdottir, S. (2006). Important needs of families in acute and palliative care settings assessed with the family inventory of needs. *Palliative Medicine*, **20**(4), 425–32.

90. Callahan, D. (1988). Families as caregivers: the limits of morality. *Archives of Physical Medicine and Rehabilitation*, 69(5), 323–8.

91. Wellisch, D., Fawzy, F., Landsverk, J. *et al.* (1989). An evaluation of psychosocial problems of the homebound cancer patient: relationship of patient adjustment to family problems. *Journal of Psychosocial Oncology*, 7, 55–76.

92. Ellifritt, J., Nelson, K.A., and Walsh, D. (2003). Complicated bereavement: a national survey of potential risk factors. *American Journal of Hospital Palliative Care*, 20(2), 114–20.

93. Kissane, D.W., McKenzie, M., McKenzie, D.P. *et al.* (2003). Psychosocial morbidity associated with patterns of family functioning in palliative care: baseline data from the Family Focused Grief Therapy controlled trial. *Palliative Medicine*, 17(6), 527–37.

94. Quinn, W. and Herndon, A. (1986).The family ecology of cancer. *Journal of Psychosocial Oncology*, 4, 45–59.

95. Kash, K.M., Holland, J.C., Breitbart, W. *et al.* (2000). Stress and burnout in oncology. *Oncology (Huntington)*, 14(11), 1621–33, discussion 1633–4, 1636–7.

96. Meier, D.E., Back, A.L., and Morrison, R.S. The inner life of physicians and care of the seriously ill. *Journal of the American Medical Association*, **286**(23), 3007–14.

97. Keidel, G.C. (2002). Burnout and compassion fatigue among hospice caregivers. *American Journal of Hospital Palliative Care*, 19(3), 200–5.

98. Akroyd, D., Caison, A., and Adams, R.D. (2002). Burnout in radiation therapists: the predictive value of selected stressors. *International Journal of Radiation Oncology Biology Physics*, 52(3), 816–21.

99. Ramirez, A.J., Graham, J., Richards, M.A. *et al.* (1995). Burnout and psychiatric disorder among cancer clinicians. *British Journal of Cancer*, **71**(6), 1263–9.

100. Whippen, D.A. and Canellos, G.P. (1991). Burnout syndrome in the practice of oncology: results of a random survey of 1,000 oncologists [see comments]. *Journal of Clinical Oncology*, **9**(10), 1916–20.

101. Grunfeld, E., Zitzelsberger, L., Coristine, M. *et al.* (2004). Job stress and job satisfaction of cancer care workers. *Psychooncology*, **14**, 61–9.

102. Shanafelt, T.D. (2005). Finding meaning, balance, and personal satisfaction in the practice of oncology. *Journal of Support Oncology*, **3**(2), 157–62, 164.

103. Cherny, N.I. and Catane, R. (2003). Attitudes of medical oncologists toward palliative care for patients with advanced and incurable cancer: report on a survery by the European Society of Medical Oncology Taskforce on Palliative and Supportive Care. *Cancer*, **98**(11), 2502–10.

104. Schaerer, R. (1993). Suffering of the doctor linked with the death of patients. *Palliative Medicine*, 7, 27–37.

105. Vachon, M.L. (1995).Staff stress in hospice/palliative care: a review. *Palliative Medicine*, 9(2), 91–122.

106. Astudillo, W. and Mendinueta, C. (1996). Exhaustion syndrome in palliative care. *Support Care Cancer*, 4(6), 408–15.

107. Harris, R., Bond, M., and Turnbull, R. (1990). Nursing stress and stress reduction in palliative care. *Palliative Medicine*, 4, 191–96.

108. Wilkes, L.M. and Beale, B. (2001). Palliative care at home: stress for nurses in urban and rural New South Wales, Australia. *International Journal of Nursing Practices*, 7(5), 306–13.

109. Newton, J. and Waters, V. (2001). Community palliative care clinical nurse specialists' descriptions of stress in their work. *International Journal of Palliative Nursing*, 7(11), 531–40.

110. van Staa, A.L., Visser, A., van der Zouwe, N. (2000). Caring for caregivers: experiences and evaluation of interventions for a palliative care team. *Patient Education and Counseling*, 41(1), 93–105.

111. Farber, S.J., Egnew, T.R., Herman-Bertsch, J.L. *et al.* (2003). Issues in end-of-life care: patient, caregiver, and clinician perceptions. *Journal of Palliative Medicine*, 6(1),19–31.

112. Redinbaugh, E.M., Baum, A., Tarbell, S. *et al.* (2003).End-of-life caregiving: what helps family caregivers cope? *Journal of Palliative Medicine*, 6(6), 901–9.

113. Limpanichkul, Y.and Magilvy, K. (2004). Managing caregiving at home: Thai caregivers living in the United States. *Journal of Cultural Diversity*, 11(1), 18–24.

114. Kristjanson, L.J., Leis, A., Koop, P.M. *et al.* (1997). Family members' care expectations, care perceptions, and satisfaction with advanced cancer care: results of a multi-site pilot study. *Journal of Palliative Care*, 13(4), 5–13.

115. Dalla-Vorgia, P., Katsouyanni, K., Garanis, T.N. *et al.* (1992). Attitudes of a Mediterranean population to the truth-telling issue. *Journal of Medical Ethics*, 18(2), 67–74.

116. Mystakidou, K., Tsilika, E., Parpa, E. *et al.* (2005). Patterns and barriers in information disclosure between health care professionals and relatives with cancer patients in Greek society. *European Journal of Cancer Care*, 14(2), 175–181.

117. Pereira, J., Hanson, J., and Bruera, E. (1997). The frequency and clinical course of cognitive impairment in patients with terminal cancer. *Cancer*, 79(4), 835–42.

118. Minagawa, H., Uchitomi, Y., Yamawaki, S. *et al.* (1996). Psychiatric morbidity in terminally ill cancer patients. A prospective study [see comments]. *Cancer*, 78(5), 1131–7.

119. Breitbart, W., Rosenfeld, B., Roth, A. *et al.* (1997). The Memorial Delirium Assessment Scale [see comments]. *Journal of Pain and Symptom Management*, 13(3), 128–37.

120. Walsh, R.A., Girgis, A., Sanson-Fisher, R.W. (1998). Breaking bad news 2: What evidence is available to guide clinicians? *Behavioral Medicine*, **24**(2), 61–72.

121. Girgis, A. and Sanson-Fisher, R.W. (1998). Breaking bad news 1: Current best advice for clinicians. *Behavioral Medicine*, **24**(2), 53–9.

122. Campbell, E.M. and Sanson-Fisher, R.W. (1998). Breaking bad news. 3: Encouraging the adoption of best practices. *Behavioral Medicine*, **24**(2), 73–80.

123. Cherny, N.I., Coyle, N., and Foley, K.M. (1994). The treatment of suffering when patients request elective death. *Journal of Palliative Care*, **10**(2), 71–9.

124. Fins, J.J., Miller, F.G., Acres, C.A. *et al.* (1999). End-of-life decision-making in the hospital: current practice and future prospects. *Journal of Pain and Symptom Management*, **17**(1), 6–15.

125. Purandare, L. (1997). Attitudes to cancer may create a barrier to communication between the patient and caregiver. *European Journal of Cancer Care (Engl)*, **6**(2), 92–9.

126. Vachon, M.L. (1998). Caring for the caregiver in oncology and palliative care. *Seminars in Oncology Nursing*, **14**(2), 152–7.

127. Karlsen, S., Addington-Hall, J. (1998). How do cancer patients who die at home differ from those who die elsewhere? *Palliative Medicine*, **12**(4), 279–86.

128. Astudillo, W. and Mendinueta, C. (1996). Exhaustion syndrome in palliative care [see comments]. *Support Care Cancer*, **4**(6),408–15.

129. Bramwell, L., MacKenzie, J., Laschinger, H. *et al.* (1995). Need for overnight respite for primary caregivers of hospice clients. *Cancer Nursing*, **18**(5), 337–43.

130. Carson, V.B. (1997). Spiritual care: the needs of the caregiver. *Seminars in Oncology Nursing*, **13**(4), 271–4.

131. Janson, L.J. and Sloan, J.A. (1991). Determinants of the grief experience of survivors. *Journal of Palliative Care*, **7**(4), 51–6.

132. Murphy, K., Hanrahan, P., and Luchins, D. (1997). A survey of grief and bereavement in nursing homes: the importance of hospice grief and bereavement for the end-stage Alzheimer's disease patient and family [see comments]. *Journal of the American Geriatric Society*, **45**(9), 1104–7.

The epidemiology of the end-of-life experience

Megan B. Sands, Michael Piza, and Jane M. Ingham

Introduction

The epidemiology of the end-of-life experience

Epidemiology has been defined as 'the study of the distribution and determinants of disease frequency'[1]. It is the study of how often, and in which populations, disease occurs. Epidemiology is central to the development of strategies for the prevention and management of disease in populations and for the planning of health services. Epidemiological data can also provide information about the nature of the progression of specific diseases and the effect of treatment options. In this chapter, we will take a broad view of the epidemiology of 'disease' and will discuss epidemiology as it relates to the human experience towards the end of life with an emphasis on diseases, symptoms, and psychosocial experiences.

Three major questions relate to the epidemiology of palliative medicine and must be addressed in relation to specific diseases.

- Which diseases do people die from, in particular when death is not unexpected, sudden, or immediate?

- What is the incidence and prevalence of symptoms and distress in individuals living with these diseases?

- What is the trajectory and time course of life threatening illness?

The answers to these questions provide an evidence base for the management of symptoms that are common in specific diseases and care settings, and for the development of services for those people living with these diseases and for their caregivers. This type of information can also provide evidence that can assist in the design of palliative care education programmes which aim to target the professional needs of those engaged in the provision of care towards the end of life.

Important definitions

The palliative care population base

The World Health Organization (WHO) defines palliative care as an 'approach which improves the quality of life of patients and their families facing life-threatening illness, through the prevention and relief of suffering by means of early identification and impeccable assessment and treatment of pain and other problems, physical, psychological, and spiritual'[2]. Definition of the palliative care population is important as it helps to articulate what palliative care is, who needs it, and who should provide it[3] (see Section 2). The type of palliative care services in demand and the needs for particular clinical skills and knowledge required by a patient living with a life-threatening disease are largely affected by the type of disease as well as the socioeconomic, cultural, home, and natural environments that the patient inhabits.

Incidence

'Incidence quantifies the number of new events or cases of disease that develop in a population of individuals at risk during a specified time interval'.[1] This is an estimate of the probability that a patient in a given population at risk, will develop the condition during a specified period of time. For example, the incidence of bowel obstruction in a population of patients with colorectal cancer followed for 30 months from the date of diagnosis. Incidence can be summarized as:

$$\frac{\text{Number of new cases}}{\text{Total population at risk}}$$

Prevalence

'Prevalence quantifies the proportion of individuals in a population who have the disease at a specific instant and provides an estimate of the probability (risk) that an individual will be ill at a point in time'.[1] For example, the point prevalence of patients meeting DSM-IV criteria for depression at admission to a palliative care unit. Prevalence can be summarized as:

$$\frac{\text{Number of cases}}{\text{Total population at a given point in time}}$$

Epidemiology of death worldwide

Limitations of mortality statistics

In reviewing mortality statistics, it is important to have an understanding of the limits of the existing data. Mortality statistics provide information on death rates and causes of death in populations. To obtain this data, epidemiologists must rely on diverse sources of information. The Global Burden of Disease (GBD) study initiated by the WHO provides a comprehensive set of mortality and morbidity statistics by age, sex, and region. The GBD study is based on four sources of information[4]:

1 *Death registration systems.* These provide information, not always complete[5], on the causes of death for most high-income countries as well as many countries in Eastern Europe, Central Asia, Latin America, and the Caribbean.

2 *Sample death registration systems.* These systems are used in China and India where the deaths of a large proportion of the population are not registered, in particular deaths in rural areas. To supplement death registration systems, a sample of the population in rural areas is registered and the death rate established. This rate is then extrapolated to the broader population.

3 *Epidemiological assessments.* These assessments provide estimates of deaths for major diseases, such as HIV/AIDS, malaria, and tuberculosis (TB), for countries in the regions most affected by these conditions. Epidemiological assessments deduce case fatality rates (i.e. people who have a specified disease who die as a result of that disease within a given period of time) from surveys on the incidence or prevalence of a specific disease over a specific period of time combined with knowledge of the usual mortality for that condition.

4 *Cause of death models.* These are used in regions (including most of sub-Saharan Africa) with non-existent or incomplete mortality data to estimate deaths according to broad cause groups.

Only a third of the world's population resides in regions where complete civil registration systems that provide adequate, cause-specific mortality data exist. In most of Africa, South East Asia, the Middle East, and parts of the Pacific, where over one-quarter of the world population resides, there is little or no mortality monitoring[4, 6].

In countries such as China and India, which rely on a relatively small sample of the population to determine national mortality statistics (called sample vital registration systems), death data may be unrepresentative. In China for example, death registration systems cover less than 10 per cent of the population. Furthermore, deaths are under-reported, even in regions with such registration systems in place. An assessment of China's mortality reporting system suggested that in regions covered by that system, adult deaths were under reported by 30 per cent[6].

Reporting errors relating to cause of death are a worldwide problem. The uncertainty for 'all cause' mortality is reported to range from ±1 per cent in high-income countries to around ±20 per cent for sub-Saharan Africa. Uncertainty intervals are even greater in estimates of mortality by specific cause. For example, the uncertainty intervals for deaths from ischaemic heart disease were estimated to range from ±12 per cent for high-income countries to ±30 per cent for sub-Saharan Africa[7]. Even in countries where deaths are reasonably consistently reported, for example, in high-income countries, significant proportions of reported deaths have been evaluated as containing errors ranging from 'unacceptable' or 'inaccurate statements' through to 'major errors'[5]. Reporting errors are more frequent in those regions where deaths occur without the involvement of medical practitioners. In these regions, mostly low- and middle-income countries, mortality data collection relies on family members for information on the cause of death[6].

It has also been suggested that regions with sub-optimal mortality monitoring systems are at added risk of reporting bias[8]. One example

is where death rate estimates are drawn from data provided by 'groups in competition for scarce resources that are acting as advocates for affected populations'[7] or groups that are responsible for both—for data collection and reporting to funding bodies[7]. Potential conflicts of interest, financial incentives, and pressures must therefore also be considered when assessing the validity of epidemiological data[9]. Along with the issues stated earlier, there is the problem that mortality data is reported by single cause of death (for reasons of complexity) despite the fact that co-morbidities and health risks may significantly contribute to cause of death. This may introduce further biases.

The comprehensive nature of the death and morbidity information captured is also a product of the coding and reporting systems in use. The electronic recording of death data and the increasing adoption of reporting systems such as the International Classification of Diseases version 10 (ICD 10) by the majority of countries (from four countries in 1994 to 75 countries in 2003) have brought about improvements in 'real-time' availability and interpretation of death data[7]. There are, however, limitations with regard to the comprehensiveness of the information gathered.

In many instances, the principal causes of death included in mortality reports exist within a spectrum of conditions that vary in severity—from conditions where disease-modifying therapy can provide a cure or substantially improved survival–to those with a universally poor prognosis[9].

TB, one of the leading causes of death globally provides an example of the complexity that occurs where multiple co-morbidities contribute to a death. This disease can present in various entities including highly morbid stains such as, multidrug-resistant tuberculosis (MDR-TB). TB may also present in a variety of clinical contexts (e.g. with no co-morbidities vs. with significant co-morbidities e.g. HIV/AIDS). The documented mortality rates due to MDR-TB in studies from high-income nations range between 50 to 100 per cent in HIV infected men to between 31 to 44 per cent in HIV-negative men[10]. Most global mortality data do not therefore report type and clinical context of TB contributing to the overall TB death rate. Disease-reporting systems such as the ICD 10 provide the opportunity to overcome these kind of limitations.

In summary, when interpreting mortality data, it is important to be aware of its limitations. Despite these limitations, however, the increasing availability of population data from different sources and regions provides the opportunity to reduce sampling biases and to gain a more complete representation of the causes and experiences of death in different parts of the world. Over time, developments in information systems will provide the potential for further improvements in the comprehensiveness and accuracy of mortality statistics.

Life expectancy

Life expectancy and cause of death vary greatly worldwide and may be associated with demographic characteristics and other factors such as socioeconomic status[11][12]. Differences in life expectancy are greatest when the lowest income countries are compared with the highest income countries (Fig. 3.2.1 and Fig. 3.2.2). Factors such as occupational, political, cultural, and lifestyle risks as well as ethnicity, gender, and genetics also influence these data. For example, worldwide females have a predicted additional 5 years in life expectancy, in comparison to males (70 years in women compared to 65 in men, for the period 2005 to 2010)[13].

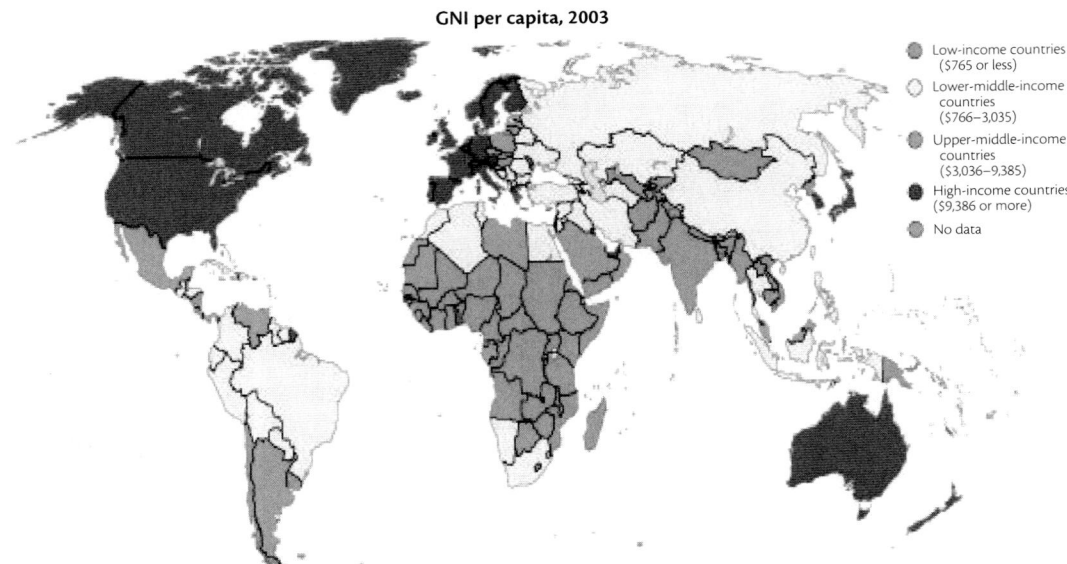

Figure 3.2.1 Countries of the world grouped by Gross National Income (GNI), 2003.
Source: reprinted with permission from the World Bank Group, 2009 World Bank Atlas: Income Per Person. http://go.worldbank.org/7ETAD6CKO0[11].

Leading causes of death

The leading reported causes of death vary between regions at different levels of economic development. The World Bank classifies the countries of the world into three income groups: low, middle, and high. In 2002, an estimated 57 million people died in the world and, of these deaths, 85 per cent occurred in low- and middle-income countries[14]. Table 3.2.1 presents the 10 leading causes of death worldwide. Among these, three major categories emerge: cardiovascular diseases (ischaemic heart and cerebrovascular diseases are the most common in this category), infectious and parasitic diseases (lower respiratory tract infections, AIDS, diarhoeal diseases, TB, and malaria are the most common), and cancers (cancers of trachea/lung are the most common cause of

cancer death)[14]. Table 3.2.2 describes the causes of death in relation to the income group of countries.

In high-income countries the leading 10 causes of death by disease group are cardiovascular diseases, followed by all cancers (lung, colorectal, breast, and stomach are included in the top 10) and other chronic diseases which include chronic obstructive pulmonary disease (COPD), dementias and diabetes (Table 3.2.2). Death rates from most infectious and parasitic diseases in high-income countries are low most (<5 per cent) and except for lower respiratory infections, these diseases do not feature as leading causes of death in this income group.

Table 3.2.1 Leading causes of death in the world, 2002.

Cause	Deaths (×1000)	Deaths (%)
All	57027	1000
Ischaemic heart disease	7208	12.6
Cerebrovascular disease	5500	9.7
Lower respiratory infections	3884	6.8
HIV/AIDS	2777	4.3
Chronic obstructive pulmonary disease	2748	3.9
Diarrhoeal diseases	1796	3.2
Tuberculosis	1566	2.7
Malaria	1777	2.7
Cancer of trachea/bronchus/lung	1243	2.2
Road traffic accidents	1192	2.1
All cardiovascular diseases	16666	29.2
All infectious and parasitic diseases	11122	19.5
All cancers	7106	12.5

Source: data reproduced with permission from World Health Organization, World Health Report, 2003. http://www.who.int/whr/2003/en/

Figure 3.2.2 Population life expectancy worldwide, 2006.
Source: United Nations, World Population Prospects, 2007. Reprinted with permission from Institute National d'Etudes Demographique. http://www.ined.fr/en/teaching kits/length of life death mortality/world life expectancy/[12].

Life expectancy worldwide, in years, in 2006

Source : ONU, World Population Prospects, 2007

Teaching Kit, INED, www.ined.fr

More than 80   60 – 69   Less than 40
75 – 79   50 – 59
70 – 74   40 – 49

Table 3.2.2 Leading causes of death in the world 2002, by broad income groups.

High-income countries			Middle-income countries			Low-income countries		
Cause	Deaths (x10 000)	Deaths %	Cause	Deaths (x10 000)	Deaths %	Cause	Deaths (x10 000)	Deaths %
All causes	789	100	All causes	2068	100	All causes	2870	100
Ischaemic heart disease	134	17.1	Cerebrovascular disease	302	14.6	Ischaemic heart disease	310	10.8
Cerebrovascular disease	77	9.8	Ischaemic heart disease	277	13.4	Lower respiratory infections	286	10.0
Cancer of trachea/bronchus/lung	46	5.8	Chronic obstructive pulmonary disease	157	7.6	HIV/AIDS	214	7.5
Lower respiratory infections	34	4.3	Lower respiratory infections	69	3.3	Perinatal conditions	183	6.4
Chronic obstructive pulmonary disease	30	3.9	HIV/AIDS	62	3.0	Cerebrovascular disease	172	6.0
Colon and rectal cancers	26	3.3	Perinatal conditions	60	2.9	Diarrhoeal diseases	154	5.4
Alzheimer's and other dementias	22	2.7	Stomach cancer	58	2.8	Malaria	124	4.4
Diabetes mellitus	22	2.7	Cancer of trachea/bronchus/lung	57	2.7	Tuberculosis	110	3.8
Breast cancer	15	1.9	Road traffic accidents	55	2.6	Chronic obstructive pulmonary disease	88	3.1
Stomach cancer	14	1.8	Hypertensive heart disease	54	2.6	Road traffic accidents	53	1.9
*All cardiovascular	–	38.1	*All cardiovascular	–	37.0	*All cardiovascular	–	23.0
*All cancer	–	26.2	*All cancer	–	16.0	*All cancer	–	7.0

Source: Data reproduced with permission from;

(1) World Health Organization; The 10 leading causes of death (2002) by broad income group, fact sheet N310/February 2007[14].

(2) *The World Bank, Mathers, C.D., Lopez, A., and Murray, C.J.L. (2006). The burden of disease and mortality by condition: data, methods, and results for 2001 In: *Global Burden of Disease and Risk Factors*, (eds. Lopez, A.M.C., Ezzati, M., Jamison, D., Murray, C.) pp. 46–93. New York: Oxford University Press[7].

The leading cause of death in high-income countries varies between demographic groups (socioeconomic class, gender, age, and ethnicity). For example, more males than females die of cancer and injuries and more females die from cardiovascular conditions and other chronic diseases such as dementias and diabetes (Table 3.2.3).

There are key differences observed between the different age groups. Among people aged 15 to 59 from high-income countries, cancers are the leading cause of death, (32.3 per cent)[7]. Injuries (21.3 per cent) and cardiovascular diseases (21.6 per cent) rank second and third in this age group[7]. In the 60-and-over age group, cardiovascular diseases (42.1 per cent) are by far the most common cause of death followed by cancers (25.3 per cent)[7]. Deaths due to injuries (2.9 per cent) are significantly lower in this group, compared to the younger age groups. Deaths from lower respiratory infection (5.0 per cent) and chronic diseases such as COPD (4.3 per cent), and dementias including Alzheimer's (3.7 per cent) are all higher in people aged 60 and over.

In children (0–14 age group) from high-income countries, perinatal conditions and congenital anomalies are the leading causes of death (Table 3.2.3). Perinatal conditions include diseases related to low birth-weight and prematurity (31 per cent of perinatal deaths) as well as birth asphyxia and trauma (34 per cent of perinatal deaths). Injury is the third leading cause of death among children under 14 in this income group (17 per cent of all deaths). The most common injuries result from road traffic accidents, which accounted for 5.9 per cent of deaths in this income group in 2001.

Marked differences in health status, life expectancy, and cause of death also exist between ethnic groups in some high-income countries; in particular between indigenous and non-indigenous people. For example, data from Australia for the period 2005–2007, shows that male indigenous Australians had a life expectancy at birth 11.5 years below that of the non-indigenous Australian population; for female indigenous Australians, the difference was 9.7 years[15]. Indigenous groups from other high-income countries also have comparatively higher rates of death and morbidity from cancer, respiratory disease, stroke, injury, and diabetes[16,17].

The leading causes of death in middle-income countries are cardiovascular diseases (37.0 per cent) followed by cancers (16.0 per cent), and chronic diseases (>8 per cent; in particular COPD). However, in contrast to high-income countries, HIV/AIDS (3.0 per cent) and perinatal conditions (2.9 per cent) feature among the leading causes of death (Table 3.2.2).

Populations from low-income countries have not experienced the rising life expectancy observed in the rest of the world, and in several countries of sub-Saharan Africa, life expectancy has declined to 40 years or below[18]. The leading causes of death among populations from low-income countries are infectious and parasitic diseases (>45 per cent; lower respiratory infections, HIV/AIDS, diarrhoeal diseases, malaria, and TB are included in the top 10). Infections and parasitic disease account for about half of all causes of deaths, therefore constitute a significant proportion of the total deaths each year for the whole world. See Table 3.2.2 for more detail about causes of death in low-income countries.

In both low- and middle-income countries there is little variation in the leading causes of death between males and females, with the exception of all types of injury and TB both of which are higher among

Table 3.2.3 Leading causes of death in high-income countries by gender and age for 2001.

Male (4 002 000)		Female (3 890 000)		Age 0–14 (96 000)		Age 15–59 (1 213 000)		Age 60+ (6 584 000)	
*Cause	%	*Cause	%	**Cause	%	**Cause	%	**Cause	%
Ischaemic heart diseases	17.9	Ischaemic heart diseases	16.7	All perinatal conditions	33.9	All injuries	21.3	Ischaemic heart disease	18.7
Other cardiac diseases	9.3	Other cardiac diseases	13.4	All congenital anomalies	20.0	Ischaemic heart disease	10.8	Other cardiac diseases	12.4
Cerebrovascular disease	8.1	Cerebrovascular disease	11.8	All injuries	17.0	Other cardiac diseases	5.4	Cerebrovascular disease	11.0
Cancer of trachea/ bronchus/lung	7.8	Lower respiratory infections	4.8	All infectious and parasitic (excl. LRI)	5.2	Cancer of trachea/ bronchus/lung	6.8	Cancer of trachea/ bronchus/lung	5.7
All injuries	7.8	All injuries	4.0	All cardiovascular	4.2	Cerebrovascular disease	4.4	Lower respiratory infections	5.0
Chronic obstructive pulmonary disease	4.3	Breast cancer	4.0	All neuropsychiatric	4.2	Cirrhosis of the liver	4.4	Chronic obstructive pulmonary disease	4.3
Lower respiratory infections	4.0	Cancer of trachea/ bronchus/lung	3.7	Lower respiratory infections	2.5	Breast cancer	4.0	Alzheimer's and other dementias	3.7
Colon and rectal cancers	3.3	Alzheimer's and other dementias	3.7	All endocrine disorders	2.0	Colon and rectal cancers	3.1	All injuries	2.9
Gastric and oesophageal cancer	3.3	Colon and rectal cancers	3.2	Leukaemia	2.0	Gastric and oesophageal cancer	3.0	Diabetes mellitus	2.7
Prostate cancer	2.9	Chronic obstructive pulmonary disease	3.2	Other cancer	2.0	Diabetes mellitus	2.1	Gastric and oesophageal cancer	2.5

Source: Data from

(1) *Western Europe only. Reproduced with permission from World Health Organization R Becker, J Silvi, D Ma Fat, AL'Hours and R Laurenti (2006). A method for deriving leading causes of death. *Bulletin of the World Health Organization*, 84 p 297–304.

(2) **All 'high income countries'. Reproduced with permission from The World Bank. Mathers, C.D., Lopez, A., and Murray, C.J.L. (2006). The burden of disease and mortality by condition: data, methods, and results for 2001 In: *Global Burden of Disease and Risk Factors*, (eds. Lopez, A.M.C., Ezzati, M., Jamison, D., Murray, C.) pp. 46–93. New York: Oxford University Press[7].

males (Table 3.2.4). Amongst children (0–14 years) in low- and middle-income countries, infectious and parasitic disease followed by perinatal conditions are the most common causes of death[7]. With regard to infectious causes of death in these children, lower respiratory infections (17 per cent), diarrhoeal diseases (13.4 per cent), malaria (9.2 per cent), measles (6.2 per cent), AIDS (3.7 per cent), whooping cough (2.5 per cent) and tetanus (1.9 per cent) are the most common infections accounting for these deaths (Table 3.2.4).

The median neonatal mortality rate (NMR) in low- and middle-income countries combined is 33 per 1000 live births accounting for almost 4 million deaths. This is several times higher than the NMR in high-income countries (4 per 1000 live births accounting for 42 000 deaths). The highest NMRs are in countries of sub-Saharan Africa (in some the NMR rate is up to 65 deaths per 1000 live births)[19]. In these regions, death statistics for people aged 60 and over are not dissimilar to those in high-income countries. Death in those people surviving to the sixth decade in low- and middle-income countries is predominantly due to cardiac and vascular diseases (48.7 per cent), followed by cancer (14.5 per cent, the leading tumour types are gastro-oesophageal and lung)[7]. In this income group, death from chronic diseases (especially COPD and diabetes) is significantly more frequent and death from injuries are less frequent in the over 60-year-olds than among younger age groups.

Projections for the future: leading causes of death

Mortality projections represent potential future occurrences. For these projections current data are used to estimate future events to provide a 'forecast'. Projections do however provide indicators useful in the planning of health services at both the global and local levels[20]. These projections also furnish palliative care providers with some insight into future palliative care needs of specific populations.

Worldwide projections for 2030, based on 2002 data, predict an overall increase in life expectancy (from 65 to 70) and a decreasing rate of infant deaths (Table 3.2.5). In some regions, however, life expectancy will continue to remain far behind the rest of the world. This is particularly the case for sub-Saharan Africa (remaining below 55 in 2030) largely as a consequence of AIDS, war, and poverty[21]. The rate of global death from communicable disease is expected to decrease from 41 per cent in 2002 to 31 per cent; however, deaths due to AIDS are expected, by contrast, to continue to rise.

Other causes of death that are expected to increase further by 2030 worldwide are: circulatory diseases, COPD, diabetes mellitus, and lung, stomach, liver, and colorectal cancers[22]. It is expected that potentially-modifiable lifestyle risks such as smoking, will continue to be a major contributor to premature deaths globally[20]. By 2015, deaths attributed to smoking will account for 10 per cent of all global deaths (6.4 million)[22]. This projected rise in smoking related death assumes a predicted increase in smoking rates in low- and middle-income countries as well as in younger women across the world[22].

For high-income countries, mortality projections for 2030 predict that the cardiovascular diseases will be the most common cause of death (Table 3.2.5). Cancers (with lung cancer expected to

Table 3.2.4 Leading causes of death in low and middle income countries by gender and age for 2001.

Male (25 554 000)		Female (22 797 000)		Age 0–14 (12 001 000)		Age 15–59 (14 547 000)		Age 60+ (21 802 000)	
Cause	**%**	**Cause**	**%**	**Cause**	**%**	**Cause**	**%**	**Cause**	**%**
All injuries	12.4	Ischaemic heart disease	11.8	Perinatal conditions	20.7	All injuries	21.7	Ischaemic heart disease	20.7
Ischaemic heart disease	11.8	Cerebrovascular disease	10.7	Lower respiratory infections	17.0	HIV/AIDS	14.1	Cerebrovascular disease	17.8
Cerebrovascular disease	8.5	Other cardiac diseases	7.4	Diarrhoeal diseases	13.4	Ischaemic heart disease	8.1	Other cardiac diseases	10.2
Lower respiratory infections	6.7	Lower respiratory infections	7.4	Malaria	9.2	Tuberculosis	7.1	Chronic obstructive pulmonary disease	9.4
Perinatal conditions	5.4	All injuries	6.8	Measles	6.2	Cerebrovascular disease	4.9	Lower respiratory infections	4.7
HIV/AIDS	5.4	HIV/AIDS	5.2	All injuries	5.9	Other cardiac diseases	4.9	All injuries	3.9
Other cardiac diseases	4.9	Chronic obstructive pulmonary disease	5.1	HIV/AIDS	3.7	Lower respiratory infections	2.3	Gastric and oesophageal cancer	3.4
Chronic obstructive pulmonary disease	4.7	Perinatal conditions	4.9	Congenital anomalies	3.7	Gastric and oesophageal cancer	2.2	Diabetes mellitus	2.5
Tuberculosis	4.1	Diarrhoeal diseases	3.7	Whooping cough	2.5	Cirrhosis of the liver	2.2	Cancer of trachea/ bronchus/lung	2.5
Diarrhoeal diseases	3.6	Malaria	2.8	Tetanus	1.9	Chronic obstructive pulmonary disease	2.2	Tuberculosis	2.2

Sources: Data reproduced with permission from The World Bank. Mathers, C.D., Lopez, A., and Murray, C.J.L. (2006). The burden of disease and mortality by condition: data, methods, and results for 2001 In: *Global Burden of Disease and Risk Factors*, (eds. Lopez, A.M.C., Ezzati, M., Jamison, D., Murray, C.) pp. 46–93. New York: Oxford University Press[7].

remain the tumour type responsible for the largest proportion of deaths) and chronic diseases including COPD, diabetes mellitus and dementias are the predicted leading causes of death in this income group[22].

In middle-income countries, cardiovascular disease is predicted to continue as the leading cause of death into 2030. Death from chronic non-cancer and non-cardiovascular disease is also expected to increase; AIDS, COPD, and diabetes are amongst the causes of death expected to rise in this income group. Death from AIDS is expected to increase dramatically to become the fourth most common cause of death in middle-income countries. Deaths from cancers, particularly cancer of the lung, stomach, and liver, are also expected to increase[22]. Population increases in regions with high prevalence of diseases such as gastric cancer, and the growing prevalence of lifestyle risks such as smoking, may contribute to an increase in deaths from these cancers.

In low-income countries, infectious and parasitic diseases (HIV, lower respiratory infections, diarrhoeal diseases, and malaria) are expected to continue to be among the leading causes of mortality in 2030. Deaths from AIDS, estimated to increase by 76 per cent are expected to contribute significantly to this increase[22]. Cardiac, vascular and other chronic diseases are also projected to be among the leading causes of death in this income group[22]. The cardiovascular group of diseases is expected to continue as the most common cause of death. Of all cardiac and vascular diseases in this income group, ischaemic heart disease is projected to be the leading

cause of death.[22] Diabetes is expected to appear for the first time among the top 10 causes of death in low-income countries, while deaths from COPD also are expected to increase (by 77 per cent) (Table 3.2.5). By 2030 TB (ranked eighth in low-income countries in 2002) is expected to drop out of the top 10 causes of death in this income group.

Projections like these are useful for the purpose of long-term planning for nationally-based palliative care services. It should be acknowledged that such projections are based on predictive models. Although acknowledged important variables that impact mortality are factored into these models, there is nonetheless uncertainty related to this process. That is; *projections* of future mortality may not match *actual* future mortality if, for example important changes in lifestyle, economic, and social factors evolve in a way that has not been adequately accounted for. Three such factors that are currently included in mortality models are; the relationship between economic and social development, known disease patterns, and tobacco and obesity risks. These may change in unpredictable ways. Similarly, unexpected health improvements related to treatment and disease prevention strategies, may also affect future mortality trends.

Place of care: where are palliative care services and support needed?

One aim of palliative care is to provide services, where possible, in a location of patient choice.[23] Preferred place of death (often the wish

Table 3.2.5 Projected leading causes of death in 2030 (predictions based on 2002 data).

High-income countries		Middle-income countries		Low-income countries	
Cause	**%**	**Cause**	**%**	**Cause**	**%**
Ischaemic heart disease	15.8	Cerebrovascular disease	14.4	Ischaemic heart disease	13.4
Cerebrovascular disease	9.0	Ischaemic heart disease	12.7	HIV/AIDS	13.2
Cancer of trachea/bronchus/lung	5.1	Chronic obstructive pulmonary disease	12.0	Cerebrovascular disease	8.2
Diabetes mellitus	4.8	HIV/AIDS	6.2	Chronic obstructive pulmonary disease	5.5
Chronic obstructive pulmonary disease	4.1	Cancer of trachea/bronchus/lung	4.3	Lower respiratory infection	5.1
Lower respiratory infections	3.6	Diabetes mellitus	3.7	Perinatal conditions	3.9
Alzheimer's and other dementias	3.6	Stomach cancer	3.4	Road traffic accidents	3.7
Colon and rectal cancers	3.3	Hypertensive diseases	2.7	Diarrhoeal diseases	2.3
Stomach cancer	1.9	Road traffic accidents	2.5	Diabetes mellitus	2.1
Breast cancer	1.8	Liver cancer	2.2	Malaria	1.8

Source: Mathers, C.D. and Loncar, D. (2006). Projections of global mortality and burden of disease from 2002 to 2030. *PLoS Medicine*, **3**(11), e442[22].

to die at home) has been an item solicited in clinical settings and collected in research and clinical audit. Preferred 'place of care' may however be a more appropriate focus of enquiry.[25,26] Increasingly, preferred place of care is being studied and there is an acknowledgement that this preference may change along the illness experience[27]. Preferred 'place of care' is expected to vary over an individual's disease trajectory and should therefore be ascertained longitudinally over the course of the illness experience. Data about changes in preferred place of care over time help inform planning and support flexibility in service provision up until and including death[24].

Data collected on 'place of death' are for the most part, from only high-income nations. In general, hospital care is scarce in low-income countries, which would suggest that the vast majority of people in these regions die outside the hospital setting[28]. The opposite is true in some high-income countries. The available data suggest that more than 50 per cent of deaths in England, the United States, Germany, Switzerland, and France take place in the hospital[23]. Significant variations in place of death exist among

high-income countries, with lower rates of hospital death reported in the Netherlands (35 per cent), Ireland (30 per cent), and Italy (35 percent)[23]. When asked to project a location of choice, the overwhelming majority of patients indicate a preference for care at home up until, and including, the time of death[29–31].

Reasons why many people die in the hospital despite a projected desire to be cared for at home until death, and why preferred place of death may vary over time, are complex and potentially interdependent (see Fig. 3.2.3)[32,33]. With disease progression, priorities often change and care planning at the end of life must accommodate these changes[34]. Also, as diseases progress, there are differences between patients and their carers regarding the experience of an illness and the expectations of care[35,36]. Generally, palliative care services attempt to support care in the location of choice and provide flexibility to accommodate changes overtime. Still, for many patients at the end of life 'care at home' is not a practical option and admission to inpatient care ought not to be viewed as 'failure'[37].

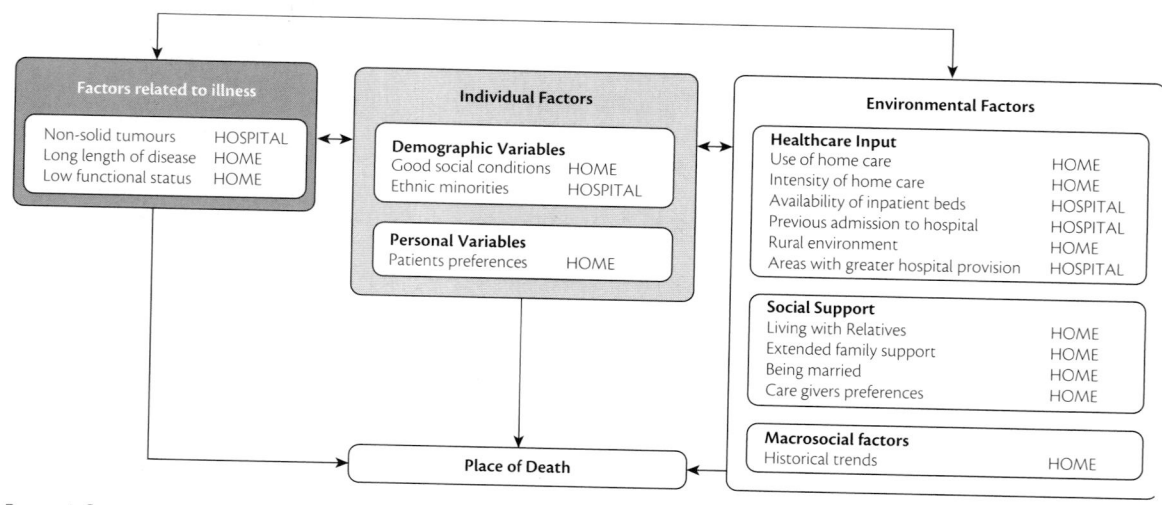

Figure 3.2.3 Factors influencing place of death.
Source: redrawn from Higginson IJ, Costantini M (2008). Dying with cancer, living well with advanced cancer. *The European Journal of Cancer*, **44**(10), 1414–24, with permission from Elsevier[32].

Gomes and Higginson carried out a systematic review of the risk factors influencing place of death[38]. The authors report data drawn from 58 original studies from 13 countries, totalling over 1.5 million patients. In this population more than 80 per cent had a cancer diagnosis. Factors found to be strongly associated with patients dying at home included; poor functional status, extended family support, patient preference, living with relatives, and availability and intensity of home care. Factors associated with dying in the hospital included: previous admission to hospital, suffering from non-solid tumours such as leukaemia and lymphoma, residing in an area with available hospital beds, and being from an ethnic minority (Fig. 3.2.3). Others have identified the availability of hospital care as a principal determinant of place of death[39,40]. It has also been suggested that the capacity for inpatient palliative care services to provide care at short notice, often without the need to attend an emergency department, may allow patients to stay at home longer and facilitate shorter duration hospitalizations. Further research may shed more light on this matter.

The few studies that provide projections of where people from high-income populations are likely to die, suggest the rate of death at home will decline further over time. One study, using data collected by the British Office of National Statistics, found that the proportion of deaths at home in England and Wales had fallen from 31.1 per cent in 1974 to 18.1 per cent in 2003. Epidemiological models predict that deaths at home in the same region, will fall further, to 9.6 per cent by 2030[27]. These predictions should be considered in context of the more immediate factors that influence place of death including patients' wishes and the availability of home and caregiver support.

The availability of, and access to, palliative care expertise: are palliative care experts available if needed?

Appropriate assessment and symptom management is indicated for all dying people, regardless of setting[41,42]. Competencies in symptom management at the end of life and knowledge about the referral process to appropriate palliative care services are required to some degree from all generalist and most specialist health practitioners. A core aspect of end-of-life care involves facilitating a patient's transition across settings (home, hospital or inpatient setting) and across levels of specialist care according to the need of individual patients[43]. In addition to providing consultation or direct care for patients at the end of life, specialist palliative care professionals can play a significant role in terms of education, policy, and planning for generalist and non-palliative care specialist health professionals[44].

Palliative care consultation and referral is available in most high-income countries through mainstream health services in community, inpatient, and acute hospital settings but availability is much more limited in middle- and low-income countries (Fig. 3.2.4)[45]. In high-income countries, many tertiary-referral centres accommodate integrated consultative, specialist palliative care services within acute and sub-acute settings[46–50]. Despite the availability of these services, a significant proportion of

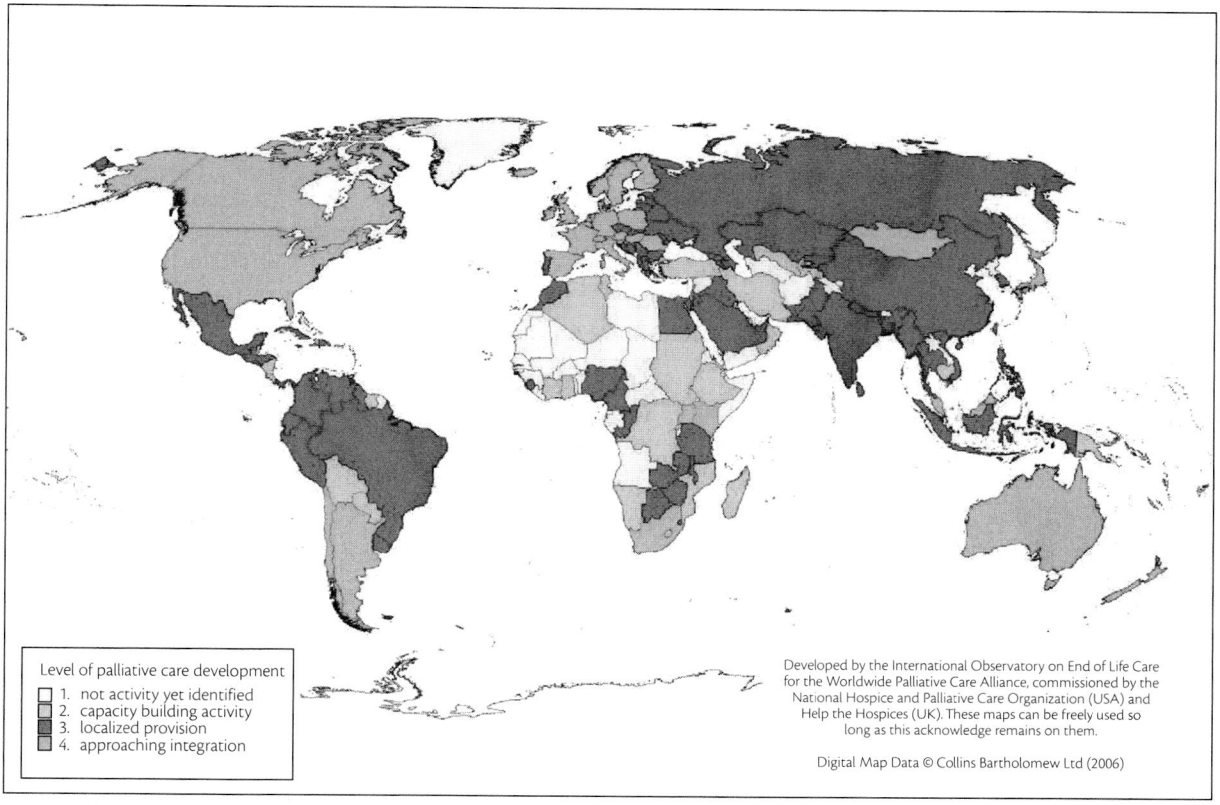

Figure 3.2.4 Levels of palliative care development: all countries.
Source: reprinted from the International Observatory on End of Life Care. Wright, M., Wood, J., Lynch, T., *et al.* Mapping levels of palliative care development: A global view (2006). Lancaster University. http://www.eolc-observatory.net/global/pdf/world map.pdf[45].

patients with far advanced disease in these countries, still have limits on their access to symptom management and end-of-life care[51].

An Italian longitudinal survey of 2000 cancer patients, with follow up until death, found that of those who died who were admitted to hospital, 20 per cent received palliative care support. While among those who died cared for at home, the rate was even lower—14 per cent[29]. In the United Kingdom, estimates from national and regional data suggest that between 25 per cent and 65 per cent of those dying from cancer in one year received specialist palliative care, and 15–25 per cent received inpatient hospice care[52]. A comprehensive population based study from Western Australia, with data from 27 971 deaths, identified that 68 per cent of individuals dying from cancer received specialist palliative care[53].

There are epidemiological data to support the claim that patients dying from illnesses other than cancer are less likely than those with cancer to receive specialist palliative care[54,55]. This disparity is well illustrated in the Western Australian population-based study mentioned earlier. In that study, only 8 per cent of patients dying from selected non-malignant conditions (heart failure, renal failure, COPD, Alzheimer's disease, liver failure, Parkinson's disease, motor neuron disease, HIV/AIDS, and Huntington's disease) were shown to have received specialist palliative care in the 12 months prior to death[53]. That stated, not receiving specialist palliative care cannot be assumed in every case to represent inadequate care, but where, disparities exist and/or access is not clearly defined as needs based, it does raise the possibility of the presence of unmet needs. Local needs assessments, using defined criteria may allow further comparison and benchmarking in relation to palliative care access[56,57].

As shown in Fig. 3.2.4[45], some middle-income countries (e.g. Argentina, Chile, Cuba, South Africa, and Malaysia), have specialist palliative care provided through mainstream health services[45]. It has however been suggested that palliative care services in these countries are inequitably distributed, and are mostly limited to individuals from higher-income groups living in urban areas[42]. It is estimated that only 5–10 per cent of the population of South America in need of palliative care, receive it[58]. Furthermore, palliative care services in middle-income regions, like their high-income region counterparts, have largely evolved in the context of providing care for people with specific diseases, in particular AIDS and cancer[45]. In summary, palliative care services in most middle-income countries are available for only some of the patients in need, and are frequently unavailable for the poor and those living in rural and remote regions.

In low-income countries, three main areas of palliative care need have been identified—symptom management, counselling, and financial assistance[59]. The majority of dying people in low-income countries are cared for at home and in communities by family and/or neighbours. In general terms, there are few palliative care services and those that exist reach only a small proportion of the people in need.

Uganda is a case in point where, despite attempts to integrate palliative care within public-health services, access is still a problem due to the fact that only an estimated 41 per cent of the population has access to any basic health care[59]. The disparities in palliative care service provision in India illustrate the disparities that exist in most low and many middle-income countries. For example, a study from 2001 reports that 16 states or territories had some hospice or palliative care service provision, including one with up to 90 per cent coverage. Another 19 states or union territories, however, had no specialist or planned palliative care services[60]. Many palliative care services in low-income countries (e.g. Guatemala) focus on the care of people with specific conditions, especially HIV/AIDS[60]. Even if these services are taken into account, half of the deaths in low-income countries are due to advanced, progressive, chronic diseases such as cardiovascular disease and cancer, and while these diseases have a known symptom burden amenable to palliative intervention, there is little specialist palliative care available.

Whether a region has a high, middle, or low income, palliative care services are not always available to meet the needs of all dying patients. An emphasis on needs-based, rather than diagnosis or prognosis-based, provision of care has been advocated by many[23,61]. Accurate and comprehensive population-based data are fundamental to identifying the needs of patients with far advanced disease, so that the available general and specialist palliative care services can be appropriately and equitably managed.

Despite significant advances, the data suggest that unmet healthcare needs amenable to palliative care interventions persist. This will be further explored in the following paragraphs, but, for example, The Study to Understand Prognosis and Preferences for the Outcomes and Risks of Treatment (SUPPORT), which followed 9105 adults hospitalized in the United States with at least one of nine life-threatening diagnoses, found that proxies reported inadequate pain control in 50 per cent of conscious patients during the last 3 days of life[51]. Epidemiological studies of cancer patients from other countries reveal similar rates of inadequate pain control[63,64] and unmet needs are also evident for patients with non-malignant, life-threatening conditions[65].

The epidemiology of symptoms experienced towards the end of life

Symptom data and health-care needs in palliative care: which health-care needs are relevant to palliative care?

Healthcare needs at the end of life, and not only at the end of life, have a direct relationship with symptom experience during that time. Debate about the definition of what constitutes a health-care need is not new, it echoes centuries of Western philosophical discourse which has attempted, in one way or another, to address the question—what life befits a human being? Contemporary liberal philosophers such as Rawls and Sen, draw on the traditions of Aristotle as well as Kant in considering a healthcare need to be; that which is required for a person to fulfil his or her potential with vitality while preserving dignity, justice, and equity.[66,67]

This philosophical perspective sits well with the principles of biomedical ethics (autonomy, beneficence, non-malfeasance and justice; see Section 5). Importantly this philosophical perspective carries with it not only justification for symptom management at the end of life, but an ethical imperative for it.[41] Clinical epidemiology, the focus of this chapter, is indispensable to this task, for in order to meet individual and group needs equitably across a population, these needs must first be systematically identified. Epidemiology is a tool that can provide the data to fulfil this task; it can identify the spectrum of needs that exist and assess the efficacy of interventions on a population basis.

The definition of a health-care need in the context of palliative care generally[57,68,69], and in relation to many specific diseases at the end of life, has been addressed in the peer reviewed literature[70,71]. Recently, clinicians and researchers have focused on developing and describing appropriate epidemiological processes that can be used to identify, compare, and contrast the palliative care needs of different people and populations.[57,73]

Barriers to defining population needs and identifying appropriate intervention and management strategies exist. Barriers include the increased focus on curative treatments due to medical advances in the modern era and the increasing information load associated with contemporary medicine. These factors, among others, have been associated with diminished focus on approaches essential for palliative care assessment and management. This is seen also in the comparatively sparce attention paid to palliative, compared to curative measures in the modern medical literature[74]. Some quality epidemiological studies, however, have begun to address the symptom experience of patients at the end of life. This type of data can be used to identify needs that may then be addressed through evidence-based management strategies, inform service planning and provide general hypotheses for research. Importantly, these data are also needed to provide adequate answers to questions that come from individuals in clinical settings such as 'am I likely to have pain that cannot be managed?' Finally, such data help to establish a health-care system's success in addressing symptom-related needs.

Methodological issues and limitations of epidemiological symptom data: what does the data mean for those within the palliative care population?

When reviewing and interpreting symptom-related epidemiological data there are a number of important aspects that must be considered. For a detailed overview readers are referred to the review of symptom assessment methodology that is available in Chapter 7.7. A summary of the key points in symptom assessment, as they relate to the epidemiology of symptoms at the end of life follows.

1. *Defining the population from which data are obtained is of utmost importance.* Care must be exercised when interpreting findings and translating the results of research into clinical practice[75]. For the most part, extrapolation beyond the source population is best avoided. Heterogeneity in patient characteristics such as primary disease, disease stage, and access to care, may render generalizations about the symptom-experience itself or the factors contributing to the nature of the experience inappropriate[75,76]. For example, some studies of patients with far-advanced disease have been conducted in the last year of life, others in the last days of life, and in others, 'time to death' is not presented. Some symptom reports may reflect pooled data from patients at various disease stages, for example, a cancer report may include patients undergoing adjuvant treatment for cancer, and/or those with early- and late-stage metastatic disease. Lastly, a major problem in the symptom-related literature is that 'cancer' without further detail (e.g. lung, colon etc.) has been the unifying 'diagnosis' that has identified the subjects in many symptom-related studies. These studies, therefore, include diverse populations and interpreting data in relation to a particular malignancy can therefore present significant problems.

In the setting of non-malignant disease, it is also common to find wide variability in the reporting of data related to stage of illness. The palliative care literature has evolved largely in the absence of standardized data points. Across local and national borders studies, instruments for data collection, reporting standards approaches (subjective, observer-related etc), and populations vary. Although for each symptom a number of studies can be identified, the heterogenous target populations and a poverty of characteristics defining populations, can mean that it is very difficult to compare studies or pool data in meta-analyses.

2. *The patient experience is personal and subjective:* a patient's lived experience is, by definition, subjective and cannot be wholly known by another, it is the complex interaction of sense perception, cognitive functions, and the unique domain of each individual. Accurate symptom data can nevertheless be recorded and relies on disclosure and faithful recording of subjective information. A common concern regarding data relating to the experience of individuals at the very end of life is that patients may be unable to report on the symptom experience due to the incapacity of illness (due to, e.g. delirium or unconsciousness) in the last days to hours of life. Other concerns that may arise, especially when chart reviews are the source of data, are that a patient may have withheld, or simply not reported, information about his or her symptom experience.

3. *The accuracy of data is dependent on the efficacy of communication* between subject and researcher. The factors mentioned earlier can influence this and, clearly, in studies where the medical record is reviewed for the collection of data, the quality of documentation in the clinical record will influence the validity of the report. There are validated tools to facilitate the collection and recording of symptom data directly from patients and also tools to record proxy symptom ratings[77–79] (see Chapter 7.7). No matter which tool is used within a study, when reviewing the validity of the epidemiological data being reported, the validity of the tool must be determined along with whether a particular tool was chosen with the target population in mind, and whether a report documents a tool's limitations[79,80].

4. *The symptom experience changes over time* and the burden imposed by a particular symptom may change over time[81,82]. The isolated nature of prevalence data does not reflect the dynamic changes of the symptom experience over time. Point prevalence data reports on the symptom status at a specific point in time. Period prevalence reports on symptom status during a period of time in the recent past (e.g. 'right now', 'in the last 2 weeks', or 'in the last year'). Other theories describe the complex changes in symptom experience over time including, for example, 'coping'[83–85], adaptation[86], resilience[32,87], and 'response shift'[82]. Each of these serve to help shape our understanding of the relationship of epidemiological data to symptom experience[82].

5. *The symptom experience is multidimensional, inter-relates with the bio-psychosocial spiritual and cultural domains and may have characteristics linked with particular populations.* Given the limits of prevalence and incidence data in illuminating the symptom experience towards the end of life, investigations that explore symptom burden are important in the provision of robust insights into the epidemiology of the end-of-life experience. An approach to this on an individual level is found in studies that address symptom burden or distress in addition to symptom prevalence and/or incidence[81,88–91].

The overall effects of symptom burden may be characterized using tools designed to capture the multidimensional nature of symptoms and the inter-relationship of different aspects of symptom experience[81,91–93]. Through the use of these types of tools, a symptom may be studied in relation to its phenomenology and its impact as well as in relation to domains of function including a variety of family, social, financial, spiritual, and existential issues.

Finally, it has increasingly been recognized that the study of the *distress* generated by the symptom experience is as important, if not more, than prevalence. Unfortunately, although data in relation to all of these constructs would contribute to a more complete picture of the epidemiology of the end-of-life experience, for many conditions, such epidemiological data are sparse or unavailable.

The characterization of the patient population, together with information about tools used, is very important in allowing for the interpretation of data and for understanding the limits of the generalizability of a study. A good example of key elements of comprehensive characterization is the following:

> *Inpatients and outpatients with prostate, colon, breast or ovarian cancer were evaluated using the Memorial Symptom Assessment Scale and other measures of psychological condition, performance status, symptom distress and overall quality of life. The mean age of the 243 evaluable patients was 55.5 years (range 23–86 years); over 60% were women and almost two-thirds had metastatic disease. The Karnofsky Performance Status (KPS) score was < or = 80 in 49.8% and 123 were inpatients at the time of assessment.*[91]

6. *In considering the overall experience of symptom burden towards the end of life, questions still exist as to which symptoms are the most common and/or most burdensome in the context of particular conditions or within particular health systems, and whether the common symptoms were appropriately assessed in a given study.* Certainly, more studies exist for pain, fatigue, and nausea than for other symptoms, but investigations are often limited by loose or varied use of definitions for the symptoms themselves. Approaches to this problem include using validated tools to capture the full array of symptoms experienced[94]. Meta-analyses have also been used to address the problem of small sample size. However, the heterogeneity of studies included in meta-analyses is also problematic[76].

Collaborative[56], multi-centre studies with attention to inclusion criteria that carefully define the population reported, can go a long way towards improving case recruitment as well as maximizing the homogeneity of data[95]. In addition, electronic data linkage has proven to be a powerful tool in palliative care services research in areas such as estimating patient needs, service utilization, cost, and place of care[53,96,97].

7. *Finally, it is crucial to consider symptom-related epidemiological data in the context of the availability of effective symptom management.* This is especially important for patients and caregivers. For example, a prevalence figure of 70 per cent for severe pain may reflect true point prevalence but may also reflect the under-treatment of a very manageable condition. Such data may reflect a 'moment in time' and not a prolonged experience. Such figures can be alarming for patients and caregivers unless linked with explanations and evidence about the potential for palliative treatments to alleviate distress. Such figures, stated alone, do not serve to clarify that most pain can be treated, nor clarify that, of the 10–20 per cent of patients, who respond poorly to initial pain management, standard multi-disciplinary approaches

are available to improve even refractory pain, suffering, and symptom burden[98].

The aim of this section has been to illustrate the relationship of empirical data and the symptom experience, and the uses, limitations, and challenges inherent in the interpretation of symptom-based epidemiological data. The following sections review symptoms at the end of life in the light of their incidence and prevalence, severity, frequency, associated distress; and in relation to impact on function and global burden for patients as well as caregivers. The important relationship between symptom burden and outcomes related to patient experience (such as distress) will also be expanded[81].

Symptom occurrence by cause of death: what symptoms can be expected over time?

Until recently, symptom prevalence studies in the palliative care setting have focused predominantly on patients with cancer diagnoses. There are now a number of good studies that have explored the prevalence of symptoms in patients with life-threatening and far-advanced chronic lung disease[70,89] and cardiovascular disease[55,61,88,99]. Two recent meta-analyses have also provided excellent overviews of this area of study[55,100].

Although generalizing is problematic, the available evidence suggests there is a core group of symptoms experienced across disease states in the last days, and probably the last year of life. In the last year of life, for example, symptoms reported to have high prevalence in cancer include fatigue (including lack of energy and weakness), pain, depression, anxiety, and loss of appetite[55]. Table 3.2.6 represents the data from a meta-analysis, which included 64 studies across progressive cancer and non-cancer illnesses[55]. One can see from this table that the ranges for symptoms are very variable, largely due to the heterogeneous populations and varying methodologies that have been used in the studies included in meta-analysis[55]. In this table, Solano *et al.* illustrate that a similar spectrum of symptoms has been identified as prevalent in cancer, heart disease (with fatigue, dyspnoea, anxiety, pain, and insomnia, appearing among the top six symptoms), and COPD (with dyspnoea, fatigue, pain, insomnia, and anxiety among the top six symptoms)[55].

Another extensive recent meta-analysis studied symptoms in cancer alone and included 46 studies including reports from 26 223 patients. In this meta-analysis, Teunissen *et al.* analysed separately those studies conducted 'in the last 1–2 weeks of life' and 'other' studies[100]. Table 3.2.7 presents the information from this study that summarizes the presence of symptoms in advanced cancer from studies that *did not* focus solely on the last 1–2 weeks of life. In this investigation, five symptoms (fatigue, pain, lack of energy, weakness, and appetite loss) occurred in more than 50 per cent of the patients in the pooled group of studies that was studied in the period before the last 2 weeks of life[100].

It should be noted that, despite these two meta-analyses, studies that focus on symptoms experience within the context of specific diseases in the palliative care setting remain somewhat scarce, and samples sizes are frequently small. Another frequent limitation is the common absence of the identification of the 'time interval between study and death', performance status, and disease stage. In addition, a major concern relating to these studies is that 'cancer' reflects many diagnoses and more data are needed in relation to specific cancers.

While common symptoms occur across different diseases, the nature of the symptom experience may vary across and among

Table 3.2.6 Symptom prevalence in specific life threatening diseases, summarized from 'grid' in original paper.

Symptom prevalence, summarized from the palliative symptom grid

Symptoms	Cancer	AIDS	HD	COPD	RD
Pain	35–96%[7,8,11,19,33–47]	63–80%[48–50]	41–77%[22,34,51,52]	34–77%[4,22,53]	47–50%[54,55]
	N = 10 379[a]	N = 942	N = 882[a]	N = 372	N = 370
Depression	3–77%[7,11,19,20,33,36,41,43,45,47,56–63]	10–82%[50,61,64,65]	9–36%[52,66]	37–71%[4,53]	5–60%[67–72]
	N = 4378[a]	N = 616[a]	N = 80[a]	N = 150	N = 956[a]
Anxiety	13–79%[19,33,36,41,45,47,58,62,63]	8–34%[12,64,73]	49%[52]	51–75%[74]	39–70%[67,68]
	N = 3274	N = 346[a]	N = 80	N = 1008	N = 72[a]
Confusion	6–93%[7,19,20,34,36,39,42–47,60,75–81]	30–65%[76,82]	18–32%[22,34,52]	18–33%[4,22]	—
	N = 9154[a]	N = ?[a]	N = 343[a]	N = 309	
Fatigue	32–90%[8,24,35,41–43,45,47,63,83]	54–85%[50,84]	69–82%[8,22,52]	68–80%[22,53]	73–87%[71,85]
	N = 2888[a]	N = 1435	N = 409	N = 285	N = 116
Breathlessness	10–70%[7,8,11,19,33–36,39–47,61,86–88]	11–62%[50,88]	60–88%[8,22,34,51,52,61]	90–95%[4,22,53,61]	11–62%[55,89]
	N = 10 029[a]	N = 504	N = 948[a]	N = 372[a]	N = 334
Insomnia	9–69%[7,8,11,19,33,39,41–43,45,47]	74%[50]	36–48%[8,52]	55–65%[4,53]	31–71%[55,85,90]
	N = 5606	N = 504	N = 146	N = 150	N = 351
Nausea	6–68%[8,11,19,33–36,39–47,61,91–93]	43–49%[50,94]	17–48%[8,34,52]	—	30–43%[85,95,96]
	N = 9140[a]	N = 689	N = 146[a]		N = 351
Constipation	23–65%[7,11,19,33–35,39–45,47,50,93]	34–35%[50,94]	38–42%[34,52]	27–44%[4,53]	29–70%[97]
	N = 7602[a]	N = 689	N = 80[a]	N = 150	N = 483
Diarrhoea	3–29%[11,33,39–41,43,44,47,61,92,93,98]	30–90%[50,61,98,99]	12%[52]	—	21%[71]
	N = 3392[a]	N = 504[a]	N = 80		N = 19
Anorexia	30–92%[7,8,11,19,33,35,39–46,92,93,100]	51%[50]	21–41%[8,52]	35–67%[150]	25–64%[89,96]
	N = 9113	N = 504	N = 146	N = 150	N = 395

1. Minimum–maximum range of prevalence (%) is shown.

2. HD = Heart Disease; COPD = Chronic Obstructive Pulmonary Disease; RD = Renal Disease.

3. N refer to the total number of patients involved in the studies found for each symptom in a given disease (e.g. there are 372 patients involved in the three studies on pain prevalence in COPD patients).

4. Superscripted numbers relate to the reference sources [cited in the original paper by Solano] and indicate the number of studies for each symptom in a given disease (e.g. there are three studies on pain prevalence in COPD patients). On two occasions, a single study reported a prevalence range rather than a single point prevalence-anxiety for COPD and constipation for renal failure. '—' was displayed when no data were found for a specific symptom and condition (e.g. confusion for renal failure).

[a] The number of patients is underestimated or unknown because prevalence figures given by textbooks were considered (for which the number of patients was not provided).

Source: reprinted from Solano, J.P., Gomes, B., and Higginson, I.J. (2006). A comparison of symptom prevalence in far advanced cancer, AIDS, heart disease, chronic obstructive pulmonary disease and renal disease. *Journal of Pain and Symptom Management*, **34**(1), 58–69, with permission from Elsevier[55].

disease states. For example, dyspnoea in lung cancer versus dyspnoea in congestive cardiac failure or dyspnoea in chronic lung disease, may have different levels of intensity and burden as well as different time courses. These conditions also may be accompanied by differing co-morbidities. All of these variables clearly may result in differing lived experiences in relation to specific symptoms. For example, data comparing dyspnoea in chronic lung disease with dyspnoea in lung cancer suggests that, although the number of symptoms experienced in the last year and week of life are similar in the two groups the duration of dyspnoea was longer in patients with chronic lung disease[71]. Studies such as these help to define symptom experience over time and illustrate the comparative symptom burden in patients with cancer and non-cancer diagnoses.

For all disease states, significant population-based studies of symptoms with excellent methodology can provide examples of the potential for epidemiology to inform service planning and clinical management[53,101–103]. Also, studies that use population databases that may be linked state- or region-wide may help to provide an accurate denominator for prevalence studies and for characterizing population-based needs.

Physical symptoms during the last year of life 'what will it be like?'

Fatigue, pain, lack of energy, weakness, and appetite loss are all highly prevalent in cancer patients in the last year of life[100]. In the non-cancer settings of chronic lung disease, heart failure, and AIDS, pain, breathlessness, and fatigue are also pre-eminent[55]. All of these symptoms may result in burden for patients and carers and imply demands on clinical skills and service provision. Distress and functional limitations are important to recognize. Constipation, nausea, vomiting, lack of appetite, and confusion are also frequently reported. These symptoms, while distressing, are eminently treatable. Many chapters in this textbook are dedicated to symptoms and

Table 3.2.7 Summary of symptom prevalence in cancer **prior** to the last 1–2 weeks of life[*].

Symptom prevalence in group 1

	Number of studies	Number of patients	Pooled prevalence (%)	95% CI (%)
N	40	25074		
Fatigue	17	6727	74	(63; 83)
Pain	37	21917	71	(67; 74)
Lack of energy	6	1827	69	(57; 79)
Weakness	18	14910	60	(51; 68)
Appetite loss	37	23112	53	(48; 59)
Nervousness	5	727	48	(39; 57)
Weight loss	17	13167	46	(34; 59)
Dry mouth	20	6359	40	(29; 52)
Depressed mood	19	8678	39	(33; 45)
Constipation	34	22437	37	(33; 40)
Worrying	6	1378	36	(21; 55)
Insomnia	28	18597	36	(30; 43)
Dyspnoea	40	24490	35	(30; 39)
Nausea	39	24263	31	(27; 35)
Anxiety	12	7270	30	(17; 46)
Irritability	6	1009	30	(22; 40)
Bloating	5	626	29	(20; 40)
Cough	24	11939	28	(23; 35)
Cognitive symptoms	9	1696	28	(20; 38)
Early satiety	5	1639	23	(8; 52)
Taste changes	11	3045	22	(15; 31)
Sore mouth/stomatitis	8	2172	20	(8; 39)
Vomiting	24	9598	20	(17; 22)
Drowsiness	16	11634	20	(12; 32)
Oedema	13	3486	19	(15; 24)
Urinary symptoms	15	12011	18	(15; 21)
Dizziness	12	3322	17	(11; 25)
Dysphagia	25	16161	17	(14; 20)
Confusion	17	11728	16	(12; 21)
Bleeding	5	8883	15	(11; 20)
Neurological symptoms	11	10004	15	(10; 23)
Hoarseness	5	1410	14	(7; 26)
Dyspepsia	7	3028	12	(9; 15)
Skin symptoms	7	9177	11	(6; 20)
Diarrhoea	22	16592	11	(7; 16)
Pruritus	14	6676	10	(7; 15)
Hiccup	7	3991	7	(3; 15)

[*]Referred to as; 'Group1' in original study.

Source: reprinted from Teunissen, S.C., Wesker, W., Kruitwagen, C. *et al.* (2007). Symptom prevalence in patients with incurable cancer: a systematic review. *Journal of Pain and Symptom Management*, **34**(1), 94–104, with permission from Elsevier.

review in more detail, some of the prevalence data in relation to specific symptoms. We have selected several common symptoms in the following paragraphs to highlight some issues regarding prevalence and methodology.

Pain

Bonica's landmark review that indicated a pain prevalence of 71 per cent for patients with advanced and far-advanced cancer is widely quoted[104,105]. This seminal work paved the way for future studies. A comprehensive systematic review by Higginson and Hearn 2003 reported that an overall prevalence of pain in advanced disease could not be derived due to heterogeneity of methodologies amongst studies in the review[76]. A meaningful summary was nevertheless provided as a 'combined weighted mean prevalence of pain' of 74 per cent (range 53–100 per cent) in metastatic and far advanced disease[76]. A 2007 meta-analysis reported a pooled prevalence of 64 per cent (CI 58–69 per cent) in advanced and far-advanced cancer and more than one-third of subjects reported their pain as moderate or severe[106]. Pain in non-cancer settings is also common. In the Solano meta-analysis (Table 3.2.6), for example the prevalence of pain in chronic obstructive pulmonary disease was 34–77 per cent ($n = 372$) and in heart failure it was 41–77 per cent ($n = 882$)[55]. When dimensions other than prevalence are explored, pain is not only among the most common symptoms in terms of incidence, but it ranks highly with regard to distress[81,91,107,108].

As alluded to above, studies rarely describe the use of palliative interventions and although pain is prevalent, distressing and, at times, under-treated, studies in cancer patients have reported good or satisfactory pain management when standard analgesic approaches, such as the WHO Pain Management guidelines, or standard palliative care assessment and management are followed[109,110] (see Chapter 10.1).

Fatigue

Fatigue is frequently listed among the most prevalent symptoms in a number of advanced illnesses (Table 3.2.6). In the Solano meta-analysis fatigue was reported to have a prevalence of 32–90 per cent in cancer patients ($n = 2888$), 69–82 per cent ($n = 409$) in those with heart disease, and 68–80 per cent ($n = 285$) in COPD[55]. Studies limited to patients with lung cancer identify fatigue among the top 3 symptoms in terms of prevalence, intensity, and symptom distress[111]. In other studies, data on fatigue are made conspicuous by their absence. This may result from the intentional or unintentional omission of a particular symptom from a symptom list or tool and highlights the need for the use of tools that have been validated in a population that is representative of the population being studied (see Chapter 7.7).

Breathlessness

Breathlessness is highly prevalent in chronic lung disease. In a meta-analysis by Solano *et al.*, a prevalence of 90–95 per cent ($n = 372$) was reported[55] (Table 3.2.6). A similar prevalence of 98 per cent is reported in a data linkage study of 209 proxy informants out of a total of 399 deaths from COPD in four London health authorities[70]. For cancer patients, the prevalence of dyspnoea in the Solano study was 10–70 per cent among 10029 patients, an extraordinarily wide range reflecting the heterogeneity of study populations with cancer as well as varying methodological approaches to collecting this data. The pooled prevalence for dyspnoea was 35 per cent in the meta-analysis conducted by Teunissen *et al.*[100] (Table 3.2.7).

Breathlessness is also prevalent in patients with heart failure, although often it occurs later in the trajectory of heart failure and lung cancer when compared with its onset in chronic lung disease. A well-designed longitudinal cohort study compared a group of patients with heart failure to a group of patients with chronic lung disease and revealed that both groups experienced common symptoms[89]. Patients with chronic lung disease reported breathlessness at base line and at final interview, whereas fatigue and depression increased over time—indicating a relatively long duration of severe (potentially burdensome) dyspnoea in chronic lung disease. In the heart failure group, severe dyspnoea was more prevalent in the final interview than in the initial interview, but as was the case with chronic lung disease, physical discomfort, fatigue, and depression increased over time. As is the case with pain, little data is provided in these studies about palliative interventions.

Psychological symptoms and neuropsychiatric disorders during the last year of life

Psychological symptoms, neuropsychiatric disorders, and psychosocial distress have been investigated in the setting of life-threatening cancers and in some life-threatening non-cancer diagnoses[88,99,112–114]. The evidence suggests that neuro-psychiatric symptoms and syndromes are particularly common (occurring in up to one in two patients)[115], and that under-recognition, misdiagnosis, and under-treatment persist[116,117] (see Chapter 15.5). For instance, Fallowfield and co-investigators assessed the ability of 143 doctors to establish the psychological status of 2297 oncology outpatient consultations in 34 centres in the United Kingdom. Doctor assessments had a sensitivity of 28.87 per cent for identifying distress indicative of psychiatric morbidity. The misclassification rate was 34.7 per cent. The investigators found that the data indicated a predominant tendency for doctors to assess patients as not distressed[117]. This leads to a conclusion that epidemiologic studies which assess the prevalence of, and distress linked with, psychological symptoms or neuropsychiatric conditions must be prospective and use validated assessment methods if they are to accurately quantify the problem.

Of note, there are two general approaches to characterizing a psychosocial concern—either as a neuropsychiatric disorder—or as a psychological symptom[118]. Some studies do not include formal mental state or psychiatric assessment (of a syndrome) and instead record the patient or proxy's report of a symptom. Both 'symptoms' and 'diagnoses' are important epidemiologically. From an epidemiological point of view it is important to note that they are different entities. Epidemiological data in this realm can be difficult to interpret and compare, for instance if thresholds for what constitutes a case are not clearly defined, or if 'symptoms' and 'syndromes' are used interchangeably. For example, depressed mood is a symptom i.e. one identified by a patient report 'I feel depressed'—or may be one, among a number of criteria that leads to a diagnosis of a major depressive disorder.[119,120]

The presence of neuropsychiatric syndromes and psychiatric disorders is significant across the course of cancer illness from prediagnosis (familial cancers, worried well, etc.) through diagnosis, treatment, survivorship, or relapse, advanced, far advanced disease and bereavement. Problems in this domain are common especially in advanced cancer. In the setting of far advanced cancer depression,[121] anxiety,[122] delirium,[123] sleep disorders,[124]

post-traumatic stress disorder (PTSD),[118] demoralization syndrome,[125] and suicidal ideation have all been identified as prevalent and distressing neuropsychiatric syndromes. Many, if not all, of these have also been described in advanced life-threatening non-cancer diagnoses.[55,126–128] Although treatment strategies exist for all of these syndromes, research suggests that psychological, neuropsychiatric and spiritual/existential concerns and symptoms may be more prevalent and/or more burdensome than physical symptoms in both cancer and non-cancer settings,[129] (see also Chapter 15.5).

Again, importantly when prevalence figures are cited in studies it is rare to find data about what palliative interventions may have been used for these problems. The prevalence figures therefore could be alarming to patients and carers. As discussed in relation to the physical symptoms above, other chapters in this textbook are dedicated to these conditions and addresses their prevalence and treatment strategies. We have selected two common psychological symptoms to discuss some prevalence and methodological matters.

Delirium

Delirium is highly prevalent in advanced illness.[131] Its prevalence is reported to be 12–18 per cent in cancer patients in general,[132,133] and 28–48 per cent in populations with advanced cancer.[134] Delirium prevalence has been reported to be even higher in the last weeks of life with prevalence reports of 25–85 per cent.[135] Delirium also carries with it the phenomenon of distressed recall.[136] Although the prognosis of delirium worsens with repeated occurrence delirium is often reversible. A prospective series of consecutive admissions to a palliative care ward in a tertiary referral hospital for example, reported 49 per cent reversibility.[135] The incidence of delirium increases with medical morbidity and co-morbidity and a multivariate analysis identified risk factors for development of delirium in 145 cancer patients admissions including: advanced age, cognitive impairment, low albumin level, bone metastases, and the presence of haematological malignancy.[137]

Delirium is also prevalent in non-cancer progressive illnesses. Solano reports a prevalence of confusion of up to one-third of patients with progressive cardiac failure and COPD patients and up to two-thirds of patients with AIDS (Table 3.2.6)[55].

The study of delirium has proved difficult in clinical and research settings[138]. To assess this syndrome, staff or carer observations must be relied upon, repeat cognitive testing may be perceived as burdensome to patients and carers,[139] and, importantly, the gaining of informed consent for studies in confused patients has posed practical and ethical difficulties. As a result of these difficulties, especially the difficulties with proxy reports and consents, some investigators have excluded patients with cognitive impairment from studies of symptoms present at the end of life. [79, 100] Importantly, this issue of methodological bias must be considered when interpreting epidemiological reports relating to this problem.

Anxiety

Anxiety is commonly reported by patients with cancer and non-cancer diagnoses. Importantly, it has been identified as a major cause of psychological morbidity in COPD, and although important wherever it causes symptom distress, it is thought to be more prevalent among elderly patients with COPD than in populations of elderly patients with cancer or heart failure.[112] Anxiety has a multifactorial aetiology, and confounding factors exist; for example patient characteristics predisposing smoking are possibly independently associated with anxiety in COPD.[113]

As an example of the spectrum of concerns that can be associated with anxiety, a review article by Hill *et al.* reported prevalence ranges of anxiety-related symptoms and disorders in far advanced COPD as being 2–96 per cent for reports of feeling anxious, 10–33 per cent for diagnosis of generalized anxiety disorder, and 8–67 per cent for diagnosis of panic attack and panic disorder.[113]

In the meta-analysis by Solano *et al*, presented in Table 3.2.6, the prevalence of anxiety was 51–75 per cent based on the sample of

Table 3.2.8 Summary of symptom prevalence in the **last** 1–2 weeks of life[**].

Symptom prevalence in group 2: patients in the last 1–2 weeks of life				
	Number of studies	Number of patients	Pooled prevalence (%)	95% CI (%)	p*
N	6	2219			
Fatigue	2	120	88	(12; 100)	0.506
Weight loss	2	1149	86	(77; 92)	0.023
Weakness	3	477	74	(50; 89)	0.262
Appetite loss	3	2008	56	(15; 92)	0.460
Pain	3	1626	43	(32; 39)	0.004
Dyspnoea	6	2219	39	(20; 62)	0.695
Drowsiness	3	894	38	(14; 70)	0.303
Dry mouth	4	1010	34	(10; 70)	0.794
Neurological symptoms	1	176	32	(26; 40)	0.500
Anxiety	2	256	30	(11; 62)	0.923
Constipation	6	2219	29	(16; 48)	0.747
Confusion	4	1070	24	(6; 62)	0.410
Depressed mood	3	850	19	(9; 36)	0.104
Nausea	6	2219	17	(8; 31)	0.047
Skin symptoms	1	593	16	(14; 20)	0.750
Dysphagia	4	1070	16	(6; 37)	0.825
Insomnia	4	889	14	(3; 44)	0.094
Cough	4	829	14	(3; 43)	0.291
Vomiting	3	799	13	(9; 18)	0.313
Bleeding	1	176	12	(8; 18)	0.667
Oedema	1	90	8	(4; 16)	0.286
Dizziness	2	653	7	(5; 9)	0.264
Irritability	1	90	7	(3; 14)	0.671
Diarrhoea	5	2129	6	(2; 19)	0.258
Urinary symptoms	3	850	6	(5; 8)	0.017
Dyspepsia	2	804	2	(1; 4)	0.111

*Comparison of median percentages, Group 2 versus Group 1, Mann-Whitney test.
** Referred to as 'Group 2' in original study.

Source: reproduced from Teunissen, S.C., Wesker, W., Kruitwagen, C. *et al.* (2007). Symptom prevalence in patients with incurable cancer: a systematic review. *Journal of Pain and Symptom Management*, **34**(1), 94–104 with permission from Elsevier.

1008 hospitalized COPD patients and 49 per cent in the sample of advanced stage heart failure patients (n=80)[55]. In the meta-analysis of cancer-related symptoms, Tuenissen *et al.* reported that 'worry' had a prevalence of 35 per cent and anxiety of 30 per cent (Table 3.2.7)[100]. As discussed earlier, the distinction between a 'symptom' and a 'psychiatric diagnosis' is also important in anxiety. For example, in an analysis of data from a United Kingdom (Tafford) database, an anxiety disorder was present in 7 per cent of patients when DSM-IIIR criteria were used,[140] and Grabsch *et al.* reported that 6 per cent of patients with advanced breast cancer had an anxiety disorder according to a structured liaison psychiatry in interview. This is in marked contrast to the high prevalence of 'worry' identified by Portenoy *et al.* in 81 per cent of the 60 patients with colorectal cancer, 56 per cent of patients with prostate cancer, and 75 per cent of patients with breast cancer.[91]

Finally, it should be noted that in cancer and non-cancer settings anxiety and breathlessness often co-exist. In addition, anxiety scores relying on somatic symptoms (e.g. shortness of breath) may result in false positives for anxiety.[112] These data also serve to highlight some complex aspects of study methodology and reporting that must be considered when interpreting symptom reports in epidemiological studies.

Distress in the setting of advanced illness

Distress, as described in relation to the 'bothersomeness' associated with a specific symptom or experience has been discussed earlier. Another global concept of distress exists and has been defined as:

> *'a multi-factorial, unpleasant emotional experience of a psychological (cognitive, behavioural, emotional), social, and/or spiritual nature that may interfere with the ability to cope effectively with cancer, its physical symptoms and its treatment. Distress extends along a continuum, ranging from common, normal feelings of vulnerability, sadness, and fears to problems that can become disabling, such as depression, anxiety, panic, social isolation, and existential and spiritual crisis'*[141].

Attempts to measure this construct have been undertaken by some investigators, and the 'routine' use of the 'distress thermometer' and an associated checklist to detect distress in cancer patients in the clinical setting has also been encouraged, particularly by the National Comprehensive Cancer Network in the United States[141,142]. Over time it will be most interesting to see whether epidemiological data about the distress thermometer or checklist further illuminate the advanced cancer experience, particularly in relation to the items on the checklist. At this time it appears that the thermometer scores themselves correlate with psychological distress[142]. Of note, data related to the distress checklist may be useful for identifying common concerns and needs, rather than for identifying specific diagnoses.

Symptom occurrence in the last days of life: what symptoms can be expected in the very last days of life?

Much has been written in the recent decade about the mandate for impeccable care for all dying patients at the end of life. Recently, health-funding bodies, locally and nationally, have invested in comprehensive programmes to assist generalist and specialist clinicians in caring for patients in the last days of life, regardless of setting or diagnosis[58,143,144] (see Section 19). The problems relating to epidemiologic reports about the last days of life have both similarities and differences to those discussed earlier in relation to reports about advanced, progressive disease. Fatigue/weakness/lack of energy are high on the prevalence list for symptoms in the last days of life with dyspnoea and pain also highly prevalent[100].

Table 3.2.8 provides pooled prevalence data reviewed in a comprehensive meta-analysis of cancer-related symptoms in the last 1–2 weeks of life[100]. Symptoms during the last days or weeks of life have also been captured by other studies. Data for this time, especially the very final days of life, are however limited, and in addition, in these settings, proxy reports become more common in the methodology of studies.

A major study—The SUPPORT study from the United States—reported that in interviews conducted after a patient died, surrogates indicated that 50 per cent of all conscious patients who died in the hospital experienced moderate or severe pain during their last 3 days of life[51]. Others have reported similar high-prevalence figures for the presence of transient proxy-reported pain and shortness of breath [145]. These data exist in the context of other studies which report that the dying process is most commonly peaceful although with the possibility, indeed likelihood, of the presence of some transient, treatable distress. That stated, these studies and others highlight the importance of investigation at this time of life by addressing and defining distress with specific individual and system based assessments.

Reports from hospice programmes and pain studies suggest that most deaths can be peaceful[146–148]. For example, the late Dame Cicely Saunders recorded data regarding 100 consecutive deaths at St Christopher's Hospice in the United Kingdom and described 98 out of the 100 patients as dying peacefully. In this population, 60 patients were reported as peaceful for the whole of the last 24 hours and transient distress was experienced by the rest of this group. Unfortunately, the details of the duration of transient distress are unclear from the report[146].

More work is needed on this subject but of note, one of the first studies in this area was a study that utilized nurse reports of patient comfort and was conducted by Osler[149,150]. This survey included 486 deaths occurring between 1900 and 1904 and was not confined to cancer patients. Most patients were described as dying comfortably with 'no sign of death one way or another, … like their birth, death was a sleep and a forgetting'. That stated, transient distress was reported in approximately one-fifth of patients with 'bodily pain or distress' reported in 90 patients, 'mental apprehension' in 11, 'positive terror' in two and 'bitter remorse' in one. Unfortunately, not unlike present-day studies, the study did not describe the palliative interventions used to treat this distress, the impact of those interventions, or the duration of distress.

Further illuminating the experience of patients in the last hours of life are studies that relate to the management of symptom distress and the indications for sedation at the end of life. Several studies have addressed the rate of sedation in the last days of life. Barriers to interpretation of these data exist because of different impressions of what constitutes 'sedation' versus the use of medications with some sedative effects for the management of a symptom. Ventafridda and Kohara report palliative sedation was required for 52.5 per cent and 50.3 per cent of patients in Italy and Japan, respectively[151,152]. Elsayem and Fassinger report rates

of 15 per cent and 18 per cent from M.D. Anderson in the United States and Edmonton in Canada, respectively[153,154]. Notably, the M.D. Anderson study reports 41 per cent of dying patients received 'sedation'[153]. The variability of rates of sedation may be related to sample bias or different definitions of what constitutes 'sedation'. Fainsinger[154], reported 'physician intention to sedate' and the Kohara[152] study included 'mean sedative dose', both of which can help to characterize the clinical situation. This important area requires more investigation.

Finally, with regard to the last days of life, some symptoms (such as dyspnoea, anorexia, difficulty in swallowing) have been noted to be associated with a poor prognosis[155]. Readers are referred elsewhere in this text for a discussion of the relevance of symptoms and functional status to prognosis (see Chapter 3.3).

Communication, consciousness, and mental acuity have been rated as highly important by cancer patients at the end of life[156]. Level of consciousness has been reported in few studies; however, the National Mortality Followback Study, a large epidemiological study in the United States, addressed many aspects of health care including the end-of-life experience and presented reports of consciousness at the end of life [157]. In the 1986 investigation, the next of kin of 18 733 deceased patients were surveyed with an impressive 87.3 per cent response. Proxies reported on the deceased persons' 'trouble understanding where he or she was during the last year of life'. Over the last year of life, the proxy reports indicated that 15 per cent of decedents had this difficulty for the 'last few hours or days', 13 per cent for 'some of the time', and 8 per cent for 'all or most of the time'. The data that pertain to cancer suggest that, in the very last days and hours of life, most people are able to communicate until close to the end of life. A survey of 100 cancer patients who died at St. Christopher's Hospice in the United Kingdom described 10 per cent as alert, 67 per cent as drowsy or semiconscious, and 23 per cent as unarousable or unconscious during the 24 hours before death[179].

The prevalence of delirium also can be viewed as a marker for consciousness being 'at risk' towards the end of life. Delirium is characterized in part by a disturbed level of consciousness and the prevalence, up to 85 per cent in the end-of-life setting, has been discussed above. Other observations that may be relevant to this aspect of the experience include reports of 'confusion' which, in the Teunisen meta-analysis, was found to have a prevalence of 24 per cent in the last 1–2 weeks of life[100]. In the same sample, 'drowsiness', was reported in 38 per cent (see Table 3.2.8)[100]. Conill reports a prevalence of confusion of 68 per cent among 176 patients in the last week of life[158]. Delirium is also reported to accompany the last hours of life for patients with non-cancer-related illnesses, but data on the non-cancer illness experience in the very last hours or days of life are patchy.

Cultural experiences and the existential context

Death is highly laden with emotional, social, and cultural significance. There are two aphorism in the English vernacular that serve to illustrate one cultural perspective on this subject 'Only two things are certain in life: death and taxes'[159] and 'there are only two themes in literature sex and death'. A diverse spectrum of beliefs about the spiritual/existential and cultural aspects of death and the period prior to, and after, it exist. Despite the fact that much is published in popular media and the fact that many hold

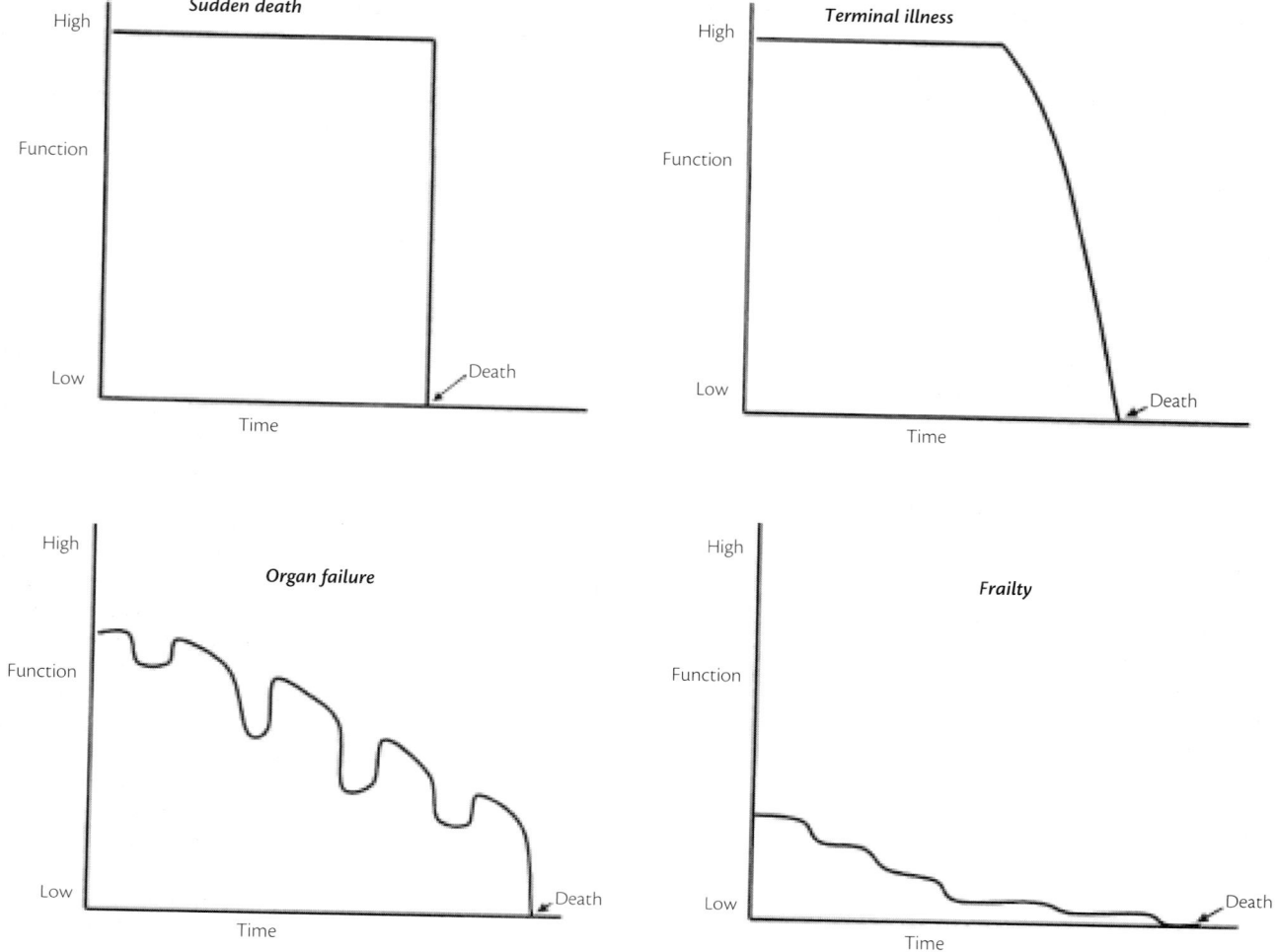

Figure 3.2.5 Functional trajectories at the end of life.
Source: reproduced from Lunney, J.R., Lynn, J., Hogan, C. (2002). Profiles of Older Medicare Decedents. *Journal of the American Geriatric Society*, **50**(6), 1108–12, with permission from Wiley-Blackwell Publishing.

strong beliefs relating to this time of life, and the time before and after death, there exists extremely little in terms of epidemiological data concerning the 'metaphysical' domains of experience at the end of life. As is the case within western philosophical debate generally, public debate frequently focuses on whether experiences (for example 'the near death experience')can be accounted for by metaphysical explanations alone, whether there are metaphysical explanations for phenomena, and the relationship between brain, mind, and consciousness. Occasionally scientific reports about 'metaphysical' aspects of experience at the end of life are published in the peer reviewed literature. When this happens they are frequently reported by the popular media. The near death experience is an example of the fascination which surrounds limited empirical information[160, 161].

Cultural factors are also important in relation to symptom experience, distress, and communication at the end of life (see Chapter 3.7). More well-designed epidemiological studies looking at culture as a variable in symptom experience are needed.

Trajectories of functional decline towards the end of life: 'what can I expect over time?'

Functional decline in the months before death is described in several studies, including one by Glaser and Strauss in 1968 that described the trajectories of dying[163]. More recently, Lunney *et al.* have described the general pattern of functional decline as following four possible trajectories, depending on the type of disease—the cancer trajectory, the chronic organ failure trajectory, the dementia/frailty trajectory, and the sudden or unexpected death trajectory (Fig. 3.2.5)[164].

Illness trajectories are concepts that map functional ability in activities of daily living (ADLs), these include walking, bathing, grooming, dressing, eating, transfer from bed to chair, using toilet, etc.[164]. While these trajectories are empirically based, they do not provide a description that can be applied to individuals by diagnosis[164,165]. Rather, they are models, which have proven useful in describing patterns of patient need and patient experience towards the end of life. In addition, while general trends exist, some patients living with cancer may have an illness experience more similar to the chronic organ failure trajectory than to the 'classic' cancer trajectory, while others may deteriorate more precipitously.

Lunney *et al.* undertook a United States-based study that interviewed 4190 patients and caregivers before death in the Established Populations for Epidemiologic Studies of the Elderly (EPESE)[164]. In this study, mean function declined across all cohorts. Cancer decedents were most frequently well functioning early in their final year but were less functionally able in the 3 months prior to death. Patients with organ failure experienced a fluctuating pattern of functional decline over the year before death with substantially poorer functioning during the last 3 months before death. Frail decedents were relatively more functionally disabled throughout their final year. In a study of 1271 cancer deaths in Italy, caregiver reports about patient function before death were collected at a mean of 234 days after bereavement. In this study, the probability of patients being described as 'free from a functional disability, was 94 per cent one year before death and this remained stable until 18 weeks before death. At 12 weeks this probability then fell to 63 per cent and again to 49 per cent at 6 weeks. The pattern of decline for these cancer patients, which may have been expected to differ significantly among cancer types, was somewhat consistent across sub-groups, except for patients with central nervous system tumours, who differed from those with other cancers in that they tended to experience a longer, slower decline in function towards death[165].

On a national, regional, or institutional level it is important for health-care planning to accommodate needs implicit in functional trajectories. For instance, there are specific biological, financial, practical, and emotional implications for patients with differing functional trajectories. In considering the implications of symptoms and disability from illness, The National Mortality Followback Survey undertaken in the United States in 1993 provided some insights into the functional and practical impact of illness at the end of life[102]. For this 1993 survey a sample of 22 957 death certificates were assessed and linked with survey data provided by proxy respondents; frequently next of kin. There was an 83 per cent response rate and this allowed for the assessment of data on over 18 000 deaths.[102]. With regard to functional impairment during the last year of life, the survey reported 37 per cent of decedents had some trouble with preparing meals, 54 per cent with walking, and 34 per cent with eating. Unfortunately, there was no information reported on the 'trajectory' of these needs over the final year; rather the survey report documented the existence of a need for assistance at some time during the year. Addington-Hall reviewed data from 2074 cancer deaths in the United Kingdom and reported that relatives were the primary caregivers in 81 per cent but district nurse assistance was needed for at least 60 per cent, home help in 20 per cent, and 'meals on wheels' in 9 per cent[177]. Further information about the trajectories of these needs would be helpful for service planning.

On an individual level, epidemiological information about performance status and function can assist in facilitating discussion about an individual's projected symptom experience and can help in answering such questions as: 'Is it likely I will have months lying in bed unable to speak or get up?', 'Is it likely I will need someone to look after me?', or 'Is it likely I will be able to stay at home?' As an example, it may appear almost redundant to many clinicians, to state the general differences between the functional decline and care needs of a patient with Alzheimer's disease and the needs of a patient with acute myeloid leukaemia. For patients and carers this is often not obvious, and individuals may benefit from information about functional trajectories rather than being left to draw their own conclusions based on what they have observed in others, in the literature and/or the media.

Caregiver concerns

A single death affects many others in terms of informal caregiving and grief. The epidemiology of the caregiver experience towards the end of life is therefore an important aspect of the epidemiology of the end–of-life experience. We will briefly summarize some aspects of this area in the following paragraphs, and readers are referred for more detail to Chapters 6.1 and 15.3.

A major study from the United States using data drawn from the 1999 National Long Term Care Study (NLTCS) revealed that of the adult deaths among participants in that study, 72 per cent of decedents had received help from an informal caregiver during the last year of life[178]. Moreover, the survey of 1149 caregivers, aged 65 years and older (The Informal Caregivers Survey—with participants identified from among the participants in the NLTCS study), reported that on average caregivers provided 43 hours per week of 'end-of-life care' to disabled community-dwelling adults and that 84 per cent provided that care on a daily basis[178]. The SUPPORT study, which targeted hospitalized patients found that 'considerable assistance' was given by a family member for 34 per cent of patients[166].

While many caregivers willingly provide care, and indeed find care rewarding and an important part of a family experience, research has tended to focus on the significant demands and burdens that arise from caring for patients with life-threatening illnesses and such research has been conducted across diagnoses and in various countries. Caregiving has been shown to affect both the physical and psychological health[167,168] and the social and financial[169] situation of caregivers.

With regard to the impact of caring on caregiver health, higher rates of mortality have been identified among spousal caregivers when their mortality is compared with mortality figures from population data[170]. Of note, it has been suggested that enrolment in a palliative care/hospice programme may be protective of caregiver morbidity and mortality[167]. In addition to the impact on physical health there is an impact of caregiving on psychological well-being. For example, a large United States study reported 34 per cent of caregivers of patients with high care needs had depressive symptoms[171]. In addition to depression, other forms of psychological morbidity are common and, for example, caregivers have been shown to be at increased risk of anxiety and other mental health disorders[168,172].

From a societal and epidemiological perspective, the financial and social impact of caregiving is also significant. As an example, in the SUPPORT study, in which care in the United States was investigated, it was reported that 31 per cent of families caring for patients near the end of life lost most or all family savings and, in 20 per cent of cases, the caregiver had to resign from work or make another major life change to continue to provide care[166].

Informal carers and their households are certainly at risk of suffering loss of income, and indeed epidemiological data has demonstrated the significant impact that caregiving has on workforce participation[169,173].

Certainly, awareness exists among palliative care researchers about the importance of the analysis of the impact of caregiver-interventions on carer burden beyond financial and health concerns. Studies have identified that carers regard information, emotional support, practical care, and patient comfort as most important, while information about ways to manage fatigue and depression is also important[174,175].

The epidemiological data reporting needs and experiences of caregivers from high-income countries contrasts with the paucity of data relating to this from low-income countries. While less research has been done in the latter areas, an interesting study by Murray *et al.* described the experiences and needs of two groups of patients and carers with advanced cancer—one group in Scotland and the other in Kenya[176] The authors of this study reported that 'the emotional pain of facing death was the prime concern of Scottish patients and their carers, while physical pain and financial worries dominated the lives of Kenyan patients and their carers'. In Scotland, where many services were available these were described as 'sometimes underused', and in Kenya, pain relief and essential equipment, food, and assistance were reported as 'often inaccessible and unaffordable'. While more data are needed to illuminate the epidemiology of the caregiver experience worldwide, the overlapping needs of caregivers, as well as the contrasting needs, reported in this study provide some insight into the spectrum of needs and the disparities that exist worldwide for caregivers.

Conclusion

The study of the epidemiology of the end-of-life experience is an evolving and important field with an increasing number of studies being published that shed light on the experience of individuals, who are nearing the end of life, and their caregivers. The use of validated tools, carefully designed studies, and data-linkage will, it is hoped, shed more light on this important area over time. It will be important for this area to be a subject of focused study throughout the world if health policy is to truly reflect the needs of the spectrum of individuals who are near to the end of life.

Acknowledgements

The research for this chapter was undertaken, in part, thanks to funding from the Cancer Institute NSW Palliative Care Academic Leaders Program.

References

1. Hennekens, C.H. Buring.J. (1987). *Epidemiology in Medicine.* Boston: Little, Brown and Company.
2. Sepúlveda, C., Marlin, A., Yoshida, T. *et al.* (2002). Palliative Care: the World Health Organization's global perspective. *Journal of Pain and Symptom Management,* **24**(2), 91–6.
3. McNamara, B., Rosenwax, L.K., and Holman, C.D. (2006). A method for defining and estimating the palliative care population. *Journal of Pain and Symptom Management,* **32**(1), 5–12.
4. Lopez, A.D., Mathers, C.D., Ezzati, M. *et al.* (2006). Global and regional burden of disease and risk factors, 2001: systematic analysis of population health data. *Lancet,* **367**(9524), 1747–57.
5. Maudsley, G., Williams, E.M. (1996). "Inaccuracy' in death certification–where are we now? *Journal of Public Health Medicine,* **18**(1), 59–66.
6. Rao, C., Lopez, A.D., Yang, G. *et al.* (2005). Evaluating national cause-of-death statistics: principles and application to the case of China. *Bulletin of the World Health Organization,* **83**(8), 618–25.
7. Mathers, C.D., Lopez, A.D, and Murray, C.J.L. (2006). The Burden of Disease and Mortality by Condition: Data, Methods, and Results for 2001 In: *Global Burden of Disease and Risk Factors,* (eds. Lopez, A.M.C., Ezzati, M., Jamison, D., Murray, C.) pp. 46–93. New York: Oxford University Press.
8. Mathers, C.D., Salomon, J.A., Ezzati, M., Begg, S. *et al.* (2006). Sensitivity and uncertainty analyses for burden of disease and risk factor estimates In: *Global Burden of disease and risk factors,* (eds. Lopez, A. M.C., Ezzati, M., Murray, C., Jamison, D.) pp. 399–426. New York: Oxford University Press.
9. Murray, C., Lopez, A., and Wibulpolprasert, S. (2004). Monitoring global health: Time for new solutions. *British Medical Journal,* **329**, 1096–100.
10. Ormerod, L.P. (2005). Multidrug-resistant tuberculosis (MDR-TB): epidemiology, prevention and treatment. *British Medical Bulletin,* **73–74**(1) 2005, 17–24.
11. The World Bank (2009). World Bank Atlas: Income Per Person available at http://go.worldbank.org/7EIAD6CKO0. (accessed 9 June, 2009).
12. Institut National d'Etudes Demographique. (2008).World life expectancy Teaching Kit. http://www.ined.fr/en/teaching_kits/length_of_life_death_mortality/world_life_expectancy/ (accessed 9 June, 2009).
13. United Nations. (2007). World Population Prospects: The 2006 Revision, Highlights, Working Paper No. ESA/P/WP.202.: Department of Economic and Social Affairs, Population Division.
14. World Health Organization. (2007). The 10 leading causes of death by broad income group for 2002. Fact sheet No 310. http://www.who.int/mediacentre/factsheets/fs310.pdf. (Accessed 5 June, 2009).
15. Australian Bureau of Statistics 2009, *Experimental Life Tables for Aboriginal and Torres Strait Islander Australians, 2005–2007* (cat.no. 3302.0.55.003). Available at:http://www.abs.gov.au/AUSSTATS/abs@.nsf/Lookup/3302.0.55.003Main+Features12005%E2%80%932007?OpenDocument (accessed 24 July 2009).
16. Hornton, R. (2006). Indigenous peoples: time to act now for equity and health.(Comment)(outcome of UN Permanent Forum on Indigenous Issues). *Lancet,* **367**(9524), 1705.
17. Stevenson, M.R. W.L., Harrison, J., Moller, J. *et al.* (1998). At risk in two worlds: injury mortality among indigenous people in the US and Australia, 1990-92. *Australian and New Zealand Public Health,* **22**(6), 641–4.
18. World Health Organization. (2006). World Health Report 2006: working together for health. *World Health Report*: World Health Organization. pp. 168–76.
19. Lawn, J., Zupan, J., Begkoyian, G., Knippenberg, R. (2006). New born survival. In: *Disease Control Priorities in Developing Countries,* (eds. Jamison, D., Brenan, J., Measham, A., *et al.*) New York: The World Bank and Oxford University Press. pp. S31–49.
20. Strong, K., Mathers, C., Epping-Jordan, J. *et al.* (2008). Preventing cancer through tobacco and infection control: how many lives can we save in the next 10 years? *European Journal of Cancer Prevention,* **17**(2), 153–61.
21. US Census Bureau. (2004). The AIDS Pandemic in the 21st Century. *International Population Reports.* Washington, DC. p. 20.
22. Mathers, C.D. and Loncar, D. (2006). Projections of global mortality and burden of disease from 2002 to 2030. *PLoS Medicine,* **3**(11), e442.
23. Davies, E. and Higginson, I.J. (2004). *Palliative Care. The solid facts.* World Health Organization.

24. Agar, M., Currow, D.C., Shelby-James, T.M. *et al.* (2008). Preference for place of care and place of death in palliative care: are these different questions? *Palliative Medicine*, **22**(7), 787–95

25. Munday, D., Dale, J., and Murray, S. (2007). Choice and place of death: Individual preferences, uncertainty, and the availability of care. *Journal of the Royal Society of Medicine*, **100**(May 2007), 211–15.

26. Storey, L., Pemberton, C., Howard, A. *et al.* (2003). Place of death: Hobson's Choice or patient choice. *Cancer Nursing Practice*, **2**(4), 33–8.

27. Gomes, B. and Higginson, I.J. (2008). Where people die (1974–2030): past trends, future projections and implications for care. *Palliative Medicine*, **22**(1), 33–41.

28. English, M, Lanata F.C., Ngugi, I, and Smith, P.C., (2006). The district hospital. In Jamison T, Breman J, Measham R, et al (eds). *Disease Control Priorities in Developing Countries*. 2nd edition. pp. 1211–28. Oxford University Press. New York.

29. Beccaro, M., Costantini, M., Giorgi Rossi, P. *et al.* (2006). Actual and preferred place of death of cancer patients. Results from the Italian survey of the dying of cancer (ISDOC). *Journal of Epidemiology and Community Health*, **60**(5), 412–6.

30. Foreman, L.M., Hunt, R.W., Luke, C.G. *et al.* (2006). Factors predictive of preferred place of death in the general population of South Australia. *Palliative Medicine*, **20**(4), 447–53.

31. Higginson, I.J. and Sen-Gupta, G.J. (2005). Place of care in advanced cancer: a qualitative systematic literature review of patient preferences. *Journal of Palliative Medicine*, **3**(3), 287–300.

32. Higginson, I.J. and Costantini, M. (2008). Dying with cancer, living well with advanced cancer. *European Journal of Cancer*, **44**(10), 1414–24.

33. Gomes, B. and Higginson, I. (2008). Where people die (1974–2030): past trends, future projections and implications for care. *Palliative Medicine*, **22**(1), 33–41.

34. Tang, S.T., McCorkle, R. (2003). Determinants of congruence between the preferred and actual place of death for terminally ill cancer patients. *Journal of Palliative Care*, **19**(4), 230–7.

35. Krishnasamy, M., Wells, M., and Wilkie, E. (2007). Patients and carer experiences of care provision after a diagnosis of lung cancer in Scotland. *Supportive Care in Cancer*, **15**(3), 327–32.

36. Maguire, P., Walsh, S., Jeacock, J. *et al.* (1999). Physical and psychological needs of patients dying from colo-rectal cancer. *Palliative Medicine*, **13**, 45–50.

37. Wheatley, V. and Baker, I. (2007). "Please I want to go home": ethical issues raised when considering choice of place of care in palliative care *Postgraduate Medical Journal*, **83**, 643–8.

38. Gomes, B. and Higginson, I. (2006). Factors influencing death at home in terminally ill patients with cancer: systematic review. *British Medical Journal*, **332**(7540), 515–21.

39. Pritchard, R., Fisher, E., Teno, J. *et al.* (SUPPORT Investigators). (1998). Influence of patient preferences and local health system characteristics on the place of death: Study to understand prognoses and preferences for outcomeds and risks of treatment. *Journal of American Geriatric Society*, **46**, 1242–50.

40. Young, H.Y., Min, K.L., Kui-Son, C. *et al.* (2006). Predictors associated with the place of death in a country with increasing hospital deaths *Palliative Medicine*, **20**, 455–61.

41. Brennan, F. (2007). Palliative care as an international human right. *Journal of Pain and Symptom Management*, **33**(5), 494–9.

42. Singer, P. and Bowman, K. (2002). Quality of end life care: A global perspective. *BMC Palliative Care*, **1**(4).

43. Dudgeon, D.J., Knott, C., Eichholz, M. *et al.* (2008). Palliative Care Integration Project (PCIP) quality improvement strategy evaluation. *Journal of Pain and Symptom Management*, **35**(6), 573–82.

44. Shipman, C., Gysels, M., White, P. *et al.* (2008). Improving generalist end of life care: national consultation with practitioners, commissioners, academics, and service user groups. *British Medical Journal*, **337**, a1720.

45. Wright, M., Wood, J., Lynch, T. *et al.* (2006). *Mapping levels of palliative care development: A global view.* International Observatory on end of life care, Lancaster University. Available at http://www.eolc-observatory.net/global/pdf/world_map.pdf (Accessed 5 June 2009).

46. Gelfman, L.P., Meier, D.E., Morrison, R.S. (2008). Does palliative care improve quality? A survey of bereaved family members. *Journal of Pain and Symptom Management*, **36**(1), 22–8.

47. Mercadante, S., Intravaia, G. *et al.* (2008). Clinical and financial analysis of an acute palliative care unit in an oncological department. *Palliative Medicine*, **22**(6), 760–7.

48. Morrison, R.S., Penrod, J.D., Cassel, J.B. *et al.* (2008). Cost savings associated with US hospital palliative care consultation programs. *Archives of Internal Medicine*, **168**(16), 1783–90.

49. Goldsmith, B., Dietrich, J., Du, Q. *et al.* (2008). Variability in Access to Hospital Palliative Care in the United States. *Journal of Palliative Medicine.* **11**(8), 1094–102.

50. Glare, P.A., Auret, K.A., Aggarwal, G. *et al.* (2003). The interface between palliative medicine and specialists in acute-care hospitals: boundaries, bridges and challenges. *Medical Journal of Australia*,179 (6 suppl) S29–31.

51. SUPPORT Principal Investigators. (1995). A controlled trial to improve care for seriously ill hospitalized patients. The study to understand prognoses and preferences for outcomes and risks of treatments (SUPPORT), *Journal of the American Medical Association*, **274**(20), 1591–8.

52. Higginson, I.J. (1997). Palliative care and terminal care. In Stevens A, Raftery J, and the Wessex Institute for Health Research and Development (eds). *Palliative and Terminal Care Health Care Needs Assessment.* (2nd edition), pp. 1–77. Radcliffe Medical Press.

53. Rosenwax, L.K. and McNamara, B.A. (2006). Who receives specialist palliative care in Western Australia–and who misses out. *Palliative medicine*, **20**(4), 439–45.

54. Murray, S.A. and Sheikh, A. (2008). Palliative Care Beyond Cancer: Care for all at the end of life. *British Medical Journal*, **336**(7650), 958–9.

55. Solano, J.P., Gomes, B., and Higginson, I.J. (2006). A comparison of symptom prevalence in far advanced cancer, AIDS, heart disease, chronic obstructive pulmonary disease and renal disease. *Journal of Pain and Symptom Management*, **34**(1), 58–69.

56. Kaasa, S., Loge, J., Fayers, P. *et al.* (2008). Symptom Assessment in Palliative Care: A Need for International Collaboration. *Journal of Clinical Oncology*, **26**(23), 3867–73.

57. Higginson, I.J., Hart, S., Koffman, J. *et al.* (2007). Needs assessments in palliative care: an appraisal of definitions and approaches used. *Journal of Pain and Symptom Management*, **33**(5), 500–5.

58. World Health Organization. (2007). *Cancer Control: Knowledge into Action.* Palliative Care. Geneva: World Health Organization.

59. Kikule, E. (2003). A good death in Uganda: survey of needs for palliative care for terminally ill people in urban areas. *British Medical Journal*, **327**(7480), 192–4.

60. Wright, M., Wood, J., Lynch, T. *et al.* (2008). Mapping levels of palliative care development: a global view. *Journal of Pain and Symptom Management*, **35**(5), 469–85.

61. Young, A.J., Rogers, A., and Addington-Hall, J.M. (2008). The quality and adequacy of care received at home in the last 3 months of life by people who died following a stroke: a retrospective survey of surviving family and friends using the Views of Informal Carers Evaluation of Services questionnaire. *Health and Social Care in the Community*, **16**(4), 419–28.

62. Seely, J., Scott, J., and Mount, B. The need for specialized training programs in palliative medicine. *Canadian Medical Association Journal*, **157**(10), 1395–7.

63. Larue, F., Colleau, M.S., Brasseur, L. *et al.* (1995). Multicentre study of pain and its treatment in France. *British Medical Journal*, **310**(6986), 1034–7.

64. Okuyama, T., Wang, X., Akechi, T. *et al.* Adequacy of cancer pain management in a Japanese cancer hospital. *Japanese Journal of Clinical Oncology*, **34**(1), 37–42.

65. Rustøen, T., Stubhaug, A., Eidsmo, I. *et al.* (2008). Pain and Quality of Life in Hospitalized Patients with Heart Failure. *Journal of Pain and Symptom Management*, **36**(5), 497–504.

66. Freeman, S. (2007). 'Rawls'. New York: Routledge.

67. Sen, A. (1993). *The Quality of life*. In (ed. A. Nussbaum and A. Sen). United Nations University.

68. Franks, P., Salisbury, C., Bosanquet, M. *et al.* (2000). The level of need for palliative care: a systematic review of the literature. *Palliative Medicine*, **14**(2), 93–104.

69. Mirando, S. (2004). Palliative care needs assessment. *International Journal of Palliative Nursing*, **10**(12), 602–5.

70. Elkington, H., White, P., Addington-Hall, J. *et al.* (2005). The healthcare needs of chronic obstructive pulmonary disease patients in the last year of life. *Palliative Medicine*, **19**(6), 485–91.

71. Edmonds, P., Karlsen, S., Khan, S. *et al.* (2001). A comparison of the palliative care needs of patients dying from chronic respiratory diseases and lung cancer. *Palliative Medicine*, **15**(4), 287–95.

72. Davies, E. (2004). What are the palliative care needs of older people and how might they be met? *Health Evidence Network Report*. Copenhagen: WHO Regional Office for Europe. Available at http://www.euro.who.int/HEN/Syntheses/palliative/20040722_3 (accessed 24 July 2009).

73. Currow, D.C., Abernethy, A.P., and Fazekas, B.S. (2004). Specialist palliative care needs of whole populations: a feasibility study using a novel approach. *Palliative Medicine*, **18**(3), 239–47.

74. Christakis, N.A. (1997). *The ellipsis of prognosis in modern medical thought*. Social Science and Medicine **44**(3), 301–15.

75. Currow, D.C., Wheeler, J., Glare, P. *et al.* (2009). A framework for generalizability in palliative care. *Journal of Pain and Symptom Management*, **37**(3), 373–86.

76. Higginson, I.J., Hearn, J. (2003). Cancer pain epidemiology a systematic review. In: Portenoy R.K., (ed.) *Cancer Pain: assessment and management* pp. 19–37, New York: Cambridge University Press.

77. Hearn, J. and Higginson, I.J. (1997). Outcome measures in palliative care for advanced cancer patients: a review. *Journal of Public Health*, **19**(2), 193.

78. Kristjanson, L., Nikoletti, S., Porock, D. *et al.* (1998). Congruence between patients' and family caregivers' perceptions of symptom distress in patients with terminal cancer. *Journal of Palliative Care* **14**(3), 24–32.

79. McPherson, C.J., Addington-Hall, J.M. (2003). Judging the quality of care at the end of life: can proxies provide reliable information? *Social Science and Medicine*, **56**(1), 95–109.

80. Addington-Hall, J. (2001). Measuring quality of life: Who should measure quality of life? *BMJ*, **322**(7299), 1417–20.

81. Hwang, S.S., Chang, V.T., Fairclough, D.L. *et al.* (2003). Longitudinal quality of life in advanced cancer patients: pilot study results from a VA medical cancer center. *Journal of Pain and Symptom Management* **25**(3), 225–35.

82. Sharpe, L., Butow, P., Smith, C. *et al.* (2005). Changes in quality of life in patients with advanced cancer: evidence of response shift and response restriction. *Journal of Psychosomatic Research*, **58**(6), 497–504.

83. Lazarus, R., Folkman, P.S. (1984). *Stress, Appraisal, and Coping*: Springer.

84. Henoch, I., Bergman, B., Gustafsson, M. *et al.* (2007). The impact of symptoms, coping capacity, and social support on quality of life experience over time in patients with lung cancer. *Journal of Pain and Symptom Management*, **34**(4), 370–9.

85. Hesselink, A.E., Penninx, B.W., Schlösser, M.A. *et al.* (2004). The role of coping resources and coping style in quality of life of patients with asthma or COPD. *Quality of Life Research*, **13**(2), 509–18.

86. Lethborg, C., Aranda, S., Cox, S. *et al.* (2007). To what extent does meaning mediate adaptation to cancer? The relationship between physical suffering, meaning in life, and connection to others in adjustment to cancer. *Palliative and Supportive Care*, **5**(4), 377–88.

87. Rutter, M. Resilience in the face of adversity. (1985). Protective factors and resistance to psychiatric disorder. *The British Journal of Psychiatry*, **147**, 598–611.

88. Blinderman, C.D., Homel, P., Billings, J.A. *et al.* (2008). Symptom distress and quality of life in patients with advanced congestive heart failure. *Journal of Pain and Symptom Management*, **35**(6), 594–603.

89. Walke, L.M., Byers, A.L., Tinetti, M.E. *et al.* (2007). Range and severity of symptoms over time among older adults with chronic obstructive pulmonary disease and heart failure. *Archives of Internal Medicine*, **167**(22), 2503–8.

90. Potter, J., Hami, F., Bryan, T. *et al.* (2003). Symptoms in 400 patients referred to palliative care services: prevalence and patterns. *Palliative Medicine*, **17**(4), 310–4.

91. Portenoy, R.K., Thaler, H.T., Kornblith, A.B. *et al.* (1994). Symptom prevalence, characteristics and distress in a cancer population. *Quality of Life Research*, **3**(3), 183–9.

92. Dunlop, G.M. (1990). A study of the relative frequency and importance of gastrointestinal symptoms and weakness in patients with far advanced cancer. *Palliative Medicine*, **4**(1), 37–43.

93. Welch, J.M., Barlow, D., and Richardson, P.H. (1991). Symptoms of HIV disease. *Palliative Medicine*, **5**, 46–51.

94. Hearn, J. and Higginson, I. (1999). Development and validation of a core outcome measure for palliative care: the palliative care outcome scale. *Quality and Safety in Health Care*, **8**(4), 219–27.

95. Currow, D.C., Agar, M., Tieman, J. *et al.* (2008). Multi-site research allows adequately powered palliative care trials; web-based data management makes it achievable today. *Palliative Medicine*, **22**(1), 91–2.

96. McNamara, B. and Rosenwax, L. (2007). Factors affecting place of death in Western Australia. *Health and Place*, **13**(2), 356–67.

97. Fassbender, K., Fainsinger, R., Brenneis, C. *et al.* (2005). Utilization and costs of the introduction of system-wide palliative care in Alberta, 1993–2000. *Palliative Medicine*, **19**(7), 513–20.

98. Hanks, G.W. and Justins, D.M. (1992). Cancer pain: management. *Lancet*, **339**(8800), 1031–6.

99. Addington-Hall, J.M., Fakhoury, W., and McCarthy, M. (1998). Specialist palliative care in nonmalignant disease. *Palliative medicine*, **12**(6), 417–27.

100. Teunissen, S.C., Wesker, W., Kruitwagen, C. *et al.* (2007). Symptom prevalence in patients with incurable cancer: a systematic review. *Journal of Pain and Symptom Management*, **34**(1), 94–104.

101. Canada Go. (2008). *Statstics Canada*. Ottawa, Ontario.

102. National Center for Health Statistics. National Mortality Followback Survey provisional data (1993). Availble at: http://www.cdc.gov/nchs/nvss/nmfs/healcond.htm (accessed 24 July 2009).

103. Addington-Hall, J. and McCarthy, M. (1995). Dying from cancer: results of a national population-based investigation. *Palliative Medicine*, **9**, 295–305.

104. Bonica, J. (1985). Treatment of cancer pain: current status and future needs. In *Advances in Pain Research and Therapy* (ed. Fields, H.L.), pp. 589–616. New York: Raven Press.

105. Portenoy, R.K. and Lesage, P. (1999). Management of cancer pain. *Lancet*, **353**(9165),1695–700.

106. van den Beuken-van Everdingen, M.H., de Rijke, J.M., Kessels, A.G., *et al.* (2007). Prevalence of pain in patients with cancer: a systematic review of the past 40 years. *Annals of Oncology*, **18**(9), 1437–49.

107. Bruera, E., Kuehn, N., Miller, M.J. *et al.* (1991). The Edmonton Symptom Assessment System (ESAS): a simple method for the assessment of palliative care patients. *Journal of Palliative Care*, **7**(2), 6–9.

108. Chang, V.T., Hwang, S.S., Feuerman, M. *et al.* (2000). Symptom and quality of life survey of medical oncology patients at a veterans affairs medical center: a role for symptom assessment. *Cancer*, **88**(5), 1175–83.

109. Meuser, T., Pietruck, C., Radbruch, L. *et al.* (2001). Symptoms during cancer pain treatment following WHO-guidelines: a longitudinal follow-up study of symptom prevalence, severity and etiology. *Pain*, **93**(3), 247–57.

110. Higginson, I.J. and Hearn, J. (1997). A multicenter evaluation of cancer pain control by palliative care teams. *Journal of Pain and Symptom Management*, **14**(1), 29–35.

111. Tishelman, C., Petersson, L.M., Degner, L.F. *et al.* (2007). Symptom prevalence, intensity, and distress in patients with inoperable lung cancer in relation to time of death. *Journal of Clinical Oncology*, **25**(34), 5381–9.

112. Hynninen, K.M., Breitve, M.H., Wiborg, A.B. *et al.* (2005). Psychological characteristics of patients with chronic obstructive pulmonary disease: a review. *Journal of Psychosomatic Research*, **59**(6) 429–43.

113. Hill, K., Geist, R., Goldstein, R.S. *et al.* (2008). Anxiety and depression in end-stage COPD. *European Respiratory Journal*, **31**(3), 667–77.

114. Averill, A.J., Kasarskis, E.J., and Segerstrom, S.C. (2007). Psychological health in patients with amyotrophic lateral sclerosis. *Amyotrophic Lateral Sclerosis*, **8**(4), 243–54.

115. Derogatis, L.R., Morrow, G.R., Fetting, J, et al. (1983). The prevalence of psychiatric disorders among cancer patients. *Journal of the American Medical Association*, **249**(6): 751–7.

116. Lloyd-Williams, M. (2003). Psychosocial care: setting the research agenda. *Palliative Medicine*, **17**(1), 78–80.

117. Fallowfield, L., Ratcliffe, D., Jenkins, V. *et al.* (2001). Psychiatric morbidity and its recognition by doctors in patients with cancer. *British Journal of Cancer*, **84**(8), 1011–5.

118. Breitbart, W., Bruera, E., Chochinov, H. *et al.* (1995). Neuropsychiatric syndromes and psychological symptoms in patients with advanced cancer. *Journal of Pain and Symptom Management*, **10**(2), 131–41.

119. World Health Organization. (2004). *International Classification of Diseases and Health related Problems (ICD)*. 10th Revision, 2nd edition. Geneva, WHO.

120. Reeve, J., Lloyd-Williams, M., and Dowrick, C. (2007). Depression in terminal illness: the need for primary care-specific research. *Family Practice*, **24**(3), 263–8.

121. Ly, K., Chidgey, J., Addington-Hall, J. *et al.* (2002). Depression in palliative care: a systematic r eview. *Palliative Medicine*, **16**(4), 279–84.

122. Roth, A.J. and Massie, M.J. (2007). Anxiety and its management in advanced cancer. *Current Opinion in Supportive and Palliative Care*, **1**(1), 50–6.

123. Leonard, M., Agar, M., Mason, C. *et al.* (2008). Delirium issues in palliative care settings. *Journal of Psychosomatic Research*, **65**(3), 289–98.

124. Mercadante, S., Girelli, D., and Casuccio, A. (2004). Sleep disorders in advanced cancer patients: prevalence and factors associated. *Supportive Care in Cancer*, **12**(5), 355–9.

125. Kissane, D.W., Clarke, D.M., and Street, A.F. (2001). Demoralization syndrome–a relevant psychiatric diagnosis for palliative care. *Journal of Palliative Care*, **17**(1), 12–21.

126. Murtagh, F.E., Addington-Hall, J., and Higginson, I.J. (2007). The prevalence of symptoms in end-stage renal disease: a systematic review. *Advances in Chronic Kidney Disease*, **14**(1), 82–99.

127. Curtis, J.R. (2008). Palliative and end-of-life care for patients with severe COPD. *European Respiratory Journal*, **32**(3), 796–803.

128. Selman, L., Beynon, T., Higginson, I.J. *et al.* (2007). Psychological, social and spiritual distress at the end of life in heart failure patients. *Current Opinion in Supportive and Palliative Care*, **1**(4), 260–6.

129. Chochinov, H.M. (2006). Dying, dignity, and new horizons in palliative end-of-life care. *CA: A Cancer Journal for Clinicians*, **56**(2), 84–103.

130. Lloyd-Williams, M., Shiels, C., Taylor, F. *et al.* (2008). Depression - An independent predictor of early death in patients with advanced cancer. *Journal of Affective Disorders*, **113**(1–2), 127–32.

131. Lawlor, P.G., Fainsinger, R.L., Bruera, E.D. (2000). Delirium at the end of life: critical issues in clinical practice and research. *Journal of the American Medical Association*, **284**(19), 2427–9.

132. Ljubisavljevic, V. and Kelly, B. (2003). Risk factors for development of delirium among oncology patients. *General Hospital Psychiatry*, **25**(5), 345–52.

133. Doriath, V., Paesmans, M., Catteau, G. *et al.* (2007). Acute confusion in patients with systemic cancer. *Journal of Neurooncology*, **83**(3), 285–9.

134. Portenoy, R.K., Thaler, H.T., Kornblith, A.B. *et al.* (1994). The Memorial Symptom Assessment Scale: an instrument for the evaluation of symptom prevalence, characteristics and distress. *European Journal of Cancer*, **30A**(9), 1326–36.

135. Lawlor, P.G., Gagnon, B., Mancini, I.L. *et al.* (2000). Occurrence, causes, and outcome of delirium in patients with advanced cancer: a prospective study. *Archives of Internal Medicine*, **160**(6), 786–94.

136. Breitbart, W.G. and C Tremblay, A. (2002). The delirium experience: delirium recall and delirium-related distress in hospitalized patients with cancer, their spouses/caregivers, and their nurses. *Psychosomatics*, **43**(3), 183–94.

137. Ljubisavljevic, V. and Kelly, B. (2003). Risk factors for development of delirium among oncology patients. *General Hospital Psychiatry*, **25**(5), 345–52.

138. Inouye, S.K. (1994). The dilemma of delirium: clinical and research controversies regarding diagnosis and evaluation of delirium in hospitalized elderly medical patients. *American Journal of Medicine*, **97**(8), 278–88.

139. Davis, M.P. and Walsh, D. (2001). Clinical and ethical questions concerning delirium study on patients with advanced cancer. *Archives of Internal Medicine*, **161**(2), 296–9.

140. American Psychiatric Association. (2000). *Diagnostic and statistical manual of mental disorders*, Fourth edition, Text revision, Washington DC, American Psychiatric Association.

141. Holland, J.C., Andersen, B., Breitbart, W.S. *et al.* (2007). The NCCN guideline for distress management: a case for making distress the sixth vital sign. *Journal of the National Comprehensive Cancer Network*, **5**(1), 66–98.

142. Jacobsen, P.B., Donovan, K.A., Trask, P.C. *et al.* (2005). Screening for psychologic distress in ambulatory cancer patients. *Cancer*, **103**(7), 1494–502.

143. National Institute for Clinical Excellence (2004). *Improving Supportive and Palliative care for Adults with Cancer*. London: National Institute for Clinical Excellence. Reference NO475.

144. Ellershaw, J., Smith, C. *et al.* (2001). Care of the dying: setting standards for symptom control in the last 48 hours of life. *Journal of Pain and Symptom Management*, **21**, 12–7.

145. Foley, D.J., Miles, T.P., Brock, D.B. *et al.* (1995). Recounts of elderly deaths: endorsements for the Patient Self-Determination Act. *The Gerontologist*, **35**(1), 119–21.

146. Cicely, M. and Saunders, D.C. (2006). Pain and Impending death. *Cicely Saunders: Selected Writings* 1958-2004, 187–8.

147. Lichter, I. and Hunt, E. (1990). The last 48 hours of life. *Journal of Palliative Care*, **6**(4), 7–15.

148. Hinkka, H., Kosunen, E., Kellokumpu-Lehtinen, P. *et al.* (2001). Assessment of pain control in cancer patients during the last week of life: comparison of health centre wards and a hospice. *Supportive Care in Cancer*, **9**(6), 428–34.

149. Osler, W. (1904). The Ingersoll Lecture. *Science and Immortality*. Houghton, Mifflin, Boston, MA.

150. Hinohara, S. (1993). Sir William Osler's Philosophy on Death. *Annals of Internal Medicine*, **118**(8), 638–42.

151. Ventafridda, V., Ripamonti, C., De Conno, F. *et al.* (1990). Symptom prevalence and control during cancer patients' last days of life. *Journal of Palliative Care*, **6**(3), 7–11.

152. Kohara, H., Ueoka, H., Takeyama, H. *et al.* (2005). Sedation for terminally ill patients with cancer with uncontrollable physical distress. *Journal of Palliative Medicine*, **8**(1), 20–5.

153. Elsayem, A., Curry Iii, E., Boohene, J. *et al.* (2009). Use of palliative sedation for intractable symptoms in the palliative care unit of a comprehensive cancer center. *Supportive Care in Cancer*, **17**(1), 53–9.

154. Fainsinger, R., Miller, M.J., Bruera, E. *et al.* (1991). Symptom control during the last week of life on a palliative care unit. *Journal of Palliative Care*, **7**(1), 5–11.

155. Stone, P.C. and Lund, S. (2007). Predicting prognosis in patients with advanced cancer. *Annals of Oncology*, **18**(6), 971–6.

156. Steinhauser, K.E., Christakis, N.A., Clipp, E.C. *et al.* (2000). Factors considered important at the end of life by patients, family, physicians, and other care providers. *Journal of the American Medical Association*, **284**(19), 2476–82.

157. Seeman, I. (1992). National Mortality Followback Survey: 1986 Summary, United States. *Vital and Health Statistics*. Hyattsville, Maryland: National Center for Health Statistics.

158. Conill, C., Verger, E., Henríquez, I. *et al.* (1997). Symptom prevalence in the last week of life. *Journal of Pain and Symptom Management*, **14**(6), 328–31.

159. Speake, J. (2008). The Oxford Dictionary of Proverbs 5th ed. Oxford University Press, Oxford, New York.

160. Gosline, A. (2007). Death Special: How does it feel to die? *New Scientist*, 2365, 53–57.

161. Williams, D. (2007). At the hour of our death. *TIME* Sydney Australia: TIME Australia Magazine, 30–7.

162. Seale, C., Addington-Hall, J.M., and McCarthy, M. (1997). Awareness of dying: prevalence, causes and consequences. *Social Science and Medicine*, **45**(3), 477–84.

163. Glaser, B, Strauss, A. (1968). *Time for Dying*. Chicago: Aldine Publishing Co.

164. Lunney, J.R., Lynn, J., Foley, D.J. *et al.* (2003). Patterns of functional decline at the end of life. *Journal of the American Medical Association*, **289**(18), 2387–92.

165. Costantini, M., Beccaro, M., and Higginson, I.J. (2008). Cancer trajectories at the end of life: is there an effect of age and gender? *BMC Cancer*, **8**, 127.

166. Covinsky, K.E., Landefeld, C.S., Teno, J.M. *et al.* (1996). Is economic hardship on the families of the seriously ill associated with patient and surrogate care preferences. SUPPORT Investigators. *Archives of Internal Medicine*, **156**(15), 1737–41.

167. Christakis, N.A. and Iwashyna, T.J. (2003). The health impact of health care on families: a matched cohort study of hospice use by decedents and mortality outcomes in surviving, widowed spouses. *Social Science and Medicine*, **57**(3), 465–75.

168. Zivin, K. and Christakis, N.A. (2007). The emotional toll of spousal morbidity and mortality. *The American Journal of Geriatric Psychiatry*, **15**(9), 772–9.

169. Carmichael, F. and Charles, S. (1998). The labour market costs of community care. *Journal of Health Economics*, **17**(6), 747–65.

170. Christakis, N.A. and Allison, P.D. (2006). Mortality after the hospitalization of a spouse. *New England Journal of Medicine*, **354**(7), 719–30.

171. Emanuel, E.J., Fairclough, D.L., Slutsman, J. *et al.* (2000). Understanding economic and other burdens of terminal illness: the experience of patients and their caregivers. *Annals of Internal Medicine*, **132**(6), 451–9.

172. Aoun, S.M., Kristjanson, L.J., Currow, D.C. *et al.* (2005). Caregiving for the terminally ill: at what cost? *Palliative Medicine*, **19**(7), 551–5.

173. Berecki-Gisolf, J., Lucke, J., Hockey, R. *et al.* (2008). Transitions into informal caregiving and out of paid employment of women in their 50s. *Social Science and Medicine* (1982), **67**(1), 122–7.

174. Addington-Hall, J.M., Lay, M., Altmann, D. *et al.* (1998). Community care for stroke patients in the last year of life: results of a national retrospective survey of surviving family, friends and officials. *Health and Social Care in the Community*, **6**(2), 112–9.

175. Osse, B.H., Vernooij-Dassen, M.J., Schadé, E. *et al.* (2006). Problems experienced by the informal caregivers of cancer patients and their needs for support. *Cancer Nursing*, **29**(5), 378–88.

176. Grant, E., Murray, S.A., Grant, A. *et al.* (2003). A good death in rural Kenya? Listening to Meru patients and their families talk about care needs at the end of life. *Journal of Palliative Care*, **19**(3), 159–67.

177. Addington-Hall, J. and McCarthy, M. (1995). Dying from cancer: results of a national population-based investigation. *Palliat Med*, **9**(4), 295–305.

178. Wolff J., Sydney D., Frick K., Kasper J. (2007). End-of-Life care: Findings From a National Survey of Informal caregivers. *Arch Intern Med*, **167** (1), 40–46.

179. Saunders, C. (1984) Pain and impending death. In: Wall P, Melzack R, eds. *Textbook of Pain*. New York: Churchill Livingstone, 472–8.

3.3

Predicting survival in patients with advanced disease

Paul Glare, Christian Sinclair,
Michael Downing, and Patrick Stone

Introduction

The importance of prognosis in palliative care

Diagnosis, treatment, and prognosis have long been recognized as the three great clinical skills in medicine[1]. Prior to the turn of the 20th century, prognosis was more prominent than today because few effective treatments were available. Over the past 100 years, prognosis gradually gave way to treatment as the core clinical skill accompanying diagnosis: increasingly successful therapies made details of the natural history of illness progression become less relevant to the clinician[2].

The growth of palliative medicine led to a renaissance of prognostication as a clinical skill. But unlike in the 19th century when prognosis most often involved acute illness in young adults, in contemporary palliative medicine prognosis relates to chronic progressive and ultimately fatal diseases and co-morbidities across all age groups.

Palliative care clinicians need to be proficient at prognosis for various reasons:

- to provide patients and their families with information so they can set their goals, priorities, and expectations of care[3–7];

- to help patients develop insight in to their dying[6];

- to assist clinicians in their decision-making[8,9];

- to compare like patients with regard to outcomes[10];

- to establish patients' eligibility for care programmes, including timely referral to hospice programmes[8,11];

- for the design and analysis of clinical trials;

- for policy making with respect to appropriate resource utilization and allocation of support services, e.g. frequency of contacts if home care is proposed[6–8]; and

- to provide a common language for health-care professionals involved in end-of-life care.

While some of these reasons are relevant before referral to palliative care services (e.g. eligibility criteria), others become more relevant after referral. A key role for palliative care services is to initiate discussions on prognosis and goals of care[12], as these are often neglected prior to the consultation[13]. An audit of 325 consecutive referrals to a palliative care service in a US academic teaching hospital indicated that discussions on prognosis and goals of care were the most common function performed by the service, occurring in almost 95 per cent of cases[14].

Domains of prognostication

Prognosis is defined as the 'relative probabilities of the various outcomes of the natural history of a disease'[15]. To address the various issues requiring physicians to utilize prognostic skills, Fries and Ehrlich coined the 'the 5Ds of prognostication'[16]:

1   disease progression/recurrence;

2   death;

3   disability/discomfort;

4   drug toxicity; and

5   dollars (costs of health care).

All five 'Ds' are relevant to palliative care and using this framework, examples of some typical day-to-day prognostic questions for palliative care practitioners are shown in Table 3.3.1. Indeed, the US survey of the information needs of patients with advanced cancer found that almost all wanted predictions of response rates and side effects to chemotherapy, while a smaller proportion (65–85 per cent) wanted predictions of survival[17].

Clinician attitudes to prognosis

Despite the importance of prognosis as a clinical skill in palliative care, many clinicians do not like performing it. A survey of

Table 3.3.1 5Ds: examples from palliative care.

'D'	Example
Disease progression/recurrence	How quickly will the ascites reaccumulate?
Death	How long have I got?
Disability	Will I walk again?
Drug toxicity	Will I get addicted to morphine?
Dollar cost	Is conventional care more expensive than palliative care?

approximately 700 US physicians found that although prognostication was a frequent act (performed 100 times a year by the 'typical' oncologist responding to the survey), nearly 60 per cent of respondents felt poorly trained in the task[18]. They reported difficulty in formulating and communicating a prognosis. Reasons for the stressfulness of prognostication included perceiving patients as desiring too much certainty and accuracy from the prediction. Surveyed physicians were intimidated by being judged by patients and other clinicians if the prognosis was wrong—though admittedly not as badly as for getting the diagnosis wrong. They claimed to avoid prognostication, generally waiting to be asked rather than volunteering a prediction, especially if the clinical situation was atypical and the course seemed more uncertain than usual. Almost all physicians surveyed said they would be optimistic, and a majority stated if the patient were optimistic about the prognosis then they would reinforce that viewpoint. Finally, almost all the surveyed physicians said they would try to avoid being specific when giving a prediction. These attributes have been referred to as the 'norms' of prognostication (see Table 3.3.2)[19]. The results emphasize the need to improve education in prognosis.

Prognosis in 'terminal' disease

The majority of research on prognosis in cancer has been done on early stage disease and concerns factors influencing the probability of cure. In the case of breast cancer, for example, these factors include TNM stage, oestrogen receptor status, HER2 status, age, menopausal status, and, more recently, genetic signature[20]. These data are used to predict not only overall survival but also response to treatment, progression-free survival, and short-term survival (1 and 5 years).

The key difference between prognosis in early and late stage cancer is that the diagnostic, pathological, and treatment-related factors determining survival in early stage cancer are typically less relevant in patients with incurable advanced disease. Moreover, because patients with cancer are a very heterogeneous group with respect to tumour type, these factors are replaced by different clinical and treatment factors which are not related to the principal diagnosis but to broader manifestations of terminal illness: functional status, the anorexia–cachexia syndrome, lymphopoenia, poor quality of life (QOL), and psychosocial factors.

Some authors have tried to make a distinction between advanced cancer (when disease is widespread but there is still some realistic hope of controlling it, if not curing it) and terminal cancer (when disease is widespread and there is no realistic way of controlling it) and to thereby determine the length of the so-called 'terminal phase'. Durations of the 'terminal phase' have been calculated (Table 3.3.3)

Table 3.3.2 'Norms' of prognostication (see reference 263).

- Do not make predictions
- Keep what predictions you do make to yourself
- Do not communicate predictions to patients unless asked
- Do not be specific
- Do not be extreme
- Be optimistic

Table 3.3.3 Durations of the terminal phase.

Author	Country	Year	Survival (days)	
			Mean	Median
McCusker[5]	USA	1984	94	45
Vigano[21]	Canada	2000	175	107
Llobera[22]	Spain	2001	99	59
Yun[23]	Korea	2001	–	54

Using this data, the median duration of the terminal phase of cancer could be considered to be approximately 2–4 months, but how this impacts on patient understanding and clinical decision-making is unclear.

In other eventually fatal non-cancer illnesses, like chronic obstructive pulmonary disease (COPD) and cardiac failure, the depth of research focused on prognosis is less comprehensive. Disease-specific factors like arterial blood gas levels and left ventricular function often form the basis of current prognostic tools. Non-specific factors like symptoms (e.g. dyspnoea at rest), functional level, and QOL are still very relevant nevertheless, and with further research may prove to have a greater role in prognostication in these conditions.

Illness trajectories

The concept of a trajectory prototype is often referenced for understanding a patient's course of illness in a broader context than the immediate clinical situation[24,25]. The immediate functionality for this idea is in teaching palliative care concepts and discussing a patient's understanding of his or her illness experience. The extent to which such hypothesized death trajectories actually occur is neither fully understood at present, nor is it clear what fraction of patients with each of several different kinds of illness show each of these, or other possible, trajectories. The four basic trajectories proposed include sudden death, progressive decline with accelerated end, progressive decline punctuated with exacerbations, and long gradual decline. Often these trajectories are labelled with a disease to define the prototype, but as mentioned before the accuracy of these hypothetical models has not been well studied.

Trauma and sudden cardiac death are examples of the sudden death trajectory. Although the role for palliative care is limited by a short time frame in this model, palliative care may be useful in offering advice on appropriate treatment withdrawal, comfort care, immediate family support, and bereavement follow-up. The proposed course of a cancer illness involves a gradual decline in health status over a period of months or years, with an accelerated decline over a period of weeks to months. Traditional palliative care services such as hospices are widely designed for this pattern of illness. The causes of death in cancer patients are quite diverse and may ultimately result from acute problems such as infection, but in most cases the underlying tumour precipitates the cause of death with anorexia–cachexia syndrome and eventually coma as the final common pathway[26,27].

Another model trajectory is the progressive decline punctuated by acute crises from which the individual recovers to—or close to—the prior health state until the final crisis occurs which cannot be, or is not, treated. The AIDS-related death and most end-organ failure deaths (e.g. COPD, congestive heart failure (CHF)) are typical of this pattern. The last proposed course is the long gradual decline demonstrated by a very poor health state culminating in death at some unpredictable time following an acute infection or possibly no obvious event, typical of the post-stroke or Alzheimer's death. Some critiques of these models are the lack of evidentiary support beyond anecdotal report, the inadequate accounting for individual variation and uncertainty, and the primary usefulness limited to a retrospective or conceptual manner.

The accuracy of survival predictions

One criticism of using prognosis for clinical decision-making is that survival predictions are inherently inaccurate and therefore are not worth making. Of course, there are many uncertainties when predicting future outcomes, especially when considering the complex dynamic of the human body and the multiple interactions between the human body and illness. Despite frequent jokes about predicting the weather, meteorological forecasting has advanced greatly in the last 200 years and saved countless lives with technological improvements (i.e. early warning systems), and in many ways weather forecasting resembles the complex variable conditions of the human body. Survival predictions and other predicted outcomes can be accurate depending on the type of prediction being made[3,28–30]. There are two major classes of medical predictions: temporal predictions (the patient will live a certain amount of time), expressed either as a continuous or categorical variable, and probabilistic predictions (the percentage chance of surviving to a certain time).

Most studies of subjective prognostic judgement have looked at temporal predictions, whereas most prognostic tools provide probabilistic predictions. The accuracy of probabilistic predictions is of the order of 50–75 per cent[29,31,32]; the accuracy of temporal predictions is only around 25 per cent (an accurate prediction being defined as the observed survival being ±33 per cent of the predicted survival)[3]. When analysing prediction research, it is important to understand the terminology of measurement, particularly the terms *accuracy, precision, discrimination,* and *calibration*[29, 32]. *Accuracy* measures the difference between measured (or estimated) values and the true value. This difference between the mean estimates for a population and the true survival allows one to discover if any optimistic or pessimistic biases exist. *Precision* defines how closely all estimates are to each other with repeated measurement. *Discrimination* is the correct allocation of individuals from two or more discrete populations to the correct sub-population without mismatch. *Calibration* is the adjustment of an instrument (or observer) so the distribution of its measurements matches a standard. Clinicians can be said to be discriminate if their probabilistic predictions are accurate and precise. They are well calibrated if their temporal predictions are accurate and precise.

Cultural aspects of prognostication at the end of life

The importance physicians place on predicting survival at the end of life will also be strongly influenced by sociocultural factors. In *Nature of Suffering*, Cassell highlights that in Hippocrates' day, the physician who was a good prognosticator was most highly esteemed among his colleagues[33]. By contrast, many religious traditions insist only God knows the hour of an individual's death. This deferral by patients, family, and staff to the idea that 'God only knows' is a way to culturally identify the acknowledged uncertainty of prognostication. In liberal, pluralist Western societies physicians are generally willing to discuss the prognosis of a life-threatening illness, when asked directly. In many non-English speaking cultures, such discussions have traditionally been avoided, although this situation may be gradually changing. It is important when considering communication of prognostic information to consider the willingness of the patient and family to participate in such conversations.

Inquiring how much the patient and family want to hear is a good strategy for respecting individual differences in prognostic discussions[34]. When working with paediatric patients, it is important to be aware of the patient's medical knowledge and maturity as well as the wishes of the parents, before discussing prognosis. Details on how to best communicate prognosis are covered later in this chapter.

The current palliative medicine approach to prognostication

There are two components to the clinical act of prognostication. The first is formulating the prediction (i.e. foreseeing). The second is communicating the prediction to the patient, family, or other medical professionals (i.e. foretelling). Both foreseeing and foretelling can be studied and improved upon[35].

Both foreseeing and foretelling have been largely ignored in formal general medical education. At most, prognostic issues may be covered in a class on 'Breaking Bad News' which typically uses disclosure of a poor prognosis as an example of difficult physician–patient communication. A particular emphasis of specialty training in palliative medicine is good clinical decision-making in the context of far-advanced disease. Stress is placed on accounting for the natural history of eventually fatal illnesses and predicting the future consequences of a therapeutic act/omission. As the patient's goals, priorities, and expectations (as opposed to disease-related issues) drive this decision-making, patients and families will often ask for a prognosis. For both these reasons, communication and formulation of prognosis should be elevated to a critical part of the curriculum.

Palliative medicine trainees are typically taught not to formulate a prognosis in terms of a specific amount of time[36], but rather to offer a meaningful time-frame to the patient/family: namely hours rather than days, days rather than weeks, weeks rather than months, and so on. Much prognostic importance is attached to interpreting how quickly the disease seems to have been progressing. While this approach is laudable, it is unclear how trainees are being taught to make such predictions, nor what the time-frame is meant to represent: the predicted actual survival of the individual, the median survival of other patients like them, the best case scenario, or the worst case scenario. In terms of disclosing the prognosis, trainees are taught both explicitly and implicitly to only disclose the formulated prognosis when it is requested and then to give a frank disclosure[19]. Much more attention to training palliative care specialists in the best way to formulate a prognosis is needed to complement the focus on the communication aspect.

A common palliative care topic when discussing prognostication in the last few hours or days, is addressing the phenomenon of individuals very close to death 'hanging on' until they achieve 'closure' or see a close family member or friend. Despite not being supported by research, this concept is widely disseminated among hospice and palliative personnel. The 'special reason' or 'closure' theory of affecting a life expectancy may be a psychological construct to help with coping among family and staff, although this may occasionally cause more psychological distress when the patient continues to live despite all possible closure opportunities being exhausted. The evidence for patients waiting for symbolically meaningful occasions such as birthdays and holidays is limited and conflicting, although there was evidence for increased mortality around Christmas and New Year in one cardiac study[37–41].

Formulating a prognosis in advanced cancer

Prognosis is often understood as a static phenomenon as evidenced from multiple research studies focusing on one point in time (e.g. admission to hospital or hospice). This is reinforced culturally as explicit discussions about prognosis usually happen only a few times in the course of a patient's illness. The illness trajectories conceptualized change over time, so that as the illness evolves new issues must be considered and the prognosis should be revised.

Originating with Mackillop[42], is a useful paradigm for conceptualizing prognostication. Clinical and pathological findings such as tumour histology, grade, and site/number of metastases lead to the diagnosis of the individual's disease. There is a general prognosis associated with this diagnosis, induced from the clinician's experience of previous patients with the same disease (expressed as 5-year survival rate, median survival, etc.). The diagnosis leads to the implementation of various therapies, which may alter the general prognosis from the natural disease course. Co-morbidities may alter the general prognosis, for example, the impact of CHF on renal patients on haemodialysis. The general prognosis is customized to the entire clinical situation revealing an individual prognosis, but needs to be modified according to other clinical findings such as performance status, symptoms, metabolic problems, and QOL scores or other psychosocial variables. In patients with advanced/terminal cancer, clinical findings and psychosocial factors (solid lines) appear to be more important than the other factors (broken lines). Hauser also highlights these differential impacts in a conceptual model for incorporating different aspects over time into a prognostic model[43]. Clinical judgement and prognostic factors in patients with advanced cancer can be conceptualized as attributes of the host, tumour, treatment and interactions between the three reflected in symptoms, QOL performance status, and laboratory tests. Factors due to the host, tumour, or treatment are seen conceptually as more important early in the course of disease, whereas in the advanced stages better indicators relate to patient performance status, symptom burden, and laboratory tests.

The two approaches to constructing a prognosis are the clinical prediction of survival (CPS) and the use of validated prognostic tools. The two approaches are not mutually exclusive and can both be used in a clinical situation to reduce uncertainty.

Clinical prediction of survival (CPS)

In daily clinical practice, the clinical prediction of survival is often used to formulate a prognosis. The main advantage of CPS is the flexibility to the immediate clinical situation, as the validated prognostic tools may not be appropriate for one's patient. To construct a prognosis using CPS, one relies on experience, but this depends on having seen a lot of similar cases and having a reliable memory. Unfortunately, CPS is subject to many cognitive biases including the framing effect (selecting a different prognosis depending on how the information is obtained), anchoring (attributing too much weight to one piece of information), confirmation bias (seeking information that only reinforces the initial choice), and selective recall (remembering only the significant and outlier cases) among others[44,45]. Consulting an 'expert' is not always feasible and is subject to the expert's own biases.

As with all research, the quality of the methodology and reporting of prognostic studies is variable, especially with concern to clinical application and relevancy. Several authors have attempted to review the literature on prognostication in patients with terminal illness and each has commented on the methodological weaknesses—and difficulties interpreting—of the studies, especially the older ones[3,26,27]. Well-designed studies to evaluate the association of prognostic factors with survival need the characteristics shown in Table 3.3.4.

The classic paper on clinicians' CPS in terminal cancer was published in the *British Medical Journal* in 1972 (it is perhaps the ultimate irony that, according to the footnote at the end of the paper, the study was planned and initiated by the late Dr. Ronald Welldon shortly before his own unexpected death in 1969)[46]. Referring doctors, and hospice medical and nursing staff made survival predictions (in weeks) at admission for patients with a cancer diagnosis admitted to St. Christopher's Hospice for 'terminal care'. Although most patients died within 12 weeks, the predictions of survival showed little relation to actual length of survival. Moreover, >80 per cent of the erroneous predictions were overestimated (often incorrect by a factor of two or more).

Subsequently, there have been multiple studies of CPS in advanced cancer with varying types of predictions by doctors and other health-care professionals of varying experience in terminal care[6,7,21–22,47–55]. Table 3.3.5 highlights some of the key studies comparing clinical estimates of survival with actual survival. The diversity of study designs impedes the certainty of clinical prediction accuracy. Most series used temporal predictions of survival, expressed as a continuous variable (i.e. actual number of days or, more usually, weeks). The use of ordinal temporal variables

Table 3.3.4 Characteristics of well-designed studies to evaluate the association of prognostic factors with survival [135].

- A well-defined study population
- Inception cohort design
- Prognostic factors selected are appropriate and clearly defined
- Sample size is adequate for sufficient statistical power
- Clearly defined end point
- Complete follow-up of all patients
- Data analysis is appropriate to test associations between the study factors and survival
- The definition of accuracy is explicit and appropriate
- The prediction tested mirrors clinical language or practice (i.e. not hazard ratios)

(e.g. <3 weeks, <6 months, >1 year) does not always reflect clinical practice, and therefore, it is hard to estimate whether this research is a true reflection of the accuracy of CPS.

Other studies have expressed survival duration as a probability, asking the clinician to estimate the probability of a patient surviving to a certain time point (e.g. what are the chances the patient will survive 2 months or less; 6 months or more; 1 year or more?). These studies hint that physicians may be less prone to error if prognosis is elicited this way[6,21,29,48,51,52,54]. For example, when asked to decide if individual patients had more or less than a year to live, doctors and nurses assigned >1000 hospitalized cancer patients to the correct survival category in >75 per cent of cases, and were as likely to overestimate as underestimate survival[51]. In another study, two physicians had an accuracy of 60 per cent in predicting whether hospice patients would survive 4 weeks or not[52].

Others have asked clinicians to provide upper and lower estimates of survival, or to give the smallest interval that would include 90 per cent of deaths of similar patients. Still others have asked estimators to put patients into temporal groups. Table 3.3.6 provides some illustrative ways that prognoses might be elicited from estimators, with answers that are denominated in different units.

The inaccuracy of temporal prognostication has been confirmed in a systematic review evaluating more than 1500 temporal-prediction

Table 3.3.5 Association of Clinicians' estimates of survival and actual survival in 12 studies.

Author, country	Year	Prognosticator/s	Type of prediction	n	Median predicted survival (weeks)	Median actual survival (weeks)	Percentage of predictions that were accurate	Percentage of predictions that were over-optimistic	Correlation coefficient (where applicable)
Parkes, UK	1972	Hospice doctors	Actual survival (weeks)	74	4.5	~3	8	66	0.28
Scotto, USA	1972	Oncologists	Actual survival (months)	178	NS	NS	NS	52	NA
Evans, UK	1985	Terminal care support team	Upper and lower limits (days)	45	NA	~7	54	37	0.44 (initial prediction)
Heyse-Moore, UK	1987	Referring doctor	Actual survival (weeks)	50	8	2	4	88	<0.001
Forster, USA	1988	University oncologist	Interval of likely death (weeks–months)	101	NA	3.5	NS	1*	0.41
Addington-Hall, UK	1990	Doctors and nurses	Live more or <1 year	1128	NA	17.5	75–83	12	NA
Bruera, Canada	1992	Hospice physicians	Live more or <4 weeks	47	NA	4 (mean)	60	26–34	NA
Maltoni, Italy	1994	Palliative care MD	Actual survival (weeks)	100	6	5	15	63	0.51
McKillop, Canada	1997	Attending physicians	Likely survival (months)	39		~52	75	NS	NA
Oxenham, UK	1998	Palliative care senior registrars	Date of death	30	NS	2.5	NS	NS	0.72
Vigano, Canada	1999	Oncologists	Actual survival (weeks–months)	233	15.3	14.5	52	NS	0.47
Christakis, USA	2000	GPs, internists, oncologists	Actual survival (weeks–months)	468	18	3.5	20	63	0.28
Llobera, Spain	2000	Oncologists, GPs	NS	200	NS	7.5	22–27	55–63	0.18–0.54

NA = not applicable NS = not stated.

*'Seriously' over-optimistic, according to authors.

Table 3.3.6 Ways in which prognoses might be elicited, with answers denominated in different units.

♦ 'What is your best estimate of how long this patient has to live?'

♦ 'What is your best estimate of this patient's percentage chance of surviving for 7/30/90/180/360 days or more?'

♦ 'Of 100 such patients, how long would it typically be before 20/50/80 died?'

♦ 'How likely is this patient to live for 7/30/90/180/360 days or more?'

♦ 'Into which of the following categories is the patient's survival most likely to fall: 0–7, 8–30, 31–90, 91–180, or 181–365 days?'

---

actual survival dyads[56]. The heterogeneity of the studies makes formal meta-analysis impossible but the pooled results demonstrates CPS consistently overestimates survival by 45 per cent. CPS was correct to within 1 week of actual survival in only 25 per cent cases, and overestimated actual survival by at least 4 weeks in 27 per cent. With longer clinical estimates, there was a wider range of actual survival. Nevertheless, although the level of agreement between CPS and actual survival was low (weighted kappa 0.36), they were highly correlated, with R2 = 0.51 for log transformations of both. Data from a study of more than 500 terminally ill patients (median survival 24 days) referred to hospices, suggests the extent of prognostic error varied depending on both observed and predicted survival[47]. Because physicians generally overestimated, the longer the observed survival, the lower the error. Conversely, the longer the predicted survival, the greater the error[57].

Different aspects of CPS have been studied to see if any identifiable variables in accuracy are present apart from the clinical factors influencing prognosis. Repeated estimates are thought to be more accurate as more clinical information is obtained and the rate of change is observed, which reflects the dynamic nature of prognosis. In the original Parkes study, doctors were actually less accurate a week later. Subsequently, several investigators found doctors' ensuing predictions on the same patients correlate more strongly with survival than their initial ones[6,55,58]. The accuracy of CPS in patients within the last few months of life has only been studied to a limited extent. In one study where patients had a median survival of 15 weeks, physicians were most likely to be correct (positive predictive value 74 per cent) when predicting a short survival (<2 months), but they only predicted this in a small number (31 per cent) of the patients who actually survived <2 months[21]. Other studies have found worse accuracy with predicting the survival of those closest to death[9,31,59] when compared with predictions of those more likely to survive. This perceived pessimism could have impacts on determining futility arguments and in counselling patients and families appropriately about their probabilities of survival.

In the Parkes paper, no significant differences were found among the accuracy of predictions made at referral by GPs, hospital doctors, hospice doctors, ward sisters, and senior nurses[46]. Several subsequent studies have mostly found no differences in the prognostic abilities of health-care workers from different disciplines, although the numbers of prognosticators were usually small [6,21,22,47,50]. One recent British study found that while doctors were the best initial predictors, nurse auxiliaries became very accurate in the last few days of life (r = 0.98), presumably because of the amount of time they spend with the patient[55].

In one study, the correlation between CPS by palliative care specialists and actual survival increased with clinician experience, and as a group these prognosticators made errors (using the Parkes criterion, i.e. predicted survival = actual survival ± 100 per cent) in only 30 per cent cases, although most errors were overestimates[7]. Another recent study demonstrated that only 20 per cent of the doctors' predictions were accurate (predicted survival = actual survival ± 33 per cent), 63 per cent were overestimates (predicted survival > actual survival + 33 per cent), and 17 per cent were underestimates (predicted survival < actual survival –33 per cent)[47]. Multivariate modelling shows most types of doctors are prone to error in most types of patients, although the greater the experience of the doctor the greater their prognostic accuracy; however, the stronger the doctor–patient relationship, the lower prognostic accuracy. The foundations of these correlations has yet to be explored and detailed comprehensively, although the leading hypothesis is the avoidance of the pessimistic predictions by the physician because of being close to the patient. This suggests that the dispassionate, experienced physician is likely to be the more accurate prognosticator and raises the concept of seeking a 'second opinion' when a definitive prognosis is required.

Despite the limitations of CPS, it has been retained as anindependent predictor of survival on multivariate analysis of a range of possible prognostic variables by several different investigators[48,60]. Understanding clinicians' reasoning behind their estimates of life expectancy might provide useful insights into consideration and valuation of select clinical and social information[61]. Only one study has explored what prognostic factors are used for CPS in advanced cancer[62]. The Italian oncologists who were surveyed mainly relied on tumour-related factors when formulating their predictions. This finding may partly explain the inaccuracy of CPS.

Statistical estimate of survival

Other ways of predicting survival duration have been investigated, primarily in patients with cancer. Using tables with data from multiple patients and their outcomes, these statistical tables and tools can be helpful in obtaining a general prognosis. The main advantage of these objective estimates is the elimination of some of the cognitive biases of CPS. Research commencing within the field of clinical psychology has shown statistical methods are superior to clinical judgement in predicting human behaviour and other outcomes[63]. Statistical estimates use empirically established relationships between data and the condition or event of interest.

Throughout the clinical medicine, simple scoring systems such as the Glasgow Coma Scale and the Killip class of myocardial infarction have proved useful. In cancer medicine, both physiological and psychological factors have been investigated for their ability to compare the accuracy of estimation of survival time. Several attempts have been made to combine one or more of the factors known to predict for survival in the terminally ill (performance status, symptoms, QOL, and biological parameters) into a parsimonious mathematical model that can be used at the bedside to improve clinicians' estimates of survival. Although there are data supporting the accuracy of these models, the clinical use is limited by availability and awareness, especially as most research of any of these models is often done only at the originating institution. In addition, there can be difficulties with inter-rater reliability limiting their wide use, but this can often be overcome with training[64].

Performance status

Various factors have been associated with survival, including demographics (age, gender, and marital status), tumour-associated factors (primary site, histology, and stage), performance status, symptoms, and psychological well-being: almost 150 different variables that have been evaluated for their ability to predict survival (see Table 3.3.7)[65-67]. Of all of them, performance status has been studied the most extensively and consistently shows an association with survival duration. The major performance scales for palliative care will be covered.

Karnofsky Performance Status (KPS)

Ever since the development of the KPS scale in the 1940s to assess the effects of chemotherapy on functional level, performance status has been recognized as a predictor of oncological outcomes, including survival (see Table 3.3.8). The first study to evaluate clinical variables as predictors of survival in advanced cancer evaluated the KPS[68]. The authors aimed to comprehensively establish the statistical properties of the KPS scale. In order to demonstrate its validity, the association of KPS score with other clinical variables including duration of survival was evaluated. The study found a poor performance status (KPS score <50 per cent) was associated with a short survival. Many other authors have subsequently confirmed this association between KPS score and survival in advanced cancer[6,7,22,26,64,65].

The National Hospice Study (USA) in the early 1980s involved over 1000 patients referred to hospice programmes, with an overall median survival of 37 days[64]. The KPS score accounted for only a small amount of the variability in survival, but was highly statistically significant. In general, each increase in KPS level (e.g. from 10 to 20) accounted for approximately 2 weeks of the remaining life span in this study. Furthermore, the KPS scores were used to group patients into survival risk classes (KPS score 10–20 per cent: median survival 2 weeks; KPS score 30–40 per cent: 7 weeks; KPS score ≥50 per cent: 12 weeks).

It is unclear whether the KPS is a better prognostic indicator than the clinician's prediction of survival and neither has much positive predicative value for individual survival to a certain time point. One group found that KPS score was more strongly correlated with survival than the clinician's estimate made at the initial visit[6], while others came to the opposite conclusion. The latter study showed that the clinician's estimate and KPS score were closely correlated(r = 0.61)[69], and it is possible that that experienced clinicians have trained themselves to base their CPS on performance status score when formulating the prognosis, so that it is like an 'intervening variable', to borrow an epidemiological concept. Patient-rated KPS scores provide independent prognostic information in addition to physician-rated KPS scores [26]. As such, it may be that experienced clinicians have trained themselves to base CPS on performance status when formulating a prognosis. An additional problem with KPS relates to the wording used at lower performance scores where it indicates that hospitalization is necessary, something common in the 1950s but not necessarily so with the development of home hospice programmes, or that special care is required. Two modifications have attempted to address these wording issues[70,71].

Palliative Performance Scale (PPS)

The PPS was developed in Canada to address the limitations of KPS and to add categories for oral intake and conscious levels (see Table 3.3.9)[72]. Initial testing of PPS showed that performance status in terminal cancer could be used for predicting various outcomes including short-term survival. For example, all patients admitted to a hospice unit with a PPS of 10 per cent died in the unit, with an average survival of 1.9 days, while 56 per cent of those with a PPS of 40 per cent on admission died in the unit, with an average survival of 10 days.

Similar results have been obtained for inpatients admitted to an Australian palliative care unit[73], while PPS scores were highly correlated with KPS scores (Spearman's ρ = 0.94) in Japanese patients admitted to a palliative care unit and an overall median survival of approximately 1 month, stratifying them into three homogenous survival groups (PPS 10–20 per cent, median survival 6 days; PPS 30–50 per cent, median survival 41 days; and PPS 60–70 per cent, median survival 108 days)[74]. This grouping was also seen in a community-based hospice[75].

Another study of 733 Canadian patients showed admission PPS score as a strong predictor of survival in patients already identified as palliative, along with gender and age, but diagnosis was not significantly related to survival[76]. Further, PPS scores from PPS 10 per cent through to PPS 50 per cent demonstrated distinct survival curves, rather than three PPS bands. Such differences are likely to be attributed to the size and characteristics of the patient populations involved. PPS performs well as a predictor of prognosis in a heterogeneous hospice population, and performs particularly well for nursing home residents and for patients with non-cancer diagnoses[77]. A study of 396 patients admitted to a community-based hospice programme confirmed its predictive ability for PPS scores and length of survival with negative-change scores predictive of patient decline toward death, while stable PPS ratings over time resulted in discharge consideration[75]. Similar associations have been demonstrated in an acute tertiary hospital consultation programme[78]. When these four studies are combined in a meta-analysis, each PPS level is distinct and without grouping[79] (see Fig. 3.3.1).

PPSv2, a minor wording clarification, is emerging as a strong predictor of survival in palliative patients. An inter- and intra-rater

Table 3.3.7 Physicians' overestimates of patient survival, by observed and predicted survival[47].

	Per cent overestimate in survival (mean)	n
Observed duration of survival (days)		
1–30	795	251
31–90	288	130
91–180	136	49
>180	71	38
Overall	526	468
Predicted duration of survival (days)		
1–30	192	150
31–90	382	144
91–180	501	119
>180	1872	55
Overall	526	468

Table 3.3.8 Karnofsky Performance Scale[264,265].

Percentage of normal performance status	Karnofsky definitions
100	Normal; no complaints; no evidence of disease
90	Able to carry on normal activity; minor signs or symptoms of disease
80	Normal activity with effort; some signs or symptoms of disease
70	Cares for self; unable to carry on normal activity or do active work
60	Requires occasional assistance, but is able to care for most of his needs
50	Requires considerable assistance and frequent medical care
40	Disabled; requires special care and assistance
30	Severely disabled; hospitalization is indicated although death not imminent
20	Very sick; hospitalization necessary; active supportive treatment necessary
10	Moribund; fatal process progressing rapidly
0	Dead

Table 3.3.9 Palliative Performance Scale v2[72].

PPS level	Ambulation	Activity level	Evidence of disease	Self-care	Intake	Conscious level
100	Full	Normal activity	No evidence of disease	Full	Normal	Full
90	Full	Normal activity	Some evidence of disease	Full	Normal	Full
80	Full	Normal activity with effort	Some evidence of disease	Full	Normal or reduced	Full
70	Reduced	Unable normal job/work	Some evidence of disease	full Full	Normal or reduced	Full
60	Reduced	Unable hobby/house work	Significant disease	Occasional assistance necessary	Normal or reduced	Full or confusion
50	Mainly sit/lie	Unable to do any work	Extensive disease	Considerable assistance necessary	Normal or reduced	Full or drowsy or confusion
40	Mainly in bed	Unable to do any work	Extensive disease	Mainly assistance	Normal or reduced	Full or drowsy or confusion
30	Totally bed bound	Unable to do any work	Extensive disease	Total care	Reduced	Full or drowsy or confusion
20	Totally bed bound	Unable to do any work	Extensive disease	Total care	Minimal sips	Full or drowsy or confusion
10	Totally bed bound	Unable to do any work	Extensive disease	Total care	Mouth care only	Drowsy or coma
0	Dead	–	–	–	–	–

Instructions: PPSv2 level is determined by reading left to right to find a 'best horizontal fit.' Begin at left column reading downwards until current ambulation is determined, then, read across to next and downwards until each column is determined. Thus, 'leftward' columns take precedence over 'rightward' columns. Also, see definitions of terms to interpret PPSv2 accurately. With permission from Victoria Hospice Society.

reliability study of 53 physicians and nurses showed a high intra-class correlation coefficient 0.96 (CI 0.864, 0.886) and was found useful for prognostication, transitional-point disease monitoring, care planning, communication, resource allocation, administrative planning, and research[80].

Other performance status scales

Other performance status ratings have not been investigated as extensively as KPS score. The Eastern Cooperative Oncology Group-Performance Status (ECOG-PS) scale has been shown to be predictive of survival in advanced cancer[26,81,82]. Activity of daily living scores have also been associated with survival of cancer patients[83].

Symptoms

The onset of various symptoms is associated with poor survival in patients with advanced cancer. Classic work on this topic was first published by Alvin Feinstein in the mid-1960s, wherein it was argued that symptoms are a more robust indicator of cancer progression/prognosis than alternative pathology-based systems[66]. Weight loss has long been identified as an indicator of adverse outcomes in oncology[81].

The National Hospice Study was re-examined to determine if symptom profile could supplement the accuracy of KPS score in accurately predicting survival[84]. This study showed that 5 of 14 symptoms evaluated were predictive of survival, i.e. anorexia,

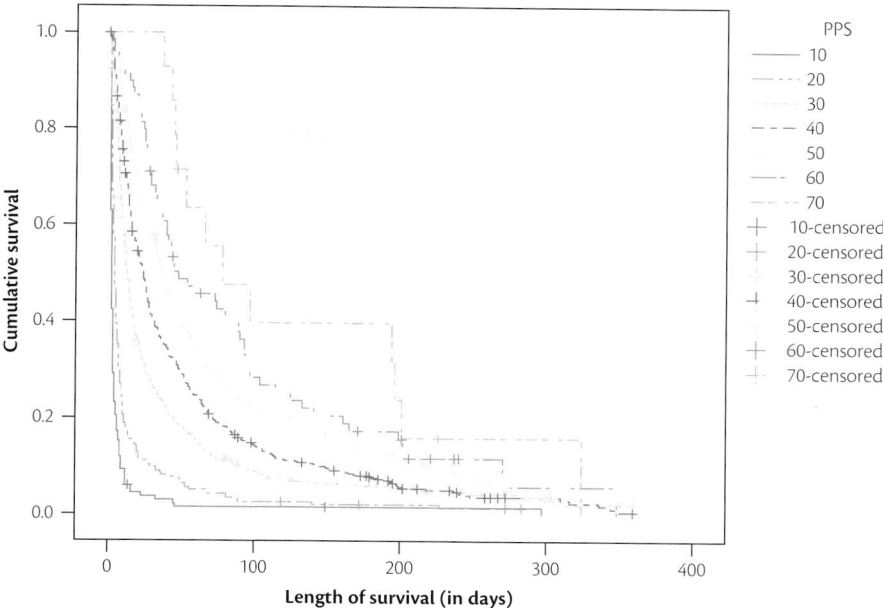

Figure 3.3.1 Kaplan–Meier plot of survival by PPS score.

weight loss, xerostomia, dysphagia, and dyspnoea. For example, patients with a KPS score >50 per cent and none of the five key symptoms had a median survival of approximately 6 months and a small (10 per cent) chance of living for 1.5 years; on the other hand, patients with similar performance status and all five symptoms had a median survival of only 2 months and a 10 per cent chance of living for 9 months. In patients with poor performance status, symptoms had less of an absolute impact on survival: those with a KPS score of 10–20 per cent and no symptoms had a median survival of 8 weeks, while those with the lowest KPS scores and all the symptoms had a median survival of 2 weeks.

The strongest association between a symptom and survival is for anorexia–cachexia. Generalized debility and weakness may be the terminal syndrome or pathway, prompting some to call cachexia the 'final common pathway' in patients dying from cancer[26,85–87]. Subsequent to the National Hospice Study, several other authors have also found dyspnoea to be significant for predicting survival[8,60,82,88,89]. Although not evaluated in the NHO study, there is also compelling evidence for cognitive failure/confusion as a predictor of a poor survival in far advanced cancer, and a small study of patients admitted to a Canadian PCU was one of the first to explore this link between cognitive failure and poorsurvival. Patients with a Mini-Mental State examination score of <24, weight loss, and dysphagia had an increased risk of surviving <4 weeks[52]. Somewhat surprisingly, neither anorexia nor dyspnoea were predictive of a short survival in that study. A number of others since[22,53,88,90]—but not all[82]—have confirmed the adverse prognostic import of confusion in advanced cancer.

Even though episodes of severe, uncontrollable pain and breathlessness have been reported to be more common in the last few weeks of life[91], pain is not usually considered to be predictive of poor survival[52,84]. This may reflect a lead-time bias in the studies, most of which have not involved an inception cohort—as pain is often a trigger for palliative care referral. Similarly, treatment with opioids does not have any impact on survival rate according to several groups of investigators[82,92,93]. Sustained tachycardia ≥100/min,

tachypnoea ≥24/min, and PPS ≤50 per cent were shown to be independent predictors of survival (median 32 days to death) in a study of 98 cancer patients followed at home[94].

Quality of life (QOL)

The relationship between symptoms and survival may be broadened to include the prognostic implications of measures of 'QOL', in part because various symptom checklists have been proposed as QOL measures. A Canadian study of 434 patients with cancer who were within the first 6 months of diagnosis and had a median survival after enrolment of 300 days found that Symptom Distress Scores (SDS) were highly correlated with survival ($r = -0.49$)[95]. Fatigue, insomnia, frequent pain, and 'outlook' were the symptoms most commonly attributed as high distress, but not anorexia, (and notably, weight loss, dysphagia, and dry mouth are not included in the SDS). Similar to performance status, low symptom distress scores did not guarantee long-term survival, but in patients with high symptom distress virtually all had short survival times. There were significant differences in levels of symptom distress according to disease site. The physical symptom subscale scores of the Rotterdam Symptom Checklist[96] and the Memorial Symptom Assessment Scale[97] have been identified as QOL measures to independently predict survival in selected populations.

The role of psychological factors in cancer survival has been controversial for more than two decades. A well-known study of over 350 newly diagnosed cancer patients conducted in the 1980s by Cassileth *et al.* found that 'the inherent biology of the disease [cancer] alone determines the prognosis'[98], and others have confirmed this finding more recently[99]. On the other hand, equally well-known studies like those by Greer, Pettingale, and Speigel have identified psychosocial aspects of cancer survivors, such as the 'fighting spirit'[100–102]. Qualitative research of 'terminally ill' cancer patients who were exceptionally long survivors showed that they adopted an 'active coping stance', characterized by belief in recovery, positive intentionality, a meaningful relationship with one doctor, and an intense desire to stay alive[103]. Recently, a prospective study of psychosocial issues and breast cancer survival by Greer and colleagues found a significantly increased risk of death from all causes by 5 years in women with high scores for depression and helplessness/hopelessness but there were no significant results found for 'fighting spirit'[104]. Despite these previous studies, a 2002 systematic review of 26 studies on psychological coping strategies in cancer has demonstrated little consistent evidence and at most weak associations in methodologically flawed studies[105].

The relationship between survival and patient-related QOL has been examined for advanced cancer in the oncology literature, and there is some evidence of an association. A significant association has been reported between patient-rated well-being and survival time in women receiving treatment for advanced breast cancer[106], and patients' perception of well-being, measured by the Functional Living Index-Cancer (FLIC) instrument (a patient self-rated, cancer-specific QOL questionnaire) is more important in predicting survival in advanced lung cancer than other predictors like KPS score or weight loss[107]. Patients with high FLIC scores lived twice as long (6 months) as those with low scores (3 months). In patients with metastatic melanoma, various measures of QOL (Spitzer QLI, VAS for mood, appetite, and global QOL) have also been shown to be independent predictors, along with KPS score and liver secondaries, of survival[108]. Global QOL scores measured using the EORTC QLQ C30, along with weight loss, have been shown to be a strong prognostic indicator in a study of patients with inoperable lung cancer[109]. In the univariate analysis, a number of QOL subscales, symptoms (anorexia, fatigue, and dyspnoea), and performance status were also significant, but they all dropped out in the multivariate analysis.

The Spitzer Quality of Life Index (SQLI) has been evaluated for its ability to reduce prognostic uncertainty[51]. In patients estimated to live <1 year, there was a trend for those with a low SQLI score to be more likely to die within 6 months than those with a high SQLI. However, the individual patients' scores were not strong predictors of 6-month survival. For example, while 86 per cent of patients who died within 6 months had a SQLI score <7, 65 per cent of those with a SQLI <7 were still alive at 6 months.

Measuring QOL in patients with terminal cancer is fraught with difficulties: (1) the usual QOL definitions and tools are not very applicable in dying patients; (2) short survival and poor cognitive function makes QOL data difficult to collect; and (3) the use of ratings by proxies has only limited value[110]. A validated Italian QOL questionnaire designed for use in hospice/palliative care, the Therapeutic Impact Questionnaire (TIQ) uses four-point Likert scales to rate four major components of QOL—physical symptoms, function, psychological state, and family, and social relationships. Global well-being is also evaluated. Of all the data provided by TIQ, only the patient-rated perception of cognitive function and global well-being showed independent prognostic value. Patients had median survivals of 137, 50, and 17 days for impairment of neither, one, or both scales, respectively[90].

The association between QOL and survival raises the same issues as with any other statistical association: what is the causality? Does the patient's QOL actively influence the natural history of the disease and therefore the survival, or is the QOL merely a reflection of the severity of the illness, progressing inexorably towards death? This issue has been controversial for more than two decades, and needs well-designed clinical trials of interventions that improve quality of life to answer it. Other non-medical factors that influence survival include marital status and socio-economic status[18]. Marital status has been shown to modify the effect of QOL on survival in cancer patients[107].

Biological parameters

Biological parameters are associated with survival of patients with early-stage cancer undergoing treatment. This observation includes both complex biological parameters, such as pathological grade and tumour receptor status, and simple biological parameters such as sodium, albumin, and lymphocyte levels[111]. Hyponatremia has been recognized as a predictor of a poor outcome in lung cancer for >20 years and was the first biological variable to be evaluated with respect to advanced cancer[50].

Interest in simple biological parameters as prognostic markers in advanced cancer has gradually increased in the past decade. An Australian study in the early 1990s found a single biological parameter—elevated serum bilirubin—to be one of only four diverse predictors for survival on admission to a palliative care unit[82]. An Italian group undertook the first large multi-centre study of simple biological factors in advanced cancer[112]. They collected blood and urine from 530 patients in 22 palliative care centres who had a median survival of 32 days. Univariate analysis of survival found the following were all associated with reduced survival: high total white blood cells (WBC), high neutrophil percentage, low lymphocyte percentage, low serum pseudocholinesterase, low serum albumin, and elevated proteinuria. On multivariate analysis, only high total WBC and low lymphocyte percentage retained independent prognostic significance.

The pro-inflammatory cytokines such as interleukin-6 have been recently implicated in the genesis of the anorexia–cachexia syndrome[113]. C-reactive protein (CRP) is a readily available marker for inflammation and several simple objective prognostic scores incorporating CRP scores have been developed in advanced cancer, of which the B12/CRP index is highlighted below. Other parameters that have been evaluated include elevations of serum alpha-1-acid glycoprotein, alkaline phosphatase, lactate dehydrogenase, and pseudocholinesterase.

Prognostic tools and models in advanced cancer

There is the potential to combine various simple clinical and laboratory factors which are easily evaluated and measured in terminally ill cancer patients to provide physicians with accurate information about prognosis (e.g. 'x per cent chance of surviving y days'). Yet caution is needed in interpreting any studies or systematic reviews on survival prediction and prognostic models. First, it is important to distinguish those based on the general population at large from ones within a defined palliative or hospice population. A strong consideration must be given for the 'zero-time' issue, which is the analytic impact of the selection of the time at which measurements of survival begins[114–116]. Second, even in a defined palliative population, attempting to compare published data with one's own palliative programme requires attention to the demographics and included/excluded criteria. There is often a difference between patients admitted directly to an acute tertiary palliative care unit compared with those cared for at home or admitted to a hospice facility. The former admissions are usually for urgent symptom assessment and management and as such, may have shorter survival data due to patient complications and difficult symptoms.

Some hospice residences will have a somewhat more stable population at least on admission. Third, prognostic scores with statistical significance will follow a Kaplan–Meier curve for the subset analysed but the location on that graph for each individual's death is less obvious, in fact indeterminate without other factors being taken into consideration.

A recent systematic review of survival prediction tools for use in a palliative population focused on those where some validation was evident[117].

Of an original screening of 975 citations, 28 studies met the inclusion criteria and were reviewed. Fifteen studies with adequate quality assessment ratings were selected for synthesis[118–133]. Ten prognostic tools were featured and grouped into four non-disease-specific tools (PaP, PPS, PIMOA, and MRIS), four disease-specific tools in cancer (PPI, CPS, ICMRM, and LCPM), and two disease-specific tools in non-cancer (HFRSS and DMI). Many of these are described in the sections above and below.

Attempts to develop prognostic models for advanced cancer have been based on similar models in early stage cancer where, for example, 61 biological variables were assessed for their prognostic value prior to commencement of chemotherapy in 400 patients with small cell lung cancer[111]. Multiple regression analysis revealed that only tumour stage, KPS score, and four biochemical variables (serum sodium, bicarbonate, alkaline phosphatase, and lactate dehydrogenase levels) were important. Combining these six factors into a simple scoring system (the 'Manchester Index'), the authors were able to accurately distinguish patients belonging to three different prognostic groups, the best of which contained all long-term survivors whereas the poor prognostic group contained no patient surviving >1 year.

In patients with advanced cancer, many studies have developed multiple regression models to determine the association between prognostic factors and survival, but few have tested the predicative accuracy of their final models, a key step in prognostic model building[63,134,135]. Ten of the better developed ones are discussed in more detail here, five of which have been developed since the last edition of this textbook.

Australian study[82]

The Australian study of patients with far advanced cancer requiring inpatient care was the first tool to apply various clinical and physiological variables to predict survival in patients with advanced cancer. Multivariate analysis of 19 variables identified four that were independently prognostic:

1 poor performance status (ECOG-PS);

2 hyperbilirubinemia;

3 hypotension; and

4 need for hospice admission at first clinic visit.

Patients were then categorized into 16 groups depending on which combination of these factors was present or not, and then these groupings were used to stratify patients into three survival groups: <1 month, 1–3 months, or >3 months. The positive predicative value of the 16 groups for the stratification was low, ranging from 0.41 to 0.79 (median 0.5).

SUPPORT study[136]

This study was designed to identify deficiencies in the care of patients with eventually fatal illnesses (only some of who had cancer) and

who were hospitalized, making it difficult to compare with the other data about terminal cancer. Nevertheless, this study is relevant because it aimed to use accurate prognostic information as the cornerstone of improved decision-making about end-of-life care in hospitals. Based on the APACHE system for prognostication in critically ill patients in ICUs, individuals' clinical and physiological parameters were utilized in a complex algorithm that was computer-generated and gave a probability for the hospitalized patient being alive in 2 and 6 months' time[136–138]. While the mathematical model is complex and not suitable for routine use by the clinician at the bedside and the information provided (chance of being alive in 6 months) is relevant to only a small minority of cancer patients referred to hospice/palliative care, it shows that application of epidemiological methodology has the potential to provide the clinician with accurate prognostic data.

Palliative Prognostic (PaP) score[60]

The Italian group who have identified elevated white cell count and low lymphocyte percentage as predictive of a poor survival have looked at combining these laboratory values with other parameters to develop a simple model for predicting survival that is useful for the palliative care/hospice clinician. As a result of multivariate analysis of more than 30 parameters, performance status, symptoms, and the haematological parameters are included with the clinician's estimate of survival in the final mathematical model. Points are allocated for each of these factors, and these sub-scores are then summed to give a final score, known as the PaP score which predicts for short-term survival, as shown in Table 3.3.10.

In developing the PaP Score system, the investigators found that this model is highly predictive of short-term survival and is able to split a heterogeneous sample of patients with far advanced cancer (median survival around 30 days) into three groups, i.e. those with a high (>70 per cent), intermediate (30–70 per cent), and low (<30 per cent) chance of still being alive in 30 days. The range of PaP scores, readily calculable at the bedside at the time of first contact with the patient, is 0–17.5, higher scores representing worse survival. Cut points of 5.5 and 11 for the three groups (i.e. 0–5.5 for the high probability group, 6–11 for the intermediate and 11.5–17.5 for the low probability group) have been identified.

The PaP score has been subsequently validated by the investigators in almost 500 Italian patients, the overwhelming majority of whom were being visited by community care teams[92], and independently in 100 hospitalized terminally ill patients in Australia[139] and hospitalized oncology patients[140].

Palliative Performance Index (PPI)

The PPI was developed from an earlier Simple Indicator[88] and is defined by functional status (using PPS), oral intake, oedema, dyspnoea at rest, and delirium with points scored to a maximum of 15 points. Three risk groups are calculated Group A (<2.0), Group B (2.0–4.0), and Group C (>4.0)[141] (see Table 3.3.11).

Cancer prognostic score

This Taiwanese study of 356 terminal cancer patients is used to predict short-term survival of 1 and 2 weeks using a seven-item scale including liver and lung metastases, functional performance status, weight loss, oedema, cognitive impairment, tiredness, and ascites which were all independently associated with shorter survival[128].

Table 3.3.10 How to compute PaP score[60].

	Partial score
Dyspnoea	
No	0
Yes	1
Anorexia	
No	0
Yes	1.5
Karnofsky performance status	
≥30 per cent	0
10–20 per cent	2.5
Clinician's estimate of survival (weeks)	
>12	0
11–12	2
7–10	2.5
5–6	4.5
3–4	6
1–2	8.5
Total white cell count	
≤8.5	0
8.6–11.0	0.5
>11	1.5
Lymphocyte percentage	
20–40 per cent	0
12–19.9 per cent	1
<12 per cent	2.5
Risk groups:	**Total score**
A (30-day survival probability >70 per cent)	0–5.5
B (30-day survival probability 30–70 per cent)	5.6–11
C (30-day survival probability <30 per cent)	11.5–17.5

Table 3.3.11 Calculation of the Palliative Performance Index.

Factor	Partial score
PPS 10–20 per cent	4
PPS 30–50 per cent	2.5
PPS >50 per cent	0
Delirium	4
Dyspnoea at rest	3.5
Oral intake mouthfuls or less	2.5
Oral intake reduced but more than mouthfuls	1
Oral intake normal	0
Oedema	1

Total score (sum of partial scores) and expected survival

◆ Group A (total score <2.0): >6 weeks
◆ Group B (2.0–4): 3–6 weeks
◆ Group C (>4.0): <6 weeks

Manchester Index, GBU has little relevance to the palliative care population, but it helps to further this interesting concept.

Poor prognostic indicator[52]

In a Bruera study, poor prognosis was considered to exist in any patient who demonstrated weight loss of 10 kg or more plus cognitive failure (Mini-Mental State Questionnaire >24) plus dysphagia to solids or liquids, with a probable survival of >4 weeks.

Scores based on biological makers

Several prognostic scores based on serum CRP levels and other biological markers have been developed in advanced cancer in the last 5 years. One is the so-called Glasgow Prognostic Score that combines CRP and albumin and has been shown to predict survival in recently diagnosed patient with advanced lung or upper gastrointestinal malignancies[143,144], even though the evidence for hypoalbuminemia as a prognostic marker is conflicting[82,145]. Another is the product of B-12/CRP index (BCI)[146]. The BCI is the product of serum vitamin B12 level (pmol/l) and serum CRP level (mg/l). In one study, 329 patients with advanced cancer were stratified into three groups based on the BCI. Those patients with a BCI > 40 000 had a median survival 29 days and had a significantly ($p < 0.01$) worse survival than patients with a BCI between 10 001 and 40 000 (median survival 43 days) and patients with a BCI 10 000 (median survival 71 days).

Most recently, the accuracy of 2-month survival predictions based on performance status and fatigue alone have been shown to be improved by including albumin, LDH, and lymphocyte percentage to the model[147]. Another group has developed a prognostic model in a population with advanced cancer who a median survival of approximately 6 months that includes brain metastases, performance status, dyspnoea, morphine use, WBC, and LDH as adverse prognostic factors (and colorectal and breast primary sites as protective)[31].

Intra-Hospital Cancer Mortality Risk Model (ICMRM)

This could be a useful tool for clinicians to predict the likelihood of dying of cancer following hospital admission. It uses ECOG-PS level 4, short duration of illness, emergency admission, low haemoglobin, and high LDH. It had a ROC area of 0.82–0.88 in the derivation and the validation cohort with a median survival of 8 days[129].

GBU index[142]

Over the past 10 years, the North Central Cancer Treatment Group (USA) has also identified performance status and nutritional factors as being predictive of short-term survival in patients enrolled in chemotherapy trials. Recently, this group has reported the 'GBU' (i.e. good, bad, or uncertain) Index which, like the Australian model and the 'Simple Indicator', uses combinations of four factors to stratify patients into three prognostic groups (good, bad, or uncertain chance of surviving 1 year). The GBU Index is most useful in patients with performance status scores ECOG 0–1. Like the

Formulating a prognosis in non-cancer diagnoses

Palliative care services often have a broader scope than oncology patients and therefore prognostication in non-malignant conditions is becoming a larger area of focus. Referral to specialist palliative care services may be prompted by any number of triggers (including symptom burden, psychosocial factors, and patient preference). However, one of the factors that will be relevant is the estimated prognosis [148–151]. Difficulty with formulating an accurate prognosis in patients with non-malignant disease has been hypothesized to be one of the barriers to such patients accessing palliative care services[152]. Predicting survival in patients with non-malignant disease is complicated by the different (often slower and/or more unpredictable) 'death trajectories' experienced by such patients compared with patients with advanced cancer. This can mean, for instance, that patients with advanced but 'stable' chronic obstructive airways disease or heart failure may suddenly succumb to an infective exacerbation or an arrhythmia. The risk of dying can fluctuate widely, soaring during acute exacerbations of illness and receding if the process can be stabilized[153]. For example, ER physicians identified 17 per cent of patients admitted for acute exacerbations of heart failure as having <10 per cent chance of surviving 90 days, when in fact 67 per cent did not survive[154]. Clinician's survival estimates for hypothetical COPD patients with respiratory failure revealed marked variability in estimates[155]. It can also mean that patients with advanced Alzheimer's dementia may appear to be very close to death because of poor functional status and loss of independence in the activities of daily living (ADL) but may 'linger' for many months or years before succumbing to a final fatal event.

Most studies of prognosis in terminally ill cancer patients suggest that clinicians' estimates are systematically over-optimistic[56]. However, less research has been undertaken with regard to the accuracy of clinician estimates in non-malignant diseases. Christakis et al.[3] reported that clinicians were more likely to overestimate prognostic assessments for cancer patients than they were for AIDS or other non-cancer patients, although on multiple regression analysis this association did not persist. Lynn et al.[156] found physicians overestimated when predicting 2 month survival in lung cancer patients when compared with predicting 2-month survival in end-stage heart failure. Wildman et al.[59] reported that clinicians underestimated survival when making prognostic estimates in patients with severe acute exacerbations of obstructive lung disease. Thus, although clinician estimates are prone to error in non-cancer patients it is possible that such errors can be inaccurate in either direction.

Formulating a prognosis in these illnesses may be more complicated than with cancer because of the difference in the death trajectories. Many of these illnesses may have precipitous declines that may not be reversible due to acute exacerbations. Nevertheless, there are some similarities with advanced cancer in terms of how one formulates a prognosis in the patient who is terminally ill with a non-cancer diagnosis. Firstly, model of prognostication used in cancer presumably remains relevant: pathology, clinical features, and environmental factors all contribute to the general and individual diagnoses as they do in cancer[35,157,158]. Secondly, performance status seems to be a useful global measure of survival in both types of conditions. Thirdly, the emotional and mental status of the patient and family influences the length of survival. Fourthly, the rate of disease progression is important in both, the rate of hospitalization and the rate of development of new complications being especially important in non-cancer diagnoses.

There are general and specific indicators of the terminal stage of non-cancer diagnoses[148,159,160]. The general indicators are impaired performance status and impaired nutritional status. As for cancer, impaired performance status plays an important role in prognostication; it has been shown to predict mortality in the elderly in several studies[161], and is the basis for the current (USA) National Hospice Organization (NHO) guidelines on prognostication in non-cancer illnesses[162]. Nutritional status is also significant; patients who experience a >10 per cent weight loss over 6 months have been shown to have an increased risk of dying. Decreased serum albumin is also associated with mortality, especially if it is <25 g/dl[163]. When impaired performance status and impaired nutritional status occur together, they are highly predictive of short-term mortality.

Unfortunately, in the SUPPORT study, predictions of having <6 month survival in the subset of patients with CHF, COPD, and chronic liver disease (CLD) but without malignancy, multi-organ system failure or acute respiratory failure were inaccurate[123]. Not only were 70 per cent of individuals who were identified as being expected to die in 6 months still alive at the end of that period, but also 54 per cent of those not expected to die in the period did so. Most strikingly, 41 per cent of patients given <10 per cent chance of surviving 6 months survived beyond this time frame. Even in the last 2–3 days of life, patients with CHF and COPD were given an 80 per cent and 50 per cent chance of surviving 6 months. There has been progress in the development of prognostic models for some non-cancer diseases in the last 5 years.

Guidelines for predicting survival in non-cancer patients

National Hospice and Palliative Care Organization (NHPCO) guidelines

Medicare in the USA provides insurance coverage for patients with advanced disease who opt for palliative care and who agree to forgo further curative treatment. The attending physician must attest that the patient has a prognosis of <6 months 'if the disease follows its usual course'. In 1996, the NHPCO (USA) published guidelines for determining prognosis in non-cancer patients to aid this process[164] and these have been recently updated to reflect subsequent changes in clinical practice[165]. The guidelines suggest that patients should be eligible for hospice care if they have a life-limiting illness, opt for palliative rather disease-modifying care and have either:

1 Documented evidence of progressive disease which may include recent declines in performance status, or

2 Documented decline in nutritional status, either in terms of weight loss of >10 per cent in previous 6 months or a serum albumin <25 g/l.

In addition, the guidelines provide specific advice about prognosticating in heart disease, pulmonary disease, dementia, HIV disease, liver disease, renal failure, stroke, and coma. For example, the guidelines on end-stage pulmonary disease suggest the following prognostic markers:

- dyspnoea at rest, fatigue, decreased functional ability;

- right heart failure;

- hypoxemia at rest on supplemental oxygen;

- hypercapnia (pCO_2 > 50 mmHg);

◆ weight loss >10 per cent body weight in last 6 months; and

◆ resting tachycardia >100/min

Although the NHPCO guidelines are widely disseminated and frequently referenced, relatively few studies have tested the validity of the recommendations. Fox and colleagues[123] undertook a study to assess how well the guidelines worked for patients with advanced heart, liver, or lung disease. In a prospective study of 2607 patients over 36 months, they evaluated whether application of broad, intermediate, or narrow referral criteria would accurately identify patients suitable for hospice admission with an estimated prognosis of <6 months. They found that if a very strict application of NHPCO criteria were used only 19 patients would have been deemed eligible for hospice care, of which 53 per cent would have survived > 6 months. If a very broad interpretation of NHPCO guidelines were used then 923 patients would have been considered eligible for hospice care of which 70 per cent would have survived > 6 months. The authors concluded that the current guidelines were ineffective at identifying patients with heart, lung, or liver failure with a prognosis of <6 months.

A number of studies have assessed the utility of the NHPCO dementia prognostic guidelines (or approximations thereof). One aspect of the dementia guidelines is that patients who reach stage 7c on the Functional Assessment Staging (FAST) system[166] may be considered eligible for enrolment in a hospice programme. In order to reach stage 7c (severe dementia with loss of ambulatory activity) it is necessary to progress through the other stages in order (e.g. loss of self-care abilities and incontinence). Two small studies[167,168] have reported that the NHPCO guidelines did appear to identify patients at higher risk of dying within 6 months. However, the authors commented that since many patients did not follow the progressive (or 'ordinal') decline in functional abilities set out in the guidelines, that sole reliance on this measure would potentially exclude the majority of dementia patients who would benefit from hospice care. In a large retrospective cohort study, Mitchell[169] reported that using stage 7c of the FAST had a predictive ability 'no better than chance' and developed a new prognostic scoring system with a better area under the receiver operating curve. Schonwetter and colleagues have assessed the NHPCO dementia guidelines in two separate studies[132,170] and have found them not to be valid indicators of survival in this population.

National Health Service (NHS) Gold Standards Framework (GSF) Prognostic Indicator Guidance (PIG)

The GSF is a UK, general practice-based, initiative with the aim of improving the quality of care for patients and their carers in the last year of life[171]. In order to improve the care of such patients, the first priority is to identify which patients are expected to live <12 months. To facilitate this process, the GSF central team[172] has produced PIG. The PIG was developed following wide consultation of special interest groups, national disease associations, and reference works. The PIG is similar to the NHPCO guidelines in that there are some general 'triggers' for identifying patients and then some more specific guidance for individual diseases. The general triggers are:

◆ The surprise question—'Would you be surprised if this patient were to die in the next 6–12 months?'

◆ Patient choice for comfort care only, or patient is in special need of supportive/palliative care.

◆ General clinical indicators of poor prognosis—multiple co-morbidities, weight loss >10 per cent, general physical decline, serum albumin <25 g/l, and KPS score <50 per cent.

In addition to these general triggers the PIG includes some specific clinical indicators for patients with cancer, heart disease, COPD, renal failure, Parkinson's disease, motor neuron disease, multiple sclerosis, frailty, dementia, and stroke. Although widely disseminated (over one-third of general practices in the UK are using the GSF) the PIG has never been formally validated and its usefulness as a prognostic guide is therefore is uncertain.

Prognostic scoring systems in non-cancer diagnoses

As with non-cancer patients, attempts have been made to improve clinicians' predictive accuracy by developing or applying prognostic scales. Such scales may broadly be categorized as 'non-disease specific' tools which can be applied in patients with any type of advanced, terminal disease and 'disease specific' tools for use in particular populations (e.g. patients with end-stage heart failure or chronic obstructive airways disease)[117,173].

Non-disease specific tools
Palliative Performance Scale (PPS)

Performance status is an important predictor of survival in some non-cancer populations[161], and PPS scores have been shown to predict survival in patients with non-cancer diagnoses referred to palliative care services[75–78,174]. A prospective cohort study of 466 hospice admissions of whom the majority had diseases other than cancer found that the PPS was a useful guide to prognosis and was most accurate at predicting short survival times (i.e. <1 week)[77]. Patients with an admission PPS 10–20 per cent had a 72 per cent risk of dying within 1 week, whereas patients with a PPS 50–70 per cent only had a 6 per cent risk of death within 1 week. As a 'routine' clinical or nursing assessment for palliative care patients the PPS also lends itself to repeated use. In this context, a decreasing PPS score was predictive of decline or death in hospice patients, while stable PPS scores were predictive of discharge[75].

Studies consistently show that low PPS scores are associated with a poor short-term prognosis, but some uncertainty still exists about how to interpret mid-range scores (PPS 30–60 per cent). Very few palliative care patients will have a PPS score >60 per cent. Another potential problem with the PPS is the difficulty in accurately scoring a patient at one point in time. Although the PPS comes with instructions that clarify some of the ambiguities around classification, in clinical practice there is scope for variation in how individual patients are scored. This ambiguity led nurses in one study[75] to score some patients as 'half-fits' (i.e. scores of PPS 25, 35, or 45 per cent, etc.), a practice not sanctioned by the tool's originators.

Palliative Prognostic (PaP) score

The PaP score has also been used in heterogeneous patient groups[130,175]. One prospective validation study of the PaP score in 100 terminally ill patients—of whom 9 per cent had non-cancer diagnoses—referred to a hospital-based palliative care team found that the three risk groups were broadly replicated[130]. A separate study involving only patients with non-cancer diagnoses (n = 65)[175], reported that patients in Group A had an 86 per cent chance of surviving 30 days (median survival 266 days), patients in Group B had a 56 per cent chance of survival (median = 18.5 days) and

Group C only had a 9 per cent 30-day survival (median = 5 days). However, these validation studies in non-cancer patients have involved very few patients and larger, independent validation studies are required.

Disease specific tools

In addition to these general prognostic scoring indices, other scales have been produced for specific 'advanced' non-cancer diagnoses. Recent systematic reviews[117,173] have identified prognostic scales for heart failure[127], dementia[132,169] and COPD[176–178].

Heart disease

The spectrum of treatment modalities for advanced cardiac disease is illustrated by Dzan and Braunwald[179]. Within this continuum, the role of palliative care finds itself located primarily at end-stage and decreased function. Heart failure is gradually changing from having an unpredictable outcome to one for which there is now a range of easily used prognostic tools[180]. Lee and colleagues[127] undertook a retrospective cohort study of patients newly admitted to hospital with heart failure. Clinical and demographic data were obtained relating to the first 24 h after hospital admission. During the development phase (n = 2624) predictive models were developed for both 30-day and 1-year survival.

As with cancer, biological markers are discussed earlier. For example, BNP[180–184] is showing promise in predicting sudden death[62] either alone or combined with troponin levels and possibly C-reactive protein. In 44 patients dying suddenly of 89 other patients who died more slowly within 3 years of first diagnosis of heart failure and EF <35 per cent, multivariate analysis showed that log BNP level was the only independent predictor of sudden death ($p = 0.0006$) with a cut-off point of log BNP < 2.11 (130 pg/ml)[185].

National Hospice Palliative Care Organization (NHPCO) criteria for heart failure

Age >64 years, New York Heart Association (NYHA) Class, left ventricular ejection fraction <20 per cent, dilated cardiomyopathy, uncontrolled arrhythmias, and systolic hypotension and chest X-ray signs of left heart failure are all associated with poor short-term survival in congestive heart failure. The NHPCO criteria for a prognosis of <6 months are: (1) NYHA Class IV (chest pain and/or breathless at rest/minimal exertion) and (2) already optimally treated with diuretics and vasodilators. Yet, in one study among 282 elderly patients (age 79 ± 6 years) hospitalized with heart failure, median survival was about 2.5 years. However, there is considerable heterogeneity in survival, with 25 per cent of patients dying within 1 year and 25 per cent surviving for more than 5 years. A simple seven-item risk score, based on data readily available at the time of admission, provides a reliable estimate of prognosis[186].

The increased use and value of devices such as left ventricular assist devices (LVAD)[187,188] as a 'bridge to transplant' has migrated into the palliative field. Interestingly in the USA, insertion of LVAD is being used in some hospice patients as a bridge and also for non-eligible transplant patients and known as 'destination therapy,' i.e. until death. These can be placed one time and last for approximately 1 year. Other high-tech devices such as pacemakers and intra-cardiac defibrillators (ICDs) make prognostication challenging.

Seattle heart failure model

Work by Levy et al.[189,190] is seen in a web-based algorithm for chronic heart failure. It was developed and validated in 9942 patients in 6 cohorts and provides an accurate estimate of 1-, 2-, and 3-year survival with the use of easily obtained clinical, pharmacological, device, and laboratory characteristics. The web model is dynamic and shows changes in Kaplan–Meier survival curves as various parameters are inserted. It can be used by clinicians and patients. The tool can be accessed at www.seattleheartfailuremodel.org.

Heart failure risk scoring system (HFRSS)[127,191,192]

Another algorithm is from the Enhanced Feedback for Effective Cardiac Treatment (EFFECT), a Canadian consortium's design. It is web-based (see www.ccort.ca) and designed from a retrospective study of 4031 community-based patients presenting with heart failure at multiple hospitals in Ontario, Canada. Factors identifiable within hours of hospital admission include age, physical (low BP, high RR), laboratory measures (low sodium, high BUN), and several comorbidities. These are used to predict 30-day and 1-year mortality risk. A risk-index stratified the probability of death and identifies low- and high-risk individuals. Patients with very low-risk scores ≤60) had a mortality rate of 0.4 per cent at 30 days and 7.8 per cent at 1 year. Patients with very high-risk scores (>150) had a mortality rate of 59.0 per cent at 30 days and 78.8 per cent at 1 year.

Chronic obstructive pulmonary disease (COPD)

Advanced age, forced expiratory volume at 1 sec (FEV_1) of <30 per cent and pulmonary hypertension with cor pulmonale/right heart failure are poor prognostic signs. The NHPCO criteria include (1) dyspnoea at rest; (2) on 24-h home oxygen with pO_2 <50 mmHg and/or $pCO_2 > 55$ mmHg; (3) documented evidence of cor pulmonale. A recent study of clinician's predictions in COPD found underestimation of survival after admission to the ICU. For example, the quintile of patients with the lowest expected prognosis (10 per cent probability to survive 6 months) had a group survival of 40 per cent at 6 months[59]. The reason for the underestimate is not elucidated in this study but the issue is important for further study as it may impact decisions to admit to the ICU that may be over-weighted towards futility arguments.

Coventry's systematic review[173] of survival prediction in older adults with non-malignant conditions identified three studies[176–178] concerned with prognostication in COPD. These studies suggested that FEV1, VO2max, severity of dyspnoea, quality of life scores, age, and mid-thigh cross-sectional area are all predictive of survival in this population. However, the subjects in these studies had a generally better prognosis than patients who would usually be considered for specialist palliative care programmes. In the Marquis study[176] 82.4 per cent of patients survived more than 41 months and in the Nishimura[177] and Oga[178] studies the 5-year survival was 73 and 78 per cent, respectively. The relevance of these studies to palliative care practice is therefore unclear and more work is required to identify prognostic indicators in advanced COPD.

MRC Dyspnoea Scale[193,194]

The MRC Dyspnoea Scale (grades I–V, Table 3.3.10) appears a better predictor of survival in COPD than FEV_1 staging endorsed by the American Thoracic Society. Of 227 patients enrolled in a 5-year study, 73 per cent survived. The level of dyspnoea was significantly correlated to the 5-year survival rate (p < 0.001). The Cox proportional hazards model revealed that the level of dyspnoea had a more significant effect on survival than disease severity based on FEV_1. They concluded that dyspnoea should be included as one of the variables, in addition to airway obstruction, for evaluating patients with COPD in terms of mortality (see Table 3.3.12)[177,178].

Factors determining in-hospital mortality and long-term survival of patients hospitalized with acute exacerbations of chronic obstructive pulmonary disease (AECOPD) are not precisely understood. A study of 205 patients related to in-hospital mortality and long-term survival after hospitalization revealed that in-hospital mortality was significantly associated with lower arterial oxygen tension (PaO_2), higher carbon dioxide arterial tension, lower arterial oxygen saturation, and longer hospital stay. The overall 6-month mortality rate was 24 per cent, with 1-, 2- and 3-year mortality rates of 33, 39, and 49 per cent, respectively. Cox regression analysis revealed that long-term mortality was associated with longer disease duration (relative risk [RR] = 1.158), lower albumin (RR = 0.411), lower PaO_2 (RR = 0.871), and lower body mass index (RR = 0.830). These findings show patients hospitalized with AECOPD have poor short- and long-term survival and survival prediction may be enhanced by considering arterial oxygen tension, albumin, body mass index, disease duration and time elapsed since the first hospitalization[195].

The characteristics of COPD patients most likely to die within 6–12 months include severe, irreversible airflow obstruction, severely impaired and declining exercise capacity and performance status, older age, concomitant cardiovascular or other co-morbid disease, and a history of recent hospitalizations for acute care[196]. More specifically, the profile of COPD patients at risk for death from acute respiratory failure[196]:

♦ severe airflow obstruction (e.g. FEV_1 <40 per cent predicted);

♦ poor functional status (e.g. MRC 4–5);

♦ poor nutritional status (e.g. BMI < 19 kg/m^2);

♦ older age; and

♦ recurrent acute exacerbation of COPD (especially requiring hospitalization and mechanical ventilation).

Guidelines for management can be found at several websites (http://www.copdguidelines.ca/), (http://www.brit-thoracic.org.uk/copd/consortium.html), and GOLD (http://www.goldcopd.org/)

Elderly patients including nursing facilities

Advanced Illness Index (AII). Brody describes a prognostic indicator to identify persons who have a higher than expected likelihood for death within 3 years developed from a retrospective cohort study[197]. AII is correct in 74.3 per cent for aged adults older than 65 years. It targets a dimension of risk different than frailty alone utilizing 11 variables of gender (female), poor general health, use of oxygen, organ conditions (heart, lung, pancreas), cancer, more than five drug prescriptions, help with ADLs, independently active, smoking, proxy-assisted Health Status Questionnaire, and age.

Prognostic Index for 1-Year Mortality in Older Adults (PIMOA). Few prognostic indices have focused on predicting post-hospital mortality in older adults. PIMOA was developed to assess 1-year mortality of adults 70 years or older after hospital discharge using information readily available at discharge. It uses six risk factors known at discharge and a simple additive point system as follows:

1 male gender (1 point);

2 number of dependent ADLs at discharge (1–4 ADLs, 2 points; all 5 ADLs, 5 points);

3 congestive heart failure (2 points);

4 cancer (solitary, 3 points; metastatic, 8 points);

5 creatinine level higher than 3.0 mg/dl (265 μmol/l) (2 points);

6 low albumin level (3.0–3.4 g/dl, 1 point; <3.0 g/dl, 2 points).

The 1-year mortality rate was 13 per cent with 0–1 points, 20 percent with 2–3 points, 37 per cent with 4–6 points, and 68 per cent with >6 points. Discrimination and calibration was good with area under ROC for the point system on 0.79.

Mortality Risk Index Score (MRIS). The MRIS was designed to predict 1-year mortality in nursing home patients. In a retrospective cohort study Flacker and co-workers[125] extracted data on newly admitted and long-stay residents in US nursing homes. In the development stage (n = 60 341), they produced an 11-item predictive model. This was then validated in a separate cohort (n = 40 328). The MRIS score varied between 0 and 19 and divided patients into 10 iso-prognostic groups. Residents with the best prognostic scores had a 1-year mortality of 11.4–11.8 per cent and those in the worst prognostic category were all dead within 1 year. As with the PIMOA, there is the potential for scores such as MRIS to identify patients 'at risk' of death within the next year and who thus might be suitable for 'flagging' on palliative care registers. However, further validation of the MRIS is required before its usefulness in palliative care practice can be determined.

Alzheimer disease (AD). Schonwetter et al.[132] undertook a study to assess the validity of the NHPCO dementia prognostic guidelines (discussed above) and found them to be of no value at predicting 6-month survival in hospice patients with dementia. However, as part of the same study the authors attempted to identify better predictors of survival in this population. They developed a Dementia Prognostic Model (DMP) which consisted of four variables (age, marital status, anorexia, and an interaction between nutritional status and performance status) that was able to predict 6-month survival significantly better than the NHPCO guidelines. The DMP was reliably able to identify patients with a survival of <6 months (median survival 22.5 days) compared with those patients who could be expected to survive more than 6 months (median survival 271.5 days).

Mitchell et al.[169] also found the NHPCO guidelines to be unhelpful at predicting 6-month survival in dementia patients admitted to nursing homes. They developed a prognostic model in a retrospective cohort study (n = 6799) and validated it in an independent sample (n = 4631). The total prognostic score was

Table 3.3.12 Medical Research Council (MRC) Dyspnoea Scale[193].

Grade	Degree of breathlessness related to activities
1	Not troubled by breathlessness except on strenuous exercise
2	Short of breath when hurrying or walking up a slight hill
3	Walks slower than contemporaries on level ground because of breathlessness, or has to stop for breath when walking at own pace
4	Stops for breath after walking about 100 m or after a few minutes on level ground
5	Too breathless to leave the house, or breathless when dressing or undressing

derived by summing the hazard ratios associated with 12 risk factors; ADL, gender, cancer diagnosis, need for oxygen therapy, heart failure, dyspnoea, reduced food intake, unstable medical condition, bowel incontinence, bed-bound, age, and day-time conscious level. After addition of the partial scores, the result was rounded to the nearest integer. The total score could range between 0–19. Patients in the best prognostic category had a 6-month survival of 91.1–98.5 per cent and patients in the worst prognostic category had a 6 month survival of 19.9–30 per cent.

Both of these scoring systems have undergone a thorough development and testing phase, but both scales require further validation in independent populations before their wider use can be recommended. Given the inherent difficulty of predicting survival in this group, it is possible that one or other of these prognostic tools will eventually have a useful role in the planning and delivery of palliative care services.

The difficult trajectory for AD follows a generally predictable decline in functional and cognitive status. The onset of inability to walk unaided indicates entering the final phase of the protracted illness. In one study, 30 per cent of patients with dementia who were >90 years of age and referred to a US hospice programme were still alive 3 years later[198]. The NHPCO general criteria include:

(1) advanced disease (unable to walk independently and/or hold a meaningful conversation), and (2) onset of medical complications (e.g. aspiration pneumonia, UTI, decubitus ulcers).

A small study of 42 patients with probable Alzheimer's disease were tested by Drachman *et al.* for prognostic value at subsequent follow-up 54 ±25 months later[199]. Potential prognostic features were of three types: degree of severity features (e.g. MMSE/IQ scores); variable clinical features (e.g. extrapyramidal signs); and individual historical features (e.g. gender, education, and age). The degree of severity predicted subsequent dependence but neither historical factors nor clinical signs influenced prognosis. They concluded initial degree of severity (how far) rather than variation in the rate of progression (how fast) best predicts prognosis in the early to intermediate stages of Alzheimer's disease.

Program of All-Inclusive Care for the Elderly (PACE) tool. A multi-dimensional prognostic index was developed and validated using age, sex, functional status, and comorbidities that effectively stratifies frail, community-living elderly people into groups at varying risk of mortality[200]. Eight independent risk factors of mortality were identified and weighted, using Cox regression, to create a risk score (see Table 3.3.13). In the development cohort, respective 1- and 3-year mortality rates were 6 per cent and 21 per cent in the lowest-risk group (0–3 points), 12 per cent and 36 per cent in the middle-risk group (4–5 points), and 21 per cent and 54 per cent in the highest-risk group (>5 points). The 1- and 3-year mortality rates were 7 per cent and 18 per cent in the lowest-risk group, 11 per cent and 36 per cent in the middle-risk group, and 22 per cent and 55 per cent in the highest-risk group.

Dementia Mortality Index. The DMI (132) was developed in a community hospice for predicting 6-month mortality. Significant multivariate predictors of shorter survival include greater age ($p = 0.02$) and anorexia ($p < 0.001$), as well as a combination of anorexia and greater functional impairment ($p = 0.005$). It is however only a single study and needs further validation.

Functional Assessment Staging Tool (FAST). FAST is currently used by the US NHPCO as one criteria in determining eligibility

Table 3.3.13 Programme of all-inclusive care for the elderly (PACE) tool

Factor	Points
Male sex	2
Age 75–84	2
Age ≥85	3
Dependence in toileting	1
Dependence in dressing, partial	1
Dependence in dressing, full	3
Malignant neoplasm	2
Congestive heart failure	3
Chronic obstructive pulmonary disease	1
Renal insufficiency	3

for hospice benefits[201]. It has seven stages with stage 7c as the cut-point. A prospective, follow-up, observational study was undertaken in a cohort of 67 community-based patients aged 65 years or older with dementia defined by DSM-IV and FAST stage 7a or above. A clinical event occurred in 52 (77.6 per cent) patients during the previous year (pneumonia, urinary infection, stroke, pressure sore, dehydration, sepsis, or others). The mean survival was 676 days (95 per cent CI, 600–752 days). Cox proportional hazards model showed that independent prognostic factors for mortality were having pneumonia within the previous year (RR: 3.7; $p = 0.001$), a permanent nasogastric tube (RR: 3.5; $p = 0.003$) and serum albumin values below 3.5 g/dl (RR: 2.9; $p = 0.028$). They concluded that in patients with advanced dementia, hypoalbuminemia and pneumonia are strongly and positively associated with mortality. Artificial nutrition via a nasogastric tube reduces survival in these patients[202].

Luchins *et al.* studied 47 patients enrolled in home hospice and institutional hospice settings. FAST scores and mobility ratings were significantly related to survival time. However, 41 per cent could not be scored on the FAST as their disease progression was not ordinal. Among patients who could be scored on the FAST and who had reached stage 7c, mean survival time was 3.2 months compared with 18 months among those who could be scored and had not reached this stage and 8.6 months among patients whose disease progression was not ordinal ($p < 0.001$). Using NHPCO criteria relying on the FAST allows the identification of a subgroup with very high mortality and a short time until death. Although the FAST can identify a subgroup of appropriate candidates for hospice, sole reliance on this measure might decrease access to hospice care for many dementia patients[167].

RAI-MDS changes in health, end-stage disease and symptom and signs (CHESS)

Although not exclusive for dementia, the Resident Assessment Instrument Minimum Data Set (RAI-MDS) is listed here as an international database developed initially for frail elderly nursing home residents[203,204]. Used for several purposes, subsets called CHESS[205], and Probability of Death[206] have predictive survival significance. These tools have not been validated with other palliative prognostic tools discussed here. MDS is complex and time consuming for staff to complete. A further subset for palliative care

MDS-PC is in draft development and remains unclear for utility in this population.

Only a small proportion of dementia patients get admitted to hospices, in part because of the difficulty in predicting survival. An RAI-MDS study of 11 430 newly admitted nursing home residents with advanced dementia was conducted in order to identify factors associated with 6-month mortality and to create a practical risk score to predict 6-month mortality in this population[169]. MDS factors were determined in the derivation group, and the resulting mortality risk score was evaluated in the validation cohort. Risk score performance was compared with the cut point of 7c on the FAST scale. In the time frame, 28.3 per cent of residents died within 6 months of nursing home admission in the derivation cohort; 35.1 per cent died in the validation cohort. The 6-month mortality rate increased across risk scores (possible range, 0–19): 0 points, 8.9 per cent mortality; 1 to 2, 10.8 per cent; 3 to 5, 23.2 per cent; 6 to 8, 40.4 per cent; 9 to 11, 57.0 per cent; and at least 12, 70.0 per cent in the validation cohort. The area under the receiver operating characteristic (AUROC) curve for predicting 6-month mortality was 0.74 and 0.70 in the derivation and validation cohorts, respectively. This risk score based on 12 variables demonstrated better discrimination to predict 6-month mortality (AUROC, 0.64 for a cut-off of ≥6 points versus 0.51 for FAST stage 7c).

Milan Overall Dementia Assessment (MODA). Ninety-one patients affected by Alzheimer's disease were assessed twice with the MODA scale at an interval of 12 months (53 patients) or 24 months (38 patients). Patients with a slow progression rate in the early stage were unlikely to show a subsequent fast progression rate, and vice versa for patients with a fast early progression. A tool is provided for predicting the speed of cognitive decline of patients from a single MODA assessment[207].

HELP Survival model. The HELP study developed a nomogram for estimating the length of life in the hospitalized elderly (>80 years of age) using a limited amount of clinical information, but has not been widely validated[208] Gender, duration of illness, age at onset, Mini-Mental State Examination score and extrapyramidal or psychotic features were combined in a validated model that predict time to nursing home placement or death for patients with Alzheimer's disease[209].

Amyotrophic lateral sclerosis (ALS)

Prognosis varies widely, but median survival from diagnosis is 3–5 years with a range of 6 months to >20 years[210]. Mandrioli studied 123 patients and noted that Kaplan–Meier survival curves dipped sharply in the first 3 years from diagnosis, followed by a flattening trend, with 50 per cent dying within 2.5 years, and 89 per cent over 7 years. The clinical form with lower limb onset was associated with longer survival than the upper limb onset and bulbar forms (median survival: 39, 27, and 25 months, respectively). Survival was also affected by age at onset (median survival: 34, 27, and 23 months for onset <60, 60–75, and >75 years, respectively), area of residence (median survival: 24 months in mountainous areas, 32 elsewhere), and type of work (median survival: 25 months in agricultural workers, 33.5 in others). Gender did not influence survival, whereas percutaneous endoscopic gastrostomy placement and invasive ventilation did influence survival[211,212].

The Amyotrophic Lateral Sclerosis Functional Rating Scale-revised (ALSFRSr) may have reasonable predictive value. Patients with a total ALSFRSr score below the median of 38 points had a 4.4-fold increased risk of death or tracheostomy compared with those who scored above the median (HR: 4.38, 95 per cent CI: 2.79 to 6.86, $p < 0.001$). Both the total ALSFRSr score at baseline (HR: 0.94, 95 per cent CI: 0.91 to 0.98, $p < 0.001$) and forced vital capacity at baseline (HR: 0.99, 95 per cent CI: 0.98 to 1.00, $p = 0.02$) were associated with death or tracheostomy. It appears that an ALSFRSr score at baseline is a strong predictor of death or tracheostomy independently of forced vital capacity[213].

Clinically relevant easily-identifiable objective information and clinical milestones could have potential prognostic significance when applied to individual patients. In 151 patients, the incidence of respiratory complications included infectious pneumonia 13 (9 per cent), venothromboembolism 9 (6 per cent), and tracheostomy and mechanical ventilation 6 (4 per cent). For 139 patients with serial measurements of forced vital capacity (FVC), median values for calculated rate of decline in FVC was 97 ml/30 days (2.4 per cent predicted/30 days); 25 per cent of patients had FVC rates of decline less than 52 ml/30 days (1.4 per cent predicted/30 days) and 25 per cent had rates of decline >170 ml/30 days (4.4 per cent predicted/30 days). Stratifying patients into two distinct clinical subgroups based upon rates of decline in FVC less than or greater than the median value of 97 ml/30 days identified an apparent twofold increase in survival duration for ALS patients with slower rates of pulmonary physiology deterioration when referenced to either date of dyspnoea onset or time from bi-level positive airway pressure (BiPAP) initiation (2.0 ± 1.4 versus 1.0 ± 0.8 years; 1.9 ± 1.5 versus 1.0 ± 0.9 years, respectively). The correlation between clinically defined milestones, most importantly onset of dyspnoea, and the calculated rate of decline in FVC represent obtainable and objective measurements provide important prognostic information in relation to individual patient survival duration[214].

Several common treatment interventions, enteral feeding, assisted ventilation, and drug therapy are discussed in relation to prognosis. In a prospective 7-month study of 55 ALS patients, malnutrition occurred in 16.4 per cent. Survival was worse for malnourished patients ($p < 0.0001$), with a 7.7-fold increased risk of death. The degree of malnutrition was independent of forms of ALS onset[215].

The use of artificial feeding is common but there is a question about whether a survival benefit exists. Ninety-eight ALS patients (49 male, 49 female; median age 61 years, range 26–86 years) received enteral feeding with either radiological-inserted gastrostomy (RIG), percutaneous endoscopic gastrostomy (PEG) or nasogastric tube (NG). Median survival (95 per cent C.I.) following RIG, PEG, and NG was 6.31 months (4.58–8.04 months), 7.13 months (4.81–9.45 months), and 0.95 months (0.00–2.77 months), respectively. The survival advantage between RIG and PEG was not statistically significant ($p = 0.50$), but for NG versus RIG and PEG groups combined, there was a significant difference ($p = 0.03$). It was concluded that RIG and PEG are equivalent in terms of survival[216].

A systematic review in older persons after PEG tube placement of 5 cohort studies compared survival with and without feeding tubes in nursing homes, but none demonstrated a survival benefit. Another study reported increased survival for tube-fed patients with ALS. The pooled proportion of all subjects surviving after PEG placement was: 1 month = 0.81 (95 per cent CI, 0.74–0.88), 2 months = 0.70 (95 per cent CI, 0.65–0.74), 6 months = 0.56 (95 per cent CI, 0.20–0.92), and 12 months = 0.38 (95 per cent CI, 0.26–0.49). Advanced age and malignancy were the factors most often reported to be associated with poorer survival among subjects with PEG tubes[217]. A Cochrane review concluded the 'best' evidence to date, based on controlled prospective cohort studies, suggests an advantage for survival in all people with ALS/MND, but these conclusions are tentative[218].

Sorenson reported aspiration pneumonia occurred in 13 per cent of ALS cases. There was a mean survival of 2 months following aspiration pneumonia. The strongest risk factor for aspiration pneumonia was nursing home residence with a relative risk of 7.1 ($p = 0.02$)[219].

Another common treatment that may affect survival is the use of non-invasive positive pressure ventilation (NIPPV). A literature review of 12 studies, four retrospective, seven prospective and one randomized, showed that in seven of the 12, NIPPV was associated with prolonged survival in patients tolerant for NIPPV, and five studies reported an improved QOL[220]. NIPPV significantly improved survival compared with those who did not use NIPPV in a study by Shoesmith. This study also showed that ALS patients with respiratory onset do not necessarily follow a rapidly progressive course[221].

Kleopa further assessed the utility of BiPAP in prolonging survival in ALS in 122 patients. All patients were offered BiPAP when their forced vital capacity (FVC) dropped below 50 per cent of predicted value. Group 1 (n = 38) accepted BiPAP and used it more than 4 h/day. Group 2 (n = 32) did not tolerate BiPAP well and used it <4 h/day. Group 3 (n = 52) refused to try BiPAP. There was a statistically significant improvement in survival from initiation of BiPAP in Group 1 (14.2 months) compared with Group 2 (7.0 months, $p = 0.002$) or Group 3 (4.6 months, $p < 0.001$), respectively. In concluding that BiPAP can significantly prolong survival and slow the decline of FVC in ALS, they suggest that all patients with ALS be offered BiPAP when their FVC drops below 50 per cent, at the onset of dyspnoea, or when a rapid drop in per cent FVC is noted[222].

Riluzole was tested in a French study of 2069 patients along with over 100 demographic, biological, clinical, and quality-of-life variables for their effect on survival. Thirteen variables were found to affect survival independently and were used to construct a survival prediction score, RL401. These included age, disease duration, slow vital capacity, intensity of tiredness (visual analogue scale), number of body levels with spasticity, atrophy, and/or fasciculations, cough, distal muscle strength, household income, depression and two biological parameters, plasma creatinine levels and neutrophil counts. A simplified score, RL401S, was constructed, designed to be easy to use and interpret. The predictive powers of the two scores were similar[223].

In another study of 841 patients with ALS seen over a 10-year period, riluzole therapy was an independently significant prognostic factor (relative risk of death 0.48, $p < 0.0001$, model chi(2) 297, $p < 0.0001$)[224]. Further Miller et al. concluded that riluzole 100 mg daily is reasonably safe and probably prolongs survival by about 2 months in ALS patients[225].

Although nearly a third of the patients with ALS showed evidence of cognitive impairment in a pattern consistent with fronto-temporal lobar dementia, such cognitive performance was not related to site of onset or survival[226].

Chronic kidney disease and end-stage renal disease

Non-dialytic treatment (NDT) has become a recognized and important modality of treatment in end-stage renal disease (ESRD)

in certain groups of chronic kidney disease (CKD) patients. Patients approaching end-stage CKD who chose not to dialyse were classified in a study by Wong[227] according to age band (<70 years, 71–80 years, and >80 years), estimated glomerular filtration rate (eGFR) (<10 ml/min, 11–20 ml/min, and >20 ml/min) according to the Modified Diet In Renal Disease formula and Stoke comorbidity grade (SCG). The SCG is a validated scoring system for the survival of patients on renal replacement therapy. Forty-three patients (60 per cent) had no admissions at all while 30 patients required admission, but 53 per cent of these were for a non-renal cause. Median overall survival was 1.95 years with 65 per cent surviving 1 year. SCG was an independent prognostic factor in predicting survival ($p = 0.005$), the hazard ratio being 2.53, for each incremental increase in the SCG. At 1 year, the survival for comorbidity grade 0, 1, and 2 were 83, 70, and 56 per cent, respectively. It appears that is SCG as an independent prognostic factor in NDT patients[227].

Survival in ESRD patients recently starting dialysis was reviewed in a retrospective cohort study of 272 024 Medicare/Medicaid patients. Cox regression was used to calculate adjusted hazard ratios for risk for death after initiation of dialysis for patients whose dementia was diagnosed before the initiation of dialysis. The average time to death for patients with dementia was 1.09 versus 2.7 years ($p < 0.001$) with an adjusted hazard ratio of 1.87 (95 per cent CI 1.77–1.98). The 2-year survival for patients with dementia was 24 per cent versus 66 per cent for patients without dementia ($p < 0.001$ via log rank test). Dementia diagnosed before initiation on dialysis is an independent risk factor for subsequent death. Such patients should be considered for time-limited trials of dialysis and careful discussion in choosing whether to pursue initiation of dialysis or palliative care[228].

Despite ongoing technological advances, ESRD patients have a mortality rate of approximately 23 per cent per year, and co-morbid cardiovascular, cerebrovascular, and peripheral vascular disorders often make life on dialysis an ordeal[229]. One study of patients discontinuing dialysis reported median time to death was 7 days (range 0–17 days)[230].

HIV/AIDS

The decrease in AIDS mortality over the past decade, along with an increase in prevalence due to longer survival, has been attributed primarily to the successful use of highly active antiretroviral therapy (HAART). HAART regimens, however, can also produce both short-term adverse effects and long-term complications. The prognostic model developed by Brechtl to identify potential predictive variables of death within 6 months may be useful in guiding treatment decisions in patients with advanced AIDS for whom a more palliative care plan may be sought. Of the 152 patients, 61 patients (40 per cent) died within 6 months from date of admission. Serum albumin, percent deviation from ideal body weight, and number of co-morbidities at the time of admission proved to be the best combination of predictors of death within 6 months[231].

Data from another study of 140 consecutive hospitalizations of 83 AIDS patients included demographic, clinical, and biological variables were collected within 48 hours of admission. Probable ($p < 0.10$) or definite ($p < 0.05$) factors contributing to a higher mortality included type of opportunistic infections, serum albumin level, total lymphocyte count, weight, CD4 cell count, and neurological manifestations. In the multivariate proportional hazards model, two factors were significantly and independently predictive of lower survival: body weight < 90 per cent of ideal body weight and neurologic manifestations. The probability of survival was significantly affected by the number of predictive factors present on admission, and patients were significantly more likely to die when these latter two factors were present concomitantly[232].

A large collaborative analysis of 20 379 adults who started HAART used parametric survival models to predict the cumulative incidence at 5 years of a new AIDS-defining event or death, and death alone, first from the start of HAART and second from 6 months after the start of HAART. Data were analysed by intention-to-continue-treatment, ignoring treatment changes and interruptions. During 61 798 person-years of follow-up, 1005 patients died and an additional 1303 developed AIDS. A total of 10 046 (49 per cent) patients started HAART either with a CD4 cell count of <200 cells/microl or with a diagnosis of AIDS. The 5-year risk of AIDS or death (death alone) from the start of HAART ranged from 5.6 to 77 per cent (1.8–65 per cent), depending on age, CD4 cell count, HIV-1-RNA level, clinical stage, and history of injection drug use. From 6 months the corresponding figures were 4.1–99 per cent for AIDS or death and 1.3–96 per cent for death alone. Prognostic models with high discriminatory power over 5 years were developed for patients starting HAART in industrialized countries. A risk calculator that produces estimates for progression rates at 1–5 years after starting HAART is discussed below[233].

Future developments in prognostic tools

Risk calculators

There is growing usage and evidence in a number of diseases for the use of survival prediction risk calculators or prognostic models. Several examples are briefly covered here.

Heart failure models

Heart failure models include EFFECT Heart Failure Risk Scoring Scale[127] and the Seattle Heart Failure model[189] algorithms discussed above. Visit www.seattleheartfailuremodel.org and www.ccort.ca

Prognostat

Based on work of the Victoria Palliative Research Network with the Palliative Performance Scale (PPS) and other tools, the Prognostat is being developed as a web-based tool for survival prediction in palliative care patients and includes calculator, survival tables and nomogram. It is being built for cancer and non-cancer patients from multiple palliative programmes and located via http://web.his.uvic.ca/research/NET2/index.php or a link at www.victoriahospice.org

Adjuvant!

This is a web-based algorithm database from the BC Cancer Agency, Canada. It is used for 10-year morbidity/mortality outcome prediction in breast and lung cancer[234]. Predicted and observed outcomes were within 2 per cent for most subgroups. It can be located at www.adjuvantonline.com

Memorial Sloan Kettering Cancer Center (MSKCC)

Another cancer example is based on the US National Cancer Institute's Surveillance and Epidemiology End Results Program (SEER) cancer registry. MSKCC has developed a number of survival risk calculators for several cancers. For example, the prostate cancer nomogram for hormone refractory stage is derived from age,

Karnofsky score, PSA, haemoglobin, ALK, LDH, and albumin levels. It then calculates survival probability for 1, 2 years and median survival in months. It may be located at http://www.mskcc.org.

HIV/AIDS

As discussed above, the ART (Antiretroviral) Cohort Collaboration risk calculator estimates the probability of experiencing a new AIDS defining disease or death by 1, 2, and 3 years [235]. It includes five parameters of age, CD4 count, HIV-1 RNA copies/ml, CDC stage, and whether HIV transmission was via drug use[233].

There is a computer simulation model of expected survival accounting for baseline CD4 cell count, progressive HAART treatment failure, progressive risk of HAART on treatment mortality, and age-associated mortality. Time to treatment failure for each of three rounds of HAART and risk of mortality on-treatment were estimated using parametric survival models with censoring of follow-up fit to CHORUS data. Median projected survivals stratified by baseline CD4 cell count subgroups were CD4 >200 cells/mm³, 15.4 years; CD4 ≤ 200 cells/mm³, 8.5 years; and CD4 ≤ 50 cells/mm³, 5.5 years. These values are 4–6 years longer than pre-HAART cohorts[236].

Sentinel events

The prognostic models above can provide improved clarity, but still within such general classes derived from Kaplan–Meier curves and analyses. Clarification of sentinel events may provide more individualized focus on prognosis as illness progresses and complications occur. What factors happen to palliative patients, who are otherwise stable, that 'turns the corner' resulting in significant decline, or improvement, or even death? If identified, can the above prognostic tools provide information for the clinician, patient, and family? Sentinel event examples include end-stage renal disease (bacteremia, amputation, acute myocardial event) or dementia (dysphagia, decubitii, aspiration pneumonia)[237] and various biological markers noted above.

When viewed from a Kaplan–Meier curve, as seen in Fig. 3.3.2, one may designate those who die more quickly than anticipated as the 'nose' issue in the first quartile or quintile, and the 'tail' issue for those in the fourth quartile/quintile who die much later than thought. These are common stress points for families and for clinicians responding to 'I thought you said it would be . . . long'.

Research to better identify these two areas will improve prognostication. For example, Caraceni et al. has shown a significant downward shift in each of the 3 PaP groups if delirium occurs[238]. Preliminary PPSv2 analysis by Lau et al.[239] of 6038 cases identified women, younger age, and brain cancer patients as significant factors in the 'tail' of PPS 10 per cent and 20 per cent levels. Further, this study reports a highly significant decline in survival if a '2-increment drop' (a 20 per cent decline in PPS within a 7-day interval) occurs.

Communicating a prognosis (see Chapters 5.3 and 6.1)

While foreseeing is the formulation of a prognosis by a clinician, foretelling is the specialized form of doctor–patient communication of a prognosis. The issue here is not merely whether and how physicians formulate prognoses, but also whether and how they might communicate them.

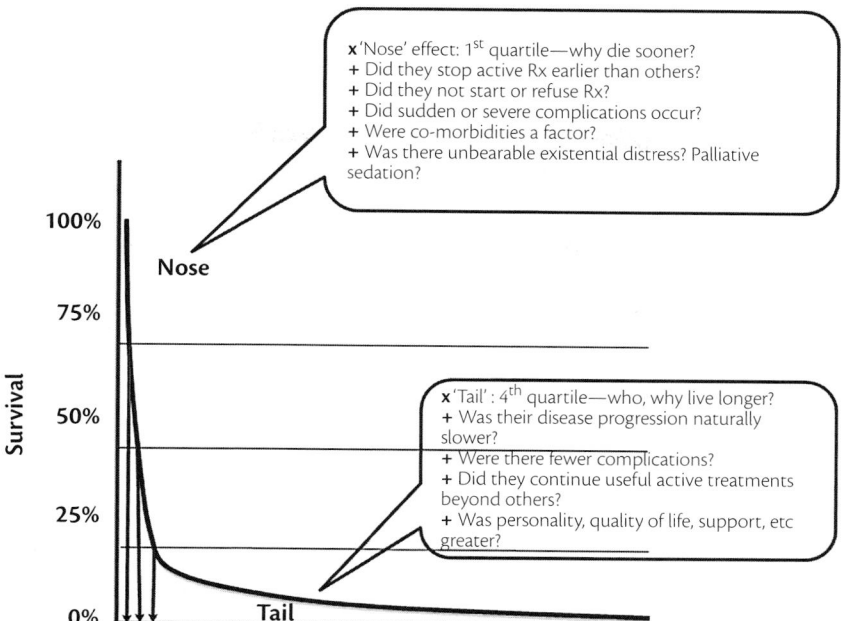

Figure 3.3.2 'Nose' and 'tail' factors in survival prediction. *Source:* M. Downing.

Talking to patients about prognosis is difficult and the evidence suggests that clinicians are poor at this type of communication. Hancock and co-workers[240] recently undertook a systematic review of the literature relating to patients', caregivers', and clinicians' perceptions about end-of-life communication. They found large discrepancies between patients' and health-care professionals' perceptions about how much information was needed, how much information had been given, and what such information meant. Clinicians tended to underestimate patients' information needs and overestimate how much they had understood about their illness and its likely outcome. In one study of patients with locally advanced or metastatic cancer only 31 per cent (correctly) believed that their cancer was incurable, 42 per cent were uncertain, and 27 per cent believed that their cancer was curable[241]. This misapprehension may have been because the clinicians failed to communicate the information correctly or clearly, because patients failed to understand the information that was given or because they chose to 'deny' the bad news.

One study sought to shed light on these possibilities[242]. It involved asking physicians to formulate prognoses in specific patients and then asking them to state what they would communicate to these patients if the patients insisted on being told their prognosis. The formulated prognosis (median 75 days) was overly optimistic by a factor of three (median actual survival 26 days). The authors reported the doctors would give a frank disclosure of their prognosis to 37 per cent, not offer any prognosis to 23 per cent of patients, and a discrepant prognosis in 40 per cent, with the majority (70 per cent) of the discrepant prognoses in the over-optimistic direction. The authors concluded many patients were thus 'twice removed' from reality, because not only was the prognosis not formulated accurately but also it was then communicated even more optimistically. This may help to explain the discrepancy between doctors and patient's perspectives on their illness.

Communicating about prognosis is clearly a difficult task for doctors to perform and a difficult thing for patients to hear. In a qualitative ethnographic study in patients with small-cell lung cancer, researchers found that doctors and patients seemed, to some extent, to enter into a level of collusion about avoiding any discussion of prognosis[243]. Consultations between patients and doctors in this study often seemed to involve 'false optimism' about the prospects of recovery. This optimism was fostered both by doctors' reluctance to give clear information about prognosis and patients' avoidance of asking direct questions. Consultations tended to focus on treatment options and the results of investigations rather than on questions of prognosis.

Why communicate the formulated prognosis to the patient?

Most patients with cancer want information about their prognosis[244–246]. Indeed, in many countries patients have a right to such information. Patients may want information about prognosis so that they can make the most of the time remaining, finish uncompleted tasks, and prepare for their own deaths. In one study, 81 per cent of patients with recently diagnosed metastatic cancer wanted information about average survival times[247]. Parker and colleagues[248] have undertaken a systematic review of studies relating to end-of-life communication in patients with advanced disease. In general, the authors reported most patients want a high level of information about prognosis. However, there did appear to be some evidence of cultural differences between English-speaking/Northern European countries and other countries. There was a tendency for patients from other countries to want less detailed information.

Giving prognostic information to patients is also important in terms of the effects that it can have on patient outcomes. Aabom and colleagues[249] found that giving patients an 'explicit terminal diagnosis' reduced admission rates to hospital and increased the chances of dying at home. Advance care planning for patients at the end of life requires frank disclosure about prognosis. Without such explicit prognostic information patients may find themselves being managed in the acute-care setting at the end-of-life rather than a more appropriate environment. Other studies have found that patients with unrealistic or inaccurate expectations of their own survival are more likely to undergo aggressive and probably futile treatments[250,251].

What prognostic information do patients want?

In general, cancer patients want to have all available information about their cancer and their chances of cure[252]. In this respect patients with advanced cancer are little different from other cancer patients. Fallowfield et al.[253] undertook a large study of 2850 heterogeneous cancer patients, 1046 of whom were undergoing treatment with palliative intent. They reported that 84.9 per cent of palliative patients wanted as much information as possible 'both good and bad news'. Slightly more palliative patients than patients being treated curatively wanted more information 'only if it was good news' (7.3 per cent versus 3.9 per cent), but the absolute numbers of patients were small.

In order to explore precisely what sort of information patients undergoing palliative care want to be told, Kirk and co-workers[254] undertook a qualitative interview study with 72 advanced cancer patients. They reported two themes repeatedly emerged: prognosis and maintenance of hope. Patients seemed to prefer more specific prognostic information and reported that when the information given was too general or vague it caused more distress. Patients felt prognostic information enhanced their communication with their families. They stated a preference for prognostic information to be given by someone whom they perceived to be an expert, and reported that inconsistent information or evasiveness on the part of the professional was distressing and unhelpful. Patients also wanted hopeful messages, even when they accepted the terminal phase of the illness. Wanting to maintain hope in the face of poor prognostic information was not necessarily a sign of denial and patients reported that having their hope crushed by an insensitive professional was extremely negative. The authors reported several strategies patients and clinicians could use to maintain hope; needing to believe in miracles, living parallel realities (acknowledging the terminal illness and still hoping for a cure), leaving the door open (health professionals allowing room for hope), retaining professional honesty (the need for professionals to acknowledge their own difficulties about prognostication), pacing of information, and respecting patients' need to follow alternative paths/treatments.

Kutner et al. [245] have also undertaken qualitative interviews in patients with advanced cancer (n = 22), and have followed this up with semi-structured interviews/questionnaires (n = 56). Like Kirk et al. they found that most patients (58.9 per cent) want to know about life expectancy. They also found that all patients wanted doctors to 'be honest', and that 91.1 per cent also wanted doctors to be 'optimistic'. In the context of communication about prognosis in terminal cancer, this is clearly a challenging demand. In both Kirks's[254] and Kutner's[245] studies, patients seemed to acknowledge this difficulty themselves and were caught between wanting to know what was going on and fearing the answers they might receive.

Many studies have stressed the importance of individualizing the content of prognostic discussions. Patients have different needs from one another and individual patients' information needs can change during the course of their illness. In one study 126 patients with metastatic cancer were surveyed about their preferences for communication about prognosis[247]. Fifty-nine percent of patients

wanted to discuss prognosis when they were first diagnosed with metastatic disease and 48 per cent wanted to negotiate with the clinician about when such issues were discussed. Depressed patients were more likely to want to know 'average survival' and 'shortest time to live without treatment'. Those with the shortest estimated survival, and the highest anxiety levels were the least likely to want to know the 1-year survival. Meredith et al.[255] found that patients undergoing palliative treatment wanted less information than those being given curative treatment (although all patients' information needs were high). In a study comparing patients undergoing first- or second-line chemotherapy for advanced breast cancer, Grunfeld et al.[256] reported that although women undergoing second-line treatment were less likely to ask for 'more information' they were more likely to take an 'active' role in decision making. Butow has also reported that patients whose condition has recently deteriorated were less likely to want to be involved in decision making[257]. Other studies have found that in general women want more information than men[253] and that older patients request less information than younger patients[252,258].

How to communicate the formulated prognosis to the patient?

Although patients generally indicate that they want information about prognosis, it is not always clear what is the best way to communicate such information. In Kirk's qualitative study[254], the authors identified six important attributes relating to the process of information-giving:

1 Playing it straight (the need for clinicians to be honest and direct).

2 Making it clear (providing information in an understandable format).

3 Showing you care (the use of empathetic words and non-verbal communication).

4 Giving time (allowing patients not to feel rushed).

5 Pacing information (providing information at a rate appropriate to the individual).

6 Staying the course (the need for clinicians to convey the message that they will not abandon the patient as the illness progresses).

Similar (although not identical) themes were identified in Butow's smaller qualitative study[244] of 17 women with metastatic breast cancer and 13 health-care professionals. These patients also stressed the importance of communication occurring within the context of a caring, trusting long-term relationship, consistency of information within the multi-professional team and the need to communicate prognostic information to other members of the family.

Although patients indicate that they want a straightforward and clear presentation of prognostic information, it is not apparent what is the best format to present such information. One survey of heterogeneous cancer patients[258] has suggested that patients prefer to receive 'qualitative' (i.e. framed using verbal descriptors) rather than 'quantitative' (i.e. framed using numbers) estimates of survival. Similarly a study in patients with early stage breast cancer found that most patients preferred prognostic information to be delivered using words rather than numbers[259]. In contrast, Hagerty and co-workers[247] reported that words and numbers were equally well understood by patients with metastatic cancer, and both formats were preferred to 100-person diagrams, pie-charts, or graphs. They also found that patients seemed to prefer to endorse more optimistic or positively-framed statements. Thus, patients preferred to know the 'chance of living for 5 years' and the 'longest survival without treatment' rather than the 'chance of living for 1 year' or the 'shortest survival without treatment'.

Just as there is a need to individualize the content of prognostic discussions, so is there a need to individualize the process of communicating such information. Patients' requirements for information are not uniform and very few patient characteristics are able to predict how much information patients want or how such information should be delivered[245]. There is also a poor correlation between patients' and doctors' perceptions of decision-making preferences[260]. In Haggerty's study of patients with metastatic cancer[247] 53 per cent of patients wanted specialists to initiate discussions about prognosis, but 21 per cent only wanted specialists to tell them about survival 'if asked', and 9 per cent of patients never wanted to discuss likely duration of survival. Moreover, although most patients preferred words and numbers to diagrams and pie-charts, older patients were significantly more likely to prefer 100-person diagrams and patients with more years of education were more likely to prefer pie-charts.

The National Health and Medical Research Council of Australia have recently produced and published evidence-based guidelines on communicating prognosis to adults with advanced life-limiting illnesses[261]. The guidelines were produced following a systematic review of the literature[248] and a review of previously published guidelines. They were then refined by an expert panel consisting of health professionals and consumers. The guidelines cover eight processes and can be remembered by use of the acronym PREPARED.

1 Prepare for the discussion
   a. Check facts
   b. Ensure appropriate environment.

2 Relate to the person
   a. Develop rapport and show empathy.

3 Elicit patient and care-giver preferences
   a. Clarify baseline understanding
   b. Check what patient wants to know.

4 Provide information
   a. Pace the information
   b. Use clear language
   c. Explain uncertainty, limitations and unreliability of prognostic estimates
   d. Ensure consistency of information.

5 Acknowledge emotions and concerns
   a. Acknowledge and respond to distress.

6 (Foster) Realistic hope
   a. But avoid giving unrealistic or false information.

7 Encourage questions
   a. Check patient's understanding
   b. Be prepared for further discussions in the future.

8 Document
   a. Write a clear summary in the medical notes
   b. Communicate with other professionals.

Both formulating and communicating prognoses to patients with advanced diseases are complex and difficult processes. Episodes of poor communication are often vividly remembered. However, communication is a skill and can be learnt. It is incumbent on all health professional to ensure that they are adequately trained to break this prototypical example of 'bad news'.

Cultural issues and communicating prognosis

The systematic review of studies relating to end-of-life communication in patients with advanced disease referred to previously[248] found some evidence of cultural differences with regard to patients' information needs. The subject of communication between palliative care physicians and their patients regarding their diagnosis and prognosis has not been extensively researched, but the attitudes and beliefs of culturally diverse palliative care specialists regarding communication with the terminally ill were compared a decade ago[262]. Almost 200 palliative care specialists in Europe, South America, and Canada responded to a survey (80 per cent response rate). Respondents from all three regions believed that cancer patients should be informed of their diagnosis and the terminal nature of their illness, and that the proportions of patients who knew this information were similar in the three regions. Likewise, respondents from all regions agreed that 'do not resuscitate' orders should be present and should be discussed with the patient in all cases. Differences were found, however with regard to the proportions of palliative care phsyicians who believed that most of their patients wanted to know about the terminal stage of their illness—more than 90 per cent of Canadians compared with 18 per cent of South American, and 26 per cent of European physicians. Similar results were found when the physicians were asked the percentage of families who want patients to know the terminal stage of their illness. However, almost all of the physicians agreed that if they had terminal cancer they would like to know. There was a significant association between patient-based decision-making and female sex, older age, and being a physician in Canada or South America. Finally, in their daily decision making, South American physicians were significantly more likely to support beneficence and justice as compared with autonomy. Canadian physicians were more likely to support autonomy as compared with beneficence. This survey suggests that major regional differences in the attitudes and beliefs of physicians regarding communication at the end of life exist. Much more research is needed on this topic, but in the meantime palliative medicine physicians need to be aware of their personal attitudes towards discussing diagnosis, prognosis, and any other sensitive issue (e.g. sexuality, spirituality) and endeavour not to impose their own values on those of the patient.

Conclusion

Prognostication remains a challenging topic in palliative care. In the past 20 years, much research has been undertaken to identify ways of improving the accuracy and precision of clinicians' estimates and as presented here many tools are now available to improve prognsotication.

While we are now in a better position to give the patient 'x per cent chance of surviving for y weeks/months', we are not yet able to posit any of the existing tools as the ideal one to be recommended for widespread use. Most of the existing tools focus on performance status, symptoms and simple laboratory markers; while these are helpful, they are no more accurate than the subjective judgements of experienced clinicians. Novel objective prognostic factors need to be identified, and biomarkers such as CRP and the proinflammatory cytokines are the main focus of current research.

Clinical judgement remains important, in our opinion. The clinical data needed to use a tool to calculate the prognosis (e.g. recent laboratory parameters) may not be available, tools may not provide the prognostic information required, and they may not have been validated in the population to which the individual patient belongs. Clinical judgement alone may be sufficient if the issue is acknowledging a probability of dying from an illness in the foreseeable future. The SUPPORT study showed that patients will change their planning behaviour once they understand that the chance of surviving beyond 6 months is small. Furthermore, models predicting survival should be thought of like any diagnostic test, i.e. they should not be interpreted in isolation but as a way of improving the pre-test probability of survival, which is based on clinical judgement.

Even if precise and accurate predictions of survival duration become available, this alone should never drive treatment plans. What ultimately is needed is not so much an accurate prediction of time but an acknowledgement of the possibility of dying, communicated carefully by the compassionate and skilful physician.

A continuously updated web page with the links contained in this chapter will be available at Pallimed (http://www.pallimed.org/2007/05/prognosis-links.html).

Summary

- Prognostication is important in end-of-life care.

- The precision of the survival estimate depends on the reason for prognosticating.

- Studies of doctors (and other health-care professionals) demonstrate inaccuracy when making temporal estimates in individual patients, although this may be improving.

- Experience improves prognostication accuracy, but this is modified by the closeness of the doctor–patient relationship.

- Probabilistic predictions appear more accurate then temporal predictions.

- The clinical estimate of survival remains a powerful independent prognostic indicator.

- In general, patients with a poor performance status live for shorter periods than those who are more functional.

- Symptoms like anorexia, breathlessness, and confusion are important predictors that an individual is rapidly approaching the end of life.

- QOL scores may be more powerful than performance scores or symptom reports in predicting survival.

- Simple, reliable, and valid prognostic models have been developed and can be readily used at the bedside of terminally ill cancer patients.

- Predicting survival in patients dying of diseases other than cancer is only recently being studied.

- Communicating survival predictions is an important part of cancer care.

References

1. Hutchinson, R. (1934). Prognosis. *Lancet*, **i**, 697.
2. Christakis, N.A. (1997). The ellipsis of prognosis in modern medical thought. *Social Science and Medicine*, **44**(3), 301–15.
3. Christakis, N.A. and Lamont, E.B. (2000). Extent and determinants of error in doctors' prognoses in terminally ill patients: prospective cohort study. *BMJ*, **320**(7233), 469–72.
4. Den Daas, N. (1995). Estimating length of survival in end-stage cancer: A review of the literature. *Journal of Pain and Symptom Management*, **10**(7), 548–55.
5. McCusker, J. (1984). The terminal period of cancer: definition and descriptive epidemiology. *Journal of Chronic Diseases*, **37**(5), 377–85.
6. Evans, C. and McCarthy, M. (1985). Prognostic uncertainty in terminal care: can the KPS help? *Lancet*, **1**, 1204–6.
7. Maltoni, M., Pirovano, M., Nanni, O. *et al.* (1994). Prognostic factors in terminal cancer patients. *European Journal of Palliative Care*, **1**(3), 122–5.
8. Hardy, J.R., Turner, R., and Saunders, M. (1994). Prediction of survival in a hospital-based continuing care unit. *European Journal of Cancer*, **30A**(3), 284–8.
9. Zahuranec, D.B., Brown, D.L., Lisabeth, L.D. *et al.* (2007) Early care limitations independently predict mortality after intracerebral hemorrhage. *Neurology*, **68**(20), 1651–7.
10. Covinsky, K.E., Justice, A.C., and Rosenthal, G.E. (1997). Measuring prognosis and case mix in hospitalized elders. The importance of functional status. *Journal of General Internal Medicine*, **12**(4), 203–8.
11. Smith, J.L. (2000). Commentary: why do doctors overestimate? *BMJ*, **320**(7233), 472–3.
12. Weissman, D.E. (1997). Consultation in palliative medicine. *Archives of Internal Medicine*, **157**(7), 733–7.
13. Homsi, J., Walsh, D., Nelson, K.A. *et al.* (2002). The impact of a palliative medicine consultation service in medical oncology. *Support Care Cancer*, **10**(4), 337–42.
14. Manfredi, P.L., Morrison, S., Morris, J. *et al.* (2000). Palliative care consultations: how do they impact the care of hospitalised patients? *Journal of Pain and Symptom Management*, **20**(3), 166–73.
15. Sackett, D.L., Haynes, R.B., Guyatt, G.H. *et al.* (1991). *Clinical epidemiology. A basic science for clinical medicine*, 2nd edition. Little, Brown and Company, Boston, MA.
16. Fries, J.F. and Ehrlich, G.E. (1981). *Prognosis. Contemporary outcomes of disease*. The Charles Press Publishers, Bowie, MD.
17. Steinhauser, K., Christakis, N.A., Clipp, E. *et al.* (2000). Factors considered important at the end of life by patients, family, physicians, and other care providers. *JAMA*, **284**(19), 2476–82.
18. Christakis, N.A. and Iwashyna, T.J. (1998). Attitude and self-reported practice regarding prognostication in a national sample of internists. *Archives of Internal Medicine*, **158**(21), 2389–95.
19. Christakis, N. (1999). *Death foretold: prophecy and prognosis in medical care*. Chicago University Press, Chicago, IL.
20. Sotiriou, C., Neo, S.Y., McShane, L.M. *et al.* (2003). Breast cancer classification and prognosis based on gene expression profiles from a population-based study. *Proceedings of the National Academy of Sciences of the United States of America*, **100**(18), 10393–8.
21. Vigano, A., Dorgan, M., Bruera, E. *et al.* (1999). The relative accuracy of the clinical estimation of the duration of life for patients with end of life cancer. *Cancer*, **86**(1), 170–6.
22. Llobera, J., Esteva, M., Rifa, J. *et al.* (2000). Terminal cancer: duration and prediction of survival time. *European Journal of Cancer*, **36**, 2036–43.

23. Yun, Y.H., Heo, D.S., Heo, B.Y. *et al.* (2001). Development of terminal cancer prognostic score as an index in terminally ill cancer patients. *Oncology Report*, **8**(4), 795–800.

24. Field, M., and Cassel, C. (eds.) (1997). *Approaching death: improving care at the end of life*. Committee on care at the end of life, National Academy Press, Division of Health Care Services, Institute of Medicine.

25. Lynn, J. (2001). Helping patients who may die soon and their families. The role of hospice and other services. *JAMA*, **285**, 925–32.

26. Loprinzi, C.L., Laurie, J.A., Wieand, H.S. *et al.* (1994). Prospective evaluation of prognostic variables from patient-completed questionnaires. North Central Cancer Treatment Group. *Journal of Clinical Oncology*, **12**(3), 601–7.

27. Inagaki, J., Rodriguez, V., and Bodey, G. (1974). Causes of death in cancer patients. *Cancer*, **33**(2), 568–73.

28. Brannen, A.L., II, Godfrey, L.J., and Goetter, W.E. (1989). Prediction of outcome from critical illness. A comparison of clinical judgment with a prediction rule. *Archives of Internal Medicine*, **149**(5), 1083–6.

29. Mackillop, W.J. and Quirt, C.F. (1997). Measuring the accuracy of prognostic judgments in oncology. *Journal of Clinical Epidemiology*, **50**(1), 21–9.

30. Poses, R.M. and Anthony, M. (1991). Availability, wishful thinking, and physicians' diagnostic judgments for patients with suspected bacteremia. *Medical Decision Making*, **11**(3), 159–68.

31. Gripp, S., Moeller, S., Bolke, E. *et al.* (2007). Survival prediction in terminally ill cancer patients by clinical estimates, laboratory tests, and self-rated anxiety and depression. *Journal of Clinical Oncology*, **25**(22), 3313–20.

32. Last, J.M. (2001). *A dictionary of epidemiology*. 4th edition, Oxford University Press, Oxford.

33. Cassell, E.J. (1991). Recognizing suffering. Hastings Center Report, (May–June), 24–31.

34. Sinclair, C.T. (2006). Communicating a prognosis in advanced cancer. *Journal of Support Oncology*, **4**(4), 201–4.

35. Lamont, E.B., and Christakis, N.A. (1999). Some elements of prognosis in terminal cancer. *Oncology* **13**(8), 1165–70.

36. Rich, A. (1999). How long have I got?—prognostication and palliative car. *European Journal Palliative Care*, **6**, 179–82.

37. Brown, J.K. and Knapp, T.R. (1995). Do people with cancer postpone death to celebrate special occasions? *Cancer Practitioner*, **3**(6), 351–5.

38. Phillips, D.P., Jarvinen, J.R., Abramson, I.S. *et al.* (2004). Cardiac mortality is higher around Christmas and New Year's than at any other time: the holidays as a risk factor for death. *Circulation*, **110**(25), 3781–8.

39. Young, D.C. and Hade, E.M. (2004). Holidays, birthdays, and postponement of cancer death. *JAMA*, **292**(24), 3012–6.

40. Phillips, D. and Smith, D. (1988). Postponement of death until symbolically meaningful occasions. *JAMA*, **263**, 1947–51.

41. Phillips, D.P. and King, E.W. (1988). Death takes a holiday: mortality surrounding major social occasions. *Lancet*, **2**(8613), 728–32.

42. Mackillop, W. (2001). The importance of prognosis in cancer medicine. In Gospodarowicz, M. (ed.). *Prognostic factors in cancer*, 2nd edition. Wiley-Liss, New York.

43. Hauser, C.A., Stockler, M.R., and Tattersall, M.H. (2006). Prognostic factors in patients with recently diagnosed incurable cancer: a systematic review. *Support Care Cancer*, **14**(10), 999–1011.

44. Tversky, A. and Kahneman, D. (1974). Judgment under uncertainty: heuristics and biases. *Science*, **185**(4157), 1124–31.

45. Groopman, J.E. (2007). *How doctors think*. Houghton Mifflin, Boston, MA.

46. Parkes, C. (2000). Commentary: Prognoses should be based on proved indices not intuition. *BMJ*, **320**, 469–73.

47. Christakis, N.A. and Lamont, E.B. (2000). Extent and determinants of error in doctors' prognoses in terminally ill patients: prospective cohort study. *BMJ*, **320**(7233), 469–72.

48. Scotto, J. and Schneiderman, M. (1972). Predicting survival in terminal cancer. *BMJ*, **4**, 50.

49. Heyse-Moore, L. and Johnson-Bell, V. (1987). Can doctors accurately predict the life expectancy of patients with terminal cancer? *Palliative Medicine*, **1**, 165–6.

50. Forster, L. and Lynn, J. (1988). Predicting life span for applicants to inpatient hospice. *Archives of Internal Medicine*, **148**, 2540–3.

51. Addington-Hall, J.M., MacDonald, L.D., and Anderson, H.R. (1990). Can the Spitzer quality of life index help to reduce prognostic uncertainty in terminal care? *Cancer*, **62**, 695–9.

52. Bruera, E., Miller, M.J., Kuehn, N. *et al.* (1992). Estimate of survival of patients admitted to a palliative care unit: a prospective study. *Journal of Pain and Symptom Management*, **7**(2), 82–6.

53. Maltoni, M., Pirovano, M., Scarpi, E. *et al.* (1995). Prediction of survival of patients terminally ill with cancer. Results of an Italian prospective multicentric study. *Cancer*, **75**(10), 2613–22.

54. Mackillop, W.J. and Quirt, C.F. (1997). Measuring the accuracy of prognostic judgments in oncology. *Journal of Clinical Epidemiology*, **50**(1), 21–9.

55. Oxenham, P. and Cornbleet, M.A. (1998). Accuracy of prediction of survival by different professional groups in a hospice. *Palliative Medicine*, **12**, 117–8.

56. Glare, P., Virik, K., Jones, M. *et al.* (2003). A systematic review of physicians' survival predictions in terminally ill cancer patients. *BMJ*, **327**(7408), 195.

57. Brandt, H.E., Deliens, L., Ooms, M.E. *et al.* (2005). Symptoms, signs, problems and diseases of terminally ill nursing home patients. *Archives of Internal Medicine*, **165**, 314–20.

58. Poses, R.M., Bekes, C., Copare, F. *et al.* What difference do two days make? The inertia of physicians' sequential prognostic judgments for critically ill patients. *Medical Decision Making*, **10**, 6–14.

59. Wildman, M.J., Sanderson, C., Groves, J. *et al.* (2007). Implications of prognostic pessimism in patients with chronic obstructive pulmonary disease (COPD) or asthma admitted to intensive care in the UK within the COPD and asthma outcome study (CAOS): multi-centre observational study. *BMJ*, **335**, 1132–4.

60. Pirovano, M., Maltoni, M., Nanni, O. *et al.* (1999). A new palliative prognostic score: a first step for the staging of terminally ill cancer patients. Italian Multicenter and Study Group on Palliative Care. *Journal of Pain and Symptom Management*, **17**(4), 231–9.

61. Perlman, R. (1988). Inaccurate predictions of life expectancy. Dilemmas and opportunities. *Archives of Internal Medicine*, **48**, 2538–9.

62. Tannenberger, S., Malavasi, I., Mariano, P. *et al.* (2002). Planning palliative or terminal care: the dliemma of doctors' prognoses in terminally ill cancer patients. *Annals of Oncology*, **13**, 1319–23.

63. Steyerberg, E., and Harrell, F. (2002). Statistical models for prognostication In (eds. Max, M., and Lynn, J.). *Symptom research: methods and opportunities*. Retrieved from http://symptomresearch. nih.gov on 16 May 2002.

64. Mor, V., Laliberte, L., Morris, J.N. *et al.* (1984). The Karnofsky Performance Status Scale. An examination of its reliability and validity in a research setting. *Cancer*, **53**(9), 2002–7.

65. Vigano, A., Dorgan, M., Buckingham, J. *et al.* (2000). Survival prediction in terminal cancer patients: a systematic review of the medical literature. *Palliative Medicine*, **14**(5), 363–74.

66. Feinstein, A. (1966). Symptoms as an index of biological behaviour and prognosis in human cancer. *Nature*, **209**, 241–5.

67. Justice, A., Covinsky, K., and Berlin, J. (1999). Assessing the generalizability of prognostic information. *Annals of Internal Medicine*, **130**(6), 515–24.

68. Yates, J., Chalmer, B., and McKegney, F.P. (1980). Evaluation of patients with advanced cancer using the Karnofsky performance status. *Cancer*, 2220–4.

69. Maltoni, M., Nanni, O., Derni, S. *et al.*(1994). Clinical prediction of survival is more accurate than the Karnofsky performance status in

estimating life span of terminally ill cancer patients. *European Journal of Cancer*, **30A**(6), 764–6.

70. Abnernathy, A., Shelby-James, T., Fazekas, B. *et al.* (2005). The Australia-modified Karnofsky Performance Status (AKPS) scale: a revised scale for contemporary palliative clinical practice. *BMC Palliative Care*, **4**, 7.

71. Nikoletti, S., Porock, D., Kristjanson, L. (2000). Performance status assessment in home hospice patients using a modified form of the Karnofsky Performance Status Scale. *Journal of Palliative Medicine*, **3**(3), 301–11.

72. Anderson, F., Downing, G.M., Hill, J. *et al.* (1996). Palliative performance scale (PPS): a new tool. *Journal of Palliative Care*, **12**(1), 5–11.

73. Virik, K. and Glare, P. (2002). Validation of the palliative performance scale for inpatients admitted to a palliative care unit in Sydney, Australia. *Journal of Pain and Symptom Management*, **23**(6), 455–7.

74. Morita, T., Tsunoda, J., Inoue, S. *et al.* (1999). Validity of the palliative performance scale from a survival perspective. *Journal of Pain and Symptom Management*, **18**, 2–3.

75. Head, B., Ritchie, C.S., and Smoot, T.M. (2005). Prognostication in hospice care: can the palliative performance scale help? *Journal of Palliative Medicine*, **8**(3), 492–502.

76. Lau, F., Downing, G.M., and Lesperance, M. (2006). Use of Palliative Performance Scale in end-of-life prognostication. *Journal of Palliative Medicine*, **9**(5), 1066–75.

77. Harrold, J., Rickerson, E., Carroll, J.T. *et al.* (2005). Is the palliative performance scale a useful predictor of mortality in a heterogeneous hospice population? *Journal of Palliative Medicine*, **8**(3), 503–9.

78. Olajide, O., Hanson, L., Usher, B.M. *et al.* (2007). Validation of the palliative performance scale in the acute tertiary care hospital setting. *Journal of Palliative Medicine*, **10**(1), 111–7.

79. Downing, G.M., Lau, F., Lesperance, M. *et al.* (2007). Meta-analysis of survival prediction with the Palliative Performance Scale. *Journal of Palliative Care*, **23**, 245–52.

80. Ho, F., Lau, F., Downing, G.M. Reliablity and validity of PPS in survival prediction for palliative care patients. In preparation.

81. Dewys, W.D., Begg, C., Lavin, P.T. *et al.* (1980). Prognostic effect of weight loss prior to chemotherapy in cancer patients. Eastern Cooperative Oncology Group. *American Journal of Medicine*, **69**(4), 491–7.

82. Rosenthal, M., Gebski, V., Kefford, R. *et al.* (1993). Prediction of life-expectancy in hospice patients: identification of novel prognostic factors. *Palliative Medicine*, **7**, 199–204.

83. Bennett, M. and Ryall, N. (2000). Using the modified Barthel index to estimate survival in cancer patients in hospice: observational study. *BMJ*, **321**(7273), 1381–2.

84. Reuben, D.B., Mor, V., and Hiris, J. (1988). Clinical symptoms and length of survival in patients with terminal cancer. *Archives of Internal Medicine*, **148**(7), 1586–91.

85. Wachtel, T., Masterson, S., Reuben, D. *et al.* (1989). The end stage cancer patient: terminal common pathway. *Hospice Journal*, **4**(4), 43–80.

86. Ma, G. and Alexander, H. (1998). Prevalence and pathophysiology of cancer cachexia. In *Topics in palliative care*. (eds. Bruera, E., Portenoy, R.), pp. 91–129. Oxford University Press, New York.

87. Vigano, A., Dorgan, M., Bruera, E. *et al.* (1999). Terminal cancer syndrome: myth or realtiy. *Journal of Palliative Care*, **15**(4), 32–9.

88. Morita, T., Tsunoda, J., Inoue, S. (1999). Survival prediction of terminally ill cancer patients by clinical symptoms: development of a simple indicator. *Japanese Journal of Clinical Oncology*, **29**(3), 156–9.

89. Escalante, C., Martin, C., Elting, L. *et al.* (2000). Identifying risk factors for imminent death in cancer patients with acute dyspnea. *Journal of Pain and Symptom Management*, **20**(5), 318–25.

90. Tamburini, M., Brunelli, C., Rosso, S. *et al.* (1996). Prognostic value of quality of life scores in terminal cancer patients. *Journal of Pain and Symptom Management*, **11**, 32–41.

91. Ventafridda, V., Ripamonti, C., Tamburini, M. *et al.* (1990). Unendurable symptoms as prognostic indicators of impending death in terminal cancer patients. *European Journal of Cancer*, **26**(9), 1000–1.

92. Maltoni, M., Nanni, O., Pirovano, M. *et al.* (1999). Successful validation of the palliative prognostic score in terminally ill cancer patients. Italian Multicenter Study Group on Palliative Care. *Journal of Pain and Symptom Management*, **17**(4), 240–7.

93. Portenoy, R.K., Sibirceva, U., Smout, R. *et al.* (2006). Opioid use and survival at the end of life: a survey of a hospice population. *Journal of Pain and Symptom Management*, **32**(6), 532–40.

94. de Miguel Sanchez, C., Elustondo, S.G., Estirado, A. *et al.* (2006). Palliative performance status, heart rate and respiratory rate as predictive factors of survival time in terminally ill cancer patients. *Journal of Pain and Symptom Management*, **31**(6), 485–92.

95. Degner, L. and Sloan, J. (1995). Symptom distress in newly diagnosed ambulatory cancer patients and as a predictor of survival in lung cancer. *Journal of Pain and Symptom Management*, **10**(6), 423–31.

96. Earlam, S., Glover, C., Fordy, C. *et al.* (1996). Relation between tumor size, quality of life, and survival in patients with colorectal liver metastases. *Journal of Clinical Oncology*, **14**(1), 171–5.

97. Chang, V.T., Thaler, H.T., Polyak, T.A. *et al.* (1998). Quality of life and survival: the role of multidimensional symptom assessment. *Cancer*, **83**(1), 173–9.

98. Cassileth, B.R., Lusk, E.J., Miller, D.S. (1985). Psychosocial correlates of survival in advanced malignant disease. *New England Journal of Medicine*, **312**, 1551–5.

99. Ringdal, G.I., Gotestam, K.G., Kaasa, S. *et al.* (1996). Prognostic factors and survival in a heterogeneous sample of cancer patients. *British Journal of Cancer*, **73**, 594–9.

100. Greer, S., Morris, T., and Pettingale, K.W. (1979). Psychological response to breast cancer: effect on outcome. *Lancet*, **2**, 785–7.

101. Pettingale, K.W., Morris, T., Greer, S. *et al.* (1985). Mental attitudes to cancer: an additional prognostic factor. *Lancet*, **1**(8431), 750.

102. Spiegel, D., Bloom, J.R., Kraemer, H.C. *et al.* (1989). Effect of psychosocial treatment on survival of patients with metastatic breast cancer. *Lancet*, **2**, 888–91.

103. Roud, P.C. (1987). Psychosocial variables associated with the exceptional survival of patients with advanced malignant disease. *Journal of National Medical Association*, **79**(1), 97–102.

104. Watson, M., Haviland, J.S., Greer, S. *et al.* (1999). Influence of psychological response on survival in breaest cancer: a population-based cohort study. *Lancet*, **354**, 1331–6.

105. Petticrew, M., Bell, R., and Hunter, D. (2002). Influence of psychological coping on survival and recurrence in people with cancer: systematic review. *BMJ*, **325**(7372), 1066.

106. Coates, A., Gebski, V., Signorini, D. *et al.* (1992). Prognostic value of quality-of-life scores during chemotherapy for advanced breast cancer. Australian New Zealand Breast Cancer Trials Group. *Journal of Clinical Oncology*, **10**(12), 1833–8.

107. Ganz, P., Lee, J.J., and Siau, J. (1991). Quality of life assessment: An independent prognostic variable for survival in lung cancer. *Cancer*, **67**(12), 3131–5.

108. Coates, A., Thomson, D., McLeod, G.R.M. *et al.* (1993). Prognostic value of quality of life scores in a trail of chemotherapy with or without interferon in patients with metastatic malignant melanoma. *European Journal of Cancer*, **29A**(12), 1731–4.

109. Langendijk, H., Aaronson, N., de Jong, J. (2000). The prognostic impact of quality of life assessed with the EORTC QLQ—C30 in inoperable non-small cell lung carcinoma treated with radiotherapy. *Radiotherapy and Oncology*, **55**, 19–25.

110. Paci, E., Miccinesi, G., Toscani, F. *et al.* (2001). Quality of life assessment and outcome of palliative care. *Journal of Pain and Symptom Management*, **21**(3), 179–88.

111. Cerny, T., Blair, V., Anderson, V. et al. (1987). Pretreatment prognostic factors and scoring system in 407 small-cell lung cancer patients. International Journal of Cancer, 39, 146–9.

112. Maltoni, M., Pirovano, M., Nanni, O. et al. (1997). Biological indices predictive of survival in 519 Italian terminally ill cancer patients. Italian Multicenter Study Group on Palliative Care. Journal of Pain and Symptom Management, 13(1), 1–9.

113. Lee, B.N., Dantzer, R., Langley, K.E. et al. (2004). A cytokine-based neuroimmunologic mechanism of cancer-related symptoms. Neuroimmunomodulation, 11(5), 279–92.

114. Feinstein, A.R., Pritchett, J.A., and Schimpff, C.R. (1969). The epidemiology of cancer therapy. II. The clinical course: data, decisions, and temporal demarcations. Archives of Internal Medicine, 123(3), 323–44.

115. Feinstein, A.R., and Spitz, H. (1969). The epidemiology of cancer therapy. I. Clinical problems of statistical surveys. Archives of Internal Medicine, 123(2), 171–86.

116. Lamont, E.B. (2005). A demographic and prognostic approach to defining the end of life. Journal of Palliative Medicine, 1, (8 Suppl) S12–21.

117. Lau, F., Cloutier-Fisher, D., Kuziemsky, C. et al. (2007). A systematic review of prognostic tools for estimating survival time in palliative care. Journal of Palliative Care, 23(2), 93–112.

118. Head, B., Ritchie, C.S., and Smoot, T.M. (2005). Prognostication in hospice care: can the palliative performance scale help? Journal of Palliative Medicine, 8(3), 492–502.

119. Harrold, J., Rickerson, E., Carroll, J.T. et al. Is the palliative performance scale a useful predictor of mortality in a heterogeneous hospice population? Journal of Palliative Medicine, 8(3), 503–9.

120. Olajide, O., Hanson, L., Usher, B.M. et al. (2007). Validation of the palliative performance scale in the acute tertiary care hospital setting. Journal of Palliative Medicine, 10(1), 111–7.

121. Morita, T., Tsunoda, J., Inoue, S. et al. (1999). Survival prediction of terminally ill cancer patients by clinical symptoms: development of a simple indicator. Japanese Journal of Clinical Oncology, 29(3), 156–9.

122. Maltoni, M., Nanni, O., Pirovano, M. et al. (1999). Successful validation of the palliative prognostic score in terminally ill cancer patients. Journal of Pain and Symptom Management, 17(4), 240–7.

123. Fox, E., Landrum-McNiff, K., Zhong, Z. et al. (1999). Evaluation of prognostic criteria for determining hospice eligibility in patients with advanced lung, heart, or liver disease. SUPPORT Investigators. Study to Understand Prognoses and Preferences for Outcomes and Risks of Treatments. JAMA, 282(17), 1638–45.

124. Walter, L.C., Brand, R.J., Counsell, S.R. et al. (2001). Development and validation of a prognostic index for 1-year mortality in older adults after hospitalization. JAMA, 285(23), 2987–94.

125. Flacker, J.M., and Kiely, D.K. (2003). Mortality-related factors and 1-year survival in nursing home residents. Journal of the American Geriatrics Society, 51(2), 213–21.

126. Glare, P.A., Eychmueller, S., and McMahon, P. (2004). Diagnostic accuracy of the palliative prognostic score in hospitalized patients with advanced cancer [erratum appears in Journal of Clinical Oncology, 23(1), 248]. Journal of Clinical Oncology, 22(23), 4823–8.

127. Lee, D.S., Austin, P.C., Rouleau, J.L. (2003). Predicting mortality among patients hospitalized for heart failure: derivation and validation of a clinical model. JAMA, 290(19), 2581–7.

128. Chuang, R.B., Hu, W.Y., Chiu, T.Y et al. (2004). Prediction of survival in terminal cancer patients in Taiwan: constructing a prognostic scale. Journal of Pain and Symptom Management, 28(2), 115–22.

129. Bozcuk, H., Koyuncu, E., Yildiz, M. et al. A simple and accurate prediction model to estimate the intrahospital mortality risk of hospitalised cancer patients. International Journal of Clinical Practionar, 58(11), 1014–9.

130. Glare, P., and Virik, K. (2001). Independent prospective validation of the PaP score in terminally ill patients referred to a hospital-based palliative medicine consultation service. Journal of Pain and Symptom Management, 22(5), 891–8.

131. Morita, T., Tsunoda, J., Inoue, S. et al. (1999). The Palliative Prognostic Index: a scoring system for survival prediction of terminally ill cancer patients. Support Care Cancer, 7(3), 128–33.

132. Schonwetter, R.S., Han, B., Small, B.J. et al. (2003). Predictors of six-month survival among patients with dementia: an evaluation of hospice Medicare guidelines. American Journal of Hospice and Palliative Care, 20(2), 105–13.

133. Schonwetter, R.S., Robinson, B.E., and Ramirez, G. Prognostic factors for survival in terminal lung cancer patients. Journal of General Internal Medicine, 9(7), 366–71.

134. Koss, N., and Feinstein, A.R. (1971). Computer-aided prognosis. II. Development of a prognostic algorithm. Archives of Internal Medicine, 127(3), 448–59.

135. Altman, D. (2001). Systematic reviews of studies of prognostic variables. In Systematic reviews in health care: meta-analysis in context (eds. Egger, M., Smith, G., Altman, D.), 2nd edition. BMJ, London.

136. Knaus, W.A., Harrell, F.E., Jr., Lynn, J. et al. (1995). The SUPPORT prognostic model. Objective estimates of survival for seriously ill hospitalized adults. Study to understand prognoses and preferences for outcomes and risks of treatments. Annals of Internal Medicine, 122(3), 191–203.

137. Knaus, W.A., Draper, E.A., and Wagner, D.P. (1991). Utilizing findings from the APACHE III research to develop operational information system for the ICU—the APACHE III ICU Management System. Proceedings—the Annual Symposium on Computer Applications in Medical Care, pp. 987–9.

138. Lynn, J., Harrell, F., Jr., Cohn, F. et al. (1997). Prognoses of seriously ill hospitalized patients on the days before death: implications for patient care and public policy. New Horizon, 5, 56–61.

139. Glare, P., Virik, K. (2001). Independent prospective validation of the PaP score in terminally ill patients referred to a hospital-based palliative medicine consultation service. Journal of Pain and Symptom Management, 22(5), 891–8.

140. Glare, P.A., Eychmueller, S., and McMahon, P. (2004). Diagnostic accuracy of the palliative prognostic score in hospitalized patients with advanced cancer. Journal of Clinical Oncology, 22(23), 4823–8.

141. Morita, T., Tsunoda, J., Inoue, S. et al. (1999). The Palliative Prognostic Index: a scoring system for survival prediction of terminally ill cancer patients. Supportive Care in Cancer, 7(3), 128–33.

142. Sloan, J., Loprinzi, C.L., Laurine, J.A. et al. (2001). A simple stratification factor prognsotic for survival in advanced cancer: the good/bad/uncertain index. Journal of Clinical Oncology, 19(15), 3539–46.

143. Forrest, L.M., McMillan, D.C., McArdle, C.S. (2003). Evaluation of cumulative prognostic scores based on the systemic inflammatory response in patients with inoperable non-small-cell lung cancer. British Journal of Cancer, 89(6), 1028–30.

144. Elahi, M.M., McMillian, D.C., McArdle, C.S. et al. (2004). Score based on hypoalbuminemia and elevated C-Reactive protein predicts survival in patients with advanced gastrointestinal cancer. Nutrition and Cancer, 48(2), 171–3.

145. Vigano, A., Bruera, E., Jhangri, G.S. et al. Clinical survival predictors in patients with advanced cancer. Archives of Internal Medicine, 160(6), 861–8.

146. Kelly, L., White, S., and Stone P. (2007). The B12/CRP index as a simple prognostic indicator in patients with advanced cancer: a confirmatory study. Annals of Oncology, 18, 1395–9.

147. Kikuchi, N., Ohmori, K., Kuriyama, S. et al.(2007). Survival prediction of patients with advanced cancer: the predictive accuracy of the model based on biological markers. Journal of Pain and Symptom Management, 34(6), 600–06.

148. Fries, J.F., and Ehrlich, G.E. (eds) (1981). Prognosis. Contemporary outcomes of disease. The Charles Press Publishers, Bowie, MD.

149. McKellar, D., Reiling, R., and Eiseman, B. (1998). *Prognosis and outcomes in surgical disease.* Quality Medical Publishing, St. Louis, MO.

150. Kapoor, A., and Singh, B. (1993). *Prognosis and risk assessment in cardiovascular disease.* Churchill Livingstone, New York.

151. Schonwetter, R., and Jani, C. (2000). Survival estimation in non-cancer patients with advanced disease. In *Topics in palliative care.* (eds. Portenoy, R., and Bruera, E.). Oxford University Press, Oxford.

152. Field, D., and Addington-Hall, J. (1999). Extending specialist palliative care to all? *Social Science and Medicine*, **48**(9), 1271–80.

153. Finucane, T. (1999). How gravely ill becomes dying. *JAMA*, **282**(17), 1–7.

154. Poses, R.M., Smith, W.R., McClish, D.K. *et al.* (1997). Physicians' survival predictions for patients with acute congestive heart failure. *Archives of Internal Medicine*, **157**(9), 1001–7.

155. Perlman, R. (1987). Variability in physician estimates of survival for acute respiratory failure in chronic obstructive pulmonary disease. *Chest*, **91**, 515–21.

156. Lynn, J., Harrell, F.E., Cohn, F. (1996). Defining the "terminally ill": insights from SUPPORT. *Duquesne Law Review*, **35**(1), 311–36.

157. Lamont, E.B., and Christakis, N.A. (1789). Some elements of prognosis in terminal cancer. *Oncology (Huntington)*, 13(8), 1165–70, discussion 72–4.

158. Chye, R. Predicting prognosis in palliative care—a five year retrospective analysis Annual Scientific Meeting, Royal Australasian College of Physicians. Sydney, Australia; May 2001.

159. von Gunten, C.F. and Twaddle, M.L. (1996). Terminal care for noncancer patients. *Clinics in Geriatric Medicine*, **12**(2), 349–58.

160. Stuart, B. (1999). Advanced cancer and comorbid conditions: prognosis and treatment. *Cancer Control*, **6**(2), 168–74.

161. Reuben, D.B., Rubenstein, L.V., Hirsch, S.H. *et al.* (1992). Value of functional status as a predictor of mortality: results of a prospective study [erratum appears in *American Journal of Medicine* 1993 **94**(2), 232]. *American Journal of Medicine*, **93**(6), 663–9.

162. Standards & Accreditation Committee—Medical Guidelines Taskforce. (1996). *Medical guidelines for determining prognosis in selected non-cancer disease.* 2nd edition. National Hospice Organization, Arlington, VA.

163. Corti, M.C., Guralnik, J.M., Salive, M.E. *et al.* (1994). Serum albumin level and physical disability as predictors of mortality in older persons. *JAMA*, **272**(13), 1036–42.

164. Council on Scientific Affairs, American Medical Association. (1996). Good care of the dying patient. *JAMA*, **275**, 474–8.

165. Lynn, J. (2001). Perspectives on care at the close of life. Serving patients who may die soon and their families: the role of hospice and other services. *JAMA*, **285**(7), 925–32.

166. Reisberg, B. Functional assessment staging (FAST) (1988). *Psychopharmacol Bulletin*, **24**(4), 653–9.

167. Luchins, D.J., Hanrahan, P., and Murphy, K. (1997). Criteria for enrolling dementia patients in hospice. *Journal of the American Geriatrics Society*, **45**(9), 1054–9.

168. Hanrahan, P., Raymond, M., McGowan, E. *et al.* (1999). Criteria for enrolling dementia patients in hospice: a replication. *American Journal of Hospice and Palliative Care*, **16**(1), 395–400.

169. Mitchell, S.L., Kiely, D.K., Hamel, M.B. *et al.* (2004). Estimating prognosis for nursing home residents with advanced dementia. *JAMA*, **291**(22), 2734–40.

170. Schonwetter, R.S., Soendker, S., Perron, V. *et al.* (1998). Review of Medicare's proposed hospice eligibility criteria for select noncancer patients. *American Journal of Hospice and Palliative Care*, **15**(3), 155–8.

171. The gold standards framework. Retrieved from http://www.goldstandardsframework.nhs.uk/ on 5 December 2007.

172. Prognostic Indicator Guidance. Retrieved from http://www.goldstandardsframework.nhs.uk/content/gp_contract/Prognostic%20Indicators%20Guidance%20Paper%20v%2025.pdf. on 5 December 2007.

173. Coventry, P.A., Grande, G.E., Richards, D.A. (2005). Prediction of appropriate timing of palliative care for older adults with non-malignant life-threatening disease: a systematic review. *Age Ageing*, **34**(3), 218–27.

174. Virik, K., and Glare, P. (2002). Validation of the palliative performance scale for inpatients admitted to a palliative care unit in Sydney, Australia. *Journal of Pain and Symptom Management*, **23**(6), 455–7.

175. Glare, P., Eychmueller, S., and Virik, K. The use of the palliative prognostic score in patients with diagnoses other than cancer. *Journal of Pain and Symptom Management*, **26**(4), 883–5.

176. Marquis, K., Debigare, R., Lacasse, Y. *et al.* (2002). Midthigh muscle cross-sectional area is a better predictor of mortality than body mass index in patients with chronic obstructive pulmonary disease. *American Journal of Respiratory Critical Care Medicine*, **166**(6), 809–13.

177. Nishimura, K., Izumi, T., Tsukino, M. *et al.* (2002). Dyspnea is a better predictor of 5-year survival than airway obstruction in patients with COPD. *Chest*, **121**(5), 1434–40.

178. Oga, T., Nishimura, K., Tsukino, M. *et al.* (2003). Analysis of the factors related to mortality in chronic obstructive pulmonary disease: role of exercise capacity and health status. *American Journal of Respiratory Critical Care Medicine*, **167**(4), 44–9.

179. Dzau, V. and Braunwald, E. (1991). Resolved and unresolved issues in the prevention and treatment of coronary artery disease: a workshop consensus statement. *American Heart Journal*, **121**(4 Pt 1), 1244–63.

180. Lehman, R. (2006). Prognosis in advanced heart failure—a team approach. In *Heart Failure and Palliative Care—a team approach* (eds. Johnson, M., Lehman, R.), pp. 44–59. Radcliffe Publishing Ltd, Abingdon.

181. Koglin, J., Pehlivanli, S., Schwaiblmair, M. *et al.* (2001). Role of brain natriuretic peptide in risk stratification of patients with congestive heart failure. *Journal of the American College of Cardiology*, **38**(7), 1934–41.

182. Ralli, S., Horwich, T.B., and Fonarow, G.C. (2005). Relationship between anemia, cardiac troponin I, and B-type natriuretic peptide levels and mortality in patients with advanced heart failure. *American Heart Journal*, **150**(6), 1220–7.

183. Fonarow, G.C. and Horwich, T.B. (2003). Combining natriuretic peptides and necrosis markers in determining prognosis in heart failure. *Reviews in Cardiovascular Medicine*, **4**(Suppl 4), S20–S28.

184. Gardner, R.S., Ozalp, F., Murday, A.J. *et al.* (2003). N-terminal pro-brain natriuretic peptide. A new gold standard in predicting mortality in patients with advanced heart failure. *European Heart Journal*, **24**(19), 1735–43.

185. Berger, R., Huelsman, M., Strecker, K. *et al.* (2002). B-type natriuretic peptide predicts sudden death in patients with chronic heart failure. *Circulation*, **105**(20), 2392–7.

186. Huynh, B.C., Rovner, A., and Rich, M.W. (2006). Long-term survival in elderly patients hospitalized for heart failure: 14-year follow-up from a prospective randomized trial. *Archives of Internal Medicine*, **166**(17), 1892–8.

187. Frazier, O.H., Rose, E.A., Oz, M.C. *et al.* (2001). Multicenter clinical evaluation of the HeartMate vented electric left ventricular assist system in patients awaiting heart transplantation. *Journal of Thoracic and Cardiovascular Surgery*, **122**(6), 1186–95.

188. Miller, L.W., Pagani, F.D., Russell, S.D. *et al.* (2007). Use of a continuous-flow device in patients awaiting heart transplantation. *New England Journal of Medicine*, **357**(9), 885–96.

189. Levy, W., Mozaffarian, D., Linker, D. *et al.* (2006). The Seattle Heart Failure Model: prediction of survival in heart failure. www.seattleheartfailuremodel.org. *Circulation*, **113**(11), 1424–33.

190. Mozaffarian, D., Anker, S., Anand, I. *et al.* (2007). Prediction of mode of death in heart failure: the Seattle Heart Failure Model. www.seattleheartfailuremodel.org. *Circulation*, **116**(4), 360–2.

191. Greipp, P.R., San Miguel, J., Durie, B.G. *et al.* (2005). International staging system for multiple myeloma. *Journal of Clinical Oncology*, **23**(15), 3412–20.

192. Ko, D.T., Tu, J.V., Masoudi, F.A. *et al.* (2005). Quality of care and outcomes of older patients with heart failure hospitalized in the

United States and Canada. *Archives of Internal Medicine*, **165**(21), 2486–92.

193. Fletcher, C.M., Elmes, P.C., Fairbairn, A.S. (1959). The significance of respiratory symptoms and the diagnosis of chronic bronchitis in a working population. *British Medical Journal*, **2**(5147), 257–66.

194. O'Donnell, D., Aaron, S., Bourbeua, J. *et al.* (2007). Canadian Thoracic Society recommendations for management of chronic obstructive pulmonary disease—2007 update. *Canadian Respiratory Journal*, **14**(Suppl.B), 5B–32B.

195. Gunen, H., Hacievliyagil, S.S., Kosar, F. *et al.* (2005). Factors affecting survival of hospitalised patients with COPD. *European Respiratory Journal*, **26**(2), 234–41.

196. Hansen-Flaschen, J. (2004). Chronic obstructive pulmonary disease: the last year of life. *Respiratory Care*, **49**(1), 90–7; discussion 7–8.

197. Brody, K.K., Perrin, N.A., and Dellapenna, R. (2006). Advanced illness index: Predictive modeling to stratify elders using self-report data. *Journal of Palliative Medicine*, **9**(6), 1310–9.

198. Aguero-Torres, H., Fratiglioni, L., Guo, Z. (1998). Prognostic factors in very old demented adults: a seven-year follow-up from a population-based survey in Stockholm. *Journal of the American Geriatrics Society*, **46**(4), 444–52.

199. Drachman, D.A., O'Donnell, B.F., Lew,R.A. *et al.* The prognosis in Alzheimer's disease. 'How far' rather than 'how fast' best predicts the course. *Archives of Neurology*, **47**(8), 851–6.

200. Whalen, C.C., Antani, M., Carey, J. *et al.* (1994). An index of symptoms for infection with human immunodeficiency virus: reliability and validity. *Journal of Clinical Epidemiology*, **47**, 537–46.

201. Olson, E. (2003). Dementia and neurodegenerative diseases. In *Geriatirc palliative care*, (eds. Morrison, R., Meier, D., Capello, C.), pp. 160–74. Oxford University Press, New York.

202. Alvarez-Fernandez, B., Garcia-Ordonez, M.A., Martinez-Manzanares, C. *et al.* (2005). Survival of a cohort of elderly patients with advanced dementia: nasogastric tube feeding as a risk factor for mortality. *International Journal of Geriatric Psychiatry*, **20**(4), 363–70.

203. Gilgen, R. and Garms-Homolova, V. (1995). Resident Assessment Instrument (RAI): System zur Klientenbeurteilung und Dokumentation in der Langzeitpflege—eine Ubersicht. *Zeitschrift fur Gerontologie und Geriatrie*, **28**(1), 25–8.

204. Hawes, C., Morris, J.N., Phillips, C.D. *et al.* (1997). Development of the nursing home Resident Assessment Instrument in the USA. *Age and Ageing*, **26**(Suppl 2), 19–25.

205. Hirdes, J.P., Frijters, D.H., and Teare, G.F. (2003). The MDS-CHESS scale: a new measure to predict mortality in institutionalized older people. *Journal of the American Geriatrics Society*, **51**(1), 96–100.

206. Fleck, A., Raines, G., Hawker, F. *et al.* (1985). Increased vascular permeability: a major cause of hypoalbuminaemia in disease and injury. *Lancet*, **1**, 781–4.

207. Capitani, E., Cazzaniga, R., Francescani, A. *et al.* (2004). Cognitive deterioration in Alzheimer's disease: is the early course predictive of the later stages? *Neurological Sciences*, **25**(4), 198–204.

208. Teno, J.M., Harrell, F.E., Jr., Knaus, W. *et al.* (2000). Prediction of survival for older hospitalized patients: the HELP survival model. Hospitalized Elderly Longitudinal Project. *Journal of the American Geriatrics Society*, **48**(5 Suppl), S16–24.

209. Cherny, N.I., Ripamonti, C., Pereira, J. *et al.* (2001). Strategies to manage the adverse effects of oral morphine: an evidence-based report. *Journal of Clinical Oncology*, **19**(9), 2542–54.

210. Hudson, A. (1990). Amyotrophic lateral sclerosis: clinical evidence of differences in pathogenesis and etilogy. In *Amyotrophic lateral sclerosis: concepts in pathogenesis and etiology*, (ed. Hudson, A.), pp. 108–43. University of Toronto Press, Toronto.

211. Mandrioli, J., Faglioni, P., Nichelli, P. *et al.* (2006). Amyotrophic lateral sclerosis: prognostic indicators of survival. *Amyotrophic Lateral Sclerosise*, **7**(4), 211–20.

212. Jablecki, C.K,. Berry, C., and Leach, J. (1989). Survival prediction in amyotrophic lateral sclerosis. *Muscle and Nerve*, **12**(10), 833–41.

213. Kaufmann, P., Levy, G., Thompson, J.L. *et al.* (2005). The ALSFRSr predicts survival time in an ALS clinic population. *Neurology*, **64**(1), 38–43.

214. Vender, R.L., Mauger, D., Walsh, S. *et al.* (2007). Respiratory systems abnormalities and clinical milestones for patients with amyotrophic lateral sclerosis with emphasis upon survival. *Amyotrophic Lateral Sclerosise*, **8**(1), 36–41.

215. Bachmann, P., Marti-Massoud, C., Blanc-Vincent, M.P. *et al.* (2003). Summary version of the Standards, Options and Recommendations for palliative or terminal nutrition in adults with progressive cancer (2001). *British Journal of Cancer*, **89**(Suppl 1), S107–S110.

216. Shaw, A.S., Ampong, M.A., Rio, A. *et al.* (2006). Survival of patients with ALS following institution of enteral feeding is related to pre-procedure oximetry: a retrospective review of 98 patients in a single centre. *Amyotrophic Lateral Sclerosise*, **7**(1), 16–21.

217. Mitchell, S.L. and Tetroe, J.M. (2000). Survival after percutaneous endoscopic gastrostomy placement in older persons. *Journals of Gerontology Series A-Biological Sciences & Medical Sciences*, **55**(12), M735–M739.

218. Langmore, S.E., Kasarskis, E.J., Manca, M.L. *et al.* (2006). Enteral tube feeding for amyotrophic lateral sclerosis/motor neuron disease. *Cochrane Database of Systematic Reviews*, **4**, CD004030.

219. Sorenson, E.J., Crum, B., and Stevens, J.C. (2007). Incidence of aspiration pneumonia in ALS in Olmsted County, MN. *Amyotrophic Lateral Sclerosise*, **8**(2), 87–9.

220. Piepers, S., van den Berg, J.P., Kalmijn, S. *et al.* (2006). Effect of non-invasive ventilation on survival, quality of life, respiratory function and cognition: a review of the literature. *Amyotrophic Lateral Sclerosise*, **7**(4), 195–200.

221. Shoesmith, C.L., Findlater, K., Rowe, A. *et al.* (2007). Prognosis of amyotrophic lateral sclerosis with respiratory onset. *Journal of Neurology, Neurosurgery and Psychiatry*, **78**(6), 629–31.

222. Kleopa, K.A., Sherman, M., Neal, B. *et al.* (1999). BiPAP improves survival and rate of pulmonary function decline in patients with ALS. [see comment]. *Journal of the Neurological Sciences*, **164**(1), 82–8.

223. Paillisse, C., Lacomblez, L., Dib, M. *et al.* (2005). Prognostic factors for survival in amyotrophic lateral sclerosis patients treated with riluzole. *Amyotrophic Lateral Sclerosis and Other Motor Neuron Disorders*, **6**(1), 37–44.

224. Turner, M.R., Bakker, M., Sham, P. *et al.* (2002). Prognostic modelling of therapeutic interventions in amyotrophic lateral sclerosis. *Amyotrophic Lateral Sclerosis and Other Motor Neuron Disorders*, **3**(1), 15–21.

225. Miller, R.G., Mitchell, J.D., Lyon, M. *et al.* (2002). Riluzole for amyotrophic lateral sclerosis (ALS)/motor neuron disease (MND). [update of *Cochrane Database of Systematic Reviews* 2001 **4**, CD001447; PMID: 11687111]. *Cochrane Database of Systematic Reviews*, **2**, CD001447.

226. Rippon, G.A., Scarmeas, N., Gordon, P.H. *et al.* (2006). An observational study of cognitive impairment in amyotrophic lateral sclerosis. *Archives of Neurology*, **63**(3), 345–52.

227. Wong, G.Y., Schroeder, D.R., Carns, P.E. *et al.* (2004). Effect of neurolytic celiac plexus block on pain relief, quality of life, and survival in patients with unresectable pancreatic cancer: a randomized controlled trial. *JAMA*, **291**(9), 1092–9.

228. Rakowski, D.A., Caillard, S., Agodoa, L.Y. *et al.* (2006). Dementia as a predictor of mortality in dialysis patients. *Clinical Journal of The American Society of Nephrology*, **1**(5), 1000–5.

229. Poppel, D.M., Cohen, L.M., and Germain, M.J. (2003). The renal palliative care initiative. *Journal of Palliative Medicine*, **6**(2), 321–6.

230. Low, J.A., Liu, R.K.Y., Strutt. R. *et al.* (2001). Specialist community palliative care services—a survey of general practitoners' experience in Eastern Sydney. *Supportive Care in Cancer*, **9**, 474–6.

231. Brechtl, J.R., Breitbart, W., Galietta, M. *et al.* (2001). The use of highly active antiretroviral therapy (HAART) in patients with advanced

HIV infection: impact on medical, palliative care and quality of life outcomes. *Journal of Pain and Symptom Management*, **21**(1), 41–51.

232. Gerard, L., Flandre, P., Raguin, G. *et al.* (1996). Life expectancy in hospitalized patients with AIDS: prognostic factors on admission. *Journal of Palliative Care*, **12**(1), 26–30.

233. May, M., Sterne, J.A., Sabin, C. *et al.* (2007). Prognosis of HIV-1-infected patients up to 5 years after initiation of HAART: collaborative analysis of prospective studies. *AIDS*, **21**(9), 1185–97.

234. Olivotto, I.A., Bajdik, C.D., Ravdin, P.M. *et al.* (2005). Population-based validation of the prognostic model ADJUVANT! for early breast cancer. *Journal of Clinical Oncology*, **23**(12), 2716–25.

235. Altman, D.G., Egger, M., Davey, S. *et al.* (2000). Systematic reviews of studies of prognostic variables. In *Systematic Reviews in Health Care* (eds. Egger, M., Davey Smith, G., and Altman, D.G.). London, BMJ Books.

236. King, J.T., Jr., Justice, A.C., Roberts, M.S. *et al.* (2003). Collaboration in HIVOR-USPT. Long-term HIV/AIDS survival estimation in the highly active antiretroviral therapy era. *Medical Decision Making*, **23**(1), 9–20.

237. Holley, J.L. (2007). Palliative care in end-stage renal disease: illness trajectories, communication, and hospice use. *Advance Chronic Kidney Disorder*, **14**(4), 402–8.

238. Caraceni, A., Nanni, O., Maltoni, M. *et al.* (2000). Impact of delirium on the short term prognosis of advanced cancer patients. Italian Multicenter Study Group on Palliative Care. *Cancer*, **89**(5), 1145–9.

239. Lau, F., Karlson, N., Downing, G.M. *et al.* 13-year survival trajectory analysis of the Palliative Performance Scale (PPSv2) in prognostication for palliative care patients. In preparation.

240. Hancock, K., Clayton, J.M., Parker, S.M. *et al.* (2007). Discrepant perceptions about end-of-life communication: a systematic review. *Journal of Pain and Symptom Management*, **34**(2), 190–200.

241. Beadle, G.F., Yates, P.M., Najman, J.M. *et al.* (2004). Beliefs and practices of patients with advanced cancer: implications for communication. *British Journal of Cancer*, **91**(2), 254–7.

242. Lamont, E.B. and Christakis, N.A. (2001). Prognostic disclosure to patients with cancer near the end of life. *Annals of Internal Medicine*, **134**(12), 1096–105.

243. The, A.M., Hak, T., Koeter, G. *et al.* (2000). Collusion in doctor-patient communication about imminent death: an ethnographic study. *BMJ*, **321**(7273), 1376–81.

244. Butow, P.N., Dowsett, S., Hagerty, R. *et al.* (2002). Communicating prognosis to patients with metastatic disease: what do they really want to know? *Support Care Cancer*, **10**(2), 161–8.

245. Kutner, J.S., Steiner, J.F., Corbett, K.K. *et al.* (1999). Information needs in terminal illness. *Social Science and Medicine*, **48**(10), 1341–52.

246. Hagerty, R.G., Butow, P.N., Ellis, P.M. (2005). Communicating prognosis in cancer care: a systematic review of the literature. *Annals of Oncology*, **16**(7), 1005–53.

247. Hagerty, R.G., Butow, P.N., Ellis, P.A. *et al.* (2004). Cancer patient preferences for communication of prognosis in the metastatic setting. *Journal of Clinical Oncology*, **22**(9), 1721–30.

248. Parker, S.M., Clayton, J.M., Hancock, K. *et al.* (2007). A systematic review of prognostic/end-of-life communication with adults in the advanced stages of a life-limiting illness: patient/caregiver preferences for the content, style, and timing of information. *Journal of Pain and Symptom Management*, **34**(1), 81–93.

249. Aabom, B., Kragstrup, J., Vondeling, H. *et al.* (2005). Defining cancer patients as being in the terminal phase: who receives a formal

diagnosis, and what are the effects? *Journal of Clinical Oncology*, **23**(30), 7411–6.

250. Murphy, D.J., Burrows, D., Santilli, S. *et al.* (1994). The influence of the probability of survival on patients' preferences regarding cardiopulmonary resuscitation. *New England Journal of Medicine*, **330**(8), 545–9.

251. Weeks, J.C., Cook, E.F., O'Day, S.J. *et al.* (1998). Relationship between cancer patients' predictions of prognosis and their treatment preferences [erratum appears in *JAMA* 2000, **283**(2)], 203. *JAMA*, **279**(21), 1709–14.

252. Jenkins, V., Fallowfield, L., and Saul, J. (2001). Information needs of patients with cancer: results from a large study in UK cancer centres. *British Journal of Cancer*, **84**(1), 48–51.

253. Fallowfield, L.J., Jenkins, V.A., and Beveridge, H.A. (2002). Truth may hurt but deceit hurts more: communication in palliative care. *Palliative Medicine*, **16**(4), 97–303.

254. Kirk, P., Kirk, I., and Kristjanson, L.J. (2004). What do patients receiving palliative care for cancer and their families want to be told? A Canadian and Australian qualitative study. *BMJ*, **328**(7452), 1343.

255. Meredith, C., Symonds, P., Webster, L. *et al.* (1996). Information needs of cancer patients in west Scotland: cross sectional survey of patients' views. *BMJ*, **313**(7059), 724–6.

256. Grunfeld, E.A., Maher, E.J., Browne, S. *et al.* (2006). Advanced breast cancer patients' perceptions of decision making forpalliative chemotherapy. *Journal of Clinical Oncology*, **24**(7), 1090–8.

257. Butow, P.N., Maclean, M., Dunn, S.M. (1997). The dynamics of change: cancer patients' preferences for information, involvement and support. *Annals of Oncology*, **8**(9), 857–63.

258. Kaplowitz, S.A., Campo, S., and Chiu, W.T. (2002).Cancer patients' desires for communication of prognosis information. *Health Communication*, **14**(2), 221–41.

259. Lobb, E.A., Kenny, D.T., Butow, P.N. *et al.* (2001). Women's preferences for discussion of prognosis in early breast cancer. *Health Expect*, **4**(1), 48–57.

260. Bruera, E., Sweeney, C., Calder, K. *et al.* (2001). Patient preferences versus physician perceptions of treatment decisions in cancer care. *Journal of Clinical Oncology*, **19**(11), 2883–5.

261. Clayton, J.M., Hancock, K.M., Butow, P.N. *et al.* (2007). Clinical practice guidelines for communicating prognosis and end-of-life issues with adults in the advanced stages of a life-limiting illness, and their caregivers. *Medical Journal of Australia*, **86**(12 Suppl), S77, S83–108.

262. Bruera, E., Neumann, C.M., Mazzocato, C. *et al.* (2000). Attitudes and beliefs of palliative care physicians regarding communication with terminally ill cancer patients. *Palliative Medicine*, **14**(4), 287–98.

263. Christakis, N. (1999). *Death foretold*. University of Chicago Press, Chicago, IL.

264. Karnofsky, D.A. (1950). Nitrogen mustards in the treatment of neoplastic disease. *Advanced Internal Medicine*, **4**, 1–75.

265. Yates, J., Chalmer, B., and McKegney, F. (1948). Evaluation of patients with advanced cancer using the Karnofsky Performance Status. *Cancer*, **45**, 2220–24.

266. Lamont, E.B., and Christakis, N.A. (2001). Prognostic disclosure to patients with cancer near the end of life. *Annals of Internal Medicine*, **134**(12), 1096–105.

Palliative medicine and modern cancer care

Nathan I. Cherny and Raphael Catane

The division of cancer care into systems that deliver primary anti-tumour therapies during the period of active treatment and systems that deliver hospice or palliative care for patients who have advanced disease is anachronistic[1]. The goals of medical oncology extend beyond reducing tumour burden and prolonging life. The care of patients with cancer includes a quality-of-life dimension, and there is need for a continuum inpatient care in which both primary therapies and palliative interventions are integrated according to the clinical circumstances of the patient. For most patients, it is the medical oncologist who assumes the role of the physician primarily responsible for the provision and coordination of cancer care. This role is enormously challenging and it demands a wide range of cognitive, clinical, and interpersonal skills (Table 3.4.1).

Traditionally, the study and practice of medical oncology has focused on the development and implementation of anti-cancer therapies. By virtue of these endeavours, along with measures to provide for early diagnosis, substantial improvements in long- and short-term survival have been achieved for a number of cancers, such as the germ cell tumours, lymphomas, early-stage breast and colorectal cancer, and the leukaemias. More sobering, however, is the cure rate for cancer overall, which remains less than 50 per cent; cancer continues to account for more than 25 per cent of all adult deaths[2]. For many patients, cancer is a chronic progressive illness, and for this population, the issues surrounding the quality of their remaining time are critical, irrespective of the clinical course of their illness or the duration of survival.

Recommendations on the integration of palliative medicine and medical oncology

An expert committee of the World Health Organization has emphasized the need for the integration of efforts directed at maintaining the patient's quality of life during all stages of cancer treatment[1]. The committee's report noted that factors causing patient distress exist from the time of diagnosis, and that supportive and palliative interventions are needed concurrently with efforts to control the underlying cancer. This holds true for patients undergoing both curative and palliative anti-cancer treatments, and is a model that has been widely endorsed by numerous national and professional bodies[3,4].

In the USA, the National Comprehensive Cancer Network (NCCN) guidelines emphasize the importance of palliative care as part of comprehensive cancer care:

All cancer patients should be screened for palliative care needs at their initial visit, at appropriate intervals, and as clinically indicated. Patients and families should be informed that palliative care is an integral part of their comprehensive cancer care. Palliative care should be delivered based upon clinical practice guidelines. Educational programs should be provided to all healthcare professionals and trainees so that they can develop effective palliative care knowledge, skills, and attitudes. Skilled, palliative care specialists and interdisciplinary, palliative care teams should be readily available to provide consultative or direct care to patients/families that request or require their expertise. Medical care contracts should include appropriate reimbursement for palliative care. Clinical health outcomes measurement should include palliative care domains. Quality of palliative care should be monitored by institutional quality improvement programs[5].

Terminology: supportive or palliative care

There has been much confusion regarding the definitions of supportive care and palliative care. The European Society of Medical Oncology (ESMO) has adopted pragmatic definitions that distinguish these two types of care and emphasizes the discrete sub-entity of end-of-life care. According to these definitions, supportive care aims to optimize the comfort, function, and social support of the patient and their family at all stages of the illness. Palliative care is care that aims to optimize the comfort, function, and social support of the patient and their family *when cure is not possible*. Although the clinical scenarios suggested by these definitions obviously overlap, it is the context of incurability, with all of its implications, that grounds palliative care. Supportive care is needed by every patient continuously; palliative care focuses on the special needs of patients who are either incurable or who have a very low likelihood of cure, and from this perspective, 'end-of-life care' or 'terminal care' is defined as palliative care when death is imminent (Fig. 3.4.1). End-of-life care acknowledges that the intensity of physical, psychological, existential, spiritual, and family issues may be magnified by the patient's approaching death.

This distinction between supportive care and palliative care is semantic in part, and it should be emphasized that the terms are used differently by various specialists across countries. Some

Table 3.4.1 The clinical roles of the medical oncologist.

Preventative oncology	Counselling
	◆ Diet
	◆ Cigarette smoking
	◆ Alcohol
	◆ Environmental
	Screening
Diagnostic evaluation	Primary evaluation of the patient with suggestive clinical findings
	Cancer staging
	Physiological staging
	Goals of care appropriate to tumour type and stage and patient physiological staging
Communication	Disclosure full and partial
	Treatment counselling
	Prognostic counselling
	Eliciting advanced directives
	Patient and family support
	Psychological support
	Advanced directives
Anti-tumour therapies	Indications
	Selection of optimal therapeutic modality
	Safe administration
	Prevention and management of adverse effects
Symptom control	Physical symptoms
	Psychological symptoms
	Complications of cancer
	Complications of treatment
Social	Optimization of social supports
Care of the dying patient	Physical symptoms
	Psychological symptoms

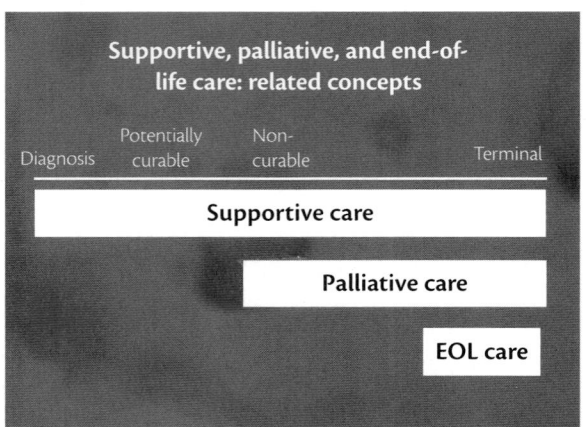

Figure 3.4.1 Schema of the European Society of Medical Oncology definitions of supportive care, palliative care and end of life care[10].

authors appear to apply these labels interchangeably and others consider supportive care to be any intervention that specifically targets complications or side effects related to anti-cancer therapy, whereas palliative care refers to a broader set of strategies that target all quality of life concerns experienced by patients with life-threatening illnesses and their families.

Regardless of the definition, the fundamental reality is that patients with cancer, and their families, may express unmet physical, psycho-social, or spiritual needs at any point during the course of the illness. These needs require specific interventions that aim to reduce suffering, enhance coping, or otherwise improve the individual's quality of life.

Oncology, hospice, and palliative medicine—the division of labour

The integration of oncologic care and palliative care requires familiarity with a range of therapeutic options, appropriate patient evaluation, and a collaborative therapeutic relationship with the patient and other members of an interdisciplinary care team. Care planning and goal setting may be facilitated by considering the natural history of cancer in five phases (Table 3.4.2). The changing status of the patient along this continuum influences the coordination and implementation of palliative interventions.

The medical oncologist is almost always the coordinating health-care provider during the first three phases: the diagnostic workup, attempts at curative therapy, and the phase of ambulatory palliative care, during which the patient continues to attend the cancer clinic. During the latter phase, community-based nursing and medical providers are often introduced to provide additional services outside of the health-care institution and in anticipation of diminished mobility.

During the fourth phase, when the patient has advanced illness and may not be ambulatory, and during the fifth, end-of-life care, new decisions often are required about the site of care and level of help required by the patient and family. Patients may be treated at home, in a nursing home, in an inpatient palliative care facility such as a hospice residence, or if indicated, an acute care hospital. The decisions about care are influenced by the nature and severity of the prevailing clinical problems, the extent of home-based medical and nursing resources, the availability of community facilities, the goals of care, and patient preference[6,7]. The role of the oncologist during these latter phases is determined by similar considerations. In some instances, the oncologist will remain the primary provider of palliative care until the patient dies. In other instances, there should be a smooth transition of care as other, usually community-based, services play a progressively greater role and the oncologist becomes a supportive figure. By maintaining continuity in care, the oncologist can ensure that cancer-related issues are adequately addressed and also can limit concerns about abandonment that can magnify patient and family distress[8].

Where oncologic palliative care is delivered

Comprehensive cancer care integrates supportive end palliative care, anti-cancer therapy, and other medical interventions from the time of diagnosis onward. Typically, care must be delivered at varying times in an ambulatory clinic, an inpatient ward, and in the patient's home (including nursing home residence). End-of-life

Table 3.4.2 Five phase in the natural history of cancer.

1	Diagnostic: ambulatory or inpatient
2	Curative primary therapy
3	Ambulatory palliative therapy
4	Sedentary palliative therapy—interactional
5	Sedentary palliative therapy—non-interactional

care can be provided in an ambulatory outpatient clinic, through an inpatient consult service, on a geographically-based unit, or in the patient's home.

Organization of services can affect the ability to deliver care in an efficient and timely manner. As most patients with advanced cancer receive a trial of therapy in an ambulatory office-based setting or radiotherapy centre, this provides an excellent opportunity to assess the need for palliative interventions, and to address concrete needs or physical or psychosocial issues. When problems are identified, onsite staff with appropriate expertise can be mobilized to assist. This approach emphasizes the need for strategic placement of services.

A large majority of cancer patients live at home during most of the course of the illness. Programmes to extend palliative-care services into the home may be available to augment the care available through ambulatory settings and community services, such as visiting nurses. Oncologists must become knowledgeable about the existing programmes, refer patients appropriately, and provide continuity of care as services are enhanced. In the USA, home-based end-of-life care often is provided by a certified hospice programme. In the US version of hospice, the oncologist can choose to remain the physician of record throughout the period of end-of-life care, or can become a consultant as appropriate.

With the changing patterns of oncologic care delivery, oncology inpatient wards increasingly are occupied by patients needing symptom control or terminal care. Thus delivery of palliative care has become a major part of inpatient oncology care.

In some inpatient and outpatient settings, palliative care consultation services can help deliver specialist palliative care in a manner similar to other consultation services. When a patient is admitted to the hospital, this service can assist oncologists by providing expert back-up in the management of difficult cases. Back-up of this type may take the form of advice, direct participation in management, or sometimes in the transfer of case management. It is through consultation that most oncologists learn about new developments outside the focus of their clinical specialty.

Dedicated palliative care units, if available, can provide a high level of expertise in palliative interventions, such as symptom control, and comprehensive end-of-life care. Oncologists can admit patients to acute palliative care units in hospitals for symptom evaluation and management, respite, management of treatment complications, or terminal care.

The oncologist's role in palliative care

Both the American Society of Clinical Oncology (ASCO)[9] and the European Society of Medical Oncology (ESMO)[10] have policy statements outlining the responsibilities of medical oncologists in the care of patients with incurable cancer. ASCO states that it is the

Table 3.4.3 ESMO policy regarding the role of the oncologist in the provision of supportive and palliative care

1. The medical oncologist must be skilled in the supportive and palliative care of patients with cancer and in end-of-life care

2. The oncologist must address the need for an appropriate medical nursing and para-medical infrastructure to address the special needs of these patients and their families

3. It is the responsibility of the medical oncologist to assess and evaluate physical and psychological symptoms of patients under their care and to ensure that these problems are adequately addressed

4. The delivery of high quality supportive and palliative care requires cooperation and coordination with physicians of other disciplines (including radiotherapy, surgery, rehabilitation, psychoncology, pain medicine and anaesthesiology, palliative medicine etc.) as well as with paramedical clinicians (including nursing, social work, psychology, physical and occupational therapy, chaplains, and others)

5. In the care of dying patients the medical oncologist must:

- Respect the dignity of both patient and caregivers

- Be sensitive to and respectful of the patient's and family's wishes

- Use the most appropriate measures that are consistent with patient choices

- Make alleviation of pain and other physical symptoms a high priority

- Recognize that good care for the dying person requires quality medical care, but also entails services that are family- and community-based to address, for example, psychological, social, and spiritual/religious problems

- Offer continuity (the patient should be able to continue to be cared for, if so desired, by his/her primary care and medical oncology providers)

- Advocate access to therapies which are reasonably expected to improve the patient's quality of life and ensure that patients who choose alternative and non-traditional treatments not be abandoned

- Provide access to palliative care and hospice care

- Respect the patient's right to refuse treatment, as expressed by the patient or an authorized surrogate

- Respect the physician's professional responsibility to discontinue some treatments when appropriate, with consideration for both patient and family preferences

- Promote clinical and evidence-based research on providing care at the end of life

Adapted from: Cherny et al.[10].

oncologist's responsibility to care for their patient along a continuum that starts at the moment of diagnosis and extends throughout the course of the illness. In addition to appropriate anti-cancer treatment, this includes symptom control and psychosocial support during all phases of care, including the last phase of life[9]. The ESMO policy statement reiterates these points and defines the role of the oncologist in palliative care (Table 3.4.3).

The oncologic management of advanced cancer

Medical oncologists have expertise in the appropriate use of anti-tumour therapies. They should appreciate the use of these strategies as palliative techniques that can both potentially prolong survival and improve comfort and function. The specific issues of palliative chemotherapy and radiotherapy are discussed in Chapters 9.1 and 9.2. As treatment options become more varied, complex, and expensive, the balancing of benefits and burdens in considering these primary treatment options is becoming increasingly challenging. Decision making must take into account a range of relevant issues, including goals of care, likelihood of benefit, likelihood of harm, and the desires, beliefs, and understanding of the patient and family. Addressing the relative roles of disease-modifying approaches requires familiarity with key concepts of patient benefit, quality of life, and risk/benefit analysis. When the therapeutic index of anti-tumour therapies is diminished and the likelihood of benefit is outweighed by either the risk or the burden of the treatments, it is the oncologist who must help steer the patient and the family to a care programme that focuses on symptom palliation and other efforts to reduce suffering, help coping, maintain quality of life, and prepare for the end of life (see below).

Communication with patients and family members

Given the complexity of the goals of care, patient and family expectations, and the range of therapeutic options, communication with patients and their families is a critical element of the oncologist's role in caring for patients with incurable cancer. Communication is challenging and requires patience and refined interpersonal and counselling skills to facilitate effective, informed decision making.

A variety of communication tasks usually are undertaken by the oncologist. The diagnosis, prognosis, and treatment options must be explained and this may involve discussions about the potential risks and benefits of treatment options, the role of palliative care, and the necessity for discontinuing anti-tumour therapies when appropriate. In performing these tasks, oncologists need the skills to deal with intense emotions, highly distressed patients, and family members with fears, anger, and anticipatory grief.

The management of the complications of cancer

Oncologists must be expert in the evaluation and management of the complications of cancer and anti-cancer therapies. Some common complications are listed in Table 3.4.4.

Evaluation and management of physical, psychosocial, and spiritual disturbances

Patients with advanced cancer commonly have multiple symptoms and other sources of suffering. To address their needs, oncologists must be expert in the evaluation and management of the common physical symptoms, including pain, dyspnoea and cough, fatigue, nausea and vomiting, constipation, diarrhoea, insomnia, and itch. In addition, psychological and existential distress is common[11], and oncologists must be prepared to assess and help manage the varied sources of these concerns. There is extensive evidence suggesting that cancer patients' informational and emotional needs are commonly underestimated and that depression, in particular, is often undetected or undertreated[12–14]. Many patients who develop psychological distress do not spontaneously disclose these problems[15]. There is a notion that 'good patients' do not complain. Furthermore, cancer patients may believe their emotional response to be an inevitable reaction to having a cancer diagnosis. Paradoxically, the most distressed patients may be least likely to acknowledge or discuss their emotional concerns[16], and these patients may be the ones most dissatisfied with their care.

Oncologists are not expected to be expert psycho-oncologists but they are expected to be familiar with the assessment of common psychological problems, such as anxiety, depression, delirium, suicidality and desire for death, death anxiety, and anticipatory grief. Where possible, they should be familiar with anxiolytic and antidepressant pharmacotherapy and they should work closely with mental-health clinicians to help address these issues.

Ensuring a care continuum

Abandonment and discontinuity of care are a cause of great distress to cancer patients. As the physician typically responsible for the primary care of the major medical problems faced by the patient, the oncologist must ensure that the patient has an ongoing and adequate care plan, particularly as the role for anti-tumour therapies diminishes and the patient approaches the end of life.

Interdisciplinary cancer care

The needs of patients with advanced cancer are too complex to be cared for by any one person. In the setting of advanced cancer, the oncologist must work with an interdisciplinary team to build a care plan around the individual needs of the patient and family. In addition to other oncologic and medical sub-specialists, interdisciplinary cancer care often will involve collaboration with social workers, mental health professionals, chaplains, physical therapists, occupational therapists, speech therapists, palliative care clinicians, and others.

Palliative care research

Quality-of-life research has had important impact on the evaluation of oncologic interventions and the quality of life is a now widely accepted clinical outcome worthy of evaluation. Oncologists should be familiar with some of the methodologies involved in the measurement of pain and other physical and psychological symptoms, such as dyspnoea, fatigue, nausea and vomiting, depression and anxiety, and desire for death. Though most oncologists will not conduct palliative care research, appreciation for the strategies used to study quality of life and its component domains is important, if only to assist in judging the level of evidence for the interventions that may be applied to address sources of distress.

Ensuring sound ethical practice

Patients with advanced and incurable illness are in a vulnerable position and there are multiple ethical issues that arise in their care. Medical oncologists must be familiar with common ethical problems that arise (Table 3.4.5) and the ethical principles that assist in their resolution.

Transitioning oncology patients to palliative care

In the setting of far advanced and refractory cancer, one of the most challenging aspects of the oncologist's role is to help patients and their families deal with the transitioning to care that is increasingly focused on palliation rather than disease modification[17]. Talking to patients and families about dying and palliative care is not easy, especially when patients and/or families want to continue aggressive therapy[18,19]. This transition to care that is not focused on disease control but palliative care alone is a stressful experience; for

Table 3.4.4 Complications of cancer.

Neurologic		
Tumour infiltration	Peripheral nerve	
	Cranial nerve	
	Nerve plexus	
	Spinal cord	
	Leptomeninges	
	Brain	
Paraneoplastic		
Pulmonary	Airway obstruction	
	Pleural effusion	
	SVC compression	
	Diffuse pulmonary metastases	
	Haemoptysis	
Musculoskeletal		
	Bone pain	
	Pathological fractures	
Gastrointestinal		
Obstruction	Oropharyngeal	
	Oesophageal	
	Gastric outlet	
	Small bowel	
	Large bowel	
	Pancreatic duct	
	Bleeding	
	Ascites	
Hepatobiliary		
	Obstruction	
	Infiltration	
Genitourinary		
Obstruction	Ureteric	
	Bladder outlet	
Bleeding		
Metabolic	Hypercalcaemia	
	Hyponatraemia	
	Cachexia	
	Anasarca	
Vascular		
Obstruction	Venous	
	Lymphatic	
Thrombosis		
Ischaemia		
Haemorrhage		

many patients it implies impending death and it often triggers fears of helplessness and abandonment by the medical profession. One can diminish the trauma of this process by gradually introducing palliative care as a legitimate and important focus of care at an earlier stage of the disease trajectory, alongside efforts to modify the natural history of the disease. This approach recognizes that with disease progression, treatment goals will evolve from seeking a cure, to control of disease and its complications while reducing sources of suffering and maintaining quality of life, and ultimately, to the latter goals alone.

When to raise the issue

In general, it is preferable to introduce the concept of palliative care as care focused on optimizing the quality of life and introducing the multi-disciplinary team early after the diagnosis of advanced cancer[20]. This approach is widely supported by data derived from patients and their family members[21,22]. Discussions of this kind need to include a review of the information needs and desires of the patient.

The setting

When possible, sensitive discussions should be held in a quiet, comfortable, and private location, and adequate uninterrupted time should be available for questions and discussion. Patients should be encouraged to invite their significant others to be present[23,24].

Assess patients' information needs

As a starting point, it is important to evaluate the patient's understanding of his/her illness and the goals of the treatments that they have undergone until this point. Open-ended questions can be used to evaluate how the patient is coping physically and emotionally. Patients' information needs vary greatly and one wants to find the balance between delivering information necessary for understanding and decision making and between an 'assault of truth' where by patients are given more information than they want or desire.[25] A small proportion of patients do not want much information[22,25,26]. A survey of 126 metastatic cancer patients[22] found that 33 per cent wanted to discuss 'dying and palliative care services' when first told cancer had spread; 19 per cent said that they would want this discussion during the next few consultations; and 33 per cent said later, upon (their) request. Eleven per cent of these patients indicated that they never wanted to discuss dying and palliative care services, and 10 per cent were unsure. Almost half wanted the oncologist to initiate the discussion; 20 per cent wanted the oncologist to check first if the patient wanted to know; and 24 per cent wanted the oncologist to address the issue only if the patient asked. For some patients, there will be a 'necessary collusion' in which these issues will not be addressed forthrightly, but rather, may emerge with the passage of time and evolution of the disease[27,28].

Talking about prognosis

It is common for patients to ask questions about prognosis. The motivation underlying queries about prognosis are not always clear. Whereas many patients want information about their anticipated future so they can plan accordingly, others are seeking reassurance that things are not so serious or hopeless. It is important to try to understand the patient's motive in seeking this information.

Table 3.4.5 Common ethical issues in the care of patients with advanced cancer.

Ethical issues related to disclosure of diagnosis and prognosis
Ethical issues in decision making: paternalism, autonomy, informed consent
Ethical issues relating to conflicts of interest
Ethical issues when patients refuse or demand treatment
The right to adequate relief of physical and psychological symptoms and its implications
Consent: informed, uninformed
Ethical issues at the end of life
Sedation for refractory symptoms
Hydration and nutrition at the end of life
DNR
Use of invasive palliative approaches, i.e. nephrostomy or dialysis
Foregoing treatment
Euthanasia, assisted suicide

In discussing prognosis, clinicians often describe median survival data or 5-year survival data. Median survival information can be particularly misleading, as it is a point descriptor that does not describe interindividual variability, which may be great. Similarly, 5-year survival data may not give adequate information about true anticipated likelihood of survival. If, indeed, prognostic information is required, the following principles are useful.[29,30]

◆ *Be honest.* If you do not know, say so. It may be useful to describe a worst case and a best case scenario.

◆ *Use averages.* 'One-third of people will still be doing well a year from now and half will live about 6 months. However, you are unique and I do not know exactly what course this disease will take'.

◆ *Emphasize the limits of predictions.* 'No one can really be sure what this will mean for you as an individual. We cannot predict surprises and it is prudent to make plans both for the best, but also to cover options if things do not go well'.

◆ *Commit to non-abandonment.* Reassure the patient you will continue to care for him or her, whatever happens.

◆ *Caution patients and their families that unexpected events can happen.* Suggest that it is worth while to get their affairs in order so they won't be totally unprepared if something unexpected does happen. 'Let's hope and work for the best but, at the same time, prepare for things in case the situation does not go as well as what we hope for'.

◆ *Avoid nihilism.* Never tell a patient 'There's nothing more that can be done'. or 'Do you want everything done?' There is *always* something to be done. Even if chemotherapy or other anti-neoplastic treatments are not indicated because the risk of harm exceeds any likelihood of benefit, there is still much that must be done to help the patient live well during the remainder of his or her life, and prepare for the end of life. Discuss what can be done to make it better (and what might make it worse).

◆ *Initiate end-of-life planning.* Sensitively bring up the important subject of advance care planning.

Discussing anti-tumour therapies when cure is not possible

It is intrinsically difficult to tell a patient and their family that there is no treatment that offers the possibility of cure. Despite progress in non-curative anti-tumour therapies in some conditions, the potential benefit of these therapies in many diseases is small, and when benefit is derived, it is often of short duration. Many patients in this setting undertake sometimes burdensome treatments based on exaggerated expectations of potential treatment benefits[31]. In counselling patients, it is important to outline treatment options, including those that do not involve potentially burdensome anti-tumour treatments. In presenting the potential benefits of anti-tumour therapies, it is appropriate to discuss both the likelihood of help and the likelihood of harm.

Situations in which cure is not possible are heterogeneous. In some instances, such as metastatic breast, colorectal cancer, ovarian or small-cell lung cancer, there may be a moderate to high likelihood of prolonging survival. In other situations, such as gastric or pancreatic cancer and most of the soft tissue sarcomas, survival prolongation is unlikely. In the latter situation, informed consent requires that patients understand the limited likelihood of benefit and should almost always be offered the options of palliation without chemotherapy or the option of participating in an experimental therapy (if one is available).

These recommendations are supported by the findings of a recent study of the recordings of the initial oncologic consultations of 118 cancer patients with incurable disease. Analysis of these consultations found that 84.7 per cent of patients were informed about the aim of anti-cancer treatment, 85 per cent were told that their disease was incurable, and 58 per cent were told about life expectancy, but only a minority of consultations included discussion of an alternative to anti-cancer treatments (44 per cent), discussion on the impact of anti-cancer treatment on quality of life (36 per cent), or an offer of management choice (30 per cent).[32] In only 10 per cent of consultations did the oncologist check a patient's understanding.

Introducing palliative care options

After indicating that further curative treatment has a low chance of being effective and that the aims of the treatment are disease control and optimizing quality of life, the clinician should introduce the option of effective palliative treatment options to help improve the quality of life. If disease-modifying treatments are available and accepted by the patient, the discussion should present anti-tumour treatment and palliative care together, emphasizing that this is not an 'either or' choice, but rather a situation in which the best care will incorporate a balanced approach between the two parallel strategies.

Maintaining hope (see Chapter 15.1)

Being told that a cancer cannot be cured is devastating for most people. It is crucial that doctors help patients find ways of maintaining hope, as well as giving them honest information about their disease[33]. Indeed, many patients and their families avoid discussions about prognosis or curability for fear that the discussion may undermine or destroy hope.

Hope has been defined as an expectation that there will be a positive outcome in the future[34]. Commonly, however, it is associated with unrealistic expectations. Magical thinking, with hope for miracles, is a trans-cultural phenomenon, and in the context of a poor prognosis, it is not necessarily inappropriate for a patient to hope for a cure even if it is highly unlikely. Nonetheless, messages about hope from health professionals should focus on more realistic events, such as periods of remission, response to treatments, and excellent symptom control. Deliberately fostering false hope of a cure, when a cure is not possible, may hinder patients and their family from making appropriate treatment and lifestyle decisions in order to make the best use of their remaining time together. Hence, it is critical that the messages of hope provided to patients are appropriate. Strategies that successfully promote appropriate hope may make a critical contribution to discussing the transition from curative care to palliative care.

In a recent survey of 156 patients with advanced and incurable illness[35], doctor behaviours that augmented hope included offering the most up-to-date treatment (90 per cent), appearing to know all there is to know about the patient's cancer (87 per cent), and saying that pain will be controlled (87 per cent). The majority of patients indicated that the doctor appearing to be nervous or uncomfortable (91 per cent), giving the prognosis to the family first (87 per cent), or using euphemisms (82 per cent) would not facilitate hope.

Qualitative data derived from interviews with patients and their caregivers[33] revealed several hope enhancing themes: (1) emphasize what can be done (particularly control of physical symptoms, emotional support, care, and dignity and practical support), (2) explore realistic goals, and (3) discuss issues related to day-to-day living. According to one experienced practitioner, hope may be enhanced by making seven (overt or implicit) commitments to patients[36]:

- You will have the best of medical treatment, aiming to prevent exacerbation, improve function and survival, and ensure comfort.

- You will never have to endure overwhelming pain, shortness of breath, or other symptoms. Symptoms will be anticipated and prevented when possible, evaluated and addressed promptly, and controlled effectively. Severe symptoms—such as shortness of breath—will be treated as emergencies. Sedation will be used when necessary to relieve intractable symptoms near the end of life.

- Your care will be continuous, comprehensive, and coordinated. You and your family can count on having certain professionals to rely upon at all times and on an appropriate and timely response to your needs. The transitions between services, settings, and personnel will be minimized in number and made to work smoothly.

- You and your family will be prepared for everything that is likely to happen in the course of your illness. If necessary you will receive supplies and training needed to handle predictable events.

- Your wishes will be sought and respected, and followed whenever possible. You will be given information about the available choices and you will be encouraged to be an active participant in decision making. You will have the right to refuse treatments.

- We will help you and your family consider your personal and financial resources, and we will respect your choices about the use of your resources.

- We will do all we can to see that you and your family will have the opportunity to make the best of everyday. We are committed to treat you as a person, not a disease. What is important to you is important to us as part of the care team. We will endeavour to respond to your physical, psychological, social, and spiritual needs as well as those of your family. Indeed, we will be there to support your family throughout this period and after your death.

Care delivery models

Integration of oncology with palliative care

There is no one best way for oncologists and specialist palliative care services to work together. Rather a number of different models have been developed.

Sequential care model

In this model, the patients are cared for by the oncology service as long as there is potential benefit in disease-modifying treatment. When it is clear that there is no further benefit to be derived from this treatment, the responsibility for the patient's ongoing care is transferred to the palliative care service. Of course, the palliative care service may be consulted earlier, when the patient is under primary oncologic management, and similarly, should anti-tumour interventions be required (such as palliative radiotherapy) when the patient is being followed primarily by the palliative-care services, expert oncologic consultation is available. In this model of care, end-of-life care is coordinated by the palliative care service.

The advantages of this model of care are that it is characterized by clear delineation of responsibility. It enables the oncologist to focus on the dominant aspects of his/her professional tasks and allows him/her to fulfil his obligations to provide palliative care and continuity of care by a process of benevolent transfer of primary responsibility to a palliative care team. Successful implementation of this model requires close cooperation between the oncology and palliative care services, good communication to minimize patient feelings of abandonment, and timely referral of patients.

Oncologist-based palliative care

In this model, the oncologist assumes the role of coordinating care and providing both anti-cancer and palliative care services, thus seeing the patient through from diagnosis until death. This approach emphasizes the importance of the oncologist/patient relationship and the notions of continuity of care and non-abandonment. Oncologists undertaking this approach need to be highly skilled in palliative care and in interdisciplinary care, including interaction with a palliative care support team. Even oncologists who are highly skilled in palliative care may sometimes benefit from expert input and this should be sought when difficult problems arise.

The major advantage of this approach is its emphasis on continuity of care. The success of this model is dependant on the level of palliative care skills and sophistication of the oncologist, and his/her ability to balance competing intellectual and practical interests. This approach is augmented by having a strong relationship with a care team, including a palliative medicine expert for backup in difficult cases.

Concurrent model

In this model, patients with advanced cancer are jointly cared for by both oncology and palliative medicine specialists in a similar way that medical, surgical, and radiation oncologists traditionally work together. The relative role of the oncology or palliative medicine physician is determined by the prevailing problems and, indeed, case management responsibilities may be handled by either and are usually determined by the circumstances of the patient.

This model emphasizes the duality of advanced cancer care and the need for continuity of care, both with regard to disease modification and palliative care. Successful implementation of this approach requires close cooperation and open communication between oncology and palliative medicine clinicians.

Palliative care delivery in major cancer centres

In the most recent survey of the best cancer hospitals in the USA, 49 of the 50 highest ranking hospitals had palliative care programmes as part of their clinical services[37]. Although this penetration is also seen in Canada, the UK, and Australia, integration of palliative care and oncology is the exception rather than the rule in many other parts of the world.

Beyond minimal requirements (Table 3.4.6), ESMO has developed an incentive programme to recognize centres that demonstrate a high level of integration between medical oncology and palliative care. To be eligible for accreditation as a 'designated centre' 13 criteria must be met (Table 3.4.7). These criteria set a gold standard for integration. As of 2008, 48 centres across Europe had been accredited with achieving this level of care.

The development of palliative care services requires appropriate resource allocation for staffing, physical space, and necessary supports. Thought should be given to the development of processes such as joint meetings to facilitate good integration between oncology and palliative care services. Tumour boards for patients with advanced cancer, radiology conferences, and interdisciplinary psychosocial conferences to discuss challenging cases, afford excellent opportunities to forge collaborative working relationships and balanced discussion.

Barriers to coordination between oncology and palliative care

Different cultures of care

Palliative care and oncology have substantially different histories and cultures of care[38]. These differences may account for some of the difficulties encountered in integration of these approaches. Whereas palliative care grew out of the hospice movement, which tends to the physical and emotional needs of patients and their families rather than focusing on the diseases themselves; modern oncology has developed out of the specialist biomedical model with a strong emphasis on addressing the disease processes, with view to cure patients or to prolong their lives. Whereas interdisciplinary care is inherent to palliative care, the concept of the 'patient care team' has not yet been universally adopted in oncology. Indeed, the ESMO survey of oncologist practice in the management of incurable cancer patients indicates that it is relatively underdeveloped and uncommon[39].

Delays in referral for palliative care consultations

Very often, the timing of referrals to specialized palliative care s ervices, including palliative care units, inpatient hospices, and home-based palliative care programmes, is delayed until patients have severe symptom burden or are close to death[40–42]. In a survey of bereaved family members of cancer patients[42], half of the

respondents regarded the timing of referrals as late or very late. Indeed, the median admission period was less than 1 month (22 days), and approximately 20 per cent of the patients died within 1 week. The reasons for this are complex: oncologist and patient reluctance to address issues implying incurability, fears that a palliative care referral will undermine hope or shorten the patient's life, and insufficient in-advance discussion about preferred end-of-life care with physicians[42]. Oncologists sometimes express reluctance about palliative care referrals for fear that anti-tumour treatment strategies will be challenged, or that the patient will be 'stolen'[39,41].

Another reason for delayed referral is the oncologist's failure to recognize the deterioration in the patient's clinical course. There are data to suggest that oncologists are commonly overoptimistic and overestimate survival substantially[43]. Indeed, a meta-analysis of the 13 available studies showed that cancer physicians tended to overestimate prognosis by at least 30 per cent.[44] To add to this, when patients request information about prognosis, many physicians consciously overstate the prognosis even beyond their own (inflated) estimate[45].

Abandonment

Unfortunately, when a patient's disease reaches an advanced stage, a point at which symptom management becomes more necessary, some oncologists relinquish their role in the care of the patient because radiotherapy and chemotherapy have nothing more to contribute[46]. Sadly, it is not uncommon to hear patients relate that the oncologist said that 'there is nothing further can be done'. In many cases, not only is there no continuity of care, but palliative care options are not presented. For some patients, this undermines hope and the desire to live[47].

Territoriality

There is anecdotal evidence that professionals in various disciplines looking after patients with cancer may never meet one another, and oncologists, family physicians, and palliative care specialists often

Table 3.4.6 Proposed minimal requirements for palliative care in cancer centres.

1. Cancer patients receiving active therapy in cancer centres, especially those with advanced cancer, should be routinely assessed regarding the presence and severity of physical and psychological symptoms and the adequacy of social supports
2. When inadequately controlled symptoms are identified they must be evaluated and treated with the appropriate urgency (depending on the nature and severity of the problem)
3. Cancer centres must provide skilled emergency care of inadequately relieved physical and psychological symptoms
4. Cancer centres must ensure an ongoing programme of palliative and supportive care for patients with advanced cancer who are no longer benefited by anti-tumour interventions
5. Cancer centres should incorporate social work and psychological care as part of routine care
6. When patients require inpatient end-of-life care, the cancer centre staff either provide the needed inpatient care or arrange adequate care in an appropriate hospice or palliative care service

Table 3.4.7 Thirteen criteria for optimal supportive and palliative care in a cancer centre.

1. The centre provides closely integrated oncology and palliative care clinical services

2. The centre is committed to a philosophy of continuity of care and non-abandonment

3. The centre provides high-level home care with expert back-up and coordination of home care with primary cancer clinicians

4. The centre incorporates programmatic support of family members

5. The centre provides routine patient assessment of physical and psychological symptoms and social supports and has an infrastructure that responds with appropriate interventions in a timely manner

6. The centre incorporates expert medical and nursing care in the evaluation and relief of pain and other physical symptoms

7. The centre incorporates expert care in the evaluation and relief of psychological and existential distress

8. The centre provides emergency care of inadequately relieved physical and psychological symptoms

9. The centre provides facilities and expert care for inpatient symptom stabilization

10. The centre provides respite care for ambulatory patients for patients unable to cope at home or in cases of family fatigue

11. The centre provides facilities and expert care for inpatient end-of-life care and is committed to providing adequate relief of suffering for dying patients

12. The centre participates in basic or clinical research related to the quality of life of cancer patients

13. The centre is involved in clinician education to improve the integration of oncology and palliative care

do not appreciate the challenges other physicians face[38,48]. The survey of European oncologists revealed that many oncologists do not feel that their palliative care colleagues understand cancer care at a level sufficient to render informed advice, and a small proportion of oncologists feel that palliative care physicians will divert patients who may otherwise still derive benefit from anti-tumour therapies[39].

Palliative care education for oncologists

Current shortcomings in oncologist education

In 1998, the American Society of Clinical Oncology (ASCO) performed a large-scale survey of US oncologists about their experiences in providing palliative care[49,50]. The survey questionnaire consisted of 118 questions. A total of 3227 oncologists responded. There were no significant differences between the percentages of medical, radiation, surgical, or paediatric oncologists who responded as a proportion of their representation in ASCO. In this survey, the most frequent sources of palliative care education were: trial and error during clinical practice (90 per cent); from colleagues during clinical practice (73 per cent); from a role model during oncology fellowship training (71 per cent); and from a traumatic experience with a patient. The ASCO survey found that the oncologists did not obtain adequate information from their colleagues and role models,

despite reporting these people as the most frequent educational resource: 81 per cent said they had inadequate mentoring or coaching in how to discuss poor prognosis; 65 per cent said they received inadequate information about controlling symptoms; and <10 per cent thought all of their formal training during medical school, internships, residency and fellowship combined was 'very helpful'.

In a 2004 survey, ASCO trainees rated end-of-life education less highly than their general fellowship training. They viewed their attendings as more expert in non-end-of-life than end-of-life care. Of those who had performed bone marrow biopsy, feedback on this technique was more likely to have occurred than feedback on an end-of-life discussion (73 per cent versus 56 per cent; $p = 0.0006$). Regarding pain management, 94 per cent of fellows felt prepared to manage pain in the dying; 75 per cent assessed pain in their patient who died most recently; 41 per cent were explicitly taught when to rotate opioids; and only 30 per cent performed an opioid conversion correctly[51].

In a recent survey of ESMO members regarding their involvement in palliative care, 42 per cent of respondents reported that they had not received adequate training in palliative care during their residency. This finding is consistent with previously published data regarding the training of medical oncologists in the management of cancer pain[52–54], communication skills[55,56], and palliative care[54,57]. In response to the statement 'most medical oncologists I know *are* expert in the management of the physical and psychological symptoms of advanced cancer', more respondents disagreed (41.8 per cent) than agreed (37.5 per cent). This finding suggests that most oncologists have a low assessment of their colleagues' readiness to manage the physical and psychological symptoms of advanced cancer, a perception that is consonant with the findings regarding training. The survey further demonstrated wide discrepancies between oncologists' positive attitudes and their actual practice patterns. Whereas 88.4 per cent of respondents agreed that medical oncologists should coordinate the care of cancer patients at all stages of disease, including end-of-life care, actual practice was found to be much less: only 43 per cent commonly coordinated the care of cancer patients at all stages of disease; fewer than 50 per cent collaborated commonly with any supportive/palliative care clinician (including social workers); only 39 per cent commonly coordinated meetings with the family of dying patients; and only 11.8 per cent commonly managed delirium (despite the high prevalence of this problem among patients with far advanced cancer). Whereas 70.4 per cent responded that they have a close working relationship with the palliative care (or hospice) services in their region, the levels of collaboration with palliative care and hospice services was actually low: only 37.8 per cent often collaborated with a home hospice (palliative care) team, and only 35.1 and 33.3 per cent often collaborated with a palliative care medical specialist or nursing specialist, respectively. The ESMO study also found that that 15–20 per cent of the responding medical oncologists had have pervasively negative views regarding the oncologist's role in the supportive/palliative care of patients with advanced cancer and end-of-life care.

A survey of burnout among 598 oncologists found that 56 per cent of medical oncologists felt some degree of burnout and that feelings of frustration and a sense of failure are commonplace[58]. The stress of providing palliative care for incurable and terminal patients was cited a major contributing factor. These data prompted an editorial in the *Journal of Clinical Oncology* by the then president of ASCO, which called for better preparation of medical oncologists for this aspect of clinical responsibility[59].

Curricular requirements of ASCO and ESMO

There is universal recognition for the need to provide training in palliative care for all oncologists. This has been incorporated into the 'Global Core Curriculum in Medical Oncology: that was developed and endorsed by ASCO and ESMO [60,61] (Table 3.4.8). ASCO has also published a curriculum for oncologists in the assessment and management of cancer pain[62].

In 2003, ESMO as part of its Palliative and Supportive care programme, published a document describing nine core elements of oncology training in palliative and supportive care[10] (Table 3.4.9). The ESMO palliative care training programme recognized that an oncologist does not need to be expert in all aspects of palliative care. Rather, the curriculum distinguishes between three levels of desired proficiency:

1 *Expert*. This refers to a high level of academic and practical knowledge. At the completion of training, oncology graduates should be expert in: the oncologic management of advanced cancer, the management of complications of cancer, and the evaluation, and management of physical symptoms of cancer and cancer treatment.

2 *Skilled*. This refers to effective clinical competence. This level of proficiency is required for communication with patients and family members

Table 3.4.8 Summary of the 'Global Core Oncology Curriculum' regarding palliative care.

Supportive and palliative measurements. Trainees should know what supportive therapy during anticancer therapy is, and should be able to use supportive therapy. They should know the indications of the different supportive treatments and their limitations and side-effects. Trainees should know what palliative therapy is and should be able to determine when palliative care is indicated.
Supportive measures, evaluation and management of:
1. Nausea and vomiting
2. Infections and neutropoenia
3. Anaemia
4. Thrombocytopoenia
5. Organ protection
6. Mucositis
7. Malignant effusions
8. Extravasation
9. Oncologic emergencies
10. Paraneoplastic syndromes
11. Nutritional support
Palliative care and end-of-life care: evaluation and management of:
1. Pain
2. Other physical symptoms
3. Communication
4. Rehabilitation

3 *Familiar*. This is the lowest level of required competence. It refers to familiarity with core concepts to the level of being able to adequately evaluate the patient, initiate basic therapy, and communicate with clinical experts. At the completion of training, oncology graduates should be familiar with: evaluation and management of psychological and existential symptoms of cancer, interdisciplinary care of patients with advanced cancer, palliative care research principles, ethical issues in the management of patients with cancer and strategies to identify and prevent burnout.

Educational materials for oncologists

Remarkably, despite the frequent role as primary care provider to cancer patients with advanced illness, oncologists are not a regular target audience for educational materials on palliative care. Nonetheless, special educational materials have been developed and should be widely promoted. Among these materials are the following:

ESMO Handbook of Advanced Cancer Care. This is a small practical handbook developed and distributed by ESMO, written by oncologists and clinicians working with cancer patients, outlining major issues in palliative care as they apply to the cancer patient. It addresses a wide range of issues in decision making, physical, and psychological management issues.

Evidence-based clinical guidelines. In the USA, both the National Cancer Center Network (NCCN, www.nccn.org) and the National Cancer Institute (NCI, www.cancer.gov/cancertopics/pdq/supportivecare) have developed online resources to deliver up-to-date, evidence-based guidelines for elements of palliative care. The NCI's supportive care subsection of the PDQ includes monographs covering common physical and psychological symptoms in patients with advanced cancer.

EPEC-O. ASCO, in collaboration with the National Cancer Institute and EPEC (Education for Physicians in End-of-Life Care), has developed a curriculum in end-of-life care specific to oncologists. This well-developed programme aims to equip oncologists with the attitudes, knowledge, and skills to provide the best possible palliative care for their patients. The educational materials, which are available on DVD includes three plenary sessions and 32 PowerPoint® presentations with background information for the instructors. The multimedia materials make excellent use of trigger films to stimulate discussion and to highlight important points.

Optimizing Cancer Care—The Importance of Symptom Management Vols I and II. These are curricular materials that have been published and marketed by ASCO. This is a well-developed (but expensive) educational resource that covers 29 supportive care topics, including effective communication, and physical and psychological symptom assessment and management. It uses an array of teaching tools—treatment scenarios, annotated slides, algorithms, and a table of medications.

Initiatives to improve oncologist understanding and involvement in palliative care

Oncology conferences

There is an encouraging trend to greater incorporation of palliative care content in major oncology meetings. Additionally, many of the international and national oncology organizations now organize conferences and workshops on palliative and supportive care issues.

Table 3.4.9 ESMO's nine core skills for supportive and palliative care training for medical oncologists.

1	**The oncologic management of advanced cancer**	Medical oncologists **must be expert** in the appropriate use of anti-tumour therapies as palliative techniques when cure is no longer possible. This includes specific familiarity with key concepts of patient benefit, quality of life and risk/benefit analysis
2	**Communication with patients and family members**	Medical oncologists **must be skilled** in effective and compassionate communication with cancer patients and their families. Specific skills include: ◆ Explaining diagnosis and treatment options ◆ Disclosure of diagnosis ◆ Explaining issues relating to prognosis ◆ Explaining the potential risk and benefits of treatment options ◆ Counselling skills to facilitate effective, informed decision making. ◆ Explaining the role of palliative care ◆ The care of distressed family members: fear, anticipatory grief, and bereavement care ◆ Convening of family meetings
3	**The management of complications of cancer**	Medical oncologists **must be expert** in the evaluation and management of the complications of cancer including: ◆ Bone metastases ◆ CNS metastases: brain and leptomeningeal metastases ◆ Neurological dysfunction: primary, metastatic, paraneoplastic, and iatrogenic ◆ Liver metastases and biliary obstruction ◆ Malignant effusions: pleural, peritoneal, and pericardial ◆ Obstruction of hollow viscera: oesophagus, airways, gastric outlet, small and large bowel, and ureters ◆ Metabolic consequences of cancer ◆ Anorexia and cachexia ◆ Haematologic consequences: anaemia, neutropoenia, thrombocytopoenia, and clotting diathesis ◆ Sexual dysfunction
4	**Evaluation and management of physical symptoms of cancer and cancer treatment**	Medical oncologists **must be expert** in the evaluation and management of the common physical symptoms of advanced cancer including: ◆ Pain ◆ Dyspnoea and cough ◆ Fatigue ◆ Nausea and vomiting ◆ Constipation ◆ Diarrhoea ◆ Insomnia ◆ Itch
5	**Evaluation and management of psychological and existential symptoms of cancer**	Medical oncologists **must be familiar** with the evaluation and management of the common psychological and existential symptoms of cancer including: ◆ Anxiety ◆ Depression ◆ Delirium ◆ Suicidality and desire for death ◆ Death anxiety ◆ Anticipatory grief
6	**Interdisciplinary care**	Medical oncologists **must be familiar** with the roles of other professions in the care of patients with cancer and with community resources to support the care of these patients.
7	**Palliative care research**	Medical oncologists **must be familiar** with research methodologies that are applicable to patients with cancer including: ◆ Quality of life research ◆ Pain measurement and research ◆ Measurement of other physical and psychological symptoms: dyspnoea, fatigue, nausea and vomiting, depression and anxiety, and desire for death ◆ Needs evaluation ◆ Decision making research ◆ Palliative care audit

(continued)

Table 3.4.9 (Continued) ESMO's nine core skills for supportive and palliative care training for medical oncologists.

8	**Ethical issues in the management of patients with cancer**	Medical oncologist **must be familiar** with common ethical problems that arise in the management of advanced cancer and ethical principles that assist in their resolution:
		◆ Ethical issues related to disclosure of diagnosis and prognosis
		◆ Ethical issues in decision making: paternalism, autonomy, informed consent
		◆ The right to adequate relief of physical and psychological symptoms and its implications
		◆ Consent: informed, uninformed
		◆ Ethical issues at the end of life: sedation for refractory symptoms, hydration and nutrition at the end of life, DNR, use of invasive palliative approaches
		◆ Foregoing treatment
		◆ Euthanasia, assisted suicide
9	**Preventing burnout**	Medical oncologist **must be familiar** with the symptoms of burnout, the factors that contribute to burnout and strategies to prevent its development

Adapted from: Cherny et al.[10].

Incorporation of palliative care issues in major oncologic journals

Journal content of the major oncologic journals reflects, to some degree, professional priorities. Although all of the major oncologic journals cover palliative care issues to some degree, they remain marginalized issues in most of the journals. Of the major oncology journals, the outstanding exception is the *Journal of Clinical Oncology*. In addition to publishing more than 600 reports of clinical trials in the area of palliative care and quality of life, it created a new section in 2000, which is entitled 'The Art of Oncology: When the Tumor Is Not the Target' and focuses on issues of patient–physician communication, ethical decision-making, and symptom control in the management of advanced cancer.

Research

Oncologist-initiated research in palliative care

As the landmark publication of the Australian breast cancer study comparing the continuous versus intermittent chemotherapy using a quality-of-life outcome in addition to survival[63], the prevalence of such studies has grown exponentially. Quality of life assessment has become a routine part of oncology clinical trials.

Oncologists have played a major role in the development of improved strategies in the prevention and management of chemotherapy-induced nausea and vomiting. Additionally, a smaller number of medical oncologists have involved themselves in projects addressing the management of other specific physical and psychological symptoms, oncologist–patient communication, and cancer-related complications such as hypercalcaemia and malignant effusions.

Chemotherapy versus 'best supportive care'

Since 1988, 30 trials have been published in relatively resistant solid tumours, ostensibly comparing cytotoxic treatment to 'best supportive care' by evaluating outcomes of quality of life, time to progression and survival. The almost universal result of thee studies had been the conclusion that patients receiving treatment had better outcomes than those receiving 'best supportive care'. Unfortunately, these studies do not usually describe the specific interventions included in a 'best supportive care' model, nor did they incorporate the involvement of experts in palliative care. As a

result, this is a flawed literature and the term 'best supportive care' has been has been criticized[64]. A more accurate description would be 'standard palliative care'.

Working toward the future

The furtherance of medical oncologist awareness, knowledge, practice, and research in palliative medicine will require an elevation of the relative priority of palliation as a goal of cancer care. This, in turn, will need to be reflected in resources allocation, programme development, and clinical practice.

Palliative medicine as an oncologic sub-specialty

There is a need for more oncologists with advanced training in palliative medicine. The prevalence of patients in need of this sort of specialty service suggests that each department would benefit from at least one oncologist with palliative medicine expertise. For the medical oncologist, an enhanced familiarity with palliative medicine can extend the clinician's therapeutic repertoire, diminish the stress of caring for patients who have incurable cancer, improve patient outcomes, and provide new avenues for clinical research and reward. Palliative medicine is clinically and intellectually challenging. It is an interface between the disciplines of oncology (medical, surgical, and radiation), psychiatry, clinical ethics, and clinical pharmacology. It encourages and, indeed, necessitates interdisciplinary practice, and it defines a scope of basic and clinical research that may elucidate symptom pathogenesis and improve management strategies.

Elevating the priority of palliation

This process requires a paradigm shift at all levels of the cancer medicine infrastructure. The groundswell of interest in palliative medicine and hospice facilities has made limited inroads into the routine care of cancer patients. Given the current infrastructure for career development and resource allocation for clinical and research programmes in medical oncology, initiatives such as those undertaken by ESMO are needed to raise the priority of palliative medicine.

Development of clinical programmes

Individual institutions must be encouraged to develop expert services to provide a clinical service and role models, and to conduct clinical and basic research in the palliative care of cancer patients. Services should incorporate clinical resources to address problems related to physical and psychological symptoms.

Research

Palliative medicine opens a vast array of potential research questions. Symptom palliation, ethics, communication, coping needs, emotional, and spiritual care, and the palliative effects of primary anti-neoplastic therapy are all valid research directions. The clinical trials expertise that currently exists in the oncology community should be used to address specific symptom control problems (such as dyspnoea, nausea, delirium) or complications of cancer (such as neoplastic plexopathies, or bowel obstruction).

The individual clinician

Every oncologist can focus their attention on the palliative needs of their own patients. Practice guidelines, journals, consultants, and other resources are available to help the oncologist address these issues. Physicians can remind themselves, their colleagues, and students to think about physical and psychological symptom control and patient supports at all stages of the illness and not just in the terminal phase. Oncologists can develop relationships with local hospice organizations to ensure close cooperation and smooth transition with continuity of care for patients referred for hospice care. Those involved with teaching can emphasize the evaluation and management of physical and psychological symptoms, communication skills, attitudes, and the care of dying patients.

Conclusion

The fusion of palliative medicine and medical oncology, in practice and in education, can provide a better standard of patient care, reduce the risk of oncologist burnout, and increase the likelihood of patient, family, and physician satisfaction. There need be no gulf between these disciplines and only together do they represent truly comprehensive cancer care. The realization of this fusion will require the participation of individual clinicians; programme directors; and the policy makers for cancer centres, professional organizations, and the health-care regulatory authorities. It is a logical next step in the evolution of medical oncology.

References

1. World Health Organization (1990). *Cancer pain relief and palliative care*. World Health Organization, Geneva.
2. Jemal, A., Murray, T., Samuels, A. *et al.* (2003). Cancer statistics. CA: *a Cancer Journal for Clinicians*, **53**(1), 5–26.
3. National Institute for Clinical Excellence (NICE) (2004). *Improving supportive and palliative care for adults with cancer*. NICE London.
4. Foley, K. and Gelband, H. (2001). *Improving palliative care for cancer: Summary and recommendations*. National Academies Press, Washington, DC.
5. National Comprehensive Cancer Network (2006). *Palliative Care*, http://www.nccn.org.
6. Hinton, J. (1994). Which patients with terminal cancer are admitted from home care? *Palliative Medicine*, **8**(3), 197–210.
7. Hinton, J. (1994). Can home care maintain an acceptable quality of life for patients with terminal cancer and their relatives? *Palliative Medicine*, **8**(3), 183–96.
8. Quill, T.E. and Cassel, C.K. (1995). Nonabandonment: a central obligation for physicians [see comments]. *Annals of Internal Medicine*, **122**(5), 368–74.
9. Smith, T.J. and Schnipper, L.J. (1998). The American Society of Clinical Oncology Program to Improve End-of-Life Care. *Journal of Palliative Medicine*, **1**(3), 221–30.
10. Cherny, N.I., Catane, R., and Kosmidis, P. (2003). ESMO takes a stand on supportive and palliative care. *Annals of Oncology*, **14**(9), 1335–7.
11. Wright, E.P., Kiely, M.A., Lynch, P. *et al.* (2002). Social problems in oncology. *British Journal of Cancer*, **87**(10), 1099–104.
12. Breitbart, W., Rosenfeld, B., Pessin, H. *et al.* (2000). Depression, hopelessness, and desire for hastened death in terminally ill patients with cancer. *JAMA*, **284**(22), 2907–11.
13. Pereira, J. and Bruera, E. (2001). Depression with psychomotor retardation: diagnostic challenges and the use of psychostimulants. *Journal of Palliative Medicine*, **4**(1), 15–21.
14. Hotopf, M., Chidgey, J., Addington-Hall, J. *et al.* (2002). Depression in advanced disease: a systematic review Part 1. Prevalence and case finding. *Palliative Medicine*, **16**(2), 81–97.
15. Maguire, P. (2002). Improving the recognition of concerns and affective disorders in cancer patients. *Annals of Oncology*, **13**(Suppl 4), 177–81.
16. Greenley, J.R., Young, T.B., and Schoenherr, R.A. (1982). Psychological distress and patient satisfaction. *Medical Care*, **20**(4), 373–85.
17. Schofield, P., Carey, M., Love, A. *et al.* (2006). 'Would you like to talk about your future treatment options'? Discussing the transition from curative cancer treatment to palliative care. *Palliative Medicine*, **20**(4), 397–406.
18. Neff, P., Lyckholm, L., and Smith, T. (2003). Truth or consequences: what to do when the patient doesn't want to know. *Journal of Clinical Oncology*, **21**(9 Suppl), 17–9.
19. Matsuyama, R., Reddy, S., and Smith, T.J. (2006). Why do patients choose chemotherapy near the end of life? A review of the perspective of those facing death from cancer. *Journal of Clinical Oncology*, **24**(21), 3490–6.
20. Morita, T., Akechi, T., Ikenaga, M. *et al.* (2004). Communication about the ending of anticancer treatment and transition to palliative care. *Annals of Oncology*, **15**(10), 1551–7.
21. Hagerty, R.G., Butow, P.N., Ellis, P.M. *et al.* (2005). Communicating with realism and hope: incurable cancer patients' views on the disclosure of prognosis. *Journal of Clinical Oncology*, **23**(6), 1278-88.
22. Hagerty, R.G., Butow, P.N., Ellis, P.A. *et al.* Cancer patient preferences for communication of prognosis in the metastatic setting. *Journal of Clinical Oncology*, **22**(9), 1721–30.
23. Ptacek, J.T. and Eberhardt, T.L. (1996). Breaking bad news. A review of the literature [see comments]. *JAMA*, **276**(6), 496–502.
24. Butow, P.N., Kazemi, J.N., Beeney, L.J. *et al.* (1996). When the diagnosis is cancer: patient communication experiences and preferences. *Cancer*, **77**(12), 2630–7.
25. Clayton, J.M., Butow, P.N., and Tattersall, M.H. (2005). When and how to initiate discussion about prognosis and end-of-life issues with terminally ill patients. *Journal of Pain and Symptom Management*, **30**(2), 132–44.
26. Sapir, R., Catane, R., Kaufman, B. *et al.* (2008). Cancer patient expectations of and communication with oncologists and oncology nurses: the experience of an integrated oncology and palliative care service. *Supportive Care in Cancer*, **8**(6), 458–63.
27. Helft, P.R. (2005). Necessary collusion: prognostic communication with advanced cancer patients. *Journal of Clinical Oncology*, **23**(13), 3146–50.
28. Groopman, J.E. (2005). A strategy for hope: a commentary on necessary collusion. *Journal of Clinical Oncology*, **23**(13), 3151–2.
29. *The Michigan Physician Guide to End-of-Life Care*. (2001) Michigan Department of Community Health, MI.

30. Clayton, J.M., Butow, P.N., Arnold, R.M. *et al.* (2005). Discussing life expectancy with terminally ill cancer patients and their carers: a qualitative study. *Supportive Care in Cancer*, **13**(9), 733–42.

31. Weeks, J.C., Cook, E.F., O Day, S. *et al.* (1998). Relationship between cancer patients' predictions of prognosis and their treatment preferences [see comments]. *JAMA*, **279**(21), 1709–14.

32. Gattellari, M., Voigt, K.J., Butow, P.N. *et al.* (2002*)*. When the treatment goal is not cure: are cancer patients equipped to make informed decisions? *Journal of Clinical Oncology*, **20**(2), 503–13.

33. Clayton, J.M., Butow, P.N., Arnold, R.M. *et al.* (2005). Fostering coping and nurturing hope when discussing the future with terminally ill cancer patients and their caregivers. *Cancer*, **103**(9), 1965–75.

34. Nunn, K.P. (1996). Personal hopefulness: a conceptual review of the relevance of the perceived future to psychiatry. *British Journal of Medical Psychology*, **69**(Pt 3), 227–45.

35. Hagerty, R.G., Butow, P.N., Ellis, P.M. *et al.* (2005). Communicating with realism and hope: incurable cancer patients' views on the disclosure of prognosis. *Journal of Clinical Oncology*, **23**(6), 1278–88.

36. Lynn, J. (2000). Sick to death and not going to take it any more. In *Promises to keep: Changing the way we provide care at the end of life: The national coalition for health care*, (ed. Schoeni, P.Q.), pp. 1–4. The Insititute for Health Care Improvement, Boston, MA.

37. US News and World Report. (2006). Best Cancer Hospitals 2006.

38. McKenzie, M.R. (1998). Oncology and palliative care: bringing together the two solitudes. *CMAJ*, **158**(13), 1702–4.

39. Cherny, N.I. and Catane, R. (2003). Attitudes of medical oncologists toward palliative care for patients with advanced and incurable cancer: report on a survery by the European Society of Medical Oncology Taskforce on Palliative and Supportive Care. *Cancer*, **98**(11), 2502–10.

40. Cheng, W.W., Willey, J., Palmer, J.L. *et al.* (2005). Interval between palliative care referral and death among patients treated at a comprehensive cancer center. *Journal of Palliative Medicine*, **8**(5), 1025–32.

41. Ferrell, B.R. (2005). Late referrals to palliative care. *Journal of Clinical Oncology*, **23**(12), 2588–9.

42. Morita, T., Akechi, T., Ikenaga, M. *et al.* (2005). Late Referrals to Specialized Palliative Care Service in Japan. *Journal of Clinical Oncology*, **23**(12), 2637–44.

43. Christakis, N.A. and Lamont, E.B. (2008). Extent and determinants of error in doctors' prognoses in terminally ill patients: prospective cohort study [see comments]. *JAMA*, **283**(6), 771–8.

44. Glare, P., Virik, K., Jones, M. *et al.* (2003). A systematic review of physicians' survival predictions in terminally ill cancer patients. *BMJ*, **327**(7408), 195.

45. Lamont, E.B. and Christakis, N.A. (2001). Prognostic disclosure to patients with cancer near the end of life. *Annals of Internal Medicine*, **134**(12), 1096–105.

46. Dias, L., Chabner, B.A., Lynch, T.J., Jr. *et al.* (2003). Breaking bad news: a patient's perspective. *Oncologist*, **8**(6), 587–96.

47. Kissane, D.W., Street, A., and Nitschke, P. (1998). Seven deaths in Darwin: case studies under the Rights of the Terminally Ill Act, Northern Territory, Australia. *Lancet*, **352**(9134), 1097–102.

48. McKenzie, M.R. (1995). BC network to improve palliative care. *CMAJ*, **152**(9), 1378.

49. Emanuel, E.J., Fairclough, D., Clarridge, B.C. *et al.* (2000). Attitudes and practices of U.S. oncologists regarding euthanasia and physician-assisted suicide. *Annals of Internal Medicine*, **133**(7), 527–32.

50. Hilden, J.M., Emanuel, E.J., Fairclough, D.L. *et al.* (2001). Attitudes and Practices Among Pediatric Oncologists Regarding End-of- Life Care: Results of the 1998 American Society of Clinical Oncology Survey. *Journal of Clinical Oncology*, **19**(1), 205–12.

51. Buss, M.K., Lessen, D.S., Sullivan, A.M. *et al.* (2005). Survey of oncology fellows' end-of-life training. ASCO Annual Meeting Proceedings. *J Clin Oncol*, **23**(Suppl 1): abstract 8032.

52. Sapir, R., Catane, R., and Cherny, N.I. (1999). Cancer pain: knowledge and attitudes of physicians in Israel. *Journal of Pain and Symptom Management*, **17**, 266–76.

53. Larue, F., Colleau, S.M., Fontaine, A. *et al.* (1995). Oncologists and primary care physicians' attitudes toward pain control and morphine prescribing in France [see comments]. *Cancer*, **76**(11), 2375–82.

54. Gerrard, G., Kiltie, A.E., and Macdonald, R.G. (1999). Training to treat cancer: future developments. *Hospital Medicine*, **60**(7), 519–21.

55. Fallowfield, L., and Jenkins, V. (1999). Effective communication skills are the key to good cancer care. *European Journal of Cancer*, **35**(11), 1592–7.

56. Baile, W.F., Lenzi, R., Kudelka, A.P. *et al.* (1997). Improving physician-patient communication in cancer care: outcome of a workshop for oncologists. *Journal of Cancer Education*, **12**(3), 166–73.

57. Gilewski, T. (2001). The art of medicine: teaching oncology fellows about the end of life. *Critical Reviews in Oncology/Hematology*, **40**(2), 105–13.

58. Whippen, D.A. and Canellos, G.P. (1991). Burnout syndrome in the practice of oncology: results of a random survey of 1,000 oncologists [see comments]. *Journal of Clinical Oncology*, **9**(10), 1916–20.

59. Abeloff, M.D. (1991). Burnout in oncology–physician heal thyself [editorial; comment]. *Journal of Clinical Oncology*, **9**(10), 1721–2.

60. Hansen, H.H., Bajorin, D.F., Muss, H.B. *et al.* (2004). Recommendations for a Global Core Curriculum in Medical Oncology. *Annals of Oncology*, **15**(11), 1603–12.

61. Hansen, H.H., Bajorin, D.F., Muss, H.B. *et al.* (2004). Recommendations for a global core curriculum in medical oncology. *Journal of Clinical Oncology*, **22**(22), 4616–25.

62. American Society of Clinical Oncology Ad Hoc Committee on Cancer Pain (1992). Cancer Pain Assessment and Treatment Curriculum Guidelines. The Ad Hoc Committee on Cancer Pain of the American Society of Clinical Oncology. *Journal of Clinical Oncology*, **10**(12), 1976–82.

63. Coates, A., Gebski, V., Bishop, J.F. *et al.* (1987). Improving the quality of life during chemotherapy for advanced breast cancer. A comparison of intermittent and continuous treatment strategies. *New England Journal of Medicine*, **317**(24), 1490–5.

64. Cullen, M. (2001). 'Best supportive care' has had its day. *Lancet Oncology*, **2**(3), 173–5.

3.5

Barriers to the delivery of palliative care

Fiona Graham, Suresh Kumar, and David Clark

At present, palliative care reaches only a small fraction of those who could benefit from it. Why this should be so is a complex and multi-factorial matter.

According to projections carried out by the World Health Organization (WHO) and published in early 2006[1], the world will experience a substantial shift in the distribution of deaths from younger age groups to older age groups, and from communicable diseases to non-communicable diseases during the next 25 years. Large declines in mortality are projected to occur between 2002 and 2030 for all of the principal communicable, maternal, perinatal, and nutritional causes, with the exception of HIV/AIDS. Global deaths from HIV/AIDS are projected to rise from 2.8 million in 2002 to 6.5 million in 2030 under a somewhat optimistic baseline scenario that assumes antiretroviral drug coverage reaches 80 per cent by 2012. Although age-specific death rates for most non-communicable diseases are projected to decline, the ageing of the global population will result in significant increases in the total number of deaths caused by most non-communicable diseases. Overall, non-communicable conditions will account for almost 70 per cent of all deaths in 2030 under the baseline scenario. The implications of all this for palliative care are enormous; if appropriate palliative care is to be made available to all who need it, then it becomes vital to address the key barriers to wider coverage that currently exist.

The total number of deaths in the world each year is around 56 million. The great majority of these, some 44 million, occur in the developing countries. It has been estimated that around 60 per cent of those dying would benefit from palliative care[2].

Methods now exist that are acceptable and maintainable at community level and which can ensure the relief of end-of-life suffering on a large scale[3,4,5]. The WHO has promoted these through public-health policies and advice for the rational implementation of pain relief and palliative care[6,7] Despite this, palliative care is not available in many settings where it has a vital contribution to make to the relief of suffering. There are many barriers to the efficient and effective delivery of high quality palliative care and these vary with factors such as geographical setting, economic resources, and the availability of education and training. In this chapter, we provide an overview of these issues beginning with a global perspective, progressing through societal, social, and organizational issues, to professional and, finally, individual barriers.

Key points

- Global indifference to the need for palliative care;
- societal problems relating to public health, culture, education, attitudes, demography, social exclusion, religion, and social class;
- organizational factors including service configuration, access and availability, sustainability, funding, and workforce capacity;
- professional concerns relating to levels of palliative care delivery, education, training, and attitudes; and
- individual issues including disease status and intellectual disability.

Global, societal, and policy barriers

There have been a number of efforts in recent times to highlight aspects of the global development of palliative care and to overcome the endemic resistance to it that is so widespread (see Chapter 2.1). Several major international palliative care organizations have a role in these efforts: the Asia Pacific Hospice Palliative Care Network[8], the African Palliative Care Association[9], the European Association for Palliative Care[10], the International Association of Hospice and Palliative Care[11] as well as some leading national associations such as the National Hospice and Palliative Care Organization (USA)[12] and Help the Hospices (UK)[13] Since 2005, World Hospice and Palliative Care Day has been used as focus for publicity and advocacy[14]. The World Wide Palliative Care Alliance is a coalition of national associations dedicated to a world with universal access to quality palliative care, and harnessing the efforts of national hospice and palliative care associations to that goal[15]. In addition, the International Observatory on End of Life Care at Lancaster University, UK has mapped the development of palliative care around the world in a series of country reports and regional studies as an information resource for global improvement[16]. One way in which the global problem is being addressed is through attempts to define access to pain relief and palliative care as basic human rights, though this concept presents many challenges and is at an early stage of formulation[17,18] Despite attempts by national and international groups working in palliative care, very few countries at present have national policies to promote it. There is a great need to ensure that cancer control policies at the national level include palliative care content and guidance on how appropriate services can be developed[19]. A strong support for this issue has been expressed by the World Health Assembly, which in a 2005 resolution called on members states to set national priorities for cancer control and palliative care and to facilitate appropriate research[20]. In 2006, the European Association for Palliative Care also highlighted the need for more research to improve service development and quality in palliative care[21].

Drug availability

Lack of access to essential medicines is a problem for a large percentage of the world population. WHO estimates that roughly two billion people—one-third of all people on the planet—lack regular access to essential medicines[22]. Much of this 'access gap' is attributable to fundamental economic, social, and educational factors that lie beyond the health sector. In the case of access to analgesics, the issue is further complicated by legal and attitudinal issues.

Inadequate access to pain-relieving analgesia and drugs for the control of other symptoms remains one of the chief barriers to global palliative care development. The majority of pain can be controlled with careful management, addressing psychological and social factors and using relatively inexpensive oral medicines; yet good pain control is still not available to millions who need it. Two-thirds of those with advanced cancer and a third of those undergoing active treatment, suffer pain[23]. Since 1986, the WHO three-step analgesic ladder has provided a simple framework for the progressive treatment of malignant pain[24]. Its originators hoped it would lead to a world free of cancer pain. This has not yet happened, for several reasons: reluctance on the part of physicians to prescribe strong opioids, fear among health-care professionals and the public about addiction and abuse, lack of state and national government engagement with the issue of cancer pain, and a lack of availability of essential drugs due to stringent regulation and economic factors.

Recognition of these issues led the WHO to develop its concept of 'foundation measures' to promote the implementation of cancer pain-relief programmes. These highlight the importance of four key factors essential if cancer pain is to be overcome: education, government policy, drug availability, and implementation of palliative care services throughout the society[25]. To work effectively in this environment, health-care professionals require training in the appropriate and safe use of analgesic drugs, particularly opioids, and this can be difficult if the dominant culture in the workplace is to view these as dangerous substances of misuse. Policy makers, drug regulators, and the general public also need to be more aware that opioid drugs such as morphine have an essential place in the management of pain—one that cannot be sacrificed because of any potential for diversion and misuse.

Key to the effective implementation of the WHO analgesic ladder is the availability of the medication necessary at each of the three steps. Economic factors can sometimes limit the availability of analgesics recommended on the first two steps of the ladder but, in reality, it is the lack of the step-three analgesics, principally morphine, which results in the most suffering. The major reason for this is regulation and its interpretation. The Single Convention on Narcotic Drugs is an international treaty that seeks to ensure that all United Nations (UN) member countries take steps to prevent the abuse of narcotic drugs whilst ensuring adequate availability for medical and scientific use. A key issue is one of securing 'balance' between the regulation

of drugs and their availability for medical purposes[26]. Because of the potential for abuse, regulation is necessary, but this *can* exist in harmony with adequate supplies for medical need and the International Narcotics Control Board (INCB), created to implement the single convention, is committed to assisting governments to achieve a more balanced approach and to reducing barriers to opioid availability for pain relief[27]. A global survey by the INCB in 1995 found that just 10 countries accounted for some 80 per cent of worldwide morphine consumption (with 16 g/per 1000 population); the next 60 countries averaged 2 g/per 1000 and in 120 countries there was no evidence of morphine consumption at all[28]; similarly 29 African countries reported no morphine use at all during 2000–2002[29] The Center for Pain and Policy Studies in Wisconsin has a leading role in tackling this issue around the world and its website is a crucial source of up-to-date information, guidelines, and practical assistance[30].

Funding and economic issues

Rapidly increasing costs and the commercialization of health-care services are making basic health care less accessible to many[31–34]. Finding adequate resources to support palliative care activities can be a major problem in such a context, especially in resource-poor settings. The increased burden of chronic diseases in most of the developing countries—those countries that also have a high infectious disease burden—is a major strain on health services. In many instances, government expenditure on health care has an inverse relationship with wealth. It has been observed that with a few exceptions, such as Cuba, developing countries generally spend proportionately less money on health care than the developed countries. The total money spent on health care rises from around 2–3 per cent of gross domestic product (GDP) at low incomes (<US$1000 per capita) to typically 8–9 per cent at high incomes (>US$7000 per capita)[35]. This results in many poor regions of the world with high palliative-care service requirements competing for resources with equally needed basic health-care services. It has also been shown that pain-relieving medication costs a greater proportion of monthly household income in the developing countries than is the case in the rich world[36].

To date there has been little systematic analysis of the funding barriers which impede the development of palliative care. In the USA, the achievement of Medicare recognition for hospice programmes has been judged as only a partial success, as it is confined to patients in the last 6 months of life[37]. In the UK, hospice provision remains heavily dependent upon charitable subvention, and despite increased government funding, the hospice sector continues to be dependent on fund-raising endeavour for some two-thirds of its costs[38]. The recognition of hospice and palliative care by insurance companies and managed care organizations for reimbursement purposes remains patchy and varied in many countries. Accordingly, the involvement of third-party donors continues to be a powerful feature of palliative care development and delivery, especially in many of the world's developing economies[39].

Most of the countries in the world with minimal or no palliative care services are also characterized by low per capita income, low scores on the UN Human Development Index, and poor or basic services in education, primary health care, drinking water, and sanitation[40]. Acute problems, such as certain infectious diseases and maternal and child care, have been the principal focus of health-care systems in the developing world[41]. In most poor countries, chronic and incurable disease remain low priorities for limited government funding, though to ignore such issues will undoubtedly add in time to the health burdens of these countries[42]. In contexts where health budgets are <US$10 per person per year, adequate care cannot be delivered, even when the finances are used prudently. Yet exceptions do exist, for example, in Uganda[43] and in Kerala (South India) where there are well-developed networks of palliative care despite low socioeconomic status. Social experiments in Kerala have shown that collaborative efforts by the community and local government can generate exceptionally good results in the area of palliative care[44].

Affordability is an important barrier to care for the poor and manifests itself in two key ways: the cost of medicines and also of transport to the treatment facility. In most low-income countries, 50–90 per cent of medicines are paid for by patients themselves. Medicines are typically the largest out-of-pocket household health expenditure in low-income countries, consuming, for example, 73 per cent of the household health budget in Bangladesh[45]. The poor often live in areas that are sparsely covered by basic health facilities and trained staff, involving expensive and arduous travel to clinics and inpatient facilities. It has also been shown that travel is a large portion of the costs of accessing health care in Africa and that the poor are less likely to use more distant facilities[46,47].

Social barriers

There are a number of social factors that must be taken into account when examining barriers to palliative care services. These pose particular problems for service providers. They may appear intractable and beyond the power of clinicians to influence. Yet, they are important dimensions that shape how palliative care is perceived by specific social groups and the type of access to palliative care that they experience. At the very least, those responsible for palliative care services must be aware of these social and cultural barriers, and should strive to address and overcome them.

Ethnicity, culture, and religion

The influence of ethnicity on accessing palliative care is complex and only partially understood. In a study in the USA, Born et al.[48], investigated factors that affect hospice use and found that lack of awareness of services was common both to those from Latino and African American backgrounds, whilst language problems were cited more by Latino people and mistrust of the system by African Americans. Ethnic minority patients use palliative care services proportionately less than the white population,[49] partly because they have lower rates of cancer (overall and because they tend to be a younger population) and also because of lower rate of referrals. A study in the UK found that patients from ethnic minorities were less likely to be referred to inpatient hospice and day care but were as likely as their white counterparts to be referred to homecare. This was explained by the referring doctors (physicians and family doctors) as a perception that the ethnic minority communities were more motivated to care for people at home than the white population, where the extended family system had all but broken down. This perception, however, may not be wholly accurate and some doctors in the study seemed to recognize this, reflecting that their belief was not based on empirical evidence[50]. There is evidence, however, to show that cancer patients in higher socioeconomic groups are more likely than others to access palliative home care[51].

Access to, and the delivery of, high quality palliative care requires excellent communication and when patients, professionals, and providers speak different first languages, this can be fundamentally compromised. The involvement of interpreters as part of the caring team is essential in these situations and clarity about their role is needed: are they there to provide straightforward language interpretation or 'cultural brokering'[52]—thereby promoting cultural understanding and insight? Many developed nations are now 'multi-cultural' in their composition, with the palliative care needs of aboriginal peoples[53,54], indigenous ethnic minorities[55], and various generations of immigrants, requiring consideration. In South Australia, efforts are being made to provide and deliver culturally sensitive palliative care to aboriginal peoples, often in remote communities, and also to a diverse wider population that speaks some 20 languages. Beginning with the five major groups (Italian, Greek, Vietnamese, Chinese, and Polish) and in consultation with these communities about issues such as the role of family and friends in care and attitudes to disclosure of diagnosis, information brochures were produced, followed by those in the 15 other languages. Experienced in this area, the authors provide a word of caution for those trying to provide transcultural palliative care: these resources can only act as guidelines because norms, even within ethnic groups, can vary between generations and individuals. The project team notes: 'Health professional and others working with people with life threatening illness and their families should always be prepared to ask their advice on how they should be treated'[56].

A study of 146 African Americans and Latinos enrolled in an outpatient palliative care unit of an inner city hospital found that 57 per cent were receiving palliative care for cancer. Compared with other patients, those with a religious affiliation did not differ regarding pain medication stress. Uninsured patients with a religious affiliation reported *more* hopeful pain and symptom attitudes, while patients with a religious affiliation covered only by Medicaid reported *less* hopeful pain and symptom attitudes. The authors took the view that *more* hopeful pain and symptom attitudes by religious-affiliated, uninsured patients may reveal adequate coping, yet also conceal problem domains. Conversely, *less* hopeful attitudes by religious-affiliated patients covered only by Medicaid served as clues to coping difficulties and problem domains. The authors concluded that palliative care programmes should carefully consider how to integrate religious support networks as pipelines for programme referrals and potential partners for care[57].

The perception that palliative care is a sequestered field with no areas of linkage to curative services has caused many professionals and policy makers to perpetuate the false dichotomy of 'palliative' versus 'curative' care. This is partly due to the early hospice focus on people who are dying. Over time, the focus of palliative care has moved to holistic care throughout the disease process, as evidenced by programmes proposed by various international bodies like WHO. Such an evolution has opened up opportunities for the integration of palliative care into the mainstream of health care. Yet this remains limited in scope. Inadequacies of the health-care system like shortages of person power, lack of training in palliative care, limitations in procuring and dispensing certain types of medication all contribute to this situation. Hospices have in turn been criticized for being a highly selective service, offering care to very few people, predominantly to cancer patients, and for being very labour intensive[58].

Excluded groups

Several groups can be identified as having problematic access to palliative care on the grounds of the wider experience of social exclusion that they encounter.

Older people

It has been observed that elders, like many marginalized groups and those with limited resources (such as income and transport) may find most health service provisions inadequate[59–61]. With the rapidly aging world population and the associated increase of multiple non-communicable diseases, the need for palliative care will rise dramatically over the next 50 years[62] By 2025, there will be 1200 million people of 60 years of age or older in the world; by 2050, the number will increase to 2000 million[63]. Yet elderly people are less likely to access palliative care and there is increasing recognition that these problems exist because the conceptual framework for palliative care as applied to older people has certain limitations. The prolonged, unpredictable process of the last phase of life faced by many older people and the wide variation in the point in time when patients, families, and doctors agree death is approaching contribute to this[64]. In the USA, the '6 months or less' prognosis requirement for enrolment to hospice can exclude many older patients with ongoing palliative care needs but less certain prognoses.

Homeless people

The palliative care needs of homeless people have only been recognized in recent times. Barriers to homeless people receiving appropriate health care, in general, and palliative care, in particular, include:

- discrimination on the grounds that they may be anti-social, violent, or have addiction problems;
- difficulty with health-care systems such as appointments and opening hours; and
- financial disincentives for practitioners[65].

Homeless populations have a higher rate of serious morbidity and premature mortality[66] yet they often live in settings where it is difficult to provide high quality palliative care. They are at risk of dying alone in public places, in hospital emergency departments, or after a prolonged period of hospitalization[67]. In a study undertaken in Canada, Podymow *et al.* describe an innovative approach to these issues based on providing palliative care based in a homeless shelter[68]. The Ottawa Inner City Health Project created a 15-bed shelter-based hospice with specialist nursing staff, client care worker, general medical input from the programme's physicians, and specialist medical support from a palliative care physician. Therapist and diatetic needs were accommodated, most users of the project received religious support and a policy of harm reduction was employed, where cigarettes, alcohol, and clean needles were available. Case review of 28 patients concluded that symptom management was much improved, without any apparent increase in substance use, and that it was likely that the costs of care were competitive. It was estimated that 68 per cent of those served would not have accessed palliative care otherwise, and would have died homeless and without pain or symptom management. In addition, there were outcomes that were difficult to quantify: many developed trust in their carers and felt a sense of security; others gave permission for long-estranged family members to be contacted, with most receiving visits.

Homeless people are an often neglected group in planning for end-of-life care, though they share many concerns with the general population about the importance of open communication with health-care professionals and relationship-centred care, where respect and compassion are features; as well as feeling their opinions are valued and that their spiritual and emotional needs are acknowledged[69]. To address such issues, it has been shown that clinical services and education must 'step outside of the box' and 'return to the community' if they are adequately to serve the needs of socially marginalized people near the end of life[70].

Prisoners

There is now a body of experience on the development of hospice and palliative care programmes for persons who are incarcerated and it has been acknowledged that the dying individual also has every one of the common needs of 'free' hospice patients[71]. An US study from 2003 found evidence of a growing effort to provide palliative care to dying inmates, grouped into five key components: (1) adjustment of hospice to the prison environment; (2) the presence of a multi-disciplinary team; (3) inmate volunteer involvement; (4) comfort care (including counselling, special privileges, contact with family, relaxed visitation rules, and appropriate funeral or memorial services for dying inmates); and (5) appropriate end-of-life care eligibility criteria and DNR arrangements[72]. There remain, however, key barriers to adequate cancer pain relief for inmates, with fears of misuse and diversion of drugs and a lack of inmate credibility cited as the key problems in a 2005 study conducted in Texas[73]. One possible approach is to designate a limited number of prison units for care of cancer patients and those terminally ill, allowing a body of expertise to build up in a small number of locations. In the UK, prison nurses have been targeted for special support in the care of those with terminal illnesses[74].

Organizational barriers

Palliative care services, like any other health-care service, should be locally appropriate, acceptable in terms of methods and technology, and affordable to the local community. This is particularly important to palliative care which requires a combination of socio-economic, cultural, and medical solutions if it is to be improved and extended. It cannot be assumed that Western models of hospice or palliative care are universally applicable. Indeed, within these models there are factors that can inhibit appropriate access to care. Promotion and marketing of inappropriate models of care by well-meaning experts from outside can become a major barrier to the development of palliative care in the developing world. Some of the palliative care initiatives in resource poor regions are aware of this. A successful community initiative in palliative care in India has in its position statement, stated that:

'Neighbourhood Network in Palliative Care (NNPC) appreciates the dedication of the external faculty, the efforts that they take and the personal sacrifices they make in coming over to teach in India. We are also aware that care that is offered to the patient should be culturally appropriate and affordable to the community. Trainers from a different socio-economic and cultural background, though well experienced in the clinical specialty, can sometimes convey wrong messages to the trainees. NNPC strongly believes that external faculty should take extra care to learn about the local culture and socio-economic situation before planning to teach. Whenever possible, the policy should be to ensure active involvement of the local faculty along with the trainers from abroad'[75].

The NNPC in Kerala, India is an attempt to develop a sustainable community-owned service capable of offering comprehensive long-term care and palliative care to the needy. In this programme, volunteers from the local community are trained to identify problems of the chronically ill in their area and to intervene effectively, with active support from a network of trained professionals. Essentially, NNPC aims to empower local communities to look after chronically ill and dying persons in the community. Over time, this network has replaced the earlier hierarchical doctor-led structure in palliative care in northern Kerala with a network of community, volunteer-led, autonomous initiatives[76]. A further evolution of this programme involving greater integration into the existing health-care system has been the development of the comprehensive home-care programme called *Pariraksha*. This project aims to look after all the bed-ridden patients in a district with 4 million population and is the result of collaborative efforts between local government in the district of Malappuram, National Rural Health Mission (Kerala) and all the local non-governmental organizations in palliative care in the district[77].

Ensuring community participation is not an easy task. Public participation is a complex social and political phenomenon which involves redefining power relationships in the community. Meaningful community participation in palliative care will require transformation of existing power relationships both in the palliative care team and also in the wider society.

Professional barriers

There are many factors related to the practices of health- and social-care professionals that impact on the quality of end-of-life care and referral to appropriate palliative care services. These can be reduced to two key elements: attitudes and knowledge.

Attitudes

Doctors are sometimes accused of being 'death denying', where this failure to come to terms with the reality and universality of death prevents the best care for their patients. Doctors are, of course, a product of the society from which they come and this lack of acceptance may reflect prevailing views within the wider social context[78]. In addition, doctors are specifically trained to preserve life and a clinical process of 'changing gear'[79] which involves placing the emphasis on care and comfort rather than cure may not come naturally to some, who may feel they have failed as a result.

'Handing over' the care of a patient who is coming towards the end of life may also pose professional difficulties. For example, a family practitioner or physician who may have looked after a patient and family for months, or even years, may feel disinclined to relinquish that role—pointing to very positive reasons (in-depth knowledge of the patient's condition, social, and psychological circumstances; genuine concern for an individual they know well; achieving closure—supporting their patient to the end). Miller et al.[80], in a study of family physicians, found that concern about loss of control was decreased with experience of hospice and palliative care, which resonates with other studies that show that the most experienced practitioners are more satisfied with hospice care[81]. In some health-care systems, such as in the USA, it has been suggested that there is a disincentive to refer to hospice and palliative care, despite government funding, because it is not in the physician's best financial interests to move away from curative care[82]. Interestingly, this has also resulted in some physicians working in not-for-profit health maintenance organizations hesitating to make referrals to hospice, lest they be accused of trying to save money[83].

There are practitioners who simply do not value hospice and palliative care or see its relevance. Few, however, are prepared to openly admit this given that 'hospice benefits from a positive social bias'[84], but nevertheless the affirmative attitudes expressed in surveys may not translate into day-to-day clinical practice. Part of the history of hospice and palliative care is a struggle to gain acceptance among doubting medical colleagues, and this may remain a barrier to access for some patients.

Knowledge

Lack of knowledge among health-care practitioners about palliative care is a potent barrier to its effective delivery. This may relate to:

◆ who to refer;

◆ how to refer; and

◆ when to refer.

The reasons for this can include a lack of convincing evidence or impaired access to convincing evidence. Also a lack of guidelines or criteria for determining appropriate care can cause uncertainty with regard to decision making in individual cases.

Health-care practitioners, such as family doctors and community nurses, often care for patients effectively at home at the end of their lives, particularly with 'uncomplicated' dying and where the symptom burden is manageable. Knowing *who* and *how* to refer to specialist palliative care depends on knowledge of local services, admission policies (e.g. whether the services only care for people with certain diseases such as cancer) and referral procedures (e.g. whether specific forms and assessments are needed). These factors can vary widely between different palliative care providers and busy practitioners may feel that they do not have the time to familiarize themselves with what can sometimes be rather complicated guidelines for referral. Barriers can exist *within* the routines of daily clinical practice, but they can also be exacerbated by service procedures that are opaque or confusing.

Knowing *when* to refer to specialist palliative care services can be challenging. A practitioner may simply be unaware of the benefits of early referral or believe that the role of specialist palliative care is to provide terminal care. It can also be very difficult to prognosticate accurately and thus refer at the optimal time. In the USA, only one-fifth of patients thought to be eligible for specialist palliative care under Medicare Hospice Benefit (MHB) receive hospice care, possibly because referring doctors need to certify that they believe the patient has <6 months to live and lack the certainty to do so[85].

Professional groups can also differ in their identification of palliative care needs. In a study carried out in a large UK teaching hospital, nursing staff were more likely than doctors to identify palliative care needs in non-cancer patients, possibly reflecting a greater awareness of the psychosocial aspects of palliative care. With proximity to death, the two professions were increasingly likely to agree about palliative care needs, again suggesting the belief that palliative care is focused on the 'actively dying'[86] Within professions, differences can also exist. Studies have shown that physicians in some specialities (e.g. oncology) are more likely to be aware of, and use, palliative care services appropriately than others (e.g. cardiology)[87] and that there can be differences between hospital doctors' and family physicians' perceptions as to a patient's requirements for palliative care[88].

Addressing the issues

Overcoming these barriers involves a multi-faceted approach to education and the dissemination of information. Palliative care services need clear, accessible referral policies, procedures, and documentation. They need open, inclusive communication between themselves and the communities in which they are based and specifically with the practitioners who can initiate referral. Subsequently, maintaining good communication with the referrer during the patient's journey can build confidence and knowledge that facilitates future appropriate referral, enhances the work of extended teams, and helps allay fears about loss of clinical involvement. Palliative care providers should maintain a high profile and regularly reinforce and update their information on the services they provide, the type of patients who may benefit, and the referral procedures that apply.

Education of health and social care professionals is also essential if these barriers are to be addressed and two key areas predominate:

1 the *formal* curriculum, and
2 the *informal* curriculum[89].

Each of these aspects has been described in relation to the training of doctors in end-of-life care, where it was noted that the *formal* curriculum had many weaknesses such as: inadequate palliative care content; lack of exposure to high-quality palliative care; and a dearth of information in medical texts. Addressing these issues without adequate attention to the *informal* curriculum can only be expected to produce partial improvement, as the latter can strongly influence attitudes. For example, in the case of trainee doctors, observing senior clinicians ignoring patients at the end of their lives or concentrating on cure even very close to death[90], is unlikely to promote insight to the possibilities of palliative care. Using these concepts, Susan Block has suggested an approach to the education of physicians that might be expected to break down specific barriers to palliative care. The approach consists of eight categories as follows:

1 leadership for change;
2 curriculum improvement and guidelines;
3 evaluation/certification/licensure;
4 enhancing educational resource quality and availability;
5 faculty development;
6 improving textbooks; and
7 Palliative care fellowships.

These interventions aim to provide excellent role models and quality education, training, and experience of palliative care that promotes a holistic approach and emphasizes the importance of good communication and multi-disciplinary team-working. The approach seeks to improve the quality of resources and facilitate

their use, in addition to promoting certification, accreditation, and academic development, thus underlining the credibility and relevance of high quality end-of-life and palliative care.

Professional barriers: final considerations

Barriers to palliative care can still exist even when a patient receives an appropriate and timely referral to specialist palliative care. Factors such as lack of staff (e.g. not enough qualified practitioners emerging from specialist training), poor multi-disciplinary team-working, professional jealousies, and staff 'burnout'[91] can all potentially contribute to less than optimal care.

Individual barriers

There are also many factors at the individual level that can create barriers to the delivery of effective and appropriate palliative care. In common with health- and social-care professionals, patients themselves may lack the necessary knowledge of palliative care services needed to access them. Similarly, they may feel that palliative care is not for people with their illness or that it is only for the dying. A survey of attitudes to hospice among primary care physicians revealed that they considered patient and family unwillingness to discuss hospice a significant barrier to referral[92]. In contrast, a study canvassing the views of the bereaved about barriers to hospice care identified physician factors, such as lack of recognition of changes in a patient's status and discomfort in discussing death, as major barriers to referral[93].

Diagnosis

In the European context, and especially in the UK, palliative care has strong associations with the care of cancer patients[94]. This is less marked in the USA and also in parts of the developing world. But in many places the continued perception that palliative care is only for those with a malignancy remains a potent barrier to the referral of those with other diseases such as chronic cardiac failure (CCF), chronic obstructive pulmonary disease (COPD), and HIV/AIDS.

Several barriers have been identified relating to the extension of palliative care services to non-cancer patients[95]. These include:

◆ lack of skills among palliative care experts;

◆ difficulties in identifying proper candidates for care;

◆ lack of information on the acceptability of palliative care services to non-cancer patients;

◆ resource implications; and

◆ vested interests in present arrangements.

Chronic cardiac failure

Heart failure is a major public health problem with around 550 000 new cases each year in the USA[96]. Mortality is high, with 40 per cent dying within a year of diagnosis[97]. Symptom burdens are similar to those with advanced cancer or HIV/AIDS[98] and in countries with established palliative care provision there is interest and debate, clinically and strategically, in the most appropriate way of providing palliative care to these patients. Yet, some specialist palliative care services refuse to accept CCF patients: in a survey of English palliative care services in 1994, 11 per cent stated that they would not accept such referrals, citing lack of resources, implications for staff training, and organizational reasons[99]. There are examples, however, of palliative care services working effectively in collaboration with cardiology specialists, clinical nurse specialists, and generalists to provide appropriate, high quality palliative care[100], and where fears of being 'overwhelmed' by CCF patients have not materialized[101].

Chronic obstructive pulmonary disease

COPD is a major cause of morbidity and mortality which is continuing to increase. Patients with COPD are more likely to die on intensive care units with ventilatory support than patients with lung cancer, despite the fact that they are as likely to prefer supportive care as those with carcinoma[102]. When compared with those with lung cancer, patients with COPD have been shown to have greater impairment of their physical, social, and emotional functioning, as well as in their activities of daily living, yet they are significantly less likely to receive palliative care[103]. The reasons for this are complex, but include difficulty with accurate prognostication in COPD and a lack of effective communication between patients and health-care professionals about the end-of-life issues. Nevertheless, a profile is emerging from the literature of the type of patient with COPD where discussion of these issues is essential and where consideration of referral to, or support and advice from, specialist palliative care may be indicated. This profile includes[104]:

- forced expiratory volume (FEV_1) of <30 per cent of predicted;
- more than one admission to hospital in the preceding year;
- increasing dependence;
- co-morbidities such as heart failure;
- depression; and
- single status.

HIV/AIDS

Patients with HIV/AIDS face some similar difficulties to those coping with CCF and COPD, in that prognostication is difficult and communication with professionals involved in care may not be well enough developed to encompass end-of-life issues in a meaningful way. In addition, the stigma of the disease can act as a barrier to effective palliative care,[105] as can negative attitudes to homosexuality or substance abuse. Patients with HIV/AIDS often have a heavy, heterogeneous symptom burden which even experienced palliative care practitioners may feel ill equipped to manage[106] and patients may prefer specialist HIV/AIDS services for this reason. Others, in contrast, may prefer the involvement of generic palliative care, thereby disguising the reality of their condition[107]. Patients with HIV/AIDS may also belong to disadvantaged groups such as prisoners, the homeless, and the poor that further negatively influence their chances of accessing appropriate palliative care. In the developing world, where the burden of HIV/AIDS is greatest, even more fundamental barriers exist, with many countries simply having no identifiable palliative care. The HIV/AIDS pandemic has become a huge burden for Africa, the world's most affected region, and more than 20 million African deaths have so far been linked to the disease. In 2003, among an estimated 34–46 million people living with HIV infection worldwide, some 26.6 million were in sub-Saharan Africa—an area which also has the highest estimated adult prevalence rate of 7.5–8.5 per cent[108] The scale and character of these problems create particular difficulties in offering palliative care for people with HIV infection: during critical

opportunistic infections, often in deeply impoverished circumstances, and up to the end of life. There are also major issues involved in the care of those bereaved and orphaned[109].

The case of HIV/AIDS care emphasizes the need for palliative care to sit alongside active treatment with highly active retroviral therapy (HAART) which can itself cause pain and other symptoms. If palliative care in HIV/AIDS is to be equitable and effective, services need to minimize discrimination, facilitate ongoing improvement in palliative care knowledge and skills for health-care professionals, produce clear referral criteria for specialist palliative care services, and ensure that high quality palliative care is available whatever the setting[110].

Other infectious diseases

Across the world each year, it is estimated that 3 million people die from tuberculosis, 3 million from malaria and 40 000–100 000 from rabies[111]. Most are in the developing world and few receive palliative care, despite often debilitating symptoms. The fact that these diseases are preventable and treatable can act as a barrier to the delivery to palliative care, with limited available resources often focused on curative measures[112]. While many continue to die of these conditions, efforts need to be made to recognize the extent of the problem and to address their palliative care needs.

Neurological diseases

Access to appropriate palliative care can also be challenging for those with neurological conditions such as amyotrophic lateral sclerosis (ALS), multiple sclerosis (MS), and stroke. The relevance of palliative care for ALS has long been established[113] but it has taken longer for its potential in the care of MS[114] and stroke[115] to be recognized, probably because the chronic, sometimes fluctuating, course of these conditions causes difficulty with prognostication. Finally, palliative care in dementia[116] can be particularly challenging to access, where sometimes a coexisting cancer is the factor that makes it possible to access appropriate support and care at the end of life.

Intellectual disabilities

People with intellectual disabilities are among the most disadvantaged in society in general and from the perspective of access to, and benefit from, appropriate palliative care. Communication can be challenging with respect to diagnosis and prognosis and when obtaining informed consent for any interventions, often leaving the patient with fewer treatment options[117]. In addition, palliative care professionals may feel they lack the skills to care for these persons[118] or may respond negatively to those with mild impairment whose behaviour they misinterpret. Overcoming these barriers begins with an awareness of the particular difficulties those with intellectual disabilities face and with acknowledging the wide spectrum of disability that exists. Those with mild to moderate disability need health education, support, and straightforward information whilst those at the severe and profound end of the spectrum need multi-professional collaboration and support to identify and meet their palliative care needs, with further research in this area essential[119]. In the UK, the National Network for the Palliative Care of People with Learning Disabilities (NNPCPLD) was set up in 1998 and aims to link people working in this area, to develop good practice through regional networks and provide resources for professionals, carers and those with intellectual disabilities, as well as project development support[120].

Conclusions

Despite many achievements in its short history, modern palliative care is still struggling to gain recognition within public health policies and national disease control programmes. It remains low on the agenda of many international health agencies and is even viewed with suspicion in some quarters[121]. If palliative care is to be made available to all who need it, then numerous barriers must be overcome. These range from impediments within global health policy to factors which inhibit appropriate care at the individual level because of disease status, age, or social position. In between, there are many organizational factors that stand in the way of easy and universal access to appropriate palliative care. Taken together, this produces a complex mixture of barriers and problems. Within the field of palliative care, various types of expertise are needed to overcome these difficulties. Good quality information is required about the global state of palliative care development. At the same time, those who plan and deliver services must tackle the key obstacles that stand in the way of palliative care for all who need it. For clinicians, there are daily challenges in matching expertise and interventions to the individual needs of patients and their companions and family members. This chapter has highlighted the many difficulties and problems that exist, but it has also shown some of the innovative approaches that are being adopted in overcoming barriers to palliative care—from the global to the local.

Acknowledgements

The authors are grateful for the assistance given by Dr. Bethan Evans in the preparation of this chapter.

References

1. Mathers, C.D. and Loncar, D. (2006). Projections of global mortality and burden of disease from 2002 to 2030. *PLoS Medicine* [online journal] 3(11), e442. Retrieved from http://www.who.int/whosis/whostat2007_10highlights. pdf on 24 December 2007.

2. Stjernsward, J. and Clark, D. (2003). Palliative medicine - a global perspective. In *Oxford textbook of palliative medicine* (eds. Doyle, D., Hanks, G., Cherny, N.I., *et al.*), 3rd edition. Oxford, Oxford University Press.

3. World Health Organization (1990). *Cancer pain relief with a guide to opioid availability*, 2nd edition. WHO, Geneva.

4. World Health Organization (1998). *Symptom relief in terminal illness*. WHO, Geneva.

5. World Health Organization (1998). *Cancer pain relief and palliative care in children*. WHO, Geneva.

6. Stjernswärd, J., Colleau, S., and Ventafridda, V. (1996). The World Health Organization cancer pain and palliative care program: past, present and future. *Journal of Pain and Symptom Management,* 12(2), 65–72

7. Foley, K., Aulina, F., and Stjernswärd, J. (2002). Palliative care in resource-poor settings. In *A guide to supportive and palliative care of people with HIV/AIDS.* (eds. J. O'Neil and P. Selwyn), HRSA, HIV/AIDS Bureau, Rockville, MD, USA.

8. http://www.aphn.org/, accessed 17 December 2007.

9. http://www.apca.co.ug/, accessed 17 December 2007.

10. http://www.eapcnet.org/index.html, accessed 17 December 2007.

11. http://www.hospicecare.com/, accessed 17 December 2007.

12. http://www.nhpco.org/templates/1/homepage.cfm, accessed 17 December 2007.

13. http://www.helpthehospices.org.uk/ accessed 17 December 2007.

14. http://www.worldday.org/, accessed 26 November 2007.

15. http://www.wwpca.net/index.asp, accessed 26 November 2007.

16. http:// www.eolc-observatory.net, accessed 8 January 2008.

17. Harding, R. (2006). Palliative care—a basic human right. *Id21 Insights Health* 8, February. Sussex, Institute of Development Studies.

18. Brennan, F. (2007). Palliative care as an international human right. *Journal of Pain and Symptom Management,* 33(5), 494–9.

19. Sloan, F. and Gelband, H. (eds.) (2007). *Cancer control opportunities in low- and middle-income countries.* The National Academies Press, Washington, DC.

20. Fifty-eight World Health Assembly WHA58.22; Agenda item 13.12 25 May 2005 Cancer prevention and control.

21. Declaration of Venice (2006). Adoption of a declaration to develop a global palliative care research initiative. *Progress in Palliative Care,* 14(5), 1–3.

22. Quick, J.D. (2003). Essential medicines twenty-five years on: closing the access gap. *Health Policy and Planning,* 18(1), 1–3

23. World Health Organization (1996). *Cancer pain relief with a guide to opioid availability*, 2nd edition. WHO, Geneva.

24. Meldrum, M. (2005). The ladder and the clock: cancer pain and public policy at the end of the twentieth century. *Journal of Pain and Symptom Management,* 29(1), 41–54.

25. Stjernswärd, J., Foley, K.M., and Ferris, F.D. (2007). The public health strategy for palliative care. *Journal of Pain and Symptom Management,* 33(5), 486–93.

26. Joranson, D.E. and Dahl, J.L. (1989). Achieving balance in drug policy: the Wisconsin model. In *Advances in pain research and therapy* (eds. Hill, C.S. Jr., and Fields, W.S.), Vol. 11, Raven Press, New York.

27. Pain and Policy Studies Group (2006). *Improving availability of essential pain medicines for cancer and HIV/Aids: Report for 2005.* University of Wisconsin Comprehensive Cancer Centre, Madison, WI.

28. International Narcotics Control Board (2000). *Annual report.* Vienna, United Nations.

29. Clark, D., Wright, M., Hunt, J. *et al.*(2007). Hospice and palliative care development in Africa: a multi-method review of services and experiences. *Journal of Pain and Symptom Management,* 33(6), 698–710.

30. http://www.painpolicy.wisc.edu/, accessed 16 December 2007.

31. Hsiao, W.C.L. and Liu, Y. (1996). Economic reform and health—lessons from China. *New England Journal of Medicine,* 335, 430–432.

32. Zhang, X. (2004). Economic growth and human development in china *UNDP Occasional Paper 28* Retrieved from http://hdr.undp.org/docs/publications/ocational_papers/oc28a.htm.

33. Trumper, R. and Phillips, L. (1997). Give me discipline and give me death: neoliberalism and health in Chile. *International Journal of Health Services,* 27(1), 41–55.

34. Hung, P.M., Dzung, T.V., Dahlgren, G. *et al.* (2001). Vietnam: efficient, equity-oriented financial strategies for health. In *Challenging inequalities in health. From ethics to action* (eds. T. Evans, Whitehead, M., Diderichsen, F. *et al.*). Oxford, Oxford University Press.

35. World Health Organization (2002). *Bulletin of the World Health Organization,* 80(2), 134–46.

36. de Lima, L., Sweeney, C., Palmer, J.L. *et al.* (2004). Potent analgesics are more expensive for patients in developing countries: a comparative study. *Journal of Pain and Palliative Care Pharmacotherapy,* 18(1), 59–70

37. Lynn, J. (2001). Serving patients who may die soon and their families. The role of hospice and other services. *Journal of the American Medical Association,* 285, 925–32.

38. http://www.helpthehospices.org.uk/policy/index.asp?submenu=2, accessed 7 January 2008.

39. Wright, M., Lynch, T., and Clark, D. (2007). *A review of donor organizations that support palliative care development in five world regions.* International Observatory on End of Life Care, Lancaster.

40. United Nations (2005). *UNDP Report 2005.* United Nations, New York.

41. World Health Organization (2002). *Innovative care for chronic conditions: building blocks for action*. World Health Organization, Geneva.

42. Unwin, N. Satel, P. Rashid, S. *et al*. (2001). Non-communicable diseases in Sub-Saharan Africa: where do they feature in the health research agenda? *Bulletin of the World Health Organization*, **79**, 947–53.

43. Jagwe, J. (2002). The introduction of palliative care in Uganda. *Journal of Palliative Medicine*, **5**(1), 159–163.

44. Shabeer, C. and Kumar, S. (2005). Palliative care in the developing world: a social experiment in India. *European journal of Palliative Care*, **13**(2), 76–9.

45. Doorslaer, E.V., O'Donnell, R.P., and Rannan-Eliya, A. (2005). Paying out-of-pocket for health care in Asia: Catastrophic and poverty impact *EQUITAP Project: Working Paper, 2* May 2005.

46. Dor, A., Gertler, P., and van der Gaag, J. (1987). Non-price rationing and the choice of medical care providers in rural Cote D'Ivoire *Journal of Health Economics*, **6**(4), 291–305.

47. Gertler, P. and van der Gaag, J. (1990). *The willingness to pay for medical care: Evidence from two developing countries*. Johns Hopkins University Press, Baltimore, MD. Published for The World Bank.

48. Born, W., Greiner, K.A., Sylvia, E. *et al*. (2004) Knowledge, attitudes and beliefs about end-of-life care among inner-city African Americans and Latinos. *Journal of Palliative Medicine*, **7**(2), 247–56.

49. Koffman, J., and Higginson, I.J. (2001). Accounts of carer satisfaction with health care at the end of life: a comparison of first generation black Caribbeans and white patients with advanced disease. *Palliative Medicine*, **14**. 337–45.

50. Karim, K., Bailey, M., Tunna, K. (2000) Non white ethnicity and the provision of specialist palliative care services: factors affecting doctors' referral patterns. *Palliative Medicine*, **14,** 471–8.

51. Grande, G.E., Addington-Hall, J., and Todd, C.J. (1998). Place of death and access to home care services: are certain patient groups at disadvantage? *Social Science and Medicine*, **47**(5), 565–79.

52. Norris, W.M., Wenrich, M.D., Nielsen, E.L. *et al*. (2005). Communication about end-of life care between language-discordant patients and clinicians: insights from medical interpreters. *Journal of Palliative Medicine*, **8**(5), 1016–24.

53. Hotson, K.E., Macdonald, S.M., and Martin, B.D. (2004) Understanding death and dying in select first nation communities in northern Manitoba: issues of culture and remote service delivery in palliative care. *International Journal of Circumpolar Health*, **63**(1), 25–8.

54. Canadian Hospice Palliative Care Association (2007). National inventory of hospice and palliative care resources and tools for aboriginal peoples. Retrieved from www.chpca.net/interest_groups. htm on 7 January 2008.

55. McQuillan, R. and van Doorslaer, O. (2007). Indigenous ethnic minorities and palliative care: exploring the views of Irish travellers and palliative care staff. *Palliative Medicine*, **21**, 635–41.

56. www.pallcare.asn.au.mc.mccontents.html, accessed 16 November 2007.

57. Francouer, R.B., Payne, R., Raveis, V.H. *et al*. (2007). Palliative care in the inner city: patient religious affiliation, underinsurance, and symptom attitude. *Cancer*, **109** (Suppl 2), 425–34.

58. James, N. and Field, D. (1992) The routinization of hospice: charisma and bureaucratization. *Social Science and Medicine*, **34**(12), 1363–75.

59. Beck, R.W., Jijon, C.R., and Edwards, J.B. (1996). The relationships among gender, perceived financial barriers to care and health status in a rural population. *Journal of Rural Health*, **12**, 188–96.

60. Mooney, C., Zwanziger, J., Phibbs, C.S. *et al*. (2000). Is travel a barrier to veterans' use of VA hospitals for medical surgical care? *Social Science and Medicine*, **50**, 1743–55.

61. Nemet, G.F. and Bailey, A.J. (2000). Distance and health care utilization among the rural elderly. *Social Science and Medicine*, **50**, 1197–208.

62. World Health Organization (1990). *Cancer pain relief and palliative care*. Technical report series 804, World Health Organization, Geneva.

63. Stjernswärd, J., Foley, K.M., and Ferris, F.D. (2007). The public health strategy for palliative care. *Journal of Pain and Symptom Management*, **33**(5), 486–93.

64. Committee on Care at the End of Life, Institute of Medicine (1997). *Approaching death: improving care at the end of life*. National Academy Press, Washington, DC.

65. Wright, N.M.J. and Tomkins, C.N.E. (2005). How can health care systems deal with the major healthcare needs of homeless people? World Health Organization Regional Office for Europe *Health Evidence Network Report*. Retrieved form http://www.euro.who.int/ Document/E85482. pdf on 7 January 2008.

66. Nordentoft, M. and Wandall-Holm, N. (2003). 10 year follow up study of mortality among users of hostels for homeless people in Copenhagen. *British Medical Journal*, **27**(7406), 81.

67. Salit, S.A., Kuhn, E.M., Hartz, A.J. *et al*. (1998). Hospitalisation costs associated with homelessness in New York City. *New England Journal of Medicine*, **338**, 1734–40.

68. Podymow, T., Turnbull, J., and Coyle, D. (2006). Shelter-based palliative care for the homeless terminally ill. *Palliative Medicine*, **20**(2), 81–6.

69. Tarzian, A.J., Neal, M.T., O'Neil, J.A. (2005). Attitudes, experiences and beliefs affecting end-of-life decision making among homeless individuals. *Journal of Palliative Medicine*, **8**(1), 36–48.

70. Moller, D.W. (2004) *Dancing with broken bones*. Oxford University Press, New York.

71. Maddocks, I. (2003). Prisoners with advanced disease – a truly marginalised population. *Journal of Pain and Palliative Care Pharmacotherapy*, **17**(3/4), 139–40.

72. Yampolskaya, S. and Winston, N. (2003) Hospice care in prison: general principles and outcomes. *American Journal of Hospice and Palliative Care*, **20**(4), 290–6.

73. Lin, J. and Mathew, P. (2005). Cancer pain management in prisons: a survey of primary care practitioners and inmates. *Journal of Pain and Symptom Management*, **29**(5), 466–73.

74. Wilford, T. (2001). Developing effective palliative care within a prison setting. *International Journal of Palliative Nursing*, **7**(11), 528–30.

75. Kumar, S. (2007). India. In *Education in palliative care. building a culture of learning* (eds. Wee, B. and Hughes, N.), Oxford University Press, Oxford.

76. Kumar, S. (2007). Kerala, India: a regional community-based palliative care model. *Journal of Pain and Symptom Management*, **33**(5), 623–7.

77. Sallnow, L., Kumar, S., and Chenganakkattil, S. (2007). Pariraksha— For those most in need. *Hospice Information Bulletin*, July, 1–2

78. Berger, A. (2006). How to have a good death. *British Medical Journal*, **322**, 799

79. National Council for Palliative Care (2006). *Changing gear—guidelines for managing the last days of life in adults—reviewed and updated November 2006*. National Council for Palliative Care, London.

80. Miller, K., Miller, M., and Single, N. (1997). Barriers to hospice care: family physicians perceptions. *Hospice Journal*, **12**(4), 29–41.

81. Wakefield, M., Beilby, J., and Ashton, M. (1993). General practitioners and palliative care. *Palliative Medicine*, **7**, 117–26.

82. Friedman, B.T., Harwood, M.K., and Sheilds, M. (2002). Barriers and enablers to hospice referrals: an expert overview. *Journal of Palliative Medicine*, **5**, 73–84.

83. Brickner, L., Scannell, K., Marquet, S. *et al*. (2004). Barriers to hospice care and referral: survey of physicians' knowledge, attitudes and perceptions in a Health Maintenence Organization. *Journal of Palliative Medicine*, **7**(3), 411–8.

84. Ogle, K., Mavis, B., and Wang, T. (2003). Hospice and primary care physicians: attitudes, knowledge and barriers. *American Journal of Hospice and Palliative Care*, **20**(1), 41–50.

85. Brickner, L., Scannell, K., Marquet, S. *et al.* (2004). Barriers to hospice care and referral: survey of physicians' knowledge, attitudes and perceptions in a Health Maintenence Organization. *Journal of Palliative Medicine*, **7**(3), 411–8.

86. Gott, C.M., Ahmedzai, S.H., and Wood, C. (2001). How many inpatients at an acute hospital have palliative care needs? Comparing the perspectives of medical and nursing staff. *Palliative Medicine*, **15**, 451–60.

87. Bradley, E.H., Fried, T.R., Kasl, S.V. *et al.*(2000). Referral of terminally ill patients for hospice: frequency and correlates. *Journal of Palliative Care*, **16**, 20–6.

88. Farquhar, M., Grande, G., Todd, C. *et al.* (2002). Defining patients as palliative: hospital doctors' versus general practitioners' perceptions. *Palliative Medicine*, **16**, 247–50.

89. Block, S. (2002) Medical education in end-of-life care: the status of reform *Journal of Palliative Medicine*, **5**(2), 243–8.

90. Meier, D.E., Morrison, R.S., and Cassel, C.K. (1997). Improving palliative care. *Annals of Internal Medicine,* **12**(3), 225–30.

91. Keidel, G.C. (2002) Burnout and compassion fatigue among hospice caregivers. *American Journal of Hospice and Palliative Care*, **19**(3), 200–5.

92. Ogle, K., Mavis, B., and Wang, T. (2003). Hospice and primary care physicians: attitudes, knowledge and barriers. *American Journal of Hospice and Palliative Care*, **20**(1), 41–50.

93. Wyatt, G.K., Ogle, K.S., and Given, B.A. (2000). Access to hospice: a perspective from the bereaved. *Journal of Palliative Medicine*, **3**(4), 433–440.

94. Clark, D. (2007). From margins to centre: a review of the history of palliative care in cancer. *The Lancet Oncology*, **8**(5), 430–8.

95. Field, D., and Addington-Hall, J. (1999). Extending specialist palliative care to all? *Social Science and Medicine*, **48**, 1271–80.

96. Levy, D., Kenchaiah, S., Larson, M.G. *et al.* (2002). Long-term trends in the incidence of and survival with heart failure. *New England Journal of Medicine*, **347**(18), 1397–402.

97. Dayer, M. and Cowie, M. (2004). Heart failure: diagnosis and healthcare burden. *Clinical Medicne*, **4**, 13–8.

98. Solano, J.P., Gomes, B., and Higginson, I.J. (2006). A comparison of symptom prevalence in far advanced cancer, AIDS, heart disease, chronic obstructive pulmonary disease and renal disease. *Journal of Pain and Symptom Management*, **31**, 58–9.

99. Gibbs, L.M.E., Khatri, A., and Gibbs, G.S.R. (2006). A survey of specialist palliative care in heart failure: September 2004. *Palliative Medicine*, **20**, 603–9.

100. Selman, L., Harding, R., Beynon, T. *et al.* (2007). Modelling services to meet the palliative care needs of chronic heart failure patients and their families: current practice in the UK. *Palliative Medicine*, **21**, 385–90.

101. Johnson, M.J. and Houghton, T. (2006). Palliative care for patients with heart failure: description of a service. *Palliative Medicine*, **20**, 211–4.

102. Claessens, M.T., Lynn, J., Zhong, Z. *et al.* (2000). Dying with lung cancer or chronic obstructive pulmonary disease: insights from SUPPORT. *Journal of the American Geriatric Society*, **48**, S146–S153.

103. Gore, J.M., Brophy, C.J., and Greenstone, M.A. (2000). How well do we care for patients with end stage chronic obstructive pulmonary disease (COPD)? A comparison of palliative care and quality of life in COPD and lung cancer. *Thorax*, **55**, 1000–6.

104. Curtis, J.R. and Rocker, G. (2006). Chronic obstructive pulmonary disease. In: *Textbook of palliative medicine* (eds. Bruera, E., Higginson, I.J., Ripamonti, C., *et al.*), Hodder Arnold, London.

105. Rondahl, G., Innala, S., and Carlsson, M. (2003). Nursing staff and nursing students' attitudes toward HIV-infected and homosexual HIV infected patients in Sweden and the wish to refrain from nursing. *Journal of Advanced Nursing*, **41**, 454–61.

106. Salt, S., Wilson, L., and Edwards, A. (1998). The use of specialist palliative care services by patients with human immunodeficiency virus-related illness in the Yorkshire Deanery of the northern and Yorkshire region. *Palliative Medicine*, **12**, 152–60.

107. Armes, P.J., Higginson, I.J. (1999). What constitutes high quality HIV/AIDS palliative Care? *Journal of Palliative Care*, **15**, 5–12.

108. UNAIDS/World Health Organization (2003). *AIDS Epidemic Update.*

109. Clark, D., Wright, M., Hunt, J. *et al.* (2007). Hospice and palliative care development in Africa: a multi-method review of services and experiences. *Journal of Pain and Symptom Management*, **33**(6), 698–710.

110. Harding, R., Easterbrook, P., Higginson, I.J. *et al.* (2005). Access and equity in HIV/AIDS palliative care: a review of the evidence and responses. *Palliative Medicine*, **19**, 251–8.

111. Marsden, S. (2006). Other infectious diseases: malaria, rabies and tuberculosis. In *Textbook of palliative medicine* (eds. Bruera, E., Higginson, I.J., Ripamonti,, C., *et al.*), Hodder Arnold, London.

112. Wenk, R. and de Lima, L. (2006). Practical aspects of palliative care delivery in the developing world. In *Textbook of palliative medicine.* (eds. Bruera, E., Higginson, I.J., Ripamonti, C., *et al.*), Hodder Arnold, London.

113. O'Brien, T., Kelly, M. and Saunders, C. (1992). Motor neurone disease: a hospice perspective. *British Medical Journal*, **304**, 471–3.

114. Kumpfel, T., Hoffman, L.T., Pollmann, W. *et al.* (2007). Palliative care in patients with severe multiple sclerosis: two case reports and a survey among German MS neurologists. *Palliative Medicine*, **21**, 109–14.

115. Stevens, T., Payne, S.A., Barton, C. *et al.* (2007). Palliative care in stroke. *Palliative Medicine*, **21**, 323–31.

116. Small, N., Froggatt, K., and Downs, M. (eds.) (2007). *Living and dying with dementia: Dialogues about palliative care.* Oxford University Press, Oxford.

117. Northfield, J., Turnbull, J. (2001). Experiences from cancer services. In *Cancer and people with learning disabilities: the evidence from published studies and experiences from cancer services* (eds. Hogg, J., Northfield, J., Turnbull, J.), BILD Publications, Kidderminster.

118. Bycroft, L. (1994). Care of a handicapped woman with metastatic breast cancer. *British Journal of Nursing*, **3**, 126–33.

119. Tuffrey-Winje, I. (2003). The palliative care needs of people with intellectual difficulties: a literature review. *Palliative Medicine*, **17**, 55–62.

120. www.helpthehospices.org.uk/NPA/learningdisabilities/index.asp, accessed 27 November 2007.

121. Farmer, P. (2006). From "marvelous momentum" to health care for all: success is possible with the right programs *Foreign Affairs* **86**(2). http://www.foreignaffairs.org/20070301faresponse86213/paul-farmer-laurie-garrett/from-marvelous-momentum-to-health-care-for-all-success-is-possible-with-the-right-programs.html, accessed 7 January 2008.

Defining a 'good death'

Karen E. Steinhauser and James A. Tulsky

Introduction

'I don't mind dying, I just don't want to be there when it happens.' This quote from Woody Allen is emblematic of our society's ambivalence toward the notion of a 'good death'[1,2]. Its inherent irony is instructive for palliative-care clinicians. While death may be inevitable, for patients, it is rarely the goal. Therefore, naming deaths 'good' or 'bad' should be met with caution.

There is a long historical and literary tradition discussing the 'good death'. In some of the best known work on evolution in Western attitudes toward death, social historian Philippe Aries uses cemetery iconography, notary records, wills, and art and literature to explore changing patterns in cultural norms of dying and death over the last 1500 years[3]. For example, we learn that contemporary preferences for sudden death or death during sleep stand in contrast to previous eras in which populations literally prayed, in the Anglican Great Litany, not to die, 'suddenly and unprepared'[3,4]. Aries work demonstrates the plasticity of how we view circumstances of death and the relativism of the terminology 'good' and 'bad'.

Extraordinary variation exists in the social construction of the meaning of dying and death and the social organization and cultural norms surrounding end of life[3,5–11]. Recent work describing end-of-life activities in Japan, North America, the Netherlands, and Papau New Guinea, among others and spanning contemporary, classical, and biblical times[12] finds that, though variable, humans create and enact cultural scripts which traditionally we have described as making death either 'good' or 'bad'[12].

While these cited works provide in-depth sociocultural and historical exploration of how we define the meaning of death, the focus of this chapter is on the reappearance in the last 40 years of attempts to define a 'good death' in the medical context, the empirical investigation of the construct, the clinical implications of using the terminology 'good death', and an alternative framework for language defining preferences at end of life.

Context of contemporary exploration of 'good death'

In 1908, William Osler conducted a study of 486 deaths at Johns Hopkins reporting that 90 patients experienced pain, 11 anxiety, and for the majority, death was 'nothing more than falling asleep'[13]. Deaths in this era occurred all across the life course spectrum and were the result of either old age or catastrophic illness with limited medical intervention capable of extending life.

Despite the site of Osler's investigation, the majority of deaths at that time did not happen in the hospital.

Rather, deaths in the 19th and early 20th centuries occurred primarily at home with support of family, church, and community[3,6,14]. However, by the second half of the 20th century the primary site of death had shifted to the hospital. Moreover, by the 1960s, the landscape of death in Western culture had changed dramatically as medicine had experienced a variety of therapeutic and technological revolutions resulting in the capacity to extend life, including antibiotic therapies, artificial nutrition, and cardiopulmonary resuscitation. In this latter 20th century hospital setting, death's meaning was narrowed primarily to a physiological event. As such, death was defined less as an expected and natural part of the life course and more as a failure of medical technology and intervention[15].

By the 1950s, social reformers, such as Cicely Saunders, began to critique conventional medical care for dying patients, arguing hospitals lacked both the specific expertise in palliation of symptoms as well as the multi-disciplinary perspective that attended to social, psychological, and spiritual aspects of care[16]. By 1963, after returning to medical school to supplement her nursing, social work, and divinity training, she opened St. Christopher's Hospice as a multi-disciplinary care centre that emphasized palliative versus curative therapies and promoted quality of life over quantity of life.

Amidst this social reform movement, in-depth inquiry of death and dying began to appear in the medical, nursing, and social science literatures. Seminal qualitative accounts were published in the few years following the opening of St. Christopher's. Prominent sociologists Glaser, Strauss, and Sudnow were among the first to refocus study on end of life and conceptualize trajectories of dying experience[14,17]. Emerging from a tradition of grounded theory, Glaser and Strauss became participant observers in hospital settings and described four 'contexts of awareness surrounding the dying experience: Closed awareness, suspicious awareness, mutual pretense, and open awareness'[17]. Their conceptualization reflected an era during which patients often were not directly informed of terminal diagnoses or poor prognoses. Their sociological critiques were heavily counter-cultural in their scrutiny of the power dynamics of the paternalistic hospital culture.

A few years following these works, Elizabeth Kubler-Ross called further attention to the unmet needs of patients and the concept of personal and emotional evolution over the course of coming to terms with a terminal diagnosis[18]. Though the stages of grief—denial, anger, bargaining, depression, and acceptance—were never tested empirically, her theory of dying and death is perhaps the best known and most frequently cited to this day. In fact, after her work, investigation of death and dying would receive scant attention until the 1990s.

The subtext of many of these investigations was that conventional medical-care settings often played host to 'bad' deaths, typified by excessive use of technology, with patient and family wishes ignored, lack of patient knowledge and autonomy in decision making, the patient reduced to a physiological system versus whole person, and quality of life devalued.

The hospice movement, both in its British foundations and its importation to the USA, arose within this context and was part of a larger 'good death' or 'death with dignity' movement of the 1960s and 1970s. Those involved in hospice and early palliative care worked to reclaim the experience of dying and death beyond a biomedical event. In this context, a 'good death' was the obverse of the previously described situations. The goals were to increase awareness of end of life as a part of a natural life course and to acknowledge dying patients as whole persons in the context of fuller lives lived, as well as family and community nexus. 'good death' connoted a model of care more closely matching patient and family preferences, with the terminology designed to serve as a vision of improved experience for dying persons.

Empirical investigations of a 'good death'

Despite the popularity and growth of the hospice movement, widespread, systematic attempts to define a 'good death' empirically did not appear in the medical literature until after the publication of the SUPPORT (Study to Understand Prognosis and Preferences for R Treatment) findings. This large multi-site study documented poor care of dying patients and their families in five top US medical centres and redefined the landscape of end-of-life and palliative care[19]. We learned that hospitalized patients were dying in pain, without their wishes known, and in isolation. The results provided empirical evidence of what was wrong with hospital deaths.

As a result, care of dying patients became a priority in the USA, as organizations such as the American Medical Association, the Veterans Health Administration, and The Robert Wood Johnson foundation committed funding to improving education and quality of care[20]. Efforts to develop and evaluate hospice and palliative care became expanded in US and international journals. However, if clinicians and administrators were to provide quality of care and quality of life at the end of life, they must first define quality. If SUPPORT had given empirical evidence of 'bad' deaths, what was the empirical evidence regarding the definition of a 'good death'?

In the 13 ensuing years, approximately 250 Medline articles include the construct 'good death'. A smaller subset of independent studies has attempted to define the construct through analyses of qualitative and quantitative data gathered from patients, family members, and health-care providers. Recently, these have been reviewed systematically in both the medical and nursing literatures[4,5,7–9,13,21–52]. While each study lends a unique population or conceptual nuance, some common features exist among attempts to define a 'good death'.

Mutli-dimensionality

The social reformers propelling the 'good death' movement of the 1960s and 1970s were responding to the narrowing of the patient experience to the biomedical realm. Recent empirical investigation suggests that perhaps the most important feature of attempting to define a 'good death' is its multi-dimensional nature.

In 2008, Hales *et al.* reviewed 17 studies defining quality at end of life (using search terms: 'good death', bad death, quality of death, and quality of dying)[52]. Five of the studies were conducted with health-care providers only; five were conducted among only patient populations; three/four were studies of non-patient, non-health-care provider populations; and the remaining included both patients and or families, and providers. Seven common broad domains were found: physical, psychological experience, social, and spiritual or existential experience, the nature of health care, life closure and death preparation, and circumstances of death. The individual studies may have used unique language that, the authors argue, falls within these common domains.

Expectedly, pain and symptom management was the most commonly identified theme. Yet, even within the consensus endorsement, qualitative study reveals variation in individual preference for how this domain may be addressed. For example, some patients may wish to balance analgesia with lucidity to allow meaningful personal interactions, and thus may tolerate some pain to achieve a higher state of alertness, if necessary. More recent studies suggest that physical dimensions include not only pain and symptoms but also attention to functional status, which is highly correlated with continued independence and quality of life[53].

This body of work confirms that the physiological aspects of end-of-life experience are only a point of departure in overall definitions of a 'good death' or quality at end of life[49]. Attention to emotional or psychological and social well-being are crucial. Patients experience their illness living a variety of roles and interrelationships that need to be sustained as part of whole person care. Interestingly, earlier sociological theory proposed that dying patients, and older adults, in general, experienced a natural 'disengagement' as end of life loomed. However, this theory has been debunked by empirical evidence showing the desire for and power of continued role engagement. Although dying patients usually experience physical decline or limitation, they may experience growth in social and emotional areas.

Similarly, attention to spiritual or transcendent aspects of experience are reported as central to quality experience and hold opportunity for growth[15,24,54]. This domain may be expressed in traditional religious terms, via connection with nature or as overall sense of meaning and purpose in life. There is some evidence of it increasing in importance as end of life nears[15]. Of note, the absence of this domain in traditional quality of life measures was a main factor limiting their reliability and validity when applied to the context of dying.

While physical, social, psychological, and spiritual domains had been predicted by some of the pre-empirical literature, several new domains emerged from empirical investigation. These include preparation for death or end of life, nature of health care, and life completion. In contrast to settings of 'closed awareness' reported as common in the 1960s, 'good death' investigations of the 1990s and early 2000s suggested many patients with advanced serious illness wanted an opportunity to know what to expect about the course of their illness, to put personal affairs in order, to make financial arrangements and personal business, to not be a burden to family, to prepare their families for the future, and, for some, to plan one's own funeral. It is important to note the contradiction found in the literature whereby populations within the same study report valuing 'dying in their sleep', 'dying suddenly', and 'being prepared'[4].

These studies show that preparation is not limited to patients. Families also need to be prepared for what to expect about the course of illness and decision making.

> I can't tell you how many times, working in the emergency room, [that I saw] families [take a patient home]; this patient was going to die at home. And, when the last breath came, the families panicked. They brought the patient into the emergency room and went through the whole process [rescuscitation]. Preparing the family, assessing what they actually know, and figuring out what you have to teach them is essential. – Nurse[50].

Finally, some have also described the importance of provider preparation, coming to terms with their own fears about mortality and the emotions generated in caring for those who die[2].

Another less-expected domain revealed in the 'good death' studies was the nature of health care. This domain focused on issues such as the appropriateness of level of technological intervention—levels in keeping with patient and family wishes, as well as communication with health-care providers, knowing how and where to get answers to questions, and overall relationship with the provider[49,50,55]. The latter issue of relationship included maintaining patient dignity and treating patients as whole persons rather than as diseases.

Finally, the domain of life completion has been central to many investigations conceptualizing a 'good death'[4,7,47,50]. Attributes of completion include life review, closure, coming to peace, resolving conflicts, contributing to others, spending time with family and friends, and saying good-bye. Completion may involve personal reflection or individual spiritual practice, or may be more explicitly communal including family or a wider social circle. Of course, many organized religions denote particular rites of spiritual completion for both the dying and the mourner. As with all domains, cues regarding specific expression should come from the patient or family. Within this domain, the attribute of contributing to others, reminds family members and providers the importance not only of what patients may need to receive but also what they need to give to experience wholeness as they face the end of their lives.

Importance of role

Studies attempting to define a positive end-of-life experience reveal the importance of role in perception of what constitutes 'good'. For example, studies show that physician perspectives tend to be more narrowly biomedical. And the data suggest a discrepancy in physician versus family and patient ratings of the importance of spirituality and completion attributes such as prayer[15,24]. In one survey asking participants to rank order nine attributes of end of life, families and patients rankings of being at peace and freedom from pain were statistically equal in importance[49]. In contrast, physicians rated coming to peace as a distant third. Patients also were more likely to rate higher the importance of mental alertness and a desire not to be a burden to family or society.

In this same study, non-physician providers were more likely than patients to rate as important, 'talking about the meaning of dying'. Family members were more likely than patients to rate the importance of discussing personal fears or meeting with clergy. Again, it is instructive to take cues from patients about how they want to discuss this issue. Qualitative findings suggest patients may wish to discuss purpose and life more than meaning of death.

In a survey of hospice nurses definitions of 'good death' McNamara found that definitions of 'bad' deaths included those in which the patient did not internalize hospice philosophy, leaving staff frustrated[42]. Non-internalization included not accepting the imminence of death, allowing non-palliative therapies to continue, and the family wanting 'everything done' despite terminal diagnoses. Such circumstances were thought to compromise a peaceful 'natural' death.

Importance of culture

In addition to individual and family variation in preferences for end of life, cultural scripts also predominate. While this is expanded upon more fully elsewhere in this textbook, studies relating to minority and majority population variation suggest a desire for clinician awareness of cultural issues, particularly heightened attention to the role spiritual beliefs play in decision making, and attention to individual interpretation of minority culture scripts[51]. Within the US population, a growing literature has demonstrated increased preference for life sustaining therapies among Latino and African American populations[56]. However, in one study, African Americans were more likely to 'want all available treatments' but less likely than Caucasian participants to want to be 'connected to machines'[49]. These varying responses among groups sensitized providers to patient and family differential interpretation of medical jargon, true variation in preferences for treatment. As many sources have noted, when working with populations of patients traditionally denied access to care, withdrawing and withholding treatments are met with understandable apprehension.

Finally, much of the empirical work defining a 'good death' has involved English-speaking Western populations in which individual decision making and autonomy is culturally rewarded. More familial or communal decision-making models, though prevalent, are less well represented in the research literature, and therefore deserving of future study. For example, Asian cultures with normative scripts including notions of filial piety will display markedly different preferences for treatment and communication on the part of patients and families.

Importance of timing

In addition to cultural variation, clinicians must take note of the importance of time frame in patient and family preferences. The literature reveals little consensus on what time frame constitutes the end of life. Furthermore, preferences will likely differ by stage of illness and evolve over time with definitions of 'good experience' while living with advanced serious illness being distinct from 'good dying', as distinct from a 'good death'. For example, immediately after a diagnosis of metastatic disease preparation may include discussions of possible courses of treatment, the combination of curative and palliative therapies and helping patients remain integrated with normal work and social roles. As illness progresses, preparation may include discussions of decreasing the use of curative therapies and increasing palliative approaches, discussion of hospice, and increased attention to issues of completion. As dying becomes imminent, preparation may involve working with the family about expectations of care, location of care, and education regarding the very end of life.

Opportunity for growth

Ira Byock has described the benefit of adopting a life-cycle model of end of life[15]. He notes that the medical model begins assessment and treatment by generating a problem list. From the time a patient presents with symptoms, the clinical interviews and choice of diagnostic testing is determined by these problems. While this approach brings focus and efficiency to diagnostic testing and treatment, it is best suited to acute medicine and has limitations when applied to the context of care of incurably ill patients. Incurably ill patients surely are met with the daunting challenges of physical symptom exacerbation and functional decline; however, a purely problem-based approach offers less guidance in helping patients navigate areas of experience in which they may experience improvement or growth. A life-cycle model assumes death is the natural end of a life course. And, building on the work of human development by Erikson, Bulter, and Cassell, Byock notes the expected developmental tasks associated with this phase of life[15,57-59]. These tasks include attention to life review, resolution of conflict, forgiveness, acceptance, and generativity. Most importantly, this framework allows one to conceptualize end of life, like other phases of the life course, as holding opportunity for growth rather than only the decline predicted by the medical model. Growth will most likely occur in emotional and spiritual domains (and areas like preparation and completion) and is hypothesized to account for discrepancies in patient versus observer ratings of quality of life.

Thinking outside the biopsychosocial/spiritual model

The seven domains listed above often are referred to under the general rubric of the biopsychosocial and spiritual model of care. The model, as just described, enjoys significant empirical support. In addition, two recent studies expand the notion of elements that contribute to the quality of end of life for patients and families. Casarett et al. highlighted advanced cancer patients' preferences for 'supportive services' even over traditional hospice services[60]. Supportive services included: vouchers for practical assistance at home, transportation, peer support, meal delivery, case management, and family care. Perkins et al. emphasizes additional supportive services such as emergency contacts and case management[55]. While much of the 'good death' literature was built on investigation into improving care of hospitalized patients, we must recognize that a majority of care in the dying trajectory occurs in the outpatient, home, and community setting. Therefore, newer models of good end-of-life experience must expand beyond the individual inpatient model of care.

Clinical implications of the term 'good death'

In this article, we have reported on research which sought to define a 'good death'. Yet, it is important to discuss the clinical implications of using such language. In one of our studies, 'In search of a 'good death': observations of patients, families, and providers' we concluded that there is no one 'good death'[50]. Rather, each end-of-life experience is a process to be negotiated and renegotiated in the context of that patient and families values, preferences, and life course. We were strongly cautioned by nurses, for example, that it was important to know there was 'no one right way to die' and warned against implying to patients that 'you're not dying the right way, because you're not dying the way we think you should'.

While early hospice founders used language of a 'good death' to rally reformers to a new vision of care, in recent years the language of a 'good death' often has taken on a denotation of specific expectations of what should occur at the end of life. The zeal driving the early movement has risked imposing a sense of a 'right way' to die. Its components include being free of pain, surrounded by family, free of conflict, acceptance of death, stopping curative treatment, being at peace, and preferably dying at home. While those may be components many or most would define as positive, the implication is that one can define a 'good death', and should achieve it. Unfortunately, though propelled by positive intentions, such definition risks imposing an unintended paternalism. Furthermore, data of patient and family preferences at end of life exhibit far more nuance and variation.

For example, a national survey we conducted revealed that only about 50 per cent of respondents ranking dying at home as important[49]. In related qualitative research linked to the survey, while many valued dying at home, other patients and families described circumstances of caregiver frailty, superstition, or fear of bad memories as dissuading them from wanting the death to occur at home. As we noted, family members and non-physician healthcare providers were significantly more likely than patients to identify 'talking about the meaning of dying' as important. And though coming to peace often is highly valued by patients, working to resolve conflicts can be complex and contain periods of great uncertainty, for patients, families, and providers hoping to guide them. And, by the time of death, everything is not always resolved. Again, there is caution to clinicians and all working with dying patients, that these uncertainties and lack of resolution do not represent failures on the parts of patients and families, but merely illustrates the rich variation in the way people live their entire lives.

Alternative language—defining goals at end of life

Therefore, rather than promoting a construct of a 'good death', we favour the language of helping patients and families define and meet goals at the end of life. This paradigm has several advantages. First, in the medical context, we expect that goals vary between individuals. Second, we expect that they may change over time. Therefore, they require ongoing communication and negotiation. Third, the language of goals allows patient as active participant. Drawing from the self-management literature, the clinician may be the expert on the disease process, but the patient is the expert on their life. Fourth, it acknowledges a future orientation and ongoing contributions. Fifth, for the clinician, it is action oriented and moves beyond the idea (not common in palliative care) of having nothing more to offer. There are always additional goals.

Although we favour the paradigm in general, it does have some disadvantages and points of caution. First, the language of goals may imply achievement and productivity, and risk imposing such expectations on patients. This would be counterproductive.

Second, culturally we may think of goals as 'doing'. Yet, we do not want to understate the importance of offering a sense of presence to patients and simply 'being' with them in their illness.

Being with patients and families may involve offering assurance, through words and actions, that the provider will be present through the course of treatment and illness. It may involve deep listening and necessary silences, in the presence of powerful emotions. And, it may involve assurance of commitment to negotiating and renegotiating preferences for care that attend to domains of physical, social, emotional, and spiritual well-being as well as issues of preparation and life completion. Together, acknowledging that the quality of end-of-life experience is dependent upon attending to the multiple dimensions of whole persons facing illness in the context of an entire lifetime of values and choices within the web of family and community.

References

1. Rousseau, P. (1997). Hope and the terminally ill. *Clinical Geriatrics*, **5**(13), 15.
2. Steinhauser, K.E., Christakis, N.A., Clipp, E.C. *et al.* (2001). Preparing for the end of life: preferences of patients, families, physicians, and other care providers. *Journal of Pain and Symptom Management*, **22**(3), 727–37.
3. Aries, P. (1980). *The hour of our death*. Knopf Publishers, New York.
4. Vig, E.K. and Pearlman, R.A. (2004). Good and bad dying from the perspective of terminally ill men. *Archives of Internal Medicine*, **164**(9), 977–81.
5. DelVecchio Good, M.J., Gadmer, N.M., Ruopp, P. *et al.* (2004). Narrative nuances on good and bad deaths: internists' tales from high-technology work places. *Social Science and Medicine*, **58**(5), 939–53.
6. Hart, B., Sainsbury, P., and Short, S. (1998). Whose dying? A sociological critique of the "good death". *Mortality*, **3**(1), 65–77.
7. Hirai, K., Miyashita, M., Morita, T. *et al.* (2006). Good death in Japanese cancer care: a qualitative study. *Journal of Pain and Symptom Management*, **31**(2), 140–7.
8. Kim, S. and Lee, Y. (2003). Korean nurses' attitudes to good and bad death, life-sustaining treatment and advance directives. *Nursing Ethics*, **10**(6), 624–37.
9. Long, S.O. (2004). Cultural scripts for a good death in Japan and the United States: similarities and differences. *Social Science and Medicine*, **58**(5), 913–28.
10. Radley, A. (2004). Pity, modernity and the spectacle of suffering. *Journal of Palliative Care*, **20**(3), 179–84.
11. Seale, C. (1998). Theories in health care and research: theories and studying the care of dying people. *BMJ*, **317**(7171), 1518–20.
12. Seale, C. and van der Geest, S. (2004). Good and bad death: introduction. *Social Science and Medicine*, **58**(5), 883–5.
13. Kring, D.L. (2006). An exploration of the good death. *ANS Advances in Nursing Science*, **29**(3), E12–24.
14. Sudnow, D. (1967). The social organization of dying. Prentice Hall, Englewood Cliffs, NJ.
15. Byock, I.R. (1996). The nature of suffering and the nature of opportunity at the end of life. *Clinics in Geriatric Medicine*, **12**(2), 237–52.
16. Saunders, C. (1978). Hospice care. *American Journal of Medicine*, **65**(5), 726–8.
17. Glaser, B. and Strauss, A. (1965). *Awareness of dying*. Aldine, Chicago, IL.
18. Kubler-Ross, E. (1969). *On death and dying*, Macmillan Publishing New York.
19. Investigators SP. (1995). A controlled trial to improve care for seriously ill hospitalized patients: The study to understand prognosis and preferences for outcomes and risks of treatments (SUPPORT). *JAMA*, **274**, 1591–8.
20. Field, M. and Cassel, C. (1997). *Approaching death: Improving care at the end of life*. Institute of Medicine, Washington, DC.
21. Asch, D.A., Hansen-Flaschen, J., Lanken, P.N. (1995). Decisions to limit or continue life-sustaining treatment by critical care physicians in the United States: conflicts between physicians' practices and patients' wishes. *American Journal of Respiratory and Critical Care Medicine*, **151**(2 Pt 1), 288–92.
22. Borbasi, S., Jones, J., Lockwood, C. *et al.* (2006). Health professionals' perspectives of providing care to people with dementia in the acute setting: toward better practice. *Geriatric Nursing*, **27**(5), 300–8.
23. Borbasi, S., Wotton, K., Redden, M. *et al.* (2005). Letting go: a qualitative study of acute care and community nurses' perceptios of a "good" versus "bad" death. *Australian Critical Care*, **18**(3), 104–13.
24. Cohen, S. and Leis, A. (2002). What determines the quality of life in terminally ill cancer patients from their own perspectives? *Journal of Palliative Care*, **18**, 48–58.
25. Curtis, J.R., Patrick, D.L., Engelberg, R.A. *et al.* (2002). A measure of the quality of dying and death: Initial validation. *Journal of Pain and Symptom Management*, **24**, 17–31 .
26. Ellington, S. and Fuller, J. (1998). A good death?: finding a balance between the interests of patients and caregivers. *Generations*, **22**(3), 87–91.
27. Emanuel, E.J., and Emanuel, L.L. (1998). The promise of a good death. *Lancet*, **351** (Suppl 2), SII21-29.
28. Ferrell, B.R. (2005). Overview of the domains of variables relevant to end-of-life care. *Journal of Palliative Medicine*, **8** (Suppl 1), S22-29.
29. Ganzini, L., Goy, E.R., Miller, L.L. *et al.* (2004). Nurses' experiences with hospice patients who refuse food and fluids to hasten death. *New England Journal of Medicine*, **349**(4), 359–65.
30. Goldsteen, M., Houtepen, R., Proot, I.M. *et al.* (2006). What is a good death? Terminally ill patients dealing with normative expectations around death and dying. *Patient Education and Counseling*, **64**(1–3), 378–86.
31. Hanson, L.C., Henderson, M., and Menon, M. (2002). As individual as death itself: a focus group study of terminal care in nursing homes. *Journal of Palliative Medicine*, **5**(1), 117–25.
32. Hopkinson, J. and Hallett, C. (2002). Good death? An exploration of newly qualified nurses' understanding of good death. *International Journal of Palliative Nursing*, **8**(11), 532–9.
33. King, D. and Bushwick, B. (1994). Beliefs and attitudes of hospital inpatients about faith healing and prayer. *J Fam Practice*, **39**(4), 349–52.
34. Kristjanson, L.J., McPhee, I., Pickstock, S. (2001). Palliative care nurses' perceptions of good and bad deaths and care expectations: a qualitative analysis. *International Journal of Palliative Nursing*, **7**(3), 129–39.
35. Layde, P.M., Beam, C.A., Broste, S.K. *et al.* (1994). Surrogates' predictions of seriously ill patients' resuscitation preferences. *Archives of Family Medicine*, **4**(6), 518–23.
36. Leichtentritt, R.D. (2004). The meaning that young Israeli adults ascribe to the least undesirable death. *Death Studies*, **28**(8), 733–59.
37. Low, J.T. and Payne, S. (1996). The good and bad death perceptions of health professionals working in palliative care. *European Journal of Cancer Care (England)*, **5**(4), 237–41.
38. Lynn, J., Teno, J.M., Phillips, R.S. *et al.* (1997). Perceptions by family members of the dying experience of older and seriously ill patients. SUPPORT Investigators. Study to understand prognoses and preferences for outcomes and risks of treatments. *Annals of Internal Medicine*, **126**(2), 97–106.
39. Mak, M.H. (2001). Awareness of dying: an experience of Chinese patients with terminal cancer. *Omega (Westport)*, **43**(3), 259–79.
40. Masson, J. (2002). Non-professional perceptions of " good death": a study of the views of hospice care patients and relatives of deceased hospice care patients. *Mortality*, **7**(2), 191–209.

41. McNamara, B. (2004). Good enough death: autonomy and choice in Australian palliative care. *Social Science and Medicine*, **58**(5), 929–38.

42. McNamara, B., Waddell, C., and Colvin, M. (1994). The institutionalization of the good death. *Social Science and Medicine*, **39**(11), 1501–8.

43. Miyashita, M., Sanjo, M., Morita, T. *et al.* (2007). Good death in cancer care: a nationwide quantitative study. *Annals of Oncology*, **18**(6), 1090–7.

44. Morris, J., Suissa, S., Sherwood, S. *et al.* (1986). Last days: a study of the quality of life of terminally ill cancer patients. *Journal of Chronic Diseases*, **39**, 47–62.

45. Payne, S.A., Langley-Evans, A., and Hillier, R. (1996). Perceptions of a 'good death': a comparative study of the views of hospice staff and patients. *Palliative Medicine*, **10**(4), 307–12.

46. Pierson, C.M., Curtis, J.R., and Patrick, D.L. (2002). A good death: a qualitative study of patients with advanced AIDS. *AIDS Care*, **14**(5), 587–98.

47. Rietjens, J.A., van der Heide, A., Onwuteaka-Philipsen, B.D. *et al.* (2006). Preferences of the Dutch general public for a good death and associations with attitudes towards end-of-life decision-making. *Palliative Medicine*, **20**(7), 685–92.

48. Singer, P.A., Martin, D.K., and Kelner, M. (1999). Quality end-of-life care: patients' perspectives. *JAMA*, **281**(2), 163–8.

49. Steinhauser, K.E., Christakis, N.A., Clipp, E.C. *et al.* (2000). Factors considered important at the end of life by patients, family, physicians, and other care providers. *JAMA*, **284**(19), 2476–82.

50. Steinhauser, K.E., Clipp, E.C., McNeilly, M. *et al.* (2000). In search of a good death: observations of patients, families, and providers. *Annals of Internal Medicine*, **132**(10), 825–32.

51. Tong, E., McGraw, S.A., Dobihal, E. *et al.* (2003). What is a good death? Minority and non-minority perspectives. *Journal of Palliative Care*, **19**(3), 168–75.

52. Hales, S., Zimmermann, C., and Rodin, G. (2008). The quality of dying and death. *Archives of Internal Medicine*, **168**(9), 912–918.

53. Walke, L.M., Byers, A.L., Gallo, W.T. *et al.* (2007). The association of symptoms with health outcomes in chronically ill adults. *Journal of Pain and Symptom Management*, **33**(1), 58–66.

54. Daaleman, T.P., and Nease, D.E., Jr. (1994). Patient attitudes regarding physician inquiry into spiritual and religious issues. *Journal of Family Practice*, **39**(6), 564–8.

55. Perkins, P., Booth, S., Vowler, S.L. *et al.* (2008). What are patients' priorities for palliative care research? – a questionnaire study. *Palliative Medicine*, **22**(1), 7–12.

56. Tulsky, J.A., Cassileth, B.R., and Bennett, C.L. (1997). The effect of ethnicity on ICU use and DNR orders in hospitalized AIDS patients. *Journal of Clinical Ethics*, **8**(2), 150–7.

57. Butler, R.N. (1974). Succesful aging and the role of the life review. *Journal of the American Geriatrics Society*, **22**(12), 529–35.

58. Butler, R.N. (1980). The life review: an unrecognized bonanza. *International Journal of Aging and Human Development*, **12**(1), 35–8.

59. Cassell, E.J. (1973). Learning to die. *Bulletin of the New York Academy of Medicine*, **49**(12), 1110–8.

60. Casarett, D., Fishman, J., O'Dwyer, P.J. *et al.* (2008). How should we design supportive cancer care? The patient's perspective. *Journal of Clinical Oncology*, **26**(8), 1296–301.

3.7

Ethnic and cultural aspects of palliative medicine

Jonathan Koffman and LaVera Crawley

Introduction

The goal of this chapter is to identify 'differences that make a difference'[1] among individuals and groups when they negotiate institutions and practices for palliative and end-of-life care. Culture is but one of several typologies of difference that has been used to signify diversity among individuals and groups. If narrowly defined from an anthropological perspective, culture can be thought of as that which refers to the '… patterns, explicit and implicit, of and for behaviour acquired and transmitted by symbols,' language, and rituals[2]. Seen as a 'recipe' for living in the world, this conceptual framework for culture explains the means of transmitting these 'recipes' to the next generation[3]. However, this is a limited understanding of culture that, if used here, risks minimizing discussions of cultural aspects of palliative medicine to an interpretive list of end-of-life beliefs and practices from a range of so-called 'cultural' groups. This has also been referred to as the 'fact-file' or 'checklist'[4] approach that, while informative in regards to interpreting behaviours, symbols, rituals, and other cultural practices of certain ethnic or religious groups that may be important and meaningful at the end of life, it runs the risk of encouraging generalizations about individuals and groups based on cultural identity. This in turn may then lead to the development of stereotypes, prejudices, and misunderstandings.

Culture is neither a static nor an intrinsic property of some cultural other. It is not static because identity, be it cultural, ethnic, religious, or other categories, is in a constant process of adaptation and change, often in response to interactions with yet 'others' who are different in multitudes of ways. Culture is not the sole possession of those who are considered 'ethnic' minority groups. All persons, the health-care practitioner included, brings his or her own cultural self into the medical or nursing encounter—a self that holds assumptions about the world and engages in practices and behaviours learned from their family and society of origin and, in the case of the health practitioner, from Western scientific and professional ideologies. Cross-cultural or intercultural interactions are not merely interpretative where each party needs only to translate language, signs, behaviours, or practices of the other. Ideally, these exchanges are also dialogic and relational. All parties enter into some transformational 'third space'[5] where meaning is negotiated and new understandings emerge. Therefore, programmes in 'cultural competency' that merely utilize an interpretive approach, emphasizing technical competencies utilized during the clinical encounter (such as communication skills) may miss the opportunity to teach skills needed for attitudinal transformations (such as sensitivity and humility) that are critical for 'developing mutually beneficial and non-paternalistic … partnerships' with patients and families'[6].

Understanding identity

In addition to culture, self or group identification may be based on race, ethnicity, tribal or clan affiliation, nativity, generational status, citizenship, gender, religion, politics, sexual orientation, social and economic class, and other categories[7]. Race, a rather contentious category of identity, has its roots in social Darwinism, and relies heavily on an expectation of perceived (versus real) biological differences between people and populations[8]. Historically, race has been used to describe geographically separated populations (such as the African race), cultural groups (Jews), nationality (the English race), and mankind in general (the human race). Racialized research in science has a long and inglorious history[9,10]. In the mid-19th century, the cephalic index, a method for describing the shape of the skull, became a popular way of describing and dividing races. Under the influence of phrenology, a hierarchy of races was devised with white Europeans at the top and black Africans at the bottom. Intelligence, physique, culture, and morality were all placed in an order, the so-called 'Great Chain of Being' philosophy used to justify slavery, imperialism, anti-immigration policy, and the social status quo[11]. Biological determinism also became prominent in medicine and medical practitioners frequently contributed to racialized science[12] with the theory of racial hygiene in Nazi Germany being a horrific and notorious example. However, differences that do exist between peoples and populations are very minor and largely reflect superficial physical characteristics such as facial features, hair, or skin colour. Many researchers have therefore now discredited race as being inaccurate and misleading[13].

Less controversial, but equally misunderstood is the concept of ethnicity[14,15]. As a category of identity, it reflects the social grouping of persons on the basis of historical or territorial identity or by shared cultural patterns and traditions maintained between generations[16,17]. One's ethnicity can be defined by language, such as Spanish language that unites Hispanic peoples in Central and

South America and the Caribbean who are otherwise separated by geography, history, and politics. It can also be defined by shared ancestry, such as subgroups of diasporic blacks who are descendants of slaves from West and Central Africa. There are also subcategories used in identifying certain ethnic groups. For example, among ethnic blacks, further delineations can be made by nativity and citizenship: African Americans who are descendants of slaves and of multiple generations born in and holding citizenship in the USA may be ethnically distinct (for example, in language or culture) from black Haitians, Cubans, Jamaicans, or other descendants of African slaves who reside in the Caribbean, South America, the UK, or other diasporic locations. Other ways in which people express their identity include kinship by tribal or clan affiliation which can be extremely influential (and potentially volatile) in intergroup dynamics.

Identity is both internally (self-) defined and externally (structurally) imposed[18] which has bearing not only in how an individual or group sees oneself but also in how they are treated by society. Needless to say, the politics and social science of identity is complex. Furthermore, semantic confusion is very common when the concepts of identity are used in clinical and research settings. Race, ethnicity, and culture are often used interchangeably, subject to misuse, or confused with other social metrics, for example, social class or education[19]. The manner in which these concepts are used may change due to prevailing fashions and politics[20].

Structural factors, defined as rules, roles, and institutions derived from dynamic social, economic, political, and historical processes, may play an important role in creating and maintaining cultural, racial, and/or ethnic identities themselves, or various aspects associated with those identities. An example can be seen with the conflation of ethnic identity with class: in places or situations where institutional racism or other forms of discrimination constrain freedom and development for certain segments of a population, say on the basis of racial or ethnic visibility, these structural factors may produce patterns (e.g. poverty, poor education, crime) that become erroneously attached to the identity of that group[18]. The same can be said for structural factors that privilege other segments of the populations.

To compound the confusion, there is no uniformity in how persons are classified across national boundaries. For example, the National Health Service and census in the UK identify five different categories of 'ethnicity' (white, mixed, Asian, black, or Chinese) that are further broken down into different sub-groups based on countries of origin (e.g. Indian, Pakistani, Bangladeshi, or other for Asian; Caribbean, African, or other for blacks.)[21]; while the USA census collapses many distinct populations into one dichotomous category of 'ethnicity' (Hispanic or non-Hispanic) and five single broad categories of 'race', (white, black or African American, American Indian or Alaska Native, Asian, and Native Hawaiian or Other Pacific Islander)[22]. The South African census uses five population categories based on self-classification (Black African, Coloured, Indian or Asian, White, or Other)[23]. Canada collects census data based on ethnic origins (defined by ancestry) and on a category called 'visible minority' status, defined as 'persons other than Aboriginal persons who are not white in race or colour'[24]. Lastly, there is evidence that many people change their assigned identity over time, as is their prerogative[25]. US-based research has shown that at least 35% of respondents altered their self-assignment over a year and in the validation study following the 1991 British

census 12% of 'black' people altered their ethnic group, as did 22% of 'other' category[26].

This mutability attests to the fact that persons inhabit multiple identities which are expressed or perceived differently as need and circumstance change[16,18]. The relevance of this discussion for palliative care is to caution the clinician and researcher to be mindful of the difficulties in interpreting events at the bedside or reports in the literature related to culture, race, ethnicity, or other identifiers. Employing clearly and rationally defined demographic categorizations of identity in studying epidemiologic patterns of morbidity and mortality has usefulness for policy implications, such as determining what systems of care are needed or measuring inequities in quality of care delivered across population groups. However, employing essentialized notions of preferences or behaviours at the bedside runs the risk of compromising an individual's 'needs and concerns [that] may not conform to preconceived or stereotyped patterns'[16]. What best serves the needs of all patients is knowledge of the particular individual's beliefs, values, preferences, and practices—knowledge gained by asking the patient or family directly or by utilizing resources that promote patient-centred and relationship-centred care.

The special case of immigration

Throughout human history, individuals, families, and groups have emigrated from their native homes to other places for many reasons: the prospect of education, economic, or social advantage; the need to escape war, political torture, or other conflicts; or the desire to reunite with other family members. Globalization has brought with it an unprecedented increase in the numbers of persons who have migrated to developed countries. In 2005, there was an estimated 191 million immigrants worldwide: approximately 64 million of these immigrants arrived in Europe and 44 million in North America—a tripling of the immigrant populations in these regions compared with 20 years earlier. This trend is expected to continue and to increase. In the USA, for example, it is estimated that by the year 2050, nearly two-thirds of the population will be immigrants.

The International Observatory on End-of-Life Care that monitors the global development of hospice and palliative care services around the world report that such services are unavailable or are uneven at best in under-developed and medium-developed countries as compared with Europe and English-speaking countries[27]. Subsequently, the immigrant may not have had much exposure to or knowledge of palliative care services provided by hospices or other health-care institutions in their home countries. For example, the Observatory documented misperceptions about and stigmas regarding palliative care in Mexico[28]. As such, expectations for palliative care may thus be lowered among Mexican immigrants who bring from their country of origin misperceptions or lowered priorities for this type of care[29]. In addition, some immigrants may find accessing quality care and finding funds for hospice, palliative care, and other end-of-life heath services to be a complex and potentially confusing process that may be compounded by unfamiliarity with laws and regulations of the host country. The immigrant's knowledge of and preference for palliative or other health care may be influenced by factors related to immigration, itself. For example, refugees and asylum seekers who have experienced violence or who may have been exposed to torture or other state-sanctioned or war-related trauma may be mistrustful of health care or social service institutions and authorities[30,31]. They may also face fears and uncertainties that accompany their experiences as an immigrant within a polarized political climate. In a report on immigration issues and end-of-life care in California, investigators identified the unique concerns of undocumented immigrants—those who have entered the USA illegally or who have overstayed their visas[29].

Over 27% of the US undocumented population reside in California, the most ethnically and culturally diverse state in that country. Greater than 25% of these undocumented persons are between ages 15 and 44 years and come to the USA primarily looking for work or other opportunities. While this younger, healthier cohort may not represent the typical patient in need of palliative care services, mortality data shows that a disproportionate number of these workers are at risk of dying from trauma and accidents. The implications of these patterns include the need to increase expertise in palliative care practices and services in emergency departments (including end-of-life decision-making and bereavement services for families and loved ones) and to support education and training programmes on unique issues of death and dying in emergency room settings for emergency personnel. This report also found that among patients for whom hospice would be appropriate (deaths following terminal illness or chronic disease trajectories), few immigrants and other ethnically diverse persons in California utilized hospice for their end-of-life care needs. The range of reasons included: barriers due to lack of eligibility for state or federal funding benefits; lack of cultural acceptance of hospice and palliative care practices; and lack of referral by health providers. In addition, the 'Salmon effect' where immigrants return home to their native countries to die, partially explained lower use of hospice[32]. Immigration also impacts the workforce that provides care-giving for those who are dying. Foreign health-care workers are motivated to leave their native countries for reasons general to all immigrants—education, economic, or social advantage; or they may leave due to inadequate health-care infrastructures and technologies[33]. The result in some receiving countries is a growing immigrant workforce who bring their own unique cross-cultural issues to health-care delivery systems. On the one hand, an increasingly diverse health-care workforce may help improve outreach to diverse communities, particularly in areas of language barriers and other access issues. On the other hand, these workers will represent a spectrum of acculturation or assimilation of the language, customs, values, and perspectives of the host country. Just as there can be native providers who lack cultural competency and sensitivity toward immigrant patients, there can be those immigrant providers who lack these skills with native patients. Central to this issue is communication capability.

Cultural versus moral relativism

Cultural relativism or multi-culturalism is defined as 'a social-intellectual movement that promotes the value of diversity as a core principle and insists that all cultural groups be treated with respect as equals'[34]. In social, economic, and political arenas, this is a laudable, albeit narrow, goal (narrow only in the sense of applying limited or narrow definitions of culture or identity as discussed above). Efforts for ensuring equitable access to societal goods across all populations, including quality care for the seriously ill and dying, requires attention to salient differences within and among groups. However, blindly embracing this principle does carry an inherent risk of mistaking cultural relativism with moral relativism. Respect for diversity does not mean one should tolerate actions that violate another's human rights. A case example is warranted: a young adult immigrant from Yemen with advanced metastatic cancer required large doses of opioids to control his pain. The patient described his pain as unbearable and requested relief from his physician. The patient's family, traditional Muslims, strongly objected to the prescribing and administering of opioids required to relieve the patient's pain and suffering, quoting scriptures that held that pain was to be endured as test of faith[35].

Cultural relativism indeed requires us to respect the role that religious and other cultural beliefs and practices hold; however, it may be difficult to be tolerant of practices if doing so forces us to violate moral principles such as non-maleficence (to avoid doing harm) or beneficence (serving what is in the patient's benefit). If the patient, rather than his family, acknowledged this preference to forego treatment of his pain, then the moral dilemma between the doctor and patient may need to be addressed. In this case, however, the patient did request relief and thus the provider might feel the *prima facie* obligation to address the patient's request for pain relief as a respect for his autonomous right for health-care decision-making. The moral dilemma then, is truly between the patient and his family.

However, one may counter argue that such moral principles are not culturally neutral to begin with and, rather, reflect a Western bias of what counts as right or wrong. Respect for individual autonomy is a Western ideal. Among other populations, the family or community is thought to be the unit of autonomy. For example, among some Asian or Hispanic populations, it is believed that the family should be the decision maker and in some cases patients should be shielded from information deemed potentially disturbing. This is a classic dilemma brought to ethics committees or consultations for deliberation and an example of why cross-cultural or intercultural interactions should be seen as dialogic and relational. The goal for all parties in such interactions is not to condone or to condemn the 'other' but rather to seek understanding and to co-create resolutions that are mutually acceptable. Understanding goes beyond interpretation of beliefs and values; it also means looking at the structural aspects of a practice: what purpose it serves in the cultural group or society. If a group values family autonomy over individual autonomy while the physician or medical system values the reverse, then a mutually acceptable solution might entail asking the patient if he or she would autonomously prefer the family to make decisions, thereby autonomously relinquishing autonomy. In summary, as ethicist Ruth Macklin has written, blind tolerance, which she calls 'extreme ethical relativism', is not useful. However, Macklin reminds us that neither is Western cultural imperialism. The middle ground is the following: cultural, religious, and ethnic groups should be treated as equals—conforming to the principle of justice as equality—while at the same time this should be balanced with intolerance of practices that are unjust and oppressive[34].

Differences that make a difference

How we understand the influence of diversity in patterns of advanced disease, illness experiences, responses to treatment, and the use of specialist palliative care services is important given increasing evidence that we are not all equal in death and dying[4,36–40]. Race or ethnic-based disparities in mortality and in diagnosis, quality of care, referral patterns to specialist palliative care, and treatments for pain and other physical symptoms have been documented in many developed countries[16,18,38,41–51]. In the USA, a comprehensive review of evidence of unequal treatment commissioned by the US congress and produced by its Institute of Medicine (IOM) documented race- or ethnic-based inequities in pain and chronic disease management, cancer care, and other clinical care settings and suggested that inequities may be due to patient-level, provider-level, and/or health system-level variables, alone or in combinations[48]. Patient-level factors would include ethno-cultural, social, or other beliefs, preferences, or knowledge about health options. According to the IOM study, patient-level factors were thought to be the least likely contributor to disparities. On the other hand, both provider stereotyping and bias and how health-care systems are organized as well as the degree to which persons have access to care were shown to more likely influence on health outcomes for minority patients.

The existence of prejudice and stereotyping from a provider's side of the exchange may difficult for many non-minority providers to accept, as we all presume to consciously abhor such discriminatory attitudes and behaviours. The important contribution of the IOM report in thinking about this issue was its suggestion that it is not conscious attitudes that drive discrimination but rather those unconscious or implicit attitudes that may compel us when we are under duress. As Fyodor Dostoyevsky stated:

In every man's memories there are such things as he will reveal not to everyone, but perhaps only to friends. There are also such as he will reveal not only to friends, but only to himself, and that in secret. Then finally, there are such as a man is afraid to reveal even to himself, and every decent man will have accumulated quite a few things of this sort. That is, one might even say: the more decent a man is, the more of them he will have.[52]

Health system level factors such as poor access to health-care services have been reported by black and minority ethnic groups in the USA and UK[44,53]. This is also an issue for end-of-life care where the impact of ageing on the black and minority ethnic groups now means larger numbers of older members within these communities will require health services for advanced disease. A limited number of reports have levelled criticism of care at the end of life for these communities and poor access to appropriate care. Low rates of cancer were seen as one explanation to account for low up-take of service provision, but the figures were likely to have been inaccurate because of inadequate ethnic monitoring[54]. The authors concluded 'some black and Asian patients and their carers are very disadvantaged, as they do not know what they are entitled to, and hence what to ask for by way of benefits and services'[55]. Most recently, a study in an inner London health authority demonstrated that African Caribbean patients with advanced disease experienced restricted access to some specialist palliative care services compared with white British patients[39], yet an analysis of local provision revealed no lack of palliative care services[56]. This example of under-utilization of palliative care services by the black Caribbean community at the end of life supports other recent research among minority ethnic communities[42,57]. The explanations to account for this, all of which may operate in combination, are highlighted in Box 3.7.1. Identifying and eliminating health inequities in the delivery of quality palliative care is a critical mandate. Institutional standards for monitoring and ensuring the cultural sensitivity and competency of the palliative medicine workforce should be employed, as should strategies to increase community-based partnerships.

Box 3.7.1 Black and minority ethnic social exclusion at the end of life: why does it occur?	
Social and economic deprivation Low socio-economic status has been positively linked to an increased likelihood of hospital deaths although this would apply equally to all population groups[88–90].	**Attitudes to palliative care** Barriers to health care that the poor and the disenfranchised have traditionally encountered may influence their receptivity to palliative[43].
Knowledge of specialist palliative care services and poor communication There is a growing body of evidence that black and ethnic minorities are not adequately aware of specialist palliative care services available to them[82,90–92].	**Dissatisfaction with health care** Uptake of health and social services among certain minority ethnic communities has revealed lower utilization of services due to dissatisfaction of services[93].
	Cultural mistrust Evidence from USA to support the contention that black and minority ethnic groups as less likely than white patients to trust the motivations of doctors who discuss end-of-life care with them[94].
Ethno-centralism Demand for services may be influenced by the 'ethnocentric' outlook of palliative care services, discouraging black and minority ethnic groups from making use of relevant provision[82].	**Gatekeepers** Some health-care professionals 'gatekeepers' to services among minority ethnic groups contributing to lower referral rates[82].

Providing equitable, culturally appropriate palliative care

The World Health Organization definition of palliative care specifies two goals: (1) improving quality of life (QOL) of patients and families, and (2) preventing and relieving suffering. It identifies three strategies for meeting those goals: early identification; impeccable assessment; and [appropriate] treatment. Lastly, the definition addresses four domains of care: (1) problems related to pain; (2) physical conditions; (3) the psychosocial; (4) and the spiritual. The remaining chapter addresses these goals, strategies, and domains in relation to delivering quality palliative care in cross- or multi-cultural settings.

Goals of palliative care in cross-cultural contexts

Quality of life

The World Health Organization defines QOL as 'an individual's perception of their position in life in the context of the culture and value systems in which they live and in relation to their goals, expectations, standards, and concerns'[58]. When applied to palliative medicine, the focus is on maximizing the quality versus the quantity of time remaining in a patient's life. Because quality should be subjectively defined by patients and their families, cultural factors relevant to the individual and their family need to be addressed when assessing their QOL preferences and requirements.

Many QOL assessment instruments include broad areas representing key domains such as physical symptoms, functional status, interpersonal relations, emotional well-being, and the experience of spiritual or existential transcendence. However, the subjective nature of the concept of QOL and instruments used to measure it must also consider variations in meanings of these domains across cultural groups. Recognizing the need to address cultural components in assessing quality, the World Health Organization initiated the WHOQOL project to 'develop an international cross culturally comparable QOL assessment instrument'[59].

The psychometric properties of the WHOQOL instrument were tested in several stages and across multi-cultural field sites to ensure cross-cultural validity including: agreement on the definition of QOL; standardization of questions or items and of scale construction; and field testing final instruments. Both the 100-item instrument (WHOQOL-100) and the shorter 26-item version (WHOQOL-BREF) are available in many languages and can be used clinically for individual patients and well as in cross-cultural research for inter- and intra-group comparisons[58]. The initial field sites, located in Australia, Croatia, France, India, Israel, Japan, the Netherlands, Panama, Russia, Spain, Thailand, the UK, the USA, and Zimbabwe, each adapted the standardized instrument to their population-based needs. To date there are now over 30 sites worldwide and more continue to field test and adapt the instrument to the unique cultural needs of their countries.

Preventing and relieving suffering:

Cultural factors mediate the ways in which symptoms associated with advanced disease are identified and interpreted, the appropriate modes of expression of pain and other symptoms and associated suffering, whether an illness and symptoms are stigmatized, and whether the dependency needs that accompany advanced disease are considered an acceptable part of the normal life cycle or marginalized. The evidence of the influence of cultural and ethnic factors on symptom interpretation is fascinating and frequently raises more questions than it answers. In the 1950s, Zborowski demonstrated differences among old American, Irish, and other migrant communities' perceptions of their pain[60]. Most recently, Koffman et al. observed significantly higher levels of symptom-related-distress among black Caribbean compared with native-born white UK patients with advanced cancer living in south London. This finding was only partly explained by simple variations in treatment levels between the two groups[46] (see Fig. 3.7.1). Along with other researchers[61,62], the authors suggest that the language of expressing symptom-related distress may be reinforced by cultural expectations[46]. Expressions of suffering have been shown to serve a purpose. It has been observed in some African Americans communities that suffering is redemptive, bringing those who experience it closer to God[37].

In other communities the actual language used to describe distress and suffering has implications for the delivery of palliative care. Krause revealed that the expression in Panjabi, 'Dil me girda hai' used by Panjabis in Bedford often translates as the 'sinking heart' to reflect a range of psychological and somatic conditions[63]. In addition, she suggests that the 'generalized hopelessness' which characterizes depressive disorders in women living in London would not be regarded as abnormal among Hindu, Muslim, and Buddhist women who would regard 'hopelessness' as an aspect of life which can only be overcome on the path to salvation. Ahmed takes the view that while South Asian patients may be well aware of their own psychosomatic symptoms, GPs (including Asian GPs) tend only to acknowledge physical symptoms but do not recognize psychological distress[64]. The ongoing challenge is for health-care professionals to explore and acknowledge culturally determined understandings and expressions associated with advanced disease that do not mirror their own.

Strategies of palliative care in cross-cultural settings

Early identification

Problems with late referrals to hospice or for palliative care in general are a concern for all populations. To avoid the appearance of medical abandonment, it is important to integrate the goals of hospice and of palliative care early in the disease process, particularly for those illnesses that are predictably fatal. This is particularly important for immigrants or members of ethnic or cultural communities who may already feel marginalized or vulnerable due to their minority status. Myths or misunderstandings about the goals of palliative care should be addressed early on through culturally effective communication—which can also enable the palliative care team to learn about and incorporate the unique perspectives of the patient into the multi-disciplinary management of their care.

Identifying preferences for medical care in advance of untoward or terminal circumstances can be a difficult and emotional process. The decision-making model of advance care planning derived from bioethics practices assumes that choices made by the individual can be arrived at through rational processes that are unchanged by time, shifting social consequences, or disease and illness progression.

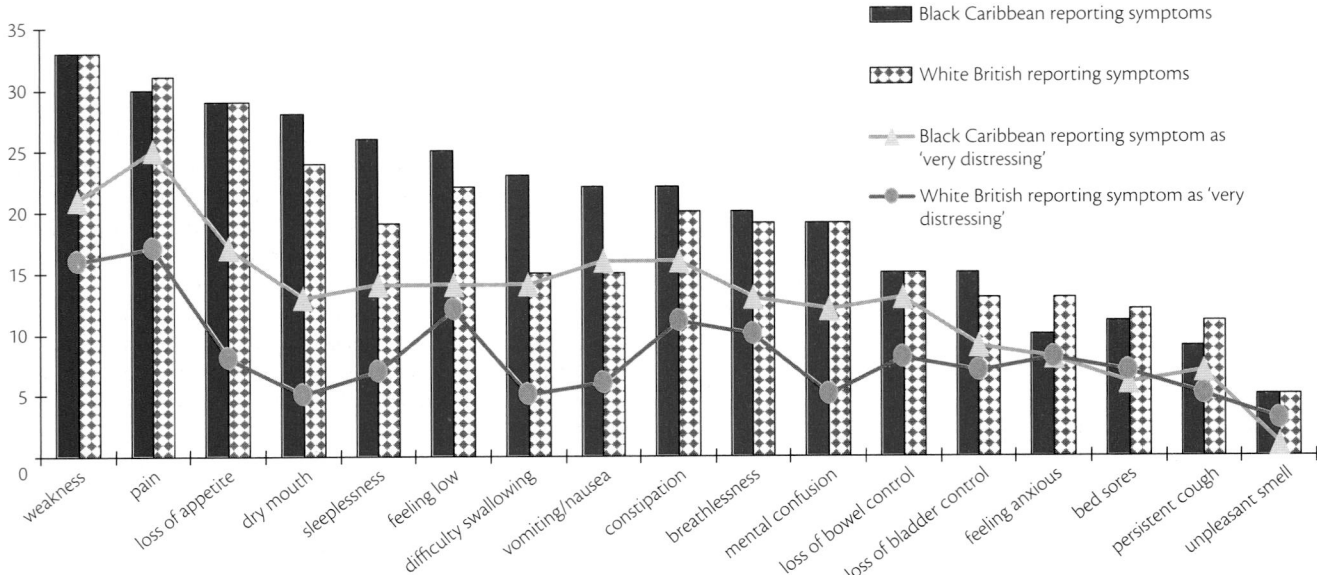

Figure 3.7.1 Reported symptoms and symptom related distress associated with advanced cancer among first-generation black Caribbean and white British-born patients with advanced cancer in the UK[46].

Such a model may only appeal to certain subsets of groups, thus limiting the utility of instruments used for advance planning (living wills or durable powers of attorney for health care). For some groups, speaking about the dying process or planning for death may represent a transgression of a strong cultural taboo and could create additional distress. Other patients, unfamiliar with or mistrustful of the legal system may misconstrue the purpose or nature of formal advance care planning documents. In all cases, rather than abandon the goals of advance care planning, strategies should be sought that facilitate understanding. For example, a generic discussion to identify a health-care proxy need not be cast as a discussion of death, but rather an opportunity to determine desired roles of various family members and support persons. Discussions about patient preferences for end-of-life care should be culturally and linguistically appropriate and reflect sensitivity to patient values and beliefs.

Impeccable assessment

Critical to assessing and monitoring palliative care needs is the ability to communicate clearly and effectively. The inability to do so not only affects access to palliative care services but also has been shown to be a source of serious problems in clinical consultations and the cause of misunderstandings among patients, family members, and health-care providers[39,65].

Important communication difficulties arise where there is an over reliance on patient's relatives acting on their loved one or dependants' behalf. While this may well be simpler than accessing an interpreter, it can potentially disadvantage both the doctor and the patient[37].

The family interpreter may filter, abbreviate, or omit very important information, or inform the doctor, or the patient what he or she thinks the doctor and patient needs to know. Important medical information may not be understood adequately or conveyed in full. Further, the use of children as interpreters is considered inappropriate. Details about an illness may be very intimate and it places an unfair burden on them, who, depending on their age, may be less likely to understand adult conversations in English, or even their own language[66]. Using friends or untrained lay interpreters from the local community can be even more problematic as there can be issues of confidentiality and fear of gossip in the wider community[67]. Moreover, communication is not only an issue of spoken language. It also involves body language, cultural rules as to what is courteous (such as not looking the professionals—especially opposite gender—in the eye) and appropriate behaviours in an unequal gender and power relationship[36]. People who speak English with a different accent or dialect, can also judged to be less intelligent or fail to be understood or understand what is being said to them[67].

Appropriate treatment

It is widely acknowledged that management of physical and psychological symptoms associated with advanced disease can be difficult in monocultural interactions between clinicians and patients because of differences in perspective between Western biomedicine and lay health beliefs and practices. However, the design and assessment of effective health care for culturally diverse patients, both long-term residents and new immigrants and refugees, is even more complicated. New immigrants increasingly come to the USA and the UK among other countries from regions such as Southeast Asia, Latin America, and Africa, and are even more heterogeneous than their European predecessors[61]. Within the same ethnic group, individuals come from all walks of life with differing educational, occupational, and economic status, ties to their country of origin, and geographical background. All these factors affect their ethnic identity and their cultural responses to health and illness. Understand and controlling patients' symptoms in a health-care system where the dominant imperative is for economic efficiency represents an overwhelming challenge. When clinicians look to published research to acquaint themselves with the ways in which ethnicity or culture may impinge upon the experience of symptoms, their expression, pain behaviours, or coping responses, they find a vast array of disciplinary lenses, diverse theoretical approaches that are often not made explicit, inconsistent findings, and methodological weaknesses. Upon closer reading, however, one can see that varied disciplines are starting to speak to each other and that a biological and social model of pain is attainable.

Domains of palliative care for culturally diverse populations

Pain and other symptoms

Investigators in a range of health-care settings in the USA have reported on disparities in the assessment and management of pain in ethnic minority groups as compared with white patients. In a qualitative study of nursing home residents, black residents consistently reported more incidents of prolonged and untreated moderate to severe pain as compared with white residents. Studies in emergency room settings similarly found inequities in pain treatment of Hispanic and black patients as compared with whites[68,69]. Surprisingly, studies in cancer centres documented similar patterns[62,70,71]. These disparities cannot be explained by cultural differences in the expression of pain, although such differences do exist. Pain and other physical symptoms are experienced, understood, and expressed by patients in ways that are mediated by culture, gender, age, social role, personality, and other factors. One's learned response for the expression and reactions of pain or other physical distress may range from the vocally or physically demonstrative to the passive or quietly stoic, with all possible forms between. Studies that explore different meanings, that can be defined as perceived relationships between the individual and his/ her world that is developed within the context of specific events[72], and forms of expression across cultures may be useful for increasing awareness of variability in patient presentation of pain and for

assessment of its subjective manifestations. For example, meanings ascribed to pain could be viewed positively as a challenge to overcome or negatively as the accompaniment to profound loss[73,74]. In a recent study exploring and comparing cancer-related pain among African Caribbeans and white British patients, pain was understood by both ethnic groups as a challenge and an enemy, and by African Caribbean patients as a test of religious faith or as a divine punishment[75]. These findings are supported by others who suggest that enduring pain is encouraged within African American where struggle and survival are considered noble[37].

Fig. 3.7.2 illustrates that health-related outcomes are not only contingent on access to services and available treatment but also on subtle yet critical social and cultural influences that are more challenging to operationalize. The clinical implications of this are messy yet fascinating.

Comparative studies on pain thresholds across populations groups—identifying which group experiences more or less pain under given conditions—are potentially racist and without clear clinical value. However, what would be clinically relevant is individual patient assessment of pain levels. Like QOL measures, a range of cross culturally validated instruments for assessing pain can be employed at the bedside. Pain intensity scales and multi-dimensional tools have been translated into several languages; however, mere translation of standardized instruments into the language of a given patient may not ensure its efficacy for that patient's cultural group. The selection of a scale or tool should be based on the patient's literacy and ability to understand numerical ratings, images, or sensory, affective and evaluative descriptors used in numerical rating, visual analogue, or multi-dimensional scales.

Symptoms of anxiety, depression, and delirium, common in advanced and terminal stages of death, may be expressed and understood differently across various ethnic and cultural groups. Symptom formation can be influenced by sociopolitical factors in conjunction with biological and environmental variables. For example, paranoia expressed by persons from oppressed groups may actually represent a healthy, protective response. Other behaviours

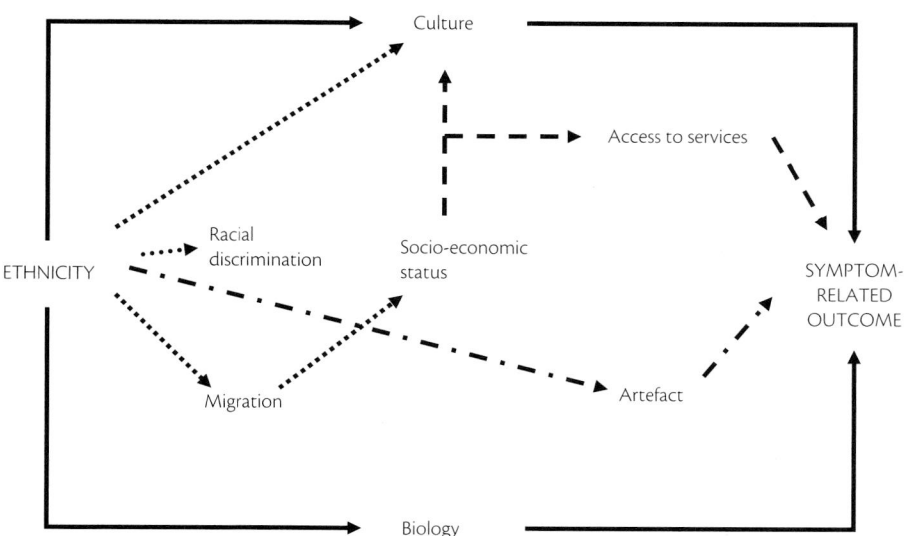

Figure 3.7.2 Possible mediation between ethnicity and the experience of symptoms associated with advanced disease.

considered normative within the psycho-spiritual belief systems of a given culture (e.g. spirit possession, visions of spirits or ghosts, etc.) may be considered delusional or otherwise pathological within a Western biomedical model. Conversely, certain culture-specific patterns of anxiety or distress that do not fit medical classifications (so-called culture bound syndromes) may be missed in evaluating the mental health of patients and their families.

Psychosocial and spiritual domains

Social support networks are crucial factors in the psychological well-being of the seriously ill and the dying patient. Within those networks, caregivers perform an essential role for both the patient and for the health delivery system. The emphasis on care in the community rather than institutions, and the growing awareness that in some comities, people would prefer to die at home given the choice[76] means that informal caregivers are indispensable partners of health- and social-care professionals. Many assume responsibilities of care that were previously confined to specialist inpatient settings and community hospitals[77]. Caring for family members is regarded as an important obligation in many ethnic communities[78]. Further, for many ethnic minority families, caring for dying relatives at home when possible is considered a matter of honour and integrity as well as a means of ensuring the death occurs in a holy place[79]. Karim *et al.* refer to the stigma and loss of face from not caring for close family relatives[80]. In the Hindu tradition, the concepts of karma and sacred duty may place the family of a loved one or dependant under additional stress in order to do the right thing[67]. Spruyt found that east London Bangladeshi children became actively involved in the care of dying patient and in interactions with professionals, and had to act as interpreters. This had a negative impact on them subsequently. A number of children were required to give up formal schooling and older sons gave up work to help with care of their dependants. When there is home care the burden often falls upon one person, but without ready access to outside support[79]. For example, in the UK, multi-generational Pakistani and Bangladeshi families who wish to provide traditional support may also be in situations with high unemployment and poverty, and large families of young children[81]. Home care is also not without problems when outside help is needed, because many ethnic minorities would regard this as a sense of failure in the eyes of the community, and it may also be regarded as an invasion of privacy[36]. Smaje and Field also point out the tensions which can arise when an elderly person needs and demands care from a female relative who may have quite different expectations, especially if the carer also has children born in the host country[82]. However, it is important to bear in mind that expectations of care from family relatives may change in coming years as patterns of family life and social networks evolve through a process of acculturation.

The experience of advanced disease can have a profound effect on patients and their family and friends. Indeed, during their illness many patients may raise questions that relate to their identity and self-worth as they seek to find the ultimate meaning in their life. Some patients attempt to answer these questions by examining their religious or spiritual beliefs. Formal religion is a means of expressing an underlying spirituality, but spiritual belief, concerned with the search for existential or the ultimate meaning in life, is a broader concept and may not always be expressed in a religious way.

Most of the published literature on role of religious faith at the end of life are descriptive and focus on 'factfile' approaches to manage the experience of death and dying across different faiths[83–85]. As discussed earlier, this approach is not without criticism as it has a tendency to over-categorize religious and cultural groups[4]. The lack of serious study of the religious and spiritual needs of ethnic minority communities may be partly due to an assumption that faith communities will provide their own religious and spiritual care. Anecdotal evidence from specialist palliative care nurses suggests that it is often assumed that ethnic minority patients have no spiritual problems because 'they have their own beliefs and rituals'—and once again, 'they look after their own'[36]. While some models of palliative and supportive care have not included mention of the role of spiritual care at the end of life others have begun to acknowledge the important role of spirituality[86]. Dein and Stygall suggest the lack of interest by health-care professionals in patients' religious concerns may be due to the discomfort created by the discussion of personal matters, that they associate religion with 'superstition, intolerance, and persecution, or that religion may be seen as a kind of consolation, a last resort, which is offered when all else fails'[87].

Conclusions

The palliative care movement has assumed a leading role in addressing the health and social care needs of patients and families facing the inevitability of death. It has only been recently that attention has focused on the importance of providing care to particular groups within increasingly diverse societies, including in the USA, UK, Australia, and New Zealand. This has now become a demographic imperative. This chapter has shown that the language of understanding difference is complex yet fascinating. When considering its influence in the provision of care at the end of life and during bereavement, perhaps we should hold a double lens: one that applies a framework of equity to understand and serve population needs of specific communities; and another that never loses sight of the individuals and families before us—those with clinical, psychosocial, and spiritual needs and concerns that may not conform to preconceived or stereotyped patterns. And always we should be mindful that an individualized approach to palliative care with a focus on quality is paramount for any patient, regardless of their ethnic or cultural background.

Further reading

Engle, V.F., Fox-Hill, E., Graney, M.J. (1998). The experience of living-dying in a nursing home: self-reports of black and white older adults. *J Am Geriatr Soc.* **46**(9), 1091–6.

References

1. Parens, E. (1998). What differences make a difference? *Cambridge Quarterly of Health Care Ethics*, **7**(1), 1–6.
2. Kroeber, A.L. and Kluckholn, C. (1952). *A critical review of concepts and definitions.* Vol **47**, The Peabody Museum of Archaeology and Ethnology, Harvard University, Cambridge, MA.
3. Donovan, J. (1986). *We don't buy sickness, it just comes.* Gower, Aldershot.
4. Gunaratnam, Y. (2003). Culture is not enough. In *Death, gender and ethnicity* (eds. Field, D., Hockey, J., and Small, N.), 1st edition, p. 166–86. Routledge, London.

5. Bhabha, H.K. (1988). The commitment to theory. *New Formations*, **5**, 5–23.

6. Tervalon, M. and Murray-Garcia, J. (1998). Cultural humility versus cultural competence: a critical distinction in defining physician training outcomes in multicultural education. *Journal of Health Care for Poor Underserved*, **9**(2), 117–25.

7. Koffman, J. (2006). The language of diversity: controversies relevant to palliative care research. *European Journal of Palliative Care*, **11**(1), 18–21.

8. Collins (2001). *Collins concise dictionary*. HarperCollins Publishers, Glasgow.

9. Gould, S.J. (1981). *The mismeasure of man*. Penguin, Harmondsworth.

10. Stepan, N. (1982). *The idea of race in science*. MacMillan Press, London.

11. Singh, S.P. (1997). Ethnicity in psychiatric epidemiology: need for precision. *British Journal of Psychiatry*, **171**, 305–8.

12. Ahmad, W.I.U. (1993). *"Race" and health in contemporary Britain*, Open University Press, London.

13. Karlesen, S. and Nazroo, J.Y. (2002). Relation between discrimination, social class and health among ethnic minority groups. *American Journal of Public Health*, **92**(4), 624–31.

14. Afshari, R. and Bhopal, R.S. (2002). Changing pattern of the use of 'ethnicity' and 'race' in scientific literature. *International Journal of Epidemiology*, **31**, 1074–6.

15. Chaturvedi, N. (2001). Ethnicity as an epidemiological determinant—crude racist or crucially important? *International Journal of Epidemiology*, **30**, 925–7.

16. Crawley, L.M. (2005). Racial, cultural, and ethnic factors influencing end-of-life care. *Journal of Palliative Medicine*, **8**(1), ss58–ss69.

17. Senior, A. and Bhopal, R. (1994). Ethnicity as a variable in epidemiological research. *BMJ*, **309**, 327–30.

18. Karlsen, S. and Nazroo, J.Y. (2002). Agency and structure: the impact of ethnic identity and racism on the health of ethnic minority people. *Sociology of Health and Illness*, **24**(1), 1–20.

19. Hillier, S. and Kelleher, D. (1996). Considering culture, ethnicity and the politics of health. In *Researching cultural differences in health,* (eds. Hillier, S., and Kelleher, D.) Routledge, London.

20. Gunaratnam, Y. (2003). Researching 'race' and ethnicity: methods, knowledge and power. Sage, London.

21. Office of National Statistics. (2003). *Ethnic group statistics: A guide for the collection and classification of ethnicity data*. Newport, Her Majesty's Stationery Office.

22. Federal Register Notice. (2004). Revisions to the Standards for the Classification of Federal Data on Race and Ethnicity.

23. Lehohla, P. (2003). *Census 2001: Census in brief*. Statistics South Africa, Pretoria.

24. Statistics Canada. 2001 Census Dictionary: Visible Minorities. Statistics Canada.

25. Bhopal, R. (1995). *Ethnicity, race, health and research: racist, black box, junk or enlightened epidemiology?* Department of Epidemiology and Public Health, University of Newcastle.

26. Pringle, M. and Rothera, I. (1995). *Ethnic group data collection in primary care: problems and solutions*. University of Nottingham Medical School, Nottingham.

27. Centeno C., Clark D., and Lynch T. *et al.* (2007). Facts and indicators on palliative care development in 52 countries of the WHO European region: results of an EAPC task force. *Palliative Medicine*, **21**, 463–71.

28. Clark, D. (2006). *Palliative Care Service Provision: Reimbursement and Funding for Services in Mexico*. http://www.eolc-observatory.net/global_analysis/mexico_reimburse.htm. Accessed October, 2008.

29. Crawley, L.M. and Chaudhary, S. (2006). *The state of the knowledge of the impact of racial, cultural, and ethnic factors on quality of end-of-life care in California: immigrant issues at the end of life*. California Healthcare Foundation, Oakland, CA.

30. Gavagan, T. and Brodyaga, L. (1998). Medical care for immigrants and refugees. *American Family Physician*, **57**(5), 1061–8.

31. Gavagan, T. and Martinez, A. (1997). Presentation of recent torture survivors to a family practice center. *Journal of Family Practice*, **44**(2), 209–12.

32. Palloni, A. and Arias, E. (2004). Paradox lost: explaining the Hispanic adult mortality advantage. *Demography*, **41**(3), 385–415.

33. Crawley, L.M., Kagawa-Singer, M. *et al.* (2007). *Racial, cultural, and ethnic factors on quality of end-of-life care in California: findings and recommendations*. California Healthcare Foundation, Oakland, CA.

34. Macklin, R. (1998). Ethical relativism in a multicultural society. *Kennedy Institute Ethics Journal*, **8**(1), 1–22.

35. Al-Jeilani, M. (1987). Pain: points of view of Islamic theology. *Acta Neurochir Suppl*, **38**, 132–5.

36. Firth, S. (2001). *Wider horizons: Care of the dying in a multi-cultural society*. National Council for Hospices and Specialist Palliative Care Services, London.

37. Crawley, L., Payne, R., Bolden, J. *et al.* (2000). Palliative and end-of-life care in the African American community. *JAMA*, **284**, 2518–21.

38. Karim, K., Bailey, M., Tunna, K. *et al.* (2000). Nonwhite ethnicity and the provision of specialist palliative care services: factors affecting doctors' referral patterns. *Palliative Medicine*, **14**(6), 471–8.

39. Koffman, J. and Higginson, I.J. (2001). Accounts of carers' satisfaction with health care at the end of life: a comparison of first generation black Caribbeans and white patients with advanced disease. *Palliative Medicine*, **15**(4), 337–45.

40. Oliviere, D. (1999). Culture and ethnicity. *European Journal for Palliative Care*, **6**, 53–6.

41. Berthoud, R. and Modood, T. (1997). Ethnic minorities in Britain: diversity and disadvantage. In *The Fourth National Survey of Ethnic Minorities*, (ed. R.Berthoud). p. 159–60, Policy Studies Institute, London.

42. Farrell, J. (2000). *Do disadvantaged and minority ethnic groups receive adequate access to palliative care services?* Glasgow University, United Kingdom.

43. Gibson, R. (2001). Palliative care for the poor and disenfranchised: a view from the Robert Wood Johnson Foundation. *Journal of the Royal Society of Medicine*, **94**, 486–9.

44. Harding, S. and Maxwell, R. (1997). Difference in mortality of migrants. In *Health Inequalities:* (eds. Drever, F., Whitehead, M.). *Decennial supplement Series DS no.15*, The Stationery Office, London.

45. Department of Health (1998). *Inequalities in Health: Report of an Independent Inquiry Chaired by Sir Donald Acheson*. The Stationery Office, London.

46. Koffman, J., Higginson, I.J., and Donaldson, N. (2003). Symptom severity in advanced cancer, assessed in two ethnic groups by interviews with bereaved family members and friends. *Journal of the Royal Society of Medicine*, **96**(1), 10–6.

47. Koffman, J., Donaldson, N., Hotopf, M. *et al.* (2005). Does ethnicity matter? Bereavement outcomes in two ethnic groups living in the United Kingdom. *Palliative and Supportive Care*, **3,** 183–90.

48. Smedley, B.D., Stith, A.Y., and Nelson, A.R. (2003). *Unequal treatment: confronting racial and ethnic disparities in healthcare*, National Academies Press, Washington, DC.

49. Casas-Zamora, J.A. and Ibrahim, S.A. (2004). Confronting health inequity: the global dimension. *American Journal of Public Health*, **94**(12), 2055–8.

50. Paradies, Y. (2006). A systematic review of empirical research on self-reported racism and health. *International Journal of Epidemiology*, **35**(4), 888–901.

51. Mooney, G. (2003). Inequity in Australian health care: how do we progress from here? *Australian and New Zealand Journal of Public Health*, **27**(3), 267–70.

52. Dostoyevsky, F. (2003). *Notes from the underground*. Everyman's Library, New York.

53. O'Neill, J., and Marconi, K. (2001). Access to palliative care in the USA: why the emphasize vulnerable groups? *Journal of the Royal Society of Medicine*, **94**, 452–4.

54. Aspinall, P.J. (1999). Ethnic groups and Our healthier nation: whither the information base? *Journal of Public Health Medicine*, 21, 125–32.

55. Hill, D. and Penso, D. (1995). *Opening doors: Improving access to hospice and specialist palliative care services by members of the black and ethnis minority communities.* Occasional Paper 7, National Council for Hospice and Specialist Palliative Care Services, London.

56. Eve, A., Smith, A.M., and Tebbit, P. (1997). Hospice and palliative care in the UK 1994–5, including a summary of trends 1990-5. *Palliative Medicine*, 11(1), 31–43.

57. Skilbeck, J., Corner, J., Beech, N. *et al.* (2002). Clinical nurse specialists in palliative care. Part 1. A description of the Macmillan Nurse caseload. *Palliative Medicine*, 16(4), 285–96.

58. World Health Organization. WHO Quality of Life-BREF (WHOQOL-BREF). 2006. http://www.who.int/substance_abuse/research_tools/whoqolbref/en (accessed October 2008).

59. Murphy, B., Herrman, H., Hawthorne, G. *et al.* (2000). *Australian WHOQoL instruments: User's manual and interpretation guide.* Australian WHO QoL Field Study Centre, Melbourne.

60. Zborowski, M. (1952). Cultural components in response to pain. *Journal of Society Issues*, 8, 16–30.

61. Lasch, K.E. (2002). Culture and Pain. *Pain: Clinical Updates*, X(5).

62. Cintron, A. and Morrison, R.S. (2006). Pain and ethnicity in the United States: A systematic review. *Journal of Palliative Medicine*, 9(6), 1454–73.

63. Krause, I. (2005). The sinking heart, a Panjabi communication of distress. *Social Science and Medicine*, 29(4), 563–75.

64. Ahmed, T. (1998). The Asian experience. In *Assessing health needs in people from minority ethnic groups.* (eds. Salman, R. and Bahal, V.). Royal College of Physicians London.

65. Nazroo, J.Y. (1997). *Ethnicity and mental health.* Policy Studies Institute, London.

66. Yee, B.W.K. (1997). The social and cultural context of adaptive aging among Southeast Asian elders. In *The Cultural Context of Aging,* (ed. Sokolovsky, J.), pp. 293–303. Greenwood, New York.

67. Firth, S. (1997). *Dying, death and breavement in the British Hindu community.* Peeters, Leuven.

68. Todd, K.H., Deaton, C., D'Adamo, A.P. *et al.* (2000). Ethnicity and analgesic practice. *Annals of Emergency Medicine*, 35, 11–6.

69. Todd, K.H. (2001). Influence of ethnicity on emergency department pain management. *Emergency Medicine*, 13, 274–8.

70. Cleeland,C.S., Mendoza, T.R., Wang, X.S. *et al.* (2000). Assessing symptom distress in cancer patients: the M.D. Anderson Symptom Inventory. *Cancer*, 89(7), 1634–46.

71. Bernabei, R., Gambassi, G., Lapane, K. *et al.* (1998). Management of pain in elderly patients with cancer. SAGE Study Group. Systematic Assessment of Geriatric Drug Use via Epidemiology.[see comment] [erratum appears in *JAMA* 1999, 281(2)136]. *JAMA*, 279(23), 1877–82.

72. Fife, B. (1994). The conceptualization of meaning in illness. *Social Science and Medicine*, 38(2), 309–16.

73. Lipowski, Z.J. (1970). Physical illness, the individual and the cancer. It may, in fact, be counterproductive to channel coping processes. *Psychiatry in Medicine*, 1, 91–102.

74. Lipowski, Z.J. (1983). Psychosocial reaction to illness. *Canadian Medical Association Journal*, 128, 1069–73.

75. Koffman, J., Morgan, M., Edmonds, P., and Speck P & Higginson, I.J. (2008). Cultural meanings of pain: a qualitative study of Black Caribbean and White British patients with advanced cancer, *Palliative Medicine*, 22, 349–59.

76. Gomes, B., Higginson, I.J. (2006). Factors influencing death at home in terminally ill patients with cancer: systematic review. *British Medical Journal*, 332, 515–21.

77. Rhodes, P. and Shaw, S. (1999). Informal care and terminal illness. *Health and Social Care in the Community*, 7, 39–50.

78. Koffman, J. and Higginson, I.J. (2003). Fit to care? A comparison of informal caregivers of first-generation Black Caribbeans and White dependants with advanced progressive disease in the UK. *Health and Social Care in the Community*, 11(6), 528–36.

79. Spruyt, O. (1999). Community-based palliative care for Bangladeshi patients in east London: accounts of bereaved carers. *Palliative Medicine*, 13, 119–29.

80. Karim, K., Bailey, M., and Tunna, K. (2000). Non white ethnicity and the provision of specialist palliative care services: factors affecting doctors referral patterns. *Palliative Medicine*, 14, 471–8.

81. Blakemore, K. (2000). Health and social care needs in minority communities: an over problemitized issue? *Health and Social Care in the Community*, 8(1), 22–30.

82. Smaje, C. and Field, D. (1997). Absent minorities? Ethnicity and the use of palliative care services. In *Death, gender and ethnicity*. (eds. Hockey, J., and Small, N.), pp. 142–65. Routledge, London.

83. Katz, J.S. (2001). Jewish perspectives on death, dying and bereavement. In *Death, dying and bereavement.* (eds. Dickerson, D., and Johnson, M.). 39th edition, p. 207. Sage Publications, London.

84. Koffman, J. (2001). Rituals surrounding death and dying within the black Caribbean community. *Palliative Care Today*, 10, 7.

85. Neuberger, J. (1994). *Caring for dying people in different faiths.* Mosby, London.

86. Ellershaw, J., Smith, C., Overhill, S. *et al.* (2001). Care of the dying: setting standards for symptom control in the last 48 hours of life. *Journal of Pain and Symptom Management*, 21, 12–7.

87. Dein, S. and Stygal, J. (1997). Religion. Coping with chronic illness: palliative medicine. *Palliative Care*, 11(4), 291–98.

88. Higginson, I.J., Astin, P., and Dolan, S. (1999). Do social factors affect place of death? Analysis of 10 years data in England. *Journal of Public Health Medicine*, 21, 22–8.

89. Higginson, I.J., Astin, P., and Dolan, S. (1998). Where do cancer patients die? Ten-year trends in the place of death of cancer patients in England. *Palliative Medicine*, 12, 353–63.

90. Koffman, J., Burke, G., Dias, A. *et al.* (2007). Demographic factors and knowledge of palliative care and related services. *Palliative Medicine*, 21, 145–53.

91. Harron-Iqbal, H., Field, D., Parker, H. *et al.* (1995). Palliative care services in Leicester. *International Journal of Palliative Nursing*, 1, 114–116.

92. Kurent, J.E. (2003). Case presentation: medical decision-making in hopeless situations: the long-lost son.[see comment]. *Journal of Pain and Symptom Management,* 25(2), 191–2.

93. Lindsay, J., Jagger, C., Hibbert, M. *et al.* (1997). Knowledge, uptake and the availability of health and social services among Asian Gujarati and white persons. *Ethnicity and Health*, 2, 59–69.

94. Caralis, P.V., Davis, B., Wright, K. *et al.* The influence of ethnicty and race on attitudes toward advanced directives, life-prolonging treatments, and euthanasia. *Journal of Clinical Ethics*, 4, 155–65.

3.8

The economic challenges of palliative medicine

Thomas J. Smith and J. Brian Cassel

Introduction: the reasons to do palliative care

Palliative care has grown dramatically as a specialty. More than 60 per cent of US hospitals with over 100 beds have palliative care programs (www.capc.org)[1,2], and in UK, the national cancer plan has endorsed full palliative care as part of every cancer network. Palliative care has been endorsed by the National Institute for Health and Clinical Excellence (NICE), and 65 per cent of hospitals had palliative care programmes by 2000[3]. In the USA, the National Cancer Institute (NCI) has mandated some form of palliative care at all NCI-designated centres. The documented reasons for growth in palliative care have been to provide better symptom management, allow better advanced care planning and medically appropriate goal setting, and continue transitions to hospice care[4].

In 2003–2204, researchers suggested that dramatic cost savings could be ascribed to palliative care of hospitalized inpatients, with up to 60 per cent savings in per day costs compared with usual care[5,6,7]. As shown in Fig. 3.8.1, costs fell by more than half after palliative care consultation, and reimbursement was higher than costs for patients who died in the hospital or who were discharged. The *Wall Street Journal* reported on the front page that there was a new and 'Unlikely way to cut hospital costs: comfort the dying'[8] and a different audience was introduced to palliative care. Prior to that article, visitors to the six Palliative Care Leadership Centres (http://www.capc.org/palliative-care-leadership-initiative) were usually clinicians who could not interest their chief executive officers (CEOs) in palliative care; overnight, CEOs were sending cobbled-together groups of clinicians and financial data analysts to 'go learn how to save money with palliative care'. Administrators and politicians hoped to save money by moving people to hospice care earlier, thus foregoing expensive treatments in the last year of life[9].

Of all the imperatives and outcomes for palliative care, one would hope that humanitarian, moral, ethical, and clinical imperatives would be more important than costs and reimbursement. In the modern world, however, financial solutions are crucial for the success of palliative care regardless of the country, system of health care, institutional values, and personal commitments of those involved.

Health economists have a different perspective than health-care professionals 'in the trenches'. Palliative care is just one more use of limited societal resources and does not get any preferential treatment for its social good, unless that good can be quantified. One applies the same criteria to palliative care as to a new cardiac imaging suite. Quality data are highly prized, but unlike biomedicine, health-care finances usually cannot be measured in terms of confidence intervals and p-values, and business decisions cannot be made on the basis of experiments with patients randomly assigned to treatment conditions. Most internal assessments of program successes are not documented and failures are rarely published. For these reasons, much of the existing data relevant to the financial outcomes of palliative care, especially concerning the potential for cost avoidance, ranges from anecdotal to correlational; most is based on non-scientifically designed data analyses.

In this chapter, we will define the various types of cost and clinical studies, the available data about the economic challenges of palliative care, how to apply the available data, how to collect and present some useful and useable data, and new directions for research. We have summarized the key learning points in Table 3.8.1.

Types of cost studies and how they are used in decision making

Although sometimes it is possible to make decisions about medical care just based on 'what works', the dramatically increasing costs associated with health care force the question today: 'does it work at a cost society can afford?'[10,11]. While most palliative medicines that cost $3500 per dose are in cancer treatment[12], there are now similarly expensive palliative drugs for macular degeneration, dementia, pain and arthritis, and expensive devices for congestive heart failure. In the past 40 years, the USA has progressed from spending 6 per cent of the gross national product on health care and education, to 16 per cent for health care alone in 2006, which is projected to top 20 per cent in 2015 (*New York Times*, 2006); education spending has stabilized at 7.5 per cent with no projected increase (http://www.oecd.org/dataoecd/51/20/37392850.pdf.). This shift is likely not in the long-term public good and health-care costs must stabilize[13]. The traditional ways of balancing cost and health outcomes are reviewed briefly in Table 3.8.2.

Clinical outcomes alone

When a drug is much better than any other treatment, for instance, imatinab mesylate (Gleevec™) in the treatment of chronic

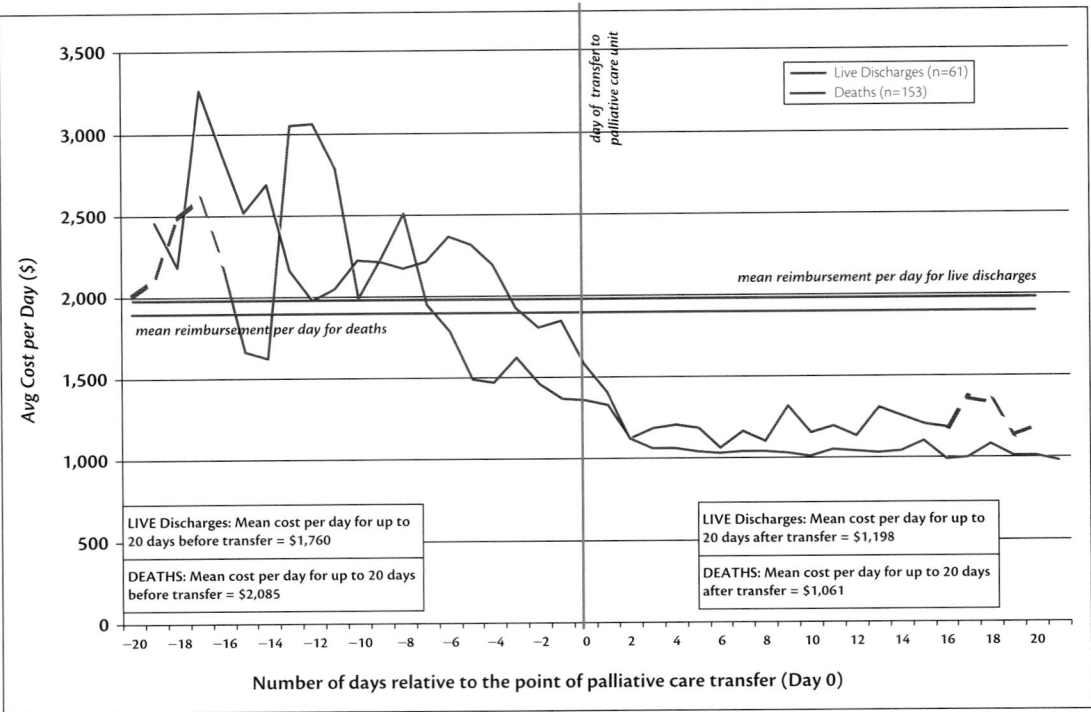

Figure 3.8.1   Representative total cost/day for patients before and after palliative care consultation, for patients who died in the hospital (deaths) or were discharged. The vertical line is the day of transfer. The horizontal line is the average reimbursement/day; after transfer, the reimbursement is higher than the cost so the patient makes a profit for the health system. Data Source: VCU Health System, Richmond, Virginia.

myelogenous leukaemia, medical care decisions are clear cut. The improvement in clinical symptoms, disease response, and survival of this revolutionary drug has made it the product of choice. The only real question is how to pay for it when resources are limited, as the cost for 30 tablets is approximately $2910, or $35 000 per year.

Cost alone

Very few, if any, new drugs cost less than the treatment they replace. Knowing that a drug or treatment is inexpensive does not help decision makers without some indication that a treatment actually works. For example, generic drugs without proof of equivalent efficacy would cost less but have some risk.

Table 3.8.1   Key learning points about palliative care finances

The imperatives for palliative care include financial issues, but the main goal is better patient care
The evidence for cost savings or cost avoidance in hospice is mixed
The evidence for cost savings and cost avoidance in acute palliative care is stronger, particularly in integrated health systems such as a national health insurance or a larger hospital
The economic outcomes of palliative care programmes include cost savings, profit, best use of scarce resources such as the operating room, good will, and are not limited to cost avoidance
Data that illustrate good care and positive financial impact on the institution are relatively simple to collect

Cost-minimization

The simplest way to combine clinical effectiveness with cost is cost-minimization. Two equally effective strategies are compared, and the one that has the least total cost is preferred. An example is drugs which are designed to simply replace expensive drugs with equivalent ones. In palliative care, Bruera and colleagues showed that methadone was equal to sustained release morphine in the relief of pain[14]; the choice should depend on which minimizes cost.

This approach is not without flaws. The initial drug cost may only be part of the picture; a less expensive drug that causes expensive complications such as hospitalizations for late recurrences may result in total higher disease management costs. There may not be comparative clinical data and assumptions must be made about equal efficacy. Comparative studies of drugs are rarely done, because most controlled trials are funded by industry and companies perceive themselves to be in a 'prisoner's dilemma': neither is willing to risk their own market share by being shown to be inferior, even though the gains associated with being a 'winner' could be much larger[15]. For instance, the second commercially available antibody to the epidermal growth factor receptor, panitunimab, was released at a price 20 per cent less than its competitor, cetuximab. While most experts in the field expect that the two drugs would have equal palliative efficacy against colon cancer, they have never been directly compared. In this case, the manufacturer is betting that most oncologists and payers will perform an informal cost-minimization analysis and choose the least costly drug.

Table 3.8.2 Types of studies and application to palliative care.

Type of study	Advantages and disadvantages	Application to palliative care
Clinical outcomes alone	Easy to perform. Ignores costs.	Traditional way to make decisions, e.g. imitinab mesylate (Gleevec™) works for chronic myelogenous leukemia CML. Find a way to pay for it.
Cost alone	Ignores clinical outcomes.	Rarely used to make decisions, unless the medical outcomes are similar (cost-minimization, below).
Costs and clinical outcomes together		
Cost-minimization: assumes two strategies are equal; lowest cost strategy is preferred.	Easy to do if there are direct comparisons.	For instance, if methadone gives equivalent pain relief to sustained release morphine, then use the least expensive option.
Cost-effectiveness: compares two strategies; assigns $ per additional year of life (LY) saved by strategy.	Requires a trial that directly compares strategies, and economic analysis alongside that trial. 'Only accept treatments that gain a year of life for under $100 000/life year.'	Palliative care usually adds no additional life years, so rarely applicable. May be most appropriate in chemotherapy or other interventions that prolong life.
Cost-utility: assigns $ per additional year of life (LY) saved by strategy, then estimates the quality of that benefit in $/quality adjusted (QALY).	Compares two strategies, with their quality of life comparisons converted to Utility, or the value placed on time in a health state, e.g. time spent on chemotherapy = 0.7 compared with a healthy individual whose Utility = 1.0	There are few interventions that make a large difference in utility. Also, there is rarely one simple yardstick of Utility that covers all health states.
Cost-benefit: compares two strategies but converts the clinical benefits to money, e.g. a year of life is worth $100 000.	Possible but rarely done due to difficulty in assigning $ value to human life.	Would almost certainly be unfavourable to most palliative interventions, as patients rarely work or generate income.
Special considerations		
Cost avoidance: measure the costs saved by not doing procedures, or by moving from an expensive place of care to a less expensive place.	Can be easy to calculate (moving from ICU bed to regular or hospice bed) or difficult (avoided CAT scans, for which there is no financial record)	Hospital-based programmes routinely show cost savings to the health system. Important to know who is avoiding the cost and who may be absorbing the cost. For instance, if palliative care transfers sick patients to hospice, it will save the hospital money but cost the hospice money[42].
Opportunity cost: the cost of performing one action rather than another. For instance, the opportunity cost of a patient staying in the ICU when appropriate for palliative care end of life is the high cost of that day plus the lost revenue of the ICU day plus the lost opportunity if a potential patient did not get appropriate trauma or ICU care.	Harder to calculate	Familiar concept to most CEOs. They may quickly realize that gaining 200 ICU bed days a year by transferring appropriate patients 1 day sooner would generate $1100/day×200 days, and prevent the hospital from being on ER diversion.

Cost-effectiveness

This method compares two known strategies in both effectiveness (for example, years of additional life gained) and cost, then assigns a cost per additional year of life (LY) saved by the best (dominant) strategy. For instance, adjuvant chemotherapy for a 45-year-old woman with early stage breast cancer would be expensive, but would add 5.1 months of additional life at a cost of about $15 000 per year[16]. Expensive therapies can be 'cost effective' too if they provide substantial benefit. For instance, trastuzamab (Herceptin™) for adjuvant treatment of breast cancer patients is expensive (over $50 000 in all countries), but the 50 per cent relative reduction in recurrence risk and 1.5 additional years for the average woman makes the cost effectiveness ratio of $14 000/LY to $40 000 acceptable[17].

There are several assumptions about this method that make it difficult to apply in the real world. First, it implies a limit to resources, such that there must be some 'cap' on the cost-effectiveness ratio.

The World Health Organization has defined 'reasonable' cost-effectiveness as interventions with a cost-effectiveness ratio that is less than the per capita gross domestic product (GDP)[18,19]. Second, it assumes that a single week of added life for 52 persons equals one full year of life for another person. Third, it assumes that all people are somehow in the same health system and share a single set of values. Fourth, it requires someone to fund these difficult studies to generate cost-effectiveness data when patients are only interested in cure, doctors are only interested in benefit, and drug companies are interested in profit, not social justice.

Palliative care brings an additional challenge in that very few palliative treatments make people live longer, with the exception of palliative chemotherapy, and therefore, additional life-years are not saved. A single study of real versus sham splanchnic nerve block appeared to show that pancreas cancer patients with pain lived longer with pain relief[20], but a more and recent better designed trial showed no difference in survival[21]. A single study of comprehensive medical management for refractory cancer pain patients versus comprehensive medical management plus an implantable intraspinal drug delivery system showed improved survival of about 2 months, at a reasonable cost effectiveness, but the *p*-value was only 0.06[22]. A randomized trial of usual oncology care versus usual oncology care plus concurrent hospice care showed a small improvement in survival, but it was not significantly different [23]. Other reports about improved pain control, or about better survival with hospice [24] or palliative care, have significant methodological problems in identifying appropriate controls.

Cost-utility adds adjustments for quality of life

In cost-utility analysis, the quality of life in a given state of disease or treatment (health state), is converted to a Utility ratio, where 1 equals perfect health and 0 equals death. For example, a patient whose pain has been relieved may have a Utility range of 0.90 of 1.00, whereas a patient with continued pain may have a utility range of 0.50. The Utility ratio converts 'cost-effectiveness' into cost per quality adjusted life year (QALY). For example, an intervention that costs $100 000 per year of life gained would be converted to $50 000 per quality adjusted life year if the treatment doubled the patient's utility score from 0.5 to 1.0. This intervention, however welcomed, would not save money but would cost an additional $50 000 to save an additional QALY with the intervention.

There are several difficulties with the cost-utility method. One is assigning proper utility ratios to the various health states. Controversy exists as to the most appropriate source of values: patients, health-care workers, or the general population (society) due to differences in perspective. Patients and clinicians place greater emphasis on the issues (such as life, morbidity, expense) that matter most to them. For example, patients are more likely than clinicians to accept toxic treatments in exchange for minor clinical benefits, and a 1 per cent chance of cure or 10 per cent chance of symptom relief may be sufficient for them to choose treatment over supportive care[25]. The most objective source is probably lay people (jurors) whose money is being used[26,27]; the difficulty lies in properly educating them in all aspects of a patient's experience, e.g. emotional turmoil, treatment toxicity, inconvenience, and other physical and psychosocial stressors.

A second problem is the magnitude of palliative care interventions, which is usually not enough to change overall (global) quality of life or utility values. For instance, intraspinal pain management compared with conventional medical management improved pain scores by 50 per cent and lowered drug toxicity by 52 per cent, but had minimal impact on global quality of life or caregiver quality of life[28]. Despite dramatic improvements in pain, there were so many other issues that quality of life, and subsequent calculated utility scores[29], did not improve by a detectable amount. Megestrol acetate helped appetite[30], but did not have enough impact on global quality of life scores to change utility values. We have been unable to find a palliative care intervention with enough impact on global quality of life to substantially change utility scores.

Several recent cost-effectiveness or cost-utility studies have produced results that will be of use to decision makers. Abernethy *et al.* used a spreadsheet-based model to compare the cost-effectiveness of three strategies for treating cancer pain: guideline-based care, oncology consultation-based care, and usual care. Treatment strategies included medications and procedure-based interventions.

The effectiveness unit used was 'additional patient relieved of cancer pain', rather than the typical additional year of life gained. Guideline-based care (GBC) was more effective at relieving cancer pain compared with oncology-based care (OBC) or usual care (UC): 80 per cent versus 55 per cent and 30 per cent, respectively. The incremental cost-effectiveness for GBC compared with OBC was $452 per additional patient relieved of cancer pain, while the cost-effectiveness of OBC compared with UC was $601 per additional patient relieved of cancer pain[31]. Single fraction radiation for painful bone metastases, instead of the usual six treatments, was as effective and cost substantially less[32]. Shorter fraction regimens for palliative treatment of lung cancer, 2×8-Gy versus 3×10-Gy, showed the opposite effect; the cost-utility ratio for the 3×10-Gy schedule versus the 2×8-Gy schedule was acceptable at $40 900/QALY. The longer regimen had an acceptable cost effectiveness ratio because people lived longer with the 3×10-Gy treatment, offsetting the higher treatment cost[33]. In other situations, the high cost of the intervention prevents it from having a cost effectiveness ratio within accepted bounds. Respite day care for frail elders was not consistently better than usual care, because it had minimal measurable impact and was at least as costly[34]. In the palliative treatment of dementia with donepezil, rivastigmine, memantine, and galantamine, the estimated cost-effectiveness (£8–68 000/QALY) was above that generally considered acceptable by NHS policy makers, as the cost savings associated with reducing the mean time spent in full-time care do not offset the cost of treatment[35].

Cost-benefit

This method compares two interventions then assigns a monetary value to the added clinical benefit of the best strategy, based on the overall economic productivity of an individual. Therefore, a treatment that costs $50 000 to prolong life by 1 year would be acceptable if the person could produce $50 000 of economic worth in that year, but not if the person only produced $10 000 that year. This kind of analysis, while useful in business decisions, is rarely used in clinical studies because of the difficulties in assigning a monetary value to a human life, especially if that value is tied to an individual's socioeconomic status. As palliative care patients rarely produce income, even if their symptoms are well-controlled, palliative care interventions would be at a distinct disadvantage.

Cost avoidance

This relatively new concept has been widely used as an economic argument for palliative care. If a patient can be moved from a $3500/day intensive care unit bed to a $1000/day palliative care bed, with equal or better care that meets the patient's goals, a $2500 cost will have been avoided each day for each patient. Taken in aggregate, these costs can be substantial and more than offset palliative care programme costs. For instance, palliative care programmes have reported only a small profit, but annual savings of over US $1 million due to cost-avoidance[1,5,8]. Similarly, not doing 50 CAT scans each year by careful matching of the goals of care with the diagnostic tests[1] could save up to $2500×50 = $125 000. In a cost-based system such as national health insurance or diagnosis-related group (DRG) payment system, this would be a desired outcome;

---

1   Bodurtha's Rule of Diagnostic Testing: doing a diagnostic test is liking picking one's nose in public. Before doing, ask what one with will do with the results if one finds something. Dr Joann Bodurtha, Richmond, Virginia.

however, in a profit-based system this could represent substantial lost profit.

Cost avoidance is relatively easy to measure from usual databases if there are comparable patients to match before the intervention, because billing systems record what was actually done. A simple historical analysis would show that more patients receive comfort care once a palliative care programme is established than under standard care. Sometimes the simplest way to collect data about cost savings is a notebook of 'avoided tests' after palliative care consult, e.g. for the first 50 palliative care consult patients, 50 planned CATs or similar procedures were cancelled. A within-patient analysis (e.g. Fig. 3.8.1) shows what happens to costs among palliative care patients displayed as a daily cost. A between-patient analysis comparing palliative care patients with non-palliative care patients shows that non-palliative care patients receive different care and have higher subsequent costs in their last days; in most cases, palliative care patients use about 60 per cent fewer resources and have about 50 per cent fewer costs [5,8]. The difference in the resources used and the subsequent costs is illustrated in Fig. 3.8.2 that compares palliative care unit patients who died in the hospital with similar patients who died other places in the hospital.

It is critically important to realize that all the above studies are retrospective correlational studies, not randomized clinical trials with an economic analysis. Whether the change in resources and costs is due to the palliative care consult by itself, or the underlying reasons for the palliative care consult (change in medical goals, change in family or patient perspective, and change in physician perspective) cannot be answered from the available data. As these studies have now been replicated in numerous settings, it seems unlikely that the reduction in resources and costs is unrelated to palliative care consultation; but one cannot ascribe all the change to the consultation itself.

Additional considerations

There are a few important other considerations in the economics of palliative care. The first is *perspective*: whose money is being spent, and on whom? In general, health economists take the societal viewpoint; that is, society has limited resources and wants to spend it to gain the most health for the most people. This runs directly counter to the individual viewpoint that only one person's health—mine—matters. The societal impact would also take into account work and time lost, and all the additional costs of care that are absorbed by families. As studies often cannot take all these into account, a common compromise is to take the view of a health system, e.g. the National Health Service in the UK or Canada or a large insurer in the USA. As an example, a palliative care programme that accepts patients from the hospital will lower the hospital costs; if however, that palliative care programme transfers these patients to a hospice, and the patients continue to use more care (IVs, pain medicines, diagnostic tests) then the hospice budget will be stretched.

A second concern is *opportunity cost*, simply defined as the additional revenue that could be gained if money had been used in a different way. For instance, an intensive care bed that is filled with someone who is not getting better may force the hospital to refuse admission of medical or surgical patients who would provide more revenue if admitted into the occupied bed. In a natural experiment, Oregon Health Center found that every hour during which the hospitals Emergency Department refused patients due to lack of capacity cost the hospital system over $1100 in profit, the opportunity cost of patient diversion from the Emergency Department. Transferring patients from the intensive care unit (ICU) to a more appropriate venue may give cost avoidance of $2500/day, and open that bed for an additional patient[36]. The opportunity cost of filled ICU beds is a sound financial concept that is understandable to most CEOs; if a palliative care programme assists in the transfer of

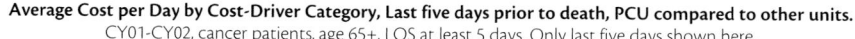

Average Cost per Day by Cost-Driver Category, Last five days prior to death, PCU compared to other units.
CY01-CY02, cancer patients, age 65+, LOS at least 5 days. Only last five days shown here.

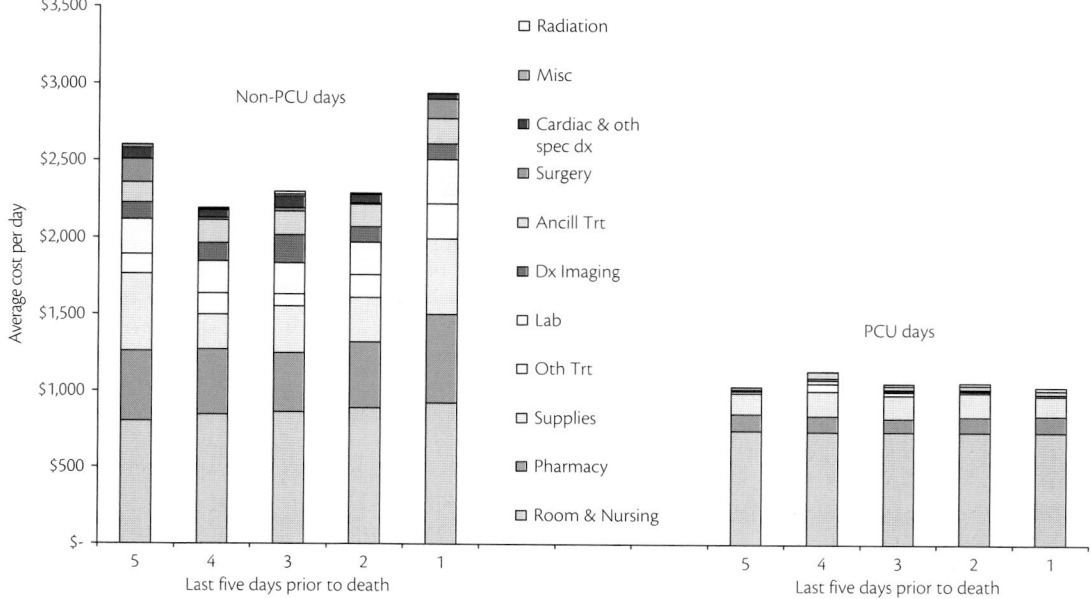

Figure 3.8.2 Changes in the types of costs and actual costs, PCU compared with other units, for patients who died in the hospital.

Table 3.8.3 Randomized trials of palliative care effectiveness with an impact on economics.

Study	Conclusions	Comments/conclusion
Raftery et al. 1994[43]	Randomized trial of care coordinator versus usual care for terminally ill patients.	No substantive difference in effectiveness. However, costs were 41 per cent lower in the coordinated care arm, due to fewer hospitalizations. Choose the least costly programme.
Grande et al. 1999[44]	Randomized trial of hospital at home palliative care versus usual care	No difference. Choose the least costly programme.
Jourdhoy et al. 2000[45]	Randomized trial of palliative care intervention and death at home.	No difference. Choose the least costly programme.
Finn et al. 2002[23]	Randomized oncology patients to standard care or standard care plus hospice/palliative care consultation. The intervention group had longer preserved quality of life, fewer symptoms, and non-significantly better survival. Although no difference was noted in symptom control (increasing symptoms over time), there was a significant reduction in the decrease of quality of life in the intervention group. The intervention cost over $1.5 million, or >$17 800 per each patient served, but was associated with cost savings of over $2500 per person by avoided hospitalizations. Final results are in process. (John Finn, personal communication, January 2004)	The only randomized controlled trial shows some improvement in symptoms, but no major difference in survival, at increased cost due to the high cost of interdisciplinary hospice services when used for palliative care.
Hanks 2002[38]	A randomized controlled trial in a 400 bed acute care hospital assessed a hospital Palliative Care Team (PCT) versus limited telephone advice ('telephone-PCT', the control group) in a teaching hospital. Highly significant improvements in symptoms, health-related quality of life, mood and 'emotional bother' in 'full-PCT' at 1 and 4 weeks; a smaller effect was seen in 'telephone-PCT'.; but, there were no significant differences between the groups when the baseline levels of symptoms were considered. There was no difference between the groups in LOS, readmission rates, or resource utilization.	Telephone consultation was just as effective as full palliative care consultation. With no impact on health care resource utilization, there will not be any impact on costs. The study should caution researchers that randomized trials sometimes do not confirm single institution trials.
Rabow et al.[39]	This randomized trial of a palliative care consult team versus usual care in the outpatient clinic showed minor effects on pain, anxiety, and insomnia. No significant effect was seen in the major clinical symptoms, resource utilization, or projected costs. Only about half the recommendations were followed.	The trial was underpowered to detect small but potentially meaningful differences in symptoms and resource utilization.

200 patients 2 days earlier, then the medical staff will have 400 more ICU bed days available.

The available clinical and economic data

The available data may be organized into studies of clinical effectiveness, cost, and both effectiveness and costs (Table 3.8.3).

Clinical effectiveness

The effectiveness data for palliative care and hospice care is mixed, with few randomized, controlled trials. Prior editions of this book noted the lack of substantive data and that prior randomized trials have shown small if any benefits[37]. The recent imPaCT study[38] showed no differences between a telephone-only palliative care consult strategy and a full palliative care consult team presence. A heartening fact was that palliative care was already fully integrated into the hospital culture so that the sickest patients were seen without randomization, and that care was good across the health system, perhaps as successful diffusion from prior palliative care consults. While alternative explanations exist, the main conclusion is that full palliative care was no better than the telephone version, or that the telephone version is sufficient. Rabow and colleagues randomized about 50 patients in the outpatient clinic to usual care versus usual care plus a palliative care consultation team and showed only minor effects; however, the study was underpowered to detect small but meaningful clinical differences[39].

The impact of hospice and palliative care on cost of care

In general, the impact of hospice on costs of care has been small. The original Medicare hospice benefit was developed with the intent to improve care, not to save money, but was required to be 'revenue neutral' (or, not cost Medicare any additional money). Some recent studies have shown that hospice does not save money when the whole terminal illness is considered. The impact of clinical symptoms has not been studied recently, but very few question that hospice provides the best available care for those at the end of life. In fact, even in the absence of randomized clinical trial data or economic data, all major US cancer organizations suggest that hospice is the most appropriate end-of-life care for dying cancer patients[40].

In contrast, data from hospital-based palliative care consult teams strongly suggest substantial cost savings when palliative care is involved. Smith et al. reported over 60 per cent cost savings when patients died under the care of the palliative care team, both in a cohort analysis matched to other patients who died in the hospital, and a pre-post analysis[5,8]. The same group subsequently reported substantial reductions in all symptoms measured, if present, within 48 h, thereby suggesting that the care was equal or better to usual care[41]. Elsayem and colleagues at M. D. Anderson Cancer Center reported good symptom control accompanied by dramatic decrease in costs[6]. Brumley et al. showed improved care outcomes, fewer

Table 3.8.4 Non-randomized trials of palliative care effectiveness with an impact on economics.

Study	Conclusions	Comments
Hospice		
Campbell et al.[46]	They carefully matched Medicare patients who did or did not use hospice, using regression analysis to discern the impact of hospice itself while adjusting for other confounding factors. 'Adjusted mean expenditures were 4.0 per cent higher overall among hospice enrolees than among non-enrolees. Adjusted mean expenditures were 1 per cent lower for hospice enrolees with cancer than for patients with cancer who did not use hospice. Savings were highest (7–17 per cent) among enrolees with lung cancer and other very aggressive types of cancer diagnosed in the last year of life. Expenditures for hospice enrolees without cancer were 11 per cent higher than for non-enrolees, ranging from 20 per cent to 44 per cent for patients with dementia and 0 per cent to 16 per cent for those with chronic heart failure or failure of most other organ systems.'	However, the economic conclusion is that hospice care in the USA saves money for young patients with cancer (by avoiding expensive treatments and complications) but does not save money overall, and for some patients costs more. This only captures direct medical care costs—what Medicare paid—so may miss important economic impacts on families. It also does not capture any impact on quality of life or bereavement.
Emanuel et al.[47]	The authors matched Medicare patients in Massachusetts and California who did or did not use hospice. 'During the last year of life, expenditures for all patients in a hospice were slightly more than expenditures for patients not in a hospice in Massachusetts, and only slightly less in California. Among patients with cancer, in the last year of life, expenditures were about 13 per cent lower for decedents receiving hospice care in Massachusetts and nearly 20 per cent lower in California.' Hospital costs were 40 per cent lower for cancer patients in hospice.	Both Emanuel et al and McCarthy [48] have reported markedly increased use of hospice by patients who are enrolled in Medicare Managed Care plans. Whether this is due to patient, physician, or health-plan characteristics is not known. Despite higher enrollment, the strategy does not save money for society.
Pyenson et al.[49]	They compared patients enrolled in the Medicare hospice benefit, or not, for 16 life ending conditions. For most conditions, mean and median cost was lower for patients who chose hospice but despite the large sample size cost saving was significant ($p < 0.05$) only for CHF, liver cancer and pancreatic cancer. Costs were higher for patients with prostate cancer, and significantly higher for patients with stroke. No summary results are given for the full impact on Medicare or society.	The impact of hospice on total care costs will be small. The impact on other important measures such as symptom control, quality of life, bereavement was not available from the data.
Passik et al.[42]	Studied the impact of palliative care on a well-established hospice. They compared direct with hospice patients with palliative care to hospice patients. The palliative care hospice patients were sicker, had shorter length of stay in hospice (median of 9 versus 17 days), pharmacy costs in the first 2 weeks of $230 versus $94/patient; higher ancillary costs ($413 versus 332/patient); and fewer designated gifts to the hospice (39 per cent versus 47 per cent) and none to the palliative care centre.	Perspective is key to understanding this study. From a societal and patient–family viewpoint, integrated care makes perfect sense. From a hospital viewpoint, palliative care will generate savings in cost avoidance and shorter length of stay. From the hospice viewpoint, sicker and more expensive patients transferred from hospice are a significant burden. Under the current financing system, this schema of care will not be financially viable. For integrated or national health systems, the costs and savings can be shared fully. The Hospice of Bluegrass saves between $1 and $2 million each year for the two hospitals in Lexington.
Palliative care programmes		
Brumley et al.[6]	At Kaiser Permanente health maintenance organization, 161 were enrolled in the palliative care programme and 139 in the comparison group. Palliative care patients had significantly fewer emergency department visits, hospital days, skilled nursing facility days, and physician visits and a 45 per cent decrease in costs as compared with usual care patients.	While not a randomized study, this well-designed study showed better clinical outcomes and lower costs by matching the resources needed to the goals of care. It has been adopted by many other Kaiser Permanente groups.
Elsayem et al.[7]	For patients at a comprehensive cancer centre referred to palliative care, there was severe distress on admission and significant improvement in symptoms. Average reimbursement rate for all palliative care charges was approximately 57 per cent, and the mean daily charges in the PCIS were 38 per cent lower than the mean daily charges for the rest of the hospital.	This was the first published demonstration of better symptom control and lower costs for patients at a tertiary comprehensive cancer centre.

(continued)

Table 3.8.4 (Continued) Non-randomized trials of palliative care effectiveness with an impact on economics.

Study	Conclusions	Comments
Cuny et al.[50]	The University Healthcare Consortium (UHC) did 40 chart reviews each from 35 member institutions, for a total of 1596 cases. For those 10 per cent of inpatients receiving palliative care, palliative care is correlated with higher quality and lower cost. The more palliative care benchmarks were reached, the lower the cost and length of stay. About one-half of the difference in cost can be accounted for by the shorter LOS, while the remainder was due either to lower intensity or less use of ancillary services.	
Guest[51,52]	The most striking finding is that opioids account for only up to 17 per cent of total cost of care, with hospitalization 71 per cent.	Economics should not interfere with pain relief since total costs are low. Only a third of all patients who received sustained release opioids also received 4-hourly morphine as part of their initial treatment[52].
Fassbender[53]	Alberta started a palliative care consult program with dispersed centers in 1993. Use of palliative care increased from 45 to 81 per cent of cancer patients 1993–2000. The costs of the programme were more than offset by the savings from fewer hospital days. The cost to society did not change, but shifted from acute care to home and community care beds.	In this fully integrated provincial health system total costs actually fell during this time period. The cost savings from avoided hospital days could be directly applied to the other needs of the health system.
Smith et al.[5]	For 237 patients during first 6 months, 52 per cent had cancer followed by vascular events, immunodeficiency, or organ failure. Daily charges and costs were reduced by 66 per cent overall and 74 per cent in 'other' (medications, diagnostics, etc.) after transfer to the PCU ($p < 0.0001$ for all). Comparing the 38 contemporary control patients who died outside the PCU to similar patients who died in the PCU, daily charges were 59 per cent lower (0.005), direct costs 56 per cent lower ($p = 0.004$), and total costs 57 per cent lower ($p = 0.009$).	This showed a 60 per cent reduction in the cost of patients who died with palliative care compared with those who did not. The reductions came from medically appropriate goal setting, and matching resource use to the goal of care.
Naik[8]	For cancer patients 65+year-old, who died in the hospital, after an admission of at least 5 days, PCU patients' pharmacy costs were $511 during those 5 days, compared with $2267 for non-PCU patients; lab costs were $56 versus $1134; and radiology was $29 versus $615. Supplies and other treatment costs showed similar differences. There was little difference in the room costs, as they were almost all in acute medical-surgical beds.	The total cost for cancer patients dying on the PCU was about one third of those who died outside the PCU. The reductions came from medically appropriate goal setting, and matching resource use to the goal of care.
Serra-Prat[54]	This comparative but not randomized study found that costs in the last month of life were lower in the patients who were co-managed by the palliative care team Programa d'Atenció Domiciliària i Equips de Suport (PADES). The PADES group had fewer hospitalizations (7/44 versus 79/111) and LOS of 8 days versus 12 days. The PADES group had 410 home visits. The average cost per patient was 101 700 versus 174 354 (standard care €437 or 71 per cent higher.)	The reductions came from medically appropriate goal setting, and matching resource use to the goal of care.
Cowan[55]	Evaluated and charges for the first 164 inpatient palliative care consultations performed by the Advanced Illness Assistance team at a community hospital. Mean daily charges were 414$ less than the charges for the 5 days prior to palliative care consultation ($p = 0.04$, t-test). There was a significant decrease in laboratory and imaging charges during AIA follow-up ($p = 0.04$, t-test). Comparable patients not seen by AIA had significantly greater mean daily charges. The estimated savings for AIA cost avoidance was >$1 801 930 dollars per year.	The reductions came from medically appropriate goal setting, and matching resource use to the goal of care.
Ireland Cancer Center and Hospice of Western Reserve[56]	Project Safe Conduct gave modified hospice consultations for all lung cancer patients starting treatment at this comprehensive cancer centre. After the programme 75 per cent died in hospice care compared with 13 per cent before, with a median length of stay in hospice of 36 days versus 10 before. At the completion of the project, The Safe Conduct Team (Advanced Practice Nurse, Social Worker and Spiritual Care Counsellor) became full time employees of the Ireland Cancer Center. The patient population has expanded to include advanced cancers specifically lung, GI (pancreatic, colon, rectal), and head and neck.	If the proof of value is in continuation, Project Safe Conduct has been sustained, is highly successful, and well received with demand for more 'Safe Conduct Teams' at the Ireland Cancer Centre. (Elizabeth Pitorak, personal communication, 2 February 2004)

hospitalizations and doctor visits, and a 45 per cent savings to the insurer[7] (Table 3.8.4).

How to use the available data

A key question before collecting data is to decide beforehand on its use. Are the data to be used in passing accreditation, improving market share, improving patient satisfaction, reducing health system costs, or increasing profits? Based on recent examples of visitors to our programme, organizations may have as a goal 'increasing intensive care bed capacity 10 per cent by increasing transfers to palliative care', 'make annual profit of $2 000 000 on home health care, home palliative care, and hospice', or 'save 25 per cent of hospital end-of-life care costs'. The goal will dictate what data to collect and how to present it.

In general, most palliative care programmes have not been asked to collect much data. In our experience, the clinicians are among the best in the health system, are inter-disciplinary by nature, and administrators assume that there will be good care. When administrators do ask for data, it is usually 'structure' (how many practitioners, office space and costs, etc.) or 'process' (how many patients were seen last year? What were the costs of the programme?) data. Increasingly, though, administrators are asking for more complex 'outcomes' data (what impact did the programme have on length of stay? What was the impact on pain scores after the programme was in operation for 1 year? Did the cost-avoidance of the programme offset the salaries and administrative costs?)

In collecting and presenting the data, the simplest approach is the most effective. Most administrators want to know that the program is successful, defined as providing good care, keeping busy, and not losing too much money.

How to collect and present useable data

To evaluate the global impact of a palliative care programme on a health system, the Center to Advance Palliative Care website tool, http://www.capc.org/impact_calculator_basic/, allows calculation of important metrics, such as length of stay and cost avoidance. For instance, in our 750-bed hospital with a 90 per cent occupancy rate, if palliative care saw 50 per cent of the eligible patients and reduced hospital length of stay by just 0.5 days, we could save over 3800 days and $2 500 000 annually (Fig. 3.8.2). This represents an important benchmark for projections and comparison to actual performance. While not all experts agree that palliative care reduces length of stay, this programme allows one to enter local projections based on shorter length of stay and lesser cost per day.

We counsel programmes to collect useful data that is being requested, and no more. Some common metrics are listed in Table 3.8.5. To collect more data than is actually used takes time, effort, and money that would be better spent doing clinical care or research.

Presentation of the data should be as simple as possible. We have found that a simple 'Improved care at no extra cost' approach, as shown in Table 3.8.6, is well received. Again, most administrators will not be expecting palliative care to make a large profit. The goal of this report is to fairly and accurately reflect the activity and impact of the program.

New directions

Better data are needed to reduce the uncertainty about the true impact of palliative care, both clinical and economical data. Ideally, patients would be randomized between usual care and palliative care, but such trials are incredibly difficult to perform. Meier and colleagues have begun a 5-year multi-centre trial that prospectively collects health and economic data on cancer patients admitted to the hospital (1R01CA116227-01A2: Palliative care for hospitalized cancer patients.) Patients who receive palliative care consults will be matched to those who do not receive consults based on their propensity scores for palliative care consultations. This trial should be sufficient to establish the impact of palliative care consultation in usual care.

More data are needed on the impact of palliative care programmes on the whole health system, not on individual silos. Traditionally, most business analyses in health care treat each department and programme as a financial silo that must produce sufficient revenues to cover the costs of its treatments. Palliative care programmes will have two populations of patients: the first comprises those admitted directly to the palliative care units or services, for whom a 'silo' analysis is appropriate. The second includes those transferred to palliative care from intensive upstream services such as Neuroscience, Oncology, and Cardiology, who have often been in the hospital for days. What cost differential does the palliative care programme achieve for each day these patients are under its care, rather than standard care? What would have happened with those patients had the palliative programme not existed? Because the goals and nature of the care on the palliative care unit are dramatically different than those elsewhere in the hospital, the costs are generally much lower. It costs less to care for those who are not responding to curative or life-extending care (e.g. in ICUs), undergo a clarification of the goals of care, and then subsequently receive care that focuses mostly or entirely on palliation, comfort and perhaps life closure. Such decisions may not be achievable in some patients and families.

The field would benefit from more research designs that assess inputs and outputs at a patient level or population level (rather than at an admission level), such as that employed by Brumley et al.[7]. Also, prospective and longitudinal studies are needed to determine at which point and for which patients palliative care is presented as an option and actually implemented. Multi-centre studies are needed that can assess whether consultative services have the same kind and degree of clinical and financial impact (for the same kinds of patients) as dedicated units. Studies are necessary to clarify whether other aspects of programme design are important, such as the degree of clinical control that the palliative care team has after their initial consultation. In all such studies, financial outcomes should be studied with as much rigor and interest as clinical effects. Another research approach that will become more important in the next 5–10 years is whether incentives and disincentives provided by payers (e.g. extra payments for better symptom management or for institutional cost savings) have an impact on the field of palliative care. These kinds of research designs are especially important as the maturing movement of palliative care begins to address care from diagnosis forward, and not just a few hours or days before death.

White fields are changeable. Grey fields are auto-generated.

INPUTS		RESULTS	
Average length of stay in your hospital (ALOS)	4.8 days	Total discharges per year	51,328
Average total cost per day (hospital-wide)	1600 dollars	Estimated deaths per year	1,283	2.5 % of annually discharged patients
Number of staffed beds	750 beds	Estimated number of potential palliative care patients	2,566	5 % of annually discharged patients
Average hospital occupancy rate (in %)	90	**Direct Costs	$960	60 Calculated as % of average total cost
Average Length-Of-Stay Savings Per Case	0.5 days	Estimated average cost savings per day on "impact days"	$384	40 Calculated as % of direct
Average Remaining Length-Of-Stay days per case after referral to palliative care (Impact Days)	3 days		

Assumed % of potential patients referred:	20	30	40	50
Estimated number of referred palliative care patients	513	770	1027	1283
**LOS Savings: (avg. total cost X number referred X avg LOS savings per case)	$410,400	$616,000	$821,600	$1,026,400
Total Impact Days: (avg. post ref. LOS days X number referred)	1,539 days	2,310 days	3,081 days	3,849 days
Cost Per Day Savings: (avg. cost savings during impact days X total impact days)	$384	$887,040	$1,183,104	$1,478,016
TOTAL SAVINGS: (LOS Savings + Cost Per Day Savings)	$410,784	$1,503,040	$2,004,704	$2,504,416

CLEAR VALUES

Figure 3.8.3 Impact calculator for new palliative care programmes. Adapted, with permission, from www.capc.org. Developed by Lynn Spragens, MBA, CPA. NOTES & DEFINITIONS:** Total Cost versus Direct Costs—The direct costs most accurately reflect real savings, as they vary the most with the number of patients and days. **LOS—'length-of-stay days saved', however, beds are in fact being made available for—and the associated overhead expenses can be borne by—new patients. Average Length of stay: National average is approximately 4.6–4.8 days. Average Total Cost per day: Range is usually $900–$1800, depending on costs and methodology. Staffed beds: Number of staffed beds is often less than the number of licensed beds.'; Occupancy Rate: 75 per cent and higher is 'pretty full' because key beds and services are full on certain days of the week. Average Length-Of-Stay Savings: This will be none on some, and a lot on others; determined by 'gaps' in current performance. Average Remaining Length-Of-Stay days: Note that an assumed estimate of 3 days is probably conservative, with an impact in the range of 3.6–5.7 days more likely (about 4.5 days on average). Total Discharges per Year: (Staffed beds×Occupancy rate×365 days)/ALOS. Estimated Deaths per Year: National average (assuming average patient mix) is 2.5–2.7 per cent of discharges. Annually Discharged Patients: Estimated Based on an estimated percentage of annual discharges. (1) Determining potential patients. 'Potential patients' are defined here as those who are likely to need palliative care and who could benefit from it. Based on experience, a suggested starting point for estimating the potential number of patients that might be helped by a mature palliative care programme is about 5 per cent of total discharges. One could vary this assumption, based on practice style, demographics, gaps in current performance, etc. Per cent Total Discharges per Year palliative Care: Note that actual percentage of discharges that could benefit from palliative care may be lower or higher. Estimated Palliative Care Patients: Based on an estimated percentage of annual discharges. Estimated Referred Patients: 'Potential patients' are defined here as those who are likely to need palliative care and who could benefit from it, about 5 per cent of total discharges. Calculated as Direct Costs: Assumed cost savings of about 40 per cent of average direct costs. Actual savings experienced may not only depend on program performance but also on how hospital allocates costs.

Table 3.8.5 Practical palliative care measures and how to collect them.

Measure	Data source	Units	Comment
Clinical			
Pain scores	Symptom assessment scale	Visual or linear scale in common use	Use what is in common use at the institution, so that palliative care scores can be compared with other unit scores.
Other symptom scores, e.g. fatigue, dyspnoea	Symptom assessment scale	Edmonton, Memorial or similar symptom assessment scale	Most other units will not collect data, so palliative care can accelerate change by showing benefit.
Patient and family satisfaction	Survey instruments		Most commercial patient satisfaction firms do not survey decedent families.
Stories of patient and family satisfaction	Collected thank you notes and letters		Stories are really important to catch someone's attention. Insert in text boxes in all newsletters. Copy and send to CEO monthly.
Economic and other			
Profit margin	Health system financials	Amount contributed to the health system	Most palliative care programmes will not generate profit, but it is important to be 'cost neutral' to the health system. If the loss is small, it can be made up by contributions.
Cost avoidance	$/day saved by transfer to palliative care team or unit, with resources matched to goals of care	Amount saved for the health system	Each day of transfer from a high cost to low cost venue may save $1500 or more. In addition, it will free up the high cost ICU beds or ED space.
Referrals	By month and year	New patients to the service	Documents the amount of work done in understandable terms
		New patients referred specifically to palliative care	May document new patients brought to system by palliative care (new business)
		Recurring patients	
Length of stay	Inpatient LOS for those patients seen by palliative care team	Days	There may not be much difference. It is important to show that LOS is not increased by palliative care compared with usual care, in most health care systems.
ICU transfers	All transfers, and LOS before/after	Measure all transfers from ICU after PC consultation	This frees valuable ICU time.
Direct ED admissions	All consultations and direct admissions	Measure the LOS, costs of ED consults and admissions	May show a shorter LOS and lower cost than similar patients who are admitted to general service then later to palliative care.
Research grants and funds	Report all submissions and successful requests	All, including $ requested and received	This is a common measure of success for many programmes housed in academic programmes.
Scholarly works		Papers, abstracts, presentations	This is the most understandable measure of academic success.
Charitable contributions			This may offset losses. Most palliative care programmes work well with their institutional development officers for fund raising.

Table 3.8.6 Model presentation for palliative care.

Clinical	Economic
All symptoms improved from day 1 to day 3	1. 1800 consultations done hospital-wide fiscal year 2006
	2. 7–8/11 palliative care beds filled daily
	3. Profit overall $20 000
	4. Profit on direct admissions from ER, clinic, hospice $250 000; losses on transfer cases $230 000.
	5. Cost avoidance $900 000
	6. Additional ICU capacity of 250 bed days
	7. Charitable contributions $250 000
	8. Grant funding $375,000
	9. Two papers; five abstracts; two regional/national presentations
	10. Two awards for exemplary service

Further reading

Inter-Institutional Collaborating Network on End-of-Life Care (IICN) web site www.growthhouse.org/palliative/. Chapter 6: Financing and Reimbursement for Palliative Care. Financial models for palliative care programmes. Gives good models for collecting data, and for helping reimbursement. Palliative Care Leadership Center Curriculum – Center to Advance Palliative Care. The PCLC curriculum addresses issues relevant to each stage of palliative care programme development: Structural, Organizational, and Financial. See Module 3: Making the Financial Case. WSJ.comonline.wsj.com/article/0,,SB1078874123576650717,00.html. 'Unlikely Way to Cut Hospital Costs: Comfort the Dying' Front page of the *Wall Street Journal* detailed the cost avoidance and cost savings of palliative care. www.capc.org/palliative-care-leadership-initiative/curriculum/This curriculum shows a programme how to build a financial case for palliative care, alongside the clinical case.

References

1. White, K.R., Stover, K.G., Cassel, B. *et al.* (2006). Nonclinical Outcomes of Hospital-Based Palliative Care. *Journal of Healthcare Management*, **51**(4), 260–74.

2. Morrison, R.S., Maroney-Galin, C., Kralovec, P.D. *et al.* (2005) The growth of palliative care programs in United States hospitals. *Journal of Palliative Medicine*, **8**(6), 1127–34.

3. Department of Health (2000). *The NHS Cancer Plan. A plan for investment. A plan for reform.* London: Department of Heath. Higginson IJ, Finlay I, Goodwin DM, *et al.*(2002) Do hospital-based palliative teams improve care for patients or families at the end of life? *Journal of Pain and Symptom Management* **23**(2), 96–106.

4. Morrison, R.S., and Meier, D.E. (2004). Clinical practice. Palliative care. *New England Journal of Medicine*, **350**(25), 2582–90.

5. Smith, T.J., Coyne, P., Cassel, J.B. *et al.* (2003). A high volume specialist palliative care unit and team may reduce in-hospital end of life care cost. *Journal of Palliative Medicine*, **6**, 699–705.

6. Elsayem, A., Swint, K., Fisch, M.J. *et al.* (2004). Palliative care inpatient service in a comprehensive cancer center: clinical and financial outcomes. *Journal of Clinical Oncology*, **22**(10), 2008–14.

7. Brumley, R.D., Enguidanos, S., and Cherin, D.A. (2003). *Journal of Palliative Medicine*, **6**(5), 715–24.

8. Naik, G. (2004). Unlikely way to cut costs: Comfort the dying. *Wall Street Journal*, **A1**.

9. Koroukian, S.M., Beaird, H., Madigan, E. *et al.* (2006). End-of-life expenditures by Ohio Medicaid beneficiaries dying of cancer. *Health Care Financial Review*, **28**(2), 65–80.

10. Smith, T.J., Hillner, B.E., and Desch, C.E. (1993). Efficacy and cost-effectiveness of cancer treatment: rational allocation of resources based on decision analysis. *Journal of National Cancer Institute*, **85**(18), 1460–74.

11. Earle, C.C., Chapman, R.H., Baker, C.S. *et al.* (2000). Systematic overview of cost-utility assessments in oncology. *Journal of Clinical Oncology*, **18**(18), 3302–17.

12. Schrag, D. (2004). The price tag on progress—chemotherapy for colorectal cancer. *New England Journal of Medicine*, **351**(4), 317–9.

13. Bodenheimer, T. and Fernandez, A. (2005). High and rising health care costs. Part 4: can costs be controlled while preserving quality? *Annals of Internal Medicine*, **143**(1), 26–31.

14. Bruera, E., Palmer, J.L., Bosnjak, S. *et al.* (2004). Methadone versus morphine as a first-line strong opioid for cancer pain: a randomized, double-blind study. *Journal of Clinical Oncology*, **22**(1), 185–92.

15. Bennett, C.L., Smith, T.J., George, S.L. *et al.*(1995). Free-riding and the prisoner's dilemma: problems in funding economic analyses of phase III cancer clinical trials. *Journal of Clinical Oncology*, **13**(9), 2457–63.

16. Hillner, B.E. and Smith, T.J. (1991). Efficacy and cost effectiveness of adjuvant chemotherapy in women with node-negative breast cancer. A decision-analysis model. *New England Journal of Medicine*, **324**(3), 160–8.

17. Hillner, B.E. and Smith, T.J. (2007). Do the large benefits justify the large costs of adjuvant breast cancer trastuzumab? *Journal of Clinical Oncology*, **25**(6), 6113.

18. Kievit, W., Bolster, M.J., van der Wilt, G.J. *et al.* (2005). Cost-effectiveness of new guidelines for adjuvant systemic therapy for patients with primary breast cancer. *Annals of Oncology*, **16**, 1874–81.

19. World Health Organization (2001). *Macroeconomics and health: investing in health for economic development: report of the Commission on Macroeconomics and Health.* World Health Organization, Geneva.

20. Lillemoe, K.D., Cameron, J.L., Kaufman, H.S. *et al.* (1993). Chemical splanchnicectomy in patients with unresectable pancreatic cancer. A prospective randomized trial. *Annals of Surgery*, **217**(5), 447–55.

21. Wong, G.Y., Schroeder, D.R., Carns, P.E. *et al.* (2004). Effect of neurolytic celiac plexus block on pain relief, quality of life, and survival in patients with unresectable pancreatic cancer: a randomized controlled trial. *JAMA*, **291**(9), 1092–9.

22. Smith, T.J., Coyne, P.J., Staats, P.S. *et al.* (2005). An implantable drug delivery system (IDDS) for refractory cancer pain provides sustained pain control, less drug-related toxicity, and possibly better survival compared with comprehensive medical management (CMM). *Annals of Oncology*, **16**(5), 825–33.

23. Finn, J., Pienta, K., and Parzuchowski, J. (2002). Bridging cancer treatment and hospice care. ASCO [Abstract]. 2002 ASCO Annual Meeting.

24. Connor, S.R., Pyenson, B., Fitch, K. *et al.* (2007). Comparing hospice and nonhospice patient survival among patients who die within a three-year window. *Journal of Pain and Symptom Management*, **33**(3), 238–46.

25. Matsuyama, R., Reddy, S., and Smith, T.J. (2006). Why do patients choose chemotherapy near the end of life? A review of the perspective of those facing death from cancer. *Journal of Clinical Oncology*, **24**(21), 3490–6.

26. Russell, L.B., Gold, M.R., Siegel, J.E. *et al.* (1996). The role of cost-effectiveness analysis in health and medicine. Panel on Cost-Effectiveness in Health and Medicine. *JAMA*, **276**(14), 1172–7.

27. Siegel, J.E., Weinstein, M.C., Russell, L.B. *et al.* (1996). Recommendations for Reporting Cost-effectiveness Analyses. *JAMA*, **276**(16), 1339–41.

28. Smith, T.J., Staats, P.S., Deer, T. *et al.* (2002). Implantable Drug Delivery Systems Study Group. Randomized clinical trial of an implantable drug delivery system compared with comprehensive medical management for refractory cancer pain: impact on pain, drug-related toxicity, and survival. *Journal of Clinical Oncology*, **20**(19), 4040–9.

29. O'Leary, J.F., Fairclough, D.L., Jankowski, M.K. *et al.* (1995). Comparison of time-tradeoff utilities and rating scale values of cancer patients and their relatives: evidence for a possible plateau relationship. *Medical Decision Making*, **15**(2), 132–7.

30. Tchekmedyian, N.S., Hickman, M., Siau, J. *et al.* (1990). Treatment of cancer anorexia with megestrol acetate: impact on quality of life. *Oncology (Williston Park)*, **4**(5), 185–92, discussion 194.

31. Abernethy, A.P., Samsa, G.P., and Matchar, D.B. (2003). A clinical decision and economic analysis model of cancer pain management. *American Journal of Managed Care*, **9**(10), 651–64.

32. van den Hout, W.B., van der Linden, Y.M., Steenland, E. *et al.*(2003). Single- versus multiple-fraction radiotherapy in patients with painful bone metastases: cost-utility analysis based on a randomized trial. *Journal of National Cancer Institute,* **95**(3), 222–9.

33. van den Hout, W.B., Kramer, G.W., Noordijk, E.M. *et al.* (2006). Cost-utility analysis of short- versus long-course palliative

radiotherapy in patients with non-small-cell lung cancer. *Journal of National Cancer Institute*, **98**(24), 1786–94.

34. Mason, A., Weatherly, H., Spilsbury, K. *et al.* (2007). A systematic review of the effectiveness and cost-effectiveness of different models of community-based respite care for frail older people and their carers. *Health Technology Assessment*, **11**(15), 1–176.

35. Loveman, E., Green, C., Kirby, J. *et al.* (2006).The clinical and cost-effectiveness of donepezil, rivastigmine, galantamine and memantine for Alzheimer's disease. *Health Technology Assessment*, **10**(1), iii-iv, ix-xi, 1–160.

36. McConnell, K.J., Richards, C.F., Daya, M. *et al.* (2006). Ambulance diversion and lost hospital revenues. *Annals of Emergency Medicine* **48**(6), 702–10. E-pub 2006 Jul 11.

37. Robbins, M.A. (1998) The economics of palliative care. In *Oxford textbook of palliative medicine*, (eds. Doyle, D., Hanks, G.W.G., MacDonald, N.) 2nd edition, **2**(5).

38. Hanks, G.W. (2002). The imPaCT study: a randomised controlled trial to evaluate a hospital palliative care team. *British Journal of Cancer*, **87**(7), 733–9.

39. Rabow, M.W., Dibble, S.L., Pantilat, S.Z. *et al.* (2004). The comprehensive care team: a controlled trial of outpatient palliative medicine consultation. *Archives of Internal Medicine*, **164**(1), 83–91.

40. Smith, T.J. and Schnipper, L.J. (1998). The American Society of Clinical Oncology program to improve end-of-life care. *Journal of Palliative Medicine*, **1**(3), 221–30.

41. Khatcheressian, J., Cassel, J.B., Lyckholm, L. *et al.* (2005). Improving palliative and supportive care in cancer patients. *Oncology (Williston Park)*, **19**(10), 1365–76; discussion 1377–8, 1381–2, 1384 passim.

42. Passik, S.D., Ruggles, C., Brown, G. *et al.* (2004). Is there a model for demonstrating a beneficial financial impact of initiating a palliative care program by an existing hospice program? *Palliative Support Care*, **2**(4), 419–23.

43. Raftery, J.P., Addington-Hall, J.M., MacDonald, L.D. *et al.* A randomized controlled trial of the cost-effectiveness of a district co-ordinating service for terminally ill cancer patients. *Palliative Medicine*, **10**(2), 151–61.

44. Grande, G.E., Farquhar, M.C., Barclay, S.I. *et al.* Caregiver bereavement outcome: relationship with hospice at home, satisfaction with care, and home death. *Journal of Palliative Care*, **20**(2), 69–77.

45. Jordhøy, M.S., Fayers, P., Saltnes, T. *et al.* (2000). A palliative-care intervention and death at home: a cluster randomised trial. *Lancet*, **356**(9233), 888–93.

46. Campbell, D.E., Lynn, J., Louis, T.A. *et al.* (2004). Medicare program expenditures associated with hospice use. *Annals of Internal Medicine*, **140**, 269–77.

47. Emanuel, E.J., Ash, A., Yu, W. *et al.* (2002). Managed care, hospice use, site of death, and medical expenditures in the last year of life. *Archives of Internal Medicine*, **162**(15), 1722–8.

48. McCarthy, E.P., McCarthy, E.P., Burns, R.B. *et al.* (2003). Hospice use among Medicare managed care and fee-for-service patients dying with cancer. *JAMA*, **289**(17), 2238–45.

49. Pyenson, B., Connor, S., Fitch, K. *et al.* (2004). Medicare cost in matched hospice and non-hospice cohorts. *Journal of Pain and Symptom Management*, **28**, 200–10.

50. Cuny, J. *et al.* J Pall med Maxwell T, Cuny, J (2005). *The UHC palliative care benchmarking project*. Annual Assembly of the American Academy of Hospice and Palliative Medicine, New Orleans, LA.

51. Guest J.F., Ruiz, F.J., Russ, J., *et al.* (2005). A comparison of the resources used in advanced cancer care between two different strong opioids: an analysis of naturalistic practice in the UK. *Current Medical Research and Opinion*, **21**(2), 271–80.

52. Guest, J.F. (2006). Palliative care treatment patterns and associated costs of healthcare resource use for specific advanced cancer patients in the UK. *European Journal of Cancer Care (England)*, **15**(1), 65–73.

53. Fassbender, K. *et al.* (2005). Utilization and costs of the introduction of system-wide palliative care in Alberta, 1993-2000. *Palliative Medicine*, **19**(7), 513–20.

54. Serra-Prat, M., Gallo, P., and Picaza, J.M. (2001). Home palliative care as a cost-saving alternative: Evidence from Catalonia. *Palliative Medicine*, **15**, 271–8.

55. Cowan, J.D. (2004). Hospital charges for a community inpatient palliative care program. American *Journal of Hospital Palliative Care*, **21**, 177–90.

56. Pitorak, E.F., Armour, M., and Sivec, H.D. (2002). Project safe conduct integrates palliative goals into comprehensive cancer care: An interview with Elizabeth Ford Pitorak and Meri Armour. *Innovations in End-of-Life Care*, 4(4): www.edc.org/lastacts

SECTION 4

The interdisciplinary team

The core team and the extended team

Dagny Faksvåg Haugen,
Friedemann Nauck, and Augusto Caraceni

Introduction

Teamwork is an essential component of palliative care. Living with advanced incurable disease can affect all aspects of life, creating psychological, spiritual, and existential challenges as well as demands for symptom control and physical care. It is therefore rarely—if ever—possible for any one professional to meet all the needs of a patient or family. This chapter gives a short overview of the positive aspects along with the challenges of teamwork, and presents and discusses the interdisciplinary palliative care team.

A team may be defined simply as two or more people working together. However, working together is not sufficient to make a pair or a group of people into a team. A widely used definition describes a team as *a small number of people with complementary skills who are committed to a common purpose, performance goals, and approach for which they hold themselves mutually accountable*[1]. Team members work in an interdependent manner. This means that they have to know each other and what every team member can contribute to the common goal.

Many groups perceived as teams are not real teams, but crews. The typical crew is the group of people working on and operating an aircraft. Each member of the crew knows and performs his assigned duties and communication between the crew members can often be kept to a minimum. Crew members may be substituted easily by other persons with the same training. In a team, however, each member is picked to complement the group because of his/her special skills and knowledge, and adjustment is always needed to integrate new members[2]. A football team starts out as a crew. It usually takes hours of practice to transform the crew into an efficient team.

Teams have become increasingly popular in various fields of health care, making it possible for health-care professionals to work closely together. *Multi-professional* teams are frequently employed in areas where patients have extensive and complex needs. Multi-professional simply means that team members have different professional backgrounds. A multi-professional team may be multi-disciplinary or interdisciplinary.

In a *multi-disciplinary* team, each team member contributes his/her expertise independent of the others, and all team members have their own clearly defined place[3,4]. Although each professional may provide vital information toward decision-making, generally only one person, usually a physician or nurse, makes the treatment decisions. A common decision-making process demands an *interdisciplinary* approach.

The interdisciplinary team

An interdisciplinary health-care team is described as an *identified collective in which members share common team goals and work interdependently in planning, problem solving, decision-making, and implementing and evaluating team-related tasks*[5]. The team is characterized by a high degree of cooperation and communication to ensure that all relevant issues are addressed.

The description above will be valid for most interdisciplinary teams, but they still differ with respect to[6]:

◆ size;

◆ professions;

◆ the degree of integration or closeness of working between team members;

◆ the extent of collective responsibility, i.e. the extent to which the team as a collective is responsible and held accountable for providing the service;

◆ membership of the team—who is and who is not a member, and what membership means;

◆ the patient pathway through the team—time and process;

◆ decision-making; and

◆ management and leadership.

All these aspects are important when describing and evaluating a team and will be addressed in this chapter.

A number of studies have shown that health-care teams are more effective than single practitioners and may improve both the quality and quantity of services[7–9]. Teamwork improves communication and coordination and allows for maximal diversity of professional expertise. These factors can lead to organizational benefits like reduced hospitalization time and costs, reduced unanticipated admissions, and better accessibility for patients.

Through the combined approach a team may achieve more together than the sum of individual team members operating on their own. In fact, successful teams may possess combinations of skills that no single individual may demonstrate on his or her own[4]. The type and diversity of clinical expertise involved in team decision-making has been shown to be a major factor accounting for teams' improvements in patient care and organizational effectiveness[9,10]. This diversity also makes teamwork rewarding and stimulating.

The interdisciplinary team tries to achieve the following objectives:

- an accurate and speedy assessment;
- effective, integrated treatment and care;
- efficient communication with the patient and the family, with other professionals, institutions, and within the team itself; and
- audit of the team's activities and outcomes.

Team members may give each other valuable feedback and support. The team is usually felt as a safe environment for sharing stresses and problems, as well as successes. On the other hand, working closely together may precipitate conflicts more easily.

Team performance

Team performance is influenced by factors relating to the *structure* of the team and to *processes* involved in team functioning (Table 4.1.1)[9-12]. The structural factors include organizational aspects as well as characteristics of the group and the individual team members.

By definition, a team is a small number of people, usually no more than 15, and often between five and 10. A team of five or six full-time members has been suggested as ideal[1,2]. Unresolved differences are better tolerated in larger teams, but rules and procedures need to be more formalized and it takes more time to reach decisions. Around 20 seems to be the maximum number of team members consistent with efficient team work[2,9,13].

Membership defines the team's boundaries. The most common membership distinction is between *core* and *associated members*, the latter belonging to the extended team[6,7]. Core members are usually full-time members governed by the team policy and managed by the team leader. Associate can mean part-time in the team, not governed by team policy and having managers outside the team, possibly with fewer or no voting rights on team decisions.

Table 4.1.1 Characteristics of effective teamwork.

Organizational structure	Individual contribution	Team process
Clear purpose	Self knowledge	Coordination
Appropriate culture	Trust	Communication
Specified task	Commitment	Cohesion
Distinct roles	Flexibility	Decision-making
Suitable leadership		Conflict management
Relevant members		Social relationships
Adequate resources		Performance feedback

© Copyright 2000. Australian Health Review – reproduced with permission from Mickan and Rodger[11]

Specific implications of these terms in palliative care teams will be discussed later.

A team is dependent on organizational support and adequate resources and staffing. An organizational culture supportive of teamwork will have a positive influence on team performance[9,14].

Team members

Teams require the appropriate mix and diversity of task and interpersonal skills among its members. Each team member must have a distinct and necessary role within the team[8].

All team members have to be specialists in their own fields to be valid 'instruments' in the interdisciplinary 'orchestra'. This includes having the necessary self-confidence and trust in their own skills to represent their professional area in the group. However, it is also necessary to have a clear understanding of the other team members' expertise and contributions. Each health-care discipline has its own 'cognitive map' consisting of its conceptual basis, terminology, observational approaches, and theoretical framework. Working together in a team requires understanding the 'maps' of the other team members to some degree[10,15]. In other words, a team needs a certain amount of shared knowledge and understanding to be able to communicate efficiently.

Even more important than getting a grasp of each other's professional knowledge are the attitudes of the team members—both towards each other and towards the work on the team[4,15]. The tendency to believe that one's own way of framing problems or solutions is the best is a common obstacle to good teamwork[10]. Team members may fear that teamwork will threaten their professional role, authority, and status. They may fear pressure to take on tasks outside their professional role, or on the contrary, to give up tasks that they have performed and enjoyed because other team members are more formally competent.

Attitudes towards team work are rooted in each team member's understanding of what teamwork really means and their belief in how it should be performed. In fact, team members' interpretations of teamworking have been shown to be just as important as organizational and group dynamic constraints[16]. Freeman *et al.* identified three philosophies of teamwork:

1 The *directive* philosophy is based on the assumption of hierarchy in the team. One person takes the lead by virtue of status and power and directs the actions of the other team members.

2 The *integrative* philosophy assumes that each professional's contribution has equal value. All team members are seen as team players and communication and discussions within the team are given vital importance.

3 The *elective* philosophy of team work is held by professionals who prefer clear and distinct team roles to operate autonomously and only relate briefly to other team members when they see a need for it themselves.

The conflicting attitudes stemming from team members consciously or unconsciously holding different team philosophies may easily compromise effective teamwork. Task clarity and role clarification are imperative if this is to be addressed. Fifteen multi-professional psychiatric teams in the USA were studied to find factors influencing the efficiency of the teams[17]. Clarity of objective was found to be one of the most important determinants for efficient interdisciplinary work. This means that the team's mission or charge must be described clearly, understood, and accepted by all the team members. This serves as a starting point and a vital foundation in guiding priorities, problem solving, and decision-making[12].

Team processes

Team processes describe how the team handles tasks and interpersonal dynamics to produce the desired outcome (Table 4.1.1)[11]. Team processes start when a new team is formed. Research on group processes have shown that teams often go through typical phases in their development[1,19,20].

Forming is the first phase when the group constitutes itself and faces its task for the first time. The team members feel insecure and test out behaviour in the group. The group is dependent on a formal leader. In this phase it is important to establish rules and develop ways of working, defining the tasks for each team member.

Storming is the characteristic phase of turbulence, critical opposition, and power struggle which often follows once the team is established. Conflicts arise among subgroups, differing opinions and competition between team members emerge.

Norming characterizes the next phase when the team players finally agree on rules and adapt to common norms. The members resist conflicts and develop a sense of belonging together. There is an open exchange of opinions and feelings, along with the development of cooperation.

Performing or *adjourning* should be the final, lasting stage of team development. By now the team has developed functional processes for problem solving. The team members know their roles, support each other, and devote their energy to fulfilling the team's objectives[19].

This simplified, schematic description is not valid for every team and the order of the phases may vary[5]. In addition, many health-care teams are not formed from scratch and will already include people who are accustomed to teamwork. Still, these common steps might be a help to understand team dynamics and guide your team in the right direction.

Roles of team members

A role is understood as the expectations the individual has of his/her work. It also centres on what others expect from the person[10]. The role is tightly linked to professional identity and gives the owner certain duties and privileges. Role ambiguity and role conflicts threaten teamwork and must be resolved[2]. Clarification of roles first of all concerns the *professional roles* in the team. Who should take on which tasks? Role overlap might lead to competition or repetition where several team members perform the same task. Should the nurse, the social worker, or the pastoral worker talk to bereaved family members? Some roles will by necessity overlap. This may be beneficial and actually increase the team's effectiveness, but should first be agreed upon by all team members[4,15].

In addition to the professional role, other roles will be cultivated. Every team member has a *personal role* rooted in his/her persona[2]. In addition, there will be *formal roles* such as team leader or supervisor.

Informal roles reflect the individual team member's personality and style which have given him/her a certain position in the group. These informal roles may not be fully articulated, but roles like 'mother', 'clown', 'messy head', or 'saviour' may be familiar.

The power and influence of each team member is often linked to his or her role in the group. Ideally, all members of a team should have equal influence on the teamwork. However, research has shown that a person's influence in a small group tends to be associated with expertise, high external status for the person and high degree of participation in the group[15]. In this respect, part-time employment can be a drawback for team members.

In many settings, the physician has the final (legal) responsibility for the patient's medical treatment and this may lead to an increased influence by the physician on the team's decision-making.

Leadership

Team leadership concerns three aspects: management, handling of professional challenges, and motivation and policy. *Management* (administration) is important, but not necessarily a job for the team leader. Although the physician will be responsible for the medical treatment, *professional, task-centred leadership* in the interdisciplinary team should vary from case to case, depending on the nature of the needs of the individual patient and family[3]. The *team leader* should guide the team in the right direction by:

◆ keeping purpose, goals, and approach both relevant and meaningful;

◆ building commitment and confidence;

◆ strengthening the mix and level of skills;

◆ managing external relations, removing obstacles;

◆ creating opportunities for others; and

◆ doing real work.

Leadership is a combination of goal-orientated and interpersonal skills[2,7,21]. Kane suggests that the team leader should be chosen on the basis of his/her understanding of group processes and skills in using them to reach team goals.

Øvretveit states that the quickest way to establish close and effective teamwork is to start with a clearly defined team leader role:

> I do not know of any teams which have close teamwork and have survived changes of membership without a clear team leader position. One of the biggest mistakes is to believe that interprofessional and interagency conflicts, rivalries, and protectionism can be avoided by not defining a team leader role[7].

Communication and cohesion

Communication, in all its forms, is the means through which the team members interact and the work gets done. Communication is equally important both within the team and between the team and the organization: patients, family members, other health-care professionals, and managers[2,11,22].

Ongoing communication requires commitment of time and energy[2]. It is enhanced through physical proximity of offices, common records, and frequent, structured meetings. Meetings provide the main forum and structure within which a team works. Multi-disciplinary team meetings for assessment, planning, and evaluation of patient care should be held at least weekly, and should be structured carefully, incorporating time for reflection and review[14].

Cohesion is a feeling of belonging which gives the team members shared enjoyment and pride in their achievements and a wish to remain within the team[11,12]. This commitment and involvement is generated by working together over time and is supported by good performance feedback, success in adversity, good communication, and conformity to norms[11,17]. In their study of Australian health-care teams, Mickan and Rodger found communication and cohesion as two of the main categories most able to distinguish effective teams. The other four categories highlighted were mutual respect, goals, purpose, and leadership[12].

Decision-making and conflict solving

Decision-making skills are a basis for effective teamwork and a main responsibility of the leader[2]. Although the degree of involvement will vary from task to task, all team members need to contribute to the team's decisions.

Decision-making includes describing the problem, presenting and discussing potential solutions, prioritizing, and choosing among the alternatives assigning responsibility and deciding upon an appropriate time frame. In the palliative care team, agenda setting as well as decision-making must ultimately be guided by the patient's and family's needs, wishes, and preferences[13,18]. The needs of the patient and carers should remain the focus of the team's efforts.

Any work group may be subject to stresses and conflicts. In a team, diversity of professional backgrounds presents an additional challenge[3,4,15]. All aspects of teamwork discussed so far may give rise to conflicts which may impact on the function and work of the team. In addition, external factors—scarcity of resources, organizational changes, and work-related strain may increase stress. The ability to resolve conflict is clearly an important feature of any successful team[2,9].

Any conflict arising in the team should be taken seriously and identified as soon as possible. What is the nature of the conflict and how serious is it? What has caused or is causing the conflict? Investigating the root of the problem is usually more productive than focusing just on the symptoms. Possible solutions must be discussed and the necessary steps taken to reach the desired outcome, including clarifying who must be involved in the process[23].

Clinical supervision is recognized as a valuable tool for professional growth and support and should be available to the interdisciplinary team. Supervision has an important role in preventing and solving team conflicts[23,24]. The style of supervision such as one-to-one versus group supervision is often dependent on organizational resources rather than specific benefits.

Team building

Teams are dynamic. Appropriate team structures facilitate the development of team processes, but as teams evolve, team processes often shape the structures within which they have optimum function[11]. Accordingly, both team structure and processes should be considered when building effective teams (Table 4.1.1).

Shared learning and getting to know each other by spending time together are the core aspects of 'team building' activities[20]. A work climate characterized by good social relationships, personal recognition, feedback, and humour can positively influence team members' psychological well-being, organizational commitment, and belief in the team's effectiveness[11].

Many health-care teams work in complex fields. Members of palliative care teams experience emotional strain and continuous exposure to death and dying[24,25]. Teams demand strong support mechanisms in order to cope with these stressors and remain physically and psychologically robust[18,20,23,24,26]; this is discussed in Section 15.

The palliative care team

Teamwork is an inherent feature of palliative care. The palliative care team is an interdisciplinary health-care team with its own characteristics and challenges. In the next section, the different clinical settings, functions, staffing requirements, and operational requirements for palliative care teams will be discussed.

A palliative care team is usually understood to be a clinical team, although many teams are also are engaged in teaching, service development, and research. The typical palliative care team is the hospital consult team serving the hospital wards and possibly the nearby communities. However, the multi-professional staff of an inpatient specialist palliative care unit or hospice also forms a team. The palliative care team should be found in any setting providing specialist palliative care.

The palliative care team: defined and flexible

To be a team, the team members need to be defined[5,9]. This is vital for the communication and collaboration within the team and for the organization served by the team. A palliative care team should be identified by the name of the team or the programme, and its members should be outlined clearly. This is usually the case for palliative care consult teams. In other settings, team boundaries are often more vague and it is not always clear who is inside and who is outside the team. Are all nursing staff part of the team? What about part-time staff and volunteers?

While efficient teamwork demands a defined core team, palliative care also needs to be flexible[13]. Ideally, the team should be tailored to suit the needs of the individual patient, family, and situation. This extended 'team' may consist of some members from the palliative care staff team or consult team in addition to family members, hospital physician, general practitioner, home care nurse, volunteer, etc. This group of care providers may over time function more like a network or a 'virtual team'. The 'team' may not even meet, but they communicate and work towards common care goals.

In this way, a palliative care team is not static. Addressing the patient's and family's needs may require involvement from all or just a few team members—and a varying number of people outside the team. In the same way, members of the palliative care team are part of other more or less formalized teams, e.g. members of the consult team joining the patient's primary care team. However, although flexibility is needed, loose team boundaries may lead to drifting team members working in a multi-disciplinary rather than an interdisciplinary way.

The palliative care solo practitioner

Some authors have advocated that a palliative care consult service consisting of a single physician or specialist nurse may also be named a team. This solo practitioner model may offer an inexpensive way to introduce a minimum palliative care support service into a hospital[4,27]. The model demands close cooperation with other departments and services, relying on the individual's ability (availability) to respond to referrals as needed. However, this is not a true interdisciplinary or team approach. The model also holds dangers of professional isolation and work overload.

The core team

Most recommendations for the organization of palliative care services define a core palliative care consult team consisting of a physician, preferably a consultant in palliative medicine, and a specialist nurse[28,29]. The UK recommendations specify the physician being supported by other medical staff including junior staff who may be on (training) rotations and also include secretarial/administrative support in the core team[28]. Guidelines from the USA include a social worker in the core team[30]. The IAHPC manual recognizes physician, nurse, social worker, pastoral worker, and therapist as the core team, but accepts a core team with only nurse and doctor if resources are limited and services from the three other professions are readily available on the hospital wards being served[29].

In a specialist palliative care unit, usually more team members will be defined as core members than on a consult team (see below)[28,31].

The nurse and physician are placed at the core of the palliative care team simply to reflect that these are the two professions most often making the clinical decisions needed by people with advanced, life-threatening disease. Accordingly, the nurse and the physician usually work full-time on the team, while other team members often will be part-time or attached staff.

The extended team

The extended palliative care team should ideally be designed to be able to address all the needs of the patients and families served by the team. The team should include psychology, social work, and chaplaincy expertise and access to specialist pain management, physiotherapy, occupational therapy, and dietetics[18,28,30–32]. Pharmacy expertise is included in some countries and likely to be increasingly important. A number of other health-care providers and therapists may be included as needed[14,29]. The team must be skilled in care of the patient population to be served[32]. For example, when working mainly with cancer patients, expertise in oncology and cancer nursing and a physiotherapist and social worker specialized in cancer care should be found on the team.

Are the patient and the family team members?

User involvement is becoming increasingly popular in health care. Palliative care populations have natural limitations in this respect, but palliative medicine as a specialty has always been patient-centred. All treatment must be given with the patient's consent and in accordance with his/her wishes. The patient may thus be considered a member of the extended team, even if he/she does not take part in all team conferences[29].

Likewise, the members of the patient's family can be considered members. They have an important role in the overall care of the patient and their opinions should be included when formulating plans for treatment and care[29].

The specialist palliative care unit

Inpatient palliative care is provided in hospices and palliative care units. Palliative care units may be found in very different settings, ranging from academic, tertiary acute care hospitals to nursing homes, and residential homes. The common purpose for all these units is to provide comprehensive, specialist palliative care by means of their interdisciplinary team. The palliative care staff team is usually fully responsible for the treatment and management of the patients admitted to their unit.

The establishment of St. Christopher's Hospice in London by Dame Cicely Saunders in 1967 is regarded as the foundation of the modern hospice movement[33]. Hospice was designed to relieve suffering at the end of life, by addressing the 'total pain' of patients and their families—their physical, emotional, social, and spiritual needs—and by addressing the needs for research and teaching in symptom control and end-of-life-care. Multi-professional teamwork was regarded an essential cornerstone of holistic hospice care. Since the 1960s, the hospice movement has grown and spread worldwide. Hospice care can be established and implemented in many settings and cultures and in countries with widely different resources[33].

The dramatic change of focus made it necessary to establish the first hospices outside the acute hospital setting[34,35]. Gradually, the pendulum has swung back. Deficiencies in terminal care for hospital patients prompted the surgeon Balfour Mount to establish a palliative care unit at the Royal Victoria Hospital in Montreal in 1975[36]. Establishing a unit within the hospital was seen as a good way to promote palliative care philosophy and skills in the acute care setting and to fit into the Canadian official health-care system.

Recent years have seen a considerable growth in the number of inpatient palliative care units across the world. In some countries, inpatient hospices are very different from hospital palliative care units in terms of funding, length of patient stay, and main task of care (end-of-life care versus crisis intervention and symptom control), while in others they are more alike. Some countries have chosen not to have 'hospice' as an organizational element—either because of the term's historical associations, or because it is not specific for the contents or quality of the service provided[31].

Staff teams in hospices and palliative care units

Most members of the palliative care staff team will be defined as core members[28]. This is necessary to provide comprehensive care addressing all the patients' and families' needs. While the number of professionals involved in each case may vary, the great advantage of the staff team is to have all professions available in the same physical area, with possibilities for daily meetings and interactions.

The staff team of an inpatient unit must relate to an extended 'team' including community or hospital personnel referring patients or receiving patients upon discharge[13,22]. Discharge planning may be time consuming, however, it is an important task for the unit.

Members of the interdisciplinary team on an inpatient unit may also staff a day-care centre, outpatient unit, or consult team. Often the nurses are linked to one particular branch of the service, while team members from other professions cover several parts. The nursing staff must make room for and include team members from other professions in day-to-day decision-making and patient care, in particular ward nurses.

Recommendations for staffing

The high complexity of problems and the extensive nursing needs combined with the quality of care delivered, demand a high ratio of staff per patient in hospices and palliative care units. Staffing levels are also influenced by disease panorama and needs for specialist skills:

◆ patients with advanced neurological disease like motor neuron disease are generally very resource-intensive;

◆ demographics (younger people and families with children often require more support);

◆ number of admissions and rate of turn-over; and

◆ cultural factors (e.g. need for interpreters and more time-consuming conferences)[32].

Recommendations for staffing vary among countries[18,28–32]. An example is given in Table 4.1.2, quoting the estimated minimum staffing levels from the Palliative Care Australia Planning Guide[37]. For comparison, the German Association for Palliative Medicine (DGP) has recommended a hospice or palliative care unit core team consisting of nurses (1.4 registered nurses per patient), physicians (1.2 palliative medicine consultants for 8–10 beds), social worker(s), psychologist(s), and physiotherapist(s). The latter professions and—if possible—art therapist and volunteers should altogether be available at least 6 h per patient per week. All members of the staff team should be specialized or at least sub-specialized in palliative care. In addition, DGP recommends all units should have good liaisons to chaplaincy and music therapy, and consult other medical specialties as needed. Further training and education on a regular basis for team members are considered as essential as team supervision (Recommendations of the German Association for Palliative Medicine for staffing of palliative care units, as of 23 February 2007).

The extended interdisciplinary medical team

Specialist palliative care may be advanced medical treatment, highlighted in academic palliative medicine units in tertiary hospitals, admitting the most complex cases[38]. These units need an extended interdisciplinary medical team to handle any emergencies or complications that may arise. The core staff team should include all relevant professions, including nurses with experience in different specialties. A number of medical specialties must be linked to the team and readily available for consult at short notice. Relevant specialties include orthopaedics, infectious diseases,

Table 4.1.2 Estimated minimum staffing levels for professional support of interdisciplinary palliative care in the community, acute-care settings, and palliative care units by discipline, expressed as full-time equivalent staff.

Discipline/staff category	Community-based services*	Acute-care hospital consultative service[†]	Designated palliative care beds[‡]
Palliative care specialist[§]	1.5	1.5	1.5
Registrar[§]	1.0	1.0	1.0
Resident medical officer	0	0	0.25
Liaison psychiatry	0.25	0.25	0.25
Clinical nurse consultant[§]	1.0	0.75	0
Registered and enrolled nurses[§]	0	0	6.5 h per patient per day
Discharge liaison	0	0.25	0
Psychology	0.25	0.1	0.1
Social work	0.5	0.25	0.25
Bereavement support	0.25	0.1	0.1
Pastoral care	0.25	0.25	0.25
Speech pathology	0.2	0.2	0.2
Dietitian	0.2	0.2	0.2
Physiotherapy	0.4	0.2	0.2
Occupational therapy	0.4	0.2	0.2
Pharmacist	0	0.25	0.1
Other therapies[¶]	0.5	0	0.25

* Full-time equivalent staff per 100 000 population served.

[†] Full-time equivalent staff per 125 hospital beds.

[‡] Full-time equivalent staff per 6.7 beds, whether in an acute-care setting or in a freestanding palliative care unit or hospice (6.7 palliative care beds per 100 000 population would be needed).

[§] Assumes that these roles in the community are consultative, with well resourced primary clinical care (general practitioners and community nurses).

[¶] Includes combinations of music, art, complementary, narrative and diversional therapies.

advanced pain medicine, oncology, urology, gastrointestinal surgery, and psychiatry.

Palliative care units in nursing homes and residential homes

Even though it is undisputed that palliative care should be provided in the settings of care for older people, this field is poorly developed[39]. In many countries, hardly any palliative care is provided in nursing homes or residential homes. However, some European countries (e.g. Belgium, the Netherlands, Sweden, Norway, and certain areas of Spain) have an active policy to establish palliative care units in nursing homes[31,40]. Many of the patients admitted to these units have palliative care needs related to chronic diseases typical of old age. This places additional demands on staff, for example, pain assessment and symptom control in demented patients and knowledge of a broad variety of chronic diseases. When setting up the team, expertise in geriatrics/nursing home medicine and geriatric nursing should be included.

The palliative care consult team

As hospice practice developed in the UK, many patients admitted to hospices for symptom control were able to be discharged back to their own home. This fact precipitated the need for hospices to develop their own home care teams. From the end of the 1970s, palliative care started to come full circle back into acute care with the formation of hospital palliative care teams[41].

The palliative care consult team seeks to influence and improve the care for patients with advanced, incurable disease by giving advice to the health professionals in charge of their care. The typical consult team is found in acute care hospitals, but teams may operate in different settings and are particularly important as links between the different levels of the health-care system.

Hospital-based palliative care teams

The move of hospice care to acute care hospitals started with the consult teams at St. Luke's Hospital in New York (1974), the Royal Victoria Hospital, Montreal, and St. Thomas's Hospital in London (1977)[42]. At that time, 50–60 per cent of all deaths occurred in hospitals, as is still the case in many developed countries today. Palliative care services in the UK now include more than 300 hospital palliative care teams.

Team composition and tasks

Team composition depends on the purpose and goals for the service. These are influenced by the hospital characteristics, the patient populations to be served, additional palliative care services inside or outside the hospital, financial issues, and existing national standards.

The team will have core and extended members as described earlier. Useful advice on team development and composition may be found in manuals and national standards[28–32] (Table 4.1.2). It should be noted that some countries do not have advanced palliative care nursing practitioners and some of their functions can in that case only be covered by physicians.

Palliative care consult teams may be linked to a palliative care unit or may operate in hospitals not having palliative care inpatient facilities[31,36,38,42].

No palliative care team can function without its own clear objectives. However, the following aims are common for most consult teams[34,35]:

◆ to work alongside the hospital ward team by advising on symptom control and psychosocial/spiritual issues;

◆ to support relatives in difficult situations;

◆ to support staff in difficult decisions and grief;

◆ to educate staff in palliative care; and

◆ to liaise with hospice / other palliative care services and home care services.

Consult teams usually have several levels of intervention:

1 Advice and guidance to professionals on the ward team without direct contact with the patient.

2 Single visit for assessment and advice on further plans for care, preferably with referrer. Further contacts specifically at referrer's request.

3 Short-term interventions with patients and families for specific problems.

4 Ongoing contact due to multiple, complex problems requiring regular specialist assessment and interventions. In this case the team might temporarily take over patient responsibility.

Consultations are also provided for cancer patients still receiving disease-modifying treatment and patients with non-malignant conditions. This gives the palliative care team a unique opportunity to be the interface between palliative medicine and other medical specialties[43]. In terms of teams, the consultant, advanced nurse practitioner, or other members of the consult team will be part of the extended medical team in the intensive care unit, the department of oncology, and other hospital wards.

Most palliative care patients want to spend time at home, but the majority have a number of hospital admissions during the disease trajectory. Access to specialist palliative care should be based on need and given in an outpatient or inpatient setting as appropriate[32,38]. The palliative care consult team has a crucial role in assessing the needs and priorities of patients and families and in helping to set goals of care and further plans for care[27]. Whether the hospital team also has outreach provision or whether it liaises with community teams, the consult team must have an overview of all relevant services and facilitate care transitions. In many cases, team members work across hospital and community settings, making the consult service a 'hub' for combined services.

Community teams

St. Christopher's Hospice pioneered the first palliative home care team in 1969. Today the UK has around 360 community support services and about 100 hospice-at-home services[41]. Home-care support teams provide specialist advice and work alongside the community personnel in charge of the patient's care[28]. Although these teams most often support general practitioners (family doctors), and district nurses, other team members such as physiotherapists or occupational therapists may have equally important roles guiding their respective community colleagues. Home-care teams must have clear objectives and guidelines for the level of intervention, which are both acceptable and agreed with the primary care team.

Services providing extended specialist palliative nursing, medical, social, and emotional support, and care in the patient's home, are often known as 'hospice-at-home'[28,41]. Care may be provided as crisis management or for longer periods of time. There are many different models of hospice-at-home, varying from rapid response teams offering a high level of specialist support (e.g. hospital connected home-care services), to those providing less intensive ongoing support. By establishing a full range of hospice at home support, the team assumes full control of the patient and works like a staff team. In such cases, responsibility must be clearly defined and assigned, both within such a team and between the team and primary care services.

Specific challenges for palliative care consult teams

Consult teams face specific challenges related to potential disagreements and conflicts with referring staff and the primary care team. Late referrals mean that the team has to be particularly adaptable, innovative, and thoughtful to ensure optimum patient care. This often leads to team compromises, however, late effective communication and management relating to late referrals can be very influential in changing practice[27,34,35,43].

Although there is a need for greater and better quality research in palliative care, palliative care teams have been shown to improve symptom control, increase patient and carer satisfaction, and have an impact on communication and psychosocial aspects of care[27,43–48]. In a recent German survey, hospital specialists thought more teams were necessary[49].

Planning the team

The majority of palliative care teams have started from an enthusiastic individual convinced of the need for and the usefulness of specialist palliative care. Although probably no team may come into being without at least one such committed person, a structured planning process will be frustration-saving and time-saving[34].

The size and composition of the team should be based on a thorough needs assessment which in turn leads to clear task objectives and careful job descriptions. In many cases, the team will be formed from practitioners already employed by the institution, brought together from different departments and grouped into a team. This situation is not ideal and calls for a dedicated team leader, well-defined roles for the team members and strong support from the institution's management and organization.

A careful selection process is warranted to build a new team or recruit new members to an 'old' team. In the palliative care consult team every team member is a specialist in an advisory position and must have specialist expertise founded in broad clinical experience[34]. However, being personally suited for the job and fitting into the team is probably even more important. If a secure professional basis is in place, further competence and expertise may be acquired through additional education and training, but a non-team player may severely disrupt a team. Specific team skills may be difficult to develop outside a team, but the ability to respect, trust, support, and work closely together with colleagues is a fundamental requirement for team members. A sense of humour is also a great advantage as a potent means to resolve conflicts at an early stage.

Evaluating the team

Audit of the team's activities and outcomes is one of the objectives of interdisciplinary team work[50]. This demands clearly defined, attainable, and measurable goals[9]. Keeping good records and compiling statistics are the first steps in evaluating the service.

Clinical and organizational audit is described in Section 7. Audit and quality measurement may be applied to three levels of teamwork, and palliative care teams should regularly formulate goals within these three domains:

1 structure;

2 processes; and

3 outcomes.

Structural factors include having job descriptions, systems for referral and feedback, telephone access, symptom assessment tools, and other organizational elements in place.

Processes refer to how the structural elements are used and the teamwork is performed:

◆ The patient pathway through the team—number of referrals, referral time, time expenditure, use of symptom assessment tools, family meetings, etc.

◆ Communication and documentation—record keeping, discharge summaries, network meetings.

◆ Internal processes of teamwork—team functioning, performance, and effectiveness—which may be measured by a number of validated tools[51].

Outcomes relate to results obtained through the team's efforts, auditing the effects of actual interventions in changing ward practice, improving symptom control, patient and family satisfaction, patient and family understanding of disease progression, etc. A large number of questionnaires and outcome scales have been developed to this end[50] (Section 7).

The interdisciplinary teaching team

Every health-care practitioner is a life-long learner, and every palliative care team should provide an environment for learning and development for its members. Equally important, everyone acting as a specialist practitioner automatically becomes a teacher and a role model.

The palliative care team should convey the attitudes and skills of teamwork as well as the knowledge, skills, and attitudes of palliative care. Optimally, these two aspects of the team's educational role should be highly integrated.

Palliative care education and training are dealt with in Section 20. The following paragraphs highlight a few aspects of the team's teaching role.

Informal teaching and support

The advisory role of the palliative care consult team makes it easy to turn almost all clinical contacts into teaching opportunities. The first visit for comprehensive assessment provides an ideal situation to demonstrate communication techniques and involve the junior doctor and ward nurse or GP and district nurse in discussions on assessment and treatment[27,34]. Case discussions, ward rounds and staff meetings provide similar opportunities. Changes in medication or other treatments should always be discussed with the staff and practical procedures should be carried out by them— whether setting up a syringe driver, applying for aids in the home, or broadening the range of physiotherapy techniques applied. These are extremely important steps to ensure provision of basic palliative care in all the services the team comes into contact with, inside or outside the hospital.

Attitudes are usually the most difficult area to change. The members of the palliative care team are important role models when demonstrating the interdisciplinary approach, when including family members in the care, and when showing that they are comfortable working with loss, grief, and dying. The support of colleagues who want to implement a palliative-care approach in their routine work is an important part of the team's role.

Working with terminally ill patients and their families can be very demanding (see Section 15). The palliative care team is a resource for individual professionals struggling with professional stressors or patient and family demands. Sometimes the whole ward team needs support, especially when dealing with complicated medical problems or ethical challenges[34]. Members of the palliative care team—the social worker, psychologist, or chaplain may organize support groups for ward staff (Section 15). If possible, two team members should run a group, both to support and complement each other and to give a practical example of team work.

Inpatient palliative care units and hospices are equally important arenas for role modelling and informal teaching. These units are continuously used for pre- and postgraduate education and practice by a number of different professions. Visiting practitioners are usually very motivated and eager to learn, but need to relate their observations and experiences to their own working practice.

Formal teaching

To fulfil the objective to pass on expertise, every palliative care team must also engage in formal educational sessions. This means that 'teaching the teachers' must be included in the team training.

Depending on the topic and situation, a variety of scenarios (seminar, study day, course, orientation programme) and methods (lecture, workshop, journal club, small group discussion, role play, gold fish bowl, sculpting, etc.) apply to the team's engagement in formal education[52,53] (Section 20). As a general rule, no team member should run a session on his/her own. Interdisciplinary educational sessions facilitate shared learning for professional groups working together. Separate teaching for each professional group within the team is also needed, but even so the interdisciplinary approach should be emphasized, e.g. in case presentations[18,52].

When teaching peers in the hospital or community setting, principles of adult learning should be applied. To learn from an educational activity, adults need to find it relevant for their own daily practice and engage actively in it. Clear goals and objectives must be set for each session and ample use of cases and clinical examples, discussion, feedback, and time for reflection are needed (see Section 20).

Education on teamwork always needs a practical base. Experience with a well-functioning, effective team delivering relevant services is the most efficient way to learn team skills. Learning team skills in practice is not only relevant for teamwork, but for all levels of interaction within the complex health-care system.

The interdisciplinary research team

Every palliative care team should strive to improve its work through research and development. Unfortunately, research often has to give way to pressing clinical demands and, in addition, there is a lack of funding, and academic units. Nevertheless palliative care research is increasing, including some exciting international collaborations.

The core clinical palliative care research team often consists of a palliative medicine specialist with research experience and qualifications together with a research nurse and one or more research fellows. The clinical palliative care team needs to be committed to supporting the research team and should never undermine the research team's work. All palliative care teams should be fully supportive of the palliative care research agenda which is necessary, to ultimately improve patient care. Translational research which attempts to answer questions originating in the clinical as well as in the molecular setting by combined approaches is an example of truly advanced interdisciplinary work[54] (Section 7).

Further reading

Dunlop, R.J., and Hockley, J.M. (1998). *Hospital-based palliative care teams. The hospital-hospice interface*, 2nd edition. Oxford University Press, Oxford.

Katzenbach, J.R., and Smith, D.K. (1992). *The wisdom of teams*. Harvard Business School Press, Boston, MA.

Speck, P. (ed.) (2006). *Teamwork in palliative care. Fulfilling or frustrating?* Oxford University Press, Oxford.

References

1. Katzenbach, J.R. and Smith, D.K. (1992). *The wisdom of teams*. Harvard Business School Press, Boston, MA.
2. Kane, R.A. (1975). The interprofessional team as a small group. *Social Work in Health Care*, **1**, 19–32.
3. Cummings, I. (1998). The interdisciplinary team. In *Oxford textbook of palliative medicine*, (eds. Doyle, D., Hanks, G.W.C., MacDonald, N.). 2nd edition, pp. 19–30, Oxford University Press, Oxford.
4. Crawford, G.B. and Price, S.D. (2003). Team working: palliative care as a model of interdisciplinary practice. *Medical Journal of Australia* **179**, S32–S34.
5. Drinka, T.J.K. (1994). Interdisciplinary geriatric teams: approaches to conflict as indicators of potential to model teamwork. *Educational Gerontology*, **20**, 87–103.
6. Øvretveit, J. (1996). Five ways to describe a multidisciplinary team. *J Interprof Care*, **10**, 163–71.
7. Øvretveit, J. (1990). Making the team work! *Journal of Professional Nursing*, **5**, 284–8.
8. Mickan, S.M. (2005). Evaluating the effectiveness of health care teams. *Aus Health Rev*, **29**, 211–7.
9. Lemieux-Charles, L. and McGuire, W.L. (2006). What do we know about health care team effectiveness? A review of the literature. *Med Care Res Rev*, **63**, 263–300.
10. Blomqvist, S. (2004). *Ju mer vi är tillsammans. Mångprofessionellt teamarbeta i vården*. FOG-report No. 50. Department of Behavioural Sciences (IBV), Linköping University, Linköping.
11. Mickan, S. and Rodger, S. (2000). Characteristics of effective teams: a literature review. *Australian Health Review*, **23**, 201–8.
12. Mickan, S.M. and Rodger, S.A. (2005). Effective health care teams: a model of six characteristics developed from shared perceptions. *J Interprof Care*, **19**, 358–70.
13. Maddocks, I. (2006). Communication—an essential tool for team hygiene. In *Teamwork in palliative care. Fulfilling or frustrating?* (ed. Speck, P.), pp. 137–52. Oxford University Press, Oxford.

14. MacMillan, K., Emery, B., and Kashuba, L. (2006). Organization and support of the interdisciplinary team. In *Textbook of palliative medicine* (eds. Bruera, E., Higginson, I., von Gunten, D., *et al.*), pp. 245–50. Oxford University Press, Oxford.

15. Reese, D.J. and Sontag, M.-A. (2001). Successful interprofessional collaboration on the hospice team. *Health and Social Work*, **26**, 167–75.

16. Freeman, M., Miller, C., and Ross, N. (2000). The impact of individual philosophies of teamwork on multi-professional practice and the implications for education. *Journal of Interprofessional Care*, **14**, 237–47.

17. Vinokur-Kaplan, D. (1995). Treatment teams that work (and those that don't): Application of Hackman's group effectiveness model to interdisciplinary teams in psychiatric hospitals. *Journal of Applied Behavioural Science*, **31**, 303–27.

18. Recommendation Rec (2003). 24 of the Committee of Ministers to member states on the organization of palliative care and explanatory memorandum (2003). Council of Europe Committee of Ministers.

19. Tuckman, B.W. (1965). Developmental sequences in small groups. *Psychological Bulletin*, **63**, 384–99.

20. Payne, M. (2006). Team building: how, why and when. In *Teamwork in palliative care. Fulfilling or frustrating?* (ed. Speck, P.), pp. 117–36. Oxford University Press, Oxford.

21. Barczak, N.L. (1996). How to lead effective teams. *Critical Care Nursing Quarterly*, **19**, 73–82.

22. Müller, M. and Kern, M. (2006). Kommunikation im Team. In *Lehrbuch der Palliativmedizin*, (eds. Aulbert, E., Nauck, F., and Radbruch, L.), 2nd edition, pp. 81-93. Schattauer, Stuttgart.

23. Speck, P. (2006). Maintaining a healthy team. In *Teamwork in palliative care. Fulfilling or frustrating?* (ed. Speck P.), pp. 95–115. Oxford University Press, Oxford.

24. Van Staa, A.L., Visser, A., and van der Zouwe, N. (2000). Caring for caregivers: experiences and evaluation of interventions for a palliative care team. *Patient Education and Counseling*, **41**, 93–105.

25. Nauck, F., Radbruch, L., Ostgathe, C., *et al.* (2002). Kerndokumentation für Palliativstationen. Strukturqualität und Ergebnisqualität. *Zeitschrift für Palliativmedizin*, **3**, 41–9.

26. Jünger, S., Pestinger, M., Elsner, F. *et al.* (2007). Criteria for successful multiprofessional cooperation in palliative care teams. *Palliative Medicine*, **21**, 347–54.

27. Cintron, A. and Meier, D.E. (2006). The palliative care consult team. In *Textbook of palliative medicine* (eds. Bruera, E., Higginson, I., von Gunten, D., Ripamonti, C.), pp. 259-65. Oxford University Press, Oxford.

28. National Council for Hospice and Specialist Palliative Care Services (1999). *Palliative Care 2000—Commissioning Through Partnership.* NCHSPCS, London.

29. Palliative care delivery in acute hospitals: hospital palliative care teams. In *Getting started: guidelines and suggestions for those considering starting a hospice/palliative care service.* (Doyle, D., Chan K.S., Mosoin, D., *et al.*) IAHPC, www.hospicecare.com

30. National Consensus Project for Quality Palliative Care (2004). *Clinical practice guidelines for quality palliative care.* National Consensus Project for Quality Palliative Care, New York.

31. Norwegian Association for Palliative Medicine (2004). *Norwegian Standard for Palliative Care.* English translation 2006. Norwegian Medical Association, Oslo. http://www.palliativmed. orgasset/32504/1/32504_1.pdf.

32. Palliative Care Australia (2002). *Palliative care. Service provision in Australia: a planning guide.* PCA, Canberra.

33. Saunders, C. (2000). The evolution of palliative care. *Patient Education and Counseling*, **41**, 7–13.

34. Dunlop, R.J., and Hockley, J.M. (1998). *Hospital-based palliative care teams. The hospital-hospice interface.* 2nd edition. Oxford University Press, Oxford.

35. Hockley, J. (1999). Specialist palliative care within the acute hospital setting. *Acta Oncologica*, **38**, 491–4.

36. Mount, B.M. (1976). The problem of caring for the dying in a general hospital; the palliative care unit as a possible solution. *CMA Journal*, **115**, 119–21.

37. Currow, D.C. and Nightingale, E.M. (2003). "A planning guide": developing a consensus document for palliative care service provision. *Medical Journal of Australia*, **179**, S23–S25.

38. El Osta, B. and Bruera, E. (2006). Models of palliative care delivery. In *Textbook of palliative medicine* (eds. Bruera, E., Higginson, I., von Gunten, D., Ripamonti, C.), pp. 266–76. Oxford University Press, Oxford.

39. Davies, E. and Higginson, I.J. (Eds.) (2004). *Better palliative care for older people. A WHO collaboration project.* WHO, Geneva.

40. Francke, A.L. and Kerkstra, A. (2000). Palliative care services in the Netherlands: a descriptive study. *Patient Education and Counseling*, **41**, 23–33.

41. Hospice information (2005). *Hospice and palliative care: Facts and figures 2005.* Hospice Information, London. www.hospiceinformation.info

42. O'Neill, W.M., O'Connor, P., and Latimer, E.J. (1992). Hospital palliative care services: three models in three countries. *Journal of Pain and Symptom Management*, **7**, 406–13.

43. Glare, P.A., Auret, K.A., Aggarwal, G. *et al.* (2003). The interface between palliative medicine and specialists in acute-care hospitals: boundaries, bridges and challenges. *Medical Journal of Australia*, **179**, S29–S31.

44. Ellershaw, J.E., Peat, S.J., and Boys, L.C. (1995). Assessing the effectiveness of a hospital palliative care team. *Palliative Medicine*, **9**, 145–52.

45. Higginson, I.J., Finlay, I., Goodwin, D.M. *et al.* (2002). Do hospital-based palliative teams improve care for patients or families at the end of life? *Journal of Pain and Symptom Management*, **23**, 96–106.

46. Hearn, J., Higginson, I.J. (1998). Do specialist palliative care teams improve outcomes for cancer patients? A systematic literature review. *Palliative Medicine*, **12**, 317–32.

47. Jack, B., Hillier, V., Williams, A., *et al.* (2004). Hospital based palliative care teams improve the insight of cancer patients into their disease. *Palliative Medicine*, **18**, 46–52.

48. Vernooij-Dassen, M.J.F.J., Groot, M.M., van den Berg, J. *et al.* (2007). Consultation in palliative care: the relevance of clarification of problems. *European Journal of Cancer*, **43**, 316–22.

49. Schneider, N., Ebeling, H., Amelung, V.E. *et al.* (2006). Hospital doctors' attitudes towards palliative care in Germany. *Palliative Medicine*, **20**, 499–506.

50. Hunt, J., Keeley, V.L., Cobb, M. *et al.* (2004). A new quality assurance package for hospital palliative care teams: the Trent Hospice Audit Group model. *British Journal of Cancer*, **91**, 248–53.

51. Fulmer, T., and Hyer, K. (1998). Evaluating the effects of geriatric interdisciplinary team training. In *Geriatric interdisciplinary team training* (eds. Siegler, E.L., Hyer, K., Fulmer, T., *et al.*), pp. 115–46. Springer, New York.

52. Lawrie, I., and Lloyd-Williams, M. (2006). Training in the interdisciplinary environment. In (ed. Speck, P.) *Teamwork in palliative care. Fulfilling or frustrating?* pp. 153-65. Oxford University Press, Oxford.

53. Jeffrey, D. (ed.) (2003). *Teaching palliative care: A practical guide.* Radcliffe Medical Press Ltd, Oxon.

54. Kaasa, S., and Dale, O. (2005). Building up research in palliative care: an historical perspective and a case for the future. *Clinics in Geriatric Medicine*, **21**, 81–92.

4.2

Nursing and palliative care

Deborah Witt Sherman

Although nursing is one of the oldest of the arts, it is one of the youngest of the professions. The origin of the word nursing is derived from the Latin word nutrire which means 'to nourish' and the word nurse has its roots in the word nutrix which means 'nursing mother'. Over the centuries, the meaning of these terms have broadened to encompass the training and education of a person who cares not only for the sick and dying but also who cares for humanity[1].

Nursing has long been defined as both an art and a science. Nursing has moved beyond knowledge gained by reliance on tradition, trial and error, or authoritative statements of experts, to the generation of knowledge based on logical analysis and scientific inquiry. As a humanistic science, the purpose of nursing is to describe, explain, predict, and control phenomenon central to its concern, that of people and our world. The art of nursing is the creative use of the science of nursing for human betterment[2].

Nursing has been an integral part of societal movements involved in the existing culture, while shaping and being shaped by the culture[1]. Although the experience of dying and death is part of the human condition, illness and death often can be delayed by science and medical technology. Life prolonging therapies have assisted individuals to live longer with life-threatening illness, although death ultimately occurs. It has been understood that the care of those with life-threatening illness requires the best of modern science with an appreciation of emotional, social, and spiritual needs and ways of alleviating associated suffering.

The hospice model of care was developed in 1967 from this understanding of the holistic needs of the dying. Yet, as individuals are living longer with life-threatening illness, practitioners have realized that patients and families have needs and concerns that begin at the time of diagnosis and that such comprehensive care is needed from the time of diagnosis forward. Furthermore, care must be extended to families during the illness experience through the death of the patient and into the bereavement period. It also has become apparent that this type of care is needed by patients with all types of life-threatening illnesses and not only by those with cancer.

Although hospice care and palliative care are viewed as synonymous by some authors, palliative care also may be understood as evolving from the original model of hospice care and more explicitly endorsing the need to provide a combination of disease-modifying and supportive therapies intended to prevent and alleviate the suffering experienced by patients with any type of life-threatening illness and their families. Palliative care focuses on pain and symptom control, while addressing the emotional, social, cultural, and spiritual needs of patients and families experiencing progressive illness. The goal of palliative care is to support the best possible quality of life of patients and their families[3].

Nurses, who are educated in palliative-care nursing, 'facilitate the caring process through a combination of science, presence, openness, compassion, mindful attention to detail, and teamwork[4] As members of the interdisciplinary palliative-care team, nurses, physicians, social workers, and other health professionals each bring their own specialized competence and expertise gained through education, credentialling, and experience. Through interdisciplinary collaboration, an effective and compassionate plan of care is developed based on the best scientific evidence available, clinical judgement, and a recognition of the wishes and preferences of the patient and family, known as evidence-based practice.

As the largest number of health-care professionals, nurses have a tremendous potential to change the care of dying of patients and their families by capitalizing on the individual's need for control and emphasizing the patients' and families' active participation in decision making. Nurses' discussions with patients and families can 'replace uncertainty with certainty, hopelessness with faith and despair with empowerment. Palliative-care nursing is an exquisite blend of aggressive management of pain and symptoms associated with disease and its treatment, coupled with holistic, humanistic caring'[5]. Palliative-care nursing requires the integration of empirical, aesthetic, personal, and ethical knowledge in providing patient- and family-centered holistic care. [6] This integration of nursing knowledge assists nurses in reshaping societal perspectives regarding dying and death from that of fear to the possibilities of dying as an opportunity for healing and continued growth for patients, families, and all who bear witness.

Integration of knowledge in palliative-care nursing

The statement 'I failed to care for him properly because I was ignorant[4]' speaks to the need for health professionals, including nurses, to be educated in palliative care. Coyle[4] states that 'Clinicians cannot practice what they do not know'. The knowledge of a discipline includes information, facts, principles, and theories that are organized according to the beliefs of the discipline. A body of knowledge is derived from the focus or unique perspective of the discipline and provides an organizing framework for the discipline's practice. The development of nursing knowledge supports expert practice and provides professional identity, which conveys to others what nursing contributes to health care.

Throughout nursing history, knowledge has been obtained through tradition, expert opinion, borrowed knowledge from other disciplines, and role modelling. As nursing has developed as a profession, it has been recognized that nursing practice must be based on empirical knowledge, or the science of nursing, which involves problem solving, logical reasoning, and scientific inquiry. Empirical knowledge draws upon a reality that can be observed and measured, and therefore verified by others[6]. Qualitative and quantitative research builds and tests nursing theories and provides important insights regarding the phenomena of interest to nursing, specifically the lives of people situated in particular environments who have diverse ways of promoting health, preventing illness, and managing disease, all with the hope of improving quality of life. The development and testing of theories through research provides the evidence that informs evidence-based practice. As a new specialty in medicine and nursing, all levels of evidence from expert opinion to meta-analyses of randomized controlled trials provide the empirical knowledge needed to guide practice in palliative care. The combination of evidence-based medicine and humanistic and compassionate care represents the imperative to couple the science of nursing with the art of nursing.

Aesthetic knowledge or the art of nursing involves a deep appreciation of the meaning of a situation. Aesthetic knowing is made visible through the actions, conduct, attitudes, narrative, and interactions of the nurse in relation to others. It involves participating in or experiencing another's feelings and the ability to envision valid ways of helping in relation to desired outcomes. Aesthetic knowledge enables a nurse to envision the possibilities and to know what to do and how to be in the moment. Aesthetic knowledge supports the dynamic integration of parts into a whole[6] In the care of those with life-threatening or chronic illness, aesthetic knowledge enables the nurse to see the entire situation related to the interplay of physical, emotional, social, cultural, and spiritual needs and to develop a plan of care that focuses on the whole person within the context of their family and community. Evidence-based practice involves not only empirical knowledge but also an understanding of the meaning of the situation, which further informs clinical judgement. In addition to the integration of empirical and aesthetic knowledge, the clinician also integrates their personal and professional experiences in the form of personal knowledge.

Personal knowledge refers to the inner experience of becoming a whole and genuine person. Personal knowing encompasses knowing one's own self and others[6]. Empiric theories can be learned, but their meaning for the individual comes from personal reflection and experience. Personal knowing occurs through entering the world of the person being cared for, understanding their world, and responding to them. Personal knowledge is therefore concerned with the quality of interpersonal contacts, promoting therapeutic relationships, and providing individualized care. Personal knowledge also involves personal integrity and honesty, as well as enthusiasm, courage, and imagination[6]. As palliative-care clinicians, nurses reflect on their own or their families' experience of illness, loss, and grief, or those of patients for whom they have cared. With personal knowledge, nurses respond in loving, and supportive ways to the suffering of patients and families. Lastly, ethical knowledge must be integrated in palliative care.

Ethical knowledge or the moral component of nursing is concerned with the right action within a situation. It includes voluntary actions that are deliberate and subject to judgement as right or wrong.

Ethical knowing in nursing requires both experiential knowledge and knowledge of the formal principles, ethical codes, and theories of the discipline and society. It involves advocating for the patient. Ethical knowledge provides insight about which choices are possible and why. It provides direction toward choices that are good, sound, responsible or just[6]. In palliative-care nursing, ethical knowledge is very important in assisting patients and families in making end-of-life decisions. Palliative-care nurses are often members of ethics committees and grapple with ethical dilemmas in clinical situations.

Each individual pattern of knowing is necessary but insufficient alone for achieving the goals of nursing. All of the ways of knowing are important in defining the whole. This is illustrated by considering the response to a common question: 'Which nursing intervention is best to relieve pain?' An *empirical* study can test hypothetical relationships among methods of pain management, each of which is influenced by *aesthetic* meanings of relieving pain, *personal* meanings concerning the experience of pain, and *ethical* values that influence how and when pain relief is given and received. Failure to integrate knowledge within all of the patterns of knowing leads to uncritical acceptance, narrow interpretation, and partial utilization of knowledge. When this occurs, the ways of knowing are used in isolation from one another and the potential for synthesis of the whole is lost. When removed from the context of the whole of knowing, empirics produces control and manipulation; aesthetics produces indulgence in self-serving expressions and lack of appreciation for the meaning in a context; personal knowing produces isolation and self-distortion, and ethics produces rigid doctrine and insensitivity to others[6]. Palliative-care nursing, therefore, involves the integration of all patterns of knowing in alleviating suffering and creating an opportunity in which illness, dying and death may be a time of healing or being made whole. Whether through formal education or continuing education of nurses in palliative care, it is important to recognize the integration of empirical, aesthetic, personal, and ethical knowledge so that nurses can 'practice what they know' and provide a holistic plan of care that is effective and compassionate.

Evolutionary persective of hospice and palliative nursing

Hospice nursing, which began in the early 1970s, predated the development of the current model of palliative-care nursing, which is now established in many countries. In the USA, the impetus for this change were the publications arising from the landmark SUPPORT study during the late 1990s. This study highlighted an urgent need for health-care professionals who are prepared and committed to improving the quality of life for seriously ill and dying patients, and their families[7]. The national attention regarding palliative care also resulted from an interest in death and dying; increasing integration of pain and symptom management into conventional care; concern about the high cost of dying; greater attention to the role of medicine in caring rather than curing; and national debates on physician-assisted suicide and euthanasia[8]. Furthermore, it was recognized that patients and families have been left on their own to decide how to achieve a 'peaceful death' and how to live with maximum quality and comfort given the existence of an incurable, life-threatening disease. In the USA, this distress was increased by the public's and professional's lack of knowledge about how to access related services and to secure reimbursement, both of which were potential contributors to ineffective end-of-life care[8].

Based on the United States' Institute of Medicine's study on end-of-life care, Field and Cassel[9] reiterated 'the urgent need for consensus and action to improve care for those approaching death'. It was noted that Americans now live far longer than they did in the 19th century, with an average life expectancy in the USA of nearly 77 years and more than 70 per cent of the population dying after the age of 65, and that the leading causes of death during the past 100 years have changed from primarily infectious processes to chronic illnesses experienced by an aging population. This demographic shift, which is shared by all developed countries, means that the dying process for a large and growing proportion of the population has been extended with some individuals facing a steady and fairly predictable decline, such as those with cancer, while others have long periods of chronic illness punctuated by crises that are often fatal[9]. The result is a national increase in the number of individuals who require palliative care. While hospice/palliative care has been delivered mainly to patients with cancer, other patients with incurable diseases are candidates for these services, including the growing number of elderly, and those suffering from chronic diseases[10].

The evolution of the field of palliative care has been a response to the changing profile of illness, dying, and death in the 20th century. The expanding purview of this model of care, which has extended 'upstream' from end-of-life care, and the growing number of patients with life-threatening illnesses, together presage a steady increase in the need for palliative-care services during the decades to come. In the USA, the rise in the number of patients and families accessing hospice care supports this projection of future needs for palliative care and hospice services[11].

In meeting the needs of patients with life-threatening illness, there has been concern about the educational preparation of nurses. In the USA, the education of nurses in end-of-life care has been inconsistent at best, and neglected for the most part, in both undergraduate and graduate nursing curricula[12]. In accordance with the International Council of Nurses' mandate that nurses have a unique and primary responsibility for ensuring the peaceful death of patients, the American Association of Colleges of Nursing convened a round table of expert nurses to identify the precepts underlying hospice and palliative care. They concurred that these precepts be foundational to the educational preparation of nurses. Based on these precepts, the document, entitled 'Peaceful Death', was developed, which outlined baccalaureate competencies for palliative/hospice care and content areas where competencies can be taught[12].

At the same time, the American Nurses Association formulated a position statement regarding the promotion of comfort and relief of pain of dying patients, reinforcing nurses' obligation to promote comfort and ensure aggressive efforts to relieve pain and suffering. National, state, and local indicators also pointed to the need for all nurses to have generalist-level knowledge of palliative care. Since 2000, initiatives in the USA have been underway to include palliative-care content in nursing textbooks; integrate palliative-care content in associate degree and baccalaureate programmes; and provide practising nurses with training through the project known as ELNEC (End-of-Life Nursing Education Consortium). Furthermore, nursing textbooks regarding palliative-care nursing have been published, the first of which were the *Textbook of Palliative Nursing*[13] and *Palliative-care Nursing: Quality Care to the End of Life*[14], which are both in their second editions.

An interdisciplinary approach is a core element of palliative and hospice care, and it has been recognized that advanced practice nurses (APNs) must have the appropriate educational preparation to assume responsibility for health-care decisions and to be acknowledged as equal members of the palliative-care team. In the USA, the first Advanced Practice Palliative Care Nurse Practitioner Program was begun at New York University, NY in 1998, and the first Palliative Care Clinical Nurse Specialist Program was begun at Ursuline College, Ohio. Today, several nursing programmes are either offering a master's degree in palliative-care nursing or combining palliative care with other master's programmes such as an adult health master's programme. Advanced Practice Palliative Master's Programs have also begun recently in other countries, such as at Tenshi College in Sapporo, Japan.

Advanced Practice Palliative Care Nurses who have advanced knowledge and skill in palliative care play a vital role by assessing, implementing, coordinating, and evaluating care throughout the disease trajectory, as well as counselling and educating patients and families, and facilitating continuity of care between hospital and home. APNs also obtain knowledge about ethical issues facing individuals and families, and develop strategies to assist them in defining expected goals of care, as well as accessing and coordinating appropriate care. In addition to clinical expertise, APNs may assume leadership roles in practice, education, research, and administration, which further advances palliative and hospice care as a nursing specialty.

The evolution of hospice nursing in the USA has been supported by the Hospice Nurses Association, which was incorporated in 1987 as the first professional organization committed to promoting excellence in hospice nursing. Certification in hospice nursing was a critical focus of the Association, particularly given the increased demand for hospice nurses. In 1992, the Board of Directors of the Hospice Association appointed the National Board for the Certification of Hospice Nurses (NBCHN). In March of 1994, the NBCHN offered the first certification examination and the credential of Certified Registered Nurse Hospice (CRNH).

During the first decade of the Hospice Nurses Association, the members largely worked in certified hospice programmes, which in the USA, have focused on patients with short life expectancies. By 1997, however, the Association realized the need to embrace palliative-care nursing as a part of the continuum of care. The results of the 1998 generalist hospice and palliative nurse Role Delineation Study, commissioned by the NBCHN, demonstrated that only minor differences in practice activity existed between end-of-life care offered by nurses who worked in hospice programmes and nurses working with seriously ill patients in non-hospice settings. These differences correlated with requirements of the role or practice setting. The association's name was thereby changed to the Hospice and Palliative Care Nurses Association (HPNA). The mission of HPNA includes:

- promoting the highest professional standards of hospice and palliative nursing;

- studying, researching and exchanging information, experiences, and ideas that improve nursing practice;

- encouraging nurses to specialize in palliative care and hospice nursing;

- fostering professional development;

- responding to the changing needs of HPNA members and the populations they represent; and

◆ promoting recognition of palliative and hospice nursing as essential components within the health-care system[15].

In 1999, the NBCHN became the National Board for the Certification of Hospice and Palliative Nurses (NBCHPN), offering a new designation to recognize basic competence in hospice and palliative nursing, specifically the title of Certified Hospice and Palliative Nurse (CHPN). Since 2000, more than 1000 new members have joined the organization each year. The current membership is more than 7500, and by early 2001, the number of nurses credentialed at the basic level rose to over 7000[15].

The development of palliative nursing as a specialty practice also continued to evolve in the USA. In 2000, the NBCHPN began discussions with New York University, which was awarded a grant by the Soros Foundation to initiate development of an advanced practice palliative care credentialling examination under the leadership of Dr. Deborah Witt Sherman. NBCHPN developed an examination in collaboration with the American Nursing Credentialing Center. In 2002, a role delineation study was conducted which examined the roles of advanced practice palliative-care nurse practitioners (NPs) and clinical nurse specialists (CNSs). The results indicated that palliative-care NPs and clinical specialists in the USA have the same knowledge and skills, but the percentage of time spent in the various domains of practice differed. For example, the CNS may spend more time educating colleagues than the NP, although both may provide palliative-care education. These findings supported the development of a single advanced practice palliative-care certification exam, which could be taken by both groups of APNs. Following the development of the scope, standards, and competencies of advanced practice palliative-care nursing, an advanced practice palliative-care certification exam was developed in 2002. This certification examination is now owned exclusively by NBCHPN.

Committed to the certification of all levels of nurses, NBCHPN also developed a certification exam for licensed practical nurses in hospice and palliative care, which was funded through the Fan Fox and Leslie R. Samuels Foundation. As of 2005, an examination for nursing assistants in hospice and palliative care has been developed, making NBCHPN the first organization to offer certification to all levels of caregivers in a specific specialty and to assure their competency in providing palliative and hospice care.

Certification in Hospice and Palliative Care Nursing is valued because the individual nurse:

◆ has a tested and proven competency across the spectrum of hospice and palliative-care nursing care;

◆ has access to a national network of experienced and knowledgeable hospice and palliative-care nurses;

◆ has demonstrated a commitment to his or her specialty practice by pursuing certification;

◆ has demonstrated dedication of professional development in his or her nursing career; and

◆ is an asset to his or her employer in an atmosphere of increasing awareness regarding quality in health care[15].

The scope of hospice and palliative-care nursing

The scope of palliative and hospice nursing continues to evolve as the art and science of palliative care develop. The philosophical precepts of palliative and hospice care emphasize the importance of holistic care offered to patients and families across the life span and in diverse health-care settings. As such, palliative and hospice nurses provide evidence-based care that addresses the physical, emotional, social, and spiritual/existential needs of patients and their families, with the primary goal of promoting quality of life through the relief of suffering along the illness trajectory.

Relief of suffering and the possibility of improved quality of life for individuals and families are enhanced by:

◆ providing effective pain and symptom management;

◆ addressing psychosocial and spiritual needs of patient and family;

◆ incorporating cultural values and attitudes in developing a plan of care;

◆ creating a healing environment to promote a peaceful death;

◆ supporting those who are experiencing loss, grief, and bereavement;

◆ promoting ethical and legal decision making;

◆ advocating for personal wishes and preferences;

◆ utilizing therapeutic communication skills in all interactions;

◆ facilitating collaborative practice;

◆ insuring access to care and community resources through influencing/developing health and social policy;

◆ contributing to improved quality and cost effective services;

◆ creating opportunities and implementing initiatives for palliative-care education for patients, families, colleagues, and community; and

◆ participating in the generation, testing, and/or evaluation of palliative-care knowledge and practice[16].

Palliative-care nursing is provided to patients and families in acute care hospital units; inpatient palliative-care units; inpatient, home, or residential hospices; ambulatory palliative-care clinics; long-term care facilities and assisted living facilities; prisons; and private practices[16].

By articulating the scope and standards of professional nursing practice, the specialty defines its boundaries, informs society about the parameters of nursing practices, and develops the regulations for the specialty. As in all nursing specialties, nurses must practice within the scope of their specialty, as outlined by regulation, a professional code of ethics, and professional practices standards[16]

Nursing practice is differentiated according to the nurses' educational preparation and level of practice, which ranges from basic through advanced level of competency. Certified at the basic level of competency, the nurse may be licensed as a licensed practical nurse or registered professional nurse who has gained competencies in palliative and hospice care through their general educational programmes, professional work experiences, and ongoing continuing education. For nurses certified with advanced practice competencies, the title APN is used as an inclusive term to describe the common core of knowledge, skills, and attitudes of both the CNS and NP. In many practice settings, a blended role exists, which combines the strengths of the CNS and NP; the primary care education as an NP is blended with the specialty focus of the CNS into a position that includes research, education, and systems change[17]. By virtue of graduate education and related clinical expertise, the advanced practice palliative-care nurse demonstrates greater depth and breath of knowledge and skill in theory, research, and practice reflected in the standards of care of palliative care and hospice nursing[16].

The standards of care of hospice and palliative-care nursing

The standards of care reflect the values and priorities of palliative-care nursing and provide a framework to evaluate practice[16]. Standards are authoritative statements, written in measurable terms, which define the palliative-care nurses' responsibilities and their accountability to the public regarding patient/family outcomes. The nursing process includes clinical decision-making and encompasses all actions of the nurse in the care of patients and families. Although the standards, which express the philosophical beliefs of palliative-care nursing, remain stable over time, the criteria related to each standard changes as scientific knowledge and technology are advanced. The standards of care are written both at the basic and advanced practice levels and reflect the nursing process, involving assessment, diagnosis, outcomes identification, planning, implementation, and evaluation. Foundational to the standards of care are the following tenets:

- care should be age appropriate and culturally sensitive;
- a safe environment is to be maintained;
- education of patients and families is essential;
- coordination and continuity of care across settings and caregivers must occur; and
- communication and the management of information must be effective[16].

Standard I: assessment

At the basic level of competence, the palliative-care nurse collects individual and family data. At the advanced practice level, the alliative-care nurse conducts in-depth and comprehensive assessment based on a synthesis of individual and family health data. The immediate needs of patients and families determine the priority for data collection. Data collection involves information from multiple sources, obtained through various assessment techniques, including the use of standardized instruments. Assessment is systematic and ongoing. Assessment includes a comprehensive health history, review of systems, physical examination, determination of functional status, information from laboratory data or diagnostic tests, identification of goals of care, and determination of patients' and families' emotional status, spiritual well-being, coping techniques, and resources. The assessment data are prioritized and documented[16].

Standard II: diagnosis

At the basic level of competence, the palliative-care nurse analyses the assessment data in determining nursing diagnoses. At the advanced practice level, the palliative-care nurse utilizes an accepted framework that supports palliative-care nursing knowledge. Clinical judgement is used in critically analyzing data in the formulation of differential medical diagnoses and nursing diagnoses. Diagnoses are derived from multi-dimensional sources of data; are validated with the patient, family, and interdisciplinary team; identify actual or potential responses to alterations in health; identify problems that may be prevented, resolved or diminished by nursing interventions; and are communicated and documented in the medical record[16].

Standard III: outcome identification

The palliative-care nurse educated at the basic level identifies expected outcomes relevant to the patient and family in collaboration with the interdisciplinary team. The palliative-care nurse educated at the advanced level identifies outcomes based on the critical analyses of both complex assessment data and diagnoses. Expected outcomes are mutually formulated with the patient, family, interdisciplinary team, and other health-care providers, when appropriate. Outcomes are culturally sensitive and reflect the patient and families values, beliefs, and preferences. Expected outcomes are realistic in accordance with the goals of care and evidence-based practice. Expected outcomes reflect continuity of care across all settings from admission through family bereavement. At the advanced practice level, the palliative-care nurse also determines risks, benefits, and costs, as well as modifying the outcomes based on changes in the patients' and families' health status[16].

Standard IV: planning

At the basic level of competency, the palliative-care nurse develops a plan of care that includes interventions and treatments to attain the expected outcomes. At the advanced practice level, the palliative-care nurse develops a comprehensive plan of care that prescribes evidence-based interventions and reviews with individuals the risks and burdens. The plan of care is individualized to the needs, desires and resources of the patient and family, and is developed in collaboration with members of the interdisciplinary team. The plan is dynamic and is updated regularly, yet provides continuity of care. At the advanced practice level, the palliative-care nurse develops strategies that promote quality of life through independent clinical decision-making and provides direction and guidance to other members of the interdisciplinary team[16].

Standard V: implementation

At the basic level, the palliative-care nurse implements the interventions ordered by the physician or APN. At the advanced level, the palliative-care nurse prescribes, orders or implements medical and nursing interventions. Interventions are evidence-based, implemented in a safe, timely and ethical manner, and modified based on continual assessment of the patients' or families' response. The interventions are documents in a format that is related to the patient and family outcomes, accessible to the interdisciplinary team, and retrievable for future data analysis and research. At the basic level of practice, the interventions involve the provision of direct care, which facilitate self-care; maximize, restore, or maintain function; enhance well-being; support healthy patterns of living; and provide emotional support and the relief of symptoms. At the advanced practice level, palliative-care nurses supplement interventions at the basic level with sophisticated skills in data synthesis; they may negotiate health-related services and additional specialized care, provide consultation, employ complex strategies, oversee interventions and teaching modalities to promote and maintain health, and makes appropriate referrals[16].

Standard VI: evaluation

The palliative-care nurse educated at the basic level evaluates the patients' and families' progress in attaining expected outcomes. At the advanced level, the palliative-care nurse critically appraises and comprehensively evaluates all relevant data related to attainment of expected outcomes. Evaluation is systematic, criterion-based, ongoing, and reviewed with other members of the interdisciplinary team. Revisions in the diagnosis, expected outcomes, and the plan of care are documented and communicated to the patient, family, and other members of the team to ensure continuity of care. At the advanced practice level, palliative-care nurses incorporate advanced knowledge, practice, and research into the evaluation process and assume responsibility for the process[16].

Achieving the standards of professional performance in palliative- and hospice-care nursing

The standards of professional performance describe the competent professional role behaviours of palliative and hospice nurses, including activities related to quality of care, performance appraisal, education, collegiality, ethics, collaboration, research, and resource utilization[16]. The palliative-care nurse participates in quality-care activities appropriate to the individual's position, education, and practice environment. Performance appraisal occurs as nurses at the basic and advanced level of competency evaluate their nursing practice in relation to the professional practice standards and standards of care. Palliative-care nurses' professionalism is enhanced through membership in professional organizations and certification in their specialty. Acting in a collegial manner, the palliative-care nurse contributes to the professional development of peers and other health-care providers. At the advanced practice level, the palliative-care nurse also serves as a leader and role model. Ethical behaviour is demonstrated as the palliative-care nurse makes decisions and acts on behalf of the patient and family. At the advanced practice level, the nurse demonstrates moral discernment, critical reasoning, and discriminating judgement in integrating ethics into palliative practice. Palliative-care nurses at the basic level of competency collaborates with other team members, while the advance practice nurse promotes an interdisciplinary approach to care. Furthermore, palliative-care nurses use research findings in practice. At the advanced practice, palliative-care nurses utilize research to identify, examine, validate, and evaluate knowledge and develop creative approaches to health care. Lastly, palliative-care nurses at both the basic and advanced levels of practice consider factors related to resource utilization such as safety, efficacy, and cost in the planning and delivery of comprehensive care.

Generalist level and specialist level palliative-care nursing

The current expectation is that all registered nurses have a basic level of knowledge regarding palliative care at the generalist level. This includes a holistic approach to care including pain and symptom assessment and management, cultural competence, effective communication skills, recognition of ethical and legal aspects of care, and knowledge regarding care of the imminently dying patient. At the specialist level, nurses have specific education related to hospice and palliative-care nursing at a basic or advanced level of competency and related clinical experience. This is accomplished through continuing education initiatives, such as attendance at conferences, or through independent learning. Advanced practice specialist level preparation is accomplished through enrolment in palliative care master's or post-master's programmes. Through clinical experience and continuing education in palliative care, APNs in other specialties are also eligible to sit for the advanced practice palliative-care certification examination.

Several studies have examined the role of the APN in palliative care, yet the majority of these studies have been conducted outside of the USA. Based on a study conducted in Switzerland, Hurlimann, Hofer and Hirter [18], reported that CNSs in palliative care influence patient care by direct care, bedside teaching, and case reviews. Jack, Oldham, and Williams [19] conducted a qualitative study to investigate the role of the CNS within a palliative-care team in an acute care hospital setting in the UK. The results, based on interviews of 23 nurses and physicians, indicated that palliative-care NPs offer support and advice to colleagues, and education, which improves the quality care. Corner *et al.*[20] conducted a longitudinal study in England, which enrolled 76 patients and assigned them to 12 Macmillan palliative-care nurses over a 28-day period. Based on the EORTC Quality of Life Questionnaire, significant improvements in emotional and cognitive functioning and in patient anxiety scores, measured by the Palliative Care Outcomes Scale, were reported from baseline to day 7. Patient records further indicated overall positive outcomes of care from Macmillan specialist palliative care interventions in 42 (55 per cent) of cases.

Quaglietti, Blum, and Ellis[21] propose that APNs are uniquely positioned to 'bridge' the gaps in health care based on their independent practice, varied practice sites, and improving reimbursement patterns. Studies have also been conducted regarding the effectiveness of specific roles of nurses in improving the quality of life of patients with life-threatening diseases. Aiken *et al.*[22] conducted a randomized trial comparing the PhoenixCare demonstration programme of palliative care and coordinated care/case management for serious chronically ill patients with chronic heart failure (n = 130) and chronic obstructive pulmonary disease (n = 62), with an equal number of controls who received active treatment from the managed care organizations. Intensive home-based case management was provided by RN case managers to address disease and symptom management, preparation for end of life, physical and mental functioning, and utilization of medical services. The results indicated that patients in the intervention group had lower symptom distress, greater physical function, higher self-rated health, and better outcomes on self-management of illness. This novel model of patient care, which combined greatly enhanced palliative care with ongoing managed care organization treatment, was associated with improved quality of life for patients with serious chronic illness. Further studies are warranted to provide evidence regarding the patient and family outcomes and cost effectiveness of care offered by hospice and palliative-care nurses, particularly those at the advanced practice level.

Visions for palliative and hospice nursing

Nursing is a way of being in the world which involves a desire to support, and care for others and the intention to heal. Nurses witness the suffering of people and are drawn towards them very often in informal caregiving roles as family members, friends, or members of a community, as well as in professional roles. In witnessing suffering and death, there is often an awakening of nurses' own sense of mortality. Nurses learn of the preciousness of each day, the struggles to find meaning in life and death, as well as the opportunities to transcend the mundane and realize a connection to something larger than self. Though nurses may view living and dying through different lenses because of different cultural or spiritual perspectives, nurses' intentions remain focused on doing good, preventing harm, and being fair and just as they care competently and compassionately for others. As nurses mature as people and in their role as nurses, the egocentric 'I' shifts to a 'We'. The pain or joys of others are felt in a nurses' heart and their intellect strives to gain the knowledge and skills necessary to offer care to the whole person—mind, body, and spirit. Nurses seek to understand the world not only through formal education, but also through their life experiences as they learn about themselves and observe others. Indeed, patients and families often demonstrate a sense of resiliency in the face of adversity and teach others how to die with grace and dignity.

Nurses strive to understand the societal changes occurring at international, national, regional, and local levels that influence health and well-being. Nurses seek to make a difference in the lives of their patients, families, and communities as they work towards human betterment and goals that promote the greater good.

The future vision for hospice and palliative-care nursing rests on the belief that nurses are a valuable resource in national efforts to improve care and quality of life for patients and their families living with advanced, life-limiting illness. It is through collaborative efforts that the roles of hospice and palliative-care nurses will be fully actualized. Professional organizations in nursing, medicine, hospice, and palliative are called upon to engage in dialogue about the role of APNs, and opportunities and strategies to advance the role. Nursing educators must become knowledgeable about palliative care and develop continuing education programs which support hospice and palliative-care nursing competencies.

Payers of health-care services are called upon to recognize the specialty of palliative care and provide APNs with adequate and consistent compensation that is commensurate with APNs scope of practice, authority, and responsibility, regardless of practice setting. Regulatory agencies, such as State Boards of Nursing in the USA, are called upon to work collaboratively and consistently to recognize the scope and standards of advanced practice palliative-care nursing. Health-care Systems or Health Service Providers are asked to develop or expand practice opportunities for APNs in all settings that care for patients who may experience life-threatening illness. who practice in hospice and palliative care are called upon to document and disseminate the outcomes of their practice experience and roles, engage in interdisciplinary research and translate research findings into practice[23].

The vision for hospice and palliative-care nursing will be actualized through the collective efforts and commitment of nurses at all levels of practice. Nurses' full potential in health care will be fulfilled by a combination of exceptional knowledge in nursing, technical skill, sensitivity, originality, ambition, desire, and self-respect. Nurses must continue to nurture their intellect, creativity, and souls; rely on their authority and not others; value the integrity of human wholeness by offering care which integrates empirical, aesthetic, personal, and ethical knowledge; and have faith and confidence in their own ability. Indeed, a universe of infinite potentials arise for hospice and palliative care nurses as they 'Dream Big' and create a reality which improves the quality of care and quality of life of patients with life-threatening illness and their families.

References

1. Donahue, M. (1985). *Nursing: The finest art*. The C. V. Mosby Company, St Louis, MO.
2. Rogers, M.E. (1992). Nursing science and the space age. *Nursing Science Quarterly*, **5**, 27–34.
3. National Consensus Project (2004). *National consensus guidelines for quality palliative care*. retrieved from http://www.national.consensusproject.org on 7 March 2006.
4. Coyle, N. (2006). Introduction to palliative care nursing. In *The textbook of palliative nursing* (eds. Ferrell, B.R. and Coyle, N.). Oxford University Press, New York.
5. Sherman, D.W., and Matzo, M. (2006). Preface. In *Palliative care nursing: quality care to the end of life* (eds. Matzo, M. and Sherman, D.W.). Springer Publishers, New York.
6. Carper, B.A. (1978). Fundamental patterns of knowing in nursing. *Advances in Nursing Science*, **1**, 13–23.
7. SUPPORT principal investigators (1995). A controlled trial to improve care for seriously ill hospitalized patients. *JAMA*, **274**, 1591–636.
8. Billings, J.A., and Block, S. (1997). Palliative care in undergraduate medical education. *JAMA*, **278**, 733–6.
9. Field, M., and Cassel, C. (1997). *Approaching death: Improving care at the end of life*. National Academy Press, Washington, DC.
10. Doyle, D., Hanks, G., Cherny, N. *et al*. (eds.) (2004). *Oxford textbook of palliative medicine*. Oxford University Press, Oxford.
11. National Hospice and Palliative Care Organization (2003). NPCPO national data set summary report. Retrieved from http://www.nhpco.org/files/members/2003 national dataset.pdf on 5 May 2003.
12. American Association of Colleges of Nursing (1997). *Peaceful death document*. Round table discussion on palliative care, Washington, DC.
13. Ferrell, B.R., and Coyle, N. (2006). *The textbook of palliative nursing*, 2nd edition. Oxford University Press, New York.
14. Matzo, M., and Sherman, D.W. (2006). *Palliative care nursing: Quality care to the end of life*, 2nd edition. Springer Publishers, New York.
15. Lentz, J., and Sherman, D.W. (2006). Professional organizations and certifications in hospice and palliative care. In *Palliative care nursing: Quality care to the end of life* (eds. Matzo, M., and Sherman, D.W.), 2nd edition, pp. 117–32. Springer Publishers, New York.
16. Hospice and Palliative Care Nurses Association (2002). *Competencies for advanced practice hospice and palliative care nurses*. Kendall/Hunt Publishing Company, Dubuque, Iowa.
17. Skalla, K. (2006). Blended role advanced practice nursing in palliative care of the oncology patient. *Journal of Hospice and Palliative Care*, **8**, 155–63.
18. Hurlimann, B., Hofer, S., and Hirter, K. (2001). The role of the clinical nurse specialist. *International Nursing Review*, **48**, 58–64.
19. Jack, B., Oldham, J., and Williams, A. (2003). A stakeholder evaluation of the impact of the palliative care clinical nurse specialist upon doctors and nurses within an acute hospital setting. *Palliative Medicine*, **17**, 283–8.
20. Corner, J., Halliday, D., Haviland, J. et al. (2003). Exploring nursing outcomes for patients with advanced cancer following intervention by Macmillan specialist palliative care nurses. *Journal of Advanced Nursing*, **41**, 561–74.
21. Quaglietti, S., Blum, L., and Ellis, V. (2004). The role of the adult nurse practitioner in palliative care. *Journal of Hospice and Palliative Nursing*, **6**, 209–14.
22. Aiken, L., Butner, J., Lockhart, C. *et al*. (2006). Outcome evaluation of a randomized trial of the PhoenixCare Intervention: Program of case management and coordinated care for the seriously chronically ill. *Journal of Palliative Medicine*, **9**, 111–26.
23. Promoting Excellence in End of Life Care (2002). *Advanced practice nursing: Pioneering Practices in palliative care*. National Program Office of the Robert Wood Johnson Foundation.

4.3

Social work in palliative medicine

Barbara Monroe

Introduction

Social work is a necessary and appropriate part of palliative care. Palliative care starts with specific physical symptoms but it can only be completed by consideration of the patient's feelings, family and friendship networks, and social circumstances. This requires a variety of skills and roles, including the social work skills and roles considered in this chapter. The chapter describes the forces that shape the social work role in palliative care, examines the social work task, provides a practical illustration, looks at the work that social workers do, and considers the social worker's contribution to extending the resources and values of palliative care.

Shaping the social work role

Three forces shape the social work role: the non-medical social goals that palliative care teams set themselves; the teamwork and multi-professional skills required to meet these social goals; and the expectations of patients, carers, relatives, and friends, and the various palliative-care professionals, of social work and social workers.

Non-medical social goals

Relieving a patient's physical symptoms reveals their and their families' emotional, spiritual, and practical needs. Because doctors and nurses can often release patients from the horror of a physically painful and unpleasant death, palliative-care teams are able to set themselves non-medical social goals aimed at these non-medical needs.

The patient's first non-medical need is to express emotional pain. Terminal illness frightens people, may make them angry, sad, or guilty, and often distances them from those to whom they are close. Helping patients to express their feelings can reduce their fear and anguish and put them back in touch with their partners, families, and friends[1]. It allows patients to say a proper goodbye and gives them the opportunity to heal rifts and complete unfinished business.

The second need is the exploration of spiritual pain[2]. Dying people want to explore 'why'; why me, why now, for what purpose? Helping them in this journey will alleviate their isolation and give them the comfort of knowing that their concerns, even if unanswered, are real, important, and valid.

The third need is for practical help. Dying people are often reduced to passive patienthood; however, they need to make decisions and exercise choice, both for practical reasons and in order to maintain their own sense of dignity and worth. For instance, they may need to make a will or to discuss and influence a child's future care. They may need the most basic assistance in order to pay a bill or obtain appropriate housing.

Patients' partners, families, and friends will experience the same three needs and ensuring that their needs are also met is a proper goal for palliative care. They may also feel frightened or angry. They too will ask 'why', and they too may have practical needs, such as some relief from a 24-h caring role. They will need to feel involved in the processes of dying and that they did what they could to help the patient. Research indicates that whether or not these needs are met can have a profound impact on their health in bereavement and their ability to cope with future crises. For example, the work of Kissane and colleagues emphasizes the importance of an assessment of family functioning during terminal illness as it influences subsequent grief outcomes[3]. A randomized controlled trial of their Family Focused Grief Therapy model demonstrated significant reduction in distress at 13 months post-death for families completing treatment, with further improvements for the 10 per cent of individuals most distressed at baseline[4].

Teamwork

The non-medical goals permitted by good symptom control require different and extra skills beyond those traditionally accruing to the doctor and nurse. In addition, patients may want to discuss emotional, spiritual, or practical problems with someone who is not involved in their physical care, or someone wearing a different label, such as a minister of religion or a social worker. As a result, good palliative care is delivered by multi-professional teams. Each member of the team will have a range of overlapping roles, some medical and some non-medical, each focused on a specific set of patient, family, or carer needs. Whilst medical needs will be met from the medical disciplines, no one discipline has the monopoly in fulfilling the non-medical roles. Patients' other needs do not come in neat boxes with discreet professional labels. Doctors, nurses, social workers, and ministers will all have to respond to patients' emotional, spiritual, and practical concerns. What matters is the definition and delivery of the social work task, and not the allocation of a role or task to the social worker or any other non-medical discipline. All disciplines will do some social work, and patients and those close to them will expect a consistent, careful, and effective approach to be adopted by all of them.

The social work profession does, however, bring its own perspective and approaches, and the exposition and demonstration of these is an important part of the contribution that a social worker should make within a palliative care team[5]. Gwyther and Terry define the necessary social work competencies[6]. These perspectives come in three forms: the first reflects what social workers cannot do. They cannot cure pain, dress wounds, or offer the appropriate religious rituals. Their professional starting point has to be that defined by the patient and his or her family, not that defined by their professional role. It is clear from a recent participatory research study of what service users want from specialist palliative care social workers that listening, seeing the real person, respecting people's need to stay 'in control' and being able to provide a wide range of helping interventions are of particular value to patients and those close to them[7].

The second perspective is that of the patient as part of a family and friendship network with a past and a future and a social and cultural context. For the social worker, the patient is not just an individual with problems but part of a whole social network, which has a variety of strengths and resources that can be marshalled to cope with the consequences of the individual's illness and death and reflects attitudes that may impact on the possibilities available. For example, cultural expectations within the immediate circle of the family about the rights and responsibilities of individual members may affect decisions about caregiving and beliefs about health care and death can affect access to services[8,9].

Lastly, the social worker will have a perspective of how the patient and their family will be affected by the law and other social institutions. For instance, the social worker will understand the implications of family and mental health legislation in particular cases. He or she will know what community services might be applicable and what social welfare provision may be available. He or she may have to balance individual needs and wishes against a social control and protection function as in adult and child protection work[10]. Bransden's literature review[11] examines the roles and activities of social work in end-of-life care, and underlines Payne's more general description of social work as balancing three objectives; 'maintaining social order and providing social welfare services effectively, helping people attain personal fulfilment and power over their lives, and stimulating social change'[12].

Expectations and attitudes

The role of the social worker is also shaped by expectations and attitudes of society, of colleagues, and of patients and families.

People in Western economies expect the welfare state to provide a safety net when things go wrong; a residential care home for the elderly disabled widow whose carer has died or foster parents for the children of a dying single parent. Society sees the social worker as an agent for the welfare state, able to manipulate its institutions to the patient's advantage. For example, social workers may be expected to negotiate financial benefits from government agencies or organize child care from a statutory agency. Palliative care colleagues expect social workers to provide them with a safety net for managing difficult social work tasks. Palliative care teams will frequently meet situations that are emotionally exhausting and difficult to deal with. A young dying mother or a suicidal relative

may need both extra time and specialist social work skills that are best provided by a separate resource.

Patients and their families will also have specific expectations from organizations that provide palliative care. They increasingly expect access to professional counselling services in order to help them manage emotional difficulties. They will expect expert advice on personal family matters, such as how much should a young child know about and be involved with a parent's death and how they should be told what they need to know[13].

The core social work task

The core social work task concerns the social and psychological health of the patient, family, friends, and carers, before and after death. It has two parts: assessment and intervention.

Assessment

The assessment of the patient at home or in an inpatient setting will often start with a medical or nursing 'clerking-in' procedure and the formulation of a care plan. This initial assessment should identify any need for further assessment, for coordination between disciplines, and for specialist help. Sometimes the process by which the patient has arrived in a service will have already identified problems that require a more detailed psychosocial assessment. For instance, in admitting the mother of a dependent adult with a learning disability the normal inpatient admission routine might be expanded to involve the social worker as well as the doctor and the nurse. There may be immediate care needs and the patient's adult child may need particular help to become involved in and to understand their mother's impending death[14].

In an important text on ethics in palliative care, Randall and Downie[15] question the potential intrusiveness of assessments in the psychosocial domain. They raise significant ethical concerns about the sensitive issues that may be touched upon. However, effective assessment creates a working partnership among the professional, the patient, and those close to them. Professionals should explain the reasons for their enquiries, establish consent, and check on it regularly: 'If there is something I ask that you would rather not discuss, please let me know.' The assessment process can never be a one-off event as circumstances alter and people change their minds. A failure to assess may diminish the options available to the patient and their family or mean that those at risk remain unidentified.

Assessments will vary in their formats and formality but will usually cover four perspectives: the individual, the family, physical resources, and social resources.

The individual

There is substantial evidence that psychological distress is a vital factor in the individual's experience of illness and interacts with physical distress[16]. It is influenced by perceptions of family and social support[17], of personal control, and attributions of meaning[18] and hope[19]. There is also evidence for links between the experiences of the dying individual and family functioning[20].

In assessing the individual, we need to establish what changes their illness has wrought, as well as who they are. We need to know how their life has changed since the illness and who or what currently supports them. We need to understand their reaction to the illness and its implications for them. We need to identify any practical or emotional unfinished business they may have. Assessing practical issues will lead us on to values and beliefs. What are their aims now that they have entered palliative care; do they, for instance, want to die at home or in a hospital or hospice? If such preferences are not assessed, documented and reviewed they are much less likely to be met[21]

The family

The individual should be placed in the context of his family and friendship network. The family can be regarded as a complex system that changes over time. In order to assess the strengths and difficulties of a family and its members, we need to understand how it works, and attempt to discover the normal patterns of communication, support, and conflict in the family, and the extent to which they have been disrupted by the illness.

The history of the current family and their individual experiences within their previous families will be significant factors in their ability to cope with the present crisis. For example, a wife who watched her own mother nurse her father through a protracted, exhausting, and painful terminal illness will in consequence approach her husband's death with reduced confidence and may value additional support. We need to understand the family's methods of coping with crisis and whether they are facing any additional change at the moment such as a redundancy or a pregnancy. Lastly, we should enquire about the existence of other vulnerable individuals within the family such as children, dependent elderly, or disabled relatives. The terminal illness of a family member can be the final burden that topples a delicately balanced system of nurture and support and it may be necessary to provide additional external help.

Whatever the place of care immediately prior to death, most palliative care takes place at home and most care is provided by informal, related carers. They may also become clients in their own right. Numerous studies attest to the burden of caring with reports of increased risk of physical and psychological morbidity running alongside a recognition of the importance of the social and practical support provided to patients by those close to them[22]. A systematic review of the factors influencing home deaths in cancer patients indicated that two strong determinants were living with relatives and having extended family support[23].The literature is clear about the needs of informal carers for information, education, and support[24,25]. Recent changes in the structure of families—geographical distance, divorce, split, and reconstituted families—may add to carers' difficulties. It is also important to emphasize that many carers see caring as a natural extension of existing relationships and report satisfaction and fulfilment in undertaking caring tasks[26].

Physical resources

The assessment should cover the family's physical resources, such as money and housing. We need to know about unmet physical needs because they may become the patient's biggest concern, and our expertise may be able to unlock money from charities or the state to relieve the problem. Social workers often play a key role in this vital activity[27]. For instance, a washing machine for the exhausted carer of a patient with night sweats and incontinence may be of more value than extra counselling or nursing support. A patient's physical resources may also affect how we care for them. Adaptations to their home or the provision of domestic help may avoid or delay the need for inpatient care.

Social resources

Finally, the family themselves must be placed within the context of their community and social network and the laws and values of the particular society. The team should attempt to understand the family's ethnic, cultural[28], and religious background and the potential impact of these influences on the individual and his illness. This means enquiring about informal and formal helping systems available to the family within their community such as churches, social groups, and schools.

Field has argued that the use of the portmanteau word 'psycho-social', rather than 'psychological and social', has diminished the understanding and importance of social factors in people's lives[29]. He also points out that not all palliative-care services have a social worker on the team 'and where they do these may well be part-time and marginal to decision-making processes.'

An assessment made with the individual, their family, and friends, of the emotional, spiritual, physical, and social resources available to them will lead to decisions. At one end of the spectrum, the decision will be to do nothing. Assessment may reveal adequate coping mechanisms in the patient and their family and community. The result of the assessment may, however, be a decision to intervene in order to support the patient and family in managing the situation facing them.

Interventions

Interventions will be aimed at patients and families who need help in order to cope with their situation[30]. They will typically want support because: they do not have the information they need; they cannot communicate sufficiently with each other to reach a solution; they lack the confidence to act; or they do not have the resources they need. In addition, an intervention may be addressed at the needs of bereaved individuals or families after the patient has died.

Information

Sometimes patients or families cannot manage simply because they lack information, leaving them at the mercy of their fears and fantasies. For instance, many patients and their relatives will be very frightened of the moment of death because they do not know how it will happen. They need information about what normally happens and what their options are. Patients may want to know how their illness will progress to death and how difficult symptoms will be treated[31]. Parents will want to know what to expect from their child in bereavement and what options they should consider for involving their child in the death. Relatives may want information about arranging funerals and registering the death.

Communication

The second objective for intervention is to help patients and their families communicate. Communication is particularly difficult at the time of bereavement, and a family that cannot share information and feelings cannot easily resolve the problems that death brings. The immediate barrier to communication is likely to be the strong, unfamiliar, and often conflicting feelings that each family member may experience in relation to the forthcoming death. These may disrupt their normal approach to communicating with each other. In addition, death and crisis often encourage people to protect one another. Loyalty and a conventional dislike of emotional display and upset may inhibit discussion of what is going on both emotionally and practically. Many carers will also be struggling with rapid and anxiety provoking changes in the physical capacities and needs of the ill person.

More specific barriers to communication may reflect the redistribution of roles within the family; a husband may be assuming unfamiliar parenting roles and responsibilities just as his dying wife is experiencing their loss. Communicating both the practical and emotional material within this transaction will be difficult. Similarly, the different perspectives of family members will reduce their ability to communicate; the husband's experience of his wife's impending death may be very different from his father-in-law's pain in losing a much loved daughter and this new difference may not be understood by the daughter, the husband, or the father. Old relationship difficulties will be placed under even greater strain and the progression of the illness may have disrupted comforting routines of interaction at work and leisure for all involved.

Intervention will be aimed at overcoming these barriers and ensuring that the family and patient can communicate effectively. The intervention will work because a skilled outsider can often provide the security and sense of control that family members may need to release their emotions. The outsider will ensure that every member of the family hears a shared story that is as complete as possible and that all understand how each one reacts to it. Most families will manage well with just a little help. Most want to support each other, to say important things, to plan for the future, it is just that they do not know where to begin or what to say in a situation with so many uncertainties, that many will be facing for the first time. Working with families where relationships are more seriously disrupted will require more structured approaches.[4,32]

Improving a family's communication can be a very powerful tool, releasing the existing strengths within the family, allowing them to solve their own problems and to establish new roles and relationships. For some families, a bereavement may provide an opportunity for resolving historic arguments. The crisis of impending bereavement can loosen the glue surrounding gummed-up communication patterns. Equally, professionals must respect people's capacity to choose. Forgiveness and reconciliation cannot be imposed, but support can always be offered.

Communicating with individuals and couples about issues of body image, sexuality, and intimacy can be particularly challenging to professionals in palliative care. However, discussion of these topics is important to quality of life. Life-threatening illness can deeply affect intimate relationships and self concepts. For example, partners may find that physical changes in the patient or their own change of role to carer alters their feelings or desires. Professional anxieties about the subject area may mean that the issues are seldom addressed in practice. In addition, there is evidence that most patients will not ask for help spontaneously. Whilst it would clearly be inappropriate to expect all professionals in palliative care to have specialist skills in psychosexual counselling, all should be able to offer and respond to cues about a wish to discuss sexuality and know how to refer on for specialist support where appropriate.[33,34] Sensitive support may involve finding questions that can be responded to at a variety of levels: 'In what ways has your illness changed how you can get close to people you particularly care about?' Generalizing can create a sense of permission: 'People often have questions they would like to ask about the sexual side of life.'

The confidence to act

The dying patient and those close to them will often believe that they have no influence on events and may lack the confidence to take decisions. Physical disability may be reinforcing their emotional conclusion. For patients to have the confidence to act they may need to be reminded of the resources available to them and about how they have coped with crises in the past. They may need help to segment their problems and to set realistic goals focusing on one or two difficulties that can be tackled out of a chaos that threatens to overwhelm. They may simply want the comforting presence of a concerned outsider as they think each stage through. For instance, the individual will often already know who or what can help them; the sympathetic teacher who can assist their child, the local church group who can mobilize a rota of supplementary carers.

The resource to act

Patients and families may have the information they require, the ability to discuss and resolve their problems, and the confidence to do what is needed. Ultimately, however, they may simply not have the resources to do what needs to be done. If you are threatened with eviction for rent arrears because your dying husband cannot work, it may be difficult to focus on other needs. More prosaically, patients may not have access to the resources they need; what aids to daily living or housing adaptations are available and who will supply them? A raised toilet seat may help the patient to continue using the lavatory rather than a commode, a ramp may allow access to the garden for a wheelchair user.

Families need information about financial resources and sources of social support. These services should not be imposed but must be provided in a way that allows families to obtain the kind of help that they decide they need. Effectiveness in this role requires advocacy and influence with social services departments, government agencies, and charities. It is important to recognize that the task of the palliative care institution is to manipulate whatever is already available in society, rather than rushing to set up specialist services, expending time and energy that should be devoted to direct patient and family care. One of the most important components of the social work task is to act on behalf of the patient in order to get other agencies to do their job properly[35].

After the death

Further interventions may be necessary following the death of the patient. The normal process of providing palliative care should include efforts to identify those individuals at special risk in bereavement[36]. Loss and the grief that follows it are normal human experiences, but some people may need additional support with their grief either because of their previous experiences and relationships or because of the particular circumstances of their bereavement. Complicated and unresolved responses to grief may result in physical symptoms, obsessive behaviours, and can precipitate individual or family breakdown[37].

Bereavement services aiming to respond to these needs can take many forms. A brief and possibly routine intervention following the immediate bereavement can offer relatives, including children, the opportunity to view the body, to say a final farewell, to ask questions about the illness and death, and to begin the necessary but painful process of remembering. It may be important to offer longer-term help, perhaps from a bereavement support volunteer who represents the community from which the patient came and to which the relative or friend is returning. Specialist help may be required when circumstances are more extreme, such as the widower who plans to commit suicide so that he can avoid what he sees as a pointless life by joining his dead wife.

Social work methods

Interventions can provide information, increase communication, give confidence, provide resources, or help the bereaved. There are three traditional methods for making these interventions: one-to-one meetings, meetings with families or couples, or groups involving unrelated individuals with shared circumstances or problems. For all forms of intervention adolescents[38] and young children will often represent a challenging and draining group, and palliative care teams will typically want to take extra care in these cases. All interventions will be made by listening and talking and here too there are particular skills and particular responsibilities.

Listening and talking

Listening and talking to patients is one of the key tasks in palliative care. Most dying patients are not looking to carers, professional, or family, for solutions to their situation. They want someone to share the problems with; what helps people who are grieving is someone trustworthy who will listen to their experiences and help them explore the depths of their pain without offering false reassurance.

People facing loss awaken powerful feelings in the professionals who meet them. We cannot listen properly to the loss of others if our own losses, actual or feared, are unexplored and unresolved. Work with the dying often makes us worry about not coping or about becoming over-involved. We do not know what to say; we do not know how to 'make things better'. We have to learn how to share what we do not know as well as our knowledge, and above all, how to listen accurately.

Silence is an important part of listening. Professionals often misinterpret and feel uncomfortable with silence. They may interrupt too readily rather than allowing the patient to express his concern for himself. Silence is a necessary part of the individual's exploration of his thoughts and feelings. Prompts should be gentle and open— 'You have been quiet for a long time now. I wonder if it would help you to share some of your thoughts.'

The professional must use language sensitively. Questioning should be direct but unassertive: 'What is the worst thing for you at the moment?' The use of clear, simple, feeling words such as 'sad, angry, death, guilty' helps in the expression of emotions. Body language can be both observed and used. 'You say you are feeling fine, but you look so very tense and anxious.' Appropriate touch can convey understanding and comfort when words seem inadequate.

For some people and some circumstances talking and listening may be ineffective[51]. Ritual is an alternative way of reaching feelings. Familiar rituals can offer great comfort, such as a cup of tea or the rites of prayer and religious observance. New rituals can be created to meet new needs. A team member may encourage a whole family to hold hands or to spend a moment in silence remembering their love for one another. A bereaved daughter may finally be able to express her ambivalent feelings towards her dead mother and to forgive her, by writing a letter to her and burying it at the grave.

One-to-one help

Any member of the team may find themselves talking to the patient or a family member with therapeutic intent. There are no solutions to the emotional anguish experienced by dying people but they can be helped by being heard. It is not necessary to approve what the patient says or does; it is important to show understanding of the feeling behind his words and actions. Staff may fear being overwhelmed by the intensity of emotion they release in the patient and more particularly that in talking about things they may have made them worse. However, it is often through tears or the expression of anger that individuals become more aware of the nature and origin of their pain and more able to decide how to cope with it[39].

Life review work and narrative therapy can also provide opportunities to leave a legacy[40].

Meeting the patient or members of the family on a one-to-one basis may be an important precursor to work with the whole family. It ensures that we understand individual perspectives and problems. For example, the loving wife of a dying patient may need privacy to begin acknowledging her resentment at the exhausting task of caring. She may want to rehearse the exposure of her conflicting feelings with a sympathetic outsider before seeking a reconciliation between her resentment and grief with her husband. It should be remembered that dying people and their carers cannot act as proxies for one another's needs and feelings[41]. The dying individual and those close to them will have different needs at different times, may require different types of support and often have conflicting agendas.

Family meetings

Meeting with a family group can be a powerful tool for change and the resolution of problems[42]. It is important to prepare properly for such meetings, and to decide, usually with the patient, who should be there and which members of staff will be the most appropriate facilitators. It is often helpful for the team to work in pairs; for example, the doctor might begin with an overview of the illness and its history, to be followed by the social worker exploring the family's reaction to it. The family should do most of the talking. The aim is to help them resolve the issues that they identify as significant in a way that feels reasonably comfortable for them, not to assume responsibility for solving all the problems for them. The family may need to experience new ways of relating to one another. For example, they may need to be prompted to allow each other to talk without interruption; a child may need to be invited to speak for herself/himself. They may need help to address painful issues: 'I think everyone in this family is wondering what will happen when Mum is not here to look after you all.'

Groups

Group work will normally involve people who share similar problems or experiences, but who are otherwise strangers to each other. For instance, bereaved fathers may meet to share the practical and emotional problems of bringing up their children alone. Patients may use a group to explore feelings about their illness. Bereaved children and adults may gain increased confidence from the normalization of grief that group work permits in contrast to their social communities where they may feel excluded or misunderstood[43].

Such groups have many benefits[44]. Members will hear others express the difficulties they felt too embarrassed, guilty, or frightened to share. Individuals within the group will increase their self-esteem by giving support as well as receiving it. Group work does not represent a 'cheap' alternative in terms of manpower or time. Groups are often more effectively run by two leaders who will need time for preparation before a session and time for assessment and discussion after it. Leaders themselves will need supervision, training, and support.

Working with children

Children facing bereavement have similar needs and emotions to adults. However, they may be expressed differently, for example, through behaviour rather than words. Many studies make clear the cost of inadequate support and involvement for children facing the death of someone close to them[45]. Children may respond with emotional and behavioural disturbance both at the time, throughout childhood, and on into adulthood. Significant factors influencing the outcome of bereavement include the relationship of the child with the ill person before the death, the openness of family communication, the availability of peer and community support, and most importantly, the extent to which the child's parenting needs have continued and will continue to be met[46]. Palliative care professionals have a responsibility to ensure that potential difficulties for children are minimized and social workers possess specialist skills in this area. Christ's work demonstrates their role and gives clear pointers for helping based on developmental observations[47].

It is impossible not to communicate with children. Terminal illness causes enormous changes within the family and children quickly sense when something so serious is happening. They pick up the emotions around them, read body language, overhear conversations, piece together chance remarks by neighbours and school friends, and see the evidence of physical deterioration. However, children's apparent vulnerability often evokes an impulse in both parents and professionals to protect children from the truth. The difficulties of deciding what level of information is appropriate and what words to use, added to the fear that saying the wrong thing will make matters worse, often lead to an excluding silence. Exclusion leads to isolation, leaving children unprotected from their fantasies and unsupported in their feelings. Like adults, children need appropriate involvement, an opportunity to ask questions and to receive information and reassurance, a chance to express and share their feelings in safety and help to remember. This support needs to be delivered in ways that are appropriate to their age and individual level of understanding and this can only be determined by asking them about their experiences.

Help for children has to start with their parents and families who will be around long after the professionals have disappeared. The task of professionals is to help parents to help their children. Parents may have good reasons for their reluctance to share information about illness and death with their children. They will be struggling to maintain some control in an uncertain situation. They themselves will be grieving and they may want to protect their children from this pain. The child may also want to protect its parents by trying to pretend that nothing is happening. It is often necessary to work with parents on their own before children's needs can be addressed. For example, a couple who cannot openly acknowledge impending death between themselves are not well placed to help their children.

We do not help parents by taking over from them—they know their children best, but we can offer them support, encouragement, and practical help. We can begin by creating environments that release parents from the expectation that children should not be involved. We can invite their presence in an inpatient unit, perhaps with a designated area with small chairs and a toy box. Equipment, such as dolls in beds and toy medical kits can help children to act out their concerns and to ask questions. Drawing can help them to express and control powerful emotions that they lack the vocabulary to voice. There are many specially designed drawing and creative workbooks available for this purpose[48]. Parents may appreciate advice about their child's likely understanding of death, their needs as they face bereavement, and the kinds of explanation and vocabulary appropriate to their developmental needs at different ages. Professionals must, of course, respect the family's own belief system. Lists of books and leaflets for parents to read for themselves or to read with their children[49] will often be appreciated. For many

parents this will be sufficient and they will then want to speak to their children alone. Others may welcome sharing the task with a professional.

Parents may be reassured by the suggestion that a professional meet them and their children to discuss changes in the family and to answer questions about the illness. Just being part of one such direct conversation can help parents to feel confident enough to continue for themselves. Children facing the death of a parent need reassurance about their own continuing care and assistance in managing their inevitable separation anxieties. Whether we raise it or not they will be wondering who will look after them and perform the familiar activities such as taking them to school. It can be an enormous relief to them and their parents when these painful issues are addressed. This is particularly important when a single parent is dying. Children also need explicit reassurance about the illness itself, for example, whether it is contagious, and to know that their own thoughts or behaviour could not have caused the death. Parents may need encouragement to widen their child's support network by involving other adults close to them such as teachers, clergy, or friends and relatives. Parents sometimes need assistance to anticipate and understand altered or difficult behaviour in their grieving children.

Children learn to grieve by observing others and families can be encouraged to understand that sharing feelings often helps, as does involvement in important rituals such as viewing the body, attending the funeral, or being given something that belonged to the dead person. Such activities help children to feel included and act as tangible reminders of the existence of the dead person and their importance. Professionals help parents by giving them information so that they and their children can decide together about what they feel comfortable with. Klass and Silverman's work on 'continuing bonds' emphasizes the importance of memories and shared remembering[50].

Sharing information

Personal information received from patients and families places particular responsibilities on team members. All palliative care professionals will operate within a professional framework requiring respect for the individual's privacy and autonomy. However, confidentiality can sometimes suffer unnecessarily in the particular atmosphere of the multi-professional team. The need to pass on personal information must always be questioned; it is neither right nor necessary that every team member should know everything a patient or relative shares with an individual within that team. Patients choose who they talk to. Wherever possible the permission of the patient or family member should be sought explicitly: 'Thank you for telling me such an important and difficult thing. Would you mind if I tell other members of the team looking after you?' No one needs to know more than will enable them to fulfil their own role in caring for the patient. A volunteer car driver, for example, does not need to know details of the patient's diagnosis but will need to know that he uses a walking frame.

Within teams we must be clear about why we want information. Often, in the rapidly developing environment engendered by terminal illness, the emotional truth perceived and expressed by patient or family is more important than amassing painstaking details about the past. The desire for more information can represent power, confirmation of inclusion in the 'inner circle', or just inquisitiveness. A test of the trust necessary for teams to function well is the willingness of members to accept that another may hold confidential information and use it appropriately.

Recording of information also demands great care. What is written, particularly if it is subjective opinion, can easily assume the status of objective truth. Recording should always be undertaken with regard to the possibility of patient and family access. Good recording can assist coordinated care and avoid duplication of enquiry.

Case study

Introduction

This case study is intended to illustrate the most demanding form that the social work task takes. Janet Skinner (no real names are used here) and her family faced a series of difficult and interconnected medical and social problems associated with Janet's death. These concerned her attempted suicide, her marriage, her children, and the threat of breast cancer in succeeding generations. The scale and breadth of her problems are untypical but they illustrate clearly the sequence of assessment and intervention, and the value of a competent and thoughtful professional approach.

Janet was 36 when she was admitted to St Christopher's Hospice. She had been married to her husband Rob for 12 years and they both knew her illness could no longer be cured. She had two children, Susan aged 7 and Paul aged 5. Her breast cancer had been diagnosed 5 years previously and was at that time treated with surgery, radiotherapy, and chemotherapy. She remained well and disease-free for 2.5 years when evidence of metastatic disease in the lung and liver was discovered. She received further chemotherapy which she tolerated very poorly.

Three months later, she presented with multiple brain metastases and an enlarged liver, and was again treated with chemotherapy and cranial irradiation, despite her previous low tolerance of the treatment and her poor prognosis. She developed a left-sided weakness, walking became increasingly difficult, and she began to use a wheelchair. She was cushingoid. She became depressed and cancelled a hospital appointment. On the evening, before her rescheduled appointment, she took an overdose of drugs and cut her wrists whilst her husband was busy getting tea for the children. Janet was admitted to the hospice from the local hospital who had treated her following the suicide attempt.

The assessment

Individual

Janet expressed sadness and anger about the many losses she was facing; she had lost her role as mother, involvement in and a sense of security about her children's future, her physical attractiveness, a normal family life, and her faith in a caring God. She was also angry about the treatment she had endured, given its eventual futility. She felt she had been trapped into continuing with active treatment and on the day of her admission said that she 'just wanted to die'.

Janet experienced her pain as total and unendurable but she also desperately wanted to live to be a mother for her children. She described them being shunted between friends and neighbours and told us that it was her son's birthday next week and that she would be useless to him. Janet felt very guilty about her suicide attempt and asked about the possibility of having further chemotherapy at the hospice. Above all, she felt completely powerless.

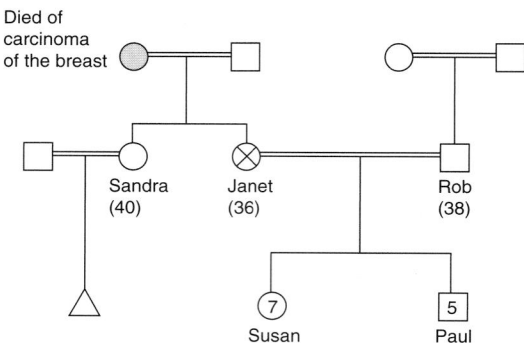

Figure 4.3.1 Family structure[52].

Family

Everyone in the family was affected by Janet's illness. It emerged that Janet's mother had also died of breast cancer when Janet was the same age as her own daughter was now (Fig. 4.3.1). Her father was reliving the loss of his wife in the loss of his daughter.

Janet's older sister, Sandra, was pregnant. She had been trying to conceive for many years. Amniocentesis the previous week had confirmed that the fetus was both healthy and female. Sandra and Janet knew what it was like to lose a mother. Sandra felt that giving birth while her sister was dying was 'obscene'.

Janet's husband, Rob, concerned the team by his noticeable reticence. He was silent throughout the procedures of his wife's admission, merely expressing concern that he might be late collecting the children from school.

The team was informed that the children had not been told about their mother's specific illness or prognosis, just that she was 'ill'. The family said that they had become clinging and difficult to get to bed at night.

Physical

Money was not a problem for this family. However, concerns were expressed about how Janet could manage at home, even on a visit, in her wheelchair with increasing weakness making transfers difficult.

Social

Janet and Rob had had a wide circle of friends and an active social life. However, the stresses and upheaval of her illness and treatment had caused them to become isolated. The consequences of this isolation were that Janet and Rob were no longer getting emotional support or sufficient practical help from their friends, family, and community network. Janet was refusing visitors and had stopped attending the local church or seeing the vicar. The children's teachers were not fully informed about Janet's illness. Rob was relying on a series of temporary arrangements with neighbours to care for his children while he tried to continue with his job. Janet's and Rob's parents wanted to help but they were uncertain both about how to offer help, and what help they could best give.

Intervention

This family were perceived to be in emotional crisis, unable to cope with the problems facing them. They did not appear to be able to communicate with one another. They were all stunned by Janet's suicide attempt. The team thought that if this pain and guilt was not addressed, Janet's wider family, and in particular her husband, would be unable to offer both Janet and her children the support and care they needed so badly. However, at this stage it was impossible to assess the problem fully and it was clear that there were many potentially conflicting individual needs. The team therefore decided to see the family individually, both to allow them to express their emotional pain and in order to understand what was going on.

Individual meetings

Rob and Janet both individually revealed that a major source of anguish and anger was a love affair of Rob's which had resulted in a child. The love affair had ended but Rob knew that Janet had not forgiven him for his betrayal of her, particularly whilst she was ill. Rob felt guilty and wanted to repair his relationship with Janet, yet felt trapped by his past. Janet feared that once she was dead he would create a new family for his daughters by marrying his former girlfriend.

Janet's sister was uncertain about continuing her pregnancy. Both she and Janet had lost their mother; Janet's children were now losing theirs. Sandra was wondering whether the same would happen to her unborn child. Janet and Sandra both feared that their daughters would repeat the same cycle of events.

Although the team had decided that the social worker needed to have a prominent and coordinating role in these meetings, the variety of team members involved allowed significant later interventions. For example, an early meeting with the chaplain paved the way for a later service in the hospice chapel focusing on peace and forgiveness with the laying on of hands. This ritual was profoundly helpful to Janet.

The data from these initial, individual meetings seemed to predict an even more hopeless future. It did, however, pinpoint some important issues for joint meetings. The team began to create a series of specific objectives against known problems.

Having met Janet and Rob individually, we were aware of their conflict and the source of the distance between them. We needed to try to achieve a sufficient reconciliation between them for them at least to address their children's needs together. Sandra needed to talk to her husband about her fears and her pregnancy. The children needed information and support.

Joint meetings

Rob and Janet voiced a wish to be seen together, although neither of them was hopeful about the outcome. They expressed enormous and vociferous anger towards one another. It was necessary to confront them very directly: 'Is this really how you want things to end?' The turning point was Rob's open expression of anguish at his inadequacies as a father. He wept at his inability to iron his daughter's dress for her brother's birthday party. He and Janet began to share their pain as well as their anger, and their common purpose in loving and caring for their children.

Sandra, Janet's sister, was seen with her husband and told him for the first time of her anxieties. He had felt excluded and he had not known why. Sharing their fears enabled him to support Sandra and together they decided that the pregnancy should continue.

Family meetings and the children

Susan and Paul joined their parents in a series of meetings with the social worker and the doctor. They were encouraged to ask questions: 'What is wrong with Mummy?' 'Why hasn't Mummy got any hair?' 'Why does her breathing sound funny?' They expressed their feelings: 'I try hard not to cry because I'm scared I'll upset Daddy.' They gradually came to a realization of the gravity of their mother's illness and it was Rob who Susan finally asked: 'Is Mummy going to die?'. He was able to answer her directly and began to express more confidence in his role of father. Janet was very upset by these meetings but also reassured and moved by the children's expression of love for her: 'I love you Mummy, I want you to come home.'

These meetings and meetings with other family groupings succeeded in creating a calmer and more positive atmosphere in which Janet and her husband could set goals for the future. The couple began to request and share appropriate information and take control. During the family meetings, and subsequently, they took a number of decisions and actions.

Janet decided against further active treatment.

Janet's family and her sister's family had a meeting with a consultant who specialized in genetic cancer counselling.

Janet planned her own funeral and had special watches engraved for the children to keep after her death. She had not been given any proper explanation of her mother's death nor attended the funeral, and wanted things to be different for her children.

The family as a whole discussed the approach they would take towards the children's needs as they faced bereavement. With Janet's help they planned an advertisement for a nanny.

The headmaster of the children's school came to the hospice to discuss future options for their education with Janet and Rob.

Janet and Rob's parents and friends arranged a rota for visiting and helped Janet to get home most weekends and to go out to the theatre and restaurants.

With the help of a nurse escort from the hospice, Janet and Rob planned and successfully completed a short holiday abroad with the children. It was important to Janet that the children had one last family memory involving her that was fun.

After death

The social worker saw Rob and the children on three occasions. Together they discussed the impact of the death, the funeral, the children's behaviour at school and home, and the family's grief. With Rob's permission the social worker again contacted the children's class teachers to discuss the help that might be offered in school. A bereavement support volunteer was in touch with the parents of Janet and Rob.

Difficulties

Helping this family posed many difficulties for the team. It was difficult not to become personally involved with the intensity of their pain. We certainly neglected this area for the nurse who accompanied them on holiday. As a social worker, I can remember how difficult it was to say good-bye to Janet when I went on annual leave knowing she might well be dead on my return. Janet herself solved this for me: 'I want to say good-bye. I probably won't be here when you get back.'

We had to grapple with setting boundaries for Janet and her family, boundaries that they sometimes could not set for themselves. Rob needed us to tell Janet when he and she could no longer cope with the visits home. However, we also needed to remember that we were not part of the family and that they needed to make their own decisions and to experience their own pain. Janet died peacefully 8 weeks after her admission to the hospice. Rob and her father were present.

The wider role of the social worker

So far, we have examined the social work task to which all members of a palliative care team will contribute, including the social worker. Next we examine the wider and more specific roles of the social worker within palliative care. The components of the social worker's task are likely to include internal consultancy, community liaison, user involvement, equality of access, training and the development of social work practice, and staff support and management.

Internal consultancy

The basic component of a typical social worker's role will be the support of nurses and doctors in carrying out the social work task. At one extreme, the support will be simple advice; at the other it will be taking a leadership role in the management of a specific patient and their family. In effect the social worker will operate as an internal consultant and as such must understand the major concerns of the other professionals. In fulfilling this role the social worker should be involved in the day-to-day decisions about how best to manage individual patients. He or she will not be an effective resource if they are only summoned from their office when someone thinks they are needed. Social workers will also contribute to policy advice within the palliative care team: how to respond to suicide threats; what facilities should be provided for children; how and when to work with interpreters.

Community liaison

Social workers will normally assume responsibility within the palliative care team for liaison with the community and its non-medical resources. This task requires both routine general contact and specific action on behalf of individual patients and their families. The specific action will be to create a 'package of care' for the patient in question perhaps involving both the resources of the social worker's institution and those of the wider community. For example, these might include domestic help, adaptations to the home, meals on wheels, childminders, and nightsitters. The community resources which may be available for tapping include money from government agencies or charities, or the time and attention of community social workers or local voluntary groups. Help may also be available from or through school teachers, community nurses, and family doctors.

User involvement

Any assessment of the role of social work in palliative care is incomplete without the opinions of the users of the services provided[7]. Social workers may also play an important part in developing user involvement not just in commenting on existing services but as active partners in the design and development of new ones[53]. For example, two parent users of a children's bereavement service drew attention to the particular needs of bereaved adults who had become single parents through the death of a partner rather than divorce or separation. They established and led a new service, supervised by a social worker[54].

Equality of access

The training and community experience of social workers mean that they should be key resources in responding to the challenge of delivering equity in palliative care. Many palliative care services operate in multi-cultural, multi-ethnic communities and are increasingly seeking to improve access to their services. If services are to become truly available, thought needs to be given to the different groups in any given population and the different ways in which they may use health services. This process operates at every level, from the efforts to extend primarily cancer-centred palliative care services to those patients with progressive non-malignant disorders[55], to the consideration of ways of improving knowledge of palliative care services and access to them by people from ethnic minority communities. Issues of disability, gender, race, and sexual orientation represent challenges to develop anti-discriminatory practice both for staff responding to patients and families and for institutions in their plans for training and recruitment of those staff, both paid and voluntary[56]. For example, do the volunteer supporters in a bereavement service represent a cross-section of the communities they seek to serve? Social workers should assist their services to develop equal opportunity strategies including clear and well-publicized codes of conduct and complaints procedures. They should also be available to help with the training needs of other staff.

Culture affects us all. The crisis of death may make an individual's relationship with his or her culture and spiritual roots deeper and closer, or may reveal conflicts, with generations in transition between their family's culture and local cultural practices.[57] The dying who have experienced previous persecution as a result of political, racial, or religious differences will often have special needs as they re-experience traumatic losses[58]. Everyone deserves respect for their individual cultural values and expectations. It is important, therefore, to clarify individual preferences about cultural and religious practices as well as improving general knowledge about the likely needs of specific groups.

In 2001, in a report for the National Council for Palliative Care in the United Kingdom, Firth commented on inadequate ethnic monitoring, an exclusive cancer focus, insensitivity, racism, and lack of cultural awareness[59]. However, she also noted progress in studies and fieldwork on patient and carer needs; for example, research on black Caribbean carers[60]. Simplified fact files about cultural practices are criticized as de-skilling by Gunaratnam[61]. Firth comments that what is 'missing in much of the culture/ethnicity discourse is an empathetic appreciation of the importance of faith to many individuals from religious communities.' Others note on the limited understanding of languages of distress, beliefs about pain and disclosure and criteria for a 'good death'[62,63].

Training and the development of social work practice

Social workers should lead the development of social work practice within their institutions[64]. This should include both the development of the service provided and the development of the skills required to support the service. Service development activities might include setting up a multi-professional group to examine potential improvements in the care offered to relatives immediately after the death. They will also include individual activity; for example, social workers should ensure that their colleagues have access to good written material such as booklists for a bereaved child or leaflets explaining how to claim state benefits. Social workers will want to develop and write their own publications, particularly where these need to be tailored to their institutions or their local community.

Development of social work practice within the institution should extend naturally into skills training and development.

Sharing and passing on skills should also flow from the internal consultancy role; all joint work with patients is an opportunity to learn new skills and understand new perspectives, both for the social worker and his or her colleagues. More formal contributions to the development of skills might include, for example, training sessions for nurses, preferably integrated into the nursing profession's own training and development programmes.

In many countries, palliative care can also form a substantial part of formal social work training at both qualifying and post-graduate levels[65].

Staff support and management

Social workers who successfully involve themselves in service and skill development are likely to find themselves also involved in staff support. Palliative care workers can enrich their work from their experience of the death of their own friends or relatives; however, the commonality between their own experience and those for whom they care is also a potential difficulty with which they may need help. For instance, the ethics of sedation and the proper response to relatives' questions such as 'Why can't you put Dad out of his misery?' may arise both as practice issues and as personal issues for those involved. Social workers who take some leadership in the service development of their institution will, in setting policy on ethical questions, also need to take some leadership on ethical questions in training and in response to the personal concerns raised by staff. They may also become members of clinical ethics committees and contribute to national ethical debates[66].

Occupational stress is increasingly seen as the result of a dynamic interaction between the person holding an individual job and the environment in which he or she is employed[67]. It is now generally recognized that an effective support system will include both personal and organizational mechanisms. Papadatou's studies examine the impact of culture and inter-professional differences[68,69]. She notes that meaning making is a social as well as a personal process and that individual values and assumptions may be supported or undermined by the explicit and implicit rules and values of the working environment. Social workers are well placed to examine the unconscious processes of projection and denial that can exist in palliative care.[70] Social work's insistence upon the value of clinical supervision is beginning to be recognized by other professional groups[71]. Sheldon's study of the specialist social worker in palliative care also emphasizes the value of recognizing limits and the importance of working creatively within them[72].

Social workers should also have a role in managing the wider issues within their institution. They should be involved in setting policy on patient care, as well as decisions on individual patients. They are likely to be involved in admissions, staff recruitment, quality control, clinical governance, and education and training services, both internal and external. They will specifically manage their own responsibilities such as welfare services and volunteer bereavement services. They may be called upon to initiate and manage innovative inter-professional practice[73]. Ideally, social workers will also be able to influence and take part in the management process of the institution itself.

Extending the service

The wider values and goals of palliative care are often under-resourced and poorly acknowledged. Support is improving; for instance, in many countries specific bereavement support is now normally established after major disasters. However, the extent to which the community provides resources or acknowledges the need for such services depends on how those in the field spread their message and how they demonstrate their effectiveness and value. Social workers have a particular duty in this area as they are the professional group in palliative care that claims to have the strongest links into the community. The social worker's response to under-resourcing and poor acknowledgement may take two forms: the use of volunteers and spreading the word.

The use of volunteers

Appropriately utilized volunteers can extend enormously the variety and scope of services offered to patients and families. Volunteers also have the advantage of representing the community from which patients come and therefore have the ability to educate and influence that community about loss, bereavement, and palliative care values. Volunteers can be used in many areas, for example, as nursing aides or car drivers. Social workers in palliative care will frequently want to provide support for bereaved relatives. One social worker might supervise a team of eight volunteers, each supporting several people, thus providing a considerable volume of service at reasonable cost. The use of volunteers should not be a reason for reduced quality; an effective volunteer bereavement service should select its volunteers rigorously and provide appropriate training[74]. Volunteers can increase community confidence about ordinary individuals' capacity to help one another thereby reducing the risk of care becoming a 'commodity'[75].

Spreading the word

The message of palliative care is relevant in many settings within the wider community, and the resources that the community devotes to palliative care depend upon effective advocacy of both our work and our message. Social workers within palliative care should be involved in a broad spectrum of activities that serve to spread the message. At one end of the spectrum, these will be an extension of the normal liaison with other local organizations concerned with the care of patients, at the other it may include political lobbying and direct attempts to influence decisions in favour of palliative care as well as public education and health promotion in end-of-life care[76].

The direct task of liaising with other local caring organizations for the benefit of individual patients may broaden in a number of ways. For example, a social worker may become involved in lecturing to staff in a general hospital about the care of dying patients, or in helping a local health centre to develop its approach to terminal care in the community. Other contacts, such as with school teachers, funeral directors, community social workers, or welfare workers in large public or commercial organizations, may turn into opportunities to offer training or support to other professionals who have to deal with the consequences of death[77]. For instance, a social worker in palliative care may be the most experienced resource within the community to advise a school on how to cope after the murder of a pupil. The Social Work Department at St Christopher's Hospice in the UK ran a series of training sessions for the Metropolitan Police Force on breaking bad news, in particular, informing relatives of a sudden death. This involvement eventually led to the development of a new community based service offering support to children and families bereaved through sudden death[78].

In addition to influencing attitudes locally, social workers should participate in the development of palliative care regionally, nationally, and internationally[79]. By the nature of their work, social workers in palliative care are widely dispersed, and it is important that this fragmentation does not cause the social work perspective to be lost. Social workers should seek roles on advisory committees and offer their expertise and advice both to specialist groups, such as the specialist disease charities, and to government. When appropriate, social workers should be prepared to lobby actively for change. For instance, in the UK the Association of Hospice Social Workers spearheaded a successful campaign to change welfare benefit rules so that terminally ill patients could claim a special attendance allowance more quickly. They are also active in campaigning for the palliative care needs of those with serious mental health problems and those with learning disabilities[14].

Finally, social workers must be involved in defining the future of palliative care. We have come to understand more and more about the medical aspects of palliative care, but we still know little about the long-term impact of terminal illness on family members and even less about what helps them. Social workers should be involved in developing a better understanding of the psychosocial aspects of palliative care, and in the implementation of new ways of caring for patients and their families[80]. It is vital that social work's unique perspectives remain integrated with the mainstream provision of palliative care[81]. These perspectives offer reminders of the importance of the patient's relationship with society and its institutions and community attitudes, cultural beliefs, and values. In a health-care environment in which most professionals are still only trained in one-to-one communication skills, the skills of working effectively with the relationships, groups, and systems in which most of life is lived and dying takes place, must not be ignored. In our increasingly resource constrained health-care environments the very concept of a 'family focus' may be under threat. Randall and Downie recently suggested that, 'The central aspect of palliative care is symptom control delivered humanely with adequate information …' They question what they see as an 'undue emphasis on attending to families', suggesting that 'such attention is demanding of resources which might be better devoted to a wider population of patients'[82]. We must all engage with the realities of health economics and the challenge to improve cost-effectiveness so that we can deliver good enough care to more. We should also remember that death, dying and bereavement are primarily social experiences, in which good symptom control is profoundly important. A necessary focus on problems and pathologies can blind us to the extraordinary things that ordinary people (even those with pre-existing vulnerabilities and deprivation) can achieve at the end of life given a little support. Patients and their families grow through such experiences[83]. At its best, palliative care is also preventive health care, helping the next generation and beyond to be less afraid of the loss and death that we shall all experience.

References

1. Earnshaw-Smith, E. (1982). Emotional pain in dying patients and their families. *Nursing Times*, **78**, 865–7.
2. Dane, B., and Moore, R. (2005). Social workers' use of spiritual practices in palliative care. *Journal of Social Work in End-of-Life and Palliative Care*, **1**(4), 63–82.
3. Kissane, D.W., and Bloch, S. (2002). *Family focused grief therapy. A Model of family-centred care during palliative care and bereavement.* Open University Press, Buckingham.
4. Kissane, D.W., Lichtenthal, W.G., and Zaider, T. (2007). Family care before and after bereavement. *OMEGA*, **56**(1), 21–32.
5. Oliviere, D., Hargreaves, R., and Monroe, B. (1997). *Good practices in palliative care: A psychosocial perspective.* Ashgate, Aldershot.
6. Gwyther, L.P., Altilio, T., Blacker, S. *et al.* (2005) Social work competencies in palliative and end of life care. *Journal of Social Work in End-of-Life. Palliative Care*, **1**(1), 87–120.
7. Beresford, P., Adshead, L., and Croft, S. (2007). *Palliative care, social work and service users: making life possible.* Jessica Kingsley Publishers. London.
8. Colon, M. (2005). Hospice and latinos: a review of the literature. *Journal of Social Work in End-of-Life and Palliative Care*, **1**(2), 27–44.
9. Gunaratnum, Y. (2006). *Ethnicity, older people and palliative care.* National Council for Palliative Care, London.
10. Payne, M. (2005). Adult Protection cases in a hospice: an audit. *Journal of Adult Protection*, **7**(2), 4–12.
11. Brandsen, C.K. (2005). Social work and end of life care: Reviewing the past and moving forward. *Journal of Social Work in End-of-Life and Palliative Care*, **1**(2), 45–70.
12. Payne, M. (2006). *What is professional social work?* 2nd edition, p. 58. Policy Press, Bristol.
13. Monroe B. (1995). It is impossible not to communicate—helping the grieving family. In *Interventions with bereaved children* (eds. Smith, S.C., and Pennells, M.), pp. 87–106. Jessica Kingsley, London.
14. McEnhill, L. (2004). Disability. In *Death, dying and social differences* (eds. Oliviere, D., and Monroe, B.), pp. 97–118. Oxford University Press, Oxford.
15. Randall, F., and Downie, R.S. (1999). *Palliative care ethics. A companion for all specialties*, 2nd edition. Oxford University Press, Oxford.
16. Vachon, M., Kristjanson, L., and Higginson, I.J. (1995). Psychosocial issues in palliative care: The patient, the family and the process and outcome of care. *Journal of Pain and Symptom Management*, **10**, 142–50.
17. Zaza, C., and Baine, N. (2002). Cancer Pain and Psychosocial Factors: A Critical Review of the Literature. *Journal of Pain and Symptom Management*, **24**(5), 526–42.
18. Barkwell, D.P. (1991). Ascribed meaning: a critical factor in coping and pain attenuation in patients with cancer-related pain. *Journal of Palliative Care*, **7**, 5–14.
19. Herth, K. (1989). The relationship between level of hope and level of coping response. *Oncology Nursing Forum*, **16**(1), 67–72.
20. Hodgson, C., Higginson, I.J., McDonnell, M. *et al.* (1997). Family anxiety in advanced cancer: a multicentre prospective study in Ireland. *British Journal of Cancer*, **76**, 1211–14.
21. Pemberton, C., Storey, L., and Howard, A. (2003). The preferred place of care document: an opportunity for communication. *International Journal of Palliative Nursing*, **9**(10), 439–41.
22. Payne, S., Smith, P., and Dean, S. (1999). Identifying the concerns of informal carers in palliative care. *Palliative Medicine*, **13**, 37–44.
23. Gomes, B., and Higginson, I.J. (2006). Factors influencing death at home in terminally ill patients with cancer: systematic review. *British Medical Journal*, **332**, 515–21.
24. Kristjanson, L.J., Leis, A., Koop, P.M. *et al.* (1997). Family members care expectations, care perceptions, and satisfaction with advanced cancer care. *Journal of Palliative Care*, **1**, 5–13.
25. Harding, R., Higginson, I.J., Leam, C. *et al.* (2004). Evaluation of a short-term group intervention for informal carers of patients attending a home palliative care service. *Journal of Pain and Symptom Management*, **27**(5), 396–408.
26. Payne, S. (2004). Carers and caregivers. In *Death, dying and social differences* (eds. Oliviere, D., and Monroe, B.), pp. 181–98. Oxford University Press, Oxford.
27. Gallagher, D. (2004). Finances. In *Death, dying and social differences* (eds. Oliviere, D., and Monroe B), pp. 165–80. Oxford University Press, Oxford.

28. Oliviere, D. (2004). Cultural issues in palliative care. In *Management of advanced disease* (eds. Sykes, N., Edmonds, P., and Wiles, J.), pp. 438–49. Arnold, London.

29. Field, D. (2000). *What do we mean by psychosocial?* National Council Briefing Paper, No. 4, London.

30. Sheldon, F. (1997). *Psychosocial palliative care. Good practice in the care of the dying and bereaved*. Stanley Thornes, Cheltenham.

31. Gallagher, D., and Monroe, B. (2000). Psychosocial care. In *Palliative care in amyotrophic laterel sclerosis* (eds. Oliviere, D., Borasio, B.G., and Walsh, D.), pp. 83–103. Oxford University Press, Oxford.

32. King, D.A., and Quill, T. (2006). Working with families in palliative care: One size does not fit all. *Journal of Palliative Medicine*, **9**(3), 704–15.

33. Monroe, B. (1998). A sexual-sensitive approach to palliative care. In *Good practices in palliative care: A psychosocial perspective* (eds. Oliviere, D., Hargreaves, R., and Monroe, B.), pp. 96–111. Ashgate, Aldershot.

34. Cort, E., Monroe, B., and Oliviere, D. (2004). Couples in palliative care. *Sexual and Relationship Therapy*, **19**(3), 337–54.

35. Levy, J., and Payne, M. (2006). Audit of welfare benefits advocacy in a palliative care setting. *European Journal of Palliative Care*, **13**(1), 15–7.

36. Sheldon, F. (1998). ABC of palliative care. Bereavement. *British Medical Journal*, **316**, 456–8.

37. Department of Health and Ageing (Australia) (2006). A systematic review of the literature on complicated grief. Retrieved from http://www.health.gov.au/internet/wcms/publishing.nsf/content/palliativecare-pubs-rsch-grief.

38. Bremner, I. (2000). Working with adolescents. *Bereavement Care*, **19**(1), 6–7.

39. Stedeford, A. (1994). *Facing death: patients, families and professionals*. Sobell Publications, Oxford.

40. Lester, J. (2005). Life Review with the terminaly ill—narrative therapies. In *Loss, change and bereavement in palliative care* (eds. Firth, P., Luff, G., and Oliviere, D.), pp. 66–79. Open University Press, Maidenhead.

41. Field, D., Douglas, C., Jagger, C. *et al.* (1995). Terminal illness: views of lay patients and their carers. *Palliative Medicine*, **9**, 45–54.

42. Monroe, B., and Sheldon, F. (2004). Psychosocial dimensions of care. In *Management of advanced disease* (eds. Sykes, N., Edmonds, P., Wiles, J.), pp. 405–37. 4th edition. Edward Arnold, London.

43. Monroe, B., and Kraus, J. (eds.) (2005). *Brief Interventions with Bereaved Children*. Oxford University Press, Oxford.

44. Oliviere, D., Hargreaves, R., and Monroe, B. (1998). Working with groups. In *Good practices in palliative care: a psychosocial perspective*. pp. 71–93. Ashgate, Aldershot.

45. Silverman, P.R. (2000) *Never too young to know. Death in children's lives*. Oxford University Press, Oxford.

46. Worden, W.J. (1996) *Children and grief. When a parent dies*. Guilford Press, New York.

47. Christ, G.H. (2000). *Healing children's grief. Surviving a parent's death from cancer*. Oxford University Press, Oxford.

48. Social Work Department (1989). *My book about*. St Christopher's Hospice, London.

49. Social Work Department. (1989). *Someone special has died*. St Christopher's Hospice, London.

50. Klass, D., Silverman, P., and Nickman, S.L. (eds.) (1996). *Continuing bonds*. Taylor and Frances, Philadelphia.

51. Kearney, M. (1992). Image work in a case of intractable pain. *Palliative Medicine*, **6**, 152–7.

52. McGoldrick, M., and Gerson, R. (1985). *Genograms in family assessment*. Norton, New York.

53. Oliviere, D. (2006). User involvement- the patient and carer as team members. In *Teamwork in palliative care—Fulfilling or frustrating?* (ed. Speck, P.), pp. 41–64. Oxford University Press, Oxford.

54. Sinclair S. (2005). Crossing the great barrier grief. In *Brief interventions with bereaved children* (eds. Monroe, B., and Kraus, F.), pp. 227–240. Oxford University Press, Oxford.

55. Addington-Hall, J.M., and Higginson, I.J. (eds.) (2001). *Palliative care for non-cancer patients*. Oxford University Press, Oxford.

56. Field, D., Hockey, J., and Small, N. (eds.) (1997). *Death, gender and ethnicity*. Routledge, London.

57. Parkes, C.M., Laungani, P., and Young, B. (1997). *Death and Bereavement across cultures*. Routledge, London.

58. Blanche, M., and Endersby, C. (2004). Refugees. In *Death, dying and social differences* (eds. Oliviere, D., Monroe, B.), pp. 149–64. Oxford University Press, Oxford.

59. Firth, S. (2001). *Wider horizons: Care of the dying in a multicultural society*. National Council for Palliative Care. London.

60. Koffman, J, and Higginson, I.J. (2001). Accounts of carers' satisfaction with health care at the end-of-life: a comparison of first generation black Caribbean and white patients with advanced disease. *Palliative Medicine*, **15**, 337–45.

61. Gunaratnam Y. (1997). Culture is not enough: a critique of multi culturalism in palliative care. In *Death, gender and ethnicity* (eds. Field, D., Hockey, J., and Small, N.), pp. 166–86, Routledge, London.

62. Koffman, J., and Higginson, I.J. (2001). Accounts of symptom severity and control during advanced disease: a comparison of first generation black Caribbean and white patients with advanced disease. *Palliative Medicine*, **16**(6), 539–540.

63. Payne, S., Chapman, A., Holloway, M. *et al.* (2005). Chinese community views: Promoting cultural competence in palliative care. *Journal of Palliative Care*, **21**(2), 111–6.

64. Walsh, K., Corbett, B., and Whitaker, T. (2005). Developing practice tools for social workers in end-of-life care. *Journal of Social Work in End of Life and Palliative Care*, **1**(2), 3–10.

65. Walsh-Burke, K., and Csikai, E.L. (2005). Professional social work education in end-of-life care: Contributions of the Project on Death in America's Social Work Leadership Development program. *Journal of Social Work in End-of-Life and Palliative Care*, **1**(2), 11–26.

66. Miller, P.J., and Hedlund, S.C. (2005). "We just happen to live here". Two social workers share their stories about Oregon's death with dignity law. *Journal of Social Work in End-of-Life and Palliative Care*, **1**(1), 71–86.

67. Vachon, M. (1995). Staff stress in hospice/palliative care: a review. *Palliative Medicine*, **9**, 91–122.

68. Papadatou, D. (2001). The grieving healthcare provider. Variables affecting the professional response to a child's death. *Bereavement Care*, **20**(2), 26–9.

69. Papadatou, D., Martinson, I., and Chung, B. (2001). Caring for dying children: a comparative study of nurses' experience in Greece and Hong Kong. *Cancer Nursing*, **24**(5), 402–12.

70. Speck, P. (2006). Maintaining a healthy team. In *Teamwork in palliative care: fulfilling or frustrating?* (ed. Speck, P.) pp. 95–115. Oxford University Press, Oxford.

71. Gilmore, A. (1999). *Review of UK evaluative literature on clinical supervision in nursing and health visiting*. UKCC, London.

72. Sheldon, F. (2000). Dimensions of the role of the social worker in palliative care. *Palliative Medicine*, **14**, 491–8.

73. Monroe, B. (1997). The Development of a Hospice Consultancy Service. *Proceedings of the 5th Congress of the European Association of Palliative Care, London*.

74. Payne, S., Horn, S., and Relf, M. (1999). The application of models of loss in clinical and community settings. In *Loss and bereavement*. pp. 90–128. Open University Press, Buckingham.

75. Silverman, P.R. (2004) *Widow to widow*, 2nd edition. Brunner-Routledge, Hove.

76. Kellehear, A. (2005). *Compassionate Cities. Public health and end-of-life care*. Routledge, Milton Park.

77. Shipman, C., Kraus, F., and Monroe, B. (2001). Responding to the needs of schools in supporting bereaved children: a questionnaire survey. *Bereavement Care*, **20**(1), 6–7.

78. Stokes, J., Pennington, J., Monroe, B. *et al.* (1999). Developing services for bereaved children: a discussion of the theoretical and practical issues involved. *Mortality*, **4**(3), 291–307.

79. Christ, G., and Blacker, S. (2005). Setting an agenda for social work in end-of-life and palliative care: an overview of leadership and organizational initiatives. *Journal of Social Work in End-of-Life and Palliative Care*, **1**(1), 9–22.

80. Kramer, B.J., and Christ, G.H. (2005). A national agenda for social work research in palliative and end-of-life care. *Journal of Palliative Medicine*, **8**(2), 418–31.

81. Berzoff, J., and Silverman, P.R. (eds.) (2004). *A handbook for end-of-life healthcare practitioners*. Columbia University Press, New York.

82. Randall, F., and Downie, R. (2006). *The Philosophy of palliative care—critique and reconstruction*. Oxford University Press, Oxford.

83. Monroe, B., and Oliviere, D. (2006). Resilience in palliative care. *European Journal of Palliative* Care, **13**(1), 22–5.

The role of the chaplain in palliative care

Rev. James M. Harper III and
Rabbi Jonathan E. Rudnick

Introduction

A chaplain is a people-person in the fullest sense, one whose role is to connect to people and care for them in their health and healing experiences, and to accompany them on their life journeys in this health and healing context— taking primary responsibility for providing spiritual care to patients, family and friends, and staff colleagues who are part of the health-care team. We open here with two central questions that constantly need to be considered when relating to the role of the chaplain. The first question is: 'What is a person?' And the second question is: 'What is spiritual care?' Since a chaplain is charged with relating to individuals by virtue of their humanness, their personhood, or as Dr. King called it, their 'somebodiness', the question of what constitutes a person is critical to understanding the chaplain's role in relating to each person as a person[1].

What is a person?

In the same spirit as the chaplain asks all of the time, 'Who is this person— who are you in the deepest and fullest sense?', we ask here, 'What is a person?'. We believe a person to be a multi-dimensional creature—one who is created in a divine/holy image. Being multi-dimensional means that there are physical, psychological, social, and spiritual elements (and even others) that make up a person, and these different dimensions of a person are constantly interacting with one another in a very dynamic way. In other words, a person is best understood as a psychosomatic unity of body, mind, and spirit that are vitally related.

Psychosomatic unity refers to the holistic understanding of the human as a unity of body, mind, and spirit. This unity assumes that aspects are synergistic, creating outcomes in mutuality with respect to their integrity as a whole. This understanding differs from a trichotomist view that sees body, mind, and spirit as distinct and substantial alone, and from a dichotomist understanding that sees persons as body and spirit. We assume all functions of living persons are organically related and mutually conditioned. A problem in any aspect affects all of the others. Thus, illness is a whole-person experience.

Persons are made for relational encounter distinguished by profound love and unconditional acceptance. Such encounter calls something into being that formerly did not exist. In the Judeo-Christian tradition, there is a teaching that it is not good that the creature be alone (Book of Genesis, the Bible). Living in relationship is the point of departure and ultimate goal of created existence, and the impact of relationship is holistic. It follows, then, that personality is the exercise of personal, willful choice in combination with influences embedded from one's social matrix of relations. Caring incorporates nurture of individuals and their community of significant others. Persons live as individuals, families, groups, communities, and organizations in diverse, multi-cultural societies. Therefore, holistic care focuses on human experiences and the meanings, patterns, and themes that emerge in human living, including nodal factors like gender, sexuality, generation, and culture. So in order to provide holistic care to someone, we must relate to the different dimensions of their humanness, and we must include here the spiritual dimension. As the professional responsible for spiritual care, the chaplain is called to focus on the spiritual dimension, while being aware of the interaction between the spiritual dimensions and the others that are at play in every human being.

The person as maker of meaning

We assume human beings are dynamic organisms who find meaning and purpose by relational connection, the *sine qua non* of human existence. Persons live inter-subjectively in relation with others and the world and are meaning-makers and interpreters of their experiences. Victor Frankl concluded from observation of concentration camp victims during the Holocaust that survival itself depended on seeking and finding meaning. He wrote based on his experience, including his observation of others: 'Suffering ceases to be suffering at the moment it finds a meaning...(we need) meaning in our life… (we are) even ready to suffer, on the condition, to be sure, that suffering has a meaning'. Thus, Frankl is suggesting that we are not destroyed by suffering; we are destroyed by suffering without meaning[2].

Honouring human dignity requires discovery of what persons hold as sacred, defining, ultimate concerns. They are often accessible in patients' descriptions concerning quality of life and inform decisions given in advanced health-care directives. Existential questions about life, its meaning and values in health, may be voiced and considered in terms that are vernacular, psychological, philosophical, or existential, as well as religious. Quality-of-life instruments used in towards-death care measures often include an existential domain, which measures purpose, meaning in life, and capacity for self-transcendence. Three items were found to correlate with good quality of life for patients with advanced disease: if the patient's personal existence is meaningful, if the patient finds fulfillment in achieving life goals, and if life to this point has been meaningful[3]. This finding corresponds well to the conclusions of significant research on understanding will-to-live in patients nearing death. One such study reports that the three most significant factors here are feeling of dignity, sense of hope (for finding meaning in whatever time is left), and the perception of being a burden to others[4]. From both perspectives, the role of the chaplain intersects all three areas.

Spirituality plays a critical role, because the relationship with a transcendent being or concept can give meaning and purpose to people's lives, to their joys, and to their sufferings. In dying, for example, healing or restoration of wholeness could involve a transcendent set of meaningful experiences while very ill and in a peaceful death[5]. In chronic illness, healing may be experienced as acceptance of limitations.

In general, chaplains engage questions of ultimate meaning or purpose that arise from the experience of persons. They help others narrate and make sense of their life story. Vital in this process is reminiscence, gaining from the foundation of what has been, the richness of what is, and the hope of what shall be through life's transition, towards death.

Spirituality and spiritual care

The second question, then, is what is spiritual care? In order to delve into this question, we must open up the word 'spiritual'. We may acknowledge here that spiritual is how we describe the feeling or experience of spirituality, something that is highly subjective and usually very personal, varying greatly with the diversity of people in the world and in many societies. Due to the individual and subjective nature of spirituality, it is impossible to agree on one definition that fits all people and all situations. There is a plethora of different definitions that have been offered for explaining spirituality. While there is no one right definition, this question of spirituality is critical to consider in order to understand the role of the chaplain. Ideally, each person could be asked to write their own definition of spirituality as pertains to them as a person. In a sense, part of the role of the chaplain is to contemplate the definition of spirituality for each person being given care and even help the person come to a conscious recognition of their individual spirituality. We offer here one definition of spirituality that by its very nature attests to the broad, accepting, and inclusive character of spirituality as a concept. It is not coincidental that the source of this definition is a nursing textbook, being that the role of the nurse is one whose roots connect the physical healing with spiritual healing:

> Spirituality is my being; my inner person. It is who I am – unique and alive. It is my body, my thinking, my feelings, my judgments, and my creativity. My spirituality motivates me to choose meaningful relationships and pursuits. Through my spirituality I give and receive love; I respond to and appreciate God, other people, a sunset, a symphony, and spring. I am driven forward, sometimes because of pain, sometimes in spite of pain. Spirituality allows me to reflect on myself. I am a person because of my spirituality – motivated and enabled to value, to worship and to communicate with the holy, the transcendent[6].

Freedom to do spiritual work is critical. Supporting spiritual reminiscence as exploration of life meanings, caregivers adapt to the world of a patient, connecting to such core values as sanctity of life, respect for human dignity, desire for meaningful existence, and alleviation of pain and suffering. This is the hallmark of compassionate care, beyond cure. Convinced that there exists a spiritual dimension inherent to being a person and with a sense of what the spiritual realm can include, we are ready to introduce the field of spiritual care. Let us do so by considering the professional spiritual caregiver, whose primary role is to focus on and provide this dimension of care. It is in this context that we meet the chaplain. What is a chaplain? We have found that a dictionary definition along with a homiletic commentary is very helpful in understanding the role of the chaplain. The dictionary rightly tells us that a chaplain is one who serves in a chapel, and according to Webster's Dictionary, there are two definitions of chapel: (1) a small church; and (2) a private worship place[7]. Building on the second definition, we come to an understanding that a chaplain is one who's primary responsibility is to help create a personal spiritual space for a patient—a space that is safe for the individual where they are, as well as open to include family and friends and even staff who are giving care and support to the patient. The chaplain has unique skill and capacity to manage the task of helping to build and support around those in his or her care, sacred space, which includes the community or the milieu of significant others. The chaplain aims to furnish those served, personally and in the rally of community, a creative mixture of being and doing that delivers the emotional, dynamic experience of chapel, that personal, private, spiritual space where love, healing, and the potential for lasting wholeness, mindfulness, and peace abide and endure.

In the general atmosphere of health care, and specifically in a hospital setting, where so much emphasis is placed on the physical dimension of a person, trying to heal by fixing the situation, the chaplain is focused on and involved with connections. The role of the chaplain in palliative care includes the provision of loving, compassionate, person-centered contact that delivers spiritual, religious, and existential care. Care as contact is characterized by empathetic listening, a capacity to suspend personal bias, attunement to otherness that acknowledges uniqueness, provides attention, support, compassion, all meaningful in experiences of vulnerability and helplessness. This can involve simple, mundane acts of embodiment (like holding hands), or complex and profound acts of ritual or religion (such as prayer, anointing, reading of holy texts, rituals of blessing, or sacrament of the sick) by a chaplain or other significant faith tradition representative (priest, rabbi, imam, lopon). The overall aim of the role of the chaplain in palliative care is to furnish for those served a congruous, quality of presence, through which is communicated meaningful connection to them on this journey. The chaplain promotes belonging, supports connection, and uses linkages to community. The chaplain does this not to 'fix' things but rather to sustain and uphold dignity and trust individual potential for healing. This assisting of people to access their spirituality as part of the healing process can be referred to as ministry of presence, encompassing a variety of skills invoked by the chaplain to release the spiritual power of the patient and facilitate the healing process[8].

The chaplain must begin by connecting to and with the patient and family (and staff when relevant), and furthermore helping those in their care connect with the spiritual resources that can help them deal with their health and healing challenges. In the dialectic of care and cure, the chaplain stands for the commitment to care based on each person's inherent value as a human being. This basic character of the chaplain's professional identity is most pronounced in the context of palliative care, where the general medical approach recognizes the reality in terms of lack of cure and focuses primarily on the care and easing of suffering, rather than fixing the medical problem. It is this common commitment to connections (rather than repairs) that brings the chaplain so close to the health-care staff in the palliative care setting. As two doctors at the George Washington University Center to Improve Care of the Dying write: 'If you are in a hospital or hospice program, a chaplain can offer support, prayer, and spiritual guidance ... They come from various religious backgrounds, but provide care regardless of religious affiliation ... Many, but not all, hospitals have chaplains whose job it is to counsel and support the very sick and their families' (see[9], p. 33).

We understand palliative care as an integrated approach to enhance the quality of life of patients and their families facing problems associated with life-threatening illness and pain. It is achieved by prevention and relief of suffering through early identification, accurate assessment, and mobilization of treatment addressing associated physical, psychosocial, religious, and spiritual needs. After medical cure is no longer possible, palliative care continues to address the underlying aim of healing. By healing, we mean addressing needs by providing relational presence attuned to matters of integrity, wholeness, and meaning—all in support of an optimal quality of life. While we understand that caregivers do not heal the patient per se (in terms of cure), we believe palliative care facilitates a processes to create a secure environment of connectedness for the patient, beneficial also for family and significant others. We understand connectedness here as the quality of 'I/Thou' engagement defined by Martin Buber[10]. It involves relational reciprocity characterized by respect, love, and compassion in honor of the sanctity of life. The role of a chaplain in palliative care requires awareness of its comprehensive features. However, its chief aim is furnishing encounter and care for persons at the point of their perceived religious and/or spiritual need. This care is person-specific, discerning, and never proselytizing.

Doing spiritual assessment is preface for actually shaping a spiritual care plan and actualizing it. Chaplains assess then address spiritual care needs. Actions or resources applied address proactively the spiritual needs of patients and their families with profound respect for their religion, faith group, statement of belief and convictions, including those who are atheists, agnostic, or estranged. A spiritual care plan represents studied outcomes and discernment that convey respect and meet the cultural, spiritual, and religious needs, traditions, and practices of the patient and those in his/her sacred circle. Done artistically, this would include non-traditional gestures for those who do not value conventional expressions of faith. This would include, but not be limited to, plans that address those who find spirituality through profound connection to nature, music, the arts, or a philosophy or other set of values and principles, or a particular way of seeking scientific truth. The role of the chaplain is

to shape interventions cognizant that persons may have sundry feelings and experience with religious organizations on a spectrum from extremely positive to extremely negative. Again, the abiding principle is meeting others at the point of their perceived need[11].

Who is a chaplain?

Chaplaincy embodies wide spiritual and religious concern about the general welfare of all people. In the deepest sense, chaplaincy is a humanitarian movement, distinguished by its unbridled commitment to meet people compassionately in the crises of their lives in the world, where they are at the point of their perceived need. Chaplains are pastoral care practitioners with the personal depth and maturity to cultivate and delve into encounters, supporting in others the freedom to inquire about their meaning of life.

Although by education, a chaplain is most often an ordained clergy person, this is not exclusively the case, and as the field of spiritual care spreads and develops internationally, there will likely be cultural variances as far as background and training are concerned. It follows that usually a chaplain will have a graduate education in theology or religion, an education that comes out of a particular spiritual/religious tradition of practice with a rigorous academic grounding in the relevant texts and sister disciplines. In addition to this educational background that is most commonly specific to a certain spiritual/religious tradition and even denomination within that tradition, a chaplain will likely have some professional training in pastoral care/spiritual care. In the international community of pastoral caregivers, these standards of professional training are included in the post-graduate educational framework known as Clinical Pastoral Education (CPE).

In terms of qualification, chaplains in palliative care need professional training. Being a competent chaplain in palliative care requires faith group and ecclesial endorsement, evidence of practised faith and good standing in one's context of faith or philosophy, possession of relevant knowledge in the field that is critically purchased, clinical skills, capacity to engage and encounter others at profound depth, mindful ability to use one's self in the care of others, ability to meet others at the point of their need, emotional maturity, and good mental health, comfort with authority (one's own and another's), and considerable accredited training in a clinical setting by certified experts in the field of clinical pastoral education. Chaplains are bound by a code of professional ethics. All palliative care chaplains must have evidence of demonstrated competence to work respectfully with patients with different religious or spiritual beliefs.

In the United States, palliative chaplains are typically educated through the Association for Clinical Pastoral Education and, as part of this educational track of professional chaplaincy training, can be certified by one of the following professional chaplaincy organizations: The Association of Professional Chaplains, The National Association of Catholic Chaplains, or The National Association of Jewish Chaplains. In Canada, they may be certified by the Canadian Association for Pastoral Practice and Education. Certification typically requires a Masters of Divinity degree (or other relevant graduate degree), faith group ordination or commissioning, faith group endorsement, and four units (1600 hours) of Clinical Pastoral Education.

A chaplain is often employed by a specific health-care institution, such as a hospital or hospice service or hospice house, but the chaplain can also be sponsored by a particular spiritual/religious denomination that actively supports the presence and work of the chaplain in a given health-care setting. However, in general (as expressed in the 'White Paper' on professional chaplaincy), 'professional chaplains reach across faith group boundaries and do not proselytize. Acting on behalf of their institutions, they also seek to protect patients from being confronted by other, unwelcome, forms of spiritual intrusion'[12].

Beyond understanding and know-how, a chaplain must be the type of person who can provide others a private, sacred space for their unique spiritual needs for religious and spiritual growth and development. This includes the intrapersonal and interpersonal awareness that allows one to be present emotionally to others with caring acceptance, a non-judgemental stance, balance, attunement to their agenda, and physical and emotional availability. This stance respects autonomy in the relationship. It is grounded compassion as segue to be present to persons in the midst of their suffering. Chaplains have the skills and heart to connect with persons as individuals through common humanity that helps provide hope and comfort.

Functions and activities of chaplains

We will begin this section with a look at and differentiation between spiritual/pastoral care and counselling. Both of these modes of spiritual support raise the issues of orientation of a chaplain as well as the clinical nature of the chaplain as spiritual caregiver to the recipient of spiritual care (patient, family, staff). Both realms of activity are often referred to as part of the chaplaincy role[13]. We can understand pastoral care as the function of providing a spiritual, religious, or faith-oriented presence and support. Pastoral counselling, then, can be understood as the process of providing spiritual guidance through the use of insights and principles from the disciplines of theology and the behavioural sciences. These terms provide a conceptual framework or context for understanding the activity of the chaplain.

Chaplains serve aware that a comprehensive loving response in treating illness or in palliative care must involve interdependency among all providers including, but not limited to, physicians and nurses, family, friends, and communities of faith. Value for the interdependency of all providers in healing is an understanding inherent to trained chaplains. In recent years, the chaplain has become a vital member of the health-care team. Beyond former roles like administering particular prayers and rites specific to a patient's religion, the role of a chaplain today is more comprehensive. For example, the chaplain can act as an extension of the patient's personal and community support system, as well as be a source of spiritual support for the patient, to ensure care is provided for others.

Professional chaplains serve as members of patient care teams by: (1) participation in medical rounds and patient care conferences, offering perspectives on the spiritual status of patients; (2) participation in inter-disciplinary education; and (3) charting spiritual care interventions in medical charts. A chaplain in palliative care identifies and addresses spiritual and religious needs as part of a multi-disciplinary team that meets with meaningful regularity. This role requires in the chaplain capacity to articulate findings. Further, it includes achieving all associated documentary requirements regarding keeping confidential records in the patient information systems. These patient notes benefit the community of professionals who share in care giving process on

a comprehensive basis. Professional chaplains also lead or participate in health-care ethics programmes by:

◆ assisting patients and families in completing advance directives;

◆ clarifying value issues with patients, family members, staff and the organization;

◆ participating in Ethics Committees and Institutional Review Boards;

◆ consulting with staff and patients about ethical concerns;

◆ pointing to human value aspects of institutional policies and behaviours;

◆ conducting in-service education.

In an ethics consultation, the chaplain is helpful in promoting ethical reflection and decision making.

In a recent survey of American health care focusing on administrators' views on the importance of various chaplain roles, the following 11 chaplain roles were mentioned as important: providing end-of-life care; providing emotional support to patients; providing emotional support to family and friends; providing emotional support to staff; being the point-person for integrating spirituality into overall institutional care; praying with patients or relatives; providing ethical consultation; serving as liaison to local clergy; serving as the patient's advocate; performing religious rituals; conducting religious services (worship)[14]. Chaplains must have exceptional communication skills and a working grasp of different faith traditions to help persons deal with how their world works, spiritually and religiously.

There is a broad spectrum of functions and activities in which chaplains engage in the context of palliative care. Whatever the spiritual tradition, when stated in explicit language of belief/faith (including but not limited to religion), effective care requires proficiency, comfort, and confidence, using unique spiritual language, symbolism, story, and ritual. Throughout the course of treatment, chaplains meet persons in their suffering, honour and explore their spiritual values, and support them as they affirm and wrestle with conflicts of meaning. At its core, palliative care recognizes occasions for spiritual healing occur until we die. Though terminal illness disrupts a person's life, it holds opportunity for persons to comprehend life differently. In serious and terminal illness, persons often experience richness and fullness in life that were hidden or absent before. Some people find new priorities, gain unexpected appreciation for aspects of life once unnoticed, or reach resolution with self, others, and God-resolution, previously thought impossible or irrelevant.

Spiritual assessment

With regard to the many key roles the chaplain assumes specific to pastoral ministry in a palliative care context, in the United States, the Joint Commission on Accreditation of Healthcare Organizations (JCAHO) requires spiritual assessment. Spiritual assessment intersects the role of the Chaplain. The Joint Commission specifies a minimum of what constitutes spiritual assessment. One must 'determine the patient's denomination, beliefs, and what spiritual practices are important to the patient ... (to) assist in determining the impact of spirituality, if any, on the care/services being provided and ... if any further assessment is needed'[15].

JCAHO furnishes examples of elements that could be part of a spiritual assessment, including the following questions directed to the patient or the patient's family:

◆ Who or what provides the patient with strength and hope?

◆ Does the patient use prayer in their life?

◆ How does the patient express their spirituality?

◆ How would the patient describe their philosophy of life?

◆ What type of spiritual/religious support does the patient desire?

◆ What is the name of the patient's clergy/minister/chaplain/pastor/rabbi?

◆ What does suffering mean to the patient?

◆ What does dying mean to the patient?

◆ What are the patient's spiritual goals?

◆ Is there a role of church/synagogue in the patient's life?

◆ How does faith help the patient cope with illness?

◆ How does the patient keep going day after day?

◆ What helps the patient get through this health-care experience?

◆ How has illness affected the patient and his/her family?

Professional chaplains do spiritual assessment to discern and understand the complex spiritual and religious needs and concerns of patients, their families, and significant others, including members of their religious community and circle of significant others. The chaplain looks for spiritual distress or spiritual crisis in which individuals are unable to find sources of meaning, hope, love, peace, comfort, strength, and connection in life. This includes paying special attention to conflicts that occur between professed belief and what is actually happening in their life. Spiritual anguish can be detrimental to physical and mental health. Medical illness and impending death often activate spiritual distress in patients and family members. Pivotal to the role of the chaplain is accurate recognition and fitting response to the various expressions of spirituality encountered in patients, families, and their significant others.

Five dimensions of spiritual care

The ideological foundation of chaplaincy sets an agenda for pastoral care that is indeed a commitment to providing spiritual care to patients, family/friends, and staff. The chaplain is often in contact with all of these people, facilitating communication and conflict resolution among them. Beyond this declaration of purpose, it is important, especially in the context of palliative care, to differentiate between these groups of people as regards the provision of spiritual care by a chaplain.

It is often emphasized that one of the unique aspects of the role of the chaplain, in general as well as, specifically, in the context of palliative care, is that pastoral care is meant to be provided for these three different groups (patients, family and friends, and staff) in the health-care setting, as opposed to focusing on just one group. Therefore, it is appropriate here to describe the role of the chaplain with respect to each of these groups. There are many different expressions of spiritual care and after outlining five such areas in general, we will focus on the expressions of spiritual care for each of the above three groups of people. The different expressions of spiritual care include:

◆ Presence—based on active and empathetic listening.

◆ Prayer—a broad spectrum of spiritual practice, including traditional liturgy, meditation, song, guided imagery, and others.

◆ Ritual—including facilitating traditional religious ceremonies as well as designing contemporary spiritual ceremonies, incorporated into blessings, holiday worship and observance, life cycle transition events, memorial services, and funerals.

◆ Learning texts as spiritual resources—including traditional scriptures, such as the Bible, Torah, Koran, Book of Buddha, and others, as well as contemporary prose and poetry. Often this will lead to theological reflection or more general 'spiritual work', whereby a chaplain can facilitate a person's opportunity to bring their own faith/belief to their current experience.

◆ Advocacy—including facilitation of communication with all staff members as well as referral and linkage to internal and external resources that include other health-care professionals, as well as to complementary spiritual therapies (including music, art, relaxation training, guided imagery, healing touch, and others).

As it is axiomatic that spiritual care is expressed differently from person to person, we can expect unique elements of spiritual care when it is provided as a service to the different groups of people mentioned earlier.

Spiritual care for patients

By definition, the palliative care patient has a physical malady, and therefore the initial expression of spiritual care by the chaplain can be referred to as ministry of presence—physically being present with the patient. This being 'there' includes being in that unique place of experiencing an ultimate health crisis and subsequent challenge (by definition the context of palliative care), the place that is distinct from person to person, even if the diagnosis and prognosis are similar. To be 'there', a chaplain must try to connect to the patient where they are, specifically in the spiritual dimension and generally as a whole person. This presence begins with the creation of an empathetic connection with the patient, a connection which is established largely through active and empathic listening. The chaplain listens to what the patient is going through—both in the immediate sense as well as from a broader perspective of how their present situation fits into the rest of their life—the patient's story as the patient tells it.

Prayer is a spiritual/ritual act of sacred attention through articulation that is profoundly mindful and respectful of a patient's given condition and personally expressed needs. Prayer must be offered with artful, passionate, sincere understanding, wonder, and care, based on expressed concerns of the patient and those from experiential wisdom furnished to promote comfort, courage, reassurance, understanding, and faith. By offering the patient the opportunity to pray, the chaplain is helping to create a personal and relevant opportunity for the patient to voice (or to voice in the patient's name) the hopes, fears, desire for forgiveness (giving as well as receiving), recognition of blessings (giving thanks). The prayer can be voiced to the patient themselves, to the family, to God, or to the universe in a very general non-religious but spiritual way. It is important to mention here the particularly powerful and calming effect of music—melody and song—on the patient's feeling of deeply connecting to 'something greater' (beyond the here and now of human physical existence). The more personal the prayer (whether specifically religious from a particular faith tradition or more open and broad spiritually), the more the chaplain succeeds in focusing on the particular patient in that moment.

Ritual refers to the initiation of an act of spiritual significance—with some aspect of 'doing' as well as saying or being—either a traditional ceremony that is familiar to the patient from their faith tradition or a formal act of special meaning that is created by the patient or for the patient. Some examples of the former in the context of religion would be confession, communion, anointing, sanctifying the Sabbath (*Kiddush*) and use of religious articles and icons. Some examples of the latter might include lighting candles, writing a letter (ethical will), donning a garment of religious/spiritual significance, eating a significant food, washing the hands, telling stories in a family circle, and many others.

Learning text (Biblical, liturgical, poetry, prose—from ancient to contemporary) together in a spiritual context (one that involves the patient in searching and making meaning of life) can be a tremendous experience of significant connection. A chaplain can offer such an experience by introducing the possibility of such study to a patient. With the establishment of content and connection, meaning can flow from these spiritual resources. As study partners, the potential arises for the health-care situation to become much more symmetrical, as there is an equalizing effect on the patient, as teacher as well as student. This equalizing dynamic can occur precisely because the patient knows something (or some things) that others, including the chaplain, do not know. The patient knows the 'other side' of palliative care, not just in general, but their particularly unique experience as an individual patient (following from their distinct value and being as a person). When the patient brings themselves to a text in the context of spiritual care, they have the opportunity of placing their story into a larger story of life—of the history of humanity and thus human being-ness. Often the chaplain's contribution to this experience happens through choosing of a text or two to offer for the patient's consideration.

Being that the hospital, and health care in general, tends to focus on the physical (in some sense easier to comprehend but in many senses lacking in relation to relating to the patient as a whole person), the patient as a person is often stripped of personhood through the experience of illness. With this emphasis often comes the metaphorical losing of voice by the patient. In this place of a silenced patient voice, the chaplain can act, if needed, as an advocate for the patient. With all due respect to the medical staff, when a chaplain asks a patient what the patient needs and what it is important for the staff to know about them as a person, there is often 'new material' brought to the fore that can be and often needs to be brought to the attention of the members of the care team.

The chaplain is a part of the professional caregiving team and must take responsibility for helping the patient in any way possible (including physical comfort to the extent that the chaplain is capable of providing that) as part of the essence of good palliative care. Like any professional health-care specialist, and certainly in the context of palliative care with the accompanying ultimate meaning to one's life as they encounter and then near death, a chaplain may well need to refer a patient to other health-care professionals (a social worker, a psychologist, a physical therapist, in addition to the doctors and nurses) as well as to complementary modes of spiritual care in which the chaplain has not necessarily been trained. This role may involve acting as liaison with a patient's chosen clergy, ecclesiastical leader, or other identified meaningful others, making critical interfaith and community building connections.

Spiritual care for family and friends

The patient as a person is always part of a family system, and as such this system is inherently relevant and significant to living one's life[16]. Therefore, the chaplain is present for family and friends of the patient no less than for the patient, understanding clearly that there must be care for the caregiver. From the outset, the family and friends of the patient are considered by the chaplain as an integral part of any health-care story, and all the more so in the context of palliative care. Central to this is the chaplain's responsibility to cultivate and solidify the type of trust it takes to enter a family's life relationships with patients, family, and significant others.

The spiritual space that the chaplain tries to create around and for the patient must include family and friends. Part of the challenge of the chaplain's job is to be present for family and friends, listening actively and empathetically to their story (or stories) as well. While the family and friends are seen by the chaplain as possible recipients of spiritual care, they are also significant resources of support for the patient. The chaplain is uniquely positioned to help make these connections significant and relevant to what is happening medically, emotionally, and spiritually.

In the realm of prayer, the family (and friends) often needs a voice for their hopes and feelings, as they are being experienced uniquely by family members, distinct from the experience of the patient. In addition, since family and friends are often people who are very close to the patient, they should be included in the spiritual space created by the chaplain, being invited to be part of any prayer experience that is offered. For example, as a chaplain considers singing to a patient, it is certainly appropriate for the chaplain to invite the family and friends to participate. This facilitation of communication seems almost unnecessary, as all of the 'players' are already there together, but in actuality this chaplain role of facilitating communication can be critical and far from simple.

With respect to ritual, a ceremony as an act of 'doing' that has spiritual significance, this realm of spiritual care can be no less important for a family (or friends) than for a patient. Sometimes, such ritual can be done with both the patient and the family together, but it might also be relevant for the chaplain to focus the ritual primarily on family members or friends. When death does come, there will often be much ritual that is part of the death and dying traditions of different faith traditions and communities, so the exploration of ritual as significant spiritual experience for families of patients receiving palliative care can be an important focus of the chaplain's activity.

Texts, as described earlier, can be important spiritual resources for family members and friends. Similarly to what we have explained about prayer and ritual, there are at least two modes of text study with relation to family and friends: (1) a family member as a study partner together with the chaplain and (2) including the family in such a text discussion with the chaplain and patient. These two modes can be described in terms of need: (1) when the family needs to be focused on separately from the patient and (2) when the family needs to be included in the relating to the patient as part of a family or broader social circle.

While the patient is the primary object of medical attention and care, the family (and friends) often have their own different and special concerns and experiences of health and healing challenges. As such, they also often need advocates in the context of palliative care. Whereas the patient is the 'boss' as far as the medical staff is concerned, the chaplain can act in good faith as an advocate for the family members as well. This advocacy can include facilitating communication between the family and the rest of the professional health-care staff, as well as referring family members to additional health-care professionals and complementary spiritual therapies for themselves.

Spiritual care for staff

The chaplain's role in palliative care includes furnishing accurate, timely, and genuine support for staff. Providing care at, and through, death is rewarding, but can be concomitantly hard-hitting. Sometimes, the strike is unexpected, perhaps unearthing cumulative feelings and thoughts as unattended internal impacts accumulated over time. Particular patients constellate our unresolved sorrow from loss, past and anticipated. This can lead to personal crises of belief and philosophy. Such events can become points of ongoing engagement that yields deeper trust and greater strength in the team as a caring community.

Being present for the staff, the chaplain provides support and care to foster growth and restoration. Occasionally, staff members turn confidentially to the chaplain and share unexpected or unusual personal challenges, troubles, or ordeals in life. The role of chaplain includes knowing and strengthening the morale of the caregiver team. This may include raising issues for group discussion without breaking individual confidence or expressing personal concern. Caring for the caregivers is a crucial role of the chaplain in palliative care.

There are two levels of relationship between a chaplain and the staff: (1) in relation to the provision of spiritual care to staff members and (2) in relation to care provided to the patient. The need for support by staff members, while not necessarily obvious in the general health-care setting, is understood by the chaplain as crucial and basic. Although it is not always clear how to go about lending support, and even spiritual support, to staff members, the chaplain understands that the staff is part of the responsibility of providing spiritual care in the health-care setting. This understanding is all the more evident in the context of palliative care, in which mortality is ever-present with the accompanying emotional and often spiritual impact on the individual staff members.

The chaplain can be a significant resource for the staff, both on an individual basis as well as in the group setting. For the staff who understand their roles as being there, present, for the patients (and, in turn, for family and friends of the patient), the question 'who is present for the staff?' is rarely voiced. The need for support, however, a deeply human need for people tending to other people in the context of life-threatening illness and death, is often felt in varying degrees by different people. Therefore, the presence of the chaplain for the staff, listening to what they are experiencing and their reactions to loss, can be most profound.

This staff support can be related to personal crises (after all each staff member has their own life outside of the health-care context) as well as to work stress (including relating to spiritual/existential questions which often arise for staff working in the context of high mortality among their patients). In addition, prayer, ritual, offering and opening of texts as spiritual resources for study, and advocacy are all modes of chaplaincy activity, which are relevant and often welcomed by staff, both as individuals as well as a group.

In the context of palliative care the chaplain is a part of a multi-disciplinary health-care team and is enmeshed with the rest of the staff (as all of the staff are related to one another) in connection to the care provided for the patient. The multi-disciplinary approach expects input by different parts of the team, and the palliative care chaplain understands that input from the perspective of spiritual care is often expected to be presented by the chaplain, as this perspective is recognized as an integral piece of the palliative care puzzle. It is normative practice that the chaplain will be invited to participate in psychosocial staff meetings, in addition to individual consultations as the need arises with particular patients. The chaplain is often adept at identifying ethical issues that may or may not be specific religious perspectives, giving a voice to these issues from a different perspective, and helping to facilitate understanding and appropriate resolution for the patient, family, and the treating staff members.

Moreover, the chaplain may try actively to include staff in the spiritual care of a patient and family. This inclusion could take place in the context of prayer with a patient and/or family in which the staff are invited to participate (even just by being present), and it could also mean involving staff in a spiritual care conversation with the patient/family (or sharing some highlights and insights from these interactions with staff to add to their view of the patient and how they relate to the patient). An additional element of shared activity in relation to care for patient/family is spiritual assessment, an evaluation of the spiritual needs and available resources, an assessment to which all of the staff can make a contribution as they get to know the patient and their family and friends.

Self-care for the chaplain

The role of the chaplain in palliative care involves loving and caring for oneself. As rewarding as service can be, we face an associated high cost of caring for others in physical and emotional pain. Merely observing painful emotional responses in others who suffer has a contagious parallel effect and can promote 'compassion fatigue'[17]. Further, the lack of personal care due to unchecked professional immersion, leads to professional burnout, including the loss of idealism, energy, and purpose due to work conditions. Lacking proper self-care can lead to excessive cynicism, a loss of interest in work, and a mechanical approach of just 'going through the motions'. Further, burnout can lead to fatigue, difficulty concentrating, depression, anxiety, insomnia, irritability, and the inappropriate use of drugs or alcohol.

Without proper self-care and recreation, consequences can show professionally. This includes avoiding assigned families, unduly blaming them for glitches in care plans, impatience and shows of anger or unbridled criticism, failures to aptly assess and rally needed resources, and more.

It is incumbent upon a chaplain in palliative care to set and keep good boundaries, to take steps that ensure relaxed awareness in the present, garner healthy stress tolerance and impulse control, and promote self-awareness, mindfulness, and clarity. Strengthening self-care taps many theological roots and traditions, including, but not limited to, personal renewal, regular prayer and meditation, journalling, healing, transformation, empowerment, discipline, cure of the soul, contemplative living, and Sabbath support.

All these, and others, at best, provide the type of support we need to remind us of who we really are, what we really desire, and how to live faithfully.

Facing death as part of life

As the physical health of a person diminishes, the importance of emotional and spiritual health is often more pronounced. Therefore, as people near death, their facing of death will often make a significant difference to how they die, to how their family (and friends and staff) experience their death, and to how the family (and friends and staff) continues living after the patient has died. The chaplain can be a spiritual companion in one's search for meaning, and as we face death this search is often more immediate in importance and significantly accelerated.

In their *Handbook for Mortals*, Drs. Lynn and Harrold focus on what they call the 'four Rs for the spirit': Remembering, Reassessing, Reconciling, and Reuniting (see[9], p. 30). This approach to understanding the spiritual search for meaning informs strongly the role of the chaplain in palliative care, towards death. The chaplain often accompanies (even guiding sometimes) a process that can include review of one's life and reflection on that life, finishing undone business and forgiveness for things left undone and/or unfulfilled, reconciliation with oneself, one's life, and one's loved ones, and reconnecting with a greater spiritual source and sense of meaning (God, a higher Being, the universe, and other ways of relating to what is bigger than we are). In this context, the chaplain helps explore and facilitate spiritual and emotional healing, including closure and release of all into caring and loving hands, be they the hands of loved ones, of nature, of God, of the Universe. As VandeCreek and Burton remind us (and their statement can be taken to the broader spiritual realm): 'When religious beliefs and practices are tightly interwoven with cultural contexts, chaplains constitute a powerful reminder of the healing, sustaining, guiding, and reconciling power of religious faith' (see[12], p. 86).

The chaplain tries to help the patient and family (and staff when appropriate) not only to find meaning at this stage in life, but also to express this meaning to themselves and to others. This expression of meaning by people (a patient as well as family members) can be very empowering as death is approached. The elements of hope, dignity, and sense of burden as experienced by a patient are especially important issues to which the chaplain must be sensitive and relate. One area of expressing found meaning in life can be referred to as leaving a legacy or passing on the tradition. Sometimes this can take the shape of an 'ethical will', the sharing (written or oral) of values, hopes, insights, beliefs, and life wisdom, that is left to and for loved ones. The chaplain can be a key person in raising this possibility as a relevant and appropriate opportunity for a patient and family.

Saying goodbye is a critical part of facing death, and every person can be offered the opportunity to say goodbye before they die. Sometimes this is referred to as grief and loss care. As hard as it is to talk about saying goodbye while one is still alive, it obviously becomes a much more difficult task after one has died. The chaplain can broach this very sensitive issue with a patient and family, as well as with staff. Of course, as with all aspects of palliative care, we all take our direction from the patient (and sometimes the family when appropriate) as we are all present as health-care professionals to serve others. In Old English, the word 'goodbye' is rooted in the wish or prayer that 'God be with you'. It is not coincidental that in Hebrew (and similarly in Arabic) the word *Shalom* is used for hello and goodbye. The root of this word has to do with wholeness, and therefore peace. Saying goodbye, then, is a parting prayer and wish for peace and wholeness—a potentially extremely meaningful, if difficult, transition from life to death.

It is important to note here that communication with the patient in the context of palliative care becomes more intricate when the patient is no longer capable of communicating with us. However, we do know from medical experience that in such cases the patient might well be capable of hearing what is said, even though they cannot respond in a clear way. It is in this context that the chaplain can serve as a role model by offering an example of sitting next to such a person, taking hold of their hand (if appropriate), speaking with them, singing to them, and praying for them. These actions and accompanying explanation on the part of the chaplain recognize the overarching significance of family communication with the patient before their loved one dies. The chaplain knows well the healing effect of such communication on the process of reconciliation before death as well as the grieving process after death (sometimes the difference between telling a dying person 'what needs to be said' while they are living and feeling deep regret over the lost opportunity to convey these deep sentiments is a matter of minutes) and can convey this message effectively to the family and friends.

The time of death itself is often very difficult for medical staff, as there is often the (unfortunate) feeling that 'nothing more can be done'. Usually in the case of palliative care, much has been done, and the presence of the health-care staff is welcome and meaningful for all involved. Indeed, these moments are often when the patient and family need the most support. The chaplain, knowing and believing that the 'physical' is not all there is, is motivated by the privilege of stepping into this holy space, where the delicate depth of life and love can often be felt so strongly.

From the time of death and into the period after death, there is often not a always a natural continuation of health care, as death is often seen as the logical endpoint as far as health care is concerned. In general with palliative care, and specifically with regard to spiritual care, there is a clear understanding that care is indeed appropriate and often needed after death. The family and friends and staff members are the ones left living in this world after a person has died, and the chaplain will see these people as those for whom spiritual care can continue to be provided. The relevant chaplaincy interventions here might include funeral consultations, accompanying the family through the funeral and possibly participating in a memorial service, grief and bereavement counselling, and periodic communication with the patient's family to check how they are doing and to show care and compassion as a continuation of the commitment of palliative care to ease the pain associated with life-threatening illness. This pain can be physical, emotional, and spiritual, and it can continue for families (and others) after the patient has died.

Conclusion

Findings from current opinion polls and research support the wisdom of involving chaplains in health care. A 1997 Gallup survey showed that persons overwhelmingly want their spiritual needs addressed when they are close to death. George H. Gallup, Jr., explained, 'The overarching message that emerges from ... study is … people want to reclaim and reassert the spiritual dimensions in dying'[18]. Other studies identify spirituality as an important factor in coping with pain, in dying, and in bereavement. Patients with advanced cancer who found comfort from their spiritual beliefs were, for example, more satisfied with their lives, were happier, and had diminished pain compared with those without connection to spiritual beliefs.

In health care, the urgent need of regimens to cure like invasive procedures, medicine, and therapies often proceed without giving parallel attention to impacts on mind and soul. Even when medical results are good, persons still experience unmet needs for healing of mind and soul. When attempts to cure fail, persons often remain ill, are incapacitated, and may be dead or bereaved. Chaplains continue to address the spirituality dimension of a person's life, especially when he or she is dealing with chronic illness and suffering. In the palliative care context, chaplains join medical care as a resource that can bring alleviation of pain and suffering. It is possible for all human beings to seek and find meaning in life, and thus heal, until the moment they take their last breath. Where chaplains serve in health-care systems, the impacts have the potential to transform and re-humanize them. Together healing and care are enjoined to community. As such, chaplaincy can fulfill the need for interpreting the interface between spirituality and health for the health-care institution as well as for the community at large.

References

1. Chinula, D.M. *Building King's Beloved Community: Foundations for Pastoral Care and Counseling with the Oppressed.* Cleveland: United Church Press, 1997.

2. Frankl, V.E. (1984). *Man's Search for Meaning*, p.117. Simon and Schuster, New York.

3. Cohen, S.R., Mount, B.M., Strobel, M.G. *et al.* (1995). The McGill Quality of Life Questionnaire: a measure of quality of life appropriate for people with advanced disease. A preliminary study of validity and acceptability. *Palliative Medicine*, **9**, 207–19.

4. Chochinov, H.M., Hack, T., Hassard, T. *et al.* (2005). Understanding will to live in patients nearing death. *Psychosomatics*, **46**, 7–10.

5. Chochinov, H.M. and Cann, B.J. (2005). Interventions to enhance the spiritual aspects of dying. *Journal of Palliative Medicine*, **8**(Supp 1), s103–15.

6. Stoll, R.I. (1989). The Essence of Spirituality. In *Spiritual Dimensions of Nursing Practice* (ed. Carson, V.B.), pp. 14–23. W.B. Saunders, Philadelphia.

7. *Webster's New Collegiate Dictionary*. (1980). G. & C. Merriam Co., Massachusetts.

8. Van Katwyk, P.L. (2002). Pastoral counseling as a spiritual practice: an exercise in a theology of spirituaity. *The Journal of Pastoral Care and Counseling*, **56**(2), 109–19.

9. Lynn, J. and Harrold, J. (1999). *Handbook for Mortals: Guidance for People Facing Serious Illness.* Oxford University Press, New York.

10. Buber, M. (1958). *I and Thou* (translated by Ronald Gregor Smith). Charles Scribner's Sons, New York.

11. Wise, C. A. (1966). *The Meaning of Pastoral Care.* Harper and Row, New York.

12. Van de Creek, L. and Burton, L., (eds.). (2001). Professional chaplaincy: Its role and importance in health care: A White Paper. *The Journal of Pastoral Care and Counseling*, **55**(1), 81–97.

13. Hunter, R.J., (ed.). (1990). *Dictionary of Pastoral Care and Counseling.* Abingdon, Tennessee.

14. Flannelly, K.J., Weaver, A.J., Handzo, G.F. *et al.* (2005). A national survey of health care administrators' views on the importance of various chaplain roles. *The Journal of Pastoral Care and Counseling*, **59**(1–2), 87–96.

15. Website of Joint Commission on Accreditation of Healthcare Organizations (JCAHO). Address (revised January 1, 2004): http://www.jointcommission.org/AccreditationPrograms/HomeCare/Standards/FAQs/Provision+of+Care/Assessment/Spiritual_Assessment.htm

16. Friedman, E.H. (1985). *Generation to Generation: Family Process in Church and Synagogue.* The Guilford Press, New York.

17. Figley, C.R. (1995). *Compassion fatigue: coping with secondary traumatic stress disorder in those who treat the traumatized.* Brunner/Mazel, New York.

18. Gallup, G., Jr. (1998). *The Gallup Poll, public opinion 1997.* Scholarly Resources, Inc., Delaware.

4.5

The contribution of occupational therapy to palliative medicine

Jennifer Miller and Jill Cooper

Introduction

Occupational therapy aims to optimize the individual's participation in their valued activities of daily living through specific interventions that will promote health and well-being[1]. Central to occupational therapy is the term occupation, which refers to the activities and roles one assumes that are both purposeful and meaningful[2]. In day-to-day use the term 'occupation' refers to an individual's job but in the context of occupational therapy, the word means much more than that and includes for example self-maintenance occupations such as toileting, washing, and dressing as well as paid employment, studying, or shopping and engaging in leisure pursuits. The literature discusses the daily activities that occupation incorporates, noting that they are not only goal-directed in nature, but also grounded in the individual's culture[3]. Thus 'occupation' goes much further than merely describing a particular job and instead extends to all the activities that contribute to a unique and individualized pattern of daily activities[4].

Within palliative care, occupational therapists work in a variety of settings including the hospital, community, and hospice and form a significant part of the multi-professional team[5]. Such a team generally includes occupational therapy, dietetics, chaplaincy, physiotherapy, psychology, specialist nurses, medics, pharmacy, social work, and speech and language therapy[6] and should be coordinated so as to avoid duplication while still enabling the patient and their carers access to a broad range of services. As patients may access the occupational therapist at different points during their illness, communication between the different disciplines is imperative to ensure that the patients' ongoing and changing needs are met, and it may be necessary to establish protocols at a local level to ensure good communication between professions in the voluntary, health, and social sectors.

Although occupational therapy has in many contexts moved away from its craft roots, it has remained inextricably linked with the notion of activity. Occupational therapy interventions are underpinned by the following core skills:

- *Collaboration with the client*: building a collaborative relationship with the client that will promote reflection, autonomy, and engagement in the therapeutic process.

- *Assessment*: assessing and observing functional potential, limitations, ability and needs, including the effects of physical and psychosocial environments.

- *Enablement*: enabling people to explore, achieve, and maintain balance in their activities of daily living in the areas of personal care, domestic, leisure, and productive activities.

- *Problem solving*: identifying and solving occupational performance problems.

- *Using activity as a therapeutic tool*: using activities to promote health, well-being, and function by analysing, selecting, synthesizing, adapting, grading, and applying activities for specific therapeutic purposes.

- *Group work*: planning, organizing, and leading activity groups.

- *Environmental adaptation*: analysing and adapting environments to increase function and social participation.[7]

These core skills are based firmly upon the adoption of a client and carer-centred approach, which appreciates the worth of establishing a partnership with the client based on the premise that clients are autonomous and value should be placed on their need to make occupation-related decisions[8]. Such a client-centred approach encourages the team to focus their knowledge and skills on the patient's, and carer's needs and requires a certain amount of flexibility to reflect the changing needs of the patient, e.g. as a patient becomes more fatigued and dependent, occupational therapy intervention may move away from teaching strategies to manage washing and dressing, and instead focus on liaising with social work or community colleagues to organize a package of care.

Rehabilitation in palliative care

The traditional definition of the profession describes the occupational therapist as enabling the individual to achieve independent function, and even though the nature of palliative care will limit the proportion of patients who could achieve this, a rehabilitative approach can still be implemented. In fact, the ethos of occupational therapy complements the World Health Organization's key principles of palliative care:

- relief from pain and other distressing symptoms;
- psychological and spiritual care;
- a support system to help patients live as actively as possible in the face of impending death; and
- a support system to sustain patients' friends and families during illness and bereavement[9].

Dietz (1980)[10] describes rehabilitation in cancer care as comprising four distinct aspects:

1 *Preventative rehabilitation*—this may include information giving and demonstration of equipment so that the patient is aware of what may occur and strategies and aids for preserving function. It may also incorporate advice on positioning.

2 *Restorative rehabilitation*—the goal of this type of rehabilitation is to regain some level of physical and emotional functioning, and may be particularly appropriate following exacerbation of symptoms.

3 *Supportive rehabilitation*—in addition to supporting individuals with new impairments, supportive rehabilitation can help educate people about long-term symptoms and also support them as their health declines.

4 *Palliative rehabilitation*—often, this involves assisting with symptom control and providing comfort and support to patients with advanced disease. The focus continues to be on optimizing independence.

Within the palliative care setting, it is essential that the occupational therapist maintains a flexible approach in view of the varying symptoms that the patient may exhibit as a result of advanced disease, and appreciates that the rehabilitative approach which predominates at any particular time may continually change.

Performance areas within activities of daily living and their components

Occupations can be broadly divided into the three main areas: *self-care*, also referred to as personal care, which applies to all activities one carries out in order to look after oneself; *productivity* which incorporates work-related roles and domestic activities; and finally, *leisure* which refers to hobbies, sports, and general interests[11].

Assessment and treatment is implemented within the following performance components:

- *Motor skills*—this relates to the functional use of muscle strength and tone, range of movement, endurance, and fine and gross motor skills. Disease-related symptoms might result in prolonged periods of inactivity leading to muscle wastage, weight loss, generalized weakness, or even weight gain as a result of long-term steroid use.
- *Sensory skills*—this involves identification and interpretation of external and internal sensory stimuli, for example, pain, altered sensation, balance deficits, and visual disturbances.
- *Cognitive skills*—deficits within this performance component may occur for a number of reasons, including tumour growth if the primary is situated within the brain, cerebral metastases

and side effects of drugs used for symptom control. The individual may present with altered levels of arousal or exhibit impairment of memory, planning, problem-solving, and communication.

- *Intrapersonal skills*—advanced disease may adversely affect an individual's self-image and self-identity, which in turn may affect how the individual participates in occupation.
- *Interpersonal skills*—individuals may experience a loss of control and may feel they are unable to fulfil their existing roles such as mother, breadwinner, or employee. This can have an enormous impact on self-esteem.
- *Self-maintenance occupations*—this refers to the activities that one regularly carries out to take care of oneself. Examples include toileting, washing, dressing, feeding and sleeping. Under normal circumstances, and with the exception of feeding and maybe sleeping, these activities are generally performed with a certain amount of privacy. Additionally, individuals are likely to have individualized methods and routines for executing the activities and so it is important to take this into account when providing assistance. Some people may place enormous value and meaning on performing these activities independently and may in some circumstances decline additional help, and therefore the focus will instead be on risk assessment, provision of equipment and education in compensatory strategies.
- *Productivity occupations*—through performance of these occupations, the individual contributes to supporting themselves, their family and society as a whole. Included here are tasks such as paid employment, studying, housework, food preparation, and shopping.
- *Leisure occupations*—these relate to all activities performed for pleasure, and enjoyment. Often the possibility of engaging in such occupations is limited due to deficits within the aforementioned performance components and so it is essential that meaningful leisure pursuits are identified and adapted to enable greater participation.

Occupational therapy and dysfunction

It is important to note that the occupational therapists' work is symptom-led as opposed to disease-led, and, although crisis cannot always be avoided, the occupational therapist will work with the patient and their carers to anticipate problems that may arise and provide carers with a point of contact as and when the patient deteriorates. Occupational therapy within the area of palliative care not only relates to oncological disease, but any life-limiting disease including cardiac and neurological disease, and mental health.

The occupational therapy process

For each new patient, the occupational therapist follows a four-stage process: gathering and analysing information; intervention planning; intervention implementation; and evaluating outcomes. Particularly within palliative care where the impairments are likely to increase due to progressive disease, the intervention implementation stage is cyclical. Within the occupational therapy process, there are three important considerations: the effect of the environment; the use of goal-setting; and graded activity.

Goal setting

Goal setting is a vital component of therapeutic interventions and its value has been demonstrated within the palliative care setting as a means of focusing the multi-professional team[12]. A goal-oriented approach can assist in optimizing outcome[13], and so through collaboration with the patient and their carers, the occupational therapist sets specific, realistic, achievable, and measurable goals relating to occupational performance.

Grading

By applying grading techniques to an activity, the occupational therapist can increase or decrease the demands of the activity according to the patient's presentation. This may be particularly appropriate to facilitate continued participation in an activity or in order to adjust to a decline in functional ability[14]. Examples of grading techniques include manipulation of one or more of the following factors: environment, position of objects required to complete the task, and level of support from another individual. Additionally, backward and forward chaining methods may be applied. In backward chaining, the therapist completes all necessary steps of an activity with exception of the last step which the patient is encouraged to do whereas in forward chaining, the patient is encouraged to complete the first step and the therapist completes the remainder of the activity. Both methods enable the patient to gradually increase the number of steps they carry out until they can perform the task independently.

Environment

Occupational function can be significantly affected by the patient's physical, social, and emotional environment and so these are of prime concern to the occupational therapist. Physical environment refers to inanimate and natural objects[15] which the individual may have to confront if routine is interrupted. For example, the patient's bedroom may be upstairs, but generalized weakness as a result of advanced disease may mean that the stairs present the patient with a challenge that they are unable to overcome and so environmental changes such as the patient being based on one level would have to be implemented. However, the social and emotional aspects of the environment are just as vital in order to achieve truly client-centred practice. The value the patient places on their environment must be considered when making changes, within the context of altering roles and self-perception[16].

Specific roles of the occupational therapist

The role of the occupational therapist in the management of symptom clusters

Within the literature, there has been increasing emphasis on symptom clusters, which are defined as three or more related symptoms that may interact with each other consequently having a significant effect on the patient's quality of life[17]. The combination of fatigue, breathlessness, and anxiety results in such a symptom cluster, and there is evidence to suggest that the management of anxiety has a positive impact on both breathlessness and fatigue[18]. The occupational therapist can contribute to the management of all the elements of this particular symptom cluster as described below.

Anxiety

It is normal for everyone to experience some degree of anxiety, and in fact by its very existence, it aids everyday survival and performance in certain situations. This natural response is referred to as the fight or flight response which when activated releases catecholamines and enables us to confront and fight the danger or run away from it. Symptoms and signs of anxiety can be divided into psychological, motor, and autonomic and can include: psychological, for example, difficulty relaxing, negative patterns of thinking, altered sleep patterns, and short-temperedness; motor, such as aching muscles, fatigue, and restlessness; and autonomic, including dyspnoea, palpitations, nausea, and sweating.

When people exhibit anxiety that impacts significantly on their participation in their chosen occupations, the fight and flight response is frequently activated as a result of negative thoughts as opposed to in response to any specific danger. Although anxiety may be viewed as an entirely appropriate reaction to advanced disease, it is important to be aware of symptoms and signs of anxiety[19] and that it is subjective and may vary from individual to individual. Precipitating factors to anxiety may include: pre-existing psychiatric conditions, poorly-controlled pain, medication toxicities, and psychological and spiritual issues[20].

Relaxation is one of the main strategies occupational thraphists use for managing anxiety. Such interventions promote a client-centred and educational approach that facilitates the individual's recognition of potential stressors and equips them with the skills required to manage such stressors[21]. A review of the literature demonstrated that relaxation has been found to be effective in managing both distressing side effects of cancer treatment[22] and common symptoms associated with the advanced stages[23]. The aims of such a programme are described by Cooper[24]:

- to understand and recognize your level of anxiety;
- to understand the need for relaxation and recognize certain situations that may trigger tension;
- to experience a variety of relaxation techniques thus enabling you to choose the most appropriate one;
- to appreciate the importance of planning time for relaxation as part of your daily activities and lifestyle;
- to improve quality of sleep;
- to lessen pain caused by inappropriate muscle tension;
- to encourage peace of mind;
- to improve performance of physical skills;
- to increase self-esteem and confidence;
- to ease relationships with others;
- to channel and control effects of anxiety; and
- to avoid unnecessary fatigue.

Relaxation programmes may vary depending on resources available and therapists' experience; however, a basic outline would include education and practise using techniques such as slow, deep breathing, or imagery.

If the patient presents with breathlessness as a result of over-breathing, the occupational therapist in collaboration the physiotherapy can advise on breathing techniques to optimize inhalation and minimize hyperventilation which can commonly occur as a result of a panic attack. It is necessary to educate the patient and carers if possible about the mechanisms underlying overbreathing in terms of causing an imbalance of oxygen and carbon dioxide within the blood stream. Controlling overbreathing involves three stages: stopping overbreathing by applying techniques such as ceasing an activity, making postural adjustments, and focusing on either a point of reference or calming thoughts; encouraging carbon dioxide back into the lungs by using a paper bag or breathing in through the nose and out through the mouth into cupped hands; and finally, regaining a control pattern of breathing by breathing gently in through the nose and out through the mouth while imagining making a candle light flicker on the exhalation and breathing from the stomach instead of the chest.

Negative thought patterns may occur especially if the patient senses a loss of control and independence in functional activities and these are likely to impact greatly on the level of anxiety the patient experiences. By encouraging the patient and their carers to omit words such as 'must', 'ought', and 'should' and replace them with more positive words like 'choose' and 'could' less demands are being imposed on the individual. Other negative thought patterns which may be exhibited include: personalizing, where the patient feels responsible for unpleasant circumstances which are out of their control; and all or nothing thinking whereby the individual considers them as hopeless if they fail in a task. In these situations, the occupational therapist can work with the patient in identifying the negative thought patterns, challenging them by considering how reasonable they are and then producing a plan for changing these thoughts to more positive ones.

The use of positive phrases may be implemented as an adjunct to addressing such negative thought patterns. The use of positive phrases before, during and after an activity can assist the patient in minimizing the physical symptoms which may occur by interrupting the fight and flight response as early in the activity as possible.

Breathlessness

Although breathlessness (dyspnoea) is obviously a common symptom in lung cancer patients, it also affects approximately a third of the palliative-care population[25]. Breathlessness is a subjective sensation and the overall physical and psychological implications are immeasurable. Multi-professional input is vital to effectively manage the breathless patient and consideration must be given to the individualized nature of the symptom. With this in mind, the occupational therapist has three main aims in the management of this symptom. They are to:

1 explore meaning of the symptom to the patients and their carers and families;

2 enable activity so that they can achieve optimum independence and control despite their debilitating symptom; and

3 help patients manage any anxiety and panic attacks, including teaching relaxation techniques as part of the management programme[26].

Meaning of breathlessness

Breathlessness can exist on a prolonged basis or be exacerbated by stress, participation in activity, and progressive disease. It is important that the occupational therapist works with the patient in identifying triggers so that activities may be adapted as necessary, for example, the patient's breathlessness may be aggravated by getting in and out of the bath and so the occupational therapist

may look at equipment options if the individual enjoys having a bath or may explore alternative options such as showering. Anxiety can result in breathlessness, whereas breathlessness may be associated with extreme fear and panic within the patient. It may also represent relinquishment of roles and both these aspects have enormous implications for the carers, family and friends as well as the patient.

Enabling activity

The implementation of energy conservation principles can assist in enabling optimal participation in valued occupations. Energy conservation has been defined as 'the deliberate planned management of one's personal energy resources in order to prevent their depletion'[27]. Approaches may include:

- *Pacing*—scheduling frequent breaks and not rushing activities.
- *Planning*—considering the best time of day and making use of this time. Also includes avoiding unnecessary exertion.
- *Prioritizing*—identifying most valued tasks.
- *Permission*—delegating to others.
- *Posture*—avoiding excessive bending and twisting and adjusting position regularly.
- *Equipment*—equipment needs may be identified through discussion with the patient and observation during personal and domestic activities.

Although care must be taken to not provide the patient with excessive amounts of equipment, examples of pieces which may assist include: wheelchairs for accessing the community, perching stools to minimize bending, twisting and standing when performing personal and domestic activities of daily living, and a commode if the patient lives in a house with a bathroom on one floor only.

Breathlessness management

Breathlessness is an anxiety-provoking symptom for both the patient and those who witness it, such as carers, friends, and family, and education is the key to maximize the ability to cope[28]. Personal plans can be an effective means of assisting the patient to regain control during an episode of breathlessness and may include techniques and methods which facilitate shoulder and upper chest relaxation, promote lower chest breathing, and provide a means of relaxation. Such a personal plan is flexible and may be adapted as the patient's needs change.

The occupational therapist, in conjunction with other members of the multi-professional team, may explore with the patient positions that they may choose to use when they are breathless. A supine position commonly exacerbates the sensation of breathlessness so high-side lying may be used as an alternative. The main aim of positioning is to avoid chest and abdomen compression[29], and other positions may include sitting forwards leaning onto a table supported by pillows, sitting backwards, or standing leaning forwards or backwards.

Breathing re-education can often form part of the comprehensive management of breathlessness and centres on breathing control. This method encourages use of the lower chest when breathing instead of using the upper chest which is extremely inefficient and energy consuming. During inhalation, the patient many be advised to place their hand on their stomach in an attempt to feel the lower ribs and stomach expanding. Upon exhalation, the patient should be encouraged to breath out slowly, sometimes the image of flickering a candle may be used. At all times the patient should be prompted to maintain shoulder and upper chest relaxation.

Additional means of regaining control following a breathless episode may include using positive phrases, relaxation techniques such as imagery, or obtaining support from a carer friend or family member.

Fatigue

Cancer-related fatigue is experienced by a high proportion of patients, and is cited within the literature as one of the most frequently experienced symptoms[30], affecting more than 70 per cent of patients in palliative care[31]. Fatigue presents as exhaustion and a lack of energy and can impede the individual's participation in occupation[32] with may manifest itself in the following functional ways:

◆ difficulty participating in activities that one is usually able to undertake independently;

◆ insomnia or disturbed sleep patterns;

◆ cognitive deficits—memory difficulties, reduced attention span; and

◆ affected psychological well-being—lability, impatience[33].

The role of the occupational therapist within fatigue management centres on educative, rehabilitative, and compensatory interventions[34] and uses many of the principles already discussed within the anxiety and breathlessness sections. Fatigue is a multidimensional symptom affecting the patient's physical, social, cognitive, and emotional well-being.

Fatigue diaries may be used to identify the patient's current level of functioning, highlight which occupations they most value, and establish goals and priorities. Educating the patient and carers about the nature of fatigue symptoms and means of management can alleviate anxiety and help them to understand this common side effect. In particular, patients and carers can be taught the energy conservation strategies as discussed within the *enabling activity* section of breathlessness. Patients should be encouraged to use goal setting as a means of setting realistic goals by breaking down tasks into smaller and more manageable components, thus enhancing the patient's perception of control.

If patients are experiencing unrefreshing or non-restorative sleep, modification to the sleep environment and application of sleep hygiene principles may be of benefit. Poor sleep can affect both the patient and their carers, and reasons for its occurrence include anxiety, medications, cognitive impairment, and depression[35]. The occupational therapist can teach relaxation techniques, in addition to addressing issues with posture and positioning, particularly if the patient is unable to lie flat and so requires equipment such as a mattress variator or pillow raise to maintain a more upright position. Advice can be given regarding optimizing comfort when in bed and this may be assisted by the provision of certain aids and adaptations such as pillow raises. The sleeping environment should be a comfortable temperature with minimum light and noise distraction. Sleep hygiene principles can be identified and discussed with the occupational therapist, and this is likely to include establishing a bedtime routine which can incorporate relaxation exercises, going to bed and getting up at the same time each day, a warm bath, or listening to quiet music. Avoidance of exercise, heavy meals, and stimulants such as caffeine, alcohol, and nicotine may also contribute to a more restorative sleep as can

minimizing the number of naps taken throughout the day. Finally, if patients are unable to sleep they should be advised, if at all possible, to get up as not being able to sleep when in bed may reinforce the pattern.

Fatigue can have consequences for cognition and carers, or patients themselves, may identify that the patient is exhibiting short-term memory loss, impaired attention and planning, and problem solving deficits[36]. This can impact on the patient's ability to maintain independence within valued occupations and also potentially affect the relationships they have with others. Occupational therapists can advise the patient and carers about minimizing too much distraction when participating in an activity, assess the implication of such cognitive deficits upon safety, and collaboratively investigate simplifying activities so as to minimize cognitive demand. Alternatively, the cognitive aspect may be something the patient wishes to address and in this case the occupational therapist may explore the possibility of engaging the patient in activities that specifically focus on the area of deficit[34].

The emotional symptoms that may feature within fatigue include heightened emotional reactivity, lability, and decreased motivation and interest in activities. Relaxation techniques as described within the anxiety section may assist in alleviating fatigue-related anxiety and stress. Additionally, the occupational therapist may identify that the patient would potentially benefit from counselling or having the opportunity to talk with somebody about how they feel and so, once consent is obtained, may refer on to another member of the multi-professional team.

The role of the occupational therapist in the management of other symptoms

Nausea and vomiting

Within palliative care, nausea and vomiting can be distressing symptoms which can have serious implications for the patient's quality of life. From an occupational perspective, these symptoms may be exacerbated by fatty and spicy foods, large portions, and prolonged exposure to odours such as cooking, smoking, and perfume.

In addition to antiemetic drugs, relaxation interventions have also been shown to be effective[37]. The occupational therapist is ideally placed to:

◆ work with other members of the multi-professional team, such as the speech and language therapist, nurse, and physiotherapist to assist the patient in obtaining the most effective position if they present with dysphagia;

◆ address alternatives for meal preparation, such as the use of ready meals;

◆ provision of equipment to use during meal and drink preparation to minimize fatigue; and

◆ educate and support carers about the symptom[38].

Cognitive and perceptual impairments

Cognitive and perceptual deficits may manifest themselves in a number of ways, and can be as a result of a number of causes, for example, brain tumour, infection, medication side effects, metastases of the central nervous system, or chemical imbalance[39]. They may result in either temporary or permanent dysfunction. Although there are numerous standardized assessments which can be completed to identify deficits within areas such as memory, planning, and problem-solving, their use may be deemed inappropriate in this setting particularly as they are so time-consuming and re-assessment may only confirm to the patient that they are deteriorating. Instead, the occupational therapist may observe the patient during functional activities such as meal preparation and personal care to identify any deficits and pre-determine any implications for safety and independence, for example, poor safety when cooking with gas or remembering to take medication. Fluctuating or deteriorating cognitive levels can be extremely distressing for both patients and carers and so the aim of occupational therapy is to assist the carers in coping with this and maximize the time the patient can be maintained at home. Practical strategies such as the use of memory aids may be explored, and advice may be necessary about the level of supervision the patient may require and whether they would be safe to be left alone within the home environment.

Physical deficits

Musculoskeletal symptoms such as spinal cord compression, pathological fractures, contractures, and weakness may result in increased dependence and compromise safety for both the patient and their carers. This may be further complicated by other problems such as cognitive deficits or ascites. With background knowledge of anatomy, physiology, and normal functioning, the occupational therapist can analyse where functional loss may occur as a result of such physical deficits while acknowledging the impact this activity has upon the lives of the patient and their carers.

Clients and carers may require education in appropriate handling strategies and this may include demonstration and instruction on the use of moving and handling aids such as hoists and sliding boards. Additionally, it is imperative to take a 24-hour approach to palliative-care patients in terms of positioning either within the bed or in alternatives such as a wheelchair or armchair. The occupational therapist should liaise with the nursing staff if exploring seating options to ensure suitable pressure relieving cushions are provided to the patient. Equipment such as riser recliner chairs, toileting aids, and bathing aids may also be appropriate.

The occupational therapist is skilled in assessing and prescribing equipment to meet a patient's complex seating needs, in addition to identifying the need for standard wheelchairs and pressure cushions. Provision of a wheelchair can increase the patient's independence, for example, the patient who is unable to mobilize but can self-propel. Also it can enable patients and their carers to participate in valued occupations that may not necessarily be possible if the patient is confined to their bed, and maintain roles within the family environment.

The role of the occupational therapist in discharge planning

The occupational therapists has an essential role within discharge planning for the palliative-care patient[40], and it may be deemed feasible to perform a home visit either prior to discharge, or following discharge in the situation of a decline in the patient's general health and occupational functioning. The home visit may be carried out according to the following aspects:

1 *Access.* It may be increasingly difficult for the patient to access their environment and so the occupational therapist will take measurements of door widths and steps to identify the needs for rails or ramps. It is vital to establish who owns the property, as it can be problematic and lengthy gaining consent for alterations if the patient or their carers do not own the property. Other issues may include discussing installation of a personal alarm should the patient need to summon help if they are at home alone and whether a key safe is necessary if carers from community agencies are to visit but the patient is unable to get to the door.

2 *Living areas.* Patients who are unable to ascend and descend the stairs may need to consider being based on one level, and if they require equipment such as a hospital bed, many community agencies stipulate that this should be on the ground floor and so this should be discussed with the patient and carers. Weakness, fatigue, and breathlessness may mean that the patient is unable to transfer on and off of existing furniture, and so the occupational therapist will take measurements of chairs and issue equipment as appropriate. Additionally, wheelchairs require a certain amount of turning space and a minimum door width and these need to be assessed.

3 *Toileting, showering, and bathing.* By measuring the height of the toilet, bath, and or shower, the occupational therapist can identify equipment needs to enable the patient to transfer on and off safely and as independently as possible. If it is not feasible to use such facilities, a discussion with the patient and carers will be necessary to establish alternative toileting and washing facilities, and this may be the use of a commode or bedpan and washing at, or in, the bed.

4 *Equipment.* Although equipment and adaptations can optimize quality of life and independence of the patient and carers, if inappropriately provided or inadequately installed, safety may be severely compromised. Additionally, people may be unrealistic about their future and may be vulnerable to the sales techniques within the open market, particularly related to the purchase of expensive items of equipment such as riser recliner chairs, bath lifts and stair lifts. Although anyone may purchase such equipment, the occupational therapist should offer advice on its appropriateness and explore where possible provision of more standard pieces of equipment through community agencies. The purpose of such equipment is to:

◆ facilitate safe transfers;

◆ optimize energy resources;

◆ avoid exacerbating symptoms such as pain and dyspnoea; and

◆ ensure patients and carers are aware of how to use the equipment safely and correctly.

Table 4.5.1 identifies some of the equipment that the occupational therapist may assess to be necessary.

If equipment is no longer required, potentially due to deterioration in the patient's condition or death, a sensitive approach should be applied and the community agencies that provided the equipment advised as necessary to arrange collection.

Higginson[41] reports that of the 56 per cent of palliative-care patients who identify home as their preferred place of death, only 26 per cent achieve this. Enabling patients to die at home invariably involves a number of members of the multi-professional team, including the discharge coordinator, occupational therapist, ward staff, district nurse, and community support agencies. It is essential that the patient experiences a seamless transition from hospital or hospice to home and that requires communication with the patient and their carers in the first instance to confirm this

Table 4.5.1 Equipment and aids available following occupational therapy assessment and education on their use and provision.

Difficulty with:	Possible aids and adaptations
Bed transfers	◆ Back rest to support patient in a sitting position ◆ Mattress variator to assist lying to sitting ◆ Leg lifter to enable the patient to lift legs into bed ◆ Blocks to raise bed height ◆ Specialist hospital bed, electrically operated and generally required if nursing care is required
Toilet transfers	◆ Toilet seats of varying height and design that are easily fitted and removed ◆ Frames to fit around the toilet and provide patients with something to push up from ◆ Strategically positioned grabrails ◆ Other equipment such as commodes, male and female urinals
Bath or shower transfers	◆ Range of bathboards that can be easily fitted to assist with getting in and out of bath ◆ Hydraulically operated baths seats which lift patients in and out of the bath ◆ Strategically placed grabrails ◆ Shower seats, either free-standing or wall-fixed
Chair transfers	◆ Range of blocks to raise chairs and settees ◆ High back, orthopaedic chair with firm armrests and of an appropriate height ◆ Riser recliner arm chair enabling patient to sit with legs elevated and sometimes with an option to help them stand from sitting
Transferring in and out of the car	◆ Sliding boards may be appropriate here but require assessment and full training
Mobility	◆ Wheelchairs with detachable sides aid sliding board transfers, and the wheelchair should have appropriately fitted footrest heights, seat dimensions, and pressure cushions
Manual handling	◆ Hoists, electric, or manual may be required ◆ Additional equipment includes sliding sheets and transfer boards
Walking aids during functional activities	◆ If patients use a frame or stick, they may benefit from a caddy that fits to the frame to enable them to move items within the environment or a kitchen trolley
Managing stairs	◆ Installation of additional hand rails may assist the patient in ascending and descending the stairs safely and independently ◆ Stairlifts can be hired or bought privately but this can be expensive and the carer and patient may require guidance as to the appropriateness of it ◆ Through-floor lifts may enable those in wheelchairs to move from lower to upper floors but are expensive and require upheaval. Grants may be available from social services but the time this requires is generally in excess of a year
Meal preparation	◆ Kitchen aids including jar openers, non-slip matting, specialist cutlery, spiked chopping boards to maintain safety within the kitchen environment
Personal care	◆ Long-handled equipment such as shoehorns and sponges may help the patient reach their lower limbs. Other equipment includes button hooks, elastic shoelaces, Velcro fastenings instead of buttons

is their wish, and then liaison with community teams when organizing practicalities such as equipment and packages of care.

It is important for the occupational therapist to be aware that an enormous amount of time and effort may be put into a complex intervention, for example, discharge planning, when ultimately the patient is unable to go home.

Outcome measures

The utilization of outcome measures enables the occupational therapist to measure changes that have occurred as a direct result of intervention although it must be acknowledged that the patient is often seen by a number of members of the multi-professional team and so change cannot be attributed solely to occupational therapy input. Whilst there is a paucity of literature concerning the use of occupational therapy specific outcome measures in palliative

care, it is acknowledged that their application to this area of practise is problematic. Therapists must be precise about the rationale underpinning the use of outcome measures and be aware of both the administrative burden and the fact that they would likely highlight the patient's deterioration. The implementation of goal setting as a means of directing intervention can be used as an outcome measure as long as goals are SMART (specific, measurable, attainable, realistic, and time bound). One example of an occupational therapy-specific outcome measure is the *Canadian Occupational Performance Measure* (COPM) which is a client-centred, individualized measure of the impact of physical, socio-cultural, mental, and spiritual aspects of occupational functioning. The patient identifies areas of difficulty within the areas of self-care, productivity, and leisure and rates them on a scale of 1–10. Five of these functional problems then become the focus for rehabilitation and determine rehabilitation goals which are then evaluated over a period of time.

Conclusion

Occupational therapy aims to enhance the patients' and carers' quality of life through facilitating participation in valued occupations, whether it be by means of education or equipment or adaptations. This enables the patient to achieve optimum control and choice throughout the advanced stages of disease. Safety is also an important issue which must not be treated complacently and it may be appropriate for the patient and carers to be aware of equipment which may be available in the event of deterioration in the patient's condition so that they can contact the occupational therapist. Although the occupational therapist's role is unique, they are a vital member of the multi-professional team when striving to deliver holistic care for the patient and carer during the final stages of their illness.

References

1. World Federation of Occupational Therapists (2004). *What is occupational therapy?* Retrieved from http://www.wfot.com/information.asp on 1 March 2007.
2. Christiansen, C. (1991). Occupational therapy: intervention for life performance. In *Occupational therapy: overcoming human performance deficits* (eds. Christiansen, C., Baum, C.), pp. 3–43. Slack, New Jersey.
3. Yerxa, E., Clark, F., Jackson, J. *et al.* (1990). An introduction to occupational science, A foundation for occupational therapy in the 21st century. *Occupational Therapy in Health Care*, **6**(4), 1–17.
4. Kielhofner, G. (1998). *Model of human occupation*. 2nd edition, Lippincott, Williams and Wilkins, Baltimore, MD.
5. National Council for Hospice and Specialist Palliative Care Services (1995). *Statement of definitions*. NCHSPCS, London.
6. Brennan, M.J., DePompolo, R.W., and Garden, F.H. (1996). Cardiovascular, pulmonary, and cancer rehabilitation. 3. Cancer rehabilitation. *Archives of Physical Medicine and Rehabilitation*, **77**(Suppl 3), S52–S58.
7. Creek, J. (2003). *Occupational therapy defined as a complex intervention*. COT, London.
8. Law, M., Baptiste, S., and Mills, J. (1995). Client-centred practice: What does it mean and does it make a difference. *Canadian Journal of Occupational Therapy*, **62**, 250–7.
9. National Council for Hospice and Specialist Palliative Care Services (2000). *Fulfilling lives. Rehabilitation in palliative care*. NCHSPCS, London.
10. Dietz, J.H. (1981). *Rehabilitation in oncology*. John Wiley, New York.
11. Canadian Association of Occupational Therapists (1997). *Enabling occupation: an occupational therapy perspective*. CAOT Publications, Ottawa.
12. Needham, P.R., and Newbury, J. (2004). Goal setting as a measure of outcome in palliative care, *Palliative Medicine*, **18**(5), 444–51.
13. Wade, D. (1998). Editorial: Evidence relating to goal planning in rehabilitation. *Clinical Rehabilitation*, **12**, 273–5.
14. Foster, M., and Pratt, P. (2002). Activity analysis. In *Occupational therapy and physical dysfunction: principles skills and practices* (eds. Turner, A., Foster, M., and Johnson, S.E.), pp. 145–63. Churchill Livingstone, London.
15. Hagedorn, R. (1992). *Foundations for practice in occupational therapy*. Churchill Livingstone, London.
16. Doman, C., Rowe, P., Tipping, L. *et al.* (2002). Tools for living. In *Occupational therapy and physical dysfunction: principles skills and practices* (eds. Turner, A., Foster, M., Johnson, S.E.), pp. 165–209. Churchill Livingstone, London.
17. Esper, P., and Heidrich, D. (2005). Symptom clusters in advanced illness. *Seminars in Oncology Nursing*, **21**(1), 20–8.
18. Wrede-Seaman, D. (2001). Management of emergent conditions in palliative care, *Primary Care*, **28**, 317–28.
19. Barraclough, J. (1997). ABC of palliative care: Depression, anxiety, and confusion. *BMJ*, **315**, 1365–8.
20. Breitbart, W.. Chochinov, H. and Passik, S. (2004). Psychiatric symptoms in palliative medicine. In *Oxford textbook of palliative medicine* (eds. Doyle, D., Hanks, G., Cherny, N.I. *et al.*), 3rd edition, pp. 746–71. Oxford University Press, New York, NY.
21. Ewer-Smith, C., and Patterson, S. (2002). The use of an occupational therapy programme within a palliative care setting. *European Journal of Palliative Care*, **9**(1), 30–3.
22. Leubbert, K., Dahme, B., and Hasenbring, M. (2001). The effectiveness of training in reducing treatment-related symptoms and improving emotional adjustment in acute non-surgical cancer treatment, a meta-analysis. *Psychooncology*, **10**, 490–502.
23. Hanratty, J., and Higginson, I. (1994). *Palliative care in terminal illness*. EPL Pub, Northampton.
24. Cooper, J. (2006). OT in anxiety management and relaxation. In *Occupational therapy in oncology and palliative care* (ed. Cooper, J.), pp. 40–50. Whurr Publishers, Chichester.
25. Potter, J., Hami, F., Bryan, T. *et al.* (2003). Symptoms in 400 patients referred to palliative care services: prevalence and patterns. *Palliative Medicine*, **17**(4), 310–4.
26. Cooper, J. (2006). Occupational therapy in the management of breathlessness. In *Occupational therapy in oncology and palliative care* (ed. Cooper, J.), pp. 51–60. Whurr publishers, Chichester.
27. Barsevick, A.M., Whitmer, K., Sweeney, C. *et al.* (2002). A pilot study examining energy conservation for cancer treatment-related fatigue, *Cancer Nursing*, **25**(5), 333–41.
28. Cox, C. (2002). Non-pharmacological treatment of breathlessness. *Nursing Standard*, **16**(24), 33–6.
29. Davis, C.L. (1997). ABC of palliative care: Breathlessness, cough, and other respiratory problems. *BMJ*, **315**(7113), 931–4.
30. Lane, I. (2005). Managing cancer-related fatigue in palliative care. *Nursing Times*, **101**(18), 38–41.
31. Ahlberg, K.M., Ekman, T., Gaston-Johansson, F. *et al.* (2003). Assessment and management of cancer-related fatigue in adults. *Lancet*, **362**(9384), 640–50.
32. Richardson, A., and Ream, E. (1996). Fatigue in patients receiving chemotherapy for advanced cancer. *International Journal of Palliative Nursing*, **2**(4), 199–204.
33. Wagner, L.I., and Cella, D. (2004). Fatigue and cancer: Causes, prevalence and treatment approaches. *British Journal of Cancer*, **91**, 822–8.
34. Lowrie, D. (2006). Occupational therapy and cancer-related fatigue. In *Occupational therapy in oncology and palliative care* (ed. Cooper, J.), pp. 61–81. Whurr publishers, Chichester.
35. Sateia, M., and Santulli, R. (2004). Sleep in palliative care. In *Oxford textbook of palliative medicine* (eds. Doyle, D., Hanks, G., Cherny, N., Calman, K.), pp. 731–46. Oxford University Press, New York.
36. Winningham, M.L. (2001). Strategies for managing cancer-related fatigue syndrome: a rehabilitation approach. *Cancer*, **92**(4), 988–97.
37. Carty, J.L. (1997). Relaxation to reduce nausea, vomiting, andanxiety chemotherapy in Japanese patients. *Cancer Nursing*, **20**, 342–9.
38. HOPE (HIV/AIDS, Oncology and Palliative Care Education) (2004). *Occupational therapy interventions in cancer: guidance for professionals, managers and decision-makers*. College of Occupational Therapists, London.
39. Cooper, J. (2006). OT in symptom control. In *Occupational therapy in oncology and palliative care* (ed. Cooper, J.), pp. 27–39. Whurr Publishers, Chichester.
40. Cheville, A. (2001). Rehabilitation of patients with advanced cancer. *Cancer*, **92**(4), 1039–48.
41. Higginson, I. (2003). *Priorities and preferences for end of life care*. National Council for Hospice and Specialist Palliative Care Settings, London.

The contribution of music therapy to palliative medicine

Clare O'Callaghan

Music therapists ... bring relief to so many whose existential suffering, in the midst of the chaos of a life threatening illness, has eclipsed their soul.

Prof J. R. Zalcberg[1]

Introduction

Music therapists aim to improve comfort and ease the distress experienced by patients with life-threatening illnesses and their families by offering a range of creative musical experiences in a therapeutic relationship. The power of music to 'move', relieve, inspire, touch one's sense of the individual and the universal, and transcend cognitive forms of knowing, is fundamental to music therapy's (MT's) impetus as a treatment modality. After delineating historical origins and defining MT in palliative care, varying aims and methods will be described. Research findings will also highlight the profession's quest to evaluate MT's role in 'total patient care'.

Historical considerations

Egyptian papyri show that various diseases were treated with drug and music therapies over 4000 years ago. In ancient Greek mythology, the God Apollo presided over music and medicine, and the philosopher Pythagoras asserted that daily music performance enabled emotional catharsis and health. In the European Middle Ages, music was prescribed for healing and believed to influence character and behaviour[2]. Music helps Australian Aborigines to socially and spiritually accept ailing people into their communities and deal with loss[3] and, in shamanic tribal cultures, ritualized music often contributes to health restoration, one's trajectory into the next life if death occurs, and adjustment in the bereaved[4].

To some extent, the emergence of biomedical treatment models in industrialized Western societies displaced music's significance in health care. These treatment models have limitations, however, which may be especially apparent in end-of-life care. Accordingly, music therapists are now reawakening interest in music's relevance to help those encountering life-threatening conditions.

In 1973, Lucanne Magill brought live music to patients at the Memorial Sloan-Kettering Cancer Center, New York. Soon after, in 1977, Susan Munro and Balfour Mount introduced MT into Royal Victoria Hospital's Palliative Care Unit, Montreal[5,6]. Munro and Magill have since inspired the expansion of palliative MT

throughout the world, a movement that has been particularly evident in four international symposia held between 1989 and 2004[7–10]. Music therapists are accredited by national registration committees and have received extensive university training in MT methods, performance skills, music history and theory, psychotherapeutic theories, counselling techniques, and biopsychosocial knowledge. Music therapists work to contribute to holistic patient care as members of multi-disciplinary health-care teams.

Definition

MT can be defined as the creative and professionally informed use of music in a therapeutic relationship with people identified as needing physical, psychosocial, or spiritual help, or with people aspiring to experience further self-awareness, enabling increased life satisfaction and quality. Numerous definitions and descriptions of MT in palliative care with patients, families, visitors, and carers exist[5–11], and these include a range of aims (see Table 4.6.1) and methods (see Table 4.6.2). The musical elements (melody, harmony, rhythm, tempo, instrumentation, and volume), lyrics, and evolving therapeutic relationship provide a creative context and foundation for improved psychosocial adjustment and symptom alleviation. The focus is on the therapeutic process rather than musical products.

Verbal reflections arising from the music experience may helpfully extend self awareness. When caring holistically for people with advanced illnesses, however, attending to cognitive and physical components may not be enough for improved well-being. Through creatively experiencing music, one's non-discursive (nonverbal) level of awareness may be accessed and experienced as a 'felt', mindful, or symbolic sensation, possibly enabling a transcendental experience and transformation. Initiating verbal reflection then may unhelpfully shift the patient's focus from a 'feelingful' to 'thinking' mode. The balance of music and counselling, therefore, is monitored and variable in sessions.

MT is suitable for patients, and those close to them, who want to explore whether varying kinds of musical experiences can help them to encounter their illness experiences. Participants do not have

Table 4.6.1 Palliative care aims that can be addressed by music therapy.

Supportive validation	One's feelings and thoughts
	A life having been and still being lived
	One's relevance; self worth; spiritual way of being
	Contemplation; a time to 'be'
Increased self-awareness to aid adaptation	Self-discovery
	Reawakening or reworking of an earlier awareness
Symptom relief and relaxation	Including pain, tension, dyspnoea, nausea, insomnia, restlessness
Connection with others, reduced isolation	Those with cognitive impairment
	Those with language barriers and communication difficulties
	Expanded opportunities for interactions with family members, friends, other patients, staff
Aesthetic experience	Pleasure
	Diversion; normalcy
	Creative expression
	Transcendence
Support expression of grief, bereavement	Dealing with loss: acceptance of one's own way; reframing regret; helpful catharsis
	Increasing confidence and strength for moving forward

to have 'musical backgrounds' to benefit. While MT may provide opportunities for patients to meet goals indicative of what is professionally considered to be a 'better way to die', the patient and family ultimately decide whether and how they will be involved.

Scope of music therapy and contextual aspects

While MT palliative care services have expanded considerably over the past 30 years, growth has been ad hoc, likely affected by the availability of music therapists and funding. In 2003, Australian music therapists were employed in 23 paediatric and adult cancer treatment and palliative care contexts[12]. A US survey in 2001 found that 22 adult hospices had MT[11], and in the UK in 2006, 13 adult hospices and a Cancer Help Centre included music therapists[13]. Jessie's Fund, a UK charity, had also established MT at 24 children's hospices by 2006. Japan has 26 hospice programmes with MT (personal communication, Rika Ikuno and Akiko Niikura, 8th November 2006) and palliative care music therapists also work in Norway, Denmark, South Africa, Canada, Argentina, Sweden, Korea, and (sporadically) New Zealand.

Many music therapists work to improve life quality when lives are threatened. This is true of the discipline overall, not just those working in palliative focussed settings. Styles of practice vary according to educational and personal backgrounds and clinical

contexts, which can include home-based palliative programmes, day hospices, cancer treatment settings, neurological units, and nursing homes. Referrals may come via staff, the patients themselves or others who care for them. Often patients' conditions and moods fluctuate and visitors appear unpredictably, thus irregularly scheduled treatments may be required. Therapists often offer sessions at flexible times, adapting MT methods to suit participants' abilities and desires. Session lengths can range from 10 min to over 1 h, and patients may receive sessions from occasionally to almost daily.

Therapists may visit patients at their bedsides in hospitals and homes bringing accompanying instruments, sheet music, or recorded music. The author, for example, often brings sheet music with up to 7000 songs and classical pieces that she can spontaneously play on a 6.5 octave electric piano. Some MT departments incorporate extensive recorded music libraries, audio equipment, and tuned and untuned instruments.

Music therapy assessment, methods, and effects

Upon meeting a patient, the music therapist may offer music for a specific purpose (e.g. relaxation or pain control). Assessment includes determining the patients' music preferences and the relevance of music throughout their lives. This is typically followed by an invitation to experience methods (Table 4.6.2), which may be used at any stage of the illness.

The following vignettes and descriptions convey examples of methods and clinical outcomes. Approaches for more specific populations will follow.

Replaying the music of one's life

Our musical life stories are often profoundly integrated within our entire being. Revisiting 'their' music in MT can elicit 'non-patient' identities and expressions of whole historically situated selves. Through 're-sounding' the music from one's earlier life, one can rethink what one thought, and rediscover who one was, at both verbal and non-verbal levels of consciousness. The invigorating and life affirming properties of music can help people live until they die.

Table 4.6.2 Music therapy methods (individual and group work; patients and significant others).

Replaying the Music of One's Life
Live performance, by therapist and/or patients and significant others
Music listening (recorded or live; chosen by patient or therapist)
Music and life review (includes reminiscence, 'memento' creation)
Word substitution in known songs
Exploring 'New' Music (instrumental and computerized)
Music improvisation
Song writing
Unfamiliar pre-composed music (recorded or live)
Music and Imagery (with live or recorded music)
Free association
Guided

Luigi, who was in a cancer hospital receiving palliative radiotherapy, leapt out of bed as the author played Reginella Campagnola; he conducted, sang, danced, and invited other patients to request songs. Luigi had conducted a local Italian choir for 25 years. Nine months later, Luigi arrived in the hospice (where the author also worked) and, again, requested further songs, conducting from his bed, whispering the lyrics and inviting others to request songs. This time his sister danced and Luigi laughed. In the final session, days before he died, Luigi could not talk but still conducted the author with one finger, while his palm rested on his sheets. He also used eye contact and head movements to invite a nearby patient to choose a song, and smiled happily as it was played.

Rather than 'prescribing' music, therapists help patients to explore what they may find helpful. One's preferred music is most associated with relaxation[14]. Hence, music therapists do not advocate the indiscriminate use of 'piped' music in palliative care settings: what one person finds helpful may be aggravating for another.

Through choosing music that they wish to hear, patients have some control over their experienced memories, emotions, and messages. One may feel validated and supported when lyrics are actual or metaphorical expressions of one's experience. In research on the relevance of oncologic MT, a young (20- to 44-year-old) female patient anonymously wrote, *'Any experience like this reminds me that I am much more than a "cancer patient", I am a person with all sorts of needs, like everyone around me, who happens to have cancer'*[15].

Music and life review

While patients often spontaneously reminisce in sessions, others are actively encouraged to do a musical life review. Patients' life stories and musical selections or performances may be placed on an audio- or digital recorder which can be left as a legacy for loved ones. Through computerized 'music scrapbooking', young cancer patients have also arranged meaningful song fragments into new musical works which validate and express important sentiments (Robyn Booth, personal communication).

Reported benefits of using music for reminiscence in palliative care include improved communication between patients and those close to them, the validation of patients' lives, enhanced insight, ethnic and cultural affirmation, and improved self-esteem, sense of worth and identity[16].

Working with families and groups

MT can provide an intimate context for patients and those close to them to express supportive and validating messages about the role each has had in the others' lives. In shared sessions, patients and families have opportunities to choose music to enjoy and relax with together, and often indirectly communicate special messages through lyric identification and shared memories. Thoughts may remain private, but are indirectly expressed through 'knowing' looks and smiles, hand-holding, massaging touch, embraces, shared singing, and even dancing.

After describing relationship issues, two children asked if the social worker could get their father to tell their unconscious and dying mother that he loved her. The music therapist later invited the family to choose music for their wife and mother. The father requested two songs, 'If I Loved You' and 'An Affair to Remember'. He then moved from the end of his wife's bed, took her hand, sat down and sang; witnessed by his children.

Shared sessions among patients on wards also offer forums where seemingly isolated patients can discover shared interests and offer mutual support. When considering supportive care initiatives in inpatient palliative contexts, organizations should consider providing opportunities for people to engage in spontaneous and helpful interactions in their ward settings. MT in public ward settings can inspire the involvement of surrounding patients, visitors, and staff in uplifting ways, uniting and acknowledging each person's value. Even 'overhearing' public MT sessions can inspire. One cancer patient's anonymously written reaction to an overheard session was, 'One of the tunes was a favorite of mine (+ my husband's) … a reminder I have a lot to live for!'[15]'.

Concerts

Bringing concert performances into palliative-care contexts, and including patients and families as performers, can also offer joyful and 'normalized' experiences for the patients, visitors and staff, inspiring interesting topics for communication and positive memories.

John, a 53-year-old man with a left parietofrontal glioblastoma, was expressively dysphasic and struggling with living in the hospice after expecting to die months earlier. However, he discovered that he could fluently sing when reading the lyrics of well known songs. Theo, a 59-year-old man with advanced metastatic disease, accompanied John's singing on the guitar and, with the author, prepared a half hour evening concert for their family, friends, and hospice inpatients. Nine songs were selected and arranged in suitable keys and styles. The final song was (I did it) 'My Way'. This celebratory concert delighted, surprised and moved many.

Exploring 'new' sounds and songs

Improvisation

The therapist and client can improvise together, vocally and on various tuned and untuned instruments, creating the development of a musical relationship. Within this relationship, the client musically expresses aspects of oneself, and the therapist's musical response contains comparable and varied musical elements. The ongoing musical dialogue potentially affirms that the client has been heard and is known, inspiring further creativity, which may lead to further adaptive self awareness. This was eloquently illustrated in Salmon's work with a gentleman with motor neuron disease[17] and Hartley's work with HIV-positive men[18].

Song writing

In MT sessions, people of all ages have found substituting personal lyrics in well-known songs, and composing new songs, an enjoyable, cathartic, and safe form of self-expression. Patients have used songs to describe thoughts and feelings that were otherwise too difficult to verbalize. During song writing, patients and significant others may be invited to 'brainstorm' ideas on a specific issue; assisted to transform the ideas into song lyrics; and offered a variety of musical styles, melodies and harmonies for its accompaniment. They may then be recorded. Patients with advanced neurological conditions have written many songs in group and individual sessions, ranging from the celebration of receiving a home-brew kit, to the expression of feelings about the death of a fellow patient. Thematic and content analyses were used to examine the lyrics of 64 songs written by these patients, and others with advanced cancer (39 patients in total), in individual and group MT sessions over 7 years. The themes that emerged, and the frequency with which they recurred in the songs, were: messages (87%), self reflections (66%), compliments (50%), memories (45%), reflections upon significant others, including pets (31%), self expression of adversity (25%), imagery (17%), and prayers (11%)[19].

> Six weeks before her death, a mother wrote songs for her four young children which included memories of their birth and childhood, and statements about who they could turn to in the future. A dying father also included lyrics describing his baby daughter as his 'greatest legacy' and thanked her and his wife '… for making my whole world complete'.

These songs, as parting gifts, may also help the bereaved. While patients can find it helpful to express important sentiments in verbal form only, adding music to lyrics may extend the cathartic properties of verbal expressions. Sometimes the structural form of song can inspire the succinct expression of ideas when people 'don't know where to start'. One hospice patient had always wanted to write a book but felt it was too late. Offered song writing, she chose to describe the story of preparing to marry her new boyfriend 2 years after being informed that her husband was 'killed in action'. She was then informed that her husband was found alive. Opening the song with, 'Was it real or my imagination?', the final lyrics were, 'I made the right choice'.

O'Brien, who is a music therapist and opera singer, has also used a 'guided original lyrics and music' method with four cancer patients to create an opera. Their cancer experience was expressed in a libretto and musical form, and performed in public by professional singers. Patients reported that the experience helped them to express fears and grief, feel calm, soothed, proud, and healed, and put a 'face on the cancer making it easier to deal with'[20].

Music and imagery

Selected music may be used to direct or encourage patients' spontaneous imagery, to distract from symptoms and enable an aesthetic experience. Guided imagery and music (GIM) is a specialist form of MT training directed at eliciting a client's imagery, enabling increased self-understanding and personal growth. GIM has helped to alleviate fear in terminally ill patients, and spiritually prepare them for death, but is not usually helpful for people with cognitive impairment and limited attention spans[21].

The relevance of the music therapist accompanying the music

The potency of MT results from both the patients' experience of the music and their relationship with the music therapist. The therapist's supportive presence may be conceptualized as providing a 'sounding board' or a musical 'human mirror'. Winnicott suggested that in psychotherapy the therapist 'reflects back' aspects about the patient, enabling the person to exist 'as an expression of I AM, I am alive, I am myself'[22]. In MT, the patient may be 'reflected back' in a multi-sensorial manner, that is, musically, verbally and non-verbally, expanding the potential for creative reintegration and helpful new awareness. Improvisations and known music from one's lifetime are, therefore, always experienced anew, creatively perceived and expressed, potentially transducing

into new and helpful ways of viewing their current situation[15]. Hence, while electronic media may enable easy access to many musical requests, the added therapeutic impetus encapsulated in live musical involvement with a trained music therapist cannot be underestimated.

As patients move closer to death, it may not be appropriate to expect significant psychotherapeutic changes. Nonetheless, the validation of people's experiences through reflective listening and playing their selected music may still support self-acceptance, leading to 'spiritual renewal', hope, peace and, faith affirmation[23].

Working with other therapists

Combining music with allied therapies may broaden the therapeutic benefits. Music therapists can assist in the music selection to accompany exercises; relax muscles to assist feeding when dysphagic; and support treatment delivery, such as palliative radiotherapy.

Conjoint family sessions with a music therapist and social worker successfully promoted supportive communication among young children and their parents, when one of the parents was dying. Children substituted lyrics in known songs, or composed new ones, to express significant messages to their parents before their deaths[24].

The author's interaction with creative art pastoral carer (Joan Ryan) has also helped patients' multi-sensory awareness development and expressions of personal meaning in the final days of their lives.

> Ella, who was 51 years old with end-stage cancer, said that she had always wanted to play a musical instrument. Ella imagined that she was in a Sri Lanken rain forest while improvising on the metallophone (metal xylophone) and 'learnt' to play the recorder. Although very breathless, Ella was delighted as she played individual notes. Ella was also creating a china painted mandala, integrating her significant emotions and life stories. Four days before her death, Ella realized that music was a significant part of her life and wanted it included. While sitting with her mandala and softly playing sustained sounds on her recorder, Ella decided that she wanted to create a musical image that captured rest, slowness and fast movement (stillness and life), integrating her Eastern spirituality. Electing to integrate representative western musical notation into the mandala, Ella chose the following: semibreve rest, 'adagio', 'presto' and 'la' (representing 'om'). Other images reflected her love of learning (books, flower of knowledge), spirituality (lotus, Buddha), and tensions (colour contrasts).

Specific populations

Music therapy with children and adolescents

Aims and methods in Tables 4.6.1 and 4.6.2 are often relevant in MT with young people with advanced illnesses, as well as the children of dying patients. Developmental levels are considered as therapists tailor interventions to participants' cognitive abilities and emotional states. While children and adolescents may not be able to discuss their feelings, or wish to, they may symbolically express aspects about their condition and find self-understanding through MT methods. This was illustrated through Daveson and Kennelly's work with a 'miserable and depressed' 8-year-old child who eventually expressed her sadness and grief, and a message to her best friend, through song writing shortly before her death[25].

Validating experiences of being 'heard' through the supportive medium of music may alleviate anxiety and instigate changes identified as a healthier response to the illness. This was evident in the reduction of pharmacological anxiolytics in two 13-year old-patients with brain tumors while undergoing radiotherapy, after experiencing improvisation, song writing, or therapeutic music lessons[26].

MT also provides opportunities for dying young patients and their families to have normalized and 'fun' experiences.

> The day before he died, Peter, a 4-year-old boy lying quietly with his mother nearby, requested, 'The blanket!' Aasgaard sang 'Hocus pocus' (a jack-in-the-box song in which the child is hidden under a cover) and a short smile was evident when the blanket was gently pulled from Peter's face as the Swedish song finished[27].

Hilliard described teaching the trumpet to a 12-year-old-boy with AIDS. His grandmother reported that the happiest she had seen him was when he received the trumpet from the hospice. The therapeutic music lessons also provided a supportive context where the boy finally expressed grief over his parents' deaths, through describing dreams, memories, and songwriting[28].

Brain impairment

Cerebral areas and neural systems activated during some musical activities are 'relatively independent from the areas used for verbal tasks'[29]. Furthermore, long-term memories, especially familiar lyrics and melodies, are relatively preserved in people with cognitive impairment. Therefore, the therapeutic use of both language and music are more likely to activate preserved neural function in these people than the use of language alone, thereby expanding opportunities for encountering aesthetic experiences and communicating meaningfully.

Many patients who had language expression and/or comprehension difficulties due to advanced cancer or other degenerative neurological conditions have sung shared songs with families, knowingly laughed at musically inspired reminiscences, and have even written songs in MT sessions.

Improvisation and familiar music also provides a highly interactive medium for working with patients in low awareness states, following profound brain injury, who display minimal and inconsistent spontaneous responses. The diagnosis of 'vegetative state' in one patient, who experienced severe anoxic brain injury following a cardiac arrest, was revised to a 'minimally conscious state' following her purposeful, non-verbal responses to MT. Her family, who 'knew she was in there', then worked with the music therapist to find ways that they could leisurely share music with her[30]. (This work has been described as 'neuropalliative rehabilitation'.)

Ethnic minorities

Music therapists attempt to offer a wide variety of musical styles from many cultures. Patients who have difficulties with the dominant language in their ward culture may experience reduced isolation, validation and joy as they experience songs from their language of origin. Furthermore, culturally significant music can help patients to reconfirm their identity within their wider sociohistorical and ethnic heritage, assisting their expression of pain, grief, and memories; supporting their preparation for death and their family members' grieving[16].

Bereavement

Many bereaved relatives have stated that the memories of, and the songs written in, patients' sessions have ameliorated their distress following the death.

> After the author accompanied one teenage daughter, who sang her mother's MT song composition at her funeral, she said that knowing that she had sang well helped her to believe that she had the strength to get on and 'do something with my life'. The song was called, 'You are my Strength'.

Group MT sessions for bereaved young people were found to significantly reduce grief symptoms and behavioural problems in 18 children (6–11 years)[31] and also help six adolescents to creatively express pent up feelings[32]. Roberts also described varying ways that six bereaved children wrote songs to play and sing their story, aiding their self esteem, acceptance of the loss, expression of emotions and memories, and connectedness to their loved one[33].

Staff support

MT can indirectly support staff as they witness and occasionally participate in public ward sessions. In the author's study on the relevance of oncologic MT, 56% of the 61 staff respondents' anonymously written responses informed the theme: MT elicited a range of helpful emotions and self-awarenesses, improving individual and team work life and the ward environment. One nurse's response informing this inductively derived theme was that MT: '… Alters the environment, it softens and humanizes … It brings joy, especially when staff become actually involved, singing—playing instruments, laughing. … Music selection by a patient may help nurses understand more about the patient.'[15].

Adverse effects

As long as participants have control over the music experienced in sessions, adverse effects are rare. Music therapists avoid conducting sessions in public locations where others find them disturbing. People tend to choose music that elicits memories and affective responses that they wish to experience (consciously or unconsciously) and can usually shift the emotional evocations by requesting or performing different music. Therefore, MT is a non-intrusive, albeit potentially transformative, form of therapy.

Neural damage, however, can occasionally result in distorted and unpleasant musical perception. Music therapists should also be wary of patients with musicogenic epilepsy (when music can directly trigger an epileptic seizure) and musically induced catastrophic reactions (heightened distress triggered occasionally in people with dementia when hearing specific music)[34].

Research

Palliative care MT research, as found in hospice care, neurology, and oncology, incorporates both positivist and interpretative (qualitative) designs, and both traditions provide multi-faceted insights into the area.

Positivist tradition

Hilliard's detailed review of 11 empirical research studies found that six supported MT's helpful effect on symptom alleviation and well-being in palliative care[35]. In two studies using pre-post test designs with at least 80 hospice patients, MT significantly reduced patients' pain sensation[36,37] and anxiety[36], and improved comfort and relaxation levels[37]. Anxiety, pain, tiredness, and drowsiness were also significantly reduced in the experimental group in a randomized controlled trial with 25 hospice patients[38]. Two studies also found significant effects from single MT sessions, substantiating the value of 'one off' sessions[37,38].

Life quality also significantly improved in home hospice-care patients who received MT in a randomized controlled trial comprising 80 patients[39]. Furthermore, in another randomized controlled trial of 62 patients receiving autologous stem cell transplants for haematological malignancies, the MT group scored significantly lower on the anxiety/depression and total mood distrubance score than the control standard care group[40].

Theoretical rationales for pain reduction in MT include direct physiological response to music stimuli that alter neural components of pain sensation, as well as cognitive and emotional changes aligned with increased self-awareness. These changes presumably alter one's sense of the meaning, and thus perception, of pain[34,41].

Interpretive tradition

While it is suggested that more randomized controlled trials are needed in MT and palliative care, where designs include larger samples and statistical testing to enable (predictive) generalizations[35], others have used interpretive designs which enable logical generalizations[15]. As positivist designs are derived from the physical sciences, they can be problematic when examining human relationship therapies, and in multi-disciplinary contexts focused on individualized need[42]. Limitations inherent in randomized controlled trials include: (a) patients cannot be blinded to group allocation; (b) the variations in patients' diagnoses, medications, and life histories mean that randomization is not likely to evenly distribute confounders between groups; (c) MT is not a standardized treatment as therapists' approaches vary and patients often choose how they wish to participate; and (d) researcher-devised standardized measurements do not necessarily capture what participants find valuable. This was evident in one study in which oncologic patients' positive verbal feedback about MT sessions contradicted statistical findings from validated scales completed by the same patients[43]. Therefore, research designs based on the social science tradition have been encouraged in palliative care[42].

Interpretive research methods can collect patients' and carers' idiosyncratic voices, identifying what they find important. Hogan first examined nine hospice patients' MT experiences in a phenomenological study using semi-structured interviews. Responses were condensed into a final statement indicating that MT was a positive, emotional experience that could elicit social interaction, inspire improved well-being and coping mechanisms, and elicit spiritual reflections and memories[44].

The constructivist and grounded theory paradigms informed the author's already mentioned research, which compared patients', visitors', staff, and her own views about oncologic MT's relevance in a hospital setting. Anonymous, open-ended questionnaire feedback was received from 257 people. Predominantly positive experiences were characterized by revisited memories and their 'transportation' to new places or thoughts and physical sensations. Staff and visitors also reported that MT helped them while they were with the patients[15].

An interpretive arts-informed methodology was used to explore the meaning of a MT cancer support group for 10 participants in a community setting. The group, who selected various MT methods, described their experiences as a profound, non-verbal connection to themselves, each other and something beyond themselves. Improvised music-making provided empowerment, feelings of control, and other positive effects (e.g. decreased pain, elevated mood) that were long-lasting[45].

Another study analysed interview responses from 20 hospice multi-disciplinary team members who described their perceptions of MT. MT was a valued and supportive modality, which addressed holistic patient care needs, and encouraged favourable environmental effects, spiritual support, and bereavement assistance. Concern was expressed, however, that occasional patients found elicited emotions distressing.[13]

Grounded theory also informed a study conducted with six patients with chronically progressive multiple sclerosis. MT provided opportunities for the patients to challenge their disabled identities. Improvisation either validated or reminded them of physical loss and songs supported coping strategies to deal with the condition's emotional impact[46].

Mixed designs

Increasingly, oncologic MT research has incorporated mixed quantitative and qualitative designs. Findings indicate that MT has enabled people with cancer to identify and express emotions, develop group cohesion and new awareness[47], experience improved well-being, energy, immunological response[48], mood and life quality[49], and reduced tension and energetic arousal[48].

Closure

A hospice patient receiving MT stated: 'The music is so beautiful it hurts my heart'. Music therapists and participants recreate melodies, rhythms, harmonies, and lyrics which resonate with sounds carried from life times. Music's sonic components can alleviate physical distress and mnemonic components can validate one's life and be a reminder of nurturance. The aesthetic components can inspire transcendental experiences. Some of the most profound moments in MT are when people express simultaneous 'joy' and 'sadness' as they 'relive' images, memories, and thoughts. The sadness, perhaps, expresses the loss in knowing what will not be recaptured or lived as mortal life closes. However, the joy may reflect one's experience of feeling understood by their musical encounter and, therefore, known.

O Music.
In your depths we deposit our hearts and souls.
Thou hast taught us to see with our ears.
And hear with our hearts.
                              Kahlil Gibran (1883–1931)[50].

As music can enable one to see and hear in new ways, it is an obvious companion for aiding one's transition from corporeal life.

[Of Music:] Nothing among the utterances allowed to man is felt to be so divine. It brings us near to the Infinite.

Thomas Carlyle (1795–1881)[50].

Acknowledgement

The author wishes to thank the colleagues who provided information about international MT programmes and helpful feedback on this chapter.

References

1. Zalcberg, J. (2006). Introduction. In O'Callaghan C, Guest ed. Special section on music therapy. *Journal of the Society for Integrative Oncology*, **4**(2), 57–81.

2. Rebollo Pratt, R. (1989). A brief history of music and medicine. In *Rehabilitation, music and human well-being* (ed. Lee, M.H.), pp. 1-12: Ann Arbor: MMB, St Louis, MO.

3. Ellis, C.J. (1985). *Aboriginal music: Education for living*. University of Queensland Press, St Lucia.

4. Laderman, C., and Roseman, M. (ed.) (1996). *The performance of healing*. Routledge, New York.

5. Munro, S., and Mount, B.M. (1978). Music therapy in palliative care. *Canadian Medical Association Journal*, **119**, 1029–34.

6. Munro, S. (1984). *Music Therapy in palliative/hospice care*. Magnamusic-Baton, St Louis, MO.

7. Martin, J.A. (Ed.) (1989). *The next step forward: Music therapy with the terminally ill*. Calvary Hospital, New York.

8. Lee, C.A. (ed.) (1995). Lonely waters: Proceedings of the international conference, Music therapy in palliative care, Oxford, 1994. Sobell Publications, Oxford.

9. Rykov, M., and Salmon, D. (2001). Guest Eds. Moments musicaux: Music therapy in palliative care (special issue), *Journal of Palliative Care*, **17**(3), 133–192.

10. Dileo, C., and Loewy, J. (eds.) (2006). *Music therapy at the end of life*. Jeffrey Books, Cherry Hill, NJ.

11. Hilliard, R.E. (2005). *Hospice and palliative care music therapy: A guide to program development and clinical care*. Jeffrey Books, Cherry Hill, NJ.

12. Hogan, B., and Cockayne, M. (2003). Striking a chord: Implications for music therapists working in palliative care. *Australian Journal of Music Therapy*, **14**, 50–62.

13. O'Kelly, J. (2006). Multi disciplinary perspectives of music therapy in adult palliative care. Unpublished Masters Dissertation. Kings College, London.

14. Stratton, V.N., and Zalanowski, A.H. (1984). The relationship between music, degree of liking and self-reported relaxation. *Journal of Music Therapy*, **21**(4), 184–192.

15. O'Callaghan, C., and McDermott F. (2004). Music therapy's relevance in a cancer hospital researched through a constructivist lens. *Journal of Music Therapy*, **41**(2), 151–85.

16. Forrest, L.C. (2000). Addressing issues of ethnicity and identity in palliative care through music therapy. *Australian Journal of Music Therapy*, **11**, 33–7.

17. Salmon, D. (1995). Music and emotion in palliative care: assessing inner resources. In *Lonely waters: Proceedings of the international conference, Music therapy in palliative care*, (ed. Lee, C.A.) Oxford, 1994, pp. 71–84. Sobell Publications, Oxford.

18. Hartley, N. (1999). Music therapists' personal reflections on working with those who are living with HIV/AIDS. In *Music therapy in palliative care: New voices* (ed. Aldridge, D.), pp. 105–25. Jessica Kingsley Pub Ltd, London.

19. O'Callaghan, C. (1996). Lyrical themes in songs written by palliative care patients. *Journal of Music Therapy*, **33**(2), 74–92.

20. O'Brien, E. (2006). Opera therapy: Creating and performing a new work with cancer patients and professional singers. *Nordic Journal of Music Therapy*, **15**(1), 89–103.

21. Marr J. (1998–1999). GIM at the end of life: Case studies in palliative care. *Journal of the Association for Music and Imagery*, **6**, 37–54.

22. Winnicott, D.W. (1971). *Playing and reality p.56*. Routledge, London.

23. Magill, L. (2006). Music therapy: Enhancing spirituality at the end of life. In *Music therapy at the end of life* (eds. Dileo, C. and Loewy, J.), pp. 3–18. Jeffrey Books, Cherry Hill.

24. Slivka, H.H., and Magill, L. (1986). The conjoint use of social work and music therapy with children of cancer patients. *Music Therapy*, **6A**(1), 30–40.

25. Daveson, B., and Kennelly, J. (2000). Music therapy in palliative care for hospitalised children and adolescents. *Journal of Palliative Care*, **16**(1), 35–8.

26. O'Callaghan, C., Sexton, M., and Wheeler, G. (2007). Music therapy as a non-pharmacological anxiolytic for paediatric radiotherapy patients. *Australasian Radiology*, **51**(2), 159–62.

27. Aasgaard, T. (2001). An ecology of love: Aspects of music therapy in the pediatric oncology environment. *Journal of Palliative Care*, **17**(3), 177–81.

28. Hilliard, R. (2003). Music therapy in pediatric palliative care: Complementing the interdisciplinary approach. *Journal of Palliative Care*, **19**(2), 127–32.

29. Sergent, J., Zuck, S., Tenial, S. *et al.* (1992). Distributed neural network underlying musical sightreading and keyboard performance. *Science*, **257**, 106–9.

30. Magee, W.L. (2005). Music therapy with patients in low awareness states: assessment and treatment approaches in multidisciplinary care. *Neuropsychological Rehabilitation*, **15**(3–4), 522–36.

31. Hilliard, R. (2001). The effects of music therapy-based bereavement groups on mood and behaviour of grieving children: A pilot study. *Journal of Music Therapy*, **38**(4), 291–306.

32. McFerran-Skewes, K., and Erdonmez Grocke, D. (2000). Group music therapy for young bereaved teenagers. *European Journal of Palliative Care*, **7**(6), 227–9.

33. Roberts, M. (2006). "I want to play and sing my story": Home-based song writing for bereaved children and adolescents. *Australian Journal of Music Therapy*, **16**, 18–24.

34. O'Callaghan, C. (1996). Pain, music creativity and music therapy in palliative care. *American Journal of Hospice and Palliative Care*, **13**(2), 43–9.

35. Hilliard, R.E. (2005). Music therapy in hospice and palliative care: A review of the empirical data. *Evidence-Based Complementary and Alternative Medicine*, **2**(2), 173–8.

36. Gallagher, L. (2001). Developing and using a computerised database for music therapy in palliative medicine. *Journal of Palliative Care*, **17**(3), 147–54.

37. Krout, R.E. (2001). The effects of single-session music therapy interventions on the observed and self-reported levels of pain control, physical comfort, and relaxation of hospice patients. *American Journal of Hospice and Palliative Care*, **18**(6), 383–90.

38. Horne-Thompson, A. (2006). *The use of music therapy with terminally ill patients experiencing anxiety*. Unpublished Master's Thesis. University of Melbourne, Australia.

39. Hilliard, R.E. (2003). The effects of music therapy on the quality and length of life of people diagnosed with terminal cancer. *Journal of Music Therapy*, **40**(2),113–37.

40. Cassileth, B.R., Vickers, A.J., and Magill, L.A. (2003). Music therapy for mood disturbance during hospitalization for autologous stem cell transplantation. *Cancer*, **98**(12), 2723–9.

41. Magill-Leverault, L. (1993). Music therapy in pain and symptom management. *Journal of Palliative Care*, **9**(4), 42–8.

42. Aoun, S.M., and Kristjanson, L.J. (2005). Challenging the framework for evidence in palliative care research. *Palliative Medicine*, **19**, 461–5.

43. Hanser, S.B., Bauer-Wu, S., Kubicek, L. *et al.* (2005). Effects of a music therapy intervention for women with metastatic breast cancer [abstract]. *Oncology Nursing Forum*, **32**, 184–5.

44. Hogan, B. (1999). A phenomenological research project. In *Music Medicine* (ed. Rebollo Pratt, R., and Erdonmez Grocke, D.), pp. 242–52. University of Melbourne, Melbourne.

45. Rykov, M.H. (2006). *Music at a time like this: Music therapy cancer support groups.* PhD Dissertation. University of Toronto, Toronto.

46. Magee, W.L., and Davidson, J.W. (2004). Music therapy in multiple sclerosis: results of a systematic qualitative analysis. *Music Therapy Perspectives*, **22**(1), 39–51.

47. Bunt, L, and Marston-Wyld, J. (1995). Where words fail, music takes over: A collaborative study by a music therapist and a counselor in the context of cancer care. *Music Therapy Perspectives,* **13**, 46–50.

48. Burns, S.J., Harbuz, M.S., Hucklebridge, F. *et al.* (2001). A pilot study into the therapeutic effects of music therapy at a cancer help center. *Alternative Therapies in Health and Medicine,* **7**(1), 48–56.

49. Bonde, L.O. (2005). The Bonny method of guided imagery and music with cancer survivors. A psychosocial study with focus on the influence of music therapy on mood and quality of life. *PhD Dissertation.* Aalborg University. Available as a pdf at http://www.mt-research.aau.dk/guided-imagery-music-resource-center Accessed 18th October, 2008.

50. *The Wordsworth dictionary of musical quotations* (1994).Wordsworth Editions Ltd, Ware, Hertfordshire.

Further reading

Music therapy chapters in previous editions of this textbook.

Abad, V. (2003). A time of turmoil: Music therapy interventions for adolescents in a paediatric oncology ward. *Australian Journal of Music Therapy,* **14**, 20–37.

Bailey, L. (1983). The effects of live versus tape recorded music in hospitalized cancer patients. *Music Therapy*, **3**(1), 17–28.

Baker, F., and Wigram, T. (2005). *Songwriting: Methods, techniques and clinical applications for music therapy clinicians, educators and students.*Jessica Kingsley Publishers, London.

Beggs, C. (1991). Life review with a palliative care patient. In *Case studies in music therapy* (ed. Bruscia, K.), pp. 611–16. Barcelona, Phoenixville PA.

Dalton, T.A., and Krout, R.E. (2005). Development of the grief process scale through music therapy song writing with bereaved adolescents. *Arts in Psychotherapy*, **32**, 131–43.

Forinash, M. (1990). The phenomenology of music therapy with the terminally ill. Doctoral Dissertation, New York University. *Dissertation Abstracts International,* **51**(09), 2915A.

Gallagher, L.M., Huston, M.J., Nelson, K.A. *et al.* (2001). Music therapy in palliative medicine. *Supportive Care Cancer,* **9**, 156–61.

Lee, C. (1996). *Music at the edge: The music therapy experiences of a musician with AIDS.* Routledge, London.

Magee, W. (1995). Case studies in Huntingtons's Disease: Music therapy assessment and treatment in the early to advanced stages. *British Journal of Music Therapy*, **9**(2), 13–9.

Mandel, S.E. (1991). Music therapy in the hospice: 'Musicalive'. *Journal of Palliative Care*, **9**(4), 42–8.

Murrant, G.M., Rykov, M., Amonite, D. *et al.* (2000). Creativity and self-care for caregivers. *Journal of Palliative Care,* **16**(2), 44–9.

O'Kelly, J. (2002). Music therapy in palliative care: Current perspectives. *International Journal of Palliative Nursing,* **8**(3), 130–6.

Pavlicevic, M. (Ed.) (2005). *Music therapy in children's hospices. Jessie's fund in action.* Jessica Kingsley Publishers, London. www.jessiesfund.org.uk Accessed 16th October, 2008

Rykov, M. (1999). Sometimes there are no reasons: Marco's song. In *Inside music therapy: Client experiences* (ed. Hibben, E.), pp. 202–7. Barcelona, Gilsum NH.

Steele, M. (2005). Coping with multiple sclerosis: A music therapy viewpoint. *Australian Journal of Music Therapy*, **16**, 70–87.

The contribution of the dietitian and nutritionist to palliative medicine

Rosemary Richardson and Isobel Davidson

Nutritional management of patients receiving palliative care has not, until recently, been considered an explicit element of care[1]. The features of cachexia such as anorexia are often considered by health-care professionals as milestones of disease progression. Traditionally, the input from palliative care specialists relating to nutrition is one of ethics and centres on the withdrawal of food and fluids. Nevertheless, many patients present with and are distressed by the presence of symptoms that affect their ability to eat 'normally' i.e. dysphagia, taste changes, xerostomia, and dementia. The deterioration and alteration in nutritional intake which results promotes weight loss, is accompanied by fatigue and often a distressing alteration in body image.

The futility of approaches that merely seek to improve patients' nutritional intake (either enterally or parenterally) and replete body mass has redirected the focus of nutritional intervention to maintenance and symptom control. (see Chapter 10.3.2) Our improved understanding of the metabolic sequelae of disease and an appreciation of nutritional strategies that may be used to ameliorate or manage symptoms (see Table 4.7.1) has resulted in the recognition of nutrition as a component of holistic palliative care. Embedding nutritional care in palliative medicine must be paralleled by formal and rigorous evaluation (i.e. randomized controlled trials) of practice. To a large part this remains to be addressed and it would be naïve not to appreciate the inherent difficulties of conducting nutritional research in the palliative-care environment. The challenge for practitioners is to strike a balance between the application of research evidence with the practical nutritional needs of the individual.

Approaches to increase nutritional intake

Dietary counselling

Dietary counselling should serve to provide the dietitian with an understanding of the patient's nutritional problems, their needs and an appreciation of limitations and barriers to complying with nutritional advice/prescriptions. Dietary counselling is a time consuming process and an initial interview, which may or may not involve the informal carer, can last about an hour. In light of this, the atmosphere in which the interview is to be conducted should be relaxed and conducive to frank and open discussion.

Developing a relationship of trust between the dietitian, patient, and their support network is central to evaluating nutritional intervention. Patients are surprisingly good at providing information the dietitian wants to hear and whilst patients may verbally confirm their compliance to nutritional treatment on careful and sensitive questioning adherence may be limited or non-existent. This may account for the disappointing results of one of the few randomized controlled trials that examined the effect of dietary counselling on food intake, body weight, and quality of life in cancer patients[2]. Patients (n = 57) were randomized to receive nutritional counselling (twice a month for 5 months) and offered nutritional supplemental drinks. The control group (n = 48) ate ad libitum and had no counselling. Results showed that when compared with the controls, 5 months of dietary counselling increased total energy intake by 15 kcal/day and 0.6 g protein/day and not surprisingly no differences in body weight or quality of life were observed. No details of the structure of the counselling interview were provided other than its aim was for patients to achieve recommended intakes. Similarly, a study[3] in patients with advanced colorectal and non-small-cell lung cancer showed no differences in intake in patients receiving and not receiving dietary counselling.

There remains a paucity of studies that have examined the effect of dietary counselling in palliative care. Evaluation of counselling determined not only by quantitative parameters such as intake or change in body weight but also qualitative elements should be considered, for example, determining patients and their carers understanding of nutritional advice/prescription, patient satisfaction (i.e. is the counselling process itself too onerous), and level of symptom relief from dietary advice.

Many dietitians undertake additional training to develop their counselling skills but further quantitative work that evaluates current practice is required. In conducting and evaluating patient interviews the interviewer may find it helpful to construct a template of 'probes' that forms the structure of the interview and facilitates the patient/carer taking the lead in discussion (Table 4.7.2). Prior to interview construction the dietitian should be fully cognizant of the patient's medical history.

Table 4.7.1 Nutritional strategies to improve symptom control.

Symptom	Causes of decrease in dietary intake	Management
1. Psychological stress/depression	◆ Poor appetite	◆ Antidepressant, complementary therapies (i.e. aromatherapy, reflexology) small frequent meals
2. Altered taste and smell	◆ Food aversions	◆ Dietary counselling and identification of food aversions/preferences
3. Oral thrush/ulceration	◆ Blunting of taste	◆ Pharmacological treatment of symptoms (i.e. nystatin, lignocaine)
		◆ Increase use of nutrient dense cold fluids
		◆ Optimize oral hygiene
4. Reduced flow and altered consistency of saliva	◆ Induce gagging and nausea	◆ Use of artificial saliva
		◆ To encourage flow of saliva—chew gum or suck on boiled sweets
		◆ Optimize oral hygiene
5. Nausea and vomiting	◆ Radio/chemotherapy	◆ Pharmacological treatment that is effective at mealtimes
	◆ Drugs, e.g. opioids	◆ Small frequent meals
	◆ Physical obstruction	◆ Avoidance of food aversions
		◆ Consume fluids after meals
6. Dysphagia	◆ Physical obstruction/constriction	◆ Altered consistency of food semi solid → puree
		◆ Use of nutrient-dense supplements
		◆ Consider initiating PEG feeding
7. Respiratory distress	◆ Focus on breathing rather than food intake	◆ Medication before mealtimes
		◆ Ensure patient wearing loose clothing
		◆ Relaxation exercises
		◆ Small meals and presentation foods that do not require a lot of chewing
8. Early satiety	◆ Cytokine mediated	◆ Maximize availability of food
		◆ Small frequent meals
		◆ Encourage food consumption when patient feels at their best/less agitated
9. Altered bowel function (i). Constipation (ii). Diarrhoea	◆ Feeling bloated ◆ Abdominal discomfort ◆ Abdominal discomfort ◆ Fear of symptom leads to food avoidance	◆ Mild laxatives ◆ Encourage fluid intake ◆ Encourage consumption of dietary fibre ◆ If possible optimize mobility ◆ Antidiarrhoeal drugs ◆ Temporarily avoid dairy products ◆ Increase intake soluble fibre (i.e. bananas, oranges, oatmeal)
10. Fatigue/lethargy	◆ Neurological ◆ Loss of muscle mass	◆ Maximize intake when patient feels at their best ◆ Avoid foods that require a lot of chewing

Often patients and their informal carer have high expectations of nutritional intervention and have themselves made a clear but inappropriate choice of treatment (i.e. total parenteral nutrition (TPN))[4,5]. Thoughtful counselling will improve patient management and by putting the patient at the centre of care allows them to make choices and identify realistic goals. It should be remembered that the Internet is a source of dietary information accessed by many patients and their carers. This may result in alternative therapies being used, for example, macrobiotic diets, supra-dosing of vitamins and homeopathy and should be reviewed but ultimately the decision to follow such regimens rests with the patient.

Nutritional supplements

Oral nutritional supplements normally provide 1.5 kcal/ml and 0.6 g/ml of protein presented in 200–250-ml cartons and are central to the dietetic management of this vulnerable patient group. However, compliance with oral nutritional support regimens is often poor[6,7]

and may prohibit primary dietetic outcomes being achieved. One reason for this may be the patients' limited understanding of the rationale for dietetic intervention. Another may be inappropriate encouragement of patients to consume these supplements after meals. Identification of a more appropriate time for ingestion of these supplements may improve quantitative intake and thus compliance.

Timing of consumption

Recent work in the understanding of the physiology of energy intake and of the pathophysiology of cachexia has permitted traditional approaches of nutritional support to be revisited. It is well recognized that the control of ingestive behaviour in cachexia profoundly influences nutritional intake. Many patients may have amplification of the satiety cascade (neural and humoral) thereby prolonging the inter meal interval and reducing post-prandial consumption. One strategy to address this would be to offer energy and protein dense supplements before meals (1 h) when feelings of

Table 4.7.2 Effective dietary counselling.

Suggestions for constructing patient interview

- ◆ What changes in your diet had there been over the last few months?
  - Quantity
  - Food aversion/taste changes
  - Consistency
  - Diet history
- ◆ Do you think nutrition is an important part of your care?
- ◆ Any symptoms around mealtimes that are troublesome?
  - Pain
  - Respiratory distress
- ◆ How are you managing with nutritional supplemental drinks?
  - Compliance
  - Change prescription
  - Taste fatigue
- ◆ Is there anytime of the day when you feel at your best?
  - Opportunity to optimize intake.
- ◆ How is your informal carer (if patient interviewed)?
  - Pressure for patient to eat (alone)
  - Anxiety of carer
  - Identify home enteral feeding problems
- ◆ Are you happy that your nutritional status is monitored?
  - Objectives

If the patient cannot be interviewed then the carer becomes the source of dietary information

hunger are strongest. In addition, patients should be discouraged from consuming low nutritive fluids at the beginning of meals i.e. soups. The rationale for this is to minimize the volume effect of fluids on satiety. In cachexia, alteration of the signalling of the afferent nerves may explain the early perception of fullness at relatively low gastric volume. This theoretical approach, based on our understanding of the pathophysiology remains to be evaluated in the clinical situation[8].

There are some concerns that consumption of supplements before meals would result in energy compensation at mealtimes. Interestingly, in a study[9] that examined the effect of nutritive pre-loads (high fat, high carbohydrate) on meal consumption in elderly subjects and younger controls found the elderly subjects did not compensate for the pre-load. These results are encouraging given that the majority of patients in palliative care are elderly but no subject in this study had metabolically active disease.

Nutritional modulation

A characteristic feature of cachexia, despite its primary cause, is the presence of systemic inflammation. A consequence of this is reduced motivation to eat and the ineffective utilization of nutrients. Thus in conditions where the inflammatory response is more profound the associated anorexia may be more resistant to intervention strategies and the accretion of lean body mass becomes an impossible goal. In recent years, there has been considerable interest in the use of nutrients with putative anti-inflammatory properties that attenuate cachexia and promote anabolism to improve body composition. The primary aim of this treatment is to improve survival and quality of life where functional ability is a key component.

Work in patients with advanced pancreatic cancer[10] examined the effect of a fish oil enriched supplement (eicosapentaenoic acid—EPA, energy, and protein dense) on total dietary intake. Nutrient intake (meals and supplement) was significantly greater in those patients receiving the fish oil than in the group randomized to energy and protein supplements alone. In addition, results from a study of 200 patients with pancreatic carcinoma supplemented with 2 g EPA revealed net gain of weight and lean tissue. However, disappointingly a more recent study[11] of a randomized controlled trial of over 500 cachectic patients (gastrointestinal and lung cancer) supplemented with either 2 or 4 g/day EPA indicated no significant treatment benefit in terms of weight or survival. This is supported by other work[12] in a more heterogeneous cachectic group showing EPA had no significant benefits on energy intake and nutritional status.

Whilst this evidence has served to inform practice it is not sufficiently strong to warrant the indiscriminate prescribing of EPA-enriched supplements to patients with cachexia in order to improve nutritional status. However, it may have a role in maintaining nutritional status but further studies in homogeneous patient groups are required.

Patient acceptance

Taste and smell

Physiological stimulation of gustation and olfaction by food in healthy individuals appears primarily to be a positive influence on intake, so long as the food itself is palatable. Hence, alterations in taste and smell, which accompany advanced disease have a significant impact on the quantity and quality of nutrients. This may also be a factor in the poor acceptance and compliance with nutritional supplements.

Factors that contribute to aberrations in taste and smell are associated with treatment (chemotherapy, radiotherapy) but also and much less understood in the disease process itself[13,14]. Specific changes in primary tastes or enhanced sensory perception will influence nutrient intake, the former inducing qualitative changes the latter quantitative changes in dietary intake. Perceived changes in taste and smell reported by patients in palliative care are not uniform. Therefore, patients should be offered a range of flavours and this applies to 'normal' diet as well as supplements. This strategy may prevent the development of sensory-specific satiety[15].

Promoting dietary intake

Health-care professionals should appreciate that mealtimes can be a stressful event for patients and the family. For example, the food presented may be modified in consistency, there may be too much food on the plate; coping with symptoms such as pain and eating can all reduce intake. In addition the pressure that the informal carer can put on the patient to eat often goes unrecognized.

'My husband is doing his best he cooks my favourite foods and brings it to me on a tray. It's too much, I just can't eat it so I scoop half of it into a bag'—Cancer patient

'At first cooking was difficult; since developing Parkinson's we have radically changed what we eat'—Parkinson's patient

These issues should be explored during dietary counselling.

Attention to detail is important in encouraging dietary intake and many issues are addressed in Table 4.7.1. It is important to make sure the patient is comfortable, i.e. correctly positioned for eating, toileting facilities and the environment conducive to eating with any catheter bag covered, and the table/tray attractively presented.

Dysphagia

Patients who may develop dysphagia include those with motor neuron disease, Alzheimer's disease, progressive multiple sclerosis, and Parkinson's disease as well as cancer patients. The severity of dysphagia varies considerably. Some patients may have mild swallowing problems requiring minor food modification (texture modification). It should be remembered that the liquid content of modified diets tends to be high and acts to dilute the nutrient content, so macronutrient and micronutrient fortification is often required. Whereas others with severe dysphagia maybe unable to tolerate very little oral diet. For those patients who are unable to swallow enough to maintain hydration or nutrition, endoscopic placement of a percutaneous gastrostomy (PEG) may be considered but long-term treatment goals must be identified.

Home artificial nutrition

The majority of palliative care patients on home feeding are prescribed enteral nutrition (naso-gastric and percutaneous endoscopic gastrostomy). Implementation of home artificial nutrition support requires significant education and training of patient and/or their carer. Meticulous discharge planning, communication between care team and a structured monitoring process are key elements to making home enteral nutrition an acceptable treatment modality. The informal carer is most likely to take responsibility for maintaining patency of the feeding tube, feed administration and routine monitoring.

Prior to starting feeding or sending patients home on feeding the patient's home should be visited to assess practical issues such as:

- What storage space is available to stock feed and related consumables, i.e. giving sets?
- Can a drip stand be moved freely round the house? Steps and loose carpets may increase the patient's risk of tripping.
- Communication support issues.

Nutritional assessment

Evaluation of nutritional intervention in palliative care relies on nutritional assessment. This not only involves determination of nutrient intake (dietary and/or artificial nutritional support) a procedure generally well accepted by the patient but should also include sequential monitoring of patients' nutritional status. The latter provides information relating to the progression or attenuation of loss of body mass. Sensitivity to the patient when undertaking the assessment is paramount. If a patient is in the terminal stage of their disease or is immobile and/or severely demented a nutritional assessment may be clearly inappropriate.

Body weight

An individual's body weight can be compared with tables[16] which provide 'normal' values for individuals of the same sex, age, and height. However, consideration of recent weight loss (over past 3 months) allows an insight into the magnitude and rate of progression of weight loss. It is important to respect patient wishes in that some might not wish their weight to be monitored and of course their wishes should be respected.

Weight loss as per cent of 'usual' body weight:

$$\text{Percentage of weight loss} = \frac{\text{usual body weight (kg)} - \text{current weight} \times 100}{\text{usual body weight}}$$

This approach allows patient to provide their own reference value. An unintentional weight loss of 10 per cent in 3 months is indicative of significant weight loss and 20 per cent of protein energy undernutrition[17].

Body mass index

Another method of using weight as a nutritional parameter is to express height as a power index of weight.

$$\text{Body mass index (BMI) units (kg/m}^2) = \frac{\text{weight (kg)}}{\text{height}^2 \text{ (m)}}$$

- A BMI <20 is indicative of mild undernutrition
- A BMI <18 is indicative of moderate undernutrition
- A BMI <16 is indicative of severe undernutrition

The assessor should be aware that the presence of oedema or ascites may mask the degree of undernutrition and care in interpretation of weight data is required.

Arm anthropometry

Triceps skinfold thickness provides an indication of fat reserves. This measurement is taken using skinfold callipers at the mid-point between the acromial process and the olecranon and results are compared with standard values[18].

An indication of skeletal muscle mass may be obtained from subtracting the skinfold thickness from the mid-upper arm circumference. This technique assumes the upper arm circumference is a perfect circle.

$$\text{Arm muscle circumference} = \text{mid-upper arm circumference} - (\text{triceps skinfold} \times (\text{pi}))$$

The upper arm is easily accessible and less prone to oedema. Information on arm anthropometry should be considered with weight data.

Hand-grip dynamometry

Weakness, asthenia, and fatigue are common symptoms of palliative care patients. Whilst weight and arm anthropometry provide quantitative information relating to body mass, hand-grip dynamometry is a functional marker of mass and in end-of-life patients correlates with body weight (Fig. 4.7.1). If one aim of nutritional intervention is to improve lean body mass it is important that both the quantity and quality of this tissue increases. Hand-grip dynamometry is a non-invasive technique which involves determination of patients' maximal grip strength[19].

It should be remembered that in the presence of a systemic inflammatory response improvements in body mass are not achievable. The overriding component of nutritional management in palliative care is ensuring the wishes of the patient and

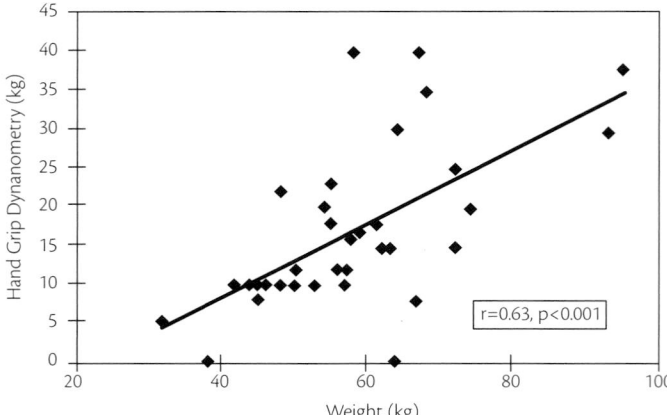

Figure 4.7.1 Association between weight and grip strength in patients in hospice.

family are fulfilled. Today patients and relatives are more informed than ever before and actively seek information relating to disease and management. This means that the boundaries of practice for health-care professionals has shifted and this is a continuous dynamic process. There is now a need for professionals to integrate their understanding of clinical science and current research to inform their practice.

References

1. Finlay, I. (2001). UK Strategies for palliative care. *Journal of the Royal Society of Medicine*, **94**, 437–41.
2. Ovensen, L. *et al.* (1993). Effect of dietary counselling on food intake, body weight, response rate, survival and quality of life in cancer patients undergoing chemotherapy: a prospective, randomised study. *Journal of Clinical Oncology,* **13**, 2043–9.
3. Evans, W.K. *et al.* (1987). A randomised study of oral nutritional support versus ad lib nutritional intake during chemotherapy for advanced colorectal and non-small cell lung cancer. *Journal of Clinical Oncology*, **5**, 113–24.
4. McCann, R., Hall, W., Groth-Juncker, A. (1994). Comfort care for terminally ill patients. The appropriate use of nutrition and hydration. *Journal American Medical Association*, **272**, 1263–6.
5. Plaisance, L. (1997). The litany of the last meal. *American Journal of Nursing*, **97**, 60–1.
6. Bruce, D., Laurance, I., McGuiness, M. *et al.* (2001). Nutritional supplements after hip fractures poor compliance effectiveness. *Clinical Nutrition*, **22**, 497–500.
7. Akner, G. and Cederholm, T. (2003). Treatment of protein-energy malnutrition in chronic non-malignant disorders. *American Journal of Clinical Nutrition*, **74**, 6–24
8. Bell, E.A., Roe, L.S., and Rolls, B.T. (2003). Sensory specific satiety is affected more by volume than energy content of a liquid food. *Physiology and Behaviour*, **78**, 593–60
9. Rolls, B.J., Kim, S., McNelis, A.L. *et al.* (1991). Time course of effects of preloads high in fat or carbohydrate on food intake and hunger ratings in humans. *American Journal of Physiology*, **260**, 756–63.
10. Richardson, R., Ferguson, M., Moses, A. *et al.* (2001). A protein and energy dense, n-3 fatty acid enriched oral nutritional supplement improves dietary intake and weight in patients with cancer cachexia. *Proceedings of the Nutrition Society*, **61**, 27a.
11. Fearon, K.C.H., Barber, M., Moses, A. *et al.* (2006). Double-blind, placebo-controlled, randomized study of eicosapentaenoic acid diester in patients with cancer cachexia. *Journal of Clinical Oncology*, **24**, 3401–7.
12. Bruera, E., Strasser, F., Palmer, J.L. *et al.* (2003). Effect of *fish oil* on appetite and other symptoms in patients with advanced cancer and anorexia/cachexia: a double-blind, placebo-controlled study. *Journal of Clinical Oncology*, **21**, 129–34.
13. Vance, D., and Burrage, J. (2006). Chemosensory declines in older adults with HIV: identifying interventions. *Journal of Gereontological Nursing*, **32**, 42–8.
14. Lennie, T.A., Moser, D.K., Heo, S. *et al.* (2006). Factors influencing food in take in patients with heart failure. *Journal of Cardiovascular Nursing*, **21**, 123–9.
15. Rolls, E.T., and Rolls, J.H. (1996). Olfactory sensory-specific satiety in humans *Physiology and Behaviour*, **61**(3), 461–73.
16. Metropolitan height and weight tables (1983). Metropolitan Life Foundation. *Statistical Bulletin*, **64**, No 1.
17. Kinney, J.M. (1988). The influence of calorie and nitrogen balance on weight loss. *British Journal of Clinical Practice*, **12**, 114–20.
18. Jelliffe, D.B. (1996). *The assessment of nutritional status in the community*. WHO Monograph, **53**, WITO, Genera.
19. Windsor, J.A., and Hill, G.L. (1988). Grip strength: a measure of the proportion of protein loss in surgical patients. *British Journal of Surgery*, **75**, 880–2.

Physiotherapy in palliative care

Diane Robinson and Anne English

Introduction (see Section 16)

Palliative care and rehabilitation both focus on the concept of helping people to maximize their potential and live as well as they can, given their circumstances. Physiotherapy is defined as 'a health-care profession concerned with human function and movement and maximizing potential'[1], and the physiotherapist's outlook is moulded by acquired knowledge of how the physical sciences (physics, hydrodynamics, biomechanics, ergonomics, and exercise science) inform the understanding and analysis of movement and function.

Physiotherapy

◆ Uses physical approaches to promote, maintain, and restore physical, psychological, and social well-being.

◆ Is science-based, committed to extending, applying, evaluating, and reviewing the evidence that underpins and informs its practice and delivery.

◆ Has the exercise of clinical judgement and informed interpretation at its core.

Physiotherapists

Physiotherapists:

◆ Have autonomy and ability to act as first-contacts, as well as accepting referrals from other health-care professionals.

◆ Through partnership and negotiation, work with people to optimize their functional ability and potential.

◆ Address problems of impairment, activity, and participation and manage recovering, stable, and deteriorating conditions.

◆ Treat a wide range of physical conditions across the life span and in patients with varying health status (both relating to physical and mental health)[1].

The physiotherapist brings to the interdisciplinary team a unique perspective, which facilitates the creation of a match between people and their activities, the environment in which they operate, and the equipment that they use.

The physiotherapist's role in palliative care

The physiotherapist's role includes:

Assessment and planning

◆ Assessment of psychological, emotional, and social needs.

◆ Assessment of physical function.

◆ Realistic, patient-centred, goal-setting.

◆ Assessment and management of disorders of communication and swallowing.

◆ Assessment of activities of daily living and support required.

◆ Assessment of home environment.

Symptom control

◆ Respiratory care.

◆ Pain management.

◆ Lymphoedema management.

Function and rehabilitation

◆ Exercise.

◆ Gait re-education and provision of walking aids.

◆ Provision of equipment to enhance function (e.g. splints, collars, wheelchairs, aids for daily living).

◆ Practising safe methods of transfer mobility.

Psychological aspects of care

◆ Retraining of cognitive and perceptual dysfunction.

◆ Relaxation training.

Prevention

◆ Assessment of pressure risk and necessary provision.

◆ Assessment of activities of daily living and support required.

Education and communication

- ◆ Education of patients, carers, students, and health-care professionals.
- ◆ Manual handling advice to professionals and carers.
- ◆ Lifestyle management.
- ◆ Advice on pacing and energy conservation.
- ◆ Liaising with other professionals and with carers.

Working alongside the patient in a one-to-one relationship provides the opportunity for the physiotherapist to explore further the patient's misconceptions and hesitantly voiced fears (e.g. because wasted muscles 'shake' on effort, does not mean that the patient has developed Parkinson's disease). The patient can be taught, using appropriate language, how their body works and helped to understand their disease processes. Understanding the physical processes involved can reduce the patient's anxiety and distress. The provision of management strategies empowers the patient to regain control over aspects of their condition, at a time when they are often experiencing helplessness and loss of independence. It is also the physiotherapist's role to equip the patient's 'significant others' to play an active part in caregiving.

Assessment and communication

Patient assessment identifies problems, enables the patient and physiotherapist to agree on realistic goals, formulate a treatment plan, and decide on appropriate outcome measures. All goals must be patient-centred, measurable, and achievable. They may be simple (e.g. 'to stand from sitting') or complex (e.g. 'to attend my grandson's Christening'). Reassessment and redefining of goals may be necessary on a daily basis as the patient's condition can alter in a short space of time.

Early referral is important to allow anticipation of problems so that coping strategies can be put in place. For example, it is preferable to prevent a hip fracture through gait training, than to treat the pain of a fracture with surgery or analgesics. However, physiotherapy is equally important in the last week or so of life if, for example, a patient's functional status can be maintained to enable that person to eat independently or to sit on the edge of the bed to use a urine bottle.

Challenging and complex problems

Patients with palliative care needs present multifactorial problems[2] associated with an increasing range of underlying pathologies in a wide range of care settings. There has recently been a welcome increase in numbers of designated specialist palliative care physiotherapists appointed to community rehabilitation teams. In all settings, the physiotherapist is involved in the treatment of patients with active and progressive conditions, which may include cancer, HIV/AIDS, neurological, cardiac, rheumatological, chronic respiratory, and endocrine diseases.

Difficult questions

Good communication skills are vitally important in this field. The physiotherapist works closely with the patient, often performing simple and sometimes repetitive tasks in a one-to-one, non-threatening situation. Time is made available to listen sensitively. In such circumstances, the patient may voice the question they have been struggling with for sometime, e.g. 'I'm not going to get home, am I?'[3] Thus the physiotherapist needs to be an informed member of the interdisciplinary team with the knowledge and skill to make the appropriate honest response in each individual situation. A discussion of ways in which to respond to such questions and some guidance is given elsewhere in this textbook.

Patients with respiratory problems

Dyspnoea

Breathlessness is a common problem in patients, experienced by 50–70 per cent of those admitted to palliative care units[2] and the physiotherapist is frequently involved in their management. Breathlessness is often a difficult symptom to deal with, and successful treatment requires an approach, based on the best available evidence, being able to modify physiotherapy techniques and take a holistic and problem-solving approach to patient care. In palliative care, the skill is in knowing when not to treat, as patients present frequently with complex and challenging symptoms.

Restrictive disorders, for example, primary and secondary lung cancers, mesothelioma, interstitial lung disease, HIV, AIDS, and neuromuscular diseases are characterized by reduced lung volume, poor compliance, and increased work of breathing. Obstructive disorders, for example, chronic obstructive pulmonary disease (COPD), bronchiectasis, and cystic fibrosis, cause increased work of breathing and airflow resistance[4].

Breathlessness is a frightening and unpleasant sensation experienced by many patients with various diagnoses. The effectiveness of breathlessness clinics for treatment of lung cancer, using a combination of physiotherapy techniques, is well documented[5,6]. These techniques include breathing control, positioning, anxiety management, pacing (controlling breathing while walking or climbing stairs), and prioritizing (choosing the most important activities that need to be done), relaxation, and education. Interventions can be used in any setting, giving the patient a choice of venue. Auscultation, pulse oximetry, a thorough history of the patient's medication, including inhalers, nebulizers, and the use of oxygen, are all important. It is essential to allow the patient time to give a history and to answer questions. Patients may be too breathless to speak for long periods, and therefore it may be necessary to assess over several visits. Breathless patients automatically adopt positions that ease their breathing. Some examples are sitting upright in a chair, forward lean sitting (i.e. sitting with feet on the floor, leaning forward from the hips with the upper chest and head supported on pillows piled on a table) and high side lying (i.e. lying on the side with knees slightly bent, rolled slightly forward, using 3–4 pillows to raise the shoulders, one pillow to fill the gap between the axilla and waist, the top pillow to support the head and neck). Efficacy of breathing is poorest in supine and slumped sitting or lying positions frequently assumed by patients in hospital beds[4]. Simple position changes can reduce the work of breathing and the sensation of breathlessness. Breathing control aims to increase lung volume, the focus being on diaphragmatic breathing (Fig. 4.8.1) and facilitating shoulder girdle and upper-chest relaxation.

Depth of breathing is gradually increased as the patient becomes more proficient. Different methods of relaxation are well documented and have been shown to reduce heart rate, respiratory rate, and blood pressure[7]. Regular practice enables the patient to recall the technique and recreate the feeling of relaxation.

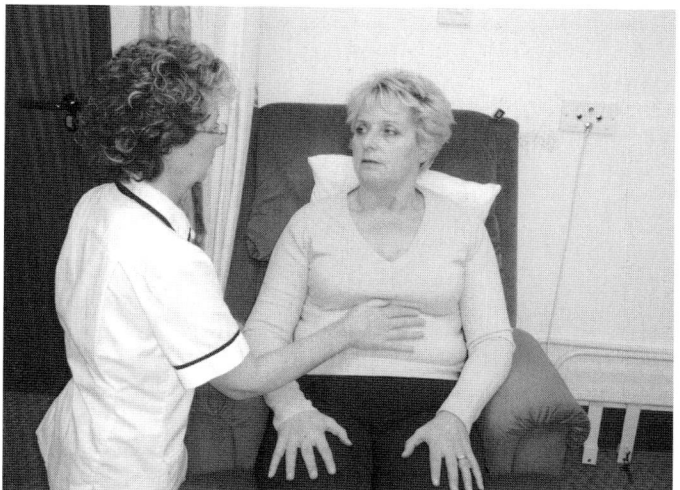

Figure 4.8.1 Diaphragmatic breathing.

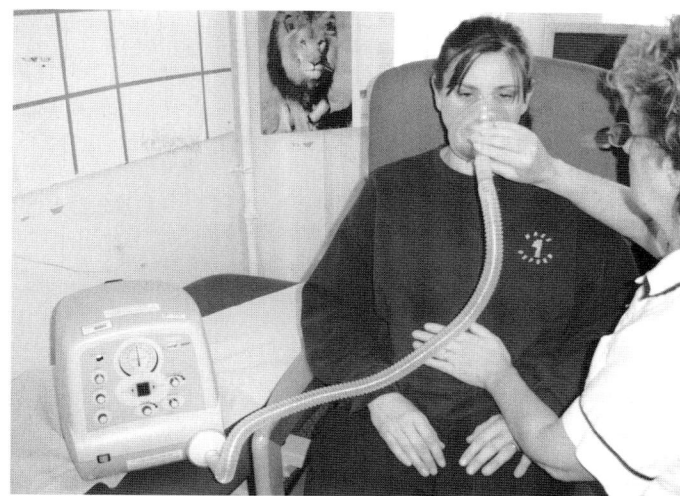

Figure 4.8.2 Using the 'cough assist'.

Pursed-lip breathing is often helpful to the breathless patient as it maintains positive pressure during expiration, stenting the smaller airways. One disadvantage is that the work of breathing is increased and may tire the patient.

Management of respiratory secretions

Traditional physiotherapy techniques (e.g. clapping, shaking, and vibrations) are used with caution in palliative care, mainly with patients with COPD and heart failure. For patients with osteoporosis, bone metastases and haemoptysis, for example, these interventions could cause damage and would be contraindicated[8]. Active cycle of breathing, forced expiratory technique ('huffing'), assisted cough, and positioning are used on a regular basis by physiotherapists. Active cycle of breathing consists of deep breathing, relaxed breathing, and 'huffing', which may mobilize secretions from the distal airways, facilitating expectoration[4]. Adequate humidification and hydration is essential to encourage secretion clearance. Postural drainage (use of gravity to assist secretion clearance), may have to be modified as certain positions may distress the patient.

The use of respiratory suction, especially at the end of life, is a controversial subject[4,9]. Suction should always be carried out with extreme caution, using a soft catheter[9] and causing as little distress as possible to the patient. Alternatives may include regular positional changes and mouth care. Relatives at the bedside may find the end stage of life distressing, and the physiotherapist must be mindful of ethical implications of treatment before deciding on the most appropriate management.

Cough

In patients with neuromuscular disorders (e.g. motor neuron disease—MND), clearance of secretions is hindered by weak inspiratory muscles and inability of the patient to cough. The cough assist (Fig. 4.8.2) or mechanical in-exsufflator assists sputum clearance by the use of both positive and negative pressure. Gradual application of positive pressure to the airways is quickly changed to a negative pressure. This pressure change produces a high expiratory flow rate and stimulates a cough[10].

Physiotherapy techniques combined with this, enable secretions to come into the mouth and be wiped or suctioned away.

Non-invasive positive pressure ventilation (NIPPV) is being used more often in patients with neuromuscular disorders and evidence shows it may prolong life[11]. Patients with COPD may also benefit from domiciliary NIPPV[12].

Anxiety management

Anxiety and emotions are closely associated with breathlessness and impact negatively on a wide range of other symptoms. The physiotherapist should give the patient opportunity to express their fears and worries. Distraction techniques, the use of a handheld fan[13], and a Calming Hand[14] may help to reduce feelings of panic and breathlessness (Fig. 4.8.3).

This uses the patient's hand as an aide memoire to remember the main points of a taught technique for the control of breathlessness,

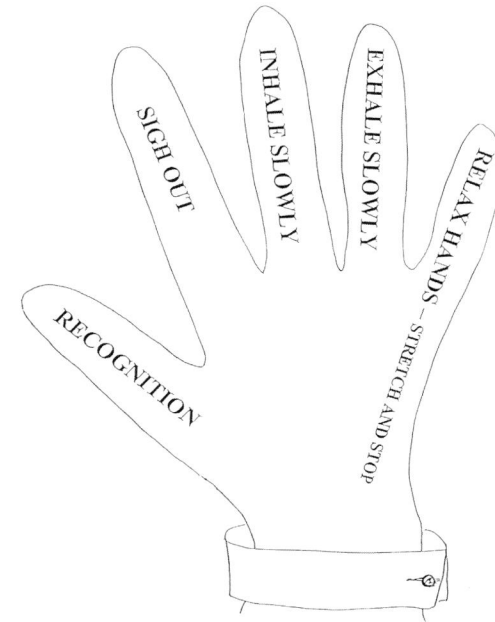

Figure 4.8.3 The calming/panic hand. *Source*: Marjorie Coulthard Dorothy House Hospice Care (1999). Adapted from anonymous.

which begins with recognition of the signs of breathlessness/panic and the need to put learned strategies into practice.

Cardiac failure

Cardiac failure is becoming more prevalent as people live longer[15], and breathlessness is one of the early symptoms patients experience[16]. Patients often demonstrate more impairment, both physically and socially, compared to other chronic conditions, and are often more interested in changes in physical symptoms, emotional states, and social roles, than what is objectively changing within their heart[17]. Palliative care plays an important role in improving the quality of life of patients with heart failure[18], and therefore presents a challenge to physiotherapists to develop future services for these patients. Interventions may include combinations of aerobic or resistive exercise[18], breathing techniques, anxiety and fatigue management, and advice on lifestyle changes.

Practical help in minimizing disability, impact on daily life, and provision of aids and equipment have been identified as a prime need of people living with heart failure[19].

Patients with neurological problems

Patients may present with a wide range of different conditions, such as spinal cord compression (SCC), peripheral neuropathies, and cerebral tumours. Patients with long-term neurological conditions (Multiple sclerosis [MS], Parkinson's disease, MND, and muscular dystrophies) also come under the palliative care umbrella, and recent guidance emphasizes the importance of controlling symptoms and offering social, psychological, and spiritual support[20]. These patients may have similar symptoms to cancer patients but, due to longer illness trajectories and slower disease progression, will experience these symptoms over a greater period of time.

Physiotherapists have a wide knowledge base and expertise in movement analysis and functional assessment, enabling them to develop individual treatment plans and agree with the patient the most appropriate interventions.

Active assisted exercises and passive movements are helpful in maintaining joint range, preventing muscle shortening and contractures, and reducing spasticity and pain. Patients are encouraged to maintain good posture when sitting and mobilizing. The physiotherapist assists with normal movement patterns, balance, gait analysis, and movement control. Training is given in use of appropriate mobility aids and often the use of a tilt-table is helpful to enable standing where this ability has been lost. The tilt-table is a sophisticated standing frame which allows the patient, lying upon and securely strapped to the horizontal surface, to be rotated through 90° to the erect position (Fig. 4.8.3).

The benefits of standing include: improved ventilation, digestion, bowel and bladder function[21], and most importantly, psychological benefits.

Introduction of a wheelchair may be difficult for the patient to accept as it represents changes in lifestyle and dependency. Instructions given to the patient and carer must be clear and supported by written information. This should include advice on transfers into, rising from, and sitting in the wheelchair, and maintenance of cushions, and safety for both patient and carer when manoeuvring the chair.

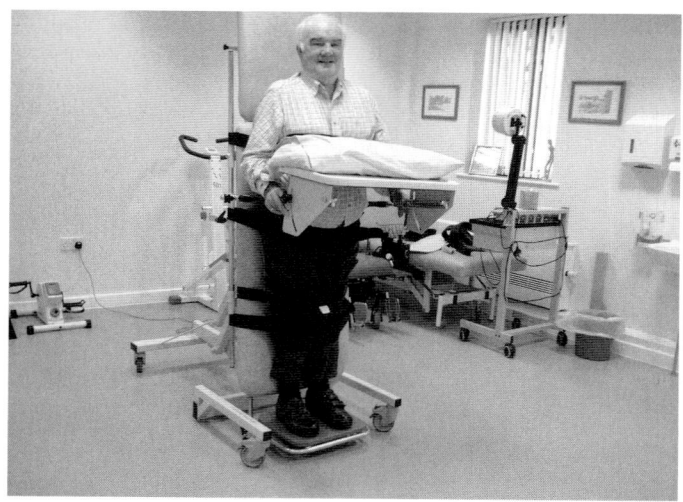

Figure 4.8.4 The tilt-table.

Spinal cord compression

Bone metastases can occur with many different types of cancer. Long bones and the spinal column are particularly vulnerable. Patients are at risk of pathological fractures which, if they occur, lead to instability. The physiotherapist is often ideally placed to note the early signs of SCC and alert the team concerned with the management of this oncological emergency. SCC occurs in 3 per cent of patients with advanced cancer, and cancers of breast, bronchus, and prostate account for 40 per cent of this number. Most others are associated with renal cell cancer, lymphoma, myeloma, melanoma, sarcoma, and cancers of the head and neck[22].

Surgery may be indicated to maintain spinal function and stability, allow weight bearing and improve quality of life[23]. The physiotherapist will be involved in respiratory care and rehabilitation both pre- and post-surgery. If SCC occurs, it results in loss of varying degrees of motor, sensory, and autonomic function below the level of compression. The patient will need help and support in adapting to a drastic reduction in functional ability and in developing future coping strategies. This may involve balance training, development of upper-body strength, instruction in transfers and use of a wheelchair. Relatives and carers will also require instruction in passive movements and positioning of limbs, use of wheelchairs, and in moving and handling techniques. Provision of braces, splints, and walking aids may enable the patient to be as independent and comfortable as possible. Interdisciplinary team communication is important as there may be difficulties in determining a patient's level of activity, and how much pain they experience. The physiotherapist, with specialist knowledge in non-pharmacological pain management, will have a central role in advising the team.

Fatigue

The many complex symptoms of the patient may lead to inactivity or to spending long periods in bed. Over-anxious carers may encourage 'PIP' (pyjama-induced paralysis), encouraging the patient to 'rest' in bed or chair. This immobility can lead to cardiovascular and muscular deconditioning[24]. Circulatory changes due to inactivity may lead to the development of deep vein thrombosis.

The effects of cancer-related fatigue are well documented, affecting between 70–100 per cent of patients[25]. Fatigue is the most common and stressful symptom experienced by patients, and will impact greatly on quality of life[2,25]. It is described by many patients as an overwhelming tiredness, which is not relieved by rest[25]. Psychological components include anxiety, depression, and loss of self-esteem and fatigue may continue for years after completion of cancer treatment. Current evidence favours individualized exercise programmes as an effective intervention for the management of cancer-related fatigue. Programmes should be of low or moderate intensity, aerobic, and progressive (three or more times per week)[25]. Education by the physiotherapist enables patients to understand their fatigue, and explain the symptom to family and friends who often have difficulty understanding why the patient feels constantly tired.

Exercise

Exercise is known to have many physiological and psychological benefits[2] and is a well-established intervention in palliative care. Exercise may be individual or group, must be safe, have known benefits, and take into account the patient's age, condition, past medical history, and nutritional status. Exercise can be incorporated into daily life and be practised in any environment. Positive effects include improvement in muscle strength, balance, endurance, joint range, functional capacity, and reduction in anxiety and depression. Patients presenting with conditions such as anaemia, bone metastases, respiratory insufficiency, and musculoskeletal problems must be carefully assessed, as exercise may be contraindicated.

Pain

Total pain encompasses the physical, psychological, social, and spiritual aspects of suffering[22], and the physiotherapist has a role in assessing and managing all facets of pain. Pain avoidance is an important part of pain management. Appropriate positioning of patients helps reduce stress on weakened joints and muscles and prevent development of pressure ulcers. Fracture sites, weakened muscles, and deformities may be immobilized and braced by provision of splints, collars, and various supports. This permits comfortable movement during nursing procedures and facilitates activities of daily living. Chronic pain may arise where there is no injury and no healing. This causes the patient to avoid certain activities and movements, resulting in stiff joints and muscles, eventually shortening muscle groups and causing joint contractures. This in turn increases pain.

Gentle and regular exercise is thus an important factor in managing pain. Massage and exercise-therapy are core skills of physiotherapists. Touch is probably the oldest method of relieving pain and discomfort. Therapeutic massage using stroking (effleurage) and gentle kneading (petrissage) may be used to reduce muscle spasm, relieve pain, and aid relaxation. Maintenance of joint range is important in the management of pain.

Bone pain and neuropathic pain are two of the most difficult pains to manage but relief may be obtained by the use of

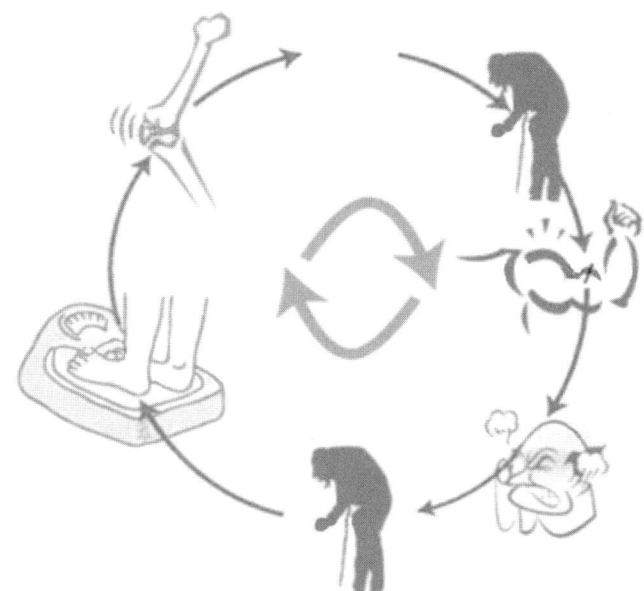

Figure 4.8.5 The pain cycle. © Napp Pharmaceuticals. Used with permission.

transcutaneous electrical nerve stimulation (TENS). TENS is the only electrical modality currently recommended for use in the presence of active neoplastic disease[26]. Used over normal tissue, and for non-cancer patients, therapeutic ultrasound, interferential or pulsed shortwave diathermy may relieve pain and muscle spasm. Where skin sensation is normal, local applications of heat and ice may also be used for pain relief.

Nausea, loss of appetite, and constipation

TENs and acupuncture may be used to relieve nausea using the Neiguan antiemetic acupuncture point[27]. These modalities are further discussed in Section 10. It has been demonstrated that patients receiving regular physiotherapy of more than 10 min daily, experience a significant reduction in appetite disturbance[28].

Evidence also suggests that there is an increased risk of constipation in people walking less than 0.5 km daily and a squatting position has been shown to facilitate efficient funnelling of the pelvic floor favouring defaecation[29]. This can be simulated by provision of a simple step on which to rest the feet, when the patient is seated on the toilet or commode. This intervention, raising knees above the level of the hips, combined with relaxed deep breathing and a gentle rocking motion may help ease the process of bowel evacuation and relieve constipation.

Chronic oedema (see Section 10)

Physiotherapy skills contribute to the team management of lymphoedema, and physiotherapists may choose to train to graduate diploma level in the management of this distressing symptom. A swollen limb is a heavy limb, placing stresses on weakened muscles and joints, affecting both posture and mobility. Gravitational oedema may develop in an immobile, dependent limb. Failure of the muscle pump will reduce venous return and increase the load on a struggling, one-way, lymphatic drainage system.

Self-management, using the four cornerstones of lymphoedema treatment:

- meticulous skin-care;
- exercise and movement (including advice on positioning and muscle work to avoid);
- compression, either in the form of hosiery, specialized garments or bandaging; and
- a modified massage technique which encourages lymph drainage.

is taught to patients and/or carers[30]. This may offer the patient some degree of control but they must be empowered to accept such control. In advanced disease, bandaging is used to control lymphorrhoea and to support the affected tissues.

Lymphoedema management includes breathing exercises. Inspiration has a major effect on thoracic lymphatic drainage and sudden increases in intra-abdominal pressure, e.g. coughing, sighing, and laughing will greatly increase abdominal drainage and empty the cisterna chyli[31].

Conclusions

Physiotherapists require a level of palliative care competency relevant to the requirements of their posts[2]. Many work as sole practitioners and need to bring to the post a broad range of knowledge, skill, and experience, and be given supervision, which includes peer support, plus ample opportunities for continuing professional development. Membership of the Association of Chartered Physiotherapists in Oncology and Palliative Care is recommended. Physiotherapists working in this speciality may choose to extend their practice to include other skills, e.g. counselling, acupuncture, hydrotherapy, reflex therapy, and there are increasing opportunities for post-graduate palliative care education. Undergraduate education in this field, however, remains patchy, but anecdotal evidence suggests that physiotherapy students on palliative care placements have benefited because of the range of skills, teamworking experience and holistic patient management demonstrated. This experience can be transferred to a wide range of physiotherapy specialities and settings.

Time is an important factor in palliative care. A recent study has shown that palliative patients receiving prompt physiotherapy referral and considerably more than 10 minutes of physiotherapy contact time per day were more likely to be discharged home, to achieve higher functional scores, and to die at home, than a control group receiving 'standard' physiotherapy (less than 10 minutes per day). This paper recommends a physiotherapy staff to patient ratio of 1:12[28].

The need for research remains. However, there is already a significant body of evidence to support the unique contribution of the physiotherapist to the management of palliative care patients, as an essential member of the interdisciplinary team[2].

References

1. Chartered Society of Physiotherapy. (2002). *Curriculum framework for qualifying programmes in physiotherapy*. CSP, London.
2. The Allied Health Professions Palliative Care Project Team. (2004). *Allied Health Professional Services for cancer related palliative care: An Assessment of Need* www.palliativecareglasgow.info/pdf/AHPreport.pdf
3. Crook, K. (2004). Responding to difficult questions *Journal of the Association of Chartered Physiotherapists in Women's Health*, **94**, 39–41.
4. Hough, A. (2001), *Physiotherapy in Respiratory Care, An Evidence based approach to respiratory and cardiac management*, 3rd edition. Nelson Thornes, United Kingdom.
5. NICE (2005). *The Diagnosis and Treatment of Lung Cancer*, NICE, London.
6. Hateley, J., Laurence, V., Scott, A. *et al.* (2003). Breathlessness clinics within specialist palliative care settings can improve quality of life and functioning in patients with lung cancer. *Palliative Medicine*, **17**, 410–17.
7. Salt, V.L. and Kerr, K.M. (1997). Mitchell's simple physiological relaxation and jacobson's progressive relaxation techniques: a comparison. *Physiotherapy*, **83**, 4.
8. Pryor, J.A, and Webber, B.A. (1998). *Physiotherapy for Respiratory and Cardiac Problems*, 2nd edition. Churchill Livingstone, Edinburgh.
9. Watts, T., Jenkins, K., and Back, I. (1997). Problem and management of noisy, rattling breathing in dying patients. *International Journal of Nursing*, **3**(5), 245–52.
10. Whitney, J., Harden, B., Keilty, S. (2002). Assisted cough, a new technique. *Physiotherapy*, **88**(4), 201–7.
11. Turkington, P.M. and Elliot, M.W. (2000). Rationale for the use of non invasive ventilation in chronic ventilatory failure. *Thorax*, **55**, 417–22.
12. Cuvelier, A. and Muir, J.F. (2001). Non-invasive ventilation and obstructive lung diseases. *European Respiratory Journal*, **17**(6), 1271–81.
13. Schwartstein, R.M., Lahive, K., Pope, A., Weinberger, S. *et al.* (1987). Cold facial stimulation reduces breathlessness induced in normal subjects. *American Review of Respiratory Diseases*, **136**(1), 58–61.
14. Burnett, J. and Blagbrough, M. (2007). *Breathlessness Management Toolbox*, Dorothy House Hospice Care.
15. McMurray, J. and Stewart, S. (2000). Epidemiology, aetiology, and prognosis of heart failure *Heart*, **83**(5), 596–602.
16. Nicholas, M. (2004). Heart failure: pathophysiology, treatment and nursing care. *Nursing Standard*, **19**(11), 46–51.
17. Hobbs, F.D.R., Kenkre, J.E., Roalfe, A.K. *et al.* (2002). Impact of heart failure and left ventricular systolic dysfunction on quality of life: a cross-sectional study comparing common chronic cardiac and medical disorders and a representative adult population. *European Heart Journal*, **23**, 1867–76.
18. National Institute of Clinical Excellence(NICE) (2003). *Chronic Heart Failure, Management of chronic heart failure in adults in primary and secondary care, Clinical Guideline 5*. NICE, London.
19. Boyd, K.J., Murray, S.A., Kendall, M. *et al.* (2004). Living with heart Failure: a prospective, community based study of patients and their carers. *European Journal of Heart Failure*, **6**(5), 585–91.
20. Department of Health, (2005). *National Service Framework for Long Term Conditions*. Department of Health, London.
21. Sainsby, K. and Thornton, H. (1999). Justifying the provision of a standing frame for home use – a good case to quote. *Journal and Newsletter of the Association of Chartered Physiotherapists interested in Neurology*, Spring (ACPIN).
22. Twycross, R. (1997). *Symptom Management in Advanced Cancer*, 2nd Edition. Radcliffe Press, Oxon.
23. Al-Hakim, W.I., Jagiello, J.M., Mannan, K. *et al.* (2006). The palliative role of orthopaedics. *British Medical Journal*, **332**(7552), 1227–8.
24. Packel, L., Claghorn, K.V.B., and Dekerlegand, J. (2006).Cancer related fatigue and deconditioning: a programme evaluation. *Rehabilitation Oncology*, **24**(2), 3–6.
25. Watson, T. and Mock, V.(2004). Exercise as an intervention for cancer related fatigue. *Physical Therapy*, **84**(8), 736–43.

26. Joliffe, J. and Bury, T. (2002). *The Effectiveness of physiotherapy in the palliative care of older people*. CSP, London.
27. McMillan, C.M. and Dundee, J.W. (1991). The role of transcutaneous electricalstimulation of Neiguan anti-emetic acupuncture point in controlling sickness after cancer chemotherapy. *Physiotherapy, 77*(7), 499–502.
28. Laakso, E.L., McAuliffe, A.J., and Cantlay, A. (2003). The impact of physiotherapy intervention on functional independence and quality of life in palliative patients. *Cancer Forum,* **27**(1), 15–20.

29. Kyle, G. (2007). Constipation and palliative care – where are we now? *International Journal of Palliative Nursing,* **13** (1), 6–15.
30. Mortimer, P. and Todd, J. (2007). *Lymphoedema Advice on self-management and treatment,* 3rd Edition. Beaconsfield Publishers Ltd., Bucks.
31. Twycross, R., Jenns, K., and Todd, J. (eds.). (2000). *Lymphoedema* Radcliffe Press, Oxon.

The contribution of speech and language therapy to palliative medicine

Alison MacDonald and Linda Armstrong

Introduction

This chapter will address the problems of people with impaired communication and/or related oral and pharyngeal stage swallowing difficulties (dysphagia and saliva control), and will focus on a description of the role in their care of the speech and language therapist.

Speech and language therapists assess and treat both communication and swallowing difficulties. Palliative care would not usually be considered as a routine care-group within acute hospitals or community-based speech and language therapy services, however, the speech and language therapist can make a valuable contribution within multi-disciplinary care of people with terminal illness, whether that is a result of, for example, head and neck cancer or progressive neurological disease[1].

General weakness, fatigue, and the effects of drugs may cause a range of communication and swallowing difficulties for many patients in palliative care, for example, reduced breath control, mobility of the speech musculature, memory, attention, and word recall. An altered level of consciousness will clearly affect a person's ability to communicate effectively. Indeed, significant speech and language deviations in a study of 12 hospice patients with cancer have been recorded[2]. It is also recognized that radiation therapy to the head and neck area may lead to transient voice changes[3]. There are, however, a significant number of terminally ill patients who, as part of their condition, will have specific speech, language, and/or swallowing difficulties. A retrospective study of hospice records identified communication disorders in 27 per cent of a group of 335 patients[4]. Several of these patients had speech production difficulties as a direct consequence of the physical symptoms of their disease, while others showed language or cognitive changes arising from their neurological deterioration. In Hunt and Burne's study, 31 per cent of the children had difficulty in swallowing their saliva and 27 per cent were tube-fed as a result of swallowing difficulty[5].

The principles of speech and language therapy intervention

The Royal College of Speech and Language Therapists' service delivery standards[6] suggest the following principles for individuals with life-threatening disease:

- A responsive and flexible service, to ensure that individuals can access them where and when required, without undue delay.
- Assessment only as required to provide the answers to plan management.
- Minimum intervention for maximum gain.
- Maintenance of function where possible. Improvement of function if appropriate and realistic.
- Utilization of compensatory strategies, diet modifications, and safe swallow strategies.
- Work as a member of the multi-disciplinary team.
- Provision of holistic, individual-centered care.
- Facilitation of communication between the individual and the team.
- Provision of education and information.
- Advice on risk-benefit evaluation.

Communication disorders

There are many ways in which communication may be affected and it is important to recognize that difficulties in the use of language as well as in speech production may be evident within the one person, that is, there may be linguistic and/or motor elements contributing to communication problems.

Speech production and voice

Impairment in motor functioning may affect speech intelligibility by reducing control at different levels of the vocal tract, that is, respiratory, laryngeal, velo-pharyngeal, and oral mechanisms. The causes may be local, as in the case of oral or laryngeal cancer, or neurological in origin (dysarthria). The ability to articulate clearly may be affected by anatomical alterations caused by surgical excision or malignant growth, but also by neuro-motor impairment of function of the lips, tongue, jaw, or velum. Reduced or asynchronous velo-pharyngeal closure will cause abnormalities in nasal resonance. Disturbance to the nerve supply to, or restricted movement of the vocal cords will affect the ability to produce a normal voice quality, resulting in whispery, gravelly, or overloud voice and possibly in abnormal pitch. Altered airstream pathways, as in tracheostomy or laryngectomy, will result in a complete absence of voice (aphonia). Rhythm and rate may also be affected in some conditions, particularly those of basal ganglia or cerebellar origin, for example, Parkinson's disease, Friedreich's ataxia.

Language

Impairment in the ability to use language effectively (aphasia or dysphasia) takes many forms depending on the site of the brain damage and on the level(s) of linguistic processing that has been affected. The ability to follow spoken language or to interpret written material, the ability to recall words, to formulate grammatical sentences, to pronounce words or to spell, may be affected separately or in combination and to a varying extent, producing mild to severe impairments. Aphasia is most commonly associated with cerebrovascular accident. However, it may equally arise from space occupying lesions or traumatic brain injury. A subtle decline in language use may also be evident in some deteriorating conditions, particularly in the later stages, for example, Parkinson's disease and Huntington's disease[7]. Cognitive deterioration or confusional states may also affect the effective use of language. Short-term memory deficit and disorientation can, for example, significantly reduce a person's ability to participate in conversations or to make informed choices.

Children with deteriorating conditions may have particular communication difficulties depending on the time of onset of their condition. For example, in Hunt and Burne's cohort of 127 children with neurodegenerative diseases, nearly all the children had impaired or no speech[5]. Where onset has been in infancy the child may have had difficulty in developing language. Such children may be taught some basic manual signs or picture symbols with which to communicate (see also the section on 'Augmentative and alternative communication').

Table 4.9.1 summarizes the effects that different medical diagnoses can have on communication, cognition, access to communication aids, and swallowing.

Non-verbal communication

The extent to which we rely on non-verbal signals (e.g. facial expression, body movements, or gesture) to support our spoken output is not often fully recognized. The patient who is seriously ill, weak, or in pain, may find these non-verbal signals difficult to produce; and the person with severe motor impairment, particularly if this affects the facial muscles, may unintentionally give signals that are misinterpreted. It may, therefore, be important for the speech and language therapist to discuss this with the patient and his/her family and to look at possible options for circumventing this potential breakdown in communication.

For others, where verbal communication is reduced through aphasia or cognitive changes, the non-verbal channel can provide an alternative and effective main mode of both message-receiving and giving. The suggestions that follow (for the person with severe dementia) can be used as a model for other patients who present with severe linguistic difficulty in terminal illness, and serve to demonstrate ways in which some degree of interpersonal communication can be preserved through non-verbal channels:

- maintain social communication (helps to maintain dignity);
- keep talking (some of the non-verbal aspects may be understood);
- use touch judiciously;
- use non-verbal communication (gestures, pictures, etc.);
- assume the person understands;
- look for signs of comfort or discomfort;
- encourage attempts to communicate; and
- provide other types of stimulation[13].

The speech and language therapist's role in the management of communication impairment

A model of care to describe in outline the pathway of a patient (child or adult, with whatever pathology) through an episode of care with speech and language therapy is shown in Fig. 4.9.1.

Timely referral

Timely referral will allow the speech and language therapist to carry out baseline assessments and monitor changes in language use and to advise other staff and relatives on how to facilitate communication. It may be necessary to alert staff and relatives to changes in verbal comprehension and to suggest ways of simplifying language input.

In the early stages of their illness, people may have difficulty in accepting or even in being aware of their speech deterioration so that referral to a speech and language therapist may be postponed. While it is important to be sensitive to each individual's level of acceptance of their illness, delayed referral unfortunately means that, particularly where cognitive changes are taking place, the ability to adapt and learn new techniques may become progressively more difficult. If compensatory strategies can be introduced or a communication aid explained and training given while the person is still able to cope with new learning, then their ability to use this effectively may be greatly extended. In a study of the use of augmentative and alternative communication (AAC) by people with Parkinson's disease speech and language therapists, patients and carers agree that earlier referral would be beneficial[35].

Communication impairment of sudden onset

Voice loss, speech, and/or language breakdown may be of sudden onset following a cerebrovascular accident or surgery. Where this

Table 4.9.1 Communication and swallowing problems associated with various medical diagnoses

Medical diagnosis	Communication difficulties	Communication aids/AAC	Swallowing difficulties	Sources
Degenerative neurological conditions				
MND/ALS	Spastic and/or flaccid dysarthria: first signs often early	Need to adapt rapidly to deterioration: VOCA (keyboard → switch) → eye/body movements; yes/no system	Often early, rate of deterioration linked to speech deterioration	(7,8)
Parkinson's disease	Hypokinetic dysarthria: weak voice, imprecise articulation, monotone, possible language processing deficits	Pacing board → first letter cueing → VOCA (introduce before cognitive changes affect learning)	Variable onset, often in later stages, tongue pumping and inefficient peristalsis	(7–10)
Huntington's disease	Hyperkinetic dysarthria, onset variable, language comprehension affected by cognitive deterioration, reduced output	Cognitive deterioration may affect usefulness of AAC: large display; phrases; memory aids; yes/no system	Variable onset—oral stage co-ordination problems prominent	(7)
Multiple sclerosis	Mixed spastic/ataxic dysarthria, may be mild, impaired control of loudness, and harsh voice quality	Less frequently required	Variable, not common, possible medication side-effects, e.g. dry mouth	(7,8)
Dementias				
Alzheimer's disease	Speech production and grammar usually spared until later in the disease, meaning and interpersonal aspects of communication affected earlier	Difficult to implement because of short-term term memory deficit but improvements have been documented	Memory-related eating problems (e.g. forgetting to swallow or how to use utensils), oral, and pharyngeal stage changes	(11–16)
Vascular dementia	Depends on location of infarcts, may include dysarthria, and dysphasia	Difficult to implement because of short-term memory deficit	Depends on location of infarcts, may have oral and pharyngeal problems at any stage of the illness	(11,17)
Pick's disease	Increasing dysphasia, often with eventual mutism	May be possible in the early stage in the light of relatively intact memory and other cognitive abilities	No known literature but may have eating problems related to reduced judgement, e.g. putting too much food in at once	(17,18)
(v)CJD	Often rapid deterioration in speech and language functioning	Difficult to implement because of rapid change and cognitive problems	Can present at oral and/or pharyngeal stage	(12,17,19)
Lewy body dementia	Variability with fluctuations in cognition, communication affected by hallucinations, dysarthria possible (as yet little available literature)	Fluctuating ability would affect AAC implementation	No known literature, but likely to be affected by altered consciousness, memory difficulties and concomitant parkinsonism if present	(18,20,21)
Other neurological conditions				
Acute confusion	Dysarthria, dysgraphia and some naming errors as well as confabulation and perseveration may be present	Not strongly indicated because of fluctuating cognitive status and short time-span for training	Swallowing may be affected by reduced attention	(17,22)
Brain tumour	Language impairment usually relatively mild in cerebral tumour compared to post-stroke, anomia common. Varies with tumour type and location	No known research literature	Oral and/or pharyngeal problems dependent on cranial nerves affected	(8,23)
Stroke	Dysarthria, dyspraxia, and/or dysphasia	Effectiveness influenced by language comprehension and reading ability. Communication book: photographs, pictures, personal word lists/topics; and VOCA	Oral and/or pharyngeal problems common especially early post-onset	(24,25)

(continued)

Table 4.9.1 (Continued) Communication and swallowing problems associated with various medical diagnoses

Medical diagnosis	Communication difficulties	Communication aids/AAC	Swallowing difficulties	Sources
HIV and AIDS	Wide range of problems documented, either primary or secondary: voice disorder, interaction problems, dysarthria, dyspraxia, dysphasia. In children, language development can be negatively affected	May provide useful communication support—little evidence in this area as yet	Problems result from AIDS dementia complex	(26–29)
Head and neck surgery				
Laryngectomy	Aphonia: no voice	Electrolarynx; writing; and VOCA	Occasional pharyngeal/oesophogeal stricture; aspiration following hemi-laryngectomy or supraglottal laryngectomy	(30,31)
Tracheostomy; ventilator dependent patient; paralysed vocal cords	Aphonia: no voice	Tracheostomy tube with speaking valve; talking tracheostomy tube; writing; VOCA; and yes/no system	Possibility of compromise due to restricted laryngeal elevation or cuff inflation.	(30,32)
Oropharyngeal tumours glossectomy	Restricted articulation	Writing or gesture supplement if necessary	Restricted tongue, jaw, lip movement; pharyngeal inefficiency, or obstruction	(8, 31, 33, 34)

Key: AAC, augmentative and alternative communication; VOCA, voice output communication aid

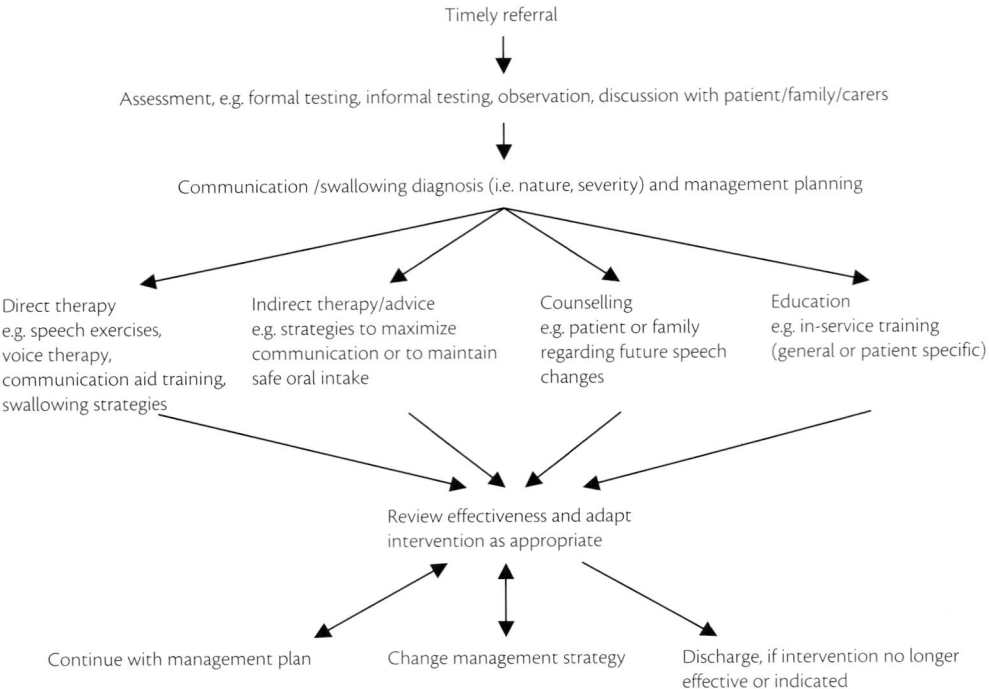

Figure 4.9.1 A model of care for speech and language therapy

can be anticipated, for example, following laryngectomy, it is good clinical practice that the speech and language therapist is called in before the event takes place[36]. This allows support to be offered to both the patient and relatives, questions to be answered, communication strategies planned, and also allows the speech and language therapist to assess the level of preoperative communication. Those who receive instruction on the use of a communication board prior to mechanical ventilation, score higher on patient satisfaction ratings than those whose communication support was unplanned.[25]

Deteriorating communication

The speech and language therapist's contribution to the support of the patient with a progressive disease may initially be for assessment and counselling only. The patient and their relatives may wish to discuss early speech changes that they notice and to consider the implications of further deterioration (see the stages described below). It may be important for the speech and language therapist to carry out baseline assessments and to monitor change. Exercises to facilitate breath control, voice use, articulatory precision, and to reduce alterations to nasal resonance may be effective in the early stages. Compensatory speech techniques may help to maximize intelligibility as speech becomes less clear. The speech and language therapist may also be able to discuss and introduce augmentative back-up in a gradual and acceptable way as speech continues to deteriorate. Augmentative and alternative communication is described more fully later.

The rate of deterioration in speech production in diseases such as MND, Parkinson's disease, Friedreich's ataxia, or Huntington's disease is variable and in some cases may fluctuate.

The type of support given by the speech and language therapist will be influenced by the stage in the progression of speech production difficulties[37].

Stage 1: no detectable speech disorder. No alterations in speech production are noted.

Stage 2: obvious speech disorder with intelligible speech. Some signs of speech deterioration are evident, particularly when the person is tired or stressed. Mild slurring or alterations in voice quality, intonation, loudness, and speech breathing coordination may be noted. Speech is intelligible but compensations may include slowing rate, careful articulation, etc. Amplifiers may be useful in cases of reduced loudness, for example, associated with Parkinson's disease.

Stage 3: reduction in speech intelligibility. Articulation, rate, and resonance are impaired and speech may be difficult to understand. Strategies to increase intelligibility need to be developed. Some people may begin to require back up to speech, for example, pointing to key words, topic headings, or initial letters on a board, or the use of a pacing board to regulate speaking rate.

Stage 4: natural speech supplemented with augmentative communication. Only highly predictable messages, for example, greetings or expected responses to questions are understood. Speech may be supplemented by writing/typing messages on a communication aid or spelling out words on a letter board.

Stage 5: no useful speech. Some individuals may be able to vocalize to indicate emotional expression and 'yes' or 'no' but speech cannot be understood. Support may include establishing eye-gaze systems, yes/no signals, memory aids, and more elaborate communication systems where appropriate (see the following section).

Augmentative and alternative communication (AAC)

'Because maintenance of optimum communication is critical to quality of life, AAC management is central to palliative care,(38). This field, which offers a range of strategies and communication devices to support the person with poor intelligibility or no speech, has expanded considerably in recent years. There are now more flexible options to offer the person at different stages in their illness (see previous section on stages in the progression of speech production difficulties). Many speech and language therapists have some experience in this field(9), and in many areas referral can be made to a communication aids centre with a team of specialist therapists and technicians.

Careful assessment by the speech and language therapist will be required in order to ensure that the most appropriate communication support is given to each individual. Visual, motor, linguistic, and cognitive impairments will influence the selection. Some may reject or fail to make much use of the communication systems offered, possibly due to increasing passivity and lack of motivation to communicate, but every person should be provided with the opportunity to try relevant aids to communication.

High-tech aids

Despite the terminal nature of their condition, some people will remain cognitively able and alert and will retain a fairly sophisticated level of communication. A range of voice output communication aids (VOCA) is available. See Fig. 4.9.2 for an example.

Many of these offer features such as banks of stored phrases, which can be triggered by one or two presses of a key or switch, or word prediction in which a choice of words appears on the screen as the individual types, predicted from the initial letters and from the grammar of the preceding words. These features greatly reduce the effort required by the user. There may also be a range of options for inputting text, from enlarged keyboards and special key guards to letter displays operated by a single switch. This allows the communication aid to be adapted to the user's abilities as motor control deteriorates.

Low-tech aids

This term refers to less technologically sophisticated support systems, for example, a chart with letters, words, or phrases, to which

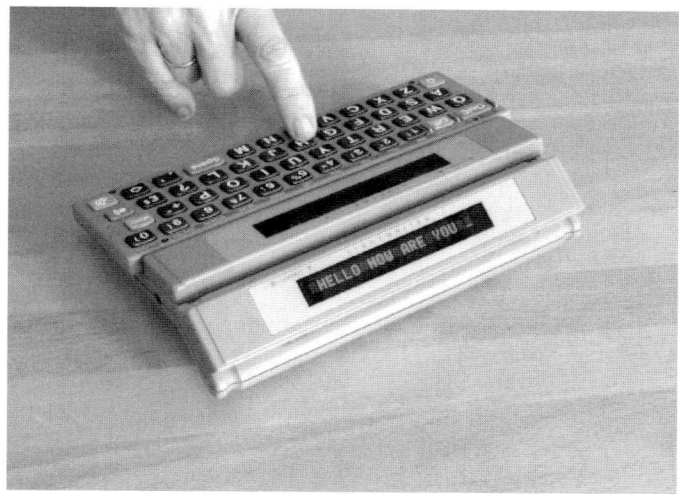

Figure 4.9.2 A Lightwriter: an example of a high-tech communication aid..

the individual can point. For weak or very physically disabled people, a display with a selection of messages to which the user can direct their eye gaze can be constructed. Where spelling or recognition of the written word is difficult, small pictures or symbols can be used as message signifiers. In Fig. 4.9.3, an eye-pointing frame is shown and explained.

Yes/no systems

For people who are in the very final stages of their illness, weakness, fatigue, and confusion may make even a simple system of communication difficult. It may, however, be possible to find a way for them to signal 'yes' and 'no' successfully. This may involve the use of some small body movement or eye signal, for example eye gaze up = 'yes', eye gaze down = 'no', or directing the eyes to the words 'yes' and 'no' mounted on either side of the bed. This allows the individual to continue to experience some level of control and involvement in everyday activities and decision-making.

Case study

A case described in *RCSLT Bulletin* (October 2000, p. 4) exemplifies the significance of having a yes–no response when no other

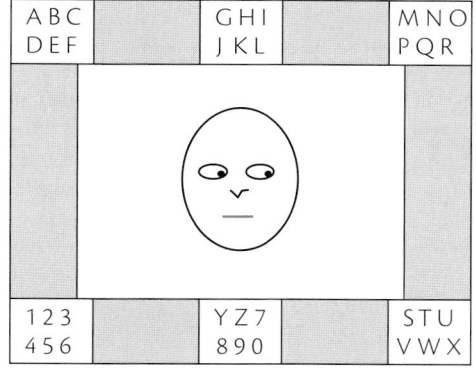
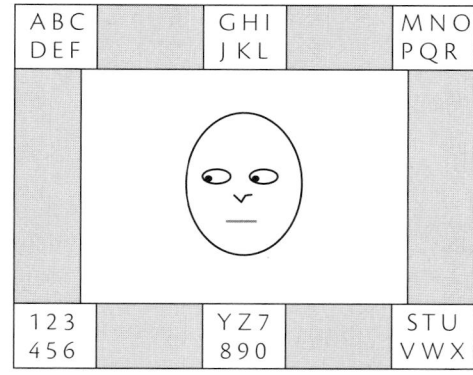

Figure 4.9.3 Eye-pointing frame: an example of a low-tech communication aid. The user first points to the block of letters containing the target letter (in this example 'S'), then to the block corresponding to the position of that letter within the first block, i.e. top left...

form of communication is possible. A ventilated 19-year-old with MND has been allowed through High Court agreement to have the ventilator switched off when he loses the ability to blink with his left eyelid.

Special considerations for children

Preliterate children will require specific considerations and assessment for appropriate communication support. For some children with well-maintained hand function, manual signs (usually taken from the sign language used by the deaf community) may prove the most effective means of communication. Other children may be taught to use either a high-tech communication aid or a low-tech communication chart. In either case, the speech and language therapist will work in close consultation with family and educational staff in selecting and teaching a set of pictorial symbols with which the child can communicate. These will either be displayed on a chart or communication aid screen or on the overlay or keys of some communication aids. Symbol communication systems and manual signs are also widely used by people of all ages with learning disabilities.

Aids to oral communication

Patients who have undergone surgical procedures that interfere with voice production and/or speech intelligibility, may be offered a range of prostheses or mechanical aids. These include speaking tracheostomy valves, artificial larynxes, and prostheses to assist velo-pharyngeal closure (palatal lift), to lower the palate in order to facilitate articulatory contact or to supply missing contact surfaces[30]. The speech and language therapist should be included in assessment for these aids, in conjunction with the medical team and possibly an orthodontist. Intensive training will probably be required once the device is available. Those with weak, low voice volume but relatively precise articulation may be helped by the use of a speech amplifier. There are several lightweight head mountable models available.

Swallowing problems

Drugs prescribed to alleviate one aspect of a patient's condition may adversely affect the ability to swallow or the amount of saliva produced. Oral tumours and glossectomy will restrict tongue movement, and tumours in the pharynx will affect the efficiency of the swallowing mechanism[33]. Radiotherapy to the head and neck may cause changes to tissue and muscle function, alterations to taste, reduced saliva flow, and possibly diminished swallow reflex both during and after radiotherapy. Dysphagia is common in non-head and neck malignancy[39]. Dysphagia is also a symptom of many of the deteriorating neurological conditions (see Table 4.9.1).

The symptoms may vary. Chewing may be affected by the lack of graded jaw movement or by muscle weakness or rigidity. Poor control of the glossal, buccal, and labial musculature will reduce the ability to manipulate food within the oral cavity and cause delayed transit towards the pharynx or disintegration of the food bolus interfering with the co-ordination and timing of the swallow. Weak or asyncronous triggering of the pharyngeal swallow, decreased or slowed laryngeal elevation, or reduced pharyngeal peristalsis, may result in pooling in the valleculae and pyriform sinuses and risk of aspiration[8].

Dysphagia can result in difficulty in swallowing food, fluid, saliva, and medication.

The speech and language therapist's role in the management of swallowing difficulties

Many professional disciplines will be involved in supporting the person with eating and swallowing difficulties. The specialist speech and language therapist is trained to assess and advise on the oral control of food, liquid, and oral secretions (saliva), and the safety of the swallowing mechanism, particularly at the pharyngeal level. Problems at the oesophageal level lie outside the remit of speech and language therapy intervention. The specialist speech and language therapist will assess the quality and safety of a patient's swallow. They may suggest head postures or alternative positioning for safer swallowing and/or different food and liquid consistencies, for example, the addition of thickener to liquids or the pureeing of solid food may be appropriate depending on the findings, as well as possible exercises to improve the swallow[8]. The speech and language therapist may request referral for videofluoroscopy (modified barium swallow) or other instrumental investigations, e.g. fibreoptic endoscopic evaluation of swallowing (FEES)[8]. These procedures not only help to determine whether the patient is aspirating but will also guide the therapist in appropriate management. However, in locations where radiological or instrumental evaluations are not readily accessible (e.g. in rural communities), dependence on bedside assessment may be necessary.

It is important that a person exhibiting even early signs of chewing or swallowing difficulty, for example, occasional coughing or choking when eating or drinking, chestiness, or a 'wet', gurgly voice after swallowing or poor saliva control, should be referred to the speech and language therapist as soon as possible. For people with degenerative conditions, small changes in posture and food/liquid consistency may be effective at first. If the patient appears to be at risk of aspiration then this will need to be carefully monitored and if necessary non-oral feeding considered by the medical team.

Eight factors will influence best practice in dysphagia management (particularly for people with degenerative diseases, but also more widely applicable to people with terminal illness):[10]

- cognitive/communicative and comprehension ability during interaction with caregivers for purposes of self-determination;

- cognitive/communicative and comprehension ability during execution of a plan of care;

- dependence–independence levels during execution of compensatory manoeuvres and therapeutic plans;

- matching changes in treatment plans to changes in the physiology of swallowing;

- establishing realistic expectations and goals for advancing conditions;

- determining appropriate times for surgical intervention and/or medication;

- developing sensitivity to personal, cultural, and familial wants, needs, and desires of patients/clients; and

◆ deciding when to terminate swallowing treatment and when to initiate palliative or supportive treatment.

Case studies

The swallowing of a child with Tay–Sachs disease was assessed and found to be a 'non-functional oral feeder' by the speech and language therapist. From this information, the medical team recommended enteral feeding[40]. In contrast, assessment of an adult with longstanding dementia, made without full knowledge of the team's perspective on what would be appropriate management, resulted in conflicting patient care recommendations[41].

Factors influencing speech and language therapy effectiveness

Apart from disease progression, there are many other factors which clinical experience shows will affect the effectiveness of speech and language therapy. These include:

◆ the patient's right to choose to decline speech and language therapy intervention;

◆ the patient's attitude to their communication and/or swallowing problem;

◆ the effect of the communication or swallowing problem in relation to other medical symptoms as perceived by the individual;

◆ the level of alertness (related to medication, fatigue, pain);

◆ family and health carer attitudes; and

◆ family/staff training, for example, in AAC, swallowing problems.

Conclusion

In this chapter, the role of the speech and language therapist for patients with communication and/or swallowing problems has been discussed. We stress the importance of timely referral for initial assessment so that appropriate intervention (support, counselling, advice, or therapy) can be offered.

References

1. Eckman, S., and Roe, J. (2005). Speech and language therapists in palliative care: what do we have to offer? *International Journal of Palliative Nursing*, **11**, 179–81.

2. Salt, N., and Robertson, S. (1998). A hidden client group? Communication impairment in hospice patients. *International Journal of Language & Communication Disorders*, **33** (Suppl.), 96–101.

3. Stoicheff, M. (1991). Post-radiotherapy voice. In *Voice Disorders and their Management* (ed. M. Fawcus), 2nd edition, pp. 333–6. Chapman and Hall., London.

4. Jackson, P., Robbins, M., and Frankel, S. (1996). Communication impediments in a group of hospice patients. *Palliative Medicine*, **10**, 79–80.

5. Hunt, A. and Burne, R. (1995). Medical and nursing problems of children with neurodegenerative disease. *Palliative Medicine*, **9**, 19–26.

6. Royal College of Speech and Language Therapists. (2006). *Communicating quality 3*. Royal College of Speech and Language Therapists, London.

7. Yorkston, K.M., Miller, R., and Strand, E. (1995). *Management of speech and swallowing in degenerative diseases*. Communication Skill Builders, Tucson, AZ.

8. Logemann, J. (1998). *Evaluation and treatment of swallowing disorders*, 2nd edition. Pro-Ed, Austin, TX.

9. Armstrong, L., Jans, D., and MacDonald, A. (2000). Parkinson's disease and aided AAC: some evidence from practice. *International Journal of Language & Communication Disorders*, **35**, 377–89.

10. Sonies, B. (2000). Patterns of care for dysphagic patients with degenerative neurological diseases. *Seminars in Speech and Language*, **21**, 333–45.

11. Bayles, K.A. and Kaszniak, A.W. (1987). *Communication and cognition in normal aging and dementia*. Taylor & Francis Ltd, London.

12. Lubinski, R., (ed.) (1991). *Dementia and communication*. BC Decker, Philadelphia.

13. Rau, M.T. (1993). *Coping with communication challenges in Alzheimer's disease*. Singular, San Diego, CA.

14. Priefer, B.A. and Robbins, J. (1997). Eating changes in mild-stage Alzheimer's disease: a pilot study. *Dysphagia*, **12**, 212–21.

15. Boylston, E.W. and O'Day, C.P. (1999). *Successful eating: Dementia swallowing assessment*. Imaginart, Bisbee.

16. Bourgeois, M. *et al.* (2001). Memory aids as an augmentative and alternative communication strategy for nursing home residents with dementia. *AAC*, **17**, 196–210.

17. Cummings, J.L. and Benson, D.F. (1992). *Dementia: A clinical approach*, 2nd edition. Butterworth-Heinemann, Boston, MA.

18. Bryan, K. and Maxim, J. (ed.) (1996). *Communication disability and the psychiatry of old age*. Whurr, London.

19. Collyer, V. (2001). Behind the headlines. B*ulletin of the Royal College of Speech and Language Therapists*, **589**, 12–14.

20. McKeith, I. *et al.* (1992). Neuroleptic sensitivity in patients with senile dementia of Lewy body type. *British Medical Journal*, **305**, 673–8.

21. Azuma, T. and Bayles, K.A. (1997). Memory impairments underlying language difficulties in dementia. *Topics in Language Disorders*, **18**, 58–71.

22. Wallesch, C.W. and Hundsalz, A. (1994). Language function in delirium: a comparison of single word processing in acute confusional states and probable Alzheimer's disease. *Brain and Language*, **46**, 592–606.

23. Thomson, A.-M. Communication Disorders in Patients with Hemispheric Intracranial Neoplasm. PhD Thesis, University of Edinburgh, 1997.

24. Chapey, R. (ed.) (1994). *Language intervention strategies in adult aphasia*, 3rd edition. Williams & Wilkins, Baltimore, MD.

25. Beukelman, D., Yorkston, K. and Reichle, J. (eds.) (2000). *Augmentative and alternative communication for adults with acquired neurologic disorders*. Paul Brookes, Baltimore, MD.

26. O'Keefe, C. *et al.* (1993). Developments in HIV/AIDS. *Bulletin of the Royal College of Speech and Language Therapists*, **473**, 12.

27. Vogel, D. and Carter, J.E. (1995). *The effects of drugs on communication disorders*. Singular, San Diego, CA.

28. Davis-McFarland, E. (2000). Language and oral-motor development and disorders in infants and young toddlers with human immunodeficiency virus. *Seminars in Speech and Language*, **21**, 19–36.

29. McNeilly, L.G. (2000). Communication intervention and therapeutic issues in pediatric human immunodeficiency virus. *Seminars in Speech and Language*, **21**, 63–78.

30. Dikeman, K.J. and Kazandjian, M.S. (1995). *Communication and swallowing management of tracheostomized and ventilator-dependent adults*.Singular, San Diego, CA.

31. Forbes, K. (1997). Palliative care in patients with cancer of the head and neck. *Clinical Otolaryngology*, **22**, 117–22.

32. Tippet, D.C. (ed.) (2000). *Tracheostomy and ventilator dependency: management of breathing, speaking and swallowing*. Thieme, New York.

33. Saunders, C. and Sykes, N. (1993). *The management of terminal malignant disease*, 3rd edition, Edward Arnold, London.

34. Lazarus, C. (2000). Management of swallowing disorders in head and neck cancer patients: optimal patterns of care. *Seminars in Speech and Language*, **21**, 293–309.

35. Armstrong, L., Jans, D., and MacDonald, A. (1999). Parkinson's disease and the use of AAC: looking for some evidence. *Communication Matters*, **13**(3), 5–6.

36. Patterson, J. (2005). Head and neck cancer dysphagia. *Speech and Language Therapy in Practice*. Autumn, 12–13.

37. Yorkston, K.M. and Beukelman, D.R. (2000). Decision making in AAC intervention. In *Augmentative and Alternative Communication for Adults with Acquired Neurologic Disorders* (eds D. Beukelman, K. Yorkston, and J. Reichle), pp. 55–82. Paul Brookes, Baltimore, MD.

38. Klasner, E.R. and Yorkston, K.M. (2000). AAC for Huntington disease and Parkinson's disease: planning for change. In *Augmentative and Alternative Communication for Adults with Acquired Neurologic Disorders* (eds. D.R. Beukelman, K.M. Yorkston, and J. Reichle), pp. 237–70. Paul Brookes, Baltimore, MD.

39. Roe, J. (2005). Oropharyngeal dysphagia in advanced non-head and neck malignancy. *European Journal of Palliative Care*, **12**, 229–32.

40. Sharp, H.M. and Geneson, L.B. (1996). Ethical decision-making in dysphagia management. *American Journal of Speech-Language Pathology*, **5**, 15–22.

41. Pollens, R. (2004). Role of the speech-language pathologist in palliative hospice care. *Journal of Palliative Medicine*, **7**, 694–702.

4.10

The contribution of art therapy to palliative medicine

Michèle J.M. Wood

In Britain, art therapy is a state-registered health-care profession and its practitioners complete a postgraduate training for 2 years full-time or equivalent. The training encompasses models of psychotherapy, psychiatry, psychology, and the role and function of aesthetics and creativity in health-care. Art therapy training consists of three core elements: the theoretical underpinnings of the practice, experiential engagement in artistic and interpersonal activities (so that trainees develop their capacity for self-reflection and insight and continue to engage in their own art-making), and clinical placements. Clinical placements or internships are central to the training of art therapists, and in this way, practitioners also learn about the roles of other health professionals, the function of interdisciplinary teamwork, and art therapy's contribution to this. State registration[1] of art therapists ensure that practitioners continue to maintain the standards of proficiency and professional practice established on qualification. In some other European countries such as Canada, Australia, and the USA, art therapy is also a recognized profession taught at the postgraduate level and practised within a wide range of settings.

In UK, art therapy had its beginnings in the tuberculosis sanatoria of the 1940s, but quickly developed within psychiatric and educational settings. Integrated with other care, it has since been widely incorporated into the fields of mental health and learning disabilities. However, there is a growing interest in art therapy with the medically and terminally ill[2–5] and one survey[6] indicated that just over 6 per cent of all art therapists in UK have worked in palliative care.

What is art therapy?

Art therapy provides a supportive psychotherapeutic relationship within which a person may explore personal issues. It involves the use of art materials for this exploration so that thoughts, feelings, and other issues of personal significance can be expressed. As such it is an alternative to spoken language, providing a means of communication and symbolic representation. The art therapist's task is to facilitate the patient's expressive capacities and to help him or her reflect upon what they have produced, including their chosen media and style of working. The ultimate aim of art therapy is to enable the patient to change and develop on a personal level. Art therapy does not aim to distract or divert a person from their

difficulties; but through encouraging an experience of creativity, these difficulties can be perceived and worked with in a new way.

An important aspect of art therapy is that it provides an opportunity to express emotions that may feel unacceptable to the patient. The patient may have repressed feelings of anger, envy, and sadness for fear of upsetting their family or staff. In art therapy, pounding clay, pouring paint, and scribbling violently on paper gives the patient permission to express strong feelings, and the presence of the therapist ensures the patient is not left alone with their distress. Art therapy also allows for the development and expression of more positive feelings such as tenderness, hope, or beauty. The breadth of emotional expression possible through art therapy demands a working environment that provides confidentiality and in which the patient can feel free to be vulnerable. A separate therapy or quiet room designated for art therapy sessions is ideal.

The loss of control in many areas of patients' lives is an inevitable consequence of illness, and one that art therapy aims to address. The physicality of art therapy, where an individual must actively engage with the materials to produce a picture or object, provides an experience that reinforces the person's ability to make choices and their sense of their own vitality. The artwork represents not only something of the patient's mental state but also, by capturing in its marks and traces the movement and pressure of the patient's pencil, brush, or finger, it represents something of their physical condition too. This articulation through the artwork of the mind–body relationship is intrinsic to art therapy. It has been suggested that art therapy's potency resides in this link[7,8] and thus art therapy is ideally placed to respond to the psychological effects of physical trauma. The developments in psychoneuroimmunology appear to be providing exciting explanations for the links between imagery and improvements in physical health. This is an area of increasing investigation[2,4].

Art therapy and creative art: similarities and differences

It is important to distinguish art therapy from creative arts activities[9]. Although there are some areas of overlap, art therapy and creative arts projects have different yet complementary functions within palliative care. Both engage the patient in actively using art media and provide a focus and sense of purpose. Both result in an increased sense of control, self-confidence, and make a positive contribution to patients' quality of life. Creative arts projects may aim to help the patient produce artwork for sale, or to bequeath to relatives. Although the artwork produced in art therapy may on occasion have a similar outcome, its focus is different. As patients strive to express and explore their inner emotional landscape through their art, there is no expectation that work should be aesthetically 'good' in a conventional sense, or that it will be viewed outside the therapy space. Consequently, the artwork may have a rough undeveloped quality to it. The process by which the artwork is made offers an additional level for expression and communication and contributes to the material with which the therapist and the patient engage. The need to witness the patient's process is one reason for the therapist's presence in the art therapy sessions. Although the primary aim of art therapy is to facilitate psychological adjustment by the patient to their changed health through this multi-faceted communication, the permanent nature of the artwork means that it can continue to communicate from session to session and outside of the therapeutic relationship. Patients have been known to use their pictures to communicate with friends, family[10], other patients in similar situations[3], and their doctors and other members of the multi-disciplinary team.

Art therapists, artists in residence, and art tutors can work alongside each other in many establishments; their combination of skills is particularly effective where their differences are understood. While both encourage the patients' creativity and improve the overall milieu of the health-care environment, art therapy works with the psychological and emotional needs of the patient, which includes their barriers to creativity and their difficulties with self-expression. It can be hard for a patient or a professional to know whether art therapy or recreational art is more appropriate. Most art therapists provide assessment sessions in which the patients' needs may be discerned. A good example of a setting where both art therapy and art activities are offered alongside each other is described in Kennett's phenomenological study of a creative arts project[11] at St Christopher's Hospice in London. The following case history describes the dual functioning of art-making in a palliative care setting showing the different roles played by art therapy and art activity for a woman with motor neuron disease.

Case 1: 'Rosemary' by Jackie Coote, art therapist

Whilst working in a large London hospice, I was introduced to Rosemary, who had recently been diagnosed with motor neuron disease. Having become paralysed down one side of her body and rapidly losing the power of speech, she had expressed a wish to 'paint her feelings'. She was, by the time I met her, using an electronic writer to communicate and only had the use of her right arm. Anything she 'said' was through the writer. Although unfamiliar with the use of art materials, she engaged in the process very quickly, allowing herself to paint freely. She began to look forward to 'the unexpected', which presented itself to her in each session, like the painting she referred to as her 'Devastated Woodland–half dead, struggling for survival' (Fig. 4.10.1). She was able to relate the image to her feelings about her own situation. Her 'fun' painting became a way to address serious issues around her encroaching illness. Through it she began to express her thoughts and feelings about the adjustments she had to make, not

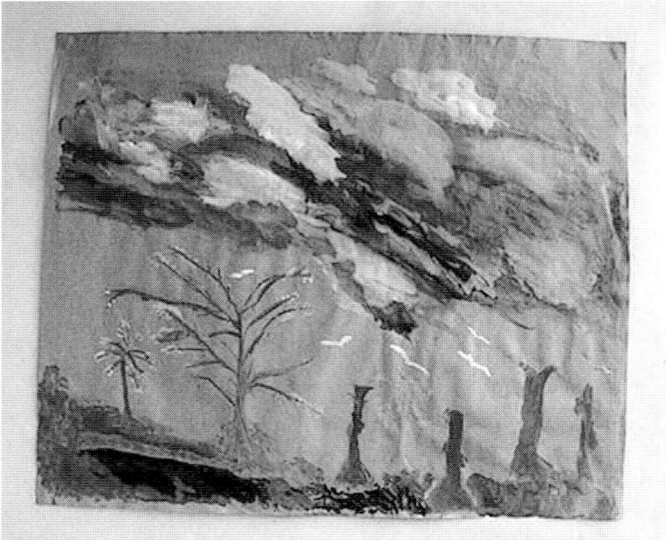

Figure 4.10.1 Devastated woodland.

just physically, but psychologically. Through her images, she was able to express her painful recognition of change and loss. With the loss of spontaneity and inflexion in speech, Rosemary's painting became her 'voice'. Her choice of materials would often indicate her tone and mood. On one occasion, she chose bright, cheerful colours, but the black paper she used reflected her underlying melancholy, and the resulting picture helped her to recognize the tendency to 'put on a cheerful front' when all behind it was not well.

In the course of using art therapy to express difficult and painful feelings, Rosemary discovered another side to her image making. She began to paint alone in her room. This work took on a 'painterly' quality. She painted gardens resembling images from 'The Arabian Nights' that contained a sense of richness and fertility. Staff and other patients would come and see what she had been doing each day, and her self-esteem increased considerably. Her images enabled her to become empowered at a time of increasing powerlessness and dependency. With the increase in Rosemary's use of her newly found creative skills, it became important to differentiate between her 'public art' and her 'private art'. She needed reassurance that she still had a private and safe space in the art therapy sessions, where she could pour out what she called her 'madness'. She seemed at this point to have moved into a third and what was to be the final phase of the art therapy sessions, where as her body deteriorated, the emotional floodgates opened. Fear, grief, anger, hatred, and despair appeared in the images before us. Her art therapy sessions provided the container necessary to hold the overwhelming grief which she poured out in torrents. It was the coping strategy which she needed in order to carry on throughout the rest of the day.

Who would benefit from art therapy?

Art therapists work in a range of settings: patients' own homes[12], prisons[13], day care units[14–16], specialist inpatient units[17,18], hospices[14], and private practice[19]. Examples showing the variety of recent art therapists' practices and research projects are given in Table 4.10.1. People with a wide range of conditions including HIV/AIDS, rheumatoid illness, multiple sclerosis, cancer, dementia, and Niemann Pick's disease have been reported as benefiting from art therapy.[20] The range of conditions and variety of settings in which art therapy is offered indicate something of the multiple contributions art therapy can make to patients' care.

Indications for art therapy?

While recognizing this breadth of application, is it possible to discern which conditions or types of patients would benefit the most? Since art therapy is a means of facilitating communication, it is particularly useful for patients, their family, or carers, who are having difficulty with other modes of communication. Such difficulties can be physical, cognitive, emotional, or even spiritual in origin, and thus provide different starting points and ways of working for the therapist. Case 1 clearly illustrates how art therapy can extend a patient's capacity to communicate when this has been curtailed for physical reasons. Similarly, the person with AIDS dementia may no longer be able to coherently discuss their fears and anxieties but may be able to use the qualities available in art to express themselves and relieve their frustrations. In this case, the art therapist may not focus on discussion or interpretation.[22] By contrast, where there are emotional difficulties, the therapist may well explore in depth the patient's associations to their image and their behaviour. Coote[29] illustrates this in her work with an attention-seeking patient where art therapy allowed an expression of bitterness and resentment, unrecognized aspects of the patient's inner self. Connell[3] gives an example of how art therapy was used to address and work through a patient's spiritual struggles. Trauger-Querry and Haghighi[27] describe an approach using art therapy and music therapy in the reduction of pain.

Young children, whose developing capacities for verbal expression limit their use of talking therapies, are an obvious group

Table 4.10.1 Examples of art therapists' practice and research with life-threatening and terminal illnesses.

Diagnosis/reason for referral to art therapy	Location of therapy	Relevant details of intervention	Evaluation/presentation of material	Reference
AIDS	UK, hospice	Single session where patient presents himself as the art work	Case study	Wood[21]
AIDS dementia	UK, hospice	Seven years analysed	Qualitative analysis	Wood[22]
AIDS/HIV	UK, prison	Closed art therapy group	Description of practice	Beaver[13]
Bone marrow transplant	USA	Individual sessions with patients in isolation	Description of practice and some qualitative analysis	Gabriel et al.[18]
Cancer	UK, patients' homes	Individual and family art therapy	Description of practice	Bell[12]
Cancer	UK, specialist cancer hospital	Art therapy—individual and group sessions; group notebook	Descriptions of a range of practices using patients' pictures	Connell[3]
Breast cancer	Undergoing radiotherapy	Sweden		Brief individual art therapy programme
Randomized controlled study	Oster et al.[16]	Cancer	USA	In-patients
One hour art therapy intervention	Quasi-experimental design	Nainis et al.[23]	Breast cancer	Canada and USA
Study exploring how art therapy and art-making were used to address psychosocial needs	Narrative research methodology	Collie et al.[7]	Cancer	USA
Inpatients	Body outline template	Thematic analysis of patients responses	Luzzatto et al.[10]	Cancer
USA	Mindfulness-based art therapy	Randomized controlled trial		Monti et al.[24]
Cystic fibrosis	USA, private practice	Art therapy with young people	Description of practice	Farrell Fenton[19]
Dementias	UK, day centres	Art therapy groups	A control group study	Sheppard et al.[25]
Melanoma	UK	Patient reports on art therapy and other resources used	Personal account	Morley[26]
Pain control	USA, hospice with adults	Art and music therapy	Theoretical discussion illustrated by case material	Trauger-Querry and Haghighi[27]
Palliative care	UK inpatients and patients' homes	Group art therapy	Description and case vignettes	Jones[28]
Post-treatment cancer	USA, outpatients	Short-term structured art therapy group work	Qualitative analyses using questionnaires and follow-up interviews	Luzzatto and Gabriel[17]

for art therapy, as art and drawing are more familiar means of self-expression. Farrell Fenton[19], who works with children and young people who have cystic fibrosis, suggests that art therapy works on two levels simultaneously, providing a means of emotional catharsis, while at the same time, harnessing the young person's coping strategies.

Many factors including class, educational level, and ethnic background influence the patient's comfort in expressing and addressing their emotional responses to illness. In my experience of serving an ethnically diverse population, art therapy can be a welcome tool for patients who have to negotiate their experiences of illness and treatment through a language and in a cultural setting that is not their own. Art therapy can strengthen their own 'voice' and validate their own experiences. The value of art as a tool for cultural communication can be seen in the project described by Fried[30], where Aboriginal artists were commissioned to paint about end-of-life issues. Although this is not an example of art therapy, it illustrates the need to find more culturally relevant modes of communication for people needing palliative care services. It also indicates the value of non-verbal and symbolic levels of expression.

Art therapists as part of the palliative care team

Art therapists usually work under the auspices of the counselling or psychosocial team and as part of the wider multi-professional palliative care team. Referrals to art therapy arise from a close consideration of patients' needs by the team, and in cases where a patient requires emotional support but is unable to access counselling for reasons such as those given above art therapy may be suggested. Referrals can be made by a variety of agencies from within the multi-professional hospital setting, the community palliative care teams or by the patient or family member themselves, and referrals come directly to the art therapist or to their team or line manager. For example, I work as part of the psychosocial team in a specialist palliative care unit alongside counsellors, social workers, chaplains, and family therapists. Referrals can be made to anyone of us, or to our psychosocial team itself for further assessment of the patients' psychosocial needs. Like many members of the palliative care team art therapists are often employed on part-time or sessional contracts, with the result that they may not always be able to attend team meetings. However, their contributions to patients' care should be conveyed to colleagues in written form in patients' records, in case reports and summaries. Where staff time is limited art therapists, counsellors and social workers do represent each other in team discussions about the emotional aspects of their patients care. In UK, specific guidelines have been written to enhance an understanding of the role of sessional arts therapies staff[9]. Sadly, when there are constraints on funding for palliative care services, these will often be felt by art therapists, whose contribution may be more readily considered disposable and 'value-added' rather than core to patient care. This issue of funding is probably the main challenge for art therapy in palliative care, since it can confine art therapists to fractional contracts which limit their work, and prohibits access to the sorts of research and continuing professional development opportunities enjoyed by their medical, nursing and allied health professional colleagues. However, the support provided by art therapists is important; often patients who may not otherwise access

hospice services, or who are wary of them for whatever reason, do go on to develop good relationships with the wider palliative care team because of their involvement with art therapy[31].

Any hazards of art therapy?

The hazards due to art therapy are minimal but the following pitfalls are worth mentioning. There can be a concern from some staff that the expression of feelings through image-making may unleash a flow of emotion that will overwhelm the patient and those around them. Usually, these concerns dissipate when it is realized that the processes and boundaries of art therapy provide a safe container that prevents this from happening. The patient never fully relinquishes control, but through the manipulation of the art materials, their usual defences can give way to more symbolic expressions of feeling states (see Case 2). The therapist's skill in keeping the boundaries of therapy ensures that these feelings are contained and that both the patient and themselves are kept safe.

The therapeutic value of art therapy may be undermined if the position of the art therapist in relation to the interdisciplinary team is not respected or clearly understood. One example of this can be seen when art therapy sessions are interrupted for procedures or questions that can be done at another time. Another example is where the art therapist is placed at the periphery of the team working without reference to colleagues. This can lead to unnecessary replication of work, or of the art therapist's important perspective on the patient being lost to the team.

Another hazard of therapeutic work, and indeed of all work in palliative care, relates to the emotional well-being of staff. Therapists need to ensure that they themselves are adequately supported through the use of supervision, supportive teamwork, and possibly their own personal therapy. All these strategies have proved to be beneficial in guarding against staff burnout and inappropriate behaviour. Art therapy itself is often used for staff support and can facilitate a valuable level of creativity, communication, and expression in tired staff teams[32].

On a practical level, the hazard posed to patients by the art materials does need to be considered. Most materials used in art therapy are non-toxic, but where materials could pose a risk (e.g. fixative), therapists ensure that usual precautions are taken. In cases where cross-infection between patients may be an issue, it is standard practice that separate sets of equipment are used.

Outcomes of art therapy

Summarizing the literature outlined in Table 4.10.1, the following outcomes of art therapy have been identified:

- development of a creative attitude by the patient towards their circumstances;
- an increased sense of control;
- better communication;
- wider range of expressive capabilities;
- increased insight into patient's own behaviour;
- body image issues addressed;
- a cathartic release of emotive issues;
- increased self-esteem and self-efficacy;

◆ increased ability to confront existential questions and relieve spiritual distress;

◆ development of positive coping strategies and an increase in coping resources;

◆ reduction in experiences and reports of physical pain;

◆ increased quality of life.

Adjusting to multiple losses (purpose, health, and social position), and facing one's own mortality, is equally central to care of the elderly. There has been much work done by art therapists with this population who are often cared for outside of palliative settings. One UK-based study[25] evaluated art therapy with people suffering from dementia using a control group design where the control situation was a standard day-centre mixed activity social group. The researchers found that there was a significant difference between the patients participating in art therapy and those in the control group.

Evaluating art therapy

The list of benefits of art therapy given above is extensive and there is widespread acceptance of its clinical value. However, systematic research in art therapy is only just emerging as practitioners and academics begin to investigate what it is that is unique to art therapy and how best to harness its therapeutic efficacy. Small-scale projects using both quantitative and qualitative research approaches are being undertaken and add to the already extensive anecdotal reports and single-case studies that are the evidence base for art therapy in supportive and palliative care (See Table 4.10.1). For example, a randomized, controlled study of art therapy among women with breast cancer has shown an improvement in their coping resources[16], and another quasi-experimental study has documented a reduction in tiredness as a result of art therapy[23]. A randomized controlled trial of a mindfulness based art therapy group intervention found a decrease in symptom distress and an increase in quality of life measures[24]. The use of art therapy to address psychosocial needs in women with breast cancer has been explored through narrative analysis[7], highlighting the value of research that utilizes the patients' knowledge as part of the research process. Innovative schemes are also being developed whereby art therapy is being embedded within more comprehensive psychosocial interventions such as the use of telecommunications technologies to deliver support to women with cancer[33], and the use of an art gallery space rather than a medical one as a location for an art therapy programme[34].

How quickly can the benefits of art therapy be seen?

Patients are referred to art therapy for a variety of reasons and at differing stages of their journey from diagnosis to terminal care. What is clear from many practitioners' reports is that patients with life-threatening and terminal illnesses are motivated to make the most of the time they have left. There is an evidence[21,23,29] that even a single session can be of value, as shown in Case 2.

Case 2: 'Robert'

Robert, a man in his early thirties, was diagnosed with AIDS and was in hospital for respite care and symptom control. He had a detached and objective approach to his diagnosis and liked to be informed of all medical facts. When we met he had announced to staff that he no longer wished to discuss his condition.

Robert began the art therapy session by being somewhat surprised by the range of art materials available, and that we had a whole hour together. He said he was unsure about what to do, and I invited him to experiment with the materials to see what marks they made, and what he liked using. Robert said he was anxious about making a fool of himself and of making a mess; he wanted to do things properly. We talked about this initially in relation to his life outside the hospital, and then how he felt about making an image with me watching. Once we had acknowledged these concerns Robert began to draw.

Robert worked with some skill and concentration. As he worked he began to cry. Initially he was embarrassed, but did not stop himself. In fact he was glad to cry. He said that he had not realized he could still feel the things the drawing had brought to mind. He allowed himself to cry freely as he continued with his picture (Fig. 4.10.2). His starting point had been to draw an image of the leaves on the tree outside his bedroom window. However, despite attempts to draw autumn leaves he found himself only able to make them green. He noticed that he concentrated on the veins of the leaves, and made a link with his constant examination of his own veins, which he did to monitor his health. We talked about his green leaves being separate from the tree in the background, and his feelings of being plucked from the tree of life before his autumn years.

The tree he had drawn was beginning to blossom, and Robert felt very positive about it. The scene in the background was one that he

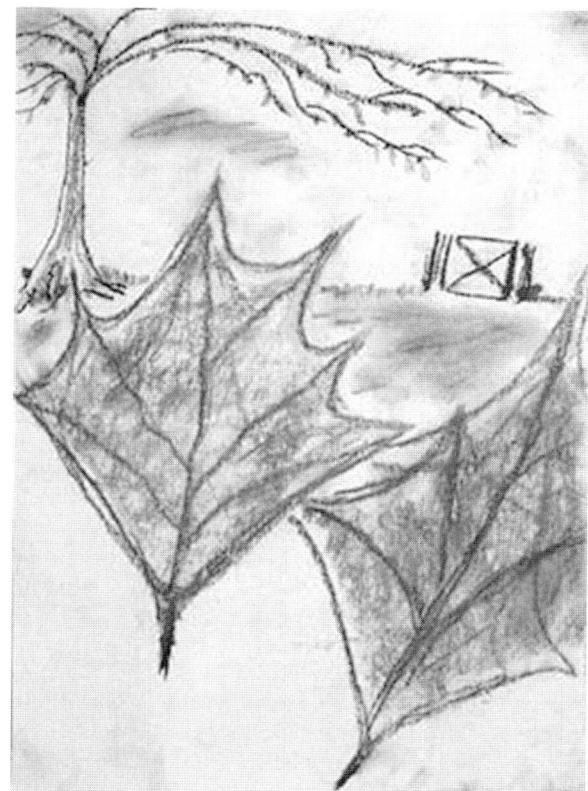

Figure 4.10.2 Case 2: Robert's image.

had drawn several times before when he was a schoolboy. He remembered growing up in the countryside and talked of the dreams he had then for his adult life. Aspirations he regretted that would never now be fulfilled. Robert noticed that he had omitted a fence, which meant that the gate was useless. There seemed to be nothing separating him from the unknown place that lay beyond this field.

At the end of the session, Robert reported feeling exhausted but light inside as though a burden had been lifted. This session had enabled Robert to connect with the grief he felt about having AIDS. Although we talked about some of the issues raised in the picture, the main focus was allowing him to feel and to cry. His announcement to staff indicated that he had gone as far as he could with words. This one-off session prompted a positive change in Robert that was noticed by hospital staff and his partner.

Art therapy and other therapies

There is growing recognition from outside palliative care circles that its fundamental principle of integrated care (based upon good interdisciplinary team work) leads to positive benefits for the patient. How the different disciplines of the palliative care team work together is a matter for consideration and in particular art therapy's part in this. For example, should a patient have art therapy at the same time as counselling or other emotional/psychological therapies? Art therapy works at verbal and non-verbal levels and therefore it can be possible for an art therapist to work in conjunction with a counsellor or psychologist. On these occasions, good communication between staff is crucial to avoid splitting staff or confusing the patient. Art therapy has also been known to work well alongside more body-based therapies such as aromatherapy and massage. In some cases art therapy may evoke issues that can be further explored in work with another discipline such as music therapy or chaplaincy. However, the principle of patients' choice is central in this matter—the patient's own wishes must be the guide by which members of the palliative care team are actively involved. After all the patients are the ones who must (together with our support) make sense of all that is happening to them. Morley describes her own journey with illness in which she used art therapy to integrate her experiences of the doctors, surgery, prayer, and her changing body[26].

Art therapy and bereavement work

Palliative care aims to support not only the patient but also those who are close to them. Support is often provided at hospices for partners, spouses, children, and other significant family members and friends while the patient is ill and after the patient has died. Art therapy with the bereaved has been well documented over the past 20 years and in some settings has become an integral part of bereavement services[35].

Conclusion

Art therapy is being practised in many parts of the world with adults and children living with life-threatening and terminal illnesses. There is a continuing recognition that art therapy does positively benefit patients, their carers and the professional team. The flexibility of art therapy to address a wide scope of issues ranging from pain to a patient's search for meaning makes it a valuable aspect of palliative care. To ensure that the benefits of art therapy are more clearly understood and that its efficacy is maximized there needs to be an increasing investment in research into this discipline.

Recommended reading[1–4] and references

1. Solomons, D. (2008). *An art therapy journey*. Limited Edition Private Publication. http://www.mariecurie.org.uk/aboutus/news/news_archive/news_archive_2008/art-therapy-book-news.htm
2. Pratt, M. and Wood, M.J.M. (eds.) (1998). *Art therapy in palliative care: the creative response*. Routledge, London.
3. Connell, C. (1998). *Something understood*. Wrexham Publications, London.
4. Malchiodi, C. (1999). *Medical art therapy with adults*. Jessica Kingsley, London.
5. Waller, D. and Sibbett, C. (eds.) (2005). *Art therapy and cancer care*. Open University Press, Buckingham.
6. Bint, J. (2000). *A report on the exploration of arts therapies in palliative care, cancer, AIDS and bereavement*. The Omega Foundation.
7. Collie, K., Bottorff, J.L., and Long, B.C. (2006). A narrative view of art therapy and art making by women with breast cancer. *Journal of Health Psychology*, **11**(5), 761–75.
8. Zammit, C. (2001). The art of healing: a journey through cancer: implications for art therapy. *Art Therapy: Journal of the American Art Therapy Association*, **18**(1), 27–36.
9. Pratt, M. and Thomas, G. (2007). *Guidelines for the arts therapies and the arts in palliative care settings*. Hospice Information, London.
10. Luzzatto, P., Sereno, V., and Capps, R. (2003). A communication tool for cancer patients with pain: the art therapy technique of the body outline. *Palliative and Supportive Care*, **1**, 135–42.
11. Kennett, C. (2000). Participation in a creative arts project can foster hope in a hospice day centre. *Palliative Medicine*, **14**, 419–25.
12. Bell, S. (1998). Will the kitchen table do? Art therapy in the community. In *Art therapy in palliative care: the creative response* (eds. M. Pratt and M.J.M. Wood), pp. 88–101. Routledge, London.
13. Beaver, V. (1998). The butterfly garden: art therapy with HIV/AIDS. In *Art therapy in palliative care: the creative response* (eds. M. Pratt and M.J.M. Wood), pp. 127–39. Routledge, London.
14. Wood, M.J.M. (2005). Shoreline: the realities of working in Cancer Care. In *Art therapy and cancer care* (eds. Waller, D. and Sibbett, C.). Open University Press, Buckingham.
15. Wilson, A. and Morris, F. (2003). Evaluation of art therapy intervention as an aid in the elevation of patients psychological and emotional distress following a diagnosis of advanced cancer. *Lung Cancer ISLAC*, **41** (Suppl. 2 August), 48–9.
16. Oster, I., Svensk, A., Magnusson, E. *et al.* (2006). Art therapy improves coping resources: a randomized, controlled study among women with breast cancer. *Palliative and Supportive Care*, **4**, 57–64.
17. Luzzatto, P. and Gabriel, B. (2000). The creative journey: a model for short term group art therapy with post-treatment cancer patients. *Art Therapy: Journal of the American Art Therapy Association*, **17**, 265–9.
18. Gabriel, B., Bromberg, E., Vandenbovenkamp, J. *et al.* (2001). Art therapy with adult bone marrow transplant patients in isolation: a pilot study. *Psycho-Oncology*, **10**(2), 114–23.
19. Farrell Fenton, J. (2000). Cystic fibrosis and art therapy. *The Arts in Psychotherapy*, **27**(1), 15–25.
20. Wood, M.J.M. (2004). The contribution of art therapy to palliative medicine. In *Oxford textbook of palliative medicine*, (eds. D. Doyle, G. Hanks, N. Cherny and K. Calman) 3rd edition. Oxford University Press, Oxford.
21. Wood, M.J.M. (1998). The body as art: individual session with a man with AIDS. In *Art therapy in palliative care: the creative response* (eds. M. Pratt and M.J.M. Wood), pp. 140–52. Routledge, London.

22. Wood, M.J.M. (2002). Researching art therapy practice with people suffering from AIDS-related dementia. *The Arts in Psychotherapy*, **29**, 207–19.

23. Nainis, N., Paice, J.A., Ratner, J. *et al.* (2006). Relieving symptoms in cancer: innovative use of art therapy *Journal of Pain and Symptom Management*, **31**, 162–9.

24. Monti, D.A., Peterson, C., Shakin Kunkel, E.J. *et al.* (2006). A randomized, controlled trial of mindfulness-based art therapy (MBAT) for women with cancer. *Psycho-Oncology*, **15**(5), 363–73.

25. Sheppard, L., MacInally, F., Rusted, J. *et al.* (1998). *Evaluating the use of art therapy for people with dementia: a control group study*. A report commissioned by the Brighton Branch of the Alzheimer's Disease Society.

26. Morley, B. (1998). Sunbeams and icebergs, meteorites and daisies: a cancer patient's experience of art therapy. In *Art therapy in palliative care: the creative response* (eds. M. Pratt and M.J.M. Wood), pp. 176–85. Routledge, London.

27. Trauger-Querry, B. and Haghighi, K.R. (1999). Balancing the focus: art and music therapy for pain control and symptom management in hospice care. *The Hospice Journal*, **14**(1), 25–37.

28. Jones, G. (2000). An art therapy group in palliative cancer care. *Nursing Times*, **96**(10), 42–3.

29. Coote, J. (1998). Getting started: introducing the art therapy service. In *Art therapy in palliative care: the creative response* (eds. M. Pratt and M.J.M. Wood), pp. 53–63. Routledge, London.

30. Fried, O. (1999). Many ways of caring: reaching out to aboriginal palliative care clients in Central Australia. *Progress in Palliative Care*, **7**(3), 116–9.

31. Website for Health Professionals Council in UK www.hpc-uk.org/

32. Belfiori, M. (1994). The group takes care of itself: art therapy to prevent burnout. *The Arts in Psychotherapy*, **12**(2), 119–26.

33. Collie, K., Bottorff, J.L., Long, B.C. *et al.* (2006). Distance art groups for women with breast cancer: guidelines and recommendations. *Supportive Care Cancer*, **14**, 849–58.

34. Deane, K., Carman, M., and Fitch, M (2000). The cancer journey: bridging art therapy and museum education. *Canadian Oncology Nursing Journal*, **10**(4), 140–2.

35. Pratt, M. (1998). The invisible injury: adolescent griefwork group. In *Art therapy in palliative care: the creative response* (eds. M. Pratt and M.J.M. Wood), pp. 153–68. Routledge, London.

The contribution of the stoma nurse specialist to palliative care

Jane Ellen Barr

Introduction

A poorly managed ostomy, draining wound/tube, or fistula has a tremendous impact on a patient and their family. Inadequate management of these problems can have devastating effects on both the patient who is approaching the end of life, and the family and professional caregivers who seek to ease the patient's suffering and maintain as good a quality of life as possible. Stoma nurse specialists have a significant role in caring for dying patients and their families. The goals of the stoma nurse specialist are consistent with the palliative care team as identified by the National Consensus Project's Clinical Practice Guidelines for Quality Palliative Care[1]. The stoma nurse specialist promotes quality of life, being supportive by focusing on managing and controlling patients symptoms to achieve the best possible quality of life for patients and families facing life-threatening illnesses. Care is holistic, focusing on physical, psychosocial, and spiritual problems of the patient.

Role of the stoma nurse specialist in palliative care

The stoma nurse specialist is an important member of the palliative care team across the continuum of care—acute care, long-term care, home care, and hospice—in managing patients with complex ostomies, draining wounds, tubes, and fistulas. The roles of the stoma nurse specialist vary from expert clinician, consultant, educator, and case manager[2].

At an administrative level, the stoma nurse specialist assists facilities/agencies that provide palliative care in developing care maps/pathways, establishing policies, procedures, and protocols, and developing product formularies for patients at or near the end of life. As an expert clinician and consultant, the stoma nurse specialist assesses and develops complex management strategies for patients with difficult to manage stomas, draining wounds/tubes, and fistulas. Nursing staff, families, and patients are assisted in problem-solving strategies, pouch fitting and selection, management of potential or actual impaired skin integrity, and maximum utilization of resources. As educator, the stoma nurse specialist educates patients, families/caregivers, and various members of the health-care team. The stoma nurse specialist acknowledges the importance of having patient participate in self-care for as long as possible. Promoting self-care, such as applying dressings or pouch changes and encouraging activities of daily living, can improve a patient's sense of dignity, wholeness, and quality of life[3].

The stoma nurse specialist may serve as the case manager. In so doing, he or she can coordinate the care provided by a wide diversity of team members, including the physicians, staff nurses, nursing assistants, dieticians, and discharge planners as they plan for the care of patients with complex problems secondary to ostomies, wounds, tubes, and fistulas.

Stoma management

Surgery continues to play a significant role in the palliative care provided to those with malignancies, fistulae, or complications after treatment, such as those that occur after pelvic radiation. For example, gastrointestinal malignancy may result in the need for emergency ostomy surgery for relief of intestinal obstruction or perforation secondary to tumour, or a stoma may be created to decompress an obstructed bowel or to divert stool from rectovaginal, rectovesical, or enterocutaneous fistulas.

The patient who is to have palliative ostomy surgery sees the stoma nurse specialist for stoma site marking, pre- and post-operative teaching, and pouch selection and fitting. Because of their compromised health status, the patient with advanced illness is at increased risk for stomal complications and impaired wound healing. This often necessitates a consult with the stoma nurse specialist for management of postoperative stomal and peristomal skin complications.

The stoma nurse specialist also is often called to see patients some time after initial evaluation and treatment, in response to stoma changes or complications secondary to clinical manifestations of their progressive disease. These changes or complications result in an poorly fitting pouching systems, changes in bowel function such as constipation or diarrhoea, impaired peristomal skin integrity secondary to a leaking pouching systems, and/or patient's and family's emotional and psychological coping difficulties.

The most common reason for a nurse on the palliative care team to consult with a stoma nurse specialist is to seek help in obtaining an effective pouching system seal. An ineffective pouching system seal results in need for frequent pouch changes, impairment in peristomal skin, pain secondary to impaired skin integrity, odour, embarrassment, and patient's further altered self-image.

Stoma pouching problems may occur secondary to stoma or abdominal changes. These changes usually relate to either weight loss or abdominal distention. Weight loss can result in stoma retraction below skin level or the creation of new abdominal folds or creases. Abdominal distention changes the contour of the abdomen. Whatever the aetiology, changes in either the level of stoma protrusion or contour of the abdomen can result in a poorly fitting pouching system or a wrong size faceplate (skin barrier opening). Both of these changes result in leakage of effluent onto the peristomal skin with resultant peristomal skin irritation.

The stoma nurse specialist adjusts the pouching system based on an assessment of the stoma, contour of abdomen, and type of effluent. They may change a two-piece system into a one-piece system that is more flexible and that will fold into the abdominal folds and creases. If the stoma has retracted below the abdominal surface and the output leaks under the flange, use of a pouching system with convexity may resolve the problem. A patient who is using a two-piece appliance whose abdomen becomes distended may not be able to maintain a good seal because the rigid flange cannot mould to the contour of their abdomen. A good seal may be obtained by using a one piece or flexible two-piece pouching

system. An algorithm for stoma faceplate selection (see Fig. 4.11.1) may be a useful resource to assist the physician or nurse on the palliative care team in selecting a pouching system's faceplate that is appropriate for the patient with stomal problems[4].

Stomal and peristomal complications, such as prolapse, hernia, and mucocutaneous separation, are the more common complications seen after emergency surgery near end of life. When emergency surgery is indicated for intestinal obstruction, often a transverse loop colostomy is performed. A transverse loop colostomy is an uncomplicated, simple surgical procedure that is performed for what is often perceived as a short-term measure to relieve symptoms of intestinal obstruction. However, this type of procedure places the patient at risk for post-operative complications of stoma prolapse and hernia[5].

Stoma prolapse of the transverse colostomy requires careful assessment and management using an effective pouching system. Prolapse is the telescoping of the bowel through the stoma, a change that often causes the stoma mucosa to become oedematous. The enlarged prolapsed stoma is susceptible to trauma and makes pouching a challenge. Conservative management is preferred and involves selection of a pouching system that can accommodate the length and width of the stoma. Flexible flanges are chosen to prevent stoma trauma from a rigid faceplate. The faceplate (skin barrier) of the pouching system opening needs to accommodate the stoma at its largest size. If this enlarged opening in the faceplate results in exposed peristomal skin, solid skin barriers, pastes or sealants are applied over the exposed skin to

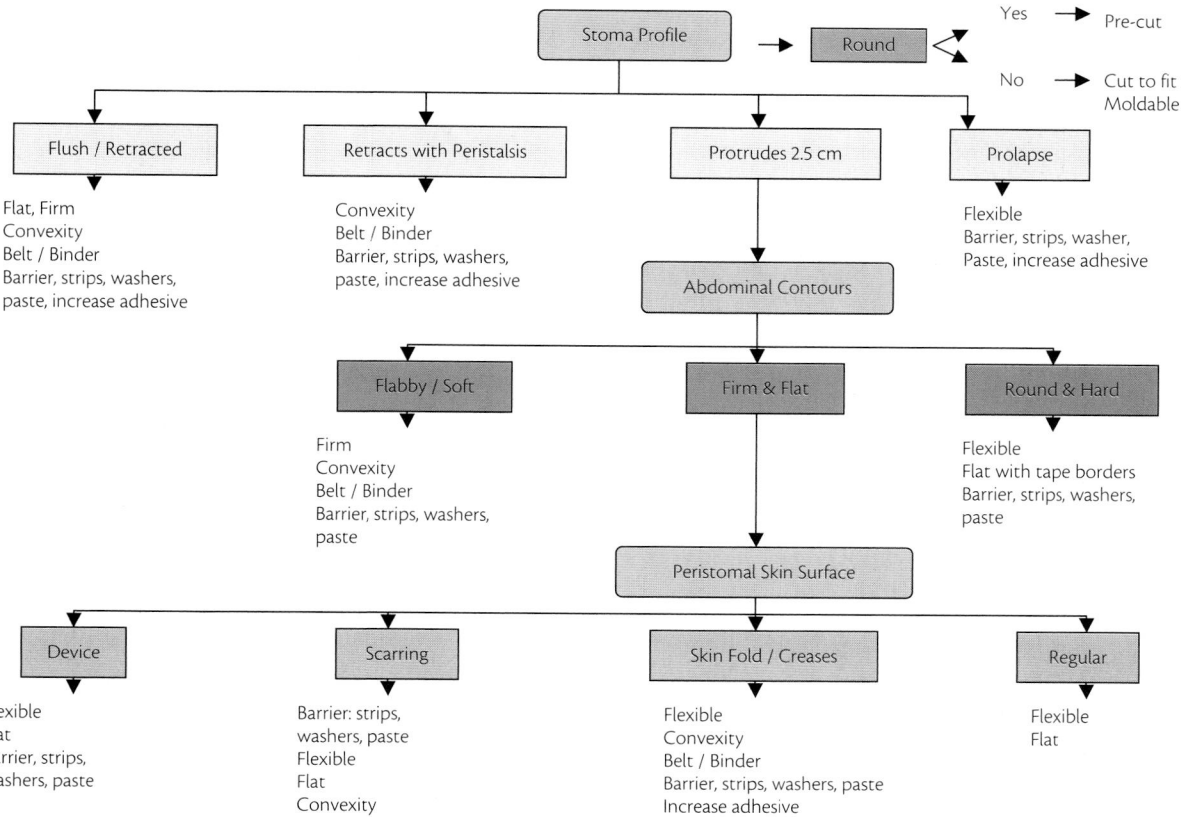

Figure 4.11.1 Algorithm: stoma faceplate selection.

protect it from maceration caused by stomal mucosal discharge or from excoriation secondary to leakage of effluent onto the skin. When possible, the patient or caregiver is taught how to reduce the prolapse stoma. With the patient in the supine position, a cold pack is applied to the pouch over the stoma (never directly on the stoma) to reduce the oedema, and then light pressure is gently applied to reduce the stoma. If the stoma can be reduced, the pouching system is applied after this is done[6].

Hernia is another complication often seen after emergency transverse loop colostomy surgery. During surgery, when the stoma is fashioned, an incision is made in the fascia to allow the intestine to be brought up to the skin level. Hernia results when loops of intestine protrude into this area of facial weakness.

A paracolostomy hernia may compromise a good pouching system seal for two reasons. First, the skin over the hernia relaxes and stretches, shifting the pouch seal. Second, the pouching system being used may not be flexible enough to mould around the abdominal bulge caused by the hernia. The end result of obtaining a poor seal is leakage of effluent and peristomal irritation. Hernia also causes some patient's discomfort in the area related to stretching of the hernia ring.

The stoma nurse specialist first confirms the presence of hernia by clinical presentation and a digital examination of the stoma. Imaging studies usually are not necessary to confirm the diagnosis, particularly in the setting of advanced illness. Conservative, non-surgical symptom management is recommended, including use of flexible pouching systems and support belts or binders. A hernia belt or binder can support the parastomal hernia and decrease the bulge, and in doing so, help to maintain pouching system seal. Irrigation, if used for colostomy regulation, is discontinued once the hernia is confirmed. The patient and caregivers are taught about the need to prevent constipation by proper diet, fluids, and when possible, exercise.

Another postoperative complication that requires the expertise of a stoma nurse specialist is mucocutaneous separation. Mucocutaneous separation, the detachment of the stoma from the skin, results from poor healing in patients who are malnourished, are receiving corticosteroids, or have varied disease-related or treatment-related complications in the region of the stoma.

The stoma nurse will assess the area of mucocutaneous separation by gently probing the area to determine its depth and circumference. If the defect is large, the base will be assessed for tissue type, such as necrotic or granulation tissue, and concurrently evaluated for the presence of a fistula.

Mucocutaneous separation is managed conservatively, if possible. The separation is filled with an appropriate dressing, either to maintain a moist environment or to absorb drainage. The goal is to facilitate granulation tissue formation and re-epithelization of the defect. The skin barrier of the pouching system fits over the filled area to provide protection from the effluent. The pouching system needs to be changed at least every 3 days to assess healing status.

Impaired skin integrity related to the leakage of effluent onto peristomal skin is the most common complication of poor fitting pouching system. The first goal in the management of this problem is to obtain a good pouching system seal for an established length of time. This allows the pouching system to be changed on a schedule rather than for leakage. The established length of time will depend on type of effluent and abdominal contour. Correctly sizing the pouching system's faceplate opening is crucial to obtaining a good seal. The standard rule is to cut the faceplate's opening size 1/8 inch larger than the stoma. The correct sizing of the faceplate opening helps prevent skin exposure to effluent, undermining of the seal, and trauma to the stoma. Skin barrier wafers, rings, and pastes are often used to improve the pouch seal by filling in scars, creases, or any uneven abdominal surfaces prior to the application of the faceplate. Skin barrier powders, wafers, and skin sealants are used to create an environment that facilitates healing of the damage peristomal skin by improving adherence of the faceplate; these may be applied prior to the pouching system. Perhaps the most traditional management of impaired peristomal skin includes cleansing with soap and water, dusting the impaired skin with a skin barrier powder, and then applying an alcohol-free skin sealant. Hydrocolloids may also used to treat the irritated peristomal skin.

The stoma nurse specialist also may assist the palliative care team in establishing a differential diagnosis or determining the aetiology of impaired skin integrity that appears unrelated to enzymatic damage from effluent or is poorly responsive to standard therapy. Peristomal skin abnormalities may include fungal infections, bacterial infections, and inflammatory conditions such as pyoderma gangrenosum. These peristomal skin conditions are more likely to occur near the end of life if the patient is immunosuppressed.

Continent diversions

Stoma nurse specialists also are consulted to manage problems associated with continent diversions, both urinary and faecal, when the patient is no longer able to be independent in self-care.

Patients with continent urinary diversions may no longer be able to independently catheterize the urinary reservoir as they become debilitated near the end of life. Therefore, caregivers need to be taught as how to do this procedure. The caregivers are taught to intubate the reservoir on a regular schedule, usually every 4 h throughout the day, and once at night. Taking into consideration the health-care needs of the caregiver, the intubation schedule may be adjusted by intubating the reservoir just before the caregiver goes to bed and on arising in the morning instead of during the night to allow for an uninterrupted sleep.

Another strategy to manage a continent urinary diversion is to place and maintain a catheter into the reservoir to facilitate drainage. The catheter is attached to a bedside drainage collector. This eliminates the need for scheduled intubation of the reservoir by caregivers. If leakage occurs from the continent urinary diversion, it can be pouched similar to a conventional urinary diversion.

If it is noted that there is an increase in mucous in the urinary output from the continent urinary diversion, the caregiver is taught to irrigate the reservoir once or twice daily with water, with or without acetylcysteine, or with normal saline. If the patient is able to participate in care, he or she is encouraged to keep the mucus thin by maintaining adequate fluid intake and by drinking 1–2 glasses of cranberry juice daily.

Similar management strategies may be needed for faecal continent diversion when the patient is no longer able to be independent in care. Caregivers are taught how to intubate a faecal continent pouch by inserting a large bore, #28–#30, lubricated French catheter through the nipple valve of the continent diversion using a gentle pressure and a slight twisting motion. Intubation is usually done four times daily and before bedtime. Water may be instilled into the internal pouch if the stool is too thick to facilitate pouch emptying with intubation. If intubation is difficult for the caregiver, the large bore catheter may be left in the internal pouch and connected to bedside drainage. To help maintain patency of the catheter, the patient is placed on a low residue diet, and irrigations with water or normal saline are performed on schedule and as needed. The continent faecal diversion can be pouched similar to a conventional faecal diversion if leakage from the internal faecal pouch occurs.

The stoma nurse specialist assists the caregiver with problem solving if the faecal output is too thick to facilitate drainage from the internal pouch. If possible, the patient is encouraged to increase fluid intake. Instillation of lukewarm water into the pouch may help to thin out the stool. Flushing the pouch once or twice daily may be necessary to prevent pouchitis caused by bacterial overgrowth secondary to faecal residue.

Management of gastrointestinal symptoms in a patient with a stoma

The development of either constipation or diarrhoea may complicate the management of a patient with an ostomy, and greatly increase the anxiety of the patient or caregiver. Both constipation and diarrhoea are common disorders in populations with advanced illness and strategies must be available for effective management when a stoma is part of the clinical picture.

Constipation is defined as a reduced frequency of bowel movements and an increased stool consistency often accompanied by feelings of cramping, bloating, and distention. Patients and their caregivers become very anxious when a stoma does not function secondary to constipation.

The prevalence of constipation among patients receiving palliative care services ranges from approximately 20 per cent to more than 50 per cent[7]. The most common cause presumably is the use of opioids for pain management. There are numerous other causes, however, including many non-opioid prescription and over-the-counter medications; metabolic conditions such as hypercalcaemia, hypokalaemia, or uraemia; partial bowel obstruction related to intraluminal tumour or extrinsic tumour or scarring; a variety of neurological disorders; immobility; impaired intake of adequate fibre and fluid; and psychosocial concerns[8]. Assessment of the patient who is constipated includes review of patient's medications, a history of stoma functioning and bowel habits, and an abdominal assessment. The patient or caregiver should be asked about frequency of stoma functioning, stool output, the appearance and consistency of stool, use of bowel medications, and any previous occurrences of constipation. A digital examination of the stoma may help identify faecal impaction. Physical examination of the abdomen for tenderness, distention, and bowel sounds is necessary to rule out intestinal obstruction. Radiographic imaging of the abdomen such as flat plate of the abdomen or computerized tomography to confirm a bowel obstruction is generally not necessary unless a surgical intervention for the bowel obstruction is being considered[9]. Serum electrolytes levels will identify hypercalcaemia or hypokalaemia.

In caring for a patient who has a stoma, the goal is to have the stoma function or for the patient to have a bowel movement every 1–2 days. Prevention of constipation is the key and both pharmacological and non-pharmacological strategies should be considered. Pharmacological management includes many types of laxatives, the most common types of which are stimulants or osmotic agents. There is little research to support the selection of laxatives in the setting of advanced illness. Empirically, the characteristics of the patient's constipation should be considered when selecting the laxative: hard stool requires a stool softener while soft but difficult to pass stool requires a stimulant. Patients receiving opioids therapy often require the routine use of a combination of stimulant and softening laxatives.

Non-pharmacologic approaches should be considered unless contraindicated by the patient's debility. These include planning a diet with adequate fibre and fluid, and encouraging activity, even if it must be limited to passive range of motion and isometric exercises to maintain some muscle strength for patients unable to get out of bed. Warm fluids with or after meals stimulate the bowel. Foods high in natural fibre include bran, oatmeal, shredded wheat, root vegetables, fruits, and whole wheat breads. Patients and families need to be educated relative to the need for increased fluid intake if the diet is high in fibre or if fibre supplements or bulk laxatives are taken. Without adequate fluid, constipation may worsen with these measures. Although it may be necessary to encourage fibre and fluids, it must always be remembered that the dietary emphasis in palliative care is on identifying patient's likes and desires.

Special issues arise in a patient who has a stoma when constipation occurs. If the patient is unable to take oral medications, suppositories via the colostomy may be helpful to relieve constipation. Glycerin suppositories may be placed in the stoma but must be held in place for 20 min to allow them to dissolve and prevent premature expulsion. If faecal impaction is a problem, an oil enema may be instilled via the colostomy at bedtime. The patient should be positioned on right side to allow the oil to penetrate across the transverse colon and down the ascending colon. Colostomy irrigation may be necessary after the use of oil enema for faecal impaction to facilitate emptying the colon; irrigation should be performed by the stoma nurse specialist, if possible[10].

Diarrhoea is defined as the frequent passage of loose, watery stools. At the end of life, diarrhoea can further compromise quality of life by leading to fatigue, insomnia, anorexia, dehydration, and electrolyte imbalance. Diarrhoea is a less common problem for patients with a stoma than constipation. Approximately 5–10 per cent of patients with advance cancer report diarrhoea[11]. The most common causes are laxative overdose, faecal impaction with overflow diarrhoea, and partial bowel obstruction. Other causes are radiation enteritis, medications such as chemotherapeutic drugs for colorectal cancer or antibiotics, steatorrhoea, graft versus host disease, and microbial infection of the bowel.

Assessment of an ostomy patient who has diarrhoea includes obtaining a history related to onset of diarrhoea, dietary habits, food intolerances, medications, and the frequency, colour and consistency of bowel movements. Abdominal assessment includes auscultation of bowel sounds and palpation for faecal or tumour mass. A stool specimen should be evaluated to determine the presence of any pathogens causing diarrhoea. The effectiveness of the pouching system needs to be evaluated in terms of changes in wear time, leakage, and any excoriation of peristomal skin.

Management of diarrhoea involves treatment of the underlying cause, preventing complications, and promoting comfort. Pharmacologic management includes the use of opioids or bulk-forming laxatives, and for severe or refractory diarrhoea, a trial of the somatostatin analogue, octreotide. Antibiotics are used to treat bacteria-induced diarrhoea.

The patient with a stoma who develops diarrhoea should be advised to avoid gas forming and bulky foods, hot spices, fats, alcohol, and milk until the diarrhoea resolves. Gradually adding foods such as white cooked rice, rice water, stewed apples or apple-sauce, bananas, and smooth peanut butter may help to manage the diarrhoea. Hydration status needs to be monitored. Beverages with added electrolytes, glucose, and water, like sport drinks, can help maintain fluid and electrolyte balance. The patient needs to be encouraged to drink fluids to prevent dehydration. The patients pouching system also may need to be adjusted. If the loose watery stools contain an increased concentration of enzymes, the skin barrier may disintegrate more easily. The patient may need to use extra skin barriers, e.g. washers, pastes, change to extended-wear skin barriers, or may need to change their pouching system more frequently. It is imperative to provide good peristomal skin care.

Draining wounds

Wounds that may be managed by the stoma nurse specialist include those with excessive drainage that cannot be contained with conventional dressings, or if contained with conventional dressing, those that require frequent dressing changes, with over-utilization of caregiver's time and resources. Moderate-to-high output draining wounds are best managed by pouching systems. There are numerous commercial wound drainage pouching systems available that contain self-adhesive skin barriers that can be cut to the size of the wound opening, providing protection for the periwound skin, and a pouch to collect and contain drainage. The pouch is often connected to bedside drainage to extend wear time of the pouching system and ease the management for the patient and caregivers. Suction can be applied to the pouching system to even further extend its wear time.

Percutaneous tubes

For the stoma nurse specialist, percutaneous tubes present the challenges of tube stabilization to prevent displacement and dilata-tion of the insertion site, and management to maintain or restore skin and tissue integrity.

Percutaneous tubes are often placed in the gastrointestinal tract, biliary system, and genitourinary tract or in an abscess cavity. Their function may be for the instillation of feedings or medications, irri-gations, or for drainage. Percutaneous gastrointestinal tubes are identified for the body part they enter, such as oesophagostomy, gastrostomy, jejunostomy, caecostomy, and biliary tubes. Percutaneous genitourinary devices include nephrostomy, ureter-ostomy, and vesicostomy tubes. Percutaneous tubes or drains can be placed in abscesses within or near the pancreas, peritoneal, pleura, or within the abdominal cavity to promote drainage of either serous or purulent exudates[12].

Each type of percutaneous tube has different potential cause of peritubular leakage. Potential leakage from enteral tubes includes functional problems such as gastric retention or distention, decreased gastrointestinal function, and mechanical problems of an overinflated or underinflated balloon. Gastric, biliary and urinary peritubular leakage may be secondary to mechanical problems of obstruction, inward or outward tube migration, tube displacement, or dilatation of insertion site secondary to tube size, tension of the tube, poor stabilization, or impaired peritubular skin healing. The level of risk for impaired skin or tissue integrity depends on the amount and type of peritubular leakage. Drainage that includes active enzymes from saliva, gastric, small bowel,

pancreas, or biliary system is caustic and has great potential to cause impaired peritubular skin integrity. Even minimal gastric leakage contains hydrochloric acid, gastric intrinsic factor and mucus that damage peritubular skin. Leakage around percutaneous genitourinary tubes also pose the risk for maceration.

Protocols can be established to maintain or restore skin integ-rity, and assure tube stabilization, in a number of ways. Pre-tube insertion, the stoma nurse specialist may discuss with the surgeon the optimal site for percutaneous tube insertion. Gastric tubes are best placed in a site approximately 5 cm to the left of the midline and 5 cm below the left costal margin and clear of the umbilicus. The site of insertion for all percutaneous tubes should be clear of bony prominences and creases. The correct tube size needs to be inserted, determined by location and purpose for insertion. Routine percutaneous tube site care includes assessing peritubular skin and insertion site for redness, tenderness, swelling, irritation, purulent drainage, or leakage; checking for tube position and patency; cleansing the site with soap and water or antiseptic of choice; and stabilizing the tube.

Percutaneous tube stabilization prevents tube migration, dislodgement, dilatation of the site, and peritubular leakage[13]. The physician or nurse should mark the tube with indelible ink at the tube entry site on placement. The nurse then assesses the tube placement daily by checking that the mark on the tube has not migrated inward or outward. Stabilization can be achieved by use of silicone discs, attachment or stabilization devices, or taping. Sutures are discouraged to prevent stitch granuloma.

When there is leakage around the tube, it is necessary to check the tube patency. Irrigation procedures depend on the type of tube. A percutaneous nephrostomy tube that is inserted directly into the renal pelvis should be irrigated with a maximum of 10 cc of sterile normal saline and only to check patency in the absence of urinary output, blood in the urine, or flank pain[14]. Irrigation of biliary tubes are discouraged unless absolutely necessary because of risk of causing a cholecystitis. If irrigated, they should be irrigated with 8–10 cc sterile normal saline. When irrigating a percutaneous nephrostomy or biliary tube, the irrigant should never be aspirated back. Gastrostomy and vesicostomy tubes that are inserted into the stomach or bladder, respectively, can be irrigated with larger amounts of saline because of the larger capacity of these organs.

Percutaneous tube stabilization and absorption of drainage from peritubular leakage can be achieved by combining products such as dressings for absorption (foams), use of silicones discs for tube stabilization, and adhesive dressing (tape) to hold the disc and dress-ing in place. If there is no leakage around the tube and skin integrity is intact, silicone disc to stabilize the tube and solid skin barrier wafers to hold the disc in place can be used. Commercial devices are also available to stabilize the tube. Tubes should be stabilized both proximally and distally. Proximally, stabilization should be close to the tube insertion site, to maintain correct tube position and prevent tube migration. Distally, stabilization should be at the free end of the tube. In this way, the tube is stabilized to prevent excessive tension or pulling on the tube, accidental tube dislodgement, or unnecessary tube rotation. Often, tape is used for this distal stabilization site.

When drainage around the tube becomes excessive and dressings cannot hold the amount of drainage or requires too frequent dressing changes, the tube can be pouched. Often, pouches with drainable spouts (urostomy or high output drainage pouches) are used to drain liquid or the less viscous exudate. If the exudate is viscous, open-ended pouches may be necessary. If it is necessary to use the tube for feeding, irrigation, or medication administration, the tube must be accessible outside the pouching system. The stoma nurse specialist helps develops protocols for pouching these tubes and allowing access by establishing systems that pull the tube out of the pouching system. One such technique is to pull the tube through hand-made hydrocolloid discs placed on either side of the pouch. A hole is made in the centre of the hydrocolloid disc and the tube is pulled through using a haemostat. The site of the tube that exits from the pouch is then sealed with a hydrocolloid/or skin barrier paste corking. Commercial exit ports are also available that allows for tubes/drains to be pulled out of pouch and still maintain a closed system to collect drainage.

The stoma nurse specialist also may be consulted to assist with management of peritubular complications known as hypertrophic granulation tissue formation. Hypergranulation tissue results from chronic inflammation secondary to a high bioburden and/or moisture at the site of tube insertion. Treatment involves the removal of the hypertrophic tissue by cauterization with silver nitrate sticks. Cauterization causes necrosis of the superficial granulation tissue that can then be rinsed or rubbed off. Selection of dressing in the peritubular area is significant in prevention and management of peritubular hypergranulation. Silicone gel dressings have preventative potential, and polyurethane foam type dressing reduce hypergranulation. Occlusive moisture retentive dressings should be avoided around tubes since they enhance the development of hypergranulation tissue[15].

Fistulas

Fistulas are abnormal connections between an organ and the skin or between two organs. Fistulas that communicate between an organ and the skin are called external fistula and, like tubes, are identified by the involved organs, e.g. colocutaneous, enterocutaneous, and vesicocutaneous. Fistulas that communicate between two internal organs are called internal fistulas; examples include-colovesical, colovaginal, vesicocolonic, and vesicovaginal. Often the internal fistulas drain through an anatomic opening in the perineal area. Fistulas are also defined by the volume of output: low volume output is <200 cc/24 h, moderate output is 200–500 cc/24 h, and high output is >500 cc/24 h[16].

Advanced abdominal cancers resulting in small bowel obstruction, abdominal sepsis, anastomotic leaks, or post-pelvic radiation complications may possibly result in formation of complex enterocutaneous fistulas for patients near the end of life[17]. These fistulas are often associated with high-volume output, abscess, and multiple organ involvement; they can open into the base of a disrupted wound. Similar to tubes/drains, fistulas present risks for the development of impaired skin and tissue integrity. The location of the fistula determines the type of effluent produced. Fistulas near the gastric, biliary, pancreatic, or small bowel areas drain corrosive effluent. Colonic fistulas output is less damaging to the skin. Fistulas place already compromised patients at further risk for sepsis, malnutrition, electrolyte disturbance, dehydration, and changes in body image.

The stoma nurse specialist can assist nurses and caregivers in management of various types of complex internal or external fistulas. The goals are to restore and protect peri-fistula skin, contain and quantify fistula output, control odour, promote patient comfort, and optimize the patient's physical functioning.

Providing a barrier over the peri-fistula skin to prevent skin contact with the fistula output provides skin protection. Using products such as solid skin barriers, liquid skin sealants, skin barrier powders, or pastes create the skin barrier. Solid skin barriers have an adhesive seal and are often integrated into a pouching system. Fistulas that are high output and have drainage corrosive to the skin require extended wear skin barriers to maintain protection and extend wear time of a containment system. The solid skin barrier needs to be extended 1.5 inches (~4cm) beyond the fistula edge. Fistulas that have small outputs can often be managed with skin barriers and gauze dressings.

A pouching system with an integrated skin barrier may manage a fistula that has a moderate to large volume of effluent that is irritating to the skin. The size and shape of the pouching system depends on the size and shape of the fistula, and the surrounding skin. The skin barrier opening must be cut large enough so that it rests flat on the skin surface. This means that skin folds, creases, and depressions are filled with skin barrier powders, pastes, and/or wafers, creating a flat surface prior to applying the pouching system. If it is not possible to create a flat surface and the pouching system must be cut (allowing skin to be exposed to the effluent), skin barrier pastes, washers, and powders can be used to protect the exposed skin. These are reapplied as necessary. An effective pouching system protects the peri-fistula skin, contains the fistula effluent, and directs the effluent to a bedside drainage collector. There are no standard intervals for changing a fistula pouch. Some systems will require changing every 24 h, and others will remain secure for up to 7 days. The changing schedule will depend on the ability to maintain a good seal and protect the peri-fistula skin.

If the volume of the fistula drainage overwhelms the pouching system and loosens the seal, connecting the pouching system to suction can extend the wear time. The pouch end can be connected to low continuous suction, or an opening can be made into the pouch, the suction catheter placed into the pouch, and the pouch opening around the suction catheter sealed using waterproof tape or products especially designed for this purpose, such as access ports.

Creation of a closed suction system is used when a high volume fistula is within a disrupted wound. A solid skin barrier is placed around the skin edge of the peri-wound-fistula, a layer of moistened saline gauze dressing is placed over the wound-fistula base to protect the tissue from desiccation, a suction catheter or suction drain is placed over the gauze and attached to low continuous suction, and finally the entire area is covered with a transparent film dressing to create an airtight seal. Skin barrier paste can be used over the site where the suction catheter or drain leaves the dressing to further secure an airtight seal. Additional methods of drainage containment include troughing procedures, saddle bagging, and bridging used in combination with pouching. More recently, negative pressure wound therapy has been used for management of fistulas within disrupted wounds[18].

The stoma nurse also may assist in the management of internal fistulas that need a system to collect drainage and protect skin, often from the rectal or vaginal areas. The goal again is to collect drainage and prevent skin from becoming excoriated from enzymes in stool or macerated from urine output. Pouches can be applied over either vaginal or anal orifices. Commercial rectal or vaginal pouches are available. These commercial pouching systems contain self-adhesive skin barriers to protect skin, a pouch to contain or collect output, and a spout that can be connected to bedside drainage if output is liquid. Clips are available for the pouching system if the output is more viscous. Several commercial faecal collection devices are also available.

Psychological issues

The care of the patient who has a stoma, a wound, or a fistula should include efforts that extend beyond the alleviation of the physical problems to specific strategies that address the emotional and spiritual needs of patients and caregivers near or at the end of life. These needs may revolve around changes in body image or involve depressed or anxious mood, various concerns and worries, or changes in relationships with family and others.

As a member of the treatment team, the stoma nurse can identify and characterize these needs, and attempt to help the patient and caregivers adapt to the challenges posed by the stoma, draining tubes, wounds, or fistulas. The patient is assisted through the grieving and adaptation process by supportive counselling. The stoma nurse assists the patient to explore feelings, identify major concerns, and problem solve in ways that will preserve the quality to their life.

The stoma nurse and the palliative care team must be careful not to mistakenly diagnose expected sadness when the patient is actually experiencing clinical depression. Depression needs to be identified and treated. The normal criteria used to diagnose depression of patients may not be valid near the end of life. Many dying patients normally experience weight loss, loss of energy, loss of appetite, and changes in sleep patterns, as well as think about death since death is actually approaching. Feelings of hopelessness, helplessness, worthlessness, guilt, and suicidal ideation are better indicators of depression in the terminally ill[19]. Optimal care for depression usually involves both supportive therapy and antidepressant medication.

It is normal for patients to have many concerns and worries near the end of life. The more common concerns include loss of independence, worries about family, concerns about the physical symptoms and problems, and feeling like a burden[20]. The stoma nurse may assist the rest of the team by addressing the physical symptoms and providing education to patient and caregivers related to stomas, tubes, and draining wounds and fistulas. Emotional support and education facilitates adaptation and makes an ostomy, tube, or fistula more manageable and less anxiety-producing. While caring for the physical needs of the patient, emotional support is provided to help the patient maintain control, dignity and a sense of purpose or meaning.

Psychological adjustment is required following surgery for a stoma, placement of a permanent percutaneous tube, or development of a draining wound or fistula. These procedures or pathologies can have a profound effect on the patient's physical appearance and ability to function; the experience may be traumatic and perceived as a violation of body integrity. No matter where a patient is on the health-illness continuum, body image reflects the way a patient sees and feels about himself or herself. For each patient, coming to terms with a stoma, tube, wound, or fistula is a deeply personal experience. How the patient reacts depends on his or her feelings, attitudes, and experiences toward their body. The patient's self-perception will influence their behaviour, opinion, and mental health and well-being[21]. An unacceptable body image may influence how the patient interacts with their caregivers and the palliative care team. Patients who endure significant changes in body image, self-concept, and self-esteem may experience grief and loss. The stoma nurse may help by providing education, assisting with identification of ineffective coping mechanisms, and promoting effective coping skill and stress management techniques. Patients view effective coping as a strategy that increases hope and improves ability to handle problems. Coping styles that have shown to be most effective and used by patients are those that are optimistic and self reliant in nature[22].

Special attention needs to be given to the psychological support and counselling of caregivers, including the family. The stoma nurse needs to assess the patient's support system and determine the caregivers' emotional status and ability to provide care for the patient. In a study done to evaluate how relatives of patients with an ostomy rated the various aspects of care, information and counselling offered to relatives was judged to be unsatisfactory[23]. The patient's caregivers and families need to be treated as part of the team and be given the opportunity to participate in consultations and in the decision-making process regarding the patient's care. The stoma nurse specialist must talk to the caregivers and families directly and determine how they are managing and coping with the situation. It is critical to provide supportive counselling for caregivers and families, as well as for the patient.

Cultural issues

When caring for patient near the end of life, it is important not to understand patients and their caregivers only through their clinical descriptions, as seen through the eyes and culture of medicine and nursing. The cultural background of patients needs to be understood in order to provide quality care. Although it is important to address cultural variables such as language, religion, family roles, sick care, and death practices, simply identifying this type of information runs the risk of stereotyping patients and their caregivers. Cultural beliefs are fluid and changeable. The stoma nurse should collaborate with the palliative care team in providing care that is both culturally competent and sensitive. Cultural competency requires knowledge of the cultural and ethnic values, beliefs, and behaviours held by each patient and family. Cultural sensitivity requires the nurses' awareness and respect for patient's cultural values, beliefs, and views[24].

Summary

The presence of an ostomy, draining wound, tubes, or fistula has a great impact on the everyday life of the patient and their caregivers. The stoma nurse specialist can make major contributions to the palliative care provided to patients and caregivers by encouraging a variety of important outcomes, including:

◆ Development and implementation of strategies to prevent and/or manage complications related to stoma leakage, draining wounds/tubes, and fistulas, such as, impaired skin integrity and infection.

◆ Prevention or management of pain secondary to impaired skin integrity or removal of dressings and tapes.

◆ Containment, and when necessary, measurement of exudate/drainage.

◆ Control of odour.

- Promotion of increased comfort and rest for patient and caregivers secondary to proper use of pouching/containment systems which result in need for minimal dressing or pouch changes in the presence of excessive drainage.

- Enhancement of patient and caregivers independence.

- Reduction of emergency room visits and hospitalizations for management of stomal, tubes, draining wounds, and fistulas complications.

- Increased staff, patient, and caregiver satisfaction.

- Improvement or restoration of body image and acceptability of self-concept near or at the end of life.

There is little research available on the impact of the treatments championed by the stoma nurse specialist in palliative care. A palliative care programme needs to be developed for the illness-specific population—those with ostomies, tubes, draining wounds/fistulas. Such a programme would identify the specific services offered; provide algorithms to manage specific symptoms experienced by patient with ostomies, tubes, draining wounds and fistulas; educate the health care community about the services offered; and contribute to the evidence–base relative to the treatment of these disorders.

References

1. (2004). Clinical practice guidelines for quality palliative care. *National Consensus Project for Quality Palliative Care*, **1**, 3.

2. Boarini, J., Colwell, J.C., Lovejoy, L. *et al.* (2004). Roles of the ostomy nurse specialist: historical perspective, role potential. In *Fecal & urinary diversions management principles* (ed. J.C. Colwell), pp. 18–29. Mosby, Inc., St Louis, MO.

3. Dirkson, S.R. (1995). Search for meaning in long-term cancer survivors. *Journal of Advanced Nursing*, **21**(4), 628–34.

4. Barr, J.E. (2003). *Selection of stoma faceplate.* Presentation at WOCN National Conference.

5. Vasilevsky, C.A. and Gordon, P.H. (2004). Gastrointestinal cancers: surgical management. In *Fecal & urinary diversions management principles* (eds. J.C. Colwell, M.T. Goldberg, and J.E. Carmel), p. 132. Mosby, Inc., St Louis, MO.

6. Wound, Ostomy and Continence Nurses Society (2003). *Stoma complications: a best practice document for clinicians.*

7. Conill, C., Verger, E., Henriquez, I. *et al.* (1997). Symptom prevalence in the last week of life. *Journal of Pain and Symptom Management*, **14**(6), 328–31.

8. Alexander, L.L. MTPW, ELS. (2006). *Pain management, palliative care and treatment of the terminally ill.* Continuing Education Medical Resource. Course #9727, 41–6.

9. Heidrich, D.E. (2002). Diarrhea. In *End of life care: clinical practice guidelines* (eds. K.K. Kuebler, P.H. Berry, and D.E. Heidrich), p. 292. Saunders, Philadelphia, PA.

10. Black, P.K. (2000). Assessment and management of stomas, fistulas, catheters, and drainage tubes in palliative care. In *Holistic stoma care*. Harcourt Publishers, London, pp. 111–5.

11. Waller, A. and Caroline, N.L. (2000). *Handbook of palliative care in cancer*. Butterworth-Heinemann, Boston, MA.

12. Faller, N.A., Beitz, J.M., and Orkin, B.A. (2007). When a wound is not a wound: tubes, drains, fistulas, and draining wounds. In *Chronic wound care: a clinical source book for healthcare professionals*, 4th edition (eds. D.L. Krasner, G.T. Rodeheaver and G. Sibbald), pp. 735–42. HMP Communications, Malvern, PA.

13. O'Brien, B., Davis, S., and Erwin-Toth, P. (1999). G-tube site care: a practical guide. *RN*, **62**(2), 52–6.

14. Cofield, V.A. (1995). Percutaneous nephrostomy tubes: nursing care. *Urologic Nursing*, **15**(4), 128–30.

15. Sussman, C. (2007). Assessment of the skin and wound. In *Wound care a collaborative practice manual* (eds. C. Sussman and B. Bates-Jensen), p. 114. Lippincott William & Wilkins, Philadelphia, PA.

16. Berry, S.M. and Fischer, J.E. (1996). Classification and pathophysiology of enterocutaneous fistulas. *Surgical Clinics North America*, **76**, 1009–18.

17. Rolstad, B.S. and Bryant, R.A. (2000). Management of drains sites and fistulas. In *Acute and chronic wounds: nursing management* (ed. R.A. Bryant), pp. 317–39. Mosby Inc., St Louis, MO.

18. Cro, C., George, K.J., Donnelly, J. *et al.* (2002). Vacuum-assisted closure system in the management of enterocutaneous fistulas. *Postgraduate Medical Journal*, **78**, 364–5.

19. Roth, A.J. and Breitbart, W. (1996). Psychiatric emergencies in terminally ill cancer patients. *Hematology/Oncology Clinics of North America*, **10**, 235–59.

20. Heaven, C. and Maguire, P. (1998). The relationship between patient's concerns and psychological distress in a hospice setting. *Psycho-Oncology*, **7**, 502–7.

21. Borwell, B. (1997). Psychological considerations of stoma care nursing. *Nursing Standard*, **11**(48), 49–55.

22. Reynaud, S.N. and Meeker, B.J. (2002). Coping styles of older adults with ostomies. *Journal of Gerontological Nursing*, **28**(5), 30–6.

23. Persson, E., Gustavsson, B., Hellstrom, A.L. *et al.* (2005). Information to the relatives of people with ostomies: is it satisfactory and adequate? *JWOCN*, **32**(4), 238–45.

24. Crawley, L.M., Marshall, P.A., and Koenig, B.A. (2001). Respecting cultural differences at the end of life. In *Physician's guide to end-of-life care, American College of Physicians-American Society of Internal Medicine End-Of Life Consensus Panel* (eds. L. Synder and T.E. Quill), pp. 38–42. American College of Physicians, Philadelphia, PA.

The contribution of clinical psychology to palliative care

Fiona Cathcart

Introduction

During the last two decades, clinical psychologists have increasingly participated in the care of populations with acute and chronic medical illnesses, including those that are life-limiting. People with cancer and other life-threatening disease often experience significant psychosocial distress. Although the psychological literature focuses predominantly on the care of patients newly diagnosed or those receiving curative treatment, recently more has been published on psychological assessment and intervention in palliative care specifically. Studies of patients receiving specialist palliative care have focused on the needs of those with cancer, despite the evidence of unmet psychological needs in patients with other conditions, such as heart failure and advanced chronic obstructive pulmonary disease[1,2]. This may reflect the challenges of research in palliative care, as well as the relative lack of clinical psychologists available to undertake this work.

Psychological models

Psychological interventions use the evidence-base of modern psychology. Specifically, interventions are based on research into how individuals learn, think, feel, and interact, both with their environment and the people within it. A psychologist may suggest that a problem could be tackled more effectively by changing an aspect of the care system or the physical environment, rather than working with the person directly. Clinical psychologists may direct their efforts to improve care at the level of the individual; groups of individuals such as a family, patient group, or staff group; or at an organizational level. The choice of intervention will be influenced also by the setting in which it is delivered. This may be the person's home in the community, a palliative care ward in a large general hospital, or a specialist unit.

Psychological assessment

Many people access specialist palliative care services after having had a long history of interventions while experiencing gradually deteriorating health. Although they may have had opportunities to acknowledge their increasing frailty, they may or may not have done so. Others will have progressed rapidly from apparent good health to a poor prognosis, and may be experiencing a sense of shock and confusion.

Family members or others who care for the person who is ill may suffer psychological problems and physical ills themselves. Some neglect their own health to care for dependants. A recent case is illustrative: an elderly man visited his wife daily and spent hours by her bedside, occasionally rubbing his painful back. After her death, he attended his physician and discovered the pain was caused by bone metastases from an unsuspected primary tumour. His shock was compounded by his recent bereavement. In specialist palliative care, the unit of care is the family, and assessment strategies for psychological distress and its potential implications should include primary caregivers and others as appropriate.

Communicating bad news is a significant challenge at the time of diagnosis and repeatedly thereafter, as issues must be addressed as the disease progresses, other health professionals no longer maintain follow-up, or interventions which had been helpful are no longer effective. The person who adjusted well initially to the life-threatening diagnosis may experience greater distress subsequently and require more support. Leaflets, audiotapes, and videotapes have been developed in an effort to reduce the sense of confusion and loss of control, and to facilitate informed decision-making[3]. These are helpful, but should not obscure the importance of addressing the emotional component of communication as well as the need for factual information. Innes cautioned that the provision of comprehensible information is important but may not be sufficient to address the concerns prioritized by the patient[4]. Patients may not prioritize the same issues for research either; the authors of one small study, for example, comment that patients focused less on symptoms than anticipated and more on communication skills, despite the increase in communication training for doctors in recent years[5]. Other authors suggest that patients are looking for information which acknowledges the serious nature of the illness but conveys hope and potential gains, such as revised values in relationships[6].

Although a variety of valid tools is available to assist in the evaluation of psychological distress, busy clinicians are more likely to use a brief screening instrument and refer to specialist help if necessary. Screening for psychological or other sources of distress can be done effectively with a unidimensional screening tool, such as the so-called 'Distress Thermometer'. This simple screening measure, a picture of a vertical thermometer on which the patient is asked to indicate the severity of distress, was developed to reflect distress across a number of areas of potential concern, including the physical, practical, family, emotional, and spiritual. It has been incorporated into a clinical pathway intended to guide the follow-up assessment and management of the sources of distress[7]. Other brief screening methods for distress are available and could be adapted to various clinical uses[8].

Simple screening approaches also may be helpful in the assessment of more specific problems, such as depression. The question.'Are you depressed?' was as effective in detecting depressed patients as a more lengthy assessment in a Canadian population, but was less sensitive and specific with a UK population[9].

A willingness to explore patients' distress is fundamental to palliative care and can be effective in itself. Clinicians may be more willing to elicit psychological problems if they believe that there are effective psychological interventions. Staff may need to ensure, however, that the assessment does not become limited to those domains that produce the least discomfort to the clinician. The dialogue between staff and patients can be steered to those problems that the clinician believes can be solved by intervention or through consultation[10]. Although this is understandable and may help the clinician maintain an important sense of professional optimism, it also may leave the patient with unresolved problems.

The methodological problems in evaluating the outcome of psychosocial interventions in patients with advanced disease are formidable. Studies have faced the challenge of recruitment, attrition, the selection of appropriate psychometric measures and precise description of the intervention used[11]. Frequently, the intervention combines several treatment strategies. A range of strategies is described below.

Interventions with the individual patient

The types of interventions are as follows:

1 *Goal-setting.*

2 *Problem-solving.*

3 *Relaxation and hypnosis.*

4 *Cognitive behaviour therapy.*

5 *Counselling and psychotherapy.*

6 *Behavioural strategies.*

Goal-setting

Early in the development of palliative care, it was argued that palliative care would be improved by goal-setting rather than by eliciting problem lists[12]. This process does not deny the limits set by the disease, but keeps the focus of care on what might still be achieved. Generating a problem list can be a demoralizing exercise for both patient and carer, whereas identifying simple goals informs the direction of care and enables short-term targets to be negotiated. Goal-setting is used extensively in rehabilitation services and could assist patients with advanced illness, and those caring for them, maintain a sense of purpose when efforts seem futile.

Goal-setting is most effective when certain conditions are met. The goals should be realistic, time limited, and specific. They also should be patient-centred, in that the goal is valued by the patient rather than imposed by another. They must be reviewed and modified over time as appropriate.

A case example illustrates a potential approach to goal-setting: A woman with advanced cancer hopes to enjoy her first grandchild, who is due in 2 months. She is no longer mobile and it is uncertain if she will live long enough. Small steps are negotiated, each of which would help her achieve her ultimate goal, if her illness progresses slowly, but which have intrinsic value if not. She may decide to perform simple daily exercises to maintain strength in the arms with which she hopes to hold the baby; she may speak into an audiocassette for a few minutes each day to record bedtime stories or favourite recipes for the future grandchild. By identifying the component parts of a larger goal, patients can learn to pace themselves and benefit from small and meaningful successes. Pacing reduces the sense of powerlessness that can occur when patients face many losses.

Focus on overactivity/rest cycle, which is a familiar concept to those working with patients with chronic pain, is another strategy for pacing in populations with advanced illness. Many patients feel too fatigued to accomplish activities and try to compensate by doing as much as possible when feeling a little stronger. The ensuing exhaustion confirms the erroneous belief that all energy is being drained by the disease, thereby increasing distress. A more realistic explanation may be that the fatigue is a combination of the limits set by the disease and the way of responding to it, and patients taught to pace themselves can learn to appreciate the difference between avoidable and unavoidable fatigue and regain some sense of control.

Problem-solving

Teaching problem-solving can help reduce the sense of being overwhelmed and help regain lost confidence. One study of cancer patients with a good prognosis[13] indicated lower distress at a 1-year follow-up if a significant other had participated in the intervention also. A small pilot study in which problem-solving skills were taught to patients indicated that this approach is feasible in the palliative care setting[14].

Relaxation and other interventions

The use of relaxation in the management of anxiety is widely accepted. It is practised both with individuals and within groups. Even a frail and bed-bound patient may be able to use a small audio device with earphones to access this type of intervention. Patients should be assessed on an individual basis and the rationale for using relaxation explained carefully. A small minority of patients experience an increase in anxiety or panic attacks when practising relaxation. This paradox may be caused by feelings of vulnerability and loss of control. Identifying the reasons for this and modifying the approach may be necessary.

A meta-analysis concluded that relaxation training reduced treatment-related symptoms and improved emotional adjustment in patients receiving acute non-surgical cancer treatments[15]. The SIGN Guidelines for the control of cancer pain stated there was enough evidence to recommend that services should offer training in some form of relaxation appropriate to the individual patient as an additional strategy to pharmacological pain management[16].

Specific advice tailored to the individual's needs may be necessary also. A case exemplifies this tailoring: a woman who was anxious during radiotherapy tried to practise the deep relaxation she had learned at antenatal classes but found the noise of the treatment equipment interfered. It was suggested that incorporating the extraneous sound into her imagery would be more effective than trying to block the sound out. Her chosen imagery was relaxing in a cornfield and she successfully incorporated the sound as agricultural machinery working nearby.

Teaching patients to transform an image can be a potent intervention itself. There is an evidence from the mental health setting that recurrent nightmares and intrusive imagery can be alleviated by rehearsing alternative positive endings. A case illustrates this: a woman with breast cancer had distressing dreams of her body being devoured by snakes. This was discussed and she created alternative images successfully herself. At the next session, she recounted a dream in which the menacing snakes were being devoured by jewelled serpents and her nightmare ceased.

Other cognitive techniques may be considered in this setting as well. A recent systematic review of guided imagery as a sole adjuvant therapy reported that there seemed to be some benefit, but the poor quality of trials prevented firm conclusions[17]. There is debate as to whether hypnosis is a distinct state or not[18], and although there is experience that suggests the value of hypnosis in alleviating pain and distress in palliative care[19], a systematic review reported that the poor quality of studies limits any conclusions about its efficacy in this setting[20]. The use of imagery is a key component in many of these interventions, but in practice, a combination of strategies may be best to achieve the desired effect, which is a sense of calm and focused attention. The best approach usually is guided by the preferences of the patient.

Cognitive behaviour therapy

Cognitive behaviour therapy teaches patients to challenge habitual ways of thinking or behaving which may exacerbate emotional distress. Cognitive behavioural interventions have been used successfully in oncology and palliative care[21,22]. Although fatigue, poor concentration and increasing frailty near the end of life may limit cognitive exploration, targeted interventions may be possible even in those who are very ill. Santos and Greer, for example, describe a patient who was able to benefit within days of his death but acknowledge the intervention may have successful because of the goal-setting component and the opportunity to discuss his fears, rather than through an understanding of the way in which his cognitions influenced his mood[23].

Counselling and individual psychotherapies

Counselling may be part of the care provided by members of the palliative care team, or may be offered by referral to other specialists or agencies. A study of an independent cancer counselling service in London indicated that it was positively viewed by those who completed evaluations[24]; it is not clear from this report, however, how many of those using this service were newly diagnosed and what proportion had advanced disease. The authors comment on the gender and social class bias of those who choose to use such a service and whether or not it would meet the needs of other sectors of the population.

A psychodynamic model of psychotherapy has been influential[25], but interest is growing in existential psychotherapy. The latter approach emphasizes strategies that assist patients in constructing meaning from their lives and impending death. Loss of meaning in life may be experienced by those with progressive illnesses and parallel the experiences reported by those bereaved traumatically when their assumptions of order and predictability are destroyed by a natural or manmade disaster[26]. Patients who feel unable to make sense of their lives or impending deaths may experience suffering which is unrelated to physical symptoms.

Chochinov and colleagues have developed an intervention, Dignity Therapy, to address this type of suffering by enabling patients to reflect on their lives a structured way[27]. Participants are invited to consider their varied roles and accomplishments, what has been important to them, and what they would most want remembered. If they wish, this is transcribed and edited with them to give to a significant other. Early studies in Canada and Australia indicate that this intervention is beneficial and there is current research into its feasibility in a Scottish hospice. Dignity Therapy is similar to life review, which has a long history in palliative care. A recent Japanese study suggested that life review was beneficial but patient selection was important[28].

Behavioural strategies

As people live longer with advanced illness, including cancer, some issues that are relevant in the management of chronic disease care become relevant in the management of life-limiting illness. For example, the disability that occurs in the context of chronic pain may have parallels in populations with serious medical illness, and as a result, the approaches used to minimize disability can have relevance for palliative care. Although it can be difficult to assess whether a new complaint relates to factors other than disease progression, careful observation may reveal an association with other factors, such as visiting time or an adjacent patient receiving care. A clinical unit may be busy for staff, but lacking in stimulation for patients. Patients may learn that staff attention is given only for symptom complaints, and this may unintentionally reinforce patterns of patient behaviour focused on symptoms. Similarly, health complaints may have been used to control the behaviour of relatives for many years, and it is unlikely that these dynamics change at the door of the palliative care unit.

Redd describes interventions in oncology and a palliative care setting in which symptoms that were troublesome to the patient or disruptive to the care of other patients were modified successfully by changing the staff response to them[29,30]. This type of approach does not appear to have been used often for a number of reasons. There are difficulties in using a behavioural programme consistently in a busy unit, where few staff have training or experience in operant methods[31]. Also, staffs who are attracted to palliative care may find it difficult to redirect their attention, and even when staff have found a behavioural approach helpful, they hesitate to use it again (R. Hillier, personal communication).

Case examples

In practice, it is often useful to consider the concurrent application of several types of psychological intervention. This is illustrated by the following case: a patient with advanced disease receiving palliative care was referred to the clinical psychologist for bereavement support and advice on managing the psychological component of her breathlessness. Additional issues emerged including the significance of past sibling dynamics, which caused friction among the current carers and a tense relationship with her adult child. Intervention required anxiety management, bereavement counselling, ventilation of past and present frustrations and family therapy. Sufficient progress was made that, when she died peacefully a few weeks later, her daughter was present and there was no conflict at the bedside.

Another case similarly demonstrates the combined use of several strategies to address multiple sources of distress: A young woman was diagnosed with advanced cancer. She was withdrawn, angry and complained frequently of pain which was difficult to assess and manage. She refused psychological intervention initially, but at the third attempt she agreed and thereafter used the sessions constructively. She distrusted health professionals, attributing this to her mother's unexpected death after a routine procedure some years before. The senior physician suggested she contact him directly with any concerns and see only him. This was interpreted as confirming the basis for her fears rather than reassurance that her needs would be met. She challenged the clinical team by demanding more help while rejecting all their efforts as useless. Her way of thinking about her pain exacerbated it, in that she catastrophized her sensations. The psychological intervention targeted her pain cognitions and helped her develop other strategies for coping with it. The relevance of her anger at her mother's death to her own situation was explored. Modest goals were negotiated, which gave her another focus and enabled the staff to engage in a more rewarding interaction. The prepubertal daughter was a close observer who modelled on her mother. She was frequently present and witnessed her mother's distress and hostility. The girls's own understanding and expectations of health care were being shaped by her interpretation of events. When efforts to engage the mother were successful, the girl interacted more positively with staff. This countered the developing family myth that all health professionals are untrustworthy. Two days before her death, the patient was enjoying visitors in the hospice garden. In this case, the effective care given has not only made the daughter's memories of her mother's dying less distressing but also been an investment for the future when the girl may need health care herself.

These two examples illustrate that pain and symptoms are not experienced in an interpersonal vacuum. Pharmacological and physical interventions are important, but are less effective unless psychological issues are addressed also.

Interventions with groups

Groups may be viewed as a more cost-effective way of delivering the same intervention to large numbers, or as having intrinsic worth because of the group dynamics. Spiegel and his colleagues reported that weekly psychological support meetings for women with metastatic breast cancer provided psychological benefits and also increased survival time[32]. Subsequent research has not confirmed a survival advantage, but has demonstrated benefits on mood and pain perception[33]. Cunningham and associates argue that a correlative approach, which relates the survival of individuals to their psychological work, as measured by qualitative data, does suggest a relationship between intervention and outcome[34], but a discussion of the structure and themes of Supportive-Expressive Group Therapy concurs that there is psychological gain but no apparent gain in survival[35]. The most recent critical review of the evidence for cancer support groups concluded there were no survival benefits but worthwhile gains in quality of life[36].

Further research should be undertaken before it can be assumed that the benefits in one country can be generalized to other cultures. A group therapy intervention was undertaken with women with metastatic breast cancer living in northeast Scotland. The psychometric scores did not show significant changes but the process analysis revealed that the group was helpful to some participants.

The authors concluded there was not strong evidence for this type of support in this particular cultural context[37].

The family

Psychological interventions may be focussed on couples, rather than individuals. McWilliams argues that there is a dual nihilism about creating psychological change in elderly people who also have palliative care needs, but describes successful psychotherapy with a married couple in their eighties based on the theoretical foundation of attachment theory[38]. Many families are able to offer emotional and practical support to the patient and work with the team. Others are distrustful of staff and both demanding and challenging of any care given.

Jenkins and Bruera cite the 'Daughter from California syndrome'[39], which depicts the tensions that arise when an absent relative returns to be confronted with a deteriorating patient and decisions being made by others. One explicit way to demonstrate concern and assert one's presence is to question the care given; a high standard of care may mean more vigorous attempts to fault-find. In this situation, it may be helpful to engage the relative in practical tasks so there is less need to use criticism of care to prove concern.

In some situations, the distress and problematic behaviours of family members have other, deeper causes, and a more rigorous assessment is needed to clarify the nature of the problem and develop a plan to address it. A case is illustrative: a daughter was making increasingly frantic attempts to communicate with her unresponsive dying mother. She persistently asked if her mother could hear or understand. On interview, it emerged the daughter had been sexually abused by the father and it was her last chance to resolve this with her mother and confirm whether she had known. Support through this crisis and subsequent referral to the community psychologist was arranged.

The contribution of clinical psychology to the team

◆ Helping staff formulate a problem in a psychological way.

◆ Teach a specific skills and interventions, for example, relaxation, cognitive behaviour therapy.

◆ Supervise specific cases.

◆ Joint working.

◆ Support team decision-making and cohesiveness.

Patients face a psychological challenge when living with life-limiting illness but this does not mean that all patients need to see a psychologist. The skills of the clinical psychologist may be more appropriately used in developing the psychological skills of other staff. The concept of triage is familiar in medicine when there is a need to deploy limited resources effectively. This principle applies to psychological care also. If a palliative care unit has access to a weekly session with the clinical psychologist, then it would be misguided to fill that time solely with direct patient care. More patients could benefit from psychological expertise if some or all of this time were spent in staff training and supervision. The Supportive and Palliative Care Guidance for England and Wales suggests a four-level model of delivery of support based on psychological need and practitioner training[40].

Raise psychological awareness

General medical and nursing staff work hard to achieve pain and symptom control and may feel bewildered or angry when these attempts fail. Raising awareness of psychological issues can lead to more useful interventions and less wasted effort. A relevant analogy is the person running faster but up the wrong ladder. Given the scarcity of clinical psychologists in general medical settings, the model of psychologist as consultant/trainer to staff can be an effective way of ensuring that more patients benefit from psychological knowledge.

Teach a specific skill

There is a clear advantage in making psychological treatments available to more patients by teaching them to staff. Doctors and nurses in oncology who were trained in behavioural treatments were as effective as clinical psychologists in reducing chemotherapy-induced nausea and vomiting[41]. Palliative care practitioners may have been trained in the techniques of cognitive behaviour therapy, but follow-up supervision is needed to maintain skills and the confidence to use them[42].

Supervision with specific cases

Supervision with specific cases can improve the care provided by front-line staff and encourage the use of specific psychological interventions. Jones *et al.*[43] describe team members feeling increasingly helpless in the face of the increasing distress and deterioration of a woman they had known over a period of months. The clinical psychologist was unable to see the patient but was able to supervise an intervention which enabled her existing carers to maintain their relationship and relieve some of her distress. This not only helped the immediate situation but also developed their future clinical skills.

Joint working

Joint working can enable each professional to achieve desired outcomes more easily. A case illustrates this process: a man with advanced lung cancer was referred to the clinical psychologist because of low mood and anxiety. There were many issues, but it emerged that the main focus of his sadness was his fear that he would be forgotten by his young son, who lived with his estranged wife. This fear was explored, and after some discussion, the man decided to make a gift for his son and future grandchildren, which he could leave in safekeeping with his own parents. The feasibility of this project was discussed with the occupational therapist, who enabled the patient to complete the task despite the limits of his concentration and fatigue.

Another case demonstrates another type of joint working: an elderly woman with a disfiguring facial tumour and limited mobility experienced anxiety and low self-esteem. A cognitive-behavioural intervention helped her leave the confines of her room and become more confident in social situations. Nurses and other staff were primed for her early ventures and praised any attempts to extend her range. Finally, she used her wheelchair expeditions to purchase items from the craft department which she used as gifts for visitors. This enabled her to regain her sense of herself as a giver rather than a passive receiver of care and helped her overcome her sense of self-worth.

Support team decision-making and cohesiveness

Some patients or families may have interacted in an aggressive or manipulative way for many years with the people and the organizational systems they encounter. They have the potential to disrupt the team, behaviours that can mirror past angry or rejecting relationships[44]. Personal relationships are highly valued by palliative care staff and they can find it challenging to work with those do not or cannot share this. The realistic role of the mental health professional in this situation may be one of limiting damage by these patients to themselves and others[45].

There can be barriers to organizing team support in a large system such as a general hospital. Cull describes a practical way of eliciting and addressing staff problems when it is not possible for group discussion to take place[46]. A forum for ventilating concerns can help staff feel that problems have been identified and the lesson incorporated into practice. There may be no new lesson to be learned but simply a need to express sadness or anger.

A reflection group is less intimidating for some team members, but more intimidating for others. Support groups are not necessarily helpful and can deteriorate into a 'grouse group'. When functioning well, however, they can be an effective resource for the team. Individual professional supervision can help junior staff manage challenging situations. Having seniority does not confer emotional immunity, although it can help understand what is happening[47].

Palliative care staff tend to dismiss the efforts of those staff in other specialities who seek 'a cure' and who abandon patients when their efforts fail. These staff may themselves then pursue the goal of a 'good death' and may feel equally frustrated when they cannot alleviate distress. This can lead to criticism of oneself, the team or the patient. There is a need to find a balance between complacency and accepting fallibility. Unrealistic goals lead to low morale and dissatisfaction. A high degree of self-criticism was found to be linked to professional stress in a study of general practitioners[48]. More training may increase professional knowledge, but professional maturity can remain elusive. Bennet discusses the doctor's loss in surrendering idealistic illusions but argues they are exchanged for more rewarding realities[49].

Caring for the patient with cognitive and sensory impairments

Cognitive impairment is prevalent in many patients receiving palliative care. Confusion may mild or profound, and may or may not be reversible. Short screening measures are available, and unless used routinely, there is a risk that cognitive problems will not be detected[50].

A formal cognitive assessment is relevant in determining the need for specific medical interventions and in clarifying the psychological plan of care. It also is important to support decision-making. Conflicts or concerns about whether the person is competent to give informed consent must be resolved.

When the patient is cognitively impaired, psychological consultation may need to address specific behaviours. For example, a patient may attempt to assault staff. In some circumstances, this challenging behaviour can be reduced by increasing the patient's sense of control and predictability over the immediate environment. For example, the patient could have a personal box which contains prompts for routine procedures. A person with visual and auditory impairments could touch items which would help anticipate the planned interaction, such as a toothbrush, a cup, a dosette tube, lavatory paper, or a piece of dressing material.

A patient with impaired sensory or cognitive abilities may require specific assistance to support the attempt to function as independently as possible. As a reaction against the impersonal clinical surrounding of a hospital ward, hospices create a home-like atmosphere. Unfortunately, neither a clinical environment nor a home-like environment may be helpful to the elderly person trying to reach the toilet independently but unable to find the correct door in time. Units which have been designed for the care of people with cognitive impairments address the need for a 'prosthetic environment'. The judicious use of colour and shape can facilitate orientation by attracting attention to some areas and minimizing others. One unit for people with multiple disabilities used sections of floor textured with a rippled effect to signal to anyone in a wheelchair when one area was being left and another area entered. Guidelines on corridor walls at shoulder height may help a disoriented person. A sailing ship for people with disabilities had ropes at wheelchair height leading along gangways with markers set at intervals to indicate in which direction the person was moving. If an ocean-going sailing ship can do this, is it unrealistic to expect a health unit to make efforts to maintain a person's failing abilities as long as possible? These ideas cost a fraction of a unit's drug bill and little time for preparation, yet are rarely used in palliative care. There is a danger that the lessons learned in one speciality are ignored as new specialties develop. There is a wealth of relevant clinical experience in the care of people with learning disabilities and neurorehabilitation units, but the boundaries between specialities lead to lost opportunities for the transfer of these skills.

The vulnerable patient

Patients who have been sexually abused in the past may begin to experience intrusive imagery and fear physical touch when helpless. The loss of body hair caused by chemotherapy can evoke a sense of being a child again, with powerful others inflicting pain. The patient may not want to disclose the previous abuse to other team members. It can be helpful to negotiate ways of interacting to enhance the person's sense of control. For example, someone who was frightened at the prospect of being handled when unable to see or speak was reassured by a preparing a short list of personal care instructions with the psychologist, which was added to the case notes before admission. These were based simply on good practice in dealing with the semi-conscious patient, such as using the patient's name and stating staff identity before touching. Nursing staff accepted them readily and the patient died a peaceful death after several weeks of accepting care.

Palliative care is practised in a social context and has to adapt to its changing society The closure of large institutions for people with learning disabilities or severe mental illness, and the subsequent integration of their former residents into the community, has challenged mainstream services to deliver an equitable service. Palliative care staff may have had little training and experience, and may share the same prejudices and fears of their community. A study of the experiences of people with learning disabilities in general hospitals revealed that basic needs for comfort and information were unrecognized[51].

Patients with severe mental illness or learning disabilities, especially those who were previously institutionalized may have had years of being told to 'behave properly' and not be a nuisance. Communication difficulties require staff to be proactive in their assessment of pain and symptom control[52]. People who have lived on the edges of their community may die there, with little understanding of their needs when facing death or bereavement[53].

A different type of challenge is faced by the team caring for the patient who is a health professional. It may be assumed that this patient understands fully everything that is happening. Staff must recognize that familiarity with the jargon of medicine and intellectual knowledge is not the same as psychological comfort. The patient may adopt the familiar and comfortable role of 'expert' and present a heroic front, which can make it more difficult to acknowledge fears or uncertainties. The more eminent the patient, the harder it can be for the team members to give support because they feel professionally intimidated. Consultations may focus on laboratory results, as natural expressions of warmth or empathy are inhibited by rank. Another danger lies in the temptation of colleagues to take short-cuts through the health-care system, which can have unforeseen and negative consequences[54].

Summary

Patients with cancer and other life-threatening disease have complex psychological and emotional needs, and may experience significant psychological distress. The psychologist can bring specialist skills to the direct care of individual patients or patient groups, or provide training, supervision and support to other professionals engaged in palliative care. In this way, psychology can make a contribution to the organization and delivery of health-care provision, in addition to providing care at the individual level. This contribution may be enhanced through recognition that the psychological issues faced by professionals in chronic disease and rehabilitation services are relevant in palliative care, and lessons could be learned from other specialities.

References

1. Murray, S.A., Boyd, M., Kendall, M. et al. (2002). Dying of lung cancer or cardiac failure: prospective qualitative interview study of patients and their carers in the community. British Medical Journal, **325**, 929–32.

2. Elkington, H., White, P., Addington-Hall, J. et al. (2005). The healthcare needs of chronic obstructive pulmonary disease patients in the last year of life. Palliative Medicine, **19**, 485–91.

3. Gysels, M. and Higginson, I.J. (2007). Interactive technologies and videotapes for patient education in cancer care: systematic review and meta-analysis of randomised trials. Supportive Care Cancer, **15**, 7–20.

4. Innes, J. (1977). Does the professional know what the client wants? Social Science and Medicine, **11**, 635–8.

5. Perkins, P., Barclay S., and Booth, S. (2007). What are patients' priorities for palliative care research? Focus group study. Palliative Medicine, **21**, 219–25.

6. Sardell, A. and Trierweiler, S. (1993). Disclosing the cancer diagnosis. Cancer, **72**, 3355–65.

7. Holland, J. (1999). Update: National Comprehensive Cancer Network guidelines for the management of psychosocial distress. Oncology, **13**(11A), 459–507.

8. Kelly, B., McClement, S., and Chochinov, H.M. (2006). Measurement of psychological distress in palliative care. Palliative Medicine, **20**, 779–89.

9. Lloyd-Williams, M., Dennis, M., Taylor, F., and Baker, I. (2003). Is asking patients in palliative care, 'Are you depressed?' appropriate: prospective study. British Medical Journal, **327**, 372–3.

10. Rogers, M. and Todd, C. (2000). The right kind of pain: talking about symptoms in outpatient oncology consultations. Palliative Medicine, **14**, 299–307.

11. Steinhauser, K.E., Clipp, E.C., Hays, J.C. et al. (2006). Identifying, recruiting and retaining seriously ill patients and their caregivers in longitudinal research. Palliative Medicine, **20**, 745–54.

12. Hillier, E.R. and Lunt, B. (1980). Goal-setting in terminal cancer. In The continuing care of terminal cancer patients (eds. R.G. Twycross and Ventafridda), pp. 271–8. Pergamon Press, Oxford.

13. Nezu, A.M., Nezu, C.M., Felgoise, S.H. *et al.* (2003). Project genesis: assessing the efficacy of problem-solving therapy for distressed adult cancer patients. *Journal of Consulting and Clinical Psychology*, **71**, 1036–48.

14. Wood, B.C. and Mynors-Wallis, L.M. (1997). Problem solving therapy in palliative care. *Palliative Medicine*, **11**, 49–54.

15. Luebbert, K., Dahme, B., and Hasenbring, M. (2001). The effectiveness of relaxation training in reducing treatment-related symptoms and improving emotional adjustment in acute non-surgical cancer treatment: a meta-analytical review. *Psycho-Oncology*, **10**, 490–502.

16. SIGN Guidelines (Scottish Intercollegiate Guidelines Network). (2000). *Control of pain in patients with cancer.* Royal College of Physicians, Edinburgh.

17. Roffe, L., Schmidt, K., and Ernst, E. (2005). A systematic review of guided imagery as an adjuvant cancer therapy. *Psycho-Oncology*, **14**, 607–17.

18. British Psychological Society. (2001). *The nature of hypnosis.* BPS, Leicester.

19. Bioy, A. and Wood, C. (2006). Hypnosis: principles of use and benefits in palliative care. *European Journal of Palliative Care*, **13**, 117–20.

20. Rajasekaran, M., Edmonds, P.M., and Higginson, I.L. (2005). Systematic review of hypnotherapy for treating symptoms of terminally ill adult patients. *Palliative Medicine*, **19**, 418–26.

21. Turk, D.C. and Feldman, C.S. (2000). A cognitive-behavioural approach to symptom management in palliative care: augmenting somatic interventions. In *Handbook of psychiatry in palliative medicine* (eds. H.C. Chochinov and W. Breitbart). Oxford University Press, Oxford.

22. Moorey, S. and Greer, S. (2002). *Cognitive behaviour therapy for people with cancer.* Oxford University Press, Oxford.

23. Santos, M.J.H. and Greer, S. (1991). Adjuvant psychological therapy with a terminally ill patient; a case-report. *Behavioural Psychotherapy*, **19**, 277–80.

24. Boulton, M., Boudioni, M., Mossman, J. *et al.* (2001). Dividing the desolation: clients' views on the benefits of a cancer counselling service. *Psycho-Oncology*, **10**, 124–36.

25. Stedeford, A. (1994). *Facing death: patients, families and professionals.* Sobell Publication, Oxford.

26. Neimeyer, R.A. (ed.) (2001). *Meaning reconstruction and the experience of loss.* American Psychological Association, Washington, D.C.

27. Chochinov, H., Hack, T., Hassard, T. *et al.* (2005). Dignity therapy: a novel psychotherapeutic intervention for patients near the end of life. *Journal of Clinical Oncology*, **23**, 5520–5.

28. Ando, M., Tsuda, A., and Morita, T. (2007). Life review interviews on the spiritual wellbeing of terminally ill cancer patients. S*upportive Care Cancer*, **15**, 225–31.

29. Redd, W. (1982). Treatment of excessive crying in a terminal cancer patient; a time series analysis. *Journal of Behavioural Medicine*, **5**, 225–35.

30. Redd, W. (1982). Behavioural analysis and the control of psychosomatic symptoms of patients receiving intensive cancer treatment. *British Journal of Clinical Psychology*, **21**, 351–8.

31. Zaza, C., Sellick, S.M., Willan, A. *et al.* (1999). Health care professionals familiarity with non-pharmacological strategies for managing cancer pain. *Psycho-Oncology*, **8**, 99–111.

32. Spiegel, D., Bloom, J.R., Kraemer, H.C. *et al.* (1989). Effects of psychological treatment on survival of patients with metastatic breast cancer. *Lancet*, **334**, 888–91.

33. Goodwin, P.J., Leszcz, M., Ennis, M. *et al.* (2001). The effect of group psychosocial support on survival in metastatic breast cancer. *New England Journal of Medicine*, **345**, 1719–26.

34. Cunningham, A.J., Edmonds, C.V.I., Philips, C. *et al.* (2000). A prospective longitudinal study of the relationship of psychological work to duration of survival in patients with metastatic cancer. *Psycho-Oncology*, **9**, 323–39.

35. Kissane, D., Grabsch, B., Clarke, D.M. *et al.* (2004). Supportive-expressive group therapy; the transformation of existential ambivalence into creative living while enhancing adherence to anti-cancer therapies. *Psycho-Oncology*, **13**, 755–68.

36. Gottlieb, B.H. and Wachala, E. (2007). Cancer support groups: a critical review of empirical studies. *Psycho-Oncology*, **16**, 379–400.

37. Llewelyn, S.P., Murray, A.K., Johnston, M. *et al.* (1999). Group therapy for metastatic cancer patients; report of an intervention. *Psychology, Health and Medicine*, **4**, 229–40.

38. McWilliams, A.E. (2004). Couple psychotherapy from an attachment theory perspective: a case study approach to challenging the dual nihilism of being an older person and someone with a terminal illness. *European Journal of Cancer Care*, **13**, 464–72.

39. Jenkins, C. and Bruera, E. (1998). Conflict between families and staff; an approach. In *Topics in palliative care Vol.* 2 (E. Bruera and R. Portenoy), pp. 311–25. Oxford University Press, Oxford.

40. National Institute of Clinical Excellence. (2004). *Guidance on cancer services. Improving supportive and palliative care for adults with cancer.* NICE, London.

41. Morrow, G.R., Asbury, R., Hammon, S. *et al.* (1992). Comparing the effectiveness of behavioural treatment for chemotherapy-induced nausea and vomiting when administered by oncologists, oncology nurses and clinical psychologists. *Health Psychology*, **11**(4), 250–6.

42. Mannix, K.A., Blackburn, I.M., Garland, A. *et al.* (2006). Effectiveness of brief training in cognitive behaviour therapy techniques for palliative care practitioners. *Palliative Medicine*, **20**, 579–84.

43. Jones, K., Johnston, M., and Speck, P. (1989). Despair felt by the patient and the professional carer; a case-study of the use of cognitive-behaviour methods. *Palliative Medicine*, **3**, 39–46.

44. Bruera, E. and Portenoy, R. (1998). *Topics in palliative care, Vol.* 2. Oxford University Press, Oxford.

45. Hay, J. and Passik, S.D. (2000). The cancer patient with borderline personality disorder. *Psycho-Oncology*, **9**, 91–100.

46. Cull, A. (1991). Staff support in medical oncology: a problem-solving approach. *Psychology and Health*, **5**, 129–36.

47. Rothenberg (1974). Problems posed for staff who care for the child. In *Care of the child facing death* (ed. L. Burton), pp. 39–45. Routledge and Kegan Paul, London.

48. Firth-Cozens, J. (1997). Predicting stress in GPs: 10 year follow-up postal survey. *British Medical Journal*, **315**, 34–5.

49. Bennet, G. (1998). The doctor's losses: ideals versus realities. *British Medical Journal*, **316**, 1238–40.

50. Robinson, J. (1999). Cognitive assessment of palliative care patients, *Progress in Palliative Care*, **7**(6), 291–8.

51. Hart, S. (1998). Learning disabled people's experience of general hospitals. *British Journal of Nursing*, **7**, 670–7.

52. Tuffrey-Wyjne, I. (2003). The palliative care needs of people with learning disabilities. *Palliative Medicine*, **17**, 55–62.

53. Cathcart, F. (1995). Death and people with learning disabilities; interventions to support clients and carers. *British Journal of Clinical Psychology*, **34**, 165–75.

54. Higgs, R. (1991). Looking after yourself. In *Developing communication and counselling skills in medicine* (ed. R. Corney). Routledge, London.

The contribution of the clinical pharmacist in palliative care

Margaret Gibbs

Introduction

Drugs play a crucial role in the provision of symptom control so it seems logical for a palliative care team to include a professional whose particular expertise is in the safe and effective use of medicines. In UK, the National Institute for Health and Clinical Excellence (NICE) in its 2004 guidance 'Improving Supportive and Palliative Care for Adults with Cancer'[1] states that the expertise of pharmacists helps to provide the appropriate level of specialist palliative care to patients. This chapter reviews the role of clinical pharmacists in palliative care and is based mainly on the situation in UK. Similar practices are seen in parts of North America and Europe but there are still many parts of the world where clinical pharmacy is developing at a slower rate and has therefore yet to reach palliative care.

All hospices with inpatients require a pharmacy supply service but not all include a clinical pharmacist as part of the multi-disciplinary team. So, what is a clinical pharmacist? Clinical pharmacy has been defined as 'that area of pharmacy concerned with the science and practice of rational medication use'[2]. The traditional training and role of pharmacists started to change in the UK during the 1970s following the Noel Hall report[3], which encouraged hospital pharmacists to step outside the dispensary and become more clinically involved in the decision-making processes for prescribing. Thirty years on, the pharmacy degree is now a 4-year Masters degree and training in clinical and therapeutic subjects occupies the largest part of the curriculum[4]. Most hospital pharmacists spend the majority of their time in clinical areas, communicating with other health-care professionals and patients and in 2006, the first cohort of pharmacists qualified as independent prescribers. Many of these now run clinics in hospital and in general practice. Pharmacists in the UK emerge from their training with a different set of skills to those of previous generations and many choose to specialize in a particular therapeutic area within the hospital, primary care, community or industrial environment. Traditional supply roles associated with the practice of pharmacy have changed too, becoming more mechanized, centralized, and delegated far more to technical staff. This too has enabled pharmacists to become more fully engaged members of clinical multi-disciplinary teams.

The number of clinical pharmacists working as part of palliative care teams in UK is not currently known, although data are being collected. A study published in 2002[5] indicated that most Canadian teams included a pharmacist (59/69) whilst in Australia the proportion was lower at (42/76). The most recent survey in USA in 1991 showed that some pharmacists work as volunteer consultants in their local hospice but most are employed and regarded as full members of the inter-disciplinary team[6].

The job specification for a palliative care pharmacist can vary greatly with many spending only part of their working week within the speciality. Most UK hospices and hospital teams have a small number of beds, usually not enough to warrant the input of a full time pharmacist. Community-based services may not have any regular clinical pharmacist input but be supported formally or informally by community or Primary Care Trust (PCT) pharmacists. A study comparing practice in Australia and Canada in 2002 showed that most pharmacists in both countries worked less than 20 h per week in their service and Canadian pharmacists were more clinically involved while Australian pharmacists spent more time on administrative and supply functions. The American Society of Health Systems Pharmacists has produced a statement outlining the role and responsibilities of a hospice and palliative care pharmacist (Box 4.13.1) which indicates broad similarities in practice in Canada, Australia, and the UK[7,8].

Several studies have evaluated the effectiveness of the interventions and recommendations of clinical pharmacists working in palliative care in the hospice inpatient[8], outpatient[10], and community[11] settings. Although the methods for assessing such a nebulous term as 'effectiveness' in this context are not well developed and

---

Box 4.13.1 The pharmacist's responsibilities

1 Assessing the appropriateness of medication orders and ensuring the timely provision of effective medications for symptom control.

2 Counselling and educating the hospice team about medication therapy.

3 Ensuring that patients and caregivers understand and follow the directions provided with medications.

4 Providing efficient mechanisms for extemporaneous compounding of non-standard dosage forms.

5 Addressing financial concerns.

6 Ensuring safe and legal disposal of all medications after death.

7 Establishing and maintaining effective communication with regulatory and licensing agencies.

The American Society of Healthcare Pharmacists[9]

the response by clinicians to the recommendations varied, the majority (60–80 per cent) of the interventions were judged to have had a positive outcome on patient care.

In UK, some specialist posts for pharmacists in palliative care have been established by charities such as Macmillan Cancer Relief and Marie Curie, which supply initial pump-priming funding with the intention that local commissioners will enable the post to continue. Many of these pharmacists work jointly in oncology and palliative care and have a role in coordinating and improving services in a given locality. Disappointingly, on review, about half of these posts were not being continued so Macmillan now insists that future funding is agreed before initiating the posts.

Clinical pharmacy in the rest of Europe is in currently in an earlier stage of development but a number of European pharmacists are establishing roles in palliative care teams. Personal communications indicate that pioneering pharmacists in Japan, Africa, and India are working to improve access to opioids and become more involved in palliative care teams where these are developing.

The fundamentals of good pharmaceutical care

Pharmaceutical care has been defined as 'the responsible provision of drug therapy for the purpose of achieving defined outcomes that improve the patient's quality of life'[12]. When pharmacists review or advise on drug regimens, the patient is always at the focus. A traditional mantra for pharmacists is the provision of 'the right drug to the right patient at the right time'. Barber[13] suggests that we monitor individual prescriptions to maximize effectiveness, minimize risks and costs, and respect the patient's choices. This patient-centred approach is, of course, fundamental in palliative care so the clinical pharmacist's attention to detail on medication complements all other aspects of care. In order to provide the best care, the clinical pharmacist ensures that the following are provided:

◆ A reliable supply function and regular monitoring of prescribing, including economic reviews.

◆ An appropriate medicines management system.

◆ Advice and guidance on safe use of drugs of particular relevance to palliative care, e.g. syringe driver compatibility.

◆ The provision and dissemination of drug-related information both clinical and legislative, e.g. involving Controlled Drugs.

The following sections will look at these areas in more detail and at how they can most effectively be executed in palliative care. Most of the text refers to the input of pharmacists specifically employed to provide services to an inpatient unit, although the role of community pharmacists caring for patients at home is included where relevant.

Supply and monitoring of drug use

In UK, hospices with inpatient units are provided with a budget for their drugs and pharmaceutical services by the host Primary Care Trust (PCT) or Health Board in Scotland, who commission health services in each locality. A contract to provide pharmaceutical services may be set up with a local hospital pharmacy, a community pharmacy, or the PCT itself. If a contract is established with a

---

> **Box 4.13.2** Functions of a pharmaceutical service to a hospice inpatient unit
>
> **Essential**
>
> 1 A reliable and responsive delivery system with provision for a back-up to provide urgently needed medicines or pharmacist advice out of opening hours.
>
> 2 Regular visits from a clinical pharmacist for clinical checking of prescriptions and provision of medicines information.
>
> 3 Provision of stock drugs using a regular top-up system, ideally carried out by pharmacy technicians including a regular monitoring system for expiry checks of medicines.
>
> 4 Provision of individual patient supplies for the duration of inpatient stay and on discharge.
>
> 5 Provision of regular supply of Controlled Drugs using Standard Operating Procedures.
>
> 6 A system for reviewing and updating agreed stock supply.
>
> 7 An effective communication system for ordering, managing queries, and supplying information where necessary when the pharmacist is not present.
>
> **Desirable**
>
> 8 Inclusion of pharmacist on clinical governance, risk management, and drug and therapeutics committees within the hospice.
>
> 9 Availability of pharmacist to run teaching sessions for hospice staff.

hospital pharmacy, it is normally possible for the hospice to benefit from the advantageous, contract prices for the drugs being used in that acute trust. The service should include the functions shown in Box 4.13.2.

An effective supply function is an essential part of the pharmaceutical service and this has in most environments become an almost mechanical process with 'original pack' dispensing of blister packaged tablets or small volumes of liquid preparations. In the UK, once a pharmacist has screened a prescription for its clinical appropriateness the dispensing can be completed by suitably qualified pharmacy technicians and, in a few larger hospitals, by robotic systems. This means that a clinical pharmacist does not need to be directly involved with the supplies of drugs but needs to set up systems, be confident that they are working, and be made aware of any problems

Economic issues

The economical use of drugs is important in all health-care settings but it is especially important in hospices, as most are registered charities. The majority of drugs used for symptom management are older, relatively inexpensive generic drugs but there are some notable exceptions such as the bisphosphonates and somatostatin analogues. In a small unit, it is very easy for the symptom management for one or two 'expensive' patients to make a huge impact on the monthly budget figures. Regular pharmacy meetings to review prescribing patterns can highlight areas of concern, then audit and written guidelines can be constructive tools to ensure the appropriate use of high-cost drugs.

Establishing an agreed stock list for an inpatient unit may evolve into compiling a core formulary. This has been shown to be an effective strategy for reducing cost and improving patient outcomes in one Kentucky Hospice[14]. In another study from the US, it was shown that newer, more expensive pharmacotherapy options were not necessarily more effective than traditional agents if doses were monitored and titrated by clinical pharmacists[15].

Ideally any formulary should be evidence-based, but the evidence for much of the drug therapy used in palliative care is of a lower level than for other therapeutic areas at least partly because of the difficulties in carrying out randomized controlled trials in dying patients[16].

Evidence-based practice—definition

The judicious use of the best available evidence, moderated by patient circumstances and preferences to guide our practice to improve the quality of clinical judgements and facilitate effective health care.
Sackett and Rosenberg[17]

Many sets of therapeutic guidelines now exist in UK and on the whole, the list of drugs used for symptom control is broadly consistent. Guidance and core formularies have also been developed by Palliative and Supportive Care Networks, which were established as a model of integrated service provision alongside cancer networks in response to the NHS Cancer Plan[18] to improve coordination of cancer and palliative care. Clinical pharmacists have been involved in many of the Network subgroups coordinating drug treatment and availability. In US, the introduction of standardized, evidence-based Medication Use Guidelines is encouraged[19].

As well as the choice of drugs, the clinical pharmacist can advise on the most appropriate formulation for individual patients. With some exceptions (such as strong opioids and drugs where the avoidance of peak effects in drug blood concentrations may lead to less side effects) prescribers are now encouraged to avoid the use of slow-release preparations on economic grounds. In palliative care, our patients' tablet 'burden' can often be a real problem and so use of a more expensive once or twice-daily preparation such as slow release metoclopramide may be justified.

Managing a drug regimen for a patient who has swallowing difficulties or is being tube fed has pharmaceutical implications. Crushing tablets is to be discouraged as changing the form of a dose not only takes it outside the terms of its licence but can also be hazardous as it may change its pharmacokinetics—especially dangerous with a slow-release formulation. Liquid or soluble tablets can be very expensive, so alternative drugs may need to be substituted. The pharmacist can advise in this area.

The pharmacist may also alert colleagues to the sensitive issue of discontinuing medication. Effectiveness and tolerability of each medication will be reviewed regularly but decisions on whether a patient nearing the end of life needs to continue with such medication as statins or oral hormonal treatments, such as exemestane need normally to be negotiated with the patient and possibly their carers. The goals of care and treatment targets should be balanced against remaining life expectancy and tablet burden. Equally, initiating some drugs with a long onset of action such as antidepressants may not be appropriate if the time to benefit exceeds the patient's life expectancy. These are emotive issues but unfortunately their cost implications can be considerable[20].

It is almost inevitable that we have a degree of wastage when drugs are dispensed for patients at the end of their life and although it is a difficult moral issue to destroy what seem to be perfectly sound drugs, we have a statutory responsibility not to re-supply any drugs that have been dispensed to a particular patient for others and we are unable to guarantee their integrity. The only practical way to counter this is to minimize waste by (1) ensuring that appropriate quantities are ordered and (2) holding ward stocks on units where the stock lists and stock levels are regularly reviewed.

Nurses need also to be aware of the relative costs of dressings and skin and mouth care preparations. Wound and mouth care are often challenging areas of palliative care and there is a huge variety of products on the market. With pharmacist input, in-house policies, guidance or decision-making tools can encourage nurses to use the most appropriate and economical choices.

Drugs for hospice patients at home

The majority of dying people would prefer to remain in their own home, although currently only 20 per cent do so and many are admitted to hospices or hospitals in the last days of life[21]. Although routine symptom control medicines are prescribed and supplied in the community, the provision of drugs for unexpectedly deteriorating patients has always been complicated by legislative limits on the ability to hold 'stock' injectable drugs outside pharmacies and hospitals. In addition, many doctors no longer carry their own supply of morphine or diamorphine for security reasons. Medical and nursing cover vary from area to area but the simple lack of availability of the required drugs has led too many times to an inappropriate hospital admission, especially during the out-of-hours period, which is almost 70 per cent of the week. Out-of-hours (OOH) care in England and Wales has undergone a substantial NHS review and other reviews of practice, such as that initiated by Macmillan[22], have contributed to subsequent re-organization in recent years. The Department of Health identified palliative care as one of its priorities when it launched its OOH plan in 2005[23].

Systems for stocking small quantities of injectable drugs in designated community pharmacies have been set up in various localities. Whilst these schemes are an invaluable source of back up, they have not always been a success. This may be because they are not always well publicized to the relevant professionals but more importantly, there is an inevitable delay in getting the pharmacist and prescription to the pharmacy and back to the patient's house, making it sometimes simpler for the nurse or doctor in the house to call the emergency services. Under-use of these schemes leads to expiry of stock and eventual loss of funding but they can be best used in conjunction with immediate access to the necessary drugs by the on-call medical service. PCT commissioners and pharmacists are now responsible for ensuring that there is a safe system in place for providing all the drugs on the national out-of-hours formulary to providers of OOH medical care. A list of essential and desirable drugs is shown in Box 4.13.3. The details of the OOH arrangements need to be agreed locally to suit the geography and population. They should encompass the NICE guidance for improving supportive and palliative care[1], be supported by improved communications, facilitated by introducing the Gold Standards Framework[24] for community care of the dying and take into account the Preferred Place of Care[25] initiative.

> **Box 4.13.3** Emergency drugs for end-of-life symptom management
>
> **Essential (and now on the NHS OOH core formulary)**
>
> *Strong opioid* in injectable form—normally diamorphine or morphine
>
> *Midazolam* for sedation
>
> *Cyclizine, haloperidol or levomepromazine* for nausea and vomiting
>
> *Glycopyrronium or hyoscine* for retained secretions
>
> **Desirable**
>
> *Lorazepam* tablets for anxiety and breathlessness
>
> *Oral morphine* liquid

Clinical pharmacists have been instrumental in establishing so-called 'Just in Case' schemes where GPs prescribe a small quantity of injectable drugs for individual patients identified as nearing the end of their life. These drugs can be kept safely in the patient's home in case of a sudden deterioration. In a pilot scheme in Hertfordshire UK[26] over 6 months in 2004, 23 'just in case' boxes were issued enabling 16 patients to have their symptoms managed and to die at home, which was their expressed preference. Each pack of drugs cost only £10 and the potential saving on an admission to hospital or hospice plus the satisfaction for the patient and their family from good end of life care is immeasurable.

Medicines management

The UK Audit Commission introduced the concept of Medicines Management within its report 'A spoonful of sugar' in 2001[27]. It aimed to optimize the use of medicines in NHS hospitals to improve the quality of patient care and rationalize expenditure. Although most hospices are independent of the NHS, the national strategies are normally adopted for the sake of congruity

> **Medicines management—definition**
>
> Medicines management in hospitals encompasses the entire way that medicines are selected, procured, delivered, prescribed, administered and reviewed to optimize the contribution that medicines make to producing informed and desired outcomes of patient care
>
> *Audit Commission*[27]

Patient-centred medicines management

When patients have a planned admission to an inpatient unit in the UK, they are encouraged to bring their current medicines in with them. This has several benefits; it is essential to establish a drug 'history', particularly if symptoms are out of control. It can offer an opportunity to clarify whether the patient is actually taking the regimen as prescribed, and establish what has been used in the past and what the outcomes were. Our patients may have a number of symptoms and coexistent pathologies making it common for them to be taking a large number of medicines so this is often a time-consuming job involving rummaging through bagfuls of dispensed medicines. Although the admitting doctor or specialist nurse will normally do this as part of any admissions process, pilot studies have shown that a pharmacy-led medicines review process uncovers further issues and is highly acceptable to the patient. Unfortunately, time limitations prevent pharmacist-led drug-history taking becoming routine in most inpatient units.

Bringing in their existing medication also ensures that patients have an ongoing supply, as most units will not have an exhaustive range of stock drugs. It also prevents duplication, reduces waste and ultimately saves money. Not all patients' own drugs can be used so they must be screened for suitability using a checklist, ensuring they are blister-packed, identifiable, not time expired and labelled correctly for the patient[28]. This also forms part of an audit trail for medicines.

One of the main aims of the NHS medicines management programme is to encourage patients to keep charge of their medicines in a bedside locker and to continue to take them independently. Clearly not all patients admitted to a hospice are suited to self-administration but those whose admission is for respite or symptom control should be encouraged to do so with multi-disciplinary team agreement. The pharmacist needs to assure that patients understand their regimen and assess practical issues such as their ability to manage the containers, read labels, and appreciate their responsibility for security of their medicines. An agreed assessment process needs to be part of the hospice medicines policy. Almost all patients who are given the chance to self-administer prefer it because it gives them more control and promotes confidence in managing what may be a complex regimen[29]. This confidence can be a major contribution to a successful discharge as many admissions and re-admissions arise because patients and families are confused about medication. We know that low adherence to instructions with medication affects all self-administered treatments so the older term 'compliance' implying simply following instructions has now been replaced with 'concordance' where patients are given sufficient information to make an informed choice on the benefits and risks of a therapeutic 'alliance'[29].

Patient counselling by pharmacists promotes understanding of the purpose of each medicine and awareness of potential adverse effects[30]. It can also provide an opportunity to discuss practical issues such as the provision of medicines in concordance aids ('dosette boxes'), which may be continued on discharge. Most GP surgeries and pharmacies have a delivery system for prescriptions from surgery to pharmacy and then on to the patient at home.

Community pharmacists establish relationships with their regular patients and their families and have a wider role to play than simply drug supply. In some countries, community pharmacists are responsible for preparing pre-filled syringes for syringe drivers. In UK, groups of community pharmacists have undergone additional training in order to support palliative care patients by setting up prescription monitoring and supply services. Research in Durham[31] showed that patients regard their community pharmacist as part of the multi-professional group providing their palliative care but their input is often absent in local teams. This encouraged initiation of a project in 2001 involving 14 community pharmacists where palliative care patients were registered with one particular pharmacy and the pharmacist had access to all patient records. This enabled them to identify and improve difficulties with medication for GPs and patients and was found to be beneficial by patients, GPs and community and specialist nurses in the area.

Another important role for palliative care pharmacists is to provide 'seamless' pharmaceutical care for patients as they move from one care setting to another[30]. The NHS electronic patient record project is not yet up and running so we rely on a number of different methods of transmitting medication information, some of which are less reliable than others. A medication list will normally be drawn up on discharge and sent to the GP or other doctor looking after a patient but their community pharmacist can sometimes be left out of the loop and both may be faced with an urgent prescription for an unusual drug unless prior explanation has been provided. Where medicines management systems exist, patients' discharge medication (from the inpatient unit) will often be dispensed well before the expected discharge. This can present last-minute problems if doses or drugs have been changed in the interim. The importance of timely prescribing and supply to patients for whom time is limited needs to be communicated to all health-care professionals providing services. Pharmacists have a major educational role in fulfilling this particular objective.

Advice and guidance on drugs in palliative care

The concept of Clinical Governance was introduced into the NHS nearly 10 years ago with the aim of increasing accountability and quality of care. In common with many other NHS initiatives, it has been extended into the voluntary sector and provides a framework for decisions we make when considering new treatment options.

Clinical governance—definition

A framework through which (NHS) organizations are accountable for continually improving the quality of their services and safeguarding high standards of care by creating an environment in which excellence in clinical care will flourish.

Scally and Donaldson[32]

Pharmacists have a major role in clinical governance issues involving medicines with many sitting on their hospice Medicines Management or Drug and Therapeutics Groups. The terms of reference of these groups may vary but usually include the review of drugs coming on to the market or drugs being suggested elsewhere for symptom control as well as ensuring the correct application of new drug-related guidance or legislation.

Use of drugs outside their licence

Palliative care practice often involves using drugs outside the terms of their product licence. In order for any new drug to reach the market, the manufacturer must be able to show that it is a safe and effective treatment. Once this has been proved in a drug development programme, it will be granted a licence for the conditions it has been tested for. Licensing is both a commercial and medico-legal issue but a doctor may prescribe, a pharmacist may dispense, and a nurse may administer drugs outside the terms of their licence as long as the drug was being used in accordance with a practice accepted at the time by a responsible body of medical opinion. There is encouragement from UK authorities to discuss the use of medicines outside licence with our patients and although we aim to involve patients in all prescribing decisions, terminology such as 'outside the terms of a drug's licence' may sound more worrying than it need be. Most of the drugs we use in this way are long established with well-documented safety and adverse effect profiles so the main issue for us is ensuring that there is sufficient evidence for this use whilst the main issue for our patients is to avoid any potential confusion arising from information they may read in the Patient Information Leaflet (PIL), which must be supplied with their dispensed medicines. Hospice pharmacists have written patient information leaflets for their own establishment

and they are usually happy for such information sheets to be used by others. (An example is shown in Appendix 4.13.1 and at www.palliativedrugs.com) At a small hospice user group this was not an issue of great concern with patients saying they trusted the health-care professionals to do what they could for them (unpublished report from St Christophers Hospice).

Pharmacists regularly advise nurses on the correct methods of administration of drugs. With tube-fed patients or other patients who may find swallowing difficult it is common practice to consider crushing a tablet, opening a capsule and sprinkling the resultant powder on food or mixing it with a drink. Any of these alterations to the original product renders it outside its licence. Pharmacists have written a number of reference sources to offer advice about the best method of administration of the drug in these circumstances. This may involve changing the drug to an alternative where a licensed liquid or soluble form is available because we should always aim to use a licensed medicine where one exists.

The use of medicines without any licence is a slightly different issue. It is unlikely that a palliative care unit would wish to use an unlicensed *drug* but we often wish to mix or compound known drugs in unlicensed *formulations* to suit individual patients. Some examples of this are the use of alfentanil injection made into a cutaneous solution that can be sprayed onto the nasal or buccal mucosa and the addition of lignoocaine (lidocaine) to a thermoversible gel for the management of painful wounds. Both products are made in regional hospital pharmacies in UK. Although US pharmacists are permitted to compound individual preparations for patients, this practice has become very limited in UK and is now restricted to a few commercial 'specials' manufacturers and regional, licensed hospital pharmacy manufacturing units. Information on unlicensed medicines is limited, as products have not been subjected to the same regulatory processes as licensed medicines so we need to obtain as much evidence as possible that we are using such products appropriately and be willing to account for our practice. Prescribers and pharmacists must both be involved in the decision-making process using a committee or the clinical governance team to approve and document the rationale for using unlicensed products. Once sufficient experience has been gained in their use, specialists may start suggesting to generalists that these products be used. The production of referenced information leaflets is important in supporting this. The Brompton Hospitals and some hospices have produced their own leaflets either covering this subject in general or for specific drugs such as the use of haloperidol to treat nausea and vomiting. An example is provided in Appendix 4.13.2

Subcutaneous administration of drugs

The use of the subcutaneous route is outside the license for the majority of drugs used in symptom management. The major area of potential problems is where drugs are mixed together in the same syringe. Although the drugs used are familiar and well established, it is not necessarily in a company's financial interests to investigate the compatibility of its injections with those of others. Additionally, many of the drugs we use have lost their patent and are made by generic manufacturers who would be even less inclined to carry out such studies. Pharmacists have been largely responsible for gathering data on the mixing of drugs in syringes for subcutaneous infusions[33]. Our knowledge in this area comes from a mixture of

Appendix 4.13.1 Information leaflet on use of drugs outside their licence.

Information on your medicines

–

for St Christopher's at Home Patients

ST CHRISTOPHER'S HOSPICE

St Christopher's   Hospice

August   2001

This leaflet contains further information on your medicines

Keep this box for notes or questions you want to ask.

Information on your medicines – for St Christopher's at Home patients

When you receive your medicines from your pharmacy, you should find that each container is labelled with the instructions on how and when to take the medicine plus any extra warnings, for example 'Take with or after food'.

Many medicines are now supplied with a 'Patient Information Leaflet'. This can provide a great deal of information about the medicine, its uses and its side effects. However, most medicines have more than one effect on the body and for many years, palliative care (hospice) doctors have found that certain medicines are safe and effective for the treatment of symptoms *other* than those specified by the medicine's manufacturer. There is now plenty of written information to confirm this. In such cases, you may find the information that you have been given from the hospice does not agree with the printed information on the 'Patient Information Leaflet'. Your pharmacist may not be aware of the reason your medicines have been prescribed as this information is not provided on the prescription This could cause you and your family or carers anxiety and confusion and for this reason, we are providing you with this extra information.

You can find information on medicines used in specialist Palliative Care textbooks and your doctor, nurse and pharmacist can obtain information on a website – www.palliativedrugs.org

If you have any further questions or would like more details, please ask one of the following people:

St Christopher's Homecare nurses

020

Hospice Pharmacist

020

Community Pharmacist

....

District Nurse

....

You have been prescribed one or more of the following medicines:

- Haloperidol to treat nausea and/or vomiting. This medicine is regularly prescribed in higher doses for patients with psychiatric symptoms, however, at low doses it has been shown also to be very effective at relieving nausea and vomiting

- Carbamazepine or sodium valproate to treat nerve pain. These medicines are regularly prescribed for patients with epilepsy, however, they are also effective for many patients for the relief of nerve pain.

- Amitriptyline to treat nerve pain. This medicine is regularly prescribed at higher doses for patients suffering with depression, however, at lower doses, it has been shown to be effective in the relief of nerve pain.

- Oramorph liquid to help with your breathlessness. Oramorph liquid contains morphine and is normally used to treat pain, but it has also been shown to be effective in

reducing the feelings of breathlessness.

- Lorazepam to help with your breathlessness. Lorazepam is usually used for the treatment of anxiety, but it has also been shown to be effective in reducing the feeling of breathlessness

- Medroxyprogesterone or Megestrol to help improve your appetite. These are hormones used in the treatment of some cancers, but they have also been shown to improve the appetite and so help you gain weight

Appendix 4.13.2 Information leaflet on the use of lutrol gel with lidocaine

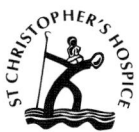

St Christopher's Hospice

51-59 Lawrie Park Road
Sydenham, London
SE26 6DZ
020 8768 4500

Lutrol gel

'Lutrol' is the registered trade name for a product widely used as a thickening or gelling agent in the pharmaceutical industry. Its viscosity depends on its concentration and temperature, making it a *thermoreversible* gel. Its viscosity increases more rapidly above 20°C and is most solid at body temperature, making it a practical preparation for providing a wound barrier. It was noted as a potentially useful carrier for other agents by MacGregor in 1994[1].

A preparation containing Lutrol 24 per cent in water with Lidocaine 2 per cent was first made at Guys and St Thomas' Hospital Pharmacy as part of an exploratory study. It proved very effective in relieving pain in malignant wounds, especially in areas where dressings are difficult to apply and keep in place[2]. This preparation has continued to be made by the licensed manufacturing unit at St Thomas' Hospital and is used within the hospice where the multi-disciplinary team decides when it is appropriate to use.

Stock may be kept at room temperature but in warmer weather and in centrally heated environments it is easier to store and use from the refrigerator. Cooling the gel by storing in the refrigerator or standing the container in ice decreases its viscosity, enabling it to be poured onto the wound. The Lutrol gel will set once it reaches body temperature, creating a protective layer whilst the lidocaine provides analgesia. It is normally applied at dressing changes but the analgesic effect normally lasts for about 6–8 h, so it may be necessary to apply more frequently to achieve prolonged analgesia. The gel can be removed from the skin quite easily using warm water.

It is also possible for GPs to prescribe Lutrol with lidocaine 2 per cent on FP10. Community pharmacists can order it from St Thomas' Pharmacy by telephoning 020 7188 7188 and it is delivered within the SE London area. *Please be aware that it takes several days to process this.*

clinical observation and laboratory tests and ongoing data collection continues to add to this[34].

Complementary medicines

The use of complementary medicines needs to be considered as a safety issue. Many patients are understandably concerned about the safety of conventional medicines but there is a perception, fuelled by marketing that if a product is herbal or marketed as 'natural' then it may be safer. There are countless products available supported by testimonials and claims that they work wonders— from improving digestion to curing cancer. When taking a drug history, pharmacists will also make specific enquiries, as patients may not mention complementary therapies because they are not regarded as 'drugs'. The quality of information on complementary medicines is in general not required to be of the same standard as that of conventional medicines, as they are not subject to the same legal controls. it This makes it difficult to unpick the evidence from the hard sell. Clinical pharmacists can critically review the information available and offer guidance on potential beneficial and adverse effects of complementary medicines as well as advising on possible contra-indications and drug interactions. Research and data collection on herbal medicines and supplements is enabling us to offer better guidance and the Medicines and Healthcare Regulatory Authority regularly releases bulletins warning us of serious safety issues with these medicines. In offering guidance on these products, pharmacists need to carefully word their findings in order to indicate the level of evidence for their statements and to take into account the patient's individual choice to continue with such products.

Practical and pragmatic guidance from the pharmacist is also required for some drug-food interactions that may impact on our patients. For example, the ingestion of excessive amounts of vitamin K-containing green vegetables can affect coagulation but a normal portion of such vegetables on a regular basis presents very low risk. Similarly, the presence of a drinks trolley on hospice wards and day centres prompts pharmacists to alert staff involved in 'administration' to the possible interaction between alcohol and drugs.

Incidents and errors with drugs

Incidents involving drugs account for about 10 per cent of all adverse events reported in NHS hospitals although over 80 per cent result in no apparent patient harm[35]. These figures are not necessarily applicable to hospices but the need to review and take appropriate action following adverse drug events is no less important. The ethos of drug error reporting has changed in recent years with a 'no blame' reporting system instigated in many hospitals and the involvement of staff in reporting 'near misses'. The focus is now on *systems* rather than individuals and we are asked to review our practice by the NHS National Patient Safety Agency in UK, which disseminates guidance and safety notices for areas of risk such as the recent alert on potential for confusion between strengths of opioid injections. Pharmacists are able to advise on systems for reporting errors and improving safety and are essential members of the group within a hospice that reviews incidents. Writing additional safety steps into policies and sending round awareness bulletins have had positive results in that incidents have not recurred (unpublished drug incident reports from St Christophers Hospice). Sharing information with other hospice pharmacists has also highlighted common areas for concern and constructive changes, such as persuading a company to improve its packaging have been achieved.

Provision and dissemination of Information

Clinical pharmacy training includes time spent in medicines information centres where pharmacists learn to source and critically appraise information and research to produce unbiased drug reviews. As palliative care expands we need to keep our teams updated on drug developments in therapeutic areas other than cancer. Pharmacists can tap into wide resources from regional medicines information services to share updates and reviews

The widespread use of Controlled Drugs (CDs) in pain and symptom management requires us to pay particular attention to legislation and regulations. We want to enable patients to make choices about their preferred place of care. If we are to facilitate this, we need to be able to supply their required medicines without delay, yet act within the law. Since the activities of Dr Harold Shipman came to light (a general practitioner who committed mass murder usually using injections of opioids), reviews on the handling of CDs have come under close scrutiny and the resulting Inquiry has made a number of valuable recommendations for, such as improved record keeping and audit as well as increasing awareness of accountability. Making patients more aware of the 'dangerous' nature of CDs by using information leaflets and asking for proof of identity on collection of prescriptions may, however be less constructive as it could be counter-productive in reducing the fear of opioids that still exists in UK. One major organization change is the introduction of an Accountable Officer for each establishment in England and Wales where CDs are used. These AOs will form a network in order to promote safety and any enable concerns to be dealt with by calling together an investigating committee to address any concerns raised within a given locality. PCT pharmacists are to lead on this and palliative care pharmacists are well placed to be the AO for their hospice unless they have day-to-day responsibilities with the drugs. A Standard Operating Procedure needs to be in place for all activities involving CDs.

The inspection body in UK for NHS and independent hospitals is the Healthcare Commission. The pharmacists working for this body are an invaluable source of information and support and if a hospice does not have a designated pharmacist, the Healthcare Commission is happy to give advice on pharmacy-related matters.

Research and audit

A number of pharmacists in different settings carry out a variety of medicines-related audit—such as creating data bases of syringe driver mixtures or reviewing the arrangements for OOH drug provision. Others have prepared or adapted guidelines for using particular therapies for palliative care patients—such as thromboprophylaxis. Some are carrying out research projects involving medicines directly and indirectly—such as the use of antisecretory agents at the end of life or the value of a training programme non-specialist pharmacists in the basics of palliative care. Many of these initiatives are modest and unpublished but in the UK we aim to collect and disseminate them as time progresses so that examples of good practice can be shared. Some of these may be in connection with a further qualification whilst others simply improve the quality of care for our patients.

Networking

Like many specialists, most palliative care pharmacists work alone so there is value in communicating with fellow pharmacists for advice and support. Regional and national groups for palliative care pharmacists exist in US, Canada, and the UK with varying levels of activity. The Scottish Palliative Care Pharmacists Association has created a benchmarking tool for staffing levels of pharmacists, coordinates research, produces guidance, and has a strategic role within the Scottish health service. As most of us work some distance from our colleagues, the Internet has become invaluable as a means of sharing information. Multi-disciplinary web-based discussion groups have been set up with pharmacists being the third largest professional group participating (after doctors and nurses) and a UK palliative care pharmacists network has now been formed.

A recent initiative in primary care is the development of Pharmacists with a Special Interest, who will provide specialist pharmaceutical care to patients with specific medical problems. To become a PhwSI, a pharmacist will have to undergo extra competency training and gain accreditation via a locally determined process based on the national framework[36]. Palliative care is one of these special interests and as most patients would prefer to be cared for at home and the NHS End of Life Strategy aims to enable this to happen more in the future in UK, more community pharmacists with expertise in palliative care will be a welcome development.

Conclusions

The role of a clinical pharmacist in a palliative care team is an especially rewarding and fulfilling one as it presents us with so many opportunities to utilize our specific skills. One needs broad outlook, a flexible and pragmatic approach and willingness to contribute to judgements based on what is best for any given patient without always having the highest level of evidence to support some decisions. As palliative care opens up to more patients with non-malignant life-limiting diseases, we need to be aware of a wider range of drug regimens and their implications and to educate as many colleagues as possible to the safe and effective use of drugs in patient-centred palliative care. It is difficult to imagine working in a more privileged environment than one where teams are dedicated to providing the best possible end-of-life care.

Further reading

Back, I. (ed.) 2001. *Palliative medicine handbook.* BPM Books, Cardiff.

Beynon, T., Laverty, D., Baxter, A. *et al.* (2003). Lutrol gel: a potential role in wounds? *Journal of Pain and Symptom Management,* **26**, 776–80.

Dickman, A., Schneider, J., and Varga (eds.) (2005). *The syringe driver.* Oxford University Press, Oxford.

MacGregor, K.J. *et al.* (1994). Symptomatic relief of excoriating skin conditions using a topical thermoreversible gel. *Palliative Medicine,* **8**, 76–7.

Margaret Gibbs Hospice Pharmacist June 2004.

Twycross, R., Wilcock, A., Charlesworth, S., and Dickman, A. (eds.) (2002). *Palliative care formulary,* 2nd edition. Radcliffe Medical Press, Oxford.

References

1. National Institute for Health and Clinical Excellence (2004). *Improving Supportive and Palliative Care for Adults with Cancer.* Available at www.nice.org.uk (accessed March 2007).
2. American College of Clinical Pharmacy (2004). Available at http://www.accp.com/clinical_pharmacy.php (accessed April 2007).
3. Report of the Working Party on the Hospital Pharmaceutical Service (1970). *Noel Hall Report.* HMSO, London.
4. Wilson, K., Jesson, J., Langley, C. *et al.* (2005). *M. Pharm. Programmes: Where are we now?* Aston University Pharmacy Practice Research Group. Available at www.rpsgb.org.uk (accessed March 2007).
5. Gilbar, P., and Stefanuik, K. (2002). The role of the pharmacist in palliative care: results of a survey conducted in Australia and Canada. *Journal of Palliative Care,* **18**(4), 287–92.

6. Arter, S., and Berry, J. (1993). The provision of pharmaceutical care to hospice patients: results of the National Hospice Pharmacist Survey. *Journal of Pharmaceutical Care in Pain and Symptom Control*, **1**, 25–9.

7. Hanif, N. (1991). Role of the palliative care unit pharmacist. *Journal of Palliative Care*, **7**(4), 35–6.

8. Lucas, C., Glare, P., and Sykes, J. (1997). Contribution of a liaison clinical pharmacist to an inpatient palliative care unit. *Palliative Medicine*, **11**, 209–16.

9. ASHP statement on the Pharmacists' Role in Hospice and Palliative Care. Available at www.ashp.org (accessed April 2007).

10. Lee, J., and McPherson, M. (2006). Outcomes of recommendations by hospice pharmacists. *American Journal of Health-System Pharmacy*, **63**, 2235–9.

11. Needham, D.S., Wong, I.C.K., and Campion, P.D. (2002). Evaluation of the effectiveness of UK community pharmacists' interventions in community palliative care. *Palliative Medicine*, **16**, 219–25.

12. Hepler, C.D., and Strand, L.M. (1990). Opportunities and responsibilities in pharmaceutical care. *American Journal of Hospital Pharmacy*, **47**, 533–43.

13. Barber, N. (1995). What constitutes good prescribing. *BMJ*, **310**, 923–5.

14. Snapp, J., Kelley, D., and Gutsgell, T.L. (2002). Creating a hospice pharmacy and therapeutics committee. *The American Journal of Hospice & Palliative Care*, **19**(2), 129–34.

15. Weschules, D.J., Maxwell, T., Reifsnyder, J. *et al.* (2006). Are newer, more expensive pharmacotherapy options associated with superior symptom control compared to less costly agents used in a collaborative practice setting? *The American Journal of Hospice & Palliative Medicine*, **23**(2), 135–149.

16. Steinhauser, K.E., Clipp, E.C., Hays, J.C. *et al.* (2006). Identifying, recruiting, and retaining seriously-ill patients and their caregivers in longitudinal research. *Palliative Medicine*, **20**(8), 745–9.

17. Sackett, D.L., Rosenberg, W.M., Gray, J.A. *et al.* (1996). Evidence-based medicine: what it is and what it isn't. *BMJ*, **312**, 71–2.

18. Department of Health. The NHS cancer plan: a plan for investment, a plan for reform. Available at www.dh.gov.uk (accessed March 2007).

19. Weschules, D. (2005). Development of guidelines for palliative care pharmacotherapy. *Journal of Pain & Palliative Care Pharmacotherapy*, **19**(4), 25–38.

20. Holmes, H., Hayley, D.C., Alexander, G.C. *et al.* (2006). Reconsidering medication appropriateness for patients late in life. *Archives of Internal Medicine*, **166**, 605–609.

21. National Council for Palliative Care. Palliative care manifesto. Available at www.ncpc.org.uk (accessed February 2007).

22. Thomas, K. (2001). *Out-of-hours palliative care in the community*. Macmillan Cancer Relief, London.

23. Department of Health Out of Hours Plans and Guidance. Available at www.dh.gov.uk.

24. Thomas, K. (2003). *Caring for the dying at home, companions on the journey*. Radcliffe Medical Press, Oxford.

25. Preferred place of care document available at http://www.cancerlancashire.org.uk/ppc.html (accessed April 2007).

26. Amass, C., and Allen, M. (2005). How a "just in case" approach can improve out-of-hours palliative care. *Pharmaceutical Journal*, **275**, 22–3.

27. The Audit Commission (2001). *A spoonful of sugar*. NHS, London.

28. Ausburn, L. (1981). Patient compliance with medication regimes. *Advances in Behavioural Medicines*, **1**.

29. Royal Pharmaceutical Society of Great Britain (1997). *Working party report; From compliance to Concordance*. London. Royal Pharmaceutical Society of Great Britain.

30. Al-Rashed, S.A., Wright, D.J., Roebuck, N. *et al.* (2000). Inpatient pharmaceutical inputs to facilitate seamless care. *The Pharmaceutical Journal*, **265** (September 16), 7114.

31. (2001). The pharmacist's role in community palliative care. *Pharmaceutical Journal*, **267**(7169), 510–25.

32. Scally, G., and Donaldson, L.J. (1998). Clinical governance and the drive for quality improvement in the new NHS in England. *BMJ*, (4 July), 61–5.

33. Wilcock, A., Jacob, J., Charlesworth, S. *et al.* (2006). Drugs given by a syringe driver: a prospective multicentre survey of palliative care services in the UK. *Palliative Medicine*, **20**, 661–4.

34. CSCI survey continuing at www.palliativedrugs.com

35. Safety in Doses: Improving the use of medicines in the NHS. NPSA 2007. Available at www.npsa.nhs.uk (accessed April 2007).

36. (2006). Pharmacists with a special interest. *The Pharmaceutical Journal*, **277**(7417), 299.

Ethical issues

5.1

Introduction

Kenneth Calman

Introduction

A discussion on ethical issues in palliative care is of particular importance. The reason should be clear, in that much of the reasoning behind making decisions with patients on how best to manage the complexity of the problems requires that judgements are made. Such judgements are based on values held by the patient, the family, and the doctor. There may well be differences in views, and almost always there will be uncertainty. It is this uncertainty which makes the whole field so difficult and one in which legitimate differences of opinion can occur.

The purpose of having an ethical view of palliative care

The purpose of this chapter is to assist the professional to be able to analyse a clinical issue from an ethical point of view, and indeed to be able to identify an ethical issue in the first place. It will also introduce a range of concepts which are helpful in understanding ethical issues, and allow a comparison to be made between the person's own values and those of others. It should also encourage a logical approach and the ability to marshal arguments in favour of one's own position and understand that others may have different views. In essence, it is about understanding one's own values and how they compare with those of others.

This chapter is designed to set the scene for the more detailed sections which follow in subsequent chapters.

Developing an ethical framework

A discussion of ethical issues in palliative care usually revolves around a series of values held by all participants, which influence the clinical decision-making process. This will always include the patient's values and almost always those of the family. The way we consider our own values is generally around a framework of concepts, some of which may even be mutually incompatible. The framework may be based on duties, rights, or a series of principles such as autonomy, and it is the balance between such principles which determines the outcome of the decision making.

The framework adopted by any individual (patient, family member, or professional) may vary on these factors (duties, right, and principles) alone. However, if one adds into this framework differences in social, cultural, and spiritual aspects of life, then the possibilities become much more complex. From this brief initial discussion certain conclusions can be drawn.

♦ There are many different ways in which framework for ethical decision making can be constructed.

♦ These variations are relevant to making decisions which will almost always be in the face of uncertainty, and thus judgements will be required.

♦ Because of this there is ample scope for disagreement on what to do.

♦ There can be no right or wrong approach, just differences between different value bases held by individuals.

These brief conclusions raise other issues such as what to do when there is a disagreement, and how such disagreements should be dealt with, and these will be discussed later.

Where do values come from?

If values are so important how are our own values formed, and where do they come from? There are a whole series of ways some of which, and for each individual, may be more important than others. These might include;

♦ *Upbringing and parental values.* These can be important in terms of early religious experiences, attitudes to discipline and the context of the family. Political influences and attitudes may also be established in this process.

♦ *Schooling is the next major factor.* The role of the teacher, school values, and subjects taught also influence our thinking.

♦ *Religious background may be critical in setting values.* Different religions have different ways of looking at issues and even within a single religious group there may be considerable variation in views. For example, within the Christian religion views on end of life decisions and abortion vary considerably.

♦ *Peer pressure.* This can be very important in setting values as the need to conform, and not have views which would be outside the context of the group, which may be seen as abnormal. This pressure occurs not only in the context of school but also at work and at play.

♦ *Role models.* We all have role models, people we look up to and admire, and whose values we espouse. For professionals these can be crucial. The 'hidden' agenda in medicine is very powerful. Doctors, and others, learn from the attitudes and behaviour of seniors. It is difficult to underestimate the importance of this, especially if there are differences of views in the clinical team.

For patients the comments of friends and loved ones, those who play a significant part in their lives, are very relevant indeed.

♦ *Professional education and experience.* As medical students and postgraduate staff learn more about the possibilities in palliative care, and lack of them, for the management of symptoms or improving quality of life, so views can change. Meeting and helping a particular patient can have a profound effect, both positive and negative.

♦ *The media.* Debates in the media, for example, about end-of-life issues, can influence public opinion and those of patients and their families. The discussions may be informative, but are sometimes unrealistic and can raise expectations about possible outcomes.

♦ *Learning about ethics.* Part of being a professional is being concerned with ethical issues. It is necessary therefore to take time to learn about the concepts which are relevant and to be able to justify one's own position. Ethics may be learned in a variety of ways: through courses, reading, and by testing experience against the concepts. As will be discussed later the use of the arts and humanities is another way in which learning can be facilitated. It should be clear, however, that having an ethical approach to palliative care is not about a 1-week lecture course, it is about attitudes and values which occur in everyday practice. It is an ongoing process and a part of continuing professional development. During the day to day work in a palliative care setting there are many opportunities to raise ethical issues as part of the normal process of clinical work. These require leadership and an ability to open up questions for discussion.

♦ *Codes of ethics.* In some cases the values which are seen to be important have been codified and written down. The most famous of these is the Hippocratic Oath, which sets out some of the ethical principles which the doctor should follow. There are many others, including the Helsinki Declaration and the Declaration of Human Rights. These provide useful checks and prompts for those practising palliative medicine.

Such influences, and there are many others, shape our feelings and our values and it is these which are tested at times of uncertainty. They guide us in what to do in difficult circumstances. This leads to a discussion on the concepts and principles, which we collectively call our values.

Some key concepts

The following section sets out some of the key concepts which may be relevant in building up a personal ethical framework. It draws from a variety of different sources over several millennia, and the reader is advised to consult the reading list at the end of this chapter for further information and greater detail.

♦ *A duty to alleviate suffering.* This is an obvious concept, but like all such concepts not as simple as it seems. Of course we should alleviate suffering, but at what cost, either clinical or financial? How far should we go to alleviate suffering? Would this include active euthanasia? What if the symptom is difficult to alleviate and we fail? Have we failed in our duty?

♦ *Respect for persons.* Once again, this is an obvious concept to consider. It is important that we consider the individual and their dignity in the palliative care setting. How we communicate,

how we show respect and courtesy, all matter. This also means respecting the wishes of patients and their values, even if they differ from our own, and this can be a source of conflict. Respect for persons is associated with the concept of confidentiality. This sets out the right of the patient to have information about them, or their condition, kept within a limited number of members of the team, and in some instances by only one of them. It is a very important principle and one which can be easily breached as teams become larger and access to information easier.

♦ *Autonomy.* This is a concept, related to respect. It states that each individual has a right to make decisions about his/her own life and as a sentient human being is capable of so doing. It is difficult to disagree with this concept but it can, like so many other issues, raise problems. These include how far we should bend to the patient's wishes, and whether we should at anytime refuse to do what the patient wants. Such issues need to be thought through and would include the patients asking for a particular treatment which might not be available, or is too expensive, or one's own ethical framework is at odds with the patient's decision. A key part of autonomy is the ability of the patient to consent to treatment or care. Their wishes should be respected and they have a right to refuse treatment offered whether or not it makes sense to the doctor.

♦ *Non-maleficence.* This at first sight seems entirely appropriate. We should not do anything which may cause a potential harm to the patient. Once again how this works in practice is more difficult. Much of what we do, for example, in cancer treatment is potentially harmful, and the benefit might not always be clear. The dictum, *primum non nocere*—first do no harm—can be difficult to live up to.

♦ *Beneficence.* This implies that we should always do the best for our patients. Difficult to disagree with. However, it also implies that we as individual professionals have the skills and expertise to deal with the problem, and the wisdom to refer the patient to someone else if we already have not.

♦ *Utility.* This is an important concept in developing our framework of ethics. In short, it makes the point that the basis for care should be for the greatest good of the greatest number. We should do what we can to alleviate the suffering of the majority. This has obvious difficulties faced with an individual patient who might fall outside of the category of 'greatest number' for whatever reason, but when resources are limited, and that includes our time, how do we rationalize this concept?

♦ *Justice.* This implies fairness for all and equity and equality of care. Clearly this is impossible to achieve in all instances. Even in the field of palliative care it is generally the case that patients with cancer have a greater chance of being looked after by a palliative care service than a patient with cardiac and respiratory disease. Is this right and fair?

♦ *Human rights.* A good case can be made for using a rights-based approach. This begins by defining what such rights are and how they can be enforced. The right to life, the right to respect, the right to education, are all part of this approach.

This brief review does no more than indicate some of the concepts that form part of the development of a framework of ethics which help each of us to make difficult decisions in the face of uncertainty.

Some examples of conflicts

The principles listed above are often in conflict with each other when it comes to dealing with individual patients, and the following examples give some indication of the complexities involved. Here are a few clinical examples to put these principles in context.

- *The right to life*. This is a fundamental principle with which few would disagree. However, in end of life situations how far should we go to keep life going? Should no expense be spared even if this means that others cannot have a service provided, either through a funding shortage or lack of clinical time? This has especial difficulty in the case of children where emotional issues are raised and these are fully discussed in Chapter 5.4.

- *Autonomy*. The patient has a right to his or her own views, but what happens if we disagree? Suppose the patient wants us to 'end it all' and asks for euthanasia as an active process and that this is against our own values? The concept of autonomy suggests that the wishes should be enacted, but it may be impossible for us to do so and agree with the patient.

- *Telling the truth*. It would be natural to tell the truth to patients about their illness and the possible treatment. Several different scenarios present themselves, however. The first is when a relative approaches the doctor and asks that the patient is not told of the diagnosis or the prognosis. The second is the converse where the patient does not wish the family to know, but what if this is an infectious disease (HIV infection) or a genetic disorder which might be transmitted to a member of the family? The issue of confidentiality, and team confidentiality, are clearly very relevant and these are dealt with in Chapter 5.2.

- In one of J.K.Rowing's Harry Potter books, *Harry Potter and the Philosopher's Stone*, Dumbledore, the Head Master, discusses the topic of truth like this; 'The truth' Dumbledore sighed, 'it is a beautiful and terrible thing, and should therefore be treated with great caution. However I shall answer your questions unless I have good cause not to, in which case I beg you to forgive me. I shall of course not lie.'

- *Issues of research*. There are many ways in which conflicts may arise in research projects and these are dealt with in detail elsewhere. One familiar example, particular to nursing staff engaged in observational research, is when the procedure being studied is being performed badly. Does one intervene and correct the process, and hence destroy the research work, or leave the situation and potentially harm the patient? More recent issues concern the use of databases or databanks which are used to collect a wide range of data on patients. The collection of specimens of tissue for research purpose has also received considerable attention particularly in relation to the consent given for removal of the tissue an the uses to which the sample will put. The development of new and potentially hazardous treatments provide another example of an are where ethical issues are of particular concern.

Making decisions

At the end of the day it is our values that are of assistance in making decisions. The issue of uncertainty and the need for judgement have already been alluded to. The section looks at some of the components of the decision-making process.

- First, what is the evidence available about the patient, the possible symptom, and how can it best be controlled? What treatments are available, including non-pharmacological methods?

- What is the usual outcome of the process? Would the treatment be better carried out elsewhere? Are all the skills and expertise required available?

- What are the views of the patient? Are they the same as that of the family, the physician, and the team?

- If the views are different, can you see a way of supporting the wishes of the patient, or do you disagree?

- Has the patient been given all the information and have they consented to the possible intervention?

Going through this process (or something similar to it) can sometimes identify ways of reconciling differences of view or identify new ways of approaching the problem. It is part of good medical practice and is not a new method.

A key part of the whole process is the issue of trust between the patient and the doctor. Such trust takes time to build and can be lost rapidly. The old proverb 'trust comes on foot and goes on horse back' feels true. How can this trust be developed? It will require getting to know the patient, being honest, and always keeping promises. Explaining the procedures, what will happen, who will be there, and what their roles will be is very much part of this. Trust means allowing someone to do something one would not normally let them do. It means giving up some autonomy. An example might help to illustrate some of these issues. Suppose you are going out for the evening and you ask a 20-year-old to look after your two children aged 5 and 7. You trust the person, though you know that something untoward may happen. You know that if it does it will not be deliberate. The baby-sitter has the interest of the children at heart. The same concept applies to patients. If they trust the doctor, then they give up some of their own control and give it to the doctor whom they know will not do anything deliberately harmful and will always be doing it in the best interests of the patient. The patient knows that they will be kept fully informed and that their views will be respected at all times.

The reason this concept is so important is that in the management of uncertainty there will always be unknowns. It will not always be possible to give all of the information because the nature of the problem may be unknown. Trust bridges the gap and allows the patient to have the most appropriate course of action. Martin Buber in his book *I and Thou* sets this out rather differently, but with the same outcome. He makes the point that some relationships are 'I and You' ones. There is respect but there is also a professional distance between the patient and the doctor. Some of the relationships however, are 'I and Thou' ones which are much closer, there is real trust, there is a 'sharing of hearts', and the depth of the relationship is considerable. Trust is part of this and those who work regularly in the palliative care field will recognize such relationships. Trust is a fundamental part of the patient–professional relationship.

Dealing with disagreements

So far there has been an assumption that everyone will agree with the outcome of the decision-making process. As the examples discussed above make clear, this is not always the case and the problem is what to do in such circumstances. There are three possible scenarios.

1 *The patient and the doctor disagree.* It is not difficult to see how such differences can come about. Poor communication, lack of trust, and differences in values, all contribute. The real issue is what to do about it? This is a situation where the doctor must not be proud and must show humility. The patient is generally right. There should be an open referral to another professional who may look at the situation from a different perspective and with a different value base. Such referrals should be made early in the process before resentment and anger build up.

2 *The patient and the family disagree.* This is a particularly tragic problem, when at a time when the family should be supportive and positive, there are family disagreements, tension, and difficulty in communicating. It requires a skilled professional to help the family come together and make the most of the remaining life of the patient.

3 *Inter-professional disputes.* These are common and the result of differing experiences in professional education and the building of values. Disagreements can be a positive and learning experience for all. The problem arises when one member of the staff has values which are different from the others' and after discussion there is no meeting of minds. This can often occur when a new member joins the team and challenges the values of others. What should be done in this instance? There can be an agreement to differ and that the group view, or that of the senior professional, prevails. The learning experience following the outcome of the decision can be very important. This may not be sufficient, however, and the member of staff still disagrees. Under these circumstances, where the ethical principles of the doctor may be compromised, it is often useful to talk the problem over with a senior colleague. It may be that the practice is unethical in the views of others and this must be shared. In extreme circumstances, the views of the individual may be so incompatible with that of the team that the staff member has to resign.

Working in other cultures

A particular subset of the differences in values which may occur relates to working in different cultures, religious faiths, or social systems. This is an area of considerable development as the world becomes smaller and more multi-cultural. Here, the differences may be very significant and the doctor may have to accept the views of the different culture, no matter how difficult it may seem. We can learn from others and their views, while challenging, may be just as relevant, they are to the individuals concerned. It is necessary for doctors and others to familiarize themselves with such differences and to be sensitive to the range of values that may be presented to them (see Chapter 3.7).

Research ethics review committees

All research to be carried out should be reviewed by an independent research ethics committee. These are set up in different ways but have as their primary function the interests of the patient and their protection. They can comment and ask questions of the research workers and ensure that patients are not disadvantaged and that the research meets ethical standards. These too may vary from country to country and from culture to culture. They are an essential safeguard for patients.

Role of the humanities

In an earlier section of the chapter, reference was made to learning about ethics and the range of methods available. One of these, covered in more depth in another chapter, is the use of the humanities, and in particular, literature. The use of novels, plays, and poems to illustrate difficult ethical issues and their complexity, can be very powerful mechanisms in assisting in the understanding of very difficult clinical problems.

Further reading

American Medical Association (1994). *Codes of Medical Ethics.* AMA, Chicago, IL.

Beauchamp, T.L. and Childress, J.F. (2001). *Principles of Biomedical Ethics,* 5th edn. Oxford University Press, Oxford.

Boyd, K.M., Higgs, R. and Pinching, A.J., ed. (1997). *The New Dictionary of Medical Ethics.* BMJ Publishing Group, London.

British Medical Association. (2001). *The Medical Profession and Human Rights.* Zed Books Ltd, London.

Buber, M. (1958). *I and Thou.* T.T. Clark, Edinburgh.

Campbell, A., Gillett, G., Jones, G. (2005). *Medical Ethics,* 4th Edition. Oxford University Press, New York.

Downie, R.S. and Calman, K.C. (1994). *Healthy Respect,* 2nd edn. Oxford University Press, Oxford.

Downie, R.S. and Macnaughton, J. (2000). *Clinical Judgement. Evidence in Practice.* Oxford Medical Publications, Oxford.

Fulford, K.W.M., Dickenson, D.L. and Murray, T., ed. (2002). *Healthcare Ethics and Human Values.* Blackwell Publishing, Oxford.

Harris, J. (2003). *The value of life. An introduction to medical ethics.* Routledge, London and New York.

Kuhse, H. and Singer, P. (2001). *A companion to bioethics.* Blackwell, Oxford.

5.2

Confidentiality

Ira R. Byock and Diane Palac

'Confidentiality is a fundamental tenet of medical care. Confidentiality is a matter of respecting the privacy of patients, encouraging them to seek medical care and discuss their problems candidly, and preventing discrimination on the basis of their medical conditions'[1].

Introduction

In the course of practice, palliative care clinicians inevitably learn private, and often intimate, details about patients' and families' lives. Palliative care and hospice practitioners share an obligation to maintain the confidentiality of information acquired through the clinician–patient relationship with all health-care professionals.

However, competing ethical and legal mandates and clinical priorities often complicate protection of patient-specific information, and there are logistical challenges to effectively protecting the privacy of patient information, most of which derive from sophisticated information systems of contemporary practice environments. The nature of palliative care, particularly its therapeutic focus on each patient with his or her family and its interdisciplinary team-based approach to care, creates tensions between ethical and clinical principles. In deciding whether, when, and with whom to share private patient-specific information, palliative care clinicians must balance the protection of patients from potential harms of disclosure against concern for the wellbeing of patients' families, close contacts, and community.

Background and context

Confidentiality refers to the protection of privacy of information about another person. An expectation of confidentiality in the relationship to one's physician or priest has roots in antiquity. Although the legal framework of an individual's right to privacy has evolved only in the last century, its justification is found in documents such as the Amendments to the Constitution of the United States of America, wherein fundamental principles of Western society and culture are expressed. Privacy and confidentiality have both legal and ethical relevancies to palliative care.

Legal and ethical textbooks from the close of the 20th century reflect complementary contemporaneous perspectives on privacy and confidentiality. In an essay on the legal history of United States privacy law, Standler quotes that 'privacy is the expectation that confidential personal information disclosed in a private place will not be disclosed to third parties, when that disclosure would cause either embarrassment or emotional distress to a person of reasonable sensitivities. Information is interpreted broadly to include facts, images (e.g. photographs, videotapes), and disparaging opinions. The right of privacy is restricted to individuals who are in a place that a person would reasonably expect to be private'[2]. Bio-ethicists Beauchamp and Childress explained that 'privacy refers to a condition of physical or informational inaccessibility'[3]. 'The right to (personal) privacy has its basis in the right to authorize or decline access, justified by the right of autonomous choice found in the principle of respect for autonomy'.

Confidentiality is a hallmark of professionalism. In the course of their service to individuals, professionals collect or otherwise have access to private information about an individual's personal life, such as the history and current status of the person's health, finances, or legal situation. Society recognizes an individual's right to keep information of this nature private and charges the professions and, by extension, individual professionals to maintain the confidentiality of such information. Confidentiality, therefore, refers to an ethical duty on the part of professionals to not divulge information collected within the confines of a professional relationship, such as the relationship of physician and patient, priest and confessor, or attorney and client.

From antiquity, medical professionals have sworn to maintain confidentiality and thereby protect the privacy of the people who became their patients. The Hippocratic Oath, originating from the era of 400 BC, has been taken by entering members of the medical profession for centuries. This oath specifically obligates physicians to guard the confidentiality of their patients.

'What I may see or hear in the course of the treatment or even outside of the treatment in regard to the life of men, which on no account one must spread abroad, I will keep to myself, holding such things shameful to be spoken about.' [Translation from the Greek by L. Edelstein. From *The Hippocratic Oath: Text, Translation, and Interpretation*, by L. Edelstein. Baltimore, MD: Johns Hopkins Press, 1943].

This ethical principle was reaffirmed in a modern version of the Hippocratic Oath published in 1964 and used by many American medical schools today:

'I will respect the privacy of my patients, for their problems are not disclosed to me that the world may know.' [Written in 1964 by Louis Lasagna, Academic Dean of the School of Medicine at Tufts University.]

A comprehensive medical history routinely inquires about a person's bodily functions, medications, habits related to use of tobacco, alcohol and non-prescription drugs, sexual orientation and history of sexually-transmitted infections. Health-care professionals are expected to restrict access to information to those who require it to assist the professional in the service of the patient. Therefore, a clinician may share patient-specific information with other members of a clinical team or consultants who require it, but must not otherwise divulge information, unless the individual extends specific permission to do so or access to such information has been accorded by law[4–7].

Clinicians advance the ethical principle of beneficence in maintaining the confidentiality of privileged patient information. Confidentiality also derives from the principle of non-malfeasance, a duty to 'do no harm', which extends to protecting patients from harms that can occur as a consequence of clinicians' actions, including the collection of private information. Breaching confidentiality in the contemporary world can expose patients to a variety of tangible threats, including losing or being denied employment or health benefits, or becoming a target of marketers and financial predators seeking vulnerable customers.

Making confidentiality a legal obligation

Societies grant self-regulating authority to professions and expect each profession to monitor and maintain a reasonable level of quality of practice by its members. Violations of confidentiality may result in imposed sanctions by a membership organization or by a professional licensing board and may even result in the revocation of an individual's license to practice resulting in de facto expulsion from the profession. However, Western societies have not been content to rely solely on the professions' capacity for self-regulation and have codified basic obligations within law. These statutes and regulations require health-care professionals to protect private information of patients with narrowly defined exceptions. These laws and rules have two complementary intentions: to protect the public from unwarranted intrusions and invasions of privacy and to protect the privileged nature of clinician–patient relationship.

In contrast to concepts of property ownership and contracts which can be found in the earliest laws, the legal right of privacy emerged in the late 19th century and gained broader recognition in statutes during the latter part of the 20th century. Writing in 1960, Prosser described privacy as 'an emerging right' that is typically delineated through 'a list of examples where the right has been recognized, instead of a simple definition'[8]. In the United States, a legal basis for privacy as non-intrusion into the lives of individual citizens by the government or other citizens, is found in the First, Fourth, Fifth and Fourteenth Amendments to the United States Constitution.

Statutory definitions of privacy vary across countries and jurisdictions. From a general legal perspective, privacy refers to the expectation that personal information disclosed in a private place will not be disclosed to third parties. Privacy is mostly addressed in law or judicial precedent through situations in which disclosure of information results in possible damage, harm or distress to a person of reasonable sensitivities. Privacy extends to situations in which people 'believe that the conversation is private and cannot be heard by others who are acting in a lawful manner' [Am. Jur. 2nd *Telecommunications* § 209 (1974)][2]. Laws and legal precedents

have specified protection of facts, images, voice recordings and the content of statements made within professional relationships. Depending on the situation in which it occurs and corresponding potential for resulting harms, the unauthorized act of divulging of private information by a professional may constitute a misdemeanour or felony under criminal law. Such violations may also constitute a civil tort. As an example, in the case of Humphers v. First Interstate Bank of Oregon, a woman successfully sued a physician for violating confidentiality in assisting the individual she had given up for adoption years earlier to identify her as the individual's biological mother[9].

In health care, natural tensions exist between the need to ensure access to patient-specific information by those serving the patient and the need to protect the sanctity of that information. These tensions can erupt into conflict and controversy when confidentiality is breached either by error or unethical behaviour.

In a well-publicized apparent error without ill intention in the United States, computer discs 'containing the names, social security numbers, and dates of birth for up to 26.5 million veterans and some spouses, as well as some disability ratings' [Office of Public Affairs Statement, Department of Veteran's Affairs, 22 May 2006] were temporarily lost, leaving their contents vulnerable to being copied. Instances of ill-intended intrusions are not hard to find and becoming almost common. Computer hackers have gained access via the Internet to medical, financial, and even Department of Defence files despite safeguards that had been considered impenetrable[10].

Legislatures in national and regional jurisdictions have responded to the changing health-care environments by requiring procedural and technological safeguards in information systems, by making unauthorized access to patient information illegal, and by imposing penalties for willfully breaching confidentiality. These laws, regulations, and formal guidelines define criteria and procedures for accessing and transferring health information and commonly rely on the concept of the 'need-to-know' as a rationale for restricting access to private patient information to personnel who require it to perform services for the patient.

A survey of Western countries' health privacy legislation reflects the rapidly evolving nature of this arena of law[4,5]. In Australia, the Privacy Act, which was adopted in 1988, encompasses protections of financial and health information, based on a set of National Privacy Principles. It has been regularly updated, most recently in June of 2006. In Britain, the Data Privacy Act was passed in 1998[11]. In Canada, the Personal Information Protection and Electronic Documents Act was enacted in 2000 and most recently updated in September 2006. The United States adopted the federal Health Insurance Portability and Accountability Act, widely referred to as HIPAA, in 1996. Due to the complexity of regulations for implementing the law and pragmatic difficulties of complying with the law's requirements, provisions for full compliance did not take effect until April of 2003 for most of the providers and insurance companies, and a year later for smaller underwriters.

The United States HIPAA statute exemplifies the practical challenges of legal approaches to confidentiality. The law applies to health-care providers, health insurance plans, and health-care clearinghouses and is intended to protect the privacy of patient-specific health information and to guarantee a patient's access to his or her own information. In addition to charging clinicians and institutions with maintaining confidentiality in their own communications and actions, HIPAA makes providers responsible for overseeing secondary users of a patient's personal health information. Despite laudable Congressional intentions, this requirement has caused considerable concern among American clinicians who generally do not have control over patients' medical information. Secondary users, including insurers, pharmacy benefit plans, and suppliers of medical equipment, can often gain access to patient-specific data independently.

Responding to problems associated with the HIPAA law's implementation, the US Department of Health and Human Services revised the regulations to allow physicians to use their judgement in disclosing to a family member or close friend information that is 'directly relevant' to that person's 'involvement with the patient's care.' If the patient is available, the physician must ascertain that the patient 'does not object to the disclosure.' Alternately, if the patient is not present or is incapacitated, the physician may 'reasonably infer based on the exercise of professional judgement' that the patient does not object or may determine that it is 'in the best interests' of the patient to make such a disclosure[12]. In a review of the early experience with this new privacy law, Lo suggests that many of the gaps in the HIPAA law's regulations would appropriately be filled by professional judgement informed by ethical guidelines. He states that 'Communication should be necessary and effective for good patient care, and the risks of a breach of confidentiality should be proportional to the likely benefit for the patient's care'[12].

Although unintended and not required in the letter of the law, the manner in which HIPAA regulations are being implemented in institutional policies and practices at times have resulted in new barriers to communication and normal human connections between people who are ill and their natural network of relatives and friends. This can increase a sense of isolation in people with serious illness. Prior to the development of hospice and palliative care in the 1970s, being terminally ill carried a stigma, and dying persons commonly remained out of sight of friends, neighbours and professional caregivers alike. The principle of 'primacy of patient welfare' must maintain its precedence, even over patient privacy[13].

Challenges to maintaining confidentiality

Technical challenges
In striving to strictly protect the privacy of patients in today's world, palliative care clinicians commonly encounter technical, cultural, and ethical complexities. The context of clinical practice continues to change rapidly. There are wide variations in the structures of health care, the modes of service delivery, and payment and the processes of clinical assessment, treatment, and documentation from one region and from country to another. In many locations, during the past two decades, clinicians have witnessed profound changes occur in their work environments, requirements of practice, and patterns of care.

In developed countries, dominant trends in health services have included increasing sophistication of medical diagnosis and treatment, increasing specialization and compartmentalization of care along with corresponding reliance on the collection, storage, and timely transfer of detailed patient-specific information. Unfortunately, this information-dependent health-care environment has greatly expanded opportunities for abuse of people's private health information.

The electronic medical record (EMR) represents a paradigmatic example of these trends. It is becoming commonplace in contemporary health-care settings and practices. The advent of the EMR is considered to be an important advance with the potential for enhancing the quality of health care and the consistency, specificity, and efficiency of health service delivery. Additionally, computerized patient records can facilitate data-driven system improvements and practice-based research. However, these expanded capacities carry concomitant risks to the confidentiality of patient information.

One of the potential advantages of the EMR is that it can be used for a range of purposes, including clinical documentation, as well as financial accounting and billing. While presumably efficient, these multiple uses of the medical record entail substantially expanded access to medical records by a range of personnel including: coders, insurers, pharmacy staff, systems analysts, and researchers. A quarter century ago, Siegler counted 76 hospital-associated personnel who had both legitimate access one person's inpatient medical record and reason to examine it[14]. The increasing use of the EMR and related developments, simultaneously make protecting private patient information more complicated and more urgent.

Ethical challenges
The value of protecting private information seems intuitive and straightforward, however, honouring the principle of confidentiality in practice can prove difficult. Bio-ethical teaching and professional guidelines make clear that confidentiality in health care is not absolute[1,3,6,7]. Ethical practice often requires clinicians to balance risks and potential benefits. Circumstances occasionally arise, for instance, in which strict adherence to protecting the confidentiality of private patient information can put other people at risk of physical or emotional harm.

Privacy laws provide protection to clinicians for breaching confidentiality in carefully defined situations and, in some instances, create legal obligations for disclosure when the safety of others is at risk.

In the United States, a landmark court case established a legal requirement for health care professionals to breach confidentiality to warn a third party when the clinician has knowledge that a particular individual may be in serious danger of physical harm from a patient [Tarasoff v. Regents of University of California]. The national laws of the United Kingdom, Canada, Australia and the United States previously referred to in this chapter each specify circumstances in which professionals may (or must) share private information with public health authorities or law enforcement. Such information typically includes knowledge of child and elder abuse or neglect, expressed homicidal intention, injuries caused by deadly weapons and positive tests for serious contagious infections. Additionally, privacy exemptions allow health information to be shared for purposes of government oversight and health-care institution accountability.

The practice of palliative care today involves myriad patient and family cultures and individual psychological and social characteristics and values. Inevitably, predicaments arise that involve questions of confidentiality that have not been anticipated by legislatures or provided for within existing laws and regulations. Ultimately, the task of weighing the extent of potential harms to the patient of disclosure and the degree of risk to others are often matters for professional judgement.

Illustrative case: a 65-year-old woman dying of advanced HIV disease with multiple opportunistic infections requests that her sister and nieces and nephews never be told about her diagnosis because of the shame she feels over her past history of IV drug abuse and prostitution. The palliative care team decides that it is able to maintain this confidence. However, when sputum tests reveal active tuberculosis, the clinicians are obligated by law to inform the family and health department of the secondary infection.

Illustrative Case: Mrs. H, a 65-year-old woman with glioblastoma multiforme, is admitted to the hospital with acute confusion. Eight months ago, she underwent surgical de-bulking of the tumour followed by whole brain radiation. Three weeks ago, she developed R hemiparesis. Mrs. H lives with her husband. The couple's daughter and two sons disagree regarding their parents' care; the sons maintain that their sister is unsupportive of their father.

In the hospital, a speech therapist reports that Mr. H repetitively kisses Mrs. H on her face in a manner that obstructs her ability to work with the patient. Nurses verbally describe Mr. H rubbing and 'groping' Mrs. H under her bed sheets, while she remains passive, seemingly confused. At times, their sons have been present, but apparently unconcerned by their father's behaviour. The patient's daughter tell the palliative care consultant that over the past few months, her mother confided that she was distressed and embarrassed by her husband touching her in this way.

In assessing Mrs. H's cognitive capacity, the consultant concludes that she is currently unable to consent to or refuse this contact. Wishing to respect the privacy of the patient and her family, the consultant is uncertain whether to discuss the matter at palliative care Interdisciplinary Team (IDT) rounds and to what extent it should be described and discussed in the medical record.

After considerable discussion with the inpatient palliative care team, the consultant concludes that the behaviour constitutes 'unconsented touching' of a sexual nature and raises concerns of abuse which must be addressed. Clinicians anticipate that any effort to modify Mr. H's behaviour will be unwelcome by him and the couple's sons. They conclude that the IDT has 'a need to know.' The IDT recommends documenting the issue in the medical record and holding a family meeting. The attending neuro-oncologist is made aware of the concerns and informs Mrs. H's family that she is unable to speak for herself and is probably dying.

A family meeting is held. The patient's sons react angrily to the palliative care team's concerns and accuse their sister of meddling. They assert that intimate contact of this nature is acceptable between a husband and wife. During the discussion, one son mentions that his father is under the care of Dr. R, a staff geriatric psychiatrist.

The palliative care clinicians discuss whether confidentiality prevents them from contacting Mr. H's psychiatrist and indirectly involving him in Mrs. H's care. The couple's sons voice no objection to a suggestion that Mr. H be re-evaluated by Dr. R, and agree to accompany their father to the appointment. The consultants communicate their concerns to Dr. R. Unfortunately, after this appointment, the sons continue to assert that their father's behaviour is appropriate and concerns are unwarranted.

The palliative care team then asks Dr. R to visit Mr. H at his wife's bedside. In the presence of the couple and their sons, Dr. R explains that Mr. H's behaviour reflects dis-inhibition due to dementia and that it is neither normal nor appropriate given the current mental status of Mrs. H. Now the sons react with sadness and agree to set limits with their father.

Dr. R enters his assessment and recommendations in Mrs. H's medical record. A plan is developed in which nursing staff is asked to monitor Mr. H's visits and set limits on the objectionable behaviours. Clinicians and the couple's children agree that this plan protects Mrs. H's rights and dignity, while supporting the couple's relationship.

Palliative medicine teams meet people at times of great vulnerability. Confidentiality is particularly pertinent to palliative care due to the intimate nature of physical care, the depth and details of a patient's personal and family history explored and the similarly sensitive range of topics routinely encompassed in counselling.

Palliative care clinicians frequently learn details of a patient's or family's current and earlier lives and relationships that have never been disclosed to others. Similarly, family members may become aware of information that is surprising and, at times, troubling. Illness often requires an individual to accept help from others in ways that entail access to their private living spaces and information. In the course of progressive decline and physical dependence, it may become difficult for an individual to maintain long-standing deceptions. Prior to HAART medications for HIV infection, the physical appearance of Kaposi's sarcoma lesions on exposed skin often made the undisclosed diagnosis of AIDS unmistakable for families. More commonly, in the course of reviewing legal or financial documents during the process of paying bills for the patient or transferring of property a spouse or adult child inadvertently uncovers information revealing a child's undisclosed adoption, parentage, religious heritage, or ethnicity. At times, the family of a recently incapacitated patient becomes aware of past instances of sexual or violent physical abuse. When revelations of this nature occur, skilful counselling is required to concurrently acknowledge the seriousness of the situations and the hurt or anger they engender, while preserving any opportunity that may exist for people (if they so choose) to reconcile these deeply wounded relationships.

Of course, not all disclosures cause harm. Palliative care teams utilize life review as a means of helping people to develop a sense of meaning about their lives. It is common practice to encourage people to tell their stories and record stories as a legacy to those they will leave behind. In the telling or retelling of old stories, hitherto private details of events or people's lives may come to light. Most often, these fresh details are not controversial, but merely enrich the histories of the individual and family.

In practice, it is rarely necessary to curtail life review over concerns about hurtful or potentially damaging private information that might be revealed within the natural network of a patient's relatives and friends. However, it is important to distinguish life review, including the recording of a person's stories, from insight therapy, in which patients explore painful times and wounded relationships for their sources and meanings. Kast suggests guiding life review by assisting individuals to create a biography of joy[15].

Internal tensions: family as a focus of palliative care

Strict confidentiality often proves difficult to maintain in the practice of palliative care due to inherent tensions with other basic tenets of the discipline.

The principle of confidentiality is intended to support the autonomy of individual patients and to advance the practice of beneficence and non-malfeasance. A fundamental principle of palliative medicine is that patients' families deserve attention to their experiences of illness, care giving, and grief. Naturally, the large majority of the time, the values and goals of a patient and his or her family are well-aligned. Occasionally, however, circumstances arise in which withholding specific information about a patient poses serious adverse consequences to the physical health or emotional well-being of a family member or close contact. While clinical ethics generally emphasizes the health and well-being of each individual, some balance must be struck between the rights of an individual and the welfare of others. Most such instances are not addressed by a specific guideline or statute and are left to the discretion and judgement of individual clinicians and palliative care teams.

Illustrative case: a 47-year-old man is dying of lung cancer. He tells his doctor that his mother died of Huntington's disease, not Alzheimer's dementia as his family has long maintained. He feels ashamed to have kept the information from his own children, who are at risk of developing the disease later in life, and of passing on the gene as they enter child-bearing age. He's worried that his 23-year-old son, who has battled depression and substance abuse, might commit suicide if he is told.

Illustrative case: a critical medicine physician and Intensive Care Unit (ICU) nurse, who were caring for Mr. R.B., a 62-year-old Native American man with sepsis and multi-system failure, needed to convene a family meeting to discuss the patient's condition, worrisome prognosis and to make treatment decisions. Entering the ICU waiting room they found it filled with nearly 30 Native Americans. They explained that they would like the patient's family to gather in the conference room for a serious discussion. A spokesman for the group took stock of those assembled and replied, 'We're almost all here; we're just waiting for two more people to arrive.'

The composition of a patient's family may not be clearly defined. The principles of palliative medicine do not restrict the definition of family to relatives by blood, formal adoption, or marriage. In practice, to the extent possible, patients and families decide for themselves whom to include in their private affairs. A range of inclusive and restrictive concepts of family membership are found across different ethnicities and cultures and may influence a family's preferences.

It is generally prudent for palliative care teams to leave the operating definition of family up to the patient, relatives, and friends involved, however, professional oversight and judgement is warranted on a case-by-case basis. In the case example of Mr. R.B., pertinent information about the patient's condition entailed a history of alcoholic liver disease, oesophageal varices and hypersplenism that contribute to the poor prognosis. In a private conversation with the physician, the patient's spouse (and power of attorney for health care) explicitly gave permission for these details to be shared with the community in hopes that it would call attention to the adverse effects of alcohol abuse. If she had wanted the details kept private, the physician and team were prepared to withhold specific details of his condition.

The challenges of cultural diversity extend beyond defining membership of a patient's family and can strongly influence the processes of communication and decision making. Caring for ethnically diverse patients often reveals value-laden assumptions that permeate Western health-care culture and influence the structures and processes of clinical practice. The assumptions and values about how decisions are made for a specific individual and family may be very different from those of western society and bioethics.

Pertinent to the principle of confidentiality, Western cultures and ethics strongly emphasize individual rights and the principles of beneficence, non-malfeasance and autonomy of the individual.

In contrast, cultures of the Middle East and Far East, as well as indigenous cultures of the West, such as Native Americans and Canadian First Nations, generally place greater emphasis on communal values. In such cultures, individuals do not possess sole moral authority for their decisions, nor by extension, to information pertinent to those decisions. Instead, an individual's family and community are seen as legitimate stakeholders in decision making. This diversity of cultural and individual preferences and patterns of decision making can be encompassed within western bioethics through the concept of delegated autonomy and legal instruments, such as the health-care directive and the power of attorney for health care. For instance, when encountered in a Canadian hospital, an elderly Chinese woman delegates her eldest son to make her decisions. On advice and with help of the palliative care social worker, she completes a power of attorney for health-care directive and specifies that it take effect immediately. Palliative care teams can honour confidentiality and support delegated decision-making styles by skilfully communicating health information to the identified decision makers and by recognizing their authority to further restrict or divulge information on the patient's behalf.

As Fins notes, the health-care ethical guidelines and decision-making tools of western societies reflect a contractual approach to decisions. Advance directives use a contractual framework for appointing a legal proxy who is expected to protect the individual's rights by adhering to the treatment choices specified in the document. Viewed from this perspective, advance directive documents are intended to protect individuals from a potentially hostile environment. Fins describes an alternative perspective and approach, based on covenantal values of fundamental trust, in which the person expects and trusts the chosen proxy to be guided by statements of preference, but ultimately, to use his or her best judgement in making decisions. In research in which people with advance directives and their actual proxies were given a series of hypothetical critical situations, many individuals make choices that are consistent with a covenantal approach[16,17].

Broadly restrictive policies and practices regarding patients' private information can impede and constrict a palliative care team's therapeutic mission. The fundamental tenet that the patient and family together be considered the focus of care is a therapeutic principle. Palliative medicine clinicians recognize that for most patients and families the experiences of illness, care giving, and grief are inextricably linked. Intimacy within most family relationships is natural, not a violation of privacy. The developmental work of completing one's relationships and life is intensely personal.

While people have an uncontested right to their privacy during such circumstances, most people gratefully accept help from extended family, friends and members of their communities. Despite common initial reluctance to burden others, many people living with progressive illness find that their connections to others and their communities become ever more important as the responsibilities and activities of their previous life fall away.

Human beings are fundamentally social animals and with rare exceptions, the quality of an individual's relationships significantly influences a person's perceived quality of life[18].

Isolation and loneliness are frequently observed causes of stress among chronically ill or frail elderly people living alone or in institutions. Contemporary philosophers, Brock and Daniels, addressing matters of national health-care policy asserted that 'We are members not only of a national community but also of many other communities that flourish within our society including religious, racial and ethnic communities, as well as the neighbourhoods, towns and cities in which people share a sense of common life. Fundamental to all these different communities is a shared concern and responsibility for one's fellow members, especially those suffering misfortune and in need of help'.

Beneficence in palliative care requires preserving for the patient the opportunities, or ethical 'goods', that derive from living in the context of one's family and community. In studies, patients with advanced illness and their families identify connections to others and achieving a sense of completion of intimate family relationships as highly important[19,20]. Including attention to the caregiver and other family members in the patient's end of life care has been found to enhance their ability to cope with the patient's death and appears to be associated with reductions in rates of depression and mortality following the patient's death[21].

These values and perspectives are resonant within the specialty of palliative medicine. However, palliative care clinicians and teams must not assume that patients and families share the values, assumptions and expectations embedded in their discipline. A straightforward way to honour confidentiality as clinicians seek to assist people in renewing, strengthening, and completing their relationships is to ask patients to set the parameters for communicating information with relatives and friends and, whenever a question arises, to ask permission before specific information is shared with another person.

Common considerations include whether a patient's clergy or congregation should be informed that the person has been admitted to the hospital and whether or not they will accept visits. Another familiar and poignant predicament arises when a patient, who hopes to get better but is becoming progressively ill, asks her clinician to speak by phone with a beloved relative or close friend who is calling from a long distance. Once, on the phone, the caller asks the clinician whether it is prudent to wait for a coming holiday, a month in the future, to visit. If in the clinician's estimation the patient is unlikely to be alive or fully responsive at the time of the planned visit, how much information should the clinician divulge?

The challenge for palliative care teams is to avoid harms to a patient's privacy while preventing isolation, diminishing loneliness and fostering connections to persons' families and communities.

Internal tensions: interdisciplinary team approach to palliative care

By definition and established principle, palliative care encompasses an interdisciplinary team approach to patients and families. This inclusive, collaborative approach to care creates natural tensions with the principle of confidentiality. Some health-care rules and regulations seek to limit access of private patient information only to physicians and nurses directly caring for the individual patient. While such restrictions seem reasonable and prudent from the perspective of confidentiality, there are important advantages to the interdisciplinary patient and family assessment, care planning and care.

Not uncommonly, in addition to their direct services to a patient, an art therapist, massage therapist, nursing aide, bath aide, or volunteer contributes a valuable insight that improves a team's ability to care for a patient and family. Similarly, in participating in discussions of an interdisciplinary case conference, a consultant pharmacist may recognize potential side effects of a patient's medication or be able to suggest an alternative medication for the team and prescribing clinicians to consider.

There is no clear consensus on the boundaries of sharing confidential information with an interdisciplinary health-care team. Palliative care teams may choose to include all the team's staff clinicians and non-professional staff members as well as volunteers in case discussions and care planning. Some teams will limit the inclusion of non-professional staff members and volunteers to those who have direct contact with the patient and family under discussion. Alternately, some teams may restrict case and care planning meetings to licensed clinicians.

Whenever ancillary professionals and non-professionals participate as members of an interdisciplinary palliative care team, they must accept and adhere to the same requirements of confidentiality that apply to the professionals involved. This obligation should be formalized by policy, included in training of all Board, management, staff and volunteers. A commitment to confidentiality applies at all levels of an organization and extends to vendors and contractors who work for the organization. The importance of confidentiality warrants periodic reminders to all personnel and contractors with access to private information. Failure to comply with rules and infractions deserves explicit attention and corrective actions. Policies can specify which individual employees or team members are responsible for training of professionals and non-professionals regarding confidentiality. Difficult instances can be seen as opportunities to review and affirm the organization's commitment to confidentiality while offering a chance for staff to debrief and problem-solve ways of implementing procedural safeguards.

Similarly, volunteers are bound by hospital or hospice confidentiality policies. The need-to-know concept can guide clinicians in judging what information is appropriate to communicate to a volunteer who is visiting a patient.

Conversely, it is not uncommon for patients or families to confide in a volunteer they have come to know and trust. And, volunteers at times may observe unguarded family interactions. Such instances include tender moments, but occasionally, volunteers witness hurtful arguments, mean-spirited statements or actions or observe what they feel is emotional abuse. At other times they may hear patients express thoughts about suicide. Without clear guidelines and professional support, the volunteer may inadvertently become enmeshed in difficult dilemmas[22].

Volunteers deserve clear education about the ethical guidelines and legal requirements that govern their volunteer activities and the legal protections accorded them in their roles. Volunteers who become aware of problematic behaviours including instances of physical abuse must have a means of reporting the information and can be assured that such disclosures are allowed and, in fact, required by law.

A hierarchy of access to information exists within the generally non-hierarchical culture of palliative care teams. This hierarchy has usually paralleled those with the highest 'need to know.' The patient's attending physician may exercise judgement to withhold specific details of a patient's history from other members of the clinical team(s), including consultants, students, or the patient's assigned volunteers. However, consultants, students, and volunteers must not withhold sensitive information from the attending physician. When there is doubt, the attending physician caring for the patient is best positioned to make assessments of what information is necessary or appropriate to share with the team and what is appropriate to hold in confidence.

Patient and family expectations of confidentiality

Limited research suggests that many people assume that their medical information is only accessible to their doctors and nurses[23]. In introducing palliative care to patients and families, it is, therefore, essential to explain and emphasize that it is a team-based approach to care. Further research is needed to examine the extent to which patients who are concerned about privacy would be reassured by learning of the technical and procedure safeguards in place and the potential advantages to them of having information about their situation and plan of care available to members of their extended clinical team.

Whenever particularly sensitive information is disclosed by the patient or a family member in the course of evaluation and treatment, it is prudent to ask explicitly whether this information can be included in the medical record. Patients need to be made aware that omitting important information from the medical record heightens the risk that it may be unavailable for clinicians later in seeking to provide sensitive and individualized patient care and family support.

These interactions offer an opportunity for clinicians to explain advantages that team-based care offers to patients and families. Policies, training, and on-going programmatic quality improvement efforts related to confidentiality can prepare clinicians to reassure individuals of the serious commitment on the part of the team to maintaining confidentiality.

In hospice programmes and palliative care practices, the large majority of patients living with serious illness accept this team-based approach, implying that the perceived advantages of a consistently informed clinical care team with multiple professionals familiar with the patient and his particular family situation outweigh the potentially negative sense of personal exposure.

Confidentiality in palliative care research

Research and quality improvement efforts involving patients commonly entail some risks, including the possibility of compromising the confidentiality of patient information. Patients with advanced and terminal disease may be uniquely vulnerable to requests to participate in research and perhaps more likely harmed by having fleeting time consumed by completing questionnaires and research survey tools. These considerations have led to assertions that no research in this patient population is ethically sound. However, the principles of Palliative Medicine call for members of the profession to engage in research to expand the evidence-base of the field and to continually improve quality of palliative care and delivery of services to this fragile population[24,25].

The ethics of research in palliative care is addressed in Chapter 7.1 of this volume.

To a large extent the general ethical principles and guidelines for clinical research apply to studies enrolling palliative care patients. Before any patient is approached to become a research subject, it is essential for the study design to minimize potential harms[26]. This must include carefully developed procedural safeguards for avoiding exposure of private patient-specific information. In prospective research, whenever possible, anonymous data should be used or pseudonymization procedures instituted in which identifying information is removed during specific phases of data collection or analysis and can be re-attached later for subsequent analyses[26].

Informed consent remains an ethical cornerstone of health-care research. Consent procedures must include an explanation of any possible risks to confidentiality and the measures taken to protect private patient-specific information. Advanced illness must not be presumed to lessen an individual's ability to give informed consent for clinical studies. However, because of the progressive nature of illness for many patients receiving palliative care, it is often advisable to obtain consent early in the course of illness and to include the patients' surrogate decision makers in the decision process. This is particularly important for studies involving patients who might be expected to develop dementia or delirium. When advance consent is obtained and decision-making ability is temporarily impaired, consent can be re-confirmed following recovery of decision-making capacity[26].

Regarding confidentiality, the general ethical guidelines for health service delivery research applies to studies involving patients receiving palliative care, including hospice care. Privacy laws typically provide exemptions for governmental social science and population-based studies for the purpose of oversight, accreditation, and quality improvement. Corresponding regulatory safeguards require de-identification of patient-specific data and in some instances and jurisdictions disallow access to data by outside researchers, eliminating studies that are not conducted within official government activities. In the United Kingdom, the Data Protection Act of 1998 imposed strict criteria for management of personal data. In recognition of the importance of health improvements to future patients and the society as a whole, the Data Protection Act allows 'sensitive personal data' to be used for medical research without consent, but requires the same level of confidentiality to be honoured by researchers as by clinicians[27].

Making matters more complex, laws are inconsistent in governing data derived from public records, including the data collected by statistical agencies. Some statutes treat such data as property in which certain rights and restrictions apply while others treat data as information in which a separate set of rights and restrictions apply[28,29].

Even statutory protection of public health data is subject to challenge. A 1998 Icelandic law, the Health Sector Database Act, which gave legal protections for a national genetic databank was later declared unconstitutional because of potential infringement of individuals' privacy[30].

Basic ethical procedures require data be stored in conditions that are physically secure and protected from electronic intrusion. Not all investigators require full access to the datasets of health information used in a study. As with health-care personnel, access to information by research staff can be allowed on a need-to-know basis.

Some oversight bodies may require that primary source data for a study be maintained for a defined period of time and then destroyed. Even the destruction of data is not free of controversy. When colleagues of a Swedish researcher destroyed years of patient-specific information with the intention of protecting the confidentiality of the information, a public outcry ensued. In Sweden, data collected with public funds are public property and must not be destroyed[31].

Human Research Committees (HRC) and Institutional Review Boards (IRB) charged with evaluating proposed studies must weigh the risk to individuals (including posthumous risk to those who have died) and to their relatives and associates of exposure of information against the potential benefits of the research. Since the emergence of health privacy laws, including the United States HIPAA statute, HRCs, and IRBs have been reluctant or unable to extend waivers of informed consent for research that requires the review of decedents' medical records of patients. In many jurisdictions, there may be no one with clear legal authority to consent to access to the decedent's health information, since it is common under prevailing statutes for the authority of an individual's power of attorney for health care to end when the individual dies.

Many studies can be conducted with a dataset from which identifying information have been excluded. When retrospective research involves extracting pre-existing data including information contained in decedents' health-care records, it may be possible for all patient identifiers and all links to publicly accessible datasets to be removed before data is analysed and reported[27,32].

A full view of the ethics of research with seriously ill people requires attention to the potential benefits to patients. Many people express the feeling that by participating in research they are contributing to others. While the patient's motivation may be selfless, the contribution may engender an enhanced sense of meaning and self-esteem. Additionally, some studies may yield valuable patient-specific information which can be communicated to the patient following completion of the study. For instance, a patient may enrol in a double-blinded cross-over study of two symptom-controlling medications and his identity may be 'pseudonymized' through key coding of individual-specific information. After the study's completion, the patient may benefit from being informed which medication was found to be the most effective. Concerns over confidentiality should not be allowed to obviate potential benefits of re-identifying patient-specific data.

Studies of activities that are illegal, morally troubling or culturally controversial may require special procedures to ensure the confidentiality of study enrollees. Such procedures might include official assurances of non-investigation from Department of Health or other governmental authorities that can be given to potential subjects during consent and enrolment. Examples include research related to assisted-suicide[33,34], as well as research into the patient's use of illicit drugs, such as marijuana for nausea or appetite enhancement or the use of psychoactive drugs such as peyote or mescaline in religious rituals and ibogaine or MDMA in spiritual explorations. Clear guidelines and protocols for the handling of information and the corresponding, thorough training of all research personnel are required.

Qualitative research is particularly valuable to palliative care. Qualitative research techniques include in-depth interviews, often recorded on audio or videotape; questionnaires; focus groups; case studies and documentary analysis. Even if all specific identifying information is removed, the narrative descriptions and direct quotes that are often integral to qualitative research can raise the possibility for a subject to be subsequently identifiable. These characteristics of qualitative research must be explained during the process of informed consent.

Patient medical records have been a major source of data for retrospective palliative care research. The analysed data from patient medical record review may include information about demographic characteristics, diagnoses, symptoms, functional levels, length of life and quality of life. Although a particular patient's data is collected, the analysis and reporting of the data are not patient specific. In the United States, the Health Insurance Portability and Accountability Act (HIPAA) Privacy Rules stipulate standards which must be met to conduct health-care research, including the use of medical records. The rules define categories of 'individually identifiable health information' and 'protected health information' collected by health plans, health-care clearinghouses or health-care providers who transmit any health information in electronic form connection with a transaction covered by the regulations that cannot be reviewed or used for research purposes without authorization from the patient, except when performed by governmental health services agencies. Institutional Review Boards may give a Waiver of Authorization if certain stringent conditions are met, including the de-identification of all patient data. Violations of the HIPAA Privacy Rule may result in criminal prosecution and sizeable fines. The institutions that maintain the medical records containing the protected health information are the subject of these legal penalties[35]. As a result, IRBs have become hesitant to grant waivers of authorization. This has resulted in an increasing percentage of research submissions requiring the much more labour-intensive full IRB review. One institution reported the impact of this more stringent requirement to be the abandonment of 77 per cent of those research projects which were declined an IRB Waiver of Exemption. The majority of these involved chart reviews[36].

Education is needed for patients and the public about the proportionate risks of disclosure of information posed by research and the potential benefits to future patients and society of research.

Reasonable international standards to protect patient privacy and simultaneously facilitate medical research would encourage collaborative studies and model respect for universal rights of individuals. Academic palliative care societies have an opportunity to lead international efforts to educate government authorities and encourage adoption of workable standards for protecting privacy of individual-specific information in research and quality improvement activities. One possible example would be advocacy to modify national privacy rules to establish guidelines to protect privacy while allowing research conducted under review and approval of a recognized Institutional Review Board[37].

Conclusions

Confidentiality of patient information is essential to establish a trusting relationship between clinicians and patients, and trust in a therapeutic relationship is essential to a patient's sense of confidence and ability to benefit from care. As health-care practice has become more complex, it has become more difficult to maintain strict confidentiality. Ethical practice in the unprecedented and rapidly changing environments of contemporary health care requires clinicians to recognize the natural tensions that exist between confidentiality and other core values and the clinical and ethical principles of palliative medicine.

Most of the challenges to maintaining confidentiality are not unique to palliative medicine. However, the vulnerable nature of patients with advanced disease and the central focus on quality of life inherently sensitizes palliative care clinicians and teams to the importance of protecting patients' privacy.

Ongoing communication with patients and their chosen proxies is essential for balancing confidentiality with the therapeutic principles and goals in the skilful practice of palliative care.

Palliative care organizations, programmes, and interdisciplinary teams would benefit from establishing clear guidelines for maintaining confidentiality of patient and family-specific information. These guidelines should address: (a) the ethical and legal basis for confidentiality; (b) procedures for determining the 'need to know' of patient-specific information by staff and volunteers; (c) consequences of breaches of policies and procedures; (d) limitations to confidentiality necessitated by interdisciplinary team care; (e) procedures for informing patients and families of the procedural safeguards and limitations related to confidentiality; and (f) opportunities for patients and families to further limit access to their private information. These programmatic and institutional policies and procedures must be supported by a robust program of training, ongoing education, monitoring, and quality improvement regarding matters of confidentiality.

Finally, while complying with prevailing rules and laws, when circumstances arise in clinical practice in which prevailing regulations cause unintended harm to patients and families or limit clinicians' abilities to provide optimal care, it is important for clinicians to lawfully minimize harms and to engage in democratic processes to amend or revise applicable laws and regulations as is fully consistent with the practice of the principles of palliative medicine[38,39].

References

1. *American College of Physicians Ethics Manual 5th edition*. American College of Physicians. April 2005.
2. Privacy Law in the USA. Ronald B. Standler. Retrieved 28 November 2006, from http://www.rbs2.com/privacy.htm.
3. Beauchamp, T.L. and Childress, J.F. (2001). *Principles of biomedical ethics*. Oxford University Press, Oxford.
4. Canadian Information Protection and Electronic Documents Act. Retrieved 28 November 2006, from http://laws.justice.gc.ca/en/P-8.6/text.html.
5. Data Protection Act 1998 (http://www.opsi.gov.uk/acts/acts1998/19980029.htm). Retrieved 28 November 2006, from British Council, http://www.britishcouncil.org/home-privacy-policy.htm.
6. Gert, B., Culver, C.M., and Clouser, K.D. (1997). *Bioethics: a return to fundamentals*. Oxford University Press, New York.
7. Randall, F. and Downie, R.S. (1999). *Palliative care ethics: a companion for all specialties*, 2nd edition. Oxford University Press, Oxford.
8. Prosser, W. (1960). Privacy, 48 Cal. L. Rev. **383**, 393–6.
9. Humphers, V. (1985). First Interstate Bank of Oregon, 696 P.2d 527.
10. Fantin, L. and Mims, B. (2006). Discarded hard drive had IHC workers' info. The woman who acquired it found over 6,000 names, Social Security numbers. *The Salt Lake Tribune* 11/04/2006.
11. British Council. Privacy Policy. Retrieved 28 November 2006, from http://www.britishcouncil.org/home-privacy-policy.htm.
12. Lo, B., Dornbrand, L., and Dubler, N.N. (2005). HIPAA and patient care: the role for professional judgment. *JAMA*, **293**(14), 1766–71.
13. (2002). Medical professionalism in the new millennium: a physicians' charter. *Annals of Internal Medicine*, **136**, 243–6.
14. Siegler, M. (1982). Sounding boards. Confidentiality in medicine – a decrepit concept. *The New England Journal of Medicine*, **307**(24), 1518–21.
15. Kast, V. (1991). *Joy, inspiration and hope*. (Trans D Whitcher). Texas A.M. University Press.
16. Fins, J.J., Maltby, B.S., Friedmann, E. *et al.* (2005). Contracts, covenants and advance care planning: an empirical study of the moral obligations of patient and proxy. *Journal of Pain and Symptom Management*, **29**(1), 55–68.
17. Fins, J.J. (1999). Commentary: from contract to covenant in advance care planning. *The Journal of Law, Medicine & Ethics*, **27**(1), 46–51.
18. Vanderpool, H.Y. (1978). The ethics of terminal care. *JAMA*, **239**(9), 850–2.
19. Steinhauser, K.E., Christakis, N.A., Clipp, E.C. *et al.* (2000). Factors considered important at the end of life by patients, family, physicians, and other care providers. *JAMA*, **284**(19), 2476–82.
20. Staton, J.S.R. and Byock, I. (2001). *A few months to live*. Georgetown University Press, Washington, D.C.
21. Ray, A., Block, S.D., Friedlander, R.J. *et al.* (2006). Peaceful awareness in patients with advanced cancer. *Journal of Palliative Medicine*, **9**(6), 1359–68.
22. Rothstein, J.M. (1994). Ethical challenges to the palliative care volunteer. *Journal of Palliative Medicine*, **10**(3), 79–82.
23. Sankar, P., Mora, S., Merz, J.F. *et al.* (2003). Patient perspectives of medical confidentiality: a review of the literature. *Journal of General Internal Medicine*, **18**(8), 659–69.
24. (1998). Last Acts Task Force. Precepts of palliative care. *Journal of Palliative Medicine*, **1**, 109–12.
25. Byock, I.R. (1992). A consensus statement by radiation oncologists regarding radiotherapy for bone metastases. *The American Journal of Hospice & Palliative Care*, **9**(5), 6–7.
26. Casarett, D.J., Knebel, A., and Helmers, K. (2003). Ethical challenges of palliative care research. *Journal of Pain and Symptom Management*, **25**(4), S3–S5.
27. Kalra, D., Gertz, R., Singleton, P., and Inskip, H.M. (2006). Confidentiality of personal health information used for research. *BMJ*, **333**(7560), 196–8.
28. Abowd, J. and Lane, J. (2006). New approaches to confidentiality protection: synthetic data, remote access and research data centers. Retrieved 17 December 2006, from http://instruct1.cit.cornell.edu/~jma7/abowd-lane-barcelona-2004.pdf.
29. Lane, J. (2006). Key issues in confidentiality research: results of an nsf workshop. Retrieved 17 December 2006, from http://www.nsf.gov/sbe/ses/mms/nsfworkshop_summary1.pdf.
30. An analysis of the Icelandic Supreme Court judgement on the health sector database act (2004). Retrieved 25 November 2005, from www.law.ed.ac.uk/ahrb/script-ed/issue2/iceland.asp.
31. White, C. (2005). Clash over public access rights and patient confidentiality sparks trial. *BMJ*, **330**, 273.
32. Department of Health and Human Services. The Caldicott Committee. Report on the review of patient-identifiable information. December 1997. Retrieved 28 November 2006, from http://static.oxfordradcliffe.net/confidential/gems/caldrep.pdf..
33. White, M. and Callahan, D. (2000). Oregon's first year: the medicalization of control. *Psychology, Public Policy, and Law*, **6**(2), 331–41.
34. Volker, D.L. (2004). Methodological issues associated with studying an illegal act: assisted dying. *ANS. Advances in Nursing Science*, **27**(2), 117–28.
35. Gostin, L.O. (2001). National health information privacy: regulations under the Health Insurance Portability and Accountability Act. *JAMA*, **285**(23), 3015–21.
36. O'Herrin, J.K., Fost, N., and Kudsk, K.A. (2004). Health insurance portability accountability act (HIPAA) regulations: effect on medical record research. *Annals of Surgery*, **239**(6), 772–6; discussion 776–8.
37. Kulynych, J. and Korn, D. (2002). The effect of the new federal medical-privacy rule on research. *The New England Journal of Medicine*, **346**(3), 201–4.
38. Gruen, R.L., Pearson, S.D., and Brennan, T.A. (2004). Physician-citizens—public roles and professional obligations. *JAMA*, **291**(1), 94–8.
39. Byock I. (2009). Principles of Palliative Medicine. In *Palliative Medicine* (ed. T.D. Walsh), pp. 33–41. Saunders Elsevier, Philadelphia.

5.3

Truth telling and consent

Martin H.N. Tattersall

Introduction

This chapter focuses on negotiating the difficult balance between truth telling and sustaining hope when seeking consent from cancer patients with a short life expectancy to invasive investigations, further palliative anti-tumour treatment, or supportive/palliative care interventions. If patients want to be involved in these decisions, they need to be adequately informed both on the interventions/treatments being considered and on their disease status and prognosis. If they prefer to accept the advice of their doctor, their consent to continuing treatment and/or additional investigations must be negotiated.

Telling the truth about a terminal illness

Cancer patients require an understanding of their disease and the potential consequences of treatment in order to be informed participants in clinical decision making. However, there are reports that many patients do not understand critical information such as the extent of their disease, the goal of therapy, and the likelihood of treatment achieving its goal. People diagnosed with cancer want information about their prognosis, but doctors have trouble estimating and talking about it. Pertinent information is essential if patients with a life-limiting illness and their caregivers are to participate in decisions about care. Clinicians need to provide information in a way that respects the individual needs of patients and their families (which may be for much or little information), enhances patient and family understanding, and assists coping and adjustment.

Research has identified deficiencies in doctors' communication regarding a short life expectancy.[1] Doctors are sometimes uncomfortable raising the topic of life expectancy with patients or their families. Oncologists are often more comfortable proposing another anticancer treatment or participation in a phase 1 clinical trial compared to ceasing anti-tumour treatment and focusing on symptom control. Issues that concern clinicians about disclosing life expectancy include how much information to give, disclosing uncertainty without increasing anxiety, reducing trust, and destroying hope. Others believe that expressing prognostic uncertainty carefully to patients is one means of sustaining hope, and that providing information decreases anxiety associated with ignorance and misunderstanding.[2] Lack of relevant training, insufficient time to attend to the patient's emotional needs, fear of upsetting the patient, and a feeling of hopelessness regarding the unavailability of curative treatment are further reasons doctors may avoid discussion of the prognosis.

Oncologists may perceive disease progression and referral to palliative care an indicator of their failure. Doctors' avoidance of a discussion about prognosis is probably caused much by doctors' uncertainty about how to think and talk about prognosis as it is by patients' reluctance to ask about it. Doctor's discomfort can lead to avoidance of such discussions altogether. Some doctors believe disclosing a prognosis likely measured in weeks or months will unnecessarily upset the patient and dispel any hope.

Patient preferences for discussing prognosis

Hagerty et al.[3,4] reported the preferences for the process of prognostic discussion among patients with incurable metastatic cancer. The vast majority (98 per cent) of 126 patients who participated in the study wanted their doctor to be realistic, provide an opportunity to ask questions, and acknowledge them as an individual when discussing prognosis. Fifty-nine per cent wanted to discuss expected survival when first diagnosed with metastatic disease. Thirty-eight and 48 per cent, respectively, wanted to negotiate when expected survival and dying were discussed. Preferred doctor behaviours included being realistic, providing an opportunity to ask questions, and acknowledging the patient as an individual while discussing the prognosis. Doctor behaviours rated the most hope giving included appearing to know all there is to know about the patient's cancer, saying that pain will be controlled and being told all the treatment options. Three factors were identified among the 30 hope items listed which accounted for approximately 54 per cent of the variance. These were (1) an expert/positive/collaborative approach (expertise, humour and inclusion of patient as part of the team); (2) avoidant behaviour (avoiding or appearing uncomfortable about discussing the cancer, using euphemisms, and giving the prognosis to others first); and (3) empathic (expressing one's own) feelings or asking the patient about their reaction to the prognosis. The most strongly endorsed hope-giving style was the expert/positive/collaborative approach.

When cancer patients are not aware of their prognosis, they are more likely to choose toxic anticancer treatments and make decisions that they later regret.[5,6] Moreover, if information about life expectancy is not provided, patients may perceive that doctors are withholding potentially frightening information. Patients who understand their prognosis are more satisfied with their care and experience less psychological morbidity.

Estimating prognosis (see Chapter 3.3)

Prognostication involves more than estimating the likely survival time of a patient. It also includes discussing symptoms that may develop as

Table 5.3.1 Steps for predicting life expectancy.[8]

1. Estimate the median survival of a group with similar characteristics.

2. Adjust the median survival from the group to account for differences with the individual.

3. Estimate the rage for the middle half of patients by taking half to double the predicted median.

4. Estimate the best and worst case scenario as ~1/6 of and three to four times the predicted median.

5. Adjust the best and worst case scenario estimates to account for any outstanding differences or biases.

the illness progresses and the likelihood of any intervention to control the symptom being successful. End-of-life discussions may also include: what the patient and their families may experience or witness leading up to and during the time of dying, preferences for place of death, general preferences for care during the terminal phase, and what may happen or need to be done after the person dies.

Prognostic factors in patients with recently diagnosed incurable cancer have been conceptualized as attributes of the host, tumour, treatment, and interactions between the three reflected in symptoms, quality of life, performance status, and laboratory tests.[7] Estimates of life expectancy are essential for rational decision-making, planning, and care of patients with advanced cancer, many of whom want information about their prognosis. Stockler *et al.*[8] have proposed describing life expectancy with approximate ranges based on simple multiples of the predicted median survival of a group of similar patients with advanced cancer (Table 5.3.1). They have also presented examples of phrases for talking about life expectancy (Table 5.3.2). There has been no examination of the effects of using these calculations or phrases in talking to incurable cancer patients.

In terminally ill patients, Christakis and Lamont[9] reported that doctors were inaccurate in their estimates of prognosis, and that their errors were systematically optimistic. The European Association for Palliative Care[10] has reviewed predictive factors in estimating survival time in palliative care patients in the last 3 months of life.

Timing of prognostic discussions

Most of the patients from Western countries prefer some information regarding prognosis when they are first diagnosed with a life-limiting illness or at least shortly after. Patients may prefer to negotiate the content and extent of this information and may change their preference over time,[11] from initially wanting much or little detail to the

Table 5.3.2 Examples of phrases for talking about life expectancy.[8]

1. The typical person with your type and stage of cancer lives X months and half the people less than X months.

2. About half the people with your type and stage of cancer live between X/2 and 2X months.

3. If we had exactly 100 million people like you, then we would expect that the 10 who did best to still be around 3–4X months, whereas the 10 who did worst would be in trouble within X/6.

4. It might be as short as a few months or as long as a few years.

reverse. Some patients never want to discuss prognosis. Most, but not all, of the patients want to have a family member or friend with them.

How to discuss prognosis

The first step is to clarify what the individual patient or family wants to know about prognosis.[12] Many studies have reported that the majority of patients (at least from Western countries) want to know their life expectancy, and be given an understanding of the likely time course of symptoms and disability. However, some patients do not want full disclosure and may experience conflict between wanting to know and fearing bad news. Some patients want to know that their lifespan will be shortened by their illness, but do not want to be given the likely time frame. Younger and more educated patients commonly want more detailed information. Patients from some cultural backgrounds prefer non-disclosure, or disclosure negotiated through the family.

Caregivers of patients may have different information needs from the patient.[13] The caregiver/family may need more detailed information than the patient about the dying process in order to provide care. It is advantageous to ask patients before the last days/weeks of life with whom the doctor is able to speak about the disease status. Seeking patient consent to permit individual discussion with family/carer allows the health professional to explore their concerns and information needs without the barrier of patient/carer protectiveness.

Balancing hope and truth telling

Patients, caregivers, and doctors have identified hope as an integral component of discussion of prognosis at the end of life.[14] These studies also emphasize the importance of balancing honesty with hope and empathy. Views of what constitutes an honest approach differ. Some studies of patients with advanced illness have found that accurate information is equated with honesty, provided this was not combined with bluntness or too much hard, factual, or detailed information. Others have defined honesty as a straightforward or direct approach.

Groopman proposed a strategy for hope rooted in the paradox of uncertainty.[2] Everybody with a severe and life threatening illness faces the fact that nothing in medicine is absolute. On the one hand, this is a source of anxiety, because there is no guarantee that a treatment/procedure will succeed 100 per cent of the time. On the other hand, the absence of absolute certainty provides a basis for hope. He advocates opening a discussion about prognosis using a general statement like 'There is a best-case scenario and a worst case scenario. We should consider both since no one can predict which will occur ....'

Recently, Eliott and Olver have reported a qualitative study of the discursive properties of hope as emerged unprompted during semi-structured interviews with 28 cancer patients in the last 3 months of their life.[15] They highlight differences between noun and verb uses of hope in dying cancer patients' speech (Table 5.3.3). They reported that when used as a noun, hope invariably referenced the medical domain, focusing either on the probability of a cure, or the subjective possession of the patient, needed to 'fight' their disease. In the former context, hope is related to the possibility of available treatments achieving cure or remission. This construction of hope has life and death implications for the patient: Presence of hope means

Table 5.3.3 Differences between noun and verb versions of hope in dying cancer patients' speech.[15]

Hope as noun	Hope as verb
Limited to medical domain	Not limited to medical domain
Typically 'No hope'	Typically 'I hope'
Negative future	Positive future
Absolutes	Possibilities
Construes the patient as *subject to*	Construes the patient as *the subject*
Limits the patient's agency	Endows the patient with agency
Construes the patient in biological terms	Construes the patient in psychological, moral and interpersonal terms
Focus on death	Focus on life

life, and absence means death. The second version of hope used as a noun saw hope as the possession of the patient, varying in amount and associated with features of patient well being. Notably, in this context, patients considered 'Not for resuscitation' discussion as eroding hope, and a justification for avoiding this discussion. Hope in this setting can be viewed not only as a patient resource but also a motivator for continuing treatment. Without hope that treatment will be effective, patient can have no reason to undertake it. This elaboration of hope as a noun illuminates some issues relevant to seeking patient consent to 'third-line' treatments and to enrolment in a phase 1 clinical trial.

Eliott and Olver[15] report that hope as a verb functions to enable patients to express themselves as the subject and to participate in life's activities. They categorize hoping in the context of an imagined positive future over which the patient has limited control. Hoping may also have interpersonal implications including outcomes in the future after their death. Hope as a verb embraces the patient's active engagement in life, identifying what was important for them. This analysis informs the question of how to nurture hope within the context of end of life care and decision making.

Several studies have addressed the question of how to provide hope within the end-of-life context. In Clayton *et al.*'s study,[14] patients identified a spectrum of hope ranging from the hope of a miracle cure to the hope of a peaceful death. It is clear that patients may simultaneously hope for a cure and acknowledge the terminal nature of the illness. Hagerty *et al.*[4] reported patients viewed the following as hope-giving behaviours: reassuring that pain will be controlled (87 per cent); appearing to know all there was to know about the patient's cancer (87 per cent); being occasionally humorous (80 per cent); offering to answer all the patient's questions (78 per cent); saying that each day the patient survives new developments are possible (75 per cent); and saying that the patient's will to live would affect the outcome (74 per cent).

Patients perceived that hope can be maintained by their doctor 'being there' and treating the patient as a whole person. Patients and caregivers perceived that doctors could communicate hope by 'leaving the door open' (communicating in ways that allow preservation of some hope); acknowledging difficulties in giving prognostic estimates and respecting alternative treatments.

Are cancer patients with incurable disease equipped to make informed decisions about their care?

People with incurable cancer confront complex and difficult treatment decisions. Their life expectancy is typically measured in weeks to months, and anticancer treatment may relieve or delay tumour-related symptoms, but these potential benefits are not guaranteed, and may be offset by side effects. An alternative may be to delay or forgo anticancer therapy and pursue symptom control with or without referral to palliative care services. The SUPPORT Investigators[5,6] reported that patients overestimated their chances of living 6 months compared with their doctors. Patients who estimated their survival as greater than 6 months were more than twice as likely to receive aggressive cancer chemotherapy instead of palliative care when compared with those who gave themselves at least a 10 per cent chance of living less than 6 months. These patients who received so-called aggressive anticancer treatment had the same survival as those who received other types of care, but were more likely to have a hospital readmission, undergo attempted resuscitation or die while receiving ventilatory assistance. Weeks *et al.*[5] recommended that doctors engage patients in an honest discussion about prognosis and treatment and ensure that patients understand this information.

The essence of informed decision-making includes two broadly defined aspects: Information disclosure and patient participation. Gattellari *et al.*[16] examined the extent to which incurable cancer patients newly referred to oncologists were enabled to make informed decisions about their treatment and determined predictors of informed decision making. They developed a coding system consisting of 12 elements to assess disclosure of information and to evaluate doctor encouragement of patient participation in decision making (Table 5.3.4). Seven elements described the content of the information disclosed to patients considered to satisfy the criteria for informed decision making. Five elements described doctor behaviours that encouraged patient participation in treatment

Table 5.3.4 Elements of Coding system.[16]

Informational components
Effect of treatment on tumour
Told aim of treatment
Told disease is incurable
Told drawbacks of treatment
Given information about life expectancy
Presented with treatment alternative
Informed of possible beneficial effect of treatment on quality of life.
Doctor facilitation of patient participation
Acknowledges uncertainty that treatment will achieve aim
Elicitation of patient values
Acknowledge trade offs
Offers treatment choice
Checks patient understanding

decision making. They reported that most patients were informed about the aim of anticancer treatment (85 per cent), that their disease was incurable (75 per cent), and about life expectancy (58 per cent). An alternative to anticancer treatment was presented to 44 per cent, 36 per cent were informed about effects of anticancer treatment on quality of life, and 29 per cent were offered a management choice. Oncologist checked patient understanding in only 10 per cent of consultations. Greater information disclosure did not elevate patient anxiety levels, but greater patient participation in the decision making was associated with increased anxiety levels which persisted over a 2-week time span. The authors concluded that gaps concerning information about prognosis and alternatives to anticancer treatment invited the question concerning whether these incurable patients were led towards anticancer treatment.

Koedoot et al.[17] determined the content and amount of information given by oncologists when proposing palliative chemotherapy. Their coding scheme comprised six categories of information given during the consultation which doctors are obliged by law in the Netherlands to present to provide to patients. The categories of information were about the disease, possible treatment options, the goals of treatment, the procedure of administration, side effects of treatment and other effects of the disease and/or treatment. Medical oncologists mentioned or explained the disease course (53 per cent), symptoms (35 per cent), and prognosis (39 per cent). Most patients were told about the absence of cure (84 per cent). Watchful waiting was mentioned to only half of the patients, either in one sentence (23 per cent) or explained more extensively (27 per cent). They stated their most prominent finding was that oncologists tell their patients hardly anything about the option of watchful waiting. They concluded that when the prospect of cure is absent, it is necessary to enable patients to decide how they would like to spend the last months of their life. Patients wishing to maintain hope and avoid the emotional impact of a full understanding of their prognosis may rather not be informed about prognosis or the goal of supportive care or forced to make an informed choice.[18] Patients with incurable metastatic disease need to be able to trust their doctor to give them all relevant information and to be aware of all available treatment options and the likely consequences.

The process by which cancer patients are informed and by which their consent are sought to participate in phase 1 trials has not been well studied. The main endpoint of a phase 1 trial is the definition of the maximum tolerated dose and of dose limiting toxicities. In a review of 213 phase 1 cancer trials, 10.3 per cent of the patients experienced serious toxicity, 0.5 per cent died of drug-related effects, and the overall tumour response rate was 3.8 per cent.[19] Cox et al.[20] reviewed 12 studies that measured phase 1 trial participants' comprehension of information given during the informed consent process. Altogether 1000 patients were surveyed in a variety of ways. Less than 50 per cent of the patients reported that the aim of a phase 1 trial was dose determination. Patients' perception of likely physical benefit from a phase 1 trial participation ranged from 20 to 90 per cent, and their perception of probability of toxicity ranged from 30–59 per cent. About 50 per cent of the patients indicated that no alternative to trial participation was discussed with them. These findings and the results of Gattellari's and Koedoot's studies[16,17] raise concerns that oncologists recruiting cancer patients to a phase 1 trial or discussing palliative chemotherapy may not adequately inform patients of options for their care. A systematic review concluded that allowing adequate time for extended discussion with a doctor, nurse, or outside educator was the most effective intervention in improving patient understanding.[21]

Provision of audio tapes or written summaries of consultations

One simple intervention to increase patients' understanding and recall of information after a consultation is the provision of audio-recordings or written summaries of the consultation. A systematic review conducted by Scott et al.[22] reported that trials consistently found that most people who received audio-recordings or written summaries of their consultations valued them. In five of nine studies, patients provided with the audio-recording had improved recall of the consultation. Patients who received an audio-recording or letter were more satisfied with the information received in four out of seven studies. There is a strong case for offering to audio-record consultations when prognosis and palliative treatment options are being discussed. Provision of the recording to patient/carer increases the opportunity for review of options and clarification of their participation preferences.

McHugh et al.[23] found that patients, who were informed of a poor prognosis at their initial oncology consultation and received an audiotape of that consultation, had less improvement in psychological distress at 6-month follow-up than those who did not receive the tape. Therefore, Scott et al.[22] advised caution in the use of audiotapes when bad news is being delivered. However, this result was found in only one study conducted at the point of initial diagnosis.

Question prompt lists

Studies of cancer patients' views have documented the high value placed on being encouraged to ask questions of their clinicians. Improved health outcomes have been reported when patients are encouraged to ask questions during general medical consultations. Some health professionals encourage patients to write down their questions and bring them to medical appointments, but patients may not know what questions to ask or how to articulate their concerns.

Butow et al.[24] explored the use of a question prompt list (QPL) given to cancer patients before their initial consultation with an oncologist. A QPL is a structured list containing examples of questions, for the patient to ask their doctor if they wish. It is designed to encourage patient participation during a medical consultation and to assist patients in acquiring information that is suited to their needs and at their own pace. This simple tool has been found to promote cancer patients to ask questions. A recent systematic review of the utility of QPL identified 15 randomized trials ($n = 2159$) and non-controlled studies ($n = 415$).[25] Use of a QPL did not consistently affect the total number of patient questions across studies. However, a closer examination of questions by categories revealed an increase in questions about diagnosis, test, with a particular emphasis on prognosis. Patient's psychological outcomes were largely unaffected by the use of a QPL, supporting the utility of the tool in opening up discussion about difficult issues such as prognosis without significant long lasting negative effects. Together, the findings indicate that the use of a QPL enhances the quality of the patient–doctor interaction by providing patients with a means of shifting the focus of the consultation towards their preferences for information.

In a recent randomized study, provided the oncologist specifically addressed questions in the QPL during the consultation, those patients who received the prompt list were significantly less anxious immediately after the consultation and had better recall and significantly shorter consultations than those in the control group.[26]

Clayton et al.[27] developed and piloted a QPL for patients being referred to a palliative care team. A series of focus groups and individual interviews with palliative care patients, their carers and palliative care health professionals were conducted to identify suitable questions for inclusion in the QPL. A wide range of issues emerged including questions about: The palliative care service, physical symptoms and treatment, lifestyle and quality of life, my illness and what to expect in the future, support, if you are concerned about your professional care, for carers, and end of life issues. Subsequently, a randomized trial of the QPL in which 174 patients participated (92 QPL, 82 control) has been reported.[28] Compared with controls, QPL patients and their caregivers asked twice as many questions ($P < 0.0001$). QPL patients asked significantly more prognostic questions and were more likely to discuss prognosis and end-of-life issues. No differences between groups were observed in anxiety or patient/physician satisfaction.

Concluding remarks

Truth telling in discussing prognosis is difficult and distressing for health professionals and patients/ families. Fears that disclosing life expectancy may erode hope is not well supported by evidence. Improved estimates of life expectancy are feasible and proposals for disclosing uncertainty while discussing prognosis merit further investigation. Accurate prediction of survival is necessary for clinical and ethical reasons, especially in helping to avoid harm, discomfort and inappropriate interventions in vulnerable patients. Providing a question prompt list and endorsing its use during consultations enhance patient's participation in management discussions. Analysis of consultation audio recordings identifies gaps in information being provided to incurable cancer patients considering palliative treatment and participation in a phase 1 clinical trial.

Recently, Matsuyama et al.[29] examined what information was available to advanced cancer patients about prognosis and treatment effectiveness and what was known about how such patients made decisions between chemotherapy and other types of supportive care. They concluded that available patient sources including the National Cancer Institute website and the American Cancer Society website give little information about prognosis in advanced disease, and how to choose between alternatives. They noted that many patients would choose chemotherapy for a small benefit in health outcomes, and that adverse effects are less a concern for patients than for their physicians. The importance of offering unbiased information about life expectancy to incurable cancer patients considering further cancer treatment is reinforced by this report.

References

1. Gysels, M., Richardson, A., and Higginson, I.J. (2004). Communication training for health professionals who care for patients with cancer: a systematic review of effectiveness. *Support Care in Cancer*, **12**, 692–700.

2. Groopman, J.E. (2005). A strategy for hope: a commentary on necessary collusion. *Journal of Clinical Oncology*, **23**, 3151–2.

3. Hagerty, R.G., Butow, P.N., Ellis, P.A. et al. (2004). Cancer patient preferences for communication of prognosis in the metastatic setting. *Journal of Clinical Oncology*, **22**, 1721–30.

4. Hagerty, R.G., Butow, P.N., Ellis, P.M. et al. (2005). Communicating with realism and hope: incurable cancer patients' views on the disclosure of prognosis. *Journal of Clinical Oncology*, **23**, 1278–88.

5. Weeks, J.C., Cook, E.F., O'Day, S.J. et al. (1998). Relationship between cancer patients' predictions of prognosis and their treatment preferences. *JAMA*, **279**, 1709–14.

6. Covinsky, K.E., Goldman, L., Cook, E.F. et al. (1994). The impact of serious illness on patients' families. SUPPORT Investigators Study to understand prognoses and preferences for outcomes and risks of treatment. *JAMA*, **272**, 1839–44.

7. Hauser, C.A., Stockler, M.R., and Tattersall, M.H.N. (2006). Prognostic factors in patients with recently diagnosed incurable cancer: a systematic review. *Support Care Cancer*, **14**, 999–1011.

8. Stockler, M.R., Tattersall, M.H.N., Boyer, M.J. et al. (2006). Disarming the guarded prognosis: predicting survival in newly referred patients with incurable cancer. *British Journal of Cancer*, **94**, 208–12.

9. Christakis, N.A. and Lamont, E.B. (2000). Extent and determinants of error in doctors' prognoses in terminally ill patients: prospective cohort study. *BMJ*, **320**, 469–73.

10. Maltoni, M., Caraceni, A., Brunelli, C. et al. (2005). Prognostic factors in advanced cancer patients: evidence-based clinical recommendations – a study by the Steering Committee of the European Association for Palliative Care. *Journal of Clinical Oncology*, **23**, 6240–8.

11. Butow, P.N., Maclean, N., Dunn, S.M. et al. (1997). The dynamics of change: cancer patients' preferences for information, involvement and support. *Annals of Oncology*, **8**, 857–63.

12. Clayton, J.M., Butow, P.N., and Tattersall, M.H.N. (2005). When and how to initiate discussion about prognosis and end-of-life issues with terminally ill patients. *Journal of Pain and Symptom Management*, **30**, 132–44.

13. Clayton, J.M., Butow, P.N., and Tattersall, M.H.N. (2005). The needs of terminally ill cancer patients versus those of their caregivers for information about prognosis and end-of-life issues. *Cancer*, **103**, 1957–64.

14. Clayton, J.M., Butow, P.N., Arnold, R.M. et al. (2005). Fostering coping and nurturing hope when discussing the future with terminally ill cancer patients and their caregivers. *Cancer*, **103**, 1965–75.

15. Eliott, J.A. and Olver, I.N. (2007). Hope and hoping in the talk of dying cancer patients. *Social Science and Medicine*, **64**, 138–49.

16. Gattellari, M., Voigt, K.J., Butow, P.N. et al. (2002). When the treatment goal is not cure: are cancer patients equipped to make informed decisions? *American Journal of Clinical Oncology*, **20**, 503–13.

17. Koedoot, C.G., Oort, F.J., de Haan, R.J. et al. (2004). The content and amount of information given by medical oncologists when telling patients with advanced cancer what the treatment options are: palliative chemotherapy and watchful waiting. *European Journal of Cancer*, **40**, 225–35.

18. De Haes, H. and Koedoot, N. (2003). Patient centred decision making in palliative cancer treatment: a world of paradoxes. *Patient Education and Counseling*, **50**, 43–9.

19. Roberts, T.G., Goulart, B.H., Squiteri, L. et al. (2004). Trends in the risks and benefits to patients with cancer participating in phase 1 clinical trials. *JAMA*, **292**, 2130–40.

20. Cox, A.C., Fallowfield, L.J., and Jenkins, V.A. (2006). Communication and informed consent in phase 1 trials: a review of the literature. *Support Care in Cancer*, **14**, 303–9.

21. Flory, J. and Emmanuel, E. (2004). Interventions to improve research participants understanding in informed consent for research: a systematic review *JAMA*, **292**, 1593–601.

22. Scott, J.T., Entwistle, V.A., Sowden, A.J. et al. (2003). Recordings or summaries of consultations for people with cancer. *Cochrane Database of Systematic Reviews*, **2**, CD001539.

23. McHugh, P., Lewis, S., Ford, S. *et al.* (1995). The efficacy of audiotapes in promoting psychological well-being in cancer patients: a randomised, controlled trial. *British Journal of Cancer*, **71**, 388–92.

24. Butow, P.N., Dunn, S.M., Tattersall, M.H. *et al.* (1994). Patient participation in the cancer consultation: evaluation of a question prompt sheet. *Annals of Oncology*, **5**, 199–204.

25. Dimoska, Tattersall, M.H.N., Butow, P.N., and Shepherd, H. Do question prompt lists help patients with cancer ask questions in consultations? A systematic review of the literature. Submitted for publication.

26. Brown, R.F., Butow, P.N., Dunn, S.M. *et al.* (2001). Promoting patient participation and shortening cancer consultations: a randomised trial. *British Journal of Cancer*, **85**, 273–9.

27. Clayton, J.M., Butow, P.N., Tattersall, M.H.N. *et al.* (2003). Asking questions can help: development and preliminary evaluation of a question prompt list for palliative care patients. *British Journal of Cancer*, **89**, 2069–77.

28. Clayton, J.M., Butow, P.N., Tattersall, M.H.N. *et al.* (2007). Helping advanced cancer patients and their caregivers to ask questions about prognosis and end-of-life care: a randomised controlled trial of a question prompt list. *Journal of Clinical Oncology*, **25**, 715–23.

29. Matsuyama, R., Reddy, S., and Smith, T.J. (2006). Why do patients choose chemotherapy near the end of life? A review of the perspective of those facing death from cancer. *Journal of Clinical Oncology*, **24**, 3490–6.

Palliative care in children: ethical and legal issues

Dilini Rajapakse and Vic Larcher

The impending death of a child poses practical, intellectual, and emotional challenges for the child, their family, and professionals. It involves an acceptance by all concerned of a change in the goal of treatment from cure to palliation and the provision of an individualized care pathway which balances, where appropriate, continuing disease-modifying and life-prolonging treatment with comfort care.

Ethical decision making is therefore central to the provision of good palliative care, and in children's palliative care, this poses unique moral and legal challenges for all concerned.

The purpose of this chapter is to explore the moral and legal arguments concerning the provision of palliative care to children when a decision has been made not to prolong life. It will outline the ethico-legal basis of such decisions as they apply to a variety of situations in childhood terminal illness. Finally, suggestions about the management of conflict will be provided, along with procedural mechanisms for dealing with the moral indeterminacy that may accompany the decision-making process. While the focus of legal analysis will inevitably be on United Kingdom law, similar principles and reasoning will apply to other national legal jurisdictions.

Background

Both technological advances and improved public health have contributed to falling death rates in infants and children. There is a greater societal expectation that the application of modern medical technology will prolong life or cure illness in circumstances where this was previously impossible, especially for children. As a result, society as a whole does not have significant experience of death in childhood and of how it differs from that in adults.

The process of dying may be sudden and unexpected (road traffic accident), involve relapses and remission with protracted periods of intensive therapy (relapsed leukaemia), or be the culmination of a slow decline in function over months and years (Batten's disease).

In children, unlike adults, this process occurs in a unique setting of continuing physical, emotional, cognitive, and social development. Therefore, family and professionals involved need to acknowledge the child's awareness of his situation, autonomy, rights and attitudes and personal decision-making abilities when confronting difficult choices.

Responses of children, parents, and professionals are as variable as the circumstances that provoke them. Some parents may want active treatment, directed at prolonging life, continued to the very moment of death. Others, seeing the pain and suffering of their child and perhaps uncertain whether they have the strength and will to support him or her, may wish for a speedy and peaceful death. There may be a sense of loss of future potential, feelings of anger, bewilderment, betrayal, and desolation at the cruel hand that an impersonal fate has dealt, coupled with a sense of injustice and perhaps depression. In these situations professionals may share many of the feelings of the child and their family and may be unsure as to how they are to fulfil their duty to protect life and health. Given children's assumed potential for growth and development, it is perhaps not surprising that paediatricians frequently give their patients more chances to recover from their illness than adults might receive. In consequence some children may receive treatments that carry greater burdens with less chances of success than those used for adults.

It is in these circumstances that palliative care assumes great importance. Since health can be defined as the absence of physical and mental disabilities that otherwise would be caused by disease, the intention to use palliative care is entirely consistent with the duty to restore health. It achieves this by attempting to relieve both pain and suffering, promoting the development of the child's emotional and cognitive abilities, and enabling the child to sustain his or her capabilities for as long as possible. In short, the aim of good palliative care is to maximize the child's potential, while acknowledging the constraints imposed by their illness. Such care also involves supporting parents and professionals in their duties and responsibilities to the child in the face of the suffering imposed by terminal illness. Seen in these terms palliative care involves far more than provision of effective pain relief and has many positive attributes, which apply throughout all life limiting illnesses, at whatever stage.

The role of child-centred palliative care is therefore integrative rather than additive and the level of involvement will vary as required throughout the illness.

Withholding and withdrawing life-sustaining treatment

The decision to withhold or withdraw potentially curative or life-sustaining treatment may be problematic for all concerned, because it involves changing the goals of care from cure to palliation. It is therefore essential to consider the circumstances, in the context of the child's illness, when it is felt that life-sustaining treatment is no longer morally or legally justified. A multi-disciplinary team, including the child (where appropriate) and family, is involved in this decision-making process, where the focus is on providing choice and support with plans to optimize comfort and dignity for the child.

Although there may be certain circumstances that are relatively straightforward, i.e. the management of a child who is actually dying, decisions not to try to prolong life can provoke self-doubt in professionals and conflict amongst team members and with parents. This is especially so in situations where death is not imminent, but there are serious moral questions about sustaining life, even though it may be technically possible to do so. It is therefore important that those who undertake palliative care have a good understanding of the ethical and legal principles that underpin such decisions, so that the basis on which decisions are made can be sensitively communicated to the child and family.

Moral arguments about not prolonging life

The first duty of clinical care is to respect the life and health of patients to an acceptable standard.[1] Individuals whose lives are at risk and can be saved, or who are suffering from illness that can be cured or effectively managed, should receive appropriate medical help that achieves these ends. For clinicians to breach this duty of care is a potentially serious offence, which may entail professional censure or exclusion and legal, possibly criminal, culpability. This is because they will have knowingly and deliberately acted in direct contravention of their duty of care.[2]

However, in some circumstances, clinicians are not only professionally and legally allowed to make decisions to withhold or withdraw life-sustaining treatment where it is clear that death is likely to result, but also do so with considerable frequency.[3,4] How can this be reconciled with their general duty of care and the potentially punitive consequences of not abiding by it? Such action can only be morally justified when providing life-sustaining treatment is no longer in the patient's best interests because it produces substantially more burdens than benefits. A decision to withhold or withdraw life-sustaining treatment cannot simply be morally justified by statements to the effect that 'nature should be allowed to take its course' or 'it would be better not to try too hard' to sustain a patient's life. Therefore, given the seriousness of the duty to protect life, there can be only one coherent justification for not doing so—that for some reason, to do so is not in the patient's best interests.

The moral justification for non-treatment decisions inevitably relates to circumstances, where it is no longer clear that patients' objective interests as humans are best served by prolonging their lives.[5] It is in this context that the benefits and burdens of medical treatment will be evaluated. Unless continued, life is in the best interests of patients, the burden of further life-prolonging treatment can have no benefit. The crucial moral question then becomes: when is it more in the interest of a patient to die than to continue to live? Generally speaking, this will be when the patient is permanently unable—or is no longer so able—to engage minimally, and with some sense of sustained self-awareness and well being, in any of the activities that uniquely characterize human life.[5,6] Such inability may occur in a range of circumstances:

◆ Patients may be so close to death and in such a physically and emotionally weakened state that they are no longer able to initiate any coherent action.

◆ Patients may be so brain damaged that they have minimal capacities to reason, to choose, to plan ahead, and thus to interact intentionally with others. It is through such interaction that individuals continue to expand their understanding of themselves, of other humans, and of the rest of the world.

Inability aside, patients may have all of the characteristic human attributes and self-awareness and be fully capable of interaction with others. However, they may themselves decide that, because of the physical and emotional impact of their terminal illness, life does not have enough sustained meaning for them to wish to continue it. They may judge the provision or continuation of life-prolonging treatment as a burden that is no longer in their best interests.

In all these circumstances, clinicians may decide that it is morally and professionally unacceptable to strive to prolong the lives of patients by medical means.[1] Against the background of poor quality of life and prospects for anything resembling a minimally fulfilled human life, the ratio of benefit to burden of treatment can no longer warrant further life-prolonging medical intervention.[6] To ignore this fact on the grounds of the 'sanctity of life' is clearly just as much a breach of the duty of care as not clinically intervening when it is in the patients best interests.[7,8]

Despite these arguments, decisions to withdraw and withhold life-sustaining treatment would be morally unacceptable if they in any way added to the suffering or indignity of the patients concerned. As has been noted, terminally ill patients who are candidates for such decisions will have often already benefited from ongoing palliative care focused on the relief of physical and psychological pain and discomfort. The palliative care team's role may expand and increase following such decisions. The knowledge that pain and other forms of suffering can be effectively managed can also be of great comfort to families and professional carers who recognize and feel the moral enormity of deciding that a patient should be allowed to die without further medical intervention.[9,10]

The legality of decisions to withhold and withdraw life-sustaining treatment

Until relatively recently, clinicians who allowed patients to die as a result of decisions to withhold and withdraw life-sustaining treatment did so within a legal environment that was potentially punitive. Prior to 1989, the only legal precedent for such decisions in the United Kingdom was a ruling by Lord Justice Templeman. In Re B (1981), he suggested that if infants—and therefore all people—had lives that were 'demonstrably awful' it might be appropriate to allow them to die without medical intervention.[11] Templeman did not specify the precise clinical meaning of this phrase, although it was clear contextually that he envisaged a level of brain damage and disability more extreme than Down's syndrome. Until the law was further clarified, therefore, clinicians who made non-treatment decisions exposed themselves to possible criminal charges.

The situation changed dramatically during the 1990s, with a series of legal cases concerning severely damaged infants. Again, these cases had consequences for all patients in that their outcome established the legality of non-treatment decisions in specific circumstances and the criteria by which such decisions could be made. These criteria directly reflect the moral arguments already outlined, in terms of their focus on best interests.

◆ Re C (89).[12] This infant was imminently and irreversibly close to death as a result of hydrocephalus and cerebral malformation.

◆ Re J (90).[13] Here, the baby was not close to death but was so brain damaged that he would never be able to engage in any form of self-directed activity. The baby had probable severe spastic quadriplegia, deafness, blindness, and very little intellectual potential or capacity to feel pain.

◆ Re J (92).[14] The child in this case was also not close to death but had severe brain damage as a consequence of microcephaly with severe cerebral palsy. The clinical decision to withhold life-sustaining treatment was legally upheld against the wishes of the child's mother. It established that clinicians cannot be forced to administer life-sustaining treatments that they believe are not in the best interests of patients with very severe brain damage, even when the patients are children and parents insist that treatment continues.

◆ Airedale NHS Trust v Bland (93).[15] As the result of severe injury, Tony Bland (an adult) was in a persistent vegetative state for over 2 years. It was held that further medical treatment would not be of any benefit to him and could be withdrawn. In a similar case from the US, but involving a 17-year-old in PVS following a motor vehicle accident, the court accepted that artificial feeding and hydration could be withdrawn taking account of the young person's known preferences and parental views.[16]

◆ Re R (96).[17] In this case, it was held that the non-provision of life-sustaining antibiotic therapy and cardio-pulmonary resuscitation was acceptable for an adult with very severe brain damage.

Since this time, further cases that have involved the proposal to withhold or withdraw life-sustaining treatment have been brought before British Courts. In all these cases, judges have balanced the principles of respect for the sanctity of life and the duty to avoid subjecting individuals to burdensome, futile and inhuman treatments from which they can expect to derive little if any benefit. In so doing they have retained the concept of best interests as the major criterion for decision-making. Although the best interests approach has been criticized by some legal commentators, it continues to inform professional and legal decision-making in this and other areas.

In effect, the cases outlined legalize what can be called passive euthanasia within the United Kingdom.[18] However, it is inconceivable that these cases would have been decided as they were without the availability of effective palliative care, since they were concerned with minimizing the long-term suffering of patients through decisions to withhold and withdraw life-sustaining treatment. This would be impossible without such care. However, it is equally clear that the judges in question did not reduce the potential interest of patients in staying alive to just the successful management of their physical and emotional discomfort. Ultimately, their judgement to legalize decisions to withhold and withdraw life-sustaining treatment was essentially moral in character, as it must be in other national legal jurisdictions where similar principles prevail. However, other jurisdictions may lay greater emphasis on the duty to preserve life and place greater weight on parental requests to continue life-sustaining treatments.

Paediatric guidelines for withholding and withdrawing life-sustaining treatment

In 1997 and 2004, these moral and legal arguments concerning withholding and withdrawal of life-sustaining treatment decisions were accepted and further developed by the Royal College of Paediatrics and Child Health (RCPCH).[19] In some cases involving children, such decisions—although traumatic—may not be too difficult for professional and parental carers (e.g. when the child is a terminally ill infant with no prospect of a future life). In others, they will raise more problems (e.g. when the terminally ill child has a fully developed personality and, on the face of it, everything to live for but no opportunity to do so).

The RCPCH guidelines address all of these different prospects and state that withholding or withdrawing curative medical treatment might be considered when:

◆ The child has been appropriately diagnosed as brain dead.

◆ The child has been appropriately diagnosed to be in a permanent vegetative state (PVS).

◆ The situation is one of 'no chance', where death is only being marginally delayed, without significant alleviation of suffering.

◆ There is 'no purpose' in keeping the child alive because of a dramatic and unacceptable degree of physical or mental impairment, such that it would be unreasonable to expect him or her to tolerate it. Either because of age or the severity of brain damage, the child will never be able to participate in 'decisions regarding treatment or its withdrawal'.

◆ The child's future life will be 'unbearable'. In the face of 'progressive and irreversible' illness, the child and/or the family believe that further treatment is more than the child can endure with any acceptable degree of human fulfilment. Such children may or may not be mentally impaired. If they are for whatever reason, the impact of such impairment on the child must be considered.

Legally, the first criterion has been long established and the second was confirmed in UK law by Airedale NHS Trust v Bland (93). The third criterion is based on Re C (89) and the fourth on Re J (90) and Re J (92), at least to the extent that it is meant to pertain to very severe brain damage. The fifth criterion—that of an 'unbearable' situation—is legally more complicated, as will be shown.

Since brain death and PVS are clinically well understood, the focus here will be on the last three criteria. Each can be illustrated as follows:[20]

◆ No chance. These are cases where there is a consensus that further clinical intervention will be futile—will not achieve the goal of significant prolongation of life. An example might be a child of 18 months who presents with meningococcal septicaemia, but who, despite intensive care, develops multiple organ failure.

◆ No purpose. Here, brain damage is so extensive that the child will develop or will regress to only minimal self-awareness and capacity for self-directed activity or interaction with others. An example might be a 3-month-old girl resuscitated at birth (weight 480 g) who required immediate ventilation and neonatal intensive care followed by further ventilation, high doses of steroids, but no significant improvement in lung function, and who also suffered severe intraventricular haemorrhages in the brain leading to a high probability of severe mental disability. Such situations might arise in any stage of childhood depending on the type of illness concerned (e.g. Tay–Sachs, Batten's, and other incurable genetic diseases associated with childhood).

◆ Unbearable. Such cases entail the necessity for repeated, dramatic, and potentially traumatic clinical interventions whose burden is deemed by parents, professional carers, and perhaps the children themselves, as being too great in light of the potential benefit. A case would be a 10-year-old boy with renal failure, with dysmorphic kidneys, moderately severe learning difficulties, but with a degree of physical independence, an attractive personality, and much love from parents and siblings. After extensive discussion with the clinical team, his school, the parents of other similarly affected children, social workers, and a chaplain, his parents decided that dialysis should not begin. Similar clinical cases may involve children who are mature enough to decide to refuse such clinical intervention themselves where their decision is supported by the family and clinical team. An example might be the child with advanced lung disease as a result of cystic fibrosis who refuses heart–lung transplantation.

With the first three criteria (i.e. brain death, PVS, and futile intervention) parental views and demands for treatment do not confer legal obligations on clinicians to provide it—as Re J (92) confirms. Yet, while the child is—and should be—the focus of the paediatric duty of care, it is equally clear that some further moral duty is owed to the parents. Their distress and concern are themselves forms of suffering that deserve support and guidance.[9] Clinical teams, especially those providing palliative care, inevitably bear the brunt of the responsibility to provide both. They must delicately negotiate with parents, helping them to understand the nature of their child's condition, prognosis, and why withholding or withdrawal of life-sustaining treatment is believed to be in the child's best interests. If done sensitively and with appropriate communication skills, such counselling can often lead to successful outcomes both for the child and the parent, however ambiguous the word 'success' must be in this context.

However, this may be impossible. For example, parents may insist on the continuation of medical intervention that will neither significantly sustain life nor confer clinical benefit (e.g. in brainstem death or PVS). Here, the clinical team must affirm their belief that the interests of the child will not be served by further active treatment, and that it is their professional duty not to provide it.[21] While courts in the United Kingdom will usually but not invariably support such clinical judgements, this picture becomes more complex in other legal national jurisdictions, where parents are deemed to have more authority. Generally, parents who reject the advice of the clinical team and wish for life-sustaining treatment to continue should:

◆ be counselled with respect and dignity;

◆ be advised that they may wish to go to court to obtain judicial intervention in their favour, but informed that this is unlikely to be the outcome;

◆ be told how to go about this and, where practical, helped to do so;

◆ be supported sympathetically with regard to the clinical and moral reasons for non-treatment; and

◆ not be engaged in adversarial conflict and debate.

These issues will often emerge in the broader context of discussions about on-going palliative care, and those responsible for such care may be actively involved in these sensitive negotiations.

The chronically deteriorating immature child

The fourth and fifth criteria of the RCPCH guidelines raise moral and legal issues more contentious than the first three.[22] Using them to justify decisions to withhold and withdraw life-sustaining treatment should therefore be approached with caution. The 'no purpose' criterion suggests that non-treatment may be acceptable in children with sufficient cognitive ability for minimal levels of self-directed activity and social interaction but overwhelming physical disability. However, the use of the term 'no purpose' suggests that the brunt of the dramatic impairment is intended to be neurodevelopmental in the context of a much reduce life expectancy—at whatever point in the child's life that this is revealed. Clinical examples of this kind have already been outlined.

This emphasis on severe neurological damage does not apply to the 'unbearable' criterion, which may include children with clear but perhaps limited cognitive and emotional development. The maturity of such children may be compromised by disability, by age, or by the effect of illness. On the one hand, through invasive treatment, their lives may be sustainable in the short to long term, perhaps even through adolescence and beyond. On the other hand, their personal experience of life under these circumstances may be terrible.

Such children may be able to experience and conceptualize bewilderment and despair about their physical disabilities and their consequent inability to achieve whatever goals they are capable of setting for themselves, albeit to a limited extent. But, it is precisely this level of awareness and understanding—and the sadness and frustration that may go with it—that can make the point of continued life-sustaining treatment and continued life itself so questionable for them, their parents, and professional carers. Such children may indeed reach a state where the prospect of further invasive and disruptive life-prolonging treatment is more than those who love and care for them believe that they can bear.

This applies to children with clinical conditions such as respiratory, cardiac, or kidney diseases that are incurable and rapidly degenerative. Equally important are childhood cancers where unpleasant treatment has been repeated, and where further treatment may extend life but with an increasingly uncertain therapeutic outcome. In these circumstances, some parents may believe that their children have such limited potential for human fulfilment that further treatment to preserve life is no longer in the child's best interest. Conversely, other parents may take the opposite view and believe that they can and should provide maximum support for their child, to continue to try to optimize their potential for as long as possible.[23]

Although cognitive impairment may vary in children in the 'unbearable' situation, case law usually only refers to circumstances where there are extreme forms of impairment. Yet, in the circumstances we have described, it may well be that continued life is not in the best interests of children who lack the maturity to make such a judgement for themselves and whose disabilities are worsening with no hope of significant improvement. If the health-care team is convinced that this is so then it is highly unlikely that a decision to withhold or withdraw life-sustaining treatment will lead to any suggestion of legal impropriety—provided that parents also agree.

A problem might arise if the team believes that life-sustaining treatment should be withdrawn and the parents disagree. Here, the wishes of the parents should be respected—unless there is some reason to believe that they are practically incapable of providing the support and resources required to optimize their child's personal potential. In the face of further dispute, a judicial ruling should be obtained.

This analysis leads to what some may regard as a disquieting conclusion. Children, with the same clinical condition, will in one situation (parental support) have their lives sustained, while in another situation (the withdrawal of parental support) will have their lives foreshortened.[5] The moral justification for this is that, since there is some indeterminacy about the child's cognitive, emotional, and physical potentials, it would be wrong to force the beliefs of the clinical team on parents who disagreed. After all, it is the parents and not the team who will have to live with either committing themselves to caring for their child or with the knowledge that they morally participated in a decision that foreshortened their child's life.

In either circumstance, effective palliative care becomes essential. In the case of the young child for whom parents and clinicians agree that continued life has become too unbearable, withholding and withdrawing life-sustaining treatment may not bring about immediate death. However such withdrawal is clinically managed, palliative measures should ensure:

- Choice in place of care and empowering the child and family in decision-making about symptom management.

- Provision of relevant information so that parental decisions can be as informed as possible.

- Proactive provision of advice and equipment for symptom management aimed at minimizing suffering and discomfort for the child.

- Facilitating maximum intimate contact between the child and family.

- Providing support for parents through their child's death and bereavement.

- Similarly, if the decision is to continue to sustain the child's life, then the inevitability of further deterioration will necessitate palliative measures designed to optimize physical and emotional functions and to minimize discomfort. Support for the parents entails the provision of appropriate information and practical help to assist them to ensure that their child will sustain the best quality of life possible.

Respect for the autonomy of the chronically deteriorating mature child

Paediatricians have a duty to act in the best interests of their patients that may result in decisions to recommend withholding or withdrawing life-sustaining treatment. They also have another, sometimes conflicting, duty to respect patients' autonomy—the right to make self determined, informed choices about their illness and its treatment—to the extent that patients have the capacity to do so.

Children with life-limiting illnesses may develop high levels of maturity before they die. Although their life expectancy may be brief and their capacity to make informed choices variable, these young people may have much that they wish to try to accomplish. The combination of life-sustaining intervention and effective palliative care is essential in assisting them to do so, and serves their best interests. Most children will want to optimize both their life expectancy and its quality as much as their parents and clinicians. As a result, they will wish to cooperate with their clinical management. Such partnership in care can be enormously rewarding for all concerned, despite the circumstances in which it occurs.

A minority of children may refuse the provision of life-prolonging care because they do not wish to continue to live with the burden that their illness imposes. Here, the duty to protect life and health comes into direct conflict with the duty to respect autonomy—to the degree that such children may be said to possess it.

The importance of respecting the autonomy of children

If the dignity of adults is abused through denying them informed choice, their capacity to return to some state of normality will probably be preserved. This is because their cognitive and emotional foundations for individual personality and personal identity are well developed. The opposite holds, however, for children. They are in the process of developing their personalities and learn through their interactive relationships with adults. Their personal identities are forged around experiencing themselves as the kinds of persons who are deemed by adults to do some things well and others not so well. Their emotional confidence and health will very much depend on their self-satisfaction with these dynamic and evolving achievements.[24]

Hence, lack of respect for a child's autonomy can severely and irretrievably undermine intellectual skills and emotional confidence, damaging the child's future potential as a person and producing psychological trauma. Yet equally, children must be protected in circumstances where they are at risk and not able to protect themselves. Finding this balance can be complex in the clinical care of children.[25]

Younger children may lack sufficient autonomy to be able to consent to or refuse medical treatment. This does not mean that it is unnecessary to consult them about their thoughts and feelings concerning their illness and its treatment. Such consultation is mandated by the United Nations Convention on the Rights of the Child and nationally in the United Kingdom by the Children Act.[26,27] Thus, the beliefs of an immature child with a chronically deteriorating life-limiting or terminal illness must be taken into account in any medical decisions made about them, even when these beliefs are ultimately rejected. Here, the balance between respect and protection weighs in favour of the latter. On the other hand, if the child satisfies the same criteria of competence as an adult (see below) the balance is in favour of respecting autonomy. In the UK, a child who is able to fully understand the nature and purpose of a medical intervention and its likely effect on themselves and their family is regarded as competent, irrespective of age.[28] In US jurisdiction, such young people are referred to as 'mature minors'. The mature minor doctrine permits a minor who exhibits the maturity of an adult to make decisions traditionally reserved for those who have attained the legal age of majority.[29] In such circumstances, their right to refuse medical treatment should be respected because they are competent.

Adults are competent to consent to and refuse treatment, including life-sustaining treatment provided they have the capacity:[30]

- to understand relevant information about treatment proposals and the consequences of refusing them;

- to remember the most important aspects of this information;

- to reason or deliberate about any clinical choices that are proposed; and

- to believe that information communicated applies to the patient who is given it and, e.g. is not being made up in order to deceive or harm.

Therefore, adults may be competent and still make choices about their medical care that clinicians deem irrational and dangerous. Provided that they are competent, the choice of such patients to embark upon a course of non-treatment that will, in effect, kill them should be respected. It is important to note that competence is essentially task-oriented and context-dependent. An adult may be incompetent to do or understand many things and still be competent to understand, remember, deliberate about, and believe basic clinical information to make crucial choices about their care.

The right of the competent child to refuse life-sustaining treatment

Why should competent children be regarded as different from adults who are often assumed to have the capacity to make informed choices? After all, if treatment is in children's best interests and they consent to it then no further moral reason (e.g. further parental consent) is required to proceed. But what if they refuse? To force unwanted treatment on such a child simply because of his/her age, when they can be shown to be competent using adult criteria seems unjust.[8] Not only may such intervention lead to the same loss of dignity that it does with adults, the loss may be compounded because competent children may be less physically and socially able to resist whatever force is administered to carry it out.

It is now widely accepted that competent children who refuse treatment that can be postponed without loss of life or serious injury should have their decision respected.[31] Not to do so may generate anger and hostility towards health professionals, placing the young person at potential risk of serious harm through their rejecting future clinical help when it is needed.

The situation when competent children or mature minors reject life-sustaining treatment is arguably more complex and compounded by the identification of an adolescent phase of brain growth and development in the areas of the brain concerned with social judgement and self-control. Although the latter may lead to theoretical reasons to doubt an adolescent's decision-making capacity, especially in times of stress, its clinical relevance remains unclear, especially in patients with long experience of illness. It seems likely that a competent child who understands that death will result from the refusal of treatment will weigh up their choice against the background of their experience of their illness and its treatment. Forced or coerced treatment can only add to a feeling of helplessness and indignity that may amount to torture, albeit well intentioned.[32]

It is therefore reasonable to argue that forcing unwanted treatment on competent young people who refuse it is immoral. Depending on the jurisdiction, however, the law does not necessarily agree.

In England, two further important cases in the early 1990s judged that age rather than competence should determine whether young people should have the same right to refuse treatment which was felt to be in their best interests.[33,34] Moreover, English Courts have authorized both blood transfusion and heart transplantation as measures to sustain the lives of young people who were otherwise competent to refuse them. As a result, English law currently appears to accept that although a competent young person may consent to such medical treatment they cannot refuse it until they are 18. It seems likely that the application of the mature minor doctrine in the US may also be constrained in such circumstances, especially when parents and clinicians believe that continuing treatment is on balance correct. Conversely, Scottish law makes no distinction between the right of a competent young person to agree or to refuse such treatment, with no apparent disastrous consequences.[35] It is possible, though not inevitable, that English Law will take more account of the wishes of competent adolescents in time as may be the case in other jurisdictions.

Procedural rules for children who refuse treatment

The only coherent justification for not giving a competent young person the right to refuse life-sustaining treatment is procedural rather than a matter of moral principle. It is reasonable to argue that it is difficult to determine whether young persons are competent to make such important decisions about their health care and its impact on their family. Life and death mistakes cannot be corrected. This underlines the importance of having clinical procedures in place to assess a child's competence to make specific decisions irrespective of their age.[36] It is vital that such clinical assessments are performed by those with sufficient professional expertise and knowledge of the child and family and their circumstances to do so.

If such procedures determine that a child is competent, then the right of choice should be with the child and no one else, although they may choose to share it with or even delegate it to others. For example, even young children suffering from leukaemia may competently decide that they do not wish to have any more chemotherapy and understand that the consequence will be that their life will be shortened. As with adults, their autonomy should be respected and should trump the duty of clinicians and/or parents to protect their life and health in ways that the latter regard as being in the child's best interests.

Conflict between such young people and parents—or between clinicians and parents—may arise under these circumstances.[37] Clinicians may continue to question the competence of such young people, even in the face of appropriate procedural steps that verify it. The stakes may just seem too high.[7] Of course, where such steps have not been taken (e.g. interviews with the duty social worker and consultant paediatric psychiatrist) the primary task is to help the child to understand their importance and in such a way that maximizes their feeling of being treated with respect and dignity. If appropriate procedural steps do confirm the competence of such children, it is the duty of their clinician to counsel the parents—and if necessary seek counselling themselves—about the harmful consequences of continuing to force life on a child for whom it has lost meaning.[38] Of course, the need for sensitivity, patience, and compassion in discussions and debates of these kinds akin to those required for shuttle diplomacy-cannot be overestimated.[39] It is precisely in these contexts that the skills and insights associated with paediatric palliative care will prove invaluable.[40]

Consequences for palliative care

Good palliative care has an important role to play in the duty to respect autonomy of children. Although children may suffer life-limiting illnesses or be terminally ill they may still want to get things done—and as competently as possible! Some children will engage in a variety of activities at home or in hospital with no clear understanding of the closeness of their death. Others will have varying amounts of understanding but will also be keen to be as active as possible. Competent children who have a full understanding of their terminal prognosis will want to do many of the things that characterize adults in such circumstances—to see and converse with people, to make some record of their experiences, to make what they believe to be important choices about a variety of matters … to reflect on their life and what it has meant to them. To be unable to do things of this kind properly because of inadequate pain relief and other support can be as harrowing as the pain and suffering themselves.

Pain and other forms of suffering may be detrimental to the exercise of competent choice. Effective palliative care can enable children to express their desires in a way that influences their clinical management. This may include a desire no longer to accept life-sustaining treatment. If such children believe that they have been able to make their views clear and that they have been listened to, this will help enormously in their ability to face their illness and its consequences. Whether or not their desires are achieved, they can at least know that they were treated with respect and dignity. For children at the very end of their lives, such feelings and beliefs will be the ones with which they die. If their deaths are peaceful and pain-free this is surely a testament to the moral worth of good palliative care.

Conclusion: palliative care and moral indeterminacy

For the purposes of exposition it has been necessary to analyse many issues as though they were more or less straightforward, when this is palpably not so. It is one thing to observe that coherent moral and legal principles dictate the boundaries of good paediatric practice. It is another thing we believe that in practice these principles will be interpreted in the same ways. They will not! Paediatricians, parents, and children will all, at times, disagree about what the correct interpretation should be.[41,42]

As regards non-treatment issues, these disagreements will be fuelled by a variety of conflicting values about, among others:

◆ the sanctity of life;

◆ the most appropriate circumstances in which to foreshorten life withholding and withdrawing life-sustaining treatment;

◆ what constitutes competence in a young person who refuses life-prolonging treatment;

◆ the amount of coercion that is acceptable in forcing treatment on semi-competent children; and

◆ how much duty is owed to protecting the well being of parents—i.e. by preserving life longer than is in a child's best interests or through not supporting a competent refusal of life-saving treatment.

It would be foolish to pretend that in such cases of moral and, perhaps, legal indeterminacy, definitively correct solutions can or will be found.

In the face of such uncertainty, it is essential that the discussions about how to proceed should take place in a form which optimizes the rationality of decision making.[43] These decisions may be a compromise, one not completely satisfying to any of the participants. It will be important, therefore, that all participants believe that the decision emerged from a rigorous and fair discussion. Given the fraught emotions that often face ethico-legal indeterminacy in paediatric decisions about the end of life, this belief should help to strengthen the realization that certainty is sometimes more than anyone can expect.

More specifically, procedural fairness dictates that relevant discussions concerning non-treatment issues are organized so that the voices of key participants are heard and respected. Thus, the traditional power of the senior personnel in the clinical team must be suspended and no single person or interest group should be allowed to dominate communication and debate. For this to be a practical reality, patients and parents involved in such discussions may need to be represented by advocates who can help them to articulate their beliefs and concerns. If they are present within the hospital, clinical ethics committees or ethics consultants may also be of help, to the degree that their advice is perceived to be objective and independent.[44]

However such ethico-legal uncertainty is procedurally approached, the most important factor in its successful resolution will be the transparency of the care and concern of the paediatric staff. Of particular importance will be their ability to reach out to patients and parents—without this necessarily entailing agreement with what they decide.[45] This is hardly surprising. Most experienced practitioners know that it is this process that constitutes the art of good medicine. Those who specialize in palliative care will have particular skills and experience in facilitating good communication and education about the material factors surrounding terminal care and death—most of them experience, in discussing with parents, the delicate balance between their concern for the interests of their children and the necessary emotional hardship brought upon them by their child's illness.[9, 10, 40] This experience can and should inform all aspects of the management of the moral indeterminacy that can surround decisions relating to withholding and withdrawing life-sustaining treatment. Indeed, without the wisdom and reassurance that such experience can provide children, parents, and professional carers, the burden of such decisions would be even more intolerable.

References

1. Chantler, C. and Doyal, L. (2000). Medical ethics: the duties of care in principle and practice. In *Clinical negligence* (eds. M. Powers and N. Harris), pp. 549–72. Butterworths, London.

2. Kennedy, I. and Grubb, A. (2000). *Medical law*. Butterworths, London.

3. van der Wal, M.E., Renfurm, L.N., van Vught, A.J. *et al.* (1999). Circumstances of dying in hospitalised children. *Intensive Care Medicine*, **158**, 560–5.

4. Balfour-Lynn, I.M. and Tasker, R.C. (1996). At the coalface—medical ethics in practice. Futility and death in paediatric medical intensive care. *Journal of Medical Ethics*, **22**, 279–81.

5. Doyal, L. (1998). When life may be too precious: the severely damaged neonate. *Seminars in Neonatology*, **3**(4), 297–382.

6. British Medical Association. (1999). *Withholding and withdrawing life-prolonging medical treatment*. pp. 1–12, BMJ Books, London.

7. Kenny, N.P. and Frager, G. (1996). Refractory symptoms and terminal sedation of children: ethical issues and practical management. *Journal of Palliative Care*, **12**(3), 40–5.

8. Levetown, M. (1996). Ethical aspects of pediatric palliative care. *Journal of Palliative Care*, **12**, 35–9.

9. Trapp, A. (1998). Support for the family. In *Care of the dying child* (ed. A. Goldman), pp. 76–92. Oxford University Press, Oxford.

10. Stein, A. and Woolley, H. Caring for the carers. In *Care of the Dying Child* (ed. A. Goldman), pp. 164–82. Oxford University Press, Oxford.

11. Re B (1981) 1 WLR 1421.

12. Re C (1989) 2 All ER 782.

13. Re J (1990) 6 BMLR 25.

14. Re J (1992) 9 BMLR 10.

15. Airedale NHS Trust v Bland (1993) 1 All ER 821.

16. Re Swan 569 A.2d.1202 (Me1990).

17. Re R (1996) 2 FLR 99.

18. Montgomery, J. (2002). *Health care law*. Oxford University Press, Oxford, pp. 437–9.

19. Royal College of Paediatrics and Child Health. (2004). *Withholding or withdrawing life saving treatment in children: a framework for practice*. Royal College of Paediatrics and Child Health, London, revised 2004.

20. Goldman, A., Burne, R., and Rees, P. (1998). Different illnesses and the problems they cause. In *Care of the dying child* (ed. A. Goldman), pp. 14–42. Oxford University Press, Oxford.

21. Jecker, N.S. and Schneiderman, L.J. (1995). When families request that 'everything possible' be done. *Journal of Medicine and Philosophy*, **20**, 145–63.

22. Doyal, L. and Larcher, V. (2000). Drafting guidelines for the withholding or withdrawing of life sustaining treatment in critically ill children and neonates. *Archive of Diseases of Childhood. Fetal and Neonatal Edition*, **83**, F60–3.

23. Pinkerton, J.A.V. *et al.* (1997). Parental rights at the birth of a near-viable infant: conflicting perspectives. *American Journal of Obstetrics and Gynaecology*, **177**, 283–8.

24. Doyal, L. and Gough, I. (1991). *A theory of human need*. Macmillan, London.

25. Kurtz, Z. (1995). Do children's rights to health care in the UK ensure their best interests? *Journal of the Royal College of Physicians of London*, **29**, 508–16.

26. General Assembly of the United Nations. (1996). *Convention on the rights of the child 1989*. The Stationery Office, London.

27. Children Act 1989, s.1(3)(a). The Stationery Office London 1989.

28. Re C (1994) 1 All ER 819 (FD).

29. Gillick v West Norfolk, and Wisbech AHA [1985] 3 All ER 402, HL.

30. Penkower, J.A. (1996). Comment. *The potential right of chronically ill adolescents to refuse life-sustaining medical treatments – fatal misuse of the mature minor doctrine* 45 DEPAUL.L REV 1165–6.

31. British Medical Association. (2001). *Consent, rights and choices in health care for children and young people*. BMJ Books, London.

32. Doyal, L. (1998). Can medicine be torture? In *Childhood abused* (ed. G. Van Bueren), pp. 155–74. Aldershott, Ashgate.

33. Re R (1991) 4 All ER 177.

34. Re W (1992) 4 All ER 627.

35. Age of Legal Capacity (Scotland) Act 1991. The Stationery Office London, 1991.

36. Dixon-Woods, M., Young, B., and Heney, D. (1999). Partnerships with children. *British Medical Journal*, **319**, 778–80.

37. Doyal, L. and Henning, P. (1994). Stopping treatment for end-stage renal failure: the rights of children and adolescents. *Paediatric Nephrology*, **7**, 768–71.

38. Dorner, S. (1976). Adolescents with spina bifida: how they see their situation. *Archives of Diseases in Childhood*, **51**, 439–44.

39. Bluebond-Langner, M., De Cico, A., and Belasco, J. (2005). Involving children with life shortening illness in discussion about participation in Clinical Research: a proposal for shuttle diplomacy and negotiation. In *Ethics and research with children: A case-based approach* (ed. Eric Kodish), pp. 323–43. Oxford University Press, New York.

40. Association for Children with Life-Threatening or Terminal Conditions and their Families. (1997). *A guide to the development of children's palliative care services*. Royal College of Paediatrics and Child Health, London.

41. Randolph, A.G., Zollo, M.B., Egger, M.J. *et al.* (1999). Variability in physician opinion on limiting pediatric life support. *Pediatrics*, **103**(4), e46.

42. Farsides, C.C.S. (1998). Autonomy and its implications for palliative care: a northern European perspective. *Palliative Medicine*, **12**, 147–51.

43. Doyal, L. (1990). Medical ethics and moral indeterminacy. *Journal of Law and Society*, **17**, 1–16.

44. Doyal, L. (2001). Clinical ethics committees and the formulation of health care policy. *Journal of Medical Ethics*, **27** (Suppl. II), 44–9.

45. Gillis, J. (1997). When lifesaving treatment in children is not the answer. *British Medical Journal*, **315**, 1246.

Euthanasia and physician-assisted suicide

Lars Johan Materstvedt and Georg Bosshard

Introduction

By far, euthanasia is the most controversial issue within end-of-life care in general and within palliative medicine in particular. The issue is extraordinarily complex because it brings up a series of difficult questions that are medical, ethical, juridical, cultural and religious of nature. Additionally, the issue is emotional and existential as it affects us at a personal level; it directly concerns our right to decide what to do with our lives.

Euthanasia: one concept, many definitions

Euthanasia stems from the Greek 'eu' = good, and 'thanatos' = death. Thus it just means a good death. Accordingly, a patient dying peacefully from natural causes would be a case of euthanasia—meaning euthanasia is widespread throughout the world. In fact, it might mean most people's deaths are instances of euthanasia. But surely this is not what the debate on euthanasia is about. So what is it about?

The first point to note is that even though euthanasia is one concept, there are many conflicting definitions of euthanasia[1]. Thus there is much debate over the definition. We cannot however enter that comprehensive debate here since it would take up too much space, space that we want to devote to clinical and empirical matters that need be dealt with in a chapter like this, in a textbook like this.

In a position paper, the European Association for Palliative Care (EAPC; www.eapcnet.org) interprets euthanasia as follows: 'a doctor intentionally killing a person by the administration of drugs, at that person's voluntary and competent request'[2]. This definition is in line with the Dutch understanding since, 'euthanasia is usually defined in the Netherlands as the administration of drugs by a physician with the explicit intention of ending the patient's life at his/her explicit request'[3]. The large-scale studies of Dutch medical end-of-life practice that have been carried out in 1990, 1995, and 2001 used the same definition[4]. The 2005 follow-up study uses a somewhat different phrasing, yet the understanding of euthanasia is exactly the same[5].

'Killing' or 'ending of life'; 'person' or 'patient'?

There are two slight dissimilarities between the EAPC definition of euthanasia and the Dutch definition. First, the former refers to 'killing', whereas the second uses the expression 'ending of life'.

But in reality they are both about the same phenomenon: the intentional (deliberate) taking of life by utilizing medicines. Dutch euthanasia guidelines recommend a sequence of coma induction with intravenous administration (preferably through a fluid drip) of sodium thiopental 20 mg/kg (2 g in a bolus of 10 ml saline), followed by neuromuscular blockers (a bolus of pancuronium hydrochloride 20 mg or vecuronium hydrochloride 20 mg), causing the paralysis of the respiratory muscles[6]. This is a procedure aimed at causing immediate and painless death. In the Netherlands, medicines used in this way are called 'euthanatics' or 'euthanatica'[6,7]. Note also that in this country it is not uncommon to name euthanasia 'killing on request'[7].

Although euthanasia is thus killing technically speaking, some deny that it is *wrongful* killing. But both definitions are descriptive not normative, and so do not address the ethical issue of whether or not euthanasia is *justified* killing. Put differently, and following the philosopher David Hume (1711–76), it is one thing to say what something 'is' (here: euthanasia) and quite another to say that this something also 'ought' to be[8]. That is, we are referring here to the fundamental, analytical divide between facts and norms. Second, the one definition speaks of 'person' whereas the other of 'patient'. Does that mean, according to the EAPC definition, that a physician taking the life of *any* person at his/her request carries out euthanasia? If so, the definition seems just too wide and thereby indefensible. But this is not the case. Like in any definition, certain things are taken for granted; otherwise a definition will become extremely long and detailed and thus impractical. It is presupposed that this concerns the doctor–patient relationship and so the person in question is, in the technical sense, a patient. Why not simply write 'patient', then? Because even though all of a physician's patients will be so in the technical sense, some will not be patients in what we may call the *traditional* sense. These might not be ill at all, or have no severe illness of a somatic or psychiatric nature, and fall within the category of persons who do not want to live anymore due to 'tiredness of life' or 'suffering through living'[9]. But again there is no real difference between the EAPC definition and the Dutch.

Physician-assisted suicide (PAS), assisted suicide, and indirect assistance

Beside euthanasia, there is the act of physician-assisted suicide (PAS), which may be defined as, 'a doctor intentionally helping a person to commit suicide by providing drugs for self-administration, at that person's voluntary and competent request'[2]. In the Netherlands, 'physician-assisted suicide is usually defined as the prescription or supply of drugs at the explicit request of the patient with the explicit intention to enable the patient to end his/her own life'[3]. This is also consistent with the understanding laid out in the Oregon Death with Dignity Act, which allows PAS but bans euthanasia[10] (Table 5.5.3). Normally, in PAS the patient digests an overdose of barbiturates that finally suppresses respiration, causing death.

All three interpretations would rule out as PAS a situation in which a patient collects medication behind the physician's back with the purpose of taking his or her own life. Even though the medication is provided by a physician, in such a setting it is not the physician's intention that the medication be so used—on the contrary, it is meant for treatment.

What if a physician suspects that a patient is collecting medication in order to be able to commit suicide, or the patient tells the physician outright that this is what is going on, but in both instances the physician turns a blind eye to it? True, the physician cannot know for sure that the patient will, eventually, go ahead with his or her plans. But is not the physician somehow implicated? It would seem that the answer is 'yes' and therefore some have called this 'indirect (unintended) assistance with suicide'. But even if it is, it still would not count as PAS as defined here because neither has the patient asked for the physician's help in taking his or her own life, nor has the physician offered such help.

In Switzerland, as opposed to in Oregon and Washington, USA[11]—as well as in the Netherlands, Belgium and Luxembourg[12] (Table 5.5.3)—lay people too may assist patients in their suicide[13,14]. Therefore there is such a thing as 'assisted suicide' only (without the 'physician' prefix).

Is there an ethical difference between euthanasia and (physician-) assisted suicide?

It is a matter of controversy whether or not the practical difference between euthanasia and (physician-) assisted suicide also amounts to an ethical difference. Philosopher Thomas Pogge argues: 'This is not a substantial moral difference when the death is, in both cases, triggered *by the patient's own voluntary and competent request*. Morally, the event is then suicide assisted by another. The extent to which the patient can physically co-operate makes no moral difference'[15].

Nevertheless, this is exactly where others detect an ethical divide between the patient being in total control up until the very moment of death—i.e. in (physician-) assisted suicide—in contradistinction to the physician having that control—i.e. in euthanasia. The patient is thus able to exercise autonomy to a lesser degree in euthanasia and *that* is ethically significant, some claim. Research in the Netherlands seems to support this point of view. The reason physicians gave most often for opting for PAS was that they wanted 'as far as possible to let the patient bear the responsibility'. Euthanasia was chosen primarily for medico-technical reasons, whereas PAS was selected primarily for moral reasons[16].

Despite these ethical concerns, in reality euthanasia is much more common than PAS in the Netherlands. The ratio was 11 to 1 in 2001; 3500 cases of euthanasia divided by 300 cases of PAS[4]. In 2005 the contrast was starker still: 23 to 1 (Table 5.5.2)[5].

Characteristics of the euthanasia definition

Several aspects stand out in the above understanding of euthanasia. To begin with, only physicians carry out euthanasia. The Dutch euthanasia law of 2002 explicitly states that euthanasia is an act that is 'reserved' for physicians (Table 5.5.3)[17]. As does the Belgian euthanasia law that entered into force the same year (Table 5.5.3)[18,19].

Euthanasia is voluntary by definition. This entails that the so-called 'euthanasia clinics' that were established even before World War II had nothing to do with euthanasia; they were about medical murder (Table 5.5.1, [f])—regardless of the fact that many of the health-care personnel involved considered what they did to be acts of mercy. Compassionate murder is a known phenomenon[20]. The EAPC definition uses the expression 'voluntary and competent request', whereas the Dutch definition formulates this point in the wording 'at his/her explicit request'. Thus individual *consent* is at the heart of the matter.

Strictly speaking, due to the possibility that an individual may explicitly ask for something without doing so freely, an explicit request need not be voluntary. Yet this is implied in the Dutch definition. Within medicine and medical research on human subjects one of the conditions for valid consent is that it be informed. However, informed consent is not a sufficient condition for voluntariness as one must also be free from various sorts of social or psychological duress coming from, say, one's relatives. As far as the topics information and voluntariness are concerned, the Dutch law requires that the physician must 'have informed the patient about his situation and his prospects', that the physician 'be satisfied that the patient has made a voluntary and carefully considered request', and 'have consulted at least one other, independent physician, who must have seen the patient'[17].

Additionally, a request may be voluntary without being 'competent' in certain clinical or psychiatric interpretations of what competence is taken to mean. Still the patient may have competence in the legal sense.

Euthanasia is also active by definition. In response to the EAPC paper[2], leading Dutch euthanasia researcher Professor Gerrit van der Wal wrote that, 'I am glad that the [EAPC] suggests, with regard to euthanasia, that the adjectives "voluntary", "active" and "passive" should no longer be used … The argumentation is valid. In the spoken and written word this will avoid many unnecessary misunderstandings'[21]. The late Dame Cicely Saunders in her comment on the same paper presents a view which is congruent with van der Wal's as far as the definition is concerned: 'as they point out, euthanasia is voluntary by definition and the term "passive euthanasia", which has led to much confusion, is certainly a contradiction in terms'[22]. 'Active euthanasia', on the other hand, is then a superfluous term—and likewise the term 'voluntary euthanasia', for reasons given in the previous paragraphs.

'Terminating' life

Quite often euthanasia is called (voluntary) 'termination' of life. Many scientific papers use this concept, so does the Dutch euthanasia law which both has it in its title and refers to a physician 'terminating' a patient's life[17]. Also, the Belgian law uses the expression 'terminating life'[18]. Yet it is implied in both laws that what is at stake is the use of lethal injections.

We recommend that the concept 'termination' not be used in connection with euthanasia. It may allude to the termination/withdrawing of life-sustaining medical treatment in the terminally ill (Table 5.5.1, [a]). In such instances, sometimes the patient dies sooner than would be the case if treatment were given. In that sense, withdrawal contributes to termination of the patient's life; death is hastened—or, the other way round, life is shortened. Ezekiel Emanuel reports that despite careful wording, US physicians frequently confound euthanasia and terminating life-sustaining treatments[23,24].

On 'passive' euthanasia

This does not mean that the above description captures what euthanasia 'really' is[1]. There have been many attempts at developing typologies that employ distinctions such as active/passive euthanasia[25,26] and direct/indirect euthanasia[7]. From a philosophical point of view, this is an important discussion that could lead to new insights and is therefore welcome. Furthermore, such discussions may alter the way we perceive the world, and hence could also impact upon legislation and medical practice.

At any given point, regardless of this discussion and for the sake of clarity, an author must however choose which wording he is going to use. Our usage in the present chapter is congruent with the Dutch understanding of euthanasia—and of PAS—as laid out above. The reasons for this choice include that the Dutch euthanasia practice is unique in the world, dating back to at least 1973[7] (Table 5.5.3). Additionally, there exists a large evidence base regarding this practice that is based upon the above interpretation of euthanasia[4,5]. Research on euthanasia and PAS in Australia, New Zealand, the USA (Oregon physicians) and in several European countries has used this Dutch framework for research[27–37]. For reasons of international comparability, then, one is well advised to take as one's point of departure the Dutch understanding.

Ethical, political, epistemological, and logical aspects of the definition

As any other normative framework, the Dutch understanding yields a number of specific moral questions. Among these are: is euthanasia something that physicians, or only physicians, ought to participate in?[19] Even if euthanasia is voluntary (by definition), is that a reason to allow the practice; is it not in flagrant violation of the longstanding Western ethical tradition that emphasizes the inviolability or sanctity of life—what bioethicist Peter Singer has called 'the old ethic'?[38]

In political and legal terms, at face value euthanasia would seem to conflict with Article 2 of the European Convention on Human Rights which states that, 'everyone's right to life shall be protected by law. No one shall be deprived of his life intentionally'[39].

A number of epistemological and logical considerations spring up also, and these include: Can we always be sure that a patient's request for euthanasia is made on an entirely voluntary basis; can we *know* this? Indeed, can requests for euthanasia at all be voluntary; does not the requirement 'unbearable suffering', like in the Dutch and Belgian laws,[17,18] actually preclude the requirement that a request must also be 'voluntary'? How can these two be reconciled if the request is really driven or determined by the experience of unbearable (or intolerable) symptoms and not by the patient's own free will—which he is no longer able to exercise because the symptoms are 'in control'?[40]

What euthanasia is not

Because the Dutch interpretation of euthanasia[3–5] is so narrow, it follows by logical implication that non-voluntary (when patients are incompetent) and involuntary (when patients are competent and made no request to die) medicalized killing by drugs fall outside its scope. Table 5.5.1 provides a categorization including these two and four other medical end-of-life decisions of which none count as euthanasia in the Netherlands.

Statistical data from around the world—and a remark on the idea of a 'slippery slope'

Table 5.5.2 displays estimated figures for medical deaths brought about by lethal drugs in the Netherlands, drawn from death certificate studies[4,5]. Percentages are of total annual deaths in the country.

In legal terms, the two types of drug-induced deaths that fall under the 'without request' heading—i.e. [e] and [f] of Table 5.5.1— are illegal in the Netherlands[7,41,42] and everywhere else[43]. Involuntary—but not non-voluntary—medicalized killing is a downright violation of patient autonomy; one fails in the most fundamental way to respect the decision-making capacities of autonomous persons[44]. That ethical observation stands firm even when the patient's life is ended by drugs with the best of intentions—as was the case with German death clinics[20]. Ethically speaking, both non-voluntary and involuntary are troubling types and one key Dutch researcher believes that although such actions in physicians are understandable, they are nevertheless indefensible in all but, possibly, certain exceptional cases[45].

It is an interesting finding that in Flanders, Belgium, the rate of unrequested administration of lethal drugs is similar to Australia, and significantly higher than in the Netherlands. The figures are 3.2 per cent (Belgium), 3.5 per cent (Australia) and 0.7 per cent (Netherlands), respectively[29]. Another comparative study carried out in 2001 found 1.5 per cent of all deaths in Flanders to fall within the unrequested category[30]. This is less than half, as compared

Table 5.5.1 Medical end-of-life decisions distinct from euthanasia.

[a] non-treatment decisions (NTDs)—i.e. withholding or withdrawing life-sustaining medical treatment that has been deemed disproportionately harmful *or* futile;

[b] alleviation of pain and other symptoms (APS)* with opioids or sedatives that have a potentially life-shortening effect;

[c] terminal/palliative sedation (PS)—i.e. the induction of a reduced level of consciousness or coma to relieve intolerable suffering in the imminently dying/in the last days of life;

[d] overtreatment and undertreatment (incorrect medical treatment) with a potentially life-shortening effect;

[e] non-voluntary medicalized killing—i.e. of patients who are incompetent/have no free will (from Latin, *'voluntas'*), e.g. severely disabled newborns, those with advanced dementia, or with severe brain damage;

[f] involuntary medicalized killing—i.e. of patients who are competent/do have a free will, but who have not requested euthanasia but are nevertheless given lethal injections.

---

* In the Dutch research, the abbreviation APS stands for 'alleviation of pain and symptoms'. But since pain is itself a symptom, in our categorization here we have added the word 'other'. This is a linguistic difference only, not one of meaning.

Table 5.5.2 Deaths caused by injection or digestion of lethal drugs, the Netherlands.

Euthanasia

1990: 2300 cases = 1.7 per cent
1995: 3200 cases = 2.4 per cent
2001: 3500 cases = 2.6 per cent
2005: 2325 cases = 1.7 per cent

Physician-assisted suicide

1990: 400 cases = 0.2 per cent
1995: 400 cases = 0.2 per cent
2001: 300 cases = 0.2 per cent
2005: 100 cases = 0.1 per cent

Without request*

1990: 1000 cases = 0.8 per cent
1995: 900 cases = 0.7 per cent
2001: 900 cases = 0.7 per cent
2005: 550 cases = 0.4 per cent

* Both non-voluntary and involuntary; [e] and [f] in Table 5.5.1, respectively.

with the earlier finding (3.2 per cent) that dates back to 1998[29]. Still, this rate in Flanders was much higher than in the other European countries included[30].

Some might take this as evidence that legalization of euthanasia and PAS works to the effect that the incidence of unrequested, drug-induced ending of life is greatly reduced. If it does, many would say this is a positive effect of legalization—perhaps even some who oppose legalization in principle. But strictly speaking, we do not know if this is so since all these data precede legalization in both the Netherlands and Belgium as well as the brief legislation in Australia's Northern Territory (Table 5.5.3). Having said that, a gradual legalization started long before the new law of 2002 in the Netherlands if one considers practice and case-by-case verdicts from the first ruling in 1973 and onwards[7,43] (Table 5.5.3). In that country, from 1990 to 1995 the number of unrequested killings dropped by 100 cases; from 1995 to 2001 it remained stable[4]. In 2005, there was a further decrease—although not significant this time either[5] (Table 5.5.2). Thus there seems to be no slippery slope from voluntary to non-voluntary and involuntary forms of killing by utilizing lethal drugs in the Netherlands—something many have feared would happen.

There is however disagreement as to what exactly the idea of a 'slippery slope' may be taken to mean. Several interpretations are possible[46]. It is therefore incorrect to speak of '*the* slippery slope', as is often done, since there is no such single phenomenon. Despite this, there have been strong claims, coming from both sides in the debate, concerning the slippery-slope issue[47–49].

In the Netherlands figures for PAS have fallen. Starting out at 400 cases in 1990, this number was the same in 1995. 2001 saw a slight reduction, whereas 2005 marks an all time low with a significant drop to 100 cases[4,5] (Table 5.5.2).

For euthanasia the picture is different: there was a significant jump upwards from 1.7 per cent in 1990 to 2.4 per cent in 1995, with a further increase to 2.6 per cent in 2001. While percentages here may seem relatively small, in actual numbers this represents an additional 1200 cases in 2001 as compared to 1990[4]. 1200 cases divided by

2300 cases in 1990 yields a very high increase of 52 per cent. The increase from 1990 to 1995 was remarkable too: up 39 per cent (900 cases). But in 2005 a distinct reversal took place and the Dutch were 'back where they started' in 1990; 1.7 per cent (Table 5.5.2)[5].

So up to now, there seems to be no 'slippery slope' in the Netherlands with regard to the volume of euthanasia either. But it must be emphasized that data from the Netherlands are from a 15-year period only and that predicting what will happen next is not easy. Apart from that, euthanasia figures in Belgium and Australia from the time before legalization in those countries are quite high. Percentages are: Flanders 1.1; Australia 1.7[29]. So the impact of a legal ban when it comes to keeping euthanasia figures low may be questioned. Indeed, in the Netherlands, the incidence of euthanasia fell markedly after the new law of April 2002[5]. Some might want to say, then, that legalization is the way ahead if one sees euthanasia as problematic. But that too would be to jump to conclusions; anyone making claims about possible, causal effects in this area is on thin ice from an empirical point of view.

Additionally, several other factors presumably play a role. There exist significant regional, national, and cultural differences in the approach to, and organization of, palliative care even within Europe. These differences are also reflected in professional practice[50]. There is reason to think that such differences also influence the frequency of all four types of drug-induced ending of life. Seale found that the proportion of these was extremely low in the UK, suggesting the impact of a palliative care approach that developed early there[37]. All of this calls for great caution when one tries to make sense of the data across countries.

In the Netherlands, the clinical criteria for euthanasia/PAS have essentially remained the same since they were given their first formulation in connection with the Postma case in 1973. Most notably, perhaps, the court back then rejected 'terminal illness' as a criterion—a condition suggested by the Medical Inspector[7] (Table 5.5.3). An important step on the way was the clarification of the criteria provided in the first official statement by the Royal Dutch Medical Association (KNMG) in 1984[7]. The most significant event in 1984 is however the Dutch Supreme Court's ruling in the Schoonheim case, through which it established the necessity defence (*force majeure*) as a ground of acquittal for physicians who perform euthanasia, due to a possible conflict of duties between preserving life and relieving intolerable suffering (Table 5.5.3). While basically still the same in 1994, the *legal interpretation* of these criteria appears to have become more liberal that year; psychiatric suffering was then accepted by the Supreme Court, in the Chabot case, as a possible justification for PAS. Even though the KNMG opened up for this in its 1984 statement, and, more importantly, the criteria in their various formulations never excluded psychiatric suffering—by the mere fact that there has never been any mention of type of suffering, nor of time left to live—the verdict in Chabot is nonetheless a watershed decision[7] (Table 5.5.3).

Whether or not this is a sign of a different type of 'slippery slope in action' is debatable[51]. Should however 'tiredness of life' or 'suffering through living'[3,9] (Table 5.5.3) also, eventually, be condoned by the courts one is perhaps justified in saying there is a *legal* slippery slope from somatic to psychiatric to existential suffering. Indeed, the KNMG itself notes that if such a development takes place, that 'would be seen internationally only to manifest proof of a slippery slope'[52].

What might explain a possible development like this? Within theory of science, a common view is that an explanation of a phenomenon is also a prediction of it—that there is symmetry between the two. This is so because an explanation can be seen as a 'backwards prediction'. The 'sliding down' towards existential suffering may be put in the form of a prediction in the following way—thereby being an explanation as well. If you open up the gates of euthanasia and PAS through legalization in a highly individualistic culture, the two main driving forces will be respect for self-determination and individual suffering. That means giving *subjectivism* the upper hand: because people's values may differ radically as to what counts as a life worth living, and since all suffering is in a fundamental way something very personal, attempts at gate keeping by setting limits to who should have access to euthanasia and PAS—types of suffering, terminal illness as criterion, etc.—will both be discriminatory and will fail.

As far as Oregon, USA is concerned, however, that very prediction of such a failure seems itself to have failed. Under its Death with Dignity Act[10] not much has changed since the law entered into force in November 1997. US researcher Barry Rosenfeld sums up: 'data from Oregon have not supported the "slippery slope" hypothesis; rates of assisted suicide have thus far been relatively stable and reassuringly low over the first 5 years of legalization. Furthermore, there has been no discussion in the USA of extending assisted suicide provisions to apply to individuals who are not terminally ill'[53]. This picture is valid as regards the next six years as well. Forty-six, 49 and 54 Oregonians died under the act in 2006, 2007 and 2008, respectively[54,55,56].

Yet there are some crucial differences between Oregon and the Netherlands that should be taken into account when speaking of a failed or false 'prediction' in this context. These include the Oregon law's requirement that the patient has (in the physician's judgement) less than 6 months left to live[10]. We have seen that in the Netherlands there has never been such a legal requirement. Terminal illness was rejected as a criterion as early as 1973; nor is there any reference to type of suffering in the 2002 law and so psychiatric suffering falls under it too[17] (Table 5.5.3). Furthermore, during the last few years, the Oregonians had reason to fear that the law would be repealed due to action taken by the US minister of justice. As a consequence, proponents of the law might have tried to walk the line as far as they could, not provoking federal authorities by trying to widen the clinical criteria or make a move from PAS to euthanasia. If the Oregon law gets firmly secured, perhaps we will then see some sort of 'sliding' in those directions.

The situation is different in Switzerland where, according to the Swiss Penal Code dating back to the first half of the last century, assisted suicide (but not euthanasia) is legal for anybody who acts without any selfish motives[57]. Against this open legal background, in the late 1980s volunteers of the Swiss right-to-die society Exit started to provide personal assistance in suicide to members suffering from a disease with 'poor prognosis, unbearable suffering, or unreasonable disability'[13]. Since then there has been a steady increase in the number of 'Exit deaths', reaching approximately one hundred cases each year in the late 1990s[58]. At present, every year Exit Deutsche Schweiz, headquartered in Zurich, accounts for about 150 assisted deaths among residents of the German-speaking part of Switzerland, and its counterpart Exit ADMD, headquartered in Geneva, is responsible for some 50 assisted deaths among residents of the French-speaking part of the country[59]. In addition, and even more controversially, since the late 1990s one has seen a rapid increase in deaths assisted by the right-to-die society Dignitas involving mainly individuals travelling to Switzerland from other countries such as Germany and the UK (so-called 'suicide tourism')[59].

Some might see the development of suicide tourism to Switzerland *per se* as another proof of a sort of slippery slope. Suicide tourism is, however, too recent a phenomenon to draw any long term conclusions from the Dignitas practice. What we know is that among the Exit assisted suicides, from the 1990s to the early 2000s the proportion of women, and the proportion of elderly people suffering from non-fatal diseases, has increased significantly[60].

The proposed, modified UK bill of 2005 is, in important respects, similar to the Oregon model[10] (Table 5.5.3). Two examples of this are that the bill is confined to PAS and requires that the patient be terminally ill[61]. It remains to be seen whether UK developments, should the bill become law, will follow those of what has been called 'the Oregon experiment'[53].

International developments 1973–2009

Most of the developments in the last three decades regarding euthanasia and PAS have taken place in the Netherlands. But there have been important incidents in other places too—and in fact the world's first law that legalized both euthanasia and PAS saw the light of day in Australia's Northern Territory[62]. Some key events during the span from 1973 through the first half of 2009 are shown in Table 5.5.3.

Table 5.5.3 Euthanasia, PAS, and assisted suicide: legislation and other key events around the world.

1973:

The *Postma* case in the Netherlands. A physician injected (in 1971) her mother with a lethal dose of medications at her request, i.e. euthanasia. Receives mild sentence by the court, which rejects 'terminal illness' as a criterion for euthanasia.

Founding of the influential Dutch right-to-die organization NVVE (www.nvve.nl).

1984:

First official statement of The Royal Dutch Medical Association (KNMG; http://knmg.artsennet.nl). Says euthanasia and PAS may be legitimate provided certain 'requirements of carefulness' are met. Also characterizes the view that the patient must be in the 'terminal phase' as medically meaningless; thereby, the chronically ill and the mentally ill are patient groups that should be sub-summed under the requirements.

The *Schoonheim* case: Dutch Supreme Court establishes the necessity defence (*force majeure*) as a ground of acquittal for physicians who perform euthanasia, due to a possible conflict of duties between preserving life and relieving intolerable suffering.

1994:

The *Chabot* case in the Netherlands. Supreme Court accepts PAS for mental/psychiatric suffering. (The case: a woman who was divorced, both her sons dead. Apparently suicidal, refused treatment.)

Table 5.5.3 (Continued) Euthanasia, PAS, and assisted suicide: Legislation and other key events around the world.

1996:

'Rights of the Terminally Ill Amendment Act 1996' becomes effective in Australia's Northern Territory; the world's first law to allow both euthanasia and PAS.

1997:

'The Oregon Death with Dignity Act' enters into force in the USA, in November; allows PAS only, euthanasia is explicitly prohibited. Patient must be terminally ill with a life expectancy of maximum 6 months.
The Australian national parliament repeals the law of 1996.

2000:

The *Brongersma* case in the Netherlands. Physician Philip Sutorius assisted (in 1998) the suicide of an old man who was tired of life—i.e. who had no severe, somatic or psychiatric illness. Sutorius is acquitted by a lower court.

2001:

Swiss parliament confirms current legal situation, which allows for assisted suicide but bans euthanasia, and rejects initiative to restrict the activities of right-to-die societies.

2002, 1 April:

Euthanasia and PAS formally legalized by statute in the Netherlands: 'Termination of Life on Request and Assisted Suicide (Review Procedures) Act 2002' (the law was enacted in 2001). Changes little, but two new elements nevertheless stand out: euthanasia according to living will/advance directive, and euthanasia and PAS for minors at the age of 12. No requirement that the patient be terminally ill, nor that he or she must suffer from a somatic illness. But the suffering must be 'unbearable', with 'no prospect of improvement'.

2002, 28 May:

Euthanasia law enacted in Belgium; enters into force 23 September the same year. No requirement that the patient be terminally ill, nor that he or she must suffer from a somatic illness. Very similar to the Dutch law, however contains many more detailed provisions. Additionally, PAS is not explicitly covered in the law.

2002, 24 December:

Sutorius (cf. the *Brongersma* case above) is given sentence by the Dutch Supreme Court. The verdict states that being tired of life/'suffering through living' is not a medical illness; hence, the criteria of the new law of April 2002 do not apply.

2004, 8 January:

Bill proposing the legalization of euthanasia and PAS for the terminally ill presented in the UK's House of Lords.

2004, 25 November:

Swiss Academy of Medical Sciences (SAMW/ASSM) revises its guidelines on the care of patients at the end of life. Avoids taking a stand on assisted dying in general, yet it rejects PAS as a part of a doctor's activity, but says doctors may face a dilemma against which they must make a conscientious decision whether to participate or not; whichever decision is arrived at, it must be respected. At the same time, the Academy is firmly opposed to euthanasia.

2004, December:

A KNMG committee's report criticises the Dutch Supreme Court's decision of 2002 in the case against Sutorius. Says the 2002 law may be interpreted as covering cases involving individuals who are tired of life/'suffer through living' in the absence of severe, somatic or psychiatric illness. The KNMG itself abstains from taking a stand on the issue, restricting itself to noting that the report represents a good point of departure for further debate.

2005, June:

The British Medical Association (BMA) gives up its longstanding opposition to euthanasia and PAS and adopts neutral position.

2005, 11 October:

KNMG says it wants further case descriptions regarding being tired of life/'suffering through living', but still avoids endorsing or opposing the conclusions of its own committee on the subject.

2006, 12 May:

The UK House of Lords rejects, by 148 votes to 100, a modified Bill on assisted dying for the terminally ill that is restricted to PAS (an 'Oregon model').

2006, June:

BMA backtracks and again opposes legalization.

2008, 4 november:

PAS law enacted in Washington, USA; similar to Oregon's law.

2008, December:

PAS for the terminally ill ruled legal in Montana, USA, however the decision is likely to be appealed.

2009, 1 April:

Euthanasia law enters into force in Luxembourg, which thereby becomes the third country of the Benelux (as Belgium, the Netherlands and Luxemburg together are called) to legalize euthanasia.

These developments have one important feature in common: they all concern the voluntary taking of life by the injection or digestion of various drugs. But this is not the whole story, as it were, since it is also possible to take life without any drugs being used at all. The big picture therefore includes this topic.

Medicalized killing by omission, and on non-treatment decisions (NTDs) (See chapter 5.6)

According to ethical theory, an ethically relevant distinction is a difference between two phenomena that *makes* a difference. Then what about the distinction between omission (passivity) and commission (activity) regularly drawn in end-of-life care? In a now classic article, philosopher James Rachels argued that this distinction *in itself* is insufficient as a means for distinguishing between what is morally acceptable and not—it cannot do that job alone[25]. In Rachels' example, there is no moral difference between (actively) drowning someone and just standing by (passively) watching that someone drown. Why? Because in both scenarios the intention is to kill. Only the method of killing is different and so any moral difference vaporizes, claims Rachels.

If a physician performs euthanasia the intention is to kill the patient[2,3], a clear instance of a commission. Suppose the same physician works in the emergency room and a patient with life-threatening hypertension is admitted and he intentionally does nothing about it when he both should and could have. The patient suffers massive brain haemorrhage and dies. Here the physician intentionally causes death through omission. Both are instances of taking life, although at different levels: using lethal medications vs doing something by doing nothing. Logically, the latter sounds like a contradiction yet practically it makes perfect sense. Rachels constructs a similar clinical case: a doctor who 'deliberately let a patient die who was suffering from a routinely curable illness'[25]. It is designed to demonstrate why we should think of letting die as sometimes even worse than euthanasia—presuming, that is, we reject euthanasia (which Rachels does not). But he misconstrues his own example: it is not a case of 'letting die' but of killing through omission.

A different case would be the physician withholding or withdrawing medically *futile* treatment in a terminally ill patient who therefore does not have 'a routinely curable illness'. Here the intention is not to kill the patient—even though the result may be shortening of life/hastening of death. Rather, the physician's intention is that the patient not suffer unnecessarily through the application of pointless and harmful medical interventions as life comes to a close. There is both a medical and an ethical duty not to harm patients in such a way. Thus the patient is allowed to die from his non-treatable illness; it is a letting die proper, if you will. Here the commission consisting in either starting or not stopping painful, ineffective treatment—i.e. overtreatment (cf. Table 5.5.1, [d])—would have been morally contestable.

Yet the concept of futility is problematic. Usually, by futile treatment is understood treatment that is unlikely or, stronger still, almost certain to be unsuccessful *in the sense* providing benefits that outweigh burdens/harms to the patient[63]. But who is to tell what treatment is worth it or not? Suppose the treatment is judged to be futile by the physician. Should the patient disagree, the physician has the final word as there is no right to futile treatment—although some claim there ought to be. To particular patients, such a decision

by a physician on behalf of them—even when the physician has discussed the matter with them—will smack of paternalism. For there are going to be situations in which a terminally ill patient would like to give futile treatment a try, for example in order to, hopefully, live a little longer so that he or she may experience the birth of a grandchild. To this patient, even highly likely burdens/harms will be outweighed by the potential extra time. In such circumstances, e.g. resuscitation in the case of cardiac arrest may be justified no matter how small the chances of its success[63]. This serves to highlight that the issue may be just as much a judgement about values as one about the 'neutral' medical judgement of the expert.

Not initiating or discontinuing futile treatment are both NTDs (Table 5.5.1, [a]). The area of NTDs is however wider than that of futile treatment. Take the example of a patient with advanced dementia who develops pneumonia. Should he be given antibiotics? Difficult question, but we cannot answer it simply by saying that giving antibiotics would be futile treatment. This patient's 'inner life' is non-accessible to outsiders. For all we know, going on living could be clearly beneficial to this patient—notwithstanding the fact that to us it looks like misery.

Another example of a difficult NTD issue is whether or not to discontinue life-sustaining treatment in a severely brain damaged adult patient. The physician may think such a life is not worth living, whereas the patient's next-of-kin may think differently and insist that their loved one would have wanted to stay alive despite being gravely handicapped.

It is important to emphasize that when life-sustaining treatment is deemed either too harmful or useless, or both—and hopefully there is agreement about this between patient and physician—providing symptom control and social, psychological and existential support is what palliative care is all about. It has been 'argued that, similar to medical futility, there is also such a thing as palliative futility'[64]—implying 'the right of patients to decide that further conventional palliative care is futile and to request and obtain physician assisted death'[64]. True, and as noted, past a certain stage life-sustaining treatment is judged to be futile in particular patients receiving palliative care. But this does not mean palliative care as such is also seen as futile. Quite the contrary, such treatment is paramount as life draws to a close. Accordingly, palliation is *never* futile and it is never discontinued; it is provided up until the very moment of death. The concept of 'palliative futility' is therefore both a misnomer and fails to mirror clinical reality.

When life-sustaining treatment is no longer given, many *other treatments* are thus still in place. Sometimes there will even be *intensified* treatment. Symptoms could become worse as death approaches and that calls for more comprehensive palliative treatment. An example of this is terminal/palliative sedation in the imminently dying (Table 5.5.1, [c]).

In conclusion, sometimes acting is right, sometimes it is wrong—and the same holds true for not acting. Which illustrates that the moral impact of the distinction can sway either way.

Intending vs wishing for death

Recently, research on end-of-life practices in six European countries has documented that physicians' withholding and withdrawing of treatment in the terminally ill in as many as 45 per cent of cases were done, 'with the explicit intention of hastening the end of the patient's life'[34].

How to interpret this finding? One possible explanation is that in carrying out these NTDs, many physicians are not actually intending the patient's death. Instead, perhaps they just *wish* some patients will die sooner rather than later so that these be spared unnecessary suffering. In such instances, physicians do not want to contribute to drawing out an overly burdensome dying process by prolonging it by medical means.

Within medicine and in medical ethics, it is essential that the concept of 'intention' be distinguished from that of a 'wish'. Intentions reflect inner mental states, including motives that *result in* particular acts of commission or omission. That is why acts are called 'intentional' in the first place. Not so with wishes, and therefore an intention should not be likened to a wish, from which there follows no acting (be it active or passive). To illustrate: if a person is in need of a heart transplant, he would wish that an appropriate donor will die shortly. Nonetheless, in no way has he thereby intended—so as to produce—that other person's death.

Symptom control and hastening of death/ shortening of life, and the 'doctrine of double effect' (DDE)

When physicians aim at APS with medicines that can have a life-shortening effect (Table 5.5.1, [b]), they are not intentionally hastening the death of patients. On the contrary, the goal is optimal symptom control. If life is nonetheless occasionally shortened/death is hastened by such action, this is normally seen as justified by the 'doctrine (or principle) of double effect' (DDE). Medical ethicist and physician Raanan Gillon presents the doctrine as shown in Table 5.5.4[65].

Table 5.5.4 The doctrine of double effect (DDE).

In the context of actions that have both good and bad effects, doing an action that has a bad effect is permissible if
(a) the action is good in itself;
(b) the intention is solely to produce the good effect;
(c) the good effect is not achieved through the bad effect; and
(d) there is sufficient reason to permit the bad effect.

Gillon notes that of these clauses, only (d) is fairly uncontroversial[65]. Furthermore, there is debate about the interpretation of all of them. Nonetheless, the DDE is widely used and accepted in medicine and in medical ethics and we cannot here discuss it further. Suffice it to say that in the context of end-of-life care, its application would mean that shortening of life, if predictable or foreseeable, is not intended but has merely to be accepted as an unavoidable side-effect of symptomatic treatment.

But even presuming the DDE is rejected the question remains: does aggressive alleviation of symptoms really shorten life? It is widely believed that it often does[66]. But in order to be able to know whether this is true or false, one would need to perform a randomized controlled trial in which one group of patients did not receive aggressive treatment while another did. Only thus could one tell for sure if the treatment shortens life[67]. But it goes

without saying that, when such treatment is available and is clinically indicated, not providing it in patients who do need it may not be justified neither medically nor ethically. Not only would such acting amount to serious undertreatment; (Table 5.5.1, [d]); it would be the intentional infliction of harm upon patients as well. Therefore, this trial cannot be carried out[67]. That kind of research has been called 'ethically impossible'[68]. It follows that it seems difficult, if possible at all, to be in a position to know the truth of the matter.

Furthermore, it is possible that *not* intervening through the application of comprehensive and competent symptom treatment when one should have may shorten life. Robert Twycross points out that, 'The correct use of morphine is more likely to prolong a patient's life … because he is more rested and pain-free'[69]. Also, Vander Stichele and colleagues note: 'High doses of opioids may not be and often are not lethal for patients who have developed tolerance. Escalating doses of opioids may in fact lengthen rather than shorten the terminal phase of dying'[6].

We stress that this does not exclude that opioids can also be used to intentionally shorten or end a patient's life. But then dosages have to be used that are clearly higher than those used for symptom treatment.

Additionally, improper (incorrect) medical treatment in the form of overtreatment with drugs may have life-shortening as an unintended side effect (Table 5.5.1, [d]). But, it has been pointed out, for example when opioids are used appropriately for pain relief, the risk of respiratory depression (that could cause death) is more myth than fact[70].

If high dosages work to the effect that the life span of a terminally ill patient is extended, the DDE does not apply i.e., it is not the case that 'the price to be paid for symptom control is premature death'. Instead, there is an entirely different sort of, and welcome, 'double effect': one *both* achieves effective relief *and* prolongs life.

Recent clinical investigations and reviews by Sykes and Thorns disclose that as far as the use of both opioids and sedatives at the end of life is concerned, it has been impossible to document that they have a life-shortening effect when their doses are titrated against the symptom response[68,71,72]. Accordingly, they attack the use of the DDE in this context, since it may act 'as a tacit admission that good symptom control is lethal'[72]. Others have argued along similar lines[73]. In conclusion, Sykes and Thorns write that 'although the doctrine is a valid ethical device, it is, for the most part, irrelevant to symptom control at the end of life. To exaggerate its involvement perpetuates a myth that satisfactory symptom control at the end of life is inevitably associated with hastening death. The result can be a reluctance to use medication to secure comfort and a failure to provide adequate relief to a very vulnerable group of patients'[68]. It might be added that because of this, perhaps it is, to put it paradoxically, ethically dubious to introduce this ethical doctrine in the context of opioid and sedative treatment at the end of life.

Death-certificate studies, i.e. studies based on large samples of death certificates in which doctors responsible at the end of life of the deceased are investigated using anonymous questionnaires, are accepted as the most exact way of assessing the incidence of different medical end-of-life decisions. From affirmative answers to the question, 'Did you use drugs to intensify the alleviation of pain and/or symptoms taking into account, but not explicitly intending, that this would hasten the patient's end of life?', these studies recently revealed an incidence of 'alleviation of pain and symptoms' with a possible or certain life-shortening effect (APS; Table 5.5.1,[b]) in about 20 per cent of all deaths not only in the Netherlands, but also in a number of other European countries; EURELD Study (medical end-of-life decisions in six European countries)[30].

These figures are surprisingly high given the fact that correct use of opioids at the end of life is not associated with any life-shortening effect. However, the meaning of these figures becomes more clear when we look at the results of an in-depth analysis of these cases described as APS in the EURELD Study: It turned out that doctors when asked about the impact of life-shortening due to APS in more than half of the cases answered that 'probably life was not shortened at all'[74]. And even when doctors did assign a life-shortening effect, the shortened life-span was estimated to be minimal, i.e. some hours or some days at most[30]. Another analysis of the type and dosage of the medication used in APS confirmed that in many cases any impact on the point in time of dying was highly unlikely[35]. Finally, an analysis of 271 Swiss EURELD cases found hardly any association between what doctors reported to be their intention and the likelihood of a death-hastening effect of administering morphine at the end of life[75]. These inconsistencies are impressive. They indicate substantial confusion amongst doctors about the effects of the opioids they use, and highlight the need for better education in palliative care.

That notwithstanding, it has been suggested that the 2005 Dutch data (Table 5.5.2) may also be read as an indication that more doctors than before now realize that the life-shortening effects of opioids are often overestimated, and that this might have contributed to the decrease in the frequency of euthanasia as assessed in this specific study design[5].

Terminal/palliative sedation (PS)

When it comes to terminal/palliative sedation (PS) in the imminently dying, the idea that this treatment strategy of last resort inevitably, or frequently, hastens death is widespread too. It has been claimed that even the very term 'terminal sedation', which was first coined by Enck in 1991[76], hints to the idea that patients' lives are shortened by the treatment[68]. The term also makes it look as if the aim of the sedation is to (intentionally) produce death[77]. Therefore, PS seems better, a term that was first introduced in a scientific paper by Materstvedt & Kaasa in 2000[78]. A year later, it was also called 'palliative sedation therapy'[79]. Since then, others have followed and defended the usage of palliative sedation (therapy) as the most appropriate term[80,81].

In the Netherlands, there is agreement among departments of health and justice and the medical association KNMG that PS is a treatment strategy. Dutch physicians have welcomed the authorities' distinction drawn between it and euthanasia, identifying the former as 'normal medical treatment' and therefore different from euthanasia[82]. This view is consistent with our categorization of PS; Table 5.5.1, [c]. Illuminating research comparing the practices of euthanasia and PS has been performed in the Netherlands[83].

This does not preclude that the treatment can be misused *as a form of* euthanasia. If a physician at the patient's voluntary and competent request deliberately increases dosages of sedatives or opioids without the existence of clear target symptoms, PS is slow euthanasia[84].

If there is no request, such overdosing would either be non-voluntary or involuntary (Table 5.5.1, [e] and [f]). A recent Dutch study showed that in 17 per cent of the cases of terminal sedation, hastening of death was the doctor's explicit intention[85].

According to the EURELD Study, between 2.5 per cent (Denmark) and 8.5 per cent (Italy) of all deaths are preceded by continuous deep sedation until death[86]. In from one-third (Italy) up to two-thirds (Denmark and the Netherlands) of these cases artificial hydration and nutrition had also been forgone.

When artificial hydration and/or nutrition is contraindicated, such forgoing is clinically sound. But what if it is, in the doctors' judgement and for some reason or other, *not* contraindicated in a particular patient, yet this patient who suffers terribly due to all other conventional treatment measures having failed, nevertheless requests that hydration and/or nutrition be withheld after he has received PS? If that request is met, he is going to die rather soon after the sedation has been induced—in particular this is true if hydration is suspended. Doctors are thereby faced with the combination of two end-of-life decisions: PS plus an NTD.

Would this be a case of slow euthanasia? We think not. This patient, being in a desperate situation, asks that he be given special treatment—not that he be killed. Next, he rejects treatment at the end of life which, to his mind, is futile (and thus unreasonable) since it would only prolong the dying process. True, the consequence may not here be all that different between euthanasia and PS since in both instances death follows in the near future. But the intention is different: ending of life vs providing treatment.

Having said that, some see 'intention' as a rather weak parameter in medical ethics, and even more so in the medical-legal field. The question will then be whether or not intention is too weak an auxiliary construction in the particular context of PS.

A systematic review of the literature performed by an international panel of 29 palliative care experts concludes that retrospective studies strongly suggest that appropriately used in the very last days of life, PS does not shorten life[81]. But PS is a relevant ethical issue even if there is no life-shortening effect, as it entails a reduction or an abruption of the patient's consciously lived life-span. It may be helpful here, following de Graeff and Dean, to distinguish between various levels of PS at the end of life[81] (see Table 5.5.5).

Table 5.5.5 Three levels of palliative sedation (PS).

- ◆ **Mild** (somnolence): the patient is awake, but the level of consciousness is lowered.

- ◆ **Intermediate** (stupor): the patient is asleep but can be woken to communicate briefly.

- ◆ **Deep** (coma): the patient is unconscious and unresponsive.

The third category is the most challenging. Sometimes there are good clinical reasons to refrain from trying to wake up a patient thus sedated[81]. In those instances, this form of PS will be both deep *and* continuous—what we, in a paper in *Lancet Oncology*, call DCPS for short[87]. Now at least from a patient's perspective it might make little difference whether one is dead, or continuously unconscious from a given point in time[88]. To take out consciousness 'for good' is a radical curtailment of personal freedom[77]. The patient is no longer able to make autonomous choices or experience the world around him, nor is there any contact with his next-of-kin. May one not say, then, that the treatment has somehow 'killed' the person he is and turned him into 'a living dead'? The answer to that question would depend on what concept of a person one subscribes to[87]. Irrespective of that philosophical topic, in DCPS the patient's life is purely biological, hence he is alive but without *a* life in the social sense of that word. Within palliative medicine, quality of life is a key value as well as paramount in all treatment measures. But in what sense could DCPS in the dying be said to promote their quality of life when they no longer have a social life?[77]. This state has also been described as 'social death'[81].

Having said that, patients who are in need of DCPS find themselves in a terrible situation. So not offering them this treatment option, when it is available and can be competently implemented, seems indefensible both clinically and ethically[77]. It therefore appears to be the lesser of two evils, intolerable suffering being the worst.

Lastly, let us, for the sake of argument, take it for granted that DCPS can shorten life—and perhaps this could somehow be demonstrated, either in individual cases or statistically. Some would say that is not such a bad thing after all. For what would be the point in keeping a constantly unconscious patient alive longer rather than shorter? On the contrary, an argument goes, such a patient's premature death should be welcomed.

The problem with this reasoning is however that the following question will stand in need of an answer: if it is considered important to get it over with as quickly as possible, then why not perform euthanasia or PAS—where legal—instead of DCPS? That solution would save a lot of health-care workers' time and energy, as well as resources, and spare family members the waiting period[87].

Physicians' attitudes, practices, and experiences regarding euthanasia/PAS

There is much information on how physicians think about euthanasia and PAS, as well as on how often they have performed these acts—both in jurisdictions where one of them or both are legal or condoned by law and in countries where both are illegal.

But there are significant issues with the evidence base. The main problem being that there is no internationally accepted gold standard for research in this area, making comparison of factual findings problematic[67]. For the same reason, even domestic comparison of data proves difficult, for example across the many studies that have been performed in the USA[23].

Thus there exist many studies that have very different designs. The methodology varies much; some ask about the legal acceptance of euthanasia, others ask about the ethics of euthanasia; medical settings and descriptions vary a lot—with regard to type of suffering, for example; there is variation in response options—yes/no only in some[67]; some are death certificate studies whereas others are structured questionnaires while still others used telephone interviews; there is a lack of consistency among questions asked[23]; and particular questions are biased[67]. Concept usage varies greatly and several studies are plagued by inappropriate and too vague definitions of crucial concepts[67]. The impact of such inappropriateness is demonstrated when, as noted, US physicians frequently confound euthanasia and terminating life-sustaining treatment[23,24].

And some do not employ the concepts euthanasia and PAS. For example, one study on attitudes, and another on both attitudes

and practices, of US oncologists replaced these concepts by descriptive phrases[89,90]. An earlier study of US oncologists that did the same revealed a significant percentage of misclassification among respondents[24]. In some studies, physicians even mistake euthanasia for PAS[23].

Another problem is that many questionnaires do not distinguish between voluntary, non-voluntary and involuntary drug-induced ending of life (cf. Table 5.5.2). Thereby it is regularly unclear both what the euthanasia figures really are, and towards exactly what physicians express their attitudes[67]. Small wonder, then, that a discussion of 30 surveys, out of which physicians were respondents in 27, found extreme differences in attitudes towards euthanasia[91]. Between 21 per cent and 78 per cent answered that ('active') euthanasia should be legalized; between 14 per cent and 51 per cent rejected this idea.

Emanuel's review of the empirical data from the USA concludes that, 'many studies indicate that a small, but definite, proportion of US physicians have performed euthanasia or PAS, despite its being illegal. Again, the data provide conflicting evidence on the precise frequency of such interventions, with reported frequencies varying more than 6-fold even among the best studies'[23]. Still, certain messages come across from the data, e.g. the fact that US physicians are significantly more opposed to euthanasia than they are to PAS[23]. It may be, writes Emanuel, that conducting a death certificate follow-back study modelled on the Dutch studies will be the best way to obtain accurate data on the frequency of euthanasia and PAS, as well as, among other things, the reasons for these interventions in the USA[23].

We have seen that in the Netherlands, in practice Dutch physicians perform euthanasia much more frequently than PAS[4,5] (Table 5.5.2). But we also noted that in theory, many of them prefer the latter for moral reasons[16]. Indeed, this is the position of the KNMG. After the new Dutch law[17] entered into force in April 2002 (Table 5.5.3), this medical association published a position paper saying that when there is a choice, PAS, not euthanasia, should be selected as it maintains the patient's proper role and responsibility[19].

As regards how Dutch physicians experience carrying out euthanasia, illuminating qualitative research was released in 2007[92]. Twenty-two primary care physicians participated. A selection of their utterances: 'If the patient [who requests euthanasia] dies of natural causes I feel very relieved.'; 'I still always have a sense of guilt. I feel as if I'm an executioner. Who am I to have the right to do this?'; 'We were crazy to do it, looking back. ... Euthanasia was put on my plate. It's a rotten job.' By contrast, another said: 'I need to care deeply for someone to be able to perform euthanasia.' And: 'I was flattered with the trust.' Others want to be able to offer both optimal palliative care and euthanasia. But one said: 'I now say clearly to everyone: I don't perform euthanasia any more. To my surprise a number of people say: "Doctor, you are so right, I understand completely." Then I thought to myself: how deep do these requests really go? I found that disconcerting to notice.'

Patients' attitudes towards, and requests for, euthanasia/PAS

We know little about euthanasia from the standpoint of patients. Hudson and colleagues reviewed papers dealing with what has been called 'desire for hastened death' in patients with advanced disease[93].

Thirty-five research studies met their inclusion criteria. The majority of research has taken place in the USA and Canada—25 studies. There is great variation in the methodology used. Most studies are surveys that utilize self report questionnaires. Qualitative studies constitute a minority. Both questionnaires and in-depth, semistructured interviews are hugely different in their design and ask different questions. Furthermore, of the 35 studies, 13 deal with patients' opinions as to why they may have a desire for hastened death in the future, 8 explore patients who had made a so-called 'desire to die statement' (DTDS), 2 reflect the views of family members, and 12 were about health professionals' opinions of patients' reason for putting forward a DTDS. It is no straightforward task, therefore, to compare findings and make sense of the data. What is fairly clear, though, is that reasons for making a DTDS are multiple and complex[93].

Despite all qualifications that must thus be made with regard to drawing general conclusions, some preliminary observations nevertheless seem to stand out. First, pain appears to be much less relevant than other factors[53]. Emanuel argues that accumulating data support what he calls the 'depression thesis'. Psychological distress, including depression and hopelessness, are significantly associated with patients' interest in euthanasia and/or PAS[94]. Wilson and colleagues performed in-depth, semi-structured interviews with 70 patients receiving palliative care for advanced cancer[95]. Eight said they would have requested euthanasia or PAS at the time of the interview if legal. These eight differed from all others on ratings of loss of interest or pleasure in activities, hopelessness, and the desire to die. They also had a higher prevalence of depressive disorders. However, they did not differ on ratings of pain severity.

Haverkate and colleagues remarked in 2000 that although studies in the USA have shown that patients with depression are more inclined than patients without depression to request PAS, whether this is the case in the Netherlands is not known[96]. In 2005, a Dutch patient-centred study was published that examines the relationship between depressed mood and incidence of euthanasia requests in cancer patients with a life expectancy of less than 3 months. The researchers' initial hypothesis was that depressed mood would show an *inverse* association with requests for euthanasia—the reason being that their clinical impression was that such requests were well-considered decisions, thoroughly discussed with health-care workers and family[97]. To their surprise, this hypothesis was falsified: the likelihood of requesting euthanasia for patients with depressed mood was 4.1 times higher than that of patients without depressed mood at inclusion.

Like the research directed at physicians, patient-centred research in this area is plagued by a terminology that is in need of clarification[93]. Also, the relationship between phenomena such as 'attitude', 'wish' and 'request' is poorly understood and very few studies address this crucial issue. Nor are these concepts satisfactorily defined in many studies[98].

One study that used semi-structured interviews explored the views of 18 cancer patients with a life expectancy of less than 9 months, all being inpatients at a palliative medicine unit in a jurisdiction where euthanasia/PAS is illegal (Norway)[98]. It was found that patients who have a positive attitude towards euthanasia/PAS—i.e. the majority—do not necessarily want these interventions for themselves. This should however come as no surprise, since there is a fundamental divide between the nature of attitudes and wishes: the hallmark of the former is that they are general whereas the latter are particular, or personal. Others have also

found that the majority of patients in a palliative care setting favours the legalization of euthanasia[95]. It would seem that these patients have a liberal bent of mind, simply: they think patients should have the legal option of euthanasia/PAS.

Furthermore, wishes were different from requests for euthanasia/PAS as well as being hypothetical and future oriented, and wishes were fluctuating and ambivalent. One patient even changed his mind during the interview, which took less than an hour. A hypothesis of this study is that desire for hastened death may serve as a coping strategy for some patients seeking some sense of control[98].

As regards clinical implications, the authors write that the obvious and most dangerous scenario is a physician responding to patients' wishes for euthanasia/PAS as if they were actual requests. But a wish for euthanasia/PAS may be something completely different from a request for it[98]. On the other hand, responding to such wishes as merely expressions of depression might lead to inadequate interventions—e.g. with antidepressants—and possibly further reinforce the patients' feelings of hopelessness. The patient may also see such a response by a physician as a violation of his autonomy. Because of the irrevocable nature of euthanasia/PAS, it is furthermore pivotal that health-care workers be aware of the apparent ambivalent nature of wishes for euthanasia/PAS[98].

Many Dutch physicians are aware of, or suspect, the possible impact of psychological factors in euthanasia requests. They turn down one out of three requests, and in 31 per cent of rejections state that the patient was depressed or had psychiatric symptoms[96].

In one study, 86 per cent of Dutch patients who died through euthanasia or PAS suffered from cancer[96]. Cardiovascular disease represents 2 per cent; disease of the nervous system 5 per cent; disease of the respiratory system 2 per cent; psychiatric disorders 0 per cent; and, other 7 per cent. Granted requests include the following reasons: 'avoiding loss of dignity' 56 per cent; 'unbearable or hopeless suffering' 74 per cent; 'weariness of life' 18 per cent; and, 'not wanting to become a burden on the family' 13 per cent.

An important limitation to this research is however that it only includes physicians' recollection of their patients' reasons for requesting euthanasia or PAS, and so the voices of the patients themselves are not heard. The same is true of the Dutch large-scale studies of 1990, 1995, 2001, and 2005[4,5] and of studies in other countries that utilized the same methodology[27–37], as well as of recent research on Dutch terminally ill patients who died after euthanasia had been performed[99]. John Griffiths sums up: 'What we know is, in effect, limited to what doctors think they know'[43].

Recently released evidence shows that the patient perspective in this field can be substantially different from that of the doctor. A Swiss study compared patients' reasons for requesting assisted suicide with doctors' reasons for granting their request. Patients and doctors largely agreed on the importance of pain and neurological symptoms, many of which are objectively accessible. By contrast, patients rated more subjective issues such as loss of dignity and being able to control the circumstances of death much higher than did their physicians. For these two categories, the numbers were 38 vs 6 per cent and 39 vs 12 per cent, respectively.[100]

It is claimed that there is no empirical evidence of pressure on vulnerable patients to cause them to ask for euthanasia[101–103]. But only looking at what *numbers* of people in which social category are given euthanasia or PAS is not an appropriate way of trying to find out whether there is pressure on vulnerable groups. It may even be that the smallest group is made up of exactly those patients who felt the heaviest pressure[104,105]. It would be most welcome if researchers would now initiate patient-centred studies concerning this very important topic in places where there are explicit euthanasia and/or PAS laws (Netherlands, Belgium, Luxembourg, Oregon, Washington), and where there is no such laws yet assisted suicide is openly practised due to its being condoned by the penal code (Switzerland). Even more, this kind of research should not be restricted to countries that have such legal regulations, since euthanasia and PAS are practised in countries where they are illegal too. There are examples of such research[106].

Palliative medicine and euthanasia/PAS: mutually exclusive or complementary?

Traditionally, there has been strong opposition against euthanasia within the hospice movement. As early as 1959, Cicely Saunders formulated her view on euthanasia in an article[107]. In a letter of the same year, she wrote: 'my whole point being that firstly euthanasia is wrong, and secondly it should be unnecessary if terminal cancer patients are properly cared for'[108]. She maintained this view throughout her life[22].

Today, the preponderant majority of health professionals within palliative care rejects euthanasia—meaning not all do[109]. Even though most palliative care providers shun euthanasia for ethical and clinical reasons, euthanasia advocates rejecting palliative care is unheard-of. On the contrary, it is not uncommon to hear praise of it coming from that 'camp': 'where high-quality palliative care is available, many terminally ill patients prefer it over PAS and euthanasia'[15].

So may euthanasia/PAS and palliative care be reconciled, or are they like fire and water? In a paper that explores both common values and contradictions of palliative care and euthanasia, Hurst and Mauron note: 'the possibility of a "good death" is an aim shared by both traditions'[110]. Thereby, both would agree that sometimes 'enough is enough'. In a recent article in the *BMJ*, which is partly a response to the EAPC's 2003 position statement[2], the Belgian model of 'integral palliative care' is introduced to an international audience[64]. In this conception, euthanasia is 'another option at the end of a palliative care pathway' if the patient so prefers and may thus be 'part of' palliative care.

Many would say that it may not, stressing that unlike palliative care, euthanasia is not medical *treatment* or *therapy* in any sense of those words—although it is a medical *act* (injection of lethal medicines by a doctor). Thereby, it literally is not, nor can be, a *part of* (palliative) care. But then what about NTDs within palliative care? *Non*-treatment appears to be just that: no treatment at all. At face value an NTD is therefore on a par with euthanasia *in this particular respect*: both represent the end of the road as far as treatment is concerned. But here appearance is deceptive. Within palliative care, as pointed out above, when life-sustaining treatment is withheld or withdrawn, *palliative* treatment does not cease.

The following difference is also of relevance as regards the relationship between palliative care and euthanasia. Palliative care providers deal with people who are seriously ill due to somatic sickness. Most are cancer patients, but some suffer from MS or ALS. Thus the life expectancy of these groups varies from a few days, weeks or months to several years, however all have life-limiting illnesses. Not necessarily so with patients that may be eligible for euthanasia/PAS. Even though the overwhelming majority here too is cancer patients[96], some are patients who would not have died from

natural causes—including patients with permanent injuries from traffic accidents and psychiatric patients. And what about those 'tired of living'?[3,9] There can be little doubt that health professionals within palliative care would reject the view that there can be such a thing as a good death for these individuals, no matter how much they 'suffer from life'. Thus the shared value 'a good death' only goes halfway.

Franz Josef Illhardt thinks that, 'Palliative caregivers must know answers to the question: What makes a terminal and perhaps miserable life important and worth living for the dying person?'[111] This question touches on the very foundation of palliative care. Yet Illhardt's demand seems quite harsh on health-care workers. And even when they are able to come up with some answers, a patient may still feel these are insufficient answers and hence euthanasia may appear as an option. And to some it obviously does.

Can optimal palliative care do away with all interest in, and all requests for, euthanasia/PAS? Would euthanasia, in the words of Cicely Saunders, be 'unnecessary if terminal cancer patients are properly cared for'?[108] The clear majority of Dutch physicians seems to think otherwise; almost two-thirds of them disagreed with the suggestion that adequate treatment of pain and terminal care make euthanasia redundant[112]. At the same time, data from 2001 display that Dutch physicians at least in some cases consider high-quality end-of-life care as an alternative to euthanasia/PAS[4]. Most interestingly, an increase in both palliative/terminal sedation and other means of aggressive symptom control took place alongside the decrease in euthanasia/PAS figures in 2005[5].

Dutch palliative care physician Zbigniew Zylicz reports that at his hospice, nearly all who bring up the issue of euthanasia at admission lose interest in the issue after having been offered good palliative care[113]. Yet about 1–2 patients each year have their mind set on euthanasia and do not stop requesting it no matter what palliative measures are taken. The main source of suffering in these patients is the loss of autonomy which they experience as extraordinarily bad, and so they are nicknamed 'control freaks'. These do not suffer in any traditional medical sense, claims Zylicz, and therefore the hospice team is unable to help.

But some 'ordinary' patients too reject palliative care and go for euthanasia or PAS instead[7]. They do not want to live through a deteriorating physical and psychological process that inevitably leads to death, even though APS may be good indeed. In the Netherlands, the law explicitly acknowledges this opportunity, stating that the attending physician must 'have come to the conclusion, together with the patient, that there is no reasonable alternative in the light of the patient's situation'[17]. So if palliative care is judged to be 'unreasonable' the green light is given for euthanasia or PAS.

This also demonstrates that euthanasia or PAS are not always last resort interventions when, alas, all other treatment attempts have failed—as if one finds oneself in an emergency situation and the injection or digestion of lethal drugs is 'the only way out'. Patients may not be forced to undergo medical treatments at the end of life and so need not give these a try in order to gain access to euthanasia/PAS[7].

It is the view of Hurst and Mauron that as regards the ethics of palliative care and euthanasia, 'the first value held in common is a focus on the importance of reducing human suffering'[110]. While true for the time preceding death, this value too may be said not to apply unrestrictedly and thus this view should be modified. Within palliative care such reduction of suffering goes on beyond the point at which euthanasia advocates would repeatedly draw the line, insisting that continuing to live is not worth it anymore. Additionally, it sounds somewhat counterintuitive that the induction of death 'reduces' suffering. In reality, it *ends* it[87].

Still, this counterargument does not fully hold true for PS when it leaves the patient in a deep and continuous coma (DCPS)[87] (Table 5.5.1, [c]). Here too, like with euthanasia, the suffering is not reduced but disappears altogether since the patient is no longer able to feel a thing. In that respect, this treatment strategy has an unclear border with euthanasia[87].

And so the term 'palliative sedation' appears to be a misnomer with regard to DCPS: To palliate means to relieve, alleviate, or ease. But when the sedation is so deep that it takes out awareness of absolutely all symptoms, palliation of symptoms is not really taking place. It is more of an *eradication* of symptoms (like in euthanasia)—a matter of 'eradicative sedation in the dying', so to speak[87].

The argument from autonomy

Griffiths and colleagues write that, 'the principle of autonomy is one of the most important arguments of those who are in favour of the legalization of euthanasia'[7]. But many have pointed out that this argument appears paradoxical, if not self-contradictory: a person uses his autonomy to eliminate autonomy itself since there can be no more autonomous acting after the performance of euthanasia or PAS. And so it would seem that for logical reasons, autonomy's scope cannot reach as far as to include its own destruction. This is a bone of contention as regards the ethics of euthanasia[110].

This counterargument in its original form is found in the philosopher Immanuel Kant (1724–1804). In one of the most influential works of ethics ever, the *Grounding for the metaphysics of morals*, Kant discusses suicide[114]. He begins by expressing great understanding towards persons contemplating killing themselves, in referring to 'a man reduced to despair [*Hoffnungslosigkeit*]', and who 'feels sick of life'. Nonetheless, Kant goes on, he is 'still so far in possession of his reason [*Vernunft*]' and can therefore 'ask himself whether his action can be consistent with the idea of humanity as an end in itself [*als Zwecks an sich selbst*]'. Now, 'if he destroys himself in order to escape from a difficult situation, then he is making use of his person merely as a means so as to maintain a tolerable condition till the end of his life. Man, however, is not a thing and hence is not something to be used merely as a means: he must in all his actions always be regarded as an end in himself. Therefore, I cannot dispose of man in my own person by mutilating [*verstümmeln*], damaging [*verderben*], or killing him'[114].

Whether or not Kant's position also has critical bite against euthanasia/PAS is a matter of controversy[115]. But presuming it has, would it not also concern patients who refuse life-sustaining treatment (when such is feasible) as they approach death? Even when the treatment is deemed futile, occasionally although rarely, abstention from it will entail premature death. And with other NTDs (Table 5.5.1, [a]), it often will. Has not the patient then contributed to extinguishing his autonomy? Put differently: is there a moral duty to stay alive as long as possible in order that one be able to exercise one's autonomy until the end?

Concluding remarks

We have seen that there is confusion as to the meaning of a key term like euthanasia, as well as regards other terms having to do with various end-of-life decisions. Clarity in this area is badly needed. Fruitful ethical and political debate depends on it; otherwise, people will be talking past each other. And research cannot do without it.

Clinically, such clarity is crucial also. For example, it is imperative that patients, and their next-of-kin alike, not believe that aggressive symptom control is 'a form of euthanasia' and therefore are fearful of it. That might lead to inadequate interventions and thereby unnecessary suffering—something that in itself could lead to a *request* for euthanasia. Physicians should make it transparently clear to patients that this is not euthanasia, and that it does not speed up the dying process. To the extent that physicians believe otherwise themselves, they need to adjust their preconception in the light of new and current scientific knowledge[68–73,81].

As shown, the evidence base on physicians' attitudes and practices is unsatisfactory. So is our knowledge about how patients relate to euthanasia/PAS. Accordingly, it is not clear what clinical conclusions may be drawn; how should health-care professionals respond to expressions of interest in these interventions in patients? Despite this, helpful recommendations in this area have recently seen the light of day[116]. However, precise, prescriptive guidelines still need to be worked out.

The KNMG is the only medical association in the world that supports euthanasia and PAS. The Belgian association has strived to come to terms with the new situation after euthanasia became legal in 2002[19]. In the UK, the British Medical Association (BMA) is now faced with the possibility that there could be a law on PAS for the terminally ill[61]. BMA first changed it longstanding opposition to euthanasia and PAS and took a neutral stance, but later backtracked[117]. Thus there is no unanimity across medical associations as to the proper role of physicians in euthanasia and PAS, let alone whether physicans should be involved at all.

Presuming some kind of involvement is recognized, exactly what ought it to consist in? The 'Swiss solution' is some kind of a middle ground approach; the Swiss Academy of Medical Sciences (SAMW/ASSM), although it rejects assistance in suicide as part of a doctor's activity, nonetheless leaves the decision to participate or not to individual physicians[14,19,118] (Table 5.5.3). In Switzerland, if they do decide to assist patients in taking their own life, physicians' involvement is reduced due to the parallel, and quite comprehensive, involvement of right-to-die societies[57]. Such is the case in Oregon too where the NGO Compassion & Choices contributes much. Yet physicians play a more crucial role there because the Oregon Death with Dignity Act explicitly requires that *only* physicians assist, as well as provide the medication[10,57].

Professor of palliative medicine, and former member of the House of Lords select committee on the UK Bill, Ilora Finlay and colleagues have suggested yet another approach. They remark that, 'a suicide service outside clinical care would not involve clinicians', and 'as prescribing is no longer the sole province of doctors … legislation could encompass a designated group of non-clinically registered individuals, able to prescribe or administer only a single lethal overdose for a patient'[119]. The way many would see it, one advantage of such an institutional arrangement is that the issue of euthanasia/PAS would be removed from the clinical-medical setting altogether. Presumably, those worrying about a possible pressure on patients that they request euthanasia or PAS should then be reassured. No inpatients need feel there is a 'duty to die'[120], but a 'right to die' would prevail on the outside. Perhaps proponents and opponents of legalization would both be happy with this compromise. As would many physicians feeling uneasy about legislative proposals that 'draw' them into a role they are inclined to strongly defy[19].

At the end of the day, each society must choose its own path. Today, no health-care worker within palliative care can avoid the issue of euthanasia/PAS. If the law prohibits one or both, they must relate to that, thinking that either that is fine or work for, or hope for, a change towards legalization. If legal, they must make up their minds about opting out of the practices or not. And some will oppose such legislation actively, whereas others will hope that euthanasia laws are eventually going to be repealed—something that happened in Australia[62] (Table 5.5.3).

The Ethics Task Force on Palliative Care and Euthanasia of the EAPC 'encourages the EAPC and its members to engage in direct and open dialogue with those within medicine and health care who promote euthanasia and physician-assisted suicide', while stressing that, 'understanding and respect for alternative viewpoints is not the same as the ethical acceptance of either euthanasia or of physician-assisted suicide'[2]. However, this statement seems to presuppose that all palliative care providers are opposed to euthanasia, something that is not the case[109]. Furthermore, not even all of the EAPC's collective members actively oppose euthanasia. The Dutch organization Netwerk Palliatieve Zorg voor Terminale Patiënten Nederland (www.nptn.nl) refrains from taking a stand on the issue, and its Swiss counterpart Schweizerische Gesellschaft für Palliative Medizin, Pflege und Begleitung (www.palliative.ch) appears not to reject assisted dying in principle[20]. The Belgian Federatie Palliatieve Zorg Vlaanderen (www.palliatief.be) states that 'palliative care and euthanasia are neither alternatives nor antagonistic'. However, it also holds the unusual (and thus radical) view that 'euthanasia may be part of palliative care'[64] that we discussed above.

It has been pointed out that although the Ethics Task Force's position paper represents 'a step in the direction of shared reflection', it nonetheless 'avoids the suggestion that palliative care providers could come to question their opposition to euthanasia'[110]. True, it does not say so explicitly, but since no one can predict the outcome of a dialogue—certainly not if it is a Socratic one—it is implied that they could.

If the result of an exchange on this extraordinarily complex issue is that some, or many, palliative care providers change their view, this might also be the case with euthanasia advocates; they too could come to reject their former position that euthanasia/PAS can be good medicine.

References

1. Taboada, P. (2003). Concepts and definitions: a source of confusion in the euthanasia debate. *Palliat Med*, **17**, 651–2.
2. Materstvedt, L.J., Clark, D., Ellershaw, J. *et al.* (2003). Euthanasia and physician-assisted suicide: a view from an EAPC Ethics Task Force. *Palliat Med*, **17**, 97–101.
3. Rurup, M.L. (2005). Setting the stage for death: new themes in the euthanasia debate. PhD thesis, VU University Medical Center, Amsterdam.
4. Onwuteaka-Philipsen, B.D., van der Heide, A., Koper, D. *et al.* (2003). Euthanasia and other end-of-life decisions in the Netherlands in 1990, 1995, and 2001. *Lancet*, **362**, 395–9.
5. Van der Heide, A., Onwuteaka-Philipsen, B.D., Rurup, M.L. *et al.* (2007). End-of-life practices in the Netherlands under the Euthanasia Act. *N Engl J Med*, **356**, 1957–65.
6. Vander Stichele, R.H., Bilsen, J.J.R., Bernheim, J.L. *et al.* (2004). Drugs used for euthanasia in Flanders, Belgium. *Pharmacoepidemiology and Drug Saf*, **13**, 89–95.
7. Griffiths, J., Bood, A., and Weyers, H. (1998). *Euthanasia and law in the Netherlands*. Amsterdam University Press, Amsterdam.
8. Hume D. (1958). *A treatise of human nature*. Selby-Bigge LA ed. Oxford University Press, Oxford.
9. Rurup, M.L., Onwuteaka-Philipsen, B.D., Jansen-van der Weide, M.C. *et al.* (2005). When being 'tired of living' plays an important role in a request for euthanasia or physician-assisted suicide: patient characteristics and the physician's decision. *Health Pol*, **74**, 157–66.
10. The Oregon Death with Dignity Act. http://oregon.gov/DHS/ph/pas/ors.shtml
11. Dyer C. (2008). Washington follows Oregon to legalise physician assisted suicide. www.bmj.com/cgi/content/full/337/nov10_1/a2480
12. Watson R. (2009). Luxembourg is to allow euthanasia from 1 April. www.bmj.com/cgi/content/full/338/mar24_1/b1248
13. Bosshard, G., Fischer, S., and Bär, W. (2002). Open regulation and practice in assisted dying. How Switzerland compares with the Netherlands and Oregon. *Swiss Med Wkly*, **132**, 527–34.
14. Bosshard, G. (2008). Switzerland. In Griffiths J, Weyers H, Adams M., eds. *Euthanasia and law in Europe*. Hart Publishing, Oxford.
15. Pogge, T.W. (2003). From New York City. *Palliat Med*, **17**, 119.
16. Onwuteaka-Philipsen, B.D., Muller, M.T., van der Wal, G. *et al.* (1997). Active voluntary euthanasia or physician-assisted suicide? *J Am Geriatr Soc*, **45**, 1208–13.
17. Termination of Life on Request and Assisted Suicide (Review Procedures) Act 2002. www.healthlaw.nl/wtlovhz_eng.pdf
18. Belgium—Euthanasia Act, 28 May 2002 (effective 23 September). www.kuleuven.ac.be/cbmer/viewpic.php?LAN=E&TABLE=DOCS&ID=23
19. Bosshard, G., Broeckaert, B., Clark, D. *et al.* (2008). A role for doctors in assisted dying? An analysis of legal regulations and medical professional positions in six European countries. *J Med Ethics* **34**, 28–32.
20. Materstvedt, L.J. (2003). Palliative care on the 'slippery slope' towards euthanasia? *Palliat Med*, **17**, 387–92.
21. Van der Wal, G. (2003). From the Netherlands. *Palliat Med*, **17**, 110.
22. Saunders, C. (2003). From the UK. *Palliat Med*, **17**, 102–3.
23. Emanuel, E.J. (2002). Euthanasia and physician-assisted suicide: a review of the empirical data from the United States. *Arch Intern Med*, **162**, 142–52.
24. Emanuel, E.J., Daniels, E.R., Fairclough, D.L. *et al.* (1998). The practice of euthanasia and physician-assisted suicide in the United States: adherence to proposed safeguards and effects on physicians. *JAMA*, **280**, 507–13.
25. Rachels, J. (1975). Active and passive euthanasia. *N Engl J Med*, **292**, 78–80.
26. Gerrard, E., and Wilkinson, S. (2005). Passive euthanasia. *J Med Ethics*, **31**, 64–8.
27. Kuhse, H., Singer, P., Baume, P. *et al.* (1997). End-of-life decisions in Australian medical practice. *Med J Aus*, **166**, 191–6.
28. Willems, D.L., Daniels, E.R., van der Wal, G. *et al.* (2000). Attitudes and practices concerning the end of life. A comparison between physicians from the United States and from the Netherlands. *Arch Intern Med*, **160**, 63–8.
29. Deliens, L., Mortier, F., Bilsen, J. *et al.* (2000). End-of-life decisions in medical practice in Flanders, Belgium: a nationwide survey. *Lancet*, **356**, 1806–11.
30. Van der Heide, A., Deliens, L., Faisst, K. *et al.* (2003). End-of-life decision-making in six European countries: descriptive study. *Lancet*, **362**, 345–50.
31. Mitchell, K., and Owens, G. (2004). End of life decision-making by New Zealand general practitioners: a national survey. *N Z Med J*, **117**, U934.
32. Miccinesi, G., Fischer, S., Paci, E. *et al.* (2005). Physicians' attitudes towards end-of-life decisions: a comparison between seven countries. *Soc Sci Med*, **60**, 961–74.

33. Bosshard, G., Nilstun, T., Bilsen, J. *et al.* (2005). Forgoing treatment at the end of life in 6 European countries. *Arch Intern Med*, **165**, 401–7.

34. Bosshard, G., Fischer, S., van der Heide, A. *et al.* (2006). Intentionally hastening death by withholding or withdrawing treatment. *Wien klin Wochensch*, **118**, 322–6.

35. Bilsen, J., Norup, M., Deliens, L. *et al.* (2006). Drugs used to alleviate symptoms with life shortening as a possible side effect: end-of-life care in six European countries. *J Pain Symptom Manage*, **31**, 111–21.

36. Onwuteaka-Philipsen, B.D., Fisher, S., Cartwright, C. *et al.* (2006). End-of-life decision making in Europe and Australia: a physician survey. *Arch Intern Med*, **166**, 921–9.

37. Seale, C. (2006). National survey of end-of-life decisions made by UK medical practitioners. *Palliat Med*, **20**, 3–10.

38. Singer, P. (1994). *Rethinking life and death: the collapse of our traditional ethics.* Oxford University Press, Oxford.

39. Council of Europe. The European Convention on Human Rights. www.hri.org/docs/ECHR50.html

40. Campbell, N. (1999). A problem for the idea of voluntary euthanasia. *J Med Ethics*, **25**, 242–4.

41. Ten Have, H., and Welie, J. (2005). *Death and medical power: an ethical analysis of Dutch euthanasia practice.* Open University Press, Maidenhead.

42. Legemaate, J. (2004). Ending a patient's life without a request: time for a good assessment procedure [in Dutch]. *Ned Tijdschr Geneesk*, **148**, 2371–4.

43. Griffiths, J., Weyers, H., and Adams, M., eds (2008). *Euthanasia and law in Europe.* Hart Publishing, Oxford.

44. Gillon, R. (2003). Ethics needs principles—four can encompass the rest—and respect for autonomy should be 'first among equals'. *J Med Ethics*, **29**, 307–12.

45. Van der Wal, G. (1993). Unrequested termination of life: is it permissible? *Bioethics*, **7**, 330–9.

46. Williams, B. (1995). Which slopes are slippery? In his *Making sense of humanity and other philosophical papers, 1982–1993*, pp. 213–23. Cambridge University Press, Cambridge.

47. Van Delden, J.J.M., Pijnenborg, L., and van der Maas, P.J. (1993). Dances with data. *Bioethics*, **7**, 323–9.

48. Jochemsen, H., and Keown, J. (1999). Voluntary euthanasia under control? Further empirical evidence from The Netherlands. *J Med Ethics*, **25**, 16–21.

49. Van Delden, J.J.M. (1999). Slippery slopes in flat countries—a response. *J Med Ethics*, **25**, 22–4.

50. Ten Have, H., and Janssens, R. (eds.) (2001). *Palliative care in Europe: concepts and policies.* IOS Press, Amsterdam.

51. Ogilvie, A.D., and Potts, S.G. (1994). Assisted suicide for depression: the slippery slope in action? *BMJ*, **309**, 492–3.

52. KNMG (2005). The debate about 'suffering from life' [in Dutch]. http:// knmg.artsennet.nl

53. Rosenfeld, B. (2004). *Assisted suicide and the right to die: the interface of social science, public policy, and medical ethics.* American Psychological Association, Washington, DC.

54. Ninth Annual Report on Oregon's Death with Dignity Act. Summary—Released March 2007. http://oregon.gov/DHS/ph/pas/docs/year9.pdf

55. Tenth Annual Report on Oregon's Death with Dignity Act. Summary—Released March 2008. http://oregon.gov/DHS/ph/pas/docs/year10.pdf

56. Eleventh Annual Report on Oregon's Death with Dignity Act. Summary—Released March 2009. http://oregon.gov/DHS/ph/pas/docs/year11.pdf

57. Ziegler, S.J., and Bosshard, G. (2007). Role of non-governmental organisations in physician assisted suicide. *BMJ*, **334**, 295–8.

58. Bosshard, G., Ulrich, E., and Bär, W. (2003). 748 cases of suicide assisted by a Swiss right-to-die organisation. *Swiss Med Wkly*, **133**, 310–7.

59. Swiss Federal Office of Justice and Police (2006). Assisted dying and palliative medicine—Federal Government due to take action? [in German]. www.dgpalliativmedizin.de/pdf/Schweiz%20EJPD%20 Sterbehilfe%20&%20Palliativmedizin.pdf

60. Fischer, S., Huber, C., Imhof, L. *et al.* (2008). Suicide assisted by two Swiss right-to-die organisations. *J Med Ethics*, **34**, 810–14.

61. Text of the Assisted Dying for the Terminally Ill Bill [HL], as ordered to be printed in the House of Lords on 9th November 2005. www. publications.parliament.uk/pa/ld200506/ldbills/036/2006036.htm

62. Rights of the Terminally Ill Amendment Act 1996. Northern Territory Government, Australia. www.nt.gov.au/lant/parliament/committees/ rotti/rottiamendmentact96.pdf

63. Ackroyd, R. (2005). Medically futile resuscitation: can it ever be justified? *Eur J Palliat Care*, **12**, 207–9.

64. Bernheim, J.L., Deschepper, R., Distelmans, W. *et al.* (2008). Development of palliative care and legalisation of euthanasia: antagonism or synergy? *BMJ*, **336**, 864–7.

65. Gillon, R. (1985). *Philosophical medical ethics.* John Wiley & Sons, Chichester.

66. Forbes, K., and Huxtable, R. (2006). Clarifying the data on double effect. *Palliat Med*, **20**, 395–6.

67. Materstvedt, L.J., and Kaasa, S. (2002). Euthanasia and physician assisted suicide in Scandinavia—with a conceptual suggestion regarding international research in relation to the phenomena. *Palliat Med*, **16**, 17–32.

68. Sykes, N., and Thorns, A. (2003). The use of opioids and sedatives at the end of life. *Lancet Oncol*, **4**, 312–8.

69. Twycross, R.G. (1982). Ethical and clinical aspects of pain treatment in cancer patients. *Acta Anaesthesiologica Scand*, **74**(Suppl), 83–90.

70. Fohr, S.A. (1998). The double effect of pain medication: separating myth from reality. *J Palliat Med*, **1**, 315–28.

71. Thorns, A., and Sykes, N. (2000). Opioid use in last week of life and implications for end-of-life decision-making. *Lancet*, **356**, 398–9.

72. Sykes, N., and Thorns, A. (2003). Sedative use in the last week of life and the implications for end-of-life decision making. *Arch Intern Med*, **163**, 341–4.

73. George, R., and Regnard, C. (2007). Lethal opioids or dangerous prescribers? *Palliat Med*, **21**, 77–80.

74. Van der Maas, P.J., van Delden, J.J., and Pijnenborg, L. (1992). Euthanasia and other medical decisions concerning the end of life. An investigation performed upon request of the commission of Inquiry into the Medical Practice concerning Euthanasia. *Health Pol*, **21**, 1–262.

75. Bosshard, G., Minder, R., de Stoutz. N. *et al.* (2006). Medical use of opioids at the end of life—intention and likelihood of a life-shortening effect. In: Sotony P, ed. *Proceedings of the XX Congress of International Academy of Legal Medicine*, pp. 221–4. Medimond, Bologna

76. Enck, R.E. (1991). Drug-induced terminal sedation for symptom control. *Am J Hosp Palliat Care*, **8**, 3–5.

77. Materstvedt, L.J. (2006). Palliative sedation—problem or obligation? [in Norwegian]. *Tidssk Nor Laegeforen*, **126**, 430.

78. Materstvedt, L.J., and Kaasa, S. (2000). Is terminal sedation active euthanasia? [in Norwegian]. *Tidssk Nor Laegeforen*, **120**, 1763–8.

79. Morita, T., Tsuneto, S., and Shima, Y. (2001). Proposed definitions for terminal sedation. *Lancet*, **358**, 335–6.

80. Broeckaert, B., and Núñez Olarte, J.M. (2002). Sedation in palliative care: facts and concepts. In Ten Have, H., and Clark, D., eds. *The ethics of palliative care: European perspectives*, pp. 166–80. Open University Press, Buckingham.

81. De Graeff, A., and Dean, M. (2007). Palliative sedation therapy in the last weeks of life: a literature review and recommendations for standards. *J Palliat Med*, **10**, 67–85.

82. Sheldon, T. (2003). 'Terminal sedation' different from euthanasia, Dutch ministers agree. *BMJ*, **327**, 465.

83. Rietjens, J.A., van Delden, J.J., van der Heide, A. *et al.* (2006). Terminal sedation and euthanasia: a comparison of clinical practices. *Arch Intern Med*, **166**, 749–53.

84. Billings, J.A., and Block, S.D. (1996). Slow euthanasia. *J Palliat Care*, **12**, 21–30.

85. Rietjens, J.A., van der Heide, A., Vrakking, A.M. *et al.* (2004). Physician reports of terminal sedation without hydration or nutrition for patients nearing death in the Netherlands. *Ann Intern Med*, **141**, 178–85.

86. Miccinesi, G., Rietjens, J.A.C., Deliens, L. *et al.* (2006). Continuous deep sedation: physicians' experiences in six European countries. *J Pain Symptom Manage*, **31**, 122–9.

87. Materstvedt, L. J., Bosshard, G. (2009). Deep and continuous palliative sedation (terminal sedation): clinical-ethical and philosophical aspects. *Lancet Oncol*, **10**, 622–7.

88. Den Hartogh, G.A. (2004). On the distinction between terminal sedation and euthanasia [in German]. *Ethik Med*, **16**, 378–91.

89. Wolfe, J., Fairclough, D.L., Clarridge, B.R. *et al.* (1999). Stability of attitudes regarding physician-assisted suicide and euthanasia among oncology patients, physicians, and the general public. *J Clin Oncol*, **17**, 1274–9.

90. Emanuel, E.J., Fairclough, D., Clarridge, B.C. *et al.* (2000). Attitudes and practices of US oncologists regarding euthanasia and physicianassisted suicide. *Ann Intern Med*, **133**, 527–32.

91. Nilstun, T., Melltorp, G., and Hermerén, G. (2000). Surveys on attitudes to active euthanasia and the difficulty of drawing normative conclusions. *Scand J Pub Health*, **28**, 111–6.

92. Van Marwijk, H., Haverkate, I., van Royen, P. *et al.* (2007). Impact of euthanasia on primary care physicians in the Netherlands. *Palliat Med* **21**, 609–14.

93. Hudson, P.L., Kristjanson, L.J., Ashby, M. *et al.* (2006). Desire for hastened death in patients with advanced disease and the evidence base of clinical guidelines: a systematic review. *Palliat Med*, **20**, 693–701.

94. Emanuel, E.J. (2005). Depression, euthanasia, and improving end-of-life care. *J Clin Oncol*, **23**, 6456–8.

95. Wilson, K.G., Scott, J.F., Graham, I.D. *et al.* (2000). Attitudes of terminally ill patients toward euthanasia and physician-assisted suicide. *Arch Intern Med*, **160**, 2454–60.

96. Haverkate, I., Onwuteaka-Philipsen, B.D., van der Heide, A., *et al.* (2000). Refused and granted requests for euthanasia and assisted suicide in the Netherlands: interview study with structured questionnaire. *BMJ*, **321**, 865–6.

97. Van der Lee, M.L., van der Bom, J.G., Swarte, N.B. *et al.* (2005). Euthanasia and depression: a prospective cohort study among terminally ill cancer patients. *J Clin Oncol*, **23**, 6607–12.

98. Johansen, S., Hølen, J.C., Kaasa, S., *et al.* (2005). Attitudes towards, and wishes for, euthanasia in advanced cancer patients at a palliative medicine unit. *Palliat Med*, **19**, 454–60.

99. Georges, J.J., Onwuteaka-Philipsen, B.D., van der Wal, G., *et al.* (2005). Differences between terminally ill cancer patients who died after euthanasia had been performed and terminally ill cancer patients who did not request euthanasia. *Palliat Med*, **19**, 578–86.

100. Fischer S, Huber CA, Furter M, *et al.* (2009). Reasons why people in Switzerland seek assisted suicide: the view of patients and physicians. *Swiss Med Wkly*, **139**, 333–8.

101. Muller, M.T., Kimsma, G.K., and van der Wal, G. (1998). Euthanasia and assisted suicide: facts, figures and fancies with special regard to old age. *Drugs Aging*, **13**, 185–91.

102. Deliens, L., and Bernheim, J. (2003). Palliative care and euthanasia in countries with a law on euthanasia. *Palliat Med*, **17**, 393–4.

103. Battin, M.P., van der Heide, A., Ganzini, L. *et al.* (2007). Legal physician-assisted dying in Oregon and the Netherlands: evidence concerning the impact on patients in "vulnerable" groups. *J Med Ethics* **33**, 591–7.

104. Materstvedt, L.J. (2003). Euthanasia: on slippery slopes and vulnerable patients. *Palliat Med*, **17**, 650–1.

105. Materstvedt, L.J. (2009). Inappropriate conclusions in research on assisted dying. *J Med Ethics*, **35**, 272.

106. Back, A.L., Starks, H., Hsu, C., *et al.* (2002). Clinician-patient interactions about requests for physician-assisted suicide. A patient and family view. *Arch Intern Med*, **162**, 1257–65.

107. Saunders, C. (1959). Care of the dying 1: the problem of euthanasia. *Nursing Times*, **9** October, 60–1.

108. Clark, D. (2002). *Cicely Saunders—founder of the hospice movement: selected letters 1959–1999*. Oxford University Press, Oxford.

109. Hermsen, M.A., and ten Have, H. (2002). Euthanasia in palliative care journals. *J Pain Symptom Manage*, **23**, 517–25.

110. Hurst, S.A., and Mauron, A. (2006). The ethics of palliative care and euthanasia: exploring common values. *Palliat Med*, **20**, 107–12.

111. Illhardt, F.J. (2001). Scope and demarcation of palliative care. In ten Have, H., Janssens. R., eds. *Palliative care in Europe: Concepts and policies*, pp. 109–16. IOS Press, Amsterdam.

112. Georges, J.J., Onwuteaka-Philipsen, B.D., van der Heide, A., *et al.* (2006). Physicians' opinions on palliative care and euthanasia in the Netherlands. *J Palliat Med*, **9**, 1137–44.

113. Zylicz, Z. (1998). Palliative care: Dutch hospice and euthanasia. In Thomasma, D.C., Kimbrough-Kushner, T., Kimsma, G.K., Ciesielski-Carlucci, C., eds. *Asking to die: inside the Dutch debate about euthanasia*, pp. 187–203. Kluwer Academic Publishers, Dordrecht.

114. Kant, I. (1981). *Grounding for the metaphysics of morals*. Ellington JW, transl. Hackett, Indianapolis.

115. Brassington, I. (2006). Killing people: what Kant could have said about suicide and euthanasia but did not. *J Med Ethics*, **32**, 571–4.

116. Hudson, P.L., Schofield, P., Kelly, B. *et al.* (2006). Responding to desire to die statements from patients with advanced disease: recommendations for health professionals. *Palliat Med*, **20**, 703–10.

117. Kmietowicz, Z. (2006). Doctors backtrack on assisted suicide. *BMJ*, **333**, 64.

118. Swiss Academy of Medical Sciences (2005). Care of patients at the end of life, medical-ethical guidelines [in German]. *Schweiz Ärztezeitung*, **86**, 172–6.

119. Finlay, I.G., Wheatley, V.J., and Izdebski, C. (2005). The House of Lords Select Committee on the Assisted Dying for the Terminally Ill Bill: implications for specialist palliative care. *Palliat Med*, **19**, 444–53.

120. Warnock, M. (2008). A duty to die? *Omsorg. Nordisk tidsskrift for palliativ medisin*. 4: 3–5. www.fagbokforlaget.no/filarkiv/Mary%20 Warnock.pdf

Withholding and withdrawing life-sustaining care

Joseph J. Fins and Elizabeth G. Nilson

Introduction (see also Chapter 10.13)

In the course of advancing illness, patients may anticipate fewer gains from medical interventions, and find the ratio of benefits to burden no longer acceptable. This may be particularly evident in the modern intensive care unit where invasive and 'heroic' measures are often employed to sustain a patient who may have little hope of recovery. Current clinical and ethical standards of care support the prerogative of patients and/or their surrogate decision-makers to withhold or withdraw life-sustaining therapies (LST) from dying patients who no longer wish to receive them.

To withhold care is a purposeful decision to forego life-sustaining medical therapies so as not to prolong life or interfere with the dying process. A decision to withhold LST typically takes the form of a Do-Not-Resuscitate (DNR) order. When a DNR order is agreed to, resuscitation (advanced cardiac life support, including endotracheal intubation and manual ventilation, chest compressions, defibrillation, and cardiac medications) is not attempted in the setting of a respiratory or cardiac arrest.

The withdrawal of LST is the removal of an intervention that is artificially sustaining life. In the case of a patient with respiratory failure for whom death is imminent, withdrawal of LST may mean the removal of a ventilator. Or for a patient with end-stage renal disease on chronic renal replacement therapy, it can mean ending dialysis.

Although the ventilator is the most commonly conceived end-of-life intervention removed, a number of other modalities—dialysis, vasopressors, blood transfusions, left ventricular assist devices as well as antibiotics and artificial nutrition—can be considered life-sustaining therapies, and can be withheld or withdrawn.

In this chapter, we will review the philosophical and ethical arguments that have advanced the right of patients and/or their surrogates to make choices about care at the end-of-life as well as the growing number of legal rulings that support these claims. We will consider under what circumstances patients make decisions about their own end-of-life care, and when the task falls to others (surrogate decision-makers). We will then offer clinical guidance on how to facilitate communication with patients and families as they consider decisions near the end of life.

Background

Ethical and philosophical considerations

Both the withholding and withdrawal of care have an ethical basis in the values of personal autonomy and self-determination—values that underlie the Western philosophical tradition and liberal democracies[1]. In the practice of medicine, these values manifest as *informed decision-making*[2,3]. For clinical medicine, informed consent and informed refusal are an integral dimension of the present-day doctor–patient relationship and shared decision making. It is the fiduciary responsibility of the physician to communicate effectively the benefits, risks, and burdens of proposed diagnostic or therapeutic interventions, so that relevant information can inform patient preferences.

A patient's right to self-determination at the end-of-life is clear and based on an autonomy principle. Just as patients can determine what should be done when they are undergoing curative treatment, they should also be allowed to decide what medical interventions to accept or refuse as they die. Self-determination is further sanctioned because the consequences of end-of-life decisions are greatest for the patient. Despite the emotional involvement of the practitioner or family member, it is the patient alone who will directly bear the physical and psychological burdens of an intervention. Because of these factors, the decision to start or continue life-sustaining interventions, *this negative right to be left alone*, should rest with the patient.

The evolution of the right to die

An evolving concern for patient self-determination has increasingly informed jurisprudence and public policy over the past 100 years. Through landmark informed consent cases early in the past century, the US legal system has recognized the centrality of patient choice in decisions about medical care. Ultimately this regard for patient choice has extended to decisions at the end of life.

These legal rulings helped transform medical decision-making from a paternalistic model to a patient-centred one, recognizing that clinical decisions are informed both by medical facts and patient values and beliefs. These legal rulings affirmed that decisions about the timing and circumstances of one's death are, de facto, personal. Formerly paternalistic judgements could neither unilaterally define what was in the patient's best interest[4], nor exclude the patient's voice in care decisions. And, with this mandate came the need for physicians to provide adequate information about clinical facts so that patients and/or their surrogates could make informed decisions to either accept or refuse medical interventions.

The legal codification of self-determination began early in the 20th century with a decision supporting a patient's right to consent to surgery. Mary Schloendorff in 1908 presented to the hospital with 'some disorder of the stomach.' She agreed to an exam under anaesthesia. While sedated, the surgeon removed a uterine fibroid. Suffering complications from the procedure, Ms. Schloendorff sued the hospital. In a landmark decision, Judge Benjamin Cardozo as a member of the New York State Court of Appeals wrote 'in the case at hand, the wrong complained of is not merely negligence. It is trespass. Every human being of adult years and sound mind has a right to determine what shall be done with his own body; and a surgeon who performs an operation without his patient's consent commits an assault, for which he is liable in damages.'[5]

Although this decision was neglected for the better half of the 20th century, it was rediscovered mid-century as the courts began to affirm an evolving doctrine of informed consent and a requisite amount of information flow. (Cardozo's eventual elevation to the US Supreme Court in 1932 and reputational standing made his 1914 ruling on informed consent especially influential as society and the legal system caught up with his prescient decision.)[6,7]

Following Schloendorff, legal rulings expanded a patient's right to decide for him- or herself what medical care to continue and what to stop. In *Salgo v Leland Stanford* (CA, 1957), the court found that Mr. Salgo had not been adequately informed of the risks associated with the aortic arteriography procedure that left him with paralysis. In *Canterbury v Spence* (DC, 1972), Jerry Canterbury suffered paralysis after a spinal procedure. He claimed that the risks of the procedure were not disclosed. In both the cases, the courts held that it is the responsibility of the physician to provide *sufficient* clinical information about the proposed treatments and expected outcomes such that a reasonable patient could make an informed decision regarding his or her care.

Perhaps the most important decision of that era was the 1976 ruling of the New Jersey Supreme Court involving Karen Ann Quinlan (*In re Quinlan*, 1976). The father of Miss Quinlan, a 22-year-old woman in a permanent vegetative state of unclear aetiology, sought legal guardianship to have her ventilator withdrawn given his daughter's grim prognosis. The right to remove life support was upheld[8], in part, because of the futility of any further interventions to improve her condition.

Despite the growing acknowledgment that dying patients can be self-determining and make decisions about LST, an ethical and legal consensus remained to be articulated for patients who could no longer speak for themselves because of decisional incapacity. When patients lose the ability to make decisions, another person or *surrogate decision-maker* may be empowered to make decisions on the patient's behalf. Surrogates are typically family members or other intimates.

Several courts expressly affirmed the rights of surrogates to make decisions about life-sustaining treatments. Beyond *Quinlan* (see above), which is generally recalled as affirming a more generic right to die, subsequent cases also recognized the standing of surrogate

decision-makers. In *the matter of Philip K. Eichner* (1980)[9], a previously healthy man (Brother Fox) suffered an intraoperative cardiac arrest, leaving him in a permanent vegetative state. Based on his previously expressed wishes to avoid 'extraordinary' care such as ventilatory support, the Court of Appeals of New York upheld his common law and Constitutional right to refuse such care. Since Brother Fox could no longer communicate, a surrogate (Father Eichner) was empowered to authorize the removal of the ventilator invoking the patient's previously expressed wishes.

These judicial rulings coalesced in the 1983 President's Commission report *Deciding to Forego Life-Sustaining Treatment*[10] and the 1987 *Hastings Center Guidelines on the Termination of Life-Sustaining Treatment and the Care of the Dying*[11]. Both articulated the ethical justifications for the refusal of unwanted medical interventions and laid the groundwork for state laws supporting an informed refusal of resuscitation (DNR orders).

Despite the emerging professional consensus on patient self-determination and the standing of surrogates to direct care when patients were unable to do so, this view was not universal. Other important legal cases questioned the role of surrogates when patients are unable to express their preferences.

Such was the case in *the matter of John Storar* (1980).[12] In Storar, a mentally retarded man with an estimated intellectual age of 18 months required frequent blood transfusions for terminal bladder cancer. Maintaining that the transfusions were causing distress and the burdens outweighed the expected benefits, Storar's mother (who was also his legal guardian) wanted them stopped. A lower court had ruled that the transfusions could cease, however, the Court of Appeals of New York reversed this decision. They ruled that the patient should be treated as a child since he was never competent and never able to articulate a preference to direct care. Thus, his mother could not withhold from him life-sustaining treatment.

Similarly, in *O'Connor* (In re Mary O'Connor, NY 1988)[13], Mrs. O'Connor's daughters were not allowed to withhold artificial nutrition and hydration in the setting of disabling strokes because they lacked 'clear and convincing' evidence that this was their mother's wish.

The US Supreme Court's rulings in *Cruzan* v. *Director* (US, 1990)[14] also invoked a reliance on prior wishes in the setting of decisional incapacity. The case involved a young woman in a permanent vegetative state and her family's request to remove artificial nutrition and hydration. The US Supreme Court held that surrogates could decide to withdraw the life-sustaining treatment, but that states could set evidentiary standards about the amount of knowledge of patient preferences necessary to permit such a decision.

Because a central question in *Cruzan* was about patient prior wishes, US Supreme Court Justice Sandra Day O'Connor suggested a role for advance care planning so patients could articulate preferences ahead of decisional incapacity[15]. This resulted in the passage of the Patient Self-Determination Act in 1990, which required health-care institutions to ask about the presence or absence of advance directives and required states to enact legislation to enable advance care planning so that patient preferences could ultimately direct end-of-life care[16].

These challenges were seemingly settled but then revisited during the struggle about the withdrawal of a feeding tube from Terry Schiavo, the Florida woman in a permanent vegetative state following anoxic injury from a prolonged cardiac arrest[17]. Mrs. Schiavo's husband, and legal surrogate, sought to remove artificial nutrition and hydration based on his knowledge of her previously expressed wishes. Despite political involvement at the highest levels in the USA, the local, state and federal courts upheld the right to die based on a patient's prior wishes and the standing of appropriate surrogates to direct care[18,19].

Although much progress has been made in expanding patient autonomy at the end-of-life, a still fragile consensus exists in the USA and Europe with respect to the role of surrogates. The societal fragility of these rights makes it especially important to develop the requisite competence to foster shared decision-making with patients and their surrogates. In the next section, we will consider how these ethical norms vary cross-culturally.

Cross-cultural perspectives

While courts and legislatures in the USA have generally affirmed a doctrine of patient self-determination at the end-of-life, the role of patient autonomy varies considerably internationally. Degrees of paternalism coexist with elements of patient self-determination. Some societies sanction end-of-life decision-making by physicians with variable degrees of patient or family input[3,20-24]. Others advocate that end-of-life practices should more closely mirror the American model of shared decision-making[21]. For instance, with respect to surrogate decision-making the broader international context remains a mosaic[3,20,22]. This appears to meet prevailing cultural norms because surrogates may desire neither this legal authority nor ethical burden. One French study, for example, found that half of families wanted the physician to decide based on patient best interest[20]. This diversity emerges from the different religious, cultural, and social backgrounds of physicians, patients, and their families[24].

There is also pluralism within cultures about beliefs and norms. For example, in the USA, African Americans are less likely on average to consent to DNR orders[25]. This refusal appears based, to some extent, on perceived disparities in the health system[26-28]. Disenfranchised minorities may think that to forego efforts to sustain life could further exacerbate differences in their care[29,30].

While we advocate an approach that values patient self-determination and choice, we also acknowledge the importance of respecting pluralism. Clinicians should recognize their patients' racial, religious, and cultural backgrounds and seek to find common ground using cultural intermediaries and trained interpreters when language barriers exist[31].

Patient and surrogate decision-making

Capacity and competence

When considering decisions regarding LST, the clinician needs to determine the appropriate decision-maker. For adult patients, the standing presumption is that the patient is capable of directing his or her own care. Such *decision-making capacity* is not a global indication of cognitive function but specific to a discrete clinical decision.

Capacity is defined as the ability to:

1 Understand the relevant information.

2 Communicate with others about the information presented.

3 Appreciate the situation and its consequences.

4 Reason about the choices in terms of personal goals and value[32-35].

Capacity should be distinguished from *competence*. To be competent a patient must have decision-making capacity and be of legal age. (In some jurisdictions an emancipated minor may be deemed competent.) A clinician determines whether a patient has medical decision-making capacity. A court empowered to deprive a patient of the ability to make choices about their care makes a legal judgement or determination about competence. Because of this possible infringement on autonomy and civil liberties, there is role sequestration between the clinical and judicial determinations of capacity and competence.

Challenges to capacity assessments

Unfortunately, the nature of severe illness and impending death often robs patients of the ability to understand and manipulate information about their diagnosis and prognosis. It is important to accurately determine when a patient no longer has decision-making capacity and can thus no longer capably participate in decisions about ongoing medical care. This inability to be self-determining marks an important transition in the patient's disease trajectory because surrogate decision-makers will need to assume increasing responsibility for care decisions.

There can be hidden challenges to the assessment of capacity in part because a patient's ability to participate in decisions can wax and wane over time. Capacity is not static in the setting of advancing illness because a number of factors can distort the patient's level of arousal, analytical abilities, memory, or emotions. Delirium and altered sensorium can be caused acutely by metabolic abnormalities like hypercalcaemia or hypoxia or by medications such as sedative agents. Chronic conditions like dementia can also progressively erode the patient's decision-making capacity.

Some psychiatric disorders may also affect decision-making capacity, although this may not be immediately apparent. For example, affective illnesses can interfere with capacity without necessarily interfering with a patient's ability to reason rationally. Patients can meet what is often termed a 'rational standard' of decision-making—what a reasonable person would want. But in the setting of depression the patient may be seemingly *decathected* from the decision, as if the consequences would accrue to some one else. In cases where affective illness is suspected, it is important to seek the consultative services of a psychiatrist for more formal capacity assessment. In addition, psychiatric assistance is often useful for finding ways to optimize a patient's participation in the decision-making process. Every effort should be made to reverse treatable causes of decisional incapacity, such as depression or delirium, in order to re-enfranchise patients in the decision-making process.

Clinicians must be especially careful to avoid mistakenly equating patient agreement with consent that is provided by a capacitated individual. In many cases, clinicians mistake mere agreement for actual consent, when the acquiescence is nothing more than *assent*. Unlike patients who engage in a process of informed consent or refusal, ones who assent merely agree to a recommendation.

Such patients do not fully appreciate the associated risks, benefits, or alternatives and can thus not defend their own interests. They are neither meaningfully informed nor able to assert independent judgement. As such they are not self-determining and require the intervention of a surrogate.

Such errors of diagnostic omission occur most typically when a patient who had been 'consenting' to procedures suddenly refuses to agree with the recommendations of treating physicians. This refusal then triggers a formal assessment of capacity that reveals that the patient in fact lacks capacity. A retrospective review of prior patient decisions, however, often reveals that this loss of decision-making capacity has been chronic and that what had been taken as consent was just assent.

Although this scenario is a common prompt to assessment of capacity, it also needs to be stressed that the mere fact that someone refuses a recommended procedure does not mean that capacity has been lost[36]. While challenging physician recommendations and authority may lead to an evaluation of capacity, a treatment refusal should not be summarily equated with loss of capacity.

Treatment refusals can be fully informed and rational. This includes decisions to forego life-sustaining treatments. In such cases, the patient makes a judgement about putative risks and benefits of life-sustaining treatments and makes a decision that 'aggressive' curative measures have become ethically disproportionate or inconsistent with personal values.

When attempting to sort out these variables it is helpful to appreciate that capacity is not a simple binary construct. Like most things in biology, the loss of this capacity falls on a continuum and is progressive. A patient may retain the ability to make simpler decisions but be unable to contribute meaningfully to more complicated or contingent ones. In order not to deprive patients of an ability to direct their own care, when they are able, many ethicists endorse a 'sliding-scale' approach to capacity assessment[37].

In this framework, what constitutes an acceptable degree of capacity is correlated with the import of the decision such that the degree of understanding and ability to justify a decision is correlated with the seriousness of the decision at hand. For example, a treatment refusal for a relatively minor problem—e.g. sutures for a superficial laceration, would require less justification and understanding than would a choice that would have implications for survival—e.g. a decision to forgo life-sustaining surgery.

Decisions by the competent patient

When a competent patient contemplates a decision to withhold cardiopulmonary resuscitation, it is important that he or she understands the benefits of this effort given his or her particular clinical circumstances. Outcomes for cardiac resuscitation vary dramatically depending on the patient's underlying disease process and co-morbidities, and well as the context of the cardiac arrest. For example, attempts at resuscitation may not work at all in patients with multi-system organ failure and sepsis. In patients with widely metastatic cancer, resuscitation may temporarily restore cardiac function but the patient's remaining days would likely be in an intensive care unit on life support. In contrast, for a hospitalized patient with an acute myocardial infarction, a witnessed cardiac arrest and resuscitation is likely to be successful, and the patient has a reasonable expectation (about 30 per cent) of discharge from the hospital in good condition.[38] Once the likely prognosis after an arrest is estimated, a patient can then make an informed decision about the utility of a DNR order in his or her plan of care.

Although the prognosis after resuscitation is intimately tied to the patient's pre-arrest clinical condition, a DNR order is not a sufficient plan for the remaining days, weeks or months of a patient's critical / terminal illness. As such, a DNR order should not be the focus of an end-of-life care discussion. Rather a DNR discussion is a small part of a much broader conversation about end-of-life preferences. The physician should undertake an informed discussion about the benefits and burdens of significant diagnostic and therapeutic choices. Depending on the clinical prognosis and the patient's values, it is quite possible that the patient will make an informed refusal to withhold other life-sustaining interventions.

However, just because a patient declines certain treatments, including cardiopulmonary resuscitation, he or she still warrants daily attention to interventions relevant to the goals of care, which might include pain and symptom management, treatment of electrolyte disturbances or infection, and nutrition.

Decisions by surrogates

Despite the ethical importance of self-determination, the nature of critical illness often means that surrogates, not patients, are called upon to make end-of-life decisions. When a patient has been found to lack decision-making capacity, the clinician should call upon a surrogate to make decisions. In this section, we will review surrogate decision-making and offer strategies to work with those who seek to represent the interests of decisionally incapacitated patients.

In one study of end-of-life care, surrogate decision-makers consented to 64 per cent of DNR orders[39]. Because of such practice patterns, the incorporation of surrogate decision-making into sound palliative care plans is often essential. To preserve the patient's voice when capacity is lost, clinicians should turn to surrogates who can robustly represent the patient's interests. The surrogate is determined from a hierarchical list of candidates[40].

The patient can, where legally sanctioned, specifically designate a surrogate decision-maker, often known as a durable power of attorney for health care (DPAHC) or health-care agent (often colloquially referred to as a proxy) who are empowered to make health-care decisions when capacity is lost. (See below for more on advance care planning.) In the absence of a proxy, there is typically a legally or culturally accepted next-of-kin ranking of decision-makers to turn to when a patient has lost capacity. A court-appointed guardian may supersede a family member, but will usually not trump a patient-appointed proxy. If there is no family, some jurisdictions allow a close friend or significant other to act as surrogate.

There are ethical standards about how surrogates should make decisions[10]. Prevailing ethical and clinical norms suggest that the surrogate should make decisions based on the patient's previously *expressed wishes*, or when these are not known, based on *substituted judgement*. Substituted judgement is an inferred opinion about what the patient would want based on the surrogate's knowledge of the patient's values and life experiences. When prior wishes are unknown and cannot be inferred, the surrogate should invoke a *best interests* standard. A best interest standard balances the benefits and burdens of the treatment options to arrive at a decision that a *reasonable person* would make[41,42]. In all of these scenarios, the clinician should work closely with surrogates to best integrate clinical developments into the surrogate's decision-making process.

There are routines that can optimize effective, shared decision-making with surrogates[43-45]. The surrogate's role is especially stressful because of the burden associated with making decisions that directly affect the manner and timing of another person's death. Take time to address questions, and acknowledge emotions, including grief and guilt[46,47]. Outline the diagnosis and prognosis, as you would with a competent patient, acknowledging that in many cases the benefits of continued LST may be hard to determine because prognostication is difficult[48].

Even though there will usually be one surrogate legally entrusted to take the lead in the decision-making process, it is helpful to involve other family members, significant others and friends since all are likely to be affected by the patient's illness. This collection of friends and intimates can help provide support to the primary surrogate and each may have important information of the patient's preferences.

Meetings should start with how the surrogate and other family members will receive clinical information, and how care decisions will be made. Since a meeting with all family members can be emotional, hold conferences in a quiet, private and comfortable room. Involve the primary care physician, when there is one, and other members of the inter-disciplinary care team. Each can make valuable contributions to deliberations, although it is important that the care team presents a cohesive picture of the patient's situation. Conflicting information can exacerbate futility disputes[49] and contribute to depression in the family[50].

Confirm that the surrogate understands information that has been shared and try to titrate difficult issues over time, if this is possible. When there is uncertainty, it may be appropriate to embark on a trial of LST to see whether or not the interventions reverse the clinical decline. Over time, a patient's prognosis may become clearer, enabling the physician and patient/surrogate to more accurately calculate whether the burdens of continued LST outweigh the benefits. With a clearer prognosis, patients/surrogates may decide that ongoing life-sustaining treatments no longer serve the goals of care. As with decisions to withhold LST, providers should similarly discuss the relevant benefits, burdens, and expected outcomes should the patient/surrogate desire to withdraw the life-sustaining treatments under discussion. The medical record should document the clinical diagnosis and prognosis and that prevailing evidentiary standards regarding prior wishes have been met.

Surrogates who are considering the withholding or withdrawing of LST may feel like they are responsible for the patient's death. Although the ethics literature asserts that there is no ethical distinction between the withholding and the withdrawal of LST[10], it can be emotionally more difficult to withdraw life-sustaining therapy than not to initiate it[51]. It is important to reassure practitioner and surrogates alike that the disease process is responsible for the patient's decline, not the withdrawal of a life-sustaining intervention.

To address these concerns, it is helpful to consider the question of causality and culpability. The withholding or withdrawal of LST is a necessary, but not sufficient to cause death in a patient dependent on that technology. Contrast this with the healthy patient who undergoes general anaesthesia. Once the patient awakens, the removal of the ventilator does not lead to respiratory failure and death. These distinctions suggest that the cause of death in dying patients is the underlying medical condition, not the withholding or withdrawal of LST, absolving those who feel culpable because they misperceived causality.

A final challenge with respect to withdrawals of care is the perception that the removal of life-sustaining therapy is akin to physician-assisted suicide. Although the distinction has warranted much ethical debate, it is possible and important to distinguish between the two[52]. Physician-assisted suicide is the wilful provision of a means to prematurely end a life. To withhold or withdraw care is a patient's informed rejection of new or ongoing treatments that are an impediment to dying. Moreover, a physician who ignores a patient's (or surrogate's) choice to decline further care and provides un-consented to care violates bodily integrity and undermines self-determination. This respect for the patient's right to be left alone is the moral warrant behind treatment refusals of life-sustaining therapies and is distinct from any affirmative physician obligation to comply with a request for assisted suicide.

Advance care planning

Many of the ethical challenges of surrogate decision-making can be mitigated through *advance care planning* in which a patient articulates his or her preferences in advance of decisional incapacity. This preventive ethic can help ease the moral and psychological burdens on the surrogate, and promote surrogate decision-making that more accurately represents patient wishes.

Patients can communicate their preferences for end-of-life care in a variety of ways. One way is through a *living will* in which a patient records in writing his or her wishes for future care, often addressing common end-of-life scenarios in a standardized fashion. Unfortunately written expressions may not foresee the actual circumstances of one's terminal condition, may be too vague about the unique conditions surrounding one's death[53], or may be too generic to extend a patient's autonomy beyond the point of incapacity. Further, a patient's written wishes may be ambiguous, such as a request for no intubation[54]. It cannot be determined if such a statement is a categorical rejection of mechanical ventilation, or rather a desire merely to avoid prolonged ventilator assistance when there is no hope for recovery. If the latter is the case, the patient might accept a trial of ventilation for a potentially treatable condition.

Given the limitations of living wills, we prefer the designation of a proxy-decision-maker or DPAHC, if the patient has identified someone to empower. This designated surrogate acts when a patient has lost decision-making ability. In some jurisdictions, a proxy may have more authority than a next-of-kin surrogate, with proxy decisions viewed as if they were the patient's. Most importantly, a proxy can use his or her knowledge of the patient's wishes, values and life experiences and apply it to the patient's changing medical circumstances.

The explicit designation of a surrogate may allow the patient to prepare the proxy for the various contingencies that might be expected when decisional capacity has been lost. So empowered, proxies can provide elegant solutions to difficult choices. In the scenario above, the proxy could consent to a ventilator for the treatable condition, and then stop the treatment should the condition worsen.

A minority of patients has executed a health-care proxy[55], and empirical studies have found variable benefits from health-care proxies, over surrogates, for end-of-life decisions[39,56]. Regrettably, most proxies are poorly prepared to assume the moral burden of making choices on behalf of another, triggering distress when decisions need to be made. Indeed, one meta-analysis of 16 studies examining the accuracy of surrogate decision-making found that surrogates predict patient's wishes in only about two-thirds of cases. This was true whether the surrogate was patient-appointed (a health-care agent) or next-of-kin[57].

Despite this lack of precision, there appears to be growing acceptance of the ethical validity of choices that emerge out of a close relationship with the patient and knowledge of a patient's values. Several empirical studies have demonstrated that patients and proxies are more interested in interpersonal relationships than philosophical arguments about patient self-determination[58,59], certainly a misnomer when the expression of a decisionally incapacitated self requires another.

Fins has argued that it is better to view the moral obligations of patient and proxy as reciprocal, or covenantal, in which the patient's choice of the proxy vests him or her with procedural moral authority[59–61]. In this framework, patient delegation of a proxy is viewed as an expression of patient autonomy. This authority needs to be weighed against knowledge of substantive patient preferences when the proxy is asked to make decisions on behalf of the patient. This mix of procedural and substantive moral authority has been seen as giving the proxy the discretion to depart from patient preferences when the patient 'wanted everything done' and the situation was grim. It did not give the proxy the discretion to override a patient preference to be left alone[60].

While the complexity of this emerging area of scholarship can not be addressed fully here, clinicians are advised to take a more expansive view of the patient–proxy relationship in order to most productively meet the needs of patients and their intimates at times of decisional incapacity.

Treatment-specific challenges

Even with the best planning, ethical challenges will emerge that force difficult choices amongst competing goals of care. In this section we review several treatment decisions that require special consideration.

Artificial nutrition and hydration

Decisions to withhold or withdraw artificial nutrition and hydration (ANH) bear special mention because many religious traditions view the provision of food and water, in whatever form, as ordinary care. While measures viewed as extraordinary by these traditions, e.g. ventilatory support or dialysis, maybe withheld or withdrawn the provision of artificial nutrition is viewed as obligatory. As an example, Pope John Paul II suggested that artificial nutrition is 'a natural means of preserving life, not a medical act'[62].

Such religious beliefs are sometimes ensconced in the legal frameworks which prohibits the removal artificial feedings or which require additional evidence of patient preferences before nutrition can be withheld or withdrawn. When deciding whether or not to initiate or withdraw ANH, it is important to address the religious traditions of patients and surrogates and determine the legal status of artificial nutrition and hydration in one's jurisdiction.

DNR and operative and sedative procedures

Decisions to not resuscitate patients who are undergoing surgery or sedative procedures is another case that can be confounding. Many operators have a difficult time bringing such patients to the operating room or endoscopy suite because they fear that they will be unable to respond to contingencies that might require resuscitation. Moreover, clinical outcomes after resuscitation in the operative setting are considerably more favourable than arrests elsewhere in the hospital. Because of this many physicians feel that patients should allow resuscitation in the operating room[63].

Despite these arguments, there is an emerging ethical consensus that patients and/or their surrogates should have the right to forgo resuscitation as they undergo procedures that have a palliative intent. Indeed some commentators have argued that a DNR order should not preclude access to procedures like a diverting colostomy for an obstructing colon cancer or the placement of a central line that will aid in the provision of opioid analgesia[64].

Philosophically, taking a patient to the operating room for a palliative procedure can be understood as preserving both the right to be left alone (the DNR) with an affirmative right to palliative care through the pain and/or symptom provided through the operative procedure. The American College of Surgeons (ACS) recommends a policy of 'required reconsideration' in the informed consent process for surgery of any pre-existing DNR as an effort to balance what may appear to be discordant goals of care[65]. This process helps to assure that decisions about resuscitation and the procedure are mutually consistent and coherent and alerts the care team about the patient's resuscitation when in the operating room.

Dialysis

Dialysis raises a number of unique challenges because it can be used acutely to reverse a transient metabolic derangement or chronically as in the case of end-stage renal disease. Understanding how dialysis is employed will help determine whether decisions constitute a withholding or withdrawing of care[66].

When employed as a temporary measure to support acute renal failure, treatments are best considered as episodic. A decision to initiate each treatment can be understood on a treatment-to-treatment basis without an ongoing expectation of need or therapeutic obligation. Conversely, in chronic renal failure, forgoing further dialysis constitutes the withholding of life-sustaining treatment.

Permanent pacemakers and automated implanted defibrillators

Another treatment that can be temporary or permanent is the implantation of permanent pacemakers (PPM) and automated implanted cardioverter defibrillators (AICD). A PPM maintains, on demand, an acceptable cardiac rate in the setting of absent or insufficient intrinsic pacemaker or atrioventricular node or in the setting of neurocardiogenic syncope or myocardial infarction. AICDs are placed for the primary or secondary prevention of serious or life-threatening arrhythmias and optimize the benefits of defibrillation treatment. While both devices continuously sense cardiac rhythm, they act only for designated abnormalities. AICDs act only when there is a need for cardioversion and may remain quiescent indefinitely. Dying patients or surrogates must consider whether the presence of these devices remain consistent the patient's goals of care[67].

Given the close relationship between internal and external defibrillation, it is reasonable to consider disabling the AICD when a patient or surrogate consents to a DNR order. This is particularly true when the goals of care are palliative and internal defibrillation would merely prolong the dying process or produce distress[68,69]. In other clinical circumstances, continued activation of the AICD may offer a survival advantage and remain consistent with patient or surrogate preferences[67].

Since AICD defibrillation activity is on stand-by waiting to respond to an arrhythmia and is not actually providing ongoing treatment, we consider the deactivation of an AICD under the rubric of a DNR order and the withholding of care. In contrast, we view the discontinuation of a continuously paced PPM as a withdrawal of care. Nonetheless, when a pacemaker is not firing regularly, and is only activated to over-drive suppress an arrhythmia, pacemaker deactivation could be considered as a withdrawal of life-sustaining therapy. In such cases, the ethical classification of deactivation as a withdrawal or withholding of LST depends upon careful analysis of the medical facts and the indications for these devices.

Futility

No consideration of decisions to withhold or withdraw LST would be complete without considering the topic of *medical futility*. Many clinical conflicts over these choices hinge, in part, over whether an intervention is viewed as being efficacious or not. In this way, these conflicts become ones over questions of utility and futility. In this section we will contextualize these disputes against the prevailing definitions of medical futility.

As might be expected for such a contentious topic, there is no single definition for futility, and this is a critical point to make in the face of conflict. Many will assert that care is futile or not, without being clear about what is meant by futile. To prevent misunderstandings over a potentially elastic term, it is important to be clear about definitions and terms that are sometimes conflated with futility. To begin with etymology, futility derives from the Latin, *futilis,* which means leaky[70]. The concept is of a vessel that is incapable of fulfilling its task, e.g. holding fluid without leaking.

Futility first needs to be distinguished from the concept of rationing. In a clinical context, rationing is best understood as making choices between interventions based on available resources. Rationing prioritizes interventions based on their relative utility and may preempt interventions which remain efficacious[71,72]. Physicians or other staff may also use the issue of medical resource utilization at the end-of-life to defend a position about withholding or withdrawing care. While just resource management is a growing imperative in hospitals, it pertains to the medical community as a whole, not to individual patients. To ensure fairness, the public should participate in decisions about how to set limits on the types and amount of care to be delivered to patients with resource-intensive clinical conditions[73]. Caregivers should not invoke resource conservation at the bedside to avoid a standoff with a patient or family about care at the end-of-life. Should a shortage occur, such as a lack of blood products or ICU beds, pre-existing policies for addressing this should be followed. If none exists, involvement of the hospital administration, ethics committee, or other uninvolved party is desirable to help ensure a fair resolution.

One definition of futility suggests that ongoing interventions are unlikely to maintain or restore *physiological* function[74]. Although sometimes difficult to determine with great certainty, because *physiological futility* is strictly focused on narrow parameters it is the least open to value judgements about the quality of the life involved. Thus, it is often the legal predicate to withhold or withdraw LST when there is no available surrogate. This definition of futility is also the principle that is invoked when efforts at resuscitation are halted after a cardiac arrest. At some point it becomes clear that further interventions will be futile because of persistent profound acidaemia or asystole. Patients who typically meet a strict definition of physiological futility are very near death. As such,

physiological futility does not help to interpret the impact of proposed therapies for patients who have a terminal illness, but who are not expected to die in the very near future.

Schneiderman offers two definitions of futility[71,76]. The first is a *quantitative* one incorporating a probability assessment based on how patients in similar clinical conditions fare. Interventions expected to produce outcomes outside a 95 per cent confidence interval are viewed as futile. While such a probabilistic framework may be useful in research, it is harder to apply to an individual because of inherent differences between people and the limited number of patients seen by any one physician.

Schneiderman's second definition of *qualitative* futility is more useful. It is invoked when clinicians feel that additional interventions are unlikely to provide a patient-centred benefit versus one that is merely physiologic. Despite this utility, defining *benefit* becomes a challenge because each of us can reach a different conclusion about such a value-laden assessment. Nonetheless, because qualitative futility is patient-centred, rather than physiologically oriented, it can be useful when trying to decide if an ongoing treatment is in keeping with a patient's goals of care. It also allows decisions to be made earlier in a patient's course before death is imminent.

Futility disputes are clinical situations in which the providers and the patient or surrogate disagree about whether or not ongoing life-sustaining care constitutes futile care. These disputes can arise when there is a discrepancy between the providers' and families' views of the dying patient's clinical situation and prognosis. Failure to adequately communicate clinical deterioration is often the root cause. When this is the case, the family labours under a misconception about the patient's likelihood of recovery, and thus continues to ask for and consent to more aggressive interventions than the care team thinks is appropriate. Communication failures can be exacerbated when clinical updates are confined to information about physiological parameters such as haemoglobin or creatinine levels. Improvement or stabilization in these numbers can be mistaken for overall recovery when this is often not the case in many critically ill patients[49]. To avoid such misunderstanding, we recommend that physicians interpret the significance of lab results and physiological parameters with respect to their impact on the overall clinical status.

Even when families are adequately informed about a patient's clinical situation, conflicts can persist over what care should be withdrawn or withheld, and who should decide[76–78]. Families may request treatments that the clinicians feel are not indicated, or which confer an undue burden on the patient. Providing such treatments may seem a violation of the practitioner's clinical discretion and the ethical imperative to avoid harming a patient.

To avoid undermining the professional integrity of its members, the American Thoracic Society in its consensus statement about withholding and withdrawing care sanctions physicians to determine futility in situations where such care can no longer help the patient[79]. In some European countries, physicians remain the final decision-maker regarding what therapies to withhold or withdraw at the end-of-life. Others maintain that the subjective nature of futility determinations renders them vulnerable to physician-imposed notions about quality of life, and thus patients and surrogates, not physicians, should have the final say about whether a treatment furthers the goals of care. The Society of Critical Care Medicine's ethics committee views as futile treatments not likely to accomplish their intended goal. Such interventions should be discussed with the patient or surrogate, recognizing that different goals of care may lead to different perspectives on the appropriateness of a particular treatment[73].

The best remedy for futility disputes is preventing them in the first place. Ongoing and effective communication from the beginning of the critical illness provides patients and families time to come to terms with the irreversibility of the illness and the inevitability of death. With realistic expectations in place, decisions to forego futile care are easier to accept. Effective communication may also reveal that the patient or family's values surrounding the meaning of life as death approaches differ from those of the healthcare providers. Caregivers should not undermine such subjective determinations, which are often informed by religious or cultural practices. To do so is unrealistic and not appropriate. However, understanding the religious and cultural values may assist the care team in negotiating a sensible course of treatment that honours the patient's beliefs and wishes.

When futility disputes are brewing or entrenched, ethics consultation and mediation may help ease the tension, realign provider and family expectations, and facilitate decision-making[80–82]. The assistance of ethics committees can help assure that patient preferences and humane goals of care, not medical technology, define life's end.

Further reading

Curtis, J.R., and Rubenfeld, G.D. (eds.) (2001). *Managing death in the ICU: The transition from cure to comfort*. Oxford University Press, New York.

Consensus statement of the Society of Critical Care Medicine's Ethics Committee regarding futile and other possibly inadvisable treatments (1997). *Critical Care Medicine*, **25**, 887–91.

Fins, J.J. (2006). *A palliative ethic of care: Clinical wisdom at life's end*. Jones and Bartlett Publishers, Sudbury.

The New York State Task Force on Life and the Law (1992). *When others must choose: deciding for patients without capacity*, pp. 21–45. The New York State Task Force on Life and the Law, New York.

References

1. Hall, M.A., Ellman, I.M., and Strouse, D.S. (1999). The law and ethics of withholding medical care and assisting suicide. In *Health Care Law and Ethics*, 2nd edition, pp. 321–2. West Group, St. Paul.

2. Salgo v. Leland Stanford Jr. University Board of Trustees, 317 P.2d 170 (Cal. App. 1957); Canterbury v. Spence, 464 F.2d 772 (DC Cir. 1972).

3. Carlet, J., Thijs, L.G., Antonelli, M. *et al.* (2004). Challenges in end-of-life care in the ICU. Statement of the 5th International Consensus Conference in Critical Care: Brussels, Belgium, April 2003. *Intensive Care Medicine*, **30**, 770–84.

4. Fins, J.J. (2006). The rise of bioethics and palliative care ethics. In *A palliative ethic of care: Clinical wisdom at life's end*, p. 23. Jones and Bartlett Publishers, Sudbury.

5. Schloendorff v Society of New York Hospital, 211 NY 125 (1914).

6. Posner, R.A. (1990). *Cardozo: A study in reputation*. University of Chicago Press, Chicago.

7. Fins, J.J. (2001). Truth telling and reciprocity in the doctor-patient relationship: a North American perspective. In *Topics in palliative care*, Volume 5. Oxford University Press, New York.

8. Re Quinlan, 355 A.2d 647 (NJ 1976); cert denied 429 US 1992, 1976.

9. Matter of Eichner (Fox), 73 A.D.2d 431, 426 N.Y.S.2d 517 (Nassau Co., 27 March 1980).

10. President's Commission for the Study of Ethical Problems in Medicine and Biomedical and Behavioral Research (1983). *Deciding to forgo life-sustaining treatment*. U.S. Government Printing Office, Washington.

11. Hastings Center (1987). *Guidelines on the termination of life-sustaining treatment and the care of the dying: A report of the Hastings Center*. Indiana University Press, Bloomington.

12. Matter of Storar, 78 A.D.2d 1013, 434 N.Y.S.2d 46 (4th Dept, 1980).

13. Matter of Westchester County Med. Center (O'Connor), 139 AD2d 344, 532 N.Y.S.2d 133 (16 August 1988).

14. Cruzan v Director, Missouri Department of Health, 110 S. Ct. 2841 (1990).

15. McCloskey, E.L. (1991). Bioethics Inside the Beltway/The Patient Self-Determination Act. *Kennedy Institute of Ethics Journal*, June, 163–9.

16. Omnibus Budget Reconciliation Act of 1990. Public Law No. 101–508.

17. Altenbernd, Chris W., Judge (for The Court). 'In re GUARDIANSHIP OF Theresa Marie SCHIAVO, Incapacitated. Robert Schindler and Mary Schindler, Appellants, v. Michael Schiavo, as Guardian of the person of Theresa Marie Schiavo, Appellee,' Case Number: 2D00-1269, Florida Second District Court of Appeal, 24 January 2001.

18. Annas, G.J. (2005). "Culture of Life" politics at the bedside – The case of Terri Schiavo. *The New England Journal of Medicine*, **352**, 1710–5.

19. Fins, J.J. (2006). Affirming the right to care, preserving the right to die: disorders of consciousness and neuroethics after schiavo. *Palliative and Supportive Care*, **4**, 169–78.

20. Moselli, N.M., Debernardi, F., and Piovano, F. (2006). Forgoing life sustaining treatments: differences and similarities between North America and Europe. *Acta Anaesthesiologica Scandinavica*, **50**, 1177–86.

21. Sprung, C.J., Cohen, S.L., Sjokvist, P. *et al.* (2003). End-of-Life Practices in European Intensive Care Units – the ETHICUS Study. *JAMA*, **290**, 790–7.

22. Yazigi, A., Riachi, M., and Dabbar, G. (2005). Withholding and withdrawal of life-sustaining treatment in a Lebanese intensive care unit: a prospective observational study. *Intensive Care Medicine*, **31**, 562–7.

23. Cardoso, T., Fonseca, T., Pereira, S. *et al.* (2003). Life-sustaining treatment decisions in Portuguese intensive care units: a national survey of intensive care physicians. *Critical Care*, **7**, R167–75.

24. Vincent, J. (2001). Cultural differences in end-of-life care. *Critical Care Medicine*, **29**, N52–5.

25. Shepardson, L.B., Gordon, H.S., and Ibrahim, S.A. (1999). Racial variation in the use of do-not-resuscitate orders. *Journal of General Internal Medicine*, **14**, 15–20.

26. Fins, J.J. (2002). Vowing to care. *Journal of Pain and Symptom Management*, **23**, 54–7.

27. Abraham, L.K. (1993). Life-sustaining technology. In *Mama might be better off dead*, pp. 213–31. The University of Chicago Press, Chicago.

28. Williams, J.F., Zimmerman, J.E., Wagner, D.P. *et al.* (1995). African–American and White patients admitted to the intensive care unit: is there a difference in therapy and outcome? *Critical Care Medicine*, **23**, 626–36.

29. Waters, C.M. (2001). Understanding and supporting African Americans' perspectives of end-of-life care planning and decision-making. *Qualitative Health Research*, **11**, 383–98.

30. Crawley, L.M. (2005). Racial, cultural, and ethnic factors influencing end-of-life care. *Journal of Palliative Medicine*, **8**(Suppl. 1), S58–69.

31. Fins, J.J. (1998). Approximation and negotiation: clinical pragmatism and difference. *Cambridge Quarterly of Healthcare Ethics*, **7**, 68–76.

32. Fins, J.J. Goals of care: when death is near. In *A Palliative Ethic of Care: Clinical Wisdom at Life's End*, p. 111. Jones and Bartlett Publishers, Sudbury.

33. Tunzi, M. (2001). Can the patient decide? evaluating patient capacity in practice. *American Family Physician*, **64**, 299–306.

34. Applebaum, P.S., and Grisso, T. (1988). Assessing patients' capacity to consent to treatment. *The New England Journal of Medicine*, **319**, 1635–8.

35. Boyle, R.J. (1997). Determining patients' capacity to share decision making. In *Introduction to clinical ethics*, (eds. J.C. Fletcher, P.A. Lombardo, M.F. Marchall, and F.G. Miller), 2nd edition. pp. 73–6. University Publishing Group, Hagerstown.

36. Zaubler, T.S., Viederman, M., and Fins, J.J. (1994). Ethical, legal and psychiatric issues in capacity, competences and informed consent: an annotated bibliography of representative articles. *General Hospital Psychiatry*, **151**, 971–8.

37. Drane, J.F. (1984). Competency to give an informed consent. a model for making clinical assessments. *JAMA*, **252**, 925–7; Lo, B. (1990). Assessing decision-making capacity. *The Journal of Law, Medicine & Ethics*, **18**, 193–203.

38. Dumot, J.A., Burval, D.J., Sprung, J. *et al.* (2001). Outcome of adult cardiopulmonary resuscitations at a tertiary referral center including results of "limited" resuscitations. *Archives of Internal Medicine*, **161**, 1751–8.

39. Fins, J.J., Miller, F.G., Acres, C.A. *et al.* (1999). End-of-life decision-making in the hospital: current practice and future prospects. *Journal of Pain and Symptom Management*, **17**, 6–15.

40. The New York State Task Force on Life and the Law (1992). *When Others must Choose: Deciding for Patients without Capacity*, pp. 21–45. The New York State Task Force on Life and the Law, New York.

41. Buchanan, A.E., and Brock, D.W. (1990). *Deciding for others: the ethics of surrogate decision making*, pp. 15–211. Cambridge University Press, New York.

42. Sachs, G.A. and Siegler, M. (1991). Guidelines for decision making when the patient is incompetent. *Journal of Critical Care Illness*, **6**, 348–59.

43. Clarke, E.B., Curtis, J.R., Luce, J.M. *et al.* (2003). Quality indicators for end-of-life care in the intensive care unit (2003). *Critical Care Medicine*, **31**, 2255–62.

44. Chaitin, E., and Arnold, R.M. (2007). Communication in the ICU: holding a family meeting. In *UpToDate* (ed. B.D. Rose). UpToDate, Waltham.

45. White, D.B., Braddock, C.H., Bereknei, S. *et al.* (2007). Toward shared decision making at the end of life in intensive care units. *Archives of Internal Medicine*, **167**, 461–7.

46. Curtis, J.R., Engelberg, R.A., Wenrich, M.D. *et al.* (2005). Missed opportunities during family conferences about end-of-life care in the intensive care unit. *American Journal of Respiratory and Critical Care Medicine*, **171**, 844–9.

47. Fins, J.J. (2006). Goals of care: end-of-life decisions. In *A palliative ethic of care: clinical wisdom at life's end*, pp. 129–32. Jones and Bartlett Publishers, Sudbury.

48. Christakis, N.A. (2001). *Death foretold: prophecy and prognosis in medical care*. The University of Chicago Press, Chicago.

49. Fins, J.J., and Solomon, M.Z. (2001). Communication in intensive care settings: The challenge of futility disputes. *Critical Care Medicine*, **29**, N10–5.

50. Pochard, F., Azoulay, E., Chevret, S. *et al.* (2001). Symptoms of anxiety and depression in family members of intensive care unit patients: ethical hypothesis regarding decision-making capacity. *Critical Care Medicine*, **29**, 1893–7.

51. Melltorp, G., and Nilstun, T. (1997). The difference between withholding and withdrawing life-sustaining treatment. *Intensive Care Medicine*, **23**, 1264–7.

52. Miller, F.G., Fins, J.J., and Snyder, L. (2000). Assisted suicide compared with refusal of treatment: a valid distinction? University of Pennsylvania Center for Bioethics Assisted Suicide Consensus Panel. *Annals of Internal Medicine*, **132**, 470–5.

53. Teno, J.M., Licks, S., and Lynn, J. (1997). Do advance directives provide instructions that direct care? *Journal of the American Geriatrics Society*, **45**, 508–12.

54. Campbell, M.L. (1995). Interpretation of an ambiguous advance directive. *Dimensions of Critical Care Nursing*, **14**, 226–32.

55. Kemp, K.R., Emmons, E., and Hayes, J. (2004). Advance directives and do-not-resuscitate orders on general medical wards versus the intensive care unit. *Military Medicine*, **169**, 443–6.

56. The SUPPORT Investigators (1995). A controlled trial to improve care for seriously ill hospitalized patients: the Study to Understand Prognoses and Preferences for Outcomes and Risks of Treatment (SUPPORT). *JAMA*, **274**, 1591–8.

57. Shalowitz, D.I., Garrett-Mayer, E., and Wendler, D. (2006). The accuracy of surrogate decision makers. *Archives of Internal Medicine*, **166**, 493–7.

58. Singer, P.A., Martin, D.K., Lavery, J.V. *et al.* (1997). Reconceptualizing advance care planning from the patient's perspective. *Archives of Internal Medicine*, **158**, 879–84.

59. Fins, J.J., Maltby, B.S., Friedmann, E. *et al.* (2005). Contracts, covenants and advance care planning: an empirical study of the moral obligations of patient and proxy. *Journal of Pain and Symptom Management*, **29**, 55–68.

60. Fins, J.J. (1999). From contract to covenant in advance care planning. *The Journal of Law, Medicine & Ethics*, **27**, 46–51.

61. Fins, J.J. (2006). Goals of care: end-of-life decisions. In *A palliative ethic of care: Clinical wisdom at life's end*, p. 131. Jones and Bartlett Publishers, Sudbury.

62. http://www.vatican.va/holy_father/john_paul_ii/speeches/2004/march/documents/hf_jp-ii_spe_20040320_congress-fiamc_en.html. Accessed 18 December 2006.

63. Clemency, M.V., and Thompson, N.J. (1993). 'Do Not Resuscitate' (DNR) orders and the anesthesiologist: a survey. *Anesthesia and Analgesia*, **76**, 394–401.

64. Cohen, C.B., and Cohen, P.J. (1991). Do-not-resuscitate orders in the operating room. *The New England Journal of Medicine*, **325**, 1879–82.

65. Statement of the American College of Surgeons on Advance Directives by Patients: 'Do Not Resuscitate' in the OR (1994). *ACS Bulletin*, September, 29.

66. Cohen, L.M., Steinman, T.I., and Robinson, W.M. (2004). Ending dialysis: new perspectives on end-of-life considerations. *Medical Ethics*, **11**, 5–8.

67. Berger, J.T. (2005). The ethics of deactivating an implanted Cardioverter Defibrillator. *Annals of Internal Medicine*, **142**, 631–4.

68. Goldstein, N.E., Lampert, R., Bradley, E. *et al.* (2004). Management of implantable cardioverter defibrillators in end-of-life care. *Annals of Internal Medicine*, **141**, 835–8.

69. Meuller, P.S., Hook, C., and Hayes, D.L. (2003). Ethical analysis of withdrawal of pacemaker or implantable cardioverter-defibrillator support at the end-of-life. *Mayo Clinic Proceedings*, **78**, 959–63.

70. Much of this section is drawn from: Fins, J.J. (2006). End-of-Life care in the hospital. In *A palliative ethic of care: clinical wisdom at life's end*, pp. 77–86. Jones and Bartlett Publishers, Sudbury.

71. Schneiderman, L.J., Jecker, N.S., and Jonsen, A. (1990). Medical futility: its meaning and ethical implications. *Annals of Internal Medicine*, **112**, 949–54.

72. Jecker, N.S., and Schneiderman, L.J. (1992). Futility and rationing. *The American Journal of Medicine*, **92**, 189–96.

73. Consensus statement of the Society of Critical Care Medicine's Ethics Committee regarding futile and other possibly inadvisable treatments (1997). *Critical Care Medicine*, **25**, 887–91.

74. Younger, S.J. (1988). Who defines futility? *JAMA*, **260**, 2094–5.

75. Schneiderman, L.J. (1994). The futility debate: effective versus beneficial intervention. *Journal of the American Geriatrics Society*, **42**, 883–74.

76. Veatch, R.M. (1994). Why physicians cannot determine if care is futile. *Journal of the American Geriatrics Society*, **42**, 871–4.

77. Tomlinson, T., and Brody, H. (1990). Futility and the ethics of resuscitation. *JAMA*, **264**, 1276–80.

78. Brody, H. (1994). The physician's role in determining futility. *Journal of the American Geriatrics Society*, **42**, 875–8.

79. American Thoracic Society guidelines: withholding and withdrawing life-sustaining therapy (1991). *The American Review of Respiratory Disease*, **144**, 726–31.

80. Schneiderman, L.J., Gilmer, T., Teetzel, H.D. *et al.* (2003). Effects of ethics consultation on nonbeneficial life-sustaining treatments in the intensive care setting. *JAMA*, **290**, 1166–72.

81. Dowdy, M.D., Robertson, C., and Bander, J.A. (1998). A study of proactive ethics consultation for critically and terminally ill patients with extended lengths of stay. *Critical Care Medicine*, **26**, 252–9.

82. Agrawal, S.K., and Fins, J.J. (2003). Ethics committees and case consultation in the hospital setting. In *A Guide to Hospitals and Inpatient Care* (eds. E. Siegler, S. Mirafzali, and J.B. Foust), pp. 256–67. Springer, New York.

SECTION 6

Communication and palliative medicine

Communication with the patient and family in palliative medicine

Lesley Fallowfield

Introduction

Talking about sad, bad, and difficult things with patients and their families is a fundamental and an inevitable part of the health-care professional's (HCPs) work, but one in which few have received sufficient help or training.[1,2] In efforts to protect patients from uncomfortable and distressing facts, doctors and nurses frequently censor their information giving in the mistaken belief that what someone does not know does not harm them. This misguided albeit well-intentioned assumption is made at all stages of the disease trajectory. Less-than-honest disclosure is apparent when a patient first reports suspicious symptoms, at confirmation of the diagnosis, when the putative therapeutic benefits of treatment are discussed, at recurrence or relapse, and towards the end of life. Most attempts by doctors to protect patients from the reality of their situation often create further problems to patients, their relatives, and their friends. Furthermore, it can lead to inconsistent messages being given by other members of the multi-disciplinary team. Economy with the truth often leads to conspiracies of silence that usually build up to a heightened state of fear, anxiety, and confusion, rather than one of calmness and equanimity. The kinds of ambiguous or deliberately misleading messages received by patients may afford them short-term benefits while things continue to go well, but it has unfortunate long-term consequences. A patient with a shortened or uncertain future needs time and space to reorganize and adapt their life towards the attainment of achievable goals. Realistic hopes and aspirations can only be generated from honest disclosure. In this chapter, evidence from research studies will be provided showing that although communicating the truth can be painful, deceit may well provoke greater problems.[3] Some suggestions will also be made about practical ways to communicate about difficult issues in palliative care.

Good palliative care presents substantial clinical, nursing, communication, and emotional challenges for all HCPs. If accomplished well, palliative care can also offer tangible, satisfying, professional and personal benefits. It might well be assumed that a speciality dealing with the care of dying people would appeal to those who possess not only good clinical and communication skills but also attitudes and beliefs compatible with an openness towards honest disclosure and truth-telling. Although the skills required for the provision of physical care may be excellent, effective communication is often less well-honed. Questionable approaches towards honest disclosure may be the consequence of poor training or may represent unawareness of the impact that dishonesty has on patients; it may also demonstrate genuine differences in cultural expectations. For example, Bruera *et al.* conducted an interesting postal survey which examined the attitudes and beliefs of palliative care specialists towards communication with the terminally ill.[4] Respondents were based in French-speaking Europe, South America (Argentina and Brazil), and Canada. Every clinician said that they would like to be told the truth about their own terminal illness. However, only 93 per cent of Canadian physicians, 26 per cent of European clinicians, and 18 per cent of South American clinicians thought that the majority of their patients would wish to know ($P = 0.001$). Similar attitudes prevailed when clinicians were asked to estimate how many relatives would want patients to know about the terminal nature of their illness. Clearly what clinicians *think* that their patients want and what the patients and their families *actually* want is often very different. The evidence for really substantial cultural differences regarding patients' actual rather than assumed information needs about prognosis is in fact rather thin or inconclusive. For example, well-conducted studies by Fielding and Hung in Hong Kong challenge the notion that Asian patients with cancer and their families want less information than their Western counterparts.[5] There are some studies however that suggest that different cultures may cope with the diagnosis of life-threatening disease in different ways. One such study showed that after being told their diagnosis Asian patients were significantly more fatalistic ($P < 0.0001$) than white Caucasian patients and had more significant hopeless/helpless scores ($P = 0.007$) on the Mental Adjustment to Cancer Scale. Asian patients were also more likely to agree with the statement 'I don't really believe that I have cancer' ($P = 0.019$). Denial was significantly related to depression and anxiety but the study did seem to suggest that Caucasian patients appear to adapt to the psychological trauma of a cancer diagnosis more successfully than Asian patients at the initial interview.[6] A vital clinical point to make is that HCPs should make concerted efforts to base their communication on an individual's expressed preference, whatever their cultural background, and not make assumptions about the needs of different ethnic groups.

Information needs of patients and their families

It is of course important to determine the information needs of patients if people are to be able to give informed consent and make educated decisions. Their future management might include further treatment options or participation in Phase I trials, but people cannot contribute to these decisions if they lack the necessary information. A recent review of studies looking at communication and informed consent in Phase I trials showed that many patients had limited understanding of the trial purpose, an unrealistic expectation of the benefits and risks of participation, and a questionable appreciation of their right to abstain or withdraw.[7] Patients desperate and hopeful for a miracle cure may not recognize that the primary aims of many Phase I studies are dose escalation and clinicians can unwittingly be somewhat ambiguous about likely therapeutic gains of participation. Good palliative and supportive care is rarely presented as a positive option, instead it can be seen by patients and their families as 'giving up' or 'giving in' rather than bravely fighting on with further active interventions. Doctors therefore need to consider carefully the manner in which options are discussed.

Truthful communication about the future is also vital if patients are to be permitted the dignity of deciding how to spend their remaining time. Unfortunately, doctors worldwide seriously underestimate not only the information needs of their patients but also their preferences about decision-making.[8] As seen in a recent systematic review,[9] some patients express a desire for more limited information at different time points during the course of their disease, but they represent the minority, most want considerably more than they are given. Research conducted in the United Kingdom by Jenkins *et al.* with a large heterogeneous sample of 2331 patients with cancer showed that 2027 (87 per cent) wanted all possible information, be that good or bad news.[10] A subsequent more recent audit by this group examining information needs and actual experiences of a different group of patients revealed multiple gaps in information provision despite a strong desire for information expressed by around 87 per cent irrespective of age, sex, tumour site, or stage of disease.[11] It interesting that the figures seem to be fairly consistent across different heterogeneous samples of patients with cancer in both these studies. Similarly, a study of the parents of children with cancer showed that 87 per cent wanted as much information as possible about prognosis.[12]

Some doctors argue that honest disclosure is reasonable in patients for whom cure is a realistic prospect but that when the outlook is bleak then they are less likely to provide full information. Results from an extension to the study by Jenkins *et al.* make this position untenable.[13] They compared the general information preferences of 1032 palliative treated patients with those of 1777 patients receiving potentially curative treatment or who were in remission. Irrespective of treatment intent, the overwhelming majority of patients expressed a preference for the doctor to give as much information as possible, be that good or bad news. Slightly more of the palliatively treated patients (7.3 per cent) than the non-palliative group (3.9 per cent) wanted additional information only if it was good news ($P < 0.001$) although the numbers of patients overall who endorsed this option were very small (144/2809). Little difference was found when the more specific information needs of palliative and non-palliative groups were compared (see Table 6.1.1), although there were some interesting sex differences. In general, women wanted more information than men for most items ($P < 0.01$), although both men and women had an equal need to know whether or not it was cancer and what the chances of cure were. Among the palliatively treated patients the sex differences disappeared, with the majority of men and women wanting the same sorts of information apart from the chances of cure, where again more women than men wanted this information ($P = 0.021$).

The effect of age was also examined; in general, younger patients under 65 years wanted more information than those over 65 ($P < 0.01$) apart from knowing their chances of cure, where needs were the same irrespective of age. Among the palliatively treated patients, more of the younger people wished to know about the specific name of the cancer they had, what all possible treatments were, and how any treatments worked ($P < 0.01$).

Appraisal of these results suggests that the intuitive censoring of information that many doctors engage in on the grounds that patients prefer not to know is unfounded. Patients may feel isolated and scared that nothing can or will be done to help them if doctors fail to give adequate information about test results, potential ways of managing symptoms, and the true therapeutic aim of different treatments. Precisely at a time when the majority of people are most in need of truthful communication and support, when

Table 6.1.1 Specific information preferences of patients with cancer.

	Absolutely need/would like to have (per cent)		Do not want information (per cent)	
	Palliative	**Non-palliative**	**Palliative**	**Non-palliative**
Specific name of the illness	87	91	13	9
Whether or not it is cancer	98	98	2	2
Week-by-week progress	90	93	10	7
Chances of cure	93	97	7	3
All possible treatments	94	95	6	5
All possible side effects	97	97	3	3
How treatment works	91	93	9	7

they have changing thoughts and feelings and need to make important decisions, a conspiracy of silence may envelop them, and the resulting anxiety and tension may hinder adjustment.

Decision-making preferences of patients in palliative care

As we have seen, patients want considerably more information than is often provided to enable them to understand the logic behind treatment recommendations made by HCPs, but how involved do they wish to be in decision-making? Desire for more information and actual participation in decision-making are not one and the same thing.[14] Certainly, in the non-palliative setting there is a large body of evidence suggesting that for women newly diagnosed with breast cancer, many wished to assume a more passive role in decision-making than a general population sample or women with benign breast disease, who tended to prefer more active or collaborative roles.[15,16] Importantly, this research has also revealed how poor doctors often are at recognizing which patients desire active or more passive roles.[17]

The iterative process of discussion and information exchange which forms the basis for shared decision-making is often somewhat lacking in early stage disease and in palliative care has received less attention.[18] In one study of 78 patients in a palliative setting, the concordance between clinicians' perceptions of their patients' preferences and patients' actual perceptions showed that only 38 per cent of the cases matched. The clinicians tended to underestimate patients' desire for more shared decision-making. Patients' age or sex had no influence on the accuracy of prediction.[8] More recently researchers examined the way 102 breast cancer patients perceived their decisions about embarking on palliative chemotherapy.[19] The medical oncologist was seen as the most important person influencing decision-making. Forty-seven per cent of women preferred a passive role, 15 per cent a shared role, and 38 per cent an active role. As with other studies age, ethnicity, education and partnership status did not predict preferences but interestingly patients discussing second-line therapy were more likely to wish for an active role. As doctors manifestly lack the skills to identify patient preferences accurately, it would seem sensible for a clinic nurse to assess this prospectively prior to the patient meeting with the doctor. Card sort techniques such as those described by Degner and Sloan are an effective means of ensuring that patient preferences are met.[15] One cautionary note, however, is that preferences may well change over time as disease progresses, thus decision-making preferences need to be checked regularly as the coping strategies employed by patients are more dynamic and adaptive than is sometimes thought.[20]

Communication and stress experienced by families

When patients become progressively sicker and increasingly dependent as they approach the end of their lives, different family members may have to assume responsibility for many of the roles fulfilled previously by their ill relative such as household tasks or caring for children. The primary carer may also have less time to spend with other family members, all of whom may also have to help out in the home or with caring for the dying person.[21] Coping with conditions such as incontinence can also be difficult for both the carers and the now dependent ill person.[22] Witnessing pain and the alterations in physical appearance or personality of a loved one can also be deeply distressing. Thus, the whole family can become stressed by the emotional burdens and extra responsibilities placed on them. The changed dynamics of family life can be exhausting, as well as upsetting. Some carers feel so worn down by the daily demands that feelings of despair, depression, and resentment are very common. In an interesting retrospective questionnaire based study of 379 relatives (spouses and children) of people who had recently died, many respondents felt that they had had limited opportunities to talk to any professional carers about the difficulties they had experienced with everyday life whilst their relative was dying.[23] Other studies have shown that the factors considered important to patients and families may differ considerably from those viewed as important by health-care professionals, hence the need to communicate well and check what is required rather than just assume needs are being met.[24]

Emotional impact of communication in palliative care on doctors and nurses

There is a wealth of evidence suggesting that a reluctance to give bad and sad news probably reflects the difficulty that doctors experience conveying this type of information as much as a desire to protect patients from the distress such knowledge provokes.[1,2,13] Some of the reasons why doctors and nurses have problems with this area can be seen in Table 6.1.2.

Inadequate communication skills

In the course of a professional career spanning perhaps 40 years, an oncologist in the United Kingdom is likely to conduct around 150 000–200 000 interviews with patients and their families. Thus, communication is a core clinical skill, yet one in which few doctors have received much useful training.[25] Many are aware that this lack of training contributes to their own stress and burnout.[26] Among palliative care physicians in the United Kingdom 32 per cent said that they felt insufficiently trained in communication.[27] The good news is that properly structured, intensive communication skills courses employing cognitive, behavioural, and affective components have been shown in a randomized trial to significantly improve cancer doctors' skills in clinics.[28] Following the course, doctors adopted a more patient-centred approach, used more open-ended questioning, displayed more empathy, responded more appropriately to patients' cues, and used fewer leading questions. Furthermore, they also changed their attitudes and beliefs about the importance of communicating in this way[29] which led to the transfer of these skills into clinics. This model of

Table 6.1.2 Some reasons for doctors' problems.

Inadequate skills due to poor training
Fear of provoking emotional distress
Not knowing how to handle an emotional outburst
Worries about containing one's own emotions
Fear of being blamed by patients and relatives for failure
Over identification with certain patients
Having to confront one's own fears about death

training has also been shown to have an enduring impact with maintenance of skills at 15 months post-training.[30]

Nurses experience similar communication difficulties to those found in doctors and also complain about inadequate training. Few, just like the doctors involved in cancer care, have received much useful formal training in basic interviewing, assessment, and counselling skills. Some find their position even more stressful when patients are given conflicting information about the diagnosis by doctors in the care team.[31,32] Research looking at the skills of hospice nurses revealed a disturbing level of blocking behaviours, especially when patients needed to talk about psychological concerns.[33,34] Nurses also appear to benefit from further communication skills training courses in terms of improved attitudes, confidence, and skills.[35,36] One interesting randomized study showed that post-training, nurses had more overt empathy with an increased use of emotionally focused communication.[37]

Fear of provoking distress and handling difficult emotions

Breaking bad news and talking about advanced disease and death will invariably provoke some emotional response from patients and whoever else is present. Most HCPs fear extreme expression of emotion and tears although some report withdrawn, stunned silence as even more challenging.[4] Some doctors assume that the nursing staff are more capable than they are in this type of situation and are therefore the best people to leave distressed patients and relatives with following a difficult interview. However, dealing with emotional reactions was perceived as the most difficult communication challenge for 46 per cent of senior oncology nurses.[31] Learning how to manage the expression of emotion by others and in ourselves is of paramount importance if HCPs are to be honest but supportive bearers of bad news.

Containing one's own emotions

Becoming emotionally close to patients is inevitable for many of us working within the so-called caring profession and has a cost. Worries about becoming upset ourselves often inhibit expression of ordinary kindness and compassion towards a distressed patient. It is not always wrong to display some emotion, in some situations it has been shown to be of value. Grieving parents just told about the death of a child appreciated those who looked moved or who shed a tear with them.[38] Nevertheless, many doctors invest considerable energy cultivating a posture of cool detachment on the grounds that it represents the more professional type of response expected of doctors. Unfortunately, patients and relatives can view this detached attitude as evasive, cold, and unsympathetic, occurring at just the time that they are in much need of empathy and support. Whilst no one would be helped by an hysterical, weeping nurse or doctor, I have yet to hear of a complaint that the doctor looked too concerned and tearful, whereas reports of cold indifference are heard frequently.

Being blamed for failure, over-identification, and confronting one's own death fears

In most Western cultures there is an inclination 'to deny death altogether and celebrate new forms of technology designed to forestall death'.[39] Not only lay populations but also doctors themselves often harbour quite unrealistic expectations about the therapeutic benefits of modern medicine, consequently anything other than cure can feel like failure. Some HCPs retreat from truthful disclosure if treatment has been less successful than was hoped; it is as though they still lived in ancient times when the bearer of the bad news that a battle had been lost would be executed. Younger, less-experienced doctors and nurses need opportunities to talk about these feelings in addition to being given training in how to deal with patients and families who react to bad news with anger and aggression, trying to find someone to blame.

Sometimes people who have difficulty accepting the inevitability of death engage in 'doing something behaviours'. For a family, this might involve dragging the hapless patient around the world in a quest to find a miracle cure. Doctors may continue with a treatment regimen that has very little prospect of alleviating symptoms or enhancing survival. As fanciful as this might seem it is a phenomenon in which the patient becomes a kind of 'talisman' for the doctor. It is a means of defying death by keeping people alive. These types of problems can influence the openness of communication in sometimes quite subtle ways and may be more obvious to an observer than to the doctor. Hoping against hope that things might just have a better outcome is more likely when the doctor identifies with the patient or the relatives. Awareness of how these issues influence and affect our communication is important.

Worldwide, most palliative care is provided by many different HCPs many of whom may not be palliative care specialists. Surgeons, medical and radiation oncologists, haematologists, chest physicians, dermatologists, and others will all see patients for whom curative treatment is not a realistic prospect, and many of these clinicians feel neither confident nor competent when communicating with patients seen as 'therapeutic failures'. Sadly, unless the cure rates for most of the common solid tumours increases considerably, a majority of oncologists will spend the bulk of their clinical careers discussing palliation with patients and their families. Thus, knowing how to pace and tailor communication about difficult issues appropriately should be a prerequisite for anyone working in the field of cancer. But, in palliation, few find this an easy or even satisfying task.

As part of a randomized trial of a communication skills training,[28] clinicians were asked to rate on a visual analogue scale, their satisfaction with their consultations immediately after patients had left the room. Mean satisfaction following 1039 palliative care consultations was significantly lower ($P < 0.0001$) than that following the 1768 consultations about active curative treatment or remission.[13]

During previous communication skills courses, informing patients about the withdrawal of active, curative treatment and discussing palliation instead was seen as a major source of stress for senior clinicians in cancer medicine.[25] Participants self-rated their confidence on a 10-cm visual analogue scale to items such as 'telling patients that you are replacing active therapy with symptomatic care only'. Mean rating was 5.76 cm and low when compared with, for example, 'telling patients they have a recurrence' (6.62 cm) or 'discussing side effects of treatment' (7.28 cm). The doctor's unease is often picked up leading to further anxiety, distress, and feelings of abandonment by patients.

Effects of minimization or ambiguity

If doctors are uncomfortable with handling transitions, then they may minimize the significance of test results or the true therapeutic aims of treatment, thus denying patients opportunities to make plans and utilize whatever time is left. Examples of this captured on audiotape and videotape in our research include the following examples: a patient with multiple myeloma who had benefited from only a few months' remission following high-dose chemotherapy, bone marrow transplantation, and maintenance interferon became very upset when told that tests confirmed relapse. In response to the patient's manifest distress the doctor said 'there's only a small amount of Bence Jones protein in your urine', thus implying that things were not really too bad. We have also heard several doctors talking about 'a few hot spots on bone scans', the significance of which was lost on patients when interviewed by us later. At times, communication is so ambiguous, oblique, or incomplete that patients are ill-prepared for the future and adjustment is impaired.[40] The following quotes reveal unfortunate examples of this. In the first a woman with metastatic breast cancer reported that her doctor had said, 'Take the tamoxifen, that'll hold it … it's quite simple to have your lung drained'. She then commented that they had talked of only 'evidence of secondaries in the lung', which she presumed meant that things were 'hopefully not too bad'. She died 9 weeks after this interview from her lung metastases.

The next example shows the interaction between a doctor and an elderly man with lung cancer before his expected third cycle of chemotherapy:

Doctor: As you may remember when we first started this chemotherapy, we told you that we would check your blood and X-rays before each cycle. I have looked at your tests today and there are signs that things are progressing so we do not think that you should have any more chemotherapy.
Patient: Oh! So what happens now then?
Doctor: Well, we just want you to come and see us if you develop any further problems with the breathing and we'll treat those symptoms.
Patient: Right then, well thank you very much doctor.

Immediately after this consultation, the patient was asked by a researcher what he remembered, he said, 'well it's good news really … the doctor thinks things are progressing so I don't need any more chemo and to just come back if my breathing starts up again … getting breathless you know'.

This scenario illustrates another problem to add to the difficulty that many have even discussing palliation, namely ambiguity. Words and phrases such as 'things are progressing' or 'positive' and 'negative' nodes have the opposite meanings when used in a lay rather than medical context.[41] It is so important to check exactly what patients have understood before the consultation ends, as studies reveal that there are often major discrepancies between what doctors think they have said and what the patient has actually heard or understood. This calls into question the veracity of any consent given for treatment.

Consultations were tape-recorded in a report from Australia in which 118 patients with incurable cancer were seeing one of nine oncologists for a first consultation about their disease.[42] Although the majority (84.7 per cent) were told about the aim of chemotherapy, 25.4 per cent were not explicitly told their cancer was incurable, and 42.4 per cent were not told their likely prognosis. Alternatives to embarking on anticancer therapy were only presented to 44.1 per cent, and only 36.4 per cent were told about side effects likely to impinge on quality of life. Choices about management were not offered to 69.3 per cent, and patient understanding was checked in only 10.2 per cent of consultations. Greater information disclosure was not related to anxiety but greater participation in decision-making was. It is interesting to speculate whether or not the decisional conflict and anxiety experienced by some patients was due to incomplete understanding about treatment. People cannot make decisions if they lack vital information about the available options.

Despite doctors' genuine lack of awareness that sometimes they have seriously misled or confused patients, others admit to using misleading and euphemistic terminology and justify this with arguments that patients do not really want to know the truth when things are bad. The data regarding patient information preferences described earlier point to the fallacy of this position.

Doctors' styles of communication

Whatever verbal communication takes place there is a necessity to ensure the congruency of this with any non-verbal messages. Facial expressions, manner, and tone of voice may reinforce or refute the intended meaning. How things are said is often as important as what is said. Doctors do have very different communication styles; some are helpful, others merely exacerbate their patients' difficulties. Patients' views about their doctors when discussing the transition from curative to palliative care were investigated in an interesting Swedish study.[43] Six categories of doctor were identified from a qualitative analysis of semi-structured interviews: the inexperienced messenger, the emotionally burdened, the rough and ready expert, the benevolent but tactless expert, the distanced doctor, and the empathic professional. The patients stressed how much their ability to cope with the information depended on their relationship with the doctor. As doctors acknowledge so many personal difficulties and barriers when communicating within this area, there is a clear need for improved training opportunities. Unless taught a patient-centred, biopsychosocial approach of relating to and talking with patients, doctors may be oblivious to the impact that their communication has on patients or feel helpless when trying to be appropriately supportive and to lessen the blow of bad news.

Discussing prognosis (see also Chapter 3.3)

We have already seen examples of less-than-honest disclosure, but problems for patients and their families are compounded further by doctors' reluctance to prognosticate; they rarely initiate discussions about prognosis and are often evasive even if the patient is brave enough to ask. No one would deny that this is a tricky topic as many cancers do have uncertain outcomes making prediction difficult. One study investigated the responses of 968 physicians to the question 'when a patient is labelled "terminal" approximately how many weeks should the patient have left to live?'. Answers ranged from 0–26 weeks with fewer than 1 per cent thinking that this was less than a week.[44] The study also highlighted differences in estimates between primary care physicians and hospital doctors which could cause further confusion for a patient and their family trying to make decisions such as when to embark on hospice care. Doctors may feel so insecure and lacking in confidence when predicting how long someone might live that they try to avoid doing it at all. Failure to talk about such important issues arises for more complex reasons than mere uncertainty and inaccuracy about the likely course of the disease. Many studies have been reported in which doctors' ability to predict survival of patients with cancer was examined. In one of the earliest, using a liberal interpretation of prediction accuracy, that is no more than twice and no less than half the actual duration of survival, 53 per cent of predictions were wrong. For the majority of these inaccuracies (90 per cent), the direction of error was for an optimistic rather than a pessimistic prediction, showing a propensity for overestimation rather than for underestimation of survival.[45]

Many more recent publications have substantiated Parkes original studies showing that things have not changed much despite better diagnostic tools, so we need to look for other reasons for this.[46–48] Over identification with patients can have negative effects and research also shows that the better the doctor knows the patient in terms of the length and intensity of their contact, the more likely they are to overestimate survival.[49] Doctors may need to hope against hope that things are better than they really are and this becomes more evident if the doctor has built up a close relationship with the patient. This also provides a partial explanation as to why doctors may promote further toxic treatment regimens for patients that have very little prospect of benefit, rather than have an honest discussion about supportive care.

Extending further the arguments first expressed by Hippocrates,[50] Lamont and Christakis[51] have described how patients may unwittingly become 'twice removed' from the truth about their illness. Disclosure of prognosis is conceptualized as comprising two distinct elements, those of foreseeing and foretelling. Foreseeing can be defined as the unexpressed cognitive estimate or prediction that a doctor may make about a patient's likely survival, which we know is inclined to be optimistic. Foretelling is the communication about this with a patient which we know may be liable to conscious and accidental ambiguity or deliberate evasion. So the 'twice removed patient' can end up with a wildly inaccurate estimation of their likely survival and consequently are unable to prepare appropriately for the future. As a systematic review argued, unless doctors can predict accurately and communicate these predictions sensitively and accurately, patients and their families cannot make sensible and appropriate decisions about therapy, phase 1 trial participation or place of death.[52]

Effect on patients of truth about prognosis

'Rare are the cases where making or offering a carefully considered and framed prognosis results in choices that are harmful to the patient … As a result of a failure to prognosticate, let alone prognosticate accurately, patients may die deaths they deplore in locations they despise. They may seek noxious chemotherapy rather than good palliative care, enrol in clinical trials of experimental therapy that offer more benefit to the researchers than to themselves, or reassure loved ones that it is not yet time to pay a visit only to lapse into a coma before there is time to say goodbye.'[49]

An argument is frequently made that most patients should not be told the truth about their prognosis as they will lose hope, become overwhelmed with an immobilizing depression, and not enjoy whatever time is left. Little hard evidence exists to support this position; in fact it is more likely that misguided evasion or frank dishonesty may add considerably to a patient's distress and prolong the necessary adjustment process.[53] If potentially distressing disclosures to patients are avoided then we give patients no opportunities to reveal their own fears and worries. This can leave them in anxiety-ridden isolation, convinced that the most unspeakably horrible fate awaits them. The uninformed patient may construct a scenario that bears little relationship to their likely demise.

Dealing with the misinformed patient

The palliative care team can find themselves dealing with a great deal of hostility and anger from patients and families who feel that they were never given honest information by HCPs involved earlier on in their care. They may feel that the choices and decisions that were made about therapeutic options were based on inaccurate or overoptimistic advice. The patient who feels very strongly that they were misled is unlikely to trust the new team members trying to offer reassurances about symptomatic care. Considerable investment in relationship-building skills is needed if the patient and relatives are going to develop the important degree of trust that will ease the physical and emotional pains that lie ahead. Discussion about why different outcomes to those hoped for have arisen is important and can sometimes be enough to correct some of the misunderstandings. However, familiarity with the official complaints procedure for the really angry person might be needed. Above all, recognition that the anger might be justified and that it may be the only way that some people have of expressing their distress and disappointment is required. Accurate documentation in hospital records about who said what to whom and when is obviously useful as are satisfactory communication channels with the multi-disciplinary team in order to provide feedback to others about what has happened and to perhaps avoid such situations in the future.

Anxiety and depression (see Chapter 15.5)

Although avoidance of communication about advanced disease does not protect patients from experiencing considerable psychological distress, palliative care patients certainly do have significantly higher psychological morbidity than other patients with curable cancer. It is a sorry fact that much of this often goes unrecognized and therefore untreated. In the United Kingdom, 2850 patients were given the General Health Questionnaire (GHQ12) and 837 (36.4 per cent) had scores suggestive of psychological morbidity.[54]

The 1046 palliative patients were more likely than other patients to have high GHQ scores ($P < 0.0001$). The ability of the clinicians to detect this probable morbidity was low overall but there were some interesting differences. The clinicians' true positive (sensitivity) rates were higher for their palliative patients than for their other patients. Unfortunately, their specificity (true negative) rates were lower and misclassification rates greater. At least 408/1046 palliative patients were either thought to have significant psychological morbidity when they did not, or were thought to be psychologically well when they needed some extra help. One interpretation of these findings is that doctors nihilistically assume that people with incurable disease will be psychologically distressed. Doctors then lack the communication skills to determine how patients are coping. Unfortunately there was very little evidence of psychosocial probing during consultations which might permit more accurate assessment and referral on to appropriate support services.

Palliation should include treatment and amelioration of all symptoms including psychological ones. There is increasing evidence from well-conducted trials that psychosocial interventions are effective with adult cancer patients.[55] Assuming that the institutions where patients are being treated have access to psychological services, it is vital that clinicians are trained in basic skills to determine which patients need help. Screening patients with validated questionnaires prior to seeing the doctor might improve detection rates.

Communication needs of the family

The most important source of psychological and physical support for most patients is likely to be a family member. Encouraging a good therapeutic alliance with partners and carers is therefore vital. Many HCPs find communicating with dying or seriously ill patients less stressful than that with relatives who can appear threatening, obstructive, and hard to deal with. However, much of the difficulty can be managed or at least understood if one steps back a pace and considers the enormous strain and stress that carers have to shoulder. Some family members can look more ill and care-worn than their dying relative as a result of the increased pressures, new roles, and expectations placed upon them.

Most HCPs will at some stage have to cope with families who wish them to conceal the truth from their dying relative on the grounds that they would not be able to take it and would suffer unnecessarily. This is always hard to manage but families need help understanding that there is little or no convincing evidence supporting the contention that terminally ill patients who have not been told the truth of their situation die happily in blissful ignorance. A dying person witnesses their deteriorating body, fatigue, and reduction in ability to function.

Concealment of the truth is rarely achievable as relatives, friends, and HCPs find it hard not to give out non-verbal clues as to what is happening. The hollow cheerfulness and feigned optimism about quite unrealistic future goals are excruciating to witness, as are the anxious and stressed expressions on faces of people trying to maintain a lie. Particularly upsetting is watching families, who have not been gently helped to confront reality, locked into stilted discussions about trivia or frozen in silence. Facilitating opportunities for partners to discuss death with each other demands tact and skill and there may occasionally be exceptional circumstances where it might not be appropriate but these exceptions are rare. Collusion with relatives of dying patients in an attempt to sustain the myth of immortality is an abrogation of our responsibility to assist patients through the stages that might be needed for people to achieve a calm acceptance and more serene and dignified death. Additionally the inability to talk through death leaves much 'unfinished business' which relatives can bitterly regret later.

Just as families may wish to stop their loved ones from learning the sad fact that they are dying, occasionally patients themselves may ask that their relatives are not told the truth. This is a tricky situation as from an ethical standpoint, if conscious, the patient does have the right of confidentiality. Family dynamics can be hard to understand but the legal next of kin may not actually be the person from whom the patient has derived most support during their life. As well as 'protecting' relatives from the hurtful news of impending death, a desire to withhold this information can be the last defiant and punitive act left to a person. The only real suggestion that can be offered in such circumstances, although this is not based on any empirical evidence, is to try and find out why the patient feels so reluctant to share the knowledge about impending death with their relative. It might help to point out that a failure to reveal the truth and to discuss the subject with relatives might mean that the patient's wishes about such things as funeral service, burial, or wishes about their estate and will are not handled appropriately. Also it might prevent reconciliation of old enmities. The services of a family therapist, social worker, or clinical psychologist might be invaluable.

Practical ways to help with information provision and communication

Assuming that HCPs accept the ethical imperative that they should at all times aim for supportive, honest disclosure, what other aids are there to assist patients and their families with the assimilation of difficult information?

Audiotapes

Many doctors provide cancer patients with tape-recordings of their consultations as an aid to improving recall and satisfaction. One group of researchers in the UK suggested that although audiotapes helped retention of information it did not reliably reduce psychological distress and could be unhelpful to some patients with a poor prognosis.[56] Another RCT conducted in North America examined the efficacy of an audiotaped recording of the consultation with a palliative care team in addition to written information for 60 patients with advanced disease. The audiocassette with written information significantly improved overall satisfaction with the clinic and recall of information given during the consultation. Patients expressed a high level of satisfaction with the tape which was also valued by family members and friends.[57]

Written material

Although verbal communication should be the primary method for transfer of information for patient education, written materials are useful adjuncts for some patients and their families. Patients can drown under a sea of paper, however, and may need guidance seeking out the most appropriate aids for them, in particular, information about reliable websites. Excellent materials in the form of booklets and leaflets are available from Cancerbackup in the United Kingdom and from their website. For individual HCPs and organizations wishing to produce more locally relevant informational aids, the Centre for Health Information Quality (CHQ) has a useful set of guides for developing readable information using a tool known as DISCERN.[58,59] The King's Fund in London also has an excellent guide called the practicalities of producing patient information (POPPI) developed with help from CHiQ and the Plain English Forum.

Prompt sheets

Some researchers have investigated the utility of prompt sheets for patients before they see the doctor in an attempt to facilitate greater participation and asking of questions. There were concerns that this would merely increase the numbers of questions asked without necessarily helping patients to discuss those topics of most concern and relevance to them. In a carefully conducted series of studies Clayton *et al.* in Australia involved 19 patients, 24 carers, and 22 palliative care professionals in the design of a question prompt list (QPL).

Interviews with participants identified 112 potential questions grouped under eight categories. After testing it was clear that patients and carers valued the QPL and that it reduced anxiety in 16/19 patients. Health-care professionals had been concerned about the inclusion of end-of-life issues but this topic was endorsed by the patients.[60] A recent randomized trial of the QPL compared communication in 92 patients and carers given the QPL with 82 controls.[61] Those in the intervention group asked significantly more questions in particular they asked for more prognostic information and about end-of-life issues. The group with the QPL had fewer unmet information needs about the future and about end-of-life issues than controls. Prompt sheets are a cheap and easy intervention in a palliative setting where patients and families may not know what to ask or be too frightened to do so.

Websites and experiences of other patients

Much confusion can be caused by unreliable websites providing information which is at best incorrect and worst downright harmful, especially dubious sources that exploit the neediness of desperate families with details about spurious, and usually expensive miracle cures. A notable exception in this confusing area is the innovative DIPEx group's website (http//:www.healthtalkonline. org). They have produced a user-friendly, easy to navigate site which shows a variety of interviews providing personal accounts of other peoples' experiences. The viewer can watch, listen to, or read these verbatims from individuals representing many different ages and backgrounds. The 'Living with dying' section contains 42 interviews with dying patients and carers. It also contains a host of other information including helpful tips about welfare benefits, community and palliative care, making wills, and talking to children.

It is worth checking with families if they have access to a computer and to help guide them to sites that offer sensible support and to monitor whether or not information on them is congruent with that given by the hospital or local palliative care team.

Conclusion

Honest communication is surely an ethical imperative for the truly caring clinician. Patients need to plan and make decisions about the place of their death, put their affairs in order, say goodbyes or forgive old adversaries, and be protected from embarking on futile therapies. All HCPs who work within an oncology or palliative care setting experience occasions when tough and distressing issues need to be discussed. Their behaviour and communication of caring and competence at this time have a major influence on the ability of patients and families to assimilate the news, consider options, and adapt and adjust to what lies ahead. Even if the news is gloomy the right touch, look, and supportive kind word always makes a difference. We know the effects that poor communication exerts but need to recognize that if patients are to receive optimal care then the training needs and emotional support required by HCPs cannot be ignored.

References

1. Fallowfield, L. (1993). Giving sad and bad news. *Lancet*, **341**(8843), 476–8.
2. Fallowfield, L. and Jenkins, V. (2004). Communicating sad, bad, and difficult news in medicine. *Lancet*, **363**(9405), 312–9.
3. Fallowfield, L. (1997). Truth sometimes hurts but deceit hurts more. *Annals of the New York Academy of Sciences*, **809**, 525–36.
4. Bruera, E., Neumann, C.M., Mazzocato, C. *et al.* (2000). Attitudes and beliefs of palliative care physicians regarding communication with terminally ill cancer patients. *Palliative Medicine*, **14**(4), 287–98.
5. Fielding, R. and Hung, J. (1996). Preferences for information and involvement in decisions during cancer care among a Hong Kong Chinese population. *Psychooncology*, **5**, 321–9.
6. Roy, R., Symonds, R.P., Kumar, D.M. *et al.* (2005). The use of denial in an ethnically diverse British cancer population: a cross-sectional study. *British Journal of Cancer*, **92**(8), 1393–7.
7. Cox, A.C., Fallowfield, L.J., and Jenkins, V.A. (2006). Communication and informed consent in phase 1 trials: a review of the literature. *Supportive Care in Cancer*, **14**(4), 303–9.
8. Bruera, E., Sweeney, C., Calder, K. *et al.* (2001). Patient preferences versus physician perceptions of treatment decisions in cancer care. *Journal of Clinical Oncology*, **19**(11), 2883–5.
9. Rutten, L.J., Arora, N.K., Bakos, A.D. *et al.* (2005). Information needs and sources of information among cancer patients: a systematic review of research (1980–2003). *Patient Education and Counseling*, **57**(3), 250–61.
10. Jenkins, V., Fallowfield, L., and Saul, J. (2001). Information needs of patients with cancer: results from a large study in UK cancer centres. *British Journal of Cancer*, **84**(1), 48–51.
11. Cox, A., Jenkins, V., Catt, S. *et al.* (2006). Information needs and experiences: an audit of UK cancer patients. *European Journal of Oncology Nursing*, **10**(4), 263–72.
12. Mack, J.W., Wolfe, J., Grier, H.E. *et al.* (2006). Communication about prognosis between parents and physicians of children with cancer: parent preferences and the impact of prognostic information. *Journal of Clinical Oncology*, **24**(33), 5265–70.
13. Fallowfield, L.J., Jenkins, V.A., and Beveridge, H.A. (2002). Truth may hurt but deceit hurts more: communication in palliative care. *Palliative Medicine*, **16**(4), 297–303.
14. Fallowfield, L. (2001). Participation of patients in decisions about treatment for cancer. *BMJ*, **323**(7322), 1144.
15. Degner, L.F. and Sloan, J.A. (1992). Decision making during serious illness: what role do patients really want to play? *Journal of Clinical Epidemiology*, **45**(9), 941–50.
16. Degner, L. (1992). Patient participation in treatment decision making. *Axone*, **14**(1), 13–4.
17. Bruera, E., Willey, J.S., Palmer, J.L. *et al.* (2002). Treatment decisions for breast carcinoma: patient preferences and physician perceptions. *Cancer*, **94**(7), 2076–80.
18. Davison, B.J., and Degner, L.F. (1998). Promoting patient decision making in life-and-death situations. *Seminars in Oncology Nursing*, **14**(2), 129–36.
19. Grunfeld, E.A., Maher, E.J., Browne, S. *et al.* (2006). Advanced breast cancer patients' perceptions of decision making for palliative chemotherapy. *Journal of Clinical Oncology*, **24**(7), 1090–8.
20. Butow, P.N., Maclean, M., Dunn, S.M. *et al.* (1997). The dynamics of change: Cancer patients' preferences for information, involvement and support. *Annals of Oncology*, **8**(9), 857–63.
21. Fallowfield, L. (1995). Helping the relatives of patients with cancer. *European Journal of Cancer*, **31A**(11), 1731–2.
22. Hinton, J. (1994). Can home care maintain an acceptable quality of life for patients with terminal cancer and their relatives? *Palliative Medicine*, **8**(3), 183–96.
23. Eriksson, E., Arve, S., and Lauri, S. (2006). Informational and emotional support received by relatives before and after the cancer patient's death. *European Journal of Oncology Nursing*, **10**(1), 48–58.
24. Steinhauser, K.E., Christakis, N.A., Clipp, E.C. *et al.* (2000). Factors considered important at the end of life by patients, family, physicians, and other care providers. *JAMA*, **284**(19), 2476–82.

25. Fallowfield, L., Lipkin, M., and Hall, A. (1998). Teaching senior oncologists communication skills: results from phase I of a comprehensive longitudinal program in the United Kingdom. *Journal of Clinical Oncology*, **16**(5), 1961–8.

26. Graham, J., Potts, H.W., and Ramirez, A.J. (2002). Stress and burnout in doctors. *Lancet*, **360**(9349), 1975–6; author reply 1976.

27. Graham, J., Ramirez, A.J., Cull, A. et al. (1996). Job stress and satisfaction among palliative physicians. *Palliative Medicine*, **10**(3), 185–94.

28. Fallowfield, L., Jenkins, V., Farewell, V. et al. (2002). Efficacy of a Cancer Research UK communication skills training model for oncologists: a randomised controlled trial. *Lancet*, **359**(9307), 650–6.

29. Jenkins, V., and Fallowfield, L. (2002). Can communication skills training alter physicians' beliefs and behavior in clinics? *Journal of Clinical Oncology*, **20**(3), 765–9.

30. Fallowfield, L., Jenkins, V., Farewell, V. et al. (2003). Enduring impact of communication skills training: results of a 12-month follow-up. *British Journal of Cancer*, **89**(8), 1445–9.

31. Fallowfield, L., Saul, J., and Gilligan, B. (2001). Teaching senior nurses how to teach communication skills in oncology. *Cancer Nursing*, **24**(3), 185–91.

32. Schulman-Green, D., McCorkle, R., Cherlin, E. et al. (2005). Nurses' communication of prognosis and implications for hospice referral: a study of nurses caring for terminally ill hospitalized patients. *American Journal of Critical Care*, **14**(1), 64–70.

33. Heaven, C.M. and Maguire, P. (1997). Disclosure of concerns by hospice patients and their identification by nurses. *Palliative Medicine*, **11**(4), 283–90.

34. Booth, K., Maguire, P.M., Butterworth, T. et al. (1996). Perceived professional support and the use of blocking behaviours by hospice nurses. *Journal of Advanced Nursing*, **24**(3), 522–7.

35. Delvaux, N., Razavi, D., Marchal, S. et al. (2004). Effects of a 105 hours psychological training program on attitudes, communication skills and occupational stress in oncology: a randomised study. *British Journal of Cancer*, **90**(1), 106–14.

36. Wilkinson, S.M., Leliopoulou, C., Gambles, M. et al. (2003). Can intensive three-day programmes improve nurses' communication skills in cancer care? *Psychooncology*, **12**(8), 747–59.

37. Razavi, D., Delvaux, N., Marchal, S. et al. (2002). Does training increase the use of more emotionally laden words by nurses when talking with cancer patients? A randomised study. *British Journal of Cancer*, **87**(1), 1–7.

38. Finlay, I. and Dallimore, D. (1991). Your child is dead. *BMJ*, **302**(6791), 1524–5.

39. Annas, G.J. (1994). Informed consent, cancer, and truth in prognosis. *The New England Journal of Medicine*, **330**(3), 223–5.

40. Dunn, S.M., Patterson, P.U., Butow, P.N. et al. (1993). Cancer by another name: a randomized trial of the effects of euphemism and uncertainty in communicating with cancer patients. *Journal of Clinical Oncology*, **11**(5), 989–96.

41. Chapman, K., Abraham, C., Jenkins, V. et al. (2003). Lay understanding of terms used in cancer consultations. *Psychooncology*, **12**(6), 557–66.

42. Gattellari, M., Voigt, K.J., Butow, P.N. et al. (2002). When the treatment goal is not cure: are cancer patients equipped to make informed decisions? *Journal of Clinical Oncology*, **20**(2), 503–13.

43. Friedrichsen, M.J., Strang, P.M., and Carlsson, M.E. (2000). Breaking bad news in the transition from curative to palliative cancer care–patient's view of the doctor giving the information. *Supportive Care in Cancer*, **8**(6), 472–8.

44. Rogg, L., Graugaard, P.K., and Loge, J.H. (2006). Physicians' interpretation of the prognostic term "terminal": a survey among Norwegian physicians. *Palliative & Support Care*, **4**(3), 273–8.

45. Parkes, C.M. (1972). Accuracy of predictions of survival in later stages of cancer. *British Medical Journal*, **2**(5804), 29–31.

46. Muers, M.F., Shevlin, P., and Brown, J. (1996). Prognosis in lung cancer: physicians' opinions compared with outcome and a predictive model. *Thorax*, **51**(9), 894–902.

47. Mackillop, W.J. and Quirt, C.F. (1997). Measuring the accuracy of prognostic judgments in oncology. *Journal of Clinical Epidemiology*, **50**(1), 21–9.

48. Christakis, N.A. and Lamont, E.B. (2000). Extent and determinants of error in doctors' prognoses in terminally ill patients: prospective cohort study. *BMJ*, **320**(7233), 469–72.

49. Christakis, N.A. (1999). *Death foretold*. University of Chicago Press, Chicago.

50. (1978). Hippocrates. Prognosis. In *Hippocratic writings* (ed. G. Lloyd), pp. 170–85. Penguin Books, London.

51. Lamont, E.B. and Christakis, N.A. (1999). Some elements of prognosis in terminal cancer. *Oncology* (Williston Park), **13**(8), 1165–70; discussion 1172–4, 1179–80.

52. Glare, P., Virik, K., Jones, M. et al. (2003). A systematic review of physicians' survival predictions in terminally ill cancer patients. *BMJ*, **327**(7408), 195.

53. Wilkinson, S., Fellowes, D., and Leliopoulou, C. (2005). Does truth-telling influence patients' psychological distress? *European Journal of Palliative Care*, **12**(3), 124–6.

54. Fallowfield, L., Ratcliffe, D., Jenkins, V. et al. (2001). Psychiatric morbidity and its recognition by doctors in patients with cancer. *British Journal of Cancer*, **84**(8), 1011–5.

55. Meyer, T.J. and Mark, M.M. (1995). Effects of psychosocial interventions with adult cancer patients: a meta-analysis of randomized experiments. *Health Psychology*, **14**(2), 101–8.

56. McHugh, P., Lewis, S., Ford, S. et al. (1995). The efficacy of audiotapes in promoting psychological well-being in cancer patients: a randomised, controlled trial. *British Journal of Cancer*, **71**(2), 388–92.

57. Bruera, E., Pituskin, E., Calder, K. et al. (1999). The addition of an audiocassette recording of a consultation to written recommendations for patients with advanced cancer: a randomized, controlled trial. *Cancer*, **86**(11), 2420–5.

58. Charnock, D., Shepperd, S., Needham, G. et al. (1999). DISCERN: an instrument for judging the quality of written consumer health information on treatment choices. *Journal of Epidemiology and Community Health*, **53**(2), 105–11.

59. Shepperd, S., Charnock, D., and Cook, A. (2002). A 5-star system for rating the quality of information based on DISCERN. *Health Information and Libraries Journal*, **19**(4), 201–5.

60. Clayton, J., Butow, P., Tattersall, M. et al. (2003). Asking questions can help: development and preliminary evaluation of a question prompt list for palliative care patients. *British Journal of Cancer*, **89**(11), 2069–77.

61. Clayton, J.M., Butow, P.N., Tattersall, M.H. et al. (2007). A randomized controlled trial of a prompt list to help advanced cancer patients and their caregivers to ask questions about prognosis and end-of-life care. *Journal of Clinical Oncology*, **25**(6), 715–23.

6.2

Talking with families and children about the death of a parent

Anna C. Muriel and Paula K. Rauch

Background

Anticipating the death of an adult who is the parent of young children is particularly distressing for families and medical providers. Concerns about the children's welfare, and impulses to protect children from the pain of parental loss create challenges to honest communication. Nonetheless, attention to children's developmental stage and specific needs can guide clinicians in helping surviving family members to support children during the end-of-life period and into bereavement.

Clinicians and families alike may fear that parental loss during childhood will necessarily create mental health problems in the future, but studies show that the majority of children do not develop psychiatric disorders. While the loss of a parent during childhood will certainly affect a person's life, individuals usually go on to have meaningful lives and loving relationships. Studies of bereaved children from the time of a parent's death reveal that even though many children may develop non-specific, sub-clinical and transient behavioural disturbances[1,2] in the year following a parent's death, only one in five children develop a psychiatric disorder.[3] Rather than the simple fact of parental loss predicting future difficulties, studies show that the quality of the surviving parent's care,[4,5] or general home life[6] are better predictors of adult depression. Other factors that may mediate depression in adulthood are reports of warmth and empathy in surviving parents, and the opportunity to participate in the mourning process.[7]

Research on normative childhood bereavement has found that children make active efforts to maintain a connection to their deceased parents, and construct a relationship that may shift with developmental stages in an effort to cope effectively with the loss.[8] The role of the surviving parent can be particularly important in providing the child with opportunities to remember and memorialize the dead parent, facilitating integration of the loss throughout different phases of growth and development.[9]

The terminal phase of parental illness may be a vulnerable time for children as they experience more anxiety and depression, lower self-esteem, fears, misconceptions, and behaviour changes.[10–12] The literature on children's coping with parental illness shows that children living with parental cancer have more anxiety associated with an inability to discuss the illness, decreased time spent in age-appropriate activities, and ongoing worries about the cancer.[13] These anxieties may be mediated by increased communication, as children given specific information about the illness have been shown to have lower rates of anxiety.[14] However, these conversations between parents and children may not happen readily; even parents who were generally rated highly as communicators by their children are no more likely to disclose the probability of death than parents with low general communication ratings.[15] Families coping with anticipated deaths may be additionally vulnerable to parent–child differences in coping due to the well parent's physical and emotional preoccupation with the dying spouse, as well as differences in cognitive understanding and therefore anticipation of the death.[16] These differences may have implications for child coping and outcomes.[17] There may also be a range of children's responses to the graphic experience of a parent's terminal illness with attendant changes in appearance, function and dependence on medical equipment, which can sometimes, but not always, be mediated by overwhelmed adult caregivers.[18]

How children understand death at different ages

In thinking about how to talk with families and children anticipating parental death, it is essential to have a sense of how children at different ages understand death itself. This will be influenced by their general level of cognitive and emotional development as well as by their exposure to death in their community. There will be individual variations in children's temperaments and development, and parents need to be respected in knowing their own children best. For clinicians, however, an understanding of basic needs at different ages provides a useful guide for recommendations for supporting children during the terminal phase of a parent's illness and death.

Infants and toddlers (0–2 years)

Infants and toddlers are working on the complex tasks of attachment, basic self-regulation, and trust in their environment and caregivers. These youngsters have no understanding of time, or of the finality of death. However, they are sensitive to separations, and will feel the absence of a familiar caregiver even with no comprehension of the permanence of death. They may be distressed by changes in regular routines, and will also likely be affected by the emotional distress of grieving adults around them.

While familiarity and structure are helpful for people of all ages during difficult times, it is even more essential for the youngest children. During the stressful months or weeks leading up to a parent's death, it is best if infants and toddlers can be cared for by a limited number of familiar caregivers who can get to know a child's routine and provide care in as consistent and predictable a way as possible. Feeding, diapering, bathing, and sleeping should have associated routines and things that help a child to feel secure: bottles and cups, stuffed animals and toys, blankets, and portable crib, etc. The closest caregivers can provide schedules and instructions for other childcare helpers to ensure that important parts of the child's day proceed in a predictable manner even when they are not available.

Pre-schoolers (3–6 years)

Pre-school children have a wider range of social interactions, and particular ways of understanding the world around them. Egocentrism, associative logic, and magical thinking have strong bearings on how they understand parental illness and death. These self-referential ideas need to be mediated in order to prevent misunderstandings and guilt about what is happening in their family. For example, a 4-year-old may believe that something they did, like jump on a parent or misbehave, caused their parent's illness. A child who yells 'Bad Mommy' during a tantrum may think that saying this, or wishing her to 'go away' can actually make someone die and go away. Children of this age do not yet have an understanding of the irreversibility of death, and so they may also offer solutions to death, and expect the person to be 'all better'. They may also attribute the grief and distress of other adults to their own behaviour and need frequent reminders that they are not the cause of everyone's upset feelings.

Pre-schoolers therefore need regular conversations about how nothing a child says or does can make a parent ill or die. Adults need to inquire about how the child thinks their parent got sick or died, and dispel misconceptions repeatedly. In addition, caregivers may need to be patient with a natural disconnection of feelings and content, such that a child might talk about the death very matter-of-factly or make up a song about it, and yet might become cranky or have trouble with routine activities or changes in schedule. Parents of pre-schoolers can also expect some regression under stress, so that fully toilet trained child may have trouble using the potty, or a child may get upset being dropped off at a previously beloved daycare centre.

In discussing death with young children it is important to be concrete and use observable examples. Descriptions of death as 'going to sleep' can create worries about bedtime or not waking up. Heaven may be conceptualized as a place that one can visit or come back from. It is therefore helpful to talk about death as meaning that 'the body doesn't work anymore,' that the person can't move or breathe or think or feel etc. Adult survivors are sometimes surprised and disturbed by how often young children need this explanation.

School-age children (7–12 years)

School-age children are immersed in mastering academic, physical, and social skills, and are working to understand cause and effect logic. They are often quite invested in fairness and are sensitive to things that set them apart from their peers. By 6 or 7 years of age, children consistently understand the permanence of death. Their conceptions may still be very concrete, though, and they may have difficulty understanding more abstract or spiritual issues. In fact, they can be preoccupied with factual, medical or physical aspects of death and dying that feel difficult for adults to discuss. The uncertainty about time that is inherent in terminal illness may be particularly hard for younger children to grasp, and so anticipating the death itself may become distorted. For example, a 10-year-old child hearing that a parent is very, very ill and 'coming home to die,' may think that the parent will die that very night. School-age children are also vulnerable to worries about their own health or the health of their surviving family members, and need reassurances about this over time.

Because so much of these children's day is spent at school, it is important that the appropriate school personnel be informed about what is happening with an ill and dying parent. Children may not want to have teachers approach them to discuss the illness at school. However, they should know to whom they can go if they are having a difficult day. Teachers might adjust some expectations for schoolwork, but it is helpful for children to still have a certain level of responsibility and routines so that they understand that life will go on even in the context of a parent's illness and death. Children may also need additional help with school tasks and activities, and families may come to rely on other families in their community in order to support their children's participation in age-appropriate activities.

Adolescents (13 years and older)

Teenagers are in the process of identity formation and separation from parents. They have more adult capacities for abstract thinking, but their brains are not fully mature until into their twenties. Adolescents understand that death is final, irreversible, and universal, and may think actively about existential and spiritual issues. They may also vacillate between abstract ideas about their parent's death, and being preoccupied with very specific and self-centred ways in which it affects their life. These young people are also likely to project forward into the future and worry about their life progressing without their parent, anticipating sadness about milestones that their parent will not be there to witness.

Surviving caregivers may need help to understand adolescent self-involvement as developmentally normal, and not attribute it to negative character flaws. In addition, adolescents will continue to need support and guidance, and be at risk for more independence than they are ready for in the context of a parental death. Families should be mindful of teenagers who are taking on too many adult responsibilities, or are engaging in risky behaviours such as substance abuse or illegal activity. Older adolescents also need specific information about a parent's illness and probability of death as they make decisions about moving away from home for employment or education. While parents may want give them as much freedom as possible, these young adults need accurate information in order to make decisions that will be most comfortable for them,

Table 6.2.1 How children understand death at different ages.

Infants and toddlers (0–2 years)

Developmental context: establishing attachment

- Have no understanding of finality of separation, but feel absence of a familiar caregiver
- May be distressed by disruptions in routines
- Will be affected by the emotional distress/grief of surviving adult caregivers

Pre-schoolers (3–6 years)

Developmental context: driven by egocentrism, magical thinking, associative logic

- Are not able to understand that death is irreversible and permanent
- May attribute death or survivors' emotional distress to own actions or attributes
- Distress and behavioural changes may be fuelled by disruption in routine

School-age children (7–12 years)

Developmental context: mastering skills, fairness, cause and effect logic, peer relationships

- Understand that death is final and irreversible
- May have difficulty with abstract/spiritual issues
- May ask factual questions that can be painful or offensive to adults
- May struggle with unfairness of loss

Adolescents (13 and above)

Developmental context: working on separation-individuation, identity formation

- Understand that death is final, irreversible and universal
- May struggle with existential issues
- May focus on personal effects of loss

and minimize the possibility of regrets about being too close or too far away during the end of a parent's life (Table 6.2.1).

An approach to talking with families

With a basic understanding of where children are developmentally, clinicians can address parental concerns about helping their children through this difficult time. This task will also be influenced by the family culture around communication in general, the adults' capacities to integrate end-of-life care, and the expected progression of disease.

Clinicians can begin by assessing the adults' understanding and expectations of the illness and death. What do they understand about the expected time course? What do they know about the expected symptomatology? What do they hope for in terms of location and likely medical circumstances of the death?

The stage is then set to explore with the parents the children's understanding of the illness to date. What language has been used? What do they expect about the outcome of the illness? What prior experiences have the children had with major life changes, or death in their community or family? How have they managed these

as a family? Do the parents have particular concerns about their children's coping with the illness so far? What are they worried about in terms of their coping with death? The answers to these questions will provide scaffolding for the discussion, and help parents to have honest conversations with their children while addressing worries and misconceptions along the way. Parents should be encouraged to use honest, straightforward and age-appropriate language, checking frequently for the children's understanding, and welcoming questions as they arise. If the children have not yet been told the specific name of the illness, i.e. 'leukaemia', 'glioblastoma', 'cardiomyopathy', it is important to do so now to minimize confusion and anxiety about illness in general.

With careful discussion with parents and adult caregivers, it may not be necessary for clinicians to meet directly with the children. In some clinical settings, it is not possible, and for most children information mediated by their parents is most easily integrated and discussed in varying iterations over time. However, when children are present during medical encounters by chance or by design, they should be welcomed into the discussion so that their questions can be addressed. Some older children may ask to participate in meetings with medical providers in order to feel more fully included in the family experience. Children often stump clinicians or parents with questions that are anxiety-provoking or out-of-the-blue. Asking a child what got them thinking about that issue can go a long way towards clarifying exactly what the child is curious or worried about, and allowing adults to provide specific answers without going into more detail than the child is interested in.

Timing of discussions with children

Families often wonder when to talk about the terminal nature of a parent's illness with the children. Sometimes it is hard for parents to talk openly, even when the children have already observed the parent's deteriorating status, or have overheard others talking about the likelihood of death. Other times, parents have trouble holding back the fact that there is a transition in care from curative to palliative treatment, even if there is no observable change in the parent's appearance or function, and death is likely many months away.

Generally, the worst way for a child to hear news is by overhearing it, and many children will experience well-intentioned protection as exclusion. A child left to their own conclusions about a parent's terminal illness may also be vulnerable to misconceptions about why the illness is progressing, or how their life will change after a parent dies. On the other hand, it is difficult for younger children to understand that a parent may live for some time even in the terminal phase, and it is confusing to be anticipating the death at every turn.

It is important to discuss the changes in a parent's appearance and functional status as they occur, and potentially use these markers to discuss the probability of death within weeks or days with children of school-age or above. Many children will ask about death directly in the context of seeing a parent getting 'sicker, or very, very sick'. For adults who feel worried about introducing the idea of death, asking, 'Do you know what could happen if Mom gets even sicker? Or different parts of her body stop working?' will allow children to articulate that they are worried about death too. For the youngest children, acknowledging the functional changes as they pertain to their interactions with the parent may be enough: 'Dad used to be able to takes walks with us and play with you, but now he can't because he is sicker, so he stays in bed a lot.' Conversations with pre-school children about death may be most meaningful after the death has occurred.

Decisions about the setting for end-of-life care in a family context

One of the most important decisions for families facing an anticipated parental death is where they would like the death to occur. There is no one answer that will suit every family, and the ill adult may have prior experience or personal wishes that will dictate whether they die at home, in the hospital or in an inpatient hospice setting. If families have choices, they might also consider the needs of the children in addition to the medical or personal needs of the dying person.

Sometimes an inpatient hospice or hospital setting makes the most sense for families. In this case, the challenge may be that the well parent will have to divide their time between the inpatient setting with their spouse, and being at home with the children. Having thoughtful, familiar adults at home can ease this strain and allow the children to continue with their usual home and school activities. Visits with children should facilitate whenever possible (see below).

If families are interested in home hospice services, and expect a parent to die at home, attention to certain physical details can make things more comfortable for children. Whenever possible, having the dying parent in a room with a door, as opposed to an open or family area, allows the children to titrate their own exposure to the ill parent and medical equipment. The advantage of having everyone at home is that the children can maintain their usual routines and likely have more access to their well parent. If there will be other adults staying in the home to help, then they should also be aware of the children's needs for privacy and daily routines. A home death also makes it even more important to talk about changes in medical status and check for questions or misconceptions about what is happening. Children may have particular fears about the death itself, and clinicians can help both adults and children who are curious by anticipating symptoms and treatments for pain, secretions, shortness of breath, etc., and explaining what the physical process of dying might look and sound like. This also allows older children to consider how much they want to be around during the final days and hours.

Visits between ill parents and children

If a parent is expected to die in an inpatient or hospice setting, visits from children should be facilitated whenever possible. Children who express reluctance may have specific worries, e.g. seeing blood, or having their parent die during the visit, and can usually be reassured with explanations and contingency plans. It is best to avoid an agitated or delirious parent who may be frightening, but a child can still visit with a sedated parent. Most importantly, children need to be prepared for the visit, with descriptions of the setting, medical equipment, roommates, as well as the physical and functional status of the parent. For younger children, these descriptions may need to be concrete comparisons to the last time they saw their parent. An additional supportive adult should accompany the child so that they can leave when the child is ready, even if the well parent would like to stay. Younger children may

only be able to tolerate brief visits, or might need structured quiet play or drawing activities to do in the room. Touching a sick parent should never be forced, but can be modelled and supported if the child is willing. After the visit, adult caregivers should take some time to debrief and ask the child what was most interesting, fun, scary, or uncomfortable, in order to reassure the child and prepare better for the next visit. When in person visits are not possible, other kinds of contact between the ill parent and child should be encouraged. Children often enjoy making cards and notes that can be used to decorate a hospital room, and if able, parents can make recordings of themselves reading books or singing songs that can go home to young children (Table 6.2.2).

When death is imminent, last visits can be meaningful for children once they have an understanding of the finality of death. Older children may have the same wishes that adults do to have a few minutes alone with a dying parent, even if comatose, to say a last 'I love you,' or share an important private moment. If possible, older school-age and teenage children should be asked about whether or not they want to be called to the bedside near the end of life or immediately after the death. For example, does a child want to be brought home from school, or woken in the middle of the night at the time of death, or not? Some children very much want to be included, while others may prefer to have healthier memories of their parent, or feel afraid and uncomfortable about seeing their parent very ill and dying. The guiding principle is to provide children with information so that they can make decisions that will help them feel that their needs and wish are considered during this important time. It is important to remind families, however, that there are many opportunities to say goodbye before the death, immediately afterwards, during memorial services and funerals, as well as during private moments of reflection or prayer.

Legacy leaving

Parents who have come to terms with a diagnosis of a terminal illness often think about specific legacies or communications that they would like to leave for their children. Even the usual family photos and memorabilia become good foundations for telling stories about a parent after they have died. Parents may choose a

Table 6.2.2 Facilitating visits to an ill or dying parent.

Explore and alleviate worries or reluctance about visiting
Prepare children for what they will see:
◆ Hospital or hospice setting
◆ Medical equipment
◆ Other patients
◆ Physical condition of parent
◆ Functional status of parent
Bring an extra supportive adult who can leave when the child is ready
Provide structure or activity for younger children
Avoid an agitated or delirious parent
Debrief after the visit
Provide alternatives to an in person visit
Remember that there are many opportunities to say Goodbye

variety of other more intentional communications, such as letters or audio recordings specifically for each child, or at particular milestones. There is little data on how these communications are received by children over time, but surviving children often look for indications from both the dead parent and surviving adults, about who the parent was as a person, their values and ideals, and what the parent saw in them, their child. Sometimes parents leave specific meaningful objects, or annotate books, music or movies that have been important to them. Children may want to choose special objects to keep themselves either before or after the death. The wider community can also be engaged in legacy-leaving, as friends and relatives attending the memorial service can be asked to write down a memory or thought about the parent that can be compiled for the children and shared when they are curious later. As described earlier, children spend a lifetime revisiting the loss of the parent, and may become interested in their parent as they themselves reach different phases in their own life.

Children's participation in funerals and memorial services

Children of pre-school age or above may participate in different aspects of funerals and memorial services. Family tradition will dictate whether there is a wake, religious service, interment, or family gathering afterwards, and children may be included for all or part of these events. As with hospital visits, it is important to prepare children for what the event will be like including the setting, who will be there, what the service will be like, what they will and won't be able to do, and that there may be a range of feelings expressed by people, from sadness to warmth and humour. Younger children will need a familiar adult to care for them throughout, and be responsive or leave when they are unable to sit still or remain quiet.

Older school-age and teenage children can be included in the planning or asked if they want to participate by reading, or playing music during the service. Many funeral homes will provide a private time for the family to have a special children's service or quiet visiting time. Children sometimes like to place a picture, note or special object in or on top of the casket. School-age children may have specific questions about the preparation of the body or cremation. Adult caregivers may want to learn about the process in advance, so that they can better answer children's questions. Alternatively, they should know whom to ask (funeral directors sometimes have age-appropriate information) about these issues during the difficult and chaotic days around the parent's death. Younger children who do not yet fully understand death may find the interment disturbing as they don't want to see their parent lowered into the cold, dark ground, and so families may consider not having them attend the burial itself, and be able to visit the gravesite at another time. For families who spread ashes or have non-traditional services that do not involve a burial site, it may still be important for the family to designate a special place to go to reflect or remember the parent.

Conclusion

The untimely death of a parent is one of the most challenging events for families and the clinicians who care for them. Attention to children's needs during this time is an important aspect of clinical care, and is much appreciated by adults in the family. A basic knowledge of child development and the ways that children understand illness and death can provide a template with which to engage families about how to help their children during this time and into bereavement. When clinicians support honest, child-centred communication, and help families anticipate common situations and questions, surviving adults are able to use their own best resources to provide thoughtful care for the children.

Further reading

Christ, G.H. (2000). *Healing children's grief: surviving a parent's death from cancer.* Oxford University Press, New York.

Harpham, W.S. (1997). *When a parent has cancer: a guide to caring for your children.* Harper Collins, New York.

Klass, D., Silverman, P.R., and Nickman, S.L. (eds.) (1996). *Continuing bonds: new understandings of grief.* Taylor & Francis, Washington DC.

McCue, K. (1994). *How to help children through a parent's serious illness.* St. Martin's Griffin, New York.

Rauch, P.R., and Muriel, A.C. (2006). *Raising an emotionally healthy child when a parent is sick.* McGraw-Hill, New York.

Worden, J.W. (1996). *Children and grief: when a parent dies.* Guilford, New York.

References

1. Black, D. (1998). Coping with loss. Bereavement in childhood. *BMJ,* **316,** 931–3.

2. Vida, S., and Grizenko, N. (1989). DSM-III-R and the phenomenology of childhood bereavement: a review. *Canadian Journal of Psychiatry,* **34,** 148–55.

3. Dowdney, L. (2000). Childhood bereavement following parental death. *Journal of Child Psychology and Psychiatry,* **41,** 819–30.

4. Bifulco, A.T., Brown, G.W., and Harris, T.O. (1987). Childhood loss of parent, lack of adequate parental care and adult depression: a replication. *Journal of Affective Disorders,* **12,** 115–28.

5. Harris, T., Brown, G.W., and Bifulco, A. (1986). Loss of parent in childhood and adult psychiatric disorder: the role of lack of adequate parental care. *Psychological Medicine,* **16,** 641–59.

6. Breier, A., Kelsoe, J.R. Jr, Kirwin, P.D. *et al.* (1988). Early parental loss and development of adult psychopathology. *Archives of General Psychiatry,* **45,** 987–93.

7. Saler, L., and Skolnick, N. (1992). Childhood parental death and depression in adulthood: roles of surviving parent and family environment. *The American Journal of Orthopsychiatry,* **62,** 504–16.

8. Silverman, P.R., Nickman, S., and Worden, J.W. (1992). Detachment revisited: The child's reconstruction of a dead parent. *The American Journal of Orthopsychiatry,* **62,** 494–503.

9. Nickman, S.L., Silverman, P.R., and Normand, C. (1998). Children's construction of a deceased parent: the surviving parent's contribution. *The American Journal of Orthopsychiatry,* **68,** 126–34.

10. Siegel, K., Karus, D., and Raveis, V.H. (1996). Adjustment of children facing the death of a parent due to cancer. *Journal of the American Academy of Child and Adolescent Psychiatry,* **35,** 442–450.

11. Christ, G.H., Siegel, K., Freund, B. *et al.* (1993). Impact of parental terminal cancer on latency age children. *The American Journal of Orthopsychiatry,* **63,** 417–25.

12. Christ, G.H., Seigel, K., and Sperber, D. (1994). Impact of parental terminal cancer on adolescents. *The American Journal of Orthopsychiatry,* **64,** 604–13.

13. Nelson, E., Sloper, P., Charlton, A. *et al.* (1994). Children who have a parent with cancer: a pilot study. *Journal of Cancer Education,* **9,** 30–6.

14. Rosenheim, E., and Reicher, R. (1985). Informing children about a parent's terminal illness. *Journal of Child Psychology and Psychiatry,* **26,** 995–8.

15. Siegel, K., Raveis, V., and Karus, D. (1996). Patterns of communication with children when a parent has cancer. In *Cancer in the family* (eds. L. Baider, C. Cooper, and A. Kaplan DeNour), pp. 109–28. John Wiley & Sons, Ltd, Chichester.

16. Saldinger, A., Porterfield, K., and Cain, A.C. (2004). Meeting the needs of parentally bereaved children: a framework for child-centered parenting. *Psychiatry*, **67**, 331–52.

17. Saldinger, A., Cain, A., Kalyter, N. *et al.* (1999). Anticipating parental death in families with young children. *The American Journal of Orthopsychiatry*, **69**, 39–48.

18. Saldinger, A., Cain, A., and Porterfield, K. (2003). Managing traumatic stress in children anticipating parental death. *Psychiatry*, **66**, 168–81.

6.3

Communication between professionals

David Jeffrey

Introduction

Patients with advanced life-threatening diseases, which are no longer curable, have a variety of complex needs which can not all be addressed by a single individual. However, an effective multi-disciplinary team can deliver a high standard of palliative care.[1] The requirement for collaborative team working of health-care professionals increases with the complexity of the patient's needs.[2]

A high quality of patient care and family support depends on sharing of information, good communication, and joint decision-making between the different professionals. In the past, there has been an emphasis on improving communication between health-care professionals and patients, but communication between health-care professionals is often inadequate.[3–5] Poor communication is not only a waste of time but also a threat to patient care and a source of staff stress.[6] It is therefore appropriate to review communication issues between the many professionals involved in the patient's care.

Barriers to effective interprofessional communication

For effective communication between health-care professionals, a number of potential barriers need to be considered:

- Palliative care is provided in a number of settings, e.g. home, community hospital, nursing home, hospice and hospital.

- Palliative care teams often work at the interface between curative and palliative care.

- Specialist palliative care teams need to liaise between groups of health-care professionals, voluntary and statutory agencies.

- Maintaining patient confidentiality in multi-disciplinary teams may be difficult.

- Health professionals may challenge communication by tending to work autonomously.

A multi-disciplinary team which is not communicating effectively will be prone to rivalries, conflict and delayed decision-making.[7] Problems of interprofessional communication can be illustrated in the context of the progress of a patient with advanced cancer. However, the principles of specialist palliative care and effective communication between professionals are as relevant in the care of patients with life-threatening non-malignant disease as in cancer care. This chapter will follow the patient, family, and carers through referral, assessment, care, discharge, death, and bereavement. Communication is emphasized in its role of maintaining effective professional relationships which foster a high standard of care. Differing communication behaviours are analysed and ways of improving communication between professionals are explored.

The patient's journey

Once cancer is diagnosed, the world is filled with uncertainty for the patient and family. Good communication among all health professionals is vital to ensure that they receive a comprehensive service with as little misunderstanding as possible.[8] Two differing clinical approaches to the same patient highlight how communication between professionals can affect the patient's quality of life.[9]

The non-collaborative approach

A 45-year-old woman with advanced pancreatic cancer and multiple liver metastases was admitted to hospital with abdominal pain. The surgeon informed that her disease was now advanced and that surgery would not help her. She was discharged from hospital and referred back to her general practitioner and district nurse. She became withdrawn and took to her bed where she died, 3 weeks later.

A collaborative approach

After seeing the patient, the surgeon requested an assessment by the specialist palliative care nurse. During this assessment, the patient revealed that she was worried: she feared that she would be in terrible pain and she did not think that her husband would cope on his own. The specialist nurse addressed each of the patient's concerns and advised her on the resources which were available. The patient was relieved to hear that her symptom control would be regularly monitored by her general practitioner and community nurse and that a specialist palliative care nurse could also be involved to support both her and her husband.

She felt confident about her discharge from hospital and died peacefully at home 3 weeks later. Three months after her death husband accepted bereavement support offered by the community specialist palliative care nurse.

These two approaches illustrate the differing quality of life which a patient with advanced cancer may experience as a result of differing communications among the health-care professionals. In both situations, the patient died 3 weeks following discharge from hospital. In the first approach, although her physical symptoms were well controlled, there was neglect of her psychosocial concerns. The opportunity was lost for the patient to resolve unfinished emotional business and her husband received no bereavement support. In contrast, in the second approach, the patient had the same short survival but was able to use this time to come to terms with her fears and to be involved in planning support for her husband.

It is now appropriate to examine the problems encountered in interprofessional communication at the various stages of the patient's journey.

Referral

The point at which the professional, either in the community or in hospital refers to specialist palliative care can present challenges.[10,11] Specialist palliative care services are often involved too late and relevant information is often lacking[12] Referrers often give relevant medical details but provide less information on the social, psychological, or spiritual aspects of the patient's history.[13] Delayed referral to specialist palliative care services may result in patients receiving inadequate care.

The reasons for delayed referral may be based on:

◆ A lack of knowledge among patients and health-care professionals of the role of the palliative care team, and of their skills and expertise.

◆ A sense of vulnerability and guilt among the primary carers that problems have not been resolved.

◆ A desire to protect professional boundaries, the 'my patient syndrome', where the professional believes that he/she can cope with all the patient's problems.

◆ A wish to protect patients from distress, since referral to specialist palliative care usually involves addressing the fact that the underlying disease is no longer curable.

Some doctors still mistakenly believe that specialist palliative care is confined to the terminal phase of the illness, when the patient is obviously dying. If patients are only referred at the terminal stage of their illness, then this belief will be reinforced both among professionals and the public.

Interdisciplinary assessment

The quality of interdisciplinary teamwork is dependent upon a complex process of sharing: the different professionals have to consider clinical, emotional, and social assessments of the patient and family. Coordinating these assessments are essential elements of effective interdisciplinary care.

There may be a problem in communicating the results of assessments from hospital to the community. For example, after attending an outpatient clinic a patient may not return to see their general practitioner but make a telephone request for the drug suggested by the consultant. The general practitioner may not have received the letter from the consultant and spend time tracing the specialist to discover what she has suggested. General practitioners want information on proposed treatment, expected outcomes and the patient's psychological concerns, information which is often omitted from the specialist's letter.[14]

Confidentiality

Communication of patient information within and among hospital, hospice and primary care teams is essential for patient well-being. Professionals may act as if they have the patient's implied consent to share information. However, a health-care professional has a duty not to divulge information about a patient to a third party without the patient's explicit consent. Without this requirement for confidentiality it would be impossible to build a trusting relationship with the patient. On the other hand, if interdisciplinary teamwork is to be effective then information about the patient has to be shared among the team. If information is judged to be highly sensitive, the patient's permission should be sought, to pass on this information to members of the team. Different levels of information about the patient can be shared with other professionals on a 'need to know' basis, in order to benefit the patient.

Continuity of care

Continuity of care is one of the essential components of high standard palliative care. Changes in the organization of primary care in the UK involving nurse triage systems for out-of-hours care have created challenges to providing continuity of care. General practitioners may lose touch with patients who are being followed up in hospital clinics and feel marginalized in their care. Implementation of European Working Time Directives in theUK has created problems in maintaining continuity in the hospital setting.

The diversity that gives the interdisciplinary team its potential for effectiveness can also make the team vulnerable if there is insufficient communication.[15] All team members have a role; the challenge is how to achieve an exchange of information. The message may not be clear, there may be misunderstanding about the goals of care which may cause patients and carers distress.

Discharge planning

There is a drive towards the rapid turnover of inpatients in National Health Service (NHS) hospitals in the UK and newly discharged patients are dependent on carefully planned care in the community. The provision of such co-coordinated care requires effective communication across the hospital-community interface.[16] However, gaps in care may cause patients frustration when they are transferred from specialist to primary care. General practitioners do not want to give conflicting messages to those of the hospital team, or to be ignorant of facts when facing patients and relatives. In the terminal phase, some patients may decide on discharge from hospital to return to their own home to die. Achieving such discharges at short notice is challenging as there may be little time available for the appropriate transfer of such frail patients.

Terminal care and bereavement support

There are a number of ethical dilemmas which may arise at the end of a patient's life. Examples include requests for euthanasia, issues surrounding withdrawal of nutrition and hydration, do not attempt resuscitation orders, and advance directives. It may be difficult for a team to reach a moral consensus when presented with such dilemmas.

The general practitioner and community nurse are the key professionals when the patient is dying at home with the specialist palliative care team available for advice. Continuity of care is important at this stage of the patient's illness to enable the patient to have a dignified death in the place of their choice.

Interprofessional communication may break down following the death of the patient: failure to inform the primary care team of the patient's death can lead to lack of support for the family or even the embarrassing error of a member of the team visiting the patient's home in ignorance of the death.

Organizational problems

Health-care systems suffer inefficiency because of a poor communication infrastructure.[17] During times of stress communication is threatened.[18] In one survey of hospital admissions, it was found that communication problems were the most common cause of preventable disability or death,[19] Despite the importance of communication in the provision and organization of health-care, there is still a need for the development of communication systems to meet clinical needs.

Although doctors and nurses may prefer face to face communication, they risk contributing to an interruptive workplace culture. Interruption may have psychological costs; diversion of attention, forgetfulness, errors, and rescheduling of work plans.[17] Doctors may not consider the effect of their telephone call or pager request might have on the other party, valuing the completion of their own tasks over that of their colleagues.

Communication and conflict

Unsatisfactory communication lies at the heart of many of the stresses experienced by professionals working in palliative care. Hospital palliative care teams may experience difficulties in integrating the collaborative approach into hospital practice; where professional boundaries are blurred and access to the patient is shared. Where role conflict exists, it can cause stress amongst the health-care professionals.

Complaints from patients can be generated by a criticism of one professional by another. Many of the stresses reported by professionals arise from difficulties with colleagues and institutional hierarchies: perhaps where there is rivalry or blocking of referral.[20]

Improving interprofessional communication

Opportunities for colleagues to meet must be created for exchanging of information, planning of interventions, and sharing of responsibility for the patient's care. This section seeks to explore ways in which the problems highlighted during the patient's journey can be addressed.

Referral

The initiation of a team approach often depends on the doctor's recognition of the need for an interdisciplinary approach to care.[1] The general practitioner is in a good position to initiate the team approach and to share knowledge with other members of the team. The primary team caring for the patient, whether in the

community or the hospital, should be adopting a palliative care approach, which involves good communication between general practitioners, community nurses, and hospital staff. The communication between these professionals forms the lynch pin of palliative care provision. However, the needs of some patients and families will exceed the resources of these teams and further support will be required from a specialist palliative care service. Patients and families need to be fully aware and in agreement with referral to the specialist palliative care team. This means that the referring doctor or nurse needs a clear understanding of the role of the palliative care team and is comfortable about discussing issues which the patient may raise as the time of this referral. The patient may ask 'Am I going to die?' or perhaps 'Am I going to get better?'

It is perhaps unusual that in specialist palliative care, teams accept referrals from a variety of health-care professionals, professions allied to medicine, patients- and carers. It is essential that the specialist team liaises with the medical team managing the patient and that the primary team has the full knowledge and agreement that the specialist palliative care team should be involved. It is a privilege for a specialist team to be invited to share care; such teams should be aware that the primary referring professional may feel threatened or guilty that pain or symptoms have not been controlled.[21]

Most patients trust their general practitioner, who facilitates the introduction of other professionals into their care. The decision to refer should be based on whether the quality of life of patients with advanced disease could be improved. Appropriate referral to a specialist team should be made whenever a health-care professional reaches the limits of their own skills. There is a need to keep up-to-date with the work of colleagues, because if the primary carer is unaware of the skills and expertise of the specialist team then he/she may fail to make appropriate referrals. The introduction of clinical governance has placed an emphasis on practitioners being sure that patients receive the right care in the right setting and at the right time.

Palliative care teams have developed referral criteria and eligibility criteria to clarify the process of referral.[22] For example, the 'Leeds eligibility criteria' emphasize that to be eligible for specialist palliative care the patient should meet three key criteria[22]

1　Progressive and advanced disease.

2　The patient has an extraordinary level of need.

3　Following referral, the patient will be assessed by a specialist palliative care service.

It is preferable that a letter or an entry in the medical notes requesting a specialist palliative care assessment should confirm verbal referrals; the reason for referral and the degree of urgency should also be specified. The specialist palliative care team needs to communicate their hours of availability and their standard of response.

The referring doctor should provide the relevant information about the patient's history, current condition, drug therapy, management plan, and any particular concerns they may have.[23]

Interdisciplinary assessment

General practitioners need to encourage interdisciplinary primary care team working as well as enlisting the skills and knowledge of the specialist palliative care team.[24] The Gold Standards

Framework recently introduced in the UK encourages regular meetings of the primary care team to discuss all palliative care patients on the practice register.[25]

Referrals to the specialist palliative care team are discussed in an interdisciplinary team meeting. These meetings are essential to plan the highest standards of care, provide an opportunity for education and to facilitate continuity of care. Effective communication between nurses and doctors is enhanced by the formation of good interpersonal relationships in a friendly supportive atmosphere.[26] The ability of nurses to communicate informally results in them being able to express their intuitions regarding their patient's condition, without fear of being ridiculed by their medical colleagues.[26] It is part of good clinical practice to ensure that everyone is given an opportunity to express their views. Doctors, nurses, and social workers have differing perspectives on the patient's problems. The doctor is skilled in diagnosis and recommending treatment options. Nurses are closer to patients and have particular insights into psychological and emotional responses to treatment. The social worker brings an yet another perspective on the patient's quality of life in a social context.[27] Sharing of ideas within the team takes time; managers need to acknowledge the need for collaborative practice and to value time spent on communication.

The specialist palliative care team assessment of the patient should be shared with the primary referring team: the patient's progress, medication, level of awareness, and needs of the family should be discussed. Joint working between different professions can be facilitated in a number of practical ways; palliative care posts exist which work across hospital and community situations.[28] Role blurring is an inevitable feature of interprofessional teamwork as the individuals making up the team depend on each other. This interdependence can result in either a competitive or a collaborative relationship.[9]

Continuity of care

It is in the patient's best interest for one doctor, usually a general practitioner, to be fully informed and responsible for continuity of the patient's medical care. The Gold Standards project also recommends the use of handover forms, and protocols for end-of-life care to improve interprofesional communication.[25]

The nursing care can similarly be best co-coordinated by the community nurse although on occasions it may be appropriate for another member of the team to be designated the key worker. Decision-making procedures need to be clear and communication regular. There is a need for regular meetings between the doctor and nurse to hand over details of the patient's progress, drug changes and any important communications between the professional and the patient or family. In all communication, whether between doctors, doctors and nurses or between nurses, it is reassuring to patients and family to hear that details are being passed between them.[10]

Communication issues to address at such meetings include:[29]

◆ What information does my colleague need?

◆ What is the management plan?

◆ Is everyone clear about his or her responsibilities?

◆ How should we communicate again?

Record keeping

Documentation is an important part of interprofessional communication which guides practice, provides information, and forms one measure of the quality of care.[30] The community nursing record, which remains with the patient, can be a helpful mechanism for communication between primary and specialist services. Patient-held records and a palliative care drug kardex may also be useful when moving from one setting to another, creating better continuity and improving interprofessional communication.[8,30] Integrated care pathways are a useful initiative which act as guidelines and multi-disciplinary case records, facilitating interprofessional communication in their preparation, implementation and review.[31] The Liverpool Care Pathway can be used in a variety of settings; home, hospital, care homes and in hospices.[31]

The oncology–palliative care interface

Specialist palliative care has become integrated with cancer care and coordinates with community care. Good communication at the oncology–palliative care interface is characterized by joint assessments. Such collaborative practice ensures patients receive expert symptom control, psychosocial care and have access to palliative anticancer treatments such as chemotherapy. Specialist palliative care teams need an understanding of oncology issues and disease-modifying options which may improve the patient's quality of life. Similarly oncologists should feel comfortable in involving the specialist palliative care team when the patient is receiving palliative chemotherapy or radiotherapy.

Advocacy

Advocacy involves representing the case of another person to a higher authority; it implies the existence of an adversary who threatens the patient's autonomy.[27] In the past, advocacy in health care has tended to be considered as a nursing issue. For example, a nurse might believe that patients need an advocate to protect them from the aggressive use of high-technology medicine; a doctor might think it was their duty to champion the needs of the individual patient against the needs of others.[27] In an ideal world advocacy would be redundant; anyone close to the patient can act as an advocate.[32] It is important that trust exists between team members so that when advocacy issues arise, the team accepts this as a way of considering the patient's interest and not as personal criticism of an individual team member. When there is a conflict in opinion between the palliative care specialist and the treating physician the doctor who has the clinical responsibility for the patient's care should make the decision whether to accept or reject the advice. These differences in medical opinion should not undermine the future working between the two specialists.

Discharge planning

General practitioners and community nurses are the professionals responsible for medical and nursing care at home; they should be the first professionals consulted when planning a discharge from hospital. This is also a good time to anticipate which other members of the team should be involved in care, such as occupational therapists, physiotherapists, and social workers. The primary care team should have detailed information on the day of discharge: they need to know the diagnosis, prognosis, aims of care, drug treatments, and details of what information has been given to the patient. The social worker is responsible for co-coordinating the package of care at home, involving the integration of home care assistance, the primary care team, specialist palliative care and non-professional voluntary support. Good communication is therefore essential if these various agencies are to be co-coordinated to provide care to meet the assessed needs of the patient and family.

Discussion with the general practitioner or community nurse by telephone or through fax or clinical e-mail may clarify the information provided in the discharge letter in more complex cases. In this way, general practitioners and community nurses are aware of their patient's medical details when facing them on their return home.

Terminal care and bereavement support

Communication within the team ensures co-coordinated care which respects the patients need for privacy. Whilst the general practitioner and community nurse are the key professionals when the patient is dying at home, the specialist palliative care team is also available for advice, some services even offer 24-h advice to professionals. Good communication between the professionals can maximize therapeutic effectiveness and create an environment in which the patient and family can feel a sense of security. Integrated care pathways are a useful tool to aid communication between professionals.[31] When there has been a difficult death arrangements can be made to review the case in a discussion facilitated by one of the specialist team.

There needs to be an efficient means of notifying the general practitioner and the primary care team of the patient's death. It is helpful to make a record of the death in the bereaved person's notes. The team will then identify an appropriate key worker who will be responsible for offering the family bereavement support and a follow up bereavement visit 3–6 months after death to assess how the family are coping.

Communication and conflict

Doctors, nurses, and other members of the team need clear ways of communicating. Mutual respect and trust between team members leads to their corporate and individual skills being employed in an optimal way. It is never helpful to be critical of colleagues in front of patients or relatives, such behaviour only serves to reduce the patient's confidence in the team. Professionals should monitor signs of stress in their colleagues and offer support when it is needed. It is sometimes easier to identify a stressed colleague than to intervene to help and support. Professionals should consider extending the support they give to patients to their colleagues. Ethical dilemmas can cause team stress, calling a family meeting or case conference to debate the issues can be a constructive way of helping to reach a team consensus.

When conflict occurs it should be acknowledged and resolved. In resolving conflict, it is vital to retain the self-respect of other individuals and to focus on specific patient-centred issues, resisting blaming individuals. Advocacy is an unhelpful concept because it implies an adversary, health-care professionals should adopt a collaborative model of care in which all disciplines work towards respecting the patient's autonomy.[27] Clinical supervision, mentoring, and peer appraisal can be methods of supporting and encouraging colleagues. Time spent building bridges or 'networking' is rarely wasted.

Communication facilities

Team members need instruction in appropriate use of communication facilities. Voice-mail, e-mail, and mobile communication can improve support, but there is a need to reassure staff that their contact has been effective.[15] Health-care professionals must consider the consequences of communication with their colleagues and possibly use alternative approaches. There is a need for dialogue between disciplines to teach health-care professionals how to design, evaluate, and set up efficient communication systems. Joint consultations may be facilitated by tele-conferencing through sound and video links without clinicians having to leave their usual work place. The Internet unites practices and hospitals, reducing paperwork and speeding access to results, referral, and discharge letters.

Education and clinical audit

Ideas of interprofessional education are central to the development of the new NHS in the UK. Learning in a clinical as well as a classroom setting may hold the key.[35] A major objective of interprofessional education is fostering of mutual respect. Interdisciplinary training programmes in communication skills also challenge working practices. While updates of clinical knowledge for individual doctors remain important, learning about multi-disciplinary working is also needed.

It could be argued that by the time doctors and nurses have undergone professional training their views may have become entrenched, making them unwilling to appreciate the others' roles and threatening the efficiency of the team. Perhaps, teaching doctors and nurses together would allow some of these barriers to be removed through an opportunity for communication.[36] Recent reforms in health provision in the UK place an emphasis on collaborative working in health, social and voluntary sectors.

Clinical audit is an integral part of clinical governance providing another mechanism for improving interprofessional communication. The General Medical Council of the UK issued guidance on maintaining good medical practice which indicated that one of the key tests of a good team is that the members can be 'open and honest about professional performance'. This requires a willingness to engage directly across professional boundaries that have long been impermeable.[37]

Conclusions

Collaborative practice involves good communication, an understanding of each other's roles and trusting interpersonal relationships. Such models of practice may be difficult to implement because they mirror the complexity of human suffering.[38] Professionals in hospital and the community need to maintain clear channels of communication, to acknowledge uncertainty and to try to reach a consensus with the patient rather than perceiving one discipline as being critical of another. Patients and families will benefit if physicians are aware both of their own abilities and limitations and are willing to enlist the skills of others. A collaborative coordinated approach is particularly important as the disease progresses, the patient becomes frailer and his/her needs become pronounced. Inevitably throughout the patient's illness more professionals become involved, making communication an essential element of a coherent care plan. A team of reliable professionals who are communicating well with each other provide patients with a sense of security and comfort.

References

1. Ingham, J.M. and Coyle, N. (1997). Teamwork in end of life care: a nurse – physician perspective on introducing physicians to palliative care concepts. In *New themes in palliative care* (eds. D. Clark, J. Hockley, and S. Ahmedzai), pp. 255–74. Open University Press, Buckingham.

2. Headrick, L.A., Wilcock, P.M., and Batalden, P.B. (1998). Interprofessional working and continuing medical education. *BMJ*, **316**, 771–4.

3. (2000). Informing, communicating and sharing decisions with people who have cancer. *Effective Health Care*, **6**, 1–8.

4. Charles, C., Gafni, A., and Whelan, T. (2000). How to improve communications between doctors and patients. *BMJ*, **320**, 1220–1.

5. Gosbee, J. (1998). Communications among health professionals. *BMJ*, **316**, 642–2.

6. Salter, R., Brettle, P., and Hobbs, F.D.R. (1998). Poor communication puts patients at risk. *BMJ*, **317**, 279.

7. Fottrell, E. (1990). Multidisciplinary functioning: will it still be of use? *British Journal of Hospital Medicine*, **43**, 253.

8. McGann, C. (1998). Communications in cancer care: introducing patient held records. *International Journal of Palliative Nursing*, **4**, 222–9.

9. Coyle, N. (1997). Interdisciplinary collaboration in hospital palliative care: chimera or goal? *Palliative Medicine*, **11**, 265–6.

10. Doyle, D. and Jeffrey, D. (2000). *Palliative care in the home*. Oxford University Press, Oxford.

11. Jeffrey, D. (2000). *Cancer from cure to care*. Hochland & Hochland, Manchester.

12. Miller, D.G., Carroll, D., Grimshaw, J. *et al.* (1998). Palliative care at home: an audit of cancer deaths in Grampian region. *British Journal of General Practice*, **48**, 1299–302.

13. Massorotto, A., Carter, H., MacLeod, R. *et al.* (2000). Hospital referrals to a hospice: timing of referrals, referrers expectation, and the nature of referral information. *Journal of Palliative Care*, **16**, 22–9.

14. McConnell, D., Burton, P.N., and Tattersall, M.H. (1999). Improving the letters we write; an exploration of doctor–doctor communications in cancer care. *British Journal of Cancer*, **80**, 427–37.

15. Mystakidou, K. (2001). Interdisciplinary working: a Greek perspective. *Palliative Medicine*, **15**, 67–8.

16. Closs, SJ. (1997). Discharge communications between hospital and community health care staff: a selective review. *Health & Social Care in the Community*, **5**, 181–97.

17. Coiera, E. and Tombs, V. (1998). Communication behaviour in a hospital setting: an observational study. *BMJ*, **316**, 673–6.

18. Cooper, J. (2000). *Stepping into palliative care*. Radcliffe Medical Press, pp. 189–96.

19. (1995). 14,000 preventable deaths in Australian hospitals. *BMJ*, **310**, 1487.

20. Vachon, M.L.S. (1995). Staff stress in hospice/palliative care: a review. *Palliative Medicine*, **9**, 91–122.

21. Smith, R. (1996). What clinical information do doctors need? *BMJ*, **313**, 1062–8.

22. Bennett, M., Adam, J., Alison, D. *et al.* (2000). Leeds eligibility criteria for specialist palliative care services. *Palliative Medicine*, **14**, 157–8.

23. General Medical Council. (2006). *Good medical practice*. GMC, London.

24. Peppiatt, R. (1998). Palliative terminal care. *British Journal of General Practice*, **48**, 1297–8.

25. Thomas, K. (2003). *Caring for the dying at home*. Radcliffe Medical Press, Oxford, p. 229.

26. Mackay, L. (1993). *Conflicts in care, medicine and nursing*. Chapman & Hall, London.

27. Shannon, S.E. (1997). The roots of interdisciplinary conflict around ethical issues. *Critical Care Nursing Clinics of North America*, **9**, 13–27.

28. Chilver, K. (2001). Joint working, joint roles: streamlining patient care. *European Journal of Palliative Care*, **8**, 112–4.

29. Buckman, R. (1998). Communication in palliative care a practical guide. In *Oxford textbook of palliative medicine*, (eds. D. Doyle, G.W.C, Hanks, N. MacDonald) 2nd edition, pp. 153–4. Oxford University Press, Oxford.

30. Anderson, E.E. (2000). Professional practice issues surrounding record keeping in district nursing practice. *British Journal of Community Nursing*, **5**, 352–6.

31. Ellershaw, J., Foster, A., Murphy, D., *et al.* (1997). Developing an integrated care pathway for the dying patient. *European Journal of Palliative Care*, **4**, 203–7.

32. Randall, F., Downie, R.S. (1996). *Palliative care ethics. a good companion*. Oxford University Press, Oxford.

33. Harrison, R., Clayton, W., and Wallace, P. (1996). Can telemedicine be used to improve communications between primary and secondary care? *BMJ*, **313**, 1377–80.

34. Willmot, M. and Sullivan, F. (2000). NHS net in Scottish primary care. Lessons for the future. *British Medical Journal*, **321**, 878–81.

35. Finch, J. (2000). Interprofessional education and team working: a view from the education providers. *BMJ*, **321**, 1138–40.

36. Keogh, K., Jeffrey, D., and Flanagan, S. (1999). The Palliative Care Education Group for Gloucestershire (PEGG): an integrated model of multidisciplinary education in palliative care. *European Journal of Cancer Care*, **8**, 44–7.

37. Department of Health. (2000). *The NHS Plan a plan for investment, a plan for reform*. Department of Health, London.

6.4

Communication with the public, politicians, and the media

Kenneth Calman

Introduction

It might well be asked why a chapter on such an issue should appear in this textbook, which is essentially concerned with issues of care, quality of life, ethical and research issues, and the delivery of a service. The answer lies precisely in that statement. Each of these areas is of direct relevance to the public (who might need the service), to politicians (who may be funding the service), and the media (who will be reporting on the service). A glance through almost any newspaper in almost any country will show how much news and political noise can be made over issues in palliative care.

Three brief examples will illustrate the kind of issues which need to be addressed

End-of-life issues

Euthanasia is a subject which is not only the province of professionals, but the public at large. The public and politicians want to know what the issues are, what discussions are taking place at the moment, what is happening in other countries, and how can their views be heard?

Resource allocation

Almost every health system is currently looking to see how palliative care can be developed and funded. It is an emotional issue and attracts publicity. Campaigns can be readily mounted to build a hospice, raise money for a post or educational purposes, and for many other reasons. But why should palliative care be funded at the expense of other services? How can the case be made to those who make the decisions? Recent discussion on children and end-of-life issues and their resource requirements have added another dimension to this topic.

Quality of care

One of the commonest complaints against health professionals is that of poor communication. Not surprisingly this becomes particularly relevant in those circumstances when patients die in inappropriate circumstances and the family is unhappy.

Another issue has been the increasing political and professional debate about choice in health care. This discussion focuses on the need for patients to be given choice (a very positive process) though at the same time raises issues of affordability and availability of expertise. These are issues which can, and will, be raised very publically.

Add to these examples other high profile issues in the press at any time, and the justification for some thinking about the topic becomes clearer. There are many more examples which could have been used; however, these should suffice to show the importance of the topic. The danger is that without thought and preparation, the doctor, the speciality, or the palliative care service may be misunderstood and under these circumstances it is much more difficult to get on top of the agenda. Better to be ahead of the game than trying to recover from a public relations disaster.

The purpose of these processes is to build up trust between the doctor and the palliative care service and the media, politicians, and the public. Trust is a key part of the process and takes time to build up and very easy to lose. The remainder of this chapter deals with the issues which arise when clinical interests in palliative care interface with the public, politicians, and the media.

The purpose of communication

The communication of an issue around palliative care to the public or the media has several different functions. First, it might be to inform the public of the scope of palliative care or give the details of a new service or treatment which is available. Second, it may be to raise the profile of the speciality or a particular service in order that funding might be approved or donations granted. It might be to assist in the patient or the public making choices, either about the services available or to raise an ethical issue such as euthanasia or other end of life issues. It might also be to encourage professional staff to consider palliative care as a career and see it as an opportunity for personal development. From the political point of view, it will partly be to raise awareness of the subject and allow opportunities to meet and talk to politicians about the ways in which palliative care can be of benefit to a wide range of people.

Part of the problem is that the response to any issue can be reactive or proactive; in so many instances it is the former—responding to a news item rather than setting the news. Both of course are relevant and can be very valuable but in reactive mode the story line is usually set and it may be difficult to change it. It is generally someone else's agenda.

Taking the lead and thus shaping the agenda sounds the right thing to do, but it can be very difficult. The media may not be interested, they tend to like 'bad news' stories where there is conflict and death, where there is controversy, or where patient lives have been put at risk. 'Good news' stories are much more difficult to get into the press though local media, as opposed the national media including print, radio, and television are often looking for news. What often matters, with media deadlines to be met, is to have a full press release available so that it can be used without much editing.

Each palliative care service must therefore hold the contact numbers of key media personnel and local politicians and invite them on a regular basis to visit the facility, meet staff, and if appropriate, patients. Such visits build up trust and a working atmosphere, which, if problems arise can allow them to be handled more readily. This inevitably takes time and in the short term there may be nothing to show for the effort. However, if the media and the public are aware of what palliative care is, and what can be offered, then they are more likely to be responsive if something new comes on the scene or a problem arises.

Communication with the public is also about providing information about health and illness, and in the palliative care setting, about death and dying. These latter two topics are still taboo in many places and the palliative care service, through a carefully developed communication strategy, can bring such topics into the public consciousness. They can help in the debate and discussion, pose questions and begin to give some of the answers, and deal with fears and misconceptions about such issues. They can help to form attitudes and ensure that when problems do arise then they know where they might get help. The provision of information is one of the services which can be provided. The use of leaflets, audio tapes, and videos can assist in this process. Notices and posters in local shops or pharmacies can be another way of disseminating information. Local seminars with other professional groups, with the public, and with the media may be another way of doing this. It is not an easy area to discuss and requires careful and sensitive writing and producing. However, if the public, the media, and the politicians can learn more and their attitudes change then a great deal will have been gained.

Mechanisms of communication

Communication with the public, the media, and the politicians is not a simple matter. However, there are some principles which have been found to be useful in assisting the process.

◆ Be clear about the message and consider the language used very carefully. Is it understandable? Is too much jargon used? Is there a single clear message? It is sometimes useful to use a non-medical colleague to check the press statement. If it is not understandable by them, then it will not be by the public.

◆ Have you considered all those who might be affected by the message? Could some of the key players be involved in the process in order that they are supportive when the message is released? For example, if a new service is being launched, local health providers and professionals might like to know this and be prepared to support the new venture rather than oppose it, a possible occurrence, if they have not been involved.

◆ Check out any possible financial implications. What does it cost? How will it be funded? Will this take resource away from other services?

◆ Make sure that you have prepared a 'question and answer' brief for the person who will be in the lead. In particular, highlight any controversial areas, or areas into which an interviewer may lead. For example, though the press launch may be to set up a new pain unit, the discussion might all be about euthanasia. Consider all aspects. Preparation is everything.

◆ Make sure you are aware of any related stories in the press which you might be asked about, and whether or not a particular politician has a special interest in some aspect of palliative care. Background information is critical if you are not to be caught out.

◆ Decide early on who will be in the lead, and that individual should be involved in the process from the beginning, not brought in at the end.

◆ Where relevant, hard-copy information should be made available for interested parties to take away and use. The use of web based information can be a rapid way of disseminating news and information. If your service does not have such a facility, consider it or link to another health provider.

◆ Where appropriate, have internal meetings of key external stakeholders to ensure that there are no surprises for them.

◆ Finally, after the event, a full de-briefing should be held to work through any of the problems and improve the presentation next time.

Some organizations find it helpful to use a checklist which is developed over the years and which fits the organization and the subject matter. Such checklists include key contacts and access to legal advice where required. Difficult issues usually occur on Friday nights when people have left the service. Make sure you are prepared. One way of doing this is to take the next public incident in palliative care and ask whether your organization could tackle it, and how. Ensure that you have available telephone numbers of staff and key personnel. There may be a rapid need to check the data, inform or meet key stakeholders, prepare a well-understood message free from jargon, and identify the individual to present the information. Audio-visual aids may be required and these should be prepared early.

Dealing with the public and the media are now regular occurrences for many palliative care services. It is worth considering staff training specifically for this purpose. It can increase confidence and ensure that important aspects of the process are not missed. This is also relevant to National Organizations and Speciality Groups. There is merit, on a regional or national basis, having a list of specialists who can be available to deal with specific issues. Once again, media training for this group is likely to be helpful. Remember that in press releases it is useful to have them checked for 'reading age' (a technique to establish its readability) and by a lay person for its comprehension and avoidance of jargon.

The broader question here relates the understanding of science by the public and the need to explain the complex processes involved in the use of a new procedure or a new drug development. Simply confusing people with scientific jargon and complex clinical issues, is not much good and will not build trust and confidence. Take time to explain, and consider the language used.

Dealing with an urgent issue

The description given above is concerned mainly with the situation in which there is a clear need to speak to the press or politicians, and which can be planned and prepared for. The alternative situation which has to be dealt with is where a problem arises and which needs immediate action or one which is a source of questioning by the public or the media. Such situations might include the use of a new and controversial treatment, an increased number of unexpected deaths, a major complaint against the hospice for poor care, a disgruntled relative (perhaps with good cause), a controversial statement made by a member of staff on an issue relevant to palliative care which might or might not have been misinterpreted, and many others.

In these situations there is much less time to prepare, and the work done before hand on the checklist—who should speak, contact numbers, etc.—will become very useful. In such situations, however, it is often clear that there has been a problem and that it might have been present for some time. This is often called the anticipatory phase of the response to an unexpected risk. Part of the function of the senior management in the hospice is to be alert to possible problems (risks), to identify them, and where possible deal with them as early as can be. Looking back, the problem may even have been detected early but no one took action. In the public presentation of the problem, whatever it is, one of the first questions usually asked is, why was this not detected earlier? Who was responsible for this, and why was no action taken? Answers to these will be needed at the press conference. Think through all possible questions and have a mock press conference with your staff who think of the difficult questions. The time to have media training is before this incident occurs. Put in another way, was this a system failure (could it have been prevented and predicted) or did it relate to an error by an individual (which again could have been prevented.) The response to these two problems may be different, though in practice they are often related.

The process during the second phase of communication of an urgent issue is similar to that described earlier, but some aspects need emphasizing.

A key contact list is essential.

◆ If other players are involved, or might have a view (e.g. the community nursing service, a pharmaceutical company, the local medical group, or health authority) then it is generally wise to inform then and meet them.

◆ The message needs to be clear, and potential questions need to be identified and answered. Hard copies of the press release should be available and checked for any errors and for language.

◆ Nothing should be held back or concealed and if the information is not known or available then this should be made public. It can be noted that more information will be made available as it becomes known.

◆ It is often helpful to enlist the views of outsiders who can put the issue into perspective and allay public fears. Such individuals

and other key groups should, if possible, be at the press conference to answer questions.

◆ When issues like this arise, the media should not be avoided or dismissed. If they have no comment or copy to use they will make it up or use other people's views. Provide them with something to take away and use.

◆ If you have a website then it can be used to provide updated information. Refer to it in the press briefing.

◆ The language used in the presentation has to be very carefully considered. The choice of words can be crucial and this is not a task which can be done without very careful presentation or rehearsal in many instances. Making comments in the press is not a trivial task as words and phrases can be so easily misconstrued.

◆ As before, the evaluation of the outcome is critical and should help to inform any other problems in the future. It is often assumed that this will be a one off and will never happen again. This is not likely to be true. Such events will continue to occur and the palliative care service needs to be able to respond.

Such communication issues are common to many different palliative care organizations and it might be useful for a local, regional, or national grouping to get together and share experience of these issues.

Media training

In a palliative care service which has regular contact with the media and the public it may be of value to have senior people trained in media skills. This allows the individual to think through some of the issues and have professional advice on presentation and on how to raise difficult issues. There are many agencies in most countries which can provide such a service. It allows confidence to be built up so that the doctor is less frightened of the media and politicians, and faces them without feeling threatened. This is of course easier if the doctor has already met the individuals and begun the process of engagement.

Evaluating the outcome—how do we know if we have been successful?

This is the final phase of the response and the one which is often neglected. Once the dust has settled and the press has gone home, what has been learned? It is easy to say that this is a one off, that it could not possibly happen again, but it might. Could the processes be tightened up? Have the basic problems been dealt with? Has a regular process of audit been set up to ensure that any further problems will be identified at the earliest possible time? If the hospice, service, or clinician is to learn from past experiences then this needs to be built into the thinking and the culture of the organization.

Interacting with politicians

Politicians, both local and national, can be of great value to a palliative care service. It is important, therefore, that efforts are made to get to know them and to ensure that they understand the work of the care service. They can be great allies. In particular, they may be of help in the following ways.

Public policy

Politicians have an important responsibility in public policy and in setting a national framework for action. They do this through the democratic process in parliament, senate, or congress. They can influence public opinion, and are influenced by it. Issues such as the use of cannabis or in the ending of life are just some of the policy issues they may deal with. They make laws and have the ability to change the way in which a service operates or is funded. They can therefore shape a palliative care service for a whole nation, and provide the resource. They will need assistance in this and are likely to turn to advisors for specialist advice. While ministers or senior politicians will generally make the running, local parliamentarians will have significant input.

Parliamentary processes

In addition to the functions described above there are other important areas to consider. There are select committees which investigate particular issues, and there are specialist parliamentary groups whose members focus on such topics as palliative care. They are usually 'All Party Associations' and thus generally free from party politics. Such groups are an important source of input into decision making. As 'Lobbying' groups they are important source of advocacy for patients and for the services they require.

International issues

There are many international bodies which have interests in palliative care and other relevant issues such as ethics. These include the World Health Organization, medical and professional organizations, and regional groupings such as the European Union and the Council of Europe. There are many others across the world and they are a useful source of information and expertise.

Conclusion

Dealing with the media is a professional task. It requires care and planning. It is a process which has been thought out and worked on with sufficient energy at a very high level in the palliative care team. Working with politicians can be very rewarding and can influence decisions about the future of the speciality. Invitations to meet senior people should be accepted with alacrity. Eating for your hospice is an occupational hazard.

Further reading

Bennett, P., and Calman, K.C. (1999). *Risk communication and public health.* Oxford University Press, Oxford.

Calman, K.C. (2001). Issues of risk. This unique opportunity. *British Journal of General Practice*, **51**, 47–51.

Calman, K.C. (2002). Communication of risk: choice, consent and trust. *Lancet*, **360**, 166–8.

Department of Health. (1997). *Communicating about risks to the public health.* HMSO, London.

National Radiological Protection Board. (2004). In terms of risk: Report of a seminar to help define important issues used in communicating about risk to the public. *NRPB*, **16**(4).

SECTION 7

Research in palliative medicine

Research in palliative care

Geoffrey Hanks, Stein Kaasa, and Karen Forbes

'Ignorance has risks, but they are largely unseen and unnoticed. Gaining knowledge has risks which are noticed, but largely unpredictable, and it is very costly (though less so than prolonged ignorance). It focuses blame, whereas ignorance dispels it. So, maintaining ignorance often seems more attractive than gaining knowledge'. Duncan Vere[1].

Introduction

Duncan Vere was Professor of Clinical Pharmacology & Therapeutics at the London Hospital and one of the key advisors to Cicely Saunders when she founded St Christopher's Hospice in 1967. Vere is an expert in clinical trials and analgesic clinical pharmacology and was one of the first people to undertake and supervise research in a hospice setting. The quotation is taken from a paper he presented at the Royal Society of Medicine in London in a debate about the ethical aspects of randomized controlled trials. He was not talking specifically about research in palliative care but making a general point that it was easy to be deterred from undertaking rigorous scientific research in a clinical setting. He went on to highlight that such research is crucial to the advance of reliable knowledge.

We have used Vere's quotation to open this chapter on research in palliative care in all three of the previous editions of this textbook because it is an apposite comment on the relatively slow progress of research in palliative care. The initial enthusiasm and urgency to gain a basic understanding of the physiology and pharmacology of the dying or severely ill patient and to evaluate the care that was provided and the treatment that was given did not grow and mature as Cicely Saunders had intended. Research in palliative care has remained in the doldrums until relatively recently in spite of wide recognition of its importance amongst palliative care practitioners. In contrast, the continued development of new clinical services has continued apace around the world.

The provision of new services has not been driven by research findings. We do not have data which demonstrate the most cost-effective model of service delivery of palliative care[2], nor, in fact, can we answer the more fundamental question of what models are effective. There remain large areas of clinical practice in palliative care that are founded on clinical experience and anecdote rather than high-quality evidence, and this has applied even to core activities such as the control of pain.

This frustrating state of affairs has changed and is changing[3]. In the 5 years since publication of the previous edition of this textbook there have been major developments in palliative care research in terms of funding and the development of infrastructure and support for academic activities of teaching and research. In the last edition of this textbook, we wrote that 'there are very few academic departments and fewer still that have sufficient core funding to allow the development of blue sky research programmes. Substantial investment in departments that have the critical mass and facilities to allow high-quality research to be undertaken would take research in palliative care a quantum leap forward. But no such investment is on the horizon ...' In fact, in the last 5 years, in different parts of the world, substantial new funding streams for palliative care research have become available.

In the United Kingdom, a report on cancer research from the National Cancer Research Institute (NCRI) drew attention to the fact that one of the most poorly funded areas in the combined research portfolios of the major cancer research funding organizations in the United Kingdom is palliative care[4]. This prompted the NCRI to set up a strategic review group to analyse the background and reasons for the relatively poor state of palliative care research and make proposals for remedying this situation[4]. As a result, two research collaboratives were funded by the NCRI in 2006 for a period of 5 years. The aim was to improve the quality and quantity of supportive and palliative care research and to develop research capacity[5].

In Canada in 2004, the Canadian Institute of Health Research (CIHR) announced funding of $16.5 million for palliative care and end-of-life research. Once more a major thrust of this initiative was to develop research capacity by attracting established researchers to move into palliative and end-of-life care and supporting the creation of interdisciplinary research teams[3]. In Europe, a consortium of 11 centres in six countries (the European Palliative Care Research Collaboration, EPCRC)[6] has been funded by the European Union within the 6th Framework Programme. The aims of this project are inter alia to identify genes and genetic variation relevant for response to opioid treatment and the development of cachexia. The emphasis of this initiative is to demonstrate the relevance of translational research to palliative care[7]. Similar funding developments have been established more recently in Australia and the United States[3]. Thus several initiatives have come to fruition simultaneously in different countries, specifically targeted towards supportive and palliative care research. All aim to develop research capacity in these areas at the same time as supporting specific research programmes. These are significant developments which will change the face of palliative care research over the coming years.

In this chapter, we briefly review the history of research in palliative care and outline some basic principles. We give some advice about practical aspects of undertaking research in palliative care and also suggest some possible ways to progress in the future. We now have the possibility of widespread collaboration and networking to really promulgate the integration of clinical research into day-to-day clinical practice in palliative care.

Research in palliative care: the beginning

Modern palliative care has its origins in the opening of St Christopher's Hospice in London in 1967. St. Christopher's was different from other long-established hospices and homes for the terminally ill because its aim was to integrate 'a scientific programme concerned with the discriminating use of drugs with the tender loving care'[8] provided within these other institutions. From the outset, research was a priority, and the studies in pain control by Twycross[9] and in the evaluation of hospice care by Hinton and later Murray-Parkes[10] had a considerable impact on the development of the specialty and widespread influence outside it. Since that time, much has been achieved and there have been many advances which are described throughout this book. However, progress has been slow, and palliative care researchers have some catching up to do. As palliative care has developed into the mainstream of health-care, research, paradoxically has tended to take a back seat. Indeed, there is still a widespread view that scientifically rigorous clinical research is incompatible with the basic tenets of palliative care: 'few people associate hospices with science-based medicine'[11]. Yet, as in any other field of health-care, practitioners have an obligation to provide the best possible treatment and care to patients at the end of their lives. The only way to ensure that high standards are established and maintained is through an understanding of the pathophysiological processes involved in patients with advanced disease and by evaluating the treatments that are employed using the most robust methodology which can be applied. Research is essential in order to be confident that current practice is best practice. We must now grasp the opportunities provided by recent developments in funding and ensure that there is strategic investment in both researchers and facilities, and infrastructure to give some substance to the often articulated exhortations for more research in palliative care.

Obstacles to research in palliative care

It has taken much time for research to become embedded in the culture of palliative care. The issues of the primacy of the individual and whole person care versus the 'greatest happiness of the greatest number' are brought sharply into focus in palliative care. The physician's obligation to keep the patient's interest paramount is a fundamental precept of medical practice and is given great emphasis in palliative care. However, the physician has another obligation, which is to promote the acquisition of scientific knowledge. These obligations constitute a real conflict and raise difficult ethical dilemmas. In daily clinical practice, patient care will always take precedence over research when time is limited.

Other members of the team will face similar dilemmas and this may be particularly acute for non-medical practitioners who are not so constrained by the biomedical model of health and ill-health and may be unsympathetic to research that is focused only or predominantly in this direction. Thus there has been a need to change the culture of palliative care so that research is seen as an integral and essential part of the discipline rather than an optional add-on for enthusiasts. Palliative care researchers need also to be eclectic in their approach to research in terms of the disciplines involved and the methodologies which are employed.

There have been problems in attracting high-quality researchers into palliative care. This is partly a consequence of the uncertain career structures and a relative lack of training opportunities (which reflects the lack of funds and investment). The need for an academic affiliation for palliative care researchers with formalized research groups within the main academic hospitals made up of a sufficient number of scientists representing a variety of disciplines working together has been highlighted in a recent topical review[12]. The research group needs to have core funding to enable it to apply for further project grants. Symptom control research is always likely to be less attractive to grant awarding bodies than molecular genetics. However, it is increasingly apparent that molecular biology may be a fertile area for exploring research questions of direct relevance to palliative care clinical practice. Pain perception, for example, is a complicated process involving the interaction of central and peripheral nervous systems and influenced by social, psychological, and cultural factors. Genetic variation may influence human pain perception through a variety of different systems including metabolic processes, nociceptors, cytokines, and membrane transporters[13]. A recent review discusses and summarizes the available evidence for the influence of human gene polymorphisms on variability in response to opioid analgesics and in terms of both analgesia and side effects[7]. There is some evidence from a study in palliative care patients that mu opioid receptor polymorphisms may be related to the need for higher doses of morphine[14] and a catechol-o-methyl transferase (COMT) may influence morphine requirements in cancer pain patients[15]. Translational research is one of the priority areas for palliative care: academic departments of palliative care may need to broaden their base to include laboratory scientists as well as social anthropologists, ethicists, and clinicians.

Palliative medicine has been a recognized speciality in the United Kingdom for 15 years but it remains the case that physicians may reach consultant status (attending, specialist) with very little experience of research. Even if they do have experience and are interested in doing research, the clinical pressures and lack of infrastructure support may make it impossible for them to engage in worthwhile studies. The situation in other countries in Europe and in the United States has been similar. However, as specialist training programmes in palliative medicine are established in different countries, some experience of research is usually requested of trainees. Research is a mandatory part of the training programme in the Nordic Curriculum in Palliative Medicine, and in the United Kingdom may take up 1 year of the 4-year higher specialist training. There is a need to encourage specialist trainees to take time out to do research. It is vital that we consolidate what has been achieved already and do not loose key posts as the first generation of palliative care researchers approach retirement. At the same time new training and substantive posts for researchers are needed together with the right sort of support for them.

National and international organizations in palliative care have a key role to play. The European Association for Palliative Care Research Network (EAPC RN) was established in 1996 by de Conno and the ideas behind it implicitly recognize that networks are essential for palliative care research[16]. The number of patients available for clinical research in any one centre is always going to be relatively small and that means that collaborative studies are necessary to recruit sufficient patients in a reasonable period of time.

It soon became clear in the mid-1990s that palliative care research activity and expertise in different countries in Europe varied considerably, and it was not feasible to launch into large multi-centre clinical trials at the outset because only a handful of centres were in a position to participate in them. This had been one of the initial ideas behind the setting up of the Research Network.

The EAPC RN decided to adopt a different strategy in those early years. Expert working groups were set up to review areas of controversy or areas that were particularly topical at the time and to draw up clinical guidelines based on the available evidence. These guidelines have generally proved to be highly influential[17] and, for the researchers, were useful in identifying gaps in the evidence base and priority areas for research. The Research Network went on to organize a cross-sectional survey of palliative care in Europe as its first collaborative study, which demonstrated the great potential of palliative care research networks to work in a coherent and collaborative fashion across many different countries and cultures. In that study, 143 centres in 21 countries provided data on more than 3000 patients[18]. The future for palliative care research lies with networks be they local, regional, national, or international.

Consolidating for future developments in palliative care research

Table 7.1.1 shows some of the recently established research collaboratives and their areas of interest formed in response to the recommendations from the previous mentioned reports in the United Kingdom and Canada: the need to establish multi-disciplinary research groups of sufficient strength and size, the need for long-term planning, and the need for international as well as national collaboration are reflected in the membership of the groups. Some of the groups individually or in collaboration with others in Table 7.1.1 are working for international consensus on patient-centred outcomes (health-related quality of life and subjective symptoms) and patient cohort classification. The long-term goal for clinical palliative care research should be to move from descriptive to intervention studies. All of these new research initiatives as well as the establishment of new chairs of palliative medicine and palliative care nursing will enable researchers to address complex research questions in the field of palliative care.

The EAPC RN needs to seek collaboration with other national and international groups/organizations in palliative care, oncology, pain, basic scientists, epidemiology, and others of relevance.

The most urgent needs for the future, which should be partly realized through the output of the new collaboratives/collaboration are that:

- Groups of sufficient size and sufficient output need to take the responsibility for further development of research.

- National and international funding needs to continue, and successful collaboratives need to receive further funding without unnecessary gaps.

- It is vital to train a sufficient number of clinicians and scientists in palliative care research.

The ethics of research in palliative care (see also Section 5)

Much progress in medicine is achieved through advances in basic science, but it also depends on clinical research which, by definition,

Table 7.1.1 Recently established palliative care research collaboratives and initiatives.

Country	Type of project	Contact address/person
UK - Supac		
A: Cancer experiences collaboratives (CECo)	Innovative approaches to complex symptoms, needs of older adults; narratives of cancer and other life-limiting illness	www.ceco.org.uk
B: COMPlex interventions: assessment, trials and implementation of services collaboratives (COMPASS)	Developing and evaluating complex interventions	www.compasscollaborative.com
Canadian - Netgrants		
Ten collaboratives were funded from 2002	Symptom management, classification of palliative care, communication, family care, end-of-life care, and pediatric care	www.cihr-irsc.gc.ca/e/36889.html
EU – European Palliative Care Research Collaborative (EPCRC)	Translational research pain, cachexia, and depression	www.epcrc.org or stein.kaasa@ntnu.no
EU – PHEA Health Information	Describe best practice in palliative care in Europe	
EU – Reflecting the positive diversities of European priorities for research and measurement in end-of life-care (PRISMA)	Coordination and supportive actions: reflecting the positive diversity of European priorities for research and measurement in end of life care	www.kcl.ac.uk/schools/medicine/depts/palliative/arp/prisma/ or irene.higginson@kcl.ac.uk
EU – Optimising Cancer Patient Care (OPCARE)	A European collaboration to optimize research and clinical care for cancer patients in the last days of life	John.Ellershaw@mariecurie.org.uk
USA – National Palliative Care Research Centre (NPCRC)	A centre to promote palliative care research	www.npcrc.org or sean.morrison@mssm.edu

means research involving patients. Serendipity continues to play a role in advancing knowledge as does astute clinical observation. But neither of these mechanisms can be relied on to ensure progress; human experimentation based on the scientific method is essential for medicine to continue to advance. This argument applies to palliative care as it does to any other area of medicine.

The Declaration of Helsinki, drawn up by the World Medical Association in 1964 (and amended in 1975 and 1983), was a response to the need for a code of ethics on human experimentation, which would be applicable to all countries and all situations where human subjects were involved in research[19]. The code acknowledges the need for guidance for physician investigators caught in the conflict between the patient's own best interests and the necessity to advance knowledge for the benefit of society as a whole.

The Declaration of Helsinki is generally accepted as an ethical code of practice for clinical research and its principles are applicable to palliative medicine. It is important that clinical research is seen to conform to these principles and that all research projects are scrutinized by independent assessors to ensure that this is the case. This function is usually undertaken by a local Research Ethics Committee and now, in many countries, there is a comprehensive network of local and multi-centre research ethics committees.

Research governance

In recent years there has been a trend towards increasingly explicit guidelines and regulations relating to research involving patients. In the United Kingdom, these guidelines are described under the heading of 'research governance'. Research can involve an element of risk regarding both the return on investment and the safety and well-being of participants. The research governance guidelines are designed to minimize risk and improve research performance and they provide a useful framework, particularly for those new to research, which has general applicability and is not only relevant in the United Kingdom.

Research governance is 'the means by which we ensure high scientific, ethical, and financial standards for the conduct of research and involves transparent decision-making processes, clear allocation of responsibilities, and robust monitoring arrangements'. The research governance framework for health and social care in the United Kingdom encompasses five domains. These are ethics (the dignity, rights, safety, and well-being of participants); science (the quality and appropriateness of research); information (the requirements for free access to research information); health, safety, and employment (of participants and research and other staff); and finance and intellectual property. The background and details of the Research Governance Framework are available at: www.doh.gov.uk/research/RD3/nhsrandd/researchgovernance.htm

In the United Kingdom the introduction of new regulations and procedures has added considerable time to the process of having an application to do research approved by various bodies involved. The changes have not been universally welcomed[20,21] because of their potential negative effects, not merely on the research process but on researchers too, particularly junior staff who may just be embarking on a research career. It is crucial that some balance is maintained in the striving to make the process as safe and as user-friendly as possible for patients and remembering that researchers too need to be supported and certainly not deterred from doing research because of the bureaucracy and inevitable delays that are involved.

Controlled clinical trials and informed consent in palliative medicine

Austin Bradford Hill set out the ethical precepts for randomized controlled trials in his Marc Daniels Lecture at the Royal College of Physicians in 1963[22]. In the United States, Henry Beecher had a similar influence on the development of ethical guidelines for clinical research[23] and the subject has been debated in many places since. It is not appropriate to discuss this subject in detail here, but the reader is referred to these reviews, which make two important points. The first is that the prospective randomized controlled trial is the most efficient, scientific way of evaluating a new treatment or of comparing alternative treatments, but the second is that it is not the only way of ensuring the advance of reliable knowledge.

Controlled clinical trials are necessary in palliative medicine, and the usual guidelines and ethical principles will apply. Some points need particular emphasis in the palliative care setting. Patients are invariably at a low ebb physically and many are elderly and frail; most have a multitude of physical and emotional and perhaps social and spiritual problems. When they come to the palliative care unit or team, many of these problems will be dealt with, and some, particularly the psychosocial issues, may receive attention for the first time. The supportive environment in palliative care may make patients particularly keen to give something back to the carers, to show their gratitude for the care they are receiving. All of these factors make patients particularly vulnerable when they are asked to participate in any sort of research project, for many will feel almost an obligation to accede to such a request. Researchers in palliative care must be on their guard not to take advantage of this situation.

In palliative care, cognitive impairment and often frank confusion is a problem encountered in many patients; when this is obvious, they will be excluded from consideration for entry to a study. However, often the impairment is mild or variable. Such patients need careful assessment, and, wherever there is any doubt that the patient is able to understand what is being asked of them, he or she should not be considered for inclusion.

There is a fine balance that needs to be achieved here. The special vulnerability of patients receiving palliative care dictates the need for special handling in obtaining consent to participate in research but at the same time the researcher must not go out of his or her way to talk the patient out of wanting to take part.

Evidence-based palliative care (see Chapter 7.2)

The principles of evidence-based medicine underpin our day-to-day clinical practice. Evidence-based medicine 'is the conscientious, explicit, and judicious use of current best evidence in making decisions about the care of individual patients. The practice of evidence-based medicine means integrating individual clinical expertise with the best available external clinical evidence from systematic research'[24].

Evidence-based medicine is not a new idea. It has always been implicit that clinical practice should be based on the best possible evidence. However, what was relatively new 10 years ago was the widespread recognition that this is not happening. The evolution of current thinking about evidence-based medicine is described in Chapter 7.2.

Evidence-based medicine is about finding ways in which to bridge the gap between the huge amount of published data and clinical practice, and encompasses a number of strategies. One of these has been the development of scientific methods (systematic reviews and meta-analyses) to combine data from a number of different randomized studies of the same or similar treatments in any particular condition. Systematic reviews differ from other types of review in that they adhere to a strict scientific design in order to make them more comprehensive, to minimize the chance of bias, and so ensure their reliability.

Taken at face value, it seems reasonable to assume that the data from several studies, which have been combined according to agreed scientific methodology, should be more meaningful than the evidence from single studies. This is not universally accepted and there is no doubt that the methodology and application of these techniques must continue to be looked at critically. However, systematic reviews and meta-analyses are powerful tools in aggregating and evaluating large amounts of data and have become an important area of research activity in palliative medicine. One function they serve is to highlight research questions and thus contribute to the research agenda by careful and comprehensive review of the available evidence.

Evidence-based medicine and the future of palliative care

Evidence-based medicine has already had a major impact on the development of health care in a time of ever-increasing demands but limited resources. It is likely that resource allocation will increasingly be based on evidence not just of efficacy but of cost effectiveness. Where proof of efficacy is lacking, funds will not be provided by government or other health-care agencies. This has particular implications for palliative care because it is an area where such research-based evidence is sparse. There are many activities within palliative care which are not amenable to investigation by randomized controlled studies. But, as noted earlier, the randomized controlled trial is not the only valid method of ensuring advances in knowledge. The recent focus on evidence-based medicine makes all the more urgent, the investment in palliative care research.

The scope of research in palliative care

One of the challenges in palliative care research is setting boundaries around the field. Because the subject and event of dying and death is at the centre of practitioners' concerns, it can be tempting to include all dimensions of scholarship related to 'death' within the field of interest. Death, as one of the major rites of passage for individuals, families, and societies, attracts research on its many ramifications, manifestations, and meanings in everyday life. The cultural context in which people present themselves as patients, come to approach death, and are cared for through their dying, is open to wide and varied interpretations drawn from historical, sociological, anthropological, theological, philosophical, and psychological perspectives; each with its own research traditions. Understanding the significance of death as a rite of passage as well as a biological or medical event is important for the skills of the practitioner when faced with the communication challenges with dying patients and their families, and so it could be argued that the field of palliative care research is in fact immense. Practically, however, the field is generally focused on a narrower range of interests, of immediate concern and relevance to practitioners and planners.

The principal questions that face palliative care professionals are those of clinical effectiveness and acceptability, service efficiency and organization, and meeting changing needs in the population. These are basic questions concerned with what palliative care practitioners do, and how they do it. The research skills to answer these questions are commonly drawn from the traditions of clinical research (medical, nursing, and allied health professional), health services research, and also epidemiology. The complexity of palliative care research and challenges to apply the most appropriate research methodology is presented and discussed in a recent special issue of *Palliative Medicine*[25].

Epidemiological research: descriptive epidemiology seeks to describe the prevalence and incidence of conditions within defined populations. Assessing the need for palliative care in different sec-tors of the population is clearly important for informing the process of service development and planning. In relation to palliative care, epidemiological research has been hampered by an absence of clearly defining population indicators linked to levels of clinical need, as well as changing perceptions within the profession of palliative care as to the appropriate 'catchment population'. The extended application of palliative care from its original main constituency of terminally ill cancer patients, to patients with any life-limiting illness, from point of diagnosis onwards, poses problems of classification. The majority of health service utilization data and measures of morbidity and mortality are based on disease categories. These do not give an indication of symptom burden or dependency levels, and thus little indication of the need for different forms of palliative care.

Clinical research: traditionally clinical research tends to focus on biochemical, microbiological, and physiological processes and the effect of pharmacological and other therapeutic agents. In palliative care, this focus is much broader because of the complexity of advanced disease and the high prevalence of psychological and existential distress. Clinical trials are based on an experimental approach and will often use outcomes from the laboratory derived from body samples (blood, tissue) or images (x-rays or scans) as well as patient responses recorded by questionnaire or structured interview. It is at the level of clinical research that trial based research methodologies are most effective and applicable. The need for access to skilled technicians and laboratory facilities will tend to limit research capacity in clinical research for researchers working in non-academic or community settings.

Health services research: research that is not strictly epidemiological or clinical can be categorized into the wider area named health services research. This kind of research is primarily focused on the evaluation of the organization and delivery of health care. Frequently, the research is applied to particular problems faced by policy-makers, managers, practitioners, and patients, and can range from questions of cost and effectiveness, policy formulation and implementation, the evaluation of new technologies, through to patient and public preferences and perceptions. Research approaches include those that underpin the social sciences as well as the more experimentally based approaches of the natural sciences. Much of the multi-disciplinary research carried out in palliative care is focused on questions of innovation and organization in services, and assessing the need for and access to different types of intervention.

Wider humanistic research: the contribution of other disciplines and research traditions to the body of research in palliative care is well recognized and valued. Concern with the ethical, moral, spiritual, and philosophical dimensions of care for the dying and bereaved from all perspectives informs a body of scholarship, which broadens out the focus of research that can be relevant to palliative care practitioners. However, lack of familiarity with disciplinary roots and epistemological theory can make the contributions from the social sciences and humanities impenetrable to practitioners schooled in the natural sciences.

Clinical and health services research: practical considerations

There are particular difficulties associated with clinical research in palliative care, in addition to the ethical constraints described earlier.

The patient population from which potential trial candidates are taken is characterized by old age, multi-system disease, generally severe illness with many symptoms, a progressive clinical condition, and limited survival time. In addition, polypharmacy is the rule, and environmental and psychological factors have a variable but potentially very great influence on physical well-being. Prospective randomized controlled studies are thus particularly difficult to carry out, because there are major problems in accrual of patients to trials, attrition, and missing data[26–29].

The choice of trial design for prospective studies will be much influenced by these characteristics of the patient population. Endpoints or outcomes are also difficult to define. Outcome measures are not generally based on hard data such as biochemical indices or survival, which are relatively easy to quantify, but on changes in symptoms and quality of life, which are much more difficult to measure. The choice of trial design and measurements will be influenced also by the need to ensure that all procedures are designed to place the least possible additional burden on patients.

Defining the patient population

A particularly complex issue is the definition of a palliative care patient population. The lack of strict criteria for defining the patient population is a threat to both the internal and external validity of research in palliative care. In this context, internal validity can be understood as the ability to define the cohort of patients included in a given study. For example, if the true patient population is more heterogeneous than the one defined, the heterogeneity might obscure, even obliterate the positive effect of a particular intervention. External validity is about the representativeness of the sample. In clinical practice, research data might be inappropriately applied if the precise characteristics of the population included in a particular research project are not accurately described. Research methods are generally predicated on the comparison of one population with another; studies of effectiveness are only meaningful when one treatment is set against another within similar or homogeneous populations. Palliative care populations are difficult to standardize however, since referral to a palliative care team is made for a wide variety of reasons, most of which will be patient-generated, but will also include reasons that involve the patient's family and professional carers, and the facilities available to the patient. Prognosis on referral is one way of categorizing patients, which is generally a matter of clinical judgement and use of dependency scores, while time from referral to death is another way; but this is only possible retrospectively. Another possibility is symptom burden—which is in most cohorts closely related to expected survival[30,31,32].

Methodology

The evaluation of the effectiveness of treatments in palliative care has either not been undertaken at all or has been conducted using poor or inadequate research methodology. This was also the case in clinical medicine generally until the late 1960s and early 1970s. Only in recent years has it become evident that properly designed and well-conducted clinical trials are needed in palliative care as much as in any other area of medicine. Most of the published studies of the effectiveness of treatments in palliative care have been related to pain and quite often the patients included have been at an early stage of their disease. Whether the results of these studies can be extrapolated to palliative care patients is open to question.

A clinical trial is any investigation that follows the principles of a scientific experiment, allowing for the evaluation of the clinical effect of an intervention in a valid and reliable way. The term 'clinical trial' is not synonymous with 'randomized controlled trial' (RCT). A clinical trial in the broadest sense of the term may mean any kind of planned experiment in patients, ranging from open descriptive studies to RCTs. The trial design will be determined by the research question.

Drawing on the experience of drug development, clinical trials are usually described in three (or four) phases. This three/four-stage process could also provide a model for research in palliative care in that it describes a sequential process requiring different experimental designs at different stages.

The choice of an appropriate study design will depend on what is already known about the particular question to be investigated. With the recent emphasis on evidence-based medicine, there has been much discussion of the need for RCTs and of the fact that the RCT is the 'gold standard' and the most robust method for evaluating new treatments. However, many research questions do not need to be answered in an RCT. Furthermore, when attempting to design a randomized study, a lack of sufficient descriptive data may make it difficult to decide upon a study design and on appropriate outcomes or to perform a valid sample size calculation. This is commonly the case in palliative care research. The choice of trial design is crucial and, in this process, collaboration between experts is essential. This is the stage at which a project group should be established, at the very beginning of the planning process of a study.

In palliative care, a pilot study (or simply a non-systematic observation of a particular intervention) could be described as 'phase I'. Such a non-systematic study is not a rigorous research experiment but is the first step in the research plan. Thus, before embarking on an RCT, it is necessary to go through a process analogous to phase I and II drug studies. This step-by-step approach highlights the fact that clinical research is a time-consuming process. Researchers and clinicians should not expect too many answers from each study.

Guidelines and books[33,34] on clinical trial methodology are widely available. The objectives and design of a study will be driven by the research questions and the resources available. This is not just about funding but also about academic and clinical resources and the availability of sufficient patients. A common problem in clinical research (not by any means unique to palliative care) is that investigators invariably and substantially overestimate the number of patients they are likely to see who would be suitable for a particular study. Changes in treatment policies might influence the availability of patients for a particular study even more if the entry criteria are based on previous policy.

A general criticism of palliative care research is that too many small studies are performed with an open non-comparative design, and thus the impact of the results in terms of changing practice will be limited. For example, in a recent systematic review of ketamine in cancer-related pain, the reviewers found 32 case series, but only two RCTs of good quality (and these involved a total of only 20 patients). This makes it impossible to draw firm conclusions about the efficacy of ketamine[35].

How to plan a clinical trial

The planning process of any clinical study often starts with new encouraging data from the laboratory or, probably more often in palliative care, from chance or non-systematic observations in the clinic.

Table 7.1.2 The evolution of a research project in palliative care.

1. Describe clearly the clinical problem or observations which prompted the idea for a study.

2. Discuss the relevance and validity of the observations with clinical colleagues.

3. Carry out a comprehensive review of the literature to find out what is already known about the topic.

4. Formulate a research question or two or three questions. These will define the aim of the study.

5. Define the patient population.

6. Decide on the appropriate study design.

7. Decide on the outcomes to be measured.

8. With these decisions made, write the protocol.

Aside from the need to collect together background information, the planning process involves a series of basic steps, which will need to

be considered to provide the framework for the study (Table 7.1.2).

Usually one will start with a literature review to see what is known about an intervention and the target condition or symptom. If the review indicates that a formal study is necessary or worthwhile, a research question or hypothesis should be formulated and this will determine the aim of the study.

A common mistake in clinical research is to bring too many ideas together and try to answer too many questions at the same time. Many studies are too complex with many research questions, which cannot be answered with a limited number of patients.

Explicit definition of the aim of the study is crucial. Many clinical research projects are undertaken without a clear and concise aim, and the consequence is a lack of precision in the subsequent steps of the planning process, and ultimately a poor study or one that is impossible to complete. The aim should be written in clear and understandable language and, ideally, it should be easily understood by a lay person. It should be formulated in a brief way in one or two sentences. It is often expressed as a general question and this is broken down into specific research questions or hypotheses.

The research questions will determine the patient population to be studied. There are several factors to take into consideration such as 'which group of patients will best give an answer to these questions?' For example, if a study was designed to examine patients' attitudes toward euthanasia and physician-assisted suicide in palliative care, the researchers would need to decide whether to ask the patient directly. In similar studies, patients themselves have not been asked, but the questions have been put to proxies or the general public. If the researchers decide to ask the patients, they must then decide how to select patients, (in this example perhaps 'not too ill, but not too far away from being confronted with death and dying'). The patient sample must also be representative of the population of patients to whom the results will be applied. In other words, if a select sub-group of the general population is recruited to a study, the usefulness and applicability of the results (the external validity or generalizability) will be compromised.

In studies evaluating the effect of adjuvant chemotherapy in breast cancer or combination therapy for HIV, the primary outcomes are easy to select, for example, tumour response or survival time[36]. However, in recent years, in oncology trials, criticisms have been made about limiting the outcomes to survival or cure and not taking account of late side effects of the treatment. During the last decade, for example. several studies have described the high prevalence of subjective side effects, such as fatigue, in Hodgkin's disease survivors[37]. These experiences emphasize that selection of outcomes, even in curative treatment studies, might be less straightforward than it at first appears. In palliative care, the number of outcomes can easily get out of hand, because of the complexity of the patient population and studies have been reported with 10 to 20 and even more outcome measures. This multiplicity of outcomes is further driven by the multi-dimensionality of the concept of health-related quality of life and the range of scales and single items found in these measures[38,39]. It is important not to fall into this trap. In general, one or two primary outcomes and perhaps two to three secondary outcomes are the most that should be included.

All of these issues should be thoroughly discussed by the researchers and the involved clinicians, together with the larger study group, before the research protocol can be finalized.

Randomization and blinding

The concept of random allocation of patients when comparing different treatments (or any other interventions) is important in the design of a clinical experiment. The purpose of randomization is to reduce selection bias. Non-randomized trials have a tendency to overestimate the effect of treatment. Randomization also provides a basis for use of standard methods of statistical analysis. When a new treatment is introduced, enthusiastic clinicians and researchers tend to overestimate its beneficial effects For example, in the early open studies of cisplatin in the treatment of non-small-cell lung cancer, the response rate was double what was found in later randomized studies[40]. The same tendency is also seen when using historical controls as a comparison group or when using other quasi-experimental designs.

In palliative care, randomized studies are particularly difficult to undertake and complete. Therefore, other types of studies might be important to consider and might be preferable. Caution needs to be taken in the analysis and in the interpretation of data from non-randomized studies. Other designs may be appropriate and may represent a slightly less robust option than an RCT but still produce persuasive data. For example, in the evaluation of palliative care programmes, cluster randomized designs have been used[41].

Unblinded trials also overestimate the effect of treatment. Blinding may be difficult to achieve and needs to be thought about early in the planning process particularly if it involves the manufacture of placebo formulations or other manufacturing processes to conceal the identity of treatments. Palliative care researchers should consult with statisticians and clinical trial methodologists early in the planning process of the study, and preferably include these advisors in the project group. There are useful texts on clinical trial methodology[33], study design[42], introduction to statistics[43], and more comprehensive textbooks on medical statistics[44]. Such texts provide useful basic background reading for researchers.

Statistical considerations

The project group will need to consult with a statistician, or preferably include a statistician. Medical statisticians have skills and expertise in several areas of clinical research, i.e. study design, sample size estimation, and in the analysis of the data. One essential step in the planning process of any clinical study is to decide how many patients will be needed to get a valid result.

The purpose of this 'sample size' calculation is to ensure that the study is large enough to detect a clinically important difference should one exist, or exclude the possibility of such a difference should none be detected. In order to estimate the sample size, the statistician will want to know how small a difference it is important to be able to detect in the main outcome measures in terms of clinical significance. For example, the number of patients treated with a new opioid, reaching a Numerical Rating Scale (NRS) score below three within 2 weeks of the initiation of treatment. In comparative studies of pain relief, the mean value of the NRS is often used as a primary outcome. The clinicians need to specify how small a difference between groups will be considered to be of clinical significance (e.g. 2 on a 0–11 NRS scale). It would also be helpful to have information about what could be expected to happen in the control group (mean and standard deviation) and this information may be derived from a pilot study or from published literature. The required number of patients is calculated according to how confident one wants to be about detecting a difference between interventions if one exists (the power of the study).

An important principle is that a statistician should be consulted early in the process of designing the study and should have continuing input through the project.

The protocol

A study cannot exist for long as an idea in researchers' minds and a few hastily written notes and memos. It has to be formalized into a protocol, which acts as the 'blue print' of the project. The protocol evolves through a series of stages to become a comprehensive document detailing the 'why', 'when', and 'how' of the study. In its final form, the protocol will describe the background to the study and its scientific relevance, the rationale behind the chosen study design, and a description of the organizational and ethical dimensions. Importantly, the protocol will include a detailed description of how the study will be carried out, from the methods of patient selection and recruitment, the procedures of data collection and handling, through to the plans for analysis. Every step along the way needs to be considered, as well as the procedures to be followed in the case of deviations. Every study will encounter unexpected consequences and unpredictable effects. In this sense, the protocol may well be added to at various points during the study to take account of unforeseen circumstances (commonly called 'protocol deviations'). Table 7.1.3 outlines a typical structure of a protocol for a clinical study.

The process of developing a rough draft of a study protocol through to a stage where all aspects of the study have been considered and piloted is a major research effort on its own. In theory, it means that short of actually carrying out the study, everything that could be done has been done. In practice, researchers who skimp on the protocol and associated development work will often find themselves faced with untenable or 'un-doable' research studies.

Access to patients

A major challenge in palliative care research involving relatively large numbers of patients is in identifying the patient population

Table 7.1.3 Writing the protocol: the headings.

1. ***Introduction***
   Current state of knowledge and literature review
   Reasons for study
   Specific aspect of problem to be investigated

2. ***Aims and objectives***

3. ***Methods***
   a) *Design of investigation*:
   Observational or experimental
   Descriptive or analytical
   Prospective (cohort)
   Retrospective (case–control)
   Control group
   Schedule with justification of design chosen
   b) *Definitions*:
   Diagnostic criteria
   Definition of terms
   c) *Populations*:
   Identification
   Sampling
   Inclusion and exclusion criteria
   Randomization (where appropriate)
   Losses and refusals
   d) *Data*:
   Study variables and extraneous variables
   Sources of data - pre-existing records
              - interview/examination
              - postal survey
   Design of survey documents - questionnaire
                      - interview schedules
                      - data abstraction forms.
   e) *Ethical and funding issues*:
   Discussion where appropriate
   f) *Analysis*:
   Indicate how each question in the objectives is to be answered
   Tabulations to be prepared and how
   Statistical tests to be used
   Sample size calculation where appropriate

4. ***Timetable and programming of the work***
   Including time to develop and pilot questionnaires if necessary

5. ***Appendices***:
   Patient information sheet
   Patient consent form
   Information sheets for: GP
                         patient's consultant
                         nursing staff
                         carers
   Data collection forms
   Questionnaires
     i) Designed for study
     ii) Validated:
         e.g. McGill pain questionnaire
         HADS
         EORTC QLQC$_{30}$ etc.

Source: reproduced with permission from *University of Bristol MSc in Palliative Medicine Handbook* 2003 (eds. Forbes, K., Davies, A.).

and gaining access to them. When research involves selected patients in a clinic, or on a ward, identifying those appropriate for research may not be problematic, especially if the clinician involved is carrying out the research. However, for non-clinical researchers, or for clinical researchers wanting to recruit patients from settings other than their own, identification and access are crucial aspects of patient recruitment. In these situations, cooperation will be needed from the other health care professionals caring for the patients. To gain access to patients may require lengthy negotiation, involving presentations at clinical meetings, permission from professional bodies, as well as strategy for communication and keeping the research project uppermost in clinicians' minds.

It can be useful to develop information sheets, specific for each professional concerned, early on in the stages of introducing a project to those who are affected. Thinking through likely questions and their answers can help to take the project off the drawing board and ground it in the reality of clinical life. Colleagues and peers will be concerned that the research is well designed and addresses a clinically important question. Justifying the purpose and value of a research project to one's peers is particularly critical in relation to palliative care research where non-palliative care colleagues may question the probity of carrying out research with this patient group. There are probably few palliative care researchers who have not, at some time, had their research intentions questioned. In addition, it will be important to listen to colleagues' concerns and offer flexibility in the carrying out of the research. Colleagues will be particularly resistant to participating in anything that involves more paperwork or disruptions to routines. The effort and time involved in securing access from professional colleagues should not be underestimated.

It is also important to feed back to practitioners who have been involved in the research through facilitating access to patients, or providing information, at the end of the research. Knowing what the findings are, and what importance they hold for future service configurations, helps make the research a collaborative experience, and can be an element in service development and change where that is indicated. This affirms the stakeholder role, which professional carers hold in the research process.

Significant others to the patient—non-professional carers: care at the end of life embraces not only the patient, but also those close to him or her. Supporting family carers in their caring role is important in relieving some of the practical difficulties and burdens that are encountered during protracted periods of high-dependency care in the home, as well as addressing the psychological distress which is associated with the loss of a close relative. Research similarly involves not only the patient but also those close to the patient in a primary caring role. Research interest may take several forms; it may focus on the long-term health of those who survive the patient (bereavement studies), but as frequently, it may focus on how patients and their home carers cope with the illness together, and the perceptions of the home carers of the professional care received by the patient. Even when research is solely concerned with patient-based indicators, those close to the patient are important in the research process by acting as intermediaries. Home or family carers can take on a number of roles in relation to patients' involvement in research and each role needs to be appreciated by the research team.

Gatekeepers/protectors: family members adopting a primary caring role also act as 'gatekeepers' to the patients. This is likely to be

increasingly critical as the patient's stamina declines, when dependency increases, and when the patient him/her self has delegated certain aspects of decision-making to a trusted family carer. When patients are approached for recruitment to a research study, it is generally advisable, therefore, to approach whoever appears to be most in contact with the patient (in hospital or at home). Research can appear threatening to those who are striving to care for the patient; primarily they may worry about the research tiring and distracting the patient, and about questions upsetting the patient—either by providing too much information or opening up areas of contemplation that may further disturb the patient. When time is perceived to be short, carers may well resent the attention of the patient being taken by people outside of the family. How family carers weigh up the benefits of participating in a research study (short-term benefits of additional monitoring and attention and long-term benefits to society) against the costs to the patient (and themselves) of time commitments and possibly extra upset will be pivotal in the recruitment process.

The family carer's role as gatekeeper is often regarded negatively by researchers, as one of the barriers to achieving adequate sample sizes. While researchers generally regard adult patients as autonomous, self-determining individuals who can decide for themselves whether they want to participate in research, the vulnerability of some palliative care patients can make this problematic. The tensions between dealing with a patient as a family member rather than as simply an individual are all too apparent. Participation in research is an intervention in itself (patients are not 'passive subjects') with consequences that cannot be wholly predicted, however meticulously procedures are followed. Family carers can be more aware of this than researchers since to them the patient is not one 'number' amongst many, he or she is a spouse, parent, sibling, or child. Being involved in research can involve the wider family context, and so the extended boundaries of the palliative care patient need to be appreciated by researchers, with procedures in place to inform and include family members.

Interpreters, substitutes, and advocates: when patients have difficulty communicating their thoughts and feelings, family members take on the role of interpreter and substitute (proxy). Interpretation can be needed for both speech and language difficulties (translation). In the face of cognitive impairment, the views of family carers can be used as a substitute for the patients' views. A number of studies have investigated the validity of proxy ratings, concluding that proxies tend to underestimate the severity of certain symptoms (pain and depression) but that in the absence of patient derived data, proxy data is valuable.

A role that sits between gatekeeper and interpreter is that of advocate. The extent to which family carers take on this role varies with their own confidence and the situations within which they find themselves. Researchers should be aware that advocacy can work in different ways; at times making sure that the best interests of the patient are promoted, at others, following an agenda that is not the patient's but that of the family member. This is another reason for extreme sensitivity to be exercised by the research team.

Significant others to the patient—professional carers: professional carers can likewise act as gate-keepers, interpreters, substitutes, and advocates, with all the cautions outlined earlier. Similarly, they are also a subject of great interest in their own right from the point of view of service/practitioner efficiency and effectiveness, and understanding the process of delivering high-quality palliative care.

There is a growing body of research on the training and educational needs of practitioners, the dynamics of inter-professional and multi-disciplinary team working, and management processes to preserve and enhance occupational health.

Finance and management

There are many sources of funding that are relevant to palliative care, but securing funds for research in this area is a competitive exercise as it is in any area of health-care. As indicated at the beginning of this chapter, palliative care research is a relatively neglected area as far as the major funders of cancer research are concerned. The great majority of patients currently being treated by palliative care services are patients with cancer so that this means that funding for studies in non-cancer patients is in even shorter supply. However, the climate is changing and this is happening in many different parts of the world. It is not possible here to give detailed information about funding sources since these will vary from country to country. This sort of information is obviously of considerable relevance to future researchers and it is one area where the scientific journals available in palliative care could play a useful role.

Finance for individual projects: the length of time between securing finance for a project and actually starting data collection is always underestimated. This period can be divided into two main phases: the time before project funds are actually drawn upon, when research staff are being recruited and when a considerable amount of planning and groundwork is being carried out; and phase two, when the funds are being disbursed and when piloting work is being undertaken. It is crucial that as much work as possible is carried out in the first phase, even though the work is essentially not funded. Efficient management of time and resources from the very start of a project are obviously key factors in its successful running.

Project group

All research projects benefit from being exposed to a group of people who have experience in the subject under research and who are interested in the project. This is particularly important for large studies. The role of a project group can vary along a spectrum of responsibilities that range from being highly involved in the administration and day-to-day concerns of the project, to being relatively distant, and receiving information about the project on a regular though infrequent basis. The value of project groups are as follows:

- They can provide peer review to the research project, thus validating the research in the eyes of external sponsors and host institutions.

- They can provide research experience and expertise, especially during the early stages of a project.

- They can provide contacts and entry to otherwise hard to access sectors.

- They can provide moral support and encouragement during the course of the project.

- They can act as a sounding board, and also participate in the understanding and analysis of data.

- They can help to disseminate the findings of the research and have a wider view of its relevance to policy and practice.

Depending on the size of the project, it can sometimes be helpful to institute a steering group of key stakeholders who are sympathetic to the research but who do not have much time to devote to it, and a management group of people who are accessible regularly and become close to project and data collection, and who report back to the steering group.

The staffing and management of major research projects will tend to be as follows:

- The researchers conducting the research and collecting data on a day-to-day basis.

- A group of researchers (including all or some of those listed in previous point) who monitor the progress of the study on a regular basis and who provide support, advice, and suggestions, and act as a sounding board.

- A wider group of interested parties who may (or may not) be formally constituted as a steering group.

At an early stage, agreement needs to be reached about decision-making (research and finance), supervision, and mentoring.

Piloting the study and study procedures

Research studies do not start off as fully formed projects. Indeed, it is impossible to anticipate all the challenges that a study will face at the planning stage. The word 'pilot' derives from the job of steering a boat on its course and the metaphor of guiding a ship through uncertain and troubled waters is an apt one. Without preliminary studies, it is difficult to steer the course of a large project. Pilot work is important for testing all aspects of research design, from the face validity and acceptability of data collection procedures, to the workability of allocation schedules, and administration tasks. Dealing with the questions and issues raised by pilot studies can be demanding at a stage when there is impatience to start the main study, not least due to the pressure on obtaining funds for research and the need to work to deadlines. However, learning the lessons from pilot work can be critical to the success of the project. For researchers working alone, the use of a research journal can encourage a reflective attitude to the pilot work, and help to refine the research design. For researchers in a team, frequent meetings at this stage, with records made of the discussions and decisions will again help to re-define and re-model the research into a workable proposition. Re-writing the protocol with the findings of the pilot work is important for the auditing of the research project.

Administration and paperwork

It will be readily appreciated that a research study will quickly develop different strands of paperwork, reflecting the different administrative tasks:

- Background work relating to the development of the study, reviews of the scientific literature, and any position papers and early proposals.

- Paperwork relating to the funding and approval of the study (sponsors, ethics committees, other professional and regulatory bodies).

- Correspondence and paperwork relating to the formation of the steering and project groups, together with the minutes and agendas of each formally convened meeting.

- A record of the protocol as it develops through successive drafts.

- Sources of information targeted at specific sectors of the study population: information sheets for patients and their professional and non-professional carers, information posters for hospital or hospice wards or other settings, information in local media about the study.

◆ Paperwork used for collecting data, ranging from consent forms, case record forms, to questionnaires and data abstraction forms. This might also include letters or cards sent by the research team to patients and carers, after data collection, to thank them for their participation, as well as any correspondence from the study population regarding the research, including letters of complaint or inquiry. Restricting access to this kind of documentation is central to preserving patient confidentiality (lockable rooms or filing cabinets).

◆ A developing account of the way the study is progressing. Most projects benefit from regular review, although this will depend on its size and timescale. Even in the absence of interim analysis, it can be important to monitor recruitment rates, protocol deviations, and any other problems with the management of the project. This can also be an opportunity for informal reflections on the study, particularly from the point of view of the day-to-day researchers.

◆ Paperwork relating to data preparation and data analysis, including any conventions used in coding data, and where the data are held and in what form. This aspect of project administration is most important for the understanding and interpretation of data in analysis.

◆ Finally, the project will be written up as a report in various formats for various audiences, and it is important to keep records of the drafts as they develop and become finalized.

Efficient administration is essential in two quite common scenarios. One is where a project is required to audit its activities and give an account of the funds that have been used, and the procedures that have been followed. This can happen as a result of a rolling programme of research audit within an institution or sector, or can happen as a result of a special investigation, triggered by a number of different concerns (perhaps unrelated to the study). Another more common scenario is where researchers move away from the project before its conclusion, which may seriously affect the smooth running of a study, but the effect can be minimized by comprehensive paperwork. Again, the role of a project group is critical to the orientation of a new researcher, mid-study, with the dangers of keeping decision-making and discussion to too small a group all too evident.

Good clinical practice

Good clinical practice or GCP relates to drug trials and evolved from FDA guidelines (the Food and Drug Administration in the USA) but are now applicable worldwide. GCP regulations were designed to ensure that reliable, verifiable, and retrievable data are obtained in a drug trial and have become essential to the drug development process. GCP guidelines explicitly outline the investigators' responsibilities: for example, in obtaining ethical approval for the study; ensuring that all patients entered into the study have given written informed consent; and in conducting the study and completing the case record forms according to the protocol. In addition, the investigator must report all adverse events; keep records of the dispensing and return of all study drugs; file all

documentation in the investigators site file; and set aside time for discussion during visits of the study monitor and the quality assurance auditor.

GCP applies to all trials on medicinal products in human beings. Usually, such studies are being carried out under the sponsorship of a commercial company and the details will be monitored by the clinical research associates employed by the company. However, clinical researchers will need to familiarize themselves with these requirements because they need to be strictly adhered to. New legislation was introduced throughout Europe to implement a European Union Directive 2001/20/EC on Good Clinical Practice in Clinical Trials. The new law significantly extends the scope of GCP to cover all clinical trials of medicinal products, including trials not directly supported by pharmaceutical companies and phase I healthy volunteer studies. One major change in the new regulations is that breach of the obligations contained in them may be, in some circumstances, a criminal offence. There were major implications in the proposals for Research Ethics Committees and for the Research Governance Framework for Health and Social care in the United Kingdom. However the widespread concerns about the potential adverse impact of the Clinical Trials Directive on academic clinical trials [45] has not been justified by subsequent experience[46].

Monitoring of study

Supporting researchers and the clinical team (keeping it going)

The initial rush of enthusiasm for a project is difficult to sustain over time without conscious management of the research team. Studies can get into difficulty quite quickly when unexpected problems start to shake the confidence of the supporting clinical teams or the front-line researchers. Encountering slow patient recruitment or high dropout rates, for example, can be disillusioning and demotivating. However, a project that is conceived as a collaborative venture, where support from others is openly valued, and where there is a commitment to teamwork, is likely to develop mechanisms for keeping the study going. Attention needs to be focused on the individual needs and group dynamics of the research team, as well as the wider group of staff who are involved in facilitating the study. Morale and support for the study can be promoted in a number of ways:

◆ For clinical staff, provision of regular feedback and direct contact with the study team to answer queries and address any concerns is desirable. This is also important considering the high turnover of clinical staff; new staff will need to be identified and inducted especially during a long-running study. Busy clinical staff anyway will also tend to forget about studies, and so an important aspect of regular contact is to remind them that the study is still running.

◆ Within the research team, time should be set aside for team-building activities (e.g. away days and social events), and to help prevent 'burn-out', the provision of mentoring, co-counselling, or debriefing should be considered.

Databases and data management

Considerable thought needs to be devoted to the system of recording and holding data early in the planning of a research study. The success of subsequent analysis will depend on the quality of the data, its reliability, and completeness. Most research data will be held in an electronic database, which is basically a way of holding, organizing, and indexing the records transferred from data capture forms (generally paper-based but can be electronic given the use of lap-top computers or palm-held devices). Many databases are used for more than their 'filing system' capacities. Records can be sorted and selected for basic ordering and counting purposes, and data held in a database can be accessed by other software packages for administrative tasks such as bulk mailings, other correspondence and automated updates. Because of the individual characteristics and requirements of each study, a certain amount of customization of the database package used is generally necessary.

Within a research study it is important to manage the data, by attending to three crucial processes:

1 How data gets onto the database.

2 How the database is maintained.

3 How data is used for analysis and report formation.

Questions of sufficient computer hardware and software should be addressed in the early stages of a study, and adequate funds made available. In addition, information and computer technology (ICT), orientation, and ongoing training should be available for all researchers engaged on the project, who are either responsible for data input, or who require access to the data. The process of inputting data during the study should be piloted for 'user-friendliness'. This would cover efficiency and ease of input, taking care not to make the process over-burdensome. The requirements of the analysis need to be borne in mind in order to avoid excessive (and costly) data recording.

However, diligent researchers are in the recording and inputting of data, mistakes happen, especially when people are rushed, tired, or distracted. Accuracy of data input can be built into data entry protocols, but it cannot always be programmed for. Regular checks of the data can show up gross inaccuracies and perhaps consistent mistakes, which becomes an important part of data management and the subsequent integrity of the data. Checking as the study progresses can also mean that omissions can be followed up quickly, rather than being left to the end when it becomes a more time-consuming task. The way that data are coded and entered needs to be written up in a manual that should sit alongside the database, allowing other researchers to understand and access the database.

The security and protection of the database is also an important aspect of data management. First, there is the necessity of adhering to national and international data protection and patient confidentiality requirements. This may determine or limit some of the data items that are actually held on the database, and may also require consent from the research subjects. Second, the database needs to be held securely, possibly by restricting physical access to it (access to computers, servers), and protecting it through the use of passwords. In addition, back-up discs of the database, which are needed in the event of computer problems, also need to be protected.

Ease of export of data to supporting software packages is clearly an important aspect of the analysis and report-writing stage of a study and warrants careful consideration of the options available, together with the adequacy of training and ongoing support for the life of the study. How the data will be used for analysis will depend partly upon who will be responsible for this, and this should be planned for at the earliest stages of the study. A statistical analysis

Table 7.1.4 Submitting abstracts for free communications at research meetings.

1. Find out the final date for submission as early as possible.

2. Read the instructions to authors carefully and follow them precisely.

3. Decide whether the data are best presented as a poster or as an oral communication. Oral communications typically are allocated 10 min plus 5 min for questions. The larger the meeting, paradoxically. the smaller the likely audience (because there are usually many parallel sessions in large meetings).

4. Follow the usual structure of Introduction, Aims, Patients/Subjects, Methods, Results, Conclusions, unless instructions say otherwise.

5. Write impeccable English (or other language if appropriate) with accurate terminology and good grammar.

6. Do not exceed the word allowance.

7. Scientific committees look for originality and interest, topicality, and sound methodology. They need some reassurance that you will have data to present (i.e. that the study has actually started or is in progress) so try to avoid submitting an abstract with no data at all.

8. Posters need to be eye-catching and succinct. However interesting the topic, poor presentation and endless detail in small print will deter people from reading it.

will involve collaboration with a statistician, and the data should be held in such a way that it is easily manipulated into files for use by a variety of statistical packages. Analysis of qualitative data also requires planning of the way textual data are collected and recorded. The CAQDAS (Computer Assisted Qualitative Data Analysis Software) Project, funded by the U.K. Economic and Social Research Council, provides practical support, training, and information in the use of a range of software programmes, which have been designed to assist qualitative data analysis. This can be accessed through their website, www. caqdas.soc.surrey.ac.uk.

Finally, questions of archiving study data and pooling or sharing data with other studies should be considered. Studies finish and researchers move on, so having a known repository for study data can be important for future researchers. More value can also be derived from a study when data is shared with other researchers working in the national or international context. The importance of this in palliative care research is particularly apt, given the many difficulties in recruiting large numbers of research participants.

Analysing and interpreting the data and presenting and publishing the results

The analysis of the data should be straightforward if all of the preceding steps have been properly adhered to and an adequate number of subjects have been recruited. The statistical methods to be used will already have been decided and the data will have been 'cleaned' and stored in files in a database, which allows easy manipulation in statistical software packages. Recruitment and attrition are major problems in palliative care research as has been discussed earlier and missing data needs careful attention and handling, but all of these problems will have been anticipated and ways of managing them agreed. As the numbers start taking shape towards one conclusion or another, there is a sense of excitement and anticipation that they will add up to a meaningful advance in knowledge.

The next step will be to present the data to colleagues and at scientific meetings to begin the process of peer review. Usually, the

Table 7.1.5 Submitting a paper for publication.

1. Decide which journal to go for. Are the data relevant to a general journal (*New England Journal of Medicine, Lancet, BMJ*) or a specialist journal (*Cancer, Journal of Clinical Oncology, Palliative Medicine*)? The general journals are much more difficult to be published in.

2. Aim high (but appropriately so) because sometimes you will catch an editor's interest and with the leading journals you will usually get a very rapid response if the paper is rejected (one of the authors had experience of acknowledgement of receipt of a paper within a week of posting, and a letter of rejection 24 h later).

3. Do not be too discouraged by rejection but try to learn from it. Usually authors will get some feedback explaining why the paper has been rejected. This should enable them to improve the paper before submitting it to another journal.

4. Before submission to any journal, study the 'Instructions to Authors' and abide by them strictly particularly in terms of length, style, and references.

5. In general, it is not worth arguing with editors if they have made it clear that they do not wish to publish your paper. However, if you believe the comments of referees or editors are unreasonable or just erroneous it is perfectly legitimate to challenge them. Occasionally the editor may change their mind!

6. Similarly, if your paper is accepted but the referees or editors suggest changes which you are not happy with, respond and explain why you feel the changes are not justified.

7. After publication, make sure you read the journal (even if it is not one you regularly take) so that you can respond to any correspondence about your paper.

first public presentation of the data will be at a scientific meeting such as the biennial Congress of the European Association for Palliative Care. Some practical advice about getting abstracts accepted, whether for poster presentation or oral communication, is outlined in Table 7.1.4.

Submitting a paper for publication

Much research is undertaken and completed and even presented at a scientific meeting but is never published in a peer-reviewed journal. There may be many reasons for this and it is not possible briefly to discuss them all here. However, Table 7.1.5 gives some advice about submitting papers for publication.

Conclusions

Research in palliative care is essential for maintaining standards and advancing knowledge and improving practice. It is challenging, sometimes frustrating, sometimes daunting, but always exciting and rewarding when a study is successfully completed whether the outcome is positive or negative. We hope that this chapter will help those who are new to research to get on and do some, and complete it and contribute to improving outcomes for patients with advanced disease, which is ultimately the aim of this endeavour.

References

1. Vere, D. (1981). Controlled clinical trials: the current ethical debate. *Journal of the Royal Society of Medicine*, **74**, 85–7.

2. Gunn, G. (2009). Palliative care in hospital and hospice. Time to put the spotlight on neglected areas of research. *Palliative Medicine* (in press).

3. Fainsinger, R.L. (2008). Global warming in the palliative care research environment – adapting to change. *Palliative Medicine*, **22**, 328–35.

4. National Cancer Research Institute. *Strategic Analysis 2002*. London, National Cancer Research Institute.

5. Payne, S., Addington-Hall, J., Richardson, A. *et al.* (2007) Supportive and palliative care research collaboratives in the United Kingdom: an unnatural experiment. *Palliative Medicine*, 21, 663–5.

6. Kaasa, S., Loge, J.H., Fayers, P. *et.al.* (2008). Symptom assessment in palliative care: A need for international collaboration. *Journal of Clinical Oncology*, **26** (23), 3867–73

7. Skorpen, F., Laugsand, E.A., Klepstad, P. *et al.* (2008). Variable response to opioid treatment: any genetic predictors within sight? *Palliative Medicine*, **22**, 310–27.

8. Saunders, C. (1978). Hospice care. *American Journal of Medicine*, **65**, 76–8.

9. Twycross, R.G. (1977). Choice of strong analgesic in terminal cancer: diamorphine or morphine? *Pain*, **3**, 93–104.

10. Murray-Parkes, C. (1985). Terminal care: home, hospital or hospice? *Lancet*, **i**, 155–7.

11. Hanks, G.W. (1985). The care of advanced cancer patients. In *Medical Perspectives in Cancer Research* (A.J.S. Davis, P.S. Rudland eds.), pp. 263–72. Chichester: Ellis Horwood.

12. Kaasa, S., Hjermstad, M.J., and Loge, J.H. (2006). Methodological and structural challenges in palliative care research: how have we fared in the last decades? *Palliative Medicine*, **8**, 727–34.

13. Diatchenko, L., Nackley, A.G., Tchivileva, I.E. *et al.* (2007). Genetic architecture of human pain perception. *Trends in Genetics*, **23**, 605–13.

14. Klepstad, P., Rakwag, T.T., Kaasa, S. *et al.* (2004). The 118 A>G polymorphism in the human micro-opioid receptor gene may increase morphine requirements in patients with pain caused by malignant disease. *Acta Anaesthesiologica Scandinavica*, **48**, 1232–9.

15. Rakwag, T.T., Lepstad, P., Baar, C. *et al.* (2005). The Val158Met polymorphism of the human catechol-o-methyltransferase (COMT) gene may influence morphine requirements in cancer pain patients. Pain, **116**, 73–8.

16. Blumhuber, H., Kaasa, S., and De Conno, F. (2002). The European Association for Palliative Care. *Journal of Pain and Symptom Management*, **24**, 124–7.

17. Hanks, G.W., De Conno, F., Ripamonti, C. *et al.* (1996). Morphine in cancer pain: modes of administration. *British Medical Journal*, **312**, 823–6.

18. Kaasa, S., Torvik, K., Cherny, N. *et al.* (2007). Patient demographics and centre description in European palliative care units. *Palliative Medicine*, **21**, 15–22.

19. Anonymous. (1964). Human experimentation: code of ethics of the World Medical Association. *British Medical Journal*, **2**, 177.

20. Jones, A.M., Bamford, B. (2004). Education and debate. The other face of research governance. *British Medical Journal*, **329**, 280–1.

21. Reid, C.M. (2004). Research bureaucracy in the United Kingdom. Ask for help. *British Medical Journal*, **329**, 624.

22. Bradford Hill, A. (1963). Medical ethics and controlled trials. *British Medical Journal*, **ii**, 1043–9.

23. New reference no 24: Sackett, D.L., Rosenberg, W.M.C., Muir-Gray, J.A., Haynes, R.B., Richardson, W.S. (1996). Evidence-based medicine: what it is and what it isn't. *British Medical Journal*, **312**, 71–72

24. Beecher, H.K. (1966). Ethics and clinical research. *New England Journal of Medicine*, **274**, 1354–60.

25. *Palliative Medicine* (2006), **20** (8). Special issue on Palliative Care Research Methodology

26. McWhinney, I.R., Bass, M.J., and Donner, A. (1994). Evaluation of a palliative care service: problems and pitfalls. *British Medical Journal*, **309**, 1340–2.

27. Rinck, G.C., van den Bos, G.A.M., Kleijnen, J. *et al.* (1997). Methodologic issues in effectiveness research on palliative cancer care: a systematic review. *Journal of Clinical Oncology*, **15**, 1697–1707.

28. Hanks, G.W., Robbins, M., Sharp, D. *et al.* (2002). The imPaCT study: a randomised controlled trial to evaluate a hospital palliative care team. *British Journal of Cancer*, **87**, 733–9.

29. Kaasa, S. and Loge, J.H. (2003). Quality of life in palliative care: principles and practice. *Palliative Medicine*, **17**, 11–20.

30. Kaasa, S., Mastekaasa, A., and Lund, E. (1989). Prognostic factors for patients with inoperable non-small cell lung cancer, limited disease. *Radiotherapy and Oncology*, **15**, 235–42.

31. Maltoni, M., Pirovano, M., Scarpi, E. *et al.* (1995). Prediction of survival of patients terminally ill with cancer. Results from an Italian Prospective Multicentric Study. *Cancer*, **75**, 2613–22.

32. Vigano, A., Bruera, E., Jhangri, G.S. *et al.* (2000). Clinical survival predictors in patients with advanced cancer. *Archives of Internal Medicine*, **160**, 861–8.

33. Pocock, S.J. (1984). *Clinical Trials: A Practical Approach*. ISBN: 0471901555.

34. Karlberg, J. and Tsang, K. (1998). *Introduction to Clinical Trials*. ISBN: 9628540513.

35. Bell, R., Eccleston, C., and Kalso, E. (2003). Ketamine as an adjuvant to opioids for cancer pain. *Cochrane Database of Systematic Review*, **1**: CD003351.

36. Early Breast Cancer Trialists' Group. (1998). Tamoxifen for early breast cancer: an overview of the randomized trials. *Lancet*, **351**, 1451–67.

37. Loge, J.H., Foss Abrahamsen, A., Ekeberg, O. *et al.* (1999). Hodgkin's disease survivors more fatigued than the general population. *Journal of Clinical Oncology*, **17**, 253–61.

38. Aaronson, N.K., Ahmedzai, S., Bergman, B. *et al.* (1993). The European Organisation for Research and Treatment of Cancer QLQ-C30: a quality of life instrument for use in international clinical trials in oncology. *Journal of the National Cancer Institute*, **85**, 365–76.

39. Cohen, S.R., Mount, B.M., Strobel, M.G. *et al.* (1995). The McGill quality of life questionnaire: a measure of quality of life appropriate for people with advanced disease: a preliminary study of validity and acceptability. *Palliative Medicine*, **9**, 207–19.

40. Kaasa, S., Thorud, E., Host, H. *et al.* (1988). A randomized study evaluating radiotherapy versus chemotherapy in patients with inoperable non-small cell lung cancer. *Radiotherapy and Oncology*, **11**, 7–13.

41. Jordhoy, M.S., Fayers, P., Saltnes, T. *et al.* (2000). A palliative care intervention and death at home: a cluster randomised trial. *Lancet*, **356**, 888–93.

42. Rothman, K.J. and Greenland, S. (1998). *Modern Epidemiology*. ISBN: 0316757802.

43. Rosner, B. (2000). *Fundamentals of Biostatistics*. 5th edition. ISBN: 053437068.

44. Altman, D.G. (1991). *Practical statistics for medical research*. ISBN: 0412276305.

45. Morice, A.H. (2003). The death of the academic clinical trials. *Lancet*, **261**, 1568

46. Berendt. L., Håkansson, C., Friis Bach, K., *et al.* (2008). Effect of European Clinical Trials Directive on academic drug trials in Denmark: retrospective study of applications to the Danish Medicines Agency 1993-2006. *British Medical Journal*, **336**. 33–35

7.2

The principles of evidence-based medicine

Henry J. McQuay, Andrew Moore, and Philip Wiffen

What constitutes evidence?

Finding and using the best available evidence should be part of our professional lives. Archie Cochrane said in 1979 'It is surely a great criticism of our profession that we have not organized a critical summary, by specialty or subspecialty, adapted periodically, of all relevant randomized controlled trials'.

There are several interlinked strands:

♦ finding the evidence;

♦ appraising the evidence;

♦ making the evidence (doing trials or systematic reviews);

♦ using the evidence.

The focus in this chapter is on randomized trials and systematic reviews of existing trials. Systematic reviews and large randomized trials constitute the most reliable sources of evidence we can muster (Table 7.2.1). Put simply, they are the best chance we have to determine what is true. We discuss how to find trials, and how to appraise their quality. Further on there is advice on how to

Table 7.2.1 Type and strength of efficacy evidence.[2]

Oxford CEBM levels of evidence (May 2001)	
Level	**Therapy/prevention, aetiology/harm**
1a	SR (with homogeneity) of RCTs
1b	Individual RCT (with narrow CI)
1c	All or none
2a	SR (with homogeneity) of cohort studies
2b	Individual cohort study (including low quality RCT; e.g. <80% follow-up)
2c	'Outcomes' research; ecological studies
3a	SR (with homogeneity) of case-control studies
3b	Individual case–control study
4	Case-series (and poor quality cohort and case–control studies)
5	Expert opinion without explicit critical appraisal, or based on physiology, bench research or 'first principles'

SR, systematic review; RCT, randomized controlled trial; CI, confidence interval

appraise the quality of systematic reviews themselves. These ideas, being critical about medical evidence as it is presented to you, have been developed at greater length as a book.[1]

Evidence-based medicine (EBM)

A current definition of EBM is that it is the conscientious, explicit, and judicious use of current best evidence in making decisions about the care of individual patients.[3,4] The practice of EBM requires the integration of individual clinical expertise with the best available external clinical evidence from systematic research. Decisions that affect the care of patients should be taken with *due weight* accorded to *all* valid, relevant information. There are many factors as well as the results of randomized controlled trials which may weigh heavily in both clinical and policy decisions, such as patient preferences and resources, and these must contribute to decisions about the care of patients (*due weight*). Valid, relevant evidence should be considered alongside these other factors in the decision-making process. No one sort of evidence should necessarily be the determining factor in a decision. *All* implies that there should be an active search for that valid, relevant information and that an assessment should be made of the accuracy of the information and the applicability of the evidence to the decision in question. i.e. information should be appraised. EBM is thus what most health-care professionals have been trying to practise all their working lives.

What is changing and what has changed over the past decade is that there is an increasing number of well-conducted randomized controlled trials and systematic reviews, and that there is a political pressure, both from those receiving care as well and from those who pay for it, to support our treatment choices with high-quality evidence. That should not be too irksome, given that professionally we would all wish to do the best for our patients. What happens is that the evidence supports some interventions and suggests that others are considerably less effective than some of us believe. This should not make palliative care health professionals paranoid. Precisely, the same message has emerged in the other areas of medicine which have received similar attention. What is clear is that very often the quality of the trials of invasive interventions is much lower than the quality of drug trials. Within the drug trials some drugs are better choices on efficacy and or safety grounds than others. The onus must be on us to do bigger and better trials if we wish to continue using some of these techniques.

Evidence-based medicine and palliative care

Palliative care has the same generic issues about evidence found in other therapeutic areas, but also has some which are specific to palliative care. One generic problem is the narrative review. The traditional narrative review, an overview of part or all of the speciality, often written by a key opinion leader, may have features which leave it open to bias. The author may select just her papers, or those of her friends, and ignore those of her competitors. This bias in the selection of the literature may not always be easy to identify, and obviously can produce a biased conclusion. The bias may be compounded by an absence of rigour in criteria for including papers, i.e. not only has the author used just her own papers, but she has included some high quality work and some of low quality. Data may not have been extracted in a logical way. The systematic review should prevent the problems of a narrative review, because the way in which the literature is searched is transparent, and so are the inclusion and exclusion criteria. The way in which data are extracted should also be crystal clear, so that the reader could repeat the search, find the papers, rule individual papers in or out and extract the data. The reader might not reach the same conclusion as the original author, but at least the starting point is the same, which is unlikely to be the case with the narrative review.

A second problem is that not all the interventions which are made in palliative care are easy to study with the gold standard randomized trial. The methods for compiling credible systematic reviews described below require credible component trials. If a topic, a particular intervention, has resisted study with high-quality trials, then it may be impossible to produce a credible review. A further level of complexity is when we want to know if a particular package of interventions is better than another package—home care versus hospital care for instance. The absence of good study methods for packages of care is obvious from parallel work in other therapeutic areas, intensive care and cognitive behavioural therapy are two examples. Until we have good study methods for individual trials it will remain difficult to draw strong evidence-based conclusions about service delivery and packages of care. The Medical Research Council (MRC) has produced a framework to help those studying complex interventions.[5]

A third problem in palliative care is that trials in palliative care are notoriously difficult to conduct, compared for instance with acute pain. Some, but not all, of the interventions in palliative care will have been studied in other settings, such as chronic non-malignant pain. The question then arises of the legitimacy of extrapolating high quality evidence derived in other therapeutic areas. The corollary is 'Is it necessary to trial an intervention in palliative care when it has been shown to work well elsewhere?'. The pragmatic answer is that this has to be context-dependent. An intervention which is safe and effective for neuropathic pain in chronic non-malignant pain will likely work well in palliative care, but may of course have additional problems in sicker patients or with different drug–drug interactions.

Where do you get the evidence?

Evidence which is both relevant and valid is necessary for effective care. The randomized controlled trial (RCT) is the most reliable way to estimate the effect of an intervention. The principle of randomization is simple. Patients in a randomized trial have the same probability of receiving any of the interventions being compared.

Randomization abolishes selection bias because it prevents investigators influencing who has which intervention. Randomization also helps to ensure that other factors, such as age or sex distribution, are equivalent for the different treatment groups. Inadequate randomization, or inadequate concealment of randomization, lead to exaggeration of therapeutic effect.[6]

To produce valid reviews of evidence, the reviews need to be systematic, and to be systematic, qualitative, or quantitative, they need to include all relevant RCTs. Identifying all the relevant trials is a 'fundamental challenge'[7] which is easily underestimated.

The first obstacle faced by any reviewer is finding out how many eligible RCTs exist. Commonly the total is unknown. Usually only for newer interventions are reviewers likely to be sure that they have found all the RCTs. Otherwise, the only way to find how many RCTs there are would be to scan every record in each of the available bibliographic databases, to search by hand all non-indexed journals, theses, proceedings, and textbooks, to search the reference lists of all the reports found, and to ask investigators of previous RCTs for other published or unpublished information.[8] In practice, constrained by time and cost, reviewers have to compromise, and then hope that what they have found is a representative sample of the unknown total population of trials. The more comprehensive the searching the more trials will be found, and any conclusions will then be stronger. Comprehensive searches can be very time consuming and costly, so again this emphasizes the necessary compromise, where the target is the highest possible yield for given resources.

Retrieval bias is the failure to identify reports which could have affected the results of a systematic review or meta-analysis.[9] This failure may be because trials are still ongoing, or completed but unpublished (publication bias) or because although published the search did not find them. Trying to identify unpublished trials by asking researchers had a very low yield,[10] and was not cheap. Registers of ongoing and completed trials are another way to find unpublished data, but such registers are still relatively rare.

Most systematic reviews use published trial results, but in some contexts the reviewer may have access to the data from individual patients. This individual patient data we all expect to produce more accurate efficacy estimates than the reviews which use published data, precisely because the reviewer has the original data rather than summary statistics from the published papers. Reassuringly it would appear that most reviews from published data produce results close to those produced by work with individual patient data,[11] but not everyone agrees.[12]

Developing a citation database for a review

This process has three phases: definition of inclusion criteria, identification of reports, and information management. The example used is for a wide search for all analgesic interventions.[13] For a particular intervention, the reviewer would follow the same path but narrow the inclusion criteria.

Inclusion criteria

A report was regarded as eligible if the following criteria were fulfilled:

◆ Allocation to the intervention was described as randomized (no precise description of the method of randomization was required) or as double-blind or as both, or if it was suggested that the interventions were given at random and/or under double-blind conditions, and

◆ Analgesic interventions with pain or adverse effects as outcomes, and/or any intervention using pain as an outcome measure, were compared.

◆ Reports were excluded which investigated analgesic effectiveness during (as opposed to after) diagnostic or surgical procedures.

Identification of reports

We use a range of databases, MEDLINE, EMBASE, the Cochrane Library, CINAHL, and PSYCHLIT as part of our standard operating procedures. The citations to the identified reports are downloaded, and stored in a reference management program. Each downloaded citation is checked on screen for definite eligibility, probable eligibility or ineligibility and coded accordingly. Hard copies of eligible and probable reports are obtained, and if necessary are translated, and eligibility is then confirmed.

Hand searching of journals

Some topics may by their nature be published in journals which are not indexed by the major databases, and these journals may need to be searched by hand to find relevant studies. These reports, either missed by MEDLINE indexing, or in non-indexed journals, are then added to the citation database if perusal of the hard copy confirms that they are indeed eligible.

Conclusions

The importance of basing systematic reviews on the highest quality evidence (randomized trials) is obvious from our experience in the pain field,[14] and from the experience of others. This means that very considerable time and effort has to be spent to gather all the relevant material for each review.

The process outlined here is a laborious task, made easier now because citations of known RCTs have been added to the Cochrane Library, so that others do not have to repeat the hand-searching process. For topics that are not mainstream the hand-searching process will still have to be done.

Judging the quality of trials

Once you have found all the reports of the trials relevant to your question there is another stage in the process. This stage is first to confirm that these reports meet certain *quality standards* and second that, even though a report may pass those quality standards, whether the trial is *valid*.

Imagine a situation where you found 40 reports of trials on your question. You then discover that 20 of the reports say that the intervention is terrific, and 20 conclude that it should never be used. Delving deeper you find that the 20 'negative' reports score highly on your quality standards scale. The 20 'positive' reports score poorly for quality. What then will you conclude? Without a quality scale you would vote for the intervention. With the quality scale you would vote against.

The quality scale should include measures of bias. Bias is the simplest explanation why poor-quality reports give more positive conclusions than high-quality reports. The quality standards which you require cannot be absolute, because for some clinical questions there may not be any RCTs. Setting RCTs as a minimum absolute standard would therefore be inappropriate for all the questions we might want to answer. In the pain world, however, there are two reasons for setting this high standard, and requiring trials to be randomized. The first reason is that we have a large number of

RCTs, particularly for drug interventions. The second is that we would argue that it is even more important to stress the minimum quality standards of randomization and double-blinding when the outcome measures are subjective.

Developing and validating a quality scale

What makes a trial worthy of the label 'high quality'? Quality could refer to the clinical relevance of the study, to the likelihood of biased results, to the appropriateness of the statistical analysis, to the presentation of the data, or to the ethical implications of the intervention or to the literary style of the manuscript. We think that quality must primarily indicate the likelihood that the study design reduced bias. Only by avoiding bias is it possible to estimate the effect of a given intervention with any confidence.

The simple scale which we developed,[15] and which is now used widely, was designed to assess the likelihood of the trial design to generate unbiased results and approach the 'therapeutic truth' (Tables 7.2.2 and 7.2.3). Other trial characteristics such as clinical relevance of the question addressed, data analysis and presentation, literary quality of the report, or ethical implications of the study are not included in our definition.

Comments on the scale

The scale is simple, short, valid, and reliable. Our results suggest that even without clinical or research experience users should be able to score the quality of research reports consistently. Chalmers suggested many years ago that the quality of clinical reports should be assessed blind.[16] We found that such blinded assessment produced significantly lower scores. This may be very important if absolute cut-off scores are imposed by systematic reviewers, and if quality scores are used to weight the results of primary studies in subsequent meta-analysis.[17,18] The results of open evaluations are

Table 7.2.2 Scale (3-point) to measure the likelihood of bias in pain research reports.

This is not the same as being asked to review a paper. It should not take more than 10 min to score a report and there are no right or wrong answers.

Please read the article and try to answer the following questions (see attached instructions):

1. Was the study described as randomized (this includes the use of words such as randomly, random, and randomization)?

2. Was the study described as double-blind?

3. Was there a description of withdrawals and drop outs?

Scoring the items

Give a score of 1 point for each 'yes' and 0 points for each 'no'. There are no in-between marks.

Give 1 additional point if: on question 1, the method of randomization was described and it was appropriate (table of random numbers, computer generated, coin tossing, etc.);

and/or: if on question 2 the method of double-blinding was described and it was appropriate (identical placebo, active placebo, dummy, etc.).

Deduct 1 point if: on question 1, the method of randomization was described and it was inappropriate (patients were allocated alternatively, or according to date of birth, hospital number, etc.);

and/or: on question 2 the study was described as double-blind but the method of blinding was inappropriate (e.g. comparison of tablet vs. injection with no double dummy).

Table 7.2.3 Advice on using the scale.

___

1. Randomization

If the word randomized or any other related words such as random, randomly, or randomization are used in the report, but the method of randomization is not described, give a positive score to this item; randomization method will be regarded as appropriate if it allowed each patient to have the same chance of receiving each treatment and the investigators could not predict which treatment was next. Therefore, methods of allocation using date of birth, date of admission, hospital numbers or alternation should not be regarded as appropriate.

2. Double-blinding

A study must be regarded as double-blind if the word double-blind is used (even without description of the method) or if it is implied that neither the caregiver nor the patient could identify the treatment being assessed.

3. Withdrawals and drop outs

Patients who were included in the study but did not complete the observation period or who were not included in the analysis must be described. The number *and* the reasons for withdrawal must be stated. If there are no withdrawals, it should be stated in the article. If there is no statement on withdrawals, this item must be given a negative score (0 points).

___

good enough for busy readers. The improved reliability with blind testing is of more relevance to journal editors for manuscript selection and to systematic reviewers. Quality scales without clinimetric evaluation have already been used in pain work to support the conclusions of systematic reviews.[16–18]

None of the items is specific to pain studies. The three items are very similar to the components of a scale used extensively to assess the effectiveness of interventions during pregnancy and childbirth,[19] and also appear in most other scales. Control of selection bias and rater bias is obviously crucial to quality.

Selection bias is best controlled by allocating patients at random to the different study groups. Each patient should have the same probability of being included in each comparison group, and the allocation should be concealed until after the patient has given consent to take part. Methods of allocation based on alternation, date of birth or hospital record number cannot be regarded as random. Failure to secure proper randomization increases the likelihood that potential participants in a 'randomized' study will be admitted to the study selectively because of prior knowledge of the group to which they would be allocated or excluded selectively before formal admission in the study.[20] Ideal methods of randomization are those in which individuals with no direct relationship to the study participants are in charge of the allocation (e.g. allocation by telephone from a central coordinating office, concealed from the investigators). Appropriate simpler alternatives are coin tossing, tables of random numbers, and numbers generated by computers, but at higher risk of selective selection.

All these methods are regarded as appropriate for the purposes of our scale, although we are aware that selective selection is still possible even if the group allocation is concealed until after consent has been obtained. We rate the randomization method as inappropriate if the potential participants did not have the same chance of being included in any of the comparison groups (methods based on date of birth, hospital number or alternation). Even with excellent randomization selection bias may still be introduced if biased and selective withdrawal and drop-outs occur after the allocations have been made.[21] This is why an adequate description of withdrawals and drop-outs is included in the scale. With that information it is possible to analyse

on an intention-to-treat basis (all those randomized whether or not they were exposed to the study interventions).[22]

Rater bias can be minimized by blinding the person receiving the intervention, the individual administering it, the investigator measuring the outcome, and the analyst. Blinding can be tested by asking the study patients and the researchers which intervention they had. This is not often done. The usual 'best' level of blinding is blinding of the study subject and those making the observations (double-blinding). Double-blinding is often achieved by using control interventions with similar physical characteristics to those of the intervention under evaluation, or by the use of dummies when two or more interventions have to be given by different routes. Sometimes, however, one of the interventions may produce effects which make blinding very difficult to sustain. Then the use of active placebos or active controls may decrease the likelihood of rater bias. All these precautions are relatively easy to achieve in drug studies. In non-drug studies testing under blind conditions is either difficult or inappropriate (e.g. surgical procedures) or impossible (e.g. acupuncture or transcutaneous electrical nerve stimulation (TENS)). The risk of rater bias limits the confidence with which conclusions can be reached. We know that studies which are not double-blind risk an average exaggeration of treatment effect of 17 per cent.[6]

Validity of trials

A study may of course be both randomized and double-blind, and describe withdrawals and dropouts in copious detail (so scoring well on this quality scale) and yet be invalid. Two examples from the pain world illustrate this point. One is from the injection of morphine into the knee joint to reduce pain after arthroscopy.[23] In some trials, this injection was made after the operation without knowledge of whether or not the patients had enough pain for the intervention to make a difference. If they had just mild pain rather than moderate or severe pain it is quite possible that the success ascribed in that trial to the intervention was actually due to the fact that they did not have any pain to begin with. The second example comes from attempts to show the efficacy of pre-emptive analgesia, where comparisons were made at multiple time points after surgery between patients receiving analgesia before pain and the group who received the same analgesia after the pain had started. A statistical difference at one of eight time points is then held up as proof that giving the analgesia before the pain is successful, when at the other seven points there was no difference. These are criticisms of the validity of the trials, and including these trials uncritically in a review will affect the conclusions. Another example is a review which proclaimed that fewer patients would die after major surgery if they had regional plus general anaesthesia.[24] The statistical significance which led the authors to this potentially important conclusion came from a number of small trials with 30 per cent mortality rates, rates so high as to make one question the validity of the trials.

How can these pitfalls be avoided? We attempted to build a checklist of validity checks,[25] hoping this would be a generic solution across all therapeutic areas. In reality, while some of the items are generic some are specific to the field, so that the reader, the author and the reviewer must all be aware of the potential problems.

Judging the quality of reviews

As professionals we want to use the best treatments and, as patients, to be given them. Knowing that an intervention works (or does not work) is fundamental to clinical decision-making. When is the evidence strong enough to justify changing practice? Some of the decisions we make are based on individual studies, often on small numbers of patients, which, given the random play of chance, may lead to incorrect decisions. Systematic reviews and large randomized trials constitute the most reliable sources of evidence we can muster (Table 7.2.1).[2] Systematic reviews identify and review all the relevant studies, and are more likely to give a reliable answer. They use explicit methods and quality standards to reduce bias. Their results are the closest we are likely to get to the truth in the absence of satisfactorily large randomized trials.

The questions a systematic review should answer for us are:

♦ How well does an intervention work (compared with placebo, no treatment, or other interventions in current use)?

♦ Is it safe?

♦ Will it work and be safe for the patients in our practice?

Clinicians need to be able to synthesize their knowledge of a particular patient in their practice, their experience and expertise, and the best external evidence from systematic review. They can then be confident that they are doing their best. But the product of systematic review and particularly meta-analysis—often some sort of statistical output—is often not interpretable or usable in day-to-day clinical practice. A common currency to help make the best treatment decision for a particular patient is what is needed. We believe that this common currency is the number-needed-to-treat (NNT). The choice of analgesic for both professional and patient will be made on the balance between efficacy and risk, where the risk may be adverse effect or drug interaction with other drugs which the patient is taking.

Quality control

Systematic reviews of inadequate quality may be worse than none, because faulty decisions may be made with unjustified confidence. Quality control in the systematic review process, from literature searching onwards, is vital. How to judge the quality of a systematic review is encapsulated in the questions:[26]

♦ Were the question(s) and methods stated clearly?

♦ Were the search methods used to locate relevant studies comprehensive?

♦ Were explicit methods used to determine which articles to include in the review?

♦ Was the methodological quality of the primary studies assessed?

♦ Were the selection and assessment of the primary studies reproducible and free from bias?

♦ Were differences in individual study results explained adequately?

♦ Were the results of the primary studies combined appropriately?

♦ Were the reviewers' conclusions supported by the data cited?

When systematic reviews of the same topic use data from different numbers of papers, reasons should be sought. Reviews can use criteria that exclude information important to individual clinicians, or may be too lax by including studies with inadequate trial design. The defence against either mistake is to read the inclusion and exclusion criteria critically to see if they make sense in your clinical circumstance.

Outcome measures chosen for data extraction should also be sensible. Usually this is not a problem, but again it is a part of the methods that needs to be read carefully to see if you agree with the outcome measure extracted. The reviewer may have used all that is available, and any problems were due to the original trials, but it is a determinant of the clinical utility of the review.

Therapeutic interventions: which study designs are admissible?

For a systematic review of therapeutic efficacy, the gold standard is that eligible studies should be randomized controlled trials (RCTs) to exclude selection bias. If trials are not randomized estimates of treatment effect may be exaggerated by an average of 40 per cent.[6] In a systematic review of TENS in postoperative pain, 17 reports on 786 patients could be regarded unequivocally as RCTs in acute postoperative pain. Fifteen of these 17 RCTs demonstrated no benefit of TENS over placebo. Nineteen reports had pain outcomes but were not RCTs; in 17 of these 19, TENS was considered by their authors to have had a positive analgesic effect.[14] When appropriate, and particularly with subjective outcomes, the gold standard for an efficacy systematic review is studies that are both randomized and double-blind (to exclude observer bias). The therapeutic effect may be exaggerated by up to 20 per cent in trials with deficient blinding.[6]

Databases can provide records of many patients who were or were not taking a particular medicine. They may record how well the patient or the health-care professional thought the medicine worked. Conclusions about the efficacy of the treatment made from databases are however necessarily subject to the selection bias and the observer bias which the randomized trial, and the systematic review which uses randomized trials to derive its efficacy estimate, are designed to minimize. Estimates of treatment efficacy from database data are likely to be overestimates unless quality and validity are good. When quality and validity are good then the database results may be similar to the trial results. A Swedish report on TNF-antagonists in rheumatoid arthritis, where the patient numbers multiplied by duration of treatment were about equal or more than that from clinical trials, showed efficacy results similar to clinical trials. The adverse events recorded confirmed those seen in clinical trials.[27]

Not all data can be combined in a meta-analysis: qualitative systematic reviews

It is often not possible or sensible to combine (pool) data, resulting in a qualitative rather than a quantitative systematic review. Combining data is not possible if there is no quantitative information in the component trials of the review. Combining data may not be sensible if trials used different clinical outcomes or followed the patients for different lengths of time. Combining continuous rather than dichotomous data may be difficult. Even if trials measure and present dichotomous data, how many patients did or did not achieve a specified outcome, if the trials are otherwise of poor quality[15] it may not be sensible to combine the data.

Making decisions from qualitative systematic reviews

Making decisions about whether or not a therapy works from such a qualitative systematic review may look easy. In the example earlier, 15 of the 17 RCTs of TENS in acute pain showed no benefit compared with control. The thinking clinician will realize that TENS in acute pain is not an effective analgesic. The problem with this simple vote counting, counting how many trials showed benefit and how many did not, is that it may mislead. It ignores the sample size of the constituent studies, the magnitude of the effect in the studies, and the validity of their design even though they were randomized.[25]

Evaluating efficacy

Combining data: quantitative systematic reviews

There are also two parts to the 'does it work?' question: how does it compare with placebo and how does it compare with other therapies? Whichever comparison is being considered, the three stages of examining a review are a L'Abbé plot, statistical testing (odds ratio or relative risk), and a clinical significance measure such as NNT.

L'Abbé plots[28]

A first stage for evaluating therapies is to look at a simple scatter plot, which can yield a surprisingly comprehensive qualitative view of the data. Even if the review does not show the data in this way, it can be done from information on individual trials presented in the review tables. Fig. 7.2.1 contains data from an updated systematic review of single-dose paracetamol in acute pain. Each point on the graph is the result of a single trial, the size of each point being proportional to the size of each trial, and what happens with paracetamol [experimental event rate (EER)] is plotted against the event rate with placebo [control event rate (CER)].

Trials in which the experimental treatment proves better than the control (EER > CER) will be in the upper left of the plot, between the y-axis and the line of equality. Paracetamol was better than placebo in all the trials; although the plot does not say how much better. If experimental was no better than control then the point would fall on the line of equality (EER = CER), and if control was better than experimental then the point would be in the lower right of the plot, between the x-axis and the line of equality (EER < CER).

Visual inspection gives a quick and easy indication of the level of agreement among trials. Heterogeneity is often assumed to be due to variation in the EER—the effect of the intervention. Fig. 7.2.1 shows that variation in the control event rate can also be a source of heterogeneity, even though the controls were all matched placebos

in relatively homogeneous acute pain conditions with single-dose treatment.

L'Abbé plots have several benefits and the simple visual presentation is easy to assimilate. They make us think about the reasons why there can be such wide variation in (especially) placebo responses, and about other factors in the overall package of care that can contribute to effectiveness. They explain the need for placebo controls if ethical issues about future trials arise. They keep us sceptical about overly good or bad results for an intervention in a single trial, where the major influence may be how good or bad was the response with placebo.

Variation in control (placebo) response rates. Variation in CER is not unusual. Similar variation was seen in trials of antiemetics in postoperative vomiting,[29] and in six trials of prophylactic natural surfactant for preterm infants, the CER for bronchopulmonary dysplasia was 24–69 per cent.[30] Such variation would not be expected in other circumstances, like use of antimicrobials. Rates of eradication of *Helicobacter pylori* with short-term use of ulcer healing drugs were 0–17 per cent in 11 RCTs (with 10 of 11 below 10 per cent).[31]

The reason for large variations in event rates with placebo may have something to do with trial design and population. The overwhelming reason for large variations in placebo rates in pain studies (and probably studies in other clinical conditions) is the relatively small group sizes in trials. Group sizes are chosen to produce statistical significance through power calculations—for pain studies, the usual size is 30–40 patients for a 30 per cent difference between placebo and active analgesic. An individual patient can have no pain relief or 100 per cent pain relief. Random selection of patients can therefore produce groups with low placebo response rate or high placebo response rate, or somewhere in between. Mathematical modelling based on individual patient data shows that while group sizes of up to 50 patients are likely to show a statistical difference 80–90 per cent of the time, to generate a close approximation to the 'true' clinical impact of a therapy requires as many as 500 patients per group (or more than 1000 patients in a trial).[32] Credible NNTs for analgesics need data from 500 patients.

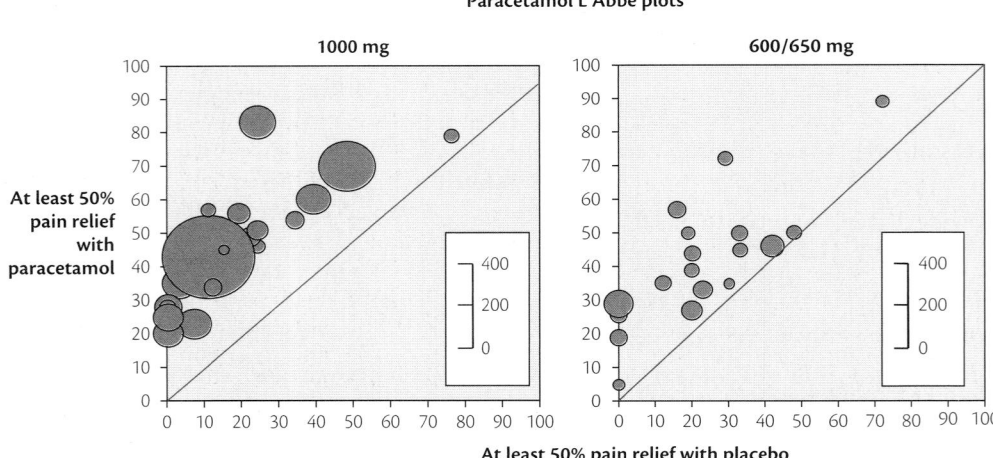

Paracetamol L'Abbé plots

Figure 7.2.1 L'Abbé plot of experimental event rate (EER; >50 per cent relief on treatment) against control event rate (CER; >50 per cent relief on placebo) for RCTs of paracetamol 1000 and 600/650 mg.

The lessons are that information from individual trials of small size should be treated with circumspection in pain and probably other therapeutic areas, and that variation in outcomes seen in trials of small size is probably artefactual.

Heterogeneity. Clinicians making decisions on the basis of systematic reviews need to be confident that apples are not being compared with oranges. The L'Abbé plot is a qualitative defence against this problem. While statistical testing ostensibly provides a quantitative way of checking for heterogeneity, the tests lack power,[33] so that while a test positive for heterogeneity suggests mixed fruits are being compared, a negative test does not provide complete reassurance that there is no heterogeneity. Heterogeneity will also appear to occur because of variations in control and experimental event rates due to the random play of chance in trials of small size. Generally trials of fewer than 10 patients per group should be omitted from systematic reviews,[28] but considerable variability will occur in group sizes below 50 patients. The crucial issues are whether the trials are clinically homogeneous and sufficiently large.

Indirect versus direct comparisons. What clinicians really need are the results of direct comparisons of the different interventions, so-called head-to-head comparisons. These are rarely available, and what we have to work with are comparisons of each of the interventions with placebo. Indeed, at present, we have no method to use the data from the direct comparisons of efficacy. The methods illustrated here tell us how fast each competitor runs against the clock, rather than who crosses the line first in a head-to-head challenge.

Statistical significance

When it is legitimate and feasible to combine data, the odds ratio and relative risk (or benefit) are the accepted statistical tests to show that the intervention works significantly better than the comparator. As systematic reviews are used more to compare therapies, clinicians need to grip these clinical epidemiological tools, which present the results in an unfamiliar way.

Odds ratios. The odds ratio can give a distorted impression when analyses are conducted on subgroups which differ substantially in baseline risk.[34] Where control event rates are high (certainly when they are above 50 per cent), odds ratios should be interpreted with caution.

Relative risk. The fact that it is the odds ratio rather than relative risk reduction that is used as the test of statistical significance for systematic reviews seems to be due to custom and practice rather than any inherent intellectual advantage.[34] Relative risk may be better than odds ratios because it is more robust in situations where control event rate is high.[35] With event rates above 10 per cent relative risk produces more conservative figures.[36] There is still considerable uncertainty and disagreement amongst statisticians and reviewers as to whether odds ratios or relative risk should be used. Importantly, odds ratios should be interpreted with caution when events occur commonly—as in treatments—and odds ratio may over-estimate the benefits of an effect when event rates are above 50 per cent. They are likely to be superseded by relative risk because it is more robust in situations where event rates are high.[4,34]

How well does the intervention work?: clinical significance

While odds ratios and relative risks can show that an intervention works compared with control they are of limited help in telling clinicians how well the intervention works—the size of the effect or its clinical significance.

Effect size

One method of estimating the amount of benefit, the effect size is to use the standardized mean difference.[37] The advantages of this approach are that it can be used to compare the efficacy of different interventions measured on continuous rather than dichotomous scales, and even using different outcome measures. The z-score output is in standard deviation units, and therefore is scale-free. The (major) disadvantage of effect size is that it is not intuitive for clinicians.

Number-needed-to-treat (NNT)

The NNT is the number of people who have to be treated for one to achieve the specified level of benefit. This concept is proving to be a very effective alternative as the measure of clinical significance from quantitative systematic reviews. It has the crucial advantage of applicability to clinical practice, and shows the effort required to achieve a particular therapeutic target.

Technically, the NNT is the reciprocal of the absolute risk reduction, and is given by the equation:

$$NNT = \frac{1}{(IMP_{act}/TOT_{act})-(IMP_{con}/TOT_{con})}$$

where:

IMP_{act} = number of patients given active treatment achieving the target;
TOT_{act} = total number of patients given the active treatment;
IMP_{con} = number of patients given a control treatment achieving the target;
TOT_{con} = total number of patients given the control treatment.

Advantage. The advantage of the NNT is that it is clinically intuitive, showing how many patients need to be treated for one to benefit. It is treatment specific. It describes the difference between active treatment and control. The level of benefit or threshold used to calculate NNT can be varied, but the NNT is likely to be relatively unchanged because changing threshold changes results for both active and control. The threshold used for the single dose analgesic data (see Fig. 7.2.2) was 50 per cent pain relief. This is a difficult target for analgesics, and, in cancer pain, patients feel a treatment is beneficial if it produces 30 per cent relief.[38] What is judged worthwhile relief may vary with the clinical context, but in terms of the NNT calculation the choice of threshold makes little impact on the relative efficacy of the different treatments, because the results for the control will improve if the threshold is lowered, and deteriorate at a higher threshold. Some patients will of course benefit from the treatment but at a lower level than the threshold.

An NNT of 1 describes an event that occurs in every patient given the treatment but in no patient in a comparator group. This could be described as the 'perfect' result in, say, a therapeutic trial of an antibiotic compared with placebo. For therapeutic benefit the NNT should be as close as possible to 1; there are few circumstances in which a treatment is close to 100 per cent effective and the control or placebo completely ineffective, so NNTs of 2 or 3 often indicate an effective intervention. For unwanted effects, NNT becomes the number-needed-to-harm (NNH), which should be as large as possible.

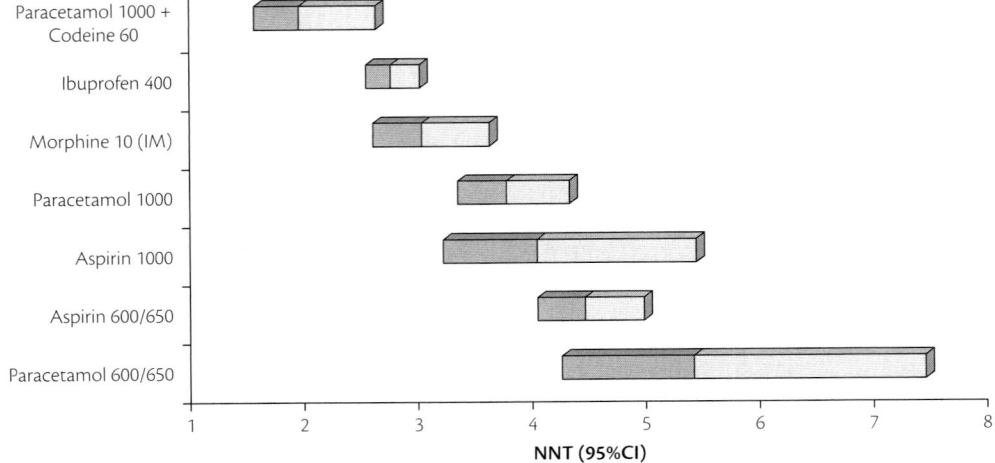

Figure 7.2.2 Numbers-needed-to-treat (NNT) for 50 per cent pain relief in postoperative pain (single dose). NNT point estimate is at the junction of the blue and white bar segments. Blue bar segment is the lower 95 per cent confidence interval, grey is the upper).

It is important to remember that the NNT is always relative to the comparator and applies to a particular clinical outcome. The duration of treatment necessary to achieve the target should be specified. The NNT for cure of head-lice at 2 weeks with permethrin 1 per cent compared with control vehicle was 1.1 (95 per cent CI 1.0–1.2).[39]

Confidence intervals. The confidence intervals of the NNT are an indication that 19 times out of 20 the 'true' value will be in the specified range. If there is inadequate or conflicting data, then the NNT may not have finite confidence intervals, and the statistical tests (odds ratio or relative risk) will not be statistically significant. An NNT with an infinite confidence interval may still have clinical value as a benchmark, but should be treated cautiously until further data permits finite confidence intervals.

Disadvantages. The disadvantage of the NNT approach—apparent from the formula—is that it needs dichotomous data. Continuous data can be converted to dichotomous for acute pain studies so that NNTs may be calculated, by deriving a relationship between the two from individual patient data.[40] Because of the way it is calculated, NNT will also be sensitive to trials with high control event rates (CER). As CER rises, the potential for treatment specific improvement decreases: higher (and apparently less effective) NNTs result. So, as with any summary measure from a quantitative systematic review, NNT needs to be treated with caution, and comparisons can only be made confidently if the pooled trials do not show major variation in their CERs.

Evaluating safety

Estimating the risk of harm is a critical part of clinical decisions. Systematic reviews should report adverse events as well as efficacy, and consider the issue of rare but important adverse events. Large RCTs apart, most trials study limited patient numbers. New medicines may be launched after trials on 1500 patients,[41] missing these rare but important adverse events. The rule of three is important here. If a particular serious event does not occur in 1500 patients given the treatment, we can be 95 per cent confident that the chance of it occurring is at most 3/1500.[42]

Much the same rules apply to harm as to efficacy, but with some important differences, the rules of admissible evidence and the NNH rather than NNT. The absence of information on adverse effects in systematic reviews reduces their usefulness.

Rules of evidence

The gold standard of evidence for harm—as for efficacy—is the RCT. The problem is that in the relatively small number of patients studied in RCTs rare serious harm may not be spotted. Therefore, study architectures of lower intrinsic quality may be admissible for an adverse effect systematic review. An extreme example is that observer blinding is superfluous if the outcome is death. Such rare and serious harm cannot and should not be dismissed just because it is reported in a case report rather than in an RCT. The 'process rules' in this area have yet to be determined.

Number-needed-to-harm (NNH)

For adverse effects reported in RCTs, NNH may be calculated in the same way as NNT. When there is low incidence it is likely that point estimates alone will emerge (infinite confidence intervals). Major harm may be defined in a set of RCTs as intervention-related study withdrawal, and be calculated from those numbers. Precise estimates of major harm will require much wider literature searches to trawl for case reports or series. Minor harm may similarly be defined in a set of RCTs as reported adverse effects. The utility of these reports is because they are reported simply as present or absent, with no indication of severity or importance to the patient.

Conclusion: using NNT and NNH to evaluate analgesics

In the ideal world, you will have three numbers for each intervention, an NNT for benefit and NNHs for minor and major harm. The thrust of this chapter is that these methods can be used to show the effectiveness or otherwise of a range of interventions, and if effective, to use the NNT as a benchmark of just how effective a particular intervention is. This then becomes the yardstick against which alternative interventions, each with its NNT for benefit, NNH for minor harm and NNH for major harm should be judged, and is the pivot for the clinical decision on whether or not to use the intervention for an individual patient. Fig. 7.2.2 ranks the analgesics by their efficacy estimate; clinical choice might be to prescribe or take a safer although marginally less effective drug.

To provide robust recommendations on choice of analgesic, prescription or over-the-counter, requires evidence of the highest quality. These methods can deliver high quality efficacy estimates if there are randomized trials of adequate size and quality, but not if the trials are deficient in number, size or quality. Safety estimates are more difficult, not least because the data from which they are derived come commonly from study designs which are nor randomized and hence more subject to bias.

Extrapolation to palliative care

More than 15 000 RCTs have been identified in the general area of pain and a few hundred systematic reviews exist.[43] The palliative care seam is much thinner with some 1200 RCTs identified, about half of which deal with palliative chemotherapy. There are just a handful of systematic reviews to inform practice. Systematic reviews by definition rely on RCTs as the raw material. Evidence-based medicine has highlighted many gaps in its pursuit of answers and this is equally true in palliative medicine. There are signs of a positive move to higher-quality research but this depends on funding, academic recognition, high-quality journals and greater coordination and collaboration between palliative care centres.[44] The US Institute of Medicine publication 'Approaching death—improving care at the end of life'[45] states 'Important gaps in scientific knowledge about the end of life need serious attention from researchers', and 'current knowledge and understanding are insufficient to guide and support the consistent practice of evidence-based medicine at the end of life'.

There is an increasing voice for promoting research in palliative medicine,[46] against a background where some considered research among this group of patients to be unethical. The limited amount of appropriate research itself limits the chances of improvements in a palliative care culture which relies primarily on clinical experience.[46] Groups such as the European Association of Palliative Care research network are seeking to change this.[47] Other developments seeking to improve training and incorporate evidence include the Project on Death in America founded in 1994 aimed at transforming the culture of dying (PDIA) and Education for Physicians on end of life care which has developed an interactive training programme.[48]

The Cochrane pain, palliative care and supportive care collaborative review group (PaPaS)

The Cochrane Collaboration[49] is an international not-for-profit organization that aims to 'prepare, maintain and disseminate *systematic reviews* of the effects of health care'. It has come about as a product of several concerns and developments:

- An awareness of the huge volume of medicine related literature and a lack of any coordinated analysis of this.

- The emergence of evidence based medicine concepts which have grown to embrace the whole of health care and health-care practitioners.

- The availability and potential of the internet. This has enabled a global research community to develop and thrive in a collaborative fashion.

Systematic reviews undertaken by the Cochrane Collaboration are published in *The Cochrane Library*[50] which is available by subscription as a CD-ROM (issued quarterly) or on-line via the Internet. A number of countries have national subscriptions for their populations. The published reviews include a full publication containing the background and methods, a detailed analysis with graphical displays where appropriate, an abstract and 100-word synopsis. In issue 4, 2008, over 3600 systematic reviews were published.

As well as Cochrane systematic reviews, other health-care databases are included in The Cochrane Library:

- The Cochrane Controlled Trials Register (a bibliographic database of controlled trials)—this contains some 550 000 references to randomized controlled trials that have been identified by the Collaboration.

- The Database of Abstracts of Reviews of Effectiveness (DARE) (structured abstracts of over 9000 systematic reviews which have been critically appraised by reviewers at the NHS Centre for Reviews and Dissemination in York and by other people, e.g. from the American College of Physicians' Journal Club and the journal Evidence-Based Medicine).

- The Cochrane Methodology Register (a bibliography of articles on the science of research synthesis) contains nearly 9000 references.

Collaborative Review Groups comprise an international multi-disciplinary group from around the world who share an interest in developing and maintaining systematic reviews relevant to a particular health area. Groups are coordinated by an editorial team who edit and assemble completed reviews for inclusion in The Cochrane Library. Each group is organized around a small team of coordinating editor and review group coordinator who are responsible for managing the group and for the quality of its output. There are currently 50 CRGs based in a number of countries, each addressing a particular health care area. The *Pain, Palliative and Supportive Care Group (PaPaS)*[51] is one such group and has its editorial base at the Pain Research Unit, Oxford, UK. PaPaS aims to generate evidence about the effectiveness of health care treatments relevant to:

- the prevention and treatment of pain;

- the relief of symptoms resulting from both the disease process, interventions used in the management of the disease, and symptom control—i.e. palliative care in its widest sense;

- the support of patients and carers through the disease process.

PaPaS has an international team of editors and peer reviewers—clinical experts, statisticians, health-care professionals, consumers—who support and advise the individuals who are preparing systematic reviews. As regards, the reviewers who are actively involved in preparing systematic reviews, there are currently more than 200 people based in 19 countries that are contributing to review production. Most reviewers are practitioners who are researching a review topic in their own time; some are researchers who have obtained funding to work full-time on a review, or are undertaking a review as part of a higher-degree qualification, others are undertaking a review as the research element of their specialist registrars training programme in palliative medicine.[51]

PaPaS is building a specialized database of all known RCTs and clinical controlled trials related to pain, palliative, and supportive care—irrespective of language of publication. This database is used as a resource by reviewers to identify trials for possible inclusion in systematic reviews.

100 completed reviews in the Cochrane Library; there are a further 50 reviews in progress.

Some examples from the palliative care field include:

- Benzodiazepines for insomnia in palliative care.
- Calcitonin for bone pain and complications secondary to bone metastases.
- Drug treatments for anxiety in palliative care.
- Drug treatments for delirium in palliative care.
- Interventions for the management of constipation in cancer patients.
- Interventions for the management of skin (and mucous membranes) before, during, and after radiation therapy.
- Ketamine as an adjuvant to opioids for cancer pain.
- Metoclopramide for chemotherapy induced nausea and vomiting.
- Pharmacological and psychological interventions for low mood in palliative care patients.
- Radionucleotides for bone pain and complications secondary to bone metastases.
- Supportive care for symptom relief in patients with gastrointestinal cancer.
- Interventions for noisy breathing.
- Acupuncture for chemotherapy-induced nausea or vomiting among cancer patients.
- Bisphosphonates for pain secondary to bone metastases.
- Cannabinoids for chemotherapy-induced nausea and vomiting.
- Cannabinoids for pain management.
- Dexamethasone for the treatment of emesis induced by cytotoxic drugs.
- Feeding regimens for bone marrow transplant patients.
- Hydromorphone for pain relief.
- Oral morphine for cancer pain.
- A range of reviews on neuropathic pain.
- Megestrol for cancer cachexia.
- Opioids for the palliation of breathlessness in terminal illness.
- Pleurodesis for malignant pleural effusions.
- Psychotherapeutic treatments for the management of chronic pain in children.
- Some complementary therapy topics are covered including music for pain relief, acupuncture, and touch therapies.

Table 7.2.4 Identified journals in palliative care.

Number of journals	31
Languages	6 (2 Asian)
Indexed in Medline	6
Indexed in EmBASE	3 (2 unique)
Handsearched by PaPaS	11

Table 7.2.4 shows the number of journals identified by the PaPaS group as containing trials relevant to palliative care, the spread of languages and the fact that many are not indexed in Medline or EmBase.

Conclusion

If there is a theme to this chapter on EBM and palliative care, it is that we know how to provide robust evidence about the efficacy of interventions. To provide that evidence, we need high-quality trials. We should not shy away from doing high quality trials in palliative care just because they are difficult. At the same time we need to acknowledge that the methodology is not adequate yet to design adequate studies of the ways in which we deliver care, either packages of care or the context in which they are delivered. The finite necessities are the fact that we know how to do some (relatively simple) trials and reviews. The infinite luxuries are all the questions to which we do not yet have the answers.

References

1. Moore, A., and McQuay, H. (2006). *Bandolier's little book of making sense of the evidence.* Oxford University Press, Oxford.
2. Oxford Centre for Evidence-based Medicine. (2006). *Levels of evidence and grades of recommendations.* 5 Feb 2005 [cited 17 Nov]; Available from: http://www.cebm.net/levels_of_evidence.asp
3. Sackett, D.L., Rosenberg, W.M.C., Muir Gray, J.A. *et al.* (1996). Evidence-based medicine: what it is and what it isn't. *British Medical Journal,* **312**, 71–2.
4. Sackett, D., Richardson, W.S., Rosenberg, W. *et al.* (1996). *Evidence based medicine.* Churchill Livingstone, London.
5. Medical Research Council. (2006). *A framework for development and evaluation of RCTs for complex interventions to improve health.* 2000 [cited 17 Nov]; Available from: http://www.mrc.ac.uk/Utilities/Documentrecord/index.htm?d=MRC003372
6. Schulz, K.F., Chalmers, I., Hayes, R.J. *et al.* (1995). Empirical evidence of bias: dimensions of methodological quality associated with estimates of treatment effects in controlled trials. *Journal of the American Medical Association,* **273**, 408–12.
7. Chalmers, I., Dickersin, K., and Chalmers, T. (1992). Getting to grips with Archie Cochrane's agenda. *British Medical Journal,* **305**, 786–7.
8. Jadad, A.R., and McQuay, H.J. (1993). A high-yield strategy to identify randomized controlled trials for systematic reviews. Online *J Curr Clin Trials* [serial online]. Feb 27; Doc No 33:3973 words, 39 paragraphs, 5 tables.
9. Simes, R.J. (1987). Confronting publication bias: a cohort design for meta-analysis. *Statistics in Medicine,* **6**, 11–29.
10. Hetherington, J., Dickerson, K., Chalmers, I. *et al.* (1989). Retrospective and prospective identification of unpublished controlled trials: lessons from a survey of obstetricians and pediatricians. *Pediatrics,* **84**, 374–80.
11. Song, F., Altman, D.G., Glenny, A.M. *et al.* (2003). Validity of indirect comparison for estimating efficacy of competing interventions: empirical evidence from published meta-analyses. *BMJ,* **326**, 1–5.
12. Ioannidis, J.P. (2006). Indirect comparisons: the mesh and mess of clinical trials. *Lancet,* **368**(9546), 1470–2.
13. Jadad, A.R., Carroll, D., Moore, A. *et al.* (1996). Developing a database of published reports of randomised clinical trials in pain research. *Pain,* **66**, 239–46.
14. Carroll, D., Tramer, M., McQuay, H. *et al.* (1996). Randomization is important in studies with pain outcomes: systematic review of transcutaneous electrical nerve stimulation in acute postoperative pain. *British Journal of Anaesthesia,* **77**(6), 798–803.

15. Jadad, A.R., Moore, R.A., Carroll, D. *et al.* (1996). Assessing the quality of reports of randomized clinical trials: is blinding necessary? *Controlled Clinical Trials*, **17**, 1–12.

16. Chalmers, T.C., Smith, H., Blackburn, B. *et al.* (1981). A method for assessing the quality of a randomized control trial. *Controlled Clinical Trials*, **2**, 31–49.

17. Fleiss, J.L., and Gross, A.J. (1991). Meta-analysis in epidemiology, with special reference to studies of the association between exposure to environmental tobacco smoke and lung cancer: a critique. *Journal of Clinical Epidemiology*, **44**, 127–39.

18. Nurmohamed, M.T., Rosendaal, F.R., Buller, H.R. *et al.* (1992). Low molecular-weight heparin versus standard heparin in general and orthopaedic surgery: a meta-analysis. *Lancet*, **340**, 152–6.

19. Chalmers, I., Hetherington, J., Elbourne, D. *et al.* (1989). Materials and methods used in synthesizing evidence to evaluate the effects of care during pregnancy and childbirth. In *Effective care in pregnancy and childbirth* (eds. I. Chalmers, M. Enkin, and M.J.N.C. Keirse), pp. 38–65. Oxford University Press, Oxford.

20. Chalmers, I. (1989). Evaluating the effects of care during pregnancy and childbirth. In *Effective care in pregnancy and childbirth* (eds. I. Chalmers, M. Enkin, and M.J.N.C. Keirse), pp. 1–37. Oxford University Press, Oxford.

21. Sackett, D.L., and Gent, M. (1979). Controversy in counting and attributing events in clinical trials. *The New England Journal of Medicine*, **301**, 1410–2.

22. Peto, R., Pike, M.C., Armitage, P. *et al.* (1976). Design and analysis of randomised clinical trials requiring prolonged observation of each patient. 1. Introduction and design. *British Journal of Cancer*, **34**, 585–612.

23. Kalso, E., Tramer, M., Carroll, D. *et al.* (1997). Pain relief from intra-articular morphine after knee surgery: a qualitative systematic review. *Pain*, **71**, 127–34.

24. Rodgers, A., Walker, N., Schug, S. *et al.* (2000). Reduction of postoperative mortality and morbidity with epidural or spinal anaesthesia: results from overview of randomised trials. *BMJ*, (Dec), **321**(7275), 1493.

25. Smith, L.A., Oldman, A.D., McQuay, H.J. *et al.* (2000). Teasing apart quality and validity in systematic reviews: an example from acupuncture trials in chronic neck and back pain. *Pain*, **86**, 119–32.

26. Oxman, A.D., and Guyatt, G.H. (1988). Guidelines for reading literature reviews. *Canadian Medical Association Journal*, **138**, 697–703.

27. Geborek, P., Crnkic, M., Petersson, I.F. *et al.* and South Swedish Arthritis Treatment Group. (2002). Etanercept, infliximab, and leflunomide in established rheumatoid arthritis: clinical experience using a structured follow up programme in southern Sweden. *Annals of the Rheumatic Diseases*, **61**, 793–8.

28. L'Abbé, K.A., Detsky, A.S., and O'Rourke, K. (1987). Meta-analysis in clinical research. *Annals of Internal Medicine*, **107**, 224–33.

29. Tramer, M., Moore, A., and McQuay, H. (1995). Prevention of vomiting after paediatric strabismus surgery: a systematic review using the numbers-needed-to-treat method. *British Journal of Anaesthesia*, **75**(5), 556–61.

30. Soll, J.C., and McQueen, M.C. (1992). Respiratory distress syndrome, Chapter 15. In *Effective care of the newborn infant* (eds. J.C. Sinclair, and M.E. Bracken), p. 333. Oxford University Press, Oxford.

31. Moore, R.A. *Helicobacter pylori and peptic ulcer. A systematic review of effectiveness and an overview of the economic benefits of implementing that which is known to be effective 1995.* [cited]; Available from: http://www.jr2.ox.ac.uk/Bandolier/bandopubs/hpyl/hpall.html

32. Moore, R.A., Gavaghan, D., Tramer, M.R. *et al.* (1998). Size is everything–large amounts of information are needed to overcome random effects in estimating direction and magnitude of treatment effects. *Pain*, **78**(3), 209–16.

33. Gavaghan, D.J., Moore, R.A., and McQuay, H.J. (2000). An evaluation of homogeneity tests in meta-analyses in pain using simulations of individual patient data. *Pain*, **85**, 415–24.

34. Sinclair, J.C., and Bracken, M.B. (1994). Clinically useful measures of effect in binary analyses of randomized trials. *Journal of Clinical Epidemiology*, **47**(8), 881–9.

35. Sackett, D.L., Deeks, J.J., and Altman, D.G. (1996). Down with odds ratios! *Evidence-Based Medicine*, **1**, 164–6.

36. Deeks, J. (1996). What the heck's an odds ratio? *Bandolier (25)*, **3**(3), 6–7.

37. Glass, G.V. (1976). Primary, secondary, and meta-analysis of research. *Educational Researcher*, **5**, 3–8.

38. Farrar, J.T., Portenoy, R.K., Berlin, J.A. *et al.* (2000). Defining the clinically important difference in pain outcome measures. *Pain*, **88**(3), 287–94.

39. van der Stichele, R.H., Dezeure, E.M., and Bogaert, M.G. (1995). Systematic review of clinical efficacy of topical treatments for head lice. *British Medical Journal*, **311**, 604–8

40. Moore, A., McQuay, H., and Gavaghan, D. (1996). Deriving dichotomous outcome measures from continuous data in randomised controlled trials of analgesics. *Pain*, **66**, 229–37.

41. Moore, T.J. (1995). *Deadly medicine.* Simon & Schuster, New York.

42. Eypasch, E., Lefering, R., Kum, C.K., *et al.*. Probability of adverse events that have not yet occurred: a statistical reminder. *British Medical Journal*, **311**, 619–20.

43. Bandolier. (2006). *Systematic reviews on pain topics.* [cited 22 November]; Available from: http://www.jr2.ox.ac.uk/Bandolier/painres/MApain.html

44. Bruera, E. (1998). Research into symptoms other than pain (Section 5.3). In *Oxford textbook of palliative medicine* (eds. D. Doyle, G. Hanks, and N. MacDonald), 2nd edition. Oxford University Press, Oxford.

45. Field, M.J.C.C. (1997) *Approaching death: improving care at the end of life.* National Academy Press, Washington DC.

46. Kaasa, S., and De Conno, F. (2001). Palliative care research. *European Journal of Cancer*, (Oct), **37**(Suppl. 8), S153–9.

47. EAPC. (2006). *European association of palliative care.* [cited 22 November]; Available from: www.eapcnet.org/home.html

48. EPEC. (2006). *Education for physicians on end of life care.* [cited 22 November]; January: Available from: www.epec.net

49. Cochrane. (2006). *The cochrane collaboration.* [cited 22 November]; Available from: www.cochrane.org

50. Cochrane Library. (2006). *The cochrane library.* [cited 22 November]; Available from: www.thecochranelibrary.org

51. PaPaS. (2006). *Pain, palliative and supportive care group, cochrane collaboration.* [cited 22 November]; Available from: www.jr2.ox.ac.uk/cochrane

Understanding clinical trials in palliative care research

John T. Farrar

Introduction

Components of the randomized, controlled trial (RCT) have been part of clinical research for several centuries but the modern concept of the importance of the random selection of a control group can be traced to one of the first studies of streptomycin for pulmonary tuberculosis conducted by the British Medical Research Council and published in 1948[1,2]. Prior to that time, the evaluation of health care relied on what today would be considered anecdotal evidence. The RCT represents the gold-standard for the evaluation of the efficacy of new medical therapies. Despite their status, several potential, scientific. and ethical difficulties continue to limit the use of RCTs in some clinical contexts such as palliative care, and hinder the generalizability of their results in others. Understanding these limitations and how to apply the results of such studies to clinical care is an important process.

By presenting the various strengths and limitations that are common to all RCTs and how they apply to trials of palliative care interventions, we will consider how decisions made regarding trial design, conduct, and analysis can influence the trial's results. Basic issues in the analysis of clinical trial data as they apply to the interpretation of RCT results will also be considered. We hope that this chapter will provide palliative care clinicians with a proper understanding of the structure and inherent problems with clinical trials. No research experiment can ever be perfect, but the information provided by RCTs is extremely useful as a basis for evidence-based approaches to clinical care. With this knowledge, the reader of science should be able to ascertain whether the results of published trials are (1) likely to be valid and (2) likely to apply to their patients.

The anatomy of a trial

Study design issues must be considered from conceptualization, through implementation and ending with the interpretation of results. Subtle flaws in a trial design or conduct may lead to inappropriate conclusions. Decisions made regarding every component of an RCT can dramatically influence the quality of the data and the outcome of a trial.

Even when a clinical trial is perfectly designed, there is no guarantee of finding the right answer to a specific research question. Because of random variation, there is always a probability of reaching a false positive or a false negative conclusion simply by chance.

A statistical analysis is conducted primarily to (1) summarize the data to estimate the size of the effect being observed that can be attributed to the treatment being tested and (2) to estimate the probability that the results obtained occurred simply by chance. The conventional selection of a p-value cut-off point of 0.05 means that we are willing to accept a 1/20 probability of getting a false positive answer by chance alone. As a result, replication of a trial's results is always preferable before clinicians can confidently make decisions about patient care, since no single trial should ever be considered definitive proof of the presence or absence of efficacy.

The question

The initial step in designing any trial or understanding the results is to define what research question is being asked. This can seem like a relatively simple process, but it is often a tremendous challenge to replicate a clinical reality in the research setting. To properly design a clinical trial requires reducing an important clinical question into a testable hypothesis. Many clinically relevant questions cannot be studied because the appropriate population is not available, the number required may be prohibitively large, or for ethical issues. This is especially true in studies of palliative care, where randomizing patients to a potentially less effective treatment may not be considered ethical.

In such situations it is often necessary to modify the research question to one that is more readily answerable. It is important to understand that getting an answer to a different question, may or may not allow its application to the original clinical scenario. Attempting to answer the right question in the setting of an RCT may result in compromises in the study design, sacrificing either precision or protection from bias. In some cases, a poor study design may reduce the value of the knowledge, and hence alter the risk–benefit calculation used to justify the research[3,4]. From the outset, an alternative design should be considered if the investigators are not clear about the clinical importance of answering the proposed question.

The choice of an appropriate outcome and the measure to be used to collect the data is an important step in ensuring that the research question can be answered with a clinically relevant primary outcome that can be measured, analysed, and the results interpreted. This must be done a priori, before the data is collected or analysed. In order to maintain acceptable limits on the probability of arriving at an incorrect result by chance, both the clinical importance of the effect of an intervention and the characteristics of the data to be collected, must be defined. Although multiple secondary outcomes are often also tested within a single trial, each should be identified at the outset, and none should subsequently replace the primary outcome after the data have been collected and analysed (a posteriori).

Choosing outcomes is often dependent on the disease area to be studied. A recently published summary of outcomes created in conjunction with the Agency for Healthcare Research and Quality (AHRQ) have specified areas, including symptom management, quality of life (QOL) including function and satisfaction, family burden, and quality-of-death measures. There are a number of evaluative tools that have been used over time or recommended by various groups, but they are beyond the scope of this chapter and well described elsewhere[5]. Almost all of the measures used for palliative care studies are patient oriented self reports, which require a careful approach to analysis and interpretation.

Types of trial

Part of the process of choosing the question is choosing the basic design of the trial. While there are many different variations on an RCT, the two basic formats are to design a trial to demonstrate an effect (either beneficial or harmful) of an exposure (or treatment) over no exposure; or to design a trial to demonstrate equivalence between two different treatments. In both cases, the goal is to demonstrate an outcome that has a less than 1/20 probability of occurring by chance.

Efficacy trials

An efficacy trial is defined by demonstrating that the two groups are not the same (i.e. that the null hypothesis is false). This trial benefits from the fact that demonstrating two things are different is substantially easier than proving that two things are the same. The calculation of sample size is based on established probability calculations that take into consideration the underlying variability of the measurement and the size of the effect to be evaluated. The majority of this chapter will focus on the issues involved in the design and interpretation of an efficacy trial.

Non-inferiority and equivalence trials

Given the concerns about the difficulties in conducting a placebo-controlled trials and the maintenance of blinding, investigators occasionally attempt to show that a new drug is either 'no worse than' (a non-inferiority trial), or 'as good as' (an equivalence trial) a treatment that is commonly accepted as effective. In evaluating therapeutics for conditions in which the risks of placebo assignment are widely regarded as too great, such as thrombolytic agents for acute myocardial infarction or stroke, active-controlled, non-inferiority trials are the standard [6, 7].

These trials are presently not considered standard for problems such as hypertension, hyperlipidaemia, and pain, because the risks of temporarily foregoing active treatment are not as obvious, and because there are several potential problems with interpreting such studies[9–13]. The first problem is that equivalence trials essentially aim to confirm the conventional null hypothesis of no treatment difference. One way to purposefully reduce the chance of showing a difference is to conduct a poorly designed study. This may create inappropriate incentives for conducting 'sloppy' research[14]. Second, such trials generally require larger numbers of participants, because equivalence or non-inferiority must be documented within relatively narrow margins. Third, demonstrating that two treatments are the same does not show that either of them works. This problem is related to 'assay sensitivity', because such trials require the assumption that the standard therapy would have proven superior to placebo had a placebo arm been included in the study design used [9]. Because of these concerns, current regulatory guidelines still call for placebo-controlled trials to evaluate treatments for problems such as pain and other symptoms[15].

Randomization

The most important feature of an experimental clinical trial is the equivalence of the comparison groups at baseline such that any differences measured at the end can be attributed to the differences between the treatments administered. Random selection of subjects from a sufficiently large single population equally distributes known and unknown factors that might otherwise influence the outcome, such as age, sex, and disease severity.

This is in contrast to, observational studies (e.g. case–control, cohort, or cross-sectional studies) which depend on nature to set up the experiment. In this type of study, there is a substantial possibility that known or unknown factors may create differences between the comparison groups at baseline, limiting our ability to attribute any subsequent changes to the treatment. Unmeasured confounding or bias can potentially leading to the wrong conclusion from the study. In experimental studies randomization is the primary mechanism used to create equivalence between the comparison groups. By minimizing the possibility of differences at baseline, an RCT enable investigators to more confidently attribute observed changes over time to the assigned treatments.

True randomization is accomplished by generating a set of random numbers, and distributing them via a mechanism that protects the integrity of the random assignment. A centrally managed randomization scheme may help to ensure consistent application of the procedure across sites and staff. Central control of the randomization will also prevent members of the study team, from knowingly or unknowingly influencing the assignment, especially if they are not be blinded to a patient's treatment allocation.

Randomization works correctly only when sufficient numbers of patients are enrolled to ensure an equal distribution of all important factors. In smaller trials, or in large, multi-centre trials with few participants from a given centre, chance alone may cause significant differences in the distributions of important demographic or disease-related characteristics between groups. In order to reduce the likelihood of such occurrences, investigators can use a block randomization scheme to ensure that selected participant characteristics will be equally distributed. For example, if investigators wished to guarantee an equal sex distribution among two treatment arms at multiple sites, they may randomize in blocks of six participants each, within which three participants would be male and three would be female.

Control group

The purpose of the control group is to provide an appropriate comparison for the treatment group, in order to be able to attribute causality to the difference between the treatments given to each group. This difference in treatment can be as specific as an individual effect of a medication, such as an opioid, or as complex as a whole system approach to care, such as inpatient versus outpatient hospice care. Assuming that the treatment groups are equivalent at baseline (through randomization), then the differences seen in outcome of the groups can be attributed to differences in the treatment. In addition, the degree to which blinding is applied to each group is important for our ability to interpret the resulting data (see following paragraphs). There are three primary types of control groups that can be used in clinical trials: (1) a no-treatment control; (2) a placebo control; and (3) an active control.

Each type provides different information in comparison to the active treatment group, and the usefulness will depend on the research question that is being explored by the study. The no-treatment control group can provide information about changes that happen based on the (1) natural history of the disease (there is a normal variation in the status of any disease state) and (2) regression to the mean (patients with severe symptoms tend to get better). The placebo-treated control group, when properly blinded, also controls for the mind–body interaction that occurs either from participating in a clinical trial or because of the subject's belief in the therapy. The mind–body response is an especially important part of many symptomatic therapy trials. An active control group is best thought of as a diagnostic test of the design and conduct of the clinical trial. By administering a drug known to be active in the disease being tested, a positive result provides evidence that the study has been properly designed and conducted. If the experimental agent then does not demonstrate an effect, the negative result is more convincing. Conversely, if the active agent does not produce an effect, the design and conduct of the trial are called into question. In this situation, a negative result with the experimental agent is as likely to be due to the problems in the design as a true lack of efficacy.

No-treatment-controlled trials

A no-treatment control group, where participants receive no intervention or a delayed intervention, is applicable in two primary situations The first situation arises when there are practical and/or ethical problems with using a placebo or sham control. For example, it is often difficult to construct an appropriate sham intervention for many trials of surgical interventions. Even if adequate shams could be constructed, some feel that assigning patients to receive an invasive, but non-active, intervention is unethical[16]. In such situations, a randomly assigned control group is clearly better than not having a control group, but the results must be viewed cautiously since there are many factors that can affect a subject's response to a treatment, when both the subject and the investigator know which group they are in. As discussed in the following paragraphs, at least the study staff that collect and record the outcome measures should be blinded to the subjects group if possible.

The second situation occurs when a goal of the trial is to determine the magnitude of the mind–body placebo effect. The placebo-treated group will have a response that is a mix of the natural history of disease and regression to the mean, along with the mind–body placebo effect. By having a no-treatment control group, the mind–body placebo effect can be estimated. In a meta-analysis of 114 trials employing both placebo- and no-treatment-controls, the placebo effect was less than might be expected, but in symptomatic relief the effect can be large[17]. In pain research, the placebo-control group patients typically have a more favourable outcome than those in no-treatment-control groups[17].

Placebo-controlled trials

A placebo control group is the best known and most widely used of the possible control groups. A placebo is defined as an inactive treatment designed to mimic as closely as possible, the characteristics of the active treatment. The purpose is to have the control group treated exactly the same as the treatment group except for the specific component being tested. The usefulness of a placebo assumes that at least the study subject will be blinded to the type of therapy they are receiving. Creating a placebo for a drug trial is relatively straight forward. An inactive substance is formulated to have similar appearance and route of administration as the active treatment. Procedure-oriented therapies are much harder to mimic and therefore, it is significantly harder to obtain true blinding (see following paragraphs). In the absence of blinding, the placebo group is equivalent to the no-treatment group.

The primary benefit of using a placebo control group, rather than a no-treatment control group, is that it enables the specific efficacy of the new intervention to be distinguished from the many non-specific effects of all therapies, including the well-known mind–body interaction (also called the placebo effect)[18,19]. The placebo control group is a group of patients who are treated with a placebo. The response measured in this group includes all three separate processes, namely: (1) natural history of the disease; (2) regression to the mean; and (3) the mind–body interaction. The mind–body interaction is a change in brain function that, at least temporarily, leads to improvement in the bodily signs or symptoms. The mind–body interaction is also sometimes know as a non-specific action, while the direct affect of the therapy on the disease is known as a specific action of the therapy.

Assuming a simple additive model of treatment effects, the magnitude of the placebo effect in a given study can be estimated by the mean (or median) response in the placebo group and subtract the response in the no-treatment group. In addition, the placebo group response can be subtracted from the mean response in the active treatment group to estimate the specific efficacy of the new intervention. Though the existence of true placebo effects across a broad range of clinical interventions can vary depending on the disease being treated, the treatment modality, and the outcome expectation of the patients, the effect is generally larger in studies of the treatment of symptoms and in the management of pain[17].

A placebo control group assumes the study will be conducted in a double-blind fashion. This helps to avoid the biases that may ensue if patients, investigators, or both, knew who would be receiving which treatment. But there are also costs to using a placebo control. The first, and most obvious, is that placebo-controlled trials require that some patients be given active treatment despite the existence of other potentially effective interventions. The ethics of placebo-controlled trials in such settings remains a hotly debated topic[8,18–20], and is considered further elsewhere in this book. The second cost to conducting placebo-controlled trials is that, while they remain the gold-standard for documenting absolute efficacy, they do not always answer a clinically relevant question. For practicing clinicians, who have several symptomatic therapies at their disposal, knowing whether another medication works better than nothing is not as important as knowing how the new therapy compares to the existing standard of care[21].

Participant selection

Another critical decision for investigators designing trials, and for clinicians who use the data, regards the selection of study participants. There are two conflicting priorities: (1) ensuring similarities between participants in the experimental and control groups and (2) testing a new treatment in a sample of patients likely to reflect all those who could benefit from using the intervention. To meet the first goal, investigators would attempt to enrol patients who are relatively homogenous so there are fewer differences to even out with randomization. Strict inclusion and exclusion criteria allow greater confidence that the observed differences in outcomes are attributable to the treatments being compared, rather than to undetected confounding variables related to the compositions of participants in each group.

By contrast, meeting the second goal requires enrolling participants from a more heterogeneous population. Because of the large interpersonal variability inherent in such a population, this approach can substantially increase the number of participants required to assure that the trial has adequate statistical power to document a treatment difference, if one exists. Despite this disadvantage, enrolling a heterogeneous sample allows sub-group analyses to be conducted, and so potential variations in a treatment's efficacy among higher- and lower-risk patients may be identified. There are thus advantages and disadvantages to enrolling more or less homogeneous participants. As a result, early investigations of efficacy are commonly conducted using a select group of participants, whereas later, more definitive trials attempt to enrol more broadly representative patient samples. Physicians should, therefore, consider the composition of a given trial's sample in order to determine the extent to which the results are generalizable to their own patients.

In palliative care populations, there is the additional issue of the frailty of the population and the potential lack of stability in their disease state over time. Finding patients who will remain relatively stable for the duration of the trial can be a difficult challenge. In addition, vulnerable populations may make choices that are not always consistent with the goals of a trial, either to participate out of desperation or to not participate because they do not want to be part of an experiment. There is frequently the additional problem of the ability of some patients to understand enough about their disease to be able to give an informed consent. When patients are cognitively challenged in addition, the process of recruitment can become a seemingly overwhelming task. The ethical issues surrounding these problems are considered elsewhere in this book.

Blinding

Over the last century, a growing understanding of the ability of the mind to influence functions of the body, along with the desire to enhance the experimental rigor of clinical trials has increased appreciation of the need for blinding. Recall that the primary goal of a clinical trial is to ensure that any changes between groups seen at the end of the trial may be attributed to a specific treatment being studied. To accomplish this, not only must all comparison groups be similar at the start, but participants in all groups should feel that they have the same probability of getting the real treatment.

Thus, the blinding of the study participants is of substantial importance, and investigators must design the study to prevent the participants from unblinding themselves. In particular, if a medication has a specific taste, common side effects, or other distinctive traits, it is important that the placebo treatment mimic these characteristics as closely as possible. Even in evaluating more invasive interventions, sham procedures have occasionally been employed such as making skin incisions[22] or burr holes in the skull[23] to mimic the real surgical procedures.

In addition to creating a suitable placebo, investigators should plan to determine whether the blinding was maintained by asking participants what treatment they think they received and why. Such questions should be posed to participants occasionally during the trial, and at the trial's completion [24]. If the blinding is successful, the participants' guesses should be no more accurate than chance (e.g. 50 per cent in a typical two-arm trial). Blinding can be difficult to maintain [24–32]. Study participants can often predict their receipt of placebo due to the absence of side effects, or their receipt of the real treatment by noting adverse effects of the intervention.

When only participants are blinded to the treatment received, the study is labelled as a single-blind trial. The standard use of the term double-blind applies when both the participants and investigators are blinded, assuming that the investigator is collecting the outcome data. If the investigator is not collecting the data, it is critical to blind the person who is, so as to minimize the chance that evaluators will more favourably rate those receiving the innovative treatment, thereby biasing the trial toward finding a benefit of that treatment. Even in studies where the subject fills out their own forms, blinding of the investigator remains essential to minimize the possibilities that they would impart different levels of enthusiasm, or prescribe different co-interventions, to patients in the different treatment groups.

Sample size

The statistical power of an RCT to show a difference between treatments is determined by: (1) the number of participants to be enrolled; (2) the effect size (treatment difference) that is deemed to be clinically important; (3) the variability of the outcomes in the two groups; and (4) the p-value (or Type I error rate, or α) chosen to connote statistical significance (typically set at 0.05). In general, the size of the sample to be tested is the variable investigators most commonly adjust to obtain adequate power (i.e. $\beta \geq 80$ per cent although some prefer 90 per cent, which equals 1 minus the Type II error rate)—that is, an adequate probability of detecting a meaningful treatment difference when one truly exists.

It is a truism that with a sufficiently large sample size, any real difference between groups, no matter how small or clinically irrelevant, can be shown to be statistically significant. The converse is also true: a large, clinically important difference between treatments can fail to reach statistical significance when inadequate numbers of participants are enrolled.

The most common method of calculating the sample size required to achieve 80 per cent power (or greater) is to first determine: (1) the size of the effect that would be considered clinically important; (2) the anticipated response in the control group; and (3) the expected variability of the outcomes in both groups. This last determination may be particularly difficult to estimate, and should, when possible, be based on evidence from prior studies of similar diseases and/or treatments.

An alternate method used when the sample size is fixed is to calculate the size of the effect that would need to be present to produce a statistically significant outcome. This approach is rarely preferable to setting the sample size to detect a specified difference but is commonly used when the available population is fixed.

Outcome measurement

Another critical decision to be made in planning an RCT involves how to measure the chosen outcome of interest. For example, if investigators are interested in studying the effects of a new antihypertensive agent on systolic and diastolic blood pressure, should they measure these values with a mercury sphygmomanometer or via an arterial line? In addition to how the outcome will be measured, investigators must further consider when and how often to measure the outcome. Are single readings once each week adequate, or should participants be equipped with ambulatory blood pressure monitors to obtain multiple readings throughout the day? Finally, investigators must consider how to account for other variables that could alter the measurement, such as body position when the blood pressure is assessed.

Regardless of what measurement technique is chosen, it should be characterized by three features. First, the measurement should be reliable—if the same measure is used repetitively in the same person under identical conditions without this person's condition changing, then the measure should produce the same results each time. Second, the measure should be valid—it should measure exactly what it is intended to measure. Third, the measure should be responsive—it should change over time if the condition being measured has truly changed. Though a full discussion of these concepts is beyond the scope of this chapter, the topics are well covered in many textbooks[33]. If the outcome measure has been not routinely used in other similar research, its reliability, validity, and responsiveness should be formally tested and documented in the intended population.

The criteria of reliability, validity, and responsiveness also depend on what form the outcome takes. For example, in pain management, the primary goal is to improve the patient's subjective sense of comfort. For this purpose, investigators might ask a simple question, such as, 'Do you feel better, yes or no?' Because such a measure has only two possible responses, it may not provide an adequately responsive measure of pain relief.

To help differentiate the level of response, investigators might ask, 'What percentage of pain relief do you get from the treatment?' However, such questions require patients to remember their previous conditions. Alternatively, investigators could use a 0–10 numerical rating scale at both the beginning and end of the study to measure the change in pain over time. Deciding which measurement is most appropriate for a given situation should be informed by considerations of how much change in the measure would be important to the patient, and the ability of the chosen scale to detect such a change.

Another measurement concerns in palliative care trials relate to the fact that a change in pain or nausea may only provide one component of an overall change in quality of life. Thus, symptomatic reports may be considered surrogate markers for changes in the more important outcome, the overall quality of life. The use of surrogate markers is a widespread practice in clinical trials. For example, investigators routinely monitor changes in serum cholesterol as a surrogate measure for the risk of myocardial infarction. However, using surrogate measures requires making the assumption that a reduction in cholesterol will lead to a reduced risk of myocardial infarction. If the use of an experimental analgesic agent relieves pain but produces substantial side effects, the patient may not consider its use as an improvement in quality of life. Therefore, if investigators wish to know an intervention's effects on both the level of pain and the overall quality of life, then they must employ tools to measure both. Since there is no single measurement strategy that is universally applicable, it is important to carefully consider whether the measured outcome is appropriate to answer the research question being posed in the clinical trial.

Analysis

Like other aspects of a clinical trial, the specific analytic strategy should be defined before commencing the study. Many different analytic approaches are possible and each will produce an answer to a slightly different research question. It is important that the chosen strategy be appropriate to evaluate the primary research question, and be compatible with the numerical distribution of the data collected. The primary role of the analysis is to summarize the data (size of the effect) and to provide an estimate of the likelihood that the result was obtained by chance alone.

Effect size

The first, and most important, result of any analysis is the summary of the size of the effect resulting from the experimental therapy. In RCTs, the size of the effect is estimated by determining a summary value for the primary outcome in each treatment groups, and then calculating the difference between these values to reveal the difference in the treatment effect. There are only two primary forms for the summary value for a set of trial data: (1) the central tendency (e.g. mean, median, or mode) of the response among participants, or (2) the proportion of participants who achieve a defined level of response.

For example, in a hypertension trial, investigators can report the mean change in diastolic blood pressure (central tendency), or the proportion of patients who achieve a diastolic blood pressures below 90 mmHg (proportion of responders). If one were interested in the effect of an intervention on hospice length of stay, it might be acceptable to report either the median time spent in the programme for each group (central tendency), or the proportion of patients in each group who die within a week or some other predefined time period. Finally, in trials of pain management, in which the outcome of reported pain symptoms is provided on a numeric scale, investigators might either report the mean response in each group, or the percentage of patients in each group reporting pain reductions of 33 per cent (or 50 per cent) or greater in pain intensity. In each case, the units of these summary values should correspond to the units of the outcome measure.

Choices regarding how to best present the summary measures should reflect the type of information that is most relevant for practicing clinicians. For most health-care providers, the question of interest is whether a given treatment will work for a given patient rather than the average change. The average change does not provide a unique answer to the question of the number of people who are likely to improve. For example, suppose investigators reported that the mean response in the active treatment group was an improvement of 10 per cent on a standard pain scale. This same result could apply to data indicating that: (1) every patient in the active treatment group improved by 10 per cent (a unimodal distribution); (2) half of the patients in the treatment group improved by 20 per cent and half had no improvement (a bimodal distribution); or (3) half of the patients in the active treatment group improved by 40 per cent, and half deteriorated by 20 per cent (a bimodal distribution in which some patients improve and other deteriorate). Because these three descriptions of the underlying data could yield strikingly different clinical decisions, it is important to present an analysis of the proportions of patients in each group who improve or deteriorate by a clinically important amount.

What is a clinically important difference?

A common concern about presenting the proportion of 'responders' in each group is the need to define a level of response to be considered clinically important. Thus, the determination of a clinically important difference (CID) in a patient's symptoms plays a key role in the interpretation of symptomatic studies. Two methods for determining the CID are 'expert opinion', and an assessment of how changes in symptom scales correspond to responses to global questions[34–36]. Regardless of the method used, however, each requires that a somewhat arbitrary decision be made in defining the scale to be considered the standard.

Recent studies of pain have adopted an alternative method of displaying response data, but graphing the proportion of responders at each possible outcome level for all the groups in a clinical trial[37]. This display is a form of a cumulative distribution and allows the readers of the published report to select the level of improvement that they feel is clinically important and then determine the difference between the various groups at that level.

Statistical considerations

Statistical significance (p values and confidence intervals)

A p-value ≥ 0.05 is the most commonly accepted statistical test of the probability that a given result occurred by chance. However, this value is strictly arbitrary and is an indication that we are willing to accept a 1/20 chance of getting the wrong answer. This traditional method of hypothesis testing, in which p-values are reported to quantify the significance of a result, is gradually being replaced by methods used to gauge the range of plausible results that are compatible with the data. The most common method for presenting this range is to report a point estimate of the effect size, along with a 95 per cent confidence interval around this estimate. A 95 per cent confidence interval will include the true population value of the effect 19 times out of 20 (95 per cent). Thus, it can help readers determine the uncertainty inherent in any result—the narrower the interval, the more precise the estimate of the true effect, and thus, the more confident readers can be that the reported result is 'right'.

Multiple comparisons

It is also important to realize that when investigators choose a p-value of 0.05 as an acceptable Type I (false positive) error rate, this value only applies to a single comparison between groups. In most clinical trials, however, performing multiple comparisons can be informative. The greater the number of comparisons, the more likely it is that at least one of them will be spuriously positive by chance alone. If an a priori decision is made to perform multiple comparisons, the p-value must be adjusted. Of the several available methods for adjusting this value, the simplest is to divide the p-value for one comparison by the number of comparisons to be performed, and to then use this new p-value as the cut-off for statistical significance across all analyses, called the Bonferroni adjustment[38]. While valid, this is a very conservative estimate, and alternative methods have been developed to deal with multiple comparisons[39].

A related issue regards the distinction between comparisons chosen a priori, and those which investigators choose to conduct post hoc, or after the data has been collected. There are times when post hoc comparisons can be informative, but the results of such analyses should never be considered conclusive because they were not explicitly planned at the outset. Rather, results of post hoc analyses may be considered exploratory, intended to guide future investigations. Authors can help highlight this distinction by reporting which comparisons were chosen a priori, and which were not.

Evidence from secondary measures

In addition to the reported effect size and statistical significance of the primary outcome results, corroborative evidence from secondary outcome analyses should be used to support a study's hypothesis. If multiple related measures are obtained, and the analyses of each show similar results, then it is less likely that any one of the positive results arose by chance. While there is no specific statistical test to document this phenomenon, showing that multiple related measures, all producing similar types of effects, lends support to the conclusions drawn from the primary outcome.

Evaluating side effects

Evaluating side effects of interventions tested in clinical trials is subject to the same considerations as those used to evaluate measures of efficacy. The major difference is that, in many cases, the side effects to be evaluated are not specified a priori, but evaluated only when they are observed to occur. Since many common side effects can occur spontaneously and independent of the treatment received, it is important to compare the relative incidence in the active treatment and control groups. Differing rates of side effect must be evaluated with caution, since clinical trials are rarely powered to detect such differences, and the large number of different side effects that are possible make it likely that one or more of the differences observed, will be due to chance. Such differences should not be ignored; but observing similar results in multiple trials can increase one's confidence that the findings may be specifically attributed to the treatment received.

Publication

Thorough presentation of methods and results

Given that many components of a trial are central to interpreting the results, it is vital that trial reports be accurate, complete, and objective in their presentation of all important aspects of the trial. In particular, the a priori hypothesis should be clearly stated, and the discovery of other findings properly identified. All randomized participants must be accounted for in the publication, and an intention-to-treat analysis of all participants is typically appropriate, even when some participants drop out early or never receive their assigned intervention. Subsequent sub-group analyses can focus on those who complete the trial, but these should not be considered as the primary result. A careful description of the randomization and blinding procedures is also important to assure readers that the trial was properly conducted. Finally, brief descriptions of the rationale behind the choice of measurement tools and analytic strategies can be helpful.

Negative studies are as important as positive ones

There is now good evidence for a publication bias against negative studies, since authors prefer to write up positive ones and editors prefer to publish the same[40,41]. This can lead to difficulties for clinicians who want a true picture of the nature of the evidence for a particular treatment.

Potential limitations of RCTs

There are several issues inherent in the design and conduct of RCTs that may threaten the internal validity of the results—that is, the likelihood that the treatment comparison is free from bias. Furthermore, even when the comparison is internally valid, the external validity, or generalizability of the results, can be limited. Finally, because the conditions in which trials are conducted only weakly approximate clinical reality, physicians must be cautious in using the results as the only guide in clinical decision making. We will briefly discuss each of these potential problems in the following paragraphs. More detailed discussions of these issues are provided by Feinstein[42] and by Kramer and Shapiro[43].

Under-enrolment

Under-enrolment occurs when too few research participants are enrolled to provide adequate statistical power to answer the study's primary research questions. The inability to recruit sufficient numbers of eligible patients is the most common cause of insufficient statistical power in RCTs[44–49]. Such under-enrolment has been attributed to characteristics of: (1) clinicians who refer their patients[50–52]; (2) patients who choose to be screened[53] or enrolled[54]; (3) investigators who design the trials[55]; and (4) institutions at which the trials are conducted[56,57].

Among the challenges to adequate participant recruitment, potential participants' reluctance to enrol in RCTs is likely to be the most formidable, especially in palliative care populations. It has been observed that patients are generally less willing to participate in RCTs than in non-randomized, observational studies[43]. In addition to yielding unacceptably high probabilities for type II errors, the resulting under-enrolment substantially reduces the trial's precision in quantifying the treatment effect.

Selective enrolment

Even when properly designed and carefully conducted, clinical trials can only provide information specific to the population from which the study participants were drawn. Selective enrolment occurs when particular sub-groups within the target population enrol in proportions greater or less than their representation in that population[58,59]. If this population does not include, for example, elderly patients, women, or children, then applying the results to these clinical populations requires extrapolation. While extrapolating results may sometimes be reasonable, it must always be done cautiously because both the beneficial and adverse effects of an intervention can vary across populations.

The level of response detected by an individual trial will depend on the patient population enrolled. For example, when first studying a novel treatment for a condition for which there is no adequately affective treatment, all patients with the condition are more likely to be willing to volunteer. By including people with relatively early or mild symptoms, the response rate may be higher than expected, although the response in the placebo group may also be larger. In contrast, when a treatment is tested in a population where an effective treatment already exists, only people who do not obtain a response to the available treatments are likely to enrol. This more recalcitrant group may have a lower response rate than expected in the total population, thereby underestimating the treatment's potential usefulness.

Poor participant adherence

In RCTs, patients often do not adhere completely to their prescribed treatment regimens[43]. Especially if patients believe they are receiving a non-preferred treatment, their enthusiasm for the trial, and subsequent adherence to their assigned treatment, may wane. This is further complicated if the patients have access to and decide to take either the experimental therapy or a concomitant additional therapy outside of the trial. This occurs more frequently in trials where patients are able to overcome the blinding. There is accumulating evidence that many study participants make concerted efforts to unblind themselves, and that participants who become aware of their treatment assignment maybe more likely to drop out of the study. For example, many patients assigned to the placebo groups in both the initial phase II trial of AZT for AIDS patients[60], and in a randomized trial of vitamin E for patients with Alzheimer's disease[61], appear to have become unblinded, and even to have obtained the active agents outside the trial[62–64]. Even more problematically, widespread unblinding in one AIDS Clinical Trial Group study[65] not only allowed approximately 9 per cent of those assigned to the placebo to receive zidovudine, but contributed to the drop-out rate in the placebo group being one-third higher than it was in the active treatment group[66].

Participant non-adherence and drop-out can substantially bias the results of a trial[67]. Though intention-to-treat analyses may mitigate this bias, if non-adherence or drop-out rates are higher in one group than in the other, such analyses may also prevent a true effect of treatment from being detected. Thus, investigators should make concerted efforts to monitor participant adherence and drop-outs. When such problems exist, the results of the trial must be interpreted cautiously.

Ethical issues in palliative care research (see also Chapter 7.6)

As with all clinical research, palliative care studies require informed consent of the participants and, when cognitive impairment is an issue, from the appropriate family member or medical surrogate. Especially in situations where curative therapies are not likely to be effective, there are a number of important issues to consider and a detailed discussion of this topic is covered in a separate chapter in this book. The most important issue is to consider the balance between the ethical issues of right of the individual to receive companionate care and the needs of the population for information on the efficacy and safety of specific therapies. When conducting clinical trials, the investigator must carefully protect the rights and well-being of the subjects in the study. One possible alternative is the use of innovative approaches for the conduct of clinical trials[68]. Although beyond the scope of this chapter, trials designs such as response-adaptive randomization procedures (e.g. 'play-the-winner' or 'drop-the-loser') may be more ethically appropriate for the testing of therapies in conditions that may have significant consequences on the quantity and/or quality of life that may result in the palliative care population. Such designs focus on minimizing the expected treatment failures while maintaining the power and randomization benefits[69]. 'Add-on' trials, where a new treatment is added to the current treatments the patient is receiving, may reduce the consequences to the individual patients from being randomized to a placebo treatment. Building in rescue strategies to the trial design can also reduce the potential risk to study participants[70]. Crossover trial designs may also be useful in studies of diseases and symptoms that are relatively stable. Using patients as their own control markedly increases the power of the study, but concerns about carryover effects between treatment periods are a serious risk to the validity of the study[71,72].

Conclusions

In this chapter, we have outlined several fundamental considerations for investigators planning clinical trials, and for clinicians attempting to discern the applicability of such trials to their practices. We have given special consideration to the nuances of clinical trials for palliative care interventions. In summary, randomized, controlled trials remain the best available means of evaluating novel palliative care interventions, and for determining how these interventions may be optimally used. Despite the strengths of the design, readers of trial reports should be mindful of the many difficulties inherent in extrapolating from the results obtained in a trial setting to the use of these same interventions in clinical practice.

References

1. Medical Research Council. (1948). Streptomycin treatment of pulmonary tuberculosis. *British Medical Journal*, **2**, 769–82.

2. Anonymous. (1998). Fifty years of randomised controlled trials. *British Medical Journal*, **317**.

3. Freedman, B. (1987). Scientific value and validity as ethical requirements for research: A proposed explication. *IRB*, **9**, 7–10.

4. Emmanuel, E.J., Wendler, D., and Grady, C. (2000). What makes clinical research ethical? *Journal of the American Medical Association*, **283**, 2701–11.

5. Mularski, R.A., Rosenfeld, K., Coons, S.J. et al. (2007). Measuring outcomes in randomized prospective trials in palliative care. *Journal of Pain and Symptom Management*, **34**(1 Suppl), S7–S19.

6. Anonymous. (1997). A comparison of continuous infusion of alteplase with double-bolus administration for acute myocardial infarction. The Continuous Infusion versus Double-Bolus Administration of Alteplase (COBALT) Investigators. *New England Journal of Medicine*, **337**, 1124–30.

7. Anonymous. (1997). A comparison of reteplase with alteplase for acute myocardial infarction. The Global Use of Strategies to Open Occluded Coronary Arteries (GUSTO III) Investigators. *New England Journal of Medicine*, **337**, 1118–23.

8. Temple, R., Ellenberg, S.S. (2000). Placebo-controlled trials and active-control trials in the evaluation of new treatments. Part 1: Ethical and scientific issues. *Annals of Internal Medicine*, **133**, 455–63.

9. Anonymous. (1999). Single-bolus tenecteplase compared with front-loaded alteplase in acute myocardial infarction: the ASSENT-2 double-blind randomised trial. Assessment of the Safety and Efficacy of a New Thrombolytic Investigators. *Lancet*, **354**, 716–22.

10. Temple, R.J. (1997). When are clinical trials of a given agent vs. placebo no longer appropriate or feasible? *Controlled Clinical Trials*, **18**, 613–20.

11. Temple, R. (1996). Problems in interpreting active control equivalence trials. *Accountability Research*, **4**, 267–75.

12. Jones, B., Jarvis, P., Lewis, J.A. et al. (1996). Trials to assess equivalence: the importance of rigorous methods. *British Medical Journal*, **313**, 36–9.

13. Fleming, T.R. (2000). Design and interpretation of equivalence trials. *American Heart Journal*, **139**, S171–6.

14. Ellenberg, S.S. and Temple, R. (2000). Placebo-controlled trials and active-control trials in the evaluation of new treatments. Part 2: Practical issues and specific cases. *Annals of Internal Medicine*, **133**, 464–70.

15. Food and Drug Administration. (2001). *Guidance for industry: E 10: Choice of control group and related issues in clinical trials*. Department of Health and Human Services, Rockville, MD.

16. Hrobjartsson, A. and Gotzsche, P.C. (2001). Is the placebo powerless? An analysis of clinical trials comparing placebo with no treatment. *New England Journal of Medicine*, **344**, 1594–602.

17. Chaput de Saintonge, D.M. and Herxheimer, A. (1994). Harnessing placebo effects in health care. *Lancet*, **344**, 995–8.

18. Freedman, B., Glass, K.C., Weijer, C. (1996). Placebo orthodoxy in clinical research II: Ethical, legal, and regulatory myths. *Journal of Law and Medical Ethics*, **24**, 252–9.

19. Freedman, B., Weijer, C., Glass, K.C. (1996). Placebo orthodoxy in clinical research I: Empirical and methodological myths. *Journal of Law and Medical Ethics*, **24**, 243–51.

20. Kleijnen, J., de Craen, A.J.M., Everdingen, J.V. et al. (1994). Placebo effect in double-blind clinical trials: a review of interactions with medications. *Lancet*, **344**, 1347–9.

21. Rothman, K.J., Michels, K.B. (1994). The continuing unethical use of placebo controls. *New England Journal of Medicine*, **331**, 394–8.

22. Halpern, S.D., Karlawish, J.H.T. (2000). Placebo-controlled trials are unethical in clinical hypertension research. *Archives of Internal Medicine*, **160**, 3167–8.

23. Cobb, L.A., Thomas, G.I., Dillard, D.H. et al. (1959). An evaluation of internal-mammary-artery ligation by double-blind technic. *New England Journal of Medicine*, **260**, 1115–8.

24. Macklin, R. (1999). The ethical problems with sham surgery in clinical research. *New England Journal of Medicine*, **341**, 992–6.

25. Freeman, T.B., Vawter, D.E., Leaverton, P.E. et al. (1999). Use of placebo surgery in controlled trials of a cellular-based therapy for Parkinson's Disease. *New England Journal of Medicine*, **341**, 988–92.

26. Morin, C.M., Colecchi, C., Brink, D. et al. (1995). How "blind" are double-blind placebo-controlled trials of benzodiazepine hypnotics? *Sleep*, **18**, 240–5.

27. Karlowski, T.R., Chalmers, T.C., Frenkel, L.D. et al. (1975). Ascorbic acid for the common cold: A prophylactic and therapeutic trial. *Journal of the American Medical Association*, **231**, 1038–42.

28. Howard, J., Whittemore, A.S., Hoover, J. et al. (1982). The Aspirin Myocardial Infarction Study Research Group. How blind was the patient blind in AMIS? *Clinical Pharmacology and Therapeutics*, **32**, 543–53.

29. Brownell, K.D. and Stunkard, A.J. (1982). The double-blind in danger: Untoward consequences of informed consent. *American Journal of Psychiatry*, **139**, 1487–9.

30. Byrington, R., Curb, D.J., and Mattson, M.E. (1985). Assessment of blindness at the conclusion of the beta-blocker heart attack trial. *Journal of the American Medical Association*, **253**, 1733–6.

31. Rabkin, J.G., Markowitz, J.S., Stewart, J. et al. (1986). How blind is blind? Assessment of patient and doctor medication guesses in a placebo-controlled trial of imipramine and phenelzine. *Psychiatry Research*, **19**, 75–86.

32. Moscussi, M., Byrne, L., Weintraub, M. et al. (1987). Blinding, unblinding and the placebo effect: An analysis of patients' guesses of treatment assignment in a double-blind clinical trial. *Clinical Pharmacology and Therapeutics*, **41**, 259–65.

33. Fisher, S. and Greenberg, R.P. (1993). How sound is the double-blind design for evaluating psychotropic drugs? *Journal of Nervous and Mental Disease*, **181**, 345–50.

34. Basoglu, M., Marks, I., Livanou, M. et al. (1997). Double-blindness procedures, rater blindness, and ratings of outcome: Observations from a controlled trial. *Archives of General Psychiatry*, **54**, 744–8.

35. Streiner, D.L. and Norman, G.R. (2003). *Health Measurement Scales: A practical guide to their development and use*, 3rd edition. New York: Oxford University Press.

36. Jaeschke, R., Singer, J., and Guyatt, G.H. (1989). Measurement of health status. Ascertaining the minimal clinically important difference. *Controlled Clinical Trials*, **10**, 407–15.

37. Jaeschke, R., Guyatt, G.H., Keller, J. et al. (1991). Interpreting changes in quality-of-life score in N of 1 randomized trials. *Controlled Clinical Trials*, **12**, 226S–33S.

38. Todd, K.H. (1996). Clinical versus statistical significance in the assessment of pain relief. *Annals of Emergency Medicine*, **27**, 439–41.

39. Farrar, J.T., Dworkin, R.H., Max, M.B. (2006). Use of the Cumulative Proportion of Responders Analysis (CPRA) Graph to Present Pain Data over a Range of Cut-off Points: Making Clinical Trial Data More Understandable. *Journal of Pain and Symptom Management*, **30**(4), 369–77.

40. Hilsenbeck, S.G., Clark, G.M. (1996). Practical p-value adjustment for optimally selected cutpoints. *Statistics in Medicine*, **15**(1), 103–12.

41. Liu, Q., Li, Y., and Boyett, J.M. (1997). Controlling false positive rates in prognostic factor analyses with small samples. *Statistics in Medicine*, **16**(18), 2095–101.

42. Begg, C.B. and Berlin, J.A. (1988). Publication bias: a problem in interpreting medical data. *Journal of the Royal Statistical Society A*, **151**, 419–63.

43. Reidenberg, M.M. (1998). Decreasing publication bias. *Clinical Pharmacology and Therapeutics*, **63**, 1–3.

44. Feinstein, A.R. (1983). An additional basic science for clinical medicine: II. The limitations of randomized trials. *Annals of Internal Medicine*, **99**, 544–50.

45. Kramer, M.S. and Shapiro, S.H. (1984). Scientific challenges in the application of randomized trials. *Journal of the American Medical Association*, **252**, 2739–45.

46. Freiman, J.A., Chalmers, T.C., Smith, H., *et al.* (1978). The importance of beta, the type II error and sample size in the design and interpretation of the randomized controlled trial: survey of 71 "negative" trials. *New England Journal of Medicine*, **299**, 690–4.

47. Altman, D.G. (1980). Statistics and ethics in medical research III: How large a sample? *British Medical Journal*, **281**, 1336–8.

48. Collins, J.F., Bingham, S.F., Weiss, D.G., *et al.* (1980). Some adaptive strategies for inadequate sample acquisition in Veterans Administration cooperative clinical trials. *Controlled Clinical Trials*, **1**, 227–48.

49. Hunningshake, D.B., Darby, C.A., Probstfield, J.L. (1987). Recruitment experience in clinical trials: Literature summary and annotated bibliography. *Controlled Clinical Trials*, **8**, 6S–30S.

50. Meinert, C.L. (1986). *Patient recruitment and enrollment. Clinical trials: Design, conduct, and analysis*, pp.149–58. New York: Oxford University Press.

51. Nathan, R.A. (1999). How important is patient recruitment in performing clinical trials? *Journal of Asthma*, **36**, 213–6.

52. Taylor, K.M., Margolese, R.G., and Soskolne, C.L. (1984). Physicians' reasons for not entering eligible patients in a randomized clinical trial of adjuvant surgery for breast cancer. *New England Journal of Medicine*, **310**, 1363–7.

53. Taylor, K.M. (1992). Physician participation in a randomized clinical trial for ocular melanoma. *Annals of Ophthalmology*, **24**, 337–44.

54. Taylor, K.M., Feldstein, M.L., Skeel, R.T., *et al.* (1994). Fundamental dilemmas of the randomized clinical trial process: results of a survey of the 1,737 Eastern Cooperative Oncology Group investigators. *Journal of Clinical Oncology*, **12**, 1796–805.

55. Greenlick, M.R., Bailey, J.W., Wild, J., *et al.* (1979). Characteristics of men most likely to respond to an invitation to be screened. *American Journal of Public Health*, **69**, 1011–5.

56. Barofsky, I. and Sugarbaker, P.H. (1979). Determinants of patient nonparticipation in randomized clinical trials for the treatment of sarcomas. *Cancer Clinical Trials*, **2**, 137–46.

57. Collins, J.F., Williford,W.O., Weiss, D.G., *et al.* (1984). Planning patient recruitment: Fantasy and reality. *Statistics in Medicine*, **3**, 435–43.

58. Begg, C.B., Carbone, P.P., Elson, P.J., *et al.* (1982). Participation of community hospitals in clinical trials. Analysis of five years of experience in the Eastern Cooperative Oncology Group. *New England Journal of Medicine*, **306**, 1076–80.

59. Shea, S., Bigger, Jr., T., Campion, J., *et al.* (1992). Enrollment in clinical trials: Institutional factors affecting enrollment in the Cardiac Arrhythmia Suppression Trial (CAST). *Controlled Clinical Trials*, **13**, 466–86.

60. Mant, D. (1999). Can randomised trials inform clinical decisions about individual patients? *Lancet*, **353**, 743–6.

61. Halpern, S.D., Metzger, D.S., Berlin, J.A., *et al.* (2001). Who will enroll? Predicting participation in a phase II AIDS vaccine trial. *Journal of Acquired Immune Deficiency Syndrome*, **27**, 281–8.

62. Fischl, M.A., Richman, D.D., Grieco, M.H., *et al.* (1987). The efficacy of azidothymidine (AZT) in the treatment of patients with AIDS and AIDS-related complex: A double-blind, placebo-controlled trial. *New England Journal of Medicine*, **317**, 185–91.

63. Sano, M., Ernesto, C., and Thomas, R.G. (1997). A controlled trial of selegiline, alpha-tocopheral, or both as treatment for Alzheimer's disease. *New England Journal of Medicine*, **336**.

64. Kodish, E., Lantos, J.D., Siegler, M. (1990). Ethical considerations in randomized controlled clinical trials. *Cancer*, **65**, 2400–4.

65. Epstein, S. (1996). *Impure science: AIDS, activism, and the politics of knowledge.* Berkeley: University of California, Berkeley Press.

66. Karlawish, J.H.T. and Whitehouse, P.J. (1998). Is the placebo control obsolete in a world after donepezil and vitamin E? *Archives of Neurology*, **55**, 1420–4.

67. Volberding, P.A., Lagakos, S.W., Koch, M.A., *et al.* (1990). Zidovudine in asymptomatic Human Immunodeficiency Virus infection: a controlled trial in persons with fewer than 500 CD4-positive cells per cubic millimeter. *New England Journal of Medicine*, **322**, 941–9.

68. Merrigan, T.C. (1990). You can teach an old dog new tricks: How AIDS trials are pioneering new strategies. *New England Journal of Medicine*, **323**, 1341–3.

69. Peto, R., Collins, R., and Gray, R. (1995). Large-scale randomized evidence: Large, simple trials and overviews of trials. *Journal of Clinical Epidemiology*, **48**, 23–40.

70. Streiner, D.L. (2007). Alternatives to placebo-controlled trials. *Canadian Journal of Neurological Sciences*, **34** (Suppl 1), S37–41.

71. Rosenberger, W.F. and Huc, F. (2004). Maximizing power and minimizing treatment failures in clinical trials. *Clinical Trials*, **1**(2), 141–7.

72. Boers, M. (2003). Add-on or step-up trials for new drug development in rheumatoid arthritis: a new standard? *Arthritis and Rheumatism*, **48**(6), 1481–3.

73. Simon, L.J. and Chinchilli, V.M. (2007). A matched crossover design for clinical trials. *Contemporary Clinical Trials*, **28**(5), 638–46.

74. Garcia, R., Benet, M., Arnau, C., *et al.* (2004). Efficiency of the cross-over design: an empirical estimation. *Statistics in Medicine*, **23**(24), 3773–80.

Qualitative research

Linda J. Kristjanson and Nessa Coyle

The nature of the clinical question is the most important guide to determining the research methodology to be used. Cohen and Mount suggest that standard quantitative research techniques are inadequate to fully explore the richness of human experience and that to learn from our teachers (patients and families) we must accompany them into their world.[1] This chapter will explore how qualitative research methods can help to address the range of complex questions encountered in palliative care and how these techniques allow the researcher to enter the multilayered subjective world of human experience.

The chapter will provide an overview of qualitative research 'scaffolding' and discuss three of the most commonly used qualitative research methods. Differences amongst these methods with examples of their application in palliative care will be outlined. Research issues that challenge palliative care clinicians and researchers when embarking upon qualitative studies will be reviewed. The chapter concludes by identifying ways in which palliative care research can be served by qualitative methods and will offer recommendations for palliative care research using these techniques.

What is qualitative research?

The term 'qualitative research' encompasses a wide domain of methods and research practices that have certain common characteristics. The most defining characteristic is that the approach to inquiry is not dependent upon statistical procedures of quantification. Words rather than numerical data are used. Qualitative research seeks meaning and understandings about processes and phenomena, with attention to narratives, personal experiences, and language.[2] Observation, interviews, focus groups, documentary analysis and case studies are all examples of qualitative research techniques.

The differences between quantitative and qualitative methods, however, are not simply research techniques. The philosophical orientations or paradigms that inform the methods are quite different. The aim of qualitative research is not to find significance in numbers but rather in themes that emerge from narratives indicative of universal human experiences. Qualitative inquiry typically focuses in depth, on relatively small numbers of participants (e.g. 5 to 30) who are selected purposefully.

Qualitative research and palliative care have common philosophical underpinnings. In both palliative care and qualitative research there is an emphasis on understanding individual experiences that may not fit into established categories of knowledge.

There is recognition that each person's perspective is unique, complex, and multifaceted. Personal experience is valued as one means of determining what is relevant to care and research. The varying ways people perceive and interpret their experiences as they construct meaning are respected. In this way, qualitative research has the power to disrupt existing assumptions and to challenge existing 'facts'. Both qualitative researchers and palliative caregivers strive to create an atmosphere of trust and mutual respect. They strive to suspend pre-determined beliefs, and to acknowledge and accept the ambiguity of multiple realities inherent in this approach to knowing the patient's world. Both recognize the need for a very flexible approach to accommodate to the particular circumstances of this population of patients, families and caregivers.

Paradigms and ways of knowing

Kuhn[3] first described the term 'paradigm' in relation to traditions of science. Kuhn argued that each scientific community has its own way of viewing what constitutes a scientific problem and consequently determines the appropriate manner in which the problems should be addressed. He used the term 'paradigm' to denote a collective view of what constitutes the nature of the world. He suggested that the set of values arising from this worldview guided the investigator in the type of research question asked and in the subsequent method that allow these questions to be best answered.

Quantitative researchers generally rely on a post-positivistic approach to gaining knowledge. This includes cause and effect thinking, reduction to specific variables and hypothesis and questions, use of measurement and observation and the test of theories.[4] Research undertaken using most quantitative research methods is *deductive* and aims to define objective reality which can be discovered, measured, and understood. Researchers are expected to be rigid in adhering to the original focus of the research question and to maintain an objective distance from the research itself.

In contrast, qualitative researchers ground their reasoning and methods in an *inductive*, interpretive approach to science and understanding. The interpretative, qualitative paradigm of the social sciences acknowledges the inherent value-laden nature of inquiry, seeking to acknowledge the ability of human beings to interpret their world and to give meaning to their subjective experiences.[2]

A simple comparison of quantitative and qualitative approaches is offered by LeCompte and Preissle:[5] 'deductive researchers hope to find data to match a theory; inductive researchers hope to find a theory that explains their data' (p. 42). Despite these apparent differences, it is becoming increasingly common for health-related research to use a mixed methods approach. Both quantitative and qualitative data is collected depending upon the nature of the research question and the scope of the study aims. For example, the researcher may want to both generalize the findings to a population and to develop a detailed view of the meaning of the phenomenon or concept for individuals.[6] Commonly in a mixed method approach there is a dominant-less dominant design mixed method design. One paradigm and its methods are dominant, while a small component of the overall study is drawn from an alternate design.[6] A sequential mixed method or two-phase design is another approach. Here the researcher conducts a qualitative phase of the study and then a quantitative phase or visa versa. Because the two study phases are clearly distinct, the paradigm assumptions behind each phase can be clearly articulated.[6]

Qualitative research questions

Research questions best informed by qualitative methods often begin with questions such as 'how', 'what', 'who', and 'why'. An example would be 'What are the meanings and uses of an expressed desire for hastened death in people living with advanced cancer?' In several types of qualitative approaches, there is an assumption that the researcher may not know the real or relevant research question until he/she is immersed in the field situation. Broad, open-ended research questions are quite acceptable, with anticipation that the research question will be refined or modified as the study proceeds. No matter how the research question is stated, the amount of time allocated for conducting the study must fit the scope of the research problem and the realities of the field situation.

Data used to answer these research questions are based upon interviews or extended periods of observation or document review. Key features include: capturing the individual's point of view; examining aspects of everyday life; and ensuring that the ensuing descriptions are full of detail. The depth of qualitative research makes it difficult to reproduce or replicate in the exact same form. The nature of the methods means that the interaction between the researcher and participant may not be something that another researcher could attain in the same depth, detail, or scope. When a person tells his/her story to someone, the story is rarely told in

exactly the same manner. However, the general themes, issues, concerns, and perceptions should endure—and it is this level of consistency that would be explored in subsequent studies. Well-crafted qualitative research can be extremely time-consuming especially during the process of analysis.

Qualitative research scaffolding

There are a number of methods within the domain of qualitative research. We will discuss three of the most commonly used methods—*ethnography, phenomenology*, and *grounded theory*. Each of these approaches has arisen from a different parent discipline, has somewhat different aims/outcomes and may use similar data collection methods, but employ different analysis techniques. Differences amongst these three methods are briefly summarized in Table 7.4.1.

The researcher is guided by the research question and the overall aim of the study in determining which qualitative method is most appropriate to use. A description of each method and an example of palliative care research undertaken using each of these methods is briefly summarized below. Rigid adherence to one particular procedure, however, is not necessary.

Ethnography: a question of culture

Ethnography is a methodology that incorporates a variety of theoretical traditions. It is more closely associated, however, with anthropological research than with sociology. Ethnography focuses on the culture of a group, the webs and patterns of meaning that make up a culture and that guide and make sense of people's actions.[4] Ethnography focuses on discovering the cultural frameworks, analysing their structure and content, and using this as a basis for explanation of particular social phenomena. Ethnography is distinct as an approach in that it attempts to interpret and present findings from a cultural perspective. Ethnography searches out the patterns of meaning and emotions that make up culture and how these make sense of actions in everyday life. At the heart of ethnography is good or 'thick' description, typically obtained through an immersion in the everyday life of the group or a given social setting.

Morales[7] used an ethnographic methodology to study the meaning of touch to hospitalized Puerto Ricans with cancer. Eight cancer

Table 7.4.1 Qualitative approaches, parent discipline, aim, and methods.

Qualitative approach	Parent discipline	Aim	Data collection techniques	Analysis methods
Ethnography	Anthropology	To understand a phenomenon from using a cultural perspective	Interviews	Language as unit of analysis
			Participant observation	Search for customs, practices, mores, and norms
			Document reviews	
Phenomenology	Philosophy	To understand the lived experience of an individual or group of individuals	Interviews	Search for meanings, essences, lived experiences, stories, and narratives
			Focus group interviews	
Ground theory	Sociology	To understand a psychosocial or social process	Interviews	Search for common themes, sub-themes, and categories
			Focus groups	
			Participant observation	Identify contexts, contrasts, co-variates, consequence

patients receiving care in a 12-bed oncology research unit in Puerto Rico participated. Data gathering methods included participant observation and several interviews during a 1-month period. Participant observation is a valuable data collection method that follows the anthropologist's research model, in which the study of people in their natural settings is undertaken using a toolkit of observation technique, with the researcher becoming immersed in the setting to a greater or lesser degree.[8] The researcher who observes human beings cannot escape, having to participate in some fashion in the experience and actions of those he/she observes. Through this type of participatory interaction, the researcher is able to see things from the people's perspectives and hence to have a deeper understanding of the people that he/she is learning from.[5] Issues of the risk of a 'Hawthorne effect' that are a concern in quantitative methods are not relevant in this type of research. In qualitative research, the researcher *is the instrument of data collection*, through use of observation, field notes, and interviews. No claim is made that the interviewer is separate from the data collection tool or process. However, it is essential that qualitative research reports include details of whether researchers are insiders or outsiders to the setting, and the relevant, existing assumption they bring to the study. Use of this technique also requires an extended period of observation so that the early influence of the observer or interviewer lessens and those observed return to their usual practices and behaviours.

Content analysis was then used to identify patterns of behaviour and meaning. Analysis of field notes and interview was undertaken to search for domains. Theme analysis was used in the search for the relationships among domains. Themes are recurrent patterns in the data that are used to connect domains. Domains are categories of meaning that refer to specific social or cultural scenes or observations.[9] In the analysis of the patient interviews, two types of touch (i.e. domains) were identified: procedural and affective. The predominant theme about perceptions of nurses' touch was that of conveying confidence (this is the recurrent pattern when examining different domains or types of touch). Confidence was related to the patient's increase in positive expectation as much as the possibility of recovery from the cancer illness. Two domains (sub-components of the theme) emerged within the confidence theme: enhancement of the patient's coping abilities and a message of acceptance of the patient as a person during their illness experience. Use of ethnographic methods for this type of study was most appropriate and provided the researcher with an opportunity to construct culturally relevant knowledge.

Phenomenology: a search for meaning

Phenomenologists study situations in the everyday world from the viewpoint of the experiencing person. In contrast to the emphasis on culture that is characteristic of ethnographers, phenomenology emphasizes the individual's construction of 'life-world'.[10] The life-world includes taken-for-granted assumptions about everyday life, such as what clothes should be worn, the way to greet someone who is dying, and how to manage embarrassing moments during personal care. The aim is to determine the meaning of an experience for the people who have had the experience and are able to provide a comprehensive description of it. Further, use of phenomenology specifies that people's actions should be explained with reference to their conscious intentions, and with references to the types or categories of understandings that people develop.

Tarzian[11] used phenomenology to study nurses' experiences of caring for dying patients who have 'air hunger'. Ten hospice, long-term care, oncology, or emergency medicine nurses who cared for air-hungry dying patients were recruited. Interviews with two family members who witnessed their dying spouses suffer from air hunger were also used to complement the nurses' accounts. Three themes were identified and provided a framework for a new vision of 'doing everything' for a dying person who suffers from air hunger. These themes included *the patient's look—panic* that beckoned them to respond, a sense of *surrendering and sharing control*, and *fine-tuning dying*. Nurses described ways they responded to relieve a patient's air hunger, including being prepared before air hunger occurs, calming patients and families, medicating patients, improvising care, attending to family members' needs, and drawing distinctions between palliating and killing. When air hunger occurs in people who are close to death, it often triggers increasing panic and breathlessness. As one home hospice nurse stated, 'He died with his eyes wide open, just gasping for breath, clearly panicked. And I just felt so bad for his wife and daughter who were at his bedside. And I felt after that, I don't ever want this to happen again to anybody' [11, p.2].

This study focused on a research question that has previously been only tangentially addressed in prior empirical work. Use of the phenomenological approach allowed the researcher to undertake this inquiry in a sensitive, systematic, and in-depth manner that resulted in articulation of new knowledge.

Grounded theory: what is the process?

Grounded theory methods are based upon the argument that theory can be built up through careful observation of the social world. A grounded theory is one that is inductively derived from the study of the phenomenon it represents. That is, it is discovered, developed, and provisionally verified through systematic data collection and analysis of data pertaining to that phenomenon.[12] The methods have their roots in symbolic interactionism. Symbolic interactionism is an analytic framework that argues that human beings construct action on the basis of the meanings of the objects they encounter. This research tradition studies the importance of meanings and symptoms to help understand human behaviour. Symbolic interactionists examine how people make sense of their experiences through a common set of symbols, emphasizing that these symbols are developed and find meaning through shared interactions. Through a process of role-taking, a person imagines how they themselves appear to others, thus becoming a symbolic object to them.

At the heart of grounded theory are two specific techniques, theoretical sampling and thematic analysis. Theoretical sampling involves a process where the representativeness of concepts, not representativeness of persons, is crucial. The aim is not simply to generalize the findings to the broader population, but to construct a theoretical explanation by specifying the conditions and processes that give rise to variations in a phenomenon. The units of analysis are concepts. Thematic analysis is used and involves a process of coding, sorting, and organizing data.

Davies[13] used grounded theory methods to examine the long-term outcomes of adolescent sibling bereavement. She conducted a series of intensive, semi-structured interviews with 12 adults who, in their early adolescence, lost a sibling. This study resulted in the development of a theoretical scheme that captured the reactions and consequences of this experience. Long-term outcomes included psychological growth, a sense of feeling different, and withdrawal from peers. Sibling who withdrew from their peers at a time when peer relationships are critical to completing developmental tasks suffered long-term feelings of sadness and loneliness.

Use of grounded theory methods was appropriate for this study question as it allowed the researcher to identify a psychosocial process, describe and theorize about the meaning and response to a traumatic life event that occurs within a complex social and developmental context. The techniques used by Davies, the reporting methods documented, and the contributions of this work to understanding long-term effects of adolescent bereavement are notable and could not have been achieved using other research methods.

These are only three of the more commonly reported methodologies in qualitative research that may be helpful in addressing research questions in the area of palliative care. Additional literature that describes these methods in greater depth or other types of qualitative methods (e.g. participatory action research, feminist analysis, critical theory, narrative analysis) is referenced [4,13–16] Although presented as separate methods, there can be overlap among methods. Research *rigor* but not rigidity is required. These terms are not synonymous when applied to qualitative research.

Trustworthiness in qualitative research

The terms reliability and validity used to evaluate quantitative research methods are not appropriate for evaluating the trustworthiness of qualitative research. The five criteria that are used to ensure that the qualitative research process is followed and emerging findings are trustworthy are: *credibility, transferability, dependability, confirmability,* and *authenticity.*[17–25]

Credibility is enhanced when researchers describe and document their experience as researchers. Self-reflection on the part of the researcher is an essential feature of qualitative research. A field journal is kept in which the content and process of interactions are noted, including reactions to various events. The journal becomes a record to these relationships and provides material for reflection. It is also considered to be one source of data that can be used to audit the study. A second way of establishing credibility is by consulting study participants themselves if feasible, and asking them to read and discuss the construction derived from the data analysis. Does it ring true to them? If reading is too burdensome for the individual but is of interest to them, then this can be done verbally. The technique is referred to as member checking.

Transferability refers to the extent to which the findings from a study might be applied to another situation. Transferability is dependent upon the degree of similarity or 'fit' between the two situations or contexts.[19] A study meets the criterion of 'fittingness' when its findings can 'fit' into contexts outside the study situation and when its audience views the findings as meaningful and applicable in terms of their own experiences.[21] In order for this to be possible, the original context must have been described adequately so that a reader can make a judgement regarding transferability.

Dependability refers to the consistency of the data. Auditability is the criterion for rigor when dealing with the consistency of data. A study and its findings can be audited when another researcher can clearly follow the decision trail used by the investigator in

the study. In addition, another researcher should arrive at the same or comparable, but not contradictory, conclusions given the researcher's data, perspective, and situation.[21]

Confirmability is concerned with assuring that data, interpretations, and outcome inquires are rooted in contexts and data collected from the study participants (subjects). Confirmability requires that the researcher clearly show the process by which interpretations of the data or study findings has been reached.[22] This requires that data can be tracked to their sources, and that the logic used to assemble the interpretations is both explicit and implicit in the narrative or case study. Both the raw products and the processes used to compress them must be available to be inspected and confirmed by an outside reviewer of the study. This data or 'paper trail' is used by study auditors.

Authenticity is the fifth criterion to evaluate the rigor of qualitative research. [23] Authenticity is demonstrated if researchers can show that they have represented a range of different realities.

Several *processes* are used to enhance trustworthiness in qualitative research studies including the use of triangulation, an audit trail, peer debriefing, prolonged engagement, member checking, and techniques to enhance reflexivity. Each of these processes is described in Table 7.4.2 as well as the methodological challenges when applied to a palliative care population.

Research challenges

Palliative care research can be especially challenging given the vulnerability of the populations to be studied, the quickly changing nature of the patient's illness, and the complexities of the phenomena to be studied. And yet, qualitative research, because of its inherent flexibility, is perhaps the approach best suited to study the needs of this population. Three particular issues that merit discussion from the perspective of qualitative methods are outlined here: methodological challenges, the range of palliative care populations to be studied, and medical and social complexities of palliative care.

Methodological challenges

Clinicians and researchers who embark upon palliative care research do so in a field that is fraught with challenges. Participant dying patients may have unpredictable illness trajectories that make longitudinal studies extremely difficult. They are frequently distressed by multiple symptoms and cognitive impairment associated with both general organ failure and the numerous medications used to relieve symptoms. Family members are also under pressure from changes in family dynamics, preparatory grief, and a desire to protect their loved one from any added burden. Health-care professionals have complex workloads, not only in the care of patients and families but also in the building and maintenance of their teams. They in turn may be protective towards adding any additional burden to 'their' patients. In addition, difficulty in recruitment and high rates of participant (subject) attrition can be very discouraging to the researcher.[26,27]

These challenges present opportunities for the use of qualitative methods, which can circumvent some of the difficulties described. For example, use of a qualitative design can allow the researcher to examine variations within an illness trajectory more closely. A more personal and flexible approach afforded by qualitative methods can facilitate patient participation and decrease the magnitude of attrition. Use of qualitative techniques can elicit

Table 7.4.2 Processes, definitions, and approaches to enhancing trustworthiness in qualitative studies.

Processes	Definitions	Approaches/variations	Methodological challenges in relation to palliative care
Triangulation	Use of multiple methods within one study[13]	Data triangulation	Patients and family members may have difficulty participating if multiple methods are used due to fatigue
		Investigator triangulation	
		Theory triangulation	
		Methods triangulation	
Prolonged engagement and persistent observation	Sufficient involvement must occur to ensure that data collected are relevant and complete[21]	Extended time in the field	Persistent observation may be difficult because of unpredictable illness trajectories and changes in cognitive status of patients
		Repeated visits to data collection site/participants	
		Rapport of researcher in study context	
Peer debriefing	Practice of involving a peer at various steps of the research process, especially in analysis phase[21]	Multiple researchers for data collection and coding	Researcher(s) may have limited access to colleagues who can serve as research peers. Palliative care clinicians may be available, but may not be able to serve in this role because of confidentiality requirements of research
		Peer-review panels to discuss challenge data collection steps, analysis process, and researchers' reflections	
Member-checking	Verification with participants that what they said has been interpreted with the meaning they ascribed[17]	Formal	Patient's cognitive status changes or meaning of the experience changes over time making member-checking unsuitable. Patients may die before member checks occur
		Informal	
		Individuals	
		Groups	
		Intermittent or final	
Audit trails	Process of research is documented in a way that can be tracked[22]	Maintenance of audit trail notes, decision points, and coding notes	Usually feasible. Volume of detailed, complex notes must be well organized for management of data analysis
Reflexivity techniques	Ways investigators use to document personal reflections on the research process, which are used in the analysis enhance transparency and construction of meanings[23]	Field notes	Usually feasible. Time consuming and emotionally demanding given the type of research undertaken and the sensitive nature of the work; however, is essential due to the above
		Journals	
		Memos	

information that would not otherwise be retrieved through surveys or paper-and-pencil questionnaires and can provide the basis for development of instruments that are more precise and appropriate for use in palliative care. And importantly, qualitative research methods allow the patient and family participants to 'give voice' to what is happening to them—they are the experts.

Use of qualitative methods, however, also present practical challenges of how to manage large amounts of complex data and the need to master qualitative data management systems (e.g. NU. DIST, IN.VITRO). These data management software programs are particularly helpful in handling large amounts of data, quickly confirming coding decisions, facilitating re-coding of data, and enhancing the transparency of the data coding and analysis process. However, time must be allowed to learn how to use these software packages so that they serve as a useful tool. It is also important to remember that these packages are only meant to manage the data; the analysis still remains the intellectual responsibility of the researcher.

It may be also difficult for qualitative researchers to know how to reduce the rich, in-depth stories that they hear from patients into categories and themes in such a way that retains the poignancy and context of the patient's experience. The intellectual prowess required to hold detail, context, variations, and similarities in one's mind at the same time whilst reviewing and analysing the data cannot be over-stated. The qualitative analysis process might be likened to the action of a high-powered camera lens. The researcher must be able to move close to the data (zoom in) and then move back to the broader context (pan the scene) with flexibility, consistency, and clarity. This analytic technique is a particular skill required for high-quality qualitative research, which may be particularly challenging to learn without experienced research consultation.

The qualitative researcher must also be alert to a potential blurring of boundaries between research and therapy. This can be particularly difficult for clinician researchers. The intent of the qualitative research interview process is not to develop a therapeutic relationship with the patient or problem-solving therapy for the patient. The intent is to describe a phenomenon or experience that the patient is fully informed of for the purpose of the research. This is not to say that participation in a qualitative interview may not be 'therapeutic'. Many participants describe the research interview as 'invigorating' and helpful. However, the primary aim of qualitative research interviews it not to offer therapy. This distinction has important ethical and methodological implications that the researcher must bear in mind. A researcher, who identifies that the participant may be requiring therapeutic support, must be alert to the need for referral (with the participant's permission) to clinicians or health professionals who may offer this assistance. Clinical researchers need to distinguish their clinical role from their research role. The line between the two can easily become blurred.

Institutional Review Board challenges

Institutional Review Boards (IRBs) may present a particular challenge to qualitative researchers because of their unfamiliarity with the philosophical underpinnings, language, and methods of this research paradigm. Quantitative research methods have long been viewed as the hall mark of evidence based medicine. IRBs are very familiar with reviewing such protocols and with the language and techniques used. Qualitative research studies, however, are still finding their place in the world of evidence-based medicine. If qualitative research techniques are new within an institution it is important that a mechanism is set in place to education IRB members on qualitative research and on how to evaluate these studies for rigor and worthiness.

Range of palliative care populations

Palliative care populations reach far beyond individuals living with cancer and their families. The needs of those with non-cancer diagnosis, elderly patients receiving care in aged care facilities, and those receiving other approaches to care (e.g. acute care, alternative therapies) in parallel with palliative care may be best studied using qualitative methods. Individuals from non-dominant cultural groups, those in lower socioeconomic groups, children requiring palliative care support, and those in rural and remote communities might all benefit from qualitative research approaches.

Individuals with non-cancer diagnoses

Palliative care research is important for patients with neurodegenerative disorders, those with end-stage cardiac or renal failure, persons living with AIDS, and children with various health conditions. To date, few studies have been undertaken to examine the palliative care needs of these populations. Use of phenomenology to understand the meaning of these illness trajectories or studies employing grounded theory techniques may reveal useful social and psychosocial processes relevant to palliative care of these groups.

Elderly individuals

Predictions for the year 2025 confirm an ageing population, with more people worldwide dying from chronic or progressive illnesses rather than acute conditions.[28] Therefore, it is quite imaginable that an array of palliative care services will be required to meet the range of needs of individuals who might benefit from palliative care. To date, little empirical work has been reported on the palliative care needs of the elderly. Qualitative methods may help to elucidate care processes, expressions of symptomatology, and issues of family caring that are unique to this population.

Individuals receiving palliative care concurrently with other types of services

Palliative care services function both integral with and adjacent to existing health-care services. Continuity of care and communication among these care systems is essential to ensure that services are coordinated and well sequenced. This interface requires that research methods and approaches take into consideration patient care needs at earlier phases of an illness trajectory or the needs of patients who may be receiving concurrent active treatments. Qualitative methods may be helpful in examining these types of interactions, illness journeys, and treatment narratives. These approaches may elucidate hypotheses or theoretical postulates concerning the effects of earlier phases of an illness on palliative care. Although health professionals may easily discern differences between palliative care and acute care treatment, patients and families may not make this distinction as crisply. Therefore, 'following' patients from one type of care service/setting to another may be helpful in understanding questions about the transition to palliative care, the history of symptomatology, and the meaning of illness experiences.

Individuals from non-dominant cultural and lower socioeconomic groups

There is also evidence that individuals in minority groups are under-served by current palliative care models. There has been little research undertaken to understand the health and caring perspectives of different cultural groups. Yet, there is a pressing need for this type of empirically-based knowledge, because cultural responses to death and dying may take on increased importance once the biomedical interventions have failed to cure. It is often at this stage of illness that patients and families turn to more culturally familiar and comforting beliefs and practices. Some reports also indicate that patients in socially deprived areas have limited access to palliative care. A family's social and cultural background may influence relationship with health-care professionals, their trust of the health-care system, access to care, and the carer roles assumed. It is clear that ethnographic methods may offer particular advantages in addressing these types of research questions, providing knowledge that takes into account the social and cultural context and meanings of illness from these perspectives.

Paediatric patients

The development of palliative care services for adults has not been paralleled in paediatrics.[29] It is not that death is less common amongst children than adults. The dying child until recently has been avoided in the literature and in practice, perhaps for emotionally charged reasons. According to Frager,[30] the provision of paediatric palliative care is patchy and inconsistent. One of the reasons may be that many of the diseases are rare and the children suffering from these diseases are distributed over a broad geographic area. Most deaths are due to uncontrollable malignant disease following unsuccessful attempts at curative treatment, and although cure rates for cancer have increased markedly in recent years, nearly one-third of childhood malignancies result in death. However, paediatric palliative care needs extend beyond cancer diagnoses and may be appropriate for a range of progressive, life-threatening illnesses (e.g. neurodegenerative and metabolic disorders, organ failure).

Qualitative methods allow investigations with smaller populations such as the paediatric population, and may provide a useful foundation for examining sensitive topics with these vulnerable patients. The methods of qualitative research are generally less intrusive (e.g. participant observation, play interviews, use of drawings) and are more context sensitive than many quantitative methods, allowing ethically sound and developmentally appropriate approaches to paediatric research.

Individuals in rural and remote communities

Health-care providers in rural and remote communities confront additional challenges associated with delivery of palliative care. They must serve as 'advanced generalists' to a wide range of patients with various health concerns with the expectation that they are able to respond equally well to these problems. Difficulties of isolation, lack of resources, and added emotional pressures associated with long-term patient–health professional relationships may challenge care providers further. The need for responsive models of palliative care appropriate to the needs of these communities is pressing. However, the issue of sample size and geographic dispersion can again be difficult. It is also important that the interventions tested and approaches to care evaluated are appropriate to the community and the social context in which they will be applied. In many instances, use of qualitative methods (e.g. ethnography, action research, grounded theory methods) are particularly useful in obtaining relevant data from a rural community and ensuring that the results obtained will be positively received and implemented.

Ethical research issues specific to the field

Palliative care research usually involves vulnerable patients, family members, and health-care professionals. The vulnerability of patients and families in palliative care settings may mean that quantitative methods using batteries of data collection tools are unsuitable.

Qualitative research approaches may in these situations be ideal methods for providing rich insights into what might otherwise be hidden areas of practice. However, patients may sometimes feel obligated to participate in research, as gratitude for the care they are receiving. Therefore, palliative care researchers (regardless of the methods chosen) must take special precautions to ensure that some distance is created in the research process between participants and their carers, to ensure that participants are not dependent on care from the researchers. Researchers must also ensure that consenting procedures are clear, open, and honest in their assessment of benefit to the patient. Participants must also be given clear opportunities to withdraw from the project. Often, this requires the researcher to be especially sensitive to signs from potential participants that they do not wish to be involved any more. Therefore, consenting procedures should be dynamic, in this way, so that there is a process of revisiting consent and renegotiation of participation.

There are also a number of consistent reports that indicate that patients and family carers who participate in qualitative studies do not report feeling burdened from their involvement. In contrast, they report feeling affirmed by the opportunity to contribute their experiences to others, may see their involvement as a type of testimony and last contribution that they offer the wider community, and may gain insights from having an opportunity to reflect on their experiences. Some participants report feeling invigorated by this participation. It seems important, therefore, to consider the potential positive benefits that occur through use of qualitative research in a palliative care context.

Summary

Qualitative research is an area of basic scientific inquiry, the fundamental description of mechanisms, processes, structures, and phenomenon. This type of basic research is needed in the area of palliative care to—among other things—help us understand what it is like to be terminally ill, what it is like for our families and friends, what we need to help us incorporate this last phase of life into our whole life's story, and what we need society and the health care system to provide for us. Qualitative methods include an ability to examine situations in depth with open-ended questions and the capacity to explore complex questions. The research approach is flexible enough for application to a wide range of palliative care patients.

Quantitative and qualitative researchers are beginning to learn each others language and to collaborate in studies. The Institutional Review Boards, long exposed to the quantitative research paradigm, are beginning to recognize the relevance of qualitative research to palliative care. Research funding for qualitative research is becoming more available and mainstream peer-reviewed journals are beginning at least to consider well done qualitative research for publication.

We conclude the chapter with a study by Yedida and MacGregor[31] to illustrate the potential for depth and breadth in qualitative research. This ethnographic study was designed to identify dominant themes characterizing patients' perspectives on death during the last months of life. The seven motifs they identified that characterized these perspectives were: struggle (living and dying are difficult), dissonance (dying is not living), endurance (triumph of inner strength), coping (finding a new balance), incorporation (belief system accommodates death), quest (seeking meaning kin death), and volatile (unresolved and unresigned). Yedidia and MacGregor found that the patients ($n = 30$, with a mean of 4.2 interviews per patient) showed a strong capacity for coherence, integrating their responses to dying with broader motifs in their life stories. The richness of this type of data and its implications for palliative care are only possible to elicit through a qualitative research approach.

References

1. Cohen, S.R., and Mount, B.M. (1992). Quality of life in terminal illness: defining and measuring subjective well-being in the dying. *Journal of Palliative Medicine*, **8**, 40–5.

2. Berglund, C.A. (eds.) (2001). *Health research*. Oxford University Press, South Melbourne.

3. Kuhn, T. (1970). *The structure of scientific revolutions*. University of Chicago Press, Chicago.

4. Rice, P.L., and Ezzy, D. (1999). *Qualitative research methods: a health focus*. Oxford University Press, South Melbourne.

5. LeCompte, M., and Preissle, J. (1993). *Ethnography and qualitative design in educational research*, 2nd edition. Academic Press Inc., San Diego.

6. Creswell, J.W. (2003). *Research design: qualitative, quantitative and mixed methods approaches*, 2nd edition. Sage Publications, London.

7. Morales, E. (1994). Meaning of touch to hospitalised Puerto Ricans with cancer. *Cancer Nursing*, **17**, 464–9.

8. Spradley, J.P. (1980). *Participant observation*. Holt, Rinchart & Winston, New York.

9. Gillis, A., and Jackson, W. (2002). *Research for nurses: methods and interpretation*. FA Davis Company, Philadelphia.

10. van Manen, M. (1990). *Researching lined experience: human science for an action sensitive pedagogy*. State University of New York, New York, pp. 30–3.

11. Tarzian, A.J. (2000). Caring for dying patients who have air hunger. *Journal of Nursing Scholarship*, **32,** 137–43.

12. Strauss, A. and Corbin, J. (1990). *Basics of qualitative research: grounded theory procedures and techniques*. Sage Publications Inc., Newbury Park.

13. Davies, B. (1991). Long-term outcomes of adolescent sibling bereavement. *Journal of Adolescent Research*, **6,** 83–96.

14. Clough, P. (1994). *Feminist thought*. Blackwell, Oxford.

15. Denzin, N. and Lincoln, Y. (eds.) (2000). *Handbook of qualitative research*. Sage Publications, Thousand Oaks.

16. Whyte, W.F. (eds.) (1991). *Participatory action research*. Sage Publications, Newbury Park.

17. Miles, M.B., and Huberman, A.M. (1994). Data management and analysis methods. In *Handbook of qualitative research* (eds. N. Denzin and Y. Lincoln), pp. 428–44. Thousand Oaks: Sage Publications.

18. Guba, E.G. and Lincoln, Y.S. (1981). *Naturalistic inquiry*. Sage, Beverly Hills.

19. Guba, E.G. and Lincoln, Y.S. (1989). *Fourth generation evaluation*. Sage Publications, Newbury Park.

20. Lincoln, Y.S. and Guba, E.G. (1985). *Naturalistic inquiry*. Sage, Beverly Hills.

21. Sandelowski, M. (1986). The problem of rigor in qualitative research. *Advances in Nursing Science, **8,** 27.

22. Koch, T. (1994). Establishing rigour in qualitative research: the decision trail. *Journal of Advanced Nursing, **19,** 976–86.

23. Guba, E.G. and Lincoln, Y.S. (1994). Competing paradigms in qualitative research. In *Handbook of qualitative research* (eds. N. Denzin and Y. Linkcon), pp. 105–17. Sage Publications, Thousand Oaks.

24. Silverman, M., Ricci, E., and Gunter, M. (1990). Strategies for increasing the rigor of qualitative methods in evaluation of health care programs. *Evaluation Review, **14,** 57–74.

25. Grbich, C. (1999). *Qualitative research in health: an introduction*. Allen & Unwin, St Leonards NSW.

26. Bruera, E. (1994). Ethical issues in palliative care research. *Journal of Palliative Care, **10,** 7–9.

27. Kristjanson, L.J., Hanson, E.J., and Balneaves, L.G. (1994). Research with palliative care populations: ethical issues. *Journal of Palliative Care, **10,** 10–15.

28. Davis, R., Wagner, E.H., and Groves, T. (1999). Managing chronic disease. *British Medical Journal, **318,** 1090–1.

29. Institute of Medicine (2003). *When children die: improving palliative and end-of-life care for children and their families*. The National Academies Press, Washington D.C.

30. Frager, G. (1996). Pediatric palliative care: building the model, bridging the gaps. *Journal of Palliative Care, **12,** 9–12.

31. Yedida, M. and MacGregor, B. (2001). Confronting the prospect of dying: reports of terminally ill patients. *Journal of Pain and Symptom Management, **22**(4), 807–19.

7.5

Research into psychosocial issues

David W. Kissane, Annette F. Street, and Erin Schweers Cornelius

Psychosocial research needs to be conducted in accordance with the core values and principles of palliative care. Patient- and family-centred care acknowledges the unique experience of each person and their family members. Key values include respect for the dignity of all, advocacy on behalf of their expressed wishes, and equity in access to services. In response, psychosocial researchers seek not only the most effective interventions, but are also concerned with the meaning such treatments have for patient and family. To do so, psychosocial researchers increasingly create multi-disciplinary teams and draw on a variety of methods.

In this chapter, we want to highlight the scope of psychosocial questions and interests by drawing on a number of different methods that have formed the basis of psychosocial research. In doing so, we have made choices. Detailed explanations of relevant methods are covered in detail in other chapters in this section on research. We highlight formative and current research, delineate the problems involved in conducting research with dying people, and make some suggestions about where future psychosocial research should be directed. A feature of the chapter is a section analysing the various instruments in use in psychosocial research. Sometimes, researchers are unaware of the potential range of validated questionnaires that can aid psychosocial research. Similarly, we have analysed a range of computer-assisted qualitative analysis programs. This chapter will serve as a most useful resource.

The scope of psychosocial research in palliative medicine

Research activity can be grouped into broad domains or themes of inquiry. Many interesting questions and controversies arise in each domain. These are listed in Box 7.5.1.

The choice of research issue is commonly determined by awareness of unmet needs, concern about the standard of care, or a desire to improve the outcomes of treatment. We illustrate pertinent issues about a number of these domains and useful methods for addressing them and return to the challenges for the future at the end of this chapter.

Literature review and meta-analysis

A comprehensive literature review is a *sine qua non* as many ideas have been considered before. Exploring the boundaries of knowledge necessitates firstly identifying what is known, what aspects remain unclear, and thinking through where the benefits of further study will lie. A formal literature search is thus crucial before the hypothesis is generated or aims and objectives of the study are delineated.

While the history of any construct and its application is of interest, the recent emphasis on a clinical approach that is evidence-based (see Chapter 7.2) requires a systematic approach to any literature review. Recently, more systematic reviews of psychosocial palliative care topics have been conducted. Systematic reviews have explored the effects of multi-disciplinary palliative care teams,[1,2] the level of need for palliative care,[3] and effective

---

Box 7.5.1 Domains of psychosocial research in palliative medicine

- Communication studies: breaking bad news and discussing prognosis and dying
- Coping and adaptation to change
- Cultural issues including those of indigenous peoples
- Dying process
- Ethics of end-of-life care
- Family studies: carers and family support
- Grief and bereavement
- Interventions: psychotherapy, pharmacological and physical
- Lived experience of illness: impact on self, the body, dignity, and burden on others
- Paediatric aspects of adaptation, coping, and care
- Psychiatric disorders: anxiety, depression, delirium, etc.
- Quality of life
- Sexuality and intimacy
- Social issues: relationships, recreation, work, and living arrangements
- Suffering, existential and spiritual distress
- Satisfaction with care

Table 7.5.1 Instruments measuring *anxiety* and *fear*.

Instrument name	Item number (response style)	Factor structure	Reliability	Validity	Comments on utility
Beck Anxiety Inventory (BAI)[6]	21 items (4-point scale)	1. Somatic 2. Panic symptoms	$\alpha = 0.92$; test–retest = 0.75	$r = 0.51$ (HAM-A)	Designed to assess anxiety in a clinical population.
Death Anxiety Scale (DAS)[7]	15 items (true/false)	1 factor	$\alpha = 0.76$; test–retest = 0.83	Well-validated	Designed to assess preoccupation with and anxiety about death.
Hamilton Anxiety Rating Scale (HAM-A)[8]	14 items (5-point scale)	1. Psychic anxiety 2. Somatic anxiety	$\alpha = 0.79–0.86$	$r = 0.56$ (BAI)	Clinician-administered measure designed to assess global anxiety.
Hospital Anxiety and Depression Scale (HADS)[9]	14 items (4-point scale)	1. Anxiety 2. Depression	$\alpha = 0.89$; test–retest $r = 0.74$	Well-validated	Designed as a rapid assessment tool in a non-psychiatric setting.
State Trait Anxiety Inventory (STAI)[10]	40 items (4-point scale)	1. State 2. Trait	$\alpha = 0.83–0.92$ on subscales	Well-validated	Designed to assess how subjects respond to psychological stress. STAI-Y (revised) available.

methods of information giving to cancer patients.[4] Meta-synthesis of qualitative studies can also inform understanding of patient experiences.[5]

Concept and construct development

The building up of a theory provides a conceptual framework on which further observations can be based and ultimately delivers an empirical basis for the development of interventions. The qualitative approach to concept development begins in grounded theory, while quantitative methodology creates instruments to measure constructs, which in turn need to be carefully validated and demonstrated to have reliability for recurrent use.

Instrument development

The commonly used rating scales used in psychosocial research in palliative medicine have been summarized in Tables 7.5.1–7.5.15. Instruments that measure distress, mood states, coping, quality of life, support, and family functioning tend to be well validated, while measures of spirituality, dignity, and existential domains warrant further work.

Rating scales can be used for screening, diagnosis, and measurement of severity and change—attention needs to be paid to the purpose for which any instrument was designed and its reliability and validity in that role. In choosing an instrument, the researcher needs to consider what they seek to measure and for what purpose. For instance, sensitivity of scales to detect small changes will vary, sometimes at the expense of specificity, and the scales' practicality and brevity will often be important when considered for use with palliative patients.

Grounded theory studies (see Chapter 7.4) have provided understanding of psychosocial concerns such as 'enduring', 'uncertainty', 'suffering', and 'hope', and then examining their interrelationships[78] or exploring how decision-making occurs at the end of life for family caregivers and health-care providers in long-term-care settings.[79]

Table 7.5.2 Instruments measuring *depression*.

Instrument name	Item number (response style)	Factor structure	Reliability	Validity	Comments on utility
Beck Depression inventory (BDI)[11]	21 items (4-point scale)	1. Cognitions 2. Somatic symptoms	$\alpha = 0.81$	$r = 0.62–0.66$ with clinician ratings	Designed to assess depressive symptoms. BDI-II and BDI-SF available.
Brief Case Find for Depression[12]	4 items		Sensitivity = 67%; Specificity = 75%	Satisfactory	Designed to screen for depression in medical patients.
Geriatric Depression Scale (GDS)[13]	30 items (yes/no)		$\alpha = 0.94$	$r = 0.84$ (Zung SDS) and 0.83 (HAM-D)	Designed to assess depression in a geriatric population. GDS-15 and GDS-5 available.
Patient Health Questionnaire (PHQ-9)[14]	9 items (4-point scale)		$\alpha = 0.86$	$r = 0.73$ (BDI); $r = 0.59$ (GHQ12)	Designed to assess depression. Self-report subscale of PRIME-MD.
Brief Zung Self Rating Scale for Depression[15]	11 items (4-point scale)	1 factor	$\alpha = 0.84$	$r = 0.92$ (SRS-D)	Designed to assess depression in the medically ill (eliminates somatic symptoms).

Table 7.5.3 Instruments measuring *distress*.

Instrument name	Item number (response style)	Factor structure	Reliability	Validity	Comments on utility
Brief Symptom Inventory[16]	18 items (5-point scale)	1. Anxiety 2. Depression 3. Somatization	$\alpha = 0.89$	$r = 0.84$ (GSI of BSI)	Designed to assess symptoms of distress. 53-item BSI available.
Distress Thermometer (DT)[17]	1 VAS + 34 items (yes/no)	Domains related to distress can be endorsed.	Sensitivity = 84%; Specificity = 61%	Well-validated in cancer studies	Designed for rapid assessment of patient distress. New variation uses an additional impact thermometer.[18]
General Health Questionnaire (GHQ 12)[19]	12 items (4-point scale)	1 factor	Split-half = 0.95	Well-validated	Designed as a distress screening measure. GHQ28 and GHQ60 available.
Impact of Events Scale Revised (IES-R)[20]	22 items (5-point scale)	1. Intrusion 2. Avoidance 3. Hyperarousal	$\alpha = 0.79{-}0.90$	$r = 0.84$ (PCL-C)	Designed to assess subjective distress and intrusive thoughts. IES available.

Cohort and longitudinal studies

Observational studies may be either retrospective or prospective. In the former, past events are studied through case notes or by interview. They may be limited by incomplete recording or biased recall, but are inexpensive and serve as a useful beginning. In contrast, prospective studies eliminate the bias of memory and permit examination of a number of associations, but may be limited by the availability of suitable subjects for recruitment within a reasonable time frame. In addition, subjects may be lost to follow-up.

Cross-sectional studies

Cross-sectional studies are both observational and descriptive, typically being used to measure the prevalence of a symptom or illness. They can be further used to identify clinical associations, well exemplified by the study of the 'desire for death' by Chochinov and colleagues in 200 Canadian hospice inpatients, which was found to be genuine and persistent in 8.5 percent and significantly associated with depressive disorder, isolation from family, and pain.[80]

Case–control studies

The case–control study is used generally to test an aetiological hypothesis, by comparing a group with a disease or specific treatment, matched with controls. The methodological challenge is in the selection criteria for the cases to ensure that they are a representative sample and similarly the variables on which matching is achieved, and whether this is by random community selection or paired match. For instance, studies of men with prostate cancer have shown global quality of life to be equivalent to community samples of similarly aged men, but urinary incontinence, impotence, and bowel symptoms to be causally related to the treatments these men have received.[81]

Cohort studies

Cohort studies are both observational and analytical in prospectively following groups of patients with key differences to assess outcome. They provide valuable information on the nature of a relationship and whether there is a causal association. Thus, the King's College cohort of women with breast cancer was followed across 15 years of illness to determine the influence of coping style on survival.[82] Women who were fatalistic, overly anxious, or hopeless/helpless in their cognitions died earlier than those using positive avoidance or fighting spirit. Time available for follow-up is an obvious limitation in palliative medicine.

Clinical case reports

Clinical reports of individual patients have always served an important function in highlighting relevant issues of presentation, diagnosis,

Table 7.5.4 Instruments measuring *pain* and *symptom management*.

Instrument name	Item number (response style)	Factor structure	Reliability	Validity	Comments on utility
Brief Pain Inventory	23 items (11-point scale)	1. Severity 2. Interference	$\alpha = 0.95$	$r = 0.71$ (VAS)	Brief measure of pain. Short form available.
Brief Pain Inventory for Ambulatory Care[21]	5 items (4-point scale)		$\alpha = 0.87{-}0.92$	$r = 0.65$ (EORTC pain)	Designed to assess pain intensity, impact, and medication doses.
Edmonton Symptom Assessment System (ESAS)[22]	9 items (11-point scale)		Satisfactory	Well-validated	Designed to assess symptoms in palliative care patients.
Memorial Symptom Assessment Scale (MSAS)[23]	32 items (4-point and 5-point scales)	1. Psychological 2. Physical	$\alpha = 0.58{-}0.88$	Well-validated	Designed to assess cancer related symptoms. MSAS-SF available.

Table 7.5.5 Instruments measuring *suffering*, *existential*, and *spiritual issues*.

Instrument name	Item number (response style)	Factor structure	Reliability	Validity	Comments on utility
Demoralization Scale (DS)[24]	24 items (5-point scale)	1. Loss of meaning 2. Dysphoria 3. Disheartenment 4. Helplessness 5. Sense of failure	$\alpha = 0.94$; 0.71–0.89 on subscales	Good concurrent validity	Designed to assess existential distress in palliative care patients.
Functional Assessment of Chronic Illness Therapy-Spiritual (FACIT-Sp)[25]	12 items (5-point scale)	1. Meaning 2. Faith	$\alpha = 0.81$–0.88	$r = -0.54$ (POMS)	Designed to assess spiritual well-being in the general population. Expanded version available.
Meaning in Life Scale[26]	15 items (5-point scale)		$\alpha = 0.78$	$r = 0.53$ (PIL)	Designed to assess sense of purpose and beliefs of hospice patients.
Posttraumatic Growth Inventory (PTGI)[27]	21 items (6-point scale)	1. Relating 2. New possibility 3. Strength 4. Spiritual 5. Appreciation	$\alpha = 0.90$	$r = 0.23$ (LOT) and $r = 0.50$ (religious participation)	Designed to assess perceived positive outcomes from traumatic events.
Sense of Coherence/ Orientation to Life[28]	29 items (7-point scale)	1 factor	$\alpha = 0.84$–0.93	$r = 0.39$ (Rotter's I-E)	Designed to assess sense of coherence/ meaningfulness.
Spiritual Involvement and Beliefs Scale[29]	26 items (5-point scale)	1. Ritual 2. Fluid 3. Existential 4. Humility	$\alpha = 0.92$	$r = 0.80$ (SWB)	Designed to assess spiritual beliefs across religions.
System of Beliefs Inventory (SBI-15)[30]	15 items (4-point scale)	1. Beliefs/practice 2. Social support	$\alpha = 0.93$	Well-validated	Designed to assess spiritual beliefs in medically ill patients.

Table 7.5.6 Instruments measuring *coping* and *adaptation*.

Instrument name	Item number (response style)	Factor structure	Reliability	Validity	Comments on utility
Brief COPE[31]	28 items (4-point scale)	1. Substance use 2. Religion 3. Humour 4. Disengagement 5. Support 6. Coping 7. Venting 8. Denial 9. Acceptance	$\alpha = 0.50$–0.90 on subscales	Well-validated	Designed to assess coping strategies of individuals. Original version available.
Life Orientation Test Revised (LOT-R)[32]	10 items (5-point scale)	1 factor	$\alpha = 0.78$; test–retest = 0.79 at 28 months	Well-validated	Designed to assess optimism.
Mini Mental Adjustment to Cancer (Mini-MAC)[33,34]	29 items (4-point scale)	1. Fighting spirit 2. Preoccupation 3. Fatalism 4. Help/hopeless 5. Avoidance	$\alpha = 0.62$–0.88 on subscales	Well-validated	Designed to assess responses to a cancer diagnosis.

Table 7.5.7 Instruments measuring *delirium*.

Instrument name	Item number (response style)	Factor structure	Reliability	Validity	Comments on utility
Confusion Assessment Method (CAM)[35]	9 items		Sensitivity = 94–100%; Specificity = 90–95%	$r = 0.82$ (VAS)	Designed to assess delirium.
Delirium Rating Scale (DRS)[36]	10 items	1 factor	$\alpha = 0.90$	$r = 0.66$ (Trailmaking)	Designed to clinically assess delirium.
Memorial Delirium Assessment Scale (MDAS)[37]	10 items (4-point scale)	1 factor	$\alpha = 0.91$	$r = 0.88$ (DRS)	Designed to assess medically ill patients for symptoms of delirium.
Mini Mental State Exam (MMSE)[38]	Interviewer administered		$\alpha = 0.82-0.84$	Well-validated	Designed as a quick standardized assessment of mental status.

Table 7.5.8 Instruments measuring *social issues*.

Instrument name	Item number (response style)	Factor structure	Reliability	Validity	Comments on utility
Bottomley Social Support Scale[39]	9 items (5-point scale)		$\alpha = 0.78$; test–retest = 0.73–0.79	$r = 0.38$ (DHD)	Designed to assess social support in cancer patients.
Duke-UNC Functional Social Support Scale[40]	8 items (5-point scale)	1. Confident 2. Affective	Test–retest = 0.66	Well-validated	Designed to assess perceived social support.
MOS Social Support Scale[41]	19 items (5-point scale)	1. Emotion/information 2. Tangible 3. Affectionate 4. Positive social interaction	$\alpha = 0.97$	$r = 0.67$ (loneliness)	Designed to assess the perceived availability of social support.
Multidimensional Scale of Perceived Social Support[42]	12 items (7-point scale)	1. Family 2. Friends 3. Significant others	$\alpha = 0.88$	Well-validated	Designed to assess the perceived availability of social support.
Short Sarason Social Support Questionnaire (SSSSQ)[43,44]	6 items (6-point scale)	1. Number 2. Satisfaction	$\alpha = 0.94-0.97$	$r = -0.52$ (loneliness)	Designed to assess the perceived availability of social support. Original version available.

Table 7.5.9 Instruments measuring *caregiving issues*.

Instrument name	Item number (response style)	Factor structure	Reliability	Validity	Comments on utility
Caregiver QOL Scale-Cancer[45]	35 items (5-point scale)	1. Burden 2. Disruptiveness 3. Positive adaptation 4. Financial concerns	$\alpha = 0.73-0.90$	$r = 0.49-0.65$ (SF36)	Designed to assess QOL of caregivers.
Caregiver Reaction Assessment (CRA)[46]	24 items (5-point scale)	1. Caregiver esteem 2. Family support 3. Finances 4. Schedule 5. Personal health	$\alpha = 0.80-0.90$ on subscales	Good construct validity (CESD, ADL)	Designed to assess reactions to caring for ill elderly patients.
Family Appraisal of Caregiving Questionnaire—Palliative Care (FACQ-PC)[47]	25 items (5-point scale)	1. Strain 2. Positive appraisals 3. Distress 4. Family well-being	$\alpha = 0.73-0.86$ on subscales	Well-validated (FRI)	Designed to assess caregivers' appraisal of the caregiving process.

Table 7.5.10 Instruments measuring *family issues.*

Instrument name	Item number (response style)	Factor structure	Reliability	Validity	Comments on utility
FAMCARE Scale[48]	20 items (5-point scale)	1. Information giving 2. Care availability 3. Psychosocial care 4. Physical care	$\alpha = 0.93$; test–retest = 0.91	$r = 0.77$–0.80 (McCusker Scale)	Designed to assess family satisfaction with advanced cancer care.
Family Crisis Oriented Personal Evaluation Scales (F-COPES)[49]	30 items (5-point scale)	1. Social support 2. Reframing 3. Spiritual support 4. Mobilizing family 5. Passive appraisal	$\alpha = 0.87$; 0.62–0.87 on subscales	Well-validated	Designed to assess family coping strategies in difficult situations.
Family Relationships Index[50]	12 items (true/false)	1. Cohesion 2. Expressiveness 3. Conflict	$\alpha = 0.56$–0.70 on subscales	Well-validated	Designed to assess family dysfunction. Subscale of the Family Environment Scale.

Table 7.5.11 Instruments measuring *paediatric aspects of advanced illness.*

Instrument name	Item number (response style)	Factor structure	Reliability	Validity	Comments on utility
Childhood Cancer Stressors Inventory[51]	18 items (true/false and 4-point scale)		$\alpha = 0.82$	$r = -0.63$ (CACI)	Designed to assess stressors in children with cancer.
Miami Pediatric Quality of Life Scale[52]	56 items (5-point scale)	1. Social competence 2. Emotional stability 3. Self competence	$\alpha = 0.89$	Good discriminant validity	Designed to assess QOL in children with cancer.
Multidimensional Anxiety Scale for Children (MASC)[53]	39 items (4-point scale)	1. Physical symptoms 2. Harm avoidance 3. Social anxiety 4. Separation anxiety	$\alpha = 0.90$; 0.74–0.85 on subscales	$r = 0.63$ (RCMAS)	Designed to assess paediatric anxiety.
Pediatric Cancer QOL Inventory (PCQL)[54]	32 items (4-point scale)	1. Disease 2. Physical 3. Psychological 4. Social 5. Cognitive	$\alpha = 0.91$ patient and 0.92 parent	Good convergent and discriminant validity	Designed to assess global QOL in paediatric cancer patients.
Pediatric Inventory for Parents (PIP)[55]	42 items (5-point scale)	1. Communication 2. Emotional functioning 3. Medical care 4. Role function	$\alpha = 0.80$–0.96	Good construct validity	Designed to assess parenting related stress in caring for an ill child.

Table 7.5.12 Instruments measuring *communication* and *satisfaction with care.*

Instrument name	Item number (response style)	Factor structure	Reliability	Validity	Comments on utility
Decisional Conflict Scale[56]	16 items (5-point scale)	1. Uncertainty about alternatives 2. Factors of uncertainty 3. Decision effectiveness	$\alpha = 0.78$–0.92; test–retest = 0.81	Well-validated	Designed to assess decisional uncertainty in patients facing a medical decision.
Decision Regret Scale[57]	5 items (5-point scale)	1 factor	$\alpha = 0.81$–0.92	Well-validated	Designed to assess decisional regret after making a medical decision.
Patient Satisfaction Index[58]	23 items (7-point scale)	1 factor	$\alpha = 0.94$; test–retest = 0.86	Well-validated	Designed to assess patient satisfaction with treatment.
Satisfaction with Decision Scale (SWDS)[59]	6 items (5-point scale)	1 factor	$\alpha = 0.85$	$r = -0.26$ (SF20)	Designed to assess patient satisfaction with medical decisions.

Table 7.5.13 Instruments measuring *sexuality* and *intimacy*.

Instrument name	Item number (response style)	Factor structure	Reliability	Validity	Comments on utility
Abbreviated Dyadic Adjustment Scale (ADAS)[60]	32 items (6-point scale)		$\alpha = 0.73–0.96$	Well-validated	Designed to assess the quality of marital relationships.
Changes in Sexual Function Questionnaire (CSFQ-14)[61]	14 items (5-point scale)	1. Pleasure 2. Frequency 3. Interest 4. Arousal 5. Orgasm	$\alpha = 0.89–0.90$	Good concurrent validity	Designed to assess change in sexual activity and satisfaction due to illness.
Female Sexual Function Index (FSFI)[62]	19 items (5-point and 6-point scales)	1. Desire 2. Lubrication 3. Orgasm 4. Satisfaction 5. Pain/discomfort	Test–retest = 0.79–0.80	Well-validated	Designed to assess sexual function in women.
International Index of Erectile Function (IIEF)[63]	15 items (5-point and 6-point scales)	1. Erectile function 2. Orgasmic function 3. Desire 4. Intercourse satisfaction 5. Overall satisfaction	$\alpha = 0.91$	Well-validated	Designed to assess erectile function in men with various medical conditions. IIEF-5 available.
Relationship Assessment Scale (RAS)[64]	7 items (5-point scale)		$\alpha = 0.86$	$r = 0.80$ (DAS)	Designed to assess relationship satisfaction in couples.

or management. One example was a series of patients who sought euthanasia under the Northern Territory of Australia's Rights of the Terminally Ill legislation, which operated for 9 months in 1996.[83] These cases exemplified non-recognition of depression, a poor standard of medical care, and disagreement over the terminal status of patients, highlighting the defective gate-keeper roles set up by the legislation. Building up collections of case reports points to the need for cohort and longitudinal studies as observational evidence is mounted. The corresponding narrative inquiry of the qualitative approach brings an equally worthwhile persepective.

Ethnographic case studies

Longitudinal ethnographic case studies draw on many of the techniques of ethnography to develop an in-depth and detailed case account to explore issues for a cultural or ethnic group. A study that identified unmet support needs of family caregivers caring for people with AIDS in Southern Thailand (Nilmanat and Street) led to a WHO-funded study to develop policy and models of care to improve the situation. An innovative study exploring the experiences of men with prostate cancer used the technique of photonovella where the men were asked to provide photos to express their experiences along with the interview texts. Some men chose to photograph themselves, others contributed photos of places or symbols that helped them make meaning from their experiences.

Narrative inquiry

Narratives constructed from research interviews mirror the social life of the person, with language forming the major cultural resource that participants draw on jointly to create meaning.[84] The seminal work of Kleinman[85] on illness narratives and Frank's[86] writings on the wounded storyteller have shaped a narrative tradition designed to offer explanatory models of the world of people experiencing life-limiting illnesses. Recent nursing work has developed individual and group narratives to explore close nurse–patient relationships in palliative care.[87]

Textual and electronic studies

Increasingly researchers are examining ways of researching palliative care practice in ways that are less intrusive to patients and allow them to write or respond at their own convenience in terms of time and place. These include the analysis of public domain texts such as published stories, media texts, and diaries or stories from the Internet. Other electronic sources include the use of online support groups.[88] Interviews and supportive therapy interventions conducted by telephone[89] and web interface are a new direction.

Controlled clinical trials

Preventive or therapeutic interventions are generally tested through controlled studies such as the randomized controlled trial (RCT), which could be double blinded, placebo-controlled, or cross-over in design.

The place of controlled trials has been much debated in palliative medicine, yet they are vital when outcome is examined as the endpoint. The study of Family Focused Grief Therapy during palliative care and bereavement delivered to 'high-risk' families selected by screening and thereafter randomized to intervention or control is

Table 7.5.14 Instruments measuring *quality of life* and *functional status*.

Instrument name	Item number (response style)	Factor structure	Reliability	Validity	Comments on utility
Assessment of Quality of Life at End of Life[65]	22 items (10-point scale)	1. Physical 2. Psychological 3. Social 4. Existential	Test–retest = 0.52–0.90	Strong correlations with CIPS	Designed to assess QOL in palliative patients.
EORTC-QLQ-C15 Palliative[66]	15 items (4-point scale)		Based on EORTC-QLQ-C30	C30 well-validated; C15 in development	Designed to assess QOL in palliative patients. EORTC-QLQ-C30 available.
Hospice Quality of Life Index Revised[67]	25 items (100-mm VAS)		$\alpha = 0.83–0.87$	Good content validity; further work needed	Designed to assess QOL in hospice patients.
McGill Quality of Life Questionnaire (MQOLQ)[68]	16 items (11-point scale)	1. Physical 2. Psychological 3. Existential 4. Support	$\alpha = 0.83$	Well-validated	Designed to assess QOL in palliative patients.
McMaster Quality of Life Scale[69]	32 items (7-point scale)		$\alpha = 0.80$	$r = 0.70$ (Spitzer QLI)	Designed to assess QOL in palliative patients.
Palliative Care Outcomes Scale[70]	12 items (4-point scale)		$\alpha = 0.70$	$r = 0.43–0.51$ (EORTC-C30)	Designed to assess outcomes in palliative patients and their families.
Palliative Care Quality of Life Inventory[71]	28 items (3-point and 5-point scales)	1. Activity 2. Self care 3. Health 4. Treatment choice 5. Support 6. Communication 7. Psychological affect	$\alpha = 0.79$	$r = 0.44–0.94$ (AQEL)	Designed to assess QOL in palliative patients.
Quality of End of Life Care and Satisfaction (QUEST)[72]	30 items (5-point scale)		$\alpha = 0.88–0.93$	$r = 0.38–0.47$ (PSI)	Designed to assess QOL and satisfaction with care in palliative patients.
Quality of Life at End of Life[73]	31 items (5-point scale)	1. Life completion 2. Provider relationship 3. Symptom management 4. Preparation 5. Social support	$\alpha = 0.68–0.87$	$r = 0.62$ (FACIT-Sp)	Designed to assess QOL in palliative patients.

another example of a carefully designed and methodologically sound study, this time a psychotherapeutic intervention.[90] Methodological difficulties experienced in controlled trials include patient refusers and withdrawals, undeclared confounding treatments, dose variations and fidelity of the treatment applied, defaults in interim assessments, and deaths prior to outcome measurements. Despite such inherent challenges, the quality of evidence achieved necessitates greater utilization of these designs in future research in palliative medicine.

Mixed methods

Increasingly, psychosocial research is being designed utilizing a combined methods approach. Mixed methods can be conducted sequentially where one method leads to another to further explore a construct or phenomena. Triangulation of different datasets can confirm and explain findings more comprehensively. Similarly a study can be designed so that two or more methods complement and inform each other. An excellent recent example of this is found in a study of coping during illness with HIV.[91] Seeking to identify the predictors of coping outcome, Folkman and colleagues began a longitudinal study in 1990 with a cohort of 253 carers of gay men dying from AIDS during the era before triple therapies became available. Bimonthly assessment occurred over 2 years, during which two-thirds became bereaved. The researchers expected to focus on negative affects, but were struck by the interviewees' desire to share positive experiences. Further analysis of 106 narratives revealed that meaning-centred coping increased self-worth, sense

Table 7.5.15 Instrument measuring the *dying process*.

Instrument name	Item number (response style)	Factor structure	Reliability	Validity	Comments on utility
Beck Hopelessness Scale (BHS)[74]	20 items (true/false)	1. Future feelings 2. Loss of motivation 3. Future expectations	$\alpha = 0.85-0.93$	$r = 0.62-0.74$ with clinical ratings	Designed to assess suicidality.
Life Closure Scale[75]	20 items (5-point scale)	1. Self reconciled 2. Self restructuring	$\alpha = 0.87$	Correlation with ABS	Designed to assess psychological adaptation at the end of life.
Needs at End of Life Screening Tool (NEST)[76]	13 items (11-point scale)	1. Financial burden 2. Access to care 3. Closeness 4. Caregiving needs 5. Psychological distress 6. Spirituality 7. Settledness 8. Sense of purpose 9. Patient clinician relations 10. Information	$\alpha = 0.63-0.85$	Well-validated	Designed to assess needs at the end of life.
Schedule of Attitudes Towards Hastened Death (SAHD)[77]	20 items (true/false)	1 factor	$\alpha = 0.83$	$r = 0.67$ (DDRS)	Designed to assess a patient's interest in a hastened death.

of resilience, wisdom, and a perspective that no longer feared death. The importance of meaning-based coping emerged to expand the earlier theory of coping (problem- or emotion-focused processes that regulate distress).

A problem with many mixed method approaches is that one or more methods may not be developed with sufficient rigor to do justice to the method or topic. Development of expertise is equally important for both qualitative and quantitative research and collaboration between such researchers generates a powerful armamentarium.

Characterization of psychological outcome can be through both form and content. Quantitative studies mostly emphasize the content through measurement of specific dimensions, which can be compared to controls over time, but usually at specific points. Qualitative studies add insight into form, with recognition of the pattern of change in outcome over time. Then, repeated measures analysis, with attention to the slope and variability of change using quantitative techniques, enriches understanding of the evaluation process.

Computer-assisted qualitative data analysis software

Computers have become an integral part of the repertoire of tools for qualitative analysis.[92] There are a number of packages available from the relative simple text retrievers that are useful to sort and manage data into categories of information, to the highly sophisticated new-generation multimedia capacities of interpretive theory building and mapping packages. Some products are free and may be all that is needed for small, straightforward projects. Complex projects usually need the facilities of commercial software, preferably with user assistance provided as part of the package. It is important to understand what capabilities are needed for the research process before deciding on a software package (Table 7.5.16).

Methodological difficulties in psychosocial research in palliative medicine

Psychosocial researchers encounter significant specific difficulties in conducting research with dying people.[93,94] The recruitment of patients, attainment of an adequate sample size,[95] attrition rates, and the variability of the patient's condition[96] create problems for researchers internationally.[97] Employment of trained data managers, adoption of several recruitment methods, and use of well-thought out inclusion criteria does assist sampling problems.[95] Moreover, ethical debates exist regarding the impact of research on patients at the end of their lives,[98] the withholding of treatment in controlled trials,[99] and the informed consent process when delirium is present.[100] Extensive interviews and use of batteries of questionnaires can be stressful and intrusive at a vulnerable and potentially poignant time in the life-cycle.[101] Despite the challenges involved in such psychosocial research, its value is beyond question and critical to our endeavours to improve the care of the dying.

Outcomes in psychosocial research and future directions

The clinical significance or utility of each study merits careful reflection so that standards of care are steadily improved. Quality assurance programmes have highlighted the importance of the feedback loop, which leads to altered practice, innovation, and change.[102] This should be a cyclical activity.

Table 7.5.16 Comparing features of computer-assisted qualitative data analysis packages.

FUNCTIONS	ATLAS.tiV5	HyperRESEARCH	MAXqda	NVivo7	QDA Miner 1.3	QUALRUS (version 2.0.4.0.)
File placement	External files	External files	Imported files	Imported files	Imported files	External files
File types	Text and multimedia	Text and multimedia	Text and multimedia	Text and multimedia	Text and multimedia	Text and multimedia
Code basis	Non-hierarchical	Non-hierarchical	Drag and drop	Non-hierarchical	Hierarchical	Non-hierarchical
Code and retrieve	Codes	Case based	Codes Weights Frequencies	Coding stripes Cases Relationships Matrixes	Variables Code margin Paragraph coding	Codes
Project management	Document families	Cases	Variables Document sets	Cases Attributes Sets	Cases Socio-demographic variables	Codes Offers code suggestions
Interrogating database	Query tool	Case selection Hypothesis tool	Matrix Frequency table	Coding query Matrix coding Compound query Relationships	Case selection Hypothesis tool	Coincidental codes Statistics tool Categorizing tool Hypothesis testing tool
Writing tools	Memo Comments	Annotations	Memos Tables Export to HTML	Memos Annotations	Annotations	Memos attached
Teamwork	Shared documents	Not direct	Merge Import	Merge Import	Multiple log-on Merge Coding agreement	Merge
Additional features	Hyperlink and mapping	Hyperlink and mapping	Mapping Additional dictionary	MS Outlook interface Hyperlink Static or dynamic mapping	Thesaurus searching Numerical and textual content analysis	Script writing tools to modify project Sophisticated tools

For palliative medicine to grow as a discipline, its research activity must be scholarly and generate the needed evidence that informs purposeful clinical activity. Psychosocial research is a cardinal component of such endeavours. It needs to grow through well-thought out national and international collaborations, utilizing integrated methodologies of the highest standards. For too long, clinicians have defensively avoided good science through flawed claims about the unsuitability of palliative patients for research. Fortunately, the specialty is maturing and recognizes the imperative for its future of excellence in research studies.

Psychosocial research in the future needs to embrace RCTs to establish a sound evidence base for its practice. Further, RCTs are needed of pharmacotherapies and particularly meaning-centred therapies to treat existential and spiritual distress. Interpersonal psychotherapy is one manualized and standardized intervention waiting to be applied in palliative care—its emphasis on grief, transitions, roles, and relationships makes it particularly suitable with this population. Interventions need to be both patient- and family-centred.

Suffering remains a cardinal domain for future research activity. Observational studies using mixed methodologies are needed to explore demoralization, dignity, shame, and unworthy dying, incorporating the experiences of patients, families and carers, doctors and nurses, and all related support staff to build a complete gestalt of the many intersecting influences on outcome. Over the next decade, such a body of work should guide future intervention studies aimed at further improving the standard of psychosocial care.

Communication studies have developed in oncology over the past decade but remain a vital research domain for palliative medicine. Discussion of prognosis and preparation for death are some of the most challenging conversations, yet there is a corresponding dearth of systematic research to guide the approach that clinicians take. Promotion of adaptive coping and maintenance of hope alongside acceptance of the reality of impending death constitute a fundamental feature of the effective communication needed in palliative medicine.

More systematic research into decision-making and informed consent in end-of-life care, that provides patient- and family-centred outcomes in terms of quality of care and satisfaction with the process, is also needed. Additionally, whilst outcomes that evaluate staff compliance with advance care planning and other decisions are required to provide empirical evidence to inform the otherwise theoretical ethical debate that abounds globally.

Finally, an urgent requirement in many countries of the world is the training of dedicated researchers who can then address many of these problems. Without solid education and experience, the pitfalls appear formidable; skill development in research methodology is crucial to respond to the many challenges emerging in this young discipline.

Further reading

Creswell, J.W., and Clark, V.L.P. (2006). *Designing and Conducting Mixed Methods Research*. Thousand Oaks: Sage Publications.
This introductory book on mixed methods takes the reader through the process of research from design of appropriate questions for mixed method studies to analytical strategies and dissemination.
Tashakkori, A., and Teddlie, C.B. (eds.) (2002). *Handbook of Mixed Methods in Social & Behavioral Research*. Thousand Oaks: Sage Publications.
In true handbook format, this collection brings together the differing approaches to mixed methods from scholars from the social and behavioural sciences.

References

1. Hearn, J., and Higginson, I.J. (1998). Do specialist palliative care teams improve outcomes for cancer patients? A systematic literature review. *Palliative Medicine*, **12**(5), 317–32(16).

2. Higginson, I.J., Finlay, I.G., Goodwin, D.M. *et al.* (2003). Is there evidence that palliative care teams alter end-of-life experiences of patients and their caregivers? *Journal of Pain and Symptom Management*, **25**(2), 150–68.

3. Franks, P.J., Salisbury, C., Bosanquet, N. *et al.* (2000). The level of need for palliative care: a systematic review of the literature. *Palliative Medicine*, **14**(2), 93–104.

4. McPherson, C.J., Higginson, I.J., and Hearn, J. (2001). Effective methods of giving information in cancer: a systematic literature review of randomized controlled trials. *Journal of Public Health Medicine*, **23**, 227–34.

5. Seymour J, Ingleton C, Payne, S. *et al.* (2003). Specialist palliative care: patients' experiences. *Journal of Advanced Nursing*, **44**(1), 24–33.

6. Beck, A.T., Epstein, N., Brown, G. *et al.* (1988). An inventory for measuring clinical anxiety: psychometric properties. *Journal of Consulting and Clinical Psychology*, **56**(6), 893–7.

7. Templer, D.I. (1970). The contruction and validation of a Death Anxiety Scale. *The Journal of General Psychology*, Apr, **82**, 165–77.

8. Hamilton, M. (1959). The assessment of anxiety states by rating. *The British Journal of Medical Psychology*, **32**(1), 50–5.

9. Zigmond, A.S., and Snaith, R.P. (1983). The hospital anxiety and depression scale. *Acta psychiatrica Scandinavica*, **67**(6), 361–70.

10. Spielberger, C.D., Gorsuch, R.L., and Lushene, R.E. (1970). *STAI manual for the state-trait anxiety inventory*. Palo Alto, p. 24.

11. Beck, A.T., Ward, C.H., Mendelson, M. *et al.* (1961). An inventory for measuring depression. *Archives of General Psychiatry*, **4**, 561–71.

12. Jefford, M., Mileshkin, L., Richards, K. *et al.* (2004). Rapid screening for depression–validation of the Brief Case-Find for Depression (BCD) in medical oncology and palliative care patients. *British Journal of Cancer*, **91**(5), 900–6.

13. Yesavage, J.A., Brink, T.L., Rose, T.L. *et al.* (1982). Development and validation of a geriatric depression screening scale: a preliminary report. *Journal of Psychiatric Research*, **17**(1), 37–49.

14. Kroenke, K., Spitzer, R.L., and Williams, J.B. (2001). The PHQ-9: validity of a brief depression severity measure. *Journal of General Internal Medicine*, **16**(9), 606–13.

15. Dugan, W., McDonald, M.V., Passik, S.D. *et al.* (1998). Use of the Zung Self-Rating Depression Scale in cancer patients: feasibility as a screening tool. *Psychooncology*, **7**(6), 483–93.

16. Zabora, J., BrintzenhofeSzoc, K., Jacobsen, P. *et al.* (2001). A new psychosocial screening instrument for use with cancer patients. *Psychosomatics*, **42**(3), 241–6.

17. Roth, A.J., Kornblith, A.B., Batel-Copel, L. *et al.* (1998). Rapid screening for psychologic distress in men with prostate carcinoma: a pilot study. *Cancer*, **82**(10), 1904–8.

18. Akizuki, N., Yamawaki, S., Akechi, T. *et al.* (2005). Development of an Impact Thermometer for use in combination with the Distress Thermometer as a brief screening tool for adjustment disorders and/or major depression in cancer patients. *Journal of Pain and Symptom Management*, Jan, **29**(1), 91–9.

19. Johnstone, A., and Goldberg, D. (1976). Psychiatric screening in general practice. A controlled trial. *Lancet*, **1**(7960), 605–8.

20. Creamer, M., Bell, R., and Failla, S. (2003). Psychometric properties of the Impact of Event Scale – Revised. *Behaviour Research and Therapy*, Dec, **41**(12), 1489–96.

21. Maunsell, E., Allard, P., Dorval, M. *et al.* (2000). A brief pain diary for ambulatory patients with advanced cancer: acceptability and validity. *Cancer*, May 15, **88**(10), 2387–97.

22. Bruera, E., Kuehn, N., Miller, M.J. *et al.* (1991). The Edmonton Symptom Assessment System (ESAS): a simple method for the assessment of palliative care patients. *Journal of Palliative Care*, **7**(2), 6–9.

23. Portenoy, R.K., Thaler, H.T., Kornblith, A.B. *et al.* (1994). The Memorial Symptom Assessment Scale: an instrument for the evaluation of symptom prevalence, characteristics and distress. *European Journal of Cancer*, **30A**(9), 1326–36.

24. Kissane, D.W., Wein, S., Love, A. *et al.* (2004). The Demoralization Scale: a report of its development and preliminary validation. *Journal of Palliative Care*, **20**(4), 269–76.

25. Peterman, A.H., Fitchett, G., Brady, M.J. *et al.* (2002). Measuring spiritual well-being in people with cancer: the functional assessment of chronic illness therapy–Spiritual Well-being Scale (FACIT-Sp). *Annals of Behavioral Medicine*, **24**(1), 49–58.

26. Warner, S.C., and Williams, J.I. (1987). The Meaning in Life Scale: determining the reliability and validity of a measure. *Journal of Chronic Diseases*, **40**(6), 503–12.

27. Tedeschi, R.G., and Calhoun, L.G. (1996). The Posttraumatic Growth Inventory: measuring the positive legacy of trauma. *Journal of Traumatic Stress*, **9**(3), 455–71.

28. Antonovsky, A. (1993). The structure and properties of the sense of coherence scale. *Social Science & Medicine* (1982), **36**(6), 725–33.

29. Hatch, R.L., Burg, M.A., Naberhaus, D.S. *et al.* (1998). The Spiritual Involvement and Beliefs Scale. Development and testing of a new instrument. *The Journal of Family Practice*, **46**(6), 476–86.

30. Holland, J.C., Kash, K.M., Passik, S. *et al.* (1998). A brief spiritual beliefs inventory for use in quality of life research in life-threatening illness. *Psychooncology*, **7**(6), 460–9.

31. Carver, C.S. (1997). You want to measure coping but your protocol's too long: Consider the brief COPE. *International Journal of Behavioral Medicine*, **4**, 92–100.

32. Scheier, M.F., Carver, C.S., and Bridges, M.W. (1994). Distinguishing optimism from neuroticism (and trait anxiety, self-mastery, and self-esteem): a reevaluation of the Life Orientation Test. *Journal of Personality and Social Psychology*, **67**(6), 1063–78.

33. Watson, M., Greer, S., Young, J. *et al.* (1988). Development of a questionnaire measure of adjustment to cancer: the MAC scale. *Psychological Medicine*, **18**(1), 203–9.

34. Watson, M., Law, M., DosSantos, M. *et al.* (1994). The Mini-MAC: Further development of the Mental Adjustment to Cancer Scale. *Journal of Psychosocial Oncology*, **12**(3), 33–46.

35. Inouye, S.K., van Dyck, C.H., Alessi, C.A. *et al.* (1990). Clarifying confusion: the confusion assessment method. A new method for detection of delirium. *Annals of Internal Medicine*, **113**(12), 941–8.

36. Trzepacz, P.T., Baker, R.W., and Greenhouse, J. (1988). A symptom rating scale for delirium. *Psychiatry Research*, **23**(1), 89–97.

37. Breitbart, W., Rosenfeld, B., Roth, A. *et al.* (1997). The Memorial Delirium Assessment Scale. *Journal of Pain and Symptom Management*, **13**(3), 128–37.

38. Folstein, M.F., Robins, L.N., and Helzer, J.E. (1983). The mini-mental state examination. *Archives of General Psychiatry*, **40**(7), 812.

39. Bottomley, A. (1995). The development of the Bottomley Cancer Social Support Scale. *European Journal of Cancer Care (Engl)*, **4**(3), 127–32.

40. Broadhead, W.E., Gehlbach, S.H., de Gruy, F.V. *et al.* (1988). The Duke-UNC Functional Social Support Questionnaire. Measurement of social support in family medicine patients. *Medical Care*, **26**(7), 709–23.

41. Sherbourne, C.D., and Stewart, A.L. (1991). The MOS social support survey. *Social Science & Medicine*, **32**(6), 705–14.

42. Zimet, G.D., Dahlem, N.W., and Zimet, S.G. (1988). The Multidimensional Scale of Perceived Social Support. *Journal of Personality Assessment*, **52**, 31–41.

43. Sarason, I.G., Levine, H.M., Basham, R.B. *et al.* (1983). Assessing social support: The Social Support Questionnaire. *Journal of Personality and Social Psychology*, **44**(1), 127–39.

44. Sarason, I.G., Sarason, B.R., Shearin, E.N. *et al.* (1987). A brief measure of social support: Practical and theoretical implications. *Journal of Social and Personal Relationships*, **4**, 497–510.

45. Weitzner, M.A., Jacobsen, P.B., Wagner, H., Jr. *et al.* (1999). The Caregiver Quality of Life Index-Cancer (CQOLC) scale: development and validation of an instrument to measure quality of life of the family caregiver of patients with cancer. *Quality of Life Research*, **8**(1–2), 55–63.

46. Given, C.W., Given, B., Stommel, M. *et al.* (1992). The caregiver reaction assessment (CRA) for caregivers to persons with chronic physical and mental impairments. *Research in Nursing & Health*, **15**(4), 271–83.

47. Cooper, B., Kinsella, G.J., and Picton, C. (2005). Development and initial validation of a family appraisal of caregiving questionnaire for palliative care. *Psychooncology*, **15**, 613–22.

48. Kristjanson, L.J. (1993). Validity and reliability testing of the FAMCARE Scale: measuring family satisfaction with advanced cancer care. *Social Science & Medicine*, Mar, **36**(5), 693–701.

49. McCubbin, H.I., Larsen, A.S., and Olson, D.H. (1996). Family Crisis Oriented Personal Evaluation Scales (F-COPES). In *Family assessment: Resiliency, coping and adaptation–inventories for research and practice* (eds. H.I. McCubbin, A.I. Thomson, and M.A. McCubbin), pp. 455–507. Madison: University of Wisconsin.

50. Edwards, B., and Clarke, V. (2005). The validity of the family relationships index as a screening tool for psychological risk in families of cancer patients. *Psychooncology*, **14**(7), 546–54.

51. Hockenberry-Eaton, M., Manteuffel, B., and Bottomley, S. (1997). Development of two instruments examining stress and adjustment in children with cancer. *Journal of Pediatric Oncology Nursing*, **14**(3), 178–85.

52. Armstrong, F.D., Toledano, S.R., Miloslavich, K. *et al.* (1999). The Miami pediatric quality of life questionnaire: parent scale. *International Journal of Cancer*, **12**, 11–7.

53. March, J.S., Parker, J.D., Sullivan, K. *et al.* (1997). The Multidimensional Anxiety Scale for Children (MASC): factor structure, reliability, and validity. *Journal of the American Academy of Child and Adolescent Psychiatry*, **36**(4), 554–65.

54. Varni, J.W., Katz, E.R., Seid, M. *et al.* (1998). The Pediatric Cancer Quality of Life Inventory (PCQL). I. Instrument development, descriptive statistics, and cross-informant variance. *Journal of Behavioral Medicine*, **21**(2), 179–204.

55. Streisand, R., Braniecki, S., Tercyak, K.P. *et al.* (2001). Childhood illness-related parenting stress: the pediatric inventory for parents. *Journal of Pediatric Psychology*, **26**(3), 155–62.

56. O'Connor, A.M. (1995). Validation of a decisional conflict scale. *Medical Decision Making*, **15**(1), 25–30.

57. Brehaut, J.C., O'Connor, A.M., Wood, T.J. *et al.* (2003). Validation of a decision regret scale. *Medical Decision Making*, **23**(4), 281–92.

58. Guyatt, G.H., Mitchell, A., Molloy, D.W. *et al.* (1995). Measuring patient and relative satisfaction with level or aggressiveness of care and involvement in care decisions in the context of life threatening illness. *Journal of Clinical Epidemiology*, Oct, **48**(10), 1215–24.

59. Wills, C.E., and Holmes-Rovner, M. (2003). Preliminary validation of the Satisfaction With Decision Scale with depressed primary care patients. *Health Expectations*, **6**(2), 149–59.

60. Spanier, G.B. (1976). Measuring dyadic adjustment: new scales for assessing the quality of marriage and similar dyads. *Journal of Marriage and the Family*, **38**, 15–28.

61. Keller, A., McGarvey, E.L., and Clayton, A.H. (2006). Reliability and construct validity of the Changes in Sexual Functioning Questionnaire short-form (CSFQ-14). *Journal of Sex & Marital Therapy*, **32**(1), 43–52.

62. Rosen, R., Brown, C., Heiman, J. *et al.* (2000). The Female Sexual Function Index (FSFI): a multidimensional self-report instrument for the assessment of female sexual function. *Journal of Sex & Marital Therapy*, **26**(2), 191–208.

63. Rosen, R.C., Riley, A., Wagner, G. *et al.* (1997). The international index of erectile function (IIEF): a multidimensional scale for assessment of erectile dysfunction. *Urology*, **49**(6), 822–30.

64. Hendrick, S.S. (1988). A generic measure of relationship satisfaction. *Journal of Marriage and the Family*, **50**, 93–8.

65. Axelsson, B., and Sjoden, P.O. (1999). Assessment of quality of life in palliative care–psychometric properties of a short questionnaire. *Acta oncologica*, **38**(2), 229–37.

66. Groenvold, M., Petersen, M.A., Aaronson, N.K. *et al.* (2006). The development of the EORTC QLQ-C15-PAL: A shortened questionnaire for cancer patients in palliative care. *European Journal of Cancer*, **42**, 55–64.

67. McMillan, S.C., and Weitzner, M. (1998). Quality of life in cancer patients use of a revised hospice index. *Cancer Practice*, **6**(5), 282–8.

68. Cohen, S.R., Mount, B.M., Strobel, M.G. *et al.* (1995). The McGill Quality of Life Questionnaire: a measure of quality of life appropriate for people with advanced disease. A preliminary study of validity and acceptability. *Palliative Medicine*, **9**(3), 207–19.

69. Sterkenburg, C.A., King, B., and Woodward, C.A. (1996). A reliability and validity study of the McMaster quality of life scale (MQLS) for a palliative population. *Journal of Palliative Care*, **12**(1), 18–25.

70. Hearn, J., and Higginson, I.J. (1999). Development and validation of a core outcome measure for palliative care: the palliative care outcome scale. Palliative Care Core Audit Project Advisory Group. *Quality in Health Care*, **8**(4), 219–27.

71. Mystakidou, K., Tsilika, E., Kouloulias, V. *et al.* (2004). The "Palliative Care Quality of Life Instrument (PQLI)" in terminal cancer patients. *Health and Quality of Life Outcomes*, **2**(1), 8.

72. Sulmasy, D.P., McIlvane, J.M., Pasley, P.M. *et al.* (2002). A scale for measuring patient perceptions of the quality of end-of-life care and satisfaction with treatment: the reliability and validity of QUEST. *Journal of Pain and Symptom Management*, **23**(6), 458–70.

73. Steinhauser, K., Clipp, E., Bosworth, H. *et al.* (2003). Measuring quality of life at the end of life: Validation of the QUAL-E. *Gerontologist*, **43**, 200.

74. Beck, A.T., Weissman, A., Lester, D. *et al.* (1974). The measurement of pessimism: the hopelessness scale. *Journal of Consulting and Clinical Psychology*, **42**(6), 861–5.

75. Dobratz, M.C. (2004). The life closure scale: Additional psychometric testing of a tool to measure psychological adaptation in death and dying. *Research In Nursing & Health*, **27**(1), 52–62.

76. Emanuel, L.L., Alpert, H.R., and Emanuel, E.E. (2001). Concise screening questions for clinical assessments of terminal care: the needs near the end-of-life care screening tool. *Journal of Palliative Medicine*, **4**(4), 465–74.

77. Rosenfeld, B., Breitbart, W., Galietta, M. *et al.* (2000). The schedule of attitudes toward hastened death: Measuring desire for death in terminally ill cancer patients. *Cancer*, **88**(12), 2868–75.

78. Morse, J., and Penrod, J. (1999). Linking concepts of enduring uncertainty, suffering and hope. *Image: Journal of Nursing Scholarship*, **31**(2), 145–50.

79. Caron, C.D., Griffith, J., and Arcand, M. (2005). Decision making at the end of life in dementia: how family caregivers perceive their interactions with health care providers in long-term-care settings. *Journal of Applied Gerontology*, **24**(3), 231–47.

80. Chochinov, H.M., Wilson, K.G., Enns, M. *et al.* (1995). Desire for death in the terminally ill. *The American Journal of Psychiatry*, **152**(8), 1185–91.

81. Litwin, M. S., Hays, R.D., Fink, A. *et al.* (1995). Quality-of-life outcomes in men treated for localized prostate cancer. *JAMA*, **273**(2), 129–35.

82. Greer, S., Morris, T., Pettingale, K.W. *et al.* (1990). Psychological response to breast cancer and 15-year outcome. *Lancet*, **335**(8680), 49–50.

83. Kissane, D.W., Street, A., and Nitschke, P. (1998). Seven deaths in Darwin: case studies under the Rights of the Terminally Ill Act, Northern Territory, Australia. *Lancet*, Oct 3, **352**(9134), 1097–102.

84. Charmaz, K. (1999). Stories of suffering: subjective tales and research narratives. *Qualitative Health Research: Keynote Address from the Fourth Qualitative Health Research Conference*, **9**, 362–82.

85. Kleinman, A. (1988). *The illness narratives: suffering, healing and the human condition*. New York: Basic Books.

86. Frank, A.W. (1995). *The wounded storyteller*. Chicago: University of Chicago Press.

87. Aranda, S., and Street, A. (2001). From individual to group: use of narratives in a participatory research process. *Journal of Advanced Nursing*, **33**(6), 791–7.

88. Høybye, M.T., Johansen, C., and Tjørnhøj-Thomsen, T. (2004). Online interaction. Effects of storytelling in an internet breast cancer support group. *Psycho-oncology*, **14**(3), 211–20.

89. Sandgren, A., McCaul, K., King, B. *et al.* (2000). Telephone therapy for patients with breast cancer. *Oncology Nursing Forum*, **27**(4), 683–8.

90. Kissane, D.W., McKenzie, M., Bloch, S. *et al.* (2006). Family focused grief therapy: a randomized, controlled trial in palliative care and bereavement. *The American Journal of Psychiatry*, **163**(7), 1208–18.

91. Folkman, S. (2001). Revised coping theory and the process of bereavement. In *Handbook of bereavement research, consequences, coping and care* (eds. M. Stroebe, R. Hansson, W. Stroebe, H. Schut), pp. 563–84. Washington: American Psychological Association.

92. Fielding, N. (2001). Computer applications in qualitative research. In *Handbook of ethnography* (eds. P. Atkinson, A. Coffey, S. Delamont, J. Lofland, L. Lofland), pp. 453–67. London: Sage.

93. Field, D., Clark, D., Corner, J. *et al.* (2001). *Researching palliative care*. Buckingham: Open University Press.

94. Glare, P. (1999). Trials in palliative care. *Cancer Forum*, **23**, 147–8.

95. Jordhoy, M.S., Kaasa, S., Fayers, P. *et al.* (1999). Challenges in palliative care research; recruitment, attrition and compliance: experience from a randomized controlled trial. *Palliative Medicine*, **13**(4), 299–310.

96. Kirkham, S.R., and Abel, J. (1997). Placebo-controlled trials in palliative care: the argument against. *Palliative Medicine*, **11**(6), 489–92.

97. Bakitas, M.A., Lyons, K.D., Dixon, J. *et al.* (2006). Palliative Care Program Effectiveness Research: developing rigor in sampling design, conduct, and reporting. *Journal of Pain and Symptom Management*, **31**(3), 270–84

98. de Raeve, L. (1994). Ethical issues in palliative care research. *Palliative Medicine*, **8**(4), 298–305.

99. Corner, J. (1996). Is there a research paradigm for palliative care? *Palliative Medicine*, **10**(3), 201–8.

100. Karim, K. (2000). Conducting research involving palliative patients. *Nursing Standard*, **15**(2), 34–6.

101. Atkinson, P., and Silverman, D. (1997). Kundera's immortality: the interview society and invention of the self. *Qualitative Inquiry*, **3**, 304–25.

102. Lawton, M.P. (1971). The functional assessment of elderly people. *Journal of the American Geriatrics Society*, **19**(6), 465–81.

7.6

Ethical issues in palliative care research

David Casarett

Introduction

The goal of good palliative care is to relieve suffering and to improve quality of life. However, it is apparent that access to palliative care is inconsistent, and standards to guide palliative care have not been established clearly. At least in part, these deficiencies exist because of a lack of solid evidence on which to base clinical decisions. Therefore, there is an urgent need for research that can provide evidence to define the standard of care and to increase access to quality care.

Recent years have seen a dramatic increase in palliative care research. This growth has created a heterogeneous field that encompasses both qualitative and quantitative techniques, and descriptive as well as interventional study designs.[1] Despite the valuable knowledge that has been produced by this research, and the promise of future important advances, its progress has been impeded by a persistent uncertainty about the ethics of these studies.[2] For instance, there have been concerns raised from several quarters about whether patients near the end of life should ever be asked to participate in any form of research,[3,4] although others have objected to this extreme position.[5,6] Nevertheless, many providers, research ethics committees, study sections, and even investigators remain uncertain about the ethical limits of research involving dying patients.

These concerns have considerable intuitive appeal, and must be taken seriously. However, overly strict limits on palliative care research can cause harm as well, by impeding the creation of new knowledge that will improve the care of future patients. Therefore, palliative care investigators and clinicians will need to consider these concerns in a fair and balanced way.

This chapter discusses five ethical aspects of palliative care research that investigators and clinicians should consider in designing and conducting palliative care research. These include: (1) the study's potential benefits to future patients; (2) the study's potential benefits to subjects; (3) the study's risks to subjects; (4) subjects' decision-making capacity; and (5) the voluntariness of subjects' choices about research participation. None of these aspects is unique to palliative care research. However, by considering each in turn, palliative care investigators can use these overarching principles to enhance the ethics of palliative care research.

Benefits to future patients: a study's validity and value

Palliative care research is designed to produce knowledge that will advance understanding of end-of-life care. Implicit in this goal is the expectation that this knowledge will eventually improve care for future patients. Therefore, the first ethical aspect of palliative care research that deserves consideration is its potential benefits for future patients. These benefits to future patients can be described in terms of validity and value.

Validity

First, palliative care research must use techniques of design and data analysis that peer reviewers can agree are appropriate. That is, they must use methods that are valid. In addition, all studies must be designed to produce knowledge that is generalizable. Indeed, generalizability is the cornerstone of one definition of research used in the United States: 'a systematic investigation, including research development, testing and evaluation, designed to develop or contribute to generalizable knowledge.'[7] (102.d) These requirements collectively describe a study's validity.[8] Validity is a threshold requirement for all research, because it is unethical to expose human subjects to risks in studies that peer reviewers agree cannot adequately answer a research question.[9] Therefore, at a minimum, investigators must routinely consider a study's validity.

Value

Above this threshold of validity, palliative care studies may offer more or less importance or 'value.' Broadly, value can be defined as the likelihood that a study's results will improve the health and well-being of future patients.[10] Like validity, value is an important measure of a study design's scientific quality, but it is also a measure of its ethical quality. Value is an essential aspect of a study's ethical design because a central goal of research is to produce knowledge that will ultimately be 'important,'[7,11] (46.111.a2) 'fruitful,'[12] or 'valuable.'[13] In fact, one reason that subjects participate in clinical research is to produce knowledge that will benefit others.[14,15] Because subjects are willing to accept risks and burdens of research at least in part in order to benefit others, investigators have an ethical responsibility to maximize the probability that a study will be able to do so. Therefore, in addition to widely accepted scientific arguments for valuable research, there are compelling ethical arguments as well.

Maximizing validity and value in palliative care research

Space does not permit a comprehensive overview of ways in which a palliative care study's validity and value can be assessed and improved. Nevertheless, several broad recommendations are possible. First, a study's sample size should be adequate to answer the research question that is posed. Problems of under-powered studies, and particularly clinical trials, are both wide-spread and well described.[16] But issues of power and sample size are particularly relevant to palliative care research, in which random variation can be quite large.[17] To minimize these problems, it may be useful to establish consortia or collaborative groups that can participate in multi-centre studies. Such arrangements have been highly effective in promoting research on rare disorders, and may be applicable as well to palliative care research, in which investigators are limited and available patients are often sparse.

Second, palliative care investigators can enhance the ethical quality of a study by taking reasonable steps to increase the generalizability of its results. These steps might include sample-size calculations that permit analysis of groups of patients that have typically not been the focus of investigation, such as patients with non-cancer diagnoses, ethnic minorities, or elderly patients. The generalizability of a study's results might also be enhanced by recruiting subjects outside the usual academic medical settings through outreach to community clinics and hospices. Researchers should also endeavour to include patients who are receiving care at home, and particularly those who are enrolled in a home care programme.

Of course, an increase in a study's generalizibility comes at a substantial cost. For instance, studies that recruit subjects from several different settings require more elaborate designs for recruit-ment and follow up. In addition, investigators who include plans for sub-group analysis in their sample size calculations face rapidly escalating sample size requirements and costs. Nevertheless, steps like these offer an important way to enhance a palliative care study's value, and therefore its ethical quality. Therefore, it will also be important that funding agencies understand the ethical importance of generalizibility, and that generalizibility comes with a financial cost.

Benefits to subjects

Palliative care investigators can also enhance the ethical rigour of a study by maximizing the benefits that it will offer to subjects. Broadly, these benefits can be considered under three categories: benefits to subjects in interventional trials, benefits from data collected during the study, and benefits to subjects after a study has ended.

Benefits to subjects during an interventional study

Investigators may have several opportunities to maximize potential benefits of research to the subjects who participate in an interven-tional study. For instance, a new intervention to be studied should have a reasonable chance of success. More important, though, if it is to offer subjects a significant potential benefit, an intervention should offer the possibility of a meaningful improvement over other interventions that are available to subjects outside the study. For instance, a pain management algorithm that is expected to reduce cancer pain[18] would only offer potential benefits if it is qualitatively or quantitatively different than those that constitute the usual standard of care. On the other hand, a comparison of two medications that are commercially available, such as topical fentanyl and sustained-release morphine would not offer subjects any potential benefit. This is true even if the study's results offer considerable clinical value.

The potential benefits of an interventional study can also be enhanced by choosing an active control design, rather than a placebo. If a placebo is used, a study's potential benefits can also be improved by altering the standard 1:1 randomization scheme in a placebo-controlled trial in a way that increases subjects' chances of receiving an active agent.[19] The potential benefits of a placebo-controlled trial can also be enhanced by using a crossover design, so that all subjects are offered potential benefits, if the medication's pharmocokinetic profile makes it possible to avoid carryover effects.

These suggestions for maximizing benefits in interventional studies should be tempered by the observation that the potential benefits of research are never certain. Indeed a trial is only ethically acceptable if there is legitimate uncertainty, or equipoise,[20] regard-ing the relative benefits of an intervention. Therefore, although investigators have an obligation to consider the benefits that a study offers to prospective subjects, this should not be interpreted as a requirement that all interventions that are evaluated in palliative care research must offer benefits.

Benefits from data collected during a study

Descriptive studies can also offer benefits to subjects who partici-pate. For instance, data gathered during a descriptive study may identify pain that is inadequately treated, dissatisfaction with pain management, or related clinical problems like depression. In antic-ipation of instances like these, investigators should design standard operating procedures that help to ensure that these problems are identified and triaged appropriately, including communication with the patient's health-care provider if appropriate.[6]

Benefits to subjects after a study has ended

Investigators should also look for ways that a study (either descrip-tive or interventional) might offer benefits to subjects after it is over. For instance, subjects in palliative care research can benefit from the study's aggregate results if they learn of those results in a timely fashion. This might be the case if a study comparing two pain medications found that one resulted in fewer side effects overall. Subjects in the study would benefit from these data because this knowledge should allow them to make a more informed choice among available medications. Although in a palliative care setting this is often not possible, it is usually possible for subjects to learn about results that are specific to them. For instance, if a subject receives two medications in a blinded crossover trial for the treat-ment of dyspnoea, and prefers one to the other, he or she would be better able to choose between these medications after the study ends, armed with the results of a blinded comparison of the two.

Finally, investigators can increase the post-study benefits of an interventional trial by ensuring that subjects have continued access to the intervention that is studied. If an intervention is not available off protocol, either due to high cost or because the intervention has not yet received regulatory approval, subjects will not benefit (immediately) from the study's results. Thus, by arranging reduced rate programmes or open label extension phases, investigators can increase a study's potential benefits for subjects by helping to ensure that subjects will benefit from the study's results.

This benefit may be particularly important in palliative care research, because mortality rates in some studies are very high. This means that subjects are unlikely to live long enough to see a study medication's approval for clinical use, or to see a study's results published and translated into improved care. For this reason, it is especially important that palliative care investigators consider mechanisms by which a study's results can be applied to the care of research subjects in a timely fashion.

Minimizing risks and burdens

Investigators can also enhance a study's ethical soundness by taking steps to minimize a study's risks and burdens. Although the distinction between risks and burdens is not always clear, a rough heuristic is useful. In general, a risk can be considered as the probability of an adverse medical event or undesirable outcome. Risks might include side effects of a medication, emotional distress caused by an interview, or increased pain during a study. The term 'burden' can be used to describe those unpleasant features of participation in a study that are more certain, and which are better thought of as inconveniences. Additional clinic visits, time spent filling out questionnaires, or time spent waiting in clinic might be described as burdens.

Identifying risks and burdens

Attention to the ethical design of pain research, and to the minimization of research risks and burdens, requires a clear agreement about how they should be defined. The criteria by which study risks and burdens are identified and evaluated uses the concept of incremental or 'demarcated' risks imposed by participation in a study.[21] For instance, in a study that compares two commonly used sustained-release opioids for relief of severe pain, patients in the study would have received one of the study medications, or a very similar medication, off protocol. Therefore, if those medications are used in the same way that they are used in clinical practice, and at similar doses, they do not present an increased ('demarcated') risk to the patient. On the other hand, in a study that evaluates a sustained-release opioid in a condition for which it is not typically used (e.g. pruritis) the risks of that opioid should be considered and justified in the study's design. In either case, however, the risks of any medication in a clinical trial should be disclosed in the informed consent process.

Minimizing risks in an interventional trial: the choice of control

Perhaps one of the most contentious and emotional questions in palliative care research,[22,23] and indeed in research generally,[24–26] is whether a placebo or sham control arm is ethically appropriate. Several general points can be made about the ethics of placebo- and sham-controlled trials. Each of these designs is discussed below.

Broadly, placebos can be defined as interventions that are 'ineffective or not specifically effective' for the symptom or disorder in question.[27 p. 12] Increased attention to the ethical issue of placebo controls in recent years has produced a growing consensus that all subjects in a clinical trial should have access to the best available standard of care.[28] Thus in infectious disease research, for instance, all subjects with meningitis would have access to an antimicrobial agent that has proven effective. However, this requirement may be difficult to apply to studies of treatment symptoms in which the placebo response can be quite substantial. These difficulties are compounded when the symptom being studied is transient, such as incident pain.

For these reasons, it is not practical to prohibit placebos in palliative care research, and a placebo control may be ethically acceptable in several situations. First, placebos are acceptable if subjects receive a placebo in addition to the standard of care. For example, subjects might be randomly assigned to receive an opioid plus an adjuvant agent for pain, or an opioid plus a placebo. Second, a placebo arm is justified if the symptom under study has no effective treatment. For example, the transient nature of incident pain often defies adequate treatment on an as-needed basis, and a placebo control might be justified in a randomized controlled trial of a novel agent for the treatment of incident pain. Third, a placebo control is justified if subjects have adequate access to breakthrough, or 'rescue' treatment. This may in turn alter a trial's endpoints. For instance, the free use of breakthrough dosing in a trial suggests the possible inclusion of these doses as a study endpoint either directly or as part of a composite endpoint.[29–31]

Concrete recommendations about sham procedures are somewhat more elusive, in part because sham procedures themselves are difficult to define. In general, though, sham procedures in palliative care research involve the use of a control procedure such as a nerve block, which is administered in a way that makes it ineffective.[32] These procedures create ethical concerns because some subjects are exposed to the risks of the procedure without any hope of its benefits.[24] Like placebo controls, though, shams also have a role in research, because the non-specific therapeutic effects of surgery may be substantial. For instance, Leonard Cobb's research in the 1950s effectively debunked a widely used cardiac procedure that, if it had been widely disseminated, would eventually have put thousands of patients at risk.

Investigators have an opportunity to reduce these concerns substantially in the design of a sham-controlled study. For instance, investigators might conduct these studies in a setting in which the procedure itself (whether sham or real) poses few if any additional, or 'incremental' risks above and beyond usual care. Investigators might insert a sham epidural catheter that would then be used for post operative analgesia.[33] When this is not possible, investigators can choose a crossover design, in which subjects are assigned to receive either the sham or the real procedure, followed by the other. This design does not decrease the incremental risks of the sham procedure. However, it does ensure that all subjects who bear the risks of the sham procedure also have access to the real procedures potential benefits. This crossover sham design has been used in other settings,[34] and might be appropriate for pain research when the risks or discomforts of the sham procedure are substantial.

Minimizing burdens

For the most part, opportunities to minimize burdens are readily apparent. For instance, it seems reasonable wherever possible to minimize surveys, interviews, and additional study visits.[35] These are all burdens that investigators routinely consider carefully in designing studies. However, there may be other needs and concerns that may be unique to, or more common in, patients near the end of life.

Although it is intuitively obvious that all research subjects would like to avoid the added time commitment and inconvenience of travel to and from additional appointment, this concern may be especially important to patients near the end of life, for whom long periods of time spent sitting in a car can exacerbate pain or fatigue. Similarly, patients may view surveys and questionnaires not only as time-consuming, but also as a drain on their energy.

Therefore, investigators who conduct palliative care research may have an added reason to minimize the burdens of extra visits and data collection procedures, and to rely on telephone data collection strategies whenever possible.

Palliative care investigators may also need to consider the burdens that a study creates for friends and family members who often take on substantial burdens as caregivers.[36–39] Although most of the burdens of research participation are borne by the subject, the requirements of time, travel, and perhaps time off from work create burdens for others. Patients may be very sensitive to these burdens and, for some patients with chronic pain, burdens to others can be influential in the decision whether or not to enrol in a study.[15] By building flexibility into a study design (e.g. use of brief telephone interviews, multiple options for timing of clinic visits) investigators may be able to reduce the burdens of research participation on others.

Ensuring decision-making capacity

Patients who consent to participate in research should have adequate decision-making capacity, which refers to subjects' ability to understand relevant information, to appreciate the significance of that information, and to reason through to a conclusion that makes sense for them.[40] These concerns parallel concerns in research involving patients with dementia,[41] psychiatric illness,[42] and patients in the intensive care setting[43] among others. However, deficits in decision-making capacity may create several additional challenges for palliative care investigators.

First, concern about capacity is reasonable given the prevalence of cognitive impairment at the end of life.[44,45] Cognitive impairment occurs in 10 to 40 per cent of patients in the final months and in up to 85 per cent of patients in the last days of life.[44,45] Cognitive impairment may be difficult to identify in palliative care research because decision-making capacity varies over time,[46] and because impairment may result from the experimental or therapeutic medications themselves, such as opioids, benzodiazepines, or corticosteroids.[47,48] Investigators who conduct trials of medications will encounter these challenges even more frequently if trials are designed to evaluate treatments for delirium, for which impairment is an inclusion criterion.[49]

Second, the effects of cognitive impairment on comprehension may be complicated by clinical depression, which occurs in between 5 and 25 per cent of patients near the end of life.[50–53] Clinically significant adjustment disorders may be even more common.[50] It is possible that these disorders may impair either comprehension or decision-making, or both,[42] but studies have not yet supported this conclusion.

Third, even in the absence of overt cognitive impairment or depression, it is possible that severe symptoms or affective disorders may impair subjects' ability to understand the risks and benefits of research participation. For some studies, particularly clinical trials, the presence of one or more of these intractable symptoms is an inclusion criterion. It is possible that severe symptoms may impair comprehension if patients are unable to concentrate on the information offered in the informed consent process.[54]

Finally, these challenges may be magnified in prospective studies that require participation over days or weeks. In these studies, even if patients have the capacity to consent at the time of enrolment, they may not retain that capacity throughout the study. Thus days or weeks after patients give consent to participate, they may be unable to understand changes in their condition clearly enough to withdraw. The result can be a 'Ulysses contract', in which research subjects find it easier to enrol than they do to withdraw.[55]

None of these challenges is easily remedied. Indeed, it is obstacles like these that lead some authors to argue that patients near the end of life should not be allowed to enrol in research.[3,4] Nevertheless, palliative care investigators have several concrete opportunities to enhance the ethical quality of palliative care research when decision-making capacity is uncertain.

First, when research involves patients near the end of life who are likely to lack decision-making capacity, a brief assessment of understanding is appropriate. Although this strategy cannot assess decision-making capacity, a few simple questions in either open-ended or multiple choice format provide a brief assessment of understanding.[56,57] In some situations, investigators may wish to assess decision-making capacity more formally using validated instruments.[58]

These sorts of safeguards need not be employed in all studies. Instead, their use should be guided by the prevalence of cognitive impairment in a study population and by the balance of risks and benefits that a study offers.[59] For instance, when palliative care research involves only interviews or behavioural interventions that pose minimal risks, informal capacity assessments are generally sufficient. When research poses greater than minimal risks, but offers potential benefits, a structured assessment of understanding may be appropriate. This research includes studies that involve a placebo or invasive interventions such as nerve blocks or epidural catheters. Finally, when a study poses greater than minimal risks but does not offer potential benefits, a formal evaluation of capacity should be considered. This research includes studies that involve a placebo when an effective agent is available, and some pharmacokinetic/pharmacodynamic studies that require blood samples and prolonged observation, without potential benefits.

If a patient does not have the capacity to give consent, a legally authorized representative may be able to give consent for research. This approach is justified by the argument that surrogate decision makers should be allowed to consent to research just as they are allowed to consent to medical therapy, using either a substituted judgement of the patient's preferences or an assessment of what would be in the patient's best interests. If a patient does not have the capacity to consent, but is still able to participate in decisions, investigators should obtain assent from the patient and informed consent from the patient's surrogate.[60,61] Futhermore 'dual consent' ensures that patients are as involved in the decision as possible, yet provides the additional protection of a surrogate's consent.

If a patient has decision-making capacity intermittently, or is expected to lose capacity, investigators may obtain advance consent. This innovative approach has been used in a study of treatment for delirium, in which informed consent was obtained from patients while they had decision-making capacity.[49] Advance consent should be obtained only for specific studies, and should be obtained close to the planned start of research (e.g. at the time of hospitalization or enrolment in a hospice or palliative care programme).

Protecting voluntariness

Another way that investigators can enhance the ethical soundness of a study's design is to examine ways in which subjects' voluntary participation can be protected. In general terms, a choice is voluntary if it is made without significant controlling influences.[62, p. 123] [63, pp. 241–68] Voluntariness can be protected by ensuring that a subject's choice to enrol is made with full knowledge of available alternatives and with the understanding that he or she can withdraw at any time. Each of these requirements is discussed below.

First, investigators should ensure that a study recruits subjects from an environment with excellent standards of palliative care. If patients generally receive excellent care, they will be best able to make a free and uncoerced choice about research participation. If, however, patients do not have access to a bare minimum of treatment options and expertise, they may view research participation more favourably, out of desperation.

Investigators can also enhance the ethics of a study's design by ensuring that subjects are able to withdraw at any time. Although a subject's ability to withdraw is a fundamental aspect of all ethical research, there may be unique barriers to withdrawal from interventional palliative care research. For instance, subjects who withdraw from a trial that involves one or more medications will usually need access to a different medication upon withdrawal. This may create barriers to withdrawal if patients do not have access to high-quality palliative care, or if palliative medications (e.g. opioids) are not readily available off protocol.

Conclusion

The field of palliative care, and the standard of care that it represents, depend upon rigorous research to provide data that will guide clinical care. Although this research raises substantial ethical questions, these questions need not curtail what promises to be a valuable, and highly productive area of research. Of course, the concerns discussed above should be taken seriously. To do otherwise risks the sorts of ethical missteps that have produced scandals in other fields. Nevertheless, these ethical questions can be addressed through careful attention to the study's consent process and scientific design.

Acknowledgements

Dr. Casarett is funded by a Health Services Advanced Research Career Development Award from the Department of Veterans Affairs, by a Beeson Physician Faculty Scholars Award in Aging Research and by a Presidential Early Career Award for Scientists and Engineers.

Further reading

Casarett, D., and Karlawish, J. (2000). Are special ethical guidelines needed for palliative care research? *Journal of Pain and Symptom Management*, **20**, 130–9.

Freedman, B. (1987). Equipoise and the ethics of clinical research. *New England Journal of Medicine*, **317**, 141–5.

Mount, B., Cohen, R., MacDonald, N., Bruera, E., and Dudgeon, D. (1995). Ethical issues in palliative care research revisited. *Palliative Medicine*, **9**, 165–70.

Temple, R.T., and Ellenberg, S.S. (2000). Placebo-controlled trials and active control trials in the evaluation of new treatments. Part 1: Ethical and scientific issues. *Annals of Internal Medicine*, **133**, 455–63.

References

1. Corner, J. (1996). Is there a research paradigm for palliative care? *Palliative Medicine*, **10**, 201–8.
2. Casarett, D., Knebel, A., and Helmers, K. (2003). Ethical challenges of palliative care research. *Journal of Pain & Symptom Management*, **25**(4), S3–5.
3. de Raeve, L. (1994). Ethical issues in palliative care research. *Palliative Medicine*, 8(4), 298–305.
4. Annas, G.J. (1998). *Some choice: law, medicine, and the market*. Oxford University Press, New York.
5. Mount, B., Cohen, R., MacDonald, N. et al. (1995). Ethical issues in palliative care research revisited. *Palliative Medicine*, **9**, 165–70.
6. Casarett, D., and Karlawish, J. (2000). Are special ethical guidelines needed for palliative care research? *Journal of Pain and Symptom Management*, **20**, 130–9.
7. Department of Health and Human Services. Protection of Human Subjects. Title 45 Part 46: Revised. Code of Federal Regulation, 1991 June 18.
8. Freedman, B. (1987). Scientific value and validity as ethical requirements for research: a proposed explication. *IRB*, **9**, 7–10.
9. Rutstein, D.R. (1970). The ethical design of human experiments. In *Experimentation with human subjects* (ed. P.A. Freund), pp. 383–401. George Braziller, New York.
10. Judson, J.A., Cant, B.R., and Shaw, N.A. (1990). Early prediction of outcome from cerebral trauma by somatosensory evoked potentials. *Critical Care Medicine*, **18**, 363–8.
11. Brody, B.A. (1998). World Medical Association, Declaration of Helsinki. In *The Ethics of Biomedical Research. An International perspective*. Oxford University Press, New York.
12. The Nuremberg Code. (1947). Reprinted in: Brody, B. *The Ethics of Biomedical Research. An International perspective*, p. 213. Oxford University Press, New York.
13. Freedman, B. (1990). Placebo-controlled trials and the logic of clinical purpose. *IRB: A review of human subjects research*, **12**, 1–6.
14. Advisory Committee on Human Radiation Experiments. (1995). *Final report*. Government Printing Office, Washington, D.C.
15. Casarett, D.J., Karlawish, J., Sankar, P. et al. (2001). Obtaining informed consent for clinical pain research: patients' concerns and information needs. *Pain*, **92**, 71–9.
16. Meinert, C.L. (1986). *Clinical trials. Design, conduct, and analysis*. Oxford University Press, Oxford.
17. Moore, R.A., Gavaghan, D., Tramer, M.R. et al. (1998). Size is everything–large amounts of information are needed to overcome random effects in estimating direction and magnitude of treatment effects. *Pain*, **78**, 209–16.
18. Du Pen, S.L., Du Pen, A.R., Polissar, N. et al. (1999). Implementing guidelines for cancer pain management: results of a randomized controlled clinical trial. *Journal of Clinical Oncology*, **17**(1), 361–70.
19. Farrar, J.T., Cleary, J., Rauck, R. et al. (1998). Oral transmucosal fentanyl citrate: randomized, double-blinded, placebo-controlled trial for treatment of breakthrough pain in cancer patients. *Journal of the National Cancer Institute*, **90**(8), 611–6.
20. Freedman, B. (1987). Equipoise and the ethics of clinical research. *New England Journal of Medicine*, **317**, 141–5.
21. Freedman, B., Fuks, A., and Weijer, C. (1992). Demarcating research and treatment: a systematic approach for the analysis of the ethics of clinical research. *Clinical Research*, **40**, 653–60.
22. Kirkham, S.R., and Abel, J. (1997). Placebo-controlled trials in Palliative care: the argument against. *Palliative Medicine*, **11**(6), 489–92.
23. Hardy, J.R. (1997). Placebo-controlled trials in palliative care: the argument for. *Palliative Medicine*, **11**(5), 415–8.
24. Macklin, R. (1999). The ethical problems with sham surgery in clinical research. *New England Journal of Medicine*, **341**, 992–6.
25. Rothman, K.J., and Michels, K.B. (1994). The continuing unethical use of placebo controls. *New England Journal of Medicine*, **331**, 394–8.
26. Temple, R.T., and Ellenberg, S.S. (2000). Placebo-controlled trials and active control trials in the evaluation of new treatments. Part 1: Ethical and scientific issues. *Annals of Internal Medicine*, **133**, 455–63.
27. Shapiro, A.K., and Shapiro, E. (1998). The placebo: is it much ado about nothing? In *The placebo effect* (eds. A. Harrington). Harvard University Press, Cambridge.

28. World Medical Association International Code of Medical Ethics. (2000). Amended by the 35th World Medical Assembly, Venice, Italy.

29. Dhaliwal, H.S., Sloan, P., Arkinstall, W.W. et al. (1995). Randomized evaluation of controlled-release codeine and placebo in chronic cancer pain. Journal of Pain and Symptom Management, 10(8), 612–23.

30. Silverman, D.G., O'Connor, T.Z., and Brull, S.J. (1993). Integrated assessment of pain scores and rescue morphine use during studies of analgesic efficacy. Anesthesia and Analgesia, 77, 168–70.

31. Broomhead, A., Kerr, R., Tester, W. et al. (1997). Comparison of a once-a-day sustained-release morphine formulation with standard oral morphine treatment for cancer pain. Journal of Pain & Symptom Management, 14(2), 63–73.

32. Polati, E., Finco, G., Gottin, L. et al. (1998). Prospective randomized double-blind trial of neurolytic coeliac plexus block in patients with pancreatic cancer. British Journal of Surgery, 85, 199–201.

33. Haak van der Lely, F., Burm, A.G., van Kleef, J.W. et al. (1994). The effect of epidural administration of alfentanil on intra-operative intravenous alfentanil requirements during nitrous oxide-oxygen-alfentanil anaesthesia for lower abdominal surgery. Anaesthesia, 49(12), 1034–8.

34. Hahn, A.F., Bolton, C.F., Pillay, N. et al. (1996). Plasma-exchange therapy in chronic inflammatory demyelinating polyneuropathy. A double-blind, sham-controlled, cross-over study. Brain, 119(Pt 4), 1055–66.

35. Bruera, E. (1994). Ethical issues in palliative care research. Journal of Palliative Care, 10, 7–9.

36. Family Caregiving: Agenda for Action, Improving Services and Support for America's Family Caregivers, National Health Council, Washington, DC; 1999.

37. Steele, R.G., and Fitch, M.I. (1996). Needs of family caregivers of patients receiving home hospice care for cancer. Oncology Nursing Forum, 23, 823–8.

38. Emanuel, E.J., Fairclough, D.L., Slutsman, J. et al. (1999). Assistance from family members, friends, paid care givers, and volunteers in the care of terminally ill patients. New England Journal of Medicine, 341, 956–63.

39. Jennett, B., and Bond, M. (1975). Assessment of outcome after severe brain damage: a practical scale. Lancet, 1, 480–4.

40. Grisso, T., and Appelbaum, P.S. (1998). Assessing competence to consent to treatment. Oxford University Press, New York.

41. Marson, D.C., Schmitt, F.A., Ingram, K.K. et al. (1994). Determining the competency of Alzheimer patients to consent to treatment and research. Alzheimer Disease & Associated Disorders, 8(Suppl. 4), 5–18.

42. Elliott, C. (1997). Caring about risks: are severely depressed patients competent to consent to research? Archives of General Psychiatry, 54, 113–6.

43. Lemaire, F., Blanch, L., Cohen, S.L. et al. (1997). Informed consent for research purposes in intensive care patients in Europe–part II. An official statement of the European Society of Intensive Care Medicine. Working Group on Ethics. Intensive Care Medicine, 23(4), 435–9.

44. Breitbart, W., Bruera, E., Chochinov, H. et al. (1995). Neuropsychiatric syndromes and psychological symptoms in patients with advanced cancer. Journal of Pain & Symptom Management, 10(2), 131–41.

45. Pereira, J., Hanson, J., and Bruera, E. (1997). The frequency and clinical course of cognitive impairment in patients with terminal cancer. Cancer, 79(4), 835–42.

46. Bruera, E., Franco, J.J., Maltoni, M. et al. (1995). Changing pattern of agitated impaired mental status in patients with advanced cancer: association with cognitive monitoring, hydration, and opioid rotation. Journal of Pain & Symptom Management, 10(4), 287–91.

47. Bruera, E., MacMillan, K., Kuehn, N. et al. (1989). The cognitive effects of the administration of narcotics. Pain, 39, 13–6.

48. Stiefel, F.C., Breitbart, W., and Holland, J.C. (1989). Corticosteroids in cancer: neuropsychiatric complications. Cancer Investigation, 7, 479–91.

49. Breitbart, W., Marotta, R., Platt, M.M. et al. (1996). A double-blind trial of haloperidol, chlorpromazine, and lorazepam in the treatment of delirium in hospitalized AIDS patients. American Journal of Psychiatry, 153(2), 231–7.

50. Derogatis, L.R., Morrow, G.R., Fetting, J. et al. (1983). The prevalence of psychiatric disorders among cancer patients. Journal of the American Medical Association, 249, 751–7.

51. Kathol, R.G., Mutgi, A., Williams, J. et al. (1990). Diagnosis of depression in cancer patients according to four sets of criteria. The Journal of the American Society for Psychical Research, 147, 1021–4.

52. Brown, J.H., Henteleff, P., Barakat, S. et al. (1986). Is it normal for terminally ill patients to desire death? The Journal of the American Society for Psychical Research, 143, 208–11.

53. Massie, M.J., and Holland, J.C. (1990). Depression and the cancer patient. The Journal of Clinical Psychiatry, 51, 12–7.

54. Kristjanson, L.J., Hanson, E.J., and Balneaves, L. (1994). Research in Palliative Care populations: ethical issues. Journal of Palliative Care, 1010–5.

55. Dresser, R. (1984). Bound to treatment: the Ulysses contract. The Hastings Center Report, 14, 13–6.

56. Miller, C.K., O'Donnell, D.C., Searight, H.R. et al. (1996). The deaconess informed consent comprehension test: an assessment tool for clinical research subjects. Pharmacotherapy, 16(5), 872–8.

57. Penman, D.T., Holland, J.C., Bahna, G.F. et al. (1984). Informed consent for investigational chemotherapy: patients' and physicians' perceptions. Journal of Clinical Oncology, 2, 849–55.

58. Grisso, T., and Appelbaum, P.S. (1995). The MacArthur Treatment Competence Study III. Law and Human Behavior, 19, 149–74.

59. Casarett, D., Kirschling, J., Levetown, M. et al. (2001). NHPCO Task Force Statement on Hospice Participation in Research. Journal of Palliative Medicine, 4, 441–9.

60. High, D.M., Whitehouse, P.J., Post, S.G. et al. (1994). Guidelines for addressing ethical and legal issues in Alzheimer disease research: a position paper. Alzheimer Disease and Associated Disorders, 8, 66–74.

61. High, D.M. (1993). Advancing research with Alzheimer Disease subjects: Investigators' perceptions and ethical issues. Alzheimer Disease and Associated Disorders, 7, 165–78.

62. Beauchamp, T.L., and Childress, J.F. (2001). Principles of biomedical ethics, 5th edition. Oxford University Press, Oxford.

63. Faden, R.R., and Beauchamp, T.L. (1986). A history and theory of informed consent. Oxford University Press, New York.

7.7

The measurement of pain and other symptoms

Jane M. Ingham, Anthoulla Mohamudally, and Russell K. Portenoy

Introduction

Medical intervention aims to eliminate disease, mitigate disease effect, and maximize quality of life (QOL). As clinicians endeavour to fulfil these goals, symptoms present both diagnostic clues and therapeutic challenges. For patients, the disease experience is inextricably linked to symptoms and the distress they produce. The assessment of symptoms and symptom distress is, therefore, a vital aspect of clinical care, particularly in advanced and incurable illnesses for which the primary goals of care may relate to comfort and quality of life.

Ideally, the management of symptoms should be guided by a comprehensive assessment that incorporates an understanding of the multi-dimensional nature of symptoms and quality of life. Symptom measurement is a part of symptom assessment and should similarly reflect the complexity of patient perceptions. This complexity can be addressed by reviewing: (1) the principles of symptom assessment and measurement; (2) the clinical and research applications of these principles; (3) the measurement instruments for several common symptoms; and (4) the challenges in the application of symptom measures in the palliative care setting.

Principles of symptom assessment and measurement

Symptoms—a general definition

The study of symptoms has been hampered to some degree by a lack of consistency in terminology. The *Shorter Oxford English Dictionary* defines symptom as 'a physical or mental phenomena, circumstance or change of condition arising from and accompanying a disorder and constituting evidence for it … specifically a *subjective* indicator perceptible to the patient and as opposed to an objective one (cf. sign)'[1]. Thus, symptoms are inherently subjective. They are perceptions, usually conveyed by language. Symptom measurement attempts to quantify aspects of these perceptions in a manner that is valid and reliable.

This definition also highlights the distinctions among symptoms, signs, and pathological processes or diagnoses. Usually, a disease process causes a spectrum of symptoms, each of which may or may not clarify disease processes and diagnoses. Symptoms are subjective physical and psychological phenomena that arise from pathological states or disorders and should never be viewed as diagnoses. In contrast, signs are clinical observations of phenomena that arise from pathological states or disorders; they, too, should not be construed as diagnoses. For example, a patient may report 'confusion'—a symptom in this instance—and the clinician may note 'signs' including poor concentration and evidence of memory loss. After eliciting a history and performing an examination, the clinician may ascertain that the diagnosis is delirium. Further evaluation may reveal that the delirium is itself causally related to a specific metabolic disturbance. The report of confusion in this case should not be used synonymously with the diagnosis of delirium, or with any of the other disease processes with which this symptom may be associated.

Defining specific symptoms

Although languages are made rich by the many nuances that are applied to words that describe human perceptions, the measurement of these perceptions is made more challenging by these nuances. The complexity of measurement is compounded when the words used to label symptoms, such as 'pain' or 'fatigue', have a plethora of meanings for patients and a wide range of implications in the medical setting.

In contrast to the generally accepted definition for 'pain' and the development of a taxonomy for the study of this symptom[2], no such definition or taxonomy has evolved to clarify other symptoms. For example, the measurement of 'fatigue', 'confusion', and even 'breathlessness', has been complicated by the slowly evolving taxonomy, absence of specific definitions, and the range of implications associated with the use of each term. Fatigue may be interpreted by some patients as sleepiness and by others as muscle weakness. The word 'confusion' may be used to refer to impaired concentration, disorganized thinking, forgetfulness, or even hallucinations.

Dyspnoea certainly provides an illustration of the complexity inherent in the varied use of language to describe symptoms and the need to understand the meaning of terms in the clinical setting to interpret distress and in the research setting to measure symptoms and related distress. A study that investigated the descriptors used by patients with dyspnoea found that 8 per cent answered 'no' to the statement 'I feel breathless' despite answering 'yes' for numerous other descriptors that are applied to dyspnoea[3]. Among healthy individuals, the descriptors of breathlessness appear to relate to different physiologic mechanisms underlying respiratory discomfort but are not simply dependent on the presence of an underlying pathophysiology or on a specific disease condition[4,5]. More recently, clusters of descriptors were found to associate with different diagnostic groups, suggesting that patients are describing qualitatively different experiences of breathlessness[6].

To further illustrate the complexity of the linguistics involved with this issue, another study explored quality of life in a population of cancer patients and found that there was instrument-to-instrument variation in the prevalence of identical symptoms (Table 7.7.1)[7–10]. In addition, items that appeared to assess similar experiences, such as 'anxiety' and 'nervousness', had differing prevalence rates. These data indicate that symptom assessment and measurement is dependent on the clarity of meanings attached to symptom descriptors. The variability of these meanings justifies the need for formal validation of symptom assessment instruments.

Subjectivity in assessment and measurement

Because symptoms are inherently subjective, patient self-report must be the primary source of information[11–17]. Numerous studies have demonstrated that observer and patient assessments are not highly correlated, and that the accuracy of a clinician's assessment cannot be assumed[11–16]. For example, a low correlation has been demonstrated between patients' visual analogue scores (VAS) for pain and those of health-care providers[11]. Clinician accuracy has been demonstrated to be especially poor even in settings where clinicians are assessing patients with the most severe pain, suggesting that inferences about subjective states may be most uncertain at a level of patient distress that is most clinically relevant. A study that concurrently assessed patients and their spouse caregivers found that, although the caregivers agreed with patients on objective measures with observable referents (e.g. ability to dress independently), they disagreed with subjective aspects of patient functioning (e.g. depression, fear of future, and confidence in treatment)[12]. Similarly, evidence from retrospective surveys completed by family members after the patient's death has suggested that assessment by family is better for symptoms that are more observable, such as dyspnoea and vomiting[17], than those that are subjective, such as psychological distress[18]. However, variability exists between family raters[19]. Studies have also demonstrated differing correlations between nurse–family, nurse–patient, and family–patient symptom reports[20,21].

The optimal approach to symptom assessment and measurement incorporates patient ratings of subjective experiences. In some cases, objective signs can be monitored to complement subjective data, but this information cannot substitute for self-report. For example, dyspnoea measurement may be complemented by measurement of oxygen saturation or the results of pulmonary function tests. Nausea measurement may be supplemented by assessment of the frequency of emesis, and pain measurement may be clarified by functional assessment.

In some populations, such as demented or obtunded patients, or pre-verbal children, it may not be possible to obtain or interpret patient self-report. Behavioural or physiologic measurements, or proxy reports, may be the only source of data. Although either family members or staff may provide useful proxy reports, these data must be interpreted cautiously when used to illuminate symptom distress and quality of life towards the end of life[21–28]. To facilitate accurate interpretation of data, investigators should always acknowledge the source of the data and describe the self-report and proxy data separately, if both are acquired[21,29].

Symptoms as measurable multi-dimensional experiences

Symptoms are multi-dimensional experiences that may be evaluated in terms of their specific characteristics and impact (Table 7.7.2). The impact of symptoms may be described in relation to spheres of functioning; any variety of family, social, financial, spiritual, and existential issues; or various global constructs such as overall symptom distress or QOL[30–32].

Symptom characteristics

Although surveys of symptoms have often assessed prevalence, or prevalence and a single descriptor (usually severity), a more detailed assessment of the characteristics of specific symptoms is often valuable. Symptom burden resulting from distress is complex and due to multiple dimensions. This may appear to be self-evident in the clinical setting, where history-taking frequently incorporates the assessment of severity, frequency, distress, and other descriptors associated with each symptom. Assessment of these characteristics has not, however, been extensively applied in

Table 7.7.1 Prevalence of selected symptoms by instrument.

Symptom	ESAS[7] (%) n=233	FACT[8] (%) n=238	MSAS[9] (%) n=232
Pain	57	61	58
Nausea	29	23	24
Depression	40	—	—
Sadness	—	42	29
Anxiety	63	—	—
Nervous feeling	—	46	37

Source: adapted from Chang, V.T., Hwang, S.S., and Feuerman, M. (2000). Validation of the Edmonton Symptom Assessment Scale. *Cancer*, **88**(9), 2164–71. With permission.

Table 7.7.2 The measurable aspects of symptoms.

Specific dimensions	Frequency
	Severity
	Distress
Symptom impact on specific factors	Other physical and psychological symptoms or diagnoses
	Function
	Family, social, financial, spiritual, and existential resources and concerns
Symptom impact on global constructs	Global symptom distress
	Health-related quality of life

research settings and studies have rarely identified the degree to which each symptom characteristic contributes to symptom burden.

The variability of symptom characteristics has been described repeatedly[9,30–36]. For example, a study of 215 patients with prostate, colon, breast, or ovarian cancer described variations in the frequency, severity, and distress (the degree to which they considered the symptom to be bothersome) associated with 32 physical and psychological symptoms[30]. Some of the symptoms were reported to be frequent or severe, but not highly bothersome or distressing, suggesting that the mere report of a symptom does not imply that it is burdensome or in need of treatment. Similar variability in the characteristics of symptoms has been demonstrated in the paediatric setting[34].

Symptom impact

The impact of symptoms can be evaluated in terms of many phenomena. In the setting of advanced medical disease, the presence of multiple symptoms and other adverse influences on QOL can complicate efforts to define the impact of a particular symptom.

Pain provides a useful example of this complexity. Pain may induce depression, exacerbate anxiety, interfere with the ability to interact socially, impair physical performance, prevent the patient from working, and decrease family income. These secondary effects can be specifically measured. The Brief Pain Inventory (BPI), for example, contains a validated subscale that assesses pain-related interference with function, mood, and enjoyment of life[37]. Surveys in the cancer population have shown that the relationship between pain severity and interference with function is non-linear and characterized by a disproportionate impairment in function above a pain severity rating of 4 on a 10-point scale[38–40]. This finding has been demonstrated to be consistent across four cultures and may ultimately be useful in research to quantify target ranges of pain severity and better assess the effectiveness of pain treatment strategies[39, 41].

The complexity of symptom impact is reflected in the many options available to measure it. Depending on the goals of measurement, symptom impact may be illuminated by the evaluation of other physical or psychological symptoms, patient function, global symptom distress, or other domains of QOL. An example of the clinical relevance of the measurement of impact is the limited mobility that may be identified in the course of measuring pain; the identification of this may prompt a clinical intervention, such as referral for physiotherapy.

Symptoms and global constructs

Some studies have explored the utility of the construct 'global symptom distress' as an indicator of overall symptom burden in the cancer population[9,35,42]. Brief measures have been validated to measure this construct (see following paragraphs)[35]. The development of these brief measures demonstrates that uni-dimensional assessment of a small group of highly prevalent physical and psychological symptoms can validly indicate global symptom distress, which correlates with both a relatively poor QOL and impairment of performance status[30,35]. A well-known example is the distress thermometer (DT)[43]. This measure is a simple, self-report, pencil-and-paper measure on which patients are asked to mark on a scale their level of distress in the previous week. Although multi-dimensional assessment probably has a greater potential for clarifying the impact of symptoms on QOL[9], the use of a brief measure like the DT, requiring limited evaluation time, can be used as a screening device in the clinic or provide clinically relevant information with minimal effort. That stated,

the diagnostic accuracy of ultra-short methods has been shown to be unclear. For example, a study that pooled results of DT studies revealed the instrument has suboptimal sensitivity and specificity, thus suggesting it cannot be used alone, but may be of some value as a first-stage distress screen[44].

The multi-dimensional construct of QOL reflects the broad influence of many positive and negative factors on perceived well-being[29,45–52]. Physical and psychological symptoms contribute to QOL, but are merely elements within a complex set of factors that increase or temper distress, or enhance well-being. This complexity is particularly apparent in the setting of advanced medical disease, which is characterized by numerous physical and psychological symptoms[30,31,34,35,53–62] and a diverse range of physical, emotional, social, ethical, and spiritual phenomena. Each of the latter concerns has the potential to independently influence QOL, and to augment or lessen the distress associated with specific symptoms.

Fig. 7.7.1 illustrates the impact that a pathophysiological process and various modifying factors may have on the perception of symptom-associated distress and overall QOL. Assessment of these complex interactions may be facilitated by the use of valid multi-dimensional measures of QOL (see Chapter 7.8).

Multi-dimensional measurement of symptoms may provide the most information about the interactions between symptoms and QOL. For example, a study of symptoms in patients with cancer provided empirical evidence that information relating to the

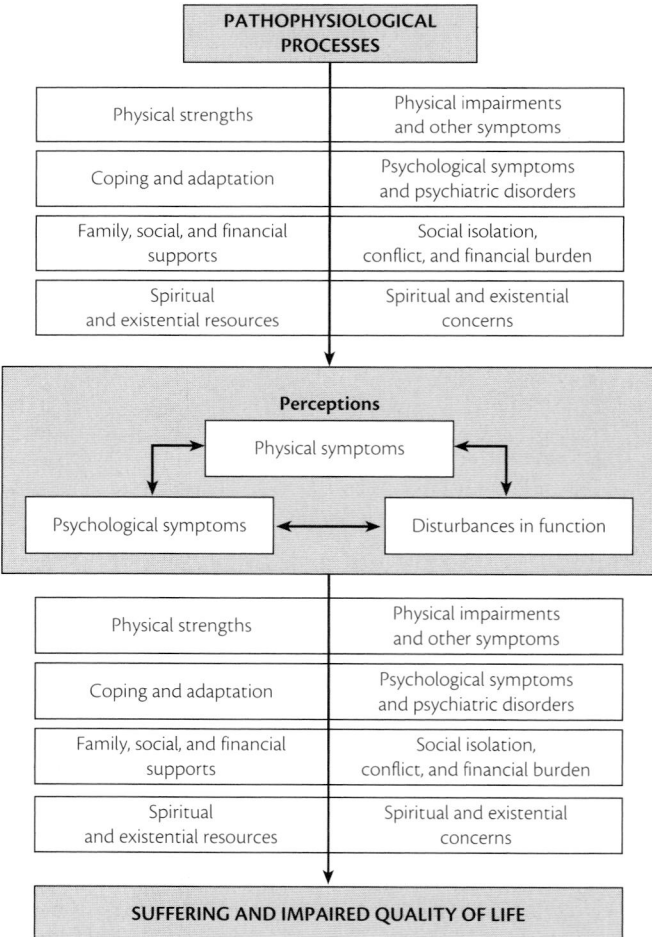

Figure 7.7.1 Interactions among pain, symptoms, and quality of life.

impact of symptoms on QOL was maximized by concurrent measurement of 'symptom distress' and either frequency or intensity[9]. Of the three dimensions assessed, distress was the most informative. These data suggest that distress, or if possible, distress and another dimension, should be assessed if the goal of the evaluation is to clarify the interaction between symptoms and QOL. Further validation of this concept was undertaken in another study, which explored the role of measurement of each of 32 symptoms with respect to distress (for physical symptoms) or frequency (for psychological symptoms) alone[35].

Symptom assessment and measurement over time

Symptoms usually change over time. Characteristics may change or the symptom itself may remit or recur. Clinically, this observation is usually addressed through repeated assessments throughout the course of disease. In the research setting, and particularly in clinical trials, the challenge of symptom measurement is to capture the relevant concerns as they evolve, using measures that are simple and brief enough to both limit patient burden and encourage compliance[63].

Numerous factors influence the changes in symptom prevalence and characteristics. Even problems that remain static, such as communication difficulty following laryngectomy, may be perceived differently as the disease, or the availability of treatment, changes, or the consequences on function or psychosocial status evolve. Although such symptoms may continue to be described by the patient as severe, the associated distress and impact on QOL may increase or decrease. These observations suggest that longitudinal measurement of multiple symptom dimensions may be essential to accurately characterize the long-term impact of symptoms, interventions, or disease-related processes on QOL.

Only recently have investigators begun to address the validity and reliability of repeated measures over time. It is well recognized that there is a risk of increasing symptom distress, and declining QOL and functional status, in the months before death. However, changes in these domains may occur at different rates and at different points along the disease trajectory[64]. When changes in functional status are subtle, findings of changes in symptom distress may be more informative. Serial accurate measurements of symptoms may help identify where patients are in the course of their disease, enhance prognostication, and be used to guide decisions regarding therapeutic intervention. Research in this area is evolving to ensure the information gathered can be applied at multiple points along the trajectory of a disease.

Clinical and research applications

Historically, symptom measurement has been used in clinical investigations to determine the positive and negative impact of disease-oriented therapies or palliative treatments. Although symptom measurement could potentially have clinical utility as a part of the routine monitoring of cancer patients in treatment settings[11,16,65–68], it has rarely been applied in this way. More recently, however, some investigators have been exploring the utility of the routine use of patient-rated QOL and other patient-reported outcomes (PROs), and successfully applied this using computer-based methodology in the clinical setting[69–75].

Symptom measurement in routine clinical management

The effective implementation of therapeutic strategies is contingent on comprehensive symptom assessment. The clinical approach to symptom assessment, which has been well described in basic medical textbooks and in specialized reviews, requires a detailed evaluation of symptom characteristics, pathogenesis, and impact (Table 7.7.3)[76–79]. Although rarely used, instruments for structured history taking and for assessment of patient needs have been developed[80–82].

Symptom measurement is one aspect of comprehensive evaluation, but the routine clinical application of symptom measures, particularly for symptoms other than pain, has not been widely explored. This is unfortunate, given the possibility of increased awareness of symptom-related distress and improved outcomes associated with careful, ongoing monitoring[68]. Systematic pain measurement may improve the understanding of health professionals of the pain status of individual hospitalized patients[83,84]. In a cancer centre, regular measurement of pain by nurses on a bedside chart has been incorporated into a continuous quality improvement strategy, and data suggest that nurse's knowledge and attitudes about pain, and patient satisfaction with pain management, improved subsequently[67]. An example of such a bedside chart is seen in Fig. 7.7.2. Guidelines from the Agency for Health Care Policy and Research[16] and the American Pain Society[66] have recommended the regular use of pain-rating scales to assess pain severity and relief in all patients who commence or change treatments. These recommendations also suggest that clinicians teach those patients who are at risk for experiencing pain, and their family members, to use assessment tools in the home to promote continuity of pain management in all settings.

The experience with pain measurement in the clinical setting could be expanded to the measurement of other symptoms. Symptom checklists, which have been developed to explore the spectrum of common physical and psychological symptoms in particular disease states, may be useful in symptom detection. Unfortunately, these simple, face-valid instruments have notable limitations, which include the lack of adequate validation and the inability to address more than one symptom dimension[7,85–88]. Although face validity, the intuitive assumption of validity based on the appearance of the items, usually is not sufficient in the research setting, it may suffice in the clinical setting, where the measurement is complemented by a full clinical evaluation. For research purposes, validated measures usually supersede simple face-valid checklists (see following paragraphs)[9,30,42,89,90].

Several simple checklists have been used routinely in palliative care units[7,86]. As discussed earlier, some investigators have utilized QOL measures in the clinic setting using computer-based touch screen methodology[69–75]. In addition to focusing staff attention on symptom assessment, such measures may be used as a means of reviewing the quality of patient care and ascertaining situation-specific barriers to symptom control[7,59,91,92]. Although comprehensive symptom assessment should query the impact of symptoms on global symptom distress and other QOL concerns, the instruments that exist for the evaluation of global distress[9,30,42] and QOL[8,52,90,93–96] have not been adapted for use in routine patient care.

A number of organizations, including those that accredit hospital organizations and national bodies such as the National Comprehensive Cancer Network (NCCN) in the United States, have recommended the implementation of routine detection methods for symptoms, in particular for pain, and the use of clinical practice guidelines for the treatment of distress and various symptoms[97–100]. To date, there is not a widely accepted methodology for the implementation of these recommendations in

Table 7.7.3 Clinical symptom assessment.

Medical history	Psychosocial issues	Current medications
Diagnosis	Family history	*Pathophysiology*
Chronology	Social resources	For each symptom:
Therapeutic interventions including operative procedures, chemo- and radiotherapy	Impact of disease and symptoms on patient and family	Inferred pathophysiology relationship to other symptoms
Patient's knowledge of current extent of disease	*Global symptom impact*	Differing pathophysiologies
Assessment	Global symptom distress	Same pathophysiology
Review of systems	Impact of overall symptom distress on quality of life	Causal pathology induced by another symptom
For each symptom:	Impact of symptoms on quality of life:	Causal factor is treatment directed at another symptom
Chronology and frequency	Physical condition	
Severity	Psychological status	
Degree of distress	Social interactions	
Impact on function	Factors that modulate global symptom distress e.g. coping strategies and family supports	
Other clinical characteristics	*Assess available laboratory and imaging data*	
Impact of each symptom on other symptoms on other symptoms		
Patient perception of aetiology		
Prior treatment modalities and their efficacy		
Other factors that alleviate or modulate distress associated with specific symptoms e.g. coping strategies and supports		
Physical examination		

Source: Ingham, J.M. and Portenoy, R.K. (1996). Symptom assessment. In *Hematology/Oncology Clinics of North America* (ed. N.I. Cherny and K.M. Foley), pp. 21–40. Philadelphia PA: WB Saunders. With permission.

the clinical setting. Increasingly it is becoming apparent that a useful contribution to this field would be the development of techniques by which such recommendations could be implemented using efficient, user-friendly (for both patients and clinicians), and valid methodologies.

Symptom measurement in clinical research

Systematic symptom measurement is important for both survey research and clinical trials. In trials, for example, assessment may clarify the toxicity profile or palliative potential of a treatment, or expose the need to alter clinical management at the time of its administration.

Numerous factors must be considered when planning methodology for symptom-related research (Table 7.7.4). A web-based resource has been developed through the National Institutes of Health in the United States to provide detailed information regarding some of these factors[101]. Interest in cancer-related patient-reported outcomes has especially grown and efforts are underway to investigate their potential to illuminate, not only symptom distress, but also various domains of function and global QOL[102].

Until recently, most cancer clinical trials included measurements of symptoms and other PROs limited to standardized toxicity scales,

such as those recommended by the World Health Organization and the National Cancer Institute in the United States[85]. These recommendations do not mandate the use of 'patient-rated' scales for the grading of severity, and data are frequently collected at relatively long intervals. Although recommendations have highlighted the importance of the documentation of side-effect duration[103], conventional side effect assessment remains limited and may not accurately assess the subjective severity and distress associated with a symptom, particularly when a symptom is transitory.

Clinical trials now frequently incorporate a QOL instrument. Validated multi-dimensional instruments that have been used for this purpose include the QLQ-C30 of the European Organization for Research and Treatment of Cancer[52], the Functional Living Index-Cancer (FLIC)[93,94], the Functional Assessment of Cancer Therapy (FACT) System[8], the Cancer Rehabilitation Evaluation System[95], and the SF-36 of the Medical Outcome Study[96]. Studies also have explored the application of modified versions of some of these and other instruments for QOL assessment in populations with symptomatic HIV infection and other illnesses[104–108]. For example, the Functional Assessment of Chronic Illness Therapy (FACIT) measurement system is an extension of the FACT scale into other chronic illnesses[109].

INSTRUCTIONS: Record numbers, letters or symbols for appropriate measure																		
TIME:																		
Temp.																		
BLOOD PRESSURE — Lying																		
BLOOD PRESSURE — Sitting																		
BLOOD PRESSURE — Standing																		
Pulse																		
Respirations																		
Pulse Ox–O_2 Sat %																		
FIO_2																		
Blood glucose																		
TIME:																		
Pain scale: 0–10 (none–most intense)																		
Key: Descriptors B = Burning, A = Aching, S = Shooting, T = Throbbing, ST = Stabbing, ✗ = No Change — Site																		
Intervention N = None, PCA = Pump, MED = Medication, COM = Comfort measures, ★ = see note — Description																		
Intervention																		
Reassessment Time 30° p IV 60° p PO																		
Reassess with Pain Scale																		

(PAIN ASSESSMENT)

Figure 7.7.2 Georgetown University Hospital observation chart. Patients are asked if there is pain 'right now', and if so, rate it on a scale where 0 = no pain and 10 = the worst pain. The hospital's policy and forms support a regular approach to assessment in which the pain score is documented, the character of the pain charted, and an assessment of any intervention administered for the pain undertaken within a 30- to 60-min time frame of the assessment and detection of pain. 'Interventions' include medications and an array of non-pharmacological 'comfort' measures, including, for example, repositioning. Reproduced with permission of Georgetown University Hospital. Copyright: Medstar-Georgetown Medical Center, Inc.

Table 7.7.4 Methodological considerations for symptom measurement in research settings.

Patient-related factors	Factors related to investigator goals and resources	Instrument-related factors
Patient's ability to provide consent and comprehend instruments	*Study aims and method*	*Validity and reliability*
Age-related factors	Which symptoms and dimensions of symptoms need to be assessed?	Validity of instrument for assessment of symptom in general and in particular population
Cognitive state	When should symptoms be assessed?	Ability of instrument to assess the dimensions and impact of symptom
Cultural and language barriers	What methodological controls are needed?	*Clinical utility and appropriateness*
Patient's descriptors for symptom	*Data management and statistical analysis*	Capacity of instrument to assess hypothesis
Presence of other symptoms	Available resources for data collection and analysis	Instrument complexity and respondent burden
Patient's willingness to participate in data collection		
Patient reluctance to participate in investigation or to report specific symptom		

All of the validated, multi-dimensional measures of health-related QOL assess a selected group of prevalent symptoms, including pain, fatigue, and anxiety[8,52,93,95]. Although this information may be clinically meaningful and sufficient for many purposes, these instruments cannot fully clarify the prevalence rates or characteristics of the diverse array of physical and psychological symptoms experienced by patients. Recent experimentation with the use of computer-assisted, real-time monitoring of QOL measures in clinical trials may improve the scope and accuracy of assessment, emphasize important patient concerns, and generate new hypotheses concerning treatment or disease management more broadly[70,74,110,111].

Although a detailed assessment of symptoms may not be required in some studies, large clinical trials or epidemiological surveys may benefit from measurement of a broad spectrum of physical or psychological symptoms. This can be accomplished by the concurrent use of a QOL instrument and an instrument that is specially designed to measure symptoms. Alternatively, a more 'tailored' approach can be used, in which a screening instrument is combined with specific supplemental measures that capture information relevant to the disease or clinical setting. The development of multi-dimensional QOL instruments with disease- or treatment-specific modules derives from this perspective[8,46,47,52]. Depending on the purpose of the assessment, the aims of the research, the anticipated outcomes and toxicities, and the resources of the investigator, tailoring can be focused on specific assessment of a single symptom or phenomenon, multiple symptoms, or any of a variety of other disease-related or treatment-specific issues (e.g. performance status or psychological function)[8,46,47,52,63].

The utility of this tailored approach to symptom and QOL assessment was demonstrated in a study that explored the importance of specific pain assessments during routine QOL evaluation[63]. It was noted in early clinical observations prior to this phase II trial of paclitaxel and recombinant human granulocyte-colony stimulating factor for breast cancer, that early frequent short-lived episodes of pain were likely to occur during this treatment regimen. To capture this information, supplemental pain measurements were included with QOL measures. The 'tailored' assessment revealed a marked disparity between the pain data obtained during a routine QOL assessment performed at 3-week intervals and those acquired through the supplemental pain evaluation obtained twice weekly. In contrast to the interval assessment, which revealed a marked decline in median pain scores, the supplemental assessment demonstrated transient acute and severe pains in almost half the patients. Clearly, such a tailored approach to measurement may be important in clarifying the usefulness of a therapy in symptom palliation, altering clinical management at the time of treatment, or determining the long-term effects of therapy on well-being. This study also illustrates the need, in all settings, for careful consideration of the optimal schedule and manner of evaluations.

Finally, in relation to 'measurement' in clinical research, consideration must not only be given to the utility of an instrument to measure a subjective effect but also to whether a reasonable presumption can be made about the extent to which a change in the measured score reflects a 'clinically relevant' change in symptom severity or distress. Statistical significance, particularly in tests of group averages, may or may not indicate that the difference is meaningful in the clinical sense. For example, a clinical trial of an analgesic with a large sample size may show that the group receiving treatment A had an average change in a pain score of 1.0 on a 0–10 scale, whereas the group that received treatment B had an average change of 1.8. This difference may be statistically significant but clinically irrelevant. Moreover, this difference reflects average scores and may hide the fact that some patients had very large changes after a treatment, whereas some did not change at all.

Measurement instruments used must not only have their conceptual framework, content validity and psychometric qualities (including reliability and validity) documented but also their responsiveness and minimal important difference (MID)[112]. Responsiveness refers to an instrument's ability to detect changes in health status while MID is used to interpret whether the observed change is important from the patient's or clinicians perspective. There are a number of 'anchor-based' and 'distribution-based' methods to determine MID. Once a MID is determined, data from a trial can be subjected to a meaning responder analysis, which is designed to determine whether a new treatment yielded a better response rate than a comparator. Longitudinal studies of each instrument are necessary to determine whether an instrument is responsive to changes or differences in health status.

In an effort to clarify clinically relevant change, a variety of strategies have been proposed[101,113]. Using pain to illustrate, the investigator can, for example, compare the number of patients who achieve pain relief greater than 50 per cent, the number of patients who must be treated to yield one patient who attains at least 50 per cent relief (known as number needed to treat, or NNT)[114], or the number of treatment days on which pain control was good[115]. Analyses of data from large pain studies suggest that change scores of 2 or more on 0–10 scale, or a 30 per cent change on an analogue scale reflect clinically meaningful change; the investigator could therefore compare the number of patients who achieve one of these criteria. An analysis of the BPI has suggested specific scores that could be interpreted as 'mild', 'moderate', or 'severe' pain[116]. A comparison of the number of patients who change from one category to another yields similar information. In the same manner, it may be possible to combine variables into an index of 'clinical benefit'. In one study of a chemotherapeutic agent, for example, a combination of changes in three variables (reduction in pain by 50 per cent, weight gain of 5 per cent, and improvement in KPS of 20 per cent), along with duration of improvement (4 weeks), was proposed a priori as an indicator of benefit[117–119].

Recent work has suggested that severity cut-off points may differ among different symptoms, at least when the object is to relate these cut-offs to physical functioning[120]. In this regard, systematic reviews may offer a method to assess the impact of symptom-related therapies by combining data through meta-analyses[121].

There continue to be many issues to be resolved through future studies[113]. Is an improvement from 2 to 1 on an 11-point numeric scale (50 per cent) as clinically significant as a change from 9 to 4.5? Can the clinical significance of a therapy be evaluated without controlling for side effects, and if not, how should these be measured and indexed? In the complex palliative care setting, can the clinical relevance of a single symptom be truly explored when most patients experience multiple distressing symptoms concurrently? The latter concern has piqued interest in the study of symptom clusters to identify pathophysiology and target therapies[122]. This approach may provide more comprehensive information on different symptoms and their interactions, though the relative contribution of each cluster component may be difficult to determine. These issues must be considered when interpreting the measurement of any symptom in clinical reports, and further research is needed to clarify methods for measuring and interpreting meaningful data.

Validated instruments for symptom assessment

Instrument selection for symptom measurement must be guided by an understanding of the goals of assessment and the practicality, applicability, and acceptability of the instrument, or instruments, in the particular patient population. Careful consideration must be given to the burden imposed on patients, clinicians, and investigators by the use of each instrument. Measurement strategies that are simple and brief may limit patient burden and encourage compliance. The effort to achieve this, however, should not preclude the assessment needed to capture complex symptom-related concerns or QOL. If the information is salient and would not be assessed otherwise, the increased burden may be warranted.

Instruments for the measurement of multiple symptoms

Historically, the spectrum of common physical and psychological symptoms has, most frequently, been explored using simple, face-valid measures, often in the form of symptom checklists(7,59,85,86). Studies have resulted in the development of new, validated measures that may supersede these simple checklists, particularly in the assessment of multiple symptoms. Readers are referred to a recent systematic review that identified 21 instruments appropriate for clinical use in the assessment of multiple symptoms in patients with cancer(123). This review highlighted the heterogeneity in design, validation, and purpose of the instruments. Some examples of the validated instruments appropriate for clinical and research uses are described below. As mentioned previously, investigators who are considering exploring research questions in populations other than the cancer population (in which many of the instruments below have been validated) should be aware of potential limitations using these instruments in other populations.

Memorial Symptom Assessment Scale (MSAS)(9,30): the MSAS is a validated, patient-rated measure that provides multi-dimensional information about a diverse group of common symptoms (Fig. 7.7.3). This instrument characterizes 32 physical and psychological symptoms in terms of intensity, frequency, and distress. The MSAS provides a Global Distress Index (MSAS-GDI), a 10-item sub-scale that reflects global symptom distress, and separate sub-scales that measure physical (MSAS-PHYS) and psychological (MSAS-PSYCH) symptom distress, respectively. The MSAS may be a useful measure in a variety of research settings. Further studies are needed to establish its reliability and validity with repeated administration, assess its utility as an outcome measure in cancer clinical trials, and confirm its value in patients with various types of cancer and disease states. Chang *et al.* have developed and validated a 'short-form' (MSAS-SF)(35) and a further 'condensed' version (CMSAS) of this instrument(124). These latter instruments are short and easily administered, and may prove useful in the clinical setting. Of note, Collins et al. have validated a paediatric version of the MSAS(34).

The Edmonton Symptom Assessment System (ESAS)(7): the ESAS evaluates eight symptoms on VAS and has been extensively used in palliative care research. The validity and reliability of this instrument has recently been explored, and in advanced cancer it is apparent that the ESAS is a valid instrument(10). Of note, a

MEMORIAL SYMPTOM ASSESSMENT SCALE

NAME: DATE:

SECTION 1:

INSTRUCTIONS: We have listed 24 symptoms below. Read each one carefully. If you have had the symptom during this past week, let us know how OFTEN you had it, how SEVERE It was usually and how much it DISTRESSED OR BOTHERED you by circling the appropriate number. If you DID NOT HAVE the symptom, make an "X" in the box marked DID NOT HAVE.

DURING THE PAST WEEK. Did you have any of the following symptoms?	DID NOT HAVE	IF YES How OFTEN did you have it?				IF YES How SEVERE was it usually?				IF YES How much did it DISTRESS or BOTHER you?				
		Rarely	Occasionally	Frequently	Almost Constantly	Slight	Moderate	Severe	Very Severe	Not At All	Alittle bit	Somewhat	Quite A Bit	Very Much
Difficulty concentrating		1	2	3	4	1	2	3	4	0	1	2	3	4
Pain		1	2	3	4	1	2	3	4	0	1	2	3	4
Lack of energy		1	2	3	4	1	2	3	4	0	1	2	3	4
Cough		1	2	3	4	1	2	3	4	0	1	2	3	4
Feeling nervous		1	2	3	4	1	2	3	4	0	1	2	3	4
Dry mouth		1	2	3	4	1	2	3	4	0	1	2	3	4
Nausea		1	2	3	4	1	2	3	4	0	1	2	3	4
Feeling drowsy		1	2	3	4	1	2	3	4	0	1	2	3	4
Numbness/tingling in hands/feat		1	2	3	4	1	2	3	4	0	1	2	3	4
Difficulty sleeping		1	2	3	4	1	2	3	4	0	1	2	3	4
Feeling bloated		1	2	3	4	1	2	3	4	0	1	2	3	4
Problem with urination		1	2	3	4	1	2	3	4	0	1	2	3	4

Continued on other side.........

DURING THE PAST WEEK. Did you have any of the following symptoms?	DID NOT HAVE	IF YES How OFTEN did you have it?				IF YES How SEVERE was it usually?				IF YES How much did it DISTRESS or BOTHER you?				
		Rarely	Occasionally	Frequently	Almost Constantly	Slight	Moderate	Severe	Very Severe	Not At All	Alittle bit	Somewhat	Quite A Bit	Very Much
Vomiting		1	2	3	4	1	2	3	4	0	1	2	3	4
Shortness of breath		1	2	3	4	1	2	3	4	0	1	2	3	4
Diarrhea		1	2	3	4	1	2	3	4	0	1	2	3	4
Feeling sad		1	2	3	4	1	2	3	4	0	1	2	3	4
Sweats		1	2	3	4	1	2	3	4	0	1	2	3	4
Worrying		1	2	3	4	1	2	3	4	0	1	2	3	4
Problems with sexual interest or activity		1	2	3	4	1	2	3	4	0	1	2	3	4
Itching		1	2	3	4	1	2	3	4	0	1	2	3	4
Lack of appetite		1	2	3	4	1	2	3	4	0	1	2	3	4
Dizzlness		1	2	3	4	1	2	3	4	0	1	2	3	4
Difficulty swallowing		1	2	3	4	1	2	3	4	0	1	2	3	4
Feeling irretable		1	2	3	4	1	2	3	4	0	1	2	3	4

Continued on other side.........

SECTION 2:

INSTRUCTIONS: We have listed 8 symptoms below. Read each one carefully. If you have had the symptom during this past week, let us know how SEVERE It was usually and how much if DISTRESSED OR BOTHERED you by circling the appropriate number. If you DID NOT HAVE the symptom, make an "X" in the box marked DID NOT HAVE.

DURING THE PAST WEEK. Did you have any of the following symptoms?	DID NOT HAVE	IF YES How SEVERE was it usually?				IF YES How SEVERE was it usually?			
		Rarely	Occasionally	Frequently	Almost Constantly	Slight	Moderate	Severe	Very Severe
Mouth sores		1	2	3	4	1	2	3	4
Change in the way food tastes		1	2	3	4	1	2	3	4
Weight loss		1	2	3	4	1	2	3	4
Hair loss		1	2	3	4	1	2	3	4
Constipation		1	2	3	4	1	2	3	4
Swelling of arms or legs		1	2	3	4	1	2	3	4
"I don't look like myself"		1	2	3	4	1	2	3	4
Changes in skin		1	2	3	4	1	2	3	4

** IF YOU HAD ANY OTHER SYMPTOMS DURING THE PAST WEEK, PLEASE LIST BELOW AND INDICATE HOW MUCH THE SYMPTOM HAS DISTRESSED OR BOTHERED YOU.

OTHER:	0	1	2	3	4
OTHER:	0	1	2	3	4
OTHER:	0	1	2	3	4

Figure 7.7.3 Revised version of the Memorial Symptom Assessment Scale(9). This article was published in *European Journal of Cancer*, **V60**, Portenoy, R.K., *et al.* The Memorial Symptom Assessment Scale: an instrument for the evaluation of symptom prevalence, characteristics, and distress, pp. 1151–8. Copyright Elsevier (1994). Published with permission from Elsevier.

validation study demonstrated that test–retest validity was better at 2 days than at 1 week, and the ESAS 'distress' score appeared to reflect physical well being. It may be patient-rated, completed with assistance, or observer-assessed and has been modified for use in the critically ill[125]. Certainly, this instrument's convenience, applicability in patients with far-advanced disease, and ease of use seem advantageous.

Rotterdam Symptom Checklist (RSCL)[89,90]: the RSCL is a validated patient-rated measure that evaluates a spectrum of common symptoms in terms of patient-rated distress. Thirty physical and psychological symptoms are included, and an additional eight items specifically attempt to define the impact of symptoms on physical activity and function. The RSCL provides quantitative information about global symptom distress and sub-scales that distinguish physical and psychological symptom distress. A validated modified version with the addition of several key physical symptoms has improved its breadth and utility[126]. This instrument does not address the issue of multi-dimensional assessment and no information is provided about potentially relevant dimensions, such as intensity or frequency. Although there are questions about pain in the head, back, abdomen, and mouth, there is no general pain item.

Symptom Distress Scale (SDS)[42]: the SDS is a 13-item patient-rated scale that evaluates 11 symptoms, nine physical and two psychological, in terms of frequency, intensity, or distress. Responses are answered on a 5-point Likert scale ranging from 1 (no distress) to 5 (extreme distress). Although the SDS provides only limited information about specific symptoms, it is a valid and useful measure of global symptom distress. The potential utility of this score has been further demonstrated in a study of lung cancer patients in which the symptom distress score was a significant predictor of survival[127].

M.D. Anderson Symptom Inventory (MDASI)[128]: the MDASI assesses the severity of multiple symptoms and their impact on daily function during the preceding 24 h. It has been developed to be self-reported, interview-assessed, or telephone-based via an interactive voice response system. The MDASI evaluates the presence and severity of 13 core symptoms and 6 symptom interference items that are rate-based on level of interference with function. The rating format is based on the BPI[37] and Brief Fatigue Inventory[129]. It has been validated in eight languages.

Instruments for the measurement of specific symptoms

Although numerous instruments have been validated for the assessment of some symptoms[101], such as pain and depression, there is a paucity of similar instruments for other symptoms that are prevalent in advanced disease, such as anorexia, dry mouth, or change in appearance. Moreover, many symptom-specific instruments have been validated in specific populations and may not be valid in others. For example, dyspnoea measurement has been developed in the disciplines of pulmonary medicine and cardiology[4,5,130–135], and there is little information specifically derived in the oncology setting[136–138]. There is an emerging focus on the development of instruments for specific disease states[139].

To illustrate the range of options available and the practical issues that may be important in selecting an instrument, the following discussion focuses on measures for four common symptoms—pain, impaired cognition, dyspnoea, and fatigue. For further detail

about specific symptoms, readers are referred to specific chapters in this text and to the web-based resource that focuses on symptom research[101].

Instruments for the assessment of pain

Uni-dimensional scales of intensity or relief, including visual analogue, numerical, and categorical scales, have been the traditional focus of pain measurement. Multi-dimensional instruments, which provide a more comprehensive evaluation of pain and its impact, include the McGill Pain Questionnaire (MPQ)[140–142] and an instrument that has been extensively validated in the cancer population, the BPI[37].

The Memorial Pain Assessment Card (MPAC)[143] is a brief, validated measure that uses 100-mm VAS to characterize pain intensity, pain relief and mood, and an 8-point verbal rating scale (VRS) to further characterize pain intensity. The mood scale correlates with measures of overall psychological distress, depression, and anxiety, and is considered to be a valid measure of global psychological distress. Although this instrument provides limited information, its brevity, simplicity, and reliability are attractive.

The BPI[37] is a self-administered, easily understood measure that provides information about pain history, intensity, location, and quality (Fig. 7.7.4). Numeric scales (range 0–10) indicate the intensity of pain in general, at its worst, at its least, and right now. A percentage scale quantifies relief from current therapies. A body figure allows localization of the pain. Seven questions evaluate the degree to which pain interferes with function, mood, and enjoyment of life. The BPI has now been translated into many languages and is commonly used in research settings.

The MPQ[140–142] is a self-administered questionnaire that evaluates the sensory, affective, and evaluative dimensions of pain, and provides global scores and sub-scale scores for each of these dimensions. The scores are derived from the adjectival pain descriptors selected by the patient. A 5-point verbal categorical scale characterizes the intensity of pain and a pain drawing localizes the pain. Additional information is collected about the impact of medications and other therapies. This instrument does not assess the impact of pain on function. To date, the predominant application of the MPQ has been in the assessment of chronic, non-malignant pain, and the utility of the sub-scale scores has not been demonstrated for cancer pain[144]. This need for validation of this instrument in other populations has been highlighted in a recent review and investigators should consider this if contemplating using the MPQ in populations with cancer and/or other advanced diseases[145].

Instruments for the assessment of impaired cognition

Instruments have been developed to specifically identify cognitive impairment and others have been developed to determine the likelihood that the impairment can be ascribed to a specific diagnosis, such as delirium.

Screening tests for cognitive impairment include the Mini Mental Status Exam[135] and the Blessed Orientation-Memory-Concentration Test[147]. These tools are sensitive indicators of impairment[92,148,149], but are not specific for the diagnosis of delirium or dementia. Further assessment with either a clinical interview or the administration of another validated instrument is necessary to clarify the diagnosis. Electroencephalography or

Brief Pain Inventory

Date: ___ / ___ / ___

Name: _____ _____ _____
 Last   First   Middle Initial

Phone: (___) _____   Sex: ☐ Female   ☐ Male

Date of Birth: ___ / ___ / ___

1) Marital Status (at present)
 1. ☐ Single   3. ☐ Widowed
 2. ☐ Married   4. ☐ Separated/Divorced

2) Education (Circle only the highest grade or degree completed)
 Grade   0   1   2   3   4   5   6   7   8   9
   10   11   12   13   14   15   16   M.A./M.S.
   Professional degree (please specify) _____

3) Current occupation_____
 (specify titles; if you are not working, tell us your previous occupation)

4) Spouse's Occupation_____

5) Which of the following best describes your current job status?
 ☐ 1. Employed outside the home, full-time
 ☐ 2. Employed outside the home, part-time
 ☐ 3. Homemaker
 ☐ 4. Retired
 ☐ 5. Unemployed
 ☐ 6. Other

6) How long has it been since you first learned your diagnosis? _____ months

7) Have you ever had pain due to your present disease?
 1. ☐ Yes   2. ☐ No   3. ☐ Uncertain

8) When you first received your diagnosis, was pain one of your symptoms?
 1. ☐ Yes   2. ☐ No   3. ☐ Uncertain

9) Have you had surgery in the past month?   1. ☐ Yes   2. ☐ No

10) Throughout our lives, most of us have had pain from time to time (such as minor headaches, sprains, and toothaches). Have you had pain other than these everyday kinds of pain during the last week?   1. ☐ Yes   2. ☐ No

IF YOU ANSWERED YES TO THE LAST QUESTION, PLEASE GO ON TO QUESTION 11 AND FINISH THIS QUESTIONNAIRE. IF NO, YOU ARE FINISHED WITH THE QUESTIONNAIRE. THANK YOU.

11) On the diagram, shade in the areas where you feel pain. Put an X on the area that hurts the most.

Front   Back

Right   Left   Left   Right

12) Please rate your pain by circling the one number that best describes your pain at its worst in the last week.
 0   1   2   3   4   5   6   7   8   9   10
 No   Pain as bad as
 Pain   you can imagine

13) Please rate your pain by circling the one number that best describes your pain at its least in the last week.
 0   1   2   3   4   5   6   7   8   9   10
 No   Pain as bad as
 Pain   you can imagine

14) Please rate your pain by circling the one number that best describes your pain on the average.
 0   1   2   3   4   5   6   7   8   9   10
 No   Pain as bad as
 Pain   you can imagine

15) Please rate your pain by circling the one number that tells how much pain you have right now.
 0   1   2   3   4   5   6   7   8   9   10
 No   Pain as bad as
 Pain   you can imagine

16) What kinds of things make your pain feel better (for example, head, medicine, rest)?
_____
_____

17) What kinds of things make your pain worse (for example, walking, standing, lifting)?
_____
_____

18) What treatments or medications are you receiving for your pain?
_____
_____

19) In the last week, how much relief have pain treatments or medications provided? Please circle the one percentage that most shows how much relief you have received.
 0%   10%   20%   30%   40%   50%   60%   70%   80%   90%   100%
 No   Complete
 Relief   Relief

20) If you take pain medication, how many hours does it take before the pain returns?
 ☐ 1. Pain medication doesn't help at all   ☐ 5. Four hours
 ☐ 2. One hour   ☐ 6. Five to twelve hours
 ☐ 3. Two hours   ☐ 7. More than twelve hours
 ☐ 4. Three hours   ☐ 8. I do not take pain medication

21) Circle the appropriate answer for each item.
 I believe my pain is due to:
 ☐ Yes   ☐ No   1. The effects of treatment (for example, medication, surgery, radiation, prosthetic device).
 ☐ Yes   ☐ No   2. My primary disease (meaning the disease currently being treated and evaluated).
 ☐ Yes   ☐ No   3. A medical condition unrelated to primary disease (for example, arthritis).

22) For each of the following words, check yes or no if that adjective applies to your pain.

Aching	☐ Yes	☐ No	Exhausting	☐ Yes	☐ No
Throbbing	☐ Yes	☐ No	Tiring	☐ Yes	☐ No
Shooting	☐ Yes	☐ No	Penetrating	☐ Yes	☐ No
Stabbing	☐ Yes	☐ No	Nagging	☐ Yes	☐ No
Gnawing	☐ Yes	☐ No	Numb	☐ Yes	☐ No
Sharp	☐ Yes	☐ No	Miserable	☐ Yes	☐ No
Tender	☐ Yes	☐ No	Unbearable	☐ Yes	☐ No
Burning	☐ Yes	☐ No			

23) Circle the one number that describes how, during the past week, pain has interfered with your:

A. General Activity
 0   1   2   3   4   5   6   7   8   9   10
 Does not   Completely
 Interfere   interferes

B. Mood
 0   1   2   3   4   5   6   7   8   9   10
 Does not   Completely
 Interfere   interferes

C. Walking ability
 0   1   2   3   4   5   6   7   8   9   10
 Does not   Completely
 Interfere   interferes

D. Normal work (includes both work outside the home and housework)
 0   1   2   3   4   5   6   7   8   9   10
 Does not   Completely
 Interfere   interferes

E. Relations with other people
 0   1   2   3   4   5   6   7   8   9   10
 Does not   Completely
 Interfere   interferes

F. Sleep
 0   1   2   3   4   5   6   7   8   9   10
 Does not   Completely
 Interfere   interferes

G. Enjoyment of life
 0   1   2   3   4   5   6   7   8   9   10
 Does not   Completely
 Interfere   interferes

Pain Research Group, Department of Neurology, University of Wisconsin-Madison

Figure 7.7.4 Brief pain inventory. Reproduced with permission from Charles Cleeland, PhD. *Source:* Daut, R.L., Cleeland, C.S., and Flanery, R.C. (1983). Development of the Wisconsin Brief Pain Questionnaire to assess pain in cancer and other diseases. *Pain*, **17**(2), 197–210. Reproduced with permission from Elsevier.

brain-imaging studies may complement clinical assessment and assist in clarifying the diagnosis.

The instruments used to diagnose delirium exemplify the utility of a tool in clarifying the existence of a phenomenon. Delirium is common in hospitalized cancer patients[61,62,92] and in the medically ill elderly[150–152]. It is also highly prevalent in those with chronic illness who are nearing the end of life[92,152–155]. Evidence suggests that this syndrome is highly distressing for patients, and their families, and professional caregivers[156]. The instruments for delirium assessment have been extensively reviewed[157,158], and although the clinical psychiatric interview using the criteria outlined by the American Psychiatric Association in the Diagnostic and Statistical Manual (DSM) IV-TR[159] remains the 'gold standard' for diagnosis, several instruments are available that facilitate the diagnosis. These include the Confusion Assessment Method[160], the Delirium Symptom Interview[161], and the Delirium Rating Scale (DRS)[162]. These instruments, which were developed based on the earlier criteria outlined in the DSM III-R[163], use an interview format to identify characteristics of the cognitive impairment. Either a score above a cut-off point or an algorithm documents the presence or absence of delirium. Although none of these measures have been adequately validated as a measure of delirium severity, they may be useful in providing a method for the monitoring of patients predisposed to delirium or receiving treatment for this condition.

The Memorial Delirium Assessment Scale (MDAS)[164] is a 10-item instrument that incorporates both diagnosis and measurement of symptom severity. It is based on criteria that are included in both the DSM III-R and the DSM IV. Scores from the MDAS and DRS have been shown in one study to be significantly correlated and, in the same study, the scores on both also correlated with a global clinical judgement of delirium severity[165]. The MDAS is intended for repeated administrations over a short time period and may prove to be useful for capturing short-term fluctuations in delirium[166]. This instrument has now been translated into Italian and Japanese[165,167], and it has been used, along with other symptom assessment instruments, for routine detection of symptoms in a French-speaking palliative care setting[168]. Specific issues surrounding assessment of delirium in the palliative care setting are further discussed by Hjermstad et al.[169].

Instruments for the assessment of fatigue

Fatigue is among the most prevalent symptoms reported by patients with advanced illness, including cancer. The definition of fatigue is evolving. Diagnostic criteria have been formulated[170,171] and initial evaluations support their validity and reliability[172]; the National Comprehensive Cancer Network in the United States has incorporated these criteria in practice guidelines for cancer-related fatigue[173]. The experience of fatigue frequently is characterized by a spectrum that includes muscular weakness, lethargy, sleepiness, mood disturbance (particularly depression), cognitive disturbances (such as difficulty concentrating), and others. Depending on the purpose of the assessment, the measurement of fatigue may need to attempt to capture this spectrum of disturbances[174–176]. Thus, fatigue provides an interesting example of the array of qualities that might be included in a multi-dimensional measurement strategy.

Although uni-dimensional scales have been used, a thorough assessment of fatigue evaluates the temporal dimensions of the symptom, its physical and psychological components, and its associated distress. The specific approach should be determined by the goals in assessment—aiming to capture severity, quality, impact, or phenomena conceptually related to fatigue[177–180]. Uni-dimensional fatigue scales include single-item scales and those that are incorporated into symptom checklists and other validated symptom assessment instruments[90,177,181,182]. The latter includes the fatigue sub-scale of the Profile of Mood States (POMS)[183] and a measure created from the EORTC QLQ-C30 as a three-item sub-scale for fatigue (Were you tired?, Have you felt weak?, Did you need a rest?—each categorized on a 4-point verbal rating scale)[184]. Scales developed in the industrial setting have also been applied to clinical assessment[175,185–188].

Several multi-dimensional fatigue assessment scales have been validated in the medically ill. These are detailed in Table 7.7.5[170,129,189–196]. As an example, the 41-item Piper Fatigue Self Report Scale (PFS) addresses the severity, distress, and impact of fatigue, and can be administered as either a series of VAS or as numeric scales[189–190]. This scale was developed to assess the multiple dimensions of fatigue in patients receiving radiation therapy and has demonstrated reliability and moderate construct validity in this population. Another example is the Visual Analogue Scale-Fatigue (VAS-F)—an 18-item, multi-dimensional patient-rated instrument. This instrument has been validated in a population with sleep disorders and has demonstrated high internal consistency and significant correlations with the POMS fatigue sub-scale and a sleepiness scale[191]. The VAS-F has not been widely used in populations with advanced medical disease, but may prove useful because of its comparative brevity.

Discussion in the literature also has focused on the measurement of various symptoms and problems that may be 'associated' with fatigue[194,195]. For example, in a series of studies evaluating psychostimulants in patients receiving opioids, investigators used a VAS to assess 'drowsiness' and other scales to evaluate cognitive status[197–200]. As an 'objective' outcome, some investigators have linked the assessment of fatigue interventions with measures of exercise capacity[201–202]. Others have evaluated sleep, and sleep efficiency in the setting of fatigue. The latter leads into an area that could relate to the impact of fatigue, or alternately could be a 'cause' of fatigue. In this category, it has been proposed that when

Table 7.7.5 Multi-dimensional fatigue questionnaires.

Piper Fatigue Scale (Piper et al., 1998)
Lee Fatigue Scale (Lee et al., 1991)
Fatigue Assessment Questionnaire (Glaus, 1996)
Functional Assessment of Cancer Therapy: Anaemia/Fatigue (Yellen et al., 1997)
Brief Fatigue Inventory (Mendoza et al., 1999)
Cancer Fatigue Scale (Okuyama et al., 2000)
Schwartz Cancer Fatigue Scale (Schwartz, 1998)
Multi-dimensional Fatigue Inventory (Smets et al., 1995)

Source: Reproduced from Portenoy National Institute of Dental and Craniofacial Research. *Available online at http://painconsortium.nih.gov/symptomresearch/Last accessed February 4, 2008.*

measuring fatigue in certain settings, it may be appropriate to measure aspects related to potential aetiologies and co-morbidities. The latter may include measurement of symptoms, sleep, psychological distress, metabolic parameters, and other factors[177].

Fatigue, in a similar manner to pain and cognitive impairment, and indeed, any symptom that is very distressing, may itself impose limitations on assessment. In the setting of fatigue, the length of a multi-dimensional instrument may be problematic in populations with advanced disease and/or severe fatigue. In the initial validation study of the PFS, for example, 24 per cent of patients experienced difficulties in responding to the scales, and almost half the patients approached for the study refused to participate. This problem compounds the challenges posed by the lack of a widely accepted definition, the complexity of the dimensions that constitute the symptom, and the paucity of instruments that are both validated and accepted. Ongoing research will hopefully clarify some of these problems and guide the development of assessment instruments.

Instruments for the assessment of dyspnoea

Instruments for the measurement of dyspnoea have, for the most part, been developed in the setting of chronic pulmonary and cardiac conditions[134,203]. Like other symptoms, numerous aspects and dimensions of dyspnoea can be assessed[204]. These include antecedents, or physiologic and psychogenic factors that precede the onset of the symptom; environmental or personal characteristics that mediate dyspnoea; subjective responses and reactions to dyspnoea; and consequences or outcomes of dyspnoea[132,204]. Instruments may assess one or more of these dimensions.

To clarify the appropriateness of the language employed in dyspnoea assessment, the descriptors used by patients have been explored using adjectival checklists[3,205,206]. These studies indicate that patients use a variety of descriptors for dyspnoea; particular descriptors, or clusters of descriptors, vary in relation to specific lung pathologies. For example, a study of patients with a spectrum of chronic lung diseases, including emphysema-bronchitis, asthma, restrictive lung disease, and vascular lung disease, demonstrated that although most patients endorsed the descriptor 'I feel short of breath', those with asthma were more likely than others to describe 'chest tightness'[205]. In a study of an outpatient population with seven different conditions, each diagnosis was associated with a unique set of clusters (e.g. asthma with 'work/effort' and 'tight', interstitial lung disease with 'work/effort' and 'rapid' breathing)[4]. The 'work/effort' cluster was common for all diagnoses. This study suggested that a questionnaire containing descriptors of breathlessness might help to establish a specific diagnosis or potentially identify mechanisms whereby a specific intervention relieves dyspnoea. In contrast, a study that compared dyspnoea descriptors used by patients with chronic non-malignant disease and those with primary or secondary lung cancer observed that those descriptor clusters linked with specific disease states did not distinguish the populations sufficiently to aid in differential diagnosis[6]. Nonetheless, the possibility of the existence of disease-specific descriptors further serves to emphasize the importance of selecting instruments for dyspnoea measurement that have been validated in the appropriate disease population.

The VAS is the most commonly utilized, uni-dimensional measures for the assessment of dyspnoea in patients with advanced disease. VAS generally have good within-subject reproducibility, particularly when dyspnoea is assessed repeatedly in a single session using a standard exercise task[207,208]. The VAS has been found to be less reliable when the same exercise task is repeated at longer intervals, such as 2 weeks[209]. In addition, considerable between-subject variation has been demonstrated[210] and, in some individuals, VAS scores are insensitive and poorly reproducible.

Verbal categorical scales and numerical scales also have been used to assess dyspnoea[130,131,206,211]. The modified Borg scale is an example of a commonly used categorical scale[212,213]. This scale, which has been validated in healthy individuals and in patients with chronic non-malignant pulmonary disease, rates the patient's perception of their dyspnoea in relation to a perceived level of exertion. For example, the dyspnoea is rated as equating with exertion that is 'very, very weak', 'very, very strong', and varying degrees in between.

The measurement of dyspnoea, unlike that of many other symptoms, frequently involves the administration of an instrument with a dyspnoea-producing task, usually standardized or graded exercise. Indeed, although the commonly used dyspnoea measures, such as the VAS and the Borg scale[212,213], have been shown to be reliable, and valid measures of dyspnoea when assessment is linked to such an exercise task, the validity and reliability of these measures have only rarely been evaluated without such a stress[136,214,215]. In addition, the work to date suggests the VAS is not appropriate for comparing dyspnoea in different patients as there are no standard principles that allow the scales to be used consistently by different subjects[204].

Because the reliability of dyspnoea assessment can be improved by the use of a standardized exercise task, both the type of task appropriate in different settings and the timing of assessments must be carefully considered. One approach involves the assessment of each subject's ability to reproduce a dyspnoea score on the VAS in response to a standard degree of exertion[207]. Other investigators have attempted to use a standardized exercise to 'calibrate' the VAS with respect to each subjects quantity and quality of breathlessness[130,131]. In such a 'calibrated' scale, the upper end of the VAS is 'anchored' to the dyspnoea associated with a specific strenuous exercise[131]. The dyspnoea at the moment that the exercise is terminated is defined as the maximum point on the VAS. This has been shown to have utility in detecting clinically significant changes in pulmonary rehabilitation of patients with chronic obstructive pulmonary disease[208].

In addition to enhancing the reliability of the assessment, an approach that incorporates an exercise task allows the assessment of therapeutic interventions that may have little impact on baseline dyspnoea but substantial effect on exercise-induced dyspnoea. When assessing dyspnoea in a population with advanced disease, it is important to define a standardized exercise that is not limited by other symptoms or disabilities. For example, in some populations, the use of short walk or treadmill exercise may be limited by pain or fatigue, whereas repetitive arm or leg lifting exercises may be feasible.

Other instruments assess the consequences of dyspnoea in relation to limitations on function. Although useful in the patient suffering from breathlessness as a single symptom, these instruments, which include the Modified Medical Research Council Dyspnoea Scale[216], the American Thoracic Society Five Level Scale of Breathlessness[217], the Baseline Dyspnoea Index[218], and the Transition Dyspnoea Index[219] have obvious limitations when function is limited by other symptoms such as pain or fatigue. Notwithstanding, it may be appropriate to measure the effects on activities of daily living for 'benchmarking' patient progress[220]. Instruments that quantify function and health-related QOL can have great utility for documenting outcomes, despite limitations in identifying treatment responsiveness for specific clinical interventions[219,220].

Of note, the complex interaction between dyspnoea and anxiety also must be considered in the measurement of dyspnoea[221]. Anxiety can be measured concurrently using a validated scale, such as the Hospital Anxiety and Depression scale. This highlights again that, as is the case in measuring fatigue, in certain settings, it may be appropriate to measure aspects of a symptom experience that could be related to the symptom's potential aetiology and/or its co-morbidity.

In summary, readers are referred to a recent systematic review of scales to measure breathlessness that highlighted the broad range available[222]. Instruments exist to measure breathlessness descriptors, severity and functional impact, with multi-dimensional measures available that have been validated in non-English speaking populations[223,224]. Additional studies are needed beyond the population with cardiopulmonary disease to evaluate the use of various measures in populations with diseases such as cancer.

Challenges in palliative medicine

There are significant challenges in bringing systematic symptom measurement to the very ill palliative care population. These include both attitudinal and conceptual barriers to the use of such measures, practical barriers, and barriers that are specific to special populations.

Conceptual and attitudinal barriers to the use of symptom measures

Conceptual and attitudinal barriers to the use of health status measures in patient care and clinical trials[225] are likely to be relevant in the clinical palliative care setting. Barriers have included skepticism about the validity and importance of self-rated health measures, preferences for physiologic and observable disease-related outcomes, and unfamiliarity of health-care providers with the scoring of measures.

Education of health professionals about measurement techniques should be viewed as a priority in efforts aimed at eliminating barriers and improving symptom management. In one survey, of physicians providing care for patients with cancer, 76 per cent stated that the single most important barrier to adequate pain management was poor pain assessment[226]. In another survey, fewer than one-half of patients with pain had a staff member ask about pain or note pain in their record during the 72-h period after their admission to the hospital[227]. The routine use of symptom assessment measures in clinical practice may be useful in approaching these difficulties[68]. Directives by accreditation organizations, such as the Joint Commission for the Accreditation of Hospital Organizations in the United States—mandating that hospitals and nursing facilities assess pain routinely—have intensified the focus on symptom assessment in 'routine' patient care settings.

Practical barriers that occur in patients with advanced disease

Although the increasing availability of validated symptom measures has been an important advance, valid measures are still lacking for many common symptoms and represents a major methodologic barrier to improving symptom measurement. As a result, many studies have used checklists to measure symptom prevalence without reference to symptom distress and impact.

Even when measures exist, a variety of factors may compromise assessment. Severe distress is likely to be an impediment, for example, and may lead to the unacceptable situation in which those patients at greatest need for symptom management are least able to provide information that could lead to treatment.

The high prevalence of delirium and fatigue in patients with advanced disease is another potential barrier. Studies have suggested that the prevalence of delirium in hospitalized medical and surgical patients is approximately 10 per cent[151,228]. A higher prevalence, ranging to 50 per cent in some studies, exists in some inpatient populations, including the elderly and patients in the post-operative period[150,151]. The prevalence of delirium in hospitalized cancer patients ranges from 8 to 40 per cent[61,62,92]. A consistently higher prevalence, up to 85 per cent, has been found in studies of cancer populations with very advanced disease, particularly those in the last week of life[92,155,229].

The difficulty that some cognitively intact individuals experience in completing VAS[130,230–231] is likely to be increased among the cognitively impaired. It has been suggested that studies should incorporate a methodology for assessing an individual's ability to consistently use measurement instruments, such as the VAS. In addition, with each study designed to assess a specific intervention, consideration should be given to the role of including cognitively impaired patients in the study and to how the assessment issue will be addressed if this population is to be included[130].

Despite the challenges, it is crucial to assess pain and other causes of distress in the cognitively impaired in the clinical setting and to develop methodologies by which distress and the impact of interventions can be assessed over time in both the clinical and research settings. Studies involving cognitively impaired elderly patients have demonstrated that many of these patients can report pain[232,233]. Those with mild to moderate cognitive impairment usually can respond to a self-report instrument[233,234]. To reduce the under-reporting of pain[233], it is important to teach patients how to use the scales and to repeat enquiries[235,236].

For non-verbal patients with severe cognitive impairment, pain assessment must rely on behavioural scales. These scales have drawbacks and should not be used if self-report is possible[237,238]. Behaviour can reflect distress caused by problems other than pain, and, complicating assessment even further, severe dementia can 'blunt' physical responses and lead to an underestimate of distress. Although behavioural measures can be useful in clinical assessment, the extent to which they can validly measure change over time has not been adequately explored[238–241]. This area is deserving of more study. Importantly, existing behavioural measures have potential to be adapted for clinical settings and incorporated into treatment protocols. For example, an 'Assessment of Discomfort in Dementia Protocol,' which is a method for addressing both physical pain and distress in patients with severe dementia[241], uses the response to 'as needed' analgesics as a part of the assessment process. As noted, the goal of this approach is to measure 'discomfort', another proxy for pain, in those with severe cognitive impairment.

Fatigue is the most common symptom in populations with advanced cancer, occurring with a prevalence of 40–70 per cent[30,31,53–55,58,242]. In addition it is also prevalent in populations with other advanced disease. The impact of fatigue on the ability of patients to complete assessment measures has not been empirically evaluated. This is another important theoretical concern deserving of additional study.

A further methodologic difficulty relates to the measurement of symptoms in patients experiencing multiple symptoms concurrently. In a study of patients with prostate, colon, breast, or ovarian cancer, the median number of symptoms per patient was 11.5 and the range was 0–25[30]. The development of instruments for the measurement of global symptom distress has provided a method by which the impact of multiple symptoms can be explored but these measures too often lack validation in populations other than the population with cancer[9,30,42].

The priorities of the patient and family may be another barrier to systematic symptom assessment in the palliative care setting. Patients may be unwilling to participate in clinical studies or provide information that requires the use of complex, time-consuming instruments. One survey demonstrated that patients in a palliative care unit gradually reduced their compliance with twice-daily VAS measures for pain, activity, nausea, drowsiness, appetite, sensation of well-being, depression, and anxiety as their disease progressed[59]. In contrast to the day of admission, when 69 per cent of the VAS were completed by the patient and 28 per cent by the nurse, only 8 per cent of the measures were completed by the patient on the day of death.

Patients' priorities for research in palliative care and the willingness or ability of patients with advanced medical disease to participate in symptom studies has only begun to be examined[243]. Clearly, this willingness will vary with the characteristics of the patient, family, disease, and study methodology. It is reassuring to note that several surveys of symptoms and QOL in patients with advanced medical illness suggest that relatively good compliance is possible. Of 1427 consecutive outpatients with recurrent or metastatic cancer who were asked to participate in a study using the BPI, only 119 patients (8.3 per cent) did not participate; of these, 68 (4.7 per cent) refused, 34 (2.4 per cent) were too ill to participate, and 17 (1.2 per cent) were unable to comprehend or complete the forms[244]. In another study of 308 patients with advanced, symptomatic HIV disease, 67 per cent participated, 15 per cent refused, and the remaining 18 per cent could not be enrolled for 'logistic' reasons[245]. The group who participated provided self-report data despite severe symptoms (mean symptom number 11) and a low performance status (41 per cent limited in self-care activities).

Concern about the response of medically ill patients to sensitive questions at a time when they are experiencing numerous physical, psychological, and emotional stressors also has not been addressed in the literature. Evidence exists, however, that sensitive areas of concern can be assessed. For example, in a survey of patients with cancer who were expected to die within a year, patients were asked to participate in interviews at bi-weekly or monthly intervals to discuss issues regarding their preferred place of death[246]. Of 98 patients approached, 84 (86 per cent) agreed to be interviewed, of whom 70 (83 per cent) died during the study. Clearly willingness to participate in such studies and to answer sensitive questions will be influenced by many factors including, among others, cultural preferences. Such confounding factors need consideration. Another potential confounding factor is the influence of the presence of a caregiver on the patient's responses. Standardization of any protocols for this would be needed.

In summary, the concerns that cognitive impairment may interfere with subjective reporting, and that fatigue and/or symptom burden may limit patient ability or willingness to provide subjective data, have important implications for clinical practice and research methodology in the palliative care population. Clinically, these issues impact on the approach to assessing patient concerns. In the research setting, these issues emphasize the importance of selection criteria, documentation of cognitive status, and recording of reasons for refusal or inability to participate in data collection.

Special populations

Symptom measurement is particularly challenging in several subpopulations. These include the paediatric population, the imminently dying, those patients whose language or culture differs from that of the health-care professionals involved in their care, and the cognitively impaired. Approaches to the symptom assessment and measurement in the cognitively impaired have been discussed earlier.

In the paediatric literature, the evolution of symptom assessment initially predominantly focused on procedural pain[247–250]. Procedural pain has been evaluated with self-report VAS and 'faces' scales[251–257], and observational scales such as the Observational Scale of Behavioural Distress[258] and the Procedure Behaviour Checklist[253]. These measures quantify the occurrence, intensity, and range of a child's pain during procedures. Although a behavioural observation scale for assessment of tumour-related pain in children aged 2–6 years has been developed[259], the 17 items in the scale lack operational definitions and demonstrated poor inter-rater reliability. Other scales have been used for the assessment of chemotherapy-related nausea and vomiting[259,260], including VAS and 'faces' scales for frequency, severity, and distress, but these have not been extensively validated.

The MSAS has been adapted for the measurement of multiple symptoms in the population aged 10–18 years[34]. This instrument can provide multi-dimensional information about symptoms experienced by children. Its use to date has been for research in the paediatric population with cancer[261]. For more detail, readers are referred to the chapters in this text that focus on paediatrics but certainly at this time it is reasonable to note that further work on paediatric symptom assessment instruments, particularly for non-cancer populations, is a priority and would serve to enhance our knowledge in this field.

The difficulties encountered in the assessment of the imminently dying population have led both clinicians and investigators to rely on observer-rated data despite concerns about the validity of this approach. As noted, cognitive impairment is highly prevalent in this population and can impede efforts to gather patient-reported data. The prevalence of cognitive impairment varies by disease and general rules cannot be proffered. For example, only 15 per cent of 16 000 decedents in the National Mortality Followback Survey had 'trouble understanding where he or she was during the last few hours or days'[262]. Although some surveys have described cancer patients with advanced disease as commonly being unable to communicate for significant periods of time towards the end of life[59,153,154,263,264], a survey of 102 inpatient and home-care cancer deaths found that significant numbers (over 50 per cent) of patients were able to interact up to 12 h before death[265]; by the hour before death, few (less than 10 per cent) were communicative. These data suggest that the majority of those who die may be able to communicate during the days immediately prior to death. Those perceived to be imminently dying should not be assumed to lack the ability to convey experience.

Significant problems relating to symptom assessment and measurement also may be encountered in patients whose culture and language differ from the professionals involved in their care[266]. Without meticulous attention to skilled translation, the nuances of the language used to describe symptoms may obscure meaning across cultures. An increasing number of instruments have been shown to be reliable and valid across cultures and languages[165,267,268], and translation and validation of other symptom measures is needed. In the clinical setting, health-care professionals may need to develop simple, face-valid symptom measures to overcome language barriers. A discussion among the clinician, the patient, and an interpreter can facilitate the construction of a simple, two-language verbal rating scale to keep by the bedside. To monitor the level of distress and impact of interventions, such scales should, at a minimum, address both symptom intensity and relief. This approach is important to ensure that symptom distress can be minimized at all times, particularly when interpreters are not freely available.

Finally, the challenges encountered in symptom assessment both in populations who are unable to express themselves and have no access to proxy assessment, and in other more cognitively intact populations, raise the question of whether alternative measurements can be considered. For the most part, efforts in this area focus on instrument development and the exploration of the validity of observational data. That stated the question of whether any bio-markers could provide useful information is one that arises frequently and has been given more attention recently. In advanced cancer, activation of the systemic inflammatory response results in high levels of cytokines and, recently, some immunomodulatory agents have been used in the treatment of malignancy. While it is accepted that cytokines contribute to anorexia and cachexia, their role in contributing to other symptoms such as pain and cognitive impairment is only now emerging[269–271]. Studies are underway in an attempt to identify these inflammatory markers as potential targets for therapy. In this context, while the subjective report remains the 'gold standard' for symptom assessment, it is possible that a role may evolve for cytokines as biological markers for symptoms, and possibly as markers of response to symptomatic treatment.

Conclusion

Systematic symptom assessment is a foundation of clinical practice and research. Instruments for the measurement of symptoms have been developed and may facilitate this process. Quantification of symptoms may be able to improve symptom management and further the goal of enhanced QOL. Clinicians and investigators should become familiar with these instruments and develop methods for their use in routine clinical practice, the research environment, and the palliative care setting.

Acknowledgements

Professor Jane Ingham's research for this chapter was undertaken, in part, thanks to funding from the Cancer Institute NSW Palliative Care Academic Leaders Program.

References

1. Stevenson, A., ed. (2007). *Shorter Oxford English Dictionary* sixth edition. Oxford University Press, Oxford.
2. IASP, Subcommittee on Taxonomy. (1980). Pain terms: a list with definitions and notes on usage. *Pain*, **8**, 249–52.
3. Elliott, M.W., *et al.* (1991). The language of breathlessness. Use of verbal descriptors by patients with cardiopulmonary disease. *American Review of Respiratory Diseases*, **144**(4), 826–32.
4. Mahler, D.A. *et al.* (1996). Descriptors of breathlessness in cardiorespiratory diseases. *American Journal of Respiratory and Critical Care Medicine*, **154**(5), 1357–63.
5. Harver, A. *et al.* (2000). Descriptors of breathlessness in healthy individuals: distinct and separable constructs. *Chest*, **118**(3), 679–90.
6. Wilcock, A., *et al.* (2002). Descriptors of breathlessness in patients with cancer and other respiratory diseases. *Journal of Pain and Symptom Management*, **23**(3), 182–189.
7. Bruera, E. *et al.* (1991). The Edmonton Symptom Assessment System (ESAS): a simple method for the assessment of palliative care patients. *Journal of Palliative Care*, **7**(2), 6–9.
8. Cella, D.F. *et al.* (1993). The Functional Assessment of Cancer Therapy scale: development and validation of the general measure. *Journal of Clinical Oncology*, **11**(3), 570–9.
9. Portenoy, R.K. *et al.* (1994). The Memorial Symptom Assessment Scale: an instrument for the evaluation of symptom prevalence, characteristics and distress. *European Journal of Cancer*, **30**A(9), 1326–36, Elsevier Science Limited.
10. Chang, V.T., Hwang, S.S., and Feuerman, M. (2000). Validation of the Edmonton Symptom Assessment Scale. *Cancer*, **88**(9), 2164–71.
11. Grossman, S.A. *et al.* (1991). Correlation of patient and caregiver ratings of cancer pain. *Journal of Pain and Symptom Management*, **6**(2), 53–7.
12. Clipp, E.C. and George, L.K. (1992). Patients with cancer and their spouse caregivers. Perceptions of the illness experience. *Cancer*, **69**(4), 1074–9.
13. Slevin, M.L. *et al.* (1988). Who should measure quality of life, the doctor or the patient? *British Journal of Cancer*, **57**, 109.
14. Kahn, S.B., Houts, P.S., and Harding, S.P. (1992). Quality of life and patients with cancer: a comparative study of patient versus physician perceptions and its implications for cancer education. *Journal of Cancer Education*, **7**, 241.
15. Osoba, D. (1994). Lessons learned from measuring health-related quality of life in oncology. *Journal of Clinical Oncology*, **12**, 608.
16. Jacox, A. *et al.* (1994). *Management of Cancer Pain. Clinical Practice Guideline*. No. 9. US Department of Health and Human Services, Public Health Service, Agency for Health Care Policy and Research.
17. Hinton, J. *et al.* (1996). How reliable are relatives' retrospective reports of terminal illness? Patients and relatives' accounts compared. *Social Science and Medicine*, **43**(8), 1229–36.
18. McPherson, C.J. and Addington-Hall, J.M. (2004). Evaluating Palliative Care: bereaved family members' evaluations of patient's pain, anxiety and depression. *Journal of Pain and Symptom Management*, **28**, 104–114.
19. Mularski, R. *et al.* (2004). Agreement among family members in their assessment of the quality of dying and death. *Journal of Pain and Symptom Management*, **28**, 306–315.
20. Bruera, E. *et al.* (2003). Perception of discomfort by relatives and nurses in unresponsive terminally patients with cancer: a prospective study. *Journal of Pain and Symptom Management*, **26**, 818–26.
21. Kutner J.S. *et al.* (2006). Symptom distress and quality-of-life assessment at the end of life: the role of proxy response. *Journal of Pain and Symptom Management*, **32**, 300–10.
22. Greer, D.S. *et al.* (1986). An alternative in terminal care: results of the National Hospice Study. *Journal of Chronic Diseases*, **39**(1), 9–26.
23. Morris, J.N. *et al.* (1986). Last days: a study of the quality of life of terminally ill cancer patients. *Journal of Chronic Diseases*, **39**(1), 47–62.
24. Reuben, D.B. and Mor, V. (1986). Dyspnea in terminally ill cancer patients. *Chest*, **89**(2), 234–6.
25. Mor, V. (1987). Cancer patients' quality of life over the disease course: lessons from the real world. *Journal of Chronic Diseases*, **40**, 535–44.

26. Mor, V. and Masterson-Allen, S. (1990). A comparison of hospice versus conventional care of the terminally ill cancer patient. *Oncology (Huntington)*, **4**(7), 85–91 (discussion 94, 96).

27. Higginson, I.J. and McCarthy, M. (1994). A comparison of two measures of quality of life: their sensitivity and validity for patients with advanced cancer. *Palliative Medicine*, **8**(4), 282–90.

28. The Support Study Investigators. (1995). A controlled trial to improve care for seriously ill hospitalized patients: SUPPORT. *Journal of the American Medical Association*, **274**, 1591–8.

29. Aaronson, N.K. (1990). Quality of life research in cancer clinical trials: a need for common rules and language. *Oncology*, **4**(5), 59–66.

30. Portenoy, R.K. *et al.* (1994). Symptom prevalence, characteristics and distress in a cancer population. *Quality of Life Research*, **3**(3), 183–9.

31. Dunlop, G.M. (1989). A study of the relative frequency and importance of gastrointestinal symptoms and weakness in patients with far advanced cancer. *Palliative Medicine*, **4**, 37–43.

32. Welch, J.M., Barlow, D., and Richardson, P.H. (1991). Symptoms of HIV disease. *Palliative Medicine*, **5**, 46–51.

33. Portenoy, R.K. and Hagen, N.A. (1990). Breakthrough pain: definition, prevalence and characteristics (see comments). *Pain*, **41**(3), 273–81.

34. Collins, J.J. *et al.* (2000). The measurement of symptoms in children with cancer. *Journal of Pain and Symptom Management*, **19**(5), 363–77.

35. Chang, V.T. *et al.* (2000). The memorial symptom assessment scale short form (MSAS-SF). *Cancer*, **89**(5), 1162–71.

36. Chang, V.T. *et al.* (2000). Symptom and quality of life survey of medical oncology patients at a veterans affairs medical center: a role for symptom assessment. *Cancer*, **88**(5), 1175–83.

37. Daut, R.L., Cleeland, C.S., and Flanery, R.C. (1983). Development of the Wisconsin Brief Pain Questionnaire to assess pain in cancer and other diseases. *Pain*, **17**(2), 197–210.

38. Daut, R.L. and Cleeland, C.S. (1982). The prevalence and severity of pain in cancer. *Cancer*, **50**(9), 1913–18.

39. Serlin, R.C. *et al.* (1995). When is cancer pain mild, moderate or severe? Grading pain severity by its interference with function. *Pain*, **61**(2), 277–84.

40. Paul, S.M. *et al.* (2005). Categorising the severity of cancer pain:further exploration of the establishment of cutpoints. *Pain*, **113**(1–2): 5–6.

41. Cleeland, C.S. *et al.* (1996). Dimensions of the impact of cancer pain in a four country sample: new information from multidimensional scaling. *Pain*, **67**(2–3), 267–73.

42. McCorkle, R. and Quint-Benoliel, J. (1983). Symptom distress, current concerns and mood disturbance after diagnosis of a life-threatening disease. *Social Science and Medicine*, **17**(7), 431–8.

43. NCCN Clinical Practice Guidelines in Oncology Distress Management V.1.2007. http://www.nccn.org/profession als/physician_gls/PDF/distress.pdf Last accessed February 4, 2008.

44. Mitchell A.J. (2007). Pooled Results From 38 Analyses of the Accuracy of Distress Thermometer and Other Ultra-Short Methods of Detecting Cancer-Related Mood Disorders. *Journal of Clinical Oncology*, **25**(29), 4670–81.

45. Till, J.E. (1994). Measuring quality of life: apparent benefits, potential concerns. *Canadian Journal of Oncology*, **4**(1), 243–8.

46. Aaronson, N.K., Bullinger, M., and Ahmedzai, S. (1988). A modular approach to quality of life assessment in cancer clinical trials. In *Recent Results in Cancer Research* (eds. H. Scheurlen, R. Kay, and M. Baum), p. 231. Berlin: Springer-Verlag.

47. Moinpour, C.M. *et al.* (1989). Quality of life end points in cancer clinical trials: review and recommendations. *Journal of the National Cancer Institute*, **81**(7), 485–95.

48. Moinpour, C.M. *et al.* (1990). Quality of life assessment in Southwest Oncology Group trials. *Oncology*, **4**(5), 79–84.

49. Cella, D.F. and Tulsky, D.S. (1990). Measuring quality of life today: methodological aspects. *Oncology*, **4**(5), 29–38.

50. Aaronson, N.K. (1991). Methodologic issues in assessing the quality of life of cancer patients. *Cancer*, **67**(Suppl. 3), 844–50.

51. Nayfield, S.G. *et al.* (1992). Report from a National Cancer Institute (USA) workshop on quality of life assessment in cancer clinical trials. *Quality of Life Research*, **1**(3), 203–10.

52. Aaronson, N.K. *et al.* (1993). The European Organization for Research and Treatment of Cancer QLQ-C30: a quality-of-life instrument for use in international clinical trials in oncology. *Journal of National Cancer Institute*, **85**(5), 365–76.

53. Curtis, E.B., Krech, R., and Walsh, T.D. (1991). Common symptoms in patients with advanced cancer. *Journal of Palliative Care*, **7**(2), 25–9.

54. Coyle, N. *et al.* (1990). Character of terminal illness in the advanced cancer patient: pain and other symptoms during the last four weeks of life. *Journal of Pain and Symptom Management*, **5**(2), 83–93.

55. Dunphy, K.P. and Amesbury, B.D.W. (1990). A comparison of hospice and homecare patients: patterns of referral, patient characteristics and predictors on place of death. *Palliative Medicine*, **4**, 105–11.

56. Brescia, F.J. *et al.* (1990). Hospitalized advanced cancer patients: a profile. *Journal of Pain and Symptom Management*, **5**(4), 221–7.

57. Grosvenor, M., Bulcavage, L., and Chlebowski, R.T. (1989). Symptoms potentially influencing weight loss in a cancer population. Correlations with primary site, nutritional status, and chemotherapy administration. *Cancer*, **63**(2), 330–4.

58. Ventafridda, V. *et al.* (1990). Quality-of-life assessment during a palliative care programme. *Annals of Oncology*, **1**(6), 415–20.

59. Fainsinger, R. *et al.* (1991). Symptom control during the last week of life on a palliative care unit. *Journal of Palliative Care*, **7**(1), 5–11.

60. Reuben, D.B., Mor, V., and Hiris, J. (1988). Clinical symptoms and length of survival in patients with terminal cancer. *Archives of Internal Medicine*, **148**(7), 1586–91.

61. Levine, P.M., Silberfarb, P.M., and Lipowski, Z.J. (1978). Mental disorders in cancer patients: a study of 100 psychiatric referrals. *Cancer*, **42**(3), 1385–91.

62. Derogatis, L.R. *et al.* (1983). The prevalence of psychiatric disorders among cancer patients. *Journal of the American Medical Association*, **249**(6), 751–7.

63. Ingham, J. *et al.* (1996). An exploratory study of frequent pain measurement in a cancer clinical trial. *Quality of Life Research*, **5**(5), 503–7.

64. Hwang S. *et al.* (2003). Longitudinal quality of life in advanced cancer patients: pilot study results from a VA medical centre. *Journal of Pain and Symptom Management*, **25**(3), 225–35.

65. Jacox, A., Carr, D.B., and Payne, R. (1994). New clinical-practice guidelines for the management of pain in patients with cancer. *New England Journal of Medicine*, **330**(9), 651–5.

66. Gordon, D.B. *et al.* (2005). American pain society recommendations for improving the quality of acute and cancer pain management: American Pain Society Quality of Care Task Force. *Archives of Internal Medicine*, **165**(14), 1574–80.

67. Bookbinder, M., Coyle, N., Kiss, M. *et al.* (1996). Implementing national standards for cancer pain management: program model and evaluation. *Journal of Pain and Symptom Management*, **12**(6), 334–47.

68. Foley, K.M. (1995). Pain relief into practice: rhetoric without reform. *Journal of Clinical Oncology*, **13**(9), 2149–51.

69. Velikova, G. *et al.* (1999). Automated collection of quality-of-life data: a comparison of paper and computer touch-screen questionnaires. *Journal of Clinical Oncology*, **17**(3), 998–1007.

70. Carlson, L.E. *et al.* (2001). Computerized quality-of-life screening in a cancer pain clinic. *Journal of Palliative Care*, **17**(1), 46–52.

71. Taenzer, P. *et al.* (2000). Impact of computerized quality of life screening on physician behaviour and patient satisfaction in lung cancer outpatients. *Psycho-oncology*, **9**(3), 203–13.

72. Cull, A. *et al.* (2001). Validating automated screening for psychological distress by means of computer touchscreens for use in routine oncology practice. *British Journal of Cancer*, **85**(12), 1842–9.

73. Velikova, G. *et al.* (2002). Computer-based quality of life questionnaires may contribute to doctor–patient interactions in oncology. *British Journal of Cancer,* **86**(1), 51–9.

74. Chang, C.H., *et al.* (2002). Real-time clinical application of quality-of-life assessment in advanced lung cancer. *Clinical Lung Cancer,* **4**(2), 104–9.

75. Davis, K., *et al.* (2007) An innovative symptom monitoring tool for people with advanced lung cancer: a pilot demonstration. *Journal of Supportive Oncology,* **5**(8), 381–7.

76. Foley, K.M. (1993). Pain assessment and cancer pain syndromes. In *Oxford Textbook of Palliative Medicine* (eds. D. Doyle, G. Hanks, and N. Macdonald), pp. 148–65. Oxford: Oxford University Press.

77. Cherny, N.I. and Portenoy, R.K. (1994). Cancer pain: principles of assessment and syndromes. In *Textbook of Pain* (eds. P.D. Wall and R. Melzack), pp. 787–823. Edinburgh: Churchill Livingstone.

78. Ingham, J.M. and Portenoy, R.K. (1996). Symptom assessment. In *Hematology/Oncology Clinics of North America* (eds. N.I. Cherny and K.M. Foley), pp. 21–40. Philadelphia PA: WB Saunders.

79. Sui, A.L., Reuben, D.B., and Moore, A.A. (1994). Comprehensive geriatric assessment. In *Principles of Geriatric Medicine and Gerontology* (ed. W.R. Hazzard *et al.*), pp. 203–11. New York: McGraw-Hill.

80. Pecoraro, R.E., *et al.* (1979). Validity and reliability of a self-administered health history questionnaire. *Public Health Reports,* **94**, 231–8.

81. Brodman, K., *et al.* (1949). The Cornell Medical Index, an adjunct to medical interview. *Journal of the American Medical Association,* **140**, 530–4.

82. Coyle, N., *et al.* (1996). Development and validation of a patient needs assessment tool (PNAT) for oncology clinicians. *Cancer Nursing,* **19**(2), 81–92.

83. Au, E., *et al.* (1994). Regular use of a verbal pain scale improves the understanding of oncology inpatient intensity. *Journal of Clinical Oncology,* **12**(12), 2751–5.

84. Bookbinder, M., *et al.* (2002). A 10-year review of quality improvement monitoring in pain management: recommendations for standardized outcome measures. *Pain Management Nursing,* **3**(4), 116–30.

85. Miller, A.B., *et al.* (1981). Reporting results of cancer treatment. *Cancer,* **47**, 207–14.

86. Donnelly, S. and Walsh, D. (1995). The symptoms of advanced cancer. *Seminars in Oncology,* **22**(No. 2, Suppl. 3), 67–72.

87. Burgess, A.P., Irving, G., and Riccio, M. (1993). The reliability and validity of a symptom checklist for use in HIV infection: a preliminary analysis. *International Journal of STD and AIDS,* **4**, 333–8.

88. Osoba, D. (1993). Self-rating symptom checklists: a simple method for recording and evaluating symptom control in oncology. *Cancer Treatment Reviews,* **19**(Suppl. A), 43–51.

89. de Haes, J.C.J.M., *et al.* (1987). Evaluation of the quality of life of patients with advanced ovarian cancer treated with combination chemotherapy. In *The Quality of Life of Cancer Patients,* (ed. N.K. Aaronson and J. Beckman), pp. 217–25. New York: Raven Press.

90. de Haes, J.C.J.M., van Kippenberg, F.C.E., and Neijt, J.P. (1990). Measuring psychological and physical distress in cancer patients: structure and application of the Rotterdam Symptom Checklist. *British Journal of Cancer,* **62**, 1034–8.

91. Bruera, E., *et al.* (1990). Palliative care in a cancer center: results in 1984 versus 1987. *Journal of Pain and Symptom Management,* **5**(1), 1–5.

92. Stiefel, F., Fainsinger, R., and Bruera, E. (1992). Acute confusional states in patients with advanced cancer. *Journal of Pain and Symptom Management,* **7**(2), 94–8.

93. Schipper, H., *et al.* (1984). Measuring the quality of life of cancer patients: The Functional Living Index-Cancer: development and validation. *Journal of Clinical Oncology,* **2**(5), 472–83.

94. Morrow, G.R., Lindke, J., and Black, P. (1992). Measurement of quality of life in patients: psychometric analyses of the Functional Living Index-Cancer (FLIC). *Quality of Life Research,* **1**, 287–96.

95. Ganz, P.A., *et al.* (1992). The CARES: a generic measure of health related quality of life for patients with cancer. *Quality of Life Research,* **1,** 19–29.

96. Stewart, A.L., Hays, R.D., and Ware, J.E. (1988). The MOS short-form general health survey: reliability and validity in a patient population. *Medical Care,* **26,** 724–35.

97. Holland, J.C. (1997). Preliminary guidelines for the treatment of distress. *Oncology (Huntington),* **11**(11A), 109–14 (discussion 115–17).

98. Mock, V., *et al.* (2000). NCCN Practice Guidelines for cancer-related fatigue. *Oncology (Huntington),* **14**(11A), 151–61.

99. Payne, R. (1998). Practice guidelines for cancer pain therapy. Issues pertinent to the revision of national guidelines. *Oncology (Huntington),* **12**(11A), 169–75.

100. Mock, V., *et al.* (2003). Cancer-related fatigue NCCN Clinical Practice Guidelines in Oncology. *Journal of the National Comprehensive Cancer Network,* **1,** 308–331.

101. Max, M.B. and Lynne, J. Symptom Research Interactive Clinical Textbook. National Institute of Dental and Craniofacial Research. http://painconsortium.nih.gov/symptomresearch/ Last accessed February 4, 2008.

102. Ganz, P.A., *et al.* (2007). Patient-reported outcomes assessment in cancer trials. *Journal of Clinical Oncology,* **25**(32), 5049–140.

103. Creekmore, S.P., Urba, W.J., and Longo, D.L. (1991). Principles of the clinical evaluation of biological agents. In *Biologic Therapy of Cancer* (eds. V.T. Devita, S. Hellmen, and S.A. Rosenberg), pp. 67–86. Philadelphia PA: Lippincott Co.

104. Kaplan, R.M., *et al.* (1989). The Quality of Well-Being Scale: applications in AIDS, cystic fibrosis, and arthritis. *Medical Care,* **27,** 35–49.

105. Wu, A.W., *et al.* (1991). A health status questionnaire using 30 items from the Medical Outcomes Study. *Medical Care,* **29**(8), 786–98.

106. Wachtel, T., *et al.* (1992). Quality of life in persons with human immunodeficiency virus infection: measurement by the Medical Outcomes Study instrument (see comments). *Annals of Internal Medicine,* **116**(2), 129–37.

107. Cleary, P.D., *et al.* (1993). Health-related quality of life in persons with acquired immune deficiency syndrome. *Medical Care,* **31**(7), 569–80.

108. Bozzette, S.A., *et al.* (1994). A Perceived Health Index for use in persons with advanced HIV disease: derivation, reliability and validity. *Medical Care,* **32**(7), 716–31.

109. Functional Assessment of Chronic Illness Therapy. www.facit.org Accessed February 4, 2008.

110. O'Brien, P. *et al.* (2001). Feasibility of computer-assisted, immediate quality of life (QOL) monitoring in lung cancer. In *Proceedings of ASCO* Vol. 20, abstract 1865. Program Proceedings American Society of Clinical Oncology. 37th Annual Meeting. Published by the American Society of Clinical Oncology, produced and printed by Lippincott, Williams and Wilkins, Philadelphia.

111. Millsopp L., *et al.* (2006). A feasibility study of computer-assisted health-related quality of life data collection in patients with oral and pharyngeal cancer. *International Journal of Oral and Maxillofacial Surgery,* **35,** 761–4.

112. Revicki D.A., *et al.* (2006). Responsiveness and minimal important differences for patient reported outcomes. *Health and Quality of Life Outcomes,,* **4,** 70.

113. Chang, V. and Ingham, J.M. (2003). Symptom control: a review. *Cancer Investigations.* **21**(4) 564-578.

114 Cook, R.J. and Sackett, D.L. (1995). The number needed to treat: a clinically useful measure of treatment effect. *British Medical Journal,* **310,** 452–4.

115. Zech, D.F., *et al.* (1995). Validation of World Health Organization Guidelines for cancer pain relief: a 10-year prospective study. *Pain,* **63,** 65–76.

116. Serlin, R.C., *et al.* (1995). When is cancer pain mild, moderate or severe? Grading pain severity by its interference with function. *Pain,* **61**(2), 277–84.

117. Rothenberg, M.L., *et al.* (1996). A rationale for expanding the endpoints for clinical trials in advanced pancreatic carcinoma. *Cancer*, **78**(3 Suppl.), 627–32.

118. Rothenberg, M.L., *et al.* (1996). A phase II trial of gemcitabine in patients with 5-FU-refractory pancreas cancer (see comments). *Annals of Oncology*, **7**(4), 347–53.

119. Burris, H.A., III, *et al.* (1997). Improvements in survival and clinical benefit with gemcitabine as first-line therapy for patients with advanced pancreas cancer: a randomized trial. *Journal of Clinical Oncology*, **15**(6), 2403–13.

120. Given, B., *et al.* (2008). Establishing Mild, Moderate, and Severe Scores for Cancer-Related Symptoms: How Consistent and Clinically Meaningful Are Interference-Based Severity Cut-Points? *Journal of Pain and Symptom Management*, **35**(2), 126–35.

121. Bandolier Library. Palliative and Supportive Care. http://www.jr2.ox.ac.uk/bandolier/booth/booths/pall.html. Last accessed February 4, 2008.

122. Walsh D. and Rybicki L. (2006). Symptom clustering in advanced cancer. *Support Care Cancer*, **14**, 831–6.

123. Kirkova J., *et al.* (2006). Cancer symptom assessment instruments: a systematic review. *Journal of Clinical Oncology*, **24**, 1459–73.

124. Chang V.T., *et al.* (2004). Shorter symptom assessment instruments: the Condensed Memorial Symptom Assessment Scale (CMSAS). *Clinical Investigation*, **22**(4), 526–36.

125. Nelson J.E., *et al.* (2001). Self-reported symptom experience of critically ill cancer patients receiving intensive care. *Critical Care Medicine*, **29**, 277–82.

126. Stein K.D., *et al.* (2003). Validation of a modified Rotterdam Symptom Checklist for use with cancer patients in the United States. *Journal of Pain and Symptom Management*, **26**, 975–89.

127. Kukull, W.A., McCorkle, R., and Driever, M. (1986). Symptom distress, psychosocial variables and survival from lung cancer. *Journal of Psychosocial Oncology*, **4**, 91–104.

128. Cleeland C.S., *et al.* (2000). Assessing symptom distress in cancer patients: The M.D. Anderson Symptom Inventory. *Cancer*, **89**, 1634–46.

129. Mendoza, T.R., *et al.* (1999). The rapid assessment of fatigue severity in cancer patients: use of the Brief Fatigue Inventory. *Cancer*, **85**(5), 1186–96.

130. Stark, R.D. (1988). Dyspnoea: assessment and pharmacological manipulation. *European Respiratory Journal*, **1**(3), 280–7.

131. Cockcroft, A., Adams, L., and Guz, A. (1989). Assessment of breathlessness. *Quarterly Journal of Medicine*, **72**(268), 669–76.

132. McCord, M. and Cronin, S.D. (1992). Operationalizing dyspnea: focus on measurement. *Heart and Lung*, **21**(2), 167–79.

133. Eakin, E.G., Kaplan, R.M., and Ries, A.L. (1993). Measurement of dyspnoea in chronic obstructive pulmonary disease. *Quality of Life Research*, **2**(3), 181–91.

134. Mahler, D.A. and Harver, A. (2000). Do you speak the language of dyspnea? *Chest*, **117**(4), 928–9.

135. Mahler D.A. (2006). Mechanisms and Measurement of Dyspnea in Chronic Obstructive Pulmonary Disease. *The Proceedings of the American Thoracic Society*, **3**, 234–8.

136. Brown, M.L., *et al.* (1986). Lung cancer and dyspnea: the patient's perception. *Oncology Nursing Forum*, **13**(5), 19–23.

137. Bruera, E., *et al.* (1993). Effects of oxygen on dyspnoea in hypoxaemic terminal-cancer patients. *Lancet*, **342**(8862), 13–14.

138. Roberts, D.K., Thorne, S.E., and Pearson, C. (1993). The experience of dyspnea in late-stage cancer. Patients' and nurses' perspectives. *Cancer Nursing*, **16**(4), 310–20.

139. Chen, L., *et al.* (2007). Psychometric validation of the Patient Symptom Assessment in Lung Cancer instrument for small cell lung cancer. *Current Medical Research and Opinion*, **23**(11), 2741–52.

140. Melzack, R. (1975). The McGill pain questionnaire: major properties and scoring methods. *Pain*, **1**, 277–99.

141. Graham, C., *et al.* (1980). Use of the McGill Pain Questionnaire in the assessment of cancer pain: replicability and consistency. *Pain*, **8**, 377–87.

142. Melzack, R. (1987). The short-form McGill Pain Questionnaire. *Pain*, **30**, 191–7.

143. Fishman, B., *et al.* (1987). The Memorial Pain Assessment Card. A valid instrument for the evaluation of cancer pain. *Cancer*, **60**(5), 1151–8.

144. DeConno, F., *et al.* (1994). Pain measurement in cancer patients: a comparison of six methods. *Pain*, **57**, 161–6.

145. Caraceni A., *et al.* (2005). Cancer pain assessment in clinical trials. A review of the literature (1999-2002). *Journal of Pain and Symptom Management*, **29**, 507–19.

146. Folstein, M.F., Folstein, S.E., and McHugh, P.R. (1975). Mini-mental state. *Journal of Psychiatric Research*, **12**, 189–98.

147. Katzman, R., *et al.* (1983). Validation of a short orientation–memory–concentration test of cognitive impairment. *American Journal of Psychiatry*, **140**(6), 734–9.

148. Bruera, E., *et al.* (1992). Cognitive failure in patients with terminal cancer: a prospective study. *Journal of Pain and Symptom Management*, **7**(4), 192–5.

149. Fainsinger, R.L., Tapper, M., and Bruera, E. (1993). A perspective on the management of delirium in terminally ill patients on a palliative care unit. *Journal of Palliative Care*, **9**(3), 4–8.

150. Lipowski, Z.J. (1987). Delirium (acute confusional states). *Journal of the American Medical Association*, **258**(13), 1789–92.

151. Levkoff, S.E., *et al.* (1992). Delirium. The occurrence and persistence of symptoms among elderly hospitalized patients. *Archives of Internal Medicine*, **152**(2), 334–40.

152. Breitbart, W. and Strout, D. (2000). Delirium in the terminally ill. *Clinics in Geriatric Medicine*, **16**(2), 357–72.

153. Exton-Smith, A.N. (1961). Terminal illness in the aged. *Lancet*, **2**, 305–8.

154. Witzel, L. (1975). Behavior of the dying patient. *British Medical Journal*, **2**, 81–2.

155. Massie, M.J., Holland, J., and Glass, E. (1983). Delirium in terminally ill cancer patients. *American Journal of Psychiatry*, **140**(8), 1048–50.

156. Breitbart, W., Gibson, C., and Tremblay, A. (2002). The delirium experience: delirium recall and delirium-related distress in hospitalized patients with cancer, their spouses/caregivers, and their nurses. *Psychosomatics*, **43**(3), 183–94.

157. Smith, M.J., Breitbart, W.S., and Platt, M.M. (1995). A critique of instruments and methods to detect, diagnose, and rate delirium. *Journal of Pain and Symptom Management*, **10**(1), 35–77.

158. Caraceni, A. and Grassi, L. (2003). *Delirium: Acute Confusional States in Palliative Medicine*. Oxford: Oxford University Press;

159. American Psychiatric Association. (2000). *Diagnostic and Statistical Manual of Mental Disorders*, 4th edition. Washington DC: American Psychiatric Association.

160. Inouye, S.K., *et al.* (1990). Clarifying confusion: the confusion assessment method. *Annals of Internal Medicine*, **113**, 941–8.

161. Albert, M.S., *et al.* (1992). The delirium symptom interview: an interview for the detection of delirium symptoms in hospitalized patients. *Journal of Geriatric Psychiatry and Neurology*, **5**(1), 14–21.

162. Trzepacz, P.T., Baker, R.W., and Greenhouse, J. (1988). A symptom rating scale for delirium. *Psychiatry Research*, **23**, 89–97.

163. American Psychiatric Association. (1987). *Diagnostic and Statistical Manual of Mental Disorders* 3rd, revised edition. Washington DC: American Psychiatric Association.

164. Breitbart, W., *et al.* (1997). The Memorial Delirium Assessment Scale (see comments). *Journal of Pain and Symptom Management*, **13**(3), 128–37.

165. Grassi, L., *et al.* (2001). Assessing delirium in cancer patients: the Italian versions of the Delirium Rating Scale and the Memorial Delirium Assessment Scale. *Journal of Pain and Symptom Management*, **21**(1), 59–68.

166. Breitbart, W., Tremblay, A., and Gibson, C. (2002). An open trial of olanzapine for the treatment of delirium in hospitalized cancer patients. *Psychosomatics*, **43**(3), 175–82.

167. Matsuoka, Y., *et al.* (2001). Clinical utility and validation of the Japanese version of Memorial Delirium Assessment Scale in a psychogeriatric inpatient setting. *General Hospital Psychiatry,* **23**(1), 36–40.

168. Mancini, I., *et al.* (2002). Supportive and palliative care: experience at the Institut Jules Bordet. *Supportive Care in Cancer,* **10**(1), 3–7.

169. Hjermstad, M., *et al.* (2004). Methods for assessment of cognitive failure and delirium in palliative care patients:implications for practice and research. *Palliative Medicine,* **18**(6), 494–506.

170. Cella, D., *et al.* (1998). Progress towards guidelines for the management of fatigue. *Oncology,* **12**(11A), 369–77.

171. Wagner, L.I. and Cella, D. (2004). Fatigue and cancer: causes, prevalence and treatment approaches. *British Journal of Cancer,* **91**, 822–8.

172. Cella, D., *et al.* (2001). Cancer-related fatigue: Prevalence of proposed diagnostic criteria in a United States sample of cancer survivors. *Journal of Clinical Oncology,* **19**, 3385–91.

173. NCCN Clinical Practice Guidelines in Oncology Management V.1.2007 http://www.nccn.org/profession als/physician_gls/PDF/ fatigue.pdf Last accessed February 4 2008.

174. Smets, E.M., *et al.* (1993). Fatigue in cancer patients. *British Journal of Cancer,* **68**(2), 220–4.

175. Glaus, A. (1993). Assessment of fatigue in cancer and non-cancer patients and in healthy individuals. *Supportive Care in Cancer,* **1,** 305–15.

176. Winningham, M.L., *et al.* (1994). Fatigue and the cancer experience: the state of the knowledge. *Oncology Nursing Forum,* **21**(1), 23–34.

177. Portenoy, R.K. (2001). Fatigue. In *Interactive Clinical Research Textbook* Chapter 9 (eds. M. Max and J. Lynn). Symptom Research Interactive Clinical Textbook. National Institute of Dental and Craniofacial Research. http://painconsortium.nih.gov/ symptomresearch/ Last accessed February 4, 2008.

178. Richardson, A. (1998). Measuring fatigue in patients with cancer. *Supportive Care in Cancer,* **6**(2), 94–100.

179. Mallinson, *et al.* (2006). Giving meaning to measure: linking self-reported fatigue and function to performance of everyday activities. *Journal of Pain and Symptom Management,* **31**, 229–41.

180. Ahlberg, K., *et al.* (2003), Assessment and management of cancer-related fatigue in adults. *The Lancet,* **362**(9384), 640–50.

181. McNair, D., Lorr, M., and Deoppleman, L.F. (1971). *Profile of Mood States Manual.* San Deigo CA: Educational and Industrial Testing Service.

182. Brunier, G. and Graydon, J. (1996). A comparison of two methods of measuring fatigue in patients on chronic haemodialysis: visual analogue versus Likert scale. *International Journal of Nursing Studies,* **33**(3), 338–48.

183. Cella, D.F., *et al.* (1987). A brief POMS measure of distress for cancer patients. *Journal of Chronic Diseases,* **40**(10), 939–42.

184. Aaronson, N.K., *et al.* (1993). The European Organization for Research and Treatment of Cancer QLQ-C30: a quality-of-life instrument for use in international clinical trials in oncology. *Journal of the National Cancer Institute,* **85**(5), 365–76.

185. Pearson, P.G. and Byars, G.E. (1956). *The Development and Validation of a Check List Measuring Subjective Fatigue.* Randolf AFB TX: School of Aviation, USAF.

186. Yoshitake, H. (1971). Relations between the symptoms and feelings of fatigue. *Ergonomics,* **14**, 175–96.

187. Haylock, P.J. and Hart, L.K. (1979). Fatigue in patients receiving localized radiation. *Cancer Nursing,* **2**(12), 461–7.

188. Kobashi-Schoot, J.A.M., *et al.* (1985). Assessment of malaise in cancer patients treated with radiotherapy. *Cancer Nursing,* **8**(6), 306–13.

189. Piper, B.F., *et al.* (1989). The development of an instrument to measure the subjective dimension of fatigue. In *Key Aspects of Comfort. Management of Pain, Fatigue and Nausea* (eds. S.G. Funk et al.), pp. 199–208. New York: Springer Publishing Company.

190. Piper, B.F., *et al.* (1998). The revised Piper Fatigue Scale: psychometric evaluation in women with breast cancer. *Oncology Nursing Forum,* **25**(4), 677–84.

191. Lee, K.A., Hicks, G., and Nino-Murcia, G. (1991). Validity and reliability of a scale to assess fatigue. *Psychiatry Research,* **36**, 291–8.

192. Glaus, A. (1998). Fatigue in patients with cancer. Analysis and assessment. *Recent Results in Cancer Research,* **145**, I–XI, 1–172.

193. Yellen, S.B., *et al.* (1997). Measuring fatigue and other anemia-related symptoms with the Functional Assessment of Cancer Therapy (FACT) measurement system. *Journal of Pain and Symptom Management,* **13**(2), 63–74.

194. Okuyama, T., *et al.* (2000). Development and validation of the cancer fatigue scale: a brief, three-dimensional, self-rating scale for assessment of fatigue in cancer patients. *Journal of Pain and Symptom Management,* **19**(1), 5–14.

195. Schwartz, A.L. (1998). The Schwartz Cancer Fatigue Scale: testing reliability and validity. *Oncology Nursing Forum,* **25**(4), 711–17.

196. Smets, E.M., *et al.* (1995). The Multidimensional Fatigue Inventory (MFI) psychometric qualities of an instrument to assess fatigue. *Journal of Psychosomatic Research,* **39**(3), 315–25.

197. Bruera, E., *et al.* (1987). Methylphenidate associated with narcotics for the treatment of cancer pain. *Cancer Treatment Reports,* **71**(1), 67–70.

198. Bruera, E., *et al.* (1989). Use of methylphenidate as an adjuvant to narcotic analgesics in patients with advanced cancer. *Journal of Pain and Symptom Management,* **4**(1), 3–6.

199. Bruera, E., *et al.* (1992). The use of methylphenidate in patients with incident cancer pain receiving regular opiates. A preliminary report. *Pain,* **50**(1), 75–7.

200. Bruera, E., *et al.* (1992). Neuropsychological effects of methylphenidate in patients receiving a continuous infusion of narcotics for cancer pain. *Pain,* **48**(2), 163–6.

201. Mock, V., *et al.* (1997). Effects of exercise on fatigue, physical functioning, and emotional distress during radiation therapy for breast cancer. *Oncology Nursing Forum,* **24**(6), 991–1000.

202. Larson, J.L., *et al.* (1996). Reliability and validity of the 12-minute distance walk in patients with chronic obstructive pulmonary disease. *Nursing Research,* **45**(4), 203–10.

203. Jadad A., *et al.* (2004). Measuring symptom response to pharmacological interventions in patients with COPD: a review of instruments used in clinical trials. *Current Medical Research and Opinion,* **20**(12), 1995–2005.

204. Dudgeon, D. (2002). Multidimensional assessment of dyspnea. In *Issues in Palliative Care Research* (eds. R. Portenoy and E. Bruera), pp. 83–96. New York: Oxford University Press.

205. Janson-Bjerklie, S., Carrieri, V.K., and Hudes, M. (1985). The sensations of dyspnea. *Nursing Research,* **35**(3), 154–9.

206. Simon, P.M., *et al.* (1989). Distinguishable sensations of breathlessness induced in normal volunteers. *American Review of Respiratory Diseases,* **140**, 1021–7.

207. O'Neill, P.A., *et al.* (1986). The effect of indomethacin on breathlessness in patients with diffuse parenchymal disease of the lung. *British Journal of Diseases of the Chest,* **80**(1), 72–9.

208. de Torres, J.P., *et al.* (2002). Power of outcome measurements to detect clinically significant changes in pulmonary rehabilitation of patients with COPD. *Chest,* **121**(4), 1092–8.

209. Wilson, R.C. and Jones, P.W. (1989). A comparison of the visual analogue scale and modified Borg scale for the measurement of dyspnea during exercise. *Clinical Science,* **76**, 277–82.

210. Stark, R.D., *et al.* (1983). Effects of codeine on the respiratory responses to exercise in healthy subjects. *British Journal of Clinical Pharmacology,* **15**(3), 355–9.

211. Eakin, E.G., Kaplan, R.M., and Ries, A.L. (1993). Measurement of dyspnea in chronic obstructive pulmonary disease. *Quality of Life Research,* **2**, 181–91.

212. Borg, G. (1970). Perceived exertion as an indicator of somatic stress. *Scandinavian Journal of Rehabilitation Medicine,* **2–3**, 92–8.

213. Borg, G. (1982). Psychophysical bases of perceived exertion. *Medicine and Science in Sports and Exercise,* **14**(5), 377–81.

214. Gift, A.G. (1989). Clinical measurement of dyspnea. *Dimensions of Critical Care Nursing,* **8,** 210–16.

215. Dhand, R., Kalra, S., and Malik, S.K. (1988). Use of visual analogue scales for assessment of the severity of asthma. *Respiration,* **54**(4), 255–62.

216. Research Council Committee on the Aetiology of Chronic Bronchitis. (1960). Standardized questionnaires on respiratory symptoms. *British Medical Journal,* **2,** 1665.

217. Thoracic Society. (1978). Recommended respiratory disease questionnaires for use with adults and children in epidemiological research. *American Review of Respiratory Diseases,* **118,** 7–53.

218. Mahler, D., *et al.* (1984). The measurement of dyspnea: contents, inter-observer agreement, and physiologic correlates of two new clinical indexes. *Chest,* **85,** 751–8.

219. Cullen, D.L. and Rodak, B. (2002). Clinical utility of measures of breathlessness. *Respiratory Care,* **47**(9), 986–93.

220. Mahler, D.A. (2000). How should health-related quality of life be assessed in patients with COPD? *Chest,* **117**(Suppl. 2), 54S–7S.

221. Smoller, J., *et al.* (1996). Panic, anxiety, dyspnea and respiratory disease. Theoretical and clinical considerations. *American Journal of Critical Care Medicine,* **154,** 6–17.

222. Dorman, S. (2007). Which measurement scales should we use to measure breathlessness in palliative care? A systematic review *Palliative Medicine,* **21,** 177–91.

223. Tanaka, K., *et al.* (2000). Development and validation of the Cancer Dyspnea Scale: a multidimensional brief self-rating scale. *British Journal of Cancer,* **82,** 800–5.

224. Henoch, I., *et al.* (2006). Validation of a Swedish version of the Cancer Dyspnea Scale. *Journal of Pain and Symptom Management,* **31,** 353–61.

225. Deyo, R.A. and Patrick, D.L. (1989). Barriers to the use of health status measures in clinical investigation, patient care, and policy research. *Medical Care,* **27**(Suppl. 3), S254–68.

226. VonRoenn, J.H., *et al.* (1993). Physician attitudes and practice in cancer pain management: a survey from the Eastern Cooperative Oncology Group. *Annals of Internal Medicine,* **119,** 121–6.

227. Donovan, M., Dillon, P., and McGuire, L. (1987). The incidence and characteristics of pain in a sample of medical–surgical outpatients. *Pain,* **30,** 69–87.

228. Lipowski, Z.J. (1990). *Delirium: Acute Confusional States.* New York: Oxford University Press.

229. Lawlor, P.G., *et al.* (2000). Occurrence, causes, and outcome of delirium in patients with advanced cancer: a prospective study. *Archives of Internal Medicine,* **160**(6), 786–94.

230. Stark, R.D., Gambles, S.A., and Chatterjee, S.S. (1982). An exercise test to assess clinical dyspnoea: estimation of reproducibility and sensitivity. *British Journal of Diseases of the Chest,* **76**(3), 269–78.

231. Ganz, P.A., *et al.* (1988). Estimating the quality of life in a clincal trial of patients with metastatic lung cancer using the Karnofsky Performance Status and the Functional Living Index-Cancer. *Cancer,* **61,** 849.

232. Selby, P. and Robertson, B. (1987). Measurement of quality of life in patients with cancer. *Cancer Surveys,* 6, 521–43.

233. Parmelee, P.A., Smith, B., and Katz, I.R. (1993). Pain complaints and cognitive status among elderly institution residents. *Journal of the American Geriatric Society,* 41(5), 517–22.

234. Ferrell, B.A., Ferrell, B.R., and Rivera, L. (1995). Pain in cognitively impaired nursing home patients. *Journal of Pain and Symptom Management,* 10(8), 591–8.

235. McCaffery, M. and Pasero, C., (eds.) (1999). *Pain Clinical Manual.* Mosby Inc., 2nd edition.

236. Sengstaken, E.A. and King, S.A. (1993). The problems of pain and its detection among geriatric nursing home residents. *Journal of the American Geriatric Society,* **41**(5), 541–4.

237. Pautex S., *et al.* (2006). Pain in severe dementia: self-assessment or observational scales? *Journal of the American Geriatrics Society,* **54,** 1040–5.

238. Pautaex, S.D., *et al.* (2006). Pain in Severe Dementia: Self-Assessment or Observational Scales? *Journal of the American Geriatrics Society,* **54,** 1040–5.

239. Baker, A., *et al.* (1996). Chronic pain management in cognitively impaired patients: a preliminary research project. *Perspectives,* **20**(2), 4–8.

240. Simons, W. and Malabar, R. (1995). Assessing pain in elderly patients who cannot respond verbally. *Journal of Advanced Nursing,* **22**(4), 663–9.

241. Kovach, C.R., *et al.* (2002). The assessment of discomfort in dementia protocol. *Pain Management Nursing,* **3**(1), 16–27.

242. McCarthy, M. (1990). Hospice patients: a pilot study in 12 services. *Palliative Medicine,* **4,** 93–104.

243. Perkins, P., *et al.* (2008). What are patients' priorities for palliative care research? -- a questionnaire study. *Palliative Medicine,* **22,** 7–12.

244. Cleeland, C.S., *et al.* (1994). Pain and its treatment in outpatients with metastatic cancer. *New England Journal of Medicine,* **330,** 592–6.

245. Cunningham, W.E., *et al.* (1995). Comparison of health-related quality of life in clinical trial and nonclinical trial human immunodeficiency virus-infected cohorts. *Medical Care,* **33**(4), AS15–25.

246. Townsend, J., *et al.* (1990). Terminal cancer care and patients' preference for place of death: a prospective study. *British Medical Journal,* **301**(6749), 415–17.

247. Karoly, P. (1991). Assessment of pediatric pain. In *Children in Pain: Clinical and Research Issues from a Developmental Perspective* (eds. J.P. Bush and S.W. Harkins), pp. 59–82. New York: Springer-Verlag.

248. Manne, S.L. and Andersen, B.L. (1991). Pain and pain-related distress in children with cancer. In *Children in Pain: Clinical and Research Issues from a Developmental Perspective* (eds. J.P. Bush and S.W. Harkins), pp. 337–72. New York: Springer-Verlag.

249. Matthews, J.R., McGrath, P.J., and Pigeon, H. (1993). Assessment and measurement of pain in children. In *Pain in Infants, Children and Adolescents* (eds. N.L. Schechter, C.B. Berde, and M. Yaster). Baltimore MD: Williams and Wilkins.

250. Gaffney, A., McGrath, F., and Dick, B. (2003). Measuring pain in children: Developmental and instrument issues. In *Pain in Infants, Children and Adolescents* (eds. N.L. Schechter, C.B. Berde, and M. Yaster), pp. 128–41. Philadelphia: Lippincott Williams and Wilkins.

251. Jay, S., *et al.* (1987). Cognitive–behavioral and pharmacologic interventions for childrens' distress during painful medical procedures. *Journal of Consulting and Clinical Psychology,* **55,** 860–5.

252. Katz, E., Kellerman, J., and Ellenberg, L. (1987). Hypnosis in the reduction of acute pain and distress in children with cancer. *Journal of Pediatric Psychology,* **12,** 379–94.

253. LeBaron, S. and Zeltzer, L.K. (1984). Assessment of pain and anxiety in children and adolescents by self-reports, and a behavior checklist. *Journal of Consulting and Clinical Psychology,* **52**(5), 729–38.

254. Kuttner, L., Bowman, M., and Teasdale, M. (1988). Psychological treatment of distress, pain and anxiety for children with cancer. *Developmental and Behavioral Pediatrics,* **9,** 374–81.

255. Manne, S., *et al.* (1990). Behavioral intervention to reduce child and parent distress during venipuncture. *Journal of Consulting and Clinical Psychology,* **58,** 565–72.

256. Jay, S. and Elliott, C. (1984). Behavioral observation scales for measuring childrens' distress: the effects of increased methodological rigor. *Journal of Consulting and Clinical Psychology,* **52,** 1106–7.

257. Elliott, C., Jay, S., and Woody, P. (1987). An observational scale for measuring childrens' distress during medical procedures. *Journal of Pediatric Psychology,* **12,** 543–51.

258. Gauvain-Piquard, A., *et al.* (1987). Pain in children aged 2–6 years: a new observational rating scale elaborated in a pediatric oncology unit—a preliminary report. *Pain,* **31,** 177–88.

259. Zeltzer, L.K., *et al.* (1988). Can children understand and use a rating scale to quantify somatic symptoms? Assessment of nausea and vomiting as a model. *Journal of Consulting and Clinical Psychology,* **56**(5), 567–72.

260. Tye, V.L., *et al.* (1993). Chemotherapy induced nausea and emesis in pediatric cancer patients: external validity of child and parent emesis ratings. *Developmental and Behavioral Pediatrics,* **14**(4), 236–41.

261. Hunt, A. (2006). Pain Assessment. In: *Oxford Textbook for Palliative Care for Children* (eds. Ann Goldman, Richard Hain, and Stephen Liben), pp. 281–303. Oxford University Press.

262. Seeman, I. (1992). National Mortality Followback Survey: 1986 Summary, United States National Center for Health Statistics. *Vital and Health Statistics,* **20**(19).

263. Saunders, C. (1984). Pain and impending death. In: Textbook of Pain (eds. P. Wall and R. Melzack), pp. 472–8. New York: Churchill Livingstone.

264. Hinton, J.M. (1963). The physical and mental distress of the dying. *Quarterly Journal of Medicine,* **32**(125), 1–21.

265. Ingham, J.M., *et al.* (1994). Pain and distress in cancer patients during the dying process. *American Pain Society Abstracts,* No. 94623, November.

266. Waxler-Morrison, N., Anderson, J.M., and Richardson, E., (eds.) (1990). *Cross Cultural Caring: A Handbook for Health Professionals in Western Canada.* University of BC Press.

267. Cleeland, C.S. and Ryan, K.M. (1994). Pain assessment: global use of the Brief Pain Inventory. *Annals of the Academy of Medicine Singapore,* **23**(2), 129–38.

268. Cleeland, C.S., *et al.* (1988). Multidimensional measurement of cancer pain: comparisons of US and Vietnamese patients. *Journal of Pain and Symptom Management,* **3**(1), 23–7.

269. Dunlop, R.J. and Campbell, C.W. (2000). Cytokines and advanced cancer. *Journal of Pain and Symptom Management,* **20,** 214–32.

270. Reyes-Gibby, C.C., *et al.* (2007). Cytokine genes and pain severity in lung cancer: exploring the influence of TNF-alpha-308 G/A IL6-174G/C and IL8-251T/A. *Cancer Epidemiological Biomarkers,* **16**(12), 2745–51.

271. Inagaki, M., *et al.* (2008). Plasma interleukin-6 and fatigue in terminally ill cancer patients. *Journal of Pain Symptom Management.* **35**(2),153–61.

7.8

Quality of life in palliative care-principles and practice

Stein Kaasa and Jon Håvard Loge

Introduction

Quality of life (QOL) is the main goal of palliative care. This is not a new idea; one of the main goals of the health-care system in ancient Greece was to improve what we might now interpret as the patients' QOL[1]. Improvement of patients' quality of life has therefore been and will be an overall goal for palliative care and health care in general.

In a sociological context, QOL is described in theories of human welfare (defined as level of education, economic, and industrial growth). Studies from the 1950s found that economic improvement did not necessarily result in greater levels of happiness, lower levels of worries, or a better outlook[2]. It was recognized that there was need for alternative indicators of welfare in addition to the economic and material indicators used at that time. On this background, indicators of human welfare, based upon subjects' perceptions, were developed. Different terminologies have been used by different groups to describe this phenomenon of subjective well-being; subjective indicators, general well-being, or QOL[3,4]. The common denominators were that the respondents' perceptions were asked for and that the information was collected by means of interviews or questionnaires.

Despite the widespread use of the term QOL as a theoretical concept, in politics and in empirical studies, no precise agreed-upon definition exists. However, in order to simplify the discussion on the content of the term, one may target two general approaches in the understanding of its meanings. Firstly, QOL may be regarded as a broad concept that encompasses 'how is your life, everything taken in consideration' and, secondly, QOL may be regarded as a more distinct health-oriented concept focusing on specific aspects of health or health care, including symptom levels and functioning. These are not mutually exclusive concepts, but rather a continuum of issues between two extremes allowing an intuitive flexibility in defining quality of life in terms of an overall general phenomenon or as a single sign or symptom, as illustrated in Fig. 7.8.1.

Overall QOL

Both in a sociological, psychological, and medical context, quality of life has been used as a broad concept. One major distinction is between QOL as a social phenomenon in which access to health care, education, etc. are seen as indicators of QOL and QOL as a subjective phenomenon in which the individual's subjective perception is the indicator of QOL. The different definitions of QOL in the latter meaning, all connect psychological, mental, and spiritual domains of a person's life. In the process of finding indicators of these phenomena satisfaction, happiness, morale, positive and negative effects have been put forward as important components of the QOL concept. In some of the literature there is an emphasis on normality, viewing QOL as fulfilment of life and the possibilities to live a normal life, while others focus more on mental capacity, to think clearly, to feel well, to love and be loved, to make decisions for oneself, to maintain contact with family and friends, to live at home and/or to be physically active. The ability to make individual decisions has also been emphasized as an important aspect of quality of life, including capacity of the individual to realize his life, which includes a perception of personal meaning.

According to these conceptualizations, QOL is strongly linked to normality, including normal function or that a minimum of human needs are met. Such a minimum of needs were also described by Maslow[5], which is often referred to as 'Maslow's needs hierarchy', consisting of biological needs, needs for close relationships, needs for meaningful occupation, and need for change. This concept has further been elaborated in a QOL context viewing quality of life as the level of a person's activity, the quality to relate to others, self-esteem, and a basic mood of happiness[6].

Inclusion of normality and biological fulfilment into the global QOL concept is strongly challenged by empirical findings of many patients with major physical and/or psychological limitations who report a high degree of global quality of life[7]. These empirical findings fit well with another theory, the so-called gap theory of Calman[8]. He described QOL as an inverse relationship to the difference between an individual's expectations and their perception

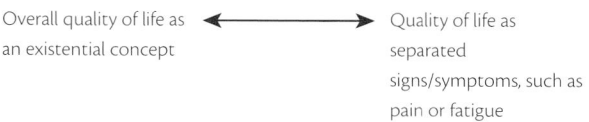

Overall quality of life as an existential concept ⟷ Quality of life as separated signs/symptoms, such as pain or fatigue

Figure 7.8.1 Quality of life as a continuum from existentiality to single symptoms.

of the given situation, 'the smaller the gap the better quality of life'. According to this gap theory, as illustrated in Fig. 7.8.2, a change in QOL from T0 to T1 can be caused by changes in both expectations and experience, case A and B report the same QOL at T0 and T1; however, the underlying causes of the change from T0 to T1 is different in the two individuals.

The gap theory may be used to explain unexpected findings between groups and within groups over time in intervention studies. In other words, one needs to explore the magnitude of all relevant factors that may contribute to changes. This is especially important to consider in non-controlled intervention studies that use subjective outcomes.

QOL in medicine

In health-care research, QOL encompasses a range of components, which are measurable and related to health, disease, illness, and medical interventions. In health care as well as in other contexts, QOL might have different meanings for different actors and take different meanings according to illness, experience, support, etc. A professional focus may also influence the perception of QOL. For example, a medical oncologist may rate tumour response after delivering combination chemotherapy to a patient with a non-Hodgkin's lymphoma as the most important achievement to improve QOL, while a nurse may focus on patients' ability to deal with daily activities. For a physician in palliative medicine, improvement of QOL for one patient may mean pain control, and for another the establishment of necessary social support. In the context of clinical trials, one is rarely interested in QOL as a global concept, but rather as a specific outcome related to the intervention in question, such as improved pain control during night time by delivery of slow-release morphine at bedtime or reduced dyspnoea after chest irradiation for a patient with lung cancer. Despite the unresolved issue about how to define QOL, most researchers and clinicians agree that QOL in palliative medicine is related to symptom control, physical function, social functioning, psychological well-being, and meaning and fulfilment (existential and spiritual issues). This multi-dimensional health-oriented concept has been named by many clinicians and researchers as health-related quality of life (HRQOL)[9–13].

As early as 1947 did the World Health Organization (WHO) by its definition of health describe health as multi-dimensional: 'Health is not only the absence of infirmity and disease, but also a state of complete physical, mental and social well-being'[14]. This definition has been identified by several researchers as the beginning of a new era in relation to health and health care. In spite of

being highly disputed, the definition includes three dimensions of health that later have been included in the HRQOL concept; physical health, mental health, and social functioning.

Another event that subsequently influenced the development of the QOL concept in health care was proposed by Karnofsky in 1948. He evaluated the palliative effects of nitrogen mustard on various malignant tumours by means of subjective improvement, objective improvement, and performance status[15]. Performance status was defined according to specific criteria, which have become widely used and known as the Karnofsky Performance status scale (Table 7.8.1). This simple scale has been shown to be a significant predictor of survival in patients with metastatic disease, as have measurers of HRQOL[16–19]. In a recent topical review it was advocated for the use of complementary prognostic factors such as indicators of cachexia, dyspnoea, delirium, and some biological factors[20].

During the 1970s standardized questionnaires were developed in cooperative groups and in academic settings. 'Linear analogue self-assessment scales' (LASAs) were used to capture the QOL of specific cancer groups, such as breast-cancer patients. These measures included a variety of subjective domains, such as general well-being, mood, anxiety, activity, pain, and social activity[10,12]. Others developed measures of health status in order to capture patients' general perceptions of health; some examples are the Sickness Impact Profile[9], Nottingham Health Profile[21], SF-36[22,23], and

Table 7.8.1 Performance status.

Definition	Percentage (%)	Criteria
Able to carry on normal activity and to work; no special care is needed	100	Normal; no complaints; no evidence of disease
	90	Able to carry on normal activity; minor signs or symptoms of disease
	80	Normal activity with effort; some signs or symptoms of disease
Unable to work; able to live at home, care for most personal needs; a varying amount of assistance is needed	70	Cares for self; unable to carry on normal activity or to do active work
	60	Requires occasional assistance; but is able to care for most of his needs
	50	Requires considerable assistance and frequent medical care
Unable to care for self; requires equivalent of institutional or hospital care; disease may be progressing rapidly	40	Disabled; requires special care and assistance
	30	Severely disabled; hospitalization is indicated although death not imminent
	20	Very sick; hospitalization necessary; active supportive treatment necessary
	10	Moribund; fatal processes progressing rapidly
	0	Dead

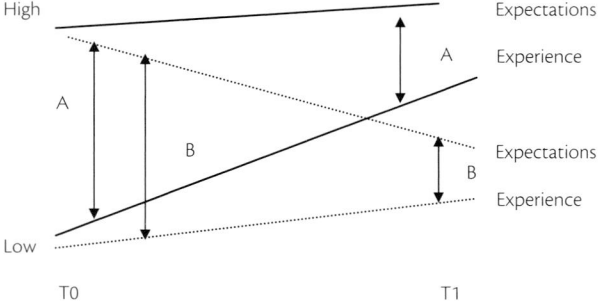

Figure 7.8.2 Quality of life as the gap between expectations and experience.

more physically oriented scales such as the Barthel index[13]. Other measures, which are also classified as QOL measures focus primarily on psychological domains, such as the General Health Questionnaire (GHQ)[11] and Profile of Mood States[24].

At the same time, a similar development of measures were seen within the area of pain assessment based upon the definition of pain launched by The International Association for the Study of Pain (IASP). IASP defined pain as 'an unpleasant sensory and emotional experience associated with actual or potential tissue damage, or described in terms of such damage'[25]. These definitions are conceptually very similar to most definitions of QOL and the WHO definition of health in that the subjective perception of the individual is recognized as the key component of health, pain, and QOL, respectively. Previously pain measurement had involved standardized external stimulants, such as radiant heat, which were used to obtain a psychophysiological standard to measure clinical pain. A 'language of pain' was developed, which is well illustrated by the McGill Pain Questionnaire (MPQ)[26]. More simple tools were also used to assess pain intensity, such as Verbal Rating Scales (VRS), Numerical Rating Scales (NRS), and Visual Analogue Scales (VAS)[27].

Most of the measurement tools for HRQOL, pain, and other aspects of subjective health are built upon the questionnaire concept, in which a standardized paper-based questionnaire is to be filled in by the patients. This approach is more or less well suited for palliative care patients. For severely ill patients, assessment by means of interviews or standardized observations may be more appropriate. Interviews are flexible and provide detailed information but are expensive and time-consuming to perform. Further, their usefulness is often limited in multi-centre trials where HRQOL is often assessed at several time points [28].

Standardized observations of behaviours or functions are alternatives to self-report questionnaires for assessment in specific groups of palliative patients such as pain assessment in cognitively impaired or assessment of functioning such as Activities of Daily Living (ADL). On a theoretical level one may dispute whether these are assessments of QOL since the observer's and not the patients' perceptions are registered. On a practical level we do not know the optimal assessment method for a given situation. For example, is physical functioning best assessed by asking the patient or by observing him/her? At what level of cognitive impairment is pain best assessed by standardized observations of behaviour and not by asking the patient? In spite of these and the other unresolved issues, assessment of QOL by use of questionnaires has become the far most commonly used approach. The questionnaires are nearly always in paper-format, but can also be administered in an electronic format[29].

Patient-reported outcomes and QOL

Another term, patient-reported outcomes (PROs), has been launched in order to improve the terminology in relation to measurement of patients' subjective health status. A PRO has been defined as a measurement of any aspect of a patient's health status that comes directly from the patient, without the interpretation of the patient's responses by a physician or anyone else. This implies that the term PROs is an umbrella that covers a wide range of measurements but is used specifically about questionnaires that are completed by the patient. Quality of life is in this context considered a broad concept referring to all aspects of a person's well-being. PROs can measure quality of life in this broad meaning of the term, but PROs can also focus more narrowly on a single symptom such as pain or on a function such as physical functioning[30,31].

The introduction of the term PROs must be understood in the context of manufacturers' claims of treatments' positive effects upon patients' QOL. Such claims should be documented by an evaluation of the impact of a given treatment on all aspects of a person's well-being since QOL in its broad meaning includes assessment of the physical aspects of disease (i.e. symptoms and function), the person's emotional state, feelings, coping behaviours, self-identity (psychological functioning), and the person's ability to interact with others (social functioning)[31]. In most cases, however, claims by manufacturer on a treatment's positive effect on QOL have not been based upon such a broad assessment. In most cases, the claims are based upon improvement in specific domains such as reduced levels of pain or less fatigue. A 'guidance for industry' on these issues published by the US Food and Drug Administration is a strong support for the relevance of outcomes based upon patients' reports but also restricts the use of the term QOL to a more clearly specified situation than has been practiced by most until now[31].

Plethora of publications and instruments

The enormous increase in publications indexed under the subject heading QOL in MEDLINE reflects the increased focus on the patients' QOL during the last 35–40 years. Seven papers were published in the period of 1966–1970 while nearly 25 000 papers were published 2001–2005 (Table 7.8.2). The rapidly increasing number of papers and newly developed questionnaires are a reminder of the ambiguity of the concept QOL but also represent a challenge for the researcher and the clinician when they shall select the most appropriate assessment tool for their purpose.

A textbook published in 1996 included more than 200 different measures of quality of life[32]. A recently established data-base on PROs and QOL Instruments (the PROQOLID®) includes descriptions of 612 instruments, 475 review copies of original instruments, review copies of 746 translations, and review copies of 161 user manuals[33].

Many of these questionnaires have not been developed based upon explicit definitions and operationalizations of the phenomena they are supposed to measure. Different wordings of the same phenomena across different questionnaires exemplified by fatigue versus vitality and psychological functioning versus mental health underline the lack of precision, both on the levels of single items (indicators), multi-item scales, as well as which domains (areas) to include in the assessment tool. On a meta-level, this increase in

Table 7.8.2 Number of papers indexed in MEDLINE under the keywords 'Quality of Life' 1961–2005.

1961–1965	1966–1970	1971–1975	1976–1980	1981–1985	1986–1990	1991–1995	1996–2000	2001–2005
0	7	205	1134	1666	3539	7299	13 573	24 707

papers and questionnaires points to a need for collaboration on development of a common nomenclature, as well as standardized and agreed-upon assessment tools. These suggestions have been put forward by several research groups for at least a decade both in HQoL-assessment in general[34] and in palliative care specifically[35,36]. Despite these suggestions, it was recently found that, in the area of pain assessment, new instruments are still developed and published[37]. Most of the instruments are rarely used in later empirical studies.

HRQOL in palliative care

The goals of palliative care are acknowledged to include HRQOL as well as spirituality, loss/grief, family involvement and coping. Many of the most common HRQOL tools have been thought inadequate by researchers for use in palliative care. The instruments have been criticized for being too narrow by only including physical, psychological, and social aspects of a patient's life. Thus outcome measures require questions that reflect the specific goals of palliative care[38], such as improving the quality of life before death, controlling symptoms, and supporting the family (Table 7.8.3). It has been proposed that also meaning should be included, as well as purpose, spirituality, and grief[39–41].

During end-stage disease, patients will often not be able to complete HRQOL instruments and proxies will be the only possible source of collection of information, either by means of interviews (open, semi-structured, or structured) or questionnaires. One possible strategy is to let the health-care provider or the family member complete the HRQOL instrument. However, many studies have shown that assessments by health-care providers or family members differ from the responses obtained from the patients. In some conditions observers overestimate the psychological burden of disease, while pain and other symptoms are often underestimated.

In summary, HRQOL is perceptions of a patient's health that are collected directly from the patient without the interpretation of others. It is a dynamic phenomenon and different dimensions might be focused, depending upon individual factors, disease factors, symptomatology, coping ability, closeness to death, etc. The content is influenced by the setting, i.e. the severity of physical symptoms, general health, spirituality, coping, existentially, etc. Still there is a general agreement to at least include symptomatology, physical, psychological, and social domains into the measures, and in many circumstances, existential and spiritual domains also seem appropriate to include.

Table 7.8.3 HRQOL measurement in palliative care.

Content of measures: dimensions:
- ◆ Symptoms
- ◆ Physical function
- ◆ Emotional function
- ◆ Existential issues (spirituality)

Proxy ratings:
- ◆ Health-care providers
- ◆ Family members

Quality of life:
- ◆ Patient and family assessment

Measurement theory

HRQOL is regarded as an 'underlying concept', which is abstract, not directly observable, individual and multi-dimensional. The experience from clinical practice can be used to better understand the practicalities related to measurement theory. In a clinical interview, specific questions are asked in order to gain knowledge about the phenomena in question. In order to communicate about an abstract phenomenon, one needs to agree upon a definition of the concept, how to explore the concept, and how to summarize the findings. In other words, an accurate description of a subjective phenomenon depends upon how the concept is defined, how data is collected, processed, and communicated.

It is well documented that reliable and valid information is best collected by standardized procedures, such as a standard clinical interview and standard clinical examination. Both include specified standards for collection of data, documentation routines, interpretation, and communication in patients' records and orally to colleagues.

For example, fatigue is generally agreed to be an important dimension of HRQOL in palliative care. A set of items or questions often based upon clinical experience in the first hand, but also based upon existing measures might be derived to measure fatigue. At present attempts to measure fatigue objectively have failed. Theoretically, as illustrated in Fig. 7.8.3, the three questions Q1, Q2, and Q3 should all contribute to measure the level of fatigue in palliative care patients. The number of items needed to measure a given concept depends upon factors such as the complexity of the phenomenon in question and how precisely we want our observations to be. Precision can be expressed as reliability, which will be improved by increasing the number of items.

Validity and reliability

Reliability is linked to the reproducibility of a measure, such as a lab test, an X-ray, or a QOL measure. The basic idea is that under different circumstances the underlying concept is constant and the measure captures the concept across contextual variations. In more technical terms, reliability is an estimate of the degree of random error of any given measurement. There are different ways to estimate reliability in QOL research. The most common procedure is to estimate the internal consistency of a uni-dimensional score. This pre-supposes that all the items address the same underlying dimension. The estimate will represent the average correlations among all of the items in the measure. Cronbach's alpha is often used as an expression of these correlations[42]. Stability or reproducibility is another estimate of reliability. This might be about the degree of agreement between observers (interobserver reliability)

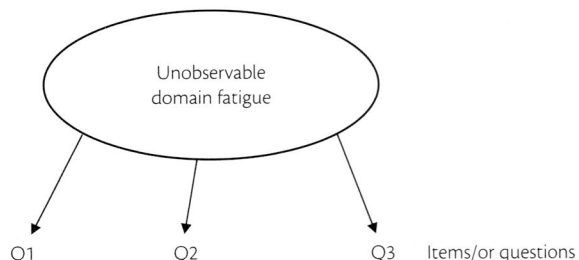

Figure 7.8.3 An unobservable domain is measured by items.

or between observations on the same patients on two different occasions (test–retest reliability).

Validity refers to whether the test measures what it is intended to measure. If there is an established instrument, which measures the underlying phenomenon, for example, anxiety, this instrument can be used as the gold standard. By comparing the new instrument to the old, estimates of validity can be calculated. However, in QOL assessments in general, no gold standard exists, which means that indirect methods must be used in order to establish the validity of the new instrument. The approach of construct validation is often used, which is based upon a theory of a given construct, for example, physical function or fatigue. Validity in this context is defined as the extent to which a method measures the underlying construct in question[43]. The validity is not a 'fixed' property of an instrument, and may change when the context and study population changes. The terminology of validity testing can be confusing. Most authors, however, agree that there are three basic types of validity: content, criterion, and construct validity (the three Cs).

Content validity

'Content validity'—or the related, 'face validity'—refers to the extent to which the scale looks reasonable. The face validity indicates whether, on the face of it, the instrument appears to assess the desired qualities, while the content validity is a judgement of whether the questionnaire samples all the relevant and important dimensions we are interested in. There is no specific technique for testing content validity; the judgement is usually based on a review and consensus by an expert panel of health-care workers and/or patients.

Criterion validity

Criterion validity is the correlation of a scale with some other measure of the dimensions under study, ideally a gold standard. It is usually divided into concurrent and predictive validity.

Concurrent validity is established by comparing a new method with the old way of assessment, with both assessments performed at the same time. In laboratory medicine a criterion or a standard is often used to calibrate a new instrument. Since there is no established gold standard for measuring patients' QOL, quite often new scales are compared with old ones, which might have sub-optimal validity. Another approach is to use indirect methods of comparisons, such as observer- or interview-based ratings. This can introduce difficulties in the interpretation of the results. If an expected association between, for example, a questionnaire and an observer rated instrument is not confirmed, it is difficult to tell whether the questionnaire or the observer-rated instrument, or both, have low validity. Predictive validity is a measure of the extent to which the questionnaire can predict an event or a test result in the future. The results from a screening instrument for psychological distress could, for example, be compared with the level of psychiatric morbidity assessed by a clinical interview at a later point in time.

Construct validity

Construct validity relates to the extent to which the instrument assesses an unobservable, hypothetical construct we are interested in, such as pain, fatigue, or anxiety. Construct validity is an ongoing process where the questionnaire and the underlying construct must be tested in various studies. However, if the test results do not support our hypotheses, it is difficult to tell whether the questionnaire has low construct validity or whether the construct is wrong or both. Pain, for example, can be defined as a uni-dimensional construct. If a pain questionnaire is found to assess several dimensions, the questions should be carefully examined and eventually revised—or alternatively the assumption of pain as a uni-dimensional construct should be re-evaluated.

Hypothesized constructs can be written as a model, and the goodness of fit can be examined by confirmatory factor analyses. The construct validity of scales such as a psychological distress scale can also be estimated by comparing results between extreme groups such as patients with or without anxiety and depression in a clinical interview. By testing the convergent validity and discriminant validity, the correlations between the new instrument and other assessment methods are reviewed. A high correlation is expected between scales assessing similar constructs such as between an anxiety scale and a mental distress scale (convergent validity). A low correlation is expected between instruments assessing different constructs such as between an anxiety scale and a scale assessing physical function (discriminant validity).

Patient population

Patient population in palliative care and compliance with QOL assessment tools

There are several issues one must take into account when assessing HRQOL in palliative care. The patients are sick and disabled. Valid and reliable data may therefore be difficult to collect, particularly in the latest stages of life. Patients have often several symptoms at the same time and physical symptoms may give raise to psychological problems (and vice versa). These relationships in palliative care in general and specifically in end-of-life care have been discussed and addressed empirically.

What is a palliative care population?

A palliative care population is not a well-defined group of patients. In some programmes most patients are dying while in others the majority of the patients have a longer life expectancy. In discussing the use of methodology to collect HRQOL data, the patient population in question should be specified. Several indicators might be used to describe the population, such as expected survival, type of tumour-directed treatment, do-not-resuscitate (DNR) status, symptom burden, type of oncological treatment, etc. Most patients in trials on palliative chemotherapy have a performance status above 60–70 and, consequently, an expected survival of more than 6 months with large variations depending upon the primary diagnosis. A second category of patients are those admitted to a palliative care programme, either as inpatients or as outpatients, but not imminently dying, often with an average survival of 1 to 3 months. And the third category may be the imminently dying patients with a Karnofsky performance status of 30–40 and lower. This latter category can be further divided into cognitively intact and cognitively impaired patients (Table 7.8.4).

The content of the assessment tools, the total length of instrument, and the use of proxy raters are some of the important issues to consider in relation to the patient population being investigated.

Table 7.8.4 Patient population in palliative care.

	A suggestion of classification	
	Expected survival	**Karnofsky**
Primary palliation	> 6 months	60–70
Early palliation	2–3 months	50–60
Late palliation	<1 month	30–0
Immediately dying	< 1–2 weeks	< 10

Compliance and patient population

Missing data can be defined as data which could be anticipated but are not returned. There are two main types of missing data: missing items (item non-response) and missing forms (unit non-response). The first relates to an uncompleted question within a QoL instrument and the second to a whole QoL assessment being missing. Missing data is a potential source of selection bias in cancer research, quality assurance programmes, and in research in palliative medicine[44]. Randomly missing data are not a problem except for some possible loss of power. Usually 1–2 per cent of the responses to a given item within a questionnaire will be missing. However, in most cases, missing data are a mixture of randomly missing data and data missing not at random[45]. When data are missing for some patients, basic questions arise as to whether the patients with missing data differ from those with complete data set. The patients in poorest health and with the shortest life expectancy are at the highest risk for both types of missing data[46]. In order to evaluate a scientific report and to compare cohorts between studies a standard reporting system of compliance, including all available information should be required. Compliance is often defined as the number of questionnaires completed as a proportion of the number expected. The issue of compliance is described in more detail in textbooks[47] and in statistical literature[48]. In this chapter, some issues relating to compliance in palliative care will be discussed.

When patients become increasingly ill with progressive disease, they will find it difficult to complete questionnaires. Acceptable compliance can be achieved with HRQOL questionnaires in palliative care, though several patients will need assistance to complete the measures. During end-of-life care, the last 1–2 months of the patient's life, more patients will need help to complete the assessment tools due to cognitive impairment, severe symptom distress, and/or emotional burdens, and consequently, compliance decreases substantially if help is not provided[49] (Fig. 7.8.4). Patients who are immediately dying will experience many distressing symptoms, but if they are excluded from not just research, but quality assurance, and in evaluating clinical practice, there is a great risk for lack of empirical knowledge needed for development of systematic treatment procedures for this fragile population[50].

Based upon these facts, there are two main strategies in relation to missing data. The first is to reduce the risk for missing data to a minimum. This will include careful consideration of the length of the questionnaire, collection of data by use of optimal procedures for the population at stake, standardized procedures for data collection, and careful observation of the data collection especially towards 'gate-keeping', which implies that the data collector for some reason want to shield the patient from participation.

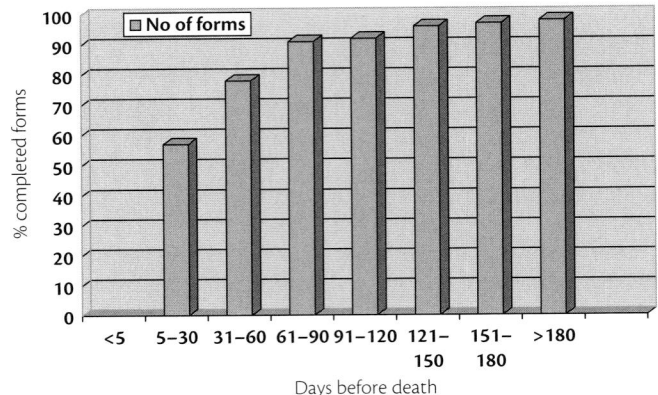

Figure 7.8.4 Number of HRQOL forms completed in proportion to those distributed within various time frames prior to patients' death.

The ethics are clear on this point, it is the eligible patient's right to choose to participate or not. The second strategy is to carefully analyse for systematic patterns of missing data (both missing forms and missing items) in order to discover a biased data set.

Proxy ratings

Proxies may be considered as an alternative or complementary source of information, especially during end-of-life care[51]. However, there has been a general negative attitude towards the use of proxy rating in the HRQOL literature because it has been repetitively demonstrated that assessment directly from the patient is the most valid way of collecting subjective data.

Review articles[52,53] and commentaries[54,55] have been written on the topic of caregivers and significant others as raters. Most of the published articles, which address this issue, relate to general cancer populations or those in 'early palliation'. The studies have been criticized because of small sample sizes, major limitations in methodology, and use of unstandardized ad hoc instruments. The findings of the published studies are not totally consistent; however, they can be summarized as follows:

- Health-care providers tend to overestimate patients' anxiety, depression, and general psychological distress.
- Agreement between health-care providers and patients' ratings was better in the absence of distress, than in the presence of distress.
- Pain and other symptoms seem to be underestimated by proxies.
- Proxy rating seems to be more accurate when the domains are concrete and observable.

There are several unanswered questions related to the use of proxy raters (Table 7.8.5): the limitation of proxy data, the content

Table 7.8.5 Limitations of proxy ratings.

- A better understanding of when and why proxy ratings and patients' ratings differ
- Simpler and shorter assessment tools
- Instruments with known psychometric properties, a clinically understandable measure, and directly comparable to a patient ratings

of proxy rating instruments and the development of a common measure.

Even with these limitations caregivers or health-care providers can be used as proxy raters and it is probably best to use one of the short validated tools in order to compare data between studies and allow for familiarity of measures for the clinicians. The COOP/WONCA chart[56], Edmonton Symptom Assessment Schedule (ESAS)[57] or EORTC QOLQ C-30[58] are examples of such instruments. Another alternative is the SF-8[59]. However, the SF-8 has not been validated in palliative care populations. This instrument has the advantage that it can be scored on the same measures as the SF-36 scales and its summary measures[23].

However, before proxy ratings can be recommended outside a methodological research setting in palliative care, measurement tools and report systems need to be further developed into a user-friendly format and the strengths and limitations of proxy ratings need to be further addressed in research settings.

Questionnaires

The rapidly increasing number of questionnaires available makes it a challenge to choose the right measure. As outlined earlier in this chapter, new instruments are developed and validated after locally or nationally initiatives without any international anchoring or consensus. For updated reviews of candidate instruments, we refer to electronic databases such as the PROQOLID®[33]. In the following, a comprehensive presentation of instruments for use in palliative medicine will not be given; instead, some principles with concrete recommendations will be outlined.

The first step in the selection procedure is to specify the overall aim of the project. This phase of the planning of the study is crucial. The overall aim needs to be followed by an outline of the specific research questions or hypotheses. For each research question, a clinical outcome should be decided upon. This will subsequently guide the selection of an assessment tool or even specific scales or items within a tool (Table 7.8.6).

It is generally recommended to assess HRQOL with multi-dimensional instruments because such measures are more comprehensive than uni-dimensional scales[60]. The HRQOL measures are commonly divided into generic, disease-specific, and domain-specific. The generic measures are not specific to any population or disease. They are therefore applicable for subjects with more than one condition, and they make comparisons across populations and conditions possible. The disease-specific measures are developed for specific groups of patients, for example, such as the EORTC-QLQ-C30 and the FACT-G[58,61] developed for cancer patients or instruments specifically developed for palliative care. Most of the instruments include various aspects of functioning such as physical, role, and social functioning and subjective appraisal of symptoms and well-being[62]. Most recent generic and disease-specific

Table 7.8.6 A generic guide for selection of outcomes.

- ◆ Step 1 Define the overall aims of the project
- ◆ Step 2 Define the research questions or hypotheses
- ◆ Step 3 Agree upon the (clinical) outcomes for each recommended question
- ◆ Step 4 Select the assessment tool or scales within a tool, guided by the clinical outcome

---

instruments also assess positive health; i.e. good health and well-being and not merely the absence of problems[63]. The domain-specific instruments assess specific domains within the overall concept of HRQOL, such as fatigue, pain, or psychological distress.

Assessments of QOL will often include combinations of generic, disease-specific, and domain-specific instruments based upon the specific purpose of the study. For example, if one wants to compare the effects of single fraction irradiation with multiple fractions in a population with painful bone metastasis, a multi-dimensional disease-specific questionnaire such as the EORTC-QLQ-C30 in combination with a domain-specific questionnaire on pain might be relevant. The number of questionnaires must fit the purpose for the assessment, but must also be balanced against the burden upon the respondents and the costs of the data collection. The increased amount of information gained by including domain-specific measures is not always obvious and is clearly dependent on the psychometric properties the content and the sensitivity of the instruments. For example, if a domain-specific instrument on fatigue does not have better measurement qualities than the fatigue scale within a generic or disease-specific instrument, it is probably best not to be included because of the increased burden to the patient.

Comparative data on different instruments measuring the same constructs are relatively scarce. The EORTC QLQ-C30 and the SF-36 were compared in patients with chronic nonmalignant pain[64]. Scales assumed to measure the same constructs were highly correlated, and for these scales, the SF-36 scales tended to have better internal consistencies. On the other hand, the EORTC QLQ-C30 includes several symptoms that are not assessed by the SF-36.

The researcher might be best off by choosing instruments that are commonly used and found relevant within similar populations and settings. By choosing commonly used instruments, one's findings can more easily be evaluated in a broader perspective. The psychometric properties of an instrument might vary across populations; therefore applying a questionnaire for the first time within a 'new population', requires testing of the psychometric properties of the instrument in that particular population. The downside of this approach is that instruments with sub-optimal measurement qualities are used repetitively due to the costs associated with the development and introduction of new instruments and possibly better instruments.

A good example of this phenomenon is the assessment of depression. Measures of depression such as the Beck Depression Inventory and Hamilton's Depression Scale was developed in the 1960s for psychiatric populations without severe physical morbidity[65,66]. These instruments include several somatic depressive symptoms, such as fatigue, weight loss, and sleeping difficulties, which confound the assessment of depression in somatically ill patients [67]. The use of these instruments in a palliative care population without testing the measurement properties in this particular population probably overestimate the prevalence of depressive symptoms by counting depressive symptoms caused by the cancer disease (i.e. the somatic symptoms) as indicators of depressive disorders. This might lead to overestimation of the prevalence of depression. Still, few attempts have been made to construct measures of depression that are less influenced by the patients' somatic status than the older instruments which are still the most commonly used[68].

In the following, some commonly used instruments are briefly discussed. This does not imply that these instruments are superior to other available instruments.

Generic instruments

The first instruments were published in the 1970s and 1980s, such as the Sickness Impact Profile (SIP)[69] and the Nottingham Health Profile[21]. For a more detailed description we refer to other reviews[32,63,70]. The first generation of instruments was generally lengthy and time-consuming to fill in.

SF-36

The Short Form 36 (SF-36) is a typical second-generation instrument, developed from a larger questionnaire[23]. Eight concepts that were not specific to any disease, age, population, or treatment group were chosen to measure health conceptualized in two main dimensions; physical and mental health (Table 7.8.7). The instrument should satisfy minimum psychometric standards necessary for group comparisons. The psychometric properties are generally very good with Cronbachs alphas in the range 0.80–0.93[22]. The instrument is available in two versions; a standard version with a time frame of 4 weeks and an acute version with a time frame of 1 week. The SF-36 has been translated into more than 80 languages, and considerable effort has been made for international harmonization of the instrument and collection of normative data through the IQOLA-project[71,72]. A revised version (Version 2) was published in 2000[73]. This version mainly differs from the first version on the two scales, measuring limitations in role functioning due to physical and emotional problems, respectively. In both these scales, the response alternatives are increased in order to reduce the floor (respondents scoring at worst possible level) and ceiling effects (respondents scoring at best possible level) which were substantial in the first version.

The SF-36 physical and mental component summary scales capture about 85 per cent of the reliable variance in the instrument[74]. On this background it was decided that a questionnaire with fewer items could be constructed. Twelve items from the SF-36 were therefore selected and the instrument labelled the SF-12[73,75], and

Table 7.8.7 Some commonly used generic and disease-specific HRQOL questionnaires.

Name	Type	Domains	No. of items	First publication.	Reference
WHOQOL	Generic	Physical Psychological Independence Social relations Environment Spirituality Overall QOL	100	1993	(76)
WHOQOL-BREF	Generic	Physical Psychological Social relations Environment	26	1998	(78)
SF-36	Generic	Health transition General health Bodily pain Physical function Role function, physical Role function, emotional Vitality Mental health Social function	36	1992	(23, 73)
SF-12	Generic	Physical Mental	12	1996	(73)
SF-8			8	2001	(59, 73)
EORTC QLQ-C30	Disease-specific (cancer)	Physical Cognitive Emotional Social + 8 symptoms	30	1993	(58, 83)
FACT-G	Disease-specific (cancer)	Physical Social/family Emotional Functional	27	1993	(61, 85)

later the even shorter SF-8[59,73]. The SF-12 reproduces the eight-scale profile of the SF-36. It yields less precise scores, as would be expected for single- and two-item scales. A revised version of the SF-12 (version 2) was published in 2002[73]. The revisions followed the same principles as used for the revision of the SF-36.

WHOQOL

The World Health Organization has developed the WHO Quality of Life Assessment Instrument (WHOQOL)[76]. The instrument was developed, according to a standardized protocol, simultaneously in several languages and cultures at 15 international centres[77]. The original instrument encompasses six domains measured by 100 items; physical health, psychological health, level of independence, social relationship, spirituality, and environment. Each domain includes several facets, in total 24. Each facet contains 4 items, and the last 4 items measure overall quality of life and general health. Because of the limitations posed upon the use of the instrument's length, a 26-item abbreviated scale has been published, primarily for use in epidemiological studies[78].

Disease-specific measures

EORTC QLQ-C30

The development of the cancer-specific questionnaires, the EORTC QLQ-C30 (European Organization for Research and Treatment of Cancer) started in 1980, and the first 30-item version was finalized in 1993[58]. Modified versions have been published and the group recommends version 3.0 of the questionnaire[79]. The questionnaire covers five functional scales (physical, role, cognitive, emotional, and social), general quality of life, three symptom scales (fatigue, pain and nausea, and vomiting), and six single items. The single items assess common symptoms in cancer patients such as dyspnoea, loss of appetite, insomnia, constipation, and diarrhoea. Two items ask for overall evaluation of health and quality of life. These two items have seven response alternatives; all the other items have four response alternatives. The scores for each functional scale, symptom scale, and single item are transformed to scales with a possible range of scores from 0 to 100. For the functional scales, a higher score means higher level of functioning. For the symptom scales/items, a higher score means a higher level of symptoms.

The timeframe for the assessment is one week, which may be of particular relevance in clinical trials. The instrument is copyrighted. The questionnaire is translated and validated in 38 languages and has been used in more than 1500 studies worldwide. The instrument has good psychometric properties including test/retest reliability[80,81]. This is an important characteristic of the instrument because it was originally developed for use in clinical trials. The instrument has also been used for other purposes such as studying the communication between patient and physician[82].

The so-called modular approach adopted by the EORTC Quality of Life Group infers that the core questionnaire can be supplemented with additional questionnaires designed for specific cancer sites [83]. By January 2008 these include disease-specific supplements for lung cancer (LC13), breast cancer (BR23), head and neck cancer (H&N35), oesophageal cancer (OES18), ovarian cancer (OV28), gastric cancer (STO22), multiple myeloma (MY20), and cervical cancer (CX24) [79]. Additionally, 15 phase-III modules are available that, among others, include modules for brain cancer, colorectal cancer, pancreatic cancer, prostate cancer, and

inpatients' satisfaction with care (EORTC IN-PATSAT32). Updates on the latest development of the EORTC questionnaires are found on the website[79].

After interviews with patients and health professionals to determine the appropriateness, relevance, and importance of the various domains and items of the QLQ-C30 for use in palliative care, a shortened version containing 15 items, the EORTC QLQ-C15-PAL, was published in 2006[84]. Item response theory methods were used to shorten scales. Pain, physical function, emotional function, fatigue, global health status/quality of life, nausea/vomiting, appetite, dyspnoea, constipation, and sleep were judged as the most important domains/items and consequently retained in the questionnaire. The EORTC QLQ-C15-PAL is a 'core questionnaire' for palliative care. Depending on the research questions or the purpose for use, it may be supplemented by additional items, modules, or questionnaires[84].

FACT-G

The Functional Assessment of Cancer – General Version (the FACT-G) was first published in 1993. In 1997 it was included as a core questionnaire in a measurement system called Functional Assessment of Chronic Illness Therapy (FACIT) intended for use in chronic diseases. Thus, FACIT is a broader, more encompassing system that includes the FACT questionnaires under its umbrella.

The FACT-G (now in Version 4) was first published in 1993 and includes 27 items arranged in subscales covering four dimensions: physical well-being, social/family well-being, emotional well-being, and functional well-being[61]. It is considered appropriate for use in patients with any type of cancer. Each of the items has five response alternatives and scores for each scale are sums of subscale scores, and a total score is also provided. The time frame is 1 week, and the psychometric properties are reported as comparable to the EORTC QLQ C30[61]. There seems to be a tendency for the FACT-G to be used more frequently in the USA than in Europe, while the EORTC QLQ-C30 is used primarily in Europe.

The FACIT measurement system has also adopted a modular approach with cancer-specific, symptom-specific, and treatment-specific subscales. Since the publishing of the first FACT-G validation paper in 1993, more than 40 questionnaires have been developed and translations to more than 45 different languages are available. These include instruments for fatigue, treatment satisfaction, spiritual well-being, HIV disease, multiple sclerosis, and other chronic conditions. An update on the complete FACIT measurement system is found at the group's website[85], http://www.facit.org/about/overview_measure.aspx.

Domain-specific measures

Generic or disease-specific instruments might not be sensitive enough for detection of differences in HRQOL. Questionnaires, also called domain-specific instruments, have been designed to assess specific symptoms, such as pain, fatigue, and anxiety. In some instances, these types of instruments might be preferable to use. For example, in a study of patients with advanced prostate cancer, the EORTC QLQ-C30 fatigue scale did not detect variations in fatigue over time whereas two fatigue-specific instruments captured group differences[86]. This finding is probably related to the so-called floor- and ceiling-effects. Numerous instruments are available and for a more comprehensive description we refer to relevant textbooks and websites[32,33,70,73,85].

Anxious and depressive symptoms

Domain-specific instruments for measurement of anxiety and depression are generally old and can be characterized as first-generation instruments. For example, the Hospital Anxiety and Depression Scale (the HADS) was constructed in 1983, but it has relatively recently been recommended for use in oncology and in palliative care[86–88]. Other commonly used instruments for measurement of depression such as the Beck Depression Inventory (BDI) and Hamilton Depression Scale (HDS) were first published as early as the 1960s[65,66].

For instruments measuring anxiety and depression in palliative care it is important to examine for somatic items (fatigue, weight-loss, loss of appetite, etc.). Such symptoms are valid symptoms of anxious and depressive conditions in psychiatric and healthy populations, and they are included in the present diagnostic criteria for these disorders[89]. However, these symptoms are not valid to measure anxiety and depression in palliative care because they may only reflect the underlying somatic disease. For example, five of the 21 items in the BDI are of a somatic nature. In spite of the relatively extensive research literature addressing this methodological challenge, many published papers do not pay attention to the consequences of including somatic items in assessments of anxiety and depression in the physically ill. The HADS is one of the most frequently used instruments for measuring anxious (seven items) and depressive symptoms (seven items) in oncology and palliative medicine. Five of the items constituting the depression subscale are about anhedonia, one item is about mood, and one is about retardation. The HADS-depression scale is probably affected by somatic status to a higher degree than previously recognized. It has been demonstrated that a total score, including both the anxiety and depression subscales is a better predictor of major depression in palliative care patients than scores on the depressive subscale[90].

A review on the prevalence of depression in palliative care identified 48 studies that used a broad spectrum of methods for assessment of depression[68]. Four studies used clinical evaluation, 14 studies used single items, 20 studies used multi-item questionnaires (15 used the HADS), and 10 studies used structured interviews and/or classified according to diagnostic criteria such as the DSM-IV[89]. If the aim of a study is to assess the prevalence of depressive disorders or to intervene, it is highly recommendable to use assessments that allow for classification according to a diagnostic system. Otherwise, the external validity of the findings can be questioned.

Fatigue

Fatigue can be defined as a subjective feeling of tiredness, weakness, or lack of energy[91]. It is the most frequent symptom in palliative care and is experienced by nearly all patients with advanced disease[92,93]. In palliative care, as opposed to healthy populations, fatigue only weakly correlates with psychological distress and probably reflects the subjective experience of being seriously ill[93].

Instruments specifically designed for measuring fatigue were first published in the late 1980s. At present several instruments are available[94–96] and most of these should be classified as first-generation instruments. A single-item with an 11-point NRS for the responses has been proposed for screening purposes[97]. The Functional Assessment of Cancer Therapy- Fatigue scale is a 13-item free-standing part of the FACT-Anaemia Scale within the FACIT measurement system[61]. The 13 fatigue items are available as a separate instrument (the FACIT-Fatigue), which is an uni-dimensional measure of physical fatigue[85]. However, most researchers agree that fatigue is a multi-dimensional phenomenon, but the number and types of dimensions is debated. All present fatigue measures include physical fatigue, which corresponds to the subjective feeling of being exhausted and lacking energy. A short (11 items) fatigue instrument (Fatigue Questionnaire (FQ)) measures fatigue in two dimensions: physical and mental fatigue[98], and is commonly used in studies of cancer-related fatigue[96]. Mental fatigue is about the subjective experience of being mentally exhausted, and the items are about concentration, memory, and speech. The FQ has good and stable psychometric properties across different populations, but the wording of the response categories might be problematic in palliative care because they ask about a comparison with what is usual. For cancer patients with active disease for several years, asking for such a comparison might be confusing.

Pain

Pain is the second-most prevalent symptom in palliative care, and for the majority of patients it is the most distressing symptom. It is well documented that pain is under-diagnosed and under-treated[99]. Pain is the aim for different interventions both clinical and for research purposes in palliative care. In most situations, pain intensity will be the main target for assessments of pain. Additional aspects such as variation in pain over time, pain triggered by physical activity, or break-through pain might be of relevance in many situations. In such cases, available instruments must be evaluated for their properties in measuring these aspects of the pain experience.

In general, pain is included as single items or as separate sub-scales in all existing generic and disease-specific instruments. In these, pain is measured as a uni-dimensional construct[100] However, it is important to underscore that pain is a complex and also a controversial area for assessment, although some of the problems are reflecting challenges for HRQOL assessments in general[100]. Some major unresolved issues in relation to pain assessments in palliative care are: to what extent shall a pain assessment include assessment of physical and emotional distress cased by pain[101] (=pain interference)? How shall pain be measured in patients receiving analgesics? How to deal with pain thresholds, which vary between individuals and with each individual's access to support? What about differentiating between specific types of pain? How to measure specific cancer pains such as break-through pain? How is pain best measured in patients with cognitive impairment who are therefore not able to respond to self-report questionnaires?

Domain-specific tools for measurement of pain such as the McGill Pain Questionnaire measure pain as a multidimensional phenomenon, but it is rather extensive and thereby difficult to apply in debilitated palliative care patients[102]. A shorter version of this instrument has been developed and validated[103]. Others, for example, the Brief Pain Inventory (BPI)[104], measure the impact of pain upon physical functioning in addition to measuring pain intensity. There is reason to question whether consequences of pain can be validly separated from functional limitations due to other factors[105]. This is of particular concern in palliative care patients due to the complexity of their diseases, the functional limitations they present, and their experience of several symptoms at the same time.

An expert working group of the European Association for Palliative Care (EAPC) recommended that selection of tools for pain assessment should be based on the study population and the specific study design[106]. The recommendations of the expert group apply to adults without cognitive impairment. For assessment of changes in pain intensity, single items with NRS were recommended while the Brief Pain Inventory short form (BPI-sf) were recommended for broader assessments[107]. The Short Form McGill Pain Questionnaire (SF-MPQ)[108] was recommended for studies of pain qualities, such as studies focusing on diagnoses and characterization of pain syndromes. For assessments in cognitively impaired, several instruments are available but not sufficiently tested for explicit recommendations[109].

Use of single items: sleeping difficulties

The use of single items either as self-constructed items or as items borrowed from a complete instrument is generally not recommended. The validity of self-constructed items is generally uncertain and moving an item from its context might affect the responses. However, if one wants to measure, for example, sleep, very few instruments include items on this important aspect of health and disease. Instead of constructing single items, it is preferable to use items that have been developed and validated as part of multi-dimensional questionnaires. The EORTC QLQ C-30 includes one item about problems with sleeping[58]. This item measures the experience of having sleeping difficulties but does not describe them in detail such as difficulties in falling asleep, frequent wakening, early wakening, or hypo- / hypersomnia. Given the importance of sleep for many patients and the high prevalence of sleep disturbances in palliative care, improved instruments for assessing sleep are required[110].

Cognitive impairment

Cognitive impairment as part of dementia, amnestic disorder, or delirium is prevalent in palliative care[111,112]. Among patients with terminal cancers, 20–40 per cent develop delirium or other neuropsychiatric conditions[113]. We are not aware of HRQOL studies in cancer patients, which have discussed their results in relation to possible cognitive impairment among the subjects. Cognitive impairment might affect completion rates, data quality, and the validity of HRQOL studies in palliative care.

Interviews conducted by health-care providers by means of specific interview guides and observation of behaviour are the appropriate methods for the detection of cognitive impairment[114]. The subjective experience of cognitive impairment is weakly related to neuropsychiatric disturbances but much stronger to psychological distress[115]. Consequently, cognitive functioning scales within HRQOL questionnaires probably measure mental fatigue rather than cognitive functioning.

The most commonly used interview-based instruments in assessments of cognitive impairment are the Mini Mental State Examination (MMSE) and the Memorial Delirium Assessment Scale (MDAS)[116,117]. Physicians or other health professionals can administer these measures without specific preparation although it is wise to compare first-time performances with more experienced personnel as part of the introduction routines into a research project or clinical practice. The MDAS is a brief, reliable tool for assessing delirium severity, while the MMSE is designed for detection of cognitive impairment irrespective of the cause or neuropsychiatric diagnosis. For the MMSE, it has been demonstrated that

the scores of selected items is equally effective as the sum-score of all the twenty items in identifying cognitive impairment in elderly patients and delirium[118,119]. However, more research is needed before such an abbreviated version can be recommended for general use.

Palliative care-specific instruments

Several instruments have been developed and validated within palliative care. A short summary of some of these will be outlined.

A short form individual quality-of-life questionnaire (SEIQOL)

The schedule for the evaluation of individual quality of life (SEIQOL) was developed in order to let the patient assess quality of life from an individual. It was designed specifically to assess three questions: what areas of life are important, how is the individual doing in each of these areas, and what is the importance of the area[120].

The SEIQOL is complex and its use in routine clinical practice may be difficult. An abbreviated form has been developed, the SEIQOL-direct weighting (SEIQOL-DW)[121] and validated in a population of advanced cancer patients[41]. It was concluded that the SEIQOL-DW seems most appropriate for routine clinical settings, while the original SEIQOL is more suitable for in-depth exploration of QOL.

Therapy-impact questionnaire (TIQ)

Therapy impact questionnaire (TIQ) is a 36-item questionnaire assessing both disease and therapy impact, and divided into four dimensions—physical symptoms, functional status, emotional and cognitive domains, and social interaction[122].

The questionnaire has been validated in a population with advanced cancer but has to our knowledge not been extensively used outside Italy.

McGill quality-of-life questionnaire (MQOL)

MQOL is a 17-item questionnaire derived from patient interviews, literature reviews, and existing instruments[123]. The instrument was designed in response to the criticism that existing HRQOL instruments in general lacked questions on existential concerns[124]. The instrument consists of five subscales, physical well-being, physical symptoms, psychological symptoms, existential well-being, and support (or relationships)[40,125]. The questionnaire was validated in a multi-centre study with patients recruited from palliative care services and later in a combined population consisting of oncology outpatients and palliative care services[126]. MQOL has been validated cross-culturally in a Hong Kong Chinese population and was found to be cross-culturally robust[127]. The reliability was satisfactory for use on a group level, but not on an individual level.

The Missoula-VITAS quality-of-life index

The subjective experience of an individual living with the interpersonal, psychological and existential, or spiritual challenges accompanying advanced diseases was used as the basic definition for the development of this instrument, focusing on the terminal phase of life[39]. The instrument includes 25 items and has been validated in a hospice setting. It covers five domains: i.e. symptoms, function, interpersonal, well-being, and spirituality. Most questions are of a global nature, including the assessment of symptoms. The instrument seems most suitable for use in the planning of care and probably in quality control.

The life evaluation questionnaire (LEQ)

The LEQ is a 45-item questionnaire developed to evaluate aspects of life that are relevant to patients with incurable cancer and that are not measured by established questionnaires[128]. The content is based upon in-depth interviews with patients and carers. The instrument consists of five main domains, freedom versus restrictions, appreciation of life, contentment, resentment, and social interaction.

McMaster quality-of-life scale (MQLS)

This measure was developed to assess QOL from the palliative care patients' perspective[129]. It is a 32-item questionnaire measuring physical, emotional, social, and spiritual domains. Each domain is subdivided into scales with low (0.09) to moderate high (0.79) internal consistencies. Each item is rated on a 7-point NRS. A parallel form is used for family and staff ratings. The inter-rater reliability was satisfactory within the patient population, while the agreement between patient and family (r = 0.64) and patient and staff (r = 0.50) was moderate.

HRQOL in the dying

Research on QOL for the dying patient is sparse—probably related to several factors, such as a lack of focus on dying patients and the dying process in general ('the battle is lost—why bother with it'). Furthermore, the dying patient is vulnerable, and the ethics related to the research is debated.

There are several methodological challenges related to HRQOL assessment in the dying, including the rapid change in most biological processes and loss of cognition, which is highly relevant to the ability to collect subjective data. As previously pointed out, there are major problems with compliance in this sub-population with the use of traditional HRQOL questionnaires. In most palliative care programmes the aim is to support the family to care for the dying at home as well as providing specialist professional care. Consequently, the team is caring for the patient in a family network. In end-of-life care, 12 important aspects of care have been identified; acceptability and continuity, team coordination and communication, communication with patients, patient education, inclusion and recognition of family, competence, pain and symptom management, emotional control, personalization, attention to patient values, respect and humanity, and support for patient decision-making[130]. Another group involved in the development of assessment tools for patients with life-limiting illness, reached similar conclusions: the outcomes should be patient focused and family-centred, clinical meaningful, administratively manageable, and psychometrically sound[131].

Quality-of-life assessment is by definition subjective in nature. In the dying patient, who is cognitively impaired, 'subjective data' needs to be collected by observers. There is a lack of validated instruments specifically designed for dying patients; however, there is a growing literature addressing measurement issues for this patient population, focusing on the development of a conceptual framework[132,133]. Recently, several attempts have been made to

develop observation-based instruments to measure pain in the cognitively impaired[109].

In summary, one may say that the patient-focused assessment recommended is very similar to the strategy developed earlier in life, focusing on symptom control and how to relieve the patient burden. However, during end-of-life care spiritual and existential issues need to be addressed in more detail in addition to family members' perception of quality of care (Table 7.8.8).

Family satisfaction, HRQOL, grief, and other domains may be used as outcomes of quality of death. A variety of instruments have been used in the published studies to examine different aspects and models of care[134–137] and no consensus on content nor on type of instruments seem to be agreed upon. In several studies a general high level of satisfaction with care has been observed and only minor differences between various palliative care programmes, which may indicate a poor ability of the existing instruments to discriminate between groups when measuring satisfaction with care and HRQOL[138–143].

Practical measurement of How to measure HRQOL during end-of-life care

The complexity, length, and content of the existing HRQOL instruments seem inappropriate for use during the dying process. Shorter and simpler instruments are needed here. To our knowledge there is no single instrument widely used for this purpose, but simple numerical rating scales (NRS) have been developed. The Edmonton symptom assessment schedule (ESAS) is a short 10-item instrument[57] and has been used extensively in several scientific reports by the Edmonton. Other symptom assessment schedules are also used, such as the Memorial Symptom Assessment Scale Short Form (MSAS-SF), which is one of the several alternatives for symptom assessment[144]. Still there is a lack of consensus on how to measure HRQOL in the dying patient. New, shorter, and more comprehensive instruments are therefore needed, which ideally could be completed by both the patient and proxy raters in sequence.

Analysis and interpretation of data

Clinical significance

What is the clinical relevance of a summary score on a single item when comparing groups of patients or individuals? This is one basic question to ask both in daily clinical practice, in interpreting clinical research and in sample size calculation in the planning process of a clinical trial. The clinical significance is related to the importance of the symptoms or the signs.

Table 7.8.8 Quality at the end of life.

Important domains
Singer: (Toronto - Canada)
◆ Symptom management
◆ Avoiding inappropriate prolongation of dying
◆ Achieving sense of control
◆ Reliving burden
◆ Strengthening of relationship between loved ones

In pain assessments, a single item on pain intensity to be answered on a numerical rating scale ranging from 0 to 10 is often used as the outcome. When discussing the clinical significance of a pain score, two important questions need to be answered. What is a relevant cut-off point in order to classify the score in need of intervention? What is the minimum difference on a pain score, say on a 0–10 scale, in a randomized trial comparing two different pain medications that is of clinical importance?

Change in any clinical variable, independent of the nature of the variable, i.e. physiological (blood pressure), psychological (anxiety), and performance (physical function), etc., needs to be interpreted in a clinical framework. It is not a methodological or statistical question whether a change of 20 on a scale from 0 to 100 is of clinical significance. In order to be able to make a valid judgement on the magnitude of a measure in order to regard it as 'clinically significant', the clinician needs at least to understand the nature of the measure, including insight into the content of the composite score, the clinical meaning of the measure and how it relates to individual patients. The discussion on clinical significance is not unique to QOL assessment. Similar discussions arise, for example, in interpreting the clinical significance of blood pressure medication, interpreting the reduction of tumour size in oncology caused by chemotherapy and the importance of change in median survival in patients with non-small-cell lung cancer admitted to a randomized chemotherapy trial.

These are some of the general problems. A more specific problem related to palliative care is the interpretation of change in several QOL estimates in the same study. QOL estimates are by nature multi-dimensional, and each estimate is often based on a summary of responses to several questions. A common metric does not apply between scales and domains (i.e. is 40 on a pain measure, similar in symptom burden to 40 on a nausea measure?). In palliative care where most patients are living with a progressive disease, improvement in overall condition cannot be expected, thus the 'improvement' expected on a single or a multiple measure may actually be nearly 'slow down' or stabilization of symptom burden. The complexity of human biology may cause increase in intensity in one symptom when another symptom is relieved. Furthermore, most patients have a mosaic of symptoms, which often needs broad interventions, and consequently one specific outcome may be difficult to identify.

Multi-dimensionality

The strength of the HRQOL concept is its multi-dimensionality; however, during analysis (see later) and in the interpretation of the outcomes, the multi-dimensionality is a challenge. Based upon a careful clinical consideration, it is recommended to identify the primary outcomes, i.e. the domains of most importance, before the study is launched. Outcomes should to be limited to two or three

Table 7.8.9 Problems related to outcome interpretation.

◆ Multi-dimensionality:	Generic
◆ Content of the measure:	Generic
◆ No common metric:	Generic
◆ Heterogenic intervention:	Palliative care-specific
◆ Multiple problems (symptoms):	Palliative care-specific
◆ Progressive disease:	Palliative care-specific

dimensions and the remaining data from the HRQOL questionnaire should be considered as additional information and can therefore not be used as indicators for change of practice.

Content of the measure

Measures may consist of multiple questions. Before any questionnaire is applied in a study, the researcher and the clinician need to investigate in detail the content of each scale. The content is the basis for a clinical understanding of the score. Without an intuitive understanding of the measure, a valid judgement of the final estimate is difficult. The use of several HRQOL instruments reduces the changes for an intuitive understanding of the outcomes. Therefore, the number of methods should be kept to a minimum both for clinical monitoring and for clinical research.

The lack of a common metric between scales within the same instrument is a problem. How much this phenomenon also influences the size of what is a clinical significant change in the instrument is still an unresolved question.

In a systematic review on HRQOL in palliative care no clear pattern was found in how various researchers address this issue[145]. In some reports a group mean change of 10 on a 0–100 scale has been proposed as a clinically significant difference[7]. Others have said that half a standard deviation is a clinically significant difference, which is close to 10 on a 0–100 scale.

Data presentation

A careful evaluation of the aims of the study is crucial in the planning process in order to determine the primary outcomes. For example, in a study of the effects of cardiocentesis for pericardial effusions in patients with advanced cancer, it is reasonable to consider pain, physical functioning, and dyspnoea as the primary outcomes and not changes on ultrasound or X-ray. The design of the study and the choice of explanatory and primary outcome variables are the main determinants in choosing the appropriate analysis strategy. The design and the variables should reflect the aims of the study, so the analytical strategy is in large parts determined before the actual analysis starts.

Lacking an important explanatory variable because it was not included in the data collection is definitely not desirable although many probably have experienced this. To avoid this, the data analyses should have been planned before the study was initiated, and ideally all tables (not the numbers) should have been constructed during the planning of the study. Clear hypotheses will definitely make this work easier and will reduce the possibilities for the researcher ending up in endless searches for significant P-values.

Still, many studies must be conducted without the possibility to perform confirmatory tests of predefined hypotheses, for example, prevalence studies. Neither can one single study support a whole series of hypotheses. It is therefore sensible to limit the number of confirmatory hypotheses, and much of the analyses therefore have to be exploratory (i.e. suggested by the data). In the latter situation it is possible to test specific hypotheses suggested by the data, but then the P-values should be used as guidelines and treated carefully.

If the limit for statistical significance is set at 0.05, then each 20th analysis will by chance reach statistical significance. Typically this occurs in univariate tests in prospective studies, where at a particular time-point a subscale demonstrates statistically significant differences between groups. This can seriously inflate the type I (false-positive) error rate. Irrespective of the possible clinical consequences, this problem makes it difficult for the researcher to distinguish between true and false-positive differences. There are several possible ways to handle this problem, although none of them are ideal, and the literature does not suggest one specific strategy. Common sense and careful consideration will always be the basis of analyses and interpretation. Possible solutions are suggested in other reviews and papers[47,146,147]. In the planning phase of a study, the problem can best be solved by stating clearly which scales within the battery of HRQOL assessments are defined as the primary outcomes (e.g. pain and fatigue). These variables will then be in the focus of the analysis, and correction for multiplicity of endpoints might perhaps be unnecessary. For the rest of the scales the number of analyses should be reduced as much as possible, and some type of correction for the multiplicity of endpoints, either by Bonferroni correction and similar methods or by the use of more conservative P-values (e.g. P<.01), must be performed. The interpretation of the latter analyses should reflect that the analyses are hypothesis generating and that the results need confirmation in later studies. For more detailed descriptions of other aspects of analyses of HRQOL-data, we refer to textbooks in medical statistics and HRQOL-assessments[32,47,148].

There is increasing focus upon a transparent presentation of research data, and we strongly advise the presentation of data in accordance with the predefined aims of the study. The CONSORT statement includes 21 items that should be presented in a paper. The essence is that the researchers shall provide enough information about the study so the reader can judge the reliability and the validity of the results[149]. In the situation described earlier, it is correct to tell the reader how the study was designed, and that the main findings were carried out as predefined secondary endpoints.

A related challenge is the treatment of criteria for statistical significance, because most HRQOL measurements include multiple endpoints and this may lead to the so-called 'multi-significance' problem. It is generally recommended to include all assessments in the presentation, but this may lead to data overload in the paper. This requires careful consideration and some pragmatism, but the presentation of the data shall always reflect the original protocol. In many instances the authors therefore end up with several endpoints, and in most cases it is therefore correct to perform some sort of adjustment for the multiplicity of endpoints, as mentioned previously.

A detailed checklist for presentation of HRQOL studies has been presented[150]. In general, this guideline is in accordance with the general rules for writing a paper. However, there are some specific points to notice for HRQOL studies apart from the points commented upon earlier. Relatively few HRQOL studies examine specific hypotheses, since observational studies are far the commonest type of study. Accordingly, the rationale for selection of HRQOL instruments should be presented. The population should be described in terms of those variables that can affect the outcome variables. These include among others, age, gender, ethnicity, educational status, functional status, timing of the assessments, compliance, data completeness, and attrition due to death[151]. In palliative care, functional status and time to death are variables that strongly influence the results of the measurements[60].

Future perspectives

Reports indicate that doctors and health professionals' recognition of subjective symptoms both in general oncology and in palliative care are suboptimal[152–154], and measurement of HRQOL has not become an integral part of clinical practice. There are probably several explanations to these shortcomings, such as the content of the measures, i.e. many of the scales may not have enough clinical relevance, clinicians do not believe in the importance of assessing subjective experience and/or the impracticalities in using comprehensive measures in daily clinical practice[155]. As an example, palliative patients' physical functioning is of central importance for clinical decisions and in clinical studies, but it was recently demonstrated that adequate measures for use in palliative care were lacking[156].

The complexity of HRQOL measures make them difficult to interpret and they are not easily accessible in the clinical decision-making process. For research purposes there are also needs for improvement of HRQOL measurements: Clinical trials often use different measures to assess the same concepts, many measures are unresponsive to changes, many represent a burden on research participants and personnel, many measures have not been validated specifically in the clinical population under study, and some/many lack adequate sufficient evidence for validity[157].

The distribution of HRQOL questionnaires in paper format has until now been the standard administration form although some studies have administered the HRQOL instruments as computer-based touch-screen programmes with promising results[29,158]. The existing measures are compromises between shortness and precision, shortness as a consequence of the paper-and-pencil format, and lack of precision because of the shortness of the questionnaire. A patient's functional capacity must be covered by relatively few items, and subjects with functional capacity at one extreme, say best possible function must answer rather irrelevant items covering the opposite extreme of the functional range. For example, a person responding that he is barely able to walk 50 m will obviously find an item about the ability to walk 2 miles irrelevant. The result is that the existing measures are somewhat imprecise and display rather large standard deviations. The latter implies that the number of participants must be high to achieve sufficient power. Most instruments also display 'floor- and ceiling-effects', which implies that a substantial number of the respondents tend towards the minimum or maximum scores of the scale, meaning that group differences will not be possible to detect. Another challenge and possible obstacle for taking fully advantage of the existing measures is the interpretation of the scores. For all published multidimensional instruments, a score of 50 on one 0–100 scale is not comparable to a numerically identical score on another scale, which is exemplified empirically in that a change in score does not relate linearly to an external criteria[75].

In palliative care measurement of symptoms may also be restricted by the patients' limited physical capacity, and even relatively short instruments are often too demanding to fill in for many patients[159]. Instruments that yield valid and reliable results with the smallest possible effort for the patients are therefore needed. Instruments that are suitable both for individual assessments (i.e. diagnosis and monitoring of individual patients) and for research have therefore obvious advantages for the clinicians, the patients, and the researchers.

Psychometric methods like the Rasch models and the Item Response Theory (IRT) have potentials to achieve precise and efficient measurement of subjective symptoms at individual patient level[160,161]. The basic idea of these methods is that a particular response to a particular item depends on the type of item (item difficulty) and on the underlying (latent) health construct. Both item difficulty and the respondent's ability are measured on the same scale or ruler. Combining IRT with a computer algorithm allows individualized selection of items to provide the most precise information for the particular patient and to score all items on a common scale. On the basis of the answer to the first question, the computer will select a new question, and in the next step, the computer will select a new question based on the answer to the second question and so forth until a pre-set level of precision is reached.

This approach can be illustrated by measurement of depression. It is demonstrated that a single question: 'Are you depressed?' is a good predictor of depression in patients with advanced cancer[162]. Assessment of depression within the IRT system could start with such a question. The next questions would then build on the answers to the first, and one will consequently achieve a precise estimation of the level of depression. CAT methodology uses a computer interface for the patient (or a computerized interview/ clinician report) that is tailored to the unique ability level of the patient. The basic notion of an adapted test is to mimic what an experienced clinician would do. A clinician learns most when he/ she directs questions at the patient's approximate level of proficiency. Administering functional items that are either too easy or too hard provides little information. An adaptive test first asks questions in the middle of the ability range, and then directs questions to an appropriate level based on the patient's responses, without asking unnecessary questions. This allows for fewer items to be administered (individual respondent, interview or clinical judgement), while gaining precise information regarding an individual's placement along a continuum of functional ability. CAT applications require a large set of items in any one functional or symptom area (item pools), items that consistently scale along a dimension of low-to-high functional proficiency, and rules guiding starting, stopping, and scoring procedures[161].

The psychometric methods that make it possible to calibrate questionnaire items on a standard metric ('ruler') also yield the algorithms necessary to run the 'engine' that powers CAT assessments. These statistical models tell how likely it is that a person at each level of health will choose each response to each survey question. This logic is reversed to estimate the probability of each health score from a particular pattern of item responses. The resulting likelihood function makes it possible to estimate each person's score, along with a person-specific confidence interval.

The computerized form will allow for more flexible ways of administering the tool, including downloading from the Internet, administration by proxies, and the employment of hand-held devices. Scores will be computed immediately and in digital form. This entire development process was strongly suggested in the *British Medical Journal* in 2001 [162]. In total, such a development can make integration with other clinical parameters easier, as patient records generally are more often stored in computerized form.

This approach to measurements of subjective symptoms and functioning has not moved outside the research laboratories although the first practical tests have been performed with success in migraine patients[161]. At present, collaboratives are working to develop PROs in health care in general[163]. For palliative care, one collaborative (EPCRC) in cooperation with European Association for Palliative Care Research Network (EAPCRN) will first develop assessment tool for pain, depression, and cachexia, based upon a stepwise approach combining systematic literature reviews with experts and patient contributions as well as empirical testings of these novel computer-based assessment tool for palliative care[35].

Summary

Quality of life is used as a term with quite differing meanings, and new terms have been suggested in order to improve the terminology. Multi-dimensional measures of HRQOL cover physical, psychological, and social aspects of life. In palliative care these measures have been criticized for not covering the existential and spiritual issues sufficiently.

A series of measures for use in health care in general (generic instruments), and for use in specific diagnostic groups, such as cancer (cancer specific) and palliative care (palliative care specific) have been developed. A third category of instruments are the domainspecific measures. The latter is developed for assessing specific symptoms or signs, such as pain, fatigue, depression, anxiety, physical function, spirituality, etc. The plethora of instruments is a challenge for the users of the instruments, the readers of scientific reports, and for the performance of meta-analyses.

Most instruments have been developed for use in research and may not be suited for use in daily clinical practice. Many instruments for measurement of the same constructs are available and validation has often been insufficient both in relation to the palliative population and on a more general level. However, ongoing efforts include multi-national research collaborations in order to develop instruments that are based upon experts' evaluations and input from patients, are computer-based with better measurement capabilities, and well suited for use in clinics and research. In the meantime, a reasonable strategy is to choose one of the most commonly used HRQOL instruments. Still, the content of a questionnaire always needs to be cautionary investigated to assure that it fits the purpose for the assessment in clinical research, in quality insurance, or in clinical practice.

References

1. Aristotle. (1975). *Nicomachean Ethics*, book 1. Harvard University Press, Cambridge, MA.
2. Bradburn, N. (1969). *The Structure of Psychological Well-Being*. Aldine, Chicago.
3. Andrews, F. and Withey, S. (1976). *Social Indicators of Well-Being: Americans Perceptions of Life Quality*. Plenum.
4. Campbell, A. (1976). *The Quality of Life Perceptions, Evaluations, Satisfactions*. Russel Sage foundation, New York.
5. Maslow, A. (1970). *Motivation and Personality*. Harper, New York.
6. Naess, S. (1987). *Methods and Applications*. Institute of Applied Social Research, Oslo.
7. Hjermstad, M.J., Evensen, S.A., Kvaloy, S.O., *et al.* (1999). Health-related quality of life 1 year after allogeneic or autologous stem-cell transplantation: a prospective study. *Journal of Clinical Oncology*, **17**, 706–18.

8. Calman, K.C. (1984). Quality of life in cancer patients–an hypothesis. *Journal of Medical Ethics*, **10**, 124–7.

9. Bergner, M., Bobbitt, R.A., Carter, W.B., *et al.* (1981). The Sickness Impact Profile: development and final revision of a health status measure. *Medical Care*, **19**, 787–805.

10. Coates, A., Dillenbeck, C.F., McNeil, D.R., *et al.* (1983). On the receiving end–II. Linear analogue self-assessment (LASA) in evaluation of aspects of the quality of life of cancer patients receiving therapy. *European Journal of Cancer and Clinical Oncology*, **19**, 1633–7.

11. Goldberg, D. and Williams, P. (1988). *A User's Guide to the General Health Questionnaire*. The NFER-NELSON Publishing Company Ltd, Windsor, UK.

12. Priestman, T.J. and Baum, M. (1976). Evaluation of quality of life in patients receiving treatment for advanced breast cancer. *Lancet*, **1**, 899–900.

13. Wade, D.T. and Collin, C. (1988). The Barthel ADL Index: a standard measure of physical disability? *International Disability Studies*, **10**, 64–7.

14. WHO (1958). The first ten years of the World Health Organization. World Health Organization, Geneva.

15. Karnofsky, D.A., Abelmann, W.H., Craver, L.F., *et al.* (1948). The use of the nitrogen mustrads in the palliative treatment of carcinoma - with particular reference to bronchogenic carcinoma. *Cancer*, **1**, 634–56.

16. Coates, A., Porzsolt, F., and Osoba, D. (1997). Quality of life in oncology practice: prognostic value of EORTC QLQ-C30 scores in patients with advanced malignancy. *European Journal of Cancer*, **33**, 1025–30.

17. Kaasa, S., Mastekaasa, A., and Lund, E. (1989). Prognostic factors for patients with inoperable non-small cell lung cancer, limited disease. The importance of patients' subjective experience of disease and psychosocial well-being. *Radiotherapy in Oncology*, **15**, 235–42.

18. Lagakos, S.W. (1983). Prognostic factors for patients with inoperable lung cancer. In: Straus MJ, eds. *Lung cancer clinical diagnosis and treatment*. Grune and Stratton, New York.

19. Maltoni, M., Pirovano, M., Scarpi, E., *et al.* (1995). Prediction of survival of patients terminally ill with cancer. Results of an Italian prospective multicentric study. *Cancer*, **75**, 2613–22.

20. Maltoni, M. (2005). Prognostic Factors in Advanced Cancer Patients: Evidence-Based Clinical Recommendations–A Study by the Steering Committee of the European Association for Palliative Care. *Journal of Clinical Oncology*, **23**, 6240.

21. Hunt, S.M. and McEwen, J. (1980). The development of a subjective health indicator. *Sociol Health and Illnesses* **2**, 231–46.

22. Ware, J.E., Jr. (1996). The SF-36 Health Survey. In *Quality of Life and Pharmacoeconomics in Clinical Trials* (ed. B.Spilker). Lippincott-Raven, Philadelphia.

23. Ware, J.E., Jr. and Sherbourne, C.D. (1992). The MOS 36-item Short-Form Health Survey (SF-36). I. Conceptual framework and item selection. *Medical Care*, **30**, 473–83.

24. McNair, D., Lord, M., and Droppleman, L. (1971). *EITS manual for the profile of mood states*. San Diego, CA.

25. IASP Task Force on Taxonomy (1994). Classification of chronic pain. IASP, Seattle.

26. Melzack, R. and Torgerson, W.S. (1971). On the language of pain. *Anesthesiology*, **34**, 50–9.

27. Jensen, M.P., Karoly, P., and Braver, S. (1986). The measurement of clinical pain intensity: a comparison of six methods. *Pain*, **27**, 117–26.

28. Kaasa, S. (1992). Measurement of quality of life in clinical trials. *Oncology*, **49**, 289–94.

29. Velikova, G., Wright, E.P., Smith, A.B., *et al.* (1999). Automated collection of quality-of-life data: a comparison of paper and computer touch-screen questionnaires. *Journal of Clinical Oncology*, **17**, 998–1007.

30. Bren, L. (2006). The importance of Patient-Reported Outcomes . . . It's all about the patients. US Food and Drug Administration; [updated 2006; cited 2006 November-December];

Available from: http://www.fda.gov/fdac/features/2006/606_patients. html.

31. Guidance for industry Patient-Reported Outcome measures: use in medical product development to support labeling claims US Food and Drug Administration; (2006) [updated 2006; cited 2006 February]; Available from: http://www.fda.gov/cber/gdlns/prolbl.pdf.

32. Spilker, B. (1996). *Quality of Life and Pharmacoeconomics in Clinical Trials*. Lippincott-Raven, Philadelphia, PA.

33. PROQOLID Patient-Reported Outcome and Quality of Life instruments database. Lyon, France: Mapi Research Institute; 2008 [updated 2008; cited 2008 April]; Available from: http://www.proqolid.org/.

34. Anderson, R.T., Aaronson, N.K., and Wilkin, D. (1993). Critical review of the international assessments of health-related quality of life. *Quality of Life Research*, **2**, 369–95.

35. Kaasa, S., Loge, J.H., Fayers, P., *et al.* (2008). Symptom assessment in palliative care: a need for international collaboration. *Journal of Clinical Oncology*, **26**, 3967–73.

36. Kaasa, S., and Radbruch, L. (2008). Palliative care research - Priorities and way forward. *European Journal of Cancer*, **44**, 1175–9.

37. Hjermstad, M.J., Gibbins, J., Haugen, D.F., *et al.* (2008). Pain Assessment Tools in Palliative Care; a call for consensus. Submitted.

38. Hearn, J. and Higginson, I.J. (1997). Outcome measures in palliative care for advanced cancer patients: a review. *Journal of Public Health Medicine*, **19**, 193–9.

39. Byock, I.R. and Merriman, M.P. (1998). Measuring quality of life for patients with terminal illness: the Missoula-VITAS quality of life index. *Palliative Medicine*, **12**, 231–44.

40. Cohen, S.R. and Mount, B.M. (1992). Quality of life in terminal illness: defining and measuring subjective well-being in the dying. *Journal of Palliative Care*, **8**, 40–5.

41. Waldron, D., O'Boyle, C.A., Kearney, M., *et al.* (1999). Quality-of-life measurement in advanced cancer: assessing the individual. *Journal of Clinical Oncology*, **17**, 3603–11.

42. Chronbach, L. (1951). Coefficient alpha and the internal structure of tests. *Psychometrika*, **16**, 297–334.

43. Streiner, D., and Norman, G. (1989). Validity. In *Health measurement scales: a practical guide to their development and use* (eds. D.Streiner D and G.Norman). Oxford University Press, Oxford.

44. Bernhard, J., Cella, D.F., Coates, A.S., *et al.* (1998). Missing quality of life data in cancer clinical trials: serious problems and challenges. *Statistics in Medicine*, **17**, 517–32.

45. Fielding, S., Fayers, P.M., Loge, J.H., *et al.* (2006). Methods for handling missing data in palliative care research. *Palliative Medicine*, **20**, 791–8.

46. Anderson, H., Hopwood, P., Stephens, R.J., *et al.* (2000). Gemcitabine plus best supportive care (BSC) vs BSC in inoperable non-small cell lung cancer--a randomized trial with quality of life as the primary outcome. UK NSCLC Gemcitabine Group. Non-Small Cell Lung Cancer. *British Journal of Cancer*, **83**, 447–53.

47. Fayers, P. and Machin, D. (2000). *Quality of Life: Assessment, Analysis and Interpretation*. John Wiley and Sons Ltd., Chichester.

48. Colton, T., Johnson, A., and Machin, D. (1998). *Statistics in Medicine*. Wiley, Chichester.

49. Jordhoy, M.S., Kaasa, S., Fayers, P., *et al.* (1999). Challenges in palliative care research; recruitment, attrition and compliance: experience from a randomized controlled trial. *Palliative Medicine*, **13**, 299–310.

50. Sneeuw, K.C., Aaronson, N.K., Sprangers, M.A., *et al.* (1997). Value of caregiver ratings in evaluating the quality of life of patients with cancer. *Journal of Clinical Oncology*, **15**, 1206–17.

51. Brunelli, C., Costantini, M., Di Giulio, P., *et al.* (1998). Quality-of-life evaluation: when do terminal cancer patients and health-care providers agree? *Journal of Pain and Symptom Management*, **15**, 151–8.

52. Higginson, I., Priest, P., and McCarthy, M. (1994). Are bereaved family members a valid proxy for a patient's assessment of dying? *Social Science and Medicine*, **38**, 553–7.

53. Sprangers, M.A. and Aaronson, N.K. (1992). The role of health care providers and significant others in evaluating the quality of life of patients with chronic disease: a review. *Journal of Clinical Epidemiology*, **45**, 743–60.

54. Lampic, C. and Sjoden, P.O. (2000). Patient and staff perceptions of cancer patients' psychological concerns and needs. *Acta Oncologica*, **39**, 9–22.

55. Sprangers, M.A. and Sneeuw, K.C. (2000). Are healthcare providers adequate raters of patients' quality of life–perhaps more than we think? *Acta Oncologica*, **39**, 5–8.

56. Van Weel, C. (1993). Functional status in primary care: COOP/WONCA charts. *Disability and Rehabilitation*, **15**, 96–101.

57. Bruera, E., Kuehn, N., Miller, M.J., *et al.* (1991). The Edmonton Symptom Assessment System (ESAS): a simple method for the assessment of palliative care patients. *Journal of Palliative Care*, **7**, 6–9.

58. Aaronson, N.K., Ahmedzai, S., Bergman, B., *et al.* (1993). The European Organization for Research and Treatment of Cancer QLQ-C30: a quality-of-life instrument for use in international clinical trials in oncology. *Journal of the National Cancer Institute*, **85**, 365–76.

59. Ware, J.E., Jr., Kosinski, M., Dewey, J., *et al.* (2001). *How to score and interpret single-item health status measures: A manual for users of the SF-8 Health Survey*. Quality Metric Incorporated, Lincoln.

60. Osoba, D. (1994). Lessons learned from measuring health-related quality of life in oncology. *Journal of Clinical Oncology*, **12**, 608–16.

61. Cella, D.F., Tulsky, D.S., Gray, G., *et al.* (1993). The Functional Assessment of Cancer Therapy scale: development and validation of the general measure. *Journal of Clinical Oncology*, **11**, 570–9.

62. Muldoon, M.F., Barger, S.D., Flory, J.D., *et al.* (1998). What are quality of life measurements measuring? *British Medical Journal*, **316**, 542–5.

63. Ware, J.E., Jr. (1995). The status of health assessment 1994. *Annual Review of Public Health*, **16**, 327–54.

64. Fredheim, O.M., Borchgrevink, P.C., Saltnes, T., *et al.* (2007). Validation and comparison of the health-related quality-of-life instruments EORTC QLQ-C30 and SF-36 in assessment of patients with chronic nonmalignant pain. *Journal of Pain and Symptom Management*, **34**, 657–65.

65. Beck, A.T., Ward, C.H., Mendelson, M., *et al.* (1961). An inventory for measuring depression. *Archives of General Psychiatry*, **4**, 561–71.

66. Hamilton, M. (1960). A rating scale for depression. *Journal of Neurology and Neurosurgical Psychiatry*, **23**, 56–62.

67. Massie, M. and Popkin, M. (1998). Depressive disorders. In (eds. J.C. Holland and W. Breitbart). *Psycho-Oncology*. Oxford University Press, New York.

68. Hotopf, M., Chidgey, J., Addington-Hall, J., *et al.* (2002). Depression in advanced disease: a systematic review Part 1. Prevalence and case finding. *Palliative Medicine*, **16**, 81–97.

69. Bergner, M., Bobbitt, R.A., Kressel, S., *et al.* (1976). The Sickness Impact Profile: conceptual formulation and methodology for the development of a health status measure. *International Journal of Health Services*, **6**, 393–415.

70. Bowling, A. (1995). *Measuring Disease*. Open University Press, Philadelphia.

71. Wagner, A.K., Gandek, B., Aaronson, N.K., *et al.* (1998). Cross-cultural comparisons of the content of SF-36 translations across 10 countries: results from the IQOLA Project. International Quality of Life Assessment. *Journal of Clinical Epidemiology*, **51**, 925–32.

72. Aaronson, N.K., Acquadro, C., Alonso, J., *et al.* (1992). International Quality of Life Assessment (IQOLA) Project. *Quality of Life Research*, **1**, 349–51.

73. Ware, J.E., Jr., SF Generic Health Surveys: SF-36® Health Survey, SF-36v2™ Health Survey, SF-12® Health Survey, SF-12v2™ Health Survey, SF-10™ Health Survey for Children, SF-8™ Health Survey, and DYNHA® Generic Health Assessment. QualityMetric; 2005 [updated 2005; cited 2008 April]; Available from: http://www.qualitymetric.com/products/sfsurveys.aspx.

74. McHorney, C.A., Ware, J.E., Jr., and Raczek, A.E. (1993). The MOS 36-Item Short-Form Health Survey (SF-36): II. Psychometric and clinical tests of validity in measuring physical and mental health constructs. *Medical Care*, **31**, 247–63.

75. Ware, J.E., Jr., and Keller, S.D. (1996). Interpreting general health measures. In *Quality of Life and Pharmacoeconomics in Clinical Trials* (ed. B. Spilker). Lippincott-Raven, Philadelphia-New York.

76. (1993). Study protocol for the World Health Organization project to develop a Quality of Life assessment instrument (WHOQOL). *Quality of Life Research*, **2**, 153–9.

77. Szabo, S. (1996). The World Health Organization Qualtiy of Life (WHOQOL) Assessment Instrument. In *Quality of Life and Pharmacoeconomics in Clinical Trials* (eds. B. Spilker). Lippincott-Raven, Philidelphia-New York.

78. (1998). Development of the World Health Organization WHOQOL-BREF quality of life assessment. The WHOQOL Group. *Psychological Medicine*, **28**, 551–8.

79. EORTC group for research into Quality of Life. Brussels: EORTC European Organization for Research and Treatment of Cancer 2008 [updated 2008; cited 2008 April]; Available from: http://groups.eortc.be/qol/index.htm.

80. Bjordal, K., and Kaasa, S. (1992). Psychometric validation of the EORTC Core Quality of Life Questionnaire, 30-item version and a diagnosis-specific module for head and neck cancer patients. *Acta Oncologica*, **31**, 311–21.

81. Hjermstad, M.J., Fossa, S.D., Bjordal, K., *et al.* (1995). Test/retest study of the European Organization for Research and Treatment of Cancer Core Quality-of-Life Questionnaire. *Joiurnal of Clinical Oncology*, **13**, 1249–54.

82. Detmar, S.B., Aaronson, N.K., Wever, L.D., *et al.* (2000). How are you feeling? Who wants to know? Patients' and oncologists' preferences for discussing health-related quality-of-life issues. *Journal of Clinical Oncology*, **18**, 3295–301.

83. Aaronson, N.K., Cull, A., Kaasa, S., *et al.* (1994). The EORTC modular approach to quality of life assessment in oncology. *International Journal of Mental Health*, **23**, 75–96.

84. Groenvold, M., Petersen, M.A., Aaronson, N.K., *et al.* (2006). The development of the EORTC QLQ-C15-PAL: a shortened questionnaire for cancer patients in palliative care. *European Journal of Cancer*, **42**, 55–64.

85. The Functional Assessment of Chronic Illness Therapy (FACIT) measurement system overview. [cited 2008 April]; Available from: http://www.facit.org/about/overview_measure.aspx.

86. Stone, P., Hardy, J., Huddart, R., *et al.* (2000). Fatigue in patients with prostate cancer receiving hormone therapy. *European Journal of Cancer*, **36**, 1134–41.

87. Maguire, P. and Selby, P. (1989). Assessing quality of life in cancer patients. *British Journal of Cancer*, **60**, 437–40.

88. Zigmond, A.S. and Snaith, R.P. (1983). The hospital anxiety and depression scale. *Acta Psychiatrica Scandinavica*, **67**, 361–70.

89. APA (1994). *Diagnostic and Statistical Manual of Mental Disorders DSM-IV*. American Psychiatric Association, Washington DC.

90. Le Fevre, P., Devereux, J., Smith, S., *et al.* (1999). Screening for psychiatric illness in the palliative care inpatient setting: a comparison between the Hospital Anxiety and Depression Scale and the General Health Questionnaire-12. *Palliative Medicine*, **13**, 399–407.

91. Radbruch, L., Strasser, F., Elsner, F., *et al.* (2008). Fatigue in palliative care patients - an EAPC approach. *Palliative Medicine*, **22**, 13–32.

92. Coyle, N., Adelhardt, J., Foley, K.M., *et al.* (1990). Character of terminal illness in the advanced cancer patient: pain and other symptoms during the last four weeks of life. *Journal of Pain and Symptom Management*, **5**, 83–93.

93. Stone, P., Hardy, J., Broadley, K., *et al.* (1999). Fatigue in advanced cancer: a prospective controlled cross-sectional study. *British Journal of Cancer*, **79**, 1479–86.

94. Loge, J.H., and Kaasa, S. (1998). Fatigue and cancer - prevalence, correlates and measurement. *Progress in Palliative Care*, **6**, 43–7.

95. Stone, P., Richards, M., and Hardy, J. (1998). Fatigue in patients with cancer. *European Journal of Cancer*, **34**, 1670–6.

96. Stone, P., and Minton, O. (2008). Cancer-related fatigue. *European Journal of Cancer*, **44**, 1097–1104.

97. NCCN Clinical practice guidelines in oncology. National Comprehensive Cancer Network; 2008 [updated 2008; cited 2008 April]; Available from: http://www.nccn.org.

98. Chalder, T., Berelowitz, G., Pawlikowska, T., *et al.* (1993). Development of a fatigue scale. *Jopuurnal of Psychosomatic Research*, **37**, 147–53.

99. Grond, S., Zech, D., Diefenbach, C., *et al.* (1996). Assessment of cancer pain: a prospective evaluation in 2266 cancer patients referred to a pain service. *Pain*, **64**, 107–14.

100. Hølen, J.C., Hjermstad, M.J., Loge, J.H., *et al.* (2006). Pain Assessment Tools: Is the Content Appropriate for Use in Palliative Care? *Journal of Pain and Symptom Management*, **32**, 567.

101. Stenseth, G., Bjornes, M., Kaasa, S., *et al.* (2007). Can cancer patients assess the influence of pain on functions? A randomised, controlled study of the pain interference items in the Brief Pain Inventory. *BMC Palliative Care*, **6**, 2.

102. Melzack, R. (1975). The McGill Pain Questionnaire: major properties and scoring methods. *Pain*, **1**, 277–99.

103. Melzack, R. (1987). The short-form McGill Pain Questionnaire. *Pain*, **30**, 191–7.

104. Daut, R.L., Cleeland, C.S., and Flanery, R.C. (1983). Development of the Wisconsin Brief Pain Questionnaire to assess pain in cancer and other diseases. *Pain*, **17**, 197–210.

105. Radbruch, L., Loick, G., Kiencke, P., *et al.* (1999). Validation of the German version of the Brief Pain Inventory. *Journal of Pain and Symptom Management*, **18**, 180–7.

106. Caraceni, A., Cherny, N., Fainsinger, R., *et al.* (2002). Pain measurement tools and methods in clinical research in palliative care. Recommendations of an expert working group of the European association of palliative care. *Journal of Pain and Symptom Management*, **23**, 239–55.

107. Brief Pain Invetory (short form). Pain Research Group; [cited 2008 April]; Available from: http://www.ohsu.edu/ahec/pain/paininventory.pdf.

108. Melzack, R. and Katz, J. (2001). The McGill Pain Questionnaire: Appraisal and Current Status. In *Handbook of pain assessment* (eds. D.Turk and R. Melzack), 2nd edition. Guilford Press, London.

109. Zwakhalen, S.M., Hamers, J.P., Abu-Saad, H.H., *et al.* (2006). Pain in elderly people with severe dementia: a systematic review of behavioural pain assessment tools. *BMC Geriatrics*, **6**, 3.

110. Savard, J. and Morin, C.M. (2001). Insomnia in the context of cancer: a review of a neglected problem. *Journal of Clinical Oncology*, **19**, 895–908.

111. Robinson, J.H. (1999). Cognitive assessment of palliative care patients. *Progress in Palliative Care*, **7**, 291–8.

112. Casarett, D.J. and Inouye, S.K. (2001). Diagnosis and Management of Delirium near the End of Life. *Annals of Internal Medicine*, **135**, 32.

113. Pereira, J., Hanson, J., and Bruera, E. (1997). The frequency and clinical course of cognitive impairment in patients with terminal cancer. *Cancer*, **79**, 835–42.

114. Hjermstad, M., Loge, J.H., and Kaasa, S. (2004). Methods for assessment of cognitive failure and delirium in palliative care patients: implications for practice and research. *Palliative Medicine*, **18**, 494–506.

115. Cull, A., Hay, C., Love, S.B., *et al.* (1996). What do cancer patients mean when they complain of concentration and memory problems? *British Journal of Cancer*, **74**, 1674–9.

116. Breitbart, W., Rosenfeld, B., Roth, A., *et al.* (1997). *The Memorial Delirium Assessment Scale*. **13**, 128–37.

117. Folstein, M.F., Folstein, S.E., and McHugh, P.R. (1975). "Mini-mental state". A practical method for grading the cognitive state of patients for the clinician. *Journal of Psychiatric Research*, **12**, 189–98.

118. Braekhus, A., Laake, K., and Engedal, K. (1992). The Mini-Mental State Examination: identifying the most efficient variables for detecting cognitive impairment in the elderly. *Journal of the American Geriatric Society*, **40**, 1139–45.

119. Fayers, P.M., Hjermstad, M.J., Ranhoff, A.H., *et al.* (2005). Which Mini-Mental State Exam Items Can Be Used to Screen for Delirium and Cognitive Impairment? *Journal of Pain and Symptom Management*, **30**, 41–50.

120. O'Boyle, C. (1994). The Schedule for the Evaluation of Individual Quality of Life (SEIQoL). *International Journal of Mental Health*, **23**, 3–23.

121. Hickey, A.M., Bury, G., O'Boyle, C.A., *et al.* (1996). A new short form individual quality of life measure (SEIQoL-DW): application in a cohort of individuals with HIV/AIDS. *British Medical Journal*, **313**, 29–33.

122. Tamburini, M., Rosso, S., Gamba, A., *et al.* (1992). A therapy impact questionnaire for quality-of-life assessment in advanced cancer research. *Annals of Oncology,* **3**, 565–70.

123. Cohen, S.R., Mount, B.M., Strobel, M.G., *et al.* (1995). The McGill Quality of Life Questionnaire: a measure of quality of life appropriate for people with advanced disease. A preliminary study of validity and acceptability. *Palliative Medicine*, **9**, 207–19.

124. Cohen, S.R., Mount, B.M., and MacDonald, N. (1996). Defining quality of life. *European Journal of Cancer*, **32A**, 753–4.

125. Cohen, S.R., Mount, B.M., Bruera, E., *et al.* (1997). Validity of the McGill Quality of Life Questionnaire in the palliative care setting: a multi-centre Canadian study demonstrating the importance of the existential domain. *Palliative Medicine*, **11**, 3–20.

126. Cohen, S.R. and Mount, B.M. (2000). Living with cancer: "good" days and "bad" days–what produces them? Can the McGill quality of life questionnaire distinguish between them? *Cancer*, **89**, 1854–65.

127. Lo, R.S., Woo, J., Zhoc, K.C., *et al.* (2001). Cross-cultural validation of the McGill Quality of Life questionnaire in Hong Kong Chinese. *Palliative Medicine*, **15**, 387–97.

128. Salmon, P., Manzi, F., and Valori, R.M. (1996). Measuring the meaning of life for patients with incurable cancer: the life evaluation questionnaire (LEQ). *European Journal of Cancer*, **32A**, 755–60.

129. Sterkenburg, C.A., King, B., and Woodward, C.A. (1996). A reliability and validity study of the McMaster Quality of Life Scale (MQLS) for a palliative population. *Journal of Palliative Care*, **12**, 18–25.

130. Curtis, J.R., Wenrich, M.D., Carline, J.D., *et al.* (2001). Understanding physicians' skills at providing end-of-life care perspectives of patients, families, and health care workers. *Journal of General Internal Medicine*, **16**, 41–9.

131. Teno, J.M., Byock, I., and Field, M.J. (1999). Research agenda for developing measures to examine quality of care and quality of life of patients diagnosed with life-limiting illness. *Journal of Pain and Symptom Management*, **17**, 75–82.

132. Singer, P.A., Martin, D.K., and Kelner, M. (1999). Quality end-of-life care: patients' perspectives. *Journal of the American Medical Association*, **281**, 163–8.

133. Stewart, A.L., Teno, J., Patrick, D.L. (1999). The concept of quality of life of dying persons in the context of health care. *Journal of Pain and Symptom Management*, **17**, 93–108.

134. Hearn, J. and Higginson, I.J. (1998). Do specialist palliative care teams improve outcomes for cancer patients? A systematic literature review. *Palliative Medicine*, **12**, 317–32.

135. Rinck, G.C., van den Bos, G.A., Kleijnen, J., *et al.* (1997). Methodologic issues in effectiveness research on palliative cancer care: a systematic review. *Journal of Clinical Oncology*, **15**, 1697–707.

136. Salisbury, C., Bosanquet, N., Wilkinson, E.K., *et al.* (1999). The impact of different models of specialist palliative care on patients' quality of life: a systematic literature review. *Palliative Medicine*, **13**, 3–17.

137. Smeenk, F.W., van Haastregt, J.C., de Witte, L.P., *et al.* (1998). Effectiveness of home care programmes for patients with incurable cancer on their quality of life and time spent in hospital: systematic review. *British Medical Journal*, **316**, 1939–44.

138. Addington-Hall, J.M., MacDonald, L.D., Anderson, H.R., *et al.* (1992). Randomised controlled trial of effects of coordinating care for terminally ill cancer patients. *British Medical Journal*, **305**, 1317–22.

139. Hughes, S.L., Cummings, J., Weaver, F., *et al.* (1992). A randomized trial of the cost effectiveness of VA hospital-based home care for the terminally ill. *Health Services Research*, **26**, 801–17.

140. Jordhoy, M.S., Fayers, P., Loge, J.H., *et al.* (2001). Quality of life in palliative cancer care: results from a cluster randomized trial. *Journal of Clinical Oncology*, **19**, 3884–94.

141. Jordhoy, M.S., Fayers, P., Saltnes, T., *et al.* (2000). A palliative-care intervention and death at home: a cluster randomised trial. *Lancet*, **356**, 888–93.

142. Kane, R.L., Wales, J., Bernstein, L., *et al.* (1984). A randomised controlled trial of hospice care. *Lancet*, **1**, 890–4.

143. Zimmer, J.G., Groth-Juncker, A., McCusker, J. (1985). A randomized controlled study of a home health care team. *American Journal of Public Health*, **75**, 134–41.

144. Chang, V.T., Hwang, S.S., Feuerman, M., *et al.* (2000). The memorial symptom assessment scale short form (MSAS-SF). *Cancer*, **89**, 1162–71.

145. Kaasa, S. and Loge, J.H. (2002). Quality-of-life assessment in palliative care. *Lancet Oncology*, **3**, 175–82.

146. Altman, D.G. (1991). *Practical Statistics for Medical Research*. Chapman and Hall, London.

147. Fairclough, D. and Gelber, R. (1996). Quality of life: Statistical issues and analysis. In: Spilker B, eds. *Quality of Life and Pharmacoeconomics in Clinical Trials*. Lippincott-Raven, Philadelphia-New York.

148. Fayers, P.M. and Martijn, P.F. (2005). *Assessing Quality of Life in Clinical Trials: Methods and Practice*. Oxord University Press, Oxford.

149. Begg, C., Cho, M., Eastwood, S., *et al.* (1996). Improving the quality of reporting of randomized controlled trials. The CONSORT statement. *Journal of the American Medical Association*, **276**, 637–9.

150. Staquet, M., Berzon, R., Osoba, D., *et al.* (1996). Guidelines for reporting results of quality of life assessments in clinical trials. *Quality of Life Research*, **5**, 496–502.

151. Hjermstad, M.J., Fayers, P.M., Bjordal, K., *et al.* (1998). Health-related quality of life in the general Norwegian population assessed by the European Organization for Research and Treatment of Cancer Core Quality-of-Life Questionnaire: the QLQ=C30 (+ 3). *Journal of Clinical Oncology*, **16**, 1188–96.

152. Cull, A., Stewart, M., and Altman, D.G. (1995). Assessment of and intervention for psychosocial problems in routine oncology practice. *British Journal of Cancer*, **72**, 229–35.

153. Passik, S.D., Dugan, W., McDonald, M.V., *et al.* (1998). Oncologists' recognition of depression in their patients with cancer. *Journal of Clinical Oncology*, **16**, 1594–600.

154. Shuster, J.L., Jr., Breitbart, W., and Chochinov, H.M. (1999). Psychiatric aspects of excellent end-of-life care. Ad Hoc Committee on End-of-Life Care. The Academy of Psychosomatic Medicine. *Psychosomatics*, **40**, 1–4.

155. Chang, C.H. (2007). Patient-reported outcomes measurement and management with innovative methodologies and technologies. *Quality of Life Research*, **16 Suppl 1**, 157–66.

156. Jordhoy, M., Ringdal, G.I., Helbostad, J.L., *et al.* (2007). Assessing physical functioning: a systematic review of quality of life measure developed for use in palliative care. *Palliative Medicine*, **21**, 673–82.

157. Garcia, S.F., Cella, D., Clauser, S.B., *et al.* (2007). Standardizing patient-reported outcomes assessment in cancer clinical trials: a patient-reported outcomes measurement information system initiative. *Journal of Clinical Oncology*, **25**, 5106–12.

158. Velikova, G., Stark, D., and Selby, P. (1999). Quality of life instruments in oncology. *European Journal of Cancer*, **35**, 1571–80.

159. Urch, C.E., Chamberlain, J., and Field, G. (1998). The drawback of the Hospital Anxiety and Depression Scale in the assessment of depression in hospice inpatients. *Palliative Medicine*, **12**, 395–6.

160. Lord, F. (1980). *Applications of Item Response Theory to Practical Testing Problems*. Erlbaum Associates, Hillsdale.

161. Ware, J.E., Jr., Bjorner, J.B., and Kosinski, M. (2000). Practical implications of item response theory and computerized adaptive testing: A brief summary of ongoing studies of widely used headache impact scales. *Medical Care*, **38**, 1173–82.

162. Higginson, I.J. and Carr, A.J. (2001). Measuring quality of life: Using quality of life measures in the clinical setting. *British Medical Journal*, **322**, 1297–300.

163. National Institutes of Health (NIH). PROMIS: Patient Reported Outcomes Measurement Information System. (2007) [updated 2007; cited 2008 April]. Available from: http://www.nihpromis.org.

Measurement of pain and other symptoms in the cognitively impaired

Keela Herr and Mary Ersek

Introduction

The focus of palliative care is to enhance the quality of life (QOL) for people with progressive, life-limiting illnesses. A key to ensuring optimal QOL is the rapid identification and management of symptoms. Clinicians recognize physiological and psychosocial symptoms through patient interview and report, and evaluation of objective clinical signs. Most end-of-life (EOL) problems that negatively affect QOL, such as pain, dyspnoea, anxiety, and depression, are most easily identified and treated when patients provide self-report of their experiences. Challenges arise when cognitive impairment hinders patients' ability to report their symptoms, leaving clinicians with no choice but to infer a patient's inner experiences through observable signs and other indicators. Alternative approaches to assessment are necessary in these circumstances.

Cognitive impairment is associated with many diseases and medical conditions (Table 7.9.1). Impairment may be temporary (e.g. during periods of delirium or hypoxia) or permanent (e.g. advance dementia, persistent vegetative state). Some type and degree of impairment occurs in most palliative care patients at some time during their illness. For example, delirium is a frequent cause of impairment, affecting 25–45 per cent of hospitalized cancer patients, and approximately 60 per cent of older (≥75 years) nursing home residents.[1] In a review of published symptom prevalence studies, Solano and colleagues reported that confusion occurs in 6–39 per cent of cancer patients, 18–33 per cent of heart disease and chronic obstructive pulmonary disease patients, and 30–65 per cent of AIDS patients.[2] Between 28–42 per cent of patients are delirious upon admission to inpatient palliative care units, and almost 90 per cent of patients experience delirium prior to death.[3]

Dementia is another frequent cause of cognitive impairment. Epidemiologists estimate that Alzheimer disease, which accounts for approximately 50 per cent of all cases of dementia, will affect as many as 14 million Americans by 2050.[4] Dementing illnesses and the severe cognitive impairment that accompanies advanced disease represent an enormous challenge for clinicians in every clinical setting but particularly those in nursing homes, which is the site for nearly 67 per cent of deaths for people with dementia.[5]

The severity of cognitive impairment is influenced by the type and stage of disease, environmental factors, and individual characteristics. If mild, cognitive impairment may not interfere with a patient's ability to report symptoms at all. More pronounced cognitive impairment may affect memory and judgement to the extent that patients can report symptoms but their report is unreliable. Conditions such as advanced Alzheimer disease, profound brain injury resulting in persistent vegetative state and severe, end-stage multi-organ system failure usually render patients completely and permanently unable to report symptoms.

Given the problems with communication, memory, and judgement that occur in cognitively impaired patients, it is not surprising that patients with decreased cognitive functioning are at risk for poor symptom assessment and management. These deficiencies in clinical care are particularly well described in older adults. For example, pain is documented less frequently for cognitively impaired nursing home residents, despite having similar numbers of painful diagnoses as less impaired residents.[6,7] In studies of older adults hospitalized with hip fracture, those with cognitive impairment received significantly less opioid analgesia than those with less or no impairment.[8,9] Less analgesic also is prescribed and administered for cognitively impaired residents, even when the impaired residents have similar numbers of painful diagnoses as cognitively intact residents.[10–12] These studies underscore an urgent need to improve methods of identifying and treating pain and other EOL symptoms in patients with cognitive dysfunction.

In addition to hindering clinical practice, patients' cognitive impairment poses serious threats to palliative care research. Lack of valid, reliable scales to measure pain and other symptoms threaten investigators' ability to describe adequately the experiences of this vulnerable group, including the effects of symptoms on QOL. The evaluation of interventions to prevent or treat symptoms also is compromised. Unreliable or missing data from impaired patients can lead to biased, inaccurate findings and conclusions because the data are not missing at random.[13]

The purpose of this chapter is to review the current state of the science for measuring symptoms in patients whose cognitive impairment hinders their ability to report physical and psychosocial distress.

Table 7.9.1 Common causes of cognitive impairment.

Neurodegenerative disorders:
* Alzheimer's disease
* Parkinson's disease
* Other dementias

Other chronic encephalopathies:
* Prolonged coma, persistent vegetative state
* Multiple sclerosis
* Cerebrovascular disease

Delirium/confusion:
* Hypoxia
* Metabolic, fluid, and electrolyte abnormalities
* Medication side effects
* Infection

Psychiatric disorders:
* Severe depression
* Psychosis

We will discuss general principles as well as specific scales to measure symptoms. Much of the research has focused on pain in older adults with dementia. However, the framework that has been developed for pain assessment in this population can be applied to other patient groups and symptoms.

Symptom assessment with pain as an example

General principles

Several challenges exist in the measurement of symptoms in the cognitively impaired patient. General principles can guide initial approaches in identifying, quantifying and monitoring symptoms in the cognitively impaired, as well as selection of specific assessment strategies. Of all EOL symptoms, pain has been the most extensively studied in cognitively impaired patients. Empirically-based models and guidelines for assessing pain in this population are available.

The American Society for Pain Management Nursing (ASPMN) recently published recommendations for a comprehensive strategy for assessing pain in non-verbal persons.[14] A hierarchical approach to identify presence of pain includes: (1) determine ability to self report; (2) investigate for possible pathologies; (3) observe for possible behaviours that may signal pain; (4) incorporate surrogate reporting, and (5) use analgesics to evaluate whether pain management causes a reduction in the behavioural indicators thought to be related to pain.[14] This process incorporates a number of strategies that present challenges to the clinician or researcher.[15]

Obtaining self-report

Self-report has been generally accepted as the most reliable source of information on an individual's subjective symptom experience, and efforts should be made to obtain patient ratings or reports even in the cognitively impaired. Studies have demonstrated that even those with mild to moderate cognitive impairment (and many

with severe dementia) can provide reliable reports of pain at some level.[16–21]

Determining the ability of the cognitively impaired patient to use a measurement instrument consistently and accurately is a challenge. Self-report impairment is often gradual and is not directly related to the stage of dementia or severity of cognitive impairment, although level of cognitive impairment is generally associated with ability to respond to a verbal pain assessment.[22–24] Although no clear method has been identified to address reliability in using self-report instruments, Buffum and colleagues[25] described one approach developed for evaluating cognitive ability to reliably complete pain intensity scales, which they called the Pain Screening Tool (PST). Respondents are asked to provide a number from 0 to 3 and a word to describe their pain. Following 1 min of distracting conversation, the respondent is asked to recall the number and word. Respondents receive one point each for being able to provide an initial number and word and one-half point each for recalling number and the word. Only respondents who score a three are identified as providing reliable pain reports. Another approach suggested involves conceptual consistency in use of the scale. Using the Brief Pain Inventory, investigators identified inconsistencies in subjects' responses to *worst*, *least*, *current* and *usual* pain. For example, if the subject rated his *worst* pain as 4/10 and his *current* pain as 7/10, the research assistant asked the subject if that's what he meant to say. If the subject again stated that his *worst* pain was less severe than his *current* pain, the response was recorded as unreliable (Ersek, personal communication).

The first step in assessing for symptoms in cognitively impaired patients with advanced disease is to maximize the patient's ability to self-report using valid and reliable scales that also address sensory and motor deficits that hinder communication. Despite these efforts, many patients' impairments will be severe enough to require alternative approaches to assessment.

Strategies for effective use of measurement instruments include scale modifications that attend to sensory impairments, careful and repeated instruction on use of the scales, and repeated reassessments focusing on current state of the symptom rather than a retrospective evaluation of past pain.[26–28] Because those with cognitive impairment have difficulty remembering prior pain in order to make a judgement of improvement, a focus on present pain is recommended to promote reliable responses.[9,29,30]

Another issue with relying on self-report in the cognitively impaired is a tendency to report less pain or to not report pain, although it may exist.[31] Although there is evidence that peripheral nociceptor responses or pain transmission is unimpaired in those with dementia, central nervous system changes may influence or diminish interpretation of the pain signals.[20,32,33] Thus, self-report of pain may not accurately represent the pain experience in this population, making pain in the cognitively impaired vulnerable to underdetection and undertreatment.

Behavioural observation

As cognitive impairment becomes more severe, reliance on external signs of pain, such as non-verbal behaviours and physiological changes, becomes a necessary approach to recognize presence of symptoms in those unable to self-report. Behavioural observation can include direct observation of behaviours or proxy or surrogate reporting of behaviour or behaviour changes. Inherent in this approach are challenges to the reliability and validity of the interpretation of the behaviours observed.

Direct observation of behaviour

Methods for observing behaviours directly provide data on specific behaviours noted during a direct encounter for a specified period; typically, these methods identify the presence or absence of behaviours consistent with pain, along with their intensity or frequency.[24,34,35] Considerations for promoting valid and reliable comparisons across raters should include whether the observation period includes patients at rest or engaged in activity that may provoke pain and the observation period between ratings. Studies have demonstrated that observation at rest is misleading and can contribute to a false judgement that pain is absent, which in turn, can lead to underrecognition and undertreatment.[9,34,36,37] Thus, observations should occur during movement or activity that is likely to elicit a pain response if pain aetiology is present. Additionally, assuring that the periods and circumstances of the behaviour observation are similar between two raters or subsequent rating episodes is essential to assure reliability of the observation conclusions.

Direct observation and measurement of physiological signs [e.g. heart rate (HR), blood pressure (BP), and respiratory rate (RR)] often is used as a non-verbal indicator of pain. Although these indicators may change with acute pain, they can also reflect a response to physiologic stress due to other disease processes or changes in condition, thus the validity can be questioned. Physiologic measures could be combined with other potential pain indicators and it should be recognized that the absence of physiological change does not indicate absence of pain.[38] However, this approach is only to a limited extent empirically verified.

A limitation of direct observation is the focus on common obvious pain behaviours, rather than *changes* occurring in behaviour, activity or mental status, which may be more sensitive indicators of pain in many patients. Reliance on the presence of pain behaviours rather than changes in behaviours would markedly influence the reliability, validity and sensitivity of the measure. A number of common behaviours observable by those unfamiliar with a person with severe dementia (e.g. facial expression, vocalizations) have been supported,[39] but the impact of focusing on a narrow set of indicators must be considered in the context of the purpose, setting and nature of the pain problem being evaluated. For example, during a painful dressing change focusing on narrow behaviours may be appropriate, while the best approach to determine the greatest number of persons with unrecognized chronic pain in the nursing home may be a more comprehensive behaviour observation approach that requires input from those familiar with the individual's usual behaviour.

Surrogate/proxy report

Proxy reports from family members, caregivers and/or health care providers are an important source of information for making judgements about symptoms. Involvement of informed surrogates is essential for completion of selected behavioural observation tools that rely on input from someone familiar with the individual's baseline behaviour and subsequent changes. However, numerous studies have documented the discrepancies between patient and proxy reports of pain severity in the cognitively impaired,[39–42]

which generally increase as cognitive impairment becomes more severe.[43] Surrogate report, whether by family caregivers or professional caregivers, is not objective given the personal interpretation involved in making judgements about the meaning of observed behaviours. Whereas professional caregivers tend to underestimate pain severity[44,45] families tend to overestimate the patient's pain intensity and level of distress.[23,46–48]

Nevertheless, surrogate reporting often is essential in recognizing pain in this population. Certified nursing assistants (CNAs) often spend more time with patients than other health-care providers, particularly in clinical settings like nursing homes; thus, their role in recognizing and measuring pain in this population needs further exploration.[45,49,50]

Observation scales attempt to provide more objectivity to the process of surrogate reporting by codifying specific behaviours to be observed and rated. The shorter pain scales tend to be direct observation focused and include items that are readily observable by trained observers (e.g. grimacing, bracing, restlessness, groaning).[34,35] For completion of longer scales that include items related to changes in activity patterns or routines, interpersonal interactions or mental status, involvement of individuals familiar with the patient's baseline or typical behaviours is essential. Asking observers to back up 'gestalt' judgements of symptom severity with objective behavioural indicators is a current approach to improving symptom measurement in this challenging population. To accurately interpret data on behaviours related to symptom presence and/or severity, it is important to note the source of the data (self vs. proxy) and evaluate separately or combine into a multidimensional assessment approach.

Presence versus severity of pain

There are significant challenges to the quantification of symptoms using a behavioural observation approach and in determining severity of symptoms based on those observations. Several studies focused on observation for pain behaviours have demonstrated that it is possible for surrogates or proxies to recognize the presence of pain, but not accurately rate its severity, particularly in those with severe dementia.[19,39,42] This may relate to the interindividual variability in the way that pain behaviours in persons with dementia may be expressed. Patient pain response can be unique and may be related to the part of the brain affected by dementia.[20,51,52] For example, some persons with severe dementia may present with agitated and aggressive physical behaviour while another presents with withdrawal and social isolation. Both may be experiencing similar pain severity although their presentations are quite different.

Data on inaccuracy of surrogate reporting makes it important that reports are interpreted cautiously and other data (e.g. physical examination, diagnoses, pathology) be considered in determining the presence of the symptom. Because ability to detect severity of a symptom from behaviour observation has been questioned, these approaches may more likely indicate presence or absence of pain reliably, but not provide accurate data on which to judge severity of the symptom being measured. Additionally, the score on a behavioural pain assessment tool is not the same as a pain intensity rating and the scores between standard pain intensity ratings or categories of pain severity should not be compared with the score on a pain behaviour tool.[53]

Behavioural observation scales

Establishing reliability and validity of behavioural scales to measure symptoms in those with cognitive impairment is an ongoing challenge. Existing scales usually have been developed to optimize clinical utility, rather than research requirements. Although important, clinical utility is not the primary emphasis in scale development and selection for use in research studies and methodology to establish scale psychometrics is in early stages for most of the available instruments.

A major issue in establishing the validity of measures for assessment of pain in non-verbal populations has been the lack of a gold standard, as it is for most symptom assessment scales in palliative care in general, by which to compare newly developed tools, since self-report has been this standard for most symptoms. Most scale developers identify expert judgement as a comparison, although limitations of this singular approach are obvious when considering the variability observed between health-care providers and patients discussed earlier. A model that combines self-reports, informant reports, and behavioural observations was proposed by Snow and colleagues[24] that attempts to address the limitations of each individual approach to pain assessment in persons with dementia.

Sensitivity versus specificity

A final consideration when evaluating scales for measuring symptoms in non-verbal patients relates to sensitivity vs. specificity of symptom recognition. Observational scales that include fewer items focused on more obvious pain behaviours are more specific, but less sensitive in detecting pain in those with less obvious pain behaviours. If the intent is to identify as many persons at risk for unrecognized pain as possible, pain assessment tools that assess a broad range of possible pain behaviours may have greater utility. Although these tools are more sensitive than shorter tools focused on common pain behaviours, the challenge is to determine those behaviours resulting from pain versus other types of distress or conditions. Behavioural indicators (e.g. irritability, agitation, breathing changes, loss of appetite, resistance to care) can be caused by problems from varying aetiologies, including pain.

An innovative clinical protocol called the Serial Trial Intervention (STI) developed by Kovach and colleagues[54] uses a systematic method for assessing and treating behaviours that may be pain-related in patients with severe dementia. A recent randomized controlled trial (RCT) involving 114 subjects residing in 14 nursing homes demonstrated that those who received this intervention had significantly less discomfort and more frequent return of behavioural symptoms to baseline than those who did not.[55] An analgesic trial is part of the STI and has been shown to be effective in increasing recognition and treatment of pain in persons with advanced dementia and is discussed below.

Evidence to support the sensitivity to change of behavioural observation and behavioural pain assessment tools is limited. The extent to which behavioural measures can be used over time to reassess and monitor response to treatment or change in pain condition remains uncertain.

Analgesic trials

One approach to address the challenge of determining if pain is indeed the cause of specific behaviours is to expose the patients to analgesics in controlled clinical trials. The underlying thesis is that changes in behaviour resulting from the pain intervention are related to improved pain control. Early unblinded studies provided initial support for this approach[56,57] and led to further controlled trials. Study outcomes using acetaminophen administered around the clock varied and may be related to the dosing provided as part of the protocols. Although Buffum et al. did not demonstrate significant changes in agitated behaviour thought to be pain-related in persons with advanced dementia, the acetaminophen dose was only 1500 mg/day.[58] In a recent RCT, Manfredi and colleagues[59] evaluated low-dose opioid (20 meq morphine sulphate per 24 h) therapy in persons with dementia. They reported decreased agitation in the over-85 age group and suggested that less response in the younger old group could be related to the low dose of the analgesic. More recently, Chibnall et al. studied patients with dementia who received 3000 mg/day of acetaminophen in a double blind, crossover RCT and demonstrated increased levels of social activity and interaction compared to times receiving placebo.[60]

This approach as a means to evaluate pain as the cause of potential pain-related behaviours requires further investigation, but is likely an important step in the process of recognizing and validating pain in those presenting with atypical pain behaviours.

Theoretical famework for measuring symptoms in cognitively impaired patients

A theoretical framework by which symptom assessment can be conceptualized in those with cognitive impairment can be very useful. Although discussion in the literature often emphasizes establishing the presence and severity of the given symptom (such as pain), it may also be important to consider broader constructs, including the impact of the symptom (e.g. functional impairment, psychological impairment), as key outcome measures. Several models currently developed with pain as the focus may be applicable when considering other symptom measurement in cognitive impairment.

Close and colleagues[49] developed a model that illustrates levels of interpretation involved in pain measurement required by the clinician/researcher as cognitive impairment advances. Although their model focuses on pain, it has utility for any symptom evaluation. As cognitive impairment advances across a continuum, types of pain cues change from proactive self-report to reactive self-report, and then to acute response behaviours and ultimately to general behaviours. The level of interpretation required is low in intact persons and becomes greater as cognitive impairment advances, making confidence in judgements more and more difficult. This model aligns well with the available data showing that many persons with advanced dementia present with more atypical, less obvious indicators of pain.[39,57,61,62] It is not clear, however, that these atypical presentations only occur in the later states of the dementia process.

A group of researchers led by Snow present a thoughtful review and framework for assessing pain in non-communicative persons with dementia. The model is a multidimensional approach to pain assessment, emphasizing the role of the external rater. The model posits that a pain stimulus leads to pain sensation, followed by pain perception, followed by exhibition of external signs of pain, and an external rater's observation and interpretation of those signs.[24] They discuss factors that influence pain sensation, pain perception and observation and interpretation of pain in persons with dementia. Two frameworks for establishing validity of pain assessments in persons with dementia based on a self-report comparison model and a known correlates model are presented.[24] These approaches evaluate expected patterns of relationships between pain assessments and between related variables using structural equation modelling to validate judgements about pain presence, severity and/or changes.[24] The proposed models to address the challenges in using external ratings to assess pain in persons with dementia merit consideration for those conducting research on measurement of pain in this population.

Finally, Kovach and colleagues present a model of discomfort in persons with dementia based on a need-driven dementia-compromised theory suggesting that failure to recognize behaviours as symptoms leads to the undertreatment of many needs, including unrecognized pain.[63] This model illustrates the importance of recognizing behavioural symptoms and using a systematic approach to examination of physical or psychological factors that could impact pain and conducting a serial assessment and treatment approach to address identified behavioural symptoms. The clinical protocol developed by Kovach et al., which is called the Serial Trial Intervention (STI), is in effect a means to validate pain as the cause of behaviour symptoms. The STI includes targeted physical and affective assessment with associated interventions, advancing from non-pharmacological comfort interventions to analgesic interventions and ultimately consultation or psychotropic trials.

The theoretical models described above can provide a framework for assessment of pain in persons with advanced dementia. A common thread in these approaches is the complexity of validating pain presence in this population, particularly using a single strategy or approach. Closs's work actually provides a conceptualization of changes in pain cues based on level of cognitive impairment that fits nicely within the multidimensional approaches proposed by Snow and Kovach. Clearly, a multifaceted approach that draws from a variety of data sources presents a stronger case on which to base judgement about the existence and severity of pain in this vulnerable population and helps to address concerns regarding validity of external raters judgements about pain. Further development of a composite approach to evaluation of pain in non-verbal persons that could provide a common measurement methodology internationally would be a significant contribution to the literature.

Recommendations for measurement of pain in cognitively impaired patients

Quantification of pain in cognitively impaired persons: using pain scales for intensity

Principles for applying pain measurement scales in studies with patients with cognitive impairment should include: (1) selecting a scale appropriate to the study design and population of interest; (2) evaluating the frequency with which a measure must be conducted to minimize burden; (3) standardizing the format and procedure applied to all patients, if possible; and (4) documenting standard demographic and clinical covariates.[64]

As noted earlier, a number of studies support the use of pain intensity scales for use with cognitively impaired older persons. Recommendations emphasize the importance of self-report measures,

if these are feasible. Self-report scales that are the simplest and most usable for cognitively impaired older adults include numeric rating scales, verbal descriptor scales or pain thermometers, and 'faces' pain scales.[9,16,17,20–22,25,65–71] Given evidence that even those with severe cognitive impairment may be capable of completing a simple pain intensity scale and reliably report their own pain, the use of observational scales should not automatically be substituted in all persons with advanced dementia.[18,19]

A European Association of Palliative Care (EAPC) Expert Working Group has recommended the use of a standard 4-point verbal rating scale (VRS) for pain measurement in cognitively impaired patients. If self-report is possible, the group has endorsed a VRS for pain present at the moment (none, mild, moderate, severe),[64] and if self-report is not possible, the recommendation calls for a similar observer rating using a 4-point VRS for pain now.[64] Although the 4-point scale is simple, it limits the sensitivity to detect change; thus, scales with more options may be superior, depending on the nature of the sample of interest and the ability of patients to respond. Certainly, self-report on a scale with fewer response options would be desired over no self report. When self-report is no longer possible and observer rating of pain intensity is not sufficient, use of behavioural observation and/or behavioural tools are an important strategy.

Quantification of pain in cognitively impaired persons: behaviour observation tools

During the past 10 years, several observational tools for assessment of pain in persons unable to self-report have been developed. The primary emphasis has been on clinically relevant tools and sound methodological evaluation has been limited. Several reviews have systematically evaluated the strengths and limitations of existing tools.[14,72–74] Although there are many promising tools now available, the limited psychometric information on each supports a consensus that no one tool can be recommended for broad use across populations and settings.[28]

Of the existing tools, two general types of measures emerge: tools with fewer items sampling more obvious pain behaviours that can be completed by observers unfamiliar with the patient, and tools with a larger number of items that screen for broader potential pain indicators and necessitate completion by a person familiar with the patient's usual behaviour/activity. The two approaches provide tools with different levels of specificity and sensitivity that are important considerations in determining the appropriate approach for a particular patient population or setting and purpose.

Atypical presentations (e.g. increased pacing, verbal abusiveness, increased confusion) and diversity in response on a given behavioural indicator (e.g. agitation and combativeness versus withdrawal/isolation) challenge the ability to identify pain presence and quantify severity using a measure of pain behaviour. Attempting to use a standardized scale with limited options may fail to identify a significant subset of patients for which pain is not recognized and/or inadequately treated.

The American Geriatrics Society (AGS)[75] has developed a synthesis of common pain behaviours in cognitively impaired older persons that includes both typical observable pain behaviours and less obvious changes in interpersonal interactions, activity patterns or routines or mental status (Table 7.9.2). This framework provides a guide for evaluating the comprehensiveness of behavioural observation indicators included in the existing tools. Most of the

Table 7.9.2 Common pain behaviours in cognitively impaired older persons.

Behaviour	Examples
Facial expressions	Slight frown, sad, frightened face
	Grimacing, wrinkled forehead, closed or tightened eyes
	Any distorted expression
	Rapid blinking
Verbalizations, vocalizations	Signing, moaning, groaning
	Grunting, chanting, calling out
	Noisy breathing
	Asking for help
	Verbal abusiveness
Body movements	Rigid, tense body posture, guarding
	Fidgeting
	Increased pacing, rocking
	Restricted movement
	Gait or mobility changes
Changes in interpersonal interactions	Aggressive, combative, resists care
	Decreased social interactions
	Socially inappropriate, disruptive
	Withdrawn
Changes in activity patterns or routines	Refusing food, appetite change
	Increase in rest periods
	Sleep, rest pattern changes
	Sudden cessation of common routines
	Increased wandering
Mental status changes	Crying or tears
	Increased confusion
	Irritability or distress

Note: some patients demonstrate little or no specific behaviours associated with severe pain

Used with permission from the American Geriatrics Society (AGS) for 'Common Pain Behaviors in Cognitively Impaired Elderly Persons' published by the AGS Panel in the 'The Management of Persistent Pain in Older Persons' from the *Journal of the American Geriatrics Society*, 2002, **5**, 205–24, Table 3. For more information visit the AGS online at www.americangeriatrics.org

available tools include a core of more obvious non-verbal indicators of pain, including facial expressions, verbalizations/vocalizations and body movements. There are greater differences between tools when considering inclusion of more subtle non-verbal indicators of pain, such as changes in interpersonal interactions, changes in activity patterns or routines and mental status changes.

Inclusion of a greater number of potential indicators increases tool sensitivity, thereby increasing the likelihood of detecting pain if present. However, including less obvious indicators in a pain assessment tool may increase the likelihood of identifying pain when it is not present (false positives) and thus result in decreased specificity. For example, the PAINAD[35] has five items, three of which are obvious pain behaviours. When behaviours are noted on this scale, it is likely the patient does have pain; however, many persons presenting with more atypical behaviours that could be pain-related will not be identified (false negatives). The PACSLAC

is a comprehensive tool with over 60 items that broadly sample common and less obvious potential pain indicators.[62] A greater number of patients may score behaviours on this tool, suggesting possible pain; however, the behaviours may be due to other causes and the specificity of this tool is likely to be relatively low. Further research is needed to establish the best composite of pain indicators for detecting pain in those unable to self-report.

Table 7.9.3 provides preliminary information on behavioural observation pain assessment tools that are available in English and can be used to assess non-verbal persons with dementia. Each tool has strengths and limitations that should be considered in determining if one is appropriate for use in the proposed study or clinical setting. A thorough critique of each scale is available at the Pain Resource Center at the City of Hope (www.cityofhope.prc/elderly.asp), as well as in the published reviews noted earlier. The following section provides a brief overview of some of the tools that have been used in multiple studies. Readers are encouraged to monitor the current literature in this area, as ongoing evaluation studies are in process or in press and additional instruments are in varying stages of development and evaluation.

Shorter observation tools that can be completed by an observer unfamiliar with patient

The Discomfort Scale-Dementia of the Alzheimer's Type (DS-DAT)[76] is well established as a reliable tool for use in research to assess discomfort in persons with dementia. It also has been used in research studies to assess pain in older adults with dementia.[30,77,78] The tool is not comprehensive in addressing the pain-related indicators identified in recent literature and includes only those pain indicators that are most common, excluding more subtle indicators related to change in behaviour, mental status change, and changes in interpersonal interactions. The tool is administered with observation at rest, which may result in non-detection of pain indicators evident only on movement. The tool has recently demonstrated strong inter-rater reliability in a RCT focused on discomfort in persons with dementia.[77]

The Checklist of Non-verbal Pain Indicators (CNPI)[34] is an itemized list designed to measure pain behaviours in cognitively impaired older adults. The tool includes six conceptually sound pain behavioural items scored on a dichotomous scale both at rest and on movement commonly observed in older adults. Preliminary tool testing provides initial support for use of the tool with older adults in acute care setting, although low reliabilities reported suggest the need for further evaluation.[34] Recent evaluation in long-term care[31] demonstrated possible support of the CNPI as a measure of pain severity, with increases in CNPI scores associated with increases in self-report of pain. However, 50 per cent of residents reporting pain had no visible indicators of pain, raising concerns about the indicators necessary to detect pain in those unable to report. Another recent study conducted in a group of Norwegian nursing homes provides evidence of acceptable test–retest and inter-rater reliabilities and concurrent validity, as well as tool practicality when administered by various categories of nursing personnel.[79] Because of the lack of subtle behaviours or change in behaviours or interaction, the ability to detect pain in those with less obvious behavioural manifestations is questioned.

Table 7.9.3 Overview of psychometric characteristics of behavioural pain assessment scales for persons with dementia.

Non-verbal pain behaviour scale	Items/scoring range	Validity	Reliability	Feasibility/utility	Summary
SHORT DIRECT OBSERVATIONAL TOOLS (can be completed by individual not familiar with the patient)					
Discomfort Scale (DS-DAT; Hurley et al., 1992)	Nine items measured for absence or presence of discomfort: noisy breathing, negative vocalizations, content facial expression, sad facial expression, frightened facial expression, frown, relaxed body language, tense body language, and fidgeting. Each item may achieve a score of 0 to 3 points (frequency, duration, intensity) yielding a total score from 0 for no observed discomfort to 27 for high level of observed discomfort	Distinguishes between discomfort and no discomfort	Moderate internal consistency Good inter-rater reliability	Requires trained observer Complex scoring	Established tool for research to differentiate discomfort in persons with dementia. Further validation as measure of pain warranted.
Checklist of Non-verbal Pain Indicators (CNPI; Feldt, 2000)	Six items including non-verbal vocalizations, facial grimacing or wincing, bracing, rubbing, restlessness, vocal complaints. Scored present or absent at rest and on movement for total score range from 0–12	Moderate construct validity differentiating pain at rest vs. on movement Weak correlations with VDS	Moderate internal consistency reliability Good inter-rater reliability	Easy to use Scoring instructions provided Interpretation not clear	Further testing in larger populations needed
Pain Assessment in Advanced Dementia (PAINAD; Warden, et al., 2003)	Five categorical items: breathing, negative vocalizations, facial expression, body language, consolability Scoring range 0–10	Moderate ability to differentiate pleasant and aversive activities and before and after pain medication	Moderate internal consistency Good inter-rater reliability	Easy to use Scoring instructions provided Requires 5-min observation period	Preliminary testing with small sample and lack of research procedures— needs further evaluation
Non-Communicating Patient's Pain Assessment Instrument (NOPPAIN; Snow et al., 2004)	Four parts including observed behaviour response to daily activities on 6-point Likert scale (words, pain faces, noises, bracing, rubbing, restlessness); pain location; pain thermometer	Good differentiation between pain conditions with video standard— needs validation with patients	No information on reliability provided	Easy to use Provides pictures and text for understanding Scoring interpretation not provided	Evidence of reliability and validity in actual patient samples needed.
COMPREHENSIVE OBSERVATIONAL TOOLS (require input from informant familiar with the patient)					
The Abbey Pain Scale (ABBEY; Abbey et al., 2004)	The tool includes six items levelled on a 4-point scale for intensity of the behaviour with a total score of intensity of pain: vocalization, facial expression, change in body language, behavioural change, physiological change, and physical change.	Overall pain impression correlated moderately with scale scores Differentiated between pre and post intervention	Moderate internal consistency Inter-rater reliability low No test–retest reported	Reported completion 1 min. Scoring interpretation provided, but relationship with self-report of pain severity of concern	Evidence of reliability and validity is not well established Conceptual issues related to items and scoring
DOLOPLUS-2 (Wary, 1999)	10 items, 3 dimensions of somatic ($n = 5$), psychomotor ($n = 2$), psychosocial ($n = 3$) Scoring range 0–30 Reflects progression of experienced pain, not current pain experience	Established in French, not in English Distinguishes between pain/no pain moderately well	Established in French, not in English Moderate inter-rater and intra-rater reliability Strong internal consistency	Translation issues and testing in English needed; Appears easy to use; estimated time 5 min	Limited information in English on psychometric qualities Needs further study

(continued)

Table 7.9.3 (Continued) Overview of psychometric characteristics of behavioural pain assessment scales for persons with dementia.

Non-verbal pain behaviour scale	Items/scoring range	Validity	Reliability	Feasibility/utility	Summary
Pain Assessment in Non-communicative Elderly Persons (PAINE; Cohen-Mansfield, 2006)	22 items rated for the past week in following categories: specific physical repetitive movements, vocal repetitive behaviours, physical signs of pain, and changes in behaviour Summary score includes mean of moaning and rigidity ratings and count based on all other variables	Moderate to good correlations with other informant ratings Low correlations with self-report and observational measures	Adequate internal consistency, inter-rater reliability, and test-retest adequate	Time to complete unknown; scoring somewhat complex	Preliminary data support need for further evaluation
Pain Assessment Checklist for Seniors with Limited Ability to Communicate (PACSLAC; Fuchs-Lacelle & Hadjistavropoulos, 2004)	60 items, 4 dimensions: facial expression (n = 13) activity/body movements (n = 20) social/personality/mood (n = 12) physiological/eating/sleeping/vocal (n = 15) Scoring range 0–60	Differentiates moderately between pain, calm and distress events based on rater memory	Moderate to good internal consistency Excellent inter-rater and good internal consistency reported recently with prospective data	Long list, but appears easy to use; Estimated time 5 min	Further refinement (factor analysis) and testing with actual patients needed
Pain Assessment in Dementing Elders (PADE; Villaneuva et al., 2003)	24 items, 3 parts: Part I, Physical, includes observable facial expression, breathing pattern and posture; Part II, Global assessment, involves proxy evaluation of pain intensity; and Part III, Functional, includes activities of daily living including dressing, feeding oneself, transfers from wheelchair to bed.	Weakly differentiates between pain and no pain groups	Low to good internal consistency Inter-rater and test-retest reliability low to good Intra-rater reliability moderate to good	Long list. Complex format with different scaling approaches Authors report 5–10 min to complete with practice No score interpretation provided	Further validation of construct validity needed. Refinement of scale parts with low reliability needed

The Pain Assessment in Advanced Dementia (PAINAD) Scale[35] was developed as a short, easy-to-use observation tool for assessing pain in individuals with advanced dementia. The PAINAD is an adaptation of the DS-DAT and the FLACC (Face, Legs, Activity, Cry, Consolability).[80] The limited number of items limits the ability of the PAINAD to detect pain in persons with dementia with more subtle behaviour changes. The use of a rating scale for pain intensity scoring of behaviours has not been substantiated in the literature. Follow-up studies conducted since initial development demonstrate strong correlations between the PAINAD and nurse-reported pain scores, but poor correlations with self-reported pain scores in the long-term care setting;[81] there was user support for the PAINAD in palliative care patients,[82] but the items of breathing and consolability were questioned. Reports of acceptable concurrent validity and reliability have been reported on an Italian version of the PAINAD when used with mildly demented subjects.[83]

The Non-Communicative Patient's Pain Assessment Instrument (NOPPAIN)[24] is an instrument that focuses on nursing assistant observation and assessment of pain in patients with dementia. Nursing assistants observe for pain-related behaviours as they perform common care tasks. Pain is assessed at rest and with movement. The NOPPAIN contains common pain behaviours and does not include comprehensive non-verbal pain behaviours. Because the NOPPAIN is conceptually grounded on validity of proxy report of pain intensity, evidence to support the validity of judgements of intensity of pain behaviours as indicators of pain severity is needed. Preliminary support for tool reliability and validity was reported based on response to video simulations, rather than actual patient observation, again suggesting the need for further testing. Although ease of administration by nursing assistants is a strength of the tool, further evaluation of their ability to use the scale with actual patients is needed.

The Abbey Pain Scale (ABBEY)[84] is an Australian tool that measures pain intensity in people with late-stage dementia. Although there is no presentation of the conceptual basis for the tool, it is apparent that the tool attempts to measure *acute pain*, *chronic pain* and *acute on chronic* in the same tool. Although the tool does include at least one cue from each of the six categories of non-verbal pain behaviour indicators from the American Geriatrics Society guidelines, the inclusion of physiological indicators is not supported in the literature to assess chronic pain. Recent evaluation of the ABBEY in palliative care patients suggested that the staff perceived the tool as a helpful in judging pain,[82] although facial expression, vocalizations and body language were considered the best and easiest pain indicators to observe. Tool revision and additional testing in well-designed studies are recommended.

The Doloplus 2[85,86] is a French tool developed for the multidimensional assessment of pain in non-verbal older adults that has been translated into several languages, including English. The Doloplus 2 is a comprehensive tool for assessing pain in non-verbal older adults and addresses many key indicators noted in the literature and the American Geriatrics Society guidelines. According to the Dolophus website, the tool developers report extensive testing in Europe; however, information in English is limited and available reports or website data do not provide sufficient detail on which to base sound judgement of the instrument. Translation issues are evident and further study or description regarding the use of Doloplus 2 in English-speaking populations is needed. Reports of translation and evaluation in Norwegian support tool validity and clinical utility.[87]

Pain Assessment for the Dementing Elderly (PADE)[88] is a tool to assess pain in individuals with advanced dementia. It was developed to assist caregivers assess patient behaviour that may indicate pain. Although the tool addresses broad areas of potential pain behaviours, the operationalization of these indicators is not clear from the published information. The tool relies on caregivers' ability to rate intensity of pain, an assumption not supported by current literature. The impact of timing differences of data collection may be a concern given that some data are retrospective and some are current. Preliminary internal consistency of the tool is not well established for all components, and the ability of the PADE to distinguish patients with and without pain conditions is not certain. Issues related to tool construction, presentation, validity, and clarity in scoring and interpretation suggest the need for revision and further testing.

The Pain Assessment Checklist for Seniors with Severe Dementia (PACSLAC),[62] developed by a Canadian team, is an observational tool for assessment of both common and uncommon pain behaviours. The PACSLAC is a potentially clinically useful behaviour checklist that appears simple to use for assessing and monitoring changes in persons with dementia and diverse presentations of pain-related behaviour. The tool is comprehensive and addresses all six pain behaviour categories included in the American Geriatrics Society guidelines. Preliminary testing of the PACSLAC used retrospective judgements and ongoing prospective evaluation is in process. The authors report recent prospective findings of excellent inter-rater reliability and good internal consistency with current long-term care residents and nurse observations (S. Fuchs-Lacelle and T. Hadjistavropolous, personal communication). Additionally, factor analysis may assist in item reduction.

Quantification of pain in intubated/unconscious: behaviour observation tools

In addition to persons with advanced dementia, intubated and unconscious patients are at risk for under-recognition and treatment of pain. The literature in this area focuses on patients in intensive care setting, rather than those in the home environment. The principles discussed earlier related to assessment of pain in those with cognitive impairment generally apply to this group as well.

Obtaining a report of pain from critically ill patients is often impeded by factors such as delirium, or other cognitive or communication limitations related to impaired level of consciousness, presence of an endotracheal tube, or treatment with sedatives and neuromuscular blocking agents.[14] As with persons with dementia, persons in the intensive care unit (ICU) may exhibit distress behaviours as a result of the fear and anxiety associated with the setting and circumstances, and careful interpretation of behaviours is necessary.

Two scales are currently available for use with adults who are unconscious/intubated and have been evaluated in the ICU setting. The Behavioural Pain Scale[89] and the Critical-Care Pain Observation Tool[90] both have preliminary psychometric evaluation that supports consideration as measurement strategies in this population. Although no single behavioural scale has been shown most effective in this population, scales from other settings also may be useful. Testing is needed to validate the appropriateness of selected scales in the environment of the ICU and with patients who are unconscious or intubated. Behavioural pain scales are not appropriate for pharmacologically paralysed adults, or those who are flaccid and cannot respond behaviourally to pain.[14] Further research is needed to refine and further validate the scales for pain assessment in these vulnerable populations.

Summary

Current methods for measuring pain in cognitively impaired patients support initial attempts at self-report, followed by measurement of observed pain-related behaviours and soliciting surrogate reports in those unable to self-report. Response to empirical therapy has been identified as a potential method to validate whether or not the presence of or changes in specific behaviours represent pain or other distressing symptoms. Tools for evaluating pain in non-verbal patients are still in early stages of development, but are finding their way into practice settings with some success. Models that provide a conceptual framework for identification and measurement of pain in cognitively impaired patients are available, but further work in refining a theoretical model that includes a composite measure for detecting and monitoring pain in this population is warranted.

Measurement of symptoms other than pain in patients with cognitive impairment

The challenges in measuring non-pain symptoms in cognitively impaired patients are similar to those confronted in the measurement of pain. However, the state of the science is not as advanced for symptoms other than pain. Instruments to measure common symptoms, such as fatigue, dyspnoea, anorexia, and nausea, in cognitively impaired patients generally are lacking. As a result,

clinicians and researchers must rely on judgements made by family and other proxies, often without data regarding the accuracy of proxies' assessments.[13,91–95] Several preliminary studies have examined the associations between physiological indicators and subjective experience of dyspnoea,[96,92] as well as behavioural indicators of mood disorders and emotional distress.[91,97] Among the common symptoms seen in palliative care, dyspnoea and depression have been examined in patients with cognitive impairment.

Dyspnoea

Dyspnoea is a common and distressing symptom at the EOL. Like pain, it is defined as a subjective experience that is influenced by multiple physiological, psychosocial and environmental factors.[98] Dyspnoea is likely to occur in many cognitively impaired or non-verbal palliative care patients, particularly those with predisposing physiological disturbances such as hypercarbia or hypoxaemia, or increased inspiratory effort.[96] Valid, reliable measures of dyspnoea that do not rely on patient self-report are necessary to identify and treat this distressing symptom.

Campbell[96] developed a model of respiratory distress in cognitively impaired, critically ill patients, which highlights the probable role of subcortical mechanisms activated in response to conditions that produce asphyxia. These mechanisms result in primitive responses such as fear and autonomic nervous system stimulation that are manifested as observable signs. Fig. 7.9.1 lists these signs, which include tachypnoea, nasal flaring, accessory muscle use, restlessness, and grunting at end-expiration. Despite the potential utility of this model in clinical practice, it has yet to be empirically validated. Moreover, it is unclear how generalizable the framework

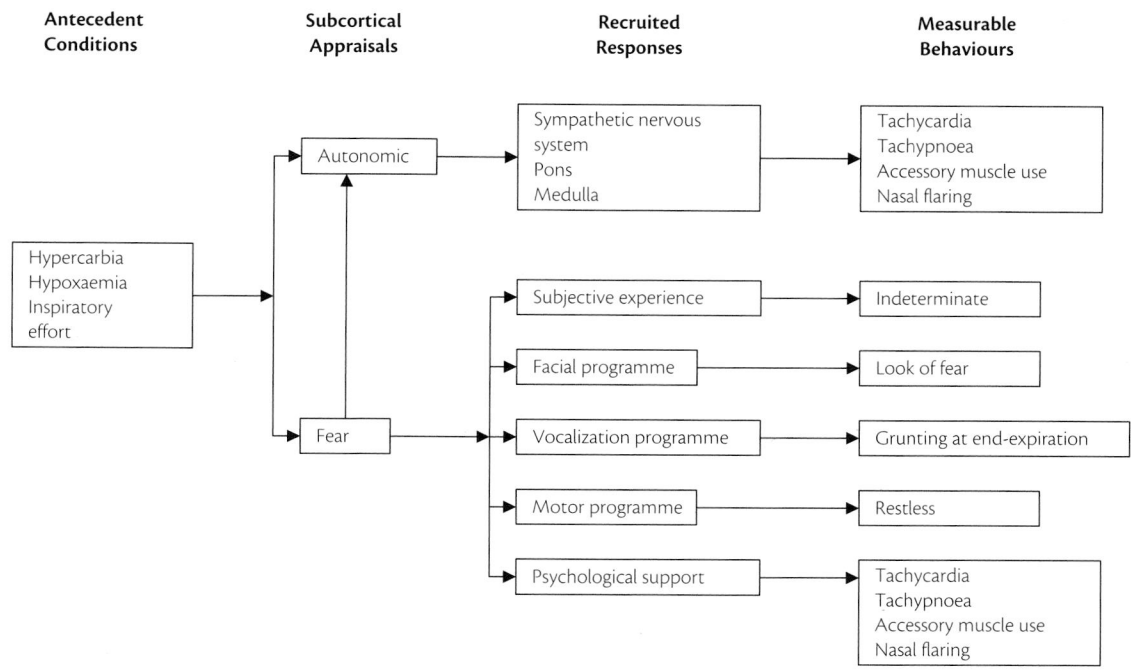

Figure 7.9.1 A model of respiratory distress in the cognitively impaired patient.
Source: Campbell, M.L. (2004). Terminal dyspnea and respiratory distress. *Critical Care Clinics*, **20**(3), 403–17, viii–ix. Printed with permission.

is to diverse patient groups such as those with dementia or in a persistent vegetative state.

Depression

The most extensive research involving depression scales in cognitively impaired patients has focused on those with dementia. Two self-report measures of depression, the Beck Depression Scale and the Adjective Mood Checklist have been examined in mildly demented patients and found to correlate well with ratings by psychiatrists.[99]

Similarly, the 15-item Geriatric Depression Scale identified depression accurately in community-dwelling patients with mild dementia;[100] however, the accuracy diminished considerably in institutionalized persons and in those with greater cognitive impairment.[100–102]

It is possible to circumvent some of the problems with self-report depression scales through the use of clinician rating scales. One widely used instrument is the Cornell Scale for Depression in Dementia (CSDD). The CSDD is a 19-item clinician-administered instrument that uses information from interviews with a caregiver (usually a nurse), as well as interviews and direct observation of the patient. Using tools with similar items, the clinician first interviews the caregiver and then the patient. If there are discrepancies among caregiver report, patient responses, and the clinician's observations, the clinician evaluator conducts a follow-up interview with the caregiver to uncover reasons for the discrepancy. The final score is based on the clinician's judgement after considering all data. Reliability and validity of the CSDD have been investigated in adults with and without dementia,[97,103] although Kurlowicz et al. questioned the validity of the scale in frail, institutionalized older adults with high levels of co-morbid medical conditions.[104] Greenberg and colleagues also cast doubt on the validity of the scale; they reported very low agreement between the CSDD and a psychiatrist's assessment of depression in nursing home residents ($K = 0.029$).[105]

The limitations of the scales and models used to assess dyspnoea and depression in cognitively impaired patients demonstrates the enormous gap that still exists in the ability of clinicians and researchers to measure non-pain symptoms using psychometrically sound and clinically useful instruments in this population. The multi-modal approaches that have been applied recently to the study of pain in cognitively impaired patients have yet to be developed for other symptoms. These comprehensive strategies, which combine self-report (when possible) observations of physiological and behavioural indicators, disease-related clues, proxy reports, and response to empirical therapy, are necessary to develop valid, reliable and sensitive instruments to measure other EOL symptoms.

Summary and recommendations for future research

Measurement of pain and other symptoms in cognitively impaired patients continues to be a major challenge. The science that undergirds symptom measurement in this population is in its infancy and many methodological hurdles must be overcome before investigators and clinicians can assess the presence, severity, and impact of symptoms in patients with limited abilities to process information and respond verbally. Despite the difficulties, improving care

to the vulnerable patients who cannot self-report their symptoms is a goal that should prompt support for research in this area.

Research teams that move the science forward will need to comprise clinicians and investigators from multiple disciplines. Since the gold standard—patient self-report—is unreliable or unavailable, developing valid, clinically sound measures will require different perspectives. Expertise in the physiological, behavioural, psychosocial, and genetic determinants of a measurable symptom will all come into play. Moreover, caregivers such as nursing assistants, who have extensive knowledge about individual patients' behaviours and history will likely provide invaluable insight about strategies to assess symptoms.

Within a research programme to develop and test instruments, several issues need to be addressed. Strategies to improve proxy reporting must be refined and applied to a variety of lay and professional caregivers. Scales need to be evaluated in rigorous, methodologically sound studies. Appropriate statistical methods should be used to determine the best composite measures that incorporate several sources of data. These measures must be evaluated to ensure that they are sensitive to treatment effects. For many existing instruments, validation studies have been conducted using small, homogeneous samples in a single palliative care setting. To the extent possible, scales should be useful in a broad range of patient and clinical settings. Another important issue is whether or not behavioural observation tools are valid for patients from diverse cultures. Finally, testable models that operationalize the antecedents, observable indicators, and consequences of symptoms should serve as the foundation of scale development.

References

1. Goy, E. and Ganzini, L. (2003). Delirium, anxiety, and depression. In *Geriatric palliative care* (eds. R.S. Morrison and D.E. Meier), pp. 286–303. New York: Oxford University Press.
2. Solano, J.P., Gomes, B., and Higginson, I.J. (2006). A comparison of symptom prevalence in far advanced cancer, AIDS, heart disease, chronic obstructive pulmonary disease and renal disease. *Journal of Pain and Symptom Management*, **31**(1), 58–69.
3. Lawlor, P.G., Fainsinger, R.L., and Bruera, E.D. (2000). Delirium at the end of life: critical issues in clinical practice and research. *JAMA*, **284**(19), 2427–9.
4. Hebert, L.E. *et al.* (2003). Alzheimer disease in the US population: prevalence estimates using the 2000 census. *Archives of Neurology*, **60**(8), 1119–22.
5. Mitchell, S.L. *et al.* (2005). A national study of the location of death for older persons with dementia. *Journal of the American Geriatrics Society*, **53**(2), 299–305.
6. Sengstaken, E.A. and King, S.A. (19931). The problems of pain and its detection among geriatric nursing home residents. *Journal of the American Geriatrics Society*, **41**(5), 541–4.
7. Williams, C.S. *et al.* (2005). Characteristics associated with pain in long-term care residents with dementia. *Gerontologist*, **45**(1), 68–73.
8. Morrison, R.S. and Siu, A.L. (2000). A comparison of pain and its treatment in advanced dementia and cognitively intact patients with hip fracture. *Journal of Pain and Symptom Management*, **19**(4), 240–8.
9. Feldt, K.S., Ryden, M.B., and Miles, S. (1998). Treatment of pain in cognitively impaired compared with cognitively intact older patients with hip-fracture. *Journal of the American Geriatrics Society*, **46**(9), 1079–85.
10. Horgas, A.L. and Tsai, P.F. (1998). Analgesic drug prescription and use in cognitively impaired nursing home residents. *Nursing Research*, **47**(4), 235–42.

11. Bernabei, R. *et al.* (1998). Management of pain in elderly patients with cancer. SAGE Study Group. Systematic Assessment of Geriatric Drug Use via Epidemiology. *JAMA*, **279**(23), 1877–82.

12. Won, A. *et al.* (1999). Correlates and management of nonmalignant pain in the nursing home. SAGE Study Group. Systematic Assessment of Geriatric drug use via Epidemiology. *Journal of the American Geriatrics Society*, **47**(8), 936–42.

13. Kutner, J.S. *et al.* (2006). Symptom distress and quality-of-life assessment at the end of life: the role of proxy response. *Journal of Pain and Symptom Management*, **32**(4), 300–10.

14. Herr, K. *et al.* (2006). Pain assessment in the nonverbal patient: position statement with clinical practice recommendations. *Pain Management Nursing*, **7**(2), 44–52.

15. Buffum, M.D. *et al.* (2007). Cognitive impairment and pain management: Review of issues and challenges. *Journal of Rehabilitation Research and Development*, **44**(2), 315–30.

16. Herr, K. and Decker, S. (2004). Assessment of pain in older adults with severe cognitive impairment. *Annals of Long-Term Care*, **12**(4), 46–52.

17. Kaasalainen, S. and Crook, J. (2003). A comparison of pain-assessment tools for use with elderly long-term-care residents. *Canadian Journal of Nursing Research*, **35**(4), 58–71.

18. Pautex, S. *et al.* (2005). Feasibility and reliability of four pain self-assessment scales and correlation with an observational rating scale in hospitalized elderly demented patients. *The Journals of Gerontology. Series A: Biological Science and Medical Science*, **60**(4), 524–9.

19. Pautex, S. *et al.* (2006). Pain in severe dementia: self-assessment or observational scales? *Journal of the American Geriatrics Society*, **54**(7), 1040–5.

20. Scherder, E.J., Sergeant, J.A., and Swaab, D.F. (2003). Pain processing in dementia and its relation to neuropathology. *Lancet Neurology*, **2**(11), 677–86.

21. Taylor, L.J. *et al.* (2005). Psychometric evaluation of selected pain intensity scales for use with cognitively impaired and cognitively intact older adults. *Rehabilitation Nursing*, **30**(2), 55–61.

22. Chibnall, J.T. and Tait, R.C. (2001). Pain assessment in cognitively impaired and unimpaired older adults: a comparison of four scales. *Pain*, **92**(1–2), 173–86.

23. Cohen-Mansfield, J. (2002). Relatives' assessment of pain in cognitively impaired nursing home residents. *Journal of Pain and Symptom Management*, **24**(6), 562–71.

24. Snow, A.L. *et al.* (2004). A conceptual model of pain assessment for noncommunicative persons with dementia. *Gerontologist*, **44**(6), 807–17.

25. Buffum, M.D. *et al.* (2001). A pilot study of the relationship between discomfort and agitation in patients with dementia. *Geriatric Nursing*, **22**(2), 80–5.

26. Herr, K. and Garand, L. (2001). Assessment and measurement of pain in older adults. *Clinics in Geriatric Medicine*, **17**(3), 457–78, vi.

27. Weiner, D., Herr, K., and Rudy, T. (2002). *Persistent pain in older adults: An interdisciplinary guide for treatment*. New York: Springer Publishing Company.

28. Hadjistavropoulos, T. *et al.* (in press) An interdisciplinary expert consensus statement on assessment of pain in older persons. *Pain Medicine*.

29. Bergh, I. *et al.* (2000). An application of pain rating scales in geriatric patients. *Aging-Clinical & Experimental Research*, **12**(5), 380–7.

30. Miller, J. *et al.* (1996). The assessment of discomfort in elderly confused patients: a preliminary study. *Journal of Neuroscience Nursing*, **28**(3), 175–82.

31. Jones, K.R. *et al.* (2005). Measuring pain intensity in nursing home residents. *Journal of Pain and Symptom Management*, **30**(6), 519–27.

32. Gibson, S.J. and Farrell, M. (2004). A review of age differences in the neurophysiology of nociception and the perceptual experience of pain. *Clinical Journal of Pain*, **20**(4), 227–39.

33. Schuler, M. *et al.* (2004). Acute and chronic pain in geriatrics: Clinical characteristics of pain and the influence of cognition. *Pain Medicine*, **5**(3), 253–62.

34. Feldt, K.S. (2000). The checklist of nonverbal pain indicators (CNPI). *Pain Management Nursing*, **1**(1), 13–21.

35. Warden, V., Hurley, A.C., and Volicer, L. (2003). Development and psychometric evaluation of the pain assessment in advanced dementia (PAINAD) scale. *Journal of the American Medical Directors Association*, (Jan/Feb), 9–15.

36. Bell, M.L. (1997). Postoperative pain management for the cognitively impaired older adult. *Seminars in Perioperative Nursing*, **6**(1), 37–41.

37. Hadjistavropoulos, T. *et al.* (2000). Measuring movement-exacerbated pain in cognitively impaired frail elders. *Clinical Journal of Pain*, **16**(1), 54–63.

38. McCaffery, M. and Pasero, C. (1999). *Pain: clinical manual*, 2nd edition. St. Louis: Mosby.

39. Manfredi, P.L. *et al.* (2003). Pain assessment in elderly patients with severe dementia. *Journal of Pain & Symptom Management*, **25**(1), 48–52.

40. Cohen-Mansfield, J. and Creedon, M. (2002). Nursing staff members' perceptions of pain indicators in persons with severe dementia. *Clinical Journal of Pain*, **18**(1), 64–73.

41. Horgas, A.L. and Dunn, K. (2001). Pain in nursing home residents. Comparison of residents' self-report and nursing assistants' perceptions. Incongruencies exist in resident and caregiver reports of pain; therefore, pain management education is needed to prevent suffering. *Journal of Gerontological Nursing*, **27**(3), 44–53.

42. Shega, J.W. *et al.* (2004). Pain in community-dwelling persons with dementia: frequency, intensity, and congruence between patient and caregiver report. *Journal of Pain and Symptom Management*, **28**(6), 585–92.

43. Cohen-Mansfield, J. (2005). Nursing staff members' assessments of pain in cognitively impaired nursing home residents. *Pain Management Nursing*, **6**(2), 68–75.

44. Cohen-Mansfield, J. and Lipson, S. (2002). Pain in cognitively impaired nursing home residents: how well are physicians diagnosing it? *Journal of the American Geriatrics Society*, **50**(6), 1039–44.

45. Fisher, S.E. *et al.* (2002). Pain assessment and management in cognitively impaired nursing home residents: association of certified nursing assistant pain report, Minimum Data Set pain report, and analgesic medication use. *Journal of the American Geriatrics Society*, **50**(1), 152–6.

46. Desbiens, N.A. and Mueller-Rizner, N. (2000). How well do surrogates assess the pain of seriously ill patients? *Critical Care Medicine*, **28**(5), 1347–52.

47. McMillan, S.C. and Moody, L.E. (2003). Hospice patient and caregiver congruence in reporting patients' symptom intensity. *Cancer Nursing*, **26**(2), 113–8.

48. Yeager, K.A. *et al.* (1995). Differences in pain knowledge and perception of the pain experience between outpatients with cancer and their family caregivers. *Oncology Nursing Forum*, **22**(8), 1235–41.

49. Closs, S.J. *et al.* (2005). Cues for the identification of pain in nursing home residents. *International Journal of Nursing Studies*, **42**(1), 3–12.

50. Mentes, J.C., Teer, J., and Cadogan, M.P. (2004). The pain experience of cognitively impaired nursing home residents: perceptions of family members and certified nursing assistants. *Pain Management Nursing*, **5**(3), 118–25.

51. Huffman, J.C. and Kunik, M.E. (2000). Assessment and understanding of pain in patients with dementia. *Gerontologist*, **40**(5), 574–81.

52. Scherder, E. *et al.* (2005). Recent developments in pain in dementia. *BMJ*, **330**(7489), 461–4.

53. Herr, K., Bjoro, K., and Decker, S. (2006). Tools for assessment of pain in nonverbal older adults with dementia: a state-of-the-science review. *Journal of Pain and Symptom Management*, **31**(2), 170–92.

54. Kovach, C.R. *et al.* (2001). Use of the assessment of discomfort in dementia protocol. *Applied Nursing Research*, **14**(4), 193–200.

55. Kovach, C.R. *et al.* (2006). The Serial Trial Intervention: an innovative approach to meeting needs of individuals with dementia. *Journal of Gerontological Nursing*, **32**(4), 18–25; quiz 26–7.

56. Douzjian, M. *et al.* (1998). A program to use pain control medication to reduce psychotropic drug use in residents with difficult behavior. *Annals of Long Term Care*, **6**(5), 174–9.

57. Kovach, C.R. *et al.* (1999). Assessment and treatment of discomfort for people with late-stage dementia. *Journal of Pain and Symptom Management*, **18**(6), 412–9.

58. Buffum, M.D. *et al.* (2004). A clinical trial of the effectiveness of regularly scheduled versus as-needed administration of acetaminophen in the management of discomfort in older adults with dementia. *Journal of the American Geriatrics Society*, **52**(7), 1093–7.

59. Manfredi, P.L. *et al.* (2003). Opioid treatment for agitation in patients with advanced dementia. *International Journal of Geriatric Psychiatry*, **18**(8), 700–5.

60. Chibnall, J.T. *et al.* (2005). Effect of acetaminophen on behavior, well-being, and psychotropic medication use in nursing home residents with moderate-to-severe dementia. *Journal of the American Geriatrics Society*, **53**(11), 1921–9.

61. AGS Panel on Persistent Pain in Older Persons (2002). The management of persistent pain in older persons. *Journal of the American Geriatrics Society*, **50**(Suppl. 6), S205–24.

62. Fuchs-Lacelle, S. and Hadjistavropoulos, T. (2004). Development and preliminary validation of the Pain Assessment Checklist for Seniors with Limited Ability to Communicate (PACSLAC). *Pain Management Nursing*, **5**(2).

63. Kovach, C.R. *et al.* (2005). A model of consequences of need-driven, dementia-compromised behavior. *Journal of Nursing Scholarship*, **37**(2), 134–40; discussion 140.

64. Caraceni, A. *et al.* (2002). Pain measurement tools and methods in clinical research in palliative care: recommendations of an Expert Working Group of the European Association of Palliative Care. *Journal of Pain and Symptom Management*, **23**(3), 239–55.

65. Briggs, M. and Closs, J.S. (1999). A descriptive study of the use of visual analogue scales and verbal rating scales for the assessment of postoperative pain in orthopedic patients. *Journal of Pain and Symptom Management*, **18**(6), 438–46.

66. Closs, S.J. *et al.* (2004). A comparison of five pain assessment scales for nursing home residents with varying degrees of cognitive impairment. *Journal of Pain & Symptom Management*, **27**(3), 196–205.

67. Krulewitch, H. *et al.* (2000). Assessment of pain in cognitively impaired older adults: a comparison of pain assessment tools and their use by nonprofessional caregivers. *Journal of the American Geriatrics Society*, **48**(12), 1607–11.

68. Manz, B.D. *et al.* (2000). Pain assessment in the cognitively impaired and unimpaired elderly. *Pain Management Nursing*, **1**(4), 106–15.

69. Taylor, L.J. and Herr, K. (2003). Pain intensity assessment: a comparison of selected pain intensity scales for use in cognitively intact and cognitively impaired African American older adults. *Pain Management Nursing*, **4**(2), 87–95.

70. Weiner, D.K. *et al.* (1998). Predictors of pain self-report in nursing home residents. *Aging: Clinical and Experimental Research*, **10**, 411–20.

71. Wynne, C.F., Ling, S.M., and Remsburg, R. (2000). Comparison of pain assessment instruments in cognitively intact and cognitively impaired nursing home residents. *Geriatric Nursing*, **21**(1), 20–3.

72. Hadjistavropoulos, T. (2005). Assessing pain in persons with severe limitations in ability to communicate. In *Pain in the elderly* (eds. S. Gibson and D. Weiner), pp. 135–51. Seattle: IASP Press.

73. Zwakhalen, S.M., Hamers, J.P., and Berger, M.P. (2006). The psychometric quality and clinical usefulness of three pain assessment tools for elderly people with dementia. *Pain*, **126**(1–3), 210–20.

74. Stolee, P. *et al.* (2005). Instruments for the assessment of pain in older persons with cognitive impairment. *Journal of the American Geriatrics Society*, **53**(2), 319–26.

75. American Pain Society (2003). *Principles of analgesic use in the treatment of acute pain and cancer pain*, 5th edition. Glenview: American Pain Society (APS), p. 73.

76. Hurley, A.C. *et al.* (1992). Assessment of discomfort in advanced Alzheimer patients. *Research in Nursing & Health*, **15**(5), 369–77.

77. Kovach, C.R. *et al.* (2006). Behaviors of nursing home residents with dementia: examining nurse responses. *Journal of Gerontological Nursing*, **32**(6), 13–21.

78. Young, D.M. (2001). Pain in institutionalized elders with chronic dementia. The University of Iowa, Ph.D., p. 169.

79. Nygaard, H.A. and Jarland, M. (2006). The Checklist of Nonverbal Pain Indicators (CNPI): testing of reliability and validity in Norwegian nursing homes. *Age Ageing*, **35**(1), 79–81.

80. Merkel, S.I. *et al.* (1997). Practice applications of research. The FLACC: a behavioral scale for scoring postoperative pain in young children. *Pediatric Nursing*, **23**(3), 293–7.

81. Leong, I.Y., Chong, M.S., and Gibson, S.J. (2006). The use of a self-reported pain measure, a nurse-reported pain measure and the PAINAD in nursing home residents with moderate and severe dementia: a validation study. *Age Ageing*, **35**(3), 252–6.

82. van Iersel, T., Timmerman, D., and Mullie, A. (2006). Introduction of a pain scale for palliative care patients with cognitive impairment. *International Journal of Palliative Nursing*, **12**(2), 54–9.

83. Costardi, D. *et al.* (2006). The Italian version of the pain assessment in advanced dementia (PAINAD) scale. *Archives of Gerontology and Geriatrics*.

84. Abbey, J.A. *et al.* (2004). The Abbey Pain Scale. A 1-minute numerical indicator for people with late-stage dementia. *International Journal of Palliative Nursing*, **10**(1), 6–13.

85. Lefebvre-Chapiro, S. and The Doloplus Group (2001). The Doloplus 2 scale – evaluating pain in the elderly. *European Journal of Palliative Care*, **8**(5), 191–4.

86. The Doloplus Group. (2003). Behavioral pain assessment scale for elderly subjects presenting with verbal communication disorders Available from: http://www.doloplus.com.

87. Holen, J.C. *et al.* (2005). The Norwegian Doloplus-2, a tool for behavioural pain assessment: translation and pilot-validation in nursing home patients with cognitive impairment. *Palliative Medicine*, **19**(5), 411–7.

88. Villanueva, M.R. *et al.* (2003). Pain assessment for the dementing elderly (PADE): Reliability and validity of a new measure. *Journal of the American Medical Directors Association*, Jan/Feb, 1–8.

89. Payen, J.F. *et al.* (2001). Assessing pain in critically ill sedated patients by using a behavioral pain scale. *Crit Care Med*, **29**(12), 2258–63.

90. Gelinas, C. *et al.* (2006). Validation of the critical-care pain observation tool in adult patients. *America Journal of Critical Care*, **15**(4), 420–7.

91. Dwyer, M. and Byrne, G.J. (2000). Disruptive vocalization and depression in older nursing home residents. *International Psychogeriatrics*, **12**(4), 463–71.

92. Hajiro, T. *et al.* (1998). Analysis of clinical methods used to evaluate dyspnea in patients with chronic obstructive pulmonary disease. *American Journal of Respiratory and Critical Care Medicine*, **158**(4), 1185–9.

93. Nekolaichuk, C.L. *et al.* (1999). A comparison of patient and proxy symptom assessments in advanced cancer patients. *Palliative Medicine*, **13**(4), 311–23.

94. Teno, J.M. *et al.* (2004). Family perspectives on end-of-life care at the last place of care. *JAMA*, **291**(1), 88–93.

95. Volicer, L., Hurley, A.C., and Blasi, Z.V. (2001). Scales for evaluation of End-of-Life Care in Dementia. *Alzheimer Disease and Associated Disorders*, **15**(4), 194–200.

96. Campbell, M.L. (2004). Terminal dyspnea and respiratory distress. *Critical Care Clinics*, **20**(3), 403–17, viii–ix.

97. Alexopoulos, G.S. *et al.* (1988). Use of the Cornell scale in nondemented patients. *Journal of the American Geriatrics Society*, **36**(3), 230–6.

98. American Thoracic Society (1999). Dyspnea. Mechanisms, assessment, and management: a consensus statement. American Thoracic Society. *American Journal of Respiratory and Critical Care Medicine*, **159**(1), 321–40.

99. Miller, N.E. (1980). The measurement of mood in senile brain disease: examiner ratings and self-reports. *Proceedings of the Annual Meeting of the American Psychopathological Association*, **69**, 97–122.

100. Muller-Thomsen, T. *et al.* (2005). Detecting depression in Alzheimer's disease: evaluation of four different scales. *Archives of Clinical Neuropsychology*, **20**(2), 271–6.

101. Gilley, D.W. and Wilson, R.S. (1997). Criterion-related validity of the Geriatric Depression Scale in Alzheimer's disease. *Journal of Clinical and Experimental Neuropsychology*, **19**(4), 489–99.

102. Montorio, I. and Izal, M. (1996). The Geriatric Depression Scale: a review of its development and utility. *International Psychogeriatrics*, **8**(1), 103–12.

103. Alexopoulos, G. (2002). The Cornell scale for depression in dementia: administration and scoring guidelines. White Plain: George S. Alexopoulos.

104. Kurlowicz, L.H. *et al.* (2002). A psychometric evaluation of the Cornell Scale for Depression in Dementia in a frail, nursing home population. *American Journal of Geriatric Psychiatry*, **10**(5), 600–8.

105. Greenberg, L. *et al.* (2004). Screening for depression in nursing home palliative care patients. *Journal of Geriatric Psychiatry and Neurology*, **17**(4), 212–8.

7.10

Clinical and organizational audit and quality improvement in palliative medicine

Irene J. Higginson

Quality of care: a worldwide concern?

Quality in health care is now centre stage in many countries. Whatever the funding system (national insurance, state, private), many countries place a high priority on 'consumer' choice, accountability, and ensuring high quality and efficient care[1]. Scandals arising from poor care, higher public expectations, increased health-care spending, and the move towards quality service in many public and private companies have all heightened the desire to introduce quality assurance, audit, and evaluation into clinical care. In response, clinicians, managers, and governments have sought to standardize clinical practice to that which is the 'best' possible practice, or which is proven to be the most effective and efficient[2,3].

Although many terms in the quality dictionary are new, many of the ideas, such as clinical review, are not[2,4–6]. The history of quality improvement and audit can be traced back as far as 1700 BC in Egypt, when King Hammurabi introduced penalties (some quite drastic) for different degrees of 'surgical incompetence' (although it is not clear who decided this incompetence). In 1518, the Charter of the Royal College of Physicians included: 'to uphold the standards of medicine both for their own honour and public benefit'. The General Nursing Council (GNC) was established in 1919 to 'monitor nurses' practice and conduct'. Florence Nightingale was one of the first clinicians to insist on measuring the outcome of care for her patients to evaluate treatment. Grand rounds, postgraduate lectures, and clinical presentations already contributed to the review of medical and nursing performance. However, the new emphasis on audit and quality improvement and governance has brought four main differences:

- Explicit criteria for good practice should be applied by all clinicians rather than those in exemplary centres.

- All patients in care and all centres should be included in quality monitoring rather than a few 'interesting' cases.

- Patients and their families should be able to seek empowerment.

- Funding or accreditation may be withheld from those units which do not comply with quality standards or which are found to be ineffective or inefficient[7].

References in the medical and nursing literature to quality assurance and clinical audit began in the late 1970s. They continue to rise, although the terms have changes over time (Fig. 7.10.1), including terms such as continuous quality improvement, clinical governance, standards, and preferred practices.

Why assess quality or audit palliative care: benefits and costs?

Even though palliative care is often neglected in general consideration of health care, particularly when it comes to assessing need or funding care, quality improvement is an essential component of good palliative care[8]. Palliative care arose out of a desire to improve the quality of care for patients with advancing disease and their families. This was based on evidence that care for people with progressive illness, and at death, was lacking[9,10]. The newness of the field coupled with scepticism or reluctance to support this form of care often resulted in many of the early evaluations of palliative services which compared hospice, home, and hospital care[11–16]. Therefore, palliative care often led the way in developing ways to examine the quality of care and sought to influence those working in oncology and other professions[17]. However, there was no cause for complacency. These evaluations were limited to a few exemplary centres[17].

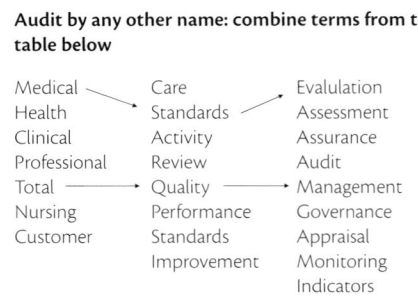

Audit by any other name: combine terms from the table below

Medical	Care	Evaluation
Health	Standards	Assessment
Clinical	Activity	Assurance
Professional	Review	Audit
Total	Quality	Management
Nursing	Performance	Governance
Customer	Standards	Appraisal
	Improvement	Monitoring
		Indicators

Figure 7.10.1 Different approaches.

Since then, palliative care has grown rapidly such that there are services in over 100 countries of the globe. With this growth have emerged many different tools and measures of the quality of palliative care and for audit, their use is now common[18–21]. National and international guides for quality are now available[22–25]. Furthermore, there is now evidence demonstrating the effectiveness of palliative care and hospice services, based on empirical studies in different sites and systematic literature reviews[26].

However, three main problems remain. First, within 'specialist palliative care' (i.e. hospice and services involving 'trained staff') the evidence reviews show a lack of comparison of different models of care[27–29].

Practice still varies from one country to another, from one part of a country to another, and from one service to another, even in simple aspects such as staffing levels and mix within a hospice or home-care team, the catchment populations, the operational policies, and the throughput[30,31]. Even today, we need to know which models of care work best and for which types of problems palliative care is most effective[32–34]. There is a need also to test some of the new treatments for symptoms, support, and counselling services or complementary therapies[35–38]. Both research and audit play complementary roles here.

Second, as the evidence base for palliative care has grown, so, in some instances, funding has followed. But there is a risk that any rapidly growing services do not follow models of best practice. Funders may be tempted to cut corners and support only the cheaper elements of palliative care, rather than all aspects. The definition of palliative care already varies among countries and this may lead to different interpretations. For this reason audit in developing, as well as developed contexts, is now not only valuable, it is essential[39–41] (see later section).

Third, in many countries, only a minority of patients and families access specialist palliative care and hospice services[42–44]. Often there is a focus on cancer patients and patients with other conditions who may have similar symptoms and problems are not referred to palliative services[45]. Therefore, to improve the quality of care for the majority of people with a progressive or terminal illness, quality improvement and audit in palliative care has spread out from specialist units to encompass general hospital wards[46–50], intensive care[51,52], geriatric care[53,54], paediatric care[55], particular diseases (e.g. heart failure[56], HIV/AIDS[41,57]), general community care[58–62], and many others. This has involved developing care pathways[50,63–65] and/or training programmes[66–70] and/or national or regional audits[71–78].

Antipathy to quality assessment and audit is based on various arguments such as:

- There is no problem since palliative care is of a high quality (I once heard of a Chief Executive who said that there was no need to measure the quality of care, because they 'knew that their care was good'.).

- Palliative care is self auditing, because staff spend time with patients and families.

- The outcomes of palliative care cannot be measured—they are too complicated or intangible.

- Measuring more simple outcomes of palliative care, such as pain or symptom control, is not enough and, until we can measure everything, audit should not be attempted.

- Resources, information, and time are not available.

- Audit looks back at practice that has gone, not the problems that lie ahead.

None of these arguments can be supported by evidence. Numerous audits and quality assessments of palliative care have helped to improve care. Audit has had a major impact in the development of hospice and palliative care in much of Europe, Canada, and Australia[79–81]. The results have been used to[24,82–93]:

- Assist the development of local and regional palliative care programmes.

- Provide outcomes information that has allowed the programme leaders to advocate for increased funding.

- Demonstrate the effectiveness of different interventions and allow for increased patient referrals.

- Review the quality of work and identify ways to improve it so that services are planned to ensure future patients and families will not suffer the same failings.

- Identify areas where care is effective and where it is not, thus allowing services to be targeted better, meaning that patients and families will receive the most up to date care

- Carry out prospective audits with systematic assessments of patients and families during care to ensure:

    a) aspects of care are less likely to be overlooked;

    b) improved communication between patients, and families and professionals, so that problems identified by patients and families are brought to the attention of staff;

    c) there is a more holistic approach to care;

    d) new staff have a clearer understanding of what they should assess and staff are helped to make appropriate assessments.

- Develop predictive models of those patients or families who may experience problems to allow for early referral.

- Improve care for most patients and families receiving palliative care, by looking at routine practice, rather than at a few 'special' cases. Quite apart from mistakes, sub-optimal care may be due to professional or administrative problems that tend to escape anecdotal case reviews.

Audit is important for education and training because the structured review allows analysis, comparison, and evaluation of individual performance; it promotes adherence to local clinical policies and offers opportunity for publication of results. Educational programmes can be constructed to meet the demonstrated needs of individuals or groups.

Increasingly, audit, clinical governance, or quality review are required for the recognition of training posts and for the revalidation of doctors. Royal colleges and faculties increasingly seek evidence of formally organized review and could withdraw recognition from departments that do not provide this.

Audit is important for those who resource palliative care, such as commissioners, primary care trusts, and health-care insurance agencies because it provides tangible evidence that the service is seeking the most effective use of existing clinical resources and aims to improve the quality of care. This is increasingly important when competing for health-care contracts[94]. Requirements for audit and the implementation of research findings may well be included in such contracts[95].

The costs of not auditing are as important as the benefits of auditing[6,95]. These include:

◆ Extra inappropriate treatment, which wastes the patients' and families' time and resources on such treatment, as well as wasting staff time and resources. Such resources could be used elsewhere where they may be more effective.

◆ Uncontrolled symptoms which may cause admission to hospice or hospital, or delay discharge. Most significantly this causes suffering to the patient, family, and staff.

◆ Extra inappropriate services, for example, unnecessary outpatient attendance.

◆ Sub-optimal services, which may be supported instead of more effective models, because they appear to be cheaper and their quality is not checked.

◆ Situations where the quality of palliative care remains the same and misses a chance to improve.

However, quality assessment and audit takes time and resources. These should not be under-estimated. Indeed, it may be impossible to undertake audit if a service is struggling, with insufficient numbers of staff to give even basic care such as washing and administering drugs. Perhaps the audit here is simply to show that the service cannot even measure and assess a patient's needs properly. Indeed, simple assessments, such as whether follow-up occurs, can be useful in assessing practice[96]. The resources needed for audit and quality assessment can include:

◆ Time from all staff to prepare for audit, to agree the standards or topic, and to review the findings.

◆ Time from some staff to carry out the audit and to analyse its results and document the findings and any recommendations.

◆ Commitment from all staff, managers, nurses, doctors, etc. to consider the results and act upon them.

◆ Resources to pay for the staff time involved, plus any other clerical, analytical, or computing support needed.

The costs of audit mean that it is important to ensure that the audit itself is as effective as possible. What is the purpose of collected audit data if the changes are not acted on? Mechanisms to review the audit and to ensure it is effective are discussed in a later section.

Computers are not necessary for audit or quality improvement. They can help if they are used to streamline the information collected and if they include ready prepared programs to make the analysis easy. A number of computer programs are available for palliative care and other services, many from commercial companies. The audit measures can be included within these programs. Increasingly, application in clinical practice can be aided by staff using palm pilot computers, or even patients completing information[24]. However, if the audit is small or in its early stages, too rigid use of computers by inexperienced staff can be a hindrance, because the need to update the computer delays the evolution of the audit.

What do we mean by quality?

Quality, as defined in many dictionaries, pertains to 'degree of excellence' or 'general excellence'. But what constitutes excellence in the context of a service, who defines it, and what components should be addressed? For example, should 'excellence' be limited to clinical skills, or should it encompass broader aspects, such as whether the service reaches all those in need? When measuring quality of a service, all the features and characteristics that bear on its ability to satisfy the stated or implied needs of the users of that service should be assessed. Quality in health care is a multi-dimensional concept and as such, a multi-dimensional approach to measurement and assessment of that quality is required[97].

Numerous authors have identified some of the dimensions that should be included when assessing the quality of a service. For example, Maxwell identifies the following as dimensions of care that need to be measured when monitoring quality[98]:

◆ effectiveness;

◆ acceptability;

◆ efficiency;

◆ access;

◆ equity;

◆ relevance.

Black agreed with all these, but added a further dimension: humanity[99], a dimension that is particularly important for palliative care services.

So how do we determine whether we are offering a good quality service if we have to consider all these dimensions? One method of assessing and ensuring service quality is to conduct a programme of review and improvement of the service; this process is what concerns clinical audit, quality assurance, and improvement.

How do we assess the quality of palliative care?

Donabedian[100] and others[6] have translated the assessment of the quality of health care into:

a) Structure/or inputs: resources in terms of manpower, equipment, and money.

b) Process: how the resources are used (such as domiciliary visits, beds, clinics, drugs, or treatments given).

c) Output: productivity or throughput (such as rates of clinic attendance or discharge, throughput—rate at which patients are seen).

d) Outcome: change in health status or quality of life that can be attributed to health care.

This model is built on the manufacturing industry and, despite limitations discussed in the following paragraphs, it has value in that it defines the steps in which health and social care are delivered.

Structural aspects influence the process of care so that its quality can be either diminished or enhanced. Similarly, changes in the process of care, including variations in its quality, will influence the output and in turn the effect of care on health status and outcomes. Thus there is a functional relationship between these in that:

$$\text{structure} \rightarrow \text{process} \rightarrow \text{output} \rightarrow \text{outcome}^{[6,100]}$$

Structure is the easiest to measure because its elements are the most stable and identifiable. However, it is an indirect measure of the quality of care and its value depends on the nature of its influence on care. Structure is relevant to quality in that it increases or decreases the probability of a good performance. Process and output are closer to changes in the health status of individuals. Their advantage is that they measure the most immediately discernible attributes of care activities. However, they are only valuable as a measure once the elements of process are known to have a clear relationship with the desired changes in health status[101]. Outcome reflects the true change in health status and thus is the most relevant for patients and society. However, it is difficult to eliminate other causes for change, such as prior care or external events. A useful approach is to focus on the difference between the desired outcome and the actual outcome. Services can then identify whether or not their goals are being achieved and investigate any failings.

Organizational audits and many quality improvement programmes assess the structure and process of care, whereas clinical audits often measure the process and outcome of care. Although structure is the easiest to measure, it is the furthest from influencing change in the patient and family. Outcome is the most difficult to measure but is of direct relevance to the patient and family. Standards of structure or process are most useful when these are of proven effectiveness, or if there is an overwhelming consensus that these are desirable. However there is a danger in measuring only structure and process, because these may not capture important failings and can lead to perverse incentives. Structure, process, and outcome measures that have been either used or advocated to assess palliative care are shown in Table 7.10.1.

Stewart et al.[102] extended the model, subdividing the 'structure' elements into: (1) personal and social environment of the patient and family and (2) the structural aspects of care. She also subdivided the outcomes into: (1) satisfaction and (2) quality and length of life. These subdivisions are consistent with the earlier model of Donabedian[100] and those proposed for palliative care audit in the United Kingdom[6]. However, Stewart's differentiation of the personal and social environment is a useful demonstration of how audit results may be different because of different settings, or with a different 'case-mix' where patients and families have differing conditions or problems.

'A rose by any other name would smell as sweet': the evolving terms—audit, quality improvement, governance?

Over the last 25 years, different terms have come in and out of vogue to describe the evolving approaches to assessing and ensuring the quality of health care. There are also differences among countries. Somewhat disappointingly, the literature in one country tends to ignore audit and quality improvement initiatives in another, thereby reducing the chance to learn. In the United Kingdom and many other European countries, clinical audit (as opposed to financial audit, concerned only with financial matters), became the initial term of choice. Later, this was accompanied by quality assurance and quality improvement (which tended to include a programme of several audits, all working together). Such a programme was similar to the development of total (or continuous) quality improvement in the United States of America and many other countries, which incorporated a cycle called Plan, Do, Study, Act[95,102].

Table 7.10.1 Aspects of care that could be measured to assess structure, process, output, or outcome in palliative care.

Type of measure	Examples
Structure	Values or aims of the service
	Financial resources
	Home care/hospital/hospice services
	Day hospice places
	Number of staff or services per cancer patient in the population
	Staffing mix, grades
	Number of staff per patient
	Drugs and equipment available
	Building design
	Physical environment (e.g. safety, pleasantness of surroundings)
Process	Number of visits
	Number of admissions
	Procedures followed
	Documentation
	Time taken in a visit
	Polices and procedures for staff training and working
	Mechanism for handling complaints and its documentation
	Adherence to ethical and legal codes
	Staff support given
Output	Rate of discharge
	Number of completed consultant episodes
	Throughput
	Rate of equipment given out
	Drugs given
	Well-coordinated care (telephone communication, etc.)
	Supply of medicines after discharge
	Completed patient management plans
	Early arrival of discharge information to GP
	Satisfaction of professionals referring to the service
Outcome	Reduction in distressing symptoms
	Improved mental health of patient and carer
	Patient and carer satisfaction
	Satisfied with place of care
	Open and honest communication as the patient wishes
	Resolved communication, fears, grief, anger
	Resolved need to plan future events (e.g. funeral or meetings)
	Good use of remaining time
	Any spiritual problems resolved or fulfilment
	Reduced carer strain
	Improved carer health
	Resolved grief after death (if appropriate)

There are various terms. Indeed, combining the one term from each of column 1, 2, and in some instances 3, in Fig. 7.10.1, will provide examples of the terms available. In that way we can form the terms clinical audit, clinical governance, total quality assessment, and so on. Some of the widely accepted definitions are shown in Table 7.10.2.

Constant concepts, which are essential, and common to all types of audit or quality review, are:

◆ Assessment is systematic.

◆ There is a cycle where care is monitored, the results reviewed, and there is a change to improve practice.

◆ Standards of care are set, either locally or nationally.

◆ The cycle is then repeated.

◆ This is part of the organization's or health-care culture.

Fig. 7.10.2 shows one cycle; most approaches are consistent with this. For the remaining part of the chapter, for simplicity, the word audit will be used, to incorporate the different approaches. Through the cycle, audit aims to improve care for patients and families by assessing whether we are doing the right thing well. Therefore, we have to: first, know what we are trying to achieve; second, have a way of observing practice to assess whether we achieve the goals or standards; and third, change practice to improve care. Standards for the delivery of care are agreed upon. Then practice is observed and compared with the standards. This often demonstrates successes,

Table 7.10.2 Common definitions: audit and quality assurance.

Term	Definition
Medical audit	The systematic critical analysis of the quality of medical care, including the procedures used for diagnosis and treatment, the use of resources, and the resulting outcome and quality of life of the patient[5].
Clinical audit	The systematic critical analysis of the quality of clinical care, including the procedures used for diagnosis and treatment, the use of resources, and the resulting outcome and quality of life of the patient.
	Clinical audit is like medical audit but involves all professionals and volunteers rather than only doctors.
Nursing audit	The methods by nurses compare their actual practice against pre-agreed guidelines and identify areas for improving their care.
Prospective audit	The standards and measures are recorded on patients and their families during their care.
Retrospective audit	This looks back at the care of patients who have been discharged or have died and the standards are applied to the information available from case notes or by asking families about the care after the patient has died.
Quality assurance	The definition of standards, the measurement of their achievement, and the mechanisms to improve performance.
	The quality assurance cycle is as for medical audit or clinical audit. However, quality assurance implies a planned programme involving the whole unit or health services. Clinical or medical audit is usually described as one part of a quality assurance programme.

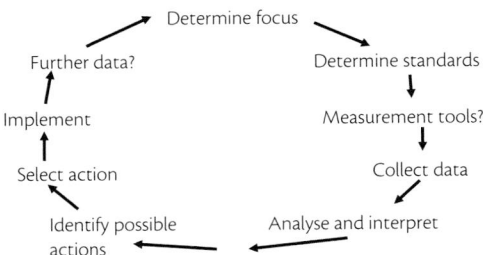

Figure 7.10.2 Cycles of quality improvement, performance measurement and audit.

but also failings and need for change. The results are then fed back and examined, so that new or modified standards can be set. The audit cycle is then repeated anew. The cycle can be entered at any point—for example, it is possible to begin by observing practice and acting on the results, and then proceed to setting standards.

Some common distinctions

Clinical audit

Clinical audit is the systematic critical analysis of the quality of clinical care, including the procedures used for diagnosis and treatment, the use of resources, and the resulting outcome and quality of life for the patient[6].

Early forms of audit involved only single professions—e.g. medical or nursing audit (Table 7.10.2). However, it is now widely accepted that audit in palliative care should be multi-professional, to reflect the multi-professional nature of care. Clinical audit is like medical and nursing audit but involves all professionals and volunteers, rather than only doctors or nurses.

The audit can be prospective, where the standards and measures are agreed at the start and are recorded on patients and families during their care, or retrospective, which looks back at the care of patients using either the clinical notes and extracting the information or by asking families.

Organizational audit, preferred practices, and peer review

A group of approaches have developed, which examine the whole organization and the practices and are often focused on accreditation. Organizational standards are developed because of evidence of organizational variation, which limits the quality of care. These include administrative delays, un-coordinated care, poor environment or sign-posting, poor staff training, etc. Organizational standards need to be straight forward enough to be monitored by an external surveyor.

The Kings Fund Centre in London originally described organizational audit as the developmental and voluntary stage towards accreditation[103] and from this developed an organizational audit system. Accreditation schemes exist in many countries and usually operate nationally. For example, Royal Colleges inspect training posts and agree where doctors can be trained. Various regions have developed their own organizational audits, for example, the Yorkshire Peer Review system or audits in the North West of the United Kingdom[104].

Organizational audit and accreditation are usually developed in three stages:

1 Development of organizational standards of the systems and process of care.

2 Implementation of the standards by the hospices, hospitals, or units included.

3 Evaluation of compliance with the standards, usually by external surveyors or auditors, sometimes called peer review.

The first stage, developing standards, can often be quite lengthy because the standards need to be agreed upon and written in clear, non-ambiguous language and then tested to determine if the standards can distinguish between good and sub-optimal practice. If the standards are able to detect only the poorest practice then they could reduce standards to just above this level, because units will not need to strive higher. Units with higher standards, which were undetected, may appear to have higher costs for the same level of practice as units with just acceptable standards.

In 2007, in the United States of America, the National Consensus Project and National Quality Forum produced a similar approach to standards of quality palliative care[105]. This report outlines a set of 'preferred practices' (equivalent to organizational standards) for palliative care, which were developed as a result of consensus among major palliative care and hospice organizations and literature review. Here, the review built on a State of the Science review on End of Life care and other major evidence appraisals[106]. There are eight domains of care and 38 preferred practices, each of which relates to a domain of care (see Table 7.10.3 for examples). The authors describe their next steps for this work as being the development, implementation, and field testing of outcome measures to assess these practices, i.e. stages 2 and 3 of above. It is hoped that the group will draw on many of the existing measures and indicators that are already validated in palliative care (see later in this chapter).

In the United Kingdom, considerable effort has gone into Peer Review in Cancer. In this process, organizational standards are developed for cancer services. These standards were developed from a combination of approaches, primarily, systematic literature reviews and appraisal commissioned by the National Institute of Health and Clinical Excellence (NICE), which sets very high standards for evidence review, and consensus work by panels of experts. Because of the NICE reviews on supportive and palliative cancer care[27,106,107], there are several chapters on different components of palliative care within the guidance. Many (but not all) of the requirements are based on good evidence, e.g. the composition of a palliative care team. However, there were several areas where evidence was not available, for which there are no standards, and other areas where the experts made recommendations, which were not really supported by evidence but seemed sensible practice at the time.

The 'performance' of an organization is determined by peer review, where other experts visit a unit and review their own documentation of how they have performed, interview staff, and inspect records. The attention is focused on structure and process components and there are potentially financial penalties for units that do not reach the standards.

Quality assurance and total quality management programmes

Although there are various definitions for quality assurance, a widely accepted one is the 'definition of standards, the measurement of their achievement and the mechanisms to improve performance'. Thus, the cycle is as clinical audit. Clinical audit lies within the frame of quality assurance: clinical audit being the review of the quality of local clinical practice on a regular basis, for example, through internal 'peer review' by practising clinicians.

Total quality management is a term which has recently entered the jargon in quality in health care and its definition is included for completeness. It has been defined as a strategy to get an organization working to its maximum effectiveness and efficiency. It has been facilitated by closer working relationships between clinicians and managers and builds on the other definitions, but switches the focus from quality practised by professionals to quality within the whole organization. Thus clinical audit would lie within a total quality management programme. It also introduces the concept of managing the quality process, such as cataloguing reports of local quality initiatives and using managers to ensure that improvements in quality occur.

Clinical governance

Clinical governance has developed recently, because of concerns about variations in clinical practice, particularly assessment, diagnosis and prescribing. This is of greater concern in modern medicine than ever in the past because of the rapid pace of developments in clinical practice, available diagnostic investigations and treatments, especially those with potentially dangerous effects if not carried out properly. Thus, clinical governance programmes assess

Table 7.10.3 Domains and some examples of preferred practice suggested in the USA National Consensus Project on Palliative Care.

Domain	Number of preferred practices	Example of preferred practice (in some instances these have been abbreviated for this chapter)
1. Structure and process of care	11	Ensure that on transfer between health-care settings there is timely and thorough communication
2. Physical aspects of care	1	Measure and document pain and symptoms using standardized scales
3. Psychological and psychiatric aspects of care	4	Manage anxiety and other psychological symptoms in a timely, effective, and safe manner, acceptable to the patient and family
4. Social aspects of care	2	Conduct regular patient and family conferences with physicians and other appropriate members of team to discuss, update, and support
5. Spiritual, religious, and existential aspects of care	2	Specialized palliative care teams should include spiritual care individuals
6. Cultural aspects of care	2	Incorporate cultural assessment into an individualized assessment
7. Care of the imminently dying	2	As part of ongoing care, planning process, routinely ascertain and document future care-planning wishes
8. Ethical and legal aspects of care	2	Document the designated surrogate or decision maker

what doctors (and most recently, nurses) do. It examines their training, continuing professional development, and all components of their practice. It aims to ensure and develop the practice of all clinicians. Participation in clinical governance is already required of many health-care services and will soon be required to ensure the revalidation of doctors in many countries[104].

Who carries out audit and what is measured?

The different approaches to audit and the assessment of quality can be categorized according to two axes: first, who carries out the audit—the local clinicians, managers, or external organization; and second, whether the audit considered the care of an individual or a few patients, or the whole organization or population. Common forms of audit according to these two axes—internal versus external and individual versus organization/population—are shown in Fig. 7.10.3. The type of appropriate audit is determined by the setting. It is extremely difficult for those resourcing services or for external bodies to assess the clinical quality of care. Instead, they are more likely to rely on organizational or environmental standards or, when determining whether the professionals are employing proven high-quality treatments, examine staff-mix and whether a clinical audit programme is in place. Thus those audits that are more orientated towards internal and individual assessment are more likely to be educational and voluntary. Those audits concerned with organizational aspects and undertaken by external experts or by inspection are more likely to be mandatory and to provide funding or accreditation (see Fig. 7.10.4).

Applying audit to palliative care

The next section reviews the steps in audit, when it is applied to palliative care.

1. Know what we are trying to achieve: goals or standards

The definitions of palliative care and palliative medicine (see Chapter 2.1 of the textbook) provide good guidance on the goals of palliative care, which might be measured in audit. These include aspects of pain and symptom control, improving the quality of life for the patient, relieving fears and anxiety, and caring for the family

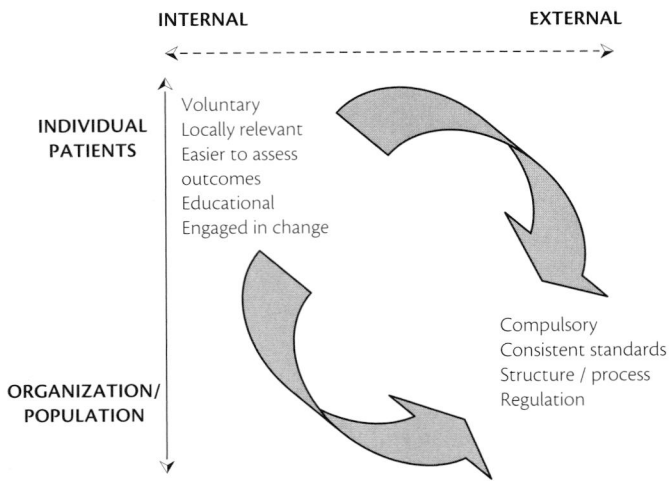

Figure 7.10.4 Effect of activities within audit.

members or carers. Therefore, in analysing the goals or standards of care, many have audited their effectiveness in controlling symptoms, such as pain or dyspnoea, their effect on a patient's quality of life or psychological well-being, or the patient's or family members' satisfaction with care, or has suggested indicators of these aspects[85,88–90,92,93,108–118]. The USA 'preferred practices[119]', the UK NICE guidance[107], and the World Health Organization (WHO) guidance on palliative care[80,81] also set out the goals of palliative care.

There are other aspects which might be included. Various work has examined the features of 'a good or appropriate' death[120], building on Weisman's definition of 'appropriate death' as 'an absence of suffering, preservation of important relationships, an interval for anticipatory grief, relief of remaining conflicts, belief in timeliness, exercise of feasible option in activities, and consistency with physical limitations, all within the scope of one's ego ideal'[121]. Kellehear described the features of a modern 'good death' as 'awareness of dying, social adjustments and personal preparations, public preparations (legal, financial, religious, funeral, medical), work or activities reduced, and farewells'[122]. Singer *et al.* identified five domains of quality end-of-life care: receiving adequate pain and symptom management, avoiding inappropriate prolongation of dying, achieving a sense of control, relieving burden and strengthening relationships with loved ones[123]. Payne also assessed different perspectives[124]. These definitions might suggest audit of aspects of patient and family awareness of the illness or their planning of personal and public preparations; such aspects have been included in some measures, such as the Support Team Assessment Schedule[125].

In many countries, the role of palliative care in supporting, advising, and educating other professions is stressed[27] (see also other chapters). Family practitioners have identified educational needs for symptom control and patient and family support[126–134]. Therefore, another form of audit could examine the educational and supportive role of palliative care services.

Poor communication is a frequent cause of stress for patients and families[135–141]. Doctors and nurses need to communicate well with patients and their families rather than withdrawing or appearing hurried or abrupt in their manner. Communication is needed between professional staff caring for the patient and family

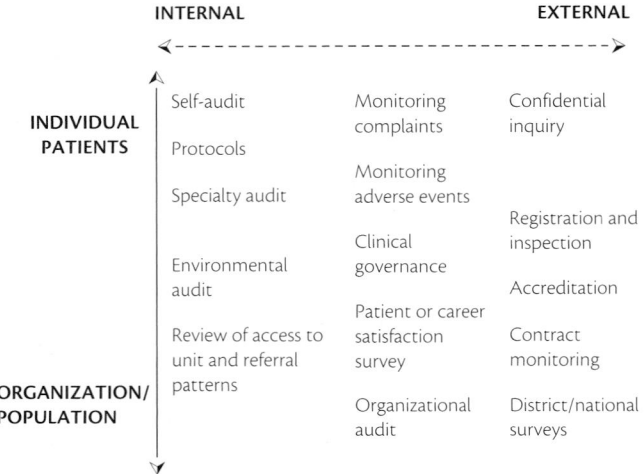

Figure 7.10.3 Range of activities possible within audit.

member, to ensure liaison and to prevent duplication or delay. These aspects are also goals suitable for audit.

Total pain has been described as including physical, emotional, social, and spiritual components. Although the earlier discussions have covered the emotional and physical aspects of palliative care, it is also important to consider audit of the spiritual and social aspects. Spiritual audit might consider whether patients are able to raise aspects of spiritual concern and find a mechanism to relieve problems or whether patients are in any form of spiritual crisis. Social aspects might include whether the patient and family have sufficient practical and financial support to remain at home.

There are also simple goals, such as place of death, or meeting other patient or family preferences, or access of certain patient groups (such as those from ethnic minorities, or non-cancer conditions)[142] that might be suitable for audit. One problem with this though, is that these goals may not reflect the wishes of all patients. For example, although around 70 per cent of patients would prefer to die at home, increasingly, patients choose hospice as a second choice, wishes are very individual, are little understood in some sections of society and are altered by experience[143]. Thus this indicator, like other process indicators, needs to be reviewed cautiously.

How can these goals be turned into standards? Any goal or standard, which is set, must be measurable, sufficiently challenging but achievable. It would be unrealistic to set a goal or standard that all patients would be free from pain, but it would be reasonable to set a goal of what proportion of patients might have pain controlled and in what circumstances pain might be uncontrolled. A baseline could be established from current practice. Standards of action when pain is uncontrolled could be audited.

2. Have a way of assessing and reassessing the quality of care

For all of the above aspects, measurement tools or indicators are needed. There are now a number of these available in palliative care, which have been validated to different degrees. The Association for Palliative Medicine of the United Kingdom established a working party to review these and subsequently published *The Which Tool Guide*[144]. The group carried out a MEDLINE search to identify potential measures and to check whether they had been used in more than one centre. Then the group provided a preliminary guide as to whether they would recommend the tools in research or clinical audit palliative care. In order to avoid conflicts of interest, the decision on awarding a research 'triangle' or clinical 'star' was made, in each case, by members of the group who had not been involved in developing that particular outcome measure. Table 7.10.4 shows some examples of the tools that were reviewed and some recent additions.

Considerable audit experience is now available with two measures, the Support Team Assessment Schedule (STAS) and the subsequent sister measure, the Palliative Care Outcome Scale (POS). The STAS is based on professional assessment of patient outcomes and includes aspects such as communication and advice, as well as symptoms (see Table 7.10.5 for details)[84,109,125,145,146]. It can easily be integrated into the clinical record and is used in over 20 different countries to assess and audit care.

The Palliative Care Outcome Scale[147,148] was developed from the STAS and other scales and sought to include only core items. It is shorter than STAS (10 items rather than 17) and has a component for patient assessment as well as professional assessment.

Its use in inpatient, home, and hospice settings is now growing rapidly and many translated validations are now being published from a range of independent units, as well as by the scale developers, in both developed and resource-poor countries[57,148–158]. A further significant development with the POS was the incorporation of open questions, so that patients can identify what problem troubles them most. This seeks to provide a patient-centred and individualized assessment, as well as a standard one. Full details of the measures are available from www.kcl.ac.uk/palliative (see Table 7.10.6).

One exciting potential future development would be to pool data from units to understand more about the mix of patients and families cared for and their needs and outcomes. The use of a common audit measure would make this more possible. Further developments include: (1) the extension of the measure, with additional items to assess particular aspects of need (e.g. symptoms); (2) the validation of a version completed by the family, and (3) the use of the measure in non-specialist settings, keeping the abbreviation POS, but renaming the scale the Patient Outcome Scale.

Most of the measures described here audit a series of key indicators, for example, pain, symptoms, and patient needs. An alternative is to audit one single symptom or problem, for example, constipation, communication, or access to care. This is called topic review. Other approaches are also possible, although seldom used. Table 7.10.7 reviews these.

Organizational audits and peer review systems have tended to develop indicators that can be used in inspections of services and concentrate on the structure and process of care, such as:

◆ Service values—a statement of service values and objectives related to the palliative care service guides the organization and delivery of high-quality care.

◆ Organization and management—the palliative care service or organization is managed efficiently to ensure patients and families receive suitable and effective multi-disciplinary care.

◆ Organizational and operational policy—organizational and operational policies reflect current knowledge and principles and are consistent with the requirements of statutory bodies, purchasing authorities, and service objectives.

◆ Physical environment for care—the physical environment is safe and accommodates individual and shared needs.

◆ Self-determination and climate for care—the caring environment for patients and families is conducive to independence, self esteem, and participation in daily life.

◆ Direct patient and family care—professional staff manage to ensure that patient and family needs are assessed, planned, implemented, and evaluated on an individual basis.

◆ Multi-disciplinary working and team work—a range of skills is available to meet service goals, and specific contributions are identified and integrated.

◆ Staffing and skill mix—good employment practices are in place and staffing levels are systematically determined in order to meet service needs.

◆ Education, training, and staff development—staff have access to education and training programmes, which reflect the different levels of activity and practice necessary to meet service goals, provide appropriate care, and respond to change.

Table 7.10.4 Review of measures and indicators that could potentially be used in audit. (As assessed by working party of the Association of Palliative Medicine, UK.)

The criteria for assessment were:

▲ Research: used in more than one centre for research in palliative care; relevant to palliative care goals.

☆ Clinical: used in more than one centre for clinical practice in palliative care; relevant to palliative care goals; short and easy to use.

Measure, scale, or tool	Used in ...	Strengths	Other issues of note	Useful for: Clinical—☆ Research—▲
CAMPAS (Cambridge Palliative Audit Schedule)[175]	Developed from STAS for use in primary care to assess palliative care	Developed for primary care team members, useful for recording assessments and monitoring care	Validation is now being published	
Edmonton Functional Assessment Tool[176]	Inpatients in palliative care units	Simple to use: 10 items, mainly function	Function alone may not be the patient's chief concern	☆
Edmonton Symptom Assessment Scale[177]	Inpatient setting	Quick and can be used either by patient or with nurse assistance	Potential bias introduced by change in the person recording the answers as care continues; patient may have concerns other than symptoms	☆
EORTC – European Organisation for Research into Treatment of Cancer – QLQ C30[178,179]	Developed for chemotherapeutic cancer trials: lung cancer patients; work of palliative module underway	Reliable and valid in research settings, broad-ranging	Functional questions may cause distress if asked repeatedly; a new shortened palliative care version is available	▲
FACT, Functional Assessment of Cancer Therapies[180,181]	General cancer settings in US, especially research studies has a palliative module	Major validation programme	Palliative care short versions now available	▲
HRCA – QL. Hebrew Rehabilitation Centre for Aged, Quality of Life Index[182]	Adapted from the Spitzer Quality of Life Index, used in the National Hospice Study, in inpatients, home care and conventional care, in elderly populations	Short and quick	Has not been revalidated and lacks responsiveness in advanced disease, completed by professionals	
Linear pain or comfort rating Scales	Forms basis of many assessment tools (e.g. post-surgical pain management evaluation)	A patient-centred approach, simple, relatively quick	Pain relief alone may not be patient's chief concern; need to look more widely, in some visual analogue scales are hard to use	☆▲
McGill Quality of Life Questionnaire[183–185]	Advanced cancer and HIV patients at home or inpatients palliative care unit	Includes an existential domain, as well as symptoms and psychological issues	Validation now in various disease groups and settings	▲
PACA – Palliative Care Assessment[186]	Hospital palliative care team and outpatient	Short and relatively simple to use	Professional completion	☆
PCCS – Palliative Care Core Standards[187,188]	Inpatients hospice	Comprehensive tool, covering structure, process, education, and training	Lengthy, expected to take 10 min to complete	
POS – Palliative Care Outcome Scale[189,190]	Used in inpatients hospice, day care, hospital support team, home care, and primary care	Simple and short, has patient completion and staff completion component; tested for validity and reliability, has items for individual patient generation	May not be sufficiently detailed; some aspects require further testing	☆▲
Proportion who die at home[191,192]	Used by health authorities to monitor overall care	Quick and easy to measure and aggregate; easy to make comparisons	Home death may not have been patient choice; may be distorted by lack of appropriate inpatients provision	
Proportion who die in their place of choice	Used by some palliative home-care and primary-care teams	Reflects patient choice and individual wishes	Difficult to get information in some circumstances, choice may change over time	
Proportion of final weeks spent at home	A proxy measure that can give some indication of the availability of community support services	Quick and easy to measure and aggregate; clear operational definitions allow valid comparisons between districts	May be distorted by lack of appropriate inpatients provision	

Table 7.10.4 (Continued) Review of measures and indicators that could potentially be used in audit. (As assessed by working party of the Association of Palliative Medicine, UK)

Measure, scale, or tool	Used in ...	Strengths	Other issues of note	Useful for: Clinical—☆ Research—▲
Spitzer Quality of Life Index[193]	Used as basis for comparison with McGill Quality of Life Scale	Short and quick	Has not been validated in palliative care and lacks responsiveness in advanced disease, completed by professionals	
Support Team Assessment Schedule (STAS)[109,125,146,194]	Used by community palliative care teams, hospital teams, day care, inpatients units, and hospital at home services	A wide-ranging checklist looking at clinical and communication issues; available in other languages and has been modified with additional specific items	Teams need actively to use this, questioning each section, not just ticking boxes; professional completion	☆▲
SEIQoL – Schedule for the Evaluation of Individual Quality of Life[195]	Inpatients palliative care	Patient-centred, the patient identifies the important areas	Can be complex and time-consuming	☆▲
VOICES – Views Of Informal Cares, Experience and Services[190,196–199]	Population based, views of bereaved carer or person who knew most about the patient's last year of life	Includes carers, and most persons irrespective of the service received, developed from questionnaire used since 1967, postal	Carers may not represent the patient's views, and are not available for some; may not get good response from minority groups	▲

- Staff support—staff support systems are in place as an integral part of the organization and a healthy working environment is promoted, which recognizes the possible physical and emotional effects of work on staff.

- Ethics and law—there is guidance and support for staff to comply with statutory requirements and use a systematic approach to decision making where ethical and legal status issues are involved.

Table 7.10.2 and Table 7.10.8 show some further examples of these, and Table 7.10.9 an example of how one of these is assessed.

3. Change practice to ensure that any deficiencies are corrected

This stage closes the audit loop in the cycle[6,95]. Any weaknesses in practice need to be considered and discussed with the whole team to determine what changes might be appropriate. This may involve a review of the literature or consulting with other individuals to determine whether they have solutions to particular problems. For example, in London, we identified that our control of dyspnoea in the last weeks of life was not reaching our targets: this was the most severe symptom in patients[159]. To decide what change was needed, we had to consult chest physicians, physiotherapists, and other colleagues about what treatment might be appropriate in the home, review the literature on effective treatment, and examine the possible causes of dyspnoea. This led us to change our practice substantially and it has led to further research into the management of dyspnoea.

In larger specialist palliative care services difficulties in implementing change have been described[160,161]. These include:

1 Inadequate cascading of the information from those present at the audit meetings to other staff.

2 Difficulties in ensuring that those with hands-on patient contact but at the end of the cascade, such as auxiliary nurses, feel ownership of any changes and therefore are willing to take part in them.

3 Difficulties if the main communicator is a resistor to change. Many health-care professionals resist change. This may be partly from fear of their deficits being revealed.[162,163].

Continuing education is important to achieve change[160,161]. It can be targeted to ensure that those to be educated feel part of the

Table 7.10.5 Example of items in the Support Team Assessment Schedule (STAS).[6,125]

Patient and family items

- Pain control
- Symptom control
- Patient anxiety
- Family anxiety
- Patient insight
- Family insight
- Spiritual
- Planning
- Predictability
- Communication between patient and family

Service items

- Practical aid
- Financial
- Wasted time
- Communication from professionals to patient and family
- Communication between professionals
- Professional anxiety
- Advising professionals

Table 7.10.6 The Palliative Outcome Scale (POS), patient completion version.

Please answer the following questions circling the answer, which you think most accurately, describes how you have been feeling.

1. Over the past 3 *days*, have you been affected by pain?

Not at all, no effect	0
Slightly: but not bothered to be rid of it	1
Moderately: pain limits some activity	2
Severely: activities or concentration markedly affected	3
Overwhelmingly: unable to think of anything else	4

2. Over the past 3 *days*, have other symptoms e.g. feeling sick, having a cough, or constipation been affecting how you feel?

No, not at all	0
Slightly	1
Moderately	2
Severely	3
Overwhelmingly	4

3. Over the past 3 *days*, have you been feeling anxious or worried about your illness or treatment?

No, not at all	0
Occasionally	1
Sometimes: affects my concentration now and then	2
Most of the time: often affects my concentration	3
Can't think of anything else: completely preoccupied	4

4. Over the past 3 *days*, have any of your family or friends been anxious or worried about you?

No, not at all	0
Occasionally	1
Sometimes: it seems to affect their concentration	2
Most of the time	3
Yes, always preoccupied with worry about me	4

5. Over the past 3 *days*, how much information have you and your family or friends been given?

Full information: always feel free to ask what I want	0
Information given but hard to understand	1
Information given on request but would have liked more	2
Very little given and some questions were avoided	3
None at all	4

6. Over the past 3 *days*, have you been able to share how you are feeling with your family or friends?

Yes, as much as I wanted to	0
Most of the time	1
Sometimes	2
Occasionally	3
No, not at all with anyone	4

7. Over the past 3 *days*, have you felt that life was worthwhile?

Yes, all the time	0
Most of the time	1
Sometimes	2
Occasionally	3
No, not at all	4

Table 7.10.6 (Continued) The Palliative Outcome Scale (POS), patient completion version.

8. Over the past 3 *days*, have you felt good about yourself as a person?

Yes, all the time	0
Most of the time	1
Sometimes	2
Occasionally	3
No, not at all	4

9. Over the past 3 *days*, how much time do you feel you have wasted on appointments relating to your health care, e.g. waiting around for transport or having the same tests repeated?

None at all	0
Up to half a day wasted	1
More than half a day wasted	2

10. Over the past 3 *days*, have any practical matters resulting from your illness, either financial or personal, been addressed?

Practical problems have been addressed and my affairs are as up to date as I would wish	0
Practical problems are in the process of being addressed	1
Practical problems exist which were not addressed	2
I have had no practical problems	3

11. If any, what have been your *main* problems in the last *three days*?

1.

2.

Note: the POS is free to use, but users must register—see www.kcl.ac.uk/palliative

There are now alternative questions (e.g. for use in Africa), or for different circumstances, including extended symptom questions, and several translated versions. The open questions can be asked first rather than last.

Table 7.10.7 Types of audit: an appraisal of their uses in palliative care.

◆ **Key indicators.**

These can be based on the structure or process of care, as in organizational audit or can be based on clinical indicators, such as in clinical audit. In organizational audit, the indicators are reviewed by inspection; in clinical audit; they are reviewed by the clinical team (see Figs. 7.10.3 and 7.10.4).

Routinely collected data, such as throughput, visits, or readmission rates can be used in some areas of health care, but in palliative care, these may not be appropriate, and the clinical records may have to be amended to include relevant items. In clinical audit, a few key indicators are chosen and recorded prospectively and examined after a period of care. In organizational audit or peer review, the survey team asks for information about the indicators and then seeks evidence of these. In clinical audit, measures such as those shown in Table 7.10.3 are used.

◆ **Topic review.**

A topic is chosen and reviewed prospectively or retrospectively. Although the latter often reveals inadequacies in the clinical records, it is often valuable in providing a baseline for later comparison. Examples of topics are: medical records and letters, referral or admission procedures, control of a particular symptom, prescribing practice, or the diagnostic procedures used.

◆ **Random case review.**

Here, notes are selected at random and critically reviewed by doctors not involved in that person's care. This method may lose direction if the aims and criteria for quality are not clear. One way to focus the audit is to develop a previously agreed checklist for use in the critical review. The method can be linked with key indicators, a random sample of notes are examined for the key indicators.

◆ **Patient or family satisfaction**.

The simplest method is to analyse patient and family complaints. However, in palliative care patients may die before they are able to complain. Surveys of patients' or families' views may be included in the overall quality improvement plan of a hospice or hospital; see Table 7.10.3 for examples of how this may be used.

◆ **Adverse patient events.**

This systematically identifies events during a patient's treatment, which may indicate some lapse in the quality of care. Patients' clinical records are reviewed retrospectively by a health professional or a ward clerk for examples of agreed adverse events. This method is of value in specialities such as surgery, where adverse events (e.g. death or post-operative infection) are usually recorded in the patients' records. However, in palliative care the method is awkward, because adverse palliative events are more difficult to identify routinely and may not be included in the patient"s records unless these are standardized.

Table 7.10.8 Example of criteria used in organizational audit and peer review systems.

Inter-disciplinary working and teamwork

Criteria

1. Systems exist for referral to the therapy professions, social workers, and ministers of religion
2. Mechanisms exist for liaison within and between disciplines, including volunteers, to ensure continuity of care
3. Staff demonstrate awareness of differing roles, relationships, and responsibilities
4. Mechanisms exist of monitoring the performance of the multi-disciplinary team
5. There are systems to inform patients and families of the range of skills and services available
6. There are arrangements of liaison and cooperations between patients and families and health-care agencies

teaching or learning process. One mechanism, which Finlay has described, asks the full team of nurses to evolve education policy themselves, facilitated by a tutor[164].

A further challenge is to make sure that policy makers adopt the quality improvement recommendations. One important strategy here is to ensure the evidence is fed back in the most appropriate way. A qualitative study of 36 such policy makers found that box plots were received more positively than league tables and qualitative information was considered more appropriate than pictorial feedback. However, quantitative data needed contextual information and the methodological assumptions of the instrument. There was also a consensus that feedback should be constructive and able to be adapted to the organizational realities in which UK health services function[165].

Audit in developing countries

As palliative medicine evolves globally, audit must be adapted to be relevant in developing as well as developed countries. Although areas

Table 7.10.9 Evidence to be considered from the standard on inter-disciplinary team work, used in organizational audits and peer review.

Inter-disciplinary working and teamwork

- For Criteria 1: Do systems exist for referral to the therapy professions, social workers/counsellors, ministers of religion, complementary therapists, dieticians, interpreters, and other specialist medical or nursing services (i.e. ostomy nurse, psychiatrist)

Documents

- Referral forms
- Response time statistics

Discussion

- How is liaison maintained?
- How are referrals made?
- How quickly are referrals met?
- Do these staff have post-qualification specialist training?

Observation

- Observe referrals and team relationship

with limited resources, such as India, Africa, South America, and Eastern Europe, have relatively few health-care professionals, with varied levels of training[93], the last few years have shown what benefits audit in these settings can bring[41,166,167]. A particular advantage is to use prospective audit systems that incorporate a form of assessment[57,168–170]. In this way nurses, doctors, and volunteers can develop their assessment and skills[171]. Because, some patients and families have high levels of illiteracy, new approaches to assessment are needed, such as using the hand and other local symbols to indicate the severity of a problem.

The burden of illness and symptom distress in patients dying of AIDS, tuberculosis, malaria, and even the cancer-related syndromes in some of these programmes is different, just as belief systems vary, and therefore, the tools may need to be adjusted to the main symptom problems in these patients[93].

On the other hand, the basic principles of documenting the results of our interventions and using them to guide our future direction are not different in these regions. It can be argued that the limited resources make it even more imperative to ensure that as the programmes evolve they are capable of serving the largest possible number of patients and families in the most effective way possible. Audit is one way to minimize the risk of failure and to learn, at an early stage, about potential problems and to identify success[93].

However, the development is not without challenges, as many programmes in developing countries have limited access to resources and technology to incorporate audit successfully. Thus, there needs to be collaboration between local programmes with specific needs and those with audit experience and methodological skills[93]. One further important development for resource-poor countries is the need to provide clear guidance on what action is needed if, for example, problems are noted for a patient or family. There is a need here and in generalist settings to provide guidance on how to manage problems, in the way that is offered with some care pathways[50,172–174], or manuals of care.

Conclusions

Audit approaches and methods are now very well advanced in palliative care, especially in clinical audit. Indeed audit approaches are now spreading out from specialist hospice and palliative care services to include audit in generalist settings. There is a good choice of possible and already tried methods and measures which we can adapt for our own needs, rather than having to undertake much of the development ourselves. Practical measures for clinical audit include the Support Team Assessment Schedule, the new shorter Palliative Outcome Scale, and the Edmonton Symptom Assessment Scale (which have either been validated or are being tested for this) and topic audits. Clinical audits, which use satisfaction surveys or surveys after bereavement, are probably more costly, but are still possible. Apart from completing the audit cycle, clinical audit should now start to explore ways of developing clinical protocols for treatment, or algorithms to predict patient problems, and the need for specialized care.

Organizational audit, peer review, and proposals for preferred practice are also now well established and different systems are available, although, in some cases, the authors need to look at the approaches available to measure their proposed practices.

Audit, or the various alternative terms that describe this assessment of the quality of care, is here to stay, and is now widely accepted.

However, it requires resources, and therefore must be of benefit to patients and families, be kept as simple and efficient as possible, and have a strong educational component. Further work is needed to evaluate the impact of different audit approaches and methods on improving care so that we know which approach is most cost-effective. In addition, there is a need to develop and test methods of audit in developing countries. If palliative approaches extend backwards to include patients earlier in care, rather than those just near to death, then the audit could become a means for clinical dialogue and education among specialties. Palliative medicine could take the lead in encouraging this, promoting methods among their medical and surgical colleagues, and presenting their own results.

References

1. Higginson, I.J. (2004). It would be NICE to have more evidence? *Palliative Medicine*, **18**, 85–6.
2. Shaw, C.D. (1993). Quality assurance in the United Kingdom. *Quality Assurance in Health Care*, **5**, 107–18.
3. Vanhaecht, K., De Witte, K., Depreitere, R. *et al.* (2006). Clinical pathway audit tools: a systematic review. *Journal of Nursing Management*, **14**, 529–37.
4. Blanchard, J., McCann, E., and Lynn, J. (2002). Quality improvement in end-of-life care. Small-scale innovations can make a dramatic difference. *Postgraduate Medicine*, **111**, 21–6.
5. Higginson, I. (1992). *Quality, Standards, Organisational and Clinical Audit for Hospice and Palliative Care Services*. London: National Council for Hospice and Specialist Palliative Care Services.
6. Higginson, I. (1993). *Clinical Audit in Palliative Care*. Oxford: Radcliffe Medical Press.
7. Shaw, C. (1989). *Medical Audit. A Hospital Handbook*. London: King's Fund Centre, p 1.
8. Higginson, I.J., Davies, E., and Tsouros, A.D. (2007). The end of life: unknown and unplanned? *European Journal of Public Health*.
9. Buckingham, R.W., III, Lack, S.A., Mount, B.M. *et al.* (1976). Living with the dying: use of the technique of participant observation. *Canadian Medical Association Journal*, **115**, 1211–5.
10. Cartwright, A., Hockey, J., and Anderson, J.L. (1973). *Life Before Death*. London: Routledge & Kegan Paul.
11. Parkes, C.M., Parkes, J. (1984). 'Hospice' versus 'hospital' care - re-evaluation after 10 years as seen by surviving spouses. *Postgraduate Medical Journal*, **60**, 120–4.
12. Parkes, C.M. (1980). Terminal care: evaluation of an advisory domiciliary service at St Christopher's Hospice. *Postgrad Medical Journal*, **56**, 685–9.
13. Brooks, C.H. and Smyth-Starvch, K. (1984). Hospice home care cost savings to third party insurers. *Medical Care*, **22**, 691.
14. Kane, R.L., Klein, S.J., Bernstein, L., *et al.* (1985). Hospice role in alleviating the emotional stress of terminal patients and their families. *Medical Care*, **23**, 189–97.
15. Mor, V., Morris, J.N., Hiris, J. *et al.* (1988). The effects of hospice care on where patients die. In *The Hospice Experiment* (Mor V, Greer DS, Kastenbaum R, eds.), pp. 133–46. Baltimore: John Hopkins University Press.
16. Ward, A.W.M. (1976). The impact of a special unit for terminal care. *Social Science and Medicine*, **10**, 373–6.
17. Higginson, I.J. (1993). Palliative care: a review of past changes and future trends. *Journal of Public Health Medicine*, **15**, 3–8.
18. Higginson, I.J. and Carr, A.J. (2003). The clinical utility of quality of life measures. In *Quality of Life* (Carr AJ, Robinson PG, Higginson IJ, eds.), pp. 63–78. London: BMJ Books.
19. Ferrell, B., Connor, S.R., Cordes, A. *et al.* (2007). The National Agenda for Quality Palliative Care: The National Consensus Project and the National Quality Forum. *Journal of Pain and Symptom Management*, **33**, 737–44.
20. Dudgeon, D., Vaitonis, V., Seow, H. *et al.* (2007). Ontario, Canada: Using Networks to Integrate Palliative Care Province-Wide. *Journal of Pain and Symptom Management*, **33**, 640–4.
21. Meier, D. (2005). Palliative care as a quality improvement strategy for advanced, chronic illness. *Journal of Healthcare Quality*, **27**, 33–9.
22. Ferrell, B., Connor, S.R., Cordes, A. *et al.* (2007). The National Agenda for Quality Palliative Care: The National Consensus Project and the National Quality Forum. *Journal of Pain and Symptom Management*, **33**, 737–44.
23. Dudgeon, D., Vaitonis, V., Seow, H. *et al.* (2007). Ontario, Canada: Using Networks to Integrate Palliative Care Province-Wide. *Journal of Pain and Symptom Management*, **33**, 640–4.
24. Higginson, I.J. and Carr, A.J. (2001). Measuring quality of life: Using quality of life measures in the clinical setting. *British Medical Journal*, **322**, 1297–300.
25. Ingleton, C., Faulkner, A. (1995). Quality assurance in palliative care - a review of the literature. *Journal of Cancer Care*, **4**, 49–55.
26. Higginson, I.J., Finlay, I.G., Goodwin, D.M. *et al.* (2003). Is there evidence that palliative care teams alter end-of-life experiences of patients and their caregivers? *Journal of Pain and Symptom Management*, **25**, 150–68.
27. Gysels, M., Higginson, I.J., Rajasekaran, M. *et al.* (2003). *Improving supportive and palliative care for adults with cancer*. National Institute for Clinical Excellence.
28. Higginson, I.J. (2004). It would be NICE to have more evidence? *Palliative Medicine*, **18**, 85–6.
29. Salisbury, C., Bosanquet, N., Wilkinson, E.K. *et al.* (1999). The impact of different models of specialist palliative care on patient's quality of life: a systematic literature review. *Palliat Medicine*, **13**, 3–17.
30. Bosanquet, N. (1999). Background and Patterns of use of service. In *Providing a Palliative Care Service: Towards an Evidence Base* (eds. N. Bosanquet and C. Salisbury), pp. 8–10, 33–42. Oxford: Oxford University Press.
31. Eve, A., Higginson, I.J. (2000). Minimum dataset activity for hospice and hospital palliative care services in the UK 1997/98. *Palliative Medicine*, **14**, 395–404.
32. Higginson, I.J. (2004). It would be NICE to have more evidence? *Palliative Medicine*, **18**, 85–6.
33. Higginson, I.J., Davies, E., and Tsouros, A.D. (2007). The end of life: unknown and unplanned? *European Journal of Public Health*.
34. Higginson, I.J., Hart, S., Koffman, J. *et al.* (2007). Needs Assessments in Palliative Care: An Appraisal of Definitions and Approaches Used. *Journal of Pain and Symptom Management*, **33**, 500–5.
35. Blanchard, J., McCann, E., and Lynn, J. (2002). Quality improvement in end-of-life care. Small-scale innovations can make a dramatic difference. *Postgraduate Medicine*, **111**, 21–6.
36. Lynn, J., Nolan, K., Kabcenell, A. *et al.* (2002). Reforming care for persons near the end of life: the promise of quality improvement. *Annals of Internal Medicine*, **137**, 117–22.
37. Lynn, J. (2004). When does quality improvement count as research? Human subject protection and theories of knowledge. *Quality Safe Health Care*, **13**, 67–70.
38. Harding, R., Higginson, I.J. (2005). Palliative care in sub-Saharan Africa. *Lancet*, **365**, 1971–7.
39. Higginson, I.J., Hart, S., Koffman, J. *et al.* (2007). Needs Assessments in Palliative Care: An Appraisal of Definitions and Approaches Used. *Journal of Pain and Symptom Management*, **33**, 500–5.
40. Logie, D.E. and Harding, R. (2005). An evaluation of a morphine public health programme for cancer and AIDS pain relief in Sub-Saharan Africa. *BMC Public Health*, **5**, 82.

41. Hardy, J.R., Haberecht, J., Maresco-Pennisi, D. *et al.* (2007). Audit of the care of the dying in a network of hospitals and institutions in Queensland. *Internal Medicine Journal,* **37**, 315–9.

42. Ahmed, N., Bestall, J.C., Ahmedzai, S.H. *et al.* (2004). Systematic review of the problems and issues of accessing specialist palliative care by patients, carers and health and social care professionals. *Palliative Medicine,* **18**, 525–42.

43. Parish, K., Glaetzer, K., Grbich, C. *et al.* (2006). Dying for attention: palliative care in the acute setting. *Australian Journal of Advanced Nursing,* **24**, 21–5.

44. Solano, J.P., Gomes, B., and Higginson, I.J. (2006). A comparison of symptom prevalence in far advanced cancer, AIDS, heart disease, chronic obstructive pulmonary disease and renal disease. *Journal of Pain and Symptom Management,* **31**, 58–69.

45. Bookbinder, M., Blank, A.E., Arney, E. *et al.* (2005). Improving end-of-life care: development and pilot-test of a clinical pathway. *Journal of Pain and Symptom Management,* **29**, 529–43.

46. Ferrell, B., Connor, S.R., Cordes, A. *et al.* (2007). The National Agenda for Quality Palliative Care: The National Consensus Project and the National Quality Forum. *Journal of Pain and Symptom Management,* **33**, 737–44.

47. Hardy, J.R., Haberecht, J., Maresco-Pennisi, D. *et al.* (2007). Audit of the care of the dying in a network of hospitals and institutions in Queensland. *Internal Medicine Journal,* **37**, 315–9.

48. Meier, D. (2005). Palliative care as a quality improvement strategy for advanced, chronic illness. *Journal of Healthcare Quality,* **27**, 33–9.

49. Veerbeek, L., van Zuylen, L., Gambles, M. *et al.* (2006). Audit of the Liverpool Care Pathway for the Dying Patient in a Dutch cancer hospital. *Journal of Palliative Care,* **22**, 305–8.

50. Clarke, E.B., Curtis, J.R., Luce, J.M. *et al.* (2003). Quality indicators for end-of-life care in the intensive care unit. *Critical Care Medicine,* **31**, 2255–62.

51. Cook, D., Rocker, G., Giacomini, M. *et al.* (2006). Understanding and changing attitudes toward withdrawal and withholding of life support in the intensive care unit. *Critical Care Medicine,* **34**, S317–S323.

52. Vandenberg, E.V., Tvrdik, A., and Keller, B.K. (2006). Use of the quality improvement process in assessing end-of-life care in the nursing home. *Journal of Amertican Medical Dir Association,* **7**, S82–S87.

53. Wu, H.Y., Malik, F.A., and Higginson, I.J. (2006). End of life content in geriatric textbooks: what is the current situation? *BMC Palliative Care,* **5**, 5.

54. Wilkinson, D.J., Fitzsimons, J.J., Dargaville, P.A. *et al.* (2006). Death in the neonatal intensive care unit: changing patterns of end of life care over two decades. *Archives of Diseases in Childhood, Fetal and Neonatal Edition,* **91**, F268–F271.

55. Horne, G. and Payne, S. (2004). Removing the boundaries: palliative care for patients with heart failure. *Palliative Medicine,* **18**, 291–6.

56. Pappas, G., Wolf, R.C., Morineau, G. *et al.* (2006). Validity of measures of pain and symptoms in HIV/AIDS infected households in resources poor settings: results from the Dominican Republic and Cambodia. *BMC Palliative Care,* **5**, 3.

57. Burt, J., Barclay, S., Marshall, N. *et al.* (2004). Continuity within primary palliative care: an audit of general practice out-of-hours co-operatives. *Journal of Public Health (Oxford),* **26**, 275–6.

58. Dudgeon, D., Vaitonis, V., Seow, H. *et al.* (2007). Ontario, Canada: Using Networks to Integrate Palliative Care Province-Wide. *Journal of Pain and Symptom Management,* **33**, 640–4.

59. Ferrell, B., Connor, S.R., Cordes, A. *et al.* (2007). The National Agenda for Quality Palliative Care: The National Consensus Project and the National Quality Forum. *Journal of Pain and Symptom Management,* **33**, 737–44.

60. Harding, R., Higginson, I.J. (2005). Palliative care in sub-Saharan Africa. *Lancet,* **365**, 1971–7.

61. Wolff, J.L., Dy, S.M., Frick, K.D., *et al.* (2007). End-of-life care: findings from a national survey of informal caregivers. *Archives of Internal Medicine,* **167**, 40–6.

62. Bookbinder, M., Blank, A.E., Arney, E. *et al.* (2005). Improving end-of-life care: development and pilot-test of a clinical pathway. *Journal of Pain and Symptom Management,* **29**, 529–43.

63. Davies, R. (2006). The potential of integrated multi-agency care pathways for children. *British Journal of Nursing,* **15**, 764–8.

64. Parish, K., Glaetzer, K., Grbich, C. *et al.* (2006). Dying for attention: palliative care in the acute setting. *Australian Journal of Advanced Nursing,* **24**, 21–5.

65. Okon, T.R., Evans, J.M., Gomez, C.F. *et al.* (2004). Palliative educational outcome with implementation of PEACE tool integrated clinical pathway. *Journal of Palliative Medicine,* **7**, 279–95.

66. Bookbinder, M., Blank, A.E., Arney, E. *et al.* (2005). Improving end-of-life care: development and pilot-test of a clinical pathway. *Journal of Pain and Symptom Management,* **29**, 529–43.

67. Byock, I., Twohig, J.S., Merriman, M. *et al.* (2006). Peer-professional workgroups in palliative care: a strategy for advancing professional discourse and practice. *Journal of Palliative Medicine,* **9**, 934–47.

68. Vandenberg, E.V., Tvrdik, A., Keller, B.K. (2005). Use of the Quality Improvement Process in Assessing End-of-Life Care in the Nursing Home. *Journal of American Medical Dir Association,* **6**, 334–9.

69. White, D.B., Braddock, C.H. III, Bereknyei, S. *et al.* (2007). Toward shared decision making at the end of life in intensive care units: opportunities for improvement. *Archives of Internal Medicine,* **167**, 461–7.

70. Burt, J., Barclay, S., Marshall, N. *et al.* (2004). Continuity within primary palliative care: an audit of general practice out-of-hours co-operatives. *Journal of Public Health (Oxford),* **26**, 275–6.

71. Byock, I., Twohig, J.S., Merriman, M. *et al.* (2006). Peer-professional workgroups in palliative care: a strategy for advancing professional discourse and practice. *Journal of Palliative Medicine,* **9**, 934–47.

72. Cook, D., Rocker, G., and Heyland, D. (2004). Dying in the ICU: strategies that may improve end-of-life care. *Canadian Journal of Anaesthesia,* **51**, 266–72.

73. Decker, S.L. and Higginson, I.J. (2006). A tale of two cities: Factors affecting place of cancer death in London and New York. *European Journal of Public Health.*

74. Morita, T., Fujimoto, K., and Tei, Y. (2005). Palliative care team: the first year audit in Japan. *Journal of Pain and Symptom Management,* **29**, 458–65.

75. Nelson, J.E., Angus, D.C., Weissfeld, L.A. *et al.* (2006). End-of-life care for the critically ill: A national intensive care unit survey. *Critical Care Medicine,* **34**, 2547–53.

76. Nelson, J.E., Mulkerin, C.M., Adams, L.L. *et al.* (2006). Improving comfort and communication in the ICU: a practical new tool for palliative care performance measurement and feedback. *Quality Safe Health Care,* **15**, 264–71.

77. Wolff, J.L., Dy, S.M., Frick, K.D. *et al.* (2007). End-of-life care: findings from a national survey of informal caregivers. *Archives of Internal Medicine,* **167**, 40–6.

78. Davies, E. and Hopkins, A. (1997). *Improving care for patients with malignant cerebral glioma.* London: Royal College of Physicians.

79. Davies, E. and Higginson, I.J. (2004). *Palliative Care: The Solid Facts.* Denmark: World Health Organization. http://www.euro.who.int/document/E82931.pdf, p 1.

80. Davies, E. and Higginson, I.J. (2004). *Better palliative care for older people.* Denmark: World Health Organization. http://www.euro.who.int/document/E82933.pdf, p 1.

81. Lynn, J. (2004).When does quality improvement count as research? Human subject protection and theories of knowledge. *Quality Safe Health Care,* **13**, 67–70.

82. Higginson, I.J., Hearn, J., and Webb, D. (1996). Audit in palliative care: does practice change? *European Journal of Cancer Care,* **5**, 233–6.

83. Higginson, I.J. (1994). Clinical audit and organizational audit in palliative care. *Cancer Surveys*, **21**, 233–45.

84. Blyth, A.C. (1990). Audit of terminal care in a general practice. *British Medical Journal*, **300**, 983–6.

85. Butters, E., Higginson, I., George, R. *et al.* (1993). Palliative care for people with HIV/AIDS: views of patients, carers and providers. *AIDS Care*, **5**, 105–16.

86. Finlay, I., Wilkinson, C., and Gibbs, C. (1992). Planning palliative care services. *Health Trends*, **24**, 139–41.

87. Glickman, M. (1997). *Making palliative care better: quality improvement, multi-professional audit and standards*. London: National Council for Hospice & Specialist Palliative Care Services.

88. Ingleton, C. and Faulkner, A. (1993). Quality assurance. Audit in palliative care: a senior nurse perspective. *Nursing Standards*, **7**, 8–9.

99. Lloyd Williams, M. (1996). An audit of palliative care in dementia. *European Journal of Cancer Care in England*, **5**, 53–5.

90. McKee, C.M., Lauglo, M., and Lessof, L. (1989). Medical Audit: A review. *Journal of the Royal Society of Medicine*, **82**, 474–8.

91. Rogers, M. (1996). Palliative care audit in primary care report: Anglia Clinical Audit and Effectiveness Team.Institute of Public Health.

92. Higginson, I.J., and Bruera, E.(2002). Do we need palliative care audit in developing countries? *Palliative Medicine*, **16**, 546–7.

93. Clark, D., Neale, B., and Heather, P. (1995). Contracting for palliative care. *Social Science Medicine*, **40**, 1193–202.

94. Lynn, J. (2001). Reforming care through continuous quality improvement. In: *Palliative Care for Non-Cancer Patients* (Addington-Hall JM, Higginson IJ, eds.), pp. 210–216. Oxford: Oxford University Press.

95. Bromberg, M.H. and Higginson, I. (1996). Bereavement follow-up: what do palliative support teams actually do? *Journal of Palliative Care*, **12**, 12–7.

96. Donabedian, A. (1980). *The Definition of Quality and Approaches to its Assessment*. Michigan: Health Administration Press.

97. Maxwell, R.J. (1992). Dimensions of quality revisited: from thought to action. *Quality Health Care*, **1**, 171–7.

98. Black, N. (1990). Quality assurance of medical care. *Journal of Public Health Medicine*, **12**, 97–104.

99. Donabedian, A. (1980). The definition of quality and approaches to its assessment. *Explorations in Quality Assessment and Monitoring*. Michigan: Health Administration Press.

100. Vachon, M.L.S., Kristjanson, L., and Higginson, I. (1995). Psychological issues in palliative care: the patient, the family, and the process and outcome of care. *Journal of Pain & Symptom Management*, **10**, 142–50.

101. Stewart, A.L., Teno, J., Patrick, D.L. *et al.* (1999). The concept of quality of life of dying persons in the context of health care. *Journal of Pain and Symptom Management*, **17**, 93–108.

102. King's Fund. (1990). *Organisational Audit (Accreditation UK): Standards for Acute Hospitals in the UK*. London: King's Fund Centre.

103. Working Party of Clinical Governance of the Quality and Clinical Governance Committee. (2002). *Clinical Governance and Quality Approaches in Palliative Care*. London: National Council for Hospice and Specialist Palliative Care.

104. Ferrell, B., Connor, S.R., Cordes, A. *et al.* (2007). The National Agenda for Quality Palliative Care: The National Consensus Project and the National Quality Forum. *Journal of Pain and Symptom Management*, **33**, 737–44.

105. Gysels, M. and Higginson, I.J. (2004). *Improving supportive and palliative care for adults with cancer: Research Evidence*. London: National Institute of Clinical Excellence.

106. National Institute of Clinical Excellence (NICE). (2004). *Improving supportive and palliative care for adults with cancer - the Manual*. London: National Institute of Clinical Excellence.

107. Bullen, M. (1995). The role of the specialist nurse in palliative care. *Professional Nursing*, **10**, 755–6.

108. Butters, E., Higginson, I., George, R. *et al.* (1992). Assessing the symptoms, anxiety and practical needs of HIV/AIDS patients receiving palliative care. *Quality of Life Research*, **1**, 47–51.

109. Finlay, I.G. and Dunlop, R. (1994). Quality of life assessment in palliative care. *Annals of Oncology*, **5**, 13–8.

110. Kristjanson, L.J. (1989). Quality of terminal care: salient indicators identified by families. *Journal of Palliative Care*, **5**, 21–30.

111. Vachon, M.L., Kristjanson, L.J., and Higginson, I. (1995). Psychosocial issues in palliative care: The patient, the family, and the process and outcome of care. *Journal of Pain and Symptom Management*, **10**, 142–50.

112. Haidet, P., Hamel, M.B., Davis, R.B. *et al.* (1998). Outcomes, preferences for resuscitation, and physician-patient communication among patients with metastatic colorectal cancer. SUPPORT Investigators. Study to Understand Prognoses and Preferences for Outcomes and Risks of Treatments. *American Journal of Medicine*, **105**, 222–9.

113. Harper, R., Ward, A., Westlake, L. *et al.* (1988). *Good practice in terminal care: some standards and guidelines for hospital inpatient units and day hospices*. Sheffield: University of Sheffield.

114. Ingleton, C. and Faulkner, A. (1993). Audit issues in palliative care: the perspective of senior nurses. *J Cancer Care*, **2**, 201–6.

115. Latimer, E. (1991). Auditing the hospital care of dying patients. *Journal of Palliative Care*, **7**, 12–7.

116. Lunt, B. and Jenkins, J. (1983). Goal-setting in terminal care: a method of recording treatment aims and priorities. *Journal of Advanced Nursing*, **8**, 495–505.

117. Teno, J.M. (2001). Quality of life and quality indicators for end of cancer care: hope for the best, yet prepare for the worst. In *Improving Palliative Care for Cancer* (eds. Foley, K.M. and Gelband, H.), pp. 96–131. Washington: National Academy Press.

118. Ferrell, B., Connor, S.R., Cordes, A. *et al.* (2007). The National Agenda for Quality Palliative Care: The National Consensus Project and the National Quality Forum. *Journal of Pain and Symptom Management*, **33**, 737–44.

119. Emanuel, E.J. and Emanuel, L.L. (1998). The promise of a good death. *Lancet*, **351**, Sii-21–Sii-29.

120. Weisman, A.D. (1988). Appropriate death and the hospice program. *Hosp Journal*, **4**, 65–77.

121. Kellehear, A. (1984). Are we a 'death-denying' society? A sociological review. *Social Science and Medicine*, **18**, 713–23.

122. Singer, P.A., Martin, D.K., and Kelner, M. (1999). Quality end-of-life care. Patients' perspectives. *Journal of the American Medical Association*, **281**, 163–8.

123. Payne, S., Smith, P., and Dean, S. (1999). Identifying the concerns of informal carers in palliative care. *Palliative Medicine*, **13**, 37–44.

124. Higginson, I.J. and McCarthy, M. (1993). Validity of the support team assessment schedule: do staffs' ratings reflect those made by patients or their families? *Palliative Medicine*, **7**, 219–28.

125. Cartwright, A. (1990). *The role of the general practitioners in caring for people in the last year of their lives*. London: King Edward's Hospital Fund for London, p 1.

126. Copperman, H. (1988). Domiciliary hospice care: a survey of general practitioners. *Journalof the Royal College of General Practitioners*, **38**, 411–3.

127. Doyle, D. (1982). Domiciliary terminal care: demands on statutory services. *Journal of the Royal College of General Practitioners*, **32**, 285–91.

128. Edgar, I. and Bytheway, A. (1988). Information exchange: the hospice nurse and the community nurse. *Nursing Times*, **84**, 42–4.

129. Finlay, I. (1992). Care of the dying in general practice. *British Medical Journal*, **291**, 179–81.

130. Grande, G.E. and Todd, C.F. (1993). Care needs at home during terminal illness: GPS', patients' and relatives' views.

131. Grande, G.E., Todd, C., Barclay, S.I.G. *et al.* (1996). What terminally ill patients value in the support provided by GPs, district and Macmillan nurses. *International Journal of Palliative Nursing*, 138–43.

132. Hjortdahl, P. and Laerum, E. (1992). Continuity of care in general practice: effect on patient satisfaction. *British Medical Journal,* **304**, 1287–90.

133. Jones, R.V.H. (1993). Teams and terminal cancer care at home: do patients and carers benefit? *Journal of Interprofessional Care,* 7, 239–45.

134. Todd, C.J. and Still, A.W. (1984). Communication between general practitioners and patients dying at home. *Social Science and Medicine,* **18**, 667–72.

135. Addington-Hall, J., Lay, M., Altmann, D. *et al.* (1995). Symptom control, communication with health professionals, and hospital care of stroke patients in the last year of life as reported by surviving family, friends, and officials. *Stroke,* **26**. 2242–8.

136. Baile, W.F., Glober, G.A., Lenzi, R. *et al.* (1999). Discussing disease progression and end-of-life decisions. *Oncology (Huntington),* **13**, 1021–31.

137. Buckman, R. (1998). Communication in palliative care: a practical guide. In *Oxford Textbook of Palliative Medicine* (eds. Doyle, D., Hanks, G.W.C., MacDonald, N.,), pp. 141–156. Oxford: Oxford University Press.

138. Buckman, R. (1988), *I don't know what to say: how to help and support someone who is dying.* London: Papermac.

139. Fallowfield, L. (1993), Giving sad and bad news [see comments]. *Lancet,* **341**, 476–8.

140. Faulkner, A., Webb, P., Maguire, P. (1991). Communication and counseling skills: Educating health professionals working in cancer and palliative care. *Patient Education and Counseling,* **18**, 3–7.

141. Koffman, J. and Higginson, I.J. (2001). Accounts of carers' satisfaction with health care at the end of life: a comparison of first generation black Caribbeans and white patients with advanced disease. *Palliative Medicine,* **15**, 337–45.

142. Higginson, I.J. and Sen-Gupta, G.J.A. (2000). Place of care in advanced cancer: a qualitative systematic literature review of patient preferences. *Journal of Palliative Medicine,* **3**, 287–300.

143. Clinical Effectiveness Working Group, Higginson, I.J., Campion-Smith, C., Miller, M., Thomas, K., Wee, B. (2002). *The Which Tool Guide.* Southampton: Association for Palliative Medicine.

144. Higginson, I.J., Wade, A.M., and McCarthy, M. (1992). Effectiveness of two palliative support teams. *Journal of Public Health Medicine,* **14**, 50–6.

145. Higginson, I.J. and McCarthy, M. (1994). A comparison of two measures of quality of life: their sensitivity and validity for patien.s with advanced cancer. *Palliative Medicine,* **8**, 282–90.

146. Hearn, J. and Higginson, I.J. (1999). Development and validation of a core outcome measure for palliative care: the palliative care outcome scale. Palliative Care Core Audit Project Advisory Group. *Quality Health Care,* **8**, 219–27.

147. Higginson, I.J. and Donaldson, N. (2004). Relationship between three palliative care outcome scales. *Health and Quality of Life Outcomes,* **2**, 68.

148. Bausewein, C., Fegg, M., Radbruch, L. *et al.* (2005). Validation and clinical application of the german version of the palliative care outcome scale. *Journal of Pain Symptom Management,* **30**, 51–62.

149. Brandt, H.E., Deliens, L., van der Steen, J.T. *et al.* (2005). The last days of life of nursing home patients with and without dementia assessed with the palliative care outcome scale. *Palliative Medicine,* **19**, 334–42.

150. Goodwin, D.M., Higginson, I.J., Myers, K. *et al.* (2003). Effectiveness of palliative day care in improving pain, symptom control, and quality of life. *Journal of Pain and Symptom Management,* **25**, 202–12.

151. Hearn, J. and Higginson, I.J. (1999). Development and validation of a core outcome measure for palliative care: the palliative care outcome scale. Palliative Care Core Audit Project Advisory Group. *Quality Health Care,* **8**, 219–27.

152. Horton, R. (2002). Differences in assessment of symptoms and quality of life between patients with advanced cancer and their specialist palliative care nurses in a home care setting. *Palliative Medicine,* **16**, 488–94.

153. Hughes, R.A., Aspinal, F., Higginson, I.J. *et al.* (2004). Assessing palliative care outcomes for people with motor neurone disease living at home. *International Journal of Palliative Nursing,* **10**, 449–53.

154. Serra-Prat, M., Nabal, M., Santacruz, V. *et al.* (2004). [Validation of the Spanish version of the Palliative Care Outcome Scale]. *Medicina Clinica (Barcelona),* **123**, 406–12.

155. Slater, A. and Freeman, E. (2004). Patients' views of using an outcome measure in palliative day care: a focus group study. *International Journal of Palliative Nursing,* **10**, 343–51.

156. Slater, A. and Freeman, E. (2005). Is the Palliative Care Outcome Scale useful to staff in a day hospice unit? *International Journal of Palliative Nursing,* **11**, 346–54.

157. Stevens, A.M., Gwilliam, B., A'hern, R. *et al.* (2005). Experience in the use of the palliative care outcome scale. *Support Care Cancer,* **13**, 1027–34.

158. Higginson, I. and McCarthy, M. (1989). Measuring symptoms in terminal cancer: are pain and dyspnoea controlled? *Jouranl of the Royal Society of Medicine,* **82**, 264–7.

159. Hayes, A. (1993). Audit experience: assessing staff's views. In *Clinical Audit in Palliative Care* (ed. Higginson, I.J.), pp. 138–143. Oxford: Radcliffe Medical Press.

160. McKee, E. (1993). Audit experience: a nurse manager in home care. In *Clinical Audit in Palliative Care* (ed. Higginson, I.). Oxford: Radcliffe Medical Press.

161. Finlay, I. and Fowell, A. (2000). A Good Death: Care pathways in Wales aims to improve care of dying patients. *British Medical Journal,* **320**, 1205.

162. McQuillan, R., Finlay, I., Branch, C. *et al.* (1996). Improving analgesic prescribing in a general teaching hospital. *Journal of Pain and Symptom Management,* **11**, 172–80.

163. Finlay, I. (1993). Audit Experience: Views of a Hospice Director. In *Clinical Audit in Palliative Care* (ed. Higginson, I.), pp. 144–149. Oxford: Radcliffe Medical Press.

164. Gysels, M., Hughes, R., Aspinal, F. *et al.* (2004). What methods do stakeholders prefer for feeding back performance data: a qualitative study in palliative care. *International Journal of Quality Health Care,* **16**, 375–81.

165. Higginson, I.J. and Bruera, E. (2002). Do we need palliative care audit in developing countries? *Palliative Medicine,* **16**, 546–7.

166. Harding, R., Stewart, K., Marconi, K. *et al.* (2003). Current HIV/AIDS end-of-life care in sub-Saharan Africa: a survey of models, services, challenges and priorities. *BMC Public Health,* **3**, 33.

167. Harding, R. and Higginson, I.J. (2005). Palliative care in sub-Saharan Africa. *Lancet,* **365**, 1971–7.

168. Higginson, I.J., Hart, S., Koffman, J. *et al.* (2007). Needs Assessments in Palliative Care: An Appraisal of Definitions and Approaches Used. *Journal of Pain and Symptom Management,* **33,** 500–5.

169. Powell, R.A., Downing, J., Harding, R. *et al.* (2007). Development of the APCA African Palliative Outcome Scale. *Journal of Pain and Symptom Management,* **33**, 229–32.

170. Powell, R.A., Downing, J., Harding, R. *et al.* (2007). Development of the APCA African Palliative Outcome Scale. *Journal of Pain and Symptom Management,* **33**, 229–32.

171. Bookbinder, M., Blank, A.E., Arney, E. *et al.* (2005). Improving end-of-life care: development and pilot-test of a clinical pathway. *Journal of Pain and Symptom Management,* **29**, 529–43.

172. Hardy, J.R., Haberecht, J., Maresco-Pennisi, D. *et al.* (2007). Audit of the care of the dying in a network of hospitals and institutions in Queensland. *Internal Medicine Journal,* **37**, 315–9.

173. Okon, T.R., Evans, J.M., Gomez, C.F. *et al.* (2004). Palliative educational outcome with implementation of PEACE tool integrated clinical pathway. *Journal of Palliative Medicine,* **7**, 279–95.

174. Rogers, M.S., Barclay, S.I., Todd, C.J. (2002). Developing the Cambridge palliative audit schedule (CAMPAS): a palliative care audit

for primary health care teams. *British Journal of Genral Practitioners*, **48**, 1224–7.

175. Kaasa, T., Loomis, J., Gillis, K. *et al.* (1997). The Edmonton Functional Assessment Tool: preliminary development and evaluation for use in palliative care. *Journal of Pain and Symptom Management*, **13**, 10–9.

176. Bruera, E., Kuehn, N., Miller, M.J. *et al.* (1991). The Edmonton Symptom Assessment System (ESAS): A simple method for the assessment of palliative care patients. *Journal of Palliative Care*, **7**, 6–9.

177. Aaronson, N.K., Ahmedzai, S., Bergman, B. *et al.* (1993). The European Organization for Research and Treatment of Cancer QLQ-C30: a quality-of-life instrument for use in international clinical trials in oncology. *Journal of the National Cancer Institute*, **85**, 365–76.

178. Aaronson, N.K., Bullinger, M., and Ahmedzai, S. (1988). A modular approach to quality-of-life assessment in cancer clinical trials. *Recent Results in Cancer Research*, **111**, 231–49.

179. Cella, D.F. and Tulsky, D.S. (1990). Measuring quality of life today: methodological aspects. *Oncology*, **4**, 29–37.

180. Cella, D. (2004). The Functional Assessment of Cancer Therapy-Lung and lung cancer subscale assess quality of life and meaningful symptom improvement in lung cancer. *Seminars in Oncology*, **31**, 11–5.

181. Morris, J.N., Suissa, S., Sherwood, S. *et al.* (1986). Last days: A study of the quality of life of terminally ill cancer patients. *Journal of Chronic Diseases*, **39**, 47–56.

182. Cohen, S.R., Mount, B.M., Tomas, J.J.N. *et al.* (1996). Existential well-being is an important determinant of quality of life: Evidence from the McGill Quality of Life Questionnaire. *Cancer*, **77**, 576–86.

183. Cohen, S.R., Mount, B.M., Strobel, M.G. *et al.* (1995). The McGill Quality of Life Questionnaire: a measure of quality of life appropriate for people with advanced disease. A preliminary study of validity and acceptability. *Palliative Medicine*, **9**, 207–19.

184. Cohen, S.R., Mount, B.M., Bruera, E. *et al.* (1997). Validity of the McGill Quality of Life Questionnaire in the palliative care setting: A multi-centre Canadian study demonstrating the importance of the existential domain. *Palliative Medicine*, **11**, 3–20.

185. Ellershaw, J.E., Peat, S.J., and Boys, L.C. (1995). Assessing the effectiveness of a hospital palliative care team. *Palliative Medicine*, **9**, 145–52.

186. Hearn, J. and Higginson, I.J. (1999). Development and validation of a core outcome measure for palliative care: the palliative care outcome scale. Palliative Care Core Audit Project Advisory Group. *Quality in Health Care*, **8**, 219–27.

187. Trent Hospice Audit Group. (1992). *Palliative care core standards.* pp. 1–32.

188. Aspinal, F., Hughes, R., Higginson, I.J. *et al.* (2002). *A user's guide to the Palliative Outcome Scale.* London: Palliative Care and Policy Publications.

189. Hughes, R., Higginson, I.J., Addington-Hall, J. *et al.* (2001). Project to impROve Management Of TErminal illness (PROMOTE). *Journal of Interprofessional Care*, **15**, 398–9.

190. Higginson, I.J., Jarman, B., Astin, P. *et al.* (1999). Do social factors affect where patients die: an analysis of 10 years of cancer deaths in England. *Journal of Public Health Medicine*, **21**, 22–8.

191. Higginson, I.J., Astin, P., and Dolan, S. (1998). Where do cancer patients die? Ten-year trends in the place of death of cancer patients in England. *Palliative Medicine*, **12**, 353–63.

192. Spitzer, W.O., Dobson, A.L., Hall, J. *et al.* (1980). Measuring the quality of life of cancer patients: a concise QL- Index for use by physicans. *Journal of Chronic Diseases*, **34**, 585–97.

193. Higginson, I.J. (1993). *Audit methods: a community schedule.* Oxford: Radcliffe, p. 34.

194. McGee, H.M., O'Boyle, C.A., Hickey, A. *et al.* (1991). Assessing the quality of life of the individual: the SEIQoL with a healthy and a gastroenterology unit population. *Psychological Medicine*, **21**, 749–59.

195. Addington-Hall, J. and Kalra, L. (2001). Measuring quality of life: Who should measure quality of life? *British Medical Journal*, **322**, 1417–20.

196. Addington-Hall, J., Walker, L., Jones, C. *et al.* (1998). A randomised controlled trial of postal versus interviewer administration of a questionnaire measuring satisfaction with, and use of, services received in the year before death. *Journal of Epidemiology and Community Health*, **52**, 802–7.

197. Addington-Hall, J.M. and McCarthy, M. (1995). Regional Study of Care for the Dying: methods and sample characteristics. *Palliat Med* **9**, 27–35.

198. Edmonds, P.M., Karlsen, S., Addington-Hall, J.M. (2000). Palliative care needs of hospital in-patients. *Palliative Medicine*, **14**, 227–8.

SECTION 8

The principles of drug use in palliative medicine

Geoffrey Hanks, Karen Forbes, and Clive J. C. Roberts

The control of distressing symptoms is central to the practice of palliative medicine. It is the foundation of 'whole patient' care in that it is not possible to deal with psychological, social, or spiritual concerns if patients have uncontrolled physical symptoms. The management of these symptoms is largely based on drug treatment, which means that effective symptom control requires some understanding of clinical pharmacology. The purpose of this chapter is to describe those principles of clinical pharmacology that are relevant to day-to-day practice in palliative medicine.

Unfortunately, symptom management is not a simple exercise of targeting a particular symptom with a specific drug. Patients with advanced disease are a vulnerable population and environmental and psychological factors have a variable but potentially very great influence on physical well-being. Sometimes, the response to drug treatment may be unpredictable for these reasons.

One hazard for palliative medicine physicians is the use of drugs for unlicensed indications or by unlicensed routes of administration, which is common in pain and symptom management. A quarter of prescriptions, affecting up to two-thirds of inpatients in specialist palliative care units in the United Kingdom, may fall into this category[1,2]. This highlights the obligation of prescribers to understand the principles of drug use, which should guide their practice and the specific limitations of the data available.

There are other complicating factors in this patient population. Patients are predominantly elderly with many co-morbidities and often with multi-system dysfunction. Polypharmacy is almost invariable, and the potential for modified or abnormal responses to drugs and drug interactions is considerable. Iatrogenic problems are common in that the prescription of one symptomatic remedy, for example, an opioid analgesic, will invariably cause other symptoms, in this case constipation, drowsiness, and possibly nausea, and dry mouth. A laxative, antiemetic, psychostimulant, and artificial saliva may all be added to the treatment regimen as a result. The skill of the palliative medicine physician is to deal effectively with each symptom without imposing a greater burden on the patient due to unwanted or intolerable drug effects or too complex a drug regimen. The principles of effective symptom control must be kept in mind: make a diagnosis of the underlying mechanism or cause of each symptom, individualize the treatment, and keep the regimen as simple as possible.

Clinical pharmacology

Clinical pharmacology may be broadly divided into pharmacokinetics ('what the body does to the drug') and pharmacodynamics ('what the drug does to the body'). It is often assumed that these are theoretical and rather esoteric disciplines that have little direct 'clinical' relevance. As we shall demonstrate, this assumption is wrong. For example, disordered handling of drugs by the body as a result of disease is common. Drugs are often used in special formulations; either modified release orally administered agents or novel forms designed for administration by other routes, and palliative care patients commonly require parenteral administration of drugs at some stage of their illness. These everyday clinical situations cannot be managed properly without some pharmacokinetic knowledge.

Pharmacodynamics is about drug action in man and, like pharmacokinetics, its measurement has become highly sophisticated; for example, in the use of imaging techniques to monitor biochemical changes in target organs. However, one of the challenges of drug use in palliative care is that often outcome measures are not easy to define and measure. In palliative care, drugs are not used to cure underlying disease but to improve comfort. Subjective symptoms such as pain, nausea, or depression are less easy to quantify than biochemical changes in the brain or even tumour size or serum calcium (although cortical responses to pain are now the subject of research because of developments in brain imaging), yet these are common targets for drug treatment in palliative medicine. Knowledge of the basic modes of action of drugs will underpin the logical selection and use of the most appropriate remedies for these symptoms.

Pharmacokinetics

Pharmacokinetics is often described under the headings of absorption, distribution, metabolism, and excretion of drugs. A number of other terms are used also to describe the way in which the body handles drugs. These terms can be defined and modelled mathematically; however, the practising clinician should not be put off by the mathematical formulae often applied to the subject. An appreciation of the physiological, pharmacological, and pathophysiological factors that influence the ultimate concentration of a drug in the blood and eventually at its site of action is invaluable

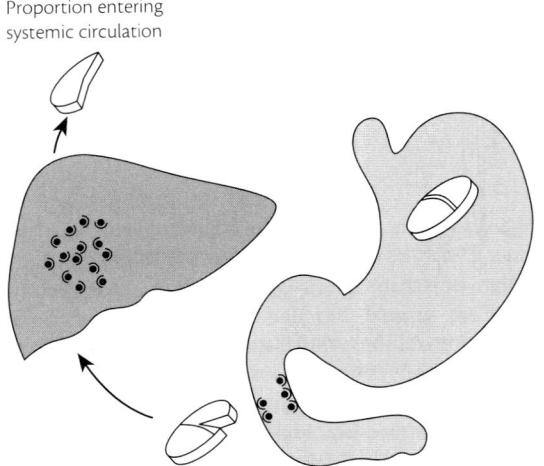

Proportion entering
systemic circulation

Figure 8.4 'First pass' metabolism may take place in the liver, and sometimes also in the intestinal mucosa, before the absorbed drug enters the systemic circulation.

in large percentage changes in bioavailability. Thus, interactions with other drugs which induce or inhibit hepatic enzymes or changes in hepatic function due to disease may have a profound effect on such drug levels after oral administration but relatively little effect when the drug is given parenterally. In patients with chronic liver disease or hepatic metastases blood may be 'shunted' from portal to systemic vessels. The drug may thus bypass hepatic enzymes, the pre-systemic metabolism will be reduced, and the bioavailability may be considerably increased. Consequently, much higher levels of drug may build up after oral administration if the enhanced bioavailability is not taken into account. The effect of pre-systemic metabolism on drug bioavailability must also be considered when calculating oral doses during conversion from parenteral regimens. The bioavailability of some drugs may also be reduced by intraluminal degradation in the gastrointestinal tract or metabolism by enzymes within the intestinal wall.

Drug absorption

In the main, the absorption of drugs is a passive process along a concentration gradient across a lipid cell membrane. As long as the drug is in solution and has a degree of lipid solubility, there is sufficient surface area for diffusion, and the drug remains in contact with the absorptive areas for long enough, then problems should not arise. Most drugs are absorbed where the greatest surface area is available, that is in the small bowel. A reduced rate of absorption may therefore occur if there is a delay in emptying of the stomach. This might arise as part of a pathological process or due to pharmacological agents that slow gastric motility, such as drugs with anticholinergic effects or opioid analgesics. Drugs must have the physicochemical characteristics to facilitate dissolution in the gut, but once presented to the vast surface area of the small bowel, their potential for full absorption should be easily achieved. Only the most severe structural gastrointestinal disease will cause problems.

Many drugs are now formulated as modified-release preparations. For them to achieve their expected absorption profile they may need to remain in the small bowel for a prolonged period of time. Usually such formulations have been tested only under ideal conditions in healthy volunteers. In patients with increased

gastrointestinal transit there is a risk that a modified-release drug will be propelled past the absorptive zone of the gut before all of the drug has been released, resulting in therapeutic failure.

Within the gut there is some potential for drug interaction, which results in reduced bioavailability. Most examples are well known and involve loose chemical binding between two drugs within the gut lumen. For example, cholestyramine binds many drugs; iron salts and tetracycline bind to each other, and sucralfate binds phenytoin. Other less obvious drug interactions may occur, involving interference with absorption. Some broad-spectrum antibiotics decrease the effectiveness of the oral contraceptive; the mechanism may be increased gastrointestinal transit caused by the antibiotic, leading to reduced absorption of the contraceptive.

Absorption and bioavailability are not the same. Morphine, for example, is more or less completely absorbed (i.e. 100 per cent). However, it undergoes extensive pre-systemic metabolism, mainly in the liver but possibly also in the wall of the gastrointestinal tract. The bioavailability of morphine is thus 20 to 30 per cent.

Drug metabolism

Drug biotransformation takes place mainly in the liver and contributes both to the rate of elimination of drug and its bioavailability. The rate at which metabolism proceeds usually determines the clearance; however, where removal is particularly rapid (high extraction ratio) the rate of delivery of drug to the liver, rather than the rate of metabolism, may determine clearance (flow-dependent kinetics). For such drugs, if liver blood flow is markedly reduced, drug accumulation will result.

The biochemical processes of drug metabolism are complex. Two phases of metabolism are usually described, involving initial oxidation or hydrolysis (phase I) followed by conjugation (phase II), but this concept can be misleading. All of the reactions involve the production of products which are more polar and, therefore, more water-soluble and amenable to excretion by the kidney. In some circumstances, phase II reactions may take place without a prior phase I reaction. Phase I reactions involve oxidation, reduction, hydrolysis, hydration, dethioacetylation, and isomerization. Such reactions may prepare the drug molecule for a phase II reaction by producing or uncovering a chemically reactive group, which then forms the substrate for a phase II reaction.

Of the phase I reactions, oxidation involving the 'mixed-function oxidase system' is the most important and its behaviour is best understood. This system of enzymes is based in hepatic microsomes and requires molecular oxygen, NADPH and cytochrome P450, and NADPH-cytochrome P450 reductase. Amongst the reactions catalysed by the mixed-function oxidase system are aromatic hydroxylation, aliphatic hydroxylation, epoxidation, N-dealkylation, O-dealkylation, oxidative deamination, N-oxidation, S-oxidation, and alcohol oxidation. Not all oxidative processes are carried out by this system; alcohol dehydrogenation is performed by a non-microsomally located enzyme which is responsible for the major pathway for alcohol detoxification (in non-enzyme induced subjects).

Phase II reactions mostly involve conjugation; glucuronidation, glycosylation, sulphation, methylation, and acetylation or conjugation with gluthatione or certain amino acids. An appreciation of these processes is necessary in developing a scientific approach to dose management.

Pharmacodynamics

Drugs produce their effects on the body by combining with receptors, by modifying enzyme processes, or by direct chemical or physical actions.

Receptors, agonists, and antagonists

Receptors are specialized areas of the cell membrane which are highly specific for certain drug or hormone molecules. A drug that combines with a receptor to 'activate' it is called an agonist; this terminology derived initially from the actions of hormones and neurotransmitters. The term agonist refers to a drug that binds to receptors to induce changes in the cell which stimulate physiological activity. Some drugs can combine with receptors without initiating any change in cell function. Such drugs are called competitive antagonists because they interfere with the action of agonists by blocking the receptor sites. Non-competitive antagonists do not compete for the same receptor as the agonist but block the effect of the agonist in some other way.

A partial agonist is a drug with low intrinsic activity (efficacy) so that its dose–response curve exhibits a ceiling effect at less than the maximal effect produced by a full agonist. The difference between a partial agonist and a full agonist is thus a difference in efficacy (Fig. 8.5). This should not be confused with potency, which is a measure of the amount of drug required to produce a given effect, and is a measure also of affinity for receptors; the more potent a drug, the greater its affinity for receptors. Thus a drug may be a partial agonist (less effective) but still more potent than a full agonist. This is the case with buprenorphine, which has limited efficacy compared with morphine but greater potency (0.3 mg intramuscular buprenorphine ≡ 10 mg intramuscular morphine[4]). However, because it is more potent it has greater affinity for μ opioid receptors and can displace morphine from them. In this way it can act as an 'antagonist' of morphine by reducing the overall μ opioid effect (see Chapter 10.1.6). Buprenorphine can therefore be classified as an 'agonist antagonist'. Other opioid analgesics, such as pentazocine, are also classified as 'agonist antagonists' but have a different profile. These drugs have both agonist and antagonist effects at receptors, but at different receptors (see following paragraphs).

There are similar examples in other therapeutic areas, and they are likely to increase as new receptors and receptor subtypes

are identified. For example, metoclopramide has been regarded primarily as a dopamine receptor blocker. This is true at low doses, however, at high doses, metoclopramide blocks (antagonizes) $5HT_3$ receptors and is a more effective antiemetic. Metoclopramide also has a prokinetic effect on the upper gastrointestinal tract and this is mediated through an agonist effect at $5HT_4$ receptors, leading to an enhancement of the effects of acetylcholine release in the gut. Metoclopramide is thus both an antagonist and an agonist at different serotonin receptors.

Morphine is an agonist at μ opioid receptors. Buprenorphine is a partial agonist at μ receptors and can, in certain circumstances, reverse (antagonize) the effects of morphine. Pentazocine is a weak competitive antagonist at μ receptors (so may also antagonize the effects of morphine but by a different mechanism) and is a partial agonist at the κ opioid receptor. Naloxone is an antagonist at the μ opioid receptor and will block the effects of μ agonists and partial agonists (but with varying efficiency).

Drugs which alter enzyme activity

Drugs affecting enzyme processes may have diverse therapeutic applications but many act by being inhibitors of enzyme actions. For example, non-steroidal anti-inflammatory drugs block the effect of the enzyme cyclo-oxygenase and thereby interfere with the synthesis of prostaglandins; this is believed to be the basis for their anti-inflammatory activity. Monoamine oxidase inhibitor antidepressants interfere with the degradation of monoamine neurotransmitters thus enhancing their effect in central synapses. Angiotensin-converting enzyme inhibitors block the conversion of angiotensin I to angiotensin II by inhibiting the relevant enzyme and are effective in the treatment of hypertension and cardiac failure.

Drugs which have a direct chemical or physical action

Antacids are an example of drugs with a direct chemical action; they are bases which neutralize gastric acid. Drugs with a physical mode of action include the bulk laxatives such as ispaghula husk. Whilst the mode of action of such drugs seems less complex than that of drugs that interact with receptors, the same attention to detail in their use and an individualized approach are necessary to maximize their benefits and reduce potential adverse effects.

Tolerance, drug dependence, and drug resistance
Tolerance

Tolerance refers to the phenomenon of decreasing response to a drug as a consequence of its continued use. It is manifest by a shift to the right in the dose–response curve; an increased dose is required to achieve a similar effect (Fig. 8.6). In contrast, sensitization refers to the phenomenon of increasing response to a drug, as a consequence of its continued use. It is manifest by a shift to the left in the dose–response curve; a decreased dose is required to achieve a similar effect (Fig. 8.6). Sensitization is a relatively uncommon phenomenon.

Tolerance may be due to:

- An alteration in the pharmacokinetic profile of a drug (pharmacokinetic tolerance). For example, tolerance to barbiturates has been linked to induction of hepatic microsomal enzymes, which results in an increased metabolism of the barbiturate.

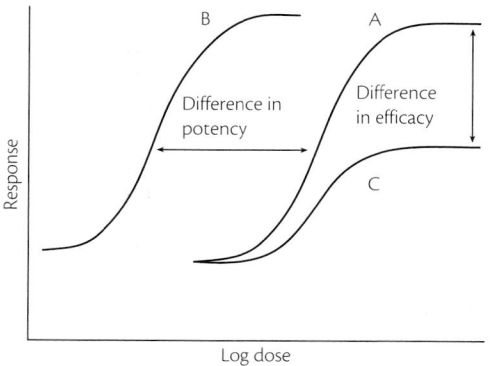

Figure 8.5 Log dose–response curves for two full agonist drugs A and B, and a partial agonist C. Drug B is more potent than drug A but no more effective. Drug A is more effective than drug C but has similar potency.

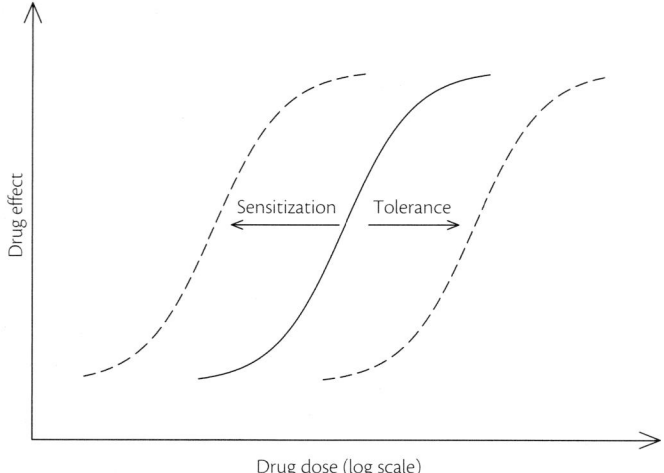

Figure 8.6 Graphical representation of drug tolerance and sensitization.

◆ An alteration in the pharmacodynamic profile of the drug (pharmacodynamic tolerance). Tolerance to opioids has been linked to uncoupling of opioid/G protein receptor complexes, which results in a decreased effect of the opioid.

Tolerance occurs at a variable time after initiation of the drug. Moreover, it may occur to some, or all, of the effects of the drug. For example, tolerance to the analgesic effects of opioids is uncommon in clinical practice. Indeed, increases in opioid requirement are invariably related to progression of disease, rather than to the development of tolerance[5]. However, tolerance to some of the adverse effects of opioids is common in clinical practice. Thus, sedation and nausea and vomiting usually settle within a few days, or a week or two. Cross-tolerance refers to a decreased response to a drug as a consequence of the use of a drug with a similar structure or function. It may occur to some or all of the effects of the drugs. The extent of cross-tolerance between opioid drugs is very variable. The practice of opioid switching relies on incomplete cross-tolerance between opioids. Thus, opioid switching will only be successful if cross-tolerance to the analgesic effects is less than cross-tolerance to the adverse effects[6].

Drug dependence

In pharmacological terms, drug dependence has been divided into two types[7]:

◆ Psychological dependence—characterized by a compulsion to continue taking the drug. This is a pathological response to the drug.

◆ Physical dependence—characterized by a withdrawal syndrome if the drug is not taken (or if an antagonist drug is taken). This is a normal physiological response to the drug.

The relationship between the two types of drug dependence is variable: patients may develop psychological dependence or physical dependence, or a combination of psychological and physical dependence. Opioid drug misusers invariably develop a combination of psychological and physical dependence.

Psychological dependence is associated with a positive (perceived) effect from taking the drug. Drugs that produce a rapid effect are more likely to induce psychological dependence than drugs producing a delayed effect. For example, a drug given intravenously is more likely to induce psychological dependence than the same drug given orally. The positive effects of the drug are often reinforced by the rituals and environment associated with drug-taking. Indeed, the treatment of psychological dependence involves measures aimed at reducing these reinforcing factor[7].

Physical dependence is associated with a negative effect from not taking the drug, i.e. a withdrawal syndrome. The features of the withdrawal syndrome are usually the opposite of the features of the drug's acute effect. The treatment of physical dependence involves trying to reduce the impact of this reinforcing factors[7]. A variety of different 'detoxification' regimens have been used, including gradual reduction of the original drug, gradual reduction of a substitute drug, and symptomatic treatment of the withdrawal syndrome. Many patients require a combination of different strategies in order to overcome their drug dependence.

Patients receiving opioids for cancer pain rarely develop psychological dependence, although they may more often develop physical dependence to the opioid[8]. The best opioid for the patient's clinical situation should be chosen, whatever its potential for abuse; a patient with difficult breakthrough pain will require an opioid with a rapid onset of action, for example, even if the patient has a history of drug misuse (see Chapter 10.1.6).

Drug resistance

Resistance refers to the phenomenon of lack of responsiveness to a drug. The expression is primarily applied to antimicrobial drugs and cytotoxic chemotherapy, but could be used for other classes of drug. Drug resistance has been sub-classified into: (1) primary or intrinsic resistance—this type of resistance develops *de novo*; and (2) secondary or acquired resistance—this type of resistance develops after exposure to the drug. Drug resistance may involve a single drug, several drugs from the same class (cross-resistance), or several drugs from different classes (also described as cross-resistance). Cross-resistance is invariably due to a common molecular mechanism.

Drug resistance is primarily related to the genetic profile of the cell. Resistance may occur in response to spontaneous mutation or, in the case of antimicrobial agents, to transfer of genetic material (involving plasmids, bacteriophages, or other mechanisms). The molecular mechanisms underlying drug resistance are shown in Table 8.1. Continuing drug usage encourages the development of resistance by suppressing the growth of sensitive cells, thereby encouraging the growth of resistant cells.

Antimicrobial drug resistance is a major clinical problem. Indeed, the Standing Medical Advisory Committee Sub-Group on Antimicrobial Resistance (UK) has described the current situation as 'looking into the abyss'[9]. Antimicrobial drug resistance involves not only antibacterial agents, but also antifungal and antiviral agents. Infections caused by resistant organisms generally result in increased morbidity, increased mortality, and increased use of resources[9].

There is relatively little information about the impact of antimicrobial resistance in palliative care, however one study from the United Kingdom reported that methicillin-resistant *Staphylococcus aureus* (MRSA) carriage was low. Only 6 per cent of patients transferred into

Table 8.1 Molecular mechanisms of drug resistance.

Molecular mechanisms of drug resistance	Specific example
Drug inactivated	Resistance to penicillin may result from the production of β lactamase
Drug prevented from entering into the cell	Melphalan resistance has been linked to deactivation of various active transport systems (e.g. system L)
Drug prevented from remaining in the cell	Fluconazole resistance has been linked to activation of various active transport systems (e.g. major facilitator efflux pump)
Pro-drug not activated	Resistance to 5-fluorouracil may result from the abnormalities of several enzymes in its metabolic pathway
Alteration of drug target	Amphotericin resistance has been linked to alteration of cell membrane
Overproduction of drug target	Methotrexate resistance has been linked to overproduction of dihydrofolate reductase
Effect of drug counteracted	Resistance to cisplatin may result from repair of damaged DNA

one large hospice from environments not known to have MRSA, and 7 per cent of patients transferred from hospital wards known to have MRSA were carriers, suggesting the burden of conventional eradication regimens in this patient group needs to be considered carefully[10]. Infections in hospices are associated with increased physical and psychological morbidity and increased use of resources[11]. Moreover, this study reported that infection control measures secondary to MRSA infections resulted in major operational problems for the hospices concerned.

Antimicrobial drugs should generally only be prescribed for cases of proven infection, and not for prophylaxis of infection. Narrow spectrum drugs should be employed, and these should be prescribed in relatively high doses, for relatively short courses[9]. Other strategies that are relevant include the use of appropriate infection-control measures (e.g. hand washing).

Cytotoxic chemotherapy drug resistance is a perennial clinical problem[12]. Many tumours are primarily resistant, whilst many other tumours become secondarily resistant.

Routes of administration of drugs in palliative care

A variety of different routes of drug administration are used in palliative care. The choice of route will depend on a combination of patient, drug, and organizational factors, including availability of drug formulations and financial and human resources. Moreover, the choice of route may vary over the course of the patient's illness.

Oral route

The oral route is the principal route of administration of drugs in palliative care. The advantages of this route are that it is simple, non-invasive, acceptable to patients, and maintains patient control. Moreover, the majority of drugs used in palliative care are available in oral forms, and often in different oral formulations (liquid and solid). The disadvantages of this route are that there are

numerous factors that can affect the absorption and bioavailability of the drug.

Modified-release formulations for oral administration

There are two theoretical benefits of modified-release oral preparations; they prolong the absorption time and thereby extend the overall duration of action of a short-acting drug (Fig. 8.7) and they attenuate peak plasma concentrations of a drug where such peak concentrations could be associated with adverse effects. The most common examples in palliative medicine are modified-release opioids. Most orally administered opioids are short-acting drugs with duration of analgesia of about 4 h. In order to maintain control of chronic pain they have to be given six times a day. Modified-release opioid tablets have a 12- or 24-h duration of effect. Reduction in the frequency of dosing has important benefits in terms of patient acceptance and compliance. The theoretical reduction in adverse effects has not been demonstrated in practice with modified-release oral opioids.

The plasma concentration profile of a modified-release preparation is different from that of a normal-release preparation; the time to peak plasma concentration is delayed and the peak is attenuated. This has implications for the use of such preparations; in general, modified-release formulations are designed for maintenance treatment. Some drugs need to be rapidly absorbed and have a relatively short duration of action if they are to achieve their intended therapeutic effect without producing significant unwanted effects. This applies, for example, to analgesics used in the treatment of acute pain. It is inappropriate, therefore, to use modified-release preparations in such situations.

Modified-release formulations prolong the absorption phase, but do not change the elimination process. For example, the elimination half-life of morphine (2–4 h) is the same whether or not a normal- or modified-release formulation is used[13].

Oral transmucosal route (sublingual, buccal)

In theory, the oral transmucosal route offers certain advantages over the oral route, particularly, increased speed of drug absorption and increased drug bioavailability for drugs that undergo first-pass hepatic metabolism. The advent of oral transmucosal and buccal preparations of opioids, usually fentanyl, has allowed more

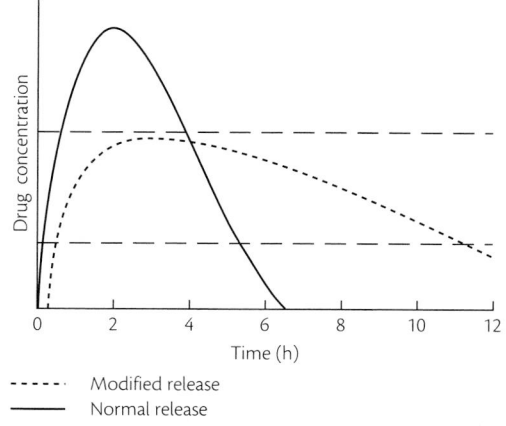

Figure 8.7 Typical plasma concentration profile for a normal-release and modified-release formulation of the same drug.

rapid management of breakthough pain than can be achieved by normal release oral preparations[14,15]. The buccal route has been used to treat epileptic seizures in children[16], and, anecdotally, this approach has also been successful for the management of seizures and terminal agitation in palliative care patients.

Nasogastric/enteral feeding tubes

The decision to use this route is dependent on a number of factors, including the availability of a suitable formulation of the drug, the compatibility of the drug and enteral feed if it is being administered, and practical issues such as the position and size of the feeding tube[17].

Ideally, liquid drug formulations should be used with feeding tubes. However, solid drug formulations can be used, though it is necessary to dissolve them or crush and suspend them in water. Occasionally, parenteral drug formulations are used in place of oral formulations. The appropriateness of crushing solid drug formulations, and of using parenteral formulations, should be verified with a reliable source of drug information.

Modified-release formulations should not be crushed, since this can affect their physical characteristics and therefore their pharmacokinetic profile, usually resulting in an increased rate of absorption or 'dose dumping'. Dose dumping may result in decreased efficacy, decreased tolerability, or sometimes even serious drug toxicity. Enteric-coated tablets should not be crushed unless the end of the feeding tube lies beyond the stomach.

Drugs should always be administered separately from the enteral feed, and the feeding tube should be flushed with water before and after the drug is given. Similarly, if several drugs are to be administered, the tube should be flushed before and after each drug. In the case of drugs that do not interact with enteral feed, the feed can be stopped immediately before and restarted immediately after the drug has been administered.

Modified-release granules of morphine are available, which can be suspended in water and given through nasogastric and enteral feeding tubes. Particular care is needed with flushing when using these preparations to avoid them blocking the tube.

Rectal route

The rectal route may be an important route for administration of drugs in palliative care, depending on the care setting. Its main advantage is that it is simple, does not require additional equipment, and non-professional carers can be taught to administer drugs via this route. Its main disadvantage is that it is not acceptable to many patients and may be inconvenient for very ill patients. A variety of drugs can be given rectally; some are formulated specifically for rectal use and, sometimes, the oral or parenteral formulation is used.

The absorption of drugs from the rectum can be very variable. Absorption is limited by the small surface area, the presence of faeces, defaecation, and involuntary expulsion of the drug. The venous drainage of the lower and middle part of the rectum is the inferior vena cava and of the upper part of the rectum the portal vein, with significant anastomoses between these two venous systems. Therefore drugs given rectally are subject to some first-pass hepatic metabolism. It is recommended that drugs are inserted one finger length into the rectum and that 10 ml of warm water is administered also to ensure dissolution if the rectum is dry[18]. Alcohol/glycol containing formulations should be avoided since they can cause rectal irritation.

Subcutaneous route

The subcutaneous route is the most commonly used parenteral route in palliative care. The advantages of the subcutaneous route are that it is simple and acceptable to patients and subcutaneous injections are less painful than intramuscular injections. A subcutaneous cannula can be inserted which allows repeated administration of intermittent boluses of drugs, or administration of a continuous subcutaneous infusion, thus reducing the need for repeated skin puncture. Whilst a number of drugs may be given subcutaneously, most will not be licensed for this route of administration.

Subcutaneous infusions can be given using infusion devices available in most hospitals, or, more commonly, using small battery-powered syringe drivers. A recent survey from the United Kingdom reported that a variety of different combinations of drugs were being given by continuous infusion; however, the stability/compatibility of only half of the drug combinations in use was known[19]. The compatibility of drug combinations is dependent on a number of factors, including the drugs used, the concentration, the diluent, and other factors such as temperature and UV light. Databases of compatible drug combinations are now available on the Internet (http://www.pallcare.info and http://palliative-drugs.com/pdi.html). It should be noted that the absence of precipitation within a drug mixture is not synonymous with compatibility between the drugs in that mixture[20].

Continuous subcutaneous infusions produce stable blood levels of drugs, which makes them suitable for the control of ongoing symptoms. Intermittent subcutaneous bolus injections of drugs are usually rapidly absorbed, which makes this route suitable for the emergency treatment of symptoms. However, the absorption of drugs may be affected if the cutaneous blood flow is compromised. Drugs given via the subcutaneous route, as for other parenteral routes, are not susceptible to first-pass hepatic metabolism and therefore tend to have a high bioavailability, generally near 100 per cent.

Intramuscular route

The intramuscular route is used infrequently in palliative care. It is generally used when the subcutaneous route is contraindicated, such as when the drug is irritant to the skin, when the drug is of large volume, and when the cutaneous blood supply is compromised.

Intravenous route

The intravenous route is used infrequently in palliative care. It is generally used in emergency situations to obtain a rapid therapeutic response and in circumstances where the other parenteral routes are contraindicated, such as where there is a bleeding diathesis or the peripheral blood supply is compromised. However, if a patient has an indwelling central venous catheter, it is often used rather than instituting another parenteral route.

Dermal route

Few drugs are reliably absorbed through the skin. Absorption is limited by the physical characteristics of the epidermis and is increased if the epidermis is damaged or destroyed. The absorption of drugs is also dependent on cutaneous hydration and blood flow—poor hydration and blood flow leading to decreased absorption. Drugs that are absorbed through the skin are not susceptible to first-pass hepatic metabolism.

Drugs are usually applied to the skin in order to achieve a local effect. Capsaicin cream is used for non-malignant neuropathic pain, and lidocaine patches are now licensed for postherpetic neuralgia; both have been used for other causes of neuropathic pain in palliative care, but experience is limited. Parenteral formulations of diamorphine and morphine (in suitable bases) have been used to treat localized pain secondary to non-malignant ulceration, tumour infiltration, and tumour fungation[21]. However, drugs can also be applied to the skin in order to achieve a systemic effect. For example, specific transdermal formulations of fentanyl and buprenorphine are available for chronic pain and are used extensively in some countries. In a European Association for Palliative Care survey of over 3000 patients in 21 countries, transdermal fentanyl accounted for 14 per cent of all opioid prescriptions[22] (see Chapter 10.1.6).

Pulmonary route

In palliative care, the pulmonary route is used primarily to administer drugs to the lungs. Drugs are given either as a fine powder or an aerosol administered via an inhaler, with or without a holding chamber or 'spacer', or a nebulizer. The addition of a spacer improves the efficiency of inhalers. A systematic review concluded that bronchodilators administered via an inhaler and spacer were as effective as bronchodilators administered via a nebulizer in acute asthma[23]. The pulmonary route of administration of drugs is discussed in more detail in Chapter 11.1.

Spinal route

The spinal route refers to administration of drugs either into the epidural space (epidural administration), or into the subarachnoid space (intrathecal administration). The spinal route of administration of drugs is discussed in detail in Chapter 10.1.9.

Other routes

Other routes of administration that have been used in palliative care include intranasal, intracavitary, and regional application of drugs. The intranasal route can be used to deliver drugs systemically, as well as locally, for instance in the management of breakthrough pain[24]. Fentanyl[25], sufentanil and diamorphine[26], have been used intranasally, although their use has largely been overtaken by the availability of oral transmucosal delivery systems. There have been several reports of the successful use of intracavitary local anaesthetics for localized pain; local anaesthetic administered into the pleural cavity has been used to manage chest wall pain[27], whilst local anaesthetic administered into the joint space has been used for bone pain secondary to pathological fracture[28]. Similarly, there have been several reports of the successful use of regional (perineural) application of local anaesthetics for neuropathic pain[29].

Variability in drug response

Wide variability in the rates of drug metabolism occurs between individuals as a result of genetic factors, pathological processes, concurrent medication, and ageing, and creates the major obstacle to matching dose to patients' requirements.

Both pharmacokinetic and pharmacodynamic factors may be responsible for therapeutic failure or adverse effects and the mechanism of each may relate to drug interaction, disease, genetics, or the effect of old age. The study of variability in drug response encompasses the whole of the science of clinical pharmacology. In this section we will merely highlight important principles and provide examples most relevant to palliative medicine.

Pharmacogenetics

Wide inter-individual variation in the rates of metabolism of drugs has been observed for many years and a combination of genetic and environmental factors is assumed to be responsible. Our understanding of the influence of genetic factors has increased rapidly with the advent of modern molecular biological techniques. For example, the rate of elimination of isoniazid within populations has been recognized to have a bimodal distribution[30]. This drug is N-acetylated and the rate of drug acetylation is under the control of two autosomal alleles, R for fast acetylation and r for slow (R being dominant and r recessive)[31]. 'Fast acetylators' of isoniazid may be more susceptible to hepatic damage caused by the drug and at the same time may be at risk of under dosage with other agents which are acetylated[32]. The high incidence of the recessive trait, which determines slow acetylation, may indicate a selective advantage for slow acetylators, which is not related to drug metabolism. There is variation in the proportion of fast and slow acetylators in different populations and ethnic groups. In most European groups, about 40 per cent, and in the United States, 45 per cent, are fast acetylators, but 80 to 90 per cent of Asian populations and nearly 100 per cent of Canadian Eskimos are fast acetylators[33]. Numerous drugs are metabolized by acetylation and the effects of genetic polymorphism have not been studied for all of these drugs. Hydralazine, some sulphonamides, and some benzodiazepines are worthy of mention but within the field of palliative medicine, where, in general, dose is titrated to patients' needs, there do not appear to be significant clinical implications of this phenomenon.

A genetic component to drug oxidation was first documented when rates of metabolism of antipyrine were shown to have a greater degree of concordance in identical rather than fraternal twins[34]. This was difficult to interpret because of the lack of any observed correlation in the rates of oxidation of different drugs between individuals. However, it was subsequently demonstrated that people who were slow oxidizers of debrisoquine were also slow metabolizers of other drugs such as sparteine, phenformin, phenytoin, metoprolol, nortriptyline, and others[35]. We now know that the enzyme system involved, cytochrome P450, can be classified into a number of sub-families each of which is probably under genetic and environmental control. The most widely studied is the debrisoquine 4-hydroxylation phenotype, which is under the control of cytochrome P450 2D6 (CYP2D6). About 90 per cent of the population are extensive metabolizers of debrisoquine and family studies have indicated this is a dominant trait[36,37]. Using kinetic tests, it has been shown that different racial groups exhibit different proportions of poor and extensive metabolizers. Egyptians show the lowest incidence of debrisoquine poor metabolizer status (about 1 per cent), whereas West Africans show the highest (about 13 per cent) and Caucasians have an intermediate incidence. CYP2D6 is involved in the methylation of codeine and failures of this drug to produce analgesia have been attributed to the inability to metabolize codeine to the active moiety, morphine[38].

There is evidence of genetic control in the metabolism of mephenytoin in which another isoform of cytochrome P450 is involved (2C19). About 3 per cent of Caucasians and 18 per cent of Japanese people are poor metabolizers of mephenytoin[39]. There is a single case report of a CYP3A5 polymorphism leading to rapid methadone metabolism in a patient with a long history of drug misuse[40]. CYP1A2, responsible for the metabolism of theophylline amongst many other drugs, is easily induced by alcohol and flavonoids found in the diet, especially cruciferous vegetables and polycyclic aromatic hydrocarbons found in barbecued food. The variation between genetically determined poor and extensive metabolism is wide and it is important therefore that the doses of susceptible drugs should be managed carefully. Recent studies in palliative care populations suggest that opioid receptor polymorphism[41] and COMT-polymorphism[42] may influence patients' requirements for opioids (see Chapter 10.1.6).

There are pharmacodynamic examples of genetic variation in drug response. These include resistance to the effects of warfarin due to increased sensitivity to vitamin K, haemolysis in patients with glucose-6-phosphate dehydrogenase deficiency in response to drugs such as sulphonamides or nitrofurantoin, and flushing in response to alcohol in patients taking chlorpropamide[43].

Disease states

A myriad of conditions, both acute and chronic, can affect the response to drugs through both pharmacokinetic and pharmacodynamic mechanisms. From the pharmacokinetic viewpoint, diseases of the two most important organs of elimination, the kidneys and the liver, are most important.

Excretion of drugs by the kidneys depends upon either filtration of drug unbound to plasma protein at the glomerulus or the active transport systems, which secrete drug at the renal tubule. The reduction in the renal clearance of any drug closely follows renal function as measured by creatinine clearance. The consequences of renal disease therefore depend upon the extent to which renal clearance contributes to total drug clearance and how critical drug concentration is in terms of toxicity. Information about the need for dose adjustment in patients with renal impairment is usually readily available in prescribing information sources. A more complex situation exists for drugs metabolized in the liver. The relevance to palliative medicine is much greater because centrally-active drugs tend to be those requiring metabolism simply because they are lipid soluble; a necessary property for penetration into the brain. The metabolic process converts them into more polar, water-soluble metabolites. The liver is also often affected in malignant disease, not least because it is a common site for metastases.

In chronic liver disease, intrahepatic and extrahepatic anastomoses ('shunts') exist between the portal and systemic circulation. This means that drugs which normally have a low bioavailability because of pre-systemic metabolism in the liver can bypass that metabolic process and thus achieve greatly increased oral bioavailability. The bioavailability of modified release morphine and tramadol are markedly increased in patients with both primary and secondary liver tumours, and clearance was reduced and elimination impaired in one study of patients with primary liver tumours[44,45]. Increased bioavailability has been shown to occur also with pentazocine, pethidine[46], chlormethiazole[47], and many other drugs not used in palliative medicine, and may be expected to occur with methadone[48], metoclopramide[49], and others. Reduced metabolite formation of several drugs in the absence of a reduction in systemic clearance in patients with hepatic metastases suggests that such shunting can also take place within tumour deposits inside the liver[50]. This has implications for the oral dosing of drugs with normally low bioavailability in malignant disease, particularly for patients with primary liver

tumours where lengthening of dose interval as well as dose reduction may be necessary[45].

In chronic liver disease, the total mass of functioning hepatocytes is reduced and therefore it is not surprising that drug metabolism is generally impaired. However, normal inter-individual variation in drug metabolism rates is so wide that an effect may only be evident when liver disease is severe. The level of serum albumin has been shown to correlate as closely as any parameter to the degree of pharmacokinetic disturbance[51]. The situation is further complicated by an apparent differential effect on the enzyme system involved. Thus, glucuronidation seems to be relatively protected from the effects of liver disease compared to oxidation and demethylation and there is also evidence of a differential effect on the subfamilies of cytochrome P450[50].

Hepatic drug metabolizing capacity is not just susceptible to local effects within that organ but widespread pathophysiological changes may affect drug clearance rates, for example, acute febrile illnesses and endocrine abnormalities may impair drug metabolism.

Some drugs rely on conversion within the liver to their active moiety, for example, prednisone, methylprednisone, and many of the angiotensin-converting enzyme inhibitors. This may render some drugs less effective than others in the presence of liver disease and influence the choice of drug in this situation[50].

In malignant disease of the liver there appears to be no overall loss of functional hepatocytes so that systemic clearance is usually unimpaired[52]. Some more detailed studies of cytochrome P450 subfamilies have emerged; it has been shown that CYP1A2 and CYP2E1 are decreased in cirrhosis but not in hepatocellular carcinoma[53] and there is evidence that cytochrome P450s of the 2C subfamily may actually be up-regulated (i.e. have increased activity) in patients with carcinoma[54].

Not only renal and hepatic failure but also other organ failures can cause changes in distribution volume either through reducing plasma proteins to which drugs bind or through a qualitative change in the binding sites. Tissue binding may also be affected and the changes in body composition in relation to organ failure, and cachexia may change a drug's distribution volume according to whether it is distributed mainly in water or in lipid tissue. Although poorly studied, the kinetic profile of many drugs is likely to be abnormal in the presence of advanced malignant disease.

In disease states, pharmacodynamic mechanisms may cause altered response. Increased sensitivity to centrally acting agents and those acting on the cardiovascular system is common. Particular care is needed when both pharmacodynamic and pharmacokinetic changes are potentially occurring in the same patient, for example, when using drugs with sedating properties in patients with hepatic impairment or respiratory insufficiency.

Ageing

Many of the changes discussed relevant to disease processes can be applied to the elderly, for after the age of about 65 years there is a gradual decline in renal and hepatic function. Body composition changes so that there is an increase in lipid in relation to total body weight and plasma albumin gradually declines. However, it should be emphasized that changes in pharmacokinetics are quite small and are only detectable in group studies. The most notable change associated with ageing is an increase in variability so that no assumptions can be made about reduced doses being required.

Titration of dose to patients' requirements must be carried out more carefully in the aged.

The effect of the ageing process on hepatic drug metabolism has been extensively studied. Total hepatic mass decreases with age, and much of the documented decline in drug metabolizing capacity has been attributed to the reduction in total functional hepatocyte mass[55]. It appears from studies with antipyrine and other agents that only microsomally-located enzyme systems decline in activity with age but the results of studies are inconsistent[56], and some authors estimate that only 3 per cent of total variance in drug metabolic rate could be attributed to ageing[57]. A further source of debate is the response of the cytochrome P450 system to enzyme inhibitors and inducers with obvious implications for drug interaction. There appears little doubt that cimetidine, and presumably other enzyme inhibitors, have a similar effect in the elderly compared to the young[58]. Earlier studies had suggested that microsomal enzymes in the elderly were incapable of being induced[59] (see following paragraphs) but this suggestion is now completely refuted[60] and it is clear that elderly patients are at risk of drug interaction through these mechanisms in the same way as the young.

Reduced cardiovascular and other homeostatic mechanisms and reduced central nervous system function in the aged make this group susceptible to excess effects from diuretics, blood pressure-lowering agents, and central nervous system depressants. The prescription of prochlorperazine for the symptom of dizziness illustrates the potential hazards, for example. The dizziness is usually due to age-related postural hypotension. However, the α-adrenergic blocking properties of the phenothiazine may cause vasodilation and worsen the symptom, the dopamine receptor blocking effect can precipitate parkinsonism and the sedating effect intellectual impairment.

Drug interaction

Patients with palliative care needs may already be receiving drugs for a variety of conditions. Some may still be required but others may not be necessary but may be continued because of possible adverse impacts of discontinuing them, physical or psychological. If drugs to relieve symptoms are added, this creates an enormous potential for drug interaction. Interaction is adverse if it causes therapeutic failure or toxicity from any one drug. It may be regarded, therefore, as simply another source of variability in drug response. Remembering all the possible drug interactions is virtually impossible; so frequent consultation with prescribing information is important. However, knowledge of the underlying mechanisms of drug interaction can put the prescriber on guard.

In broad terms, drug interactions are either pharmacokinetic or pharmacodynamic. Kinetic interaction results in a change in the total body exposure to the drug reflected in a change in blood concentration. The effect is entirely predictable from that change. However, the existence of a pharmacokinetic interaction cannot be predicted easily; every drug has to be studied before its potential for kinetic interaction can be recognized.

The site of pharmacodynamic interaction is the receptor and so it follows that the consequences of such interactions are common to pharmacological groupings of drugs and are therefore to some extent predictable from a working knowledge of each drug group. Kinetic interaction arises through alterations in the rate and extent of absorption and changes in metabolism (both pre-systemic and elimination), distribution, and renal excretion. Drugs such as metoclopramide, anticholinergics[61], and opioid analgesics[62], which alter the rate of gastric emptying, will affect the speed of absorption of other agents. The resultant effects may not be easily predictable. For example, food increases the bioavailability of morphine[63] and metoclopramide increases morphine's rate of absorption and sedative effects[64]. Some drugs bind others in the gastrointestinal tract and affect their bioavailability. Certain antacid preparations, iron salts, and cholestyramine are the worst offenders and care is necessary in the use of these drugs concurrently with others.

Of least importance are interactions due to changes in distribution. This is because volume of distribution is not a determinant of steady-state concentration, although an acute change could cause a temporary effect. In the past, much was made of interactions between drugs as a result of plasma protein-binding displacement but it is now known this is rarely a problem. Even if a drug is very heavily bound to protein, displacement will result in only a temporary rise in the free (unbound) fraction because of immediate compensatory mechanisms. There will be wider distribution throughout the distribution volume and the first-order nature of the elimination process results in increased removal of drug. Most clinically significant interactions previously ascribed to protein-binding displacement have now been explained by enzyme inhibition[65].

Drug interactions resulting from changes in the rate of metabolism by the liver will result in both changes in bioavailability for those drugs with a significant first-pass effect, and decreased clearance. Steady-state concentrations of drug may be profoundly affected. A number of drugs (particularly the barbiturates, carbamazepine, phenytoin, and rifampicin) are capable of inducing the mixed function oxidase and glucuronidase enzyme systems in the liver. The process involves hypertrophy of the endoplasmic reticulum and takes some weeks to be fully achieved. There is a myriad of substrates for this interaction, amongst them warfarin, corticosteroids, the oral contraceptive, and anticonvulsant drugs. Serum methadone levels can be reduced by the concurrent use of carbamazepine, phenobarbitone, and phenytoin[66] and by rifampicin[67]. The oestrogen component of the oral contraceptive has been shown to double the clearance of morphine by induction of glucuronyl transferase, suggesting the need for increased doses in patients on oestrogens[68]. The plasma clearance of dexamethasone can be trebled in patients receiving concurrent phenytoin, phenobarbitone, or rifampicin, and presumably other enzyme inducers, leading to a reduced bioavailability and shortened half-life[69]. This may be important clinically in the care of patients with malignancy.

Our understanding of the process of inhibition of the mixed function oxidase system by drugs increased dramatically with the identification of the subfamilies of cytochrome P450. Previously, there was no explanation as to why one drug might reduce the clearance of a second but not that of a third. It is now clear that some drugs inhibit specific sub-families whilst others, such as cimetidine, are capable of inhibiting all forms of cytochrome P450; this is why cimetidine causes interactions with so many other agents. Cimetidine has been reported to precipitate apnoea in patients taking methadone[70] and to have had a similar effect in a patient taking morphine[71]; however, others have found only a small and insignificant effect on morphine kinetics[72]. Other H_2 receptor blocking drugs have no enzyme inhibitory effect and the proton pump inhibitor omeprazole has a modest and rather unpredictable effect.

Clomipramine and amitriptyline increase the bioavailability and reduce the clearance of morphine and enhance the analgesic effect. The mechanism seems to be both kinetic, through enzyme inhibition, and pharmacodynamic, through the antidepressants' analgesic effects[73]. Enzyme inhibition tends to occur rapidly, so the full effect is seen after four or five of the newly prolonged half-lives. The list of drugs that cause interaction through enzyme inhibition is long but non-steroidal anti-inflammatory drugs, especially azapropazone[74], and some of the opioid analgesics, such as dextropropoxyphene[75], and tramadol[76], are implicated.

Interactions between drugs and foods due to hepatic enzyme induction and inhibition are now recognized. Flavonoids in cabbage and broccoli, for example, may induce some cytochrome P450 sub-families whereas a component of grapefruit juice can inhibit them. These interactions may reach clinical significance when large quantities of these products are taken.

The most important drug interactions in the kidney involve competition between agents for active tubular secretion. Active tubular secretion is used by organic acids, and the most frequent interactions are caused by the loop diuretics and some non-steroidal anti-inflammatory drugs. The renal excretion of methotrexate may be inhibited by some non-steroidal anti-inflammatory drugs through this mechanism[77]. Although renal excretion of some drugs is pH dependent, in general this has minor implications in normal therapeutics. There are a few exceptions; for example, methadone's renal clearance is considerably enhanced by concurrent use of urinary acidifiers such as acetazolamide[78]. Whilst acetazolamide is used rarely now, this interaction may be relevant with other carbonic anhydrase inhibitors, although it has not been reported.

In palliative medicine, the most important pharmacodynamic interactions involve intracerebral mechanisms. Drugs that cause sedation also have the potential to cause confusion. Not only will the effects of central nervous system depressants be additive, but if the ionic or metabolic environment is deranged by other drugs, such as diuretics, the problem may be compounded. For example, phenothiazines increase the risk of respiratory depression, sedation, and hypotension[79].

Polypharmacy

Polypharmacy is endemic in palliative medicine. A survey of 385 patients three weeks after referral to a palliative care service found that the median number of drugs per patient was five, with a maximum of 11[80]. These numbers are similar to those reported in other elderly patient populations, particularly those admitted to hospital with drug-induced illness[81]. There are several causes of polypharmacy[82]. Patients with advanced cancer invariably suffer several symptoms, many of which will be amenable to drug therapy. These symptoms may justify the use of combinations of drugs, which may lead to polypharmacy, even in leading specialist centres[80]. The overriding principle should be to avoid unnecessary duplicate prescribing and to be aware of the potential consequences of multiple drug use. Clearly, the more drugs employed at any one time the greater the likelihood of drug interaction. Sometimes, such interactions will be unpredictable, but often the adverse consequences of polypharmacy are both predictable and avoidable. The increasing availability of clinical guidelines and drug formularies should improve prescribing habits and encourage the use of the most simple effective regimens possible.

The adverse effects of one symptomatic remedy may be self-limiting, both in terms of severity and duration, so that any additional treatment introduced to deal with these adverse effects should be reviewed and stopped if possible. Nausea associated with morphine, for example, is usually an initiation side effect, if it occurs at all, and may need specific treatment only for a few days. Trials of therapy for specific symptoms should be encouraged and the treatment changed if it is ineffective rather than being continued in conjunction with a new drug.

Apart from avoiding duplicate prescribing of similar drugs, other important principles of good practice should reduce the tendency towards polypharmacy. The drug regimen should be reviewed regularly and potentially redundant treatments identified. Both patient and physician may need to be persuaded of the benefit of stopping drugs. These conversations can be difficult, since suggesting drugs taken to reduce long-term harm could be stopped requires the physician to talk about the patient's shortened prognosis.

Use of drugs for unlicensed indications

Legislation regarding the manufacture, marketing, and medical use of therapeutic drugs varies throughout the world. Pharmaceutical companies can only market drugs that have an appropriate marketing authorization or product licence. The conditions for licensed use of a drug will be laid out in the Summary of Product Characteristics, such as indications for use, patient populations, formulations, and dosages of the drug. In contrast, doctors are permitted to prescribe

Table 8.2 Factors associated with adherence to drug treatment.

Patient-related factors:
- Personality
- Health care beliefs
  - General
  - Drug therapy
- Physical impairment
- Cognitive impairment
- Social support mechanisms
- Impact of disease or symptom

Drug-related factors:
- Efficacy of drug
- Tolerability of drug
- Drug regimen
  - Formulation
  - Dose
  - Frequency
  - Duration of treatment
- Concomitant drug treatment

Prescriber-related factors:
- Information supplied
- Monitoring provided
- Prescriber–patient relationship

drugs beyond these specific criteria. This practice is known as 'unlicensed', 'off licence', or 'off label' use.

Unlicensed use of drugs is common in palliative medicine and in other fragile populations, such as children and the elderly, because the clinical research necessary for licensing is difficult to perform in these patients. In observational studies from two inpatient palliative care units in the United Kingdom about 15 per cent of all prescribed drugs were being used for an unlicensed indication[1], and 12 per cent of all prescribed drugs were being given via an unlicensed route, i.e. subcutaneously[2]. Indeed, a more recent study reports that 40 per cent of all medication prescribed for the five most common symptoms in one unit was unlicensed, and that staff were often unaware they were prescribing outside the product licence[83].

The use of unlicensed drugs has implications for clinical governance and medical litigation. Thus, the decision to use an unlicensed drug should be influenced by the:

◆ risk:benefit ratio for the patient;

◆ strength of evidence for the use of the drug;

◆ availability of alternative pharmacological therapies;

◆ availability of alternative non-pharmacological therapies;

◆ practice of other palliative medicine physicians.

It has been recommended that consent should be obtained before starting the drug, that the reasons for prescribing the drug are recorded in the clinical notes, and that these reasons are conveyed to other members of the health-care team[84]. It is important to stress, however, that prescribing of drugs off label is not poor practice or 'experimental'; the reasons no licence will have been obtained for the use of the drug in the given population will therefore need to be explained. However, a recent questionnaire survey suggested 69 per cent of paediatricians would not seek informed consent for the unlicensed use of a drug in a child[85], and it is still not routine practice to obtain consent before starting an unlicensed drug in palliative care in the United Kingdom[86]. The reasons given for this include the impracticality of obtaining consent, the potential impact on compliance, and the possibility of causing distress to patients and carers. In clinical practice there seems to be a preference for not burdening patients, carers, or parents with the information, or informing them that a drug is being used off label, rather than seeking informed consent.

Sources of drug information

There are a large number of different sources of information on the drugs used in palliative medicine, including journals, textbooks, national pharmacopoeias, drug information units, drug regulatory authorities, and pharmaceutical companies. Many sources of information are generic in nature, and provide limited information specifically about the uses of drugs in palliative medicine. However, some sources are particular to palliative medicine, such as the Palliative Care Formulary[87] and the Hospice and Palliative Care Formulary, USA. The UK Palliative Care Formulary is modelled on the British National Formulary and provides similar information such as formulations, cautions and side effects, with additional information about the uses of the drug in palliative medicine.

An increasingly important source of information is the Internet. The Internet has a number of advantages, especially ease of access, but also a number of disadvantages, particularly the lack of peer review of information[88]. The Health On the Net Foundation (http://www.hon.ch/) was set up in response to the latter problem. It provides impartial information about the quality of health-care websites; it also produces a voluntary code of conduct for the developers of health-care websites. Table 8.3 gives a list of some useful drug resources on the Internet. These websites are maintained by respected organizations, are freely accessible to health-care professionals, and have links to other relevant websites.

Clinical pharmacists can also be useful sources of drug information. A study from Australia reported that a clinical pharmacist identified potential problems with the drug regimen of 13 per cent of hospice inpatients, and that changes in the drug regimen resulted in improvements in care in the majority of instances[89]. The problems identified included inappropriate drug dose or frequency, and potential drug interactions; the problems were predominantly related to drugs being used for general medical, rather than for palliative care, indications.

Conclusions

The skilful use of drugs to palliate symptoms is essential to the practice of palliative medicine. Individualization of drug and dose and simplicity are fundamental whatever type of treatment is being prescribed. An understanding of the principles outlined in this chapter should facilitate day-to-day management of clinical problems, improve the risk:benefit ratio of drugs used in symptom control,

Table 8.3 Selected Internet sources of drug information.

Website address	Website content
http://www.bnf.org/	British National Formulary online
http://www.usp.org/USPNF/	The United States Pharmacopeia: National Formulary; public pharmacopoeial standards
http://www.allaboutmedicalsales.com/search/electronic_medicines_compendium.html	The UK electronic Medicines Compendium (eMC) provides electronic Summaries of Product Characteristics (SPCs) and Patient Information Leaflets (PILs)
http://www.palliativedrugs.com/	UK Palliative Care Formulary online
http://www.pallcare.info/	Palliative Care Matters: a generic UK website with syringe driver drug compatibility database
http://nccam.nih.gov/	National Center for Complementary and Alternative Medicine, National Institute of Health, USA.

and ultimately contribute to improving the quality of life of patients with advanced disease.

References

1. Atkinson, C.V. and Kirkham, S.R. (1999). Unlicensed uses for medication in a palliative care unit. *Palliative Medicine,* **13,** 145–52.

2. Todd, J. and Davies, A. (1999). Use of unlicensed medication in palliative medicine. *Palliative Medicine,* **13,** 446.

3. Ettinger, D.S., Vitale, P.J., and Trump, D.L. (1979). Important clinical pharmacologic considerations in the use of methadone in cancer patients. *Cancer Treatment Reports,* **63,** 457–9.

4. Bullingham, R.E.S., McQuay, H., Dwyer, D. *et al.* (1981). Sublingual buprenorphine used post-operatively: clinical observations and preliminary pharmacokinetic analysis. *British Journal of Clinical Pharmacology,* **12,** 117–22.

5. Collin, E., Poulain., Gauvain-Piquard, A., Petit, G., Pichard-Leandri, E. (1993). Is disease progression the major factor in morphine 'tolerance' in cancer pain treatment? *Pain,* **55,** 319–26.

6. Fallon, M. (1997). Opioid rotation: does it have a role? *Palliative Medicine,* **11,** 177–8.

7. Littleton, J. (1997). Drug dependence and drugs of abuse. In *Integrated Pharmacology* (eds. C.P. Page, M.J. Curtis, M.C. Sutter, *et al.*), pp. 539–51. London: Mosby.

8. Kanner, R.M. and Foley, K. (1981). Patterns of narcotic use in a cancer pain clinic. *Annals of New York Academy of Science,* **362,** 161–72.

9. Standing Medical Advisory Committee Sub-Group on Antimicrobial Resistance. (1998). *The Path of Least Resistance,* London: Department of Health.

10. Ali, S., Sykes, N., Flock, P. *et al.* (2005). An investigation of MRSA infection in a hospice. *Palliative Medicine,* **19,** 188–96.

11. Prentice, W., Dunlop, R., Armes, P.J. *et al.* (1998). Methicillin resistant *Staphylococcus aureus* infection in palliative care. *Palliative Medicine,* **12,** 443–9.

12. Souhami, R.L., Tannock, I., Hohenberger, P. *et al.* (eds.) (2002). *Oxford Textbook of Oncology,* 2nd edition. Oxford: Oxford University Press.

13. Savarese, J., Goldenheim, P.D., Thomas, G.B. *et al.* (1986). Steady-state pharmacokinetics of controlled release oral morphine sulphate in healthy subjects. *Clinical Pharmacokinetics,* **11,** 505–10.

14. Hanks, G.W., Nugent, M., Higgs, C.M. *et al.* OTFC Multicentre Study Group. (2004). Oral transmucosal fentanyl citrate in the management of breakthrough pain in cancer: an open, multicentre, dose-titration and long-term use study. *Palliative Medicine,* **18,** 698–704.

15. Portenoy, R.K., Taylor, D., Messina, J. *et al.* (2006). A randomised, placebo-controlled study of fentanyl buccal tablet for breakthrough pain in opioid-treated patients with cancer. *Clinical Journal of Pain,* **22,** 805–11.

16. Scott, R.C., Besag, F.M., Neville, B.G. (1999). Buccal midazolam and rectal diazepam for treatment of prolonged seizures in childhood and adolescence: a randomised trial. *Lancet,* **353,** 623–6.

17. Gilbar, P.J. (1999). A guide to enteral drug administration in palliative care. *Journal of Pain and Symptom Management,* **17,** 197–207.

18. Warren, D.E. (1996). Practical use of rectal medications in palliative care. *Journal of Pain and Symptom Management,* **11,** 378–87.

19. Wilcock, A., Jacob, J.K., Charlesworth, S. *et al.* (2006). Drugs given by a syringe driver: a prospective multicentre survey of palliative care services in the UK. *Palliative Medicine,* **20,** 661–64.

20. Grassby, P.F. and Hutchings, L. (1997). Drug combinations in syringe drivers: the compatibility and stability of diamorphine with cyclizine and haloperidol. *Palliative Medicine,* **11,** 217–24.

21. Krajnik, M., Zylicz, Z., Finlay, I. *et al.* (1999). Potential use of opioids in palliative care – report of 6 cases. *Pain,* **80,** 121–5.

22. Klepstad, P., Kaasa, S., Cherny, N. *et al.* and the Research Steering Committee of the EAPC. (2005). Pain and pain treatments in European palliative care units. A cross sectional survey from the European Association for Palliative Care Research Network. *Palliative Medicine,* **19,** 477–84.

23. Cates, C.J., Crilly, J.A., and Rowe, B.H. (2006). Holding chambers (spacers) versus nebulisers for beta-agonist treatment of acute asthma. *Cochrane Database of Systematic Reviews,* **19,** CD000052.

24. Zepetella, G. (2000). An assessment of the safety, efficacy, and acceptability of intranasal fentanyl citrate in the management of cancer-related breakthrough pain: a pilot study. *Journal of Pain and Symptom Management,* **20,** 253–8.

25. Borland, M., Jacobs, I., King, B. *et al.* (2007). A randomized controlled trial comparing intranasal fentanyl to intravenous morphine for managing acute pain in children in the emergency department. *Annals of Emergency Medicine,* **49,** 335–40.

26. Kendall, J.M., Reeves, B.C., Latter, V.S. Nasal Diamorphine Trial Group. (2001). Multicentre randomised controlled trial of nasal diamorphine for analgesia in children and teenagers with clinical fractures. *British Medical Journal,* **322,** 261–5.

27. Amesbury, B., O'Riordan, J., and Dolin, S. (1999). The use of intrapleural analgesia using bupivicaine for pain relief in advanced cancer. *Palliative Medicine,* **13,** 153–8.

28. Shabat, S., Stern, A., Kollender, Y. *et al.* (2001). Continous intra-articular patient-controlled analgesia in a cancer patient with pathological hip fracture. A case report. *Acta Orthopaedica Belgica,* **67,** 304–6.

29. Wang, M.Y., Teitelbaum, G.P., Loskota, W.J. *et al.* (2000). Brachial plexus catheter reservoir for the treatment of upper-extremity cancer pain: a technical case report. *Neurosurgery,* **46,** 1009–12.

30. Evans, D.A.P., Manley, K.A., and McKusick, V.A. (1960). Genetic control of isoniazid metabolism in man. *British Medical Journal,* **2,** 485–91.

31. Sim, E. and Hickman, D. (1991). Polymorphism in human N-acetyltransferase - the case for the missing allele. *Trends In Pharmacological Science,* **12,** 1211–13.

32. Ellard, G.A. and Gammon, P.T. (1977). Acetylator phenotyping of tuberculosis patients using matrix isoniazid on sulphadimidine and its prognostic significance for treatment with several intermittent isoniazid-containing regimens. *British Journal of Clinical Pharmacology,* **4,** 5–14.

33. Lunde, P.K.M., Frislid, K., Hansteen, V. (1977). Disease and acetylation polymorphism. *Clinical Pharmacokinetics,* **2,** 182.

34. Vesell, E.S. Pharmacogenetics. (1975). *Biochemical Pharmacology,* **24,** 445–50.

35. Steiner, E., Iselius, L., Alvan, G. *et al.* (1985). A family study of genetic and environmental factors determining polymorphic hydroxylation of debrisoquine in man. *Clinical Pharmacology and Therapeutics,* **38,** 394–401.

36. Eichelbaum, M. and Gross, A.S. (1990). The genetic polymorphism of debrisoquine/sparteine metabolism - clinical aspects. *Clinical Pharmacology and Therapeutics,* **46,** 377–94.

37. Gonzalez, F.J. and Meyer, U.A. (1991). Molecular genetics of the debrisoquine/sparteine polymorphism. *Clinical Pharmacology and Therapeutics,* **50,** 233–8.

38. Chen, Z.R., Somogyi, A.A., Reynolds, G. *et al.* (1991). Disposition and metabolism of codeine after single and chronic doses in one poor and seven extensive metabolisers. *British Journal of Clinical Pharmacology,* **31,** 381–390.

39. Gibson, G.G. and Skett, P. (1994). *Introduction to Drug Metabolism.* 2nd edition. Glasgow: Blackie Academic and Professional.

40. De Fazio, S., Gallelli, L., De Siena, A. *et al.* (2008). Role of CYP3A5 in abnormal clearance of methadone. *Annals of Pharmacotherapy,* **42,** 893–7.

41. Klepstad, P., Rakvag, T.T., Kaasa, S. *et al.* (2004). The 118 A > G polymorphism in the human mu-opioid receptor gene may increase

morphine requirements in patients with pain caused by malignant disease. *Acta Anaesthesiologica Scandinavica*, **48**, 1232–1239.

42. Rakvag, T.T., Klepstad, P., Baar, C. *et al.* (2005). The Val158Met polymorphism of the human catechol-O-methyltransferase (COMT) gene may influence morphine requirements in cancer pain patients. *Pain*, **116**, 73–78.

43. Anonymous. (1999). Pharmacogenetics. In *A Textbook of Clinical Pharmacology* (eds. J.M.Ritter, L.D. Lewis and T.G.K. Mant), 4th edition, pp. 108–18. London: Arnold.

44. Kotb, H.I., El-Kady, S.A., Emara, S.E. *et al.* (2005). Pharmacokinetics of controlled release morphine (MST) in patients with liver carcinoma. *British Journal of Anaesthesia*, **94**, 95–9.

45. Kotb, H.I., Fouad, I.A., Fares, K.M. *et al.* (2008). Pharmacokinetics of tramadol in patients with liver cancer. *Journal of Opioid Management*, **4**, 99–104.

46. Pond, S.M., Tong, T., Benowitz, N.L. *et al.* (1980). Enhanced bioavailability of pethidine and pentazocine in patients with cirrhosis of the liver. *Australian and New Zealand Journal of Medicine*, **10**, 515.

47. Pentikainen, P.J., Neuvonen, P.J., and Jostell, K.G. (1980). Pharmacokinetics of chlormethiazole in healthy volunteers and patients with cirrhosis of the liver. *European Journal of Pharmacology*, **17**, 275.

48. Inturrusi, C.E. and Verebely, K. (1972). Disposition of methadone in man after a single oral dose. *Clinical Pharmacology and Therapeutics*, **13**, 923–30.

49. Bateman, D.N. (1983). Clinical pharmacokinetics of metoclopramide. *Clinical Pharmacokinetics*, **8**, 523–9.

50. Morgan, D.J. and McLean, A.J. (1995). Clinical pharmacokinetic and pharmacodynamic considerations in patients with liver disease. *Clinical Pharmacokinetics*, **29**, 370–91.

51. Homeida, M., Jackson, L., and Roberts, C.J.C. (1978). Decreased first pass metabolism of labetalol in chronic liver disease. *British Medical Journal*, **2**, 1048.

52. Robertz-Vaupel, G.M., Lindecken, K.D., Edeki, T. *et al.* (1992). Disposition of antipyrine inpatients with extensive metastatic liver disease. *European Journal of Clinical Pharmacology*, **42**, 465–9.

53. Guengerich, F.P. and Turvy, C.G. (1991). Comparison of levels of several human microsomal cytochrome P450 enzymes and epoxide hydrolase in normal and disease states using immunochemical analysis of surgical liver samples. *Journal of Pharmacology and Experimental Therapeutics*, **256**, 1189–91.

54. Murray, M. (1992). P450 enzymes: inhibition mechanisms, genetic regulation and effects of liver disease. *Clinical Pharmacokinetics*, **23**, 132–46.

55. Swift, C.G., Homeida, M., Halliwell, M. *et al.* (1985). Antipyrine disposition and liver size in the elderly. *European Journal of Clinical Pharmacology*, **20**, 119–28.

56. Durnas, C., Loi, C.M., and Cusack, B.J. (1990). Hepatic drug metabolism and aging. *Clinical Pharmacokinetics*, **19**, 359–89.

57. Vestal, R.E., Norris, A.H., Tobin, J.D. *et al.* (1975). Antipyrine metabolism in man: influence of age, alcohol, caffeine and smoking. *Clinical Pharmacology and Therapeutics*, **18**, 425–32.

58. Feely, J., Pareira, I., Guy, E. *et al.* (1984). Factors affecting the response to inhibition of drug metabolism by cimetidine - dose response and sensitivity of elderly and induced subjects. *British Journal of Clinical Pharmacology*, **17**, 77–81.

59. Salem, S.A.M., Rajjayabun, P., Shepherd, A.M.M. *et al.* (1978). Reduced induction of drug metabolism in the elderly. *Age and Ageing*, **7**, 68–73.

60. Pearson, M.W. and Roberts, C.J.C. (1984). Drug induction of hepatic enzymes in the elderly. *Age and Ageing*, **13**, 313–16.

61. Nimmo, J., Heading, R.C., Tothill, P., *et al.* (1973). Pharmacological modification of gastric emptying: effects of propantheline and metoclopramide on paracetamol absorption. *British Medical Journal*, **1**, 587–9.

62. Nimmo, W.S., Heading, R.C., Wilson, J. *et al.* (1975). Inhibition of gastric emptying and drug absorption by narcotic analgesics. *British Journal of Clinical Pharmacology*, **2**, 509–13.

63. Gourlay, G.K., Plummer, J.L., Cherry, D.A. *et al.* (1989). Influence of a high fat meal on the absorption of morphine from oral solutions. *Clinical Pharmacology and Therapeutics*, **46**, 463–8.

64. Manara, A.R., Shelley, M.P., Quinn, K. *et al.* (1988). The effect of metoclopramide on the absorption of oral controlled release morphine. *British Journal of Clinical Pharmacology*, **25**, 518–21.

65. Kristensen, M.B. (1983). Drug interaction and clinical pharmacokinetics. In *Handbook of Clinical Pharmacokinetics*. (eds. M. Gibaldi and L. Prescott), pp. 242–64. Auckland: ADIS Health Science Press.

66. Bell, J., Seves, V., Bowren, P. *et al.* (1988). The use of serum methadone levels in patients receiving methadone maintenance. *Clinical Pharmacology and Therapeutics*, **43**, 623–9.

67. Bending, M.R. and Skacel, P.O. (1977). Rifampicin and methadone withdrawal. *Lancet*, **1**, 1211.

68. Watson, K.J.R., Ghabrial, H., Mashford, M.L. *et al.* (1986). The oral contraceptive pill increases morphine clearance but does not increase hepatic blood flow. *Gastroenterology*, **90**, 1779.

69. Anonymous. (1991). Dexamethasone. In *Therapeutic Drugs* (eds. C. Dollery, A.R. Boobis, D. Burley *et al.*), pp. D44–50. Edinburgh: Churchill Livingstone.

70. Dawson, G.W. and Vestal, R.E. (1984). Cimetidine inhibits the *in vitro* N-demethylation of methadone. *Research Communications in Chemical Pathology and Pharmacology*, **46**, 301–4.

71. Fine, A. and Churchill, D.N. Potential lethal interaction of cimetidine and morphine. (1981). *Canadian Medical Association Journal*, **124**, 1434.

72. Lam, A.M. and Clement, J.L. (1984). Effect of cimetidine pre-medication on morphine-induced ventilatory depression. *Canadian Anaesthetic Society Journal*, **31**, 36–43.

73. Ventafridda, V., Ripamonti, C., De Conno, F. *et al.* (1987). Antidepressants increase bioavailability of morphine in cancer patients. *Lancet*, **1**, 1204.

74. Roberts, C.J.C., Daneshmend, T.K., Macfarlane, D. *et al.* (1981). Anti-convulsant intoxication precipitated by azapropazone. *Postgraduate Medical Journal*, **57**, 191.

75. Orme, M. and Breckenridge, A. (1976). Warfarin and distalgesic interaction. *British Medical Journal*, **1**, 200.

76. Adverse Drug Reactions Advisory Committee (ADRAC), Australia. (2004). Tramadol-warfarin interaction. *ADRAC Bulletin*, **23**(4).

77. Daly, H.M., Scott, G.L., Boyle, J. *et al.* (1986). Methotrexate toxicity precipitated by azapropazone. *British Journal of Dermatology*, **114**, 733–5.

78. Bellward, G.D., Warren, D.M., Howald, W. *et al.* (1977). Methadone maintenance: effect of urinary pH on renal clearance in chronic high and low doses. *Clinical Pharmacology and Therapeutics*, **22**, 92–9.

79. Grothe, D.R., Ereshefsky, L., Jann, M.W. *et al.* (1986). Clinical implication of the neuroleptic–opioid interaction. *Drug Intelligence in Clinical Pharmacology*, **20**, 75–7.

80. Twycross, R.G., Bergl, S., John, S. *et al.* (1994). Monitoring drug use in palliative care. *Palliative Medicine*, **8**, 137–43.

81. Colt, A.G. and Shapiro, A.P. (1989). Drug induced illness as a cause for admission to a community hospital. *Journal of the American Geriatric Society*, **37**, 323–6.

82. Kroenke, K. (1985). Polypharmacy. Causes, consequences, and cure. *The American Journal of Medicine*, **79**, 149–52.

83. Verhagen, C.C., Niezink, A.G., Engels, Y.Y. *et al.* (2008). Off-label use of drugs in pain medicine and palliative care: an algorithm for the assessment of its safe and legal prescription. *Pain Practice*, **8**, 157–163.

84. Ferner, R.E. (1996). Prescribing licensed medicines for unlicensed indications. *Prescribers' Journal,* **36,** 73–8.

85. McLay, J.S., Tanaka, M., Ekins-Daukes, S. *et al.* (2006). A prospective questionnaire assessment of attitudes and experiences of off label prescribing among hospital based paediatricians. *Archives of Disease in Childhood,* **91,** 584–7.

86. Pavis, H. and Wilcock, A. (2001). Prescribing of drugs for use outside their licence in palliative care: survey of specialists in the United Kingdom. *British Medical Journal,* **323,** 484–5.

87. Twycross, R., Wilcock, A., Charlesworth, S. *et al.* (2002). *Palliative Care Formulary,* 2nd edition. Oxford: Radcliffe Medical Press.

88. Pereira, J. and Bruera, E. (1998). The Internet as a resource for palliative care and hospice: a review and proposals. *Journal of Pain and Symptom Management,* **16,** 59–68.

89. Lucas, C., Glare, P.A., and Sykes, J.V. (1997). Contribution of a liaison clinical pharmacist to an inpatient palliative care unit. *Palliative Medicine,* **11,** 209–16.

SECTION 9

Disease-modifying management in advanced cancer

The medical treatment of cancer in palliative care

Malcolm McIllmurray

The optimal management of cancer requires a multi-disciplinary team approach in which palliative care physicians and surgical, radiation, and medical oncologists play an important part. Patients may experience physical, emotional, psychological, and spiritual distress at any time during the course of the illness and involving palliative care physicians from diagnosis ensures that patients are referred for specialist palliative care when they need it. However, so that they are fully integrated members of the multi-disciplinary team, palliative care physicians should understand the respective roles of the oncologists on the team and know about the cancers that they treat and the expectations and side effects of their treatments. In addition, this knowledge should ensure that palliative care physicians are able to recognize patients in their care who might benefit from cancer treatment and refer them to an appropriate oncologist.

This chapter describes the medical treatment of cancer, which is provided by the medical oncologist in the multi-disciplinary team. In some countries, this role is shared between medical and radiation oncologists. Emphasis is placed on the treatment of advanced and incurable cancer, because palliative care physicians are more likely to be involved in that clinical setting, although patients with early and curable cancer may also need their expertise.

Background

Cancer is a disease which is derived from the mutation of a single cell. The mutation is the result of defects in the genes associated with the cell cycle and the cell signalling pathways, which control cell replication and cell death. The defects can be inherited, occur by chance, or be acquired by exposure to certain viruses or carcinogens. The mutated cell (the cancer phenotype) has various characteristics, which include the ability:

- to avoid apoptosis (programmed cell death);
- to resist the normal ageing process;
- to replicate outside normal controlling mechanisms;
- to produce chemicals, which dissolve surrounding connective tissue (matrix metalloproteinases);
- to stimulate a microvascular blood supply (angiogenesis);

- to invade and disseminate to other parts of the body (metastatic spread);
- to overcome or paralyse the immune system.

Cell signalling pathways begin with cell surface receptors which, when activated, initiate the cascade of molecular events that transfer instructions from outside the cell to the cell nucleus. Over-expression of the receptors that are activated by growth factors and which instruct the cell to divide, is also a feature of the cancer phenotype.

An understanding of the relationship between a cancer cell and its environment and of the cellular changes that produce these various biological effects has given rise to the treatment of some cancers with hormones or hormone-blocking drugs (hormone therapy) and with other receptor or protein-modifying agents (biological therapy). However, the gold standard for the medical treatment of cancer is the use of cytotoxic drugs (chemotherapy) whose effects do not depend on the genetic differences that distinguish cancer cells from their normal counterparts. This chapter considers the use of these three types of treatment in a palliative care setting and gives the reader an understanding of the principles that underlie their use. Prescribing details are omitted because this is the responsibility of the oncologist and not the palliative care physician.

Chemotherapy in palliative care

The mode of action of cytotoxic drugs

Cells divide in an orderly sequence known as the cell cycle (Fig. 9.1.1) in which DNA synthesis (S phase) is followed by mitosis (M phase) with gaps between these two events (G1 and G2), during which DNA copy defects are identified and corrected or the cell is programmed to die. Cells can leave the cell cycle and remain in a resting phase (G0) until they re-enter the cycle in response to an appropriate stimulus.

Cytotoxic drugs target cells during cell division in the cell cycle. However, some drugs only kill cells if they happen to be in a particular phase of the cycle when the drug is administered (phase-specific drugs). Prolonging the time during which a cancer is exposed to a phase-specific drug will increase the number of cells

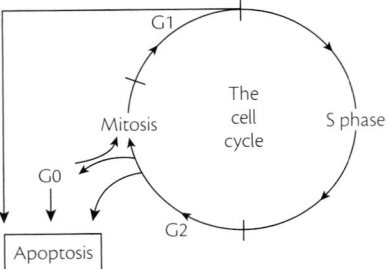

Figure 9.1.1 The cell cycle.

killed because dividing cells cycle at random and all dividing cells must pass through that phase of the cycle for maximum cytotoxic effect. Other drugs kill cells in cycle in whatever phase of division the cells have reached when the drug is administered (cycle-specific drugs), and the number of cells killed is related to the administered dose of the drug rather than the exposure time. The distinction between phase-specific and cycle-specific drugs is useful when it comes to selecting drugs and doses for combination regimens because, for example, it makes sense to avoid administering two drugs together which are specific for the same phase of the cell cycle; and when two cycle-specific drugs are administered together, the doses of each must be reduced to avoid severe toxic side effects.

Cytotoxic drugs can also be classified according to their pharmacological effects on the biological events which take place during the cell cycle as follows:

Antimetabolites interfere with the incorporation of nucleic acid bases into the DNA molecule. Their activity is greatest in the S phase of the cell cycle. Examples are 5-fluorouracil, fludarabine, methotrexate, and gemcitabine.

Alkylating drugs typically form linkages between the strands of DNA, which prevent them from separating during the M phase of the cell cycle but they also have other biochemical effects and are cycle-specific rather than phase-specific. Examples are cyclophosphamide, ifosfamide, chlorambucil, and melphalan. Other drugs with alkylating activity include the platinum compounds, cisplatin and carboplatin.

Antitumour antibiotics act through a number of different mechanisms but typically interfere with the binding of base pair molecules and prevent the separation of the DNA strands during the M phase of the cell cycle. Some drugs are phase-specific such as bleomycin and others are cycle-specific such as doxorubicin and epirubicin.

Plant alkaloids are derived from natural sources. They are phase-specific and are either mitotic spindle inhibitors such as vincristine, vinblastine, and the taxanes, paclitaxel and docetaxel, or topoisomerase inhibitors such as topotecan, irinotecan, and etoposide.

The effect of cytotoxic drugs on cancer cells

The factors that determine the greater damage inflicted by cytotoxic drugs on cancer tissues compared to normal tissues are related to two important observations. Firstly, the proportionate cell kill following treatment is generally greater in cancer tissues than in normal tissues because cytotoxic drugs only effect dividing cells and the proportion of dividing cells (the growth fraction) is generally higher in cancer tissues than in normal tissues. Secondly, after

cytotoxic damage, the processes of repair are more efficient in normal tissues than in cancer tissues. Therefore, if treatment is given intermittently and the time between treatments is just enough to allow normal tissues to recover, there is a gradual reduction in the population of cancer cells, whilst the normal cell population is maintained. In theory it should be possible to eliminate all cancer cells if treatment is continued for long enough but, in practice it is rare for cancers to be cured in this way. As cancers grow they outstrip their own blood supply, which reduces drug penetration and they contain an increasing number of mutant cell lines, some of which are sensitive to cytotoxic drugs and others which are not. The continued growth of resistant cell lines means that most cancers cannot be cured by chemotherapy alone (Table 9.1.1).

The principles that govern the use of chemotherapy in cancers are based on these pharmacokinetic and biological observations. Thus, chemotherapy is most effective when the cancer load is small and the growth fraction is high and when cytotoxic drugs with different modes of action are given together (combination chemotherapy). The drugs used in combination should be prescribed at their optimum dose and schedule and drugs should be selected with different toxicity profiles to allow as wide a range of dose as possible.

Table 9.1.1 Response of cancers to chemotherapy and hormone therapy.

Cancers that can be cured by chemotherapy (including patients with advanced disease)	
Germ cell	Hodgkin's lymphoma
Chorioncarcinoma	Acute lymphoblastic leukaemia
Non-Hodgkin lymphoma (high-grade)	

Cancers that can be cured by induction [a] or adjuvant chemotherapy [b] and/or hormone therapy [c]	
Breast [a,b,c]	Colon [b]
Non-small-cell lung (local advanced)	Osteosarcoma [b]

Cancers in which survival may be prolonged by chemotherapy [a] and/or hormone therapy [b] in patients with advanced disease	
Breast [a,b]	Small-cell lung [a]
Non-Hodgkin lymphoma (low-grade) [a]	Bladder [a]
Colon [a]	Ovary [a]
Myeloma [a]	Rectum [a]
Prostate [b]	Endometrium [b]

Cancers that may respond to chemotherapy for advanced disease with little effect on survival but with possible quality-of-life benefits	
Non-small-cell lung	Pancreas
Cervix	Stomach
Melanoma	Glioma
Oesophagus	Head/neck
Mesothelioma	Prostate

Cancers that are resistant to chemotherapy	
Renal	Endometrium

A knowledge of the effectiveness of chemotherapy in each type of cancer and of the toxicity of chemotherapy is necessary to inform the discussion, which must take place between the patient and oncologist about the decision to treat.

The effectiveness of chemotherapy

The process whereby drugs move from the laboratory to clinical practice is painstakingly slow. Extensive animal testing establishes cytotoxic efficacy and safety and is followed by three phases of clinical trials involving patients. These are designed to determine the optimum dose and schedule and the toxicity profile of the drug (phase I trials), the response of different cancers to the drug (phase II trials), and the clinical benefits, either alone or in combination with other cytotoxic drugs in the cancers that respond (phase III trials). Informed consent for treatment is mandatory for all patients recruited into clinical trials.

Clinical decisions are based on the outcome of phase III trials. A phase III trial usually takes the form of a randomized controlled trial (RCT) in which the new drug, either alone or in combination, is compared to standard treatment, which may be supportive care only. Patients selected for RCTs must meet eligibility criteria, which are clearly defined so that both treatment groups are comparable. Stratification may be necessary to control for the patient and cancer characteristics that are known to affect the outcome. Differences between treatment groups are usually small, and large numbers of patients are needed to detect a significant effect of a new drug. Many phase III trials are not large enough to detect small differences, and it is necessary to combine the data from all published trials of a particular treatment for a particular cancer to obtain proof of effectiveness. This is called a meta-analysis and is a method of evaluating new drugs and combinations in common cancers.

The effectiveness of chemotherapy in treating patients with cancer is assessed by the effect it has on:

- The survival time from commencement of treatment.
- The time from commencement of treatment to cancer progression.
- The cancer response rate, which is the proportion of treated patients whose cancer either becomes undetectable (complete remission), or reduces in size by at least 50 per cent (partial remission), or stays the same size (stable disease), or continues to grow during treatment (progressive disease).
- The quality of life.

Quality-of-life measurements have become very important in the evaluation of cytotoxic drugs since it was shown that the quality of life of cancer patients can be improved by chemotherapy, despite the associated toxicity and without there necessarily being any improvement in survival time [1,2].

The toxicity of chemotherapy

The normal tissues that are most vulnerable to the effects of chemotherapy are those which are in a constant state of regeneration and repair. It can be predicted, therefore, that the commonest toxicities will arise from the effects on the bone-marrow, gastrointestinal tract, and skin. Other toxicities such as the effects on kidneys, nervous system, lungs, and heart are less predictable and much less common.

Bone-marrow. Erythrocytes, neutrophils, and platelets are produced by haemopoeitic stem cells in the bone-marrow. Their production rate is such that new cell formation keeps pace with cell losses and in the normal steady state about 5 per cent of stem cells are undergoing cell division (in cell cycle) at any one time. These dividing stem cells are vulnerable to the effects of cytotoxic drugs. A fall in the number of circulating neutrophils, which follows a course of chemotherapy, will take several days to appear because the life span of a mature neutrophil is about 10 days. For erythrocytes the period is much longer, about 120 days, and for platelets about 5 days. Low erythrocyte counts (anaemia) and low platelet counts (thrombocytopenia) can be corrected by transfusion but any benefit is short-lived. Fortunately, platelet transfusions are rarely necessary. However, blood transfusions are commonly used to relieve the fatigue associated with anaemia, which is a significant symptom in up to 80 per cent of patients on chemotherapy. Repeated transfusions expose the patient to the combined risks of infection and disease transmission, and this method of treatment is not satisfactory in the long term. Erythropoietin, the naturally-occurring erythrocyte stem-cell growth factor is equally effective in relieving fatigue, and the newer analogues such as darbepoietin alfa, which have a long half-life and therefore require less frequent administration, provide a more precise and practical way of correcting the anaemia that occurs in these patients. Published guidelines state that treatment should be initiated at a haemoglobin level of between 9 g/dl and 11 g/dl based on the severity of symptoms, and continued to maintain a level of between 12 g/dl and 13 g/dl in patients whose symptoms improve[3,4]. Questions remain about the cost-effectiveness of this treatment however, and there are concerns that survival may be reduced in some patients.

Whilst a low erythrocyte count may not be life-threatening, a low neutrophil count exposes a patient to the risks of serious and sometimes fatal infection. This is especially dangerous for there is no symptom that will alert a patient to a falling neutrophil count and it may only be brought to their attention when infection is established. Thus in any chemotherapy service, there must be clear instructions to patients about recognizing the symptoms and signs of infection and fast-tracking them through the health-care services, so that the combination of a low neutrophil count and a fever is identified and treated without delay. Such patients must be regarded as acute medical emergencies and they require immediate admission to hospital. After obtaining samples of body fluids and secretions for culture, treatment with broad-spectrum potent antibiotics given intravenously must be initiated and continued until positive specimen cultures suggest more specific treatment, or until the fever has abated and the body temperature has been normal for at least 48 h. If the fever persists and the neutrophil count remains low ($<1.5 \times 10^6$ per cubic mm), neutrophil recovery should be stimulated by the administration of a granulocyte stem-cell growth factor (GCSF), but this is not usually necessary. Recent studies have identified low-risk patients with a low neutrophil count and a fever in whom treatment with oral antibiotics may be as safe as conventional treatment[5].

Gastrointestinal tract. The mucosal lining of the gastrointestinal tract is being shed and replaced continuously, and the clinical effects of cytotoxic drugs on the mucosal stem cells in cycle is seen within days of treatment. These include nausea, vomiting, mucositis, and diarrhoea. There is considerable variation in the severity of these symptoms amongst individuals and amongst different cytotoxic drugs, but the symptoms can be so severe that admission to hospital may be necessary for parenteral hydration and alimentation.

There are other causes for the nausea and vomiting associated with cytotoxic drugs that involve 5HT3 and dopamine receptors found peripherally and in the central nervous system. Symptoms can occur acutely (within 24 h of chemotherapy) or be delayed (from 48 h onwards) and can be abolished or diminished by the administration of 5HT3 receptor-blocking drugs such as ondansetron and granisetron, an hour or so before chemotherapy is given, and orally for several days thereafter if necessary. Dexamethasone given orally or by intravenous injection has a similar antiemetic effect, and recent evidence suggests that it may be more effective. The combination of a 5HT3-blocking drug with dexamethasone appears to have important advantages over either given alone[6]. The mechanism of action of dexamethasone is not known. These drugs have largely replaced metoclopramide, a drug that blocks dopamine receptors in the medulla of the brain (and has a variety of other receptor effects). Although effective as an antiemetic, the doses needed were frequently associated with extrapyramidal side effects. Short-acting benzodiazepines, such as lorazepam, can be useful adjuncts to antiemetic therapy in patients where anxiety is a factor. With some cytotoxic drugs, their potential for causing vomiting is so low that no prophylactic treatment is necessary although it is a sensible precaution to give an oral antiemetic such as domperidone an hour or so before chemotherapy is given.

Delayed nausea and vomiting can be prevented by oral medication such as: domperidone, dexamethasone in reducing doses, and ondansetron taken by mouth for between 5 and 10 days depending on the severity of the symptoms. There may be a psychological component to these symptoms and the phenomenon of anticipatory vomiting where patients vomit at the thought of treatment or at the sight or smell of the hospital, is well described and can be alleviated by behavioural therapy such as hypnosis.

Diarrhoea as a toxic effect of cytotoxic drugs is rarely severe and is usually self-limiting. Preventative measures are not necessary and constipating drugs can be taken as required should it arise. There are exceptions however. For example, the diarrhoea from irinotecan, a cytotoxic drug commonly used in the treatment of colorectal cancer, can be so severe that serious dehydration is a real possibility. With sensible precautions, such as subcutaneous atropine with treatment and the use of potent constipating drugs if symptoms arise, treatment with irinotecan has become safe and manageable.

Mucositis, an inflammation of the mucous membranes of the mouth, tongue, pharynx, and sometimes extending into the oesophagus, can vary from slight redness to severe ulceration which can make eating and drinking impossible. The combination of severe mucositis and a low neutrophil count is dangerous because the inflamed mucous membrane can be a portal of entry for bacteria into the systemic circulation. Mucositis settles in time and the discomfort can be relieved by local anaesthetics such as benzydamine hydrochloride as a mouthwash or spray. If mucositis is severe and prolonged, patients may need admission to hospital and strong analgesics may be required until the symptoms have resolved. Oral and oesophageal candidiasis, which is common in these patients can be indistinguishable in appearance from drug-induced mucositis. It is prudent to culture the inflamed mucosa and treat with antifungal agents where there is doubt. Similarly, the herpes simplex virus can cause mucositis for which antiviral treatment can be prescribed.

Skin. Surprisingly, skin rashes are uncommon with cytotoxic drugs. Photosensitivity, urticaria, hyperpigmentation, and dermatitis have been described. The worst effects are those associated with the hair and nails. Hair thinning or total hair loss is predictable with certain drugs and it can be seen soon after the first course of chemotherapy. Various techniques for cooling the scalp have been developed to prevent hair loss but they are not wholly satisfactory and are not in general use. The hair loss is not permanent and hair can grow again before chemotherapy has been completed. The nail changes can result in horizontal ridges of the nails, each ridge marking a course of treatment, or in complete avulsion of the nail bed. There are no effective preventative measures and eventually these changes will grow out. The hand/foot syndrome is a curious skin reaction associated with 5-fluorouracil and its orally administered precursor, capecitabine, especially with treatment by continuous infusion. It is a painful, erythematous desquamation with fissuring of the palms of the hands and soles of the feet, which recovers if the drug is withdrawn.

Kidneys. Renal damage from cytotoxic drugs is most often associated with the platinum derivatives particularly cisplatin. This is a dose-related effect and because the blood level is itself related to renal function; it is essential that renal function is determined before each course of chemotherapy is prescribed and an adjustment made to the dose as appropriate. Drugs that cause renal toxicity should not be administered unless the creatinine clearance is greater than 40 ml per min. Toxic damage can be permanent.

Nervous system. An altered mental state has been associated with methotrexate, ifosfamide and other cytotoxic drugs giving rise to confusion, depression, and drowsiness. Cerebellar disturbance can occur with 5-fluorouracil, and seizures have been described with vincristine, cisplatin and ifosfamide. A peripheral neuropathy is more common and can occur with the vinca alkaloids, platinum drugs, the taxanes, and etoposide. Symptoms include numbness and paresthesiae and if the autonomic nerves are involved, colicky abdominal pain and constipation. The platinum drugs in high doses cause nerve deafness but this is rarely seen at recommended dose levels. If it does occur recovery is slow and damage may be permanent.

Lungs. Cytotoxic drugs such as bleomycin, methotrexate, and cyclophosphamide are well-documented causes of lung toxicity. It is more likely with concomitant chest radiotherapy. Symptoms include cough and breathlessness and may occur acutely or be delayed for many years after treatment. The radiological changes in the lungs can be difficult to distinguish from pulmonary oedema, lymphangitis carcinomatosa, and infection. Trans-bronchial lung biopsy may be required to establish the diagnosis.

Heart. Cardiotoxicity is a feature of the anthracycline drugs, particularly the parent compound doxorubicin. At total cumulative doses not exceeding 450 mg/m^2 the incidence of cardiomyopathy is 2 per cent; this rises to 7 per cent at 550 mg/m^2, 15 per cent at 600 mg/m^2, and 40 per cent at 700 mg/m^2. The clinical features are those of congestive cardiac failure which typically appears 30 to 60 days after the last dose. The response to diuretic therapy, digoxin, and ACE inhibitors is disappointing, and patients may die. Cardiac ischaemia can be caused by 5-fluorouracil resulting in arrhythmias, angina, hypotension, and congestive cardiac failure. Patients at risk are the elderly with pre-existing cardiac disease and previous mediastinal radiotherapy.

A list of cytotoxic drugs commonly used in palliative chemotherapy schedules with common toxicities is shown in Table 9.1.2.

To treat or not to treat

The goal of palliative chemotherapy is cancer control, with the expectation of prolonged survival and improved quality of life including the relief or prevention of symptoms, rather than cure. It is preferable that patients participate in the treatment decision and chemotherapy should not be given without the patient's informed consent. Treatment decisions are based on a consideration of the balance between the benefits expected and the toxicity and risks of chemotherapy, which are different for each patient. Sometimes, improved quality of life is the only expected benefit and indication for treatment. Patients can share in the decision only if they are given the relevant information. The fear that imparting this information to patients with incurable cancer might leave them bereft and in a state of despair has proved unfounded[7,8]. Indeed, patients are eager for information and want to be involved in decisions about treatment[9]. They want to know the duration of treatment and the effect it may have on their working capacity and lifestyle, as well as information about their disease, the treatment options, the possible outcomes, and the toxicity of treatment.

The medical assessment of each patient should include a detailed history and examination with bidirectional measurements of any palpable masses. A histological diagnosis and staging investigations are essential. A blood count, and kidney and liver function tests are important baseline tests. Physical fitness is graded according to validated performance status scales as shown in Table 9.1.3. These are used for defining eligibility for clinical drug trials and for recording changes in physical fitness over time.

The decision to treat or not to treat is made when the oncologist can interpret these findings and place the patient's situation into a clinical context. The histological diagnosis and staging investigations will determine the chemotherapy options if any, which are based on response, survival and quality-of-life data from previous controlled clinical trials. Co-morbid conditions, blood tests, age, and performance status may affect the decision to treat or the choice of drugs and indicate the need for any dose modifications. For example, chemotherapy is usually only appropriate for patients with a performance status score of 60 or above (Karnofsky scale), because they need to be reasonably physically robust to cope with the toxicity of treatment. An exception, however, may be a patient, whose cancer can be cured by chemotherapy, when the additional risks associated with the treatment because of their poor physical condition, may be worth taking. In presenting this information to

Table 9.1.2 Common toxicity profiles of commonly used cytotoxic drugs.

Drug	Toxicity			
	Bone marrow	Hair loss	Vomiting	Other
Antimetabolites				
5-fluorouracil	++		+	M D
Methotrexate	++			N M
Gemcitabine	+		+	L
Alkylating drugs				
Cyclophosphamide	+++	+++	++	L B M
Melphalan	++			
Cisplatin	++	+	+++	N K
Carboplatin	+++		+	
Antitumour antibiotics				
Doxorubicin	+++	+++	++	H D
Epirubicin	+++	+++	++	
Bleomycin		++	+	L M
Plant alkaloids				
Vincristine	+	++	+	N C
Vinblastine	+++	+	+	N
Vinorelbine	+++	+	+	N
Paclitaxel	++	+++	+	N H
Docetaxel	++	+++	++	N
Irinotecan	++	+	+	D
Topotecan	+++	++	+	
Etoposide	++	+	+	N

Note: +=mild; ++=moderate; +++=severe; M=mucositis; D=diarrhoea; C=constipation; N=neuropathy; B=bladder; K=kidney; H=heart; L=lung.

Table 9.1.3 Performance status scales.

Karnofsky scale		ECOG[a]/WHO scale	
No complaints; No evidence of disease	100	0	Normal activity No restrictions
Able to carry on normal activity; minor signs or symptoms of disease	90	1	Restricted but ambulatory; able to carry out light work
Some signs or symptoms of disease; normal activity with effort	80		
Cares for self; unable to carry on normal activity or to do active work	70	2	Ambulatory and self-caring but unable to carry out light work; up more than 50 per cent of waking hours
Requires occasional assistance but is able to care for personal needs	60		
Requires considerable assistance and frequent medical care	50	3	Limited self-care; symptomatic, confined to bed or chair more than 50 per cent of waking hours
Disabled; requires special care and assistance	40		
Severely disabled; hospitalisation indicated although death not imminent	30	4	Completely disabled; totally confined to bed; may need hospitalization
Very sick; hospitalization necessary; requires active supportive treatment	20		
Moribund; fatal processes progressing rapidly	10		
Dead	0	5	Dead

Note: [a]ECOG = Eastern Cooperative Oncology Group.

patients, medical jargon should be avoided and understanding can be increased by the use of information leaflets, diagrams, and taped recordings of the consultation. Careful thought should be given to the way in which information is presented because this may affect the patient's choice of a treatment option, for example, outcome can be expressed as the chance of survival rather than the probability of death. Some patients find it helpful to meet other similar patients or to obtain a second opinion or to access a nurse counsellor. Chemotherapy involves a commitment to repeated hospital visits, venepunctures, cannulations, investigations, and assessments and to a risk of hospital admissions and death. It should not be taken lightly. Some patients with treatable cancer prefer to allow the disease to run its course without intervention, and this view should always be respected. Some patients with untreatable cancer may ask to be treated with chemotherapy but this can only be justified in the context of phase I or phase II clinical trials, and any pressure to administer speculative treatments should be resisted.

The elderly and chemotherapy

Ageing is associated with physiological changes, which alter the absorbtion, distribution, metabolism, and elimination of drugs. The ability of the bone marrow and the immune system to respond to the damaging effects of cytotoxic drugs and the presence of infection is also impaired. The toxicity and risks associated with chemotherapy in the elderly will be high unless these factors are taken into account. Elderly patients have been excluded from clinical trials in the past, and any guidance on the use of chemotherapy in this age group is based on the extrapolation of evidence obtained from clinical trials in younger patients. The situation is changing. Methods for assessing and recording performance status that are relevant to an elderly population have been devised and validated and the distinction between the 'fit elderly' and the 'frail elderly' is more clearly defined[10]. More elderly patients are being recruited into clinical trials, and these methods are used increasingly to evaluate the effects of chemotherapy on the quality of life in this age group. Information is slowly accumulating so that guidelines for chemotherapy in the elderly will soon be available and old age alone should no longer be a bar to treatment.

The timing of chemotherapy

Typically, chemotherapy is given to patients when there is demonstrable metastatic spread but it may be given to treat local disease when surgery or radiotherapy are either not possible or are inappropriate. Occasionally, chemotherapy is given before surgery or radiotherapy (neo-adjuvant or induction chemotherapy) to reduce the size of a cancer so that surgery or radiotherapy can be done more easily. Chemotherapy may be given after surgery (adjuvant chemotherapy) in the absence of demonstrable disease to reduce the chance of systemic relapse in patients with micrometastases. This approach has been shown to increase the 5- and 10-year survival rates in early-stage breast[11] cancer, colon[12] cancer, and some stages of lung, gastric, oesophageal, and pancreatic cancers.

The administration of chemotherapy

Chemotherapy is usually administered by intravenous injection or infusion, although increasingly oral formulations of cytotoxic drugs are being developed. Most chemotherapy regimens dictate that the drugs are given intermittently with 3 to 4 weeks between each course of treatment to allow time for normal tissues to recover. There is evidence that some chemotherapy may be better tolerated and as effective when given more frequently, say weekly in smaller doses[13], and the optimal scheduling of chemotherapy is under continuous review. A course of chemotherapy should not be administered unless the neutrophil count is greater than 1.5×10^6 per cubic mm and any drug-induced gastrointestinal symptoms have settled. Dose reductions or the addition of stem-cell growth factors (GCSF) should be considered for subsequent courses of chemotherapy after a life-threatening toxic episode.

Multiple courses of chemotherapy means repeated venepunctures and cannulations. Cytotoxic drugs are irritants and local phlebitis is common. Venous access can be a problem, unless a permanent access line is established. This is necessary anyway for continuous infusional treatment. There are various devices for securing permanent venous access. They involve the insertion of a long polymerized silicone rubber (Silastic®) catheter into the right atrium. The catheter may be single, double, or triple lumen, and some devices include a subcutaneous implantable injection port so that the whole system is concealed beneath the skin. Intravenous fluid, drugs, and blood can be administered, and blood samples can be taken through the catheter. Catheter-related deaths are rare but infection and thrombosis can occur and a pneumothorax can complicate the insertion procedure. Reasons for early withdrawal of the catheter include persistent fever and jugular or superior vena caval thrombosis.

Intra-arterial chemotherapy is occasionally considered for the treatment of localized cancer in the limbs, head and neck, and liver. Its use is experimental and confined to specialized units. Similarly, installation of cytotoxic drugs into the abdominal cavity is being evaluated for the treatment of ovarian cancer.

Chemotherapy should be administered in specialized units by staff who are properly trained and under the supervision of cancer specialists (oncologists). There should be procedures for preparing and administering treatment, which protect the staff from skin and aerosol contamination and for dealing with drug spillage and extravasation.

The monitoring of chemotherapy

Patients on chemotherapy require regular assessment, and it is normal practice to record symptoms, toxicity, and response before each course of treatment. The methods for monitoring response depend on the cancer type and the sites of disease and include repeated measurements of palpable masses, or masses identified radiologically or with scanning techniques, and serum tumour markers. Tumour markers are substances, usually proteins, which are produced by cancers and can be detected and quantified in the blood or urine. The serum tumour markers commonly used in clinical practice for monitoring as well as for diagnosis and detecting recurrence are shown in Table 9.1.4. It is not necessary to repeat the radiological investigations each time but a formal review of the disease status should be carried out after no more than three courses of treatment have been given. Chemotherapy should be with-drawn if there is evidence of progressive disease or if there are other compelling clinical reasons for doing so. Only by treating the patient and monitoring the response can the sensitivity of the cancer to chemotherapy be determined. There are, as yet no predictive tests as there are, for example, for antibiotics in the treatment of infection.

The number of courses of chemotherapy and the duration of continuous infusional chemotherapy is not fixed. Much depends on the regimen, the toxicity, the patient's condition, and the disease status. Some cytotoxic drugs have cumulative toxicities and maximum recommended doses should not be exceeded. Clearly if toxicity is minimal, and the patient's condition is improved by treatment, it is reasonable to continue until there is evidence of disease progression. However, the tolerability of some regimens is such that a maximum of 4–6 courses, or for continuous infusional chemotherapy, a maximum period of 6 months, is recommended. Patients whose cancer is resistant to one chemotherapy regimen can sometimes be treated with another. Similarly, different regimens can be given to patients with relapsed disease, although response rates become progressively less.

There are many questions about cancer chemotherapy that remain largely unanswered, such as the optimal combination of cytotoxic drugs and the optimal scheduling, timing, and duration of treatment to give the highest response with the lowest toxicity for each type of cancer. These issues can only be resolved by RCTs. It is the ambition of oncologists that as many patients as possible be treated in the context of a randomized controlled trial.

Hormone therapy in palliative care

The mode of action of hormones and hormone therapy

Hormones are polypeptides produced by the endocrine system, which influence metabolic processes throughout the body. The effects are mediated either directly by binding with specific cell surface receptors or indirectly by stimulating or inhibiting the local production of cell growth factors. Some cancers contain cells that require particular hormones to proliferate (hormone-dependent) and these are the cancers that are amenable to hormone therapy (Table 9.1.1). The therapy either blocks the binding of hormones to receptors or reduces the circulating and cellular concentrations of the hormone. The cancers most susceptible to this approach are breast cancer and prostate cancer.

Breast cancer. Hormone-dependent breast cancer cells proliferate under the influence of oestrogen. Oestrogen is produced mainly by the ovaries in pre-menopausal women and from the conversion of androgens mainly from the adrenal glands, in post-menopausal women. Androgens are converted into oestrogen by aromatase, an enzyme found in peripheral sites such as adipose tissue, skin, muscle, and liver and in up to 70 per cent of breast cancers[14]. Oestrogen production can be reduced by surgical intervention (oophorectomy, adrenalectomy, hypophysectomy), radiation of the ovaries or by gonadotrophin-releasing hormone analogues all of which have the same effect in pre-menopausal women. Aromatase inhibition is used in post-menopausal women and this can be achieved by the administration of steroidal androgen analogues such as exemestane, which inactive the enzyme irreversibly or by non-steroidal drugs such as anastrozole and letrozole, which are less specific and reversible and whose inhibitory effects depend on the continued presence of the drug. Both types of aromatase inhibitors reduce circulating oestrogen to nearly undetectable levels in post-menopausal women but the steroidal drugs may be more effective and responses are seen in patients who have progressed on treatment with non-steroidal drugs. The side effects of oestrogen depletion include hot flushes, sweats, and osteoporosis.

Anti-oestrogens, such as tamoxifen, bind to oestrogen receptors and their clinical effects in breast cancer are largely confined to

Table 9.1.4 Serum tumour markers which are used in clinical practice.

Marker	Cancer
Carcinoembryonic antigen	Colorectal, breast, lung (small cell)
CA 125	Ovary
CA15-3	Breast
CA 19-9	Pancreas
Prostate specific antigen	Prostate
Lactic dehydrogenase	Lymphoma, lung (small cell)
Alpha fetoprotein	Germ cell, hepatoma
Human chorionic gonadotrophin	Germ cell chorioncarcinoma
Thyrocalcitonin	Thyroid (medullary)
Monoclonal immunoglobulin	Myeloma, lymphoma

patients with oestrogen-receptor positive disease. Tamoxifen has other pharmacological effects and can act as an agonist when oestrogen concentrations are low. Newer drugs which are purely competitive inhibitors are being introduced into clinical practice[15]. The agonist activity of tamoxifen is thought to explain the small increased incidence of endometrial cancer in patients taking it for many years. Other side effects include hot flushes, thromboembolism, and corneal and retinal deposits. Any serious effects are rare, however, and tamoxifen is a remarkably well-tolerated drug.

Progestational drugs such as medroxyprogesterone acetate are used to treat hormone- dependent breast cancer and response rates are similar to tamoxifen. The mechanism of action is unknown but they may interfere with binding to progesterone and oestrogen receptors and with aromatisation. Side effects include weight gain, vaginal bleeding, and thromboembolism.

Prostate cancer. Hormone-dependent prostate cancer cells proliferate under the influence of androgens. Most androgen activity comes from testosterone, which is produced in the testes. Secretion is regulated by luteinizing hormone (LH) from the pituitary gland, which in turn is regulated by luteinizing hormone-releasing hormone (LHRH) from the hypothalamus. Other androgens are synthesized in the adrenal glands and are converted peripherally to testosterone. Their secretion is regulated by adrenocorticotrophic hormone (ACTH). Testosterone is metabolized to dihydro-testosterone (DHT), which drives cell proliferation and DHT receptors are found in hormone- dependent prostate cancer cells.

Testosterone production can be reduced by surgical intervention (castration) or by drugs, which inhibit LH secretion (oestrogens, cyproterone acetate, and LHRH agonists, such as goserelin and leuprolide acetate), ACTH secretion (glucocorticoids) and steroid synthesis (ketoconazole). Oestrogens are no longer used alone in the treatment of prostate cancer because of cardiovascular side effects, although in combination with nitrogen mustard (estramustine) they may have a place in second-line treatment. The LHRH agonists produce an initial rise in serum testosterone concentration followed by a fall to castration levels. The rise can produce a tumour 'flare' and a temporary worsening of symptoms, which can be blocked by a peripheral anti-androgen drug such as cyproterone acetate or flutamide. Side effects include loss of potency and hot flushes. The advantages of castration compared to LHRH agonists are the rapidity of the effect, cost-effectiveness, and the elimination of compliance as an issue. However, there are psychological consequences, which make it an unacceptable option for some patients.

Glucocorticoids and ketononazole have modest effects on serum testosterone levels and their side effects have limited their use in the treatment of prostate cancer.

Non-steroidal antiandrogens such as flutamide bind to DHT receptors in prostate cancer cells. The steroidal antiandrogen cyproterone acetate is less effective as a binding agent but has progestational activity and suppresses LH secretion as well. Total androgen blockade can be achieved by combining testosterone deprivation with an antiandrogen. Both flutamide and cyproterone acetate can cause serious liver toxicity and liver function tests must be monitored.

Miscellaneous cancers. Hormone-dependent endometrial cancer is regulated by an interaction between circulating oestrogen and progesterones. Cancer regression is seen in up to 30 per cent of patients during treatment with progestational drugs such as medroxyprogesterone acetate and megestrol acetate, and response rates are higher in progesterone-receptor positive, well-differentiated cancers.

Some ovarian cancers express oestrogen and progesterone receptors, some malignant melanomas express oestrogen receptors, some renal cancers express progesterone receptors, and some pancreas cancers express androgen receptors; but it is doubtful if hormone therapy has any part to play in the management of these cancers.

Biological agents in palliative care

Biological agents to treat cancer have been developed from an understanding of the molecular changes, which characterize the cancer phenotype and of the effects cancer cells have on their immediate surroundings and on host defence mechanisms. This is an evolving science and the reader is given an insight into some of the new targets for anti-cancer treatments and examples of agents, which are being introduced into clinical practice.

Growth factor receptors and tyrosine kinases

Cell signalling pathways are the means by which cells receive the instruction to proliferate or to die. They begin with the activation of surface receptors, which cause messages to cascade through the cytoplasm to the nucleus and to the cell cycle. Any of the genes, which code for the proteins involved in these processes (proto-oncogenes), may be abnormally expressed in a cancer cell (known then as an oncogene) and can result in either a continuous drive to cell proliferation or escape from apoptosis. Oncogenes and their protein products are potential targets for anticancer treatment. One of the pathways includes epidermal growth factor receptors (EGFRs) and a family of enzymes, the tyrosine kinases, which transfer the information from activated cell surface receptors into the cytoplasm. These receptors and enzymes are over-expressed in a number of epithelial cancers, (cancer of the breast, ovary, pancreas, stomach, colon, rectum, and non-small cell lung cancer) and probably have a part to play in their pathogenesis[16]. Several treatment strategies for targeting EGFR-expressing cancers are being pursued. These include anti-EGFR monoclonal antibodies and tyrosine kinase inhibitors, which block the transfer of signals in different ways.

Trastuzumab (Herceptin®) is a humanized monoclonal antibody (one in which specific regions of a murine antibody are inserted into the framework of a generic human IgG antibody) that binds to the EGFR-related receptor HER2, which is over-expressed in 30 per cent of breast cancers, where it is associated with a poor prognosis[17]. A number of studies have demonstrated the efficacy of trastuzumab in HER2-positive metastatic breast cancer either alone[18] or in combination with chemotherapy[19]. Similar studies are being conducted with trastuzumab in the other epithelial cancers, which over-express HER2[20].

Imatinide (Glivec®) is a small molecule that inhibits a particular tyrosine kinase, which is the protein product of the bcr-abl oncogene. This oncogene is expressed as a result of a chromosome translocation and the fusion of the bcr gene on chromosome 22 with the abl gene on chromosome 9 and is the genetic abnormality that characterizes chronic myeloid leukaemia (the Philadelphia chromosome). The continuous production of the bcr-abl tyrosine kinase is thought to drive cell proliferation. Imatinide produces complete haematological responses in most patients in the chronic and accelerated phase of the disease[21]. As well as improving symptoms and prolonging survival, it is possible that imatinide either alone or in combination with conventional treatment, will cure patients with chronic myeloid leukaemia.

The cell cycle

When the signal to proliferate reaches the cell nucleus, replication begins. The orderly progression of the cell cycle is initiated and controlled by cyclins and cyclin-dependent kinases (CDKs). Cyclins are over-expressed in a number of different cancers and together with CDKs are targets for therapeutic intervention[22].

Normally, if damaged DNA is detected during cell replication, the cell cycle is arrested at the G1/S and G2/M interfaces (known as checkpoints) whilst the damage is repaired. If repair is not possible, the cell is triggered into apoptosis (Fig. 9.1.1). In this way, mutations in proto-oncogenes, which might lead to a cancer phenotype, may be eliminated. The checkpoints are controlled by protein products of genes known as tumour suppressor genes, which have the effect of slowing or blocking progression through the cell cycle by inhibiting the formation of cyclin complexes. If tumour suppressor genes are inactivated, abnormal genetic material passes on to successive generations of the original cell. Inactivation of one tumour suppressor gene in particular, known as P53 is critical in carcinogenesis. Mutations are found in 50 per cent of cancers. The technology exists to transfer non-mutated P53 DNA into cancer cells, to raise antibodies against mutated P53 protein, and to produce vaccines that kill cells containing mutated P53[23] — three more ways of treating cancer if theoretical possibilities can be translated into clinical practice.

Matrix metalloproteinases and angiogenesis

As a cancer grows, the surrounding connective tissue matrix is reorganized through the release of metalloproteinase enzymes. This process facilitates invasion and spread of cancer cells and is an important step in allowing the migration of endothelial cells, which lead to new blood vessel formation (angiogenesis). Angiogenesis is controlled by stimulatory and inhibitory molecules released by cancer cells and by cells contained within the connective tissue. The stimulatory molecules include fibroblast growth factor, vascular endothelial growth factor (VEGF), platelet-derived growth factor, and various matrix metalloproteinases. The inhibitory molecules include interferon and angiostatin. The balance between the two determines the micro-environment and influences the growth characteristics of the cancer and its potential for metastatic spread. These discoveries provide a number of possibilities for treating cancer by inhibiting angiogenesis and the reorganization of the connective tissue stroma. Matrix metalloproteinase inhibitors, VEGF receptor inhibitors, interferon alpha, endogenous angiostation, and drugs such as thalidomide, which have anti-angiogenic properties are all being evaluated in clinical trials. Thalidomide has anti-cancer activity in multiple myeloma[24].

Host defence mechanisms

Sometimes, cancer cells express or secrete tumour associated or tumour specific proteins, which provoke an immune response. The response includes the release of cytokines by macrophages and lymphoid cells which activate cytotoxic T lymphocytes and natural killer cells and the production of antibodies by B lymphocytes, which activate antibody-dependent cell-mediated cytotoxicity. The reasons why the immune system fails to eliminate these cancer cells are unclear but enhancing the response through immunological manipulation can have anticancer effects and different methods of doing this are being evaluated in clinical practice.

Although it is not a tumour antigen as such, the CD20 antigen is a cell surface protein which characterizes the B lymphocyte. Large numbers of B lymphocytes are produced and accumulate in some forms of non-Hodgkin lymphoma. Rituximab is a humanized monoclonal antibody raised against the CD20 antigen and is a new approach to the treatment of this disease[25]. Increased survival has been reported when rituximab is included in the treatment of patients with diffuse large-cell lymphoma and other aggressive non-Hodgkin lymphomas as well as patients with indolent forms of the disease such as follicular lymphoma, which are not cured by current chemotherapy regimens alone[26].

Treatment strategies

In this section, the treatment strategies of certain cancers are outlined. Breast cancer, lung cancer, and colorectal cancer are selected because they are common, their clinical course is often protracted, and together they account for a large part of the workload of a palliative care physician. Myeloma is selected because patients are often symptomatic at the outset and may present first to a palliative care physician and it is important to recognize that myeloma responds well to medical treatment. Carcinoma from an unknown primary source (CUP) is selected because these patients present doctors with difficult diagnostic and management decisions and may be referred to palliative care physicians without a full oncology assessment. The reader is referred to text books of cancer medicine for information about the medical treatment of the other cancers listed in Table 9.1.1.

Response rates and survival data are given as an indication of the effectiveness of treatment but an improvement in quality-of-life measures may be the main expected benefit and these details are not given here. It is worth stating that an improvement in median survival of say 3 months may seem small to the reader but it may be very significant to a patient whose life-expectancy is only 6 months[27]. Certainly, patients view small gains from treatment as being much more worthwhile than the prescribing doctors[28].

Breast cancer

The management of metastatic breast cancer depends on the site or sites of disease, whether the disease is local or systemic, and if systemic, whether it is life-threatening (involving liver or lung) or not (involving bone or soft tissue). Other important factors include the patient's menopausal status, performance status and physical symptoms and the cancer's oestrogen, progesterone, and HER2 receptor status. The choice of treatment and the expected outcomes are as follows:

Hormone therapy[29]. Hormone therapy is only considered for patients with oestrogen and/or progesterone receptor-positive breast cancer. It is used rather than chemotherapy because the administration is easier, side effects are fewer, and responses are more durable. However, it is used only if the patient is not symptomatic and the situation is not life-threatening, because the response to hormone therapy is slow and a failure to respond in these circumstances would not adversely effect the patient's comfort or survival. Otherwise, chemotherapy is used first and is followed by hormone therapy. In pre-menopausal patients, hormone therapy includes any of the surgical, radiation, and medical techniques to remove or prevent oestrogen production. Drugs such as tamoxifen, anastrozole, exemestane, and progesterones are used regardless of menopausal status.

Most patients do not present with metastatic disease and will have been treated previously for early-stage breast cancer with adjuvant hormone therapy. If relapse occurs within 1 year of primary treatment, the disease is likely to be hormone-resistant, and chemotherapy is recommended. If relapse occurs after 1 year of primary treatment, with say tamoxifen or within 1 year of stopping it, the next line of hormone therapy with say anastrozole should be used. Otherwise, tamoxifen is used again. Whilst a cancer continues to demonstrate hormone sensitivity, the different hormones can be used in sequence for each episode of relapse. Sometimes, stopping hormone therapy for disease progression is followed by regression of the cancer. By contrast, the administration of hormone therapy may produce a temporary exacerbation of symptoms known as a tumour 'flare' which may result in hypercalcaemia in patients with metastatic bone disease.

The overall response to first-line hormone therapy is between 30 per cent and 40 per cent, although it can be as high as 60 per cent in patients with non-visceral disease and a long disease-free interval, factors which predict a good response. Response rates of 25 per cent and between 10 per cent and 15 per cent are seen with second and third-line hormone therapy respectively. Responses may last for several years.

Chemotherapy[30]. In addition to its use for life-threatening disease, chemotherapy is recommended for patients with metastatic breast cancer that is oestrogen-receptor negative or which is refractory or becomes resistant to hormone therapy. HER2-positive disease (between 20 per cent and 30 per cent of all patients) may also be an indication for chemotherapy because it is associated with hormone resistance in breast cancer which is also oestrogen-receptor positive. There is also an increased rate of cancer growth, an enhanced rate of metastases, a shorter disease-free interval, and a reduced overall survival in these patients.

Chemotherapy regimens have changed over the years as new drugs and combinations are introduced into clinical practice. First-line chemotherapy for metastatic disease is either one or a combination of two or three of any of the following: cyclophosphamide, methotrexate, 5-fluorouracil, doxorubicin, and epirubicin, avoiding any drugs that were used previously as adjuvant treatment. Second- and third-line chemotherapy is either one or a combination of any of the same drugs together with vinorelbine, docetaxel, and paclitaxel avoiding drugs that were used as first-line treatment.

Overall response rates to first-line treatment are between 40 per cent and 60 per cent, which includes between 10 per cent and 20 per cent complete responses. The median duration of the response is between 6 and 10 months. Response rates of 25 per cent or less are seen with second- and third-line chemotherapy. High-dose chemotherapy with GCSF to hasten bone marrow recovery has not shown a survival benefit and is not recommended[31].

Biological agents. Phase II trials have demonstrated the efficacy of trastuzumab in patients with HER2 positive disease and early phase III data have shown improvement in response rates, median time to progression and survival when trastuzumab is added to first-line chemotherapy in metastatic breast cancer[19]. The combination of trastuzumab and an anthracycline should be used with caution for increased cardiac toxicity has been reported when they are given together.

Other treatment. The bone is the commonest site for metastases in breast cancer and may be the only site of spread for several years. Metastatic bone disease can give rise to serious morbidity including pathological fractures, hypercalcaemia, and spinal cord compression, especially when the metastases are associated with increased osteoclastic activity and osteolysis. Bisphosphonates inhibit osteoclastic activation. They control hypercalcaemia and reduce the frequency of fractures and the severity of bone pain[32]. They may also reduce the incidence of bone metastases but this has not been confirmed[33] and there is no evidence of an increase in survival. Patients with metastatic bone disease and osteolysis should be treated with bisphosphonates indefinitely.

Lung cancer[34]

The management of lung cancer depends on the histological sub-type, either small-cell or non-small-cell (includes squamous, adenocarcinoma, and large-cell cancers), the stage of the disease and the performance status of the patient.

Small-cell lung cancer (20 per cent). Metastatic spread occurs early in the natural history of the disease. It may be associated with inappropriate anti-diuretic hormone secretion, ectopic ACTH secretion and a myasthaenic syndrome. The median survival of untreated patients is about 2 months. Prognostic factors include the performance status, the stage of disease (either limited to one hemithorax (30 per cent), or beyond this limit (70 per cent) and called extensive disease) and serum sodium and lactic dehydrogenase concentrations. Patients with limited disease, a good performance status and normal biochemistry respond well to systemic chemotherapy. The standard regimen is a combination of either cisplatin or carboplatin and etoposide. The response rate is between 80 per cent and 95 per cent and the median survival is 20 months. Between 50 per cent and 60 per cent are complete responders and a proportion of these patients (between 10 per cent and 20 per cent) are long-term survivors provided they have prophylactic cranial[35] and mediastinal radiation[36] therapy as well.

Patients with extensive disease and poor prognostic factors may also respond to chemotherapy[37]. The response rate is about 40 per cent but there are few complete responders. The median survival is between 7 and 10 months. Few patients live beyond 2 years.

The prognosis for patients after relapse is poor. There is no standard second-line chemotherapy regimen but the taxanes and the newer topoisomerase inhibitors (topotecan and irinotecan) are being studied and look promising.

Non-small-cell lung cancer[38] *(80 per cent),* Where possible, non-small-cell lung cancer is treated by surgical resection, which results in a 5-year survival rate of about 60 per cent in patients with early-stage disease. An additional benefit from adjuvant chemotherapy has not yet been established. Induction chemotherapy in locally advanced disease can sometimes convert an unresectable cancer to one which is resectable. Response rates of 75 per cent and resection rates of 60 per cent have been reported with up to 25 per cent of patients alive and in remission after 5 years. However, patients in these studies were carefully selected by age, performance status, and medical history and the results may not be widely applicable. Patients with locally advanced unresectable non-small-cell lung cancer (30 per cent) are treated by induction chemotherapy followed by radiotherapy, which increases median and 2-year survival compared to radiotherapy alone[39].

About 50 per cent of patients with non-small-cell lung cancer present with evidence of metastatic spread. The median survival for these patients without treatment is about 6 months and there is no prospect of cure. Several randomized trials have shown the benefit of chemotherapy in good performance status patients |compared to supportive care alone[40]. There is an overall increase in median survival of 3 months and an increase from 30 per cent to 40 per cent in the numbers of patients alive at 1 year. More importantly, there is an improvement in a range of quality-of-life measures including the relief of physical symptoms if chemotherapy is used[1]. Cisplatin or carboplatin combined with vinorelbine or docetaxel give the highest response and survival rates. Docetaxel and pemetrexid can improve survival when used as second-line treatment and there is evidence that the oral human epidermal growth factor receptor inhibitor, erlotinib may improve survival further in some patients previously treated with chemotherapy[41].

Colorectal cancer

About 60 per cent of patients with colorectal cancer have metastatic disease either at presentation or after surgical resection and adjuvant chemotherapy. The liver and lungs are the commonest sites of involvement. Until recently, chemotherapy with 5-fluorouracil modulated by the concomitant administration of folinic acid was the standard regimen giving a response rate of 30 per cent and a median survival of between 12 and 14 months, 6 months more than supportive care alone. However, the combination of these two drugs with irinotecan has increased the response rate to nearly 50 per cent, and the median survival to 17 months and has become the new gold standard regimen[42]. Other active drugs, oxaliplatin[43] (a platinum derivative) and capecitabine[44] (an orally administered precurser of 5-fluorouracil) are being evaluated. Chemotherapy is generally given for a fixed period and resumed when there is evidence of disease progression.

Promising results are emerging from studies where chemotherapy is given with cetuximab, a monoclonal antibody targeting an epidermal growth factor receptor, which is preferentially expressed on some adenocarcinomas[45] and bevacizumab a monoclonal antibody targeting a vascular endothelial growth factor receptor[46] and it seems likely that survival will be further increased by the inclusion of these agents in patients whose tumours express the appropriate receptors.

Myeloma[47]

Multiple myeloma is a cancer of bone-marrow plasma cells. A monoclonal protein (paraprotein) secreted by the cancer is found in the serum in 80 per cent of patients and free immunoglobulin light chains are often found in the urine. In 20 per cent of patients, light chains only are produced by the cancer. Symptoms include bone pain (60 per cent), and the symptoms associated with anaemia, hypercalcaemia, infection, and renal failure. Standard medical treatment is chemotherapy with melphalan and prednisolone, which gives a response rate (greater than 50 per cent reduction in the paraprotein concentration) of 50 per cent. Maintenance chemotherapy is ineffective. More aggressive chemotherapy with vincristine, doxorubicin, and dexamethasone is appropriate for patients with a good performance status and gives a response rate of between 60 per cent and 80 per cent[48]. Patients under 60 years

who have chemo-sensitive myeloma may go on to high-dose therapy supported by peripheral blood or bone-marrow stem cell transplantation[49]. This increases the median survival from 2 years to 5 years. Thalidomide gives responses in 30 per cent of patients whose myeloma is resistant to chemotherapy[24]. Other treatments include bisphosphonates which reduce bone pain, hypercalcaemia, and the frequency of pathological bone fractures[50]; blood transfusions or erythropoietin for anaemia; and plasmaphoresis for the hyperviscosity syndrome.

Carcinoma of unknown primary (CUP)[51]

About 3 per cent of cancers present with metastatic spread and the primary cancer cannot be found despite careful clinical examination and screening x-rays, CT scans, and mammography. The management of these patients is difficult because the tissue of origin of the cancer is an important factor in determining a treatment plan. In these circumstances, treatment decisions are based on additional information derived from immunochemical staining of tissue samples (Table 9.1.5) and serum tumour marker studies (Table 9.1.4) and from the distribution of the metastases which may indicate the most likely source of the cancer.

The distribution of histological sub-types in CUPs is adenocarcinoma (60 per cent), squamous cancer (5 per cent), and poorly/undifferentiated cancer (35 per cent). About two-thirds of the primary cancers can be found at autopsy and their distribution gives an indication of the range of primary sites which can present as a CUP. The commonest sites for an adenocarcinoma are lung, pancreas, stomach, and prostate; for a squamous cancer are head and neck, oesophagus, skin, and lung; and for an undifferentiated cancer are lymphoma, germ cell, melanoma, and neuroendocrine. It is essential to identify germ cell tumours and lymphomas because these cancers may be curable (Table 9.1.1). Similarly, patients with prostate cancer may have prolonged survival with hormone treatment. If the primary cancer remains unknown after a thorough evaluation, chemotherapy may be offered to patients with a good performance status with regimens that reflect the most likely source of the cancer[52]. Alternatively, vincristine, doxorubicin and cyclophosphamide in combination give a response rate of 20 per cent[53]. The median survival of these patients is only 6 months and only 20 per cent live beyond one year.

Table 9.1.5 Immunochemical markers in common use.

Marker	Cancer
Cytokeratin	Carcinoma
Vimentin	Sarcoma
Common leucocyte antigen	Lymphoma
S100	Malignant melanoma
Prostate-specific antigen	Prostate
Oestrogen receptor	Breast
Alpha fetoprotein Human chorionic gonadotrophin Placental alkaline phosphatase	Germ cell
Chromogranin	Neuroendocrine

Future directions

Further progress in the medical treatment of cancer may come from new cytotoxic drug development or modifying the schedules and combinations of the cytotoxic drugs already in use. However, this is likely to produce small incremental gains rather than a dramatic revolution in treatment outcomes. Real hope for the future comes from the increasingly detailed understanding of the molecular changes, which characterize the cancer phenotype and from the innovative ways of correcting and combating them. Treatments that target some of these changes are already being used in clinical practice and have been described (trastuzumab, rituximab, and imatinide). Many more like them are being developed and evaluated[54]. Furthermore, it is now possible to inactivate oncogenes and their products, to restore the function of damaged proto-oncogenes and tumour-suppressor genes and to target cells containing particular gene defects with cytotoxic agents, giving rise to further possibilities for specific cancer treatments in the future.

It can be predicted that these biological therapies will be most effective when they are given early in the disease process because of better drug penetration and fewer cell mutations when the cancer load is small. Thus, unless or until molecular techniques for earlier diagnosis and more sensitive screening become a reality, the need for conventional debulking procedures (surgery, radiotherapy, chemotherapy) will remain.

References

1. Anderson, H. *et al.* (2000). Gemcitabine plus best supportive care (BSC) vs BSC in inoperable non-small-cell lung cancer – a randomised trial with quality of life as the primary outcome. *Bristol Journal of Cancer,* **83**, 447–53.

2. Thatcher, N. *et al.* (1995). Symptomatic benefit from gemcitabine and other chemotherapy in advanced non-small cell lung cancer: changes in performance status and tumour-related symptoms. *Anti-Cancer Drugs,* **6** Suppl. 6, 39–48.

3. Rizzo, J.D., Lichten, A.E., Woolf, S.H. *et al.* (2002). Use of epoetin in patients with cancer: evidence-based clinical practice guidelines of ASCO and ASH. *Journal of Clinical Oncology,* **20**, 4083–107.

4. Bokemeyer, C., Aapro, M.S., Courdi, A. *et al.* (2004). EORTC guidelines for the use of erythropoietic proteins in anaemic patients with cancer. *European Journal of Cancer,* **40**, 2201–16.

5. Moores, K.G. (2007). Safe and effective outpatient treatment of adults with chemotherapy-induced neutropenic fever. *American Journal of Health-Systems Pharmacy,* **64**(1), 717–22.

6. Ioannidis, J.P.A., Hesketh, P.J., and Lau, J. (2000). Contribution of dexamethasone to control of chemotherapy-induced nausea and vomiting: a meta-analysis of randomised controlled trials. *Journal of Clinical Oncology,* **18**, 3409–22.

7. Fallowfield, L., Ford, S., and Lewis, S. (1994). Information preferences of patients with cancer. *Lancet,* **344**, 1576.

8. Ajaj, A., Singh, M.P., Abdullah, A.J.J. (2001). Should elderly patients be told they have cancer? Questionnaire survey of older people. *British Medical Journal.* **323**, 1160.

9. Meredith, C. *et al.* (1996). Information needs of cancer patients in West Scotland: cross-sectional survey of patients' views. *British Medical Journal,* **313**, 724–6.

10. Careca, I., Baloucci, L., and Extermann, M. (2005). Cancer in the older person. *Cancer Treatment Reviews,* **31**, 380–402.

11. Early Breast Cancer Trialist 5 Collaborative Group (1992). Systemic treatment of early breast cancer by hormonal, cytotoxic or immune therapy. 133 randomised trials involving 31,000 recurrences and 24,000 deaths among 75,000 women. *Lancet,* **339**, 71–85.

12. Midgley, R.S.J. and Kerr, D.J. (2000). ABC of colorectal cancer: adjuvant therapy. *British Medical Journal,* **321**, 1208–11.

13. Seidman, A.D. *et al.* (1998). Dose-dense therapy with weekly 1-hour paclitaxel infusions in the treatment of metastatic breast cancer. *Journal of Clinical Oncology,* **16**, 3353–61.

14. Millar, W.R. (1990). Endocrine treatment for breast cancers: Biological, rationale and current progress. *Journal of Steroid Biochemistry and Molecular Biology,* **37**, 467–80.

15. Howell, A. and Dowsett, M. (1997). Recent advances in endocrine therapy of breast cancer. *British Medical Journal,* **315**, 863–6.

16. Salomon, D.S. *et al.* (1995). Epidermal growth factor-related peptides and their receptors in human malignancies. *Critical Reviews in Oncology and Haematology* **19**, 183–232.

17. Klijn, J.G. *et al.* (1992). The clinical significance of epidermal growth factor receptor in human breast cancer: A review of 5232 patients. *Endocrine Review,* **13**, 3–17.

18. Cobleigh, M.A. *et al.* (1999). Multinational study of the efficacy and safety of humanized anti–HER2 monoclonal antibody in women who have HER2 – overexpressing metastatic breast cancer that has progressed after chemotherapy for metastatic disease. *Journal of Clinical Oncology,* **17**, 2639–48.

19. Slamon, D.J. *et al.* (2001). Use of chemotherapy plus a monoclonal antibody against HER2 for metastatic breast cancer that overexpresses HER2. *New England Journal of Medicine,* **344**, 783–92.

20. Scholl, S., Beuzeboc, P., and Pouillart, P. (2001). Targeting HER2 in other tumour types. *Annals of Oncology,* **12** (Suppl.1.), 81–7.

21. Mughal, T.I. and Goldman, J.M. (2001). Chronic myeloid leukaemia: STI 571 magnifies the therapeutic dilemma. *European Journal of Cancer,* **37**, 561–8.

22. Sausville, E.A. (1999). Cyclin-dependent kinases: Novel targets for cancer treatment. *Thirty-fifth Annual Meeting of the American Society of Clinical Oncology: Educational Book,* pp. 9–21.

23. Harris, C.C. (1996). Structure and function of the P53 tumour suppressor gene: clues for rational cancer therapeutic strategies. *Journal of the National Cancer Institute,* **88**, 1442–55.

24. Singhal, S. *et al.* (1999). Antitumour activity of thalidomide in refractory myeloma. *New England Journal of Medicine,* **341**, 1565–71.

25. McLaughlin, P. *et al.* (1998). Rituximab chimeric anti-CD20 monoclonal antibody therapy for relapsed indolent lymphoma: half of patients respond to a four-dose treatment programme. *Journal of Clinical Oncology,* **16**, 2825–33.

26. Cheung, M.C., Haynes, A.E., Meyer, R.M. *et al.* (2007). A systemic review and consensus practice guideline from Cancer Care Ontario. *Cancer Treatment Reviews,* **33**, 161–76.

27. Silvestri, G., Pritchard, R., and Welch, H.G. (1998). Preferences for chemotherapy in patients with advanced non-small-cell lung cancer: Descriptive study based on scripted interviews. *British Medical Journal,* **317**, 771–5.

28. Slevin, M.L. *et al.* (1990). Attitudes to chemotherapy: comparing views of patients with cancer with those of doctors, nurses and general public. *British Medical Journal,* **300**, 1458–60.

29. Goldhirsch, A. and Gelber, R.D. (1996). Endocrine therapies of breast cancer. *Seminars in Oncology,* **23**, 494–505.

30. Fossati, R. *et al.* (1998). Cytotoxic and hormonal treatment for metastatic breast cancer: A systematic review of published randomised trials involving 35,510 women. *Journal of Clinical Oncology,* **16**, 3439–60.

31. Pusztai, L. and Hortobagyi, G.N. (1998). Discouraging news for high-dose chemotherapy in high-risk breast cancer. *Lancet,* **352**, 501–2.

32. van Holten-Verzantvoort, A.T. *et al.* (1993). Palliative bone treatment in patients with bone metastases from breast cancer. *Journal of Clinical Oncology,* **11**, 491–8.

33. Kanis, J.A. *et al.* (1996). Clodronate decreases the frequency of skeletal metastases with breast cancer. *Bone,* **19**, 663–7.

34. Hoffman, P.C., Mauer, A.M., and Vokes, E.E. (2000). Lung Cancer. *Lancet*, **355**, 479–85.

35. Auperin, A. *et al.* (1999). Prophylactic cranial irradiation for patients with small-cell lung cancer in complete remission. *New England Journal of Medicine*, **341**, 476–84.

36. Perry, M.L. *et al.* (1987). Chemotherapy with or without radiation therapy in limited small-cell carcinoma of the lung. *New England Journal of Medicine*, **316**, 912–8.

37. Chute, J.P. *et al.* (1999). Twenty years of phase III trials for patients with extensive stage small-cell lung cancer. Perceptible progress. *Journal of Clinical Oncology*, **17**, 1794–1801.

38. Carney, D.N. and Hansen, H.H. (2000). Non-small-cell lung cancer – stalemate or progress? *New England Journal of Medicine*, **343**, 1261–2.

39. Pritchard, R.S. and Anthony, S.P. (1996). Chemotherapy plus radiotherapy compared with radiotherapy alone in the treatment of locally advanced, unresectable, non-small cell lung cancer: a meta-analysis. *Annuals of Internal Medicine*, **125**, 723–9.

40. Non-Small Cell Lung Cancer Collaborative Group. (1995). Chemotherapy in non-small cell lung cancer: a meta-analysis using updated data on individual patients from 52 randomised clinical trials. *British Medical Journal*, **311**, 899–908.

41. Shepherd, F., Rodrigues Pereira, J., Guleanu, T. *et al.* (2005). Erlotinib in previously treated non-small cell lung cancer, a trial of the National Cancer Institute of Canada Clinical Trials Group. *New England Journal of Medicine*, **353**, 123–32.

42. Douillard, J.Y., *et al.* (2000). Irinotecan combined with fluorouracil compared with fluorouracil alone as first-line treatment for metastatic colorectal cancer: a multicentre randomised trial. *Lancet*, **355**, 1041–7.

43. Mainfrault-Goebel, F. *et al.* (1999). High dose oxaliplatin with the simplified 48h bi-monthly leucovorin and 5-fluorouracil regimen in pre-treated metastatic colorectal cancer. *Proceedings of the American Society of Clinical Oncology*, **18**, 898.

44. Twelves, C. *et al.* (1999). A phase III trial of capecitabine in previously untreated advanced/metastatic colorectal cancer. *Proceedings of the American Society of Clinical Oncology*, **18**, 1010.

45. Folprecht, G., Lutz, MP., Schoffski, P. *et al.* (2006). Cetuximab and irinotecan/5 fluorouracil/folinic acid is a safe combination for the first line treatment of patients with epidermal growth factor receptor expressing metastatic colorectal cancer. *Annals of Oncology*, **17**, 450–6.

46. Hurwitz, H., Fehrenbacher, L., Novotny, W. *et al.* (2004). Bevacizumab plus irinotecan, fluorouracil and leucovorin for metastatic colorectal cancer. *New England Journal of Medicine*, **350**, 2335–42.

47. Samson, D. and Singer, C. (2001). Multiple myeloma, *Journal of the Royal College of Physicians of London*, **1**, 365–70.

48. Samson, D. *et al.* (1989). Infusion of vincristine and doxorubicin with oral dexamethasone as first-line therapy for multiple myeloma. *Lancet*, **2**, 882–5.

49. Attal, M. *et al.* (1996). A prospective randomised trial of autologous bone marrow transplantation and chemotherapy for multiple myeloma. *New England Journal of Medicine*, **335**, 91–7.

50. Berenson, J.R. *et al.* (1996). Efficacy of pamidronate in reducing skeletal events in patients with advanced multiple myeloma. *New England Journal of Medicine*, **334**, 488–93.

51. Le Chevalier. *et al.* (1988). Early metastatic cancer of unknown origin at presentation. A clinical study of 302 consecutive autopsied patients. *Archives of Internal Medicine*, **148**, 2035-9.

52. Mainsworth, J.D. and Greco, F.A., (1993). Treatment of patients with cancer of an unknown primary site. *New England Journal of Medicine*, **329**, 257–63.

53. Anderson, H. *et al.* (1983). VAC chemotherapy for metastatic carcinoma from unknown primary site. *European Journal of Cancer*, **19**, 49–52.

54. Schnipper, L.E. and Strom, T.B. (2001). A magic bullet for cancer – how near and how far? *New England Journal of Medicine*, **345**, 283–4.

9.2

Radiotherapy in symptom management

Peter J. Hoskin

Introduction

The majority of cancer patients will require radiation therapy at some time in the course of their disease with many having several treatment episodes. Radiotherapy has a major role in symptom control and over half of all radiation treatments are given with palliative intent for control of local symptoms.

General principles of radiotherapy

Radiobiology

Radiotherapy is treatment with ionizing radiation which causes damage to DNA. The most frequently used forms of ionizing radiation in clinical practice are x-rays produced from an x-ray machine or linear accelerator and gamma rays produced from a radioactive source. Biologically these have identical effects. Particle radiation is also sometimes used, in particular electrons for superficial treatments and beta particles from systemic radioisotopes. Proton therapy has advantages in some settings such as base of skull tumours but is not indicated in palliative treatments.

The results of radiation passing through a living cell are to cause both direct and indirect damage to the DNA of the cell. Direct damage results in base deletions and single and double strand breaks in the DNA chain. Indirect damage, which is the major component of the radiation effect, is a result of the interaction of radiation with water molecules in the cell releasing toxic free radicals. Normal cells have a large capacity to repair most of this 'sub-lethal' radiation damage but this is less efficient in malignant cells. Differences in repair capacity partly account for the variations seen in radiosensitivity. The mechanism of cell death after radiation exposure may be either reproductive failure due to DNA damage or apoptosis through its impact on the cell regulatory mechanisms.

The response of cells to radiation is affected by other factors in addition to DNA repair capacity. These include oxygenation (hypoxic cells are relatively radioresistant), the number of cells actively dividing (cells in certain phases of the cell cycle are more sensitive than others; non-cycling cells are relatively radioresistant), and the rate of repopulation within the tumour. These parameters of repair, re-oxygenation, repopulation, and redistribution within the cell cycle, are the fundamental influences on the cellular response to radiation. In clinical practice, radiation is delivered to maximize tumour cell kill whilst minimizing normal tissue damage by exploiting differences in these properties between normal and malignant cells.

Palliative compared to radical radiotherapy

The aim of radical radiotherapy is cure. This will require complete eradication of tumour cells within the treated volume which must encompass the entire extent of the tumour. An additional consideration in radical treatment is to minimize associated long-term normal tissue damage. In contrast, the aim of palliative radiotherapy is the control of symptoms with minimum associated acute radiation reaction.

These two very different aims result in different philosophies in the delivery of radiation. To minimize normal tissue damage the radiation dose is built up by delivering treatment on a daily basis over several weeks. Conventional treatment schedules deliver a single dose of radiation, often called a fraction, daily Monday to Friday. In this way, high doses of radiation close to or beyond those which surrounding normal tissues will tolerate can be given. Greater tumour damage may be achieved by *acceleration* of the treatment to reduce the opportunities for tumour repopulation. This is achieved by giving treatment two or three times a day over a relatively shorter period. The extent to which a schedule can be accelerated is limited by the increase in acute normal tissue reaction which is seen. In order to deliver higher doses with sparing of normal tissues, *hyperfractionation* may be employed in which the total dose is delivered in an increased number of fractions but given over the same period as a daily treatment by dividing the daily dose into two or three smaller doses; in this way a greater total daily dose can be delivered than when delivered as a single daily dose. This considerable investment in time by the patient can be readily justified where cure is the aim but for patients with a survival of only a few weeks or months a treatment period of 6–8 weeks will represent a major proportion of their remaining life span. In the palliative setting, therefore simpler, more pragmatic schedules are more appropriate provided they are effective in their aim of achieving local symptom control. In general, symptom control does not require complete eradication of the tumour and indeed in some scenarios, for example metastatic bone pain, symptom response appears independent of tumour shrinkage.

Table 9.2.1 Types of external beam radiotherapy.

	Energy	Source	Depth of penetration	Clinical use
Superficial x-rays	50–150 kV	X-ray tube	5–10 mm	Surface skin tumours
Orthovoltage x-rays	250–500 kV	X-ray tube	15–30 mm	Surface tumours
				Superficial bones, e.g. ribs, sacrum
Electrons	4–20 MeV	Linear accelerator	15–70 mm	Surface tumours
				Superficial bones, e.g. ribs, sacrum
				Lymph nodes
Megavoltage x-rays	4–25 MV	Linear accelerator	3–20 cm	Main source of radiation beams for sites other than above
Gamma rays	2.5 MV	Cobalt source	5–10 cm	All sites except superficial skin

A large proportion of the cells in a tumour, between 60 and 80 per cent of the total, will be killed by the first one or two radiation exposures from a course of treatment. In radical treatment, the challenge is to eradicate the remainder whilst in palliative treatment this initial effect may be more than adequate for long-term symptom control. Thus most palliative treatments can be delivered in one or two treatments and rarely is it necessary to extend a course of treatment beyond 1 week. The delivery of short relatively low dose schedules will also result in less acute reaction and a minimal risk of late damage to normal tissues within the expected life span of the patient.

Clinical radiation delivery

The aim of radiotherapy in clinical practice is to accurately deliver an effective dose of radiation with minimal side effects. There are three main types of radiation therapy:

- external beam treatment;
- brachytherapy;
- systemic radioisotope therapy.

The most common type of radiotherapy is external beam irradiation. The different modes of external beam radiation are shown in Table 9.2.1. In a modern radiotherapy department, most treatments will be given using a linear accelerator producing high energy x-ray beams or for superficial lesions an electron beam. Fig. 9.2.1 shows patient being prepared for treatment on a modern linear accelerator.

Brachytherapy is the use of a radioactive source placed directly onto or within the area to be treated so that radiation is given directly into the tumour. Examples of this are shown in Table 9.2.2.

Systemic radioisotopes are used in situations where a specific tissue or pathophysiology can be targeted for example radioiodine for thyroid cancer and strontium for bone metastases. Radiation is damaging to normal tissues and it is therefore important to ensure that it is directed as accurately as possible to the area requiring treatment whilst minimizing the amount of sensitive normal tissue within the treated area. The process of defining with accuracy the treatment volume and optimal treatment technique is called 'planning'. The steps in treatment planning are as follows:

- Immobilization: it may be necessary to immobilize the patient particularly when treating an area where small movements can result in the beam passing through critical structures for example around the eye. The patient may be immobilized using simple techniques such as sandbags or for more complex treatments a plastic shell using an individualized face mask may be necessary.

- Treatment volume localization: superficial lesions which are visible or palpable can be easily defined on clinical examination but deep-seated tumours require radiographic localization. In many common palliative scenarios such as bone metastases or a primary lung tumour plain x-ray images are sufficient for localization. A treatment simulator will be used which is an x-ray machine identical to the therapy machine in its geometric specifications and movement but which differs by emitting a diagnostic x-ray beam producing an image of the proposed therapeutic beam. For more

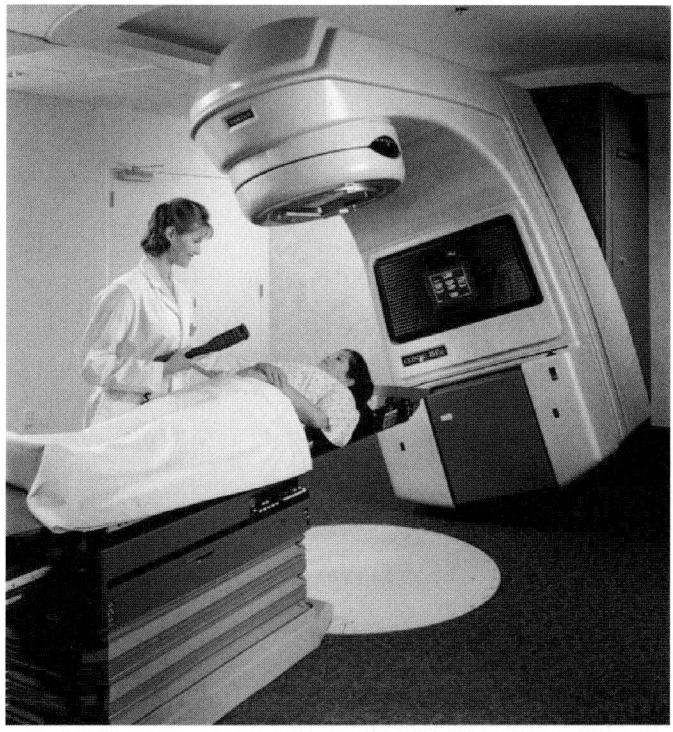

Clinac® Accelerators: Clinac 23EX with MLC-120 and PortalVision™

Figure 9.2.1 Treatment with a modern linear accelerator (courtesy Varian Medical, United Kingdom).

Table 9.2.2 Isotope use in brachytherapy.

Intracavitary	Caesium	Intrauterine
	Cobalt	Intravaginal
	Iridium	Intrauterin and intravaginal
		Endo-oesophageal
		Endobronchial
		Endorectal
Interstitial	Iridium	Tongue, floor of mouth
		Buccal mucosa
		Breast
		Anal canal
		Vulva / vagina
Surface (mould)	Iridium	Skin
		Penis

deep seated tumours localization can be enhanced by coupling the simulator process with CT scanning which is now used for most planning situations in radiotherapy. This enables accurate three-dimensional reproduction of the anatomical region of interest ensuring not only clear definition of the treatment volume but also surrounding normal tissues.

◆ Dosimetric planning: once the volume has been defined then the means of treatment delivery is determined. For simple treatments such as those to bone metastases a single beam or two opposing beams to treat a block of tissue will be all that is required; for internal volumes more complex three- or four-field arrangements may be optimal.

◆ Verification: the defined beam arrangement must be checked on the patient before treatment delivery. Beam position may be checked by imaging on the treatment machine using the megavoltage treatment beam or on modern linear accelerators integrated CT imaging. In simple superficial fields, clinical measurement and observation are adequate. Accurate documentation of the beam position with indelible marking of defined skin entry points on the patient will facilitate this and ensure accurate day to day reproducibility where more than one fraction is to be given.

A linear accelerator produces high energy radiation at a rate of around 1 Gy per minute which means that most treatments even using large single fractions in the palliative setting will last for only a few minutes. There are no accompanying symptoms during radiation exposure provided the patient is comfortable at the outset. It is important to facilitate patient compliance with the procedure to ensure that they can cooperate in achieving the required position and lying still during treatment. Unfortunately some of the constraints of accurate radiation delivery may impinge upon this, for example the need to immobilize the patient in a fixed position, the use of hard wooden flat couches and the need for staff to leave the patient isolated whilst radiation delivery is taking place.

The judicious administration of analgesia or anxiolytic drugs prior to treatment for those having significant pain or other symptoms should always be considered.

Side effects of radiotherapy

The side effects of radiotherapy are categorized into two groups based on their timing relative to the radiation exposure. Acute effects will be seen during and may persist for several weeks after radiotherapy. Late effects are rarely seen before 9 months after treatment but there is then an ongoing risk for many years if not forever that they may appear. They are therefore two distinct events with different aetiologies.

The common clinical manifestations of acute and late radiation toxicity are shown in Table 9.2.3.

Acute toxicity is due to loss of surface epithelial cells resulting in skin erythema or desquamation, mucositis in the oropharynx, oesophagitis, cystitis or gastrointestinal irritation. Repair of the denuded surface with new epithelial cells occurs once treatment is completed provided that the underlying stem cell population has not been damaged irreparably. Recovery usually occurs within a period of a few days or weeks from treatment. On rare occasions however there may be persistent damage, termed 'consequential

Table 9.2.3 Acute and late effects of radiation.

Site	Acute effect	Late effect*
Skin	Erythema	Atrophy, fibrosis
	Desquamation	Telangectasia
		Necrosis
Gastrointestinal tract	Nausea, anorexia	Stricture
	Vomiting	Telangiectasia, bleeding
	Diarrhoea	Perforation
		Malabsorption
		Chronic enteritis, colitis, proctitis
Bladder	Sterile cystitis	Reduced volume
		Telangiectasia, bleeding
		Urethral or ureteric stricture
		Fistula
Oral cavity	Mucositis	Mucosal atrophy
Pharynx	Dry mouth	Telangiectasia, bleeding
	Taste loss	Dental caries
		Mandibular necrosis
Lung	Pneumonitis	Fibrosis
Central nervous system	Transient demyelination	Myelitis
	Lhermitte's sign	Necrosis
		Local oedema
Eye	Keratitis	Cataract
		Entropion or ectropion
		Dry eye

* in most patients only minor late effects are seen. These are minimized by reducing the dose of radiation delivered to sensitive structures with the treated region to known safe 'tolerance' doses. Late effects are not expected after palliative radiotherapy.

damage' seen particularly in vulnerable sites such as the back or the lower leg where skin healing appears less efficient. Poor healing after radiotherapy may also be seen where there is secondary infection or trauma and it is these events which can predispose to the rare occurrence of radionecrosis.

Late radiation damage is the major cause of treatment related loss of function and even mortality in patients receiving radical radiotherapy. It occurs due to vascular damage with pathological changes of endarteritis obliterans resulting in progressive closure of small blood vessels. The clinical manifestations of this may be relatively minor such as the commonly observed appearance of skin atrophy or telangiectasia seen on the skin and mucosal surfaces where radiation was delivered. More serious consequences due to tissue breakdown may however occasionally be seen. Common sites for this are within the pelvis where the bowel or bladder may be damaged resulting in fibrosis and bowel perforation or fistula formation between the bladder, bowel or vagina. In the central nervous system because of its very limited ability to repair damage catastrophic necrosis will occur if dose limits are exceeded. For every tissue a 'tolerance dose' is defined up to which late normal tissue damage is not expected in the 'normal' population. One of the reasons for the complex planning systems which have evolved for radiation delivery is the strenuous effort required to avoid exceeding these doses whilst delivering effective doses to nearby tumour. Unfortunately there are genetically predisposed individuals to radiation damage where even a conventional tolerance dose may result in late damage.

Management of radiation side effects

Acute side effects may still occur, even after relatively low dose palliative radiation. Management requires no more than relief of symptoms whilst allowing the affected area to heal.

Mild skin reactions require no active treatment. Local skin irritation can be relieved by application of aqueous cream. Desquamation will rarely if ever be seen after palliative doses. The use of topical preparations such as gentian violet is to be discouraged and talcum powder and proprietary creams containing metallic salts should be avoided at all costs during treatment as these can enhance the reaction. Starch powder as found in proprietary baby powders may be helpful in keeping the surrounding skin dry and comfortable.

Nausea during irradiation to the abdomen or pelvis will usually respond to simple antiemetic therapy such as metoclopramide 10 mg 6–8 hourly or where more severe 5HT-antagonists such as granisetron or ondansetron. Where anti-emetics are ineffective then a small dose of steroid such as prednisolone 10–30 mg daily may be valuable. Single doses given for bone pain to the lumbar spine and pelvis have an exit dose of radiation to the abdomen and prophylactic antiemetics given 30 min before treatment using dexamethasone 8 mg and a 5HT-antagonist such as granisetron or ondansetron is effective in avoiding severe symptoms.

Radiation-induced acute diarrhoea usually responds to dietary advice avoiding fruit and other fibre-containing foods and where required loperamide taken with each loose stool or codeine phosphate on a regular basis three to four times daily.

Radiation cystitis is more difficult to ameliorate. The use of an alpha blocker such as tamsulosin may be effective where there is severe bladder spasm and potassium citrate or cranberry juice are time-honoured remedies which may be of supportive value.

Where there is significant dysuria or strangury then systemic analgesics are also of value and secondary infection should be excluded.

Oropharyngeal mucositis occurs within the radiation field when treating the head and neck region. It is important to maintain a high level of oral hygiene using regular chlorhexidine mouthwashes and prophylactic anti-candidal preparations with nystatin suspension or clotrimazole gel. Local relief of pain may be achieved using soluble aspirin or benzydamine mouthwashes. Radical high dose treatment to the oral cavity particularly where the salivary glands are included in the treatment volume can result in troublesome mouth dryness, loss of taste and predispose to major dental caries and osteo-radionecrosis of the jaw. For this reason formal dental assessment pre-treatment and meticulous dental hygiene using fluoride dental gel, both during radiotherapy and thereafter, is important in these patients. However where simple low dose palliative treatment is to be given for example to a metastasis in the mandible, then such measures are not required. Throughout the oral cavity and pharyngeal tract, symptoms will be made worse in those patients who smoke or take alcoholic spirits and where possible these should be avoided during treatment. If symptoms are severe and nutritional intake is compromised enteral feeding, using a nasogastric fine bore tube or more commonly a percutaneous gastrostomy, may be required.

Pneumonitis may be seen even after palliative treatment to the lungs. This will present with a dry cough and dyspnoea up to 4 months after treatment and has a classical appearance on chest x-ray shown in Fig. 9.2.2, with patchy shadowing conforming to the geometry of the radiation field. A 2- to 3-week course of systemic steroids with antibiotics for secondary infection is recommended but continuing symptoms and late radiation fibrosis may well ensue.

It is always important to anticipate probable acute side effects, explain their likelihood to the patient and encourage the prophylactic use of anti-emetics, anti-diarrhoeal drugs and mouthwashes. The patient should also be reassured that these are temporary events which will resolve following completion of radiotherapy.

Combined modality treatment

There is increasing use of combined modality treatment in which chemotherapy is given during a course of radical radiotherapy

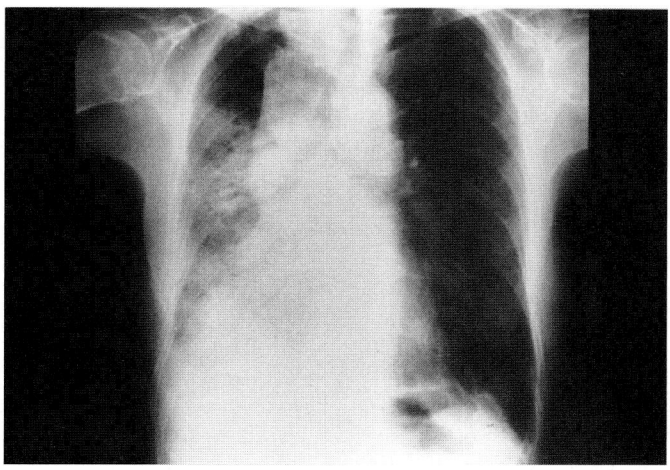

Figure 9.2.2 Interstitial pneumonitis in the right and lower zones on chest radiograph after palliative radiotherapy for carcinoma of the bronchus.

to enhance the effects. Many sites have now been shown in large randomized Phase III trials to benefit from the addition of chemotherapy to a radical course of radiotherapy. This includes treatments of cancers from the oesophagus[1], anal canal[2], uterine cervix[3], non-small-cell lung cancer[4] and head and neck region[5]. There are other instances however where chemotherapy may be given before (neo-adjuvant) or more commonly after (adjuvant) radiotherapy to provide early control of micro-metastasis whilst the radiotherapy obtains local control of the more bulky primary site. Examples are seen in the modern management of breast cancer, small cell lung cancer, colorectal cancer and lymphoma. Few if any of these treatments however fall readily within the scope of palliative medicine.

Specific indications for radiotherapy and symptom control

Radiotherapy is effective for many cancer-related symptoms particularly those due to pressure or infiltration by a tumour. A simple classification and examples of these is shown in Table 9.2.4.

Bone metastases

Radiotherapy may be indicated for bone metastases because of bone pain, pathological fracture or pressure on nerves. The majority of patients with bone metastases survive for less than 1 year and radiotherapy will achieve pain control over this period for the majority of patients. With short median predicted survival times a simple short treatment schedule is most appropriate.

Bone pain

Radiotherapy is a highly effective treatment for local metastatic bone pain. The use of radiotherapy in this setting has been subject to extensive investigation in randomized clinical trials over the past decade or more. There are now three meta-analyses including over 3000 patients all of which conclude as shown in Fig. 9.2.3 that there is no advantage for prolonged fractionated courses of radiotherapy over simple single fraction treatments delivering a dose of 8 Gy[6–8]. The results from a large randomized UK trial evaluating this shown in Fig. 9.2.4 demonstrates that this is maintained out to 12 months after treatment with response rates of around 80 per cent[9]. However, some patients still receive a more protracted fractionated course of treatment delivering 20–30 Gy over 1–2 weeks which is preferred by some centres where there is concern over possible fracture or nerve compression.

When accurate prospective assessments of pain have been used to monitor the response to the local irradiation of painful bone metastasis an increasing incidence of pain relief is seen for several weeks from the time of treatment and whilst around half of patients will respond achieving pain relief within the first 2–4 weeks others may yet experience improved pain 6–8 weeks after treatment as shown in Fig. 9.2.4.

A consistent finding from the meta-analyses is that after single dose treatments a higher proportion of patients require retreatment, accounting for around 25 per cent of patients in most trials. This is not a justification for more prolonged treatments however, since single treatments can again be used effectively for retreatment. The Dutch bone pain trial[10] has specifically looked at the impact of retreatment on outcome and confirms that even when the effect of retreatment is allowed for that single dose radiotherapy is equivalent to multifraction treatment in this setting of localized bone pain.

Table 9.2.4 Indications for radiotherapy in symptom palliation.

Symptom	Cause
Pain	
Bone pain	Bone metastases
Visceral pain	Soft tissue metastases
Neuropathic pain	Bone metastases
	Soft tissue primary or metastases
	Intrinsic tumour in nerve tissue
Local pressure	
Spinal canal compression	Extradural metastases
	Bone metastases
Cranial nerve palsies	Skull base bone metastases
	Meningeal metastases
	Intrinsic brain tumour
Obstruction	
Bronchus	Intrinsic bronchial tumour
	Extrinsic lymphadenopathy
Oesophagus	Intrinsic oesophageal tumour
	Extrinsic lymphadenopathy
Superior vena cava	Primary mediastinal tumour
	Primary lung or oesophageal tumour
	Metastatic mediastinal lymphadenopathy
Hydrocephalus	Malignant meningitis
	Primary or metastatic brain tumour
Limb swelling	Metastatic lymphadenopathy
Bleeding	
Haemoptysis	Primary bronchial tumour
	Metastatic bronchial or lung tumour
Haematuria	Primary tumour in kidney,
	Ureter, bladder, prostate
Vaginal bleeding	Primary tumours of vagina, cervix or uterus
	Metastases in vagina
Rectal bleeding	Primary anal or colorectal tumours

Re-irradiation should certainly be considered where pain returns after a previous good response but may also be of value where the initial response is unsatisfactory. The probability of response after re-treatment is around 80 per cent, similar to that after primary treatment and is not always predicted by the initial response[11].

The treatment techniques for bone metastasis are simple. Superficial bones such as the clavicle, ribs, and sacrum may be treated with a direct field using orthovoltage x-rays or electrons and other sites will be treated using a linear accelerator or cobalt beam. Under optimal conditions the site will be localized using a treatment simulator based on clinical examination and radiographic or bone scan evidence of metastatic disease. Increasingly CT simulation is used from which fields can be more accurately defined[12].

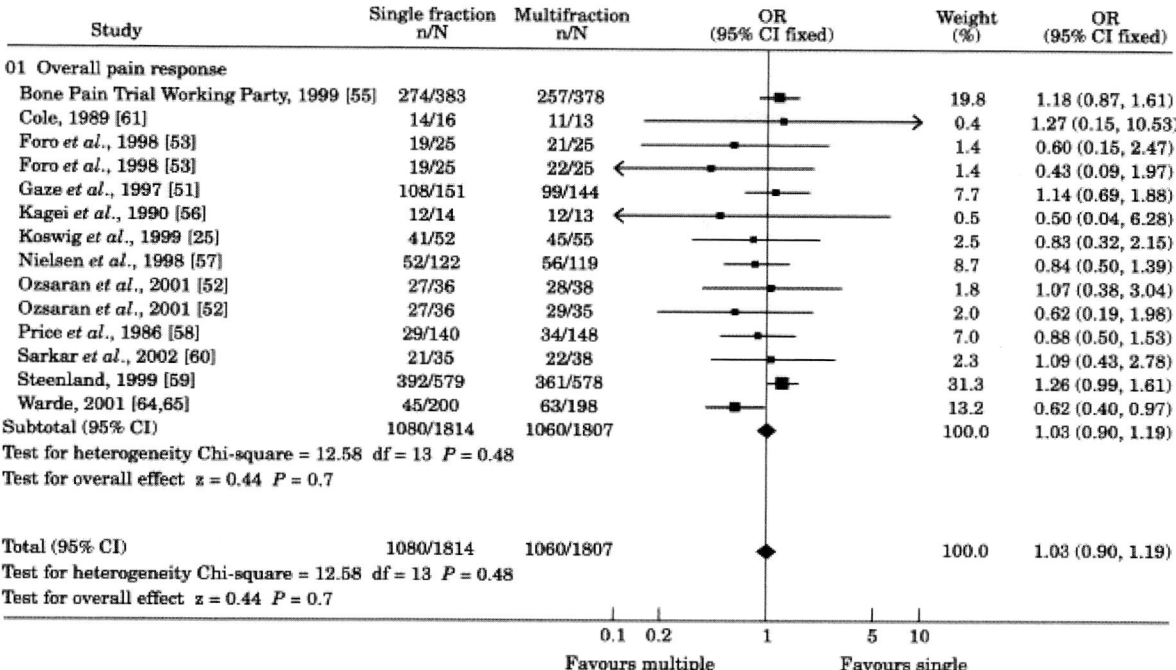

Study	Single fraction n/N	Multifraction n/N	OR (95% CI fixed)	Weight (%)	OR (95% CI fixed)
01 Overall pain response					
Bone Pain Trial Working Party, 1999 [55]	274/383	257/378		19.8	1.18 (0.87, 1.61)
Cole, 1989 [61]	14/16	11/13		0.4	1.27 (0.15, 10.53)
Foro et al., 1998 [53]	19/25	21/25		1.4	0.60 (0.15, 2.47)
Foro et al., 1998 [53]	19/25	22/25		1.4	0.43 (0.09, 1.97)
Gaze et al., 1997 [51]	108/151	99/144		7.7	1.14 (0.69, 1.88)
Kagei et al., 1990 [56]	12/14	12/13		0.5	0.50 (0.04, 6.28)
Koswig et al., 1999 [25]	41/52	45/55		2.5	0.83 (0.32, 2.15)
Nielsen et al., 1998 [57]	52/122	56/119		8.7	0.84 (0.50, 1.39)
Ozsaran et al., 2001 [52]	27/36	28/38		1.8	1.07 (0.38, 3.04)
Ozsaran et al., 2001 [52]	27/36	29/35		2.0	0.62 (0.19, 1.98)
Price et al., 1986 [58]	29/140	34/148		7.0	0.88 (0.50, 1.53)
Sarkar et al., 2002 [60]	21/35	22/38		2.3	1.09 (0.43, 2.78)
Steenland, 1999 [59]	392/579	361/578		31.3	1.26 (0.99, 1.61)
Warde, 2001 [64,65]	45/200	63/198		13.2	0.62 (0.40, 0.97)
Subtotal (95% CI)	1080/1814	1060/1807		100.0	1.03 (0.90, 1.19)

Test for heterogeneity Chi-square = 12.58 df = 13 P = 0.48
Test for overall effect z = 0.44 P = 0.7

Total (95% CI)	1080/1814	1060/1807		100.0	1.03 (0.90, 1.19)

Test for heterogeneity Chi-square = 12.58 df = 13 P = 0.48
Test for overall effect z = 0.44 P = 0.7

0.1 0.2   1   5 10
Favours multiple   Favours single

Figure 9.2.3 Results of meta-analysis of fractionation studies for metastatic bone pain (from[7] with permission).

It is particularly important to document carefully the field margin since most patients will have multiple sites of metastasis and further treatment with the potential for overlap of fields may be required. This is of particular concern in the spine where metastasis at several levels may require sequential treatment. Overlap of fields in the spine can result in overdosage to the spinal cord with the risk of subsequent radiation myelitis and irreversible neurological deterioration developing within 6–9 months from treatment. For patients with a short prognosis this may not be relevant and a positive decision to accept an overlap may be made, with the full knowledge of the patient, where it is considered that benefit from treatment in the short term outweighs any theoretical hazard of later myelitis; in others however where the expected prognosis is greater than 6 months the risks may be an issue.

Many patients have multiple sites of disease with pain that is often not well localized but presents as a diffuse symptom affecting multiple sites. Such patients should be considered for wide field radiotherapy or radioisotope therapy.

Wide field radiotherapy delivers treatment to an area which may include up to half the body as described above using doses of 6 Gy to the upper half-body where the lungs limit higher doses, or 8 Gy to the lower half-body. Again no advantage for higher doses has been seen, although a recent large randomized trial has recommended 8 Gy in two fractions as the optimum dose[13]. Inevitably wide field treatment is associated with greater toxicity than local field irradiation with around two-thirds of patients having gastrointestinal symptoms of nausea, vomiting or diarrhoea and the majority a period of bone marrow suppression following treatment. This may result in some patients requiring blood transfusions but rarely is severe enough to cause clinically relevant neutropenia or thrombocytopenia. Spontaneous recovery is to be expected and indeed sequential treatment of upper and lower half-bodies is possible given a 4- to 6-week gap for marrow recovery.

The most serious consequence of upper hemibody irradiation is the development of radiation pneumonitis, which is avoided by limiting the dose to 6 Gy through the lungs. Hemibody irradiation is a valuable tool for the treatment of widespread bone pain and response rates are consistently around 80 per cent maintained in the majority of patients until their death[13–14].

The timing of response varies between local radiotherapy to an isolated bone metastasis and wide field hemibody radiotherapy. Rapid responses are often seen after wide field radiotherapy and this contrast is illustrated in Fig. 9.2.5. Timing of response is important in considering whether alternative treatments or re-irradiation should be considered.

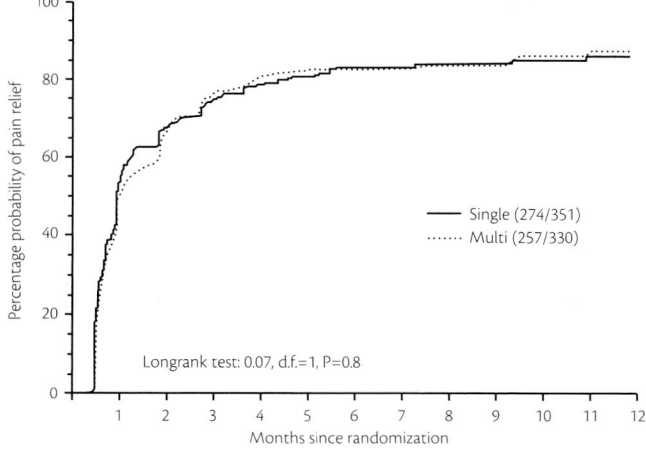

Figure 9.2.4 Probability of pain relief seen after local radiotherapy for metastatic bone pain (from[9] with permission).

Radioisotope treatment is an alternative means of delivering radiation to multiple sites of bone metastasis. Radioactive isotopes which are used to selectively concentrate at sites of bone metastasis are shown in Table 9.2.5. The ideal isotope in this setting will deliver radiation dose by the release of beta particles with a short range of only a few millimetres thereby concentrating their dose within the immediate area of uptake but also have low energy gamma release which enables imaging with a gamma camera.

In the specific case of differentiated thyroid cancer, using radio-iodine, published series reported disappointingly low response rate in terms of bone pain relief after radio-iodine and external beam therapy is considered better for painful bone metastasis in this setting[15].

The most commonly used isotopes are strontium[16] and samarium[17]. Both compounds are highly effective in achieving pain relief with similar response rates to wide field external beam irradiation and few side effects[18]. Their efficacy has been demonstrated predominantly in prostate cancer but bone metastases from other primary sites in particular breast and lung are effectively treated. Efficacy has also been demonstrated in metastases from osteosarcoma which retain an osteblastic response thereby concentrating isotope.

These agents are given as a single dose intravenous injection; strontium having no gamma release has no additional restrictions for the patient other than careful disposal of urine.

Transient bone marrow depression may be seen but is rarely of clinical significance provided patients have a normal blood count before treatment.

The radioisotope is cleared by renal excretion; patients therefore must be continent of urine to prevent contamination with radioactive urine, or be prepared to have a catheter passed for the duration of radioactive excretion. Renal impairment is also a relative contraindication causing prolonged clearance and potentially exacerbating bone marrow toxicity due to extended radiation exposure.

Despite their proven efficacy, convenience, and favourable toxicity profile radioisotope therapy for bone metastases is relatively underused, particularly in less wealthy health ecomonies due to their cost.

The mechanism by which radiation achieves pain control is not clear. A considerable proportion of malignant cells within a

Table 9.2.5 Radioisotopes available for treatment of metastatic bone pain.

Tumour specific	Bone specific	Bisphosponate conjugates
131I	89Sr	153Sm
		186Re
		188Re

tumour mass are undoubtedly killed after small single doses of radiation similar to those which result in pain relief but rapid tumour shrinkage is not routinely observed at these dose levels. Further evidence suggesting that tumour shrinkage itself may not be necessary include the observation that rapid pain relief may be seen within 24 h of treatment particularly after hemibody irradiation (Fig. 9.2.3), that no relationship has been shown between the response in terms of pain relief and different histological types of tumour correlating with variations in radiosensitivity and that no clear dose response effect above 8 Gy has been shown for the onset or duration of pain relief. Other factors may therefore be important in particular local effects upon the mechanisms involved in the pathophysiology of bone metastases. Osteoclast activation is a fundamental and universal step in establishing metastatic bone disease; hence the efficacy of bisphosphonate drugs which are potent osteoclast inhibitors. In metastatic bone pain, it has been demonstrated that changes in biochemical markers of osteoclast activity occur following radiotherapy to bone pain which can predict for response[19], supporting the hypothesis that this may also be important in the mechanism of action of radiation.

The increased understanding of the pathophysiology of metastatic bone pain has led to further developments in treatment. Current research is seeking to evaluate the role of pregabalin with radiotherapy and new agents directed at RANKL, a pivotal molecule in osteoclast activation are also under evaluation.

Prophylactic radiotherapy to bone metastases

Radiotherapy has no routine role in the prophylactic treatment of bone metastases. Inadvertent irradiation of certain sites such as the thoracic spine when a breast is irradiated has been shown to reduce the instance of subsequent bone metastases in that region of the spine. Additional hemibody irradiation at the time of presentation of localized bone pain has been evaluated and a reduction in subsequent episodes of bone pain demonstrated[20]. Similarly the use of radioactive strontium has been explored when bone metastases first presented and this also has been shown to reduce or delay the need for further treatment for bone pain[21]. The gains are relatively modest, hemibody irradiation resulting in a 16 per cent reduction in requirements for additional local radiotherapy and strontium delaying the median time to further radiotherapy for a site of bone pain by 15 weeks.

In practice the best evidence base for prophylactic treatment is for bisphosphonates which are now routinely given for myeloma and high risk patients with breast cancer where there is proven benefit[22,23]. The relative roles of radiotherapy and bisphosphonates and the interaction between them in the overall management of bone metastases have yet to be defined and is currently an active area of research[24].

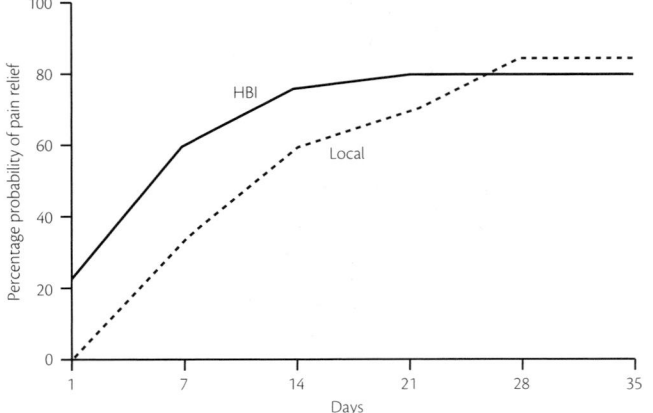

Figure 9.2.5 Comparison of onset of pain relief after hemibody radiotherapy compared to local radiotherapy (from[14] with permission).

Pathological fracture

Pathological fracture at a site of bone metastasis may occur spontaneously or as a result of minor trauma particularly in weight-bearing bones. Surgical internal fixation is the preferred management in long bones but there will be situations including vertebral collapse and fractures of the rib and girdle bones where surgery is not feasible. Surgery may also be inappropriate where a patient has fracture of a long bone but advanced disease or poor performance status. In these cases, local irradiation remains a valuable palliative tool both to achieve local pain relief and to enable bone healing. When the object of treatment is pain relief alone a single dose of 8 Gy is adequate treatment and following irradiation around two-thirds of patients with pathological fracture will achieve pain relief. There are no comparative data defining the optimal dose to achieve bone healing after pathological fracture. Remineralization is reported in one-third of patients after doses of 40–50 Gy delivered in 4–5 weeks but anecdotally is also seen after lower doses of only 20 Gy in 2 weeks. In practice, most patients will receive courses delivering 20–30 Gy in 5–10 fractions over 1–2 weeks.

Radiotherapy may also be indicated postoperatively following internal fixation to prevent further progression of the remaining metastatic tumour and enable healing of the bone around the prosthesis. There is however little published data to support this common practice although non-randomized data suggest better functional recovery when radiotherapy is given[25]. Conventionally fields covering the entire length of the prosthesis or intra-medullary nail are used because of the perceived risk of dissemination through the marrow cavity by the operative procedure. Patients with widespread metastatic disease and limited survival whose pain is controlled postoperatively gain little benefit from postoperative radiotherapy and this should be deferred unless local pain develops.

Neurological symptoms

Spinal cord and cauda equina compression

Spinal cord or cauda equina compression with loss of function of limbs and loss of sphincter control is catastrophic It occurs because of tumour compression of neurological tissue in the spinal canal. The initial events are predominantly vascular with venous engorgement and oedema followed by mechanical compression with ultimately irreversible damage to the nervous tissue. Magnetic resonance imaging (MRI) of spinal cord compression has shown around one-quarter of these cases to be due to direct encroachment of the spinal canal by tumour arising in a vertebral body with the remainder attributable to blood-borne extradural or intradural metastasis[26] as demonstrated in Fig. 9.2.6. Approximately 70 per cent of cases involve thoracic cord, 20 per cent the lumbosacral region, and 10 per cent the cervical cord.

Early diagnosis is essential in this condition and the major determinant of outcome independent of treatment. It should be considered and excluded in any patient presenting with sensory or motor changes in the limbs or urinary symptoms, in particular where there is associated backache or known vertebral metastasis. Urgent imaging of the spinal canal using MRI as the method of choice is mandatory even where recent investigations have shown no evidence of metastatic disease. Alternative but less satisfactory imaging methods of the spinal canal where MRI is unavailable or in the occasional patient where it is contraindicated because of metal implants or a pacemaker, include spinal myelography and

CT imaging. Where MRI is negative and the picture is of cauda equina involvement a lumbar puncture should be performed having excluded raised intracranial pressure, to exclude carcinomatous meningitis. Fig. 9.2.6 demonstrates spinal cord compression from direct invasion of a bone metastasis (A) and extradural tumour metastasis (B).

Histological diagnosis is essential before embarking upon definitive treatment. In many patients, there will already be an underlying diagnosis of metastatic malignancy but in one series 48 per cent of patients presenting with spinal cord compression

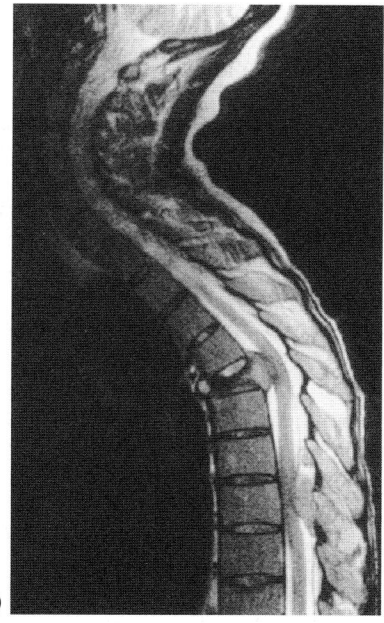

(A)

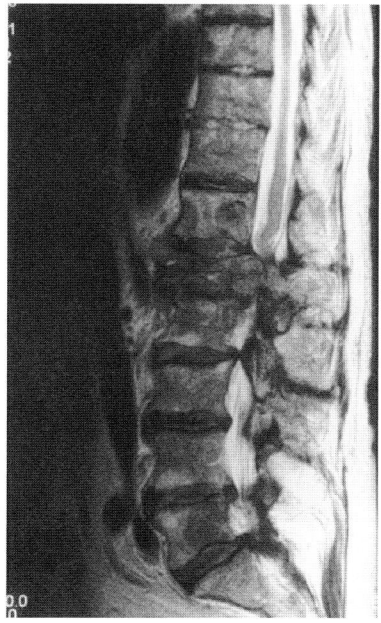

(B)

Figure 9.2.6 Magnetic resonance imaging of spinal cord compression demonstrating (A) both extradural and vertebral collapse with adjacent compression and (B) direct infiltration of the canal from bone metastases in the spine.

had no previous history of malignant disease[27]. The commonest sites for spinal cord compression are breast, lung, and prostate, each accounting for over 20 per cent of patients in most series. Most other primary sites have also been associated with spinal canal involvement the next two commonest being kidney and lymphoma. Where a patient with no metastatic disease presents with spinal cord compression it is usually reasonable to assume that this will be the same disease process unless there are atypical features to suggest a second primary. In most cases, where a histological diagnosis is not available a CT-guided fine needle aspirate cytology specimen or needle biopsy will be sufficient[28].

Initial management for most patients should include high-dose steroids (dexamethasone 4 mg 6-hourly). Certain histological types of tumour should be considered for primary chemotherapy and these include lymphoma and small-cell lung cancer.

Both radiotherapy and decompressive surgery are effective in the initial management of spinal cord compression. In patients who have extensive vertebral collapse with intrusion to the spinal canal radiotherapy is of little value in re-establishing neurological function. It is in this group of patients that surgery has its main application with the use of anterior spinal surgery involving resection and spinal stabilization. This represents a more invasive procedure than radiotherapy with significant operative morbidity and even mortality but results in series of selected patients are superior to either laminectomy or radiotherapy alone, with between 62 and 83 per cent of patients being able to walk following anterior surgery and pain relief being achieved in 71 per cent[29,30]. Many of these patients however have poor general condition as shown by a 30 per cent mortality in one series of 26 consecutive patients operated on for pain or neurological deficits, and careful selection of patients for surgical referral is therefore required[31].

One randomized trial has compared radiotherapy with decompressive surgery and postoperative radiotherapy showing a significant advantage for the group receiving initial surgery both for functional status and survival. The population in this trial was selected for those with good performance status, absent metastases elsewhere and a single level of spinal cord compression; patients falling into this category should be referred for primary surgery to be followed by postoperative radiotherapy. Whilst no randomized comparison of the two modalities of treatment with sufficient numbers to provide a true comparison has been undertaken no advantage of surgery over radiotherapy has been demonstrated in published series where patients have a previously confirmed diagnosis of malignant disease and no evidence of vertebral collapse. The role of postoperative radiotherapy has not been tested but a non-randomized comparison has suggested that better pain relief is seen after radiotherapy or where radiotherapy is given postoperatively[32].

Many patients however will fall outside these criteria and will receive primary radiotherapy. The radiation technique in most cases is simple using a single posterior field to encompass the vertebral level and a suitable margin. With accurate localization using MR one vertebral body or 3 cm above and below the area of cord compression is adequate. Problems may arise where there are multiple sites of compression particularly if anatomically distant and in some patients more than one radiation field may be required to cover for example sites in the high thoracic and lumbar region. Where there is a large para-vertebral mass more complex planning may be necessary to ensure complete coverage. Two or three angled fields to cover the tumour volume taking care to avoid sensitive para-vertebral structures, in particular the kidneys in the lower thoracic and upper lumbar regions, may be needed.

Most patients with good performance status will receive fractionated courses of treatment delivering 20–30 Gy in 5–10 fractions, however there is evidence that single doses are equally effective in terms of neurological function and survival[33]. The optimal dose fractionation schedule for metastatic spinal cord compression remains under investigation in current clinical trials. Recovery after paraplegia that has been established for more than 24 h is not to be expected and in these patients single doses of 8–10 Gy are often given for pain relief without any expectation of neurological recovery. In other selected cases, particularly those with a localized potentially curable tumour, such as a solitary plasmacytoma higher doses of up to 40 or 50 Gy over 3–5 weeks may be delivered.

The outcome of treatment depends primarily upon the speed of diagnosis and neurological status at initiation of treatment. When patients present ambulatory, 79 per cent are still ambulant following radiotherapy treatment; in contrast of those presenting with paraparesis only 42 per cent become ambulant and 20–25 per cent will suffer significant neurological deterioration during treatment by radiotherapy alone. Where pain relief is the goal of treatment, radiotherapy will achieve this in over three-quarters of patients compared with only one-third of patients following laminectomy. Histology may influence outcome, patients with myeloma and lymphoma having a better outcome than those with breast cancer who in turn respond better than those with lung or kidney primary tumours.

Since the outcome of treatment is best when diagnosis is made very early there would be considerable advantages in predicting those patients at risk of spinal cord compression and treating them prophylactically. It is possible using MRI to detect metastasis in vertebral bodies at very early stages of development and minor encroachment into the spinal canal which is often clinically asymptomatic and not detectable on plain radiographs. Other predictors for spinal canal compression reported in small cell lung cancer are local back pain associated with positive bone scan in the spine or cerebral metastasis with a positive bone scan. These situations are associated with cord compression in 36 and 25 per cent, respectively[34]. There is some evidence from the use of bisphosphonates that prophylactic treatment of subclinical bone metastasis can reduce spinal complications and similar observations have been made using early anti-androgen treatment in prostate cancer. In some centres, there is an aggressive policy of prophylactic irradiation for spinal metastasis on this basis.

The most important issue in the management of spinal cord compression remains high awareness of the condition and a low threshold for investigating relatively minor symptoms, particularly in patients with known vertebral metastasis or disease in the nervous system.

Brain metastasis

Up to 10 per cent of all cancers metastasize to the brain, the most common primary sites being the lung and breast; approximately one-third of these will be solitary deposits. Disability from brain metastasis is disproportionate to the bulk of the tumour with a very small deposit on the motor cortex having catastrophic results for the patient whilst a deposit of similar size would have little effect in the lung or liver. In many patients, therefore, brain metastases will present with a significant neurological deficit and poor performance status. The spread of malignant cells to the brain is via blood borne spread and therefore isolated brain metastatses are relatively unusual, the typical picture being in the context of more widespread metastatic disease in multiple other sites. Careful patient assessment and selection of those who may benefit from active treatment is therefore essential, recognizing that for a proportion this will herald the terminal phase of an advanced malignancy for which local treatment will have little benefit.

Initial management requires confirmation of the diagnosis by CT or magnetic resonance scanning and the introduction of steroids. This will help control raised intracranial pressure and where symptoms are due to oedema rather than tumour infiltration some initial improvement in neurological deficit is often seen. There is however also evidence that high dose steroids in this setting contribute significantly to morbidity and total doses of 4–8 mg dexamethasone daily may be adequate.

As with any other symptomatic metastatic disease it is important to have an underlying histological diagnosis. In general, whilst it is preferable to biopsy a site other than the brain if a solitary metastasis is present and this is the first manifestation of malignancy there may be no alternative.

Further management will then depend upon the general condition of the patient, underlying primary site and the distribution of the brain metastases. A simple algorithm is shown in Fig. 9.2.7[35].

Solitary metastases usually reflect a more favourable prognosis and in selected patients with no detectable systemic disease elsewhere surgical removal gives good local and long-term control. Postoperative radiotherapy is usually recommended on the basis of two randomized trials showing a statistically significant reduction in brain recurrence but because of a high incidence of death from progressive systemic disease there was no impact on overall survival. However, a third larger trial has failed to confirm this advantage for postoperative radiotherapy[35]. Localized high dose radiotherapy using radiosurgery is an alternative to surgical excision. There has been no formal comparison between the two but where surgery is limited by the site of metastasis and proximity to functionally critical structures it may be considered as an alternative. This uses either a dedicated multi-source cobalt unit (gamma knife) or a stereotactic multiple-arc radiotherapy technique from a linear accelerator. Radiosurgery is typically delivered as single doses of 15–20 Gy. The role of whole brain radiotherapy in addition to radiosurgery, analogous to the use of postoperative radiotherapy, remains uncertain but is recommended in some centres. More recent studies suggest that whilst this may reduce the likelihood of relapse outside the initial site of treatment additional whole brain radiotherapy has no survival benefit. Unfortunately despite surgery or radiosurgery achieving local control most patients still ultimately succumb to the effects of distant metastasis and careful selection and screening is required before embarking upon aggressive local therapy of this type.

Whole brain radiotherapy is well established as an effective palliative treatment for multiple cerebral metastasis. Overall headache, motor and sensory loss and confusion will respond to treatment in around 80 per cent of selected patients with a complete response of between 35 and 55 per cent[36]. However the median survival after irradiation for brain metastasis is less than 6 months reflecting the fact that brain metastasis often heralds widespread advanced metastatic disease with the majority of patients dying from the combined effect of distant metastasis rather than progressive disease in the brain alone. Twenty per-cent of patients who embark upon a course of radiotherapy for brain metastases fail to complete the course which highlights the need for careful selection in determining which patients may benefit from radiotherapy. In particular, those with multiple metastases outside the central nervous system and those with poor performance status with rapidly progressive disease are most likely to succumb within the period of treatment. Factors influencing survival after radiation are shown in Table 9.2.6.

Treatment techniques for multiple brain metastases are simple using lateral fields from each side (parallel opposed fields) covering the entire intracranial contents. A series of randomized trials have shown no benefit for doses greater than 20–30 Gy in 1–2 weeks[36] and more recent trials have shown that 12 Gy in two fractions is equivalent to 30 Gy in 10 fractions for symptom control with a small but clinically not significant improvement in survival of 7 days in the 30-Gy arm[37]. This difference was greater in a subgroup of good prognosis patients and the longer schedule may therefore be selected for this group but for patients with advanced disease and only moderate performance status a simple two fraction schedule is to be recommended.

There is usually little acute toxicity from a short palliative course of whole brain radiotherapy for multiple brain metastasis but an unfortunate and unavoidable effect is complete alopecia. Hair re-growth will occur within a period of 2–3 months but for many patients this is a particularly distressing and on occasions unacceptable cost of treatment. Mild scalp erythema may also occur particularly around the external pinnae and most patients will continue steroids through treatment, transient rises in intracranial pressure having been reported which can be troublesome if pressure is already raised when treatment starts. It is also important following completion of cranial irradiation, to reduce and if possible discontinue the steroids in order to minimize long-term side effects provided there is no neurological deterioration whilst doing so.

The majority of patients with multiple cerebral metastases will die from widespread metastatic disease outside the central nervous system but around a quarter will suffer persistent or recurrent symptomatic cerebral metastasis. Steroids may achieve short-term control of symptoms but significant side effects may occur. Re-treatment following a dose of 20–30 Gy carries a risk of radiation damage to the brain and there is often reluctance to consider

Table 9.2.6 Prognostic factors influencing survival after irradiation of brain metastases.

Increased survival	Decreased survival
◆ Brain first site of relapse	◆ Multiple lobes involved
◆ Brain sole site of relapse	◆ Meningeal disease
◆ Long disease-free interval	
◆ Performance status 0/1	
◆ Age <60 years	
◆ Prior to br ain relapse	
◆ Primary site in brain	

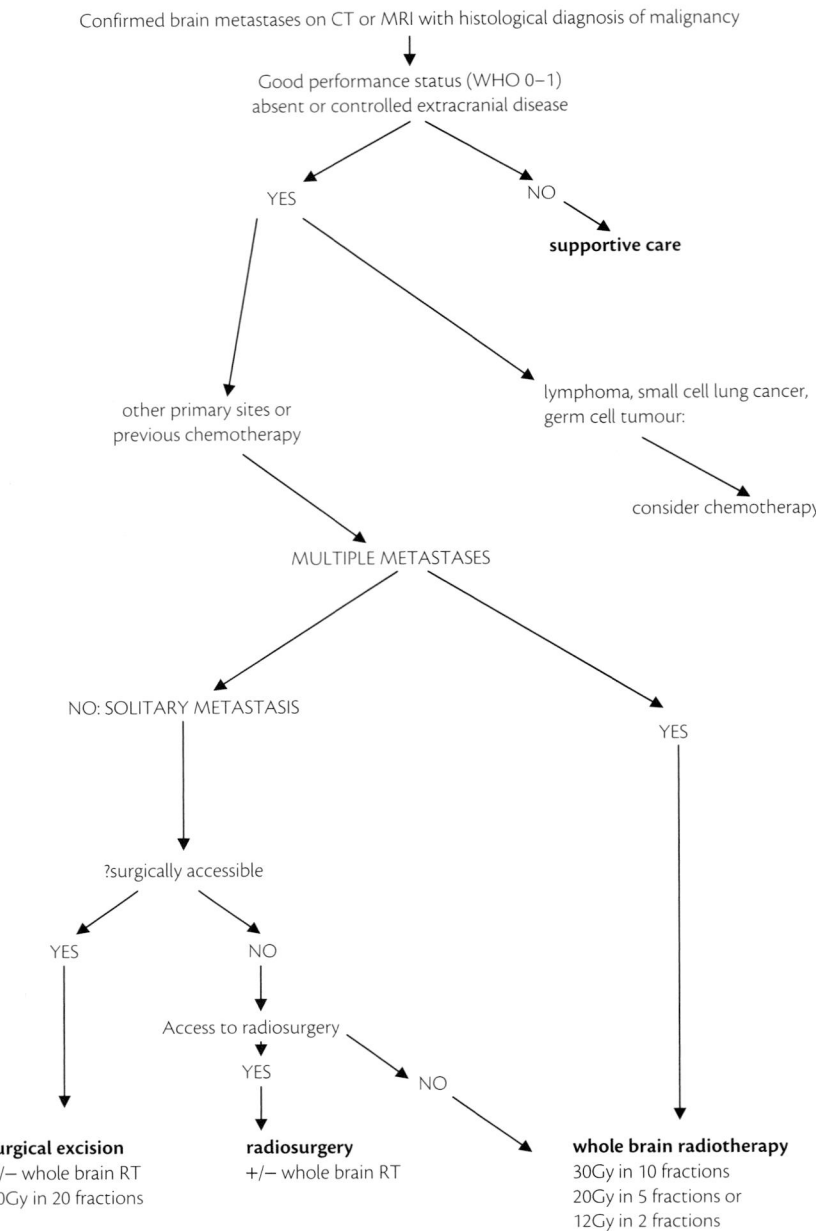

Confirmed brain metastases on CT or MRI with histological diagnosis of malignancy

Good performance status (WHO 0–1)
absent or controlled extracranial disease

YES

NO

supportive care

other primary sites or
previous chemotherapy

lymphoma, small cell lung cancer,
germ cell tumour:

consider chemotherapy

MULTIPLE METASTASES

NO: SOLITARY METASTASIS

YES

?surgically accessible

YES   NO

Access to radiosurgery

YES   NO

surgical excision
+/– whole brain RT
40Gy in 20 fractions

radiosurgery
+/– whole brain RT

whole brain radiotherapy
30Gy in 10 fractions
20Gy in 5 fractions or
12Gy in 2 fractions

Figure 9.2.7 Algorithm for the management of brain metastases[35].

re-irradiation for recurrent disease. Without treatment however progressive morbidity and ultimately death from brain metastasis will occur and neurological sequelae from radiation damage may take many months if not years to be manifest. On this basis therefore low dose re-treatment delivering a further 20–30 Gy in 2–3 weeks may be beneficial for selected patients who have a good initial response to treatment.

Primary brain tumours

Primary brain tumours (including low grade I or II astrocytoma, oligondendroglioma, ependymoma and meningioma) will in most cases be treated by surgery, radiotherapy or both with curative intent. However, high grade astrocytomas (Grade III or IV) are extremely malignant incurable tumours with untreated a prognosis of only a few months. Palliative radiotherapy may be of value in this situation for selected patients with good performance status and the best results are seen in those aged under 60 with no neurological deficits who present with only fits. High-dose treatment delivering 60 Gy in 30 fractions over 6 weeks has been shown to be superior to 45 Gy in 20 fractions over 4 weeks in this group[38] and an improvement in survival has now been demonstrated in a large randomized controlled trial for using adjuvant and concomitant temozolamide in good performance status patients with an improvement in median survival from 12.1 months to 14.6 months and 2-year survival from 10.4–26.5 per cent[39]. However, in patients with poor performance status, significant neurological defecits and aged >65 years significant benefit from a high dose treatment schedule is rarely seen and in these patients short pragmatic schedules delivering doses of 20–30 Gy over 1–3 weeks should be considered[40].

Malignant meningitis

Diffuse meningeal carcinomatosis is generally a pre-terminal event with a median survival of only a few weeks if untreated. It commonly presents with multiple spinal root symptoms and signs and multiple cranial nerve palsies. Raised intracranial pressure may occur resulting in headache and other symptoms. Common primary sites associated with malignant meningitis are carcinoma of the breast and lung. Central nervous system relapse of leukaemia also typically presents with malignant meningitis. The diagnosis can be made on MR scan and confirmed cytologically, once raised intracranial pressure has been excluded, by CSF sampling at lumbar puncture.

Intensive treatment may be indicated where there is a treatable underlying malignancy. In the case of acute leukaemia and lymphoma, sustained remissions may be achieved by the use of intrathecal chemotherapy using methotrexate and cytosine arabinoside sometimes combined with craniospinal irradiation (radiotherapy to the entire brain and spinal cord) or cranial irradiation alone. Such treatment is no small undertaking and may be associated with significant morbidity due to bone marrow depression and nausea, vomiting, and alopecia from the radiotherapy. In children, there are also the associated issues of impaired spinal growth and intellectual development after radiotherapy to the spine and brain, respectively. Furthermore it is unfortunately the case that despite initial remission, central nervous system relapse of lymphoma or leukaemia is generally associated with a poor overall prognosis and subsequent relapse with death often occurs within a few months.

The outlook for carcinomatous meningitis from solid tumours however is even worse and whilst untreated the median survival is only a few weeks even intensive therapy with intrathecal chemotherapy and craniospinal irradiation will extend this to no more than a few months, much of which may be taken up with treatment[41]. On this basis judicious local irradiation to specific sites causing symptoms such as the skull base when cranial nerves are involved or the segments of the spinal cord related to nerve root symptoms, delivering a dose of 20 Gy in five fractions offers a more pragmatic approach achieving effective palliation whilst minimizing the morbidity and duration of treatment in a universally fatal condition.

Cranial nerve palsies

Cranial nerve symptoms and signs due to metastatic cancer may arise from intrinsic metastasis in the brain stem and mid brain, infiltration of the leptomeninges, compression by extra-dural deposits, or bone involvement in the skull base. The management of intrinsic metastasis and leptomeningeal metastasis has been discussed above; results of whole brain irradiation for cranial nerve deficits due to cerebral metastasis show an overall response rate of 78 per cent and a complete response rate of 42 per cent[42]. Local irradiation of the skull base is of value where diffuse bone involvement has resulted in cranial nerve compression and symptomatic improvement is reported in between 50 and 78 per cent of patients

maintained until death in around 80 per cent. In general, patients with skull base metastasis, representing metastatic bone disease, will have a better prognosis than those with intrinsic central nervous system metastases, their median survival being between 10 and 20 months[42,43].

Peripheral nerve symptoms

Involvement of peripheral nerves will typically result in nerve root pain and loss of motor function in the distribution of that nerve. This may be due to compression of the nerve by tumour at any point from the spinal root canal to its peripheral receptors. A large randomized trial has evaluated the efficacy of local radiotherapy in neuropathic pain. An overall response rate of 57 per cent was found with 26 per cent achieving a complete response at 3 months after treatment[44]. In keeping with the experience of uncomplicated bone metastases single doses of 8 Gy were found to be not inferior to more prolonged fractionated doses. Cauda equina compression from spinal canal tumour has been discussed in the section above. Outside the spinal canal symptoms may arise because of direct tumour compression and infiltration particularly in the brachial plexus from apical lung tumours or metastatic lymph nodes and at the lumbosacral plexus from pelvic tumours of the bowel, bladder, ovary or uterus. Lumbosacral neuropathic pain will respond to palliative doses of radiotherapy with complete pain relief within 1 month reported in 85–100 per cent of patients[45]. Pelvic irradiation for pain relief for recurrent colorectal cancer is successful in up to 80 per cent of patients with no difference detected between a 3-week course of treatment delivering 45 Gy and a single dose of 10 Gy[46]. Treatment to apical lung tumours or axillary recurrence of breast cancer causing upper limb pain due to brachial plexus neuropathy is reported to be successful in up to 77 per cent of patients using typical doses of 20–30 Gy in 1–2 weeks[47].

Choroidal and orbital metastasis

Metastases to the eye are unusual but may cause distressing symptoms of proptosis, pain and visual disturbance. The most common intra-occular site is the choroid where over 50 per cent of metastases arise from primary breast cancer, 30 per cent from lung cancer and around 25 per cent are bilateral. The diagnosis is made on fundoscopy or slit lamp examination. Untreated there is progressive deterioration and ultimately loss of vision. Local treatment with radiotherapy delivering doses of 30–40 Gy in 2–4 weeks is reported to achieve stabilization and improvement of vision in up to 86 per cent of patients[48,49]. Asymptomatic lesions should also be treated as in these patients vision is invariable preserved without deterioration. Local tumour control is reported in 98 per cent of treated patients.

Metastasis at other intra-orbital sites are less common and may arise not only from blood-borne secondary spread but also as a result of direct invasion from other head and neck sites, in particular the nasopharynx, nasal cavity, and sinuses. Palliative local irradiation is again of value in preventing and relieving local symptoms from pressure and infiltration.

Radiotherapy to the eye and orbit requires meticulous attention to technique, avoiding as far as possible direct irradiation of the cornea which can result in painful keratitis. Radiation cataracts may be induced after only small doses of 5–10 Gy to the lens of the eye and wherever possible therefore this should also be shielded. In the context of palliative treatment, however, it is important to bear in mind that radiation cataracts may take many years to evolve and should not be considered a reason for avoiding radiation to the orbit where indicated.

Cerebral lymphoma

Primary lymphoma of the central nervous system is a rare extranodal site for non-Hodgkin's lymphoma but has increased in incidence considerably in recent years due to its association with HIV infection when it is often a manifestation of advanced, late stage disease. It may cause headache, fits, cranial nerve palsies or other focal neurological signs. Initial treatment with steroids will often achieve good symptom palliation and some regression. The mainstay of modern treatment in fit patients is chemotherapy typically using schedules containing high dose methotrexate which results in a median survival of 10–18 months[50]. The role of whole brain radiotherapy in addition to chemotherapy in radical treatment has been questioned, particularly in the light of late effects on cognitive function in survivors and this is currently under investigation. However whole brain radiotherapy has an important role in primary treatment for older patients unable to tolerate intensive chemotherapy when 'radical' doses of 40–50 Gy may be given[51] and also for palliation in advanced cases relapsing after chemotherapy or presenting with poor performance status or significant co-morbidity when a short treatment delivering a dose of 30 Gy in 10 fractions over 2 weeks will be used.

Obstructive symptoms

Mediastinal compression and superior vena cava obstruction (SVCO)

The syndrome of SVCO may arise due to occlusion by extrinsic compression, intraluminal thrombosis, or direct invasion of the vessel wall. The majority of cases are due to malignant tumour within the mediastinum but other rare causes which should be excluded include aortic aneurysm, chronic mediastinitis, trauma, or thrombosis following central venous catheterization. Approximately 3 per cent of patients with carcinoma of the bronchus and 8 per cent of those with lymphoma will develop SVCO and of the patients who present with this syndrome 75 per cent will have primary bronchial carcinomas (40 per cent of which will be small-cell lung cancer) and 15 per cent will have mediastinal lymphoma.

The clinical effects arise as a result of increased venous pressure above the site of obstruction. The extent to which this produces symptoms will depend on the efficiency of collateral vessels (particularly the internal mammary vessels, pulmonary veins, and the thoracic and vertebral venous plexuses) which may bypass the obstruction. Because of this obstruction above the azygos vein will have less effect than obstruction below this level. A wide variety of presenting symptoms may result including headaches, somnolence, and dizziness together with the effects of oedema and pressure within the mediastinum causing dysphagia, dyspnoea, cough, or hoarseness; more rarely convulsions may result from cerebral hypertension. Examination may reveal fixed engorgement of arm and neck veins with visible dilatation of superficial skin veins, cyanosis, and facial oedema. Management requires both alleviation of symptoms and shrinkage of intra-thoracic tumour to relieve the obstruction. SVCO, whilst potentially a hazardous condition, rarely needs emergency treatment and it is more important to have a full and accurate assessment of the underlying disease together with a histological diagnosis in order that correct effective therapy may be instigated. Presentation with SVCO is not a contraindication to radical curative treatment in patients where this is appropriate, for example mediastinal Hodgkin's disease. It is important not to compromise the management of these patients by inappropriate emergency treatment. A policy of delayed treatment until definitive tissue diagnosis can be achieved has been evaluated in a large review of 1986 patients presenting with SVCO which found only one death directly attributable to venous obstruction which occurred as a result of inhalation from an epistaxis[52].

The first approach to management therefore should always be to obtain a histological diagnosis and to fully stage the patient so that those patients eligible for radical treatment, and those for whom chemotherapy as the primary treatment will be more appropriate than radiotherapy can be identified. Whilst there are theoretical problems in performing a biopsy within a region of raised venous pressure, with an increased risk of haemorrhage, in practice bronchoscopy, mediastinoscopy, or lymph node biopsy are performed without major complications and should be undertaken unless there is life-threatening large airways obstruction. Even in this setting bronchoscopy and stenting may be the most appropriate primary treatment and similarly for severe venous occlusion the insertion of an SVC stent will be more immediately successful than radiotherapy or chemotherapy. During the acute phase of investigation steroids may also be of value in high doses such as dexamethasone 12–16 mg daily although there is no good objective data to support this practice.

On the basis of a histological diagnosis those patients with chemo-sensitive tumours, in particular small-cell lung cancer, Hodgkin's disease, non-Hodgkin's lymphoma, and germ cell tumours can be identified and treated with primary chemotherapy. For the remainder, the majority of whom will have non-small-cell lung cancer, radiotherapy to the mediastinum covering the tumour mass and adjacent lymph nodes areas where appropriate is indicated, however where there are significant symptoms then initial referral for a stent procedure is recommended[53]. This may then be followed by radiotherapy; in the palliative setting it is usual to deliver doses of 20–30 Gy in 1–2 weeks but where the primary tumour is localized and radical treatment would otherwise be indicated a radical course of radiotherapy or chemoradiation should not be denied the patient.

Symptomatic relief following irradiation for SVCO is reported in 50–95 per cent of patients within the first 2 weeks of treatment. The survival of patients presenting with SVCO is determined by their underlying disease rather than the syndrome itself with the exception of the relatively rare instance of large airway obstruction or cerebral oedema when urgent treatment is required. There is data to suggest treatment has little effect upon the obstruction to blood flow in the superior vena cava which persists in three-quarters of patients. This implies that the development of collaterals is most important in achieving the observed clinical improvement rather than the physical release of compression from the superior vena cava[52].

Lung collapse secondary to bronchial obstruction

Complete bronchial occlusion will lead to collapse of lung distal to that site. Obstruction may occur due to extrinsic compression by mediastinal lymph nodes secondary to bronchial or other epithelial cancers or lymphoma. A more common cause is intrinsic carcinoma of the bronchus. When obstruction occurs rapidly then acute dyspnoea with associated cough due to the secondary lung collapse will be the presenting symptom. Treatment is aimed at restoring the patency of the bronchus. For intrinsic tumours this may be best achieved by local treatment such as cryotherapy or laser therapy via a bronchoscope. For extrinsic tumours appropriate radiotherapy or in the case of chemosensitive tumours chemotherapy is indicated. As with SVCO, presentation with bronchial obstruction does not preclude radical treatment in those patients where that would be appropriate, for example lymphoma, limited disease small-cell lung cancer, or localized non-small-cell lung cancer. Lymphoma and small-cell lung cancer will be best treated with primary chemotherapy. Localized non-small cell lung cancer will benefit from radical doses of radiotherapy given either as an accelerated schedule such as CHART (continuous hyperfractionated accelerated radiotherapy) or within a chemoradiation programme[54]. For poor performance status patients and those with distant metastasis palliative radiotherapy is indicated. In these patients, a single dose of 10 Gy has been shown to be as effective as more prolonged schedules in large randomized trials being equivalent in terms of both symptom control and survival, with a reduced risk of acute morbidity[55,56]. There is an intermediate group of good performance status patients with advanced tumours who may have a small but significant survival advantage from higher dose radiotherapy with randomized trials comparing 17 Gy in two fractions with either 39 Gy in 13 fractions or 20 Gy in 5 fractions showing a survival advantage of around 2 months which was statistically significant, for the higher dose schedules[57,58].

An alternative method of delivering radiotherapy in the bronchial lumen is using the technique of endobronchial brachytherapy. This may be particularly appropriate for patients relapsing after previous external beam irradiation. It is performed as a day case requiring fibreoptic bronchoscopy during which a fine plastic catheter is passed through the suction channel of the bronchoscope and under direct vision left to lie alongside the tumour-bearing region of bronchus, shown in Fig. 9.2.8. This area is irradiated using brachytherapy with a high dose rate afterloading machine which passes a radioactive source, iridium 192, along the catheter to dwell within the area bearing tumour where treatment is required. This technique can be combined with either laser therapy or cryotherapy to restore the lumen where there is complete bronchial obstruction. Endobronchial brachytherapy has now been compared in a randomized controlled trial with external beam radiotherapy[59]. No difference in survival or symptom control scores for cough, haemoptysis, shortness of breath, or hoarseness was seen but external beam radiotherapy was found to be superior for symptoms of chest pain, anorexia, tiredness, and nausea. In contrast, less dysphagia was found in patients receiving endobronchial brachytherapy. The standard dose is 15 Gy at 1 cm and the major advantage of brachytherapy is that it can be given as a single procedure often possible as an outpatient day case.

It is also important to recognize that chemotherapy is the palliative treatment of choice in small-cell lung cancer and has an increasing place in the management of inoperable non-small cell-lung cancer and many patients will benefit from both chemotherapy and radiotherapy in this setting[60].

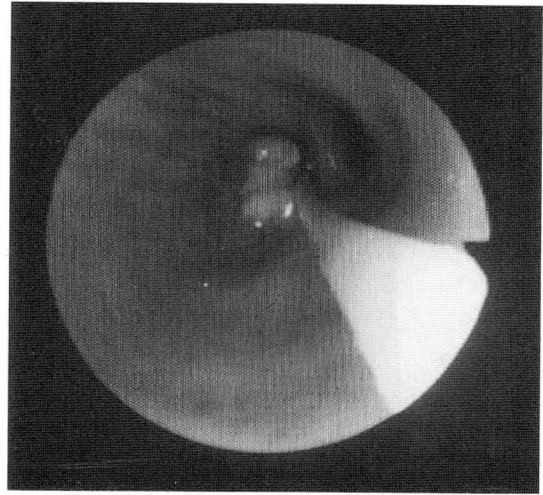

(a)

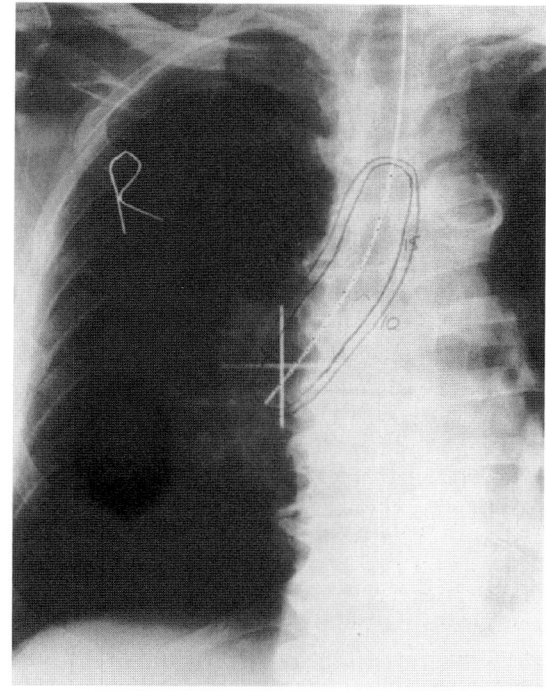

(b)

Figure 9.2.8 View of (A) endobronchial catheter being passed through fibre optic bronchoscope for endobronchial brachytherapy and (B) subsequent x-ray showing catheter position.

Dysphagia

Pain and difficulty in swallowing is a common symptom in patients with advanced cancer within the mediastinum. This may be due to intrinsic tumour arising from the wall of the oesophagus, hypopharynx (piriform fossa, post-cricoid region, and posterior pharyngeal wall), and stomach. Alternatively there may be extrinsic compression from mediastinal lymph nodes or tumours in the thymus, thyroid gland or adjacent bronchus. Post-mortem data shows that around 80 per cent of patients presenting with dysphagia have intrinsic tumour within the oesophagus and in one study multiple levels of obstruction were seen in almost a quarter of these patients[61]. Local symptoms may be alleviated with analgesia and anticholinergic drugs to reduce secretion while

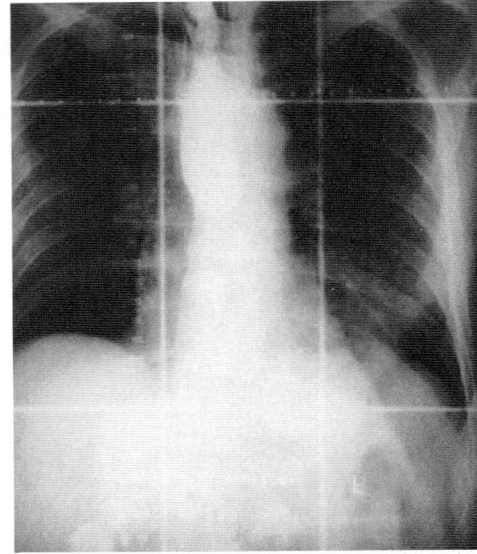

(A)

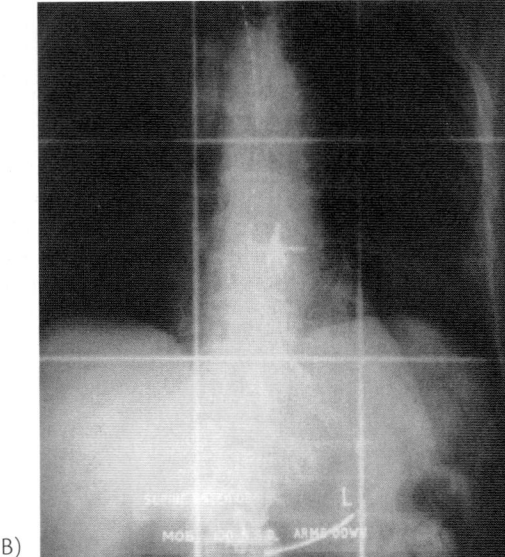

(B)

Figure 9.2.9 Planning films to treat inoperable palliative radiotherapy for dysphagia from carcinoma of oesophagus using (A) external beam fields and (B) endobronchial brachytherapy showing the treatment catheter in situ.

nutrition can be maintained by a fine bore nasogastric tube or percutaneous gastrostomy. Where there is widespread metastatic disease in poor performance patients more active treatment may be inappropriate and unsuccessful. In selected patients, however, with good performance status and limited disease surgical intervention with either radical resection or if not appropriate laser resection or stenting should be considered and has the advantage of rapid symptom relief if successful. There is however a significant morbidity and procedure-related mortality associated with these approaches and external beam irradiation should also be considered as a means of relieving dysphagia both for intrinsic tumour obstruction and where there is extrinsic compression. A typical radiation field for this is shown in Fig. 9.2.9, the usual dose delivered to such an area being 20–30 Gy in 1–2 weeks with re-established swallowing reported in over 80 per cent of patients maintained for

a mean duration of 6 months[62]. The disadvantage of radiotherapy in this setting however is that relief is not immediate, may take several weeks to occur and there may initially be a period of enhanced dysphagia because of acute oesophagitis. This should be managed with simple topical medication such as soluble aspirin.

There is some evidence that higher doses of radiotherapy delivering 50 Gy in 5 weeks or more may give a higher and more durable response rate and this should be considered for patients who have good performance status and limited disease in whom a longer prognosis may be expected[63]. Where radical treatment using radiotherapy is used, chemoradiation has been shown to be superior to radiotherapy alone using concomitant cisplatin and 5FU during the course of radiotherapy[1].

An alternative technique is endo-oesophageal radiotherapy which is similar to that of endobronchial brachytherapy. A tube is passed through the area of oesophageal constriction and a radioactive source passed along the tube shown in Fig. 9.2.8. A small diameter high dose afterloading source will pass readily through a fine catheter which itself fits inside a nasogastric tube and the procedure can be undertaken as an outpatient requiring passage of the nasogastric tube with local anaesthetic followed by x-ray verification of its position and delivery of the treatment which typically takes only a few minutes. Used alone sustained improvement in swallowing is reported in 54 per cent of patients[64]. This technique has also been used in an attempt to achieve high local doses in combination with external beam radiotherapy for radical treatment. Randomized trials suggest there may be an advantage to this approach and one series of 171 patients reports improved swallowing for 3 or more months in 90 per cent of patients with 56 per cent achieving complete restoration of normal swallowing[65].

In addition to acute toxicity there may be later changes which develop within the life span of patients with advanced disease. Of these oesophageal stricture is the most common late complication reported in 35 per cent of cases receiving combined external beam and brachytherapy[65]. In contrast after short palliative doses of 20–30 Gy stricture is unusual in the absence of tumour recurrence. After palliative doses of radiotherapy other more severe complications such as perforation and fistula are also unusual unless related to tumour progression.

Urinary tract obstruction

Urinary tract obstruction may arise because of obstruction of the renal pelvis, ureter, bladder or urethra at any point. This may be due to both benign and malignant conditions and the most satisfactory means of re-establishing renal drainage is a surgical procedure to bypass the obstruction using a nephrostomy, ureteric stents or transurethral resection of an intrinsic urethral tumour.

The role of radiotherapy in relieving urinary tract infection is restricted to those patients in whom surgery is either technically not possible or otherwise inappropriate, but it is also important to consider radiotherapy following immediate relief of obstruction to treat the underlying cause. Common clinical scenarios include locally advanced cancer of the cervix, bladder, or prostate or recurrence of colorectal tumour. It is important to ascertain the primary site of the tumour and in the setting of para-aortic lymphadenopathy obtain histological confirmation since in some instances for example lymphoma and germ cell tumour primary chemotherapy with curative intent will be appropriate. Radiotherapy for the underlying tumour should be based on the merits of the tumour and radical treatment not denied the patient. Conventionally primary tumours of the cervix, prostate, or bladder causing urinary tract obstruction in the absence of lymph node or distant metastasis will be treated with high radiation doses to achieve tumour shrinkage and re-establish urinary flow with the expectation that a proportion of patients will have long-term disease control or even cure. Doses of 50–60Gy in 5 weeks with intracavitary brachytherapy being given for cervical cancers in addition to external beam treatment will be necessary. One series of patients with carcinoma of the prostate presenting with urinary retention found that radiotherapy alone was sufficient to restore normal urinary drainage in 84 per cent with a mean time to catheter removal from completion of radiotherapy of 10 weeks[66].

In some instances intraluminal or interstitial radiotherapy may also be possible a specific example being that of a sub-urethral metastasis from through endometrial carcinoma. This is a recognized pattern of spread from sub-mucosal vaginal lymphatic invasion to the urethra meatus. An interstitial implant will enable high dose local treatment to be delivered. Techniques are also available to deliver intraluminal brachytherapy to the urethra where recurrent prostate cancer or bladder base tumours are troublesome.

Limb oedema

Limb oedema in a patient with advanced cancer may result from venous obstruction, lymphatic obstruction, or both. This may be compounded by general debility, immobility and poor nutrition with accompanying hypo-albuminaemia. In a proportion of patients, particularly those with upper limb oedema due to carcinoma of the breast, post-radiation changes may have caused lymphatic obstruction; ipsilateral arm oedema is seen in over 30 per cent of patients undergoing both axillary surgery and radiotherapy to the axilla for breast cancer.

Local radiotherapy may be of value in the treatment of limb oedema where enlarged malignant axillary, inguinal or pelvic nodes are the cause of obstruction. The best results are obtained with early treatment when the circulatory obstruction can be reversed. Relatively low doses of 20–30 Gy in 1–2 weeks are used taking care to preserve wherever possible a channel of unirradiated skin and soft tissue through which lymph drainage can be maintained despite post-radiation changes.

Hydrocephalus

Obstructive hydrocephalus is an uncommon manifestation of cancer within the central nervous system and may result from primary or secondary tumours which obstruct the cerebrospinal fluid at any point in the ventricular system. Typically it occurs when tumours of either the mid brain or the posterior fossa obstruct the aqueduct or fourth ventricle; it may also be secondary to malignant meningitis. Patients present with features of raised intracranial pressure together with focal neurological symptoms, depending upon the site of the tumour. Rapid relief of hydrocephalus may be gained by inserting an intraventricular shunt and patients with advanced disease may need no further treatment to achieve temporary symptom control. Where surgery is not feasible or where there are multiple intracerebral lesions palliative radiotherapy should be given in the same way as discussed for the management of brain metastasis in the previous section.

Advanced primary central nervous system tumours of the mid brain and posterior fossa are also treated by radiotherapy usually delivering doses of 50–55 Gy given over 6–7 weeks.

Haemorrhage

Haemoptysis

Haemoptysis is a common symptom of bronchial carcinoma occurring in around 50 per cent of patients at presentation. It may also accompany pulmonary metastasis and is distressing for the patient although rarely of haemodynamic significance. It is life-threatening only if a major vein or bronchial artery is eroded when it is usually beyond all treatment. Haemoptysis is otherwise an indication for local radiotherapy and control rates of up to 80 per cent are reported with palliative doses using either external beam treatment or endobronchial brachytherapy as discussed above. The randomized trials show that a single dose of 10-Gy external beam is as effective as other more prolonged schedules with less acute morbidity[55].

It is important to remember that haemoptysis is a presenting symptom of bronchial carcinoma and is not in itself a contraindication to radical treatment in patients having localized disease which can be radically resected or encompassed in a high dose radiation volume. Screening for this possibility should always occur prior to embarking upon palliative irradiation. Patients with non-small-cell lung cancer having Stage I or II disease, that is without involvement of mediastinal lymph nodes, should all be considered for high dose radiotherapy using either accelerated schedules such as CHART or chemoradiation[54]. Patients with good performance status and Stage III disease, that is mediastinal node involvement, may also in selected cases benefit from high dose chemoradiation. Patients with small-cell lung cancer will usually be selected for primary chemotherapy but in extensive disease palliative radiotherapy for symptoms such as haemoptysis is highly effective using the same techniques as those used for non-small-cell lung cancer.

The management of haemoptysis due to pulmonary metastasis is more difficult. Local irradiation is only of value where a specific site of haemorrhage can be identified or where there is only a solitary metastasis. Bronchoscopic confirmation of the origin of bleeding is therefore needed where there are multiple metastasis; arbitrary irradiation of the particular area of metastatic disease is not to be recommended although low dose whole lung irradiation delivering a dose of 25 Gy in 20 fractions over 4 weeks has been used in the past for widespread metastasis from radiosensitive tumours such as Ewing's sarcoma or Wilms' tumour. In general, however chemotherapy or hormone therapy is the preferred treatment in this setting and only when this has failed should palliative irradiation be explored.

There is no proven advantage in terms of survival for treating the asymptomatic patient with inoperable lung cancer but there is evidence that tumours greater than 10 cm in diameter whether primary or metastatic carry a significant risk of haemorrhage and it has been suggested that such lesions should receive prophylactic treatment.

Haematuria

Haematuria may be related to bleeding from primary or metastatic disease at any site along the urinary tract from the renal pelvis to the urethra. Thus before embarking upon palliative treatment careful localization of the site of bleeding, including intravenous urography, CT scanning or cystoscopy is vital. Haematuria in patients with advanced cancer is usually caused by bleeding from a local bladder tumour, which may be primary or secondary to local infiltration of an advanced rectal or uterine carcinoma, advanced renal cell carcinoma or urethral infiltration by carcinoma of the prostate. Other causes that may be relevant to the cancer patient are infective cystitis, chemical cystitis associated with certain chemotherapy agents such as cyclophosphamide or ifosfamide, bladder telangiectasia as a late change following high dose radiotherapy to the bladder or as a rare manifestation of thrombocytopenia or a blood coagulation defect.

The main role of radiotherapy in this setting is to achieve haemostasis in patients with inoperable or recurrent tumours. Haematuria may settle with conservative measures such as bladder irrigation, administration of antifibrinolytic drugs such as tranexamic acid and cystoscopic diathermy. Where this fails modest doses of irradiation delivered to a small volume encompassing the site of haemorrhage will often be successful.

In advanced muscle invasive bladder cancer a large randomized trial comparing 35 Gy in 10 fractions with 21 Gy given in three fractions on alternate days over 1 week has shown equivalent symptomatic improvement of bladder-related symptoms with no excess toxicity from the shorter 21-Gy schedule[67]. Haematuria was improved in 50 per cent of patients at completion of treatment and 63 per cent at 3 months after treatment. Careful localization of bladder tumours is important with CT planning. The same doses and techniques can be used for prostatic cancer causing urethral or bladder base infiltration and haemorrhage. In poor performance status, patients' single doses of 8–10 Gy may be equally effective and 17 Gy in two fractions has also been reported as a useful schedule in this setting with a 59 per cent response rate for haematuria[68].

As with other sites haematuria may be the presentation of a potentially curable primary bladder or prostatic carcinoma and full assessment of the patient both in terms of their tumour and general status is important before deciding upon palliative treatment. For advanced tumours of the bladder radical radiotherapy is appropriate delivering doses of 55 Gy in 4 weeks or 60–65 Gy in 6–6½ weeks. Radical radiotherapy to the prostate gland will deliver doses in excess of 70 Gy in 7 weeks or in selected cases brachytherapy will be preferred.

Haematuria due to locally advanced inoperable renal carcinoma may also benefit from local irradiation where a nephrectomy is not possible. The tolerance of the normal kidney to radiation is low and even with modest palliative doses it is to be expected that the kidney bearing the tumour will be damaged with loss of function. It is therefore important to ensure that renal function from the contra-lateral kidney is normal before treatment. Doses of 10 Gy as a single dose, 21 Gy in three fractions over 1 week, or 20–30 Gy over 1–2 weeks have all been used in this setting; there is little published data on the expected response rate.

Treatment of the bladder or prostate may result in diarrhoea because of the inevitable inclusion of some of the rectum in the treatment volume. In the MRC-randomized trial of palliative radiotherapy in bladder cancer, there was a 5 per cent incidence of mild diarrhoea not requiring medication and a 2 per cent incidence of moderate diarrhoea requiring medication for control[67]. Treatment of the kidney may include stomach or small bowel resulting in nausea, vomiting, and diarrhoea. Careful explanation and reassurance about these side effects together with ready availability of antidiarrhoeal agents and antiemetics is an important part of management.

Uterine and vaginal bleeding

Tumours of the uterus including endometrial and cervical cancer and uterine sarcomas frequently present with abnormal vaginal bleeding. This is rarely excessive and readily managed conservatively before embarking upon definitive treatment. Occasionally major haemorrhage may be the presenting feature of a uterine tumour requiring resuscitation and vaginal packing before urgent treatment is instigated. Haemorrhage in patients with advanced and metastatic cancer may be due to recurrent or locally advanced tumours of the cervix or uterus, local infiltration from advanced cancers of the bladder or rectum or metastatic mucosal deposits along the vaginal wall typical of the pattern of spread from endometrial cancer. Haemorrhagic mucosal deposits are also a particular feature of vulval or vaginal melanoma.

Radiotherapy is of value in obtaining control of bleeding using either external beam irradiation or intracavitary treatment as appropriate. Where vaginal bleeding represents the primary presentation of advanced cervical cancer then radical chemoradiation is often appropriate delivering external beam treatment to a dose of around 50 Gy in 5 weeks with cisplatin followed by intracavitary treatment to the cervix and para-cervical tissues. Where locally advanced bladder, rectal, or uterine tumours are the cause and previous radiotherapy has not been given palliative pelvic doses are effective using a schedule of 21 Gy in three fractions or 20–30 Gy over 1–2 weeks. Where previous radiotherapy has been given to the pelvis further low doses can often be considered and these can be effective in obtaining haemostasis although there may be risks of additional late bowel damage associated with this. These decisions must be balanced between the severity of symptoms and the anticipated life expectancy of the patient. Where thought appropriate single doses of 8 Gy or short courses of up to 20 Gy in five fractions are effective.

Where bleeding is from small volume disease such as nodules of the vaginal vault or along the vaginal mucosa intracavitary treatment may be preferable. Vaginal sources in the form of either ovoids or a vaginal tube can be introduced directly into the vagina and used to carry a radiation source in the form of caesium or iridium which whilst in position within the applicator will deliver local radiation to its surface along the vaginal wall[69]. The use of intracavitary brachytherapy in this way enables a high surface dose to be given to the mucosa but with a rapid fall off in dose away from the source so that critical structures such as bladder and rectum are relatively spared from the radiation dose. This may be of value in patients who have previously received radiotherapy to the pelvis but is also highly effective in otherwise untreated patients. This form of treatment does however have limitations in being able to treat only a depth of 5–10 mm. For larger recurrent tumours around the vulva and vaginal region and in the peri-urethral tissues an interstitial implant may be necessary. Whilst more demanding for the patient requiring a general anaesthetic and either radioactive needles or afterloading implant tubes to be placed through the tumour area, as shown in Fig. 9.2.10, it enables high dose treatment to be delivered locally within the tumour even where previous radiotherapy has been given to the pelvis and may provide highly effective palliation from an otherwise very difficult situation of progressive tumour in the vulvo-vaginal region.

Gastrointestinal haemorrhage

Symptomatic gastrointestinal haemorrhage may arise from either the upper or lower gastrointestinal tract resulting in haematemesis,

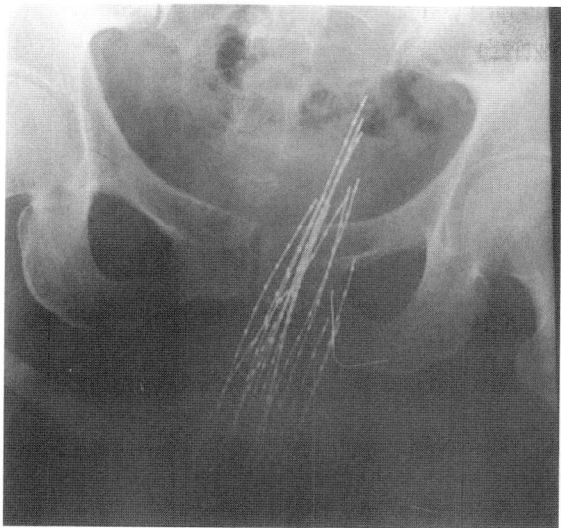
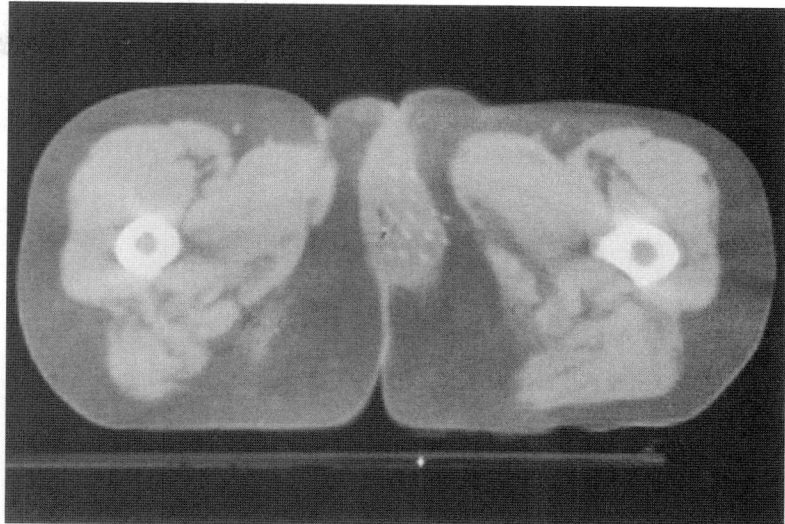

Figure 9.2.10 X-ray and CT planning films of brachytherapy catheters in situ to treat locally advanced recurrent carcinoma of the vulva. Treatment is delivered by the passage of a high dose rate iridium source along the catheters once planning procedures have been completed and verified.

melaena or rectal bleeding. The underlying tumour may be a primary neoplasm arising within the gastrointestinal tract, most commonly from the stomach, large bowel or rectum, or as a result of direct invasion by locally advanced tumour in adjacent structures such as the uterus, bladder or prostate invading the rectum. Blood-borne metastasis to the bowel are rare but metastatic malignant melanoma is a recognized cause of haemorrhagic deposits within the small bowel wall and Kaposi's sarcoma, seen with HIV infection, may cause a similar problem.

As in other sites local radiotherapy in modest doses to a site of haemorrhage within the bowel will often achieve effective and durable control of bleeding. In the lower bowel, tumours in the rectum and colon are usually readily identified and localized within a treatment volume. Treatment of the stomach may be more difficult both because it can be a relatively mobile structure and also because the sensitivity of surrounding tissues, in particular liver, small bowel, and kidneys, limits tolerance and the dose that can be delivered safely. Localization of tumours within the small bowel can be difficult because of its mobility and radiation to the stomach and small bowel can have considerable associated morbidity with nausea, vomiting, and diarrhoea.

The most common scenario will be recurrent tumours of the rectum or sigmoid colon, particularly at the site of an anastomosis where a primary has been previously resected. External beam radiotherapy for bleeding from recurrent colorectal cancer has been reported to achieve an overall response rate of 85 per cent with complete control of bleeding in 63 per cent of patients following a dose of 30–35 Gy in 10 fractions over 2 weeks[70]. An alternative approach is to use intra-luminal brachytherapy similar to the technique used for vaginal bleeding, passing a tube into the rectum through which a radioactive source can be placed to deliver a high surface dose to the rectal mucosa and associated tumour area. This approach has the advantage of being delivered as a single outpatient procedure when high dose rate afterloading brachytherapy is used, the actual technique being little different to a sigmoidoscopic examination. Control of bleeding is achieved in 64 per cent[71] It is however limited to accessible tumours in the lower sigmoid colon, rectum, and anal canal.

Chest wall and other skin lesions

Locoregional recurrence remains a significant problem in patients with breast cancer occurring in 7–10 per cent of those with early disease and up to 40 per cent of those presenting with advanced local disease. Postoperative irradiation at the time of primary treatment significantly reduces the likelihood of locoregional relapse but despite this a number of patients with recurrent metastatic breast cancer will also have progressive locoregional tumour on the chest wall which will fungate and bleed.

Where total mastectomy is possible this may be the best procedure to surgically clear recurrent tumour on the chest wall. In many cases, however the tumour will be fixed and inoperable with multiple satellite nodules across the chest, often involving the contralateral breast or extending laterally across the mid axillary line on to the back. In general, chemotherapy will be the most appropriate initial treatment but often such disease will recur and not remain chemo-sensitive. Where no previous radiotherapy has been given and there is no evidence of distant metastasis high-dose local irradiation may be appropriate delivering doses of up to 60 Gy in 6 weeks. In patients with distant metastasis and a poor prognosis, shorter schedules of 10 Gy in one fraction or longer courses of 20–30 Gy in 1–2 weeks may be more appropriate. Often it is not possible to encompass the entire extent of clinically detectable disease and in these circumstances those causing greatest symptoms may be targeted.

Where there has been recurrence despite previous irradiation further radiotherapy may be possible to a limited area of symptomatic tumour since the risks of skin necrosis are negligible compared with the effects of progressive fungating tumour within the skin. Superficial x-ray treatment or low energy electrons to fungating or bleeding chest wall nodules is often highly effective and a single dose of 8–10 Gy or a longer course delivering 20–30 Gy over 1–2 weeks is commonly used. More complex techniques using a surface mould in which radioactive sources are placed over the involved area or interstitial brachytherapy in which larger tumour masses are implanted with radioactive needles or afterloading applicator tubes can also be considered.

Skin nodules may also be a manifestation of primary tumours in other sites and once established may fungate and bleed. These will by definition reflect blood borne metastasis and therefore radical treatment is usually inappropriate but local treatment to symptomatic nodules is of value. Techniques and doses similar to those discussed above for recurrent breast cancer will be employed.

Primary skin tumours may also present with locally advanced inoperable disease. Bleeding and fungation are likely to become major problems in the management of these patients and local radiotherapy is of value in their control. In the absence of metastasis, or in the case of basal cell carcinoma which do not metastasize, high radical doses may be considered using appropriate techniques with either electrons of appropriate energy to treat to the depth of the tumour or tangential x-ray beams to cover the tumour volume. Doses of 60 Gy in 6 weeks or equivalent are given to large tumours where this is appropriate in the light of the patient's general performance status. For patients with poor performance status or metastatic disease shorter courses delivering doses of 20–30 Gy in 1–2 weeks may be considered and will be effective in achieving growth delay and stopping haemorrhage. Melanoma characteristically presents with haemorrhagic tumours and may in more advanced cases result in multiple skin nodules. Local radiotherapy delivering higher doses of 30 Gy in 5–6 fractions treating twice weekly is often used with good effect[72].

Other local tumour effects

Fungation

Fungation of a superficial tumour mass is a distressing feature of locally advanced cancer. It is seen most commonly in chest wall recurrence after breast carcinoma and with metastatic lymph nodes in the neck or groin. Local irradiation is most valuable in the prevention of fungation at a time when the overlying skin is intact. A palliative course of treatment delivering 20–30 Gy in 1–2 weeks will usually delay growth within a tumour mass sufficient to prevent fungation. In certain instances where local tumour is the sole manifestation of malignancy, higher doses may be appropriate. The most common scenario is the presence of a cervical lymph node containing squamous carcinoma from the head and neck region or inguinal lymph nodes with squamous carcinoma from the perineal region. Radical radiotherapy to malignant nodes from an unknown primary in the neck can achieve long-term control in this setting with overall 5-year survival figures of 20–30 per cent in selected series[73].

Once fungation has occurred, successful treatment is more difficult but alongside nursing care and administration of analgesics and antibiotics, local irradiation may still be of value in reducing the underlying tumour bulk, arresting surface haemorrhage and drying the surface as the process of healing is allowed to commence. This will make nursing care simpler and relieve the patient from the distress of local haemorrhage.

Kaposi's sarcoma

Kaposi's sarcoma is now most commonly seen as a feature of HIV infection. It may also be seen in sporadic cases when it typically presents in the skin of the lower limbs in European men. Multiple skin lesions are usual but extracutaneous disease is also common affecting the oral cavity and gastrointestinal tract. The characteristic purplish raised plaques may bleed and ulcerate. In contrast to other soft tissue sarcomas Kaposi's is markedly radiosensitive and small doses of irradiation will result in complete regression of lesions in up to 70 per cent of patients[74]. There is good evidence that single doses are as effective as more prolonged schedules and superficial irradiation delivering 8 Gy to symptomatic sites is recommended.

Liver metastases

In most instances the presence of liver metastasis heralds the terminal phases of advanced cancer. Clinical symptoms will include anorexia, malaise, and weight loss alongside local pain and discomfort from hepatic enlargement and stretching of the liver capsule. Pain may be acute where there is rapid expansion of the liver or haemorrhage into a metastasis. Local radiotherapy may be of value particularly in those patients with good performance status and normal bilirubin and where the primary site is other than stomach or pancreas[75]. If the primary tumour is chemosensitive this is usually the first line of approach and where there are solitary metastases, resection should be considered. High frequency ultrasound has recently introduced a further treatment option for superficial metastases but for other patients palliative low dose radiotherapy may provide valuable relief of symptoms. Two prospective randomized trials have demonstrated relief of hepatic pain in 80 per cent of patients with complete relief in 55 per cent and improvements in nausea, vomiting, fever, and night sweats in 45 per cent[75,76].

The liver has limited tolerance to radiation and so hepatic radiotherapy may be associated with side effects and when doses greater than 30 Gy are given there is a risk of inducing radiation hepatitis. Toxicity is related not only to dose but also the volume of liver included in the treatment volume and unless there is diffuse infiltration of the entire organ, uninvolved liver should be excluded from the radiation volume. With doses of 30 Gy delivered in 2–3 weeks relatively mild self-limiting toxicity is reported with lethargy and nausea being the predominant symptoms.

Splenomegaly

Symptomatic splenomegaly from malignant diseases is usually associated with haematological malignancies in particular chronic granulocytic leukaemia and certain types of non-Hodgkin's lymphoma. It is also a feature of myelodysplasia. Surgical removal of the spleen is the preferred management but in advanced disease or in patients with poor performance status this may not be appropriate and local irradiation is an effective means of palliation. Symptoms due to local bulk (causing pain and discomfort) and hypersplenism (causing consumption of red cells and platelets) benefit from treatment. Pain relief is reported in over 90 per cent of patients and durable size reduction in 60 per cent[76]. The spleen containing lymphoma or leukaemia is extremely sensitive to radiation and high doses should be avoided as these may precipitate pancytopenia and rapid tumour lysis. Single doses of 1 Gy or less delivered at weekly intervals are recommended to a total dose of between 3 and 10 Gy with weekly assessment before each treatment to evaluate the effect on the peripheral blood count and the degree of splenic shrinkage. Even at these low doses precautions should be taken against the effects of rapid tumour lysis ensuring the patient is well hydrated and giving allopurinol to prevent hyperuricaemia.

Hypercalaemia

Hypercalaemia complicates the clinical course of around 10 per cent of all patients with malignant disease particularly those with common epithelial tumours such as breast and lung cancer. Whilst it frequently occurs in patients with widespread metastatic disease no clear correlation with the extent of bone metastasis is usually demonstrated and most arise due to the production of chemical agents promoting osteoclast activating factors (OAFs) for example parathyroid hormone-related protein (PTHrP). The initial management of a patient with hypercalcaemia secondary to advanced cancer includes rehydration, diuresis, and the introduction of bisphosphonates. However whilst an initial reduction of serum calcium is usually achieved, rebound hypercalcaemia frequently follows requiring further intensive treatment and often a refractory phase is entered after several episodes. Where a potential source of the OAF can be identified such as locally advanced endobronchial carcinoma, local irradiation to reduce its production and enable stabilization of blood calcium levels may be of value. Standard palliative doses are usually delivered as described earlier and whilst anecdotally a valuable treatment in this setting no published data is available for accurate estimates of response.

Paraneoplastic phenomena

Certain conditions may be seen in patients with malignancy which are not directly related to the process of tumour growth, invasion and metastasis but are nonetheless associated with the malignant process. Their severity often mirrors the extent of the associated tumour.

It is most common is in primary carcinoma of the bronchus when neoplastic symptoms arise in around 2 per cent of patients and include neuropathies, myopathies, myasthenia (the Eaton–Lambert syndrome) and cutaneous manifestations such as acanthosis nigricans, erythema gyratum, or hairy man syndrome. It is probable that these symptoms reflect secretion of a humeral agent possibly an auto-antibody. The para-endocrine syndromes are associated with ectopic production of ACTH, ADH, human chorionic gonadotrophin (HCG), 5 hydroxytryptamine (5HT), or thyroid stimulating hormone (TSH), as well as those mentioned above in the context of hypercalcaemia. Where there is an identifiable local tumour and where surgical excision is not possible or appropriate local irradiation may result in improvement and resolution of the paraneoplastic symptoms as the tumour regresses. In advanced disease, only palliative doses may be appropriate but in localized disease the presence of a paraneoplastic syndrome should not exclude consideration of radical treatment. As with hypercalcaemia there is no good data on precise response rates to treatment in this setting.

Conclusion

Local irradiation is a valuable treatment for palliation of local symptoms with consistently high response rates in the relief and control of bone pain, neurological symptoms, obstructive symptoms, and haemorrhage. Short treatments and simple techniques can minimize disruption and acute morbidity for the patient with advanced cancer whilst enabling control of symptoms.

References

1. Herskovic, A., Martz, K., Al-Sarraf, M. *et al.* (1992). Combined chemotherapy and radiotherapy compared with radiotherapy alone in patients with cancer of the esophagus. *The New England Journal of Medicine*, **24**, 1593–8.
2. Ryan, D.P., Compton, C.C., and Mayer, R.J. (2000). Carcinoma of the anal canal. *The New England Journal of Medicine*, **342**, 792–800.
3. Thomas, G.M. (1999). Improved treatment for cervical cancer – concurrent chemotherapy and radiotherapy. *The New England Journal of Medicine*, **340**, 1198–9.
4. Komakil, R., Seiferheld, W., Curran, W. *et al.* (2000). Sequential vs. concurrent and radiation therapy for inoperable non-small cell lung cancer (NSCLC): Analysis of failures in a Phase III Study (RTOG 9410). *International Journal of Radiation Oncology, Biology, Physics*, **48**, (Suppl) 1: 113.
5. Munro, A.J. (1995) An overview of randomised controlled trials of adjuvant chemotherapy in head and neck cancer. *British Journal of Cancer*, **71**, 83–91.
6. McQuay, H.J., Carroll, D., and Moore, R.A. (1997). Radiotherapy for painful bone metastases: a systematic review. *Clinical Oncology*, **9**, 150–4.
7. Sze, W.M., Shelley, M.D., Held, I., Wilt, *et al.* (2003). Palliation of Metastatic Bone Pain: Single Fraction versus Multifraction Radiotherapy – A Systematic Review of Randomised Trial. *Clinical Oncology*, **15**, 345–52.
8. Wu, J. S-Y, Wong, R., Johnston, M., Bezjak, A., and Whelan, T. (2003). Meta-analysis of dose-fractionation radiotherapy trials for the palliation of painful bone metastases. *International Journal of Radiation Oncology, Biology, Physics*, **55**, 594–605.
9. Bone Pain Trial Working Party. (1999). 8 Gy single fraction radiotherapy for the treatment of metastatic skeletal pain: randomised comparison with a multifraction schedule over 12 months of patient follow-up. *Radiotherapy and Oncology*, **52**, 111–21.
10. van der Linden, Y.M., Lok, J.J. *et al.* (2004). Single fraction radiotherapy is efficacious: a further analysis of the Dutch Bone Metastasis Study controlling for the influence of retreatment. Dutch Bone Metastases Study Group. *Radiotherapy and Oncology,* **59**(2), 528–37.
11. Mithal, N., Needham, P.R., and Hoskin, P.J. (1994). Retreatment with radiotherapy for painful bone metastases. *International Journal of Radiation Oncology, Biology, Physics*, **29**, 1011–4.
12. Haddad, P., Wong, R.K., Levin, W. *et al.* (2004). Computed tomographic simulation in palliative radiotherapy: the Princess Margaret Hospital experience. *Clinical Oncology (Royal College of Radiologists (Great Britain))*, **16**(6), 425–8.
13. Salazar, O.M., Sandhu, T., Da Motta, N.W. *et al.* (2001). Fractionated half-body irradiation (HBI) for the rapid palliation of widespread, symptomatic, metastatic bone disease: a randomized phase III trial of the International Atomic Energy Agency (IAEA). *International Journal of Radiation Oncology, Biology, Physics*, **50**, 765–75.
14. Salazar, O.M., Rubin, P., Hendrickson, F. *et al.* (1986). Single dose hemibody irradiation in palliation of multiple bone metastases from solid tumours. *Cancer*, **58**, 29–36.
15. Brown, A.P., Greening, W.P., McCready, V.R. *et al.* (1984). Radioiodine treatment of metastatic thyroid carcinoma: The Royal Marsden Hospital experience. *The British Journal of Radiology*, **57**, 323–7.
16. Hoskin, P.J. (1994). Strontium. In *Therapeutic drugs* (ed. C. Dollery), Suppl 2, pp. 223–7. Churchill Livingstone, Edinburgh.
17. Sartor, O., Reid, R.H., Hoskin, P.J. *et al.* (2004). Samarium-153-Lexidronam complex for treatment of painful bone metastases in hormone-refractory prostate cancer. *Urology*, **63**(5), 940–5.
18. Quilty, P.M., Kirk, D., Bolger, J.J. (1994). A comparison of the palliative effects of strontium-89 and external beam radiotherapy in metastatic prostate cancer. *Radiotherapy and Oncology*, **31**, 33–40.
19. Hoskin, P.J., Stratford, M.R.I., and Folkes, L.K. (2000). Effect of local radiotherapy for bone pain on urinary markers of osteoclast activity. *Lancet*, **355**, 1428–9.
20. Poulter, C. *et al.* (1992). A phase III study of whether the addition of single dose hemibody irradiation to standard fractionated local field irradiation is more effective than local field irradiation alone in the treatment of symptomatic osseous metastases. *International Journal of Radiation Oncology, Biology, Physics*, **23**, 74–8.
21. Porter *et al.* (1993). Results of a randomised Phase III trial to evaluate the efficacy of Strontium-89 adjuvant to local field external beam

irradiation in the management of endocrine-resistant metastatic prostate cancer. *International Journal of Radiation Oncology, Biology, Physics*, **25**, 805–13.

22. Diel, I.J., Solomayer, E-F, Costa, S.D. *et al.* (1998). Reduction in new metastases in breast cancer with adjuvant clodronate treatment. *The New England Journal of Medicine*, **339**, 357–63.

23. McCloskey, E.V., MacLennan, I.C.M., Drayson, M.T. *et al.* (1998). for the MRC Working Party on Leukaemia in Adults. *British Journal of Haematology*, **100**, 317–25.

24. Hoskin, P.J. (2003). Bisphosphonates and radiation therapy for palliation of metastatic bone disease. *Cancer Treatment Reviews*, **29**, 321–7.

25. Townsend, P.W., Smalley, S.R., Cozad, S.C. *et al.* (1995). Role of postoperative radiation therapy after stabilization of fractures caused by metastatic disease. *International Journal of Radiation Oncology, Biology, Physics*, **31**, 43–9.

26. Pigott, K., Baddeley, H., and Maher, E.J. (1994). Pattern of disease in spinal cord compression on MRI scan and implications for treatment. *Clinical Oncology*, **6**, 7–10.

27. Shaw, M.D.M., Rose, J.E., and Patterson, A. (1980). Metastatic extradural malignancy of the spine. *Acta Neurochirurgica*, **52**, 113–20.

28. Findlay, G.F.G. (1988). The role of needle biopsy in the management of cervical metastases. *British Journal of Neurosurgery*, **2**, 479–84.

29. Siegal, T., and Siegal, T. (1985). Surgical decompression of anterior and posterior malignant epidural tumours compressing the spinal cord: a prospective study. *Neurosurgery*, **17**, 424–32.

30. Moore, A.J., and Uttley, D. (1989). Anterior decompression and stabilisation of the spine in malignant disease. *Neurosurgery*, **24**, 713–7.

31. Patchell, R., Tibbs, P.A., Regine, W.F. *et al.* (2005). Direct decompressive surgical resection in the treatment of spinal cord compression caused by metastatic cancer: a randomised trial. *Lancet*, **366**, 643–8.

32. Findlay, G.F.G. (1984). Adverse effects of the management of malignant spinal cord compression. *Journal of Neurology, Neurosurgery, and Psychiatry*, **47**, 761–8.

33. Rades, D., Stalpers, L.J., Veninga, T. *et al.* (2005). Evaluation of five radiation schedules and prognostic factors for metastatic spinal cord compression. *Journal of Clinical Oncology*, **23**, 3366–75.

34. Goldman, J.M. *et al.* (1989). Spinal cord compression in small cell lung cancer: a retrospective study of 610 patients. *British Journal of Cancer*, **59**, 591–3.

35. Hoskin, P.J. and Brada, M. on behalf of the participants of the Second Workshop on Palliative Radiotherapy and Symptom Control (2000), London. *Clinical Oncology*, **13**, 91–4.

36. Borgelt, B. *et al.* (1982). The palliation of brain metastases: final results of the first two studies by the Radiation Therapy Oncology Group. *International Journal of Radiation Oncology, Biology, Physics*, **6**, 1–9.

37. Priestman, T.J., Dunn, J., Brada, M. *et al.* (1996). Final results of the Royal College of Radiologists' trial comparing two different radiotherapy schedules in the treatment of cerebral metastases. *Clinical Oncology*, **8**, 308–15.

38. Bleehan, N. *et al.* (1991). A Medical Research Council trial of two radiotherapy doses in the treatment of grades 3 and 4 astrocytoma. *British Journal of Cancer*, **64**, 769–74.

39. Stupp, R., Mason, W.P., van den Bent, M.J. *et al.* (2005). Radiotherapy plus concomitant and adjuvant temozolamide for glioblastoma. *New England Journal of Medicine*, **352**, 987–96.

40. Thomas, R., James, N., Guerro, D. *et al.* (1994). Hypofractionated radiotherapy as a palliative treatment in poor prognosis patients with high grade glioma. *Radiotherapy and Oncology*, **33**, 113–6.

41. Wasserstrom, W.R., Glass, J.P., and Posner, J.B. (1982). Diagnosis and treatment of leptomeningeal metastases from solid tumours. *Cancer*, **49**, 759–72.

42. Vikram, B., and Chu, F. (1979). Radiation therapy to metastases to the base of the skull. *Radiology*, **130**, 465–8.

43. Hall, S., Buzdar, A., and Blumenschein, G. (1983). Cranial nerve palsies in metastatic breast cancer due to osseous metastases without intracranial involvement. *Cancer*, **52**, 180–4.

44. Roos, D., Turner, S.L., O'Brien, P.C. *et al.* (2005). Randomized trial of 8 Gy in 1 versus 20 Gy in 5 fractions of radiotherapy for neuropathic pain due to bone metastases. *(Trans-Tasman Radiation Oncology Group, TROG 96.05) Radiotherapy and Oncology*, **75**, 54–63.

45. Russi, E.G., Pergolizzi, S., Gaeta, M. *et al.* (1993). Palliative radiotherapy in lumbosacral carcinomatous neuropathy. *Radiotherapy and Oncology*, **26**, 172–3.

46. James, R.D., Johnson, R.J., Eddleston, B. *et al.* (1983). Prognostic factors in locally recurrent rectal carcinoma treated by radiotherapy. *British Journal of Surgery*, **70**, 469–72.

47. Ampil, F.L. (1985). Radiotherapy for carcinomatous brachial plexus plexopathy. *Cancer*, **56**, 2185–8.

48. Rudoler, S.B., Shields, C., Corn, B.W. *et al.* (1997). Functional vision is improved in the majority of patients treated with external beam radiotherapy for choroidal metastases: a multivariate analysis of 188 patients. *Journal of Clinical Oncology*, **15**, 1244–51.

49. Wiegel, T., Bottke, D., Kreusel, K-M. *et al.* (2002). External beam radiotherapy of choroidal metastases – final results of a prospective study of the German Cancer Society (ARO 95-08). *Radiotherapy and Oncology*, **64**, 13–8.

50. Laperriere, N.J., Cerezo, L., Milosevic, M.F. *et al.* (1997). Primary lymphoma of brain: results of management of a modern cohort with radiation therapy. *Radiotherapy and Oncology*, **43**, 247–52.

51. Denton, A.S., and Spittle, M.F. (1995). Leukaemia and Lymphoma. *Current Medical Literature, The Royal Society of Medicine*, **3**, 35–41.

52. Ahman, F.R. (1984). A reassessment of the clinical implications of the superior vena caval syndrome. *Journal of Clinical Oncology*, **2**, 961–8.

53. Lanciego, C., Chacon, J.L., Julian, A. *et al.* (2001). Stenting as the first option for endovascular treatment of malignant superior vena cava syndrome. *Journal of the American College of Radiology*, **177**, 585–93.

54. Timothy, A.R., Girling, D.J., Saunders, M.I. *et al.* (2001). Radiotherapy for inoperable lung cancer. *Clinical Oncology*, **13**, 86–7.

55. MRC Lung Cancer Working Party. (1991). Inoperable non-small cell lung cancer (NSCLC): A Medical Research Council randomised trial of palliative radiotherapy with two fractions or ten fractions. *British Journal of Cancer*, **63**, 265–70.

56. MRC Lung Cancer Working Party. (1992). A Medical Research Council (MRC) randomised trial of palliative radiotherapy with two fractions or a single fraction in patients with inoperable non-small cell lung cancer (NSCLC) and poor performance status. *British Journal of Cancer*, **65**, 934–41.

57. Medical Research Council Lung Cancer Working Party. (1996). Randomized trial of palliative two-fraction versus more intensive 13-fraction radiotherapy for patients with inoperable non-small cell lung cancer and good performance status. *Clinical Oncology*, **8**, 167–75.

58. Bezjak, A., Dixon, P., Brundage, M. *et al.* (2002). Randomized phase III trial of single versus fractionated thoracic radiation in the palliation of patients with lung cancer (NCIC CTG SC.15). *International Journal of Radiation Oncology, Biology, Physics*, **54**(3), 719–28.

59. Stout, R., Barber, P., Burt, P. *et al.* (2000). Clinical and quality of life outcomes in the first United Kingdom randomized trial of endobronchial brachytherapy (intraluminal radiotherapy) vs. external beam radiotherapy in the palliative treatment of inoperable non-small cell lung cancer. *Radiotherapy and Oncology*, **56**, 323–7.

60. Clegg, A., Scott, D.A., Sidhu, M. *et al.* (2001). A rapid and systematic review of the clinical effectiveness and cost-effectiveness of paclitaxel, docetaxel, gemcitabine and vinorelbine in non-small-cell lung cancer. *Health Technology Assessment*, **5**(32), 1–195.

61. Sykes, N.P., Baines, M., and Carter, R.L. (1998). Clinical and pathological study of dysphagia conservatively managed in patients with advanced malignant disease. *Lancet*, **ii**, 726–8.

62. Wara, M., Mauch, P.M., Thomas, A.N. *et al.* (1976). Palliation for carcinoma of the oesophagus. *Radiology*, **121**, 717–20.

63. Leslie, M.D. *et al.* (1992). The role of radiotherapy in carcinoma of the thoracic oesophagus: an audit of the Mount Vernon experience 1980–1989. *Clinical Oncology*, **4**, 114–8.

64. Brewster, A.E., Davidson, S.E., Makin, W.P. *et al.* (1995). Intraluminal brachytherapy using the high ose rate microselectron in the palliation of carcinoma of the oesophagus. *Clinical Oncology*, **7**, 102–5.

65. Flores, A.D. *et al.* (1990). The impact of new radiotherapy modalities in thesurgical management of cancer of the oesophagus and cardia. In *Brachytherapy HDR and LDR* (eds. A.A. Martinez, C.G. Orton, and R.F. Mould), pp. 27–43. Columbia: Nucletron.

66. Wells, P., Hoskin, P.J., Towler, J. *et al.* (1996). The effect of radiotherapy on urethral obstruction from carcinoma of the prostate. *British Journal of Urology*, **78**, 752–5.

67. Duchesne, G.M., Bolger, J.J., Griffiths, G.O. *et al.* (2000). A randomized trial of hypofractionated schedules of palliative radiotherapy in the management of bladder carcinoma: results of Medical Research Council Trial BA09. *International Journal of Radiation Oncology, Biology, Physics*, **47**, 379–88.

68. Srinivasan, V., Brown, C.H., and Turner, A.G. (1994). A comparison of two radiotherapy regimes for the treatment of symptoms from advanced bladder cancer. *Clinical Oncology*, **6**, 11–3.

69. Hoskin, P.J., and Coyle, C. (2004). *Radiotherapy in practice: brachytherapy*. Oxford University Press, Oxford.

70. Taylor, R.E., Kerr, G.R., and Arnott, S.J. (1987). External beam radiotherapy for rectal adenocarcinoma. *British Journal of Surgery*, **74**, 455–9.

71. Hoskin, P.J., de Canha, S.M., Bownes, P. *et al.* (2004). High dose rate afterloading intraluminal brachytherapy for inoperable rectal carcinoma. *Radiotherapy and Oncology*, **73**, 195–8.

72. Overgaard, J. (1986). The role of radiotherapy in recurrent and metastatic malignant melanoma: A clinical radiobiological study. *International Journal of Radiation Oncology, Biology, Physics*, **12**, 867–72.

73. Fletcher, G.H. (1990). Controversial views in the management of cervical metastases. *International Journal of Radiation Oncology, Biology, Physics*, **19**, 1101–2.

74. Munro, A.J., and Stewart, J.S.W. (1989). Aids: Incidence and management of malignant disease. *Radiotherapy and Oncology*, **14**, 121–31.

75. Leibel, S.A. *et al.* (1981). A comparison of misonidazole sensitised radiation therapy to radiation therapy alone for the palliation of hepatic metastases: results of a Radiation Therapy Oncology Group randomised study. *International Journal of Radiation Oncology, Biology, Physics*, **7**, 587–91.

76. Borgelt, B.B., Gelber, R., Brady, L.W. *et al.* (1981). The palliation of hepatic metastases: results of the Radiation Therapy Oncology Group pilot study. *International Journal of Radiation Oncology, Biology, Physics*, **7**, 587–91.

77. Paulino, A.C., and Reddy, S.P. (1996). Splenic irradiation in the palliation of patients with lymphoproliferative and myeloproliferative disorders. *The American Journal of Hospice & Palliative Care*, **13**, 32–5.

The role of general surgery in the palliative care of patients with cancer

Robert S. Krouse

Introduction

Role of surgeon in palliative care of the cancer patient

While there have been dramatic advances leading to increased survival for oncology patients, many individuals with cancer will ultimately succumb to their disease. Therefore, palliation is increasingly becoming recognized as an important component of care of the cancer patient. This includes general surgeons, who have long played a critical role in curative attempts in oncology patients, but now are increasingly recognized as important contributors in the palliative care of patients with cancer. This has been aided through advances in technology, improved surgical techniques, and a greater knowledge of the disease and its effects on anatomy and physiology. Thus, surgical procedures have become accepted as an important and common component of the comprehensive palliative care of patients with advanced cancer. In fact, in one review at a cancer centre, it was noted that 12.5 per cent of cases were done with a palliative intent[1]. Additionally, in a survey of cancer surgeons, it was estimated that 21 per cent of all surgical procedures for cancer patients are for palliation[2].

The role of the surgeon is multifactoral in the treatment of palliative issues. The diverse indications for palliative procedures include hormonal imbalance, malignant fluid re-accumulation, obstructions, tumour bleeding or other local complications, and pain[3]. The general surgeon may participate in the care of the advanced cancer patient to improve the quality of life (QOL) related to each of these indications, which may be due to the many various primary or metastatic cancers.

Primary cancers and the need for surgery

In addition to specific symptom management, the role of the general surgeon is often based on the primary disease being treated. This may be due to the complication that occurs, such as a bowel obstruction in a colorectal (CRC) cancer patient, or related to the surgeon's intimate knowledge of the normal progression of disease and surgical indications. Cancers generally associated with the general surgeon are breast, skin, gastrointestinal (including pancreas, biliary tree, and liver), and soft tissue sarcomas. The care of some primary tumours will have overlap with other specialties, such as oesophageal carcinoma (Cardiothoracic Surgery), head and neck cancers (Otolaryngologists) and skin cancers (Plastic Surgeons). The ability of General Surgeons to address these tumours is based on training, including specialty oncology training, as well as necessity (whether surgeons with greater training in these areas are available). Ultimately, the General Surgeon should have knowledge related to each of these tumours to understand surgical indications, as well as other alternatives that are available. In addition, the General Surgeon should have an understanding of the survival related to metastatic disease for these primary cancers and the likelihood an invasive procedure will have success.

Goals of surgery

Definition of success

The benefits and risks of surgical procedures are always of paramount importance, and are crystallized in the patient with advanced cancer. The benefits of palliative surgery should always focus on QOL, symptom control, and symptom prevention[3]. One must also consider that there will frequently be a secondary benefit: survival. This is clearly an important goal of patients and families and must not be forgotten, even in the setting of incurable disease. Unfortunately, the literature frequently focuses exclusively on survival as an endpoint, leaving surgeons with little information on an intervention's impact on QOL.

A major dilemma for the surgeon caring for a patient with a terminal cancer is that measures of success are unclear. The surgical literature has been a poor guide for decision-making for this population of patients. Outcome measures related to QOL are not clearly defined and documented. Historically, what little focus there is on palliation in the surgical literature has been remiss in examining appropriate QOL outcomes. In fact, from 1990 to 1996, QOL measurements have been included in only 17 per cent of reports of palliative procedures in the surgical literature and only 12 per cent examined pain[4]. This is in contrast to the more common outcome measures of physiologic response (69 per cent), survival (64 per cent), and morbidity and mortality (61 per cent). While it is imperative to understand these outcomes, they should not be the primary focus of palliative procedures, as they may not equate with an improvement in QOL. In addition, goals for palliative procedures may be broad and multifaceted. When queried about major goals of palliative procedures, in addition to the obvious aims of symptom relief and pain relief, surgeons also felt that common objectives of such procedures include maintaining independence and function, symptom avoidance, and fewer and shorter hospitalizations[2]. One specific example of the lack of a defined literature related to determining success is malignant bowel obstruction (MBO), where multiple outcomes are measured leading to no consensus for practising surgeons[5].

Pre-emptive surgical palliation

Palliative surgery is most often considered in the setting of an active symptom that needs to be addressed. Less attention has been given to the prevention of symptoms in the palliative setting, but this, too, is a goal of palliative surgery[3]. Many symptoms related to tumours are known to occur, but it is less understood if or when the symptom will actually occur. Therefore, it is not always clear when or if a procedure would be helpful. Appropriate pre-emptive palliative surgery must consider prognostication related to a particular symptom, as well as the lifespan of a patient. For example, in the setting of biliary obstruction where a surgical bypass is attempted, one must also consider a gastric bypass to alleviate the risk of a patient having a gastric outlet obstruction prior to death. Another example may be with nodal dissections in the setting of positive sentinel node mappings, especially if distant disease is noted. A nodal dissection will have little effect on long-term survival, but this procedure may alleviate the risk of nodal recurrence and the suffering this may cause. Therefore, while there is frequently no clear direction for surgeons in these settings, pre-emptive palliative procedures should be considered in settings where tumour-related morbidity can be anticipated. As always, the inherent risks of an operation must be considered, but these are more difficult to assess when the benefits are ultimately unknown.

Surgical risks

With every goal of success must be an understanding of risk. While all treatments contain risk, this is magnified related to a surgical procedure. It is further highlighted with patients who are facing the end of life. Complications will still occur even in the most fastidious care, especially if the patient is debilitated related to the cancer or underlying conditions. First, surgical morbidity may include complications unrelated to the surgical site, such as pneumonia, deep venous thrombosis, ileus, and heart failure. With meticulous care, these can often be avoided. Related to the procedure itself, pain is a major issue that occurs in the perioperative setting, and may persist throughout the patient's course. Epidural, patient controlled analgesia, and local anaesthetic pumps may improve pain control and ultimate outcomes. Related to the surgical site, wound complications must always be considered. For example, it has been noted that lymph node dissections may have quite high rates of wound problems (47 per cent for axillary node and 71 per cent after inguinal node dissections)[6]. Issues such as seromas and infections may be long-term problems that take weeks to months to heal. Patients with advanced cancers may not have time to heal these wounds. Lymphatic leaks may necessitate procedures to isolate the offending lymphatic vessel. Therefore, when considering any surgical procedure, whether for curative or palliative intent, these issues must be discussed prior to the operation. As new innovations are utilized, outcomes will continue to improve for surgical patients. Next, acceptance of major disfigurement and lifestyle changes are most pronounced in the immediate postoperative setting. For example, the shock of a permanent stoma may be overwhelming for many patients. While QOL problems related to ostomies may diminish with time[7], this may not be possible for the patient facing the end of life. It must be considered that symptoms may actually worsen after a procedure. Hospital stays may be longer if complications occur. Finally, an invasive procedure may hasten someone's death, which is the ultimate poor outcome.

There are multiple issues to consider who is a surgical candidate. These considerations may lead to a successful palliative procedure with limited morbidity and mortality. For example patient nutritional status, and specifically albumin level, is frequently an excellent tool to decide when not to operate. Related to oesophageal resections, which for many patients is a procedure whose goal is primarily the ability to swallow, albumin along with pulmonary function may be the best determiner of likely success[8]. In addition, surgeons must consider the overall status of patients, including other medical problems and how they may affect overall risk. In all, there are no defined criteria of who the surgeon should not operate on, but there are multiple clues as to who is unlikely to have a good outcome.

Surgical palliative care problems for cancer patients: indications, options, and outcomes

Hormonal control of hepatic metastases of neuroendocrine tumours

Indications

There are multiple symptoms due to metastatic endocrine tumours that may necessitate an invasive procedure. Cancers to consider that are hormonally active include carcinoid, insulinoma, gastrinoma, and VIPoma. The carcinoid syndrome may be the most common of these rare palliative care situations, but it only occurs from primary gastrointestinal carcinoid tumours when there is metastatic disease to the liver. The surgical goals of carcinoid are to limit or minimize the endocrine symptoms or to lessen the medications patients are currently taking. Non-functional endocrine tumours may lead to fatigue or pain, and it may be reasonable to attempt an intervention to relieve these symptoms.

Options

Invasive options for symptomatic endocrine tumours are based on location of the tumour, type of tumour, and alternative treatment options. For pancreatic neuroendocrine tumours, aggressive surgical treatment of the primary tumour is usually indicated[9]. For metastatic gastrinoma, total gastrectomy may also be indicated, although newer medications may alleviate the necessity for such a drastic procedure. While somatostatin analogues frequently modulate symptoms in the setting of liver metastases, it may be short-lived and necessitate increasing doses. The major invasive options for liver metastasis include surgical debulking or ablative techniques. Surgical debulking may necessitate a major hepatectomy or segmental ('wedge') resections. The major ablative technique utilized currently is radiofrequency ablation (RFA), which is associated with low morbidity and mortality[10]. RFA also allows options to perform open, laparoscopic, or radiologist-guided procedures. Finally, it has even been suggested that liver or multivisceral transplantation is a therapeutic option for metastatic neuroendocrine tumours[11].

Outcomes

In addition to minimizing treatment-related complications and shortening hospital stays, ablative techniques can also offer improved QOL in the treatment of pain and tumour hormone output. Anecdotal accounts and small series have shown RFA to be useful in treating metastatic endocrine tumours, but the long-term outcomes are not yet known. Laparoscopic RFA has been shown to achieve symptomatic improvement in patients with secreting neuroendocrine tumours[12,13]. This technique does not require an advanced skill set, but does have a learning curve to efficiently complete procedures. The laparoscopic approach should be considered for patients with symptomatic neuroendocrine liver metastases, although the procedure may be difficult to accomplish in the setting of extensive adhesions.

While ablation of metastatic neuroendocrine tumours is an option for some patients with bulky disease, radical resection with or without ablation must still be an alternative for these patients. As there is a more defined long-term history with radical resection of metastatic hepatic tumours, it should remain the first choice of care in the appropriately selected patient. The surgery must accomplish a significant reduction of tumour bulk to have a symptomatic response, although this number is difficult to quantify.[14] Nevertheless, cytoreductive surgery for selected patients with carcinoid tumours does seem to accomplish a symptomatic advantage related to relief/prevention of obstructions or relief of the carcinoid syndrome[15,16]. Resection and ablative techniques, when followed by a somatostatin analogue, can lead to extremely high rates of long-term symptom-free survival[17].

There are limited reports of liver or multivisceral transplantation in the setting of metastatic neuroendocrine tumours. A recent report has shown a 5-year survival of 90 per cent ($n = 15$)[11]. The QOL benefit is unclear. While this may be a consideration, the experience is quite small and therefore should be attempted with trepidation.

Malignant bowel obstruction

Indications

Malignant bowel obstruction (MBO) is a common problem in patients with ovarian and colorectal cancer. MBO also occurs with other abdominal (e.g. pseudomyxoma pertinoneii, peritoneal mesothelioma, primary peritoneal carcinomas, and gastric or pancreatic carcinomas) and occasionally with non-abdominal malignancies (e.g. melanoma, lung or breast cancers). MBO may be related to cancer (intraluminal or extraluminal tumour growth), its treatment (e.g. radiation enteritis), or benign aetiologies (e.g. adhesions or internal hernia). The goals of treatment include relieving nausea and vomiting, allowing oral intake, alleviating pain, and permitting the patient to return to their chosen care setting. Persistent obstructions in the face of conservative therapy (usually nasogastric decompression, hydration, and bowel rest) or evidence of complete obstructions are indications that a surgical procedure should be considered. Invasive treatment options should be contemplated for all patients with MBO except those who are actively dying.

Options

In cases where surgical management is not feasible, medical management can be very effective at relieving symptoms. The optimal procedure is that which offers the quickest, safest, and most efficacious ability to alleviate the obstruction and improve symptoms. Options include bowel resection, which may lead to the best overall outcome[18,19], bypass, or a gastrostomy. An intestinal stoma may be necessary after resection or to adequately bypass the blockage. Laparoscopic procedures may be attempted, although this approach may be difficult due to adhesions, carcinomatosis, or bowel dilatation. Cytoreductive procedures (resection of intraperitoneal tumour) frequently carry a high morbidity and usually are only considered with very low-grade tumours, such as pseudomyxoma peritonii. Many patients are deemed inoperable (6.2–50 per cent)[5], with the most frequent reasons being extensive tumour, multiple partial obstructions, and inability to correct obstructions surgically[20].

Anywhere from 3 to 48 per cent of malignant bowel obstructions presenting occur because of a benign aetiology[19]. There are a lot of potential contraindications for operation. Ascites (greater than 3 L), carcinomatosis, a patient who has multiple obstructions, palpable intraabdominal mass, overwhelming disease or poor clinical status are relatively strong contraindications for operative intervention[20].

Endoscopic approaches

Endoscopic procedures are suited for patients who are poor operative candidates or who decline an open operative intervention. They also may obviate the need for an intestinal stoma. The major approaches include stenting and percutaneous endoscopic gastrostomy (PEG) tube placement. Stenting may include procedures to initially canalize the lumen (e.g. laser or balloon dilatation). PEG tubes are generally well tolerated 'venting' procedures that can alleviate symptoms of intractable vomiting and nausea for upper GI obstructions[21]. In combination with other medical techniques, both open and percutaneous gastrostomy offer the possibility of intermittent oral intake.

Outcomes

Although it is recognized that improvement in QOL after surgery is variable (42–85 per cent)[5,22], there is no consistent parameter used to determine this clinical outcome; operations may offer an advantage of an increased survival. Surgical risks must be carefully considered prior to an operation, as morbidity (42 per cent)[23] and mortality (5–32 per cent)[5,19,23] are common, and the re-obstruction rate is high (10–50 per cent)[5,24]. Poor prognostic indicators for surgical intervention include ascites, carcinomatosis, palpable intraabdominal masses, multiple bowel obstructions, prior obstructions and very advanced disease with poor performance status.

Endoluminal wall stents have a high success rate for relief of symptoms (64–100 per cent) in complete and incomplete colorectal obstructions[25], and in over 70 per cent of upper intestinal malignant obstructions including gastric outlet, duodenal and jejunal obstructions[26]. While risks include perforation (0–15 per cent), stent migration (0–40 per cent), or re-occlusion (0–33 per cent), stents can frequently lead to adequate palliation for long periods of time[25]. Stent occlusion by tumour in-growth is usually amenable to another endoscopic intervention. Complications related to PEGs are rare, even when puncturing other organs[21]. The presence of significant ascites is a relative contraindication.

Wounds/fistulae

Indications

There are multiple different kinds of wounds related to advanced cancer that require the involvement of a General Surgeon. These are often directly related to tumours, but may be due to treatments such as surgical procedures or radiation therapy. Tumour-related wounds can be seen with primary, recurrent, or nodal manifestations of tumours. Primary cancers that frequently lead to wound problems include breast cancer, skin cancers, soft tissue sarcomas, or soft tissue manifestations of other cancers (e.g. lung cancer). Special consideration must be taken related to the primary tumour type. As treatment approaches are frequently multi-disciplinary, it is important for the surgeon to include other specialists, including medical and radiation oncologists, in the decision-making. Procedure-related wounds may be due to node dissections, local resections, or simple incisions. Radiation may lead to non-healing ulcers at resection sites. Finally, due to debilitation, patients may have pressure sores which complicate their overall course and lead to suffering. In the debilitated patient, pressure sores are more likely to occur. It is unlikely that there would be an indication for a major procedure for this complication, although minor procedures may be helpful.

Fistulae, like wound problems, may occur in patients who are facing the end of life for various reasons. Fistulae are a heterogeneous group of problems. A fistula is simply a communication of one structure to another, including bowel to bowel, bowel to skin, or pancreas to skin. Fistulae may be a complication of procedures, such as pancreatic fistulae after a resection, or due to other treatments, such as a radiation therapy leading to enterocutaneous fistulae. These problems may be extremely difficult to cure, especially in the setting near death. Indications for surgical options are rare.

Options

First, prevention is of primary importance. For example, resection of a nodal or soft tissue metastasis can simply be excised to avoid the potential wound problems that will ensue if ignored. Another preventative consideration is related to pressure wounds. This entails ensuring patients are not stationary for long periods of time. Once a pressure sore has started, it can be difficult or impossible to heal.

Many wounds, especially related to radiation injury or in the severely malnourished, may not heal. Therefore, this should not be a goal of treatment, but focus should be on control of pain, odour, and mess. Wound care is of primary importance. This may include local debridement as indicated to keep the wound as clean as possible.

One example of a chronic wound problem is chest wall complications of breast tumours. There are many articles in the nursing literature regarding local wound care. Chemotherapy, especially if the patient is chemo-naïve, is an option. Radiation therapy, although unlikely to have a great effect with a very large tumour, is possible. Of course, surgical resection is an alternative. The term 'toilet' mastectomy is used in the setting of a fungating incurable breast cancer to remove the tumour with the intent of wound control. It is always important to know the previous treatments to better understand possible success. This will also help to identify the optimal reconstruction alternatives as well as the extent of resection that is possible. The surgical literature is not very helpful in directing the extent of resection, and this must be based on surgeon judgement.

Reconstruction options include primary closure, skin grafts, and an omental flap with skin graft, musculocutaneous flaps, or free flaps. The major surgical complications that must be considered include infection, open wounds, and flap loss.

Additional morbid options are possible based on the site of the tumour and medical status of the patient. These may include amputations, limb perfusions, and major head and neck resections. While these options may seem quite radical in the setting of palliation, they may be reasonable solutions based on symptoms and if the patient can withstand a large procedure.

While treatment options for fistulae in the patient with advanced cancer may not significantly differ from those not facing the end of life, there are many issues in this population that necessitate special consideration. As with the non-advanced cancer patient, controlling fistulae is the most important treatment. For cutaneous fistulae, this may be through the utilization of stoma bags, drains, or active wound care. For internal fistulae, such as bowel communicating to bowel or bladder, the specific anatomy of the communication is paramount to decide if a surgical option is reasonable.

Outcomes

There have been many reports concerning local wound care for tumour-related wounds. Most of these are in nursing journals. This component of care is extremely important, and has been shown to have great impact on QOL. For example, controlling odour and seepage has been shown to lead to less isolation, greater comfort, and increased psychosocial well-being[27]. This straightforward approach to some wounds will lead to the best outcomes for many patients facing the end of life.

Multiple reports have focused on chest wall resections for breast cancer. These were either related to recurrent disease or an initial presentation of a fungating breast tumour. Many different reconstruction techniques have been shown to be efficacious, including myocutaneous or omental flaps. The recurrence rates in this setting may be high. In one small series it was noted to be 73 per cent[28], and 20–52 per cent in some of the larger series[29–32]. The majority of these recurrences were quite small, though, and could be locally excised or observed in patients who already had other major metastatic disease. Local wound morbidity is variable, and most are quite minor, such as local skin necrosis in a skin graft which will not have great impact on the patient's life. Importantly, if there is major local wound morbidity, this could have a profound effect on the patient for the remainder of their life.

Related to amputation, there are multiple small reports that do indicate good to excellent palliation[33]. Complications may be over 50 per cent, including flap necrosis, infection, and death. Complication rates will depend on the extent of amputation. In addition to amputation, limb perfusion most commonly utilizing melphalan with or without tumour necrosis factor-alpha (TNF-α) has been advocated in some centres for melanoma or sarcoma recurrences. Complete response rates are 45–72 per cent, usually greater if TNF-α was used[34]. Importantly, it has been shown that QOL can be excellent, with reasonable long-term function[34].

Related to fistulae, there is little evidence specific to the end-of-life patient. Therefore, non-surgical techniques are usually optimal. One can look to the non-palliative literature for guidance, but in patients with limited survival, this is unlikely to be a sufficient guide.

Biliary obstruction

Indications

Biliary obstructions are commonly from pancreatic cancer. Tumours causing obstruction of the extrahepatic bile duct may also occur all along the biliary tree, most likely at the ampulla of Vatar. Blockages must be treated expediently as this will lead to hyperbilirubinemia which may become symptomatic, leading to pruritis, bleeding diathesis, and liver failure. Surgical involvement today is mainly in the instances of a failed endoscopic retrograde cholangiography procedure (ERCP) stenting or inoperability at the time of surgical exploration for a presumed resection with a curative intent. There are multiple studies comparing methods, especially stenting versus surgery[35–39]. Stenting has been shown to have similar success rates as surgery with less morbidity. While stent recurrence may be higher, the immediate benefits outweigh this detriment. If the bile duct is entered via the ERCP but a stent could not be placed, it may necessitate a relatively urgent surgical procedure due to the potential cholangitis risk. If urgent surgery is not realistic due to patient co-morbidities, overall status, or operating room availability, a transhepatic drain placed by an Interventional Radiologist is indicated. If a laparoscopic exploration is first undertaken for a potentially resectable mass and metastatic disease is noted, it is reasonable to abort the procedure with the hope that a less morbid endoscopic stenting can be accomplished. Also, if endoscopic stenting fails or is unavailable, open or laparoscopic bypass is warranted. If at open exploration the patient is found to be unresectable, it is reasonable to proceed with a surgical intervention.

Options

There are multiple surgical options to bypass the biliary system. They include cholecystojejunostomy, choledochojejunostomy, or choledochoduodenostomy. In addition, the bypass may be performed higher along the duct to the hepatic duct (above the cystic duct). While these procedures may be undertaken with a laparoscope, few surgeons have the technical skills for this procedure[40]. Importantly, in the appropriate operative candidate, a pancreaticoduodenectomy (Whipple procedure) is an option. While the surgeon should not proceed with a Whipple procedure if there are clear signs of metastasis to the liver or other organs or invasion of major vascular structures, many surgeons will complete the procedure if there is limited local nodal disease.

Outcomes

The overall morbidity of surgical bypass is almost 20 per cent, and the recurrence rate is 0–15 per cent[35–39]. It has been shown that choledochoduodenostomy has the fewest complications at only 3 per cent[41]. Of course, the ability to mobilize the duodenum may not be possible in all patients. There have been several reports of laparoscopic biliary bypass of malignant biliary obstructions, mainly via cholecystojejunostomy, although hepaticojejunostomy also might be performed[42], though it requires expertise available in only a few centres.

Finally, a pancreaticoduodenectomy is considered by many to be a large palliative procedure. Whipple himself said that 'the considerable risk,' which certainly was considerable in 1942, 'was justified if they can be made comfortable for a year or two'[43]. It has been shown that QOL can be improved from a Whipple procedure[44], and should be considered in the appropriate surgical candidate without evidence of metastasis.

Gastric outlet obstruction

Indications

There is some controversy as to when to do a surgical procedure for gastric outlet obstruction. Typically, these procedures are considered in the setting of persistent nausea, vomiting, eructation, and early satiety. They also may be considered when there is evidence of duodenal compression on radiographic or endoscopic evaluations. With the advent of endoscopic stents, the indications for an operative approach may be less common today. Stents for gastric outlet obstruction are noted to be quite successful (approximately 90 per cent) with rare complications[45,46]. In addition, if the stent fails due to tumour in-growth or migration (around 10 per cent), another stent can often be placed[45,46]. On the other hand, few centres have gastroenterologists with the technical ability to accomplish this procedure successfully.

In the setting where a biliary bypass is planned, there is some controversy as to whether to do a pre-emptive gastric bypass (gastrojejunostomy) in the asymptomatic patient. Late gastric obstruction occurs from 9 to 23 per cent[47–49], and this must be considered at the time of biliary bypass. If the patient is of good performance status with limited disease (no or minimal metastasis), then a pre-emptive procedure may be indicated.

Options

The surgical options for gastric outlet obstruction are a bypass procedure (gastrojejunostomy) or a resection (antrectomy or pancreaticoduodenectomy). There are several technical variations of a bypass procedure, but the results are similar. The simplest method is to take a loop of jejunum and attach to the stomach. This can be achieved via open or laparoscopic techniques[50]. There might be slightly better emptying if this is done to the posterior wall of the stomach. A distal gastric tumour may also be resected with a palliative intent. As stated earlier regarding biliary obstruction, a pancreaticojejunostomy may also be an option in the optimal patient.

Outcomes

If endoscopic expertise is available, stenting is preferable for both biliary and gastric obstructions. Most institutions can offer endoscopic biliary tract stenting, but less have the ability to stent gastric outlet obstructions. If endoscopic stenting fails for the gastric outlet blockage or is unavailable, open or laparoscopic bypass is warranted. If exploration via a laparoscope reveals that the patient is unresectable, it is reasonable not to continue the procedure and then attempt an endoscopic procedure. If the expertise is unavailable, an operative bypass is warranted. If exploration via an open procedure reveals that the patient is unresectable, it is reasonable to bypass the patient.

It has been shown that symptomatic patients (vomiting prior to operation) typically have a poor outcome (approximately 90 per cent did not have relief of symptoms) to gastric bypass. In comparison, if patients were not symptomatic but had evidence of impending obstruction, only about 40 per cent had a poor outcome[51]. One consideration as to the reason for this is that symptomatic patients are potentially sicker with a greater tumour burden.

Gastric outlet obstruction has been safely treated with a laparoscopic gastrojejunostomy. In fact, for unresectable gastric cancer this technique has been shown to have less suppression of immune function, less pain, shorter hospital stays, lower postoperative morbidity, and earlier recovery of bowel movements than an open procedure[50].

Antrectomy along with gastrojejunostomy in the setting of unresectable pancreatic cancer has been shown to have excellent results until death in one small series[52]. There is limited evidence in the literature to support this procedure in the setting of gastric outlet obstruction, and a simpler bypass may be more reasonable.

Bleeding

Indications

Tumour-related bleeding is frequently difficult to treat, especially with patients who may have a coagulopathy related to illness or treatments. Bleeding may be related to superficial tumours such as recurrent breast, head and neck, or sarcomas. Symptoms related to deeper tumours include hemoptysis (e.g. primary or metastatic lung tumours), hematemasis (e.g. gastric cancer), melena or hematochezia (e.g. colorectal tumours), vaginal bleeding (e.g. cervical or endometrial carcinomas) or hematuria (e.g. renal or bladder tumours). Indications for surgical involvement will be related to location of the tumour and whether another approach is less morbid and has a reasonable chance at success. Non-surgical options include radiation therapy, arterial embolization, endoscopic procedures, and bronchoscopic techniques.

Options

Obviously there are multiple reasons for bleeding, leading to a very heterogeneous group of patients, and the optimal surgical option will depend mainly on the location and reason for bleeding. For example, if there is superficial tumour bleeding, direct suturing may be possible. It must be considered though, that the bleeding may be diffuse and simple suturing may not be efficacious. Therefore, resection may be indicated. For deeper tumours, such as colon tumours, a resection may more clearly be the best option. Rectal tumours, which necessitate larger, more complex procedures and probably an intestinal stoma, may be better served first with non-surgical attempts (e.g. radiation therapy or interventional radiology embolization). The success of alternative approaches will be based on the availability and expertise at each institution.

Outcomes

The outcomes to the treatment of bleeding depend specifically on the treatment approach and the aetiology of the bleeding. Resecting a bleeding tumour will universally stop the bleeding, but there may be added surgical morbidity and mortality than if the operation was performed in the non-emergent setting. Other options to temporize the situation or attempt to alleviate the need for an operation, such as an embolization procedure, may carry a greater risk of recurrence of bleeding but will often be less morbid than a major operation. Of course, this may be quite variable and depends on the tumour location.

Malignant ascites

Indications

Ascites may be due to overwhelming liver metastasis, cirrhotic liver disease, or carcinomatosis. It can be a difficult management problem, and treatment may be determined by the extent of ascites, condition of patient, or aetiology. If ascites is minimal, no therapy is indicated. Treatments will be necessary with larger volumes of ascites, which can lead to discomfort, fullness, or respiratory problems. Surgical options should be considered if diuretics no longer are helping or percutaneous aspirations are becoming painful and frequent. In addition to improving patient comfort, a reasonable indication for surgical interventions is to ease the burden of care. If the patient has very advanced disease, simpler approaches should be initiated. If the patient has a longer lifespan, more invasive techniques may be considered.

Options

Probably the simplest surgical techniques are the insertion of permanent intraperitoneal drainage catheters. This will allow serial drainage of fluid by the patient or their caretaker. Catheters can be placed surgically or by the interventional radiology team via computed tomography[53] or ultrasound guidance[54]. Multiple types of catheters have been used, including a pigtail catheter, peritoneal dialysis catheters (e.g. Tenckhoff catheter), pleural cavity catheters (e.g. Pleurx® catheter), fenestrated port-a-catheters, and even a Foley catheter[55–59]. The patient and/or caregiver can be trained to drain excess peritoneal fluid when the patient is symptomatic.

Another option for malignant ascites is a peritoneovenous shunt. The two most common are the LeVeen or Denver® shunt. Ascitic fluid travels from the peritoneal cavity into the venous circulation due to higher peritoneal pressures. Surgeons are often apprehensive to perform this procedure due to the historical catastrophic complications, including sepsis, disseminated intravascular coagulation (DIC), heart failure, and pulmonary embolism leading to a rapid death. In addition, patients often die within 1 month of their procedure due to their poor general condition[60].

A much more invasive surgical technique includes a major debulking of carcinomatosis followed by intraperitoneal hyperthermic chemotherapy. Improved perioperative care has allowed surgeons to utilize such approaches more often and in sicker patients. This procedure is only available at specialized institutions that have great experience with this technique.

Outcomes

The success rates for permanent intraperitoneal catheters functioning until death is quite high (90 per cent)[54,55]. There is low procedural morbidity. It has even been reported that a percutaneously placed catheter that passed through the colon did not have any adverse sequelae[61]. The major complications are obstruction and infection, and are around 17 per cent[54,55], although catheter sepsis has been reported to be 35 per cent[62]. To avoid infection there must be meticulous insertion technique, close patient follow-up, and liberal use of antibiotics. In fact many catheter-related infections can be treated with antibiotics[54,61]. Sometimes the catheters may need to be removed due to infection, occlusion or leakage around the catheter. Leakage has been reported to be alleviated by continuous drainage[55] or a suture around the drain[62].

While the incidence of major complications may be less common than previously reported for peritoneovenous shunts, the overall complication rate can be quite high (14–51 per cent)[60,63,64]. DIC is the major complication that most frequently will lead to patient death. It has been reported from 5 to 10 per cent of these procedures. Congestive heart failure is another major complication. The more common complication is shunt occlusion. The advantage of the Denver® shunt over the LeVeen shunt is that the Denver® shunt has a pump to help the shunt remain patent (26 per cent Denver® vs. 50 per cent LeVeen shunt occlusion rates)[64]. Denver® shunts have been shown to have quite high function of these shunts until death (96 per cent)[63]. The risk of infection is variable (0–18 per cent)[63], and this may lead to shunt removal if not relieved with antibiotics. Importantly, relief of symptoms can be as high as 87.5 per cent[63]. Therefore, a peritoneovenous shunt may be an excellent option in properly selected patients.

In the carcinomatosis patient, cytoreduction and intraperitoneal chemotherapy can have dramatic effects on ascites. In one report, 79 per cent of patients did not have recurrence for the remainder of their life (median survival 7.6 months)[65]. Surprisingly, their group has also shown that this procedure can lead to an acceptable QOL and return of function status for many patients[66]. Therefore, cytoreduction and intraperitoneal chemotherapy can be considered in the well-selected patient with an experienced surgical team. Further research is needed to better delineate the role of intraperitoneal chemotherapy in the setting of carcinomatosis and ascites.

Splenomegaly

Indications

Splenectomy due to splenomegaly in the palliative setting may be on an urgent/emergent basis due to injury, or in an elective setting related to symptomatic splenic hypertrophy. Splenomegaly may have profound symptoms due to a mass effect, most commonly on the stomach leading to early satiety. Large spleens may also compress other structures, such as the kidney. In addition, splenomegaly may lead to an increased chance of injury, with consideration of a prophylactic splenectomy to avoid such a complication. Related to splenic trauma, in the non-palliative setting it is common to try to preserve the spleen and avoid an operation. In the context of a patient facing the end of life, splenic preservation is less of a priority and may be more dangerous. Therefore, urgent splenectomy is usually indicated in this setting, provided the patient is an operative candidate. For symptomatic splenomegaly, the choice of treatment is usually related to the anticipated survival of the patient. If the patient is felt to have a survival of at least 3–6 months, an operation is usually the best alternative as the recurrence rate related to radiation for haematologic disorders is quite high[67]. If survival is predicted to be low, it is reasonable to attempt radiation therapy.

Options

Today, splenectomies can frequently be accomplished via laparoscopy. Some feel that laparoscopic splenectomy is the procedure of choice for elective spleen removal[68]. While massive splenomegaly may make a laparoscopic procedure difficult or impossible, most experienced surgeons can remove large spleens by this technique. Splenic tissue is removed via morcellation. This is acceptable as margin of resection is not of significance in this setting. Of course, open splenectomy is also reasonable, although it may carry a higher morbidity and mortality, especially in this sick population. In the emergency setting due to injury, a laparoscopic approach may not be reasonable.

Outcomes

Laparoscopic splenectomy has been reported to carry a complication rate of 13 per cent, and a mortality of 1 per cent[69], with decreased hospitalization and pain[69]. These rates are likely to be higher in the setting of advanced cancer. Use of a hand port (the introduction of a surgeon's hand into the peritoneal cavity to assist the procedure) may greatly facilitate the operation, and is advocated by some

surgeons especially for significantly enlarged spleens[68,70–72]. While port-site splenosis has been documented[73], this is unlikely to be an issue for patients facing the end of life. However, only a surgeon skilled in the procedure should undertake laparoscopic splenectomy in a patient with massive splenomegaly[74,75]. No matter how a spleen is removed, obstructive symptoms such as early satiety will ultimately be resolved.

Future directions

Technology

As technology improves for the surgical treatment of tumours for cure, this will also have impact on palliative care. For example, the use of RFA techniques for primary hepatomas and metastatic colorectal cancers also has a role for the less common endocrine metastases. Many other technologies, including minimally invasive techniques can effectively treat complications related to tumours or their care with less morbidity.

Education

Palliative surgery is becoming increasingly recognized as an important role of the surgeon. While education of the surgeon has been lacking, its importance is being increasingly recognized, which will lead to improved patient care. The reasons for a lack of focus on end-of-life care in surgical residency programmes are multifaceted, and are based in the culture of surgeons and the clinical dilemmas they face. First, many surgeons may not feel comfortable or competent with end-of-life issues. This is in part due to the 'cut to cure' mentality that has been passed on through the generations. Medical students over the years have been drawn to surgery because they want to 'fix' the problem. In the setting of the cancer patient with advanced disease, where cure is not an option, then QOL must be the focus as the problem to be 'fixed.'

While all medical specialties have been remiss in the teaching of palliative care, General Surgery has been especially deficient. Surgical textbooks are inferior to all others in ensuring that end-of-life topics are addressed. In fact, one investigation revealed that 71.8 per cent of all end-of-life topics were not included in the leading surgery textbooks[76]. Furthermore, in a survey by the Society of Surgical Oncology, 48 per cent of respondents said they had had no palliative care training while in medical school[2]. In fact, 30 per cent of the respondents had had no training in these issues during their residency or fellowship training. Almost 80 per cent reported 10 h or less of such instruction during all of their training. This confirms a previous report that surgical training is deficient in adequately educating residents in end-of-life care[77]. Of greatest concern, however, is the lack of postgraduate CME in end-of-life care, as shown by a study in which 23.6 per cent of surgeons with a special interest or focus in cancer said that they have had no continuing education in palliative care.

Research

As surgeons strive to improve their care of patients with palliative care issues, research will also need to follow suit. There is currently a paucity of prospective palliative studies in the surgical literature[4]. This is for many reasons, including ethical considerations in surgical palliative care studies[78]. Issues such as vulnerability of patients or the clinician as the researcher are not exclusive to palliative research, but they certainly are highlighted in the advanced cancer setting. There are matters unique to palliative research itself, such as the lack of clarity of the risk–benefit relationship. Another concern is with randomization, which can be quite difficult, especially if there is a placebo arm. A placebo arm is likely impossible in a palliative surgery trial. Finally, there are issues unique to surgical palliative research in that surgery is obviously quite invasive. In addition, once a procedure is completed it is difficult or impossible to reverse, unlike a chemotherapy trial where the medication can be stopped.

There are many barriers to surgical palliative care studies[78]. The ethical dilemma of participating in a trial for a patient with advanced cancer may be a barrier for some surgeons. There are barriers inherent to surgery such as surgeon and procedure variability. Patients and family agreement to participate in such trial may be a barrier. Funding is clearly an impediment to such studies; in 1999 it was shown that 0.9 per cent of the NCI funding was for end-of-life care[79]. The consent process can also be an obstacle, especially if there are mental status changes or no family member available. Finally, there may be an inaccessibility of patients based on referring practitioner bias or patients being in hospice care. Therefore, some of the procedures that could improve QOL are never offered. This is an issue regarding care in general and not just related to research issues.

Research in the advanced cancer patient is important to pursue to improve patient care related to treatment alternatives, but also to improve the care by the surgical team. In assessing QOL in extremity sarcoma trials, it was observed that the very act of trying to determine what QOL means to people seemed to have had a humanizing effect on the investigative team[80]. Therefore, additional importance placed on palliative care through research could lead to greater importance of QOL issues for surgeons.

Conclusions

Palliative procedures are an important component of the practice for General Surgeons who care for cancer patients. It is imperative to understand the surgical and non-surgical options afforded each patient. If a surgical procedure is considered, the patient, family, and treating teams must have a firm understanding of realistic goals of success which focus on QOL. In addition, the chances of attaining those goals must be understood. Finally, the risks of the procedure, including worsening of symptoms and death must be clearly described. As long as these criteria are met, surgical procedures may be undertaken in the setting of terminal cancer. In addition, surgeons should maintain follow-up with the patient whether they operate or not. If an alternative approach is attempted, there may be evolution of disease and surgical intervention may be subsequently indicated. Importantly, the surgeon should continue to follow their patient if at all possible, even when no surgical procedure is undertaken, especially if a relationship has been established. Care of patients by a surgeon includes much more than the operations they perform.

References

1. Krouse, R.S., Nelson, R.A., Ferrell, B.R. et al. (2001). Surgical palliation at a cancer center. Archives of Surgery, 136, 773–8.
2. McCahill, L.E., Krouse, R., Chu, D. et al. (2002). Indications and use of palliative surgery: results of Society of Surgical Oncology survey. Annals of Surgical Oncology, 2, 104–12.
3. Markman, M. (1995). Surgery for support and palliation in patients with malignant disease. Seminars in Oncology, 22, 91–4.
4. Miner, T.J., Jaques, D.P., Tavaf-Motamen, H. et al. (1999). Decision making on surgical palliation based on patient outcome data. American Journal of Surgery, 177, 150–4.
5. Feuer, D.J., Broadley, K.B., Shepherd, J.I.I. et al. (1999). Systematic review of surgery in malignant bowel obstruction in advanced gynecological and gastrointestinal cancer. Gynecologic Oncology, 75, 313–22.
6. Serpell, J.W., Carne P.W., and Bailey, M. (2003). Radical lymph node dissection for melanoma. ANZ Journal of Surgery, 73, 294–9.
7. Persson, E., and Wilde Larsson, B. (2005). Quality of care after ostomy surgery: a perspective study of patients. Ostomy Wound Manage, 51(8), 40–8.
8. Fan, S.T., Lau, W.Y., Yip, W.C. et al. (1987). Prediction of postoperative pulmonary complications in oesophagogastric cancer surgery. The British Journal of Surgery, 74, 408–10.
9. Schurr, P.G., Strate, T., Rese, K. et al. (2007). Aggressive surgery improves long-term survival in neuroendocrine pancreatic tumors. Annals of Surgery, 245, 273–81.
10. Erce, C., and Parks, R.W. (2003). Interstitial ablative techniques for hepatic tumours. The British Journal of Surgery, 90, 272–89.
11. Olausson, M., Friman, S., Herlenius, G. et al. (2007). Orthotopic liver or multivisceral transplantation as treatment of metastatic neuroendocrine tumors. Liver Transplanation, 13, 327–33.
12. Siperstein, A.E., Rogers, S.J., Hansen, P.D. et al. (1997). Laparoscopic thermal ablation of hepatic neuroendocring tumor metastases. Surgery, 122, 1147–55.
13. Berber, E., Flesher, N., and Siperstein, A.E. (2002). Laparoscopic radiofrequency ablation of neuroendocrine liver metastases. World Journal of Surgery, 26, 985–90.
14. Gronbech, J.E., Soreide, O., and Bergan, A. (1992). The role of resective surgery in the treatment of the carcinoid syndrome. Scandinavian Journal of Gastroenterology, 27, 433–7.
15. Gulec, S.A., Mountcastle, T.S., Frey, D. et al. (2002). Cytoreductive surgery in patients with advanced-stage carcinoid tumors. The American Surgeon, 68, 667–72.
16. Chamberlain, R.S., Canes, D., Brown, K.T. et al. (2000). Hepatic neuroendocrine metastases: does intervention alter outcomes? Journal of the American College of Surgeons, 190, 432–45.
17. Chung, M.H., Pisegna, J., Spirt, M. et al. (2001). Hepatic cytoreduction followed by a novel long-acting somatostatin analog: a paradigm for intractable neuroendocrine tumors metastatic to the liver. Surgery, 30, 954–62.
18. Aranha, G.V., Folk, F.A., and Greenlee, H.B. (1981). Surgical palliation of small bowel obstruction due to metastatic carcinoma. The American Surgeon, 47, 99–102.
19. Legendre, H., Vahhuyse, F., Caroli-Bose, F.X. et al. (2001). Survival and quality of life after palliative surgery for neoplastic gastrointestinal obstruction. The European Journal of Surgery, 27, 364–7.
20. Ripamonti, C. (1994). Management of bowel obstruction in advanced cancer. Current Opinion in Oncology, 6, 351–7.
21. Campagnutta, E., and Cannizzaro, R. (2000). Percutaneous endoscopic gastrostomy (PEG) in palliative treatment of non-operable intestinal obstruction due to gynecologic cancer: a review. European Journal of Gynaecological Oncology, 21, 397–402.
22. Miner, T.J., Jaques, D.P., and Shriver, C.D. (2002). A prospective evaluation of patients undergoing surgery for the palliation of an advanced malignancy. Annals of Surgical Oncology, 9, 696–703.
23. Makela, J., Kiviniemi, H., Laitinen, S. et al. (1991). Surgical management of intestinal obstruction after treatment for cancer. The European Journal of Surgery, 157, 73–7.
24. Miner, T.J., Jaques, D.P., Paty, P.B. et al. (2003). Symptom control in patients with locally recurrent rectal cancer. Annals of Surgical Oncology, 10, 72–9.

25. Harris, G.J.C., Senagore, A.J., Lavery, I.C. *et al.* (2001). The management of neoplastic colorectal obstruction with colonic endoluminal stenting devices. *American Journal of Surgery*, **181**, 499–506.

26. Soetikno, R.M., and Carr-Locke, D.L. (1999). Expandable metal stents for gastric outlet, duodenal, and small intestinal obstruction. *Gastrointestinal Endoscopy Clinics of North America*, **9**, 447–58.

27. Lund-Nielsen, B., Muller, K., and Adamsen, L. (2004). Malignant wounds in women with breast cancer: feminine and sexual perspectives. *Journal of Clinical Nursing*, **14**, 56–64.

28. Cheung, K.L., Willsher, P.C., Robertson, J.F.R. *et al.* (1997). Omental transposition flap for gross locally recurrent breast cancer. *The Australian and New Zealand Journal of Surgery*, **67**, 185–6.

29. Flook, D., Webster, D.J.T., Hughes, L.E., (1989). Salvage surgery for advanced local recurrence of breast cancer. *The British Journal of Surgery*, **76**, 512–4.

30. Sweetland, H.M., Karatsis, P., and Rogers, K. (1995). Radical surgery for advanced and recurrent breast cancer. *Journal of the Royal College of Surgeons of Edinburgh*, **40**, 88–92.

31. Downey, R.J., Rusch, V., Hsu, F.I. *et al.* (2000). Chest wall resection for locally recurrent breast cancer: is it worthwhile? *The Journal of Thoracic and Cardiovascular Surgery*, **119**, 420–8.

32. Henderson, M.A., Burt, J.D., Jenner, D. *et al.* (2001). Radical surgery with omental flap for uncontrolled locally recurrent breast cancer. *ANZ Journal of Surgery*, **71**, 675–9.

33. Paz, I.B. (2004). Major palliative amputations. *Surgical Oncology Clinics of North America*, **13**, 543–7.

34. Noorda, E.M., Vrouenraets, B.C., Nieweg, O.E. *et al.* (2006). Isolated limb perfusion in regional melanoma. *Surgical Oncology Clinics of North America*, **15**, 373–84.

35. Bornman, P.C., Harries-Jones, E.P., Tobias, R. *et al.* (1986). Prospective controlled trial of transhepatic biliary enoprosthesis versus biliary bypass surgery for incurable carcinoma of head of pancreas. *Lancet*, **I**, 69–71.

36. Shepherd, H.A., Royle, G., Ross, A.P.R. *et al.* (1988). Endoscopic biliary endoprostheses in the palliation of malignant obstruction of the distal common bile duct: a randomized trial. *The British Journal of Surgery*, **75**, 1166–8.

37. Andersen, J.R., Sorensen, S.M., Kruse, A. *et al.* (1989). Randomised trial of endoscopic endoprosthesis versus operative bypass in malignant obstructive jaundice. *Gut*, **30**, 1132–5.

38. Dowsett, J.F., Russell, R.C.G., Hatfield, A.R.W. *et al.* (1989). Malignant obstructive jaundice: a prospective randomized trial of by-pass surgery versus endoscopic stenting. *Gastroenterology*, **96**,128A.

39. Smith, A.C., Dowsett, J.F., Russell, R.C.G. *et al.* (1994). Randomised trial of endoscopic stenting versus surgical bypass in malignant low bile duct obstruction. *Lancet*, **344**, 1655–60.

40. Krouse, R.S. (2004). Advances in palliative surgery for cancer patients. *The Journal of Supportive Oncology*, **2**, 80–7.

41. Potts, J.R. III, Broughan, T.A., and Hermann, R.E. (1990). Palliative operations for pancreatic carcinoma. *American Journal of Surgery*, **159**, 72–8.

42. Gentileschi, P., Kini, S., and Gagner, M. (2002). Palliative laparoscopic hepatico-and gastrojejunostomy for advanced pancreatic cancer. *JSLS*, **6**, 331–8.

43. Whipple, A.O. (1942). Present day surgery of the pancreas. *The New England Journal of Medicine*, **226**, 515.

44. Huang, J.J., Yeo, C.J., Sohn, T.A. *et al.* (2000). Quality of life and outcomes after pancreaticoduodenectomy. *Annals of Surgery*, **231**, 890–8.

45. Kaw, M., Singh, S., Gagneja, H. *et al.* (2003). Role of self-expandable metal stents in the palliation of malignant duodenal obstruction. *Surgical Endoscopy*, **17**, 646–50.

46. Kim, J.H., Yoo, B.M., Lee, K.J. *et al.* (2001). Self-expanding coil stent with a long delivery system for palliation of unresectable malignant gastric outlet obstruction: a prospective study. *Endoscopy*, **33**, 838–42.

47. Coene, P.P.L.O., Huibregtse, K., Gulk, T.M. van *et al.* (1994). Duodenal obstruction requiring surgery following endoscopic palliation in patients with pancreatic local tumors. *The Netherlands Journal of Medicine*, **45**, A28.

48. Holbrook, A.G., Chester, J.F., and Britton, D.C. (1990). Surgical palliation for pancreatic cancer: will biliary bypass alone suffice? *Journal of the Royal Society of Medicine*, **83**, 12–14.

49. Huguier, M., Baumel, H., Manderscheid, J-C. *et al.* (1993). Surgical palliation for unresected cancer of the exocrine pancreas. *The European Journal of Surgical Oncology*, **19**, 342–7.

50. Choi, Y.B. (2002). Laparoscopic gastrojejunostomy for palliation of gastric outlet obstruction in unresectable gastric cancer. *Surgical Endoscopy*, **16**, 1620–6.

51. Weaver, D.W., Wiencek, R.G., Bouwman, D.L. *et al.* (1987). Gastrojejunostomy: is it helpful for patients with pancreatic cancer? *Surgery*, **102**, 608–13.

52. Lucas, C.E., Ledgerwood, A.M., and Bender, J.S. (1991). Antrectomy with gastrojejunostomy for unresectable pancreatic cancer-causing duodenal obstruction. *Surgery*, **110**, 583–90.

53. Mercadante, S., La Rosa, S., Nicolosi, G. *et al.* (1998). Temporary drainage of symptomatic malignant ascites by a catheter inserted under computerized tomography. *Journal of Pain and Symptom Management*, **15**, 374–8.

54. O'Neill, M.J., Weissleder, R., Gervais, D.A. *et al.* (2001). Tunneled peritoneal catheter placement under sonographic and fluoroscopic guidance in the palliative treatment of malignant ascites. *American Journal of Roentgenology*, **177**, 615–8.

55. Barnett, T.D., and Rubins, J. (2002). Placement of a permanent tunneled peritoneal drainage catheter for palliation of malignant ascites: a simplified percutaneous approach. *Journal of Vascular and Interventional Radiology*, **13**, 379–83.

56. Richard, H.M. III, Coldwell, D.M., Boyd-Kranis, R.L. *et al.* (2001). Pleurx tunneled catheter in the management of malignant ascites. *Journal of Vascular and Interventional Radiology*, **12**, 373–5.

57. Iyengar, T.D., and Herzog, T.J. (2002). Management of symptomatic ascites in recurrent ovarian cancer patients using an intra-abdominal semi-permanent catheter. *The American Journal of Hospice & Palliative Care*, **19**, 35–8.

58. Rosenblum, D.I., Geisinger, M.A., Newman, J.S. *et al.* (2001). Use of subcutaneous venous access ports to treat refractory ascites. *Journal of Vascular and Interventional Radiology*, **12**, 1343–6.

59. Kuruvillea, A., Busby, G., and Ramsewak, S. (2002). Intraoperative placement of a self-retaining Foley catheter for continuous drainage of malignant ascites. *European Journal of Gynaecological Oncology*, **23**, 68–9.

60. Smith, D.A.P., Weaver, D.W., and Bouwman, D.L. (1989). Peritoneovenous shunt (PVS) for malignant ascites. *The American Surgeon*, **55**, 445–9.

61. Kirk, I.R., Carrasco, C.H., Lawrence, D.D. *et al.* (1993). Intraperitoneal catheters: Percutaneous placement with fluoroscopic guidance. *Journal of Vascular and Interventional Radiology*, **4**, 299–304.

62. Lee, A., Lau, T.N., and Yeong, K.Y. (2000). Indwelling catheters for the management of malignant ascites. *Support Care Cancer*, **8**, 493–9.

63. Zanon, C., Grosso, M., Apra, F. *et al.* (2002). Palliative treatment of malignant refractory ascites by positioning of Denver peritoneovenous shunt. *Tumori*, **88**, 123–7.

64. Bieligk, S.C., Calvo, B.F., and Coit, D.G. (2001). Peritoneovenous shunting for nongynecologic malignant ascites. *Cancer*, **91**, 1247–55.

65. Loggie, B.W., Fleming, R.A., McQuellon, R.P. *et al.* (2000). Cytoreductive surgery with intraperitoneal hyperthermic chemotherapy for disseminated peritoneal cancer of gastrointestinal origin. *The American Surgeon*, **66**, 561–8.

66. McQuellon, R.P., Danhauer, S.C., Russell, G.B. *et al.* (2007). Monitoring health outcomes following cytoreductive surgery plus intraperitoneal hyperthermic chemotherapy for peritoneal carcinomatosis. *Annals of Surgical Oncology*, **14**, 1105–13.

67. Weinmann, M., Becker, G., Einsele, H. *et al.* (2001). Clinical indications and biological mechanisms of splenic irradiation in chronic leukaemias and myeloproliferative disorders. *Radiotherapy and Oncology*, **58**, 235–46.

68. Rosen, M., Brody, F., Walsh, R.M. *et al.* (2002). Hand-assisted laparoscopic splenectomy vs conventional laparoscopic splenectomy in cases of splenomegaly. *Archives of Surgery*, **137**, 1348–52.

69. Brodsky, J.A., Brody, F.J., Walsh, R.M. *et al.* (2002). Laparoscopic splenectomy. *Surgical Endoscopy*, **16**, 851–4.

70. Targarona, E.M., Balague, C., and Trias, M. (2001). Hand-assisted laparoscopic splenectomy. *Seminars in Laparoscopic Surgery*, **8**, 126–34.

71. Hellman, P., Arvidsson, D., and Rastad, J. (2000). Hand Port-assisted laparoscopic splenectomy in massive splenomegaly. *Surgical Endoscopy*, **14**, 1177–9.

72. Ailawadi, G., Yahanda, A., Dimick, J.B. *et al.* (2002). Hand-assisted laparoscopic splenectomy in patients with splenomegaly or prior upper abdominal operation. *Surgery*, **13**, 689–96.

73. Kumar, R.J., and Borzi, P.A. (2001). Splenosis in a port site after laparoscopic splenectomy. *Surgical Endoscopy*, **15**, 413–4.

74. Terrosu, G., Baccarani, U., Bresadola, V. *et al.* (2002). The impact of splenic weight on laparoscopic splenectomy for splenomegaly. *Surgical Endoscopy*, **16**, 103–7.

75. Targarona, E.M., Espert, J.J., Bombuy, E. *et al.* (2000). Complications of laparoscopic splenectomy. *Archives of Surgery*, **135**, 1137–40.

76. Rabow, M.W., Hardie, G.E., Fair, J.M. *et al.* (2000). End-of-life care content in 50 textbooks from multiple specialties. *JAMA*, **283**, 771–8.

77. Rappaport, W., Prevel, C., Witzke, D. *et al.* (1991). Education about death and dying during surgical residency. *American Journal of Surgery*, **161**, 690–2.

78. Krouse, R.S., Easson, A.M., and Angelos, P. (2003). Ethical considerations and barriers to research in surgical palliative care. *Journal of the American College of Surgeons*, **196**, 469–74.

79. Foley, K.M., and Gelband, H. (eds.) (2001). *Improving palliative care for cancer, summary and recommendations*. Washington, DC: National Cancer Policy Board, Institute of Medicine and National Research Council, National Academy Press.

80. Sugarbaker, P.H., Barofsky, I., Rosenberg, S.A. *et al.* (1982). Quality of life assessment of patients in extremity sarcoma trials. *Surgery*, **91**, 17–23.

The role of orthopaedic surgery in the palliative care of patients with cancer

John H. Healey and Wakenda K. Tyler

Introduction

Once cancer metastasizes to bone it is rarely curable, but always treatable. Orthopaedic surgery has an important role in the palliation of pain and disability of patients with all degrees of tumour progression. It is a powerful tool to maintain quality of life and occasionally may also extend life. Orthopaedic surgery can be effective even in far advanced disease when used judiciously. Even when the patient has been placed on 'Do not resuscitate' status, surgery can be considered, and may be the definitive method to relieve pain and maintain patient independence, or assist in terminal care. In order to guide the complex decision-making the clinician needs a broad understanding of metastatic bone disease and a specific understanding of the types of surgery that are appropriate. Good therapeutic choices can then be made. This chapter provides the context in which to evaluate patients with metastatic bone disease, and management guidelines for the common disease patterns.

Metastatic disease to the bone is a significant source of morbidity for patients diagnosed with cancer. Approximately half of the 570 000 people who died from cancer in the year 2005 had metastatic disease.[1] The most common primary carcinomas to metastasize to bone are breast, prostate, lung, kidney, and thyroid.[2] Seventy-five to 85 per cent of men and women with advanced prostate or breast cancer have boney involvement.[3] As many as 40 per cent of patients with lung cancer and 25 per cent of patients with renal cancer will have bony involvement in the course of their disease process.[3] With the tremendous improvements in treatment that have occurred over the last few decades, patients are surviving longer with advanced disease. The long-term survival of a patient with metastatic bone disease can be variable depending on the type of primary lesion. Men with metastatic prostate cancer to bone have a median survival of 40 months, while women with boney metastasis from breast cancer have a median survival of 24 months. Similarly patients with bone involvement from thyroid cancer have a median survival of 48 months. Lung, on the other hand, has a less than 6-month median survival when bone involvement is noted.[4]

Pathologic fractures in patients with bone involvement have been reported to occur in as few as 8 per cent of patients when long bone fractures only were looked at in all patients with metastatic disease.[5] One series looking at breast cancer patients with bone involvement noted a rate of pathologic fracture of 57 per cent when the entire skeleton was included in the analysis.[6] Variable life expectancies have been observed in patients with metastatic bone disease depending on the type of primary cancer and host characteristics at the time of presentation. Lung cancer patients with pathologic fractures have a median survival of approximately 4 months, while renal carcinoma patients have a median survival of 20 months.[7] Breast, prostate, and other cancers have an overall median survival of 8–12 months.[7] It has also been noted that patients with pathologic fractures with a single boney metastasis have a longer survival compared to patients with a fracture and multiple boney metastases (24 versus 6 months). Similarly, patients who present with a fracture who have a better overall performance status also do appreciably better than patients with a poor performance status (14-month median survival versus 5 months).[7]

Pathologic fractures and bone pain are just two of much morbidity associated with metastatic disease to the bone. The treatment of metastatic disease to bone requires coordination from several disciplinary teams. The orthopaedic surgeon's role is to work in conjunction with the radiation and medical oncologist, radiologists, and other surgical teams to provide stability of impending or already present pathologic fractures in order to facilitate mobility as promptly as possible in a patient with metastatic disease. The orthopaedic surgeon also has the goal of providing pain relief to patients with metastatic disease particularly in situations where surgical intervention can provide better or more prompt pain relief than available medical interventions.

Patient presentation

Aside from pathologic fractures and bone pain, metastatic bone disease can also lead to hypercalcaemia, spinal instability, and spinal cord compression. Knowledge of these potentially life-threatening complications is essential for all clinicians caring for patients with metastatic bone disease. Although a patient can present with any of these processes, the most common presenting sign or symptom of metastatic bone disease is pain.

Bone pain from cancer invasion can be the result of mechanical instability that occurs at sites of bone destruction. Bone destruction results from the stimulation of osteoclasts by the cancer cell release of cytokines and growth factors. Bone pain can also result from cancer cell stimulation of primary sensory afferent nerve fibres.[8] Sensory afferent fibres exist in abundance within the connective tissue sheath that covers the outer surface of bone, known as the periosteum. They also exist within the medullary canal of bones in close proximity to blood vessels within the haversion canals of the bone. Several neurochemical studies of protein production within the spinal cord and afferent nerve fibres have shown that cancer-induced bone pain differs from neuropathic and inflammatory type pain.[9,10] Increased protein production of specific proteins has been noted in cancer-induced bone pain, while down regulation of proteins normally seen in abundance in neuropathic and inflammatory pain has been observed in recent studies.[11] Specific changes within the spinal cord, such as astrocytosis have been observed in cancer-induced bone pain states as well.[9,12] Cancer-induced bone pain is therefore an entity in and of itself that warrants specific directed therapeutic modalities that may differ from modalities used to treat inflammatory or neuropathic type pain. This specific type of pain also differs from the mechanical pain that is seen when the structural integrity of the bone has been compromised.

Bone metastases most frequently involve the axial skeleton (spine, pelvis, and ribs). When the appendicular skeleton is involved the most common sites are the femur and humerus.[13] The further distal one moves on the appendicular skeleton, the less likely one is to see metastatic disease. In the axial skeleton, pain may be diffuse and poorly localized while in the appendicular skeleton, pain is often more discrete. In both situations, the patient will often complain of night pain or pain at rest that is the result of abnormal stimulation of afferent nerve fibres. It may also be noted that the pain is inadequately relieved with anti-inflammatory agents or traditional over the counter pain relievers. If this pain worsens with functional activities or weight bearing, it may also be associated with a mechanical component. When functional pain is present, this frequently indicates a bone at risk for fracture.

It is important for the clinician to identify and distinguish localized pain within the axial or appendicular skeleton and radicular pain that radiates most commonly from the spine. Patient with radicular pain as the result of spinal nerve root involvement from their metastatic disease will often complain of electrical shooting pain down their legs or into their arms. They may report symptoms of spinal stenosis or spinal canal compromise, such as improvement in pain with bending forward. On exam the patients will have reproduction of their symptoms with straight leg raise test in the lower extremities or a positive spurling's test in the upper extremities. Deep tendon reflexes and pathologic reflexes need to be carefully examined in these patients to rule out myelopathic symptoms as well. Radicular pain can be treated differently that impending fracture pain or cancer bone pain and often requires a referral to a spine specialist (either in neurosurgery or orthopaedic spine surgery).

Evaluation of a patient with a bone lesion

Patients who present with bone involvement from metastatic disease usually present in one of three manners: (1) with known widely metastatic disease; (2) with a known primary and a new bone lesion; and (3) with an unknown primary and a bone lesion. Each one of these scenarios must be addressed differently. To start, all patients should have a careful history and physical examination performed. A long-standing history of smoking or abnormal findings on abdominal exam may point one to source disease if one is not known. A careful history will also help to elucidate a patient's current functional status and current functional demands, which may influence the treatment options for a patient.

In a patient with known widely metastatic disease, there is usually no role for biopsy of a bone lesion. In this situation, the most important focus is to identify the location of the pain, the type of pain the patient is experiencing (mechanical versus tumour-induced) and the severity of bone involvement. In a patient with a known primary who has otherwise been disease free who now presents with a new bone lesion, the identification of other possible sites (bone and visceral) of metastases need to be undertaken. This usually requires imaging of the initial primary site as well as the chest, abdomen, and pelvis. It also requires imaging of the rest of the skeleton to look for other sites of bone involvement. In this situation a biopsy of the most easily accessible metastatic site should be undertaken to confirm recurrence of disease.

In the patient who presents with an unknown primary and a bone lesion, it is imperative to also look for the other sites of involvement in the skeletal system as well as visceral system. A CT of chest, abdomen, and pelvis allows one to look at the remaining visceral system as well as search for a primary site of involvement. A bone scan should be performed to look for other sites of bone involvement. Serum biochemical markers such as prostate specific antigen for prostate cancer, PTH for hyperparathyroidism, serum and urine protein electrophoresis for multiple myeloma, cancer antigen-125 for breast cancer, and microglobulin levels for lymphoma and myeloma should be performed. The combination of laboratory studies along with radiographic evaluation will identify 85 per cent of primary lesions in patients with unknown primaries.[14] In the remaining 15 per cent of patients a biopsy must be performed at the most accessible site of involvement. One must remember that in all of these patients with a bone lesion and no known primary cancer, a primary malignancy of bone cannot be ruled out and the biopsy should be performed in such a manner as to not compromise later definitive surgical treatment of a primary bone tumour.

Imaging of patients with metastatic bone disease

Plain radiographs

Initial evaluation of a patient with bone pain should be performed with a plain radiograph. At least two views (usually an anterior-posterior and lateral view) of the area of interest should be performed. Approximately 30 per cent loss of cortical and a 50 per cent loss of medullary bone density must occur before a lytic lesion will be detectable on plain x-ray, which makes it a very insensitive test for detecting metastatic disease.[15] However, plain films are an inexpensive way to obtain a good initial evaluation. They are especially useful in evaluating the overall structural integrity of the bone and identify the patients who need surgery and can benefit from it. They also are needed in preoperative planning for any surgical intervention and can be useful to the radiation oncologist for planning areas of treatment. There is ready access to plain radiographs in home care and hospice environments. New pain or functional loss can almost always be evaluated by plain radiographs in a practical, cost-effective way.

There are three types of boney reactions to metastatic deposits within bone. These include: osteoblastic reactions, which appear as increased density (whiter) on plain films; osteolytic reactions, which appear as less dense (blacker); and mixed osteolytic and blastic, which show a combination of patterns (Figs. 9.4.1–9.4.3). The type of pattern seen is dependent on the amount of bone formation (osteoblastic) or bone destruction (osteolytic) that occurs as a result of osteoclast and osteoblast response to the tumour cytokines. Certain patterns are often seen associated with particular primary malignancies. Prostates cancer is predominantly osteoblastic in appearance, while breast cancer can be osteolytic or mixed. Lung, thyroid, and renal carcinoma tend to be purely lytic in nature. While these patterns are general tendencies seen with these types of metastatic lesions, they are not set in stone.

The types of patterns of bone destruction seen on plain radiographs can also often be helpful to the clinician and may help guide treatment. Generally, the types of bone destruction seen can be characterized as moth-eaten, permeative, or geographic. A moth-eaten appearance is often seen with multiple myeloma and indicates a slightly more aggressive process. A permeative pattern is seen with the most aggressive bone destruction, while a geographic pattern may indicate a slow-growing tumour process.

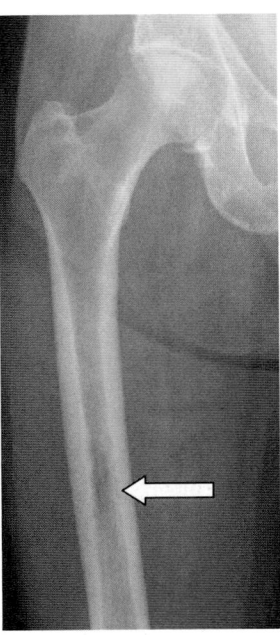

Figure 9.4.2 Multiple myeloma of the right femur. The white arrow points to the bottom of the permeative portion of the lesion, just below the pure lytic area.

Plain radiographs are an integral part of following patients with metastatic bone disease. They are a relatively inexpensive way to track response to treatment. They also allow for the monitoring of progression of disease.

Bone scintigraphy

Bone scintigraphy can be an extremely useful tool in detecting other bone lesions throughout the skeleton. It utilizes a technetium-labelled diphosphonate, which incorporates with a strong affinity into the hydroxyapatite mineral matrix of bone. New bone formation must be occurring at the site of involvement for the bone scintigraphy to detect it. The bone scintigraphy usually has three phases to it. The first part is a blood flow phase that occurs in the first few minutes after injection of the diphosphonate. It displays blood flow through the arterial system. The second phase occurs around 30 min and is the blood pool phase, which represents blood within the venous system. The final phase, and the one of greatest interest when examining patients with bone disease, is the delayed phase. It usually occurs at 1.5–2.5 h and represents the labelled diphosphonate bound to bone that is under a state of high turn over.

The bone scan is a very helpful test with sensitivity for detecting bone disease of around 72–84 per cent.[16,17] Its fallbacks are that it does not provide information about structural integrity and lacks specificity. Lesions from multiple myeloma will often be cold on bone scan, due to the lack of new bone deposition, despite bone destruction. Similarly, highly aggressive lesions that do not elicit a new bone response, such as those from lung or melanoma will not be detected by bone scintigraphy.

Computed tomography (CT)

CT is a very useful test for evaluating the structural integrity of bone. This can be very helpful in pre operative planning, particularly for

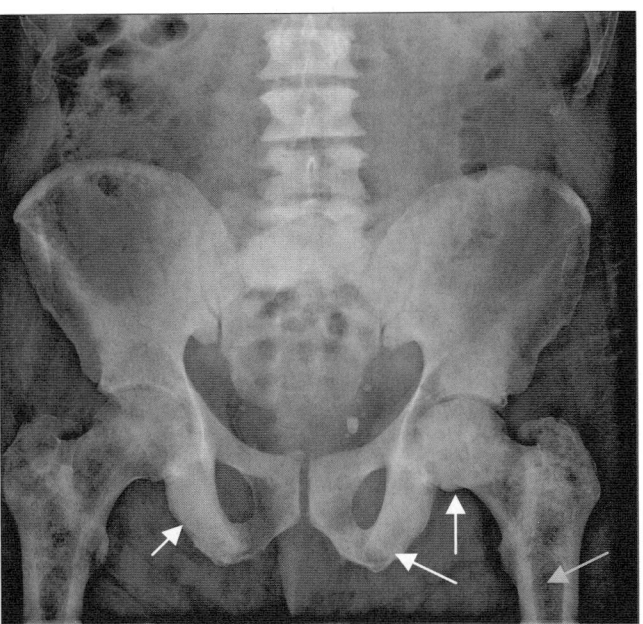

Figure 9.4.1 Osteoblastic lesion involving both sides of the pelvis as well as right and left proximal femurs. This patient has metastatic prostate cancer. Note the osteoblastic lesions of the proximal femur and pelvis (white arrows) as opposed to the normal bone density (grey arrow).

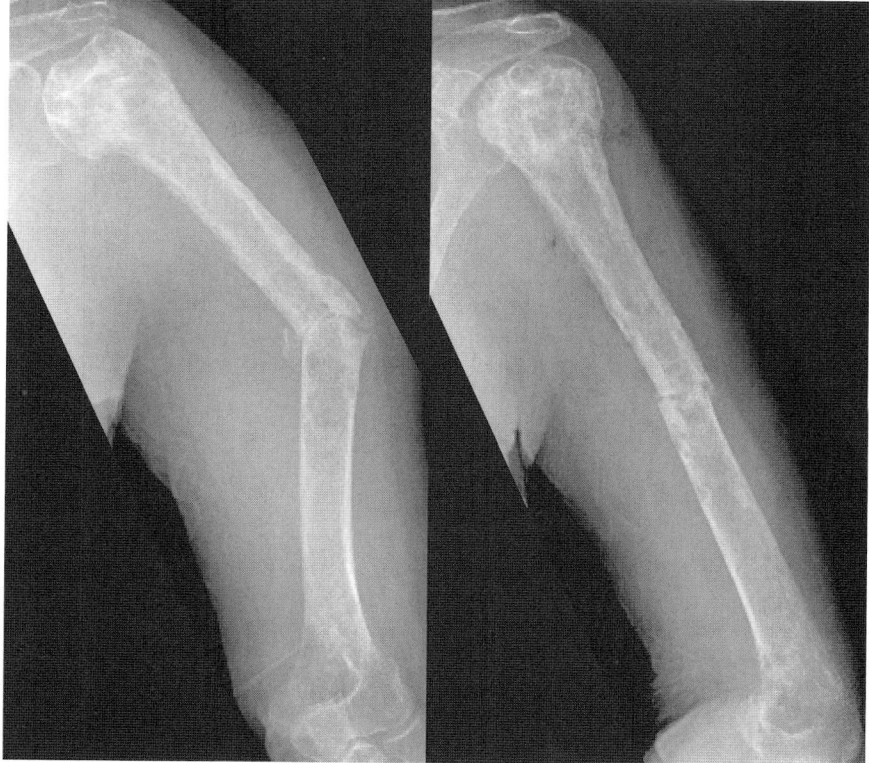

Figure 9.4.3 This is an 80-year-old female with metastatic breast cancer to the humerus. Note the bone destruction and lysis as well as diffuse pattern of involvement that permeates throughout the involved bone. Areas of sclerosis seen in the head represent the blastic component to this lesion.

pelvis and spine lesions. It also can be extremely helpful in detecting occult fractures in the setting of a metastatic lesion, which can be difficult to see on MRI because of all the marrow oedema that occurs from the tumour itself. It is useful over plain radiographs in that it better delineate bone involvement of a lesion and can be helpful in evaluating soft tissue extension. However, MRI is still superior to CT in evaluating soft tissue and marrow involvement of a lesion.

Magnetic resonance imaging (MRI)

MRI studies are capable of providing excellent contrast between normal bone marrow- and tumour-involved marrow space. MRI detects even subtle difference in water content within two adjacent tissues. It does this by utilizing the number of hydrogen atoms present in a given tissue. Normal marrow has a high fat content and relatively low water content, while tumours produce oedema within the marrow space, which will create an area of high water content. T2-weighted images will show high signal (white) in areas with high water content (Fig. 9.4.4). The normal marrow will appear dark on T2-weighted images. In the immature patient the marrow content is red haematopoietic marrow. This type of marrow lacks the fatty content of adult marrow, which will make it more difficult to distinguish tumour-infiltrated marrow from normal marrow. In this setting a gadolinium-enhanced study will amplify the tumour-involved segment of bone.

MRI is a valuable tool for studying the anatomic characteristics of a metastatic lesion to bone. However, it lacks the ability to provide detailed information about the structural integrity of the bone.

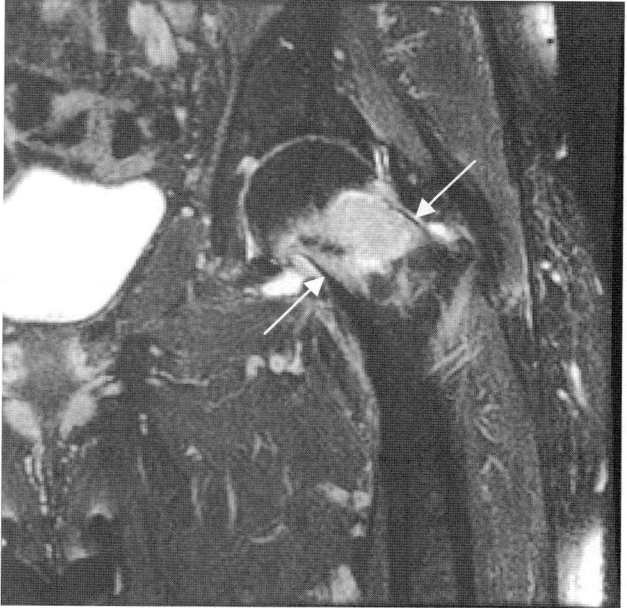

Figure 9.4.4 T2-weighted MRI of the left proximal femur showing a metastatic thyroid cancer lesion in the femoral neck (arrows). Note the increased signal intensity, indicating oedema within the bone at the site of metastatic disease. The normal marrow appears dark grey and the normal cortical bone is black in this image.

It therefore is best used in conjunction with plain films and/or CT scan, but not as a stand-alone evaluation of the bone. MRI of the entire spine with sagittal images is now fast and the most efficient way to get an overall evaluation of the patient. It helps to avoid missing a critical remote lesion that is producing neurogenic or referred pain.

Positron emission tomography (PET)

PET scan is a nuclear study that utilizes ^{18}F radioactive-labelled fluorodeoxyglucose as a tracer element. Fluorodeoxyglucose is a glucose analogue, which is taken up by metabolically active cells throughout the body. The more metabolically active a cell is, the greater the tracer uptake. The premise of this study is that tumour cells use glucose as their main source of energy and are very metabolic.

The benefit of PET scan is that it can detect both soft tissue and boney tumours, which make it a useful study for localizing other boney metastases as well as detecting unknown primary lesions. In looking at non-small-cell lung cancer, it was found to have a superior diagnostic accuracy compared to bone scan for detecting osseous metastases (96 vs. 66 per cent).[18] However, recent literature suggests that PET scan may have a lower sensitivity and diagnostic accuracy for osteoblastic lesions compared to osteolytic lesions. One study looking at PET scan versus bone scintigraphy found comparable overall specificities and sensitivities when studying metastatic breast cancer. However, when the bone lesions were broken down into type of bone process, PET scan was found to have a sensitivity of only 55 per cent for osteoblastic lesions. Bone scan was found to have a sensitivity of 100 per cent for these same lesions.[19] The sensitivity for osteolytic lesions was greater for PET compared to bone scintigraphy in this same study (94.7 and 84.2 per cent, respectively).[19]

PET scan as a diagnostic tool has potential to be helpful in the setting of metastatic bone disease. However, it is still currently in its investigational stages of use for most cancers. Much like MRI and bone scintigraphy, it also lacks the ability to provide information on the structural integrity of the bone and therefore needs to be used in conjunction with plain films or CT scan.

Therapeutic considerations in patients with metastatic bone disease

The goal of the treatment of patients with metastatic bone disease is to provide an increase in the quality of life remaining. This is accomplished through increasing mobility, improving function, and decreasing tumour burden and pain. These tasks are not solely accomplished by surgical intervention and require the coordination of multiple treatment modalities. Other treatment modalities, such as systemic bisphosphonate treatment, local and global radiation therapy, hormone and chemotherapy are discussed elsewhere in this book. The following discussion will focus mainly on orthopaedic surgical intervention as a means of palliative care in patients with cancer.

Bone pain can be the result of the tumour itself causing local environment changes that lead to the abnormal stimulation of afferent nerve fibres or it can be due to the mechanical weakening of bone. Orthopaedic stabilization of a metastatic site results in decreased mechanical pain. Orthopaedic surgical interventions can also decrease tumour-related pain by decreasing the tumour burden at a given site. The ultimate goal of almost all orthopaedic interventions in patients with metastatic disease is immediate weight-bearing as tolerated. This allows for the quickest return to normal function in patients.

Surgical intervention is mainly aimed at the treatment of impending fractures or already present pathologic fractures. In rare instances, patients who have suffered pathologic fractures or who have impending fractures who are too sick to undergo surgery or whose life expectancies are too short to benefit from surgical intervention may be candidates for non-operative treatment of these areas. In these settings, casting or splinting the areas of involvement may provide mechanical pain relief for the patient. Casting will usually not provide improved function. The cast or splint should be exceedingly well-padded and have no areas of increased pressure. This will prevent skin breakdown and ulceration. Casts should be avoided in limbs with lymphoedema, because they can lead to circumferential constriction of an area, which can lead to unintended tissue damage or compartment syndrome.

In almost all other instances, impending fractures and pathologic fractures should be surgically stabilized. The ideal time to intervene on a patient with metastatic disease is prior to pathologic fracture. Surgical intervention is more easily carried out in this setting and the patient will experience less pain if the site can be stabilized before fracture. Pathologic fractures have a very poor healing rate. Therefore, the surgeon is dependent on the surgical fixation to provide long-term stability to the area.

A factor that may influence the type of stabilization used is the estimated survival of a patient with an impending or pathologic fracture. Patients with bone metastases from thyroid cancer have the longest median survival (48 months), followed closely by prostate cancer (40 months), then beast cancer (24 months).[4] Lung cancer with metastases to bone has the shortest median survival of less than 6 months.[4] The presence of an actual pathologic fracture decreases life expectancy. The median overall survival of all patients who present with pathologic fracture is 8 months.[7] Renal carcinoma patients have a median survival after pathologic fracture of 20 months, while lung cancer patients have a median survival of only 4 months.[7]

It is important to mention that although patients with advanced cancer are at increased risk of metastatic disease to the bones and therefore pathologic fractures, not all patients with a history of advanced disease who suffer a fracture will have a pathologic tumour-related fracture. Many of these elderly patients and those who have been on androgen deprivation therapy for prostate cancer can develop osteoporotic fractures, just like the rest of the population. In one population-based study, patients with prostate cancer treated with luteinizing hormone-releasing hormone agonists had a 19 per cent incidence of non-pathologic fractures and only a 6 per cent incidence of pathologic fracture.[20] In the setting of a non-pathologic fracture basic orthopaedic trauma principles should be implemented and treatment should still be aimed at providing a durable and stable construct that the patient can immediately weight-bear on.

Classification and characterizing of impending pathologic fractures

Much research in orthopaedics has been devoted to determining factors that accurately predict the likelihood of a pathologic fracture developing from a metastatic lesion. Metastatic lesions that are at low risk for pathologic fracture are often best treated with non-surgical systemic interventions and radiation therapy. Patients with lesions not at risk for fractures treated in this manner have less morbidity and equal or better pain control. It is essential in the treatment of patients with metastases to distinguish these two groups of patients.

Unfortunately, there is no clear-cut consensus among researchers as to the exact predictive factors, nor is there any one predictive scoring system that has 100 per cent accuracy. In 1964, Snell and Beals were able to predict 58 per cent of pathologic fractures by adopting the criteria that any lesion greater than 2.5 cm in the femoral cortex or in any other bone with pain would lead to a fracture.[21] After reviewing 104 pathologic fractures, Parrish and Murray-recommended fixation of femoral shaft fractures in which greater than 50 per cent of the diameter of the cortex was destroyed and pain was present.[22] These criteria were later revised to include any lesion in the femoral cortex in which greater than 30 per cent cortical destruction was present along with pain and failure of radiotherapy.[23] Zickel and Mouradian in their retrospective review of 34 patients found that the presence of purely lytic lesions, subtrochanteric lesions, cortical involvement, and pain were all risk factors for fracture.[24] They did not find that size of lesion was correlated with risk of fracture. In one of the largest series to look at risk of pathologic fracture, 203 patients with 516 metastatic lesions were evaluated. No correlations between risk of fracture and size of lesion, presence of pain or lesion patterns were noted.[25] Even the ability of surgeons to predict fracture risk accurately has even been called into question. Hipp et al. found poor intra-observer reliability between three orthopaedic oncologists when predicting size of lesion and load bearing capacity of the bone.[26]

In 1989, Mirels published the first scoring system intended to predict likelihood of pathologic fracture in patients with metastatic lesions. Mirels described four important variables based on previous literature. Those variables were location of lesion, type of pain, lesion characteristics and size of lesion relative to the bone involved. Each variable was assigned a score of 1–3 based on the characteristics of these variables (Table 9.4.1). He then used his scoring system to analyse 78 metastatic lesions in 28 patients with various types of malignancies. All lesions were looked at prior to irradiation of the area. All patients were followed for a 6-month period of time. Mirels found that patients with a score of 7 had only a 4 per cent risk of fracture. A score of 6 or less resulted in no fractures during his study period. A score of 8 had a fracture risk of 15 per cent, with a false positive rate of 6 per cent. A score of 9 had a 33 per cent risk of fracture and a 0 per cent false positive rate. He concluded from this data that all patients with scores of 9 or greater should undergo prophylactic stabilization of the involved bone, while all patients with scores of 7 or less can be treated with irradiation and monitoring. He also noted in his data that no one risk factor alone was significantly correlated with fracture, but that by combining them and assigning a scoring system, the accuracy of predicting pathologic fracture greatly improved. The key points to Mirels work is that all of the variables listed in Table 9.4.1 are important and that the combination of clinical markers and radiographic markers are what allow a more accurate prediction of fracture.[27]

Draw backs to Mirels' work are that his rating system still leaves out factors that previous literature has found to be important in assessing risk of pathologic fracture. Such factors as greater or less than 50 per cent cortical destruction been found by several studies to be important predictors of fracture.[22,28,29] At Memorial Sloan-Kettering Cancer Center, surgery is performed in any patient with endosteal cortical destruction of greater than 50 per cent or with functional pain after radiotherapy or with cortical defects larger than the diameter of the bone or larger than 2.5 cm.

A score of 9 or greater is recommended for surgical stabilization, based on the original work of Mirels.[27]

Bone biology and biomechanics

The overall strength of bone is based on its material and structural properties. The structural properties of bone are based mainly on the shape and distribution of cortical and cancellous bone. Cortical bone is denser than cancellous bone and has a higher resistance to deformation and failure under given stresses. Therefore, the greater the amount of cortical bone present, the less likely the bone will be to fracture.

The material properties of bone are composed of an organic matrix (40 per cent total content of bone) and an inorganic matrix (60 per cent total content of bone). The organic matrix is made mostly of collagen (90 per cent), matrix proteins (10 per cent), and proteoglycans (<1 per cent). The inorganic matrix is composed mainly of calcium hydroxyapatite. The collagen present in bone provides most of the tensile strength of bone, while the calcium hydroxyapatite provides most of the compressive strength of bone. Bone is strongest in compression and weakest in shear forces. Tumour-induced osteolysis is brought about by tumour cell stimulation of osteoclasts. The osteoclasts are stimulated to reabsorb the organic and inorganic components of bone and consequently release free calcium from the calcium hydroxyapatite into the circulation. Lytic lesions result in greater removal of both the mineral and organic components of bone leading to greater loses in strength and stiffness. Blastic lesions however do not disturb the mineral content of bone and only act to disrupt the normal trabecular framework of the cancellous bone. This results in a lower likelihood of fracture with blastic lesions. Chemotherapy and radiation therapy also reduce the strength of bone by shutting down both the osteoblasts and osteoclasts. This results in decreased ability for bone repair.[30]

Metastatic bone disease can result in bone fracture in one of two ways. Smaller osteolytic defects in the cortex can lead to stress risers. Stress risers are areas of bone where stresses are concentrated around a small hole in the bone. The bone's bending strength is reduced by as much as 60 per cent when an area with a lesion diameter to bone diameter is just 0.2.[31] Smaller lesions lead to greater decreases in torsional strength than compressive or

Table 9.4.1 Mirels scoring system for pathologic fractures.[27]

Variable	Score		
	1	**2**	**3**
Site	Upper limb	Lower limb	Peritrochanteric
Pain	Mild	Moderate	Functional
Lesion	Blastic	Mixed	Lytic
Size	<1/3	1/3–2/3	>2/3

bending strength. Torsional loads to bone occur most frequently when patients are carrying out normal daily activities that involve turning or pivoting from a standing position. Also activity such as getting up from a chair to transfer can also lead to high torsional loads. Larger metastatic lesions create an open section defect where the lesion creates a hole in the bone that is greater than the diameter of the bone. In this situation the strength of the bone is reduced by 90 per cent.[32]

The location of the lesion within the skeleton greatly influences the likelihood of fracture. Lesions in the upper extremity are much less likely to fracture compared to lesions in the lower extremity. The upper extremity experiences less load as compared to the lower extremity. When fractures do occur in the upper extremity it is often the result of torsional forces or abnormal loads from a fall. With normal walking, the proximal femur experiences close to three and half times bodyweight in force. Loads can be as high as 8 N with certain activities. The proximal femur is also a majority metaphyseal area where cortical bone is thin and cancellous bone composites the bulk of the structural integrity of the bone. These are some of the reasons that the proximal femur is the most common site of pathologic fracture in the appendicular skeleton.

Metastatic lesions affect not only the strength of bone, but also the healing capacity of bone. Other factors that may also influence the ability of bone to heal in a patient with metastatic disease is the presence of radiation to the area, use of systemic chemotherapy, type of surgical fixation and histology of the lesion. Systemic chemotherapy has been shown to greatly retard the healing process of bone.[30] In a classic study by Gainor and Buchert, bone healing in the setting of pathologic fractures was looked at in 129 pathologic fractures. They found an overall fracture healing rate of 35 per cent for all cancer types.[33] Multiple myeloma was found to have the highest healing rate of 67 per cent. Renal and breast cancer were found to have healing rate of 44 per cent and 37 per cent, respectively.[33] Lung cancer patient with pathologic fractures had the poorest healing rate with all patients dying before healing had occurred. The treatment of internal fixation combined with radiotherapy resulted in the highest union rate in this study.[33] Other factors that may influence bone healing in the setting of pathologic fracture are nutritional status of the patient, use of hormone therapy and pre-existing osteoporosis.

Once surgery is chosen, the operation should be done that will last the patient's lifetime. Proper assessment of life expectancy is necessary to make the best decision. Prediction of survival is fraught with uncertainty. There are no reliable objective standards. Combining staging studies, laboratory factors, patient performance status, and experienced clinical judgement, only one-half of the variance of life expectancy can be accounted for.[9] Yet these factors should all be weighed in the equation. Despite the vagaries,

Table 9.4.2 Factors predicting life expectancy.

- Multiple bone involvement
- Parenchymal organ involvement
- Low absolute neutrophil count
- Hypoalbuminemia
- Anaemia
- Hypercalcaemia

the operation chosen should be designed to last longer than the patient's prognosis. Recent work suggests that the patient's self assessment as measured with the SF-36 provides the best across the board prediction of survival.

Types of orthopaedic surgical interventions

Impending and pathologic fractures of bone can be treated in several ways. There are advantages and disadvantages to each type of surgical treatment and specific indications for each as well. Treatment of fractures includes surgical excision, arthroplasty replacement, and intramedullary or plate fixation. Radiofrequency ablation, cryotherapy, and embolization are becoming widely accepted means for treatment or augmentation of treatment for certain types of lesions as well. An important component of treatment of metastatic bone lesions is to reduce the tumour burden at the site of involvement. This can be accomplished through curettage in conjunction with other surgical interventions or with ablation of the tumour using radiofrequency ablation. Finally, all of the above surgical interventions can be augmented with bone cement (polymethylmethacrylate). Bone cement provides both torsional and compressive strength to a construct. In the setting of poor bone healing, it may be critical to a stable limb that can tolerate immediate weight bearing and function.

Tumour excision

Reducing the tumour burden is an important part of orthopaedic treatment of metastatic lesions. This can be accomplished through either intralesional excision or extralesional. The most common form of treatment is intralesional excision. This process results in significant reduction in pain, by removing the offending tumour cells. It also results in fewer failures of fixation and reduces the likelihood of tumour progression at the involve site.

Marginal or wide excision has been advocated for certain tumours. Marginal excision removes the bulk of the tumour by excising the tumour just at the cuff of normal and abnormal tissue. Often microscopic disease still remains, but the tumour burden is greatly reduced. Marginal excision is often performed in conjunction with arthroplasty.

Rarely, wide excision of a metastatic lesion may be indicated. The situation in which this is most commonly indicated is in patients with a long projected survival time. Patients with renal, thyroid, and even breast cancer may have a protracted length of survival. Complete resection of an isolated tumour can reduce the incidence of local recurrence to the area. This can reduce the need for further surgery and improve long-term pain control in these patients.[34]

Prosthetic joint replacement (arthroplasty)

Joint arthroplasty involves resection of either one side (hemiarthroplasty) or both sides (total arthroplasty) of a joint surface with prosthetic replacement of the resected components of the joint (Fig. 9.4.5). This is most frequently performed in the knee, hip, shoulder, and elbow joints. In fractures that involve the epiphyseal surface of joints, healing is exceedingly poor. In such cases, the best treatment is resection of the lesion and prosthetic replacement of the joint. This provides the best long-term outcome for patients. If there is involvement on both sides of the joint, than total joint replacement should be strongly considered. After resection and

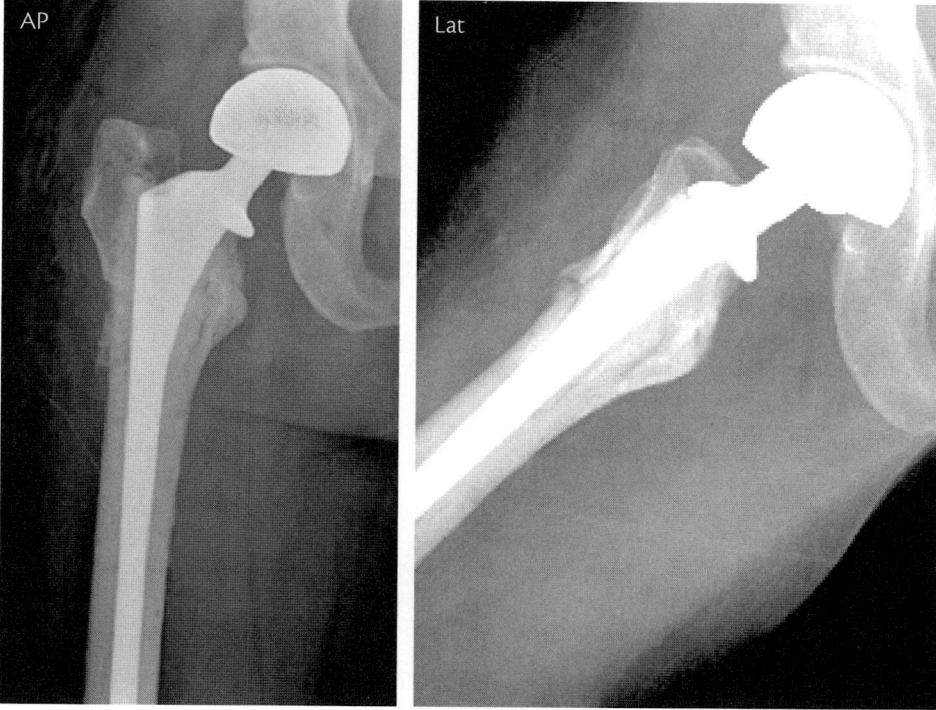

Figure 9.4.5 A hemiarthroplasty was performed on this 40-year-old female with metastatic breast cancer to the proximal femur. A cemented long stem component was used. Note that only one side of the joint was replaced with a large head that articulates with the native acetabulum.

curettage of the lesion the prosthetic components are cemented into the remaining bone. The stem of the prosthetic component should always bypass any distal lesions by at least two diameters of the bone involved to prevent later periprosthetic fracture. Cement is almost universally used because in the setting of malignancy, bone in growth that is required for a stable non-cemented component will not occur.

Plate fixation

Plate fixation provides load bearing stability to a fracture site. The plate therefore bears all of the weight transmitted through the bone until fracture union occurs. The downfall of this type of stability is that the plate is subjected to repeated stresses from weight bearing, which can lead to screw and plate breakage. If tumour progression occurs at the site of the plate, the screws used to stabilize the plate may also pull out of the bone as a result of lose of fixation. Plates are useful devices in places where bone healing is expected to occur in a relatively short period of time. Unfortunately, this is rarely the case in pathologic fractures. Plates are best used in bones that cannot accommodate intramedullary devices as in severely sclerotic medullary cavities or to augment another type of fixation (Fig. 9.4.6).

Intramedullary fixation

Intramedullary fixation usually involves a rod or nail that is placed down the centre of the medullary cavity of the bone (Fig. 9.4.7). Intramedullary devices are load sharing devices and therefore share the weight that is transmitted through the bone. Because the device is in the centre of the bone, where most forces are directed, the

device also sees less bending force as compared to plate fixation. This makes them much less likely to break is the setting of a slowly healing fracture. It also allows for more immediate weight bearing. Intramedullary devices are particularly useful in diaphyseal

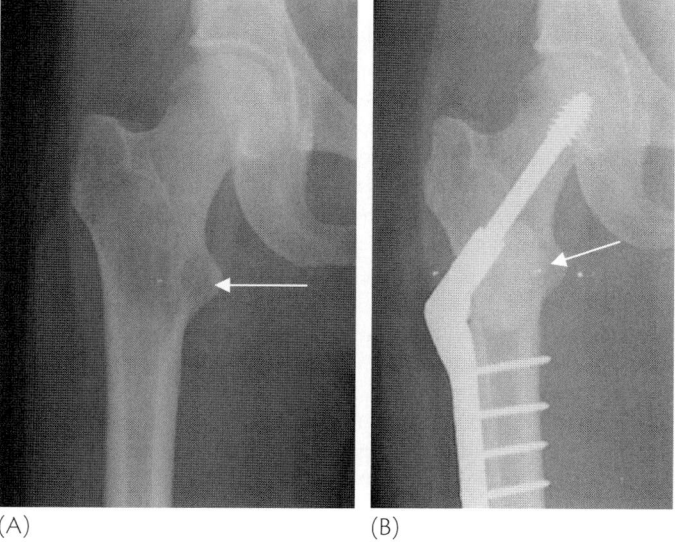

(A)   (B)

Figure 9.4.6 (A) A lytic breast cancer lesion of the intertrochanteric region of the femur (arrow). (B) This was treated with a dynamic hip screw and side plate. Treatment was augmented with curettage and cement stabilization (arrow). The cement normally appears opaque on plain radiographs.

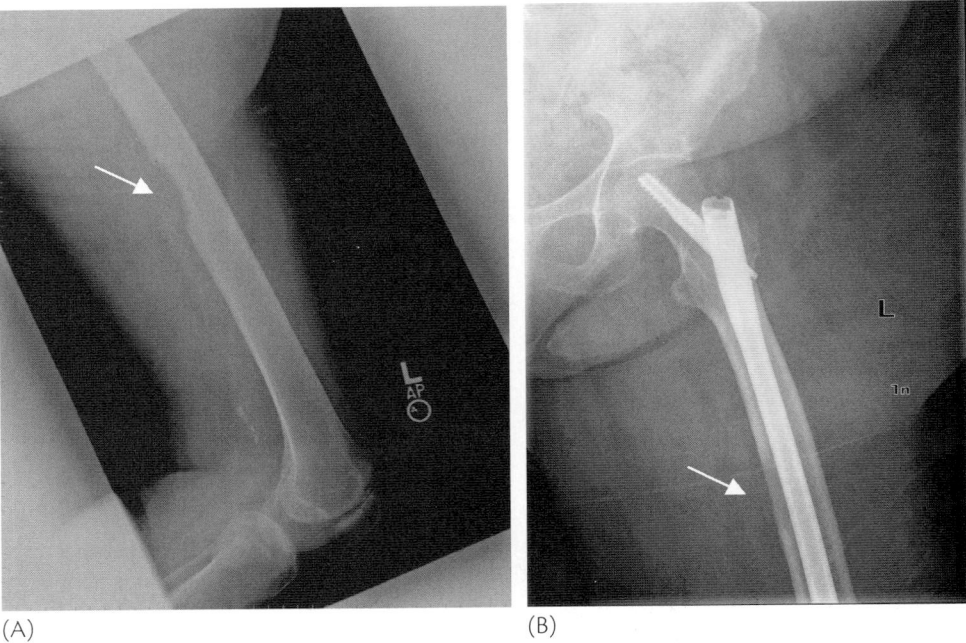

(A)   (B)

Figure 9.4.7 (A) Lytic lesion from metastatic renal carcinoma to the mid-shaft femoral region (arrow). (B) It was treated with open curettage and intramedullary nail placement.

fractures. They are fixed proximally and distally with interlocking screws to help create torsional control at the fracture site. They can also be augmented with cement to produce even more torsional stability and prevent failure in the setting of disease progression. The metastatic lesion should be curetted prior to insertion of the intramedullary device to help prevent seeding of the rest of the bone with tumour cells.

Bone cement

Bone cement is a very useful adjuvant stabilizer of a fracture site. In a well-delineated lesion the cement can fill the defect created by excision and curettage of the lesion. Bone cement has very strong compressive force resistance. It can be used in conjunction with any of the above mentioned devices to improve torsional and compressive strength of the fixation. The barium contrast that is used in the cement also makes it easy to see on plain radiograph and therefore allows for monitoring of disease progression or recurrence at the site the cement is placed. It also has the added benefit of giving off large quantities of heat as it solidifies in the bone, which can result in tumour cell death and further reduction in tumour burden.

Prior to the 1960s, conventional methods of fracture fixation without cement augmentation were used in patients with pathologic and impending pathologic fractures. The results were less than 50 per cent healing rate and even poorer rates of return to function.[22,35] In 1976, Harrington and colleagues reported on 323 patients treated with cement augmentation of conventional intramedullary fracture fixation techniques.[36] They reported 94 per cent return to function and 85 per cent satisfactory pain relief in their patient population. This study brought to light the importance of cement augmentation in the surgical treatment of pathologic lesions of bone. The authors included in this population of patients, 90 cases of just cement stabilization augmented

with rush rods for 62 humeral lesions, 27 tibial lesions, and one ulnar lesion. No failures of fixation were noted. The authors felt that the rush rods provided additional torsional strength to the already good compressive strength of the cement in these patients.[36]

Amputation

Amputation has a very limited role in the treatment of patients with metastatic disease. The current indications include a limb that is unreconstructable due to extensive disease involvement or in situations where complications of the disease leave no other options. These complications include fungating masses, recurrent infections that cannot be controlled with antibiotics and intractable pain in a limb that has failed treatment by other conventional methods. Amputation may also be indicated for acrometastases, which are metastases to the distal limb, such as the fingers or toes. Acrometastases are exceedingly rare and make up less that 0.5 per cent of all metastatic bone disease.[37] The most common malignancies to metastasize to the hands and feet are lung, renal, and oesophageal.[38] An amputation can often provide lasting pain relief for the patient with good functional outcomes.

Anatomic considerations

The type of fixation used to stabilize a fracture site or site of metastasis is dependent on the site of bone involvement. These anatomic considerations are important in choosing the correct type of stabilization in a patient.

Epiphyseal fractures

Epiphyseal fractures are those that occur at the very ends of long bones near or involving the articular surface. The most common epiphyseal fractures involve the femoral neck and head and humeral neck and head, but they can occur throughout the body. These fractures have a very poor healing rate and are not easily stabilized in the setting of malignancy. Therefore they are best treated with cemented arthroplasty. This provides a stable, pain-free joint that can tolerate immediate weight bearing.

Metaphyseal fractures

Metaphyseal fractures create quit a dilemma in orthopaedic oncology. They are frequently at sites where intramedullary fixation is difficult because there is not enough bone on the joint side of the fracture to provide adequate torsional or translational stability. Therefore, the options that remain are usually plate fixation or arthroplasty. As mentioned previously, plate fixation has a high failure rate when used alone. Failure rates have been reported around 40 per cent at 5 years.[39] Plates are better suited for patients with radiosensitive tumours that will heal after surgery with radiation treatment. The plate then functions to support the limb while the fracture is healing. Plates can also be used in patients who have estimated extended life expectancies who can tolerate partial or non-weight bearing for a period of time, while the fracture heals. Rarely can full weight bearing be allowed on a bone that is stabilized with just a plate and screws. Cement augmentation is also highly useful when plate fixation is chosen as a treatment means.

Arthroplasty can be performed for metaphyseal fractures, but is usually a more extensive surgery and requires resection of larger segments of bone. The metaphyseal region and its associated apophyses are often the sites of major tendon attachments. Examples are the greater and lesser trochanters around the hip and greater and lesser tuberosities around the shoulder. All attempts at preservation of these structures and reattachment to the prosthesis should be made. Reattachment of these structures often requires augmentation with mesh or cables. Even with good augmentation techniques these structures can later avulse off the prosthesis and lead to joint instability, muscle weakness and diminished function.

Diaphyseal fractures

Diaphyseal lesions are usually well treated with intramedullary nails. In most situations the site of malignant involvement should be opened and the tumour curetted out. This reduces tumour burden and prevents further dissemination of the tumour throughout the bone. Once curetted, the site can than be filled with bone cement after the nail is inserted to provide further compressive strength to the area. Closed nailing technique in which the site of involvement is not opened and curetted can be performed, but should only be done in select situations. Those situations include patients who have minimal survival expectancy for whom disease progression over the short time remaining is unlikely to occur. The other situation for which it may be acceptable to use closed nailing techniques is in those patients with exquisitely radiosensitive tumours in whom postoperative radiotherapy will provide the local control of tumour burden.

In bones that have both diaphyseal and epiphyseal or metaphyseal involvement, arthroplasty for the periarticular involvement should be performed and a cemented long stem device should be used. The cemented long stem component of the joint prosthetic device will provide stability to a diaphyseal lesion similar to the intramedullary nail.

Upper extremity

Upper extremity metastases comprise approximately 20 per cent of all bone metastases. The humerus is the most common bone involved, followed by the scapula and clavicle.[40] The ulna, radius, and hand together comprise less than 1 per cent of all skeletal metastases.[40] The upper extremity is thought to be less of a weight bearing structure than the lower extremity. Although in many instances, the patient is reliant on the upper extremity for weight bearing during transfers and in use of walkers or crutches if these are indicated for other reasons. The upper extremity is also critical for a person to feed him or herself and to do other necessary grooming activities. The goals of treatment for pathologic lesions of the upper extremity are to provide a limb that can assist is carrying out these basic activities of daily living and to relieve pain.

Pathologic fractures of the humerus frequently fail in torsion rather than as the result of compressive loads. Obtaining torsional stability becomes essential in treatment of humeral fractures. Fractures that involve the periarticular surfaces of the humerus can usually be treated with cemented arthroplasty. In the proximal humerus, involvement of the rotator cuff attachments at the greater

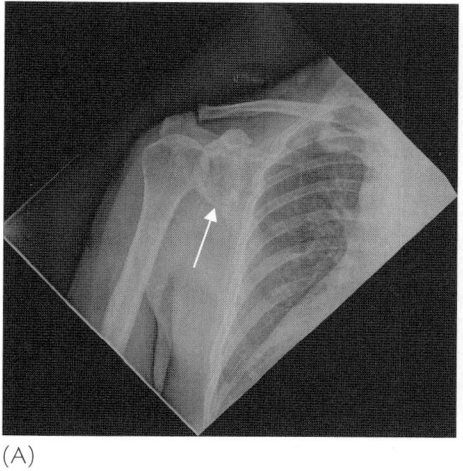
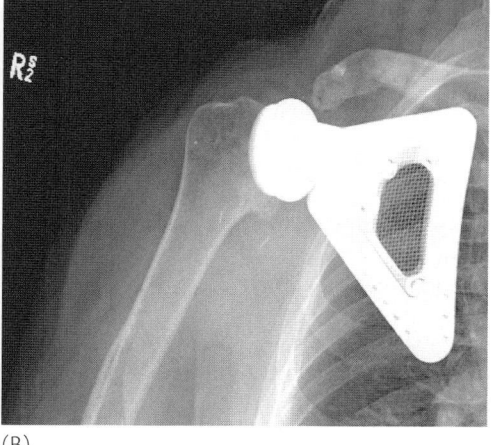

(A)   (B)

Figure 9.4.8 (A) Metastatic renal carcinoma of right scapula (arrow). Note the lytic involvement of the glenoid and entire scapula. (B) A titanium scapular replacement was used to reconstruct the area after resection of the native scapula.

and lesser tuberosities with tumour may make maintenance of rotator cuff function impossible. If the greater and lesser tuberosities cannot be spared, attempts to reattach the rotator cuff using synthetic material like mesh or Dacron® can be performed with variable success. Patients without rotator cuff function will still have a relatively pain-free arm, but may lack motion compared to those in whom the rotator cuff is maintained. Because they will still have good use of their elbow and hand, they will still be able to carry out most activities of daily living, but will likely not be able to carry out over-the-head activities.

Elbow replacement for distal humeral metastases can provide pain relief and adequate function. Terminal extension is often lost, but maintenance of flexion allows for good control of hand position for most activities. For diaphyseal lesions of the humerus, cemented intramedullary devices have the greatest success. In one series of 59 patients treated for pathologic fractures of the humerus with either cemented intramedullary nailing or prosthetic replacement, all patients had good pain relief, but patients treated with intramedullary fixation augmented with cemented had the best functional outcomes.[41] In this same series, it was noted that 95 per cent of patients treated surgically for humeral metastatic disease had 68 per cent or greater normal function on the involved side.

Most lesions of the scapula and clavicle can be treated with radiation therapy. Concern regarding dose of radiation can be an issue since the lung and other vital organs may be involved in the radiation field. In radio insensitive lesions, resection and/or reconstruction may be required. The clavicle is an expendable bone and frequently can be resected without much functional sequelae. Metal scapula replacements can be used when resection of the entire scapula, including the glenoid is necessary for tumour control (Fig. 9.4.8). Smaller portions of the scapula can be resected without the need for prosthetic reconstruction.

Lower extremity

The femur is the third most common site of skeletal metastases. Fractures of the femur account for 2/3 of all pathologic long bone fractures. The proximal femur accounts for 90 per cent of all pathologic femur fractures.[42] Forces within the proximal femur can be as high as 8 N with certain activities, which may explain why fractures to this region are so frequent.[43] Any reconstruction to this area also must be able to support significant loads.

Metastatic lesions of the proximal femur involving the femoral neck should be treated with arthroplasty. The advantage to hemiarthroplasty over total joint arthroplasty is that the operative time is shorter, there is less blood loss and less risk of postoperative dislocation. However if there is any evidence of disease within the acetabulum, then total hip replacement should be considered. More complex reconstructions of the acetabulum may be necessary if disease within this region is extensive (see discussion below). Peritrochanteric lesions can be treated with arthroplasty as well. Some have advocated treatment of pathologic peritrochanteric fractures with intramedullary nails that include cephalomedullary screws to provide further stability proximally in the neck region, but the long-term results of these constructs in this setting are still unknown and the standard of care is still joint replacement.

Lesions below the lesser trochanter should be treated like femoral shaft fractures with intramedullary nail stabilization. Lesions very distal in the femur near the knee joint should be

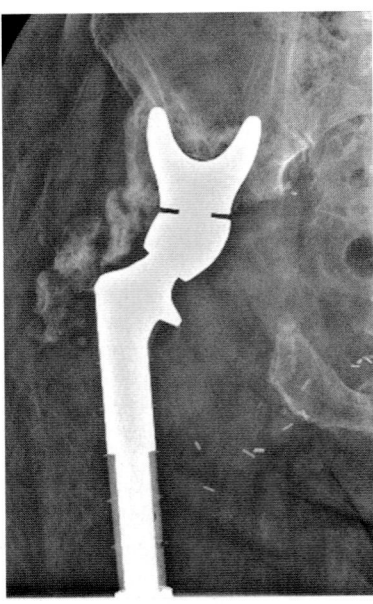

Figure 9.4.9 Saddle prosthesis used after resection of the acetabulum and portion of the ilium for large metastatic lesion to these areas.

treated with cemented total knee arthroplasty or if well contained and not involving the epiphyseal region can be treated with curettage, cement and plate fixation.

Lesions of the tibia comprise about 4.5 per cent of metastases to the skeleton.[44] In one series, 25 impending and pathologic fractures of the tibia were evaluated.[44] Twenty-three of those 25 were proximal or diaphyseal with only two distal lesions. Well-contained metaphyseal lesions not involving the epiphysis were treated with curettage, cement, and plate fixation, while diaphyseal lesions were treated with intramedullary nailing and cement augmentation. Only two endoprosthetic replacements were performed for aggressive metaphyseal lesion that extended into the epiphysis. All patients experience good pain relief and there was only a 4-per cent failure rate in this series of patients.

Pelvis and acetabulum

Metastatic disease to the pelvis and acetabulum are frequent causes of pain and disability in patients with cancer. Metastatic disease in this area can lead to significant mechanical instability. Conventional total hip arthroplasty can fail in this region if there is not adequate bone stock on the acetabular side to support the metal and polyethylene cup component of the arthroplasty. A CT scan of the pelvis and acetabulum is necessary to evaluate the bone stock in this region. Only after careful evaluation of the CT scan can the appropriate treatment option be determined. Four anatomic parts of the acetabulum are evaluated on the CT scan. The medial wall, the superior dome, the anterior column and posterior column are each evaluated for integrity.

Only in situations where there is limited disease and intact superior, medial, and anterior and posterior cortices can a conventional total hip arthroplasty be performed. In these situations, cups should be cemented into place since the disease itself and post operative radiation will prevent normal bone in growth into the conventional non-cemented cups.

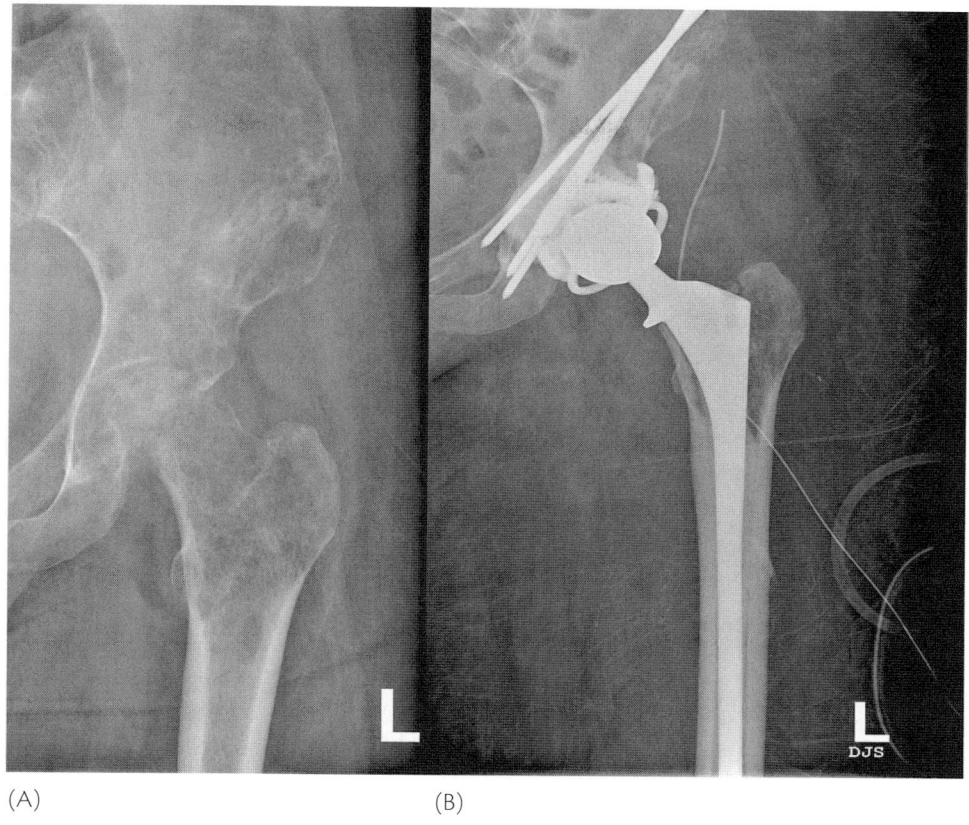

(A)   (B)

Figure 9.4.10 (A) Metastatic breast cancer involving the proximal femur, acetabulum and extending up into the ilium. (B) The patient was treated with a total hip arthroplasty that includes a Harrington reconstruction of the acetabulum. Note the large pins within the pelvis and cement surrounding them. These provide support for the cup component of the arthroplasty.

The greatest dilemma exists when there is complete destruction of the acetabular bone with significant disease involvement of the medial wall, superior dome, and anterior and posterior columns. Under these circumstances, the acetabulum either needs to be completely resected and replaced or supplemental fixation around the acetabulum needs to be provided. The saddle prosthesis is a device that was originally created for large acetabular defects following failed conventional total hip arthroplasties (Fig. 9.4.9). It has been used in the setting of pelvic reconstructions for metastatic disease as well as after resection of primary bone tumours of the pelvis. It relies on a portion of retained ilium as the weight-bearing component of the prosthesis. Although there has been some success in its use in patients with metastatic disease, it has also been noted to be fraught with complications. Any concern about disease progression into the ilium precludes use of this device, since a minimum of 2 cm of adequate bone within the ilium located close to the sacroiliac joint is required for stability of this construct. Even with adequate bone remaining, the complications of limb shortening, dislocation of device, infection, and periprosthetic fracture have been reported in high numbers.[45] This type of reconstruction should be reserved for select patients with intermediate life expectancies.

When solid iliac bone remains, pins or screws can be secured into it and the defect filled with cement and a large anti-protrusio cup (Fig. 9.4.10). This relieves mechanical pain and prevents migration of the acetabular cup. Harrington's method

was modified by Marco *et al.* who presented a series of 55 patients with extensive acetabular disease. They found that 76 per cent of the 48 patients still alive at 3 months had significant decreases in pain and 50 per cent of patient who could not walk prior to surgery regained the ability to walk after surgery. Of the patient who remained alive at 1 year, 67 per cent continued to have improved pain relief and 57 per cent retained the ability to ambulate. They had a very low rate of fixation failure suggesting that this construct is biomechanically sound in this population of patients.

Minimally invasive and adjuvant treatment options

Kyphoplasty and vertebroplasty

Vertebroplasty and kyphoplasty are both techniques used to treat painful compression fractures in the spine due either to osteoporosis or malignancy. Treatment of spinal metastatic disease will be discussed in another chapter, but a brief mention of these two techniques will be made here. Both vertebroplasty and kyphoplasty are minimally invasive techniques that are performed through percutaneus instrumentation. Both techniques involve the injection of bone cement posteriorly through the spinal pedicles into the vertebral body. The cement functions to stabilize the fractured vertebral body to prevent further collapse and reduce the mechanical pain created at the site of fracture.

Kyphoplasty differs from vertebroplasty in that a balloon is first inserted through the pedicle into the vertebral body and then inflated. The inflation of the balloon re-expands the collapsed vertebra and creates an open space for the cement to go when injected into the vertebral body. One advantage of kyphoplasty is that some of the height of the vertebral body is restored. This restores normal biomechanics to the entire spine, which prevents collapse of other weakened adjacent vertebra. The other advantage of kyphoplasty is that there is less likely to be cement extrusion into the spinal canal because the space created by the balloon allows for lower pressure during cement insertion.[46] Both techniques have been found to provide significant pain relief in patients with metastatic spinal disease and pain non-responsive to other treatments.[46]

These techniques should only be considered in patients who have no evidence of cord compromise from tumour involvement and who aside from pain have an otherwise normal neurological exam. Although these techniques are minimally invasive, they are not without risk. Cement migration and extrusion into the spinal canal, fat embolization during cement insertion, and abnormal cardiovascular response to the cement monomer are known complications of both techniques.

Cryotherapy

The technique of cryosurgery entails use of use of liquid nitrogen (stored at −197°C) to produce a fast freeze followed by slow thaw. This process results in intracellular protein denaturation, intracellular water crystallization, and cell membrane destabilization, all of which lead to cell death. Cryosurgery for the treatment of metastatic disease was reported as early as 1972 by Dr. Marcove at Memorial Sloan-Kettering Cancer Center.[47] He initially reported on four cases of metastatic renal disease and than in 1977 extended that series to include eight other patients with metastatic renal carcinoma.[48] Eleven out of the 12 patients had good pain relief that persisted until time of last follow-up or death. Today cryotherapy can be used as both the primary means of treatment of a lesion or as an adjuvant to other surgical techniques.

Isolated lesions within a bone that is easily accessible via surgical means are good candidates for open curettage and cryotherapy. A bone window is made at the site of involvement and gross tumour in curetted from the lesion. The liquid nitrogen is then introduced into the bone through the window. The result is increased zone of cell death and reduced tumour burden. The freeze–thaw process is repeated several times to improve cell death rates. The area of involvement is than packed with bone cement to improve stability to the area.

Newer percutaneous techniques have been examined in which a probe is introduced into the area of involvement and liquid nitrogen or argon beam is introduced through this probe.[49] This technique has been used in areas of soft tissue metastases with good success. The probes are difficult to insert into bone making this less useful in bone metastases. Furthermore, the probes can only cover a small area of involvement and cannot be used to treat larger lesions. With percutaneous techniques, bone cement cannot be used to stabilize the area making them even less desirable is areas where fracture is a concern.

Radiofrequency ablation

Radiofrequency (RF) ablation elicits the use of alternating electrical current operating in the same frequency as radio waves (460–480 kHz).[49] The current is emitted from a small electrode that is placed near or directly in the target tissue. The current produces ion vibration within the tissue, which leads to increased local temperatures. The increased temperature leads to thermal necrosis of the tissue and cells.

The size of the lesion influences the efficacy of RF ablation. Historically, a limitation of RF ablation used to be size of the lesion with it being only effective for lesions 1–2 cm in size. With newer technical advances tumours greater than 5 cm can be adequately treated with this technique.[49] RF ablation is a good alternative to surgical stabilization for isolated small painful lesions in the extremity, where a need for surgical stabilization is not warranted. Similarly, lesions within the flat bones of the pelvis and remaining axial skeleton may respond well to this treatment and not require further surgical intervention. A recent study looked at 43 patients treated for metastatic bone disease with RF ablation.[50] Twenty-four of the patients had sacral or pelvic lesions. All patients in this study were considered poor candidates for external beam radiation or had failed prior treatment with external radiation. The authors found clinically significant pain reduction in 95 per cent of patients, including some with larger lesions as well.[50]

The most common complications associated with RF ablation include skin necrosis, unplanned tissue damage, and fracture at the site of involvement.[49] RF ablation should not be performed in areas where impending pathologic fracture is a concern. In these areas surgical intervention is required.

Embolization

Embolization is a technique used to reduce blood flow to vascular tumours. The technique is usually performed by the interventional radiologist and involves injecting small particles or stainless steel coils into vascular pedicles feeding into tumours. The end result is diminished blood flow to the lesion and local tissue necrosis. The tumours that are most responsive to this technique are those known to be hypervascular. The two most common hypervascular tumours that metastasize to bone are renal and thyroid carcinoma. These tumours are known to produce significant haemorrhage when entered during surgery. The technique of embolization can be used as primary treatment of lesions in areas at low risk of fracture. In areas where further surgical stabilization and excision of the tumour are required, embolization can be performed prior to surgery. The procedure is usually performed 24–72 h before surgery. Several studies have shown a significant reduction in intraoperative blood lose and transfusion requirement with use of preoperative embolization.[51,52] The more complete the devascularization is, the better the bleeding control will be during the case.[51]

Conclusion

Orthopaedic surgical intervention can be exceedingly successful in reducing pain and improving function in patients with metastatic bone disease. Orthopaedic surgery is much less successful in isolation. It is best used in combination with other modalities of treatment. All bones treated with surgery for metastatic disease should be considered for postoperative radiation therapy. All patients with metastatic disease should also be considered for systemic treatment with bisphosphonates, hormone therapy, and/or chemotherapy when ever possible.[53,54] This requires the integration of all modalities of oncologic care and coordination of all teams caring for the patient.

The physician's goal when treating patients with metastatic bone disease is to cure some, help most, and provide comfort for all. Proper fracture care is fundamental to achieve this goal.

References

1. American Cancer Society. (2006). *Cancer statistics.*
2. Jaffe, H.L. (1958). *Tumor and tumorous conditions of the bone and joints*, 1st edition. Lea and Febiger, Philadelphia.
3. Coleman, R.E. (1997). Skeletal complications of malignancy. *Cancer*, Oct 15, **80**(8 Suppl.), 1588–94.
4. Rubens, R.D., and Coleman, R.E. (1995). Bone metastases. In *Clinical oncology* (eds. M.D. Abeloff, J.O. Armitage, A.S. Lichter, J.E. Niederhuber), p. 643. Churchill Livingstone, New York.
5. Higinbotham, N.L., and Marcove, R.C. (1965). The management of pathological fractures. *The Journal of Trauma*, Nov, **5**(6), 792–8.
6. Scheid, V., Buzdar, A.U., Smith, T.L., and Hortobagyi, G.N. (1986). Clinical course of breast cancer patients with osseous metastasis treated with combination chemotherapy. *Cancer*, Dec 15, **58**(12), 2589–93.
7. Nathan, S.S., Healey, J.H., Mellano, D. *et al.* (2005). Survival in patients operated on for pathologic fracture: implications for end-of-life orthopedic care. *Journal of Clinical Oncology*, Sep 1, **23**(25), 6072–82.
8. Goblirsch, M.J., Zwolak, P., and Clohisy, D.R. (2005). Advances in understanding bone cancer pain. *Journal of Cellular Biochemistry*, Nov 1, **96**(4), 682–8.
9. Honore, P., Luger, N.M., Sabino, M.A. *et al.* (2000). Osteoprotegerin blocks bone cancer-induced skeletal destruction, skeletal pain and pain-related neurochemical reorganization of the spinal cord. *Nature Medicine*, May, **6**(5), 521–8.
10. Mantyh, P.W., DeMaster, E., Malhotra, A. *et al.* (1995). Receptor endocytosis and dendrite reshaping in spinal neurons after somatosensory stimulation. *Science*, Jun 16, **268**(5217), 1629–32.
11. Honore, P., Schwei, J., Rogers, S.D. *et al.* (2000). Cellular and neurochemical remodeling of the spinal cord in bone cancer pain. *Progress in Brain Research*, **129**, 389–97.
12. Schwei, M.J., Honore, P., Rogers, S.D. *et al.* (1999). Neurochemical and cellular reorganization of the spinal cord in a murine model of bone cancer pain. *Journal of Neuroscience*, Dec 15, **19**(24), 10886–97.
13. Harrington, K.D. (1997). Orthopedic surgical management of skeletal complications of malignancy. *Cancer*, Oct 15, **80**(8 Suppl.), 1614–27.
14. Rougraff, B.T., Kneisl, J.S., and Simon, M.A. (1993). Skeletal metastases of unknown origin. A prospective study of a diagnostic strategy. *The Journal of Bone and Joint Surgery*, Sep, **75**(9), 1276–81.
15. Edelstyn, G.A., Gillespie, P.J., and Grebbell, F.S. The radiological demonstration of osseous metastases. Experimental observations. *Clinical Radiology*, Apr, **18**(2), 158–62.
16. Eustace, S., Tello, R., DeCarvalho, V. *et al.* (1997). A comparison of whole-body turboSTIR MR imaging and planar 99mTc-methylene diphosphonate scintigraphy in the examination of patients with suspected skeletal metastases. *AJR American Journal of Roentgenology*, Dec, **169**(6), 1655–61.
17. Galasko, C.S. (1969). The detection of skeletal metastases from mammary cancer by gamma camera scintigraphy. *The British Journal of Surgery*, Oct, **56**(10), 757–64.
18. Bury, T., Barreto, A., Daenen, F. *et al.* (1998). Fluorine-18 deoxyglucose positron emission tomography for the detection of bone metastases in patients with non-small cell lung cancer. *European Journal of Nuclear Medicine*, Sep, **25**(9), 1244–7.
19. Nakai, T., Okuyama, C., Kubota, T. *et al.* (2005). Pitfalls of FDG-PET for the diagnosis of osteoblastic bone metastases in patients with breast cancer. *European Journal of Nuclear Medicine*, Nov, **32**(11), 1253–8.
20. Krupski, T.L., Smith, M.R., Lee, W.C. *et al.* (2004). Natural history of bone complications in men with prostate carcinoma initiating androgen deprivation therapy. *Cancer*, Aug 1, **101**(3), 541–9.
21. Snells, W., and Beals, R.K. (1964). Femoral metastases and fractures from breast cancer. *Surgery, Gynecology & Obstetrics*, Jul, **119**, 22–4.
22. Parrish, F.F., and Murray, J.A. (1970). Surgical treatment for secondary neoplastic fractures. A retrospective study of ninety-six patients. *The Journal of Bone and Joint Surgery. American Volume*, Jun, **52**(4), 665–86.
23. Murray, J.A., Bruels, M.C., and Lindberg, R.D. (1974). Irradiation of polymethylmethacrylate. In vitro gamma radiation effect. *The Journal of Bone and Joint Surgery. American Volume*, Mar, **56**(2), 311–2.
24. Zickel, R.E., and Mouradian, W.H. (1976). Intramedullary fixation of pathological fractures and lesions of the subtrochanteric region of the femur. *The Journal of Bone and Joint Surgery. American Volume*, Dec, **58**(8), 1061–6.
25. Keene, J.S., Sellinger, D.S., McBeath, A.A., and Engber. W.D. (1986). Metastatic breast cancer in the femur. A search for the lesion at risk of fracture. *Clinical Orthopaedics and Related Research*, Feb, **203**, 282–8.
26. Hipp, J.A., Springfield, D.S., and Hayes, W.C. (1995). Predicting pathologic fracture risk in the management of metastatic bone defects. *Clinical Orthopaedics and Related Research*, Mar, **312**, 120–35.
27. Mirels, H. (1989). Metastatic disease in long bones. A proposed scoring system for diagnosing impending pathologic fractures. *Clinical Orthopaedics and Related Research*, Dec, **249**, 256–64.
28. Fidler, M. (1981). Incidence of fracture through metastases in long bones. *Acta orthopaedica Scandinavica*, Dec, **52**(6), 623–7.
29. Fidler, M. (1973). Prophylactic internal fixation of secondary neoplastic deposits in long bones. *British Medical Journal*, Feb 10, **1**(5849), 341–3.
30. Pelker, R.R., Friedlaender, G.E., Panjabi, M.M. *et al.* (1985). Chemotherapy-induced alterations in the biomechanics of rat bone. *Journal of Orthopaedic Research*, **3**(1), 91–5.
31. McBroom, R.J., Cheal, E.J., and Hayes, W.C. (1988). Strength reductions from metastatic cortical defects in long bones. *Journal of Orthopaedic Research*, **6**(3), 369–78.
32. Pugh, J., Sherry, H.S., Futterman, B. *et al.* (1982). Biomechanics of pathologic fractures. *Clinical Orthopaedics and Related Research*, Sep, **169**, 109–14.
33. Gainor, B.J., and Buchert, P. (1983). Fracture healing in metastatic bone disease. *Clinical Orthopaedics and Related Research*, Sep, **178**, 297–302.
34. Althausen, P., Althausen, A., Jennings, L.C. *et al.* (1997). Prognostic factors and surgical treatment of osseous metastases secondary to renal cell carcinoma. *Cancer*, Sep 15, **80**(6), 1103–9.
35. Koskinen, E.V., and Nieminen, R.A. (1973). Surgical treatment of metastatic pathological fracture of major long bones. *Acta orthopaedica Scandinavica*, **44**(4), 539–49.
36. Harrington, K.D., Sim, F.H., Enis, J.E. *et al.* (1976). Methylmethacrylate as an adjunct in internal fixation of pathological fractures. Experience with three hundred and seventy-five cases. *The Journal of Bone and Joint Surgery. American Volume*, Dec, **58**(8), 1047–55.
37. Morris, D.M., and House, H.C. (1985). The significance of metastasis to the bones and soft tissues of the hand. *Journal of Surgical Oncology*, Feb, **28**(2), 146–50.
38. Healey, J.H., Turnbull, A.D., Miedema, B. *et al.* (1986). Acrometastases. A study of twenty-nine patients with osseous involvement of the hands and feet. *The Journal of Bone and Joint Surgery. American Volume*, Jun, **68**(5), 743–6.
39. Dijstra, S., Wiggers, T., van Geel, B.N. *et al.* (1994). Impending and actual pathological fractures in patients with bone metastases of the long bones. A retrospective study of 233 surgically treated fractures. *The European Journal of Surgery.*, Oct, **160**(10), 535–42.

40. Clain, A. (1965). Secondary malignant disease of bone. *British Journal of Cancer*, Mar, **19**, 15–29.

41. Bickels, J., Kollender, Y., Wittig, J.C. *et al.* (2005). Function after resection of humeral metastases: analysis of 59 consecutive patients. *Clinical Orthopaedics and Related Research*, Aug, **437**, 201–8.

42. Sim, F.H. (1992). Metastatic bone disease of the pelvis and femur. *Instructional Course Lectures.*, **41**, 317–27.

43. Jacofsky, D.J., and Haidukewych, G.J. (2004). Management of pathologic fractures of the proximal femur: state of the art. *Journal of Orthopaedic Trauma*, Aug, **18**(7), 459–69.

44. Kelly, C.M., Wilkins, R.M., Eckardt, J.J. (2003). Treatment of metastatic disease of the tibia. *Clinical Orthopaedics and Related Research*, Oct, (415 Suppl.), S219–29.

45. Aljassir, F., Beadel, G.P., Turcotte, R.E. *et al.* (2005). Outcome after pelvic sarcoma resection reconstructed with saddle prosthesis. *Clinical Orthopaedics and Related Research*, Sep, **438**, 36–41.

46. Masala, S., Fiori, R., Massari, F., and Simonetti, G. (2003). Vertebroplasty and kyphoplasty: new equipment for malignant vertebral fractures treatment. *Journal of Experimental & Clinical Cancer Research*, Dec, **22**(4 Suppl.), 75–9.

47. Marcove, R.C., Sadrieh, J., Huvos, A.G. *et al.* (1972). Cryosurgery in the treatment of solitary or multiple bone metastases from renal cell carcinoma. *Journal of Urology*, Oct, **108**(4), 540–7.

48. Marcove, R.C., Searfoss, R.C., Whitmore, W.F. *et al.* (1977). Cryosurgery in the treatment of bone metastases from renal cell carcinoma. *Clinical Orthopaedics and Related Research*, **127**, 220–7.

49. Simon, C.J., and Dupuy, D.E. (2005). Image-guided ablative techniques in pelvic malignancies: radiofrequency ablation, cryoablation, microwave ablation. *Surgical Oncology Clinics of North America*, Apr, **14**(2), 419–31.

50. Goetz, M.P., Callstrom, M.R., Charboneau, J.W. *et al.* (2004). Percutaneous image-guided radiofrequency ablation of painful metastases involving bone: a multicenter study. *Journal of Clinical Oncology*, Jan 15, **22**(2), 300–6.

51. Chatziioannou, A.N., Johnson, M.E., Pneumaticos, S.G. *et al.* (2000). Preoperative embolization of bone metastases from renal cell carcinoma. *European Radiology*, **10**(4), 593–6.

52. Roscoe, M.W., McBroom, R.J., St Louis, E. *et al.* (1989). Preoperative embolization in the treatment of osseous metastases from renal cell carcinoma. *Clinical Orthopaedics and Related Research*, Jan, **238**, 302–7.

53. Hillner, B.E., Ingle, J.N., Berenson, J.R. *et al.* (2000). American Society of Clinical Oncology guideline on the role of bisphosphonates in breast cancer. American Society of Clinical Oncology Bisphosphonates Expert Panel. *Journal of Clinical Oncology*, Mar, **18**(6), 1378–91.

54. Saad, F., Higano, C.S., Sartor, O. *et al.* (2006). The role of bisphosphonates in the treatment of prostate cancer: recommendations from an expert panel. *Clinical Genitourinary Cancer*, Mar, **4**(4), 257–62.

The role of interventional radiology in the palliative care of patients with cancer

Tarun Sabharwal, Nicos I. Fotiadis, and Andy Adam

Over the past four decades, a variety of invasive diagnostic and therapeutic procedures have been developed by radiologists. The term 'Interventional Radiology' most appropriately refers to therapeutic procedures performed under imaging guidance[1]. The emergence of this specialty has been made possible by enormous technological advances in relation to catheter and instrument design and manufacture, imaging systems, and radiological expertise. Interventional radiological procedures have virtually replaced several more invasive and hazardous surgical alternatives. Other interventional techniques offer completely new therapeutic options. Some diagnostic radiological procedures are frequently followed by therapeutic manoeuvres. For example, percutaneous antegrade pyelography, performed to delineate the site and nature of renal obstruction, is usually followed immediately by the placement of a nephrostomy drainage catheter[2]. Purely diagnostic procedures, such as percutaneous biopsy, will not be discussed in any detail, as they are largely inappropriate for the patient with a known neoplastic process receiving palliative care.

All interventional procedures carry some risk, which is related to the underlying condition, the nature of the procedure, and the experience of the radiologist. Therefore, it is important in patients with advanced malignant disease receiving palliative care to contemplate only those procedures that will alleviate symptoms, and in which the potential benefits outweigh the risks[3].

Interventional radiology can make a significant contribution to the palliation of patients with irresectable malignant tumours, as many of the procedures can relieve symptoms without the need for general anaesthesia, a prolonged stay in hospital, or the discomfort associated with recovery from a surgical operation. The vast majority of procedures are performed using local anaesthesia and mild sedation. The emphasis in this chapter is on the indications, contraindications, and likely outcomes, rather than on detailed technical descriptions.

Therapeutic interventional radiological procedures

A summary of procedures that may be useful in patients undergoing palliative care is shown in Table 9.5.1.

Table 9.5.1 Interventional radiological procedures.

Procedure	Examples of indications
Drainage	Malignant obstruction of renal and biliary tract, pleural effusions, ascites
Dilation/stenting	Malignant gastrointestinal, biliary, ureteric and airway obstruction, superior or inferior vena caval obstruction, etc.
Feeding	Venous access—Hickman lines peripherally-inserted central catheter (PICC) lines
	Percutaneous gastrostomy
Extraction	Retrieval or resiting of venous lines
Infusion	Regional, selective infusion of chemotherapeutic agents
Embolization	Hormone-producing metastases, primary hepatocellular carcinoma, skeletal metastases, etc.
Neurolysis	Coeliac ganglion in pancreatic cancer
Vertebroplasty	Vertebral metastasis, osteoporosis
Tumour ablation	Liver, renal, bony, and soft tissue tumours

Percutaneous puncture and drainage procedures

Utilizing fluoroscopy, ultrasound, computed tomography (CT) or magnetic resonance imaging (MRI) guidance it is possible to image and drain obstructed renal and biliary systems, cysts, abscesses, and effusions.

Renal tract[4]

Antegrade pyelography and percutaneous nephrostomy are used in the management of a variety of situations, including malignant obstruction of the urinary tract, haemorrhagic cystitis secondary to chemotherapy (where it is desirable to divert the urine to 'rest' the bladder), and in patients with recto-vaginal or recto-vesical fistula caused by pelvic malignancy. Diversion of urinary flow may assist in healing of the fistulas, ease nursing problems, and allow patients to become 'dry'.

The pelvicalyceal system is initially punctured under ultrasound guidance with a fine gauge needle through which radiographic contrast medium is instilled to demonstrate the anatomy and determine the level of obstruction. Urine can be aspirated for microbiological and cytological examinations. Percutaneous nephrostomy entails the insertion into the collecting system of a pigtail configuration catheter with multiple, large side-holes. If drainage is to be of short duration, an external bag may be satisfactory; however, if long-term drainage is required and if it is possible to cross the area of obstruction, an internal stent is preferred[5], as it allows the patient to be free of 'bags'. It is noteworthy that, in most cases, it is possible to manipulate a catheter across an area of apparently complete obstruction. Although a contrast study may indicate total obstruction, a hydrophilic guide wire can usually be advanced through the 'obstruction', as it finds the (very narrow) lumen and follows it. The balloon catheter can then be advanced over the guide wire to dilate the stricture and restore patency before a stent is inserted.

In patients with pelvic malignancy and fistulas to the perineum it may prove necessary to combine nephrostomy with ureteric embolization using steel coils or segments of gelatine sponge to prevent any urine reaching the skin of the perineum. A catheter can be manipulated into the ureter and embolic materials, such as steel coils and sterile sponge, can be injected to occlude the ureter[6].

Biliary tract

Patients with obstructive jaundice due to irresectable malignant biliary strictures can be palliated by the insertion of an endoprosthesis (stent) (Fig. 9.5.1). Stents may be inserted endoscopically for lesions affecting the low common bile duct or percutaneously in patients with lesions at the hilum of the liver or when ERCP (endoscopic retrograde cholangiopancreatography) fails to relieve the obstruction. In most cases unilateral drainage is usually sufficient for relieving jaundice and pruritus. The procedure is usually carried out under fluoroscopic and ultrasound guidance. First a percutaneous transhepatic cholangiogram (PTC) is performed using a 22G needle. It is important to visualize the entire biliary system prior to selecting the most suitable duct for insertion of a drainage catheter. Self-expandable metallic stents are now widely available and generally preferable to the conventional plastic endoprosthesis. Such stents can be inserted using a small introducing catheter (5–7 French diameter) and yet they achieve a large internal diameter (10 mm) when released across the obstructing lesion.

The large calibre of these devices ensures that the rate of occlusion is lower than that of a plastic endoprosthesis. The overall failure rate of plastic stents is in the region of 30–40 per cent, whereas that of metallic stents is 10–15 per cent. The frequency of cholangitis is approximately 30 per cent in patients with plastic stents and approximately 10 per cent in patients with metallic endoprostheses[7]. Occluded plastic stents can be replaced using a variety of endoscopic or percutaneous techniques. Occluded metallic endoprostheses cannot be removed but their patency can be restored by the introduction of a second device inserted coaxially within the first. Unless life expectancy is very short, it is well worth considering restoring the patency of an occluded stent, as this can greatly improve the patient's quality of life[8].

Malignant pleural effusions

Malignant pleural effusions (MPEs) can produce significant respiratory symptoms and diminished quality of life in patients with terminal malignancies. A patient who presents with a MPE should

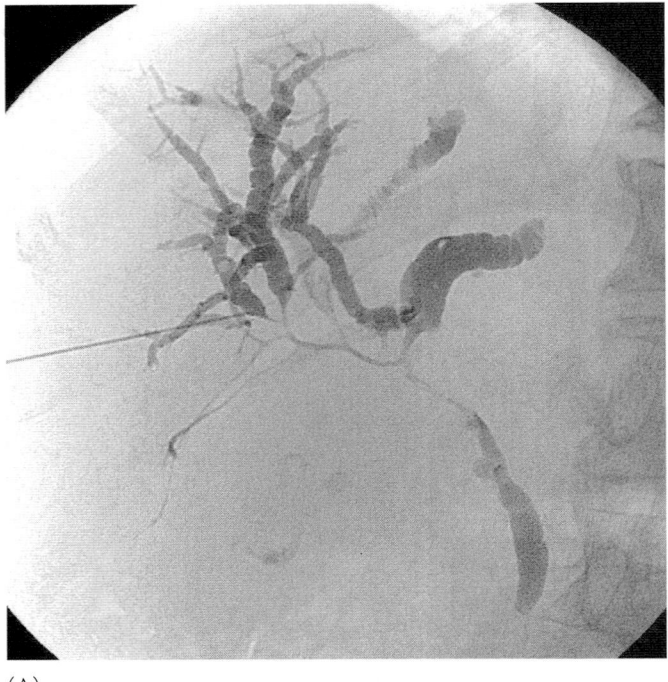

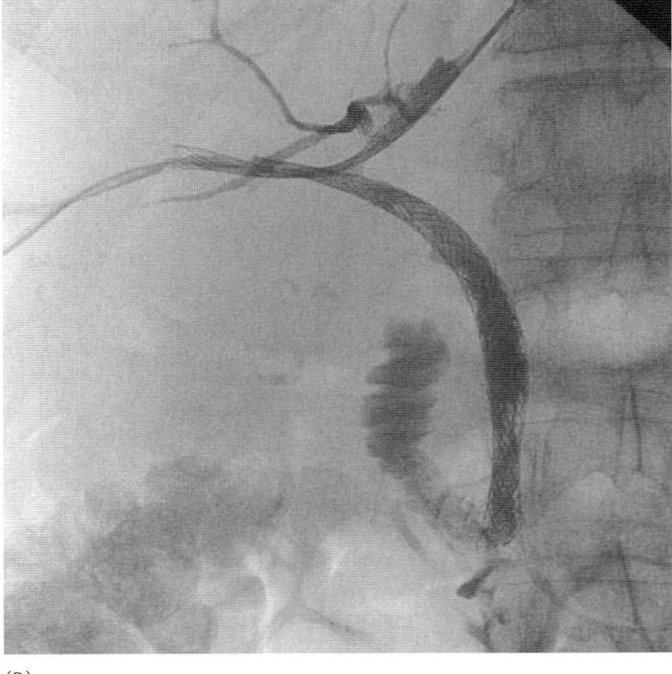

(A)   (B)

Figure 9.5.1 Percutaneous biliary drainage. (A) Percutaneous cholangiogram shows stricture of the central bile ducts and proximal common bile duct due to cholangiocarcinoma (Klatskin tumour), and dilated intrahepatic ducts. (B) Biliary drainage with two metallic endoprosthesis.

first have a diagnostic and therapeutic thoracocentesis. This can be done under ultrasound guidance. It is important to assess for symptom improvement and the ability of the lung to re-expand. The fluid will re-accumulate in almost all patients, at which time local treatment is needed. This typically consists of tube thoracostomy, usually followed by instillation of a sclerosing agent (doxycycline, bleomycin, or talc) to chemically induce pleurodesis[9]. A tunnelled pleural catheter, The Denver Pleurx® catheter (Denver Biomaterials, Inc., Golden, CO) is also available for those patients who are ineligible or fail sclerotherapy. This is a 66-cm long 15.5 French soft silicone catheter with a polyester cuff to promote fibrosis to the subcutaneous tissue and multiple side-holes to enhance drainage. A valve in its hub is opened only when a dilator is passed through it. This prevents inadvertent entry of air or leakage of fluid. The drainage system consists of a vacuum bottle with a pre-connected tube that has a dilator at its end to pass into the hub of the catheter. Drainage will typically take no longer than 15 min and should be performed at least every other day. In the outpatient setting, this can be done by a visiting nurse, family members, or the patient[10].

Malignant ascites

The accumulation of large volume ascites is a common occurrence for patients with intraperitoneal spread of tumour. These patients have a very poor prognosis, with anticipated mean survival ranging from 1 to 4 months. Patients often experience symptoms of abdominal pressure, shortness of breath, nausea, early satiety, and limited mobility because of the mass effect of the fluid. Management of symptoms is palliative and methods used include percutaneous drainage, diuretics, shunt placement, and intraperitoneal drug therapy. Paracentesis is not only the most common treatment method used by physicians, but also the most effective at relieving symptoms[11]. Unfortunately, management of recurrent ascites with paracentesis requires frequent trips to the hospital and has greater risk of complications associated with multiple needle passes into the abdomen. There are increasing number of published reports which show that a 15.5 French tunnelled draining catheter, the Pleurx® catheter, provides effective palliation with a complication rate similar to that for large volume paracentesis, while obviating the need for frequent trips to the hospital for repeated percutaneous drainage[12,13].

Dilatation/stenting techniques

Dilatation and stenting procedures are most commonly employed for the treatment of non-malignant conditions in the vascular tree (percutaneous transluminal angioplasty). However, these techniques can also be applied to benign and malignant stenoses and occlusions in other systems, including the gastrointestinal tract, renal, biliary and respiratory systems.

Gastrointestinal tract

Within the gastrointestinal tract, fluoroscopically-guided balloon dilatation has proved to be a particularly useful technique. Dilatation alone is unlikely to be effective in malignant strictures and should be followed by some form of stenting[14].

Oesophagus (see Chapter 10.2.2)

The main indication for oesophageal stenting is the alleviation of dysphagia in patients with irresectable oesophageal cancer. Rigid plastic tubes inserted endoscopically have been used for several years. More recently, self-expandable metallic endoprostheses have become available[15]. Such stents are usually covered with plastic in order to prevent ingrowth of tumour through the wall of the stent[16]. They can be introduced using fluoroscopic guidance under light sedation, unlike rigid plastic tubes that are too large to be inserted without the use of general anaesthesia in many patients. Placement of a metallic stent across a tight stricture produces a virtually immediate and substantial improvement in swallowing. With recent advances[17] and increased experience in the use of metallic stents, over 95 per cent of patients with inoperable oesophageal strictures can be palliated successfully with these devices. A commonly used device is the Ultraflex® Stent (Boston Scientific Corp., USA), which consists of a woven nitinol mesh, and is available in covered and uncovered forms. The procedure can be performed rapidly, on an outpatient basis if necessary. The quality of swallowing can be graded from 0 for normal swallowing to 4 for complete dysphagia. The mean dysphagia score of patients with oesophageal carcinoma treated with self-expandable metallic endoprostheses is 1[18]. Most patients treated with rigid plastic tubes have a dysphagia score greater than 2, and the majority can manage only a liquid or semi-liquid diet. A prospective randomized comparison has shown that although metallic stents are more expensive than rigid plastic tubes, they are cost-effective, because they minimize the rate of complications and reduce the length of hospital stay [19].

Other palliative options for relieving dysphagia in patients with oesophageal cancer include surgery, radiotherapy, chemotherapy, brachytherapy, and endoscopic laser therapy. Metallic stents relieve dysphagia more effectively than endoscopic laser therapy does, which should be reserved for special cases, such as exophytic tumours[18]. Stent insertion is a straightforward procedure with negligible mortality and low morbidity, and seldom needs to be repeated in the majority of patients.

Covered metallic stents are also very useful in the management of malignant oesophageal fistulas. Unlike fistulas associated with benign diseases, which may heal with conservative therapy, fistulas associated with malignant lesions do not heal spontaneously. Without definitive treatment, most patients succumb to malnutrition and thoracic sepsis within weeks. Radiological insertion of a covered metallic stent can result in immediate sealing of the fistula and the patient can drink fluids a few hours after the procedure, resuming a normal diet on the following day[15] (Fig. 9.5.2).

Gastroduodenal and colorectal (see Chapter 10.2.4)

Self-expanding metallic stents are playing an increasingly important role in the treatment of gastroduodenal obstruction and acute colonic obstruction[20, 21]. Patients with these conditions are often elderly and frail with dehydration and electrolyte imbalance. Self-expanding stents offer a non-surgical therapeutic alternative that rapidly relieves the obstruction and improves their clinical condition, with a high success rate and low morbidity. This may be a temporizing measure allowing stabilization of the patient prior to definitive surgery, or alternatively, for patients who are not surgical candidates, the stent may provide adequate palliation[22]. Currently the 22-mm 'enteral' Wallstent® (Schneider, Bulach, Switzerland) seems the most suitable stent because of its high longitudinal flexibility, adequate self-expanding force, and small diameter introducer system (Fig. 9.5.3).

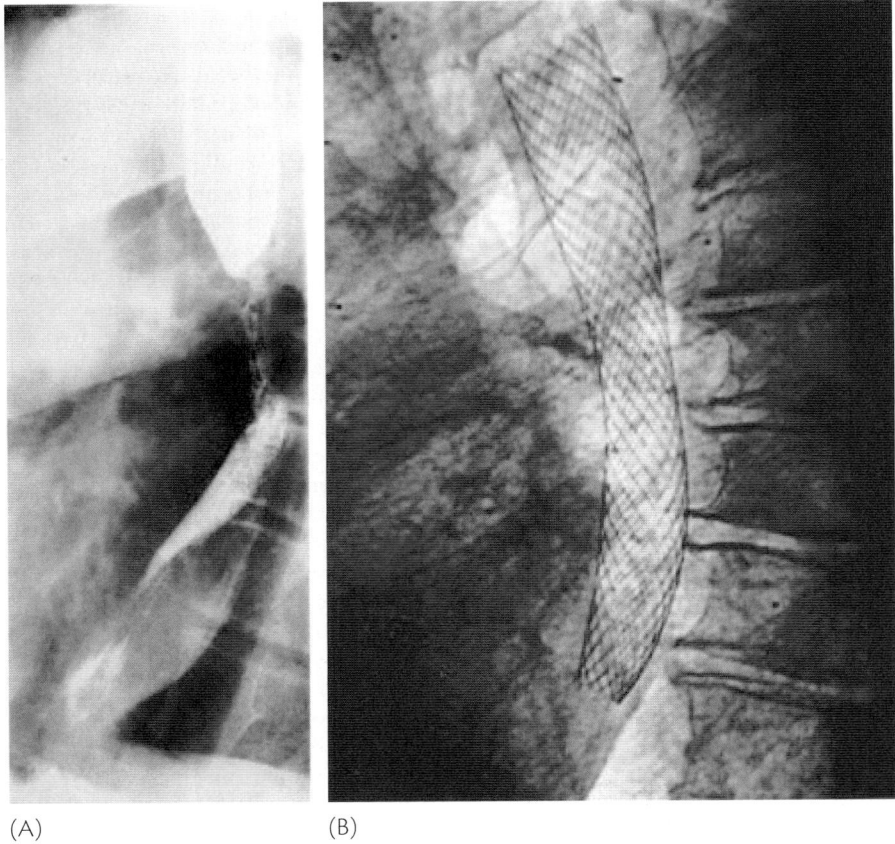

(A)   (B)

Figure 9.5.2 Oesophageal stenting.

Tracheobronchial

Malignant airways obstruction can cause considerable distress to patients. When surgical resection is not possible, self-expanding metallic stents can provide good palliation[23]. This procedure is best carried out under general anaesthesia, as a combined effort between an interventional radiologist and a bronchoscopist. Bronchoscopic visualization is used to determine the position of the stricture, the limits of which are marked with a radio-opaque marker. The stricture is then dilated under fluoroscopic guidance. Following dilatation, a self-expandable metallic stent is released across the stricture, again under fluoroscopic guidance. This can result in significant symptomatic improvement and prevent collapse and/or infection and abscess formation beyond an obstructing lesion[24]. Placement of plastic-covered metallic stents in the trachea is an effective method of managing tracheo-oesophageal fistulae unsuitable for treatment with covered oesophageal stents[25].

Venous obstruction

The superior vena cava syndrome often presents as a very distressing pre-terminal event in patients with thoracic malignancy. It is most commonly related to mediastinal neoplasia, particularly primary and secondary lung tumours and lymphoma. The obstruction, which can be partial or complete, can be caused by caval compression and/or invasion by tumour and is frequently complicated by venous thrombosis.

Superior venocavography delineates the site and extent of the obstruction. If extensive thrombosis is present, selective intravenous thrombolysis with a catheter placed within the thrombus is undertaken under local anaesthesia. Percutaneous transfemoral dilatation of the narrowed superior vena cava is followed by the insertion of a self-expandable metallic endoprosthesis. Flow is restored immediately, providing excellent and immediate palliation of symptoms[25] (Fig. 9.5.4). This procedure can be performed prior to, in conjunction with, or after therapy, including radiotherapy or chemotherapy. It can also be performed in conjunction with airway stenting (Fig. 9.5.5). Malignant involvement of the inferior vena cava can be managed in a similar fashion. All patients with malignant superior or inferior vena caval obstruction should be considered for this relatively straightforward and usually successful procedure, which can readily improve their quality of life.

Percutaneous insertion of an inferior vena cava filter is indicated in patients with recurrent pulmonary embolism refractory to or unsuitable for treatment with anticoagulation therapy and in those patients with free-floating thrombus in the inferior vena cava[26].

Feeding techniques

Venous access

Central venous access may be essential in some patients with terminal disease for feeding and the delivery of medication, palliative

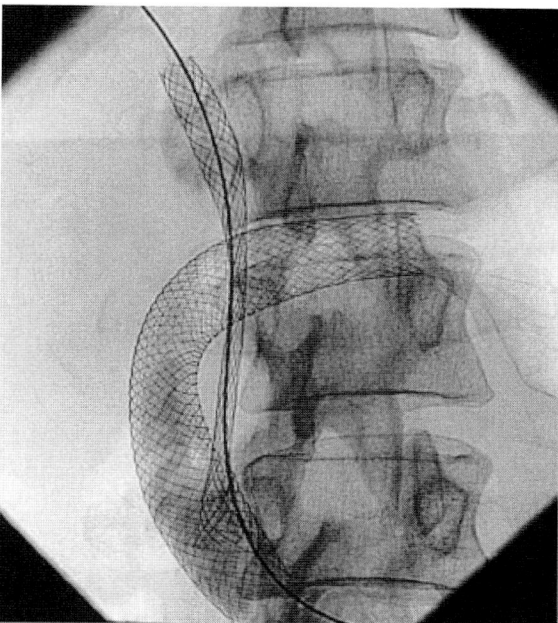

Figure 9.5.3 Concurrent percutaneous biliary (Wallstent®) and gastroduodenal (enteral) stent in patient with inoperable pancreatic cancer.

chemotherapy or analgesia. A variety of long-term venous access systems (e.g. tunnelled central venous catheters, peripherally inserted central catheters (PICCs), and venous ports), have been developed for insertion under fluoroscopic and ultrasound guidance[27,28]. The procedure is now usually performed in the radiology department under local anaesthesia and strict asepsis[29]. The main advantage over the surgical venous cut-down technique is that performing the procedure under fluoroscopic guidance ensures that the tip of the catheter is always in the correct position and virtually eliminates the need for repositioning the catheter at a later date. The procedure is rapid, well tolerated by the patient, and associated with high success and low complication rates[30]. In our

experience, it is virtually always possible to gain venous access using interventional radiological methods. The rate of occurrence of pneumothorax when using a subclavian approach is approximately 1 per cent. This complication is very rare when access is gained via the internal jugular vein. The long-term complications of occlusion and infection of the catheter are not significantly different from those observed when a surgical method of venous access is used. The traditional surgical method of placement without imaging guidance is associated with a misplacement rate of approximately 6 per cent, whereas this complication does not occur when catheter placement is performed under imaging guidance.

Percutaneous gastrostomy

Nutritional support may be required in patients with end-stage disease. This sometime raises difficult questions particularly in relation to parenteral nutrition (see Chapter 10.3.2). Enteric feeding is generally a simpler option and can be accomplished by the insertion of gastrostomy tubes. The insertion of a feeding gastrostomy tube either under fluoroscopic or endoscopic guidance and local anaesthesia can significantly improve the patient's well-being and ease of management, often avoiding the need for uncomfortable psychologically distressing nasogastric tubes and intravenous lines. A gastrostomy tube can be readily managed in the home environment by the patient's family and carers as well as by nursing staff[31,32].

Gastro-jejunostomy tubes are preferable when there is gastric outlet obstruction or in cases of gastro-oesophageal reflux.

Extraction techniques[33]

Developments in intravenous feeding therapy and monitoring techniques have led to a vast increase in the number of indwelling venous cannulas and catheters. Unfortunately, these occasionally break or become disconnected and a part or all of the catheter is 'lost' within the venous system[34]. It is important to retrieve these intravascular foreign bodies as they not only perforate vascular structures and cause dysrhythmias but also act as a seat of infection, particularly in immunosuppressed patients. Surgical retrieval of

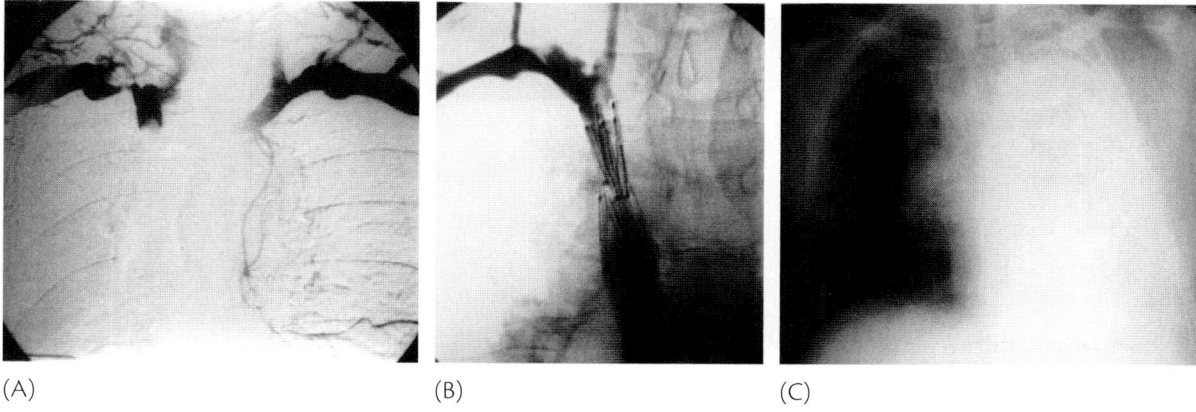

(A)   (B)   (C)

Figure 9.5.4 Superior vena caval stenting. (A) Superior venocavogram reveals extensive thrombosis and narrowing of the superior vena cava by tumour. (B) Following selective thrombolysis, metallic stents have been placed across the compressed area which was initially dilated with a balloon. A repeat venogram confirms patency of the superior vena cava. (C) A chest radiograph shows the stents in place and the extensive tumour affecting the left hemithorax and mediastinum. The patient's symptoms showed immediate improvement and had completely resolved by 24 h.

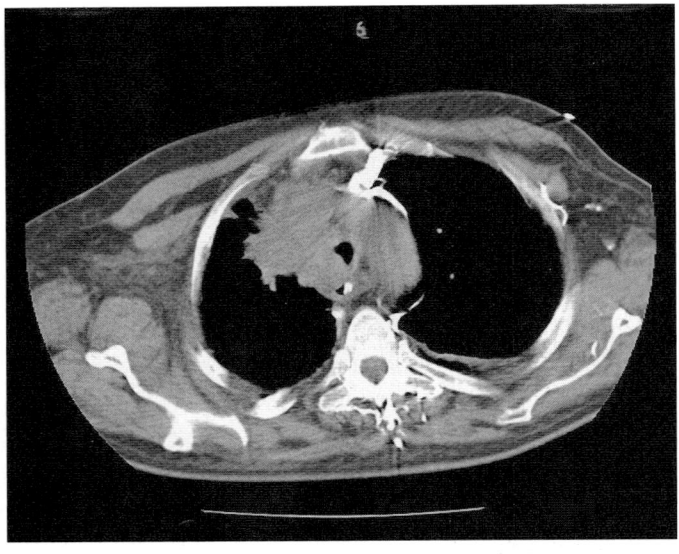

(A)

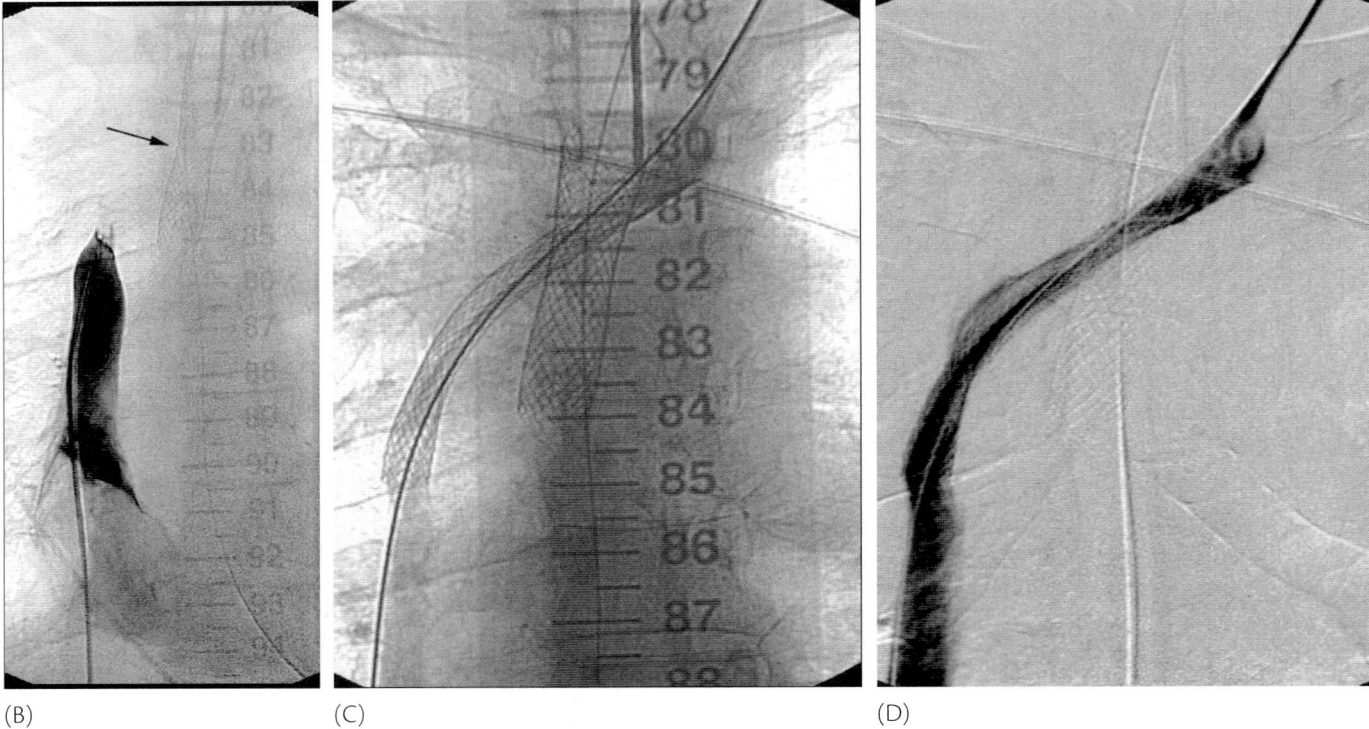

(B)   (C)   (D)

Figure 9.5.5 Tracheal and superior vena cava stenting. (A) CT shows a Pancoast tumour occluding the SVC and compromising the trachea. (B) A tracheal stent was inserted initially (arrow) and a venogram reveals the obstructed SVC. (C) A metallic Wallstent® has been placed across the obstructed SVC.
(D) Completion venogram shows patency of the SVC stent and also the widely opened tracheal stent.

catheter fragments is hazardous (and sometimes impractical), necessitating a thoracotomy. It is almost invariably possible to retrieve these catheter fragments, which usually lodge within the right side of the heart or the pulmonary arteries, percutaneously under fluoroscopic guidance. Detailed descriptions of all the retrieval techniques available are beyond the scope of this chapter but any interventional radiologist offering a comprehensive vascular

service is well advised to become acquainted with the various methods and have the necessary equipment available[35].

The ability to snare or 'catch' the end of a catheter can also be of value when the tip of an indwelling central venous catheter has become displaced into the jugular vein. It is usually possible to 'pull' such a catheter back into a correct position using a percutaneous vascular approach under local anaesthesia.

Infusion techniques

The ability of the radiologist accurately to site a catheter into virtually any blood vessel within the body has brought into play the concepts of regional infusion of chemotherapeutic agents, monoclonal antibodies and isotopes. The principle underlying these techniques is that a high dose of the therapeutic agent is delivered to the tumour(s) with minimal side effects. Recent advances include the addition of embolic materials (see 'Vascular embolization' section) and the microencapsulation of cytotoxic agents to achieve gradual and sustained release. Lipiodol is now also used in combination with cytotoxic drugs for the treatment of certain hepatic tumours; it is retained in tumour vessels and also acts as a contrast agent, thus allowing monitoring of tumour response to treatment using CT imaging.

These techniques have been used with varying degrees of success to treat primary and metastatic liver tumours[36], bone neoplasms, cerebral neoplasms, sarcomas, melanomas, and pelvic neoplasms. It is possible to insert fine catheters that can be left in place for weeks at a time[37].

Vascular embolization

The deliberate occlusion of arteries and/or veins by the injection of embolic agents through selectively placed catheters, is one of the major therapeutic applications of interventional radiology in the patient with neoplastic disease. This technique has been employed in the management of severe and disabling symptoms from a very wide variety of tumours throughout the body. Embolization, which usually involves a percutaneous technique with local anaesthesia, offers an attractive alternative to surgery under general anaesthesia and, in some situations, is the only therapeutic option available. A wide variety of embolic agents are available[38]. The broad categories of substances used include particulate emboli (sterile sponge—Spongostan®, polyvinyl alcohol—Ivalon®, and the newer clear acrylic microspheres—Embosphere®), mechanical emboli (balloons, steel coils), and liquids (50 per cent dextrose, absolute alcohol, lipiodol). The appropriate agent or combination of agents depends on the lesion to be treated and its site (with particular reference to adjacent vulnerable vascular structures).

Embolization can be used definitively to treat benign conditions and preoperatively to assist effective, safe surgery, but in many cases it is used palliatively to alleviate distressing symptoms (Fig. 9.5.6).

Palliative embolization

Embolization can be used to control pain, haemorrhage, and hormone production as well as to reduce tumour bulk. The technique may be used as the primary mode of treatment in inoperable malignancy and embolization of metastatic deposits has, in some situations, been shown to extend survival times in advanced disease[39]. Tumours in all sites have been treated in this fashion (liver, kidney, bone, lung, soft tissues, nervous system, and gastrointestinal tract). Hormone-secreting neoplasms such as metastatic APUD cell tumours show the greatest therapeutic response to arterial embolization. Appropriate pharmacological blockade is necessary during the embolization to avoid the effects of a dramatic outpouring of hormone as the tumour is deprived of its blood supply. The beneficial effects of embolization may become apparent within a

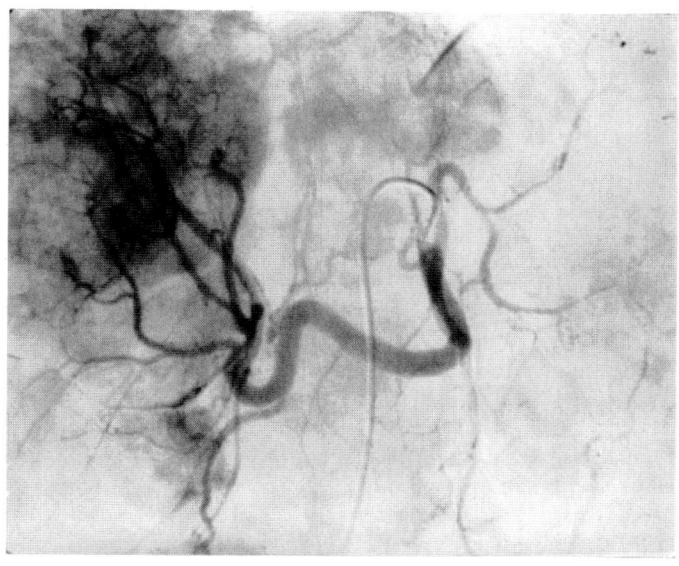

(A)

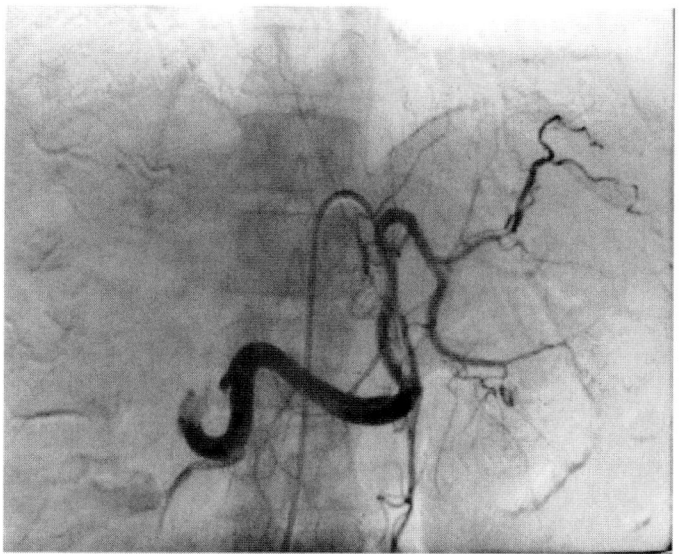

(B)

Figure 9.5.6 Hepatic embolization for metastatic carcinoid tumour. (A) The arterial parenchymal phase shows hepatic enlargement and reveals multiple tumour deposits. (B) Post-embolization arteriogram shows that the arterial supply has been obliterated. The patient's symptoms (flushing and diarrhoea) were dramatically alleviated by this procedure.

matter of hours. In embolization procedures it is important that adequate premedication is given prior to the procedure, including broad-spectrum antibiotics. In many situations, for example, liver and bone, it is necessary to continue antibiotics for 10 days after the procedure to prevent sepsis developing in the devascularized tissue.

A significant advance in tumour embolization has been the development of chemoembolization[40]. In this technique embolic materials are mixed with chemotherapeutic drugs; the emboli cause ischaemia of the tumour cells and by increasing the transit time through the tumour vascular bed, the contact time between the cytotoxic agent and the neoplastic cells is prolonged, resulting in a greater therapeutic effect. It has been discovered that vascular tumours in the liver have a particular affinity for lipiodol injected into the hepatic artery. The possibility of tagging cytotoxic agents to the lipiodol has been investigated in many centres worldwide. Mid-term results, in primary hepatoma, are very encouraging[41,42].

In patients with cirrhosis of the liver complicated by hepatocellular carcinoma it is best to avoid arterial embolization because it may lead to further deterioration in liver function. In such patients, percutaneous tumour ablation with injection of alcohol, or usage of radiofrequency probes has been shown to lead to a significant increase in life expectancy (see 'Percutaneous tumour ablation' section).

After embolization of large tumour masses, patients may experience some discomfort and pain and they may have a fever for a few days accompanied by a feeling of malaise and an elevated white cell count. This combination of signs and symptoms has been called the *post-embolization syndrome*, and is an indicator of the presence of necrotic tissue. Sustained pyrexia should alert the clinician to the possibility of abscess formation and blood cultures plus regional ultrasound should be performed. Elevated serum C reactive protein can also provide a useful indication that infection may be present[43].

Neurolysis

Alcohol injection is useful in the palliation of intractable pain which occasionally accompanies retroperitoneal malignancy. For example, certain patients with carcinoma of the pancreas experience severe pain due to infiltration of the coeliac ganglion by the tumour. In these patients the coeliac ganglion may be ablated by injecting alcohol in its immediate vicinity under CT guidance.

Percutaneous vertebroplasty/kyphoplasty

Percutaneous vertebroplasty is a therapeutic, image-guided procedure that involves injection of radio-opaque cement into a partially collapsed vertebral body, in an effort to relieve pain and provide stability[44].

This procedure is being used for patients with intractable debilitating pain due to vertebral compression fractures that is refractory to conventional therapies such as analgesic use, bed rest, and bracing. Neoplastic causes of vertebral compression fractures include bone metastases, multiple myeloma, lymphoma and aggressive haemangiomas. Up to 80 per cent of patients with pain unresponsive to

conventional medical treatment experience a significant degree of pain relief, and few serious complications have been reported[45,46].

Percutaneous vertebroplasty is usually performed under local anaesthesia with sedation, and may be carried out as an outpatient procedure or may require a short hospital stay. Local, deep, periosteal and endosteal anaesthesia is provided at the outset. CT and/or fluoroscopic guidance is used. The patient lies in the prone position, and then a large bore (10–15 gauge) needle is placed into the vertebral body, through a transpedicular route for the lumbar spine or peripedicular/transpedicular route for the thoracic spine. Access to cervical lesions is via an anterolateral approach. Once positioned in the vertebral body acrylic bone cement, usually methyl methacrylate, mixed with contrast medium, is then injected into the affected vertebra. This material is viscous to minimize leakage into adjacent structures or blood vessels. The whole procedure usually takes 1–2 h. Non-steroidal anti-inflammatory drugs can be used for 2–4 days after vertebroplasty to minimize the inflammatory reaction to the acrylic compound. Pain relief is expected within 24 h of the procedure (Fig. 9.5.7). Complication rates are <2 per cent for osteoporotic indications and <10 per cent for malignant indications and include temporary or permanent neurologic deficit, infection, bleeding from puncture site and allergic reaction[44,47,48].

Kyphoplasty is a refinement of the vertebroplasty procedure. In addition to the reduction of fracture-related pain, some or all of the height is restored to the compressed vertebral body. Normalizing the height of the fractured vertebra reduces the focally exaggerated curvature of the spine (i.e. kyphosis). This effect, in turn, results in an aesthetic improvement, improved posture, and a reduced risk of fracture of the adjacent vertebra as a result of abnormal load bearing. The restoration of a more normal appearing configuration of the vertebral body and improvement in the load-bearing physics is accomplished with the intravertebral inflation of 1 or 2 high-pressure balloon tamps (KyphX®; Kyphon) prior to the infusion of methylmethacrylate.

Percutaneous tumour ablation

Ablation refers to local (rather than systemic) methods that destroy the tumour without removing it. These techniques are usually reserved for patients with recurrent malignancy in areas of previous radiation therapy, localized metastatic disease, and primary neoplasms in patients who are poor surgical candidates. They are not always considered curative but can produce survival rates equal to

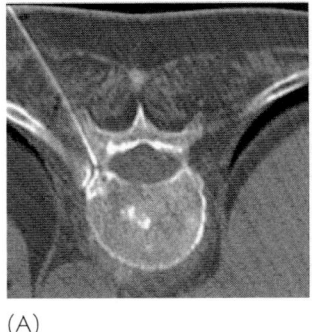 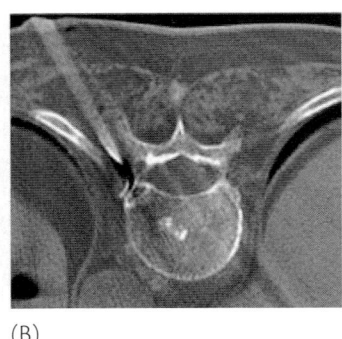 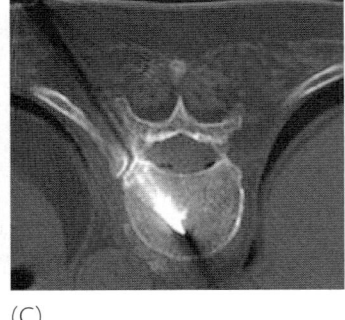 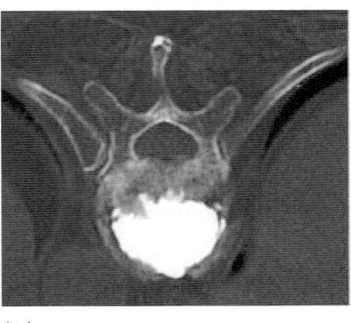

(A)　　　　　　　　　(B)　　　　　　　　　(C)　　　　　　　　　(D)

Figure 9.5.7 Percutaneous vertebroplasty. CT images. (A) 22G spinal needle in situ for local anaesthetic injection. (B) 11G vertebroplasty needle has been percutaneously positioned with tip in vertebral body using CT and fluoroscopic guidance. (C) Careful injection of cement through needle. (D) Post-cement injection. (Films reproduced with kind permission from Prof A. Gangi.)

surgery in people with small tumours. Percutaneous techniques of local tumour ablation may be categorized into three major groups: injection (ethanol, acetic acid, hot saline), heating (radiofrequency ablation [RFA][49] electrocautery, interstitial laser therapy, microwave coagulation therapy, high-intensity focused ultrasound), and freezing (cryotherapy). Advantages of the ablative therapies compared to surgical resection include reduced morbidity and mortality, low cost, and the ability to perform procedures on an outpatient basis. All these techniques induce cell death by coagulative necrosis.

Percutaneous liver tumour ablation

The liver is the organ with the greatest number of patients eligible for treatment with percutaneous tumour ablation given the large number of patients with primary or secondary hepatic malignancies and the low number eligible for surgical resection. Multiple minimally invasive techniques have been developed including percutaneous ethanol injection (PEI), interstitial laser photocoagulation, microwave, cryotherapy, focused ultrasound, and RFA. Of these the most widely used are PEI for hepatocellular carcinoma (HCC) and thermal ablation for HCC and hepatic metastasis.

Percutaneous ethanol injection therapy

Percutaneous ethanol injection therapy (PEIT) was first described in 1983. Since that time PEIT has been used extensively for treatment of unresectable HCC[50]. There is no absolute limitation to the size or number of lesions treated. However, as tumour size increases, homogeneity of ethanol diffusion diminishes at the periphery, increasing the probability that residual viable tumour cells will persist at the margin of the lesion following therapy. The limitation of diffusion radius and homogeneity is particularly relevant to metastases that have a firmer consistency than hepatocellular carcinoma, making them more resistant to ethanol diffusion at any size. The frequent need for multiple treatment sessions for each lesion, and the limited injection volume tolerated in a single session, place practical limitations on the number of lesions treated. For these reasons, as well as the documented greater effectiveness of PEIT for small, solitary tumours, many restrict the use of PEIT to nodular lesions 3 cm or less in diameter and three or fewer in number. However, PEIT is sometimes used in conjunction with thermal ablation in an effort to increase the area of tumour destruction[51].

Thermal ablation

Lesional heating techniques such as RFA and interstitial laser photocoagulation (ILP) effect tumour necrosis by hyperthermia. RF electrodes or laser fibres are inserted into the tumour under ultrasound, CT, or MRI guidance.

ILP produces thermal coagulation by conversion of absorbed light energy into heat[52]. In RFA, alternating current induces ionic agitation, which results in frictional heat production within the tissues. The size and shape of the necrotic lesion produced by RF has been shown to be a function of the probe gauge, length of the exposed tip, temperature along the exposed electrode, and duration of therapy. Strategies aiming at increasing the volume of tissue coagulation include the use of multi-probe electrodes and saline enhancement[53]. Cooling the electrode with saline during the ablation prevents charring of the liver and reduces the impedance of the tissues adjacent to the electrode. In turn, this permits dissemination of heat further out into the tumour and increases the area of coagulation. The procedure is tolerated well and causes either no or only slight and transient abnormalities of liver function

tests. Serious complications are rare and consist mainly of intraperitoneal haemorrhage and liver abscess formation.

The follow-up of patients after all forms of percutaneous tumour ablation includes a combination of imaging, tumour marker assay, and selected use of fine needle aspiration biopsy. It is useful to follow serial levels of alpha-fetoprotein or carcino-embryonic antigen, in the case of hepatocellular carcinoma or metastatic disease, respectively, only when the serum levels of these markers are elevated prior to the initiation of therapy. The immediate goal of imaging is to assess whether complete necrosis has been achieved. Ultrasound does not usually provide useful information, as the echogenicity of fibrosis and neoplastic tissue overlap. Contrast-enhanced MRI and contrast-enhanced CT are capable of demonstrating remaining viable tumour requiring treatment. However, in difficult cases, PET scanning may provide additional information.

Several clinical series using different methods of RFA have been reported. The results appear to be promising, showing a 40 per cent 5-year survival rate and 52–67 per cent complete ablation rate. RF thermal ablation is a quick, relatively safe, and highly effective technique for bulky primary and secondary malignant hepatic tumours. Also, it holds great promise as a technique for local tumour eradication. However, it is difficult to create an adequate tumour-free margin around tumours and failure to do so results in incomplete ablations and tumour recurrence. There are two factors responsible for this difficulty: (1) the differential blood flow that exists between tumours and normal hepatic parenchyma, and (2) difficulty in accurate placement of the RF electrode.

RF thermal ablation has many potential advantages over existing therapies. It is far more effective for debulking tumours than is radiation therapy or systemic chemotherapy. Unlike surgical resection or cryosurgery, it is minimally invasive and can be repeated as necessary to treat new tumours. It has far fewer complications than chemoembolization. Lastly, it has two major advantages compared to percutaneous ethanol ablation: (1) it can be used to treat primary and secondary malignant hepatic tumours, and (2) it requires fewer sessions to treat hepatocellular carcinoma.

Radiofrequency ablation of renal and adrenal masses

In patients with renal or adrenal tumours, recurrent malignancy in areas of prior radiation treatment, localized metastatic disease and primary neoplasms in patients who are poor surgical candidates RFA may be a suitable treatment option. Renal cell carcinomas are often incidental findings in older patients in which the standard of care has been total or partial nephrectomy. The growth pattern in many renal cell carcinomas can be slow and the risk of metastasis variable. VHL and hereditary RCC may also be successfully treated with RFA, which preserves kidney function[54].

Patient selection should include those with known contraindications to partial or complete nephrectomy due to cormorbid conditions or advanced age, and small tumour burden. Centrally located masses may be harder to treat and the complication rate may be higher. This is likely related to the higher blood flow in the renal hilum that prevents complete thermocoagulation due to a heat sink effect.

Complications in the kidney include haemorrhage, urinoma, abscess, paresthesias, transient haematuria, and pain. Ureteral stricture may occur with a tumour touching the ureter.

RFA has also been found to be effective for the control of persistent haematuria in patients with renal cell carcinoma[55].

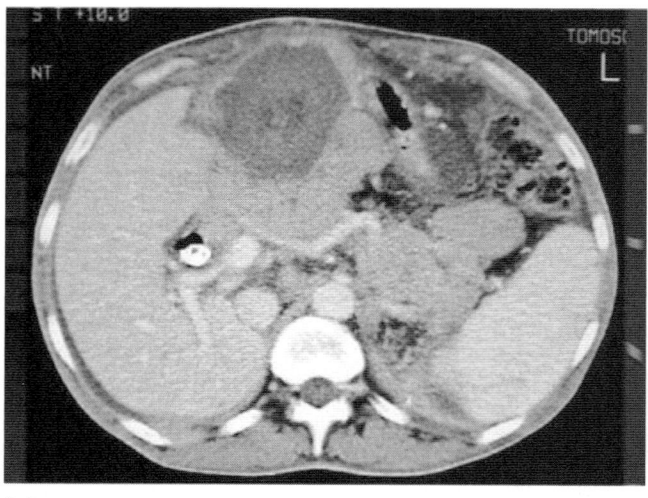

(A)

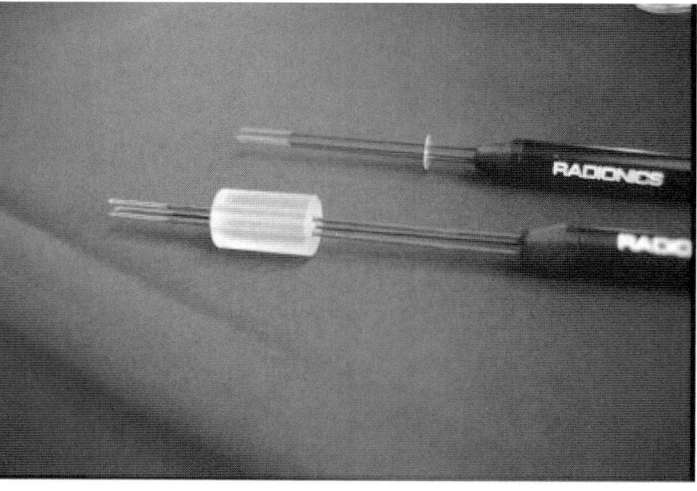

(B)

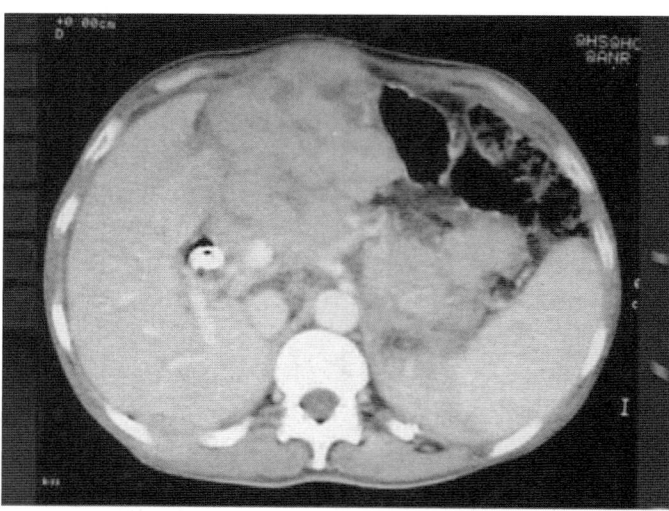

(C)

Figure 9.5.8 RFA of a pancreatic secondary tumour. Patient had inoperable disease with metastatic melanoma and suffered with symptoms of severe abdominal pain and bowel obstruction. (A) CT scan of abdomen demonstrating large tumour in the head of the pancreas thought to be responsible for current symptoms. (B) Radionics triple cooled RF probe that was used for percutaneous RFA therapy. (C) Follow-up CT scan (1 week later) showed a low attenuation area within the tumour mass that represents necrosis; the pancreatic tumour lesion is smaller and there was now less mass effect. Patient's symptoms were significantly alleviated.

Treatment options for primary and metastatic adrenal tumours are limited. For adrenocortical carcinoma, chemotherapy and radiation therapy play a limited role. However, repeat surgical resection may prolong survival. Extrapolation from these data suggests that local adrenal tumour destruction with RFA may improve survival in selected patients. Phaeochromocytoma, aldosteronoma, and metastases to the adrenal may also be treated with RFA, with the appropriate endocrine evaluation (and blockade for phaeochromocytoma)[56].

Radiofrequency ablation of lung tumours

First reported in 2000[57], RFA for primary and metastatic lung tumours is now gaining momentum. Results are encouraging particularly when palliation for pain or mass lesion is needed. Pneumothorax rates appear to be in the range of 10–20 per cent, with other complications less common, such as bleeding, fistula, haemoptysis, subcutaneous emphysema, effusions, fever, infection, and pain[58].

The surrounding air in adjacent normal lung parenchyma may provide insulation for the thermal lesion, making cooking easier or faster than in the well-vascularized liver.

Radiofrequency ablation of painful metastases

Early reports show promise for RFA of painful soft tissue tumours that are resistant to conventional radiation and pharmacological therapies. RFA has been found to be effective for short-term local control of painful soft tissue tumours and of bone metastases in multiple locations, decreasing or obviating the need for opioids[59]. Other examples of the role of RFA in palliative care include the relief of distressing symptoms of bowel obstruction, abdominal distension and pain from a large pancreatic mass[60] (Fig. 9.5.8).

Better methods of imaging guidance and more sophisticated equipment are likely to increase the importance of percutaneous tumour ablation in the future.

Gene therapy

The most rapidly evolving area in medicine is gene therapy. The underlying principle is to identify and clone a gene, and then to insert it into a vector capable of directing expression in mammalian tissues[61]. The main aim at present is to treat genetic deficiencies and malignant diseases refractory to conventional therapies. The delivery systems involved include: retroviral vectors (RNA viruses), adenoviral vectors (DNA viruses), and cationic liposomes, along with strategies that involve ultrasound-directed gene transfer, CT-guided gene transfer[62], and transcatheter gene delivery, in particular via the hepatic artery. Examples of genes being evaluated in clinical trials include: oncogenes, tumour suppressor genes, suicide genes, and antiangiogenesis factors. The liver is an ideal therapeutic target for gene therapy. Hepatic malignancies being considered for treatment include metastatic colorectal carcinoma, hepatoma, cholangio-carcinoma, lymphoma, metastatic melanoma, and haemangioma. Gene therapy strategies for managing occluded biliary stents (resulting from tumour ingrowth) and vascular transjugular intrahepatic portosystemic stents (resulting from neoendothelialization) are also under consideration. In gene delivery, angiographic guidance will be of use in localizing tumour blood supply and directing the targeted intra-arterial delivery of genes of interest, so that vector–DNA complexes can be delivered with accuracy and specificity[63]. Embolization techniques may also be of benefit, by prolonging vector contact with the target cells, thus delaying washout and further enhancing target cell uptake[64]. Radiological monitoring will be of considerable importance during gene delivery, e.g. the process of liposomal vector delivery can be monitored accurately with ultrasound because lipid vesicles are echogenic. Guided biopsy of transduced tissues for histopathological analysis after gene delivery should also improve confidence in the evaluation of gene expression.

Conclusions

This chapter was not intended to be an exhaustive list of every procedure that can be performed but to give an overall impression of the vast range of interventional techniques available. The patient undergoing palliative care should not be subjected to any unnecessary procedures or instrumentation. However, there are many readily performed, well tolerated, and safe interventional procedures which can significantly alleviate distressing symptoms, improve the quality of remaining life, and ease the nursing burden. Further detailed information can be obtained from the many reviews, journals, and books on the subject, some of which are included in the reference list.

References

1. Adam, A. (1998). The definition of interventional radiology (or, 'When is a barium enema an interventional procedure?'). *European Radiology*, **8**, 1014–5.

2. Wallace, S., and Charanangavej, C. (1987). Interventional radiology in renal neoplasms. *Seminars in Roentgenology*, **22**, 303.

3. Bogda, K. (2003). Radiological interventions: Special considerations in cancer patients. In *SIR syllabus-interventions in oncology* (eds. Ray, Hicks, and Patel), pp. 1–7. North Fairfax: Society of Interventional Radiology.

4. Papanicolaou, N. (1996). Uroradiological intervention. In *Interventional radiology, a practical guide* (eds. A. Watkinson and A. Adam), pp. 88–118. Oxford: Radcliffe Medical Press.

5. Pingoud, E.G. et al. (1980). Percutaneous antegrade bilateral ureteral dilation and stent placement for internal drainage. *Radiology*, **134**, 780.

6. Gaylord, G., and Johhsrude, I.S. (1989). Transrenal ureteral occlusion with Gianturco coils and gelatin sponge. *Radiology*, **172**, 1047–8.

7. Adam, A. et al. (1991). Self-expandable stainless steel endoprostheses for treatment of malignant bile duct obstruction. *American Journal of Roentgenology*, **156**, 321–5.

8. Davids, P.H.P. et al. (1992). Randomized trial of self-expanding metal stents versus polyethylene stents for distal malignant biliary obstruction. *Lancet*, **340**, 1488–92.

9. Patz, E.F. et al. (1996). Ambulatory sclerotherapy for malignant pleural effusions. *Radiology*, **199**(1), 133–5.

10. Pollak, J.S. et al. (2001). Treatment of malignant pleural effusions with tunneled long-term drainage catheters. *Journal of Vascular and Interventional Radiology*, **12**, 201–8.

11. Lee, C.W. et al. (1999). A survey of practice in management of malignant ascites. *Journal of Pain and Symptom Management*, **16**, 96–101.

12. Iyengar, T.D. et al. (2002). Management of symptomatic ascites in recurrent ovarian cancer patients using an intraabdominal semi-permanent catheter. *The American Journal of Hospice & Palliative Care*, **19**, 35–8.

13. Rosenberg, S. et al. (2004). Comparison of percutaneous management techniques for recurrent malignant ascites. *Journal of Vascular and Interventional Radiology*, **15**, 1129–31.

14. Sabharwal, T., Morales, J.P., Salter, R., et al. (2004). Esophageal cancer: self-expanding metallic stents. *Abdominal Imaging*, **29**, 1–9.

15. Watkinson, A.F. et al. (1995). Oesophageal carcinoma: initial results of palliative treatment with covered self-expanding endoprostheses. *Radiology*, **195**, 821–71.

16. Song, H.Y., Do, Y.S., Han, Y.M. et al. (1994). Covered, expandable esophageal metallic stent tubes: experiences in 119 patients. *Radiology*, **193**, 689–95.

17. Sabharwal, T., Morales J.P., Irani, F., et al. (2005). Quality assurance guidelines for placement of oesophageal stents. *Cardiovascular and Interventional Radiology*, **28**, 284–8.

18. Adam, A. et al. (1997). Palliation of inoperable esophageal carcinoma: a prospective randomised trial of laser therapy and stent placement. *Radiology*, **202**, 344–8.

19. Knyrim, K. et al. (1993). A controlled trial of an expansile metal stent for palliation of oesophageal obstruction due to inoperable cancer. *New England Journal of Medicine*, **329**, 1302–3.

20. De Baere, T. et al. (1997). Self-expanding metallic stents as palliative treatment of malignant gastro-duodenal stenosis. *American Journal of Roentgenology*, **169**, 1079–83.

21. Mainar, A. et al. (1996). Colorectal obstruction: treatment with metallic stents. *Radiology*, **198**, 761–4.

22. De Gregorio, M.A., Mainar, A., Tejero, E. et al. (1998). Acute colorectal obstruction: stent placement for palliative treatment – results of a multicenter study. *Radiology*, **209**, 117–20.

23. Hatrick, A., Sabharwal, T., and Adam, A. (2001). Tracheobronchial stents. *Seminars in Interventional Radiology*, **18**(3).

24. Tan, B.S., Watkinson, A.F., Dussek, J.E., et al. (1996). Metallic endoprosthesis for malignant tracheo-bronchialobstruction: initial experience. Cardiovasc. Interventional Radiology, **19**, 91–6.

25. Morgan, R. et al. (1997). Malignant esophageal fistulas and perforations: management with plastic-covered metallic endoprostheses. *Radiology*, **204**, 527–32.

26. Irving, J.D. et al. (1992). Gianturco self-expanding stents: clinical experience in the vena cava and large veins. *Cardiovascular and Interventional Radiology*, **15**, 351–5.

27. Becker, D.M., Philibrick, J.T., and Selby, J.B. (1992). Inferior vena cava filters: indications, safety, effectiveness. *Archives of Internal Medicine*, **152**, 1985–94.

28. Robertson, L.J., Mauro, M.A., and Jacques, P.F. (1989). Radiologic placement of Hickman catheters. *Radiology*, **170**, 1007–9.

29. Parkinson, R. et al. (1998). Establishing an ultrasound guided peripherally inserted central catheter (PICC) insertion service. *Clinical Radiology*, **53**(1), 33–6.

30. Adam, A. (1995). Insertion of long term central venous catheters: time for a new look. *British Medical Journal*, **311**, 341–2.

31. Page, A.C. et al. (1990). The insertion of chronic indwelling central venous catheters (Hickman lines) in interventional radiology suites. *Clinical Radiology*, **10**, 105–9.

32. Saini, S.J., Muller, P.R. et al. (1990). Percutaneous gastrostomy with gastropexy: experience in 125 patients. *American Journal of Roentgenology*, **154**, 1003–6.

33. Bell, S.D. et al. (1995). Percutaneous gastrostomy and gastrojejunostomy: additional experience in 519 procedures. *Radiology*, **194**, 817–20.

34. Rossi, P. (1982). Percutaneous removal of intravascular foreign bodies. In *Interventional radiology* (eds. R.A. Wilkins and M. Viamonte), pp. 359–69. Oxford: Blackwell Scientific Publications.

35. Gibson, R.N. et al. (1985). Major complications of central venous catheterization. A report of five cases and brief review of the literature. *Clinical Radiology*, **36**, 204–8.

36. Belli, A.M., and Hemingway, A.P. (1993). Retrieval of intravascular foreign bodies. In *Interventional radiology in the peripheral vascular system*, Vol. 4. (ed. A.M. Belli), pp. 88–92. London: Edward Arnold.

37. Balch, C.M., and Levin, B. (1987). Regional and systemic chemotherapy for colorectal metastases to the liver. *World Journal Of Emergency Surgery*, **11**, 521–6.

38. Chuang, V.P., and Wallace, S. (1987). Hepatic artery embolization in the treatment of hepatic neoplasms. *Radiology*, **140**, 51–8.

39. Hemingway A.P. (1986). Materials for embolization. *Radiology Now*, **3**, 63–4.

40. Morgan, R., Jackson, J.E., and Adam, A. (2001). Interventional techniques in the hepatobiliary system. In *Diagnostic radiology: a textbook of medical imaging*, 4th edition. (eds. R.G. Grainger, D.J. Allison, A. Adam, and A.K. Dixon), pp. 1321–6. Edinburgh: Churchill Livingstone.

41. Kato, L. et al. (1981). Arterial chemoembolization with microencapsulated anticancer drug. *Journal of the American Medical Association*, **245**, 1123–7.

42. Takaysu, K., Arii, S. et al. (2006). Prospective cohort study of transarterial chemoembolization for unresectable hepatocellular carcinoma in 8510 patients. *Gastoenterology*, **131**, 461–9.

43. Ueno, K. et al. (2000). Transcatheter arterial chemoembolization therapy using iodized oil for patients with unresectable hepatocellular carcinoma: evaluation of three kinds of regimens and analysis of prognostic factors. *Cancer*, **88**, 1574–81.

44. Hemingway, A.P., and Allison, D.J. (1986). Complications of embolization: analysis of 410 procedures. *Radiology*, **166**, 669–72.

45. Gangi, A., Sabharwal, T., Irani, F.G., et al. (2006). Quality assurance guidelines for percutaneous vertebroplasty. *Cardiovascular and Interventional Radiology*, **29**, 173–8.

46. Gangi, A. et al. (1999). Computed tomography (CT) and fluoroscopy-guided vertebroplasty: results and complications in 187 patients. *Seminars in Interventional Radiology*, **16**, 137–42.

47. Cotton, A. et al. (1998). Percutaneous vertebroplasty: state of the art. *Radiographics*, **18**, 311–23.

48. McGraw K.J., Cardella, J. et al. (2003). Society of Interventional Radiology Quality Improvement Guidelines for Percutaneous Vertebroplasty. *Journal of Vascular and Interventional Radiology*, **14**, 827–31.

49. Sabharwal, T., Salter, R., Adam, A., et al. (2006). Image-guided therapies in orthopedic oncology. *The Orthopedic Clinics of North America*, **37**, 105–12.

50. Wood, B.J. et al. (2002). Percutaneous tumour ablation with radiofrequency. *Cancer*, **94**, 443–51.

51. Castells, A. et al. (1993). Treatment of small hepatocellular carcinoma in cirrhotic patients: a cohort study comparing surgical resection and percutaneous ethanol injection. *Hepatology*, **18**(5), 1121–6.

52. Vallone, P. et al. (2006). Combined ethanol injection therapy and radiofrequency ablation therapy in percutaneos treatment of hepatocellular carcinoma larger than 4 cm. *Cardiovascular and Interventional Radiology*, **29**, 554–1.

53. Steger, A. et al. (1992). Multiple-fibre low-power interstitial laser hyper-thermia: studies in normal liver. *British Journal of Surgery*, **79**, 139–45.

54. Livraghi, T. et al. (1997). Saline-enhanced radiofrequency tissue ablation in the treatment of liver metastases. *Radiology*, **202**, 205–10.

55. Gervais, D.A. et al. (2005). Radiofrequency ablation of renal cell carcinoma: part 1, Indications, results, and role in patient management over a 6-year period and ablation of 100 tumours. *AJR*, **185**, 64–71.

56. Bradford, J.W. et al. (2001). Percutaneous radiofrequency ablation for hematuria. *The Journal of Urology*, **166**, 2303–4.

57. Bradford, J.W. et al. (2003). Radiofrequency ablation of adrenal tumours and adrenocortical carcinoma metastases. *Cancer*, **97**, 554–60.

58. Dupuy, D.E. et al. (2000). Percutaneous radiofrequency ablation of malignancies in the lung. *AJR*, **175**, 1263–6.

59. Steinke, K. et al. (2004). Pulmonary radiofrequency ablation – an international study survey. *Anticancer Research*, **24**, 339–43.

60. Callstrom, M.R. et al. (2002). Painful metastases involving bone: feasibility of percutaneous CT- and US-guided radio-frequency ablation. *Radiology*, **224**, 87–97.

61. Sabharwal, T. and Adam, A. Radiofrequency ablation treatment for the palliation of large secondary pancreatic mass. *Eurorad Database* (Case No. 678).

62. Voss, S.D. and Kruskal. J.B. (1998). Gene therapy: a primer for radiologists. *Radiographics*, **18**, 1343–7.

63. Shu, R.D., Goldin, J.G. et al. (2004). Metastatic renal cell carcinoma: CT-guided immunotherapy as a technically feasible and safe approach to delivery of gene therapy for treatment. *Radiology* **231**, 359–64.

64. Mahmood, U. (2006). Can a clinically used chemoembolization vehicle improve transgene delivery? *Radiology*, **240**, 619–20.

65. Kim, Y.I., Chung, J.W. et al. (2006). Intraarterial gene delivery in rabbit hepatic tumours: transfection with nonviral vector by using iodized oil emulsion. Radiology, **240**, 771–7.

SECTION 10

The management of common symptoms and disorders

10.1

The management of pain

Contents

10.1.1 Pathophysiology of pain in cancer and other terminal illnesses

R.M. Gordon-Williams and A.H. Dickenson

Introduction

Whereas acute pain involves a series of excitatory events at peripheral and central levels that faithfully transmit painful signals, clinically important pains are now known to have distinct altered neurophysiological and pharmacological substrates at many levels from the periphery to the central nervous system (CNS). Thus, the relation between the level of pain experienced and the noxious stimulus can become altered, and the extent of the peripheral damage, lesion, or abnormality does not always match the level of pain reported. This plasticity, the ability of the nervous system to alter in response to injury-evoked dysfunction leads to changes that can be observed throughout the pathways involved in the perception of pain. Exploitation of continually developing pharmacological, anatomical, molecular, and genomic techniques is providing a basis for understanding the molecular and cellular mechanisms that contribute to the pain that follows pathophysiology. Whereas many pains arise from damage to tissue such as that from arthritis, chronic neuropathic pains can arise from injury to both the peripheral and central nervous systems. Recent animal studies are shedding light on some of the specific mechanisms underlying cancer pain. Characteristic symptoms experienced with chronic or persistent pain, resulting from these various causes, include expanded receptive fields, increased amplitude of response to a given stimulus (hyperalgesia), pain elicited by normally innocuous stimuli (allodynia), and spontaneous pain in the absence of external stimuli. Sensory deficits can also exist in neuropathic pain. In addition, as pain persists, there are the affective and emotional responses that have to be considered along with the sensory aspects of the stimulus. It is clear that although the sensory and psychological aspects of pain are separable, the neural pathways that contribute to these aspects of pain are interlinked. Furthermore, at both peripheral and central sites, there are mechanisms that can amplify and prolong the painful stimulus so that the pain becomes greater—this can result in severe pain in the presence of relatively minor peripheral pathology. This chapter considers these signalling systems and changes therein in the context of pain in cancer.

Anatomy of pain

Primary afferents and inputs to the dorsal horn

The dorsal horn receives sensory information from somatosensory receptors in the periphery via primary afferents. The area of the dorsal horn in which these primary afferents terminate is determined by the type of primary afferent and, therefore, the nature of the information that they carry. Different sensory inputs are carried by fibres of different thickness, from thick myelinated to thin and unmyelinated and, due to the differing degrees of myelination, these different groups exhibit differing conduction velocities at which they transmit a stimulus. The largest of the afferent sensory fibres, with thick myelin sheaths are the Aβ fibres that carry information from muscle and tendons, and furthermore these are the fastest conducting. A subset of thickly myelinated fibres are the Aδ nerve fibres, carrying mostly information from cutaneous mechanoreceptors; these usually do not transmit nociceptive signals. However, the neurons considered to be mainly involved in carrying nociceptive information are the thinly myelinated Aδ nociceptors and particularly the thin unmyelinated C fibres and these are therefore pivotal in detection of potentially harmful stimuli in the external environment.

Aδ and C fibres terminate primarily in the superficial laminae of the dorsal horn, namely lamina I, which is an area intrinsically important in pain processing due to its large output to supraspinal areas. The large majority of neurons found within lamina I are nociceptive specific with small receptive fields, responding to only noxious pinch and/or heat stimulation, yet a smaller population of polymodal neurons are found that are also cold responsive[1,2]. Of late, a small population of wide dynamic range neurons that code throughout innocuous and noxious stimulus intensities have been classified in the superficial dorsal horn[3]. Other neurons that respond purely to itch-inducing stimuli or those that respond to only non-noxious heat have been noted[4,5]. Lamina I neurons have been shown to project to areas such as the periaqueductal grey (PAG), lateral parabrachial nucleus (PB), thalamus, nucleus tractus solitarius (NTS), and the medullary reticular formation[6]. A large number of projection neurons from lamina I express the receptor for substance P, NK1[7]. This group of neurons is the origin from which a spinobulbospinal loop ascends from the cord to the brain that then drives descending controls back to the cord; in this way the circuit can control dorsal horn excitability from higher centres[8].

Deep dorsal horn neurons are mostly wide dynamic range neurons and consequently have larger receptive fields than the neuronal populations of the superficial dorsal horn. Projections from the deep dorsal horn neurons have been shown to be mainly to the reticular nuclei[9] and to the thalamus in the spinothalamic pathways. These nuclei of the brain have good connections with areas concerned with primary somatosensory cortex and therefore discriminatory perception of pain.

Acute pain

Peripheral sensitization

In order to sense the external environment it is necessary to have a number of transduction molecules on the peripheral neuron that allow detection of a wide range of both exogenous and endogenous stimuli. While the full pharmacology and physiology of each of these peripheral sensory transducers falls outside the scope of this chapter, Table 10.1.1.1 illustrates a number of mechanisms through which a peripheral neuron can sense the peripheral environment. Needless to say, the actions of these transducers have a large part to play in pathological states, including cancer pain, and the next section will review a number of families of receptors that make sensory transduction possible. Transduction molecules seem to be highly preserved throughout evolution, with homology found throughout non-mammalian and mammalian species, showing the huge importance of an animal's ability to sense its surroundings[10]. Peripheral tissue damage and subsequent local inflammation can cause the release of a wide variety of chemical factors that are able to sensitize primary afferent fibres. Neurogenic inflammation, one of the mechanisms of peripheral sensitization, can further amplify the peripheral response of nociceptors. Peripheral terminations of nociceptors may arborize over a large area. Activation of peripheral afferents may cause neuromodulator release from nearby peripheral branches into peripheral tissues. These include factors such as substance P, neuropeptide Y, CGRP, ATP, and glutamate and may act on peripheral blood vessels, mast cells, and sympathetic nerve fibres. This would lead to an increase in vasodilation, vascular permeability, and therefore plasma extravasation, causing erythema and oedema. Serotonin, bradykinin, glutamate, nerve growth factor, and other cytokines in the inflammatory infiltrate can cause further activation of primary afferent fibres and help propagate nociception. TRPV1 is a ligand gated ion channel that is responsive to noxious heat and capsaicin, the pungent component of chilli peppers[10]. This channel is able to pass current at noxious heat in the normal physiological setting;

Table 10.1.1.1 Algogenic ligands, their origins and their cognate receptors.

Ligand	Origin	Receptor
H+	Tissue damage, macrophages	ASIC, TRPV1
Bradykinin	Macrophages, mast cells	B2/B1 (TRPV1)
Histamine	Mast cells	H1
Prostagandins	Mast cells, fibroblasts	Endoprostinoid (EP)
Nerve growth factor	Macrophage, fibroblasts	trkA
ATP	Platlets, Sympathetic terminals	P2X3
Adenosine	Tissue damage	A1/A2
5HT	Platelets, mast cells	5HTr
IL-1	Macrophage	IL-1r
Heat	Exogenous, inflammation	TRPV
Cold		TRPM8

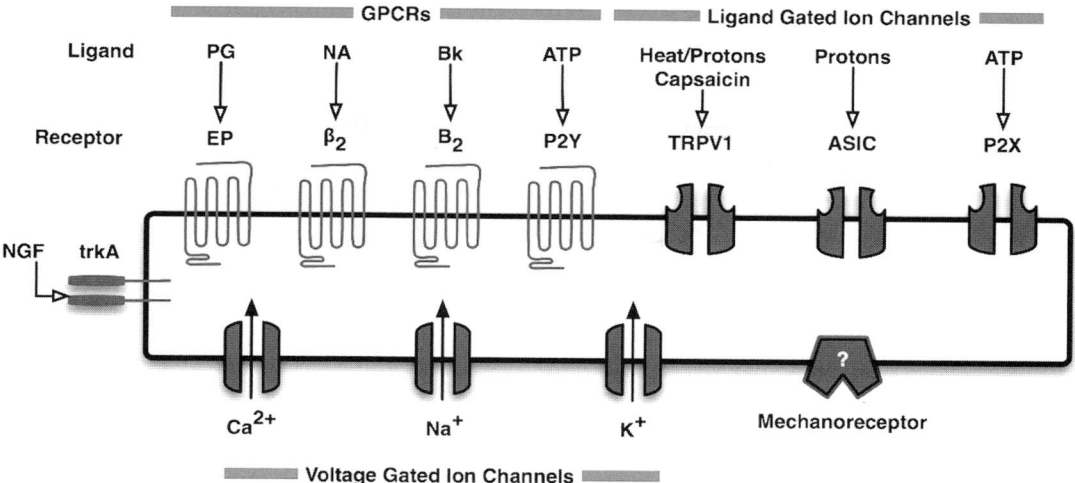

Figure 10.1.1.1 Peripheral receptors and channels involved in transduction of nociceptive stimuli in the periphery. The diagram depicts a C fibre where the polymodal nociceptor is comprised of numerous receptors, channels activated by voltage changes (voltage-gated ion channels) or chemical mediators of pain. Adenosine (acting at P2Y), bradykinin (B2), prostaglandin (endoprostinoid receptor, EP), noradrenaline (β2), Protons (acid sensing ion channel, ASIC/TRPV1), heat/capsaicin (TRPV1), ATP (P2X), NGF (trkA/p75). The precise molecular identity of a mechanoreceptor is still unclear.

however, in inflammation, a decrease in acidity can poteniate the channel's response so that it is active at temperatures nearer body temperature[10]. This is a good example of how inflammation may cause a lowering of the nociceptive threshold in peripheral fibres and allodynia. A hugely intriguing point of note is that a receptor for noxious transduction has yet to be fully elucidated. As mechanical allodynia presents such a large problem in the clinic, a cognate receptor for mechanical noxious stimuli may be of great therapeutic benefit.

Central sensitization

While peripheral sensitization may play a large role in development of pain states, a large amount of interest has been generated in the CNS's abilities to amplify the inputs it receives from the peripheral nervous system and therefore cause an increased perception of pain. One such mechanism is a process called 'wind up'. 'Winding up' of neuronal responses is made possible by the physiological properties of the N-methyl-D-aspartate (NMDA) receptor[3]. The NMDA receptor is a ligand gated ion channel whose central pore is, under normal neuronal activity, blocked by a magnesium ion. Due to this, the NMDA receptor plays little part in normal neuronal activity. However, after prolonged peripheral C fibre nociceptive drive, increased presynaptic release of neurotransmitters such as glutamate and substance P causes depolarization of the postsynaptic neurons via their actions on the AMPA and NK1 receptors, respectively[8]. This membrane depolarization allows the release of the magnesium ion blocking the pore of the NMDA receptor, and calcium to flow through the pore, further increasing postsynaptic excitability. The influx of calcium through the NMDA receptor allows short-term changes, such as phosphorylation of AMPA and NMDA receptors in the postsynaptic membrane. All these events lead to the potentiation of postsynaptic response. NMDA receptor blockers such as ketamine and MK-801 have been shown to be effective in the reduction of neuronal actions and pain behaviours in animal models of acute and

chronic pain as well as in human acute and chronic pain states. However, due to the widespread nature and important role that the NMDA receptor plays in many other physiological systems, these NMDA blockers have unacceptable neurological side effects thus limiting their ability to provide adequate analgesia. A related mechanism has also been implicated in longer-term changes. 'Long-term potentiation', a process that has been shown to be key in memory formation in the hippocampus, has been shown to lead to sustained excitability of dorsal horn pain transmission neurons of the spinal cord.

Pathophysiology of chronic cancer pain

Aetiology

Pain is a common feature in the palliative care setting, whether it be due directly to primary tumour burden (tissue or nerve destruction), treatment side effects (chemotherapy-induced neuropathic pain), or secondary metastases to bone. Of these, metastases to bone are found to be a common problem facing the palliative care team, with only the lung and liver having more frequent secondary tumours[11]. Metastatic cancer forming secondaries in bone are thought to have a prevalence of 64 to 80 per cent[12], and this metastatic spread to bone has been shown to be the most common cause of pain in cancer patients, with cancer-induced bone pain affecting 28 per cent of hospice inpatients, 34 per cent of those patients in cancer pain clinics[13] and 45 per cent of advanced cancer patients followed at home[12]. This highlights the need to find better drug therapies to combat pain in the clinical setting.

Animal models of cancer-induced bone pain

Until recent years, advancement in the treatment of malignant bone pain has been hindered by the lack of knowledge of the basic mechanisms of disease. Original attempts at modelling this pathology involved administering a systemic bolus injection of metastatic tumour cells. This, however, led to systemically unwell animals

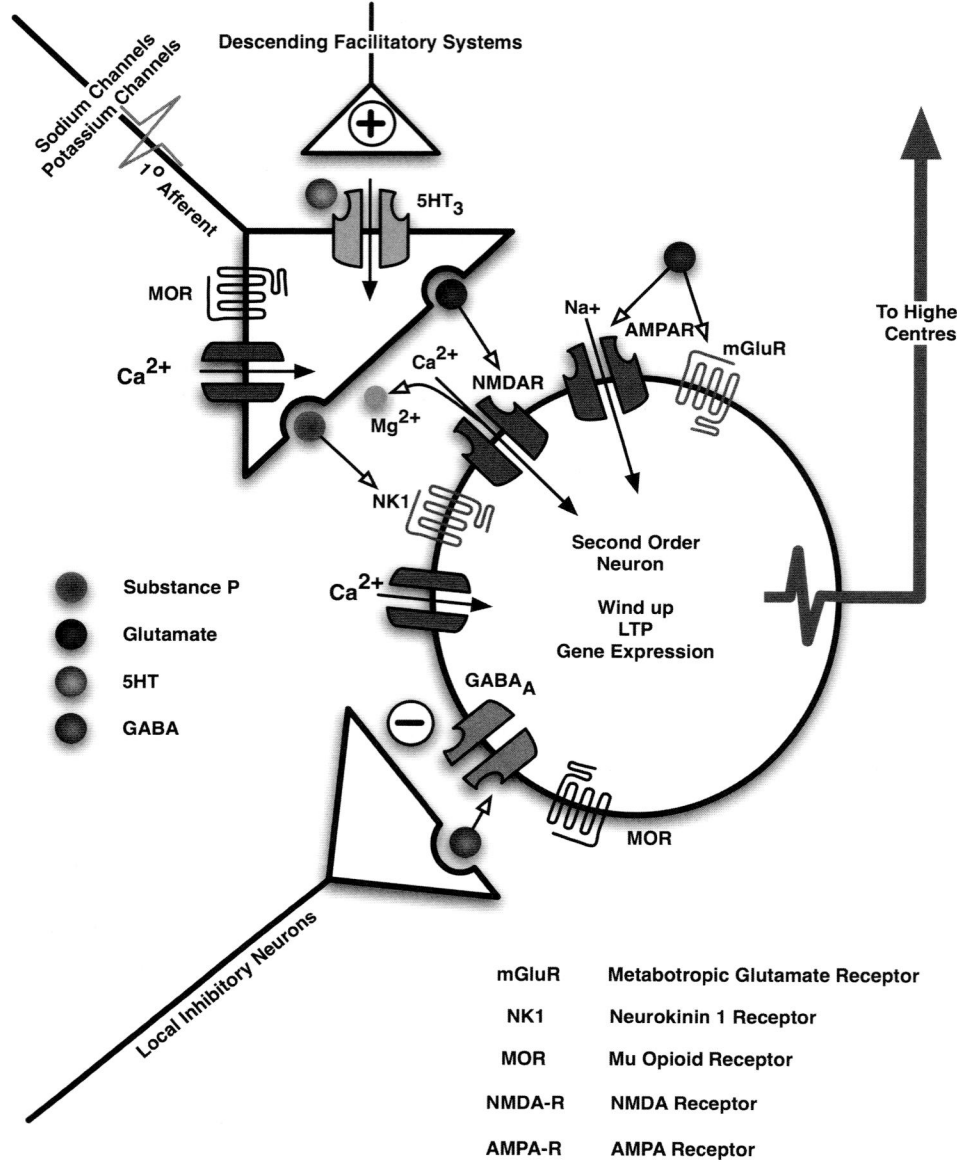

Figure 10.1.1.2 Pharmacology of a central synapse of the nociceptive pathway. For details see text.

from which it was hard to draw conclusions about underlying mechanisms specific to pain rather than those related to systemic cancer[14,15]. With no established animal model of cancer pain, any advancement regarding the treatment of cancer pain have been derived from clinical data and observations. As a consequence of these recognized deficiencies, a number of novel models have been established in recent times to elicit the mechanisms of cancer-induced bone pain related to tumour burden as well as chemotherapy-induced neuropathic pain. These new models rely on injecting a bolus of a variety of different tumour cells into either the long bones or the calcaneum of rodents. In general, this leads to the progressive and reliable development of pain-like behaviours to either mechanical or thermal stimuli in the postoperative period. Using both, a number of pharmacological and genetic manipulations as well as anatomical investigations, some basic common mechanisms have now been uncovered.

Pain arising from tumour within the bone

Originally, evidence supporting innervation of tumours was limited, and therefore the precise peripheral mechanisms underlying bone cancer pain were of great debate. While there were suspect players implicated in the generation of this particular pain state; such as primary afferents, interactions in the bone/cancer microenvironment, and tumour-associated macrophages, naming a few, none had substantial support. To this day the question remains: 'Is bone cancer pain one of neuropathic or inflammatory origin?' Answering this question will involve dissecting apart the various mechanisms implicated thus far.

Structure and innervation of bone

Before looking at the development of pain in a pathological setting, it is important to understand the structure, innervation, and physiology of bone under normal conditions. Bone is far from being simply a framework to support and protect the body's internal organs. It plays key roles as a reservoir for calcium and phosphate, as a source of blood cells from the bone marrow, and it permits moments via actions of the muscles of the body. The multitude of functions carried out by bone is reflected in its complex physiology and innervation.

Structure of bone

There are two main types of bone which differ in structure and density: cortical bone and trabecular bone. Cortical bone is the dense outer layer of all bones, representing nearly 80 per cent of all skeletal mass, and has a high resistance to torsion and bending forces. Trabecular bone is found in the epiphyseal regions of long bones and constitutes a large proportion of the bone tissue of the ribs, spine, and skull. Paradoxically, this tissue type represents 20 per cent of the skeletal mass, yet 80 per cent of its surface area. Trabecular bone has a much less dense, woven appearance, created by interspersed trabeculae (plates) and bars of bone adjacent to red marrow cavities. For these reasons, it has more of an elastic characteristic compared with cortical bone. The cavities are connected through canaliculi via which they receive their blood supply. Trabecular bone undergoes a greater amount of constitutive remodelling compared with the dense cortical bone and therefore bone pathology is often largely evident in bone of this type. The periosteum forms the fibrous sheath surrounding the outer surface of bone.

The remodelling of bone is reliant on an equilibrium of two main cell groups[16, 17]; osteoclasts and osteoblasts. Osteoblasts are derived from primitive mesenchymal cells and are responsible for bone formation through the secretion of an array of extracellular matrix proteins (Type I collagen, proteoglycans). Once osteoblasts have finished their function, they either apoptose or terminally differentiate into osteocytes, which remain viable surrounded by the bone matrix. Osteoblasts also have the interesting role of interacting with osteoclast progenitors and therefore regulate osteoclast activity.

Osteoclasts on the other hand are derived from the monocyte-macrophage lineage and are the primary bone resorption cells and are of great interest in bone pathologies such as osteoporosis and in bone cancer pain. While a specialized cell for bone degradation may seem counter-intuitive, it permits regulation of extracellular calcium, periodic bone repair, as well as remodelling in response to mechanical loads[16]. An acidic extracellular microenvironment is highly important for an osteoclast to function properly, as it is the predominant mechanism through which osteoclasts degrade the base mineral hydroxyapatite. High expression of the vacuolar-(v) type electrogenic ATP-H+ channel is found along the ruffled border of the resorptive surface of an osteoclast, permitting the required development of an acidic environment of around pH 4.0–4.5[16].

Innervation of bone

Even though it has been shown since the 1500s that nerve fibres are present in mineralized bone and the marrow cavity tracing along the paths of blood vessels, the consensus of thought had been that pain arising from bone was principally the result of dense periosteal innervations[18,19]. While the periosteum is the most densely innervated structure, Mach and colleagues[20], showed that the bone marrow space receives the highest number of sensory and sympathetic fibres. Mineralized bone also receives a high volume of sympathetic and sensory fibres, more so than that of the densely innervated periosteum. All of the bone marrow, mineralized bone,

and the periosteum receive both myelinated and unmyelinated sensory afferent fibres as well as sympathetic fibres. Interestingly, of these small diameter unmyelinated fibres (presumably C fibre population), only the CGRP trkA expressing peptidergic neurons are found to innervate bone and not the non-peptidergic IB4 labelled populations. This point may be of interest in the clinical setting and will be discussed later.

Mechanisms of cancer-induced bone pain

Pain arising from bone metastases was once thought to be only the result of structural weakness leading to mechanical distortion of the periosteum by innocuous stressors. This theory made it hard to explain pain arising from bone with little or no radiographic evidence of periosteum involvement. Models of cancer-induced bone pain have now highlighted a number of other mechanisms that may be important both in peripheral and central sites.

Peripheral mechanisms of cancer-induced bone pain
Factors released in the periphery

Changes in the periphery have been shown to cause peripheral sensitization of the primary nociceptive afferents, and this peripheral sensitization can, in turn, drive central changes and hyperexcitability. When considering a tumour seeded within a bone, it is important to recognize that this includes not only cancer cells but also an inflammatory infiltrate including macrophages, neutrophils, and T-lymphocytes[20]. The immune-mediated response to the tumour leads to the release of a plethora of factors such as cytokines, interleukins, chemokines, prostanoids, growth factors, and endothelins[21–23]. Peripheral nociceptors have an array of receptors that respond to these algogenic agents in the periphery. These factors are therefore able to sensitize and/or directly excite nociceptive fibres by acting on these peripheral receptors and lowering their threshold for activation. Pharmacological manipulation of these factors in a murine model of cancer-induced bone pain has shown promise in reducing measures of pain behaviour. Antagonism of endothelins, TNFα, and bradykinin, all reduced pain behaviours[24–28] with endothelin antagonism also reducing central neurochemical markers that have been associated with the development of cancer-induced bone pain[26]. As previously stated, the peptidergic CGRP-expressing neurons are the exclusive group of unmyelinated neurons that innervate the bone[25]. This group of neurons express the receptor for nerve growth factor (NGF), namely trkA/p75. Macrophages, tumour cells, and other immune cells associated with the tumour mass have been previously shown to express NGF[29]. The use of a NGF sequestering antibody attenuated both early and late phases of pain in the murine model of cancer-induced bone pain[30,31] and reduced central markers of this pain state. Due to the exclusivity of trkA expressing peptidergic neurons in the bone, antagonism of this fibre type means that there can be no compensatory mechanisms in a differing fibre type.

The osteoclast and acidosis

With an uncertain relationship between bone destruction and pain, a number of other mechanisms for the generation of this pain state have been studied, one of which involves the activation of osteoclasts. Osteolytic tumours have been widely studied in the animal literature and have been shown to involve the recruitment of osteoclasts within the bone, leading to bone resorption. Primary tumours in bone (i.e. osteosarcoma) and secondary tumours in bone (i.e. metastatic spread from primary lung, breast, or prostate tumours) each have a profile of effects on the remodelling of bone. While some have a mainly osteolytic profile (i.e. osteosarcoma) others have a predominately osteoblastic profile (i.e. prostate carcinoma). However, in both osteolytic and osteoblastic tumours abnormal osteoclast regulation has been proposed as both a mechanism through which tumours destroy bone and for the generation of pain in cancer patients.

Cancer-induced bone destruction has been shown to be osteoclast-mediated and, in a proportion of cases, dependent on the RANK/RANK-L regulatory axis. In the non-pathological situation, osteoblast and osteoclast activity are in equilibrium so that normal bone remodelling can occur[32]. In the presence of the growth factor colony stimulating factor-1 (CSF-1), osteoblasts expressing RANK ligand (RANKL) bind to RANK (Receptor Activator of Nuclear Factor κβ) on local osteoclasts and osteoclast progenitor cells to stimulate bone resorption. This in turn stimulates nearby osteoblast activity and local bone formation[32]. It has been shown that metastatic cancer cells release a number of factors that may disrupt this axis, importantly, parathyroid-hormone-related peptide (PTHrP). Metastatic breast cancer in bone has a higher expression of PTHrP than metastases in soft tissue[33]. In light of this, it is apparent that PTHrP causes up-regulation of RANKL on osteoblast cells, which causes terminal differentiation of osteoclast progenitor cells[34]. Activated T lymphocytes in the immune infiltrate of the tumour mass may also express RANKL and cause further osteoclast activation[35]. It is therefore unsurprising that osteoprotegerin, the soluble ligand of RANK-L, has shown efficacy in preventing cancer-induced bone destruction in animal models of osteolytic skeletal destruction[36]. Additionally, osteoprotegerin attenuates development of pain behaviours in a murine model of osteolytic sarcoma bone pain[37]. As mentioned previously, osteoclasts rely on an acidic extracellular microenvironment at the osteoclast/bone interface to facilitate resorption[38]. Moreover, increased osteoclast activation leads to a decreased extracellular pH. CGRP fibres that innervate the marrow or mineralized bone express acid sensing ion channels (ASIC)[25] as well as the capsaicin and heat responsive channels, TRPV1[39]. Both of these channels are either sensitized or excited by protons and therefore likely to cause nociceptive transmission due to a decrease in extracellular pH. The increase in osteoclast actions may not be solely responsible for the decrease in extracellular pH, as tumours themselves lower the extracellular pH in order to assist invasion into surrounding tissues[40]. Both TRPV1 antagonism and TRPV1 knockout in murine models of bone-cancer pain show attenuation of pain behaviours[41]. However, in these models, both osteoclast inhibition and TRPV1 antagonism does not completely attenuate all facets of the pain behaviours seen, even in light of the fact that osteoprotegerin almost completely prevented bone destruction and osteoclast activation[37,41]. This suggests that while osteoclast-induced acidosis and structural weakening may play an important role in the development of malignant bone pain, it is not the sole mechanism through which this pain is generated.

Structural damage to the bone and damage to nerves
Increased osteoclast activity in this setting may also cause structural weakness. Mechanical stress upon the periosteum and its distension due to tumour burden may well result in peripheral fibre activation and the sensation of pain[42]. It would be expected that the tumour growing within bone would damage the distal processes of nerves within the bone marrow, mineralized bone, and the

periosteum. Studies in animal models suggest that this is indeed the case. A marker for neuronal cell injury ATF-3, which is upregulated in the dorsal root ganglion in peripheral neuropathic pain models, is also found to be up-regulated in models of malignant cancer pain. Of interest is that gabapentin, a drug that has been shown to be efficacious in models of neuropathic pain has also been shown to be of benefit in models of cancer-induced bone pain[43,44]. This suggests that nerve injury may play a role in the development of bone cancer pain. Mechanisms underlying neuropathic pain will be discussed in greater depth later in this chapter.

Central mechanisms of cancer-induced bone pain
It is also clear that the CNS undergoes changes that aid the maintenance of this pain state. The early murine models of cancer-induced bone pain involving confinement of tumour (NCTC 2472 sarcoma cells) within the femur established the neurochemical 'fingerprint' of cancer-induced bone pain. Confinement of tumour to within the bone not only lead to development of post operative behavioural signs of pain, but increased osteoclastic bone destruction in the periphery[45]. However, of greater interest in this murine model of malignant pain were the immunohistochemical studies showing a number of central cellular and neurochemical changes in the segments of the spinal cord relating to the peripheral input. The spinal cord segments that receive afferent input from tumour-laden femur showed a massive astrocyte hypertrophy and elevation of the pro-hyperalgesic peptide dynorphin[45]. These changes were seen exclusively in the side of the spinal cord ipsilateral to the affected limb and not on the contralateral side. Glia, a family of which astrocytes are a member, are in the normal situation quiescent. Upon becoming activated, glia release a myriad of pro-inflammatory cytokines including IL-1, TNF, IL-6, reactive oxygen species, nitric oxide, prostaglandins, excitatory amino acids, and ATP[46]. This in turn can cause enhanced second-order neuron excitability within the dorsal horn and further exaggerates primary afferent neurotransmitter release. It has also been demonstrated in murine models that normally non-noxious palpation of the affected femur not only produced nocifensive behaviour but a increase in substance P receptor internalization and an increase in c-Fos expression in lamina I neurons of the dorsal horn[45]. This provides a weight of evidence showing that primary afferent fibres are sensitized following tumour growth in the periphery. This astrocyctosis, increased dynorphin expression, increased substance P internalization, and increased c-Fos expression has been shown in models of inflammatory and/or neuropathic pain. While substance P levels in primary afferent neurons have been shown to increase in inflammatory models and decrease in neuropathic models, levels remain unchanged in cancer-induced bone pain states[20]. However, the coexistence of all these features in cancer-induced bone pain provides evidence that this is a unique pain state that may have mechanisms similar to inflammation and neuropathy. Furthermore, this may well be the basis of reasoning behind why conventional treatments have failed thus far in the battle with malignant bone pain and further highlights the need for unique pharmacotherapy.

By recording second-order neurons in the dorsal horn of the spinal cord using *in vivo* electrophysiology, we can gain an idea of the supra-threshold response to peripheral stimuli that cannot be ascertained using behavioural techniques[43, 47]. Neurons can be characterized, based on their responses to mechanical, thermal, and electrically evoked stimuli. The superficial dorsal horn (SDH) is predominantly populated with nociceptive specific (NS) neurons,

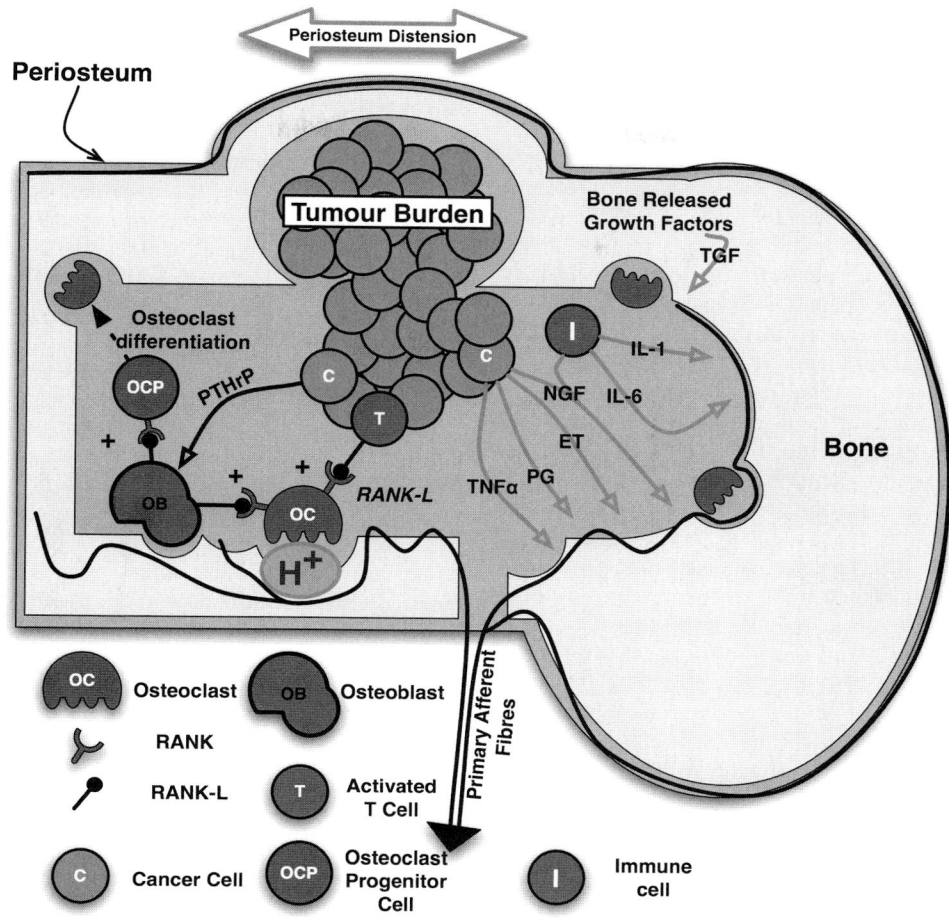

Figure 10.1.1.3 A summary of the peripheral mechanisms of cancer-induced bone pain. Increased expression of RANK-L (Ligand for RANK, receptor activator of nuclear κβ—activator of osteoclast progenitor cells, OCP), on osteoblasts (due to interaction with tumour cells via PTHrP) and activated T cells in the tumour mass causes increased activation of osteoclasts. An increasingly acidic extracellular environment may activate/sensitize peripheral neurons, by activating TRPV1 / ASIC on the peripheral neuron (see Fig.10.1.1.1). This in conjunction factors release from tumour cells, bone matrix, and tumour-associated immune cells that are known to sensitize primary afferents acting at their cognate receptors (see text) on primary afferent neurons innervating the bone. Disease progression may lead to further bone destruction and a swelling of the periosteum leading to activation of periosteal nerve fibres and the transmission of noxious stimuli.

which respond to nociceptive stimuli compared with wide dynamic range neurons (WDR), which respond to a wide range of both noxious and innocuous stimuli[3]. Establishment of cancer-induced bone pain changes the ratio of WDR: NS neurons in the SDH from the 26 per cent WDR: 74 per cent NS in a sham animal to 47 per cent WDR to 53 per cent in the pathological setting[47]. The phenotype shift seen in the superficial dorsal horn was also paralleled with the development of superficial and deep dorsal horn neuronal hyperexcitability to mechanical, thermal, and electrical stimuli, further suggesting ongoing central sensitization. Furthermore, these lamina I neurons that become hyperexcitable after cancer-induced bone pain now show a *de novo* or increased responsivity in the innocuous range[47]. Thus pain selective neurons can now be activated by innocuous stimuli. This may allow the limbic areas of the brain, concerned with affective/emotional aspects of pain, via the parabrachial pathways, to be activated by low-threshold stimuli. Plausibly, this may result in tactile stimuli being able to activate pain experience areas of the brain and so relate to the distress caused by allodynia. This hyperexcitability in lamina I also plays a role in further maintaining neuronal dorsal

horn hyperexcitability through descending facilitations. Spinal events are not only controlled by afferent input but also by descending controls from higher centres[8]. Higher-order cognitive and emotional processes such as anxiety, mood, and attention can influence perceived pain. Such phenomena are enabled by the convergence of somatic and limbic systems into such descending modulatory systems. Areas in the midbrain and brainstem such as the PAG and the rostroventral medial medulla (RVM) are key structures in the descending modulatory repertoire[8]. Such a system is important as it provides neural networks by which cognitive and emotional states can influence pain processing at the level of the spinal cord[48]. In short, these circuits allow the brain to exert some control over spinal pain events. Recent animal studies suggest that in addition to inhibitory systems, there are important descending facilitations that can be engaged by external and internal processes, and act to enhance intrinsic spinal mechanisms of pain. Lamina I neurons expressing the substance P receptor NK1 form the origin of a spinobulbospinal loop, which relays through the RVM[6,8]. The RVM has been highlighted as a key area involved with descending facilitations which are thought to be mediated through the 5HT$_3$ receptor. Blockade of spinal 5HT$_3$ receptors with intrathecal ondansetron reduces the mechanical and thermal evoked responses of superficial and deep dorsal horn neurons[8]. This suggests that descending facilitations are indeed important in amplifying nociceptive transmission from the dorsal horn to higher centres[48].

Mechanisms of cancer-induced bone pain related to treatment

Current therapies give researchers a great insight into the possible mechanisms undelying cancer pain. Opioids are the mainstay of treatment of severe malignant pain in the clinic[12]. However, while the benefits to be gained from opioid therapy are obvious, opioid treatment is associated with a large number of side effects such as nausea, vomiting, constipation, sedation, and delirium. At the high doses required to relieve intense cancer pain, these side effects become even more problematic to control and, in some cases, may be the reason for inadequate analgesia. In line with clinical evidence, opioids are effective in reducing pain-like behaviours in a number of animal models of cancer-induced bone pain. Early data from murine models suggest that higher doses of morphine were required to attenuate cancer-induced bone pain than those needed in inflammatory pain and this point was used to further highlight the mechanistic differences between these two pain states[49]. This low efficacy of acute morphine has since been further validated[12,50]; however, a situation that more closely mimicked the clinical paradigm was sought. A bi-daily injection schedule over 5 days after the establishment of the pain state has been shown to be highly effective in reducing behavioural signs of cancer-induced bone pain[51]. This regimen is also found to be more efficacious than a single acute dose[51]. However even in light of this, behavioural measurements taken pre and post the final morphine administration, at peak disease progression, indicated a significantly reduced analgesia between consecutive morphine administrations. This is not to say that the analgesia provided by morphine completely wore off between doses. Behavioural signs of pain were still, 12 h after the last dose, significantly reduced from that of the vehicle-treated animals and no different from that of the acutely treated group. However this may help to explain the requirement for escalated doses of opioids to treat severe cancer-induced bone pain.

Chronic but not acute gabapentin has also been shown to be effective in these models[43,52]. Gabapentin acts by binding to the calcium channel accessory subunit $\alpha 2\delta$. This implies a role of $\alpha 2\delta$ in the pathology underlying this pain state. Yet looking at the response of neurons in chronic morphine and chronic gabapentin regimens highlights two differing mechanisms involved in cancer-related bone pain. While chronic morphine and gabapentin administration both lead to behavioural attenuation of pain, chronic morphine treatment was unable to completely reset dorsal horn excitability and the associated phenotype shift towards the WDR neuronal population in superficial dorsal horn[51]. The bias of superficial neurons toward the WDR phenotype, even in the presence of morphine analgesia, suggests that low-threshold inputs to the spinal cord may still access areas of the brain concerned with both pain affect and perception. This is a possible physiological mechanism through which breakthrough pain may remain refractory to morphine analgesia in the clinic. In contrast, gabapentin completely attenuated dorsal horn excitability and reversed the

phenotype shift of WDR:NS ratio back towards that seen in a normal animal[43]. This suggests that while morphine may cause behavioural attenuation of pain, it is not acting on the mechanisms that are intricately involved in producing those behavioural signs. On the other hand, gabapentin is able to inhibit the mechanisms that lead to cancer-induced bone pain rather than merely blocking sensory inputs as seen with morphine. Upon the termination of gabapentin treatment, pain behaviours and dorsal horn excitability returned to their hyperexcitable 'pathological' state implicating neuronal physiological mechanisms rather than anatomical changes to be key in development of cancer-induced bone pain.

Peripheral opioids may also have a role to play in the management of malignant cancer pain, with evidence showing that loperamide, the peripheral mu opioid receptor agonist, is able to attenuate thermal hyperalgesia in a murine model of cancer-induced bone pain[53]. Non steroidal anti-inflammatory drugs (NSAIDs) are the first step on the WHO ladder for the use of analgesics for the relief of cancer pain. NSAIDs may still be of use as an analgesic additive even after increased pain severity[12], however, the clinical data supporting their efficacy is limited[54]. NSAIDs inhibit the cyclooxygenase (COX) enzyme and therefore attenuate the synthesis of prostaglandins from arachidonic acid. This ultimately prevents sensitization or activation of primary afferents by prostaglandins produced locally by tumour cells and/or the immune response. Inhibition of the COX-2 enzyme, the local inducible form of cyclooxygenase, using three different COX-2 selective inhibitors in a rat and murine models of cancer-induced bone pain has been shown to be effective in ameliorating behavioural pain signs. In both these studies, chronic COX-2 inhibition has been shown to be better at attenuating pain-like signs than a single acute dose. Chronic administration reduced tumour burden and bone destruction[55,56], suggesting that COX-2 inhibition may be acting at multiple sites rather than at a single point in a pathway.

Bisphosphonates are used widely in the clinical setting and prevent bone resorption by osteoclast inhibition. Bisphosphonates were able to reduce pain scores as well as bone and sensory nerve destruction in both rat and mouse models of cancer-induced bone pain[44,57]. However, tumour burden was found to not be affected, with both tumour burden and tumour necrosis increasing[44]. Bisphosphonates, therefore, may have a role to play in reducing bone pain in malignancy, especially if combined with other analgesics[12]. Radiotherapy of tumours within bone causes analgesia but the mechanism is still unclear. Radiotherapy in the murine model of bone cancer pain reduced tumour burden by more than 75 per cent[58]. However, it did not affect the osteoclast density, suggesting that radiotherapy causes analgesia via direct mechanisms on tumour cells themselves.

Pain arising from tumour within soft tissues

While pain arising from bone is a common clinical problem, pain arising from soft tissue can also be painful. The pathophysiology in this pain state, however, is still not clear. A novel model of pancreatic cancer pain has recently been developed to elucidate the relationship between disease progression and pain development[59]. This model uses a transgenic mouse that develops pancreatic cancer showing changes similar to that seen in the human condition. These include tumour growth, increased innervation, macrophage infiltration, weight loss, and pain. More significantly, pain was only evident at a point at which cancer progression was highly advanced.

Sensory innervation has now been quantified and models such as these will hopefully provide mechanistic insights in to the development of pancreatic cancer pain in the future.

Neuropathic pain

The International Association for the Study of Pain (IASP) defines neuropathic pain as 'pain initiated or caused by a primary lesion or dysfunction in the nervous system'. While this may not necessarily be a complete definition of neuropathic pain, the words of the definition hint towards a broad mechanism. The large-scale changes that occur within the peripheral and central nervous systems, after nerve injury, can lead to development of pain. This nerve plasticity has been heavily scrutinized and some of these plastic changes have been proposed as possible important mechanisms for the generation of pain in neuropathic states.

Mechanisms of cytotoxic neuropathy

Neuropathic pain may arise in the palliative care setting for a multitude of reasons. Nerve damage is known to occur as a result of tumour compressing a nerve, surgical resection, radiotherapy, and chemotherapy. The frequent problem of neuropathic pain has lead to a wide array of pre-clinical animal models being set up in order to pull out the basic mechanisms involved in the generation and maintenance of neuropathic pain. These include models of peripheral nerve injury (common in traumatic neuropathic pain) and chemotherapy-induced neuropathic pain. Peripheral lesions to nerves are obvious, and therefore many models of traumatic peripheral nerve injury exist. Consequently, a multitude of mechanisms have been implicated in painful peripheral nerve lesions. It would be wrong to believe that mechanisms of peripheral nerve injury are the same whether caused by chemical injury, constriction, or by the surgeon's scalpel. It is for these reasons that the pharmacotherapy of different types of neuropathic pain should differ. One only has to look at the differing responsiveness of trigeminal neuralgia to drugs such as carbamazepine, still a front line drug for this indication, compared to other peripheral neuropathies to see that mechanisms underlying these neuropathies must differ. Iatrogenic neuropathic pain caused by various drug treatments is well recognized. Theoretically, it should be of no surprise that chemotherapeutic agents and anti-retrovirals, compounds which broadly act through inhibiting cellular processes, may have neuropathic side effects.

The chemotherapy agents vincristine and paclitaxel and the nucleoside reverse transcriptase inhibitors (NRTI) such as dideoxycytidine (ddC) have a well-established history of causing painful neuropathy[60–63], with the incidence of painful neuropathies in paclitaxel-treated patients suggested to be around 22 per cent[63]. Paclitaxel binds to microtubules and promotes hyperpolymerization. This interferes with the mitotic spindle formation and promotes cellular arrest in the metaphase-anaphase transition and consequently apoptosis[64,65]. As the precise mechanism of paclitaxel-induced neuropathy is still not clear, it has been assumed that the binding of paclitaxel to microtubules of neurons, which consequently prevents anterograde and reterograde axonal transport, could lead to a neuropathic state. However, these proposed mechanisms of both tumour apoptosis and neuropathy have been questioned, and the precise mechanisms are still not clear[66,67]. Another chemotherapeutic agent vincristine is said to act via a similar mechanism, inhibiting normal polymerization of β-tubulin, leading to abnormal spindle function. Early studies showed that

epineural injection of paclitaxel caused oedema and axonal degeneration[68] along with interference of axonal transport and microtubule anomalies. However, a number of sources have doubted the theory that axonal degeneration and microtubule anomalies occur, citing the unusually high concentrations of paclitaxel in the epineural injections responsible for the local axonal reactions[69]. These local epineural injections allowed paclitaxel to bypass the liver, so that any metabolites usually involved in the development of pathology would not be present. Mitochondria have now been shown to play an important role in the establishment of some pain states, especially chemotherapy and NRTI-induced neuropathic pain. Change in mitochondrial function has been shown to be involved in the pathogenesis of neurodegenerative diseases; however, this has not previously been widely studied in pain. In patients, neuropathies solely due to disarray in mitochondrial function have been shown to have an increased incidence of developing pain[70]. Recently, models of chemotherapy-induced neuropathic pain have been developed that are more akin to the clinical scenario. Low-dose systemic injections of paclitaxel, produced mechanical hypersensitivity, yet even at the stage of peak pain-like behaviours, there were no signs of axonal degeneration, markedly altered microtubules, or impairment of axonal transport[71]. However, abnormal mitochondria in C fibres and myelinated axons were noted and this was suggested to be the cause of paclitaxel's actions. In this model, it was proposed that paclitaxel's binding to mitochondria caused opening of the mitochondria permeability transition pore (mPTP), causing calcium ion influx into the cytosol. This mitochondrial calcium efflux has been suggested to be both the cause of mitchondrial swelling as well as of primary afferent excitabilty and pain behaviour[71]. The T-type calcium channel blocker ethosuximide, $\alpha 2\delta$ calcium channel subunit ligand, gabapentin, and calcium chelators, all block neuropathic pain behaviours caused by chemotherapeutic agents[72–75]. Mitochondrial damage is also the proposed mechanism for the neuropathy seen after treatment with NRTIs for HIV/AIDs[76,77]. The mitochondrial electron transport chain (mETC) and its end product ATP have also been a suggested pathological player in the development of neuropathic pain due to both chemotherapy and antiretroviral treatment; however, the downstream targets in the pathological setting are still to be elucidated[77]. It has also been noted that both paclitaxel and vincristine-evoked painful peripheral neuropathies show a loss of innervation of the epidermal sensory fibres as well as the Langerhans cells, the skin's resident immune cells. Whether this is a causal or merely consequential finding is yet to be shown[78].

Pain associated with HIV infection

Iatrogenic neuropathic pain due to treatment with NRTIs is not the only cause of neuropathic pain in HIV/AIDS patients. Around 10–15 per cent of all HIV-1 infected patients have a symptomatic distal polyneuropathy[79], a proportion of which experience pain as a result. It has been shown that direct infection of neurons by HIV has a negligible incidence rate and it is for this reason that the attention of researchers turned to the neuroimmune system. An envelope protein of HIV-1, gp120 has been widely shown to produce hindpaw hypersensitivity to thermal and mechanical stimuli when injected into the intrathecal space[80] as well as directly to the sciatic nerve of the rat[81]. Astrocytes and microglia have been shown to bind to the virus epitope gp120, which in turn causes their activation. Milligan *et al.* showed that attenuating glial activation, ameliorates the development of behavioural hypersensitivity of animals once exposed to gp120[80]. In this study, the response of microglia and astrocytes to gp120 was blocked. As mentioned previously, activation of glia in the spinal cord by exogenous factors, such as gp120, causes the transcription and release of factors such as prostaglandins, excitatory amino acids, IL-1, and IL-6 as well as inducing nitric oxide synthetase expression in glial cells[82–84]. The release of these factors from glia in the dorsal horn may well be able to directly excite local sensory neurons and propagate the sensation of pain, even without the presence of a peripheral pathology. The development of spinal sensitization has been put forward as an explanation for why pains in HIV-1 infected patients commonly present without obvious peripheral pathologies and are vague and diffuse in nature[85,86].

Mechanisms underlying the generation of pain in neuropathy

Many changes in the periphery have been implicated in the development of neuropathic pain, but none have been more heavily studied than the role of ion channel dysregulation on peripheral nerves. Normally, tactile stimulation of sensory nerve terminals in the skin, viscera, or bone leads to the propagation of an action potential and sensory signalling. However, after nerve injury, many peripheral nerves display ectopic discharge, which may lead to an increased barrage of nociceptive signalling onto dorsal horn transmission neurons without a peripheral stimulus. Electrophysiologically, it is clear to see that neuronal responses of second-order deep dorsal horn neurons are heightened after nerve injury in rodent models, with an increase in receptive field size and an increased response to natural stimuli applied to the hindpaw. This goes hand in hand with increased spontaneous activity and hyperexcitability of these neurons.

Changes in the sodium channel populations on peripheral nerves and their subsequent aberrant activity have been of great interest due to their key role in setting neuronal excitability and therefore the development of pain states[87, 88]. Expression of sets of sodium channels on the peripheral neurons shows plasticity after nerve injury. The mRNA of $Na_V1.3$, a usually embryonic TTX-sensitive current, has been found to increase after axotomy and this may play a role in the generation of ectopic activity in peripheral nerve fibres. The sensory neuron specific sodium channel, $Na_V1.8$ is also thought to play a key role in the generation of abnormal sensory signalling following nerve injury. $Na_V1.8$ protein is markedly decreased in the dorsal root ganglion of predominantly small fibres after nerve injury. This is paralleled by an increase in immunoreactivity of the channel in the distal axons and nerve terminals, representing a redistribution of the channel to the distal sites of the neuron, where it may take part in the development of hyperexcitability and increased nociceptive transmission. Both in humans and animals, sodium channel accumulation has been shown to occur around the neuroma formed at the site of the nerve lesion. This has long been the pharmacological basis for the use of drugs such as carbamazepine, lamotrigine, and local anaesthetics in patients with neuropathic pain. After nerve injury, demyelination and abnormal trafficking of sodium channels occurs along the membrane of injured nerves and maybe in the uninjured neighbours. This may lower the threshold for activation and induce ectopic activity in the peripheral nerve. This contributes to the development of central sensitization and

amplification of peripheral events, possibly leading to the allodynia and hyperalgesia seen in patients.

Voltage-gated calcium channels (VGCC) may also play a large hand in the increased peripheral nociceptive drive in neuropathic pain. VGCCs play a key role in permitting neurotransmitter release from the presynaptic terminal and, therefore, the post-synaptic propagation of the sensory signal. As with sodium channels, there are a large number of calcium channels that play a role in neuronal excitability. As the name suggests, activation of calcium channels by peripheral electrical events causes the inward flow of calcium and allows neurotransmitter vesicle exocyctosis and thus post-synaptic depolarization. However, VGCCs not only have pre-synaptic actions but also act at the post-synaptic site, allowing activation of post-synaptic second messenger cascades. This may lead to altered gene expression, protein synthesis, and therefore long-term plastic changes. Long-term potentiation of dorsal horn neurons, caused by repetitive afferent stimulation, may be of importance in maintaining exaggerated neuronal responses for long periods after increased peripheral drive has subsided[87]. Specific targeting of these VGCCs and their accessory sub-units seems to be beneficial in the treatment of neuropathic pain, with novel drugs acting at these sites now available. Gabapentin and its newer analogue pregabalin have shown benefit to patients with neuropathic pain. Their target is thought to be the α2δ accessory subunit of calcium channels. Gabapentin has been shown to be effective in reducing neuronal responses in a model of neuropathic pain[90]. However, gabapentin's inability to reduce neuronal responses in normal animals highlights a clear state dependency of gabapentin's action and implicates a role for the α2δ subunit in neuropathic pain pathology. The α2δ subunit has been shown to up-regulate after nerve injury and this correlates not only with the development of behavioural allodynia in these animals but also with gabapentin's behavioural antiallodynic efficacy[91]. Gabapentin's actions have now been characterized in many differing animal models of neuropathic pain including a model of chemotheraputic paclitaxel-induced neuropathic pain[75].

Another target for the treatment of neuropathic pain is the N-type calcium channel. It was shown that blockade of the N-type calcium channel with ω-conotoxin-GIVA reduced dorsal horn neuronal responses in animals with neuropathic pain and that the release of substance P and CGRP from primary afferents was N-type dependant[92,93]. An analogue of ω-conotoxin-GIVA, ziconotide, has now been developed and is now licensed for the treatment of neuropathic pain.

As well as spinal changes, the higher brain centres are able to facilitate dorsal horn neuronal activity. This ascending descending facilitatory pathway seems to play a critical role in chronic pain states such as neuropathic pain. Superficial dorsal horn NK1-neurons project to higher brainstem nuclei such as the parabrachial nucleus, which receives connections from amygdala and hypothalamus and may explain the ability of emotion to affect pain processing[8]. Along with the affective implications, these brainstem nuclei form a part of a spinal-bulbo-spinal loop, which through the RVM, can facilitate dorsal horn neuronal responses. Ablation of these NK1-expressing projection neurons, using a saporin toxin conjugated to substance P, is able to attenuate dorsal horn neuronal responses to stimuli evoked in the periphery[90]. This is, to a large extent, mimicked by the spinal application of ondansetron, an antagonist of the excitatory $5HT_3$ receptor, showing that these descending facilitations are in the large part serotonergic acting at the $5HT_3$ receptor in the spinal cord. These descending facilitations contribute to maintaining central sensitization in pathological pain states and may well aid the development of tactile allodynia seen in patients with chronic pain.

Astonishingly, gabapentin's actions in reducing neuronal responses in nerve-ligated animals were blocked by both the ablation of these superficial projection neurons and by the application of ondansetron[90]. However, the activation of the 5HT$_3$ receptor allowed gabapentin to reduce neuronal responses in normal animals, suggesting that this supraspinal loop needs to be in place for gabapentin's action to be unmasked.

Conclusion

Any advances in the understanding and treatment of pain in cancer and other terminal illnesses will need to be based on a better understanding of pain mechanisms, so that existing therapies can be used with greater efficacy. Further knowledge of these mechanisms is a basis for the development of future therapeutic approaches based on controlling the pathophysiology as well as the pain itself.

This chapter illustrates how important advances in understanding the pathophysiology of pain have been made in recent years and provide a basis for improvements in the treatment of the pain, distress, and co-morbidities. We have attempted to show how a tumour growing in the periphery elicits a series of changes that run from peripheral tissue and nerve, causing profound changes in spinal cord function and that the final experience of pain involves complex circuits in the brain that link pain with affective function.

Glossary

CNS—central nervous system; PAG—periaqueductal grey; PB—lateral parabrachial nucleus thalamus; NTS—nucleus tractus solitarius; NK1—neurokinin 1, receptor for substance P; CGRP—calcitonin gene related peptide; TRPV1—transient receptor potential vanilloid receptor, heat/capsaicin receptor; ASIC—acid sensing ion channel; H1—histamine 1 receptor; A1/A2—adenosine receptors; 5HT—5 hydroxytryptamine; IL—interleukin (including 1 and 6); TRPM8—transient receptor potential menthol receptor; EP—endoprostinoid; NMDA—N-methyl-D-aspartate receptor, a glutamate receptor; ATP—adenosine triphosphate; NGF—nerve growth factor; RANK—receptor activator of nuclear factor κβ; RANKL—ligand for the receptor; PTHrP—parathyroid-hormone-related peptide; ATF-3—activating transcription factor (marker of neuronal damage); NCTC—National Collection of Type Culture; SDH—superficial dorsal horn; WDR—wide dynamic range (spinal neurons with innocuous and noxious responses); NS—nociceptive specific (spinal neurons with noxious-only responses); RVM—rostroventral medial medulla; NSAIDs—non-steroidal anti-inflammatory drugs; COX—cyclooxygenase; NRTI—nucleoside reverse transcriptase inhibitors; ddC—dideoxycytidine; mPTP—mitochondria permeability transition pore; mETC—mitochondrial electron transport chain; Na$_V$—sodium channel; VGCC—voltage-gated calcium channels.

References

1. Andrew, D. and Craig, A.D. (2002). Responses of spinothalamic lamina I neurons to maintained noxious mechanical stimulation in the cat. *Journal of Neurophysiology*, **87**(4), 1889–901.

2. Craig, A.D. and Andrew, D. (2002). Responses of spinothalamic lamina I neurons to repeated brief contact heat stimulation in the cat. *Journal of Neurophysiology*, **87**(4), 1902–14.

3. Seagrove, L.C, Suzuki, R., Dickenson, A.H. Electrophysiological characterisations of rat lamina I dorsal horn neurones and the involvement of excitatory amino acid receptors. *Pain* 2004; **108**(1–2): 76–87.

4. Andrew, D. and Craig, A.D. (2001). Spinothalamic lamina I neurons selectively sensitive to histamine: a central neural pathway for itch. *Nat Neurosci*, **4**(1), 72–7.

5. Light, A.R., Sedivec, M.J., Casale, E.J. *et al.* (1993). Physiological and morphological characteristics of spinal neurons projecting to the parabrachial region of the cat. *Somatosensory and Motor Research*, **10**(3), 309–25.

6. Todd, A.J. (2002). Anatomy of primary afferents and projection neurones in the rat spinal dorsal horn with particular emphasis on substance P and the neurokinin 1 receptor. *Experimental Physiology*, **87**(2), 245–9.

7. Todd, A.J., McGill, M.M., and Shehab, S.A. (2000). Neurokinin 1 receptor expression by neurons in laminae I, III and IV of the rat spinal dorsal horn that project to the brainstem. *European Journal of Neuroscience*, **12**(2), 689–700.

8. Suzuki, R., Morcuende, S., Webber, M. *et al.* (2002). Superficial NK1-expressing neurons control spinal excitability through activation of descending pathways. *Nature Neuroscience*, **5**(12), 1319–26.

9. Raboisson, P., Dallel, R., Bernard, J.F. *et al.* (1996). Organization of efferent projections from the spinal cervical enlargement to the medullary subnucleus reticularis dorsalis and the adjacent cuneate nucleus: a PHA-L study in the rat. *Journal of Comparative Neurology*, **367**(4), 503–17.

10. Caterina, M.J. and Julius, D. (2001). The vanilloid receptor: a molecular gateway to the pain pathway. *Annual Review of Neuroscience*, **24**, 487–517.

11. Tubiana-Hulin, M. (1991). Incidence, prevalence and distribution of bone metastases. *Bone*, **12** Suppl 1, S9–10.

12. Mercadante, S., Dardanoni, G., Salvaggio, L. *et al.* (1997). Monitoring of opioid therapy in advanced cancer pain patients. *Journal of Pain and Symptom Management*, **13**(4), 204–12.

13. Banning, A., Sjogren, P., and Henriksen, H. (1991). Pain causes in 200 patients referred to a multidisciplinary cancer pain clinic. *Pain*, **45**(1), 45–8.

14. Sasaki, A., Yoneda, T., Terakado, N. *et al.* (1998). Experimental bone metastasis model of the oral and maxillofacial region. *Anticancer Research*, **18**(3A), 1579–84.

15. Kostenuik, P.J., Orr, F.W., Suyama, K. *et al.* (1993). Increased growth rate and tumor burden of spontaneously metastatic Walker 256 cancer cells in the skeleton of bisphosphonate-treated rats. *Cancer Research*, **53**(22), 5452–7.

16. Blair, H.C. (1998). How the osteoclast degrades bone. *Bioessays*, **20**(10), 837–46.

17. Mackie, E.J. (2003). Osteoblasts: novel roles in orchestration of skeletal architecture. *International Journal of Biochemistry and Cell Biology*, **35**(9), 1301–5.

18. Foley, K.M. (2004). Treatment of cancer-related pain. *Journal of the National Cancer Institite*, Monographs, **32**, 103–4.

19. Mundy, G.R. (2002). Bisphosphonates and tumor burden. *Journal of Clinical Oncology*, **20**(15), 3191–2.

20. Mantyh, P.W., Clohisy, D.R., Koltzenburg, M. *et al.* (2002). Molecular mechanisms of cancer pain. *Nat Review Cancer*, **2**(3), 201–9.

21. Safieh-Garabedian, B., Poole, S., Allchorne, A. *et al.* (1995). Contribution of interleukin-1 beta to the inflammation-induced increase in nerve growth factor levels and inflammatory hyperalgesia. *British Journal of Pharmacology*, **115**(7), 1265–75.

22. Sorkin, L.S., Xiao, W.H., Wagner, R. *et al.* (1997). Tumour necrosis factor-alpha induces ectopic activity in nociceptive primary afferent fibres. *Neuroscience*, **81**(1), 255–62.

23. Suzuki, K. and Yamada, S. (1994). Ascites sarcoma 180, a tumor associated with hypercalcemia, secretes potent bone-resorbing factors including transforming growth factor alpha, interleukin-1 alpha and interleukin-6. *Bone Mineral*, **27**(3), 219–33.

24. Baamonde, A., Lastra, A., Fresno, M.F. *et al.* (2004). Implantation of tumoral XC cells induces chronic, endothelin-dependent, thermal hyperalgesia in mice. *Cellular and Molecular Neurobiology*, **24**(2), 269–81.

25. Davar, G. (2001). Endothelin-1 and metastatic cancer pain. *Pain Medicine*, **2**(1), 24–7.

26. Peters, C.M., Lindsay, T.H., Pomonis, J.D. *et al.* (2004). Endothelin and the tumorigenic component of bone cancer pain. *Neuroscience*, **126**(4), 1043–52.

27. Sevcik, M.A., Ghilardi, J.R., Halvorson, K.G. *et al.* (2005). Analgesic efficacy of bradykinin B1 antagonists in a murine bone cancer pain model. *Journal of Pain*, **6**(11), 771–5.

28. Wacnik, P.W., Eikmeier, L.J., Simone, D.A. *et al.* (2005). Nociceptive characteristics of tumor necrosis factor-alpha in naive and tumor-bearing mice. *Neuroscience*, **132**(2), 479–91.

29. Vega, J.A., Garcia-Suarez, O., Hannestad, J. *et al.* (2003). Neurotrophins and the immune system. *Journal of Anatomy*, **203**(1), 1–19.

30. Halvorson, K.G., Kubota, K., Sevcik, M.A. *et al.* (2005). A blocking antibody to nerve growth factor attenuates skeletal pain induced by prostate tumor cells growing in bone. *Cancer Research*, **65**(20), 9426–35.

31. Sevcik, M.A., Ghilardi, J.R., Peters, C.M. *et al.* (2005). Anti-NGF therapy profoundly reduces bone cancer pain and the accompanying increase in markers of peripheral and central sensitization. *Pain*, **115**(1–2), 128–41.

32. Boyle, W.J., Simonet, W.S., Lacey, D.L. (2003). Osteoclast differentiation and activation. *Nature*, **423**(6937), 337–42.

33. Powell, G.J., Southby, J., Danks, J.A. *et al.* (1991). Localization of parathyroid hormone-related protein in breast cancer metastases: increased incidence in bone compared with other sites. *Cancer Research*, **51**(11), 3059–61.

34. Guise, T.A. (2000). Molecular mechanisms of osteolytic bone metastases. *Cancer*, **88**(12 Suppl), 2892–8.

35. Kong, Y.Y., Feige, U., Sarosi, I. *et al.* (1999). Activated T cells regulate bone loss and joint destruction in adjuvant arthritis through osteoprotegerin ligand. *Nature*, **402**(6759), 304–9.

36. Clohisy, D.R., Ogilvie, C.M., and Ramnaraine, M.L. (1995). Tumor osteolysis in osteopetrotic mice. *Journal of Orthopaedic Research*, **13**(6), 892–7.

37. Honore, P., Luger, N.M., Sabino, M.A. *et al.* (2000). Osteoprotegerin blocks bone cancer-induced skeletal destruction, skeletal pain and pain-related neurochemical reorganization of the spinal cord. *Nature Medicine*, **6**(5), 521–8.

38. Delaisse, J-M. and Vaes, G. (1992). Mechanism of mineral solubilization and matrix degradation in osteoclastic bone resorption. In *Biology and physiology of the osteoclast* (eds. B.R. Rifkin and C.V. Gay), pp. 289–308. London: CRC Press.

39. Tominaga, M., Caterina, M.J., Malmberg, A.B. *et al.* (1998). The cloned capsaicin receptor integrates multiple pain-producing stimuli. *Neuron*, **21**(3), 531–43.

40. Stubbs, M., McSheehy, P.M., Griffiths, J.R., Bashford, C.L. (2000). Causes and consequences of tumour acidity and implications for treatment. *Molecular Medicine Today*, **6**(1), 15–9.

41. Ghilardi, J.R., Rohrich, H., Lindsay, T.H. *et al.* (2005). Selective blockade of the capsaicin receptor TRPV1 attenuates bone cancer pain. *Journal of Neuroscience*, **25**(12), 3126–31.

42. Mach, D.B., Rogers, S.D., Sabino, M.C. *et al.* (2002). Origins of skeletal pain: sensory and sympathetic innervation of the mouse femur. *Neuroscience*, **113**(1), 155–66.

43. Donovan-Rodriguez, T., Dickenson, A.H., and Urch, C.E. (2005). Gabapentin normalizes spinal neuronal responses that correlate with behavior in a rat model of cancer-induced bone pain. *Anesthesiology*, **102**(1), 132–40.

44. Sevcik, M.A., Luger, N.M., Mach, D.B. *et al.* (2004). Bone cancer pain: the effects of the bisphosphonate alendronate on pain, skeletal remodeling, tumor growth and tumor necrosis. *Pain*, **111**(1–2), 169–80.

45. Schwei, M.J., Honore, P., Rogers, S.D. *et al.* (1999). Neurochemical and cellular reorganization of the spinal cord in a murine model of bone cancer pain. *Journal of Neuroscience*, **19**(24), 10886–97.

46. Watkins, L.R., Maier, S.F. (2003). Glia: a novel drug discovery target for clinical pain. *Nat Rev Drug Discovery*, **2**(12), 973–85.

47. Urch, C.E., Donovan-Rodriguez, T., and Dickenson, A.H. (2003). Alterations in dorsal horn neurones in a rat model of cancer-induced bone pain. *Pain*, **106**(3), 347–56.

48. Suzuki, R., Rygh, L.J., Dickenson, A.H. (2004). Bad news from the brain: descending 5-HT pathways that control spinal pain processing. *Trends in Pharmacological Sciences*, **25**(12), 613–7.

49. Luger, N.M., Sabino, M.A., Schwei, M.J. *et al.* (2002). Efficacy of systemic morphine suggests a fundamental difference in the mechanisms that generate bone cancer vs inflammatory pain. *Pain*, **99**(3), 397–406.

50. Vermeirsch, H., Nuydens, R.M., Salmon, P.L. *et al.* (2004). Bone cancer pain model in mice: evaluation of pain behavior, bone destruction and morphine sensitivity. *Pharmacology, Biochemistry, and Behavior*, **79**(2), 243–51.

51. Urch, C.E., Donovan-Rodriguez, T., Gordon-Williams, R. *et al.* (2005). Efficacy of chronic morphine in a rat model of cancer-induced bone pain: behavior and in dorsal horn pathophysiology. *Journal of Pain*, **6**(12), 837–45.

52. Peters, C.M., Ghilardi, J.R., Keyser, C.P. *et al.* (2005). Tumor-induced injury of primary afferent sensory nerve fibers in bone cancer pain. *Experimental Neurology*, **193**(1), 85–100.

53. Menendez, L., Lastra, A., Hidalgo, A. *et al.* (2003). Peripheral opioids act as analgesics in bone cancer pain in mice. *Neuroreport*, **14**(6), 867–9.

54. Urch, C. (2004). The pathophysiology of cancer-induced bone pain: current understanding. *Palliative Medicine*, **18**(4), 267–74.

55. Fox, A., Medhurst, S., Courade, J.P. *et al.* (2004). Anti-hyperalgesic activity of the cox-2 inhibitor lumiracoxib in a model of bone cancer pain in the rat. *Pain*, **107**(1–2), 33–40.

56. Sabino, M.A., Ghilardi, J.R., Jongen, J.L. *et al.* (2002). Simultaneous reduction in cancer pain, bone destruction, and tumor growth by selective inhibition of cyclooxygenase-2. *Cancer Research*, **62**(24), 7343–9.

57. Walker, K., Medhurst, S.J., Kidd, B.L. *et al.* (2002). Disease modifying and anti-nociceptive effects of the bisphosphonate, zoledronic acid in a model of bone cancer pain. *Pain*, **100**(3), 219–29.

58. Goblirsch, M., Lynch, C., Mathews, W. *et al.* (2005). Radiation treatment decreases bone cancer pain through direct effect on tumor cells. *Radiation Research*, **164**(4 Pt 1), 400–8.

59. Lindsay, T.H., Jonas, B.M., Sevcik, M.A. *et al.* (2005). Pancreatic cancer pain and its correlation with changes in tumor vasculature, macrophage infiltration, neuronal innervation, body weight and disease progression. *Pain*, **119**(1–3), 233–46.

60. Berger, A.R., Arezzo, J.C., Schaumburg, H.H. *et al.* (1993). 2',3'-dideoxycytidine (ddC) toxic neuropathy: a study of 52 patients. *Neurology*, **43**(2), 358–62.

61. Cohen, J. (2002). Therapies. Confronting the limits of success. *Science*, **296**(5577), 2320–4.

62. Dougherty, P.M., Cata, J.P., Cordella, J.V. *et al.* (2004). Taxol-induced sensory disturbance is characterized by preferential impairment of myelinated fiber function in cancer patients. *Pain*, **109**(1–2), 132–42.

63. Forsyth, P.A., Balmaceda, C., Peterson, K. *et al.* (1997). Prospective study of paclitaxel-induced peripheral neuropathy with quantitative sensory testing. *Journal of Neurooncology*, **35**(1), 47–53.

64. Jordan, M.A., Wendell, K., Gardiner, S. *et al.* (1996). Mitotic block induced in HeLa cells by low concentrations of paclitaxel (Taxol) results in abnormal mitotic exit and apoptotic cell death. *Cancer Research*, **56**(4), 816–25.

65. Yvon, A.M., Wadsworth, P., and Jordan, M.A. (1999). Taxol suppresses dynamics of individual microtubules in living human tumor cells. *Molecular Biology of the Cell*, **10**(4), 947–59.

66. Fan, W. (1999). Possible mechanisms of paclitaxel-induced apoptosis. *Biochemical Pharmacology*, **57**(11), 1215–21.

67. Komiya, Y. and Tashiro, T. (1988). Effects of taxol on slow and fast axonal transport. *Cell Motility and the Cytoskeleton*, **11**(3), 151–6.

68. Roytta, M. and Raine, C.S. (1986). Taxol-induced neuropathy: chronic effects of local injection. *Journal of Neurocytology*, **15**(4), 483–96.

69. Polomano, R.C. and Bennett, G.J. (2001). Chemotherapy-evoked painful peripheral neuropathy. *Pain Medicine*, **2**(1), 8–14.

70. Finsterer, J. (2004). Mitochondriopathies. *European Journal of Neurology*, **11**(3), 163–86.

71. Flatters, S.J. and Bennett, G.J. (2006). Studies of peripheral sensory nerves in paclitaxel-induced painful peripheral neuropathy: evidence for mitochondrial dysfunction. *Pain*, **122**(3), 245–57.

72. Flatters, S.J. and Bennett, G.J. (2004). Ethosuximide reverses paclitaxel- and vincristine-induced painful peripheral neuropathy. *Pain*, **109**(1–2), 150–61.

73. Joseph, E.K. and Levine, J.D. (2004). Caspase signalling in neuropathic and inflammatory pain in the rat. *European Journal of Neuroscience*, **20**(11), 2896–902.

74. Siau, C. and Bennett, G.J. (2006). Dysregulation of cellular calcium homeostasis in chemotherapy-evoked painful peripheral neuropathy. *Anesthesia and Analgesia*, **102**(5), 1485–90.

75. Xiao, W., Boroujerdi, A., Bennett, G.J. *et al.* (2006). Chemotherapy-evoked painful peripheral neuropathy: analgesic effects of gabapentin and effects on expression of the alpha-2-delta type-1 calcium channel subunit. *Neuroscience*, **144**, 714–20.

76. Joseph, E.K., Chen, X., Khasar, S.G. *et al.* (2004). Novel mechanism of enhanced nociception in a model of AIDS therapy-induced painful peripheral neuropathy in the rat. *Pain*, **107**(1–2), 147–58.

77. Joseph, E.K. and Levine, J.D. (2006). Mitochondrial electron transport in models of neuropathic and inflammatory pain. *Pain*, **121**(1–2), 105–14.

78. Siau, C., Xiao, W., and Bennett, G.J. (2006). Paclitaxel- and vincristine-evoked painful peripheral neuropathies: loss of epidermal innervation and activation of Langerhans cells. *Experimental Neurology*, **201**(2), 507–14.

79. Verma, A. (2001). Epidemiology and clinical features of HIV-1 associated neuropathies. *Journal of the Peripheral Nervous System*, **6**(1), 8–13.

80. Milligan, E.D., O'Connor, K.A., Nguyen, K.T. *et al.* (2001). Intrathecal HIV-1 envelope glycoprotein gp120 induces enhanced pain states mediated by spinal cord proinflammatory cytokines. *Journal of Neuroscience*, **21**(8), 2808–19.

81. Herzberg, U. and Sagen, J. (2001). Peripheral nerve exposure to HIV viral envelope protein gp120 induces neuropathic pain and spinal gliosis. *Journal of Neuroimmunology*, **116**(1), 29–39.

82. Kreutzberg, G.W. (1996). Microglia: a sensor for pathological events in the CNS. *Trends in Neuroscience*, **19**(8), 312–8.

83. Koka, P., He, K., Zack, J.A. *et al.* (1995). Human immunodeficiency virus 1 envelope proteins induce interleukin 1, tumor necrosis factor alpha, and nitric oxide in glial cultures derived from fetal, neonatal, and adult human brain. *Journal of Experimental Medicine*, **182**(4), 941–51.

84. Kong, L.Y., Wilson, B.C., McMillian, M.K. *et al.* (1996). The effects of the HIV-1 envelope protein gp120 on the production of nitric oxide and proinflammatory cytokines in mixed glial cell cultures. *Cell Immunology*, **172**(1), 77–83.

85. Breitbart, W., McDonald, M.V., Rosenfeld, B. *et al.* (1996). Pain in ambulatory AIDS patients. I: Pain characteristics and medical correlates. *Pain*, **68**(2–3), 315–21.

86. Hewitt, D.J., McDonald, M., Portenoy, R.K. *et al.* (1997). Pain syndromes and etiologies in ambulatory AIDS patients. *Pain*, **70**(2–3), 117–23.

87. Cummins et al. (2007). The roles of sodium channels in nociception: Implications for mechanisms of pain. *Pain*, **131**(3), 243–57.

88. Dickenson and Ghandehari. (2007). Anti-convulsants and anti-depressants. *Handb Exp Pharmacol*, **177**, 145–77

89. Rygh, L.J., Suzuki, R., Rahman, W. *et al.* (2006). Local and descending circuits regulate long-term potentiation and zif268 expression in spinal neurons. *European Journal of Neuroscience*, **24**(3), 761–72.

90. Suzuki, R., Rahman, W., Rygh, L.J. *et al.* (2005). Spinal-supraspinal serotonergic circuits regulating neuropathic pain and its treatment with gabapentin. *Pain*, **117**(3), 292–303.

91. Luo, Z.D., Chaplan, S.R., Higuera, E.S. *et al.* (2001). Upregulation of dorsal root ganglion (alpha)2(delta) calcium channel subunit and its correlation with allodynia in spinal nerve-injured rats. *Journal of Neuroscience*, **21**(6), 1868–75.

92. Matthews, E.A. and Dickenson, A.H. (2001). Effects of spinally delivered N- and P-type voltage-dependent calcium channel antagonists on dorsal horn neuronal responses in a rat model of neuropathy. *Pain*, **92**(1–2), 235–46.

93. Santicioli, P., Giuliani, S., Bartho, L. *et al.* (1993). Tachykinin NK-1 and NK-2 receptors in the circular muscle of the guinea-pig proximal colon. *Regulatory Peptides*, **46**(1–2), 386–8.

10.1.2 Pain assessment and cancer pain syndromes

Nathan I. Cherny

Surveys indicate that pain is experienced by 30 to 60 per cent of cancer patients during active therapy and more than two-thirds of those with advanced disease[1]. Unrelieved pain is incapacitating and precludes a satisfying quality of life; it interferes with physical functioning and social interaction, and is strongly associated with heightened psychological distress. It can provoke or exacerbate existential distress, disturb normal processes of coping and adjustment, and augment a sense of vulnerability, contributing to a preoccupation with the potential for catastrophic outcomes. Persistent pain interferes with the ability to eat, sleep, think, interact with others, and is correlated with fatigue in cancer patients.

The high prevalence of chronic pain among cancer patients, and the profound psychological and physical burdens engendered by this symptom, obliges all treating clinicians to be skilled in pain management. Relief of pain in cancer patients is an ethical imperative, and it is incumbent upon clinicians to maximize the knowledge, skill, and diligence needed to attend to this task.

The undertreatment of cancer pain has many causes, among the most important of which is inadequate assessment[2,3]. In a study to evaluate the correlation between patient and clinician evaluation of pain severity, Grossman et al.[3] found that when patients rated their pain as moderate to severe, oncology fellows failed to appreciate the severity of the problem in 73 per cent of cases. In studies of pain relief among cancer patients in the United States[4] and in France[5], the discrepancy between patient and physician evaluation of the severity of the pain problem was a major predictor of inadequate relief.

Approach to cancer pain assessment

Assessment is an ongoing and dynamic process that includes evaluation of presenting problems, elucidation of pain syndromes and pathophysiology, and formulation of a comprehensive plan for continuing care. The objectives of cancer pain assessment include: (1) the accurate characterization of the pain, including the pain syndrome and inferred pathophysiology; and (2) the evaluation of the impact of the pain and the role it plays in the overall suffering of the patient.

This assessment is predicated on the establishment of a trusting relationship with the patient in which the clinician emphasizes the relief of pain and suffering as central to the goal of therapy, and encourages open communication about symptoms. Clinicians should not be cavalier about the potential for symptom underreporting; symptoms are frequently described as complaints, and there is a common perception that the 'good patient' refrains from complaining. The prevalence of pain is so great that an open-ended question about the presence of pain should be included at each patient visit in routine oncological practice. If the patient is either unable or unwilling to describe the pain, a family member may need to be questioned to assess the distress or disability of the patient.

Pain syndromes

Cancer pain syndromes are defined by the association of particular pain characteristics and physical signs, with specific consequences of the underlying disease or its treatment. Syndromes are associated with distinct aetiologies and pathophysiologies, and have important prognostic and therapeutic implications. Pain syndromes associated with cancer can be either acute or chronic. Whereas acute pains experienced by cancer patients are usually related to diagnostic and therapeutic interventions, chronic pains are most commonly caused by direct tumour infiltration. Adverse consequences of cancer therapy, including surgery, chemotherapy, and radiation therapy, account for 15 to 25 per cent of chronic cancer pain problems, and a small proportion of the chronic pains experienced by cancer patients are caused by pathology unrelated to either the cancer or the therapy.

Pain characteristics

The evaluation of pain characteristics provides some of the data essential for syndrome identification. These characteristics include intensity, quality, distribution, and temporal relationships.

Intensity

The evaluation of pain intensity is pivotal to therapeutic decision-making. It indicates the urgency with which relief is needed and

influences the selection of analgesic drug, route of administration, and rate of dose titration. Furthermore, the assessment of pain intensity may help characterize the pain mechanism and underlying syndrome. For example, the pain associated with radiation-induced nerve injury is rarely severe; the occurrence of severe pain in a previously irradiated region therefore suggests the existence of recurrent neoplasm or a radiation-induced second primary neoplasm.

Quality

The quality of the pain often suggests its pathophysiology. Somatic nociceptive pains are usually well localized and described as sharp, aching, throbbing, or pressure-like. Visceral nociceptive pains are generally diffuse and may be gnawing or crampy when due to obstruction of a hollow viscus, or aching, sharp, or throbbing when due to involvement of organ capsules or mesentery. Neuropathic pains may be described as burning, tingling, or shock-like (lancinating).

Distribution

Patients with cancer pain commonly experience pain at more than one site. The distinction between focal, multifocal, and generalized pain may be important in the selection of therapy, such as nerve blocks, radiotherapy, or surgical approaches. The term 'focal pain', which is used to denote a single site, has also been used to depict pain that is experienced in the region of the underlying lesion. Focal pains can be distinguished from those that are referred to a site remote from the lesion. Familiarity with pain referral patterns is essential to target appropriate diagnostic and therapeutic manoeuvers (Table 10.1.2.1). For example, a patient who develops progressive shoulder pain and has no evidence of focal pathology needs to undergo evaluation of the region above and below the diaphragm to exclude the possibility of referred pain from diaphragmatic irritation.

Temporal relationships

Cancer-related pain may be acute or chronic. Acute pain is defined by a recent onset and a natural history characterized by transience. The pain is often associated with overt pain behaviours (such as moaning, grimacing, and splinting), anxiety, or signs of generalized

Table 10.1.2.1 Common patterns of pain referral.

Pain mechanism	Site of lesion	Referral site
Visceral	Diaphragmatic irritation	Shoulder
	Urothelial tract	Inguinal region and genitalia
Somatic	C7–T1 vertebrae	Interscapular
	L1–L2	Sacroiliac joint and hip
	Hip joint	Knee
	Pharynx	Ipsilateral ear
Neuropathic	Nerve or plexus	Anywhere in the distribution of a peripheral nerve
	Nerve root	Anywhere in the corresponding dermatome
	Central nervous system	Anywhere in the region of the body innervated by the damaged structure

sympathetic hyperactivity, including diaphoresis, hypertension, and tachycardia. Chronic pain has been defined by persistence for 3 months or more beyond the usual course of an acute illness or injury, a pattern of recurrence at intervals over months or years, or by association with a chronic pathological process. Chronic tumour-related pain is usually insidious in onset, often increases progressively with tumour growth, and may regress with tumour shrinkage. Overt pain behaviours and sympathetic hyperactivity are often absent, and the pain may be associated with affective disturbances (anxiety and/or depression) and vegetative symptoms, such as asthenia, anorexia, and sleep disturbance.

Transitory exacerbations of severe pain over a baseline of moderate pain or less may be described as 'breakthrough pain'[6]. Breakthrough pains are common in both acute and chronic pain states. These exacerbations may be precipitated by volitional actions of the patient (so-called incident pains), such as movement, micturition, cough or defecation, or by non-volitional events, such as bowel distention. Spontaneous fluctuations in pain intensity can also occur without an identifiable precipitant (see Chapter 10.5).

Inferred pain mechanisms

Inferences about the mechanisms that may be responsible for the pain are helpful in the evaluation of the pain syndrome and in the management of cancer pain. The assessment process usually provides the clinical data necessary to infer a predominant pathophysiology.

Nociceptive pain

'Nociceptive pain' describes pain that is perceived to be commensurate with tissue damage associated with an identifiable somatic or visceral lesion. The persistence of pain is attributed to ongoing activation of nociceptors. Nociceptive pain that originates from somatic structures (somatic pain) is usually well localized and described as sharp, aching, burning, or throbbing. As previously described, pain that arises from visceral structures (visceral pain) is generally diffuse; pain characteristics may differ depending on the involved structures. From the clinical perspective, nociceptive pains (particularly somatic pains) usually respond to opioid drugs or to interventions that ameliorate or denervate the peripheral lesion.

Neuropathic pain

The term 'neuropathic pain' is applied when pain is due to injury to, or diseases of, the peripheral or central neural structures or is perceived to be sustained by aberrant somatosensory processing at these sites[7,8]. It is most strongly suggested when a dysesthesia occurs in a region of motor, sensory, or autonomic dysfunction that is attributable to a discrete neurological lesion. The diagnosis can be challenging, however, and is often inferred solely from the distribution of the pain and identification of a lesion in neural structures that innervate this region.

Although neuropathic pains can be described in terms of the pain characteristics (continuous or lancinating) or site of injury (for example, neuronopathy or plexopathy), it is useful to distinguish these syndromes according to the presumed site of the aberrant neural activity (generator) that sustains the pain. Peripheral neuropathic pain is caused by injury to a peripheral nerve or nerve root and is presumably sustained by aberrant processes originating in the nerve root, plexus, or nerve. Neuropathic pains believed to be sustained by a central 'generator' include sympathetically-maintained pain (also known as reflex sympathetic dystrophy or causalgia) and a group of syndromes traditionally known as the deafferentation pains (e.g. phantom pain). Sympathetically-maintained pain may occur following injury to soft tissue, peripheral nerve, viscera, or central nervous system, and is characterized by focal autonomic dysregulation in a painful region (e.g. vasomotor or pilomotor changes, swelling, or sweating abnormalities) or trophic changes[9].

Understanding of 'reflex sympathetic dystrophy' (RSD) and 'causalgia' and sympathetically maintained pain have undergone considerable review. The IASP has suggested classification of these syndromes as Complex Regional Pain Syndromes types I and II, indicating that sympathetically maintained pain is a frequent but variable component of these syndromes. Type I, corresponds to RSD and occurs without a definable nerve lesion, and type II, formerly called causalgia, refers to cases where a definable nerve lesion is present[10].

The diagnosis of neuropathic pain has important clinical implications. The response of neuropathic pains to opioid drugs is less predictable and generally less dramatic than the response of nociceptive pains. Optimal treatment may depend on the use of so-called adjuvant analgesics (see Chapter 10.1.8) or other specific approaches, such as somatic or sympathetic nerve block (see Chapters 10.1.9 and 10.1.10).

Idiopathic pain

Pain that is perceived to be excessive for the extent of identifiable organic pathology can be termed idiopathic unless the patient presents with affective and behavioural disturbances that are severe enough to infer a predominating psychological pathogenesis, in which case a specific psychiatric diagnosis (somatoform disorder) can be applied[11]. When the inference of a somatoform disorder cannot be made, however, the label 'idiopathic' should be retained, and assessments should be repeated at appropriate intervals. Idiopathic pain in general, and pain related to a psychiatric disorder specifically, are uncommon in the cancer population, notwithstanding the importance of psychological factors in quality of life.

A stepwise approach to the evaluation of cancer pain

A practical approach to cancer pain assessment incorporates a stepwise approach that begins with data collection and ends with a clinically relevant formulation.

Data collection

History A careful review of past medical history and the chronology of the cancer are important to place the pain complaint in context. The pain-related history must elucidate the relevant pain characteristics, as well as the responses of the patient to previous disease-modifying and analgesic therapies. The presence of multiple pain problems is common, and if more than one is reported, each must be assessed independently. The use of validated pain assessment instruments can provide a format for communication between the patient and health-care professionals, and can also be used to monitor the adequacy of therapy (see following paragraphs).

The clinician should assess the consequences of the pain, including impairment in activities of daily living; psychological, familial, and professional dysfunction; disturbed sleep, appetite, and vitality; and financial concerns. The patient's psychological status, including current level of anxiety or depression, suicidal ideation, and the perceived meaning of the pain, is similarly relevant. Pervasive dysfunctional attitudes, such as pessimism, idiosyncratic interpretation of pain, self-blame, catastrophizing, and perceived loss of personal control, can usually be detected through careful questioning. It is important to assess the patient–family interaction, and to note both the kind and frequency of pain behaviours and the nature of the family response.

Most patients with cancer pain have multiple other symptoms, and the clinician should evaluate the severity and distress caused by each of these symptoms. Symptom checklists and quality-of-life measures may contribute to this comprehensive evaluation[12,13].
Examination A physical examination, including a neurological evaluation, is a necessary part of the initial pain assessment. The need for a thorough neurological assessment is justified by the high prevalence of painful neurological conditions in this population. Physical examination should attempt to identify the underlying aetiology of the pain problem, clarify the extent of the underlying disease, and discern the relationship of the pain complaint to the disease.
Review of previous investigations Careful review of previous laboratory and imaging studies can provide important information about the cause of the pain and the extent of the underlying disease.

Provisional assessment

The information derived from these data provides the basis for a provisional pain diagnosis, an understanding of the disease status, and the identification of other concurrent concerns. This provisional diagnosis includes inferences about the pathophysiology of the pain and an assessment of the pain syndrome.

Additional investigations are often required to clarify areas of uncertainty in the provisional assessment. The extent of diagnostic investigation must be appropriate to the patient's general status and the overall goals of care. For some patients, comprehensive evaluation may require numerous investigations, some targeted at the specific pain problem and others needed to clarify extent of disease or concurrent symptoms.

The lack of a definitive finding on an investigation should not be used to override a compelling clinical diagnosis. In the assessment of bone pain, for example, plain radiographs provide only a crude assessment of bony lesions and further investigation with bone scintigrams, computed tomography (CT), or magnetic resonance imaging (MRI) may be indicated. To minimize the risk of error, the physician ordering the diagnostic procedures should personally review them with the radiologist to correlate pathologic changes with the clinical findings.

Pain should be managed during the diagnostic evaluation. Comfort will improve compliance and reduce the distress associated with procedures. No patient should be inadequately evaluated because of poorly controlled pain.

The comprehensive assessment may also require additional evaluation of other physical or psychosocial problems identified during the initial assessment. Expert assistance from other physicians, nurses, social workers, or others may be essential.

Formulation and therapeutic planning

The evaluation should enable the clinician to appreciate the nature of the pain, its impact, and concurrent concerns that further undermine quality of life. The findings of this evaluation should be reviewed with the patient and appropriate others. Through candid discussion, current problems can be prioritized to reflect their importance to the patient.

This evaluation may also identify potential outcomes that would benefit from contingency planning. Examples include evaluation of resources for home care, pre-bereavement interventions with the family, and the provision of assistive devices in anticipation of compromised ambulation.

The measurement of pain and its impact on patient well-being

Although pain measurement has generally been used by clinical investigators to determine the impact of analgesic therapies, it has become clear that it has an important role in the routine monitoring of cancer patients in treatment settings[14]. Because observer ratings of symptom severity correlate poorly with patient ratings and are generally an inadequate substitute for patient reporting[3], patient self-report is the primary source of information for the measurement of pain.

Pain measures in routine clinical management

Guidelines from the World Health Organization [15], Agency for Health Care Policy[16], and the American Pain Society [14] recommend the regular use of pain-rating scales to assess pain severity and relief in all patients who commence or change treatments. These recommendations also suggest that clinicians teach patients and families to use assessment tools in the home to promote continuity of pain management in all settings.

The two most commonly used scales for adults are a verbal descriptor scale (i.e. 'Which word best describes your pain; none, mild moderate, severe, or excruciating?') or a numerical scale (i.e. 'On a scale from 0 to 10, where 0 indicates no pain and 10 indicates the worst pain you can imagine, how would you rate your pain?')[16].

Au *et al.* demonstrated that the use of a simple verbal pain assessment tool improved the caregiver's understanding of pain status in hospitalized patients[17]. Routinely measuring pain intensity as a fifth vital sign, using a pain scale incorporated into to the bedside chart (Fig. 10.1.2.1) can help make pain a visible parameter that is monitored dynamically[18,19].

Instruments for the measurement of pain in research settings

Pain can be measured using a unidimensional or multidimensional scale. Unidimensional scales generally address intensity or relief, using visual analogue, numerical, and categorical scales. Multidimensional instruments include the Memorial Pain Assessment Card, the McGill Pain Questionnaire, and the Brief Pain Inventory.
Memorial pain assessment card (MPAC) The MPAC[20] is a brief, validated measure that uses 100-mm VASs to characterize pain intensity, pain relief, and mood, and an eight-point verbal rating scale (VRS) to further characterize pain intensity (Fig. 10.1.2.2). The mood scale, which is correlated with measures of global psychological distress, depression and anxiety, is considered to be a brief measure of global symptom distress[20]. Although this instrument does not provide detailed descriptors of pain, its brevity and simplicity may facilitate the collection of useful information while minimizing patient burden and encouraging compliance.
Brief pain inventory (BPI) The BPI (Fig. 10.1.2.3)[21] is a simple and easily administered tool that provides information about pain history, intensity, location, and quality. Numeric scales (range 1 to 10) indicate the intensity of pain in general, at its worst, at its least, and right now. A percentage scale quantifies relief from current therapies. A figure representing the body is provided

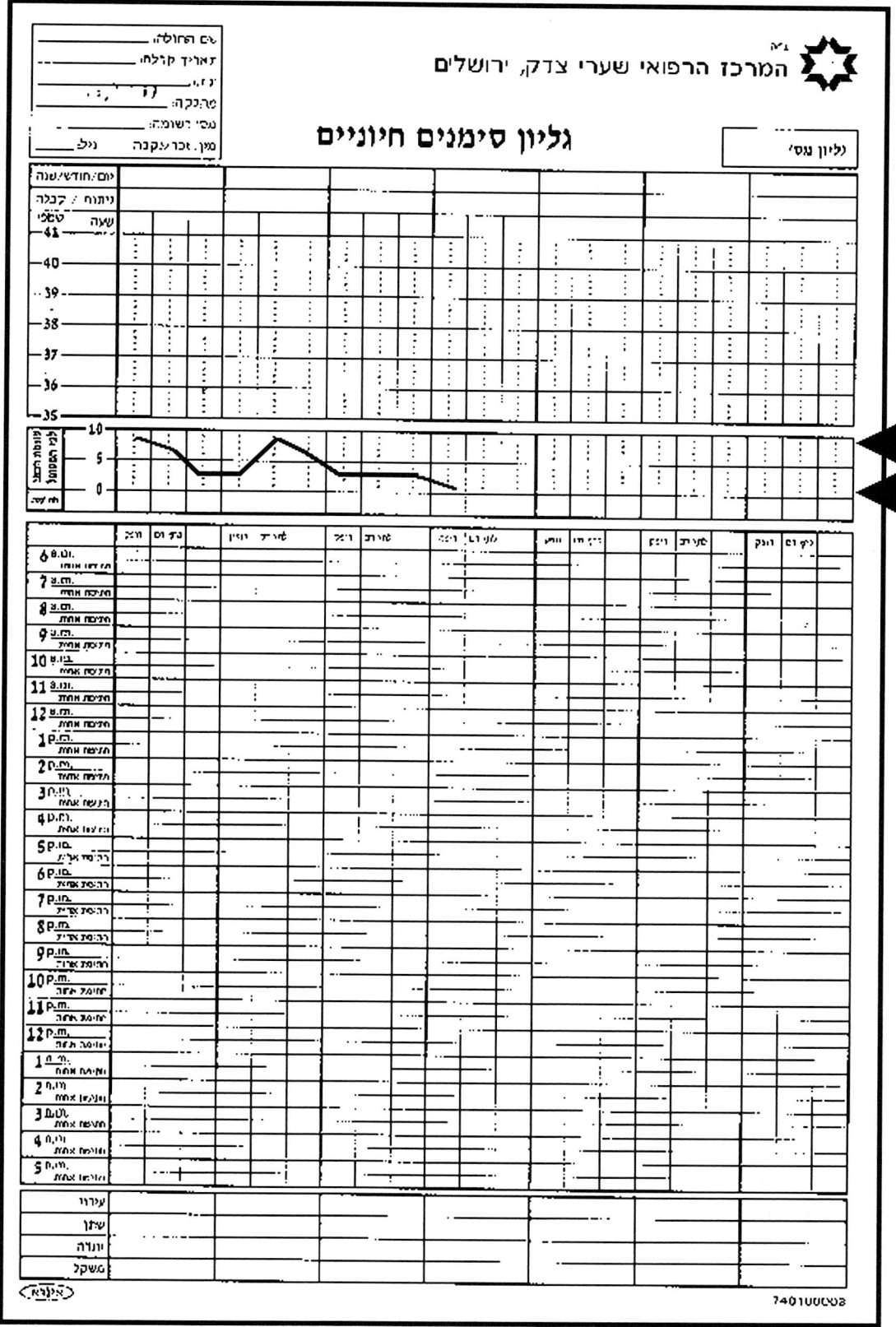

Figure 10.1.2.1 Vital signs chart incorporating 10-point pain scale.

Memorial Pain Assessment Card

4 Mood Scale

|————————————————————————|
Worst   Best
mood   mood

Put a mark on the line to show your mood.

2 Pain Description Scale

Moderate   Just noticeable

Strong   No pain

Mild

Excruciating   Severe

Weak

Circle the word that describes your pain.

1 Pain Scale

|————————————————————————|
Least   Worst
possible   possible
pain   pain

Put a mark on the line to show how much pain there is.

3 Relief Scale

|————————————————————————|
No relief   Complete
of pain   relief of
                                            pain

Put a mark on the line to show how much relief you get.

Fold page along broken line so that each measure is presented to the patient in the numbered order.

Reprinted by permission. Memorial Sloan-Kettering Cancer Center Pain Assessment Card.

Figure 10.1.2.2 Memorial pain assessment card.

for the patient to shade the area corresponding to his or her pain. Seven questions determine the degree to which pain interferes with function, mood, and enjoyment of life. The BPI is self-administered and easily understood, and has been translated into several languages[22–24]. It is suitable for periodic evaluation of pain, i.e. weekly or two-weekly.

The McGill pain questionnaire (MPQ) The MPQ[25] is a self-administered questionnaire that provides global scores and subscale scores that reflect the sensory, affective, and evaluative dimensions of pain. The scores are derived from ratings of pain descriptors selected by the patient. A 5-point verbal categorical scale characterizes the intensity of pain, and a pain drawing localizes

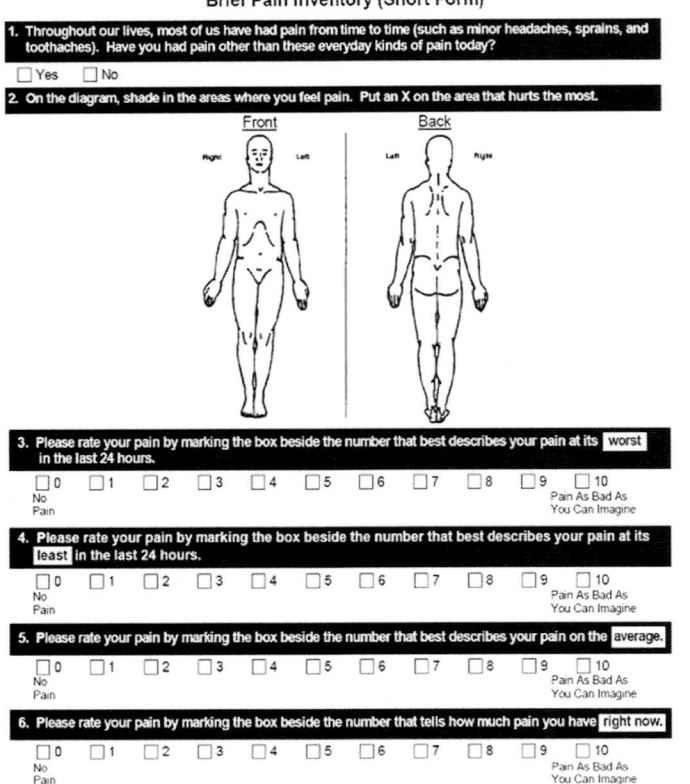

Figure 10.1.2.3 Brief pain inventory short form.

the pain. Further information is collected about the impact of medications and other therapies. The impact of pain on function is not assessed. A short form of the MPQ (SF-MPQ) (Fig. 10.1.2.4) was developed for use in research settings and has been validated in a palliative care setting[26].

Acute pain syndromes

Cancer-related acute pain syndromes are most commonly due to diagnostic or therapeutic interventions and they generally pose little diagnostic difficulty. Although some tumour-related pains have an acute onset (such as pain from a pathological fracture), most of these will persist unless effective treatment for the underlying lesion is provided.

Acute pain associated with diagnostic and therapeutic interventions

Many investigations and treatments are associated with predictable, transient pain. For those patients with a preexisting pain syndrome, otherwise innocuous manipulations can also precipitate incident pain.

Acute pain associated with diagnostic interventions

Lumbar puncture headache Lumbar puncture (LP) headache is the best-characterized acute pain syndrome associated with a diagnostic intervention. This syndrome is characterized by the delayed development of a positional headache, which is precipitated or markedly exacerbated by upright posture. The pain is believed to be related to reduction in cerebrospinal fluid volume, due to ongoing leakage through the defect in the dural sheath, and compensatory expansion of the pain-sensitive intracerebral veins[27]. The incidence of headache is related to the calibre of the LP needle (0–2 per cent with 27- to 29-gauge; 0.5–7 per cent with 25- to 26-gauge; 5–8 per cent with 22-gauge; 10–15 per cent with 20-gauge; and 20–30 per cent with 18-gauge needles)[28].

The risk of LP headache can be reduced by several strategies: When using a regular bevelled needle, longitudinal insertion of the needle bevel, which induces less trauma to the longitudinal elastic fibres in the dura, may reduce the incidence of headache. Non-traumatic, conical-tipped needles with a lateral opening are associated with a substantially lesser risk of post LP headaches than regular cannulae [28]. The evidence that recumbency after LP reduces the incidence of this syndrome is controversial[29].

LP headache, which usually develops hours to several days after the procedure, is typically described as a dull occipital discomfort that may radiate to the frontal region or to the shoulders Pain is commonly associated with nausea and dizziness. The duration of the headache is usually 1–7 days, and routine management relies on rest, hydration, and analgesics[30]. Persistent headache may necessitate application of an epidural blood patch[30]. Severe headache has also been reported to respond to treatment with intravenous or oral caffeine.

Transthoracic needle biopsy Transthoracic fine-needle aspiration of intrathoracic mass is generally a non-noxious procedure. Severe pain has, however, been associated with this procedure when the underlying diagnosis was a neurogenic tumour.

Transrectal prostatic biopsy Transrectal ultrasound-guided prostate biopsy is an essential procedure in the diagnosis and management of prostate cancer. In a prospective study 16 per cent of the patients reported pain of moderate or greater severity and 19 per cent would not agree to undergo the procedure again without anaesthesia[31]. When present, pain may persist up to 4 weeks after the biopsy. Preprostatic lidocaine infiltration and unilateral pudendal nerve block may substantially reduce the pain associated with this procedure.

Mammography pain Breast compression associated with mammography can cause moderate and rarely severe pain. The duration of the pain is generally short[32]. Unless patients are adequately counseled and treated, occasional patients will refuse repeat mammograms because of pain. In a systematic review, the only intervention to significantly reduce the pain was of patient controlled compression[33].

Acute pain associated with therapeutic interventions

Postoperative pain Acute postoperative pain is universal unless adequately treated. Unfortunately, undertreatment is endemic despite the availability of adequate analgesic and anaesthetic techniques[34]. Guidelines for management have been reviewed[34,35]. Postoperative pain that exceeds the normal duration or severity should prompt a careful evaluation for the possibility of infection or other complications.

Radiofrequency tumour ablation Radiofrequency tumour ablation is commonly used in the management of liver metastases. It is also increasingly used in other settings including adrenal metastases and renal tumours as well as in lung, bone, breast, and bone tumours. Percutaneous ablation of liver tumours may be associated with severe right-upper quadrant abdominal pain or pain radiating to the right shoulder in 5–10 per cent of patients.

Cryosurgery Cryotherapy is commonly applied in the management of skin and cervical tumours. Topical cryotherapy typically causes a local painful reaction that decreases in severity over 2–7 days. Cryosurgery of the cervix in the treatment of intraepithelial neoplasm commonly produces an acute cramping pain syndrome. The severity of the pain is related to the duration of the freeze period and it is not diminished by the administration of prophylactic non-steroidal anti-inflammatory drugs (NSAIDs).

Other interventions Invasive interventions other than surgery are commonly used in cancer therapy and may also result in predictable acute pain syndromes. Examples include the pains associated with tumour embolization techniques and chemical pleurodesis.

Acute pain associated with analgesic techniques

Local anaesthetic infiltration pain Intradermal and subcutaneous infiltration of lidocaine produces a transient burning sensation before the onset of analgesia. This can be modified with the use of buffered solutions. Other manoeuvers, including warming of the solution or slowing rate of injection do not diminish injection pain.

Opioid injection pain Intramuscular (IM) and subcutaneous (SC) injections are painful. When repetitive dosing is required, the IM route of administration is not recommended[16,34]. The pain associated with subcutaneous injection is influenced by the volume injected and the chemical characteristics of the injectant.

Opioid headache Rarely, patients develop a reproducible generalized headache after opioid administration. Although its cause is not known, speculation suggests that it may be caused by opioid-induced histamine release.

SHORT FORM McGILL PAIN QUESTIONNAIRE and PAIN DIAGRAM

(Reproduced with permission of author © Dr. Ron Melzack for publication and distribution)

Date: _____

Name: _____

Check the column to indicate the level of your pain for each word, or leave blank if it does not apply to you.____

		Mild	Moderate	Severe
1	Throbbing	___	___	___
2	Shooting	___	___	___
3	Stabbing	___	___	___
4	Sharp	___	___	___
5	Cramping	___	___	___
6	Gnawing	___	___	___
7	Hot-burning	___	___	___
8	Aching	___	___	___
9	Heavy	___	___	___
10	Tender	___	___	___
11	Splitting	___	___	___
12	Tiring-Exhausting	___	___	___
13	Sickening	___	___	___
14	Fearful	___	___	___
15	Cruel-Punising	___	___	

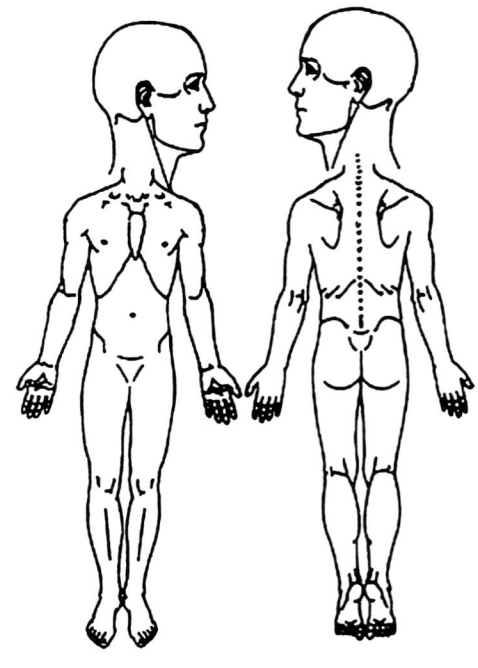

Mark or comment on the above figure where you have your pain or problems.

Indicate on this line how bad your pain is—at the left end of line mean no pain at all, at right end means worst pain possible.

No Pain	_____	Worst Possible Pain

S	/33	A	/12	VAS	/10

Figure 10.1.2.4 McGill pain questionnaire (MPQ) short form.

Spinal opioid hyperalgesia syndrome Intrathecal and epidural injection of high opioid doses is occasionally complicated by pain (typically perineal, buttock, or leg), hyperalgesia, and associated manifestations including segmental myoclonus, piloerection, and priapism. This is an uncommon phenomenon that remits after discontinuation of the infusion.

Epidural injection pain Back, pelvic, or leg pain may be precipitated by epidural injection or infusion. The incidence of this problem has been estimated at approximately 20 per cent[36]. It is speculated that it may be caused by the compression of an adjacent nerve root by the injected fluid. Similar problems have been described with intrathecal injections associated with periactheter fibrosis[37].

Acute pain associated with anticancer therapies

Acute pain associated with chemotherapy infusion techniques

Intravenous infusion pain Pain at the site of cytotoxic infusion is a common problem. Four pain syndromes related to intravenous infusion of chemotherapeutic agents are recognized: venous spasm, chemical phlebitis, vesicant extravasation, and anthracycline-associated flare. Venous spasm causes pain that is not associated with inflammation or phlebitis, and which may be modified by application of a warm compress or reduction of the rate of infusion. Chemical phlebitis can be caused by cytotoxic medications including amasarcine, decarbazine, carmustine, vinorelbine, similar to that seen with the infusion of potassium chloride and hyperosmolar solutions. The pain and linear erythema associated with chemical phlebitis must be distinguished from the more serious complication of a vesicant cytotoxic extravasation.

Vesicant extravasation may produce intense pain followed by desquamation and ulceration. Finally, a brief venous flare reaction is often associated with intravenous administration of the anthracycline, doxorubicin. The flare is typically associated with local urticaria and occasional patients report pain or stinging.

Hepatic artery infusion pain Cytotoxic infusions into the hepatic artery (for patients with hepatic metastases) are often associated with the development of a diffuse abdominal pain. Continuous infusions can lead to persistent pain. In some patients, the pain is due to the development of gastric ulceration or erosions, or cholangitis. If the latter complications do not occur, the pain usually resolves with discontinuation of the infusion. A dose relationship is suggested by the observation that some patients will comfortably tolerate reinitiating of the infusion at a lower dose[38].

Intraperitoneal chemotherapy pain A transient mild abdominal pain, associated with sensations of fullness or bloating is reported by approximately 25 per cent of patients after intraperitoneal chemotherapy[39]. A further 25 per cent of patients reports moderate or severe pain necessitating opioid analgesia or discontinuation of therapy. Moderate or severe pain is usually caused by chemical serositis or infection. Chemical serositis is a common complication of intraperitoneal of the anthracycline agents, mitoxantrone and doxorubicin, and with taxol, but it is relatively infrequent with 5-flurouracil or cis-platinum. Pain may indicate suboptimal drug distribution within the abdominal cavity. Some patients experience discomfort related to sensing abdominal distention, or from intercostal nerve irritation. Abdominal pain associated with fever and leukocytosis in blood and peritoneal fluid is suggestive of infectious peritonitis.

Intravesical chemo-or immunotherapy Intravesical bacillus Calmette-Guerin (BCG) therapy for transitional cell carcinoma of the urinary bladder usually causes a transient bladder irritability syndrome, characterized by frequency and/or micturition pain[40]. Similarly, intravesical doxorubicin, mitimycin –C and thiotepa can also cause a painful chemical cystitis. Rarely, intravesical BCG treatment may trigger a painful poly-arthritis sometimes associated with a full-blown Reiter's syndrome[41].

Acute pain associated with chemotherapy toxicity

Mucositis Severe mucositis is an almost invariable consequence of the myeloablative chemotherapy and radiotherapy that precedes bone marrow transplantation, but it is less common with standard intensity therapy. The cytotoxic agents most commonly associated with mucositis are: cytarabine, doxorubicin, etoposide, 5-FU, and methotrexate. Pretreatment oral pathology and poor denatal hygiene increase the risk of chemotherapy-induced mucositis. Younger patients have a relatively greater risk of chemotherapy-induced stomatitis, perhaps related to a higher epithelial mitotic rate. Damaged mucosal surfaces may become super infected with microorganisms, such as *Candida albicans* and herpes simplex. The latter complication is most likely in neutropenic patients, who are also predisposed to systemic sepsis arising from local invasion by aerobic and anaerobic oral flora.

Corticosteroid-induced perineal discomfort A transient burning sensation in the perineum is described by some patients following rapid infusion of large doses (20–100 mg) of dexamethasone[42]. Clinical experience suggests that this syndrome is prevented by slow infusion.

Steroid pseudoheurmatism The withdrawal of corticosteroids may produce a pain syndrome, which manifests as diffuse myalgias, arthralgias, and tenderness of muscles and joints. These symptoms occur with rapid or slow withdrawal and may occur in patients taking these drugs for long or short periods of time. Treatment consists of reinstituting the steroids at a higher dose and withdrawing them more slowly.

Painful peripheral neuropathy Chemotherapy-induced painful peripheral neuropathy, which is usually associated with vinca alkaloids, cis-platinum, oxaliplatin, and paclitaxel can have an acute course. The vinca alkaloids (particularly vincristine) are also associated with other, presumably neuropathic acute pain syndromes, including pain in the jaw, legs, arms, or abdomen that may last from hours to days. Vincristine-induced orofacial pain in the distribution of the trigeminal and glossopharyngeal nerves occurs in approximately 50 per cent of patients at the onset of vincristine treatment[43]. The pain, which is severe in about half of those affected, generally begins 2–3 days after vincristine administration and lasts for 1–3 days. It is usually self-limiting and if recurrence occurs, it is usually mild[43]. Vinorelbine is associated with mild paresthesias in about 20 per cent of patients and severe neuropathy is rare[44]. The neuropathy associated with paclitaxel is dose related, and is generally subacute in onset with resolution after the completion of therapy; however, in a proportion of cases it can be severe and persistent[45].

Headache Intrathecal methotrexate in the treatment of leukaemia or leptomeningeal metastases produces an acute meningitic syndrome in 5–50 per cent of patients. Headache is the prominent symptom and may be associated with vomiting, nuchal rigidity, fever, irritability, and lethargy. Symptoms usually begin hours after intrathecal treatment and persist for several days. Cerebrospinal fluid (CSF) examination reveals a pleocytosis that may mimic bacterial meningitis. Patients at increased risk for the development of this syndrome include those who have received multiple intrathecal injections and those patients undergoing treatment for proven leptomeningeal metastases[46]. The syndrome tends not to recur with subsequent injections.

Systemic administration of L-asparaginase for the treatment of acute lymphoblastic leukaemia produces thrombosis of cerebral veins or dural sinuses in 1–2 per cent of patients[47]. This complication typically occurs after a few weeks of therapy, but its onset may be delayed until after the completion of treatment. Headache is the most common initial symptom, and seizures, hemiparesis, delirium, vomiting, or cranial nerve palsies may also occur. The diagnosis may be established by angiography or by gradient echo sequences on MRI scan.

Trans-retinoic acid therapy, which may be used in the treatment of acute promyelocytic leukaemia (APML), can cause a transient severe headache[48]. The mechanism may be related to pseudotumour cerebri induced by hypervitaminosis A.

Diffuse bone pain Trans-retinoic acid therapy in patients with APML often produces a syndrome of diffuse bone pain. The pain is generalized, of variable intensity, and closely associated with a transient neutrophilia. The latter observation suggests that the pain may be due to marrow expansion.

Taxol-induced arthralgia and myalgia Administration of paclitaxel generates a syndrome of diffuse arthralgias and myalgia in 10–20 per cent of patients[49]. They are related to individual doses; associations with the cumulative dose and infusion duration are less clear. Diffuse joint and muscle pains generally appear 1–4 days after drug administration and persist for 3–7 days. Steroids may reduce tendency to myalgia and athralgias[50].

5-Flurouracil-induced anginal chest pain Patients receiving 5-flurouracil may develop ischemic chest pain. Although the overall risk is generally considered low (1–2 per cent), this is controversial and there is some evidence suggesting risk as high as 20 per cent[51]. Overall, the risk is higher with patients who are receiving continuous infusion than those receiving bolus therapy and patients with pre-existing ischaemic heart disease. It is widely speculated that coronary vasospasm may be the underlying mechanism[51]. There have been recent reports of similar ischaemic cardiotoxicity among patients receiving the 5-FU pro drug capecitabine.

Palmar–plantar erythrodysesthesia syndrome (also called acral erythema, hand–foot syndrome, toxic erythema of the palms and soles, and Burgdof's syndrome) This is a painful rash seen in association with continuously infused 5-fluoruracil, capecitabine, and liposomal doxorubicin. It has also been reported with paclitaxel. It is characterized by the development of a tingling or burning sensation in the palms and soles followed by the development of an erythematous rash. The pathogenesis is unknown. The eruption is self-limiting in nature and it does not usually require discontinuation of therapy. Symptomatic measures are often required[52], and treatment with pyridoxine has been reported to induce resolution of the lesions[53].

Post-chemotherapy gynaecomastia Painful gynaecomastia can occur as a delayed complication of chemotherapy. Testis cancer is the most common underlying disorder, but it has been reported after therapy for other cancers as well. Gynaecomastia typically develops after a latency of 2–9 months and resolves spontaneously within a few months. Persistent gynaecomastia is occasionally observed[54].

Chemotherapy-induced acute digital ischaemia Raynaud's phenomenon or transient ischaemia of the toes is a common complication of bleomycin, vinblastine, and cisplatin (PVB) treatment for testicular cancer[55]. Rarely, irreversible digital ischaemia leading to gangrene has been reported after bleomycin. Capecitabine and vincristine have been implicated in case reports.

Chemotherapy-induced tumour pain Pain at the site of tumour is reported to occur in some patients (7 per cent) after treatment with vinorelbine. Typically, pain begins within a few minutes of the vinorelbine infusion, is moderate to severe in intensity, and requires analgesic therapy.

Acute pain associated with hormonal therapy

Leutenizing hormone releasing factor (LHRF) tumour flare in prostate cancer Initiation of LHRF hormonal therapy for prostate cancer produces a transient symptom flare in 5–25 per cent of patients. The flare is presumably caused by an initial stimulation of leutenizing hormone release before suppression is achieved. The syndrome typically presents as an exacerbation of bone pain or urinary retention; spinal cord compression and sudden death have been reported[56]. Symptom flare is usually observed within the first week of therapy, and lasts 1–3 weeks in the absence of androgen antagonist therapy. Co-administration of an androgen antagonist during the initiation of LHRF agonist therapy can prevent this phenomenon.

Hormone-induced pain flare in breast cancer Any hormonal therapy for metastatic breast cancer can be complicated by a sudden onset of diffuse musculoskeletal pain commencing within hours to weeks of the initiation of therapy[57]. Other manifestations of this syndrome include erythema around cutaneous metastases, changes in liver function studies, and hypercalcaemia. Although the underlying mechanism is not understood, this does not appear to be caused by tumour stimulation, and it is speculated that it may reflect normal tissue response.

Aromotase inhibitor-induced arthralgias Aromotase inhibitor medications used in the hormonal therapy of breast cancer may cause a multifocal arthralgia syndrome in 10–20 per cent of patients[58]. This most commonly manisfests as early morning stiffness and hand/wrist pain. Pain intensity is variable, and in some patients, it precudes interferes in daily activities. Occasionally, it is reason to discontinue treatment due to severe symptoms. The possible mechanisms are unclear. Treatment options for arthralgia (primarily NSAIDs) are often inadequate, and areas of active research include high-dose vitamin D and new-targeted therapies to inhibit bone loss.

Acute pain associated with immunotherapy

Interferon (IFN)-induced acute pain Virtually all patients treated with IFN experience an acute syndrome consisting of fever, chills, myalgias, arthralgias, and headache. The syndrome usually begins shortly after initial dosing and frequently improves with continued administration of the drug[59]. Doses of 1–9 million units of alpha-interferon are usually tolerated, but doses greater than or equal to 18 million units usually produce moderate-to-severe toxicity[59]. Acetaminophen pretreatment is often useful in ameliorating these symptoms.

Acute pain associated with bisphosphonates

Bisphosphonate-induced bone pain Bisphosphonates are widely used in the care of patients with bony metastases[60]. Infusion of bisphosphonate is commonly associated with the development of multifocal bone pain and or myalgia. Typically, pain occurs within 24 h of infusion and may last up to 3 days. Pain intensity is variable and may be severe. Symptoms usually resolve following discontinuation of therapy and may recur with rechallenge of the same or different bisphosphonate. The condition is self-limiting and may require analgesic therapy but, rarely, pain can be persistent.

Acute pain associated with growth factors

Granulocyte-macrophage CSF (GM-CSF) and granulocyte CSF (G-CSF) commonly produce mild-to-moderate bone pain and constitutional symptoms such as fever, headache, and myalgias during the period of administration. In studies of G-CSF in dose-dense chemotherapy, the prevalence of pain is 20–30 per cent[61,62]. Pain intensity is variable and may be severe. Co-administration of dexamethasone may reduce the prevalence and severity of bone pain.

Subcutaneous administration of r-HuEPO alpha is associated with pain at the injection site in about 40 per cent of cases. Subcutaneous injection of r-HuEPO alpha is more painful than r-HuEPO beta. Alpha erythropoietin injection pain can be reduced by dilution of the vehicle with benzyl alcohol saline, reduction of the volume of the vehicle from 1.0 to 0.1 ml or addition of lidocaine.

Acute pain associated with radiotherapy

Incident pains can be precipitated by transport and positioning of the patient for radiotherapy. Other pains can be caused by acute radiation toxicity, which is most commonly associated with inflammation and ulceration of skin or mucous membranes within the radiation port. The syndrome produced is dependent upon the involved field: head and neck irradiation can cause a stomatitis or pharyngitis, treatment of the chest and esophagus can cause an oesophagitis, and pelvic therapy can cause a proctitis, cystitis-urethritis, vaginal ulceration, or radiation dermatitis.

Oropharyngeal mucositis Radiotherapy-induced mucositis is invariable with doses above 1000 cGy, and ulceration is common at doses above 4000 cGy. Although the severity of the associated pain is variable, it is often severe enough to interfere with oral alimentation. Painful mucositis can persist for several weeks after the completion of the treatment.

Acute radiation enteritis and proctocolitis Acute radiation enteritis occurs in as many as 50 per cent of patients receiving abdominal or pelvic radiotherapy. Involvement of the small intestine can present with cramping abdominal pain associated with nausea and diarrhoea. Pelvic radiotherapy can cause a painful proctocolitis, with tenesmoid pain associated with diarrhoea, mucous discharge, and bleeding. These complications typically resolve shortly after completion of therapy, but may have a slow resolution over 2–6 months. Acute enteritis predicts for an increased risk of late onset radiation enteritis (see following paragraphs).

Early onset brachial plexopathy A transient brachial plexopathy has been described in breast cancer patients immediately following radiotherapy, to the chest wall and adjacent nodal areas[63], and after mantle radiotherapy for Hodgkin's disease[64]. In retrospective studies, the incidence of this phenomenon has been variably

estimated as 1.4–20 per cent[63,65]; clinical experience suggests that lower estimates are more accurate. The median latency to the development of symptoms was 4.5 months (3–14 months) in one survey[65]. Paresthesias are the most common presenting symptom, and pain and weakness occur less frequently. The syndrome is self-limiting and is not predictive of the subsequent development of delayed onset, progressive plexopathy.

Subacute radiation myelopathy Subacute radiation myelopathy is an uncommon phenomenon that may occur following radiotherapy of extraspinal tumours[66]. It is most frequently observed involving the cervical cord after radiation treatment of head and neck cancers and Hodgkin's disease. In the latter case, patients develop painful, shock-like pains in the neck that are precipitated by neck flexion (Lhermitte's sign); these pains may radiate down the spine and into one or more extremities. The syndrome usually begins weeks to months after the completion of radiotherapy, and typically resolves over a period of 3–6 months[66].

Radiopharmaceutical-induced pain flare Strontium-89, rhenium-186 hydroxyethylidene diphosphonate, and samarium-153 are systemically administered beta-emitting calcium analogues that are taken up by bone in areas of osteoblastic activity and which may help relieve pain caused by blastic bony metastases. A 'flare' response, characterized by transient worsening of pain 1–2 days after administration, occurs in 15–20 per cent of patients[67]. This flare usually resolves after 3–5 days and most affected patients subsequently develop a good analgesic response[67].

Acute pain associated with infection

Acute herpetic neuralgia

A significantly increased incidence of acute herpetic neuralgia occurs among cancer patients, especially those with hematological or lymphoproliferative malignancies and those receiving immunosuppressive therapies. The pain, which may be continuous or lancinating, usually resolves within 2 months. Pain persisting beyond this interval is referred to as postherpetic neuralgia (see following paragraphs). Patients with active tumour are more likely to have a disseminated infection[68]. In those predisposed by chemotherapy, the infection usually develops less than 1 month after the completion of treatment. The dermatomal location of the infection is often associated with the site of the malignancy[68]. The infection also occurs twice as frequently in previously irradiated dermatomes as non-radiated areas[69].

Acute pain associated with vascular events

Acute thrombosis pain

Thrombosis is the most frequent complication and the second cause of death in patients with overt malignant disease[70]. Thrombotic episodes may precede the diagnosis of cancer by months or years and represent a potential marker for occult malignancy. Postoperative deep vein thrombosis is more frequent in patients operated for malignant diseases than for other disorders, and both chemotherapy and hormone therapy are associated with an increased thrombotic risk[70].

Possible prothrombic factors in cancer include the capacity of tumour cells and their products to interact with platelets, clotting and fibrinolytic systems, endothelial cells, and tumour-associated macrophages. Cytokine release, acute phase reaction, and neovascularization may contribute to vivo clotting activation. Data from a very large cohort of 66 329 cancer patients demonstrated that bone, ovary, brain, and pancreas cancers are associated with the highest incidence of thrombosis and distant metastases, chemotherapy, and hormonal therapy, all led to 1.5–2.5x increased risk.

Lower-extremity deep venous thrombosis Pain and swelling are the commonest presenting features of lower-extremity deep vein thrombosis. The pain is variable in severity and it is often mild. It is commonly described as a dull cramp, or diffuse heaviness. The pain most commonly affects the calf but may involve the sole of the foot, the heel, the thigh, the groin or pelvis. Pain usually increases on standing and walking. On examination, suggestive features include swelling, warmth, dilatation of superficial veins, tenderness along venous tracts, and pain induced by stretching.

Rarely, patients may develop tissue ischaemia or frank gangrene, even without arterial or capillary occlusion; this syndrome is called phlegmasia cerulea dolens. It is most commonly seen in patients with underlying neoplasm[71] and is characterized by severe pain, extensive oedema, and cyanosis of the legs. Gangrene can occur unless the venous obstruction is relieved. Intravenous thrombolytic therapy may be more effective than traditional treatments with anticoagulation and thrombectomy. Until recently, the mortality rate for ischemic venous thrombosis was about 30–40 per cent, the cause of death usually being the underlying disease or pulmonary emboli.

Upper-extremity deep venous thrombosis The three major clinical features of upper-extremity venous thrombosis are oedema, dilated collateral circulation, and pain. Approximately two-thirds of patients have arm pain. Among patients with cancer, the most common causes are central venous catheterization and extrinsic compression by tumour[72]. Although thrombosis secondary to intrinsic damage usually responded well to anticoagulation alone and rarely causes persistent symptoms, when extrinsic obstruction is the cause, persistent arm swelling and pain are commonplace.

Superior vena cava obstruction Superior vena cava (SVC) obstruction is most commonly caused by extrinsic compression by enlarged mediastinal lymph nodes[73]. In contemporary series, lung cancer and lymphomas are the most commonly associated conditions. Increasingly, thrombosis of the superior vena cava is caused by intravascular devices[74], particularly with left-sided ports, and when the catheter tip lies in the upper part of the vena. Patient usually present with facial swelling and dilated neck and chest wall veins. Chest pain, headache, and mastalgia are less common presentations.

Acute mesenteric vein thrombosis Acute mesenteric vein thrombosis is most commonly associated with hypercoaguability states. Rarely it has been associated with extrinsic venous compression by malignant lymphadenopathy, extension of venous thrombosis, or as a result of iatrogenic hypercoaguable state.

Superficial thrombophlebitis Superficial thrombophlebitis is more common among patients with cancer. It presents with the development of a palpable tender cord in the course of a superficial vein; often associated with erythema of the overlying skin. Duplex ultrasound should be considered to rule out occult DVT, particularly when the greater or lesser saphenous veins are involved.

Trousseau's syndrome or migratory thrombophlebitis is a rare condition characterized by a recurrent and migratory pattern and involvement of superficial veins, frequently in unusual sites such as the arm or chest[75].

Chronic pain syndromes

Most chronic cancer-related pains are caused directly by the tumour. Data from the largest prospective survey of cancer pain syndromes revealed that almost one-quarter of the patients experienced two or more pains. Over 90 per cent of the patients had one or more tumour-related pains and 21 per cent had one or more pains caused by cancer therapies. Somatic pains (71 per cent) were more common than neuropathic (39 per cent) or visceral pains (34 per cent)[76]. Bone pain and compression of neural structures are the two most common causes.

Bone pain

Bone metastases are the most common cause of chronic pain in cancer patients. Cancers of the lung, breast, and prostate most often metastasize to bone, but any tumour type may be complicated by painful bony lesions. Although bone pain is usually associated with direct tumour invasion of bony structures, more than 25 per cent of patients with bony metastases are pain-free[77], and patients with multiple bony metastases typically report pain in only a few sites. The pathophysiology of bone pain is reviewed in Chapter 10.1.4.

Differential diagnosis

Bone pain due to metastatic tumour needs to be differentiated from less common causes. Non-neoplastic causes in this population include osteoporotic fractures (including those associated with multiple myeloma), focal osteonecrosis, which may be idiopathic or related to chemotherapy, corticosteroids or radiotherapy (see following paragraphs), and osteomalacia. Rarely, a paraneoplastic osteomalacia, which is assocated with elevated levels of fibroblast growth factor 23, can mimic multiple metastases[78].

Multifocal or generalized bone pain

Bone pain may be focal, multifocal, or generalized. Multifocal bone pains are most commonly experienced by patients with multiple bony metastases. A generalized pain syndrome is occasionally produced by replacement of bone marrow[79]. This bone marrow replacement syndrome has been observed in hematogenous malignancies and, less commonly, in solid tumours and brain tumours. This syndrome can occur in the absence of abnormalities on bone scintigraphy or radiography, increasing the difficulty of diagnosis. It is best demonstrated on MRI imaging[80].

Vertebral syndromes

The vertebrae are the most common sites of bony metastases. More than two-thirds of vertebral metastases are located in the thoracic spine; lumbosacral and cervical metastases account for approximately 20 per cent and 10 per cent, respectively. Multiple-level involvement is common, occurring in greater than 85 per cent of patients[81]. The early recognition of pain syndromes due to tumour invasion of vertebral bodies is essential, because pain usually precedes compression of adjacent neural structures, and prompt treatment of the lesion may prevent the subsequent development of neurologic deficits. Several factors often confound accurate diagnosis; referral of pain is common, and the associated symptoms and signs can mimic a variety of other disorders, both malignant (e.g. paraspinal masses) and nonmalignant.

Atlantoaxial destruction and odontoid fracture Nuchal or occipital pain is the typical presentation of destruction of the atlas or fracture of the odontoid process. Pain often radiates over the posterior aspect of the skull to the vertex and is exacerbated by movement of the neck, particularly flexion. Pathologic fracture may result in secondary subluxation with ompression of the spinal cord at the cervicomedullary junction. This complication is usually insidious and may begin with symptoms or signs in one or more extremity. Typically, there is early involvement of the upper extremities and the occasional appearance of so-called 'pseudo-levels' suggestive of more caudal spinal lesions; these deficits can slowly progress to involve sensory, motor, and autonomic function in the[82].

C7–T1 syndrome Invasion of the C7 or T1 vertebra can result in pain referred to the interscapular region. These lesions may be missed if radiographic evaluation is mistakenly targeted to the painful area caudal to the site of damage. Additionally, visualization of the appropriate region on routine radiographs may be inadequate due to obscuration by overlying bone and mediastinal shadows. Patients with interscapular pain should therefore undergo radiography of both the cervical and the thoracic spine.

T12–L1 syndrome: A T12 or L1 vertebral lesion can refer pain to the ipsilateral iliac crest or the sacroiliac joint. Imaging procedures directed at pelvic bones can miss the source of the pain.

Sacral syndrome Severe focal pain radiating to buttocks, perineum, or posterior thighs may accompany destruction of the sacrum. The pain is often exacerbated by sitting or lying and is relieved by standing or walking. The neoplasm can spread laterally to involve muscles that rotate the hip (e.g. the pyriformis muscle). This may produce severe incident pain induced by motion of the hip, or a malignant 'pyriformis syndrome', characterized by buttock or posterior leg pain that is exacerbated by internal rotation of the hip. Local extension of the tumour mass may also involve the sacral plexus (see following paragraphs).

Back pain and epidural compression (see Chapter 10.11)

Epidural compression of the spinal cord or cauda equina is the second most common neurologic complication of cancer, occurring in up to 10 per cent of patients. In a large retrospective series, 0.23 per cent of cancer patients had epidural compression at the presentation of their disease and 2.5 per cent of patients dying of cancer had at least one admission for cord compression in the 5 years preceding death[83]. Breast, lung, and prostate cancers each account for 20–25 per cent of events[83,84]. Most epidural compression is caused by posterior extension of vertebral body metastasis to the epidural space. Occasionally, epidural compression is caused by tumour extension from the posterior arch of the vertebra or infiltration of a paravertebral tumour through the intervertebral foramen.

Untreated, epidural compression leads inevitably to neurological damage. Effective treatment can potentially prevent these complications. The most important determinate of the efficacy of treatment is the degree of neurological impairment at the time therapy is initiated. Seventy-five per cent of patients who begin treatment while ambulatory remain so; the efficacy of treatment declines to 30–50 per cent for those who begin treatment while markedly paretic, and is 10–20 per cent for those who are plegic[85]. Despite this, delays in diagnosis are commonplace.

Back pain is the initial symptom in almost all patients with epidural compression[86], and in 10 per cent it is the only symptom at the time of diagnosis. Because pain usually precedes neurologic signs by a prolonged period, it should be viewed as a potential indicator of epidural compression, which can lead to treatment at a time that a favourable response is most likely.

Back pain, however, is a non-specific symptom that can result from bony or paraspinal metastases without epidural encroachment, from retroperitoneal or leptomeningeal tumour, epidural lipomatosis due to steroid administration, or from a large variety of other benign conditions. Because it is not feasible to pursue an extensive evaluation in every cancer patient who develops back pain, the complaint should impel an evaluation that determines the likelihood of epidural compression and thereby selects patients appropriate for definitive imaging of the epidural space. The selection process is based on symptoms and signs and the results of simple imaging techniques.

Clinical features of epidural extension Some pain characteristics are particularly suggestive of epidural extension [87]. Rapid progression of back pain in a crescendo pattern is an ominous occurrence[88]. Radicular pain, which can be constant or lancinating has similar implications[87]. It is usually unilateral in the cervical and lumbosacral regions and bilateral in the thorax, where it is often experienced as a tight, belt-like band across the chest or abdomen[87]. The likelihood of epidural compression is also greater when back or radicular pain is exacerbated by recumbency, cough, sneeze, or strain. Other types of referred pain are also suggestive, including Lhermitte's sign and central pain from spinal cord compression, which usually is perceived some distance below the site of the compression and is typically a poorly localized, non-dermatomal dysesthesia.

Weakness, sensory loss, autonomic dysfunction, and reflex abnormalities usually occur after a period of progressive pain[87]. Weakness may begin segmentally if related to nerve root damage or in a multisegmental or pyramidal distribution if the cauda equina or spinal cord, respectively, is injured. The rate of progression of weakness is variable; in the absence of treatment, following the onset of weakness, one-third of patients will develop paralysis within 7 days[89]. Without effective treatment, sensory abnormalities, which may also begin segmentally, may ultimately evolve to a sensory level, with complete loss of all sensory modalities below site of injury. The upper level of sensory findings may correspond to the location of the epidural tumour or be below it by many segments[87]. Ataxia without pain is the initial presentation of epidural compression in 1 per cent of patients; this finding is presumably due to early involvement of the spinocerebellar tracts[90]. Bladder and bowel dysfunction occur late, except in patients with a conus medullaris lesion who may present with acute urinary retention and constipation without preceding motor or sensory symptoms[87].

Other features that may be evident on examination of patients with epidural compression include scoliosis, asymmetrical wasting of paravertebral musculature, and a gibbus (palpable step in the spinous processes). Spinal tenderness to percussion, which may be severe, often accompanies the pain.

Diagnosis and management of spinal cord compression is reviewed in Chapters 9.4, 9.5, and 10.11.

Pain syndromes of the bony pelvis and hip

The pelvis and hip are common sites of metastatic involvement. Lesions may involve any of the three anatomic regions of the pelvis (ischiopubic, iliosacral, or periacetabular), the hip joint itself, or the proximal femur. The weight-bearing function of these structures, essential for normal ambulation, contributes to the propensity of disease at these sites to cause incident pain with walking and weight bearing.

Hip joint syndrome Tumour involvement of the acetabulum or head of femur typically produces localized hip pain that is aggravated by weight bearing and movement of the hip. The pain may radiate to the knee or medial thigh, and occasionally, pain is limited to these structures. Medial extension of an acetabular tumour can involve the lumbosacral plexus as it traverses the pelvic sidewall. Evaluation of this region is best accomplished with CT or MRI, both of which can demonstrate the extent of bony destruction and adjacent soft tissue involvement more sensitively than other imaging techniques[91]. Important differential diagnoses include avascular necrosis, radicular pain (usually L1) or, occasionally, occult infections.

Acrometastases

Acrometastases, metastases in the hands and feet, are rare and often misdiagnosed or overlooked. In the feet, the larger bones containing the higher amounts of red marrow, such as the os calcis, or talus, are usually involved. Symptoms may be vague and can mimic other conditions, such as osteomyelitis, gouty rheumatoid arthritis, Reiter's syndrome, Paget's disease, osteochondral lesions, and ligamentous sprains.

Arthritidies

Hypertrophic pulmonary osteoarthropathy (HPOA) A paraneoplastic syndrome that incorporates clubbing of the fingers, periostitis of long bones, and occasionally a rheumatoid-like poly-arthritis[92]. Periosteitis and arthritis can produce pain, tenderness and swelling in the knees, wrists, and ankles. The onset of symptoms is usually subacute, and it may precede the discovery of the underlying neoplasm by several months. It is most commonly associated with non-small cell lung cancer. Less commonly, it may be associated with benign mesothelioma, pulmonary metastases from other sites, smooth muscle tumours of the oesophagus, breast cancer, and metastatic nasopharyngeal cancer. HPOA is diagnosed on the basis of physical findings, radiological appearance, and radionuclide bone scan. Effective anti-tumour therapy is sometimes associated with symptom regression and bisphosphonate therapy may help relieve symptoms[93,94].

Other polyarthritides Rarely, rheumatoid arthritis, systemic lupus erythematosus, and an asymmetrical polyarthritis may occur as paraneoplastic phenomena that resolve with effective treatment of the underlying disease[95,96]. A syndrome of palmar plantar fasciitis and polyarthritis characterized by palmar and digital with polyarticular painful capsular contractions, has been associated with ovarian, breast, and gastric cancers.

Muscle pain

Muscle cramps

Persistent muscle cramps in cancer patients are usually caused by an identifiable neural, muscular, or biochemical abnormality. In one series of 50 patients, 22 had peripheral neuropathy, 17 had root or plexus pathology (including 6 with leptomeningeal metastases), 2 had polymyositis, and 1 had hypomagnesemia. In this series, muscle cramps were the presenting symptom of recognizable and previously unsuspected neurologic dysfunction in 64 per cent (27 of 42) of the identified causes[97]. Cramps have been reported as an adverse effect of imatinib, goserelin, and vincristine.

Skeletal muscle tumours

Soft-tissue sarcomas arising from fat, fibrous tissue, or skeletal muscle are the most common tumours involving the skeletal muscles. Skeletal muscle is one of the most unusual sites of metastasis from any malignancy. They occur disproportionately at sites of prior muscle trauma. Lesions are usually painless but they may present with persistent ache.

Headache and facial pain

Headache in the cancer patient results from traction, inflammation or infiltration of pain-sensitive structures in the head or neck. Early evaluation with appropriate imaging techniques may identify the lesion and allow prompt treatment, which may reduce pain and prevent the development of neurological deficits[98].

Intracerebral tumour (see Chapter 10.11)

Among 183 patients with new onset chronic headache, as an isolated symptom, investigation revealed underlying tumour in 15 cases[99]. The prevalence of headache in patients with brain metastases or primary brain tumours is 60–90 per cent and headache is often the first presenting symptom of patients with brain tumours or metastases[100,101]. The headache is presumably produced by traction on pain-sensitive vascular and dural tissues. Patients with multiple metastases and those with posterior fossa metastases are more likely to report this symptom. The pain may be focal, overlying the site of the lesion, or generalized. Headache has lateralizing value, especially in patients with supratentorial lesions. Posterior fossa lesions often cause a bifrontal headache. The quality of the headache is usually throbbing or steady, and the intensity is usually mild to moderate[101].

Among children, clinical features predictive of underlying tumour include sleep-related headache, headache in the absence of a family history of migraine, vomiting, absence of visual symptoms, headache of less than 6 months duration, confusion, and abnormal neurologic examination findings[102]. The headache is often worse in the morning and is exacerbated by stooping, sudden head movement or valsalva maneuvers (cough, sneeze, or strain)[103].

Leptomeningeal metastases

Leptomeningeal metastases, which are characterized by diffuse or multifocal involvement of the subarachnoid space by metastatic tumour occur in 1–8 per cent in patients with systemic cancer[104]. Non-Hodgkin's lymphoma and acute lymphocytic leukaemia, both demonstrate predilection for meningeal metastases; the incidence is lower for solid tumours[105]. Of solid tumours, adenocarcinomas of the breast and small-cell lung cancer predominate[105].

Leptomeningeal metastases present with focal or multifocal neurological symptoms or signs that may involve any level of the neuraxis. More than one-third of patients present with evidence of cranial nerve damage, including double vision, hearing loss, facial numbness, and decreased vision[106,107]. This is particularly true among patients with underlying hematologic malignancy[107]. Less common features include seizures, papilloedema, hemiparesis, ataxic gait, and confusion.

Generalized headache and radicular pain in the low back and buttocks are the most common pains associated with leptomeningeal metastases[107]. The headache is variable and may be associated with changes in mental status (e.g. lethargy, confusion, or loss of memory), nausea, vomiting, tinnitus or nuchal rigidity. Pains that resemble cluster headache or glossopharyngeal neuralgia with syncope have also been reported. Diagnosis and treatment are reviewed in Chapter 10.11.

Base of skull metastases

Base of skull metastases are associated with well-described clinical syndromes[108], which are named according to the site of metastatic involvement: orbital, parasellar, middle fossa, jugular foramen, occipital condyle, clivus, and sphenoid sinus. Cancers of the breast, lung, and prostate are most commonly associated with this complication[108,109], but any tumour type that metastasizes to bone may be responsible. When base of skull metastases are suspected, axial imaging with CT (including bone window settings) is the usual initial procedure[108]. MRI is more sensitive for assessing soft-tissue extension, and CSF analysis may be needed to exclude leptomeningeal metastases.

Orbital syndrome Orbital metastases usually present with progressive pain in the retroorbital and supraorbital area of the affected eye. Blurred vision and diplopia may be associated complaints. Signs may include proptosis, chemosis of the involved eye, external ophthalmoparesis, ipsilateral papilloedema, and decreased sensation in the ophthalmic division of the trigeminal nerve.

Parasellar syndrome The parasellar syndrome typically presents as unilateral supraorbital and frontal headache, which may be associated with diplopia[110]. There may be opthalmoparesis or papilloedema, and formal visual field testing may demonstrate hemianopsia or quadrantinopsia.

Middle cranial fossa syndrome The middle cranial fossa syndrome presents with facial numbness, paresthesias or pain, which is usually referred to the cheek or jaw (in the distribution of second or third divisions of the trigeminal nerve)[111]. The pain is typically described as a dull continual ache, but may also be paroxysmal or lancinating. On examination, patients may have hypesthesia in the trigeminal nerve distribution and signs of weakness in the ipsilateral muscles of mastication. Occasional patients have other neurological signs, such as abducens palsy[108].

Jugular foramen syndrome The jugular foramen syndrome usually presents with hoarseness or dysphagia. Pain is usually referred to the ipsilateral ear or mastoid region and may occasionally present as glossopharyngeal neuralgia, with or without syncope[108]. Pain may also be referred to the ipsilateral neck or shoulder. Neurologic signs include ipsilateral Horner's syndrome, and paresis of the palate, vocal cord, sternocleidomastoid, or trapezius. Ipsilateral paresis of the tongue may also occur if the tumour extends to the region of the hypoglossal canal.

Occipital condyle syndrome The occipital condyle syndrome presents with unilateral occipital pain that is worsened with neck flexion[112,113]. The patient may complain of neck stiffness. Pain intensity is variable, but can be severe. Examination may reveal a head tilt, limited movement of the neck, and tenderness to palpation over the occipitonuchal junction. Neurological findings may include ipsilateral hypoglossal nerve paralysis and sternocleidomastoid weakness[114].

Clivus syndrome The clivus syndrome is characterized by vertex headache, which is often exacerbated by neck flexion. Lower cranial nerve (VI–XII) dysfunction may develop[115] and may become bilateral[116].

Sphenoid sinus syndrome A sphenoid sinus metastasis often presents with bifrontal and or retroorbital pain, which may radiate to the temporal regions[117]. There may be associated features of nasal congestion and diplopia[118]. Physical examination is often unremarkable, although unilateral or bilateral sixth nerve paresis can be present.

Painful cranial neuralgias

As noted, specific cranial neuralgias can occur from metastases in the base of skull or leptomeninges. They are most commonly observed in patients with prostate and lung cancer. Invasion of the soft tissues of the head or neck, or involvement of sinuses can also eventuate in such lesions. Each of these syndromes has a characteristic presentation. Early diagnosis may allow effective treatment of the underlying lesion before progressive neurologic injury occurs.

Glossopharyngeal neuralgia Glossopharyngeal neuralgia has been reported in patients with leptomeningeal metastases[119], the jugular foramen syndrome[108], or head and neck malignancies[120]. This syndrome presents as severe pain in the throat or neck, which may radiate to the ear or mastoid region. Pain may be induced by swallowing. In some patients, pain is associated with sudden orthostasis and syncope.

Trigeminal neuralgia Trigeminal pains may be continual, paroxysmal, or lancinating. Pain that mimics classical trigeminal neuralgia can be induced by tumours in the middle or posterior fossa or leptomeningeal metastases. Sometimes, pain may be caused by perineural spread without evidence of a discrete mass[121]. Continual pain in a trigeminal distribution may be an early sign of acoustic neuroma. All cancer patients who develop trigeminal neuralgia should be evaluated for the existence of an underlying neoplasm.

Ear and eye pain syndromes

Otalgia Otalgia is the sensation of pain in the ear, while referred otalgia is pain felt in the ear but originating from a nonotologic source. The rich sensory innervation of the ear derives from four cranial nerves and two cervical nerves, which also supply other areas in the head, neck, thorax, and abdomen. Pain referred to the ear may originate in areas far removed from the ear itself. Otalgia may be caused by acoustic neuroma and metastases to the temporal bone or infratemporal fossa. Referred otalgia is reported among patients with tumours involving the oropharynx or hypopharynx.

Eye pain Blurring of vision and eye pain are the two most common symptoms of choroidal metastases[122]. More commonly, chronic eye pain is related to metastases to the bony orbit, intraorbital structures such as the rectus muscles or optic nerve.

Uncommon causes of headache and facial pain

Headache and facial pain in cancer patients may have many other causes. Unilateral facial pain can be the initial symptom of an ipsilateral lung tumour[123]. Presumably, this referred pain is mediated by vagal afferents. Facial squamous cell carcinoma of the skin may present with facial pain due to extensive perineural invasion. Patients with Hodgkin's disease may have transient episodes of neurological dysfunction that has been likened to migraine[124]. In some cases, this may be a reversible posterior leukoencephalopathy syndrome (RPLS), which is characterized by headache, conscious disturbance, seizure, and cortical visual loss with neuroimaging finding of oedema in the posterior regions of the brain[125].

Headache may occur with cerebral infarction or haemorrhage, which may be due to nonbacterial thrombotic endocarditis or disseminated intravascular coagulation. Headache is also the usual presentation of sagittal sinus occlusion, which may be due to tumour infiltration, hypercoaguable state, or treatment with L-asparaginase therapy[126]. Headache due to pseudotumour cerebri has also been reported to be the presentation of superior vena caval obstruction in a patient with lung cancer. Tumours of the sinonasal tract may present with deep facial or nasal pain (Fig. 10.1.2.5).

Neuropathic pains involving the peripheral nervous system

Neuropathic pains involving the peripheral nervous system are common. The syndromes include painful radiculopathy, plexopathy, mononeuropathy, or peripheral neuropathy.

Painful radiculopathy

Radiculopathy or polyradiculopathy may be caused by any process that compresses, distorts, or inflames nerve roots. Painful radiculopathy is an important presentation of epidural tumour and leptomeningeal metastases (see earlier paragraphs).
Postherpetic neuralgia (PHN) The precise clinical definition of PHN has been a matter of disipute. There is agreement that acute herpetic neuralgia refers to pain preceding or accompanying the eruption of rash that persists up to 30 days from its onset. Some authorities refer to all persistent pain as PHN, others describe a subacute herpetic neuralgia that persists beyond healing of the rash, but which resolves within four months of onset, reserving the term PHN that refers to pain persisting beyond 4 months from the initial onset of the rash[127]. One study suggests that postherpetic neuralgia is two to three times more frequent in the cancer population than the general population[68].

Cervical plexopathy

Among cancer patients, cervical plexus injury is frequently due to tumour infiltration or treatment (including surgery or radiotherapy) to neoplasms in this region[128]. Tumour invasion or compression of the cervical plexus can be caused by direct extension of a primary head and neck malignancy or neoplastic (metastatic or lymphomatous) involvement of the cervical lymph nodes[128]. Pain may be experienced in the preauricular (greater auricular nerve) or postauricular (lesser and greater occipital nerves) regions, or the

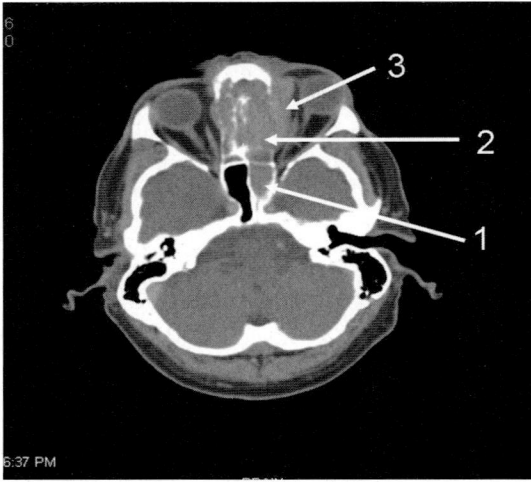

Figure 10.1.2.5 Axial CT scan of 54-year-old man with tumour arising in paranasal sinuses with extension to the orbit and nasopharynx.

anterior neck (transverse cutaneous and supraclavicular nerves). Pain may refer to the lateral aspect of the face or head, or to the ipsilateral shoulder. The overlap in the pain referral patterns from the face and neck may relate to the close anatomic relationship between the central connections of cervical afferents and the afferents carried in cranial nerves V, VII, IX, and X in the upper cervical spinal cord.

Associated features can include ipsilateral Horner's syndrome or hemidiaphragmatic paralysis. The diagnosis must be distinguished from epidural compression of the cervical spinal cord and leptomeningeal metastases. MRI or CT imaging of the neck and cervical spine is usually required to evaluate the aetiology of the pain.

Brachial plexopathy

The two most common causes of brachial plexopathy in cancer patients are tumour infiltration and radiation injury. Less common causes of painful brachial plexopathy include trauma during surgery or anesthesia, radiation-induced second neoplasms, acute brachial plexus ischaemia, and paraneoplastic brachial neuritis.
Malignant brachial plexopathy Plexus infiltration by tumour is the most prevalent cause of brachial plexopathy. Malignant brachial plexopathy is most common in patients with lymphoma, lung or breast cancer. The invading tumour usually arises from adjacent axillary, cervical and supraclavicular lymph nodes (lymphoma and breast cancer), or from the lung (superior sulcus tumours or so-called Pancoast tumours)[129,130]. Pain is nearly universal, occurring in 85 per cent of patients, and often precedes neurologic signs or symptoms by months[129]. Lower plexus involvement (C7, C8, T1 distribution) is typical, and is reflected in the pain distribution, which usually involves the elbow, medial forearm, and fourth and fifth fingers. Pain may sometimes localize to the posterior arm or elbow. Severe aching is usually reported, but patients may also experience constant or lancinating dysesthesias along the ulnar aspect of the forearm or hand.

Tumour infiltration of the upper plexus (C5–C6 distribution) is less common. This lesion is characterized by pain in the shoulder girdle, lateral arm, and hand. Seventy-five per cent of patients presenting with upper plexopathy subsequently develop a panplexopathy, and 25 per cent of patients present with panplexopathy.

Cross-sectional imaging is essential in all patients with symptoms or signs compatible with plexopathy (Fig. 10.1.2.6). Although comparative data on the sensitivity and specificity of MRI to CT in evaluating lesions of the brachial plexus is not available, the MRI is widely thought to be the best choice for evaluating the anatomy and pathology of the brachial plexus[131,132]. Limited experience has been reported for PET-CT imaging[133].

Electrodiagnostic studies may be helpful in patients with suspected plexopathy, particularly when neurological examination and imaging studies are normal[134]. Although not specific for tumour, abnormalities on electromyography (EMG) or somatosensory evoked potentials may establish the diagnosis of plexopathy, and thereby confirm the need for additional evaluation.

Patients with malignant brachial plexopathy are at elevated risk for epidural extension of the tumour. Epidural encroachment can occur as the neoplasm grows medially and invades vertebrae or tracks along nerve roots through the intervertebral foramina. In the latter case, there may be no evidence of bony erosion on imaging studies. The development of Horner's syndrome, evidence of pan-plexopathy, or finding of paraspinal tumour or vertebral damage

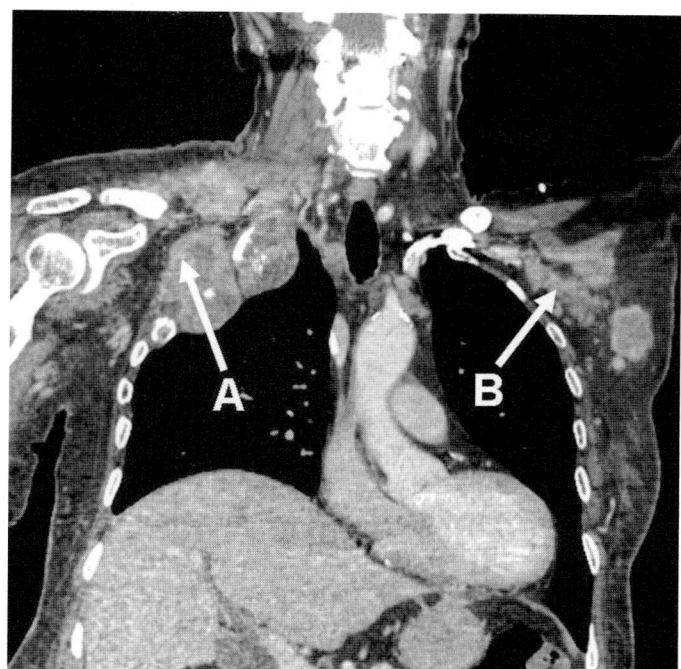

Figure 10.1.2.6 Coronal CT reconstruction of a patient with bilateral brachial plexopathy. Arrow A shows bulky metastases arisng from ribs compressing inferior right plexus. Arrow B shows tumour infiltrates deposited on left plexus.

on CT or MRI are highly associated with epidural extension and should lead to definitive imaging of the epidural tumour[128, 135].

Radiation-induced brachial plexopathy Two distinct syndromes of radiation-induced brachial plexopathy have been described: (1) early onset transient plexopathy (see earlier paragraphs) and (2) delayed onset progressive plexopathy. Delayed onset progressive plexopathy can occur 6 months to 20 years after a course of radiotherapy that included the plexus in the radiation portal. In contrast to tumour infiltration, pain is a relatively uncommon presenting symptom (18 per cent), and when present, is usually less severe[136]. After surpraclavicular node radiotherapy, there is a progressively increasing incidence over time which rises to 56 per cent after 20 years[137]. Weakness and sensory changes predominate in the distribution of the upper plexus (C5, C6 distribution). Radiation changes in the skin and lymphoedema are commonly associated.

The typical appearance of radiation fibrosis of the plexus on CT studies is a diffuse infiltration and loss of tissue planes without a mass lesion. There is often associated lymphoedema in the arm, evident on CT, and occasionally, radiation necrosis of the clavicle or rib or humeral head occurs at the adjacent level. Tumour infiltration of the plexus cannot be differentiated from radiation fibrosis by CT studies when diffuse infiltration is noted. On MRI, the most common findings observed with radiation fibrosis are thickening and diffuse enhancement of the brachial plexus without a focal mass and/or soft-tissue changes with low signal intensity on both T1- and T2-weighted images[132].

Electrodiagnostic studies in patients with radiation fibrosis have been demonstrated to show signs of fibrillation and positive waves associated with denervation. Widespread myokymia is strongly suggestive of radiation-induced plexopathy. Although a careful history,

combined with neurologic findings and the results of tomographic and electrodiagnostic studies can strongly suggest the diagnosis of radiation-induced injury, repeated assessments over time may be needed to confirm the diagnosis. Rare patients require surgical exploration of the plexus to exclude neoplasm and establish the aetiology. When due to radiation, plexopathy is usually progressive[128], although some patients plateau for a variable period of time.

Uncommon causes of brachial plexopathy Malignant peripheral nerve tumour or a second primary tumour in a previously irradiated site can account for pain recurring late in the patient's course[138]. Pain has been reported to occur as a result of brachial plexus entrapment in a lymphoedematous shoulder[139], and as a consequence of acute ischaemia many years after axillary radiotherapy[140]. An idiopathic brachial plexopathy has also been described in patients with Hodgkin's disease[141].

Lumbosacral plexopathy

In the cancer population, lumbosacral plexopathy is usually caused by neoplastic infiltration or compression. Radiation-induced plexopathy also occurs, and occasional patients develop the lesion as a result of surgical trauma, infarction, cytotoxic damage, infection in the pelvis or psoas muscle, abdominal aneurysm, or idiopathic lumbosacral neuritis. Polyradiculopathy from leptomeningeal metastases or epidural metastases can mimic lumbosacral plexopathy.

Malignant lumbosacral plexopathy The primary tumours most frequently associated with malignant lumbosacral plexopathy include colorectal, cervical, breast, sarcoma, and lymphoma[142]. Most tumours involve the plexus by direct extension from intrapelvic neoplasm; metastases account for only one-quarter of cases.

Pain is, typically, the first symptom and it is experienced by almost all patients at some point, and it is the only symptom in almost 20 per cent of patients. The quality is aching, pressure-like, or stabbing; dysesthesias are relatively uncommon. Most patients develop numbness, paresthesias, or weakness weeks to months after the pain begins. Common signs include leg weakness that involves multiple myotomes, sensory loss that crosses dermatomes, reflex asymmetry, focal tenderness, leg oedema, and positive direct or reverse straight-leg-raising signs.

A lower plexopathy is most common and accounts for just over 50 per cent of patients with malignant lumbosacral plexopathy[142]. It is usually caused by direct extension from a pelvic tumour, most frequently rectal cancer, gynaecological tumours, or pelvic sarcoma. Pain may be localized in the buttocks and perineum, or referred to the posterolateral thigh and leg. Associated symptoms and signs conform to an L4–S1 distribution. Examination may reveal weakness or sensory changes in the L5 and S1 dermatomes and a depressed ankle jerk. Other findings include leg oedema, bladder or bowel dysfunction, sacral or sciatic notch tenderness, and a positive straight-leg-raising test. A pelvic mass may be palpable.

An upper plexopathy occurs in almost one-third of patients with lumbosacral plexopathy[142]. Pain may be experienced in the back, lower abdomen, flank or iliac crest, or the anterolateral thigh. Examination may reveal sensory, motor, and reflex changes in a L1–4 distribution.

A subgroup of these patients presents with a syndrome characterized by pain and paresthesias limited to the lower abdomen or inguinal region, variable sensory loss, and no motor findings. CT scan may show tumour adjacent to the L1 vertebra (the L1 syndrome[142] or along the pelvic sidewall, where it presumably damages the ilioinguinal, iliohypogastric, or genitofemoral nerves.

Another subgroup has neoplastic involvement of the psoas muscle and presents with a syndrome characterized by upper lumbosacral plexopathy, painful flexion of the ipsilateral hip, and positive psoas muscle stretch test; this has been termed the malignant psoas syndrome[143,144]. Similarly, pain in the distribution of the femoral nerve has been observed in the setting of recurrent retroperitoneal sarcoma[145] and tumour in the iliac crest can compress the lateral cutaneous nerve of the thigh producing a pain that mimics meralgia parasthetica[146].

Sacral plexopathy may occur from direct extension of a sacral lesion or a presacral mass[147]. This may present with predominant involvement of the lumbosacral trunk, characterized by numbness over the dorsal medial foot and sole and weakness of knee flexion, ankle dorsiflexion, and inversion. Other patients demonstrate particular involvement of the coccygeal plexus, with prominent sphincter dysfunction and perineal sensory loss. The latter syndrome occurs with low pelvic tumours, such as those arising from the rectum or prostate.

A panplexopathy with involvement in a L1–S3 distribution occurs in almost one-fifth of patients with lumbosacral plexopathy[142]. Local pain may occur in the lower abdomen, back, buttocks, or perineum. Referred pain can be experienced anywhere in distribution of the plexus. Leg oedema is extremely common. Neurological deficits may be confluent or patchy within the L1–S3 distribution and a positive straight-leg-raising test is usually present.

Cross-sectional imaging, with either CT or MRI, is the preferred diagnostic procedure to evaluate lumbosacral plexopathy (Fig. 10.1.2.7). Scanning should be done from the level of the L1 vertebral body, through the sciatic notch. Limited data suggests superior sensitivity MRI over CT imaging[148]. Definitive imaging of the epidural space adjacent to the plexus should be considered in the patient who has features indicative of a relatively high risk of epidural extension including bilateral symptoms or signs, unexplained incontinence, or a prominent paraspinal mass[135,142].

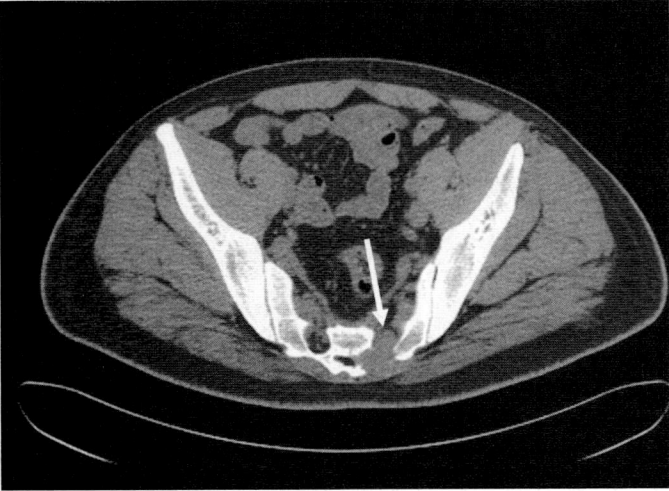

Figure 10.1.2.7 Axial CT scan image of a 29-year-old male with known renal cell cancer and pain radiating into his left buttock. CT demonstrated a soft tissue lesion in the foramen of S2 (arrowed).

Radiation-induced lumbosacral plexopathy Radiation fibrosis of the lumbosacral plexus is a rare complication that may occur from 1 to over 30 years following radiation treatment. The use of intracavitary radium implants for carcinoma of the cervix may be an additional risk factor. Radiation-induced plexopathy typically presents with progressive weakness and leg swelling; pain is not usually a prominent feature. Weakness typically begins distally in the L5–S1 segments and is slowly progressive. The symptoms and signs may be bilateral[149]. If CT scanning demonstrates a lesion, it is usually a non-specific diffuse infiltration of the tissues. Electromyography may show myokymic discharges.

Uncommon causes of lumbosacral plexopathy Lumbosacral plexopathy may occur following intra-arterialcis-platinum infusion (see following paragraphs) and embolization techniques. This syndrome been observed following attempted embolization of a bleeding rectal lesion. Benign conditions that may produce similar findings include haemorrhage or abscess in the iliopsoas muscle[150], abdominal aortic aneurysms, diabetic radiculoplexopathy, vasculitis, and an idiopathic lumbosacral plexitis analogous to acute brachial neuritis[150].

Painful mononeuropathy

Tumour-related mononeuropathy Tumour-related mononeuropathy usually results from compression or infiltration of a nerve from tumour arising in an adjacent bony structure. The most common example of this phenomenon is intercostal nerve injury in a patient with rib metastases. Other examples include the cranial neuralgias previously described, sciatica associated with tumour invasion of the sciatic notch, and common peroneal nerve palsy associated with primary bone tumours of the proximal fibula and lateral cutaneous nerve of the thigh neuralgia associated with iliac crest tumours.

Other causes of mononeuropathy Cancer patients also develop mononeuropathies from many other causes. Post-surgical syndromes are well described (see following paragraphs) and radiation injury of a peripheral nerve occurs occasionally. Rarely, cancer patients develop nerve entrapment syndromes (such as carpal tunnel syndrome) related to oedema or direct compression by tumour[151].

Painful peripheral neuropathies

Painful peripheral neuropathies have multiple causes, including nutritional deficiencies, other metabolic derangements (e.g. diabetes and renal dysfunction), neurotoxic effects of chemotherapy, and, rarely, paraneoplastic syndromes.

Paraneoplastic painful peripheral neuropathy Paraneoplastic painful peripheral neuropathy can be related to injury to the dorsal root ganglion (also known as subacute sensory neuronopathy or ganglionopathy) or injury to peripheral nerves[152]. These syndromes may be the initial manifestation of an underlying malignancy. Except for the neuropathy associated with myeloma, their course is usually independent of the primary tumour[152].

Subacute sensory neuronopathy is characterized by pain (usually dysesthetic), paresthesias, sensory loss in the extremities, and severe sensory ataxia[153]. Although it is usually associated with small-cell carcinoma of the lung, other tumour types, including breast cancer, Hodgkin's disease, and varied solid tumours, are rarely associated. The pain usually develops before the tumour is evident and its course is typically independent. Coexisting autonomic, cerebellar, or cerebral abnormalities are common[153]. An antineuronal IgG antibody (anti-Hu), which recognizes a low–molecular-weight protein present in most small-cell lung carcinomas, has been associated with the condition[154]. Recently, a number of other paraneoplastic antibodies associated with neuropathy have been identified including anti-CV2[155] and anti-Ri[156].

A sensorimotor peripheral neuropathy, which may be painful, has been observed in association with diverse neoplasms, particularly Hodgkin's disease and paraproteinemias[157]. Clinically evident peripheral neuropathy occurs in approximately 15 per cent of patients with multiple myeloma, and electrophysiologic evidence of this lesion can be found in 40 per cent of patients. The pathophysiology of the neuropathy is unknown.

Pain syndromes of the viscera and miscellaneous tumour-related syndromes

Pain may be caused by pathology involving the luminal organs of the gastrointestinal or genitourinary tracts, the parenchymal organs, the peritoneum, or the retroperitoneal soft tissues. Obstruction of hollow viscus, including intestine, biliary tract, and ureter, produces visceral nociceptive syndromes that are well described in the surgical literature[158]. Pain arising from retroperitoneal and pelvic lesions may involve mixed nociceptive and neuropathic mechanisms if both somatic structures and nerves are involved.

Hepatic distention syndrome (Fig.10.1.2.8)

Pain sensitive structures in the region of the liver include the liver capsule, blood vessels, and biliary tract[159]. Nociceptive afferents that innervate these structures travel via the coeliac plexus, the phrenic nerve, and the lower-right intercostal nerves. Extensive intrahepatic metastases, or gross hepatomegaly associated with cholestasis, may produce discomfort in the right subcostal region, and less commonly in the right mid-back or flank. Referred pain may be experienced in the right neck or shoulder, or in the region of the right scapula[160].

Occasional patients who experience chronic pain due to hepatic distension develop an acute intercurrent subcostal pain that may be exacerbated by respiration. Physical examination may demonstrate a palpable or audible rub. These findings suggest the development of an overlying peritonitis, which can develop in response to some acute event, such as a haemorrhage into a metastasis.

Midline retroperitoneal syndrome (Fig. 10.1.2.9)

Retroperitoneal pathology involving the upper abdomen may produce pain by injury to deep somatic structures of the posterior abdominal wall, distortion of pain-sensitive connective tissue, vascular and ductal structures, local inflammation, and direct infiltration of the coeliac plexus. The most common causes are pancreatic cancer and retroperitoneal lymphadenopathy, particularly coeliac lymphadenopathy[161]. The reasons for the high frequency of perineural invasion and the presence of pain in pancreatic cancer may be related to locoregional secretion and activation of growth factor (NGF) and its high-affinity receptor TrkA. These factors are involved in stimulating epithelial cancer cell growth and perineural invasion[162]. In contrast, tumours with overexpression of a low-affinity receptor, p75NGFR, are associated with less pain[163].

In some instances of pancreatic cancer, obstruction of the main pancreatic duct with subsequent ductal hypertension generates pain, which can be relieved by stenting of the pancreatic duct[164].

The pain is experienced in the epigastrium, in the low thoracic region of the back, or in both locations. It is often diffuse and poorly localized. It is usually dull and boring in character, exacerbated with recumbency, and improved by sitting. The lesion can usually be demonstrated by CT, MRI or ultrasound scanning of the upper abdomen.

Intestinal obstruction (see Chapter 10.2.4)

Abdominal pain is an almost invariable manifestation of intestinal obstruction, which may occur in patients with abdominal or pelvic cancers[165]. The factors that contribute to this pain include smooth muscle contractions, mesenteric tension, and mural ischaemia.

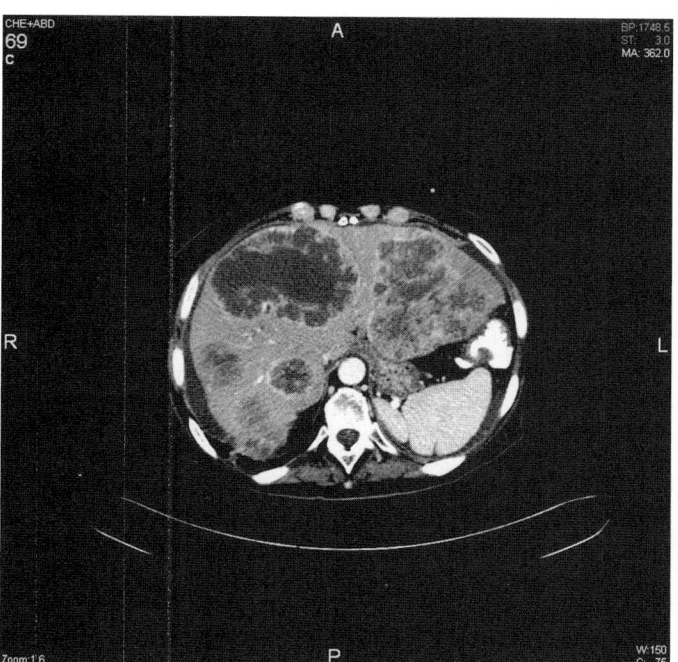

Figure 10.1.2.8 CT scan of a 53-year-old woman with right-upper-quadrant abdominal pain caused by multiple liver metsastases.

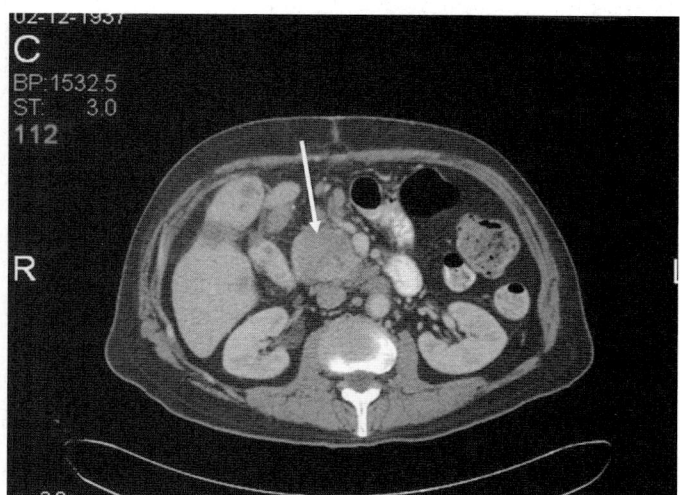

Figure 10.1.2.9 Axial CT scan of a 72-year-old man with epigastric and back pain caused by cancer in the head of the pancreas (arrowed).

Obstructive symptoms may be due primarily to the tumour, or more likely, to a combination of mechanical obstruction and other processes, such as autonomic neuropathy and ileus from metabolic derangements or drugs. Both continuous and colicky pains occur, which may be referred to the dermatomes represented by the spinal segments supplying the affected viscera. Vomiting, anorexia, and constipation are important associated symptoms.

Peritoneal carcinomatosis

Peritoneal carcinomatosis occurs most often by transcoelomic spread of abdominal or pelvic tumour; excepting breast cancer, hematogenous spread of an extra-abdominal neoplasm in this pattern is rare. Carcinomatosis can cause peritoneal inflammation, mesenteric tethering, malignant adhesions, and ascites, all of which can cause pain. Pain and abdominal distension are the most common presenting symptoms. Adhesions can also cause obstruction of hollow viscus, with intermittent colicky pain[166]. CT scanning may demonstrate evidence of ascites, omental infiltration, and peritoneal nodules[167].

Malignant perineal pain

Tumours of the colon or rectum, female reproductive tract, and distal genitourinary system are most commonly responsible for perineal pain[168–170]. Severe perineal pain following resection of pelvic tumours often precede evidence of detectable disease and should be viewed as a potential harbinger of progressive or recurrent cancer[168–170]. There is evidence to suggest that this phenomenon is caused by microscopic perineural invasion by recurrent disease[171]. The pain, which is typically described as constant and aching, is often aggravated by sitting or standing, and may be associated with tenesmus or bladder spasms[168].

Tumour invasion of the musculature of the deep pelvis can also result in a syndrome that appears similar to the so-called 'tension myalgia of the pelvic floor'[172]. The pain is typically described as a constant ache or heaviness that exacerbates with upright posture. When due to tumour, the pain may be concurrent with other types of perineal pain. Digital examination of the pelvic floor may reveal local tenderness or palpable tumour.

Adrenal pain syndrome (Fig. 10.1.2.10)

Large adrenal metastases, common in lung cancer, may produce unilateral flank pain, and less commonly, abdominal pain. Pain is of variable severity, and it can be severe. Adrenal metastases can be complicated by haemorrhage which may cause severe abdominal pain.

Ureteric obstruction (see Chapter 10.8)

Ureteric obstruction is most frequently caused by tumour compression or infiltration within the true pelvis[173]. Less commonly, obstruction can be more proximal, associated with retroperitoneal lymphadenopathy, an isolated retroperitoneal metastasis, mural metastases, or intraluminal metastases. Cancers of the cervix, ovary, prostate, and rectum are most commonly associated with this complication. Pain may or may not accompany ureteric obstruction. When present, it is typically a dull chronic discomfort in the flank, with radiation into the inguinal region or genitalia. If pain does not occur, ureteric obstruction may be discovered when hydronephrosis is discerned on abdominal imaging procedures or renal failure develops. Ureteric obstruction can be complicated by pyelonephritis or pyonephrosis, which often present with features of sepsis, loin pain, and dysuria. Diagnosis of ureteric obstruction can usually be

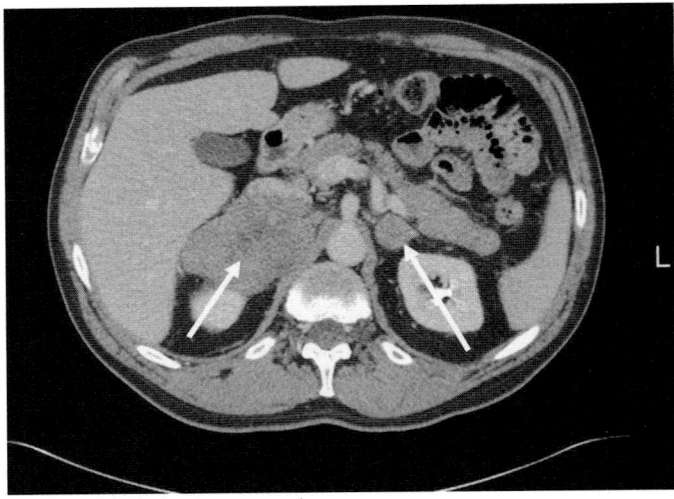

Figure 10.1.2.10 Axial CT scan image of a 62-year-old male with small-cell lung cancer and pain radiating into his right loin. CT demonstrated bilateral adrenal mestastases. The right lesion is much larger than that on the left.

confirmed by the demonstration of hydronephrosis on renal sonography. The level of obstruction can be identified by pyelography, and CT scanning techniques will usually demonstrate the cause[173].

Ovarian cancer pain

Moderate-to-severe chronic abdominopelvic pain is the most common symptom of ovarian cancer; it is reported by almost two-thirds of patients in the 2 weeks prior to the onset or recurrence of the disease[174]. Pain is experienced in the low back or abdomen. In patients who have been previously treated, it is an important symptom of potential recurrence[174].

Lung cancer pain

Even in the absence of involvement of the chest wall or parietal pleura, lung tumours can produce a visceral pain syndrome. In a large case series of lung cancer patients, pain was unilateral in 80 per cent of the cases and bilateral in 20 per cent. Among patients with hilar tumours, the pain was reported to the sternum or the scapula. Upper- and lower-lobe tumours referred to the shoulder and to the lower chest, respectively. As previously mentioned, early lung cancers can generate ipsilateral facial pain[123]. It is postulated that this pain syndrome is generated via vagal afferent neurons.

Other uncommon visceral pain syndromes

Sudden onset severe abdominal or loin pain may be caused by non-traumatic rupture of a visceral tumour. This has been most frequently reported with hepatocellular cancer[175] but also with other liver metastases[176]. Kidney rupture due to a renal metastasis from an adenocarcinoma of the colon[177], splenic ruoture in acute leukaemia[178], rupture of adrenocortical cancers[179] and metastasis-induced perforated appendicitis[180] have been reported. Torsion of pedunculated visceral tumours can produce a cramping abdominal pain.

Paraneoplastic nociceptive pain syndromes

Tumour-related gynaecomastia Tumours that secrete chorionic gonadotrophin (HCG), including malignant and benign tumours of the testis and rarely cancers from other sites[181–183], may be associated with chronic breast tenderness or gynaecomastia.

Approximately 10 per cent of patients with testis cancer have gynaecomastia or breast tenderness at presentation, and the likelihood of gynaecomastia is greater with increasing HCG level [184]. Breast pain can be the first presentation of an occult tumour.

Paraneoplastic pemphigus Paraneoplastic pemphigus is a rare mucocutaneous disorder associated with non-Hodgkin's lymphoma; chronic lymphocytic leukaemia. The condition is characterized by widespread shallow ulcers with haemorrhagic crusting of the lips, conjunctival bullae and, uncommonly, pulmonary lesions. Characteristically, histopathology reveals intraepithelial and subepithelial clefting, and immunoprecipitation studies reveal autoantibodies directed against desmoplakins and desmogleins [185].

Paraneoplastic Raynaud's syndrome Paraneoplastic is a rare manifestation of solid tumours. It has been reported with lung cancer, ovarian cancer, testicular cancer, and melanoma [186].

Chronic pain syndromes associated with cancer therapy

Most treatment-related pains are caused by tissue-damaging procedures. These pains are acute, predictable and self-limited. Chronic treatment-related pain syndromes are associated with either a persistent nociceptive complication of an invasive treatment (such as a postsurgical abscess), or more commonly, neural injury. In some cases, these syndromes occur long after the therapy is completed, resulting in a difficult differential diagnosis between recurrent disease and a complication of therapy.

Post-chemotherapy pain syndromes

Toxic peripheral neuropathy Chemotherapy-induced peripheral neuropathy is a common problem, which is typically manifested by painful paresthesias in the hands and/or feet, and signs consistent with an axonopathy, including 'stocking-glove' sensory loss, weakness, hyporeflexia, and autonomic dysfunction [187]. The pain is usually characterized by continuous burning or lancinating pains, either of which may be increased by contact. The drugs most commonly associated with a peripheral neuropathy are the vinca alkaloids (especially vincristine), cis-platinum, oxaliplatin, and paclitaxel. Procarbazine, carboplatinum, misonidazole, and hexamethylmelamine are less common causes. Data from several studies indicates that the risk of neuropathy associated with cis-platinum and oxaliplatinum can be diminished by amifostine [188], glutathione [189], and calcium and magnesium infusion at the time of treatment [190]. Recent data indicates that prophylactic vitamin E may reduce paclitaxel neuriopathy [45].

Avascular (aseptic) necrosis of femoral or humeral head Avascular necrosis of the femoral or humeral head may occur either spontaneously or as a complication of intermittent or continuous corticosteroid therapy or high-dose chemotherapy with bone marrow transplantation [191]. Osteonecrosis may be unilateral or bilateral. Involvement of the femoral head is most common and typically causes pain in the hip, thigh, or knee. Involvement of the humeral head usually presents as pain in the shoulder, upper arm, or elbow. Pain is exacerbated by movement and relieved by rest. There may be local tenderness over the joint, but this is not universal. Pain usually precedes radiological changes by weeks to months; bone scintigraphy and MRI are sensitive and complementary diagnostic procedures. For the detection of radiographically occult AVN, radionuclide bone scanning and MRI are both sensitive methods but MRI is preferred because it has greater sensitivity and a greater specificity than bone scanning. Early treatment consists of analgesics, decrease or discontinuation of steroids, and sometimes surgery. With progressive bone destruction, joint replacement may be necessary.

Plexopathy Lumbosacral or brachial plexopathy may follow cisplatinum infusion into the iliac artery or axillary artery, respectively. Affected patients develop pain, weakness, and paresthesias within 48 h of the infusion. The mechanism for this syndrome is thought to be due to small vessel damage and infarction of the plexus or nerve. The prognosis for neurologic recovery is not known.

Raynaud's phenomenon Among patients with germ cell tumours treated with cisplatin, vinblastine, and bleomycin, persistent Raynaud's phenomenon is observed in 20–30 per cent [192]. This effect has also been observed in patients with carcinoma of the head and neck treated with a combination of cisplatin, vincristine, and bleomycin. Pathophysiological studies have demonstrated that a hyper-reactivity in the central sympathetic nervous system results in a reduced function of the smooth muscle cells in the terminal arterioles [193].

Chronic pain associated with hormonal therapy

Gynaecomastia with hormonal therapy for prostate cancer Chronic gynaecomastia and breast tenderness are common complications of antiandrogen therapies for prostate cancer [194]. The incidence of this syndrome varies among drugs; it is frequently associated with diethyl stilbesterol and bicalutamide, is less common with flutamide and cyproterone and is uncommon among patients receiving LHRH agonist therapy. Gynaecomastia in the elderly must be distinguished from primary breast cancer or a secondary cancer in the breast.

Chronic post-surgical pain syndromes

Surgical incision at virtually any location may result in chronic pain. Although persistent pain is occasionally encountered after nephrectomy, sternotomy, craniotomy, inguinal dissection, and other procedures, these pain syndromes are not well described in the cancer population. In contrast, several syndromes are now clearly recognized as sequelae of specific surgical procedures. The predominant underlying pain mechanism in these syndromes is neuropathic, resulting from injury to peripheral nerves or plexus.

Breast surgery pain syndromes Chronic pain of variable severity is a common sequel of surgery for breast cancer. Although chronic pain has been reported to occur after almost any surgical procedure on the breast (from lumpectomy to radical mastectomy), it is most common after procedures involving axillary dissection. This is a common pain syndrome after axillary lymph node dissection, occurring in 30–70 per cent of patients [195].

The pain is usually characterized as a constricting and burning discomfort that is localized to the medial arm, axilla, and anterior chest wall. Pain may begin immediately or as late as many months following surgery. The natural history of this condition appears to be variable, and both subacute and chronic courses are possible [196,197]. The onset of pain later than 18 months following surgery is unusual, and a careful evaluation to exclude recurrent chest wall disease is recommended in this setting. On examination, there is often an area of sensory loss within the region of the pain. Chronicity of pain is related to the intensity of the immediate postoperative pain [198,199], postoperative complications and subsequent treatment with chemotherapy and radiotherapy[200]. In many cases, pain is chronic and persists over many years[201].

It is most commonly associated with neuropraxia of the intercostobrachial nerve during the process of axillary lymph node dissection. There is marked anatomic variation in the size and distribution of the intercostobrachial nerve, and this may account for some of the variability in the distribution of pain observed in patients with this condition. In some cases pain may be caused by haematoma in the axilla.

The risk for, and severity of, pain is correlated positively with the number of lymph nodes removed and is inversely correlated with age[202–204]. There is conflicting data as to whether preservation of the intercostobrachial nerve during axillary lymph node dissection can reduce the incidence of this phenomenon. The incidence is reduced when axillary dissection is avoided either by sentinel node excision without full dissection or when nodes are irradiated without dissection.

This syndrome must be differentiated from post mastectomy frozen shoulder, axillary web syndrome[205], and breast cellulitis[206]. In some cases of pain after breast surgery, a trigger point can be palpated in the axilla or chest wall.

Post-radical neck dissection pain Chronic neck and shoulder pain after radical neck dissection is common[207]. Shoulder pain is most often caused by damage to the spinal accessory nerve (CN XI). In other cases, it can result from musculoskeletal imbalance in the shoulder girdle following surgical removal of neck muscles[208]. Similar to the droopy shoulder syndrome, this syndrome can be complicated by development of a thoracic outlet syndrome or suprascapular nerve entrapment, with selective weakness and wasting of the supraspinatus and infraspinatus muscles.

Escalating pain in patients who have undergone radical neck dissection may signify recurrent tumour or soft tissue infection. These lesions may be difficult to diagnose in tissues damaged by radiation and surgery. Repeated CT or MRI scanning may be needed to exclude tumour recurrence. Empiric treatment with antibiotics should be considered.

Post-thoracotomy pain There have been two major studies of post-thoracotomy pain[209,210]. In the first study[210], three groups were identified. The largest (63 per cent), had prolonged postoperative pain that abated within 2 months after surgery. Recurrent pain, following resolution of the postoperative pain, was usually due to neoplasm. A second group (16 per cent) experienced pain that persisted following the thoracotomy, and then increased in intensity during the follow-up period. Local recurrence of disease and infection were the most common causes of the increasing pain. A final group had a prolonged period of stable or decreasing pain that gradually resolved over a maximum 8-month period. This pain was not associated with tumour recurrence. Overall, the development of late or increasing post-thoracotomy pain was due to recurrent or persistent tumour in greater than 95 per cent of patients. This finding was corroborated in the more recent study, which evaluated the records of 238 consecutive patients who underwent thoracotomy, which identified recurrent pain in 20 patients, all of whom were found to have tumour regrowth[209].

Patients with recurrent or increasing post-thoracotomy pain should be carefully evaluated, preferably with a chest CT scan or MRI. Chest radiographs are insufficient to evaluate recurrent chest disease. In some patients, postthoracotomy pain appears to be caused by a taut muscular band within the scapular region. In such cases, pain may be amenable to trigger point injection of local anaesthetic[211].

Postoperatve frozen shoulder Patients with post-thoracotomy or postmastectomy pain are at risk for the development of a frozen shoulder[212]. This lesion may become an independent focus of pain, particularly if complicated by reflex sympathetic dystrophy. Adequate postoperative analgesia and active mobilization of the joint soon after surgery are necessary to prevent these problems.

Phantom pain syndromes Phantom limb pain is perceived to arise from an amputated limb, as if the limb were still contiguous with the body. Phantom pain is experienced by 60–80 per cent of patients following limb amputation but is only severe in about 5–10 per cent of cases[213]. The incidence of phantom pain is significantly higher in patients with a long duration of preamputation pain and those with pain on the day before amputation. Patients who had pain prior to the amputation may experience phantom pain that replicates the earlier one.

Phantom pain is more prevalent after tumour-related than traumatic amputations, and postoperative chemotherapy is an additional risk factor[213,214]. The pain may be continuous or paroxysmal and is often associated with bothersome paresthesias. The phantom limb may assume painful and unusual postures and may gradually telescope and approach the stump. Phantom pain may initially magnify and then slowly fade over time. There is evidence that preoperative or postoperative neural blockade reduces the incidence of phantom limb pain during the first year after amputation.

Some patients have spontaneous partial remission of the pain. The recurrence of pain after such a remission, or the late onset of pain in a previously painless phantom limb, suggests the appearance of a more proximal lesion, including recurrent neoplasm[215].

Phantom pain syndromes have also been described after other surgical procedures. Phantom breast pain after mastectomy, which occurs in 15–30 per cent of patients[216], also appears to be related to the presence of preoperative pain. The pain tends to start in the region of the nipple and then spread to the entire breast. The character of the pain is variable and may be lancinating, continuous, or intermittent[216]. A phantom rectum pain syndrome occurs in approximately 15 per cent of patients who undergo abdominoperineal resection of the rectum[169]. Phantom rectal pain may develop either in the early postoperative period or after a latency of months to years. Late onset pain is almost always associated with tumour recurrence[169]. Rare cases of phantom bladder pain after cystectomy and phantom eye pain after enucleation have also been reported.

Stump pain Stump pain occurs at the site of the surgical scar several months to years following amputation[217]. It is usually the result of neuroma development at a site of nerve transection. This pain is characterized by burning or lancinating dysesthesias, which are often exacerbated by movement or pressure and blocked by an injection of a local anaesthetic.

Postsurgical pelvic floor myalgia Surgical trauma to the pelvic floor can cause a residual pelvic floor myalgia, which like the neoplastic syndrome described previously, mimics so-called tension myalgia[172]. The risk of disease recurrence associated with this condition is not known, and its natural history has not been defined. In patients who have undergone anorectal resection, this condition must be differentiated from the phantom anus syndrome (see earlier paragraphs).

Chronic post-radiation pain syndromes

Chronic pain complicating radiation therapy tends to occur late in the course of a patient's illness. These syndromes must always be differentiated from recurrent tumour.

Radiation-induced brachial and lumbosacral plexopathies
Radiation-induced brachial and lumbosacral plexopathies were described previously (see earlier paragraphs).

Chronic radiation myelopathy Chronic radiation myelopathy is a late complication of spinal cord irradiation. The latency is highly variable but is most commonly 12–14 months. The most common presentation is a partial transverse myelopathy at the cervicothoracic level, sometimes in a Brown–Sequard pattern[218]. Sensory symptoms, including pain, typically precede the development of progressive motor and autonomic dysfunction[218]. The pain is characterized as a burning dysesthesia localized to the area of spinal cord damage or below. Imaging studies, particularly MRI, are important to exclude epidural metastases and demonstrate the nature and extent of intrinsic cord pathology, which may include atrophy, swelling, or syrinx. On MRI, the signs of radiation myelitis include high-intensity signals on T2-weighted images or gadolinium enhancement of T1-weighted images. The course of chronic radiation myelopathy is characterized by steady progression over months followed by a subsequent phase of slow progression or stabilization.

Chronic radiation enteritis and proctitis Chronic enteritis and proctocolitis occur as a delayed complication in 2–10 per cent of patients who undergo abdominal or pelvic radiation therapy[219,220]. The rectum and rectosigmoid are more commonly involved than the small bowel, a pattern that may relate to the retroperitoneal fixation of the former structures. The latency is variable (3 months–30 years)[219,220]. Chronic radiation injury to the rectum can present as proctitis (with bloody diarrhoea, tenesmus, and cramping pain), obstruction due to stricture formation, or fistulae to the bladder or vagina. Small bowel radiation damage typically causes colicky abdominal pain, which can be associated with chronic nausea or malabsorption. Barium studies may demonstrate a narrow tubular bowel segment resembling Crohn's disease or ischaemic colitis. Endoscopy and biopsy may be necessary to distinguish suspicious lesions from recurrent cancer.

Radiation cystitis Radiation therapy used in the treatment of tumours of the pelvic organs (prostate, bladder, colon/rectum, uterus, ovary, and vagina/vulva) may produce chronic radiation cystitis. The late sequelae of radiation injury to the bladder can range from minor temporary irritative voiding symptoms and asymptomatic haematuria to more severe complications such as gross haematuria, contracted nonfunctional bladder, persistent incontinence, and fistula formation. The clinical presentation can include frequency, urgency, dysuria, haematuria, incontinence, hydronephrosis, pneumaturia, and fecaluria.

Lypmphoedema pain One-third of patients with lymphoedema as a complication of breast cancer or its treatment, experience pain and tightness in the arm and pain is a major part of the morbidity among affected patients[221]. In some patients, pain is caused by a secondary rotator cuff tendonitis caused by internal derangement of tendon fibres caused by impingement, functional overload, and intrinsic tendinopathy. Conservative treatment with analgesics and physiotherapy is a safe and effective treatment. Some patients develop nerve entrapment syndromes of the carpal tunnel syndrome or brachial plexus[139]. Severe or increasing pain in a lymphoedematous arm is strongly suggestive of tumour invasion of the brachial plexus[129].

Burning perineum syndrome Persistent perineal discomfort is an uncommon delayed complication of pelvic radiotherapy. After a latency of 6–18 months, burning pain can develop in the perianal region; the pain may extend anteriorly to involve the vagina or scrotum[222]. In patients who have had abdominoperineal resection, phantom anus pain and recurrent tumour are major differential diagnoses.

Post-prostate brachytherapy pelvic pain Brachytherapy patients with prostate cancer may produce a chronic radiation-related pelvic pain syndrome that is exacerbated by urination or perineal pressure. Data suggests that it may be partly related to higher central prostatic radiation doses[223].

Osteoradionecrosis Osteoradionecrosis is another late complication of radiotherapy. Bone necrosis, which occurs as a result of endarteritis obliterans, may produce focal pain. Overlying tissue breakdown can occur spontaneously or as a result of trauma, such as dental extraction or denture trauma[224]. Delayed development of a painful ulcer must be differentiated from tumour recurrence.

Conclusion

Adequate assessment is a necessary precondition for effective pain management. In the cancer population, assessment must recognize the dynamic relationship between the symptom, the illness, and larger concerns related to quality of life. Syndrome identification and inferences about pain pathophysiology are useful elements that may simplify this complex undertaking.

References

1. Goudas, L.C., Bloch, R., Gialeli-Goudas, M. *et al.* (2005). The epidemiology of cancer pain. *Cancer Investigation*, **23**(2), 182–90.
2. Von Roenn, J.H., Cleeland, C.S., Gonin, R. *et al.* (1993). Physician attitudes and practice in cancer pain management. A survey from the Eastern Cooperative Oncology Group. *Annals of Internal Medicine*, **119**(2), 121–6.
3. Grossman, S.A., Sheidler, V.R., Swedeen, K. *et al.* (1991). Correlation of patient and caregiver ratings of cancer pain. *Journal of Pain and Symptom Management*, **6**(2), 53–7.
4. Cleeland, C.S., Gonin, R., Hatfield, A.K. *et al.* (1994). Pain and its treatment in outpatients with metastatic cancer. *New England Journal of Medicine*, **330**(9), 592–6.
5. Larue, F., Colleau, S.M., Brasseur, L. *et al.* (1995). Multicentre study of cancer pain and its treatment in France. *British Medical Journal*, **310**(6986), 1034–7.
6. Portenoy, R.K. and Hagen, N.A. (1990). Breakthrough pain: definition, prevalence and characteristics [see comments]. *Pain*, **41**(3), 273–81.
7. Elliott, K.J. (1994). Taxonomy and mechanisms of neuropathic pain. *Seminars in Neurology*, **14**(3), 195–205.
8. Devor, M., Basbaum, A.I., Bennett, G.J. *et al.* (1991). Group Report: Mechanisms of neuropathic pain following peripheral injury. In *Towards a New Pharmacotherapy of Pain* (eds. A. Basbaum and J.M. Besson), pp. 417–40. John Wiley & Sons, New York.
9. Simon, D.L. (1997). Algorithm for timely recognition and treatment of complex regional pain syndrome (CRPS): a new approach for objective assessment [letter]. *Clinical Journal of Pain*, **13**(3), 264–72.
10. Stanton-Hicks, M., Janig, W., Hassenbusch, S. *et al.* (1995). Reflex sympathetic dystrophy: changing concepts and taxonomy [see comments]. *Pain*, **63**(1), 127–33.
11. American Psychiatric Association. Somatoform disorders. (1994). In *Diagnostic and Statistical Manual of Mental Disorders (DSM-IV)*, pp. 445–71, 4th edition. American Psychiatric Association, Washington.
12. Bruera, E., Kuehn, N., Miller, M.J. *et al.* (1991). The Edmonton Symptom Assessment System (ESAS): a simple method for the assessment of palliative care patients. *Journal of Palliative Care*, **7**(2), 6–9.

13. Portenoy, R.K., Thaler, H.T., Kornblith, A.B. *et al.* (1994). The Memorial Symptom Assessment Scale: an instrument for the evaluation of symptom prevalence, characteristics and distress. *European Journal of Cancer*, **30A**(9), 1326–36.

14. American Pain Society Quality of Care Committee. (1995). Quality improvement guidelines for the treatment of acute pain and cancer pain. American Pain Society Quality of Care Committee [see comments]. *Journal of the American Medical Association*, **274**(23), 1874–80.

15. *World Health Organization. Cancer Pain Relief.* (1996). 2nd edition. World Health Organization, Geneva.

16. Agency for Health Care Policy and Research. (1994). Management of cancer pain: adults. Cancer Pain Guideline Panel. Agency for Health Care Policy and Research. *American Family Physician*, **49**(8), 1853–68.

17. Au, E., Loprinzi, C.L., Dhodapkar, M. *et al.* (1994). Regular use of a verbal pain scale improves the understanding of oncology inpatient pain intensity. *Journal of Clinical Oncology*, **12**(12), 2751–5.

18. Bookbinder, M., Coyle, N., Kiss, M. *et al.* (1996). Implementing national standards for cancer pain management: program model and evaluation. *Journal of Pain and Symptom Management*, **12**(6), 334–47.

19. Coyle, N., Thaler, H., Bookbinder, M. *et al.* (1993). Implementation of the American Pain Society (APS) standards for cancer pain management: a pilot study at Memorial Sloan-Kettering Cancer Center (MSKCC) (Meeting abstract). *Proceedings of the Annual Meeting of the American Society of Clincal Oncology*, **12**.

20. Fishman, B., Pasternak, S., Wallenstein, S.L. *et al.* (1987). The Memorial Pain Assessment Card. A valid instrument for the evaluation of cancer pain. *Cancer*, **60**(5), 1151–8.

21. Daut, R.L., Cleeland, C.S., and Flanery, R.C. (1983). Development of the Wisconsin Brief Pain Questionnaire to assess pain in cancer and other diseases. *Pain*, **17**(2), 197–210.

22. Caraceni, A., Mendoza, T.R., Mencaglia, E. *et al.* (1996). A validation study of an Italian version of the Brief Pain Inventory (Breve Questionario per la Valutazione del Dolore). *Pain*, **65**(1), 87–92.

23. Cleeland, C.S. and Ryan, K.M. (1994). Pain assessment: global use of the Brief Pain Inventory. *Annals of the Academy of Medicine, Singapore*, **23**(2), 129–38.

24. Wang, X.S., Mendoza, T.R., Gao, S.Z. *et al.* (1996). The Chinese version of the Brief Pain Inventory (BPI-C): its development and use in a study of cancer pain. *Pain*, **67**(2–3), 407–16.

25. Melzack, R. (1975). The McGill Pain Questionnaire: major properties and scoring methods. *Pain*, **1**(3), 277–99.

26. Dudgeon, D., Raubertas, R.F., and Rosenthal, S.N. (1993). The short-form McGill Pain Questionnaire in chronic cancer pain. *Journal of Pain and Symptom Management*, **8**(4), 191–5.

27. Bakshi, R., Mechtler, L.L., Kamran, S. *et al.* (1999). MRI findings in lumbar puncture headache syndrome: abnormal dural- meningeal and dural venous sinus enhancement. *Clinical Imaging*, **23**(2), 73–6.

28. Lambert, D.H., Hurley, R.J., Hertwig, L. *et al.* (1997). Role of needle gauge and tip configuration in the production of lumbar puncture headache. *Regional Anesthesia*, **22**(1), 66–72.

29. Gonzalez, D.P. (2000). Lumbar puncture headache exacerbated by recumbent position [editorial]. *Military Medicine*, **165**(9), vi, 690.

30. Evans, R.W. (1998). Complications of Lumbar Puncture. *Neurology Clinics*, **16**(1), 83–105.

31. Irani, J., Fournier, F., Bon, D. *et al.* (1997). Patient tolerance of transrectal ultrasound-guided biopsy of the prostate. *British Journal of Urology*, **79**(4), 608–10.

32. Sapir, R., Patlas, M., Strano, S.D. *et al.* (2003). Does mammography hurt? *Journal of Pain and Symptom Management*, **25**(1), 53–63.

33. Miller, D., Martin, I., and Herbison, P. (2002). Interventions for relieving the pain and discomfort of screening mammography (Cochrane Review). *Cochrane Database of Systematic Reviews*, **4**, CD002942.

34. Agency for Health Care Policy and Research: Acute Pain Management Panel. Acute pain management: operative or medical procedures and trauma. Washington: U.S. Dept. of Health and Human Services; 1992.

35. Rowlingson, J.C. and Rawal, N. (2003). Postoperative pain guidelines–targeted to the site of surgery. *Regional Anesthesia Pain Med*, **28**(4), 265–7.

36. Naumann, C., Erdine, S., Koulousakis, A. *et al.* (1999). Drug Adverse Events and System Complications of Intrathecal Opioid Delivery for Pain: Origins, Detection, Manifestations, and Management. *Neuromodulation*, **2**(2), 92–107.

37. Gaertner, J., Sabatowski, R., Elsner, F. *et al.* (2003). Encapsulation of an intrathecal catheter. *Pain*, **103**(1–2), 217–20.

38. Kemeny, N. (1992). Review of regional therapy of liver metastases in colorectal cancer. *Seminars in Oncology*, **19**(2 Suppl 3), 155–62.

39. Jaaback, K. and Johnson, N. (2006). Intraperitoneal chemotherapy for the initial management of primary epithelial ovarian cancer. *Cochrane Database of Systematic Reviews*, **1**, CD005340.

40. Shelley, M.D., Court, J.B., Kynaston, H. *et al.* (2003). Intravesical bacillus Calmette-Guerin versus mitomycin C for Ta and T1 bladder cancer. *Cochrane Database of Systematic Reviews*, **3**, CD003231.

41. Pardalidis, N.P., Papatsoris, A.G., Kosmaoglou, E.V. *et al.* (2002). Two cases of acute polyarthritis secondary to intravesical BCG adjuvant therapy for superficial bladder cancer. *Clinical Rheumatology*, **21**(6), 536–7.

42. Perron, G., Dolbec, P., Germain, J. *et al.* (2003). Perineal pruritus after i.v. dexamethasone administration. *Canadian Journal of Anaesthesia*, **50**(7), 749–50.

43. McCarthy, G.M. and Skillings, J.R. (1992). Jaw and other orofacial pain in patients receiving vincristine for the treatment of cancer. *Oral Surgery, Oral Medicine, Oral Pathology*, **74**(3), 299–304.

44. Scalone, S., Sorio, R., Bortolussi, R. *et al.* (2004). Vinorelbine-induced acute reversible peripheral neuropathy in a patient with ovarian carcinoma pretreated with carboplatin and paclitaxel. *Acta Oncologica*, **43**(2), 209–11.

45. Argyriou, A.A., Chroni, E., Koutras, A. *et al.* (2006). Preventing paclitaxel-induced peripheral neuropathy: a phase II trial of vitamin E supplementation. *Journal of Pain and Symptom Management*, **32**(3), 237–44.

46. Weiss, H.D., Walker, M.D., and Wiernik. P.H. (1974). Neurotoxicity of commonly used antineoplastic agents (first of two parts). *New England Journal of Medicine*, **291**(2), 75–81.

47. Priest, J.R., Ramsay, N.K., Steinherz, P.G. *et al.* (1982). A syndrome of thrombosis and hemorrhage complicating L-asparaginase therapy for childhood acute lymphoblastic leukemia. *Journal of Pediatrics*, **100**(6), 984–9.

48. Visani, G., Bontempo, G., Manfroi, S. *et al.* (1996). All-trans-retinoic acid and pseudotumor cerebri in a young adult with acute promyelocytic leukemia: a possible disease association [see comments]. *Haematologica*, **81**(2), 152–4.

49. Garrison, J.A., McCune, J.S., Livingston, R.B. *et al.* (2003). Myalgias and arthralgias associated with paclitaxel. *Oncology (Williston Park)*, **17**(2), 271–7, discussion 281–2, 286–8.

50. Markman, M., Kennedy, A., Webster, K. *et al.* (1999). Use of low-dose oral prednisone to prevent paclitaxel-induced arthralgias and myalgias. *Gynecologic Oncology*, **72**(1), 100–1.

51. Wacker, A., Lersch, C., Scherpinski, U. *et al.* (2003). High incidence of angina pectoris in patients treated with 5-fluorouracil. A planned surveillance study with 102 patients. *Oncology*, **65**(2), 108–12.

52. Bellmunt, J., Navarro, M., Hidalgo, R. *et al.* (1988). Palmar-plantar erythrodysesthesia syndrome associated with short-term continuous infusion (5 days) of 5-fluorouracil. *Tumori*, **74**(3), 329–31.

53. Fabian, C.J., Molina, R., Slavik, M. *et al.* (1990). Pyridoxine therapy for palmar-plantar erythrodysesthesia associated with continuous 5-fluorouracil infusion. *Investigational New Drugs*, **8**(1), 57–63.

54. Trump, D.L., Pavy, M.D., and Staal, S. (1982). Gynecomastia in men following antineoplastic therapy. *Archives of Internal Medicine*, **142**(3), 511–3.

55. Aass, N., Kaasa, S., Lund, E. *et al.* (1990). Long-term somatic side-effects and morbidity in testicular cancer patients. *British Journal of Cancer*, **61**(1), 151–5.

56. Thompson, I.M., Zeidman, E.J., and Rodriguez, F.R. (1990). Sudden death due to disease flare with luteinizing hormone-releasing hormone agonist therapy for carcinoma of the prostate [see comments]. *Journal of Urology*, **144**(6), 1479–80.

57. Plotkin, D., Lechner, J.J., Jung, W.E. et al. (1978). Tamoxifen flare in advanced breast cancer. *Journal of the American Medical Association*, **240**(24), 2644–6.

58. Burstein, H.J. Aromatase inhibitor-associated arthralgia syndrome. (2007). *Breast*, **16**, 223–34.

59. Quesada, J.R., Talpaz, M., Rios, A. et al. (1986). Clinical toxicity of interferons in cancer patients: a review. *Journal of Clinical Oncology*, **4**(2), 234–43.

60. Hillner, B.E., Ingle, J.N., Berenson, J.R. et al. (2000). American Society of Clinical Oncology guideline on the role of bisphosphonates in breast cancer. American Society of Clinical Oncology Bisphosphonates Expert Panel. *Journal of Clinical Oncology*, **18**(6), 1378–91.

61. Venturini, M., Del Mastro, L., Aitini, E. et al. (2005). Dose-dense adjuvant chemotherapy in early breast cancer patients: results from a randomized trial. *Journal of the National Cancer Institute*, **97**(23), 1724–33.

62. Paciucci, P.A., Raptis, G., Bleiweiss, I. et al. (2002). Neo-adjuvant therapy with dose-dense docetaxel plus short-term filgrastim rescue for locally advanced breast cancer. *Anticancer Drugs*, **13**(8), 791–5.

63. Pierce, S.M., Recht, A., Lingos, T.I. et al. (1992). Long-term radiation complications following conservative surgery (CS) and radiation therapy (RT) in patients with early stage breast cancer [see comments]. *International Journal of Radiation Oncology, Biology, Physics*, **23**(5), 915–23.

64. Churn, M., Clough, V., and Slater, A. (2000). Early onset of bilateral brachial plexopathy during mantle radiotherapy for Hodgkin's disease. *Clinical Oncology (Royal College of Radiologists)*, **12**(5), 289–91.

65. Salner, A.L., Botnick, L.E., Herzog, A.G. et al. (1981). Reversible brachial plexopathy following primary radiation therapy for breast cancer. *Cancer Treatment and Research*, **65**(9–10), 797–802.

66. Ang, K.K. and Stephens, L.C. (1994). Prevention and management of radiation myelopathy. *Oncology (Huntingt)*, **8**(11), 71–6, discussion 78, 81–2.

67. Robinson, R.G., Preston, D.F., Schiefelbein, M. et al. (1995). Strontium 89 therapy for the palliation of pain due to osseous metastases. *Journal of the American Medical Association*, **274**(5), 420–4.

68. Rusthoven, J.J., Ahlgren, P., Elhakim, T. et al. (1988). Varicella-zoster infection in adult cancer patients. A population study. *Archives of Internal Medicine*, **148**(7), 1561–6.

69. Dunst, J., Steil, B., Furch, S. et al. (2000). Herpes zoster in breast cancer patients after radiotherapy. *Strahlentherapie und Onkologie*, **176**(11), 513–6.

70. Battinelli, E.M. and Ansell, J. (2005). Cancer and thrombosis. *Current Hematology Reports*, **4**(5), 378–84.

71. Lorimer, J.W., Semelhago, L.C., and Barber, G.G. (1994). Venous gangrene of the extremities [see comments]. *Canadian Journal of Surgery*, **37**(5), 379–84.

72. Burihan, E., de Figueiredo, L.F., Francisco Junior, J. et al. (1993). Upper-extremity deep venous thrombosis: analysis of 52 cases. *Cardiovascular Surgery*, **1**(1), 19–22.

73. Rice, T.W., Rodriguez, R.M., and Light, R.W. (2006). The superior vena cava syndrome: clinical characteristics and evolving etiology. *Medicine (Baltimore)*, **85**(1), 37–42.

74. Morales, M., Llanos, M., and Dorta, J. (1997). Superior vena cava thrombosis secondary to hickman catheter and complete resolution after fibrinolytic therapy. *Support Care Cancer*, **5**(1), 67–9.

75. Callander, N. and Rapaport, S.I. (1993). Trousseau's syndrome. *Western Journal of Medicine*, **158**(4), 364–71.

76. Caraceni, A. and Portenoy, R.K. (1999). An international survey of cancer pain characteristics and syndromes. IASP Task Force on Cancer Pain. International Association for the Study of Pain. *Pain*, **82**(3), 263–74.

77. Wagner, G. (1984). Frequency of pain in patients with cancer. *Recent Results in Cancer Research*, **89**, 64–71.

78. Edmister, K.A. and Sundaram, M. (2002). Oncogenic osteomalacia. *Seminars in Musculoskeletal Radiology*, **6**(3), 191–6.

79. Hesselmann, S., Micke, O., Schaefer, U. et al. (2002). Systemic mast cell disease (SMCD) and bone pain. A case treated with radiotherapy. *Strahlentherapie Onkologie*, **178**(5), 275–9.

80. Ollivier, L., Gerber, S., Vanel, D. et al. (2006). Improving the interpretation of bone marrow imaging in cancer patients. *Cancer Imaging*, **6**, 194–8.

81. Constans, J.P., de Divitiis, E., Donzelli, R. et al. (1983). Spinal metastases with neurological manifestations. Review of 600 cases. *Journal of Neurosurgery*, **59**(1), 111–8.

82. Sundaresan, N., Galicich, J.H., Lane, J.M. et al. (1981). Treatment of odontoid fractures in cancer patients. *Journal of Neurosurgery*, **54**(2), 187–92.

83. Loblaw, D.A., Laperriere, N.J., and Mackillop, W.J. (2003). A population-based study of malignant spinal cord compression in Ontario. *Clinical Oncology (Royal College of Radiologists)*, **15**(4), 211–7.

84. Loblaw, D.A., Perry, J., Chambers, A. et al. (2005). Systematic review of the diagnosis and management of malignant extradural spinal cord compression: the Cancer Care Ontario Practice Guidelines Initiative's Neuro-Oncology Disease Site Group. *Journal of Clinical Oncology*, **23**(9), 2028–37.

85. Prasad, D. and Schiff, D. (2005). Malignant spinal-cord compression. *Lancet Oncology*, **6**(1), 15–24.

86. Ruckdeschel, J.C. (2005). Early detection and treatment of spinal cord compression. *Oncology (Huntington NY)*, **19**(1), 81–6, discussion 86, 89–92.

87. Helweg-Larsen, S. and Sorensen, P.S. (1994). Symptoms and signs in metastatic spinal cord compression: a study of progression from first symptom until diagnosis in 153 patients. *European Journal of Cancer*, **30A**(3), 396–8.

88. Rosenthal, M.A., Rosen, D., Raghavan, D. et al. (1992). Spinal cord compression in prostate cancer. A 10-year experience. *British Journal of Urology*, **69**(5), 530–3.

89. Barron, K.D., Hirano, A., Araki, S. et al. (1959). Experience with metastatic neoplasms involving the spinal cord. *Neurology*, **9**, 91–100.

90. Gilbert, R.W., Kim, J.H., and Posner, J.B. (1978). Epidural spinal cord compression from metastatic tumor: diagnosis and treatment. *Annals of Neurology*, **3**(1), 40–51.

91 Beatrous, T.E., Choyke, P.L., and Frank, J.A. (1990). Diagnostic evaluation of cancer patients with pelvic pain: comparison of scintigraphy, CT, and MR imaging [see comments]. *AJR American Journal of Roentgenology*, **155**(1), 85–8.

92. Martinez-Lavin, M. (1997). Hypertrophic osteoarthropathy. *Current Opinion in Rheumatology*, **9**(1), 83–6.

93. Amital, H., Applbaum, Y.H., Vasiliev, L. et al. (2004). Hypertrophic pulmonary osteoarthropathy: control of pain and symptoms with pamidronate. *Clinical Rheumatology*, **23**(4), 330–2.

94. Suzuma, T., Sakurai, T., Yoshimura, G. et al. (2001). Pamidronate-induced remission of pain associated with hypertrophic pulmonary osteoarthropathy in chemoendocrine therapy-refractory inoperable metastatic breast carcinoma. *Anticancer Drugs*, **12**(9), 731–4.

95. Chakravarty, E.F. and Genovese, M.C. (2004). Associations between rheumatoid arthritis and malignancy. *Rheumatic Diseases Clinics of North America*, **30**(2), 271–84, vi.

96. Stummvoll, G.H., Aringer, M., Machold, K.P. et al. (2001). Cancer polyarthritis resembling rheumatoid arthritis as a first sign of hidden neoplasms. Report of two cases and review of the literature. *Scandinavian Journal of Rheumatology*, **30**(1), 40–4.

97. Steiner, I. and Siegal, T. (1989). Muscle cramps in cancer patients. *Cancer*, **63**(3), 574–7.

98. Vecht, C.J., Hoff, A.M., Kansen, P.J. et al. (1992). Types and causes of pain in cancer of the head and neck. *Cancer*, **70**(1), 178–84.

99. Vazquez-Barquero, A., Ibanez, F.J., Herrera, S. et al. (1994). Isolated headache as the presenting clinical manifestation of intracranial

tumors: a prospective study [see comments]. *Cephalalgia*, **14**(4), 270–2.

100. Wilne, S.H., Ferris, R.C., Nathwani, A. *et al.* (2006). The presenting features of brain tumours: a review of 200 cases. *Arch Dis Child*, **91**(6), 502–6.

101. Argyriou, A.A., Chroni, E., Polychronopoulos, P. *et al.* (2006). Headache characteristics and brain metastases prediction in cancer patients. *European Journal of Cancer Care (England)*, **15**(1), 90–5.

102. Medina, L.S., Pinter, J.D., Zurakowski, D. *et al.* (1997). Children with headache: clinical predictors of surgical space-occupying lesions and the role of neuroimaging. *Radiology*, **202**(3), 819–24.

103. Suwanwela, N., Phanthumchinda, K., and Kaoropthum, S. (1994). Headache in brain tumor: a cross-sectional study. *Headache*, **34**(7), 435–8.

104. Grossman, S.A. and Krabak, M.J. (1999). Leptomeningeal carcinomatosis. *Cancer Treatment Reviews*, **25**(2), 103–19.

105. Bruno, M.K. and Raizer, J. (2005). Leptomeningeal metastases from solid tumors (meningeal carcinomatosis). *Cancer Treatment and Research*, **125**, 31–52.

106. Wasserstrom, W.R., Glass, J.P., and Posner, J.B. (1982). Diagnosis and treatment of leptomeningeal metastases from solid tumors: experience with 90 patients. *Cancer*, **49**(4), 759–72.

107. van Oostenbrugge, R.J. and Twijnstra, A. (1999). Presenting features and value of diagnostic procedures in leptomeningeal metastases. *Neurology*, **53**(2), 382–5.

108. Greenberg, H.S., Deck, M.D., Vikram, B. *et al.* (1981). Metastasis to the base of the skull: clinical findings in 43 patients. *Neurology*, **31**(5), 530–7.

109. Hawley, R.J., Patel, A., and Lastinger, L. (1999). Cranial nerve compression from breast cancer metastasis [letter; comment]. *Surgical Neurology*, **52**(4), 431–2.

110. Yi, H.J., Kim, C.H., Bak, K.H. *et al.* (2000). Metastatic tumors in the sellar and parasellar regions: clinical review of four cases. *Journal of Korean Medical Science*, **15**(3), 363–7.

111. Lossos, A. and Siegal, T. (1992). Numb chin syndrome in cancer patients: etiology, response to treatment, and prognostic significance [see comments]. *Neurology*, **42**(6), 1181–4.

112. Moris, G., Roig, C., Misiego, M. *et al.* (1998). The distinctive headache of the occipital condyle syndrome: a report of four cases. *Headache*, **38**(4), 308–11.

113. Loevner, L.A. and Yousem, D,M. (1997). Overlooked metastatic lesions of the occipital condyle: a missed case treasure trove. *Radiographics*, **17**(5), 1111–21.

114. Capobianco, D.J., Brazis, P.W., Rubino, F.A. *et al.* (2002). Occipital condyle syndrome. *Headache*, **42**(2), 142–6.

115. Malloy, K.A. (2007). Prostate cancer metastasis to clivus causing cranial nerve VI palsy. *Optometry*, **78**(2), 55–62.

116. Fink, F.M., Ausserer, B., Schrocksnadel, W. *et al.* (1987). Clivus chordoma in a 9-year-old child: case report and review of the literature. *Pediatric Hematology and Oncology*, **4**(2), 91–100.

117. Lawson, W. and Reino, A.J. (1997). Isolated sphenoid sinus disease: an analysis of 132 cases. *Laryngoscope*, **107**(12 Pt 1), 1590–5.

118. Mickel, R.A. and Zimmerman, M.C. (1990). The sphenoid sinus--a site for metastasis. *Otolaryngology - Head and Neck Surgery*, **102**(6), 709–16.

119. Sozzi, G., Marotta, P., and Piatti, L. (1987). Vagoglossopharyngeal neuralgia with syncope in the course of carcinomatous meningitis. *Italian Journal of Neurological Sciences*, **8**(3), 271–5.

120. Metheetrairut, C. and Brown, D.H. (1993). Glossopharyngeal neuralgia and syncope secondary to neck malignancy. *Journal of Otolaryngology*, **22**(1), 18–20.

121. Boerman, R.H., Maassen, E.M., Joosten, J. *et al.* (1999). Trigeminal neuropathy secondary to perineural invasion of head and neck carcinomas. *Neurology*, **53**(1), 213–6.

122. De Potter, P. (1998). Ocular manifestations of cancer. *Current Opinion in Ophthalmology*, **9**(6), 100–4.

123. Sarlani, E., Schwartz, A.H., Greenspan, J.D. *et al.* (2003). Facial pain as first manifestation of lung cancer: a case of lung cancer-related cluster headache and a review of the literature. *Journal of Orofacial Pain*, **17**(3), 262–7.

124. Dulli, D.A., Levine, R.L., Chun, R.W. *et al.* (1987). Migrainous neurologic dysfunction in Hodgkin's disease [letter]. *Archives of Neurology*, **44**(7), 689.

125. Miyazaki, Y., Tajima, Y., Sudo, K. *et al.* (2004). Hodgkin's disease-related central nervous system angiopathy presenting as reversible posterior leukoencephalopathy. *Internal Medicine*, **43**(10), 1005–7.

126. Sigsbee, B., Deck, M.D., and Posner, J.B. (1979). Nonmetastatic superior sagittal sinus thrombosis complicating systemic cancer. *Neurology*, **29**(2), 139–46.

127. Dworkin, R.H. and Portenoy, R.K. (1996). Pain and its persistence in herpes zoster. *Pain*, **67**(2–3), 241–51.

128. Jaeckle, K.A. (1991). Nerve plexus metastases. *Neurologic Clinics*, **9**(4), 857–66.

129. Kori, S.H. (1995). Diagnosis and management of brachial plexus lesions in cancer patients. *Oncology (Huntington NY)*, **9**(8), 756–60, discussion 765.

130. Jaeckle, K.A. (2004). Neurological manifestations of neoplastic and radiation-induced plexopathies. *Seminars in Neurology*, **24**(4), 385–93.

131. van Es, H.W. (2001). MRI of the brachial plexus. *European Radiology*, **11**(2), 325–36.

132. Wittenberg, K.H. and Adkins, M.C. (2000). MR imaging of nontraumatic brachial plexopathies: frequency and spectrum of findings. *Radiographics*, **20**(4), 1023–32.

133. Luthra, K., Shah, S., Purandare, N. *et al.* (2006). F-18 FDG PET-CT appearance of metastatic brachial plexopathy in a case of carcinoma of the breast. *Clinical Nuclear Medicine*, **31**(7), 432–4.

134. Synek, V.M. (1986). Validity of median nerve somatosensory evoked potentials in the diagnosis of supraclavicular brachial plexus lesions. *Electroencephalography and Clinical Neurophysiology*, **65**(1), 27–35.

135. Portenoy, R.K., Galer, B.S., Salamon, O. *et al.* (1989). Identification of epidural neoplasm. Radiography and bone scintigraphy in the symptomatic and asymptomatic spine. *Cancer*, **64**(11), 2207–13.

136. Kori, S.H., Foley, K.M., and Posner, J.B. (1981). Brachial plexus lesions in patients with cancer: 100 cases. *Neurology*, **31**(1), 45–50.

137. Bajrovic, A., Rades, D., Fehlauer, F. *et al.* (2004). Is there a life-long risk of brachial plexopathy after radiotherapy of supraclavicular lymph nodes in breast cancer patients? *Radiotherapy and Oncology*, **71**(3), 297–301.

138. Binder, D.K., Smith, J.S., and Barbaro, N,M. (2004). Primary brachial plexus tumors: imaging, surgical, and pathological findings in 25 patients. *Neurosurgery Focus*, **16**(5), E11.

139. Vecht, C.J. (1990). Arm pain in the patient with breast cancer. *Journal of Pain and Symptom Management*, **5**(2), 109–17.

140. Gerard, J.M., Franck, N., Moussa, Z. *et al.* (1989). Acute ischemic brachial plexus neuropathy following radiation therapy. *Neurology*, **39**(3), 450–1.

141. Lachance, D.H., O Neill, B.P., Harper, C.M., Jr. *et al.* (1991). Paraneoplastic brachial plexopathy in a patient with Hodgkin's disease. *Mayo Clinic Proceedings*, **66**(1), 97–101.

142. Jaeckle, K.A., Young,D.F., and Foley, K.M. (1985). The natural history of lumbosacral plexopathy in cancer. *Neurology*, **35**(1), 8–15.

143. Stevens, M.J. and Gonet, Y,M. (1990). Malignant psoas syndrome: recognition of an oncologic entity. *Australasian Radiology*, **34**(2), 150–4.

144. Agar, M., Broadbent, A., and Chye, R. (2004). The management of malignant psoas syndrome: case reports and literature review. *Journal of Pain and Symptom Management*, **28**(3), 282–93.

145. Zografos, G.C. and Karakousis, C.P. (1994). Pain in the distribution of the femoral nerve: early evidence of recurrence of a retroperitoneal sarcoma. *European Journal of Surgical Oncology*, **20**(6), 692–3.

146. Tharion, G. and Bhattacharji, S. (1997). Malignant secondary deposit in the iliac crest masquerading as meralgia paresthetica. *Archives of Physical Medicine and Rehabilitation*, **78**(9), 1010–1.

147. Payer. M. (2003). Neurological manifestation of sacral tumors. *Neurosurg Focus*, **15**(2), E1.

148. Taylor, B.V., Kimmel, D.W., Krecke, K.N. *et al.* (1997). Magnetic resonance imaging in cancer-related lumbosacral plexopathy. *Mayo Clinic Proceedings*, **72**(9), 823–9.

149. Thomas, J.E., Cascino, T.L., and Earle, J.D. (1985). Differential diagnosis between radiation and tumor plexopathy of the pelvis. *Neurology*, **35**(1), 1–7.

150. Chad, D.A. and Bradley, W.G. (1987). Lumbosacral plexopathy. *Seminars in Neurology*, **7**(1), 97–107.

151. Desta, K., O'Shaughnessy, M., and Milling, M.A. (1994). Non-Hodgkin's lymphoma presenting as median nerve compression in the arm. *Journal of Hand Surgery [Br]*, **19**(3), 289–91.

152. Grisold, W. and Drlicek, M. (1999). Paraneoplastic neuropathy. *Current Opinion in Neurology*, **12**(5), 617–25.

153. Brady, A,M. (1996). Management of painful paraneoplastic syndromes. *Hematology/Oncology Clinics of North America*, **10**(4), 801–9.

154. Dalmau, J.O. and Posner, J.B. (1997). Paraneoplastic syndromes affecting the nervous system. *Seminars in Oncology*, **24**(3), 318–28.

155. Antoine, J.C., Honnorat, J., Camdessanche, J.P. *et al.* (2001). Paraneoplastic anti-CV2 antibodies react with peripheral nerve and are associated with a mixed axonal and demyelinating peripheral neuropathy. *Annals of Neurology*, **49**(2), 214–21.

156. Fasolino, M., Sabatini, P., Cuomo, T. *et al.* (2004). Paraneoplastic subacute sensory neuronopathy associated with anti-ri antibodies. *Journal of Peripheral Nervous System*, **9**(2), 109.

157. Kelly, J.J. and Karcher, D,S. (2005). Lymphoma and peripheral neuropathy: a clinical review. *Muscle and Nerve*, **31**(3), 301–13.

158. Silen, W. (1983). *Cope's Early Diagnosis of the Acute Abdomen*, 16th edition. Oxford, New York.

159. Coombs, D.W. (1990). Pain due to liver capsular distention. In *Common Problems in Pain Management* (ed. T. Ferrer-Brechner), pp. 247–53. Year Book Medical Publishers, Chicago.

160. Mulholland, M.W., Debas, H., and Bonica, J.J. (1990). Diseases of the liver, biliary system and pancreas. In *The Management of Pain* (ed. J.J.Bonica), pp. 1214–31. Lea & Febiger, Philadelphia.

161. Schonenberg, P., Bastid, C., Guedes, J. *et al.* (1991). Percutaneous echography-guided alcohol block of the celiac plexus as treatment of painful syndromes of the upper abdomen: study of 21 cases. *Schweizerische Medizinische Wochenschrift*, **121**(15), 528–31.

162. Zhu, Z., Friess, H., diMola, F.F. *et al.* (1999). Nerve Growth Factor Expression Correlates With Perineural Invasion and Pain in Human Pancreatic Cancer. *Journal of Clinical Oncology*, **17**(8), 2419.

163. Dang, C., Zhang, Y., Ma, Q. *et al.* (2006). Expression of nerve growth factor receptors is correlated with progression and prognosis of human pancreatic cancer. *Journal of Gastroenterology and Hepatology*, **21**(5), 850–8.

164. Tham, T.C., Lichtenstein, D.R., Vandervoort, J. *et al.* (2000). Pancreatic duct stents for "obstructive type" pain in pancreatic malignancy. *American Journal of Gastroenterology*, **95**(4), 956–60.

165. Ripamonti, C. Management of bowel obstruction in advanced cancer. (1994). *Current Opinion in Oncology*, **6**(4), 351–7.

166. Averbach, A.M. and Sugarbaker, P.H. (1995). Recurrent intraabdominal cancer with intestinal obstruction. *International Surgery*, **80**(2), 141–6.

167. Archer, A.G., Sugarbaker, P.H, and Jelinek, J.S. (1996). Radiology of peritoneal carcinomatosis. *Cancer Treatment and Research*, **82**, 263–88.

168. Stillman, M. (1990). Perineal pain: Diagnosis and management, with particular attention to perineal pain of cancer. In *Second international congress on cancer pain* (eds. K.M. Foley, J.J. Bonica, and V. Ventafrida), pp. 359–77. Raven Press, New York.

169. Boas, R.A., Schug, S.A., and Acland, R.H. (1993). Perineal pain after rectal amputation: a 5-year follow-up. *Pain*, **52**(1), 67–70.

170. Rigor, B.M. (2000). Pelvic cancer pain. *Journal of Surgical Oncology*, **75**(4), 280–300.

171. Seefeld, P.H. and Bargen, J.A. (1943). The spread of carcinoma of the rectum: invasion of lymphatics, veins and nerves. *Annals of Surgery*, **118**, 76–90.

172. Sinaki, M., Merritt, J.L., and Stillwell, G.K. (1977). Tension myalgia of the pelvic floor. *Mayo Clinic Proceedings*, **52**(11), 717–22.

173. Russo, P. (2000). Urologic emergencies in the cancer patient. *Seminars in Oncology*, **27**(3), 284–98.

174. Portenoy, R.K., Kornblith, A.B., Wong, G. *et al.* (1994). Pain in ovarian cancer patients. Prevalence, characteristics, and associated symptoms. *Cancer*, **74**(3), 907–15.

175. Miyamoto, M., Sudo, T., and Kuyama, T. (1991). Spontaneous rupture of hepatocellular carcinoma: a review of 172 Japanese cases. *American Journal of Gastroenterology*, **86**(1), 67–71.

176. Marini, P., Vilgrain, V., and Belghiti, J. (2002). Management of spontaneous rupture of liver tumours. *Digestive Surgery*, **19**(2), 109–13.

177. Wolff, J.M., Boeckmann, W., and Jakse, G. (1994). Spontaneous kidney rupture due to a metastatic renal tumour. Case report. *Scandinavian Journal of Urology and Nephrology*, **28**(4), 415–7.

178. Rajagopal, A., Ramasamy, R., Martin, J. *et al.* (2002). Acute myeloid leukemia presenting as splenic rupture. *Journal of Association of Physicians of India*, **50**, 1435–7.

179. Stamoulis, J.S., Antonopoulou, Z., and Safioleas, M. (2004). Haemorrhagic shock from the spontaneous rupture of an adrenal cortical carcinoma. A case report. *Acta Chirurgica Belgica*, **104**(2), 226–8.

180. Ende, D.A., Robinson, G., and Moulton, J. (1995). Metastasis-induced perforated appendicitis: an acute abdomen of rare aetiology. *Australian and New Zealand Journal of Surgery*, **65**(1), 62–3.

181. Forst, T., Beyer, J., Cordes, U. *et al.* (1995). Gynaecomastia in a patient with a hCG producing giant cell carcinoma of the lung. Case report. *Experimental and Clinical Endocrinology Diabetes*, **103**(1), 28–32.

182. Wurzel, R.S., Yamase, H.T., and Nieh, P.T. (1987). Ectopic production of human chorionic gonadotropin by poorly differentiated transitional cell tumors of the urinary tract. *Journal of Urology*, **137**(3), 502–4.

183. Rosenfield Darling, M.L., Chan, J. *et al.* (1999). Gynecomastia in a patient with lung cancer. *Journal of Clinical Oncology*, **17**(6), 1956.

184. Tseng, A., Jr., Horning, S.J., Freiha, F.S. *et al.* (1985). Gynecomastia in testicular cancer patients. Prognostic and therapeutic implications. *Cancer*, **56**(10), 2534–8.

185. Allen, C.M. and Camisa, C. (2000). Paraneoplastic pemphigus: a review of the literature. *Oral Diseases*, **6**(4), 208–14.

186. Wilmalaratna, H.S. and Sachdev, D. (1987). Adenocarcinoma of the lung presenting with Raynaud's phenomenon, digital gangrene and multiple infarctions in the internal organs. *British Journal of Rheumatology*, **26**(6), 473–5.

187. Ocean, A.J. and Vahdat, L.T. (2004). Chemotherapy-induced peripheral neuropathy: pathogenesis and emerging therapies. *Supportive Care in Cancer*, **12**, 619–25.

188. Penz, M., Kornek, G.V., Raderer, M. *et al.* (2001). Subcutaneous administration of amifostine: a promising therapeutic option in patients with oxaliplatin-related peripheral sensitive neuropathy. *Annals of Oncology*, **12**(3), 421–2.

189. Cascinu, S., Catalano, V., Cordella, L. *et al.* (2002). Neuroprotective effect of reduced glutathione on oxaliplatin-based chemotherapy in advanced colorectal cancer: a randomized, double-blind, placebo-controlled trial. *Journal of Clinical Oncology*, **20**(16), 3478–83.

190. Gamelin, L., Boisdron-Celle, M., Delva, R. *et al.* (2004). Prevention of oxaliplatin-related neurotoxicity by calcium and magnesium infusions: a retrospective study of 161 patients receiving oxaliplatin combined with 5-Fluorouracil and leucovorin for advanced colorectal cancer. *Clinical Cancer Research*, **10**(12 Pt 1), 4055–61.

191. Fink, J.C., Leisenring, W.M., Sullivan, K.M. *et al.* (1998). Avascular necrosis following bone marrow transplantation: a case-control study. *Bone*, **22**(1), 67–71.

192. Berger, C.C., Bokemeyer, C., Schneide, R.M. *et al.* (1995). Secondary Raynaud's phenomenon and other late vascular complications following chemotherapy for testicular cancer. *European Journal of Cancer*, **31A**(13–14), 2229–38.

193. Hansen, S.W., Olsen, N., Rossing, N. *et al.* (1990). Vascular toxicity and the mechanism underlying Raynaud's phenomenon in patients treated with cisplatin, vinblastine and bleomycin [see comments]. *Annals of Oncology*, **1**(4), 289–92.

194. McLeod, D.G. and Iversen, P. (2000). Gynecomastia in patients with prostate cancer: a review of treatment options. *Urology*, **56**(5), 713–20.

195. Poleshuck, E.L., Katz, J., Andrus, C.H. *et al.* (2006). Risk factors for chronic pain following breast cancer surgery: a prospective study. *Journal of Pain*, **7**(9), 626–34.

196. International Association for the Study of Pain: Subcommittee on taxonomy. (1986). Classification of chronic pain. *Pain*, **3**(Suppl),135–8.

197. Ernst, M.F., Voogd, A.C., Balder, W. *et al.* (2002). Early and late morbidity associated with axillary levels I-III dissection in breast cancer. *Journal of Surgical Oncology*, **79**(3), 151–5, discussion 156.

198. Tasmuth, T., von Smitten, K., and Kalso, E. (1996). Pain and other symptoms during the first year after radical and conservative surgery for breast cancer. *British Journal of Cancer*, **74**(12), 2024–31.

199. Stevens, P.E., Dibble, S.L., and Miaskowski, C. (1995). Prevalence, characteristics, and impact of postmastectomy pain syndrome: an investigation of women's experiences. *Pain*, **61**(1), 61–8.

200. Tasmuth, T., von, S.K., Hietanen, P. *et al.* (1995). Pain and other symptoms after different treatment modalities of breast cancer. *Annals of Oncology*, **6**(5), 453–9.

201. Macdonald, L., Bruce, J., Scott, N.W. *et al.* (2005). Long-term follow-up of breast cancer survivors with post-mastectomy pain syndrome. *British Journal of Cancer*, **92**(2), 225–30.

202. Hack, T.F., Cohen, L., Katz, J. *et al.* (1999). Physical and psychological morbidity after axillary lymph node dissection for breast cancer. *Journal of Clinical Oncology*, **17**(1), 143–9.

203. Warmuth, M.A., Bowen, G., Prosnitz, L.R. *et al.* (1998). Complications of axillary lymph node dissection for carcinoma of the breast: a report based on a patient survey. *Cancer*, **83**(7), 1362–8.

204. Smith, W.C., Bourne, D., Squair, J. *et al.* (1999). A retrospective cohort study of post mastectomy pain syndrome. *Pain*, **83**(1), 91–5.

205. Moskovitz, A.H., Anderson, B.O., Yeung, R.S. *et al.* (2001). Axillary web syndrome after axillary dissection. *American Journal of Surgery*, **181**(5), 434–9.

206. Hughes, L.L., Styblo, T.M., Thoms, W.W. *et al.* (1997). Cellulitis of the breast as a complication of breast-conserving surgery and irradiation. *American Journal of Clinical Oncology*, **20**(4), 338–41.

207. Dijkstra, P.U., van Wilgen, P.C., Buijs, R.P. *et al.* (2001). Incidence of shoulder pain after neck dissection: a clinical explorative study for risk factors. *Head and Neck*, **23**(11), 947–53.

208. Talmi, Y.P., Horowitz, Z., Pfeffer, M.R. *et al.* (2000). Pain in the neck after neck dissection. *Otolaryngology - Head and Neck Surgery*, **123**(3), 302–6.

209. Keller, S.M., Carp, N.Z., Levy, M.N. *et al.* (1994). Chronic post thoracotomy pain. *Journal of Cardiovascular Surgery*, *(Torino)*, **35**(6 Suppl 1), 161–4.

210. Kanner, R., Martini, N., and Foley, K.M. (1982). Nature and incidence of postthoracotomy pain. *Proceedings of the American Society of Clinical Oncology*, **1**, Abstract 590.

211. Hamada, H., Moriwaki, K., Shiroyama, K. *et al.* (2000). Myofascial pain in patients with postthoracotomy pain syndrome. *Regional Anesthesia Pain Med*, **25**(3), 302–5.

212. Maunsell, E., Brisson, J., and Deschenes, L. (1993). Arm problems and psychological distress after surgery for breast cancer. *Canadian Journal of Surgery*, **36**(4), 315–20.

213. Flor, H. (2002). Phantom-limb pain: characteristics, causes, and treatment. *Lancet Neurology*, **1**(3), 182–9.

214. Smith, J. and Thompson, J.M. (1995). Phantom limb pain and chemotherapy in pediatric amputees. *Mayo Clinic Proceedings*, **70**(4), 357–64.

215. Chang, V.T., Tunkel, R.S., Pattillo, B.A. *et al.* (1997). Increased phantom limb pain as an initial symptom of spinal-neoplasia [published erratum appears in *Journal of Pain and Symptom Management*, 1997, Sep;14(3):135]. *Journal of Pain and Symptom Management*, **13**(6), 362–4.

216. Rothemund, Y., Grusser, S.M., Liebeskind, U. *et al.* (2004). Phantom phenomena in mastectomized patients and their relation to chronic and acute pre-mastectomy pain. *Pain*, **107**(1–2), 140–6.

217. Davis, R.W. (1993). Phantom sensation, phantom pain, and stump pain. *Archives of Physical Medicine and Rehabilitation*, **74**(1), 79–91.

218. Schultheiss, T.E. and Stephens, L.C. (1992). Invited review: permanent radiation myelopathy. *British Journal of Radiology*, **65**(777), 737–53.

219. Yeoh, E.K. and Horowitz, M. Radiation enteritis. (1987). *Surg Gynecol Obstet*, **165**(4), 373–9.

220. Nussbaum, M.L., Campana, T.J., and Weese, J.L. (1993). Radiation-induced intestinal injury. *Clinics in Plastic Surgery*, **20**(3), 573–80.

221. McWayne, J. and Heiney, S,P. (2005). Psychologic and social sequelae of secondary lymphedema. *Cancer*.

222. Mannaerts, G.H., Rutten, H.J., Martijn, H. *et al.* (2002). Effects on functional outcome after IORT-containing multimodality treatment for locally advanced primary and locally recurrent rectal cancer. *International Journal of Radiation Oncology, Biology, Physics*, **54**(4),1082–8.

223. Wallner, K., Elliott, K., Merrick, G. *et al.* (2004). Chronic pelvic pain following prostate brachytherapy: a case report. *Brachytherapy*, **3**(3), 153–8.

224. Epstein, J., van der Meij, E., McKenzie, M. *et al.* (1997). Postradiation osteonecrosis of the mandible: a long-term follow-up study. *Oral Surgery, Oral Medicine, Oral Pathology, Oral Radiology, and Endodontics*, **83**(6), 657–62.

10.1.3 **Neuropathic pain**

Nanna Brix Finnerup and Troels Staehelin Jensen

Introduction

Neuropathic pain is a heterogeneous group of chronic pain conditions arising from injury or dysfunction of the peripheral or central nervous system. When due to injury, the responsible lesion may be of any type and occur at any location along the sensory transmission pathways. Syndromes that are conventionally considered to be neuropathic are commonly divided into peripheral and central groups, and further classified according to anatomical site and disease (Table 10.1.3.1)[1].

Whether directly related to a life-threatening disease, or caused by a co-morbidity, neuropathic pain may be therapeutically challenging and have a substantial impact on quality of life and mood. Treatment often is difficult and may involve interventions distinct from those typically used for nociceptive pains. Given these challenges, awareness of the various neuropathic pain syndromes and an understanding of issues related to assessment and treatment may lead to better recognition and improved outcomes.

Clinical characteristics

Neuropathic pain may develop immediately after a nerve injury or occur as a late effect, often after several months. The pain is likely to be chronic and is characterized by spontaneous and evoked types of pain perceived in areas of sensory abnormality, either hyposensitivity and/or hypersensitivity.

Table 10.1.3.1 Classification of neuropathic pain.

Peripheral	Central
Neuropathy	Multiple sclerosis
Plexopathy	Neoplasms
Radiculopathy	Spinal cord injury
Nerve injury	Syringomyelia
Amputation	Stroke
Root avulsion	
Postherpetic neuralgia	
Trigeminal neuralgia	
Neoplasms	

Spontaneous pain may be ongoing, with constant or fluctuating pain intensity, or dominated by pain paroxysms of short duration with pain-free intervals or a less intense background pain. The quality of the pain is highly variable and neuropathic pain cannot be diagnosed based on the description alone. The diagnosis may be strongly suggested when it is described in terms such as burning, pricking, sharp, cold, squeezing, or electric-shock-like. Other sensations, such as paraesthesia (abnormal sensation that is not painful or unpleasant) and dysaesthesia (unpleasant abnormal sensation) may be present spontaneously or occur only when evoked by a stimulus[2].

Allodynia is a type of evoked pain that is elicited by a non-noxious stimulation. Dynamic mechanical allodynia or touch-evoked allodynia is the most common form, but allodynia to cold, pressure, movement, and, to a lesser degree, warm stimuli may also be present. Allodynia may accompany spontaneous pain or occur in isolation; it may have little impact on the patient's daily life or be very disabling. In the latter situation, the touch from cloth or taking a shower may cause intense pain, and a gentle touch may be felt as a burning sensation. There may or may not be after-sensations, i.e. pain outlasting the time of the stimulation; after-sensation may be described, for example, as a persistent burning pain that follows touching the sensitive skin area. Hyperalgesia, which describes an increased response to a stimulus that is normally painful, also is often present but usually not described as a symptom by the patient.

In some neuropathic pain conditions, there are signs of sympathetic hyperactivity with excessive sweating, change in skin temperature and colour, and trophic changes in the skin. The presence of other neurological signs, such as focal weakness or reflex changes is variable. The pain may correspond with the entire region affected by sensory or motor dysfunction, or be focally distributed within it. For example, pain associated with spinal cord injury may be located diffusely or in any region below the level of spinal injury, pain caused by stroke may affect part of a limb or the whole hemibody, and pain due to polyneuropathy often is distributed in a stocking or glove distribution.

Definition and diagnosis of neuropathic pain

Definition of neuropathic pain

Neuropathic pain is defined as pain initiated or caused by a primary lesion or dysfunction in the nervous system[2]. To diagnose neuropathic pain, an effort must be made to demonstrate a nervous system lesion, a relevant onset of pain related to this, and a location of pain in areas of sensory disturbance that are neuroanatomically compatible with the lesion. The diagnosis cannot rely on single pain descriptors and is not always easy in the absence of clear diagnostic criteria. The diagnosis may be particularly challenging when sensory loss is masked by areas of hypersensitivity, and when neuropathic and nociceptive components to the pain occur together.

Pain assessment

A medical history including a detailed pain history and a careful medical and neurological examination is essential[1,3].

Pain history

The pain history should try to explore the course of pain, the impact, and multidimensional aspects of pain. Body charts can be useful when exploring the distribution of pain. The pain intensity can be assessed using a categorical scale, such as mild, moderate, and severe. Other unidimensional scales are often used, e.g. an 11-point numeric rating scale (NRS) from 0 to 10, where 0 indicates 'no pain' and 10 'worst possible pain' or 'most intense pain imaginable.' A visual analogue scale (VAS), which is a 100-mm long line with anchor points of 'no pain' and e.g. 'worst possible pain' also is widely used but may be difficult for the elderly patient. It may be useful to separately assess pain 'on average,' pain 'at its worst,' and pain 'at its least'[4]. The affective and motivational component of the pain experience is often neglected, and a recording of the pain unpleasantness is also recommended[3]. Pain descriptors (i.e. the quality of the pain); the impact of pain on daily life; the temporal aspects, including onset, course, and daily variation; associated symptoms; and factors that provoke or relieve the pain also should be assessed, as should the response to current and previous treatments.

Medical and neurological examination

The neurological examination is essential for the diagnosis of neuropathic pain and should include a careful sensory examination evaluating decreased or increased responses to touch, vibration, pinprick, and thermal stimuli, as well as a mapping of the distribution of the sensory dysfunction. Touch is best assessed using cotton wool. Dynamic mechanical allodynia can be assessed by brushing the skin lightly using a small brush or cotton wool. This may elicit a non-painful dysaesthesia or a burning pain sensation in patients with dynamic mechanical allodynia. Allodynia to cold and warm stimuli may be assessed using thermo rolls. Increased or decreased sensation to pinprick may be assessed using a pin or a wooden stick. In cases of pinprick hyperalgesia, the patient will report increased pain compared to the mirror site. After-sensations with continued pain long after the stimulation has ceased may be observed. Vibration can be assessed using a turning fork. Motor function including assessment of muscle strength, tone, reflexes, coordination, and gait should be tested, and the painful area should be carefully examined for signs of autonomic alteration such as skin temperature and colour changes and abnormal sweating. Additional diagnostic testing, such as imaging with CT or MRI, electromyography, and nerve conduction velocity testing, or nerve biopsy may be indicated. Electromyography and nerve conduction velocity testing only assess large-fibre function and may be supplemented with quantitative sensory testing using thermal testing to identify a small-fibre neuropathy.

Neuropathic pain questionnaires

Tools have been developed for identifying patients with neuropathic pain based on clusters of symptoms and signs. The Leeds Assessment of Neuropathic Symptoms and Signs (LANNS scale) includes questions on pain descriptors, evoked pain and autonomic changes, and a simple examination of the patient for evoked pain [5]. Pricking, electric shocks, and burning were descriptors identified to be more common in neuropathic pain. The Neuropathic Pain Questionnaire (NPQ) includes pain descriptors (burning, shooting, electric, tingling, squeezing, freezing pain, and numbness) and increased pain to touch and weather change[6]. Originally developed and validated in French, the 10-item questionnaire DN4 is a clinician-administered questionnaire with pain descriptors (burning, painful cold, electric shocks, pins and needles, tingling, numbness, and itching) and a bedside sensory examination of evoked pain[7]. Recently, validated screening tools, one in English (IDPain) and one in German (painDetect) have been published; these are simple patient-based screening questionnaires that may suggest the presence of neuropathic pain[8]. The diagnosis of neuropathic pain cannot be confirmed on the basis of these tools alone.

Neuropathic pain syndromes

Neuropathic pain may occur in many advanced progressive diseases. Any disease affecting the nervous system, including cancer, HIV/AIDS, stroke, herpes zoster, diabetic polyneuropathy, and multiple sclerosis may cause neuropathic pain. Description of all neuropathic pain syndromes are beyond the scope of this chapter and only some with special reference to palliative care will be mentioned here.

Neuropathic pain in cancer

Neuropathic pain syndromes (Table 10.1.3.2) have become an increasing problem in cancer patients, affecting up to 40 per cent of patients[9,10]. Neuropathic pain conditions may persist independently of the cancer and affect the quality of life in disease-free cancer survivors. In those with active disease, painful mononeuropathy or plexopathy often is caused by direct infiltration of peripheral nerves by the cancer. As an example, lung tumours may affect the lower brachial plexus or the intercostobracial nerve causing pain

Table 10.1.3.2 Cancer-related neuropathic pain syndromes.

Peripheral neuropathic pain	Central pain
Mononeuropathy	Brain tumour/metastasis
Brachial and lumbosacral plexopahy	Spinal cord tumour/metastatis
Paraneoplastic sensory neuropathy	
Chemotherapy-induced peripheral neuropathy	
Postradiation plexopathy	
Phantom limb pain and postmastectomy pain	
Postherpetic neuralgia	

and hypoaesthesia and/or hyperaesthesia in the territory of the affected nerves.

Painful peripheral polyneuropathy may complicate treatment with specific types of chemotherapy[10]. Chemotherapy-induced neuropathy usually has an onset early in treatment and presents with numbness in a distal stocking and glove distribution, which often progresses to pain. Evoked hypersensitivity with touch and cold allodynia may accompany spontaneous pain. In the cancer population, polyneuropathy also may occur in association with malnutrition or paraneoplastic syndromes, which may affect as many as 5 per cent of patients[10].

Radiation therapy also may cause pain syndromes. Radiation-induced fibrosis of the lumbar or brachial plexus can cause progressive sensory and motor dysfunction together with pain, which may be delayed in onset and difficult to distinguish from recurrence of the tumour or myelopathy.

Neuropathic pain may also develop after cancer surgery, including lymph node dissection. Chronic neuropathic pain is common after mastectomy with axillary node dissection, thoracotomy, and amputation, but any surgery causing nerve damage carries the risk of persistent pain[11]. Postamputation pain includes stump pain, which is pain localized at the amputated area, and may be accompanied by allodynia and phantom limb pain, which is pain felt in the amputated limb.

Neuropathic pain in AIDS

Distal sensory, predominantly axonal, polyneuropathy is the most common form of neuropathy associated with AIDS and occurs in about one-third of patients[12,13]. The symptoms begin insidiously with the onset of distal paraesthesia and burning pain in lower extremities, sometimes associated with hypersensitivity and allodynia. Immunological dysfunction secondary to the HIV infection itself and toxicity caused by nucleoside antiretroviral agents are thought to be the two most important mechanisms[12]. Mononeuritis multiplex due to cytomegalovirus or hepatitis and postherpetic neuralgia are other causes of neuropathic pain in AIDS.

Neuropathic pain due to central nervous system lesions

Central pain develops in about 8 per cent of stroke patients, 25 per cent of patients with multiple sclerosis, and 40–50 per cent of patients with spinal cord injury; brain and spinal cord tumours, and other diseases affecting the central nervous system, are other, less common, causes of central pain[14]. Central pain is characterized by ongoing pain, which may be burning, prickling, and shooting. This pain is sometimes accompanied by evoked pain, most often to touch and cold. The pain is located within areas of sensory disturbance covering various proportions of the deafferented body regions. Decreased thermal sensation, which is believed to be related to a spinothalamocortical lesion, is common and may suggest something about the pathophysiology of this pain; it is not sufficient, however, for the diagnosis of central pain[14].

Postherpetic neuralgia

Herpes zoster is due to reactivation of varicella zoster infection and occurs most often in later life and in immunocompromised patients, such as those with HIV infection. The most common and disabling complication is postherpetic neuralgia, which is characterized by steady burning and paroxysmal, lancinating pain in the affected dermatome. The dermatome often exhibits hypo-aesthesia or anaesthesia, but may have allodynia and hyperalgesia that sometimes extend to the surrounding skin, causing light touch and contact with cloth unbearable.

Mechanisms of neuropathic pain

The mechanisms involved in neuropathic pain are multiple and only incompletely understood. This chapter will not discuss mechanisms in detail but give a broad overview of mechanisms as a basis for understanding targets of drugs used in neuropathic pain. Various neuropathic pain syndromes are thought to share common underlying mechanisms[15], but in the single patient it is often impossible to determine what mechanisms are present.

Neuronal plasticity

The transmission of pain is subject to modulation at various synaptic sites at all levels along the neural systems subserving the perception of pain. Any lesion or disease affecting the nervous system may cause irreversible functional changes at these relay sites, and this plasticity may cause fundamental changes in the transmission of pain. The neurological changes after nerve damage may spread centrally in a cascade, so that multiple sources may be involved in the chronic stage of neuropathic pain.

These neuronal changes include a heightened sensitivity to sensory stimuli and a disturbed balance between excitation and inhibition. Neuronal hyperexcitability, which is considered the main cellular change responsible for neuropathic pain, may involve two main pathophysiological elements: (1) sensitization of primary afferent nociceptors and (2) central sensitization[16,17]. The clinical manifestations of this neuronal hyperexcitability are increased pain to painful stimuli, decreased pain thresholds, after-sensations, and spread of pain. Ongoing discharges in peripheral and central pain pathways are thought to cause spontaneous pain, and decreased threshold in nociceptor excitation may cause ongoing pain if the nociceptor is activated by stimuli present at physiological levels.

Peripheral sensitization

A lesion or disease affecting a peripheral nerve may result in a range of molecular changes that sensitize the nociceptor. The outcomes of this sensitization include spontaneous nociceptor activity, decreased threshold, increased response to noxious stimulation, changes in cell phenotypes, and recruitment of silent nociceptors[16,17]. The mechanisms behind such sensitization are multiple, and only some will be mentioned here.

Changes in sodium, calcium, and potassium channel expressions

Following nerve injury, sodium channels may be up-regulated in nerve sprouts, in the dorsal root ganglia supplying the affected nerves, and in neighbouring uninjured nerve fibres. At the same time, some channels may be down-regulated in some fibres and cell bodies. Accumulation of sodium channels may cause increased excitability, as well as spontaneous neuronal ectopic discharges in the peripheral nerves and dorsal root ganglia. Such ectopic activity is thought to result in spontaneous pain and dysaesthesia. Slowing of the recovery rate of voltage-gated sodium channels and inhibition of sustained high-frequency repetitive firing without affecting normal nerve conduction may underlie the efficacy of some anti-convulsants in neuropathic pain[18].

Voltage-gated calcium channels also are up-regulated in sensory neurons. Change in the $\alpha_2\delta$ protein, which modulates the voltage-gated calcium channel has been found to correlate with gabapentin sensitivity[19].

Down-regulation of potassium channels and reduction in the generation of the M current, a subthreshold potassium current that stabilizes the membrane potential and controls neuronal excitability, are also implicated in enhanced excitability and ectopic activity[20]. It is for this reason that potassium channel openers are potential targets for analgesic drug development.

Adrenergic sensitivity

Some pain syndromes respond favourably to inhibition of noradrenergic activity. This sympathetically maintained pain is believed to be most common in complex regional pain syndromes (also known as reflex sympathetic dystrophy and causalgia)[21]. This mechanism may correlate with up-regulation of α-adrenergic receptors in damaged nerve fibres and sprouting of sympathetic fibres, which form basket-like structures around cell bodies in dorsal root ganglia.

Chemical mediators

Various chemical mediators are released during inflammation and nerve injury, and may underlie the development or persistence of neuropathic pain. Nerve growth factor is released from injured nerves during Wallerian degeneration and may sensitize spared nociceptors in the vicinity[22]. Proinflammatory cytokines, such as the interleukins and tumour necrosis factor α (TNF-α), and brady-kinin are released as part of the inflammatory cascade, and may act on injured nerve to contribute to hyperalgesia and spontaneous nociceptor activity, either directly or by mediating the release of other algogenic mediators[23].

Up-regulation of receptor proteins

Injury may result in the up-regulation of proteins, which in turn, may contribute to the occurrence or characteristics of neuropathic pain. Up-regulation of receptor proteins in nerve terminals, such as the transient receptor potential vanilloid-1 (TRPV1) receptor, may be involved in heat allodynia and hyperalgesia[17].

Central sensitization

An increased afferent neuronal barrage, or an imbalance in sensory inflow resulting from primary sensory nerve degeneration, may induce secondary changes, including increased excitability in spinal cord neurons. These changes are termed central sensitization and are manifested by an increased response to synaptic inputs, decreased threshold, and expansion of receptive fields[17]. Furthermore, central sensitization may include processes by which input from low threshold Aβ mechanoreceptors gain access to pain-transmitting systems, causing normally non-painful stimuli to be perceived as painful[24]. Some of the changes involved in central sensitization are summarized in the following paragraphs.

Increased activity at glutamate receptor sites

Central sensitization involves activation of the N-methyl-D-aspartate (NMDA) receptor by release of the excitatory amino acid, glutamate, from primary afferent neurons[24]. Prolonged glutamate release from these primary afferents also may act on non-NMDA receptors, and combined with release of calcitonin gene-related peptide and substance P, may cause additional depolarization of postsynaptic neurons, leading to the displacement of magnesium from the NMDA receptor, which now becomes activated. NMDA-receptor activation, which increases the influx of calcium ions and initiates a cascade of intracellular events, is a target for drug intervention.

Imbalance between inhibition and facilitation

The ongoing activity from primary afferents may cause a degeneration of inhibitory dorsal horn interneurons containing γ-aminobutyric acid (GABA), which may contribute to increased sensitivity[25]. Also, loss of inhibition from descending pathways dependent on monoamines such as noradrenaline, serotonin (5-HT), and dopamine, as well as opioids, may further contribute to disinhibition and enhanced sensitivity. Recently, it has become clear that descending pathways can also exert excitatory influences that facilitate nociception, and studies have suggested an important role for facilitatory 5-HT pathways working via 5-HT$_3$ receptors[26].

Changes in sodium channel expression

The importance of sodium channel up-regulation following peripheral nerve injury was noted previously. After both peripheral and central nervous system lesions, sodium channel expression also may be altered in second-order dorsal horn and thalamic neurons, and this, too, may contribute to neuropathic pain[27].

Glia cells and inflammatory mediators

Peripheral and central nerve injuries have been shown to activate spinal cord glia cells. This activation leading to release of proinflammatory cytokines, which may act upon neurons and is likely to be an important mechanism of exaggerated pain and spread of pain to neighbouring healthy tissue outside the nerve injury[28].

Pharmacological treatment of neuropathic pain

Treating neuropathic pain remains a great challenge. The drugs that are commonly used for these disorders have limited response rates, and responders typically experience only partial reduction in pain at tolerable doses. Nonetheless, even a 30 per cent reduction in pain may be clinically important[29]. Today, more than 100 randomized controlled trials support decision making and provide a basis for evidence-based treatment algorithms[30]. Few comparative drug trials exist, however, and the most rational approach to comparing treatments involves calculation of the number-needed-to-treat (NNT) and the number-needed-to-harm (NNH) from clinical trials data. NNT is calculated as the number of patients needed to treat with a certain drug to obtain one patient with a defined degree of pain relief (usually 50 per cent) and is calculated as the reciprocal of the absolute risk reduction[30,31]. NNH is likewise calculated as the reciprocal of the absolute difference in risk, with risk defined as side effects or dropouts. Pharmacological agents and their principal molecular targets and related non-cancer pain syndromes for which there are consistent evidence of a clinically significant pain-relieving effect from randomized controlled trials are presented in Table 10.1.3.3.

Anticonvulsants

Anticonvulsant drugs are primarily used for the treatment of epilepsy. They have several pharmacological actions that can interfere with processes involved in neuronal hyperexcitability, either by decreasing excitatory or increasing inhibitory transmission, thereby exerting a net neuronal depressant effect. These effects may underlie the analgesic effects that some of these drugs exert in neuropathic pain states.

Gabapentin and pregabalin

Gabapentin and pregabalin are structurally related compounds. Their analgesic effect in neuropathic pain is thought to be mediated through antagonism of the α$_2$δ subunit of voltage-dependent calcium channels at presynaptic sites[32]. The subsequent reduction in calcium influx reduces the release of excitatory amino acids, attenuates postsynaptic excitability, and modulates GABAergic function—mechanisms that may be responsible for the analgesic efficacy of these drugs[32].

The effects of gabapentin and pregabalin are well established in postherpetic neuralgia, painful diabetic neuropathy, and spinal cord injury pain[30,33,34]. Both drugs seem equally effective, with a combined NNT in peripheral neuropathic pain of 4.1 (3.6–4.8) (Fig. 10.1.3.1). The pain relief is rapid, within the first or second week, and often accompanied by improvements in sleep and quality-of-life measures. The effects of gabapentin in HIV neuropathy and postamputation pain are inconclusive, but a study in cancer patients with neuropathic pain already treated with opioids was positive[35].

Both gabapentin and pregabalin are generally well tolerated. Neither drug has any known drug–drug interactions. Somnolence and dizziness are the most common side effects and peripheral oedema, weight gain, nausea, vertigo, asthenia, dry mouth, and ataxia may occur. Side effects may resolve over time or improve with dose reduction. Gabapentin is usually administered three times daily. Dosing is initiated slowly, e.g. starting with 300 mg the first day and increased by 300 mg every one to seven days. The final daily dose is between 1800 and 3600 mg, but side effects may limit dose escalation. Pregabalin may be initiated with 75 or 150 mg daily and increased every three to seven days by 150 mg, up to 600 mg in two divided doses. Both gabapentin and pregabalin undergo renal excretion and renal impairment requires dosage adjustment. Pregabalin has anxiolytic effects in patients with generalized anxiety disorders[36] and may therefore be the first drug choice in patients with anxiety. It is still unknown whether patients failing to respond to one of these drugs will benefit from the other.

Carbamazepine and oxcarbazepine

The main action of carbamazepine and its analogue oxcarbazepine is blocking of sodium channels. Slowing of the recovery rate of voltage-gated sodium channels and inhibition of sustained high-frequency repetitive firing cause a suppression of spontaneous neuronal ectopic discharges in the peripheral nerves and dorsal root ganglia, without affecting normal nerve conduction[37]. Sodium channel blockers probably also act on altered sodium channel expression in the central nervous system[27].

Carbamazepine and oxcarbazepine are first-line drugs for trigeminal neuralgia[38], based on the favourable outcomes of early randomized controlled trials. Newer trials comparing oxcarbazepine to carbamazepine have reported comparable analgesic effects, but fewer side effects during oxcarbazepine treatment[39]. Additional studies have not confirmed clinically significant effects on other neuropathic pain conditions. One trial from 1969, which may not meet current methodological standards, reported a good effect of carbamazepine in painful diabetic neuropathy[40], but

Table 10.1.3.3 Pharmacological agents and their principal molecular targets and related non-cancer pain syndromes for which there is consistent evidence of clinically significant pain-relieving effect from randomized controlled trials.

Drug/drug class	Major effect on neuropathic pain	Pain syndrome
Antidepressants		
Tricyclic antidepressants (TCAs)	Inhibition of serotonin and noradrenaline reuptake, blockade of sodium and calcium channels, and NMDA receptors	Painful polyneuropathy, postherpetic neuralgia, postmastectomy pain[a], central poststroke pain[a], multiple sclerosis[a]
Serotonin noradrenaline reuptake inhibitors (SNRIs)	Inhibition of serotonin and noradrenaline reuptake	Painful polyneuropathy
Anticonvulsants		
Carbamazepine/oxcarbazepine	Blockade of voltage-dependent sodium channels	Trigeminal neuralgia
Lamotrigine	Blockade of voltage-dependent sodium channels and inhibition of glutamate release	Trigeminal neuralgia[a], painful polyneuropathy[a], central poststroke pain[a]
Gabapentin/pregabalin	Blockade of the $\alpha_2\delta$ subunit of voltage-gated calcium channels	Painful polyneuropathy, postherpetic neuralgia, spinal cord injury pain
Opioids		
Tramadol	Opioid agonist, inhibition of serotonin and noradrenaline reuptake	Painful polyneuropathy, postherpetic neuralgia[a]
Oxycodone	Opioid agonist	Painful polyneuropathy, postherpetic neuralgia[a]
Morphine	Opioid agonist	Postherpetic neuralgia[a], phantom limb pain[a]
Topical lidocaine		
Lidocaine patch	Blockade of voltage-dependent sodium channels	Postherpetic neuralgia with allodynia, focal neuropathy with allodynia[a]
Cannabinoids		
Cannabinoids	Cannabinoid agonist	Pain in multiple sclerosis, brachial plexus avulsion[a]

[a] Only one randomized trial performed.

more recent trials of oxcarbazepine have found either a questionable effect [41] or a statistically significant effect but with a high NNT of 6.0 (3.3–41.0) [42].

Carbamazepine treatment is associated with cognitive side effects, drowsiness, dizziness, ataxia, diplopia, and, in elderly patients, confusion [43]. Other side effects include rash, nausea, weight gain, and hyponatremia. Slow titration is needed to minimize side effects. In rare cases, severe blood dyscrasia may be seen, and a complete blood count should be obtained prior to treatment and continuously throughout treatment. Carbamazepine has several drug interactions [43] and is contraindicated in patients with atrioventricular block and hepatic insufficiency. Oxcarbazepine is generally better tolerated but side-effects include drowsiness, ataxia, diplopia, dizziness, headache, hyponatremia, rash, and nausea. [44]. Serum sodium levels should be monitored during treatment. Carba- mazepine is usually initiated with 300 mg/day and increased by 100 mg every other day to a maximum dosage of 1500–2000 mg/day. The starting dose of oxcarbazepine may be 600 mg/day, increased by 150–300 mg every other day to 1500–3000 mg/day.

Other anticonvulsants

Lamotrigine acts by blocking voltage-dependent sodium channels and inhibiting pathological release of excitatory amino acid transmitters, principally glutamate, from presynaptic neurons[45,46]. Controlled studies involving limited numbers of patients found statistically significant pain-relieving effects in central poststroke pain, painful diabetic polyneuropathy, and as add-on therapy, in trigeminal neuralgia. The NNT in painful diabetic polyneuropathy based on one study is 4.0 (2.1–42)[47]. Generally, lamotrigine is well tolerated but side effects may occur and include dizziness, ataxia, diplopia, somnolence, and nausea[43]. The most serious side effects are allergic exanthema and Stevens–Johnson syndrome; the risk of these effects is diminished by slow initial dose escalation, and this approach is strongly recommended.

Valproate is a first-generation anticonvulsant with a wide range of actions, including potentiation of GABAergic functions. Its effect in neuropathic pain has only been studied in few randomized controlled trials from two centres with conflicting results, and thus its role must await further studies[48,49].

Topiramate has a pharmacologic profile that suggested a strong likelihood of analgesic effects in neuropathic pain. Results from controlled trials have been disappointing, however. It is no longer in development as a treatment for neuropathic pain after three large trials in patients with painful diabetic neuropathy failed to establish a pain-relieving effect[50].

Antidepressants

Antidepressants have a well-established beneficial effect in various neuropathic pain states. Antidepressants used in neuropathic pain

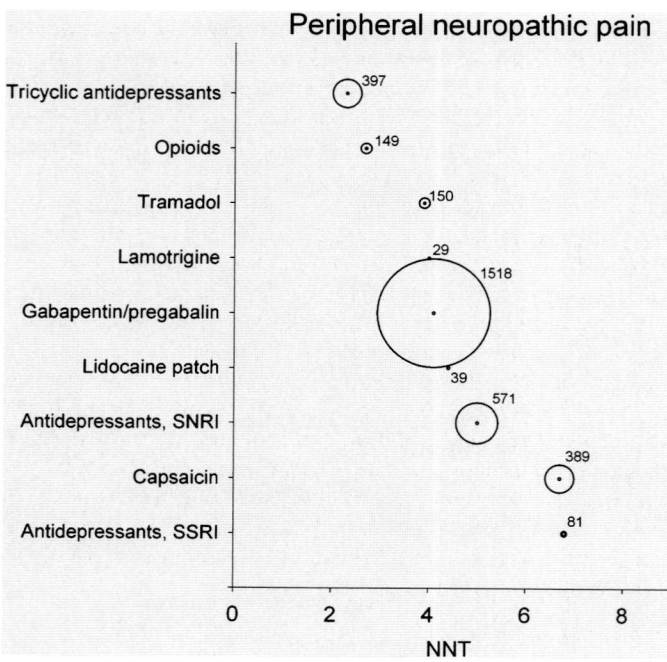

Figure 10.1.3.1 Combined numbers-needed-to-treat (NNTs) in peripheral neuropathic pain (postherpetic neuralgia, painful diabetic neuropathy, and peripheral nerve injury). Circle size and related numbers indicate the number of patients who have received active treatment. SNRIs = serotonin noradrenaline reuptake inhibitors, SSRI = selective serotonin reuptake inhibitors. (Modified from Finnerup, N.B., Otto, M., McQuay, H.J., et al. (2005). Algorithm for neuropathic pain treatment: an evidence based proposal. *Pain*, 118, 289–305.)

treatment include tricyclic antidepressants (TCAs) (e.g. amitriptyline and imipramine) and the selective serotonin noradrenaline reuptake inhibitors (SNRIs) (duloxetine and venlafaxine). The analgesic effects of the selective serotonin reuptake inhibitors (SSRIs) are less certain[51]. Antidepressants relieve pain in non-depressed patients, and it is well established that their pain-relieving effects are independent of their antidepressant effects[51]. However, because of this dual effect, antidepressants may be the first drug choice in patients with a coexisting depression.

Tricyclic antidepressants
The mechanism by which TCAs relieve neuropathic pain is thought to be mainly by blocking the reuptake of noradrenaline or serotonin, thereby augmenting endogenous pain-suppressing pathways descending from the brainstem. TCAs also have a wide range of other pharmacological actions with potential pain-relieving effects. TCAs block voltage-gated sodium channels, and it is likely that the selective block of both persistent late openings and the inactivated state of neuronal sodium channels contributes to its analgesic efficacy[52]. Also, central NMDA receptor antagonist activity and calcium channel blockade are likely to be involved[51]. TCAs also bind to opioid receptors, but their affinity for the opioid receptor is low, and this mechanism is not likely to be relevant at its therapeutic concentration[53].

Several randomized controlled trials have documented the effect of TCAs in relieving central poststroke pain, postherpetic neuralgia, and painful diabetic and non-diabetic polyneuropathy[30]. In peripheral neuropathic pain, the combined NNT is 2.3 (2.0–2.7) (Fig. 10.1.3.1). In HIV-related neuropathy, amitriptyline failed to relieve neuropathic pain in two randomized trials[54,55]. In mixed cancer patients with neuropathic pain partially controlled with opioids, amitriptyline had no pain-relieving effect and was associated with adverse effects[56]. The treatment period was, however, short (one week), and the dose was relatively low (up to 50 mg daily). Nortriptyline up to 100 mg/day was evaluated in the treatment of cis-diamminedichloroplatinum (CDDP)-induced dysaesthesia in a randomized trial[57]. Nortriptyline only provided modest relief of dysaesthesia and pain.

Anticholinergic side effects are common during TCAs therapy and include dry mouth, constipation, urinary retention, sweating, and blurred vision. The risk of somnolence and confusion may be present when initiating treatment, and the risk is increased in elderly patients and others predisposed to such side effects, including patients treated with concomitant centrally-acting drugs. Orthostatic hypotension and gait disturbances are concerns, especially in the elderly. Combination with class IC antiarrhythmics or SSRIs that are metabolized by P4502D6 may cause toxic serum levels of TCAs. TCAs are contraindicated in patients with epilepsy.

The most serious side effect of the TCAs is cardiotoxicity. TCAs are contraindicated in patients with heart failure and cardiac conduction blocks, and an ECG is needed before initiating treatment. A recent large retrospective cohort study found that TCAs in doses of 100 mg or more daily were associated with increased relative risk of sudden cardiac death, which suggests that such doses should be used cautiously, particularly in patients with an elevated baseline risk of sudden death[58]. The secondary amines (desipramine and nortriptyline) may be better tolerated than tertiary amines (imipramine, amitriptyline, and clomipramine)[59].

Initiation of TCA treatment is best done slowly, starting with 25 mg daily (10 mg in the elderly) and slowly increased (25 mg every 3–7 days) up to 50–150 mg daily. There is a large pharmacokinetic variability in the metabolic pathways of TCAs due to a genetic polymorphism of the enzymes that metabolize these drugs[60]. Some patients may therefore attain high plasma drug concentrations at doses normally used, while others may have subtherapeutic concentrations at such doses, and monitoring of serum drug concentrations may be helpful in guiding treatment.

Selective serotonin noradrenaline reuptake inhibitors
The SNRIs are inhibitors of serotonin and noradrenaline reuptake with no effect on postsynaptic receptors. Duloxetine has no effect on sodium channels, while venlafaxine has some blocking effect. Bupropion inhibits noradrenaline and serotonin reuptake as well as dopamine reuptake.

Recent randomized trials have documented the effect of venlafaxine[61,62] and duloxetine in painful polyneuropathy[63,64]. The combined NNT from these four trials of SNRIs in painful polyneuropathy was 5.0 (3.8–7.4). The effect of duloxetine was present from week 1, and the most effective dose associated with fewest side effects was 60 mg once daily. It has been shown that in patients with major depression, duloxetine significantly reduces painful physical symptoms[65].

Only one randomized trial has studied bupropion in neuropathic pain[66]. Results were positive. This drug is less sedating than other antidepressants and therefore better tolerated in patients with fatigue or sedation.

The SNRIs are generally well tolerated, and side effects tend to decrease with continued treatment[67]. The most common side effect is nausea. Other side effects include somnolence, dizziness, constipation, anorexia, and hyperhidrosis. Sexual dysfunction with decreased libido, ejaculation failure, and erectile dysfunction related to serotonergic actions has been reported for the SNRIs, as well as for the SSRIs[67]. Regular monitoring of blood pressure is recommended during venlafaxine treatment due to risk of elevated blood pressure[68]. In the two trials in neuropathic pain, duloxetine treatment was not associated with clinically significant cardiovascular changes[63,64], and a meta-analysis showed no clinically significant changes in blood pressure or ECG during treatment with duloxetine in therapeutic doses[69]. Cardiovascular side effects to venlafaxine have been reported[62,70], and further studies probably are needed to determine the risk of cardiac arrhythmias. Duloxetine should not be used in patients with hepatic dysfunction, and venlafaxine dose should be decreased in patients with renal or hepatic insufficiency. Duloxetine can be started at 30 mg once daily and increased to 60 mg once daily after one week, and venlafaxine should be initiated with 37.5 mg and increased by 75 mg weekly up to 150–225 mg daily.

Topical lidocaine

Lidocaine blocks voltage-gated sodium channels, and topical application is thought to silence ectopic discharges on small afferent fibres. Lidocaine patches are increasingly used in the treatment of postherpetic neuralgia and focal peripheral neuropathic pain. Randomized trials have shown positive effects of a lidocaine patch 5 per cent in postherpetic neuralgia and mixed peripheral focal neuropathy[71,72]. So far, only patients with concomitant allodynia have been studied in randomized trials, but lidocaine relieves non-allodynic symptoms as well[73]. Lidocaine gel 5 per cent did not relieve HIV-related painful neuropathy[74].

Side effects from the lidocaine patch are mild, usually skin irritation. Lack of systemic side effects is favourable, particularly in the treatment of the elderly and in patients prone to side effects. It also may be useful as add-on therapy due to the lack of interference with systemic treatment. Although there is minimal absorption, it should not be used in patients taking oral class I antiarrhytmic drugs[75]. A maximum of 3–4 patches should be applied for no more than 12–18 h.

Opioids in neuropathic pain

The three types of opioid receptors—μ, κ, and δ —are widely distributed in the nervous system. Opioids inhibit pain transmission mainly by interacting with these receptors at presynaptic and postsynaptic sites in the dorsal horn of the spinal cord and by increasing descending inhibition from brain to spinal cord.

Although neuropathic pain does not respond reliably to opioids[76], randomized trials have shown positive effects of various drugs (oxycodone, morphine, methadone, and levorhanol) in painful polyneuropathy, postherpetic neuralgia, phantom limb pain, and mixed neuropathic pain[30]. The combined NNT in peripheral neuropathic pain is 2.7 ((2.1–3.6), which is comparable with TCAs and $\alpha_2\delta$ agonists (Fig. 10.1.3.1). In one study conducted in a mixed population with neuropathic pain disorders, patients with central poststroke pain were least likely to report pain relief[76]. Switching from one opioid to another, e.g. from morphine to methadone, improved analgesic effects in patients with neuropathic cancer pain[77]. Studies of opioids have high rates of withdrawal due to

side-effects; increasing the dose may yield more side effects without additional beneficial effects on multidimensional pain measures, such as interference in functioning and affective distress[76].

The most common adverse effects of opioids are sedation, constipation, and nausea. In a majority of patients, the sedation decreases or resolves with continued treatment; it may persist, however, or be additive with the sedating effects of other centrally-acting drugs. Often, opioid treatment requires the additional administration of laxative and antiemetics. Other side effects include confusion, especially in elderly patients; urinary retention; dizziness; dysphoria and nightmares; and, less commonly, respiratory depression. In chronic non-cancer pain, opioids are not first-line analgesics and long-term therapy is generally considered only after other reasonable therapies have failed to provide adequate pain relief[78]. Pain relief and quality of life should be monitored during treatment, and sustained-release opioids administered at regular intervals are recommended[78]. In palliative care, oral opioids, or epidural and intrathecal opioids when indicated, may need to be supplemented with antidepressants or anticonvulsants if they do not provide adequate analgesia for neuropathic pain components.

Tramadol

The mechanism of analgesic effects produced by tramadol involves both mu-opioid agonism and monoaminergic effects, specifically inhibition of noradrenaline reuptake and stimulation of serotonin release. The opioid actions result from binding of the main metabolite to the mu receptor. The analgesia produced by tramadol is comparable to the effects produced by other opioid agonists in naïve patients, but the effects in neuropathic pain specifically have not been extensively studied[79](Fig. 10.1.3.1). Side effects include nausea, constipation, dizziness, somnolence, hyperhidrosis, and dry mouth. There is an increased risk of seizures in patients with decreased seizure threshold. Caution is needed when combining tramadol with antidepressants because of the risk of the serotonin syndrome (a potentially life-threatening syndrome ranging from mild tremors, diarrhoea, restlessness, and confusion to delirium, neuromuscular rigidity and hyperthermia)[80]. Although tramadol, like other opioid drugs, is not considered a first-line drug in non-cancer-related neuropathic pain, some patients benefit from short-term use or 'as needed' administration (usually 50 mg per dose). When long-term treatment is undertaken, the dosage can be increased up to 400 mg daily in four divided doses.

Other pharmacological agents

NMDA antagonists

NMDA antagonists given as intravenous infusions have been shown to relieve varied types of neuropathic pain, but the effects of oral NMDA antagonists, such as dextromethorphan, riluzole and memantine, have been less convincing because of low response rates and unfavourable therapeutic indices[30]. Two small studies have found a clinically relevant efficacy in painful diabetic polyneuropathy, while nine studies in postherpetic neuralgia, phantom limb pain, and mixed neuropathic pain conditions failed to find an effect. These drugs also have psychomimetic side effects and memory impairment, which limit their use in chronic pain management.

Cannabinoids

The cannabinoid system has an important role in inhibiting synaptic transmission and controlling synaptic plasticity in pain pathways.

Cannabinoids have recently been studied in a few randomized trials with positive outcomes. Central pain in multiple sclerosis[81,82], brachial plexus avulsion[83], and mixed neuropathic pain conditions[84] have been studied. Cannabinoids were generally well tolerated with gradually increasing doses. Side effects include dizziness, drowsiness, impaired psychomotor function, and dry mouth, especially during the run-in period, and other psychoactive effects like dysphoria[85]. The abuse liability associated with marijuana raises concern about abuse and addiction of all the cannabinoids, as well as the associated legal and regulatory issues. These are being addressed through appropriate pre-approval studies and risk management programmes for the post-approval period. Cannabinoids have antiemetic effects and improve appetite, and may therefore be considered for treating neuropathic pain in patients with AIDS-related wasting disease or in the palliative care of patients with nausea and decreased appetite[85].

Capsaicin

Capsaicin is thought to act by depleting substance P from primary afferent nociceptors. Capsaicin is applied topically. Evidence for the effect in neuropathic pain is not substantial and the effect size is relatively low[86]. Consistent pain-relieving effect has been found in patients with postherpetic neuralgia, but results have been contradictory in nerve injury pain and painful diabetic polyneuropathy[30].

Combination therapy

If treatment with a single drug is only partly effective, other drugs may be added.

In a randomized study, 60 patients with painful diabetic neuropathy were treated with gabapentin or placebo[87]. Gabapentin significantly relieved pain, but 12 patients treated with gabapentin had minimal or no improvement. These patients were randomized to either gabapentin and venlafaxine or gabapentin and placebo. The gabapentin/venlafaxine-treated group had significantly more pain relief than the gabapentin-treated group, but importantly, no comparison was made to venlafaxine treatment alone. Combination therapy caused more dizziness, somnolence, and nausea than gabapentin as monotherapy. In a four-way crossover trial, patients with painful diabetic neuropathy or postherpetic neuralgia received placebo (lorazepam), morphine, gabapentin, or a combination of gabapentin and morphine[88]. The combination of gabapentin and morphine resulted in better pain relief than with either treatment alone, without significantly increased adverse effects. Maximal tolerated doses were lower with the combination therapy than with treatment with a single agent.

Because very few controlled studies have evaluated the efficacy and side effects when combining two pharmacological agents, the rationale for such combination therapy is based on theory. A rational way is to try two drugs that provide partial pain relief and act on different mechanisms. Examples are gabapentin combined with TCAs, SNRIs, or opioids, and TCAs or SNRIs combined with opioids. The exception to this is the use of tramadol with drugs that increase serotonin levels such as antidepressants.

Pre-emptive treatment

Chronic postoperative pain may be limited when minimally invasive techniques are used, presumably with less risk of damaging major nerves[11]. Although pre-emptive or preventive analgesia may be able to accomplish the same result, studies that have evaluated the use of aggressive or multimodal analgesia in the perioperative period have yielded contradictory results regarding the effect on chronic pain[11].

Few studies in non-surgical neuropathic pain have evaluated the effect of early treatment in preventing or reducing pain. A study that compared low-dose amitriptyline 25 mg daily with placebo during the initial 90 days after eruption of herpes zoster found that the active drug reduced pain prevalence at 6 months by more than 50 per cent[89]. In another study[90], 39 patients received either amitriptyline titrated up to 75 mg or placebo for a period of 365 days following acute thalamic stroke; central pain developed in three patients who received amitriptyline and in four receiving placebo. With an expected 8 per cent incidence of central post-stroke pain, this sample size is probably too small to detect an effect. Neuroprotective agents may, combined with chemotherapy regimens, protect peripheral nerves from chemotherapeutic injury with preserved control of malignancy[10]. Such agents, e.g. vitamin E or sulfur-containing thiol drugs, are under investigation as neuroprotective agents preventing chronic neuropathy caused by chemotherapy or antiviral AIDS treatment.

Non-pharmacological treatment

Psychological management

When chronic pain is severe or associated with a high level of disability, concurrent treatment with multiple modalities via a multi-disciplinary approach may be preferred. Chronic pain is a complex psychological experience, which may have consequences for daily activities, sleep, cognition, emotion, behavioural, and social relations. Concomitant anxiety, depression, and psychological distress should be evaluated and treated. Explanation of the underlying mechanisms of neuropathic pain is important. The pain may be accompanied with more distress if the patient believes it represents the spread of cancer or an underlying progressive disorder, or that the pain intensity will keep progressing.

Psychological treatment is complex and lengthy, and may be difficult to access. Nonetheless, there is increasing evidence for the effect of cognitive behavioural therapy in chronic pain[91]. Cognitive behavioural therapy includes a variety of approaches[92], including cognitive reconstructuring and coping strategies, problem solving, relaxation training, attention-diversion techniques, assertiveness training, and modification in activity and exposure to feared activities.

Other non-pharmacological treatment

Physical therapy may be indicated in some patients with neuropathic pain to alleviate complications related to immobility or to other effects of the neurological disease. Nociceptive pain contributing to overall pain intensity and disability may be reduced by techniques that may include correcting poor posture, dystonia and contractures, passive mobilization, stretching and massage, and active exercise. The effect of transcutaneous electrical nerve stimulation and acupuncture in neuropathic pain also may be useful in a subset of patients, but their role and predictors for determining a positive outcome are not well established. Other non-pharmacological treatments such as sympathetic blockade, spinal cord and motor cortex stimulation, and neurosurgery may be considered in severe refractory pain, but depend on many factors such as pain type and life expectancy.

General treatment principles

A broad approach to the treatment of chronic neuropathic pain is essential. Patients may be elderly; may have concurrent medical problems and impairments, depression, sleep disturbances, or psychosocial problems; and may be treated with multiple drugs with unwanted side effects. The diagnosis of the neuropathic pain syndrome and the presumptive underlying mechanisms is the first important step and requires a thorough assessment. The diagnosis of neuropathic pain is not always easy, and often, neuropathic pain coexists with other types of pain. Whenever possible, the underlying disease should be treated. Whether or not the underlying mechanisms causing the pain can be treated, symptomatic treatment of pain and related disability should be offered. Realistic expectations for the outcome of a given treatment should be discussed with the patient, explaining that often only partial pain relief from neuropathic pain can be expected.

As analgesic therapies are applied, the effects are unpredictable, and patients with the same disease or same symptom may respond differently to the same treatment. There is little evidence to support the use of specific drugs for specific symptoms. Although sodium channel blockers like carbamazepine are the drug of choice for treating paroxysmal pain in trigeminal neuralgia, there is little evidence for choosing this drug, or other sodium channel blockers, to treat pain dominated by paroxysmal pain, or for the use of other types of drugs, such as the antidepressants, for burning and pricking ongoing pain. For example, painful paroxysms can occur with decreased small-fibre function[93], and this entity has been reported to be relieved by tricyclic antidepressants and the SNRI venlafaxine[61,94]. At the present time, treatment of neuropathic pain is a trial-and-error process. Although a mechanism-based treatment approach has been suggested, future trials will tell whether pain mechanisms can be identified in an individual patient, and whether specific symptoms and signs, or clusters, will be able to predict response to certain treatments.

Treatment algorithm

Although a general treatment algorithm may be proposed, each treatment has to be individualized to the single patient, taking into account all co-morbidities and drug interactions. Most randomized controlled trials are performed in patients with diabetic polyneuropathy and postherpetic neuralgia, and to what extent a treatment which is found effective in one neuropathic pain condition can be expected to relieve other conditions is unknown. Based on experience, it seems likely that efficacy demonstrated in one condition can be extrapolated to others[15]. There are clearly exceptions, however, and the existing studies, albeit very limited, suggest that some disorders, such as central pain and HIV-related pain, may be more difficult to treat.

During the course of pain treatment, the level and character of the pain, and side effects should be monitored. If there is no effect of a first-line drug, the treatment should be switched to another first-line drug, then ultimately to a second-line drug. In case of partial pain relief, another drug with complementary mechanisms can be added. It is important to avoid drug interference and patients should be monitored for additive adverse effects.

NNTs (Fig. 10.1.3.1) only provide rough estimates of relative effectiveness among various drugs due to differences in design and patient populations among trials. Based on the amount and consistency of evidence for efficacy in neuropathic pain and knowledge on short-term and long-term side effects, a treatment algorithm for treating neuropathic pain may be proposed[30,75,95,96].

First-line treatments

In patients with trigeminal neuralgia, carbamazepine and oxcarbazepine are the first drug choices. In other neuropathic pain conditions, tricyclic antidepressants, SNRIs (duloxetine or venlafaxine), or calcium channel $\alpha_2\delta$ agonists (gabapentin or pregabalin) are the first drug choices. In patients with focal peripheral neuropathy with allodynia, topical lidocaine patch is also a first-line drug. Antidepressants may be the first drug choice in patients with depression, and both TCAs and calcium channel $\alpha_2\delta$ agonists may be considered in patients with sleep disturbances. Pregabalin may be the first choice in patients with anxiety.

Second-line treatments

Opioids (including tramadol), lamotrigine, and cannabinoids may be considered if there is no or insufficient effect of first-line drug classes. Opioids, including tramadol, may be first line in episodic pain or in patients with cancer-related non-neuropathic pain. Switching from one opioid to another may improve pain relief. Combination therapy may be considered in patients with insufficient effect from one drug.

References

1. Jensen, T.S., Gottrup, H., Sindrup, S.H. et al. (2001). The clinical picture of neuropathic pain. European Journal of Pharmacology, 429, 1–11.
2. Merskey, H. and Bogduk, N. (1994). Classification of chronic pain: descriptions of chronic pain syndromes and definitions of pain terms. IASP Press, Seattle.
3. Cruccu, G., Anand, P., Attal, N. et al. (2004). EFNS guidelines on neuropathic pain assessment. European Journal of Neurology, 11, 153–62.
4. Dworkin, R.H., Turk, D.C., Farrar, J.T. et al. (2005). Core outcome measures for chronic pain clinical trials: IMMPACT recommendations. Pain, 113, 9–19.
5. Bennett, M. (2001). The LANSS Pain Scale: the Leeds assessment of neuropathic symptoms and signs. Pain, 92, 147–57.
6. Krause, S.J. and Backonja, M.M. (2003). Development of a neuropathic pain questionnaire. Clinical Journal of Pain, 19, 306–14.
7. Bouhassira, D., Attal, N., Alchaar, H. et al. (2005). Comparison of pain syndromes associated with nervous or somatic lesions and development of a new neuropathic pain diagnostic questionnaire (DN4). Pain, 114, 29–36.
8. Freynhagen, R., Baron, R., Gockel, U. et al. (2006). painDETECT: a new screening questionnaire to identify neuropathic components in patients with back pain. Current Medical Research and Opinion, 22, 1911–20.
9. Caraceni, A. and Portenoy, R.K. (1999). An international survey of cancer pain characteristics and syndromes. IASP Task Force on Cancer Pain. International Association for the Study of Pain. Pain, 82, 263–74.
10. Forman, A.D. (2004). Peripheral neuropathy and cancer. Current Oncology Report, 6, 20–5.
11. Kehlet, H., Jensen, T.S., and Woolf, C.J. (2006). Persistent postsurgical pain: risk factors and prevention. Lancet, 367, 1618–25.
12. Williams, D., Geraci, A., and Simpson, D.M. (2002). AIDS and AIDS-treatment neuropathies. Current Pain Headache Report, 6, 125–30.
13. Pardo, C.A., McArthur, J.C., and Griffin, J.W. (2001). HIV neuropathy: insights in the pathology of HIV peripheral nerve disease. Journal of Peripheral Nervous System, 6, 21–7.
14. Boivie, J. (2006). Central Pain. In Wall and Melzack's Textbook of Pain (eds. S.B. McMahon, and M. Koltzenburg), pp. 1057–74. Elsevier Churchill Livingstone, Edinburgh.

15. Hansson, P.T. and Dickenson, A.H. (2005). Pharmacological treatment of peripheral neuropathic pain conditions based on shared commonalities despite multiple etiologies. *Pain*, **113**, 251–4.

16. Scholz, J., Woolf, C.J. (2002). Can we conquer pain? *Natural Neuroscience*, **5** (Suppl),1062–7.

17. Woolf, C.J. (2004). Dissecting out mechanisms responsible for peripheral neuropathic pain: implications for diagnosis and therapy. *Life Sciences*, **74**, 2605–10.

18. Wood, J.N., Abrahamsen, B., Baker, M.D. *et al.* (2004). Ion channel activities implicated in pathological pain. *Novartis Found Symp*, **261**, 32–40.

19. Luo, Z.D., Calcutt, N.A., Higuera, E.S. *et al.* (2002). Injury type-specific calcium channel alpha 2 delta-1 subunit up-regulation in rat neuropathic pain models correlates with antiallodynic effects of gabapentin. *Journal of Pharmacology and Experimental Therapeutics*, **303**, 1199–205.

20. Wua, Y.J. and Dworetzky, S.I. (2005). Recent developments on KCNQ potassium channel openers. *Current Med Chem*, **12**, 453–60.

21. Baron, R., Levine, J.D., and Fields, H.L. (1999). Causalgia and reflex sympathetic dystrophy: does the sympathetic nervous system contribute to the generation of pain? *Muscle and Nerve*, **22**, 678–95.

22. Wu, G., Ringkamp, M., Hartke, T.V. *et al.* (2001). Early onset of spontaneous activity in uninjured C-fiber nociceptors after injury to neighboring nerve fibers. *Journal of Neuroscience*, **21**, RC140.

23. McMahon, S.B., Cafferty, W.B., and Marchand, F. (2005). Immune and glial cell factors as pain mediators and modulators. *Experimental Neurology*, **192**, 444–62.

24. Coderre, T.J., Katz, J., Vaccarino, A.L. *et al.* (1993). Contribution of central neuroplasticity to pathological pain: review of clinical and experimental evidence. *Pain*, **52**, 259–85.

25. Scholz, J., Broom, D.C., Youn, D.H. *et al.* (2005). Blocking caspase activity prevents transsynaptic neuronal apoptosis and the loss of inhibition in lamina II of the dorsal horn after peripheral nerve injury. *Journal of Neuroscience*, **25**, 7317–23.

26. Suzuki, R., Rahman, W., Rygh, L.J. *et al.* (2005). Spinal-supraspinal serotonergic circuits regulating neuropathic pain and its treatment with gabapentin. *Pain*, **117**, 292––303.

27. Hains, B.C., Saab, C.Y., Klein, J.P. *et al.* (2004). Altered sodium channel expression in second-order spinal sensory neurons contributes to pain after peripheral nerve injury. *Journal of Neuroscience*, **24**, 4832–9.

28. Wieseler-Frank, J., Maier, S.F., and Watkins, L.R. (2004). Glial activation and pathological pain. *Neurochemistry International*, **45**, 389–95.

29. Farrar, J.T., Young, J.P., LaMoreaux, L. *et al.* (2001). Clinical importance of changes in chronic pain intensity measured on an 11-point numerical pain rating scale. *Pain*, **94**, 149–58.

30. Finnerup, N.B., Otto, M., McQuay, H.J. *et al.* (2005). Algorithm for neuropathic pain treatment: an evidence based proposal. *Pain*, **118**, 289–305.

31. Cook, R.J. and Sackett, D.L. (1995). The number needed to treat: a clinically useful measure of treatment effect *British Medical Journal*, **310**, 452–4.

32. Sills, G.J. (2006). The mechanisms of action of gabapentin and pregabalin. *Current Opinion in Pharmacology*, **6**, 108–13.

33. Freynhagen, R., Strojek, K., Griesing, T. *et al.* (2005). Efficacy of pregabalin in neuropathic pain evaluated in a 12-week, randomised, double-blind, multicentre, placebo-controlled trial of flexible- and fixed-dose regimens. *Pain*, **115**, 254–63.

34. van Seventer, R., Feister, H.A., Young, J.P. *et al.* (2006). Efficacy and tolerability of twice-daily pregabalin for treating pain and related sleep interference in postherpetic neuralgia: a 13-week, randomized trial. *Current Medical Research and Opinion*, **22**, 375–84.

35. Caraceni, A., Zecca, E., Bonezzi, C. *et al.* (2004). Gabapentin for neuropathic cancer pain: a randomized controlled trial from the Gabapentin Cancer Pain Study Group. *Jounal of Clinical Oncology*, **22**, 2909–17.

36. Frampton, J.E. and Foster, R.H. (2006). Pregabalin: in the treatment of generalised anxiety disorder. *CNS Drugs*, **20**, 685–93.

37. Macdonald, R.L. and Kelly, K.M. (1995). Antiepileptic drug mechanisms of action. *Epilepsia*, **36** (Suppl 2), S2–S12.

38. Sindrup, S.H. and Jensen, T.S. (2002). Pharmacotherapy of trigeminal neuralgia. *Clincal Journal of Pain*, **18**, 22–7.

39. Beydoun. A. and Kutluay, E. (2002). Oxcarbazepine. *Expert Opinion in Pharmacotherapy*, **3**, 59–71.

40. Rull, J.A., Quibrera, R., Gonzalez-Millan, H. *et al.* (1969). Symptomatic treatment of peripheral diabetic neuropathy with carbamazepine (Tegretol): double blind crossover trial. *Diabetologia*, **5**, 215–8.

41. Beydoun, A., Shaibani, A., Hopwood, M. *et al.* (2006). Oxcarbazepine in painful diabetic neuropathy: results of a dose-ranging study. *Acta Neurologica Scandnavica*, **113**, 395–404.

42. Dogra, S., Beydoun, S., Mazzola, J. *et al.* (2005). Oxcarbazepine in painful diabetic neuropathy: a randomized, placebo-controlled study. *European Journal of Pain*, **9**, 543–54.

43. Adverse effects of established and new antiepileptic drugs: an attempted comparison. *Pharmacology and Therapeutics*, **68**, 425–34.

44. Carrazana, E. and Mikoshiba, I. (2003). Rationale and evidence for the use of oxcarbazepine in neuropathic pain. *Jounal of Pain and Symptom Management*, **25**, S31–S35.

45. Lees, G. and Leach, M.J. (1993). Studies on the mechanism of action of the novel anticonvulsant lamotrigine (Lamictal) using primary neurological cultures from rat cortex. *Brain Research*, **612**, 190–9.

46. Teoh, H., Fowler, L.J., and Bowery, N.G. (1995). Effect of lamotrigine on the electrically-evoked release of endogenous amino acids from slices of dorsal horn of the rat spinal cord. *Neuropharmacology*, **34**, 1273–8.

47. Eisenberg, E., Lurie, Y., Braker, C. *et al.* (2001). Lamotrigine reduces painful diabetic neuropathy: a randomized, controlled study. *Neurology*, **57**, 505–9.

48. Kochar, D.K., Rawat, N., Agrawal, R.P. *et al.* (2004). Sodium valproate for painful diabetic neuropathy: a randomized double-blind placebo-controlled study. *QJM*, **97**, 33–8.

49. Otto, M., Bach, F.W., Jensen, T.S. *et al.* (2004). Valproic acid has no effect on pain in polyneuropathy: a randomized, controlled trial. *Neurology*, **62**, 285–8.

50. Thienel, U., Neto, W., Schwabe, S.K. *et al.* (2004). Topiramate in painful diabetic polyneuropathy: findings from three double-blind placebo-controlled trials. *Acta Neurologica Scandinavica*, **110**, 221–31.

51. Sindrup, S.H., Otto, M., Finnerup, N.B. *et al.* (2005). Antidepressants in the treatment of neuropathic pain. *Basic Clinical Pharmacology and Toxicology*, **96**, 399–409.

52. Wang, G.K., Russell, C., and Wang, S.Y. (2004). State-dependent block of voltage-gated Na$^+$ channels by amitriptyline via the local anesthetic receptor and its implication for neuropathic pain. *Pain*, **110**, 166–74.

53. Hall, H. and Ogren, S.O. (1981). Effects of antidepressant drugs on different receptors in the brain. *European Journal of Pharmacology*, **70**, 393–407.

54. Kieburtz, K., Simpson, D., Yiannoutsos, C. *et al.* (1998). A randomized trial of amitriptyline and mexiletine for painful neuropathy in HIV infection. AIDS Clinical Trial Group 242 Protocol Team. *Neurology*, **51**, 1682–8.

55. Shlay, J.C., Chaloner, K., Max, M.B. *et al.* (1998). Acupuncture and amitriptyline for pain due to HIV-related peripheral neuropathy: a randomized controlled trial. Terry Beirn Community Programs for Clinical Research on AIDS. *Journal of the American Medical Association*, **280**, 1590–5.

56. Mercadante, S., Arcuri, E., Tirelli, W. *et al.* (2002). Amitriptyline in neuropathic cancer pain in patients on morphine therapy: a

randomized placebo-controlled, double-blind crossover study. *Tumori*, **88**, 239–42.

57. Hammack, J.E., Michalak, J.C., Loprinzi, C.L. *et al.* (2002). Phase III evaluation of nortriptyline for alleviation of symptoms of cis-platinum-induced peripheral neuropathy. *Pain*, **98**, 195–203.

58. Ray, W.A., Meredith, S., Thapa, P.B. *et al.* (2004). Cyclic antidepressants and the risk of sudden cardiac death. *Clinical Pharmacology and Therapeutics*, **75**, 234–41.

59. McQuay, H.J., Tramer, M., Nye, B.A. *et al.* (1996). A systematic review of antidepressants in neuropathic pain. *Pain*, **68**, 217–27.

60. Brosen, K. and Gram, L.F. (1989). Clinical significance of the sparteine/debrisoquine oxidation polymorphism. *European Journal of Clinical Pharmacology*, **36**, 537–47.

61. Sindrup, S.H., Bach, F.W., Madsen, C. *et al.* (2003). Venlafaxine versus imipramine in painful polyneuropathy: a randomized, controlled trial. *Neurology*, **60**, 1284–9.

62. Rowbotham, M.C., Goli, V., Kunz, N.R. *et al.* (2004). Venlafaxine extended release in the treatment of painful diabetic neuropathy: a double-blind, placebo-controlled study. *Pain*, **110**, 697–706.

63. Goldstein, D.J., Lu, Y., Detke, M.J. *et al.* (2005). Duloxetine vs. placebo in patients with painful diabetic neuropathy. *Pain*, **116**, 109–18.

64. Raskin, J., Pritchett, Y.L., Wang, F. *et al.* (2005). A double-blind, randomized multicenter trial comparing duloxetine with placebo in the management of diabetic peripheral neuropathic pain. *Pain Medicine*, **6**, 346–56.

65. Detke, M.J., Lu, Y., Goldstein, D.J. *et al.* (2002). Duloxetine, 60 mg once daily, for major depressive disorder: a randomized double-blind placebo-controlled trial. *Journal of Clinical Psychiatry*, **63**, 308–15.

66. Semenchuk, M.R. and Davis, B. (2000). Efficacy of sustained-release bupropion in neuropathic pain: an open-label study. *Clinical Journal of Pain*, **16**, 6–11.

67. Stahl, S.M., Grady, M.M., Moret, C. *et al.* (2005). SNRIs: their pharmacology, clinical efficacy, and tolerability in comparison with other classes of antidepressants. *CNS Spectrum*, **10**, 732–47.

68. Feighner, J.P. (1995). Cardiovascular safety in depressed patients: focus on venlafaxine. *Journal of Clinical Psychiatry*, **56**, 574–9.

69. Thase, M.E., Tran, P.V., Wiltse, C. *et al.* (2005). Cardiovascular profile of duloxetine, a dual reuptake inhibitor of serotonin and norepinephrine. *Journal of Clinical Psychopharmacology*, **25**, 132–40.

70. Pacher, P. and Kecskemeti, V. (2004). Cardiovascular side effects of new antidepressants and antipsychotics: new drugs, old concerns? *Current Pharm Des*, **10**, 2463–75.

71. Rowbotham, M.C., Davies, P.S., Verkempinck, C. *et al.* (1996). Lidocaine patch: double-blind controlled study of a new treatment method for post-herpetic neuralgia. *Pain*, **65**, 39–44.

72. Meier, T., Wasner, G., Faust, M. *et al.* (2003). Efficacy of lidocaine patch 5% in the treatment of focal peripheral neuropathic pain syndromes: a randomized, double-blind, placebo-controlled study. *Pain*, **106**, 151–8.

73. Galer, B.S., Rowbotham, M.C., Perander, J. *et al.* (1999). Topical lidocaine patch relieves postherpetic neuralgia more effectively than a vehicle topical patch: results of an enriched enrollment study. *Pain*, **80**, 533–8.

74. Estanislao, L., Carter, K., McArthur, J. *et al.* (2004). A randomized controlled trial of 5% lidocaine gel for HIV-associated distal symmetric polyneuropathy. *Journal of Acquired Immune Deficiency Syndrome*, **37**, 1584–6.

75. Dworkin, R.H., Backonja, M., Rowbotham, M.C. *et al.* (2003). Advances in neuropathic pain: diagnosis, mechanisms, and treatment recommendations. *Archives of Neurology*, **60**, 1524–34.

76. Rowbotham, M.C., Twilling, L., Davies, P.S. *et al.* (2003). Oral opioid therapy for chronic peripheral and central neuropathic pain. *New England Journal of Medicine*, **348**, 1223–32.

77. Mercadante, S., Casuccio, A., and Calderone, L. Rapid swithing from morphine to methadone in cancer patients with oor response to morphine. *Journal of Clinical Oncology*, **10**, 3307–12.

78. Kalso, E., Allan, L., Dellemijn, P.L. *et al.* (2003). Recommendations for using opioids in chronic non-cancer pain. *European Journal of Pain*, **7**, 381–6.

79. Hollingshead, J., Duhmke, R.M., and Cornblath, D.R. (2006). Tramadol for neuropathic pain. *Cochrane Database of Systematic Reviews*, CD003726.

80. Boyer, E.W. and Shannon, M. (2005). The serotonin syndrome. *New England Journal of Medicine*, **352**, 1112–20.

81. Svendsen, K.B., Jensen, T.S., and Bach, F.W. (2004). Does the cannabinoid dronabinol reduce central pain in multiple sclerosis? Randomised double blind placebo controlled crossover trial. *British Medical, Journal*, **329**, 253–61.

82. Rog, D.J., Nurmikko, T.J., Friede,T. *et al.* (2005). Randomized, controlled trial of cannabis-based medicine in central pain in multiple sclerosis. *Neurology*, **65**, 812–9.

83. Berman, J.S., Symonds, C., and Birch, R. (2004). Efficacy of two cannabis based medicinal extracts for relief of central neuropathic pain from brachial plexus avulsion: results of a randomised controlled trial. *Pain*, **112**, 299–306.

84. Karst, M., Salim, K., Burstein, S. *et al.* (2003). Analgesic effect of the synthetic cannabinoid CT-3 on chronic neuropathic pain: a randomized controlled trial. *Journal of the American Medical Association*, **290**, 1757–62.

85. Hall, W., Christie, M., and Currow, D. (2005). Cannabinoids and cancer: causation, remediation, and palliation. *Lancet Oncology*, **6**, 35–42.

86. Mason, L., Moore, R.A., Derry, S. *et al.* (2004). Systematic review of topical capsaicin for the treatment of chronic pain. *British Medical Journal*, **328**, 991.

87. Simpson, D.A. (2001). Gabapentin and venlafaxine for the treatment of painful diabetic neuropathy. *Journal of Clinical Neuromuscular Diseases*, **3**, 53–62.

88. Gilron, I., Bailey, J.M., Tu, D. *et al.* (2005). Morphine, gabapentin, or their combination for neuropathic pain. *New England Journal of Medicine*, **352**, 1324–34.

89. Bowsher, D. (1997). The effects of pre-emptive treatment of postherpetic neuralgia with amitriptyline: a randomized, double-blind, placebo-controlled trial. *Journal of Pain and Symptom Management*, **13**, 327–31.

90. Lampl, C., Yazdi, K., and Roper, C. (2002). Amitriptyline in the prophylaxis of central poststroke pain. Preliminary results of 39 patients in a placebo-controlled, long-term study. *Stroke*, **33**, 3030–2.

91. Morley, S., Eccleston, C., and Williams, A. (1999). Systematic review and meta-analysis of randomized controlled trials of cognitive behaviour therapy and behaviour therapy for chronic pain in adults, excluding headache. *Pain*, **80**, 1–13.

92. Turk, D.C. and Flor, H. (2006). The cognitive-behavioral approach to pain management. In *Wall and Melzack's Textbook of pain* (eds. S.B. McMahon and M. Koltzenburg), pp. 339–48. Elsevier Churchill Livingstone, Edinburgh.

93. Otto, M., Bak, S., Bach, F.W. *et al.* (2003). Pain phenomena and possible mechanisms in patients with painful polyneuropathy. *Pain*, **101**, 187–92.

94. Max, M.B., Culnane, M., Schafer, S.C. *et al.* (1987). Amitriptyline relieves diabetic neuropathy pain in patients with normal or depressed mood. *Neurology*, **37**, 589–96.

95. Attal, N., Cruccu, G., Haanpaa, M. *et al.* (2006). EFNS guidelines on pharmacological treatment of neuropathic pain. *European Journal of Neurology*, **13**, 1153–69.

96. Dworkin, R.H., O'Connor, A.B., Backonja, M. *et al.* (2007). Pharmacologic management of neuropathic pain: evidence-based recommendations. *Pain*, **132**, 237–251.

10.1.4 Cancer-induced bone pain

Lesley A. Colvin and Marie Fallon

Cancer-induced bone pain (CIBP) is a major clinical problem, with limited options for predictable, rapid, and effective treatment for some of the elements without unacceptable adverse effects. When treating the different components of CIBP, background pain may respond reasonably well to opioids, whereas both spontaneous and movement-evoked pain may be much more problematic. Our understanding of how current therapy acts is based mainly on studies in non-cancer pain syndromes, which are likely to be quite different, not only in clinical presentation, but also in terms of pathophysiology. It has been difficult to study the specific neurobiological changes associated with CIBP, as there were no good laboratory models of isolated bone metastases until relatively recently. Most of the previous models involved systemic disease, making it difficult to determine specifically the changes associated with CIBP. In order to evaluate our current therapies properly and direct the development of new therapies logically, it is important to understand the underlying mechanisms of CIBP.

Animal models

The laboratory models of CIBP, developed within the last decade, involve focal inoculation of tumour cells into the intramedullary cavity of a single bone in rodents. This results in the growth of an isolated bone metastasis, without any of the systemic effects associated with widespread tumour, as was seen in previous models. These models allow measurement of behavioural signs of pain as well as study of pathophysiological changes and appear to correlate well with the clinical syndrome. A range of sites, such as humerus, femur, and calcaneus have been used, with tumour cell lines varying from osteosarcoma to breast, prostate, and melanoma[1-5]. The underlying changes in nociceptive pathways are unique and quite distinct from those seen in other pain states, such as neuropathic

or inflammatory pain[6]. There is also some evidence that tumour type may have subtle changes on nociceptive processing in CIBP, with evidence that cortical destruction is not necessary for CIBP to develop[7,8].

It is clear that there are complex interactions between tumour, the tumour environment, nociceptive processing, and other factors (e.g. genetic) that will define precisely the nature of CIBP and response to treatment in any one individual[9].

Pain processing

In order to understand the pathophysiology of CIBP, it is useful to consider the neurobiology of nociception prior to the occurrence of tissue injury. Much of our understanding of this is based on basic science research, although brain-imaging techniques are providing exciting evidence of alterations in many areas of the brain. This confirms earlier laboratory work with direct clinical evidence of how pain perception is processed at a cortical level. The IASP (International Association for the Study of Pain) definition of pain 'as an unpleasant sensory and emotional experience associated with actual or potential tissue damage or described in terms of such damage' is useful in reminding us that pain is more than nociception and involves a balance between sensory, cognitive, and affective components[10]. The traditional concept of sensory input being processed in the brain, with little interaction between spinal and cortical response is incomplete, as increasing evidence from brain imaging studies indicates significant potential for bi-directional modulation between sensory input and cortical activity[11-13].

It was not until the 1960s that nociceptors were first identified and the Gate Control Theory of Pain was introduced by Melzack and Wall[14]. This theory emphasized the importance of spinal modulation, with continuous interaction between small and large diameter afferents, local spinal neurons, and descending systems from the brain.

A basic outline of the nociceptive system is shown in Fig. 10.1.4.1, showing the neuraxis (the peripheral and central nervous system) involved in sensory processing and giving a framework for understanding the changes occurring in CIBP. Importantly, this is a

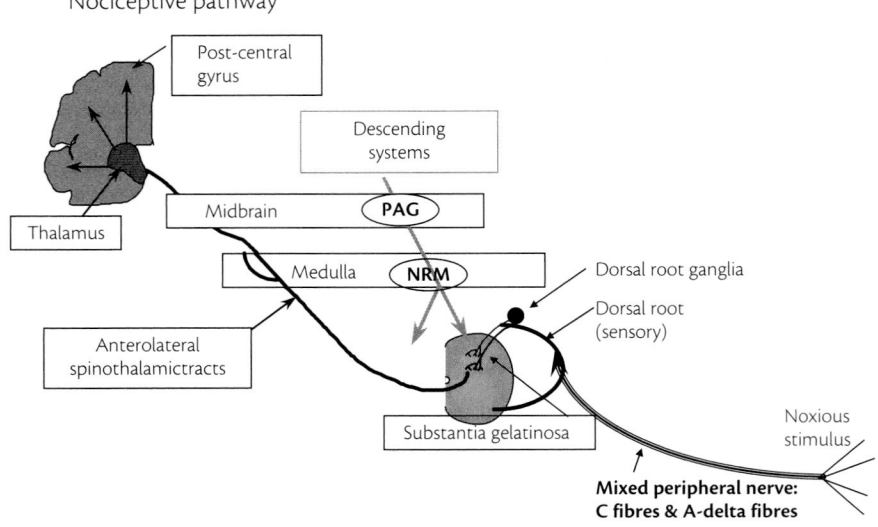

Figure 10.1.4.1 Nociceptive pathway: Peripheral noxious stimuli activate nociceptors and generate action potentials in C and A delta fibres, that may result in neuronal activity within the brain and pain perception. Descending systems from the brain modulate this process, as do local interneurons within the spinal cord.
PAG = Periaqueductal grey matter; NRM = Nucleus raphe magnus.

dynamic system, with the potential for significant alterations at all levels within the system dependent on sensory input, tumour effects, and treatment.

Peripheral processing

Painful stimuli, whether mechanical, thermal, or chemical, may activate nociceptors (non-specialized free nerve endings) on particular sensory neurons (or primary afferent fibres). Sensory neurons vary in function, size, and conduction velocity, as outlined in Table 10.1.4.1, with generation of action potentials in C and A-delta fibres in response to noxious stimuli[15].

The sensory fibres ascend towards the spinal cord in mixed nerves. Close to the spinal cord, the sensory fibres split into the dorsal root and enter the spinal cord. The cell bodies of all sensory fibres are situated close to the spinal cord, in the dorsal root ganglia. This is where the cell nucleus lies and where neurotransmitters essential for synaptic transmission are synthesized, before peripheral and central transport to axon terminals[16].

Receptors

A range of receptors has been identified on the peripheral terminations of sensory neurons. These are important in transduction of noxious mechanical, thermal, and chemical stimuli. These include mechanically gated channels and purinergic receptors, which have a role in mechanical transduction and the transient receptor potential (TRP) family of ion channels, involved in noxious heat and cold processing, in particular, the vanilloid receptor VR1 (heat) and TRPA1 nkyrin (cold). Some of these receptors may also detect alterations in pH (acid sensing ion channels—ASICs)[17–25]. In addition, there are several types of receptor-detecting noxious chemical stimuli such as prostaglandins, endothelins, nerve growth factor (NGF), and bradykinin, as may be found in response to tissue injury[26–29]. Peripheral opioid receptors are also found and may have a role in certain pain states, including CIBP[30,31].

Central processing

Spinal cord

After entering the dorsal horn, the majority of C fibres and A-delta fibres synapse, in a somatotopic manner, in laminae I and II of the superficial dorsal horn (the substantia gelatinosa), with some A-delta fibres terminating in lamina V[32–35]. The sensory fibres synapse with second-order projection neurons that ascend to the brain in specific tracts. These second-order neurons vary in their response, with, for example, nociceptive specific (NS) neurons, responding only to noxious stimuli, and wide dynamic range (WDR) neurons, responding to innocuous and noxious stimuli.

Table 10.1.4.1 Classification of sensory neurons.

Fibre type	Diameter (μm)	Conduction velocity (ms⁻¹)	Sensory modality
A-beta: large, myelinated	6–15	30–100	Light touch, proprioception
A-delta: small, myelinated	2–6	12–30	Noxious and innocuous sensory
C: unmyelinated	0.5–2	0.5–2.0	Pain, temperature; also post-ganglionic autonomic

Complex modulation of second-order activity occurs both via intrinsic spinal mechanisms and descending systems[16,36–38]. At a local level within the spinal cord, there are a range of inhibitory mechanisms at a spinal level, which may be augmented by descending inhibitory pathways from the brain (Fig. 10.1.4.1), acting to reduce nociceptive transmission[15,39,40].

Within the spinal cord, the main neurotransmitter involved in fast synaptic transmission in the spinal cord is glutamate, acting at a range of ionotropic (ion channels) and metabotropic (G-protein coupled) receptors. Normally, the alpha-amino-3-hydroxyl-5-methyl-4- isoxazole propionic acid (AMPA) receptor is involved in nociceptive transmission. The main inhibitory neurotransmitters, predominantly found in local interneurons and descending projection neurons, are glycine and gamma–amino-butyric acid (GABA)[39,41–43]. Neuropeptides, such as substance P are also released in response to noxious stimulation, with some endogenous opioid peptides acting to reduce onward transmission of noxious input[44–46].

Spinal connections and supraspinal pathways

Ascending spinal tracts

After synapsing in the dorsal horn, second-order spinal neurons mainly cross to the opposite side of the spinal cord and ascend in the spinothalamic tracts to thalamic nuclei, conveying predominantly noxious information[47,48]. There are also spinomesencephalic tracts, originating from cells in laminae I, V, and VI to the mesencephalic tegmentum region, which includes the periaqueductal grey area (PAG)[49].

Descending systems

The concept of descending inhibitory pathways, or 'descending noxious inhibitory control' first originated from Melzack and Wall's gate control theory of pain[50,51]. There are several areas within the brainstem that the descending pathways originate from, including the medullary nucleus raphe magnus (NRM) and rostral ventromedial medulla (RVM). The NRM contains endogenous opioids and has been shown to have an anti-nociceptive effect, with a major descending serotonergic input to the dorsal horn[52–54]. In the midbrain, the PAG is also involved in opioid-mediated analgesia and the locus coeruleus (LC) in modulating nociceptive transmission, via its actions on the parafascicular neurons (PF) of the thalamus[55–59].

There is accumulating evidence for the existence of both anti- and pro-nociceptive pathways from the RVM, via a mechanism that may involve the N-methyl-D-aspartate (NMDA) receptor[60].

If there is persistent noxious input, such as may occur in CIBP, this may increase activity of this system contributing to increased spinal excitability. There is also some evidence of an indirect connection of the RVM with the anterior cingulate cortex, normally associated with the affective—motivational—aspects of pain perception. Thus, alterations in the balance of inhibition and facilitation from the brainstem, which may itself be modulated by higher centres, can alter inherent excitability at the level of the spinal cord (for review, see Reference 61).

Cortical processing

Multiple areas of the brain are activated in response to pain, reflecting the complex nature of pain perception. In the clinical setting, brain imaging techniques, such as functional magnetic resonance imaging (fMRI), have been used to study the cortical response to nociceptive stimuli: the most consistently activated areas include the insular and the anterior cingulate regions[62–64]. It is clear that there are many complex bi-directional interactions between the brain and the spinal cord in pain processing[11,65].

Mechanisms of CIBP

Peripheral factors

Evidence from the animal models of CIBP demonstrates wide-ranging alterations in the peripheral environment around the site of the bony metastasis and subsequent sensory processing. The relationship between the site of bone metastasis, the sensory nerves, and the surrounding microenvironment plays a key role in CIBP.

The complex interaction between the tumour itself and the development of CIBP may be modulated by tumour type, site, and degree of bony destruction. CIBP may occur prior to evidence of bony destruction, with clear signs of pain behaviours found in animal models[7]. Other factors, both local and central, must play a role in the generation of pain in CIBP. The type of tumour clearly influences the likelihood of bony metastases occurring, although the relationship to CIBP has not been described[66,67] Fig. 10.4.1.2.

Local changes in sensory neurons

Direct pressure and compression of surrounding structures, including the sensory nerves innervating the bone and periosteum, will occur with tumour growth. Both myelinated and unmyelinated primary afferent neurons innervating the marrow and mineralized bone may be injured and sensitized in CIBP[68]. Although not examined in CIBP, a rodent bone fracture model found that the periosteum is densely innervated by a meshwork of calcitonin gene-related peptide (CGRP) containing fibres. This subgroup of C fibres is thought to be involved in nociceptive transmission and could thus contribute to the marked movement-related pain that is such a challenging component of CIBP[69]. It has also been shown that

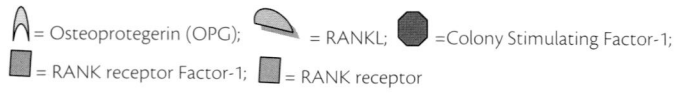

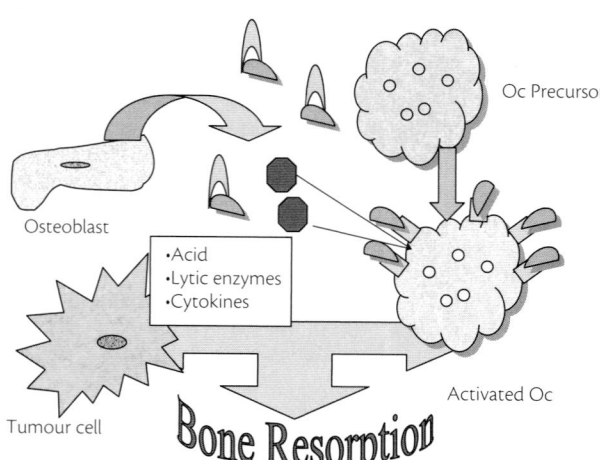

Figure 10.1.4.2 Schematic diagram of bone and tumour cell interaction. The balance between OPG and RANKL is disrupted with a relative reduction in OPG and thus an increase in osteaclast activation and hypertophy resulting in increased bone resorption. Oc = osteoclast.

purinergic receptors (P2X3) on these fibres are up-regulated in CIBP and may contribute to peripheral sensitization[70].

The capsaicin receptor, the transient receptor potential vanilloid ion channel (TRPV1), is increased on sensory neurons close to the tumour site and also within the dorsal root ganglia, preferentially in CGRP-containing neurons. TRPV1 antagonists reduce pain behaviour in CIBP models[59,71,72].

Inflammation

In the area of bony metastases, a range of pro-hyperalgesic mediators, commonly associated with inflammation, is released from the tumour and associated immune system cells, including macrophages, neutrophils, and T cells. This includes prostaglandins, endothelins, bradykinin, tumour necrosis factor-alpha and a range of growth factors, such as transforming growth factor beta (TGF-β), all of which are likely to contribute to CIBP[73–77]. These will not only sensitize peripheral nociceptors to subsequent stimuli, but also have a direct action on specific receptors on the primary sensory neurons in the area. For example, TGF-β may promote proliferation of prostate cancer cells, activate osteoclasts, and has been implicated in the development of bone metastases[78,79]. Interleukin -1(IL1) beta has been shown to be up-regulated, in a rodent model: electroacupuncture decreased this increase in IL1-beta as well as reducing pain behaviours[80]. Bradykinin antagonist may have a therapeutic role and non-steroidal anti-inflammatory drugs (NSAIDs) may also modulate CIBP. Of the growth factors, there is some evidence that NGF has a particular role in CIBP, with a potential therapeutic option in the form of an anti-NGF antibody[83–85].

CIBP, at least peripherally, seems to display a combination of neuropathic pain, either due to direct tumour compression or ischaemia, plus peripheral sensitization as is found in inflammatory pain, with release of cytokines and other mediators.

Bone microenvironment

Other factors specific to the bone, its response to tumour implantation, and the effect of the microenvironment must also be considered[86]. Within the tumour, there may be low oxygen levels, an acidic pH, and high extracellular calcium concentrations[87]. Bone turnover is altered, with an increase in bone resorption, formation of abnormal bone matrix, and disruption of the precise balance between osteoclast and osteoblast activity, such that normal regulatory mechanisms are lost[88].

An increase in osteoclasts and their activity results in increased degradation of bone matrix, by secretion of acid and lytic enzymes. Bone resorption is increased correspondingly. The receptor for activator of NF-κB (RANK) signalling pathway plays a key role in this process. The TNF-related cytokine, RANK ligand (RANK-L), expressed on osteoblasts, and colony stimulating factor (CSF)-1 combine to stimulate production of activated osteoclasts. This process is normally controlled via a negative feedback loop, involving osteoprotegerin (OPG), a secreted soluble receptor that is also a member of the TNF family. OPG acts by sequestering RANK-L, preventing osteoclast activation and reducing bone resorption[88]. This feedback loop is disrupted in CIBP, with a marked osteoblastic inflammatory response, increased secretion of a range of cytokines increasing osteoclast activity and an increased ratio of RANK-L to OPG[89,90].

Agents that interfere with osteolysis may therefore improve therapy of CIBP. This includes not only currently available agents such as bisphosphonates, but also novel agents that would alter the balance of bone metabolism to reduce CIBP. These include OPG type drugs, anti-NGF, and other agents that interfere with intracellular pathways in osteoclasts[84,91–95].

Central factors

While it is clear that peripheral changes, due to tumour effects on the bone, drive or at least initiate, central responses, it is not understood at all how much the central changes contribute to the degree of severity of the pain syndrome. It is known from other chronic pain states that changes in spinal pain processing, with central sensitization and wind up, play a major role in the development of chronic pain[96]. What has been found in animal models of CIBP is that the central changes are quite different from either inflammatory or neuropathic pain.

Glial cells

A particular feature that has been noted is an increase in glial cells, with a marked astrocytosis in the spinal cord on the side of the lesion. Interventions to reduce glial activation have been shown to correlate with reductions in pain behaviour and reduced spinal cord cytokines[1,97]. For example, local radiotherapy, at the site of CIBP, will reduce glial activity in the spinal cord, as well as reversing some of the abnormal neurochemistry[98]. There is increasing interest on the interaction between the immune system and sensory neurons in the generation of chronic pain syndromes and it seems likely that this may be particularly relevant to CIBP[99].

Glutamate and neuronal responsiveness

Metabotropic glutamate receptors are found on glial cells within the spinal cord and may contribute to pain behaviour, in addition to more well-defined glutamate receptors, such as the NMDA receptor[100].

The likely involvement of glutamate, one of the main excitatory neurotransmitters in the spinal cord, has been confirmed by the efficacy of gabapentin in CIBP models, with a pre-synaptic effect on glutamate release[101].

Gabapentin has also been found to reduce activity of a particular type of dorsal horn neuron—the WDR neuron. WDR neurons appear to alter in CIBP, with increased responsiveness to mechanical and thermal stimuli in addition to ongoing spontaneous activity[101–103]. An alteration in descending pathways from the brainstem to the spinal cord has also been found, with an increase in activity of pro-nociceptive pathways, as can occur in other chronic pain states[61,104].

Opioids

Clinically, opioids may control some elements of CIBP well, but have significant limitations in controlling aspects of breakthrough pain, common in CIBP. There may be a neurobiological basis for this, with alterations in the endogenous opioid systems found in animal models of CIBP.

Mu opioid receptors (MOR) have been found to decrease in specific subpopulations of primary afferent neurons in the dorsal root ganglia. These neurons were predominantly CGRP or TRPV1-containing neurons, known to be involved in CIBP. This reduction in MOR expression seemed to correlate to a reduced analgesic response to intrathecal morphine and was not seen in an inflammatory model[105]. The dose–response curve for morphine is shifted to the right, with greater doses needed to reduce pain behaviour compared to inflammatory pain, suggesting fundamental differences in the underlying mechanisms[106]. Prolonged morphine treatment may increase pain behaviour, associated with an increase in CGRP neurons in the dorsal root ganglia and increased osteoclast activity[107]. Conversely, another group found that chronic systemic morphine had greater efficacy than acutely administered morphine[108]. The pro-nociceptive opioid peptide, dynorphin, increases markedly in the dorsal horn of the spinal cord[109]. This may contribute to an increase in the activity of descending facilitatory systems from the brain[61,110].

Summary of pre-clinical aspects of CIBP

The advent of locally restricted bone metastases models has allowed us to begin defining the underlying mechanisms related to CIBP, separate from the systemic effects of widespread tumour. There are complex interactions between local factors at the site of tumour metastasis to bone, with inflammatory and neuropathic processes, contributing to the response that is elicited within the central nervous system. The spinal cord changes occurring in CIBP appear to be unique and distinct from other chronic pain states. Improved understanding of all these processes should aid development of novel targeted therapies that may improve our clinical armamentarium for managing this challenging clinical problem.

Clinical features

Introduction

Pain as a result of metastatic spread to bone is a significant clinical problem for patients, their care givers, and health-care professionals[111]. Bone pain can have a significant impact on physical, psychological, and social functioning (and so overall quality of life)[112]. CIBP can be difficult to manage and treatment may require the use of multiple types of interventions[113]. The optimum use of the WHO analgesic ladder is critical for successful management of CIBP. This, of course, means using the ladder as outlined in Chapter 10.1.6 but remembering that the ladder was never intended for use in isolation of other methods of cancer pain relief. CIPB provides a classical paradigm for the WHO analgesic ladder sitting within a wider context of other pain-relieving techniques (Fig. 10.1.4.3).

Epidemiology

Bone is the most common source of pain in patients with malignant disease with studies suggesting that ~ 28 per cent of hospice inpatients, 34 per cent of patients in a cancer pain clinic and 45 per cent of advanced cancer patients followed up at home, are affected by pain from bone metastases [114–117]. Studies also suggest that lesions in bone account for 30–35 per cent of all cancer pains in patients with advanced disease[114,118]. Some patients will experience multiple sites of pain due to bone metastases.

However, not everyone will have pain as a result of bone metastases. For example, one-third of patients with metastatic breast disease affecting the skeleton, do not complain of pain [119]. The mechanisms, which mediate the onset of pain in some metastases, but not others in the same patient, are poorly understood; however, the local tumour and its immediate environment must play an important role.

Clinical characteristics

Descriptors of CIBP are varied, but it is generally accepted that there is a triad of background pain, spontaneous pain at rest, and movement-related pain. Movement-related pain is a form of incident pain and along with spontaneous pain at rest, they are types of breakthrough pain[120,27].

Breakthrough pain is referred to as 'transitory exacerbation of pain experienced by the patient who has relatively stable and adequately

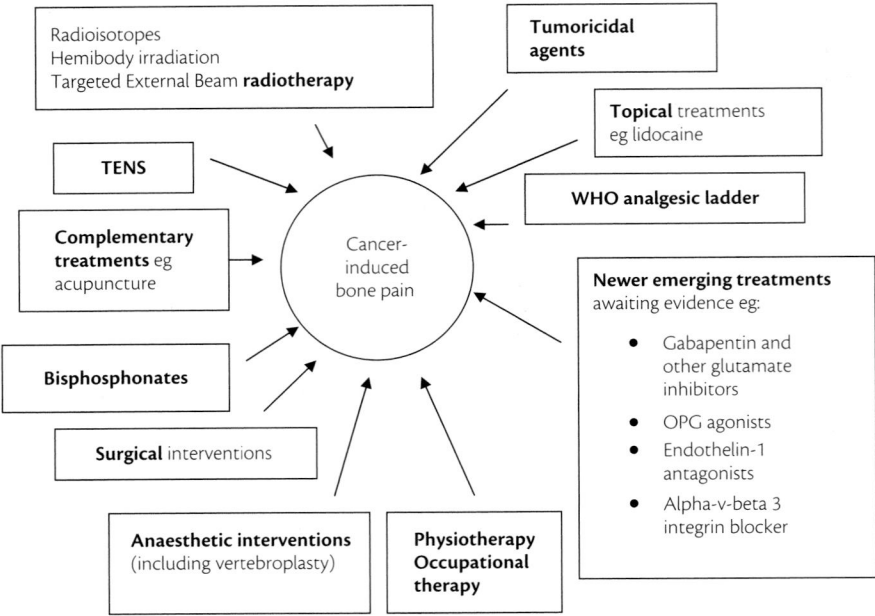

Figure 10.1.4.3 CIBP requires a multimodality approach individualized for each patient.

controlled baseline pain'[121]. Spontaneous pain refers to episodes of breakthrough pain that occur unexpectedly at rest. In contrast, movement-related pain (also known as incident pain or precipitated pain) refers to episodes of breakthrough pain that are related to specific events[122]. Movement-related pain is the more common form of incident pain in patients with CIBP; however, other types of incident pain, such as pain on coughing or breathing, associated with rib or sternal metastases, are common.

Background pain

Temporal pattern of pain

Background pain can be intermittent initially, but rapidly progresses to become constant in nature. Once established it is usually unrelenting.

Site of pain

In a study where 41 per cent of participants had pain due to neoplastic damage to bones and joints, 13 per cent had vertebral (including sacral) pain, 7.1 per cent had pelvic pain, 6.8 per cent had pain in the chest wall from rib lesion(s), 3.9 per cent had pain in the long bones, and 10.2 per cent had generalized bone pain from multiple bone metastases[123]. The skeleton was affected in slightly different patterns depending on the primary site of the tumour (Table 10.1.4.2).

Radiation of pain

Usually the pain is localized to a specific area (and frequently there is point tenderness over the affected area of bone). In other cases, pain may be referred[124]. For example, a metastatic deposit in the hip may result in pain in the knee area; a lesion in the T12/L1 site may cause pain felt in the iliac crest or sacro-iliac joint (either unilaterally or bilaterally); a cervical spine metastasis may have pain referred to the occipital region or the skull vertex[116].

Another feature which is recognized in CIBP is the phenomenon of a 'migratory pattern of pain,' where pain might appear in one area of the body at a given time, then move to a completely different part of the body with total resolution of the pain at the original site[125].

Table 10.1.4.2 Prevalence of different pain syndromes in patients with different tumours.

Cancer diagnosis	Pain syndrome					
	Skull	Vertebral	Pelvis and long bones	Generalized bone pain	Chest wall	Pathological fracture
All tumours	5.2	13.0	10.5	11.4	6.8	5.0
Breast	2.1	20.9	12.5	25.3	9.7	8.3
Lower GI tract	1.9	10.6	17.4	0	0.9	1.9
Upper GI tract	1.9	4.8	0.9	0.9	0	0
Head & neck	21.6	4.5	6.3	5.4	0.9	0.9
Leukaemia/lymphoma	0	4.7	11.9	14.2	0	0
Lung	4.6	18.0	8.8	10.4	20.7	7.7
Prostate	1.5	21.5	26.1	40.0	4.6	3.0
Uterus	0	4.2	4.2	0	2.8	0

Source: From Caraceni, A. and Portenoy, R.K. (1999). An international survey of cancer pain characteristics and syndromes. *Pain,* **82**, 263–74. With permission.

Quality (character) of pain

Background pain is often described as a dull ache[126]. However, the descriptions of the pain were variable in a study of patients with bone pain from metastatic prostate cancer[125]. Recent work has suggested that it may be more commonly associated with terms like 'sharp,', 'throbbing,' and 'tingling'[127].

Intensity (severity) of pain

The intensity of bone pain is independent of tumour type, location, number and size of metastases, gender, and age of patient[128].

In a study of patients with bone pain from metastatic prostate cancer, 60 per cent had 'severe' pain, 30 per cent had 'moderate' pain and the rest described their pain as being 'mild'[125]. Bone pain usually increases in intensity over time[124].

A study of hospitalized patients with advanced cancer demonstrated that, while 49 per cent of patients with bone metastases reported severe pain, only 31 per cent of patients without bone involvement reported a similar level of pain[129]. This concurs with the clinical impression that CIBP often presents a therapeutic challenge.

Exacerbating factors of pain

As discussed earlier, exacerbation of pain is often related to specific events (incident pain). Incident pain can be further divided into: (1) volitional pain—precipitated by a voluntary act e.g. walking; (2) non-volitional—precipitated by an involuntary act, e.g. coughing[122]. However, for practical purposes, it is the individual patient's history, which is important, as there clearly exists an overlap between these categories. We suggest always using explicit terms to describe the different categories of CIBP outlined in Fig. 10.1.4.4.

Relieving factors of pain

A variety of different non-pharmacological, pharmacological, oncological, and other types of interventions have been used to treat bone pain. These interventions are discussed in the following paragraphs and outlined in Fig. 10.1.4.3.

Other features of pain

As bone pain due to cancer becomes more established, mechanical allodynia can develop, resulting in pain from a stimulus or activity, which was normally not painful e.g. moving in bed[130]. Recent studies also suggest that cancer-related bone pain can result in paraesthesia (altered sensation), dynamic allodynia (perception of pain in response to light brushing of the skin), static allodynia (perception of pain in response to pressure), or thermal hyperalgesia (pain at normal, low, and high temperature thresholds)[3,131,132]. Interestingly, normalization of thermal hyperalgesia and hypoalgesia has been shown to be associated with successful pain relief from palliative radiotherapy[132].

Breakthrough pain: epidemiology

An International Association for the Study of Pain (IASP) survey found that breakthrough pain was present according to clinicians in 65 per cent of patients with cancer-related pain[123,133]. However, breakthrough pain was more likely to be reported in English-speaking countries, which may reflect factors more to do with the definition, than the recognition, of the phenomenon.

Bone pain is a major source of breakthrough pain and has been reported as the predominant source of incident pain[133]. In the aforementioned survey, breakthrough pain was significantly associated with certain pain syndromes, including those due to vertebral lesions and lesions in the pelvis, long bones, or joints. Thus, of the patients with vertebral pain syndrome, 85 per cent had breakthrough pain. Similarly, of the patients with pelvis and long bone lesions, 78 per cent had breakthrough pain.

The clinical features of breakthrough pain vary from individual to individual[121]. Nevertheless, breakthrough pain is often reported to be frequent in occurrence, acute in onset, short in duration, and moderate-to-severe in intensity[134–136]. Zeppetella et al. reported a mean number of four episodes per day (range 0–14 episodes per day) among hospice inpatients with pain[136]. Portenoy et al. found the median interval between onset and peak of pain to be 3 min, with a range of 1 s to 30 min[135]. In addition, Portenoy and Hagen reported a median duration of 30 min (range 1–240 min) amongst hospital inpatients with pain[134]. The clinical features of breakthrough pain often mirror the clinical features of the background pain; however, they may differ.

The clinical features of breakthrough pain may also vary within an individual. For example, patients may experience both spontaneous pain and incident pain. In the study by Portenoy et al. almost two-thirds of patients could identify a precipitant for their pain, such as weight-bearing and/or movement[135]. However, nearly half of patients also stated that their pain could be unpredictable at times.

Patients with breakthrough pain have more intense background pain that those without breakthrough pain[133,135]. Moreover, the study by Portenoy et al. confirms that patients with breakthrough pain have greater functional impairment (as measured on the interference scale of the brief pain inventory [BPI]) when compared to patients without such pain[135]. In addition, patients with breakthrough pain have significantly increased levels of depression and anxiety (as measured by the Beck Depression Inventory and the Beck Anxiety Inventory) when compared with patients without such pain.

Practical aspects of CIBP which impact on management

Our work in patients attending a Regional Cancer Centre with CIBP has shown that:

- Pain on movement or spontaneous pain at rest, have a mean visual analogue scale (VAS) score of 7/10, compared with pain at rest, which has a mean score of 3/10.
- Eighty-three per cent of patients have pain which is significantly worse on movement.
- Fifty per cent of patients with movement-related or spontaneous pain reported that the duration was less than 30 min and twenty-five per cent reported a duration of less than 15 min.
- Fifty-two per cent of patients felt that both movement-related and spontaneous pain were unpredictable[137].

While the tonic background pain is usually controlled with opioid analgesia, the other two components, spontaneous or movement-related (including incident pain, which is not movement-related) are problematic because:

- There is a mismatch between temporal onset of pain in relation to temporal onset of analgesia from opioids.

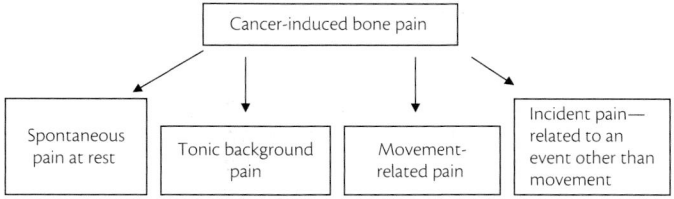

Figure 10.1.4.4 Clinical characteristics of cancer-induced bone pain.

◆ Resolution of pain in relation to duration of opioid analgesia again has a mismatch. Although immediate (normal) release morphine may have analgesic effects for up to 4 h, spontaneous and movement-related pain can resolve in less than 30 min in 50 per cent of patients, rendering the patient more susceptible to opioid side effects.

◆ There is evidence of poor opioid-responsiveness of some aspects of the underlying neurophysiology of the spontaneous and movement-related pain components[137–139]. This may mean that some patients may fail to achieve adequate analgesia with even the 'ideal' formulation of opioid.

The combination of the earlier mentioned factors indicates that opioid side effects, especially sedation, are more likely to dominate over analgesia. In any pain syndrome where there are sudden, short-lived, peaks of pain, over and above a stable background pain, the opioid side effects are more likely to be problematic. In particular, such patients may become opioid toxic.

Opioid toxicity

Opioid toxicity is a spectrum, which at one extreme may involve sleepiness, poor concentration, and vivid dreams, while at the other end of the spectrum may involve hallucinations, confusion, agitation, and even a paradoxical increase in pain known also as hyperalgesia. A survey of inpatients in a Regional Cancer Centre showed 50 per cent of patients to have some symptoms of opioid toxicity, most of which were not identified by staff[140]. Significant opioid toxicity is associated with 50 per cent mortality and it is known that in those patients who recover, the distress experienced was profound. It is therefore very important to avoid opioid toxicity and to develop treatments which minimize this risk.

Current management of CIBP

Currently, non-steroidal anti-inflammatory drugs (NSAIDs) and palliative radiotherapy form the key strategies, which complement simple or opioid analgesia in CIBP relief. The evidence base for these strategies, along with emerging newer strategies is discussed in the following paragraphs; however, a major problem with the evidence base is the lack of information on the components of CIBP, which are helped by specified treatments.

The standard approach to the management of CIBP is a combination of analgesia and radiotherapy. Fig.10.1.4.5 While it is accepted that radiotherapy is the gold standard treatment for pain relief in CIBP, there are a significant number of patients who fail to receive adequate analgesia. A systematic review showed external beam radiotherapy, whether single or multiple fractions, produced 50 per cent pain relief in 41 per cent of patients and complete pain relief at one month in 24 per cent of patients[141]. However, many patients are too frail to attend for palliative radiotherapy or it is too late to reasonably expect pain relief before death.

We know that current therapeutic regimens leave up to 45 per cent of patients with inadequate and under-managed pain control[142,143].

For such reasons, an improved understanding of the pathophysiological mechanisms underlying, in particular, spontaneous pain at rest and movement-related pain, are important. The development of effective pharmacological interventions to act as adjuvants or synergists to palliative radiotherapy to improve the degree of pain relief, in addition to providing analgesia to those too unwell to benefit from palliative radiotherapy, is an important area of research.

Opioid-based therapy does remain the basis for most analgesia in CIBP and in theory, there are two aspects to the optimisation of opioid analgesia: (1) to establish the best opioid for an individual, based on the pharmacogenomic principle of interindividual variation in balance between analgesia and side effects and (2) to assess the optimal pharmacokinetic pharmacodynamic profile from the opioids available. There is more weight given to the first aspect in relation to chronic background pain; however, more weight given to the second in relation to spontaneous pain at rest and movement-related pain. For example, a patient may use a long-acting opioid preparation, such as morphine, for background pain and a fast-acting fentanyl preparation for breakthrough pain.

A subgroup of patients experience uncontrolled CIBP only after considerable and predictable movement, such as a long walk. This group is often satisfied to use a standard opioid such as immediate (normal) release morphine, 30 min in advance of such activity. Conversely, in those patients whose pain, or the exacerbating factor, is unpredictable and of fast onset, unacceptable side effects are likely to occur with standard opioids. In such cases a faster, short-acting opioid is more appropriate. Most of the evidence for opioids with faster onset of analgesia and faster peak plasma analgesic levels is limited to fentanyl[144].

Non-steroidal anti-inflammatory drugs

The use of NSAIDs in CIBP has been questioned due to the lack of robust, clinical evidence[145–151]. The newer COX2 (an inducible isoform of cyclooxygenase [COX] enzyme involved in prostaglandin synthesis) specific inhibitors may, in theory, be of greater therapeutic potential due to their anti-tumour/antiangiogenesis properties[152,153]. In an animal model of CIBP acute treatment with a highly selective COX2 inhibitor attenuated both background and movement-related pain, whereas chronic treatment additionally reduced tumour burden and osteoclast destruction[154]. Clearly the use and availability of COX2 inhibitors has fluctuated since they were first available because of concerns with some drugs within this class. A systematic review of randomized controlled clinical trials of NSAIDs for cancer pain was published in 2004[155,156]. It included 42 trials involving 3084 patients. The review concluded that NSAIDs were effective for the short-term treatment of cancer pain and that there was no clear evidence to support a superior efficacy or safety of one NSAID over another. It included 14 trials involving patients with bone metastases, although the authors were unable to conclude from the data presented whether NSAIDs have a specific role in CIBP.

The results of this systematic review were in keeping with the results of an earlier systematic review of the literature on NSAIDs for cancer pain and a concurrent evidence-based review of the literature on the generic treatment of cancer pain[157,158]. It should be noted that many of the trials included in these reviews are single-dose studies, and few of the trials evaluate the efficacy or safety of NSAIDs beyond a few days of treatment.

In summary, therefore, despite good pre-clinical evidence, there is a lack of clinical evidence for a specific role for NSAIDs in the management of CIBP.

Clinicians do, however, still regard NSAIDs as an important part of CIBP management unless contraindications exist.

Breakthrough pain

Here we are referring to all types of breakthrough pain, other than that caused by inadequate around-the-clock analgesia to control background pain or 'end-of-dose' failure. It is a heterogeneous phenomenon, although it is typically of fast onset, short duration as previously discussed.

Despite implementation of guidelines, patients continue to have inadequate pain control and often express a variety of problems secondary to this. Breakthrough pain associated with CIBP can be particularly difficult to control[159].

Three principles have been proposed for the management of general breakthrough pain, not specifically related to bone metastases[160]:

1 Implementation of primary therapies for the underlying aetiology of the pain.

2 Optimizing around-the-clock analgesia.

3 Specific pharmacological or non-pharmacological interventions for the breakthrough pain.

It is generally agreed that one of the main problems with breakthrough pain due to bone metastases is that multiple breakthrough doses of opioid to control pain on movement and/or spontaneous pain at rest, usually leaves the patient with frank, unacceptable opioid side effects, especially sedation, or with frank opioid toxicity. However, it has been suggested that increasing around-the-clock medication may prevent or limit breakthrough pain associated with CIBP [161]. Twenty-five patients admitted to a palliative care unit with movement-related breakthrough pain were titrated with intravenous morphine to background pain relief. The morphine dose was then increased further until patients began to experience unacceptable side effects at which point the increase was either stopped, or the morphine dose reduced. Patients remained as inpatients for an average of 5 days, and the breakthrough pain intensity on a 0–10 scale fell from an average of 9.2 before titration to 4.6 at the time of discharge. Most patients tolerated the higher dose of morphine. Translation of these findings to other settings may be limited by the fact that inpatients are often less mobile, and there may be particular characteristics in this group, which are not representative of CIBP patients in general.

The commonest method of managing breakthrough pain continues to be the use of so-called 'rescue' medication (breakthrough medication). Ideally, rescue medication should have an onset/duration of action appropriate for the pain, should have a potency of effect appropriate for the pain, and be easily administered. Rescue medication should be offered soon after the pain has started in cases of unpredictable pain, and before the pain has started in cases of predictable pain.

Opioids are commonly used as rescue medication. Morphine, hydromorphon, and oxycodone are the most common oral opioids used, and a fixed proportion of the daily dose is usually advised (e.g. the 4-hourly dose equivalent)[162]. One study formally addressed the use of a fixed dose of rescue medication[163]: Forty-eight patients using oral morphine for background cancer pain, and admitted to a palliative care unit, were treated with intravenous morphine, equivalent to one-fifth of the around-the-clock dose, for management of their breakthrough pain. A total of 172 episodes of pain were assessed and most patients had a 33 per cent reduction in their pain within 18 min. Although most patients had somatic cancer pain, there was no specific reference to CIBP.

Non-opioids such as NSAIDs could have a role in the management of breakthrough pain as their mode of action suggests that they could be efficacious. However, with an onset of action of ~30 min, a relatively long duration of action and dose-limiting adverse effects, they are not ideally suited to the management of breakthrough pain. There are no studies to suggest that they are effective in this clinical scenario.

A systematic review on the use of opioids for breakthrough pain identified four studies, each concerned with the application of oral transmucosal fentanyl citrate (OTFC)[144]. These studies confirmed the efficacy of this delivery system for the management of breakthrough pain[164–167]. However, all of the studies failed to demonstrate a relationship between the effective dose of OTFC and the effective dose of around-the-clock medication and, as a result, the optimum dose of OTFC is determined by titration. This differs from usual practice of prescribing one-sixth of the 24-h opioid dose as a breakthrough dose. It is, however, hardly surprising that when an opioid dose is carefully titrated for breakthrough pain in the context of a clinical trial, the individual effective doses vary between patients and rarely work out as one-sixth of the 24-h opioid dose. Although one of these OTFC studies did describe the number of patients with CIBP[164], none of the studies distinguished between CIBP and non-CIBP in their analyses which perhaps leaves a question over the favourable efficacy of OTFC or other fentanyl equivalents over standard opioids for breakthrough pain in CIBP.

Bisphosphonates for bone pain

Over the years, a number of different bisphosphonates have been developed, with the newer agents exhibiting increased potency as compared to the original agents[168]. The data on bisphosphonates in the management of CIBP are presented here. In addition, bisphosphonates are also used to manage/prevent other skeletal complications of cancer and also to manage cancer-related hypercalcaemia[169,170].

Structure of bisphosphonates

With side chain modifications from a simple methyl group (CH_3) to progressively longer alkyl chains, successive generations of bisphosphonates have been developed, each with increasing potency to inhibit osteoclast-mediated bone resorption.

Bisphosphonates have a number of actions, which account for their anti-resorptive properties[171,172]. They inhibit dissolution of hydroxyapatite crystals, have an effect on osteoclasts and osteoblasts, and also have an effect on the underlying tumour. Different bisphosphonates have a different range of activities.

Bisphosphonates can inhibit the differentiation of stem cells to osteoclasts, affect the structure and function of osteoclasts, and cause apoptosis of osteoclasts[171]. The latter actions rely on the bisphosphonate being taken up into the osteoclast by a process of endocytosis. Bisphosphonates also affect the interaction between osteoclasts and osteoblasts via the OPG, RANK, and RANK-L axis. The normal RANK–RANK-L balance is described in the basic science section of this chapter.

In addition, bisphosphonates can inhibit the growth of tumour cells, stimulate the immune system (against the tumour), and cause apoptosis of tumour cells[171]. The inhibition of growth is achieved by a reduction in the adhesion of tumour cells to bone, a reduction in the secretion of tumour growth factors into the bone (secondary to a reduction in bone resorption), and an inhibition of tumour angiogenesis.

Bisphosphonates delay the development of skeletal events, particularly in patients with breast cancer, multiple myeloma, and prostate cancer[173,174]. A positive effect of delaying skeletal events is clearly a reduction in pain (e.g. pathological fracture).

However, bisphosphonates can also improve pain secondary to established bone lesions; many patients only respond after months of treatment, whilst other patients respond soon after treatment is initiated. The mechanism by which bisphosphonates cause long-term pain relief is likely to be due to their effect on bone resorption (and healing of the bone lesions). The mechanism by which bisphosphonates cause short-term pain relief is unclear, but is likely to be related to their effect on tumour growth factors and other nociceptive agents.

A Cochrane systematic review addressing the (acute) analgesic effect of bisphosphonates was first published by Wong and Wiffen[175]. The data were subsequently updated to create a Health Technology Report for the Canadian Coordinating Center of Health Technology Assessment[176]. The data were further updated by Wong.

Fifty-six trials fulfiled the selection criteria for the most recen analysis. The data support the fact that bisphosphonates provide moderate relief of pain within 12 weeks of therapy. The odds ratio (OR) for the best response within 12 weeks was 1.87 (95 per cent confidence interval [CI]: 1.23–2.86). The time-course of the effect was not immediate. While there was a trend towards pain relief at weeks 4 and 8, this only became statistically significant at week 12.

It is not possible to say from the studies available if there is a different analgesic effect with different primary tumour sites.

Results for different bisphosphonates

Five randomized trials provided direct comparisons between different bisphosphonates. All of them compared pamidronate against a different bisphosphonate: three compared it with clodrondate[177–179] and two against zolendronate[180,181]. Based on the limited data available, pamidronate appears to be a better choice than clodronate with a greater response rate and a greater magnitude of pain relief. Further studies are necessary to elucidate the relative merits of pamidronate and the more potent bisphosphonates, such as ibandronate and zolendronate[182].

Clinical data tolerability

Bisphosphonate side effects commonly described include flu-like syndromes and injection site reactions. Randomized trials with standard doses did not identify excessive gastrointestinal toxicities, although concern has been raised about gastrointestinal toxicities[183].

Renal toxicity is another important area. Rapid infusions may result in renal toxicity, especially in patients with renal compromise. Pamidronate infusions (90 mg) are typically delivered over a period of 2 h, while zolendronate infusions (2 mg) are typically delivered over 15 min. Ibandronate does not appear to possess the same renal toxicity concerns and can be used in patients with varying degrees of renal impairment[184,185]. Adverse ocular events including uveitis, scleritis, and conjunctivitis have been reported withamino-bisphosphonate use, particularly pamidronate use[186].

Bisphosphonate-associated osteonecrosis of the mandibular and maxillary bone has been described[187]. The pathophysiology of this condition is unknown, but the risk factors include dental extraction, local trauma, local infection, and systemic chemotherapy. The condition has been reported with pamidronate and zolendronate and usually appears after many months of treatment. Appropriate prophylactic dental assessment and management, along with antibiotic therapy if indicated, are keystone to minimizing occurrence of this complication. This is discussed in more detail in Chapter 11.2.

Summary of clinical use of bisphosphonates in CIBP

Bisphosphonates delay the development of skeletal events, particularly in patients with breast cancer, multiple myeloma, and prostate cancer. A positive effect of delaying these skeletal events is an overall reduction in pain secondary to bone resorption and its complications (e.g. pathological fracture). In addition, bisphosphonates also provide relief of bone pain, although the magnitude of the effect is modest in the short term and can take up to 12 weeks to work. Currently there are numerous small studies, which suggest a potential role for bisphosphonates in acute CIBP relief; however, the studies are very heterogeneous and all use different outcome measurements. Further work is underway to evaluate the utility of the potent bisphosphonates such as ibandronate in achieving acute pain relief.

Radiotherapy

External beam radiotherapy is by far the most commonly used radiation modality in the management of bone pain; the most common type of treatment is local field radiotherapy[188]. Wide-field radiotherapy and radioisotopes are used in treating disseminated bone metastases.

In 2000, the Cochrane group published on the use of radiotherapy for painful bone metastases. The review included data from 20 randomized controlled trials; 15 other studies were excluded for various methodological reasons. The trials were not sufficiently alike to allow pooling of data and therefore no meta-analysis was performed. Nevertheless, the authors concluded that radiotherapy provides effective analgesia for bone metastases. Over 40 per cent of patients could expect ≥ 50 per cent pain relief at 1 month and 20 per cent could expect complete relief[141]. There was no discernible difference between fractionation schedules, or between different doses using the same schedule.

The Bone Pain Trial Working Group led a study to compare treatment with an 8-Gy single fraction and a multiple-fraction regimen of either 20 Gy in five fractions or 30 Gy in 10 fractions (98 per cent of patients in the multiple-fraction arm received 20 Gy in five fractions and only 2 per cent of patients received 30 Gy in 10 fractions)[189].

There was no difference between the arms in the time to first improvement in pain, time to complete pain relief, or time to increase in pain at any time over the 12-month follow-up period. There was also no difference in the acute toxicity of a single fraction of 8 Gy and the multiple-fraction regimens. Although retreatment was more common in the single-fraction arm, this was felt to be possibly due to clinicians being more likely to retreat after a single fraction than after a multiple-fraction regimen[189]. In general, the equal efficacy, patient convenience, and lower cost should make a single 8-Gy fraction the standard treatment for palliation of pain from bone metastases.

Wide-field radiotherapy

Wide-field radiotherapy can be done in several ways, including radiation to the entire upper half of the body, radiation to the entire lower half of the body, radiation to the mid-section (from the lower chest to the upper thighs), and sequential hemi-body radiation in which half the body is irradiated in one session and the other half of the body is irradiated in a later session (4–6 weeks later). The latter procedure allows enough time for the bone marrow from the un-irradiated half of the body to re-populate the marrow cavity in the irradiated half of the body[188].

A number of radioisotopes have been used in the treatment of bone metastases (e.g. phosphorus-32, strontium-89, samarium-153, rhenium-186). Despite evidence, they are not widely used and while there are a number of potential reasons for low use of radioisotopes, cost is likely to be an issue in many countries.

Table 10.1.4.3 Chemosensitivity of primary tumours commonly metastasizing to bone.

Primary site	Sensitivity [a]
Myeloma	High
Bronchus	High
Breast	High
Rectum	Mid
Oesophagus	Mid/low
Prostate	Low
Thyroid	Low
Kidney	Low

[a] High = >50 per cent response rate; Mid = 25–50 per cent response rate; Low = <25 per cent response rate

Chemotherapy

Chemotherapy can also be of considerable value in the management of metastatic bone pain where a tumour is chemosensitive. Examples would include myeloma, both small-cell and non-small-cell lung and breast cancer, where the natural history of these tumours is for widespread dissemination including bone as a common site of metastasis (Table 10.1.4.3).

Hormone therapy

Hormone therapy is also of value in hormone-sensitive tumours and both breast and prostate cancers commonly spread to bone; in the latter this being the most common site and pattern of metastasis. Quite dramatic responses can be achieved within a few days of starting anti-androgen therapy in prostate cancer.

Response in metastatic breast cancer is generally slower, and additional measures for pain relief are usually required in the first few weeks of starting hormone therapy. Hormone therapy, as with any other treatment which may induce acute new activity in bone, may be associated with a transient flare-up of pain, which needs to be managed with appropriate manipulation of analgesia.

Physiotherapy and occupational therapy

Many of the techniques in maximizing pain control through a multi-disciplinary team approach discussed in the chapter on rehabilitation (Chapter 16) are integral to the adequate care of patients with CIBP. Life can be made infinitely easier for the patient who has difficulty mobilizing and problems in such areas as toileting and bathing, by the introduction of specific mobilizing techniques along with appropriate individualized aides.

Interventional analgesia

Vertebral cementoplasty

Instability of vertebrae due to metastatic disease can cause significant pain. Vertebral collapse causes pain per se, but structural change may also risk nerve root compression[190]. Percutaneous vertebral cementoplasty (also known as percutaneous vertebroplasty) under radiological control has been used to reduce pain and treat vertebral body collapse[191]. Access to this technique depends on local expertize.

The analgesic mechanism of this technique is not explained solely by treating collapse, since as little as 2 ml of methylmetharylate cement can achieve good pain relief[192]. Stabilization of microfractures, and subsequent reduction in mechanical forces

through the bone, has been postulated as analgesic mechanisms[193]. Analgesia could also be secondary to cytotoxic and thermal destruction of tumour cells, and interference with tumour blood supply.

A study of patients with intractable pain from vertebral myeloma found that 97 per cent of patients had at least a 'moderate' reduction in pain following percutaneous vertebral cementoplasty[194]. The improvement in pain of 36 to 37 patients in this study was unrelated to the proportion of vertebral filling, reiterating the importance of tumour destruction rather than anatomical correction[195].

Complications

Cement leak is a potential problem, which can encroach upon the epidural space, risking root or cord compression, and also chemo-thermal damage[192]. Cement embolism may also occur if there is evidence of a venous leak. In a case series of 868 percutaneous cementoplasty procedures for malignant and non-malignant vertebral body collapse, epidural leak was only observed in 15 cases (three had neuropathic pain) and asymptomatic pulmonary embolism in two cases[192].

It is interesting that injection of methylmethacrylate is not restricted to the vertebrae and has been reported to be successful in the management of bone pain involving the pelvic bones[195,196].

Spinal analgesia

Generally, where patients suffer uncontrolled CIBP despite optimal pharmacological and non-pharmacological management, then either epidural or intrathecal analgesia should be considered. This is discussed in more detail in 'Opioid analgesic therapy' (Chapter 10.1.6), however, it involves infusion of small amounts of opioid combined with local anaesthetic, sometimes in combination with clonidine.

Local anaesthetic is particularly useful for movement and other incident-related pains.

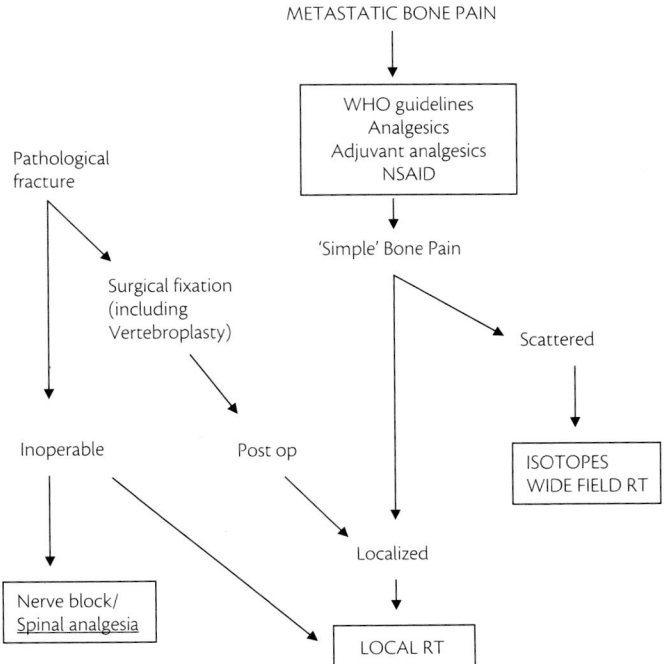

Figure 10.1.4.5 Management of metastatic bone pain. RT, Radiotherapy.

It is important that patients who have a pathological fracture but who are too unwell and close to death to consider internal fixation, are assessed urgently for an epidural or intrathecal line. Such patients often suffer extreme pain on even slight movement and their end-of-life care can be improved by interventional analgesia.

Orthopaedic interventions
Surgery for pathological fracture
The aim of fixing pathological fractures is different from that of traumatic (non-pathological) fractures[197]. Bone healing in these situations is impaired, and often the fragments do not unite together. It is, therefore, a priority that the operation involves a method of fracture fixation that can allow immediate return to normal function.

Surgery for impending fracture
Some malignant bone lesions cause symptoms in the absence of a fracture; such lesions are at risk of fracturing some time in the future (although many do not fracture and the symptoms settle with conservative measures). In general, metastases in long bones progress to fractures in 25 per cent of cases (although this rises to ~60 per cent in the proximal femur).

The criteria for operating on impending fractures vary. A widely used method is Mirel's scoring system (Table 10.1.4.4). This uses four factors related to the likelihood of a malignant bone lesion fracturing. These include:

◆ The site of the lesion.

◆ The amount of pain caused by the lesion.

◆ Whether the lesion is blastic, lytic, or a combination.

◆ The size and involvement of the lesion (defined as the maximum amount of cortex destroyed).

A score of 1–3 is given for each variable, so that the lowest total score is four and the highest total score is twelve. A score of ≤7 indicates that surgery is not needed, whereas a score of ≥9 indicates that surgery is warranted; a score of 8 means that the decision has to be taken in the context of the patient and his or her disease.

However, patients with severe pain every time they bear weight—in spite of appropriate analgesics, radiotherapy, and other appropriate measures—may benefit from surgery, no matter what their calculated score.

There is mixed evidence to support the case that the outcome for surgical management of impending pathological fractures is better

Table 10.1.4.4 Mirels' scoring system for impending pathological fracture.

Variable	Score		
	1	2	3
Site	Upper limb	Lower limb	Peritrochanteric
Pain	Mild	Moderate	Functional
Lesion	Blastic	Mixed	Lytic
Size[a]	<1/3	1/3 to 2/3	>2/3

[a]Maximum destruction of cortex in any view as seen on plain X-ray.

Source: From Mirels, H. (1989). Metastatic disease in long bones. A proposed scoring system for diagnosing impending pathological fractures. *Clinical Orthopedic Related Results*, **249**, 256–64. With permission.

than that for actual fractures. Ward *et al.* reported a significant difference in favour of patients with impending fractures in terms of perioperative blood loss, shorter hospital stay, greater likelihood of discharge home instead of temporary step-down facilities, and higher rates of unassisted ambulation[199]. In contrast, Dijkstra *et al.* reported no significant difference in outcomes such as pain relief, physical function, complications, and survival[200]. The decision about surgical intervention has to be highly individualized while taking into account the accepted, but limited, evidence base.

New approaches under evaluation
Glutamate inhibitors and NMDA antagonists
On the basis that CIBP has neuropathic and inflammatory components and clinical and laboratory evidence of central wind-up, it is not surprising that inhibitors of glutamate release have been considered and investigated. It is known that in animal studies, gabapentin reverses dorsal horn changes associated with CIBP, resulting in relief of spontaneous and movement-related pain[101]. The specific role of pregabalin as adjuvant drug therapy in CIBP is under evaluation in a double-blind randomized, placebo-controlled study on a background of standardized best supportive care[201]. This is a good example of translational research in palliative medicine and follows on from Dickenson's group pre-clinical work[101].

Inhibitors of the NMDA glutamate receptor complex may also be of interest, especially if NMDA subtype inhibitors are developed. At present the non-specific NMDA antagonist, ketamine, is used in some difficult to manage cases.

Osteoprotegerin
Osteoprotegerin (OPG) is a promising target, which may act through reduction of osteoclast function to diminish tumour-induced bone destruction. Indeed, early clinical work with OPG is interesting and may hold future promise[202]. A single SC dose of AMGN-0007 (a recombinant construct of OPG) suppressed bone resorption as indicated by a rapid, sustained, and profound decrease of urinary N-telopeptide of collagen (NTX)/creatinine in multiple myeloma and breast carcinoma patients. Changes were comparable to those with pamidronate.

Endothelin-1 antagonists
Androgen refractory prostate cancer continues to evade effective treatment. The potent vasoconstrictor endothelin-1 is produced by prostate cancer and appears to have a role in prostate cancer progression and morbidity. Based on pre-clinical and clinical trial data, the endothelin axis is emerging as potentially important in this response[203]. Drugs targeting the endothelin axis, such as the potent ET(A) receptor antagonists atrasentan, have been studied in large clinical trials and appear to have an impact on disease progression and morbidity. The role of the endothelin axis in prostate cancer deserves further investigation in the laboratory and clinic. Laboratory studies of ET(A) in CIBP have demonstrated analgesic effects on both background and movement- evoked pain[68].

Future concepts
Alphavbeta3 ($\alpha v \beta 3$) integrin blocker
The integrin $\alpha v \beta 3$ mediates cell-matrix interactions(Nelson S65-S67)[204]. Vitaxin®, a humanized monoclonal antibody that blocks human and rabbit $\alpha v \beta 3$ integrins, is in clinical trials for metastatic melanoma and prostate cancer. Vitaxin® decreases bone resorption by impairing osteoclast attachment, without affecting osteoclast multinucleation. Data also show that the inhibitory

effects of Vitaxin® on osteoclasts can be modulated by factors known to alter the conformation of αvβ3. The effects of Vitaxin® on reducingosteoclast activity may have future clinical utility in the management of CIBP.

Summary

CIBP remains a clinical challenge if we aim to achieve pain relief without unacceptable opioid side effects. An accurate assessment-followed by an individualized management plan is important. A multimodality approach is required. Standard analgesic approaches using the WHO guidelines along with palliative radiotherapy as appropriate form the basis of management; however, every patient should be assessed with all modalities in mind. Clearly the patient's general physical condition, primary tumour diagnosis, extent of bone disease, previous treatments, and treatment response, along with specific features such as the likelihood of pathological fracture, are among the factors which will influence management decisions.

It is encouraging that we are emerging into an era where, largely due to an improved pre-clinical understanding of CIBP along with new drug development, we are likely to see the emergence of an improved evidence-based armamentarium for this challenging and frequent clinical problem.

References

1. Zhang, R.X., Liu, B., Wang, L. et al. (2005). Spinal glial activation in a new rat model of bone cancer pain produced by prostate cancer cell inoculation of the tibia. *Pain*, 118, 125–36.

2. Schwei, M.J., Honore, P., Rogers, S.D. et al. (1999). Neurochemical and cellular reorganization of the spinal cord in a murine model of bone cancer pain. *Journal of Neuroscience*, 19, 10886–97.

3. Medhurst, S.J., Walker, K., Bowes, M. et al. (2002). A rat model of bone cancer pain. *Pain*, 96, 129–40.

4. Wacnik, P.W., Kehl, L.J., Trempe, T.M. et al. (2003). Tumor implantation in mouse humerus evokes movement-related hyperalgesia exceeding that evoked by intramuscular carrageenan. *Pain*, 101, 175 –86.

5. Seong, J., Park, H.C., Kim, J. et al. (2004). Radiation-induced alteration of pain-related signals in an animal model with bone invasion from cancer. *Annals of the New York Academy of Sciences*, 1030, 179–86.

6. Honore, P., Rogers, S.D., Schwei, M.J. et al. (2000). Murine models of inflammatory, neuropathic and cancer pain each generates a unique set of neurochemical changes in the spinal cord and sensory neurons. *Neuroscience*, 98, 585–98.

7. Luger, N.M., Mach, D.B., Sevcik, M.A. et al. (2005). Bone cancer pain: from model to mechanism to therapy. *Journal of Pain and Symptom Management*, 29, S32–S46.

8. Sabino, M.A., Luger, N.M., Mach, D.B. et al. (2003). Different tumors in bone each give rise to a distinct pattern of skeletal destruction, bone cancer-related pain behaviors and neurochemical changes in the central nervous system. *International Journal of Cancer*, 104, 550–8.

9. Mantyh, P.W., Clohisy, D.R., Koltzenburg, M. et al. (2002). Molecular mechanisms of cancer pain. *Nature Reviews Cancer*, 2, 201–9.

10. Merskey, H. (1986). IASP Subcommittee on Taxonomy: Classification of chronic pain. *Pain*, 3, S216–S222.

11. Tracey, I., Ploghaus, A., Gati, J.S. et al. (2002). Imaging attentional modulation of pain in the periaqueductal gray in humans. *Journal of Neuroscience*, 22, 2748–52.

12. Longe, S.E., Wise, R., Bantick, S. et al. (2001). Counter-stimulatory effects on pain perception and processing are significantly altered by attention: an fMRI study. *Neuroreport*, 12, 2021–5.

13. Ploghaus, A., Tracey, I., Gati, J.S. et al. (1999). Dissociating pain from its anticipation in the human brain. *Science*, 284, 1979–81.

14. Melzack, R. and Wall, P.D. (1965). Pain mechanisms: a new theory. *Science*, 150, 971–9.

15. Besson, J.M. and Chaouch, A. (1987). Peripheral and spinal mechanisms of nociception. *Physiological Review*, 67, 67.

16. Willis, W.D. and Coggeshall, R.E. (1991). Sensory Mechanisms of the Spinal Cord. Plenum Press, New York.

17. Bandell, M., Story, G.M., Hwang, S.W. et al. (2004). Noxious cold ion channel TRPA1 is activated by pungent compounds and bradykinin. *Neuron*, 41, 849–57.

18. Cortright, D.N., Krause, J.E., and Broom D.C. (2007). TRP channels and pain. *Biochimica et Biophysica Acta*, 1772, 978–88.

19. Fleetwood-Walker, S.M., Proudfoot, C.J., Garry, E.M. et al. (2007). Cold comfort pharm. *Trends in Pharmacological Sciences*, 28(Suppl 12), 621–8.

20. Wang,H. and Woolf, C.J. (2005). Pain TRPs. *Neuron*, 46, 9–12.

21. Sluka, K.A., Radhakrishnan, R., Benson, C.J. et al. (2007). ASIC3 in muscle mediates mechanical, but not heat, hyperalgesia associated with muscle inflammation. *Pain*, 129, 102–12.

22. Wemmie, J.A., Price, M.P., and Welsh, M.J. (2006). Acid-sensing ion channels: advances, questions and therapeutic opportunities. *Trends in Neurosciences*, 29, 578–86.

23. Welsh, M.J., Price, M.P., and Xie, J. (2002). Biochemical basis of touch perception: mechanosensory function of degenerin/epithelial Na+ channels. *Journal of Biological Chemistry*, 277, 2369–72.

24. Price, M.P., McIlwrath, S.L., Xie, J. et al. (2001). The DRASIC cation channel contributes to the detection of cutaneous touch and acid stimuli in mice. *Neuron*, 32, 1071–83.

25. Burnstock, G. and Wood, J.N. (1996). Purinergic receptors: their role in nociception and primary afferent neurotransmission. *Current Opinion in Neurobiology*, 6, 526–32.

26. Marceau, F. and Regoli, D. (2004). Bradykinin receptor ligands: therapeutic perspectives. *Nature Reviews Drug Discovery*, 3, 845–52.

27. Urch, C. (2004). The pathophysiology of cancer-induced bone pain: current understanding. *Palliative Medicine*, 18, 267–74.

28. Voilley, N. (2004). Acid-sensing ion channels (ASICs): new targets for the analgesic effects of non-steroid anti-inflammatory drugs (NSAIDs). *Current Drug Targets - Inflammation & Allergy*, 3, 71–9.

29. Kidd, B.L. and Urban, L.A. (2001). Mechanisms of inflammatory pain. *British Journal of Anaesthesia*, 87, 3–11.

30. Janson, W. and Stein, C. (2003). Peripheral opioid analgesia. *Current Pharmaceutical Biotechnology*, 4 270–4.

31. Menendez, L., Lastra, A., Hidalgo, A. et al. (2003). Peripheral opioids act as analgesics in bone cancer pain in mice. *Neuroreport*, 14, 867–9.

32. Woolf, C.J. and Fitzgerald, M. (1986). Somatotopic organization of cutaneous afferent terminals and dorsal horn neuronal receptive fields in the superficial and deep laminae of the rat lumbar spinal cord. *Journal of Comparative Neurology*, 251, 517–31.

33. Cervero, F. and Iggo, A. The substantia gelatinosa of the spinal cord: a critical review. *Brain*, 103, 717–72.

34. Handwerker, H.O., Iggo, A., and Zimmermann, M. (1975). Segmental and supraspinal actions on dorsal horn neurons responding to noxious and non-noxious skin stimuli. *Pain*, 1, 147–65.

35. Swett, J.E. and Woolf, C.J. (1985). The somatotopic organization of primary afferent terminals in the superficial laminae of the dorsal horn of the rat spinal-cord. *Journal of Comparative Neurology*, 231, 66–77.

36. Stamford, J.A. (1995). Descending control of pain. *British Journal of Anaesthesia*, 75, 217–27.

37. Biella, G. and Sotgui, M.L. (1995). Evidence that inhibitory mechanisms mask inappropriate somatotopic connections in the spinal cord of normal rat. *Journal of Neurophysiology*, 74(Suppl 2), 495–505.

38. Coghill, R.C., Mayer, D.J., and Price, D.D. The roles of spatial recruitment and discharge frequency in spinal coding of pain: a

combined electrophysiological and imaging investigation. *Pain*, **53**, 295–309.

39. Antal, M., Petko, M., Polgar, E. *et al.* (1996). Direct evidence of an extensive gabaergic innervation of the spinal dorsal horn by fibers descending from the rostral ventromedial medulla. *Neuroscience*, **73**, 509–18.

40. Dickenson, A.H. (2002). Gate control theory of pain stands the test of time. *British Journal of Anaesthesia*, **88**, 755–7.

41. Wiesenfeld-Hallin, Z., Aldskogius, H., Grant, G. *et al.* (1997). Central inhibitory dysfunctions: mechanisms and clinical implications. *Behavioral And Brain Sciences*, **20**, 420.

42. Baba, H., Ji, R.R., Kohno, T. *et al.* (2003). Removal of GABAergic inhibition facilitates polysynaptic A fiber-mediated excitatory transmission to the superficial spinal dorsal horn. *Molecular and Cellular Neurosciences*, **24**, 818–30.

43. Todd, A.J. (1996). Gaba and glycine in synaptic glomeruli of the rat spinal dorsal horn. *European Journal of Neuroscience*, **8**, 2492–8.

44. Duggan, A.W., Hendry, I.A., Morton, C.R. *et al.* (1988). Cutaneous stimuli releasing immunoreactive substance P in the dorsal horn of the cat. *Brain Res*, **451**, 261–73.

45. Allen, B.J., Rogers, S.D., Ghilardi, J.R. *et al.* (1997). Noxious cutaneous thermal stimuli induce a graded release of endogenous substance P in the spinal cord: imaging peptide action in vivo. *Journal of Neuroscience*, **17**, 5921–7.

46. Costigan, M. and Woolf, C.J. (2002). No DREAM, No pain. Closing the spinal gate. *Cell*, **108**, 297–300.

47. Giesler, G.J. Jr., Katter, J.T., and Dado, R.J. (1994). Direct spinal pathways to the limbic system for nociceptive information. *Trends in Neurological Sciences*, **17**, 244–50.

48. Todd, A.J. (2002). Anatomy of primary afferents and projection neurones in the rat spinal dorsal horn with particular emphasis on substance P and the neurokinin 1 receptor. *Experimental Physiology*, **87**, 245–9.

49. Menetrey, D., Chaouch, A., Binder, D. *et al.* (1982). The origin of the spinomesencephalic tract in the rat - an anatomical study using the retrograde transport of horseradish-peroxidase. *Journal of Comparative Neurology*, **206**, 193–207.

50. Wall, P.D. (1967). The laminar organization of dorsal horn and effects of descending impulses. *Journal of Physiology*, 188, 403–23.

51. Morgan, N.M., Gogas, K.R., and Basbaum, A.I. (1994). Diffuse noxious inhibitory controls reduce the expression of noxious stimulus-evoked fos-like immunoreactivity in the superficial and deep laminae of the rat spinal cord. *Pain*, **56**, 347–52.

52. Polgar, E., Puskar, Z., Watt, C. *et al.* (2002). Selective innervation of lamina I projection neurones that possess the neurokinin 1 receptor by serotonin-containing axons in the rat spinal cord. *Neuroscience*, **109**, 799–809.

53. Basbaum, A.I. and Fields, H.L. (1984). Endogenous pain control systems - brainstem spinal pathways and endorphin circuitry. *Annual Review of Neuroscience*, **7**, 309–38.

54. McGaraughty, S. and Heinricher, M.M. (2002). Microinjection of morphine into various amygdaloid nuclei differentially affects nociceptive responsiveness and RVM neuronal activity. *Pain*, **96**, 153–62.

55. Gray, B.G. and Dostrovsky, J.O. (1983). Descending inhibitory influences from periaqueductal gray, nucleus raphe magnus, and adjacent reticular-formation.1. effects on lumbar spinal-cord nociceptive and nonnociceptive neurons. *Journal of Neurophysiology*, **49**, 932–47.

56. Mokha, S.S., McMillan, J.A., and Iggo, A. (1985). Descending control of spinal nociceptive transmission. Actions produced on spinal multireceptive neurones from the nuclei locus coeruleus (LC) and raphe magnus (NRM). *Experimental Brain Research*, **58**, 213–26.

57. Zhang, C., Yang, S.W., Guo, Y.G. *et al.* (1997). Locus coeruleus stimulation modulates the nociceptive response in parafascicular neurons: An analysis of descending and ascending pathways. *Brain Research Bulletin*, **42**, 273–8.

58. Sonohata, M., Katafuchi, T., Yasaka, T. *et al.* (2004). Actions of noradrenaline on substantia gelatinosa neurones in the rat spinal cord revealed by in vivo patch recording. *Journal Of Physiology-London*, **555**, 515–26.

59. Men, D.S., Matsui, A., and Matsui, Y. (1996). Somatosensory afferent inputs release 5-HTand NA from the spinal- cord. *Neurochemical Research*, **21**, 1515–9.

60. Suzuki, R., Rahman, W., Hunt, S.P. *et al.* (2004). Descending facilitatory control of mechanically evoked responses is enhanced in deep dorsal horn neurones following peripheral nerve injury. *Brain Research*, **1019**, 68–76.

61. Porreca, F., Ossipov, M.H., and Gebhart, G.F. (2002). Chronic pain and medullary descending facilitation. *Trends in Neurosciences*, **25**, 319–25.

62. Berman, H.H., Kim, K.H.S., Talati, A. *et al.* (1998). Representation of nociceptive stimuli in primary sensory cortex. *Neuroreport*, **9**, 4179–87.

63. Davis, K.D. (2000). The neural circuitry of pain as explored with functional MRI. *Neurological Research*, **22**, 313–7.

64. Peyron, R., Laurent, B., and Garcia-Larrea, L. (2000). Functional imaging of brain responses to pain. A review and meta-analysis. *Neurophysiologie Clinique-Clinical Neurophysiology*, **30**, 263–88.

65. Eccleston, C. and Crombez, G. (2005). Attention and pain: merging behavioural and neuroscience investigations. *Pain*, **113**, 7–8.

66. Halvorson, K.G., Sevcik, M.A., Ghilardi, J.R. *et al.* (2006). Similarities and differences in tumor growth, skeletal remodeling and pain in an osteolytic and osteoblastic model of bone cancer. *Clinical Journal Of Pain*, **22**, 587–600.

67. Alarmo, E.L., Korhonen, T., Kuukasjarvi, T. *et al.* (2008). Bone morphogenetic protein 7 expression associates with bone metastasis in breast carcinomas. *Annals of Oncology*, **19**, 308–14.

68. Peters, C.M., Ghilardi, J.R., Keyser, C.P. *et al.* (2005). Tumor-induced injury of primary afferent sensory nerve fibers in bone cancer pain. *Experimental Neurology*, **193**, 85–100.

69. Martin, C.D., Jimenez-Andrade, J.M., Ghilardi, J.R. *et al.* (2007). Organization of a unique net-like meshwork of CGRP+ sensory fibers in the mouse periosteum: implications for the generation and maintenance of bone fracture pain. *Neuroscience Letters*, **427**, 148–52.

70. Gilchrist, L.S., Cain, D.M., Harding-Rose, C. *et al.* (2005). Re-organization of P2X3 receptor localization on epidermal nerve fibers in a murine model of cancer pain. *Brain Research*, **1044**, 197–205.

71. Niiyama, Y., Kawamata, T., Yamamoto, J. *et al.* (2007). Bone cancer increases transient receptor potential vanilloid subfamily 1 expression within distinct subpopulations of dorsal root ganglion neurons. *Neuroscience*, **148**, 560–72.

72. Ghilardi, J.R., Rohrich, H., Lindsay, T.H. *et al.* (2005). Selective blockade of the capsaicin receptor TRPV1 attenuates bone cancer pain. *Journal of Neuroscience*, **25**, 3126–31.

73. DeLeo, J.A., Colburn, R.W., and Rickman, A.J. (1997). Cytokine and growth factor immunohistochemical spinal profiles in two animal models of mononeuropathy. *Brain Research*, **759**, 50–7.

74. Wagner, R. and Myers, R.R. (1996). Schwann cells produce tumor necrosis factor alpha: expression in injured and non-injured nerves. *Neuroscience*, **73**, 625–62.

75. Woolf, C.J., Ma, Q.P., Allchorne, A. *et al.* (1996), Peripheral cell types contributing to the hyperalgesic action of nerve growth factor in inflammation. *The Journal of Neuroscience*, **16**(Suppl 9), 2716–23.

76. Sabino, M.C., Ghilardi, J.R., Feia, K.J. *et al.* (2002). The involvement of prostaglandins in tumorigenesis, tumor-induced osteolysis and bone cancer pain. *Journal of Musculoskeletal Neuronal Interactions*, **2**, 561–2.

77. Cain, D.M., Wacnik, P.W., Turner, M. *et al.* (2001). Functional interactions between tumor and peripheral nerve: Changes in excitability and morphology of primary afferent fibers in a murine model of cancer pain. *Journal of Neuroscience*, **21**, 9367–76.

78. Buijs, J.T., Henriquez, N.V., van Overveld, P.G. *et al.* (2007). TGF-beta and BMP7 interactions in tumour progression and bone metastasis. *Clinical & Experimental Metastasis*, **24**, 609–17.

79. Sato, S., Futakuchi, M., Ogawa, K. *et al.* (2008). Transforming growth factor beta derived from bone matrix promotes cell proliferation of prostate cancer and osteoclast activation-associated osteolysis in the bone microenvironment. *Cancer Science*, **99**, 316–23.

80. Zhang, R.X., Li, A., Liu, B. *et al.* (2007). Electroacupuncture attenuates bone cancer pain and inhibits spinal interleukin-1 beta expression in a rat model. *Anesthesia & Analgesia*, **105**, 1482–8.

81. Sevcik, M.A., Ghilardi, J.R., Halvorson, K.G. *et al.* (2005). Analgesic efficacy of bradykinin B1 antagonists in a murine bone cancer pain model. *Journal of Pain*, **6**, 771–5.

82. Sevcik, M.A., Luger, N.M., Mach, D.B. *et al.* (2004). Bone cancer pain: the effects of the bisphosphonate alendronate on pain, skeletal remodeling, tumor growth and tumor necrosis. *Pain*, **111**, 169–80.

83. Halvorson, K.G., Kubota, K., Sevcik, M.A. *et al.* (2005). A blocking antibody to nerve growth factor attenuates skeletal pain induced by prostate tumor cells growing in bone. *Cancer Research*, **65**(20), 9426–35.

84. Jimenez-Andrade, J.M., Martin, C.D., Koewler, N.J. *et al.* (2007). Nerve growth factor sequestering therapy attenuates non-malignant skeletal pain following fracture. *Pain*, **133**, 183–96.

85. Sevcik, M.A., Ghilardi, J.R., Peters, C.M. *et al.* (2005). Anti-NGF therapy profoundly reduces bone cancer pain and the accompanying increase in markers of peripheral and central sensitization. *Pain*, **115**(1–2), 128–41.

86. Marguiles, A., Klimberg, V., Bhattacharrya, S. *et al.* (2006). Genomics and Proteomics of Bone Cancer. *Clinical Cancer Research*, **12**, 6217s–21s.

87. Kingsley, L.A., Fournier, P.G., Chirgwin, J.M. *et al.* (2007). Molecular biology of bone metastasis. *Molecular Cancer Therapeutics*, **6**, 2609–17.

88. Boyle, W.J., Simonet, W.S., and Lacey, D.L. (2008). Osteoclast differentiation and activation. *Nature*, **423**, 337–42.

89. Kinder, M., Chislock, E., Bussard, K.M. *et al.* (2008). Metastatic breast cancer induces an osteoblast inflammatory response. *Experimental Cell Research*, **314**, 173–83.

90. Nagae, M., Hiraga, T., and Yoneda, T. (2007). Acidic microenvironment created by osteoclasts causes bone pain associated with tumor colonization. *Journal of Bone & Mineral Metabolism*, **25**, 99–104.

91. Roudier, M.P., Bain, S.D., and Dougall, W.C. (2006). Effects of the RANKL inhibitor, osteoprotegerin, on the pain and histopathology of bone cancer in rats. *Clinical & Experimental Metastasis*, **23**, 167–75.

92. Tsubaki, M., Kato, C., Manno, M. *et al.* (2007). Macrophage inflammatory protein-1alpha (MIP-1alpha) enhances a receptor activator of nuclear factor kappaB ligand (RANKL) expression in mouse bone marrow stromal cells and osteoblasts through MAPK and PI3K/Akt pathways. *Molecular & Cellular Biochemistry*, **304**, 53–60.

93. Clohisy, D.R. and Mantyh, P.W. (2004). Bone cancer pain and the role of RANKL/OPG. *Journal of Musculoskeletal Neuronal Interactions*, **4**(3), 293–300.

94. Walker, K., Medhurst, S.J., Kidd, B.L. *et al.* (2002). Disease modifying and anti-nociceptive effects of the bisphosphonate, zoledronic acid in a model of bone cancer pain. *Pain*, **100**, 219–29.

95. Medhurst, S., Bowes, M., Kidd, B.L. *et al.* (2001). Antinociceptive effects of the bisphosphonate, zoledronic acid, in a novel rat model of bone cancer pain. *British Journal of Pharmacology*, **134**, 156P.

96. Woolf, C.J. (2007). Central sensitization: uncovering the relation between pain and plasticity. *Anesthesiology*, **106**, 864–7.

97. Honore, P., Mantyh, P.W. (2000). Bone cancer pain: From mechanism to model to therapy. *Pain Medicine*, **1**, 303–9.

98. Vit, J.P., Ohara, P.T., Tien, D.A. *et al.* (2006). The analgesic effect of low dose focal irradiation in a mouse model of bone cancer is associated with spinal changes in neuro-mediators of nociception. *Pain*, **120**, 188–201.

99. Scholz, J. and Woolf, C.J. (2007). The neuropathic pain triad: neurons, immune cells and glia. *Nature Neuroscience*, **10**(11), 1361–8.

100. Saito, O., Aoe, T., Kozikowski, A. *et al.* (2006). Ketamine and N-acetylaspartylglutamate peptidase inhibitor exert analgesia in bone cancer pain. *Canadian Journal of Anaesthesia*, **53**, 891–8.

101. Donovan-Rodriguez, T., Dickenson, A.H., and Urch, C.E. (2005). Gabapentin Normalizes Spinal Neuronal Responses That Correlate with Behavior in a Rat Model of Cancer-induced Bone Pain. *Anesthesiology*, **102**, 132–40.

102. Khasabov, S.G., Hamamoto, D.T., Harding-Rose, C. *et al.* (2007). Tumor-evoked hyperalgesia and sensitization of nociceptive dorsal horn neurons in a murine model of cancer pain. *Brain Research*, **1180**, 7–19.

103. Urch, C.E., Donovan-Rodriguez, T., and Dickenson, A.H. (2003). Alterations in dorsal horn neurones in a rat model of cancer-induced bone pain. *Pain*, **106**, 347–56.

104. Donovan-Rodriguez, T., Urch, C.E., and Dickenson, A.H. (2006). Evidence of a role for descending serotonergic facilitation in a rat model of cancer-induced bone pain. *Neuroscience Letters*, **393**, 237–42.

105. Yamamoto, J., Kawamata, T., Niiyama, Y. *et al.* (2008). Down-regulation of mu opioid receptor expression within distinct subpopulations of dorsal root ganglion neurons in a murine model of bone cancer pain. *Neuroscience*, **151**, 843–53.

106. Luger, N.M., Sabino, M.A., Schwei, M.J. *et al.* (2002). Efficacy of systemic morphine suggests a fundamental difference in the mechanisms that generate bone cancer vs inflammatory pain. *Pain*, **99**, 397–406.

107. King, T., Vardanyan, A., Majuta, L. *et al.* (2007). Morphine treatment accelerates sarcoma-induced bone pain, bone loss, and spontaneous fracture in a murine model of bone cancer. *Pain*, **132**, 154–68.

108. Urch, C.E., Donovan-Rodriguez, T., Gordon-Williams, R. *et al.* (2005). Efficacy of chronic morphine in a rat model of cancer-induced bone pain: behavior and in dorsal horn pathophysiology. *Journal of Pain*, **6**, 837–45.

109. Honore, P., Schwei, J., Rogers, S.D. *et al.* (2000). Cellular and neurochemical remodeling of the spinal cord in bone cancer pain. *Prog.Brain Res.*, **129**, 389–97.

110. Vanderah, T.W., Ossipov, M.H., Lai, J. *et al.* (2001). Mechanisms of opioid-induced pain and antinociceptive tolerance: descending facilitation and spinal dynorphin. *Pain*, **92**, 5–9.

111. Fallon, M.T., McConnell, S. (2007). Clinical features. In: *Cancer-related Bone Pain OPML* (ed. A. Davies), pp. 17–26. Oxford University Press.

112. Rusteon, T., Moum, T., Padilla, G. *et al.* (2005). Predictors of quality of life in oncology outpatients with pain from bone metastasis. *Journal of Pain Symptom Management*, **20**, 234–42.

113. Clare, C., Royle, D., Saharia, K. *et al.* (2005). Painful bone metastases: a prospective observational cohort study. *Palliative Medicine*, **19**, 521–5.

114. Twycross, R.G. and Fairfield, S. (1982). Pain in far advanced cancer. *Pain*, **14**, 303–10.

115. Portenoy, R.K. and Lesage, P. (1999). Management of cancer pain. *Lancet*, **353**, 1695–700.

116. Loeser, J.D. (2000). Cancer pain: assessment and diagnosis. In *Bonica's management of pain* (eds. J.J.Bonica and J.D. Loeser), pp. 634–41. Lippincott/Williams K Wilkins, Philadelphia [AD2].

117. Banning, A., Sjogren, P., and Henriksen, H. (1991). Pain causes in 200 patients referred to a multidisciplinary cancer pain clinic. *Pain*, **45**, 45–8.

118. Grond, S., Zech, D., Diefenbach, C. *et al.* (1996). Assessment of cancer pain: a prospective evaluation in 2266 cancer patients referred to a pain service. *Pain*, **64**, 107–14.

119. Front, D., Schneck, S.O., Frankel, A. *et al.* (1979). Bone metastases and bone pain in breast cancer. *JAMA*, **242**, 1747–48.

120. Mercadante, S. and Arcuri, E. (1998). Breakthrough pain in cancer patients: pathophysiology and treatment. *Cancer Treatment Review*, **24**, 425–32.

121. Portenoy, R.K., Forbes, K., Lussier, D. *et al.* (2004). Difficult pain problems: an integrated approach. In *Oxford Textbook of Palliative Medicine* (eds. D. Doyle, G. Hanks, N. Cherny *et al.*) 3rd Edition, pp. 438–58. Oxford University Press.

122. Davies, A.N. (2006). Introduction. In *Cancer-related breakthrough pain* (ed. A.N. Davies), pp. 1–11. Oxford University Press.

123. Caraceni, A. and Portenoy, R.K. (1999). An international survey of cancer pain characteristics and syndromes. *Pain*, **82**, 263–74.

124. Mercadante, S. (1997). Malignant bone pain: pathophysiology and treatment. *Pain*, **69**, 1–18.

125. Pollen, J.J. and Schmidt, J.D.(1979). Bone pain in metastatic cancer of prostate. *Urology*, **13**, 129–34.

126. Colleau, S.M. (2002). Palliation of bone pain in cancer; facts and controversies. *Cancer Pain Release*, **15**, 1.

127. Walley, J., Colvin, L., and Fallon, M.T. (2006). Characterisation of malignant bone pain. British Pain Association, Harrogate.

128. Oster, M.W., Visel, M. and Turgeon, L.R. (1978). Pain in terminal cancer patients. *Archives of Internal Medicine*, **138**, 1801–2.

129. Brescia, F.J., Adler, D., Gray, G. et al. (1999). Hospitalized advanced cancer paints: a profile. *Journal of Pain and Symptom Management*, **5**, 221–7.

130. Clohisy, Dr. and Mantyh, P.W. (2003). Bone cancer pain. *Clinical Orthopaedics and Related Research*, (Suppl 415), S279–88.

131. Menendez, L., Lastra, A., Fresno, M.F. et al. Initial thermal heat hypoalgesia and delayed hyperalgesia in a murine model of bone cancer pain. *Brain Research*, **969**, 102–9.

132. McConnell, S., Colvin, L., and Fallon, M.T. (2007). *Features of Cancer-Induced Bone Pain (CIBP) Pre- and Post-Radiotherapy (XRT)*. British Pain Association, Glasgow.

133. Caraceni, A., Martini, C., Zecca, E. et al. (2004). Breakthrough pain characteristics and syndromes in patients with cancer pain. An international survey. *Palliative Medicine*, **18**, 177–83.

134. Portenoy, R.K. and Hagen, N.A. (1990). Breakthrough pain: definition, prevalence and characteristics. *Pain*, **41**, 273–81.

135. Portenoy, R.K., Payne, D., and Jacobsen, P. (1999). Breakthrough pain: characteristics and impact in patients with cancer pain. *Pain*, **81**, 129–34.

136. Zeppetella, G., O'Doherty, C.A., and Collins, S. (2000). Prevalence and characteristics of breakthrough pain in cancer patients admitted to a hospice. *Journal of Pain and Symptom Management*, **20**, 87–92.

137. Walley, J., Colvin, L.A., Fallon, M.T. et al. (2006). Characterisation of Cancer-induced Bone Pain. *Proceedings of NCRI*, A62.

138. Martin, C.D., Jimenez-Andrade, J.M., Ghilardi, J.R. et al.(2007). Organization of a unique net-like meshwork of CGRP+ sensory fibers in the mouse periosteum: implications for the generation and maintenance of bone fracture pain. *Neuroscience Letters*, **427**,148–52.

139. Yamamoto, J., Kawamata, T., Niiyama, Y. et al. (2008). Down-regulation of mu opioid receptor expression within distinct subpopulations of dorsal root ganglion neurons in a murine model of bone cancer pain. *Neuroscience*, **151**, 843–53.

140. Sherry, K. and Fallon, M. (2000). Opioid toxicity in cancer patients. *Research Congress in Palliative Care*.

141. McQuay, H.J., Collins, S.L., Carroll, D. et al. (2000). Radiotherapy for the palliation of painful bone metastases. *Cochrane Database of Systematic Reviews*, CD001793.

142. de Wit, R., van Dam, F., Loonstra, S. et al. (2001). The Amsterdam Pain Management Index compared to eight frequently used outcome measures to evaluate the adequacy of pain treatment in cancer patients with chronic pain. *Pain*, **91**, 339–49.

143. Meuser, T., Pietruvk, C., Radbruch, L. et al. (2001). Symptoms during cancer pain treatment following WHO-guidelines: a longitudinal follow-up study of symptom prevalence, severity and etiology. *Pain*, **91**, 247–57.

144. Zeppetella, G. and Ribeiro, M.D. (2006). Opioids for the management of breakthrough (episodic) pain in cancer patients. *Cochrane Database of Systematic Reviews*, CD004311.

145. Estape, J., Vinolas, N., Gonzalez, B. et al. (1990). Ketorolac, a new non-opioid analgesic: a double-blind trial versus pentazocine in cancer pain. *Journal of International Medical Research*, **18**, 298–304.

146. Fuccella, L.M., Conti, F., Corvi, G. et al. (1975). Double-blind study of the analgesic effect of indoprofen (K 4277). *Clinical Pharmacology and Therapeutics*, **17**, 277–83.

147. Minotti, V., de Angelis, V., Righetti, E. et al. (1998). Double-blind evaluation of short-term analgesic efficacy of orally administered diclofenac, diclofenac plus codeine, and diclofenac plus imipramine in chronic cancer pain. *Pain*, **74**, 133–7.

148. Minotti, V., Patoia, L., Roila, F. et al. (1989). Double-blind evaluation of analgesic efficacy of orally administered diclofenac, nefopam, and acetylsalicylic acid (ASA) plus codeine in chronic cancer pain. *Pain*, **36**, 177–83.

149. Stambaugh, J., Drew, J., Stambaugh, J. et al. (1988). A double-blind parallel evaluation of the efficacy and safety of a single dose of ketoprofen in cancer pain. *Journal of Clinical Pharmacology*, **28**, S34–S39.

150. Staquet, M.J. (1989). A double-blind study with placebo control of intramuscular ketorolac tromethamine in the treatment of cancer pain. *Journal of Clinical Pharmacology*, **29**, 1031–6.

151. Sunshine, A., and Olson, N.Z. (1988). Analgesic efficacy of ketoprofen in postpartum, general surgery, and chronic cancer pain. *Journal of Clinical Pharmacology*, **28**, S47–S54.

152. Sheng, H., Shao, J., Kirkland, S.C. et al.(1997). Inhibition of human colon cancer cell growth by selective inhibition of cyclooxygenase-2. *Journal Of Clinical Investigation*, **99**, 2254–9.

153. Sumitani, K., Kamijo, R., Toyoshima, T. et al. (2001). Specific inhibition of cyclooxygenase-2 results in inhibition of proliferation of oral cancer cell lines via suppression of prostaglandin E2 production. *Journal of Oral Pathology and Medicine*, **30**, 41–7.

154. Sabino, M.A.C., Ghilardi, J.R., Jongen, J.L.M. et al. (2002). Simultaneous reduction in cancer pain, bone destruction, and tumor growth by selective inhibition of cyclooxygenase-2. *Cancer Research*, **62**, 7343–9.

155. Zeppetella, J. (2007). Conventional analgesics for bone pain. In *Cancer-related Bone Pain OPML* (ed. A. Davies), pp. 53–8. Oxford University Press.

156. McNicol. E., Strassels, S., Goudas, L. et al. (2004). Non-steroidal anti-inflammatory drugs, alone or combined with opioids for cancer pain: a systematic review. *Journal of Clinical Oncology*, **22**, 1975–92.

157. Eisenberg, E., Berkey, C.S., Carr, D.B. et al. (1994). Efficacy and safety of non-steroidal anti-inflammatory drugs for cancer pain: a meta-analysis. *Journal of Clinical Oncology*, **12**, 2756–65.

158. Carr, D.B., Goudas, L.C., Balk, E.M. et al. (2004). Evidence report on the treatment of pain in cancer patients. *Journal of the National Cancer Institute, Monographs*, **32**, 23–31.

159. Banning, A., Sjogren, P., and Henriksen, H. (1991). Treatment outcome in a multidisciplinary cancer pain clinic. *Pain*, **47**, 129–34.

160. Portenoy, R.K. (1997). Treatment of temporal variations in chronic cancer pain. *Seminars in Oncology*, **5** (Suppl 16), 7–12.

161. Mercadante, S., Villari, P., Ferrera, P. et al. (2004a). Optimization of opioid therapy for preventing incident pain associated with bone metastases. *Journal of Pain and Symptom Management*, **28**, 505–10.

162. Hanks, G.W., De Conno, F., Cherny, N. et al. (2001). Morphine and alternative opioids in cancer pain: the EAPC recommendations. *British Journal of Cancer*, **84**, 587–93.

163. Mercadante, S., Villari, P., Ferrera, P. et al. (2004b). Safety and effectiveness of intravenous morphine for episodic (breakthrough) pain using a fixed ratio with the oral daily morphine dose. *Journal of Pain and Symptom Management*, **27**, 352–9.

164. Christie, J.M., Simmonds, M., Patt, R. et al. (1998). Dose-titration, multicenter study of oral transmucosal fentanyl citrate for the treatment of breakthrough pain in cancer patients using transdermal fentanyl for persistent pain. *Journal of Clinical Oncology*, **16**, 3238–45.

165. Farrar, J.T., Cleary, J., Rauck, R. et al. (1998). Oral transmucosal fentanyl citrate: randomized, double-blinded, placebo-controlled trial for treatment of breakthrough pain in cancer patients. *Journal of the National Cancer Institute*, **90**, 611–6.

166. Portenoy, R.K., Payne, R., Coluzzi, P. *et al.* (1999). Oral transmucosal fentanyl citrate (OTFC) for the treatment of breakthrough pain in cancer patients; a controlled dose titration study. *Pain*, **79**, 303–12.

167. Coluzzi, P.H., Schwartzberg, L., Conroy Jnr, J.D. *et al.* (2001). Breakthrough cancer pain: a randomized trial comparing oral transmucosal fentanyl citrate (OTFC) and morphine sulphate immediate release (MSIR). *Pain*, **91**, 123–30.

168. Wong, R. (2007). Bisphosphonates for bone pain. In *Cancer-related Bone Pain OPML* (ed. A. Davies), pp. 61–74. Oxford University Press.

169. Krempien, R., Niethammer, A., Harms, W. *et al.* (2005). Bisphosphonates and bone metastases: current status and future directions. *Expert Reviews in Anticancer Therapy*, **5**, 295–305.

170. Stewart, A.F. (2005). Clinical Practice. Hypercalcaemia associated with cancer. *New England Journal of Cancer*, **352**, 373–9.

171. Santini, D., Vaspasiani Gentilucci, U., Vicenzi, B. *et al.* (2003). The anti-neoplastic role of bisphosphonates: from basic research to clinical evidence. *Annals of Oncology*, **14**, 1468–76.

172. Green, J.R. (2004). Bisphosphonates: preclinical review. *Oncologist*, **9** (Suppl 4), 3-13.

173. Bloomfield, D.J. (1998). Should bisphosphonates be part of the standard therapy of patients with multiple myeloma or bone metastases from other cancers? An evidence-based review. *Journal of Clinical Oncology*, **16**, 1218–25.

174. Michaelson, M.D. and Smith, M.R. (2005). Bisphosphonates for treatment and prevention of bone metastases. *Journal of Clinical Oncology*, **23**, 8219–24.

175. Wong, R. and Wiffen, P.J. (2002). Bisphosphonates for the relief of pain secondary to bone metastases. *Cochrane Database of Systematic Reviews* (2), CD002068.

176. Wong, Shukla, V., Mensinkai, S. *et al.* (2004). *Bisphosphonate agents for the management of pain secondary to bone metastases: a systematic review of effectiveness and safety.* Technology Report Number 45. Canadian Coordinating Office for Health Technology Assessment, Ottawa.

177. Zhang, L., Guan, Z. and He, Y. (1997). Randomized comparative clinic trial of treatment of bone metastatic diseases by infusion of pamidronate and clodronate. *Chinese Journal of Cancer*, **16**, 340–432.

178. Diel, I.J., Marschner, N., Kindler, M. *et al.* (1999). *Continual oral versus intravenous interval therapy with bisphosphonates in patients with breast cancer and bone metastases.* (Abstract 488). Proceedings of Annual Meeting of American Society of Clinical Oncologists.

179. Jagdev, S.P., Purohit, P., Heatley, S. *et al.* (2001). Comparison of the effects of intravenous pamidraonte and oral clodronate on symptoms and bone resorption in patients with metastatic bone disease. *Annals of Oncology*, **12**, 1433–8.

180. Berensen, J.R., Rosen, L.S., Howell, A. *et al.* (2001). Zolendronic acid reduced skeletal-related events in patients with osteolytic metastases. *Cancer*, **91**, 1191–1120.

181. Rosen, L.S., Gordon, D., Kaminski, M. *et al.* (2001). Zolendronic acid versus pamidronate in the treatment of skeletal metastases in patients with breast cancer or osteolytic lesions of multiple myeloma: a phase III double-blind, comparative trial. *Cancer Journal*, **7**, 377–87.

182. Cameron, D., Fallon, M., and Diel, I. (2006). Ibandronate: Its role in Metastatic Breast Cancer. *The Oncologist*, **11** (Suppl 1), 27–33.

183. Lanza, F.L. (2002). Gastrointestinal adverse effects of bisphosphonates: etiology, incidence and prevention. *Treatments Endocrinology*, **1**, 37–43.

184. Jackson, G.H. (2005). Renal safety of ibandronate. *Oncologist*, **10** (Suppl 1), 14–8.

185. von Moos, R. (2005). Bisphosphonate treatment recommendations for oncologists. *Oncologist*, **10** (Suppl 1), 19–24.

186. Leung, S., Ashar, B.H. and Miller, R.G. (2005). Bisphonate-associated scleritis: a case report and review. *Southern Medical Journal*, **98**, 733–5.

187. Migliorati, C.A., Schubert, M.M., Peterson, D.E. *et al.* (2005). Bisphosphonate-associated osteonecrosis of mandibular and maxillary bone: an emerging oral complication of supportive cancer therapy. *Cancer*, **104**, 83–93.

188. van As, N. and Huddart, R. (2007). Radiotherapy. In *Cancer-related Bone Pain OPML* (ed. A. Davies), pp. 75–84. Oxford University Press.

189. Anonymous. (1999). 8 Gy single fraction radiotherapy for the treatment of metastatic skeletal pain: randomized comparison with a multifraction schedule over 12 months of patient follow-up. Bone Pain Trial Workshop Party. *Radiotherapy and Oncology*, **52**, 111–21.

190. Farquhar-Smith, P. (2007). Anaesthetic and interventional techniques. In *Cancer-related Bone Pain OPML* (ed. A.Davies), pp. 85–97. Oxford University Press.

191. Gangi, A., Dietemann, J.L., Schultz, A. *et al.* (1996). Interventional radiologi procedures with CT guidance in cancer pain management. *Radiographics*, **16**, 1289–304.

192. Gangi, A., Guth, S., Imbert, J.P. *et al.* (2003). Percutaneous vertebroplasty: indications, technique and results. *Radiographics*, **23**, e10.

193. Legroux-Gerot, I., Lormeau, C., Boutry, N. *et al.* (2004). Long-term follow-up of vertebral osteoporotic fractures treated by percutaneous vertebroplasty. *Clinical Rheumatology*, **23**, 310-7.

194. Cortet, B., Cotton, A., Boutry, N. *et al.* (1997). Percutaneous vertebroplasty in patients with osteolytic metastases or multiple myeloma. *Revue du Rhumatisme* (English Edn.), **64**, 117–83.

195. Cotton, A., Dewatre, F., Cortet, B. *et al.* (1996). Percutaneous vertebroplasty for osteolytic metastases and myeloma: effects of the percentage of lesion filling and the leakage of methyl methacrylate at clinical follow-up. *Radiology*, **200**, 525–30.

196. Cotton, A., Deprez, X., Migaud, H. *et al.* (1995). Malignant acetabular osteolyses: percutaneous injection of acrylic bone cement. *Radiology*, **197**, 307–10.

197. Al-Hakim,W., Jagiello, J., and Briggs, T. (2007). Orthopaedic interventions. In *Cancer-related Bone Pain OPML* (ed A. Davies), pp. 99–114. Oxford University Press.

198. Mirels, H. (1989). Metastatic disease in long bones. A proposed scoring system for diagnosing impending pathological fractures. *Clinical Orthopedics and Related Research*, **249**, 256–64.

199. Ward, W.G., Holsenbeck, S., Dorey, F.J. *et al.* (2003). Metastatic disease of the femur: surgical treatment. *Clinical Orthopedics and Related Research*, **415** (Suppl), S230-44.

200. Dijkstra, S., Wiggers, R., Van Geel, B.N. *et al.* (1994). Impending and actual pathological fractures in patients with bone metastases of the long bones. A retrospective study of 233 surgically treated fractures. *European Journal of Surgery*, **160**, 535–42.

201. Delaney, A., Fleetwood-Walker, S.M., Colvin, L.A. *et al.* (2008). Translational medicine: cancer pain mechanisms and management. *British Journal of Anaesthesia* **101**(1), 87–94.

202. Gramoun, A. *et al.* (2007). Effects of Vitaxin, a novel therapeutic in trial for metastatic bone tumors, on osteoclast functions in vitro. *Journal of Cellular Biochemistry*, **102**, 341–52.

203. Body, J.J., Greipp, P., Coleman, R.E. *et al.* (2003). A phase 1 study of AMGN-0007, a recombinant osteoprotegerin construct, in patients with multiple myeloma or breast carcinoma related bone metastases. *Cancer*, **97** (Suppl 3), 887–92.

204. Nelson JB. (2003) Endothelin inhibition: novel therapy for prostate cancer. *Journal of Urology*, **170**, S65–S67.

10.1.5 **Breakthrough pain**

Giovambattista Zeppetella

Introduction

In recent years, with the improvement in pain assessment methods, it has become evident that patients with persistent pain often report that their pain varies in clinically meaningful ways during the course of the day. Two broad patterns may be identified: background (or baseline) pain, which is present for most of the day, and breakthrough pain, which is perceived as a distinct, transitory exacerbation of pain. There is emerging evidence that breakthrough pain is associated with more severe pain, an increased risk of pain-related adverse outcomes, and greater cost of care. A systematic approach to the assessment and treatment of breakthrough pain now is viewed as an important element in a successful strategy to enhance comfort and reduce pain-related impairments and distress.

Definition of breakthrough pain

Breakthrough pain is a transient increase in pain intensity over background pain. It was first highlighted by Portenoy and Hagen as a common and distinct component of cancer pain[1]. The term itself refers to the notion that acute severe pain can 'break through' an around-the-clock (ATC) analgesic regimen. Although originally described in opioid-treated patients with cancer, who reported transient increases in pain to greater-than-moderate intensity, which occurred on a baseline pain of moderate intensity or less, it has since become clear that the definition of breakthrough pain can be broadened beyond the diagnosis of cancer or treatment with opioids.

One significant factor complicating our understanding of breakthrough pain is the lack of consensus on a formal definition, which has led to difficulties when comparing studies or recommending management strategies. The potential problem of divergence in definition and terminology was underlined when an international study noted variation in the recognition of breakthrough pain in different countries[2]. A number of definitions have appeared in the literature, some broader than others[1,3–5]. For example, some clinicians consider breakthrough pain only after background pain is adequately controlled, while others describe it as occurring irrespective of analgesic regimen or in patients with uncontrolled background pain who may experience exacerbations.

Indeed, even the term 'breakthrough pain' is not one that is universally accepted. Some clinicians prefer alternative terms, such as episodic pain, end-of-dose failure, incident pain, pain flare, transient pain, or transitory pain[6]. In this chapter, the term breakthrough pain is used and a more stringent definition is applied in an effort to identify a distinct, clinically-relevant phenomenon. In this context, breakthrough pain is considered a transitory exacerbation of pain experienced by the patient who has relatively stable and adequately controlled background pain as a result of an opioid treatment regimen[7].

Characteristics of breakthrough pain

Breakthrough pain has been characterized in a number of clinical settings, including cancer centres and pain clinics, and in patients managed in hospice inpatient units or their outpatient services. These studies have varied in their sampling procedures and their inclusion and exclusion criteria; some have specifically addressed breakthrough pain whilst others describe breakthrough pain as an incidental finding. In the more detailed reports, breakthrough pain usually is characterized according to its location, severity, temporal characteristics, relationship to the fixed-schedule analgesic regimen, precipitating factors, predictability, pathophysiology, aetiology, and palliative factors[8].

The reported prevalence of breakthrough pain has varied from 20 per cent to 95 per cent, depending on the population and survey methodology[9]. Breakthrough pain appears to be heterogeneous. In the cancer population, it is prevalent at all stages of disease[1,10], but most common among those with advanced disease and poor performance status. Cancer-related breakthrough pain appears to complicate tumour invasion of the vertebral column or brachial plexus more often than it does other types of pain syndromes[5,11,12]. Breakthrough pain usually represents a flare of the background pain and presumably results from the same mechanisms in most patients. The pathophysiology in cancer patients has been reported as nociceptive (38–74 per cent)[11,13], neuropathic (9–27 per cent)[1,11], or mixed (16–52 per cent)[11,13], and the aetiology has been observed to be directly due to cancer (65–76 per cent)[1,11], cancer treatment (11–35 per cent)[11,13], or unrelated to the cancer (0–19 per cent)[11,13]. By definition, the intensity of breakthrough pain is more severe than the background pain (usually stated as severe or excruciating)[1,4,11,13], and the reported quality and location usually are similar to the background pain[1,11,13].

Patients may have one type of breakthrough pain, or multiple types[1,11,13,14]. Some patients indicate that breakthrough pain (and use of breakthrough pain medication) varies with the time of day[4,14]; this circadian variation may be affected by a co-morbidity such as confusion[15].

The daily number of breakthrough pains varies greatly. Most studies suggest that the modal frequency is 1–4 episodes per day[1,4,13,16]. Breakthrough pain may be predictable or unpredictable, and the onset of pain is typically fast (reaching a maximum severity within 5 min). Although most breakthrough pains are relatively brief, subsiding within 30 min, variation in the duration is also large and ranges from momentary to many hours[1,13,16,17].

Three subtypes of breakthrough pain have been described—incident pain, spontaneous pain, and end-of-dose pain—and an individual patient may experience more than one type[1]. Incident pains are precipitated by voluntary actions, such as walking. The prevalence in cancer patients with breakthrough pain has been reported as between 32 per cent and 94 per cent of patients[18,19]. Although incident pains are usually predictable, their occurrence has been associated with a relatively poor response to opioid therapy[20,21]. Spontaneous pain has been reported in between 17 per cent and 59 per cent of patients[13,16]. These pains may occur in the absence of a specific trigger or may be precipitated by non-voluntary phenomena, such as fullness of the bladder, bowel movement, or cough. These pains also may be predictable or unpredictable. Finally, breakthrough pain that occurs reliably at the end of the dosing interval of an analgesic drug, or end-of-dose failure, has been reported in between 2 per cent and 29 per cent of patients[1,18]. The occurrence of these pains suggests that the prescribed dose is too low or the interval between doses is too long. Some authors consider end-of-dose failure to be a subtype of breakthrough pain, while others interpret the occurrence of these pains as evidence of uncontrolled background pain.

Despite the self-limiting nature of breakthrough pain, it can have a negative impact on quality of life by imposing a significant physical, psychological, or economic burden on patients and their caregivers. Patients with breakthrough pain are often less satisfied with their analgesic therapy[11,13], have decreased functioning because of their pain, and may experience social and psychosocial consequences, such as increased levels of anxiety and depression[11]. Breakthrough pain can be a poor prognostic indicator for the overall effectiveness of opioid therapy[20,22], and the site of breakthrough pain may predict response to treatment[16].

Inadequately relieved breakthrough pain can place a economic burden on patients and families, and on the health-care system. Patients with breakthrough pain are more likely to incur higher direct costs (e.g. prescription charges) and indirect costs (e.g. transportation)[23]. They are more likely to require health-care resources, such as emergency and medical visits, hospital admissions and longer hospital stays[24,25].

Although most published studies have described breakthrough pain in the cancer population, there are limited data suggesting that the phenomenon also is important in patients with chronic pain unrelated to cancer. A study of 67 hospice patients with advanced heart failure, multiple sclerosis, and pulmonary disease reported that 63 per cent of patients with background pain also experienced breakthrough pain[26]. A survey of 228 patients referred to pain management programmes for chronic non-cancer pain reported that 74 per cent experienced breakthrough pain[27]. The patients in both studies shared many characteristic of patients with cancer-related breakthrough pain, and it has been suggested that similar mechanisms underlie the experience of breakthrough pain in diverse populations with and without cancer[28]. Given the prevalence and impact of non-cancer background pain[29], this is an area which merits further attention.

Management of breakthrough pain

The management of breakthrough pain should aim to reduce the frequency and severity of the pain, and ultimately improve function; these goals should be realistic and meaningful to the patient. Given the heterogeneity of breakthrough pain, a highly individualized and systematic approach to its management is essential. This approach should be integrated into the overall plan of care, consider the use of both pharmacological and non-pharmacological modalities, and be appropriate for the stage of disease. Patients with multiple breakthrough pains may require more than one management option.

The basic principles of breakthrough pain management are:

◆ General assessment (e.g. pain assessment, explanation).

◆ Lifestyle changes (e.g. coping strategies).

◆ Modification of the pathological processes (e.g. anti-neoplastic therapies).

◆ Management of reversible causes (e.g. incident pain precipitants).

◆ Symptomatic management of breakthrough pain (e.g. pharmacological and non-pharmacological).

Interventions should form part of a holistic framework aimed at providing comfort, supporting the patient's sense of control over the pain, and addressing the concurrent physical and psychosocial burdens that contribute to the impaired quality of life.

General assessment of breakthrough pain

Successful management of breakthrough pain, like the pain syndrome overall, is best achieved by thorough assessment, good communication, reassurance about pain relief, and the encouragement of patients and caregivers to participate in the process of care. Unlike the background pain, which could be assessed using any of a number of valid assessment tools[30], there are currently no validated instruments for the assessment of breakthrough pain. Assessment tools are currently being developed[31].

Assessment follows the usual principles of history, examination, and relevant investigations to determine the characteristics, aetiology, and pathophysiology of the breakthrough pain, and the relation of the pain to the patients overall condition. Both unidimensional (e.g. numerical rating scales) and multidimensional instruments (e.g. brief pain inventory) may have a role to play. Ideally, patient self-report provides the details about the pain. If illness precludes this, however[13,26], assessment must rely on a proxy, such as the family or a professional caregiver. Physical examination (both general and specific to the pain) can help localize the pain and determine aetiology and pathophysiology. The examination also may confirm the importance of specific precipitating factors (e.g. movement). Investigations, such as imaging, may confirm the cause and help determine treatment options. Patients should be re-assessed regularly to determine the efficacy and tolerability of the management strategies; inadequate re-assessment may lead to continuance of ineffective and inappropriate treatment[31].

A variety of barriers to optimum pain management relating to both health-care professionals and patients have been described[32]. It is important that health-care professionals recognize the impact of breakthrough pain and that patient involvement and co-operation is best achieved through a good understanding of the management options and their possible adverse effects. Good communication and a mutual recognition of the problem is therefore essential. Without this, patents may be prescribed inadequate treatment[13,33,34] or fail to adhere to the proposed treatments[33,35]. Education is important and may benefit both patients and caregivers[36,37].

Lifestyle changes

Breakthrough pain may cause marked disability and result in the loss of social activities or an increased reliance on health professionals and medications. Patients who adopt active coping strategies may have better outcomes overall. Specific interventions that encourage this are relatively inexpensive options and may empower patients to accept responsibility for their own pain management and be more involved in their treatment. Some may be suggested by a health-care professional as a lifestyle change. For example, patients may be taught pacing to reduce activities that precipitate breakthrough pain when they are most likely to occur. They may be encouraged to use specific aids for activities of daily living (e.g. washing, dressing, and cooking), to engage in specific exercises, or to use the help provided by family in a way that maximizes benefit.

Modification of pathological processes

Interventions that modify pathological processes may result in an improvement in both background and breakthrough pain. In the cancer populations, these interventions include systemic therapies (e.g. chemotherapy, biological therapies, and hormonal therapies), radiation therapy, and surgery. Systemic therapies have diverse and characteristic antitumour activities, sites of action, and toxic effects. Drugs may be used either singly or in combination, and may be combined with surgery or radiotherapy. Relief of breakthrough pain is likely to occur only when the response to these therapies is substantial, and if the goals of care warrant consideration of primary antineoplastic therapy, consultation with an oncologist may be valuable when developing a plan of care for breakthrough pain.

Radiotherapy is often used primarily for cancer pain control and should be considered when breakthrough pain is associated with a discrete neoplastic lesion, even if the tumour type is known to be relatively radio-resistant. Radiation is particularly effective for pain associated with bone metastases, which may cause incident or spontaneous breakthrough pain[38]. Pain relief can be achieved with hypo-fractionated therapy, thereby minimizing inconvenience and cost[39].

Surgery may be used as an anti-neoplastic approach to achieve local tumour control, or may be appropriate for management of specific co-morbidities. For example, tumour excision and fixation of a pathological fracture may be highly effective in relieving severe incident pain, and surgical treatment of intestinal or urinary obstruction, if possible and appropriate, can eliminate breakthrough pains associated with these lesions. Surgery usually is considered when conservative approaches have failed, the patient's performance status is favourable, the disease is not widespread, and the patient is agreeable to this option.

Treatment of infection is another primary intervention that has the potential to improve breakthrough pain. Although infection usually is obvious, some clinical scenarios are challenging and suggest the value of empirical therapy. For example, worsening breakthrough pain in a previously irradiated region or a region adjacent to a pressure ulcer may be related to concomitant infection, the diagnosis of which may be difficult.

Management of reversible causes

Breakthrough pains may be precipitated by numerous processes[1], some of which are amenable to therapy. This therapy may be pharmacological or non-pharmacological. Pain related to cough or constipation, for example, may be effectively ameliorated by an anti-tussive or laxative, respectively. Pain related to joint movement may be addressed in some cases by an orthotic that limits the mobility of the joint. The assessment of the patient with breakthrough pain should identify all potential precipitants in the hope that primary interventions against the precipitating process can be implemented and thereby reduce reliance on symptomatic therapy.

Symptomatic management of breakthrough pain

Non-pharmacological management

Despite a lack of evidence in appropriately designed clinical trials, non-pharmacological approaches should be considered in the management of breakthrough pain. Patients often volunteer that such treatments are helpful. Some require health-care professionals, such as an occupational therapist, physiotherapist, clinical psychologist, or chronic pain nurse. The use of an orthosis to brace a painful limb, for example, or a cognitive therapy such as imagery, may be appropriately considered in selected patients. These non-pharmacologic strategies can be tried either before, or alongside, pharmacological therapy.

Patients have reported a number of helpful therapies, including massage[4,18], application of heat or cold[4,18,40], distraction therapies[8,40], and relaxation techniques[4,8]. Related cognitive behavioural strategies also might be considered, and other physical medicine or complementary strategies, such as therapeutic exercise, transcutaneous electrical stimulation, and acupuncture, also can play a role.

Despite comprehensive assessment and the careful use of systemic pharmacologic therapy, some patients fail to gain adequate analgesia. These patients may benefit from interventional techniques[45]. Injection therapy ranges from trigger-point injection to neural blockade. Neuraxial analgesia may involve epidural or intrathecal administration of an opioid, local anaesthetic, or other drug. These procedures require consultation with a physician trained in interventional pain management strategies. They typically are not considered unless less invasive strategies are ineffective and the goals of care support such a trial.

Pharmacological management: optimizing ATC medication

Pharmacological strategies for the management of breakthrough pain have been developd for the cancer population. Presumably, the principles could be applied to any patient.

Oral opioid therapy usually is the first-line in the treatment of moderate-to-severe pain in patients with cancer. Management often follows the principles of the World Health Organization's (WHO) analgesic ladder, which recommends that analgesics should be selected according to the severity of the pain and not the severity of the disease[42]. This strategy is applied to the management of breakthrough pain by optimizing both the fixed scheduled ATC regimen and providing a co-administered 'as needed' drug for the breakthrough pain[43].

In the absence of treatment-limiting side effects, an increase in the ATC opioid dose may be considered in an effort to reduce the frequency or intensity of breakthrough pains. Although the evidence for this approach is very limited, anecdotal experience suggests that it can benefit some patients. An open-label study of patients with incident pain showed that titration of the dose beyond analgesia to the point of adverse effects prevented or limited breakthrough pain[44]. Another study reported a 32 per cent to 70 per cent reduction in breakthrough pain within one week of increasing both the ATC analgesic and adjuvant analgesics[16]. However, a study of 137 oncology outpatients with pain from bone metastases appeared to show that patients using opioids only as needed had pain relief similar to patients taking opioids ATC despite using lower daily doses of opioid[45]. Adjusting the fixed-schedule opioid regimen is most clearly appropriate in patients with end-of-dose failure, for whom the usual intervention is to increase the dose. If an adjustment in the ATC dose leads to side effects between episodes of breakthrough pain, the dose should again be lowered.

Optimizing the ATC regimen by adding a non-opioid analgesic or an adjuvant analgesic also could play an important role in the management of breakthrough pain. Paracetamol and the non-steroidal anti-inflammatory drugs (NSAIDs) are widely used in the management of mild cancer pain and often obtained by patients over the pharmacy counter. The evidence for the analgesic efficacy of paracetamol is primarily in acute postoperative pain[46], and although included in a systematic review of cancer pain treatments[47], it could not be analysed separately due to insufficient data. Studies examining a possible additive analgesic effect of paracetamol during concurrent opioid therapy in cancer patients have had conflicting results[48,49]. The evidence for NSAIDs from systematic reviews suggests they are effective analgesics in cancer pain, both when studied in a single doses and with chronic dosing[48,50–52], although the heterogeneity of study designs and outcome measures make analysis difficult.

Adjuvant analgesics should be considered at all stages of the patient's illness and at each step of the WHO analgesic ladder. It is important to explain to patients that these drugs have a non-analgesic primary indication so as to avoid confusion. The most commonly used adjuvant analgesics in the cancer population are those that may be efficacious for neuropathic pain, which can present with a component of breakthrough pain. Although there are very few studies of drugs for cancer-related neuropathic pain, treatment generally is extrapolated from experience with non-cancer pain. The best-studied drugs are specific anticonvulsants and antidepressants[53,54]. Other classes, including corticosteroids and membrane-stabilizing drugs[55], are also tried for this indication. Paroxysmal neuropathic pains can be among the most challenging breakthrough pains, and the addition of one or more drugs specific for neuropathic pain to the opioid regimen often is a valuable strategy to reduce or prevent them.

Patients with metastatic bone pain also are candidates for several classes of adjuvant analgesics. The most important are the corticosteroids and the bisphosphonates[56]. The bisphosphonates are drugs that inhibit osteoclast-mediated bone resorption and are usually prescribed to reduce the incidence of skeletal complications of metastases[57]. If bone pain responds overall to these therapies, movement-related breakthrough pains may be less likely to occur.

Corticosteroids also are used as adjuvant analgesics for a variety of other syndromes. These include pain from raised intracranial pressure, obstruction of hollow viscus, and organ infiltration. Breakthrough pains associated with any of these syndromes should be considered targets for a trial of a corticosteroid co-administered with the opioid. At low doses, they also increase general well-being.

Pharmacological management: rescue medication

Rescue medication refers to the use of a symptomatic medication for breakthrough pain 'as required'. Rescue medication is prescribed in combination with the ATC opioid regimen and may be used either prophylactically for predictable pains, or more commonly, as soon as pain starts. Conventionally, rescue medication is a short-acting, normal-release formulation. Occasionally, paracetamol or a NSAID is used empirically and there have been reports of other drugs, including nitrous oxide, ketamine, midazolam, and cannabinoids[58–62]. The evidence for the latter treatments is mostly in the form of case reports or small controlled studies and is sometimes conflicting. Although one review confirmed that NSAIDs are effective analgesics for cancer pain[50], the maximal analgesic effectiveness of the non-opioid analgesics, their side effects, and the relatively slow onset of action, and long duration of effect limit their value overall in the treatment of breakthrough pain.

The ideal rescue medication should be efficacious, have a rapid onset of action, a relatively short duration of effect, and minimal adverse effects. Oral opioids have been the mainstay approach for patients who are receiving an oral or transdermal baseline opioid regimen. Recently, new formulations that deliver a lipophilic opioid, fentanyl, directly through mucous membranes have been developed in an effort to provide a more rapid onset of effect, and one or two of these formulations are now in use in some countries. Novel delivery systems for other lipophilic drugs are in development. Alternative non-oral routes also are available, including the parenteral and rectal, and these may play a role in selected populations with breakthrough pain.

Oral rescue medication

The oral route, which is often preferred because it is convenient and usually inexpensive, is commonly used to deliver rescue medication. Normal-release formulations of morphine, hydromorphone, or oxycodone are amongst those most frequently used. Occasionally, methadone is used for rescue, typically in patients receiving methadone as the baseline therapy; this approach must be undertaken cautiously because of concerns about accumulation of a long half-life drug with repeated administration.

The dose of rescue medication is often based on the patient's around-the-clock analgesia. Some suggest 5–10 per cent of the daily dose, others 5–15 per cent, whilst others recommend the rescue medication should be the same as the 4-hourly dose[42, 63–66]. The practice of using a proportionate dose is based largely on anecdotal observations and is consistent with the known relationship between plasma drug concentration and effects, which becomes linear when plotted on a log-linear scale. Given this relationship, there is a greater likelihood of a reliable change in effects when transiently increasing the dose if the increment is a percentage of the baseline dose. However, given that breakthrough pains may vary in aetiology, intensity, and duration, it also is possible that the effective dose of rescue medication varies in each individual. Recent controlled trials of transmucosal fentanyl formulations did not in fact confirm that the effective dose for breakthrough pain was proportionate to the baseline opioid dose (see following paragraphs)[67], and for this reason, the '5–15 per cent rule' should be applied cautiously to oral or parenteral rescue doses. Indeed, it has been suggested that titration of rescue medication may be a more appropriate strategy in all cases[42, 63,67].

The time–action relationship of an orally-administered opioid rescue dose, which may be characterized by an onset of meaningful analgesia up to an hour after administration and a duration that may last four hours or more, may not be ideal for breakthrough pains that peak rapidly and persist for less than an hour. Patients may therefore obtain very little or delayed relief, even when rescue medication is used prophylactically, or adverse effects may become problematic due to effects of the medication that persist long after the pain has resolved[68–71]. There is some evidence to suggest that methadone has a faster onset of action[72], but as noted, its use is complicated by complex pharmacokinetics and pharmacodynamics[73]. The mismatch between pharmacokinetics and the time course of the pain has driven the development of transmucosal opioid formulations that may have a more rapid onset of effect.

Transmucosal rescue medication

Transmucosal formulations comprise a variety of delivery systems that present the drug to the oral, nasal, bronchial, or rectal mucosa. Rectal administration has been used for many years and a number of short-acting opioids are commercially available in rectal formulations. These drugs may be useful when patients are temporarily unable to tolerate oral medication, or the parenteral route becomes compromised by a bleeding disorder or generalized oedema[74,75]. The use of rectal drugs for breakthrough pain is compromised by dose-to-dose variability in absorption and effects, and limited patient acceptance for long-term use[76].

The sublingual route of administration also has been used historically for patients with advanced disease who become unable to tolerate oral medication. It is a relatively simple route to use and offers the potential for more rapid onset of action[77]. The only drug currently licensed by this route in the United Kingdom and the United States is buprenorphine, which has a relatively slow onset and long duration of analgesia, and is therefore not ideally suited to the management of breakthrough pain. Sublingual administration of injectable formulations, including morphine and diamorphine, has been tried in the clinical setting, but the response has been variable[78,79]. The use of sublingual fentanyl and related opioids also have been reported[80,81] and sublingual formulations are in development for cancer-related breakthrough pain. Like other transmucosal formulations of fentanyl, sublingual fentanyl is likely to provide a reliable alternative for rapid-onset analgesia.

Other transmucosal formulations of fentanyl are already available in some countries, and others also are in development. These drugs, and formulations of lipophilic alternatives such as sufentanil[82], are being studied as treatments for breakthrough pain that may address an unmet need by providing a more rapid onset of effect than oral drugs. Presumably, a proportion of patients with breakthrough pain that peaks rapidly would indeed gain substantial benefit from a rapid-onset rescue-dose formulation. Given the lack of trials comparing these formulations with currently available oral rescue drugs, however, the size and characteristics of this subgroup are not known, and oral drugs are generally tried first because of cost.

Oral transmucosal fentanyl citrate (OTFC), a fentanyl-impregnated lozenge, was the first transmucosal fentanyl formulation developed specifically for the management of breakthrough cancer pain. OTFC is rapidly absorbed through the oral mucosa and may produce analgesia in minutes[83]. A number of trials have confirmed the efficacy, safety, and tolerability of OTFC, including two randomized controlled studies and a long-term follow-up study[84–86].

The second transmucosal fentanyl formulation to become commercially available is the fentanyl buccal tablet (FBT)[87]. This tablet, which has been approved in the United States for the management of breakthrough pain in opioid-treated patients with cancer, provides rapid penetration of fentanyl through the buccal mucosa by using effervescence to cause pH shifts that enhance the rate and extent of fentanyl absorption[88]. Compared to OTFC, the buccal tablet provides a larger proportion of the dose transmucosally (48 per cent versus 22 per cent) and has an earlier T_{max} (47 min versus 91 min)[89]. The efficacy of this formulation has been shown in placebo-controlled studies of both patients with cancer and non-cancer-related breakthrough pain[90,91]; as expected, the studies demonstrated an onset of effect more rapid than would be expected from oral therapy.

The controlled clinical trials of OTFC and FBT determined that the successful dose of these formulations did not correspond to the ATC dose. Accordingly, it is recommended that treatment with these formulations always start with a low dose, which should then be titrated to identify the effective dose.

The use of inhaled opioids for postoperative pain has been described in several studies[92,93] and although also described in the palliative care setting[94], there are few data relevant to the treatment of breakthrough pain[95]. Although traditional nebulizers may not be acceptable to some patients and may be an inefficient method of drug delivery[96], several newer types of systems to aerosolize opioids are now undergoing trials. Among the drugs under study is a formulation of free and liposome-encapsulated fentanyl, which can provide a more precise patient-controlled analgesia system for nebulization[97].

Nasal administration is another approach to transmucosal delivery and permits the administration of opioid by both patient and caregiver[98]. Reports describing the nasal administration of morphine, fentanyl, alfentanil, or sufentanil suggest that this route provides a rapid onset of action[99–102]. Although the relatively small volume of drug accommodated by the nose can be a disadvantage, the use of highly potent drugs such as fentanyl circumvents the problem. Nasal formulations are currently being tested[103].

Other transmucosal formulations are in development. For example, fentanyl and alfentanil bio-erodible mucoadhesive patches have been developed, which adhere to the buccal mucosa and rapidly release drug through the mucous membrane. Like most other transmucosal formulations, these systems have been designed to yield a rapid onset of effect in the hope that this profile better meets the analgesic needs of patients with breakthrough pain.

Parenteral formulations

Intravenous morphine has been shown to be effective, well-tolerated, and safe for the inpatient management of breakthrough pain[104,105], and hydromorphone has been delivered subcutaneously using a 'pain pen'[106]. In these studies, the successful rescue dose was proportionate to the ATC dose. Although the use of a parenteral rescue medication may not always be practical, as it is invasive and can be inconvenient and uncomfortable, it is commonly considered when patients are receiving long-term parenteral opioid therapy by means of continuous subcutaneous or intravenous administration, and may be considered for short-term therapy when pain is very severe and rapid titration of doses with quick peak effects would be advantageous. Indeed, when pain is severe, this route appears to be acceptable to patients[107].

Summary

Breakthrough pain is a heterogeneous phenomenon that varies in frequency, onset, duration, predictability, precipitants, pathophysiology, and aetiology. Despite the self-limiting nature of each breakthrough pain, the repeated episodes of severe pain can have a significant impact on both patients' and caregivers' quality of life. The successful management of pain depends on a comprehensive assessment, which must take into account both background and breakthrough pains, and consider whether the underlying disease, co-morbidities, or precipitating events are amenable to primary interventions. Symptomatic therapy relies on both efforts to optimize the analgesic regimen for the background pain and co-administration of a rescue dose specifically for the breakthrough pain. In some cases, treatment may require a combination of pharmacological and non-pharmacological strategies. Most of the evidence for the management of breakthrough pain is based on case studies and larger observational studies. Controlled trials have been done with rapid onset formulations containing fentanyl, but there have been no comparative trials. Guidelines remain empirical and more studies are needed to evaluate the different treatment options.

References

1. Portenoy, R.K. and Hagen, N.A. (1990). Breakthrough pain: definition, prevalence and characteristics. *Pain*, **41**, 273–81.

2. Caraceni, A. and Portenoy, R.K. (1999). An international survey of cancer pain characteristics and syndromes: IASP Task Force on Cancer Pain, International Association for the Study of Pain. *Pain*, **82**, 263–74.

3. Mercadante, S., Radbruch, L., Caraceni, A. *et al.* (2002). Episodic (breakthrough) pain: consensus conference of an expert working group of the European Association for Palliative Care. *Cancer*, **94**, 832–9.

4. Bennett, D., Burton, A.W., Fishman, S. *et al.* (2005). Consensus panel recommendations for the assessment and management of breakthrough pain. *Part 1 Assessment P & T*, **30**, 296–301.

5. Fine, P.G. and Busch, M.A. (1998). Characterisation of breakthrough pain by hospice patients and their caregivers. *Journal of Pain and Symptom Management*, **16**, 179–83.

6. Colleau, S.M. (1999). The significance of breakthrough pain in cancer. *Cancer Pain Release*, **12**, 1–3.

7. Portenoy, R.K., Forbes, K., Lussier, D. *et al.* (2004). Difficult pain problems: an integrated approach. In *Oxford Textbook of Palliative Medicine* (eds. D. Doyle, G. Hanks, N. Cherny *et al.*), pp. 438–58, 3rd edition. Oxford University Press.

8. Portenoy, R.K. (1997). Treatment of temporal variations in chronic cancer pain. *Seminars in Oncology*, **24**, S16-7–S16-12.

9. Zeppetella, G. and Ribeiro, M.D.C. (2003). Pharmacotherapy of cancer-related episodic pain. *Expert Opinion in Pharmacotherapy*, **4**, 493–502.

10. Caraceni, A., Martini, C., Zecca, E. *et al.* (2004). Breakthrough pain characteristics and syndromes in patients with cancer pain: an international survey. *Palliative Medicine*, **18**, 177–83.

11. Portenoy, R.K., Payne, D., and Jacobsen, P. (1999). Breakthrough pain: characteristics and impact in patients with cancer pain. *Pain*, **81**, 129–34.

12. Colleau, S.M. (2004). Breakthrough (episodic) pain vs. baseline (persistent) pain in cancer. *Cancer Pain Release*, **17**, 1–3.

13. Zeppetella, G., O'Doherty, C.A., and Collins, S. (2000). Prevalence and characteristics of breakthrough pain in cancer patients admitted to a hospice. *Journal of Pain and Symptom Management*, **20**, 87–92.

14. Bruera, E., Macmillan, K., Kuehn, N. *et al.* (1992). Circadian distribution of extra doses of narcotic analgesics in patients with cancer pain: a preliminary report. *Pain*, **49**, 311–4.

15. Gagnon, B., Lawlor, P.G., Mancini, I.L. *et al.* (2001). The impact of delirium on the circadian distribution of breakthrough analgesia in advanced cancer patients. *Journal of Pain and Symptom Management*, **22**, 826–33.

16. Hwang, S.S., Chang, V.T., and Kasimis, B. (2003). Cancer breakthrough pain characteristics and responses to treatment at a VA medical center. *Pain*, **101**, 55–64.

17. Gomez-Batiste, X., Madrid, F., Moreno, F. *et al.* (2002). Breakthrough cancer pain: prevalence and characteristics in patients in Catalonia, Spain. *Journal of Pain and Symptom Management*, 45–52.

18. Swanwick, M., Haworth, M., and Lennard, R.F. (2001). The prevalence of episodic pain in cancer: a survey of hospice patients on admission. *Palliative Medicine*, **15**, 9–18.

19. Banning, A., Sjøgren, P., and Henriksen, H. (1991). Treatment outcome in a multidisciplinary cancer pain clinic. *Pain*, **47**,129-34.

20. Mercadante, S., Maddaloni, S., Roccella, S. *et al.* (1992). Predictive factors in advanced cancer pain treated only by analgesics. *Pain*, **50**, 151–5.

21. Bruera, E., Scholler, T., Wenk, R. *et al.* (1995). A prospective multicentre assessment of the Edmonton staging system for cancer pain. *Journal of Pain and Symptom Management*, **10**, 348–55.

22. Bruera, E., Fainsinge, R., MacEachern, T. *et al.* (1992). The use of methylphenidate in patients with incident cancer pain receiving regular opiates: A preliminary report. *Pain*, **50**, 75–7.

23. Fortner, B.V., Demarco, G., Irving, G. *et al.* (2003). Description and predictors or direct and indirect costs of pain reported by cancer patients. *Journal of Pain and Symptom Management*, **25**, 9–18.

24. Fortner, B.V., Okon. T.A., and Portenoy, R.K. (2002). A survey of pain-related hospitalizations, emergency department visits, and physician office visits reported by cancer patients with and without history of breakthrough pain. *Journal of Pain*, **3**, 38–44.

25. Grant, M., Ferrell, B.R., Rivera, L.M. *et al.* (1995). Unscheduled readmissions for uncontrolled symptoms. A healthcare challenge for nurses. *Nursing Clinics of North America*, **30**, 673–82.

26. Zeppetella,G., O'Doherty, C.A., and Collins, S. (2001). Prevalence and characteristics of breakthrough pain in patients with non-malignant terminal disease admitted to a hospice. *Palliative Medicine*, **15**, 243–6.

27. Portenoy, R.K., Bennett. D.S., Rauck, R. *et al.* (2006). Prevalence and characteristics of breakthrough pain in opioid-treated patients with chronic noncancer pain. *Journal of Pain*, **7**, 583–91.

28. Svendsen, K., Andersen, S., Arnason, S. *et al.* (2005). Breakthrough pain in malignant and non-malignant diseases: a review of prevalence, characteristics and mechanisms. *European Journal of Pain*, **9**, 195–206.

29. Breivik, H., Collett, B., Ventafridda, V. *et al.* (2006). Survey of chronic pain in Europe:prevalence, impact on daily life and treatment. *European Journal of Pain*, **10**, 287–333.

30. Caraceni, A., Cherny, N., Fainsinger, R. *et al.* (2002). Pain measurement tools and methods in clinical research in palliative care:recommendatios of an Expert Working Group of the European Association of Palliative Care. *Journal of Pain and Symptom Management*, **23**, 239–55.

31. Laverty, D. and Davies, A. (2006). Assessment. In *Cancer-related breakthrough pain* (ed. A.Davies), pp. 23–30. Oxford University Press.

32. National Cancer Institute. Pain (PDQ®) health professional version 2005. http://www.nci.nih.goc/cancertopics/pdq/supportivecare/pain/HealthProfessional. Accessed 20th December 2006.

33. Ferrell, B.R., Juarez, G., and Borneman, T. (1999). Use of routine and breakthrough analgesia in home care. *Oncology Nursing Forum*, **26**, 1655–61.

34. Weber, M. and Huber, C. (1999). Documentation of severe pain, opioid doses, and opioid-related side effects in outpatients with cancer: a retrospective study. *Journal of Pain and Symptom Management*, **17**, 49–54.

35. Zeppetella, G. (1999). How do terminally ill patients at home take their medication?. *Palliative Medicine*, **13**, 469–75.

36. Ferrell, B.R., Rhiner, M., and Reffell, B.A. (1993). Development and implementation of a pain education programme. *Cancer*, **72**(Suppl 11), S3426–32.

37. De Wit, R., Van Dam, F., Zandbelt, L. *et al.* (1997). A pain education programme for chronic cancer pain patients: follow-up results from a randomised controlled trial. *Pain*, **73**, 55–69.

38. McQuay, H.J., Collins, S.L., Carroll, D. *et al.* (1999). Radiotherapy for the palliation of painful bone metastases. *Cochrane Database of Systematic Reviews*, **3**, CD001793.

39. Sze, W.M., Shelley, M.D., Held, I. *et al.* (2003). Palliation of metastatic bone pain: single fraction versus multifraction radiotherapy - a systematic review of randomised trials. *Clinical Oncology*, **15**, 345–52.

40. Petzke, F., Radbruch, L., Zech, D. *et al.* (1999). Temporal presentation of chronic cancer pain: transitory pains on admission to a multidisciplinary pain clinic. *Journal of Pain and Symptom Management,* **17**, 391–401.

41. Miguel, R. (2000). Interventional treatment of cancer pain: The fourth step in the World Health Organization analgesic ladder? *Cancer Control,* **7**, 149–56.

42. World Health Organization. (1996). *Cancer Pain Relief* (2nd edition). World Health Organization. Geneva.

43. Hanks, G.W., De Conno, F., Cherny, N. *et al.* (2001). Morphine and alternative opioids in cancer pain: the EAPC recommendations. *British Journal of Cancer,* **84**, 587–93.

44. Mercadante, S., Villari, P., Ferrera, P. *et al.* (2004). Optimization of opioid therapy for preventing incident pain associated with bone metastases. *Journal of Pain and Symptom Management,* **28**, 505–10.

45. Miaskowski, C., Mack, K.A., Dodd, M. *et al.* (2002). Oncology patients with pain from bone metastases require more than around-the-clock dosing of analgesia to achieve adequate pain control. *Journal of Pain,* **3**, 12–20.

46. Moore, A., Collins, S., Carroll, D. *et al.* (1998). Single dose paracetamol (acetaminophen), with and without codeine, for postoperative pain. *The Cochrane Database of Systematic Reviews,* **4**, CD001547.

47. McNicol, E., Strassels, S., Goudas, L. *et al.* (2004). Nonsteroidal anti-inflammatory drugs, alone or combine with opioids, for cancer pain: a systematic review. *Journal of Clinical Oncology,* **22**, 1975–92.

48. Axelsson, B. and Borup, S. (2003). Is there an additive analgesic effect of paracetamol at step 3? A double-blind randomized controlled study. *Palliative Medicine,* **17**, 724–5.

49. Stockler, M., Vardy, J., Pillai, A. *et al.* (2004). Acetaminophen (Paracetamol) improves pain and well-being in people with advanced cancer already receiving a strong opioid regimen: a randomized, double-blind, placebo-controlled cross-over trial. *Journal of Clinical Oncology,* **22**, 3389–94.

50. Eisenberg, E., Berkey, C.S., Carr, D.B. *et al.* (1994). Efficacy and safety of nonsteroidal anti-inflammatory drugs for cancer pain: a meta-analysis. *Journal of Clinical Oncology,* **12**, 2756–65.

51. Alkhenizan, A., Librach, L., and Beyene, J. (2004). NSAIDs: are they effective in treating cancer pain? *European Journal of Palliative Care,* **11**, 5–8.

52. Carr, D.B., Goudas, L.C., Balk, E.M. *et al.* (2004). Evidence report on the treatment of pain in cancer patients. *Journal of National Cancer Institute. Monographs,* **32**, 23–31.

53. Wiffen, P., Collins, S., McQuay, H. *et al.* (2005). Anticonvulsant drugs for acute and chronic pain. *Cochrane Database of Systematic Reviews,* **3**, CD001133.

54. Saarto, T. and Wiffen, P.J. (2005). Antidepressants for neuropathic pain. *Cochrane Database of Systematic Reviews,* **3**, CD005454.

55. Kalso, E., Tramer, M.R., Moore, R.A. *et al.* (1998). Systemic local-anaesthetic-type drugs in chronic pain: a systematic review. *European Journal of Pain,* **2**, 3–14.

56. Wong, R. and Wiffen, P.J. (2002). Bisphosphonates for the relief of pain secondary to bone metastases. *Cochrane Database of Systematic Reviews,* **2**, CD002068.

57. Djulbegovic, B., Wheatley, K., Ross, J. *et al.* (2002). Bisphosphonates in multiple myeloma. *Cochrane Database of Systematic Reviews,* **4**, CD003188.

58. Parlow, J.L., Milne, B., Tod, D.A. *et al.* (2005). Self-administered nitrous oxide for the management of incident pain in terminally ill patients: a blinded case series. *Palliative Medicine,* **19**, 3–8.

59. Enting, R.H., Oldenmenger, W.H., van der Rijt, C.C. *et al.* (2002). Nitrous oxide is not beneficial for breakthrough cancer pain. *Palliative Medicine,* **16**, 257–9.

60. Mercadante, S., Arcuri, E., Tirelli, W. *et al.* (2000). The analgesic effect of intravenous ketamine in cancer patients on morphine therapy: a randomised double-blind cross-over double-dose study. *Journal of Pain and Symptom Management,* **20**, 246–52.

61. del Rosario, M.A., Martin, A.S., Ortega, J.J. *et al.* (2001). Temporary sedation with midazolam for control of severe incident pain. *Journal of Pain and Symptom Management,* **21**, 177–8.

62. Campbell, F.A., Tramer, M.R., Carroll, D. *et al.* (2001). Are cannabinoids an effective and safe treatment option in the management of pain? A qualitative systematic review. *British Medical Journal,* **323**, 1–6.

63. Portenoy, R.K. and Hagen, N.A. (1989). Breakthrough pain: definition and management. *Oncology (Williston Park),* **3**(Suppl), 25-9.

64. Hanks, G.W. and Justins, D.M. (1992). Cancer pain: management. *Lancet,* **339**, 1031–6.

65. Cherny, N.I. and Portenoy, R.K. (1993). Cancer pain management. Current strategy. *Cancer,* **72**(Suppl), 3393–415.

66. Levy, M.H. (1996). Pharmacologic treatment of cancer pain. *New England Journal of Medicine,* **335**, 1124–32.

67. Zeppetella, G. and Ribeiro, M.D. (2006). Opioids for the management of breakthrough (episodic) pain in cancer patients. *Cochrane Database of Systematic Reviews,* **Jan 25**(Suppl 1), CD004311.

68. Collins, S.L., Faura, C.C., Moore, R.A. *et al.* (1998). Peak plasma concentrations after morphine: A systematic review. *Journal of Pain and Symptom Management,* **16**, 388–402.

69. Poyhia, R., Seppala, T., Olkkola, K.T. *et al.* (1992). The pharmacokinetics and metabolism of oxycodone after intramuscular and oral administration to healthy subjects. *British Journal of Clinical Pharmacology,* **33**, 617–21.

70. Murray, A. and Hagen, N.A. (2005). Hydromorphone. *Journal of Pain and Symptom Management,* **29**(Suppl), S57–S66.

71. Bennett, D., Burton, A.W., Fishman, S. *et al.* (2005). Consensus panel recommendations for the assessment and management of breakthrough pain. Part 2 Management. *Pharmacology and Therapeutics,* **30**, 354–61.

72. Fisher, K., Stiles, C., and Hagen, N.A. (2004). Characterization of the early pharmacodynamic profile of oral methadone for cancer-related breakthrough pain: a pilot study. *Journal of Pain and Symptom Management,* **28**, 619–25.

73. Felder, C., Uehlinger, C., Baumann, P. *et al.* (1999). Oral and intravenous methadone use: Some clinical and pharmaokinetic aspects. *Drug and Alcohol Dependence,* **55**, 137–43.

74. Cole, L. and Hanning, C.D. (1990). Review of the rectal use of opioids. *Journal of Pain and Symptom Management,* **5**, 118–26.

75. Warren, D.E. (1996). Practical use of rectal medications in palliative care. *Journal of Pain and Symptom Management,* **11**, 378–87.

76. Davis, M.P., Walsh, D., LeGrand, S.B. *et al.* (2002). Symptom control in cancer patients: the clinical pharmacology and therapeutic role of suppositories and rectal suspensions. *Supportive Care in Cancer,* **10**, 117–38.

77. Weinberg, D.S., Inturrisi, C.E., Reidenberg, B. *et al.* (1988). Sublingual absorption of selected opioid analgesics. *Clinical Pharmacology and Therapeutics,* **44**, 335–42.

78. Coluzzi, P.H. (1998). Sublingual morphine: efficacy reviewed. *Journal of Pain and Symptom Management,* **16**, 184–92.

79. McQuay, H.J., Moore, R.A., and Bullingham, R.E. (1986). Sublingual morphine, heroin, methadone and buprenorphine: kinetics and efficacy. In *Opioid analgesics in the management of clinical pain, advances in pain research therapy* (eds. K.M. Foley and C.E. Inturrisi), pp. 407–12, volume 8. Raven Press, New York.

80. Zeppetella, G. (2001). Sublingual fentanyl citrate for cancer-related breakthrough pain: a pilot study. *Palliative Medicine,* **15**, 323–38.

81. Duncan, A. (2002). The use of fentanyl and alfentanil sprays for episodic pain. *Palliative Medicine,* **16**, 550.

82. Gardner-Nix, J. (2001). Oral transmucosal fentanyl and sufentanil for incident pain. *Journal of Pain and Symptom Management,* **22**, 627–30.

83. Hanks, G. (2001). Oral transmucosal fentanyl citrate for the management of breakthrough pain. *European Journal of Palliative Care*, **8**, 6–9.

84. Farrar, J.T., Cleary, J., Rauch, R. *et al.* (1998). Oral transmucosal fentanyl citrate: randomized, double-blind, placebo-controlled trial for the treatment of breakthrough pain in cancer patients. *Journal of the National Cancer Institute*, **90**, 611–6.

85. Coluzzi, P.H., Schwartzberg, L., Conroy, J.D. *et al.* (2001). Breakthrough cancer pain: a randomized trial comparing oral transmucosal fentanyl citrate (OTFC) and morphine sulfate immediate release (MSIR) *Pain*, **91**, 123–30.

86. Payne, R., Coluzzi, P., Hart, L. *et al.* (2001). Long-term safety of oral transmucosal fentanyl citrate for breakthrough cancer pain. *Journal of Pain and Symptom Management*, **22**, 575–83.

87. Webster, L.R. (2006). Fentanyl buccal tablets. *Expert Opinion on Investig Drugs*, **15**, 1469–73.

88. Pather, S.I., Seibert, J.M., Hontz, J. *et al.* (2001). Enhanced buccal delivery of fentanyl using the oravescent drug delivery system. *Drug Delivery Technology*, **1**, 54–7.

89. Darwish, M., Kirby, M., Robertson, P. Jr. *et al.* (2006). Pharmacokinetic properties of fentanyl effervescent buccal tablets: a phase I, open-label, crossover study of single-dose 100, 200, 400, and 800 microg in healthy adult volunteers. *Clinical Therapeutics*, **28**, 707–14.

90. Portenoy, R.K., Taylor. D., Messina, J. *et al.* (2006). A randomized, placebo-controlled study of fentanyl buccal tablet for breakthrough pain in opioid-treated patients with cancer. *Clinical Journal of Pain*, **22**, 805–11.

91. Portenoy, R.K., Messina, J., Xie, F. *et al.* (2007). Fentanyl buccal tablet (FBT) for relief of breakthrough pain in opioid-treated patients with chronic low back pain: a randomized, placebo-controlled study. *Current Medical Research Opinion*, **23**, 223–33.

92. Thipphawong, J.B., Babul, N., Morishige, R.J. *et al.* (2003). Analgesic efficacy of inhaled morphine in patients after bunionectomy surgery. *Anesthesiology*, **99**, 693–700.

93. Higgins, M.J., Asbury, A.J., and Brodie, M.J. (1991). Inhaled nebulised fentanyl for postoperative analgesia. *Anaesthesia*, **46**, 973–6.

94. Ahmedzai, S. and Davis, C. (1997). Nebulised drugs in palliative care. *Thorax*, **52** (Suppl 2), S75–S77.

95. Zeppetella, G. (2000). Nebulized and intranasal fentanyl in the management of cancer-related breakthrough pain. *Palliative Medicine*, **14**, 57–8.

96. Clay, M.M. and Clarke, S.W. (1987). Wastage of drug from nebulisers: a review. *Journal of the Royal Society of Medicine*, **80**, 38–9.

97. Hung, O.R., Whynot, S.C., Varvel, J.R. *et al.* (1995). Pharmacokinetics of inhaled liposome-encapsulated fentanyl. *Anesthesiology*, **83**, 277–84.

98. Dale, O., Hjortkjaer, R., and Kharasch, E.D. (2002). Nasal administration of opioids for pain management in adults. *Acta Anaesthesiologica Scandinavica*, **46**, 759–70.

99. Zeppetella, G. (2000). An assessment of the safety, efficacy, and acceptability of intranasal fentanyl citrate in the management of cancer-related breakthrough pain: a pilot study. *Journal of Pain and Symptom Management*, **20**, 253–8.

100. Pavis, H., Wilcock, A., Edgecombe, J. *et al.* (2002). Pilot study of nasal morphine-chitosan for the relief of breakthrough pain in patients with cancer. *Journal of Pain and Symptom Management*, **24**, 598–602.

101. Fitzgibbon, D., Morgan, D., Dockter, D. *et al.* (2003). Initial pharmacokinetic, safety and efficacy evaluation of nasal morphine gluconate for breakthrough pain in cancer patients. *Pain*, **106**, 309–15.

102. Jackson, K., Ashby, M., and Keech, J. (2002). Pilot dose finding study of intranasal sufentanil for breakthrough and incident cancer-associated pain. *Journal of Pain and Symptom Management*, **23**, 450–2.

103. Sprintz, M., Benedetti, C., and Ferrari, M. (2005). Applied nanotechnology for the management of breakthrough cancer pain. *Minerva Anestiologica*, **71**, 419–23.

104. Mercadante, S., Villari, P., Ferrera, P. *et al.* (2004). Safety and effectiveness of intravenous morphine for episodic (breakthrough) pain using a fixed ratio with the oral daily morphine dose. *Journal of Pain and Symptom Management*, **27**, 352–9.

105. Mercadante, S., Villari, P., Ferrera, P. *et al.* (2006). Safety and effectiveness of intravenous morphine for episodic breakthrough pain in patients receiving transdermal buprenorphine. *Journal of Pain and Symptom Management*, **32**, 175–9.

106. Enting, R.H., Mucchiano, C., Oldenmenger, W.H. *et al.* (2005). The 'pain pen' for breakthrough cancer pain: a promising treatment. *Journal of Pain and Symptom Management*, **29**, 213–7.

107. Walker, G., Wilcock, A., Manderson, C. *et al.* (2003). The acceptability of different routes of administration of analgesia for breakthrough pain. *Palliative Medicine*, **17**, 219–21.

10.1.6 **Opioid analgesic therapy**

Marie Fallon, Nathan I. Cherny, and Geoffrey Hanks

Introduction

Treatment with analgesic drugs is the mainstay of cancer pain management[1,2]. Although concurrent use of other approaches and interventions may be appropriate in many patients, and necessary in some, analgesic drugs are needed in almost every case. Drugs whose primary clinical action is the relief of pain are conventionally classified on the basis of their activity at opioid receptors as either opioid or non-opioid analgesics. A third class, adjuvant analgesics, are drugs with other primary indications which can be effective analgesics in specific circumstances. The major group of drugs used in cancer pain management is the opioid analgesics.

During the last 30 years, there has been a dramatic increase in our knowledge of the sites and mechanism of action of the opioids. The development of analytical methods has also been of great importance in facilitating pharmacokinetic studies of the disposition and fate of opioids in patients. More recently, advances in genomic research have indicated the potential importance of pharmacogenetic factors in the response to opioid analgesics[3]. These studies have begun to offer us a better understanding of some of the sources of variation between individuals in their response to opioids and to suggest ways of minimizing some of their adverse effects. Although there are gaps in our knowledge of opioid pharmacology, the rational and appropriate use of these drugs is based on their clinical pharmacological properties demonstrated in well-controlled clinical trials. However, in order to reflect the dramatic increase in preclinical opioid research in recent years, this chapter has been divided into two; a pre-clinical and a clinical section.

Terminology

In this chapter and throughout this textbook, we have adopted the following conventions in terminology.

Opiate is a specific term that is used to describe drugs derived from the juice of the opium poppy. For example, morphine is an opiate but methadone (a completely synthetic drug) is not[4].

Opioid is a general term that includes naturally occurring, semi-synthetic, and synthetic drugs, which produce their effects by combining with opioid receptors and are stereospecifically antagonized by naloxone. In this context we refer to opioid agonists, opioid antagonists, opioid peptides, and opioid receptors.

Narcotic is commonly used to describe morphine-like drugs and other drugs of abuse. The term is derived from the Greek *narke*, meaning numbness or torpor. Since this is an imprecise and pejorative term that is not useful in a pharmacological context, its use with reference to opioids is discouraged. The term narcotic is not used in this book.

Section I: pre-clinical pharmacology

Opioid receptors

Opioid receptors were originally classified by pharmacological activity in animal preparations and later, by molecular sequence. The three main receptors were classified as μ (mu) or OP3, κ (kappa) or OP1, and δ (delta) or OP2. Another opioid-like receptor has been identified recently; the nociceptin orphanin FQ peptide receptor. Receptor nomenclature has changed several times in the last few years; the current International Union of Pharmacology (IUPHAR) classification is MOP (mu), KOP (kappa), DOP (delta), and NOP (nociceptin orphanin FQ peptide) (Table 10.1.6.1).

The formerly identified sigma receptor is not a true opioid receptor and is not included in the opioid receptor group. Opioid receptors are widely distributed in both central and peripheral nervous systems. One of the characteristics of DNA and RNA is known as sequencing and this can be an indicator of normal biologic processes, pathogenic processes, and/or response to a therapeutic or other intervention. (See Table 10.1.6.2 for definitions of key terms in the discipline of pharmacogenomics and pharmacogenetics.) The mu, delta, and kappa receptors are very similar, sharing over 70 per cent sequence homology, whilst the orphan receptor shares only 50 per cent sequence homology[5]. Extensive pre-mRNA splicing gives rise to numerous splice-variants also known as receptor subtypes. The mu receptor gene has been shown to have

Table 10.1.6.1 Classification of opioid receptors.

Receptor	Molecular classification	Endogenous ligand	Site
Mu	OP3	Beta-endorphin, Leu- and Met-enkephalin; Endomorphins	Peripheral inflammation; pre- and post-synaptic neurons in spinal cord, PAG, NRM, thalamus, cortex
Kappa	OP1	Dynorphins	Spinal cord, supraspinal, hypothalamus
Delta	OP2	Enkephalins; beta-endorphin	Olfactory centres, motor integration areas in cortex, limited distribution in nociception areas
Orphan	ORL-1 (opioid-like receptor)	Nociceptin	Spinal cord

Table 10.1.6.2 Terminology in pharmacogenomics.

GENOMIC BIOMARKER

Definition

A genomic biomarker is defined as:

A measurable DNA or RNA characteristic that is an indicator of normal biologic processes, pathogenic processes, and/or response to therapeutic or other intervention

Additional information

1. The definition for a genomic biomarker is not limited to human samples.
2. A genomic biomarker could, for example, reflect:
   - The expression of a gene
   - The function of a gene
   - The regulation of a gene
3. A genomic biomarker can consist of one or more deoxyribonucleic acid (DNA) or ribonucleic acid (RNA) characteristics
4. The definition for a genomic biomarker does not include the measurement and characterization of proteins or low-molecular-weight metabolites
5. DNA characteristics include, but are not limited to
   - Single nucleotide polymorphisms (SNPs)
   - Variability of short sequence repeats
   - DNA modification, e.g. methylation
   - Insertions
   - Deletions
   - Copy number variation
   - Cytogenic rearrangements, e.g. translocations, duplications, deletions, or inversions
6. RNA characteristics include, but are not limited to:
   - RNA sequence
   - RNA expression levels
   - RNA processing, eg splicing and editing
   - MicroRNA levels

PHARMACOGENOMICS AND PHARMACOGENETICS

Definitions
Pharmacogenomics
Pharmacogenomics (PGx) is defined as:

The investigation of variations of DNA and RNA characteristics as related to drug response

Pharmacogenetics
Pharmacogenetics (PGt) is a subset of pharmacogenomics and is defined as:

The influence of variations in DNA sequence on drug response

Additional information

1. PGx and PGt are applied to activities such as drug discovery, drug development, and clinical practice
2. Drug response includes drug disposition (pharmacokinetics, PK) and drug effect (pharmacodynamics, PD)
3. The term drug should be considered synonymous with investigational (medicinal) product, medicinal product, and pharmaceutical product (including vaccines and other biological products)
4. The definition of PGx and PGt does not include other disciplines such as proteomics and metabonomics

25 different splice variants in mice, 8 in rats, and 11 in humans. These splice variants are controlled by diverse promoters. It has been demonstrated that different splice variants exhibit differences in agonist induced G protein activation, adenylyl cyclase activity and receptor internalization or endocytosis. In addition, some differences between the splice variants can lead to modification of phosphorylation, membrane translation, scaffolding protein binding, and G protein binding[6]. The potential activation and destination

of the receptor is changed by such modifications. The different effects of currently available opioids are dependent on complex interactions at various receptors and they function as neurotransmitters, neuromodulators, and neurohormones.

The three families of endogenous opioid peptides are well characterized. They are the endorphins, enkephalins, and dynorphins, which have binding affinities to all the receptors. Each family originates from a different gene, their precursors being pro-opiomelanocortin, proenkephalin, and prodynorphin. The endogenous tetrapeptide endomorphins 1 and 2 do not have an identified precursor; however, they are potent agonists acting very specifically at the mu receptor and they play a role in modulating inflammatory pain. Peripherally they interact extensively with immune cells, primarily in inflammatory states, when beta-endorphin-containing cells as well as signalling molecules (vascular P-selectin and intercellular adhesion molecular-1), which stimulate these cells, are up-regulated[7].

The receptor family

The mu opioid receptor

This is clinically the most important of all the receptor family. It is the main opioid receptor responsible for inhibition of nociceptive pathways, and is exploited by all exogenous opioids[8]. Many of the unwanted effects of opioids are also related to activity at this receptor.

Expression

The mu receptor is expressed on central and peripheral neurons, although in the latter it is only activated in response to inflammatory stimuli. Peripherally, mu receptors are found pre- and post-synaptically, for example, in the dorsal horn; approximately 70 per cent are expressed on the primary afferent terminations (pre-synaptic) modulating afferent transmission[9]. Mu receptors are present on C and A delta fibres, the sympathetic nervous system and immune cells. Centrally, they are expressed widely including the cerebral cortex, the amygdala, and the peri-aqueductal grey. In the peri-aqueductal grey, the presence of mu receptors on inhibitory neurons seems to lead to disinhibition of descending pathways resulting in excitation, as opposed to the more usual inhibition of neural transmission. The relative contribution of each binding site to the overall analgesic effects of systemic opioids is not known. We do understand from both the pre-clinical and clinical paradigm of inflammatory pain, that the pain state itself is highly likely to have a major role in the pattern of binding. In inflammation, the receptor undergoes pre- and post-transcriptional splicing and alteration, leading to a huge variation in the activation state of the receptor[5].

The delta receptor

Evidence suggests that other opioid endogenous ligands and receptors are linked to analgesic response and to mu receptor activation. It is interesting that deletion of the delta receptor gene and pre-proenkephalins inhibits the development of morphine tolerance, but not withdrawal, in mice[10]. On the other hand, the potency of mu agonists can be increased by the co-administration of a delta agonist, and such co-administration can induce a translocation of delta receptors to the cell surface. This pre-clinical information is of interest in relation to methadone, which has strong delta, as well as mu activity.

The kappa receptor

Kappa receptors are also involved in pain, in particular, in response to inflammation (peripherally); however, activation is associated clinically with a number of unpleasant side effects such as nausea and vomiting and dysphoria, which are mediated centrally. The latter have limited the clinical development of kappa agonists for pain of gastrointestinal aetiology, which is often associated with inflammation.

The ORL-1 receptor

The ORL-1 receptor was identified because of its homology with classical opioid receptor types. Its natural ligand is 'nociceptin' or 'orphanin'. There is a suggestion that centrally ORL-1 agonists appear to antagonize mu opioids but this is not yet clearly elucidated. The ORL-1 receptor is involved in modulation of a range of biological functions including the stress response, movement, memory, cardiovascular and renal mechanisms[5].

Opioid receptor, structure, and function

The opioid receptors belong to the superfamily of seven transmembrane-spanning G-protein-coupled receptors. The three major opioid receptors (mu, delta, and kappa) originate from different genes. Each of the transcribed receptor proteins consists of an extracellular N-terminus, seven transmembrane helices, three extra and intracellular loops, and an intracellular C-terminus characteristic of G-protein-coupled receptors (GPCR). The opioid receptor belongs to the rhodopsin family of GPCR[11–13]. The extracellular regions are involved in opioid binding and intracellular domains interact with G proteins. GPCRs were originally thought to function as monomers in a 1:1 stochiometric ratio with downstream heterotrimeric G proteins[14]. Their primary function is to transmit extracellular stimuli to intracellular signals. Opioid receptors are transduced by the Gi/Go proteins which are relatively resistant to tolerance or desensitization. Transport proteins, metabolizing enzymes, opioid receptors, and second messenger molecules are all essential to the effect of opioids (Table 10.1.6.3). At a cellular level, mu receptor activation results in an overall inhibitory effect via:

- inhibition of adenylyl cyclase;
- increased opening of potassium channels (hyperpolarization of post-synaptic neurons, reduced synaptic transmission); and
- inhibition of calcium channels (decreases pre-synaptic neurotransmitter release).

Opioid receptors and the accompanying G proteins interact with a vast array of other intracellular proteins that are responsible for trafficking receptors to the cell membrane anchoring and scaffolding proteins. This combination of events alters the response of the

Table 10.1.6.3 Factors influencing opioid effectiveness.

◆ Absorption	◆ Intrinsic efficacy at receptors
	• Transport proteins
◆ Distribution	• Metabolizing enzymes
	• Opioid receptors
	• Second messenger molecules
◆ Metabolism	
◆ Excretion	

receptor to a ligand. G-protein-coupled receptors, including mu, kappa, and delta have been shown to form different configurations including, dimers, homo-, and hetero-oligomers, which have relevance in internalization and activation pathways. This is discussed further in the section 'Receptor activation versus endocytosis'. Dimerization modulates receptor pharmacology and this process could present targets for novel interventions[5].

Modulation of opioid responses

There are multiple cellular adaptations in response to chronic opioid exposure, which may lead to tolerance[10]. Tolerance to exogenous opioids is relatively easy to produce in animal studies, where repeated doses of a given opioid rapidly lead to loss of efficacy in response to noxious stimuli. Cellular processes, which occur in response to chronic ligand binding to mu receptors, include diminution of spare opioid receptors, decreased receptor density, altered coupling, activation and phosphorylation of G proteins, and alteration of downstream pathways[11]. It has been reported that chronic exposure to mu or delta agonists induces and up-regulates the proexcitatory peptides, calcitonin-gene-related peptide (CGRP), substance P and protein kinase C (responsible for phosphorylation). There is some evidence that the N-methyl-d-aspartate (NMDA) or neurokinin 1 (NK1) receptors may play a role in acute tolerance. Interactions with the orphanin (NOP) receptor may also be important. The effect of these adaptations is to lead to a pro-excitatory state and an attenuation of the inhibitory effects of opioid activation[15,16].

Endogenous peptides such as neuropeptide FF, cholecystokinin, nociceptin, and dynorphin exhibit anti-opioid actions, which in turn modulate the physiological and/or pharmacological action and outcome of opioid agonists. Chronic morphine exposure leads to little change in mu receptor expression but does seem to produce changes in the non-neuronal population of glial cells, with increased activation[12]. Glia have come under increased scrutiny in many pain states. Although previously glia were considered an inert, supporting structure, there is increasing evidence that they play a key role, particularly in central sensitization where glia may modulate chronic opioid analgesia.

It is widely accepted that clinically relevant pharmacological tolerance to opioid analgesic effects is not an issue for the majority of patients with cancer-related pain. It is, however, difficult to assess analgesic tolerance clinically[15]. There does not appear to be a simple correlation between exposure to opioids and induction of analgesic tolerance. A process of adaptation occurs, which is likely to depend on many factors, but this process cannot be explained on the basis of current knowledge of cellular mechanisms.

Receptor activation versus endocytosis

The clinical use of combinations of different opioids is increasing, and the use of more than one opioid or partial opioid substitutions have recently been reported to reduce agitated terminal delirium, opioid tolerance, and dose escalation[16–18]. The benefits have been explained on the basis of receptor activation versus endocytosis (abbreviated to RAVE). This is discussed here not because of any evidence of clinical importance, rather to give the reader a complete picture of the evolving theories around opioid function. Potent opioids that activate but do not internalize or recycle the receptor are said to have a high RAVE value. Opioids, which cause receptor endocytosis or internalization, curtail opioid signalling. Paradoxically, sustained opioid signalling

causes adenylyl cyclase superactivation and antagonizes opioid responses[10, 19–23].

The opioid receptor binding site is different for each opioid. The number of receptors needed to be activated in order to suppress adenylyl cyclase (a hallmark for analgesia) differs significantly between major opioid receptors. This difference is not related to receptor density or to the amount of intracellular G protein[13]. Opioid alkaloids (morphine, methadone, fentanyl) bind within the core of the transmembrane portion of the receptor, whereas large peptidyl ligands bind to the extracellular loops[10,24,25]. A single receptor has the ability to activate multiple G protein heterotrimers independent of receptor density. Receptor conformation changes as a result of opioid binding and subsequently determines the efficacy of receptor activation and G protein interactions. Opioid receptors oscillate naturally between active and inactive states. Full agonists stabilize the receptor in an active conformation, partial agonists favour receptor conformation between fully active and inactive states. Opioid antagonists stabilize the receptor in an inactive conformation and prevent G protein activation. Antagonists can become opioid agonists when mutations occur within the fourth membrane helix (TM4), which influences receptor conformation and G protein interactions. The efficiency by which an opioid activates the receptor is dependent on the conformation that allows G proteins to interact with certain transmembrane helices (TM1 and TM7) and the C-terminus[13].

Opioid receptor conformational changes trigger conformational changes in the alpha sub-unit of G proteins (G alpha) that dissociate GDP from the alpha sub-unit of the G protein complex and promote GTP binding to the G alpha sub-unit. The other component of the G protein (G beta-gamma) is released for downstream signalling. Receptor signalling is curtailed by regulators of G protein signalling (RGS) and certain kinases[11,26]. G protein activation inhibits cyclic AMP production by adenylyl cyclase, and also initiates counteropioid responses and receptor desensitization through the activation of G-protein-coupled receptor kinase (GRK) as well as other protein kinases such as protein kinases A and C and mitogen-activated protein kinase (MAPK)[27–29].

G-protein-coupled receptor activity is balanced by molecular signals that govern receptor desensitization and resensitization. Mechanisms by which receptors are desensitized involve GRK, RGS, kinases, and receptor endocytosis. Receptor desensitization, which is the diminution of receptor responsiveness to agonist activation over time, also represents an important mechanism that limits opioid tolerance. Desensitization prevents acute and chronic

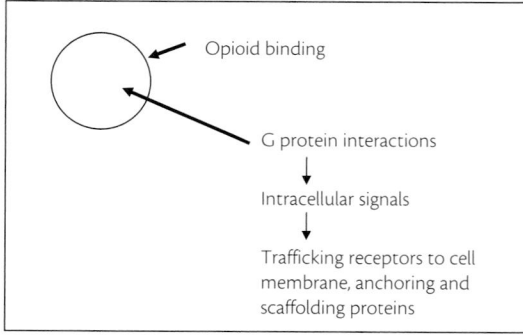

Figure 10.1.6.1 Opioid receptor which is G protein-coupled and transmits extracellular stimuli to intracellular signals.

overstimulation (or, in the case of opioids, over inhibition) by agonists[17]. Receptor mechanisms that paradoxically reduce signalling (GRK) are responsible for resensitization by directing receptor trafficking into endocytosis and resensitization[17]. These acute desensitization processes may be a protective mechanism whereby cells adapt to avoid physiological tolerance by attenuating receptor response to a new sustainable level.

Endocytosis or internalization

G protein activation (partially G beta-gamma subunits) activates GRK-2, which phosphorylates the C-terminus of the opioid receptor, as well as the second (TM2) and third transmembrane helices (TM3)[17]. Beta arrestin binds to the phosphorylated receptor, which then binds to clathrin pits within the membrane. Dynamin, a type of GTPase, causes fission of the membrane which results in the formation of small phosphorylase-rich endosomes[11,19,28,30,31]. The receptor is dephosphorylated within the endosome and returned resensitized to the membrane surface (or catabolized in the process of down-regulation)[17]. The degree of endocytosis is highly variable and depends on the opioid. Peptides and lipophilic alkaloid opioids (methadone and fentanyl) readily induce receptor endocytosis and recycling. Clinically, both methadone and fentanyl have high opioid intrinsic efficacy, and in some animal models, reduced adenylyl cyclase superactivation associated with opioid tolerance[21,23,24,31–33]. Morphine, on the other hand, is believed to activate MAPK, resulting in opioid receptor phosphorylation, which prevents internalization.

The use of combinations of opioids is becoming more common in clinical practice, clinicians citing putative differences in RAVE, the formation of dimers and oligomers and the resulting G-protein cascade reactions. Opioid combinations have also been proposed as both a preventative treatment and management of opioid-induced hyperalgesia. The evidence base for this approach is poor[16].

Given the complex, cell-specific, and multi-feedback dimension of opioid interactions, it is probably simplistic to assume that greater benefit from using such combinations might outweigh other factors such as poor patient compliance, confusion over dosing, and prescriber dosing errors along with potentially unanticipated increased side effects. At present, opioid combination therapy is without an evidence base.

Genetic modulation of the response to opioid analgesics

Pharmacogenomics is currently an intensely studied area of medicine to which great hope and expectations are attached[18]. Research, investigating the relationship between the genetic variability among individuals and susceptibility to disease, clinical symptoms, or treatment responses, has been growing exponentially.

There is considerable variability in response to opioid analgesics in clinical practice and in the balance of wanted and unwanted effects in individual patients. Pharmacogenetic factors are believed to play an important role in this variability. Possible candidates are polymorphisms in drug metabolizing enzymes, drug transporters, opioid receptors, or in the structures involved in the perception and processing of nociceptive information[19], all of which may result in the modulation of the pharmacokinetic or pharmacodynamic effects of opioid analgesics.

Candidate genetic polymorphisms are, of course, only identified on the basis of our current understanding of opioid analgesic mechanisms. Despite sufficient possible candidates with potential importance for pain therapy, evidence for a modulation of the effects of analgesics is only available for a few genes (Table 10.1.6.4). A variety of polymorphisms have been shown to be important for pain perception and processing and early work suggests that the mu opioid receptor (OPRM1) gene polymorphisms may relate to opioid dose requirements and side effects[36]. Identification of such polymorphisms in an individual patient would currently not provide an immediate individual therapeutic benefit. Benefit will only be obtained when pharmacogenetic testing provides a basis for individual drug selection or dosing. There are also polymorphisms, which affect the plasma concentrations of opioid analgesics but this does not necessarily have any direct clinical implications.

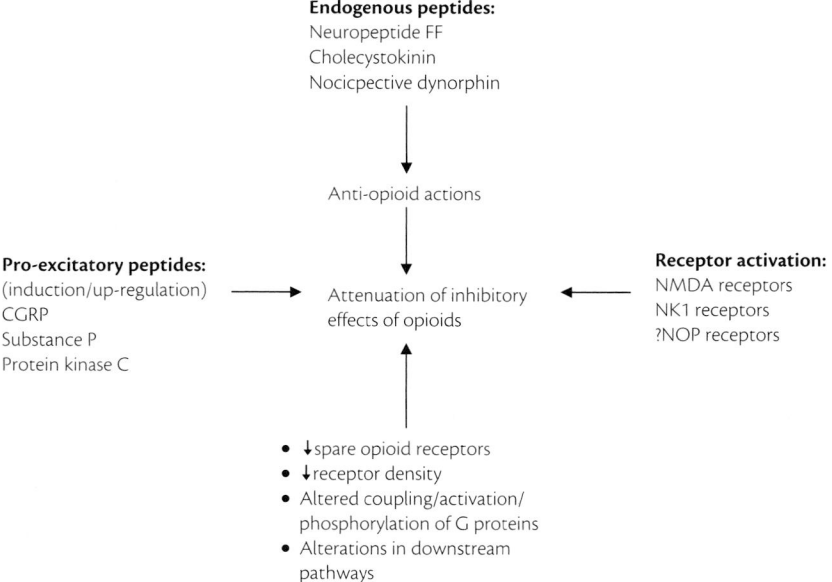

Figure 10.1.6.2 Chronic opioid exposure.

Table 10.1.6.4 Evidence for statistically significant pharmacogenetic modulation of the therapeutic effects of analgesic drugs and their consequences. The clinical significance of these effects has not been established.

Gene	Frequency of affected subjects (%)	Affected analgesics (positive available evidence)
OPRM1 (mu opioid receptor)	17.2	Morphine[20] M6G[3, 37–39]
COMT (catechol-O-methyl transferase)	46.2 (Protective to opioid central side effects)	Morphine[40, 41]
MC1R (melanocortin-1 receptor)	2[42] 4.5 4.3 3[42]	Morphine[42] M6G[42] Pentazocine[43]
CYP2D6 (cytochrome P450 2D6)	2[21] 20.7[21] 2[21] 0.9[21] 0.1[21] 0[21] 2[21]	Codeine[45,46] Tramadol[22] Codeine[23,24]
P-glycoprotein ABCB1 (adenosine triphosphate-binding cassette subfamily B member 1) ABCB1 is also known as MDR-1 (multi-drug resistance-1 gene)	47.6 (Protective to opioid central side effects)	Morphine[25] Morphine[41]

Genetic polymorphisms of relevance to opioid analgesic therapy

Mu-opioid receptor gene

The functional importance of the mu opioid receptor (OPRM1) variant N40D (with an asparagine in place of aspartate at the 40 position of the receptor protein) coded by the single nucleotide polymorphism (SNP) 118A>G of the OPRM1 gene has been suggested by several reports. In a study of patients with cancer-related pain, patients homozygous for the variant 118G allele needed significantly more morphine to achieve pain control, as compared to heterozygous and homozygous wild-type subjects[36].

Accumulated evidence suggests that the OPRM1 118G causes a decrease in opioid potency by a factor of 2 to 3, which may provide a scientific basis for increased doses for those patients. Conflicting evidence in relation to tolerance to opioid side effects has been reported; however, it mostly comes from pain studies in healthy volunteers, making the relevance to clinical practice poor[3,37,38].

Catechol-O-methyl transferase gene

In a study of patients with cancer pain, those who carried the V158M variant of the catechol-O-methyl transferase (COMT), coded by the 472G>A SNP of the COMT gene, needed less morphine than patients not carrying this variant (daily oral dose: 95 mg/day for homozygous carriers of the variant 472A allele [n=67], 117 mg/day for heterozygous carriers [n=96] and 115 mg/day for noncarriers of the variant [n=44])[26] The effect of the COMT 158M variant on opioid activity could be explained as follows: the variant leads to a low-function COMT enzyme which fails to degrade dopamine, which may cause a depletion of enkephalin resulting in compensatory up-regulation of opioid receptor expression. This has been demonstrated in human post-mortem brain tissue and *in vivo* by assessing the binding of the mu opioid receptor-selective radiolabelled [11C] carfentanil using positron emission tomography[40,51].

Melanocortin-1 receptor gene

Seventy-five per cent of people with a red-head-pale-skin phenotype carry two or more inactivating variants of the melanocortin-1 receptor gene (MC1R), among which the most important SNPs are 29insA, 451C>T coding for R151C MC1 receptors, 478>T coding for R160W MC1 receptors, and 880G>C coding for a D294H receptor protein (Table 10.1.6.4)[42]. They result in loss of functional MC1 receptors due to impaired G-protein coupling. The observation of greater analgesic effects of kappa-opioids in female carriers of MC1R non-functional variants, suggests that this neurochemical pain modulation has a gender-specific regulation when the kappa opioid system is involved[43]. However, it appears to be non-gender-specific for the mu opioid-mediated pain modulation[42].

Cytochrome P450 2D6 gene

Increased opioid effects close to opioid toxicity have been reported after oral administration of 25 mg or 60 mg of codeine and were explained by enhanced activity due to gene duplication of cytochrome P450 (CYP) 2D6, which catalyses the o-demethylation of codeine to morphine[48,49].

CYP2D6 gene multiplications are found at a frequency of 2.6 per cent in Caucasians but explain only 40 per cent of the ultrarapid metabolizer phenotype, reflecting the difficulties in identifying this phenotype by genetic testing[44,52]. On the other hand, codeine is ineffective in producing analgesia in patients with absent CYP2D6 function[27]. Codeine has a 200-times lower affinity at mu opioid receptors than morphine and, therefore, its clinical effects largely depend upon its O-demethylation to morphine, although some of its clinical effects appear to persist independently of morphine formation[53,54]. Non-functional CYP2D6 variants are coded by various CYP2D6 alleles. When present homozygously, they cause the CYP2D6 poor metabolizer phenotype, which is found in 7 per cent of Caucasian subjects[21]. In addition, there are alleles, which code for CYP2D6 with decreased function, resulting in the intermediate metabolizer.

The analgesic effect of tramadol is diminished in CYP2D6 dysfunction because the active metabolite O-demethyltramadol is not formed. However, tramadol is not completely devoid of analgesic effects in this situation because of its non-opioid analgesic activity.

P-glycoprotein gene

Genetic polymorphisms relating to opioid side effects

Central side effects such as drowsiness, confusion, and hallucinations can limit the use of opioids in clinical practice, therefore determining 'opioid-responsiveness'. In cancer pain management this is often seen as the key limiting factor to achieving pain relief.

The membrane-bound drug transporter P-glycoprotein is important in regulating drugs crossing the blood–brain barrier. It actively pumps drugs out of the central nervous system (CNS) and, therefore, may affect the frequency of opioid-induced CNS side effects[28]. Inter-individual variability in P-glycoprotein activity is well recognized, and genetic variation in the multi-drug resistance (MDR) gene MDR-1, which encodes for P-glycoprotein, alters P-glycoprotein activity[56,57].

Opioid side effects were studied in 228 patients with cancer-related pain who received morphine[29]. The control group were those who achieved adequate pain relief without unacceptable side effects, and the remaining patients were given a switch of opioid because of unacceptable side effects with morphine. Analysis confirmed that the genotypes for MDR-1 and COMT were associated independently with 'drowsiness and confusion or hallucinations'. In each instance, analyses were performed on the total population and on the Caucasian population alone to ensure that such associations held true independent of ethnicity. On univariate and multivariate analyses for the Caucasian cohort, both MDR-1 and COMT were associated significantly with reduction in central side effects. The percentage of patients with moderate or severe central side effects who had neither genetic susceptibility marker was 54 per cent. Patients who had COMT -4873G were less likely to be drowsy and confused, and the presence of the common G allele at 21/2677 in MDR-1 also was protective. The greatest proportion of patients with drowsiness and confusion were those patients with the variant A allele at COMT – 4873 and a variant T or A allele at 21/2677 in MDR-1[41]. This study is interesting as it addresses such a key area; however, it involves a very complicated clinical phenotype. More work is required with the clinical characterization of opioid side effects along with other contributory factors, which together characterize this phenotype.

Individual analgesic dosing for carriers of single or multiple functional pharmacogenetic variants

Available quantitative information may allow for a preliminary recommendation for a dose adaptation of morphine therapy based on the individual genotype with respect to OPRM1, COMT, MDR-1, and MC1R (Table 10.1.6.4). For example, carriers of the variant OPRM1 118G allele may be given double the standard morphine dose. However, the recommended dose adaptation is the arithmetic product of the dose adaptation factors for each polymorphism, which is clearly not straightforward for a variety of reasons, not least the fact that individuals may carry genotypes, which are additive or in fact cancel each other out.

Potential clinical applications

The substantial advances in the understanding of genetic polymorphisms, mutations affecting opioid receptors, activation, ligand response, and pain processing are of great interest but as yet do not have direct clinical applications The implications for clinical practice are that all known active pharmacogenetic variants would need to be identified.

One of the great challenges in translating pre-clinical and early clinical evidence to the clinic, especially concerning genetic modulation, is the undisputed complexity involved in pain perception in individual patients with a heterogenous spectrum of pain syndromes along with environmental and behavioural factors. Improved, more robust clinical phenotyping is necessary in all genetic studies to allow improved understanding and meaningful interpretation of any findings. Researchers and clinicians need to agree on well-defined measurable end-points and of course agree on how we will measure such endpoints.

Opioid structure

The structures of opioid analgesics are diverse, although for most opioids it is usually the laevorotatory (*levo*)- stereoisomer that is the active compound. The structures of some of the common agents are shown. Those in current use include phenanthrenes (e.g. morphine), phenylpiperidines (e.g. fentanyl), and diphenylpropylamines (e.g. methadone, dextropropoxyphene). Structural modification affects agonist activity and alters physicochemical properties such as lipid solubility. Tertiary nitrogen is necessary for activity, separated from a quaternary carbon by an ethylene chain. Chemical modifications that produce quaternary nitrogen significantly reduce potency, due to decreased CNS penetration. If the methyl group on the nitrogen is changed, antagonism of analgesia can be produced.

Other important positions for activity and metabolism, as seen on the morphine molecule, include the C-3 phenol group (the distance of this from the nitrogen affects activity) and the C-6 alcohol group. Potency may be increased by hydroxylation of the C-3 phenol; oxidation of C-6 (e.g. hydromorphone); double acetylation at C-3 and C-6 (e.g. diamorphine); hydroxylation of C-14, and reducing the double bond at C-7/8. Further additions at the C-3 OH group reduce activity. A short-chain alkyl substitution is found in mixed agonist–antagonists, hydroxylation or bromination of C-14 produces full antagonists, and removal or substitution of the methyl group reduces agonist activity[30].

Pharmacokinetics and physicochemical properties

Knowledge of the specific physicochemical properties and pharmacokinetics of individual agents is important in determining the optimal route of drug delivery in order to achieve an effective receptor site concentration for an appropriate duration of action. All opioids are weak bases. The relative proportion of free and ionized fractions is dependent on plasma pH and the pKa of the particular opioid. The amount of opioid diffusing to the site of action (diffusible fraction) is dependent on lipid solubility, concentration gradient, and degree of binding. Plasma protein concentrations of albumin and acid glycoprotein as well as tissue-binding determine the availability of the unbound, unionized fraction. This diffusible fraction moves into tissue sites in the brain and elsewhere; the amount reaching receptors is dependent not only on lipophilicity, but also the amount of non-specific tissue-binding, e.g. to CNS lipids.

The ionized, protonated form is active at the receptor site. This has important implications for speed and duration of activity. For example, morphine is relatively hydrophilic and penetrates the blood–brain barrier slowly. However, a large mass of any given dose eventually reaches the receptor site due to low levels of non-specific tissue-binding. This effect-site equilibration time ($t_{1/2}$ keo) is measured by assessing the effect of opioids on the EEG. The offset time may also be prolonged with resultant longer duration of action than would be expected from the plasma half-life. Most opioids have a very steep dose–response curve. Therefore, if the dose is near the minimum effective analgesic concentration (MEAC), very small fluctuations in plasma or effect-site concentrations can lead to large changes in the level of analgesia[31].

Opioids tend to have a large volume of distribution (Vd) because of their high lipid solubility. A consequence of this can be that redistribution, particularly after a bolus dose or short infusion, can have significant effects on plasma concentrations. In addition, first-pass effects in the lung can remove significant amounts of drug from the circulation, reducing the initial peak plasma concentration. However, the drug re-enters the plasma several minutes later. Plasma concentrations of opioids such as fentanyl, can be affected by this. Other lipophilic amines such as lidocaine and propranolol can be affected similarly and may reduce pulmonary uptake of co-administered opioids.

After prolonged infusion, significant sequestration in fat stores and other body tissues can occur for highly lipid soluble opioids. This is reflected in the 'context-sensitive $t_{1/2}$' i.e. the time taken for the plasma concentration to fall by 50 per cent after the infusion has stopped. The context-sensitive $t_{1/2}$ is increased after prolonged infusion for most opioids. For example, the elimination $t_{1/2}$ for fentanyl after bolus administration is 3–5 h, but increases to 7–12 hours after prolonged infusion.

Most opioid metabolism occurs in the liver (phase I and II reactions) with the hydrophilic metabolites predominantly excreted renally, although a small amount may be excreted in the bile or unchanged in the urine. As a result, hepatic blood flow is one of the major determinants of plasma clearance. Metabolism of individual drugs is shown in Table 10.1.6.5. Enterohepatic re-circulation may occur when water-soluble metabolites excreted in the gut are metabolized by gut flora to the parent opioid and then re-absorbed. Lipid soluble opioids may diffuse into the stomach, become ionized due to the low pH and then are re-absorbed in the small intestine; this results in a secondary peak in plasma concentrations.

A summary of physicochemical and pharmacokinetic properties of some opioids is shown in Table 10.1.6.6. Metabolism (including production of active metabolites), distribution between different tissues, and elimination, all interact within individual subjects to produce clinically important actions at receptor sites. The physicochemical and pharmacokinetic properties of opioids can change when used for chronic pain relief.

Factors affecting pharmacokinetics include:

◆ *Age.* Age is important due to both pharmacokinetic and pharmacodynamic factors. Metabolism and volume of distribution are often reduced in the elderly, leading to increased free drug concentrations in the plasma. Hepatic blood flow may have declined by 40–50 per cent by age 75, with reduced clearance of opioids. Increased CNS sensitivity to opioid effects is also found in the elderly.

◆ *Hepatic disease* has unpredictable effects, although there may be little clinical consequence, unless there is coexisting encephalopathy. Reductions in plasma protein concentrations will also have effects on plasma concentrations of free unbound drug.

◆ *Renal failure* may have significant effects for opioids with renally excreted active metabolites such as morphine and diamorphine.

◆ *Obesity* will result in a larger volume of distribution and prolonged elimination half-life.

◆ *Hypothermia, hypotension, and hypovolaemia* may also result in variable absorption and altered distribution and metabolism of opioids.

Agonists, antagonists, potency, and efficacy

Based on their interactions with the various receptor sub-types, opioid compounds can be divided into agonist, agonist–antagonist, and antagonist classes (Table 10.1.6.7).

Agonists

An agonist is a drug that has affinity for and binds to cell receptors to induce changes in the cell that stimulate physiological activity. The agonist opioid drugs have no clinically relevant ceiling effect to analgesia. As the dose is raised, analgesic effects increase in a log linear function, until either analgesia is achieved or dose-limiting adverse effects supervene. Efficacy is defined by the maximal response induced by administration of the active agent. In practice, this is determined by the degree of analgesia produced following dose escalation through a range limited by the development of adverse effects. Potency, in contrast, reflects the dose–response relationship. Potency is influenced by pharmacokinetic factors (i.e. how much of the drug enters the body's systemic circulation and then reaches the receptors) and by affinity to drug receptors.

The concepts of efficacy and potency are illustrated in Fig. 10.1.6.3, which shows the dose–response curves for two drugs A and B. If the logarithm of dose is plotted against response an agonist will produce an S-shaped or sigmoid curve. The efficacy of the two drugs,

Table 10.1.6.5 Metabolism and excretion of some opioids.

Drug	Metabolism	Faeces	Urine
Morphine	Glucuonidation Sulphation N-dealkylation	Trace	90% in 24 h (10% morphine; 70% glucuronides; 10% 3-sulphate; 1% normorphine; 3% normorphine glucuronide)
Codeine	O-demethylation Glucuronidation	Trace	86% in 24 h (5–10% codeine; 60& codeine glucuronide 5–15% morphine(mainly conjugated); trace normorphine)
Diamorphine	O-deacetylation Glucuronidation	Trace	80% in 24 h (5–7% morphine; 90% morphine glucuronides; 1% 6-acetylmorphine; 0.1% diamorphine)
Buprenorphine	Glucuronidation N-dealkylation	70%. Mainly unchanged	2–13% in 7 days. Mainly N-dealkylbuprenorphine (and glucuronide), buprenorphine-3-glucuronide
Meperidine (pethidine)	N-demethylation Hydrolysis	No evidence of excretion	70% in 24 h (10% meperidine; 10% normeperidine; 20% mepridinic acid; 16% meperidinic acid glucuronide; 8% normeperidinic acid; 10% normeperidinic acid glucuronide; plus small amounts of other metabolites)
Methadone	N-dealkylation	30%	60% in 24 h (33% methadone; 43% EDDP; 10% EMDP plus small amounts of other metabolites)
Fentanyl	N-dealkylation Hydroxylation	9%	70% in 4 days (5–25% fentanyl; 50% 4-N-(N-proprionylanilino-piperidine) plus other metabolites)

Table 10.1.6.6 Pharmacokinetic and physiochemical properties of some opioids.

Opioid	pKa	Protein binding (%)	Octanol: water partition coefficient	Terminal half-life (h)	Clearance (ml/kg/min)	Volume of distribution litre/kg	Duration of action (h)
Morphine	7.9	30	6	1.7–3.0	15–20	3–5	3–5
Oxycodone	8.5	45	0.7	3–4	13	2–3	2–4
Codeine	8.2	20	0.6	2–4	9–13	2.5–3.5	4–6
Meperidine	8.5	70	39	3–5	8–18	3–5	2–4
Fentanyl	8.4	90	813	2–4	10–20	3–5	1–1.5
Alfentanil	6.5	91	128	1–2	4–9	0.4–1	0.25–0.4
Remifentanil	7.3	70	18	0.1–0.2	40–60	0.3–0.4	2–5 min
Methadone	8.3	90	26–57	15–20	2	5	4–8

defined by maximum response is the same. Drug A produces the same response as B but at a lower dose, and therefore is described as more potent.

Antagonist

Antagonist drugs have no intrinsic pharmacological action but can interfere with the action of an agonist. Competitive antagonists bind to the same receptor and compete for receptor sites, whereas non-competitive antagonists block the effects of the agonist in some other way.

Opioid antagonists

Naloxone (short-acting) and naltrexone (long-acting) are opioid antagonists and block mu, delta, and kappa receptors equally. They are generally only used to reverse respiratory depression associated with opioid overdose as they will also reverse analgesia. Recently, however, a combined opioid and peripherally acting antagonist preparations such as oxycodone/naloxone has been made available for the prevention/management of opioid-induced constipation syndrome.

Agonist–antagonist

The agonist–antagonist analgesics can, in turn, be subdivided into the mixed agonist–antagonists and the partial agonists, a distinction also based on specific patterns of drug–receptor interaction. Both the partial agonist and agonist–antagonist drugs have a ceiling effect for analgesia, and although they produce analgesia in the opioid-naïve patient, in theory they can precipitate withdrawal in patients who are physically dependent on morphine-like drugs. For these reasons, they have been considered generally to have a limited role in the management of patients with cancer pain.

Mixed agonist–antagonists

The mixed agonist–antagonist drugs produce agonist effects at one receptor and antagonist effects at another. Pentazocine is the prototype agonist–antagonist: it has agonist effects at kappa receptors and weak mu antagonist actions. Thus, in addition to analgesia, pentazocine may produce κ-mediated psychotomimetic effects not seen with full or partial mu agonists. When a mixed agonist–antagonist is administered together with an agonist, the antagonist effect at the mu receptor can generate an acute withdrawal syndrome.

Partial agonists

A partial agonist has low intrinsic activity (efficacy) so that its dose–response curve exhibits a ceiling effect at less than the maximum effect produced by a full agonist. Buprenorphine is the main example of a partial agonist opioid. Increasing the dose of such a drug above its ceiling does not result in any further increase in response. This phenomenon is illustrated in Fig. 10.1.6.4 in which C is a partial agonist. C is more potent than B (in the lower part of the curve it will produce the same response at a lower dose), but is less effective than both A and B because of its ceiling effect.

Table 10.1.6.7 Classification of opioid analgesics into agonist, agonist–antagonist, and antagonist classes.

Agonists
- Morphine
- Codeine
- Oxycodone
- Dihydrocodeine
- Oxymorphone
- Pethidine
- Levorphanol
- Hydromorphone
- Methadone
- Fentanyl
- Dextropropoxyphene
- Diamorphine (heroin)
- Tramadol
- Phenazocine
- Dextromoramide
- Dipipanone

Partial agonists
- Buprenorphine

Agonist–antagonists
- Pentazocine
- Butorphanol
- Nalbuphine
- Dezocine
- Meptazinol

Antagonists
- Naloxone
- Naltrexone

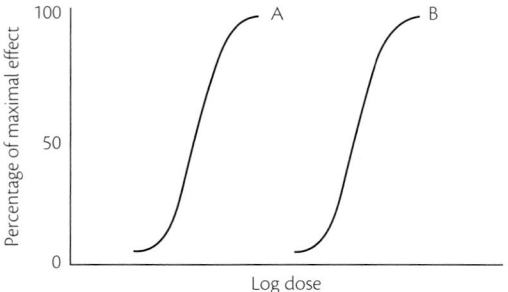

Figure 10.1.6.3 Dose–response curves for two full opioid agonists (A and B) similar in efficacy but different in potency (A is more potent than B).

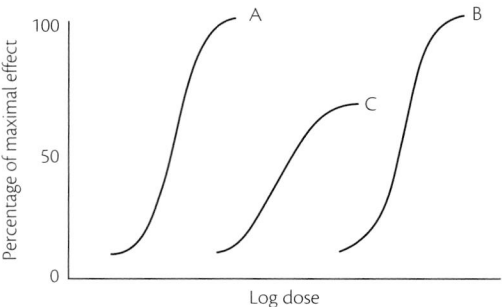

Figure 10.1.6.4 Dose–response curves for two full opioid agonists (A and B) and a partial opioid agonist C.

When a partial agonist is administered together with an agonist, displacement of the agonist can cause a net reduction in pharmacological action, which may be sufficient to generate an acute withdrawal syndrome. Whilst this is a theoretical possibility with morphine and buprenorphine, no such interaction has been reported. Similarly, it has been suggested that the effects of morphine may be blocked in a patient switched from buprenorphine, because of the prolonged action of buprenorphine and the assumption that it will 'antagonize' the effect of morphine. This has been one of the reasons why buprenorphine has not been used in cancer pain management. However, the recent development of a transdermal formulation of buprenorphine may encourage its use in chronic cancer pain (and chronic non-cancer pain). An analgesic ceiling with buprenorphine is only reached at doses of 8–16 mg or more in 24 h[32]. When used in usual recommended doses (e.g. two patches of 70 μg/h of transdermal buprenorphine, equivalent to 3–4 mg/24 h) buprenorphine can be considered a full mu agonist, since at these doses, its effect will lie on the linear part of the dose–response curve.

Relative potency and equianalgesic doses

Relative potency is the ratio of the doses of two analgesics required to produce the same analgesic effect. By convention, the relative potency of each of the commonly used opioids is based upon a comparison with 10 mg of parenteral morphine. Data from single- and repeated-dose studies in patients with acute or chronic pain have been used to develop an equianalgesic dose table (Table 10.1.6.8) that provides guidelines for dose selection when the drug or route of administration is changed. The information contained in the equianalgesic dose table does not represent standard doses, nor is it intended as an absolute guideline for dose selection. Many variables may influence the appropriate dose for an individual patient, including intensity of pain, prior opioid exposure in terms of drug, duration, and dose (and the degree of cross-tolerance that this confers), age, route of administration, level of consciousness, metabolic abnormalities (see following paragraphs), and genetic polymorphism in the expression of relevant enzymes or receptors. In particular, care should be exercised when switching from one opioid to another as part of the management of opioid toxicity. In this situation, highly conservative conversions should be used.

Dose–response relationship

As noted earlier, there is no ceiling to the analgesic effects of full agonist opioids. As the dose is raised, analgesic effects increase as a log linear function. In practice, the appearance of adverse effects, including confusion, sedation, nausea, vomiting, or respiratory depression, imposes a limit on the useful dose of an opioid agonist. Thus the efficacy of any particular drug in an individual patient will be determined by the degree of analgesia produced following dose escalation to intolerable and unmanageable side effects.

Section II: clinical aspects of opioid analgesia

The role of opioids in the management of cancer pain

Analgesic therapy with opioids, non-opioids, and adjuvant analgesics is developed for the individual patient through a process of continuous evaluation so that a favourable balance between pain relief and adverse pharmacological effects is maintained.

The analgesic ladder

An expert committee convened by the Cancer and Palliative Care Unit of the World Health Organization (WHO) proposed a structured approach to drug selection for cancer pain, which has become known as the 'WHO analgesic ladder'[2,33]. When combined with appropriate dosing guidelines, this approach is capable of providing adequate relief to 70–90 per cent of patients[63–69]. Emphasizing that the intensity of pain, rather than its specific aetiology, should be the prime consideration in analgesic selection; the approach advocates three basic steps (Fig. 10.1.6.5). This strategy should be integrated with non-pharmacological methods of cancer pain control including, radiotherapy, chemotherapy, hormone therapy, surgery, anaesthetic interventions, physiotherapy and psychological/cognitive approaches.

- Patients with mild cancer-related pain should be treated with a non-opioid analgesic, which should be combined with adjuvant drugs if a specific indication for these exists. For example, a patient with mild to moderate arm pain caused by radiation-induced brachial plexopathy may benefit when a tricyclic antidepressant is added to paracetamol (acetaminophen)[70,71].

- Patients who are relatively non-tolerant and present with moderate pain, or who fail to achieve adequate relief after a trial of a non-opioid analgesic, should be treated with an opioid conventionally used for mild to moderate pain (formerly known as a 'weak' opioid). This treatment is typically accomplished using a combination product containing a non-opioid (e.g. aspirin or paracetamol) and an opioid (such as codeine, oxycodone, or propoxyphene). This combination can also be co-administered with an adjuvant analgesic. The doses of these combination products can be increased until the maximum dose of the

Table 10.1.6.8 Opioid analgesics (pure mu agonists) used for the treatment of chronic pain.

Morphine-like agonists	Equi-analgesic doses[a]	Half-life (h)	Peak effect (h)	Duration (h)	Toxicity	Comments	Oral bioavailability (%)	Active metabolites
Morphine	10 s.c.	2–3	0.5–1	3–6	Constipation, nausea, sedation most common; respiratory depression rare in cancer patients	Standard comparison for opioids; multiple routes available	20–30	M6G
	20–60 p.o.[b]	2–3	1.5–2	4–7				
Sustained-release morphine	20–60 p.o.[b]	2–3	3–4	8–12		Twice daily administration	20–30	M6G
Sustained-release morphine	20–60 p.o.[b]	2–3	4–6	24		Once-a-day morphine approved in some countries	20–30	M6G
Hydromorphone	1.5 s.c.	2–3	0.5–1	3–4	Same as morphine	Used for multiple routes	35–80	No
	7.5 p.o.	2–3	1–2	3–4				
Oxycodone	20–30	2–3	1	3–6	Same as morphine	Combined with aspirin or paracetamol (acetaminophen), for moderate pain in USA; available orally without non-opioid for severe pain	60–90	Oxymorphone
Sustained-release oxycodone	20–30	2–3	3–4	8–12				Oxymorphone
Oxymorphone	1 s.c.	—	0.5–1	3–6	Same as morphine	No oral formulation		Glucuronides
	10 p.r.	—	1.5–3	4–6				
Pethidine (meperidine)	75 s.c.	2–3	0.5–1	3–4	Same as morphine + CNS excitation; contraindicated in those on MAO inhibitors	Not used for cancer pain due to toxicity in higher doses and short half-life	30–60	Norpethidine
Diamorphine	5 s.c.	0.5	0.5–1	4–5	Same as morphine	Analgesic action due to metabolites, predominantly morphine; only available in some countries		Morphine
Levorphanol	2 s.c.	12–16	0.5–1	4–6	Same as morphine	With long half-life, accumulation occurs after beginning or increasing dose		No
	4 p.o.							
Methadone[c]	10 s.c.	12–>150	0.5–1.5	4–8	Same as morphine	Risk of delayed toxicity due to accumulation; useful to start dosing on p.r.n. schedule	60–90	No
	20 p.o.(see text)							
Codeine	130 s.c.	2–3	1.5–2	3–6	Same as morphine	Usually combined with non-opioid	60–90	Morphine
	200 p.o.							
Propoxyphene HCl (dextropropoxyphene)	—	12	1.5–2	3–6	Same as morphine plus seizures with overdose	Toxic metabolite accumulates but not significant at doses used clinically; usually combined with non-opioid	40	Norpropoxyphene

(continued)

Table 10.1.6.8 (Continued) Opioid analgesics (pure mu agonists) used for the treatment of chronic pain.

Morphine-like agonists	Equi-analgesic doses[a]	Half-life (h)	Peak effect (h)	Duration (h)	Toxicity	Comments	Oral bioavailability (%)	Active metabolites
Propoxyphene napsylate (dextropropoxyphene)	—	12	1.5–2	3–6	Same as hydrochloride	Same as hydrochloride	40	Norpropoxyphene
Hydrocodone	—	2–4	0.5–1	3–4	Same as morphine	Only available combined with paracetamol; only available in some countries		Hydromorphone
Dihydrocodeine	—	2–4	0.5–1	3–4	Same as morphine	Only available combined with aspirin or paracetamol in some countries	20	Morphine
Fentanyl	—	3–12	—	—	Same as morphine	Can be administered as a continuous i.v. or s.c. infusion; based on clinical experience, 100 g/h is roughly equianalgesic to morphine 4 mg/h i.v.	25/buccal <2/oral	No
Fentanyl transdermal system	—	13–22	—	48–72	Same as morphine	Based on clinical experience 100 g/h is roughly equianalgesic to morphine 4 mg/h; recent study indicates a ratio of oral morphine: transdermal fentanyl of 100:1	90/transdermal	No
Effervescent fentanyl tablets	—				Same as morphine	May be twice as potent as oral transmucosal fentanyl lozenge	48	No

[a] Dose that provides analgesia equivalent to 10 mg i.m. morphine. These ratios are useful guidelines when switching drugs or routes of administration.

[b] Extensive survey data suggest that the relative potency of i.m.;p.o. or s.c.;p.o., morphine of 16 changes to 1:2–3 with chronic dosing.

[c] When switching from another opioid to methadone, the potency of methadone is much greater than indicated in this table.

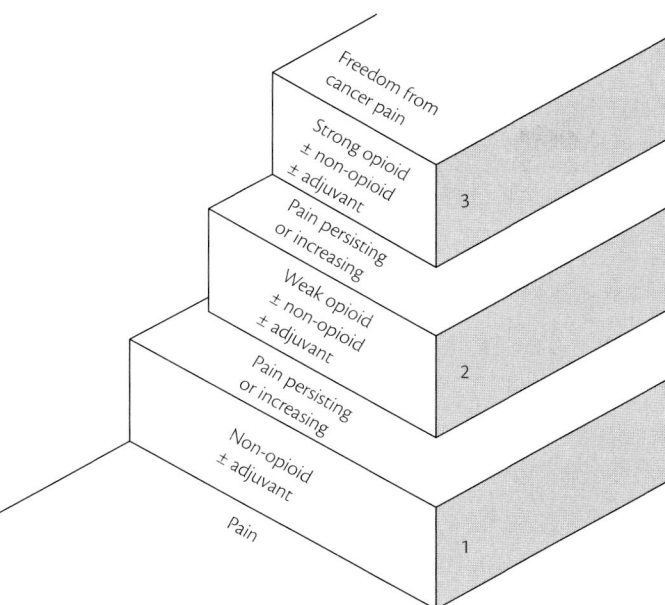

Figure 10.1.6.5 The WHO three-step analgesic ladder. (Reproduced with permission from WHO.)

non-opioid analgesic is attained (e.g. 4000–6000 mg paracetamol); beyond this dose, the opioid contained in the combination product could be increased as a single agent, or the patient could be switched to an opioid conventionally used in step 3.

♦ Patients who present with severe pain, or who fail to achieve adequate relief following appropriate administration of drugs on the second step of the analgesic ladder, should receive an opioid conventionally used for moderate to severe pain (formerly known as a 'strong' opioid). This group includes morphine, diamorphine, fentanyl, oxycodone, phenazocine, hydromorphone, methadone, levorphanol, and oxymorphone. These drugs may also be combined with a non-opioid analgesic or an adjuvant drug. Clearly, the boundary between opioids used in the second and third steps of the analgesic ladder is somewhat artificial since low doses of morphine or other opioids for severe pain can be less effective than high doses of codeine or propoxyphene.

According to these guidelines, a trial of opioid therapy should be given to all patients with pain of moderate or greater severity.

The evidence of the long-term efficacy of this approach and the evidence base underlying its recommendations has been the subject of criticism[34]. Several other developments have also contributed to a reevaluation of the WHO ladder. The introduction of low-dose formulations of opioid agonists traditionally used for severe pain, and of other agents such as tramadol has widened the repertoire of agents suitable for the management of moderate pain (step 2). Indeed, many authorities now advocate the use of the same opioid for all pains of moderate or greater intensity[73–76].

Despite these reservations, the guiding principle that analgesic selection should be primarily determined by the severity of the pain remains sound, and continues to be endorsed widely [61,73,77].

Opioid analgesics

The division of opioid agonists into 'weak' or 'strong' opioids, which was incorporated into the original analgesic ladder proposed by the WHO, was not based on fundamental differences in their pharmacology, but rather reflected the customary manner in which these drugs were used. In this chapter we will refer to opioids for mild to moderate pain and opioids for moderate to severe pain rather than 'weak' or 'strong' opioids. This terminology is now incorporated into the current version of the WHO analgesic ladder.

Opioids for mild to moderate pain
Codeine

Codeine (methylmorphine) is a naturally occurring opium alkaloid used as an analgesic, antitussive, and antidiarrhoeal agent (Fig. 10.1.6.6). Codeine is much less potent than morphine and produces its analgesic effects in part by binding to mu opioid receptors, but with low affinity and, in part, through biotransformation to morphine by cytochrome P-450 CYP2D6 (sparteine oxygenase), which exhibits genetic polymorphism. Approximately 7 per cent of Caucasians lack CYP2D6 activity (poor metabolizers) due to inheritance of two non-functional alleles and, in these individuals, codeine has a diminished analgesic effect[78,79].

Codeine phosphate is absorbed well from the gastrointestinal tract, but oral bioavailability varies considerably between individuals (from 12 to 84 per cent in one study[35]. The main metabolite is codeine-6-glucuronide, with much smaller amounts of norcodeine, morphine, and morphine 3- and 6-glucuronides also being produced[36]. The usual oral dose of codeine is 30–60 mg and its duration of action is 4–6 h.

Codeine is not generally given as a single agent when used orally as an analgesic, but is usually combined with a non-opioid and recent systematic reviews confirm that the combination of codeine and paracetamol is more effective than paracetamol alone[82,83]. A sustained-release formulation of codeine is available in some countries. When changing from regular administration of a codeine/non-opioid combination to morphine, patients receiving a total daily dose of 240–360 mg codeine are usually started on 60 mg morphine daily.

Dihydrocodeine

Dihydrocodeine is a semi-synthetic analogue of codeine that is used as an analgesic, antitussive, and antidiarrhoeal agent. When administered by mouth, dihydrocodeine is equianalgesic to codeine. However, when administered parenterally, it is approximately twice

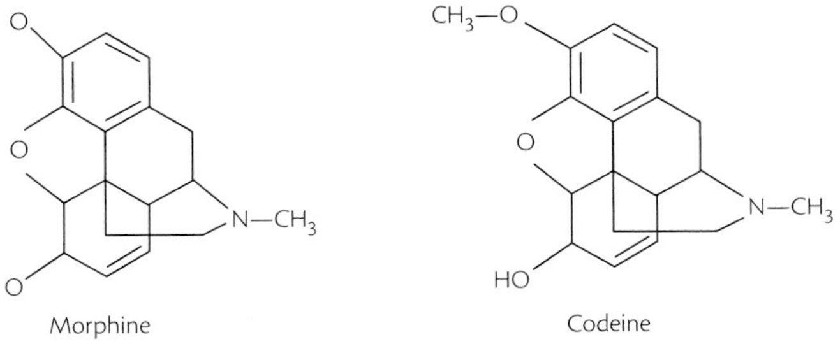

Morphine

Codeine

Figure 10.1.6.6 The chemical structures of morphine and codeine.

as potent as codeine. This may be explained by the consistently poorer bioavailability of dihydrocodeine (20 per cent), which probably results from hepatic pre-systemic metabolism[37].

The usual starting dose is 30 mg every 4–6 h (by mouth), and this may be increased to 60mg. However, dihydrocodeine appears to have a narrower therapeutic index than codeine, with a high incidence of adverse effects at the 60-mg dose. A controlled-release formulation of dihydrocodeine is available in several countries.

There have been a number of reports of severe toxicity associated with dihydrocodeine in patients with impaired renal function[85,86]. The mechanism is not clear because of the limited data available on the pharmacokinetics of this drug, although it seems most likely that the cause is accumulation of active glucuronide metabolites, as occurs with morphine.

There is confusion about the relative analgesic potency of dihydrocodeine. It seems reasonable to assume that oral dihydrocodeine is roughly equipotent to oral codeine, and to use a similar conversion ratio when changing to morphine.

Dextropropoxyphene

Propoxyphene is a synthetic derivative of methadone, and its dextrorotatory stereoisomer dextropropoxyphene is responsible for its analgesic activity. Dextropropoxyphene is a mu agonist with low receptor affinity similar to that of codeine. It is readily absorbed from the gastrointestinal tract with peak serum levels about 2 h after administration. The mean elimination half-life is about 12 h, with steady state levels being reached after 3–4 days of regular administration every 6–8 h. The half-life may be very long (over 50 h) in elderly patients[38].

Dextropropoxyphene undergoes extensive first-pass metabolism. Its principal metabolite is norpropoxyphene, which is active but penetrates the brain to a much lesser extent and has much weaker opioid effects. Norpropoxyphene has a longer half-life (about 23 h) than dextropropoxyphene itself and accumulates in plasma[39]. Norpropoxyphene accumulation is associated with excitatory effects, including tremulousness and seizures.

The analgesic efficacy and relative potency of dextropropoxyphene have been questioned. This is in part because single-dose studies comparing aspirin, paracetamol, and non-steroidal anti-inflammatory drugs (NSAIDs), including ibuprofen 400 mg, mefenamic acid 250 mg, and fenoprofen 50 mg, have shown dextropropoxyphene to be a less effective analgesic[40]. A more recent systematic review found that paracetamol alone is as effective as the combination of paracetamol with dextropropoxyphene, though the studies included were again all single-dose studies[41]. Single-dose studies may be misleading, as is the case with single-dose studies of oral morphine.

The extensive first-pass metabolism of dextropropoxyphene is dose-dependent such that the systemic availability of the drug increases with increasing oral doses[42]. Thus, with regular administration, there is enhanced bioavailability and some degree of accumulation because of the long elimination half-lives of the parent drug and its main metabolite. Both dextropropoxyphene and norpropoxyphene reach plasma concentrations in the steady state, which are five to seven times greater than those found after the first dose. There is, therefore, a pharmacokinetic basis for believing that repeated doses of dextropropoxyphene are likely to be more effective than single doses. The usual starting dose of morphine for patients receiving dextropropoxyphene–paracetamol combinations every 4–6 h (representing 260–390 mg of dextropropoxyphene daily) is 60 mg/day.

For a long time, a combination of dextropropoxyphene and paracetamol was the most commonly prescribed analgesic in the United Kingdom and some Scandinavian countries, but it received much adverse publicity because of its lethal effects in overdose and fears about its addiction potential. Part of this concern was stimulated by its very widespread use. In addition to usual opioid adverse effects, propoxyphene may rarely induce a hepatotoxic reaction[43], cardiac conduction disorder[44], and potentially dangerous drug interactions have been reported when propoxyphene has been administered along with carbamazepine[45], warfarin[46], or alcohol[47]. Currently, however, there is insufficient evidence to conclude that dextropropoxyphene is inherently more toxic than codeine, or other opioids of similar efficacy, nor is there evidence that one is more effective than another. At present, in the United Kingdom, dextropropoxyphene in combination with paracetamol has been removed from the general prescribing list because of an association with fatal drug overdose; however, dextropropoxyphene remains available in several countries.

Oxycodone

Oxycodone is a semi-synthetic congener of morphine, which has been on the market for 80 years but until relatively recently was only available in formulations which effectively circumscribed its use. In the United States of America, it has been prescribed in low-dose combination products with a non-opioid for oral administration (usually 5 mg of oxycodone with either aspirin or paracetamol) and has traditionally been used as a step 2 analgesic. Formerly in the United Kingdom and some other countries, only a rectal suppository and no oral formulations existed. Oxycodone has been more widely used by mouth as a first line step 3 opioid in Scandinavia where it has also been widely used as a postoperative opioid[48]. Recently, oxycodone has been produced as a single agent in new oral formulations, both normal release and sustained release, which has substantially improved the convenience of administration. In many countries, sustained release oxycodone is available in 5-, 10-, 20-, 40-, and 80-mg formulations with a corresponding range of normal release formulations. Oxycodone is increasingly used as a step-3 opioid, though the low-dose formulations allow its use at step 2 also. Oxycodone probably provides the best example of the overlap in efficacy between opioids at steps 2 and 3; however, other opioids now also fulfil this role (see following paragraphs).

Tramadol

Tramadol is a centrally acting analgesic that possesses opioid agonist properties and may also activate monoaminergic spinal inhibition of pain[49]. It has modest affinity with mu opioid receptors, with weak affinity to delta and kappa receptors, and its analgesic effect is reversed by naloxone. Unlike other opioids, it also inhibits the uptake of noradrenaline and serotonin, and in an animal model systemically administered yohimbine or ritanserin blocks tramadol-induced analgesia, suggesting that this effect contributes significantly to the drug's analgesic action[49].

Tramadol can be administered orally, rectally, intravenously, subcutaneously, or intramuscularly. In many countries, it is available in both normal- and sustained-release formulations. Parenterally, 50–150 mg of tramadol is equianalgesic to 5–15 mg morphine[50]. There are insufficient data for a reliable assessment of its oral-to-parenteral relative analgesic potency and estimates range from 1:4 to 1:10[103,104].

Recent studies have demonstrated the efficacy of oral tramadol in the management of chronic cancer pain of moderate severity[103–105]. Few patients with severe pain are managed adequately by tramadol[104,106]. Tramadol has a similar side effect profile to morphine, but may cause less constipation and respiratory depression at equianalgesic doses.

The second step of the analgesic ladder

As previously described, by convention, formulations combining aspirin or paracetamol with a low dose of codeine, oxycodone, or propoxyphene have been recommended for pain of moderate intensity (step 2 of the analgesic ladder). This recommendation was pragmatic rather than evidence based. It reflected the concern that in many parts of the world it would be unacceptable to use morphine or other potent opioids for moderate pain.

Some combination preparations used doses of opioid that were too low (e.g. codeine 8 or 16 mg) but, even in full doses, these drugs have limited efficacy. Indeed, in the validation studies of the WHO ladder few patients using these agents maintained adequate relief for more than a few weeks[51]. Additionally, these formulations all have a short duration of effect and require patients to use repeated doses every 3–4 h to achieve continuous analgesia in the setting of chronic pain.

The most frequently employed step 2 analgesics in cancer pain are combination preparations containing 300–500 mg paracetamol with 30 mg codeine, 32.5 mg dextropropoxyphene, or 5 mg oxycodone. The combination of dextropropoxyphene with paracetamol has been withdrawn in the United Kingdom and other parts of the world because of its lethal effects in overdose, and is much less used generally. Codeine plus paracetamol is now by far the most frequent combination at step 2.

Recent studies comparing single doses of opioid/non-opioid combinations with various NSAIDs in postoperative pain have shown advantages for the latter in terms of greater efficacy and less adverse effects[107–109]. Chronic use of NSAIDs may negate any advantage in terms of unwanted effects, although at present there are no comparative data for chronic cancer pain. NSAIDs are increasingly employed as step 2 analgesics.

Given the limitations of the conventional approach, many clinicians now use a variety of single agent opioid agonists, some previously designated as 'step 3' opioids, in an appropriate dose, for moderate pain. Over recent years, sustained-release formulations of oxycodone, tramadol, and morphine in dose formulations appropriate for pain of moderate severity, along with low-dose transdermal fentanyl, have become widely available and are now often used in this setting. This practice is supported by evidence of efficacy[99,105,110].

The partial agonist opioid buprenorphine also may be used in this setting since it has recently become available in a transdermal formulation. A low-dose formulation of transdermal fentanyl is also under development and is designed for use in patients who may be opioid naïve. There are potential dangers in the earlier use of the most potent opioids, particularly when administered in long-acting formulations and more clinical trial data are required to clarify some of the issues surrounding these trends in opioid prescriptions.

Opioids for moderate to severe pain
Morphine

Morphine is a potent mu-agonist drug that was first introduced into clinical use almost 200 years ago. It is the main naturally occurring alkaloid of opium derived from the poppy *Papaver somniferum* and is available for therapeutic use as the sulphate, hydrochloride, and tartrate. Recent evidence suggests that biosynthetic pathways for morphine exist in animal and human tissues such as liver, blood, and brain[52]. Its chemical structure is shown in Fig. 10.1.6.6. The WHO has placed oral morphine on the Essential Drug List, and preparations are available for oral, rectal, parenteral, and intraspinal administration.

Bioavailability

Morphine is available in four oral formulations: an elixir, a normal-release tablet, a modified-release tablet or capsule (of which there are now several preparations using different sustained-release mechanisms), and sustained-release suspensions. Absorption of morphine after oral administration occurs predominantly in the alkaline medium of the upper small bowel (morphine is a weak base) and is more or less complete. After oral administration, extensive pre-systemic elimination of the drug occurs predominantly in the liver. In healthy volunteers and cancer patients, the average bioavailability for oral morphine is 20–30 per cent[112–114]. Like all other pharmacokinetic parameters, bioavailability demonstrates marked inter-individual variability. In patients with normal renal function, the plasma half-life (2–3 h) is somewhat shorter than the duration of analgesia (4–6 h). The pharmacokinetics remain linear with repetitive administration, and there does not appear to be autoinduction of biotransformation even following large chronic doses[53]. Rectal morphine bio-availability is similar to the oral route.

Morphine is relatively hydrophilic and, when administered epidurally or intrathecally, it is not rapidly absorbed into the systemic circulation. This results in a long half-life in cerebrospinal fluid (90–120 min) and extensive rostral redistribution[54].

Morphine metabolism

About 90 per cent of morphine is converted into metabolites (Fig. 10.1.6.7), principally, the glucuronide conjugates morphine-3-glucuronide (M3G) and morphine-6-glucuronide (M6G); minor metabolites include codeine, normorphine, and morphine ethereal sulphate. The liver appears to be the predominant site of metabolism in humans, although, in animal models, extrahepatic metabolism has been demonstrated in the small bowel and the proximal renal tubule of rodents. These sites may become important where liver function is impaired. M3G is the major metabolite and in recent years there has been some controversy about its possible role as an opioid antagonist or in mediating some of the adverse effects of morphine.

Morphine-6-glucuronide

M6G binds to opioid receptors[55] and produces potent opioid effects in animals[117–119] and humans[117,120–122]. M6G excretion by the kidney is directly related to creatinine clearance[56]; its elimination half-life is 2–3 h in patients with normal renal function (similar to that of morphine) but becomes progressively longer with deteriorating function, resulting in significant accumulation[56]. In patients with impaired renal function, M6G may accumulate in blood and cerebrospinal fluid[57], and high concentrations of this metabolite have been associated with toxicity[120,125]. Although further studies are needed to clarify the clinical importance of M6G and other metabolites, the data available are sufficient to recommend caution when administering morphine to patients with renal impairment. Patients who are receiving regular morphine and

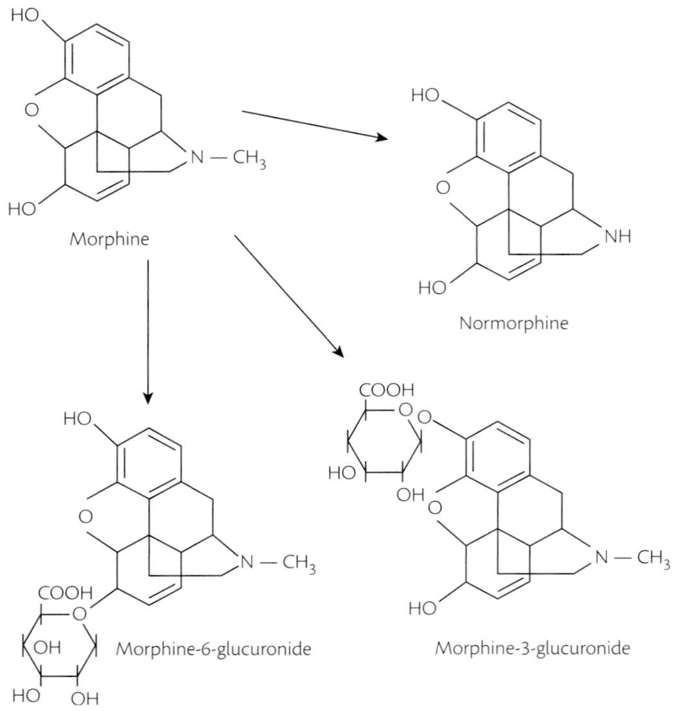

Figure 10.1.6.7 The metabolites of morphine.

develop acute renal failure in a previously stable situation (e.g. a rapidly developing obstructive uropathy in a patient with pelvic malignancy) may develop a sudden onset of signs and symptoms of opioid toxicity, necessitating temporary withdrawal of the morphine and subsequent dose reduction, and/or less frequent administration.

M6G is thought to be a potent analgesic and studies in acute postoperative pain are currently ongoing. It is not yet clear whether M6G will have fewer side effects than morphine, though it has been suggested that M6G causes less respiratory depression[126–128].

Morphine-3-glucuronide

For many years, it has been assumed that M3G is inert as is the case with most glucuronide metabolites[58]. Recent behavioural studies in rodents, however, suggested that M3G produces a functional antagonism of the analgesic effects of morphine and its active metabolite M6G[130,131]. There is also some evidence in animal models that M3G may be responsible for the CNS excitatory adverse effects seen with morphine, such as myoclonus[58,132].

It is now clear that M3G does not bind to opioid receptors. Data from electrophysiological animal models indicate no evidence of an antagonistic effect of M3G[59], and recent studies in human volunteers indicate that M3G appears to be devoid of significant activity[127,134]. In particular, there is no evidence of functional antagonism of morphine or M6G in humans and, overall, it seems that M3G plays no significant role in the pharmacodynamics of morphine.

Oral-to-parenteral relative potency

Single-dose studies of morphine in postoperative cancer patients demonstrated an oral-to-intramuscular potency ratio of 1:6[60]. However, empirical clinical practice using chronically administered oral morphine in cancer patients has generated a different ratio of 1:3 or 1:2[136,137]. The reason for the discrepancy between relative potency estimates derived from single-dose versus chronic dosing

studies is probably associated with both methodology[61] and the pharmacokinetics and pharmacodynamics of M6G[62]. It is possible that M6G accumulation relative to morphine may be greater with oral than with parenteral administration; this would lead to an increase in the relative potency of the orally administered drug when given on a chronic basis.

The important principle for clinical practice is that there is a difference in relative analgesic potency when the route of administration is changed, and that adjustment of dose is necessary in order to achieve an equivalent effect and to avoid either underdosing or toxicity. The usual practice when converting from oral morphine to subcutaneous morphine (or diamorphine) is to divide the oral dose by two or three[76].

Parenteral morphine

The inorganic salts of morphine (morphine sulphate and morphine hydrochloride) have limited solubility. Standard formulations are available up to 20 mg/ml, and morphine can be constituted from lyophilized power up to 50 mg/ml. Morphine tartrate is substantially more soluble and, in some countries, is formulated in a concentration of 80 mg/ml.

Sustained-release morphine preparations

The development of modified-release morphine preparations has had a major impact on clinical practice. These preparations, which are usually administered on a 12h schedule, provide a much more convenient means of administering oral morphine[63]. Several preparations are available worldwide with a range of dose formulations (10, 15, 30, 60, 100, and 200 mg, depending on the country), allowing considerable flexibility in their use. Some preparations allow once-daily administration and sustained-release suspensions are also available[64].

In contrast with morphine solution or normal-release tablets, where peak plasma concentrations are achieved within the first hour, followed by a rapid decline and an elimination half-life of 2–4 h, sustained-release morphine typically achieves peak plasma concentrations 3–6 h after administration, the peak is attenuated, and plasma concentrations are sustained over a 12 or 24h period[141–143]. The type and incidence of adverse effects with sustained-release morphine and normal-release oral morphine appear to be similar with the currently available formulations.

Although some clinicians advocate the use of sustained-release morphine when initiating morphine therapy in cancer patients, a normal-release preparation is generally recommended in the dose titration period[65]. Initial dose titration using sustained-release morphine is difficult because of the delay in achieving peak plasma concentrations, the attenuation of peak concentrations, and the long duration of action. In this situation, dose finding is performed more efficiently with a short-acting morphine preparation. Once the effective dose is identified using a normal-release formulation, this may be changed to a sustained-release preparation using a milligram-to-milligram conversion. For the same reasons, sustained-release morphine is not appropriate for the treatment of acute pain or 'breakthrough' pain (BTP). A normal-release morphine preparation should be provided to patients stabilized on sustained-release morphine to be used 'as required' for BTP.

Diamorphine (heroin)

Diamorphine (diacetylmorphine) is a semi-synthetic analogue of morphine and has a long tradition of use for cancer pain in the

United Kingdom. It is only available for legal medicinal use in the United Kingdom and Canada.

Following oral administration of diamorphine, the drug is rapidly deacetylated so that only morphine can be measured in the patient's blood. The use of oral diamorphine is an inefficient way of delivering morphine to the systemic circulation. There is no good basis to believe that there is any difference between these two drugs when given by mouth. Sublingual administration of diamorphine has been advocated by some but, as discussed in the following paragraphs, this route is not appropriate for either morphine or diamorphine because of poor absorption.

It has been thought that diamorphine does not itself bind to the mu opioid receptor but must be biotransformed to 6-acetylmorphine and morphine to produce its analgesic effect[66]. However, recent studies with mor-knockout mice seem to indicate that it does not produce its effects through mu receptor binding and may have effects at other receptors[67]. This may explain some of the pharmacodynamic differences between morphine and diamorphine when given parenterally.

Since diamorphine is more soluble and lipophilic than morphine, it does have some advantages for parenteral administration. When administered by subcutaneous or intramuscular injection, diamorphine is approximately twice as potent as morphine. There are also differences between diamorphine and morphine administered by intravenous injection: diamorphine has a marginally quicker onset of action, produces greater sedation, and possibly less vomiting[68]. This may be explained by different receptor binding. The greater solubility of diamorphine (shared also with hydromorphone and morphine tartrate) is of particular advantage for patients who require large doses of subcutaneous opioids.

Methadone

Methadone is a synthetic opioid with an oral-to-parenteral potency ratio of 1:2 and an oral bioavailability greater than 85 per cent. In single-dose studies, methadone is only marginally more potent than morphine; however, with repeated administration it is several times more potent. Methadone has a very long plasma half-life, averaging approximately 24h (with a range from 12 to over 150 h[69,70]. Whereas most patients can be well controlled on 8- to 12h dosing, some patients require dosing at a 4 to 8h interval to maintain analgesic effects[71]. Methadone may be a useful alternative to morphine, but its safe administration requires knowledge of its pharmacology and experience of its use.

After treatment is initiated or the dose is increased, plasma concentration rises over a prolonged period, and this may be associated with a delayed onset of side effects. Consequently, patients must be followed closely until there is reasonable certainty that a steady-state plasma concentration has been approached (approximately 1 week but may take up to 4 weeks). Serious adverse effects can be avoided if the initial period of dosing is accomplished with 'as needed' administration[72]. When steady state has been achieved, scheduled dose frequency should be determined by the duration of analgesia following each dose[73].

Oral and parenteral preparations of methadone are available. Subcutaneous infusion is possible[74] but caution is required since local skin toxicity may be a problem[75].

The equianalgesic dose ratio of morphine to methadone has been a matter of confusion and controversy. Data from cross-over studies with morphine and methadone and hydromorphone and methadone indicate that methadone is much more potent than previously described in the literature, and that the ratio correlates with the total opioid dose administered before switching to methadone[76]. Among patients receiving oral equivalent doses of morphine less than 90 mg/daily, the ratio is 4:1, a ratio of 8:1 for patients receiving 90–300 mg/day and for patients receiving more than 300mg morphine/day, a ratio of 12:1 should be used[76].

Pethidine (meperidine)

Pethidine is a synthetic opioid with agonist effects similar to those of morphine but a profile of potential adverse effects that limits its utility as an analgesic for chronic cancer pain. Intramuscular pethidine 75 mg is equivalent to 10 mg of intramuscular morphine. Pethidine has an oral bioavailability of 40–60 per cent, and its oral-to-parenteral potency ratio is 1:4. It is more lipophilic than morphine, and produces a faster onset and shorter duration of analgesia of 2–3 h.

Pethidine is N-demethylated to norpethidine, which is an active metabolite that is twice as potent as a convulsant and half as potent as an analgesic compared with its parent compound. Accumulation of norpethidine after repetitive dosing of pethidine can result in CNS excitability characterized by subtle mood effects, tremors, multifocal myoclonus, and occasionally, seizures[77,78]. Naloxone does not reverse pethidine-induced seizures, and it is possible that its administration to patients receiving pethidine chronically could precipitate seizures by blocking the depressant action of pethidine and allowing the convulsant activity of norpethidine to become manifest[79]. If naloxone is necessary in this situation, it should be diluted and slowly titrated while appropriate seizure precautions are taken. Selective toxicity of pethidine can also occur following administration to patients receiving monoamine oxidase inhibitors. This combination may produce a syndrome characterized by hyperpyrexia, muscle rigidity, and seizures which may occasionally be fatal[80]. The pathophysiology of this syndrome is related to excess availability of serotonin at the 5HT1A-receptor in the CNS.

Although accumulation of norpethidine is most likely to affect patients with overt renal disease, toxicity is sometimes observed in patients with normal renal function. These potential adverse effects and its short duration of action contraindicate pethidine for the management of chronic cancer pain. Given the availability of alternative drugs that lack these toxicities, its use in acute pain management is also not recommended[81].

Hydromorphone

Hydromorphone is another morphine congener. It is about five times more potent than morphine and can be administered by the oral, rectal, parenteral, and intraspinal routes. Its oral bioavailability varies from 35 to 80 per cent[82]. Its half-life is 1.5–3 h and it has a short duration of action. Although it is largely excreted unchanged by the kidney, it is partially metabolized in the liver to a 3-glucuronide, which is excreted by the kidneys[82,83].

Its solubility, the availability of a high-concentration preparation (10 mg/ml), and high bioavailability by the subcutaneous route (78 per cent) make it particularly suitable for subcutaneous infusion[84]. In the United States of America, it is routinely available in oral, rectal, and injectable formulations, and a sustained-release oral formulation[85]. For patients who require very high opioid doses via the subcutaneous route, hydromorphone can be constituted in concentrations of up to 50 mg/ml from lyophilized powder. It has also been administered via the epidural and intrathecal routes to manage acute and chronic pain. In fact, for newer intrathecal programmable pump devices, hydromorphone rather than morphine should be used because of device interactions with the latter. Hydromorphone is hydrophilic and, when administered via the epidural route, its pharmacokinetic profile, including its long half-life and extensive rostral distribution in cerebrospinal fluid, is similar to that of morphine[86].

The equianalgesic ratio of parenteral morphine to hydromorphone has been a matter of controversy. There is evidence that potency ratios for hydromorphone are not bidirectional. An equianalgesic ratio of 7:1 is quoted when switching from morphine to hydromorphone but ratios of 4:1–8:1 are reported when switching in the other direction. The reported oral equianalgesic ratio for morphine to hydromorphone is 7.5:1, and the parenteral analgesic ratio is 7:1; so when converting from oral to subcutaneous hydromorphone, the dose should be divided by two, presuming an oral-to-parenteral potency ratio for morphine of 1:2[87]. Although some studies suggest a more favourable side effect profile than morphine, there is conflicting evidence. It is highly likely as with all opioids that it will depend on the individual patient. A systematic review of hydromorphone in cancer pain did not find any significant differences between hydromorphone and oxycodone for acute and chronic pain[88]. A transdermal formulation of hydromorphone is in development.

Levorphanol

Levorphanol is a morphine congener with a long half-life (12–16 h)[89]. It shares a number of pharmacological properties with methadone. It is five times more potent than morphine and has an oral-to-parenteral potency ratio of 1:2[90]. Like methadone, the discrepancy between plasma half-life (12–16 h) and duration of analgesia (4–6 h) may predispose to drug accumulation following the initiation of therapy or dose escalation. Although dose titration needs to be done carefully in the opioid-Naïve patient, problems with drug accumulation appear to be less than those produced by methadone.

In the United States of America, levorphanol is generally used as a second-line agent in patients with chronic pain who cannot tolerate morphine. The possibility that this drug may be particularly useful in morphine-tolerant patients has been proposed on the basis of its additional affinity for kappa and delta receptors that are presumably not involved in morphine analgesia[91]. It seems also to have NMDA antagonist activity. It is no longer available in the United Kingdom or Canada.

Oxycodone

As previously described, oxycodone is a synthetic morphine congener that has a high oral bioavailability (60–90 per cent) and an analgesic potency 30–50 per cent greater than morphine[92,93]. Since the development of sustained-release formulations in doses suitable for severe pain, it is now widely used for this indication. The sustained release formulation is available in a wide range of dose formulations (5, 10, 20, 40, and 80 mg)[55] and has a duration of action of 8–12 h. The sustained-release formulation achieves effective therapeutic levels within an hour[94] and appears to be suitable for dose titration[95].

There has been confusion about the relative efficacy of oxycodone. It had been viewed primarily as a 'step 2' opioid because it had long been available in low dose in combination products with non-opioid analgesics. It seems clear that the relative potency of

oxycodone has been underestimated in early clinical studies in which it appeared to be less potent than morphine. As indicated earlier, more recent studies indicate that it is more potent, in a ratio of about 1.5:1[92].

There remains uncertainty also about the role of its active metabolite oxymorphone, which accounts for 10 per cent of its metabolites, in mediating the effects of oxycodone. However, current evidence suggests that the metabolites of oxycodone including oxymorphone do not contribute significantly to its pharmacological effects[96].

Oxymorphone

Oxymorphone is a lipophilic congener of morphine, formerly available as a rectal formulation. It is now available in the United States of America in oral normal and sustained-release preparations. It has a predictable dose response and linear pharmacokinetics. The injectable formulation is 10 times more potent than morphine and the oral is 3 times more potent than morphine[97]. The plasma half-life of oxymorphone is 1.2–2 h, and its duration of action is 3–5 h. It is less likely to produce histamine release than morphine[98], and may be particularly useful for patients who develop itch in response to other opioids[99]. It is not metabolized through CYP3A4 or CP2D6, which is useful for avoiding drug–drug interactions. Oxymorphone is currently not available in the United Kingdom.

Fentanyl

Fentanyl is a semi-synthetic opioid and is a highly selective mu agonist[100] that is about 80 times as potent as parenteral morphine in the non-tolerant acute pain patient. It is also extremely lipophilic and is extensively taken up into fatty tissue[101]. Its elimination half-life ranges from 3 to 12 h and is influenced by the duration of prior administration and the extent of fat sequestration. Fentanyl has been used mainly as an intravenous anaesthetic agent and continues to be used parenterally as a pre-medication for painful procedures and in continuous infusions. When used intravenously, fentanyl has a very short duration of action of 0.5–1 h. This is related to the rapid re-distribution of the drug into body tissues rather than to hepatic and renal elimination[102]. The development of a transdermal system and an oral transmucosal formulation has broadened the clinical utility of fentanyl for the management of cancer pain.

Transdermal fentanyl

The low molecular weight and high lipid solubility of fentanyl facilitate absorption through the skin and a transdermal formulation that delivers 12.5, 25, 50, 75, or 100 mcg/h is widely available[103–105]. The transdermal system consists of a drug reservoir that is separated from the skin by a copolymer membrane that controls the rate of drug delivery to the skin surface. The drug is released at a nearly constant amount per unit time along a concentration gradient from the patch to the skin. After application of the transdermal system, serum fentanyl concentration increases gradually, usually levelling off after 12–24 h, and then remaining stable for a time before declining slowly. When the patch is removed, serum concentration falls 50 per cent in approximately 17 h (range 13–22 h)[106]. The slow onset of effect after application and an equally slow decline in effect after removal are consistent with the development of a subcutaneous depot of drug that maintains the plasma concentration. There is significant inter-individual variability in fentanyl bioavailability by this route and dose titration is necessary[106]. The dosing interval for each system is usually 72 h, but inter-individual pharmacokinetic variability is large and some patients require a dosing interval of 48 h[107].

Familiarity with the kinetics of the transdermal system is essential for optimal use. Since there is a delay of 8–12 h in achieving effective analgesia after initial application of the patch, it is necessary to provide alternative analgesia for this initial period. It is prudent to apply the patch in the early hours of the day so that the patient can be observed as blood levels rise over the ensuing 12 h to minimize the risk of overdosing during sleep. Significant concentrations of fentanyl can remain in the plasma for up to 24 h after removal of the patch because of delayed release from tissue and subcutaneous depots. Neither age nor patch location appears to affect fentanyl absorption from the transdermal system[105]. There is a potential for temperature-dependent increases in fentanyl release from the system associated with increased skin permeability in patients with fever, who should be monitored for opioid side effects. Patients should also avoid exposing the patch to direct external heat.

Empirically, the indications for the transdermal route include intolerance of oral medication, poor compliance with oral medication, and occasionally the desire to provide a trial of fentanyl to patients who have reacted unfavourably to other opioids. However, there are a number of limitations. The delay in onset of analgesia and in the establishment of steady-state blood levels require the liberal use of an alternative short-acting opioid (usually morphine) for BTP during the early treatment period. Because of its 3-day duration of action, transdermal fentanyl is generally unsuitable for patients with unstable pain, and if a patient's pain goes out of control, management may be complicated because of the delay in re-establishing steady state. If dose reductions are required or discontinuation is indicated, the continuing absorption following patch removal must be taken into account. Poor patch adhesion may be a problem in some patients. Set against these considerations are the advantages in terms of convenience and compliance and there is high patient acceptability of this mode of administration. Additionally, there are experimental and clinical data to suggest that transdermal fentanyl is associated with less constipation than morphine[108].

Empirical observations suggest that a 100-mcg/h fentanyl patch is approximately equianalgesic to 2–4 mg/h of intravenous morphine (or equivalent). The relative potency ratio that is applicable when converting patients from oral morphine to transdermal fentanyl has been the subject of some controversy, but the dosing recommendations of the manufacturer seem about right. The patch should be placed in an area where skin movement is limited, such as the upper anterior chest wall or either side of the midline on the back, preferably the lower back. Studies have shown that all areas of skin absorb the drug at roughly the same rate[105]. Since the adhesive strips on these patches are less than optimal, securing the patch with non-irritant tape is often necessary.

Transdermal fentanyl is best reserved for patients whose opioid requirements are stable[65] and, in general, it is likely to be a second-line choice. However, for suitable patients it works well and they like it[109].

Oral transmucosal fentanyl citrate (OTFC)

An oral transmucosal formulation of fentanyl (which incorporates the drug in a hardened lozenge on a stick) that is absorbed across the buccal mucosa, has recently been introduced in many countries for the management of BTP. The lozenge is rubbed gently against the inside of the cheek until it has dissolved. The formulation is rapidly absorbed and achieves blood levels and time to peak effect that are comparable to parenterally administered fentanyl. Indeed, the time to onset of analgesia is 5–10 min[110–113] and studies in cancer patients suggest that it can provide rapid and very effective relief of BTP. Formulations incorporating 200, 400, 600, 800, and 1600 mcg are available. The most common adverse effects associated with this formulation are somnolence, nausea, and dizziness. One interesting observation which has emerged from the clinical trials and clinical use is that the successful dose of OTFC cannot be predicted and is not directly related to the daily dose of regular opioids being received for background pain. This raises some questions about the current management of BTP with conventional formulations of oral or parenteral opioids and, in particular, if it should be routine practice to titrate the breakthrough dose for each patient rather than adopting the standard 1/6th of 24-h opioid dose. (For detailed description and management of BTP see Chapter 10.1.5.)

Until recently, oral immediate-release (IR) formulations of opioids, also including hydromorphone, and oxycodone were the rescue medication most commonly in use. These oral IR opioids have an extensive first-pass effect and are hydrophilic in nature, which slows the onset of analgesia to approximately 30 min and more. By the time these agents reach their peak effect the pain has already resolved (Fig. 10.1.6.8).

The efficacy of OTFC; ACTIQ® in the management of cancer related BTP has been recently reviewed by Cochrane reviewers[114]. Four well-designed studies were included in the review: two studies examined dose titration of OTFC, one study compared OTFC to placebo and one study compared it to morphine sulphate immediate release (MSIR). All four studies have shown that OTFC was superior to placebo, MSIR, and the usual rescue medications in providing pain relief with a faster onset and a greater degree of relief.

Other fentanyl preparations

Effervescent tablets The second oral transmucosal fentanyl delivery system to be developed for the treatment of BTP was effervescent tablets. The effervescent tablets disintegrate rapidly in the presence of water with formation of carbon dioxide (the effervescent activity). In addition to active ingredients, it contains mixtures of acids (like citric, tartaric, malic, and fumaric acid) and carbonates such as sodium bicarbonate. The effervescent activity is the result of an acid–base chemical reaction that evolves the evolution of gas bubbles which starts in presence of water as a catalysing agent. It is suggested that the carbon dioxide (CO_2) bubbling

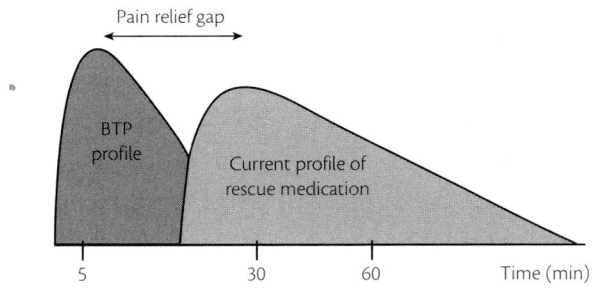

Figure 10.1.6.8 Pain relief gap (see Chapter 10.1.5).

formation induces enhanced drug permeability from this delivery system[115].

The effervescent tablet delivery system has now been licensed for use. Pharmacokinetic studies have demonstrated an absolute bioavailability of 65 per cent of which 48 per cent is the result of an initial absorption from the buccal mucosa[116]. Both absolute bioavailability (65 per cent vs. 50 per cent) and rapid transmucosal bioavailability (48 per cent vs. 25 per cent) of the effervescent tablet are higher than those obtained with the original lozenge formulation of OTFC. Moreover, fentanyl enters the systemic circulation significantly more rapidly from the effervescent tablets than from the lozenge preparation[117]. It has been demonstrated that these pharmacokinetic advantages are maintained even in patients who have developed oral mucositis[118].

There are pharmacokinetic differences between the effervescent system and OTFC. The same dose of fentanyl in two different formulations should not be viewed as equivalent and caution must be exercised when selecting an initial dose or when switching patients from one product to another. (The initial dose of the effervescent tablet should be 100 μg while that of the lozenge is 200 μg.)

The transmucosal buccal disc (TBD) The TBD dosage form refers to a flexible film that adheres to the oral mucosa and delivers a drug over a period of time. The TBD can be further divided into three types or sub-categories: (1) dissolvable matrix drug-delivery patches; (2) patches with a non-dissolvable backing; and (3) patches with a dissolvable backing[117]. The patches with dissolvable matrix or backing are designed to release drug into the oral cavity. BEMA™ (bioerodible mucoadhesive disc) Fentanyl is the first buccal patch to be developed. It consists of a small, dissolvable, polymer disc formulated with fentanyl for application to the buccal membrane. It will be available in a range of dosage strengths: 200, 400, 600, 800, and 1200 μg.

Sublingual transmucosal formulations The sublingual mucosa is relatively more permeable than the buccal mucosa[119]. Although it is constantly washed by saliva, which may disturb placement of devices like adhesive discs, its higher permeability could produce rapid onset of action and makes this an appropriate route for drugs administered for the management of BTP.

The effectiveness of sublingual fentanyl citrate (SLFC) was first investigated with the injectable solutions with positive results[120]. There are currently two commercial products of SLFC: one that has been recently approved in Europe and the other is still undergoing phase III studies.

Rapinyl™/Abstral is a transmucosal adhesive delivery system similar to BEMA™ but it adheres to the sublingual mucosa. In pharmacokinetic studies of this formulation, first detectable plasma concentration of fentanyl was observed at 8–11 min after administration and the formulation seemed to be well tolerated by the patients[121]. Phase III studies have been completed, and the formulation is scheduled to be released in Sweden in 2008 and will be in other countries in 2009. It is available in 50-, 100-, 200-, 400-, 600-, and 800-mcg dose units.

The other fentanyl preparation is a nasal spray, which is being evaluated for efficacy and safety in Phase III studies of BTP in opioid-tolerant cancer patients.

Other drugs

Drugs such as phenazocine, dextromoramide, and dipipanone are now largely obsolete in chronic pain management.

Agonist–antagonist opioid analgesics

The agonist–antagonist opioid analgesics are a heterogeneous group of drugs with moderate–to-strong analgesic activity, comparable with that of the agonist opioids such as codeine and morphine. The group includes drugs that act as an agonist or partial agonist at one receptor and as an antagonist at another (pentazocine, dezocine, butorphanol, nalbuphine)—'the mixed agonist–antagonists'—and drugs acting as a partial agonist at a single receptor (buprenorphine). These two groups of drugs can be also classified as nalorphine- or morphine-like. Meptazinol fits neither classification and occupies a separate category. The place of this group of drugs in chronic cancer pain has been limited[122]. However, the recent development of a transdermal formulation of buprenorphine may allow its more widespread use in both chronic cancer and non-cancer pain.

Mixed agonist–antagonist analgesics

The agonist–antagonists produce analgesia in the opioid-naïve patient but may precipitate withdrawal in patients who are physically dependent on morphine-like drugs. Therefore, when used for chronic pain, they should be tried before repeated administration of a morphine-like agonist drug.

Pentazocine, butorphanol, and nalbuphine are mu antagonists and kappa agonists or partial agonists. All three drugs are strong analgesics when given by injection: pentazocine is one-sixth to one-third as potent as morphine, nalbuphine is roughly equipotent with morphine, and butorphanol is 3.5–7 times as potent. The duration of analgesia is similar to that of morphine (3–4 h). Oral pentazocine is closer in analgesic efficacy to aspirin and paracetamol than the weak opioid analgesics, such as codeine. Neither nalbuphine nor butorphanol is available as an oral formulation, and butorphanol is no longer available in any form in the United Kingdom.

At usual therapeutic doses, nalbuphine and butorphanol have respiratory depressant effects equivalent to that of morphine (although the duration of such effects may be longer with butorphanol). Unlike morphine, there appears to be a ceiling to both the respiratory depression and the analgesic action.

All three drugs have a lower abuse potential than the agonist opioid analgesics such as morphine. However, all have been subject to abuse and misuse, and pentazocine (but not the others) is subject to controlled drug restrictions. In North America, the oral preparation of pentazocine is marketed in combination with naloxone (but is available without naloxone elsewhere).

Meptazinol is a synthetic hexahydroazepine derivative with opioid agonist and antagonist properties, but is unlike either the nalorphine-type agonist–antagonists or buprenorphine. Meptazinol has central cholinergic properties, which may account at least in part for its analgesic effects. Receptor-binding studies show it to be a specific μ agonist. Meptazinol is one-tenth as potent as morphine by intramuscular injection and has a duration of action of about 4 h. Some studies have shown adverse effects to be more frequent than with morphine, although respiratory depression and constipation appear to be less.

In therapeutic doses, the mixed agonists–antagonists may produce certain self-limiting psychotomimetic effects in some patients; pentazocine is the most common drug associated with these effects. These drugs play a very limited role in the management of chronic cancer pain because the incidence and severity of the psychotomimetic effects increase with dose escalation, and nalbuphine and butorphanol are only available for parenteral use.

A transnasal formulation of butorphanol is now on the market in the United States of America, but there is no reported experience of its use in the management of chronic cancer pain.

Partial agonist analgesics

Buprenorphine is a semi-synthetic derivative of thebaine and chemically closely related to the strong agonist etorphine. Buprenorphine is a true partial agonist at the mu receptor and exhibits a ceiling effect in dose response curves in various animal models. In some, a bell-shaped curve is seen, indicating that at doses above a certain level, the pharmacological effect actually decreases with increasing dose[123]. Buprenorphine has until recently only been available by injection or for sublingual administration. A dose of 0.4 mg sublingually gives similar analgesia to 0.2–0.3 mg intramuscularly, with an onset of analgesia within 30–60 min of administration and a duration of 6–9 h[124]. In contrast, if taken orally, buprenorphine is a poor analgesic due to extensive presystemic elimination[125]. The long duration of analgesia with buprenorphine may be related to its affinity for the mu-opioid receptor and an unusually slow dissociation constant for the drug–receptor complex.

Buprenorphine has been in clinical use for more than 30 years and has been evaluated in a variety of acute pain models. Direct single-dose comparisons with other analgesics such as morphine are complicated by its long duration of action, but results from a number of studies in postoperative pain suggest that single doses of 0.3 mg buprenorphine parenterally or 0.4 mg sublingually give equivalent analgesia to 10–15 mg intramuscular morphine. A ceiling effect for analgesia in humans has not been clearly demonstrated.

Buprenorphine produces typical opioid adverse effects. Overall, the available data (which is limited) suggest that the incidence of common adverse effects compared with morphine is similar. Naloxone has been reported as being relatively ineffective in reversing opioid effects due to buprenorphine[126]. Clinical experience does not necessarily agree with this. Buprenorphine was introduced in high-dose sublingual tablet formulations in 1999 for the management of drug dependence. This potential use of the drug has long been recognized[127] and it has been suggested that there is less overdose risk compared with other opioids[128].

Buprenorphine is available in a patch for transdermal administration. The drug is incorporated into an adhesive polymer matrix, which controls the release of the drug by diffusion. There are two preparations: one lasting 4 days and the other 7 days.

Three patch sizes of the 4-day preparation are available delivering 35, 52.5, and 70 mcg buprenorphine per hour. Therapeutic plasma concentrations are achieved within 11–21 h and steady state between the second and third applications of the patch. The 7-day patch also comes in three sizes, delivering 5, 10 and 20 mg buprenorphine per hour. At usual clinical doses of 3–4 mg/24 h buprenorphine functions as a pure mu agonist.

Transdermal buprenorphine has been licensed for use in both cancer pain and non-cancer pain. The lack of renal excretion (majority excreted unchanged in stool) makes this of potential use in renal dysfunction.

Principles of opioid administration

The effective clinical use of opioid analgesics requires familiarity with the different drugs available, routes of administration, dosing guidelines, and potential adverse effects.

Indications

A trial of opioid therapy should be given to all patients with pain of moderate or greater severity, irrespective of the underlying pathophysiological mechanism. As discussed in Chapter 10.1.14, the suggestion that some forms of pain, such as neuropathic pain, are intrinsically refractory to opioid analgesia has been refuted by several studies that demonstrate that pain mechanisms do not accurately predict analgesic outcome from opioid therapy[129]. Given the variability in response, all opioid trials in the clinical setting should include dose titration until adequate analgesia occurs or intolerable adverse effects supervene. This approach will identify those responders who can gain substantial clinical benefit from opioid therapy.

Patients whose pain is not easily controlled with an opioid analgesic because of troublesome adverse effects may benefit from alternative strategies and these are discussed in the following paragraphs.

Drug selection

The factors that influence opioid selection include pain intensity, pharmacokinetic considerations and available formulations, previous adverse effects, and the presence of coexisting disease.

Pain intensity

Patients who present with severe pain are usually treated with a 'step 3' opioid (morphine, hydromorphone, oxycodone, oxymorphone, fentanyl, methadone, or levorphanol). Patients with moderate pain are treated conventionally with a combination product containing paracetamol or aspirin plus a conventional step 2 opioid (codeine, dihydrocodeine, hydrocodone, oxycodone [low dose], and propoxyphene).

Pharmacokinetic considerations and type of formulation

Any of the available agonist opioids can be selected for the opioid-naïve patient without major organ failure. Short-half-life opioids (morphine, hydromorphone, oxycodone, or oxymorphone) are generally favoured because they are easier to titrate than the long-half-life drugs, which take longer to achieve steady-state plasma concentrations. Among the short-half-life opioids, the range of available formulations often influences specific drug selection. For ambulatory patients who are able to tolerate oral opioids, morphine sulphate is generally preferred since it has a short half-life and is easy to titrate in its normal-release form; it is also available as sustained-release preparations that allow 12 and 24h dosing intervals. The long-half-life opioids methadone and levorphanol are not usually considered for first-line therapy because they can be difficult to titrate and present challenging management problems if delayed toxicity develops as plasma concentrations gradually rise, following dose increments. The use of pethidine for the management of cancer pain is discouraged.

When the oral route of opioid administration is contraindicated, the available routes of administration may become an important consideration in opioid selection. Fentanyl and buprenorphine are available for administration by the transdermal route. Although most of the full agonist drugs are well absorbed by subcutaneous infusion, some (like morphine tartrate, hydromorphone, and diamorphine) are more suitable by virtue of their high solubility and low irritability. Methadone and fentanyl may produce significant local irritation when administered by the subcutaneous route. For cultural and aesthetic reasons, the subcutaneous route is often preferred to rectal administration. Subcutaneous infusion may be preferable also in patients at the end of life because it is less disruptive than using intermittent analgesic suppositories when nursing a sick patient.

Response to previous trials of opioid therapy

It is always important to review the response to previous trials of opioid therapy. If the current opioid is well tolerated, it is usually continued unless difficulties in dose titration occur or the required dose cannot be administered conventionally. If dose-limiting side-effects develop, a trial of an alternative opioid should be considered as discussed in the section on adverse effects.

Coexisting disease

Pharmacokinetic studies of pethidine, pentazocine, and propoxyphene have revealed that liver disease may decrease the clearance and increase the bioavailability and half-lives of these drugs[130,131]. These changes may result in above-normal plasma concentrations. Mild or moderate hepatic impairment has only a minor impact on morphine clearance[132]; however, advanced disease may be associated with reduced elimination[133].

Patients with renal impairment may accumulate the active metabolites of propoxyphene (norpropoxyphene), pethidine (norpethidine), morphine (M6G), codeine, and dihydrocodeine (several metabolites). Particular caution is required in the administration of these drugs to such patients[56,134–137]. Until more data are available, it may be wise to assume that other opioids with active metabolites may produce similar problems of toxicity in patients with impaired renal function. On this basis buprenorphine, fentanyl and alfentanil show potential advantages in renal impairment.

Morphine remains the standard step-3 opioid analgesic against which others are measured and is the most widely available in a variety of oral formulations[65]. It has limitations; the systemic availability of morphine by the oral route is poor (20–30 per cent) and this contributes to the sometimes unpredictable onset of action and great interindividual variability in dose requirements and response. Active metabolites may contribute to toxicity particularly in patients with renal impairment[137]. Sometimes, the pain does not respond well or completely to morphine, notably neuropathic pain. However, none of the alternatives to morphine has so far demonstrated advantages which would make it preferable in routine use as the first-line oral opioid for cancer pain. Morphine remains the standard but for reasons of familiarity, availability, and cost, rather than proven superiority. Early pilot work by Reid and Hanks comparing, standard 3-step approach with morphine versus a 2-step approach with oxycodone indicates that such a 2-step approach may be superior in terms of time to effective pain relief with all the associated secondary gains.

Routes of administration

Opioids should be administered by the least invasive and safest route capable of providing adequate analgesia. In a survey of patients with advanced cancer, more than half required two or more routes of administration prior to death, and almost a quarter required three or more[138].

Oral administration

The oral route of opioid administration remains an important route and appropriate in routine practice. Orally administered drugs have a slower onset of action, a delayed peak time, and a longer duration of effect compared with parenterally administered drugs. The time to peak effect depends on the drug and the nature of the formulation. For most normal-release oral formulations, peak effect is typically achieved within 60 min. The oral route of drug administration is inappropriate for patients who have impaired swallowing or gastrointestinal obstruction, and for some patients who require a rapid onset of analgesia. For patients who require very high doses, the inability to prescribe a manageable oral opioid regimen may be an indication for the use of a non-oral route.

When given orally, the opioids differ substantially with respect to their relative analgesic potency compared with parenteral administration. To some extent, this reflects differences in pre-systemic metabolism, that is, the degree to which they are inactivated as they are absorbed from the gastrointestinal tract and pass through the liver into the systemic circulation. As indicated in Table 10.1.6.3, morphine, diamorphine, pethidine, hydromorphone, and oxymorphone, have ratios of oral-to-parenteral potency ranging from 1:3 to 1:12. Methadone, levorphanol, and oxycodone are subject to less pre-systemic elimination and also demonstrate a lower oral-to-parenteral potency ratio of at least 1:2. Failure to recognize these differences may result in a substantial reduction in analgesia when a change from parenteral to oral administration is attempted without upward titration of the dose, or toxic effects when changing in the opposite direction.

Rectal administration

The rectal route is a non-invasive alternative to parenteral routes for patients unable to use oral opioids. Rectal suppositories containing morphine, hydromorphone, oxymorphone, and oxycodone are available. The pharmacokinetics and bioavailability of drugs given rectally may differ from that of oral administration because of delayed or limited absorption and partial bypassing of pre-systemic hepatic metabolism. In practice, however, the potency of opioids administered rectally is approximately equal to that achieved by oral dosing[139]. In contrast with morphine, rectal oxycodone appears to have a delayed absorption and prolonged duration of action.

For many patients, the rectal route is not used because it is more convenient to convert directly to a subcutaneous infusion of opioid using a portable syringe driver or similar device.

Transmucosal/buccal/nasal administration

As previously described, transmucosal, buccal, and nasal administration is possible with lipophilic opioids such as fentanyl. Advantages of this route include relatively easy self-administration, rapid absorption, and quick onset of analgesia. This is described in detail earlier and in Chapter 10.1.5 on BTP.

Parenteral administration

Bolus injections Parenteral routes of administration are considered for patients who have impaired swallowing or gastrointestinal obstruction, those who require a rapid onset of analgesia, and those who require very high doses that cannot be administered conveniently by other methods. Repeated parenteral bolus injections, which can be delivered by the intravenous, intramuscular, or subcutaneous routes, may be complicated by the occurrence of untoward 'bolus' effects (toxicity at peak concentration and/or pain breakthrough at the trough). Intravenous bolus provides the most rapid onset; the time to peak effect correlates with the lipid solubility of the opioid, ranging from 2 to 5 min for methadone and from 10 to 15 min for morphine. Although repeated intramuscular injections are commonplace in some countries, they are painful and offer no pharmacokinetic advantage, and their use is not recommended[65,81]. Repeated bolus doses, if required, can be accomplished without frequent skin punctures by using an indwelling intravenous or subcutaneous infusion device. To deliver repeated subcutaneous injections, a 25–27 gauge 'butterfly' can be left under the skin for up to a week[140]. The discomfort associated with this technique is partially related to the volume to be injected; it can be minimized by the use of concentrated formulations.

Continuous infusions Continuous infusions avoid the problems associated with the 'bolus effect' and can be administered intravenously or subcutaneously[141,142]. Continuous subcutaneous infusion using a portable battery-operated syringe driver or other similar device was originally devised to administer infusions of desferrioxamine to patients with thalassemia, but was subsequently used to deliver diamorphine to patients with advanced cancer who were unable to take oral drugs[143]. This technique is now well established in palliative care and is used to administer analgesics, antiemetics, anxiolytic sedatives, and dexamethasone.

Ambulatory infusion devices vary in complexity, cost, and ability to provide patient-controlled 'rescue doses' as an adjunct to a continuous basal infusion. A variety of devices have been employed, all designed to be lightweight and portable, and in one case disposable. Opioids suitable for continuous subcutaneous infusion must be soluble, well absorbed, and non-irritant. Extensive experience has been reported with morphine, diamorphine, hydromorphone, fentanyl, and oxymorphone[84,141,144]. Methadone[75] and fentanyl appear to be relative irritants and are best avoided by this route.

Studies suggest that dosing with subcutaneous administration can proceed in a manner identical to continuous intravenous infusion: a postoperative study comparing patients who received an identical dose of morphine by either intravenous or subcutaneous infusion found no difference in blood levels[145], and a controlled study of hydromorphone calculated a bioavailability of 78 per cent for the subcutaneous route and observed that analgesic outcome was identical during intravenous or subcutaneous infusion. To maintain the comfort of an infusion site, the subcutaneous infusion rate should not exceed 5 ml/h. Subcutaneous infusion has become the first choice when parenteral analgesia is required in palliative care patients.

Continuous intravenous infusion may be the most appropriate way of delivering an opioid for patients with a pre-existing implanted central line, when there is a need for infusion of a large volume of solution, or when using methadone. If continuous intravenous infusion must be continued on a long-term basis, a permanent central venous port is recommended.

Continuous infusions of drug combinations may be indicated when pain is accompanied by nausea, anxiety, or agitation. In such cases an antiemetic, neuroleptic, or anxiolytic may be combined with an opioid, provided that it is non-irritant, miscible, and stable in combined solution. As noted in the following paragraphs, a variety of different combinations of drugs are commonly given by continuous infusion[146]. However, the stability/compatibility of many of these combinations is not known. The compatibility of drug combinations is dependent on a number of factors, including the types of drugs, the concentrations of drugs, the diluent and temperature, and UV light. A database of compatible drug combinations is now available on the Internet (http://www.pallcare.info). Generally, infusions should contain as few drugs as possible, preferably no more than three. The absence of precipitation within a drug mixture does not necessarily mean that the drugs are chemically compatible[147].

Epidural, intrathecal, and intraventricular administration (see also Chapter 10.1.9)
The discovery of opioid receptors in the dorsal horn of the spinal cord led to the development of intraspinal opioid delivery techniques. In general, they provide a longer duration of analgesia at doses lower than required by systemic administration. The delivery of low opioid doses near the sites of action in the spinal cord may decrease supraspinally mediated adverse effects. Opioid selection for intraspinal delivery is influenced by several factors. Hydrophilic drugs, such as morphine and hydromorphone, have a prolonged half-life in cerebrospinal fluid and significant rostral redistribution[148]. Lipophilic opioids, such as fentanyl and sufentanil, have less rostral redistribution and therefore fewer prolonged adverse effects if these become a problem.

The addition of local anaesthetic such as bupivacaine to an epidural or intrathecal opioid has been demonstrated to improve analgesia without increasing toxicity[149,150]. Unlike in acute postoperative pain, where a large volume of low-concentration local anaesthetic is used, in chronic cancer pain, a small volume of high concentration of local anaesthetic is preferred and can be mixed with an appropriate dose of a small volume of opioid.

The initial conversion of opioid dose from systemic subcutaneous diamorphine or morphine is:

◆ epidural—1/10 of systemic dose;
◆ intrathecal—1/10 of epidural dose.

Thus, if a patient were on 100 mg of subcutaneous morphine or diamorphine/ day, the equivalent epidural dose would be 10 mg, and the equivalent intrathecal dose would be 1 mg/day.

The initial solution used for epidural infusion is usually:

◆ 9 ml 0.5 per cent bupivacaine;
◆ 75–150 mcg clonidine;
◆ morphine or diamorphine dose according to individual patient requirements (as calculated above). This gives a total volume of 10 ml infused over 24 h.

The initial solution used for intrathecal infusion is normally around 1/10 of the above, that is:

◆ 1 ml 0.5 per cent bupivacaine;
◆ 15 mcg clonidine;
◆ morphine or diamorphine according to individual patient requirements.

Hydromorphone is preferred to morphine for use in programmable intrathecal pumps because of incompatibility between the commonly used devices and morphine.

Should there be a major problem with pump malfunction, and the whole dose is delivered as a bolus, this should *not* result in a major, life-threatening overdose.

There are no clinical studies comparing the intrathecal and epidural routes in cancer pain. Choice of route often depends on individual patients and local practice. A combined analysis of adverse effects observed in numerous trials of epidural or intrathecal administration suggests that the risks associated with these techniques are similar (see Chapter 10.1.9). The potential morbidity associated with these procedures emphasizes the need for a well-trained clinician and long-term monitoring for individual patients.

Limited experience suggests that the administration of an opioid into the cerebral ventricles can provide long-term analgesia in selected patients. This technique has been used for patients with upper-body or head pain or with severe diffuse pain. Schedules have included both intermittent injection via an Ommaya reservoir and continual infusion using an implanted pump.

The indication for the spinal routes of administration of opioid analgesics in palliative care patients is discussed in more detail in Chapter 10.1.9.

Other routes and modes of administration

Transdermal As previously described, fentanyl and buprenorphine are available in a transdermal formulation and their use is discussed earlier. Studies with a transdermal hydromorphone preparation are currently ongoing.

Sublingual Sublingual absorption potentially could occur with any opioid, but bioavailability is very poor with drugs that are not highly lipophilic[151,152]. A sublingual preparation of buprenorphine is available in some countries, although not in the United States of America. Anecdotally, sublingual morphine has also been reported to be effective; given the poor sublingual absorption of this drug, this efficacy may be related in part to swallowing of the dose. Methadone is well absorbed sublingually. Sublingual administration has been discussed earlier.

Topical There are several case series and one very small randomized controlled trial that examine the role of topical morphine for local analgesia. The small amount of existing evidence seems to point to a role in some situations, for example, cutaneous ulcers or tumour with cutaneous inflammation. Doses of 10–40 mg of morphine are used in simple gel, saline soaks, or local anaesthetic gel[153–155]. Randomized controlled trials in non-malignant cutaneous pain, e.g. burns or photodynamic therapy, have been negative.

Changing the route of administration

As described earlier, when changing from the oral to parenteral routes, or vice versa, an adjustment in dose is required to avoid either toxic effects or a reduction in analgesia. The ratios of oral-to-parenteral relative potency given in Table 10.1.6.7 are estimates and should not be taken as precise figures but used as guidelines to achieve a roughly equianalgesic effect. There is considerable variation between patients, and upward or downward adjustment may then be required for individual patients. The slower onset of analgesia after oral administration often requires some adaptation on the part of a patient who is accustomed to the more rapid onset seen after parenteral opioid. In some patients, the problems associated with switching from the parenteral to the oral route of opioid administration may need to be minimized by slowly reducing the parenteral dose and increasing the oral dose over a 2–3-day period.

Usually, no dose adjustment is required when patients are switched from the subcutaneous to the intravenous route or vice versa.

Scheduling opioid administration

'Around-the-clock' dosing To provide the patient with continuous relief by preventing the pain from recurring, patients with continuous or frequent pain are usually scheduled for 'around-the-clock' dosing. However, clinical vigilance is required in patients with no previous opioid exposure and those administered drugs with long half-lives. With methadone, for example, delayed toxicity may develop as plasma concentration rises slowly toward steady-state levels.

Rescue doses All patients who receive an around-the-clock opioid regimen should also be offered a 'rescue dose', that is, a supplemental dose given on an as-needed basis to treat pain that breaks through the regular schedule[65]. The integration of scheduled dosing with rescue doses provides a method for safe and rational stepwise dose escalation and is applicable to all routes of opioid administration. Typically the rescue drug is identical to that administered on a continuous basis, with the exception of transdermal fentanyl and methadone; the use of an alternative short-half-life opioid is recommended for the rescue dose when these drugs are used. The frequency with which the rescue dose can be administered depends on the time to peak effect for the drug and the route of administration. Oral rescue doses can be offered up to every 60–90 min, and parenteral rescue doses can be offered up to every 15–30 min. Clinical experience suggests that the size of the rescue dose should usually be equivalent to one-sixth of the 24h baseline dose, that is, the same as the 4-hourly dose of opioid. The magnitude of the rescue dose should be individualized and some patients with low baseline pain but severe exacerbations may require rescue doses that are substantially larger. As discussed in this chapter, in the setting of clinical trials where rescue doses are individualized, the effective doses rarely calculate as one-sixth of the 24h dose.

Scheduling with sustained-release formulations Sustained-release formulations can reduce the inconvenience associated with around-the-clock administration. These formulations should not be used for rapid titration of the dose in patients with severe pain. Sustained-release oral morphine sulphate and oxycodone, and transdermal fentanyl are now widely used, and sustained-release formulations of codeine, tramadol, and hydromorphone have been introduced in various countries.

A normal-release formulation of a short-half-life opioid (usually the same drug) is generally used as the rescue medication. Sustained- and normal-release formulations of oral morphine are dose equivalent; switching from one to the other is done on a milligram-for-milligram basis after the daily dose requirement is identified using a normal-release formulation.

As-needed dosing In some limited situations, an as-needed dosing regimen alone can be recommended. This type of dosing provides additional safety during the initiation of opioid therapy in the opioid-naïve patient, particularly when rapid dose escalation is needed or a long-half-life drug is administered. This technique is strongly recommended when starting methadone therapy, and for patients with acute renal failure.

Patient-controlled analgesia Patient-controlled analgesia is a technique of parenteral drug administration in which the patient controls a pump that delivers bolus doses of an analgesic according to parameters set by the physician. Use of a patient-controlled analgesia device allows the patient to titrate the opioid dose carefully to his or her individual analgesic needs. Long-term patient-controlled analgesia in cancer patients is accomplished via subcutaneous or intravenous routes using an ambulatory infusion device[156]. The more technologically advanced of these devices have programmable variables, including infusion rate, rescue dose, and lockout interval. The option for bolus dosing is typically used in conjunction with continuous opioid infusion. There is relatively little experience of patient-controlled analgesia in chronic cancer pain; it is a technique largely confined to the management of acute postoperative pain.

Dose selection and adjustment

Initial dose selection A patient with severe pain that is not controlled with a step-2 opioid–non-opioid combination in full dose should begin one of the opioid agonists at a dose equivalent to 10 mg oral morphine sulphate every 4 h.

Dose titration Inadequate pain relief should be addressed by gradual escalation of the opioid dose until adequate analgesia is reported or intolerable side effects (that cannot be managed by simple interventions) supervene. Because analgesic response to opioids increases linearly with the logarithm of the dose, dose escalations of less than 30–50 per cent are not likely to improve analgesia significantly. Clinical experience indicates that a dose increment of this order of magnitude is safe and is large enough to observe a meaningful change in effects. In most cases, gradual dose escalation identifies a favourable balance between analgesia and side effects, which remains stable for a prolonged period. While doses can become extremely large during this process, the absolute dose is immaterial as long as the balance between analgesia and side effects remains favourable. In a retrospective study of 100 patients with advanced cancer, the average daily opioid requirement was equivalent to 400–600 mg of intramuscular morphine, but approximately 10 per cent of patients required more than 2000 mg and one patient required over 30 000 mg every 24 h. Other centres generally have reported lower doses; a median dose of 60 mg/day in one centre and 120 mg/day in another[157].

A simple method of dose titration using oral morphine is to prescribe a dose of immediate-release morphine every 4 h and the same dose for rescue (for BTP)[65]. The rescue dose can be given as often as required (e.g. every hour) and the total dose of morphine can be reviewed daily. The regular dose can then be adjusted according to how many rescue doses have been given.

Rate of dose titration The severity of the pain should determine the rate of dose titration. Patients with very severe pain can be managed by repeated parenteral dosing every 15–30 min until pain is partially relieved when an oral dosing regimen should be started.

Tolerance Patients vary greatly in the opioid dose required to manage their pain. The need for escalating doses is a complex phenomenon. Most patients reach a dose that remains constant for prolonged periods. When the need for dose escalation arises, any of a variety of distinct processes may be involved. Clinical experience suggests that true pharmacological tolerance is a much less common reason than disease progression or increasing psychological distress. Changes in the pharmacokinetics of an analgesic drug could also be implicated.

True pharmacological tolerance probably involves changes at the receptor level, and in this situation continued drug administration itself induces an attenuation of effect. Clinically, tolerance to the non-analgesic effects of opioids appears to occur commonly albeit at varying rates for different effects. For example, tolerance to respiratory depression, somnolence, and nausea generally develops rapidly, whereas tolerance to opioid-induced constipation develops very slowly, if at all. Tolerance to these opioid side effects is not a clinical problem, and indeed is a desirable outcome that allows effective dose titration to proceed.

From the clinical perspective, the concern is that tolerance to the analgesic effect of the drug will develop and that this will necessitate rapid dose escalation, which may continue until the drug is no longer useful. Induction of true analgesic tolerance which could compromise the utility of treatment can only be said to occur if a patient manifests a need for increasing opioid doses in the absence of other factors (e.g. progressive disease) that would be capable of explaining the increase in pain. Extensive clinical experience suggests that most patients who require an escalation in dose to manage increasing pain have demonstrable progression of disease. With the emergence of our understanding of opioid-induced hyperalgesia, both generalized pain and/or appearance of features of central wind-up should be assessed very carefully. This is discussed in the following paragraphs.

This conclusion has two important implications: concern about tolerance should not impede the use of opioids early in the course of the disease, and worsening pain in a patient receiving a stable dose of opioid should not be attributed to tolerance but taken as presumptive evidence of disease progression or, less commonly, increasing psychological distress.

Determination of an equianalgesic dose The overriding clinical issue with an opioid switch is that it is nearly always done because a problem exists. Assessment of appropriate dose conversion is critical when switching a patient from one opioid to another. The most common reason for a switch is an unacceptable side-effect profile often also associated with uncontrolled pain. It is clear that any deterioration in either side effects and/or pain control is disastrous for the patient, therefore a switch needs to find the right balance. In practice, this means a very conservative equianalgesic conversion should be made (no more than 75 per cent of the equianalgesic dose and clearly less in the case of drugs such as methadone) and appropriate breakthrough analgesia is prescribed in a clear and practical way to prevent any distress due to underdosing. Failure to do this can lead to the development of opioid toxicity or worsening of existing opioid toxicity.

Management of opioid adverse effects

Successful opioid therapy requires that the benefits of analgesia clearly outweigh treatment-related adverse effects. This requires understanding of adverse opioid effects, and the strategies used to prevent and manage them are essential skills for all involved in cancer pain management. The adverse effects that are frequently observed in patients receiving oral morphine and other opioids are summarized in Table 10.1.6.9. The most common are sedation, constipation, and nausea and vomiting, but there are other adverse effects including confusion, hallucinations, nightmares, urinary retention, multifocal myoclonus, dizziness, and dysphoria. The mechanisms that underlie these adverse effects, even the most common, are only partly understood and, as discussed earlier,

Table 10.1.6.9 Common opioid-induced adverse effects.

Gastrointestinal	Nausea
	Vomiting
	Constipation
Autonomic	Xerostomia
	Urinary retention
	Postural hypotension
Central nervous system	Drowsiness
	Cognitive impairment
	Hallucinations
	Delirium
	Respiratory depression
	Myoclonus
	Seizure disorder
	Hyperalgesia
Cutaneous	Itch
	Sweating

appear to depend upon a number of factors including age, extent of disease, and organ dysfunction, concurrent administration of certain drugs, prior opioid exposure, and the route of drug administration. Studies comparing the adverse effects of one opioid analgesic with another in this population are lacking. Similarly, controlled studies comparing the adverse effects produced by the same opioid given by various routes of administration are also lacking.

As a general rule, caution is required when using opioids in patients in acute pain with impaired ventilation, bronchial asthma, or raised intracranial pressure; the same caveats do not usually limit dose titration in chronic cancer pain management.

Factors predictive of opioid adverse effects

Drug-related Overall, there is very little reproducible evidence suggesting that any one opioid agonist has a substantially better adverse effect profile than any other. Pethidine is not recommended in the management of chronic cancer pain because of concerns regarding its side-effect profile. Data from controlled studies indicate that the transdermal administration of fentanyl is associated with a lesser incidence of constipation than oral morphine or codeine[144–146].

Route-related There is very limited evidence to suggest differences in adverse effects associated with specific routes of systemic administration. Compared to oral morphine administration, small studies have demonstrated less nausea and vomiting with rectal[158] and subcutaneous administration [159]. Four studies comparing transdermal fentanyl to oral morphine demonstrated less constipation among the patients receiving transdermal fentanyl. It is not clear as to whether this is a route- or drug-related effect[144,145].

Patient-related For reasons that are not well explained, there is striking inter-individual variability in the sensitivity to adverse effects from morphine and other opioid drugs. Genetic variability clearly affects the sensitivity to opioids[160], and it is reasonable to assume that the genetic background plays a similar important role in sensitivity to adverse effects[161].

Some of this variability is related to co-morbidity. Aging is associated with altered pharmacokinetics, particularly characterized by diminished clearance and volume of distribution. This has been well evaluated for morphine[162] and fentanyl [163,164]. In a study of morphine use in the management of chronic cancer pain in the elderly, overall elderly patients required lower doses than their younger counterparts without exhibiting an enhanced risk for opioid induced adverse effects[165]. In patients with impaired renal function there is delayed clearance of an active metabolite of morphine, morphine-6-glucuronide[166]. Anecdotally, high concentrations of M6G have been associated with toxicity; however, in a prospective study of patients with opioid-induced delirium or myoclonus no relationship to renal function was observed[156,157].

Other patient related factors that may enhance the risk of adverse effects include the co-administration of drugs which may have cumulative toxicity, especially sedation or other concurrent co-morbidity (Table 10.1.6.10).

Opioid initiation and dose escalation

Among adverse effects there is substantial variability in their dose response. A dose–response relationship is most commonly evident with regards to the CNS adverse effects of sedation, cognitive impairment, hallucinations, myoclonus, and respiratory depression. Even among these, however, there is very substantial interindividual variability to many of these effects. Additionally, as tolerance develops to some effects, the spectrum of adverse effects varies with prolonged use. Commonly, patients who have had prolonged opioid exposure have a lesser tendency to develop sedation or respiratory depression, and the predominant CNS effects become the neuroexcitatory ones of delirium and myoclonus. Gastrointestinal adverse effects generally have a weaker dose–response relationship. Some, like nausea and vomiting, are common with the initiation of therapy but are subsequently unpredictable with resolution among some patients and persistence among others. Constipation is virtually universal and it demonstrates a very weak dose relationship.

Some adverse effects appear transiently after starting an opioid, or after dose escalation, and spontaneously abate. This phenomenon has been well demonstrated in a prospective study on the effect of morphine dose escalation on cognitive performance[167]. This study demonstrated that opioid-induced cognitive impairment commonly improved after 7 days. This phenomenon, though often described, has not been formally studied in regards to other adverse effects.

Differential diagnosis

Adverse changes in patient well-being among patients taking opioids are not always caused by the opioid. Adverse effects must be differentiated from other causes of co-morbidity that may develop in the treated patient and from drug interactions. Common causes of co-morbidity that may mimic opioid-induced adverse effects are presented in Table 10.1.6.9.

Indeed, the appearance of a new adverse change in patient well-being that occurs in the setting of stable opioid dosing is rarely caused by the opioid, and an alternate explanation should be vigorously sought. Since polypharmacy is common among patients with advanced cancer, it is essential to scrutinize medication records and patient reports of medication administration to evaluate for possible drug interactions or some other drug-related explanation for the reported symptoms.

Table 10.1.6.10 Co-morbidity that may mimic opioid induced adverse effects.

Cause		Adverse effects
Central nervous system	Cerebral metastases	Drowsiness, cognitive impairment, nausea, vomiting
	Leptomeningeal metastases	Drowsiness, cognitive impairment, nausea, vomiting
	Cerebrovascular event	Drowsiness, cognitive impairment
	Extradural haemorrhage	Drowsiness, cognitive impairment
Metabolic	Dehydration	Drowsiness, cognitive impairment
	Hypercalcaemia	Drowsiness, cognitive impairment, nausea, vomiting
	Hyponatraemia	Drowsiness, cognitive impairment
	Renal failure	Drowsiness, cognitive impairment, nausea, vomiting, myoclonus
	Liver failure	Drowsiness, cognitive impairment, nausea, vomiting, myoclonus
	Hypoxaemia	Drowsiness, cognitive impairment
Sepsis/Infection		Drowsiness, cognitive impairment, nausea, vomiting
Mechanical	Bowel obstruction	Nausea, vomiting
Iatrogenic	Tricyclics	Drowsiness, cognitive impairment, constipation
	Benzodiazepines	Drowsiness, cognitive impairment
	Antibiotics	Nausea and vomiting
	Vinca alkaloids	Constipation
	Flutamide	Constipation
	Steroids	Agitated delirium
	Non-steroidal anti-inflammatory drugs	Nausea, drowsiness
	Chemotherapy	Nausea, vomiting, drowsiness, cognitive impairment
	Radiotherapy	Nausea, vomiting, drowsiness

Overview of the alternative approaches to treating opioid adverse effects

In general, four different approaches to the management of opioid adverse effects have been described:

1   Dose reduction of systemic opioid.

2   Specific therapy to reduce the adverse effect.

3   Opioid switching.

4   Change route of administration.

Dose reduction of systemic opioid

Reducing the dose of administered opioid usually results in a reduction in dose-related adverse effects. When patients have well-controlled pain, gradual reduction in the opioid dose will often result in the resolution of dose-related adverse effects whilst preserving adequate pain relief[168].

When opioid doses cannot be reduced without the loss of pain control, reduction in dose must be accompanied by the addition of an accompanying synergist approach. Extensive experience has been reported with four accompanying approaches:

1   The addition of a non-opioid co-analgesic.
    The analgesia achieved from non-opioid co-analgesics is additive and often synergistic with that achieved by opioids. This is supported from a number of prospective studies[160–162].

2   The addition of an adjuvant analgesic that is appropriate to the pain syndrome and mechanism (see Chapter 10.1.8).

Adjuvant analgesics (see following) may be combined with primary analgesics to improve the outcome for patients who cannot otherwise attain an acceptable balance between relief and side effects[169]. There is great inter-individual variability in the response to all adjuvant analgesics and, for most, the likelihood of benefit is limited. Furthermore, many of the adjuvant analgesics have the potential to cause side effects, which may be additive to the opioid-induced adverse effects that are already problematic. In evaluating the utility of an adjuvant agent in a particular patient setting, one must consider the likelihood of benefit, the risk of adverse effects, the ease of administration, and patient convenience.

The application of a therapy targeting the cause of the pain.
    Specific antitumour therapies, such as radiotherapy, chemotherapy, or surgery targeting the cause of cancer-related pain can provide substantial relief and thus reduce the need for opioid analgesia. Radiotherapy is of proven benefit in the treatment of painful bone metastases, epidural neoplasm, and headache due to cerebral metastases[164–166]. In other settings, there is a lack of well-established supportive data, and the use of radiotherapy is largely anecdotal. Despite a paucity of evidence concerning the specific analgesic benefits of chemotherapy[170,171], there is a strong clinical impression that tumour shrinkage is generally associated with relief of pain. Although there are some reports of analgesic value even in the absence of significant tumour shrinkage, the likelihood of a

favourable effect on pain is generally related to the likelihood of tumour response[169,170]. Surgery may have a role in the relief of symptoms caused by specific problems, such as obstruction of a hollow viscus, unstable bony structures, and compression of neural tissues[171–173].

The application of a regional anaesthetic or neuroablative intervention (see Chapter 10.1.10).

The results of the WHO 'analgesic ladder' validation studies suggest that 10–30 per cent of patients with cancer pain do not achieve a satisfactory balance between relief and side effects using systemic pharmacotherapy alone without unacceptable drug toxicity[65,67]. Anaesthetic and neurosurgical techniques may reduce or eliminate the requirement for systemically administered opioids to achieve adequate analgesia. In general, regional analgesic techniques such as intraspinal opioid and local anaesthetic administration or intrapleural local anaesthetic administration are usually considered first because they can achieve this end without compromising neurological integrity. Neurodestructive procedures, however, are valuable in a small subset of patients; and some of these procedures, such as coeliac plexus blockade in patients with pancreatic cancer, may have a favourable enough risk:benefit ratio that early treatment is warranted.

Symptomatic management of the adverse effect

Symptomatic drugs used to prevent or control opioid adverse effects are commonly employed. Most of these approaches are based on cumulative anecdotal experience. With few exceptions, the literature describing these approaches is anecdotal or 'expert opinion'. Very few studies have prospectively evaluated efficacy and no studies have evaluated the toxicity of these approaches over long term. In general, this approach involves the addition of a new medication, adding to medication burden and with the associated risks of adverse effects or drug interaction.

Opioid switching

3 Over the past 10 years there have been numerous reports of successful reduction in opioid side effects by switching to an alternative opioid[172,173]. This experience has recently been reviewed[174,175].

Improvements in cognitive impairment, sedation, hallucinations, nausea, vomiting and myoclonus are commonly reported[174,175]. This approach requires familiarity with a range of opioid agonists, and with the use of equianalgesic tables to convert doses when switching between opioids. While this approach has the practical advantage of minimizing polypharmacy, outcomes are variable and unpredictable. When switching between opioids, even with prudent use of equianalgesic tables, patients are at risk of under or overdosing by virtue of individual sensitivities.

The biologic basis for the observed intraindividual variability in sensitivity to opioid analgesia and adverse effects

The biologic basis for the observed intra-individual variability in sensitivity to opioid analgesia and adverse effects is multifactorial[176]. The pharmacokinetic and pharmacodynamic differences among the opioids and the spectrum of proteins involved in determining response create great potential for response variability.

Heterogeneity of opioid metabolism: different opioids have different metabolic and excretion pathways. Of the processes of metabolism and excretion, some are genetically determined and some reflect phenotypic changes particularly with regard to renal and hepatic functions. The genetic factors influencing metabolism

play an important role in analgesia for some opioids and similar phenomena may contribute to variability in adverse effect sensitivity[177].

Genetic influences of receptor function: the potential for genetic influences on opioid effects and tolerability is vast and understanding of this very complex system remains rudimentary[161]. Still several important findings have contributed to understanding of differences in opioid effects as outlined in Section I of this chapter.

Genetic factors influencing drug transport: the membrane-bound drug transporter P-glycoprotein influences drug absorption and drug excretion as well as transport of drugs in and out of the CNS across the blood–brain barrier[178]. Furthermore the P-glycoprotein modulation of opioid CNS levels varies substantially between different opioids[179]. To add to the potential heterogeneity of responses, these critical transporter proteins are encoded by the multi-drug resistance gene MDR-1, which has multiple genetic variations some of which are associated with differences in P-glycoprotein expression or function[180] (see Chapter 10.1.5).

Switching route of systemic administration

4 Limited data indicates that some adverse side effects among patients receiving oral morphine can be relieved by switching the route of administration to the subcutaneous route. In one small study, this phenomenon was reported for nausea and vomiting[159], in another there was less constipation, drowsiness, and nausea[181].

Initial management of the patient receiving opioids who presents with adverse effects

Among patients receiving opioid analgesic therapy there are two key steps in the initial management of adverse effects. Firstly, the clinician must distinguish between morphine adverse effects from co-morbidity or drug interactions. This step requires careful evaluation of the patient for factors outlined in Table 10.1.6.9. If present, these factors should be redressed. Metabolic disorders, dehydration, or sepsis should be treated, non-essential drugs that may be producing an adverse interaction should be discontinued. Symptomatic measures may be required until an effect is observed.

Secondly, if indeed it seems that this is a true adverse effect of the opioid, consideration should be given to reducing the opioid dose. If the patient has good pain control, reduce morphine dose by 25 per cent.

Adverse drug interactions: in patients with advanced cancer, side effects due to drug combinations are common. The potential for additive side effects and serious toxicity from drug combinations must be recognized. The sedative effect of an opioid may add to that produced by numerous other centrally-acting drugs, such as anxiolytics, neuroleptics, and antidepressants[182]. Likewise, drugs with anticholinergic effects probably worsen the constipatory effects of opioids. As noted previously, a severe adverse reaction, including excitation, hyperpyrexia, convulsions, and death, has been reported after the administration of pethidine (meperidine) to patients treated with a monoamine oxidase inhibitor[183].

Gastrointestinal side effects: the gastrointestinal adverse effects of opioids are common. In general, they are characterized by having a weak dose–response relationship.

Constipation: all opioids cause constipation and tolerance to this effect is not observed over time. Importantly, the dose–response relationship to this effect is very flat and the severity does not appear to be strongly dose-related. There is some data to indicate that the severity is less severe with fentanyl and, possibly, methadone[184,185].

The likelihood of opioid-induced constipation is so great that laxative medications should be prescribed prophylactically to most patients. In general, bulking laxatives are discouraged. Besides that, there is no firm data indicating superiority of one laxative over another and recommendations are not evidence based.

Methylnaltrexone, a quaternary derivative of naltrexone that does not cross the blood–brain barrier in humans, is a potentially important product recently licensed in Europe. It antagonizes only peripherally located opioid receptors while sparing centrally mediated analgesic effects of opioid pain medications. There is evidence of very predictable effectiveness after administration by either oral[186,187] or parenteral routes[188] with most patients achieving defecation within 90 min of administration.

Oxycodone and naloxone combined in an oral preparation is already on the market in Europe and such novel combinations are likely to come into increasing use.

Nausea and vomiting: opioids may produce nausea and vomiting through both central and peripheral mechanisms. These drugs stimulate the medullary chemoreceptor trigger zone, increase vestibular sensitivity and have effects on the gastrointestinal tract (including increased gastric antral tone, diminished motility, and delayed gastric emptying). With the initiation of opioid therapy, patients should be informed that nausea can occur. Routine prophylactic administration of an antiemetic is not necessary, except in patients with a history of severe opioid-induced nausea and vomiting, but patients should have access to an antiemetic at the start of therapy if the need for one arises. Nausea and vomiting that persists more than a few days is likely to be a chronic problem. No anti-emetic has proven superiority over another and, indeed, there is little supportive efficacy for any specific agent. Anecdotally, the use of prochlorperazine and metoclopramide or haloperidol is sometimes helpful. Additionally, there is also limited evidence supporting use of transdermal scopolamine[189]. Persistent nausea and vomiting often necessitates an opioid switch.

CNS side effects: the CNS side effects of opioids are generally dose related. The specific pattern of CNS adverse effects is influenced by individual patient factors, duration of opioid exposure, and dose.

Sedation: initiation of opioid therapy or significant dose escalation commonly induces sedation that persists until tolerance to this effect develops, usually in days to weeks. It is useful to forewarn patients of this potential, and thereby reduce anxiety, and encourage avoidance of activities, such as driving, that may be dangerous if sedation occurs[190]. Some patients have a persistent problem with sedation, particularly if other confounding factors exist. These factors include the use of other sedating drugs or coexistent diseases such as dementia, metabolic encephalopathy, or brain metastases. Limited evidence supports the potential efficacy of amphetamines and amphetamine-like agents such as dextroamphetamine; methylphenidate, donepezil, and modafinil in the treatment of opioid-induced sedation[191]. Treatment with methylphenidate or dextroamphetamine is typically begun at 2.5 mg to 5 mg in the morning, which is repeated at mid day if necessary to maintain effects until evening. Doses are then increased gradually if needed. Few patients require more than 40 mg/day in divided doses. This approach is relatively contraindicated among patients with cardiac arrhythmias, agitated delirium, paranoid personality, and past amphetamine abuse.

Confusion and delirium: mild cognitive impairment is common following the initiation of opioid therapy or increase in dose.

Similar to sedation, however, pure opioid-induced encephalopathy appears to be transient in most patients, persisting from days to a week or two. Although persistent confusion attributable to opioid alone occurs[192], the aetiology of persistent delirium is often related to the combined effect of the opioid and other contributing factors, including electrolyte disorders, neoplastic involvement of CNS, sepsis, vital organ failure, and hypoxaemia[192,193]. A stepwise approach to management (Table 10.1.6.10) often culminates in a trial of a neuroleptic drug or opioid rotation. Among the neuroleptic agents, haloperidol in low doses (0.5–1.0 mg PO or 0.25–0.5 mg IV or IM) is most commonly recommended because of its efficacy and low incidence of cardiovascular and anticholinergic effects. As an alternative strategy, there is limited anecdotal experience of the use the of acetylcholinesterase inhibitors; initiated with IV physostigmine, and then maintained with oral donepezil[194].

Respiratory depression: when sedation is used as a clinical indicator of CNS toxicity and appropriate steps are taken, respiratory depression is rare. When, however, it does occur, it is always accompanied by other signs of CNS depression, including sedation and mental clouding[195]. Respiratory compromise accompanied by tachypnoea and anxiety is never a primary opioid event. With repeated opioid administration, tolerance appears to develop rapidly to the respiratory depressant effects of the opioid drugs, consequently clinically important respiratory depression is a very rare event in the cancer patient whose opioid dose has been titrated against pain.

The ability to tolerate high doses of opioids is also related to the stimulus-related effect of pain on respiration in a manner that is balanced against the depressant opioid effect. Opioid-induced respiratory depression can occur, however, if pain is suddenly eliminated (such as may occur following neurolytic procedures) and the opioid dose is not reduced[196].

Careful observation is the best method for monitoring sedation level and respiratory status.

The University Of Wisconsin Hospital And Clinics Sedation Assessment Scale[197] (Table 10.1.6.11) is a very useful aid to assessment, particularly in the sleeping patient.

When respiratory depression occurs in patients on chronic opioid therapy, administration of the specific opioid antagonist, naloxone, usually improves ventilation[195]. This is true even if the primary cause of the respiratory event was not the opioid itself, but rather, an intercurrent cardiac or pulmonary process. A response to naloxone, therefore, should not be taken as proof that the event was due to the opioid alone and an evaluation for these other processes should ensue.

Table 10.1.6.10 A stepwise approach to the management of confusion and delirium.

1) Discontinue non-essential centrally acting medications

2) If analgesia is satisfactory, reduce opioid dose by 25%

3) Exclude sepsis or metabolic derangement

4) Exclude CNS involvement by tumour

5) If delirium persists, consider:
   - Trial of neuroleptic (e.g. haloperidol)
   - Change to an alternative opioid drug
   - A change in opioid route to the intraspinal route (± local anaesthetic)
   - A trial of other anaesthetic or neurosurgical options

Table 10.1.6.11 University Of Wisconsin Hospital And Clinics Sedation Assessment Scale.

N = Normal sleep
1 = Anxious, agitated or restless
2 = Calm, cooperative to tranquil (normal baseline without sedation)
3 = Quiet, drowsy, responds to verbal commands
4 = Asleep, brisk response to forehead tap or loud verbal stimuli
5 = Asleep, sluggish response to increasingly vigorous stimuli
6 = Unresponsive to painful stimuli
(Moderate sedation = sedation score of 4)

Naloxone can precipitate a severe abstinence syndrome and should be administered only if strongly indicated. If the patient is bradypnoeic but readily arousable, and the peak plasma level of the last opioid dose has already been reached, the opioid should be withheld and the patient monitored until improved. If severe hypoventilation occurs (regardless of the associated factors that may be contributing to respiratory compromise), or the patient is bradypnoeic and unarousable, naloxone should be administered. To reduce the risk of severe withdrawal following a period of opioid administration, dilute naloxone (1:10) should be used in doses titrated to respiratory rate and level of consciousness. In the comatose patient, it may be prudent to place an endotracheal tube to prevent aspiration following administration of naloxone.

Multifocus myoclonus: all opioid analgesics can produce myoclonus. Mild and infrequent myoclonus is common. In occasional patients, however, myoclonus can be distressing or contribute to BTP that occurs with the involuntary movement. If the dose cannot be reduced due to persistent pain, consideration should be given to either switching to an alternative opioid[198] or to symptomatic treatment with a benzodiazepine (particularly clonazepam or midazolam), dantrolene or an anticonvulsant such as gabapentin[199].

Other effects

Urinary retention: opioid analgesics increase smooth muscle tone and can occasionally cause bladder spasm or urinary retention (due to an increase in sphincter tone). This is an infrequent problem that is usually observed in elderly male patients. Tolerance can develop rapidly but catheterization may be necessary to manage transient problems.

Opioid-induced hyperalgesia

Accumulating evidence suggests that opioids may cause opioid-induced hyperalgesia. Somewhat paradoxically, opioid therapy aiming at alleviating pain may render patients more sensitive to pain and potentially may aggravate their pre-existing pain. Several recent articles have reviewed this phenomenon[202–206]. The term 'paradoxical pain' has been used in the past and associated with the now unfounded theory of morphine-3-glucuronide being antalgesic[200]. An increase in pain to noxious stimuli, or hyperalgesia, can occur in two types of syndrome. The first is part of the spectrum of opioid toxicity and also includes to variable degrees, hallucinations, vivid dreams, myoclonic jerks, confusion, agitation, and drowsiness. The second form of hyperalgesia occurs as an isolated phenomenon in patients who are taking opioid medication and in whom there are none of the classical signs of opioid toxicity. In both situations, clinical evidence suggests that opioids can elicit increased sensitivity to noxious stimuli, suggesting that the administration of opioids can activate both pain inhibitory and pain facilitatory systems. The exact mechanism of hyperalgesia with opioid toxicity and without opioid toxicity is unclear and may be very different in each of these two broad conditions. There will be a third group of patients in whom the diagnosis of opioid-induced hyperalgesia is missed and escalation of the dose of opioid results in opioid toxicity.

Classically, in opioid-induced hyperalgesia an increase in opioid dose results in worsening pain which is quite different to opioid tolerance where an increase in dose may be ineffective but not associated with acute worsening of the pain. As such patients are understandably very distressed, the problem can often be mislabelled as general distress. The general hyperalgesia and associated distress may also be labelled naïvely as 'total pain' and of course it is genuine 'total pain' according to our modern understanding of the complex underlying mechanisms of this phenomenon, and as such needs appropriate modern palliative care management. Clearly, prognosis can be shortened if an appropriate diagnosis is not made, either because the patient is offered 'palliative sedation' or is rendered opioid toxic by continuing escalation of opioid medication. Successful strategies that may decrease or prevent opioid-induced hyperalgesia include the concomitant administration of drugs like NMDA-antagonists, alpha2-agonists such as clonidine, NSAIDs, or an opioid switch[213,214]. Research in this area is underway.

Opioids and driving

The ability to continue driving is very important to maintaining the quality of life of many patients with advanced cancer. Many assume that they must stop driving whilst taking regular potent opioid analgesics, but this is not necessarily so. The usual advice to patients is that they should not drive or engage in other skilled activities such as operating machinery when they first start on morphine or a similar opioid, or when they increase the dose. However, once the initial sedative effects have resolved and both the patient and physician are confident that cognitive and psychomotor performance is no longer impaired, driving and other similar activities may restart.

This advice is based to a large extent on empirical experience and there have been few objective data to substantiate it. However, recent studies confirm, perhaps surprisingly, that morphine produces little measurable impairment of cognitive and psychomotor function, particularly in patients receiving continuous treatment with stable doses[190,201]. In one study, which used a battery of performance tests designed specifically to assess functions related to driving ability, chronic morphine use was associated with slower reaction times, more mistakes, and a slowing in ability to process visual information and perform motor sequences, but these changes were not statistically significant compared with a control group of cancer patients not taking morphine[190]. These data support the clinical impression that stable doses of morphine are unlikely to cause substantial impairment of the psychomotor skills required for driving, and allow us to continue to advise patients to this effect.

Patients, however, must be reminded of the responsibility of critical self-examination of their fitness to drive on a moment-by-moment basis before and during operating a motor vehicle and should desist if they are aware of any impairment of concentration or alertness[202].

'Allergy' and intolerance to morphine

Morphine and other opioids cause histamine release, and this is said to contribute to asthma or urticaria in allergic patients[98,203,204]. There is no published information on the incidence of this phenomenon and, in our experience, it is very uncommon.

However, it is not uncommon for patients to claim that they are 'allergic' to morphine. This usually means that they have had a bad experience with the drug but, on investigation, what they describe are its common side effects. There is no doubt that most patients experience some adverse effects when they first start regular morphine treatment. Most commonly this is sedation, nausea and, less often, vomiting. All patients must be warned about this and appropriate measures must be taken, as described earlier. If patients are not warned and experience unpleasant adverse effects they will be discouraged from continuing with the drug, and if they do not understand what is going on they may assume they that are 'allergic' to it.

The opioid-dependent patient: definitions and misconceptions

Addiction and substance abuse are social and medical problems of pandemic proportions, which are associated with major social and human costs. Commonly, opioid drugs are the preferred substances of abuse. This association, combined with the principle of non-malfeasance is the basis for concern regarding risk of addiction caused by the medical use of opioids. In recent years the relationship between the medical use of opioids and the risk of addiction has been the focus of policy makers, medical sociologists, and pain clinicians.

Overall, this body of research has demonstrated: (1) the risk of developing addictive behaviours or substance abuse as a consequence of the medical use of opioids for chronic cancer pain is low[205,206]; (2) patient, family members, members of the health-care professions and regulators commonly overestimate the risk of addiction; (3) patient, family members, members of the health-care professions and regulators often confuse physical dependence and addiction; (4) together, these concerns contribute substantially to physician reluctance to prescribe opioids and patient reluctance to use them[207,208]. Sadly, in the United States of America there is now clear evidence of an increasing problem of diversion of prescribed opioids[209,210]. This has generated much public discussion and anxiety about opioid use and underscores the need for vigilance in the storage of opioid medications and the disposal of unused drugs, and used opioid patches.

To understand these phenomena as they relate to opioid treatment of cancer pain, it is useful first to present a concept that might be called 'therapeutic dependence'. Patients who require a specific drug therapy to control a symptom or disease process are clearly dependent on the therapeutic efficacy of the drugs in question. Examples of this 'therapeutic dependence' include the requirements of patients with congestive cardiac failure for cardiotonic and diuretic medication or the reliance of insulin-dependent diabetics on insulin therapy. In these patients, undermedication or withdrawal of treatment would result in serious untoward consequences. Patients with chronic cancer pain have an analogous relationship to their analgesic therapy. This relationship may or may not be associated with the development of physical dependence, but is virtually never associated with addiction.

Psychological dependence and 'addiction'

The properties of the opioid analgesics that are most likely to lead to their being misused are effects mediated in the CNS. The term addiction refers to a psychological and behavioural syndrome characterized by a continued craving for an opioid drug to achieve a psychic effect (psychological dependence) and associated aberrant drug-related behaviours, such as compulsive drug-seeking, unsanctioned use or dose escalation, and use despite harm to self or others. Addiction should be suspected if patients demonstrate compulsive use, loss of control over drug use, and continuing use despite harm. The term addiction should never be used when physical dependence is meant.

There is a common perception that opioid use, for any reason, is associated with a high risk of iatrogenic psychological dependence and that it is best avoided or minimized. Many health-care professionals and laypersons fail to distinguish between patients with substance abuse disorder and psychologically well patients with pain, and consequently overestimate the risk of iatrogenic addiction. This skews evaluation of the therapeutic index of opioids, and impacts adversely on the likelihood of a clinician to prescribe opioids and on the patients' compliance with an opioid prescription.

Physical dependence

Physical dependence is the term used to describe the phenomenon of withdrawal when an opioid is abruptly discontinued or an opioid antagonist is administered[211]. The severity of withdrawal is a function of the dose and duration of administration of the opioid just discontinued (i.e. the patient's prior opioid exposure). The administration of an opioid antagonist to a physically dependent individual produces an immediate precipitation of the withdrawal syndrome. Patients who have received repeated doses of a morphine-like agonist to the point where they are physically dependent may experience an opioid withdrawal reaction when given a mixed agonist–antagonist. It can be shown that prior exposure to a morphine-like drug greatly increases a patient's sensitivity to the antagonist component of a mixed agonist–antagonist. Therefore, when used for chronic pain, the mixed agonist–antagonists should be tried before prolonged administration of a morphine-like agonist is initiated.

The abrupt discontinuation of an opioid analgesic in a patient with significant prior opioid experience will result in signs and symptoms characteristic of the opioid withdrawal or abstinence syndrome[212]. The onset of withdrawal is characterized by the patient's report of feelings of anxiety, nervousness, and irritability, and alternating chills and hot flushes. A prominent withdrawal sign is 'wetness' including salivation, lacrimation, rhinorrhoea, sneezing, and sweating, as well as gooseflesh. At the peak intensity of withdrawal patients may experience nausea and vomiting, abdominal cramps, insomnia, and, rarely, multifocal myoclonus. The time course of the withdrawal syndrome is a function of the elimination half-life of the opioid on which the patient has become dependent. Abstinence symptoms generally appear within 6 to 12 h and reach a peak at 24 to 72 h following cessation of a short-half-life drug such as morphine, while onset may be delayed for 36 to 48 h with methadone which has a long half-life. Therefore it is important to emphasize that, even in a patient in whom pain has been completely relieved by a procedure (e.g. a cordotomy), it is necessary to decrease the opioid dose slowly to prevent withdrawal.

Experience indicates that the usual daily dose required to prevent withdrawal is equal to 75 per cent of the previous daily dose. Following this rule of thumb, doses can be gradually titrated down until the drug is discontinued.

'Pseudoaddiction'

Some cancer patients who continue to experience unrelieved pain manifest intense concern about opioid availability and drug-seeking behaviour that is reminiscent of addiction but ceases once pain is relieved, often through opioid dose escalation. This behaviour has been termed 'pseudoaddiction'[213]. Pain relief usually produced by dose escalation eliminates this aberrant behaviour and distinguishes the patient from the true addict. Misunderstanding of this phenomenon may lead the clinician inappropriately to stigmatize the patient with the label 'addict' which may compromise care and erode the doctor–patient relationship. In the setting of unrelieved pain the request for increases in drug doses requires careful assessment, renewed efforts to manage pain, and avoidance of stigmatizing labels.

Management of cancer pain in patients with a history of drug abuse

Patients with a history of abuse of opioid analgesics may develop cancer and severe pain[214]. It is important to distinguish between the patient with a previous history of abuse and one who is currently abusing or who is in the company of active abusers.

In general, a multi-disciplinary team approach is recommended for the management of at-risk patients. Mental-health professionals who specialize in addiction therapy may be instrumental in helping palliative care team members develop strategies for management and treatment compliance.

In the setting of pain from advanced cancer, having clear treatment goals is essential. In such circumstances, complete abstinence is an unrealistic and inappropriate goal. In general, the aim of therapy is harm-reduction. Reducing the risk of harm from pain, whilst at the same time aiming to minimize risk to the patient and to his social surroundings.

There is no evidence-based experience; advice is anecdotal. Among the published literature suggestions include:

1   In all cases, one clinician should be identified as responsible for pain management.

2   For patients receiving therapy for drug abuse, with or without opioid maintenance therapy (e.g. methadone maintenance), it is essential that the issues relating to the use of opioid analgesics for pain management are discussed not only with the patient but also with his or her family and drug abuse counsellors, so that the patient's support group reaches a consensus on the utility and appropriateness of analgesic therapy. An open and supportive approach, and the use of concomitant psychotropic medication as appropriate, will aid the effective management of these patients.

3   Use of a written agreement between the team and patient provides structure to the treatment plan, establishes clear expectations, and outlines the consequences of aberrant drug-taking.

4   The inclusion of spot urine toxicology screens and pill counts to identify, and possibly address, abuse of other agents.

5   Initially dispensing only enough medication for a limited number of days to reduce the risk of diversion.

6   Regarding drug selection. If the patient is on methadone maintenance, methadone, titrated to effect may be a useful analgesic for strong cancer pain. In other circumstances, longer-acting formulations, which have a slow onset, may help reduce aberrant

drug-taking behaviours when compared with the rapid onset and increased dosage frequency associated with short-acting drugs.

7   Whenever possible, oral medication is preferred, even though patients may require very much larger doses than normal. If parenteral medication is required, continuous subcutaneous infusion remains the mode of administration of choice.

8   These patients are at high risk and they need frequent reassessment of the adequacy of pain and symptom control and of the drug-taking behaviours.

In managing these patients clinicians should be aware of several common issues that may confound therapy. Mental clouding, either as an effect of disease progression or as an iatrogenic adverse effect, commonly raises concerns about the relapse or recurrence of psychological dependence. A request for escalation of their opioid dose may be generated by increased psychological stress rather than pain alone. Aberrant drug-seeking behaviour such as acquisition of opioids from multiple sources, 'loss' of prescribed drugs or prescriptions, unsanctioned dose escalation, and prescription fraud must be recognized as suggestive of true addiction and addressed openly as such.

Conclusions

The 4th edition of this book has seen a dramtic increase in pre-clinical research in opioid analgesic therapy. This will hopefully continue to promote even further our natural curiosity about the clinical effectiveness of this remarkable group of analgesics. However, at present, in spite of the expanding pre-clinical field and some new drug development, the overarching advice about opioids in patient care remains largely unchanged. Some interesting areas of debate should be evaluated in appropriate clinical trials, such as the 2-step versus 3-step question. The optimal management of a patient with cancer-related pain remains in a comprehensive assessment of the pain, concommitent conditions, and psychosocial status of the patient as well as an understanding of the clinical pharmacology of analgesic drugs. Our evolving understanding of 'total pain' and the related pharmacology is undoubtedly going to be an area of major importance to all those managing pain associated with life-limiting illness.

References

1.   Portenoy, R. and Lesage, P. (1999). Management of cancer pain. *Lancet*, **353**(9165), 1695–700.

2.   World Health Organization. (1986). *Cancer Pain Relief*. Geneva: WHO.

3.   Lötsch, J., Zimmermann, M., Darimont, J. *et al.* (2002). Does the A118G polymorphism at the mu-opioid receptor gene protect against morphine-6-glucuronide toxicity? *Anesthesiology*, **97**(4), 814–9.

4.   Hughes, J. and Kosterlitz, H. (1983). Opioid Peptides: introduction. *British Medical Bulletin*, **39**(1), 1–3.

5.   Milligan, G. (2005). Opioid receptors and their interacting proteins. *Neuromolecular Medicine*, **7**(1–2), 51–9.

6.   Mollereau, C., Roumy, M., and Zajac, J. (2005). Opioid-modulating peptides: mechanisms of action. *Current Topics in Medical Chemistry*, **5**(3), 341–55.

7.   Zöllner, C. and Stein, C. (2007). Opioids. *Handbook of Experimental Pharmacology*, (177), 31–63.

8. Urch, C.E., Donovan-Rodriguez, T., and Dickenson, A.H. (2003). Alterations in dorsal horn neurones in a rat model of cancer-induced bone pain. *Pain*, **106**(3), 347–56.

9. Stein, C., Schafer, M., and Machelska, H. (2003). Attacking pain at its source: new perspectives on opioids. *Nature Medicine*, **9**(8), 1003–8.

10. Bailey, C. and Connor, M. (2005). Opioids: cellular mechanisms of tolerance and physical dependence. *Current Opinion in Pharmacology*, **5**(1), 60–8.

11. Ferguson, S. (2001). Evolving concepts in G protein-coupled receptor endocytosis: the role in receptor desensitization and signaling. *Pharmacological Reviews*, **53**(1), 1–24.

12. Watkins, L., Hutchinson, M., Johnston, I. *et al.* (2005). Glia: novel counter-regulators of opioid analgesia. *Trends in Neuroscience*, **28**(12), 661–9.

13. Zhang, J., Ferguson, S., Barak, L. *et al.* (1998). Role for G protein-coupled receptor kinase in agonist-specific regulation of mu-opioid receptor responsiveness. *Proceedings of the National Academy of Sciences, U S A*, **95**(12), 7157–62.

14. Rios, C., Jordan, B., Gomes, I. *et al.* (2001). G-protein-coupled receptor dimerization: modulation of receptor function. *Pharmacology and Therapeutics*, **92**(2–3), 71–87.

15. Chang, G., Chen, L., and Mao, J. (2007). Opioid tolerance and hyperalgesia. *Medicine Clinics of North America*, **91**(2), 199–211.

16. Davis, M., LeGrand, S., and Lagman, R. (2005). Look before leaping: combined opioids may not be the rave. *Support Care Cancer*, **13**(10), 769–74.

17. Trapaidze, N., Gomes, I., Bansinath, M. *et al.* (2000). Recycling and resensitization of delta opioid receptors. *DNA and Cell Biology*, **19**(4), 195–204.

18. Skorpen, F., Laugsand, E.A., Klepstad, P. *et al.* (2008). Variable response to opioid treatment: any genetic predictors within sight? *Palliative Medicine*, **22**(4), 310–27.

19. Lötsch, J. and Geisslinger, G. (2006). Current evidence for a genetic modulation of the response to analgesics. *Pain*, **121**(1–2), 1–5.

20. Skarke, C., Darimont, J., Schmidt, H. *et al.* (2003). Analgesic effects of morphine and morphine-6-glucuronide in a transcutaneous electrical pain model in healthy volunteers. *Clinical Pharmacology and Therapeutics*, **73**(1), 107–21.

21. Sachse, C., Brockmöller, J., Bauer, S. *et al.* (1997). Cytochrome P450 2D6 variants in a Caucasian population: allele frequencies and phenotypic consequences. *American Journal of Human Genetics*, **60**(2), 284–95.

22. Stamer, U., Lehnen, K., Höthker, F. *et al.* (2003). Impact of CYP2D6 genotype on postoperative tramadol analgesia. *Pain*, **105**(1–2), 231–8.

23. Dalén, P., Frengell, C., Dahl, M. *et al.* (1997). Quick onset of severe abdominal pain after codeine in an ultrarapid metabolizer of debrisoquine. *Therapeutic Drug Monitoring*, **19**(5), 543–4.

24. Gasche, Y., Daali, Y., Fathi, M. *et al.* (2004). Codeine intoxication associated with ultrarapid CYP2D6 metabolism. *New England Journal of Medicine*, **351**(27), 2827–31.

25. Campa, D., Gioia, A., Tomei, A. *et al.* (2008). Association of ABCB1/MDR1 and OPRM1 gene polymorphisms with morphine pain relief. *Clinical Pharmacology and Therapeutics*, **83**(4), 559–66.

26. Rakvåg, T., Klepstad, P., Baar, C. *et al.* (2005). The Val158Met polymorphism of the human catechol-O-methyltransferase (COMT) gene may influence morphine requirements in cancer pain patients. *Pain*, **116**(1–2), 73–8.

27. Sindrup, S., Brøsen, K., Bjerring, P. *et al.* (1990). Codeine increases pain thresholds to copper vapor laser stimuli in extensive but not poor metabolizers of sparteine. *Clinical Pharmacology and Therapeutics*, **48**(6), 686–93.

28. Thompson, S., Koszdin, K., and Bernards, C. (2000). Opiate-induced analgesia is increased and prolonged in mice lacking P-glycoprotein. *Anesthesiology*, **92**(5), 1392–9.

29. Ross, J., Riley, J., Taegetmeyer, A. *et al.* (2008). Genetic variation and response to morphine in cancer patients: catechol-O-methyltransferase and multidrug resistance-1 gene polymorphisms are associated with central side effects. *Cancer*, **112**(6), 1390–403.

30. Yaksh, T.L. (1997). Pharmacology and mechanisms of opioid analgesic activity. *Acta Anaesthesiologica Scandinavica*, **41**(1 Pt 2), 94–111.

31. Mcdonald, J. and Lambert, D. (2005). Opioid receptors. *Continuing Education in Anaesthsia Critical Care and Pain*, **5**, 22–25.

32. Johnson, R. (1997). Review of US clinical trials of buprenorphine. *Research and Clinical Forums*, **19**, 17–23.

33. World Health Organization. (1996). *Cancer Pain Relief*. Second edition. Geneva: WHO.

34. Jadad, A. and Browman, G. (1995). The WHO analgesic ladder for cancer pain management. Stepping up the quality of its evaluation. *Journal of the American Medical Association*, **274**(23), 1870–3.

35. Persson, K., Hammarlund-Udenaes, M., Mortimer, O. *et al.* (1992). The postoperative pharmacokinetics of codeine. *European Journal of Clin Pharmacology*, **42**(6), 663–6.

36. Vree, T. and Verwey-van Wissen, C. (1992). Pharmacokinetics and metabolism of codeine in humans. *Biopharmaceutics and Drug Disposition*, **13**(6), 445–60.

37. Rowell, F., Seymour, R., and Rawlins, M. (1983). Pharmacokinetics of intravenous and oral dihydrocodeine and its acid metabolites. *European Journal of Clinical Pharmacology*, **25**(3), 419–24.

38. Crome, P., Gain, R., Ghurye, R. *et al.* (1984). Pharmacokinetics of dextropropoxyphene and nordextropropoxyphene in elderly hospital patients after single and multiple doses of distalgesic. Preliminary analysis of results. *Human Toxicology*, 3 Suppl, 41S–48S.

39. Inturrisi, C., Colburn, W., Verebey, K. *et al.* (1982). Propoxyphene and norpropoxyphene kinetics after single and repeated doses of propoxyphene. *Clinical Pharmacology and Therapeutics*, **31**(2), 157–67.

40. Beaver, W. (1984). Analgesic efficacy of dextropropoxyphene and dextropropoxyphene-containing combinations: a review. *Human Toxicology*, 3 Suppl, 191S–220S.

41. Li Wan Po, A. and Zhang, W. (1997). Systematic overview of co-proxamol to assess analgesic effects of addition of dextropropoxyphene to paracetamol. *British Medical Journal*, **315**(7122), 1565–71.

42. Perrier, D. and Gibaldi, M. (1972). Influence of first-pass effect on the systemic availability of propoxyphene. *Journal of Clinical Pharmacology New Drugs*, **12**(11), 449–52.

43. Rosenberg, W., Ryley, N., Trowell, J. *et al.* (1993). Dextropropoxyphene induced hepatotoxicity: a report of nine cases. *Journal of Hepatology*, **19**(3), 470–4.

44. Hantson, P., Evenepoel, M., Ziade, D. *et al.* (1995). Adverse cardiac manifestations following dextropropoxyphene overdose: can naloxone be helpful? *Annals of Emergency Medicine*, **25**(2), 263–6.

45. Pippenger, C. (1987). Clinically significant carbamazepine drug interactions: an overview. *Epilepsia*, 28 Suppl 3, S71–6.

46. Justice, J. and Kline, S. (1988). Analgesics and warfarin. A case that brings up questions and cautions. *Postgraduate Medicine*, **83**(5), 217–8, 220.

47. Whittington, R. (1984). Dextropropoxyphene deaths: coroner's report. *Human Toxicology*, 3 Suppl, 175S–185S.

48. Kalso, E., Pöyhiä, R., Onnela, P. *et al.* (1991). Intravenous morphine and oxycodone for pain after abdominal surgery. *Acta Anaesthesiologica Scandinavica*, **35**(7), 642–6.

49. Raffa, R., Friderichs, E., Reimann, W. *et al.* (1992). Opioid and nonopioid components independently contribute to the mechanism of action of tramadol, an 'atypical' opioid analgesic. *Journal of Pharmacology and Experimental Therapeutics*, **260**(1), 275–85.

50. Lee, C., McTavish, D., and Sorkin, E. (1993). Tramadol. A preliminary review of its pharmacodynamic and pharmacokinetic properties, and therapeutic potential in acute and chronic pain states. *Drugs*, **46**(2), 313–40.

51. Ventafridda, V., Tamburini, M., Caraceni, A. *et al.* (1987). A validation study of the WHO method for cancer pain relief. *Cancer*, **59**(4), 850–6.

52. Benyhe, S. (1994). Morphine: new aspects in the study of an ancient compound. *Life Sciences*, **55**(13), 969–79.

53. Säwe, J., Svensson, J., and Rane, A. (1983). Morphine metabolism in cancer patients on increasing oral doses--no evidence for autoinduction or dose-dependence. *British Journal of Clinical Pharmacology*, **16**(1), 85–93.

54. Max, M., Inturrisi, C., Kaiko, R. *et al.* (1985). Epidural and intrathecal opiates: cerebrospinal fluid and plasma profiles in patients with chronic cancer pain. *Clinical Pharmacology and Therapeutics*, **38**(6), 631–41.

55. Paul, D., Standifer, K., Inturrisi, C. *et al.* (1989). Pharmacological characterization of morphine-6 beta-glucuronide, a very potent morphine metabolite. *Journal of Pharmacology and Experimental Therapeutics*, **251**(2), 477–83.

56. Portenoy, R., Foley, K., Stulman, J. *et al.* (1991). Plasma morphine and morphine-6-glucuronide during chronic morphine therapy for cancer pain: plasma profiles, steady-state concentrations and the consequences of renal failure. *Pain*, **47**(1), 13–9.

57. D'Honneur, G., Gilton, A., Sandouk, P. *et al.* (1994). Plasma and cerebrospinal fluid concentrations of morphine and morphine glucuronides after oral morphine. The influence of renal failure. *Anesthesiology*, **81**(1), 87–93.

58. Hanks, G. (1991). Morphine pharmacokinetics and analgesia after oral administration. *Postgraduate Medical Journal*, **67** Suppl 2, S60–3.

59. Hewett, K., Dickenson, A., and McQuay, H. (1993). Lack of effect of morphine-3-glucuronide on the spinal antinociceptive actions of morphine in the rat: an electrophysiological study. *Pain*, **53**(1), 59–63.

60. Houde, R., Wallenstein, S., and Beaver, W. (1965). Clinical measurement of pain. *Analgesics*, 75–122.

61. Kaiko, R.F. (1986). Commentary: equianalgesic dose ratio of intramuscular/oral morphine, 1:6 versus 1:3. *Advances in Pain Research and Therapy*, **8**, 87–93.

62. Hanks, G., Hoskin, P., Aherne, G. *et al.* (1987). Explanation for potency of repeated oral doses of morphine? *Lancet*, **2**(8561), 723–5.

63. Hanks, G. (1989). Controlled-release morphine (MST Contin) in advanced cancer. The European experience. *Cancer*, **63**(11 Suppl), 2378–82.

64. Forman, W., Portenoy, R., Yanagihara, R. *et al.* (1993). A novel morphine sulphate preparation: clinical trial of a controlled-release morphine suspension in cancer pain. *Palliative Medicine*, **7**(4), 301–6.

65. Hanks, G., Conno, F., Cherny, N. *et al.* (2001). Morphine and alternative opioids in cancer pain: the EAPC recommendations. *British Journal of Cancer*, **84**(5), 587–93.

66. Inturrisi, C., Max, M., Foley, K. *et al.* (1984). The pharmacokinetics of heroin in patients with chronic pain. *New England Journal of Medicine*, **310**(19), 1213–7.

67. Pasternak, G.W. and Standifer, K.M. (1995). Mapping of opioid receptors using antisense oligodeoxynucleotides: correlating their molecular biology and pharmacology. *Trends in Pharmacological Sciences*, **16**(10), 344–50.

68. Kaiko, R., Wallenstein, S., Rogers, A. *et al.* (1981). Analgesic and mood effects of heroin and morphine in cancer patients with postoperative pain. *New England Journal of Medicine*, **304**(25), 1501–5.

69. Ripamonti, C., Zecca, E., and Bruera, E. (1997). An update on the clinical use of methadone for cancer pain. *Pain*, **70**(2–3), 109–15.

70. Davis, M. and Walsh, D. (2001). Methadone for relief of cancer pain: a review of pharmacokinetics, pharmacodynamics, drug interactions and protocols of administration. *Support Care Cancer*, **9**(2), 73–83.

71. Grochow, L., Sheidler, V., Grossman, S. *et al.* (1989). Does intravenous methadone provide longer lasting analgesia than intravenous morphine? A randomized, double-blind study. *Pain*, **38**(2), 151–7.

72. Säwe, J., Hansen, J., Ginman, C. *et al.* (1981). Patient-controlled dose regimen of methadone for chronic cancer pain. *British Medical Journal*, *(Clinical Research Ed.)*, **282**(6266), 771–3.

73. Mercadante, S., Sapio, M., Serretta, R. *et al.* (1996). Patient-controlled analgesia with oral methadone in cancer pain: preliminary report. *Annals of Oncology*, **7**(6), 613–7.

74. Mathew, P. and Storey, P. (1999). Subcutaneous methadone in terminally ill patients: manageable local toxicity. *Journal of Pain and Symptom Management*, **18**(1), 49–52.

75. Bruera, E., Fainsinger, R., Moore, M. *et al.* (1991). Local toxicity with subcutaneous methadone. Experience of two centers. *Pain*, **45**(2), 141–3.

76. Ripamonti, C., De Conno, F., Groff, L. *et al.* (1998). Equianalgesic dose/ratio between methadone and other opioid agonists in cancer pain: comparison of two clinical experiences. *Annals of Oncology*, **9**(1), 79–83.

77. Szeto, H., Inturrisi, C., Houde, R. *et al.* (1977). Accumulation of normeperidine, an active metabolite of meperidine, in patients with renal failure of cancer. *Annals of Internal Medicine*, **86**(6), 738–41.

78. Eisendrath, S., Goldman, B., Douglas, J. *et al.* (1987). Meperidine-induced delirium. *American Journal of Psychiatry*, **144**(8), 1062–5.

79. Umans, J. and Inturrisi, C. (1982). Antinociceptive activity and toxicity of meperidine and normeperidine in mice. *Journal of Pharmacology and Experimental Therapeutics*, **223**(1), 203–6.

80. Sporer, K. (1995). The serotonin syndrome. Implicated drugs, pathophysiology and management. *Drug Safety*, **13**(2), 94–104.

81. Agency for Health Care Policy and Research: Cancer Pain Management Panel. Management of Cancer Pain. (1994). *Clinical Practice Guideline 9*. Washington DC: US Department of Health and Human Services.

82. Houde, R. (1986). Clinical analgesic studies of hydromorphone. In *Advances in Pain Research and Therapy* (eds K.Foley and C.Inturrisi), pp. 129–36. New York: Raven Press.

83. Sarhill, N., Walsh, D., and Nelson, K. (2001). Hydromorphone: pharmacology and clinical applications in cancer patients. *Support Care Cancer*, **9**(2), 84–96.

84. Moulin, D., Kreeft, J., Murray-Parsons, N. *et al.* (1991). Comparison of continuous subcutaneous and intravenous hydromorphone infusions for management of cancer pain. *Lancet*, **337**(8739), 465–8.

85. Hays, H., Hagen, N., Thirlwell, M. *et al.* (1994). Comparative clinical efficacy and safety of immediate release and controlled release hydromorphone for chronic severe cancer pain. *Cancer*, **74**(6), 1808–16.

86. Brose, W.G., Tanelian, D.L., Brodsky, J.B. *et al.* (1991). CSF and blood pharmacokinetics of hydromorphone and morphine following lumbar epidural administration. *Pain*, **45**(1), 11–15.

87. Anderson, R., Saiers, J., Abram, S. *et al.* (2001). Accuracy in equianalgesic dosing. conversion dilemmas. *Journal of Pain and Symptom Management*, **21**(5), 397–406.

88. Quigley, C. (2002). Hydromorphone for acute and chronic pain. *Cochrane Database of Systematic Reviews*, **1**, CD003447.

89. Dixon, R., Crews, T., Inturrisi, C. *et al.* (1983). Levorphanol: pharmacokinetics and steady-state plasma concentrations in patients with pain. *Research Communications in Chemical Pathology and Pharmacology*, **41**(1), 3–17.

90. Wallenstein, S., Rogers, A.G., Kaiko, R.F. *et al.* (1986). Clinical analgesic studies of levorphanol in acute and chronic cancer pain. In *Advances in Pain Research and Therapy* (eds. K. Foley and C. Inturrisi). New York, Raven Press.

91. Moulin, D.E., Ling, G.S., and Pasternak, G.W. (1988). Unidirectional analgesic cross-tolerance between morphine and levorphanol in the rat. *Pain*, **33**(2), 233–9.

92. Kalso, E. and Vainio, A. (1990). Morphine and oxycodone hydrochloride in the management of cancer pain. *Clinical Pharmacology and Therapeutics*, **47**(5), 639–46.

93. Poyhia, R., Vainio, A., and Kalso, E. (1993). A review of oxycodone's clinical pharmacokinetics and pharmacodynamics. *Journal of Pain and Symptom Management*, **8**(2), 63–7.

94. Kaiko, R.F., Benziger, D.P., Fitzmartin, R.D. *et al.* (1996). Pharmacokinetic-pharmacodynamic relationships of controlled-release oxycodone. *Clinical Pharmacology and Therapeutics*, **59**(1), 52–61.

95. Salzman, R.T., Roberts, M.S., Wild, J. *et al.* (1999). Can a controlled-release oral dose form of oxycodone be used as readily as an immediate-release form for the purpose of titrating to stable pain control? *Journal of Pain and Symptom Management*, **18**(4), 271–9.

96. Leow, K., Cramond, T., and Smith, M. (1995). Pharmacokinetics and pharmacodynamics of oxycodone when given intravenously and rectally to adult patients with cancer pain. *Anesthesia and Analgesia*, **80**(2), 296–302.

97. Eddy, N.B. and Lee, L.E., Jr. (1959). The analgesic equivalence to morphine and relative side action liability of oxymorphone (14-hydroxydihydro morphinone). *Journal of Pharmacology and Experimental Therapeutics*, **125**(2), 116–21.

98. Hermens, J.M., Ebertz, J.M., Hanifin, J.M. *et al.* (1985). Comparison of histamine release in human skin mast cells induced by morphine, fentanyl, and oxymorphone. *Anesthesiology*, **62**(2), 124–9.

99. Rogers, A.G. (1991). Considering histamine release in prescribing opioid analgesics. *Journal of Pain and Symptom Management*, **6**(1), 44–5.

100. Yeadon, M. and Kitchen, I. (1988). Comparative binding of mu and delta selective ligands in whole brain and pons/medulla homogenates from rat: affinity profiles of fentanyl derivatives. *Neuropharmacology*, **27**(4), 345–8.

101. Hess, R., Stiebler, G., and Herz, A. (1972). Pharmacokinetics of fentanyl in man and the rabbit. *European Journal of Clinical Pharmacology*, **4**(3), 137–41.

102. Mather, L.E. (1983). Clinical pharmacokinetics of fentanyl and its newer derivatives. *Clinical Pharmacokinetics*, **8**(5), 422–46.

103. Lehmann, K.A. and Zech, D. (1992). Transdermal fentanyl: clinical pharmacology. *Journal of Pain and Symptom Management*, **7**(3 Suppl), S8–16.

104. Varvel, J.R., Shafer, S.L., Hwang, S.S. *et al.* (1989). Absorption characteristics of transdermally administered fentanyl. *Anesthesiology*, **70**(6), 928–34.

105. Southam, M.A. (1995). Transdermal fentanyl therapy: system design, pharmacokinetics and efficacy. *Anticancer Drugs*, **6** Suppl 3, 29–34.

106. Portenoy, R.K., Southam, M.A., Gupta, S.K. *et al.* (1993). Transdermal fentanyl for cancer pain. Repeated dose pharmacokinetics. *Anesthesiology*, **78**(1), 36–43.

107. Jeal, W. and Benfield, P. (1997). Transdermal fentanyl. A review of its pharmacological properties and therapeutic efficacy in pain control. *Drugs*, **53**(1), 109–38.

108. Megens, A.A., Artois, K., Vermeire, J. *et al.* (1998). Comparison of the analgesic and intestinal effects of fentanyl and morphine in rats. *Journal of Pain and Symptom Management*, **15**(4), 253–7.

109. Payne, R., Mathias, S., Pasta, D. *et al.* (1998). Quality of life and cancer pain: satisfaction and side effects with transdermal fentanyl versus oral morphine. *Journal of Clinical Oncology*, **16**(4), 1588–93.

110. Fine, P.G., Marcus, M., De Boer, A.J. *et al.* (1991). An open label study of oral transmucosal fentanyl citrate (OTFC) for the treatment of breakthrough cancer pain. *Pain*, **45**(2), 149–53.

111. Farrar, J.T., Cleary, J., Rauck, R. *et al.* (1998). Oral transmucosal fentanyl citrate: randomized, double-blinded, placebo-controlled trial for treatment of breakthrough pain in cancer patients. *Journal of the National Cancer Institute*, **90**(8), 611–6.

112. Christie, J.M., Simmonds, M., Patt, R. *et al.* (1998). Dose-titration, multicenter study of oral transmucosal fentanyl citrate for the treatment of breakthrough pain in cancer patients using transdermal fentanyl for persistent pain. *Journal of Clinical Oncology*, **16**(10), 3238–45.

113. Egan, T.D., Sharma, A., Ashburn, M.A. *et al.* (2000). Multiple dose pharmacokinetics of oral transmucosal fentanyl citrate in healthy volunteers. *Anesthesiology*, **92**(3), 665–73.

114. Zeppetella, G. and Ribeiro, M. (2006). Opioids for the management of breakthrough (episodic) pain in cancer patients. *Cochrane Database of Systematic Reviews*, **1**, CD004311.

115. Eichman, J. and Robinson, J. (1998). Mechanistic studies on effervescent-induced permeability enhancement. *Pharmaceutical Research*, **15**(6), 925–30.

116. Darwish, M., Kirby, M., Robertson, P.J. *et al.* (2007). Absolute and relative bioavailability of fentanyl buccal tablet and oral transmucosal fentanyl citrate. *Journal of Clinical Pharmacology*, **47**(3), 343–50.

117. Darwish, M., Tempero, K., Kirby, M. *et al.* (2006). Relative bioavailability of the fentanyl effervescent buccal tablet (FEBT) 1,080 pg versus oral transmucosal fentanyl citrate 1,600 pg and dose proportionality of FEBT 270 to 1,300 microg: a single-dose, randomized, open-label, three-period study in healthy adult volunteers. *Clinical Therapeutics*, **28**(5), 715–24.

118. Darwish, M., Kirby, M., Robertson, P. *et al.* (2007). Absorption of fentanyl from fentanyl buccal tablet in cancer patients with or without oral mucositis: a pilot study. *Clinical Drug Investigation*, **27**(9), 605–11.

119. Shojaei, A. (1998). Buccal mucosa as a route for systemic drug delivery: a review. *Journal of Pharmacy and Pharmaceutical Science*, **1**(1), 15–30.

120. Zeppetella, G. (2001). Sublingual fentanyl citrate for cancer-related breakthrough pain: a pilot study. *Palliative Medicine*, **15**(4), 323–8.

121. Lennernas, B., Hedner, T., Holmberg, M. *et al.* (2005). Pharmacokinetics and tolerability of different doses of fentanyl following sublingual administration of a rapidly dissolving tablet to cancer patients: a new approach to treatment of incident pain. *British Journal of Clinical Pharmacology*, **59**(2), 249–53.

122. Hoskin, P.J. and Hanks, G.W. (1991). Opioid agonist-antagonist drugs in acute and chronic pain states. *Drugs*, **41**(3), 326–44.

123. Rance, M.J. (1979). Animal and molecular pharmacology of mixed agonist-antagonist analgesic drugs. *British Journal of Clinical Pharmacology*, **7** Suppl 3, 281S–286S.

124. Bullingham, R.E., McQuay, H.J., and Moore, R.A. (1983). Clinical pharmacokinetics of narcotic agonist-antagonist drugs. *Clinical Pharmacokinetics*, **8**(4), 332–43.

125. Bullingham, R.E., McQuay, H.J., Dwyer, D. *et al.* (1981). Sublingual buprenorphine used postoperatively: clinical observations and preliminary pharmacokinetic analysis. *British Journal of Clinical Pharmacology*, **12**(2), 117–22.

126. Gal, T.J. (1989). Naloxone reversal of buprenorphine-induced respiratory depression. *Clinical Pharmacology and Therapeutics*, **45**(1), 66–71.

127. Mello, N.K. and Mendelson, J.H. (1980). Buprenorphine suppresses heroin use by heroin addicts. *Science*, **207**(4431), 657–9.

128. Hammersley, R., Cassidy, M.T., and Oliver, J. (1995). Drugs associated with drug-related deaths in Edinburgh and Glasgow, November 1990 to October 1992. *Addiction*, **90**(7), 959–65.

129. Portenoy, R.K., Foley, K.M., and Inturrisi, C.E. (1990). The nature of opioid responsiveness and its implications for neuropathic pain: new hypotheses derived from studies of opioid infusions. *Pain*, **43**(3), 273–86.

130. Neal, E.A., Meffin, P.J., Gregory, P.B. *et al.* (1979). Enhanced bioavailability and decreased clearance of analgesics in patients with cirrhosis. *Gastroenterology*, **77**(1), 96–102.

131. Giacomini, K.M., Giacomini, J.C., Gibson, T.P. *et al.* (1980). Propoxyphene and norpropoxyphene plasma concentrations after oral propoxyphene in cirrhotic patients with and without surgically constructed portacaval shunt. *Clinical Pharmacology and Therapeutics*, **28**(3), 417–24.

132. Patwardhan, R.V., Johnson, R.F., Hoyumpa, A., Jr. *et al.* (1981). Normal metabolism of morphine in cirrhosis. *Gastroenterology*, **81**(6), 1006–11.

133. Hasselstrom, J., Eriksson, S., Persson, A. *et al.* (1990). The metabolism and bioavailability of morphine in patients with severe liver cirrhosis. *British Journal of Clinical Pharmacology*, **29**(3), 289–97.

134. Osborne, R., Joel, S., and Slevin, M. (1986). Morphine intoxication in renal failure: the role of morphine-6-glucuronide. *British Medical Journal (Clinical Research Ed.)*, **292**(6535), 1548–9.

135. Chan, G.L. and Matzke, G.R. (1987). Effects of renal insufficiency on the pharmacokinetics and pharmacodynamics of opioid analgesics. *Drug Intelligence and Clinical Pharmacy*, **21**(10), 773–83.

136. McQuay, H. and Moore, R. (1997). Antidepressants and chronic pain. *British Medical Journal*, **314**(7083), 763–4.

137. Dean, M. (2004). Opioids in renal failure and dialysis patients. *Journal of Pain and Symptom Management*, **28**(5), 497–504.

138. Coyle, N., Adelhardt, J., Foley, K.M., and Portenoy, R.K. (1990). Character of terminal illness in the advanced cancer patient: pain and other symptoms during the last four weeks of life. *Journal of Pain and Symptom Management*, **5**(2), 83–93.

139. Warren, D.E. (1996). Practical use of rectal medications in palliative care. *Journal of Pain and Symptom Management*, **11**(6), 378–87.

140. Coyle, N., Cherny, N.I., and Portenoy, R.K. (1994). Subcutaneous opioid infusions at home. *Oncology (Williston Park)*, **8**(4), 21–7; discussion 31–2, 37.

141. Oliver, D.J. (1985). The use of the syringe driver in terminal care. *British Journal of Clinical Pharmacology*, **20**(5), 515–6.

142. Portenoy, R.K. (1987). Continuous intravenous infusion of opioid drugs. *Medicine Clinics of North America*, **71**(2), 233–41.

143. Russell, P.S. (1979). Analgesia in terminal malignant disease. *British Medical Journal*, **1**(6177), 1561.

144. Bruera, E., Brenneis, C., Michaud, M. *et al.* (1988). Patient-controlled subcutaneous hydromorphone versus continuous subcutaneous infusion for the treatment of cancer pain. *Journal of the National Cancer Institute*, **80**(14), 1152–4.

145. Waldmann, C.S., Eason, J.R., Rambohul, E. *et al.* (1984). Serum morphine levels. A comparison between continuous subcutaneous infusion and continuous intravenous infusion in postoperative patients. *Anaesthesia*, **39**(8), 768–71.

146. O'Doherty, C.A., Hall, E.J., Schofield, L. *et al.* (2001). Drugs and syringe drivers: a survey of adult specialist palliative care practice in the United Kingdom and Eire. *Palliative Medicine*, **15**(2), 149–54.

147. Grassby, P.F. and Hutchings, L. (1997). Drug combinations in syringe drivers: the compatibility and stability of diamorphine with cyclizine and haloperidol. *Palliative Medicine*, **11**(3), 217–24.

148. Moulin, D.E., Inturrisi, C.E., and Foley, K.M. (1986). Cerebrospinal fluid pharmacokinetics of intrathecal morphine sulfate and D-Ala2-D-Leu5-enkephalin. *Annals of Neurology*, **20**(2), 218–22.

149. Du Pen, S.L. and Williams, A.R. (1992). Management of patients receiving combined epidural morphine and bupivacaine for the treatment of cancer pain. *Journal of Pain and Symptom Management*, **7**(2), 125–7.

150. Hogan, Q., Haddox, J.D., Abram, S. *et al.* (1991). Epidural opiates and local anesthetics for the management of cancer pain. *Pain*, **46**(3), 271–9.

151. Weinberg, D.S., Inturrisi, C.E., Reidenberg, B. *et al.* (1988). Sublingual absorption of selected opioid analgesics. *Clinical Pharmacological Therapeutics*, **44**(3), 335–42.

152. Ripamonti, C. and Bruera, E. (1991). Rectal, buccal, and sublingual narcotics for the management of cancer pain. *Journal of Palliative Care*, **7**(1), 30–5.

153. Stein, C. (1995). The control of pain in peripheral tissue by opioids. *New England Journal of Medicine*, **332**(25), 1685–90.

154. Back, I.N. and Finlay, I. (1995). Analgesic effect of topical opioids on painful skin ulcers. *Journal Pain and Symptom Management*, **10**(7), 493.

155. Krajnik, M., Zylicz, Z., Finlay, I. *et al.* (1999). Potential uses of topical opioids in palliative care--report of 6 cases. *Pain*, **80**(1–2), 121–5.

156. Citron, M.L., Kalra, J.M., Seltzer, V.L. *et al.* (1992). Patient-controlled analgesia for cancer pain: a long-term study of inpatient and outpatient use. *Cancer Investigation*. **10**(5), 335–41.

157. Brooks, D.J., Gamble, W., Ahmedzai, S. (1995). A regional survey of opioid use by patients receiving specialist palliative care. *Palliative Medicine*, **9**(3), 229–38.

158. Babul, N., Provencher, L., Laberge, F. *et al.* (1998). Comparative efficacy and safety of controlled-release morphine suppositories and tablets in cancer pain. *Journal of Clinical Pharmacology*, **38**(1), 74–81.

159. McDonald, P., Graham, P., Clayton, M. *et al.* (1991). Regular subcutaneous bolus morphine via an indwelling cannula for pain from advanced cancer. *Palliative Medicine*, **5**, 323–9.

160. Somogyi, A.A., Barratt, D.T., and Coller, J.K. (2007). Pharmacogenetics of opioids. *Clinical Pharmacology and Therapeutics*, **81**(3), 429–44.

161. Stamer, U.M., Bayerer, B., and Stuber, F. (2005). Genetics and variability in opioid response. *European Journal of Pain*, **9**(2), 101–4.

162. Baillie, S.P., Bateman, D.N., Coates, P.E. *et al.* (1989). Age and the pharmacokinetics of morphine. *Age and Ageing*, **18**(4), 258–62.

163. Holdsworth, M.T., Forman, W.B., Killilea, T.A. *et al.* (1994). Transdermal fentanyl disposition in elderly subjects. *Gerontology*, **40**(1), 32–7.

164. Bentley, J.B., Borel, J.D., Nenad, R.E., Jr. *et al.* (1982). Age and fentanyl pharmacokinetics. *Anesthesia and Analgesia*, **61**(12), 968–71.

165. Rapin, C.H. (1989). The treatment of pain in the elderly patient. The use of oral morphine in the treatment of pain. *Journal of Palliative Care*, **5**(4), 54–5.

166. Osborne, R., Joel, S., Grebenik, K. *et al.* (1993). The pharmacokinetics of morphine and morphine glucuronides in kidney failure [see comments]. *Clinical Pharmacology and Therapeutics*, **54**(2), 158–67.

167. Bruera, E., Macmillan, K., Hanson, J. *et al.* (1989). The cognitive effects of the administration of narcotic analgesics in patients with cancer pain. *Pain*, **39**(1), 13–6.

168. Fallon, M. and O'Neill, B. (1998). Substitution of another opioid for morphine. Opioid toxicity should be managed initially by decreasing the opioid dose. *British Medical Journal*, **317**(7150), 81.

169. Portenoy, R.K. (1996). Adjuvant analgesic agents. *Hematological Oncology Clinics of North America*, **10**(1), 103–19.

170. Rubens, R.D., Towlson, K.E., Ramirez, A.J. *et al.* (1992). Appropriate chemotherapy for palliating advanced cancer. *British Medical Journal*, **304**(6818), 35–40.

171. Queisser, W. (1984). Chemotherapy for the treatment of cancer pain. *Recent Results in Cancer Research*, **89**, 171–7.

172. Ripamonti, C., Groff, L., Brunelli, C. *et al.* (1998). Switching from morphine to oral methadone in treating cancer pain: what is the equianalgesic dose ratio? *Journal of Clinical Oncology*, **16**(10), 3216–21.

173. Ashby, M.A., Martin, P., and Jackson, K.A. (1999). Opioid substitution to reduce adverse effects in cancer pain management. *Medical Journal of Australia*, **170**(2), 68–71.

174. Mercadante, S. and Bruera, E. (2006). Opioid switching: A systematic and critical review. *Cancer Treatment Review*, **32**(4), 304–15.

175. Quigley, C. (2004). Opioid switching to improve pain relief and drug tolerability. *Cochrane Database of Systematic Review*, **3**, CD004847.

176. Ross, J.R., Riley, J., Quigley, C. *et al.* (2006). Clinical pharmacology and pharmacotherapy of opioid switching in cancer patients. *Oncologist*, **11**(7), 765–73.

177. Poulsen, L., Brosen, K., Arendt-Nielsen, L. *et al.* (1996). Codeine and morphine in extensive and poor metabolizers of sparteine: pharmacokinetics, analgesic effect and side effects. *European Journal of Clinical Pharmacology*, **51**(3–4), 289–95.

178. Hennessy, M. and Spiers, J.P. (2007). A primer on the mechanics of P-glycoprotein the multidrug transporter. *Pharmacology Research*, **55**(1), 1–15.

179. Dagenais, C., Graff, C.L., and Pollack, G.M. (2004). Variable modulation of opioid brain uptake by P-glycoprotein in mice. *Biochemical Pharmacology*, **67**(2), 269–76.

180. Hoffmeyer, S., Burk, O., von Richter, O. *et al.* (2000). Functional polymorphisms of the human multidrug-resistance gene: multiple sequence variations and correlation of one allele with P-glycoprotein expression and activity in vivo. *Proceedings of the National Academy of Sciences, U S A*, **97**(7), 3473–8.

181. Drexel, H., Dzien, A., Spiegel, R.W. *et al.* (1989). Treatment of severe cancer pain by low-dose continuous subcutaneous morphine. *Pain*, **36**(2), 169–76.

182. Pies, R. (1996). Psychotropic medications and the oncology patient. *Cancer Practice*, **4**(3), 164–6.

183. Browne, B. and Linter, S. (1987). Monoamine oxidase inhibitors and narcotic analgesics. A critical review of the implications for treatment. *British Journal of Psychiatry*, **151**, 210–2.

184. Staats, P.S., Markowitz, J., and Schein, J. (2004). Incidence of constipation associated with long-acting opioid therapy: a comparative study. *Southern Medical Journal*, **97**(2), 129–34.

185. Pappagallo, M. (2001). Incidence, prevalence, and management of opioid bowel dysfunction. *American Journal of Surgery*, **182**(5A Suppl), 11S–18S.

186. Yuan, C.S. and Foss, J.F. (2000). Oral methylnaltrexone for opioid-induced constipation. *Journal of the American Medical Association*, **284**(11), 1383–4.

187. Yuan, C.S., Foss, J.F., Osinski, J. *et al.* (1997). The safety and efficacy of oral methylnaltrexone in preventing morphine-induced delay in oral-cecal transit time. *Clinical Pharmacology and Therapeutics*, **61**(4), 467–75.

188. Yuan, C.S. (2004). Clinical status of methylnaltrexone, a new agent to prevent and manage opioid-induced side effects. *Journal of Support Oncology*, **2**(2), 111–7, discussion 119–22.

189. Ferris, F.D., Kerr, I.G., Sone, M. *et al.* (1991). Transdermal scopolamine use in the control of narcotic-induced nausea. *Journal of Pain and Symptom Management*, **6**(6), 389–93.

190. Vainio, A., Ollila, J., Matikainen, E. *et al.* (1995). Driving ability in cancer patients receiving long-term morphine analgesia. *Lancet*, **346**(8976), 667–70.

191. Reissig, J.E. and Rybarczyk, A.M. (2005). Pharmacologic treatment of opioid-induced sedation in chronic pain. *Annals of Pharmacotherapy*, **39**(4), 727–31.

192. Gaudreau, J.D., Gagnon, P., Roy, M.A. *et al.* (2007). Opioid medications and longitudinal risk of delirium in hospitalized cancer patients. *Cancer*, **109**(11), 2365–73.

193. Centeno, C., Sanz, A., and Bruera, E. (2004). Delirium in advanced cancer patients. *Palliative Medicine*, **18**(3), 184–94.

194. Slatkin, N. and Rhiner, M. (2004). Treatment of opioid-induced delirium with acetylcholinesterase inhibitors: a case report. *Journal of Pain and Symptom Management*, **27**(3), 268–73.

195. Dahan, A. (2007). Respiratory depression with opioids. *Journal of Pain Palliative Care Pharmacotherapy*, **21**(1), 63–6.

196. Wells, C.J., Lipton, S., and Lahuerta, J. (1984). Respiratory depression after percutaneous cervical anterolateral cordotomy in patients on slow-release oral morphine [letter]. *Lancet*, **1**(8379), 739.

197. Gordon, D., Deeren, S., Ford, M. *et al.* (2000). *Epidural Analgesia*. 3rd ed. University of Wisconsin Hospital & Clinics.

198. Cherny, N.J., Chang, V., Frager, G. *et al.* (1995). Opioid pharmacotherapy in the management of cancer pain: a survey of strategies used by pain physicians for the selection of analgesic drugs and routes of administration. *Cancer*, **76**(7), 1283–93.

199. Mercadante, S., Villari, P., and Fulfaro, F. (2001). Gabapentin for opiod-related myoclonus in cancer patients. *Support Care Cancer*, **9**(3), 205–6.

200. Penson,R,. Joel, S., Gloyne, A. *et al.* (2005). Morphine analgesia in cancer pain: role of the glucuronides. *Journal of Opioid Management*, **1**(2), 83–90.

201. Byas-Smith, M.G., Chapman, S.L., Reed, B. *et al.* (2005). The effect of opioids on driving and psychomotor performance in patients with chronic pain. *Clinical Journal of Pain*, **21**(4), 345–52.

202. Brandman, J.F. (2005). Cancer patients, opioids, and driving. *Journal of Support in Oncology*, **3**(4), 317–20.

203. Katcher, J. and Walsh, D. (1999). Opioid-induced itching: morphine sulfate and hydromorphone hydrochloride. *Journal of Pain and Symptom Management*, **17**(1), 70–2.

204. Warner, M.A., Hosking, M.P., Gray, J.R. *et al.* (1991). Narcotic-induced histamine release: a comparison of morphine, oxymorphone, and fentanyl infusions. *Journal of Cardiothoracic and Vascular Anesthesia*, **5**(5), 481–4.

205. Hojsted, J. and Sjogren, P. (2007). Addiction to opioids in chronic pain patients: a literature review. *European Journal of Pain*, **11**(5), 490–518.

206. Passik, S., Kirsh, K., McDonald, M. *et al.* (2000). A Pilot Survey of Aberrant Drug-Taking Attitudes and Behaviors in Samples of Cancer and AIDS Patients. *Journal of Pain and Symptom Management*, **19**(4), 274–86.

207. Ward, S.E., Goldberg, N., Miller-McCauley, V. *et al.* (1993). Patient-related barriers to management of cancer pain. *Pain*, **52**(3), 319–24.

208. McCaffery, M. (1992). Pain control. Barriers to the use of available information. World Health Organization Expert Committee on Cancer Pain Relief and Active Supportive Care. *Cancer*, **70**(5 Suppl), 1438–49.

209. Joranson, D.E. and Gilson, A.M. (2007). A much-needed window on opioid diversion. *Pain Medicine*, **8**(2), 128–9.

210. Epstein, R.H., Gratch, D.M., and Grunwald, Z. (2007). Development of a scheduled drug diversion surveillance system based on an analysis of atypical drug transactions. *Anesthesia and Analgesia*, **105**(4), 1053–60, table of contents.

211. Jasinski, D.R. (1981). Opiate withdrawal syndrome: acute and protracted aspects. *Annals of the New York Academy of Science*, **362**, 183–6.

212. Rogers, A.G. (1991). Prevention of the withdrawal syndrome in an opioid-dependent one-year-old child with decreasing pain. *Journal of Pain and Symptom Management*, **6**(3), 129.

213. Weissman, D.E. and Haddox, J.D. (1989). Opioid pseudoaddiction-- an iatrogenic syndrome. *Pain*, **36**(3), 363–6.

214. Passik, S.D. and Kirsh, K.L. (2005). Managing pain in patients with aberrant drug-taking behaviors. *Journal of Support in Oncology*, **3**(1), 83–6.

10.1.7 **Non-opioid analgesics**

Per Sjøgren, Frank Elsner, and Stein Kaasa

Introduction

Non-opioid analgesics encompass the non-steroidal anti-inflammatory drugs (NSAIDs), acetylsalicylic acid (ASA, aspirin), and paracetamol (acetaminophen). Advantages of non-opioid analgesics include their wide availability, familiarity to patients, effectiveness for milder pain conditions, ease of administration, additive analgesia when combined with other analgesics, and relatively low cost. In most Western societies patients use them off-prescription to treat minor ailments. In palliative medicine, they represent the first step of the analgesic ladder with or without adjuvant analgesics as well as an important supplement to opioids and adjuvant analgesics at higher steps of the ladder[1]. Non-opioid analgesics are widely used in mild-to-moderate pain and NSAIDs and ASA seem to be particularly efficient in inflammatory pain conditions such as bone pain, while paracetamol has very limited anti-inflammatory effects. All non-opioids have antipyretic properties. Disadvantages of non-opioid analgesics include a ceiling for analgesic effect versus dose, risk of side effects, including gastrointestinal bleeding and renal toxicity (NSAIDs and ASA), and hepatotoxicity (paracetamol).

Dipyrone and nefopam are also characterized as non-opioid analgesics, however, due to their limited use they will not be considered in this chapter.

Anti-inflammatory mechanisms

Only 36 years ago Vane postulated that an inhibitory influence on prostaglandin (PG) synthesis was the main effect of analgesics such as ASA[2]. Subsequently, this led to the development of different types of drugs, which aimed at inhibiting the synthesis of PGs. A large number of NSAIDs were designed, and after the discovery of the two isoforms of cyclooxygenase (COXs), specific COX-inhibitors became the focus of NSAID development. The COX-2-specific

NSAIDs (coxibs) are the latest group to emerge from these activities. The expression of COX-1 produces PGs, which are responsible for the protection of gastric mucosa, maintenance of normal kidney function, and platelet aggregation, and COX-2 expression produces more specifically PGs involved in inflammation, fever, and pain. Conventional NSAIDs inhibit both COX-1 and COX-2, whereas coxibs inhibit COX-2. Thus, the inhibition of PG synthesis using NSAIDs or ASA reduces inflammation and relieves pain, however, as PG synthesis takes place in many different organs of the body inhibition of this pathway may cause many other effects[3–5]. Other substances like bradykinin and cytokines also induce nociception as well as stimulate the synthesis of PGs, which, in turn together with mediators such as substance P and calcitonin gene-related peptide cause further nociception[6].

The antipyretic action of NSAIDs is still not fully understood. In animal studies, endothelial cells expressed COX-2-mRNA in response to systemic interleukin-1 beta. The resulting production of PGs in the hypothalamus area may play an important role in producing fever[7].

Arachidonic acid as the precursor of PGs is produced by cell-membrane phospholipids. PGs are lipid-soluble, short-lived molecules, which are not stored in the body, but will be produced in response to noxious stimuli. The different actions of the PGs are indicated in Fig. 10.1.7.1. In addition to COX-1 and COX-2, a COX-3 has been proposed as a variation expressed by the COX-1-gene[8]. Current opinion, however, is that COX-3 does not exist in humans, and the discussions regarding COX variants are still ongoing[9–12].

Mediators of the inflammatory process—especially the cytokines—induce the production of COX-2 within hours. The induction of COX-2 does not only take place in injured tissues, but also in the CNS. In CNS, high concentrations of COX-2 cause increasing concentrations of PGs, which, in turn, induce central sensitization and consequently more pain[13,14]. However, under normal physiological conditions, COX-2 is found only at very low concentrations in the body including brain tissue[15,16].

Not only PGs, but also leukotrienes are responsible for and involved in anaphylactic reactions, broncho-constriction, chemotaxis, as well as vascular permeability and inflammation[6]. PG synthesis inhibitors such as NSAIDs and ASA do not inhibit the production of leukotrienes, which to some extent may explain the limited efficacy of NSAIDs and ASA, when treating pain of inflammatory origin.

COX-1 is constitutive, which means that it exists and acts continuously in many different tissues (Fig. 10.1.7.1). Especially in gastric epithelial cells COX-1 predominates and is responsible for the production of the protective PGI_2 (prostacyclin). Multiple actions of PGI_2 are involved in the protection of gastric mucosa: maintenance of mucosal blood flow, mucus production, secretion of bicarbonate, and also a positive influence on epithelial cell regeneration in order to provide a well-protected gastric mucosa. Thus, the inhibition of the production of PGI_2 by NSAIDs can upset this protective equilibrium[17].

COX-1 is also responsible for the synthesis of PGE_2, which in addition to vasodilatation during inflammatory processes counteracts vasoconstriction in the kidneys. Under normal physiological conditions, the PG synthesis activity in the kidney is low and its role in modifying renal blood flow is not of major importance[18]. However, if renal blood flow is critically lowered, glomerular filtration rate may be partly restored by vasodilatatory effects of PGE$_2$. If PGE$_2$ production is reduced due to the use of NSAIDs or ASA, volume depletions of different aetiologies may aggravate the reduction of renal blood flow. Moreover, inhibition of PGs may also result in a higher extra-cellular concentration of electrolytes such as sodium, which may cause water retention and oedema. In 10 to 25 per cent of the patients treated with NSAIDs, sodium retention can be found[6].

Tromboxane A$_2$ (TXA$_2$) and PGI$_2$ are produced in platelets. PGI$_2$ prevents aggregation of platelets, but does not influence endothelial adherence, whereas TXA$_2$ is mainly responsible for coagulation. When NSAIDs reduce inflammation by COX-2 inhibition, they inhibit temporarily platelet aggregation by decreasing TXA$_2$ synthesis via incomplete and reversible inactivation of COX-1. The anti-thrombotic action of ASA is mainly due to inhibition of TXA$_2$-mediated platelet aggregation related to a complete and irreversible inactivation of COX-1 in platelets by acetylation of the enzyme[19].

Recently, epidemiological surveys studying users and non-users of NSAIDs and ASA have shown that NSAIDs could be of benefit against the development and growth of malignancies. Clinical trials in patients with familial adenomatosis polyposis have shown the efficacy of NSAIDs in reducing the number as well as the size of colorectal polyps. However, a primary chemo-preventive effect has not yet been demonstrated. NSAIDs are also supposed to have a preventive and growth inhibitory effect in extra-colonic epithelial malignancies. Pre-clinical studies show promising results with combination treatments of either chemotherapy or radiotherapy with NSAIDs. However, NSAID effects in cancer cells are mediated not only by COX enzymes, but also by interactions with downstream effectors of inflammation[20].

NSAIDS have also been proposed to be effective in the treatment of cancer-induced cachexia. The effect can be explained through the 'cytokine pathway' in the development of cachexia and consequently the blocking effect of NSAIDS on cytokines may slow down the development of cancer cachexia.

The pharmacology of NSAIDs

Absorption, distribution, metabolism, and excretion

Most important NSAIDs are administered orally, and absorption takes place mainly in the upper gastrointestinal tract; however, stomach mucosa may also absorb substantial parts of the NSAID, especially at low pH. If administered as suppositories, most of the NSAID crosses the mucosal membrane easily. Recommended maximum doses and pharmacokinetic data of widely used NSAIDs are shown in Table 10.1.7.1.

If administered orally pain relief will be achieved within 30 min and a peak concentration will be reached within 120 min with most of the NSAIDs. Depending on the half-life of each NSAID, a continuous decline of the drug's concentration can be observed.

There is evidence that topical administration of NSAIDs can be an effective way of treating pain in special indications. However, the pharmacology of topical NSAIDs is not completely understood[21].

Intravenous and intramuscular injections are also possible routes of administration. There are only a few publications which compare possible advantages and disadvantages of the parenteral and oral routes[22].

In general, plasma protein binding of NSAIDs ranges from 90 per cent to 99 per cent. NSAIDs are predominantly metabolized in the liver by conjugation to sulphate and glucuronide compounds. Conjugation in a quite small and insignificant percentage may also take place in other tissues of the body. Hepatic metabolism by the CYP system may be subject to circadian differences. However, the potential clinical relevance of this phenomenon remains unclear[6].

Most of the NSAIDs are rapidly distributed in all tissues of the body. The more lipid-soluble a NSAID is, the more CNS effects can be expected. However, the very high plasma protein binding will retain most of the drug within the plasma compartment[6].

NSAIDs are eliminated in the urine in free and conjugated forms. The relative amounts of free and conjugated compounds in the

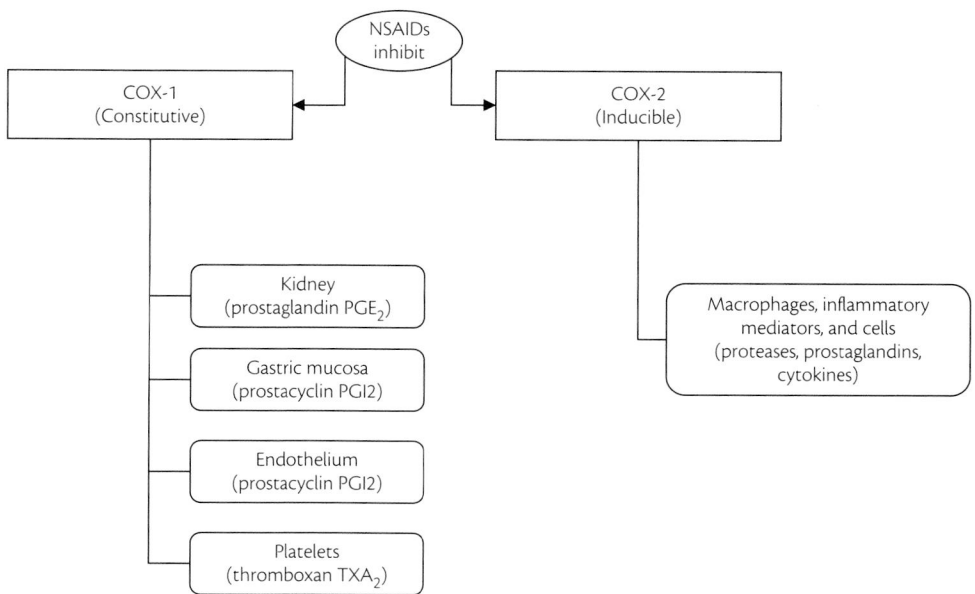

Figure 10.1.7.1 Simple diagram of NSAIDs' influence on prostaglandin synthesis.

Table 10.1.7.1 Choice of oral NSAIDs.

	Pharmacokinetics		Dosage
NSAID			
Ibuprofen	◆ Peak Cp	◆ 15–30 min	400–800 mg 3–4 times/day
	◆ Protein binding	◆ 99 per cent	
	◆ Half-life	◆ 2–4 h	
Diclofenac	◆ Peak Cp	◆ 2–3 h	50–75 mg 3 times/day
	◆ Protein binding	◆ 99 per cent	
	◆ Half-life	◆ 1–2 h	
Naproxen	◆ Peak Cp	◆ 1 h	500 mg Twice/day
	◆ Protein binding	◆ 99 per cent	
	◆ Half-life	◆ 14 h	
Flurbiprofen	◆ Peak Cp	◆ 1–2 h	200–300 mg/day Resp. 100 mg 3 times/day
	◆ Protein binding	◆ 99 per cent	
	◆ Half-life	◆ 6 h	
Indomethacin	◆ Peak Cp	◆ 1–2 h	25 mg 2–3 times/day
	◆ Protein binding	◆ 90 per cent	
	◆ Half-life	◆ 2.5h	
Meloxicam	◆ Peak Cp	◆ 5–10 h	7.5–15 mg Once/day
	◆ Protein binding	◆ 99 per cent	
	◆ Half-life	◆ 24 h	
COX-2-inhibitors			
Celecoxib	◆ Peak Cp	◆ 2–4 h	200–400 mg Twice/day
	◆ Protein binding	◆ 97 per cent	
	◆ Half-life	◆ 6–12 h	
Valdecoxib	◆ Peak Cp	◆ 2–4 h	20 mg Twice/day
	◆ Protein binding	◆ 98 per cent	
	◆ Half-life	◆ 7–8 h	
Etoricoxib	◆ Peak Cp	◆ 1 h	60–120 mg Once/day
	◆ Protein binding	◆ 92 per cent	
	◆ Half-life	◆ 20–26 h	

Note: Cp: Plasma concentration; half-life: is the amount of time it takes before half of the active elements are either eliminated or broken down.
Source: World Health Organization. (1996). *Cancer pain relief: with a guide to opioid availability.* Geneva: World Health Organization.

urine is highly dependent on its pH. Higher pH-values favour more acidic forms of elimination products. A small percentage of the drug can be found in the bile as well, which indicates that excretion also takes place via the intestines into the faeces[6].

Clinical efficacy of NSAIDs alone and in combination with opioids

Using systematic reviews, a useful measure of the relative efficacy of a treatment is the number-needed-to-treat (NNT), which is the number of patients that need to be treated before one benefits from a specific drug compared to placebo[21]. The degree of efficacy can be defined for instance as 30 per cent or 50 per cent pain relief for a certain period of time. NNT data regarding the use of NSAIDs alone in patients suffering from pain of malignant origin do not exist. Assessing efficacy of NSAIDs alone during long-term treatment of cancer patients by defining NNT is quite difficult as very

few patients are treated solely with NSAIDs for a prolonged period of time. However, data on NNT exist regarding the different NSAIDs in postoperative settings aiming at 50 per cent pain relief for a period of 6 h after having received a single dose of the drug. NNTs for diclofenac 50 mg and ibuprofen 400 mg were between 2 and 3, which may be considered an effective intervention. In comparison, a single-dose 10 mg intramuscular morphine injection had a slightly higher NNT value[23].

The efficacy of NSAIDs alone or in combination with opioids has been reviewed systematically[24]. The authors did not to calculate NNT for the analysed studies, because of few reported dichotomous data. Based on limited data, they cautiously concluded, that NSAIDs seem to be more effective than placebo for cancer-related pain. There seems to be no evidence that might show superior efficacy or safety of one NSAID in comparison to another. Furthermore, the efficacy of NSAIDs in different cancer-related pain mechanisms could not be established.

In 2001, the Agency for Health Care Research and Quality (AHRQ) in the United States published a report on the management of cancer pain. They concluded that NSAIDs or opioids individually reduced cancer-related pain. They also concluded that the analysed studies neither could separate the analgesic efficacy of the individual NSAIDs and opioids, nor could they show that NSAIDs were specifically effective for bone pain[25].

Side effects and toxicity of NSAIDs

NSAIDs administered alone or in combination with other analgesics should be used carefully. Especially, during chronic use, the potential side effects have to be weighed carefully against potential advantages. Generally, side effects can occur widely in the body, where prostaglandin synthesis plays a role in modifying physiological mechanisms.

Gastrointestinal side effects

The most common symptoms associated with the intake of NSAIDs are gastrointestinal side effects (Table 10.1.7.2). Symptoms like these may be associated with gastric and/or intestinal erosions followed by ulcerations and can be observed in up to 30 per cent of users of NSAIDs. The degree of erosive or ulcerative changes of the mucosa may vary widely and haemorrhage may range from harmless to life threatening. *Helicobacter pylori* seems to lead to more serious lesions and bleeding. On the whole, the likelihood of serious gastrointestinal adverse events is three times higher in persons taking NSAIDs than in non-users[6].

Coxibs have been shown to be less likely to cause gastric ulcers than traditional NSAIDs[26,27]. Whether the outcome was complicated by bleeding events, symptomatic ulcers, or both, the gastrointestinal risks with coxibs was consistently about half of that with traditional NSAIDs. In randomized trials, coxibs had significantly lower rates for upper gastrointestinal bleeding, symptomatic ulcers, endoscopic ulcers, anaemia, and withdrawal due to gastrointestinal symptoms. Coxibs combined with low-dose ASA demonstrated the same frequency of endoscopic ulcers as traditional NSAIDs[26,28–32]. Regarding lower gastrointestinal bleeding the evidence, however, is weaker. Most studies indicate a significant reduction of these events (by about 50 per cent) with coxibs compared with traditional NSAIDs. How far these effects are only related to COX-2-selectivity is still unclear. Gastrointestinal toxicity does not only depend on the effects of NSAIDs alone, but is related to other risk factors such as age above 65 years, *Helicobacter pylori* infection, peptic ulceration

Table 10.1.7.2 Side effects of NSAIDs in general.

Where	What
◆ Gastrointestinal tract	◆ Pain
	◆ Nausea
	◆ Gastric erosion: ulceration
	◆ Bleeding
	◆ Perforation
◆ Kidney	◆ Water and sodium retention
	◆ Oedema
	◆ Hyperkalaemia
	◆ Decreased effectiveness of
	• Antihypertensive agents
	• Diuretics
◆ Central nervous system	◆ Dizziness
	◆ Headache
	◆ Confusion
	◆ Vertigo
	◆ Depression
◆ Platelet function	◆ Inhibition of activation
	◆ Increased risk of haemorrhage
◆ Special areas of hypersensitivity	◆ Rhinitis
	◆ Bronchial asthma
	◆ Urticaria
	◆ Flushing
	◆ Hypotension
	◆ Shock

Source: Modified from Goodman and Gilman's. (2006). *The Pharmacological Basis of Therapeutics,* 11th edition. McGraw-Hill Medical Publishing Division. With permission.

within the last year, simultaneous intake of corticosteroids, low-dose ASA and/or anticoagulants, far-advanced disease, cardiovascular disease, renal and hepatic impairment, diabetes mellitus, smoking, and excessive alcohol use[33].

Of the traditional NSAIDs, ibuprofen seems to be the least harmful drug in terms of the risk of upper gastrointestinal bleeding. In comparison to non-users of NSAIDs, patients taking coxibs seem to have a low relative risk of gastrointestinal bleeding followed by ibuprofen and diclofenac. A medium risk seems to be present for flurbiprofen, indomethacin, and naproxen, and a high risk has been proposed for ASA and ketorolac[34].

Due to the high risks of gastrointestinal side effects of traditional NSAIDs in frail patients, the use of gastro-protective strategies prevails, although the evidence is still limited[32]. Proton pump inhibitors (PPIs) and misoprostol, both reduce the incidence of gastric and duodenal ulcers, as well as recurrence in patients receiving traditional NSAIDs. Although misoprostol is slightly more effective in preventing gastric ulcers, PPIs are better tolerated as misoprostol often causes diarrhoea[35,36]. Upper gastrointestinal bleeding, endoscopic ulcers and withdrawal from treatment were significantly reduced by the combination of traditional NSAIDs and a PPI compared to traditional NSAIDs alone[37]. Randomized trials have directly compared coxibs with traditional NSAIDs plus PPI in patients with previous ulcer bleeding, and who needed NSAIDs for

arthritis. Serious gastrointestinal complications were of no difference for coxibs and traditional NSAIDs plus PPI (4.2 per cent vs. 6.0 per cent), withdrawal from treatment due to side effects were of a similar magnitude in the groups (4.5 per cent vs. 3.8 per cent), however, dyspepsia was significantly more common with coxibs than traditional NSAIDs plus PPI[32,38,39].

There is only weak evidence for beneficial effects of histamine antagonists with traditional NSAIDs as only one study has shown reduction of endoscopic ulcers compared with traditional NSAIDs alone[37]. The potential preventive effects histamine antagonists on NSAID induced peptic ulcers have not been proven.

The duration of the use of NSAIDs and the risk of developing gastrointestinal bleeding seem to be weakly associated, whereas the incidence of haemorrhage is highly associated with high doses[34].

Nephrotoxicity and hypertension

With acute- and chronic-use NSAIDs, both coxibs and traditional NSAIDs can cause acute renal failure and hypertension[40]. Especially, in patients with renal failure, NSAIDs may reinforce impairment by suppressing PG synthesis. In contrast, NSAIDs only marginally influence renal function and blood pressure in healthy humans.

Patients with chronic heart or kidney diseases, liver cirrhosis, dehydration, or any other condition causing activation of the sympatico-adrenergic and/or renin–angiotensin system depend very much on a normal PG status for maintaining adequate function of the kidneys[41]. Probably, the production of PGE2 and PGI2 depends on the activity of COX-2[42]. This may indicate that there is no difference in side effects of traditional NSAIDs and COX-2-inhibitors with regard to the induction of nephrotoxicity and hypertension. Furthermore, long-term treatment may significantly increase the risk of developing and maintaining renal failure, as may the use of NSAIDs with a long half-life[43].

Renal papillary necrosis induced by non-specific NSAIDs is well recognized, however, recent case reports have also described this complication with the COX-2-specific inhibitors[44,45]. The vascular supply within the renal papillae is dependent on local renal prostagladin production. Clinical conditions resulting in volume depletion or decreased renal blood flow in association with NSAID ingestion may lead to elevated concentrations of NSAIDs and their metabolites within the papillae, which inhibit the vasodilatatory effect of the PGs and can lead to renal papillary necrosis.

Congestive heart failure, coronary heart disease, and thrombosis

In frail and elderly patients, congestive heart failure may result from treatment with NSAIDs. In patients who were admitted to hospital diagnosed with congestive heart failure, a higher percentage (17 per cent) had recently used NSAIDs than in a control group of patients not suffering from congestive heart failure (use of NSAIDs only in 12 per cent). The risk of congestive heart failure increased with an additional history of heart disease[46,47].

As mentioned earlier, TXA_2 is a potent vasoconstrictor, which promotes platelet aggregation. TXA_2 is induced by the activity of COX-1 and in effect it acts as a prothrombotic agent. On the other hand, PGI_2 causes vasodilatation, and thereby inhibits the aggregation of platelets. Selective inhibition of COX-2 increases the relative activity of TXA_2, which subsequently may facilitate the formation of thromboses. Thus, in patients with coronary heart disease, a reduction of COX-2 activity by using coxibs may increase the risks for acute cardiovascular events such as strokes, thromboses, and myocardial infarction[27,48–50]. However, recent findings have also showed that celecoxib does not increase cardiovascular risks[50], and a recent meta-analysis of randomized trials including coxibs and traditional NSAIDs of a treatment length greater than 4 weeks showed that coxibs were associated with a moderate increase in the risk of vascular events (defined as myocardial infarction, stroke, or vascular death), as were high-dose regimens of ibuprofen and diclofenac. However, high-dose naproxen was not associated with such events[51]. Another recent systematic review confirmed that the relative risk of myocardial infarction varied with the individual NSAIDs. An increased risk was observed for diclofenac and rofecoxib, the latter with a clear dose–response trend: the risk elevation was higher for doses greater than 25mg/day (78 per cent) than for lower doses (18 per cent)[52]. Rofecoxib was withdrawn from the market in September 2004.

Contraindications and drug interactions

Gastrointestinal haemorrhage within the last year, renal failure, a specific history of NSAID-induced asthma, a specific incident of an allergic reaction to NSAIDs are contraindications to using NSAIDs. Specific contraindications for coxibs are a history of stroke or coronary heart disease. Following recommendations of the European Agency for the Evaluation of Medicinal Products (www.emea. europa.eu/pdfs/human/epar/Etoricoxib.pdf) etoricoxib is additionally contraindicated in cases of hypertension, severe hepatic dysfunction, inflammatory bowel disease, and congestive heart failure. In general, NSAIDs should be used with caution in patients suffering from hypertension, hyperlipidaemia, diabetes mellitus, and peripheral arterial obstructions as well as in patients who smoke.

Increasing age and declining health contribute to cardio-vascular co-morbidity for some patients, which, in turn, may lead to the use of anticoagulant therapy. Warfarin is a commonly used drug in this situation. NSAIDs may attenuate the metabolism of warfarin and thus increase its effect.

NSAIDs may reduce renal function which during concomitant lithium, methotrexate, and amino-glycoside therapy can give rise to increased plasma concentrations. Furthermore, the high plasma protein binding of NSAIDs can displace phenytoin from plasma proteins resulting in overdosing of phenytoin.

One should take into consideration that most of the studies of patients with advanced disease and short life expectancy typically involve small numbers of patients. Therefore, the studies investigating side effects are probably underestimating the frequency of such symptoms and signs. As a general rule in old and/or frail patients, polypharmacy should be avoided if possible. Indications for the use of all drugs should be carefully considered by evaluating the probability of effect versus the probability of side effects. These considerations seem to be of utmost importance when using NSAIDS.

ASA

ASA and its derivatives are the prototypes of NSAIDs and have been known since ancient times. In the mid-18th century Edward Stone, an English clergyman, wrote the first scientific description of the effects of willow bark.

ASA inhibits covalently and irreversibly both COX-1 and COX-2. This is an important feature of ASA, as the duration of the effects are related to the turnover rate of COX in the different tissues.

Particularly, platelets are susceptible to ASA-mediated irreversible inhibition of COX, because they have limited capacity for protein synthesis and thus cannot regenerate COX enzymes. This means, that a single and small dose of ASA will inhibit the COX enzymes for the lifetime of the platelets[19]. An important issue is the prevalent low-dose use of ASA for cardio-protection in patients also treated with traditional NSAIDs, coxibs, or paracetamol. The combination of traditional NSAIDs and low-dose ASA may increase the risk of gastrointestinal toxicity and attenuate the anti-thrombotic effects of ASA. The combination of coxibs and low-dose ASA may reduce the gastrointestinal protection of the coxibs, and this benefit may decrease after 6 months of treatment. However, the combination of paracetamol and low-dose ASA does not interfere with the inhibition of platelet aggregation procuced by ASA[53].

The results of systematic reviews of single-dose studies confirm ASA's efficacy as a postoperative analgesic. Analysis of the analgesic dose–response tells us that higher doses give more analgesia, and comparing ASA with paracetamol the analgesia produced by the two drugs are very similar. One gram of ASA gives the same analgesia as one gram of paracetamol[54,55]. Furthermore, significant benefit of ASA over placebo was shown for ASA 600–650 mg, 1000 mg, and 1200 mg, with NNT values for at least 50 per cent pain relief of 4.4, 4.0, and 2.4, respectively. However, in single-dose studies even low doses of ASA 600/650 mg produced significantly more gastric irritation and drowsiness than placebo[55].The gastrointestinal side effects of ASA are the main reason for the limited use of ASA in palliative care.

Paracetamol (acetaminophen)

Paracetamol (acetaminophen; N-acetyl-p-aminophenol) is one of the most commonly used analgesic antipyretic drugs worldwide, and it is widely available by prescription and over the counter. Paracetamol, a so-called coal-tar analgesic, was discovered by accident as an active metabolite of phenacetin. The site of action seems to be in the brain, however, the mechanism of action is still poorly understood. In a double-blind, placebo-controlled study in healthy volunteers, Piletta and his colleagues obtained some evidence for a central analgesic action of paracetamol. Application of a transcutaneous electrical stimulus to the sural nerve caused a flexion reflex and a subjective sensation of pain. In contrast to ASA, paracetamol raised the threshold to both types of pain, indicating an analgesic action both at the spinal cord level and in higher centres[56].

There is a considerable overlap in the actions of paracetamol, NSAIDS, and ASA regarding inhibition of COX, nevertheless, *in vitro* studies show that paracetamol is not a highly potent inhibitor of COX-1 and COX-2[57]. As mentioned earlier, a third form of COX has been proposed, which has been referred to as COX-3[58]. However, cloning studies have failed to confirm the existence of COX-3 in humans and the search for a convincing mechanistic explanation of the therapeutic activity of paracetamol continues[59].

Paracetamol possesses also antipyretic activity and being an inhibitor of COX within the brain, this is likely to be the site of its antipyretic effects. The antipyretic activity of the compound resides in its aminobenzene structure. Paracetamol is the antipyretic drug of choice in children, and the antipyresis seems to be caused by inhibition of COX-2 or a variant of this enzyme[60]. Because of the association between ASA and Rey's syndrome in children, most of the interest has been toward paracetamol, which, when used in recommended doses, has few side effects and is remarkably well tolerated.

Pharmacokinetics and metabolism

Paracetamol is commercially available in a considerable number of products both alone and in combination with other drugs. Alone it can be administered orally as tablets (conventional, sustained release, effervescent), capsules, powders, and elixirs and rectally as suppositories. Paracetamol is rapidly and almost completely absorbed from the gastrointestinal tract. Gastric emptying rate rather than the diffusion across the intestinal mucosa is the rate-limiting step in paracetamol absorption after oral administration. Therefore, any drug, disease, or other condition, which alters the rate of gastric emptying will influence the rate of absorption. Although paracetamol is rapidly absorbed from the gastrointestinal tract, it is incompletely available to the systemic circulation due to hepatic first-pass metabolism accounting for a 10 per cent loss in therapeutic doses. Intestinal metabolism also contributes to decreased bioavailability[61]. In adults, the bioavailability of paracetamol after administration of suppositories is approximately 60 per cent[62]. After oral administration of therapeutic doses, the concentration in plasma reaches a peak in 30 to 60 min, and the half-life in plasma is about 2 h. Paracetamol is relatively uniformly distributed throughout most body fluids[63]. The proportion of paracetamol bound to plasma proteins is small and varies from 5–20 per cent[64]. Biotransformation takes place primarily in the liver and the oxidative reactions via the cytochrome P-450 system are followed by conjugation. After therapeutic doses, 90 to 100 per cent of the drug may be recovered in urine within the first day, primarily after hepatic conjugation with glucuronic acid (about 60 per cent), sulphuric acid (about 35 per cent), or cysteine (about 3 per cent); small amounts of hydroxylated and deacethylated metabolites also have been detected[65].

Pharmacodynamics

Generally, in systematic reviews the lack of dichotomous data—a prerequisite for calculations of NNTs for non-opioids in cancer pain—excludes meaningful assessment of efficacy, especially during long-term treatment[24]. However, regarding the first step of the ladder, the management of mild pain, the evidence strongly suggests the use of non-opioids alone is superior to placebo, at least during short-term treatment[24,25]. The efficacy of paracetamol compared to NSAIDS has not been thoroughly investigated[66] and the combination of paracetamol and NSAIDS has not been investigated in cancer-related pain. Most studies have assessed paracetamol in combination with other analgesics, and these studies do not give any information on the analgesic effect that paracetamol provides on its own[67,68]. Only one randomized, double-blind, placebo controlled study indicated that the addition of paracetamol to ongoing oral opioid therapy improved pain relief and general well-being in cancer patients[69].

Side effects and toxicity

At therapeutic doses side effects are rare, and the clinical advantage during long-term treatment is that the side effects are less severe than with the NSAIDS. Allergic reactions have been described and during long-term treatment; chronic headache may occur[70]. Despite the safety of paracetamol when used in doses up to a maximum of 4 g daily, however, toxicity can occur, due to either accidental or deliberate overdose (>10 g). A small proportion of paracetamol undergoes P450-mediated N-hydroxylation to form N-acetyl-benzoquinoneimine, a highly reactive intermediate metabolite. This metabolite normally reacts with sulfhydryl groups in glutathione. At large doses of paracetamol, the metabolite is formed in sufficient amounts to deplete liver cells completely of glutathione, which seems to trigger hepato-toxicity and a prolonged rise in liver-derived transaminase and alkaline phosphatase levels in the serum. Intervention to sustain hepatic glutathione is an effective treatment for paracetamol overdose and administration of N-acetyl-L-cystein, which replenishes glutathione stores, remains the treatment of choice[71].

Conclusions and recommendations

A cautious approach should be taken to the use of all types of NSAIDs in high-risk patients, including patients aged 65 years and above; those with *Helicobacter pylori* infection; peptic ulceration within the last year; patients being treated with corticosteroids or low-dose ASA and/or anticoagulants; those with advanced disease including cancer, cardiovascular disease, renal and hepatic impairment, diabetes mellitus, smoking, and excessive alcohol use. Some of these risks factors are nearly always in play in palliative medicine and gastro-protective strategies as well as the cardiovascular risks should always be considered thoroughly.

Regarding the gastrointestinal risks, strategies should include interventions that should precede oral NSAID use such as paracetamol, topical NSAIDs, adjuvant analgesics, and opioids. When treatment with NSAIDs is indicated and effective, it is strongly recommended to use the lowest effective dose for the shortest period of time and combine the treatment with a gastro-protective agent (PPI or histamine antagonists), or if not contraindicated for other reasons, choose a COX-2-inhibitor. Palliative care patients are often at high risk and either lowest effective dose of an NSAID combined with PPI or the lowest effective dose of a coxib should be considered.

The cardiovascular risks have to be considered carefully, and it seems increasingly likely that these are related to individual NSAIDs or coxibs rather than coxibs versus NSAIDs. Generally, coxibs are associated with a moderate increase in the risk of vascular events (defined as myocardial infarction, stroke, or vascular death). However, celecoxib seems not to increase cardiovascular risks, whereas an increased risk is observed for rofecoxib with a clear dose–response trend. High-dose regimens of ibuprofen and diclofenac are also associated with cardiovascular risks, whereas high-dose naproxen is not associated with such events. Thus, the relative risk of cardiovascular events seems to vary with the type of NSAID and coxib and drugs with a higher COX-2/COX-1 effect ratio should be avoided when cardiovascular risks are present. Furthermore, the dose level as well as treatment duration seems to increase the cardiovascular risks. However, if we are to estimate the risk–benefit ratio of individual coxibs versus traditional NSAIDs, the cardiovascular toxicity would have to be balanced against the gastrointestinal safety benefits within groups of patients where, for instance, the gastrointestinal risk is high and the cardiovascular risk is low. In such cases, the benefits of coxibs may outweigh the potential risks in properly selected and informed patients (i.e. patients at a low cardiovascular risk). However, based on current evidence, palliative care patients at high cardiovascular risks should be treated with either naproxen (plus PPI) or celecoxib. Finally, the lowest effective dose for the shortest possible duration of time should be used.

Generally, the efficacy and side effects of NSAIDs should be monitored and evaluated during long-term treatment and, in case of doubtful effects and/or side effects, the treatment should be discontinued.

Future trends

There remains a need for a substantial increase in the number of high-quality trials of non-opioid analgesics in patients with cancer. Studies that specifically address the question of whether addition of an opioid to a non-opioid analgesic regimen actually increases efficacy and/or reduces side effects are required. In addition, the safety and efficacy of chronic use of traditional NSAIDs and coxibs in cancer patients needs to be established. Emerging questions especially regarding coxibs, such as their role in treating cancer pain and their beneficial anti-angiogenic properties, remain unanswered[72]. Translation of emerging preclinical insights into distinct mechanisms for cancer-related pain of different aetiologies (e.g. bone metastases) would be another step towards more rational pharmacotherapy[73].

Due to the many cardiovascular, gastrointestinal, and renal adverse effects encountered with both traditional NSAIDs and coxibs, combined with a very economically lucrative market, this is an area of continuing major investment in research. The COX-inhibiting nitric oxide donors (CINODs) are a new class of agents designed for the treatment of pain and inflammation. CINODs have a multi-pathway mechanism of action that involves COX-inhibition and nitric oxide donation. The anti-inflammatory and analgesic effects of COX-inhibition are reinforced through inhibition of caspase-1 regulated cytokine production, while nitric oxide donation provides multi-organ protection. The CINODs are devoid of hypertensive effects in animal models and their mechanism of action suggests that they may not cause oedema. CINODs also have other renal-sparing effects, being better tolerated than NSAIDs in models of kidney failure. CINODs have been shown to prevent platelet activation *in vitro* and exhibit anti-thrombotic activity *in vivo*. In animal models of ischaemia/reperfusion treatment with CINODs results in improved recovery of heart contractility and reduced left ventricular end-diastolic pressure, in contrast to the effects of NSAIDs and ASA. The combination of improved analgesia, reduced gastrointestinal toxicity, and cardio-renal protection has been established in animal models; however, results from clinical studies in humans are awaited[74]. Furthermore, combined inhibition of the biosynthesis of both prostaglandins (COX) and leukotrienes (LOX), has emerged as a possibility to attenuate anti-inflammatory/analgesic effects and avoid side effects related to COX-inhibition. Animal research and *in vitro* studies are currently being undertaken with agents with dual COX/LOX inhibition[75,76].

References

1. World Health Organization. (1996). *Cancer pain relief: with a guide to opioid availability*. Geneva: World Health Organization.
2. Vane, J.R. (1971). Inhibition of prostaglandin synthesis as a mechanism of action for aspirin-like drugs. *Nature New Biology*, **231**(25), 232–5.
3. Abramson, S., Korchak, H., Ludewig, R. *et al.* (1985). Modes of action of aspirin-like drugs. *Proceedings of the National Academy of Science, USA*, **82**(21), 7227–31.
4. McCormack, K. (1994). Non-steroidal anti-inflammatory drugs and spinal nociceptive processing. *Pain*, **59**(1), 9–43.
5. Richardson, C.E. and Emery, P. (1995). Innovative treatment approaches for rheumatoid arthritis. New cyclo-oxygenase and cytokine inhibitors. *Baillieres Clinical Rheumatology*, **9**(4), 731–58.
6. Burke, A., Smyth, E.M., and FitzGerald, G.A. (2006). *Analgesic-Antipyretic Agents; Pharmacotherapy of Gout*, 11th edition. New York: McGraw-Hill.
7. Cao, C., Matsumura, K., Yamagata, K. *et al.* (1996). Endothelial cells of the rat brain vasculature express cyclooxygenase-2 mRNA in response to systemic interleukin-1 beta: a possible site of prostaglandin synthesis responsible for fever. *Brain Research*, **733**(2), 263–72.
8. Chandrasekharan, N.V., Dai, H., Roos, K.L. *et al.* (2002). COX-3, a cyclooxygenase-1 variant inhibited by acetaminophen and other analgesic/antipyretic drugs: cloning, structure, and expression. *Proceedings of the National Academy of Science, USA*, **99**(21), 13926–31.
9. Kis, B., Snipes, A., Bari, F. *et al.* (2004). Regional distribution of cyclooxygenase-3 mRNA in the rat central nervous system. *Brain Research Molecular Brain Research*, **126**(1), 78–80.
10. Kis, B., Snipes, J.A., Isse, T. *et al.* (2003). Putative cyclooxygenase-3 expression in rat brain cells. *Journal of Cerebral Blood Flow and Metabolism*, **23**(11), 1287–92.
11. Snipes, J.A., Kis, B., Shelness, G.S. *et al.* (2005). Cloning and characterization of cyclooxygenase-1b (putative cyclooxygenase-3) in rat. *Journal of Pharmacology and Experimental Therapeutics*, **313**(2), 668–76.
12. Warner, T.D. and Mitchell, J.A. (2002). Cyclooxygenase-3 (COX-3): filling in the gaps toward a COX continuum? *Proceedings of the National Academy of Science, USA*, **99**(21), 13371–3.
13. Baba, H., Kohno, T., Moore, K.A. *et al.* (2001). Direct activation of rat spinal dorsal horn neurons by prostaglandin E2. *Journal of Neuroscience*, **21**(5), 1750–6.
14. Samad, T.A., Moore, K.A., Sapirstein, A. *et al.* (2001). Interleukin-1beta-mediated induction of Cox-2 in the CNS contributes to inflammatory pain hypersensitivity. *Nature*, **410**(6827), 471–5.
15. Seibert, K., Zhang, Y., Leahy, K. *et al.* (1997). Distribution of COX-1 and COX-2 in normal and inflamed tissues. *Advanced Experimental Medical Biology*, **400**A, 167–70.
16. Breder, C.D., Dewitt, D., Kraig, R.P. (1995). Characterization of inducible cyclooxygenase in rat brain. *Journal of Comparative Neurology*, **355**(2), 296–315.
17. Scarpignato, C. (1995). Nonsteroidal anti-inflammatory drugs: how do they damage gastroduodenal mucosa? *Digestive Diseases*, **13** (Suppl 1), 9–39.
18. Ruilope, L.M., Garcia Robles, R., Paya, C. *et al.* (1986). Effects of long-term treatment with indomethacin on renal function. *Hypertension*, **8**(8), 677–84.
19. Patrono, C., Coller, B., FitzGerald, G.A. *et al.* (2004). Platelet-active drugs: the relationships among dose, effectiveness, and side effects: the Seventh ACCP Conference on Antithrombotic and Thrombolytic Therapy. *Chest*, **126**(3 Suppl), 234S–264S.
20. Meric, J.B., Rottey, S., Olaussen, K. *et al.* (2006). Cyclooxygenase-2 as a target for anticancer drug development. *Critical Reviews in Oncology/Hematology*, **59**(1), 51–64.
21. Mason, L., Moore, R.A., Edwards, J.E. *et al.* (2004). Topical NSAIDs for chronic musculoskeletal pain: systematic review and meta-analysis. *BMC Musculoskeletal Disorders*, **5**, 28.
22. Tramer, M.R., Williams, J.E., Carroll, D. *et al.* (1998). Comparing analgesic efficacy of non-steroidal anti-inflammatory drugs given by

different routes in acute and chronic pain: a qualitative systematic review. *Acta Anaesthesiologica Scandinavica*, **42**(1), 71–9.

23. Eisenberg, E., Berkey, C.S., Carr, D.B. *et al.* (1994). Efficacy and Safety of Nonsteroidal Antiinflammatory Drugs for Cancer Pain: A Meta-Analysis. *Journal of Clinical Oncology*, **12**, 2756–65.

24. McNicol, E., Strassels, S., Goudas, L. *et al.* (2004). Nonsteroidal anti-inflammatory drugs, alone or combined with opioids, for cancer pain: a systematic review. *Journal of Clinical Oncology*, **22**(10), 1975–92.

25. Goudas, L., Carr, D.B., Bloch, R. *et al.* (2001). Management of cancer pain. *Evid Reports Technology Assessment*, (Summ) (35), 1–5.

26. Deeks, J.J., Smith, L.A., and Bradley, M.D. (2002) Efficacy, tolerability, and upper gastrointestinal safety of celecoxib for treatment of osteoarthritis and rheumatoid arthritis: systematic review of randomised controlled trials. *British Medical Journal*, **325**(7365), 619.

27. Bombardier, C., Laine, L., Reicin, A. *et al.* (2000). Comparison of upper gastrointestinal toxicity of rofecoxib and naproxen in patients with rheumatoid arthritis. VIGOR Study Group. *New England Journal of Medicine*, **343**(21), 1520–8, 2 p following 1528.

28. Laine, L., Harper, S., Simon, T. *et al.* (1999). A randomized trial comparing the effect of rofecoxib, a cyclooxygenase 2-specific inhibitor, with that of ibuprofen on the gastroduodenal mucosa of patients with osteoarthritis.Rofecoxib Osteoarthritis Endoscopy Study Group. *Gastroenterology*, **117**(4), 776–83.

29. Lanza, F.L., Rack, M.F., Simon, T.J. *et al.* (1999). Specific inhibition of cyclooxygenase-2 with MK-0966 is associated with less gastroduodenal damage than either aspirin or ibuprofen. *Alimentary Pharmacology and Therapeutics*, **13**(6), 761–7.

30. Hawkey, C., Laine, L., Simon, T. *et al.* (2000). Comparison of the effect of rofecoxib (a cyclooxygenase 2 inhibitor), ibuprofen, and placebo on the gastroduodenal mucosa of patients with osteoarthritis: a randomized, double-blind, placebo-controlled trial. The Rofecoxib Osteoarthritis Endoscopy Multinational Study Group. *Arthritis and Rheumatism*, **43**(2), 370–7.

31. Moore, R.A., Derry, S., Makinson, G.T. *et al.* (2005). Tolerability and adverse events in clinical trials of celecoxib in osteoarthritis and rheumatoid arthritis: systematic review and meta-analysis of information from company clinical trial reports. *Arthritis Research Therapy*, **7**(3), R644–65.

32. Moore, R.A., Derry, S., Phillips, C.J. *et al.* (2006). Nonsteroidal anti-inflammatory drugs (NSAIDs), cyxlooxygenase-2 selective inhibitors (coxibs) and gastrointestinal harm: review of clinical trials and clinical practice. BMC *Musculoskeletal Disorders*, **7**, 79.

33. Hawkins, C. and Hanks, G.W. (2000). The gastroduodenal toxicity of nonsteroidal anti-inflammatory drugs: a review of the literature. *Journal of Pain and Symptom Management*, **20**(2), 140–51.

34. Hernandez-Diaz, S. and Rodriguez, L.A. (2000). Association between nonsteroidal anti-inflammatory drugs and upper gastrointestinal tract bleeding/perforation: an overview of epidemiologic studies published in the 1990s. *Archives of Internal Medicine*, **160**(14), 2093–9.

35. Dubois, R.W., Melmed, G.Y., Henning, J.M. *et al.* (2004). Risk of Upper Gastrointestinal Injury and Events in Patients Treated With Cyclooxygenase (COX)-1/COX-2 Nonsteroidal Antiinflammatory Drugs (NSAIDs), COX-2 Selective NSAIDs, and Gastroprotective Cotherapy: An Appraisal of the Literature. *Journal of Clinical Rheumatology*, **10**(4), 178–89.

36. Rostom, A., Dube, C., Wells, G. *et al.* (2002). Prevention of NSAID-induced gastroduodenal ulcers. *Cochrane Database of Systematic Reviews*, **4**, CD002296.

37. Hooper, L., Brown, T.J., Elliott, R. *et al.* (2004). The effectiveness of five strategies for the prevention of gastrointestinal toxicity induced by non-steroidal anti-inflammatory drugs: systematic review. *British Medical Journal*, **329**(7472), 948.

38. Chan, F.K., Hung, L.C., Suen, B.Y. *et al.* (2002). Celecoxib versus diclofenac and omeprazole in reducing the risk of recurrent ulcer bleeding in patients with arthritis. *New England Journal of Medicine*, **347**(26), 2104–10.

39. Lai, K.C., Chu, K.M., Hui, W.M. *et al.* (2005). Celecoxib compared with lansoprazole and naproxen to prevent gastrointestinal ulcer complications. *American Journal of Medicine*, **118**(11), 1271–8.

40. Cheng, H.F. and Harris, R.C. (2004). Cyclooxygenases, the kidney, and hypertension. *Hypertension*, **43**(3), 525–30.

41. Patrono, C. and Dunn, M.J. (1987). The clinical significance of inhibition of renal prostaglandin synthesis. *Kidney International*, **32**(1), 1–12.

42. Qi, Z., Hao, C.M., Langenbach, R.I. *et al.* (2002). Opposite effects of cyclooxygenase-1 and -2 activity on the pressor response to angiotensin II. *Journal of Clinical Investigation*, **110**(1), 61–9.

43. Henry, D., Page, J., Whyte, I. *et al.* (1997). Consumption of non-steroidal anti-inflammatory drugs and the development of functional renal impairment in elderly subjects. Results of a case-control study. *British Journal of Clinical Pharmacology*, **44**(1), 85–90.

44. Whelton, A. (1999). Nephrotoxicity of nonsteroidal anti-inflammatory drugs: physiologic foundations and clinical implications. *American Journal of Medicine*, **106**(5B), 13S–24S.

45. Akhund, L., Quinet, R.J., and Ishaq, S. (2003). Celecoxib-related renal papillary necrosis. *Archives of Internal Medicine*, **163**(1),114–5.

46. Page, J. and Henry, D. (2000). Consumption of NSAIDs and the development of congestive heart failure in elderly patients: an underrecognized public health problem. *Archives of Internal Medicine*, **160**(6), 777–84.

47. Merlo, J., Broms, K., Lindblad, U. *et al.* (2001). Association of outpatient utilisation of non-steroidal anti-inflammatory drugs and hospitalised heart failure in the entire Swedish population. *European Journal of Clinical Pharmacology*, **57**(1), 71–5.

48. Bresalier, R.S., Sandler, R.S., Quan, H. *et al.* (2005). Cardiovascular events associated with rofecoxib in a colorectal adenoma chemoprevention trial. *New England Journal of Medicine*, **352**(11), 1092–102.

49. Fitzgerald, G.A. (2004). Coxibs and cardiovascular disease. *New England Journal of Medicine*, **351**(17), 1709–11.

50. McGettigan, P. and Henry, D. (2006). Cardiovascular risk and inhibition of cyclooxygenase: a systematic review of the observational studies of selective and nonselective inhibitors of cyclooxygenase 2. *Journal of the American Medical Association*, **296**(13), 1633–44.

51. Kearney, P.M., Baigent, C., Godwin, J. *et al.* (2006). Do selective cyclo-oxygenase-2 inhibitors and traditional non-steroidal anti-inflammatory drugs increase the risk of atherothrombosis? Meta-analysis of randomised trials. *British Medical Journal*, **332**(7553), 1302–8.

52. Hernandez-Diaz, S., Varas-Lorenzo, C., and Garcia Rodriguez, L.A. (2006). Non-steroidal anti-inflammatory drugs and the risk of acute myocardial infarction. *Basic Clinical Pharmacology and Toxicology*, **98**, 266–74.

53. Gaziano, J.M. and Gibson, C.M. (2006). Potential for drug-drug interactions in patients taking analgesics for mild-to-moderate pain and low-dose aspirin for cardioprotection. *American Journal of Cardiology*, **97**(9A), 23–9.

54. McQuay, H.J. and Moore, R.A. (2007). Dose-response in direct comparisons of different doses of aspirin, ibuprofen and paracetamol (acetaminophen) in analgesic studies. *British Journal of Clinical Pharmacology*, **63**(3), 271–8.

55. Edwards, J.E., Oldman, A.D., Smith, L.A. *et al.* (1999). Oral aspirin in postoperative pain: a quantitative systematic review. *Pain*, **81**(3), 289–97.

56. Piletta, P., Porchet, H.C., and Dayer, P. (1991). Central analgesic effect of acetaminophen but not of aspirin. *Clinical Pharmacology and Therapeutics*, **49**(4), 350–4.

57. Ouellet, M. and Percival, M.D. (2001). Mechanism of acetaminophen inhibition of cyclooxygenase isoforms. *Archives of Biochemistry and Biophysics*, **387**(2), 273–80.

58. Ayoub, S.S., Colville-Nash, P.R., Willoughby, D.A. et al. (2006). The involvement of a cyclooxygenase 1 gene-derived protein in the antinociceptive action of paracetamol in mice. *European Journal of Pharmacology*, **538**(1–3), 57–65.

59. Qin, N., Zhang, S.P., Reitz, T.L. et al. (2005). Cloning, expression, and functional characterization of human cyclooxygenase-1 splicing variants: evidence for intron 1 retention. *Journal of Pharmacology and Experimental Therapeutics*, **315**(3), 1298–305.

60. Simmons, D.L. (2003). Variants of cyclooxygenase-1 and their roles in medicine. *Thrombosis Research*, **110**(5–6), 265–8.

61. Tone, Y., Kawamata, K., Murakami, T. et al. (1990). Dose-dependent pharmacokinetics and first-pass metabolism of acetaminophen in rats. *Journal of Pharmacobiodynamics*, **13**(6), 327–35.

62. Beck, D.H., Schenk, M.R., Hagemann, K. et al. (2000). The pharmacokinetics and analgesic efficacy of larger dose rectal acetaminophen (40 mg/kg) in adults: a double-blinded, randomized study. *Anesthesia and Analgesia*, **90**(2), 431–6.

63. Prescott, L.F. (1996). *Paracetamol (acetaminophen). A critical bibliographic review*. London: Taylor and Francis.

64. Milligan, T.P., Morris, H.C., Hammond, P.M. et al. (1994). Studies on paracetamol binding to serum proteins. *Annals of Clinical Biochemistry*, **31** (Pt 5), 492–6.

65. Steventon, G.B., Mitchell, S.C., and Waring, R.H. (1996). Human metabolism of paracetamol (acetaminophen) at different dose levels. *Drug Metabolism and Drug Interaction*, **13**(2), 111–7.

66. Ventafridda, V., De Conno, F., Panerai, A.E. et al. (1990). Non-steroidal anti-inflammatory drugs as the first step in cancer pain therapy: double-blind, within-patient study comparing nine drugs. *Journal of International Medical Research*, **18**(1), 21–9.

67. Carlson, R.W., Borrison, R.A., Sher, H.B. et al. (1990). A multiinstitutional evaluation of the analgesic efficacy and safety of ketorolac tromethamine, acetaminophen plus codeine, and placebo in cancer pain. *Pharmacotherapy*, **10**(3), 211–6.

68. Chary, S., Goughnour, B.R., Moulin, D.E. et al. (1994). The dose-response relationship of controlled-release codeine (Codeine Contin) in chronic cancer pain. *Journal of Pain and Symptom Management*, **9**(6), 363–71.

69. Stockler, M., Vardy, J., Pillai, A. et al. (2004). Acetaminophen (paracetamol) improves pain and well-being in people with advanced cancer already receiving a strong opioid regimen: a randomized, double-blind, placebo-controlled cross-over trial. *Journal of Clinical Oncology*, **22**(16), 3389–94.

70. Meskunas, C.A., Tepper, S.J., Rapoport, A.M. et al. (2006). Medications associated with probable medication overuse headache reported in a tertiary care headache center over a 15-year period. *Headache*, **46**(5), 766–72.

71. Josephy, P.D. (2005).The molecular toxicology of acetaminophen. *Drug Metabolism Reviews*, **37**, 581–94.

72. Steinbach, G., Lynch, P.M., Phillips, R.K. et al. (2000). The effect of celecoxib, a cyclooxygenase-2 inhibitor, in familial adenomatous polyposis. *New England Journal of Medicine*, **342**(26), 1946–52.

73. Davar, G. (2002).What causes cancer pain. *Pain Clinics*, **10**, 1–4.

74. Muscara, M.N. and Wallace, J.L. (2006). COX-inhibiting nitric oxide donors (CINODs): potential benefits on cardiovascular and renal function. *Cardiovascular Hematological Agents Medicine Chemistry*, **4**(2), 155–64.

75. Ulbrich, H., Soehnlein, O., Xie, X. et al. (2005). Licofelone, a novel 5-LOX/COX-inhibitor, attenuates leukocyte rolling and adhesion on endothelium under flow. *Biochemical Pharmacology*, **70**(1), 30–6.

76. Marcouiller, P., Pelletier, J.P., Guevremont, M. et al. (2005). Leukotriene and prostaglandin synthesis pathways in osteoarthritic synovial membranes: regulating factors for interleukin 1beta synthesis. *Journal of Rheumatology*, **32**(4), 704–12.

10.1.8 Adjuvant analgesics in pain management

David Lussier and Russell K. Portenoy

The term 'adjuvant analgesic' has been defined as any drug that has a primary indication other than pain, but is analgesic in some painful conditions. As drugs in this category have begun to be used in the treatment of diverse chronic pain disorders, the term itself, and its definition, have become outmoded. There are now drugs in this category that are approved in many countries as primary analgesics for selected pain disorders. The evolution of this group of non-traditional drugs has been rapid and a strongly positive development in the search for a more effective pharmacological armamentarium for chronic pain.

In the palliative care literature, the term 'adjuvant analgesic' also is often used synonymously with 'co-analgesic'. These labels refer to drugs that may be administered with a primary analgesic, usually an opioid, to enhance pain relief, treat pain that is refractory to the analgesic, or allow reduction of the analgesic dose for the purpose of limiting side effects. In this context, adjuvant analgesics should be distinguished from other adjuvant drugs that are co-administered with analgesics for the specific purposes of treating side effects produced by the analgesic or managing symptoms other than pain. In the latter sense, laxatives and antiemetics are adjuvant drugs.

Given this imprecise terminology and the expanding use of adjuvant analgesics as non-traditional primary analgesics, it is important to understand the pharmacology of these drugs and their therapeutic role in varied patient populations. In this way, the use of the adjuvant analgesics can be optimized, both as 'add-on' therapy to an opioid regimen and as distinct, primary therapy in those painful disorders that are likely to demonstrate a good response.

General considerations

Several principles guide the administration of all adjuvant analgesics. These emphasize the importance of a comprehensive patient assessment and a broad foundation in analgesic pharmacotherapy.

Comprehensive assessment

The selection of a drug and optimal dosing regimen depends on a systematic assessment of the patient. This assessment requires a careful history and review of records, physical examination, and appropriate laboratory and imaging studies. The information obtained includes the following:

1 Characteristics of the pain, including severity, location, temporal features, quality, and syndrome.

2 Aetiology of the pain and its relationship to the underlying disease.

3 Inferences about the predominating type of pain pathophysiology, for example, nociceptive or neuropathic.

4 Impact of pain on function and quality of life.

5 Presence of associated factors (comorbidities), including physical and psychological symptoms, functional impairments, psychiatric disorder, family or social disruption, financial problems, and spiritual or religious concerns, and their effects on quality of life.

The need for systematic assessment continues during the course of therapy with an adjuvant analgesic. Over time, changes in pain, side effects, or any of the broader quality of life concerns may impel a shift in therapeutic strategy. The use of adjuvant analgesics in the management of pain may be a 'labour intensive' endeavour, which requires frequent contact with the patient to ensure continuous, appropriate administration of the drug.

Positioning of treatment

Extensive experience in the cancer population indicates that the adjuvant analgesics are, as a group, less reliable analgesics than opioids. This characteristic may be determined by a smaller proportion of treated patients who respond adequately, a higher likelihood of troublesome side effects, or a slower onset of analgesic effect for most drugs (perhaps due to the need to initiate therapy at low doses to avoid side effects). For example, in contrast to survey data that demonstrate a favourable outcome within days for 70 to 90 per cent of cancer patients who receive opioid therapy[1, 2], studies of the tricyclic antidepressants show that these drugs require treatment for weeks to obtain optimal results and offer 50 per cent, or greater, relief to 50 to 75 per cent of patients with neuropathic pain[3,4].

This observation suggests that most patients with moderate or severe pain related to serious medical illness who have no relative contraindications to opioid therapy should not receive an adjuvant analgesic until opioid therapy has been optimized. Although some clinicians attempt to improve patient response by initiating therapy with an opioid and an adjuvant analgesic concurrently, this approach increases the risk of additive toxicity. Unless another indication for an earlier trial exists (e.g. a co-morbidity that may also respond to the drug, a history of problems with opioids, or a type of pain that may be particularly responsive to a specific adjuvant), the safest and most efficient approach usually involves the addition of an adjuvant analgesic to an opioid regimen that is yielding inadequate analgesia despite dose escalation to limiting side effects. This positioning of the adjuvant analgesics must be understood in relation to the other options that exist in this situation (Table 10.1.8.1). In the absence of data from comparative clinical trials, the decision to use an adjuvant analgesic drug instead of an alternative therapy, such as a trial of spinally administered opioids or a nerve block, is usually a matter of clinical judgement.

The selection of a specific adjuvant analgesic may be suggested by the characteristics of the pain (see following paragraphs) or, in some instances, by the existence of another symptom concurrent with pain that may be amenable to a non-analgesic effect of the drug. In many situations, multiple options exist, and priorities for therapeutic trials must also be developed on the basis of a comprehensive assessment of the patient and best clinical judgement.

Pharmacological characteristics

To select and properly administer an adjuvant analgesic, the clinician must be familiar with the drug's actions, approved indications,

unapproved indications accepted in medical practice, likely side-effects and potential serious adverse effects, usual time–action relationship, pharmacokinetics, specific dosing guidelines for pain, and interactions with other drugs. Very few of the adjuvant analgesics have been studied in the palliative care setting and the information used to develop dosing guidelines is usually extrapolated from other patient populations.

Caution is usually appropriate as adjuvant analgesics are used in a medically ill population. Low initial doses and gradual dose escalation may avoid early side effects and identify dose-dependent analgesic effects that can be explored to optimize the balance between pain relief and adverse effects. The use of low initial doses and dose titration may delay the onset of analgesia, however, and patients must be forewarned of this possibility to improve adherence with the therapy.

Inter-individual and intra-individual variability

There is great variability in the response to all adjuvant analgesics. Although specific patient characteristics, such as advanced age or coexistent major organ failure, may increase the likelihood of some (usually adverse) responses, it is nonetheless true that neither favourable effects nor specific side effects can be reliably predicted in the individual patients. Additionally, there is remarkable intra-individual variability in the response to different drugs, including those within the same class. Implicit in both these observations is the potential utility of sequential trials of adjuvant analgesics. The process of sequential drug trials, like the use of low initial doses and dose titration, should be explained to the patient at the start of therapy to enhance adherence and reduce the distress that may occur as treatments fail.

Risks and benefits of polypharmacy

Adjuvant analgesics are typically administered to patients who are receiving several other drugs. Although this is widely regarded as appropriate, the potential for additive side effects and unpredictable adverse effects must be anticipated by the practitioner whenever an adjuvant is added to an existing drug regimen. The decision to add, or continue, a therapy must be based on a careful assessment of outcomes and a clear understanding of the goals of care.

Table 10.1.8.1 Therapeutic options when opioid therapy regimen fails due to dose-limiting toxicity.

Approach	Therapeutic options
I. Pharmacological techniques to reduce systemic opioid requirement	Use of adjuvant analgesics Use of spinal opioids
II. Identifying an opioid with a more favourable balance between analgesia and side effects	Sequential opioid trials
III. Improving the tolerability of the opioid regimen to allow further dose escalation	More aggressive side-effect management (e.g. psychostimulants for opioid-induced somnolence)
IV. Non-pharmacological techniques to reduce the systemic opioid requirement	Anaesthetic approaches Surgical approaches Rehabilitative approaches Psychological approaches

If a treatment yields demonstrable benefit without serious risk, and without cumulative side effects that otherwise impair function or quality of life, there is ample justification for continuing. Additional pain relief at the price of somnolence or mental clouding is not acceptable for patients whose goals include restoration of function, but may be completely appropriate for those who seek comfort as the only goal.

The risks of additive toxicity from polypharmacy derive from both pharmacokinetic and pharmacodynamic changes. For example, the addition of a tricyclic antidepressant to a morphine regimen may produce somnolence due to an increase in morphine plasma concentration or a pharmacodynamic interaction independent of changes in drug concentration.

Adjuvant analgesics

The adjuvant analgesics comprise an extraordinarily diverse group of drug classes (Table 10.1.8.2). A generally useful, broad classification distinguishes those that may be considered non-specific, multi-purpose analgesics from those used for more specific indications. A review of the evidence supporting the analgesic efficacy of agents in each class provides the foundation for the development of clinical guidelines.

Multi-purpose analgesics

The data supporting the analgesic efficacy of some drug classes derive from numerous studies of very diverse syndromes. The range of positive outcomes for these drugs suggests that they can be considered multi-purpose analgesics, fundamentally similar in this respect to the opioid and non-opioid analgesics (Table 10.1.8.3). This designation is appropriate even if these drugs are used only for selected indications in the palliative care setting.

Antidepressant drugs

There is compelling evidence that the tricyclic antidepressants are analgesic in a variety of chronic pain syndromes[5]. The efficacy of the tertiary amine compounds has been demonstrated in a large number of controlled and uncontrolled trials. Amitriptyline was effective in migraine and other types of headache[6], arthritis[7], chronic low-back pain[8], postherpetic neuralgia[9,10], fibromyalgia[11], painful diabetic polyneuropathy[3,12,13], central post-stroke pain[14], spinal cord injury pain[15], post-amputation and phantom limb pain[16], chronic facial pain[17], and cancer-related neuropathic pain[18]. Imipramine was useful for painful diabetic neuropathy[19] and idiopathic chest pain[20]. Doxepin relieved coexistent pain and depression[21]. Topical doxepin applied to skin has been shown to decrease neuropathic pain in a controlled trial[22]. Oral topical doxepin rinse can be effective in pain from radiation-induced mucositis[23,24] and the analgesic effect can last up to 4 h[24], which is longer than the anaesthetic effect and suggests that pain relief is due to an analgesic rather than anaesthetic effect[25]. Clomipramine was analgesic in various neuropathic pains and idiopathic pain[26,27], and dothiepin was effective in fibromyalgia and psychogenic pain[28].

Analgesic efficacy has also been demonstrated for the secondary amine tricyclic antidepressants. In controlled trials, desipramine was analgesic in painful diabetic neuropathy[12] and postherpetic neuralgia[4,29], for which it might be more effective and less expensive than gabapentin and pregabalin[30]. Nortriptyline was effective

in mixed neuropathic pains[26] and, combined with fluphenazine, in painful diabetic polyneuropathy[31]. For postherpetic neuralgia, it has been shown to be as effective as amitriptyline, with fewer intolerable side effects[10].

Table 10.1.8.2 Adjuvant analgesics: major classes.

Multipurpose adjuvant analgesics
- Antidepressants
- Corticosteroids
- Alpha-2 adrenergic agonists
- Neuroleptics

Adjuvant analgesics used for neuropathic pain
- Anticonvulsants
- Oral and parenteral sodium channel blockers
- N-methyl-D-aspartate receptor blockers
- Cannabinoids
- Miscellaneous
  - Baclofen
  - Calcitonin
  - Drugs used for sympathetically-maintained pain
  - Anticholinesterase drugs

Topical analgesics
- Capsaicin
- Local anaesthetics
- Tricyclic antidepressants
- NSAIDs

Adjuvant analgesics used for bone pain
- Calcitonin and bisphosphonates
- Radiopharmaceuticals

Adjuvant analgesics used for bowel obstruction
- Anticholinergics
- Octreotide

Adjuvant analgesics used for musculoskeletal pain

Table 10.1.8.3 Multi-purpose adjuvant analgesics.

Class	Examples
Antidepressants	
- Tricyclic antidepressants	- Amitriptyline, nortriptyline, desipramine, doxepin, imipramine, clomipramine
- Serotonin/norepinephrine reuptake inhibitors	- Venlafaxine, duloxetine
- Selective serotonin reuptake inhibitors	- Paroxetine, citalopram, fluoxetine, sertraline, fluvoxamine, trazodone
- Monoamine oxidase inhibitors	- Phenelzine
- Others	- Maprotiline, bupropion
Alpha-2-adrenergic agonists	- Clonidine Tizanidine
Corticosteroids	- Dexamethasone, prednisone, methylprednisolone
Neuroleptics	- Methotrimeprazine

Among the newer antidepressants, the noradrenaline and serotonin reuptake inhibitors (SNRIs) are the most promising analgesics, with established efficacy and a better side-effect profile that the tricyclic drugs. Venlafaxine has been shown to increase experimental pain tolerance[32] and, in a recent study of patients with neuropathic pain, this drug reduced hyperalgesia and temporal summation but did not affect pain intensity and pain detection thresholds[33]. A case series support analgesic effects in chemotherapy-induced neuropathy[34]. Randomized studies showed analgesic efficacy in painful diabetic neuropathy[35], atypical facial pain[36], fibromyalgia[37], and painful polyneuropathy, where it was as effective as imipramine[38]. In patients with breast cancer, it can also prevent the development of chronic post-mastectomy pain when started the night before surgery and admistered for 2 weeks[39].

Duloxetine is newer than venlafaxine, but already has impressive scientific evidence of a good analgesic effect, with randomized controlled trials done in painful diabetic neuropathy[40], depression-associated pain[41,42], and fibromyalgia[43]. Effectiveness, tolerability, and safety appear to be maintained during long-term use[44]. In older depressed patients, it can improve mood, cognition and pain[42].

Milnacipran is another SNRI currently available only in a few countries, but should be available more widely in the next few years. Antiallodynic and antihyperalgesic effects have been observed in animal models of neuropathic pain[45], where it potentiates the effecs of tramadol[45]. In humans, efficacy has only been shown by one randomized trial in fibromyalgia[46].

Although some studies have reported positive results with selective serotonin reuptake inhibitors (SSRIs), randomized controlled trials and clinical experience have yielded mixed outcomes. Paroxetine has been shown to be effective in a study of painful diabetic neuropathy[47], where it relieved both steady and lancinating pain. Citalopram seems effective in painful diabetic neuropathy[48] and in somatoform pain disorder, in which the analgesic and antidepressant effects are not correlated[49]. Fluvoxamine decreases pain perception in healthy volunteers[50] and might be useful for the treatment of central post-stroke pain when used early after stroke[51]. A controlled trial performed in patients with cancer pain suggested benefits with trazodone[18]. Limited evidence suggests that fluoxetine might have a role in the treatment of fibromyalgia[52]. A controlled trial in patients with diabetic neuropathy, however, failed to demonstrate benefit from this drug[12]. The latter study demonstrated that a SSRI was less likely to be analgesic than a tricyclic antidepressant.

Several other non-tricyclic antidepressant drugs may have utility as analgesics. The efficacy of the norepinephrine reuptake blocker maprotiline has been established in controlled comparisons against clomipramine in idiopathic pain[27] and against amitriptyline in postherpetic neuralgia[9].

Bupropion specifically inhibits neuronal norepinephrine reuptake and, less potently, dopamine reuptake. A randomized study[53] reported substantial pain relief in patients with neuropathic pain. A more recent, randomized controlled trial, however, did not find any pain relief in non-neuropathic chronic low back pain[54]. Bupropion has a low risk of somnolence and sexual dysfunction, side effects that may be limiting with other antidepressants. Anecdotally, patients may report increased energy that appears to be unrelated to mood effects, which has led to empirical use for fatigue.

These favourable characteristics suggest that a trial of bupropion as an adjuvant analgesic should be considered for selected patients.

Nefazodone also inhibits serotonin and norepinephrine reuptake. Unlike other antidepressants, however, it also has a direct postsynaptic serotonin antagonist effect. This drug has been reported to potentiate morphine analgesia in animals[55] but there have been no controlled human trials confirming efficacy. For this reason, and because of its association with serious and potentially life-threatening liver failure, nefazodone should rarely be used as an adjuvant analgesic.

Monoamine oxidase inhibitors (MAOIs) have been evaluated in limited clinical settings. Given the lack of scientific evidence of their analgesic activitiy and the risk of acute cardiovascular toxicity following ingestion of monoaminergic foods or drugs during treatment with the MAOIs, these drugs are rarely considered.

Very few clinical trials have specifically evaluated the efficacy of antidepressants as analgesics for cancer pain. Nonetheless, a few partially controlled trials[18,56,57] confirm the analgesic potential of the tricyclic antidepressants in the cancer population. A recent review of US health insurance claims showed that 14 per cent of cancer patients were using tricyclic antidepressants and that amitriptyline is the most commonly prescribed drug[58].

In summary, there is very substantial evidence that antidepressant drugs have analgesic effects in diverse types of chronic pain. Given the range of pain syndromes that are potentially responsive, it is appropriate to classify these drugs as non-specific, multi-purpose analgesics. The strongest evidence of analgesic efficacy is found in the numerous controlled trials of the tertiary amine tricyclic drugs, the best studied of which has been amitriptyline. Although less abundant data support the efficacy of the secondary amine tricyclic drugs, desipramine and nortriptyline have been carefully studied and have clear analgesic potential. The latter drugs have a better side-effect profile than the tertiary amine drugs and often are considered first in the medically ill for this reason. Drugs with more selective actions at specific monoaminergic synapses are also analgesic, and recent data strongly support the efficacy of SNRI compounds which, given their relatively good side-effect profiles, might be considered early when selecting an analgesic antidepressant for a patient with a serious or advanced illness. There is far weaker support for the efficacy of the SSRIs. Comparative trials of the various analgesic antidepressants are badly needed.

Mechanism of action

Although effective treatment of concurrent depression can contribute to a favourable outcome from antidepressant therapy in patients with chronic pain, the analgesic effect of these drugs is not dependent on their antidepressant activity. Many of the controlled studies of the tricyclic drugs cited previously have demonstrated that the usually effective analgesic dose is generally lower than that required to treat depression, and that the onset of analgesia typically occurs much sooner than the antidepressant effect, usually within one week. More important, studies have shown that non-depressed patients can experience analgesia and depressed patients can report pain relief without a change in mood[3,4,12,14]. Finally, single-dose studies of amitriptyline in animal models have demonstrated dose-dependent antinociception[59], further suggesting an independent analgesic effect from these drugs.

Presumably, the antidepressants interact with the complex array of endogenous anti-nociceptive systems that involve monoaminergic neurotransmission[60]. An experimental study of fluvoxamine in healthy volunteers suggests that there are interactions between these somatosensory systems and systems involved in the affective and integrative components of pain, and the latter also may be affected by antidepressant drugs[50]. Animal studies have also demonstrated that the acute antinociceptive effects produced by various classes of antidepressants can be partially blocked by the specific opioid antagonist, naloxone[61], suggesting that antidepressant analgesia also may involve activation of the opioid systems.

The tricyclic antidepressants are not highly selective and they also interact with other types of receptors (e.g. acetylcholine, histamine, GABA) that may be important in the development of analgesia[62]. Further elucidation of these mechanisms awaits additional investigations using more selective drugs.

Adverse effects

Although serious adverse effects are uncommon at the doses of antidepressants usually administered for pain, side effects are frequent. Dose-related side effects can occur even at low doses, particularly in patients who may be predisposed to adverse effects due to major organ dysfunction, use of multiple other drugs, or advanced age. Moreover, some patients who receive low doses of the tricyclic antidepressant actually attain relatively high plasma drug concentrations[63], and this pharmacokinetic variability may also account for some cases of toxicity.

Among the antidepressants, the tricyclic drugs are most likely to produce side effects, and the incidence of side effects is highest with the tertiary amine drugs. Although the most serious adverse effect, cardiotoxicity, is very uncommon, patients who have significant heart disease, including conduction disorders, arrhythmia, or heart failure, should not be treated with a tricyclic. Overdose of a tricyclic antidepressant can be lethal due to cardiac toxicity.

Orthostatic hypotension is far more common during treatment with a tricyclic antidepressant and is more likely in the elderly. Combined with the central nervous system effects of these drugs, orthostasis may predispose to an increased risk of hip fracture in this population[64]. Patients who are predisposed to orthostasis, such as those with autonomic neuropathy, usually are considered better candidates for an antidepressant in an alternative class.

Tricyclic antidepressants, particularly the tertiary compounds, can cause somnolence, mental clouding and, less commonly, delirium. All of these effects are more likely in the elderly and those with predisposing factors, such as dementia, brain metastases, prior cranial radiotherapy, or concurrent use of other centrally-acting drugs. A recent study demonstrated that driving ability may be impaired when treatment is initiated, but that tolerance to this effect often develops within a few weeks, at least when a relatively low dose (25 mg) is administered to otherwise healthy chronic pain patients[65].

Most of the minor side effects produced by the tricyclic antidepressants are related to their anticholinergic properties. These include dry mouth, blurred vision, and constipation. These problems usually are tolerated or effectively managed. Rarely, more serious anticholinergic toxicity can occur, including precipitation of acute angle closure glaucoma, tachycardia, severe constipation, or urinary retention. Male patients with a history of prostatism should be given a secondary amine tricyclic or considered for an alternative drug class. Due to the risk of precipitating acute intra-ocular hypertension, the tricyclics are contraindicated in those with a known history of a narrow anterior chamber of the eye or prior attacks of acute glaucoma; monitoring of eye pressures should be considered in those with open-angle glaucoma.

The secondary amine tricyclic drugs, desipramine and nortriptyline, are less anticholinergic than the tertiary amine drugs, and also are less likely to cause orthostatic hypotension, somnolence, and cognitive impairment. Nortriptyline has been shown to be as effective and better tolerated than amitriptyline in patients with postherpetic neuralgia[10]. Patients who are predisposed to the side effects associated with the tricyclics, or who have distressing side effects during a trial of a tertiary amine drug, should be considered for a trial of desipramine or nortriptyline.

Both the SNRIs and the SSRIs have a more favourable side-effect profile than the tricyclic drugs. The most common adverse events are nausea, headache, sedation, insomnia, weight gain, impaired memory, sweating, tremor, and sexual dysfunction. Clinical experience and several case reports suggest that SSRIs can induce or worsen akathisia and parkinsonian symptoms, but the evidence is conflicting. Rapid discontinuation of the SNRIs or SSRIs, can cause a discontinuation syndrome characterized by both somatic (dizziness, light-headedness, nausea, fatigue, lethargy, sleep disturbances) and psychological (anxiety, agitation, crying, irritability) symptoms. A gradual tapering should avoid these symptoms. Of the SNRIs, duloxetine and milnacipran appear better tolerated than venlafaxine. Venlafaxine can cause a dose-related hypertension, and if appropriate, blood-pressure monitoring should be done during initiation of treatment.

Bupropion can cause dry mouth, insomnia, nausea, headache, rash, and agitation/excitement. It also decreases seizure threshold, and is relatively contraindicated in patients with factors predisposing to seizures, such as sedative–hypnotic withdrawal states, co-administered drugs with seizure-lowering potential, and central nervous system pathology. The main advantages of bupropion are the absence of sexual side effects and its propensity to be activating rather than sedating, which can be very helpful in depressed or sedated patients.

Pharmacology

The tricyclic antidepressants are metabolized by several isozymes of cytochrome P450. The tertiary amines are metabolized by CYP1A2 and CYP2C19, whereas the secondary amines are cleared by the CYP2D6. There is large inter-individual variation in these metabolic pathways. For example, the extensive metabolizers of desipramine and nortriptyline clear the drug up to seven times faster than poor metabolizers, who require a 2-week period before achieving a steady state[66].

Tricyclic antidepressants may be co-administered with nontricyclic antidepressants (SNRIs, SSRIs, or bupropion) during treatment for depression or pain. This combination therapy should be informed by knowledge of potential drug–drug interactions. SSRIs may produce a reduction in the clearance of the tricyclics and, therefore, result in a significantly higher plasma level[67]. This potential interaction suggests that the tricyclic dose should be lowered initially when adding a SSRI.

Most SSRIs, especially paroxetine and fluoxetine, inhibit CYP2D6, which could produce interactions with other medications metabolized by this isozyme[67]. Clinically significant drug interactions with paroxetine seem to be limited, however[67]. As their effect on CYP2D6 is less, sertraline and citalopram are less likely to interact with other drugs[67]. Due to the presence of an active metabolite, fluoxetine has a much longer half-life than the other SSRIs and is more prone to drug–drug interactions.

Venlafaxine also is highly metabolized by CYP2D6 and can interact with other drugs affected by this isozyme. Although unexpected adverse effects can occur with such drug combinations, the clinical significance of these interactions in practice appears to be limited. The dose of venlafaxine should be reduced in patients with several renal disease or cirrhosis, due to lower clearance. Dose adjustments are not required in the setting of advanced age alone. Like venlafaxine, the dose of bupropion should be reduced in patients with severe renal or liver disease. Drug interactions are uncommon.

Indications and dosing guidelines

The antidepressant drugs are multi-purpose analgesics and potentially could be considered for the treatment of any chronic pain syndrome. The available evidence does not support their use as analgesics for acute pain[68] despite the demonstrated efficacy of selected tricyclic antidepressants in animal models of acute nociception[59] and human experimental pain[69].

As discussed previously, treatment with an adjuvant analgesic, such as an antidepressant drug, is usually considered in the palliative care setting when a favourable balance between analgesia and side effects cannot be attained with an opioid. There are many potential reasons for a poor response to an opioid, among which is a 'neuropathic' pathophysiology[70]. Given the established benefit of the antidepressants in patients with diverse types of neuropathic pains[3,4,9,12,14], these drugs may be particularly valuable in any painful condition related to such mechanisms. A broad consensus suggests that the first-line drugs for neuropathic pains in populations that do not have advanced medical illness are either antidepressants or specific anti-epileptic drugs, which act via modulation of the alpha-2-delta-1 protein of the N-type calcium channel (gabapentin or pregabalin, see following paragraphs)[5]. The antidepressants should be considered first if neuropathic pain is accompanied by a comorbid depression.

Given the very extensive data supporting the analgesic efficacy of the tricyclic antidepressants, especially amitriptyline, it is reasonable to consider whether one of these drugs should be administered first if a trial of an analgesic antidepressant is indicated. Amitriptyline usually is appropriate only if a patient is relatively young and has no significant factors predisposing to anticholinergic, sedative, or cardiovascular side effects. Medically ill patients seldom meet this criterion, and usually, a trial with a secondary amine drug, specifically desipramine or nortriptyline, is more appropriate. If tricyclic antidepressants have not been tolerated, or are expected to yield problematic effects, a trial of a drug in an alternative class should be considered. The SNRIs are then preferred and data supporting analgesic efficacy is most abundant for duloxetine.

It is now common practice to combine antidepressants in different classes as a strategy to address treatment-refractory depression. Anecdotally, the same approach may be useful when pain is the indication for these drugs. A combination of a tricyclic (amitriptyline) and a SSRI (fluoxetine) has been shown to be more effective than either drug alone in relieving pain from fibromyalgia[52]. In patients with medical illness, this approach usually is considered in the setting of severe neuropathic pain that has not responded to more conservative pharmacotherapy.

Anecdotal observations suggest that there is substantial variability in the analgesic response to the different antidepressants. Failure of a drug due to inefficacy, therefore, might reasonably be followed by a trial of an alternative drug. There are no guidelines for drug selection during these sequential trials, and the process usually proceeds by trial and error.

The starting dose of the tricyclic antidepressants should be low, 10 mg in the elderly or the medically ill, and 25 mg in younger patients. The initial dosing increments are usually the same size as the starting dose until a daily dose of 50 mg is reached. Dose increments above this typically are approximately 50 per cent of the baseline dose. Doses can be increased every few days. The usual effective dose range for amitriptyline or desipramine is 50 to 150 mg; some patients will benefit from doses below or above this range. Although most patients can be treated with a single night-time dose, some patients have less morning 'hangover' and some report less late afternoon pain if doses are divided.

Venlafaxine can be started at 37.5–75 mg daily. The dose can be increased as tolerated, up to a usual maximum dose of 225–375 mg/day. Duloxetine can be started at 30 mg once daily and increased to 60 mg once daily, which is the effective dose in clinical trials. Milnacipran should be started at 25 mg twice daily, and progressively titrated up to a target dose of 200 mg/day. The doses of venlafaxine, duloxetine, and milnacipran should be reduced by 25 per cent in mild–moderate renal function impairment and by 50 per cent in dialysis patients. As noted, dose tapering is important when planning to discontinue these drugs, particularly if treatment has continued for more than 6 weeks; tapering over 2 weeks reduces the risk of any withdrawal phenomena.

The SSRIs, like the SNRIs, are administered for pain in a manner similar to recommended approaches for depression. In the elderly and those with advanced illness, it is prudent to initiate therapy at a relatively low dose. In these populations, treatment with bupropion, similarly, may be initiated at a relatively low dose of 100–150 mg/day, and dose titration can target a maximum daily dose of 300–450 mg/day.

Given evidence of dose-dependent analgesic effects, at least for the tricyclic antidepressants, it is reasonable to continue upward dose titration beyond the usual analgesic doses in patients who fail to achieve benefit and have no limiting side effects. This course is clearly justified in patients with a coexistent depression, but should be considered even in patients without evidence of this disorder. There is currently no justification for increasing doses beyond the levels associated with antidepressant effects.

Plasma drug concentrations may be followed during dose titration of the tricyclic antidepressants. Although current data are insufficient to define concentration–effect models for analgesia, it is useful to monitor concentrations during therapy, if feasible, in order to determine whether a lack of response may be related to a low plasma drug concentration. An unexpectedly low concentration indicates either poor adherence to treatment or rapid metabolism; in the latter case, doses can be increased while repeatedly monitoring the plasma drug level. Likewise, non-responders whose plasma concentration is not very low, but is lower than the antidepressant range, should be considered for a trial of higher doses if side effects are not a problem. For patients who are benefiting from therapy, plasma levels provide a baseline for comparison should pain recur in the future.

Changes in pain, mood, cognitive status, sleep pattern, and other clinical effects must be carefully monitored during initiation of antidepressant therapy. There are limited, anecdotal observations that suggest the existence of a therapeutic window for analgesia during dose escalation with some tricyclic drugs, a phenomenon defined by the decline of favourable effects as the dose is increased above some threshold. This potential for a therapeutic window has not been confirmed in trials, but nonetheless, emphasizes the importance of careful monitoring during dose escalation.

A favourable analgesic effect is usually observed within a week after achieving an effective dosing level and, in some patients, maximal effect appears to evolve over days or weeks thereafter. This delay, combined with the many days required to increase the dose to a therapeutic level, may result in a prolonged period during which patients experience unsatisfactory effects from the therapy, and sometimes experience uncomfortable side effects. Unless the patient is well informed about this potential, non-compliance is likely.

Corticosteroids

Corticosteroid drugs have many potential indications in the palliative care setting. Numerous studies have suggested that these drugs may improve appetite, nausea, malaise, and overall quality of life[71–75]. Although concern about toxicity has generally limited the primary analgesic use of these drugs to patients with advanced disease and short life expectancies, there is a substantial anecdotal experience with both short-term and long-term administration for a variety of clinical problems, including pain.

Data from controlled trials and clinical series support the classification of corticosteroids as multi-purpose analgesics. Efficacy has been suggested in reflex sympathetic dystrophy, a type of neuropathic pain[76], and diverse types of cancer pain, including bone pain, neuropathic pain from infiltration or compression of neural structures, headache due to increased intracranial pressure, arthralgia, and pain due to obstruction of a hollow viscus (e.g. bowel or ureter)[74,77].

Analgesic effects have been described for a variety of corticosteroids and a broad range of doses. A placebo-controlled trial in patients with far-advanced cancer demonstrated that relatively low doses of methylprednisolone (16 mg twice daily) were analgesic but that these effects waned over a 20-day evaluation period[75]. A randomized trial showed that dexamethasone was profoundly analgesic in spinal cord compression but could not identify any difference between a high (10 mg) and low (10 mg) initial dose[78]. Symptoms related to bowel obstruction have been shown to respond to dexamethasone 8 to 60 mg/day[77] and methylprednisolone 30 to 50 mg/day[72]. Although a recent randomized controlled study of low-dose oral dexamethasone (8 mg daily) combined with an opioid failed to show any benefit on pain or most other symptoms in a sample of patients with far advanced illness[79], gastrointestinal side effects of the opioid were diminished and the drug produced short-lasting improvement of weakness, drowsiness, and well-being.

Mechanism of action

The mechanism of analgesia produced by corticosteroids is unknown. Any of several processes may be involved. Compression of pain sensitive structures may be relieved by reduction of peritumoural oedema or, in the case of steroid-responsive neoplasms, by shrinkage of tumour masses themselves. Activation of nociceptors may be lessened by reduced tissue concentrations of some inflammatory mediators, including prostaglandins, leukotrienes, and cytokines[80]. Aberrant electrical activity in damaged nerves may also be tempered by these agents[81].

Adverse effects

Well-recognized adverse effects are associated with short-term and long-term administration of corticosteroids, and with the withdrawal of these drugs following chronic use. The risk of serious toxicity increases with the dose of the drug, the duration of therapy, and predisposing factors associated with the medical condition of the patient.

Although acute toxicity is possible, transitory corticosteroid therapy is usually well tolerated. The potential toxicities include adverse neuropsychological effects, hyperglycaemia, fluid retention (which can lead to hypertension or volume overload in predisposed patients), and gastrointestinal disturbances ranging from dyspepsia to frank ulceration. A study of a high-dose dexamethasone regimen for epidural spinal cord compression (96 mg intravenously, followed by 96 mg orally for 3 days, then a taper for 10 days) noted three cases of serious toxicity among the 27 patients randomized to the steroid therapy (11 per cent); one patient became hypomanic, one developed a confusional state, and one developed a perforated gastric ulcer[82].

The neuropsychological toxicity associated with corticosteroid therapy ranges from delirium to relatively isolated changes in mood, cognitive functioning, or perception. Mood disturbances can themselves vary from euphoria to depression. In another study of patients who received a high-dose dexamethasone regimen for epidural spinal cord compression (100 mg followed by 24 mg every 6 h), the overall rate of psychiatric disorders was no greater than a comparison group, but there was a greater incidence of major depressive disorders and a trend toward a greater incidence of delirium in the steroid-treated group; those who received steroids also had more depressive and anxious symptomatology[83]. Although neuropsychological toxicity is usually observed early during treatment and when relatively high doses are administered, these adverse effects can complicate a steroid regimen at any time. There is no proven association with any specific drug and the occurrence of acute toxicity during one course of therapy does not predict a similar response during subsequent courses.

Chronic administration of a corticosteroid can produce a cushingoid habitus; changes in integument, subcutaneous tissues, and connective tissues; weight gain; hypertension; severe osteoporosis; myopathy; increased risk of infection; hyperglycaemia; gastrointestinal toxicity; and late neuropsychological effects. Long-term treatment with relatively low doses is generally well tolerated, however, even among patients with advanced illness. A study of advanced cancer patients chronically administered prednisolone or dexamethasone at varying doses observed oropharyngeal candidiasis in approximately one-third of patients and oedema or cushingoid habitus in less than one-fifth; dyspepsia, weight gain, neuropsychological changes, and ecchymoses occurred in 5 to 10 per cent and the incidence of other adverse effects, such as hyperglycaemia, myopathy, and osteoporosis, was even lower than this[75].

Chronic administration of a corticosteroid approximately doubles the risk of peptic ulcer and gastrointestinal perforation, even during short-term therapy[84]. This risk is increased further by co-administration of a non-steroidal anti-inflammatory drug, which contraindicates the combined use of a corticosteroid and a non-steroidal anti-inflammatory drug in the palliative care setting.

Steroid withdrawal following chronic therapy can produce a syndrome of myalgia and arthralgia known as steroid 'pseudorheumatism'. Withdrawal may also produce other symptoms, such as malaise, headache, and mood disturbance, or yield a flare of the symptoms for which steroid therapy had been initiated previously. Following a reduction to low doses, patients also may be at risk for disturbances associated with adrenal insufficiency, particularly during a period of intercurrent stress such as systemic infection. The symptoms associated with steroid withdrawal can occur with either dose reduction or discontinuation of therapy. In some cases, symptoms appear after a relatively modest decline in a relatively high baseline dose. Escalation of the steroid dose can provide relief, and a slower, more gradual taper may avoid recurrence.

Pharmacology

Dexamethasone is metabolized by the hepatic isozyme CYP3A4[85]. It can also induce or inhibit this isozyme, thereby increasing or decreasing the metabolism of other drugs metabolized by CYP3A4, including the tertiary tricyclics, methadone, carbamazepine, venlafaxine, and dextromethorphan[85]. Phenytoin and nefazodone, which are inhibitors of CYP3A4, can theoretically increase the effect of dexamethasone but the clinical significance of this interaction remains unknown[67].

Indications

Corticosteroids are used acutely in the management of epidural compression, raised intracranial pressure, and superior vena cava syndrome. Pain may accompany each of these syndromes and symptomatic relief is one of the goals of therapy.

On the basis of anecdotal experience, corticosteroids are also administered for many other painful syndromes, including metastatic bone pain, neuropathic pain due to compression or infiltration of peripheral nerves or nerve plexus, painful lymphoedema, pain due to obstruction of a hollow viscus, and pain due to organ capsule distension. Like other adjuvant analgesics, corticosteroids are usually added to an opioid regimen following dose escalation to limiting toxicity. Patients who present with these pain syndromes commonly have other symptoms that could potentially be improved by steroid therapy, such as nausea or malaise, and corticosteroid therapy may be considered earlier if primarily indicated by these other symptoms.

Dosing guidelines

The relative risks and benefits of the various corticosteroids are unknown. In the United States, dexamethasone is usually selected, a choice that gains theoretical support from the relatively low mineralocorticoid effects of this drug. Prednisone and methylprednisolone have also been used.

On the basis of clinical experience, corticosteroids are usually administered either in a high-dose regimen or a low-dose regimen. A high-dose regimen (e.g. dexamethasone 100 mg followed initially by 96 mg per day in divided doses) has been used for patients who experience an acute episode of very severe pain that cannot be promptly reduced with opioids, such as that associated with a rapidly worsening malignant plexopathy. This regimen has been widely used in the setting of emerging spinal cord or cauda equina signs related to epidural metastasis and may also be appropriate when treating other oncological emergencies, such as superior vena cava syndrome. Following the loading dose, the fixed-dose regimen can be tapered over weeks, concurrent with the initiation of other analgesic approaches such as radiotherapy.

A low-dose corticosteroid regimen (e.g. dexamethasone 1–2 mg once or twice daily) has been used for patients with advanced medical illness who continue to have pain despite optimal dosing of opioid drugs. In most cases, long-term therapy is planned. Although the risks associated with prolonged steroid use in this setting are more than balanced by the need for enhanced comfort, repeated assessments are required to ensure that benefits are sustained. Ineffective regimens should be tapered and discontinued, and in all cases, the lowest dose that yields the desired results should be sought.

Alpha-2 adrenergic agonists

Classification of the alpha-2 adrenergic agonists as multi-purpose analgesics is supported by both animal and human studies. Strong antinociceptive effects in animals can be produced by clonidine, a partial agonist at the alpha-2 adrenergic receptor[86] and by both medetomidine, a full alpha-2 agonist[87], and dexmedetomidine, the active d-isomer of medetomidine[88]. These effects can be observed in a variety of experimental models, including models of neuropathic pain[86,88]. In humans, analgesic effects in diverse pain syndromes have been established in controlled studies of systemic dexmedetomidine[89], and both systemic and intraspinal clonidine[90,91]. These and other reports suggest that clonidine can be beneficial in pain syndromes that may be relatively less opioid-responsive, including chronic headache, non-malignant neuropathic pains[90], and some cancer pain syndromes (including neuropathic cancer-related pain)[91,92].

Two controlled trials have illuminated the role of clonidine as an analgesic. The first study used an 'enriched enrolment' design, in which an open-label phase was used to identify patients with painful diabetic polyneuropathy who might be potential clonidine responders. These patients were then tested in a controlled trial of transdermal clonidine, which demonstrated that fewer than one-quarter of patients are potential responders, but that those who do respond can experience analgesia that is both substantial and sustained[90].

The second study compared a 14-day epidural infusion of clonidine (30 mcg/h) with an epidural placebo infusion in patients with cancer pain who were receiving titrated intraspinal opioids via epidural morphine patient-controlled analgesia[91]. Overall, clonidine reduced pain but not opioid consumption. Therapeutic success, defined as either reduced opioid requirement or pain reduction, occurred in 45 per cent of those who received clonidine and 21 per cent of those who received placebo. Remarkably, most of this difference in success rates was due to the response of patients with neuropathic pain; in this subgroup, success was achieved by 56 per cent of those who received clonidine and only 5 per cent of those who received placebo.

These data provide evidence that clonidine is a multi-purpose analgesic that may be particularly useful in the management of neuropathic pain. Both systemic administration, by the oral or transdermal route, and epidural administration can yield favourable effects. Although a minority (fewer than one-quarter during systemic administration) are likely to respond, those that do can experience clinically meaningful effects.

Tizanidine is another centrally acting alpha-2 agonist and is commercially available in the United States as an antispasticity agent, with established efficacy in hypertonicity associated with multiple sclerosis, acquired brain injury, and spinal cord injury[93]. Its antinociceptive properties have been observed in animal studies[94] and a few open-label studies have revealed some analgesic effect in myofascial pain syndrome[95]. Although the evidence of analgesic efficacy is limited, the mechanism of this drug and a favourable clinical experience has supported its use as a multi-purpose analgesic.

Mechanism of action

The mechanism of analgesia produced by the alpha-2 adrenergic agonists has not been established and is likely to be complex. Noradrenergic receptors are clearly important in the modulation of nociceptive processing and it is possible that interaction with alpha-2 receptors in the spinal cord or brainstem activates endogenous systems that reduce nociceptive input to the central nervous system, possibly via sodium and potassium channels[96]. Presumably, these systems may be relatively more or less involved in the processing of different types of noxious stimuli or the development of different types of pain syndromes[96]. It is also possible that the alpha-2 adrenergic agonists produce analgesia in some cases through interference with the mechanisms that perpetuate so-called sympathetically-maintained pain, a subtype of neuropathic pain.

Adverse effects

In placebo-controlled trials, the most common adverse effects associated with systemic or epidural clonidine administration have been somnolence, hypotension (usually orthostatic), and dry mouth[90,91]. The controlled trial of epidural clonidine in cancer pain demonstrated that the drug produced a sustained hypotensive effect in almost one-half of the patients and six of the 38 patients (16 per cent) who received clonidine experienced serious blood pressure changes associated with dizziness, hypotension, or rebound hypertension[91].

The most frequent side effects associated with tizanidine are somnolence and dry mouth. This drug has less affinity for the alpha-1 adrenergic receptor and, therefore, produces hypotension less often than clonidine.

Pharmacology

Clonidine is metabolized by the liver to inactive metabolites, which are renally excreted. The drug interactions are minimal and mainly concern potentiation of the effects of other hypotensive medications[97].

Indications

Like other multi-purpose analgesics, clonidine and tizanidine can be considered for a therapeutic trial in any chronic pain state. In the medically ill, however, anecdotal experience has generally been limited to patients with opioid-refractory neuropathic pains. Although the data in support of analgesic effects is better for clonidine, a trial of tizanidine may be favoured because of concern about hypotension. Both drugs are usually avoided in patients who are haemodynamically unstable, predisposed to serious hypotension (e.g. by autonomic neuropathy, intravascular volume depletion, or concurrent therapy with potent hypotensive agents), or markedly somnolent from other causes. Given limited experience with the adrenergic agonists in those with advanced illness, trials of these drugs are usually considered after other adjuvant analgesics, such as the antidepressants and anticonvulsants, have failed.

Dosing guidelines

When administered systemically for pain, clonidine is typically initiated at a relatively low dose, 0.1 mg/day orally or one-half of a TTS-1 patch transdermally. Given its delivery characteristics, the transdermal system can be safely cut into pieces to change the dose. Tizanidine can be initiated at a dose of 1–2 mg/day.

Monitoring of both pain and adverse effects is necessary during gradual dose escalation. Neither dose-dependent effects nor the potential for a ceiling dose has been evaluated during systemic clonidine therapy. Consequently, gradual dose escalation should continue until significant side effects occur or blood pressure declines to a degree that is worrisome. Anecdotally, some patients have benefited from relatively high doses, and it is reasonable to continue upward dose titration until dose-limiting toxicity is encountered.

Neuroleptics

The demonstration of antinociceptive effects in animal models[98,99] and the favourable results of several controlled clinical trials in diverse pain syndromes[100–102] suggest that some neuroleptics might be considered non-specific, multi-purpose analgesics. Nonetheless, there is relatively little evidence of analgesic activity for most neuroleptic compounds and their role as adjuvant analgesics is limited by this lack of definitive data and the potential for adverse effects[102].

Controlled trials have yielded mixed results. The strongest evidence of analgesic efficacy has been acquired in older studies of the phenothiazine methotrimeprazine in cancer pain and chronic pain states[100]. A controlled comparison of pimozide (4–12 mg/day) and carbamazepine in patients with trigeminal neuralgia demonstrated that pimozide has analgesic efficacy in this lancinating neuropathic pain syndrome[101]. Unfortunately, a very high incidence of disturbing side effects, including physical and mental slowing, tremor, and parkinsonian symptoms, limited the value of this therapy.

A recent systematic review suggested that the second-generation 'atypical neuroleptics' may have analgesic properties[102]. A case series suggests that olanzapine decreases pain in opioid-unresponsive cancer pain by potentiating the effect of opioids, thereby allowing a significant decrease of the opioid dose[103].

Mechanism of action

The mechanism of neuroleptic analgesia is unknown, but may involve the effect of dopaminergic blockade on endogenous pain-modulating systems. Dopamine receptors, specifically the D_2 subtype, are represented among the numerous pathways that subserve pain modulation. Studies in animals have suggested that selective dopamine antagonists can potentiate morphine analgesia[98] and controlled clinical trials have demonstrated that metoclopramide, a relatively selective blocker of the D_2 receptor, is analgesic in humans[104]. This evidence does not confirm that a dopaminergic mechanism underlies the analgesic effects of neuroleptic drugs, however, because all these drugs interact with other receptors that could potentially mediate analgesic effects. Indeed, it has been suggested that the atypical neuroleptics might differ in their mechanisms of analgesia, since clozapine seems to act as an opioid agonist and olanzapine acts via its alpha-adrenergic effects[99].

Adverse effects

Common side effects of neuroleptic drugs include sedation, orthostatic dizziness, and anticholinergic effects. Some patients experience mental clouding or confusion. Phenothiazines, such as chlorpromazine and fluphenazine, are more likely to produce these effects than other subclasses, such as the butyrophenones (e.g. haloperidol). The sedation produced by the neuroleptics can be additive to other central nervous system depressants. Rare, idiosyncratic reactions include blood dyscrasias, dermatoses (including photosensitivity), and hepatic damage.

The possibility of extrapyramidal side effects is perhaps the greatest concern in the clinical use of neuroleptic drugs. The incidence of these disorders varies with the drug, duration of therapy, and dose. Compared to other neuroleptics, both fluphenazine and haloperidol are relatively more likely to produce these effects, whereas the newer 'atypical' neuroleptics are less likely to induce them.

The most serious extrapyramidal reaction is the neuroleptic malignant syndrome, which is characterized by rigidity, autonomic instability, and encephalopathy. Successful management requires prompt diagnosis, discontinuation of the neuroleptic, and intensive supportive measures. The use of dantrolene and bromocriptine has been suggested in severe cases.

Indications

In the palliative care setting, neuroleptics are used commonly in the management of delirium or nausea. Their specific use as analgesics has been limited by concerns about toxicity and the availability of alternative, safer drugs. Methotrimeprazine is difficult to obtain, but if available, may be useful in bedridden patients with advanced illness, who are experiencing pain associated with anxiety, restlessness, or nausea. For patients with advanced disease, the sedative, anxiolytic, and antiemetic effects of this drug can be favourable, and side effects, such as orthostatic hypotension, are less of an issue.

Use of the newer atypical neuroleptics as adjuvant analgesics may evolve should studies provide more evidence of analgesia and confirm a favourable risk:benefit ratio in the medically ill. Experience is so limited at this time that they, like their older counterparts, generally are not considered for pain unless treatment with many other drugs has proved unsuccessful.

Dosing guidelines

With known dose-related toxicity and no confirmation of dose-dependent efficacy, the neuroleptics are prudently dosed to some arbitrary ceiling based on published reports, then discontinued if no analgesia ensues. Methotrimeprazine has been administered by intramuscular or subcutaneous bolus, by continuous subcutaneous infusion, and brief intravenous infusion (administration over 20–30 min). Dosing usually begins with 5 mg every 6 h, or a comparable dose delivered by infusion, which is gradually increased as needed. Most patients will not require more than 20 mg every 6 h to gain desired effects. Olanzapine can be started at a dose of 2.5–5 mg, used at bedtime or twice daily. Its sedative effects can be useful in terminally ill patients presenting with restlessness, agitation, or insomnia.

Adjuvant analgesics used for neuropathic pain

As noted previously, the focus on neuropathic pain as a target for the adjuvant analgesics in the palliative care setting derives from the observation that pains of this type may be relatively less responsive to opioid drugs than other pains[70,105,106]. A recent survey revealed that the appropriate use of both opioid and adjuvant analgesics

can yield analgesic outcomes in cancer-related neuropathic pain that mirror those obtained during treatment of nociceptive or mixed pain syndromes[2]. As described previously, many of the multi-purpose analgesics are among the first-line adjuvant analgesics for neuropathic pain. Numerous other drugs also are conventionally used, however, selected anticonvulsants are similarly considered first-line drugs for these conditions.

Anticonvulsant drugs

The analgesic potential of anticonvulsant drugs has been recognized for decades for the management of neuropathic pains. The older drugs, such as phenytoin and carbamazepine, are now complemented by a rapidly increasing number of newer agents. Among the newer drugs, the alpha-2-delta-1 modulators (gabapentin or pregabalin) have garnered compelling evidence of analgesic efficacy, are approved in many countries for diverse types of neuropathic pain, and are generally considered first-line agents—along with selected antidepressants and the corticosteroids—in neuropathic pain associated with medical illness.

The analgesic efficacy of carbamazepine has been established by controlled studies in patients with trigeminal neuralgia[107], postherpetic neuralgia (in which an effect against lancinating but not continuous pains was demonstrated)[107], and painful diabetic neuropathy[108]. These data, along with uncontrolled trials in other types of neuropathic pain, suggest that carbamazepine has analgesic efficacy in neuropathic pain, regardless of the specific pathology that induces it. This drug continues to be considered the first-line agent for the treatment of trigeminal neuralgia[5].

Support for the analgesic activity of phenytoin is limited to an older controlled trial in painful diabetic neuropathy[109], and to surveys and case reports in other non-malignant neuropathic pains or cancer pain[110].

The role for anticonvulsants in neuropathic pain expanded greatly with the advent of gabapentin, a modulator of the alpha-2-delta-1 protein of the N-type calcium channel. The analgesic efficacy of this drug has been established through randomized trials in several types of neuropathic pain, including diabetic neuropathy[111,112], postherpetic neuralgia[113,114], acute herpes zoster[115], spinal cord injury[116], post-thoracotomy pain[117], lumbar spinal stenosis[118], and fibromyalgia[119]. Open label trials and surveys suggest its efficacy in complex regional pain syndrome[120], HIV neuropathy[121], neuropathic cancer pain[122], and diverse pains from multiple sclerosis[123]. According to a pilot randomized controlled study, gabapentin might decrease the incidence of postoperative delirium in older patients, probably via an opioid-sparing effect[124]. Two studies comparing gabapentin and amitriptyline in diabetic neuropathy yielded conflicting results. In one trial, amitriptyline was more effective than gabapentin (difference not statistically significant) and the occurrence of adverse events was similar[13]; the other trial revealed gabapentin to be superior to amitriptyline in relieving pain and paresthesias, and better tolerated[112]. A comparison of gabapentin and nortriptyline for postherpetic neuralgia also showed gabapentin to be equally effective and better tolerated[125]. In a sample with neuropathic pain, the combination of gabapentin with an opioid (e.g. morphine) provided beter analgesia at lower doses of each drug than each drug alone[126].

Evidence of an analgesic efficacy of gabapentin for cancer-related neuropathic pain has been accumulating, with a few positive randomized controlled[127,128] and open label[122,129,130] trials. One study failed to demonstrate any benefit in chemotherapy-induced peripheral neuropathy[131]. The addition of gabapentin to an opioid provides better relief of neuropathic cancer pain than opioid monotherapy[127,129]. Treatment with gabapentin and local anaesthetics in the wound decreased both acute and chronic pain after breast surgery for cancer[128] and one case report suggests successful use as a co-analgesic to relieve pain from cancer wound dressing care[132].

Pregabalin is a newer gabapentinoid drug, with a similar mechanism of action as gabapentin, but different pharmacokinetics. It has been extensively studied in several types of non-malignant neuropathic pain, including painful diabetic neuropathy[133,134], postherpetic neuralgia[135], and central pain from spinal cord injury[136]. It is also analgesic in the non-neuropathic conditions fibromyalgia[137] and irritable bowel syndrome[138]. When administered prior to surgery, pregabalin decreased the postoperative use of opioids[139]. A 15-month open-label trial suggests that it may provide long-term benefit in neuropathic pain refractory to other adjuvant (e.g. gabapentin and antidepressants) and opioid analgesics[140]. Studies also have demonstrated that pregabalin can reduce pain-related sleep interference[135] and treat generalized anxiety disorder, as well as a few other conditions including pruritus[141] and restless leg syndrome[142]. The onset of analgesic activity is faster with pregabalin (significant difference in pain on second day) than with gabapentin[135]. Although there is currently no evidence of pregabalin's analgesic efficacy in cancer-related neuropathic pain, its pharmacological properties and clinical experience support its use.

With extensive evidence of analgesic efficacy in diverse neuropathic pains, generally good tolerability and a paucity of drug–drug interactions, gabapentin and pregabalin have been recommended as first-line agents for the treatment of neuropathic pain of diverse etiologies[5]. Gabapentin is also the most commonly used adjuvant analgesic in cancer patients with neuropathic pain[8], and on palliative care units[143].

Lamotrigine has been shown in randomized trials to relieve pain from trigeminal neuralgia[144], HIV neuropathy[145], and central post-stroke pain[146]. Studies on painful diabetic neuropathy yielded conflicting results[147,148], and the addition of lamotrigine to either a nonopioid analgesic, gabapentin, or a tricyclic antidepressant did not increase the analgesic response[149]. Only one case report suggested that lamotrigine could be beneficial in neuropathic cancer pain, providing pain relief and allowing a decrease of the opioid doses[150].

The analgesic effect of topiramate has been assessed in several studies. Randomized trials were positive in diabetic neuropathy[151], chronic lumbar radicular pain[152], and chronic low-back pain[153]. In the latter study, it also improved anger, subjective disability, and health-related quality of life. One case report suggested that topiramate could be analgesic for chemotherapy-induced peripheral neuropathy[34].

Tiagabine is a GABA agonist and also has antinociceptive action in animal models[154]. In humans, an open-label study suggests that it is as effective as gabapentin for chronic pain of different etiologies, and has a better effect on sleep quality[155]. Felbamate has been used anecdotally to treat hemifacial spasm and trigeminal neuralgia, but given its association with myelosuppression and hepatotoxicity, it is very rarely considered for pain. Levetiracetam is antinociceptive in an animal model[156]; in experimental human pain models, it increased the pain tolerance and the pain detection thresholds[157]. In a small open-label trial, adding levetiracetam, following a poor response to gabapentin, provided good or excellent relief in 60 per cent of patients[158]. A case series of seven patients with neoplastic plexopathies suggests an analgesic and opioid-sparing effect[159]. These limited observations suggest the need for additional trials. Zonisamide has been shown to be effective in one randomized controlled trial of painful diabetic neuropathy[160]. These limited data also support the need for further evaluation of this drug. Oxcarbazepine is a metabolite of carbamazepine and has a similar spectrum of effects, with better tolerability. It seems to be effective in painful diabetic neuropathy[161], including in some patients who were refractory to gabapentin[162].

Several older anticonvulsants are widely used as analgesics for neuropathic pain despite limited data from clinical trials. There is a large clinical experience with both clonazepam and valproate. Clonazepam often is considered for an early trial if co-morbid anxiety is a substantial problem. Results of more recent randomized controlled trials of valproate for peripheral neuropathy are conflicting[163,164].

In summary, selected anticonvulsant drugs may be effective for diverse types of neuropathic pain. Gabapentin and pregabalin are now recommended as first-line drugs for all types of neuropathic pain due to their proven efficacy and good tolerability. Based on more limited observations, it is likely that individual patients vary in their response to these two gabapentinoids. Patients with neuropathic pain who do not respond to these anticonvulsants, and have not responded favourably to selected antidepressant analgesics or corticosteroids, can be considered for trials of other anticonvulsant drugs, particularly those for which clinical trials data are supportive of efficacy.

Mechanism of action

With a few exceptions, the specific mechanisms that result in the analgesia produced by the varied anticonvulsant drugs are not known[165]. Nonetheless, it can be postulated that the aberrant electrical activity at different levels of the neuraxis that has been recorded in patients with chronic neuropathic pains reflect pain-related neural dysfunction (such as sensitization of neurons), which can be favourably affected by actions of anticonvulsants on specific receptors or channels.

The analgesia produced by gabapentin and pregabalin results from binding to the alpha-2-delta-1 sub-unit of the voltage-sensitive N-type calcium channel[166]. This action inhibits the release of several neurotranmitters such as glutamate.

Other anticonvulsants have one or more than one action on other receptors or channels, which presumably also impact favourably on mechanisms sustaining the pain or pain-modulating processes that attenuate these mechanisms. For example, some anticonvulsants, such as carbamazepine, oxcarbazepine, lamotrigine, and valproate, produce effects on voltage-gated sodium channels; some, such as lamotrigine, act on glutamate receptors; and some, such as tiagabine, are GABAergic[165].

Adverse effects

Carbamazepine commonly causes sedation, dizziness, nausea, and unsteadiness. These effects can be minimized by low initial doses and gradual dose titration. The intensity diminishes in most patients maintained on the drug for several weeks. Of much greater concern is that carbamazepine causes leucopenia and/or thrombocytopenia in approximately 2 per cent of patients; aplastic anaemia is a rare complication. Other rare adverse effects of carbamazepine include hepatic damage, hyponatremia due to inappropriate secretion of antidiuretic hormone, and congestive heart failure. Baseline liver and renal function tests should be obtained prior to therapy.

Most of the common side effects of phenytoin are dose-dependent. These include sedation or mental clouding, dizziness, unsteadiness, and diplopia. These effects usually occur at plasma concentrations above the therapeutic range for seizure control. Occasional patients experience toxicity at lower concentrations. Ataxia, progressive encephalopathy, and even seizures can occur at toxic levels. Of the idiosyncratic effects, the most serious are hepatotoxicity and exfoliative dermatitis. The occurrence of a maculopapular rash, which can be the harbinger of the more severe cutaneous reactions, should lead to discontinuation of the drug.

At usual therapeutic doses, the side effects of valproate are usually mild, consisting of sedation, nausea, tremor, and sometimes increased appetite. Hepatotoxicity, encephalopathy, dermatitis, alopecia, and a rare hyperammonaemia syndrome are among the reported idiosyncratic reactions. The hyperammonaemia syndrome can occur in the absence of abnormal liver function tests; patients who become confused during valproate therapy should have serum ammonia measured.

The newer anticonvulsant drugs, including gabapentin, pregabalin, lamotrigine, topiramate, and oxcarbazepine, are generally associated with a favourable side-effect profile[111,112,133,144]. The most common side effects are non-specific central nervous system complaints of somnolence, mental clouding, dizziness, fatigue, or unsteadiness. Gabapentin and pregabalin also may cause oedema and weight gain. The most serious adverse effect associated with lamotrigine is an exfoliative rash, which occurs in approximately 0.3 per cent of treated patients. All types of rash, which affect more than 4 per cent of treated patients, are more likely to occur with high initial doses and in younger patients. For this reason, the drug should be started at a low initial dose (25–50 mg/day) and titrated over one month; patients younger than 15 years should not be treated in the usual circumstances. If any rash occurs, the drug must be stopped immediately.

Pharmacology

Carbamazepine is highly bound to serum proteins. It induces liver enzymes responsible for its metabolism, which shortens its half-life with repetitive administrations. Serum concentrations can be monitored as the dose is increased in order to determine where the concentration falls relative to the therapeutic range for seizures. Conventionally, doses for pain are not increased above those associated with a concentration at, or just above, the upper limit of this range.

Phenytoin also is highly bound to serum proteins. Its clearance is highly variable, and is dependent on intrinsic hepatic function and dose administered. At higher doses, the elimination kinetics transition to zero-order, which means that a relatively small increment in dose can result in a large increase in plasma concentration. It is therefore important to increase the dose by small increments at the upper therapeutic range (for example, above 200 mg/day) and to monitor the serum levels. This will reduce the risk of toxicity and indicate whether continued upward titration is likely to be safe. In order to get the active form of phenytoin, the level should be corrected depending on the albumin level.

Phenytoin is an inducer of the isozymes CYP2D6 and CYP3A4, and is a substrate of CYP2C9[97]. It increases clearance of other drugs metabolized by CYP3A4, including methadone, midazolam, and imipramine[67], which may necessitate upward dose adjustment of these drugs if phenytoin is added. It may decrease serum concentrations of lamotrigine, warfarin, corticosteroids, cyclosporin, theophylline, rifampin, quinidine, mexiletine, dysopyramide, dopamine, and several muscle relaxants[97]. Phenytoin levels themselves may be decreased by erythromycin, and increased by fluoxetine and sertraline, via a competitive inhibition of the enzyme system. Acute ingestion of alcohol decreases phenytoin levels and chronic administration may increase levels. Interaction with valproic acid is complex and can cause both an increase and a decrease of the phenytoin level.

Gabapentin and pregabalin are minimally protein-bound and are excreted unchanged in the urine. They are not metabolized by the liver and have no known pharmacokinetic drug–drug interactions[97]. Due to a saturable absorption process in the gastrointestinal tract, gabapentin's bioavailability varies from 60 per cent for a single 300-mg dose to 35 per cent for 1600 mg three times daily[167]. This declining oral bioavailability at higher doses may contribute to the ceiling effect observed clinically. Pregabalin does not require active transporters to be absorbed and has linear pharmacokinetics through the effective dose range; this characteristic, which means that a dose increase leads to a proportionate increase in serum concentration, simplifies dose titration (e.g. by reducing the number of dose changes necessary to theoretically explore the therapeutic range of serum concentrations).

Other anticonvulsants have similarly complex pharmacologies[97]. Lamotrigine undergoes both hepatic and renal metabolism and elimination. Its serum concentration is decreased by carbamazepine and phenytoin, and is increased by valproate. Topiramate has minimal protein-binding and hepatic metabolism, and is excreted unchanged in the urine. Its serum concentration can be decreased by phenytoin, carbamazepine, and valproate. Tiagabine is highly protein-bound and undergoes significant hepatic metabolism, mainly by the CYP3A4 isozyme. Its half-life is decreased by co-administration of carbamazepine and phenytoin. Like gabapentin, levetiracetam is not metabolized in the liver and has a low potential for drug interactions. Oxcarbazepine has low protein-binding and is mainly metabolized by noninducible enzymes. Although its minimal metabolism by the cytochrome P450 diminishes its potential for drug interactions, it can nevertheless interact with some medications, including phenytoin and oral contraceptives.

Indications

Anticonvulsant drugs are now widely considered for all types of neuropathic pain. There is a broad consensus that one of the gabapentinoids, gabapentin or pregabalin, may be considered first-line therapy unless co-morbid depression suggests the value of an analgesic antidepressant, such as desipramine or duloxetine[5]. The principle of drug selection based on existing co-morbidities implicit in the latter guideline is extended further in the setting of advanced medical illness, where first-line treatment of neuropathic pain with a corticosteroid often is considered in the hope that concurrent symptoms, such as malaise or anorexia, will be improved. If an anticonvulsant is selected, the only commonly accepted exception to the current consensus supporting the first-line use of a gabapentinoid is the use of carbamazepine as first-line treatment for trigeminal neuralgia[5].

Patients who do not respond to first-line therapy for neuropathic pain may undergo sequential trials of many drugs, including other anticonvulsants. Given the limited data and lack of comparative trials, the selection of second-line analgesic anticonvulsants is empirical. There is some evidence supporting the use of lamotrigine, oxcarbazepine, and topiramate, and it is reasonable on this basis to try these drugs next.

Dosing guidelines

Dosing guidelines when treating neuropathic pain with an anticonvulsant are typically extrapolated from those recommended for the treatment of seizures. When treating older patients or those with multiple medical illnesses, lower initial doses and more gradual upward dose titration are prudent to increase tolerability and compliance.

In the medically ill, it is prudent to initiate therapy with gabapentin or pregabalin using relatively low starting doses. Although starting doses as high as 300—900 mg/day for gabapentin and 150 mg/day for pregabalin have been used, it is safer to begin gabapentin treatment at 100—300 mg/day and pregabalin treatment at 25–50 mg/day, usually starting with a single bedtime dose. The dose can be increased by an amount equal to the starting dose every few days, dividing the doses. The effective dose range is very broad for gabapentin. Some patients report benefit at 300 mg/day, whereas others require more than 3600 mg/day; the usual effective dose range is 900–2700 mg/day in two to four divided doses. For pregabalin, the usual effective dose range is 150–300 mg daily in two divided doses. Some patients with co-morbid insomnia appear to benefit from imbalanced dosing, with a relatively larger dose at bedtime to assist with sleep. Patients with severe renal insufficiency should receive a low initial dose of these drugs (100 mg of gabapentin or 25 mg of pregabalin) and dose titration should be performed cautiously.

Low initial doses and dose titration also are appropriate for other anticonvulsants. Given experience with phenytoin loading doses, however, this drug may be initiated at the presumed therapeutic dose (e.g. 300 mg/day) or with a cautious oral loading regimen (e.g. 500 mg twice, separated by hours). Regardless of the drug, dose escalation typically is tried until favourable effects occur, intolerable side effects supervene, or drug concentrations (for those, like phenytoin, valproate and carbamazepine, with widely available monitoring) has reached the upper end of the therapeutic range for seizures.

Carbamazepine usually is started at 100–200 mg twice daily. The dose can be increased gradually at intervals of days to weeks depending on the clinical situation. The usual therapeutic dose is 600–1600 mg daily in 2–4 divided doses.

To reduce the risk of dermatitis, lamotrigine should be started at a low initial dose of 25–50 mg/day, and the initial few weeks of dosing should incorporate slow titration. An initial dose of 25 mg/day can be increased after one week to 25 mg twice daily, and then increased by 25-mg increments each week for another two weeks. Alternatively, a starting dose of 25 mg twice daily can be used, and then increased to 50 mg twice daily after two weeks. After the dose reaches 100 mg/day, further increments can be performed more quickly, and in larger amounts. The usual effective dose is between 200 mg and 500 mg per day. The need for a slow initiation of dosing may be problematic in those with severe pain and in the medically ill with limited life expectancies.

Topiramate can be initiated at 25 mg daily and titrated gradually up to 400 mg daily, in two divided doses. The usual effective dose range is 100–300 mg/day in two divided doses. Tiagabine should be initiated with a dose of 4 mg at bedtime and increased gradually. The maximum dose studied has been 12 mg daily, in three divided doses. Levetiracetam can be initiated at 500–1000 mg daily, and then gradually increased; the effective dose range appears to be as high as several grams per day in divided doses. The initial daily dose of oxcarbazepine should be 75–150 mg twice daily; doses can be gradually increased to a usual maximum of 2400 mg/day in divided doses. Zonisamide is usually titrated from a starting dose of 100–200 mg/day and has an effective dose range that appears to be as high as 400 mg/day.

Oral and parenteral sodium channel blockers

As noted, some of the anticonvulsants presumably affect pain through actions involving sodium channels. Other classes of sodium channel blockers, including anaesthetics and anti-arrhythmics, also are used in the treatment of pain. Athough studies suggest that these drugs may be multi-purpose analgesics, a large clinical experience has focused on their use for neuropathic pain.

Controlled trials have demonstrated that a brief intravenous infusion of lignocaine (lidocaine) can relieve acute postoperative pain and pain due to burns[168] and have provided strong evidence of efficacy for neuropathic pain, including central pain[169,170], postherpetic neuralgia[171], and painful diabetic neuropathy[172]. There have, however, been several negative studies of local anaesthetics in neuropathic cancer pain[173,174].

Prolonged relief of pain following a brief intravenous infusion of a local anaesthetic may be possible. If pain recurs, long-term subcutaneous administration of lignocaine also has been used anecdotally to yield sustained relief of refractory neuropathic pain in cancer patients[175].

Oral formulations of sodium channel blockers similar to the local anaesthetics are available and long-term systemic therapy can be accomplished simply using these drugs. A survey of cancer patients suggested that flecainide can be effective in the treatment of pain due to tumour infiltration of nerves[176]. In controlled trials, tocainide was effective for trigeminal neuralgia[177] and mexiletine lessened the pain of diabetic neuropathy[178]. These data establish the analgesic potential of systemically administered drugs that block sodium channels and suggest that diverse types of pain can potentially respond. Controlled trials have emphasized the value of this therapy in neuropathic pain, and this is the use that has been pursued in clinical practice.

Mechanism of action

Animal studies reveal that intravenous lidocaine reduces hyperalgesia[179], and a clinical trial observed an isolated effect on mechanical allodynia and hyperalgesia[170].

These effects presumably reflect a reduction in sensitization or ectopic electrical activity in nociceptive neurons, which in turn, presumably relates to a non-depolarizing conduction block of the action potential produced by sodium channel blockade. In regional anaesthesia, this conduction block is induced in axons by local instillation of a drug. This type of peripheral effect does not explain the analgesia produced by systemic administration, however; non-toxic systemic doses do not block the peripheral action potential, although amplitudes are decreased to a degree. Rather, systemic administration probably suppresses activity in dorsal horn neurons that are activated by C fibre input, as well as the spontaneous firing of neuromas and dorsal root ganglion cells[180].

Adverse effects

The major dose-dependent toxicities associated with this drug class affect the central nervous system and the cardiovascular system. The central nervous system effects generally occur at a lower concentration than cardiac changes. Dizziness, perioral numbness, and other paraesthesias, and tremor usually occur first; at higher plasma concentrations, progressive encephalopathy develops and seizures may occur. There is a correlation between the local anaesthetic potency and the dose required to produce this central nervous system toxicity.

Toxic concentrations of local anaesthetic drugs can produce cardiac conduction disturbances and myocardial depression. The effect on the conduction system is first observed as prolongation of the PR interval and the QRS duration. At higher concentrations, bradycardia and other arrhythmias occur. If severe enough, the depression of myocardial contractility can result in pump failure. Similar to the central nervous system effects of these drugs, the likelihood of cardiovascular toxicity with relatively low doses is correlated with local anaesthetic potency.

These toxicities also characterize the oral formulations, such as mexiletine, tocainide, and flecainide. In the United States, flecainide has not been used commonly due to an association with sudden death during a trial of therapy for patients immediately post-myocardial infarction[181]. Neither the general applicability of this risk of sudden death to other medical settings nor the degree to which it reflects a specific effect of flecainide is known. Nonetheless, flecainide does have relatively potent local anaesthetic effects and greater negative inotropic effects than the other oral local anaesthetics, and these pharmacological actions, combined with the association with sudden death, has tended to place it in a negative light as a therapy for chronic pain. In the absence of comparative safety data, it is reasonable to consider flecainide less preferred as a potential adjuvant analgesic than other oral sodium channel blockers.

Rare serious reactions to local anaesthetics include interstitial pneumonitis, severe encephalopathy, blood dyscrasia, hepatitis, and dermatological reactions.

Pharmacology

Lidocaine is metabolized by the liver and is a substrate of CYP3A4. It can therefore interact with other substrates and inhibitors of this isozyme. Its active metabolites can accumulate and cause neurological toxicity[97]. Mexiletine is a substrate of CYP2D6 and an inhibitor or CYP1A2. Phenytoin can decrease mexiletine plasma concentrations, whereas SSRIs can increase it. Its half-life is increased in elderly and patients with liver or heart failure[97].

Indications

Data from controlled trials and clinical experience suggest that any type of neuropathic pain can be considered a potential indication for systemic therapy with a sodium channel blocker. A survey of patients treated with a brief lignocaine infusion found that neuropathic pains related to disorders of the peripheral nervous system are more likely to respond than pains related to a central nervous system lesion, but some patients with central pain do attain at least partial relief[182].

There have been no comparative clinical trials to help define the appropriate use of these drugs in relation to the many other adjuvant analgesics that may be used for neuropathic pain. Based on the potential for serious cardiovascular and central nervous system toxicity, and the limited data available concerning long-term efficacy, it is appropriate to position the systemically administered sodium channel blockers as second-line drugs for neuropathic pain. Specifically, a trial with one or more of these drugs usually is considered after antidepressant and anticonvulsant drugs have been tried.

The potential utility of brief intravenous local anaesthetic infusions has not been adequately explored in the medically ill and it is possible that a larger role for this approach should be considered. Some patients experience immediate analgesia with this technique and favourable effects have been observed to continue for some period in a minority. On the basis of clinical experience, a trial of a brief local anaesthetic infusion is sometimes implemented in patients with severe neuropathic pain that has not responded promptly to an opioid and requires immediate relief. Repeated infusions with escalating doses can be performed over a period of hours and may be a useful approach to the acute management of severe neuropathic pain even in those with advanced illness. One study showed that the response to an intravenous infusion of lidocaine is a good predictor of the response to oral mexiletine treatment[182], and although this trial was limited by a very small sample size, it may be useful to consider brief infusion as a means to guide the selection of an oral therapy after trials of anticonvulsants and antidepressants have proved unhelpful.

Dosing guidelines

On the basis of the limited data available, mexiletine appears to be the drug least likely to produce serious toxicity. Although intra-individual variability in the response to different drugs in this class has not been systematically assessed, such variability has been observed commonly with other drug classes and is likely to exist. Thus, if mexiletine does not yield benefit to the patient with severe neuropathic pain that has already proved refractory to other adjuvant analgesics, trials with tocainide or flecainide may be justified.

There have been no controlled comparisons of the analgesic effects produced by brief intravenous infusions of the various parenteral anaesthetics. The published experience is greatest with procaine and lignocaine, and it is reasonable to consider these drugs first.

All these drugs must be used cautiously in patients with pre-existing heart disease. It is prudent to avoid this therapy in those patients with cardiac rhythm disturbances, those who are receiving antiarrhythmic drugs, and those who have cardiac insufficiency. Patients who have significant heart disease should undergo cardiac evaluation before local anaesthetic therapy is administered.

Low initial doses and dose titration may reduce the likelihood of adverse effects. In the absence of contrary information, dosing strategies should conform to those employed in the treatment of cardiac arrhythmias. For example, mexiletine should usually be started at 150 mg once or twice per day. This and subsequent doses are better tolerated when taken with food. If intolerable side effects do not occur, the dose can be increased by a like amount every few days until the usual maximum dose of 300 mg three times per day is reached. Plasma drug concentrations, if available, can provide useful information as described previously for the tricyclic antidepressants.

There has been no systematic evaluation of the safety or efficacy of a systemically-administered sodium channel blocker and other adjuvant drugs, such as a tricyclic antidepressant or an anticonvulsant. Based on clinical experience, trials of such combinations, undertaken with close clinical monitoring, can be justified in patients with refractory neuropathic pain. If administration of the local anaesthetic has yielded meaningful partial analgesia, it should be continued as a trial while another drug is initiated. If there is a risk of drug interactions, or additive toxicities, dosing must be very cautious and monitoring must be intensified.

Dosing guidelines for local anaesthetics infusion are derived from the large clinical experience with this approach and a limited number of trials in patients with neuropathic pain. Lignocaine infusions have been administered at varying doses, typically within a range of 2 to 5 mg/kg infused over 20 to 30 min[169]. In the medically frail patient, it is prudent to start at the lower end of this range and provide repeated infusions at successively higher doses. For example, an initial infusion of 1 mg/kg over 30 min can be followed by an infusion of 2 mg/kg over 30 min, which in turn, can be followed by an infusion of 3 mg/kg or 4 mg/kg over 30 min.

N-methyl-D-aspartate receptor blockers

Excitatory amino acids, such as glutamate and aspartate, are released by primary afferent neurons in response to noxious stimuli and are important in the central processing of the pain-related information. Interactions at the N-methyl-D-aspartate (NMDA) receptor are involved in the development of central nervous system changes that may underlie chronic pain and modulate opioid mechanisms—specifically tolerance[183]. Preclinical studies have established that the NMDA receptor is involved in the sensitization of central neurons following injury and the development of the 'wind-up' phenomenon, a change in the response of central neurons that has been associated with neuropathic pain[184].

Although there is evidence that antagonists at the NMDA receptor may be multi-purpose analgesics, which could potentially ameliorate acute pain[185] and diverse types of chronic pain[186], the most intense interest has focused on their role as new therapies for neuropathic pain. At the present time, there are four commercially available drugs in the United States that have primary effects at the NMDA receptor and have been explored as potential analgesics: ketamine, dextromethorphan, memantine, and amantadine.

There is strong evidence that ketamine, a so-called dissociative anaesthetic, is analgesic. Intravenous or subcutaneous ketamine has been shown to be effective in reducing pain from fibromyalgia[186] and diverse neuropathic pains including postherpetic neuralgia[187], phantom limb pain[188] and pain after spinal cord injury[189]. Intranasal ketamine provides good relief from breakthrough pain in patients with chronic pain[190] and the addition of ketamine to an opioid regimen after surgery reduced pain in the postoperative period[191]. Although an open-label study suggested positive effects from topical amitriptyline 2 per cent/ketamine 1 per cent cream[192], these were not confirmed in a randomized controlled trial[193].

Numerous case reports and open-label trials support the potential utility of ketamine in the medically ill. Two randomized trials[194,195] have reported effectiveness of ketamine in relieving cancer pain or reducing opioid requirements. The use of ketamine has also been reported in children or adolescents with severe cancer pain or near the end of life, or as a means to induce palliative sedation also has been reported[196].

Ketamine therapy for pain management in the medically ill typically involves the delivery of sub-anaesthetic doses. Several different regimens have been recommended, most of which provide the equivalent of 0.1–1.5 mg/kg/h or an equivalent dose per day. Low initial doses must be titrated against effects. Treatment may involve continuous intravenous or subcutaneous infusion starting at the low end of the aforementioned dose range, repeated intravenous boluses (typically 0.25–0.50 mg/kg), intravenous 'burst' doses (100–500 mg/day for 3–5 days), or oral doses (e.g. 0.3–0.5 mg/kg three times daily). Some clinicians recommend an initial test dose of 5–10 mg to determine the patient's response and tolerance, and many clinicians will use a loading dose to initiate a low-dose continuous infusion. Epidural and intrathecal administration also seem to provide analgesia but have been linked to neurotoxicity with severe histological abnormalities of the spinal cord and nerve roots[197].

The side-effect profile of ketamine can be daunting, particularly in the medically frail. Ketamine may cause dysphoria, nightmares, and restlessness; hallucinosis or frank delirium can occur at any point during the treatment. Concurrent treatment with a benzodiazepine or a neuroleptic commonly is used to blunt or prevent these adverse effects. Ketamine also can cause tachycardia and hypertension, which may be a concern depending on the goals of care. It does not depress respirations.

As described in the many published cases, these side effects are unlikely to be problematic when low sub-anaesthetic doses are used. In the palliative care setting, ketamine may be a valuable strategy for severe refractory pain, particularly neuropathic pain, for pain emergencies and for pain that occurs in the context of a decision to offer sedation.

Evidence in favour of analgesic efficacy for the other commercially-available NMDA receptor antagonists is less compelling. In controlled trials, the antitussive dextromethorphan has been demonstrated to be analgesic in patients with painful diabetic neuropathy[198], phantom pain[199], and facial neuralgias[200]. In another randomized trial, a single high dose of dextromethorphan (270 mg) was analgesic in neuropathic pain of traumatic origin, but there was a significant inter-individual variability[201]; extensive metabolizers had a better analgesic effect, suggesting that the metabolite dextrorphan plays an important role in the analgesic activity. There also is substantial evidence supporting the analgesic and opioid-sparing effects of dextromethorphan in the immediate postoperative period[185].

In contrast to these positive findings, dextromethorphan was not efficacious in postherpetic neuralgia[198], and although a mixture of morphine and dextromethorphan initially seemed to be more effective than morphine alone in both non-cancer and cancer pain, three randomized trials yielded negative results[202].

Low-dose dextromethorphan has been widely used for cough and is very well tolerated. At the higher doses needed for pain, approximately one-third of patients report uncomfortable symptoms, including dysarthria, light-headedness, nystagmus, gastrointestinal disturbances; more serious but less common adverse events include memory loss, depression, unsteady gait, and decreased coordination[202].

A trial of dextromethorphan for refractory neuropathic pain generally is initiated at a dose of 45 to 60 mg divided into three or four doses daily. This starting dose can be gradually escalated until favourable effects occur, side effects supervene, or a conventional maximal dose of 1 g is achieved. One study suggested that analgesia following an intravenous dose of ketamine can predict response to oral dextromethorphan[203] and further investigation of this possibility is warranted.

Amantadine and memantine are also non-competitive oral NMDA antagonists and limited data support their analgesic potential in neuropathic pain. Amantadine was effective in chronic neuropathic pain, surgical neuropathic cancer pain, and painful diabetic neuropathy[204]. Perioperative oral amantadine has been suggested to reduce postoperative pain and opioid consumption[205] but it does not prevent the development of postmastectomy neuropathic pain[206]. Memantine, which like amantadine may be relatively well tolerated, has been used for refractory neuropathic pain, including complex regional pain syndrome[207]. When administered concomitantly with a continuous brachial plexus blockade, it reduced the prevalence and intensity of phantom limb pain following acute traumatic upper limb amputations[208].

Despite these very limited data, an empirical trial of amantadine or memantine sometimes is undertaken in refractory neuropathic pain. Common adverse events are somnolence, dizziness, or mood changes. These drugs deserve further studies to confirm efficacy and determine whether benefits outweigh the risk of toxicity in the medically ill.

The d-isomer of the opioid methadone also blocks the NMDA receptor[209]. In most countries where methadone is commercially available, a racemate containing 50 per cent of the D-isomer is used. The contribution of this nonopioid molecule to the analgesia produced by methadone is uncertain, but the greater-than-anticipated potency of methadone in patients who undergo a switch to this drug from another mu agonist suggests that it can play a clinically important role. There are no data, however, to support the conclusion that methadone is better than other opioids for the treatment of neuropathic pain.

Other adjuvant analgesics used for neuropathic pain

Cannabinoids

It is now known that exogenous cannabinoid molecules interact with an endogenous system that includes cannabinoid-like molecules—the endocannabinoids—and multiple receptors in both the periphery and central nervous system; as demonstrated in animal models, this system mediates antinociception[210]. As a result of this expanding knowledge of cannabinoid pharmacology, the potential for the clinical use of these compounds as analgesics is undergoing empirical reassessment. Although the abuse potential of these compounds is undisputed, they may be important analgesics that can be made available to patients, as opioids are, by appropriately managing the risk of abuse, addiction, and diversion.

There are several cannabinoids now available and others in development. Clinical trials have established the analgesic efficacy of some of these drugs. The oral synthetic cannabinoid nabilone has been shown to be analgesic in spasticity-related pain from chronic upper motor neuron syndrome[211] and fibromyalgia[212]. A recent observational study of nabilone in patients with advanced

cancer used propensity scoring to demonstrate significant benefit for pain and other symptoms[213].

In other trials, pain and other symptoms from multiple sclerosis have responded to oral delta(9)-tetrahydrocannabinol (THC)[214] and to plant extracts containing mixtures of various alkaloids[215]. An oromucosal spray containing tetrahydrocannabinol plus cannabidiol (and smaller concentrations of other compounds) is undergoing worldwide development, has already been approved in several countries for pain due to multiple sclerosis or cancer pain, and has been demonstrated to be efficacious in clinical trials involving opioid-refractory cancer pain, pain due to peripheral nerve lesions, and pain due to rheumatoid arthritis[216].

The most common side effects associated with the cannabinoids are dizziness, omnolence, and dry mouth. An older study of THC for cancer pain, noted a narrow therapeutic window and a relatively low efficacy, comparable to codeine at conventional doses[217]. Studies of the plant extracts suggest that better outcomes occur with drugs that include a combination of cannabinoid compounds. Additional studies will provide new agents for clinical use and hopefully clarify the relative benefits and burdens.

The existing data suggest that the newer cannabinoid drugs, such as the oromucosal spray containing THC and cannabidiol, ultimately will be characterized as multi-purpose analgesics, potentially appropriate for a trial in the medically ill whenever pain is refractory to opioid therapy. At this point, however, both experience and available agents are limited, and most of the data in relation to this class has been collected in neuropathic pain populations. A trial of a commercially-available cannabinoid usually is considered only in those patients who are refractory to opioids and other appropriate adjuvant analgesics; most of these patients will have neuropathic pain. Nabilone should be started at 0.5–1 mg at night and titrated up to 3 mg twice daily, or higher if tolerated. THC usually is started at a dose of 2.5 mg once or twice daily, and titrated. The oromucosal spray containing THC and cannabinol has been initiated with an 'as needed' schedule and effectively titrated by the patient to an effective dose.

Baclofen

Baclofen is an agonist at the gamma aminobutyric acid type B ($GABA_B$) receptor and has been conclusively demonstrated to have efficacy in trigeminal neuralgia[218]. On the basis of these data and a positive clinical experience, it generally is considered to be a second-line treatment for diverse types of neuropathic pains (Table 10.1.8.4)[219]. This conclusion gains support from a positive clinical experience in the use of intrathecal baclofen to treat challenging central pains[220]. Intrathecal baclofen also is very effective in relieving pain related to spasticity. Although there have been a few observations that suggest a broader analgesic potential for systemically-administered baclofen, the data are too limited to recommend a trial for non-neuropathic pain.

The administration of baclofen for pain is undertaken in a manner similar to the use of the drug for its primary indication, spasticity. A starting dose of 5 mg two to three times per day is gradually escalated until positive effects occur, side effects supervene, or doses above the conventionally-accepted range are reached. In those who experience neither benefit nor side effects, it is appropriate to continue dose escalation until doses are greater than 200 mg per day. The common side effects (dizziness, somnolence, and gastrointestinal distress) are minimized by low starting doses and gradual

Table 10.1.8.4 Adjuvant analgesics used for neuropathic pain.

Class	Examples
First line	
Antidepressants	See Table 10.1.8.3
Anticonvulsants	Gabapentin, pregabalin, topiramate, carbamazepine, phenytoin, valproate, oxcarbazepine, lamotrigine, levetiracetam
Other drugs	
Topical agents	Capsaicin, lidocaine patch, EMLA
Oral sodium channel blockers	Mexiletine, tocainide, flecainide
Alpha-2 adrenergic agonists	Clonidine, tizanidine
N-methyl-D-aspartate receptor antagonists	Dextromethorphan, ketamine
GABA agonists	Baclofen
Cannabinoids	Tetrahydrocannabinol (THC), nabilone, THC:cannabidiol mixture
Miscellaneous	Calcitonin

dose escalation. The potential for a serious withdrawal syndrome, including delirium and seizure, exists with abrupt discontinuation following prolonged use; doses should always be tapered before discontinuation of the drug.

Calcitonin

Calcitonin is an interesting drug that may have several pain-related indications in the palliative care setting. Its potential role in bone pain is discussed in the following paragraphs. There is some evidence that calcitonin also may have efficacy in neuropathic pain states. Favourable controlled trials have been reported in populations with complex regional pain syndrome[221] and acute phantom pain[222]. Although the mechanisms that may be responsible for these analgesic effects are unknown, these observations may justify a trial of calcitonin in refractory neuropathic pain of diverse types.

Other drugs for sympathetically-maintained pain

Sympathetically-maintained pain refers to a subtype of neuropathic pain believed to be sustained by efferent activity in the sympathetic nervous system. The disorders characterized as complex regional pain syndromes (older terms include reflex sympathetic dystrophy and causalgia), are believed to be relatively more likely to include this mechanism than other types of neuropathic pain. When a complex regional pain syndrome is suspected because of the existence of a regional pain associated with focal autonomic dysregulation (e.g. swelling, vasomotor disturbances, and sweating abnormalities), focal motor disturbances (e.g. tremor or dystonia), or trophic changes (e.g. focal osteoporosis, atrophy of skin or subcutaneous tissues, and changes in nail or hair growth), sympathetic nerve blocks and trials of specific drug therapy may be considered.

Although any of the drugs used for neuropathic pain may be used to treat a suspected complex regional pain syndrome (with its potential sympathetically-maintained pain), therapy also may focus on trials of drugs that either influence sympathetic function or have been specifically studied in this condition. In addition to clonidine,

these drugs include phenoxybenzamine, prazosin, propranolol, or nifedipine.

Anticholinesterase drugs

Anecdotal reports have described the successful use of a variety of anticholinesterase drugs in patients with diverse types of neuropathic pain[223], and to improve cognition and delirium in an opioid-treated patient with advanced cancer[224]. The mechanism of the putative benefits produced by these drugs is not established and treatment is associated with the potential for serious adverse effects, such as bradycardia. A trial of one of these drugs should only be considered for medically stable patients with severe refractory pain.

Topical analgesics

Topical therapies have the potential to deliver analgesic compounds directly to a site that presumably is responsible, at least in part, for the persistence of pain. As a result, relatively low doses can be applied and the likelihood of systemic toxicity is reduced. Although topical analgesics largely have been used for neuropathic pains, they have the potential for broader application. Commercially available topical therapies include capsaicin preparations, formulations of aspirin or non-steroidal anti-inflammatory drugs, creams, and patches containing local anaesthetics, and preparations containing tricyclic preparations. Other formulations in clinical use are compounded by pharmacies and may include opioids, selected anticonvulsants, or other drugs.

Capsaicin is the naturally-occurring constituent of the chili pepper that produces its pungent taste. When applied topically, it inhibits function in polymodal primary afferent nociceptive neurons by binding to the transient receptor potential vanilloid type 1 (TRPV1) receptor and inhibiting the release of substance P and other compounds. Regular use eventually leads to depletion of substance P from the terminals of afferent C-fibres and this presumably is the analgesic mechanism of the low-dose creams that are now commercially available[225].

Low-dose topical capsaicin has been demonstrated to be effective in both painful mononeuropathies and polyneuropathies, as shown by controlled trials conducted in populations with postherpetic neuralgia[226], painful diabetic neuropathy[227], and peripheral painful mononeuropathies following cancer surgery (post-mastectomy, post-thoracotomy, post-amputation)[228]. A controlled trial in HIV-associated painful peripheral neuropathy failed to show any analgesic effect[229].

Other controlled trials suggest that some painful somatic disorders also may be amenable to topical capsaicin therapy. A controlled trial demonstrated benefit in the pain associated with osteoarthritis of the finger joints[230] and a meta-analysis confirmed the benefit of topical capsaicin in painful diabetic neuropathy and osteoarthritis, as well as one non-painful condition, psoriasis[231].

The concentrations of capsaicin available commercially and tested in the aforementioned trials have been low, specifically less than 0.75 per cent. There also is evidence that much higher doses of capsaicin (7.5–10 per cent), which presumably rapidly deplete substance P and may destroy C-fibres, may be effective and provide relief that persists for a prolonged period after a single application for several months after a single capsaicin exposure[225]. Application of this high concentration formula is accomplished using general or regional anaesthesia to reduce the acute pain. The safety and efficacy of this approach remains to be clarified in future studies.

Notwithstanding the evidence that low-dose capsaicin cream 0.025 per cent to 0.075 per cent is analgesic, clinical use has been limited. This may relate to the relatively common side effect of local burning and to the inconvenience of administration. Guidelines call for application to the painful area four times a day by rubbing it in until it vanishes. A trial of several weeks is needed to adequately judge effects. Hands must be washed thoroughly immediately after each application (to reduce the risk of unintentional contact with the eyes or with mucous membranes, which is associated with intense burning), even as burning at the application site gradually decreases over a few days of regular use. Some patients tolerate the cream better if a local anaesthetic is applied to the site before the capsaicin.

A trial of capsaicin cream (typically the 0.75 per cent) should be considered for patients with focal areas of neuropathic pain or arthropathy if these application challenges can be met with limited burden. The concurrent use of capsaicin with topical doxepin might also pose an opportunity for a trial with less burning pain[232].

Numerous anti-inflammatory drugs have been investigated for topical use. Like capsaicin, there is some evidence that diverse types of pain may respond favourably. Data from controlled trials of populations with musculoskeletal pain are conflicting[233,234]. NSAID-containing (e.g. diclofenac) patches and creams are commercially available in many countries and there is sufficient evidence of effectiveness and safety to warrant trials in patients with small areas of pain related to neuropathic or nociceptive mechanisms.

Evidence on the analgesic efficacy of a cream containing a tricyclic antidepressant is conflicting. There are favourable clinical observations pertaining to the topical administration of amitriptyline 2 per cent cream, given alone or in combination with ketamine 1 per cent, for the treatment of neuropathic pain[192]. Randomized trials, however, failed to confirm the efficacy of topical amitriptyline[193,235]. Nonetheless, given the mixed evidence and the safety of the topical formulations, a trial of topical doxepin or some other tricyclic drug is justified in patients with focal areas of neuropathic pain.

A commercially available mixture of local anaesthetics, which contains a 1:1 mixture of prilocaine and lignocaine, is capable of penetrating the skin and producing a dense local cutaneous anaesthesia; this product, known as eutectic mixture of local anaesthetics, is widely used to prevent the pain of needle puncture or incision, as well as pain from debridement of leg ulcers. A limited study in patients with postherpetic neuralgia suggests its utility in the management of some chronic neuropathic pains[236]. Surveys of relatively high concentrations of topical lignocaine and a controlled trial of 5 per cent lignocaine gel[237] have also been positive in patients with postherpetic neuralgia. Although there is a very remote risk of toxicity from systemic absorption of a topical local anaesthetic, careful monitoring is needed if the anaesthetic is applied repeatedly to mucous membranes or open wounds.

Guidelines for a trial of topical local anaesthetic are ill defined. To create an area of dense sensory loss using the eutectic mixture of lignocaine and prilocaine, a relatively thick application must remain in contact with the skin under an occlusive dressing for at least 1 h. This mode of administration may be difficult if the painful area is large or adjacent to the face or a mobile region of the body. There is no evidence in populations with chronic pain that cutaneous anaesthesia is necessary to gain benefit from a topical local anaesthetic and, anecdotally, some patients seem to respond favourably to a thin application applied without a dressing. In the absence of any systematic evaluation of dosing techniques, the patient should be encouraged to try various modes of administration in an effort to identify a salutary approach. If possible, one of these trials should include an occlusive dressing of some type and a duration of application of at least 1 h.

Topical application of local anaesthetics recently has been facilitated by the development of a lidocaine 5 per cent patch. There is evidence that the lidocaine patch reduces pain and allodynia from postherpetic neuralgia[238], and it is now commonly used for this indication. Analgesia also has been demonstrated in open-label trials in painful diabetic neuropathy[239], moderate-to-severe knee osteoarthritis[240], and non-neuropathic low back pain[240]. It can provide further relief when response to gabapentin and other systemic analgesics is only partial[241].

Given these data, a trial of the lidocaine patch should be considered in all patients with relatively small areas of pain unrelated to local skin injury. Although the lidocaine patch was studied with use limited to 12 h/day, continuous application is common in the clinical setting and multiple patches are often used. There are limited data that indicate a high level of safety with up to three patches for periods up to 24 h[242]. Application of more than three patches may be useful for some patients, but this approach should be accompanied by initial monitoring for lidocaine toxicity. An adequate trial may require several weeks of observation and two weeks of regular use. The most frequently reported adverse event is mild-to-moderate skin redness, rash, or irritation at the patch application site, which seems to be related to the vehicle rather than to lidocaine. Cost also may be prohibitive.

Adjuvant analgesics used for bone pain

Bone pain is a common problem in the palliative care setting. Radiation therapy is usually considered when bone pain is focal and poorly controlled with an opioid, or is associated with a lesion that appears prone to fracture on radiographic examination. Anecdotally, multifocal bone pain has been observed to benefit from treatment with a non-steroidal anti-inflammatory drug or a corticosteroid. Other adjuvant analgesics that are potentially useful in this setting include calcitonin, bisphosphonate compounds, gallium nitrate, and selected radiopharmaceuticals (Table 10.1.8.5). There have been no comparative trials of these adjuvant analgesics for bone pain and the selection of one over another is usually based on convenience, patient preference, and the clinical setting.

Calcitonin and bisphosphonates

Calcitonin and the bisphosphonate compounds inhibit osteoclast activity and may be useful adjuvant drugs for the treatment of bone pain. Calcitonin provides significant analgesia in acute osteoporotic vertebral compression fractures, allowing earlier mobilization[243]. Although not studied, benefits also may be seen in those with other types of lesions, such as pelvic fracture.

In cancer patients, calcitonin may relieve pain from bone metastases[244–246]. The most frequent routes of administration are subcutaneous or intranasal. One trial also described benefit from the use of a high intravenous dose administered daily for five consecutive days[247]. If subcutaneous boluses are used, they should be preceded by skin testing with 1 IU to screen for hypersensitivity reactions, especially in patients with a history of reactions to salmon or seafood; a trial may be initiated at a relatively low dose, then gradually increased to 200 IU, if tolerated, and sometimes higher. Continuous subcutaneous administration also has been described[245]. The intranasal formulation avoids the need for subcutaneous injections. It is administered once daily, with an initial dose of 200 IU in one nostril, alternating nostrils every day. Although the potential for better efficacy with higher doses has not been studied, an inadequate response can be followed by a trial of two sprays per day (400 IU), and even more in some cases.

Apart from infrequent hypersensitivity reactions, the main side-effect of calcitonin is nausea. The likelihood and severity of this effect may be reduced by gradual escalation from a low starting dose. According to clinical experience, nausea usually subsides after a few days and is less frequent with the intranasal form. Periodic monitoring of calcium and phosphorus is prudent during treatment.

Although calcitonin inhibits osteoclast activity, the relationship between this effect and analgesia is unclear. The drug can increase endorphin levels in the central nervous system[245] and possibly can interact with the serotonergic system[248].

Although calcitonin may be considered as an adjuvant analgesic for metastatic bone pain, the evidence in favour of this compound is far less than for the bisphosphonates, and one of the latter drugs typically is used first. The bisphophonates are analogues of inorganic pyrophosphate and inhibit osteoclast activity. They are mainstay approaches in the treatment of osteoporosis, Paget's disease, and tumour-induced hypercalcemia. Several controlled trials also have established the analgesic efficacy of these compounds.

Although the data are not uniformly positive, the analgesic effect of clodronate has been shown in several studies of breast cancer[249], prostate cancer[250], multiple myeloma[251] and various neoplasms[252]. It appears more effective when used soon after diagnosis[250]. An intravenous dose of 600 mg weekly provides analgesia and decreases the use of analgesics[253]. In terminally ill elderly patients, 300 mg administered subcutaneously every other day improved pain and quality of life[252]. The main advantage of clodronate over pamidronate is its good oral bioavailability, which avoids the need of an intravenous administration. An oral dose of 1600 mg daily resulted in moderate analgesic effect and seems to be the optimal dose[253].

Pamidronate has been extensively studied in populations with bone metastases. It has been proven to have good analgesic effect in

Table 10.1.8.5 Adjuvant analgesics used for malignant bone pain.[a]

- ◆ Corticosteroids
- ◆ Calcitonin
- ◆ Bisphosphonates
  - • Clodronate
  - • Pamidronate
- ◆ Radionuclides
  - • Strontium-89 (^{89}Sr)
  - • Rhenium-186 (^{186}Re)
  - • Samarium-153 (^{153}Sm)
- ◆ Gallium nitrate

Note: [a] Anecdotal data suggests that non-steroidal anti-inflammatory drugs are also useful in bone pain.

several studies of breast cancer[254] and multiple myeloma[255]. Although different doses have been used, the usual recommendation calls for the administration of 60–90 mg intravenously every 3–4 weeks. This dose benefits approximately 50 per cent of patients[253]. There are dose-dependent effects, and a poor response at 60 mg can be followed by a trial of 90 mg; doses of 120 mg are sometimes used. Doses may be repeated monthly.

The newer third-generation bisphosphonates, such as zoledronic acid and ibandronate, also are analgesic. An intravenous infusion of 4 mg of zoledronic acid given in 15 min every 3 weeks can decrease bone pain from breast, prostate, and lung metastases, as well as multiple myeloma[256,257]. This treatment also has been shown to decrease opioid consumption and improve quality of life[257]. Benefits seem greater when it is administered in a community rather than a hospital setting[257] and are present even in patients who have previously received other bisphosphonates[256].

Ibandronate has been effective for bone pain in both intravenous and oral formulation. An intravenous 6-mg infusion, given in 1–2 h every 3–4 weeks, decreases pain and analgesic use in patients with bone metastases from breast cancer[258–260]. It is beneficial in opioid-resistant bone pain[259] and long-term safety has been assessed for up to 4 years[258]. An oral daily dose of 50 mg improves bone pain, decreases opioid use, and preserves quality of life in metastatic breast cancer[260].

The bisphosphonates also reduce other skeletal morbidity, including pathological fractures, need for bone radiation or surgery, spinal cord compression, and hypercalcaemia[254,255,261].

The commercially-available bisphosphonates have different toxicity profiles. The most common adverse effects associated with bisphosphonates are renal toxicity, acute-phase (flu-like) reactions, gastrointestinal toxicity, and osteonecrosis of the jaw (ONJ). The incidence of these adverse events varies significantly between bisphosphonates. Renal toxicity is a potentially serious event and characterizes both zoledronic acid and pamidronate. Renal function should be checked prior to administration of these drugs and monitored during the course of therapy. Gastrointestinal effects occur only with oral agents and may be avoided by adhering to dosing instructions. Acute-phase reactions are transitory and usually are tolerated well with acetaminophen or an NSAID. ONJ is a very uncommon, yet worrisome toxicity, the true incidence of which is not yet known. It does not reverse with discontinuation of the offending drug, appears to be associated with the dose and duration of treatment, can occur even with oral bisphosphonate therapy, and is far more likely to occur in the setting of significant dental disease or procedures. If appropriate given the context of the patient's medical illness, the risk in those with dental disease may be sufficient to suggest dental evaluation before treatment and meticulous dental follow-up care during treatment.

Radiopharmaceuticals

Radionuclides that are absorbed at areas of high bone turnover have been evaluated as potential therapies for metastatic bone disease. The first radionuclide introduced into clinical practice was phosphorus-32 orthophosphate. Although it is often effective in relieving bone pain, bone marrow is a major toxicity, and the desire for a compound with a better therapeutic index has spurred the development of several new radionuclides.

Many newer radionuclides have been advocated as potential therapies for bone pain. Strontium chloride-89, rhenium-186 hydroxyethylenediphosphonic acid, and samarium-153 ethylene-diaminetetramethylenephosphonic acid have been most promising thus far. Surveys of patients with bone metastases from a variety of tumour types have provided strong evidence that these compounds can reduce bone pain without undue risk to bone marrow or other vital structures.

Strontium-89 and samarium-153, which are commercially available in the United States of America, have been most extensively evaluated as a treatment for bone pain. Like other radiopharmaceuticals, they are potentially effective in the treatment of pain due to osteoblastic bone lesions or lesions with an osteoblastic component. An osteoblastic component should be confirmed by positive bone scintigraphy before treatment with this drug.

Strontium-89 has been most studied, with the favourable effects noted in numerous surveys confirmed in placebo-controlled trials[262], and the available data provide a foundation for the use of all these drugs. These studies revealed that treatment reduced the need for both radiotherapy and analgesic drugs, and compared favourably with hemibody irradiation in a randomized trial[262].

The data suggest that treatment with a radiopharmaceutical yields meaningful pain relief in approximately 80 per cent of patients, 10 per cent of whom attain complete relief[263]. Initial clinical response occurs in 7 to 21 days and peak response may be delayed for a month or more. Approximately 5 to 10 per cent of patients experience a transitory pain flare immediately after treatment. The usual duration of benefit is 3 to 6 months, after which retreatment may regain a favourable effect. Following treatment, clinically significant leucopenia or thrombocytopenia peak a few weeks after treatment and occurs to a clinically significant degree in approximately 10 per cent and 33 per cent of patients, respectively. Bone marrow effects usually wane by 12 weeks after treatment.

Given the delayed onset and peak effects, treatment with a radiopharmaceutical should not be considered unless a patient has a life expectancy of greater than 3 months. This delay also implies that treatment should not be considered as the sole approach for patients with severe pain. Due to the potential for bone marrow toxicity, treatment should not be considered unless adequate bone marrow reserve has been documented. In the case of strontium-89, this is usually considered to be a platelet count above 60 000 and a white blood cell count above 2400[263]. Patients who continue to be candidates for myelosuppressive chemotherapy should not be treated because the effects on bone marrow may worsen the toxicity of later cytotoxic therapy or limit the ability to rebound after therapy.

Adjuvant analgesics used for bowel obstruction

The management of symptoms associated with malignant bowel obstruction may be challenging. If surgical decompression is not feasible, the need to control pain and other obstructive symptoms, including distension, nausea, and vomiting, becomes paramount. The use of opioids may be problematic due to dose-limiting toxicity (including gastrointestinal toxicity) or the intensity of breakthrough pains. Anecdotal reports suggest that anticholinergic drugs, the somatostatin analogue octreotide, and corticosteroids may be useful adjuvant analgesics in this setting. The use of these drugs may also ameliorate non-painful symptoms and minimize the number of patients who must be considered for chronic drainage using nasogastric or percutaneous catheters.

Anticholinergic drugs

Anticholinergic drugs could theoretically relieve the symptoms of bowel obstruction by reducing propulsive and non-propulsive gut motility and decreasing intraluminal secretions. Some patients appear to benefit from the administration of hyoscine (scopolamine)[264]. In some countries, hyoscine is only commercially available as the hydrobromide salt, which readily crosses the blood–brain barrier. Although this formulation can be delivered via a transdermal system, which simplifies treatment in patients with bowel obstruction, it is likely to be associated with a relatively higher incidence of central nervous system side effects, such as somnolence and confusion, than an anticholinergic drug with less penetration through the blood–brain barrier. Hyoscine butylbromide, which is less likely to pass the blood–brain barrier due to low lipid solubility, can be effective for obstructive symptoms, including pain[265]. Glycopyrrolate has a pharmacological profile similar to hyoscine butylbromide, but has not been systematically evaluated in a population with symptomatic bowel obstruction. In medically ill patients who are predisposed to central nervous system toxicity, a trial of one of the latter drugs may be warranted on theoretical grounds.

Octreotide

The somatostatin analogue octreotide inhibits the secretion of gastric, pancreatic, and intestinal secretions and reduces gastrointestinal motility. These effects probably underlie the analgesic effects that have been reported in case series of symptomatic treatment of bowel obstruction[265]. The benefits of this drug may occur more rapidly than hyoscine[266]. Octreotide has also been used to manage severe diarrhoea due to enterocolic fistula, high output jejunostomies or ileostomies, or secretory tumours of the gastrointestinal tract. A newer long-acting formulation, administered intramuscularly once monthly, can provide sustained reduction of bowel obstruction symptoms[267].

Octreotide has a good safety profile but is expensive. In some settings, however, the cost may be balanced by an excellent clinical response or the avoidance of the costs involved in the use of a gastrointestinal drainage procedure.

Corticosteroids

As discussed previously, the symptoms associated with bowel obstruction may improve with corticosteroid therapy. The mode of action is unclear and the most effective drug, dose, and dosing regimen are unknown. A broad range of doses have been described anecdotally. For example, dexamethasone has been used for this indication in a dose range of 8 to 60 mg/day[77], and methylprednisolone has been administered in a dose range of 30 to 50 mg/day[72]. The potential for complications during long-term therapy, including an increased risk of bowel perforation, may limit this approach to patients with short life expectancies.

Adjuvant analgesics used for musculoskeletal pain

Although pains that originate from injury to muscle or connective tissue are prevalent in the medically ill, there has been no systematic evaluation of analgesic therapies for this problem. In the management of acute traumatic sprains or strains in the non-medically ill, non-opioid and opioid analgesics are commonly supplemented by treatment with so-called muscle relaxant drugs or benzodiazepines. The role of the latter drugs for opioid-refractory musculoskeletal pains in populations with advanced medical illness remains ill defined.

Muscle relaxants

The so-called muscle relaxants include drugs in a variety of classes, all of which are marketed for the treatment of acute musculoskeletal pain. In the United States of America, this group includes drugs that are also administered as antihistamines (e.g. orphenadrine), tricyclic compounds structurally similar to the tricyclic antidepressants (e.g. cyclobenzaprine), and other types of drugs (e.g. carisoprodol, chlorzoxazone, metaxalone, and methocarbamol).

The efficacy of the muscle relaxant drugs in common musculoskeletal pains has been established in placebo-controlled studies[268,269]. Some studies have demonstrated analgesic effects that are superior to either aspirin or acetaminophen, and others have shown that the combination of a muscle relaxant and one of the latter drugs provides better analgesia than does aspirin or acetaminophen alone. There have been no controlled comparative trials or studies that have directly compared the efficacy and side-effect profiles of these drugs with either non-steroidal anti-inflammatory drugs or opioids.

Although muscle relaxant drugs can relieve musculoskeletal pains, these effects may not be specific and do not depend on relaxation of skeletal muscle. The label 'muscle relaxant' notwithstanding, there is actually no evidence that these drugs relax skeletal muscle in the clinical setting. They do inhibit polysynaptic myogenic reflexes in animal models, but the relationship between this action and analgesia is not known. Thus, the muscle relaxant drugs are best viewed as alternatives to the anti-inflammatory drugs and opioids, which may be indicated in musculoskeletal pains because of the evidence of analgesic efficacy in these conditions. These drugs should not be administered in the mistaken belief that they relieve muscle spasm.

The muscle relaxant drugs are generally well tolerated, but have sedative effects that may be additive to other centrally acting drugs, including the opioids. Anecdotally, some patients report differences among drugs in analgesic efficacy or sedative side effects, and it is reasonable to switch to an alternative drug if treatment is initially ineffective. Although the dose–response relationships of the muscle relaxant drugs have not been systematically explored, there are probably dose-dependent effects and the use of a low initial dose followed by gradual dose escalation can be recommended as a means to identify the most salutary balance between analgesia and side effects. Experience with these drugs is too limited to pursue dose escalation beyond the usual recommended range.

If the muscle spasm is believed to be related to the pain, it may be justifiable to consider a trial of a drug with established effect on skeletal muscle. Treatment with diazepam or another benzodiazepine, the alpha-2 adrenergic agonist tizanidine, or the $GABA_B$ agonist baclofen could be tried. A trial of one of the muscle relaxants might be considered, but not as a drug with specific efficacy, and the potential for side effects and withdrawal phenomenon should elicit caution in selecting drugs of this class.

Other adjuvant analgesics

Many other drugs have analgesic effects, but are not usually administered for pain in the palliative care setting. Some, such as the psychostimulants, are given for alternative indications; others have been disappointing in clinical practice or are yet too new to confirm safety and efficacy in the medically ill population.

Psychostimulants

There is substantial evidence, mostly from controlled, single dose studies, that psychostimulant drugs have analgesic effects, including in postoperative pain (dextroamphetamine), in pain associated with Parkinson's disease (methylphenidate) and in headache, sore throat, and oral surgery pain (caffeine)[270]. Although pain is not considered a primary indication for these drugs, this potential for analgesic effects may influence the decision to recommend a trial in the medically ill.

The pychostimulant drugs usually are considered for the treatment of opioid-induced somnolence, cognitive impairment, fatigue or depression. Surveys and clinical trials provide strongest support for the efficacy of methylphenidate and modafinil for these conditions[271–273]. The management of central nervous system side effects is an important issue, and, accordingly, the practical use of psychostimulants in the palliative care setting has focused on this indication, rather than the treatment of unrelieved pain.

Although these drugs are generally well tolerated, the potential for tremulousness, anorexia and weight loss, insomnia, and tachycardia or hypertension should be recognized and monitored during therapy. Treatment with methylphenidate or dextroamphetamine is typically begun at 2.5 to 5 mg in the morning and again at mid-day, if necessary, to keep the patient alert during the day and not interfere with sleep at night. The second dose usually is needed. Doses are increased gradually until efficacy is established. Although few patients require more than 40 mg/day in divided doses, occasional patients benefit from higher doses. Some patients require dose escalation later in the course of therapy. Modafinil is usually started at 100 mg daily and then increased. Maximal doses have not been defined.

Antihistamines

As noted previously, some antihistamine drugs are marketed as muscle relaxants. Controlled trials have demonstrated that many of these agents, including diphenhydramine, hydroxyzine, orphenadrine, phenyltoloxamine, and pyrilamine, can exert analgesic effects[274,275]. These data suggest that antihistaminic drugs are non-specific, low-efficacy analgesics. Clinical experience in medically ill populations is limited and a small survey yielded disappointing outcomes. This experience suggests that treatment should be considered only for patients who have primary indications other than pain, such as anxiety, nausea, or itch, in the hope that analgesia will be augmented while these other symptoms are relieved. The use of these agents must also be tempered by the potential for side-effects (e.g. somnolence) that add to those produced by other centrally acting drugs, including the opioids.

Conclusions

Although the use of adjuvant analgesics in palliative care remains largely guided by anecdotal experience, controlled clinical trials have begun to provide a scientific rationale for many therapies. Future investigations of nociceptive processes and pain pathophysiology will undoubtedly lead to the development of novel drugs.

For example, the adjuvant analgesics may one day include drugs that modulate peripheral nociceptive processes, such a substance P or bradykinin antagonists, or drugs that alter central processing by interacting with gangliosides or second messenger systems activated by excitatory amino acids. Although opioid drugs continue to be the major approach to the treatment of pain in the palliative care setting, adjuvant analgesics offer opportunities for improved outcomes in the substantial group of patients who cannot attain an acceptable balance between pain relief and side effects.

References

1. Schug, S.A., Zech, D., and Dorr, U. (1990). Cancer pain management according to WHO analgesic guidelines. *Journal of Pain and Symptom Management*, **5**, 27–32.

2. Grond, S., Radbruch, L., Meuser, T. *et al.* (1999). Assessment and treatment of neuropathic cancer pain following WHO guidelines. *Pain*, **79**, 15–20.

3. Max, M.B., Culnane, M., Schafer, S.C. *et al.* (1987). Amitriptyline relieves diabetic neuropathy pain in patients with normal or depressed mood. *Neurology*, **37**, 589–96.

4. Kishore-Kumar, R., Max, M.B., Schafer, S.C. *et al.* (1990). Desipramine relieves postherpetic neuralgia. *Clinical Pharmacology and Therapeutics*, **47**, 305–12.

5. Dworkin, R.H., O'Connor, A.B., Backonja, M. *et al.* (2007). Pharmacologic management of neuropathic pain: evidence-based recommendations. *Pain*, **132**, 237–51.

6. Couch, J.R., Ziegler, D.K., and Hassannin, R. (1976). Amitriptyline in the prophylaxis of migraine: effectiveness and relationship of antimigraine and antidepressant effects. *Neurology*, **26**, 121–7.

7. Frank, R.G., Kashani, J.H., Parker, J.C. *et al.* (1988). Antidepressant analgesia in rheumatoid arthritis. *The Journal of Rheumatology*, **15**, 1632–8.

8. Ward, N.G. (1986). Tricyclic antidepressants for chronic low back pain: mechanism of action and predictors of response. *Spine*, **11**, 661–5.

9. Watson, C.P.N., Chipman, M., Reed, K. *et al.* (1992). Amitriptyline versus maprotiline in postherpetic neuralgia: a randomized double-blind, crossover trial. *Pain*, **48**, 29–36.

10. Watson, C.P.N., Vernich, L., Chipman, M. *et al.* (1998). Nortriptyline versus amitriptyline in post-herpetic neuralgia: a randomized trial. *Neurology*, **51**, 1166–71.

11. Carette, S., Bell, M.J., Reynolds, W.J. *et al.* (1994). Comparison of amitriptyline, cyclobenzaprine, and placebo in the treatment of fibromyalgia: a randomized, double-blind clinical trial. *Arthritis and Rheumatism*, **37**, 32–40.

12. Max, M.B., Lynch, S.A., Muir, J. *et al.* (1992). Effects of desipramine, amitriptyline, and fluoxetine on pain in diabetic neuropathy. *New England Journal of Medicine*, **326**, 1250–6.

13. Morello, C.M., Leckband, S.G., Stoner, C.P. *et al.* (1999). Randomized double-blind study comparing the efficacy of gabapentin with amitriptyline on diabetic peripheral neuropathy pain. *Archives of Internal Medicine*, **159**, 1931–7.

14. Leijon, G. and Boivie, J. (1989). Central post-stroke pain: a controlled trial of amitriptyline and carbamazepine. *Pain*, **36**, 27–36.

15. Rintala, D.H., Holmes, S.A., Courtade, D. *et al.* (2007). Comparison of the effectiveness of amitriptyline and gabapentin on chronic neuropathic pain in persons with spinal cord injury. *Archives of Physical Medicine and Rehabilitation*, **88**, 1547–60.

16. Robinson, L.R., Czerniecki, J.M., Ehde, D.M. *et al.* (2004). Trial of amitriptyline for relief of pain in amputees: results of a randomized controlled study. *Archives of Physical Medicine and Rehabilitation*, **85**, 1–6.

17. Sharav, Y., Singer, E., Schmidt, E. *et al.* (1987). The analgesic effect of amitriptyline on chronic facial pain. *Pain*, **31**, 199–209.

18. Ventafridda, V., Bonezzi, C., Caraceni, A. *et al.* (1987). Antidepressants for cancer pain and other painful syndromes with deafferentation component: comparison of amitriptyline and trazodone. *Italian Journal of Neurological Sciences*, **8**, 579–87.

19. Sindrup, S.H., Bach, F.W., Madsen, C. *et al.* (2003). Venlafaxine versus imipramine in painful polyneuropathy: a randomized, controlled trial. *Neurology*, **60**, 1284–9.

20. Cannon, R.O., Quyyumi, A.S., Mincemoyer, R. *et al.* (1994). Imipramine in patients with chest pain despite normal coronary angiograms. *New England Journal of Medicine*, **330**, 1411–17.

21. Ward, N.G., Bloom, V.L., and Friedel, R.P. (1979). The effectiveness of tricyclic antidepressants in the treatment of coexisting pain and depression. *Pain*, **7**, 331–41.

22. McCleane, G. (2000). Topical application of doxepin hydrochloride, capsaicin and a combination of both produces analgesia in chronic human neuropathic pain: a randomized, double-blind, placebo-controlled study. *British Journal of Clinical Pharmacology*, **49**, 574–9.

23. Epstein, J.B., Truelove, E.L., Oien, H. *et al.* (2001). Oral topical doxepin rinse: analgesic effect in patients with oral mucosal pain due to cancer or cancer therapy. *Oral Oncology*, **37**, 632–7.

24. Epstein, J.B., Epstein, J.D., Epstein, M.S. *et al.* (2006). Oral doxepin rinse: the analgesic effect and duration of pain reduction in patients with oral mucositis due to cancer therapy. *Anesthesia and Analgesia*, **103**, 465–70.

25. Epstein, J.B., Truelove, E.L., Oien, H. *et al.* (2003). Oral topical doxepin rinse: anesthetic effect in normal subjects. *Pain Research and Management*, **8**, 195–7.

26. Panerai, A.E., Monza, G., Movillia, P. *et al.* (1990). A randomized, within-patient crossover, placebo-controlled trial on the efficacy and tolerability of the tricyclic antidepressants chlorimipramine and nortriptyline in central pain. *Acta Neurologica Scandinavica*, **82**, 34–8.

27. Eberhard, G., von Knorring, L., Nilsson, H.L. *et al.* (1988). A double-blind randomized study of clomipramine versus maprotiline in patients with idiopathic pain syndromes. *Neuropsychobiology*, **19**, 25–34.

28. Caruso, I., Sarzi Putini, P.C., Boccassini, L. *et al.* (1987). Double-blind study of dothiepin versus placebo in the treatment of primary fibromyalgia syndrome. *Journal of International Medical Research*, **15**, 154–7.

29. Rowbotham, M.C., Reisner, L.A., Davies, P.S. *et al.* (2005). Treatment response in antidepressant-naïve postherpetic patients: a double-blind, randomized trial. *Journal of Pain*, **6**, 741–6.

30. O'Connor, A.B., Noyes, K., and Holloway, R.G. (2007). A cost-effectiveness comparison of desipramine, gabapentin, and pregabalin for treating postherpetic neuralgia. *Journal of the American Geriatrics Society*, **55**, 1176–84.

31. Gomez-Perez, F.J., Riell, J.A., Dies, H. *et al.* (1985). Nortriptyline and fluphenazine in the symptomatic treatment of diabetic neuropathy. A double-blind crossover study. *Pain*, **23**, 395–400.

32. Enggaard, T.P., Klitgaard, N.A., Gram, L.F. *et al.* (2001). Specific effect of venlafaxine on single and repetitive experimental painful stimuli in humans. *Clinical Pharmacology and Therapeutics*, **69**, 245–51.

33. Yucel, A., Ozyalcin, S., Koknel Talu, G. *et al.* (2005). The effect of venlafaxine on ongoing and experimentally induced pain in

neuropathic pain patients: a double blind, placebo controlled study. *European Journal of Pain*, **9**, 407–16.

34. Durand, J.P., Alexandre, J., Guillevin, L. *et al.* (2005). Clinical activity of venlafaxine and topiramate against oxaliplatin-induced disabling permanent neuropathy. *Anticancer Drugs*, **16**, 587–91.

35. Rowbotham, M.C., Goli, V., Kunz, N.R. *et al.* (2004). Venlafaxine extended release in the treatment of painful diabetic neuropathy: a double-blind, placebo-controlled study. *Pain*, **110**, 697–706.

36. Forssell, H., Tasmuth, T., Tenovuo, O. *et al.* (2004). Venlafaxine in the treatment of atypical facial pain: a randomized controlled trial. *Journal of Orofacial Pain*, **18**, 131–7.

37. Sayar, K., Aksu, G., Ak, I. *et al.* (2003). Venlafaxine treatment of fibromyalgia. *Annals of Pharmacotherapy*, **37**, 1561–5.

38. Sindrup, S.H., Bach, F.W., Madsen, C. *et al.* (2003). Venlafaxine versus imipramine in painful polyneuropathy: a randomized, controlled trial. *Neurology*, **60**, 1284–9.

39. Reuben, S.S., Makari-Judson, G., and Lurie, S.D. (2004). Evaluation of efficacy of the perioperative administration of venlafaxine XL for the prevention of postmastectomy pain syndrome. *Journal of Pain and Symptom Management*, **27**, 133–9.

40. Wernicke, J.F., Pritchett, Y.L., D'Souza, D.N. *et al.* (2006). A randomized controlled trial of duloxetine in diabetic peripheral neuropathic pain. *Neurology*, **67**, 1411–20.

41. Brecht, S., Courtecuisse, C., Debieuvre, C. *et al.* (2007). Efficacy and safety of dulozetine 60 mg once daily in the treatment of pain in patients with major depressive disorder and at least moderate pain of unknown etiology: a randomized controlled trial. *Journal of Clinical Psychiatry*, **68**, 1707–16.

42. Raskin, J., Wiltse, C.G., Siegal, A. *et al.* (2007). Efficacy of duloxetine on cognition, depression, and pain in elderly patients with major depressive disorder: an 8-week, double-blind, placebo-controlled trial. *American Journal of Psychiatry*, **164**, 900–9.

43. Arnold, L.M., Rosen, A., Pritchett, Y.L. *et al.* (2005). A randomized, double-blind, placebo-controlled trial of duloxetine in the treatment of women with fibromyalgia with or without major depressive disorder. *Pain*, **119**, 5–15.

44. Wenicke, J.F., Wang, F., Pritchett, Y.L. *et al.* (2007). An open-label 52-week clinical extension comparing duloxetine with routine care in patients with diabetic peripheral neuropathic pain. *Pain Medicine*, **8**, 503–13.

45. Onal, A., Parlar, A., and Ulker, S. (2007). Milnacipran attenuates hyperalgesia and potentiates antihyperalgesic effect of tramadol in rats with mononeuropathic pain. *Pharmacology, Biochemistry and Behavior*, **88**, 171–8.

46. Gendreau, R.M., Thorn, M.D., Gendreau, J.F. *et al.* (2005). Efficacy of milnacipran in patients with fibromyalgia. *Journal of Rheumatology*, **32**, 1975–85.

47. Sindrup, S.H., Gram, L.F., Brosen, K. *et al.* (1990). The selective serotonin reuptake inhibitor paroxetine is effective in the treatment of diabetic neuropathy symptoms. *Pain*, **42**, 135–44.

48. Sindrup, S.H., Bjerre, U., Dejgaard, A. *et al.* (1992). The selective serotonin reuptake inhibitor citalopram relieves the symptoms of diabetic neuropathy. *Clinical Pharmacology and Therapeutics*, **52**, 547–52.

49. Aragona, M., Bancheri, L., Perinelli, D. *et al.* (2005). Randomized double-blind comparison of serotonergic (citalopram) versus noradrenergic (reboxetine) reuptake inhibitors in outpatients with somatoform, DSM-IV-TR pain disorder. *European Journal of Pain*, **9**, 33–8.

50. Nemoto, H., toda, H., Nakajima, T. *et al.* (2003). Fluvoxamine modulates pain sensation and affective processing of pain in human brain. *Neuroreport*, **14**, 791–7.

51. Shimodozono, M., Kawahira, K., Kamishita, T. *et al.* (2002). Reduction of central poststroke pain with the selective reuptake inhibitor fluvoxamine. *International Journal of Neuroscience*, **112**, 1173–81.

52. Goldenberg, D., Mayskiy, M., Mossey, C. *et al.* (1996). A randomized, double- blind crossover trial of fluoxetine and amitriptyline in the treatment of fibromyalgia. *Arthritis and Rheumatism*, **39**, 1852–9.

53. Semenchuk, M.R., Sherma, S., and Davis. B. (2001). Double-blind, randomized trial of bupropion SR for the treatment of neuropathic pain. *Neurology*, **57**, 1583–8.

54. Katz, J., Pennella-Vaughan, J., Hetzel, R.D. *et al.* (2005). A randomized, placebo-controlled trial of bupropion sustained release in chronic low back pain. *Journal of Pain*, **6**, 656–61.

55. Pick, C.G., Paul, D., Eison, M.S. *et al.* (1992). Potentiation of opioid analgesia by the antidepressant nefazodone. *European Journal of Pharmacology*, **211**, 375–81.

56. Walsh, T.D. (1986). Controlled study of imipramine and morphine in chronic pain due to advanced cancer. *Proceedings of the American Society of Clinical Oncology*, **5**, 237.

57. Breivik, H. and Rennemo, F. (1982). Clinical evaluation of combined treatment with methadone and psychotropic drugs in cancer patients. *Acta Anaesthetica Scandinavica*, **74**, 135–40.

58. Berger, A., Dukes, E., Mercadante, S. *et al.* (2006). Use of antiepileptics and tricyclic antidepressants in cancer patients with neuropathic pain. *European Journal of Cancer Care (England)*, **15**, 138–45.

59. Spiegel, K., Kalb, R., and Pasternak, G.W. (1983). Analgesic activity of tricyclic antidepressants. *Annals of Neurology*, **13**, 462–5.

60. Bingel, U., Schoell, E., and Büchel, C. (2007). Imaging pain modulation in health and disease. *Current Opinion in Neurology*, **20**, 424–31.

61. Gray, A.M., Spencer, P.S.J., and Sewell, R.D.E. (1998). Then involvement of the opioidergic system in the antinociceptive mechanism of action of antidepressant compounds. *British Journal of Pharmacology*, **124**, 669–74.

62. Charney, D.S., Menkes, D.B., and Heninger, F.R. (1981). Receptor sensitivity and the mechanism of action of antidepressant treatment. *Archives of General Psychiatry*, **38**, 1160–80.

63. Preskorn, S.H. and Irwin, H.A. (1982). Toxicity of tricyclic antidepressants—kinetics, mechanism, intervention: a review. *Journal of Clinical Psychiatry*, **43**, 151–6.

64. Ray, W.A., Griffin, M.R., Schaffner, W. *et al.* (1987). Psychotropic drug use and the risk of hip fracture. *New England Journal of Medicine*, **316**, 363–9.

65. Veldhuijzen, D.S., van Wijck, A.J., Verster, J.C. *et al.* (2006). Acute and subchronic effects of amitriptyline 25mg on actual driving in chronic neuropathic pain patients. *Journal of Psychopharmacology*, **20**, 782–8.

66. Nordin, C., Siwers, B., Benitez, J. *et al.* (1985). Plasma concentrations of nortriptyline and its 10-hydroxy metabolite in depressed patients: relationship to the debrisoquine hydroxylation metabolic ratio. *British Journal of Clinical Pharmacology*, **19**, 832–5.

67. Bernard, S.A. and Bruera, E. (2000). Drug interactions in palliative care. *Journal of Clinical Oncology*, **18**, 1780–99.

68. Kerrick, J.M., Fine, P.G., Lipman, A.G. *et al.* (1993). Low-dose amitriptyline as an adjunct to opioids for postoperative orthopedic pain: a placebo-controlled trial trial. *Pain*, **52**, 325–30.

69. Poulsen, L., Arendt-Nielsen, L., Brosen, K. *et al.* (1995). The hypoalgesic effect of imipramine in different human experimental pain models. *Pain*, **60**, 287–93.

70. Portenoy, R.K., Foley, K.M., and Inturrisi, C.E. (1990). The nature of opioid responsiveness and its implications for neuropathic pain: new hypotheses derived from studies of opioid infusions. *Pain*, **43**, 273–86.

71. Ettinger, A.B. and Portenoy, R.K. (1988). The use of corticosteroids in the treatment of symptoms associated with cancer. *Journal of Pain and Symptom Management*, **3**, 99–103.

72. Farr, W.C. (1990). The use of corticosteroids for symptom management in terminally ill patients. *American Journal of Hospice Care*, **7**, 41–6.

73. Bruera, E., Roca, E., Cedaro, L. *et al.* (1985). Action of oral methylprednisolone in terminal cancer patients: a prospective randomized double-blind study. *Cancer Treatment Report*, **69**, 751–4.

74. Tannock, I., Gospodarowicz, M., Meakin, W. *et al.* (1989). Treatment of metastatic prostatic cancer with low-dose prednisone: evaluation of pain and quality of life as pragmatic indices of response. *Journal of Clinical Oncology*, **7**, 590–7.

75. Hanks, G.W., Trueman, T., and Twycross, R.G. (1983). Corticosteroids in terminal cancer. *Postgraduate Medical Journal*, **59**, 702–6.

76. Kozin, F., Ryan, L.M., Carerra, G.F. *et al.* (1981). The reflex sympathetic dystrophy syndrome (RSDS). III. Scintigraphic studies, further evidence for the therapeutic efficacy of systemic corticosteroids, and proposed diagnostic criteria. *American Journal of Medicine*, **70**, 23–9.

77. Fainsinger, R.L., Spanchynski, K., Hanson, J. *et al.* (1994). Symptom control in terminally ill patients with malignant bowel obstruction. *Journal of Pain and Symptom Management*, **9**, 12–8.

78. Vecht, Ch.J., Haaxma-Reiche, H., van Putten, W.L.J. *et al.* (1989). Initial bolus of conventional versus high-dose dexamethasone in metastatic spinal cord compression. *Neurology*, **39**, 1255–7.

79. Mercadante, S.L., Berchovich, M., Casuccio, A. *et al.* (2007). A prospective randomized study of corticosteroids as adjuvant drugs to opioids in advanced cancer patients. *American Journal of Hospice Palliative Care*, **24**,13–9.

80. Reeve, A.J., Patel, S., Fox, A. *et al.* (2000). Intrathecally administered endotoxin or cytokines produce allodynia, hyperalgesia and changes in spinal cord neuronal responses to nociceptive stimuli in the rat. *European Journal of Pain*, **4**, 247–57.

81. Devor, M., Govrin-Lippman, R., and Raber, P. (1985). Corticosteroids reduce neuroma hyperexcitability. In *Advances in Pain Research and Therapy* (eds. H.L. Fields, R.Dubner, F.Cervero), pp. 451–5,volume 9. Proceedings of the Fourth World Congress on Pain. New York: Raven Press.

82. Sorensen, P.S., Helweg-Larsen, S., Mouridsen, H. *et al.* (1994). Effect of high-dose dexamethasone in carcinomatous metastatic spinal cord compression treated by radiotherapy: a randomized trial. *European Journal of Cancer*, **30A**, 22–7.

83. Breitbart, W., Stiefel, F., Kornblith, A.B. *et al.* (1993). Neuropsychiatric disturbance in cancer patients with epidural spinal cord compression receiving high dose corticosteroids: a prospective comparison study. *Psycho-oncology*, **2**, 233–45.

84. Messer, J., Reitman, D., Sacks, H.S. *et al.* (1983). Association of adrenocorticosteroid therapy and peptic ulcer disease. *New England Journal of Medicine*, **309**, 21–4.

85. Lussier, D., Huskey, A.G., and Portenoy, R.K. (2004). Adjuvant analgesics in cancer pain management. *The Oncologist*, **9**, 571–91.

86. Kayser, V., Desmeules, J., and Guilbaud, G. (1995). Systemic clonidine differentially modulates the abnormal reactions to mechanical and thermal stimuli in rats with peripheral mononeuropathy. *Pain*, **60**, 275–85.

87. Pertovaara, A., Kauppila, T., and Tukeva, T. (1990). The effect of medetomidine, an alpha-2 adrenoceptor agent in various pain tests. *European Journal of Pharmacology*, **179**, 323–8.

88. Puke, M.J.C. and Wiesenfeld-Hallin, Z. (1993). The differential effects of morphine and the alpha 2 adrenoceptor agonists clonidine and dexmedetomidine on the prevention and treatment of experimental neuropathic pain. *Anesthesia and Analgesia*, **77**, 104–9.

89. Aho, M.S., Erkola, O.A., Scheinin, H. *et al.* (1991). Effect of intravenously administered dexmedetomidine on pain after laparoscopic tubal ligation. *Anesthesia and Analgesia*, **73**, 112–18.

90. Byas-Smith, M.G., Max, M.B., Muir, H. *et al.* (1995). Transdermal clonidine compared to placebo in painful diabetic neuropathy using a two-staged 'enriched enrollment' design. *Pain*, **60**, 267–74.

91. Eisenach, J.C., Du Pen, S., Dubois, M. *et al.* and the Epidural Clonidine Study Group. (1995). Epidural clonidine analgesia for intractable cancer pain. *Pain*, **61**, 391–400.

92. Tumber, P.S. and Fitzgibbon, D.R. (1998). The control of severe cancer pain by continuous intrathecal infusion and patient controlled intrathecal analgesia with morphine, bupivacaine and clonidine. *Pain*, **78**, 217–20.

93. Nance, P.W., Bugaresti, J., Shellenberger, K. *et al.* (1994). Efficacy and safety of tizanidine in the treatment of spasticity in patients with spinal cord injury. North American Tizanidine Study Group. *Neurology*, **44** (Suppl 9), S44–52.

94. Kameyama, T., Nabeshima, T., Matsuno, K. *et al.* (1986). Comparison of alpha-adrenoceptor involvement in the antinociceptive action of tizanidine and clonidine in the mouse. *European Journal of Pharmacology*, **125**, 257–64.

95. Malanga, G.A., Gwynn, M.W., Smith, R. *et al.* (2002). Tizanidine is effective in the treatment of myofascial pain syndrome. *Pain Physician*, **5**, 422–32.

96. Wolff, M., Heugel, P., Hempelmann, G. *et al.* (2007). Clonidine reduces the excitability of spinal dorsal horn neurones. *British Journal of Anaesthesia*, **98**, 353–61.

97. Semla, T.P., Beizer, J.L., and Higbee, M.D. (1998). *Geriatric Dosage Handbook*, pp. 238–40, 4th edition. Hudson, OH: Lexi-Comp.

98. Yjritsy-Roy, J.A., Standish, S.M., and Terry, L.C. (1989). Dopamine D-1 and D-2 receptor antagonists potentiate analgesic and motor effects of morphine. *Pharmacology Biochemistry and Behavior*, **32**, 717–21.

99. Schreiber, S., Getslev, V., and Backer, M.M. (1999). The atypical neuroleptics clozapine and olanzapine differ regarding their antinociceptive mechanisms and potency. *Pharmacology Biochemistry and Behavior*, **64**, 75–80.

100. Beaver, W.T., Wallenstein, S., Houde, R.W. *et al.* (1966). A comparison of the analgesic effects of methotrimeprazine and morphine in patients with cancer. *Clinical Pharmacology and Therapeutics*, **7**, 436–46.

101. Lechin, F., van der Dijs, B., Lechin, M.E. *et al.* (1989). Pimozide therapy for trigeminal neuralgia. *Archives of Neurology*, **9**, 960–2.

102. Fishbain, D.A., Cutler, R.B., Lewis, J. *et al.* (2004). Do the second-generation "atypical neuroleptics" have analgesic properties? A structured evidence-based review. *Pain Medicine*, **5**, 359–65.

103. Khojainova, N., Santiago-Palma, J., Kornick, C. *et al.* (2002). Olanzapine in the management of cancer pain. *Journal of Pain and Symptom Management*, **23**, 346–50.

104. Rosenblatt, W.H., Cioffi, A.M., Sinatra, R. *et al.* (1991). Metoclopramide an analgesic adjunct to patient-controlled analgesia. *Anesthesiology and Analgesia*, **73**, 553–5.

105. Cherny, N.I., Thaler, H.T., Friedlander-Klar, H. *et al.* (1994). Opioid responsiveness of cancer pain syndromes caused by neuropathic or nociceptive mechanisms. *Neurology*, **44**, 857–61.

106. Mercadante, S., Maddaloni, S., Roccella, S. *et al.* (1992). Predictive factors in advanced cancer pain treated only by analgesics. *Pain*, **50**, 151–5.

107. Killian, J.M. and Fromm, G.H. (1968). Carbamazepine in the treatment of neuralgia. Use and side effects. *Archives of Neurology*, **19**, 129–36.

108. Rull, J.A., Quibrera, R., Gonzalez-Millan, H. *et al.* (1969). Symptomatic treatment of peripheral diabetic neuropathy with carbamazepine (Tegretol): double-blind cross-over trial. *Diabetologia*, **5**, 215–8.

109. Chadda, V.S. and Mathur, M.S. (1978). Double-blind study of the effects of diphenylhydantoin sodium in diabetic neuropathy. *Journal of the Association of Physicians of India*, **26**, 403–6.

110. Yajnik, S., Singh, G.P., Singh, G. *et al.* (1992). Phenytoin as a coanalgesic in cancer pain. *Journal of Pain and Symptom Management*, **7**, 209–13.

111. Backonja, M., Beydoun, A., Edwards, K.R. *et al.* (1998). Gabapentin for the symptomatic treatment of painful neuropathy in patients with diabetes mellitus: a randomized controlled trial. *Journal of the American Medical Association*, **280**, 1831–6.

112. Dallocchio, C., Buffa, C., Mazzarello, P. *et al.* (2000). Gabapentin vs. amitriptyline in painful diabetic neuropathy: an open-label pilot study. *Journal of Pain and Symptom Management*, **20**, 280–5.

113. Rowbotham, M., Harden, N., Stacey, B. *et al.* (1998). Gabapentin for the treatment of postherpetic neuralgia: a randomized controlled trial. *Journal of the American Medical Association*, **280**, 1837–42.

114. Rice, A.S.C. and Maton, S. (2001). Gabapentin in postherpetic neuralgia: a randomised, double blind, placebo controlled study. *Pain*, **94**, 215–24.

115. Berry, J.D. and Petersen, K.L. (2005). A single dose of gabapentin reduces acute pain and allodynia in patients with herpes zoster. *Neurology*, **9**, 444–7.

116. Levendoglu, F., Ogün, C.O., Ozerbil, O. *et al.* (2004). Gabapentin is a first line drug for the treatment of neuropathic pain in spinal cord injury. *Spine*, **29**, 743–51.

117. Solak, O., Metin, M., Esme, H. *et al.* (2007). Effectiveness of gabapentin in the treatment of chronic post-thoracotomy pain. *European Journal of Cardiothoracic Surgery*, **32**, 9–12.

118. Yaksi, A., Ozgönenel, L., and Ozgönenel, B. (2007). The efficiency of gabapentin therapy in patients with lumbar spinal stenosis. *Spine*, **32**, 939-42.

119. Arnold, L.M., Goldenberg, D.L., Stanford, S.B. *et al.* (2007). Gabapentin in th treatment of fibromyalgia: a randomized, double-blind, placebo-controlled, multicenter trial. *Arthritis and Rheumatism*, **56**, 1336–44.

120. Mellick, G.A. and Mellick, L.B. (1995). Gabapentin in the management of reflex sympathetic dystrophy. *Journal of Pain and Symptom Management*, **10**, 265–6.

121. La Spina, I., Porazzi, D., Maggiolo, F. *et al.* (2001). Gabapentin in painful HIV-related neuropathy: a report of 19 patients, preliminary observations. *European Journal of Neurology*, **8**, 71–5.

122. Caraceni, A., Zecca, E., Martini, C. *et al.* (1999). Gabapentin as an adjuvant to opioid analgesia for neuropathic cancer pain. *Journal of Pain and Symptom Management*, **17**, 441–5.

123. Solaro, C., Lunardi, G.L., Capello, E. *et al.* (1998). An open-label trial of gabapentin treatment of paroxysmal symptoms in multiple sclerosis patients. *Neurology*, **51**, 609–11.

124. Leung, J.M., Sands, L.P., Rico, M. *et al.* (2006). Pilot clinical trial of gabapentin to decrease postoperative delirium in oler patients. *Neurology*, **67**, 1251–3.

125. Chandra, K., Shafiq, N., Pandhi, P. *et al.* (2006). Gabapentin vrsus nortriptyline in post-herpetic neuralgia patients: a randomized, double-blind clinical trial – the GONIP trial. *International Journal of Clinical Pharmacology and Therapeutics*, **44**, 358–63.

126. Gilron, I., Bailey, J.M., Tu, D. *et al.* (2005). Morphine, gabapentin, or their combination for neuropathic pain. *New England Journal of Medicine*, **352**, 1324–34.

127. Caraceni, A., Zecca, E., Bonezzi, C. *et al.* (2004). Gabapentin for neuropathic cancer pain: a randomized controlled trial from the Gabapentin Cancer Pain Study Group. *Journal of Clinical Oncology*, **22**, 2909–17.

128. Fassoulaki, A., Triga, A., Melemeni, A. *et al.* (2005). Multimodal analgesia with gabapentin and local anesthetics prevents acute and chronic pain after breast surgery for cancer. *Anesthesia and Analgesia*, **101**,1427–32.

129. Keskinbora, K., Pekel, A.F., and Aydinli, I. (2007). Gabapentin and an opioid combination versus opioid alone for the management of neuropathic cancer pain: a randomized open trial. *Journal of Pain and Symptom Management*, **34**, 183–9.

130. Ross, J.R., Goller, K., Hardy, J. *et al.* (2005). Gabapentin is effective in the treatment of cancer-related neuropathic pain: a prospective, open-label study. *Journal of Palliative Medicine*, **8**, 1118–26.

131. Rao, R.D., Michalak, J.C., Sloan, J.A. *et al.*, North Central Cancer Treatment Group. (2007). Efficacy of gabapentin in the management of chemotherapy-induced peripheral neuropathy: a phase 3 randomized, double-blind, placebo-controlled, crossover trial (N00C3). *Cancer*, **110**, 2110–8.

132. Devulder, J., Lambert, J., and Naeyaert, J.M. (2001). Gabapentin for pain control in cancer patients's wound dressing care. *Journal of Pain and Symptom Management*, **22**, 622–6.

133. Freeman, R., Durso-Decruz, E., and Emir, B. (2008). Efficacy, safety and tolerability of pregabalin treatment of painful diabetic peripheral neuropathy: findings from 7 randomized, controlled trials across a range of doses. *Diabetes Care*, **31**, 1448–54.

134. Rosenstock, J., Tuchman, M., LaMoreaux, L. *et al.* (2004). Pregabalin for the treatment of painful diabetic peripheral neuropathy: a double-blind, placebo-controlled trial. *Pain*, **110**, 628–38.

135. Sabatowski, R., Gálvez, R., Cherry, D.A. *et al.*; 1008-045 Study Group. (2004). Pregabalin reduces pain and improves sleep and mood disturbances in patients with post-herpetic neuralgia: results of a randomised, placebo-controlled clinical trial. *Pain*, **109**, 26–35.

136. Siddall, P.J., Cousins, M.J., Otte, A. *et al.* (2006). Pregabalin in central neuropathic pain associated with spinal cord injury: a placebo-controlled trial. *Neurology*, **67**, 1792–800.

137. Crofford, L.J., Rowbotham, M.C., Mease, P.J. *et al.*; Pregabalin 1008-105 Study Group. (2005). Pregabalin for the treatment of fibromyalgia syndrome: results of a randomized, double-blind, placebo-controlled trial. *Arthritis Rheumatism*, **52**, 1264–73.

138. Houghton, L.A., Fell, C., Whorwell, P.J. *et al.* (2007). Effect of a second-generation alpha2delta ligand (pregabalin) on visceral sensation in hypersensitive patients with irritable bowel syndrome. *Gut*, **56**, 1218–25.

139. Jokela, R., Ahonen, J., Tallgren, M. *et al.* (2008). A randomized controlled trial of perioperative administration of pregabalin for pain after laparoscopic hysterectomy. *Pain*, **134**, 106–12.

140. Stacey, B.R., Dworkin, R.H., Murphy, K. *et al.* (2008). Pregabalin in thet treatment of refractory neuropathic pain: Results of a 15-month open-label trial. *Pain Medicne*, **9**, 1202–8.

141. Porzio, G., Aielli, F., Verna, L. *et al.* (2006). Efficacy of pregabalin in the management of cetuximab-related itch. *Journal of Pain and Symptom Management*, **32**, 397–8.

142. Sommer, M., Bachmann, C.G., Liebetanz, K.M. *et al.* (2007). Pregabalin in restless legs syndrome with and without neuropathic pain. *Acta Neurologica Scandinavica*, May, **115**, 347–50.

143. Oneschuk, D., and al-Shahri, M.Z. (2003). The pattern of gabapentin use in a tertiary palliative care unit. *Journal of Palliative Care*, **19**, 185–7.

144. Zakrzewska, J.M., Chaudhry, Z., Nurmikko, T.J. *et al.* (1997). Lamotrigine (Lamictal) in refractory trigeminal neuralgia: results

from a double-blind placebo controlled crossover trial. *Pain*, **73**, 223–30.

145. Simpson, D.M., Olney, R., McArthur, J.C. *et al.* (2000). A placebo-controlled trial of lamotrigine for painful HIV-associated neuropathy. *Neurology* **54**, 2115–9.

146. Vestergaard, K., Andersen, G., Gottrup, H. *et al.* (2001). Lamotrigine for central poststroke pain: a randomized controlled trial. *Neurology*, **56**, 184–90.

147. Jose, V.M., Bhansali, A., Hota, D. *et al.* (2007). Randomized double-blind study comparing the efficacy and safety of lamotrigine and amitriptyline in painful diabetic neuropathy. *Diabetes Medicine*, **24**, 377–83.

148. Vinik, A.I., Tuchman, M., Safirstein, B. *et al.* (2007). Lamotrigine for treatment of pain associated with diabetic neuropathy: results of two randomized, double-blind, placebo-controlled studies. *Pain*, **128**, 169–79.

149. Silver, M., Blum, D., Grainger, J. *et al.* (2007). Double-blind, placebo-controlled trial of lamotrigine in combination with other medications for neuropathic pain. *Journal of Pain and Symptom Management*, **34**, 446–54.

150. Devulder, J.E.R. (2000). Lamotrigine in refractory cancer pain: a case report [letter]. *Journal of Clinical Anesthesia*, **12**, 574–5.

151. Thienel, U., Neto, W., Schwabe, S.K. *et al.* Topiramate Diabetic Neuropathic Pain Study Group. (2004). Topiramate in painful diabetic polyneuropathy: findings from three double-blind placebo-controlled trials. *Acta Neurologica Scandinavica*, **110**, 221–31.

152. Muehlbacher, M., Nickel, M.K., Kettler, C. *et al.* (2006). Topiramate in treatment of patients with chronic low back pain: a randomized, double-blind, placebo-controlled study. *Clinical Journal of Pain*, **22**, 526–31.

153. Khoromi, S., Patsalides, A., Parada, S. *et al.* (2005). Topiramate in chronic lumbar radicular pain. *Journal of Pain*, **6**, 829–36.

154. Ipponi, A., Lamberti, C., Medica, A. *et al.* (1999). Tiagabine antinociception in rodents depends on GABA(B) receptor activation: parallel antinociception testing and medial thalamus GABA microdialysis. *European Journal of Pharmacology*, **368**, 205–11.

155. Todorov, A.A., Kolchev, C.B., and Todorov, A.B. (2005). Tiagabine and gabapentin for the management of chronic pain. *Clinical Journal of Pain*, **21**, 358–61.

156. Ardid, D., Lamberty, Y., Alloui, A. *et al.* (2003). Antihyperalgesic effect of levetiracetam in neuropathic pain models in rats. *European Journal of Pharmacology*, **473**, 27–33.

157. Enggaard, T.P., Klitgaard, N.A., and Sindrup, S.H. (2006). Specific effect of levetiracetam in experimental human pain models. *European Journal of Pain*, **10**, 193–8.

158. Ward, S., Jenson, M., Royal, M., Movva, V. *et al.* (2002). Gabapentin and levetiracetam in combination for the treatment of neuropathic pain. *Journal of Pain*, **3** (2 Suppl. 1), 38 (abstract 750).

159. Dunteman, E.D. (2005). Levetiracetam as an adjunctive analgesic in neoplastic plexopathies: case series and commentary. *Journal of Pain and Palliative Care Pharmacotherapy*, **19**, 35–43.

160. Atli, A. and Dogra, S. (2005). Zonisamide in the treatment of painful diabetic neuropathy: a randomized, doubled-blind, placebo-controlled pilot study. *Pain Medicine*, **6**, 225–34.

161. Dogra, S., Beydoun, S., Mazzola, J. *et al.* (2005). Oxcarbazepine in painful diabetic neuropathy: a randomized, placebo-controlled study. *European Journal of Pain*, **9**, 543–54.

162. Criscuolo, S., Auletta, C., Lippi, S. *et al.* (2005). Oxcarbazepine monotherapy in postherpetic neuralgia unresponsive to carbamazepine and gabapentin. *Acta Neurologica Scandinavica*, **111**, 229–32.

163. Kochar, D.K., Rawat, N., Agrawal, R.P. *et al.* (2004). Sodium valproate for painful diabetic neuropathy: a randomized

double-blind placebo-controlled study. *Quarterly Journal of Medicine*, **97**, 33–8.

164. Otto, M., Bach, F.W., Jensen, T.S. *et al.* (2004). Valproic acid has no effect on pain in polyneuropathy: a randomized, controlled trial. *Neurology*, **62**, 285–8.

165. Johannessen Landmark, C. (2008). Antiepileptic drugs in non-epilepsy disorders: relations between mechanisms of action and clinical efficacy. *CNS Drugs*, **22**, 27–47.

166. Dooley, D.J., Taylor, C.P., Donevan, S. *et al.* (2007). Ca2+ channel alpha2delta ligands: novel modulators of neurotransmission. *Trends in Pharmacological Sciences*, **28**, 75–82.

167. Perucca, E. (1999). The clinical pharmacokinetics of the new antiepileptic drugs. *Epilepsia*, **40** (Suppl. 9), S7–13.

168. Cassuto, J., Wallin, G., Hogstrom, S. *et al.* (1985). Inhibition of postoperative pain by continuous low dose infusion of lidocaine. *Anesthesia and Analgesia*, **64**, 971–4.

169. Backonja, M. and Gombar, K. (1992). Response of central pain syndromes to intravenous lidocaine. *Journal of Pain and Symptom Management*, **7**, 172–8.

170. Attal, N., Gaudé, V., Brasseur, L. *et al.* (2000). Intravenous lidocaine in central pain: a double-blind, placebo-controlled, psychophysical study. *Neurology*, **54**, 564–74.

171. Rowbotham, M.C., Reisner-Keller, L.A., and Fields, H.L. (1991). Both intravenous lidocaine and morphine reduce the pain of postherpetic neuralgia. *Neurology*, **41**, 1024–8.

172. Kastrup, J., Petersen, P., Dejgard, A. *et al.* (1987). Intravenous lidocaine infusion—a new treatment for chronic painful diabetic neuropathy. *Pain*, **28**, 69–75.

173. Bruera, E., Ripamonti, C., Brenneis, C. *et al.* (1992). A randomized double- blind crossover trial of intravenous lidocaine in the treatment of neuropathic cancer pain. *Journal of Pain and Symptom Management*, **7**, 138–40.

174. Chong, S.F., Bretscher, M.E., Mailliard, J.A. *et al.* (1997). Pilot study evaluating local anesthetics administered systemically for treatment of pain in patients with advanced cancer. *Journal of Pain and Symptom Management*, **13**, 112–7.

175. Brose, W.G. and Cousins, M.J. (1991). Subcutaneous lidocaine for treatment of neuropathic cancer pain. *Pain*, **45**, 145–8.

176. Dunlop, R., Davies, R.J., Hockley, J. *et al.* (1989). Letter to the Editor. *Lancet*, **1**, 420–1.

177. Lindstrom, P. and Lindblom, U. (1987). The analgesic effect of tocainide in trigeminal neuralgia. *Pain*, **28**, 45–50.

178. Oskarsson, P., Ljunggren, J.G., Lins, P.E. (1997). Efficacy and safety of mexiletine in the treatment of painful diabetic neuropathy. *Diabetes Care*, **20**, 1594–7.

179. Koppert, W., Ostermeier, N., Sittl, R. *et al.* (2000). Low-dose lidocaine reduces secondary hyperalgesia by a central mode of action. *Pain*, **85**, 217–24.

180. Woolf, C.J. and Wiesenfeld-Halli, Z. (1985). The systemic administration of local anesthetic produces a selective depression of C-afferent evoked activity in the spinal cord. *Pain*, **23**, 361–74.

181. CAST (Cardiac Arrhythmia Suppression Trial) Investigators. (1989). Preliminary report: effect of encainide and flecainide on mortality in a randomized trial of arrhythmia suppression after acute myocardial infarction. *New England Journal of Medicine*, **321**, 406–12.

182. Galer, B.S., Harle, J., and Rowbotham, M.C. (1996). Response to intravenous lidocaine infusion predicts subsequent response to oral mexiletine: a prospective study. *Journal of Pain and Symptom Management*, **12**, 161–7.

183. Mao, J., Price, D.D., and Mayer, D.J. (1995). Experimental mononeuropathy reduces the antinociceptive effects of morphine: implications for common intracellular mechanisms involved in morphine tolerance and neuropathic pain. *Pain*, **61**, 353–4.

184. Dickenson, A.H. and Sullivan, A.F. (1987). Evidence for a role of the NMDA receptor in the frequency dependent potentiation of deep dorsal horn nociceptive neurons following C fibre stimulation. *Neuropharmacology*, **26**, 1235–8.

185. Weinbroum, A.A., Bender, B., Bickels, J. *et al.* (2003). Preoperative and postoperative dextromethorphan provides sustained reduction in postoperative pain and patient-controlled epidural analgesia requirement: a randomized, placebo-controlled, double-blind study in lower body bone malignancy-operated patients. *Cancer*, **97**, 2334–40.

186. Graven-Nielsen, T., Aspegren Kendall, S., Henriksson, K.G. *et al.* (2000). Ketamine reduces muscle pain, temporal summation, and referred pain in fibromyalgia patients. *Pain*, **85**, 483–91.

187. Eide, K., Stubhaug, A., Oye, I. *et al.* (1995). Continuous subcutaneous administration of the N-methyl-D-aspartic acid (NMDA) receptor antagonist ketamine in the treatment of post-herpetic neuralgia. *Pain*, **61**, 221–8.

188. Eichenberger, U., Neff, F., Sveticic, G. *et al.* (2008). Chronic phantom limb pain: the effects of calcitonin, ketamine, and their combination on pain and sensory thresholds. *Anesthesia and Analgesia*, **106**, 1265–73.

189. Kwarnström, A., Karlsten, R., Quiding, H. *et al.* (2004). The analgesic effect of intravenous ketamine and lidocaine on pain after spinal cord injury. *Acta Anaesthesiologica Scandinavica*, **48**, 498–506.

190. Carr, D.B., Goudas, L.C., Denman, W.T. *et al.* (2004). Safety and efficacy of intranasal ketamine for the treatment of breakthrough pain in patients with chronic pain: a randomized, double-blind, placebo-controlled, crossover study. *Pain*, **108**, 17–27.

191. Michelet, P., Guervilly, C., Hélaine, A. *et al.* (2007). Adding ketamine to morphine for patient-controlled analgesia after thoracic surgery: influence on morphine consumption, respiratory function, and nocturnal desaturation. *British Journal of Anaesthesia*, **99**, 396–403.

192. Lynch, M.E., Clark, A.J., Sawynok, J. *et al.* (2005). Topical amitriptyline and ketamine in neuropathic pain syndromes: an open-label study. *Journal of Pain*, **6**, 644–9.

193. Lynch, M.E., Clark, A.J., Sawynok, J. *et al.* (2005). Topical 2% amitriptyline and 1% ketamine in neuropathic pain syndromes: a randomized, double-blind, placebo-controlled trial. *Anesthesiology*, **103**, 140–6.

194. Lauretti, G.R., Lima, I.C.P.R., Reis, M.P. *et al.* (1999).Oral ketamine and transdermal nitroglycerin as analgesic adjuvants to oral morphine therapy for cancer pain management. *Anesthesiology*, **90**, 1528–33.

195. Mercadante, S., Arcuri, E., Tirelli, W. *et al.* (2000). Analgesic effect of intravenous ketamine in cancer patients on morphine therapy: a randomized, controlled, double-blind, crossover, double-dose study. *Journal of Pain and Symptom Management*, **20**, 246–52.

196. Anghelescu, D.L. and Oakes, L.L. (2005). Ketamine use for reduction of opioid tolerance in a 5-year-old girl with end-stage abdominal neuroblastoma. *Journal of Pain and Symptom Management*, **30**, 1–3.

197. Vranken, J.H., Troost, D., Wegener, J.T. *et al.* (2005). Neuropathological findings after continuous intrathecal administration of S(+)-ketamine for the management of neuropathic cancer pain. *Pain*, **117**, 231–5.

198. Nelson, K.A., Park, K.M., Robinovitz, E. *et al.* (1997). High-dose oral dextromethorphan versus placebo in painful diabetic neuropathy and postherpetic neuralgia. *Neurology*, **48**, 1212–8.

199. Ben Abraham, R., Marouani, N., Kollender, Y. *et al.* (2002). Dextromethorphan for phantom pain attenuation in cancer amputees: a double-blind crossover trial involving three patients. *Clinical Journal of Pain*, 282–5.

200. Gilron, I., Booher, S.L., Rowan, J.S. *et al.* (2000). A randomized, controlled trial of high-dose dextromethorphan in facial neuralgias. *Neurology*, **55**, 964–71.

201. Carlsson, K.C., Hoem, N.O., Moberg, E.R. *et al.* (2004). Analgesic effect of dextromethorphan in neuropathic pain. *Acta Anesthesiologica Scandinavica*, **48**, 328–36.

202. Galer, B.S., Lee, D., Ma, T. *et al.* (2005). MorphiDex (morphine sulfate/dextromethorphan hydrobromide combination) in the treatment of chronic pain: three multicenter, randomized, double-blind, controlled clinical trials fail to demonstrate enhanced opioid analgesia or reduction in tolerance. *Pain*, **115**, 284–95.

203. Cohen, S.P., Chang, A.S., Larkin, T. *et al.* (2004). The intravenous ketamine test: a predictive response tool for oral dextromethorphan treatment in neuropathic pain. *Anesthesia and Analgesia*, **99**, 1753–9.

204. Pud, D., Eisenberg, E., Spitzer, A. *et al.* (1998). The NMDA receptor antagonist amantadine reduces surgical neuropathic pain in cancer patients: a double blind, randomized, placebo-controlled trial. *Pain*, **75**, 349–54.

205. Snijdelaar, D.G., Koren, G., and Katz, J. (2004).Effects of perioperative oral amantadine on postoperative pain and morphine consumption in patients after radical prostatectomy: results of a preliminary study. *Anesthesiology*, **100**, 134–41.

206. Eisenberg, E., Pud, D., Koltun, L. *et al.* (2007). Effect of early administration of the N-methyl-d-aspartate receptor antagonist amantadine on the development of postmastectomy pain syndrome: a prospective pilot study. *Journal of Pain*, **8**, 223–9.

207. Sinis, N., Birbaumer, N., Gustin, S. *et al.* (2007). Memantine treatment of complex regional pain syndrome: a preliminary report of six cases. *Clinical Journal of Pain*, **23**, 237–43.

208. Schley, M., Topfner, S., Wiech, K. *et al.* (2007). Continuous brachial plexus blockade in combination with the NMDA receptor antagonist memantine prevents phantom pain in acute traumatic upper limb amputees. European *Journal of Pain*, **11**, 299–308.

209. Davis, A.M. and Inturrisi, C.E. (1999). d-methadone blocks morphine tolerance and N-methyl-D-aspartate-induced hyperalgesia. *Journal of Pharmacology and Experimental Therapeutics*, **289**, 1048–53.

210. Pascual, D., Goicoechea, C., Suardíaz, M. *et al.* (2005). A cannabinoid agonist, WIN 55,212-2, reduces neuropathic nociception induced by paclitaxel in rats. *Pain*, **118**, 23–34.

211. Wissel, J., Haydn, T., Muller, J. *et al.* (2006). Low dose treatment with the synthetic cannabinoid Nabilone significantly reduced spasticity-related pain: a double-blind placebo-controlled cross-over trial. *Journal of Neurology*, **253**, 1337–41.

212. Skrabek, R.Q., Galimova, L., Ethans, K. *et al.* (2008). Nabilone for the treatment of pain in fibromyalgia. *Journal of Pain*, **9**, 164–73.

213. Maida, V., Ennis, M., Irani, S. *et al.* (2008). Adjunctive nabilone in cancer pain and symptom management: a prospective observational study using propensity scoring. *Journal of Supportive Oncology*, **6**, 119–24.

214. Svendsen, K.B., Jensen, T.S., and Bach, F.W. (2004). Does the cannabinoid dronabinol reduce central pain in multiple sclerosis? Randomised double blind placebo controlled crossover trial. *British Medical Journal*, **329**, 253.

215. Rog, D.J., Nurmikko, T.J., Friede, T. *et al.* (2005). Randomized, controlled trial of cannabis-based medicine in central pain in multiple sclerosis. *Neurology*, **27(65)**, 812–9.

216. Russo, E.B., Guy, G.W., and Robson, P.J. (2007). Cannabis, pain, and sleep: lessons from therapeutic clinical trials of Sativex, a cannabis-based medicine. *Chemistry and Biodiversity*, **4**, 1729–43.

217. Noyes, R., Brunk, S.F., Avery, D.H. *et al.* (1976). The analgesic properties of delta-9-tetrahydrocannabinol and codeine. *Clinical Pharmacology and Therapeutics*, **18**, 84–9.

218. Fromm, G.H., Terrence, C.F., and Chattha, A.S. (1984). Baclofen in the treatment of trigeminal neuralgia: double-blind study and long-term follow-up. *Annals of Neurology*, **15**, 240–4.

219. Fromm, G.H. (1994). Baclofen as an adjuvant analgesic. *Journal of Pain and Symptom Management*, **9**, 500–9.

220. Sadiq, S.A. and Poopatana, C.A. (2007). Intrathecal baclofen and morphine in multiple sclerosis patients with severe pain and spasticity. *Journal of Neurology*, **254**, 1464–5.

221. Gobelet, C., Waldburger, M., and Meier, J.L. (1992). The effect of adding calcitonin to physical treatment on reflex sympathetic dystrophy. *Pain*, **48**, 171–5.

222. Jaeger, H. and Maier, C. (1992).Calcitonin in phantom limb pain: a double blind study. *Pain*, **48**, 21–7.

223. Schott, G.D. and Loh, L. (1984). Anticholinesterase drugs in the treatment of chronic pain. *Pain*, **20**, 201–6.

224. Slatkin, N. and Rhiner, M. (2004). Treatment of opioid-induced delirium with acetylcholinesterase inhibitors: a case report. *Journal of Pain and Symptom Management*, **27**, 268–73.

225. Knotkova, H., Pappagallo, M., and Szallasi, A. (2008). Capsaicin (TRPV1 Agonist) therapy for pain relief: farewell or revival? *Clinical Journal of Pain*, **24**, 142–54.

226. Watson, C.P.N., Tyler, K.L., Bickers, D.R. *et al.* (1993). A randomized vehicle-controlled trial of topical capsaicin in the treatment of postherpetic neuralgia. *Clinical Therapeutics*, **15**, 510–26.

227. Capsaicin Study Group. (1991). Treatment of painful diabetic neuropathy with topical capsaicin. A multicenter, double-blind, vehicle-controlled study. *Archives of Internal Medicine*, **151**, 2225–9.

228. Ellison, N., Loprinzi, C.L., Kugler, J. *et al.* (1997). Phase III placebo-controlled trial of capsaicin cream in the management of surgical neuropathic pain in cancer patients. *Journal of Clinical Oncology*, **15**, 2974–80.

229. Paice, J.A., Ferrans, C.E., Lashley, F.R. *et al.* (2000). Topical capsaicin in the management of HIV-associated peripheral neuropathy. *Journal of Pain and Symptom Management*, **19**, 45–52.

230. McCarthy, G.M. and McCarty, D.J. (1992). Effect of topical capsaicin in the therapy of painful osteoarthritis of the hands. *Journal of Rheumatology*, **19**, 604–7.

231. Zhang, W.Y., Li Wan Po, A. (1994). The effectiveness of topically applied capsaicin: a meta-analysis. *European Journal of Clinical Pharmacology*, **46**, 517–22.

232. McCleane, G. (2000). Topical application of doxepin hydrochloride, capsaicin and a combination of both produces analgesia in chronic human neuropathic pain: a randomized, double-blind, placebo-controlled study. *Journal of Clinical Pharmacology*, **49**, 574–9.

233. Lin, J., Zhang, W., Jones, A. *et al.* (2004). Efficacy of topical non-steroidal anti-inflammatory drugs in the treatment of osteoarthritis: meta-analysis of randomised controlled trials. *British Medical Journal*, **329**, 324.

234. Mason, L., Moore, R.A., Edwards, J.E. *et al.* (2004). Topical NSAIDs for chronic musculoskeletal pain: systematic review and meta-analysis. *BMC Musculoskeletal Disorders*, **5**, 28.

235. Ho, K.Y., Huh, B.K., White, W.D. *et al.* (2008). Topical amitriptyline versus lidocaine in the treatment of neuropathic pain. *Clinical Journal of Pain*, **24**, 51–5.

236. Stow, P.J., Glynn, C.J., and Minor, B. (1989). EMLA cream in the treatment of post herpetic neuralgia: efficacy and pharmacokinetic profile. *Pain*, **39**, 301–5.

237. Rowbotham, M.C., Davies, P.S., and Fields, H.L. (1995). Topical lidocaine gel relieves postherpetic neuralgia. *Annals of Neurology*, **37**, 246–53.

238. Galer, B.S., Rowbotham, M.C., and Perander, J. (1999). Topical lidocaine patch relieves postherpetic neuralgia more effectively than a vehicle topical patch: results of an enriched enrollment study. *Pain*, **80**, 533–8.

239. Barbano, R.L., Herrmann, D.N., Hart-Gouleau, S. *et al.* (2004). Effectiveness, tolerability, and impact on quality of life of the 5% lidocaine patch in diabetic polyneuropathy. *Archives of Neurology*, **61**, 914–8.

240. Gammaitoni, A.R., Galer, B.S., Onawola, R. *et al.* (2004). Lidocaine patch 5% and its positive impact on pain qualities in osteoarthritis: results of a pilot 2-week, open-label study using the Neuropathic Pain Scale. *Current Medical Research and Opinion*, **20**(Suppl 2), S13–9.

241. Meier, T., Wasner, G., Faust, M. *et al.* (2003). Efficacy of lidocaine patch 5% in the treatment of focal peripheral neuropathic pain syndromes: a randomized, double-blind, placebo-controlled study. *Pain*, **106**, 151–8.

242. Gammaitoni, A.R. and Davis, M.W. (2002). Pharmacokinetics and tolerability of lidocaine patch 5% with extended dosing. *Annals of Pharmacotherapy*, **36**, 236–40.

243. Lyritis, G.P., Ioannidis, G.V., Karachalios, T. *et al.* (1999). Analgesic effect of salmon calcitonin suppositories in patients with acute pain due to recent osteoporotic vertebral crush fractures: a prospective double-blind, randomized, placebo-controlled clinical study. *Clinical Journal of Pain*, **15**, 284–9.

244. Szanto, J., Ady, N., and Jozsef, S. (1992). Pain killing with calcitonin nasal spray in patients with malignant tumors. *Oncology*, **49**, 180–2.

245. Mystakidou, J., Befon, S., Hondros, J. *et al.* (1999). Continuous subcutaneous administration of high-dose salmon calcitonin in bone metastasis: pain control and beta-endorphin plasma levels. *Journal of Pain and Symptom Management*, **18**, 323–30.

246. Hindley, A.C., Hill, A.B., Leyland, M.J. *et al.* (1982). A double-blind controlled trial of salmon calcitonin in pain due to malignancy. *Cancer Chemotherapy Pharmacology*, **9**, 71–4.

247. Tsavaris, N., Kopterides, P., Kosmas, C. *et al.* (2006). Analgesic activity of high-dose intravenous calcitonin in cancer patients with bone metastases. *Oncology Report*, **16**, 871–5.

248. Ormazabal, M.J., Goicoechea, C., Sanchez, E. *et al.* (2001). Salmon calcitonin potentiates the analgesia induced by antidepressants. *Pharmacology, Biochemistry and Behavior*, **68**, 125–33.

249. Paterson, A.H.G., Powles, T.J., Kanis, J.A. *et al.* (1993). Double-blind controlled trial of oral clodronate in patients with bone metastases from breast cancer. *Journal of Clinical Oncology*, **11**, 59–65.

250. Dearnaley, D.P., Sydes, M.R., Mason, M.D. *et al.* (2003). A double-blind, placebo-controlled, randomized trial of oral sodium clodronate for metastatic prostate cancer (MRC PR05 Trial). *Journal of the National Cancer Institute*, **95**, 1300–11.

251. McCloskey, E.V., MacLennan, I.C.M., Kanis, J.A. *et al.* (2001). Effect of clodronate on progression of skeletal disease in multiple myelomatosis. *British Journal of Haematology*, **113**, 1035–43.

252. Santangelo, A., Testai, M., Barbagallo, P. *et al.* (2006). The use of bisphosphonates in palliative treatment of bone metastases in a terminally ill, oncological elderly population. *Archives of Gerontology and Geriatrics*, **43**, 187–92.

253. Fulfaro, F., Casuccio, A., Ticozzi, C. *et al.* (1998). The role of bisphosphonates in the treatment of painful metastatic bone disease: a review of phase III trials. *Pain*, **78**, 157–69.

254. Hortobagyi, G.N., Theriault, R.L., Porter, L. *et al.* (1996). Efficacy of pamidronate in reducing skeletal complications in patients with breast cancer and lytic bone metastases. *New England Journal of Medicine*, **335**, 1785–91.

255. Berenson, J.R., Lichtenstein, A., Porter, L. *et al.* (1996). Efficacy of pamidronate in reducing skeletal events in patients with advanced multiple myeloma. *New England Journal of Medicine*, **334**, 488–93.

256. Vogel, C.L., Yanagihara, R.H., Wood, A.J. *et al.* (2004). Safety and pain palliation of zoledronic acid in patients with breast cancer, prostate cancer, or multiple myeloma who previously received bisphosphonate therapy. *Oncologist,* **9,** 687–95.

257. Wardley, A., Davidson, N., Barrett-Lee, P. *et al.* (2005). Zoledronic acid significantly improves pain scores and quality of life in breast cancer patients with bone metastases: a randomised, crossover study of community vs hospital bisphosphonate administration. *British Journal of Cancer,* **92,** 1869–76.

258. Pecherstorfer, M., Rivkin, S., Body, J.J. *et al.* (2006). Long-term safety of intravenous ibandronic acid for up to 4 years in metastatic breast cancer: an open-label trial. *Clinical drug investigation,* **26,** 315–22.

259. Mancini, I., Dumon, J.C., and Body, J.J. (2004). Efficacy and safety of ibandronate in the treatment of opioid-resistant bone pain associated with metastatic bone disease: a pilot study. *Journal of Clinical Oncology,* **22,** 3587–92.

260. Body, J.J., Diel, I.J., Bell, R. *et al.* (2004). Oral ibandronate improves bone pain and preserves quality of life in patients with skeletal metastases due to breast cancer. *Pain,* **111,** 306–12.

261. Rosen, L.S., Gordon, D., Kaminski, M. *et al.* (2003). Long-term efficacy and safety of zoledronic acid compared with pamidronate disodium in the treatment of skeletal complications in patients with advanced multiple myeloma or breast carcinoma: a randomized, double-blind, multicenter, comparative trial. *Cancer,* **98,** 1735–44.

262. Quilty, P.M., Kirk, D., Bolger, J.J. *et al.* (1994). A comparison of the palliative effects of strontium-89 and external beam radiotherapy in metastatic prostate cancer. *Radiotherapy and Oncology,* **31,** 33–40.

263. Robinson, R.G., Preston, D.F., Schiefelbein, M. *et al.* (1995). Strontium-89 therapy for the palliation of pain due to osseous metastases. *Journal of the American Medical Association,* **274,** 420–4.

264. Baines, M., Oliver, D.J., and Carter, R.L. (1985). Medical management of intestinal obstruction in patients with advanced malignant disease: a clinical and pathological study. *Lancet,* **2,** 990–3.

265. Ripamonti, C., Mercadante, S., Groff, L. *et al.* (2000). Role of octreotide, scopolamine butylbromide, and hydration in symptom control of patients with inoperable bowel obstruction and nasogastric tubes: a prospective randomized trial. *Journal of Pain and Symptom Management,* **19,** 23–34.

266. Mercadante, S., Ripamonti, C., Casuccio, A. *et al.* (2000). Comparison of octreotide and hyoscine butylbromide in controlling gastrointestinal symptoms due to malignant inoperable bowel obstruction. *Supportive Care in Cancer,* **8,** 188–91.

267. Massacesi, C. and Galeazzi, G. (2006). Sustained release octreotide may have a role in the treatment of malignant bowel obstruction. *Palliative Medicine,* **20,** 715–6.

268. Bercel, N.A. (1977). Cyclobenzaprine in the treatment of skeletal muscle spasm in osteoarthritis of the cervical and lumbar spine. *Current Therapeutic Research,* **22,** 462–8.

269. Gold, R.H. (1978). Treatment of low back pain syndrome with oral orphenadrine citrate. *Current Therapeutic Research,* **23,** 271–6.

270. Dalal, S. and Melzack, R. (1998). Potentiation of opioid analgesia by psychostimulant drugs: a review. *Journal of Pain and Symptom Management,* **16,** 245–53.

271. Wilwerding, M.B., Loprinzi, C.L., Mailliard, J.A. *et al.* (1995). A randomized, crossover evaluation of methylphenidate in cancer patients receiving strong narcotics. *Supportive Care in Cancer,* **3,** 135–8.

272. Macleod, A.D. (1998). Methylphenidate in terminal depression. *Journal of Pain and Symptom Management,* **16,** 193–8.

273. Sarhill, N., Walsh, D., Nelson, K.A. *et al.* (2001). Methylphenidate for fatigue in advanced cancer: a prospective open-label pilot study. *American Journal of Hospice and Palliative Care,* **18,** 187–92.

274. Campos, V.M. and Solis, E.L. (1980). The analgesic and hypothermic effects of nefopam, morphine, aspirin, diphenhydramine and placebo. *Journal of Clinical Pharmacology,* **20,** 42–9.

275. Stambaugh, J.E. and Lance, C. (1983). Analgesic efficacy and pharmacokinetic evaluation of meperidine and hydroxyzine, alone and in combination. *Cancer Investigation,* **1,** 111–17.

10.1.9 Injections, neural blockade, and implant therapies for pain control

Robert A. Swarm, Menelaos Karanikolas, and Michael J. Cousins

Introduction

Severe, uncontrolled pain remains one of the most common problems in cancer and palliative care. Despite optimized use of systematic analgesics[1], 10–30 per cent of persons with advanced cancer still have inadequate pain control[2] and require further treatment (Fig. 10.1.9.1). Although interventional pain therapies often have marked analgesic efficacy for otherwise intractable pain, these therapies are often underutilized or withheld until the very end of life. Interventional pain therapies include local anaesthetic (LA) and/or steroid injections, neurolytic neural blockade, and the regional administration of agents that modify neural transmission (Fig. 10.1.9.2). Because pain associated with advanced cancer or other terminal illness often has multiple components, these treatments are best used as components of a multimodal approach for pain and symptom management, along with appropriate utilization of non-pharmacological and psychosocial therapies[3]. They should certainly be considered whenever pain that appears to be intractable is encountered in palliative care.

Generally accepted indications for interventional pain therapies include:

◆ Pain not controlled with systemic analgesics.

◆ Unacceptable adverse effects from systemic analgesic.

Because conventional practice dictates that the dose of a systemic analgesic should be increased until pain is adequately controlled or treatment-limiting adverse effects occur, adverse effects are the most common indication for interventional therapies. Interventional approaches generally are not indicated in sepsis, coagulopathy, or if there is localized infection in the region of the proposed injection. Increasingly, these therapies are considered as options to optimize pain control and/or allow opioid dose reduction as a specific treatment goal.

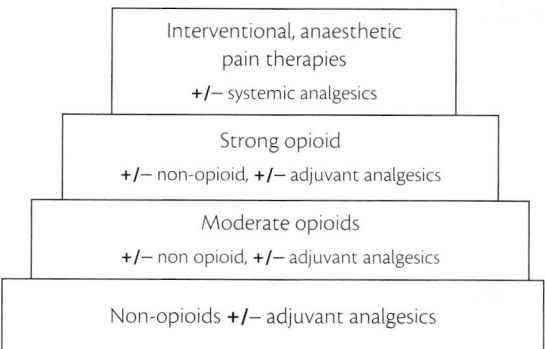

Figure 10.1.9.1 Four-step analgesic ladder for stratified use of analgesic therapies. The lower three steps indicate the World Health Organization's algorithm for use of oral analgesics for cancer pain. When pain is not adequately controlled, or systemic analgesics are associated with unacceptable adverse effects, patients should be considered for step 4—interventional pain therapies, which include injections, neural blockade, and implant therapies. (Modified from World Health Organization. 1990. *Cancer pain relief and palliative care: Report of a WHO expert committee. Rep. 804,* World Health Organization. With permission.)

Disease and patient characteristics limiting the effectiveness of systemic analgesics should be recognized as risk factors for inadequate pain control and possible indications for interventional pain therapies. Neuropathic pain may be less responsive to opioid analgesics than other types of pain, and many resistant cancer pain syndromes include a neuropathic component due to compression or invasion of nervous tissue by tumour (e.g. brachial plexopathy in Pancoast tumour). Sharp, severe somatic pain, as with pathologic fracture or wound debridement, may be so intense as to surpass the efficacy of systemic analgesic therapies and require a more potent 'anaesthetic' approach to block nociceptive transmission. Pain that fluctuates markedly (e.g. pain exacerbation with weight bearing or movement) is difficult to control, because an opioid dose sufficient to control pain at peak intensity may be excessive when pain subsides. Patients' susceptibility to analgesic adverse effects varies widely, but there are rare individuals who cannot tolerate opioids despite optimal use of strategies to manage nausea, constipation, or sedation. Patients with risk factors for ineffective pain control from systemic analgesics should be identified early so that interventional pain therapies can be given timely consideration.

Although the World Health Organization analgesic ladder promises 'freedom from cancer pain'[1], the systemic opioid treatment recommended in this guideline is not ideal in clinical practice[4]. Opioids often fail to provide adequate relief of severe pain, have adverse effects (respiratory depression, sedation, constipation, pruritis, urinary dysfunction), and can be abused[5]. Hormonal abnormalities[6], immune suppression[7], and opioid-mediated facilitation of pain signal transmission[8,9] are further worrisome opioid consequences. Increased awareness of limited efficacy and adverse effects has reduced enthusiasm for chronic opioid therapy, and palliative care clinicians must be aware of adverse opioid effects to optimize management.

Opioid facilitation of pain signal transmission resulting in increased pain (opioid-induced hyperalgesia) is of great clinical concern. Although the principal opioid effect is pain signal inhibition, opioids have widespread effects including activation of processes that enhance pain signal transmission, similar to those identified in neuropathic pain[8,10]. Animal[11] and human[9] data indicate that even short-term, acute opioid administration may produce significant hyperalgesia. Chronic opioid use also appears to induce clinical hyperalgesia: methadone maintenance patients have reduced tolerance to noxious stimuli[12], and patients on chronic opioid experience more intense postoperative pain despite higher analgesic doses[9].

Although the clinical implications of these phenomena during long-term opioid therapy for chronic pain are uncertain, clinicians should carefully evaluate patients with refractory pain and consider therapeutic strategies that would lead to a reduction of the opioid dose. For example, severe opioid toxicity occasionally may occur in patients with advanced disease, severe pain, and a pronounced need for opioid dose escalation[13]. In such cases, escalating opioid dose may be associated with a paradoxical increase in pain, which occurs in tandem with myoclonus and other signs of encephalopathy. This syndrome has been described after systemic[13] or spinal[14] administration of high opioid doses. Opioid toxicity of this type is managed by reducing opioid dose through opioid rotation, interventional pain therapies, and/or alternative systemic therapies, such as lignocaine (lidocaine)[15] or ketamine infusion[16].

In the setting of relatively high-dose opioid therapy, clinical concerns about the development of tolerance and opioid-induced hyperalgesia may lead to consideration of strategies intended to limit the need for opioid-dose increases. Optimized use of non-opioid pain therapies, including interventional pain therapies, may result in improved pain control with a reduced reliance on opioids. LA and neurolytic conduction blockade limit nociceptive input, and thereby may limit facilitation of pain transmission, and hyperalgesia. Spinal co-administration of opioid with non-opioid analgesics may enhance pain control, even in the presence of significant opioid tolerance[10,17]. To the extent that interventional techniques allow opioid dose reduction, tolerance, and opioid toxicity may be reduced or avoided.

Interventional pain therapies, in addition to their role in chronic pain, may also be used to control acute pain or exacerbations of chronic pain so that patients can tolerate diagnostic or therapeutic procedures. For example, regional anaesthetic techniques such as epidural blockade may allow patient positioning for radiographic imaging, radiation therapy, or other palliative procedures such as neurolytic coeliac plexus block or vertebroplasty.

Interventional pain techniques comprise a range of therapies that differ widely in indication, technical complexity, invasiveness, and cost. While systemic analgesics have broad indications, interventional techniques have narrow, specific indications; for this reason, accurate clinical and radiologic assessment is essential to guide their use. Peripheral soft tissue and joint injections are appropriate for most physicians to use, but complex interventions, such as neurolytic blockade, vertebroplasty, or spinal analgesic administration, require special training and expertise. Interventional pain therapies for cancer pain require particular caution, as prior surgery, radiation therapy, and/or tumour mass may alter local anatomy and preclude some procedures or necessitate technique modification.

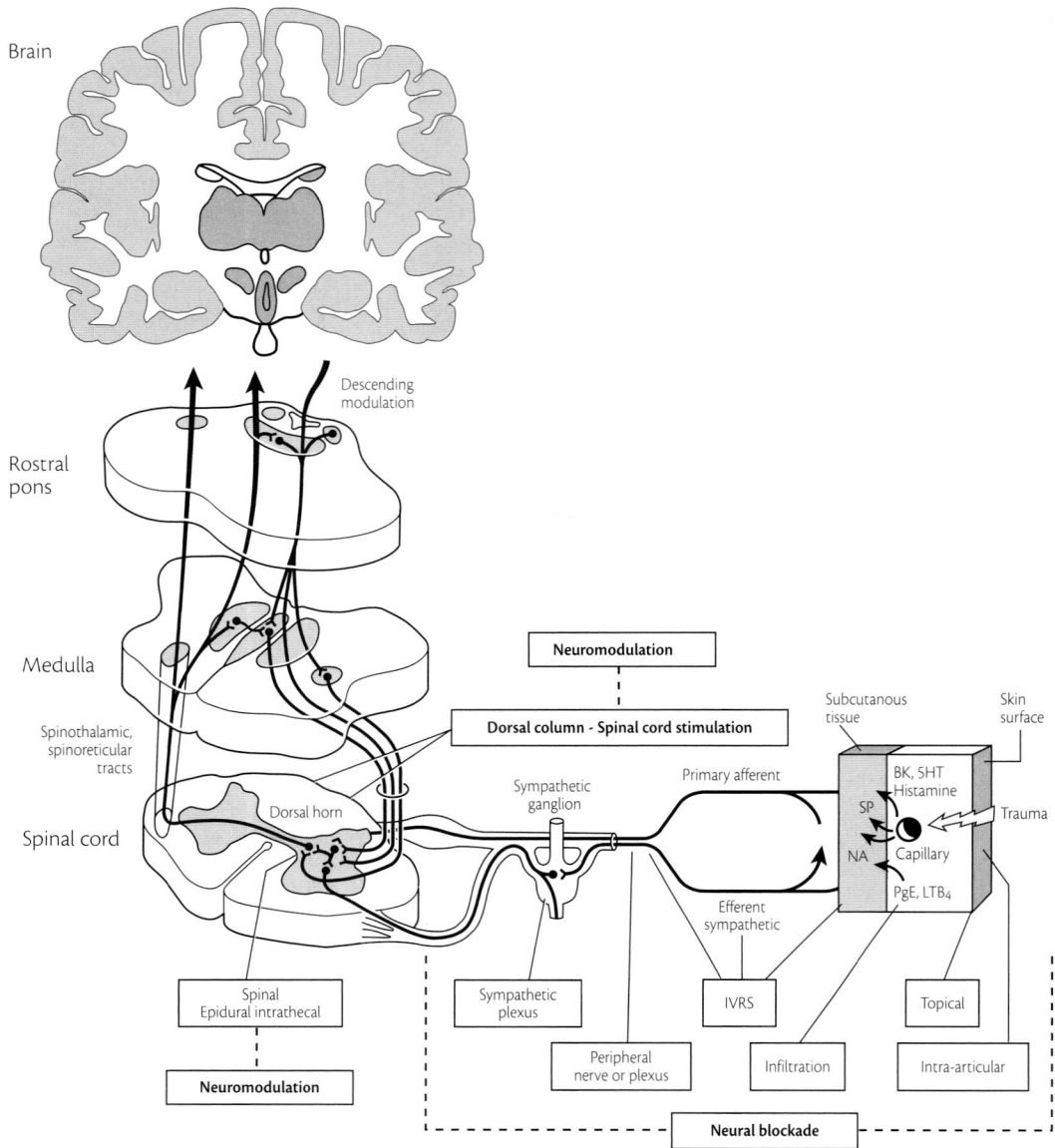

Figure 10.1.9.2 Anatomic sites for injections, neural blockade, and implant therapies for pain control. Peripheral tissues: topical analgesics; regional injection of local anaesthetics, BTXs, and/or corticosteroid. Peripheral nerves: local anaesthetic blockade (including catheter techniques for long-term administration); neurolytic techniques rarely used. Sympathetic ganglia: local anaesthetic and/or neurolytic techniques for neuropathic, ischaemic, and/or visceral pain. Spinal cord: a wide ranage of analgesic and (rarely used) neurolytic interventional pain therapies. Electrical stimulation techniques target the spinal cord (or peripheral nerves) for control of localized neuropathic or ischaemic pain. BK=bradykinin; IVRB = intravenous regional block; LTB4 = leukotriene B4; NA = norepinephrine; PgE = prostaglandin E; SP = substance P. (Reproduced with permission from Murphy, P. and Cousins, M.J. [2005]. Neural blockade and neuromodulation. In *The Paths of Pain* [eds. H. Mersky, J.D. Loeser, and R. Dubner], p. 448. IASP Press, Seattle.)

Agents used in injection and neural blockade techniques

Local anaesthetics

Local anaesthetic (LA) agents are widely used to control pain through topical application, peripheral infiltration, intra-articular injection, and both peripheral and central neural blockade[18] (Fig. 10.1.9.2). Lignocaine (lidocaine) and bupivacaine are the most frequently used LAs for chronic pain. At excessive systemic doses, all LAs can cause cardiac and/or CNS toxicity, including arrhythmias and seizures; therefore, physicians must be familiar with dosing limits. Newer LAs, ropivacaine and levobupivacaine, may have less cardiac toxicity than bupivacaine.

Systemically-administered LAs (e.g. intravenous lignocaine [lidocaine]) or their congeners (e.g. oral mexiletine) can sometimes help in neuropathic pain management[15]. Pain relief from systemic LA had been thought solely to be due to sodium channel blockade in nervous tissue, but LAs also have broad impact on the inflammatory cascade associated with tissue injury and neuropathic pain[19]. For example, LAs inhibit leukocyte migration and inflammatory mediator release. Given the central role of inflammatory mediators in modulation of pain signal transmission[20], systemic LA administration (or the systemic and regional effects of regionally administered LAs) may have important effects in limiting hyperalgesia[19].

Corticosteroids

Corticosteroids are widely used for pain control through injections directly to peripheral lesions, joints, or nerves. Typically, the use of corticosteroid is considered when inflammation is felt to contribute significantly to pain. Sustained-release steroid formulations, such as methylprednisolone (Depo-medrol®), triamcinolone (Kenalog®, Adcortyl®), and betamethasone (Celestone Chronodose®) often are used to prolong treatment effect. Steroid analgesic action has been generally attributed to peripheral anti-inflammatory effects; however, steroids also have analgesic efficacy in settings where there is little acute inflammation (e.g. spinal steroid injection in chronic spinal stenosis due to spondylosis). Inflammatory mediators, including prostaglandins and cytokines, are important in the establishment and maintenance of neuropathic pain[20], and therefore, some of the analgesic effect of corticosteroids also may be related to inhibition of CNS pain facilitation[21].

Corticosteroids have numerous adverse effects associated with chronic administration, including immunosuppression, osteoporosis, hyperglycaemia, and impaired wound healing. These adverse effects may raise less concern in populations with advanced illness, and therefore steroids also are widely used systemically in palliative care.

Neurolytic agents: thermal and chemical

Radiofrequency neural ablation

Radiofrequency (RF) neurotomy is the destruction of neural tissue with heat generated within tissue by a high-frequency electrical current[22,23]. Carefully-controlled RF energy is delivered via a wire probe placed adjacent to the neural tissue to be destroyed. Because RF lesions are limited in size, the area of tissue damage may be more predictable than with neurolytic injections. When a focused lesion is needed, as is the case in the treatment of trigeminal neuralgia, RF has clear advantages over neurolytic injection techniques; however, injection techniques using chemical agents continue to be the neurolytic technique of choice when the tissue target is large and diffuse (e.g. coeliac plexus). RF has been used for pain control in many clinical settings, including trigeminal ganglion ablation; spinal facet denervation; dorsal root ganglion ablation; and sympathetic chain lesioning at different levels (thoracic and lumbar sympathetic ganglia). The use of spinal medial branch nerve RF for control of chronic neck or low-back pain due to facet arthropathy has been supported in a randomized controlled trial (RCT)[23]. There is also extensive experience with RF for trigeminal neuralgia in patients not responding to appropriate analgesics. RF of somatic nerves with cutaneous sensation has a high risk of generating neuropathic pain and thus is rarely used.

Cryoablation

Cryoanalgesia is the destruction of neural tissue by the application of extreme cold. The cryo needle is chilled to -50° to -70°C by the rapid expansion of carbon dioxide or nitrous oxide gas within the needle tip. Although the cold injury is associated with a lesser risk of neuritis or dysaesthesias compared to other neuroablative techniques[22], neuralgia can still occur[24] and the technique must be used with caution. Partial nerve regeneration after cryoanalgesia may result in return of pain a few months later. Cryoanalgesia has

a limited role in palliative care, including control of pain from rib fractures.

Chemical agents

Phenol and ethyl alcohol (ethanol) are the neurolytic agents most frequently used[25]. Phenol has both LA and neurolytic effects, resulting in nearly painless injection. Phenol dose should be limited to 1–10 ml of 6–10 per cent solution for peripheral or sympathetic blocks, and 1–3 ml for subarachnoid injection. Excessive systemic doses or accidental intravascular phenol injection may cause convulsions, CNS depression, or cardiovascular collapse. In contrast, ethanol is associated with few significant adverse effects from systemic absorption of doses used in neurolytic injection techniques, but may cause pain on injection. There are few comparative data on which to base a choice of neurolytic agent.

Peripheral injections for muscular and arthritic pain

As many pain problems in palliative care are localized to regions of the body or a limb, local injections are often a reasonable consideration. Injections can be carried out at various sites, such as skin, muscles, joints, soft tissues, or close to peripheral nerves. The agents most often used for peripheral injections are LAs and/or steroids, or botulinum toxin (BTX).

Intramuscular injections

Intramuscular (IM) injections can be used to parenterally deliver systemic medications or as targeted treatment for muscular pain. For systemic drug delivery, IM injections provide bioavailability comparable to intravenous administration, but they can be painful, and rarely result in haematoma, nerve injury, or infection. Enteral medication administration is preferred in palliative care, and most medications that cannot be delivered enterally can be delivered subcutaneously. Although IM injections are generally not recommended for systemic medication administration, LA injections into trigger points (TPs) is a relatively simple and effective treatment for myofascial pain problems and BTX injections are useful in management of chronic, painful muscle spasm.

Trigger-point injections

Myofascial pain syndromes (MPS) potentially involve any skeletal muscle. MPS may be the primary problem, or may be a secondary manifestation of underlying pathology, such as infection, intervertebral disc disease, vertebral compression fracture, or bone metastasis. MPS may complicate cancer-related pain, but are also common in palliative care patients without malignancy.

MPS diagnosis requires a thorough physical examination for muscular TPs. A TP is a hyperirritable spot in skeletal muscle that is associated with a hypersensitive nodule that may be palpable, is painful on compression, and may cause characteristic referred pain and/or autonomic phenomena[26]. The pathophysiology of MPS is not fully understood, but it is thought that cycles of sustained muscle contraction, impaired metabolic activity, and ischaemia cause nociceptor sensitization and receptive field changes, which account for the complex referred pain patterns that complicate MPS. TPs often arise from tissues affected by injury, which perhaps then become susceptible to further injury.

Management of MPS depends on severity and chronicity. Physical therapy is often adequate. When pain persists, local anaesthetic TP injections and other therapies (i.e. dry needling, vasocoolants, acupuncture, spray and stretch, analgesics) should be combined with interventions addressing the underlying or perpetuating factors (i.e. physical therapy for postural or muscular abnormalities, orthotic devices for structural abnormalities).

Botulinum toxin injections

Botulinum toxin (BTX) is a potent neuroparalytic agent produced by the bacterium *Clostridium botulinum*, an important cause of food poisoning. There are at least two commercial BTX A preparations for clinical use (Botox®, Allergan; Dysport®, Ipsen), and one BTX B preparation (Myobloc®, Elan [US]; Neurobloc®, Elan [Europe]). These products have different doses, efficacy, and safety profiles, and are not interchangeable generic equivalents. BTX irreversibly inhibits acetylcholine release at the neuromuscular junction, thereby blocking neurotransmission. At recommended doses, BTX injections cause localized chemodenervation at the target organ (e.g. muscle, glands), with minimal risk of systemic adverse effects. Evidence suggests that BTX-A also may block peripheral sensitization and indirectly reduce central sensitization[27]. BTX effects start approximately 1 week after injection, last 3 to 4 months, and subsequently fade.

BTX is used to treat pathologically increased muscle activity, such as spasticity, movement disorders, and chronic myofascial pain[28,29]. BTX is generally safe and well tolerated (there are no reported cases of permanent organ damage), and BTX injections may be repeated if needed. To limit development of neutralizing antibodies, which render subsequent BTX use ineffective, an interval of at least 12 weeks between injections is recommended. BTX must be used with caution to avoid systemic effects from excessive dose and/or excessive or unintended muscle weakness.

The role of BTX in palliative care is not well defined, and high cost limits its use. Patients who may benefit from BTX include those with spasticity from traumatic brain injury, multiple sclerosis, or spinal cord injury. By relieving spasticity, BTX may improve motor function (ability to stand and walk, improved upper-extremity movement) and facilitate care (personal hygiene in patients with hipadductor spasticity; self-care and dressing in patients with arm spasticity)[30]. BTX also may be beneficial in myofascial painmanifesting as chronic headache, neck, or back pain, as well as chronic joint pain[31] and certain neuropathic pain conditions (post-herpetic neuralgia[32], trigeminal neuralgia[33], allodynic stump pain[34], and spinal cord pathology[35]). Adjunctive physical therapy is important to maximize BTX benefit.

Intra-articular injections

Arthritis and joint-related pain is common in palliative care patients. Intra-articular injection of corticosteroids, hyaluronic acid[36], or newer investigational agents, such as tropisetron[37], tumour necrosis factor alpha (TNF-a) antagonists (etanercept)[38], and BTX [31] have been used with some success in severe arthritis. Corticosteroids are commonly used for intra-articular injections and different steroid preparations seem to have similar efficacy. Outcome data are very limited, but joint injections potentially result in significant pain relief for months. Potential complications of these injections include nerve injury, bleeding, infection, and joint destruction.

Neural blockade and spinal injections

Local anaesthetic versus neurolytic injections

Regional blockade is best used for pain localized to the distribution of a peripheral nerve or plexus. Regional blockade provides dense block of sensory neurons, thereby relieving even intense pain (anaesthesia), but sometimes at the expense of numbness (complete sensory blockade) and weakness (motor blockade). LA blocks are typically of short duration, but placement of a catheter close to the targeted nerve may overcome this shortcoming by allowing repeated injection or a continuous infusion[39,40].

Neurolytic blocks can provide long-term relief of well-localized pain, but they are used less frequently than in the past due to improved utilization of systemic analgesics and widespread use of spinal analgesics. Neurodestructive techniques are most appropriately viewed as complements to, rather than a replacement for, systemic opioids, adjuvant analgesics, or other pain therapies.

Neurolytic techniques must only be used in selected patients and with meticulous technique. These techniques are useful only to the extent that they provide pain relief without unacceptable numbness or weakness, or subsequent tissue damage to the denervated (and hence unprotected) part of the body.

Patients who survive for months or longer often experience pain recurrence after neurolysis as a result of nerve regeneration. Neurolysis itself may produce neuralgic pain, which presumably occurs because the neural destruction is incomplete. Equally troubling, somatic neurolytic block-induced denervation may result in deafferentation pain in up to 30 per cent of patients undergoing peripheral neurolytic block. This deafferentation pain is less common after subarachnoid neurolysis. Regardless of the mechanism, post-neurolysis neuropathic pain may be worse than the original pain. If it occurs, it usually is best treated with centrally acting analgesics or electrical stimulation techniques (transcutaneous, spinal cord, or peripheral nerve stimulation), rather than with further attempts at neurolysis[22]. Because of limited duration of effect and significant incidence of neuritis, neurolytic blocks are generally reserved for patients with life expectancy less than 3 months.

LA block may have prognostic value, potentially foretelling the degree of pain relief and potential complications from a proposed neurolytic block[22]. However, LA blocks cannot reliably predict the results of neurolytic block: systemic LA absorption, analgesic and sedative medications given during the procedure, LA spread to adjacent neural structures, neural plasticity, and placebo response may all contribute to a misleading temporary success from LA blocks[41]. If the combination of a prognostic LA block plus a separate procedure for neurolysis exceeds a terminally ill patient's willingness or ability to undergo additional procedures, it is reasonable to omit the prognostic block and proceed directly to neurolysis.

Peripheral nervous system blockade

LA blockade can provide dramatic but temporary relief of severe acute pain with relatively simple interventions. These approaches may be very helpful in acute pains caused by tumour, including pathological fractures, ischaemia, or infection. Almost any somatic nerve can be blocked, and imaging technology, such as fluoroscopy, CT, or ultrasound, may improve success rates. A variety of catheter techniques have been developed to prolong the analgesic effect through continuous LA infusion[39,40]. Regional block catheter techniques may be used either as a means to help patients tolerate therapy (e.g. surgery for fracture stabilization, radiation therapy), or may serve as the primary analgesic modality. Examples of successful continuous peripheral block are brachial plexus block for upper-extremity pain, suprascapular nerve block for shoulder pain, thoracic paravertebral nerve block for breast pain, and sciatic and femoral nerve block for lower-extremity pain. Long-term peripheral nerve catheter use may be complicated by infection[42], LA toxicity, catheter displacement, or technical difficulties such as catheter knotting; however, with good care and strict attention to sterility, it may be possible to maintain peripheral nerve catheters for up to several weeks[39].

Most nerves in the head and neck region can be blocked by an interventional pain specialist with expertise in regional anaesthesia, or an oral-maxillofacial surgeon, otolaryngologist, or neurosurgeon with expertise in pain management. Neurolytic blocks in the head and neck can be done percutaneously or endoscopically. Neurolytic blocks are rarely applied in the head and neck, due to risk of significant complications related to close proximity of these nerves to critical structures. In addition, if targeted nerves are close to the skin, cutaneous ulceration may complicate neurolytic injections.

Brachial plexus blockade

Brachial plexus blockade[39] can be accomplished with several approaches (interscalene, supraclavicular, axillary etc.), either as injections or as infusions using various catheter techniques. Because neurolytic brachial plexus blockade carries significant morbidity (due to proximity to critical structures, such as the lung, carotid artery, phrenic nerve, recurrent laryngeal nerve, and subarachnoid space), it is rarely used. Alternatives include dorsal root entry zone (DREZ) lesioning for pain due to brachial plexus avulsion, or spinal analgesics (especially if the tip of the spinal catheter can be placed at the cervicothoracic junction).

Intercostal nerve blocks

Intercostal nerve blocks have been used for a variety of pain problems, including chest-wall pain from rib fractures, chest- and abdominal-wall pain from tumour infiltration, herpes zoster pain, and post-herpetic neuralgia. Intercostal blocks are a relatively simple procedure with significant potential benefits, but can rarely result in significant complications, including pneumothorax, high spinal anaesthesia, and bleeding. Although intercostal blocks typically last a few hours, reports suggest that combining LA with steroid[43], or using high concentrations of LAs such as tetracaine, can result in long-lasting pain relief[44]. Due to risk of post-neurolysis neuropathic pain, neurolytic intercostal nerve blocks should only be considered for intractable chest wall pain in terminally ill patients.

Thoracic paravertebral nerve blocks

Thoracic paravertebral nerve blocks can be helpful in severe thoracic pain from trauma. In patients with a poor prognosis, neurolytic thoracic paravertebral blocks may provide some benefit when pain is limited to a few thoracic dermatomes[45]. Neurolytic paravertebral blocks should be done with great attention to technique, because unintended spread of neurolytic solution could cause spinal damage. In addition, as with neurolytic intercostal block, there is significant risk of post-neurolysis neuralgia with neurolytic thoracic paravertebral block.

Femoral nerve blocks

Femoral nerve blocks have been used for pain from femoral neck fracture, but are more often used for postoperative pain control following knee surgery. Femoral nerve catheters can extend the block duration, but also have been associated with complications, including infection, psoas abscess, femoral nerve injury, catheter knotting, and technical failures[42].

Motor points neurolysis

Control of spasticity through somatic neurolytic blockade[46,47], or motor points neurolysis, can be of significant benefit in patients with spasticity due to central nervous system disease. These techniques are generally reserved for situations in which subarachnoid baclofen infusion has been ineffective or is contraindicated. The risk of neuralgia after peripheral neurolysis for spasticity control should limit its use to palliative care patients with short life expectancy.

Sympathetic nervous system blockade

Sympathetic nervous system blockade, with LA or neurolytic solutions, is important for managing a variety of pain problems, including neuropathic, ischaemic, and/or visceral pain, as well as complex regional pain syndrome (CRPS)[48]. LA sympathetic block may also be helpful in managing pain from acute processes (e.g. renal colic or ischaemic crises in Raynaud's disease or other obliterative arteriopathies)[49]. LA sympathetic block is ineffective in established post-herpetic neuralgia, but often provides significant relief of pain from acute or subacute (less than 2 months' duration) herpetic neuralgia[50]. It is uncertain if LA sympathetic block for acute or subacute herpetic neuralgia decreases the risk of chronic post-herpetic neuralgia[51]. LA sympathetic block is sometimes used to predict a given patient's response to sympathetic neurolysis, but the response to LA blockade should be interpreted with caution because of the analgesic effect of absorbed (systemic) LA and/or placebo response[41].

In advanced malignancy, various neurolytic blocks of sympathetic ganglia are used for management of abdominal (coeliac plexus block), pelvic (superior hypogastric plexus block), and perineal (ganglion impar block) pain of visceral origin (Table 10.1.9.1). These blocks may work by reducing input from visceral afferent nerves that travel through these plexuses. Patients with mixed somatic and visceral pain, perhaps due to tumour invasion of somatic structures or distant metastases, may experience incomplete relief following sympathetic ganglion block; however, even partial relief through neural blockade may improve overall pain control and allow reduction of opioid dose and opioid-related side effects.

Stellate ganglion and upper-thoracic sympathetic blocks

LA cervicothoracic sympathetic blockade (CTSB) may be of benefit in neuropathic or ischaemic pain involving the head, neck, upper extremities, or thorax, including CRPS[48], ischaemic crises (e.g. Raynaud's or other vasculopathy), or intractable angina[52]. Neurolytic solutions (phenol, alcohol) are rarely used for CTSB due to risk of injury to nearby somatic nerves, but surgical sympathectomy (increasingly done as a transthoracic, video-assisted, endoscopic procedure) appears to be an effective alternative. Percutaneous radiofrequency ablation of upper-thoracic sympathetic ganglia has been suggested as a minimally invasive and effective

Table 10.1.9.1 Neurolytic sympathetic blockade by location and clinical indication.

Location	Clinical use	Results
Stellate ganglion block [a]	Angina, inoperable coronary artery disease	Rarely indicated[a]
	Upper-extremity pain:	Upper-thoracic (T2–T3) paravertebral sympathectomy (surgical or radiofrequency ablation) is the preferred technique of cervicothoracic sympathectomy when needed
	Complex regional pain syndrome	
	Peripheral vascular disease	
	Raynaud's disease	
	Brachial plexus infiltration by tumour	
	Herpes zoster	
	Phantom pain	
Coeliac plexus block[b]	Visceral pain from:	Partial to complete pain relief in 90% of patients alive after 3 months
	Pancreatic cancer	Results similar for pancreatic cancer and other abdominal malignancies[56]
	Other upper-abdominal tumours	
Lumbar sympathetic block[b]	Kidney pain (including 'phantom kidney pain')	Variable, depending on pain condition
	Intractable lower-extremity pain:	Peripheral vascular disease: 50–80% of patients experience partial or complete relief of pain at rest[49,63]
	Inoperable peripheral vascular disease	
	Chronic painful leg ulceration	
	Complex regional pain syndrome	
	Phantom pain	
	Herpes zoster	
	Diabetic neuropathy	
	Testicular pain	
Superior hypogastric plexus block[b]	Pelvic visceral pain from gynaecological, colorectal, or genitourinary cancer	Long-lasting relief in 72% of patients with positive response to diagnostic block[65]
Ganglion impar block[b]	Intractable perineal pain	Case series suggest efficacy but little data available[22]

[a] Neurolysis of the Stellate Ganglion is controversial, due to risk of complications. In some cases persistent relief can be achieved from a series of local anaesthetic blocks[22].

[b] Some clinicians do a local anaesthetic block before proceeding with neurolytic block to assess the effect of neurolysis.

sympathectomy technique[53]. There are no published trials comparing the safety and efficacy of different cervicothoracic sympathectomy techniques, but endoscopic surgical techniques require general anaesthesia and have been associated with rare life-threatening complications and post-sympathetic hyperhydrosis[54]. Cervicothoracic spinal analgesic administration and spinal cord stimulation are alternative techniques for cases in which cervicothoracic sympathectomy is considered.

Patients with intractable angina may have less pain and better quality of life after local anaesthetic CTSB. In an uncontrolled, prospective trial, the majority of patients reported complete relief of angina for at least 2 weeks after a single local anaesthetic CTSB, responders most frequently reported 2–4 weeks of pain relief, and repeat blocks provided similar periods of pain relief[52]. Advantages of local CTSB include low cost, low morbidity, and widespread availability. Patients with intractable angina should be offered local anaesthetic CTSB, with injections repeated as needed or utilized as a temporizing intervention until longer-lasting interventions (radio-frequency or surgical CTSB neurolysis, spinal analgesics, or spinal cord stimulation) are implemented[55].

Neurolytic coeliac plexus and splanchnic nerve blocks

Neurolytic coeliac plexus block (NCPB) or neurolytic splanchnic block (NSB) is most commonly used for upper-abdominal pain related to pancreatic cancer or other upper-abdominal malignancies[22]. NCPB has been consistently reported to be highly effective for pain from pancreatic or other abdominal malignancies, with good to excellent relief in 85–90 per cent of patients, and pain relief persisting until death in 70–90 per cent of responders[56]. Massive tumours or other anatomic abnormalities limiting the spread of injected neurolytic solution may limit effectiveness of NCPB or NSB. NCPB or NSB typically provides pain relief for a few months, but repeat injection is rarely needed due to the short life expectancy associated with advanced upper-abdominal malignancy.

There are numerous approaches to accomplish a NCPB. The most commonly used approaches involve the injection of alcohol directly into the region of the ganglion. Posterior injection through two needles placed on either side of the spine was the most common historically, but more recently has been complemented by a single needle posterior transaortic approach, a single needle anterior approach, and an ultrasound-guided endoscopic approach. There have been no comparative trials and the decision to use one or the other typically relates to the experience of the physician, the appearance of the tumour on imaging, and the ability of the patient to assume positions comfortably. Retrocrural neurolysis of splanchnic nerves also can accomplish this block and is used occasionally.

In an RCT of patients with pancreatic cancer, NCPB provided equivalent pain relief with fewer adverse effects, compared to systemic analgesics[57]. In another RCT, patients found during operation to have unresectable pancreatic cancer received intraoperative NCPB or placebo block[58]; patients receiving NCPB had less pain, and those with significant preoperative pain survived longer. Although a subsequent study failed to confirm a survival benefit[59], it is clear that NCPB is effective for upper-abdominal pain related to malignancy.

Immediately following NCPB, many patients have diarrhoea (due to increased gastrointestinal motility) and/or orthostatic hypotension. These typically transient symptoms are expected consequences of interrupting sympathetic innervation to abdominal viscera. NCPB usually can be done on an outpatient basis; however, frail patients or those living far from the facility, where the block is performed, may be best served by overnight observation. Patients may rarely need oral ephedrine (30 mg three times daily) to control orthostatic hypotension or an oral opioid to control diarrhoea. In patients who have had constipation due to chronic opioid therapy, modest diarrhoea may be a welcome change.

Major, catastrophic complications occur rarely after NCPB. A survey of 2730 patients treated with NCPB[60] reported 4 cases of paraplegia, for an incidence of 1:683. It is postulated that paraplegia following NCPB is due to injury or vasospasm of the artery of Adamkiewicz, resulting in ischaemic spinal cord injury. Other serious NCPB complications include aortic dissection, generalized seizures, and circulatory arrest[22]. Because it is unclear if complication risk is affected by the technique or imaging used, it is prudent to assume that all NCPB and NSB techniques carry risk of serious complications. Even paralysis has been described after open, intraoperative NCPB[61]. Potential benefits and risks must be assessed in each situation, but in abdominal pain due to malignancy, NCPB provides 70 per cent to 90 per cent of patients with good to excellent pain relief, with risks comparable to other palliative therapies (chemotherapy, radiation therapy, or surgical intervention) offered to patients with advanced malignancy.

Lumbar sympathetic block

Intractable lower-extremity ischaemic pain due to inoperable peripheral vascular disease is the most common indication for neurolytic lumbar sympathetic block (NLSB). In such settings, NLSB appears to increase cutaneous blood flow, reduce ischaemic rest pain, and enhance healing of chronic ischaemic ulceration[62,63]. It may also be useful in neuropathic lower-extremity pain, especially in some cases of CRPS[48]. Less common indications are visceral pain from lower-abdominal and pelvic structures, such as renal pain, testicular pain, and tenesmus[49]. Serious complications from NLSB are rare when radiographic imaging is used to verify appropriate needle placement and neurolytic solution spread.

Lumbar sympathectomy can be done by NLSB or surgery with comparable results: the majority of peripheral vascular disease patients experience partial or complete relief of pain at rest, and the mean duration of effect is approximately 6 months. Compared to surgical sympathectomy, NLSB is less invasive; has lower morbidity, mortality, and cost; and can be repeated[62]. Percutaneous radiofrequency lumbar sympathectomy has been suggested as an alternative to NLSB[64] but further comparative data are needed.

Hypogastric plexus and ganglion impar block

Neurolytic superior hypogastric plexus block appears to be effective for pelvic visceral pain from gynaecologic, colorectal, or genitourinary cancer[65]. Patients with pelvic pain from tumour

invasion of the pelvic wall may have incomplete relief after superior hypogastric plexus block, presumably because the somatic component is unlikely to respond to block of the ganglion. Extensive retroperitoneal disease may interfere with neurolytic agent spread and also contribute to poor results.

The ganglion impar (or ganglion of Walther) is the terminal sympathetic ganglion of the paravertebral sympathetic chain, located in the retroperitoneal space at the sacrococcygeal junction. Neurolytic ganglion impar block may be used for relief of intractable rectal or perineal pain, but published data are limited[22].

Neuraxial injections and neural blockade

A wide range of spinal injection techniques are commonly used for pain management, including injections into the epidural space or the subarachnoid (intrathecal) space (Table 10.1.9.2). Spinal LA injections can be used to quickly control acute or severe pain (e.g. pain from pathologic hip fracture) to allow time for necessary diagnostic evaluations or more definitive treatments. Various catheter techniques allow repeated or continuous spinal analgesic administration (see spinal analgesic techniques in following paragraphs). Epidural and transforaminal epidural (or selective nerve root) steroid injections are widely used for control of back, neck, and radicular pain syndromes. Spinal neurolytic injections of phenol or ethanol are now rarely used but remain useful techniques in carefully selected patients.

Spinal corticosteroid injection

The use of spinal corticosteroid injections is prevalent in populations with acute and chronic, non-cancer-related neck and back pain. Given the high prevalence of back pain among the elderly and the frequency with which the spine is involved in disease-related processes, these approaches also are important in palliative care.

Table 10.1.9.2 Terms used to describe sites for neuraxial or spinal analgesics and injection techniques.

Spinal	Broadly used to refer to any injection or routes of administration near or within the spinal meninges ('spinal anaesthesia' is generally used to indicate subarachnoid administration of local anaesthetic)
Epidural	Immediately outside the dura mater, within the vertebral spinal canal. Injections typically done via a posterior approach with needle entering the epidural space between the posterior lamina (i.e. interlaminar epidural injection)
Transforaminal epidural injections	Needles placed with radiographic imaging to intervertebral neural foramen. Injected solution often tracks along nerve root into the epidural space
Intrathecal	Inside the thecal sac or dura mater. Intrathecal is often used synonymously with subarachnoid, but anatomically also includes the subdural space
Subdural	Between the dura mater and arachnoid mater
Subarachnoid	Inside the arachnoid mater. This space contains the cerebrospinal fluid

The specific techniques include epidural injections[66] via a 'routine' posterior, interlaminar approach; the more recently described transforaminal epidural injections (or selective nerve root injections) through an oblique approach to the intervertebral foramen[67]; caudal epidural injections; and rarely, subarachnoid steroid injections. Epidural steroid injections can provide temporary relief from axial spine or radicular pain due to spinal metastasis or primary spine tumours; chronic spinal administration of analgesics (opioid, LA, clonidine, etc.) is more likely to provide long-term benefit. As with any spinal injection in the setting of spinal malignancy, care must be taken to avoid placing needles into friable, haemorrhagic tumours, which could lead to spinal haematoma.

Although the effectiveness of spinal injections has not been conclusively proven in any clinical disorder, broad experience suggests that selected patients with chronic, non-cancer-related neck, back, and/or spinal radicular pain benefit from epidural and/or transforaminal steroid injections[68]. While the LA may provide temporary relief, the injected steroid may provide longer-term relief, perhaps through local anti-inflammatory effects. Although surgery may be the most effective approach in some settings[69], spinal steroid injections are commonly tried to provide symptom relief and potentially obviate the need for surgery. In patients with chronic spine disease, epidural steroid injections are perhaps best used to provide periods of relief to facilitate physical therapy and rehabilitation.

The most common unsatisfactory outcome following epidural steroid injections is inadequate pain relief. However, although epidural steroid injections are considered reasonably safe, numerous serious complications have been reported, including anaphylaxis, epidural haematoma, paraplegia (due to spinal cord infarction, direct injection into the cord, or transverse myelitis), transient blindness, and pneumocephalus. Injections should be avoided in very severe stenosis, due to concern about neural injury. Concern about toxicity from inadvertent subarachnoid steroid injection has contributed to widespread use of fluoroscopy with injection of radiographic contrast to confirm appropriate steroid spread into the epidural space.

Spinal cord and brain infarction are rare complications following transforaminal epidural steroid injections. These devastating complications may arise from inadvertent injection of particulate steroid suspension into radicular arterioles adjacent to spinal nerve roots within the spinal neural foramen, with subsequent embolization to the spinal cord or brain, resulting in vascular occlusion and infarct[70]. Although most commonly associated with cervical transforaminal steroid injections, spinal cord infarct has also been described following lumbar transforaminal steroid injections[71]. Complications from transforaminal injections might be minimized by avoiding particulate steroid suspensions (perhaps at the cost of reduced efficacy)[72] and injecting radiographic contrast under real-time fluoroscopic imaging to detect rapid vascular uptake of injectate[70].

Despite limited data suggesting efficacy, subarachnoid steroid injection for intractable pain remains controversial because of concern about neurotoxicity. Animal data suggest that subarachnoid water-soluble methylprednisolone may reverse nerve-injury-induced hypersensitivity to mechanical and heat stimuli[21], perhaps due to inhibition of spinal glia, and case series suggest that some patients with metastatic cancer and intractable pain have significant relief following subarachnoid betamethasone injection[73,74]. An RCT of subarachnoid depot methylprednisolone in lignocaine (lidocaine) indicated significant, long-lasting pain relief from chronic post-herpetic neuralgia[75]; however, this study has not been replicated, and the technique has not gained broad acceptance. Although debate continues over the significance of reported toxicity and whether toxicity is related to the steroid per se or to added preservatives[76], subarachnoid steroid injections should be considered experimental pending further investigation of safety and efficacy.

Spinal neurolytic injection techniques

Spinal neurolytic blocks are used less frequently now than in the past, likely reflecting improved use of systemic and other analgesic therapies, increased awareness of potential complications from neurolytic techniques, and the lack of RCTs confirming efficacy. Nevertheless, available evidence supports use of these techniques in selected cases of advanced cancer[22,77].

Subarachnoid neurolysis is an effective analgesic technique, but should be restricted to patients with advanced malignancy whose pain is limited to only a few dermatomes[77]. The aim is to produce a chemical posterior rhizotomy, thereby interrupting pain signal transmission. It should be avoided when the pain is widespread or of undiagnosed etiology.

Subarachnoid neurolysis is best used for perineal pain in patients with colostomy and permanent bladder catheter, or in relatively localized (unilateral) somatic chest wall or trunk pain[22]. Particular care must be taken to avoid increasing disability through motor weakness, incontinence, sexual dysfunction, or loss-of-position sense. Available data indicate that carefully selected patients are likely to get a period of good to excellent pain relief following subarachnoid neurolysis[77], which in some patients extends for 6–12 months[22]. In skilled hands, results are similar regardless of the agent (alcohol vs. phenol) used to effect neurodestruction. With appropriate patient selection and meticulous attention to technique, complication rates range between 1–14 per cent, which is acceptable to some patients. For example, if a bladder catheter is already in use, the risk of incontinence may be of no consequence, whereas a continent patient might find this risk unacceptable.

Subarachnoid neurolysis also has a limited role in palliation of intractable lower-extremity spasticity. Although most spasticity problems can be managed with systemic medications or spinal baclofen, there are individuals with extreme spasticity in whom these therapies are ineffective or unacceptable[78]. Neurolytic blockade of motor pathways to the lower extremities may produce flaccid lower-extremity paralysis, which can facilitate wheelchair mobility and nursing care and relieve spasm-related pain. This technique should be considered for control of spasticity only in non-ambulatory and incontinent individuals.

Standard spinal neurolysis techniques may be insufficient in rare, extreme cases of lower-body and/or lower-extremity pain, e.g. in bed-bound, terminally ill patients with significant nerve root or spinal cord tumour involvement. In such situations, chemical spinal cord transection at the upper-lumbar or lower-thoracic dermatomal level may be a reasonable alternative to palliative sedation or continuous spinal anaesthesia. This intervention is rarely used, but may offer high-quality relief of otherwise intractable pain and/or spasticity, in the appropriate setting[22].

Epidural neurolysis typically is considered only when pain has been refractory to subarachnoid neurolysis and other interventions, such as spinal analgesics or sympathetic neurolytic blockade, have been ineffective or are not appropriate. Epidural neurolysis is typically accomplished over a few days, with daily injections of small volumes of neurolytic solution via a temporary percutaneous catheter, so that the extent of neurolysis is titrated to the degree required[22]. While improving the accuracy of neurolysis, repeated injections over several days may be unacceptable due to delayed pain relief and/or the burden of repeated procedures. Pain relief from epidural neurolysis may not be as profound as with subarachnoid injection, and scarring of the epidural space from the neurolytic solution may preclude repeat epidural neurolysis if pain returns in the future.

Spinal analgesics: epidural and subarachnoid

Although a relatively recent development, spinal opioid administration has an established, increasingly significant role in severe pain. After the first clinical reports in 1979, spinal opioid use quickly spread to various settings of acute, non-cancer chronic, and cancer-related pain[10]. Today, spinal analgesic administration is the most commonly used interventional pain therapy for patients whose pain from advanced malignancy cannot be controlled with systemic analgesics. In this context, 'spinal' includes both epidural and subarachnoid (or intrathecal) routes of administration (Table 10.1.9.2).

Compared to systemic administration, spinal administration delivers analgesic drugs directly to the regions of the neuraxis in which cells that are relevant to nociception or pain modulation reside, in the hope of producing better analgesia and fewer adverse effects than systemic drug administration[79]. A recent RCT suggests that, compared to comprehensive medical pain management in advanced cancer, subarachnoid analgesic administration via an implantable delivery system may result in reduced pain and anxiety, and may even be associated with increased 6-month survival[80].

Morphine is, worldwide, the most frequently used spinal analgesic for chronic pain. Other opioids for spinal administration include hydromorphone, fentanyl, and sufentanil[17]. Clinical experience shows that adverse spinal opioid effects are predictable, and therefore should be anticipated and managed. When spinal opioid monotherapy no longer suffices, opioids can be combined with non-opioid analgesics, especially LAs (bupivacaine, ropivacaine) and/or clonidine, as the addition of non-opioid analgesics decreases opioid requirements (opioid-sparing effect) and enhances analgesia. A Polyanalgesic Consensus Conference, updated in 2007, formulated guidelines for spinal analgesic drug use based on expert opinion[17].

Very few analgesics have been extensively studied and approved for spinal administration. Morphine (epidural and subarachnoid), clonidine (epidural), baclofen (subarachnoid), and ziconotide (subarachnoid) are the only drugs approved for chronic spinal administration by the US Food and Drug Administration. As the approval process differs significantly among countries, practitioners in different locales must be familiar with the national approval status of each spinal analgesic.

Due to the concern about neurotoxicity[17], great caution should be used when considering analgesics not approved for spinal administration. Non-approved agents reported to have analgesic efficacy following spinal administration include midazolam, ketamine, and neostigmine[17]. In addition to concerns regarding toxicity from the analgesic agent itself, using 'non-approved' agents requires independently compounded 'custom' preparations, which are not produced with the same high standards as commercial pharmaceuticals[81]. Even with 'approved' analgesics, it should not be assumed that non-standard drug preparations, concentrations, doses, or multiple-drug combinations will be devoid of significant neurotoxicity[17].

Spinal opioid administration

Spinal administration delivers opioid close to the opioid receptors within the dorsal horns of the spinal grey matter, where opioid binding inhibits synaptic transmission between primary afferent nociceptors and second-order spinal neurons (Fig. 10.1.9.3). By their presence on both presynaptic (peripheral afferent nociceptor) and postsynaptic (second-order spinal neuron) nerve terminals, spinal opioid receptors are strategically positioned to inhibit nociceptive transmission. Studies in humans have documented that cerebrospinal fuid (CSF) opioid concentrations following spinal administration are far in excess of plasma concentrations, and the time course of analgesia correlates with CSF opioid concentration rather than with plasma concentrations[10].

Pharmacokinetic model of spinal opioids

There is considerable pharmacokinetic variation between different spinally-administered opioids, and this variation can be largely explained by differences in lipid solubility[82,10]. Following epidural administration, opioids must cross the dura, spread within the CSF, and penetrate into the spinal cord to reach spinal opioid receptors; therefore, vascular uptake and absorption reduce the quantity of drug available to opioid receptors. Morphine has favourable pharmacokinetic characteristics for chronic epidural administration, because it is hydrophilic and highly ionized. The movement of the non-ionized morphine moiety across the dura, as well as in and out of the spinal cord, is a slow process produced by small concentration gradients (Fig. 10.1.9.4). From the CSF, hydrophilic morphine moves slowly into the lipid-rich spinal cord. Morphine reaching spinal receptors has a long-lasting effect, as egress from the spinal cord is inhibited by the prolonged presence of morphine in the CSF [10]. Spinal hydromorphone is very similar to morphine with regard to CSF pharmacokinetics and efficacy.

Epidural administration of a less ionized, lipophilic opioid (e.g. fentanyl) results in more rapid drug transfer across the dura than occurs with morphine. From the CSF, lipophilic opioids pass readily into the lipid-rich spinal cord, resulting in rapid onset of analgesia. Egress from spinal receptors is enhanced by rapid systemic redistribution due to vascular uptake and by opioid binding to various tissue sites. This model explains the rapid onset, short analgesia duration, and limited cephalad migration of lipophilic opioids such as fentanyl[82].

Intrinsic efficacy, the fraction of opioid receptors that must be occupied to produce a given effect, also influences the effects produced by spinal opioids. Compared to morphine, sufentanil needs to occupy a smaller fraction of opioid receptors to produce a comparable effect. Use of such high-efficacy agonists may reduce tolerance and increase spinal analgesia potency. On this basis,

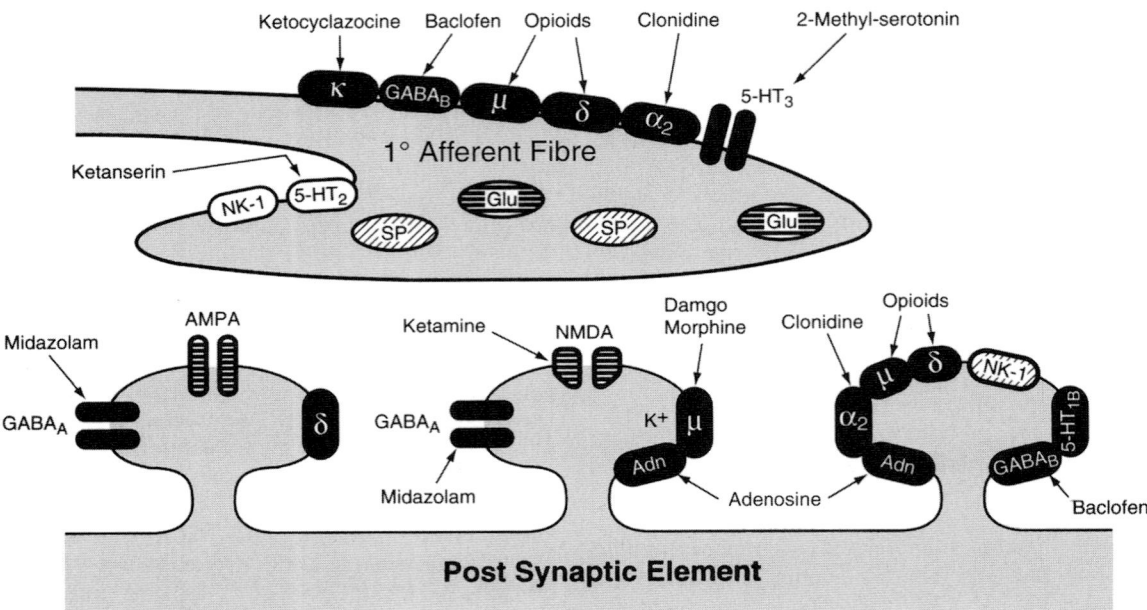

Figure 10.1.9.3 Summary of neurotransmission from primary afferent sensory fibres to second-order spinal neurons (postsynaptic element) in the spinal dorsal horns. Neurotransmitters (open circles) include the excitatory amino-acid transmitters (e.g. glutamine = Glu) and neurokinins (e.g. substance P = SP). Activation of postsynaptic, excitatory amino-acid receptors (classified by their response to *N*-methyl-D-aspartate [NMDA] and α-amino-3-hydroxy-5-methyl-4-isoxazoleproprionic acid [AMPA]), as well as neurokinin receptors (NK-1), results in depolarization of the postsynaptic membrane. Excitatory receptors (open ovals) are also located presynaptically, where activation results in enhanced transmitter release (5-HT$_2$ = excitatory serotonin receptors). Activation of inhibitory receptors (filled ovals), located both pre- and postsynaptically, decreases the release and effectiveness of transmitters (κ, μ, δ, opioid; GABA, γ-aminobutyric acid; 5-HTβ, inhibitory serotonin receptor; α$_2$, α$_2$-adrenergic; Adn = adenosine). The drugs shown affect pain transmission, at least experimentally, and are believed to be active at the sites indicated (arrows). (Reproduced with permission from Carr, D.B. and Cousins, M.J. [1998]. Spinal route of analgesia: opioids and future options. In *Neural Blockade in Clinical Anesthesia and Management of Pain* [eds. M.J. Cousins and P.O. Bridenbaugh], p. 923. 3rd Edition. J. B. Lippincott, Philadelphia.)

sufentanil may be selected as a second-choice agent when tolerance or insufficient effect limits spinal morphine analgesia[17].

Subarachnoid opioid administration avoids initial uptake by the epidural vasculature and tissue-binding sites. As a result, subarachnoid doses are generally only 10 per cent of the equianalgesic epidural doses. Compared to epidural administration, a subarachnoid bolus of morphine has a shorter time to onset of analgesia and a longer duration of effect[10].

Due to the CSF circulation, morphine migrates from the spinal level of epidural or subarachnoid injection to other spinal segments, and to supra-spinal or brain structures. This extends the level of analgesia and increases the utility of spinal morphine in chronic pain. Unless CSF circulation is blocked, (e.g. tumour, congenital malformation, or arachnoiditis), spinal morphine need not be administered at the segmental level of pain. If there is pathologythat may restrict CSF flow, consideration should be given to administering intrathecal morphine above the level of spinal canalobstruction[83].

Adverse effects of spinal opioids

Adverse effects and complications that occur during spinal opioid administration are related to spinal opioid pharmacology or the devices and techniques employed for spinal delivery (see following technical considerations). The most common adverse effects are those of opioid therapy in general[84]. Fortunately, respiratory depression, nausea and vomiting, dysphoria, urinary retention, and pruritus are not common when spinal opioids are used in palliative

care, because these patients usually have developed tolerance to opioid adverse effects through prior systemic opioid administration. In this setting, adverse effects usually are self-limiting or can be successfully managed by opioid dose adjustment. Constipation is a problem, which should be anticipated and managed with laxative therapy.

Cephalad morphine migration within the CSF may explain the delayed respiratory depression (onset 3–20 h) reported in opioid-naive acute pain patients following spinal morphine administration[10]. Clinically significant respiratory depression from spinal opioid is particularly rare in patients who have previously received chronic systemic opioid therapy. If respiratory depression or other serious opioid toxicity occurs, small naloxone doses may be used to reverse the effects, often without reducing analgesia. In this setting, naloxone is best administered initially as an intravenous loading dose, given in 40-mcg increments, followed by intravenous infusion (approximately 1–5 mcg/kg·h) titrated to effect.

Endocrine abnormalities, sweating, and peripheral oedema are adverse effects associated with both systemic and spinal chronic opioid therapy. In one study of spinal opioid for non-malignant pain[84], most male and all female patients developed hypogonadotropic hypogonadism, and other endocrine abnormalities were also common. Peripheral oedema associated with chronic spinal opioid, related to opioid anti-diuretic effect, is usually manageable with diuretics.

As with systemic opioid[13], very high spinal opioid doses may cause myoclonus and hyperalgesia[14]. Allodynia has also been

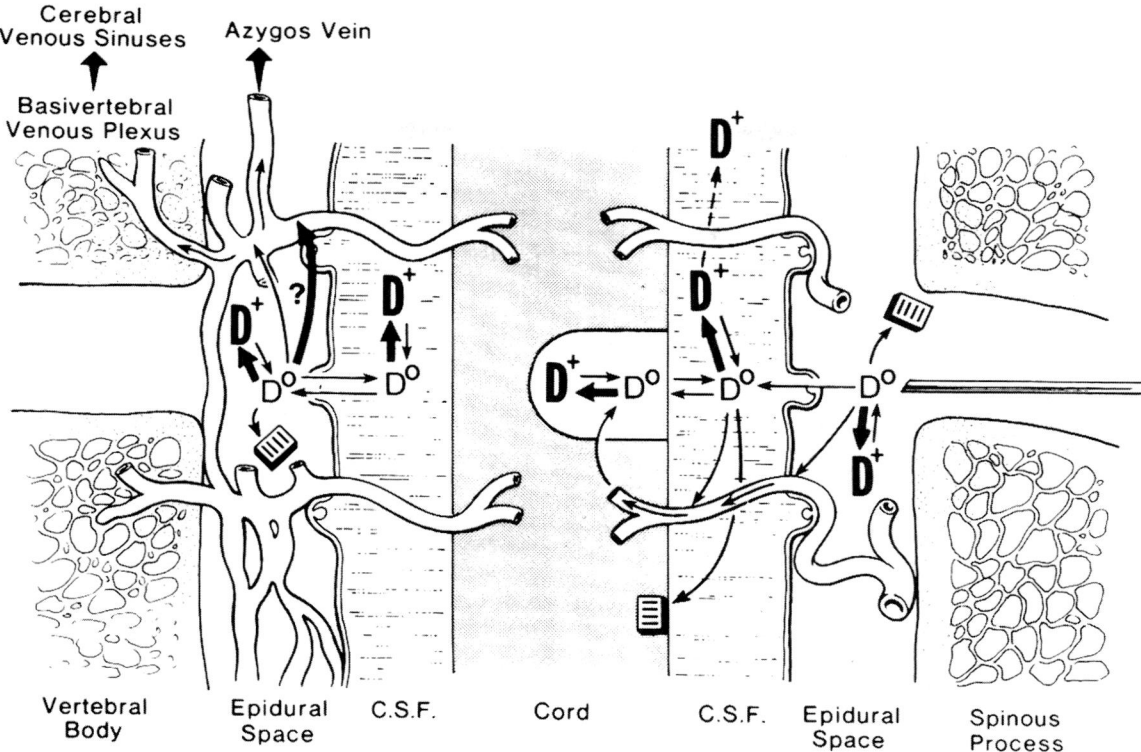

Figure 10.1.9.4 Pharmacokinetic model of spinal opioid administration. An epidural needle (right) is shown delivering a hydrophilic opioid, such as morphine, to the epidural space. Within the epidural space, CSF, and spinal cord equilibria of D^0 (non-ionized moiety of drug) and D^+ (ionized, hydrophilic moiety) are shown. Nonspecific lipid-binding sites are indicated by the shaded squares. The role of spinal arteries, in proximity to arachnoid granulations, in drug delivery is speculative. Epidural veins are the major point of clearance of epidural drugs. (Reproduced with permission from Carr, D.B. and Cousins, M.J. [1998]. Spinal route of analgesia: opioids and future options. In *Neural Blockade in Clinical Anesthesia and Management of Pain* [eds. M.J. Cousins and P.O. Bridenbaugh], p. 943. 3rd Edition. J. B. Lippincott, Philadelphia.)

described after subarachnoid administration of low morphine doses in a patient with neuropathic pain from spinal cord injury[85]. Opioid-induced hyperalgesia should be suspected when individuals on high-dose opioid (e.g. subarachnoid morphine greater than 20 mg per day) develop generalized hyperalgesia, especially if associated with myoclonus[86]. Opioid toxicity may be managed with opioid rotation, dose reduction, or addition of non-opioid spinal analgesics.

If systemic opioid is suddenly discontinued when subarachnoid administration begins, patients may experience opioid withdrawal. Similarly, withdrawal symptoms also may develop if chronic epidural opioid is replaced with subarachnoid opioid, typically at 10 per cent of the epidural dose. Withdrawal symptoms in these settings are readily managed with tapering doses of systemic opioid, whilecontinuing to control pain with spinal opioid.

Non-opioid spinal analgesics

Local anaesthetics

When spinal opioids do not provide adequate analgesia, addition of spinal LA may be indicated[17,87]. In addition to the direct analgesic effect produced by LA spinal conduction blockade, decreasing the nociceptive input to the spinal dorsal horns may decrease spinal sensitization, and the ability to subsequently reduce the opioid dose may limit the development of tolerance [88]. Bupivacaine is the most commonly used LA for long-term spinal administration.

Chronic spinal lignocaine (lidocaine) and tetracaine are increasingly avoided due to concern for neurotoxicity.

Low-dose epidural LA administration[10,17] can generally achieve good pain relief without significant motor or sensory impairment. Analgesia without loss of sensory or motor function may be more readily obtained with epidural than with subarachnoid LA use, and is one of the main advantages of the epidural route. Subarachnoid LA may also provide good analgesic effects without significant sensory or motor block, if doses are low (less than 20–30 mg bupivacaine per day) and carefully adjusted. Long-term subarachnoid LA, alone or with spinal opioid, can successfully control intractable pain in a variety of settings[17,89,90]. In extreme cases, when pain is intractable and the patient is non-ambulatory and has advanced illness, continuous spinal anaesthesia with dense sensory and motor block from intentional infusion of high subarachnoid LA doses (greater than 2 mg per h bupivacaine) may be acceptable[91].

Clonidine

Clonidine is well accepted as a second-line spinal analgesic[17], with efficacy demonstrated in RCTs of cancer and spinal cord injury pain[83]. Epidural clonidine is approved by the US Food and Drug Administration for cancer pain. Clonidine analgesia appears to be mediated by the inhibitory effects of α_2-adrenergic receptors on spinal nociceptive transmission (Fig. 10.1.9.3). Adverse effects, including hypotension, bradycardia, and sedation, are dose-related and generally manageable. Given its apparent safety and efficacy, spinal clonidine is likely to remain an important spinal analgesic, often combined with opioid and/or local anaesthetic, especially in neuropathic pain. However, a recent report of spinal cord injury, after 3 years of uneventful subarachnoid clonidine-bupivacaine administration, raises concern about possible toxicity[92].

Subarachnoid baclofen

Baclofen binds to presynaptic $GABA_B$ receptors on afferent neurons and inhibits release of excitatory neurotransmitters, which in turn, inhibits spinal motor reflexes and reduces spasticity from upper-motor neuron lesions. Oral baclofen usually is more effective and better tolerated that other spasticity agents (benzodiazepines, dantrolene, tizanidine), but sedation and other adverse effects may limit tolerance (especially at doses greater than 60 mg daily). Subarachnoid baclofen may be useful for severe spasticity in patients unresponsive to, or intolerant of, oral baclofen[93]. Subarachnoid baclofen results in significantly higher CSF concentrations compared to oral administration, even though subarachnoid doses are 100 to 1000 times lower. It is well tolerated and no significant neurotoxicity has been identified. Baclofen can be analgesic when musculoskeletal pain is related to spasticity, and also may be a useful second-line spinal analgesic for CRPS or other types of neuropathic pain[17]. Chronic subarachnoid baclofen administration is achieved with a fully implanted infusion pump identical to those used for subarachnoid opioid.

The effectiveness of subarachnoid baclofen is evaluated with a test dose before spinal pump implantation. Finding the appropriate test dose is critical: too little drug could lead to erroneous conclusion of ineffectiveness, while excess can cause generalized muscle weakness or hypotonia. Accidental overdose may result in respiratory arrest through generalized weakness and/or CNS depression. With appropriate support, however, no long-term complications have been reported.

Ziconotide

Ziconotide, the synthetic analog of the omega-conotoxin derived from the marine snail *Conus magus*, has analgesic effect through blockade of N-type calcium channels in the superficial dorsal horn of the spinal cord. Subarachnoid ziconotide is a potent analgesic and is approved for chronic severe pain; it is typically considered for patients who cannot tolerate or do not respond to systemic analgesics, adjunctive therapies, or subarachnoid morphine. The safety and analgesic efficacy of subarachnoid ziconotide has been demonstrated in large case series and placebo-controlled RCTs[94–96]. Dosing starts from ≤2.4 mcg/day and is slowly titrated to a maximum of 21.6 mcg/day, with an average dose of 7 mcg/day[95]. Ziconotide has a narrow therapeutic window, and neuropsychiatric adverse events, including depression, cognitive impairment, hallucinations, and depressed level of consciousness have been described[97]. In addition, it has also been associated with creatine kinase level elevation and meningitis (perhaps due to microinfusion device contamination). When initiating ziconotide therapy, inadequate pain control and adverse effects can limit patient acceptance; therefore, slow ziconotide titration and avoidance of opioid withdrawal are necessary to achieve analgesia without excessive adverse effects[17].

Other spinal analgesics: ketamine and midazolam

NMDA receptor-linked calcium channels (Fig. 10.1.9.3) appear to play a significant role in spinal neural transmission and

sensitization[8], and ketamine (along with other experimental NMDA-receptor antagonists) is a potent analgesic in settings of hyperalgesia. Spinal ketamine has analgesic efficacy[17], especially as a co-analgesic with opioid, but concerns about psychotropic adverse effects and neurotoxicity limit its use. Although not a consistent finding, spinal neuron vacuolization has been identified followingsubarachnoid preservative-free ketamine in animals[98], andneuron vacuolization with marked neurological deficit has been described in a clinical case[99]. Other reports describe the addition of ketamine to spinal opioid resulting in improved pain control without neurological deficit [100]. In selected patients with advanced illness, the risk of ketamine spinal neurotoxicity may be acceptable in return for control of intractable pain; however, the paucity of published, clinically evident neurologic deficit should not beinterpreted as proof that subarachnoid ketamine is withoutsignificant neurotoxicity.

γ-Aminobutyric acid (GABA) is a neurotransmitter that inhibits synaptic transmission in the spinal dorsal horn through activation of inhibitory GABA receptors (Fig. 10.1.9.3). Similar to other benzodiazepines, midazolam inhibits neuronal transmission by enhancing GABA effect at (inhibitory) $GABA_A$ receptors. Animal studies demonstrate analgesic efficacy of spinal midazolam but some animal models suggest neurotoxicity[101]. Several clinical trials demonstrate improved control of acute obstetrical and postoperative pain when midazolam is added to spinal anaesthetic agents[101] and epidural analgesia[102], but there is little safety or efficacy data on long-term spinal midazolam administration. Because of concerns about neurotoxicity[17,98], the role of spinal midazolam is under debate[101,103]. Recent data from animals [104], and humans[105], including one case report of subarachnoid midazolam administration for over 5 years[106], provide some reassurance that subarachnoid midazolam may not be as neurotoxic as initially feared. Similar to ketamine, the unresolved questions about spinal midazolam neurotoxicity suggest that this agent should be considered as a therapeutic option only in the setting of intractable pain related to advanced illness.

Indications for spinal analgesics in palliative care

The nature of the underlying diseases and the character of pain are important factors when considering spinal analgesic therapy. Limited life expectancy is a factor in selecting among spinal administration systems, but should not deter consideration of spinal analgesia. Spinal opioids work best for deep, constant somatic pain, but other types of pain (cutaneous, intermittent somatic [pathologic fracture], intermittent visceral [intestinal obstruction], and coexistent cancer and non-cancer pain) are variably responsive. In the past, it was felt that neuropathic, central, or deafferentation pains were not responsive to opioid therapy, so that patients with such pain were not offered spinal opioids. It is now evident that spinal opioid has some efficacy in these settings, but neuropathic pain that is not adequately controlled with spinal opioid is an indication for trial of non-opioid spinal analgesics (e.g. ziconotide, clonidine, local anaesthetic, or baclofen). Patients with extreme opioid tolerance are unlikely to have good pain control with spinal opioid alone, and will likely require non-opioid spinal analgesic co-administration. If the benefit of spinal analgesics is uncertain, a spinal analgesic trial through a temporary catheter is recommended before permanent spinal delivery system implantation.

Ongoing chemotherapy or radiation therapy is not a contraindication to initiation of spinal analgesic therapy. Adequate analgesia, perhaps with spinal medications, may help patients with intractable pain tolerate needed anti-tumour therapies. Radiation therapy may interfere with surgical wound healing in or near irradiated areas; therefore, it is advisable to avoid spinal analgesic system (epidural ports, spinal infusion pumps) implantation around the time of radiation therapy, if radiation portals would include surgical sites. Instead, simple percutaneous spinal catheters may be used if spinal analgesics and radiation therapy need to be initiated simultaneously. With appropriate sterile technique, percutaneous spinal catheters have been utilized for prolonged periods[87,89,90,107].

Although the use of spinal analgesics in the palliative care setting has largely occurred in the population with cancer pain, numerous other types of intractable pain have been targets for this approach [108,109]. Among the syndromes that have been treated are severe, inoperable peripheral vascular disease with ischaemic rest pain or intractable myocardial ischaemic pain[90,110]; pain due to vertebral compression fractures (not suitable for vertebroplasty or kyphoplasty) or stress rib fractures; neuropathic pain due to spinal cord injury[83] or postherpetic neuralgia[111], and other chronic pain conditions such as nonoperable spinal stenosis, other types of chronic back and neck pain, and other neuropathic pains.

Contraindications to spinal therapy are similar to those for any regional anaesthetic technique, with a few additional concerns related to the spinal analgesic itself. Bleeding diathesis increases the risk of spinal haematoma and neurologic deficit from spinal cord or nerve root compression. The increasing use of anticoagulants, including warfarin and newer anti-platelet agents in cardiovascular disease, is posing an additional set of problems when spinal analgesia is considered. It is clear that anticoagulation therapy should be modified or withheld before implementing spinal analgesic techniques, but recommendations vary depending on the specific agent and the indication for its use. The consensus statement on Neuraxial Anesthesia and Anticoagulation[112] by the American Society of Regional Anesthesia is a useful guide in dealing with questions about anticoagulation and interventional pain therapies.

Septicaemia is another important contraindication to spinal analgesia, due to the risk of spinal delivery system infection. Local, cutaneous infection is a contraindication if a site free of infection cannot be found for spinal catheter system implantation. Although the risk of infection may be higher in immunosuppressed patients, immunosuppression is only a relative contraindication and must be evaluated in each patient.

The presence of epidural or spinal metastasis deserves special consideration. Spinal metastasis might be considered a contraindication for spinal anaesthetic or analgesic techniques, yet patients with such lesions may have severe pain and therefore benefit from spinal analgesia. The concern is that trauma to a friable tumour mass during catheterization could result in haemorrhage, spinal haematoma, and neural compression. Severe spinal stenosis, including stenosis caused by tumour invasion, also increases the risk of neural injury from needle or catheter placement into the spinal canal. To avoid such trauma, catheters should be inserted away from spinal metastases, under fluoroscopy. Furthermore, the potential for interruption of CSF circulation, by an expanding tumour should encourage catheters placement cephalad to known (or suspected) epidural or spinal metastases.

Although spinal analgesics are potent, it is not realistic to expect elimination of pain. Patients considered for spinal analgesic therapies generally have severe pain problems, which were previously resistant to systemic analgesics. Case series of patients with cancer[89] and non-cancer pain[113,114] indicate that 50–87 per cent of carefully selected patients receive significant relief from spinal analgesic therapy.

Technical considerations and complications in spinal drug administration

Various technical considerations are important for successful long-term spinal analgesia. Dependable catheter access to the subarachnoid or epidural space is required: the catheter may be a simple, percutaneous catheter for intermittent injection or part of a totally implanted, computer-controlled infusion pump system[10]. No single system is appropriate for all cases, and any system can result in complications such as infection, catheter dislodgement, or other technical failure[115]. Before initiating long-term spinal analgesia, it is essential to ensure the availability of necessary nursing and social support to assist with maintenance of the spinal analgesic system.

'Low tech' versus 'high tech' spinal implant therapies

Spinal implant therapies generally involve one of two types of systems: low-cost, low tech, versus high-cost, high-tech. Low-cost systems, consisting of percutaneous catheters, perhaps combined with an external infusion pump, can be used for epidural or subarachnoid analgesic administration, whereas high-cost, high-tech systems consist of completely implantable electronic programmable infusion systems suitable only for subarachnoid administration.

'High-tech' spinal administration systems have a long battery life, need refills at regular intervals, and with good care and aseptic technique, can last for years. Because of the high costs involved with the purchase and implantation of the pump, these systems are generally reserved for patients with life expectancy of at least a few months. An important limitation of implanted pumps is the small medication-reservoir volume (18–50 ml), which makes use of commercial bupivacaine and/or clonidine preparations difficult and may necessitate use of custom-compounded solutions. Use of non-standard solutions is a potential source of neurotoxic contaminants or infection, but is done with increasing frequency worldwide[17].

In contrast, 'low tech' spinal infusion systems cost significantly less, and usually consist of an implanted epidural or subarachnoid catheter connected to an implanted or externalized injection port. Spinal analgesics are then administered by intermittent injection or external pump. Infection, the principal concern regarding these systems, is a serious complication, because it can cause meningitis, epidural abscess, or encephalitis[115,116]. Although the risk of infection is real, it should not preclude low-tech system use. Experience has shown that with aseptic technique during placement, followed by careful maintenance and medication administration, these systems can provide significant relief in cancer (and even in carefully selected chronic non-cancer) pain patients for weeks to months, with a low risk of infection.

A percutaneous epidural catheter, as may be used for epidural anaesthesia or analgesia, is the simplest means of providing long-term analgesia. Epidural catheters are widely available, inexpensive, and may be used for days to weeks. However, even with careful technique, these devices carry a risk of epidural infection and abscess. For longer-term use, an implanted epidural catheter (epidural Port-A-Cath®, Deltec; Du Pen® catheters, Bard) is preferred; these devices are less likely to become dislodged and may have a lower infection rate[107,117]. The routine use of bacterial filters (0.2 micron) may help decrease the risk of infection[107], but epidural abscess remains a concern even when bacterial filters are used[116].

The efficacy of epidural analgesia during long-term therapy may be limited by epidural fibrosis, i.e. formation of scar tissue around the catheter within the epidural space[118]. Epidural fibrosis is a variable process, may develop as early as two weeks after epidural catheter placement, and limits analgesic solution spread. The result may be pain on injection and/or loss of analgesic effect. Management of epidural fibrosis requires repositioning the epidural catheter or replacing it with a subarachnoid catheter.

In recent years, percutaneous subarachnoid catheters have been used increasingly in the palliative care of terminally ill persons. The concern of infection and meningitis appears to be reasonably managed by the use of bacterial filters (0.2 micron) and a sterile technique that strictly minimizes the changing of external infusion pump reservoirs and tubing[87,107,115]. Advantages of subarachnoid analgesia are its efficiency and potency, which may translate into improved pain control with lower drug cost.

Regardless of the spinal system used, adequate skilled nursing assistance and/or physician evaluation is essential. After implantation, implanted infusion pumps only require refill every few weeks, but refills require physician or skilled nursing personnel. Percutaneous catheters or implanted injection port systems, with or without external infusion pumps, may be managed by some patients and/or family members, but still require periodic nursing support. It is possible to initiate and maintain percutaneous subarachnoid analgesia at home for terminally ill, homebound patients[89], if physician home visits can be arranged. In general, follow-up for spinalanalgesic systems can be accomplished through office evaluations, home visits, or institutionalization, depending on other patient care needs[115].

Infections of spinal catheter systems are among the most concerning problems associated with long-term spinal analgesia (Table 10.1.9.3)[87,107,115,119]. As a rule, an infected spinal analgesic administration system must be removed to prevent infection spread to CNS structures. In end-of-life care, however, an attempt to contain the infection with antibiotics is reasonable in an effort to avoid removal of the spinal administration system and continue spinal analgesia.

Infections are usually superficial, localized to skin at the catheter insertion or implantation site. Cultures of any drainage, followed by antibiotics, are necessary[107,115]. Epidural abscess and meningitis are rare, but must be treated aggressively because they may cause permanent neurological deficit or death. Epidural systems should be removed as part of epidural abscess management, yet the catheter may temporarily serve as an epidural space drainage conduit[107]. Antibiotics may also be delivered via the epidural catheter[107], but if infection does not rapidly improve, the catheter should still be removed. Meningitis associated with subarachnoid catheter systems should be treated with intravenous antibiotics, but treatment may also include antibiotics delivered via the subarachnoid system (only antibiotics suitable for subarachnoid administration, such as vancomycin, should be administered through the spinal catheter). If the infection does not rapidly clear with antibiotics, the subarachnoid catheter system should be removed[115].

Spinal catheter system malfunction can cause deterioration of previously satisfactory analgesia (Table 10.1.9.3) or opioid withdrawal symptoms. As long-term use of spinal delivery systems increases, complications and technical failures related to spinal delivery systems will likely increase, and physicians caring for patients receiving spinal analgesia must be aware of such problems to provide prompt intervention. Loss of analgesia may be abrupt (e.g. infusion pump malfunction) or gradual (e.g. epidural fibrosis), perhaps making it difficult to distinguish between system malfunction and disease progression. In such cases, infusion device function must be evaluated: epidurography or myelography (only with appropriate myelographic contrast) may be used to verify spinal catheter location and patency, and plain radiographs may be used to confirm structural integrity of the spinal system. Compared to the risk of scar tissue formation around chronic epidural catheters (epidural fibrosis), the risk of scarring around subarachnoid catheters is small; however, subarachnoid catheter systems are associated with various technical problems, including catheter migration and formation of catheter-tip granulomas.

Subarachnoid catheter catheter-tip granulomas are thought to develop slowly over several weeks, and can present with loss of pain control or neurological symptoms or signs related to spinal cord or nerve root compression. The vast majority of reported analgesic catheter-tip granulomas have been described following spinal administration of opioid[119]. These granulomas are thought to be related to concentrated opioid from the subarachnoid catheter activating opioid receptors on inflammatory cells[120]. Recently, a catheter-tip mass on CT-myelogram (similar in appearance to previously reported catheter-tip granulomas) has been reported after baclofen administration without opioid[121], suggesting that etiologic factors in addition to opioid receptor activation may contribute to catheter-tip granuloma formation.

Consideration should be given to evaluating for catheter-tip granuloma when a patient reports worsening pain control or new onset of sensory or motor abnormalities. Few patients eventually found to have a catheter-tip granuloma actually present with new back or radicular pain, but many experience loss of spinal analgesic efficacy before neurologic deficit becomes evident. With careful follow-up, patients with catheter-tip granulomas are often identified while sensory or motor symptoms are still modest. Spine MRI is the preferred imaging technique[122] (patients with implanted-spinal pumps can undergo MRI), but CT myelography is a good alternative. Surgical granuloma resection is only indicated if significant neurologic deficit is present. In other cases, discontinuation of the spinal analgesics without surgical intervention is often associated with resolution of the granuloma. Careful monitoring is required over subsequent days to weeks to ensure ongoing improvement. The apparently low incidence of catheter-tip granulomas should not discourage use of necessary spinal analgesic palliative therapies, but should encourage careful follow-up, so that necessary interventions can be undertaken promptly.

Management of pain when spinal analgesia systems malfunction may be difficult because inadequate analgesia from systemic medications is the most common indication for starting spinal analgesics

Table 10.1.9.3 Evaluation and management of spinal catheter complications.

Catheter system	Symptoms	Complication	Prevention	Evaluation	Management
Epidural	Back pain Paraesthesias on injection Loss of analgesic effect No signs of infection	Epidural fibrosis[118]	Unknown	Epidurography	Replace epidural or insert subarachnoid catheter
	Back and extremity pain Weakness Sensory abnormalities Fever, leucocytosis	Epidural infection or abscess[107]	Sterile technique, bacterial filters[107]	Catheter aspirate for Gram stain, culture; Spine MRI	Catheter aspiration for decompression Intravenous antibiotics Remove catheter
Epidural or Subarachnoid	Loss of analgesic effect Opioid withdrawal	Catheter dislodgement or disconnection	Implanted rather than percutaneous system Subarachnoid catheter anchored to fascia	Plain radiographs with contrast injection via catheter	Revise or replace catheter
		Pump malfunction	Pump maintenance Utilize low volume and low battery alarm	Pump analysis Technical support from manufacturer	Revise or replace pump
	Erythema, tenderness at catheter insertion point or incision site	Infection at catheter insertion site	Sterile technique Catheter care	Culture: catheter exit site catheter aspirate	Antibiotics Local site care Remove catheter system if no rapid improvement
Subarachnoid	Meningeal irritation: Severe headache Cervical stiffness Photophobia, fever	Meningitis	Sterile technique[87] Bacterial filters for pump refill or on percutaneous catheters	Catheter aspirate (CSF) for cell count, gram stain, glucose, culture	Systemic (and possibly subarachnoid) antibiotics Remove catheter system if no rapid improvement
	Spinal cord compression: Paraesthesias Weakness	Subarachnoid granuloma[122]	Unknown Avoid excessive doses, concentrations of spinal opioid	Spine imaging: CT myelogram or MRI	Discontinue spinal analgesics Surgical consultation if significant sensory or motor deficits present

in the first place. Nonetheless, such patients will require systemic analgesics to relieve pain and prevent opioid withdrawal. If an epidural catheter has malfunctioned due to epidural fibrosis, the patient's pain can likely be adequately managed with systemic opioids at a similar dose, because epidural fibrosis would have prevented spinal absorption, and the medication would have provided analgesic effect through systemic absorption anyway. On the other hand, if the epidural system were functioning well and opioids were efficiently delivered to spinal receptors, equal doses of systemic opioid will likely not suffice for pain control, but should at least prevent opioid withdrawal.

Effective subarachnoid morphine doses are approximately 10 per cent of epidural doses, and as low as 1 per cent of systemic (parenteral) doses, but these estimations are just starting points for analgesic titration, and must be used cautiously in order to prevent significant under or over-dosing (Table 10.1.9.4). If spinal local anaesthetic had been previously added due to lack of efficacy of spinal opioid alone, it is unlikely that systemic opioids will provide adequate analgesia should the spinal delivery system fail. Additional interventional pain management techniques may be necessary if the spinal system cannot be repaired. An intravenous or subcutaneous infusion of a non-opioid analgesic, such as lignocaine (lidocaine), 50–100 mg/h, or ketamine 10–20 mg/h, may temporarily control intractable pain unresponsive to opioids[15]. If systemic ketamine is utilized, a benzodiazepine also should be administered to control possible dysphoric hallucinations.

Intracerebroventricular opioid administration

Catheter techniques similar to those for spinal opioid administration also are used for opioid administration directly into the cerebral ventricles. Data suggest that intracerebroventricular opioid is a reasonable option for intractable pain (usually cancer-related) in the following settings:

- inadequate analgesia through conventional techniques;
- inaccessible spinal epidural and subarachnoid spaces;
- known obstruction of spinal CSF circulation;
- intractable head and neck pain.

A recent Cochrane review[123] based on case series, concluded that intracerebroventricular opioid may have similar efficacy with

Table 10.1.9.4 Equivalent morphine dose by administration route.

Administration route	Morphine dose approximate (mg)	Dosing interval (h)
Oral	300	4
Intravenous	100	4
Epidural	10	6–8
Subarachnoid	1	12–24

Note: Doses are approximate and must be applied to individual patients with caution. These ratios do not apply to other opioids. Conversion factors used to estimate equipotent doses for systemic administration of opioids should not be used to predict equipotency of opioid doses for spinal administration due to variations in spinal pharmacokinetics.

a lower incidence of complications compared to spinal analgesics, but no comparative studies are available.

Miscellaneous techniques for pain control

Vertebroplasty and kyphoplasty

Vertebral compression fracture (VCF) remains an important source of pain and morbidity. VCFs are most commonly related to osteoporosis in postmenopausal women, but also may be caused by spinal neoplasm, including metastatic cancers and multiple myeloma. Percutaneous vertebroplasty (PV) and kyphoplasty (PK) are similar image-guided, minimally invasive procedures in which a compressed vertebra is stabilized by injection of polymethylmethacrylate bone cement into the vertebral body via large bore needles[124,125]. Both PV and PK are effective and provide good to excellent pain relief to 80–90 per cent of persons with painful VCF due to osteoporosis, and 50–60 per cent of those with painful neoplastic VCF.

In PV, bone cement is injected through needles into the interstices of the vertebral body marrow space. PK is similar to PV, but with the addition of steps to include temporary placement of a high-pressure balloon into the vertebral body. Inflation of the PK balloon creates a cavity within the vertebral body which is subsequently filled with bone cement. The PK balloon expansion may partially restore vertebral height, but the degree of height restoration may be modest and is of unclear clinical significance. There are no comparative studies between PV and PK[124].

Serious complications related to PV or PK are rare, but can be devastating[126]. Bone cement can extrude outside the vertebral body into the spinal canal, resulting in serious neural compromise. Furthermore, venous cement embolism can result in symptomatic pulmonary embolism or even cardiovascular collapse[125]. Because the risk of serious adverse effects is low, and the likelihood of providing good to excellent pain relief is reasonably high, PV and PK are good options for management of painful VCFs.

PV or PK planning requires neuraxial imaging (MRI or CT scan) to evaluate VCF anatomy, with attention to possible extension of bone fragments or tumour into the spinal canal. PV and PK are more likely to provide pain relief when used for acute VCFs. MRI is the most useful imaging modality for detecting acute VCFs, because vertebral marrow oedema (indicating acute fracture) is readily identified. Bone scan is less useful because it will identify increased activity in VCF for up to 2 years, long after the fracture may have

spontaneously stabilized. Neither PV nor PK need delay treatment of spinal metastases with radiation therapy, but instead may provide rapid onset of pain relief, which may improve patient tolerance of needed antitumour therapies.

Spinal cord stimulation

Spinal cord stimulation (SCS) involves placing stimulating electrode arrays in the epidural space overlying the posterior aspect of the spinal cord, at a spinal level corresponding to the site of pain (e.g. T_8–T_{10} vertebral level for lower-lumbar pain). Stimulation paraesthesias from SCS are delivered to the area of pain and are generally perceived as warm, soothing sensations associated with significant pain relief. Electrical current is provided by an implanted battery-powered pulse generator, or an external pulse generator electromagnetically linked to the implanted stimulating electrodes[127]. Most SCS currently implanted are powered by an internal, battery-powered pulse generator that is periodically recharged transcutaneously, with an electromagnetically-linked external recharging device.

SCS is thought to provide pain relief by interrupting nociceptive afferents through activation of CNS endogenous inhibitory systems, but the analgesic mechanism of SCS has not been fully elucidated[128]. SCS is most effective for moderate to moderately severe neuropathic pain limited to a single body region, especially the extremities. Most often used for low-back and radiating lower-extremity pain (especially post-lumbar laminectomy syndrome), SCS also has been widely used for intractable angina[129] and ischaemic pain from inoperable peripheral vascular disease[130]. Clinical data[127,131] also support SCS use in CRPS, peripheral neuropathic pain (e.g. diabetic or chemotherapy-induced neuropathy), and abdominal visceral pain[132]. Diffuse and/or sharp somatic pain (e.g. wound pain or arthritis pain) often do not respond to SCS.

The main drawbacks to SCS include high cost (US$15 000–25 000) and difficulty in predicting which patient will gain lasting benefits. Because only 20–80 per cent of patients treated with SCS experience long-term pain control[131], permanent SCS implantation is preceded by a temporary SCS trial to help predict its benefit. (In the authors' experience, 80 per cent of SCS trials in which patients have successful pain control are followed by long-term pain control from implanted SCS.) Analgesic failures may be due to technical difficulties, placebo response during initial trial, development of tolerance to SCS, or progression of underlying pathology. Despite its high cost, SCS may be cost-effective in cases where resultant pain control reduces need for other health care services[129,133].

SCS has an important role in palliation of inoperable ischaemic peripheral vascular disease (PVD), with improvements attributed to enhanced microvascular blood flow[130]. An RCT in inoperable PVD indicates that SCS is associated with improved pain control and reduced risk for major amputation [130]. Case reports also describe pain and ischaemia improvement in patients with severe ischaemia and threatened digit loss due to intractable Raynaud's disease[134] or thromboangiitis obliterans (Buerger's disease)[135]. Although clinical reports suggest that SCS is a promising treatment option, there are no studies comparing SCS with neurolytic lumbar sympathetic block in inoperable lower-extremity ischaemic PVD. SCS electrodes can also be implanted next to peripheral nerves. Peripheral nerve stimulation has been anecdotally reported to be valuable in treatment of neuropathic post-surgical pain and occipital neuralgia.

The management of intractable pain: when all else fails

Despite recent palliative care advances, a few patients still experience distressing end-of-life symptoms, which cannot be adequately controlled even with optimized standard therapies. For example, pain from a pathologic fracture may be so intense that no amount of opioid, by any route of administration, can provide relief. Instead, surgical fracture stabilization (if feasible) is the method of choice; otherwise, anaesthetic or neurodestructive techniques likely will be required. Therefore, a few palliative care patients will need 'anaesthetic,' rather than 'analgesic' interventions for symptom control, in the same way that a patient undergoing surgery requires 'anaesthesia,' rather than simple 'analgesia.' Such 'anaesthetic' interventions include spinal (epidural or subarachnoid) anaesthesia, peripheral neural blockade, or deep palliative sedation. Spinal or regional anaesthesia should be considered when localized pain is so intense that it can no longer be adequately controlled with analgesic techniques[91], whereas palliative sedation should be considered for patients with diffuse, intractable pain or other intractable symptoms[136].

Before initiating palliative sedation, it is important to distinguish symptoms merely difficult to control from symptoms truly refractory to standard palliative interventions (including interventional pain therapies). This distinction will protect patients with refractory symptoms from unnecessary, futile interventions, and also avoid unnecessary sedation in patients with difficult but controllable symptoms[137]. Obtaining 'second opinion' consultation, perhaps from a pain specialist or multi-disciplinary palliative care team, may help determine if effective symptom management therapies are yet available.

Recent advances and future direction

The need for improved pain management techniques is clear: uncontrolled pain is a maleficent force with significant adverse effects, and sometimes 'pain can kill'[138]. At the same time, opioids, the mainstay of analgesic therapy, are imperfect drugs with significant adverse effects. Pain may be resistant to treatment due to neuronal sensitization from tissue injury/inflammation, nerve injury, and/or opioid tolerance; there is a potential for opioid-induced hyperalgesia. Fortunately, extensive research in recent years has yielded new insight into pain pathophysiology and identified new targets for analgesic therapies. Recent advances suggest that neurotrophins and sodium channels on sensory neurons may be useful targets to block hyperalgesia associated with injury, inflammation, and/or neuropathic pain. Improved neural blockade techniques, including pulsed radiofrequency treatment, are under investigation in an effort to identify therapies with improved risk–benefit profiles. For the sake of persons with uncontrolled pain, progress in such research is urgently needed to identify new analgesic therapies.

Nerve growth factor (NGF) and other neurotrophins are potential targets for analgesic therapies. Originally identified as an essential factor for normal growth and survival of peripheral neurons in the developing nervous system, it is now apparent that NGF plays a major role in pain signal facilitation in tissue injury and neuropathic pain. Techniques to reduce peripheral tissue NGF levels, with anti-NGF monoclonal antibody, for example, have proven effective in reducing pain behaviour in animal models of inflammatory pain, and clinical studies of these types of compounds are underway[139]. In addition to peripheral effects, neurotrophins are now recognized to have a role in CNS pain signal regulation. Spinal or regional administration of agents to limit neurogenic facilitation of pain signal transmission could be potent analgesic treatments.

Other research has identified that CNS microglia significantly contribute to allodynia, hyperalgesia, and opioid tolerance[140], in addition to neuronal mechanisms of sensitization. Because current analgesic therapies exclusively target neuronal components of pain, development of neuraxial analgesic therapies targeting microglia could dramatically alter clinical pain management.

Because sodium channels play a central role in propagation of neuronal action potentials, sodium channel blockers could be potential analgesics. Local anaesthetics are non-selective sodium channel blockers, acting on both sensory and motor neurons. Several different voltage-gated sodium channels have been identified in mammals, but a small subset known as $Na_v1.8$ channels are present only in sensory neurons. A large majority of $Na_v1.8$ channels are present on nociceptors and data implicate $Na_v1.8$ channels as significant in tissue-injury and neuropathic pain[20]. A search to identify a sensory neuron-specific sodium channel blocker successfully identified μO-conotoxin MrVIB, which selectively blocks $Na_v1.8$ sodium channels [141]. Testing in animal neuropathic and inflammatory pain models suggests that subarachnoid MrVIB administration has analgesic effect without significant effect on motor neurons. Although more research is needed to determine if MrVIB or a similar conotoxin is an effective clinical analgesic, the identification of a selective $Na_v1.8$ blocker highlights the potential analgesic utility of therapies focused on nociceptor-specifictargets.

Peripheral nerve destruction to control pain is often avoided because resultant nerve injury may lead to more severe neuropathic pain. Notable exceptions include the use of thermal RF ablation for trigeminal neuralgia, or for neck or back pain due to facet arthropathy[142]. Efforts to expand the utility of RF techniques, while avoiding neural injury, led to development of pulsed RF treatments. In this approach, brief RF energy pulses are applied to neural structures. Pulsed RF does not create heat lesions, and may provide pain relief without neurolysis. Case series show analgesic effect following pulsed RF to peripheral nerves[143] and spinal dorsal root ganglia[144]. Pulsed RF often yields modest and temporary results, and there is concern that reported benefits may represent placebo effect[142,145]. Recently, an RCT in a small and highly selected patient group suggested that cervical dorsal root ganglion pulsed RF may have efficacy in chronic cervical radiculitis[146]. Although further evaluation of pulsed RF is needed, a non-destructive analgesic intervention providing even a few months of pain relief could have tremendous utility in palliative care.

Ongoing research continues to present improved understanding of familiar pain problems and opportunities for better analgesic therapies. Translation of recent pain science advances into clinical medicine will eventually improve the efficacy of pain therapies. Fortunately, although a few pain problems cannot be adequately controlled with current therapies, the vast majority of patients need not wait for future developments to have adequate pain control. A diverse array of effective techniques, including a wide range of injections, neural blockade, and implant therapies is already available. For the vast majority of persons with pain, the management of severe pain poorly responsive to routine systemic analgesic therapy does not need to wait for future developments, but must only await the consistent application of available pain management strategies.

Further reading

Cousins, M.J., Carr, D.B., Horlocker, T., et al. 2008. *Neural blockade in clinical anesthesia and management of pain*, 4th Edition. Lippincott. Williams & Wilkins, Philadelphia.

Deer, T., Krames, E.S., Hassenbusch, S.J. et al. (2007). Polyanalgesic consensus conference 2007: Recommendations for the management of pain by intrathecal (intraspinal) drug delivery: Report of an interdisciplinary expert panel. *Neuromodulation*, **10**, 300–28.

Hassenbusch, S., Burchiel, K., Coffey, R.J. et al. (2002). Management of intrathecal catheter-tip inflammatory masses: a consensus statement. *Pain Medicine*, **3**, 313–23.

Ossipov, M.H., Lai, J., King, T. et al. (2005). Underlying mechanisms of pronociceptive consequences of prolonged morphine exposure. *Biopolymers*, **80**, 319–24.

References

1. World Health Organization. 1990. *Cancer pain relief and palliative care: Report of a WHO expert committee. Rep. 804*, World Health Organization.

2. Hoskin, P.J. (2006). Cancer pain: treatment overview. In *Wall and Melzack's Textbook of Pain* (eds. S.B. McMahon and M. Koltzenburg), pp. 1141–57, 5th edition. Elsevier Churchill Livingstone.

3. National Comprehensive Cancer Network. (2007). Clinical Practice Guidelines in Oncology: Adult Cancer Pain. *http://nccn.org/ professionals/physician_gls/PDF/pain.pdf*.

4. Ballantyne, J.C. and Mao, J. (2003). Opioid therapy for chronic pain. *New England Journal of Medicine*, **349**, 1943–53.

5. Ballantyne, J.C. and LaForge, K.S. (2007). Opioid dependence and addiction during opioid treatment of chronic pain. *Pain*, **129**, 235–55.

6. Rajagopal, A., Vassilopoulou-Sellin, R., Palmer, J.L. et al. (2004). Symptomatic hypogonadism in male survivors of cancer with chronic exposure to opioids. *Cancer*, **100**, 851–58.

7. Budd, K. (2006). Pain management: is opioid immunosuppression a clinical problem? *Biomedicine and Pharmacotherapy*, **60**, 310–17.

8. Ossipov, M.H., Lai, J., King, T. et al. (2005). Underlying mechanisms of pronociceptive consequences of prolonged morphine exposure. *Biopolymers*, **80**, 319–24.

9. Angst, M.S. and Clark, J.D. (2006). Opioid-induced hyperalgesia: a qualitative systematic review. *Anesthesiology*, **104**, 570–87.

10. Carr, D.B. and Cousins, M.J. (1998). Spinal route of analgesia: opioids and future options. In *Neural Blockade in Clinical Anesthesia and Management of Pain* (eds. Cousins, J. Michael, and Bridenbaugh, O.Phillip), pp. 915–83, 3rd edition. Lippincott-Raven, Philadelphia.

11. Van Elstraete, A.C., Sitbon, P., Trabold, F. et al. (2005). A single dose of intrathecal morphine in rats induces long-lasting hyperalgesia: the protective effect of prior administration of ketamine. *Anesthesia and Analgesia*, **101**, 1750–56.

12. Compton, P., Charuvastra, V.C., Kintaudi, K. et al. (2000). Pain responses in mehadone-maintained opioid abusers. *Journal of Pain and Symptom Management*, **20**, 237–45.

13. Bruera, E. and Pereira, J. (1998). Recent developments in palliative cancer care. *Acta Oncologica*, **37**, 749–57.

14. De Conno, F., Caraceni, A., Martini, C. et al. (1991). Hyperalgesia and myoclonus with intrathecal infusion of high-dose morphine. *Pain*, **47**, 337–9.

15. Tremont-Lukats, I.W., Challapalli, V., McNicol, E.D. et al. (2005). Systemic administration of local anesthetics to relieve neuropathic pain: a systematic review and meta-analysis. *Anesthesia and Analgesia*, **101**, 1738–49.

16. Mercadante, S., Arcuri, E., Tirelli, W. et al. (2000). Analgesic effect of intravenous ketamine in cancer patients on morphine therapy: a randomized, controlled, double-blind, crossover, double-dose study. *Journal of Pain and Symptom. Management*, **20**, 246–52.

17. Deer, T., Krames, E.S., Hassenbusch, S.J. et al. (2007). Polyanalgesic consensus conference 2007: Recommendations for the management of pain by intrathecal (intraspinal) drug delivery: Report of an interdisciplinary expert panel. *Neuromodulation*, **10**, 300–28.

18. Catterall, W.A. and Mackie, K. (2006). Local anesthetics. In *Goodman and Gilman's The Pharmacological Basis of Therapeutics* (ed. L.L. Brunton), pp. 369–86, 11th edition. McGraw-Hill Companies, Inc., New York.

19. Cassuto, J., Sinclair, R., and Bonderovic, M. (2006). Anti-inflammatory properties of local anesthetics and their present and potential clinical implications. *Acta Anaesthesiologica. Scandinavica*, **50**, 265–82.

20. Okuse, K. (2007). Pain signalling pathways: from cytokines to ion channels. *International Journal of Biochemistry and Cell Biology*, **39**, 490–96.

21. Takeda, K., Sawamura, S., Sekiyama, H. et al. (2004). Effect of methylprednisolone on neuropathic pain and spinal glial activation in rats. *Anesthesiology*, **100**, 1249–57.

22. Patt, R.B. and Cousins, M.J. (1998). Techniques for neurolytic neural blockade. In *Neural Blockade in Clinical Anesthesia and Management of Pain* (eds. M.J. Cousins, and P.O. Bridenbaugh), pp. 1007–61, 3rd edition. Lippincott-Raven, Philadelphia.

23. Niemisto, L., Kalso, E., Malmivaara, A. et al. (2003). Radiofrequency denervation for neck and back pain: a systematic review within the framework of the cochrane collaboration back review group. *Spine*, **28**, 1877–88.

24. Conacher, I.D., Locke, T., Hilton, C. (1986). Neuralgia after cryoanalgesia for thoracotomy. *Lancet*, **1**, 277.

25. Myers, R.R. (1998). Neuropathology of neurolytic agents. In *Neural Blockade in Clinical Anesthesia and Management of Pain* (eds. M.J. Cousins and P.O. Bridenbaugh), pp. 985–1006, 3rd edition. Lippincott-Raven, Philadelphia.

26. Simons, D.G., Travell, J.G., and Simons, L.S. (1999). *Myofascial Pain and Dysfunction: The Trigger Point Manual*. Williams & Wilkins, Baltimore.

27. Aoki, K.R. (2005). Review of a proposed mechanism for the antinociceptive action of botulinum toxin type A. *Neurotoxicology*, **26**, 785–93.

28. Foster, L., Clapp, L., Erickson, M. et al. (2001). Botulinum toxin A and chronic low back pain: a randomized, double-blind study. *Neurology*, **56**, 1290–93.

29. Gobel, H., Heinze, A., Heinze-Kuhn, K. et al. (2001). Evidence-based medicine: botulinum toxin A in migraine and tension-type headache. *Journal of Neurology*, **248** (Suppl 1), 34–8.

30. Reichel, G. (2001). Botulinum toxin for treatment of spasticity in adults. *Journal of Neurology*, **248** (Suppl 1), 25–7.

31. Mahowald, M.L., Singh, J.A., and Dykstra, D. (2006). Long term effects of intra-articular botulinum toxin A for refractory joint pain. *Neurotoxicology Research*, **9**, 179–88.

32. Liu, H.T., Tsai, S.K., Kao, M.C. et al. (2006). Botulinum toxin A relieved neuropathic pain in a case of post-herpetic neuralgia. *Pain Medicine*, **7**, 89–91.

33. Allam, N., Brasil-Neto, J.P., Brown, G. et al. (2005). Injections of botulinum toxin type a produce pain alleviation in intractable trigeminal neuralgia. *Clinical Journal of Pain*, **21**, 182–84.

34. Kern, U., Martin, C., Scheicher, S. et al. (2003). Botulinum toxin type A influences stump pain after limb amputations. *Journal of Pain and Symptom Management*, **26**, 1069–70.

35. Jabbari, B., Maher, N., and Difazio, M.P. (2003). Botulinum toxin a improved burning pain and allodynia in two patients with spinal cord pathology. *Pain Medicine*, **4**, 206–10.

36. Hochberg, M.C. (2000). Role of intra-articular hyaluronic acid preparations in medical management of osteoarthritis of the knee. *Seminars in Arthritis and Rheumatism*, **30**, 2–10.

37. Samborski, W., Stratz, T., Mackiewicz, S. *et al.* (2004). Intra-articular treatment of arthritides and activated osteoarthritis with the 5-HT3 receptor antagonist tropisetron. A double-blind study compared with methylprednisolone. *Scandivian Journal of Rheumatology Supplement*, 51–54.

38. Bliddal, H., Terslev, L., Qvistgaard, E. *et al.* (2006). Safety of intra-articular injection of etanercept in small-joint arthritis: an uncontrolled, pilot-study with independent imaging assessment. *Joint Bone Spine*, **73**, 714–7.

39. Vranken, J.H., van der Vegt, M.H., Zuurmond, W.W. *et al.* (2001). Continuous brachial plexus block at the cervical level using a posterior approach in the management of neuropathic cancer pain. *Regional Anesthesia Pain Medicine*, **26**, 572–5.

40. Boezaart, A.P. (2006). Perineural infusion of local anesthetics. *Anesthesiology*, **104**, 872–80.

41. Hogan, Q.H. and Abram, S.E. (1997). Neural blockade for diagnosis and prognosis. A review. *Anesthesiology*, **86**, 216–41.

42. Cuvillon, P., Ripart, J., Lalourcey, L. *et al.* (2001). The continuous femoral nerve block catheter for postoperative analgesia: bacterial colonization, infectious rate and adverse effects. *Anesthesia and Analgesia*, **93**, 1045–9.

43. Waldman, S.D., Feldstein, G.S., Donohoe, C.D. *et al.* (1988). The relief of body wall pain secondary to malignant hepatic metastases by intercostal nerve block with bupivacaine and methylprednisolone. *Journal of Pain and Symptom Management*, **3**, 39–43.

44. Doi, K., Nikai, T., Sakura, S. *et al.* (2002). Intercostal nerve block with 5% tetracaine for chronic pain syndromes. *Journal of Clinical Anesthesia*, **14**, 39–41.

45. Antila, H. and Kirvela, O. (1998). Neurolytic thoracic paravertebral block in cancer pain. A clinical report. *Acta Anaesthesiologica Scandinavica*, **42**, 581–5.

46. Viel, E.J., Perennou, D., Ripart, J. *et al.* (2002). Neurolytic blockade of the obturator nerve for intractable spasticity of adductor thigh muscles. *European Journal of Pain*, **6**, 97–104.

47. Chua, K.S. and Kong, K.H. (2001). Clinical and functional outcome after alcohol neurolysis of the tibial nerve for ankle-foot spasticity. *Brain Injury*, **15**, 733–9.

48. Sharma, A., Williams, K., and Raja, S.N. (2006). Advances in treatment of complex regional pain syndrome: recent insights on a perplexing disease. *Curent.Opinion in Anaesthesiology*, **19**, 566–72.

49. Breivik, H., Cousins, M.J., and Lofstrom, B.J. (1998). Sympathetic neural blockade of upper and lower extremity. In *Neural Blockade in Clinical Anesthesia and Management of Pain* (eds. M.J. Cousins and P.O. Bridenbaugh), pp. 411–45, 3rd edition. Lippincott-Raven, Philadelphia.

50. Wu, C.L., Marsh, A., and Dworkin, R.H. (2000). The role of sympathetic nerve blocks in herpes zoster and postherpetic neuralgia. *Pain*, **87**, 121–9.

51. Opstelten, W., van Wijck, A.J., and Stolker, R.J. (2004). Interventions to prevent postherpetic neuralgia: cutaneous and percutaneous techniques. *Pain*, **107**, 202–6.

52. Moore, R., Groves, D., Hammond, C. *et al.* (2005). Temporary sympathectomy in the treatment of chronic refractory angina. *Journal of Pain and Symptom Management*, **30**, 183–91.

53. Wilkinson, H.A. (1996). Percutaneous radiofrequency upper thoracic sympathectomy. *Neurosurgery*, **38**, 715–25.

54. Ojimba, T.A. and Cameron, A.E. (2004). Drawbacks of endoscopic thoracic sympathectomy. *Brain Journal of Surgery*, **91**, 264–9.

55. Mannheimer, C., Camici, P., Chester, M.R. *et al.* (2002). The problem of chronic refractory angina; report from the ESC Joint Study Group on the Treatment of Refractory Angina. *European Heart Journal*, **23**, 355–70.

56. Eisenberg, E., Carr, D.B., and Chalmers, T.C. (1995). Neurolytic celiac plexus block for treatment of cancer pain: a meta- analysis. *Anesthesia and Analgesia*, **80**, 290–5.

57. Mercadante, S. (1993). Celiac plexus block versus analgesics in pancreatic cancer pain. *Pain*, **52**, 187–92.

58. Staats, P.S., Hekmat, H., Sauter, P. *et al.* (2002). The effects of alcohol celiac plexus block, pain, and mood on longevity in patients with unresectable pancreatic cancer: A double-blinded, randomized, placebo-controlled study. *Pain Medicine*, **2**, 28–34.

59. Wong, G.Y., Schroeder, D.R., Carns, P.E. *et al.* (2004). Effect of neurolytic celiac plexus block on pain relief, quality of life, and survival in patients with unresectable pancreatic cancer: a randomized controlled trial. *Journal of the American Medical Association*, **291**, 1092–9.

60. Davies, D.D. (1993). Incidence of major complications of neurolytic coeliac plexus block. *Journal of R.Social Medicine*, **86**, 264–6.

61. Abdalla, E.K. and Schell, S.R. (1999). Paraplegia following intraoperative celiac plexus injection. *Journal of Gastrointestinal Surgery*, **3**, 668–71.

62. Walsh, J.A., Glynn, C.J., Cousins, M.J. *et al.* (1985). Blood flow, sympathetic activity and pain relief following lumbar sympathetic blockade or surgical sympathectomy. *Anaesthesia and Intensive Care*, **13**, 18–24.

63. Alexander, J.P. (1994). Chemical lumbar sympathectomy in patients with severe lower limb ischaemia. *Ulster Medicine Journal*, **63**, 137–43.

64. Noe, C.E. and Haynsworth, R.F., Jr. (1993). Lumbar radiofrequency sympatholysis. *Journal of Vascular Surgery*, **17**, 801–6.

65. Plancarte, R., de Leon-Casasola, O.A., El-Helaly, M. *et al.* (1997). Neurolytic superior hypogastric plexus block for chronic pelvic pain associated with cancer. *Reg Anesthesia*, **22**, 562–8.

66. Abram, S.E. (1999). Treatment of lumbosacral radiculopathy with epidural steroids. *Anesthesiology*, **91**, 1937–41.

67. Riew, K.D., Yin, Y., Gilula, L. *et al.* (2000). The effect of nerve-root injections on the need for operative treatment of lumbar radicular pain. A prospective, randomized, controlled, double-blind study. *Journal of Bone and Joint Surgery American Volume*, **82-A**, 1589–93.

68. Fanciullo, G.J., Hanscom, B., Seville, J. *et al.* (2001). An observational study of the frequency and pattern of use of epidural steroid injection in 25,479 patients with spinal and radicular pain. *Regional Anesthesia Pain Medicine*, **26**, 5–11.

69. Buttermann, G.R. (2004). Treatment of lumbar disc herniation: epidural steroid injection compared with discectomy. A prospective, randomized study. *Journal of Bone and Joint Surgery. American Volume*, **86-A**, 670–9.

70. Huntoon, M.A. (2005). Anatomy of the cervical intervertebral foramina: vulnerable arteries and ischemic neurologic injuries after transforaminal epidural injections. *Pain*, **117**, 104–11.

71. Houten, J.K. and Errico, T.J. (2002). Paraplegia after lumbosacral nerve root block: report of three cases. *Spine Journal*, **2**, 70–5.

72. Dreyfuss, P., Baker, R., and Bogduk, N. (2006). Comparative effectiveness of cervical transforaminal injections with particulate and nonparticulate corticosteroid preparations for cervical radicular pain. *Pain Medicine*, **7**, 237–42.

73. Inada, T., Kushida, A., Sakamoto, S. *et al.* (2007). Intrathecal betamethasone pain relief in cancer patients with vertebral metastasis: a pilot study. *Acta Anaesthesiologica Scandinavica*, **51**, 490–4.

74. Taguchi, H., Oishi, K., Sakamoto, S. *et al.* (2007). Intrathecal betamethasone for cancer pain in the lower half of the body: a study of its analgesic efficacy and safety. *British Journal of Anaesthesia*, **98**, 385–9.

75. Kotani, N., Kushikata, T., Hashimoto, H. *et al.* (2000). Intrathecal Methylprednisolone for Intractable Postherpetic Neuralgia. *New England Journal of Medicine*, **343**, 1514–9.

76. Nelson, D.A. and Landau, W.M. (2001). Intraspinal steroids: history, efficacy, accidentality, and controversy with review of United States Food and Drug Administration reports. *Journal of Neurology, Neurosurgery and Psychiatry*, **70**, 433–43.

77. Candido, K. and Stevens, R.A. (2003). Intrathecal neurolytic blocksfor the relief of cancer pain. *Best Pract.Res Clin Anaesthesiol*, **17**, 407–28.

78. Jarrett, L., Nandi, P., and Thompson, A.J. (2002). Managing severe lower limb spasticity in multiple sclerosis: does intrathecal phenol have a role? *Journal of Neurology, Neurosurgery and Psychiatry*, **73**, 705–9.

79. Burton, A.W., Rajagopal, A., Shah, H.N. *et al.* (2004). Epidural and intrathecal analgesia is effective in treating refractory cancer pain. *Pain Medicine*, **5**, 239–47.

80. Smith, T.J., Coyne, P.J., Staats, P.S. *et al.* (2005). An implantable drug delivery system (IDDS) for refractory cancer pain provides sustained pain control, less drug-related toxicity, and possibly better survival compared with comprehensive medical management (CMM). *Annals of Oncology*, **16**, 825–33.

81. Jones, T.F., Feler, C.A., Simmons, B.P. *et al.* (2002). Neurologic complications including paralysis after a medication error involving implanted intrathecal catheters. *American Journal of Medicine*, **112**, 31–6.

82. Gourlay, G.K., Murphy, T.M., Plummer, J.L. *et al.* (1989). Pharmacokinetics of fentanyl in lumbar and cervical CSF following lumbar epidural and intravenous administration. *Pain*, **38**, 253–59.

83. Siddall, P.J., Molloy, A.R., Walker, S. *et al.* (2000). The efficacy of intrathecal morphine and clonidine in the treatment of pain after spinal cord injury. *Anesthesia and Analgesia*, **91**, 1493–8.

84. Winkelmuller, M. and Winkelmuller, W. (1996). Long-term effects of continuous intrathecal opioid treatment in chronic pain of nonmalignant etiology. *Journal of Neurosurgery*, **85**, 458–67.

85. Parisod, E., Siddall, P.J., Viney, M. *et al.* (2003). Allodynia after acute intrathecal morphine administration in a patient with neuropathic pain after spinal cord injury. *Anesthesia and Analgesia*, **97**, 183–6.

86. Portenoy, R.K. and Savage, S.R. (1997). Clinical realities and economic considerations: special therapeutic issues in intrathecal therapy--tolerance and addiction. *Journal of Pain and Symptom Management*, **14**, S27–S35.

87. van Dongen, R.T., Crul, B.J., and De Bock, M. (1993). Long-term intrathecal infusion of morphine and morphine/bupivacaine mixtures in the treatment of cancer pain: a retrospective analysis of 51 cases. *Pain*, **55**, 119–23.

88. van Dongen, R.T., Crul, B.J., and van Egmond, J. (1999). Intrathecal coadministration of bupivacaine diminishes morphine dose progression during long-term intrathecal infusion in cancer patients. *Clinical Journal of Pain*, **15**, 166–72.

89. Mercadante, S. (1994). Intrathecal morphine and bupivacaine in advanced cancer pain patients implanted at home. *Journal of Pain and Symptom Management*, **9**, 201–7.

90. Dahm, P., Nitescu, P., Appelgren, L. *et al.* (1998). High thoracic/low cervical, long-term intrathecal (i.t.) infusion of bupivacaine alleviates "refractory" pain in patients with unstable angina pectoris. Report of 2 cases. *Acta Anaesthesiologica Scandinavica*, **42**, 1010–7.

91. Berde, C.B., Sethna, N.F., Conrad, L.S. *et al.* (1990). Subarachnoid bupivacaine analgesia for seven months for a patient with a spinal cord tumor. *Anesthesiology*, **72**, 1094–6.

92. Perren, F., Buchser, E., Chedel, D. *et al.* (2004). Spinal cord lesion after long-term intrathecal clonidine and bupivacaine treatment for the management of intractable pain. *Pain*, **109**, 189–94.

93. Burchiel, K.J. and Hsu, F.P. (2001). Pain and spasticity after spinal cord injury: mechanisms and treatment. *Spine*, **26**, S146–S160.

94. Staats, P.S., Yearwood, T., Charapata, S.G. *et al.* (2004). Intrathecal ziconotide in the treatment of refractory pain in patients with cancer or AIDS: a randomized controlled trial. *Journal of the American Medical Association*, **291**, 63–70.

95. Rauck, R.L., Wallace, M.S., Leong, M.S. *et al.* (2006). A randomized, double-blind, placebo-controlled study of intrathecal ziconotide in adults with severe chronic pain. *Journal of Pain and Symptom Management*, **31**, 393–406.

96. Wallace, M.S. (2006). Ziconotide: a new nonopioid intrathecal analgesic for the treatment of chronic pain. *Expert Reviews in Neurotherapy*, **6**, 1423–28.

97. Lynch, S.S., Cheng, C.M., and Yee, J.L. (2006). Intrathecal ziconotide for refractory chronic pain. *Annals of Pharmacotherapy*, **40**, 1293–300.

98. Hodgson, P.S., Neal, J.M., Pollock, J.E. *et al.* (1999). The neurotoxicity of drugs given intrathecally (spinal). *Anesthesia and Analgesia*, **88**, 797–809.

99. Karpinski, N., Dunn, J., Hansen, L. *et al.* (1997). Subpial vacuolar myelopathy after intrathecal ketamine: report of a case. *Pain*, **73**, 103–5.

100. Sen, S., Aydin, O.N., and Aydin, K. (2006). Beneficial effect of low-dose ketamine addition to epidural administration of morphine-bupivacaine mixture for cancer pain in two cases. *Pain Medicine*, **7**, 166–9.

101. Yaksh, T.L. and Allen, J.W. (2004). The use of intrathecal midazolam in humans: a case study of process. *Anesthesia and Analgesia*, **98**, 1536–45.

102. Nishiyama, T., Matsukawa, T., and Hanaoka, K. (2002). Effects of adding midazolam on the postoperative epidural analgesia with two different doses of bupivacaine. *Journal of Clinical Anesthesia*, **14**, 92–7.

103. Lavand'homme, P. (2006). Lessons from spinal midazolam: When misuse of messages from preclinical models exposes patients to unnecessary risks. *Reg Anesth Pain Medicine*, **31**, 489–91.

104. Johansen, M.J., Gradert, T.L., Satterfield, W.C. *et al.* (2004). Safety of continuous intrathecal midazolam infusion in the sheep model. *Anesthesia and Analgesia*, **98**, 1528–35.

105. Tucker, A.P., Lai, C., Nadeson, R. *et al.* (2004). Intrathecal midazolam I: a cohort study investigating safety. *Anesthesia and Analgesia*, **98**, 1512–20.

106. Canavero, S., Bonicalzi, V., and Clemente, M. (2006). No neurotoxicity from long-term (>5 years) intrathecal infusion of midazolam in humans. *Journal of Pain and Symptom Management*, **32**, 1–3.

107. Du Pen, S. (1999). Complications of neuraxial infusion in cancer patients. *Oncology (Huntington, NY)*, **13**, 45–51.

108. Nitescu, P., Dahm, P., Appelgren, L. *et al.* (1998). Continuous infusion of opioid and bupivacaine by externalized intrathecal catheters in long-term treatment of "refractory" nonmalignant pain. *Clinical Journal of Pain*, **14**, 17–28.

109. Dahm, P., Nitescu, P., Appelgren, L. *et al.* (1998). Efficacy and technical complications of long-term continuous intraspinal infusions of opioid and/or bupivacaine in refractory nonmalignant pain: a comparison between the epidural and the intrathecal approach with externalized or implanted catheters and infusion pumps. *Clinical Journal of Pain*, **14**, 4–16.

110. Blomberg, S.G. (1994). Long-term home self-treatment with high thoracic epidural anesthesia in patients with severe coronary artery disease. *Anesthesia and Analgesia*, **79**, 413–21.

111. Tsai, Y.C., Wang, L.K., Chen, B.S. *et al.* (2000). Home-based patient-controlled epidural analgesia with bupivacaine for patients with intractable herpetic neuralgia. *Journal of the Formosan Medical Association*, **99**, 659–62.

112. Horlocker, T.T., Wedel, D.J., Benzon, H. *et al.* (2003). Regional anesthesia in the anticoagulated patient: defining the risks (the second ASRA Consensus Conference on Neuraxial Anesthesia and Anticoagulation). *Reg Anesth.Pain Medicine*, **28**, 172–97.

113. Anderson, V.C. and Burchiel, K.J. (1999). A prospective study of long-term intrathecal morphine in the management of chronic nonmalignant pain. *Neurosurgery*, **44**, 289–300.

114. Kumar, K., Kelly, M., and Pirlot, T. (2001). Continuous intrathecal morphine treatment for chronic pain of nonmalignant etiology: long-term benefits and efficacy. *Surgical Neurology*, **55**, 79–86.

115. Mercadante, S. (1999). Problems of long-term spinal opioid treatment in advanced cancer patients. *Pain*, **79**, 1–13.

116. Smitt, P.S., Tsafka, A., Teng-van de Zande, F. *et al.* (1998). Outcome and complications of epidural analgesia in patients with chronic cancer pain. *Cancer*, **83**, 2015–22.

117. de Jong, P.C. and Kansen, P.J. (1994). A comparison of epidural catheters with or without subcutaneous injection ports for treatment of cancer pain. *Anesthesia and Analgesia*, **78**, 94–100.

118. Cherry, D.A. and Gourlay, G.K. (1992). CT contrast evidence of injectate encapsulation after long-term epidural administration. *Pain*, **49**, 369–71.

119. Coffey, R.J. and Burchiel, K. (2002). Inflammatory mass lesions associated with intrathecal drug infusion catheters: report and observations on 41 patients. *Neurosurgery*, **50**, 78–86.

120. Yaksh, T.L., Hassenbusch, S., Burchiel, K. *et al.* (2002). Inflammatory masses associated with intrathecal drug infusion: a review of preclinical evidence and human data. *Pain Medicine*, **3**, 300–12.

121. Murphy, P.M., Skouvaklis, D.E., Amadeo, R.J. *et al.* (2006). Intrathecal catheter granuloma associated with isolated baclofen infusion. *Anesthesia and Analgesia*, **102**, 848–52.

122. Hassenbusch, S., Burchiel, K., Coffey, R.J. *et al.* (2002). Management of intrathecal catheter-tip inflammatory masses: a consensus statement. *Pain Medicine*, **3**, 313–23.

123. Ballantyne, J.C. and Carwood, C.M. (2005). Comparative efficacy of epidural, subarachnoid, and intracerebroventricular opioids in patients with pain due to cancer. *Cochrane Database of Systematic Reviews* CD005178.

124. Hulme, P.A., Krebs, J., Ferguson, S.J. *et al.* (2006). Vertebroplasty and kyphoplasty: a systematic review of 69 clinical studies. *Spine*, **31**, 1983–2001.

125. Burton, A.W., Reddy, S.K., Shah, H.N. *et al.* (2005). Percutaneous vertebroplasty–a technique to treat refractory spinal pain in the setting of advanced metastatic cancer: a case series. *Journal of Pain and Symptom Management*, **30**, 87–95.

126. Nussbaum, D.A., Gailloud, P., and Murphy, K. (2004). A review of complications associated with vertebroplasty and kyphoplasty as reported to the Food and Drug Administration medical device related web site. *Journal of Vascular and Interventional Radiology*, **15**, 1185–92.

127. Mailis-Gagnon, A., Furlan, A.D., Sandoval, J.A. *et al.* (2004). Spinal cord stimulation for chronic pain. *The Cochrane Database of Systematic Reviews*.

128. Oakley, J.C. and Prager, J.P. (2002). Spinal cord stimulation: mechanisms of action. *Spine*, **27**, 2574–83.

129. Yu, W., Maru, F., Edner, M. *et al.* (2004). Spinal cord stimulation for refractory angina pectoris: a retrospective analysis of efficacy and cost-benefit. *Coronary Artery Diseases*, **15**, 31–7.

130. Ubbink, D.T. and Vermeulen, H. (2005). Spinal cord stimulation for non-reconstructable chronic critical leg eschaemia. *The Cochrane Database of Systematic Reviews*.

131. Cameron, T. (2004). Safety and efficacy of spinal cord stimulation for the treatment of chronic pain: a 20-year literature review. *Journal of Neurosurgery*, **100**, 254–67.

132. Tiede, J.M., Ghazi, S.M., Lamer, T.J. *et al.* (2006). The use of spinal cord stimulation in refractory abdominal visceral pain: case reports and literature review. *Pain, Pract*, **6**, 197–202.

133. Taylor, R.S., Taylor, R.J., Van Buyten, J.P. *et al.* (2004). The cost effectiveness of spinal cord stimulation in the treatment of pain: a systematic review of the literature. *Journal of Pain and Symptom Management*, **27**, 370–8.

134. Sibell, D.M., Colantonio, A.J., and Stacey, B.R. (2005). Successful use of spinal cord stimulation in the treatment of severe Raynaud's disease of the hands. *Anesthesiology*, **102**, 225–7.

135. Swigris, J.J., Olin, J., and Mekhail. N.A. (1999). Implantable spinal cord stimulator to treat the ischemic manifestations of thromboangiitis obliterans (Buerger's disease). *Journal of Vascular Surgery*, **29**, 928–35.

136. Lo, B. and Rubenfeld, G. (2005). Palliative sedation in dying patients: "we turn to it when everything else hasn't worked". *Journal of the American Medical Association*, **294**, 1810–6.

137. Cherny, N.I. and Portenoy, R.K. (1994). Sedation in the management of refractory symptoms: guidelines for evaluation and treatment. *Journal of Palliative Care*, **10**, 31–8.

138. Liebeskind, J.C. (1991). Pain can kill. *Pain*, **44**, 3–4.

139. Hefti, F.F., Rosenthal, A., Walicke, P.A. *et al.* (2006). Novel class of pain drugs based on antagonism of NGF. *Trends in Pharmacological Sciences*, **27**, 85–91.

140. Watkins, L.R., Hutchinson, M.R., Ledeboer. A. *et al.* (2007). Norman Cousins Lecture. Glia as the "bad guys": implications for improving clinical pain control and the clinical utility of opioids. *Brain, Behaviour, and Immunity*, **21**, 131–46.

141. Ekberg, J., Jayamanne, A., Vaughan, C.W. *et al.* (2006). muO-conotoxin MrVIB selectively blocks Nav1.8 sensory neuron specific sodium channels and chronic pain behavior without motor deficits. *Proceedings of the National Academy of Science U.S.A*, **103**, 17030–5.

142. Bogduk, N. (2006). Pulsed radiofrequency. *Pain Medicine*, **7**, 396–407.

143. Rozen, D. and Parvez, U. (2006). Pulsed radiofrequency of lumbar nerve roots for treatment of chronic inguinal herniorraphy pain. *Pain Physician*, **9**, 153–6.

144. Cohen, S.P., Sireci, A., Wu, C.L. *et al.* (2006). Pulsed radiofrequency of the dorsal root ganglia is superior to pharmacotherapy or pulsed radiofrequency of the intercostal nerves in the treatment of chronic postsurgical thoracic pain. *Pain Physician*, **9**, 227–35.

145. Gallagher, R.M. (2006). Pulsed radiofrequency treatment: what is the evidence of its effectiveness and should it be used in clinical practice? *Pain Medicine*, **7**, 408–10.

146. Van Zundert, J., Patijn, J., Kessels, A. *et al.* (2007). Pulsed radiofrequency adjacent to the cervical dorsal root ganglion in chronic cervical radicular pain: a double blind sham controlled randomized clinical trial. *Pain*, **127**, 173–82.

10.1.10 The role of surgical neuroablation for pain control

Nicholas Park and Nik K. Patel

The management of cancer pain represents a difficult diagnostic and therapeutic problem for the clinician. Pain is present in up to 90 per cent of patients in the terminal stages of malignancy[1]. In a multi-disciplinary approach to the management of cancer pain, neurosurgical methods are an essential part of the therapy.

Neurosurgery for the relief of persistent pain began in the 19th century with root sections and later cordotomy. Pain relief was dominated by these methods until the second half of the 20th century, when the paradigm shifted predominantly to pharmacotherapy. This occurred in tandem with advances in the pharmacology of analgesics and the development of pain clinics and hospices. There was then a virtual cessation in the practice of neurosurgery for pain relief.

Despite the many advances in analgesic drug therapy, it is estimated that 10–20 per cent of cancer patients fail to obtain adequate analgesia with pharmacological treatments. These patients must be considered for alternative strategies, among which are surgical approaches. These treatments historically have been destructive or ablative techniques involving intracranial and spinal targets. In the last 20 years, however, with advances in knowledge of cancer pain mechanisms and technological developments, such as microsurgical and stereotactic techniques, implant technology, and computed tomography (CT) and magnetic resonance imaging, older methods have been replaced by more precise, safer, and presumably more effective techniques. These include percutaneous and minimally invasive ablative methods and non-destructive or augmentative techniques such as electrical stimulation or the implantation of sophisticated devices for intrathecal drug delivery.

The distinction between destructive and non-destructive procedures is important. Destructive procedures are most appropriate for the treatment of persistent pain due to malignancy, when life expectancy is limited; they are rarely used for non-malignant pains. The reasons are relapse rates are high after destructive procedures, there is a risk of neurological deficit and therefore disability, and new syndromes (particularly dysaesthetic type pains) may arise after destruction of the nervous system at either peripheral or central levels, though more particularly after peripheral lesions. This is due to the plasticity of the central nervous system—the same type of phenomena responsible for prolonged pain and hyperalgesia.

For most of the pain syndromes occurring in patients who may be candidates for neuroablation, there are potentially several ablative techniques which could be employed. The use of a given technique should depend on a thorough assessment of its likelihood to yield adequate analgesia, the duration of its effect, potential adverse consequences, and the likely life expectancy of the patient. It should be remembered that[2]:

- ablative techniques should be deferred until non-ablative modalities have the opportunity to yield adequate analgesia,

- the most efficacious therapy should be selected but if there is a choice, the one with fewest side effects is preferred,

- the aim of a single neuroablative procedure should be to reduce the pain to a level manageable with safe doses of pharmacological agents because complete eradication of cancer pain is rarely possible due to its multifocal nature, and

- the choice of a specific operation is based on the type of pain, severity, location and primary cause of the painful sensation.

Ablative strategies can be classified according to the anatomical location of the target. The broadest distinction is between peripheral nervous system and central nervous system targets (Figs. 10.1.10.1 and 10.1.10.2).

Peripheral procedures

Peripheral neurectomy

Although peripheral nerve injury pain is usually associated with trauma to a sensory or mixed nerve, invasion of nerves by tumour, entrapment syndromes, and polyneuropathies also can give rise to peripheral nerve pain. The pain may be felt at the site of the injury, or in the distribution of the affected nerve, but remote from the site of injury. Presumably, pain at the injured site is mediated by local nociceptive afferents, whereas pain experienced in the territory of the affected nerve relates to intrinsic damage within the nerve. This intrinsic damage may be caused by:

- neuroma formation, in which an injured nerve sprouts unmyelinated fibres, which are unusually sensitive to stimuli (pain caused by neuroma can be eliminated by resection of this lesion); and

- ephaptic transmission, in which abnormal electrical connections may develop between fibres at the site of injury, such that nociceptive afferents may be activated by normally innocuous stimuli.

Prior to embarking on an ablative strategy, the patient should undergo peripheral nerve root blocks. If satisfactory analgesia is not achieved with an appropriate block, surgery is not appropriate. If analgesia is achieved, then the patient may undergo exploration of the injured nerve with the intention of peripheral neurectomy (in the case of a non-critical sensory nerve) or excision of any identified neuroma and nerve repair for larger nerves.

Technique

The technique of peripheral neurectomy involves adequate exposure of the nerve followed by ligation and surgical cautery. The proximal stump should then be buried deep within adjacent muscle to prevent neuroma formation.

Results

Even with complete analgesia from local anaesthetic nerve blocks, the success rate for peripheral neurectomy is no greater than 50–60 per cent[3]. Given these results and the unusual occurrence of pain in the distribution of a specific, surgically amenable peripheral nerve, peripheral neurectomy is rarely useful in the palliative care setting.

Ablative techniques directed towards spinal targets

Surgery can be targeted to several locations to interrupt nociceptive pathways transiting the spinal cord. These approaches chiefly comprise lesions in the dorsal root entry zone (DREZ), the midline posterior column visceral pathway, and the spinothalamic tracts.

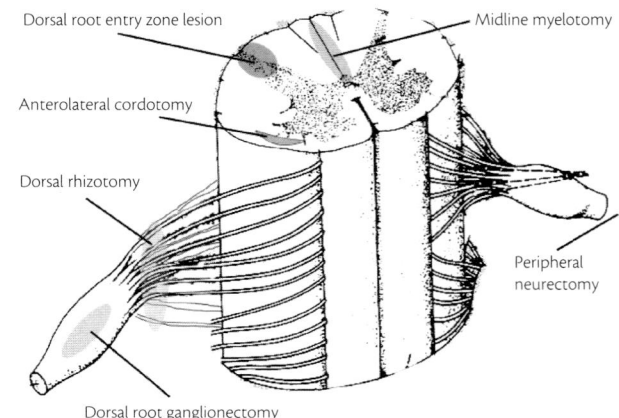

Figure 10.1.10.1 Peripheral and spinal ablative targets.

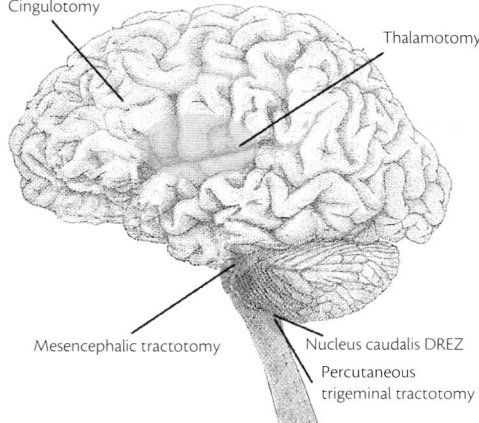

Figure 10.1.10.2 Central ablative targets.

Interruption of the spinothalamic tracts tends to abolish pain and temperature sensation on the contralateral side below the level of the lesion. In contrast, DREZ lesions tend to produce a segmental pattern of analgesia. Lesions of the midline posterior column visceral pathway prevent transmission of pelvic and visceral pain.

Dorsal root entry zone (DREZ) lesioning

The dorsal horn serves as the first site of modulation for pain sensation. The dorsal root entry zone is an anatomical entity comprising the proximal extensions of the dorsal roots, Lissauer's tract, and Rexed's laminae 1–5 (Fig. 10.1.10.3). Upon entering the dorsal horn, most of the small diameter nociceptive fibres are located laterally and the larger diameter lemniscal fibres are located medially. The axons of the small nociceptive afferents enter Lissauer's tract, run up and down the spinal cord's 1 or 2 segments, and then synapse on the cells of the substantia gelatinosa, a region of the dorsal horn grey matter situated in the superficial lamina. In addition, the larger diameter lemniscal fibres, en route to the dorsal columns, also synapse in the substantia gelatinosa. This enables the substantia gelatinosa to exert a strong modulating influence on the nociceptive input[4]. The objective of DREZ lesioning is to interrupt the lateral part of the dorsal root entry zone and Lissauer's tract. The placement of the lesion attempts to preserve the lemniscal fibres reaching the dorsal horn medially.

Technique

The open microsurgical approach involves bipolar coagulation at the ventrolateral entry of the roots into the dorsal horn. The lesions are 2 mm deep and made at a 45° angle, as shown by the hatched area in Fig. 10.1.10.4[5]. This methodology aims to prevent abolition of tactile and proprioceptive modalities by preserving the larger fibres medially. It also seeks to avoid deafferentation pain, thought to arise from loss of inhibitory control that may follow sectioning of these lemniscal fibres. Nashold has described a technique using radiofrequency electrocoagulation instead of bipolar cautery[6]. The use of CO_2 and argon lasers also has been advocated[7,8].

Results

The success of DREZ lesioning depends on the ability to select the appropriate level for ablation. In 70 patients with cancer pain due to focal lesions, Sindou's group obtained effective analgesia in 87.5 per cent and 78.5 per cent of patients operated on at cervical and lumbosacral levels, respectively, using bipolar lesioning[5]. The mortality rate in this series was 2.5 per cent and the rate of pyramidal and dorsal column injury was very low. This contrasts with radiofrequency and laser lesioning, in which the complication rate from pyramidal and dorsal column injury appears to be substantially higher, perhaps 5–10 per cent[9]. Sindou et al. series also included neurogenic chronic pains, for example, brachial plexus injury and post-radiation plexopathies, and long-term benefit was obtained in 87 per cent of 87 patients[5].

Possible indications for DREZ lesioning include refractory pain related to a thoracic apex syndrome (e.g. due to a Pancoast

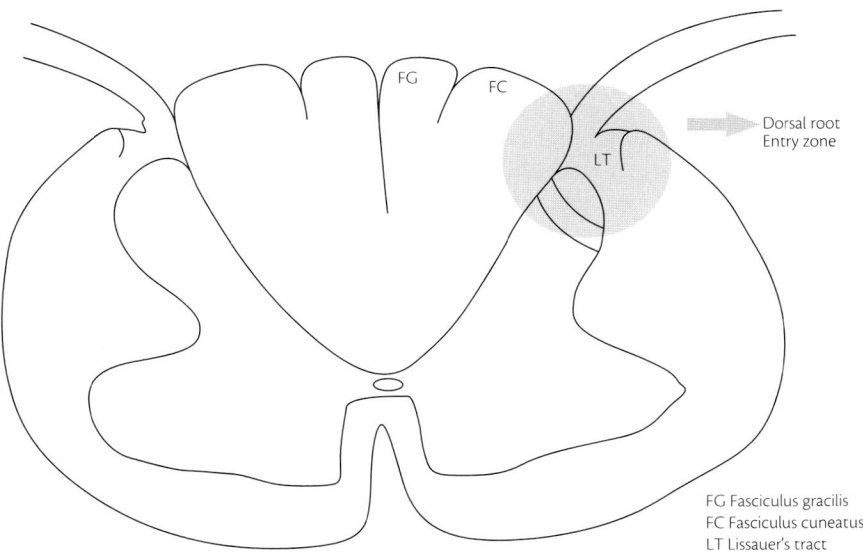

Figure 10.1.10.3 Cross-section of spinal cord showing dorsal root entry zone and adjacent fibre tracts.

tumour), which would require a C7–T2 ablation, circumscribed invasion of the thoracic wall, and limited involvement of lumbar and sacral roots or plexuses. In summary, DREZ lesioning can be particularly useful to manage topographically limited pain caused by well-localized lesions. It is not indicated for more diffuse pain.

Midline commissural myelotomy and punctate myelotomy

Section of midline fibres posterior to the central canal, which cross in the anterior commissure, can be accomplished by midline commissural myelotomy. This target was first identified by Armour in 1927 and aimed to divide the decussating spinothalamic fibres from both sides of the body[10]. On this basis, the myelotomy would require rostral extension from the painful territory due to the extension of the fibres in Lissauer's tract, and this necessitates an extended laminectomy. A potential benefit over anterolateral cordotomy is the ability to abolish bilateral pain with a single procedure.

More recently, Al-Chaer et al. has produced evidence of a tract in the anterior part of the medial borders of the dorsal columns[11–14]. This tract is thought to mediate abdominal and pelvic visceral pain, with afferents relaying to the ventroposterolateral nucleus of the thalamus. Disruption of this region can be achieved with a much more limited laminectomy, using the technique of punctate midline myelotomy [15]. The lesions, which usually are created at the thoracolumbar level for abdominal and pelvic pain, can be made using a knife, a blunt instrument, or CO_2 laser to incise the cord between the two gracilis tracts.

Technique

As shown in Fig. 10.1.10.5, commissural myelotomy requires a midline transection of the commissure. Punctate myelotomy requires 2 incisions in the gracilis tracts, each around 1 mm from the midline, to a depth within the cord of about 5 mm.

Results

Sindou et al. reviewed 445 cases of midline commissural myelotomy in 17 literature series. Early adequate analgesia was obtained in 75 per cent but remained long-lasting in only 50 per cent.

Persistent lemniscal sensory disturbances were present in 10 per cent, and related postoperative dysaesthesias were very frequent (55 per cent) in the early postoperative period, but remained chronic in only 6.4 per cent[9]. The number of patients who have currently undergone punctate myelotomies is small, but the rate of effective analgesia seems comparable to midline myelotomy and the morbidity appears to be lower. Hwang et al. performed punctate midline myelotomy in six patients with hepatobiliary carcinoma and achieved immediate analgesia in all, with no complications[16].

Due to the low rate of long-lasting analgesia, midline myelotomy is generally reserved for pain due to advanced terminal malignancies. The technique of punctate midline myelotomy appears particularly well suited for abdominal and pelvic visceral pain.

Anterolateral cordotomy

Anterolateral cordotomy was first performed by Spiller in 1911 at the cervicothoracic level via an open posterolateral approach[17]. Later, Collis (1963) and Cloward (1964) described the open anterior cervical approach[18,19]. The percutaneous method was pioneered by Mullan et al. in 1963, utilizing bipolar cautery[20]. In 1965, Rosomoff et al. described a technique using radiofrequency ablation[21]. More recently, Kanpolat et al. have described a percutaneous CT-guided technique[22,23].

The aim of anterolateral cordotomy is to disrupt the spinothalamic tract just below the medulla oblongata. Because 80 per cent of the entering nociceptive fibres decussate over 2–5 segments prior to entering the spinothalamic tract, the cordotomy must be performed on the side contralateral to the pain. It is important to note that the fibres are somatotopically arranged, with sacral fibres located posterolaterally and cervical fibres located anteromedially (Fig. 10.1.10.6). Thus, pain that is located at a site mediated by sacral or inferior lumbar fibres must be addressed by sectioning of the tract more posteriorly.

Technique

In the open posterior approach, access to the spinal canal is gained via a laminotomy. The dura is opened and the anterolateral surface of the cord viewed. An avascular area is selected for the incision, anterior to the pial insertion of the dentate ligament, as shown in Fig. 10.1.10.7. A smooth hook is then introduced to ablate the tract, minimizing damage to surrounding structures, most notably the anterior spinal artery. In a study of 146 patients, it was found

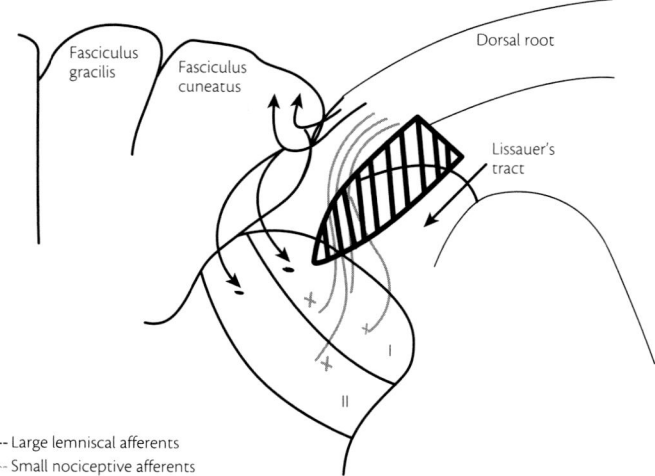

Figure 10.1.10.4 Technique of open microsurgical DREZ lesioning.

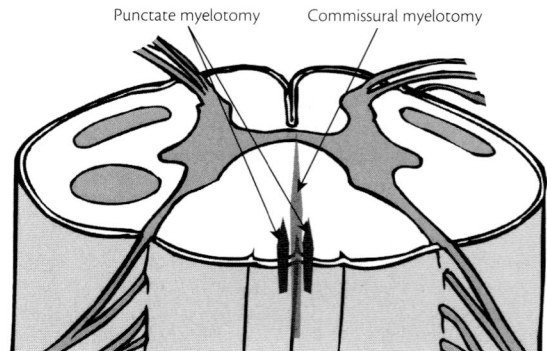

Figure 10.1.10.5 Dorsal view of spinal cord demonstrating myelotomy techniques.

that optimum analgesia was only achieved if pin-prick sensation was abolished in the affected territories. Preservation of this sensory modality was associated with a high rate of early recurrent pain[24].

An open anterior approach also is possible. This approach is via discectomy and has the advantage of direct visualization of the anterior spinal artery. It cannot be used at high cervical levels, however, and restricted access via the disc space makes dural closure difficult.

The percutaneous approach using radiofrequency ablation has gained popularity since its inception in the 1960s. X-ray fluoroscopy, CT-guidance[22] or MRI-guidance[25] is used to insert the radiofrequency electrode at the level of the C1–C2 interspace into the anterolateral spinothalamic tract. Confirmation of needle placement is obtained by stimulation and simultaneous questioning of the patient regarding sensory changes. Due to the somatotopic organization within the spinothalamic tract (Fig. 10.1.10.6), image-guided techniques have enabled selective lesioning using radiofrequency ablation.

Results

Kanpolat *et al.* utilized selective lesioning and reported adequate analgesia in 97 per cent of patients, with preservation of pain and temperature sensation in territories subserved by the remainder of the spinothalamic tract. Early recurrence of pain was significant and often was amenable to a repeated ablation[22]. Sindou and Daher[9] combined their personal cases with 37 published series of anterolateral cordotomy. In patients with cancer pain (*n*=2022), effective analgesia was achieved in 75 per cent at 6 months and 40 per cent after 1 year. More recently, Crul *et al.* analysed the results of 43 patients with terminal cancer causing unilateral pain; they observed early effective analgesia in 95 per cent, which fell to 70 per cent by the end of the patients' lives (mean survival duration 118 days)[26].

Adverse effects caused by cordotomy relate primarily to disruption of adjacent fibre tracts. At high cervical levels, the respiratory pathways lie just lateral to the ventral horn of grey matter. Most of the early mortality associated with anterolateral cordotomy (around 3 per cent), is caused by respiratory failure. For this reason, preoperative assessment of suitability should incorporate pulmonary function tests to evaluate the likely risk. Bilateral high

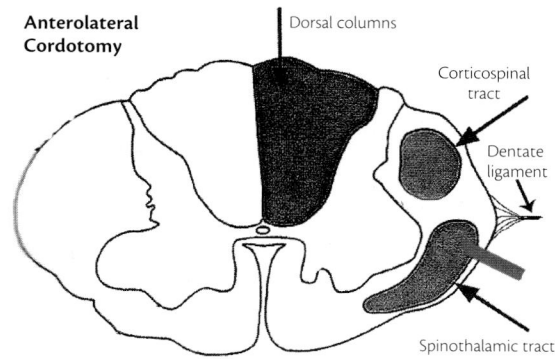

Figure 10.1.10.7 Cross-section of spinal cord demonstrating technique of percutaneous anterolateral cordotomy.

cervical cordotomy carries a high risk of sleep apnoea, due to a loss of automonic respiratory drive when asleep, a function ordinarily mediated by the spinothalmic tracts. This usually occurs within 5 days of the procedure, and has a high mortality when unrecognized. Because to the high incidence of sleep apnoea, bilateral high cervical cordotomy is now rarely performed.

The descending autonomic fibres for vasomotor and bladder control are intermingled with the lumbosacral spinothalamic fibres. In one case series, urinary retention occurred in 6 per cent of patients[27]; hemiparesis due to damage of the adjacent corticospinal tract was seen in 8 per cent. The complication rate rose to 28 per cent after bilateral cordotomy, strongly suggesting that cordotomy be confined to unilateral pain[27].

Another common complication following cordotomy is dysaesthetic pain and unmasking of pain on the contralateral side. If pain is present bilaterally preoperatively, the unmasking effect may be profound, much reducing the analgesic benefit. In Nagoro *et al.*'s series of 45 patients, 73 per cent developed new pains postoperatively[28]; in most cases, these were less severe than the original pain, and tended to settle with time.

In summary, the evidence suggests that anterolateral cordotomy can provide effective, immediate pain relief in the vast majority of selected patients. The incidence of adverse effects is acceptably low, but the effects of the therapy only last for longer than 1 year in about 40 per cent. This makes it particularly suitable for treatment of persistent unilateral cancer pain in terminally ill patients.

Ablative techniques directed against intracranial targets

Ablation of intracranial targets differs substantially from spinal targets because nociceptive processing may be significantly affected while preserving the basic pain pathways. This has the advantage of failing to induce deafferentation phenomena. As techniques progress, intracranial ablative targets, which had previously been abandoned due to unacceptable associated morbidity, are being re-examined, especially with the advent of radiosurgical procedures. Radiosurgical ablations are accurate and associated with few complications. However, they lack electrophysiological confirmation of the lesion placement[29], an advantage of open procedures. In future, this may be counterbalanced by improvement in functional magnetic resonance imaging or PET scanning.

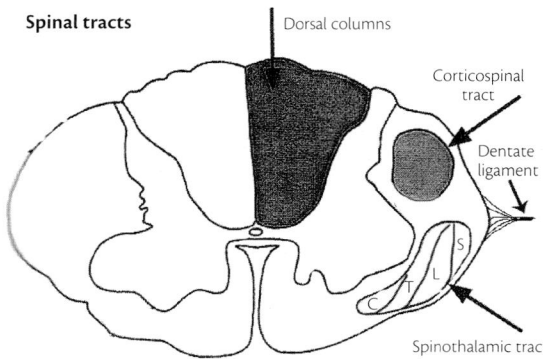

Figure 10.1.10.6 Cross-section of the cervical spinal cord showing position of major fibre tracts and somatotopic organization of the spinothalamic tract.

Percutaneous trigeminal tractotomy

The trigeminal nerve supplies sensation to most of the head and neck, in addition to subserving motor function of the muscles of mastication. The nuclei of the trigeminal nerve comprise the mesencephalic, motor, primary sensory, and spinal. The spinal nucleus extends from the medulla oblongata to the level of C2 and is histologically identical to the grey matter of the dorsal horn of the spinal cord. The most caudal portion of the spinal nucleus is termed the nucleus caudalis. It is to here that nociceptive afferents from the head and neck project. Somatotopic organization is present within the nucleus caudalis such that fibres from the ophthalmic division of the trigeminal nerve project to more caudal regions of the nucleus caudalis, whereas nociceptive fibres from the circumoral region project more rostrally.

Percutaneous trigeminal tractotomy is used for refractory pain in the head or neck and has replaced the open trigeminal tractotomy technique in clinical practice. The trigeminal tract descends in the brainstem, conveying second-order fibres to their synapses with the trigeminal nucleus. Ablations here cause ipsilateral analgesia in all three divisions of the trigeminal nerve.

Technique

Previously, tractotomy was performed via a suboccipital craniotomy. This invasive technique was associated with considerable morbidity and has been superseded by stereotactic radiofrequency lesioning under local anaesthesia, which was first performed by Crue et al. in 1967[30]. The tract is ablated in the medullary region, and as it lies in close proximity to the spinocerebellar tract, ataxia is a common complication. Electrophysiological localization prior to ablation is mandatory, and stimulation produces a dysaesthesia in the appropriate anatomical territory.

Results

Percutaneous trigeminal tractotomy may be effective in cancer-related facial pain. It may provide immediate relief in 85–100 per cent of patients, although long-term results often demonstrate relapse [31].

Nucleus caudalis DREZ lesioning

Another approach to pain in the head or neck is nucleus caudalis DREZ lesioning. This approach uses an open microsurgical procedure.

Technique

The procedure is performed under general anaesthesia and somatosensory evoked potential monitoring. The patient is positioned prone in a Mayfield 3-pin head fixator. A midline suboccipital craniotomy is fashioned, and the posterior arch of C1 is removed to gain access to the lower brainstem and cervicomedullary junction. The dura is opened, and the dorsal columns are identified, with the trigeminal tract and nucleus located laterally. In order to precisely localize that portion of the nucleus corresponding to the pain, the appropriate division of the trigeminal nerve is peripherally stimulated, and recordings are made from the exposed neural elements. At the site of maximal signal intensity, lesioning can be performed with radiofrequency current.

Results

In a study of 58 patients undergoing nucleus caudalis DREZ, the mean preoperative pain score of 9 was reduced to a mean of 5.2 over a 2-year follow-up. The use of opioid analgesics fell from 100 per cent to 37 per cent[32].

It is easier to control pain in the ophthalmic division of the trigeminal nerve than in the circumoral region, as ophthalmic division trigeminal fibres extend more caudally in the nucleus, and are also located more laterally. As only nociceptive fibres are lesioned, nucleus caudalis DREZ avoids complications such as corneal anaesthesia and anaesthesia dolorosa, which may occur with more peripherally denervating procedures. The spinocerebellar tract overlies the spinal trigeminal tract and nucleus, and can be damaged during nucleus caudalis DREZ, causing ataxia.

In summary, nucleus caudalis DREZ has a role in the management of facial pain refractory to other therapies, but it is a major neurosurgical procedure with associated morbidity and mortality rates. As a result, mesencephalic tractomy remains the mainstay of neurosurgical ablative strategies for head and neck cancer pain.

Mesencephalic (midbrain) tractotomy

Mesencephalic tractotomy is the intracranial equivalent of cordotomy, and is the procedure of choice for cancer-related pain which extends above the C5 dermatome. It aims to interrupt fibres carrying somatic pain to the thalamus and higher centres. Lesioning of the mesencephalon was first described by Spiegel et al. in 1948 and the target was the spinothalamic, trigeminothalamic, and spinoreticular tracts[33]. Within the mesencephalic tegmentum, the periaqueductal grey, trigeminothalamic tract, and spinothalamic tract are located from medial to lateral, thus enabling specific targetting of the spinothalamic tract.

Technique

This procedure is performed under local anaesthetic, and stereotactic localization is achieved using magnetic resonance imaging. The target lies at a level between the superior and inferior colliculi, in the same coronal plane as the aqueduct, and 5–10 mm from the midline on the contralateral side of the symptoms. Most commonly, it is performed for unilateral pain, but lesions can be made bilaterally, as it avoids the risk of respiratory depression associated with bilateral anterolateral cordotomy. Intraoperative electrophysiological confirmation of electrode position is mandatory to avoid damage to adjacent structures, including the colliculi and lemniscal tracts. Stimulation of the target should cause a well-localized sensation of pain or temperature in the contralateral face or body. Following surgery, the patient should be closely monitored for several hours. The development of hypertension may be an early indicator of a postoperative haematoma.

Results

Mesencephalic tractotomy is useful in pain originating in the face, neck, or shoulder. Frank et al. treated 109 cancer patients with rostral pain, and found that 83.5 per cent were pain-free until death, up to 7 months later[34]. Shieff and Nashold reported few complications and effective analgesia in 67 per cent of patients studied[35]. Complications include disorders of ocular mobility (transient diplopia affects over 50 per cent of patients, resulting from injury to the ocular nuclei, medial longitudinal fasciculus, or superior colliculus) and anaesthesia dolorosa (medial lemniscal injury). Fountas et al. recently described a technique using high-resolution MRI guidance and a side-searching intraoperative electrode to enable topographic mapping of the spinothalamic tract[36]. These advances in technology may enable mesencephalic tractotomy to be performed more effectively and with a lower incidence of side effects.

Hypophysectomy

Destruction of the pituitary gland was a procedure used in the 1970s and 1980s for treatment of cancer-related pain. Although relief is perhaps greater in cases of pain caused by hormonally dependent cancer, relief also occurs in non-hormone-dependent disease. It has recently undergone resurgence with the use of radiosurgical hypophysectomy.

The mechanism by which pituitary lesions mediate analgesia is unclear. It seems likely that pituitary ablations cause alterations in hypothalamic–pituitary interactions. Following ablation, there are morphological changes in the posterior medial hypothalamus, particularly the supraoptic and paraventricular nuclei. These areas are known to project to anti-nociceptive brain regions[37].

Technique

The commonest method in use involves insertion of a needle into the sellar via a transnasal, transphenoidal route under image intensification. Once in position, 1–2ml of absolute alcohol is instilled. Other techniques include open or endoscopic transphenoidal hypophysectomy or percutaneous stereotactic methods, again using alcohol or radiofrequency electrodes.

Results

Corssen et al. used alcohol adenolysis in 100 patients and found excellent analgesia in approximately 60 per cent. The mean duration of analgesia was 3 months and repeated injections were frequently required. Complications include a 2–5 per cent mortality rate, diabetes insipidus (5–20 per cent), CSF leaks (10 per cent), and visual fields defects (10 per cent but usually temporary)[38].

Other studies have also demonstrated that pain relief is usually short-term, lasting less than 3 to 4 months. In one review[39], 41 per cent to 95 per cent of patients with hormone-dependent cancer reported relief, in comparison with 69 per cent of patients with non-hormone-dependent cancer; 67 per cent to 84 per cent of patients probably enjoyed short-term relief[39].

Recently, radiosurgical ablation of the pituitary gland has been reported to be effective in the treatment of cancer pain. Hayashi et al. took 9 patients with bony metastases and performed radiosurgical ablation, taking care to minimize the dose to the optic nerve. Within several days of the procedure, analgesia was obtained in all 9 patients. The duration of efficacy was up to 2 years and there were no adverse effects[40]. It seems likely that radiosurgical hypophysectomy may become an important option for cancer pain in the future.

Medial thalamotomy and pulvinotomy

The thalamus is the termination site of the spinothalamic tract. The lateral thalamus is principally involved with sensory discrimination aspects of pain, and its nuclei include the ventral posteromedial and posterolateral nuclei and the ventral anterior nuclei. The medial thalamus mediates affective responses, and its nuclei comprise the large dorsomedial nuclei and the smaller parafascicular and centromedian nuclei.

The output of the medial thalamus is mainly directed to the cingulate gyrus (Brodmann area 24). Neurons located within the medial thalamic nuclei have large, usually bilateral receptive fields, suggesting that they cannot localize pain. Primate studies have suggested that these neurons can distinguish between different stimulus intensities, implying a role in the perception of pain intensity[41].

The pulvinar is part of the lateral group of thalamic nuclei situated at the posterior aspect of the thalamus. The pulvinar seems involved in appreciation of painful stimuli. It has interconnections with other thalamic nuclei and also connects to the temporal lobe and post-central gyrus.

Technique

The technique of thalamotomy and pulvinotomy involves the use of stereotactic frames, which are affixed to the patient's skull using local anaesthesia. Fine-cut axial CT or MR images are then obtained for lesion placement. In the operating theatre, a burr hole is then planned and drilled, again using local anaesthesia. A thermal electrode is then introduced and electrophysiological testing performed to determine the site prior to definitive lesioning. More recently, the Leksell gamma knife has been increasingly used to perform destructive thalamotomies. It is an excellent radiosurgical target because it is large and devoid of specific eloquent contents.

Results

Young et al. reported 24 unilateral gamma knife thalamotomies, with 27 per cent abolition of pain and a further 33 per cent rate of reduction of pain to half of its original intensity[42]. Jeanmonod et al. found that medial thalamotomy produced adequate analgesia in 67 per cent of 69 patients with widespread body pain, without complications[43]. Whittle and Jenkinson performed combined anteromedial pulvinotomy and medial thalamotomy for malignant intractable pain in 2 patients, both of whom were afforded significant amelioration of their symptoms in the weeks before death[44]. Sweet also suggested that combination lesioning of the medial thalamus with the pulvinar may produce better results[45]. Davis et al. found that both medial and lateral lesions of the thalamus provide around 60 per cent pain relief for cancer pain, but lesions of the lateral thalamus have a higher risk of adverse effects; these include hemiparesis, cognitive disorders, seizures, and speech disturbances[46].

In conclusion, lesions of the medial thalamus, especially when combined with pulvinar lesioning, appear to provide effective analgesia with minimal side effects. The analgesia obtained is generally short-lived, its effects waning after 3 to 6 months [47]. It is therefore ideally suited to patients in the terminal stages of malignancy.

Cingulotomy

The anterior cingulate gyrus incorporates motor, affective, memory, and nociceptive functions, and has extensive connections with the basal ganglia, insular, somatosensory, and motor cortices. Nociceptive stimuli produce bilateral activation of the cingulate gyrus [48]. A series of stereotactic lesions of the cingulate gyrus were first described by Foltz and White in 1962 and it was noted that such lesions did not abolish pain but rather modified the affective response of the patient [49].

Technique

Several recent studies have used MRI-guided techniques to lesion the cingulate gyrus bilaterally. A stereotactic frame is attached to the head of the patient and then MR imaging is performed. The patient is transferred to the operating theatre, where the lesioning is performed accurately via a twist-drill hole. The target is classically 20–30 mm posterior to the anterior tip of the lateral ventricles, 1.5 mm lateral to the midline, and 15 mm superior to the roof of the lateral ventricles [50]. A radiofrequency ablation also is commonly used. Owing to the low morbidity of these techniques, there is no role for an open surgical ablation of the cingulate gyrus.

Results

In a series by Wilkinson and colleagues, 28 patients with severe chronic pain underwent bilateral cingulate gyrus ablation. He reported a 72 per cent improvement in pain, with a 40 per cent incidence of subsequent seizures. Fifty-six per cent of the patients felt that the cingulotomy was beneficial overall[51]. Hassenbusch *et al.* took four patients with advanced malignancy refractory to all treatments except high-dose intravenous morphine. The diffuse nature of the pain precluded other techniques of neurosurgical ablation. They underwent bilateral cingulotomy, and all four patients noticed immediate pain relief. In each, the persistent analgesia over the ensuing months enabled a reduction in morphine dosage, with a consequent improvement in their cognition[52].

Complications of cingulotomy include seizures, hemiparesis from intracerebral haematomas, neuropsychiatric disturbances, and a low mortality risk. However, recent studies have shown that bilateral cingulate gyrus lesion result in only mild cognitive impairment[53]. Cingulotomy tends to produce deficits of focus and sustained attention, with self-initiated response being the most impaired modality.

In summary, bilateral cingulotomy remains a valuable option for the palliation of diffuse pain in advanced malignancy. It appears to work by modulating the affective response to painful stimuli. Potential side effects include seizure activity and the induction of a mild level of executive dysfunction.

References

1. Sundaresan, N., DiGiacinto, G.V., and Hughes, J.E. (1989). Neurosurgery in the treatment of cancer pain. *Cancer*, **63** (Suppl 11), 2365–77.

2. Cherny, N.I., Arbit, E., and Jain, S. (1996). Invasive techniques in the management of cancer pain. *Hematology/Oncology Clinics of North America*, **10**(1), 121–37.

3. Burchiel, K.J., Johans, T.J., and Ochoa, J. (1993). The surgical treatment of painful traumatic neuromas. *Journal of Neurosurgery*, **78**(5), 714–9.

4. Wall, P. (1964). Presynaptic control of impulses at the first central synapse in the cutaneous pathway. In *Physiology of Neurons* (ed. J. Eccles), pp. 92–118. Elsevier.

5. Sindou, M., Jeanmonod, D., and Mertens, P. (1990). Ablative neurosurgical procedures for the treatment of chronic pain. *Neurophysiologie Clinique*, **20**(5), 399–423.

6. Nashold, B.S., Jr. (1981). Modification of DREZ lesion technique. *Journal of Neurosurgery*, **55**(6), 1012.

7. Levy, W.J. *et al.* (1983). Laser-induced dorsal root entry zone lesions for pain control. Report of three cases. *Journal of Neurosurgery*, **59**(5), 884–6.

8. Powers, S.K. (1984). Laser-induced dorsal root entry zone lesions for pain control. *Journal of Neurosurgery*, **60**(4), 871–2.

9. M Sindou, A.D. (1988). Spinal cord ablation procedures for pain. In *Proceedings of the Fifth World Congress on Pain* (ed. A. Dunber), pp. 477–95. Elsevier.

10. Armour, D. (1927). Surgery of spinal cord and its membranes. *Lancet*, **ii**, 691–7.

11. Al-Chaer, E.D. *et al.* (1996). Visceral nociceptive input into the ventral posterolateral nucleus of the thalamus: a new function for the dorsal column pathway. *Journal of Neurophysiology*, **76**(4), 2661–74.

12. Al-Chaer, E.D. *et al.* (1996). Pelvic visceral input into the nucleus gracilis is largely mediated by the postsynaptic dorsal column pathway. *Journal of Neurophysiology*, **76**(4), 2675–90.

13. Al-Chaer, E.D. and Traub, R.J. (2002). Biological basis of visceral pain: recent developments. *Pain*, **96**(3), 221–5.

14. Al-Chaer, E.D., Westlund, K.N., and Willis, W.D. (1997). Nucleus gracilis: an integrator for visceral and somatic information. *Journal of Neurophysiology*, **78**(1), 521–7.

15. Nauta, H.J. *et al.* (2000). Punctate midline myelotomy for the relief of visceral cancer pain. *Journal of Neurosurgery*, **92**(Suppl 2), 125–30.

16. Hwang, S.L. *et al.* (2004). Punctate midline myelotomy for intractable visceral pain caused by hepatobiliary or pancreatic cancer. *Journal of Pain and Symptom Management*, **27**(1), 79–84.

17. Spiller, W. (1912). The treatment of persistent pain of organic origin in the lower part of the body by division of the antero-lateral column of the spinal cord. *Journal of American Medical Association*, **58**, 1489–90.

18. Collis, J.S., Jr. (1963). Anterolateral Cordotomy by an Anterior Approach: Report of a Case. *Journal of Neurosurgery*, **20**, 445–6.

19. Cloward, R.B. (1964). Cervical Chordotomy by the Anterior Approach. Technique and Advantages. *Journal of Neurosurgery*, **21**, 19–25.

20. Mullan, S. *et al.* (1963). Percutaneous Interruption of Spinal-Pain Tracts by Means of a Strontium 90 Needle. *Journal of Neurosurgery*, **20**, 931–9.

21. Rosomoff, H.L., Brown, C.J., and Sheptak, P. (1965). Percutaneous radiofrequency cervical cordotomy: technique. *Journal of Neurosurgery*, **23**(6), 639–44.

22. Kanpolat, Y. *et al.* (1995). CT-guided pain procedures for intractable pain in malignancy. *Acta Neurochirurgie Supplement*, **64**, 88–91.

23. Kanpolat, Y. (2007). Percutaneous destructive pain procedures on the upper spinal cord and brain stem in cancer pain: CT-guided techniques, indications and results. *Advances and Technical Standards in Neurosurgery*, **32**, 147–73.

24. Lahuerta, J. *et al.* (1994). Percutaneous cervical cordotomy: a review of 181 operations on 146 patients with a study on the location of "pain fibers" in the C-2 spinal cord segment of 29 cases. *Journal of Neurosurgery*, **80**(6), 975–85.

25. McGirt, M.J. *et al.* (2002). MRI-guided frameless stereotactic percutaneous cordotomy. *Stereotactic and Functional Neurosurgery*, **78**(2), 53–63.

26. Crul, B.J. *et al.* (2005). The present role of percutaneous cervical cordotomy for the treatment of cancer pain. *Journal of Headache and Pain*, **6**(1), 24–9.

27. Sanders, M. and Zuurmond, W. (1995). Safety of unilateral and bilateral percutaneous cervical cordotomy in 80 terminally ill cancer patients. *Journal of Clinical Oncology*, **13**(6), 1509–12.

28. Nagaro, T. *et al.* (2001). New pain following cordotomy: clinical features, mechanisms, and clinical importance. *Journal of Neurosurgery*, **95**(3), 425–31.

29. Romanelli, P., Esposito, V., and Adler, J. (2004). Ablative procedures for chronic pain. *Neurosurgery Clinics of North America*, **15**(3), 335–42.

30. Crue, B.L. *et al.* (1967). Percutaneous trigeminal tractotomy. Case report-utilizing stereotactic radiofrequency lesion. *Bulletin of Los Angeles Neurological Society*, **32**(2), 86–92.

31. Osenbach. Nontrigeminal Craniofacial Pain Syndromes. In *Neurosurgical Pain Management* (ed. K. A.Follett), p. 92. Elsevier.

32. Gorecki, J.P. *et al.* (1995). The Duke experience with nucleus caudalis DREZ coagulation. *Stereotactic and Functional Neurosurgery*, **65**(1–4), 111–6.

33. Spiegel, E.A., Wycis, H.T. *et al.* (1948). Stereoencephalotomy. *Transactions of the American Neurological Association*, **73**(73 Annual Meet), 160–3.

34. Frank, F., Fabrizi, A.P., and Gaist, G. (1989). Stereotactic mesencephalic tractotomy in the treatment of chronic cancer pain. *Acta Neurochirurgica (Wien)*, **99**(1–2), 38–40.

35. Shieff, C. and Nashold, B.S., Jr. (1990). Stereotactic mesencephalotomy. *Neurosurgery Clinics of North America*, **1**(4), 825–39.

36. Fountas, K.N. *et al.* (2004). MR-based stereotactic mesencephalic tractotomy. *Stereotactic and Functional Neurosurgery*, **82**(5–6), 230–4.

37. Takeda, F. *et al.* (1983). Alterations of hypothalamopituitary interaction and pain threshold following pituitary neuroadenolysis–a clinical

investigation of the mechanism of cancer pain relief. *Neurologia Medico-Chirurgica (Tokyo)*, **23**(7), 551–60.

38. Corssen, G. *et al.* (1977). Alcohol-induced adenolysis of the pituitary gland: a new approach to control of intractable cancer pain. *Anesthesia and Analgesia*, **56**(3), 414–21.

39. Gybels, J.M. and Sweet W.H. (1989). Neurosurgical treatment of persistent pain. Physiological and pathological mechanisms of human pain. *Pain Headache*, **11**, 1–402.

40. Hayashi, M. *et al.* (2002). Gamma knife surgery for cancer pain-pituitary gland-stalk ablation: a multicenter prospective protocol since 2002. *Journal of Neurosurgery*, **97**(Suppl 5), 433–7.

41. Bushnell, M.C. and Duncan, G.H. (1987). Mechanical response properties of ventroposterior medial thalamic neurons in the alert monkey. *Experimental Brain Research*, **67**(3), 603–14.

42. Young, R.F. *et al.* (1995). Technique of stereotactic medial thalamotomy with the Leksell Gamma Knife for treatment of chronic pain. *Neurological Research*, **17**(1), 59–65.

43. Jeanmonod, D., Magnin, M., and Morel, A. (1994). Chronic neurogenic pain and the medial thalamotomy. *Schweizerische Rundschau Fur Medizin Praxis*, **83**(23), 702–7.

44. Whittle, I.R. and Jenkinson, J.L. (1995). CT-guided stereotactic antero-medial pulvinotomy and centromedian-parafascicular thalamotomy for intractable malignant pain. *British Journal of Neurosurgery*, **9**(2), 195–200.

45. Sweet, W.H. (1980). Central mechanisms of chronic pain (neuralgias and certain other neurogenic pain). *Res Publ Assoc Res Nerv MentDis*, **58**, 287–303.

46. Davis, K.D. *et al.* (1998). Brain targets for pain control. *Stereotactic and Functional Neurosurgery*, **71**(4), 173–9.

47. Laitinen, L.V. (1988). Psychosurgery today. *Acta Neurochirurgica. Supplementum (Wien)*, **44**, 158–62.

48. Vogt, B.A., Derbyshire, S., and Jones, A.K. (1996). Pain processing in four regions of human cingulate cortex localized with co-registered PET and MR imaging. *European Journal of Neuroscience*, **8**(7), 1461–73.

49. Foltz, E.L. and White, L.E., Jr. (1962). Pain "relief" by frontal cingulumotomy. *Journal of Neurosurgery*, **19**, 89–100.

50. Ballantine, H.T., Jr. *et al.* (1987). Treatment of psychiatric illness by stereotactic cingulotomy. *Biological Psychiatry*, **22**(7), 807–19.

51. Wilkinson, H.A., Davidson, K.M., and Davidson, R.I. (1999). Bilateral anterior cingulotomy for chronic noncancer pain. *Neurosurgery*, **45**(5), 1129–34, discussion 1134–6.

52. Hassenbusch, S.J., Pillay, P.K., and Barnett, G.H. (1990). Radiofrequency cingulotomy for intractable cancer pain using stereotaxis guided by magnetic resonance imaging. *Neurosurgery*, **27**(2), 220–3.

53. Cohen, R.A. *et al.* (2001). Emotional and personality changes following cingulotomy. *Emotion*, **1**(1), 38–50.

10.1.11 Treating pain with transcutaneous electrical nerve stimulation

Michaela Bercovitch and Nathan I. Cherny

Transcutaneous electrical nerve stimulation (TENS) is a way of controlling pain through the 'gate' theory, where it is believed, selective electrical stimulation of certain nerve fibres block signals carrying pain impulses to the brain. It is usually administered by physiotherapists, upon referral by a physician. However, it is also employed directly by some physicians and in some hospital settings. Though it is commonly employed, and advocated by enthusiasts, firm evidence supporting its efficacy is scant.

The historical use of electricity to relieve pain

Pain has always been part of the human experience, and humans have always endeavoured to alleviate it[1]. One of the earliest records of pain relief, from the fifth dynasty in Egypt (2500 BC), depicts the use of Malapterurus Electricus, a fish with electrical properties, to relieve pain. Electricity as treatment for pain was also found during the Hippocratic era (400 BC).

The first written record of treating pain with electricity was attributed to Scribonius Largus (AD 46)[2]. In 1759, John Wesely[3] described the use of electrotherapy for pain of sciatica, headache, gout, and kidney stones. Two centuries later, Sarlandiere used the effect of electrical stimulus on acupuncture points in treating pain of rheumatism, gout, neuralgia, and migraine headaches[4]. During the 18th and 19th centuries, galvanic sources were also used to relieve pain. In the 20th century, electroanalgesia therapy became very popular, and was applied, in such diverse situations as dental extraction, labour pain, or amputation[5,6].

Theoretical basis of TENS analgesia

Pain is defined as a sensory and emotional experience associated with total or partial tissue damage, or described in terms of such damage[7]. To better understand the mechanism of pain relief with TENS, a short description of pain mechanisms is useful.

The anatomy of pain transmission is described in Fig. 10.1.11.1.

The Gate Control Theory, proposed in 1965 by Melzack and Wall, emphasized the modulation of inputs in the spinal dorsal horn and the dynamic role of the brain in processing pain[8]. The proposed mechanism of pain transmission is based on the existence of a 'barrier' between A delta fibres and C fibres that project to the substantia gelatinosa of the dorsal horn and synapses with the first central transmission cell—T-cell. The T-cell receives the impulses from peripheral fibres and activates the response and perception system. According to this theory, high-level stimulation of A delta fibres has an inhibitory influence effectively 'closing the gate' of the T-cells of the ascending spinothalamic tract. Opening the gate is a result of high levels of activity from the C fibres producing excitation of T-cells and of biophysical mechanisms that lead to the perception of pain (Fig. 10.1.11.2).

Based on the gate control theory, it was postulated that using a low-level electrical stimulus will preferentially activate larger A-delta fibres. These fibres have a relatively low electrical threshold and may subsequently activate the small inhibitory interneurons of the substantia gelatinosa to effectively reduce the small fibre nociceptive input[9].

In 1968, Melzack and Casey introduced a new concept to the basic gate theory— 'the central control trigger.' According to this theory, dorsal column stimulation and spinothalamic stimulation may activate descending inhibitory pathways from the reticular and limbic systems which, subsequently, modify the sensory input at the level of the dorsal horn[10]. Thus TENS may act, at least in part, through the stimulation of large afferent fibres acting on the central control trigger, to modulate the input through descending pathways.

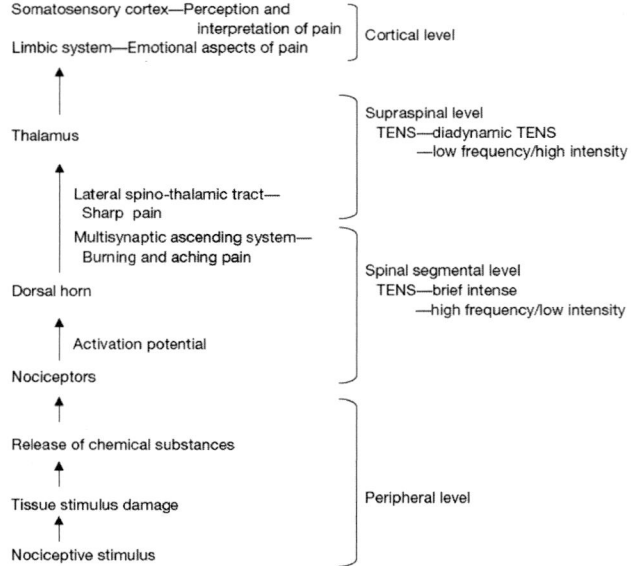

Figure 10.1.11.1 The anatomy of pain transmission.

Electrical stimulation may also modulate the activity of the opioid-mediated descending inhibitory pathways. Basbaum and Fields described opioid-mediated inhibitory descending pathways from the nucleus reticularis gigantocellularis (RGC) through periaqueductal grey (PAG) nuclei are transmitted to the dorsal horn via the nucleus raphe magnus and the nucleus magnocellularis[11]. According to this theory, afferent input from small fibres is transmitted through ascending pathways to the thalamus and nucleus RGC. By the stimulation of PAG it is possible to generate analgesia, and it is hypothesized that TENS may act by excitation of the brain stem nuclei.

Activation of the sympathetic nervous system to produce changes in tissue chemistry is another mechanism proposed for relieving pain. Electricity used on the painful area produces vasodilatation via cholinergic receptors. Blood flow to the damaged tissues increases, and this may help dissipate pain-producing substances.

Based on work in animal models it has recently been proposed that TENS can reduce hyperalgesia via an effect on opioid receptors

and this effect is frequency dependent. Using antagonist studies in cats, researchers demonstrated that high-frequency TENS activates the μ opioid receptors, and that low frequencies activate delta receptors[12].

Early development of TENS

Two years after the Gate Theory was published, Shealy and his colleagues tried, and succeeded, to manage intractable back pain by stimulating the dorsal column in cats. In 1967, they implanted the first spinal cord stimulator in a patient's dorsal column. This procedure takes into consideration that this region of the medulla is rich in ascending collaterals of the large efferent A-delta fibres. Following this success he began evaluating patients for dorsal column stimulator implantation[9]. As part of his evaluations, patients were tested for their tolerance of electrical stimulation using a TENS prototype. Many of the patients reported so much relief from the TENS itself that they never returned for the implant! In 1974, he took out a patent on TENS and thus began the development of TENS as a modality of pain treatment.

Structure of a TENS unit and principle of action

A simple TENS unit consists of a hand-held, battery-operated, electrical pulse generator and electrodes (Fig. 10.1.11.3). The common commercial apparatus has three different pulse patterns: continuous, pulsed (burst), and modulated (ramped). These provide a cyclic variation of pulse duration, frequency, or amplitude that may offer the patient more comfort.

Electro-therapeutic devices used for pain treatment may be low frequency (LF)—1 to 4 Hz—or high frequency (HF)—120 to 150 Hz. Some brands use low-frequency, high-intensity currents via electrodes applied to the skin over an 'acupuncture point', thus producing 'acupuncture-like TENS'.

Since the 1980s, a large number of such electrical stimulators have been developed, and along with them, a variety of techniques for chronic and even acute pain management. TENS models range from single-channel devices to multi-channel ones, with the single and dual models being battery operated (V battery). The multi-channel unit requires an electrical outlet connection.

The type of TENS unit is individualized to suit the patients prevailing condition. Mobile patients use a small single- or dual-channel unit (e.g., Unitouch® or the British Tenscare), which are as small as 5.5 cm and weigh 60 g, and are equipped with clips, which attach them to clothing. These units are less powerful, and are recommended for chronic pain such as arthritis. Most TENS apparatus today are constructed to offer variable intensity, pulse duration, and frequency[13]. Moreover, they offer a choice as to type of output: continuous, burst, or modulation (Fig.10.1.11.4).

Types of TENS administration

Conventional tens

The conventional apparatus contains electrodes made of electroconductive material (carbon-filled vinyl sheets). Electrodes are applied to designated areas on the skin called 'dermatomal points.' These dermatomal points are areas that receive their nerve supply from a specified spinal nerve. Activation of the TENS unit results in transmission of electrical pulses in the selected dermatomal nerves.

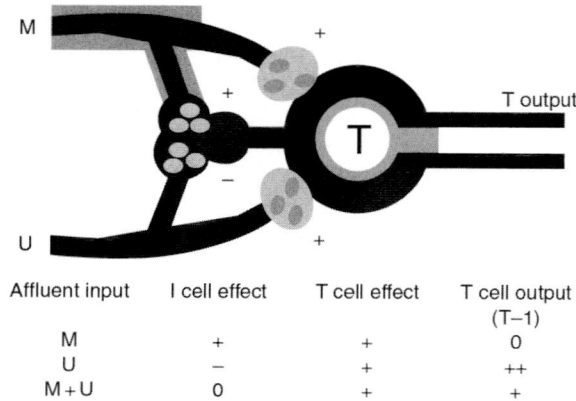

Figure 10.1.11.2 Schematic diagram of the components of the 'gate' in the dorsal horn of the spinal cord.

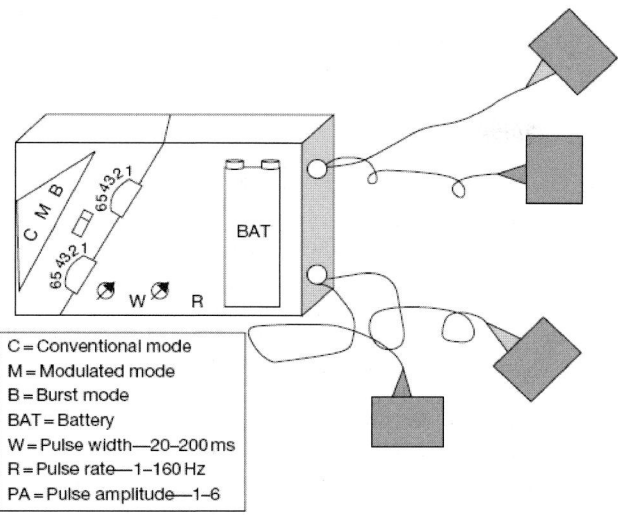

Figure 10.1.11.3 Transcutaneous electrical stimulation system.

There are four categories of anatomical sites to which the electrodes can be applied:

1 Close to the painful area. This stimulates the afferent sensory nerves that lead from the spinal cord to the painful area[14–16].

2 Over a peripheral nerve with cutaneous distribution in the painful area (e.g. radial nerve, ulnar nerve, peroneal nerve). In these cases, the electrodes should be placed along the more superficial course of the nerve[17]. This approach has been reported in the management of peripheral nerve injury and peripheral neuropathy[18–20].

3 Spinal nerve routes. Placing the electrodes paraspinally for stimulating the appropriate roots of spinal nerves, which supply a specific dermatomal or myotomal painful area[21].

4 Motor or trigger point placement. For stimulation of a specific group of skeletal muscles, tendons, joints, ligaments, periosteum[22,23].

Variants of conventional TENS

H-wave therapy (HWT)

HWT is a form of TENS designed to produce a localized effect on the conduction of underlying peripheral nerves, using a very specific pattern of stimulation. Stimulation is delivered using a fixed-pulse duration, a low-frequency range 2–60 Hz, and a biphasic exponentially decaying waveform[24]. In 1998, Julka *et al.* used HWT in patients with diabetic neuropathic pain, and reported reduced pain in 76 per cent of patients[25].

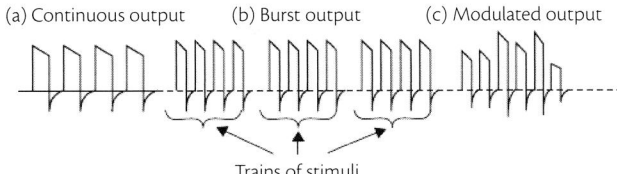

Figure 10.1.11.4 Illustration of (a) continuous, (b) burst, and (c) modulated types of output available on most TENS units. (Adapted with permission from Walsh, D.M. (1997). TENS modes available. In *TENS Clinical Applications and Related Theory*, 1st edition, p. 38. Churchill Livingstone, Edinburgh.)

Interferential current therapy (ICT)

ICT is a variation of TENS that incorporates amplitude modulation to decrease the discomfort of stimulating deeper tissues (e.g. muscle). Based on summation of two alternating current signals of slightly different frequency, resultant current consists of cyclical modulation of amplitude, based on the difference in frequency between the two signals. The current that is generated with modulating amplitude is alleged to more effectively penetrate the soft tissues while producing less discomfort at the skin surface[24].

Acupuncture-like TENS

This technique employs a low-frequency, high-intensity stimulus administered to 'acupuncture points' over the skin, without using needles (see Chapter 10.1.12). The stimulus produces paraesthesia and muscle contraction. It is hypothesized that it acts via the descending inhibitory pain pathways. The onset of analgesia is delayed, and lasts longer than using conventional TENS[25].

Percutaneous electrical nerve stimulation (PENS)

PENS involves the use of electrically stimulated acupuncture needles at 'acupuncture points' or at 'dermatomal points.' In a small anecdotal series, PENS has been reported to have an analgesic effect in cancer patients with bone metastases. In this case, the electrode needles are placed in the soft tissue and muscle surrounding bones, thus bypassing the resistance of the coetaneous barrier and delivering the electrical stimulus closer to nerve endings located in the soft tissue, muscles, and periosteum of the involved dermatomes[26]. Ahmed *et al.* report that two of three patients with bone pain who used PENS reported benefits from this technique[27]. Two patients with bone metastases reported significant pain relief, with a decreased need for analgesic drugs.

Efficacy of TENS therapy in cancer pain

The efficacy of TENS remains controversial. Beyond anecdotes and testimonials, there are very little data to support its utility in cancer pain. At best, it is advocated as an adjuvant approach to routine therapy[28]; at worst, it is an ineffectual therapy, no more effective than placebos[29].

The recent literature on TENS in cancer pain is sparse and anecdotal; it provides little substantive support for the effectiveness of this technique for this indication. In 1996, Khor *et al.* described a 39-year-old man with intractable metastatic femoral bone pain who received adjuvant therapy with TENS in addition to opioids[30]. In a survey of 20 patients with head and neck cancers, Chiarini *et al.* found that 60 per cent may have benefited from TENS, but only when the pain intensity is moderate or low[31]. As described earlier, Ahmed *et al.* reported their experience with percutaneous electrical stimulation in management of three patients with metastatic bone[28]. Finally, in a survey of analgesic techniques used in a sample of 593 cancer patients, 13 per cent received TENS as supportive therapy to systemic analgesia for nociceptive (1 per cent), neuropathic (6 per cent), and mixed (6 per cent) cancer pain[32].

While there is no good evidence of efficacy for chronic pain, some of the alternative long-term analgesic approaches often involve either similarly limited efficacy or serious adverse effects.

To its credit, TENS is unlikely to cause harm. If it is to be considered, TENS therapy should be undertaken with a realistic expectation of the results, and only continued after demonstrating a beneficial effect in that particular patient.

Efficacy of TENS in other chronic pain settings

Two Cochrane systematic reviews have addressed the use of TENS for 'chronic pain' and for 'chronic low-back pain.' Both of these systematic reviews found that the evidence for efficacy was somewhat suggestive of limited efficacy but, ultimately, inconclusive. Both reviews highlight the need for further evaluation of this approach in well-designed randomized studies[33,34].

Administration of TENS

The treating physician will select the appropriate device based on the patient's needs and on availability. Stimulation sites are selected as described earlier.

Selection of TENS parameters

After the optimal site has been found, the next step is to determine the best combination TENS electrical stimulation parameters to provide significant pain relief.

The output current of the TENS electrodes are characterized by:

* Frequency—the rate of change or the number of pulses delivered per second (measured in Hz).

* Amplitude (intensity)—the magnitude of current (measured in mA) and voltage (measured in V) applied by the TENS unit.

* Pulse duration (width)—measured in microseconds.

* Continuity—generated continuously or in bursts (trains of pulses or single pulses).

* Modulation—frequency, pulse duration, and amplitude change periodically.

* Current flow direction.

The TENS 'work modes' are combinations of these parameters. Common work modes include high-frequency continuous (50–200 Hz), low-frequency continuous (1–4 Hz), and high-frequency bursts in which the unit delivers brief bursts of high-frequency stimulation at a low frequency, i.e. 2 Hz. The selection of the most appropriate work mode is largely empirical.

Frequency The signal frequency for conventional TENS is in the range of 50 to 200 Hz. This gives the optimum presynaptic inhibition through the gate mechanism[9]. Theoretically, high-frequency TENS is used to stimulate the large A-delta nerve fibres (which feature fast conduction rates and short refractory periods) and low frequencies are used to stimulate Aδ and C fibres (which have slower conduction rates and longer refractory periods, lower-frequency pulses should be used). A study conducted by Gopalkrishnan et al.[35] indicated a significant relief of primary and secondary heat and mechanical hyperalgesia when using high-frequency TENS signals.

Intensity The conventional TENS uses low-intensity signals. In practice, intensity is adaptively set to a value that best fits the patient needs. While applying an incremental intensity TENS stimulus, the patient will be asked to report his or her sense of it. 'Vibration,' 'tapping,' and 'buzzing' are terms usually used by the patient in

relation with low-intensity stimulation. In general, the intensity should be set just below the pain threshold (when the patient reports discomfort) so that paraesthesiae are felt in the painful region. Sometimes discomfort appears after a variable time interval from starting the treatment. Therefore the patient's condition should be checked after about 10 min.

Current flow direction, pulse duration, and continuity In some TENS units the current flow between the TENS electrodes may be constant or change in a periodical or pulsed manner. Direct current (DC) describes a current constantly flowing in one direction, Alternating current (AC) flows continuously but periodically changes its direction and pulsed current is periodic rather than constant. Pulsed current may be monophasic with current flows in one direction or biphasic with two phases of opposite flowing current.

Modulation A periodical change in amplitude, frequency, or duration may have a positive effect on a patient's comfort and treatment efficiency. Some TENS units offer a continuous change programme that is said to overcome the nerve fibre adjustment to the stimulus, maintaining its 'alertness' to the treatment[36].

Guidelines for the application of TENS

1 Explain the technique to the patient.

2 Clean skin and hair and dry well.

3 Fix the electrode to the site of pain using hydrogel pads.

4 Assess the patient's sensation after 5 min and then again after 10 min of treatment and readapt the stimulus frequency and amplitude until pain threshold is reached such that the patient has sensation of paraesthesias are felt in the painful region.

5 Reassess the pain 30 min after beginning of treatment; if there is no analgesic effect, reevaluate placement of the electrodes.

6 If satisfactory analgesia is obtained, establish duration of daily treatment period for a trial of therapy.

7 Observe the appearance of the skin throughout treatment.

Once a successful strategy is identified, this treatment should be followed by a trial of therapy at home. If the response to the treatment is favourable, patients should then rent or purchase their own unit. TENS treatments may be used as long as it is effective. In some settings it is used on a fixed schedule, i.e. for 10–60 min three times per day. Other patients may use it on an 'as needed' basis.

Pain indications

Indications There is no evidence-based indication for the use of TENS in cancer patients. Given the lack of data, it is reasonable to consider a trial of therapy in patients who have achieved suboptimal outcomes from other evidence-based approaches. There are no data to indicate higher or lower likelihood of effect for different pain syndromes or mechanisms.

Contraindications TENS has minimal side effects and there are few contraindications. Documented contraindications include:

* Severe allodynia.

* Incompetent patient.

* Cardiac pacemakers.

◆ Allergic reactions of the skin to the tape or electrode gel.

◆ Patients suffering from epilepsy.

◆ During driving or operating machinery.

◆ During pregnancy.

Additionally, electrodes placement on the anterior aspect of the neck, over the carotid sinuses, and eyes is contraindicated.

The use of TENS for other indications

Since the early 1900s, the use of electro analgesia has undergone a long sequence of changes. Initially used only for pain management, TENS has also come to be used for its non-analgesic effects.

Chemotherapy-induced nausea and vomiting Beginning in 1989, the late Prof. Dundee demonstrated that electrical stimulation of the P6 acupuncture point has an antiemetic effect[37]. In 1991, McMillan et al. investigated the antiemetic effect of TENS applied to the P6 acupuncture point, in addition to ondansetron in a group of 16 cancer patients receiving chemotherapy. Results showed significantly less nausea and vomiting when TENS was added to the antiemetic drugs[38]. In the same year Dundee and colleagues compared the use of TENS and acupuncture as adjuvant treatment before cytotoxic treatment. They found benefits with TENS application in 77 per cent of administrations, with best results achieved by two-hourly self-administered treatments of 15-Hz TENS[37]. Furthermore, in 1999, Cancer Nursing published a randomized double blind study by Pearl et al. that demonstrated once again the use of a miniaturized portable TENS as an adjuvant to standard antiemetic therapy for control of nausea and vomiting induced by cisplatin-based chemotherapy in 42 gynaecology patients[39].

In 2003, Treish et al. used the Reliefband, a device that delivers electrical pulses in a slow and weak manner, to the P6 point for treatment of nausea and vomiting due to chemotherapy and other medical causes. The Reliefband incorporates two metallic electrodes into a wristband device, and the electrical output may be controlled by the patient up to 10–35 mA/pulse. Treish et al. proposed a randomized, prospective, double-blind, placebo-controlled study to demonstrate the efficacy of the device when used as an addition to standard antiemetic treatment[40].

Lymphoedema In 1995, Waller and Bercovitch used TENS for pain control in a patient after mastectomy for breast cancer who presented with painful lymphoedema. A considerable reduction in the degree of lymphoedema was observed after 2 days of systematic application. Two subsequent studies demonstrated the effectiveness of TENS application on lymphoedematous limbs (arms and legs). In 1996, TENS was used for the relief of facial pitting oedema of one patient, using one channel and two electrodes. After 24 h there was a substantial reduction in the facial oedema. Further methodological research is needed[41].

Wound healing—ulcers In recent decades, many proponents have used electrical stimulation as a technique to promote wound healing, based on the theory that electrical stimulation may: increase ATP concentration in the skin; increase DNA synthesis; attract epithelial cells and fibroblasts to wound sites; accelerate the recovery of damaged neural tissue; reduce oedema; increase blood flow; or inhibit pathogenesis. The evidence for efficacy is scant[42–45] and it is not an approved indication.

Conclusions

Accumulated anecdotal evidence suggests that TENS may have a role in relieving pain in general and cancer pain in particular. There is, however little substantiated evidence to support this belief. Given the potential for patient benefit and its low intrinsic morbidity, it can be adopted as a trial of therapy for patients with chronic pain. When it is considered, TENS therapy should be undertaken with a realistic expectation of the results, and only continued after demonstrating a beneficial effect in that particular patient.

References

1. Meryl, R.G. (2000). Electrotherapy in rehabilitation. In *TENS for management of pain and sensory pathology*, pp. 149–196. FA Davis Company, Philadelphia.

2. Schonoch, W. (1912–1913). Die rezept sammlung des Scribonius. Jena: Baken museum of electricity in life. Mineaplis, MN.

3. Wesley, J. (1760). *The desideratum: or electricity made plain and useful.* W Flexney, London.

4. Sarlandiere, J.B. (1825). *Memoires sur l'electro-puncture.* Delaunay, Paris.

5. Burton, C. (1975). Dorsal column stimulation: optimization of application. *Surgical Neurology*, **4**, 169–77.

6. Burton, C. and Maurer, D.D. (1997). An assessment of the efficacy of physical therapy and physical modalities for the control of chronic musculoskeletal pain. *Pain*, **71**, 5–23.

7. Merskey et al. (1979). Lecture delivered at the IASP Convention. Proceedings of IASP.

8. Melzack, R. (1993). Past, present and future pain. *Canadian Journal of Experimental Psychology*, **47**, 615–29.

9. Shealy, C.N., Mortimer, J.T., and Reswich, J.B. (1967). Electrical inhibition of pain by stimulation of the dorsal column: preliminary clinical reports. *Anesthesia and Analgesia*, **45**, 489.

10. Melzack, R. and Casey, K.L. (1968). Sensory motivational and central control determinants of pain. In *The skin senses* (ed. D.R. Kenshalo). Charles C Thomas, Springfield, [Il].

11. Basbaum, A.I. and Fields, H.L. (1978). Endogenous pain control mechanisms: review and hypothesis. *Annual Journal of Neurology*, **4**, 451.

12. Kalra, A., Urban, M.O., and Sluka, K.A. (2001). Blockade of opioid receptors in rostral ventral medulla prevents antihyperalgesia produced by transcutaneous electrical nerve stimulation (TENS). *Journal of Pharmacology and Experimental Therapeutics*, **298**, 257–63.

13. Stux, G. and Pomeranz, B. (1995). *Basics of acupuncture.* 3rd edition. Spinger-Verlag, Berlin.

14. Ebersold, M., Laws, E., Stonnington, H. *et al.* (1976). Transcutaneous electrical nerve stimulation for treatment of chronic pain: A preliminary report. *Surgical Neurology*, **4**, 96.

15. Linzer, M. and Long, D.M. (1976). Transcutaneous neural stimulation for relief of pain. *IEEE Trans Biomedical Engineering*, **23**, 341.

16. Loesor, J.D., Black, R.G., and Christman, A. (1975). A relief of pain by transcutaneous stimulation. *Journal of Neurosurgery*, **42**, 308.

17. Berlandt, S.R. (1984). Method of determining optimal stimulation sites for transcutaneous nerve stimulation. *Physical Therapy*, **64**, 924.

18. Picaza, J.A., Cannon, B.V., Hunter, S.E. *et al.* (1975). Pain supression by peripheral stimulation, Part I. Observation with transcutaneous stimuli. *Surgical Neurology*, **4**, 105.

19. Sweet, W.H. and Wepsic, J.G. (1968). Treatment of chronic pain by stimulation of Primary afferent neuron. *Transactions of the American Neurological Association*, **93**, 103.

20. Mannheimer, J.S. (1978). Electrode placements for transcutaneous electrical nerve stimulation. *Physical Therapy*, **58**, 1455.

21. Melzack, R., Stillwell, D.M., and Fox, E.J. (1977). Trigger points and accupuncture points for pain:correlations and implications. *Pain*, **3**, 3–23.

22. Laitinen, J. (1976). Acupuncture and transcutaneous electrical stimulation in the treatment of chronic sacrolumbalgia and ischialgia. *American Journal of Chinese Medicine*, **4**(2), 169–75.

23. Walsh, D.M. (1997). *TENS Physiological Principles and Stimulation Parameters. The clinical application of TENS and Related theory*, pp. 25–40. Churchill Livingstone, Edinbrough.

24. White, P.F., Li, S., and Kiu, J.W. (2001). Electroanalgesia: its role in acute and chronic pain management. *Anesthesia and Analgesia*, **92**, 505–13.

25. Julka, I.S., Alvaro, M., and Kumar, D. (1998). Beneficial effects of electrical stimulation on neuropathic symptoms in diabetic patients. *Journal of Foot and Ankle Surgery*, **37**, 191–4.

26. Paul, F.W., Philips, J., Thimoty, B.S. *et al.* (1999). *Bulletin of the American Pain Society*, 9.

27. Ahmed, H.E., Craig, W.F., White, P.F. *et al.* (1998). Percutaneous electrical nerve stimulation (PENS) a complementary therapy for the management of pain secondary to bone metastasis. *The Clinical Journal of Pain*, **14**, 320–3.

28. Wall, P.D. and Sweet, W.H. (1967). Temporary abolition of pain in man. *Science*, **155**, 108–9.

29. Lewis, B., Lewis, D., and Cumming, G. (1994). The comparative analgesic efficacy of transcutaneous electrical nerve stimulation and a non-steroidal anti-inflamatory drug for pain osteoarthritis. *British Journal of Rheumatology*, **33**, 455–60.

30. Khor, K.E. and Dittor, J.N. (1996). Femoral nerve blockade in the mutlidisciplinary management of intractable localized pain due to metastatic tumor. A case report. *Journal of Pain and Symptom Management*, **11**(1), 56–7.

31. Chiarini, L., Stacca, R., Bertoldi, C. *et al.* (1997). Management of facial pain resulting from cancer in oral and maxillofacial surgery. *Minerva-Stomatologica*, **46**(1–2), 27–38.

32. Grond, S., Radbruch, L., Meusner, T. *et al.* (1999). Assessment of treatment of neuropathic cancer pain following WHO guidelines. *Pain*, **79**(1), 15–20.

33. Carroll, D., Moore, R.A., McQuay, H.J. *et al.* (2001). Transcutaneous electrical nerve stimulation (TENS) for chronic pain. *Cochrane Database of Systematic Reviews*, **3**, CD003222.

34. Khadilkar, A., Milne, S., Brosseau, L. *et al.* (2005). Transcutaneous electrical nerve stimulation (TENS) for chronic low-back pain. *Cochrane Database of Systematic Reviews* **3**, CD003008.

35. Gopalkrishnan, P. and Sulka, K.A. (2000). Effect of varying frequency, intensity and pulse duration of TENS on primary hyperalgesia in inflamed rats. *Archives of Physical Medicine and Rehabilitation*.

36. Johnson, M.I., Ashton, C.H., Bousfeld, D.R. *et al.* (1991). Analgesic effects of different pulse patterns of transcutaneous electrical nerve stimulation on cold-induced pain in normal subjects. *Journal of Psychosomatic Research*, **35**(2/3), 313–21.

37. Dundee, J.W., Ghaly, R.G., Bill, K.M. *et al.* (1989). Effect of stimulation of the P-6 anti-emetic point on post operative nausea and vomiting. *British Journal of Anaesthesia*, **63**, 612–8.

38. McMillan, C., Dundee, J.W., and Abraham, W.P. (1991). Enhancement of the antiemetic action of ondasetron by Transcutaneous Electical Stimulation of the P6 anti-emetic point in patients having highly anti-emetic citotoxic drugs. *British Journal of Cancer*, **64**, 971–2.

39. Pearl, M.L., Fisher, M., McCauley, D.L. *et al.* (1999). Transcutaneous electrical nerve stimulation as an adjunct for controlling chemotherapy induced nausea and vomiting in gynecologic oncology patients. *Cancer Nursing*, **22**(4), 307–11.

40. Treish, I., Shord, S., Valgus, J. *et al.* (2003). Randomized double-blind study of the Reliefband as an adjunct to standard antiemetics in patients receiving moderately-high to highly emetogenic chemotherapy. *Supportive Care in Cancer*, **11**(8), 516–21.

41. Waller, A. and Bercovitch, M. (2000). *Treatment of lymphoedema with TENS. Lymphoedema*, pp. 27–184. Radcliffe Medical Press, Oxford.

42. Kaada, B. (1983). Promoted healing of chronic ulceration by Transcutaneous Nerve Stimulation (TNS). *VASA*, **12**, 262–9.

43. Feedar, J.A., Kloth, L.C., and Gentzkow, G.D. (1992). Chronic dermal ulcer healing enchanced with monophasic pulsed electrical stimulation. *Physical Therapy*, **71**(9), 639–49.

44. Huoghton, P.E., Kincaid, C.B., Lowell, M. *et al.* (2003). Effect of electrical stimulation on chronic leg ulcer size and appearance. *Physical Therapy*, **83**(1), 17–28.

45. Wood, J.M., Evans, P.E. 3rd, Schallreuter, K.U. *et al.* (1993). A multicenter study on the use of pulsed low intensity direct current for healing chronic stage II and stage III decubitus ulcers. *Archives of Dermatology*, **129**(8), 999–1009.

10.1.12 **Acupuncture**

Jacqueline Filshie and John W. Thompson

Introduction

Medical historians and anthropologists have described numerous ways in which painful conditions have been managed by sensory modulation[1]. One common feature in such folklore techniques such as cupping, scarification, cauterization, and acupuncture, is that a painful stimulus is applied to abolish the pain.

The exact timing of the origin of acupuncture is unclear, with reports that it may have been as early as the 21st century BC[2] with stone and bone needles having been used. One of the earliest and most elegantly written texts about this ancient Chinese system of healing was 'The Yellow Emperor's Classic of Internal Medicine'[3]. 'Celestial Lancets' by Lu and Needham[4] provide the reader with a colourful description of historical and traditional Chinese acupuncture. More recently in 1991, Ötzi, the European ice man was discovered in the Alps, having been preserved for 5200 years[5]. Imaging revealed widespread arthritis of the spine and lower legs and many of the numerous tattoos found on his body corresponded with acupuncture points currently used for arthritis.

Traditional Eastern style acupuncture involves an elaborate system of diagnosis based on 'energy flow' round the body with subsequent selection of acupuncture points for stimulation by the insertion of fine needles in order to effect any benefit or 'cure.' It is unlike our modern medical concepts of health and disease[4,6]. Western practitioners use acupuncture, following orthodox Western diagnosis and is a neurophysiologically-based method of point selection, which includes traditional points.

Acupuncture has an increasing role in the treatment of cancer pain and symptom management and is increasingly integrated in primary care as well as pain management services in many countries.

Techniques of acupuncture

The techniques employed by an individual acupuncturist vary enormously, not only in the selection of acupuncture points but also in the mode and length of stimulation (Table 10.1.12.1).

Traditional chinese acupuncture

The traditional Chinese view included appreciation of the intimate relationship between man and his environment, much like

Taoist philosophy. Historically, the Chinese described a circulation of vital energy Qi, which circulates the body in deep channels and along numerous meridians, which are invisible lines joining a series of acupuncture points on the surface of the body (Fig. 10.1.12.1).

Numerous 'laws' are utilized to guide the traditional acupuncturist to make the correct diagnosis, including the need to balance Yin and Yang, forces of opposite polarities, and 'five elements.' After taking a history, and a complex tongue and pulse diagnosis, disease can theoretically be diagnosed in 12 distant 'organs'. The validity of this approach and pulse diagnosis in particular has been seriously challenged in recent years[7]. Chosen acupuncture points are manually stimulated with a needle until the patient feels a needling sensation or 'De Qi,' a feeling of aching, numbness, tingling, heaviness, and fullness. Intriguingly, less than one per cent of patients experience a propagated sensation from the needle point, which often follows the pathway of a meridian[8]. No convincing theory to support the existence of meridians has emerged, although a plausible theory of conduction via collagen intersections and planes has been postulated[9].

Many acupuncture points are slightly tender to palpation in health and many more become tender in disease. These points

Table 10.1.12.1 Techniques of acupuncture.

Traditional Chinese acupuncture	Energetic diagnostic system—disease due to imbalance of Qi or flow of vital energy
	'De Qi' or needling sensation elicited with vigorous stimulation up to 30 min ± moxibustion (thermal stimulus)
	The forces of opposite polarities Yin and Yang need to be balanced in health
	Pulse and tongue diagnosis and several laws utilized for traditional diagnosis
Western acupuncture	Manual acupuncture
	Minimal stimulation up to 20 min
	Maximal stimulation intermittently up to 20 min or longer
	Electroacupuncture
	2–4 Hz low frequency
	50–200 Hz high frequency
	2–100 Hz modulated frequency
Acupuncture analgesia	Vigorous manual stimulation or EA
	Used for operations in China
	Now as sole anaesthetic in < 6% operations but often used with general anaesthetic
Acupressure	Massage treatment of acupuncture points
	No needles—less effective than needling
Auricular acupuncture	Needles inserted in tender regions or 'recipe' points
Ryodoraku	Reduced skin impedance on electrodermal testing – treatment a form of electroacupuncture
Laser therapy	No needles – advantage paediatrics (not strictly acupuncture)
Veterinary	± EA Unlikely to be a placebo!

appear commonly in 'recipes' for treatment of various conditions. Moxibustion involves a thermal stimulus applied to the needle or held above acupuncture points.

Western medical acupuncture

Western-trained doctors rely on orthodox history taking, examination, and appropriate investigations before making a diagnosis. Such abstract concepts as Qi and Yin and Yang are unacceptable to many Western trained doctors and have contributed to the scepticism with which many still view acupuncture. However, if the balance of Yin and Yang represents autonomic balance, and circulation of Qi represents the circulation of oxygen, blood etc., then the ancient system appears to be quite advanced for its time.

Recent neuropharmacological and neurophysiological advances have provided acupuncture with a sound scientific basis and far more clinical credibility. Acupuncture releases multiple endogenous substances that no single drug treatment could attempt to mimic. Acupuncture's actions are blocked by pre-treatment with injection of local anaesthetic[10,11]. It releases β-endorphin, metenkephalin, and dynorphins, which activate mu, delta, and kappa (OP3, OP1, and OP2) opioid receptors[12-15]. It releases serotonin which has both analgesic and mood-enhancing properties[13]. Oxytocin is released which is anxiolytic and analgesic[16]. It releases endogenous steroids[17] and produces widespread autonomic effects[18,19]. Acupuncture up-regulates endogenous opioid gene production[20,21], which, in part, may explain why 'top-ups' are required to maintain the analgesic gene expression in a 'switched on' mode. For further information, see neurophysiology section at the end of this chapter.

As increasing neurophysiological evidence for its actions accumulates, it seems likely that acupuncture works more through

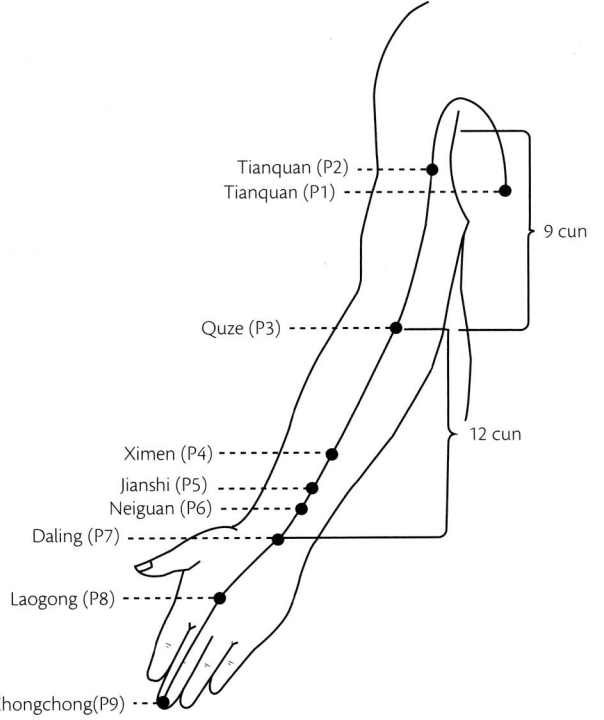

Figure 10.1.12.1 The 'pericardium' meridian, in traditional Chinese acupuncture.

neurophysiological modulation of multiple endogenous homeostatic mechanisms and less likely via energetic principles, or in a metaphysical way.

Clinical approaches

In practice, a pragmatic approach is taken using a mixture of segmental points appropriate to the disordered region, trigger points, tender points, plus selected 'strong' traditional points. Trigger points are hyperirritable spots in taut bands of muscle, which are painful on compression and can elicit a characteristic 'jump' sign that may be accompanied by a twitch response and by autonomic changes[22]. Referral patterns of discomfort often resemble the meridian lines and it is possible that the meridian theory developed as observations of the referral pattern from trigger points or the coalescence of several trigger point patterns[23] (see Fig. 10.1.12.2). There is considerable overlap between acupuncture points and trigger points[24,25]. Needling trigger points can successfully treat pain of myofascial origin[26], which is very common in both cancer patients and non-cancer patients with musculoskeletal problems. Trigger points are exacerbated by stress, which is extremely common in cancer patients.

The 'dose' of acupuncture used varies widely amongst practitioners with stimulation of needles from 5 s to 20 min with no attempt to elicit 'De Qi'. Some use minimal and others more vigorous manual stimulation of the needles to deliberately elicit 'De Qi'. Other factors which influence the overall 'dose' of treatment include the number of needles used, diameter of the needles, depth of insertion, and degree of stimulation, manual or electrical. There is no consensus on optimal 'dosage' for different conditions to date. Cancer patients can be more sensitive to acupuncture than others, and these 'strong reactors'[27] require shorter gentle treatments.

In general, patients are treated somewhat empirically with treatment intensified or reduced on a trial and error basis, depending on individual progress. The treatment schedules are usually weekly for 6 weeks or twice weekly for 3 weeks. 'Top-ups' are subsequently given at increasing intervals depending on the patient, their response, and state of advancement of the disease.

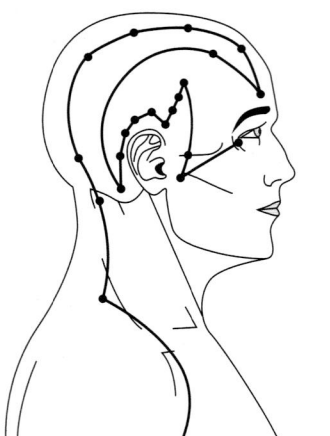
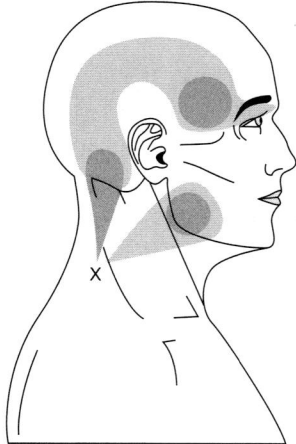

Figure 10.1.12.2 This figure shows the close correlation between the referral pattern from a trigger point in upper trapezius and the path of the gallbladder meridian. The trigger point is anatomically co-incident with the acupuncture point GB21.

A wide variety of techniques are both available and effective. These range from a traditional approach on the one hand[28,29], to the other extreme, in which some respected Western practitioners no longer believe in the special properties associated with formal traditional acupuncture points, and who teach a simplified yet effective system of needling[27,30]. Many use an eclectic mix of traditional points, trigger points, and segmental points.

Electroacupuncture (EA)

EA was first established as a substitute for the vigorous manual stimulation required for perioperative acupuncture or acupuncture analgesia[31]. This is stronger than transcutaneous electrical nerve stimulation (TENS), as the electrical stimulus is transmitted through the skin via needles. Low-frequency EA 2–4 Hz stimulates the release of enkephalins and cortisol whereas high frequency 50–200 Hz releases serotonin (5-HT) and dynorphin. EA is used to treat acute pain following surgery, chronic pain, and complex pain problems such as fibromyalgia[31].

Acupuncture analgesia

Acupuncture performed in a vigorous manner with or without electrical stimulation can raise pain tolerance to experimental and surgically induced pain[32,33]. Acupuncture analgesia was introduced in 1958 and became popular in China for perioperative analgesia with dramatic reports and video clips of patients having major surgery, for example pneumonectomy, with seemingly only acupuncture as analgesia. James Reston, a journalist in the party accompanying President Nixon to China in 1973, benefited from acupuncture analgesia following an appendicectomy and was instrumental in the dissemination of knowledge about acupuncture in the West.

White summarizes important aspects of acupuncture analgesia[31]. The lengthy induction time, coupled with inadequate analgesia in many cases, requiring opioid supplementation, understandably diminished its popularity yet it remains particularly useful as an adjunct to modern anaesthesia to diminish postoperative analgesic requirements and can enhance the quality of postoperative recovery[34].

Laser therapy

Laser stimulation at acupuncture points (often described as laser acupuncture) is not strictly acupuncture because no needles are involved[35]. It is associated with changes in blood flow[36]. One Cochrane review of laser therapy for osteoarthritis was equivocal[37], and another review on short-term relief in patients with rheumatoid arthritis was positive[38]. There are anecdotal reports that laser therapy reduces mucositis following bone marrow transplantation, but there have been no formal studies as yet. Laser therapy, as it is painless, is more acceptable to paediatric patients, needle-phobic patients, and veterinary subjects. Optimal parameters for treatment have yet to be elucidated.

Acupressure

Acupressure is the massage of traditional acupuncture points, e.g. when applied for treatment of chronic obstructive pulmonary disease (COPD)[39]. Acupressure is a weaker stimulus than acupuncture with needles and 'Tuina' is a form of massage used especially on children in China.

Auricular acupuncture

In traditional Chinese acupuncture, the ear is deemed to be closely connected by channels to internal organs. Nogier in France, in the 1950s, further developed auricular acupuncture[40] suggesting that different parts of the external helix might represent different parts of the body, as though the external helix represented an upside down fetus. Treatment of tender points on the pinna that represent the points on the body with pain was found to be helpful. Whilst sounding improbable, one study showed some effect when needling tender sites in this way[41]. The hypothesis of somatotopic representation of the body on the ear requires further testing. Because the pinna is richly innervated by multiple nerves including the vagus, it is not surprising that strong sensory stimulation has far-reaching effects. The importance of point specificity on the ear has been challenged for the treatment of addictions[42].

Ryodoraku

This is a Japanese form of EA where skin impedance is measured by electrodermal testing, which, if abnormal, can be modified electrically by a form of EA[43].

Veterinary acupuncture

Acupuncture and EA are used increasingly for domestic, farm animals, and racing stock[44]. The effectiveness of treatment in animals lends some credence to the view that acupuncture is more than merely a placebo.

Equipment

Numerous wall charts and models are available, which depict traditional acupuncture points for accurate localization purposes. Acupuncture needles are usually made of surgical stainless steel and are predominantly disposable. As the quality control of sterilization techniques is variable, it is safest and should be mandatory to use disposable needles. The size, length, and gauges of needles vary according to practitioner preferences. Many use a plastic introducing guide tube to facilitate a quick and relatively painless insertion.

There is an enormous selection of electrical and laser equipment available. It is beyond the scope of this book to include this topic in any depth; so the reader is advised to consult suppliers for further details.

Indications

In China, acupuncture is first-line treatment for hundreds of minor and major complaints[28], and there is an increasing base of evidence accumulating on its use in the Western literature[45,46]. It is steadily gaining popularity in the West because of its success in treating a host of common ailments, in many cases obviating the need for medication, or at least reducing the dosage of drugs and the risk of side effects.

Clinical research

Efficacy, effectiveness, safety, and cost-effectiveness need to be examined objectively in acupuncture, as they should be in all aspects of modern health care. The results of clinical trials of acupuncture have been conflicting and this has been partly due to the complex issues surrounding the methodology of acupuncture trials[47].

The generally accepted method of testing the efficacy of a new treatment is to subject it to a randomized, double blind, controlled trial.

Whilst randomization should not be a problem in any study, blinding the therapist is difficult, though not impossible or indeed desirable in most cases! However blinding of the patient, independent observer, and statistician involved in the study are feasible. The choice of a control is more problematic. Many studies have employed needling of non-traditional acupuncture points as the control treatment, but this procedure is now known to produce neurophysiological effects and is thus not truly inactive. Moreover, sham needling in the same segment as the 'correct needles' is much less likely to show a difference than when correct needling is compared with extrasegmental control points[48]. Conversely, non-needling placebos are not sufficiently credible. Recently, 'placebo needles' have been devised with retractable handles, which do not penetrate the skin, operating on the 'stage dagger' principle, although this causes some degree of stimulation. Acupuncture was found to be superior using this sham control in a trial for rotator cuff problems[49].

Acupuncture is an invasive form of treatment and undoubtedly causes strong non-specific effects. Placebo analgesia works in part via stimulation of endogenous opioids[50,51], as does acupuncture, so it is difficult to delineate one effect from the other. Thomas et al. 1991[52] showed superiority of superficial and deep needling and diazepam over a placebo diazepam tablet for neck pain, measuring pain scores, but all four treatments improved the affective, emotional component of pain. Key research challenges remain for acupuncture. Indeed, neuroimaging can show that expectation of a therapeutic effect influences cerebral activity[53].

Early systematic reviews on acupuncture for pain control were inconclusive in their results[54,55] but were based on pooled heterogeneous data often with flawed methodology. Ezzo et al. 2000[56], examining much of the same evidence was similarly inconclusive, but did show superiority of acupuncture over patients on a waiting list.

More recently, several positive systematic reviews have shown the efficacy of acupuncture for postoperative nausea and vomiting[57,58], and for nausea and vomiting due to chemotherapy[59], for dental pain[60], for headache[61], for fibromyalgia[62], EA for experimental pain[33], back pain[63], and osteoarthritis of the knee[64,65]. The evidence remains inconclusive for asthma[66], stroke[67], and is negative for weight loss[68] and smoking cessation[69], although results of the latter are no worse than nicotine patches. Some feel any effects in aiding nicotine withdrawal may be useful in the short term.

Pain

Acupuncture has been found to help a wide variety of pain conditions with between 40 per cent and over 80 per cent symptomatic improvement in primary care[70–72]. The shorter the duration of the problem, the better the response. Old age and multiple illnesses reduce the benefit. Ross in 2001 showed a dramatic reduction in referrals from primary to secondary care, by extensively integrating its use in primary care[73].

Cancer pain and symptom control

Acupuncture can be used to treat acute postoperative pain as well as chronic or intractable pain associated with cancer and its treatment.

Acute pain

Many aspects of acupuncture analgesia have been reviewed by White[31]. Acupuncture is infrequently used as a sole anaesthetic because it is time consuming, requires lengthy counselling and a prolonged induction period before surgery. It does not give adequate muscle relaxation for abdominal surgery or mechanical ventilation and only the minority achieve sufficient analgesia to remain comfortable during surgery. Awareness can be a problem so it is risky as an *alternative* to general anaesthesia. Acupuncture as an adjuvant to anaesthesia is a different matter, decreasing analgesic requirement pre- and postoperatively and improving postoperative recovery characteristics. Poulain showed this in 1997 in a series of 250 cancer patients having gynaecological surgery for cancer[74]. Kotani showed efficacy in reducing postoperative pain and analgesic requirements following major gastrointestinal surgery, using paravertebral semi-permanent needles for several days versus a control group[34]. Vickers has shown this to be a feasible treatment to reduce post-thoracotomy pain[75].

The optimal choice of dose, points, duration, timing of treatment before, during, or postoperatively, and mode of stimulation (EA or manual), have yet to be defined for different types of surgery.

Cancer pain and cancer-related pain

The failure of pharmacological means to singly control pain has led many to use non-drug treatments, including acupuncture and TENS. Pain can be caused by cancer, cancer treatment, or it may be completely unrelated to the cancer diagnosis. It is often due to a combination of causes. It may include nociceptive and/or neuropathic components. Acupuncture can improve pain control sufficiently to permit a decrease in dosage and side effects of analgesics and co-analgesics. Acupuncture can help patients who are oversensitive to normal doses of analgesics as well as those who have pain despite appropriate titration of analgesics and co-analgesics[76,77].

Treatment is usually given for 10–20 min, with a total of six treatments planned in the initial course. In clinical practice, results of treatment are undoubtedly due to the combination of any specific effects of the treatment, and the opportunity for reflective listening, and support given to the patient during the treatment at a very crucial time in their lives. Acupuncture is relaxing and can facilitate a catharsis in patients who find difficulty in coming to terms with their disease (Filshie, unpublished observation).

At the initial visit, gentle stimulation is given to assess whether the patient is a 'strong reactor' or not. Then the treatment is subsequently tailored to the individual response. Appropriate segmental points are chosen, plus trigger points and strong analgesic points, which may or may not be segmental. Fig. 10.1.12.3A shows a combination of paravertebral segmental points and trigger points used for a patient with neck pain. The traditional point LI4 (Fig. 10.1.12.3B) is also often used, which has been shown to raise the pain threshold in numerous experimental studies[33]. Paravertebral points at C7, T1, and T2 are particularly useful for pain and vascular problems in the head and neck, arm, and breast regions, and appear to be interchangeable with sympathetic blockade[76]. The paravertebral points L1–L5 are used for pain in the abdomen, low back, and lower leg, ± vascular problems (Fig. 10.1.12.3C). Sacral points are added for perineal pain.

Wen, in 1977[78] used several EA sessions a day, reducing to once or twice per day in a series of 29 patients whose pain was inadequately

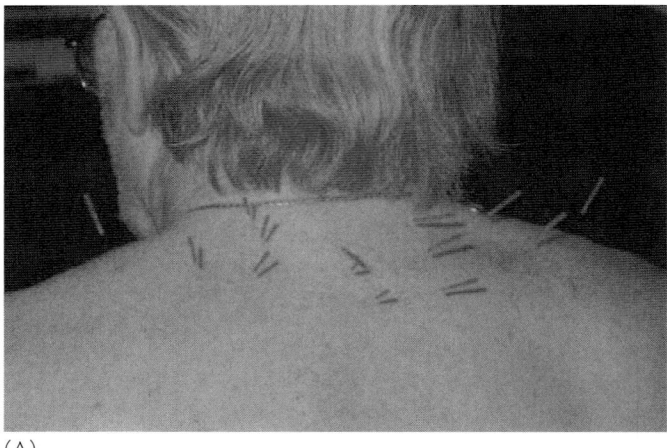

(A)

Figure 10.1.12.3A This shows a combination of segmental and trigger points for a patient with neck pain.

controlled in advanced disease and who were suffering from excessive side effects from opioids. Though time consuming, analgesia improved significantly enabling pain medication to be significantly reduced.

Following the successful use in a series of 80 patients with advanced cancer-related pain, brief summaries of two extensive retrospective audits were published on 339 patients[76,77]. These patients had a heterogeneous collection of pain symptoms, which had failed to respond to conventional analgesics and co-analgesics. Over 50 per cent of patients obtained worthwhile analgesia after three weekly treatments and enabled it to be a useful outpatient-based treatment[76,77]. Yet, the more advanced the disease, the shorter the response to treatment. Many patients experienced a significant improvement in mobility. Treatment-related pain such as post-surgical or post-irradiation pain often responded better. Muscle spasm, bladder spasm, and vascular problems were also significantly helped. When the initial course of treatment was increased from three to six treatments, a small but significant number of these initial non-responders obtained benefit, as found

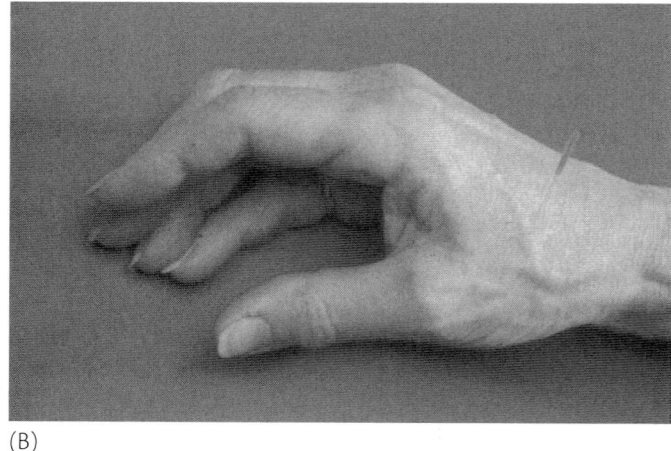

(B)

Figure 10.1.12.3B This shows the traditional acupuncture point Large Intestine 4 (LI4), which raises the pain threshold.

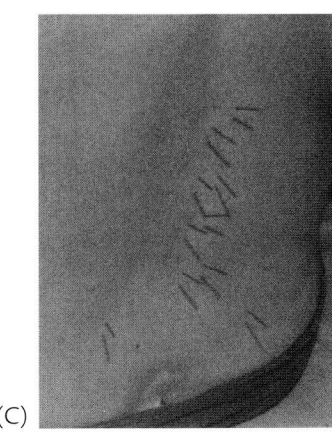

(C)

Figure 10.1.12.3C This shows segmental acupuncture in a patient with low back pain.

by others[56]. Further 'top ups' could be given as necessary. Aung 1994[79] and Leng[80] describe similar results. A further audit of 89 patients with pain and xerostomia showed similar results with 86 per cent of patients considering it 'very important' to continue to provide an acupuncture service[81].

Another audit detailing the psychological profile in 67 patients with breast cancer and related pain showed a statistically significant drop in pain, pain behaviour, interference with lifestyle, distress, and depression, after one month of weekly acupuncture treatments[82]. Any improvement in symptoms and depression scores may be important because depression has been linked to a significantly decreased chance of survival[83]. Another study of patients in the two-week period following breast surgery with axillary dissection showed improvement in pain and increased arm abduction compared with a control group having no acupuncture[84].

Lee *et al.* conducted a systematic review of acupuncture treatment for cancer pain but included only one high-quality randomized controlled trial (RCT), which was positive[85]. Methodological problems were outlined and the results overall were inconclusive, and further RCTs were recommended for this patient population.

Phantom limb pain

Acupuncture can alleviate phantom limb pain (PLP)[86], especially in those patients who have a cold leg stump, when needling the paravertebral upper-lumbar sympathetic blocking points (Fig. 10.1.12.3B) warms the limb through sympathetic blockade. Acupuncture causes sympathetic stimulation followed by blockade[18,87], and this is often evident clinically. Upper-thoracic paravertebral points are helpful for upper-limb PLP. Mirror sites on the opposite limb are usually treated together with paravertebral points plus strong 'traditional points.' Although pain relief can be instant and dramatic in selected patients, most are not helped and only short case series are described[88].

Auriculoacupuncture for cancer pain

Dillon and Lucas 1999[89] treated 28 hospice patients, including five with motor neuron disease, and showed a significant improvement in pain over a 4-week period. In another pilot study of 20 cancer patients, auriculoacupuncture produced a significant

reduction in pain intensity[90]. The same group compared acupuncture in an RCT with two control treatments and showed significant relief at 30 days and 2 months over the control interventions[91].

Percutaneous electrical nerve stimulation (PENS)

PENS is reported as a 'novel treatment' but is simply EA under a new title! Cummings (2001) has reviewed the literature and found nothing to distinguish it from EA and no substantial justification to call it 'novel'[92].

Acupuncture and TENS

TENS is often used as a backup for acupuncture, especially if the acupuncture effect wears off between outpatient visits. The therapies are not interchangeable, some patients responding to acupuncture alone and others to TENS (see following section 'Neuroanatomy and neuropharmacology of acupuncture').

Tolerance

It is interesting to note that cancer patients with advanced disease need multiple and continuing 'top up' treatments to maintain adequate analgesia and, over time, some patients exhibit a reduced response to acupuncture. In fact, an almost inverse relationship was noted between tumour size and longevity of acupuncture response[76,77]. The larger the tumour burden, or the more active the disease, the shorter the analgesic benefit of acupuncture. Any sudden tolerance in a patient who has previously responded well to acupuncture is considered to be a sinister sign. When this occurs, the patient should be referred to the oncologists for further investigation; 17 out of 27 patients audited had developed further metastases[77]. Furthermore, when metastatic disease was found and treated successfully, the patient reverted to being acupuncture responsive again. Tolerance has been observed in animal models when the opioid antagonists, angiotensin II[93], and CCK[94], had been released by prolonged EA. It is tempting to hypothesize that in patients with cancer, the output of endogenous opioids is already homeostatically increased to near maximum, thereby preventing them from achieving any greater response when treated with acupuncture.

Methods of overcoming acupuncture tolerance in late-stage disease include increasing the frequency of treatments. In terminal patients, Wen[78] used multiple acupuncture treatments daily, initially, to good effect such that the patients could reduce opioid medication with its attendant side effects, though this is very labour intensive. Semipermanent needles have also been used to prolong analgesia and patients can massage them as required to improve pain and symptom control.

Shortness of breath

In an RCT of patients with COPD, the acupuncture-treated group showed significant benefit in subjective breathlessness and six-minute walking distance[95] compared with a control group. Acupressure has also been used to assist pulmonary rehabilitation in patients with COPD[96] as did Wu[39]. Neumeister also showed acupuncture to improve pulmonary function in COPD[97].

One pilot study on the short-term effects of acupuncture in 20 patients with advanced cancer-related dyspnoea[98] using two sternal needles (Fig. 10.1.12.4A), and LI4 (Fig. 10.1.12.3B) showed

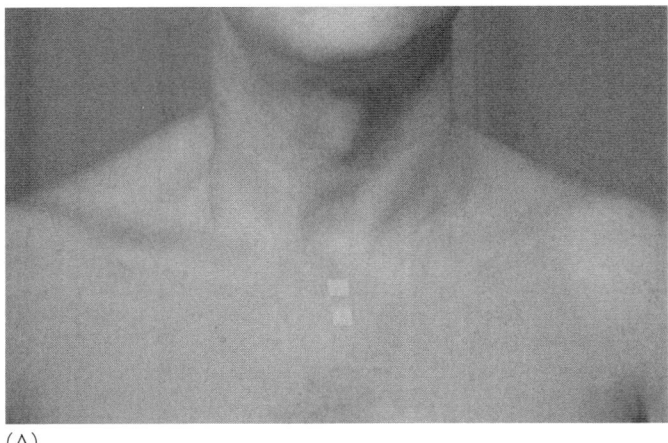

(A)

Figure 10.1.12.4A This illustrates two needles inserted at the top of the sternum for treatment of dyspnoea.

significant improvement in subjective scores of breathlessness, relaxation, and anxiety at 90 min. There was also a reduction in the respiratory rate, sustained for the treatment period. Ongoing relief was maintained by the use of two indwelling studs inserted into the sternal points in an attempt to prolong the response as in Fig. 10.1.12.4B. A clear plastic dressing was used to secure the needles. This gave patients control by instructing them to massage the studs during breathless 'panic attacks' or prior to any even trivial exercise. It was successful in patients who had failed to respond to multiple treatments for dyspnoea including steroids, opioids, nebulizers, and oxygen. The two upper-sternal semipermanent needles are used extensively in palliative care units in the United Kingdom and are named 'ASAD' points —anxiety, sickness, and dyspnoea points. After appropriate skin cleansing, these studs are inserted and covered by a clear plastic dressing and can remain in place for up to 4 weeks at a time. Vickers *et al.*, in a subsequent study, failed to show a difference between acupuncture and acupressure[99].

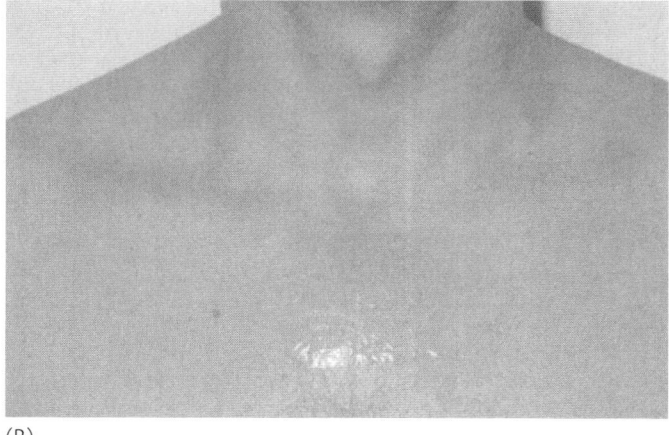

(B)

Figure 10.1.12.4B This shows two indwelling acupuncture needles covered by a clear plastic dressing which can be massaged to give relief in panic attacks or prior to activity.

Yet, the placebo treatment included one real acupuncture needle, which possibly might have been a confounding influence. A further RCT is in progress comparing acupuncture with morphine for advanced cancer-related breathlessness.

The mechanisms of action of acupuncture for dyspnoea remain speculative, but the sedative and central actions of endogenous opioid peptide release may be contributory. The profound sense of relaxation and relief of anxiety experienced using sternal points[98] may have been due to the release of oxytocin.

Nausea and vomiting

The late Professor John Dundee conducted numerous studies on acupuncture using a single needle placed at the point PC6 on the pericardium meridian (Fig. 10.1.12.1). He found PC6 a clinically useful antiemetic treatment for postoperative nausea and vomiting, morning sickness, and chemotherapy-induced emesis. McMillan has summarized his findings[100]. Benefit, correlated with the intensity of the stimulus and manual needling and EA gave greater effects than acupressure. A systematic review by Vickers showed acupuncture to be superior to a control group for nausea and vomiting in 27 out of 33 RCTs[101]. One high-quality RCT showed benefit for nausea and vomiting associated with high-dose chemotherapy for breast cancer[102]. Subsequently Ezzo *et al.* have reviewed 11 trials using acupuncture point stimulation for chemotherapy-induced nausea and vomiting[59]. A significant reduction of acute vomiting was found with both needling and electro stimulation. Acupressure reduced the mean severity of acute nausea but not acute vomiting. The non-invasive electro stimulation tested did not benefit any outcome. Acupressure, though insufficient to prevent vomiting, was thought to be convenient for self-administration to reduce acute nausea at low cost. Delayed vomiting and nausea following chemotherapy remain a significant challenge and methods to prolong any antiemetic effects should be explored.

In late-stage palliative care, nausea and vomiting is often multifactorial with contributory causes that include opioid and other medication, metabolic and electrolyte imbalance, anorexia, gastrointestinal symptoms, and dehydration often contributing to the cause. In these cases, treatment of the cause or causes would be the ideal, if feasible. The addition of strong gastrointestinal points such as CV12, ST25, and ST36 can help. Acupuncture will not work in cases with established gastrointestinal obstruction but might help ameliorate symptoms if that obstruction is only partial. Indwelling ASAD points can be helpful on occasions. As to the possible mechanisms of action of acupuncture for nausea and vomiting, there are, as yet, no clear-cut explanations.

Xerostomia

Several studies have shown acupuncture to help xerostomia of different aetiology[103,104]. Blom *et al.* 1996[104], in an RCT on 38 patients with xerostomia following radiotherapy, compared classical with superficial acupuncture. Both groups showed a significant increase in salivary flow. In those patients who had had all the salivary gland irradiated, 50 per cent in both groups had increased flow rates at a one-year follow up. Thus the superficial acupuncture was by no means an inactive treatment. Wong *et al.* showed acupuncture-like TENS to be also effective for xerostomia[105].

Patients post-radiotherapy for head and neck cancer with pilocarpine-resistant xerostomia, benefited from acupuncture[106].

Acupuncture was also useful for patients in late-stage cancer with additional dysphagia and articulation problems[107]. Therefore acupuncture may have a significant role in palliation of this common and unpleasant symptom in palliative care.

Lundeberg[19] discusses several studies and describes the mechanisms by which acupuncture is effective. These include stimulation of both parasympathetic (volume effect) and sympathetic (viscosity effect) nervous systems and the release of the vasodilator calcitonin gene-related peptide (C-GRP), which also increases salivary secretion.

Vascular problems

Vascular problems can be helped by acupuncture, including ischaemic skin flaps[19]. Two radionecrotic ulcers (which classically never heal) healed completely using acupuncture[108].

Cancer-related hot flushes

Wyon et al. (1995)[109] demonstrated that acupuncture could decrease hot flushes in the natural climacteric. Acupuncture has been found to reduce hot flushes associated with cancer treatment in women[110,111]. An algorithm has been developed for treatment with the effects of the initial course of treatment maintained for up to 6 years by weekly self-needling at SP6 or by using semipermanent needles. For self-needling, patients need clear instructions for cleansing, insertion, and safe disposal[110,112]. (See 'Cautions and contraindications' for the insertion of semipermanent needles.) Acupuncture also helped control vasomotor symptoms in men due to treatment of prostate cancer[113].

Miscellaneous

Acupuncture has helped radiation rectitis following radiotherapy for carcinoma of the cervix[114], experimentally induced itch[115], and uraemic pruritus[116]. Anecdotally, one of the authors (J.F.) has had several unexpected dramatic successes in the short-term rehabilitation of patients with intracranial tumours, and this observation may merit further testing.

AIDS

Greene et al. (1999)[117] showed that 48 per cent of 1016 HIV-infected participants used needle acupuncture to treat their symptoms. Individualized acupuncture treatment was found helpful for treatment of sleep disturbance[118]. One RCT, comparing acupuncture with amitriptyline and placebo, failed to show any benefit of acupuncture or amitriptyline over placebo for peripheral neuropathy[119] though a subsequent small observational study in a group setting was positive[120]. Some preliminary work has shown promise for reduction of HIV/AIDS-related diarrhoea[121]. Possible infection with HIV reinforces the need for all practitioners to use disposable needles, as patients may not know their diagnosis, or fail to reveal it when seeking advice.

Immunological considerations

There is limited evidence, mainly from studies in experimental animals, to suggest that acupuncture produces immunomodulating effects, similar to moderate exercise[19,122]. Much further study is required before recommending acupuncture wholeheartedly for any immuno-enhancing effects.

Anxiety and depression

The upper-sternal 'ASAD' (Fig. 10.1.12.3b) points are used in the United Kingdom extensively for control of anxiety. Patients can give themselves a burst of anxiolysis by gently massaging the studs for 1–2 minutes. This can give the added benefit of a sense of control over this distressing symptom. Acupuncture was helpful for depression, though a systematic review on this topic showed most studies were of low quality[123].

Complications and contraindications

Complications

Lazarou and Pomeranz (1998) estimated that drugs are between the fourth and sixth commonest causes of death in the United States[124]. By contrast, acupuncture is a safe method of treatment with low side effects, and White, in a cumulative review of the significant adverse events associated with acupuncture, has shown a very low incidence worldwide, which is in contrast with conventional treatment[125].

Acupuncture's adverse effects have been classified as the following:

♦ Delayed or missed diagnosis of the condition treated.

♦ Negative reactions e.g. sweating, vertigo, syncope.

♦ Bacterial and viral infections (hepatitis B, hepatitis C, and HIV).

♦ Trauma of tissues and organs.

The safety aspects of acupuncture in palliative care have been reviewed[126] and guidelines for safe practice in cancer patients published[112]. Acupuncture can mask cancer and disease progression, for example, the pain of bone metastases. The disease must therefore be monitored continuously by oncology and palliative care teams. Furthermore, acupuncture treatment should be given by (or closely supervised by) a physician who has full knowledge about the stage and clinical condition of the patient.

Two recent prospective studies including 66 000 acupuncture treatments concluded that there is a 13–14 per 10 000 chance of a significant minor adverse event such as a forgotten needle or fainting following treatment[127,128]. Concordance between the studies was remarkably high, reporting respectively, a low incidence of minor adverse events such as bleeding and bruising $\cong$ 3 per cent; pain $\cong$ 1 per cent; and aggravation of symptoms < 3 per cent.

Table 10.1.12.2 outlines some of the contraindications and cautions for treatment of cancer patients. Cancer patients appear to be more sensitive to acupuncture than other patients and may become excessively sleepy during the treatment so that it is advisable to arrange for nursing assistance, particularly during the first treatment. Cachectic patients should be needled superficially with particular care.

Bacterial infection, including bacterial endocarditis, has been described, and the most serious viral infections include hepatitis B, and hepatitis C[125]. For safety of both patients and acupuncturists, it should be mandatory for all needles to be single use and disposable.

Although rare, serious anatomical damage to most organs and structures have been reported, including lungs (unilateral and bilateral pneumothorax), heart, liver, spleen, kidney, vessels, and nerves[129]. Some traditional textbooks include diagrams with alarmingly deep needling techniques, which are more likely to cause damage due to the failure of basic anatomical knowledge. Burns from moxibustion and faulty electrical apparatus have also been described.

Semipermanent needle use

Semipermanent needles are now used extensively to prolong the effects of acupuncture for treatment of cancer-related pain, dyspnoea, anxiety, and hot flushes, so that their possible contraindications and cautions should be considered, as summarized in Table 10.1.12.2[112].

Needles that 'fall out' can represent a sharps hazard and it is not necessarily clearly described what happens to the needles after they have fallen out[89–91]. When kits for self-needling are given to a patient for self-treatment of symptoms, for example, hot flushes, these should include clear instructions on how to clean the skin and use the needles; and a sharps box should be supplied to be returned to the hospital for safe disposal[112].

An unusual complication in one patient with rheumatoid arthritis and thyroid cancer was due to indwelling gold needles, which caused artifacts in the bone I[131] scan, similar to metastases[130].

Contraindications

Acupuncture needling is contraindicated in the area of an unstable spine due to metastatic disease, especially in a patient with good neurological function below that level. There is the serious theoretical danger of removal of protective muscle spasm around the unstable area, with ensuing danger of further cord compression or transection[77]. TENS is a useful alternative for pain relief in these cases. Table 10.1.12.2 outlines further important cautions and contraindications.

Patients should not be given unrealistic expectations about the likely benefits of acupuncture (or any other complementary therapy). Finally, many patients receiving acupuncture for pain describe *positive* side effects[128,131] with coincidental improvement of a variety of other conditions including migraine, hay fever, and psoriasis. These side effects are generally most welcome!

Neuroanatomy and neuropharmacology of acupuncture

Great progress has been made recently with the study of the neuroanatomy and neuropharmacology of nociceptive systems including the possible mechanisms of both acupuncture and TENS. Fig. 10.1.12.5 shows a diagram of the neuroanatomical and neuropharmacological basis of pain and the way in which this is modified by acupuncture and also by TENS. The diagram is based on the writings of Duggan and Foong[132], Bowsher[133,134], Han and Terenius[13], Le Bars *et al.*[135], Fields and Basbaum[136], Jones *et al.*[137], and Dickenson[138]. So-called 'first', 'rapid', or 'aversive' pain is due to the activation of small myelinated A delta fibres, whereas 'second,' 'slow,' or 'tissue damage' pain is due to activation of mostly unmyelinated C fibres with activation of some A delta fibres[133].

There are four conditions to be considered:

1 **Pathways for tissue damage pain**: Peripheral polymodal nociceptor afferents (C) respond, via a wide variety of channels and receptors, to mechanical, thermal, and chemical stimuli[139], for example, as in a painful scar as depicted in Fig. 10.1.12.5.

Table 10.1.12.2 Contraindications and cautions.

Acupuncture is contraindicated:

- In patients who refuse, e.g. in cases of extreme needle phobia
- In patients with severe clotting dysfunction or who bruise spontaneously

Semipermanent needles are contraindicated:

- In patients with valvular heart disease—risk of sub-acute bacterial endocarditis
- In neutropenic patients—risk of infection
- In patients after splenectomy—risk of infection

Electroacupuncture is contraindicated:

- In patients with an intracardiac defibrillator

Needling should be avoided:

- Directly onto a tumour nodule or into an area of ulceration
- In lymphoedematous limbs or limbs prone to lymphoedema
- In the ipsilateral arm in patients who have undergone axillary dissection, as there is a risk of development of swelling and lymphoedema after insertion of any needle
- In areas of spinal instability due to potential risk of cord compression due to acupuncture's muscle relaxing properties
- Into a prosthesis as this could cause leakage of saline/silicone
- Over intracranial deficits following neurosurgery

Cautions:

- Cancer patients may be very sensitive to acupuncture, so close supervision is advised especially at the first treatment
- Take extra care with all patients who are 'strong reactors' to acupuncture
- Care should be taken not to needle too deeply over the chest wall in cachectic patients
- Disease progression should always be considered in those who become suddenly tolerant to acupuncture having previously responded well
- Patients prone to keloid scar formation
- Pregnancy
- Epilepsy—patients need to be accompanied
- Confused patients
- Electroacupuncture in a patient with a cardiac pacemaker

The C fibre afferents terminate in the substantia gelatinosa (SG) (lamina II) where their axon terminals release the fast excitatory transmitters glutamate (GLU) and C-GRP, and the slow excitatory transmitters substance P(SP) or vasoactive intestinal peptide (VIP), according to whether these arise from skin or viscera, respectively. The SG indirectly excites transmission cells (T) deep in the spinal grey matter whose axons form the spinoreticular tract and which constitutes one component of the crossed anterolateral funiculus, which ascends to the brain. The spinoreticular tract sends collaterals to the hypothalamus (triggering autonomic responses to pain) and then synapses in the thalamus. In the latter, it excites other neurons, which are

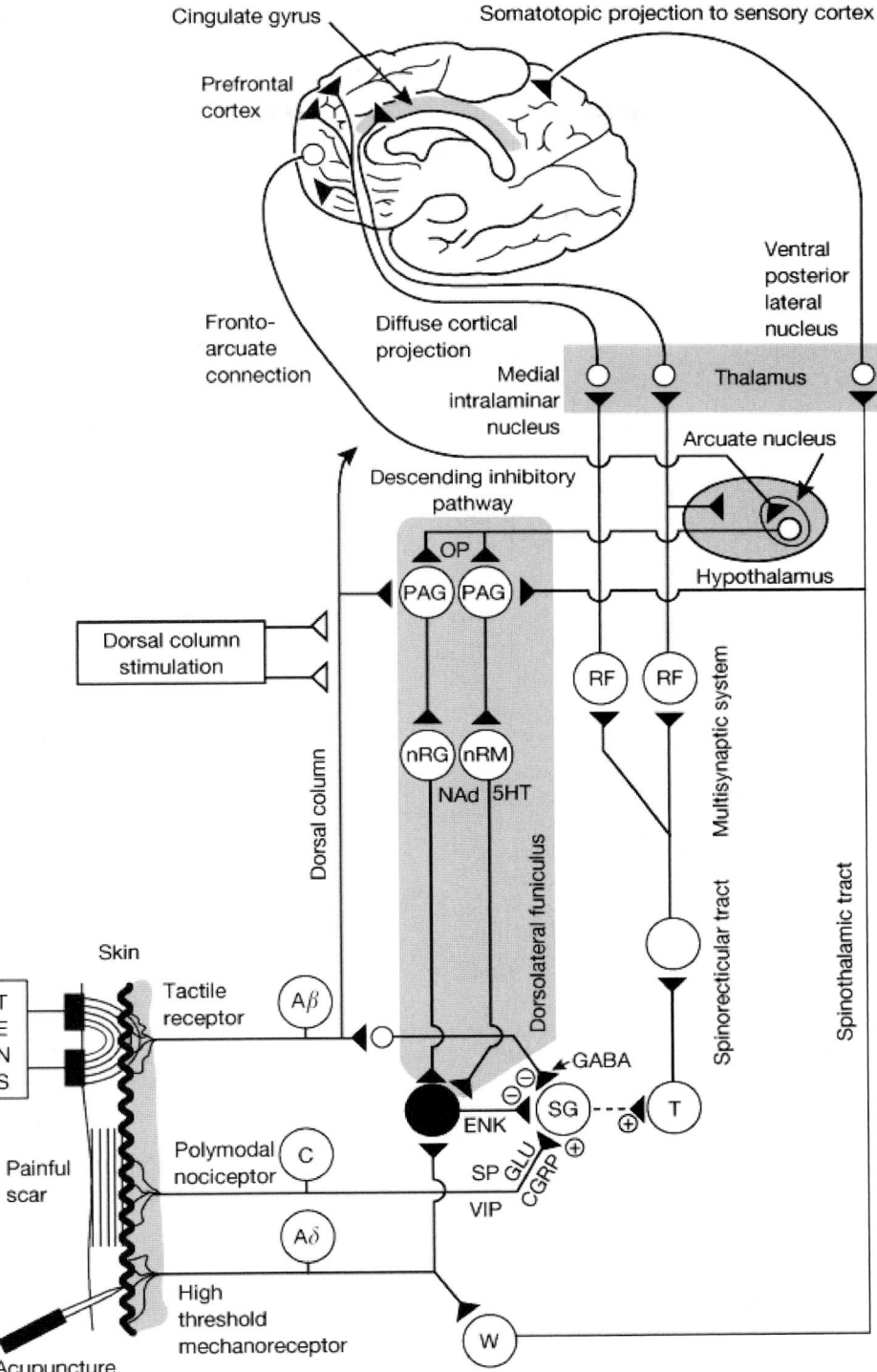

Figure 10.1.12.5 Diagram to show neuronal circuits involved in acupuncture and TENS analgesia. The afferent pathways involved in transmitting nociceptive information from a painful scar to the higher centres via the dorsal horn, the ascending tracts and the thalamus are shown. The connections to the descending inhibitory pathways which descend in the dorsolateral funiculus are also shown. The connections to the hypothalamus are indicated. Abbreviations: Ab, C, and Ad represent the posterior root ganglion cells of Ab , C, and Ad fibres, respectively; CGRP = calcitonin gene- related peptide; ENK = enkephalinergic neuron; GABA = g-amino-butyric acid; GLU = glutamate; 5HT = 5-hydroxytryptamine , serotonin; Nad = noradrenaline = norepinephrine; nRG = nucleus raphé gigantocellularis; nRM = nucleus raphé magnus; OP = opioid peptides; PAG = periaqueductal grey; RF = reticular formation; SG = cell in the substantia gelatinosa; SP = substance P; T = transmission cell; VIP = vasoactive intestinal polypeptide; W = Waldeyer cell; + stimulant effect; − inhibitory effect.

distributed widely over the cerebral cortex including the frontal cortex and also the limbic system, which give rise to the conscious sensation and emotional experience of tissue-damage (second) pain.

2 **Segmental acupuncture:** High-threshold mechanoreceptors connected to small myelinated primary afferents (A delta) are activated by acupuncture. One central branch of the A delta afferent excites the inhibitory enkephalinergic interneuron (on the borders of laminae I and II), releasing enkephalin (Enk), which produces post-synaptic block of the SG cell. This prevents the onward transmission of noxiously generated information. This mechanism would explain segmental acupuncture. Recent work suggests that a second opioid peptide (orphanin FQ/nociceptin [OFQ]) may also be involved[140].

3 **Extra-segmental acupuncture:** Waldeyer cells (W) in lamina I of the spinal grey matter are excited by acupuncture via another central branch of A delta primary afferents. The axons of the Waldeyer cells constitute another component (spinothalamic tract) of the crossed anterolateral funiculus and convey pin-prick information to consciousness through the ventral poster-olateral nucleus of the thalamus and thence to the somatosensory cortex (where there is somatotopic representation). Collaterals excite the periaqueductal grey (PAG), which in its turn projects to the nucleus raphe magnus (nRM) situated in the midline of the lower brainstem reticular formation.

Serotinergic (5HT) and adrenergic (Nad) axons of nRM cells descend through the dorsolateral funiculus of the spinal cord to synapse eventually with the cells described earlier and so block the onward transmission of noxiously generated information in the same manner as does segmental acupuncture. However, this descending inhibitory pathway gives off these connections *at all levels of the spinal cord* thereby explaining the extra-segmental effect of acupuncture.

4 **TENS:** By contrast with acupuncture, high-frequency low-intensity electrical stimulation excites A beta afferents connected to tactile receptors. After entering the spinal cord, these afferents ultimately ascend in the dorsal columns. At spinal cord level, these A beta afferent fibres give collaterals, which synapse with short interneurons, the endings of which end in proximity to the terminations of the C fibres as the latter synapse with SG cells. The evidence available suggests that these interneurons release gamma-amino butyric acid (GABA), which causes pres-ynaptic blockade of the C afferents thereby preventing them from exciting the SG cells and so blocking the onward transmission of nociceptive information. The elegant demonstration by Garrison and Foreman[141] that TENS decreases the activity of spontaneous and noxiously evoked dorsal horn cells is in accord with this explanation. Subsequently, it was discovered that analgesia produced by low-frequency high-intensity TENS is attenuated by a mu opioid-blocker, such as naloxone, suggesting that an opioid mechanism is involved[142].

Recent work on TENS, using an animal model of inflammatory joint pain[140] has confirmed that the analgesic mechanism is frequency dependent and involves several neurotransmitters. Thus, high-frequency stimulation involves both gabaergic and delta opioid mechanisms (with delta opioid linked inhibition of glutamate release), whereas low-frequency stimulation involves mu opioid and also serotoninergic ($5HT_2$ & $5HT_3$) mechanisms[140]. In addition, part of TENS analgesia may involve peripheral $alpha_{2A}$ noradrenergic receptors, irrespective of stimulation frequency[143]. In future, the therapeutic implications of all these mechanisms need to be taken into account.

Duration of analgesia: A striking and puzzling difference between analgesia produced by acupuncture and TENS is the duration of pain relief. Whereas TENS usually produces analgesia for minutes or hours, acupuncture can, and often does, produce analgesia for weeks. The mechanisms discussed previously cannot account for the prolonged analgesia commonly seen after acupuncture and so some additional mechanisms must be involved. One suggested by Professor Jisheng Han of Beijing Medical University postulates that acupuncture sets up a so-called Meso-Limbic Loop of Analgesia[144] formed by the PAG, the nucleus Accumbens and the Habenula. Han and his colleagues have suggested that acupuncture may set in motion this particular loop of neuronal activity which, whilst it is in motion, blocks the upward transmission of nociceptive impulses from the spinal cord to the thalamus and cortex. Furthermore, Han and his colleagues[145] have shown that acupuncture analgesia can be blocked by injecting naloxone into any one of the main neuronal stations on the loop. Presumably, once the loop has been set in motion, it takes some time to slow down, and it is during this time that analgesia occurs and so explains its prolonged effect. Support for involvement of the limbic system comes from recent functional MRI (fMRI) studies in humans, which show that acupuncture causes prominent decreases (deactivation) in the signals detected in the nucleus accumbens, amygdala, hippocampus, parahippocampus, hypothalamus, ventral tegmentum, anterior cingulate gyrus, caudate and putamen areas[146]. The cerebellum may also form a part of the pain neuromatrix affected by acupuncture[147,148].

The sustained effects of acupuncture may also be due to up-regulation in analgesic gene expression and 'top-ups' are required to maintain the analgesic genes in a 'switched-on' mode[21]. Most recently, Sandkühler[149] has proposed a cellular mechanism in the spinal dorsal horn that may underlie the long-lasting analgesia that follows EA, or *deliberately painful* TENS (intense TENS), of sufficient strength to stimulate Aδ nerve fibres.

Acupuncture, neurotransmitters, and clinical effects

Many of the analgesic (and other) effects of acupuncture are due to the action it has on various neurotransmitter systems (see Table 10.1.12.3). Furthermore, the effects of real and placebo acupuncture studied with positron emission tomography (PET) suggest that both specific and non-specific factors are involved in the analgesic actions and that these can be modulated by expectancy and belief[53]. A further complication is that most controlled clinical trials of acupuncture have used minimal, superficial, sham, or placebo acupuncture. Recent work has shown that light touch of the skin stimulates mechanoreceptors coupled to slow-conducting unmyelinated C afferents that activate the insular, but not the somatosensory, cortex[150]. It is suggested that this activates the limbic region thereby resulting in emotional and hormonal reactions, effects that alleviate the affective component of pain[151].

Table 10.1.12.3 Some neurotransmitters and the effects of acupuncture upon them.

	References
5-Hydroxytryptamine (5HT), serotonin	(13)
Stimulates release of this 5HT agonist which acts centrally and peripherally via descending pain inhibitory pathways → analgesia and elevation of mood	
Noradrenaline (Nad), norepinephrine	(13)
Stimulates release of this α receptor agonist which acts centrally and peripherally via descending pain inhibitory pathways → analgesia	
Noradrenaline as transmitter in sympathetic nervous system	(18, 19)
Stimulates the hypothalamus to activate efferent sympathetic pathways and so causes the release of this α receptor agonist from postganglionic adrenergic nerve endings → circulatory and metabolic effects; normalizes blood flow and skin temperature	
met-Enkephalin	(14, 153)
δ opioid agonist (DOR) released preferentially by low-frequency (2 Hz) EA → analgesia. Action blocked by naloxone	
β-Endorphin	(14, 153)
μ opioid agonist (MOR) released preferentially by low-frequency (2 Hz) EA → analgesia. Action blocked by naloxone	
Dynorphin A & B	(14, 153)
κ opioid agonist (KOR) released preferentially by high-frequency (100 Hz) EA → analgesia. Action not blocked by normal doses of naloxone	
Orphanin OFQ, nociceptin	(140, 154)
Stimulates release of this opioid which acts on receptor LC132/ORL1 as an agonist but antagonizes the action of morphine. Role not clear, but may operate as a modulator of opioid systems. Analgesic effects of acupuncture may be antagonized by orphanin	
Adrenocorticotrophic hormone (ACTH)	(17)
Stimulates release of this pituitary peptide [co-released with β-endorphin (*qv*)] → anti-inflammatory, modulates stress and immune responses	
Substance P (SP)	(138, 155)
An excitatory agonist (slow action) released from presynaptic endings of C fibres (somatic afferents) that stimulates NK1 receptors of substantia gelatinosa (SG) cells in the process of nociceptive transmission. Acupuncture-induced release of opioid peptides (*qv*) block post-synaptically the action of SP thereby blocking nociception → analgesia	
Vasoactive intestinal peptide (VIP)	(138)
An excitatory agonist (slow action) released from presynaptic endings of C fibres (visceral afferents) that stimulates NK1 receptors of substantia gelatinosa (SG) cells in the process of nociceptive transmission. Acupuncture-induced release of opioid peptides (*qv*) block post-synaptically the action of VIP thereby blocking nociception → analgesia	
Cholecystokinin (CCK)	(94)
Stimulates release of this endogenous opioid antagonist that may contribute to the development of tolerance to acupuncture (and opioids)	
Angiotensin II (AII)	(93)
Stimulates release of this endogenous opioid antagonist (cf. cholecystokinin)	
AII may contribute to development of tolerance to acupuncture (and possibly opioids)	
Calcitonin gene-related peptide (CGRP)	(19, 138)
An excitatory neurotransmitter released from presynaptic endings of C fibres in the process of nociceptive transmission. Acupuncture-induced release of opioid peptides (*qv*) block post-synaptically this agonist and thereby blocks nociception. Also powerful vasodilator	
Nerve growth factor (NGF)	(19)
Stimulates release of NGF → CGRP & VIP (*qv*) influencing sensory and autonomic activity	
Oxytocin	(16)
Stimulates release of oxytocin from posterior pituitary gland → analgesia and sedation	
γ-Amino butyric acid (GABA)	(141)
TENS releases this inhibitory neurotransmitter from gabaergic neurons → presynaptic inhibition of C fibre endings so blocking nociceptive transmission → segmental analgesia	

(continued)

Table 10.1.12.3 (Continued) Some neurotransmitters and the effects of acupuncture upon them.

	References
Aspartate (ASP) and Glutamate (GLU)	(138)
Excitatory neurotransmitters (fast action) released from presynaptic endings of C fibres during nociceptive transmission. Acupuncture-induced release of opioid peptides (qv) block ASP & GLU post-synaptically and thereby block nociception → analgesia	
Pre-prometenkephalin, pre-prodynorphin (opioid precursors)	(21)
Electroacupuncture (EA) modulates mRNA molecules coding for opioid precursors. EA 2 Hz induces the expression of preprometenkephalin and EA 100 Hz induces the expression of preprodynorphin. Thus, EA may increase the distribution and amount of opioid peptides	
A possible mechanism by which acupuncture induces analgesia of long duration	

This may well explain why control interventions in clinical trials are found to be as effective as acupuncture and from which it is incorrectly deduced that acupuncture has had no real effect.

Whatever the cause, the assessment and evaluation of perceived pain in an individual patient represents a difficult challenge because pain is a subjective, multidimensional experience that can only be based on the individual's own report[152]. In the absence of a standard pain measure, the clinician is obliged to fall back on available rating scales, questionnaires, and other methods, but ensuring that these are relevant to the patient's specific needs. In palliative care, when the decision to use acupuncture has been reached, it is important to keep in mind the possible mechanisms that may or may not operate in an individual patient because this may have important implications for the best regimen to be used. For example, in patients with advanced cancer, the frequency of acupuncture therapy required to maintain analgesia often needs to be increased beyond that used in patients without cancer. It is likely that this is the result of neurotransmitter and immune systems (see Table 10.1.12.3), which are operating at reduced efficiency. This may well account for the different responses observed within and between patients and should be anticipated.

Epilogue

Acupuncture is not only of importance in its own right, but also because it has acted as a powerful catalyst in the study of the neurophysiology and neuropharmacology of pain. Acupuncture continues to help lead to a better understanding of the mechanism of pain and analgesia and also to the development of better analgesic agents. Acupuncture has an increasing role in the palliation of non-pain syndromes. Although some of the mechanisms of action for these remain uncertain, the success in using a non-drug treatment with minimal side effects is surely appealing for symptom management in palliative care.

Acknowledgements

The authors wish to acknowledge, with grateful thanks, the dedication, secretarial skills and long suffering efforts of Mrs Jane Brooks during the preparation of this chapter.

Reference

1. Melzack, R. (1994). Folk Medicine and the Sensory Modulation of Pain. In *Textbook of Pain* (eds. R. Melzack and P.D. Wall), pp.1209–17, 3rd edition. Churchill Livingstone, Edinburgh.

2. Ma, K.W. (1992). The roots and development of Chinese Acupuncture: from prehistory to early 20th century. *Acupuncture in Medicine*, **10** (Suppl), 92–9.

3. Veith, I. (1972). *The Yellow Emperor's Classic of Internal Medicine.* University of California Press, Berkeley.

4. Lu, G.D. and Needham, J. (1980). *Celestial lancets, a history and rationale of acupuncture and moxa.* Cambridge University Press.

5. Dorfer, L., Mose, M., Bahr, F. *et al.* (1999). A medical report from the stone age? *Lancet*, **354**(9183), 1023–5.

6. Kaptchuk, T.J. (2000). *Chinese Medicine: The Web That Has No Weaver.* Ryder, London.

7. Vincent, C.A. (1992). Acupuncture research: why do it? *Complementary Medical Research*, **6**(1), 21–4.

8. MacDonald, A.J. (1989). Acupuncture Analgesia and Therapy. In *Textbook of Pain* (eds. R. Melzack and P.D. Wall), pp. 906-19, 2nd edition. Churchill Livingstone.

9. Langevin, H.M. and Yandow, J.A. (2002). Relationship of acupuncture points and meridians to connective tissue planes. *Anatomical Record*, **269**(6), Dec 15, 257–65.

10. Chiang, C.Y., Chang, C.T., Chu, H.L. *et al.* (1973). Peripheral afferent pathway for acupuncture analgesia. *Scientia Sinica*, **16**(2), 210–7.

11. Dundee, J.W. and Ghaly, G. (1991). Local anesthesia blocks the antiemetic action of P6 acupuncture. *Clinical Pharmacology and Therapeutics*, **50**, 78–80.

12. Clement-Jones, V., McLoughlin, L., Tomlin, S. *et al.* (1980). Increased beta-endorphin but not met-enkephalin levels in human cerebrospinal fluid after acupuncture for recurrent pain. *Lancet*, **2**(8201), Nov 1, 946–9.

13. Han, J.S. and Terenius, L. (1982). Neurochemical basis of acupuncture analgesia. *Annu Rev Pharmacology and Toxicology*, **22**, 193–220.

14. Han, J.S., Chen, X.H., Sun, S.L. *et al.* (1991). Effect of low- and high-frequency TENS on Met-enkephalin-Arg-Phe and dynorphin A immunoreactivity in human lumbar CSF. *Pain*, **47**(3), Dec, 295–8.

15. Han, J.S. (2004). Acupuncture and endorphins. *Neuroscience Letters*, **361**(1–3), May 6, 258–61.

16. Uvnas-Moberg, K., Bruzelius, G., Alster, P. *et al.* (1993). The antinociceptive effect of non-noxious sensory stimulation is mediated partly through oxytocinergic mechanisms. *Acta Physiologica Scandinavica*, **149**(2), Oct, 199–204.

17. Roth, L.U., Maret-Maric, A., Adler, R.H. *et al.* (1997). Acupuncture Points have Subjective (Needling Sensation) and Objective (Serum Cortisol Increase) Specificity. *Acupuncture in Medicine*, **15**(1), 2–5.

18. Ernst, M., Lee, M.H. (1985). Sympathetic vasomotor changes induced by manual and electrical acupuncture of the Hoku point visualized by thermography. *Pain*, **21**(1), Jan, 25–33.

19. Lundeberg, T. (1999). Effects of sensory stimulation (acupuncture) on circulatory and immune systems. In *Acupuncture: a scientific appraisal* (eds. E. Ernst and A.White), pp. 93–106. Butterworth-Heinemann, Oxford.

20. Lee, J.H. and Beitz, A.J. (1993). The distribution of brain-stem and spinal cord nuclei associated with different frequencies of electroacupuncture analgesia. *Pain*, **52**(1), Jan, 11–28.

21. Guo, H.F., Tian, J., Wang, X. *et al.* (1996). Brain substrates activated by electroacupuncture of different frequencies (I): Comparative study on the expression of oncogene c-fos and genes coding for three opioid peptides. *Brain Research. Molecular Brain Research*, **43**(1–2), Dec 31, 157–66.

22. Travell, J.G. and Simons, D.G. (1983). *Myofascial Pain and Dysfunction. The Trigger Point Manual*. Williams and Wilkins, Baltimore.

23. Filshie, J. and Cummings, M. (1999). Western medical acupuncture. In *Acupuncture: a scientific appraisal* (eds. E. Ernst and A. White), pp. 31–59. Butterworth-Heinemann, Oxford.

24. Melzack, R., Stillwell, D.M., and Fox, E.J. (1977). Trigger points and acupuncture points for pain: correlations and implications. *Pain*, **3**(1), Feb, 3–23.

25. Dorsher, P.T. (2004). Poster 196 Myofascial Pain: Rediscovery of a 2000-Year-Old Tradition. *Archives of Physical Medicine and Rehabilitation*, **85**(9).

26. Baldry, P.E. (2004). *Acupuncture, Trigger Points and Musculo-Skeletal Pain*. 3rd edition. Churchill Livingstone, Edinburgh.

27. Mann, F. (2000.). *Reinventing Acupuncture*. 2nd edition. Butterworth Heinemann.

28. *Essentials of Chinese Acupuncture* (1980). Foreign Languages Press, Beijing.

29. Stux, G. and Hammerschlag, R. (2001). *Clinical Acupuncture: Scientific Basis*. Springer-Verlag, Berlin and Heidelberg.

30. Campbell, A. (2001). *Acupuncture in Practice*. Butterworth Heinemann.

31. White A. (1998). Electroacupuncture and acupuncture analgesia. In *Acupuncture: A Western Scientific Approach* (eds. J. Filshie and A. White), pp.153–75. Churchill Livingstone, Medical Edinburgh.

32. Brockhaus, A. and Elger, C.E. (1990). Hypalgesic efficacy of acupuncture on experimental pain in man. Comparison of laser acupuncture and needle acupuncture. *Pain*, **43**, 181–5.

33. White A. (1999). Neurophysiology of acupuncture analgesia. In *Acupuncture: A Scientific Appraisal*. (eds. E. Ernst and A. White), pp. 60–92. Butterworth-Heinemann, Oxford.

34. Kotani, N., Hashimoto, H., Sato, Y. *et al.* (2001). Preoperative intradermal acupuncture reduces postoperative pain, nausea and vomiting, analgesic requirement, and sympathoadrenal responses. *Anesthesiology*, **95**(2), Aug, 349–56.

35. Pontinen, P.J. (1992). *Lower Level Laser Therapy as a Medical Treatment Modality: a Manual for Physicians, Dentists, Physiotherapists and Veterinary Surgeons*. Art Upo Ltd, Tampere.

36. Litscher, G. (2006). Bioengineering assessment of acupuncture, part 2: monitoring of microcirculation. *Critical Reviews in Biomededical Engineering*, **34**(4), 273–94.

37. Brosseau, L., Welch, V., Wells, G. *et al.* (2002). Low Level Laser Therapy (Classes I, II & III) for Treating Osteoarthritis (Cochrane Review). The Cochrane Library [1]. Oxford, Update Software.

38. Brosseau, L., Welch, V., Wells, G. *et al.* (2002). Low Level Laser Therapy (Classes I, II & III) for Treating Rheumatoid Arthritis (Cochrane Review). The Cochrane Library [1]. Oxford, Update Software.

39. Wu, H.S., Wu, S.C., Lin, J.G. *et al.* (2004). Effectiveness of acupressure in improving dyspnoea in chronic obstructive pulmonary disease. *Journal of Advanced Nursing*, **45**(3), Feb, 252–9.

40. Nogier, P.F.M. (1972). *Treatise of Auriculotherapy*. Maisonneuve, France.

41. Oleson, T.D., Kroening, R.J., and Bresler, D.E. (1980). An experimental evaluation of auricular diagnosis: the somatotopic mapping of musculoskeletal pain at ear acupuncture points. *Pain*, **8**, 217–29.

42. White, A. and Moody, R. (2006). The effects of auricular acupuncture on smoking cessation may not depend on the point chosen - an exploratory meta-analysis. *Acupuncture in Medicine*, **24**(4), Dec, 149–56.

43. Nakatari, Y. and Yamashita, K. (1977). *Ryodoraku Acupuncture*. Ryodoraku Research Institute Ltd.

44. Lindley, S. and Cummings, T.M. (2006). *Essentials of Western Veterinary Acupuncture*. Blackwell Publishing, Oxford.

45. *Medical Acupuncture: A Western Scientific Approach*. (1998). Churchill Livingstone, Edinburgh.

46. *Acupuncture: A Scientific Appraisal*. (1999). Butterworth-Heinemann, Oxford.

47. White, A.R., Filshie, J., and Cummings, T.M. (2001). Clinical trials of acupuncture: consensus recommendations for optimal treatment, sham controls and blinding. *Comparative Ther Med*, **9**(4), Dec, 237–45.

48. Sanchez Aranjo, M. (1998). Does the Choice of Placebo Determine the Results of Clinical Studies on Acupuncture? *Forsch Komplementarmed*, **5** (Suppl), S1:8–11.

49. Kleinhenz, J., Streitberger, K., Windeler, J. *et al.* (1999). Randomised clinical trial comparing the effects of acupuncture and a newly designed placebo needle in rotator cuff tendinitis. *Pain*, **83**(2), Nov, 235–41.

50. ter Riet, G., de Craen, A.J., de Boer, A. *et al.* (1998). Is placebo analgesia mediated by endogenous opioids? A systematic review. *Pain*, **76**(3), Jun, 273–5.

51. Levine, J.D., Gordon, N.C., and Fields, H.L. (1978). The mechanism of placebo analgesia. *Lancet*, **23**, 2(8091), Sep, 654–7.

52. Thomas, M., Eriksson, S.V., and Lundeberg, T. (1991). A comparative study of diazepam and acupuncture in patients with osteoarthritis pain, a placebo controlled study. *American Journal of Chinese Medicine*, **19**, 95–100.

53. Pariente, J., White, P., Frackowiak, R.S. *et al.* (2005). Expectancy and belief modulate the neuronal substrates of pain treated by acupuncture. *Neuroimage*, **25**(4), May 1, 1161–7.

54. Patel, M., Gutzwiller, F., Paccaud, F. *et al.* (1989). A meta-analysis of acupuncture for chronic pain. *International Journal of Epidemiology*, **18**(4), Dec, 900–6.

55. ter Riet, G., Kleijnen, J., and Knipschild, P. (1990). Acupuncture and chronic pain: a criteria-based meta-analysis. *Journal of Clinical Epidemiology*, **43**(11), 1191–9.

56. Ezzo, J., Berman, B., Hadhazy, V.A. *et al.* (2000). Is acupuncture effective for the treatment of chronic pain? A systematic review. *Pain*, **86**(3), Jun, 217–25.

57. Lee, A. and Done, M.L. (1999). The use of nonpharmacologic techniques to prevent postoperative nausea and vomiting: a meta-analysis. *Anesthesia Analgesia*, **88**(6), Jun, 1362–9.

58. Lee, A. and Done ML. (2004). Stimulation of the wrist acupuncture point P6 for preventing postoperative nausea and vomiting. *Cochrane Database of Systematic Review*, **3**, CD003281.

59. Ezzo, J., Vickers, A., Richardson, M.A. *et al.* (2005). Acupuncture-point stimulation for chemotherapy-induced nausea and vomiting. *Journal of Clinical Oncology*, **23**(28), Oct 1, 7188–98.

60. Ernst, E. and Pittler, M.H. (1998). The effectiveness of acupuncture in treating acute dental pain: a systematic review. *British Dental Journal*, **184**(9), May 9, 443–7.

61. Melchart, D., Linde, K., Fischer, P. *et al.* (2001). Acupuncture for idiopathic headache. *Cochrane Database Syst Rev*, **1**, CD001218.

62. Berman, B., Ezzo, J., Hadhazy, V. *et al.* (1999). Is acupuncture effective in the treatment of fibromyalgia? *Journal of Family Practice*, **48**, 213–8.

63. Manheimer, E., White, A., Berman, B. *et al.* (2005). Meta-analysis: acupuncture for low back pain. *Annals of Internal Medicine*, **142**(8), Apr 19, 651–63.

64. Ezzo, J., Hadhazy, V., Birch, S. *et al.* (2001). Acupuncture for osteoarthritis of the knee: a systematic review. *Arthritis and Rheumatism*, **44**(4), Apr, 819–25.

65. White, A., Foster, N.E., Cummings, M. *et al.* (2007). Acupuncture treatment for chronic knee pain: a systematic review. *Rheumatology (Oxford)*, **46**(3), Mar, 384–90.

66. Linde, K., Jobst, K., and Panton, J. (2000). Acupuncture for chronic asthma. *Cochrane Database of Systematic Reviews*, **2**, CD000008.

67. Park, J., Hopwood, V., White, A.R. *et al.* (2001). Effectiveness of acupuncture for stroke: a systematic review. *Journal of Neurology*, **248**(7), Jul, 558–63.

68. Ernst, E. (1997). Acupuncture/acupressure for weight reduction? A systematic review. *Wien Klin Wochenschr*, **109**(2), Jan 31, 60–2.

69. White, A.R., Rampes, H., and Ernst, E. (2002). Acupuncture for smoking cessation. *Cochrane Database of Systematic Reviews*, **2**, CD000009.

70. Cummings, M. (1996). Audit in Acupuncture Practice: A Computerised Audit of Acupuncture in Two Populations: Civilian and Forces. *Acupuncture in Medicine*, **14**(1), 37–9.

71. Stellon, A. (2001). An Audit of Acupuncture in a Single-Handed General Practice Over One Year. *Acupuncture in Medicine*, **19**(1), 36–42.

72. Freedman, J. (2002). An Audit of 500 Acupuncture Patients in General Practice. *Acupuncture in Medicine*, **20**(1), 30–4.

73. Ross, J. (2001). Audit of the impact of introducing microacupuncture into primary care. *Acupuncture in Medicine*, **19**(1), 43–5.

74. Poulain, P., Pichard Leandri, E., Laplanche, A. *et al.* (1997). Electroacupuncture Analgesia in Major Abdominal and Pelvic Surgery: A Randomised Study. *Acupuncture in Medicine*, **XV**(1), 10–3.

75. Vickers, A.J., Rusch, V.W., Malhotra, V.T. *et al.* (2006). Acupuncture is a feasible treatment for post-thoracotomy pain: results of a prospective pilot trial. *BMC Anesthesiology*, **6**, 5.

76. Filshie, J. and Redman, D. (1985). Acupuncture and malignant pain problems. *European Journal of Surgical Oncology*, **11**(4), Dec, 389–94.

77. Filshie, J. (1990). Acupuncture for Malignant Pain. *Acupuncture in Medicine*, **8**(2), 38–9.

78. Wen, H.L. (1977). Cancer pain treated with acupuncture and electrical stimulation. *Modern Medicine in Asia*, **13**(2), 12–6.

79. Aung, S. (1994). The clinical use of acupuncture in oncology: Symptom control. *Acupuncture in Medicine*, **12**(1), 37–40.

80. Leng, G. (1999). A year of acupuncture in palliative care. *Palliative Medicine*, **13**, 163–4.

81. Johnstone, P.A.S, Polston, G.R., Niemtzow, R.C. *et al.* (2002). Integration of acupuncture into the oncology clinic. *Palliative Medicine*, **16**, 235–9.

82. Filshie, J., Scase, A., Ashley, S. *et al.* (1997). *A study of the acupuncture effects on pain, anxiety and depression in patients with breast cancer* (abstract). Pain Society Meeting.

83. Watson, M., Haviland, J.S., Greer, S. *et al.* (1999). Influence of psychological response on survival in breast cancer: a population-based cohort study. *Lancet*, **354**, 1331–6.

84. He, J.P., Friedrich, M., Ertan, A.K. *et al.* (1999). Pain-relief and movement improvement by acupuncture after ablation and axillary lymphadenectomy in patients with mammary cancer. *Clinical and Experimental Obstetrics and Gynecology*, **26**(2), 81–4.

85. Lee, H., Schmidt, K., and Ernst, E. (2005). Acupuncture for the relief of cancer-related pain - a systematic review. *European Journal of Pain*, **9**(4), Aug, 437–44.

86. Monga, T.N. and Jaksic, T. (1981). Acupuncture in phantom limb pain. *Archives of Physical Medicine Rehabilitation*, **62**(5), May, 229–31.

87. Ernst, E. and Lee, M.H.M. (1986). Sympathetic effects of manual and electrical acupuncture of the tsusanli knee point: comparison with the hoku hand point sympathetic effects. *Experimental Neurology*, **94**, 1–10.

88. Filshie, J. and Cummings, M. (2000). *Acupuncture. Management of Phantom Limb Pain.* The First International Consensus Meeting, Oxford University.

89. Dillon, M. and Lucas, C.F. (1999). Auricular stud acupuncture in palliative care patients: an initial report. *Palliative Medicine*, **13**(3), 253–4.

90. Alimi, D., Rubino, C., Leandri, E.P. *et al.* (2000). Analgesic effects of auricular acupuncture for cancer pain. *Journal of Pain and Symptom Management*, **19**(2), Feb, 81–2.

91. Alimi, D., Rubino, C., Pichard-Leandri, E. *et al.* (2003). Analgesic effect of auricular acupuncture for cancer pain: a randomized, blinded, controlled trial. *Journal of Clinical Oncology*, **21**(22), Nov 15, 4120–6.

92. Cummings, M. (2001). Percutaneous electrical nerve stimulation–electroacupuncture by another name? A comparative review. *Acupuncture in Medicine*, **19**(1), Jun, 32–5.

93. Wang, K. and Han, J.S. (1990). Accelerated synthesis and release of angiotensin II in the rat brain during electroacupuncture tolerance. *Science in China*, **33**(6), 686–93.

94. Zhou, Y., Sun, Y.H., Shen, J.M. *et al.* (1993). Increased release of immunoreactive CCK-8 by electroacupuncture and enhancement of electroacupuncture analgesia by CCK-B antagonist in rat spinal cord. *Neuropeptides*, **24**(3), Mar, 139–44.

95. Jobst, K., Chen, J.H., McPherson, K. *et al.* (1986). Controlled trial of acupuncture for disabling breathlessness. *Lancet*, **2**(8521–2), Dec 20, 1416–9.

96. Maa, S-H., Gauthier, D., and Turner, M. (1997). Acupressure as an Adjunct to a Pulmonary Rehabilitation Program. *Journal of Cadiopulmonary Rehabilitation*, **17**, 268–76.

97. Neumeister, W., Kuhlemann, H., Bauer, T. *et al.* (1999). Effect of acupuncture on quality of life, mouth occlusion pressures and lung function in COPD. *Medizinische Klinik*, **94**(1 Spec No), Apr, 106–9.

98. Filshie, J., Penn, K., Ashley, S. *et al.* (1996). Acupuncture for the relief of cancer-related breathlessness. *Palliative Medicine*, **10**(2), Apr, 145–50.

99. Vickers, A.J., Feinstein, M.B., Deng, G.E. *et al.* (2005). Acupuncture for dyspnea in advanced cancer: a randomized, placebo-controlled pilot trial [ISRCTN89462491]. *BMC Palliative Care*, **18**, Au, 4–5.

100. McMillan, C.M. (1998). Acupuncture for nausea and vomiting. In *Medical Acupuncture: A Western Scientific Approach* (eds. J. Filshie and A. White), pp. 295–317. Churchill Livingstone, Edinburgh.

101. Vickers, A.J. (1996). Can acupuncture have specific effects on health? A systematic review of acupuncture antiemesis trials. *Journal of the Royal Society of Medicine*, **89**, 303–11.

102. Shen, J., Wenger, N., Glaspy, J. *et al.* (2000). Electroacupuncture for control of myeloablative chemotherapy-induced emesis: A randomized controlled trial. *JAMA*, **284**(21), Dec 6, 2755–61.

103. Blom, M., Dawidson, I., and Angmar-Mansson, B. (1992). The effect of acupuncture on salivary flow rates in patients with xerostomia. *Oral Surgery, Oral Medicine, Oral Pathoogyl*, **73**(3), Mar, 293–8.

104. Blom, M., Dawidson, I., Fernberg, J.O. *et al.* (1996). Acupuncture treatment of patients with radiation-induced xerostomia. *European Journal of Cancer B Oral Oncology*, **32B**(3), May, 182–90.

105. Wong, R.K., Jones, G.W., Sagar, S.M. *et al.* (2003). A Phase I-II study in the use of acupuncture-like transcutaneous nerve stimulation in the treatment of radiation-induced xerostomia in head-and-neck cancer patients treated with radical radiotherapy. *International Journal of Radiation Oncology, Biology, Physics*, **57**(2), Oct 1, 472–80.

106. Johnstone, P.A.S., Peng, Y.P., May, B.C. *et al.* (2001). Acupuncture for Pilocarpine-Resistant Xerostomia Following Radiotherapy for Head and Neck Malignancies. *International Journal of Radiation Oncology, Biology, Physics*, **50**(2), 353–7.

107. Rydholm, M. and Strang, P. (1999). Acupuncture for patients in hospital-based home care suffering from xerostomia. *Journal of Palliative Care*, **15**(4), 20–3.

108. Filshie, J. (1988). The non-drug treatment of neuralgic and neuropathic pain of malignancy. *Cancer Surveys*, **7**(1), 161–93.

109. Wyon, Y., Lindgren, R., Lundeberg, T. *et al.* (1995). Effects of Acupuncture on Climacteric Vasomotor Symptoms, Quality of Life, and Urinary Excretion of Neuropeptides Among Post Menopausal Women. *Menopause*, **2**(1), 3–12.

110. Filshie, J., Bolton, T., Browne, D. *et al.* (2005). Acupuncture and self acupuncture for long-term treatment of vasomotor symptoms in cancer patients--audit and treatment algorithm. *Acupuncture Medicine*, **23**(4), Dec, 171–80.

111. de Valois, B. (2006). *Using Acupuncture to Manage Hot Flushes and Night Sweats in Women Taking Tamoxifen for Early Breast Cancer: Two Observational Studies.* Thames Valley University.

112. Filshie, J. and Hester, J. (2006). Guidelines for providing acupuncture treatment for cancer patients - a peer-reviewed sample policy document. *Acupuncture in Medicine*, **24**(4), Dec, 172–82.

113. Hammar, M., Frisk, J., Grimas, O. *et al.* (1999). Acupuncture Treatment of Vasomotor Symptoms in Men with Prostatic Carcinoma: A Pilot Study. *The Journal of Urology*, **161**, 853–6.

114. Zhang, Z.H. (1987). Effect of acupuncture on 44 cases of radiation rectitis following radiation therapy for carcinoma of the cervix uteri. *Journal of Traditional Chinese Medicine*, **7**(2), Jun, 139–40.

115. Lundeberg, T., Bondesson, L., and Thomas, M. (1987). Effect of acupuncture on experimentally induced itch. *British Journal of Dermatology*, **117**(6), Dec, 771–7.

116. Duo, L.J. (1987). Electrical needle therapy of uremic pruritus. *Nephron*, **47**(3), 179–83.

117. Greene, K.B., Berger, J., Reeves, C. *et al.* (1999). Most frequently used alternative and complementary therapies and activities by participants in the AMCOA study. *Journal of the Association of Nurses in AIDS Care*, **10**(3), May, 60–73.

118. Phillips, K.D. and Skelton, W.D. (2001). Effects of individualized acupuncture on sleep quality in HIV disease. *Journal of the Association of Nurses in AIDS Care*, **12**(1), Jan, 27–39.

119. Shlay, C.J., Chaloner, K., Max, M.B. *et al.* (1998). Acupuncture and amitriptyline for pain due to HIV-related peripheral neuropathy. *JAMA*, **280**, 1590–5.

120. Phillips, K.D., Skelton, W.D., and Hand, G.A. (2004). Effect of acupuncture administered in a group setting on pain and subjective peripheral neuropathy in persons with human immunodeficiency virus disease. *Journal of Alternative and Complementary Medicine*, **10**(3), Jun, 449–55.

121. Anastasi, J.K. and McMahon, D.J. (2003). Testing strategies to reduce diarrhea in persons with HIV using traditional Chinese medicine: acupuncture and moxibustion. *Journal of the Association of Nurses in AIDS Care*, **14**(3), May, 28–40.

122. Jonsdottir, I.H. (1999). Physical exercise, acupuncture and immune function. *Acupuncture in Medicine*, **17**(1), 50–3.

123. Mukaino, Y., Park, J., White, A. *et al.* (2005). The effectiveness of acupuncture for depression – a systematic review of randomised controlled trials. *Acupuncture in Medicine*, **23**(2), Jun, 70–6.

124. Lazarou, J., Pomeranz, B.H., and Corey, P.N. (1998). Incidence of adverse drug reactions in hospitalized patients: a meta- analysis of prospective studies. *JAMA*, **279**(15), Apr 15, 1200–5.

125. White, A. (2004). A cumulative review of the range and incidence of significant adverse events associated with acupuncture. *Acupuncture in Medicine*, **22**(3), Sep, 122–33.

126. Filshie, J. (2001). Safety aspects of acupuncture in palliative care. *Acupuncture in Medicine*, **19**(2), Dec, 117–22.

127. White, A., Hayhoe, S., Hart, A. *et al.* (2001). Survey of adverse events following acupuncture (SAFA): a prospective study of 32,000 consultations. *Acupuncture in Medicine*, **19**(2), Dec, 84–92.

128. MacPherson, H., Thomas, K., Walters, S. *et al.* (2001). A prospective survey of adverse events and treatment reactions following 34,000 consultations with professional acupuncturists. *Acupuncture in Medicine*, **19**(2), Dec, 93–102.

129. Peuker, E. and Grönemeyer, D. (v). Rare But Serious Complications of Acupuncture: Traumatic Lesions. *Acupuncture in Medicine*, **19**(2), 103–8.

130. Otsuka, N., Fukunaga, M., Morita, K. *et al.* (1990). Iodine-131 uptake in a patient with thyroid cancer and rheumatoid arthritis during acupuncture treatment. *Clinical Nuclear Medicine*, **15**, 29–31.

131. Odsberg, A., Schill, U., and Haker, E. (2001). Acupuncture treatment: side effects and complications reported by Swedish physiotherapists. *Complementary Therapeutic Medicine*, **9**(1), Mar, 17–20.

132. Duggan, A.W. and Foong, F.W. (1985). Bicuculline and spinal inhibition produced by dorsal column stimulation in the cat. *Pain*, **22**(3), Jul, 249–59.

133. Bowsher, D. Sensory Mechanisms. (1985). In *Clinical Neuropsychology* (ed. J.A.M. Frederiks), p. 45. In *Handbook of Clinical Neurology* (eds. P.J. Vinken, G.W. Bruyn and H.L. Klawans), pp. 227–44. Elsevier, Amsterdam.

134. Bowsher, D. (1987). The physiology of acupuncture. *Journal of the Intractable Pain Society of Great Britain and Ireland*, **5**(1), 15–8.

135. Le Bars, D., Dickenson, A.H., and Besson, J.M. (1979). Diffuse noxious inhibitory controls (DNIC). II. Lack of effect on non-convergent neurones, supraspinal involvement and theoretical implications. *Pain*, **6**(3), Jun, 305–27.

136. Fields, H.L. and Basbaum, A.I. (1994). Central nervous system mechanisms of pain modulation. In *Textbook of Pain*. (eds. P.D. Wall and R. Melzack), pp. 243–57, 3rd edition. Churchill Livingstone, Edinburgh.

137. Jones, A.P.K., Brown, W.D., Friston, K.J. *et al.* (1991). Cortical and subcortical localization of response to pain in man using positron emission tomography. *Proceedings of the Royal Society of London, Series B*, **244**(1309), Apr 22, 39–44.

138. Dickenson, A.H. (1996). Pain mechanisms and pain syndromes. In *Pain-an updated review*. Seattle: International Association for the Study of Pain (ed. J.N.Campbell), pp. 113–21.

139. Dickenson, A. and Suzuki, R. (2005). Targets in Pain and Analgesia. In *The Neurobiology of Pain* (eds. S.P. Hunt and M. Koltzenburg), pp. 149–63. Oxford University Press.

140. Sluka, K.A., Wu, G-C., and Chung, J.M. (2006). Recent Insights into Analgesic Mechanisms of Acupuncture and TENS. In *Proceedings of the 11th World Congress on Pain.Seattle: International Association for the Study of Pain* (eds. H. Flor, E. Kalso, and J.O. Dostrovsky)

141. Garrison, D.W. and Foreman, R.D. (1994). Decreased activity of spontaneous and noxiously evoked dorsal horn cells during transcutaneous electrical nerve stimulation (TENS). *Pain*, **58**(3), Sep, 309–15.

142. Sjölund, B. and Eriksson, M. (1979). Endorphins and Analgesia Produced by Peripheral Conditioning Stimulation. In *Advances in Pain Research and Therapy 3.Seattle: International Association for the Study of Pain* (eds. J.J.Bonica, J.C. Liebeskind, and D.G. Albe-Fessard), pp. 587–92.

143. King, E.W., Audette, K., Athman, G.A. *et al.* (2005). Transcutaneous electrical nerve stimulation activates peripherally located alpha-2A adrenergic receptors. *Pain*, **115**(3), Jun, 364–73.

144. Han, J.S., Yu, L.C., and Shi, Y.S. (1986). A Mesolimbic Loop of Analgesia. III A Neuronal Pathway from Nucleus Accumbens to Periaqueductal Grey. *Asian Pacific Journal of Pharmacology*, **1**, 7–22.

145. Zhou, Z.F., Du, M.Y., Wu, W.Y. *et al.* (1981). Effect of intracerebral microinjection of naloxone on acupuncture and morphine analgesia in the rabbit. *Scientia Sinica*, **24**(8), Aug, 1166–78.

146. Hui, K.K., Liu, J., Makris, N. *et al.* (2000). Acupuncture modulates the limbic system and subcortical gray structures of the human brain: evidence from fMRI studies in normal subjects. *Human Brain Mapp*, **9**(1), 13–25.

147. Yoo, S.S., Teh, E.K., Blinder, R.A. *et al.* (2004). Modulation of cerebellar activities by acupuncture stimulation: evidence from fMRI study. *Neuroimage*, **22**(2), Jun, 932–40.

148. Hui, K.K., Liu, J., Marina, O. *et al.* (2005). The integrated response of the human cerebro-cerebellar and limbic systems to acupuncture stimulation at ST 36 as evidenced by fMRI. *Neuroimage*, **27**(3), Sep, 479–96.

149. Sandkühler, J. (2000). Long-Lasting Analgesia Following TENS and Acupuncture: Spinal Mechanisms Beyond Gate Control. In *Proceedings of the 9th World Congress on Pain - Progress in Pain Research and Management. Seattle: International Association for the Study of Pain* (eds. M. Devor, N.C. Rowbotham, and Z. Wiesenfeld-Hallin), pp. 359–69.

150. Olausson, H., Lamarre, Y., Backlund, H. *et al.* (2002). Unmyelinated tactile afferents signal touch and project to insular cortex. *Nature Neuroscience*, **5**(9), Sep, 900–4.

151. Lund, I. and Lundeberg, T. (2006). Are minimal, superficial or sham acupuncture procedures acceptable as inert placebo controls? *Acupuncture in Medicine*, **24**(1), Mar, 13–5.

152. Lund, I. and Lundeberg, T. (2006). Aspects of pain, its assessment and evaluation from an acupuncture perspective. *Acupuncture in Medicine*, **24**(3), Sep, 109–17.

153. Han, J.S. and Sun, S. (1990). Differential release of enkephalin and dynorphin by low and high frequencies electroacupuncture in the central nervous system. *Acupuncture: The Scientific International Journal (New York)*, **1**(1), 19–27.

154. Tian, J. (1997). Involvement of endogenous orphanin FQ in electroacupuncture-induced analgesia. *Neuroreport*, **8**, 497–500.

155. Han, J.S. (1984). Progress in the pharmacological studies of acupuncture analgesia. In *9th International Congress of Pharmacology*. London: Macmillan Proceedings, vol 1(ed. S.W. Paton)

10.1.13 Psychological and psychiatric interventions in pain control

William Breitbart, Steven D. Passik, and David J. Casper

Introduction

Effective management of pain in patients with advanced illness requires a multi-disciplinary approach, enlisting expertise from a wide variety of clinical specialties including neurology, neurosurgery, anaesthesiology, and rehabilitation medicine[1–3]. The utilization of psychiatric and psychological interventions in the treatment of pain and distress is an integral part of such a comprehensive approach[4–6].

The scope of the problem

Pain is a common problem in populations with advanced illness and has been best characterized in those with cancer or AIDS. Approximately 70 per cent of cancer patients experience severe pain at some time in the course of their illness[2] and that nearly 75 per cent of those with advanced cancer have pain[7]. Overall, approximately 50 per cent of terminally ill patients are in moderate to severe pain[8]. It also has been estimated that 25 per cent of cancer patients die in severe pain[9].

There is considerable variability in the prevalence of pain among different types of cancer. For example, approximately 5 per cent of leukemia patients experience pain during the course of their illness, as compared to 50–75 per cent of patients with tumours of the lung, gastrointestinal tract, or genitourinary system. Patients with cancers of the bone or cervix have been found to have the highest prevalence of pain, with as many as 85 per cent of patients experiencing significant pain during the course of their illness[1].

Despite the high prevalence of pain in populations with advanced illness, there is evidence that pain is frequently under-diagnosed and inadequately treated[9,10]. This phenomenon presumably has multiple causes, one of which is the complex presentation of pain in these populations. It is important to remember that pain is frequently only one of multiple concurrent symptoms. In one survey, cancer patients were found to suffer from an average of three additional troubling physical symptoms[11]. With disease progression, the number of distressing physical symptoms increases. Another study observed that patients with advanced disease reported a median of 11 symptoms[12]. A global evaluation of the symptom burden allows for a more complete understanding of the impact of pain[13].

Pain is a significant and often neglected problem in patients with AIDS. Estimates of the prevalence of pain in AIDS generally range from 30 per cent to 90 per cent, with prevalence increasing as the disease progresses[14,15]. The incidence of disturbing pain in AIDS may be as high as 88 per cent, and 69 per cent of patients may suffer from pain that results in moderate to severe impairment in activities of daily living[16]. A retrospective chart review of hospitalized patients with AIDS revealed that more than 50 per cent required treatment for pain; pain was the presenting complaint in 30 per cent (second only to fever)[17]. In the latter study, chest pain occurred in 22 per cent, headache in 13 per cent, oral cavity pain in 11 per cent, abdominal pain in 9 per cent, and peripheral neuropathy in 6 per cent. Another retrospective review of pain in an AIDS population reported abdominal pain, peripheral neuropathy, and Kaposi's sarcoma as the three most frequent pain problems, which together affected 15 per cent of patients[18]. Other reviews report that between 5 per cent and 30 per cent of AIDS patients have painful peripheral neuropathy[19–22]. In a hospice setting, Schofferman and Brody[22] described pain in 53 per cent of patients with far-advanced AIDS; the main diagnoses were peripheral neuropathy, abdominal pain, headache, and Kaposi's sarcoma (skin pain). In an ambulatory AIDS population, 43 per cent of patients reported pain of at least 2 weeks duration[23]; painful neuropathy accounted for 50 per cent of pain diagnoses and lower-extremity pain related to Kaposi's sarcoma was found in 45 per cent. While pains of a neuropathic nature are an important clinical problem that has attracted a great deal of attention, the evolving literature on AIDS pain syndromes suggests that somatic and visceral pain syndromes are more prevalent in this population. Recent work suggests that of the pains experienced by ambulatory patients with AIDS, approximately 33 per cent are somatic, 35 per cent are visceral, and 33 per cent are neuropathic. In addition, somatic, visceral, and neuropathic pains often occur concurrently, and neuropathic pain is not often the predominant pain[24].

Multi-dimensional concept of pain in terminal illness

Pain is not a purely physical experience, but involves complex aspects of human functioning, including personality, affect, cognition, behaviour, and social relations[25]. A more enlightened description of the pain resulting from a terminal illness coined by Cecily Saunders[26] is 'total pain', a label that attempts to describe the all-encompassing nature of this type of pain. This description helps explain the observation that the use of analgesic drugs alone does not always lead to pain relief[27] and that that psychological factors play a modest but important role in pain intensity[28]. The interaction of cognitive, emotional, socio-environmental, and nociceptive aspects of pain shown in Fig. 10.1.13.1 illustrates the multi-dimensional nature of pain in terminal illness and suggests a model for multimodal intervention[3]. The challenge of untangling and addressing both the physical and psychological issues involved in pain is essential to developing rational and effective management strategies. Psychosocial therapies directed primarily at psychological variables have an impact on nociception, while somatic therapies directed at nociception have beneficial effects on the psychological aspects of pain. Ideally, such somatic and psychosocial therapies are used simultaneously in a multi-disciplinary approach to pain management in the terminally ill[4].

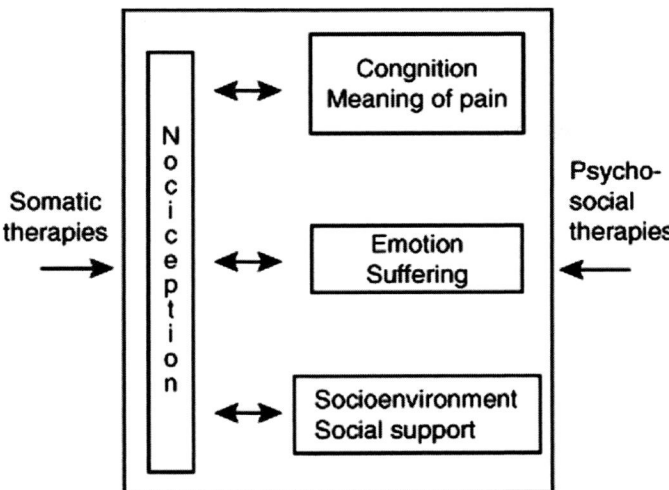

Figure 10.1.13.1 The multi-dimensional nature of pain in terminal illness.

Psychological factors in pain experience

Among the many stressors faced by patients with advanced disease are dependency, disability, and fear of painful death. Such fears are universal; however, the level of psychological distress is variable and depends on medical factors, social supports, coping capacities, and personality. Pain has profound effects on psychological distress, and psychological factors such as anxiety, depression, and the meaning of pain can intensify pain. Daut and Cleeland[29] showed that cancer patients who attributed a new pain to an unrelated benign cause reported less interference with their activity and pleasure than cancer patients who believed that their pain represented progression of disease. Spiegel and Bloom[30] found that women with metastatic breast cancer experienced more intense pain if they believed that their pain represented spread of their cancer, and if they were depressed. Beliefs about the meaning of pain and the presence of a mood disturbance are better predictors of level of pain than is the site of metastasis.

In an attempt to define the potential relationships between pain and psychosocial variables, Padilla et al.[31] found that there were pain-related quality-of-life variables in three domains: (1) physical well-being; (2) psychological well-being (consisting of affective factors, cognitive factors, spiritual factors, communication, coping, and meaning of pain or cancer); and (3) interpersonal well-being (focusing on social support or role functioning). Patients who feel that their pain is related to their cancer report pain of greater intensity, coupled with greater affective distress[32]. The perception of marked impairment in activities of daily living has been shown to be associated with increased pain intensity[33,34]. Measures of emotional disturbance have been reported to be predictors of pain in late stages of cancer, and cancer patients with less anxiety and depression are less likely to report pain[35,36]. Patients with higher overall levels of pain express significantly more existential concerns, including fears about the future[37], and both cancer patients and AIDS patients who report negative thoughts about their personal or social competence report increased pain intensity and emotional distress[34,35]. In a prospective study of cancer patients, it was found that maladaptive coping strategies, lower levels of self-efficacy, and

distress specific to the treatment or disease progression were modest but significant predictors of reports of pain intensity[28], and another survey reported that cancer patients with unpredictable episodes of pain reported greater psychological distress[38].

Rather than a homogeneous presentation, studies of patients with cancer-related pain reveal broad interpersonal variation in the response to pain. The classifications of 'dysfunctional', 'interpersonally distressed', and 'adaptive coping', categories used in chronic non-malignant pain also apply to patients with cancer pain. These different styles of adaptation to pain further suggest the importance of psychosocial evaluation of patients[39]. A strong association exists between numbers of concerns that patients endorse and their psychological distress. Concerns about pain and treatment were particularly associated with depression[40].

Most of the studies that illuminate the relationships between pain and psychosocial factors in the medically ill have been performed in the cancer population. The findings of these studies are complemented by research in the AIDS population, which also shows that psychological variables—such as the amount of control people believe they have over pain, emotional associations and memories of pain, fear of death, depression, anxiety, and hopelessness—contribute to the experience of pain and can increase suffering[41]. The negative thoughts related to pain are associated with greater pain intensity, psychological distress, and disability in ambulatory patients with AIDS[33]. Pain appears to have a profound impact on levels of emotional distress and disability. In a study of the impact of pain on ambulatory HIV-infected patients[42], depression was significantly correlated with the presence of pain. In addition to being significantly more distressed and depressed, those with pain were twice as likely to have suicidal ideation (40 per cent) than those without pain (20 per cent). HIV-infected patients with pain were more functionally impaired and functional interference was highly correlated with levels of pain intensity and depression. Those who felt that pain represented a threat to their health reported more intense pain than those who did not see pain as a threat. Patients with pain were more likely to be unemployed or disabled, and they reported less social support. Singer and colleagues[43] also reported an association among the frequency of multiple pains, increased disability, and higher levels of depression.

Although these data underscore the importance of psychological variables as factors that may help explain continued pain or lack of response to therapy, it also is important to emphasize the need for an accurate pain diagnosis as a foundation for treatment. Often, the psychiatrist is the last physician to consult on a patient with pain. An essential element of this role is the assessment of the medical evaluation of the pain and the adequacy of the analgesic management provided. Moreover, psychological distress in terminally ill patients with pain must initially be assumed to be the consequence of uncontrolled pain and pain treatment often is prerequisite to both the assessment and management of other sources of distress. Indeed, personality factors may be quite distorted by the presence of pain, and relief of pain often results in the disappearance of a perceived psychiatric disorder[10,44].

Psychiatric disorders and pain in the terminally ill

There is an increased frequency of psychiatric disorders in cancer patients with pain. In the Psychosocial Collaborative Oncology

Group Study[45] on the prevalence of psychiatric disorders in cancer patients, 39 per cent of the patients who received a psychiatric diagnosis (Table 10.1.13.1), reported significant pain, whereas only 19 per cent of patients without a psychiatric diagnosis had significant pain. The psychiatric disorders in cancer patients with pain primarily included adjustment disorder with depressed or anxious mood (69 per cent) and major depression (15 per cent). This finding of increased frequency of psychiatric disturbance in cancer pain patients also has been reported by other investigators[46,47].

The incidence and patterns of psychiatric disorders may vary systematically in subgroups of patients. For example, Breitbart *et al.*[48] described the psychiatric complications seen in cancer patients undergoing treatment for epidural spinal cord compression, which may include high-dose dexamethasone (as much as 96 mg a day for up to a week, followed by a tapering course for up to 3 or 4 weeks). Twenty-two per cent of patients with ESCC had a major depressive syndrome diagnosed as compared to 4 per cent in the comparison group. Also, delirium was much more common in the dexamethasone-treated patients with ESCC, with 24 per cent diagnosed with delirium during the course of treatment as compared to only 10 per cent in the comparison group.

Although there is limited information about patterns of disorders in other subpopulations, it is apparent that advanced disease itself, at least among patients with cancer, is associated with a relatively high prevalence of depression and delirium[49]. Approximately 25 per cent of all cancer patients experience severe depressive symptoms, with the prevalence increasing to 77 per cent in those with advanced illness. The prevalence of organic mental disorders (delirium) among cancer patients requiring psychiatric consultation has been found to range from 25 per cent to 40 per cent, and to be as

Table 10.1.13.1 Rates of DSM-III psychiatric disorders and prevalence of pain observed in 215 cancer patients from three cancer centres.

Diagnostic category	Number in diagnostic class	Percentage of psychiatric diagnoses	Number with significant pain[a]
Adjustment disorders	69	32	68
Major affective disorders	13	6	13
Organic mental disorders	8	4	8
Personality disorders	7	3	7
Anxiety disorders	4	2	4
Total with psychiatric diagnosis	101	47	39 (39%)
Total with no psychiatric diagnosis	114	53	21 (19%)
Total patient population	215	100	60 (28%)

Note: [a] Score greater than 50 mm on a 100-mm VAS pain severity.

high as 85 per cent during the terminal stages of illness[50]. Opioid analgesics and many other drugs can cause confusional states, particularly in the elderly and terminally ill[51].

Rosenfeld, Breitbart, and colleagues[23] described the psychological impact of pain in an ambulatory AIDS population. AIDS patients with pain reported significantly greater depression and functional impairment than those without pain. Psychiatric disorders, in particular the organic mental disorders such as AIDS dementia complex, can occasionally interfere with adequate pain management. The use of an opioid in this setting may worsen dementia or cause treatment-limiting sedation, confusion, or hallucinations, and has suggested the judicious use of psychostimulants to diminish sedation and neuroleptics to clear confusional states. Other psychiatric disorders that have an impact on pain management in the AIDS population include substance abuse and personality disorders.

Pain and suicide

Uncontrolled pain is a major factor in suicide and suicidal ideation in the medically ill[52-54]. Cancer is perceived by the public as an extremely painful disease compared with other medical conditions. A US study revealed that 69 per cent of the public agreed that cancer pain could cause a person to consider suicide[55]. Although relatively few cancer patients commit suicide, they are at increased risk[55,57], and the majority of suicides involve patients who have severe, inadequately controlled or tolerated poorly, pain[56]. Patients with advanced illness, who are most likely to have pain, depression or delirium, are at highest risk.

Psychiatric disorders also are frequently present in cancer patients who attempt suicide. A review of the psychiatric consultation data at Memorial Sloan-Kettering Cancer Center (MSKCC) showed that one-third of hospitalized cancer patients who were seen for evaluation of suicide risk received a diagnosis of major depression; approximately 20 per cent met criteria for delirium and more than 50 per cent were diagnosed with an adjustment disorder[52].

Thoughts of suicide probably occur quite frequently, particularly in the setting of advanced illness[58]. For many patients, these thoughts actually may be reassuring, acting as a 'steam valve' for feelings: 'If it gets too bad, I always have a way out'. Work with terminally ill cancer patients has revealed that, once a trusting and safe relationship develops, patients almost universally note that they occasionally have thoughts of suicide as a means of escaping the threat of being overwhelmed by pain. Nonetheless, recent reports suggest that persistent suicidal ideation is relatively infrequent in the cancer population and is limited to those who are significantly depressed. Silberfarb *et al.*[59] found that only three of 146 breast cancer patients had suicidal thoughts, whereas none of the 100 cancer patients interviewed in a Finnish study expressed suicidal thoughts[13]. A study conducted at St Boniface Hospice in Winnipeg, Canada, demonstrated that only 10 of 44 terminally ill cancer patients were suicidal or desired an early death, and all 10 were suffering from clinical depression[60]. At MSKCC, suicide risk evaluation accounted for 8.6 per cent of psychiatric consultations, usually requested by staff in response to patients verbalizing suicidal wishes[52]. In the 71 cancer patients who had suicidal ideation with serious intent, significant pain was a factor in only 30 per cent. In striking contrast, virtually all 71 suicidal cancer patients had a psychiatric disorder (mood disturbance or organic mental disorder) at the time of evaluation[52].

In the cancer population, pain has been associated with the desire for hastened death, and both the severity of clinical depression and the experienced of hopelessness were significantly associated with suicidal ideation. In multivariate analyses, depression and hopelessness provided independent and unique contributions to the prediction of the desire for hastened death, while social support and physical functioning added significant but smaller contributions[61]. In a study performed by the Pain and Psychiatry Services at MSKCC, 17 per cent of 185 patients with pain expressed suicidal ideation, with the majority reporting suicidal ideation without intent to act[62] Interestingly, in this population of cancer patients who had significant pain, suicidal ideation was not directly related to pain intensity but was strongly related to degree of depression and mood disturbance. Pain was related to suicidal ideation indirectly in that patients' perception of poor pain relief was associated with suicidal ideation. Perceptions of pain relief may have more to do with aspects of hopelessness than pain itself.

These data suggest that pain plays an important role in vulnerability to suicide in the population with advanced cancer; however, associated psychological distress and mood disturbance seem to be essential cofactors in raising the risk of suicide. Pain has adverse effects on patients' quality of life and sense of control, and impairs the family's ability to provide support. Factors other than pain, such as mood disturbance, delirium, loss of control, and hopelessness, also contribute to cancer suicide risk[56]. Frequency of suicidal ideation in one study was associated with poor well-being, depression, anxiety, and shortness of breath but not with other somatic symptoms such as pain, nausea, and loss of appetite[63].

Although work in other populations has been limited, studies of patients with advanced AIDS also have found complex and variable relationships among pain, depression, hopelessness, and suicidal ideation, and suggest that the findings in cancer studies may be more universal. A study of men with AIDS in New York City[64] demonstrated a relative risk of suicide 36 times greater than that of males in the general population. Many of these patients had advanced AIDS, with Kaposi's sarcoma and other potentially painful conditions. However, the role of pain in contributing to increased risk of suicide was not specifically examined. In a study at MSKCC[65], suicidal ideation in ambulatory AIDS patients was found to be highly correlated with the presence of pain, depressed mood (as measured by the Beck Depression Inventory), and low T4 lymphocyte counts. While 20 per cent of ambulatory AIDS patients without pain reported suicidal thoughts, more than 40 per cent of those with pain reported suicidal ideation. Only two of the 110 patients in this study reported suicidal intent. One of these two men was in the pain group; both scored highly on measures of depression. No correlations were observed between suicidal ideation and pain intensity or pain relief. The mean visual analogue scale measure of pain intensity for the group overall was 49 mm (range 5–100 mm), thus falling predominantly in the moderate range. As with cancer pain patients, suicidal ideation in AIDS patients with pain is more likely to be related to a concomitant mood disturbance than to the intensity of pain experienced. Although AIDS patients are frequently found to have suicidal ideation, these thoughts are more often context-specific, occurring almost exclusively during exacerbations of the illness, when pain is severe, or at times of bereavement[65].

Inadequate pain management

The adequacy of pain management can be best judged when there is consensus about best practice and data that illuminate the likelihood of satisfactory pain control when treatment is optimal. From this perspective, studies in the cancer population and AIDS population may illuminate the prevalence and causes of undertreatment and suggest the seriousness of the problem in other medically ill groups. Recent studies suggest that pain in cancer is undertreated[66] and pain in AIDS is dramatically undertreated[67–69]. In one study of a cohort of AIDS patients treated in New York City[69], only 6 per cent of patients reporting pain in the severe range(8–10 on a numerical rating scale) received a strong opioid, such as morphine. This degree of undermedication far exceeds published reports of undermedication of pain in cancer populations[66]. Similar to the cancer population, undertreatment of AIDS-related pain may be more likely in women, those with limited education or a substance abuse history, and those who express a variety of patient-related barriers to opioid treatment[69,70]. It is also clear that adjuvant agents such as the antidepressants are also dramatically underused[67–69]. Only 6 per cent of patients in a sample of AIDS patients reporting pain received an adjuvant analgesic drug (i.e. an antidepressant).

Inadequate management of pain often is due the inability to properly assess pain in all its dimensions[2,4,9]. Psychological variables may be ignored, or contrariwise, may be proposed to explain pain when in fact medical factors have not been adequately appreciated. Other causes of inadequate pain management include: lack of knowledge of current pharmacy or psychotherapeutic approaches; focus on prolonging life rather than alleviating suffering; lack of communication between doctor and patient; limited expectations of patients to achieve pain relief; limited capacity of patients impaired by organic mental disorders to communicate; unavailability of opioid drugs; doctors' fear of opioid toxicity; and doctors' fear of amplifying addiction and substance abuse. In advanced cancer, several related factors have been noted to predict the undertreatment of pain, including a discrepancy between physician and patient in judging the severity of pain; the presence of pain that physicians did not attribute to cancer, better performance status, age of 70 or over; and female sex[66].

The pharmacological risks associated with opioid drugs, including respiratory depression, is too often overestimated and also can limit appropriate use of opioid analgesics. Investigators have demonstrated that morphine can improve dyspnoea without causing a significant deterioration in respiratory function, even in patients with far-advanced cancer[71].

The adequacy of cancer pain management also can be adversely influenced by discordance between patient ratings or complaints and those made by caregivers. Persistent cancer pain is often ascribed to a psychological cause when it does not respond to treatment attempts. Clinical observation suggests that the complaint of 'severe' pain is relatively more likely to be viewed as having a psychological contribution. Indeed, staff members' ability to empathize with a patient's pain complaint may be limited by the report of high intensity. Grossman et al.[72] found that while there is a high degree of concordance between patient and staff ratings of patient pain intensity at the low and moderate levels, this concordance broke down at high pain levels; specifically, the clinicians' ability to assess a patient's level of pain became unreliable when pain intensity was greater than 7 on a 0 to 10 scale. Physicians must be educated about the limitations of their ability to objectively assess the severity of a subjective pain experience. Additionally, patient education often is a useful intervention in such cases. Patients are more likely to be believed and adequately treated if they are taught to request pain relief in a non-hysterical, business-like fashion.

A history of drug abuse has been repeatedly is associated with the undertreatment of pain. The prevalence of drug abuse in populations with serious medical illness may be overestimated by clinicians. At MSKCC, for example, only eight (1.7 per cent) of 468 inpatient referred for cancer pain had a history of intravenous drug abuse, and none had been actively abusing drugs during the previous year. All eight of these patients were intentionally under-medicated because of concern by staff that drug abuse was active or would recur, and adequate pain control was ultimately achieved in these patients by using appropriate analgesic dosages and intensive staff education. Although populations in other settings may have far higher prevalences of substance use disorders—for example, the base rate of substance use disorders is clearly higher in the younger HIV population[74]—clinicians should be able to reassure colleagues and others through knowledge of the true prevalence rates. Derogatis et al.[45] assessed 215 ambulatory cancer patients for psychiatric diagnoses and found that fewer than 5 per cent met the criteria for a substance use disorder.

Limited knowledge about the presentation, assessment and management of drug abuse most likely contributes to an overestimation of risk, which may, in turn, discourage the appropriate use of opioids to treat pain[3,9,73,75]. Studies of populations with cancer pain suggest that abuse and addiction are rare among those with no prior history of drug abuse[76]. The need for opioid dose escalation during the treatment of cancer pain usually is linked to observable progression of disease and cannot be ascribed either to addiction or to other pharmacological phenomena, such as addiction or tolerance. Although tolerance, a biological adaptation to a drug characterized by the need for a higher dose to maintain an effect, presumably occurs during the treatment of pain, most patients benefit from stable doses for prolonged periods. Similarly, physical dependence, which is defined as the potential for abstinence if the dose is abruptly reduced or an antagonist is administered, is not a clinical problem if withdrawal is avoided. In contrast, addiction should be understood as a neurobiological disease with a strong genetic basis, which is defined by the occurrence of craving, loss of control over drug use, compulsive use, and continuing use despite harm. Understanding these definitions, and acknowledging the key differences between tolerance and physical dependence, which are presumably activated whenever opioids are used therapeutically, and the disease of addiction, is essential to accurately judge the true risks associated with opioid.

Patients who require pain treatment with opioids or other potentially abusable drugs and who have a history of significant alcohol or drug abuse, or meet criteria for true addiction, do pose a challenge for clinicians. This is exemplified by the management of pain in the growing segment of the AIDS population that is actively abusing intravenous drugs[74]. Active drug use, particularly intravenous opioid abuse, may predispose to several difficulties including: (1) high tolerance to opioid analgesics needed for disease-related pain; (2) drug-seeking and manipulative behaviour; (3) lack of adherence or reliability of patient history; and (4) the risk of spreading HIV. Because subjective report may be the only indication of the presence

and intensity of pain, or the degree of pain relief achieved by an intervention, patients who are assumed to lie as an element of addictive disease are at high risk to generate concern among clinicians, whose reluctance to believe the patient may lead to anger and limited pain therapy. Undertreatment is clearly a risk in this context.

Most clinicians experienced in working with medically ill patients with substance abuse history recommend clear and direct limit setting. To the extent possible, clinicians should attempt to eliminate the issue of drug abuse as an obstacle to pain management by dealing directly with the problems of opioid withdrawal and drug abuse treatment. Often, specialized substance abuse consultation services are available to help manage such patients and initiate structured drug administration, or other elements of drug treatment, at the same time that pain management is occurring. If analgesic drugs are the focus of a battle for control between the patient and physician, therapy will be compromised, especially in terminal stages of illness. In this setting, it is appropriate for clinicians to err on the side of believing patients when they complain of pain, and present a bias toward treatment, as long as three is no clear evidence of self-destructive behaviours or drug diversion to the illicit market.

Psychiatric and psychological management of pain in advanced disease

Optimal treatment of pain associated with advanced disease may require a multimodality strategy, including pharmacological, psychotherapeuticrehabilitative and interventional approaches. Psychiatric participation in pain management involves the use of psychotherapeutic, cognitive behavioural, and psychopharmacologic interventions, usually in combination.

Psychotherapy and pain

The goals of psychotherapy with medically ill patients with pain are to provide support, knowledge, and skills (Table 10.1.13.2). Utilizing short-term supportive psychotherapy, focused on the crisis created by the medical illness, the therapist provides emotional support, continuity, and information, and assists in adaptation. The therapist has a role in emphasizing past strengths, supporting previously successful coping strategies, and teaching new coping skills, such as relaxation, cognitive coping, use of analgesics, self-observation, documentation, assertiveness, and communication skills. Communication skills are of paramount importance for both patient and family, particularly around pain and analgesic issues. The patient and family is the unit of concern, and there is a need to support a more general, long-term supportive relationship within the health-care system, in addition to providing specific psychological approaches.

Psychotherapy with the patient who has advanced illness and pain consists of active listening with supportive verbal interventions and the occasional interpretation[77]. Despite the seriousness of the patient's plight, it is not necessary for the psychiatrist or psychologist to appear overly solemn or emotionally restrained. Often, the relationship is strengthened by the ability of the psychotherapist to converse lightheartedly and allow the patient to talk about his or her life and experiences, rather than focus solely on impending death. The patient who wishes to talk or ask questions about death and pain and suffering should be allowed to do so freely, with the therapist maintaining an interested, interactive stance. This work may ensue in parallel with discussions between the patient or family and other members of the treatment team, including the chaplain.

Table 10.1.13.2 Goals and forms of psychotherapy for pain in patients with advanced disease.

Goals	Form
Support: provide continuity	Individuals: supportive/crisis intervention
Knowledge: provide information	Family: patient and family are the unit of concern
Skills: relaxation cognitive coping use of analgesics communication	Group: share experiences identify successful coping strategies

As illness progresses, psychotherapy with the individual patient may become limited by cognitive or speech deficits. It is at this point that the focus of supportive psychotherapeutic interventions shifts primarily to the family. As common issue for the family at this point is the level of alertness of the patient. Attempts to control pain are often accompanied by sedation that can limit communication between patient and family. This can sometimes become a source of conflict, with family members disagreeing among themselves or with the patient about what constitutes an appropriate balance between comfort and alertness. It can be helpful for the physician to clarify the patient's preferences as they relate to these issues early so that conflict can be avoided and work related to bereavement can begin.

Group interventions with individual patients (even in advanced stages of disease), spouses, couples, and families are a powerful means of sharing experiences and identifying successful coping strategies. The limitations of using group interventions for patients with advanced disease are primarily pragmatic. The patient must be physically comfortable enough to participate and have the cognitive capacity to be aware of group discussion. It is often helpful for family members to attend support groups during the terminal phases of the patient's illness.

Family caregivers can play an effective role in assisting in pain management. In an novel intervention, Keefe et al.[78] tested the efficacy of a partner-guided cancer pain management protocol consisting of a three-session intervention conducted in patients' homes that integrated educational information about cancer pain with systematic training of patients and partners in cognitive and behavioural pain coping skills (see section in following paragraphs on cognitive behavioural approaches); this approach produced significant increases in partners' ratings of their self-efficacy for helping the patient control pain and self-efficacy for controlling other symptoms.

Psychotherapeutic interventions that have multiple targets may be most useful. Based upon a prospective study of cancer pain, cognitive behavioural and psychoeducational techniques based upon increasing support and self-efficacy, and providing education, may help patients deal with increased pain[79]. Distress related to the illness, self-efficacy, and coping may be associated with pain and be specifically addressed by these interventions.

Utilizing psychotherapy to diminish symptoms of anxiety and depression, factors that can intensify pain, empirically has beneficial effects on cancer pain experience. In a randomized controlled study, Spiegel and Bloom[80] demonstrated that both supportive group therapy and training in hypnotic pain-control exercises benefited patients with pain related to metastatic breast cancer. The supportive group focused not on interpersonal processes or self-exploration, but rather on a series of themes related to the practical and existential problems of living with cancer.

While psychotherapy in populations with advanced illness is primarily non-analytical and focuses on current issues, exploration of reactions to illness often involve insights into earlier, more pervasive life issues. Some patients choose to continue a more exploratory psychotherapy during extended periods of stable disease, or during survivorship.

Cognitive-behavioural techniques

Cognitive-behavioural techniques can be useful as adjuncts to the management of pain in the setting of serious medical illness (Table 10.1.13.3). The goal of these techniques is to guide the patient towards a sense of control over pain. Some of the specific interventions are primarily cognitive in nature, focusing on perceptual and thought processes, and others are directed at modifying patterns of behaviour that may help patients cope with pain. Specific strategies include passive relaxation with mental imagery, cognitive distraction or focusing, progressive muscle relaxation, biofeedback, hypnosis, and music therapy[44,81–83]. Behavioural techniques may seek to modify physiologic pain reactions, respondent pain behaviours, or operant pain behaviours (see Table 10.1.13.4 for definitions).

The cognitive interventions that are used to reduce pain intensity or associated distress may attempt to modify the thoughts about the pain, introduce more adaptive coping strategies, or provide instruction in various types of relaxation techniques. Cognitive

Table 10.1.13.3 Cognitive behavioural techniques used by pain patients with advanced disease.

Psychoeducation
- Preparatory information
- Self-monitoring

Relaxation
- Passive breathing
- Progressive muscle relaxation

Distraction
- Focusing
- Controlled by mental imagery
- Cognitive distraction
- Behavioural distraction

Combined techniques (relaxation and distraction)
- Passive/progressive relaxation with mental imagery
- Systematic desensitization
- Meditation
- Hypnosis
- Biofeedback
- Music therapy

Cognitive therapies
- Cognitive distortion
- Cognitive restructuring

Behavioural therapies
- Modelling
- Graded task management
- Contingency management
- Behavioural rehearsal

Table 10.1.13.4 Cognitive behavioural techniques: definitions and descriptions.

Behavioural therapy	The clinical use of techniques derived from the experimental analysis of behaviour, i.e. learning and conditioning for the evaluation, prevention, and treatment of physical disease or physiological dysfunction
Cognitive therapy	A focused intervention targeted at changing maladaptive beliefs and dysfunctional attitudes; the therapist engages the client in a process of collaborative empiricism, where these underlying beliefs are challenged and corrected
Operant pain	Pain behaviours resulting from operant learning or conditioning; pain behaviour is reinforced and continues because of secondary gain, i.e. increased attention and caring
Respondent pain	Pain behaviours resulting from respondent learning or conditioning; stimuli associated with prior painful experiences can elicit increased pain and avoidance behaviour
Cognitive restructuring	Redefinition of some or all aspects of the patient's interpretation of the noxious or threatening experience, resulting in decreased distress, anxiety, and hopelessness
Self-monitoring (pain diary)	Written or audiotaped chronicle that the patient maintains to describe specific agreed-upon characteristics associated with pain
Contingency management	Focusing of patient and family member responses that either reinforce or inhibit specific behaviours exhibited by the patient; method involves reinforcing desired 'well' behaviours
Grade task assignments	A hierarchy of tasks, i.e. physical, cognitive, and behavioural, are compartmentalized and performed sequentially in manageable steps ultimately achieving an identified goal
Systematic desensitization	Relaxation and distraction exercises paired with a hierarchy of anxiety-arousing stimuli presented through mental imagery, or presented in vivo, resulting in control of fear

modification (cognitive restructuring) is an approach derived from cognitive therapy for depression or anxiety and is based on how one interprets events and bodily sensation. It is assumed that patients have dysfunctional automatic thoughts that reflect underlying assumptions and beliefs. In both cancer and AIDS populations, negative thoughts about pain have been shown to be significantly related to pain intensity, degree of psychological distress, and level of interference in functional activities[33,34]. By identifying and challenging dysfunctional automatic thoughts and underlying beliefs by restructuring or modifying thought processes, a more rational response to pain can occur[81]. Examples of such automatic thoughts that have been shown to worsen pain experience are: 'The intensity of my pain will never diminish' or 'Because my pain limits my activities, I am completely helpless'. Patients can be taught to recognize and interrupt such thoughts and proceed to develop a view of the pain experience as time limited and themselves as functional despite periods in which they are limited.

The use of cognitive restructuring may shift as the goals change in the palliative care context. In the setting of advanced illness, the goal may not be to change the patient's maladaptive thoughts, but rather, to utilize techniques designed to diminish the patient's frustration, anxiety, and anger. Helping patients to employ more adaptive coping strategies and thereby avoid catastrophizing and increase problem-solving skills, may be helpful at this stage[84–86].

Aside from modifying dysfunctional thoughts and attitudes, the most fundamental behavioural technique is self-monitoring. The development of the ability to monitor one's behaviours allows a person to notice their dysfunctional reactions to the pain experience and learn to control them.

Another approach, systematic desensitization (see Table 10.1.13.4), may be useful in extinguishing the anticipatory anxiety that can lead to avoidant behaviours, and in remobilizing inactive patients. Graded task assignment may be viewed as a type of systematic desensitization, by which function is improved by teaching patients to take small steps gradually and thereby avoid the anxiety associated with specific task. Finally, contingency management

is a method of reinforcing 'well' behaviours only; thus modifying dysfunctional operant pain behaviours associated with secondary gain[82,83].

The range of cognitive behavioural interventions that may be useful in the setting of advanced illness is very broad[87] and there is some evidence that all methods are not equally effective. Cognitive strategies, including relaxation, suggestion, and distracting imagery appear to hold the greatest promise, although research on the usage of these techniques to control pain is scant[88,89]. Notwithstanding, the recommendation to consider a combined non-pharmacological and pharmacological pain management strategy is common, and is especially promoted with paediatric populations[90].

The mechanisms by which these cognitive and behavioural techniques relieve pain are not known; however, they all seem to share the elements of relaxation and distraction. Distraction or redirection of attention helps reduce awareness of pain, and relaxation reduces muscle tension and sympathetic arousal[82]. These interventions may be a particularly attractive part of a multi-modality approach because they produce no side effects. Importantly, they should be considered a substitute for aggressive pharmacotherapy and a favourable response to a psychological technique must not be viewed as evidence that pain is psychogenic.

Patient selection for cognitive behavioural interventions for pain

The selection of patients with advanced illness and pain for trials of cognitive behavioural strategies should take into account the intensity of pain and the mental clarity of the patient. Ideal candidates have mild to moderate pain, either at baseline or as a result of analgesic drug therapy. Confusional states interfere dramatically with a patient's ability to focus attention and thus limit the usefulness of these techniques[83]. Occasionally, however, these techniques can be modified so as to include mildly impaired patients. This may involve the therapist taking a more active role by orienting the patient, creating a safe and secure environment, and evoking a conditioned response to the therapist's voice or presence.

Barriers to engaging patients in cognitive behavioural therapies can be divided into physician/nurse-based barriers and patient-based barriers. The health-care provider who works with patients with advanced illness may have particular difficulty in becoming comfortable with the use of behavioural therapies. Pharmaco-therapy is highly effective in the management of pain and seems simpler and easier to use than labour-intensive and time-consuming non-pharmacological interventions. Physicians and nurses have typical concerns about the practice of behavioural interventions such as: 'What if the patient laughs, doesn't buy it?' or 'It seems too theatrical, unscientific, non-medical; too New Age!' Overcoming such obstacles will be greatly rewarded. It is imperative that physicians working with patients with advanced illness be aware of the effective non-pharmacological interventions and be able to make appropriate referrals to practitioners who can provide them.

Patients themselves may be uncertain about the utility of these therapies. Some may ask, 'How can breathing take away my pain?' They may be frightened by the word 'hypnosis' and its connotations. Although hypnosis is often associated with powerful and magical properties, some patients become frightened at the prospect of losing control or being under the influence of someone else. It generally is best to introduce cognitive behavioural interventions after some rapport has been established with a patient. Although some patients may benefit from a discussion of the theoretical basis of these interventions, it is important to stress that an understanding of the mechanism is not needed for effectiveness and the outcome is most important. Apprehensions must be affirmed and dealt with. Patients must also feel in control of the process at all times and be reassured that they can stop at any time.

Practical considerations in the use of cognitive behavioural approaches

A general approach to using cognitive behavioural interventions with patients with advanced illness and pain involves the following: (1) assessment of the symptom; (2) choosing a cognitive behavioural strategy; and (3) preparing the patient and the setting.

The main purpose of conducting a cognitive behavioural assessment of pain is to determine what, if any, interventions are indicated[76]. One must initially engage the patient and establish a therapeutic alliance. A history of the pain symptom must be taken. One should review previous efforts to treat the patient's pain, and collect data regarding the nature of the pain and its impact on the patient and their family. Choosing the appropriate behavioural strategy should consider the patient's medical condition, physical and cognitive limitations, time constraints, and practical matters. For instance, patients with cognitive impairment or delirium will probably be unable to keep a pain diary or employ techniques that involve cognitive manipulation.

Muscular tension, autonomic arousal, and mental distress exacerbate pain[82,83], and a variety of techniques can be used to achieve a state of relaxation. These include: (1) passive relaxation through the focusing of attention on sensations of warmth and decreased tension in various parts of the body; (2) progressive muscle relaxation involving active tensing and relaxing of muscles; and (3) meditation. Other techniques that employ relaxation and other cognitive techniques include hypnosis, biofeedback, and music therapy (see following paragraphs). A review of relaxation studies cannot confirm a positive effect on chronic pain but indicates that relaxation training can reduce some pain scores and more clearly has a positive effect on anxiety[91–93].

Passive relaxation, focused breathing, and passive muscle relaxation exercises involve the focusing of attention systematically on one's breathing, on sensations of warmth and relaxation, or on release of muscular tension in various body parts. Verbal suggestions and imagery are used to help promote relaxation. Muscle relaxation is an important component of the relaxation response and can augment the benefits of simple focused breathing exercises, leading to a deeper experience of relaxation and self-control.

Progressive or active muscle relaxation involves the active tensing and relaxing of various muscle groups in the body, focusing attention on the sensations of tension and relaxation. Clinically, in the hospital setting, relaxation is most commonly achieved through the use of a combination of focused breathing and progressive muscle relaxation exercises. Once patients are in a relaxed state, imagery techniques can then be used to induce deeper relaxation and facilitate distraction from or manipulation of a variety of cancer-related symptoms.

Script for passive relaxation (focused breathing)

The following script is a generic relaxation exercise, utilizing passive relaxation or focused breathing, that is based on and integrates the work of Erickson[94], Benson[95], and others[83].

'Why don't you begin by finding a comfortable position. Slowly allow your body to unwind and just let it go. That's it … I wonder if you can allow your body to become as calm as possible … just let it go, just let your body sink into that bed (or chair) … feel free to move or shift around in any way that your body needs to, to find that comfortable position. You need not try very hard, simply and easily allow yourself to follow the sound of my voice as you allow your body to find itself a safe, comfortable position to relax in.

If you like, you can gently allow your eyes to close, just let the lids cover your eyes … allow your eyes to sink back deeply into their sockets … that's it, just let them go, falling back gently and deeply into their sockets as your lids begin to feel heavier and heavier. As you allow your head to fall back deeply into the pillow, feeling the weight of your head sinking into the pillow as you breathe out, just breathe out, one big breath. Slowly, if you can begin to turn your attention to your breathing. Notice your breath for a few moments, how much air you take in, how much air you let out, and just breathe evenly and naturally, and with the sound of my voice I wonder if you can begin to take in more air, breathing in and out, in and out, that's it, gradually breathing in and out … in and out … breathing in calmness and quietness, breathing out tiredness and frustration, that's it … let it go, it's not important to you now … breathing in quietness and control, breathing out fear and tension … breathing in and out … in and out … you can enjoy breathing in this relaxed way for as long as you need to. You are peaceful now as you continue to observe your even and steady breathing that is allowing you to feel gentle and calm, breathing that is allowing you to feel a gentle calm, that's it, breathing relaxation in and tension out … in and out … breathing in quietness and control, breathing out tiredness and tension … that's it (patient's name here) as you continue to notice the quietness and stillness of your body, Why don't you take a few quiet moments to experience this process more fully.'

It may be helpful for the clinician to mark the end of an exercise by increasing the pace, raising the volume of voice, and shifting position. Additionally, it is helpful for the clinician to both pace and model for the patient. This includes positioning yourself as similarly to the patient as possible (e.g. closing eyes, assuming a position of relaxation, and breathing at the same rate). If the patient exhibits any visible anxiety or agitation, this can be briefly explored verbally, and then, if appropriate, the exercise can be continued.

Script for active or progressive muscle relaxation

This exercise involves the patient actively tensing and then relaxing specific body parts. Once again, it may be helpful if the clinician paces and models for the patient.

'Now, I wonder if you can tense up every muscle in your body … that's it, squeeze in the muscles … hold it, and then just let it go … once more, tense up your muscles … make them very tight and tense, hold it, hold it … and then breathe out, and let your muscles relax, just let them go … Now, as your body begins to feel more and more relaxed, clench your jaw, squeeze it tight, clench it and then let it go … now open your mouth wide, as wide as it will go, stick out your tongue, stick it way out, hold it and then let it go. Feel your head becoming more and more relaxed, as it sinks down into the pillow, allowing all the tension and tightness to drift out of it … Now, I wonder if you can lift up your shoulders, lift them up, up to your ears, hold them there, squeezing them tightly, squeeze, and then let them drop down, just let them go … and then once more lift them up … hold it … then let them go … as you feel all the tightness and tension in your shoulders begin to drain away … Now, I wonder if you can clench your hands into a fist, make a tight fist as your whole arm tightens, tense your arms as you squeeze in your fingers tighter and tighter … and now just let them go, once more now make a fist, a tight fist, hold it, and then let it go.'

As with passive muscle relaxation, the clinician guides the patient through the exercise, requesting the patient to tense and release specific muscles in a progressive order.

Imagery/distraction techniques

Clinically, relaxation techniques are most helpful in managing pain when combined with some distracting or pleasant imagery. The use of distraction or focusing involves control over the focus of attention and can be used to make the patient less aware of the noxious stimuli[96]. One can employ imaginative inattention by picturing oneself on a beach. Mental distraction can be used and is similar to the practice of counting sheep to aid sleep. Keeping oneself busy is a form of behavioural distraction. Imagery, that is, using one's imagination while in a relaxed state, can be used to transform pain into a warm or cold sensation. One can also imaginatively transform the context of pain; for example, one could imagine oneself in battle on the football field instead of the hospital bed. Dissociated somatization can be employed by some patients whereby they imagine that a painful body part is no longer part of their body[3,4,81,83]. It is important to note that not every patient finds these techniques acceptable, and the therapist must try out a number of approaches to determine which are consistent with the patient's style.

Imagery (often referred to as guided imagery) is most effective when the specific image is obtained from the patient. The clinician may ask the patient to close his or her eyes and think of a place, an activity, or an experience where the patient felt most safe and secure. The clinician may provide suggestions for the patient such as a favourite beach scene, or a room in a house, or riding a bicycle in a state park. Once the patient identifies the scene, the clinician may ask the patient to elaborate upon the scene, asking for specific details such as the temperature, season, time of day, type of ocean (calm, or with big waves), etc. The clinician then utilizes this information and

describes an image for the patient in detail. The skill is for the clinician to be as flexible and as creative as possible, and to elaborate upon the scene, utilizing all aspects of the senses and bodily sensations such as 'feel the suns rays touch your skin, allow your skin to feel warm and tingly all over …'or, 'breathe in the fresh, clear air, allow it to fill your lungs with its freshness …' or, 'feel the fresh dew of the grass under your feet'. The clinician can focus on 'aromas in the garden' or the 'sounds of birds singing' always reminding the patient to breathe evenly and steadily as he or she feels more and more relaxed and more and more in control. If possible, the clinician should avoid volunteering an image or scene for the patient because the clinician is unaware of the association or meaning the image may have for the patient. For example, a patient may have a fear of the water, and therefore a beach scene may invoke feelings of fear and loss of control.

Script for pleasant distracting imagery

The following script is a generic script for an imagery exercise.

'Once you are in a comfortable position, I wonder if you can continue lying there with your eyes closed, continuing to breathe in out … in and out to the sound of my voice. Let your mind wander … just let it go … and if any unwanted thoughts come into your mind, you can allow then to pass out as easily as they came in … You don't need them now … they are not important to you now. You have the ability to control your thoughts. You have the ability to be in control.'

Slowly, I wonder if you can allow your mind to travel … to travel far away to your favourite beach. The beach that you have many fond memories of. I wonder if you can imagine that it's almost the end of the day and the beach is deserted … and the sun, while setting, is still warm, as it beats down … and makes your skin feel tingly and warm all over. As you begin to walk on the sand, you can feel the granules underneath your feet. Step evenly and steadily along the sand. As you look around, you can see the different colors in the sky. You can see for miles off into the distance and you feel exhilarated and free because no one is around you. You are alone and in control. As you walk closer to the edge of the ocean the sand is becoming a little damp and you can feel the dampness underneath your feet—it feels refreshing. As you continue walking, you may notice a few odds and ends on the sand maybe something that the ocean brought in … some shells perhaps. They may be broken from being knocked against the rocks … or there may be a few bits of seaweed or some jellyfish. You stop to notice them as you walk past … marvelling at the wonders of nature. As you get to the edge of the ocean, you can feel the tiny little ripples of water washing over your feet … bouncing over your feet making you feel light and fresh. The water is warm—it soothes your feet. Washing back and forth … back and forth. As you keep walking you see your rubber raft. This is your old dependable rubber raft. You get to the raft and you secure it in your hands and lie down on it letting your whole body sink into the raft—just let it go … that's it. Slowly you kick off as the raft begins to take you away. The ocean is very calm and very gentle. Your whole body begins to unwind and sink deeper and deeper into the raft as you feel more and more relaxed. This raft allows you to drift off … and underneath you can feel the ripples of the ocean … rocking back and forth … back and forth as you continue to float away evenly and gently. You can become aware of the sun beating down in your skin. You are aware of the sounds around you—you can hear the ocean washing against the rocks as the waves rock back and forth … back and forth. You can hear the gulls crying in the distance. There is a very tiny protected bay that you are floating away in. It is a very calm and peaceful day, and you are feeling more and more relaxed. You are in control now … and as you continue to sail away, all your troubles and problems wash right out of you. They're not important to you now. You don't need them now. What's important is that your whole body, from the tip of your toes all the way up to the top of your head, is relaxed and calm in this very safe and private place that is your own. You can continue to lie here as you rock back and forth … back and forth for as long as you need to.

When you are ready, you can slowly readjust yourself to the sound of my voice and I am going to count slowly backwards from ten and with each count backwards, you can become more and more familiar with where you are. Perhaps when I get to number five you may want to open your eyes or you can keep then closed for as long as you need to. Ten, nine …—become aware of the sounds around you … eight, seven … become aware of the temperature of the room—how does it feel?, how does your body feel? … six, five …—you can open your eyes now if you want to or you can keep them closed … four, three, two, one. You can stay in this relaxed position for as long as you need to. When you feel ready you may slowly prepare to sit up.'

Hypnosis

Hypnosis can be a useful adjunct in the management of pain[80, 97–102], including pain associated with invasive procedures[88]. In a controlled trial comparing hypnosis with cognitive behavioural therapy in relieving mucositis following a bone marrow transplant, patients utilizing hypnosis reported a significant reduction in pain compared to patients who used cognitive behavioural techniques[79]. The hypnotic trance is essentially a state of heightened and focused concentration, and thus it can be used to manipulate the perception of pain. The depth of hypnotizability may determine the effectiveness as well as the strategies employed during hypnosis. One-third of patients are not hypnotizable, and it is recommended that other techniques be employed for them. Of the two-thirds of patients who are identified as being less, moderately, and highly hypnotizable, three principles underlie the use of hypnosis in controlling pain[96]: (1) use self-hypnosis; (2) relax, do not fight the pain; and (3) use a mental filter to ease the hurt in pain. Patients who are moderately and highly hypnotizable can often alter sensations in a painful area by changing temperature sensation or experiencing tingling. Less hypnotizable patients can often utilize an alternative focus by concentrating on a sensation in a non-affected body part or on a mental image of a pleasant scene. The main disadvantage of hypnosis for cancer patients is that the technique frequently requires more attentional capacity than these patients generally have. For paediatric patients, hypnosis and cognitive–behavioural skills are effective in managing the pain associated with procedure related pain[103].

Biofeedback

Fotopoulos et al.[104] noted significant pain relief in a group of cancer patients who were taught electromyographic (EMG) and electroencephalographic (EEG) biofeedback-assisted relaxation. Only two of 17 were able to maintain analgesia after the treatment ended. A lack of generalization of effect can be a problem with biofeedback techniques. Although physical condition may make a prolonged training period impossible, especially for the terminally ill, most cancer patients can often utilize EMG and temperature biofeedback techniques for learning relaxation-assisted pain control[90].

Music, aroma, and art therapies

Munro and Mount[105] have written extensively on the use of music therapy with cancer patients, documenting clinical examples and suggesting mechanisms of action. Music can often capture the focus of attention like no other stimulus, offers patients a new form of expression, and helps patients distract themselves from their perception of pain, while expressing themselves in meaningful ways[106,107]. Music therapy can be helpful in managing the discomfort associated with procedures[108].

Aromas have been shown to have innate relaxing and stimulating qualities. Utilizing the scent, heliotropin, Manne et al.[109] reported that two-thirds of the patients found the scent especially pleasant and reported much less anxiety than those who were not exposed to the scent during MRI. As a general relaxation technique, aroma therapy may have an application for pain management, but this is as yet unstudied.

Art therapy has been shown to help with pain, tiredness, anxiety, and overall well-being[110]. In addition, art therapy allows the less verbally skilled adult or children to express the fears and concerns that they have in a more comfortable fashion. The creative experience can be used as both a important means of providing support and also as an avenue for providing patients with psychological insights into their experience[111].

Psychotropic adjuvant analgesics for pain in the patient with advanced illness

The patient with advanced disease and pain has much to gain from the appropriate and maximal utilization of psychotropic drugs. Psychotropic drugs, particularly the tricyclic antidepressants, are useful as adjuvant analgesics in the pharmacological management of cancer pain and neuropathic pain (see Chapter 10.1.8). Table 10.1.13.5 lists the various psychotropic medications with analgesic properties, their routes of administration, and their approximate daily doses. These medications are not only effective in managing symptoms of anxiety, depression, insomnia, or delirium that commonly complicate the course of advanced disease in patients who are in pain, but also potentiate the analgesic effects of the opioid drugs and have innate analgesic properties of their own[112]. A common use of adjuvant analgesics is to manage neuropathic pain. In this population, non-opioid adjuvant drugs that are neuroactive or neuromodulatory may be needed to complement opioid therapy. The primary adjuvant analgesics are anti-convulsant and antidepressant medications but a variety of other drugs are used[113].

Antidepressants

The current literature supports the use of antidepressants as adjuvant analgesic agents in the management of a wide variety of chronic pain syndromes, including cancer pain[114–121]. While clinically useful as adjuvant analgesics in managing AIDS-related pain (e.g. HIV neuropathies), there are no published controlled clinical trials of antidepressants as analgesics[74,122]. Amitriptyline is the tricyclic antidepressant most studied, and proven effective as an analgesic, in a large number of clinical trials, addressing a wide variety of chronic pains[123–127]. Other tricyclic antidepressants that have been shown to have efficacy as analgesics include

Table 10.1.13.5 Psychotropic adjuvant analgesic drugs for pain in patients with advanced disease.

Generic name	Approximate daily dosage range (mg)	Route
Tricyclic antidepressants		
Amitriptyline	10–150	PO, IM, PR
Nortriptyline	10–50	PO
Imipramine	12.5–150	PO, IM
Desipramine	12.5–150	PO
Clomipramine	10–150	PO
Doxepin	12.5–150	PO, IM
Non-cyclic antidepressants		
SSRIs		
Fluoxetine	20–60	PO
Paroxetine	20–60	PO
Citalopram	10–40	PO
Escitalopram	10–20	PO
Sertraline	50–100	PO
NSRIs		
Venlafaxine	37.5–450	PO
Duloxetine	20–90	PO
Others		
Trazodone	50–60	PO
Mirtazapine	7.5–60	PO
Psychostimulants		
Methylphenidate	2.5–20 b.i.d.	PO
Dextroamphetamine	2.5–20 b.i.d.	PO
Modafinil	50–200	PO
Phenothiazines		
Fluphenazine	1–3	PO, IM
Methotrimeprazine	10–20 q6h	PO, IM, IV, SC
Butyrophenones		
Haloperidol	1–3	PO, IM, IV, SC
Pimozide	2–6 b.i.d.	PO
Atypical antipsychotics		
Atypical neuroleptics		
Olanzapine	2.5–20	PO
Risperidone	5–6	PO
Quetiapine	50–200	PO
Ziprazidione	20–80 q 12h	PO, IM
Aripiprazole	10–20	PO
Antihistamines		
Hydroxyzine	50 q4–6h	PO, IM, IV
Benzodiazepines		
Alprazolam	0.25–2.0 t.i.d.	PO
Clonazepam	0.5–4 b.i.d.	PO

Note: PO, per oral; IM, intramuscular; PR, parenteral; IV, intravenous; q6 h, every 6 h; q4–6h, every 4 to 6 h; t.i.d., three times a day; b.i.d., two times a day.

imipramine[128–130], desipramine[131,132], nortriptyline[133], clomipramine[134,135], doxepin[136], and sertraline[137]. In a placebo-controlled double-blind study of imipramine in chronic cancer pain, Walsh[138] demonstrated that imipramine had analgesic effects independent of its mood effects and was a potent co-analgesic when used along with morphine. In another effort to apply an antidepressant to the control of symptoms, sertraline was shown to reduce hot flashes in early stage breast cancer patients taking tamoxifen, but the reduction was not significant[139].

In general, the antidepressants are combined with opioid drugs when used to treat pain in populations with advanced illness; the are rarely used as primary analgesics[119,138,140]. Ventafridda *et al.*[119] reviewed a multi-centre clinical experience with antidepressant agents (trazodone and amitriptyline) in the treatment of chronic cancer pain that included a neuropathic component. Almost all of these patients were already receiving opioids and experienced improved pain control with the antidepressant. A subsequent randomized, double-blind study showed both amitriptyline and trazodone to have similar therapeutic analgesic efficacy[119]. Magni *et al.*[120] reviewed the use of antidepressants in Italian cancer centres and found that a wide range of antidepressants were used for a variety of cancer pain syndromes, with amitriptyline being the most commonly prescribed, for a variety of cancer pains. In nearly all cases, antidepressants were used in association with opioids. There is some evidence that patients respond differentially to the various antidepressants, and should one fail to relieve pain, an alternative may be tried[140]. The antidepressants may be effective for pain through a number of mechanisms, including: (1) antidepressant activity[114]; (2) potentiation or enhancement of opioid analgesia[141–143]; (3) direct analgesic effects[144].

The heterocyclic and non-cyclic antidepressant drugs, such as trazodone, mianserin, maprotiline, and the newer serotonin-specific reuptake inhibitors, fluoxetine and paroxetine, may also be useful as adjuvant analgesics; however, clinical trials of their efficacy as analgesics have been equivocal[145–149]. There are several case reports that suggest that fluoxetine may be a useful adjuvant analgesic in the management of headache[150], fibrositis[151], and diabetic neuropathy[152]. In a recent clinical trial, fluoxetine was shown to be no better than placebo as an analgesic in painful diabetic neuropathy[153]. Paroxetine is the first serotonin-specific reuptake inhibitor shown to be analgesic in the treatment of neuropathic pain[154]. Although it has not been tested as an analgesic in medically ill populations, this drug, or other SSRIs such as citalopram[155], might be considered for trials if other antidepressants are ineffective. Escitalopram, a yet newer SSRI, may have advantages over other SSRIs in that it has the highest selectivity in its class, no active metabolites, and does not significantly affect the CYP450 isoenzyme[156]; it lessens both depression and anxiety[157] and also might be considered for a trial as an adjuvant analgesic. SSRIs may offer greater benefit to these patients as evidenced by greater improvements in quality-of-life measures[158].

Newer antidepressants such as sertraline, venlafaxine, nefazodone, and duloxetine also may be clinically useful as adjuvant analgesics. Duloxetine, a dual reuptake inhibitor of serotonin and norepinephrine, has been shown to be an effective treatment for depression and for neuropathic pain[159]. This drugs is approved in the United States of America for painful diabetic neuropathy. Nefazodone has been demonstrated to potentiate opioid analgesics in an animal model[160]; and venlafaxine, has been shown by

Tasmuth et al.[161] to decrease the maximum pain intensity following treatment of breast cancer.

At this point, it is clear that many antidepressants have analgesic properties, and although there are very few comparative trials, it is likely that the most studied drugs, the tricyclic antidepressants, have the greatest analgesic effects overall. There is extensive experience with amitriptyline, but the side-effect liability of this drug may be excessive for many patients with serious illness; an alternative tricyclic with fewer side effects, such as desipramine, may be preferred. There is limited evidence that the therapeutic analgesic effects of amitriptyline are correlated with serum levels, just as the antidepressant effects are, and analgesic treatment failure during a treatment trial with a tricyclic antidepressant may be due to low serum levels[123,124,162]. Although both pain and depression may respond to lower doses, titration of the dose is suggested if effects are unsatisfactory, and may be complemented by monitoring of serum drug concentrations[126,163]. There may be a biphasic time course of effects when these drugs are used, with early analgesic effects that occur within hours or days[135,141,144] and later, longer analgesic effects that peak over a 4- to 6-week period[123–125].

All of the antidepressant analgesics should be started at a relatively low dose in populations with pain complicating serious medical illness. Maximal effect as an adjuvant analgesic may require continuation of drug for 2–6 weeks. The choice of drug often depends on the side-effect profile, existing medical problems, the nature of depressive symptoms, if present, and past response to specific antidepressants. Sedating drugs like amitriptyline are helpful when insomnia complicates the presence of pain and depression on a cancer patient. Occasionally, in patients who have limited analgesic response to a tricyclic, potentiation of analgesia can be accomplished with the addition of lithium augmentation[164]. Tricyclic antidepressants have been shown to be effective as analgesics for mucositis when compared to opioids and for patients for whom opioids are contra indicated tricyclic antidepressants may be used[165].

In a small sample, mirtazapine has been shown to improve, though not statistically significant, pain, nausea, appetite, insomnia, and anxiety. Gains were small, but one must consider that patients left untreated are likely to show decline in these symptoms, not improvement[166]. Freynhagen et al.[167] has shown that in a large sample of 594 patients, from baseline to endpoint (a 6-week period), mirtazapine significantly improves pain, sleep disturbances, irritability, and exhaustion. This study also showed that the adverse side effects are minimal (<7 per cent), and the AE's side effects were overall mild to moderate. Of those who did leave the study (18 per cent), the main motivation was lack of efficacy, potentially a result of the antidepressant component of mirtazapine.

Monoamine oxidase inhibitors (MAOIs) are less useful in the cancer setting because of dietary restriction and potentially dangerous interactions between MAOIs and meperidine. Among the MAOI drugs available, phenelzine has been shown to have adjuvant analgesic properties in patients with atypical facial pain and migraine[168,169].

Psychostimulants

The psychostimulants dextroamphetamine and methylphenidate are useful antidepressant agents prescribed selectively for medically ill cancer patients with depression[170,171]. Psychostimulants are also useful in diminishing excessive sedation secondary to opioid analgesics, and are adjuvant analgesics. Bruera et al.[172–174]

demonstrated that a regimen of 10 mg methylphenidate with breakfast and 5 mg with lunch significantly decreased sedation and potentiated the analgesic effect of opioid drugs in patients with cancer pain. Dextroamphetamine has also been reported to have additive analgesic effects when used with morphine in postoperative pain[175]. In a relatively low dose, psychostimulants stimulate appetite, promote a sense of well-being, and improve feelings of weakness and fatigue in cancer patients. Treatment with dextroamphetamine or methylphenidate usually begins with a dose of 2.5 mg at 8:00 a.m. and at noon. The dosage is slowly increased over several days until a desired effect is achieved or side effects (overstimulation, anxiety, insomnia, paranoia, confusion) intervene. Typically, a dose greater than 30 mg/day is not necessary although occasionally patients require up to 60 mg/day or higher. Tolerance may develop to the beneficial effects of the stimulants and adjustment of dose may be necessary.

Modafinil is a wakefulness agent, which is approved in the United States of America for the treatment of excessive daytime sedation secondary to sleep disorders (e.g. narcolepsy, sleep apnoea). It is often utilized clinically in the palliative care setting as a mild psychostimulant[176]. A study by DeBattista et al.[177] tested modafinil on subjects with major depression and partial response to antidepressants, and found that adjunctive treatment with modafinil significantly improved fatigue and depressive symptoms. Furthermore, modafinil was found to increase attention, concentration, and cognitive functioning. Fatigue is a common symptom of cancer and cancer treatment, and modafinil has been shown to improve fatigue in patients with multiple sclerosis and in cancer populations[178,179]. Modafinil, in doses ranging from 50–400 mg, is used in the palliative care settings to treat fatigue as well as to counteract the sedation caused by opioids in the setting of pain management. Modafinil is not a sympathomimetic agent, and its mechanism of action is distinct from classic psychostimulants, suggesting that issues of dependence, tolerance, and abuse may be significantly less of a concern with modafinil than with agents such as dextroamphetamine or methylphenidate[176].

Neuroleptics

Methotrimeprazine is a neuroleptic drug with limited commercial availability, but a long history of use as an adjuvant analgesic. It presumably produces analgesia through alpha-adrenergic blockade[180]. It is a dopamine blocker and so has antiemetic as well an anxiolytic effects. Methotrimeprazine can produce sedation and hypotension and should be given cautiously by slow intravenous infusion. Other phenothiazines, such as chlorpromazine and prochlorperazine are useful as antiemetics, but probably have limited use as analgesics[181]. Fluphenazine in combination with a tricyclic antidepressant has been shown to be helpful in neuropathic pains[134]. Haloperidol is the drug of choice in the management of delirium or psychoses in cancer patients, and has clinical usefulness as a co-analgesic for cancer pain[181]. Pimozide, a butyrophenone that also has limited availability, has been shown to be effective as an analgesic in the management of trigeminal neuralgia, at doses of 4–12 mg/day[182].

Atypical antipsychotics, such as olanzapine, risperidone, quetiapine, apiprazole, and ziprasidone are primarily used to treat delirium in the palliative care setting[183]. Boettger and Breitbart[183] suggest that olanzapine and risperidone are the atypical antipsychotics with the most demonstrated efficacy for managing the symptoms of delirium, however smaller studies and case series reports suggest potential benefit for quetiapine[184], ziprasidone[185], and apiprazole[186]. Olanzapine has been used to treat unmanaged pain in the context of anxiety and mild cognitive impairment[187]. Patients received 2.5–7.5 mg of olanzapine daily. Daily pain scores decreased; anxiety and cognitive impairment resolved. Aripiprazole has been shown to be potentially beneficial in reducing bone pain[188].

Anxiolytics

Hydroxyzine is a mild anxiolytic with sedating and analgesic properties that are useful in the anxious cancer patient with pain[189,190]. This antihistamine has antiemetic activity as well. One hundred milligrams of parenteral hydroxyzine has analgesic activity approaching 8 mg of morphine, and has additive analgesic effects when combined with morphine. Benzodiazepines have not been felt to have direct analgesic properties, although they are potent anxiolytics and anticonvulsants[191]. Some authors have suggested that their anticonvulsant properties make certain benzodiazepine drugs useful in the management of neuropathic pain. Fernandez *et al.*[192] showed that alprazolam, a unique benzodiazepine with mild antidepressant properties, was a helpful adjuvant analgesic in cancer patients with phantom limb pain or deafferentation (neuropathic) pain. Clonazepam also may be useful in the management of neuropathic pains[193,194]. With the use of midazolam by IV in a patient-controlled dosage, there was no reduction in the use of postoperative morphine requirements or in the patient's perception of pain[195]. Intrathecal midazolam in animal models, however, has been shown to potentiate morphine analgesia[196].

Placebo

A mention of the placebo response is important in order to highlight the misunderstandings and relative harm that may ensue if this phenomenon is misused. The placebo response is common, and at least in part, probably mediated through endogenous opioids. The deceptive use of a placebo in an effort to distinguish psychogenic pain from 'real' pain is misguided, unscientific, and should not be condoned.

References

1. Foley, K.M. (1975). Pain syndromes in patients with cancer. In *Advances in Pain Research and Therapy*, (eds. V.V. J.J. Bonica, R.B. Fink, L.E. Jones, J.D. Loeser), pp. 59–75. Raven Press: New York.
2. Foley, K.M. (1985). The treatment of cancer pain. *New England Journal of Medicine*, **313**, 845.
3. Breitbart, W.A.H., J. (1990). Psychiatric aspects of cancer pain. In *Advances in Pain Research and Therapy*, (ed. K.M.F. *et al.*), pp. 73–87. Raven Press: New York.
4. Breitbart, W. (1989). Psychiatric management of cancer pain. *Cancer*, **63**, 2336–42.
5. Breitbart, W. (1990). Psychiatric aspects of pain and HIV disease. *Focus: A Guide to AIDS Research and Counseling*, **5**, 1–2.
6. Massie, M.J.A.H., J.C. (1987). The cancer patient with pain: psychiatric complications and their mangement. *Medical Clinics of North America*, **71**, 243–58.
7. Fitzgibbon, D.R. (2001). Cancer pain: management. In *Bonica's Management of Pain* (ed. J.D.L. *et al.*), pp. 659–703. Lippincott Williams & Wilkins: Philadelphia.
8. Weiss, S.C., Emanuel, L.L., Fairclough D.L. *et al.* (2001). Understanding the experience of pain in terminally ill patients. *Lancet*, **357**, 1311–5.
9. Twycross, R.G.A.L., S.A. (1983). *Symptom Control in Far Advanced Cancer: Pain Relief*. London: Pitman Brooks.
10. Marks, R.M.A.S., E.J. (1973). Undertreatment of medical inpatients with narcotic analgesics. *Annals of Internal Medicine*, **78**, 173–81.
11. Grond, S., Zech, D., Diefenbach, C. *et al.* (1994). Prevalence and pattern of symptoms in patients with cancer pain: a prospective evaluation of 1635 cancer patients referred to a pain clinic. *Journal of Pain and Symptom Management*, **9**, 372–82.
12. Walsh, D., Donnelly, S., and Rybicki, L. (2000). The symptoms of advanced cancer: relationship to age, gender, and performance status in 1000 patients. *Support Care Cancer*, **8**(3), 175–9.
13. Achte, K.A.A.V., M.L. (1971). Cancer and the psych. *Omega*, **2**, 46–56.
14. Breitbart, W., McDonald, M.V., Rosenfeld, B. *et al.* (1196). Pain in ambulatory AIDS patients. I: Pain characteristics and medical correlates. *Pain*, **68** (2–3), 315–21.
15. Norval, D. (2004). Symptoms and sites of pain experienced by AIDS patients. *South African Medical Journal*, **94**, 450–4.
16. Frich, L.M.A.B., F.M. (2000). Pain and pain treatment in AIDS patients: a longitudinal study. *Journal of Pain and Symptom Management*, **19**(5), 339–47.
17. Lebovits, A.H., Lefkowitz, M., McCarthy, D. *et al.* (1989). The prevalence and management of pain in patients with AIDS. A review of 134 cases. *The Clinical Journal of Pain*, **5**, 245–8.
18. Newshan, G., Wainapel, S., and Schmitz, D. (1989).Pain related syndromes and their treatment in persons with AIDS (Abstract). In *Eighth Annual Scientific Meeting of the American Pain Society*. Phoenix, AZ.
19. Levy, R.M., Bredesen, D.E., and Rosenblum, M.L. (1985). Neurological manifestations of the AIDS experience at UCSF and review of the literature. *Journal of Neurosurgery*, **62**, 475–95.
20. Snider, W.D. *et al.* (1983). Neurological complications of AIDS; analysis of 50 patients. *Annals of Neurology*, **14**, 403–18.
21. Cornblath, D.R.A.M., I.C. (1988). Predominantly sensory neuropathy in patients with AIDS and AIDS-related complex. *Neurology*, **38**, 794–6.
22. Schofferman, J.A.B., R. (1990). Pain in far advanced AIDS. In *Advances in Pain Research and Therapy*, (ed. e.K.M.F. *et al.*), pp. 379–86. Raven Press: New York.
23. Rosenfeld, B., Breitbart, W., McDonald, M. *et al.* (1996). Pain in ambulatory AIDS patients - II: Impact of pain on psychological functioning and quality of life. *Pain*, **68**, 323–8.
24. Hewitt, D., McDonald, M., Portenoy, R.K. *et al.* (1997). Pain syndromes and etiologies in ambulatory AIDS patients. *Pain*, **70**, 117–23.
25. Breitbart, W., Stiefel, F., Kornblith, A. *et al.* (1993). Neuropsychiatric disturbances in cancer patients with epidural spinal cord compression receiving high dose corticosteroids: A prospective comparison study. *Psycho-oncology*, **2**, 233–45.
26. Saunders, C.M. (1967). *The Management of Terminal Illness*. London: Hospital Medicine Publications.
27. Hanks, G.W. (1991). Opioid responsive and opioid non-responsive pain in cancer. *British Medical Bulletin*, **47**, 718–31.
28. Syrjala, K.A.C., M. (1995). Evidence for a biopsychosocial model of cancer treatment-related pain. *Pain*, **61**, 69–79.
29. Daut, R.L.A.C., C.S. (1982). The prevalence and severity of pain in cancer. *Cancer*, **50**, 1913–8.
30. Spiegel, D.A.B., J.R. (1983). Pain in metastatic breast cancer. *Cancer*, **52**, 341–5.
31. Padilla, G., Ferrell, B., Grant, M. *et al.* (1990). Defining the content domain of quality of life for cancer patients with pain. *Cancer Nursing*, **13**, 108–15.
32. Smith, W.B., Gracely, R.H., and Safer, M.A. (1998). The meaning of pain: cancer patients' rating and recall of pain intensity and affect. *Pain*, **78**(2), 123–9.

33. Payne, D., Jacobsen, P., Breitbart, W. *et al.* (1994). Negative thoughts related to pain are associated with greater pain, distress, and disability in AIDS pain. In *Presentation at the American Pain Society*, Miami, Florida.

34. Payne, D. (1995). *Cognition in Cancer Pain*, In unpublished dissertation.

35. McKegney, F.P., Bailey, C.R., and Yates, J.W. (1981). Prediction and management of pain in patients with advanced cancer. *General Hospital Psychiatry*, **3**, 95–101.

36. Bond, M.R.A.P., I.B. (1969). Psychological aspects of pain in women with advanced cancer of the cervix. *Journal of Psychosomatic Research*, **13**, 13–9.

37. Strang, P. (1997). Existential consequences of unrelieved cancer pain. *Palliative Medicine*, **11**(4), 299–305.

38. Portenoy, R.K., Payne, D., and Jacobsen, P. (1999). Breakthrough pain: characteristics and impact in patients with cancer pain. *Pain*, **81**(1–2), 129–34.

39. Turk, D.C., Sist, T.C., Okifuji, A. *et al.* (1998). Adaptation to metastatic cancer pain, regional/local cancer pain and non-cancer pain: role of psychological and behavioral factors. *Pain*, **74**(2–3), 247–56.

40. Heaven, C.M.A.M., P. (1998). The relationship between patients' concerns and psychological distress in a hospice setting. *Psychooncology*, **7**(6), 502–7.

41. Breitbart, W., Passik S., Rosenfeld, B. *et al.* (1994). Pain intensity and its relationship to functional interference in patients with AIDS (Poster). In *American Pain Society*.

42. Rosenfeld, B., Breitbart, W., McDonald, M. *et al.* (1996). Pain in ambulatory AIDS patients - II: Impact of pain on psychological functioning and quality of life. *Pain*, **68**, 323–8.

43. Singer, E.J., Zorilla, C., Fahy-Chandon, B. *et al.* (1993). *Painful symptoms reported for ambulatory HIV-infected men in a longitudinal study*. *Pain*, **54**, 15–9.

44. Cleeland, C.S.a.T., B.H. (1986). Behavioral control of cancer pain, In *Pain Mangement* (ed. D.H.a.D. Turk). pp. 93–212. Pergamon Press: New York.

45. Derogatis, L.R. *et al.* (1983).The prevalence of psychiatric disorders among cancer patients. *Journal of the American Medical Association*, **249**, 751–7.

46. Ahles, T.A., Blanchard, E.B., and Ruckdeschel, J.C. (1983). *The multi-dimensional nature of cancer related pain*. *Pain*, **17**, 277–88.

47. Woodforde, J.M.A.F., J.R. (1970). Pain and cancer. *Journal of Psychosomatic Research*, **14**, 3648.
    Stiefel, F.C., Breitbart, W., and Holland, J.C. (1989). Corticosteroids in cancer: neuropsychiatric complications. *Cancer Investigation*, **7**, 479–91.

48. Breitbart, W., Stiefel, F., Kornblith, A. *et al.* (1993). Neuropsychiatric disturbances in cancer patients with epidural spinal cord compression receiving high dose corticosteroids: A prospective comparison study. *Psycho-oncology*, **2**, 233–45.

49. Bukberg, J., Penman, D., and Holland, J. (1984). Depression in hospitalized cancer patients. *Psychosomatic Medicine*, **43**, 199–212.

50. Massie, J.M., Holland, J.C., and Glass, E. (1983). *Delirium in terminally ill cancer patients*. *American Journal of Psychiatry*, **140**, 1048–50.

51. Bruera, E. *et al.* (1989). The cognitive effects of the administration of narcotics. *Pain*, **39**, 13–6.

52. Breitbart, W. (1987). Suicide in cancer patients. *Oncology*, **1**, 49–53.

53. Breitbart, W. (1990). Cancer pain and suicide. In *Advances in Pain Research and Therapy*, (ed. K.M.F. *et al.*), pp. 399–412., Raven Press: New York.

54. Sison, A., Eller, K., Segal, J. *et al.* (1991). Suicidal ideation in ambulatory HIV-infected patients: the roles of pain, mood, and disease status (Abstract). In *Current Concepts in Psycho-oncology IV*. New York.

55. Levin, D.N., Cleeland, C.S., and Dan, R. (1985). Public attitudes toward cancer pain. *Cancer*, **56**, 2337–9.

56. Bolund, C. (1985). Suicide and cancer: II. Medical and care factors in suicide by cancer patients in Sweden, 1973-1976. *Journal of Psychosocial Oncology*, **3**, 17–30.

57. Farberow, N.L., Schneidman, E.S., and Leonard, C.V. (1963), *Suicide among general medical and surgical hospital patients with malignant neoplasms*. US Veterans Administration: Washington D.C.

58. Massie, M., Gagnon, P., and Holland, J. (1994). Depression and suicide in patients with cancer. *Journal of Pain and Symptom Management*, **9**(5), 325–31.

59. Silberfarb, P.M., Manrer, L.H., and Cronthamel, C.S. (1980). Psychological aspects of neoplastic disease, I: Functional status of breast cancer patients during different treatment regimens. *American Journal of Psychiatry*, **137**, 450–5.

60. Brown, J.H., Henteleff, P., Barakat, S. *et al.* (1986). Is it normal for terminally ill patients to desire death. *American Journal of Psychiatry*, **143**, 208–11.

61. Breitbart, W., Rosenfeld, B., Pessin, H. *et al.* (2000). Depression, hopelessness, and desire for hastened death in terminally ill patients with cancer. *Journal of the American Medical Association*, **284** (22), 2907–11.

62. Saltzburg, D. *et al.* (1989).The relationship of pain and depression to suicidal ideation in cancer patients (Abstract). In *ASCO Annual Meeting*. San Francisco.

63. Suarez-Almazor, M.E., Newman, C., Hanson, J. *et al.* (2002). Attitudes of terminally ill cancer patients about euthanasia and assisted suicide: predominance of psychosocial determinants and beliefs over symptom distress and subsequent survival. *Journal of Clinical Oncology*, **20**(8), 2134–41.

64. Marzuk, P., Tierney, H., Tardiff, K. *et al.* (1988). Increased risk of suicide in persons with AIDS. *Journal of the American Medical Association*, **259**, 1333–7.

65. Rabkin, J., Remien, R., Katoff, L. *et al.* (1993). Suicidality in AIDS long-term survivors: what is the evidence? *AIDS-Care*, **5**(4), 401–11.

66. Cleeland, C., Gonin, R., Hatfield, A. *et al.* (1994). Pain and its treatment in outpatients with metastatic cancer. *New England Journal of Medicine*, **330**, 592–6.

67. Lebovits, A.K., Lefkowitz, M., and McCarthy, D. (1989). The prevalence and management of pain in patients with AIDS. A review of 134 cases. *The Clinical Journal of Pain*, **5**, 245–8.

68. McCormack, J.P., Li, R., Zarowny, D. *et al.* (1993). Inadequate treatment of pain in ambulatory HIV patients. *The Clinical Journal of Pain*, **9**, 279–83.

69. Breitbart, W., Rosenfeld B., Passik S.D. *et al.* (1996). The undertreatment of pain in ambulatory AIDS patients. *Pain*, **65**, 243–9.

70. Breitbart, W., Passik, S., McDonald, M. *et al.* (1998), Patient-related barriers to pain management in ambulatory AIDS patients. *Pain*, **76**, 9–16.

71. Bruera, E., MacMillan, K., Pither, J. *et al.* (1990). Effects of morphine on the dyspnea of terminal cancer patients. *Journal of Pain and Symptom Management*, **5**, 341–4.

72. Grossman, S.A., Sheidler, V.R., Sweden, K. *et al.* (1991). Correlations of patient and caregiver ratings of cancer pain. *Journal of Pain and Symptom Management*, **6**, 53–7.

73. Macaluso, C., Weinberg, D., and Foley, K.M. (1988).Opiod abuse and misuse in a cancer pain population (Abstract). In *Second International Congress on Cancer Pain*. Rye, New York.

74. Breitbart, W. Pain in HIV Disease. (2003). In *A Clinical Guide to Supportive & Palliative Care for HIV/AIDS* (ed. J. O'Neil), pp. 85–122. U.S. Dept. of Health and Human Services, Health Resources and Services Administration (HRSA) HIV/AIDS Bureau.

75. Charap, A.D. (1978). The knowledge, attitudes, and experience of medical personnel treating pain in the terminally ill. *Mt Sinai Journal of Medicine*, **45**, 561–80.

76. Kanner, R.M.A.F., K.M. (1981). Patterns of narcotic use in a cancer pain clinic. *Annals of the New York Academy of Science*, **362**, 161–72.

77. Cassem, N.H. (1987). They dying patient. In *Massachusetts General Hospital Handbook of General Hospital Psychiatry*, (ed. T.P.H.a.N.H. Cassem), pp. 332–52. PSG Publishing Co. Inc.: Littleton, MA.

78. Keefe, FJ. (2005). Partner-Guided Cancer Pain Management at the End of Life: A Preliminary Study. *Journal of Pain and Symptom Management*, **29**, 263–72.

79. Syrajala, K., Cummings, C., and Donaldson, G. (1992). Hypnosis or cognitive behavioral training for the reduction of pai and nausea during cancer treatment: a controlled trial. *Pain*, **48**, 137–46.

80. Spiegel, D.A.B., J.R. (1983). Group therapy and hypnosis reduce metastatic breast carcinoma pain. *Psychosomatic Medicine*, **4**, 333–9.

81. Fishman, B.A.L., M. (1987). Cognitive-behavioral interventions in the management of cancer pain: principles and applications. *Medical Clinics of North America*, **71**, 271–87.

82. Cleeland, C.S. (1987). Nonpharmacologic management of cancer pain. *Journal of Pain and Symptom Control*, **2**, 523–8.

83. Loscalzo, M.A.J., P.B. (1990). Practical behavioral approaches to the effective management of pain and distress. *Journal of Psychosocial Oncology*, **8**, 139–69.

84. Turk, D.A.F., E. (1990). On the Putative Uniqueness of cancer pain: do psychological principles apply? *Behaviour Research and Therapy*, **28**(1), 1–13.

85. Fishman, B. (1990). The treatment of suffering in patients with cancer pain. In *Advances in Pain Research and Therapy*, (ed. J.B.a.V.V. K. Foley), pp. 301–16. Raven Press: New York.

86. Jensen, M., Turner, J., Romano, J. *et al.* (1991). Coping with chronic pain: a critical review of the literature. *Pain*, **47**, 249–83.

87. Breitbart, W.A.H., J.C. (1988). Psychiatric complications of cancer. In *Current Therapy in Hematology Oncology* (ed. M.C.B.a.P.P. Carbone), pp. 268–74. B.C. Decker, Inc: Toronto and Philadelphia.

88. Montgomery, G.H., Weltz, C.R., Seltz, M. *et al.* (2002). Brief presurgery hypnosis reduces distress and pain in excisional breast biopsy patients. *International Journal of Clinical and Experimental Hypnosis*, **50**(1), 17–32.

89. Sellick, S.M.A.Z., C. (1998). Critical review of 5 nonpharmacologic strategies for managing cancer pain. *Cancer Prevention and Control*, **2**(1), 7–14.

90. Kazak, A.E., Penati, B., Brophy, P. *et al.* (1998). Pharmacologic and psychologic interventions for procedural pain. *Pediatrics*, **102** (1 Pt 1), 59–66.

91. Carroll, D.A.S., K. (1998). Relaxation for the relief of chronic pain: a systematic review. *Journal of Advanced Nursing*, **27**(3), 476–87.

92. Wallace, K.G. (1997). Analysis of recent literature concerning relaxation and imagery interventions for cancer pain. *Cancer Nursing*, **20**(2), 79–87.

93. Luebbert, K., Dahme, B., and Hasenbring, M. (2001). The effectiveness of relaxation training in reducing treatment-related symptoms and improving emotional adjustment in acute non-surgical cancer treatment: a meta-analytical review. *Psycho-oncology*, **10**(6), 490–502.

94. Erickson, M.H. (1959). Hypnosis in painful terminal illness. *American Journal of Clinical Hypnosis*, **1**, 1117–21.

95. Benson, H. (1975). *The Relaxation Response*.

96. Broome, M., Lillis, P., McGahhe, T. *et al.* (1992). The use of distraction and imagery with children during painful procedures. *Oncology Nursing Forum*, **19**, 499–502.

97. Spiegel, D. (1985). The use of hypnosis in controlling cancer pain. *CA-A Cancer Journal for Clinicians*, **4**, 221–31.

98. Levitan, A. (1992). The use of hypnosis with cancer patients. *Psychiatry and Medicine*, **10**, 119–31.

99. Tan, S.Y.A.L., C.A. (1997). Cognitive-behavioral therapy for clinical pain control: a 15-year update and its relationship to hypnosis.

International Journal of Clinical and Experimental Hypnosis, **45**(4), 396–416.

100. Douglas, D.B. (1999). Hypnosis: useful, neglected, available. *American Journal of Hospice and Palliative Care*, **16**(5), 665–70.

101. Rajasekaran, M., Edmonds, P.M., Higginson, I.L. (2005). Systematic review of hypnotherapy for treating symptoms in terminally ill adult cancer patients. *Palliative Medicine*, **19**(5), 418–26.

102. Montgomery GH, D.K., Redd WH. (2000). A meta-analysis of hypnotically induced analgesia: how effective is hypnosis? *International Journal of Clinical and Experimental Hypnosis*, **48**(2), 138–53.

103. Liossi, C.A.H., P. (1999). Clinical hypnosis versus cognitive behavioral training for pain management with pediatric cancer patients undergoing bone marrow aspirations. *International Journal of Clinical and Experimental Hypnosis*, **47**(2), 104–16.

104. Fotopoulos, S.S., Graham, C., and Cook, M.R. (1979). Psychophysiologic control of cancer pain, in *Advances in Pain Research and Therapy* (ed. J.J.B.a.V. Ventafridda), pp. 231–44. Raven Press: New York.

105. Munro, S.M.A.M., B. (1978). Music therapy in palliative care. *Canadian Medical Association Journal*, **119**, 1029–34.

106. Schroeder-Sheker, T. (1993). Music for the dying: a personal account of the new field of music thanatology-history, theories, and clinical narratives. *Advances*, **9**, 36–48.

107. Magill, L. (2001). The use of music therapy to address the suffering in advanced cancer pain. *Journal of Palliative Care*, **17**(3), 167–72.

108. Chlan, L., Evans, D., Greenleaf, M. *et al.* (2000). Effects of a single music therapy intervention on anxiety, discomfort, satisfaction, and compliance with screening guidelines in outpatients undergoing flexible sigmoidoscopy. *Gastroenterology Nursing*, **23**(4), 148.

109. Manne, S., Redd, W., Jacobsen, P. *et al.* (1991). *Aroma for treatment of anxiety during, MRI scans (Abstract)*. in *Symposium on New Trends in the Psychological Support of the Cancer Patient, American Psychiatric Association Annual Meeting*. New Orleans, LA.

110. Nainis, N., Paice, J. A., Ratner, J. *et al.* (2006). Relieving Symptoms in Cancer: Innovative Use of Art Therapy. *Journal of Pain and Symptom Management*, **31**(2), 162–9.

111. Connell, C. (1992). Art therapy as part of a palliative cancer program. *Palliative Medicine*, **6**, 18–25.

112. Breitbart, W. (1992). Psychotropic adjuvant analgesics for cancer pain. *Psycho-Oncology*, V, p. 133-45.

113. Farrar, J.T.A.P., R.K. (2001). Neuropathic cancer pain: the role of adjuvant analgesics. *Oncology*, **15**(11), 1435–42, 1445, 1450–3.

114. France, R.D. (1987). The future for antidepressants: treatment of pain. *Psychopathology*, **20**, 99–113.

115. Getto, C.J., Sorkness, C.A., and Howell, T. (1987). Antidepressants and chronic nonmalignant pain: a review. *Journal of Pain and Symptom Control*, **2**, 9–18.

116. Walsh, T.D., *Antidepressants and chronic pain*. Clinical Neuropharmacology, 1983. **6**, p. 271–95.

117. Walsh, T.D. (1990). Adjuvant analgesic therapy in cancer pain. In *Second International Congress on Cancer Pain*, New York: Raven Press.

118. Butler, S. (1986). *Present status of tricyclic antidepressants in chronic pain therapy*, in *Advances in Pain Research and Therapy* (ed. C.B.e. al.,), pp. 173–96, Raven Press: New York.

119. Ventafridda, V., Bonezzi, C., Caraceni, A. *et al.* (1987). Antidepressants for cancer pain and other painful syndromes with deafferentation component: comparison of Amitriptyline and Trazodone. *Italian Journal of Neurological Sciences*, **8**, 579–87.

120. Magni, G., Arsie, D., and DeLeo, D. (1987). Antidepressants in the treatment of cancer pain. A survey in Italy. *Pain*, **29**, 347–53.

121. Onghena, P.A.V.H., B. (1992). Antidepressant-induced analgesia in chronic non-malignant pain: a meta-analysis of 39 placebo-controlled studies. *Pain*, **49**, 205–19.

122. Lefkowitz, M.A.B., W. (1992).Chronic pain and AIDS. *Innovations in Pain Medicine*, **36**(2–3), 18.

123. Max, M.B., Culnane, M., Schafer, S.C. *et al.* (1987). Amitriptyline relieves diabetic-neuropathy pain in patients with normal and depressed mood. *Neurology*, **37**, 589–96.

124. Max, M.B., Schafer, S.C., Culnane, M. *et al.* (1982). Amitriptyline, but not lorazepam, relieves postherpetic neuralgia. *Neurology*, **38**, 427–32.

125. Pilowsky, I., Hallett, E.C., Bassett, D.L. *et al.* (1982). A controlled study of amitriptyline in the treatment of chronic pain. *Pain*, **14**, 169–79.

126. Sharav, Y., Singer, E., Schmidt, E. *et al.* (1987). The analgesic effect of amitriptyline on chronic facial pain. *Pain,* **31**, 199–209.

127. Watson, C.P., Evans, R.J., Reed, K. *et al.* (1982). Amitriptyline versus placebo in post herpetic neuralgia. *Neurology,* **32**, 671–3.

128. Kvindesal, B., Molin, J., Froland, A. *et al.* (1984). Imipramine treatment of painful diabetic neuropathy. *Journal of the American Medical Association*, **251**, 1727–30.

129. Young, R.J.A.C., B.F. (1985). *Pain relief in diabetic neuropathy: the effectiveness of imipramine and related drugs.* Diabetic Medicine, **2**: p. 363-6.

130. Sindrup, S.H. *et al.* (1989). Imipramine treatment in diabetic neuropathy: relief of subjective symptoms without changes in peripheral and autonomic nerve function. *European Journal of Clinical Pharmacology*, **37**, 151–3.

131. Max, M.B. *et al.* (1991). Efficacy of desipramine in painful diabetic neuropathy: a placebo-controlled trial. *Pain*, **45**, 3–10.

132. Gordon, N., Heller, P., Gear, R. *et al.* (1993). Temporal factors in the enhancement of morphine analgesic by desipramine. *Pain*, **53**, 273–6.

133. Gomez-Perez, F.J. *et al.* (1985). Nortriptyline and fluphenazine in the symptomatic treatment of diabetic neuropathy. A double-blind cross-over study. *Pain*, **23**, 395–400.

134. Langohr, H.D., Stohr, M., and Petruch, F. (1982). An open and double-blind crosover study on the efficacy of clomipramine (anafranil) in patients with painful mono- and polyneuropathies. *European Neurology*, **21**, 309–15.

135. Tiegno, M., Pagnoni, B., Calmi, A. *et al.* (1987). Chlorimipramine compared to pentazocine as a unique treatment in post-operative pain. *International Journal of Clinical and Pharmacological Research*, **7**, 141–3.

136. Hammeroff, S.R. *et al.* (1982). Doxepin effects on chronic pain, depression and plasma opioids. *Journal of Clinical Psychiatry*, **2**, 22–6.

137. Lee, R.A., West, R.M., and Wilson, J.D. (2005). The response to sertraline in men with chronic pelvic pain syndrome. *Sexually Transmitted Infections*, **81**(2), 147–9.

138. Walsh, T.D. (1986). Controlled study of imipramine and morphine in chronic pain due to advanced cancer (Abstract). In *ASCO*. May 4–6, Los Angeles.

139. Kimmick, G.G. *et al.* (2006). Randomized, double-blind, placebo-controlled, crossover study of sertraline (Zoloft) for the treatment of hot flashes in women with early stage breast cancer taking tamoxifen. *Breast Journal*, **12**(2), 114–22.

140. Watson, C., Chipan, M., Reed, K. *et al.* (1992). Amitriptyline versus maprotiline in postherpetic neuralgia: a randomized double-blind crossover trial. *Pain*, **48**, 29–36.

141. Botney, M.A.F., H.C. (1983). Amitriptyline potentiates morphine analgesia by direct action on the central nervous system. *Annals of Neurology*, **13**, 160–4.

142. Malseed, R.T.A.G., F.J. (1979). Enhancement of morphine analgesics by tricyclic antidepressnts. *Neuropharmacology*, **18**, 827–9.

143. Ventafridda, V. *et al.* (1990). Studies on the effects of antidepressant drugs on the antinociceptive action of morphine and on plasma morphine in rat and man. *Pain*, **43**, 155–62.

144. Spiegel, K., Kalb, R., and Pasternak, G.W. (1983). Analgesic activity of tricyclic antidepressants. *Annals of Neurology*, **13**, 462–5.

145. Davidoff, G. *et al.* (1987). Trazodone hydrochloride in the treatment of dysesthetic pain in traumatic myelopathy: a randomized, double-blind, placebo-controlled study. *Pain*, **29**, 151–61.

146. Costa, D., Mogos, I., and Toma, T. (1985). Efficacy and safety of mianserin in the treatment of depression of woman with cancer. *Acta Psychiatrica Scandinavica*, **72**, 85–92.

147. Eberhard, G. *et al.* (1988). A double-blind randomized study of clomipramine versus maprotiline in patients with idiopathic pain syndromes. *Neuropsychobiology*, **19**, 25–32.

148. Feighner, J.P. (1985). A comparative trial of fluoxetine and amitriptyline in patients with major depressive disorder. *Journal of Clinical Psychiatry*, **46**, 369–72.

149. Hynes, M.D. *et al.* (1985). Fluoxetine, a selective inhibitor of serotonin uptake, potentiates morphine analgesia without altering its descriminative stimulus properties or affinity for opioid receptors. *Life Sciences*, **36**, 2317–23.

150. Diamond, S.A.F., F.G. (1989). The use of fluoxetine in the treatment of headache. *Clinical Journal of Pain*, **5**, 200–1.

151. Geller, S.A. (1989). Treatment of fibrositis with fluoxetine hydrochloride (Prozac). *American Journal of Medicine*, **87**, 594–5.

152. Theesen, K.A.A.M., W.R. (1989). Relief of diabetic neuropathy with fluoxetine. *DICP, The Annals of Pharmacotherapy*, **23**, 572-4.

153. Max, M.B., Lynch, S.A., Muir, J. *et al.* (1992). Effects of desipramine, amitriptyline, and fluoxetine on pain in diabetic neuropathy. *New England Journal of Medicine*, **326**, 1250–6.

154. Sindrup, S.H., Gram, L.F., Brosen, K. *et al.* (1990). The selective serotonin reuptake inhibitor paroxetine is effective in the treatment of diabetic neuropathy symptoms. *Pain*, **42**, 135–44.

155. Sindrup, S.H. *et al.* (1992). The selective serotonin reuptake inhibitor citalopram relieves the symptoms of diabetic neuropathy. *Clinical Pharmacology and Therapeutics*, **52**(5), 547–52.

156. Sidney H. Kennedy, H.F.A., Raymond W. Lam. (2006). Efficacy of escitalopram in the treatment of major depressive disorder compared with conventional selective serotonin reuptake inhibitors and venlafaxine XR: a meta-analysis. *Journal of Psychiatry and Neuroscience*, **31**(2), 122–131.

157. Thase, M.E. (2006). Managing depressive and anxiety disorders with escitalopram. *Expert Opinion on Pharmacotherapy*, **7**(4), 429–440.

158. Holland, J.C., Romano, S.J., Heiligenstein, J.H. *et al.* (1998). A controlled trial of fluoxetine and desipramine in depressed women with advanced cancer. *Psychooncology*, **7**(4), 291–300.

159. Goldstein, D.J. *et al.* (2004). Duloxetine in the treatment of depression: a double-blind placebo-controlled comparison with paroxetine. *Journal of Clinical Psychopharmacology*, **24**(4), 389–99.

160. Pick, C.G., Paul, D., Eison, M.S. *et al.* (1992). Potentiation of opioid analgesia by the antidepressant nefazodone. *European Journal of Pharmacology*, **211**, 375–81.

161. Tasmuth, T., Hartel, B., and Kalso, E. (2002). Venlafaxine in neuropathic pain following treatment of breast cancer. *European Journal of Pain*, **6**, 17-24.

162. McQuay, H., Carroll, D., and Glynn, C. (1993). Dose-response for analgesic effect of amitriptyline in chronic pain. *Anesthesia*, **48**, 281–5.

163. Watson, C.P.A.E., R.J. (1985). A comparative trial of amitriptyline and zimelidine in post-herpetic neuralgia. *Pain*, **23**, 387–94.

164. Tyler, M.A. (1974). Treatment of the painful shoulder syndrome with amitriptyline and lithium carbonate. *Canadian Medical Association Journal*, **111**, 137–40.

165. Ehrnrooth, E., Grau, C., Zachariae, R. *et al.* (2001). Randomized trial of opioids versus tricyclic antidepressants for radiation-induced mucositis pain in head and neck cancer. *Acta Oncologica*, **40**(6), 745–50.

166. Theobald, D.E. *et al.* (2002). An open-label, crossover trial of mirtazapine (15 and 30 mg) in cancer patients with pain and other distressing symptoms. *Journal of Pain and Symptom Management*, **23**(5), 442–7.

167. Freynhagen, R. *et al.* (2006). The effect of mirtazapine in patients with chronic pain and concomitant depression. *Current Medical Research Opinion*, **22**(2), 257–64.

168. Lascelles, R.G. (1966). Atypical facial pain and depression. *British Journal of Psychology*, **122**, 651.

169. Anthony, M.a.L., J.W. (1969). MAO inhibition in the treatment of migraine. *Archives in Neurology*, **21**, 263.

170. Fernandez, F. *et al.* (1987). Methylphenidate for depressive disorders in cancer patients. *Psychosomatics*, **28**, 455–61.

171. Kaufmann, M.W., Murray, G.B., and Cassem, N.H. (1982). Use of psychostimulants in medically ill depressive patients. *Psychosomatics*, **23**, 817–19.

172. Bruera, E., Chadwick, S., Brennels, C. *et al.* (1987). Methylphenidate associated with narcotics for the treatment of cancer pain. *Cancer Treatment Reports*, **71**, 67–70.

173. Bruera, E., Brenneis, C., Paterson, A.H. *et al.* (1989). Use of methylphenidate as an adjuvant to narcotic analgesics in patients with advanced cancer. *Journal of Pain and Symptom Management*, **4**, 3–6.

174. Bruera, E., Fainsinger, R., MacEachern, T. *et al.* (1992). The use of methylphenidate in patients with incident cancer pain receiving regular opiates: a preliminary report. *Pain*, **50**, 75–7.

175. Forrest, W.H. *et al.* (1977). Dextroamphetamine with morphine for the treatment of post-operative pain. *New England Journal of Medicine*, **296**, 712–15.

176. Kingshott, R.N. *et al.* (2001). Randomized, double-blind, placebo-controlled crossover trial of modafinil in the treatment of residual excessive daytime sleepiness in the sleep apnea/hypopnea syndrome. *American Journal of Respiratory and Critical Care Medicine*, **163**(4), 918–23.

177. DeBattista, C. *et al.* (2004). A prospective trial of modafinil as an adjunctive treatment of major depression. *Journal of Clinical Psychopharmacology*, **24**(1), 87–90.

178. Morrow, G.R. *et al.* (2005). Management of cancer-related fatigue. *Cancer Investigation*, **23**(3), 229–39.

179. Rammohan, K.W. *et al.* (2002). Efficacy and safety of modafinil (Provigil) for the treatment of fatigue in multiple sclerosis: a two centre phase 2 study. *Journal of Neurology Neurosurgical Psychiatry*, **72**(2), 179–83.

180. Beaver, W.T. *et al.* (1966). A comparison of the analgesic effect of methotrimeprazine and morphine in patients with cancer. *Clinical Pharmacology and Therapeutics*, **7**, 436–46.

181. Maltbie, A.A. *et al.* (1979). Analgesia and haloperidol: a hypothesis. *Journal of Clinical Psychiatry*, **40**, 323–6.

182. Lechin, F. *et al.* (1989). Pimozide therapy for trigeminal neuralgia. *Archives in Neurology*, **9**, 960–4.

183. Boettger, S. and W. Breitbart. (2005). Atypical antipsychotics in the management of delirium: a review of the empirical literature. *Palliative Support Care*, **3**(3), 227–37.

184. Sasaki, Y. *et al.* (2003). A prospective, open-label, flexible-dose study of quetiapine in the treatment of delirium. *Journal of Clinical Psychiatry*, **64**(11), 1316–21.

185. Leso, L. and T.L. Schwartz. (2002). Ziprasidone treatment of delirium. *Psychosomatics*, **43**(1), 61–62.

186. Alao, A.O. *et al.* (2005). Aripiprazole in the treatment of delirium. *International Journal of Psychiatry Medicine*, **35**(4), 429–33.

187. Khojainova, N., Santiago-Palma, J., Kornick, C. *et al.* (2002). Olanzapine in the management of cancer pain. *Journal of Pain and Symptom Management*, **23**(4), 346–50.

188. Wilson, M.S., 2nd. (2005). *Aripiprazole and bone pain*. Psychosomatics, **46**(2), 187.

189. Beaver, W.T.a.F., G. (1976). Comparison of the analgesic effects of morphine, hydroxyzine and their combination in patients with post-operative pain. In *Advances in Pain Research and Therapy*, (ed. J.J.B.a. Albe-Fessard), pp. 533–57. Raven Press: New York.

190. Rumore, M.a.S., D. (1986). *Clinical efficacy of antihistamines as analgesics*. Pain, **25**, 7–22.

191. Coda, B., Mackie, A., and Hill, H. (1992). Influence of alprazolam on opioid analgesia and side effects during steady-stage morphine infusions. *Pain*, **50**, 309–16.

192. Fernandez, F., Adams, F., and Holmes, V.F. (1987). Analgesic effect of alprazolam in patients with chronic, organic pain of malignant origin. *Journal of Clinical Psychopharmacology*, **3**, 167–9.

193. Caccia, M.R. (1975). Clonazepam in facial neuralgia and cluster headache: clinical and electrophysiological study. *European Neurology*, **13**, 560–3.

194. Swerdlow, M.a.C., J.G. (1981). Anticonvulsant drugs used in the treatment of lancinating pains: a comparison. *Anesthesia*, **36**, 1129–34.

195. Egan, K., Ready, L., Nessly, M. *et al.* (1992). Self administration of midazolam for post-operative anxiety: a double blinded study. *Pain*, **49**, 3–8.

196. Liao, J.a.T., A. (1990). Quantitative assessment of antinociceptive effects of midazolam, amitriptyline, and carbamazepine alone and in combination with morphine in mice. *Anesthesiology*, **73**, A753.

10.2

Gastrointestinal symptoms

Contents

10.2.1 Palliation of nausea and vomiting

Kathryn A. Mannix

Introduction

Nausea and vomiting are unpleasant symptoms that are reported as highly distressing by sufferers[1,2]. The symptoms are separate, but related, and arise in many conditions including cancer, AIDS, and hepatic or renal failure[3,4]. Nausea and vomiting commonly cause misery for people with advanced cancer (up to 70 per cent patients) and despite major advances in antiemetic drug development in the last two decades, the incidence and severity of these symptoms is largely unchanged[1,2,5,6].

The neurophysiology of the vomiting reflex is well established in experimental animals[7,8], and is becoming better understood in man[9,10]. Intervention aimed at reducing nausea and vomiting must take into account the cause of the symptoms and the central emetogenic pathways involved. Thus, treatment requires knowledge of these pathways, careful assessment of the patient, and prescribing tailored to the cause of the symptoms and to the patient's individual needs.

The distress caused by the experience of nausea and, to a lesser extent, vomiting, is less well understood. The physiological processes can be partly extrapolated from animal models but the management of a nauseated patient also demands empathy, supportive care, and attention to the patient's concerns, in addition to any pharmacological intervention deemed appropriate.

Pathways involved in emesis

Central pathways involved in emesis

Emesis is mediated centrally by two separate 'centres'. Whilst these are anatomically distinct in experimental animals, in man the pathways are more diffuse (see Fig. 10.2.1.1).

The chemoreceptor trigger zone (CTZ) is located in the area postrema, in the floor of the fourth ventricle, where there is effectively no blood–brain barrier. Chemosensitive nerve cell projections are bathed by cerebrospinal fluid (CSF), which is in chemical equilibrium with blood in the fenestrated local capillaries. The nature of the chemoreceptors in the CTZ remains obscure. Neural pathways project from the CTZ to the nucleus of the tractussolitarius and the reticular formation in the medulla oblongata: these structures are the location of the 'vomiting centre'[7,8,11].

There may be a central antiemetic tone sustained by medullary neurons, inhibition of which potentiates the CTZ[12]. An enkephalinergic pathway has been hypothesized: displacement of enkephalins from their receptors by naloxone[10] or opioids[13] may reduce antiemetic tone, as may inhibition of enkephalin synthesis by chemotherapy[14]. This interesting hypothesis would help to explain, for example, the different emetogenic potentials of chemotherapeutic agents according to the point at which they interrupt cellular protein synthesis. The presence of medullary antiemetic tone and its influence on the CTZ remains speculative.

The vomiting centre (VC) is a diffuse, interconnecting neural network that integrates emetogenic stimuli with parasympathetic and motor efferent activity to produce the vomiting reflex. This is a complex reflex with respiratory, salivary, vasomotor, and somatic motor components: the VC acts as a central pattern generator. It has been proposed that sequential activation of various components of the VC, with amplification at each step, is required to

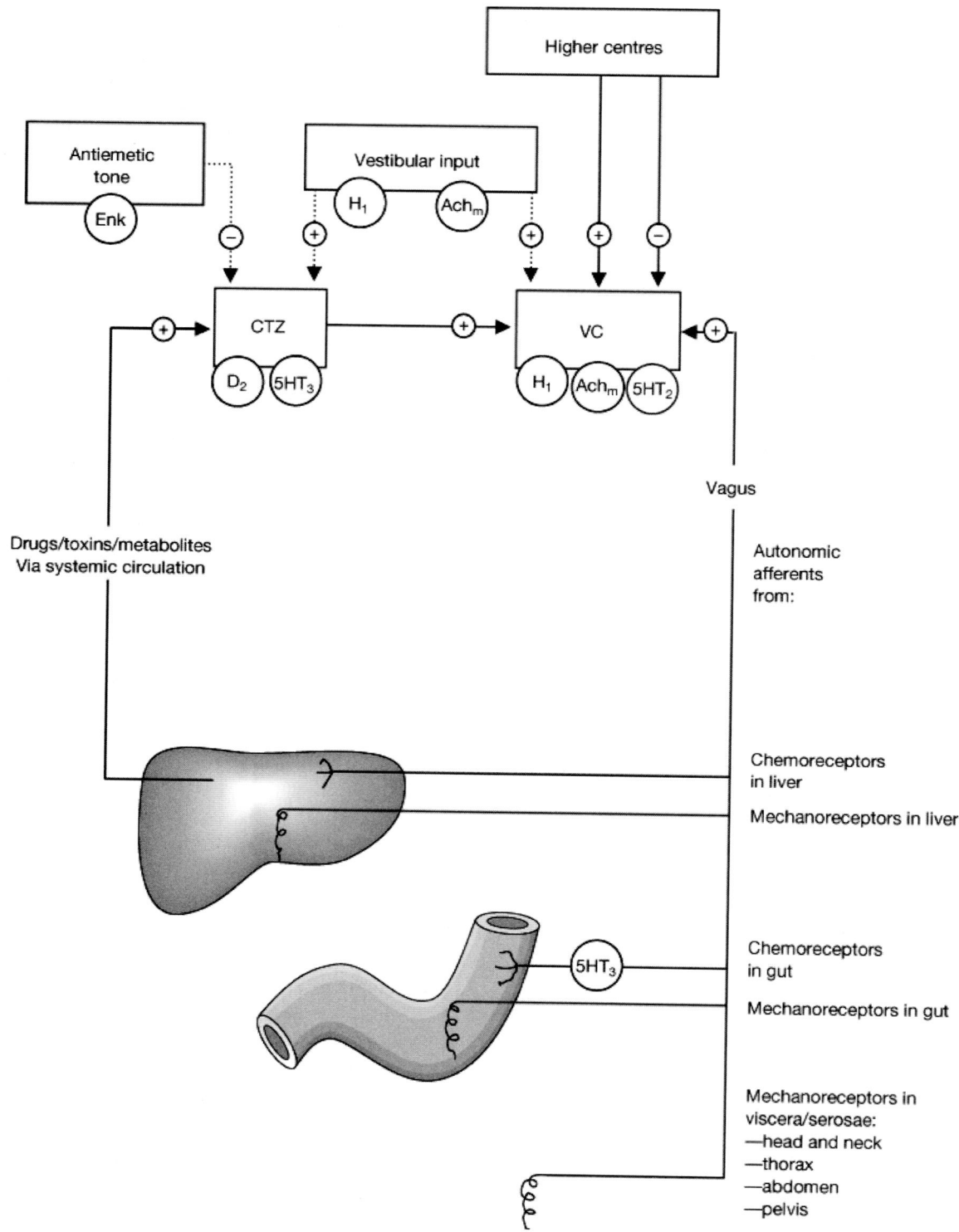

Figure 10.2.1.1 The interrelationship between CTZ, VC, and their afferent inputs. —, established connections; ----, postulated connections; CTZ, chemoreceptor trigger zone; VC, vomiting centre; Enk, enkephalinergic pathways. *Receptors*: D_2, dopamine type 2; $5HT_{2,3}$, serotonin types 2,3; Ach_m, muscarinic cholinergic; H_1, histamine type 1.

trigger vomiting[11]. Nausea in the absence of vomiting may arise from stimuli that excite the VC without sufficient amplification to trigger the vomiting cascade[7,15]. Thus, nausea usually accompanies the prodromal autonomic effects that precede vomiting. However, the degree of nausea cannot be predicted by the accompanying autonomic changes, for example, the relative reduction in gastric contraction[7]. Also, nausea is not always relieved by vomiting: this usually indicates continuing excitation of the central emetogenic pathway.

The VC receives afferents from the cerebral cortex and higher brainstem, thalamus and hypothalamus, the vestibular system, and via the vagus and splanchnic nerves, the pharynx, gastrointestinal tract, and serosae. There is also input from the CTZ, which can only initiate vomiting via the VC (Fig. 10.2.1.1)[7,16,17].

At least 17 potential neurotransmitters or receptors have been identified in the CTZ and nucleus of the tractus solitarius. These include dopamine, serotonin, histamine, opioid, cannabinoid, and neurokinin receptors. The principal receptors at the CTZ are dopamine type 2 (D_2); at the VC the principal receptors are muscarinic cholinergic (Ach_m) and histamine type 1 (H_1). Both sites exhibit serotonin type 3 ($5HT_3$) receptors, and serotonin type 2 ($5HT_2$) receptors appear to be important in the VC[12]. Neurokinin type 1 (NK_1) receptors are widely distributed in the central nervous system, and particularly in those areas of the brainstem involved in emesis[15].

Nausea is reported as a highly distressing symptom; the link between nausea and mood has not yet been explained, but recent research suggests some possibilities. A preliminary report of involvement of the inferior frontal gyrus of the human cerebral cortex in the sensation of nausea is intriguing[18]. This area is association cortex, and such cortical involvement would help to explain the highly aversive nature of nausea. NK_1 receptors, distributed widely in the brain and associated with regulation of mood, are also implicated in emesis. Blockade of NK_1 receptors is associated with both anti-depressant[19] and antiemetic[20,21] activity. Thus, the link between nausea and dysphoria may be biochemical or structural.

Afferent pathways involved in emesis

The interrelationship between CTZ, VC, and their various afferent inputs is summarized in Fig. 10.2.1.1. The major afferent neural pathway from the body to the central structures is the vagus, with additional input via the splanchnic nerves, sympathetic ganglia, and the glossopharyngeal nerve. The vagus itself is stimulated via mechanoreceptors and chemoreceptors in the gastrointestinal tract, serosae, and viscera.[12,17,22,23]

The VC receives descending fibres from higher centres, which may stimulate or inhibit activation of the emetic cascade. Most vagal afferents terminate at the VC, but there is some vagal input to the CTZ.

Projections from the vestibular nuclei, which mediate emesis, are incompletely understood; the CTZ may be involved, although D_2 antagonists are not particularly effective in motion sickness[24]. H_1 and Ach_m antagonists are more effective: they are thought to act on first-order vestibular neurons. Opioids can increase sensitivity of the labyrinth[25].

Choosing an antiemetic

Before prescribing drugs, care should be taken to reduce the stimulus to nausea from the patient's environment. This includes avoidance of cooking smells, attention to unpleasant odours (e.g. from an infected, necrotic tumour), and presentation of small, attractive meals. Cool, fizzy drinks are more palatable than still or hot drinks. Many patients experience a taste change so that previously innocuous foods taste nauseating.

Selection of an appropriate antiemetic strategy involves seven steps, namely:

1 identify the likely cause(s) of nausea and/or vomiting;

2 identify the pathway by which each cause triggers the vomiting reflex (Fig. 10.2.1.1);

3 identify the neurotransmitter receptor involved in the identified pathway;

4 choose the most potent antagonist to the receptor identified—the binding affinity of a particular antagonist predicts its antiemetic efficacy[26,27] (Table 10.2.1.1);

5 choose a route of administration that ensures that the drug reaches its site of action—this often excludes the oral route;

6 titrate the dose carefully, review the patient frequently, give the antiemetic regularly;

7 if symptoms persist, review the likely cause(s): additional treatment may be required for an overlooked cause, or alternative treatment may be suggested by a different cause becoming apparent.

If several different receptors are involved, use of a potent antagonist for each receptor is preferable to use of one drug that weakly antagonizes several receptors.

Antiemetic drugs available

A wide variety of antiemetic drugs is available. Those that have potent, receptor-specific action are summarized in Table 10.2.1.1. The antiemetic efficacy and side effects of a drug can be predicted by its binding affinity for particular receptors[26,27].

Drugs with receptor-specific action

Dopamine (D_2) antagonists

Of the dopamine (D_2) antagonists, haloperidol is the most potent at the CTZ.[26] Metoclopramide and domperidone, whilst having some CTZ anti-dopaminergic activity, act in the gut to antagonize D_2 and stimulate $5HT_4$ receptors. Local acetylcholine release, mediated by the $5HT_4$ receptor, appears to play an important role in reversing gastroparesis and bringing about normal peristalsis in the upper gastrointestinal tract. At high doses, metoclopramide blocks $5HT_3$ receptors in the CTZ and gut; extra-pyramidal side-effects are common and this mode of use has been superseded by development of specific $5HT_3$ antagonists for cancer chemotherapy-induced emesis[28].

Any agent that is prokinetic may induce colic in an obstructed intestine.

Table 10.2.1.1 Receptor-specific antiemetics of use in palliative care.

Drug	Receptor and site (see text)		Indications	Dosage and routes	Side effects	Notes
Butyrephenones Haloperidol	D2	-CTZ	Opioid induced N; chemical/ metabolic N	1.5–5.0 mg/day; PO, SC (occ up 20mg/ day)	Dystonias Dyskinesia Akathisia	Side effects unusual at low doses
Prokinetic agents Metoclopramide	D_2 D_2 5-HT$_4$ (potentiation)	-CTZ -GIT -GIT	Gastric stasis; ileus	10–30mg 2–4 hourly PO, SC, IV	Dystonias Akathisia Oesophagealspasm; Colic in GI obstruction	Prolonged half-life in renal failure
	5-HT$_3$ 5-HT$_3$ (at high doses)	-CTZ -GIT	Chemotherapy	N/A	Frequent at high doses	Superseded by 5HT$_3$ antagonists
Domperidone	D_2 D_2	-CTZ -GIT	Gastric stasis ileus	10–30mg PO 4–8 hrly; 30–90mg PR4–8 hrly	Colic if GIT obstructed; oesophageal pain	Extrapyramidal side effects are rare
Cisapride	5-HT$_4$ (potentiation) Ach	-GIT -GIT	Gastric stasis ileus	0mg PO 6–8 hourly 30mg PR 6–8 hourly	Abdominal cramps; diarrhoea; cardiac arrhythmias particularly with systemic azole antifungals	Prokinetic throughout GIT
Phenothiazines (including Prochlorperazine chlorpromazine, thiethylperazine)	D_2 D_2 H$_1$ Ach α_1 Ad	-CTZ -GIT -VC -CNS -GIT -CVS		Prochlorperazine: 5–20mg PO, 12.5–25mg IM, 25mg PR 6–8 hrly Chlorpromazine: 25–50mg IM 4–6 hourly	Vary according to spectrum of receptor blockade: see text	Not recommended for routine use, but see text
Levomepromazine	5HT$_2$ H$_1$ D$_2$ α_1 Ad	-VC -VC -CTZ -GIT -CVS -CNS	Intestinal obstruction: peritoneal irritation; nausea of unknown aetiology; vestibular causes; raised ICP	5–12.5mg/24 hourly PO, SC	Drowsiness at higher doses	Long half-life: once daily injection may suffice
Antihistamines Cyclizine Cinnarizine Diphenylhydramine Promethazine	H$_1$	-VC -vestibular afferents -brain substance		Cyclizine: 25–50mg 8 hrly PO/SC/PR Only cyclizine is tolerated by SC injection	Dry mouth; blurred vision (rare); sedation Cyclizine: skin irritation at SC injection sites in some patients	Cyclizine is least sedative therefore the drug of choice
Diphenylhydramine Promethazine	Ach$_m$	-VC				
Anticholinergics Hyoscine (scopolamine) Hydrobromide	Ach$_m$	-VC -GIT	Intestinal obstruction; peritoneal irritation; raised ICP; excess secretions	200–400mcg 4–8 hourly subling/SC 500–1500mcg/72h transdermal patches	Dry mouth; ileus urinary retention; blurred vision; occasionally agitation	Useful if N & V coexist with colic

(continued)

Table 10.2.1.1 (Continued) Receptor-specific antiemetics of use in palliative care.

Drug	Receptor and site (see text)		Indications	Dosage and routes	Side effects	Notes
5-HT₃ antagonists Granisetron Ondansetron Tropisetron	5-HT₃	-GIT -CTZ -(VC)	Chemotherapy; abdominal radiotherapy; postoperative nausea and vomiting	Granisetron: 3mg slowly IV up to 8 hourly; Odansetron: 8mg PO or slowly IV 8 hourly; Tropisetron: 5mg PO or slowly IV daily	Headache in 30%; constipation; diarrhoea	Effectiveness increased by combination with dexamethasone
NK₁ antagonist Aprepitant	NK₁	Widespread	Late onset chemotherapy-related N&V	125mg 1 hour prior to chemotherapy; then 80mg od for the next 2 days		Only available PO

CTZ = chemoreceptor trigger zone; VC = vomiting centre; GIT = gastrointestinal tract; ICP = intracranial pressure; N = nausea v = vomiting; PO = by mouth; PR = by rectum; SC = by subcutaneous injection; IV = by intravenous injection; IM = by intramuscular injection; occ = occasionally; OD = once daily.

Phenothiazines

The phenothiazines are less potent D_2 antagonists. They have varying antagonist activity at other receptors which predicts their side effects (e.g. chlorpromazine—α_1 adrenergic receptor—may cause hypotension and sedation; diphenhydramine, a phenothiazine antihistamine—Ach_m receptor—may cause sedation and dry mouth). Extra-pyramidal reactions occur with all of the D_2 antagonists, although the incidence with domperidone is extremely low[27]. Levomepromazine blocks a wide spectrum of receptors at higher doses; it is highly sedative and causes hypotension but it is a useful antiemetic at lower doses (5–12.5 mg per 24 h by mouth or subcutaneous infusion). Circumstantial evidence suggests that $5HT_2$ blockade may mediate levomepromazine antiemetic activity[29]. The binding affinity of low-dose levomepromazine for the $5HT_2$ receptor suggests that it is likely to be an effective antiemetic at the VC; its lower affinity for D_2 receptors may nevertheless make it a broad-spectrum antiemetic. Comparative clinical trials are awaited.

Antihistamines and anticholinergics

The antihistamines act on H_1 receptors in the VC and on vestibular afferents[24,25]. Only cyclizine is suitable for subcutaneous injection. Cyclizine is less sedating than the anticholinergic hyoscine (scopolamine) hydrobromide, which blocks Ach_m receptors in the VC and peripherally[24,27]. Hyoscine hydrobromide can be given sublingually, subcutaneously, and transdermally. Its side effects are those of parasympathetic blockade, which may be beneficial (drying of secretions, reduction of colic) or troublesome (dry mouth, ileus, urinary retention, blurred vision). Drowsiness is not uncommon.

Hyoscine butylbromide does not have central antiemetic action. In the gut, however, its anticholinergic properties reduce peristalsis and inhibit exocrine secretions, thus contributing to the palliation of colic and nausea in intestinal obstruction.[30] Glyopyrrolate, a powerful peripheral anticholinergic drug with similar potency to atropine but little penetration into the central nervous system, may be used as an alternative to hyoscine butylbromide.

5HT₃ receptor antagonists

The discovery of selective $5HT_3$ receptor antagonists caused a revolution in antiemetic prescribing in oncology and a massive drive for the perfect antidote to chemotherapy-induced emesis. The initial early promise of this class of drugs in the 1980s has proved successful for acute-onset emesis in chemotherapy, although later-onset nausea remains a problem[13,22,28,31–35] which may be amenable to NK1 receptor blockade (see below).

Although extremely effective for cancer chemotherapy-induced radiotherapy-induced emesis, no place has been demonstrated for $5HT_3$ antagonists in the management of nausea and vomiting from other causes. They do not reverse nausea mediated by dopamine pathways (e.g. opioid induced) and they remain largely untested in the nausea and vomiting syndromes associated with advanced cancer and AIDS. Some role in postoperative emesis is claimed for them and ondansetron is licensed in the United Kingdom for this indication. Benefit is probably only to be expected in 25 per cent of patients, and is no greater than with droperidol or metoclopramide[37].

$5HT_3$ receptors have been demonstrated in the CTZ and VC centrally, and on terminals of vagal afferents in the gut peripherally. The bulk of human serotonin is located within enterochromaffin cells in the gut wall; this serotonin is released and metabolized locally in response to various insults including direct abdominal irradiation and highly emetogenic chemotherapy[9,17,38,39]. Release appears to be by active secretion, although it is not blocked by octreotide[9]. The emetogenic action of serotonin derived from enterochromaffin cells appears to be by direct stimulation of local vagal $5HT_3$ receptors: high abdominal vagotomy abolishes emesis induced by abdominal irradiation, and blood serotonin levels are rarely raised during emesis, although raised urinary levels of the serotonin metabolite 5-hydroxindole acetic acid reflect the timing and severity of emesis after chemotherapy[22,38]. $5HT_3$ antagonists block vagal afferent activity. A reflex increase in vagal efferent activity may be caused, and this has been shown to give rise to temporary (and inconsequential) bradyarrhythmias in patients receiving repeated doses of these drugs, although not in healthy volunteers[40,41].

Several 5HT$_3$ antagonists are currently available (see Table 10.2.1.1). Of these, dolasetron and its major metabolite, and granisetron are the most specific 5HT$_3$ receptor antagonists, ondansetron and tropisetron both showing some affinity for other receptors including α-adrenergic, other 5HT and opioid μ receptors. In clinical trials that have compared granisetron, ondansetron, and tropisetron, there appears to be little to choose between them, although patients who expressed a preference consistently preferred granisetron. All are licensed for use in children, and adverse effects are few. Evidence-based antiemetic guidelines issued by the American Society of Clinical Oncology make no distinction between the different agents available, suggesting that cost should dictate local practice. They also recommend the use of cheaper oral preparations rather than intravenous treatment as first line[28].

NK1 receptor antagonists

These drugs show great promise in control of late emesis from chemotherapy[34–36], and elegant analysis of the timing of their effect demonstrates differential stimulation of 5HT$_3$ receptors during the first 8 h following emetogenic chemotherapy, followed by onset of stimulation of NK$_1$ receptors and loss of response to 5HT$_3$ antagonists[42]. The first commercial NK$_1$ receptor antagonist antiemetic is available as an oral preparation; its role in palliative care settings is yet to be explored. There is also a suggestion of benefit for postoperative nausea and vomiting[43]. NK$_1$ receptor antagonists appear to have a broad spectrum of action for diverse causes of emesis in animals, but similar studies have not been undertaken in man.

Other antiemetic drugs

Corticosteroids

Corticosteroids are known to possess intrinsic antiemetic properties and to enhance the effect of other antiemetics[28,44]. Their mechanism of action is unclear and may be multiple. Corticosteroids may enhance antiemetic tone in the medulla by:

- reducing the permeability of the blood–brain barrier to chemicals that antagonize medullary antiemetic tone, such as chemotherapy agents;

- depleting the inhibitory amine γ-aminobutyric acid (GABA) in medullary antiemetic neurons;

- reducing leu-enkephalin release in the brainstem[13].

In addition, the anti-inflammatory effects of corticosteroids can reduce tumour mass, thereby reducing the stimulus to emesis from peripheral autonomic stretch receptors or from intracranial tumours.

Cannabinoids

Anecdotal reports of a lower incidence of chemotherapy-induced emesis amongst marijuana smokers led to clinical trials of cannabinoids. Synthetic cannabinoids with and without psychotropic effects are antiemetic, although cannabis may be more effective than its synthetic analogues[45].

The identification of a brain-stem cannabinoid receptor suggests a site of action of these compounds[46]; cerebral ligands for this receptor are arachidonic congeners, dubbed anandamides[47]. However, some antiemetic effects of synthetic cannabinoids are reversed by naloxone, raising the possibility that some of their mechanism of action is via opioid μ receptors[13].

The use of the currently licensed cannabinoids is limited by psychotomometic side effects, particularly dysphoria in the elderly. This effect can be reduced by low-dose phenothiazines but the resulting drowsiness may undermine any therapeutic advantage of the cannabinoids[48]. Euphoria is more common than dysphoria in younger patients, and there are reports of the successful use of nabilone for intractable nausea in AIDS patients, who tend to be younger than adults with cancer, and in children receiving chemotherapy[49–51]. Larger studies are needed to assess the value of cannabinoids for emesis in advanced disease.

Benzodiazepines

Benzodiazepines have been used in chemotherapy antiemetic combinations. Although they have little antiemetic activity per se, in drug combinations they reduce anxiety and akathisia, and reduce the likelihood of anticipatory nausea. These drugs are sedative and sometimes amnesic when used in effective doses, which limits their usefulness for patients with chronic nausea[52,53].

Octreotide

Octreotide is a long-acting somatostatin analogue that exerts wide-ranging potent inhibition of endocrine and exocrine secretions and promotes reabsorption of electrolytes in the gut; there is clinical evidence of both inhibition and restoration of normal gastrointestinal transit[54,55]. Its combination of effects can be useful in palliating emesis caused by intestinal obstruction: inhibition of exocrine secretion in the gut reduces distension, thus diminishing the stimulus to nausea and to colic[56–58]. Subcutaneous infusion is useful during titration to establish the effective dose; for patients with a longer prognosis, a long-acting depot injection may be an alternative.

Propofol

Propofol, an intravenous anaesthetic agent, has been noted to protect against postoperative emesis[59,60]. Recent work shows that subhypnotic doses of propofol have antiemetic action in post-anaesthetic and chemotherapy-induced emesis[61–63]. The duration of antiemetic action of an intravenous low-dose bolus outlasts the very short duration of hypnosis that would be introduced by a far larger dose, suggesting that hypnosis or anxiolysis are not the mechanisms of antiemetic action. Propofol has a widespread central nervous system depressant effect and it is possible that its antiemetic action is at a subcortical level, in either the CTZ or within the VC complex. The observation that propofol is less successful as an antiemetic following vagal-stimulating abdominal surgery suggests that its site of action may be the CTZ.

Opioids

Opioids can induce or block emesis in experimental models; both actions can be antagonized by naloxone. It has been proposed that δ and/or κ opioid receptors are emetogenic, whilst μ receptors are antiemetic. Experimentally, intravenous fentanyl in subanaesthetic doses abolishes emesis due to morphine, cisplatin, and copper sulphate, an effect which is reversed by naloxone[64]. In clinical practice, the nauseating properties of the opioids are well known: it remains to be seen whether more μ-specific drugs can be developed, and whether these may have any role as antiemetics.

Non-drug measures of palliation of nausea and vomiting

Psychological techniques

Most of the authoritative research on psychological techniques for palliation of emesis has been conducted amongst chemotherapy patients, which is not analogous to the situation of nauseated patients with disease which is not amenable to chemotherapy. However, these studies have shown that patients can learn techniques such as progressive muscle relaxation and guided mental imagery, and use these during the stress of chemotherapy with good effect[65–67]. Cognitive therapy has been used to help relieve the psychological morbidity arising from physical symptoms in advanced cancer[68]. The possibility of adapting such techniques for the needs of nauseated patients with advanced diseases warrants further exploration (see Chapter 10.1.13).

Transcutaneous electrical nerve stimulation (see Chapter 10.1.11)

Transcutaneous electrical nerve stimulation (TENS) has been shown to enhance the effect of antiemetic drugs: the TENS effect is blocked by naloxone, suggesting that it is mediated by endogenous opioid peptides[69].

Acupuncture and acupressure (see Chapter 10.1.12)

Acupuncture and acupressure have been shown to augment the effect of antiemetics during chemotherapy, and to reduce postoperative nausea and vomiting. The benefit of acupuncture is lost if administered under general anaesthetic[70]. Acupressure prolongs the effect of acupuncture, and the use of TENS in place of traditional acupuncture needles at the P6 acupuncture point is a practical technique for self-use by patients, being only slightly less effective than the use of traditional needles[71,72]. The P6 (Neiguan) acupuncture point is located in the midline of the palmar aspect of each wrist, approximately 3 cm from the palmar crease.

Clinical syndromes associated with nausea and vomiting

Table 10.2.1.2 summarizes some common or important causes of nausea and vomiting in palliative care patients. They are grouped according to the pathway that mediates emesis, and are similarly grouped in the following discussion.

It must be emphasized, however, that in advanced disease nausea and vomiting may have more than one cause, stimulating symptoms via more than one pathway. Sometimes, apparently appropriate treatment fails to relieve symptoms, necessitating a search for additional and less obvious causes. Sometimes, a cause cannot be identified: into this category are likely to fall those with cancer-associated autonomic failure. Growth factors and other tumour products may be emetogenic; their actions are still only partly understood, but it is likely that such factors would act via the CTZ.

Tumours arising outside the areas described in the table may generate emesis via the same pathways, for example, head and neck tumours cause pressure effects which trigger autonomic relays to the VC. The key to good management of nausea and vomiting is a high index of suspicion, an understanding of the pathways involved, and the setting of realistic goals.

Chemical causes of emesis

Drug-induced nausea may arise by chemical action at the CTZ, by serotonin release in the gut, through gastrointestinal irritation or gastric stasis, or a combination of these (Table 10.2.1.3).

Transient nausea mediated by the CTZ accompanies the introduction or increase of morphine in about one-third of patients;[73] these patients will benefit from haloperidol, a central D_2 antagonist, during this period. In the United Kingdom and New Zealand, haloperidol is used with good effect; in Northern America metoclopramide is often used as an alternative although it has weaker central anti-D_2 activity. The appearance of nausea with other opioid toxicity manifestations (small pupils, drowsiness, myoclonic jerks) in a patient taking morphine who was previously tolerant of the same dose of morphine may herald the onset of renal insufficiency: the opioid should be reduced in dose and/or frequency. An alternative opioid may be prescribed, at equinalgesic dose, provided it does not rely on renal excretion of active metabolites (Chapter 10.1.6). A proportion of patients experience opioid-induced gastric stasis. Tolerance to this does not develop; a prokinetic agent is required, sometimes in high doses, if change to a different opioid is ineffective or not possible.

Cytotoxic-induced nausea is mediated by the CTZ and by $5HT_3$ receptors on vagal gut afferents. Selective blockade of $5HT_3$ receptors in the gut is highly effective for immediate-onset emesis;[27] these drugs may also act as the CTZ. Adding antiemetics that work at other sites enhances the effectiveness of treatment, particularly for delayed-onset emesis. Combinations of $5HT_3$ antagonist with a corticosteroid and/or benzodiazepine have been particularly effective, with 65–89 per cent complete control of symptoms in patients receiving cisplatin[28,32]. Addition of an NK1 receptor antagonist to granisetron plus dexamethasone significantly reduced cisplatin induced emesis over a 5-day observation period[42].

Metabolic causes of nausea include organ failure and hypercalcaemia, which may progress insidiously. Nausea can be controlled using a central D_2 blocker: higher doses of haloperidol may be required (5–20 mg daily) with a consequently higher incidence of extrapyramidal side effects. These respond to antimuscarinic drugs such as procyclidine and benztropine, which may be given by slow intravenous injection for relief of acute dystonias.

Gastrointestinal causes of emesis

Pharyngeal irritation may cause retching, nausea, or cough-induced vomiting. The oropharynx is richly innervated by the glossopharyngeal nerve and vagus, and is highly sensitive to touch. Tenacious sputum or candida overlying the pharyngeal mucosa can stimulate the VC via these afferents; AIDS patients may also have mucosal lesions of cytomegalovirus or herpes simplex. Appropriate antimicrobial therapy is indicated for infections of mouth, pharynx, oesophagus, or respiratory tract. Sticky sputum may be loosened by inhalations, and irritating nocturnal cough causing retching and disturbed sleep may be palliated by application of local anaesthetic

Table 10.2.1.2 Common syndromes involving nausea and vomiting in patients requiring palliative care.

Syndrome	Causes	Key features	Pathway and receptors	Treatment possibilities
Chemically induced nausea	◆ Drugs: opioids, digoxin, anticonvulsants, antibiotics, cytotoxics ◆ Toxins: food poisoning, ischaemic bowel, e.g. gut obstruction, ? tumour products ◆ Metabolic: organ failure, hypercalcaemia, ketoacidosis	Of drug toxicity or of underlying disease, plus constant nausea, variable vomiting	Chemical action stimulates D_2 ($\pm 5HT_3$) in CTZ Chemotherapy → serotonin release in GI tract → $5\text{-}HT_3$ receptors on vagus Chemotherapy → NK_1 receptor activation in brain	◆ Stop or reduce the offending drug ◆ Treat the underlying cause ◆ Haloperidol ◆ $5HT_3$ antagonists for chemotherapy or direct abdominal irradiation ◆ NK_1 antagonist for delayed emesis with chemotherapy
Gastric stasis	◆ Anticholinergic drugs, opioids ◆ Ascites ◆ Hepatomegaly ◆ Peptic ulcer ◆ Gastritis 　• Stress 　• Drugs 　• Radiotherapy ◆ Autonomic failure	Epigastric pain, fullness, nausea, early satiety, flatulence, acid reflux, hiccup, large volume vomits, (possibly projectile) gastric regurgitation, other features of autonomic failure	Gastric mecho-receptors ↓ Vagal afferents ↓ VC H1; Achm	◆ Treat the underlying causes ◆ Prokinetic agents ◆ Reduce gastric secretions: 　• H_2 blocker 　• Omeprazole 　• Octreotide ◆ Aid eructation: dimeticone
Stretch/distortion of GI tract	◆ Constipation ◆ Intestinal obstruction ◆ Mesenteric metastases	Altered bowel habit, nausea, vomiting, may be faeculent, colic	Gut/serosal Mechanoreceptors ↓ Vagal afferents ↓ VC	◆ Treat underlying cause ◆ Active bowel management ◆ Corticosteroids may reduce the size of tumour mass
Serosal stretch/irritation	e.g.: ◆ Liver metastases ◆ Ureteric obstruction ◆ Retroperitoneal cancer	Of underlying condition, nausea, occasional vomiting	H_1; Ach_m	◆ Cyclizine ◆ Hyoscine hydrobromide if bowel paralysis is acceptable
Irritation of GI tract	◆ e.g. cryptospordiosis	Profuse diarrhoea, nausea, occasional vomiting.		
Raised intracranial pressure/meningism	◆ Cerebral oedema ◆ Intracranial tumour ◆ Intracranial bleeding ◆ Meningeal infiltration by tumour ◆ Skull metastases ◆ Cerebral infections (AIDS)	Headache, (diurnal); papilloedema, photophobia may be absent. Nausea may be diurnal; neurological signs may be absent	May be direct stimulation of cerebral H_1 Meningeal mechanoreceptors ↓ VC H_1; Ach_m	◆ Treat underlying cause ◆ High-dose corticosteroids may reduce cerebral oedema/mass size ◆ Cyclizine ◆ Levomepromazine
Movement-associated emesis	◆ Opioids (more common in ambulant patients) ◆ Gut distortion ◆ Gastroparesis → passive regurgitation	Nausea and/or sudden vomits on movement/turning in bed	Opioid-induced sensitivity of vestibular afferents H_1; Ach_m Gut mechanoreceptors ↓ vagal afferents ↓ VC H_1;Ach_m	◆ Treat the underlying cause ◆ Nasogastric aspiration in terminal gastroparesis ◆ Cyclizine ◆ Cinnarizine ◆ Hyoscine hydrobromide

(continued)

Table 10.2.1.2 (Continued) Common syndromes involving nausea and vomiting in patients requiring palliative care.

Syndrome	Causes	Key features	Pathway and receptors	Treatment possibilities
Anxiety-induced emesis	◆ Anxiety 　• About self 　• About others 　• About disease 　• About symptoms ◆ Anticipatory emesis 　with cytotoxics	'Waves' of nausea, ± vomiting, reminders trigger nausea; may be relieved by distraction	Cortex ↓ VC H_1; Ach_m	◆ Address the anxiety ◆ Psychological techniques ◆ Relaxation ◆ Benzodiazepines may 　be useful

D2 = dopamine type 2 receptor; 5-HT3 = serotonin type 3 receptor; H1 – histamine type 1 receptor; Achm – muscarinic cholinergic receptor; CTZ = chemoreceptor trigger zone; VC = vomiting centre; GI = gastrointestinal.

spray to the pharynx (with appropriate caution about eating and drinking for the next few hours).

Delayed gastric emptying may arise from physiological abnormalities or mechanical resistance to emptying. Mechanical resistance includes ascites, hepatomegaly, prepyloric inflammation, duodenal ulceration or tumour, and pancreatic cancer. Resistance may be partial or there may be complete obstruction. Physiological abnormalities include anticholinergic effects of drugs (Table 10.2.1.3), and autonomic failure. The symptoms are listed in Table 10.2.1.2; they may not all occur and the diagnosis can easily be missed.

Complete gastric outlet obstruction is managed as high intestinal obstruction (see Chapter 10.2.4). Other causes of delayed emptying are managed by attention to:

◆ *Anxiety:* listening to concerns, explanation of cause of vomiting and plan of treatment.

◆ *Optimizing gastric emptying:* the prokinetic agents metoclopramide and domperidone normalize the rate of gastric and upper intestinal peristalsis, increase lower oesophageal tone (thus reducing reflux), and relax the pylorus; gastric and upper intestinal transit time is shortened. The prokinetic agent cisapride increases the rate of peristalsis throughout the gastrointestinal tract. It was withdrawn in the United Kingdom because of concerns about cardiotoxicity, but remains available on a named-patient basis.

◆ *Reducing stimulus to gastric stretch:* reduction in volume of meals and drinks and inhibition of gastric secretion using H_2 blockers, proton-pump inhibitors, or octreotide will reduce gastric stretch,

Table 10.2.1.3 Causes of drug-induced nausea.

Mechanism	Drugs	
Activation of chemo-receptor trigger zone	Opioids Digoxin Anticoagulants	Cytotoxics Imidazoles Antibiotics
Gastrointestinal irritation	Non-steroidal anti-inflammatory drugs Iron supplements	Antibiotics Cytotoxics
Gastric stasis	Tricyclics Phenothiazines	Opioids Anticholinergics

thus reducing both the diaphragmatic irritation which gives rise to hiccup and the vagal stimulation which gives rise to nausea and pain.

Two adverse effects of the prokinetic agents are noteworthy. In a partially obstructed intestine, prokinetic agents may induce colic. Gastric colic may have a long periodicity mimicking ulcer or tumour-related pain. Action of prokinetic agents in the lower oesophagus may provoke oesophageal spasm; typically, this is retrosternal and may mimic angina pectoris. Oesophageal spasm may be relieved by sublingual glyceral trinitrate (which may give rise to further suspicions of cardiac pain).

Stretch and distortion of the gastrointestinal tract activates mechanoreceptors in the bowel wall; similar receptors are present in visceral capsules and in parietal serosal surfaces. Their afferent input is to the VC via the vagus and splanchnic nerves. Mechanoreceptors may be triggered by tumour distorting an organ, stretching or directly invading serosa or mesentry, or by increased transmural pressure in a hollow viscus proximal to a site of obstruction, for example, ureter or colon. This is, therefore, a common complication of advanced intra-abdominal, retroperitoneal, or pelvic malignancy. Local inflammation may potentiate afferent nerve receptors in the gastrointestinal tract, mediating emesis in bowel infections such as cryptosporidiosis in AIDS patients.

If reversal of the cause of emesis is not possible, nausea may be palliated by using antiemetics active at the VC. Control of vomiting may be more difficult to achieve with obstruction in the gastrointestinal tract: this is discussed in more detail in Chapter 10.2.4.

Constipation with resultant colonic stretch is assumed to be a common cause of nausea and anorexia in advanced disease, although there are no studies to prove this. Management is of the constipation, although antiemetics acting at the VC may help to reduce the nausea. Anticholinergic agents should be avoided as they will exacerbate the constipation.

Cranial causes of emesis

Raised intracranial pressure may present with nausea and vomiting before headache is apparent. Meningeal irritation can also trigger emesis. Clinical associations are with intracerebral tumours (primary and secondary), bone metastases to skull (base of skull metastases may give rise to cranial nerve symptoms and signs), intracranial bleeding, and cerebral oedema. High-dose corticosteroids are the treatment of choice; an antiemetic acting at the VC may be necessary in addition. Palliative radiotherapy, chemotherapy or surgery should be considered.

Other causes of emesis

Movement-associated emesis may be triggered by distorted or distended viscera exerting increased traction upon their mesentery during movement. Movement-associated nausea may also occur as a side effect of opioids, related to increased vestibular sensitivity. Centrally-mediated emesis must be distinguished from passive regurgitation of gastric contents during movements of a terminally ill patient, which is usually related to gastroparesis; temporary passage of a nasogastric tube to aspirate the stomach dry of fluid and gas may be necessary to relieve this symptom.

Anxiety-induced emesis is a common experience in health. The patient with advanced disease may be able to identify anxiety as the trigger to nausea, or carers may notice an association between symptoms and stressful situations or conversations. Other causes of emesis must be excluded as far as possible before attributing nausea and vomiting to anxiety. Treatment is by identifying anxiety as a trigger and then working collaboratively with the patient to increase relaxation, identify and manage anxiety-provoking thoughts, and establishing workable coping strategies[66,68]. Benzodiazepines may be useful as short-term adjuvants: it is preferable to select a benzodiazepine with a longer half-life given as a single, evening dose (e.g. diazepam) to prevent as required use of anxiolytics, which is unlikely to be helpful. Some patients benefit from tricyclic antidepressants with secondary anxiolytic properties, for example, amitriptyline. All these drugs reduce a patient's ability to concentrate and can therefore reduce a patient's ability to learn or practise psychotherapeutic techniques[65].

Anticipatory emesis is a conditioned response in some patients who have suffered nausea and/or vomiting provoked by cytotoxic drugs. Any reminder of their previous experience may trigger emesis, including television pictures of hospitals, hospital smells, or visits by hospital personnel. It can be refractory to treatment and is best avoided by control of emesis from the first cycle of chemotherapy. Management is as for anxiety-induced emesis. Systematic desensitization has also been used successfully in these patients[65,66].

Intractable nausea

As with pain, the pathways of emesis are probably incompletely documented. Identification of triggers and administration of receptor-specific antiemetics was successful in 93 per cent of patients in a well-conducted study[22], but a minority remain for whom nausea continues unabated. There are few published data about these patients. Amongst cachexic patients with chronic nausea, Bruera's group have identified a high incidence of autonomic failure[74].

Appropriate goal-setting is important. It is unwise to expect or to promise total relief of nausea and vomiting. Most patients will be content with major relief of nausea, even if intermittent vomiting continues, provided they have been led to expect this as a possible outcome. It may be helpful to grade emesis or to use a tool to measure change, in order to assess response to treatment. Patients' perceptions are different from those of nurses observing them, and there is a need for an agreed tool for measurement of nausea and vomiting[75,76].

When apparently appropriate measures have failed to relieve symptoms, and combinations of antiemetics directed at different receptors have proved ineffective, empirical use of levomepromazine may offer relief to some patients. Good clinical trials of therapy for such patients are necessary.

Future developments

Progress has been made in the recognition of nausea as an important symptom that must be evaluated separately from vomiting. This has improved the quality of the data emerging from chemotherapy-related emesis and postoperative nausea and vomiting studies. The development of tools for self-evaluation of symptoms by patients, and the identification of biological markers for emesis, would enhance the evaluation of antiemetic strategies. A comprehensive review of available tools for rating nausea and vomiting in palliative care concluded that an ideal measurement tool for the assessment of nausea, vomiting and retching has not yet been developed[77]. However, the authors point out a variety of tools that may be reliable measures of change in a single symptom in a palliative care population.

Good, controlled trials of therapy are still awaited, including further outcome studies of receptor-based prescribing to expand earlier work.

The potential for the development of broad spectrum antiemetics is intriguing, particularly levomepromazine and the NK_1 receptor antagonists. Multicentre studies will be necessary to produce sufficient numbers of patients for robust studies of clinical outcomes in a palliative care population.

References

1. Dunlop, G.M. (1989). A study of the relative frequency and importance of gastrointestinal symptoms, and weakness in patients with far advanced cancer. *Palliative Medicine*, **4**, 37–43.

2. Meuser, T. *et al.* (2001). Symptoms during cancer pain treatment following WHO guidelines: a longitudinal follow-up study of symptom prevalence, severity and etiology. *Pain*, **93**, 247–57.

3. Bliss, J.M., Robertson, B., and Selby, P.J. (1992). The impact of nausea and vomiting upon quality of life measures. *British Journal of Cancer*, **66**, S14–23.

4. Coates, A. *et al.* (1983). On the receiving end—patient perception of the side-effects of cancer chemotherapy. *European Journal of Cancer*, **19**, 203–8.

5. Grond, S., Zech, D., Diefenbach, C. *et al.* (1994). Prevalence and pattern of symptoms in patients with cancer pain: a prospective evaluation of 1635 cancer patients referred to a pain clinic. *Journal of Pain and Symptom Management*, **9**, 372–82.

6. Fainsinger, R., Miller, M., Bruera, E. *et al.* (1991). Symptom control during the last week of life on a palliative care unit. *Journal of Palliative Care*, **7**, 5–11.

7. Borison, H.L. and Wang, S.C. (1953). Physiology and pharmacology of vomiting. *Pharmacological Reviews*, **5**, 192–230.

8. Wang, S.C. (1965). Emetic and antiemetic drugs. In *Physiological pharmacology: a comprehensive treatise* (eds. W.S. Root and F.G. Hofman), Vol. II, pp. 255–328. New York: Academic Press.

9. Cubeddu, L.X., Hoffman, I.S., Fuenmayor, N.T. *et al.* (1992). Changes in serotonin metabolism in cancer patients: its relationship to nausea and vomiting induced by chemotherapeutic drugs. *British Journal of Cancer*, **66**, 198–203.

10. Costello, D.J. and Borison, H.L. (1972). Naloxone antagonises narcotic self-blockade of emesis in the cat. *Journal of Pharmacology and Experimental Therapeutics*, **203**, 222–30.

11. Davis, C.J., Harding, R.K., Leslie, R.A. *et al.* (1986). The organisation of vomiting as a protective reflex. In *Nausea and vomiting: mechanisms and treatment* (eds. C.J. Davis, G.V. Lake-Bakaar, and D.G. Grahame-Smith), pp. 65–75. Berlin: Springer-Verlag.

12. Lang, I.M. (1999). Noxious stimulation of emesis. *Digestive Diseases and Sciences*, **44** (Suppl), 58S–63S.

13. Harris, A.L. and Cantwell, B.M.J. (1986). Mechanisms and treatment of cytotoxic-induced nausea and vomiting. In *nausea and vomiting: mechanisms and treatment* (eds. C.J. Davis, G.V. Lake-Bakaar, and D.G. Grahame-Smith), pp. 78–93. Berlin: Springer-Verlag.

14. Harris, A.L. (1982). Cytotoxic therapy-induced vomiting is mediated via enkephalin pathways. *Lancet*, **i**, 714–16.

15. Edwards, C.M. (1988). Chemotherapy induced emesis—mechanisms and treatment. A review. *Journal of the Royal Society of Medicine*, **81**, 658–62.

16. Lichter, I. (1993). Which antiemetic? *Journal of Palliative Care*, **9**, 42–50.

17. Willems, J.L. and Lefebvre, R.A. (1986). Peripheral nervous pathways involved in nausea and vomiting. In *Nausea and vomiting: mechanisms and treatment* (eds. C.J. Davis, G.V. Lake-Bakaar, and D.G. Grahame-Smith), pp. 56–64. Berlin: Springer-Verlag.

18. Miller, A.D., Rowley, H.A., Roberts, T.P.L. *et al.* (1996). Human cortical activity during vestibular and drug-induced nausea detected using M.S.I. In *New directions in vestibular research* (eds. S.M. Highstein, B. Cohen, and J.A. Büttner-Ennever), pp. 670–2. Ann NY Acad Ser 781.

19. Kramer, M.S. *et al.* (1998). District mechanism for antidepressant activity by blockade of central substance P receptors. *Science*, **281**, 1640–5.

20. Navari, R., M. (2004). Role of neurokinin-1 receptor antagonists in chemotherapy-induced emesis: summary of clinical trials. *Cancer Investigation*, **22**, 569–76.

21. Gobbi, G. and Blier, P. (2005). Effect of neurokinin-1 receptor antagonists on serotoninergic, noradrenergic and hippocampal neurons: Comparison with antidepressant drugs. *Peptides*, **26**, 1383–93.

22. Lichter, I. (1993). Results of antiemetic management in terminal illness. *Journal of Palliative Care*, **9**, 19–21.

23. Andrews, P.L.R., Davis, C.J., Bingham, S. *et al.* (1990). The abdominal visceral innervation and the emetic reflex: pathways, pharmacology and plasticity. *Canadian Journal of Physiology and Pharmacology*, **68**, 325.

24. Stott, J.R.R. (1986). Mechanisms and treatment of motion illness. In *Nausea and vomiting: mechanisms and treatment* (eds. C.J. Davis, G.V. Lake-Bakaar, and D.G. Grahame-Smith), Berlin: Springer-Verlag.

25. Gutner, L.B., Gould, W.J., and Batterman, R.C. (1952). The effects of potent analgesics upon vestibular function. *Journal of Clinical Investigation*, **31**, 259–66.

26. Peroutka, S.J. and Snyder, S.H. (1982). Antiemetics: neurotransmitter binding predicts therapeutic actions. *Lancet* **ii**, 658–9.

27. Ison, P.J. and Peroutka, S.J. (1986). Neurotransmitter receptor binding studies predict antiemetic efficacy and side effects. *Cancer Treatment Reports*, **70**, 637–41.

28. Kris, M.G. *et al.* (2007) American Society of Clinical Oncology guideline for antiemeticsin oncology: update 2006 *Journal of Clinical Oncology*, **24**, 1–16

29. Twycross, R., Barkby, G.D., and Hallwood, P.M. (1997). The use of low dose levomepromazine (methotrimeprazine) in the management of nausea and vomiting. *Progress in Palliative Care*, **5**, 49–53.

30. DeConno, F., Caraceni, A., Zecca, E. *et al.* (1992). Continuous subcutaneous infusion of hyoscine butylbromide reduces secretions in patients with gastrointestinal obstruction. *Journal of Pain and Symptom Management*, **6**, 484–6.

31. Roberts, J.J. and Priestman, T.H. (1993). A review of ondansetron in the management of radiotherapy-induced emesis. *Oncology*, **50**, 173–9.

32. Yarker, Y.E. and McTavish, D. (1994). Granisetron: an update of its therapeutic use in nausea and vomiting induced by antineoplastic therapy. *Drugs*, **48**, 761–93.

33. Gardner, C.J. *et al.* (1995). The broad-spectrum anti-emetic activity of the novel non-peptide tachykinin NK$_1$ receptor antagonist GR 203040. *British Journal of Pharmacology*, **116**, 3158–63.

34. Navari, R.M. *et al.* (1999). Reduction of cisplatin-induced emesis by a selective neurokinin 1 receptor antagonist. L-754,030 Antiemetic Trials Group. *New England Journal of Medicine*, **340**, 190–5.

35. Rizk, A.N. and Hesketh, P.J. (1999). Antiemetics for cancer chemotherapy-induced nausea and vomiting. A review of agents in development. *Drugs in Research and Development*, **2**, 229–35.

36. Hesketh, P.J. *et al.* (1999). Randomised phase II study of the Neurokinin 1 receptor antagonist CJ-11, 974 in the control of cisplatin induced emesis. *Journal of Clinical Oncology*, **17**, 338–43.

37. Tramer, M.R., Moore, R.S., Reynolds, D.J.M. *et al.* (1997). A quantitative systematic review of ondansetron in established post-operative nausea and vomiting. *British Medical Journal*, **314**, 1088–92.

38. Cubeddu, L.X., O'Connor, D.T., and Parmer, R.J. (1995). Plasma chromogranin A: a marker of serotonin release and of emesis associated with cisplatin chemotherapy. *Journal of Clinical Oncology*, **13**, 681–7.

39. Scarantino, C.W., Ornitz, R.D., Hoffman, L.G. *et al.* (1994). On the mechanisms of radiation-induced emesis: the role of serotonin. *International Journal of Radiation Oncology, Biology and Physics*, **30**, 825–30.

40. Watanabe, H., Hasegawa, A., Shinozaki, T. *et al.* (1995). Possible cardiac side effects of granisetron, an antiemetic agent, in patients with bone and soft-tissue sarcomas receiving cytotoxic chemotherapy. *Cancer Chemotherapy Pharmacology*, **35**, 278–82.

41. Upward, J.W., Archbold, B.D.C., Link, C. *et al.* (1990). The clinical pharmacology of granisetron (BRL 43694), a novel specific 5HT$_3$ antagonist. *European Journal of Cancer*, **26**, S12–15.

42. Hesketh, P., J., van Belle, S., Aapro, M. *et al.* (2003). Differential involvement of neurotransmitters through the time course of cisplatin-induced emesis as revealed by therapy with specific receptor antagonists. *European Journal of Cancer*, **39**, 1074–80.

43. Diemmunsch, P. (1999). Antiemetic activity of the NK$_1$ receptor antagonist GR 205171 in the treatment of established postoperative nausea and vomiting after major gynaecological surgery. *British Journal of Anaesthesia*, **82**, 274–6.

44. Aapro, M.S. (1991). Present role of corticosteroids as antiemetics. In *Recent Results in Cancer Research*. Vol. 121, pp. 91–100. Berlin: Springer-Verlag.

45. Doblin, R.E. and Kleiman, M.A.R. (1991). Marijuana as antiemetic medicine: a survey of oncologists' experiences and attitudes. *Journal of Clinical Oncology*, **9**, 1314–19.

46. Devane, W.A. *et al.* (1992). Isolation and structure of a brain constituent that binds to the cannabinoid receptor. *Science*, **258**, 1946–9.

47. Feldman, R.S., Meyer, J.S., and Quenzer, L.F. *Principles of Neuropsycho-pharmacology*. Sunderland MA: Sinauer, 1997.

48. Cunningham, D. *et al.* (1985). Nabilone and prochlorperazine: a useful combination for emesis induced by cytotoxic drugs. *British Medical Journal*, **291**, 864–5.

49. Flynn, J. and Hanif, N. (1992). Nabilone for the management of intractable nausea and vomiting in terminally staged AIDS. *Journal of Palliative Care*, **8**, 46–7.

50. Green, S.T., Nathwani, D., Goldbery, D.J. *et al.* (1989). Nabilone as effective therapy for intractable nausea and vomiting in AIDS. *British Journal of Clinical Pharmacology*, **28**, 494–5.

51. Dalzell, A.M., Bartle, H.M., and Lylleyman, J.S. (1986). Nabilone: an alternative antiemetic for cancer chemotherapy. *Archives of Disease in Childhood*, **61**, 502–5.

52. Potanovich, L.M. *et al.* (1993). Midazolam in patients receiving anticancer chemotherapy and antiemetics. *Journal of Pain and Symptom Management*, **8**, 519–24.

53. Gordon, C.J. *et al.* (1989). Metoclopramide vs metoclopramide and lorazepam: superiority of combined therapy in the control of cisplatin-induced emesis. *Cancer*, **63**, 578–82.

54. Fallon, M.T. (1994). The physiology of somatostatin and its synthetic analogue, octreotide. *European Journal of Palliative Care*, **1**, 20–2.

55. Soudah, H.C., Hasler, W.L., and Chung, O. (1991). Effect of octreotide on intestinal motility and bacterial overgrowth in scleroderma. *New England Journal of Medicine*, **325**, 1461–7.

56. Riley, J. and Fallon, M. (1994). Octreotide in terminal malignant obstruction of the gastrointestinal tract. *European Journal of Palliative Care*, **1**, 23–5.

57. Mercadante, S. *et al.* (1993). Octreotide in relieving gastrointestinal symptoms due to bowel obstruction. *Palliative Medicine*, **7**, 295–9.

58. Khoo, D., Riley, J., and Waxman, J. (1992). Control of emesis in bowel obstruction in terminally ill patients. *Lancet*, **339**, 375–6.

59. Raftery, S. and Sherry, E. (1992). Total intravenous anaesthesia with propofol and alfentanyl protects against postoperative nausea and vomiting. *Canadian Anaesthetists' Society Journal*, **39**, 37–40.

60. Barst, S. *et al.* (1990). Anesthesia for pediatric cancer patients: ketamine, etomidate, or propofol? *Anaesthesiology*, **73**, A1114.

61. Borgeat, A., Wilder-Smith, O., Forni, M. *et al.* (1994). Adjuvant propofol enables better control of nausea and emesis secondary to chemotherapy for breast cancer. *Canadian Journal of Anaesthetists*, **41**, 117–19.

62. Scher, C.S. and McDowall, R.H. (1992). Use of propofol for the prevention of chemotherapy-induced nausea and emesis in oncology patients. *Canadian Anaesthetists' Society Journal*, **39**, 170–2.

63. Ewalenko, P., Janny, S., Dejonckheere, G.A. *et al.* (1996). Anti-emetic effect of subhypnotic doses of propofol after thyroidectomy. *British Journal of Anaesthesia*, **77**, 463–7.

64. Baines, N.M., Bunce, K.T., Naylor, R.J. *et al.* (1991). The actions of fentanyl to inhibit drug-induced emesis. *Neuropharmacology*, **30**, 1073–83.

65. Burish, T.G. and Tope, D.M. (1992). Psychological techniques for controlling the adverse side effects of cancer chemotherapy: findings from a decade of research. *Journal of Pain and Symptom Management*, **7**, 287–301.

66. Fallowfield, L.J. (1992). Behavioural interventions and psychological aspects of care during chemotherapy. *European Journal of Cancer*, **28A**, S39–41.

67. Contach, P.H. (1991). Use of nonpharmacological techniques to prevent chemotherapy-related nausea and vomiting. *Recent Results in Cancer Research*, **121**, 101–7.

68. Moorey, S. and Greer, S. (2002). *Cognitive Behaviour Therpary for People with Cancer*. Oxford University Press, Oxford, UK.

69. Saller, R., Hellenbrecht, D., Bühring, M. *et al.* (1986). Enhancement of the antiemetic action of metoclopramide against cisplatin-induced emesis by transdermal electrical nerve stimulation. *Journal of Clinical Pharmacology*, **26**, 115–19.

70. Vickers, A.J. (1996). Can acupuncture have specific effects on health? A systematic review of acupuncture antiemesis trials. *Journal of the Royal Society of Medicine*, **89**, 308–11.

71. Dundee, J.W. and Yang, J. (1991). Prolongation of the antiemetic action of P6 acupuncture by acupressure in patients having cancer chemotherapy. *Journal of the Royal Society of Medicine*, **83**, 360–2.

72. Dundee, J.W., Yang, J., and McMillan, C. (1991). Noninvasive stimulation of the P6 (Neiguan) antiemetic acupuncture point in cancer chemotherapy. *Journal of the Royal Society of Medicine*, **84**, 210–12.

73. Compora, E. *et al.* (1991). The incidence of narcotic-induced emesis. *Journal of Pain and Symptom Management*, **6**, 428–30.

74. Bruera, E. *et al.* (1987). Chronic nausea and anorexia in advanced cancer patients: a possible role for autonomic dysfunction. *Journal of Pain and Symptom Management*, **2**, 19–21.

75. Olver, I.N., Matthews, J.P., Bishop, J.F. *et al.* (1994). The roles of patient and observer assessments in antiemetic trials. *European Journal of Cancer*, **30A**, 1223–7.

76. Herrstedt, J. (1994). We still need common criteria for the assessment of nausea and vomiting. *European Journal of Cancer*, **30A**, 1217.

77. Saxby, C. *et al.* (2007). How should we measure emesis in palliative care? *Palliat Med*, **21**, 369–83

10.2.2 Dysphagia, dyspepsia, and hiccup

Claud Regnard

Dysphagia

Definition

Dysphagia is difficulty in transferring liquids or solids from the mouth to the stomach.

Prevalence

The prevalence of dysphagia in a palliative care patient population varies considerably depending on the cause and stage of disease. In a large series of nearly 7000 patients at St Christopher's Hospice, London, the overall prevalence was 23 per cent[1], although in a later series of 800 patients dysphagia occurred in only 12 per cent[2]. Some patients with other pre-existing disease start from a high baseline. For example, up to a third of patients with mental health problems suffer from dysphagia[3]. The prevalence of dysphagia in patients with head and neck cancer depends on the site of the problem, being as low as 4 per cent with anterior oral lesions, rising to 100 per cent with postcricoid lesions[4,5]. Laryngeal and hypopharyngeal tumours produce most severe problems[6]. In motor neuron disease the prevalence of dysphagia is about 60 per cent[7], but, despite its progressive nature, it is a fallacy that aspiration is a common cause of death in this condition[8]. Sixty-three per cent of patients with Parkinson's disease and 47 per cent of patients with multiple sclerosis have objective evidence of swallowing difficulty[9,10]. Stroke can result in dysphagia in up to 87 per cent of patients[11,12]. Swallowing becomes slower with age[13]. Older people may therefore be more vulnerable to disturbances of swallowing, which may explain why 55 per cent of a group of nursing home patients had swallowing problems[14].

Anatomy and physiology

Although the path taken by fluids and food to the stomach is direct, the mechanism to achieve a smooth and easy passage is complex. It requires intact anatomy, normal mucosa, normal functioning of five cranial nerves and the brainstem and the co-ordination of the cortex, limbic system, basal ganglia, cerebellum, and brain stem centres involved in respiration, salivation and motor function. Thirty-four skeletal muscles are involved. This complexity reflects the biological necessity for respiration and nutrition, with respiration taking priority. Swallowing comprises four distinct phases[15]. The first two are voluntary; the latter two automatic:

1 *Oral preparatory phase:* food is mixed with saliva and chewed to break down larger particles.

2 *Oral swallowing phase:* the lips are closed to prevent leakage and the anterior tongue retracts and elevates in a wave that pushes the bolus into the oropharynx.

3 *Pharyngeal phase:* this is triggered by the bolus reaching the posterior tongue. The larynx closes, breathing stops, and the larynx elevates to seal with the epiglottis and vocal cords to pro-tect the airway and prevent aspiration. A peristaltic wave moves the bolus into the oesophagus in under 1 s. These complex actions are necessary to protect the airway because the pharynx is a shared passage for air and food.

4 *Oesophageal phase:* reflex peristalsis carries the bolus down the oesophagus, the lower oesophageal sphincter relaxes and the bolus enters the stomach.

Mechanisms and causes

Any disruption of normal anatomy and physiology may result in dysphagia and consequently there are many causes, sometimes with several present together (Table 10.2.2.1). Mechanical obstruc-tion is usually caused by cancer. Tumours of the mouth and upper pharynx cause early symptoms, while those of the lower pharynx and oesophagus are often silent at first. Food will collect proximally and may spill over into an unprotected airway (Fig. 10.2.2.1). Stricture formation may occur following surgery[16], radiotherapy or because of gastro-oesophageal reflux disease.

In the absence of mechanical obstruction, severe dysphagia due to functional disturbance can occur. For example, inability to raise the posterior tongue because of tumour infiltration may allow food to trickle into the pharynx and into an unprotected airway. Fibrosis following surgery or radiotherapy can also seriously disrupt the swallowing phases, but radiation dosage and volume is not related to the incidence, onset, or severity of dysphagia[17]. Nerve damage is another factor and perineural spread of head and neck cancers can be demonstrated at autopsy in nearly 90 per cent of patients at post-mortem[18]. In life, this is often associated with dysaesthesia and pain, particularly in the territories of cranial nerves 5 and 9. Damage to cranial nerves 7, 9, 10, and 12 disturbs the pharyngeal phase of swallowing, often accompanied by aspiration[19]. Perineural vagal and sympathetic invasion combined with local fibrosis and tumour infiltration can cause severe functional dys-phagia, which is indistinguishable from gross mechanical obstruction[18]. Pharyngeal and laryngeal sensory loss caused by cancer-related damage of the superior laryngeal nerve will cause silent aspiration. Other neurological and neuromuscular disorders listed in Table 10.2.2.1 can cause severe dysphagia, including the motor neuron diseases[6,7], Parkinson's disease[8,20], multiple sclerosis[10], and Huntingdon's disease. The mechanisms causing

Table 10.2.2.1 Causes of dysphagia related to advanced disease

Caused by disease process

Obstruction by mass lesion in mouth, pharynx, or oesophagus

Infiltration or fibrosis of walls of mouth, pharynx, or oesophagus causing reduced motility ± damage to nerve plexus

External compression (e.g. mediastinal tumour)

Perineural tumour spread

Upper motor neuron damage (cerebral tumour or infarction)

Lower motor neuron damage (motor neuron disease, multiple sclerosis, cranial nerve palsy)

Motor or sensory cranial nerve palsy (tumour at base of skull, leptomeningeal infiltration, brainstem metastases or infarction)

Cerebellar damage (infarction, surgery, tumour, paraneoplastic)

Neuropathy (paraneoplastic)

Neuromuscular dysfunction (myasthenic-myopathic syndrome, polymyositis, dermatomyositis, Parkinsonism, Huntingdon's disease)

Cerebral cortex damage (stroke, tumour, dementia)

Caused by treatment

Surgery (loss of structure, motor loss, sensory loss, fibrosis, fistula)

Radiotherapy (fibrosis, reduced saliva, mucosal inflammation)

Chemotherapy (mucosal inflammation)

Drugs, by causing abnormal motility or dry mouth (e.g. neuroleptics, metoclopramide, anticholinergic drugs)

Associated with advanced disease

Dry mouth

Mucosal infection of mouth, pharynx, or oesophagus (candidiasis, apthous ulceration, herpes simplex, herpes zoster, cytomegalovirus)

Dental caries

Extreme weakness

Hypercalcaemia (rare cause of dysphagia)

Concurrent disease

Benign stricture

Reflux oesophagitis (hiatus hernia, gastric stasis, GORD)—see Dyspepsia section in this chapter

Functional (non-ulcer) dysmotility dyspepsia—see Dyspepsia section in this chapter

Pain (mucosal, soft tissue, dental, bone)

Brain injury (trauma, infection, hypoxia)

Factors that may compromise swallowing

Old age

Lack of time to eat

Missing teeth

Poor environment

Uninteresting, tepid food

Insufficient staff to help

Drowsiness

Withdrawal (depression, fear)

Dry mouth (anxiety, drugs)

Mental health problems, including intellectual disability

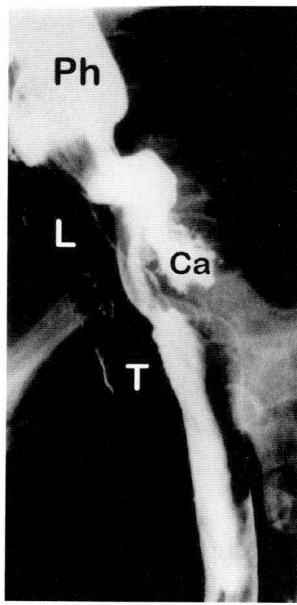

Figure 10.2.2.1 Lateral view of barium swallow showing an ulcerating squamous cell carcinoma of the upper oesophagus (Ca) with poor pharyngeal emptying demonstrated by the presence of a fluid level in the pharynx (Ph). Laryngeal (L) and tracheal (T) aspiration of barium can be seen.

dysphagia in such conditions are complex. Mechanisms suggested in Parkinson's disease, for example, include a defect in a non-dopaminergic pathway from the medulla causing laryngeal dysmotility[21,22], and disturbance of the oral phase due to bradykinesia[23], resulting in a delay in triggering the swallowing reflex, with slowed elevation of the larynx and a slow oesophageal phase[24].

Loss of structures through surgery has varying effects. For example, hemilaryngectomy will rarely cause swallowing problems if the epiglottis is preserved, and yet a unilateral supraglottic laryngectomy is likely to result in a chronic swallowing disability[25]. Oesophageal spasm causes functional obstruction and, if intense, can cause severe central chest pain indistinguishable from ischaemic cardiac pain[26]. Spasm of the lower oesophageal sphincter or the cricopharyngeal muscle can be caused by anxiety[27], but there is no evidence that dysphagic patients without obvious physical cause have psychological profiles that are different from patients with physical causes of dysphagia[28]. Drugs are another cause of dysphagia[29,30], while severe functional dysphagia can occur as a rare complication of hypercalcaemia[31].

Mucosal inflammation due to infection, radiotherapy, or chemotherapy may cause painful dysphagia (odynophagia). Candida may affect the mouth, pharynx, and oesophagus and may present as a reddened mucosa, angular stomatitis, pale patches of chronically infected epithelium, or the classical white patches that leave an erythematous area when rubbed away. Oral candida is found in only 50 per cent of patients with oesophageal candidiasis[32]. The 'moth-eaten' appearances of oesophageal ulceration on barium swallow are characteristic of candida, herpes simplex, or cytomegalovirus infection. Infection in advanced cancer is usually mild, but can be severe and extensive in patients with AIDS. Painful swallowing for

any reason can disrupt one or more swallowing phases sufficiently to reduce oral intake.

A number of factors can worsen or precipitate swallowing difficulties. Concurrent disease causing pain or dry mouth will cause difficulties. Brain injury can cause dysphagia and this is well recognized in stroke where anterior or periventricular white matter damage is more likely to result in aspiration[33]. Excessive drowsiness, disinterest and weakness will result in a poor oral preparatory phase with leakage of food from the mouth, drooling and possibly aspiration because of delayed or absent triggering of the swallowing reflex. Ageing affects swallowing; for example, missing teeth make the oral preparation phase more difficult[34], swallowing is slower[13], and there is reduced sensitivity in the mouth and pharynx[35,36]. Inadequate staffing can increase the risk of dehydration in dysphagic patients[37], while the urge to swallow can be greatly diminished by a poor environment, tepid food temperatures or uninteresting food.

Evaluation

History
The patient's description can provide useful information (Table 10.2.2.2). Difficulty with certain food consistencies provides some information but is far less specific than is commonly believed[38]. For example, although obstructing lesions generally produce dysphagia for solids initially with progression to liquids later, neuromuscular disorders may well cause dysphagia for both solids and liquids more or less simultaneously. In contrast to information about food consistency, localization by the patient of an obstruction is very accurate and in one series of 1000 patients, 99 per cent of patients accurately localized the anatomical site of the problem[15]. The level is important as it determines the next stage of the evaluation (Table 10.2.2.2). A detailed treatment history is essential, especially for current drugs, previous surgery and past radiotherapy. A number of assessment tools, scales and questionnaires have been developed to assess dysphagia[39–46].

Examination
A basic evaluation can be carried out by the doctor and nurse but if abnormalities are found or suspected, this should be carried out by a professional qualified in dysphagia assessment and management. This is most usually a role fulfiled by a speech and language therapist[48,49]. A non-specialist examination can be done at the bedside (see Table 10.2.2.3). Examination includes evaluation of the relevant cranial nerves, looking for evidence of muscle weakness (e.g. drooling or leakage of food, food collecting on palate, or lateral sulci), checking for stridor, observing any jaw misalignment during chewing, assessing lip closure, and checking the condition of the teeth and mucosa. Anterior tongue movement is observed easily and posterior tongue movement can be checked by rapidly repeating the syllable 'ka'. Tongue strength and tone can be assessed by asking the patient to push against the examiner's gloved finger and it is generally possible to differentiate between lower motor neuron (bulbar) lesions and upper motor neuron (pseudobulbar) lesions. A laryngeal mirror can be used when checking for mucosal sensation and then used to look for food debris or a pathological condition. The oropharyngeal transit time is measured from the first tongue movement to the last laryngeal movement. Times of more than 1 s are abnormal and in two studies this

Table 10.2.2.2 Evaluation of dysphagia: history.[15,47]

Information provided	Possible interpretation(s)
Dysphagia at level of chest or abdomen	
Abnormality on barium swallow (if aspiration suspected order small volume gastrograffin swallow)	Oesophageal abnormality requiring referral to gastroenterologists for endoscopy
Dysphagia at level of mouth or throat Examples:	NB. Requires swallowing assessment, best done by a speech and language therapist specializing in swallowing problems
Oral stage	
Food loss from the mouth	Weak lip closure, reduced tongue control
Food pocketing in the cheeks	Reduced tone in cheeks, reduced tongue control, weak tongue movements
Food sitting in the mouth	Reduced tongue control, weak and/or reduced tongue movements
Food coming down the nose	Reduced movement of the soft palate
Pharyngeal stage	
Coughing/choking before the swallow	Weak, reduced or uncoordinated movements of the base of the tongue, larynx and pharynx.
Coughing/choking during the swallow	Reduced elevation of the larynx, or difficulties with the movement of the valleculae
Coughing/choking after the swallow	Reduced, weak and/or uncoordinated movements of the tongue base, larynx and pharynx, or poor opening of upper oesophageal sphincter

screening test gave a sensitivity of 80 per cent and a specificity of 54 per cent in stroke patients, and a specificity of 86 per cent in general medical patients[50,51]. It is sensitive enough to identify patients with a simple, viral sore throat[52]. Coughing or choking indicates that fluid or food may have penetrated the larynx, although the absence of coughing does not exclude penetration, while its presence does not imply that laryngeal contents have been aspirated into the airway[53]. Similarly, a 'gargle' quality to the voice after swallowing suggests penetration but not aspiration, while its absence does not exclude either penetration or aspiration[54]. If oxygen saturation (SpO$_2$) is monitored during swallowing using pulse oximetry, a reduction in SpO$_2$ after a swallow may indicate that fluid or food has been aspirated[55,56]. Contrary to popular belief, the presence or absence of the gag reflex does not reflect on the patient's ability to swallow[15,57,58]. In the motor neuron disorders the pharyngeal response is brisk rather than depressed[59].

Investigation

Although examination may uncover the cause of dysphagia in the oral preparatory phase, accurate evaluation of the remaining phases is best done radiologically. For example, aspiration will be missed on clinical evaluation in 40 per cent of patients[15]. Videofluoroscopy under the direction of a swallowing therapist has become the gold standard of assessing dysphagia, but weakness, immobility and cognitive impairment can prevent its use[57,60], while differing protocols can limit its value[61]. Fibreoptic endoscopic evaluation of swallowing (FEES) is an alternative that can be used at the bedside and is particularly good at identifying laryngeal penetration, overspill into the larynx/pharynx pre swallow, the timing and coordination of events, anatomical abnormalities and cranial neuropathies[62–64]. It can also be used to test the sensitivity of the structures involved in swallowing and may be used to assess dry swallows where patients are too unstable to assess using food or fluid.

Management

Clinical decisions for dysphagia[65]

1 Is there doubt about the need for hydration and/or feeding?

2 Is a complete obstruction present?

3 Is aspiration causing troublesome symptoms?

4 Is mucosal infection or a dry mouth present?

5 Could drugs be a cause?

6 Is pain affecting swallowing?

7 Is the dysphagia persisting?

1. Is there doubt about the need for hydration and/or feeding?

Those patients with a very short prognosis (day to day deterioration or faster) are unlikely to need or want feeding and hydration by any route. If it is clear that hydration and feeding are unnecessary (e.g. the patient is comatose and comfortable in the last hours or days), then the aim is comfort or pleasure and often all that is needed at the end of life is to moisten the mouth. If the family or partner feels a need to continue hydration or feeding, they will need help to understand that hunger is not usually a problem at the end of life[66,67], and that unwanted feeding by any route may increase distress[68]. Dehydration causes few symptoms at the end of life[69], but occasionally it can contribute to an agitated (hyperalert) delirium which will need non-oral hydration[70,71]. If the dysphagia is due to exhaustion or fatigue caused by cancer, non-oral hydration and feeding are only appropriate if active cancer treatment is planned with the anticipation of full or partial recovery.

In cases of doubt it is often possible to delay for several days. It is easier not to start a treatment than to stop it a short time later.

Table 10.2.2.3 Non-specialist evaluation of dysphagia: some examples of observations and interpretations.

Observation	Possible interpretation
Stridor—'rough' wheeze from upper airway	Airway narrowing—needs urgent treatment
Abnormal mucosa (dry, ulcerated, or infected) or teeth (missing or damaged)	Mucosal dryness/pain or dental problems causing dysphagia
Leakage from mouth, drooling	Poor lip closure, reduced lip sensation, abnormal tongue movement, or reduced/absent swallowing reflex
Bites cheeks or tongue	Reduced lip or tongue sensation
Food collecting in mouth	Poor lip, buccal, or tongue control
Prolonged chewing or food collecting in vallecula or pyriform fossae	Reduced/absent swallowing reflex
Patient washes food down with a drink or pushes food in with finger	Reduced tongue control
Coughing, choking before swallowing	Laryngeal penetration due to poor tongue control or delayed or absent swallowing reflex
Coughing, choking during swallowing	Laryngeal penetration due to reduced airway protection
Poor or absent laryngeal elevation on swallowing	Poorly protected airway
Coughing, choking after swallowing	Laryngeal penetration due to reduced pharyngeal emptying, reduced laryngeal elevation, cricopharyngeus dysfunction, pharyngeal or oesophageal obstruction, or tracheooesophageal fistula
Voice changes	
Inability to say 'pa'	Poor lip closure
Inability to say 'ta'	Poor movement of anterior tongue
Inability to say 'ka'	Poor movement of posterior tongue
'Hot potato' voice	Vallecular tumours
'Breathy' voice or hoarseness	Recurrent laryngeal nerve palsy
Nasal escape speech	Lower motor neuron lesion
'Donald Duck' speech	Upper motor neuron lesion
Flaccid, fasciculating tongue	Lower motor neuron lesion
Small, spastic tongue	Upper motor neuron lesion
Bedside swallowing test	
Oropharyngeal transit time >1 s	Dysphagia present
'Gargle' type voice or 'bubbling' heard through stethoscope on neck	Penetration or aspiration of food/fluid into larynx
Drop in SaO_2 on pulse oximetry	Aspiration below vocal cords into airway
Unable to feel cold mirror	Sensory loss in area tested

2. Is a complete obstruction present? (see Chapter 10.2.4)

In malignancy, and in the absence of infection, corticosteroids may offer the possibility of easing dysphagia by reducing luminal obstruction, extramural compression, or nerve compression. Patients with dysphagia related to head and neck tumours may respond in the short term to dexamethasone[72]. This will occur only if oedema is present, but since there is no simple way of assessing this, treatment is often empirical. Dexamethasone 8 mg daily orally or parenterally is a typical starting dose and can be given as a single oral or subcutaneous dose. Any beneficial effect may be present only for a few days or weeks but this is helpful, for example, in a patient awaiting radiotherapy.

If hydration or nutrition are needed, but there is complete obstruction, the use of a non-oral route will be required. Endoscopic dilatation of the obstruction relieves dysphagia in over half of patients but, in malignant obstructions, improvement generally lasts less than 2 weeks[73]. Endoscopic dilatation is therefore used mostly as a short-term measure before radiation, intubation, laser resection, or local injection of alcohol or cisplatin. Single-dose intra-luminal radiation (brachytherapy) of oesophageal cancer has a similar initial response rate to endoscopic dilatation, but improvement is maintained for a median of about 4 months[74]. However, patients with stenotic tumours who previously had chemotherapy will need higher doses of brachytherapy or will need stenting[75]. Endoscopic stenting provides another option (see Chapter 9.5) and self-expanding metal stents are now preferred to plastic stents as they are easier to insert, stay patent for longer and have fewer complications[76–79]. Covered expandable prostheses are better if

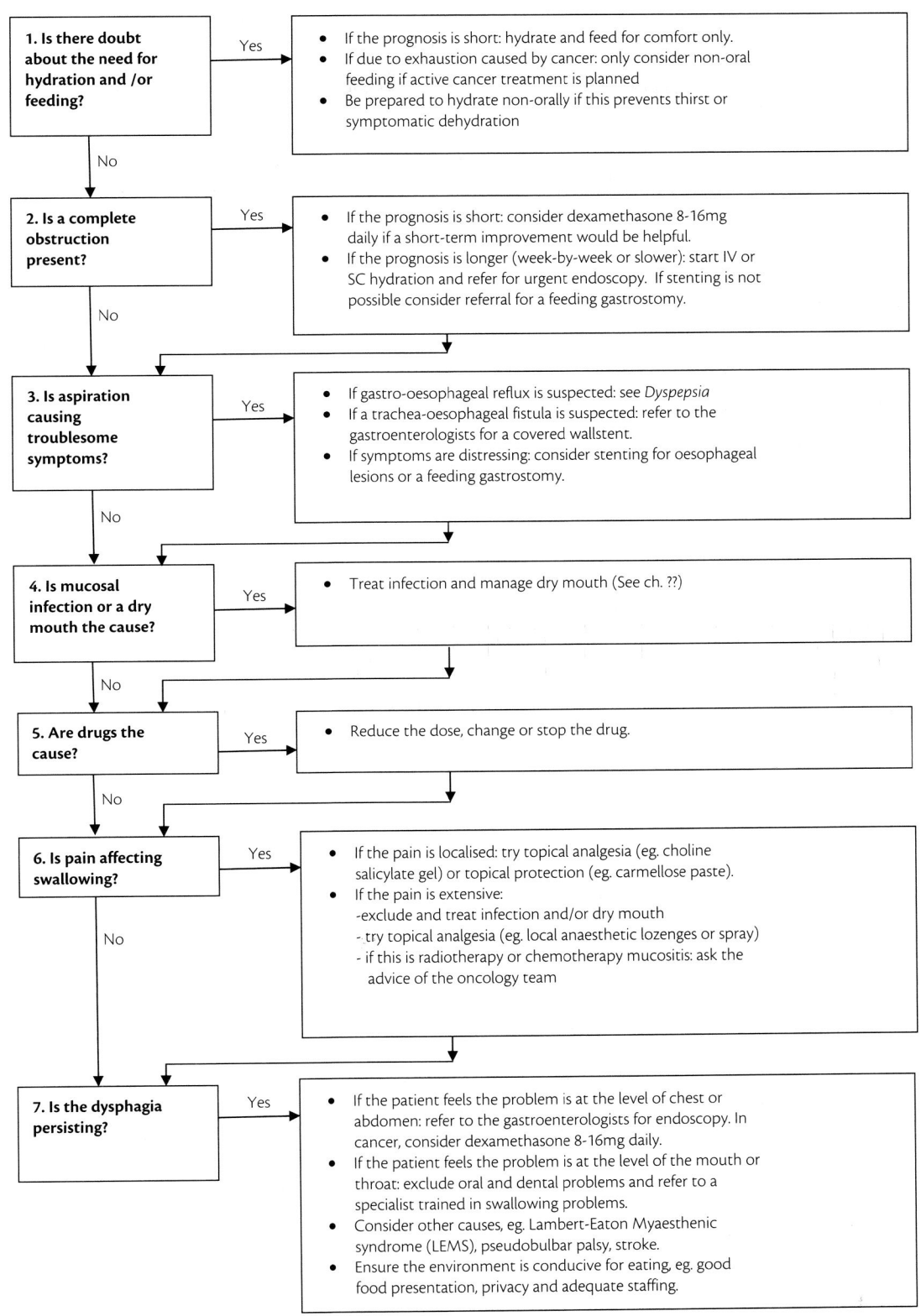

Figure 10.2.2.2 Clinical decision algorithms for dysphagia (adapted with permission from Regnard C, Dean M, Harris J-D. *A Guide to Symptom Relief in Palliative Care, 6th ed.* Oxford: Radcliffe Press, in press)

palliating a fistula or perforation[80]. Such stents can provide effective palliation with median survival times of 4 months (range 1–24 months) when combined with laser therapy to remove any recurrent over-growing tumour[81], although survival is less if the stent projects into the stomach[82], and only 17 per cent are alive at 12 months[83]. However, troublesome complications from stents can occur in up to half of patients and include pain, bleeding, blockage by food, stent migration, and increased oesophageal reflux[82–84]. Endoscopic laser therapy produces better relief of dysphagia than stenting[72,85], but the median survival of 4 months is the same as with brachytherapy and metal stents[86]. Photodynamic therapy (using a laser directed at tumour previously sensitized by a systemic injection of photosensitizer) in one series of 65 patients resulted in relief of dysphagia in all patients and a similar median survival of 6 months[87]. If laser is not available, then an alternative method is to cause tumour necrosis by local injection of ethanol[88,89], or cisplatin[90].

3. Is aspiration causing troublesome symptoms?

Penetration of small amounts of food or fluid into the larynx commonly occurs in dysphagia and is also seen in some people who are not dysphagic[91]. In contrast, aspiration of food or fluid past the vocal cords into the airway is not seen in healthy people, but is seen in dysphagic patients, occurring in 33 per cent of stroke patients with dysphagia[91,92]. Even in patients who aspirate, however, 40 per cent do so without clinical signs or symptoms, their aspiration only being visible with videofluoroscopy or nasal endoscopy[15]. This challenges the commonly held view that aspiration is always dangerous and life-threatening and suggests that the airways can cope with small amounts of aspirated material. This view is supported by the observation that dysphagia is only a modest risk factor for aspiration pneumonia and that other factors, such as oral hygiene, smoking, tube feeding and immobility are more important[93–95]. Consequently, in advanced disease aspiration need only be of concern if it is causing symptoms such as coughing, respiratory embarrassment, or repeated chest infections.

4. Is mucosal infection or a dry mouth present? (see Chapter 10.9)

The commonest mucosal infection is candidiasis and may present as white plaques, a red tongue, stomatitis, or angular chelitis. All candida species are sensitive to nystatin and some resistance to systemic antifungals is appearing[96]. Alternatives to nystatin are ketoconazole 200 mg once daily for 5 days, or a single dose of 150 mg fluconazole, the latter being useful when compliance is difficult[97]. Extensive herpes simplex or zoster infections should be treated promptly with systemic acyclovir 200 mg every 4 h for 5 days. The cause of apthous ulceration is still unclear but can be helped by topical analgesia (e.g. Antacid plus oxetacaine local anaesthetic), topical steroid[98] or tetracycline 250 mg as a 2-min mouthwash three times a day[99]. Thalidomide may be an alternative for persistent apthous ulceration[100]. Chlorhexidine has been

Table 10.2.2.4 Types and examples of specialist swallowing therapy.[109]

Type of therapy	Brief description	Example(s)
Facilitation techniques		
Postural changes	Alter angle of head to encourage gravity to alter the flow of food or fluid	Tilting head down to prevent premature spilling of bolus into pharynx
		Tilting head to the stronger side to direct bolus away from a unilateral pharyngeal paralysis
Swallowing manoeuvres	Altering the natural pattern of swallowing to facilitate a safer swallow	Multiple swallows to clear residue from laryngeal opening
		Supraglottic swallow (breath hold before and during swallow, followed by immediate cough or forceful exhalation of breath) to clear residue from laryngeal opening
Indirect techniques		
Strengthening and manipulation exercises	Range of motion and resistance exercises to improve muscle function	Prevention of muscle fibrosis after surgery or radiotherapy
Direct techniques		
Sensory stimulation	Used to enhance sensory input (temperature, taste, and pressure) prior to swallowing	Used in patients with reduced sensation or coordination
Compensatory treatment		
Food characteristics	Alteration of texture, taste, temperature, and amount of food and fluid	Adjusting textures and amounts to individuals, whilst maintaining taste, variation, and attractiveness of food and drink
Time and environment	Ensuring an environment appropriate for the individual	Providing time, whilst ensuring variety of temperatures in an environment that is dedicated to feeding
Positioning and help	Ensuring posture is suitable and sufficient help is available	Stabilizing the head with pillows if head control is poor
		Ensuring sufficient staff to help patients who cannot feed themselves

recommended to improve oral hygiene[101], but chlorhexidine causes taste alteration, stains teeth and can damage oral mucosa[102].

If the cause of a dry mouth cannot be reversed, local measures are helpful, for example, petroleum jelly to the lips, iced drinks, or semi-frozen fruit juices (e.g. pineapple or cranberry) and regular mouth care. Artificial salivas (methylcellulose or porcine mucin) can help if used several times every hour. Glycerin or lemon should be avoided as the former dehydrates the mucosa and the latter soon exhausts the salivary glands. Chewing gum has been suggested as a way of stimulating saliva.[101] Pilocarpine stimulates salivation but doses need to be kept low to minimize adverse effects. When patients in one study were given a choice, they felt pilocarpine was no better than a mucin-based saliva substitute[103]. Previous work has shown that porcine mucin was felt by patients to be no better than water[103]. It seems that what patients find most helpful are sprays containing water or cool, pleasant drinks.

5. Could drugs be a cause?

Drugs can cause a dry mouth (anticholinergic drugs, opioids) and, occasionally, oesophageal spasm (neuroleptic drugs, metoclopramide). In these circumstances, the dose should be reduced, if possible, or an alternative drug prescribed. For patients who already have a feeding tube, drugs can cause tube blockages either by using an incorrect preparation, a physical interaction with enteral feed or by inadequately flushing the tube[104,105].

6. Is pain affecting swallowing?

Mucosal pain in the mouth can be eased by topical analgesics such as choline salicylate gel or benzydamine mouthwash, which are topical non-steroidal anti-inflammatory drugs with a mild local anaesthetic action. Increased local anaesthesia can be obtained with local anaesthetic lozenges or spray 15 min before eating or drinking. This is also helpful if there is oesophageal pain on swallowing. Having excluded or treated mucosal infection, the soft tissues need to be considered, particularly in patients with head and neck cancer. The rapid onset of pain over a few hours in such patients may well be caused by infection, but with little or no outward signs. Treatment with oral flucloxacillin and metronidazole resolve the infection and the pain within 24 h. Other causes of pain affecting bone, soft tissues, or nerve are treated as described elsewhere. Despite 30 years of research and products, radiotherapy or chemotherapy induced mucositis remains a difficult problem, relying on coating agents, local anaesthetics and topical or systemic analgesics[102,106–108].

7. Is dysphagia persisting?

If the problem persists then a swallowing therapist can advise on a wide range of treatments[109]. Table 10.2.2.4 gives examples of the different types of therapy that can be offered. Direct, indirect and facilitation techniques need to be managed by a swallowing therapist. Imaginative food preparation and presentation are vital and even soft diets can be transformed with care and imagination (Table 10.2.2.5). Chilled foods are pleasant and patients with neurological dysfunction find them easier to swallow. Someone with poor muscular control of the head can be helped by stabilizing the head with pillows or a lightweight chin support[110]. Patients may need help with feeding, allowing them to concentrate on swallowing, while the helper concentrates on positioning and transferring the

Table 10.2.2.5 Tomato bavrois with yellow pepper coulis.

Contents	
Beef tomatoes	5
Caradom	1
Whipped cream	140 ml
Beaten egg whites	2
Chopped fresh basil leaves	5
Sheets of leaf gelatine	4
Maxijul powder	60 g
Yellow peppers	2
Butter	30 g
Pinch of salt and pepper	

Nutritional content: 169 kcal, 3 g protein, 11 g fat

Instructions

1. Remove the inside of the tomato
2. Puree the inside of the tomato with caradom, Maxijul, and chopped basil
3. Warm the pureed tomato and basil in a pan; then add gelatine
4. When the mixture is nearly set, add whipped cream and beaten egg whites
5. Gently mix without beating, and then pipe into the tomato skin
6. To make the yellow pepper coulis:
   - chop the yellow pepper
   - place in a pan with the butter
   - place the lid on the pan
   - cook gently for 1–2 min until tender
7. Place the tomato on the yellow pepper coulis, and then garnish with fresh basil leaves

David Taylor and Neil Bosomworth, St Oswald's Hospice, Newcastle-upon-Tyne, United Kingdom, 1994.

food from plate to mouth[111]. The patient needs to be helped into a comfortable position and allowed to pause for a few minutes before eating. Spectacles and hearing aids should be in place and in good working order. Dentures should also be in place, even if chewing is not required. The helper should face the patient so that they can see each other. Small amounts of food or drink should be given slowly. The technique advised by the swallowing therapist is then followed and its effect observed.

Non-oral hydration and feeding

Choosing a route

The indications and contraindications for non-oral feeding are shown in Table 10.2.2.6.

Nasogastric route: standard nasogastric tubes are uncomfortable for more than a few days, whereas fine bore tubes are well tolerated for a week or more but are more difficult to replace if displaced. Contrary to common belief, nasogastric tubes do not protect patients from aspiration[112,113]. Nasogastric tubes may even worsen aspiration by markedly increasing oropharyngeal secretions[114].

Table 10.2.2.6 Indications and contraindications for choosing a non-oral feeding route.

All non-oral routes	Intravenous route	Nasogastric tube	Subcutaneous	Gastrostomy
Indications				
Oral + pharyngeal transit time >10 s Failure to modify swallowing technique during treatment to improve muscle control Nutritional support for surgery or chemotherapy	Complete pharyngeal or oesophageal obstruction Short term use for hydration (<1 week) (peripheral vein) Long-term use for nutrition (central venous line) Anatomical or functional bowel loss	Medium-term use (1–3 weeks)	Medium term use (1–3 weeks) Hyperactive delirium due to dehydration	Long-term use (4 weeks or more)
Contraindications				
Rapid deterioration Cachexia Psychological need of staff or family to provide 'active treatment'	Hyperactive delirium Presence of sepsis Limited or no access to biochemical monitoring Limited or no access to a parenteral nutrition team Poor home circumstances Superior vena caval obstruction	Hyperactive delirium Nasal, pharyngeal, or oesophageal obstruction Cosmetic appearance Long-term use (4 weeks or more)	Extensive skin disease	Hyperactive delirium Intra-abdominal tumour

This may explain why survival was no better in patients receiving nasogastric tube feeding in a study of 1386 patients over 65 years with cognitive impairment[112]. In contrast, another large study suggested that tube feeding did modestly increase survival in nursing home residents, but patients were not all cognitively impaired and initially less disabled than in the previous study[115]. In MND nasogastric tube feeding does not improve survival or distressing symptoms and sometimes causes new problems[114]. This suggests that early use of non-oral feeding can be helpful, but when patients suffer from multiple clinical problems nasogastric feeding offers few advantages.

Pharyngostomy: a pharyngostomy is probably the simplest to insert and maintain[116], but has never been widely accepted, cannot be used in luminal obstructions of the pharynx or oesophagus and is unsatisfactory for patients with motor neuron disease[117].

Subcutaneous or rectal route: these are useful routes for a few weeks' hydration, but cannot be used for feeding[118]. The subcutaneous route has a role in hyperactive delirium due to dehydration since accidental removal of the infusion cannula is much less of a problem than in the intravenous or enteral routes.

Gastrostomy: a tube can be inserted either endoscopically under sedation and local anaesthetic (percutaneous endoscopic gastrostomy—PEG)[119,120], or percutaneously under fluoroscopic control after distending the stomach with air or carbon dioxide through a temporary nasogastric tube (percutaneous fluoroscopic gastrostomy—PFG)[121,122]. Gastrostomies are usually well tolerated and feeding and hydration through a gastrostomy improves nutrition more effectively than the nasogastric route[123], with less aspiration[124]. Major complications of PEG are low (<3 per cent) but minor problems (blockage, leakage, local infection) occur in up to one-third[125,126]. PEG insertion can be done as a day case[127], but it is common practice for patients to remain in hospital for a few days until their bowels are coping with the increased nutrition and the patient and carers are confident of managing feeds. The support of a PEG team is invaluable in ensuring success and

providing follow-up. Patients with a gastrostomy are easily managed at home[128].

The use of non-oral feeding in progressive neurological disease

For the reasons outlined above, the nasogastric route is not acceptable as a medium or longterm solution in any patient. However, there remains considerable controversy about PEG feeding, especially in dementia. A common view is that the current evidence fails to show that PEG feeding has a favourable outcome[129]. The criticisms are based on work in patients with dementia (mainly Alzheimer's type) showing that there is:

- a failure of PEG feeding to lengthen survival[130,131];
- a worsening of prognosis after PEG insertion[132];
- a higher complication rate with PEGs than without PEGs[133];
- a higher complication rate, poorer quality of life and survival in malnourished patients receiving tube feeding.[134]

However there remain many unanswered questions:

Is survival a relevant outcome measure? It should not be surprising that survival is unchanged against the background of a progressive, untreatable condition. Although the survival curves for PEGs in dementia are less favourable than the survival curves for PEG in the general population, the two curves are parallel[132], suggesting it is the dementia that reduces survival, not the insertion of a PEG.

When does dysphagia become an issue? In many progressive neurological conditions, including Alzheimer's dementia, dysphagia occurs early in the disease process and may not be a terminal symptom as is often believed[135].

Is early dysphagia being identified? Dysphagia is often missed because of poor screening, so that when it becomes obvious it is already at an advanced stage[136].

Are PEGs being inserted too late? The delay in identification of dysphagia means that PEGs are inserted when nutritional deficiency has already developed. There is evidence that dementia patients with low albumin levels who have PEGs inserted do much less well than those with normal albumin levels[137].

Is the refeeding syndrome being recognized? There is nothing in the PEG-dementia literature about the refeeding syndrome in malnourished patients. This syndrome occurs when malnourished patients are fed carbohydrates too early which results in severe electrolyte imbalances and a risk of death[138,139].

Is gastric stasis being treated? This is common in patients with malnutrition, advanced disease and many neurological conditions. Its presence will reduce the feed rate and increase the risk of aspiration. There is no mention of this problem in PEG-dementia literature.

Are the most appropriate outcomes being assessed? There is very little data on outcomes more relevant to palliative care. Examples are patient distress; the shift from struggling to eat for survival with dysphagia, to eating for pleasure with supplementary feeding through a PEG; avoiding symptoms of malnutrition (taste changes, fatigue, poor wound healing, increased pressure sores, gastric stasis); reducing hospital admissions for respiratory infections (since the intravenous route is not needed with a PEG); and the ease of administration of medications, especially at the end of life.

These questions need to be answered before the issue of PEGs in progressive neurological disease can be clarified. The current view that PEGs are contraindicated in dementia is based on incomplete data. Until these data can be obtained, each patient with persistent dysphagia should be assessed individually for non-oral feeding and a decision made on the:

- speed of deterioration;
- patient's present opinion (or a decision made in their best interests if they do not have capacity for this decision);
- potential advantages of feeding and/or hydration;
- feasibility of an alternative route;
- potential disadvantages of the route chosen.

Other considerations

Psychological issues: the psychological impact of dysphagia can be profound. This is not surprising because from childhood we are taught that we must eat if we are to keep well and strong, making dysphagia a tangible threat. Anxiety, anger, fear, and depression may result or be exacerbated and will need support and management. Non-oral hydration and feeding can cause additional problems for the patient and family—both resistance to starting or distress at stopping. Problems with deciding on the right treatment are usually either due to uncertainty about prognosis or a failure of communication.

Respiratory problems: troublesome and repeated aspiration will produce recurrent chest infections which cause distress with pyrexia, fatigue, breathlessness, purulent sputum and may be life-threatening.

Dysphagia: key points

- Swallowing problems are common in advanced disease.
- Severe dysphagia at the level of the chest or abdomen needs assessment by a gastroenterologist.
- Severe dysphagia at the level of the mouth or throat needs assessment by a specialist trained in swallowing problems.
- Non-oral feeding and hydration should be considered in all patients who will benefit.

- In the last days or weeks of life hydration and feeding should be for comfort and pleasure, but non-oral feeding is usually unnecessary.

Coping with saliva: if the patient cannot swallow saliva adequately, drooling is likely to be an embarrassing and troublesome problem. Anticholinergic drugs are helpful and transdermal hyoscine hydrobromide (scopolamine) is convenient, but delivers a low dose (500 mcg over 3 days). Radiation of the salivary glands also helps, with no adverse effects, although to avoid excessive (and permanent) dryness the treatment is given in two stages—2–6 Gy are given initially, repeated if necessary 3 weeks later. In practice, however, radiation treatment is rarely indicated.

Nutritional deficiencies: there is little information on the effect of nutritional deficiencies in patients with terminal illness. Consequently, we do not know which specific deficiencies need to be corrected. Until more data are available, it is necessary to rely on advice from a dietician/nutritionist. It is important, however, to avoid a rigid approach which places major burdens on the patient in terms of nutritional demands and/or financial cost.

Dyspepsia

Definition

The Greek term dyspepsia means bad (dys) digestion (peptin) and is often linked with the Latin-derived term indigestion, an equally vague term. Over the past 25 years, new definitions of dyspepsia have emerged at the rate of almost one each year[140]. This reflects the difficulty of defining a term that describes a syndrome whose symptoms share very different pathologies. There is now agreement that dyspepsia is *not* air swallowing, biliary pain, chronic pancreatitis, or irritable bowel disease—all conditions that in the past have been given a 'dypepsia' label. Some believe that gastro-oesophageal reflux disease (GORD) should not be considered as dyspepsia, but this view is not so clear in other classifications[141].

The current view is that dyspepsia is a syndrome whose symptoms arise in the upper gastrointestinal tract and are unrelated to defaecation[140]. Dyspepsia encompasses a range of symptoms that vary in intensity and onset and are not present in every patient or in every episode, although upper abdominal pain is the commonest feature (see Table 10.2.2.7)[141]. There is still disagreement about what should be included in a classification of dyspepsia, but from studies of patients' symptoms there are two distinct types of dyspepsia (Table 10.2.2.7) to which can be added gastro-oesophageal reflux:

1 *Structural (organic) dyspepsia* for which a structural change can be demonstrated, for example, a gastric ulcer. This type of dyspepsia is due to acid-related disease of the upper gastrointestinal tract.

2 *Functional dysmotility (non-ulcer dyspepsia)* which is due to dysmotility of the upper gastrointestinal tract, of which there are two distinct types:
   - gastric/duodenal dysmotility;
   - oesophageal dysmotility.

3 *Gastro-oesophageal reflux disease (GORD)* due to reflux of gastric contents into the oesophagus sufficient to cause mucosal damage and symptoms[142].

Table 10.2.2.7 Symptoms of structural and functional dyspepsia (correlation of symptoms with three types of dyspepsia).

Structural acid-related dyspepsia	Functional dysmotility, (non-ulcer) dyspepsia	
Acid-related dyspepsia	Gastric/duodenal dysmotility dyspepsia	Oesophageal dysmotility dyspepsia
High positive correlations, i.e. symptom likely to be present (%)		
Symptoms listed in descending order of correlation score, i.e. from highest to lowest		
Epigastric pain (63%)	Nausea (32%)	Pain after meals (36%)
Pain relieved by antacids (37%)	Morning vomiting (5%)	Dysphagia (3%)
Acid regurgitation (42%)	Pain relieved by vomiting (13%)	
Heartburn (26%)		
Pain in the night (41%)		
High negative correlations, i.e. symptom likely to be absent (%)		
Other abdominal pain (25%)	—	Pain relieved by food (29%)
Low correlations, i.e. symptom likely to be present for reasons other than dyspepsia (%)		
Symptoms listed in descending order of correlation score, i.e. from highest to lowest		
Pain relieved by food (29%)	Pain in the morning (17%)	Weight loss (4%)
Upper abdominal pain (36%)	Weight loss (4%)	Heartburn (26%)
Pain relieved by stool or flatus (25%)	Loose stools (23%)	Nausea (32%)
Pain relieved by vomiting (13%)	Heartburn (26%)	Pain relieved by antacids (37%)
Loose stools (23%)	Pain relieved by antacids (37%)	Pain in the night (41%)
Bloating (42%)	Pain in the night (41%)	Loose stools (23%)

Percentages are from a survey of 7270 unselected patients presenting to general practitioners with dyspepsia[142].

Prevalence

Dyspepsia is common[142], but the incidence depends on the criteria used to define this syndrome. In one survey, 42 per cent of patients attending a community clinic were identified as having dyspepsia by their general practitioners, but a validated dyspepsia questionnaire agreed with the general practitioner's opinion in little more than half of cases[144]. When dyspeptic patients were selected using a questionnaire this gave a prevalence of 12 per cent[145]. In the general population, of those fully investigated, about one-third had a peptic ulcer, one-third had no obvious abnormality, and one-third had a variety of other diagnoses[146]. Chronic duodenal ulceration occurs in 10–15 per cent of the general population[147]. The risk of ulcer complications among all non-steroidal anti-inflammatory drug (NSAID) users is between 25 and 35 per cent with 1200 deaths each year in the United Kingdom from non-aspirin NSAIDs[148], with up to 44 per cent developing symptoms of dyspepsia[149]. Functional dyspepsia (i.e. *Dysmotility non-ulcer cause*) is seen in about 25 per cent of the normal population and is therefore common in patients with advanced disease. It may account for up to 70 per cent of patients presenting with symptoms of dyspepsia[150].

Mechanisms and causes

There are many causes of dyspepsia in advanced disease (Table 10.2.2.8).

Structural (acid-related) dyspepsia

The end-result in this type of dyspepsia is mucosal damage, because of *Heliobacter pylori* infection, direct damage (e.g. radiotherapy), compromised mucosal protection (e.g. NSAIDs), or delayed mucosal healing (e.g. corticosteroids).

Non-steroidal anti-inflammatory drugs

NSAIDs are the most widely reported drug-cause of adverse effects and they have been described as representing a major health problem[148]. The mechanism of NSAID damage to the gastric and duodenal mucosa is inhibition of the enzyme cyclo-oxygenase-1 (COX-1) that synthesizes prostaglandins E_2 and I_2 that are normally protective of the mucosa[148,151]. There is also some evidence that NSAIDs may slow the healing of existing ulcers[152], and this may be mediated by inhibition of cyclo-oxygenase-2 (COX-2)[153]. Most NSAIDs inhibit both enzymes, although some such as diclofenac preferentially inhibit COX-2, while newer NSAIDs are specific COX-2 inhibitors. These actions are a systemic, not a local effect, so that remote administration of an NSAID does not reduce the risk[154]. A paradoxical and potentially dangerous effect is that the anti-inflammatory action of NSAIDs can mask ulcer pain, delaying diagnosis and treatment. There is a linear increase in the risk of ulcer complications as the dose of NSAID increases[155], and a difference in risk among NSAIDs, with ibuprofen and diclofenac having approximately one-quarter of the risk of piroxicam and ketoprofen[156]. In contrast, age and *H. pylori* infection appear to be independent and less important risk factors. The newer, selective COX-2 NSAIDs produce fewer clinically significant ulcers[157], but still share some of the adverse effects of non-selective NSAIDs, such as salt and water retention, renal failure and delayed ulcer healing[152,158]. The discovery of the risk of NSAID-related vascular event has cast a yet another

Table 10.2.2.8 Causes of dyspepsia in advanced disease.

Caused by the disease process	Associated with advanced disease
Acid related	*Acid related*
Mucosal damage, e.g. gastric carcinoma	Mucosal damage, e.g. oesophageal candidiasis or CMV
Excessive acid production (→ ulceration), e.g. gastrinoma in Zollinger–Ellison syndrome	
Dysmotility	*Dysmotility*
Small stomach capacity, e.g. large stomach cancer or massive ascites	Minimal food and fluid intake
Gatroparesis (e.g. paraneoplastic autonomic neuropathy)	Depression/anxiety
Caused by treatment	**Concurrent disease**
Acid related	*Acid related*
Physical irritant (→ gastritis), e.g. iron, metronidazole, tranexamic acid	Chronic peptic ulcer disease
Loss of mucosal protection (→ gastropathy), e.g. NSAIDs	*H. pylori* infection
Delayed mucosal healing, e.g. corticosteroids, NSAIDs	Gastro-oesophageal reflux disease (GORD)
Radiotherapy to lumbar spine or epigastrium (→ mucosal damage)	Dysmotility
Dysmotility	Functional (non-ulcer) dyspepsia
Postsurgical, e.g. gastrectomy	Alcoholism
Delayed gastric emptying, e.g. anticholinergics, opioids, cisplatin	Uraemia
Reduced tone of lower oesophageal sphincter	Diabetes mellitus

shadow over this surprisingly widely used group of drugs (see Chapter 10.1.7)[159].

Corticosteroids
Evidence suggests that the conventional view that corticosteroids cause ulceration can be attributed to the risks due to concurrent use of NSAIDs[160,161]. Although this is a view that is still considered uncertain and controversial[162], the concurrent use of an NSAID and a corticosteroid in doses equivalent to 10 mg or more of prednisolone per day increases the risk of ulcer haemorrhage by a factor of nearly 15[160].

Peptic ulcer disease
Although NSAIDs can cause acute ulceration, there is much less evidence of their role in chronic ulceration. The strongest causal link with peptic ulceration is *H. pylori* infection which is associated with 95 per cent of duodenal ulcers and 70 per cent of gastric ulcers[163,164].

Functional dysmotility (non-ulcer) dyspepsia
This type of dyspepsia has a low frequency of *H. pylori* infection[163,165], but there is evidence of a weak association with oesophageal and gastric transit delay[166,167]. Most cases of cancer associated dyspepsia syndrome[168] are probably examples of dysmotility exacerbated by opioid-induced delayed gastric emptying and/or gross hepatomegaly and/or gross ascites. A few cancer patients complain of marked early satiety (a sensation that the stomach is full soon after eating) and/or other dyspeptic symptoms without any obvious predisposing cause[169]. In cancer, this probably relates to paraneoplastic visceral autonomic neuropathy[170], but it may also be a mechanism in non-cancer patients[171]. There is often associated evidence of impaired autonomic control of the cardiovascular system manifesting, for example, as postural hypotension. Many drugs have an adverse effect on lower oesophageal sphincter tone and the use of morphine and other opioids may lead to reflux secondary to delayed gastric emptying. Lower oesophageal tone can be decreased by alcohol, nicotine, caminatives

(mint, anise, dill), anticholinergics, pethidine (meperidine), benzodiazepines, nitrates and calcium channel blockers; and can be increased by antacids, prokinetic drugs (metoclopramide, domperidone), and parasympathomimetics (e.g. bethanechol). Psychiatric disorders, mainly depression and anxiety, have been observed in over half of patients with functional oesophageal dysmotility dyspepsia, rising to nearly 80 per cent if pain was absent as a feature, suggesting the possibility that long-term distress, anxiety and depression can influence functional dyspepsia symptoms[172]. Chronic alcoholism and uraemia are two further conditions that have been shown to reduce gastric activity[173,174], and both are known to be associated with dyspepsia.

Gastro-oesophageal reflux disease (GORD)
While some reflux is normal, repeated exposure of the lower oesophagus to gastric contents has been considered to be reflux disease once mucosal damage occurs that can be visualized on endoscopy[143]. Most reflux occurs after food during the day, but the change to severe oesophagitis is accelerated by nocturnal reflux of acidic gastric contents. However, the symptoms of GORD do not equate with endoscopic evidence of oesophagitis[175], and this may explain the disagreement over its inclusion as a cause of dyspepsia. GORD therefore seems to be a syndrome consisting of classic symptoms of heartburn (especially on bending and lying flat) and epigastric pain, with atypical symptoms of vomiting, dental enamel erosion, cardiac pain, respiratory symptoms (e.g. nocturnal postprandial asthma), and ear, nose and throat problems (e.g. hoarseness). GORD occurs in up to 75 per cent of neurologically impaired children[176,177].

Evaluation
A study in 7270 patients with abdominal symptoms showed three distinct symptom patterns relating to dyspepsia (Table 10.2.2.7)[141]. Structural, acid-related dyspepsia was most likely to be accompanied by pain restricted to the epigastrium, pain relief with antacids, acid regurgitation, heartburn and pain at night.

Two functional (non-ulcer) types of dysmotility were identified. Gastric and/or duodenal dysmotility had nausea, together with vomiting that occurred in the morning and relieved any pain. Oesophageal dysmotility had pain after meals (but not relieved by food) and dysphagia as the main features. Other symptoms were present, but showed a low correlation with any one type of dyspepsia. GORD was not included in this study, but its main features of heartburn, regurgitation and, occasionally, dysphagia (due to a stricture or mucosal oedema) overlap with the symptoms of structural dyspepsia and oesophageal dysmotility dyspepsia[143].

It is important to differentiate between these conditions because the treatment differs. Careful history-taking and clinical examination generally indicate which type is predominant. Investigations are now reserved for patients who have not responded to initial treatment with antacids or antisecretory drugs[178]. The most important investigation is to test for *H. pylori* infection by laboratory serum immunoabsorbant assay, stool antigen test, or the urea breath test. Endoscopy is needed if alarm symptoms are present (i.e. symptoms that should prompt referral for investigation), symptoms persist, or the *H. pylori* test is positive. Barium studies are necessary only in a few patients.

Management

General

As always, treatment begins with explanation. There may be a need for advice on diet, smoking and alcohol. The causal role, if any, of medication should be discussed. Some patients keep over-the-counter proprietary 'indigestion' tablets or mixture in the home. The use of these for occasional dyspepsia can be supported provided the discomfort is relieved.

Clinical decisions for dyspepsia

1   Are there any alarm symptoms?
2   Could this be acid-related dyspepsia?
3   Could this be a functional (dysmotility or non-ulcer) dyspepsia?
4   Could this be gastro-oesophageal reflux disease (GORD)?
5   Is the dyspepsia persisting?

1. Are there any alarm symptoms?

A number of symptoms should prompt urgent referral for investigation[164]:

- chronic gastrointestinal bleeding;
- unintentional weight loss;
- dysphagia;
- persistent vomiting;
- iron deficiency anaemia;
- epigastric mass;
- suspicious findings after a barium meal;
- patients over 55 years with recent, persistent or unexplained dyspepsia.

Some patients will be too ill from their advanced disease to benefit from hospital admission, while others will choose not to be treated. These patients will require adequate analgesia, antiemetics, comfort and company for their last days and hours.

2. Could this be structural (acid-related) dyspepsia?

If bleeding: intravenous fluid or blood should be given if this is needed or appropriate. Sucralfate 2 g every 4 h is also an efficient haemostatic agent that will reduce or stop gastric bleeding[179].Some patients will be fit enough to be referred for urgent endoscopy.

Check if H. pylori infection is present: the two most accurate diagnostic methods are the urea breath test and the stool antigen test, but antibiotics should have been stopped for 4 weeks, proton pump inhibitors for 2 weeks, and H_2 inhibitors for 1 day before the investigations. Drugs do not have to be stopped before a serology test, but it has a high false positive rate[164]. Patients with a positive result should be treated with a 7-day, twice daily course of a full dose proton pump inhibitor plus either (a) metronidazole 400 mg + clarithromycin 250 mg, or (b) amoxicillin 1 g + clarithromycin 500 mg[180].

Treat mucosal damage: any existing ulceration or mucosal damage needs to be treated with a proton pump inhibitor[181]. Omeprazole 20 mg or lansoprazole 30 mg once daily are both effective in treating chronic peptic ulceration and NSAID ulceration. Higher doses can be used for resistant ulceration. Sucralfate is a mucosal protective agent that is effective at both preventing and healing peptic ulceration[182], including NSAID-induced dyspepsia and ulceration[183]. Of the two commonly available antisecretory H_2-receptor antagonists, ranitidine is preferable to cimetidine because the likelihood of drug interactions is much less. For example, cimetidine (but not ranitidine) inhibits methadone metabolism and on occasion this has resulted in respiratory depression and coma[184]. An initial dose of ranitidine 300 mg at bedtime for 2 weeks followed by 150 mg at bedtime is generally sufficient.

Stop irritant drugs: drug medication needs to be reviewed to stop or change the formulation of physical irritants such as iron.

For patients on an NSAID: for many palliative care patients who develop dyspepsia with an NSAID, the safest solution is to stop the NSAID and find an alternative method of analgesia. However, if the NSAID has been the only method offering good pain relief then the alternatives are:

- *Start a protective agent:* omeprazole 20 mg once daily has been shown to be more effective than misoprostol 400 mcg 12-hourly in preventing NSAID ulceration[185]. However, the same study showed that for gastric erosions, misoprostol was more effective. Misoprostol sometimes causes diarrhoea, but this has the advantage that it can be used as a 'co-laxative' in constipated patients. H_2-receptor antagonists prevent NSAID-related duodenal ulceration, but they do not prevent NSAID-related gastric ulceration[186].

- *Change NSAID:* using a non-selective NSAID with a proton pump inhibitor provides greater protection than switching to a COX-2 selective NSAID alone[187].

3. Do the symptoms suggest a functional (dysmotility) dyspepsia?

If the features for dysmotility dyspepsia in Table 10.2.2.7 are present then a prokinetic drug needs to be started[188]. Tumour-related gastroparesis also benefits from a prokinetic[189,190]. The choice lies between metoclopramide (dopamine antagonist and 5-HT_4 agonist) and domperidone (dopamine antagonist)[191]. Both trigger the cholinergic system in the myenteric plexus. Despite its dual mechanism of action, metoclopramide is not more potent than domperidone when used in standard doses, that is,

10 mg 6–8 hourly[192,193]. Domperidone has the advantage of being very unlikely to cause extrapyramidal symptoms. In the initial phase of treatment the prokinetic should be given by a non-oral route (e.g. subcutaneous for metoclopramide, rectal for domperidone).

A review of the drugs taken may reveal causes of reduced motility.

If dyspepsia is associated with a small stomach capacity, patients should be advised to separate their main fluid from their main solid intake, and to eat 'small and often', that is, take five or six small meals/snacks during the day rather than two or three big meals. Patients with a small stomach capacity may benefit from a defoaming agent after meals to separate fluid and air, and so allow the air to be brought up, thus clearing space in a relatively overfull stomach. An example of a defoaming agent is silica activated dimethicone/simethicone (as in Asilone®)[194].

4. Could this be GORD?

An antacid containing simethicone is superior to a plain antacid in the management of reflux oesophagitis[195]. Proton pump inhibitors are effective for treatment and maintenance of acid reflux[196]. If bile salts are being refluxed then hydrotalcite (magnesium aluminium carbonate hydrate) is a naturally occurring antacid that reversibly binds bile acids but needs an acid medium, so would be much less effective in combination with proton pump inhibitors or after gastrectomy[197]. At higher bile acid concentrations, cholestyramine is more efficacious than hydrotalcite[198]. No dose regimen for this condition has been established but it is suggested that 2 g cholestyramine (half a sachet) four times a day (after meals and at bedtime) might be tried[199]. There is a likelihood of steatorrhoea and, if treatment is long continued, supplements of fat-soluble vitamins A, D, E, and K should be considered.

5. Is the dyspepsia persisting?

Other causes of mucosal damage need to be considered. Malignant ulceration will cause pain and may either need a mucosal protective agent such as sucralfate, or a local anaesthetic such as oxetacaine mixed with an antacid. Mucosal damage due to infection such as candida, CMV or herpes can be extensive and will need specific antimicrobial treatment. If dysmotility persists, consider using the prokinetic erythromycin 100–250 mg 12 hourly, a potent motilin agonist[200–202].

Key points on dyspepsia

◆ Dyspepsia is an imprecise term, but the current view is that there are two types: acid-related causes visible on endoscopy and disordered motility of the upper gastrointestinal tract.

◆ GORD is now considered to be a separate condition, but its symptoms overlap those of dyspepsia.

◆ NSAIDs are a major cause of dyspepsia.

◆ Alarm symptoms (clinical deterioration, bleeding, severe dysphagia, or persistent pain) should prompt urgent admission, unless the patient is too ill from their advanced disease or they choose not to receive further treatment.

◆ Acid-related dyspepsia is best treated with a proton pump inhibitor.

◆ The risk of NSAID ulceration is reduced most effectively by proton pump inhibitors—H$_2$ antagonists do not prevent gastric ulceration. There is little to be gained by switching to a COX-2 selective NSAID and stopping the NSAID is the most effective strategy.

◆ Dysmotility dyspepsia is best treated by a prokinetic drug.

◆ If dyspepsia persists consider mucosal ulceration, mucosal infection, or gastro-oesophageal reflux.

Hiccup

Definition

Hiccup is a pathological respiratory reflex characterized by spasm of one or both sides of the diaphragm, resulting in sudden inspiration and closure of the glottis. Accessory muscles of respiration (anterior scalene, intercostal, abdominal) are occasionally involved[203].

Prevalence

Occasional hiccup is such a common human experience that it only warrants designation as a symptom when it is severe and intractable[204]. Over a 28-year period at the Mayo Clinic, 220 patients reported hiccup lasting for more than 2 days[205]. The prevalence of troublesome hiccup in terminal disease is not known. Children are more prone to hiccups than adults and in one series of 200 children premedicated with midazolam prior to minor surgery, 22 per cent developed hiccups[206]. It shows a circadian rhythm, being more common in the evening[207].

Mechanisms and causes

In the Mayo clinic series 82 per cent of those with hiccups were men[207]. Of the 220 patients with hiccup, 66 per cent had medical problems, 22 per cent were diagnosed as having a psychological cause and 18 per cent were postoperative. Specific diagnoses included cerebrovascular and coronary heart disease (20 per cent), hiatus hernia (15 per cent), duodenal ulcer (5 per cent), and metabolic disturbances (mainly diabetes mellitus and uraemia) (5 per cent). Many had two concurrent disorders. In terminal disease, clinical experience suggests that gastric distension is the commonest cause. Other relatively common causes include diaphragmatic irritation and toxicity (uraemia or infection). Less common causes include phrenic nerve irritation and CNS tumour. Hiccup is occasionally the presenting symptom of neoplasms of the brain stem and oesophagus[208,209]. Persistent hiccup occurs, therefore, in association with one or more of many diseases (Table 10.2.2.9). In addition, a wide variety of drugs have been reported as causing hiccup, with some of the same drugs being reported to cure hiccup (Table 10.2.2.10).

Persistent hiccup is generally considered to be pathological because it appears to serve no useful function[210]. Because of an association with eating, it has been suggested that hiccup may serve to shift food lodged in the oesophagus[211]. The relationship of hiccup to gastric distension, however, probably explains this association. Hiccup appears to be a reflex that is not under direct cortical control and there is evidence that it penetrates all stages of sleep, although it is modified by different sleep stages[209,212]. The fact that the pharynx is the cross-over point for both air and food/fluid suggests powerful mechanisms exist to favour only one at a time. This 'singleness of action' was proposed over 75 years ago[213] and more recently it has been suggested that a failure of this control is the cause for hiccup[209]. This theory suggests that the brainstem

Table 10.2.2.9 Selected causes of hiccups in advanced disease.[206]

Caused by the disease process	Associated with advanced disease
Irritation of the vagus nerve	
Hepatomegaly	Pneumonia
Intra-abdominal tumour	Bowel obstruction
Oesophageal tumour	Oesophageal irritation (e.g. infection, stent)
Prostatic cancer	Gastrointestinal bleeding
	Hydronephrosis
	Urinary tract infection
Irritation of the phrenic nerve	
Mediastinal tumour or sarcoid	Pleurisy or empyema
Tumour involving diaphragm	
Cervical tumour	
Central nervous system	
Intracranial tumours	Encephalitis
Brainstem lesions (tumour, infarct, multiple sclerosis)	Toxic (renal failure)
	Hyponatraemia
	Psychological
Caused by treatment	**Concurrent disease**
Irritation of the vagus nerve	
Surgery	Pancreatitis
Gastric distension	Oesophageal reflux
Gastritis	Oesophageal obstruction
	Coronary occlusion
Irritation of the phrenic nerve	
Surgery	Subphrenic abscess
Central nervous system	
Drugs (see Table 10.2.2.10)	Basilar arterial insufficiency
Hypocalcaemia (e.g. due to bisphosphonates)	Head injury
	Meningitis
Hypocapnia	Toxic (alcohol)
	Multiple sclerosis

Table 10.2.2.10 Drug causes and treatments of hiccup.

Reported drug causes of hiccup	Reported drug treatments of hiccup
Corticosteroids (dexamethasone, prednisolone, methylprednisolone)	Anticonvulsants (carbamazepine, gabapentin, valproate)
Chemotherapeutic drugs (cisplatin, etoposide)	Calcium channel blockers (nifedipine, nimodipine)
Dopamine antagonists (perphenazine)	Corticosteroids (dexamethasone, prednisolone, methylprednisolone)
Megestrol acetate	Dopamine antagonists (chlorpromazine, haloperidol, droperidol)
Methyldopa	Ketamine
Nicotine	Marijuana
Opioids (diamorphine, hydrocodone)	SSRI antidepressants (sertraline)
Skeletal muscle relaxants (chlordiazepoxide, diazepam, midazolam)	Skeletal muscle relaxants (chlordiazepoxide, baclofen, midazolam)
	Methylphenidate

connections to the phrenic nerve nuclei, reticular formation, and hypothalamus.

◆ *From centre to periphery (efferent pathway)*: primarily the phrenic nerve to diaphragm. Occasional patients continue to hiccup despite surgical section of both phrenic nerves[207]. In these patients, the efferent pathway will involve the accessory muscles of respiration.

The receptors involved in this reflex arc are not known, but the nature of the drugs that both cause and treat hiccups (Table 10.2.2.10) suggest that dopamine, serotonin, opioid, calcium channel, and GABA pathways may be involved[218].

Evaluation

There is no difficulty recognizing the presence of persistent hiccups, although only the patient can decide how troublesome it is to them. Rarely, hiccup is a major cause of distress[219], interrupting talking, eating, and sleeping, and resulting in weight loss, exhaustion, anxiety, and depression. In such situations treatable causes need to be found. Knowing the past surgical history and the current extent of any tumour from examination or recent scans can help identify the possibility of local pressure or damage to the vagus nerve, phrenic nerve or to the lower medulla. Symptoms of acid-related dyspepsia (Table 10.2.2.7) may identify a gastritis or symptoms suggesting GORD. A history of dysphagia, or pain on swallowing (odynophagia), may suggest oesophageal mucosal damage (infection, tumour), oesophageal dysmotility dyspepsia, or physical obstruction. Gastric hypomotility is suggested by feeling full after only a little food (early satiety), epigastric fullness, heartburn or vomiting with brief or little nausea (together with relief after vomiting). Chest examination and a bedside urine test will check for chest or urine infections, while testing for faecal occult blood in the faeces will check for upper gastrointestinal bleeding. An electrocardiogram will help to identify cardiac ischaemia. Blood biochemistry will check for causes such as hyponatraemia, hypocalcaemia, uraemia, and myocardial infarction. In advanced

complex which closes the glottis is never activated at the same time as the brainstem complex which stops respiration—one is inhibited while the other is activated and vice versa. In pathological situations the two are activated together. This hypothesis is supported by two observations: (1) the two complexes are next to each other in the dorsal part of the lower medulla;[209] and (2) damage to the part of the medulla containing these two complexes can result in severe and intractable hiccup[214–216]. The reported benefits of drugs that reduce CNS excitation such as benzodiazepines and anticonvulsants suggest that they are suppressing an abnormal signal bouncing back and forth between the two centres[209]. The reflex arc for hiccup is more extensive however[209,217]:

◆ *From periphery to centre (afferent pathway)*: vagus nerve, phrenic nerve, or thoracic sympathetic fibres.

◆ *The central connections*: the inspiratory and glottis control centres in the posterior lower medulla. In addition, there may be disease, it is unusual to carry out more complex investigations for hiccup.

Management

Clinical decisions for hiccup

1 Are the hiccups troublesome to the patient?

2 Is infection present?

3 Is a drug the cause?

4 Is a biochemical cause present?

5 Is peritumour oedema a likely cause?

6 Are the hiccups persisting?

1. Are the hiccups troublesome to the patient?

Hiccups can be mild and intermittent and may respond to simple physical treatments, but more severe hiccups are distressing[220]. Stimulation of the pharynx with a plastic or rubber suction catheter was successful in the treatment of hiccup in 84 out of 85 patients, 65 of whom were anaesthetized[221]. Stimulation of the pharynx by an oral catheter is equally effective. The nasal route is better tolerated in conscious patients[222]. Nebulized saline every 4 h has been used successfully in one patient whose hiccup failed to respond to various drugs[223]. Palatal massage is also successful in stopping hiccup[224]. A cotton-wool 'bob' is inserted into the mouth and used to massage the anterior soft palate in the midline for about 1 min. Other 'folk' remedies involve pharyngeal stimulation such as the rapid ingestion of two heaped teaspoons of granulated sugar, the rapid ingestion of two glasses of liqueur, swallowing dry bread, swallowing crushed ice, drinking from the wrong side of a cup, or a cold key dropped down the collar of the shirt or blouse[225]. Other remedies such as breath holding and rebreathing into a bag are also physiological since the resultant hypercapnia has a central depressant effect and blocks the central component of the reflex[226]. Deep breathing and chest physiotherapy also may disrupt the repetitive diaphragmatic spasms.

2. Is infection present?

Infections in the chest, urine, or affecting the oesophageal mucosa (e.g. candida, herepes zoster, hereps simplex, CMV) are treated conventionally with appropriate antimicrobials. For oesophageal mucosal damage, pain can be helped with a mixture of antacid and local anaesthetic (e.g. oxetacaine) 15 min before eating or drinking.

3. Is a drug the cause?

The onset of hiccups after starting a new drug (taking into account the time for that drug to reach a steady blood level—usually 5 half-lives) suggests that drug as a cause and a therapeutic trial of stopping the drug is worthwhile. Some drugs have been reported to both cause and treat hiccups (corticosteroids, dopamine antagonists, and benzodiazepines) suggesting that if these drugs are suspected, rather than being stopped, their dose should be reduced.

4. Is a biochemical cause present?

Renal failure may be irreversible unless stenting or haemodialysis is possible. Hypocalcaemia after treatment with bisphosphonates is unusual, but is easily treated with 10 ml (2.25 mmol) calcium gluconate 10 per cent solution followed by a continuous infusion of 40 ml (9 mmol) daily. Hyponatraemia severe enough to cause

hiccups needs to be investigated. If it is due to inappropriate ADH secretion, democycline can be used.

5. Is peritumour oedema a likely cause?

If tumour is compressing surrounding structures, the use of dexamethasone may reduce peritumour oedema and so relieve pressure. Doses of 8 mg orally or subcutaneously once in the morning is a reasonable starting dose. Higher doses are only needed if very urgent oedema reduction is needed or lower doses have failed.

6. Are the hiccups persisting?

Unusual causes such as brainstem lesions need to be considered, but treatment is needed to relieve the hiccups. If gastric distension is suspected, a 2-day trial of a defoaming agent (e.g. silica activated dimethicone/simethicone) before or after meals and at bedtime should be considered, together with a prokinetic. With more troublesome hiccup, a combination of simethicone and a prokinetic drug (metoclopramide, domperidone) should be used. At some centres, peppermint water is used as first-line treatment. Although this facilitates belching by relaxing the lower oesophageal sphincter, it does not have a defoaming action on the gastric contents. It is therefore probably less effective than a defoaming agent, although no controlled trials have been reported. The concurrent use of metoclopramide and peppermint should be discouraged since there is little sense in deliberately combining two drugs with opposing actions on the lower oesophageal sphincter. A defoaming agent and enhanced belching is preferable to a permanently relaxed oesophageal sphincter.

Drug treatments that have been tried are:

- *Baclofen:* there is now increasing evidence of the effectiveness of baclofen, although the numbers of patients in studies is small[227,228]. It is effective in doses as small as 5–10 mg twice a day, although occasionally 20 mg three times a day have been necessary.

- *Gabapentin* 300–600 mg orally 8-hourly alone[229]; or in addition to baclofen.[230]

- *Nifedipine* 10–20 mg orally or sublingually 8-hourly.[231]

- *Haloperidol* 3 mg orally at bedtime, but other regimens have been suggested.[232]

- *Methylphenidate* 10 mg orally.[233]

- *Midazolam:* starting with 1 mg intravenously or 2.5 mg subcutaneously and repeated at 2-min intervals for the intravenous route and 15-min intervals for the subcutaneous route until the hiccups settle, but short of producing sedation[234]. The midazolam can be continued as a continuous subcutaneous infusion using doses of 30–120 mg/24 h.

Although widely used in the past, chlorpromazine can no longer be recommended because of its adverse effects. Although destroying the efferent arc of the hiccup reflex by crushing one or both phrenic nerves might seem an attractive option for resistant cases, this has never been necessary in the author's experience. Phrenic nerve stimulation is another possible option[235].

Key points for hiccup

- Hiccup may be due to an abnormal reciprocating circuit between inspiratory and swallowing centres in the lower medulla, caused by stimulation or damage to the vagus nerve, the phrenic nerve, or the brainstem.

◆ A wide variety of diseases and conditions can cause hiccup—reversible causes need to be considered.

◆ Simple physical treatments are often effective.

◆ In persistent hiccup, baclofen is the drug of choice, with parenteral midazolam being used for intractable cases of distressing hiccup.

Acknowledgements

The author would like to recognize and thank Dr Robert Twycross who co-authored earlier editions of this chapter, and on which this updated chapter is based. Particular thanks go to Hannah Crawford, Speech and Language Therapist, Tees, Esk and Wear Valleys NHS Trust, and Sue Clark, Head Speech and Language Therapist, Royal Victoria Hospital, Newcastle upon Tyne for their invaluable advice on the dysphagia section.

References

1. Twycross, R.G. and Lack, S.A. (1986). *Control of alimentary symptoms in far advanced cancer*. Churchill Livingstone, Edinburgh.

2. Sykes, N.P., Baines, M., and Carter, R.L. (1988). Clinical and pathological study of dysphagia conservatively managed in patients with advanced malignant disease. *Lancet*, **2**, 726–8.

3. Regan, J., Sowman, R., and Walsh, I. (2006). Prevalence of Dysphagia in acute and community mental health settings. *Dysphagia*, **21**(2), 95–101.

4. Robertson, M.S. and Hornibrook, J. (1982). The presenting symptoms of head and neck cancer. *New Zealand Medical Journal*, **95**, 337–41.

5. Aird, D.W., Bihari, J., and Smith, C. (1983). Clinical problems in the continuing care of head and neck cancer patients. *Ear Nose and Throat Journal*, **62**, 10–30.

6. Stenson, K.M., MacCracken, E., List, M. *et al*. (2000). Swallowing function in patients with head and neck cancer prior to treatment. *Archives of Otolaryngology and Head and Neck Surgery*, **126**, 371–7.

7. Saunders, C., Walsh, T.D., and Smith, M. (1981). *A review of 100 cases of motor neuron disease in a hospice*. Edward Arnold, London.

8. O'Brien, T., Kelly, M., and Saunders, C. (1992). Motor neuron disease: a hospice perspective. *British Medical Journal*, **304**, 471–3.

9. Fuh, J.L., Lee, R.C., Lin, C.H. *et al*. (1997). Swallowing difficulty in Parkinson's disease. *Clinical Neurology and Neurosurgery*, **99**, 106–12.

10. Thomas, F.J. and Wiles, C.M. (1999). Dysphagia and nutritional status in multiple sclerosis. *Journal of Neurology*, **246**, 677–82.

11. Martino, R., Foley, N., Bhogal, S. *et al*. (2005). Dysphagia after stroke: incidence, diagnosis, and pulmonary complications. *Stroke*, **36**(12), 2756–63.

12. Terre, R. and Mearin, F. (2006). Oropharyngeal dysphagia after the acute phase of stroke: predictors of aspiration. *Neurogastroenterology & Motility*, **18**(3), 200–5.

13. Rademaker, A.W., Pauloski, B.R., Colangelo, L.A. *et al*. (1998). Age and volume effects on liquid swallowing function in normal women. *Journal of Speech, Language and Hearing Research*, **41**, 275–84.

14. Kayser-Jones, J. and Pengilly, K. (1999). Dysphagia among nursing home residents. *Geriatric Nursing*, **20**, 77–82.

15. Logemann, J.A. (1998). *Evaluation and treatment of swallowing disorders*. Pro-ed., Austin.

16. Duranceau, A., Jamieson, G., and Hurwitz, A.L. (1976). Alteration in esophageal motility after laryngectomy. *American Journal of Surgery*, **131**, 30–5.

17. Wu, C.H., Hsaio, T.Y., Ko, J.Y. *et al*. (2000). Dysphagia after radiotherapy: endoscopic examination of swallowing in patients with nasopharyngeal carcinoma. *Annals of Otology, Rhinology and Laryngology*, **109**, 320–5.

18. Carter, R., Pittam, M., and Tanner, N. (1982). Pain and dysphagia in patients with squamous carcinomas of the head and neck: the role of perineural spread. *Journal of the Royal Society of Medicine*, **75**, 598–606.

19. Perie, S., Coiffier, L., Laccourreye, L. *et al*. (1999). Swallowing disorders in paralysis of the lower cranial nerves: a functional analysis. *Annals of Otology, Rhinology and Laryngology*, **108**, 606–11.

20. Logemann, J., Blonsky, R.E., and Boshes, B. (1975). Dysphagia in parkinsonism. *Journal of the American Medical Association*, **231**, 69–70.

21. Leopold, N.A., and Kagel, M.C. (1997). Laryngeal deglutition movement in Parkinson's disease. *Neurology*, **48**, 373–6.

22. Hunter, P.C., Crameri, J., Austin, S. *et al*. (1997). Response of parkinsonian swallowing dysfunction to dopaminergic stimulation. *Journal of Neurology, Neurosurgery and Psychiatry*, **63**, 579–83.

23. Nagaya, M., Kachi, T., Yamada, T. *et al*. (1998). Videoflurographic study of swallowing in Parkinson's disease. *Dysphagia*, **13**, 95–100.

24. Potulska, A., Friedman, A., Krolicki, L. *et al*. (2003). Swallowing disorders in Parkinson's disease. *Parkinsonism & Related Disorders*, **9**(6), 349–53.

25. Weaver, A.W. and Fleming, S.M. (1978). Partial laryngectomy: analysis of associated swallowing disorders. *American Journal of Surgery*, **136**, 486–9.

26. Vantrappen, G., Janssens, J., and Ghillebert, G. (1987). The irritable oesophagus—a frequent cause of angina-like pain. *Lancet*, **1**, 1232–4.

27. Rogers, A.I., Abrams, K.S., and Presley, D. (1980). Can emotional stress induce esophageal spasm in man? *Gastroenterology*, **78**, 1246.

28. Kim, C.H., Hsu, J.J., Williams, D.E. *et al*. (1996). A prospective psychological evaluation of patients with dysphagia of various etiologies. *Dysphagia*, **11**, 34–40.

29. Schechter, G. (1998). Systemic causes of dysphagia. *Otolaryngologic Clinics of North America*, **31**(3), 525–35.

30. Sokoloff, L.G. and Pavlakovic, R. (1997). Neuroleptic-induced dysphagia. *Dysphagia*, **12**, 177–9.

31. Grieve, R. and Dixon, P. (1983). Dysphagia: a further symptom of hypercalcaemia. *British Medical Journal*, **286**, 1935–6.

32. Trier, J.S. and Bjorkman, D.J. (1984). Esophageal, gastric and intestinal candidiasis. *American Journal of Medicine*, **77**, 39–43.

33. Daniels, S.K. and Foundas, A.L. (1999). Lesion localization in acute stroke patients with risk of aspiration. *Journal of Neuroimaging*, **9**(2), 91–8.

34. Hildebrandt, G.H. Dominguez, L., Schork, M.A. *et al*. (1997). Functional units, chewing, swallowing and food avoidance among the elderly. *Journal of Prosthetic Dentistry*, **77**, 588–95.

35. Caruso, A.J. and Max, L. (1997). Effects of aging on neuromotor processes of swallowing. *Seminars in Speech and Language*, **18**, 181–92.

36. Aviv, J.E. (1997). Effects of aging on sensitivity of the pharyngeal and supraglottic areas. *American Journal of Medicine*, **103**(5A), 74S–6S.

37. Kayser-Jones, J. Schell, E.S., Porter, C. *et al*. (1999). Factors contributing to dehydration in nursing homes: inadequate staffing and lack of professional supervision. *Journal of the American Geriatrics Society*, **47**, 1187–94.

38. Logemann, J.A. (1985). Aspiration in head and neck surgical patients. *Annals of Otology, Rhinology and Laryngology*, **94**, 373–6.

39. McHorney, C.A., Bricker, D.E., Kramer, A.E. *et al.* (2000). The SWAL-QOL outcomes tool for oropharyngeal dysphagia in adults: I. Conceptual foundation and item development. *Dysphagia*, **15**, 115–21.

40. McHorney, C.A., Bricker, D.E., Robbins, J. *et al.* (2000). The SWAL-QOL outcomes tool for oropharyngeal dysphagia in adults: II. Item reduction and preliminary scaling. *Dysphagia*, **15**, 134–5.

41. Salassa, J.R. (1999). A functional outcome swallowing scale for staging oropharyngeal dysphagia. *Digestive Diseases*, **17**, 230–4.

42. Dray, T.G., Hilliel, A.D., and Miller, R.M. (1998). Dysphagia caused by neurologic deficits. *Otolayngologic Clinics of North America*, **31**(3), 507–24.

43. O'Neil, K.H., Purdy, M., Falk, J. *et al.* (1999). The dysphagia outcome and severity scale. *Dysphagia*, **14**, 139–45.

44. Logemann, J.A., Veis, S., and Colangelo, L. (1999). A screening procedure for oropharyngeal dysphagia. *Dysphagia*, **14**, 44–51.

45. Wallace, K.L., Middleton, S., and Cook, I.J. (2000). Development and validation of a self-report symptom inventory to assess the severity of oral-pharyngeal dysphagia. *Gastroenterology*, **118**, 678–87.

46. O'Loughlin, G. and Shanley, C. (1998). Swallowing problems in the nursing home: a novel training exercise. *Dysphagia*, **13**, 172–83.

47. Crawford, H. (2007). Dysphagia in people with profound and multiple learning disability. In *Profound and Multiple learning disabilities: nursing complex needs* (eds. J. Pawlyn and S. Carnaby). Blackwells, Edinburgh.

48. Eckman, S. and Roe, J. (2005). Speech and language therapists in palliative care: what do we have to offer? *International Journal of Palliative Nursing*, **11**(4), 179–81.

49. Pollens, R. (2004). Role of the speech-language pathologist in palliative hospice care. *Journal of Palliative Medicine*, **7**(5), 694–702.

50. DePippo, K.L., Holas, M.A., and Reding, M.J. (1994). The Burke dysphagia screening test: validation of its use in patients with stroke. *Archives of Physical and Medical Rehabilitation*, **75**, 1284–6.

51. Smithard, D.G. and Crockford, C. (1997). The swallow test. *RCSLT Bulletin*, January, 7–8.

52. Hughes, T.A. and Wiles, C.M. (1996). Measurement of swallowing in patients with sore throats. *Clinical Otolaryngology and Allied Sciences*, **21**, 305–7.

53. Logemann, J.A. (1999). Do we know what is normal and abnormal airway protection? *Dysphagia*, **14**, 233–4.

54. Warms, T. and Richards, J. (2000). 'Wet voice' as a predictor of penetration and aspiration in oropharyngeal dysphagia. *Dysphagia*, **15**, 84–8.

55. Sherman, B., Nisenboum, J.M., Jesberger, B.L. *et al.* (1999). Assessment of dysphagia with the use of pulse oximetry. *Dysphagia*, **14**, 152–6.

56. Collins, M.J. and Bakheit, A.M. (1997). Does pulse oximetry reliably detect aspiration in dysphagic stroke patients? *Stroke*, **28**, 1773–5.

57. Farell, Z. and O-Neill, D. (1999). Towards better screening and assessment of oropharyngeal swallow disorders in the general hospital. *Lancet*, **354**, 355–6.

58. Hughes, T.A. and Wiles, C.M. (1996). Palatal and pharyngeal reflexes in health and in motor neuron disease. *Journal of Neurology, Neurosurgery and Psychiatry*, **61**, 96–8.

59. Leder, S.B. (1996). Gag reflex and dysphagia. *Head and Neck*, **18**, 138–41.

60. Bastian, R.W. (1998). Contemporary diagnosis of the dysphagic patient. *Otolaryngologic Clinics of North America*, **31**, 489–506.

61. O'Donaghue, S. and Bagnall, A. (1999). Videofluoroscopic evaluation in the assessment of swallowing disorders in paediatric and adult populations. *Folio Phoniatrica et Logopedica*, **51**, 158–71.

62. Tohara, H., Saitoh, E., Mays, K. *et al.* (2003). Three tests for predicting aspiration without videofluroscopy. *Dysphagia*, **18**, 126–34.

63. Mathers-Schmidt, B.A. and Kurlinski, M. (2003). Dysphagia evaluation practices: inconsistencies in clinical assessment and instrumental examination decision-making. *Dysphagia*, **18**, 114–25.

64. Broniatowski, M., Sonies, B.C., Rubin, J.S. *et al.* (1999). Current evaluation and treatment of patients with swallowing disorders. *Otolaryngology—Head and Neck Surgery*, **120**, 464–73.

65. Regnard, C. and Hockley, J. (2004). Dysphagia. In *A Guide to symptom relief in palliative care*, 5th edition (eds. C. Regnard, and J. Hockley), pp. 91–5.

66. McCann, R.M., Hall, W.J., and Groth-Juncker, A. (1994). Comfort care for terminally ill patients. The appropriate use of nutrition and hydration. *JAMA*, **272**(16), 1263–6.

67. Parkash, R. and Burge, F. (1997). The family's perspective on issues of hydration in terminal care. *Journal of Palliative Care*, **13**(4), 23–7.

68. Winter, S.M. (2000). Terminal nutrition: framing the debate for the withdrawal of nutritional support in terminally ill patients. *American Journal of Medicine*, **109**(9), 723–6.

69. Dunphy, K., Finlay, I., Rathbone, G. *et al.* (1995). Rehydration in palliative and terminal care: if not-why not? *Palliative Medicine*, **9**(3), 221–8.

70. Fainsinger, R.L. and Bruera, E. (1997). When to treat dehydration in a terminally patient? *Supportive Care in Cancer*, **5**, 205–11.

71. Lawlor, P.G., Gagnon, B., Mancini, I.L. *et al.* (2000). Occurrence, causes, and outcome of delirium in patients with advanced cancer: a prospective study. *Archives of Internal Medicine*, **160**(6), 786–94.

72. Carter, R., Smith, J.S., and Anderson, J.R. (1992). Laser recanalization versus endoscopic intubation in the palliation of malignant dysphagia: a randomized prospective study. *British Journal of Surgery*, **79**, 1167–70.

73. Aste, H., Munizzi, F., Martines, H. *et al.* (1985). Esophageal dilation in malignant dysphagia. *Cancer*, **11**, 2713–15.

74. Brewster, A.E., Davidson, S.E., Makin, W.P. *et al.* (1995). Intraluminal brachytherapy using the high dose rate microselectron in the palliation of carcinoma of the oesophagus. *Clinical Oncology*, **7**, 102–5.

75. Homs, M.Y., Steyerberg, E.W., Eijkenboom, W.M., Siersema, P.D., and Dutch SIREC Study Group. (2006). Predictors of outcome of single-dose brachytherapy for the palliation of dysphagia from esophageal cancer. *Brachytherapy*, **5**(1), 41–8.

76. Sanyka, C., Corr, P., and Haffejee, A. (1999). Palliative treatment of oesophageal carcinoma—efficacy of plastic versus self-expandable stents. *South African Medical Journal*, **89**, 640–3.

77. Birch, J.F., White, S.A., Berry, D.P. *et al.* (1998). A cost–benefit comparison of self-expanding metal stents and Atkinson tubes for the palliation of obstructing esophageal tumours. *Diseases of the Esophagus*, **11**, 172–6.

78. Ell, C., Hochberger, J., May, A. *et al.* (1994). Coated and uncoated self-expanding metal stents for malignant stenosis in the upper GI tract: preliminary clinical experiences with wallstents. *American Journal of Gastroenterology*, **89**, 1496–500.

79. Tytgat, G.N.J. and Tytgat, S. (1994). Esophageal endoprosthesis in malignant stricture. *Journal of Gastroenterology*, **29**, 80.

80. Bartelsman, J.F., Bruno, M.J., Jensema, A.J. *et al.* (2000). Palliation of patients with esophagogastric neoplasms by insertion of a covered expandable, modified Gianturico-Z endoprosthesis: experiences in 153 patients. *Gastrointestinal Endoscopy*, **51**, 134–8.

81. Singhvi, R., Abbasakoor, F., and Manson, J.M. (2000). Insertion of self-expanding metal stents for malignant dysphagia: assessment of a simple endoscopic method. *Annals of the Royal College of Surgeons of England*, **82**, 243–8.

82. Elphick, D.A., Smith, B.A., Bagshaw, J. *et al.* (2005). Self-expanding metal stents in the palliation of malignant dysphagia: outcome analysis in 100 consecutive patients. *Diseases of the Esophagus*, **18**(2), 93–5.

83. Thompson, A.M., Rapson, T., Gilbert, F.J. *et al.* (2004). Endoscopic palliative treatment for esophageal and gastric cancer: techniques, complications, and survival in a population-based cohort of 948 patients. *Surgical Endoscopy*, **18**(8), 1257–62.

84. Neale, J.C., Goulden, J.W., Allan, S.G. *et al.* (2004). Esophageal stents in malignant dysphagia: a two-edged sword? *Journal of Palliative Care,* **20**(1), 28–31.

85. Lewis-Jones, C.M., Sturgess, R., and Ellershaw, J.E. (1995). Laser therapy in the palliation of dysphagia in oesophageal malignancy. *Palliative Medicine,* **9**, 327–30.

86. Savage, A.P., Baigrie, R.J., Cobb, R.A. *et al.* (1997). Palliation of malignant dysphagia by laser therapy. *Diseases of the Esophagus,* **10**, 243–6.

87. Moghissi, K., Dixon, K., Thorpe, J.A. *et al.* (2000). The role of photodynamic therapy (PDT) in inoperable oesophageal cancer. *European Journal of Cardio-Thoracic Surgery,* **17**, 95–100.

88. Nwokolo, C.U., Payne-James, J.J., and Silk, D.B.A. (1994). Palliation of malignant dysphagia by ethanol induced tumour necrosis. *Gut,* **35**, 299–303.

89. Carazzone, A., Bonavina, L., Segalin, A. *et al.* (1999). Endoscopic palliation of oesophageal cancer: results of a prospective comparison of Nd:YAG laser and ethanol injection. *European Journal of Surgery,* **165**, 351–6.

90. Monga, S.P., Wadleigh, R., Sharma, A. *et al.* (2000). Intratumoral therapy of cisplatin/epinephrine injectable gel for palliation in patients with obstructive esophageal cancer. *American Journal of Clinical Oncology,* **23**, 386–92.

91. Robbins, J.A., Coyle, J., Rosenbek, J. *et al.* (1999). Differentiation of normal and abnormal airway protection during swallowing using the penetration-aspiration scale. *Dysphagia,* **14**, 228–32.

92. Ramsey, D., Smithard, D., and Kalra, L. (2005). Silent aspiration: what do we know? *Dysphagia,* **20**(3), 218–25.

93. Langmore, S.E., Terpenning, M.S., Schork, A. *et al.* (1998). Predictors of aspiration pneumonia: how important is dysphagia? *Dysphagia,* **13**, 69–81.

94. Loeb, M., McGeer, A., McArthur, M. *et al.* (1999). Risk factors for pneumonia and other lower respiratory tract infections in elderly residents of long-term care facilities. *Archives of Internal Medicine,* **159**, 2058–64.

95. Marik, P.E. (2001). Aspiration pneumonitis and aspiration pneumonia. *New England Journal of Medicine,* **344**, 665–71.

96. Davies, A., Brailsford, S., Broadley, K. *et al.* (2002). Resistance amongst yeasts isolated from the oral cavities of patients with advanced cancer. *Palliative Medicine,* **16**(6), 527–31.

97. Regnard, C. (1994). Single dose fluconazole versus five day ketoconazole in oral candidiasis. *Palliative Medicine,* **8**, 72–3.

98. Kerr, A.R. and Ship, J.A. (2003). Management strategies for HIV-associated aphthous stomatitis. *American Journal of Clinical Dermatology,* **4**(10), 669–80.

99. Graykowski, E.A. and Kingman, A. (1978). Double-blind trial of tetracycline in recurrent aphthous ulceration. *Journal of Oral Pathology,* **7**(6), 376–82.

100. Youle, M., Clarbour, J., and Farthing, C. (1989). Treatment of resistant apthous ulceration with thalidomide in patients positive for HIV antibody. *British Medical Journal,* **298**, 432.

101. Lucas, V.S., Roberts, G.J., Dixon, J.M. *et al.* (1998). Mouth care and skin care in palliative medicine. *British Medical Journal,* **316**, 1246–7.

102. Potting, C.M.J., Uitterhoeve, R., Scholte op Reimer, W. *et al.* (2006). The effectivenss of commonly used mouthwashes for the prevention of chemotherapy-induced mucositis: a systematic review. *European Journal of Cancer Care,* **15**, 431–9.

103. Davies, A.N., Daniels, C., Pugh, R. *et al.* (1998). A comparison of artificial saliva and pilocarpine in the management of xerostomia in patients with advanced cancer. *Palliative Medicine,* **12**, 105–11.

104. Gilbar, P.J. (1999). A guide to enteral drug administration in palliative care. *Journal of Pain & Symptom Management,* **17**(3), 197–207.

105. Charlesworth, S. (2007). Appendix 10: Administering drugs via feeding tubes. In *Palliative care formulary* (R.G. Twycross, A. Wilcock, S. Charlesworth, and A. Dickman). On www.palliativedrugs.com (accessed Feb 2007).

106. Wong, P.C., Dodd, M.J., Miaskowski, C. *et al.* (2006). Mucositis pain induced by radiation therapy: prevalence, severity and use of self-care behaviours. *Journal of Pain & Symptom Management,* **32**(1), 27–39.

107. Barasch, A., Elad, S., Altman, A. *et al.* (2006). Antimicrobials, mucosal coating agents, anesthetics, analgesics, and nutritional supplements for alimentary tract mucositis. *Supportive Care in Cancer,* **14**(6), 528–32.

108. Dodd, M.J. *et al.* (1996). Randomized clinical trial of chlorhexidine versus placebo for prevention of oral mucositis in patients receiving chemotherapy. *Oncology Nurse Forum,* **23**, 921–7.

109. Poertner, L.C. and Coleman, R.F. (1998). Swallowing therapy in adults. *Otolaryngologic Clinics of North America,* **31**, 561–79.

110. Unsworth, J. (1994). *Coping with the disability of established disease.* Chapman & Hall Medical, London.

111. Hargrove, R. (1980). Feeding the severely dysphagic patient. *Journal of Neurosurgical Nursing,* **12**, 102–7.

112. Mitchell, S.L., Kiely, D.K., and Lipsitz, L.A. (1997). The risk factors and impact on survival of feeding tube placement in nursing home residents with severe cognitive impairment. *Archives of Internal Medicine,* **157**, 327–32.

113. Finucane, T.E. and Bynum, J.P.W. (1996). Use of tube feeding to prevent aspiration pneumonia. *The Lancet,* **348**, 1421–4.

114. Scott, A.G. and Austin, H.E. (1994). Nasogastric feeding in the management of severe dysphagia in motor neuron disease. *Palliative Medicine,* **8**, 45–9.

115. Rudberg, M.A., Egleston, B.L., Grant, M.D. *et al.* (2000). Effectiveness of feeding tubes in nursing home residents with swallowing disorders. *Journal of Parenteral and Enteral Nutrition,* **24**, 97–102.

116. Meehan, S.E., Wood, R.A.B., and Cuschieri, A. (1984). Percutaneous cervical pharyngostomy: a comfortable and convenient alternative to protracted nasogastric intubation. *American Journal of Surgery,* **148**, 325–30.

117. Leighton, S.E.J., Burton, M.J., Lund, W.S. *et al.* (1994). Swallowing in motor neuron disease. *Journal of the Royal Society of Medicine,* **87**, 801–5.

118. Fainsinger, R.L., MacEachern, T., Miller, M.J. *et al.* (1994). The use of hypodermoclysis for rehydration in terminally ill cancer patients. *Journal of Pain and Symptom Management,* **9**, 298–302.

119. Ashby, M., Game, P., Devitt, P. *et al.* (1991). Percutaneous gastrostomy as a venting procedure in palliative care. *Palliative Medicine,* **5**, 147–50.

120. Boyd, K.J. and Beeken, L. (1994). Tube feeding in palliative care: benefits and problems. *Palliative Medicine,* **8**, 156–8.

121. Laing, B., Smithers, M., and Harper, J. (1994). Percutaneous fluoroscopic gastrostomy: a safe option? *Medical Journal of Australia,* **161**, 308–10.

122. Myssiorek, D., Siegel, D., and Vambutas, A. (1998). Fluoroscopically placed gastrostomies in the head and neck patient. *Laryngoscope,* **108**, 1557–60.

123. Norton, B., Homer-Ward, M., Donelly, M.T. *et al.* (1996). A randomised prospective comparison of percutaneous endoscopic gastrostomy and nasogastric tube feeding after dysphagic stroke. *British Medical Journal,* **312**, 13–16.

124. Dwolatzky, T., Berezovski, S., Friedmann, R. *et al.* (2001). A prospective comparison of the use of nasogastric and percutaneous endoscopic gastrostomy tubes for long-term enteral feeding in older people. *Clinical Nutrition,* **20**(6), 535–40.

125. Kimber, C.P. and Beasley, S.W. (1999). Limitations of percutaneous endoscopic gastrostomy in facilitating eneteral nutrition in children: review of the shortcomings of a new technique. *Journal of Paediatric and Child Health,* **35**, 427–31.

126. Keeley, P. (2002). Feeding tubes in palliative care. *European Journal of Palliative Care*, **9**(6), 229–31.

127. Mandal, A., Steel, A., Davidson, A.R. *et al.* (2000). Day-case percutaneous endoscopic gastrostomy: a viable proposition? *Postgraduate Medical Journal*, **76**, 157–9.

128. Campos, A.C.L., Butters, M., and Meguid, M.M. (1990). Home enteral nutrition via gastrostomy in advanced head and neck cancer patients. *Head and Neck*, **12**, 137–42.

129. Dharmarajan, T.S., Unnikrishnan, D., and Pitchumoni, C.S. (2001). Percutaneous endoscopic gastrostomy and outcome in dementia. *American Journal of Gastroenterology*, **96**(9), 2556–63.

130. Swaroop, V.S. and Bergstrom, L.R. (2003). Percutaneous endoscopic gastrostomy in clients with dementia. *American Journal of Gastroenterology*, **98**(8), 1904.

131. Murphy, L.M. and Lipman, T.O. (2003). Percutaneous endoscopic gastrostomy does not prolong survival in clients with dementia. *Archives of Internal Medicine*, **163**(11), 1351–3.

132. Sanders, D.S., Carter, M.J., D'Silva, J. *et al.* (2000). Survival analysis in percutaneous endoscopic gastrostomy feeding: a worse outcome in clients with dementia. *American Journal of Gastroenterology*, **95**(6), 1472–5.

133. Abuksis, G., Mor, M., Segal, N. *et al.* (2000). Percutaneous endoscopic gastrostomy: high mortality rates in hospitalized clients. *American Journal of Gastroenterology*, **95**(1), 128–32.

134. Hoffer, L.J. (2006). Tube feeding in advanced dementia: the metabolic perspective. *BMJ*, **333**, 1214–5.

135. Priefer, B.A. and Riobbins, J.A. (1997). Eating changes in mild-stage Alheimer's disease: a pilot study. *Dysphagia*, **12**, 212–21.

136. McHorney, C.A., Bricker, D.E., Kramer, A.E. *et al.* (2000). The SWAL-QOL outcomes tool for oropharyngeal dysphagia in adults: i. Conceptual foundation and item development. *Dysphagia*, **15**, 115–21.

137. Nair, S., Hertan, H., and Pitchumoni, C.S. (2000). Hypoalbuminemia is a poor predictor of survival after percutaneous endoscopic gastrostomy in elderly clients with dementia. *American Journal of Gastroenterology*, **95**(1), 133–6.

138. Kraft, M.D., Btaiche, I.F., and Sacks, G.S. (2005). Review of the refeeding syndrome. *Nutrition in Clinical Practice*, **20**(6), 625–33.

139. Crook, M.A. and Panteli, J.V. (2005). The refeeding syndrome and hypophosphataemia in the elderly. *Journal of Internal Medicine*, **257**(5), 397–8.

140. Chiba, N. (1998). Definitions of dyspepsia: time for a reappraisal. *European Journal of Surgery Supplement*, **583**, 14–23.

141. Meinechie-Schmidt, V. and Christensen, E. (1998). Classification of dyspepsia. *Scandinavian Journal of Gastroenterology*, **33**, 1262–72.

142. de Caestecker, J. (2001). ABC of the upper gastrointestinal tract. Oesophagus: heartburn. *British Medical Journal*, **323**, 736–9.

143. Grainger, S.L., Klass, H.J., Rake, M.O. *et al.* (1994). Prevalence of dyspepsia: the epidemiology of overlapping symptoms. *Postgraduate Medical Journal*, **70**, 154–61.

144. Moayyedi, P., Duffett, S., Braunholtz, D. *et al.* (1998). The Leeds Dyspepsia Questionnaire: a valid tool for measuring the presence and severity of dyspepsia. *Alimentary Pharmacology and Therapeutics*, **12**, 1257–62.

145. Woodward, M., Morrison, C.E., and McColl, K.E. (1999). The prevalence of dyspepsia and use of antisecretory medication in North Glasgow: role of *Helicobacter pylori* vs. lifestyle. *Alimentary Pharmacology and Therapeutics*, **13**, 1505–9.

146. Editorial (1986). Non-ulcer dyspepsia. *Lancet*, **1**, 1306–7.

147. Misiewicz, J.J. and Pounder, R.E. (1996). Peptic ulceration. In *Oxford textbook of medicine*, 3rd edition. on CD-ROM (eds. D.J. Weatherall, J.G.G. Ledingham, and D.A. Warrell), pp. 1877–91. Oxford University Press, Oxford.

148. Hawkey, C.J. (2000). Non-steroidal anti-inflammatory drug gastropathy. *Gastroenterology*, **119**, 521–35.

149. Hollenz, M., Stolte, M., Leodolter, A. *et al.* (2006). NSAID-associated dyspepsia and ulcers: a prospective cohort study in primary care. *Digestive Diseases*, **24**(1–2), 189–94.

150. Lambert, R. (1999). Digestive endoscopy: relevance of negative findings. *Italian Journal of Gastroenterology and Hepatology*, **31**, 761–72.

151. Hull, M.A., Brough, J.L., and Hawkey, C.J. (1999). Expression of cyclooxygenase-1 and -2 by human gastric endothelial cells. *Gut*, **45**, 529–36.

152. Schmassmann, A., Peskar, B.M., Stettler, C. *et al.* (1998). Effects of prostaglandin endoperoxide synthetase-2 in chronic gastrointestinal ulcer models in rats. *British Journal of Pharmacology*, **123**, 795–804.

153. Horie-Sakata, K., Schimida, T., Hiraishi, H. *et al.* (1998). Role of cyclooxygenase 2 in hepatocyte growth factor-mediated gastric epithelial restitution. *Journal of Clinical Gastroenterology*, **27**(Suppl. 1), **S40–6.**

154. Kelly, J.P., Kaufman, D.W., Jurgelon, J.M. *et al.* (1996). Risk of aspirin-associated major upper-gastrointestinal bleeding with enteric-coated or buffered product. *Lancet*, **348**, 1413–16.

155. Wolfe, M.M., Lichtenstein, D.R., and Sing, G. (1999). Gastrointestinal toxicity of non-steroidal anti-inflammatory drugs. *New England Journal of Medicine*, **340**, 1888–99.

156. Henry, D., Lim, L.L.-Y., Garcia Rodriquez, L.A. *et al.* (1996). The ability in risk of gastrointestinal complications with individual non-steroidal anti-inflammatory drugs: results of a collaborative meta-analysis. *British Medical Journal*, **312**, 1563–6.

157. Langman, M.J., Jensen, D.M., Watson, D.J. *et al.* (1999). Incidence of upper gastrointestinal perforations, symptomatic ulcers and bleeding (PUBS). Rofecoxib compared to NSAIDs. *Journal of the American Medical Association*, **282**, 1929–33.

158. Hippisley-Cox, J., Coupland, C., and Logan, R. (2005). Risk of adverse gastrointestinal outcomes in patients taking cyclo-oxygenase-2 inhibitors or conventional non-steroidal anti-inflammatory drugs: population based nested case-control analysis. *BMJ*, **331**, 1310–2.

159. Vonkeman, H.E., Brouwers, R.B.J., and van de Laar, M.A.F.J. (2006). Understanding the NSAID related risk of vascular events. *BMJ*, **332**, 895–8.

160. Piper, J.M., Ray, W.A., Daugherty, M.R. *et al.* (1991). Corticosteroid use and peptic ulcer disease: role of nonsteroidal anti-inflammatory drugs. *Annals of Internal Medicine*, **114**, 735–40.

161. Hochain, P., Berkelmans, I., Czernichow, P. *et al.* (1995). Which patients taking non-aspirin non-steroidal anti-inflammatory drugs bleed? A case–control study. *European Journal of Gastroenterology and Hepatology*, **7**, 419–26.

162. Weil, J., Langamn, M.J.S., Wainwright, P. *et al.* (2000). Peptic ulcer bleeding: accessory risk factors and interactions with non-steroidal anti-inflammatory drugs. *Gut*, **46**, 27–31.

163. Childs, S., Roberts, A., Meineche-Scmidt, V. *et al.* (2000). The management of *Helicobacter pylori* infection in primary care: a systematic review of the literature. *Family Practice*, **17**(Suppl 2), S6–11.

164. Shah, R. (2006). Dyspepsia and *Heliobacter pylori*. *BMJ*, **334**, 41–3.

165. Talley, N.J., Janssens, J., Lauritson, K. *et al.* (2000). Eradication of *Helicobacter pylori* in functional dyspepsia: randomised double blind placebo controlled trial with 12 month's follow up. The Optimal Regimen Cures Helicobacter Dyspepsia (ORCHID) Study Group. *British Medical Journal*, **318**, 833–7.

166. Chaudhuri, S., Santra, A., Dobe, P.B. *et al.* (2000). Esophageal and gastric dysmotility. *Indian Journal of Gastroenterology*, **19**, 109–11.

167. Talley, N.J., Locke, G.R. 3rd, Lahr, B.D. *et al*, (2006). Functional dyspepsia, delayed gastric emptying, and impaired quality of life. *Gut*, **55**(7), 933–9.

168. Nelson, K., Walsh, T., O'Donovan, P. *et al.* (1993). Assessment of upper gastrointestinal motility in the cancer-associated dyspepsia syndrome (CADS). *Journal of Palliative Care,* 9, 27–31.

169. Armes, P.J., Plant, H.J., Allbright, A. *et al.* (1992). A study to investigate the incidence of early satiety in patients with advanced cancer. *British Journal of Cancer,* 65, 481–4.

170. Bruera, E., Catz, Z., Hooper, R. *et al.* (1987). Chronic nausea and anorexia in advanced cancer patients: a possible role for autonomic dysfunction. *Journal of Pain and Symptom Management,* 2, 19–21.

171. Muth, E.R., Koch, K.L., and Stern, R.M. (2000). Significance of autonomic nervous system activity in functional dysyepsia. *Digestive Diseases and Sciences,* 45, 854–63.

172. Handa, M., Mine, K., Yamamoto, H. *et al.* (1999). Esophageal motility and psychiatric factors in functional dyspepsia with or without pain. *Digestive Diseases and Sciences,* 44, 2094–8.

173. Pfaffenbach, B., Adamek, R.J., Hagemann, D., Scaffstein, J., and Wegener, M. (1998). Gastric emptying and antral myoelectrical activity in chronic alcoholics with dyspepsia. *Hepato-Gastroenterology,* 45, 1165–71.

174. Ko, C.W., Chang, C.S., Lien, H.C. *et al.* (1998). Gastric dysrhythmia in uremic patients on maintenance hemodialysis. *Scandinavian Journal of Gastroenterology,* 33, 1047–51.

175. Dent, J. (1996). Diseases of the oesophagus. In *Oxford textbook of medicine,* 3rd edition. on CD-ROM (eds. D.J. Weatherall, J.G.G. Ledingham, and D.A. Warrell), pp. 1865–76. Oxford University Press, Oxford.

176. Sullivan, P.B. (1997). Gastro-intestinal problems in the neurologically-impaired child. *Bailliere's Clinical Gastroenterology,* 11(3), 529–46.

177. Martinez, D.A., Ginn-Pease, M.E., and Caniano, D.A. (1992). Recognition of recurrent gastroesophageal reflux following antireflux surgery in the neurologically disabled child: high index of suspicion and definitive evaluation. *Journal of Pediatric Surgery,* 27(8), 983–8.

178. Logan, R. and Delaney, B. (2001). ABC of the upper gastrointestinal tract. Implications of dyspepsia for the NHS. *British Medical Journal,* 323, 675–7.

179. Regnard, C.F.B. and Mannix, K. (1990). Palliation of gastric carcinoma haemorrhage with sucralfate. *Palliative Medicine,* 4, 329–30.

180. NICE (National Institute for Health and Clinical Excellence). (2005). *Managing dyspepsia in adults in primary care.* NICE, London. www.nice.org.uk.

181. Delaney, B., Ford, A.C., Forman, D. *et al.* (2005). Initial management strategies for dyspepsia. *Cochrane Database of Systematic Reviews,* 4, CD001961.

182. Lam, S.K. (1990). Why do ulcers heal with sucralfate? *Scandinavian Journal of Gastroenterology,* 25 (Suppl 173), 6–16.

183. Caldwell, J.R., Roth, S.H., Wu, W.G. *et al.* (1987). Sucralfate treatment of nonsteroidal anti-inflammatory drug-induced gastrointestinal symptoms and mucosal damage. *American Journal of Medicine,* 83 (Suppl 3B), 74–82.

184. Sorkin, E. and Ogawa, C. (1983). Cimetidine potentiation of narcotic action. *Drug Intelligence and Clinical Pharmacy,* 17, 60–1.

185. Hawkey, C.J., Karrasch, J.A., Szcepanski, L. *et al.* for the Omeprazole vs Misoprostol for NSAID-Induced Ulcer Management (OMNIUM) Study Group (1998). Omeprazole compared with misoprostol for ulcers associated with non steroidal anti inflammatory drugs. *New England Journal of Medicine,* 338, 727–34.

186. Koch, M., Capurso, L., Dezi, A. *et al.* (1995). Prevention of NSAID-induced gastroduodenal mucosal injury: meta-analysis of clinical trials with misoprostol and H$_2$ antagonists. *Digestive Diseases,* 1, 62–74.

187. Spiegel, B.M., Farid, M., Dulai, G.S. *et al.* (2006). Comparing rates of dyspepsia with Coxibs vs NSAID+PPI: a meta-analysis. *American Journal of Medicine,* 119(5), 448.e27–36.

188. Twycross, R.G. (1995). The use of prokinetic drugs in palliative care. *European Journal of Palliative Care,* 4, 141–5.

189. Shivshanker, K., Bennett, R.W., and Haynie, T.P. (1983). Tumor-associated gastroparesis: correction with metoclopramide. *American Journal of Surgery,* 145, 221–5.

190. Kris, M.G., Yeh, S.D.J., Gralla, R.J. *et al.* (1985). Symptomatic gastroparesis in cancer patients. A possible cause of cancer-associated anorexia that can be improved with oral metoclopramide. *Proceedings of the American Society of Clinical Oncology,* 4, 267.

191. Sanger, G.J. and King, F.D. (1988). From metoclopramide to selective gut motility stimulants and 5HT3 receptor antagonists. *Drug Design and Delivery,* 3, 273–95.

192. Loose, F.D. (1979). Domperidone in chronic dyspepsia: a pilot open study and a multicentre general practice crossover comparison with metoclopramide and placebo. *Pharmatheripeutica,* 2(3), 140–6.

193. Moriga, M. (1981). A multicentre double blind study of domperidone and metoclopramide in the symptomatic control of dyspepsia. In *Progress with domperidone. a gastrokinetic and anti-emetic agent* (eds. G. Touse), pp. 77–9. Royal Society of Medicine, London.

194. Bernstein, J. and Kasich, M. (1974). A double-blind trial of simethicone in functional disease of the upper gastrointestinal tract. *Journal of Clinical Pharmacology,* 14, 614–23.

195. Ogilvie, A.L. and Atkinson, M. (1986). Does dimethicone increase the efficacy of antacids in the treatment of reflux oesophagitis? *Journal of the Royal Society of Medicine,* 79 (10), 584–7.

196. Jasperson, D., Diehl, K.L., Schoeppner, H. *et al.* (1998). A comparison of omeprazole, lansoprazole and pantoprazole in the maintenance treatment of severe reflux disease. *Alimentary Pharmacology and Therapeutics,* 12, 49–52.

197. Watters, K.J., Murphy, G.M., Tomkin, G.H. *et al.* (1979). An evaluation of the bile acid binding and antacid properties of hydrotalcite in hiatus hernia and peptic ulceration. *Current Medical Research Opinion,* 6, 85–7.

198. Llewellyn, A.F., Tomkin, G.H., and Murphy, G.M. (1977). The binding of bile acids by hydrotalcite and other antacid preparations. *Pharmaceutica Acta Helvetiae,* 52, 1–5.

199. Keeckner, F.S., Stahler, E.J., Hartzell, G. *et al.* (1972). Esophagitis and gastritis secondary to bile reflux. *Gastroenterology,* 62, 890.

200. Berne, J.D., Norwood, S.H., McAuley, C.E. *et al.* (2002). Erythromycin reduces delayed gastric emptying in critically ill trauma patients: a randomized, controlled trial. *Journal of Trauma-Injury Infection & Critical Care,* 53(3), 422–5.

201. Booth, C.M., Heyland, D.K., and Paterson, W.G. (2002). Gastrointestinal promotility drugs in the critical care setting: a systematic review of the evidence. *Critical Care Medicine,* 30(7), 1429–35.

202. Costalos, C., Gounaris, A., Varhalama, E. *et al.* (2002). Erythromycin as a prokinetic agent in preterm infants. *Journal of Pediatric Gastroenterology & Nutrition,* 34(1), 23–5.

203. Nathan, M.D., Leshner, R.T., and Keller, A.P. (1980). Intractable hiccups. *Laryngoscope,* 90, 1612–18.

204. Launois, S., Bizec, J., Whitelaw, W. *et al.* (1993). Hiccup in adults: an overview. *European Respiratory Journal,* 6, 563–75.

205. Souadjian, J.V. and Cain, J.C. (1968). Intractable hiccup: etiologic factors in 220 cases. *Postgraduate Medicine,* 43, 72–7.

206. Marhofer, P., Glaser, C., Krenn, C.G. *et al.* (1999). Incidence and therapy of midazolam induced hiccups in paediatric anaesthesia. *Paediatric Anaesthesia*, **9**, 295–8.

207. Askenasy, J.J.M. (1992). About the mechanism of hiccup. *European Neurology*, **32**, 159–63.

208. Stotka, V.L., Barclay, S.J., Bell, H.S. *et al.* (1962). Intractable hiccough as the primary manifestation of brain stem tumor. *American Journal of Medicine*, **32**, 313–5.

209. Kaufman, H.J. (1982). Hiccups: an occasional sign of esophageal obstruction. *Gastroenterology*, **82**, 1443–5.

210. Fodstad, H. and Nilsson, S. (1993). Intractable singultus: a diagnostic and therapeutic challenge. *British Journal of Neurosurgery*, **7**, 255–62.

211. Wagner, H.S. and Stapczynski, J.S. (1982). Persistent hiccups. *Annals of Emergency Medicine*, **11**, 24–6.

212. Askenasy, J.J. (1988). Sleep hiccup. *Sleep*, **11**, 187–94.

213. Liddell, E.G.T., and Sherrington, C. (1925). Further observations on myotatic reflexes. *Proceedings of the Royal Society of London (Biology)*, **97**, 267–83.

214. Moretti, R., Torre, P., Antonello, R.M. *et al.* (2000). Gabapentin as a drug therapy of intractable hiccup due to vascular lesion. *Nuova Rivista di Neurologica*, **10**, 58–62.

215. Ward, B.A. and Smith, R.R. (1994). Hiccups and brainstem compression. *Journal of Neuroimaging*, **4**, 164–5.

216. Musumeci, A., Cristofori, L., and Bricolo, A. (2000). Persistent hiccup as presenting symptom in medulla oblongata cavernoma: a case report and review of the literature. *Clinical Neurology and Neurosurgery*, **102**, 13–17.

217. Rousseau, P. (1994). Hiccups in terminal disease. *American Journal of Hospice and Palliative Care*, **11**(6), 7–10.

218. Lauterbach, E.C. (1999). Hiccup and apparent myoclonus after hydrocodone: review of the opiate-related hiccup and myoclonus literature. *Clinical Neuropharmacology*, **22**, 87–92.

219. Mukhopadhyay, P., Osman, M.R., Wajima, T. *et al.* (1986). Nifedipine for intractable hiccups. *New England Journal of Medicine*, **314**, 1256.

220. Phillips, R.A. (2005). The management of hiccups in terminally ill patients. *Nursing Times*, **101**(31), 32–3.

221. Howard, R.S. (1992). Persistent hiccups. *British Medical Journal*, **305**, 1237–8.

222. Salem, M.R., Baraka, A., Rattenborg, C.C. *et al.* (1967). Treatment of hiccups by pharyngeal stimulation in anesthetized and conscious subjects. *Journal of the American Medical Association*, **202**, 126–30.

223. De Ruyssche, D., Spaas, P., and Specenier, P. (1996). Treatment of intractable hiccup in a terminal cancer patient with nebulized saline. *Palliative Medicine*, **10**, 166–7.

224. Goldsmith, A. (1983). A treatment for hiccups. *Journal of the American Medical Association*, **249**, 1566.

225. Lamphier, T.A. (1977). Methods of management of persistent hiccup (singultus). *Maryland State Medical Journal November*, 80–1.

226. Saitto, C., Gristina, G., and Cosmi, E.V. (1982). Treatment of hiccups by continuous positive airway pressure (CPAP) in anesthetized subjects. *Anesthesiology*. **57**, 345.

227. Guelaud, C., Similowski, T., Bizec, J.L. *et al.* (1995). Baclofen therapy for chronic hiccup. *European Respiratory Journal*. **8**, 235–7.

228. Ramirez, F.C. and Graham, D.Y. (1992). Treatment of intractable hiccup with baclofen: results of a double-blind randomized, cross-over study. *American Journal of Gastroenterology*, **87**, 1789–91.

229. Petroianu, G., Hein, G., Syegmeier-Petroianu, A. *et al.* (2000). Gabapentin 'add-on therapy' for idiopathic chronic hiccup (ICH). *Journal of Clinical Gastroenterology*, **30**, 321–4.

230. Smith, H.S. and Busracamwongs, A. (2003). Management of hiccups in the palliative care population. *American Journal of Hospice & Palliative Care*, **20**(2), 149–54.

231. Lipps, D.C., Jabbari, B., Mitchell, M.H. *et al.* (1990). Nifedipine for intractable hiccups. *Neurology*, **40**, 531–2.

232. Ives, T.J., Fleming, M.F., Weart, C.W. *et al.* (1985). Treatment of intractable hiccups with intramuscular haloperidol. *American Journal of Psychiatry*, **142**, 1368–9.

233. Marechal, R., Berghmans, T., and Sculier, P. (2003). Successful treatment of intractable hiccup with methylphenidate in a lung cancer patient. *Supportive Care in Cancer*, **11**(2), 126–8.

234. Wilcock, A., and Twycross, R. (1997). Midazolam for intractable hiccup. *Journal of Pain and Symptom Management*, **12**, 59–61.

235. Aravot, D.J., Wright, G., Rees, A., Maiwand, O.M. *et al.* (1989). Non-invasive phrenic nerve stimulation for intractable hiccups. *Lancet*, **2**, 1047.

10.2.3 **Constipation and diarrhoea**

Nigel Sykes

Constipation

Definition

Constipation is the passage of small, hard faeces infrequently and with difficulty. Individuals vary in the weight they give to the different components of this definition when assessing their own constipation and may introduce other factors, such as flatulence, bloating, or a sensation of incomplete evacuation.

Less than 1 per cent of a healthy British population[1] or 5 per cent of a North American one[2] fail to defecate at least three times a week. These findings have informed what are sometimes referred to as the 'Rome criteria'[3], which are often used to define constipation for research or drug regulatory purposes; the presence of two or more of the following symptoms for at least 3 months:

♦ straining at least 25 per cent of the time;

♦ hard stools at least 25 per cent of the time;

♦ incomplete evacuation at least 25 per cent of the time;

♦ two or fewer bowel movements per week.

In practice, the bowel frequency criterion is often given most importance, but the validity of this in a palliative care or general population is doubtful. There is evidence that many people feel constipated when still not meeting the Rome criteria[4,5].

Prevalence of constipation

The first National Health and Nutrition Examination Survey in US found that 8 per cent of men and 21 per cent of women reported themselves to be constipated[6]. In a British survey, 10 per cent overall said they were constipated[1], and more women than men reported themselves to be constipated. Both self-reported constipation and laxative consumption increase with ageing.

Physical illness is a risk factor for constipation: 63 per cent of elderly people in hospital have been found to be constipated, compared with 22 per cent of the same age group living at home[7]. Constipation is more common in people terminally ill with cancer than in those dying of other causes[8], and about 50 per cent of patients admitted to British hospices complain of it. This is an underestimate of the problem, as some patients will already be receiving effective laxative therapy.

Constipation has been reported to rival or exceed pain as a cause of distress. Depression is a risk factor for constipation in population surveys[6], but results of a depression rating scale used on British hospice patients do not correlate with indices of constipation.

Intestinal motility

The small and large intestines each have their own characteristic motility patterns. Throughout the gut, most muscle movements mix the contents rather than propel them. This facilitates enzymatic and bacterial breakdown of food and absorption of the resulting nutrients and of water.

Bursts of propagated motor activity occur in the small gut every 90–120 min. This activity is associated with increased gastric, pancreatic, and biliary secretion and is suggested to represent a cleansing mechanism for the small intestine. Feeding abolishes the regularity of this pattern, resulting in an increased variability of the rate of transit of luminal contents. Motor activity in the fed state is apparently random and presumably performs the function of mixing the gut contents in order to allow digestion and absorption of nutrients. Resumption of regular propagated activity correlates closely with the end of gastric emptying; both are delayed by larger or more fatty meals[9], again suggesting that adequate facilities for digestion are being provided.

The colon shows much less frequent episodes of forward peristalsis, which result in mass movements of gut contents. Manometry suggests this activity occurs about six times per day, but is grouped into two peaks, a larger one associated with wakening and breakfast and a smaller one associated with midday meal[10]. The frequency is reduced by inactivity[11].

Food residues normally spend 1–2 h in the small intestine, but 2–3 days in the colon. In constipation, colonic transit may be greatly prolonged: nearly half of a hospice population had transit times of between 4 and 12 days[12].

Gut muscle layers form a syncytium through which depolarization spreads from pacemaker areas. The myenteric nerve plexus coordinates motility, which is also under external neuronal influence, particularly via the parasympathetic system. High spinal cord transection mainly abolishes the motility response to food, but low cord or pelvic outflow lesions produce colonic dilation and slowing of transit in the descending and distal transverse colon.

Autonomic neuropathy has been implicated in some cases of chronic constipation and in constipation related to diabetes mellitus. Autonomic neuropathy can occur as a non-metastatic manifestation of malignancy, particularly in association with small cell carcinoma of the lung and carcinoid tumours. The resulting neural damage most commonly causes gastroparesis, but can also be associated with severe constipation[13].

Immunocytochemical work in animals has revealed multiple putative transmitter peptides and amines in myenteric neurons. The two principal neurotransmitters involved in the control of peristalsis appear to be acetylcholine (ACh) and vasoactive intestinal peptide (VIP). Peristalsis movements have two components, ascending contraction and descending relaxation; ACh mediates the first of these and VIP the second. Anti-cholinergic drugs tend to constipate because they control part of the peristaltic complex. Both ACh and VIP neurons are modulated by other agents of which endogenous opioids are one group.

Fluid and electrolytes

About 7 litres of fluid enter the jejunum daily from gastric, salivary, pancreatic, and biliary secretions, to which is added a further 1.5 l of dietary fluid. Approximately 75 per cent of the total volume is absorbed in the small intestine and all but about 150 ml of the remainder in the colon. The difference between constipation and diarrhoea in terms of fluid excretion is around 100 ml/day, implying a remarkably precise control of water absorption in the colon. Because maximal colonic absorptive capacity is 4.5–5 l/day, the colon can tolerate wide fluctuations in ileal output; diarrhoea can result, however, from relatively small variations in colonic absorption. There is no evidence that constipation is accompanied by increased water absorption save by virtue of the extended time contents remain in the gut.

Gut fluid absorption is an active process, chiefly dependent on electrogenic Na^+ transport by the Na^+/K^+-ATPase system at the basolateral surface of the enterocytes. Fluid also follows neutral absorption of Cl^- in exchange for HCO_3, and of NaCl. Na^+ is also co-transported with glucose and amino acid molecules. At the mucosal surface, a cyclic AMP-dependent system mediates Cl^- and consequently fluid, secretion.

Non-absorbed solutes retain water in the lumen by osmosis, but luminal factors can also influence active transport. Short-chain fatty acids increase absorption and bile acids, prostaglandins, bacterial toxins, and some laxatives stimulate secretion. Accordingly, diarrhoea can sometimes be relieved by a bile acid-binding resin or a prostaglandin inhibitor.

Electrolyte, and hence, water, transport is under neuronal control. The basic secretory condition of intestinal epithelium is cholinergic, mediated through changes in intracellular calcium concentrations. Anti-cholinergic agents and hypercalcaemia tend to constipate and hypocalcaemia tends to cause diarrhoea.

Lipophilic agents, such as bile salts, could stimulate villous nerve endings directly, but it has been proposed that epithelial 'receptor' cells mediate a defence response of increased secretion and peristalsis to dilute water-soluble toxins[14]. Endogenous opioids inhibit this defence response experimentally, and although the physiological significance of such modulation is unclear, it may be a component of exogenous opioids' action in infective and perhaps other forms of diarrhoea (Table 10.2.3.1).

Defaecation

During defecation, abdominal pressure is raised by contraction of the abdominal muscles against a closed glottis, a process facilitated by assuming a squatting position. This pressure is

Table 10.2.3.1 Opioid effects on the gut.

Increased tone in ileocaecal and anal sphincters
Reduced peristaltic component of motility in small intestine and colon
Increased electrolyte and water absorption in small intestine, and colon during induced diarrhoea
Restoration of colonic capacitance after intracaecal fat infusion
Impaired defecation reflex
Reduced sensitivity to distention
Increased internal anal sphincter tone

transmitted to the rectum and tends to expel a stool positioned in the rectal ampulla. However, once defecation has been initiated, stools from the length of the descending colon can be expelled without abdominal contraction. Such effortless expulsion is probably due to an anocolonic reflex that produces distal colonic contraction in response to anal contact with passing stool. The effort required to pass a stool is inversely proportional to its size, accounting for the straining involved in passing a small, constipated stool[15].

Normal defecation depends on the ability of upper anal canal receptors to detect the presence of stool, and on the relaxation of the involuntary internal anal sphincter and of puborectalis, which also exerts a sphincter function. These actions are abolished by lower motor neuron lesions to produce loss of rectal sensation, decreased rectal tone, and inability to defecate. Upper motor neuron lesions also destroy rectal sensation, but leave intact both reflex relaxation of the internal sphincter and the anocolonic reflex. Hence, many patients with high spinal lesions learn to initiate defecation by digital stimulation of the anal canal.

Mechanisms of the contribution of opioids to constipation

Opioid analgesics, specifically morphine, are probably the largest single identifiable constipating influence in palliative care patients. Sixty-three per cent of such patients *not* taking morphine required laxatives, a figure similar to that found in the ill elderly[7], but 87 per cent of those receiving morphine needed them and used a higher average dose[16]. There appeared to be the type of dose–response relationship between morphine and constipation that might be expected from a drug–receptor interaction, although with considerable scatter.

Exogenous opioids are well known to constipate, not by relaxing intestinal muscle but by suppressing forward peristalsis and raising sphincter tone (Table 10.2.3.1). These effects are apparent in both the small and the large intestines. If sufficiently severe, the clinical results on the gut of opioid analgesia produce functional colonic obstruction, a situation whose symptoms have been called the 'narcotic bowel syndrome'[17], but which appears simply to represent severe constipation.

Opioid receptors are present on gut smooth muscle and at all levels of nervous input to the intestine, mu- and delta-receptors apparently being the most important in motility, the former predominating in the myenteric plexus and the latter in the submucous plexus. In animals, gut opioid effects involve both central and peripheral receptors, but only peripheral opioid activity has been confirmed in man. This does not imply that parenterally-administered opioids are not constipating: it has been shown in man that subcutaneous morphine slows transit and reduces stool frequency[18]. No doubt opioid receptors in the gut wall can be reached not just by opioids in the lumen but also in the circulation.

Endogenous opioids have been shown to be involved in the modulation of other neurotransmitters, notably ACh and VIP, which are involved in control of peristalsis. Human studies using naloxone suggest that endogenous opioids may exert a basal control of gut motility[18] and, clinically, oral naloxone has been reported to improve idiopathic constipation[19] and constipation in geriatric patients[20]. Although these results are in line with some animal data, they require confirmation and further work with more specific antagonists to clarify the contribution of different opioid receptor populations.

Experimentally, mu$_2$-receptor-mediated opioid actions such as delaying of intestinal transit show less development of tolerance than mu$_1$-mediated analgesia does[21]. The development of clinical tolerance to morphine-induced constipation remains to be quantified: 28 palliative care patients followed up for over 2 months did not differ significantly from 470 shorter-lived patients in morphine or laxative consumption, but did have higher stool frequencies and somewhat lower use of enemas and suppositories. Their median laxative dose had risen over the review period but by much less than had their median morphine dose[16]. In a smaller study, 12 patients survived for 6 months. Among them were four who required no laxatives despite taking morphine, sometimes in substantial amounts. It is not clear whether these four patients had never needed laxatives or whether they had at some point been able to give them up, that is, whether they had become tolerant to the constipating effect of morphine or whether they lay at one extreme of a morphine dose–response curve for constipation[22].

Opioids may vary in their constipating potency. There is now reasonable evidence that transdermal fentanyl is somewhat less constipating than morphine[23], possibly because of the smaller doses that have to be given in order to achieve CNS penetration. Reduction in laxative use has also been reported after changing from morphine to methadone, but to date only on a case history basis[24], and lower laxative requirements have been observed with the use of methadone as compared to morphine or hydromorphone[25].

A physiological role for endogenous opioids in defecation has yet to emerge, but exogenous opioids inhibit anorectal sphincteric relaxation and diminish anorectal sensitivity (Table 10.2.3.1). Both actions exacerbate constipation. As anorectal sensitivity decreases with age, the constipating effects of opioid therapy are likely to be more pronounced in the elderly.

Causes of constipation in palliative medicine

Constipation in patients with progressive disease is usually multifactorial; for instance, an ill person with poor food intake, impaired mobility, and a requirement for opioid analgesia has three reasons

Table 10.2.3.2 Causes of constipation in palliative medicine.

Malignancy
Directly due to tumour
Intestinal obstruction due to (i) tumour in the bowel wall; (ii) external compression by abdominal or pelvic tumour
Damage to lumbosacral spinal cord, cauda equina or pelvic plexus
Hypercalcaemia
Due to secondary effects of disease
Inadequate food intake
Low fibre diet
Dehydration
Weakness
Inactivity
Confusion
Depression
Unfamiliar toilet arrangements
Drugs
Opioids
Drugs with anti-cholinergic effects:
Hyoscine
Phenothiazines
Tricyclic anti-depressants
Anti-parkinsonian agents
Antacids (calcium and aluminium compounds)
Diuretics
Anti-convulsants
Iron
Anti-hypertensive agents
Vincristine
Concurrent disease
Diabetes
Hypothyroidism
Hypokalaemia
Hernia
Diverticular disease
Rectocoele
Anal fissure or stenosis
Anterior mucosal prolapse
Haemorrhoids
Colitis

to be constipated. A list of the constipating factors most relevant to palliative medicine is given in Table 10.2.3.2. Of these, the most important are the secondary effects of disease and the use of opioids.

Clinical manifestations and diagnostic considerations in constipation

History

It is important to clarify a complaint of constipation by a careful history. The degree to which constipation pre-dated the present illness should be established, as this may justify wider investigations. Whether it was construed by the patient as constipation or not, the prior stool pattern should be elicited as a basis for comparison. Some necessary questions for taking a constipation history are suggested in Table 10.2.3.3.

Occasionally, the patient reports a trick that aids defecation: a finger inserted in the vagina implies the presence of a rectocoele, a finger in the rectum to push away a flap suggests a solitary rectal ulcer, and pressure exerted behind the anus assists defecation if the levator muscles are weak. All these are distinct from the digital rectal evacuation to which many constipated patients are forced to resort.

Such symptoms as abdominal pain, bloating, flatulence, nausea, malaise, headache, and halitosis are associated by some patients with constipation, but are non-specific and mostly can occur also with diarrhoea. It is the frequency and difficulty of defecation that are the basis for the diagnosis of constipation.

Assessment tools for constipation

In palliative care, constipation is important as a symptom, and hence it is the patient's perspective that is most valid. However, the widely accepted 'Rome criteria'[3] invite the measurement of objective outcomes that are taken to be indicators of the severity of constipation. Whether they also reflect the impact of disordered bowel function upon the patient is much less clear (Table 10.2.3.4). The correlation of the objective assessment of stool appearance with bowel transit time has been validated in a palliative care population[12], and is a non-invasive, technology-free method of assessing this key indicator of intestinal function.

An objective indicator of the presence of constipation is a plain abdominal radiograph. A scoring system to describe the amount of stool present was described and tested in a in a palliative care population by Bruera *et al*[26]. Similar systems of more or less

Table 10.2.3.3 History-taking in constipation.

When were the bowels last opened?
What were the characteristics of the last stool, e.g. loose or formed; thin and ribbon-like or small, hard pellets?
Was straining necessary for defecation?
Was defecation painful?
How characteristic of recent bowel actions was the last stool?
What is the usual stool frequency now?
Does the patient feel a need to defecate but is unable to do so (suggests hard stool or rectal obstruction)?
Is the urge to defecate largely absent (suggests colonic inertia)?
Does the stool emerge part way through a bulging anal outlet after significant straining (suggests haemorrhoids)?
Is there blood or mucus in the stool (suggests tumour obstruction or haemorrhoids or both)?

Table 10.2.3.4 Methods of objective assessment of constipation.

Parameter	Test	Comments
Bowel frequency	Counting episodes of defecation	Patient diary recording or clinical observation are more accurate than recall. Often only 'satisfactory' episodes of defecation are counted, but who decides
	Stool-free interval	72-h periods without defecation are counted.[57] May be more clinically relevant than simple bowel frequency
Whole intestinal transit time	Radio-opaque markers	Requires minimal specialized equipment, but cumbersome[28] (Fig. 10.2.3.1)
	Scintigraphy	Specialist facilities required
	Radio-telemetry	Can demonstrate regional contributions to transit time
	Stool consistency	Non-invasive, quick. Shape of stools can be graded, and can be estimated reliably either by patients or staff. Shown to correlate well with transit time in palliative care patients[12]
Small bowel transit time	Lactulose-hydrogen breath test	More rapid than any direct measure of whole intestinal transit
Extent of faecal loading	Radiography	Rapid. Gives only a static measure of intestinal function. Scoring methods have been devised, but show poor correlation with other tests

complexity have been described by Barr[27] and others, and are claimed to show high inter-observer reliability and good correlation with stool frequency. Radiographs are of course a static measure of current faecal loading and give no information about the speed of transit or about performance of different colonic segments. In a large paediatric study, Barr scores showed poor correlation with transit time and too great a variability to be reliable in diagnosing chronically constipated subjects[28]. On the other hand, scoring of pre- and post-intervention radiographs could aid objectivity of assessment in the badly needed trials of the efficacy of suppositories and enemas in palliative care.

Subjective measures of constipation, which assess patients' reports of their bowel function without externally measurable criteria, take the form of visual analogue (VAS) or adjectival scales, or of questionnaires. A discrete response modification of the VAS and an adjectival scale have each been found to have validity and to be easy to use in a palliative care setting[29]. Since up to about 10 per cent of palliative care patients have diarrhoea, whose commonest cause in this setting is an excess of laxatives, it is appropriate that any subjective measure includes the ability to assess not only constipation but also diarrhoea as well. This is easily arranged with VAS and adjectival scales, but is lacking in the questionnaires that have been validated for the assessment of constipation.

Perhaps the best-established constipation questionnaire is the Constipation Assessment Scale (CAS) of McMillan and Williams[30]. This is an eight-item scale validated in the cancer population, although not specifically patients receiving specialist palliative care. Completion time averages 2 min. The Constipation Scoring System also has eight items, and when tested on 50 constipated and 50 non-constipated patients, it predicted the presence of constipation correctly in 96 per cent of cases[31]. Unlike the CAS, it has not been shown to distinguish among varying severities of constipation, although it seems likely that it would do so.

The PAC-SYM and PAC-QOL are related questionnaires directed at the patient's perspective on constipation[32]. The PAC-SYM has three subscales related to stool symptoms, rectal symptoms and abdominal symptoms, and has been validated on a large ($n = 216$)

sample of chronically constipated subjects, but not a cancer or palliative care population. The PAC-QOL is a constipation-specific quality of life measure. The PAC-SYM contains no assessment of diarrhoea, although the PAC-QOL has a bowel frequency rating. Several other bowel function rating scales exist but are either derived from one of those already mentioned or are not specific to constipation.

Examination

Abdominal examination and, unless there has been a recent full evacuation, rectal examination, are vital, and will help to avoid

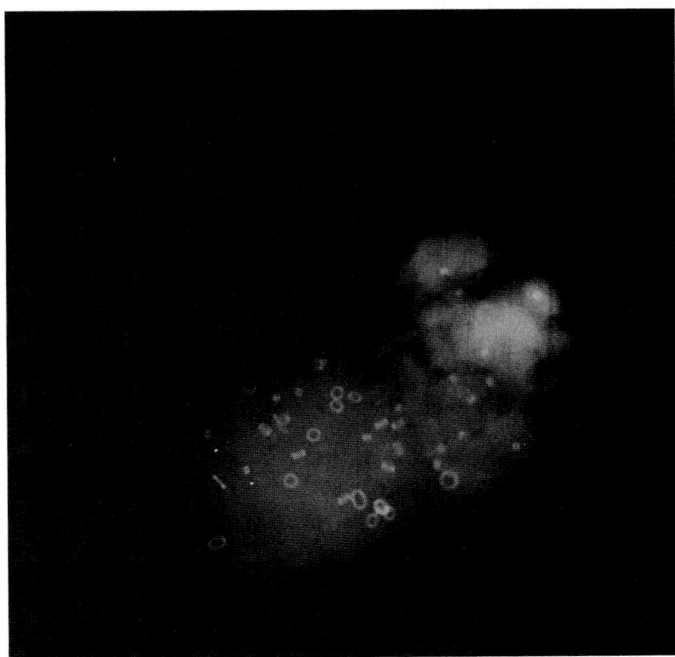

Figure 10.2.3.1 Radiograph of stool taken during the estimation of transit time, showing different sizes of radio-opaque markers.

the major pitfalls in the diagnosis of constipation in palliative medicine. These are:

Impaction, presenting as diarrhoea, often with incontinence. This occurs characteristically in elderly patients in whom inattention to the need to defecate, confusion, or rectal insensitivity leads to the formation of a large faecal mass that is impossible to pass spontaneously. Faecal material higher in the colon is broken down into semi-liquid form by bacterial action and seeps past the mass, appearing as diarrhoea. If the closing pressure of the anal sphincters has been exceeded by the mass, faecal leakage or incontinence occurs. Ninety-eight per cent of faecal impactions are said to occur in the rectum and although it is probable that opioid analgesia alters this distribution, rectal examination will diagnose the great majority.

Intestinal obstruction by tumour or adhesions. Known intra-abdominal malignant deposits, previous intestinal surgery, alternating constipation and diarrhoea, gut colic, and nausea and vomiting combine to suggest the presence of intestinal obstruction. A similar picture can occur, however, in severe constipation, of which the 'narcotic bowel syndrome' following use of opioid analgesia is probably one manifestation. The distinction is important, as attempts to clear 'constipation' using stimulant laxatives can cause severe pain when the underlying cause is obstruction.

Nausea. Some patients rapidly experience nausea, with or without vomiting, in the presence of intestinal hold-up[33]. Unexplained nausea or vomiting should prompt enquiry and examination for constipation.

Abdominal pain. The effort of colonic muscle to propel hard faeces commonly leads to abdominal pain, frequently colicky in nature. History and examination usually suggest the cause of the pain, but constipation is still sometimes 'treated' with an opioid. Such pain may be particularly marked—and difficult to diagnose—when abdominal or pelvic tumour exists, presumably as a result either of pressure on the tumour from distended gut or because of partial intestinal obstruction.

Palpation of the abdomen may reveal faecal masses in the line of the descending colon and even that of the more proximal colon and caecum. The distinction between tumour and faecal masses can be hard to make. Faeces will usually indent, if the patient will tolerate sufficiently firm pressure, and may give a crepitus-like sensation because of entrained gas. They also move, given time. Sometimes, an abdominal radiograph is needed to distinguish tumour from stool, but this is uncommon (Fig. 10.2.3.2).

Digital examination of the rectum may reveal a hard mass of impacted faeces. The clinical picture, however, may be of faecal leakage. Alternatively, the complete absence of stool implies colonic inertia. Rectal examination may also uncover rectal tumour, a rectocoele, solitary rectal ulcer, or anal stenosis. A lax anal sphincter may indicate spinal cord damage associated with colonic hypotonia. If a rectocoele or compression from pelvic tumour masses is suspected, vaginal examination may be justifiable.

Examination of the stool can be useful. Small, hard pellets suggest slow colonic transit, ribbon-like stools suggest stenosis or haemorrhoids, and blood or mucus suggests tumour, haemorrhoids, or coexisting colitis.

Urinary incontinence. Faecal impaction is well-recognized as a precipitant of urinary incontinence in the elderly, and the recent onset of incontinence should indicate abdominal and rectal examination as the first investigative steps.

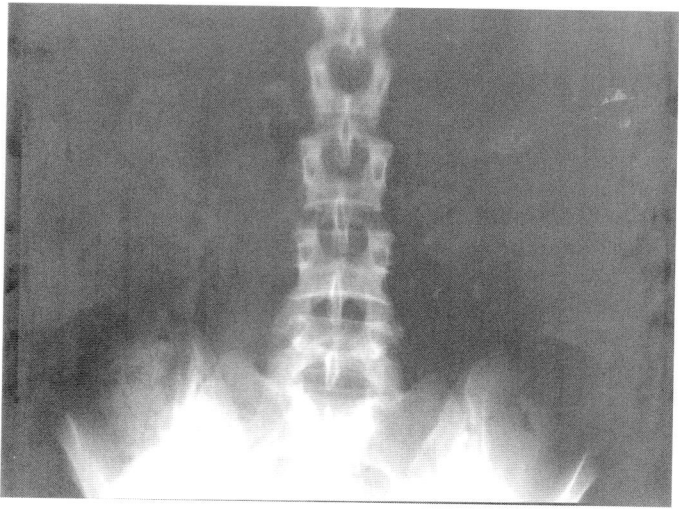

Figure 10.2.3.2 Abdominal radiograph of constipation, showing extensive faecal loading of all colonic segments.

Investigations

Investigations are rarely needed in the assessment of constipation in palliative medicine. Abdominal radiography may distinguish between constipation and obstruction if there is persisting doubt, but is rarely necessary and should certainly not be a standard procedure.

Blood tests are confirmatory rather than a screening procedure, but if the clinical picture is suggestive, corrected calcium levels and thyroid function tests should be performed.

Management approaches

Prophylaxis

The aetiologies of constipation in patients with progressive disease (Table 10.2.3.1) suggest several prophylactic measures (Table 10.2.3.5). First of all, there should be good general symptom control, without which no other measures are possible. A key stimulus to colonic peristalsis and defecation is activity[11] and hence patients should be encouraged and enabled to be as mobile as their physical limitations allow.

Constipated stools have relatively low water content, rendering them hard and difficult to pass. This tendency will be exacerbated if the individual is dehydrated. Adequate fluid intake is therefore helpful in the management of constipation. The overall comfort of the person must be considered, however, and constipation does not justify the use of parenteral infusions. Rather, the policy must be to enhance oral intake by encouragement and the provision of

Table 10.2.3.5 Prophylaxis of constipation.

Maintain good general symptom control
Encourage activity
Maintain adequate oral fluid intake
Maximize the fibre content of the diet
Anticipate constipating effects of drugs, altering treatment or starting a laxative prophylactically
Create a favourable environment

drinks the patient likes—men frequently identify beer as a laxative in its own right.

Ill people have small appetites and what food they do eat tends to be low in fibre. Dietary fibre deficiency has been linked with constipation in Western society, but individuals with severe constipation are not fibre deficient and their gut function responds poorly to added fibre[34]. Work with radiotherapy patients in Oxford suggested that an increase in stool frequency of 50 per cent would require an approximately 450 per cent mean increase in dietary fibre, well beyond the tolerance of most subjects[35]. Hence, although opportunities should be taken to raise the fibre content of patients' diets, this alone will not correct severe constipation and the priority remains that food should be as attractive as possible to the person who is expected to eat it.

Doctors should know which drugs are likely to cause constipation (Table 10.2.3.2) and either avoid them or make a laxative available at the time of first prescription, without waiting until constipation is established.

Institutional lack of privacy for defecation and the use of bed pans, which impose an inappropriate posture and greatly increase the pressure required to expel a stool, create an environment conducive to constipation. There is evidence that practised patients adapt to such indignities, but it should be a priority to allow patients privacy and the use of a lavatory, or at least a commode, for defecation.

Use of oral laxative agents

Despite prophylaxis, the majority of patients with advanced disease require laxatives. Nearly 80 per cent of hospice cancer patients need laxatives, including 63 per cent of those who do not receive an opioid and 87 per cent of those who do. The former figure is similar to the reported prevalence of constipation in a hospitalized, elderly population with non-malignant disease[7].

Laxative agents may be divided into those that predominantly soften the stool and those that predominantly stimulate gut peristalsis (Table 10.2.3.6). However, any drug that softens stool also increases its bulk and thus reflexly stimulates colonic peristalsis. Agents that directly stimulate gut muscle contraction are known also to enhance intestinal fluid secretion and so improve stool consistency. There is evidence that the combination of softener and stimulant is effective at a lower total dose than a predominantly softening agent alone and causes fewer adverse effects than a predominantly peristalsis-stimulating agent given singly[36].

The acceptability of laxative therapy will be maximized if previously satisfactory drugs are not changed unnecessarily and if the patient's preference regarding the choice of a solid or liquid laxative, sweet or less sweet, is heeded. Clinical criteria guide the selection of the class of laxative, but within most classes there are options that can reflect the patients' wishes.

The aim of laxative therapy is comfortable defecation, not any particular frequency of evacuation. No single laxative dose is adequate for everyone, and many patients are subjected to both rectal interventions and an inadequate oral dose of laxative. The dose needs to be titrated against the response and the advent of adverse effects, remembering the latent period of action of the drug concerned. The dose should be increased prophylactically if, say, opioids are introduced or their dose is being substantially increased.

As in chronic pain, so in chronic constipation, therapy should be regular, not intermittent. Low doses of laxative are best given at night, but higher doses will need to be divided, usually morning and evening, but sometimes more often. Diarrhoea usually settles promptly by suspending therapy for 24 h and resuming one dose level down.

Lubricant laxatives
Preparation: liquid paraffin.
  Starting dose: 10 ml daily.
  Mechanism: liquid paraffin lubricates the stool surface and softens the stool by penetration allowing easier passage.
  Latency of action: 1–3 days.
  Uses: liquid paraffin has been blamed for many adverse effects. Most relevant to palliative medicine are the lipoid pneumonia, which may follow paraffin inhalation, and the propensity to cause leakage of oily faecal material with consequent embarrassment and perianal irritation.

There seems no justification for reliance on liquid paraffin as the sole laxative. However, its emulsion with magnesium hydroxide, which contains only 25 per cent paraffin, has not been associated with the above adverse effects and has been recommended as an effective and cheap laxative preparation[37].

Surfactant laxatives
Preparations: docusate sodium, poloxamer.
  Starting dose: docusate sodium 300 mg daily.
  Mechanism: surfactant laxatives act as detergents to increase water penetration, and hence softening, of the stool. Docusate also promotes water, sodium, and chloride secretion in the jejunum and colon[38]; there is a clinical impression that at higher doses it may stimulate peristalsis.
  Latency of action: 1–3 days.
  Use: docusate is available alone or in combination with danthron (codanthrusate) or bisacodyl. Poloxamer is marketed only in combination with danthron (codanthramer). Docusate's ability as a laxative has been questioned, as it failed to increase colonic output of solids or water in healthy volunteers [39]. However, docusate has been found to be more effective than placebo in clinical trials in elderly or chronically ill patients[40]. Poloxamer has been claimed to be an effective laxative, but in clinical practice there is no opportunity to separate its benefits from those of the danthron with which it is combined. Docusate alone has failed to win popularity in British hospice practice.

Bulk-forming agents
Preparations: bran, methyl cellulose, ispaghula.
  Starting doses: bran 8 g daily, others 3–4 g daily.

Table 10.2.3.6 Oral laxative classification.

Predominantly softening ↓	Liquid paraffin
	Bulk-forming laxatives, e.g. methyl cellulose, ispaghula
	Polyethylene glycol
	Lubiprostone
	Docusate sodium
	Lactulose
	Saline laxatives, e.g. magnesium hydroxide
Predominantly peristalsis-stimulating	Anthracenes, e.g. senna, danthron
	Polyphenolics, e.g. bisacodyl, sodium picosulfate

Mechanism: these agents increase stool bulk partly by providing material that resists bacterial breakdown and hence remains in the gut, and partly by providing a substrate for bacterial growth and gas production. The balance between these mechanisms varies from agent to agent. Non-digestible polythene particles will enhance stool bulk and shorten transit time, presumably by a reflex response to stretch or direct mechanical irritation. However, it appears that transit is speeded especially as a result of fermentation and is to some degree independent of stool bulking action[41].

Latency of action: 2–4 days.

Use: bulking agents are 'normalizers' rather than true laxatives: they will soften a hard stool but make firmer a loose one. Effective in mild constipation, they are less helpful in palliative medicine for three main reasons. First, they need to be taken with ample water (at least 200–300 ml); this and their consistency are unacceptable to many ill patients. Second, if taken with inadequate water, a viscous mass may result, which can complete an incipient malignant obstruction. Third, their effectiveness in severe constipation is doubtful.

Osmotic laxatives

Preparations: lactulose, mannitol, and sorbitol.

Starting dose: 15 ml bd.

Mechanism: osmotic laxatives are not broken down or absorbed in the small gut, where they exert an osmotic influence to retain water in the lumen. Bacterial degradation in the colon produces short-chain organic acids, which lower the intestinal pH, possibly stimulating peristalsis, and increasing stool bulk by enlargement of the microbial mass. These acids are absorbed and so the osmotic effect does not extend throughout the colon. Lactulose and its relatives are now among the oligosaccharides characterized as prebiotics, for which a range of health benefits are claimed, including avoidance of constipation[42].

Latency of action: 1–2 days.

Use: lactulose is the most popular single laxative in British hospices and probably in British general hospitals too, where its expense has caused concern. It significantly increases faecal weight, volume, water, and frequency but if used alone in opioid-induced constipation often requires to be given in doses that result in bloating and colic. Flatulence is a problem for about 20 per cent of patients. Its sweet taste is sickly to some. There are suggestions that tolerance to its laxative effects may occur, presumably through changes in bacterial flora. Mannitol and sorbitol are less used as oral preparations, but sorbitol has been reported to be as effective as lactulose, cheaper and less nauseating[43].

Saline laxatives

Preparations: magnesium hydroxide or sulphate, sodium sulphate.

Starting doses: 2–4 g daily.

Mechanism: these agents are poorly absorbed and, unlike lactulose, exert an osmotic influence throughout the gut. They also increase intestinal water secretion and appear directly to stimulate peristalsis. Magnesium and sulphate ions are the most potent. It has been suggested that saline laxatives' actions are mediated by cholecystokinin (CCK)[44] but other releasers of CCK, such as calcium, lack a purgative effect.

Latency of action: 1–6 h (dose dependent).

Use: saline laxatives, especially magnesium sulphate, can produce an undesirably strong purgative action. They are generally considered a last resort in ill patients. Magnesium hydroxide is less potent than the sulphate and, either alone or as an emulsion with liquid paraffin, deserves re-evaluation as a cheaper alternative to lactulose and other more popular preparations[37].

Polyethylene glycol (PEG)

Starting doses: for constipation, two sachets daily, dissolved in 250 ml water. For faecal impaction, eight sachets per day in 1 l of water.

Latency of action: higher doses 1–3 days, longer for lower doses.

Mechanism: PEG is a non-absorbed, non-degraded polymer prepared in an iso-osmotic solution (with sodium bicarbonate and sodium and potassium chlorides) to avoid electrolyte disturbance. It, therefore, provides a source of non-absorbed fluid, which can then exert a softening effect on the bowel contents. Stool weight is increased in proportion to the total mass of PEG ingested[45]. It accelerates gut transit and can provide an oral treatment for faecal impaction[46] and chronic constipation[47]. However, large volumes may be needed. Culbert et al[46]. used 500 ml bd of 110 g/l PEG solution for up to 3 days in impacted elderly patients. The full dose was managed by 12 out of 16 patients on day 1, six out of eight on day 2, and one out of two on day 3. Fifteen of the 16 passed a good volume of stool with ease. The PEG solution was consumed in an average of 143 (75–300) min. Corazziari's 'small volume' approach used a total of 500 ml daily over 4 weeks[47]. PEG has been reported to be effective in a palliative care population although, not surprisingly, the best results were obtained by combining it with a stimulant laxative[48].

Use: for those patients who can tolerate the volumes involved, PEG can be either their routine laxative or, at higher doses, can relieve faecal impaction without recourse to suppositories or enemas. Trial evidence of the effectiveness and acceptability of PEG in palliative care is pending.

Lubiprostone

Starting doses: 24 mcg bd. There is no evidence for a dose response beyond this.

Latency of action: within 24 h.

Mechanism of action: lubiprostone, a bi-cyclic fatty acid, is a locally acting type 2 chloride channel activator that is claimed to stimulate fluid secretion into the gut without disturbing serum sodium or potassium concentrations[49]. There is said to be a corresponding increase in intestinal motility, but this would appear to be an indirect effect mediated through gut wall distension as a result of increased fluid volume. Lubiprostone itself is only minimally absorbed but there is appreciable absorption of its only known active metabolite, which is then principally eliminated renally. In trials in chronically constipated patients the principal adverse effects were nausea (31 per cent) and diarrhoea (13 per cent). Lubiprostone has recently been introduced in USA but is not currently available in UK.

Uses: although not evaluated in palliative care, lubiprostone appears to be an alternative to other laxative agents that soften stool by increasing its fluid content. No comparative studies have been reported and so it is not known if it has any advantages.

Anthracene and polyphenolic laxatives

Preparations: anthracenes: senna, danthron; polyphenolics: bisacodyl, sodium picosulphate.

Starting doses: senna 15 mg daily, danthron 50 mg daily, bisacodyl 10 mg daily, and sodium picosulphate 5 mg daily.

Mechanism: these drugs directly stimulate the myenteric plexus to induce peristalsis; their action can be abolished by local anaesthetic infiltration of the mucosa. Colonic electromyography in man following oral senna shows an increase in myoelectrical activity of the type seen in diarrhoea. Net absorption of water and electrolytes in the colon is reduced, partly through inhibition of Na^+, K^+-ATPase and probably also by stimulation of cAMP, prostaglandin E_2, and perhaps serotonin synthesis. The effects on water and electrolyte transport may be relatively more important for polyphenolic agents than for the anthraquinones[50].

Senna contains anthraquinone glycosides, which are almost inactive as laxatives but are converted by colonic bacteria to the active aglycone forms. In consequence, activity is concentrated almost entirely in the colon. The aglycones are absorbed to a limited degree and secreted in the bile, but this circulation is more important for dantron and the polyphenolic agents, which undergo glucuronidation and can then be reconverted in the gut to active drug, prolonging the agents' action.

Latency of action: 6–12 h (bisacodyl suppository 15–60 min).

Uses: senna is the most popular laxative in British hospices after lactulose, and the two drugs are often used in combination. This is a logical practice, lactulose providing a relatively greater stool softening effect and senna a relatively greater peristalsis-stimulating effect. Danthron (not available in US as either a single agent or in combination products) is available in combination with a surfactant agent, either docusate (codanthrusate) or poloxamer (codanthramer, which is available in two strengths with differing proportions of the constituents, the higher strength containing three times as much danthron as the lower but five times as much poloxamer). Both codanthrusate and codanthramer are available as a capsule or a suspension. It should be noted that in the standard strength of codantramer one capsule is equal to 5 ml suspension, but in the higher strength one capsule is the equivalent of only 2.5 ml of the suspension. Equal proportions of senna liquid and lactulose are significantly more potent than standard codanthramer, but are probably less potent than higher strength codanthramer[51]. Sodium picosulphate is formulated as a single strength elixir.

Any of the anthraquinones or polyphenolics can cause severe purgation, with colicky abdominal pains. This can generally be avoided by dose titration and combined use of a more specific stool-softening agent. They are valuable where there is evidence of colonic inertia.

Morphine is known to antagonize the water and electrolyte effects of senna[52] and it has been suggested that there is a relatively fixed relationship between a dose of codeine and that of senna, which will counteract the resulting constipation[53]. This may be true for a given individual taking relatively low doses of opioid analgesia, but increase of opioid dosage does not proportionately increase constipation[16]. Also, effective doses of polyphenolic laxatives show four- to eightfold variation between individuals[54] and the same seems true of the anthraquinones.

Both the anthraquinones and polyphenolics have been implicated in causing myenteric plexus damage[55], but neither this nor danthron's unconvincing association with carcinogenicity in rats is sufficient to influence their use in palliative medicine. Patients should, however, be warned of the pink discoloration of the urine that danthron can cause and care should be taken to avoid the perianal rash it may precipitate, especially in incontinent patients.

Use of rectal laxatives

The use of rectal laxatives is undignified for the patient and may be unpleasant for staff, but their short latency of action is satisfying for both parties, who may in consequence come to rely heavily on them.

Rectal laxatives may be given either as suppositories or enemas, the latter usually being used as second-line therapy or for rectal impaction. Any rectal intervention may precipitate defecation by stimulation of the ano-colonic reflex, but more specific mechanisms of action parallel those of oral agents.

Lubricant rectal laxatives
Enemas: arachis oil, olive oil.

Use: these agents are normally used as retention enemas overnight to allow evacuation or manual removal of hard faeces impacted in the rectum. Naturally, their efficacy depends on the patient's ability to retain the oil.

Osmotic rectal laxatives
Suppositories: glycerine.
Enema: sorbitol.

Use: glycerine softens stools by osmosis and is also lubricant. Any stimulation of colonic contraction is presumably mechanical. Sorbitol is a constituent of several proprietary micro-enemas.

Surfactant rectal laxatives
Enemas: sodium docusate, sodium lauryl sulphoacetate, sodium alkyl sulphacetate.

Uses: docusate elixir can be used as an enema, but all the above agents are included in different proprietary mini-enemas to aid stool softening by aiding water penetration of the faecal mass.

Saline rectal laxatives
Suppositories: sodium phosphate.
Enemas: sodium phosphate, sodium citrate.

Uses: in rectal use, the saline laxatives are claimed to release bound water from faeces, but as with oral saline laxatives, these agents also may stimulate rectal or distal colonic peristalsis, an action that is presumably aided when an extended enema tube is used to place the liquid as high as possible in the rectum. Use of phosphate enemas can cause hypocalcaemia and hyperphosphataemia in ill patients or those with renal impairment[56]. Phosphate enemas can also produce rectal gangrene in ill patients with a history of haemorrhoids[57]. Hence, care should be taken in their use.

Sodium phosphate is available in an effervescent base as a suppository (Carbalax®). The resultant production of gas is intended to assist defecation, although as rectal distension by gas is readily distinguishable from that by stool the rationale is unclear.

Polyphenolic rectal laxative
Suppositories: bisacodyl suppositories, 5 mg (paediatric), 10 mg (adult).

Use: alone among rectal laxative preparations, bisacodyl suppositories act principally by promoting colonic peristalsis. Their latency of action is claimed to be 15–60 min, compared with 6–12 h orally. The difference is probably due to bisacodyl's immediate conversion to its active desacetyl form by colonic flora in the rectum. As activity depends on bisacodyl reaching the rectal mucosa[58], care should be taken so that stool does not separate the suppository from the rectal wall.

Bisacodyl suppositories are sometimes inserted in an empty rectum to 'bring the stool down'. A plausible rationale exists for this practice but its efficacy relative to use of oral laxatives, or even a high phosphate enema, is untested.

Selection of rectal laxatives

As with oral laxatives, there are few data on the comparative efficacy of rectal laxatives. One study showed the following percentages of patients achieving defecation within an hour of the rectal intervention: phosphate enema 100 per cent, mini-enema (Micralax®) 95 per cent, bisacodyl suppository 66 per cent, and glycerine suppository 38 per cent[59]. The approximately equal effectiveness of phosphate and mini-enemas[60], the speed of action of mini-enemas[61], and the superiority of bisacodyl suppositories over glycerine suppositories[62] have been confirmed elsewhere. The volume (about 130 ml) and potential adverse effects of phosphate enemas mean that, if an enema is required, the much smaller (5 ml), rather cheaper, and nearly as effective mini-enema, of which various proprietary products are available, is preferable. If a constipated patient simply requires assistance with an initial evacuation, suppositories may be adequate if only moderate softening is required. A combination of a bisacodyl and a glycerine suppository is often used, as is that of an enema followed by suppositories. Both practices are logical, but no data yet exist to show what advantages they may hold or which categories of patient may benefit.

If none of the rectal laxatives mentioned proves adequate to remove impacted faeces, rectal lavage with normal saline can be performed. This is cumbersome and messy, requiring about 8 l of (preferably) warmed saline. Tap water should not be used because of the risk of circulatory overload and neither should soap and water, which is irritant to the rectal mucosa and can cause hyperkalaemia if a potassium-based soap is employed. In practice, most units will prefer in these circumstances to follow the softening action of an oil retention enema with a manual removal of faeces, under cover of diazepam sedation if necessary.

Whenever rectal laxatives have been needed, the doses and types of oral laxatives being taken by the patient should be reappraised and if possible modified to obviate further rectal measures.

A guideline for laxative therapy

It would be desirable to produce an evidence-based guideline for the use of laxatives in palliative care, and a European Consensus group has recently produced clinical practice recommendations in this area.[62A] However, to date only three randomized controlled trials of laxatives appear to have been conducted in this patient group, together with another carried out in healthy volunteers using a model of opioid-induced constipation[36]. Of the clinical trials, one claimed to find a difference in effectiveness[51] and the others did not[63,64]. Because of differing designs and end-points, it is not possible to make a synthesis from these studies. The volunteer study found that all the preparations tested could relieve constipation, but the most favourable combination of medication burden and adverse effects arose from a combination of stimulant and softening types.

We are therefore still in the position of extrapolating evidence from other fields of medicine. Three possibly relevant systematic reviews of laxatives have been published: one looks at trials in chronic constipation[65] and the second, which is an extension of it, focuses on constipation in the elderly[66]. Seventeen out of 36 admissible trials in the first review and 9 out of 20 in the second

involved fibre-based preparations, which may be inappropriate for routine use in patients with advanced cancer. Both reviews conclude that laxatives and fibre improve bowel frequency by about 1.5 bowel movements per week compared with placebo. Neither was able to find evidence that any particular group of laxatives was more effective than another. The third review[67] addresses the effectiveness of laxatives in adults generally and reaches similar conclusions, although it draws attention to the cost implications of the lack of comparative data, that is, start with the cheapest laxative as there is no evidence that expensive ones are any better.

There is therefore no single correct way of selecting and employing laxatives, but one rational approach is summarized below. Naturally these situations may succeed one another.

1 *Exclude intestinal obstruction:* If in doubt, use only laxatives with a predominantly softening action, for example, lactulose or sodium docusate, in order to avoid causing colic. Do not use bulking agents.

2 *If the rectum is impacted with hard faeces* spontaneous evacuation is unlikely to be possible without local measures to soften the faecal mass, for example, glycerine suppositories, olive, or arachis oil enema. It still may be necessary to perform a manual rectal evacuation, for which sedation or additional analgesia is often required. Alternatively, saline rectal lavage can be given.

3 *If the rectum is loaded with soft faeces*, a predominantly peristalsis-stimulating laxative, for example, senna, may be effective alone. If there is rectal discomfort, a mini-enema may assist the initial defecation. Frequent review is essential, as there is a likelihood that a stool-softening laxative will be required later as well, given either separately, for example, lactulose, or as in combination preparation, for example, codanthrusate, codanthramer.

4 *If there is little or no stool in the rectum*, a peristalsis-stimulating laxative is the drug of choice, for example, senna, but the stools are likely to be hard and it is a reasonable policy to use a stool-softening laxative in addition, for example, lactulose, or a combination preparation, for example, codanthrusate, codanthramer.

New developments and alternative approaches

An important recent development is the availability for the first time of a specific antagonist to opioid-induced constipation, with the approval early in 2008 of methylnaltrexone by subcutaneous injection (Relistor®) for this indication. Methylnaltrexone is formed by N-methylation of the basic naltrexone molecule, which restricts its ability to cross the blood-brain barrier. Hence methylnaltrexone antagonises opioid actions at gastrointestinal mu-opioid receptors without impairing analgesia mediated by opioids in the central nervous system. In a double-blind randomised controlled trial conducted in 133 palliative care patients, methylnaltrexone was significantly superior to placebo in stimulating laxation without evidence of exacerbation of pain or precipitation of withdrawal.[67B] Initially the therapeutic role of methylnaltrexone is likely to be the treatment of opioid-induced constipation that has been resistant to conventional laxative interventions.

Meanwhile, among non-specific agents there is interest in the use of prokinetic agents to accelerate intestinal transit. Cisapride, which acts by enhancing acetylcholine release from myenteric neurons through $5HT_4$ receptor agonism, is better than placebo in improving stool consistency and frequency in idiopathic constipation[68]. It has, however, been withdrawn from the market in UK. A similar drug, tegaserod, is available in the US, where it is marketed for the relief of symptoms of irritable bowel syndrome including constipation[69]. Metoclopramide, which also increases gastrointestinal motility by interaction with gut $5HT_4$ receptors, has been shown to be effective in the so-called 'narcotic bowel syndrome' when given by continuous subcutaneous infusion[70]. Oral metoclopramide has not found a place in routine laxative treatment and is less potently prokinetic than cisapride.

As an antibiotic, oral erythromycin causes diarrhoea on about 50 per cent of occasions[71]. Apart from altering the balance of the gut flora, erythromycin acts as an agonist at motilin receptors, which are responsible for initiating the migrating motor complex in the small bowel. Motilin receptors are also present elsewhere in the gut and erythromycin reduces transit time in the right colon in healthy humans[72]. However, colonic activity was not stimulated in a group of chronically constipated individuals[73].

Morphine-induced constipation can be counteracted by an opioid antagonist given orally, because a major part of the opioid effect on the human gut is mediated peripherally rather than centrally. Naloxone has shown success experimentally in patients receiving strong opioid analgesia., but its variable systemic absorption poses too much risk of release of pain or opioid withdrawal symptoms for it to be marketed for this indication[74] Oral naloxone has a systemic availability of under 1 per cent, due to first pass hepatic metabolism, allowing a laxative effect without reversal of analgesia or generalized withdrawal. However, although non-controlled studies have shown response rates of 67–82 per cent, opioid withdrawal or return of pain has occurred in 13–30 per cent of people. Quaternary derivatives of opioid antagonists, which do not cross the blood–brain barrier, have proved to be a more secure alternative to naloxone. Alvimopan is a potent orally active mu-opioid antagonist that does not enter the central nervous system even when administered intravenously. Trials of the oral formulation in patients who were either on methadone maintenance or taking long-term opioids for chronic non-malignant pain have shown siginficant laxative effects compared to placebo[75]. Phase 3 trials that confirm these earlier findings have now been reported and alvimopan is likely to be marketed in the relatively near future. Methylnaltrexone, the quaternary derivative of the opioid antagonist naltrexone, has been trialed extensively in fairly small studies and usually in parenteral form. However, the results consistently show that methylnaltrexone can relieve opioid-induced constipation, including in a series of hospice patients in whom it showed a dose-related effect when given subcutaneously[76]. Attempts are being made to bring the drug to market.

Herbal medicine knows of many plants with laxative properties. Chrysanthemum stems and rhubarb have both been investigated recently as they contain anthraquinones, similar to the constituents of senna [77]. Patients may prefer such treatments to pharmaceutical laxatives

Diarrhoea

Definition

Diarrhoea is the passage of frequent loose stools with urgency. Objectively, it has been defined as the passage of more than three unformed stools within a 24-h period. Patients, however, may describe as 'diarrhoea' a single loose stool, frequent small stools of normal or even hard consistency, or faecal incontinence. As with constipation, therefore, a complaint of diarrhoea requires careful clarification.

Prevalence

Diarrhoea is a complaint of 7–10 per cent of cancer patients on admission to a hospice and 6 per cent of similar patients in hospital. It is, therefore, a far less common problem in palliative medicine than constipation when cancer patients are being considered, but 27 per cent of symptomatic HIV-infected patients have been reported to suffer diarrhoea[78]. (For management of HIV-related diarrhoea, see Chapter 12.2.)

Clinical manifestations and diagnostic considerations

Diarrhoea persisting for over 3 weeks is said to be chronic and is often linked to serious organic disease. Most diarrhoea is acute, lasting only a few days, and is generally the result of gastrointestinal infection (Table 10.2.3.7), possibly including overgrowth by *Candida*. In populations with advanced illness, however, the most common cause of diarrhoea is an imbalance of laxative therapy[79]. This particularly occurs when laxative doses have been increased to address an episode of severe constipation. The diarrhoea normally settles within 24–48 h if laxatives are temporarily stopped, after which they should be reinstated at a lower dose. Meanwhile the diarrhoea may be distressing, especially if it leads to faecal incontinence.

A variety of other common drugs can also precipitate diarrhoea, either commonly, as in the case of antacids and antibiotics, or idiosyncratically, as in the case of non-steroidal anti-inflammatory agents or iron preparations. Sorbitol, used as a sweetener in some 'sugar-free' elixirs, is easily overlooked as a cause of diarrhoea in sensitive patients. Those receiving enteral feeding appear particularly prone, sorbitol being more than twice as likely to be the cause of diarrhoea as the feed itself[80].

Malignant intestinal obstruction and faecal impaction are the next most common causes of diarrhoea in this patient group. Complete intestinal obstruction produces intractable constipation, but partial obstruction may present with either diarrhoea or alternating diarrhoea and constipation. This clinical picture can also result from severe constipation caused by opioid analgesia, where it has been dubbed the 'narcotic bowel syndrome'[17]. Faecal impaction results in fluid stool leaking past the mass, often with anal leakage or incontinence. In elderly patients hospitalized for non-malignant disease, faecal impaction can account for 55 per cent of instances of diarrhoea[81], emphasizing the need for careful attention to regular laxative therapy in any ill, relatively immobile population.

Certain cytotoxic chemotherapy agents, notably 5-fluorouracil (5FU) and irinotecan, can cause severe diarrhoea. The mechanism involves epithelial necrosis and inflammation, leading to a loss of absorptive surface and an imbalance between absorptive and secretory cells[82].

Radiotherapy involving the abdomen or pelvis is liable to cause diarrhoea, with a peak incidence in the second or third week of therapy and continuing for some time after cessation of the course. Damage to intestinal mucosa by radiation results in the release of prostaglandins and the malabsorption of bile salts, both of which increase peristaltic activity. Chronic radiation enteritis rarely presents as diarrhoea.

Table 10.2.3.7 Causes of diarrhoea in palliative medicine.

Drugs
Laxatives
Antacids
Antibiotics
Chemotherapy agents, esp. 5-fluorouracil, irinotecan
NSAID, esp. mefenamic acid, diclofenac, indomethacin
Mitomycin
Iron preparations
Disaccharide-containing elixirs
Radiation
Obstruction
Malignant
Faecal impaction
Narcotic bowel syndrome
Malabsorption
Pancreatic carcinoma
Gastrectomy
Ileal resection
Colectomy
Tumour
Colonic or rectal carcinoma
Pancreatic islet cell tumours
Carcinoid tumours
Concurrent disease
Diabetes mellitus
Hyperthyroidism
Inflammatory bowel disease
Irritable bowel syndrome
Gastrointestinal infection
Diet
Bran
Fruit
Hot spices
Alcohol

Uncommonly, another iatrogenic cause of diarrhoea relevant to palliative care is coeliac plexus blockade, which can be associated with the onset of profuse, long-lasting watery diarrhoea. This possibly results from anatomical variations in the innervation of the gut so that in certain individuals interruption of the coeliac plexus has an excessive influence on bowel activity[83].

Malabsorption sufficient to cause diarrhoea may occur in carcinoma of the head of the pancreas, or after gastrectomy or ileal resection. Failure of pancreatic secretion leads to reduced fat absorption and consequent steatorrhoea. Gastrectomy can also produce steatorrhoea, presumably as a result of poor mixing of food with pancreatic and biliary secretions. However, the accompanying vagotomy causes increased faecal secretion of bile acids in some patients, resulting in increased water and electrolyte secretion in the colon and hence a chologenic diarrhoea, compounding the problem.

A different type of malabsorption that can be seen in palliative care patients treated with antibiotics, or as a complication of gut infection such as *Clostridium difficile*, is lactose intolerance secondary to changes in the intestinal flora. Although this gradually resolves on its own, a lactose-free diet can produce prompt resolution of the diarrhoea[84].

Ileal resection reduces the gut's ability to reabsorb bile acids, of which up to 97 per cent are normally recirculated, again producing chologenic diarrhoea. This diarrhoea is characteristically watery and explosive. If less than 100 cm of terminal ileum is removed, fat malabsorption generally does not occur, as the liver can compensate for the increased biliary loss. A resection of over about 100 cm results in relative bile acid deficiency and hence fat malabsorption, exacerbating the diarrhoea. Ileal resection produces a disaccharidase deficiency proportional to the length of removed; this may result in an osmotic diarrhoea due to carbohydrate malabsorption.

Partial colectomy produces little, if any, persistent diarrhoea. However, total or almost total colectomy results in a high volume of liquid effluent that rapidly diminishes over 7–10 days but still remains at 400–800 ml/day owing to the small intestine's inability to compensate fully for the loss of the colon's water absorbing capacity. For this reason an ileostomy is normally fashioned. Such patients require an average of an extra litre of water per day and about 7 g of extra salt to compensate, with special care needed in hot weather. Iron and vitamin supplementation is also indicated. Similar symptoms can also result from an enterocolic fistula, caused either by cancer or as a result of operation[85]. Alteration of gut anatomy by surgery may also promote diarrhoea through bacterial overgrowth.

A colonic or rectal tumour can precipitate diarrhoea through causing partial intestinal obstruction, or loosen stools through increased mucus secretion. Rarely, endocrine tumours cause a secretory diarrhoea. The WDHA syndrome (watery diarrhoea hypokalaemia achlorhydria) is associated with tumours of the pancreatic islet cells and of the sympathetic nervous system, including the adrenal glands, and can occur with bronchogenic carcinomas. VIP is thought to be the causative hormone both here and in the diarrhoea of the Verner–Morrison syndrome encountered in childhood ganglioneuroblastoma. Diarrhoea occurs also in the Zollinger–Ellison syndrome, seen with pancreatic islet cell tumours secreting gastrin, and in carcinoid tumours, where serotonin, prostaglandins, bradykinin, and VIP secretions have all been implicated[86].

Apart from concurrent gastrointestinal disease (Table 10.2.3.6), the ability of dietary factors to cause diarrhoea should be remembered. Excessive dietary fibre may produce diarrhoea and fruits may do so both by this means and by their content of specific laxative factors.

Assessment

A complaint of diarrhoea demands a careful history, detailing first of all the frequency of defecation, the nature of the stools, and the time course of the problem. Together, these often indicate the diagnosis. Defecation described as 'diarrhoea', which occurs only once or twice a day, suggests anal incontinence. Profuse watery stools are characteristic of colonic diarrhoea, whereas the pale, fatty, offensive stools of steatorrhoea indicate malabsorption due to a pancreatic or small intestinal cause. The sudden advent of diarrhoea following a period of constipation, perhaps with little warning of impending defecation, should raise the suspicion of faecal impaction.

Both current and recent medication should be sought. If laxatives are to blame, the error may be of insufficiently regular therapy, resulting in alternating constipation and diarrhoea, or an excessive dose. Too much of a predominantly peristalsis-stimulating laxative tends to produce colic and urgency, and too much of a predominantly stool-softening agent may cause faecal leakage, although at high doses lactulose and docusate have the ability to produce colic and watery diarrhoea in some patients.

Examination and investigations

Examination should exclude the possibilities of faecal impaction and intestinal obstruction, and should therefore include rectal examination and abdominal palpation for faecal masses. If there is doubt, an abdominal radiograph will make the distinction, but this is rarely necessary.

Steatorrhoea is generally clearly suggested in the history and readily confirmed on examination of the stool. Persistent watery diarrhoea, without systemic upset, which would suggest an infective cause, may be more difficult to diagnose. If in doubt, the stool osmolality and sodium and potassium concentrations should be measured. The anion gap, the difference between the stool osmolality and double the sum of the cation concentrations, is over 50 mmol/l in osmotic diarrhoea, because of the presence of an additional non-absorbed solute, for example, a disaccharide from a medicinal elixir. An anion gap of below 50 mmol/l shows secretory diarrhoea, resulting from active secretion of fluid and electrolytes, as in the WDHA syndrome. Ileal resection gives rise to a mixed picture, which will become purely secretory if the patient can be fasted.

In any persistent diarrhoea, haematology and blood chemistry should be checked. Diarrhoea occurring within 3 days of inpatient admission may be due to community-acquired bacterial enteric pathogens such as *Salmonella*, *Shigella*, or *Campylobacter*, or to viral infection. After this point, the infection is likely to have originated in the inpatient unit and stool culture is usually unrewarding; repeating the culture does not improve the diagnostic yield[87]. *Clostridium difficile* is the most commonly detected cause of

nosocomial diarrhoea, most commonly the result of treatment with quinolone or cephalosporin antibiotics, and is identified by immunoassay of its toxins. In UK, its frequency in hospitals is increasing and strains are appearing that have higher yields of toxin[88].

Management approaches

Supportive treatment

Other than in HIV infection, diarrhoea in palliative medicine is rarely of sufficient degree or duration to cause significant risk through dehydration. If rehydration *is* needed the oral route is superior to the intravenous. Proprietary rehydration solutions, containing appropriate electrolyte concentrations and a source of glucose to facilitate active electrolyte transport across the gut wall, are adequate for all but the most severe diarrhoea. Any diarrhoea will benefit from a diet of clear liquids, such as flat lemonade or ginger ale, and simple carbohydrates, as in toast or crackers. Some infective causes of diarrhoea cause transient lactase deficiency and so milk should be avoided in these circumstances[84]. Protein and, later, fats are reintroduced gradually to the diet as the diarrhoea resolves.

Specific treatment

Specific treatments exist for several causes of diarrhoea (Table 10.2.3.8). Pancreatin is a combination of amylase, lipase, and protease, which is available in several forms for pancreatic enzyme replacement. The effective dose varies widely between individuals and it may be more effective if gastric acidity is reduced with an H_2-receptor antagonist, in which case enteric-coated preparations should not be used.

Cholestyramine is a bile acid-binding resin that is effective in controlling cholologenic diarrhoea provided ileal resection has not been too extensive. It is often found unpalatable. Both cholestyramine[89] and aspirin[90] have been claimed to be effective in radiation-induced diarrhoea.

Carcinoid syndrome diarrhoea often responds to general anti-diarrhoeals, but peripheral serotonin antagonists, such as methysergide or the less toxic cyproheptadine, have been claimed to be effective against more severe diarrhoea and, sometimes, the accompanying malabsorption[86]. $5HT_3$ antagonists may also have a role in this type of diarrhoea[91].

Metronidazole is the recommended antibiotic for *Clostridium difficile* diarrhoea, and can reasonably be tried also in situations where diarrhoea is suspected to be due to bacterial overgrowth, where it may produce a prompt resolution.

General treatment

Non-specific anti-diarrhoeal agents are numerous, and are either absorbent, adsorbent, mucosal prostaglandin inhibitors, opioids, or somatostatin derivatives. These agents may make illness due to *Shigella* and *Clostridium difficile* worse and so should be used with caution if these organisms are known to be present, or if there is blood in the stool or fever.

Absorbent agents

Preparations: bulk-forming agents, for example, methyl cellulose; pectin.

Mechanism: these agents absorb water to form a gelatinous or colloidal mass that gives a thicker consistency to loose stools. Water is held between the fibres in the case of bulk-forming agents,

Table 10.2.3.8 Specific treatments for diarrhoea in palliative medicine.

Fat malabsorption: pancreatin (may be more effective if H_2 antagonist given before meals)
Chologenic diarrhoea: cholestyramine, 4–12 g tds
Radiation diarrhoea: cholestyramine 4–12 g tds, or aspirin
Zollinger–Ellison syndrome: H_2-antagonist, e.g. ranitidine, initially 150 mg tds
Carcinoid syndrome: cyproheptadine, initially 12 mg daily; methysergide, 12–20 mg/day
Pseudomembranous colitis: vancomycin 125 mg qds; metronidazole 400 mg tds
Ulcerative colitis: mesalazine 1.2–2.4 g/day steroids

which are better regarded as 'stool normalizers than either laxative or anti-diarrhoeal preparations'. Pectin produces a viscous colloidal solution with both absorbent and adsorbent properties.

Uses: bulk-forming agents may have a delay of up to 48 h in onset of anti-diarrhoeal action and are poorly tolerated in ill patients. They have proved useful in the management of colostomies but exacerbate electrolyte loss from ileostomies.

The use of pectin against diarrhoea is time-honoured. It can be prepared simply from grated raw apple, but is sometimes combined with the adsorbent kaolin in proprietary anti-diarrhoeal mixtures. There is some evidence of effectiveness in children[92].

Adsorbent agents

Preparations and dose: kaolin, 2–6 g 4 hourly; chalk, 0.5–5 g 4 hourly; attapulgite, 1.2 g stat, 1.2 g after each loose stool up to 8.4 g/day.

Mechanism: adsorbents non-specifically take up dissolved or suspended substances, such as bacteria, toxins, and water, on to their surfaces. All are naturally occurring minerals, kaolin being hydrated aluminium silicate and attapulgite a hydrated magnesium aluminium silicate. The adsorptive capacity of a molecule depends on its surface area and attapulgite, having a three-layered crystalline structure, is claimed in consequence to have 33 times the adsorbent capacity of kaolin. How this translates into relative therapeutic efficacy is unknown.

Uses: attapulgite is used alone, but both kaolin and chalk are available in mixtures with morphine, the British Pharmacopoeia formulation of chalk with opium mixture containing considerably more morphine (5 mg/10 ml) than that of kaolin with morphine (0.7 mg/10 ml). Any difference in anti-diarrhoeal effectiveness between the mixtures is surely due to this factor. Indeed, there is no evidence, despite their popularity, of any significant anti-diarrhoeal effectiveness of either kaolin or chalk apart from that of the opiate with which they may be combined. Kaolin is also available in combination with pectin; there is the same dearth of evidence for efficacy. Attapulgite has, however, been shown to be better than placebo in acute diarrhoea although significantly less effective than loperamide[93].

Adsorbents may be appropriate for mild, non-specific acute diarrhoea in a healthy population. Their at best modest effectiveness, and the quite large volumes of a rather unattractive liquid that may have to be taken, make them unsuitable for general use in palliative medicine.

Mucosal prostaglandin inhibitors

Preparations and doses: aspirin, 300 mg 4 hourly, up to 4 g/day; mesalazine, 1.2–2.4 g/day; bismuth subsalicylate, 525 mg half-hourly up to 5 mg/day.

Mechanism: prostaglandins increase intestinal water and electrolyte secretion, and prostaglandin inhibitors (with exceptions such as mefenamic acid and indomethacin) reduce secretion. Bismuth subsalicylate is said to have a direct antimicrobial effect on enterotoxigenic *Escherichia coli*[94]. The active constituent of mesalazine is 5-amino-salicylic acid.

Uses: apart from bismuth subsalicylate, which is used for treatment of non-specific acute diarrhoea, these agents are used as specific anti-diarrhoeal treatments, aspirin for radiation-induced diarrhoea, and mesalazine in ulcerative colitis. All these agents are contraindicated in patients sensitive to salicylate, and the bismuth

compound in its upper dose range can produce toxic blood salicylate levels.

Anti-cholinergic agents

Any drug with anti-cholinergic actions will have a constipating effect, but the wider effects beyond the bowel make these drugs unattractive as routine anti-diarrhoeal management. However, more recently-developed selective muscarinic anti-cholinergic drugs have been shown to reduce small and large bowel motility in humans with significantly fewer general anti-cholinergic adverse effects than older agents, and in animals to reduce secretory and stress-related diarrhoea[95]. Although darifenacin and zamifenacin have been identified as having a role in controlling colic and diarrhoea in irritable bowel syndrome, darifenacin is marketed (Enablex®: not in UK) primarily for the relief of overactive bladder.

Opioid agents

Preparations and doses: codeine, 10–60 mg 4 hourly, duration of action: 4–6 h. Diphenoxylate, 10 mg stat, then 5 mg 6 hourly, duration of action 6–8 h. Loperamide, 4 mg stat, then 2 mg after each loose stool up to 16 mg per day, duration of action 8–16 h.

Mechanism: the opioids act via specific gut opioid receptors to reduce peristalsis in the colon. They also preserve the fasting pattern of motility in the small intestine after food intake. Their effects on water and electrolyte secretion in man at therapeutic doses are unconvincing. Loperamide is capable of reducing ileal calcium fluxes by a mechanism that is not inhibited by naloxone, but the contribution of this effect to its clinical activity is undetermined. Opioids increase anal sphincter pressure and loperamide and codeine have been shown to improve continence in patients with diarrhoea suffering from faecal incontinence[96]; diphenoxylate is less effective, even at the same stool frequency.

Alone of the three, loperamide given orally does not reach or cross the blood–brain barrier significantly. In animal studies the relative specificity for anti-diarrhoeal as opposed to analgesic effects for codeine, diphenoxylate, and loperamide was 5.24, 23.7, and greater than 552, respectively. The specificity for morphine was 6.45[97]. Although the recommended maximum daily dose of loperamide is 16 mg, volunteers have received 54 mg/day without ill-effects. Below its recommended maximum of 20 mg/day, diphenoxylate rarely gives significant systemic opioid effects, but does so at doses of 40 mg/day or more. As a result, it is available only in combination with atropine in order to limit its abuse potential.

In man, approximate equivalent anti-diarrhoeal doses are 200 mg/day of codeine, 10 mg/day of diphenoxylate, and 4 mg/day of loperamide[79].

Uses: the opioids are the mainstay of general anti-diarrhoeal treatment in palliative medicine. A requirement for morphine analgesia may obviate the need for any additional anti-diarrhoeal medication. Loperamide is the opioid anti-diarrhoeal of choice, being significantly more effective than diphenoxylate or codeine and with few adverse effects in adults. In children, it has been reported to cause ileus-like conditions, irritability, drowsiness, and signs of opioid toxicity, and more caution is therefore required in its use. For persistent diarrhoea, regular therapy can be given, the dose being titrated against the clinical response. The drug's duration of action means that administration can often be twice daily. Loperamide 8–12 mg/day significantly reduces ileostomy output[98], but in some severe chronic diarrhoeas, the required dose may need to be higher than usually recommended.

Codeine is prone to cause systemic opioid effects, but has the merit of cheapness, which encourages some units to use it for mild diarrhoea. In addition, despite the research evidence, clinical experience suggests that the individual response to opioids for diarrhoea can be as idiosyncratic as that for pain, and in some patients, codeine has superior anti-diarrhoeal properties than the other opioids without causing excessive nausea or drowsiness.

Diphenoxylate is at least as expensive as loperamide in equi-effective doses and appears to hold no advantages.

Somatostatin analogues

Preparations: octreotide: 300–600 mcg/24 h by subcutaneous infusion (British National Formulary recommendation—see notes below). Lanreotide: 30 mg intramuscularly every 14 days.

Mechanism: somatostatin is produced in intestinal D cells and acts on gut epithelial receptors to inhibit secretion and peristalsis. The native form has a short half-life but analogues have been created that are capable of extended activity.

Uses: octreotide has been shown to be effective in cryptosporidial diarrhoea and diarrhoea due to the carcinoid, Zollinger–Ellison, and Verner–Morrison syndromes as well as to ileostomy[99] or enterocolic fistula[85]. Subcutaneous injection of octreotide may be painful, but continuous subcutaneous infusion is generally well tolerated and the drug can be combined with morphine, diamorphine, haloperidol, midazolam, or hyoscine without apparent loss of efficacy[99]. Mixing with cyclizine may cause precipitation.

Although it is still not licensed in UK for the indication, octreotide is now established as an effective therapy for severe secretory diarrhoea, particularly that related to HIV infection, where doses up to 1500 mcg/24 h have been found necessary[100]. It also improves symptoms of malignant intestinal obstruction in up to 85 per cent of cases at doses that are usually within the range of 300–600 mcg/24 h. Although this principally relates to the incidence of vomiting, partial obstruction may produce diarrhoea and a trial of octreotide for this symptom is appropriate in these circumstances. However, expert consensus has recommended octreotide dose titration as high as 2400 mcg/24 h for chemotherapy-induced diarrhoea[101].

Lanreotide has a far more prolonged duration of action which, while being a valuable quality for stable conditions such as the acromegaly which is its primary indication, makes it inflexible for use in the continually changing clinical situations of palliative care. However, it has the advantage of requiring neither frequent injections nor an infusion device.

New developments

Calcium carbonate 3.6 g/day reduced stool frequency by a mean of 49 per cent and faecal wet weight by 50 per cent over 12 weeks in 15 post-gut-resection patients. No change in plasma calcium concentrations was found[102]. Results in healthy subjects have been variable. Oral calcium supplements precipitate free bile acids and fatty acids in the colon. As bile acids and fatty acids inhibit colonic absorption and stimulate fluid and electrolyte secretion, this may be calcium's mode of action.

There is increasing interest in the use of probiotics, or beneficial micro-organisms, for the management of diarrhoea, among other conditions. *Lactobacillus* spp. are the most commonly used.

To date there is limited evidence that they can be effective in infective diarrhoea in adults[103] and in the management of acquired lactose intolerance[84].

The pathogenesis of diarrhoea frequently involves neurohumoral mechanisms controlling water secretion, with a notable role for 5-hydroxytryptamine (5-HT), substance P, and VIP[104]. Antagonists to 5-HT and substance P may prove clinically useful in the future and peptide YY, which reduces intestinal fluid secretion, has been used experimentally in humans[105].

Further reading

Derby, S. and Portenoy, R.K. (1997). Assessment and management of opioid-induced constipation. In *Topics in palliative care*, Vol. 1 (eds. R.K. Portenoy and E. Bruera), pp. 95–112. Oxford University Press, New York.

Mancini, I. and Bruera, E. (2002). Constipation. In *Gastrointestinal symptoms in advanced cancer patients* (ed. C. Ripamonti), pp 193–206. Oxford University Press, Oxford.

Mercadante, S. (2002). Diarrhoea and malabsorption. In *Gastrointestinal symptoms in advanced cancer patients* (ed. C. Ripamonti), pp. 207–22. Oxford University Press, Oxford.

References

1. Connell, A.M., Hilton, C., Irvine, G. *et al.* (1965). Variation in bowel habit in two population samples. *British Medical Journal*, **ii**, 1095–9.
2. Drossman, D.A., Sandler, R.S., McKee, D.C. *et al.* (1982). Bowel patterns among subjects not seeking health care. *Gastroenterology*, **83**, 529–34.
3. Thompson, W.G., Longstreth, G.F., Drossman, D.A. *et al.* (1999). Functional bowel disorders and functional abdominal pain. *Gut*, **45**(Suppl. 2): 1143–7.
4. Herz, M.J., Kahan, E., Zalevski, S. *et al.* (1996). Constipation: a different entity for patients and doctors. *Family Practice*, **13**, 156–9.
5. Ashraf, W., Park, F., Lof, J. *et al.* (1996). An examination of the reliability of reported stool frequency in the diagnosis of idiopathic constipation. *American Journal of Gastroenterology*, **91**, 26–32.
6. Everhart, J.E., Go, V.L., Johannes, R.S. *et al.* (1989). A longitudinal survey of self-reported bowel habits in the United States. *Digestive Diseases and Sciences*, **34**, 1153–62.
7. Wigzell, F.W. (1969). The health of nonagenarians. *Gerontologia Clinica*, **11**, 137–44.
8. Cartwright, A., Hockey, L., and Anderson, J.L. (1973). *Life before death*. Routledge and Kegan Paul, London.
9. Madsen, J.L. and Dahl, K. (1990). Human migrating myoelectric complex in relation to gastrointestinal transit of a meal. *Gut*, **31**, 1003–5.
10. Bassotti, G. and Gaburri, M. (1988). Manometric investigation of high-amplitude propagated contractile activity of the human colon. *American Journal of Physiology*, **255**, G660–4.
11. Holdstock, D.J., Misiewicz, J.J., Smith, T. *et al.* (1970). Propulsion (mass movements) in the human colon and its relationship to meals and somatic activity. *Gut*, **11**, 91–9.
12. Sykes, N.P. (1990). Methods of assessment of bowel function in patients with advanced cancer. *Palliative Medicine*, **4**, 287–92.
13. Sykes, N.P. (2006). The pathogenesis of constipation. *J Supportive Oncol*, **4**, 213–8.
14. Lundgren, O. (1988). Nervous control of intestinal transport. *Baillieres Clinical Gastroenterology*, **2**, 85–106.
15. Read, N.W. and Timms, J.M. (1986). Defaecation and the pathophysiology of constipation. *Clinics in Gastroenterology*, **15**, 937–65.

16. Sykes, N.P. (1998). The relationship between opioid use and laxative use in terminally ill cancer patients. *Palliative Medicine*, **12**, 375–82.

17. Sandgren, J.E., McPhee, M.S., and Greenberger, N.J. (1984). Narcotic bowel syndrome treated with clonidine. *Annals of Internal Medicine*, **101**, 331–4.

18. Kaufman, P.N., Krevsky, B., Malmud, L.S. *et al.* (1988). Role of opiate receptors in the regulation of colonic transit. *Gastroenterology*, **94**, 1351–6.

19. Kreek, M.J., Schaefer, R.A., Hahn, E.F. *et al.* (1983). Naloxone, a specific opioid antagonist, reverses chronic idiopathic constipation. *Lancet*, **i**, 261–2.

20. Kreek, M.J., Paris, P., Bartol, M.A. *et al.* (1984). Effects of short term oral administration of the specific opioid antagonist naloxone on fecal evacuation in geriatric patients. *Gastroenterology*, **86**, 1144.

21. Ling, G.S., Paul, D., Simontov, R. *et al.* (1989). Differential development of acute tolerance. *Life Sciences*, **45**, 1627–36.

22. Fallon, M. and Hanks, G. (1999). Morphine, constipation and performance status in advanced cancer patients. *Palliative Medicine*, **13**, 159–60.

23. Radbruch, L., Sabatowski, R., Loick, G. *et al.* (2000). Constipation and the use of laxatives: a comparison between transdermal fentanyl and oral morphine. *Palliative Medicine*, **14**, 111–19.

24. Daeninck, P.J. and Bruera, E. (1999). Reduction in constipation and laxative requirements following opioid rotation to methadone. *Journal of Pain and Symptom Management*, **18**, 303–9.

25. Mancini, I.L., Hanson, J., Neumann, C.M. *et al.* (2000). Opioid type and other predictors of laxative dose in advanced cancer patients: a retrospective study. *J Pall Med*, **3**, 49–56.

26. Bruera, E., Suarez-Almazor, M., Velasco, A. *et al.* (1994). The assessment of constipation in terminal cancer patients admitted to a palliative care unit. *Journal of Pain and Symptom Management*, **9**, 515–19.

27. Barr, R.G., Levine, M.D., Wilkinson, R.H. *et al.* (1979). Occult stool retention: a clinical tool for its evaluation in school aged children. *Clinical Pediatrics*, **18**, 674–9.

28. Benninga, M.A., Buller, H.A., Staalman, C.R. *et al.* (1995). Defaecation disorders in children, colonic transit time versus the Barr score. *European Journal of Paediatrics*, **154**, 277–84.

29. Sykes, N.P. (2001). Methods for clinical research in constipation. In *Symptom research: methods and opportunities. An interactive textbook* (eds. M. Max and J. Lynn). National Institutes of Dental and Craniofacial Research, Bethesda. Available at www.symptomresearch. com/chapter_3/index.htm (accessed 18 July 2003).

30. McMillan, S.C. and Williams, F.A. (1989). Validity and reliability of the Constipation Assessment Scale. *Cancer Nursing*, **12**, 183–8.

31. Agachan, F., Chen, T., Pfeifer, J. *et al.* (1996). A constipation scoring system to simplify evaluation and management of constipated patients. *Diseases of the Colon and Rectum*, **39**, 681–5.

32. Frank, L., Kleinman, L., Farup, C. *et al.* (1999). Psychometric validation of a constipation assessment questionnaire. *Scandinavian Journal of Gastroenterology*, **34**, 870–7.

33. Twycross, R.G. and Lack, S.A. (eds) (1986). Constipation. In *Control of alimentary symptoms in far advanced cancer*, pp. 166–207. Churchill Livingstone, London.

34. Muller-Lissner, S.A. (1988). Effect of wheat bran on weight of stool and gastrointestinal transit time: a meta-analysis. *British Medical Journal*, **296**, 615–17.

35. Mumford, S.P. (1986). Can high fibre diets improve the bowel function in patients on a radiotherapy ward? Cited in: Twycross, R.G., and Lack, S.A. *Control of Alimentary Symptoms in Far Advanced Cancer*, p. 183. Churchill Livingstone, Edinburgh.

36. Sykes, N.P. (1997). A volunteer model for the comparison of laxatives in opioid-induced constipation. *Journal of Pain and Symptom Management*, **11**, 363–9.

37. Bateman, D.N. and Smith, J.M. (1988). A policy for laxatives. *British Medical Journal*, **297**, 1420–1.

38. Moriarty, K.J., Fairclough, P.D., Clark, M.L. *et al.* (1982). Inhibition of glucose and water absorption in the human jejunum by dioctyl sodium sulphosuccinate: a prostaglandin-mediated phenomenon? *Gut*, **23**, A443.

39. Chapman, R.W., Sillery, J., and Saunders, D.R. (1984). Dioctyl sodium sulphosuccinate, 300 mg daily, does not increase human ileal or colonic output. *Gut*, **25**, A1156.

40. Hyland, C.M. and Foran, J.D. (1968). Dioctyl sodium sulphosuccinate as a laxative in the elderly. *Practitioner*, **200**, 698–9.

41. Read, N.W. (1990). Motility: functional diseases. *Current Opinion in Gastroenterology*, **6**, 9–13.

42. Gibson, G.R. and Roberfroid, M.B. (1995). Dietary modulation of the human colonic microbiota: introducing the concept of prebiotics. *Journal of Nutrition*, **125**, 1401–12.

43. Lederle, F.A., Busch, D.L., Mattox, K.M. *et al.* (1990). Cost-effective treatment of constipation in the elderly: a randomised double-blind comparison of sorbitol and lactulose. *American Journal of Medicine*, **89**, 597–601.

44. Harvey, R.F. and Read, N.W. (1975). Mode of action of the saline purgatives. *American Heart Journal*, **89**, 810–13.

45. Hammer, H.F., Santa Ana, C.A., Schiller, L.R. *et al.* (1989). Studies of osmotic diarrhea induced in normal subjects by ingestion of PEG and lactulose. *Journal of Clinical Investigation*, **84**, 1056–62.

46. Culbert, P., Gillett, H., and Ferguson, A. (1998). Highly effective new oral therapy for faecal impaction. *British Journal of General Practice*, **48**, 1599–600.

47. Corazziari, E., Badiali, D., Habib, F.I. *et al.* (1996). Small volume isosmotic polyethylene glycol electrolyte balanced solution (PMF-100) balanced solution in treatment of chronic non-organic constipation. *Digestive Diseases and Sciences*, **41**, 1636–42.

48. Wirz S. and Klaschik E. (2005). Management of constipation in palliative care patients undergoing opioid therapy: is polyethylene glycol an option? *American Journal of Hospice and Palliative Care*, **22**, 375–81.

49. Camilleri M., Bharucha A.E., Ueno R. *et al.* (2006). Effect of a selective chloride channel activator, lubiprostone, on gastrointestinal transit, gastric sensory, and motor functions in healthy volunteers. *American Journal of Physiology Gastrointestinal and Liver Physiology*, **290**, G942–7.

50. Leng-Peschlow, E. (1989). Effects of sennosides A + B and bisacodyl on rat large intestine. *Pharmacology*, **38**, 310–8.

51. Sykes, N.P. (1991). A clinical comparison of laxatives in a hospice. *Palliative Medicine*, **5**, 307–14.

52. Verhaeren, E.H., Geeraerts, V.C., and Lemli, J. (1987). The antagonistic effect of morphine on rhein-stimulated fluid, electrolyte and glucose movements in guinea-pig perfused colon. *Journal of Pharmacy and Pharmacology*, **39**, 39–44.

53. Maguire, L.C., Yon, J.L., and Miller, E. (1981). Prevention of narcotic-induced constipation. *New England Journal of Medicine*, **305**, 1651.

54. Brunton, L.L. (1985). Laxatives. In *The pharmacological basis of therapeutics*, 7th edition (eds. A.G. Gilman, L.S. Goodman, T.W. Rall, and F. Murad), pp. 994–1003. Macmillan, New York.

55. Joo, J.S., Ehrenpreis, E.D., Gonzalez, L. *et al.* (1998). Alterations in colonic anatomy induced by chronic stimulant laxatives: the cathartic colon revisited. *Journal of Clinical Gastroenterology*, **26**, 283–6.

56. Woo Y.M., Crail S., Curry G. *et al.* (2006). A life threatening complication after ingestion of sodium phosphate bowel preparation. *British Medical Journal*, **333**, 589–90.

57. Sweeney, J.L., Hewett, P., Riddell, P. *et al.* (1986). Rectal gangrene: a complication of phosphate enema. *Medical Journal of Australia*, **144**, 374–5.

58. Flig E., Hermann T.W., and Zabel M. (2000). Is bisacodyl absorbed at all from suppositories in man? *International Journal of Pharmaceutics*, **196**, 11–20.

59. Sweeney, W.J. (1963). The use of disposable microenema in obstetrical patients. *Proceedings of a Symposium on the Clinical Evaluation of a New Disposable Microenema*, New Brunswick, June, pp. 7–8.

60. Postlethwait, R.W. (1965). Microenema as evacuant before proctoscopy. *Current Therapeutic Research*, **7**, 7–9.

61. Lieberman, W. (1964). Rapid patient preparation for sigmoidoscopy by microenema. *American Journal of Proctology*, **15**, 138–41.

62. Mandel, L. and Silinsky, J. (1960). Bisacodyl (Dulcolax): an evacuant suppository. A controlled therapeutic trial in chronically ill and geriatric patients. *Canadian Medical Association Journal*, **83**, 384–7.

62A. Larkin PJ, Sykes NP, Centeno C, Ellershaw JE, Elsner F, Eugene B, Gootjes JR, Nabal M, Noguera A, Ripamonti C, Zucco F, Zuurmond WW. The management of constipation in palliative care: clinical practice recommendations. *Palliative Medicine*, 2008; **22**, 796–807.

62B. Thomas, J., Karver, S., Cooney, G.A. *et al.* (2008). Methylnaltrexone for opioid-induced constipation in advanced illness. *New England Journal of Medicine*, 358, 2332–43.

63. Agra, Y., Sacristan, A., Gonzalez, M. *et al.* (1998). Efficacy of senna versus lactulose in terminal cancer patients treated with opioids. *Journal of Pain and Symptom Management*, **15**, 1–7.

64. Ramesh, P.R., Suresh Kumar, K., Rajagopal, M.R. *et al.* (1998). Managing morphine-induced constipation: a controlled comparison of an Ayurvedic formulation and senna. *Journal of Pain and Symptom Management*, **16**, 240–4.

65. Tramonte, S.M., Brand, M.B., Mulrow, C.D. *et al.* (1997). The treatment of chronic constipation in adults: a systematic review. *Journal of General Internal Medicine*, **12**, 15–24.

66. Petticrew, M., Watt, I., and Sheldon, T. (1997). Systematic review of the effectiveness of laxatives in the elderly. *Health Technology Assessment*, **1**, 1–52.

67. NHS Centre for Reviews and Dissemination (2001). Effectiveness of laxatives in adults. *Effective Health Care*, **7**(1), 1–12.

67A. Thomas, J., Karver, S., Cooney, G.A. Methylnaltrexone for opiod-induced constipation in advanced illness. *New England Journal of Medicine 2008*. **358**, 2332–2343.

68. Muller-Lissner, S.A. (1987). Treatment of chronic constipation with cisapride and placebo. *Gut*, **28**, 1033–8.

69. Evans, B.W., Clark, W.K., Moore, D.J. *et al.* (2005). Tegaserod for the treatment of irritable bowel syndrome. *Cochrane Review*. In: The Cochrane Library, 2.

70. Bruera, E., Brenneis, C., Michand, M. *et al.* (1987). Continuous subcutaneous infusion of metoclopramide for treatment of narcotic bowel syndrome. *Cancer Treatment Reports*, **71**, 1121–2.

71. Shanson, D.C., Akash, S., Harris, M. *et al.* (1985). Erythro-mycin stearate 1.5g, for the oral prophylaxis of streptococcal bacteraemia in patients undergoing dental extraction: efficacy and tolerance. *Journal of Antimicrobial Chemotherapy*, **15**, 83–90.

72. Hasler, W., Heldsinger, A., Soudah, H. *et al.* (1990). Erythromycin promotes colonic transit in humans: mediation via motilin receptors. *Gastroenterology*, **98**, A358.

73. Bassotti, G., Chiaroni, G., Vantini, I. *et al.* (1998). Effect of different doses of erythromycin on colonic motility in patients with slow transit constipation. *Zeitschrift fur Gastroenterologie*, **36**, 209–13.

74. Sykes, N.P. (2005). Using oral naloxone in management of opioid bowel dysfunction. In *Handbook of opioid bowel dysfunction* (ed. C.-S. Yuan), pp. 175–95. Haworth, New York.

75. Foss, J.F. and Schmidt, W.K. (2005). Management of opioid-induced bowel dysfunction and postoperative ileus: potential role of alvimopan. In *Handbook of opioid bowel dysfunction* (ed. C.-S.Yuan), pp. 223–49. Haworth, New York.

76. Thomas, J., Portenoy, R.K., Moehl, M. *et al.* (2003). A phase II randomized dose-finding trial of methylnaltrexone for the relief of opioid-induced constipation in hospice patients. *Proceedings of the American Society of Clinical Oncology*, **22**, 2933.

77. Sykes, N. and Gibbs, M. (2006). Constipation. In *Textbook of complementary and alternative medicine* (eds. C.S. Yuan, E.J. Bieber, and B.A. Bauer), pp. 471–8. Informa, London.

78. Rolston, K.V., Rodriguez, S., Hernandez, M. *et al.* (1989). Diarrhoea in patients infected with HIV. *American Journal of Medicine*, **86**, 137–8.

79. Twycross, R.G. and Lack, S.A. (1986). Diarrhoea. In *Control of alimentary symptoms in far advanced cancer*, pp. 208–29. Churchill Livingstone, London.

80. Edes, T.D., Walk, B.E., and Austin, J.L. (1990). Diarrhoea in tube-fed patients: feeding formula not necessarily the cause. *American Journal of Medicine*, **88**, 91–3.

81. Kinnunen, O., Janhonen, P., Salokannel, J. *et al.* (1989). Diarrhoea and faecal impaction in elderly long-stay patients. *Zeitschrift Gerontologie*, **22**, 321–3.

82. Kornblau S., Benson A.B., Catalano R. et al. (2000). Management of cancer treatment-related diarrhea: issues and therapeutic strategies. *Journal of Pain and Symptom Management*, **19**, 118–29.

83. Dean, A.P. and Reed, W.D. (1991). Diarrhoea—an unrecognised hazard of coeliac plexus block. *Australian and New Zealand Journal of Medicine*, **21**, 47–8.

84. Noble, S., Rawlinson, F., and Byrne, A. (2002). Acquired lactose intolerance: a seldom considered cause of diarrhea in the palliative care setting. *Journal of Pain and Symptom Management*, **23**, 449.

85. Mercadante, S. (1992). Treatment of diarrhoea due to enterocolic fistula with octreotide in a terminal cancer patient. *Palliative Medicine*, **6**, 257–9.

86. Norton, J.A., Doppman, J.L., and Jensen, R.T. (1989). Cancer of the endocrine system. In *Cancer: principles and practice of oncology*, 3rd edition (eds. V.T. DeVita, S. Hellman, and S.A. Rosenberg), pp. 1269–344. Lippincott, Philadelphia.

87. Chitkara, Y.K., McCasland, K.A., and Kenefic, L. (1996). Development and implementation of cost-effective guidelines in the laboratory investigation of diarrhea in a community hospital. *Archives of Internal Medicine*, **156**, 1445–8.

88. Health Protection Agency. (2005). Management, prevention and surveillance of *Clostridium difficile*: interim findings from a national survey of NHS acute trusts in England. Commission for Healthcare Inspection and Audit, London.

89. Condon, J.R., South, M., Wolveson, R.L. *et al.* (1996). Radiation diarrhoea and cholestyramine. *Postgraduate Medical Journal*, **54**, 838–9.

90. Mennie, A.T., Dalley, V.M., Dinneen, L.C., and Collier, H.O. (1975). Treatment of radiation-induced gastrointestinal distress with acetylsalicylate. *Lancet*, **ii**, 942–3.

91. Saslow, S.B., Scolapio, J.S., Camilleri, M. *et al.* (1998). Medium-term effects of a new 5HT3 antagonist, alosetron, in patients with carcinoid diarrhoea. *Gut*, **42**, 628–34.

92. de la Motte, S., Bose-O'Reilly, S., Heinisch, M. *et al.* (1997). Double-blind comparison of an apple pectin-chamomile extract preparation with placebo in children with diarrhoea. *Arzneimittel-Forschung*, **47**, 1247–9.

93. DuPont, H.L., Ericsson, C.D., DuPont, M.W. *et al.* (1990). A randomized, open-label comparison of nonprescription loperamide and attapulgite in the symptomatic treatment of acute diarrhoea. *American Journal of Medicine*, **88**(Suppl. 6A), 205–35.

94. Graham, D.Y., Evans, M.K., and Gentry, L.O. (1983). Double-blind comparison of bismuth subsalicylate and placebo in prevention and treatment of ETEC-induced diarrhoea in volunteers. *Gastroenterology*, **85**, 1017–22.

95. Callahan, M.J. (2002). Irritable bowel syndrome neuropharmacology: a review of approved and investigational compounds. *Journal of Clinical Gastroenterology*, **35**(1) (Suppl), S58–67.

96. Palmer, K.R., Corbett, C.L., and Holdsworth, C.D. (1980). Double-blind cross-over study comparing loperamide, codeine and diphenoxylate in the treatment of chronic diarrhoea. *Gastroenterology*, **79**, 1272–5.

97. Awouters, F., Niemeegers, C.J.E., and Janssen, P.A.J. (1983). Pharmacology of antidiarrhoeal drugs. *Annual Review of Toxicology and Pharmacology*, **23**, 279–301.

98. Ruppin, H. (1987). Review: loperamide—a potent antidiarrhoeal drug with actions along the alimentary tract. *Alimentary Pharmacology and Therapeutics*, **1**, 179–90.

99. Riley, J. and Fallon, M.T. (1994). Octreotide in terminal malignant obstruction of the gastrointestinal tract. *European Journal of Palliative Care*, **1**, 23–5.

100. Romeu, J., Miro, J.M., Sirera, G. et al. (1991). Efficacy of octreotide in the management of chronic diarrhoea in AIDS. *AIDS*, **5**, 1495–9.

101. Harris, A.G., O'Dorisio, T.M., Woltering, E.A. et al. (1995). Consensus statement: octreotide dose titration in secretory diarrhea. Diarrhea Management Consensus Development Panel. *Digestive Diseases and Sciences*, **40**, 1464–73.

102. Steinbach, G., Lupton, J., Reddy, B.S. et al. (1996). Calcium carbonate treatment of diarrhoea in intestinal bypass patients. *European Journal of Gastroenterology and Hepatology*, **8**, 559–62.

103. D'Souza A.L., Rajkumar C., Cooke J. et al. (2002). Probiotics in the prevention of antibiotic associated diarrhea: meta-analysis. *British Medical Journal*, **324**, 1361–6.

104. Farthing, M.J. (2000). Novel targets for the pharmacotherapy of diarrhoea: a view for the millenium. *Journal of Gastroenterology and Hepatology*, **15**(Suppl), G38–45.

105. Playford, R.J., Domin, J., Beacham, J. et al. (1990). Preliminary report: role of peptide YY in defence against diarrhoea. *Lancet*, **335**, 1555–7.

10.2.4 **Pathophysiology and management of malignant bowel obstruction**

Carla Ripamonti and
Sebastiano Mercadante

Introduction

Malignant bowel obstruction (MBO) is a complex problem occurring particularly in cancer patients with advanced gynaecological and gastrointestinal cancer. Although it may develop at any time in the disease, it occurs most frequently at the advanced stage, with the highest incidence ranging from 5.5 to 42 per cent in ovarian carcinoma. Bowel obstruction occurs in 4.4–24 per cent of patients with colorectal cancer[1–7]. Breast and lung cancer and melanoma are the most frequent extra-abdominal primaries causing bowel obstruction, ranging from 3–15 per cent of cases. Different clinical settings, variation in admission criteria of individual palliative care units or diagnosis parameters, or clinical evaluation may explain the difference in incidence[8–10].

MBO may be a presenting feature of intra-abdominal malignancy or a feature of recurrent disease or other pathology in patients with a history of malignancy. The aetiology may be benign in 10–48 per cent of cases at operation, caused by adhesions or radiation enteritis, or malignant with single site, multiple site, or diffuse disease. MBO can be at a single site or multiple sites, partial or complete, and occurs in the small intestine more commonly than the large intestine.

Primary cancer, relapse after surgery, chemotherapy or radiotherapy, associated pathologies, and diffuse carcinomatosis may cause bowel obstruction with different mechanisms[11]. Such phenomena are often concomitant. The enlargement of the primary tumour or recurrence of abdominal masses, fibrosis, or adhesions may produce extrinsic occlusion of the lumen. Polypoidal lesions or annular narrowing due to dissemination may cause an intraluminal occlusion of the lumen. Infiltration of the intestinal muscles or superimposed inflammation may produce intramural occlusion of the lumen. Intestinal motility disorders due to a deranged extrinsic neural control of viscera may produce delay in intestinal transit, resulting in a clinical picture similar to bowel obstruction, namely, pseudo-obstruction. Concomitant diseases, such as diabetes, paraneoplastic syndromes, or previous gastric surgery, may contribute to dysmotility of this kind.

Constipation, due to illness and/or to drugs such as anticholinergics and opioids, is a frequent concomitant factor, as pain due to opioid-induced constipation, wrongly treated with increased doses of opioids, may result in faecal impaction producing signs of bowel obstruction[12].

Pathophysiology

A state of bowel obstruction is defined as an occlusion of the lumen or a functional dysfunction due to damage of structures that activate the propulsion of the intestinal contents. A delay in intestinal transit is responsible for the accumulation of non-absorbed secretions, which produces abdominal distension and a colicky activity to surmount the obstacle in an early stage. This early stage—a 'sub-obstructive' stage—may be still reversible. The bowel continues to contract with increased uncoordinated peristaltic activity, becomes distended, stimulating intestinal fluid secretion, thus creating a vicious cycle of distension and secretion, further stretching the bowel wall. An increased production of gases in the small intestine, due to an abnormally increased flora, may also contribute to the distension[13].

The consequence is the creation of a hypertensive state in the lumen, inducing mucosal damage and a reactive inflammatory response. This inflammatory response involves activation of the cycloxygenase pathway and the release of prostaglandins, which are potent secretagogues, either by a direct effect on enterocytes or via the enteric nervous reflex[13]. Hypoxia, caused by the reduction in venous drainage from the obstructed segment interfering with oxygen consumption, is the primary stimulus for vasoactive intestinal polypeptide (VIP) release, as well as intraluminal bacterial overgrowth. VIP is released into the portal and peripheral circulation and mediates local intestinal and systemic pathophysiological alterations as hyperaemia and oedema of the intestinal wall and an accumulation of fluid in the lumen thanks to its stimulating effects[14,15]. Experimental studies have shown that higher VIP content is present in duodenal tissue when compared to colonic tissue. High portal levels of VIP are known to cause hypersecretion and splanchnic vasodilatation[16]. These effects result in changes in redistribution of blood flow between the obstructed segment and the distal sites. Alterations of the auto-regulatory local and neuro-humoral control mechanisms of the splanchnic flow lead to the production of a third space for fluids and electrolytes in the gut wall and in its lumen[17]. The hypovolaemic state may induce functional renal failure due to a decrease in the renal blood flow and, as a consequence, a reduction in glomerular filtration. Oliguria, azotaemia, and haemoconcentration may accompany dehydration. Metabolic disorders in intestinal obstruction depend on the site and duration of the obstruction and are caused by dehydration, electrolyte losses, and disorders of acid–base balance[18]. The respiratory pattern will depend on the level of obstruction. The increased abdominal distension reduces the venous return and may impair pulmonary ventilation as a result of elevation of the diaphragm. With a high-level obstruction, a prevalent loss of gastric secretions will produce metabolic alkalosis, hypochloraemia, and hypokalaemia, whereas in the presence of a low-level obstruction, intestinal stasis of biliary, pancreatic, intestinal, as well as gastric secretions will induce deficiencies of chloride, sodium, potassium, and bicarbonates[11,19]. Sepsis will occur in the late stages of bowel obstruction, probably as a result of bacterial action. The increase in endoluminal pressure, stasis, intestinal ischaemia and gangrene, and perforation, progressively observed in the late stages of bowel obstruction, facilitate the passage of toxins through the intestinal wall into the lymphatic and systemic circulation. The time course of these events is variable, occurring over several days in malignant mechanical bowel obstruction.

Symptoms and diagnosis

The level of obstruction will determine the pattern of symptoms. The progression may be slow or fast, from partial obstruction to complete occlusion, each producing a different spectrum of symptoms, differing intensity of suffering, and ultimate outcome. Accumulation and increased production of secretions cause the principal symptoms, namely abdominal pain and distension, vomiting, and constipation (Fig. 10.2.4.1). In the presence of a high level of obstruction, such as in the stomach, duodenum, pancreas, or jejunum, vomiting develops early and in larger volumes, whereas in large bowel obstruction, symptoms occur progressively and abdominal distension is more pronounced. Distension may be minimal in both jejunal involvement and fixed tumours extensively infiltrating the small bowel and abdominal wall. Nausea is persistent or occasionally subsides temporarily after an episode of vomiting. Continuous pain is due to an enlarging visceral mass compressing the intestine, intestinal distension, or hepatomegaly. Severe superimposed colic above the obstruction in the small or large intestine may worsen the distress. This symptom is variable in intensity and site and is due to distension proximal to the obstruction.

Dry mouth is invariably associated with the other symptoms, and is the consequence of severe dehydration and metabolic alterations, as well as the use of anticholinergic drugs. No evacuation of

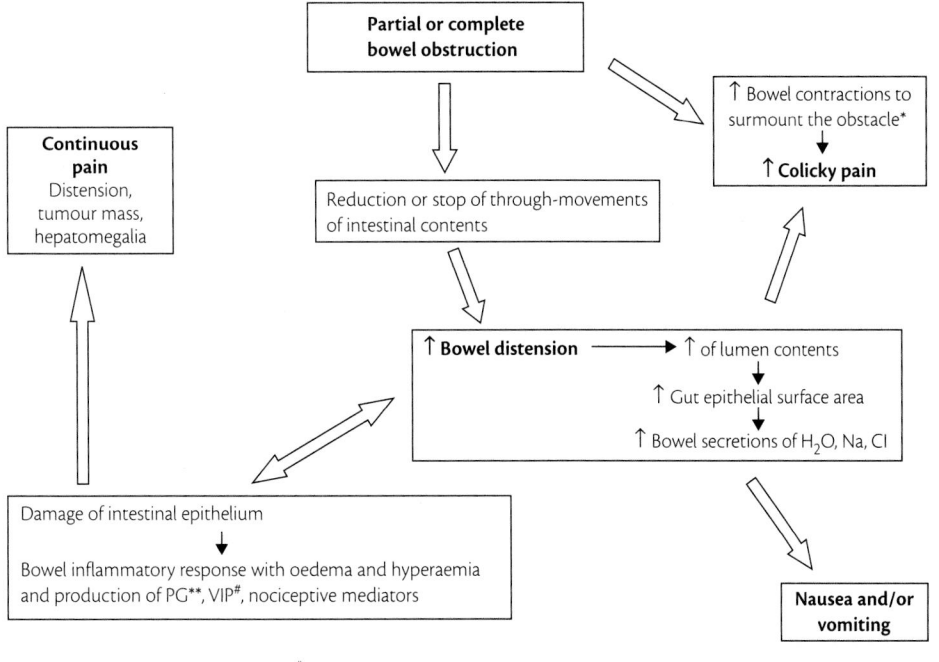

*Mechanical obstruction. **Prostaglandins. #Vasoactive intestinal polypeptide

Figure 10.2.4.1 Causes of symptoms in malignant bowel obstruction.

faeces and no passing of flatus are typical features of complete obstruction. The eventual appearance of paradoxical diarrhoea results from leakage of faecal fluid from faecal impaction due to bacterial overgrow, generally in large bowel obstruction.

The diagnosis of intestinal obstruction is established or suspected on clinical grounds and usually confirmed with plain abdominal radiography demonstrating fluid levels. Contrast radiography may help in defining the site and the extent of obstruction. Barium is not absorbed and may interfere with subsequent diagnostic studies; so it is contraindicated. Gastrografin offers a good radiological definition and may be useful in restoring intestinal transit in reversible obstruction. Abdominal CT scan is useful in evaluating the global extent of disease, which may be important for a surgical decision. It is often very difficult to differentiate between complete and partial bowel obstruction[20].

Management of intestinal obstruction

The management of patients with MBO is one of the greatest challenges facing physicians who care for cancer patients. While surgery should be always considered first for MBO, it is now recognized that many patients with advanced disease, who are in a poor general condition, are unfit for surgery and require alternative management to relieve distressing symptoms. Thus, significant patient discomfort and suffering must be balanced by the need to simplify the care of those patients with a short time to live. Self-expanding metallic stents are increasingly used as an option in the management of MBO at the level of the gastric outlet, proximal small bowel, and colon. (see Chapter 9.5) Medical treatment by parenteral administration of analgesics, antisecretory drugs, and/or antiemetics has been shown to be an effective approach for controlling pain, nausea, and vomiting in patients with inoperable MBO. Nasogastric suction or percutaneous gastrostomy may be considered for the patients with refractory symptoms or upper MBO who do not respond satisfactorily to pharmacological measures[20].

Surgery (see also Chapter 9.3)

The role of surgery remains controversial because of the lack of clear information evaluating outcome measures appropriately. Surgical treatment that palliates symptoms of MBO includes bypass procedures such as entero–entero anastomosis, enterocolon anastomosis, or the creation of an external stoma. The surgical technique used depends on the type and site of obstruction[21]. Surgical intervention should be considered when relief of obstructive symptoms is not achieved with 48–72 h of conservative, medical management[22,23].

The guidelines for conservative versus surgical treatment in patients with advanced cancer are still conflicting[20,24]. In the surgical literature, benefit from surgery is commonly defined as at least 60 days of survival after operation. However, outcome assessment, quality of life, symptom control, and patient comfort have been never assessed appropriately. In the study by Lund et al.[2], Forthy-three per cent of fifty-six per cent of patients who survived 60 days after operation manifested intermittent symptoms of incomplete and complete intestinal obstruction until death. In a large percentage of cases, surgery can lead to further complications.

Table 10.2.4.1 reviews the operative mortality rate (defined as death from any cause within 30 days of the operation), the morbidity, and the length of survival after surgery for bowel obstruction, according to publications from 1989 to 1997. Published data show that, in advanced cancer, the operative mortality is 9–40 per cent; with complication rates varying from 9–90 per cent[1,2,18,24–34].

Table 10.2.4.1 Complications and survival time after surgery for bowel obstruction.

Authors (reference)	No. of patients	Primary cancer	30-day mortality (%)	Other operative complications (%)	Survival (months)
Lund et al.[2]	25	Ovary	32	32.0	2.0 median
Rubin et al.[25]	43	Ovary	9	11.5	6.8 mean
Beattie et al.[1]	11	Ovary	9	9	7.0 mean
van Oojen et al.[26]	20	Ovary	30	90	1.0 median
Jong et al.[27]	53	Ovary	—	42[a]	3.0 median
Sun et al.[32]	57	Ovary	9	39[b]	3.0 median
Turnbull et al.[28]	89	Abdominal	13	44	4.5 mean
Butler et al.[29]	25	Various	24	50	2.5 median
Chan et al.[18]	10	Various	40	80	2 median
Lau et al.[30]	30	Colorectal	37	27	6.1 median
Tang et al.[31]	43	Abdominal	12	—	—
Yazdi et al.[33]	17	Various	41	—	—
Woolfson et al.[34]	32	Abdominal	22	48[b]	7.0 mean

Note: — not reported.
[a] Died with signs and symptoms of persistent or recurrent bowel obstruction.
[b] Continued to have some obstructive symptoms or recurrence of intestinal obstruction.

Table 10.2.4.2 Prognostic indicators of low likelihood of clinical benefit from surgery of MBO[a].

1	Obstruction secondary to cancer[29]
2	[b]Intestinal motility problems due to diffuse intraperitoneal carcinomatosis[5,7,26,28,37]
3	[c]Widespread tumour[4]
4	[c]Patients over 65[4] in association with cachexia[6,37]
5	[b]Ascites requiring frequent paracentesis[4–7,26,33,38]
6	[c]Low serum albumin level[6] and low serum pre-albumin level[39]
7	[c]Previous radiotherapy of the abdomen or pelvis[3,4]
8	Patients with nutritional deficits[40,41]
9	[b]Diffuse palpable intra-abdominal masses[6,26] and liver involvement
10	[c]Distant metastases, pleural effusion, or pulmonary metastases[4,35,38]
11	[b]Multiple partial bowel obstruction with prolonged passage time on X-ray examination[6,38]
12	[c]Elevated blood urea nitrogen levels, elevated alkaline phosphatase levels, advanced tumour stage, short diagnosis to obstruction interval[6,38]
13	[c]Poor performance status[42]
14	[b]A recent laparotomy which demonstrated that further corrective surgery was not possible[20]
15	[b]Previous abdominal surgery which showed diffuse metastatic cancer[20]
16	[b]Involvement of proximal stomach[20]
17	[c]Extra-abdominal metastases producing symptoms which are difficult to control (e.g. dyspnoea)[20]

Note: [a] Data from retrospective studies.
[b] Absolute contraindications = each is a 'stand-alone'.
[c] Relative contraindications (Ripamonti *et al.*[20]).

Surgical outcomes

The most frequent complications are wound infections and/or wound dehiscence, sepsis, enterocutaneous fistula, further obstruction, peritoneal abscess, anastomosis dehiscence, gastrointestinal (GI) bleeding, pulmonary embolus, and deep venous thrombosis.

The type of obstruction (partial vs. complete) and the surgical procedure used (bypass vs. resection and re-anastomosis) have no significant effect on the outcome[35,36]. In the series of Piver *et al.*[36], the survival was primarily related to the response to postoperative chemotherapy rather than the type of surgery performed.

Of interest, recently published results are no better than those published in the past; improvements in surgical techniques and peri-operative care appear not to have influenced the outcome (Table 10.2.4.1). However, the fact that outcomes have not improved may be because of changes over time in the severity of the presenting condition of the patients, as opposed to how they are managed. In the non-randomized study of Woolfson *et al.*[34], there was no difference in survival after hospital discharge, between the patients being operated on and those receiving conservative treatment. Long-term survival rates in both groups of patients were poor (median 1 month). The grade of the primary tumour and genitourinary cancers seemed to be associated with a more

acceptable outcome whereas operative treatment generally was not correlated with a good outcome. The authors conclude that the value of operative intervention for MBO in patients with cancer is primarily to exclude a benign cause and deal with it rather than allow alleviation of the consequences of carcinomatosis.

Since surgical palliation in advanced cancer patients is a complex issue, the decision to proceed with surgery must be carefully evaluated for each individual patient. The decision should be made by the doctors together with the patient and family members. In patients with known intra-abdominal recurrence of disease, however, operative intervention must be carefully weighed in the light of the limited survival, prolonged hospitalization necessary, the high morbidity and mortality, and the possibility that surgery may fail to resolve the obstruction.

In cancer patients, bowel obstruction is rarely an emergency and strangulation is uncommon; thus, there is time to monitor the clinical situation, undertake appropriate radiological investigations, and consider the prognostic indicators associated with the poor outcome from surgical intervention before deciding for or against surgery. Table 10.2.4.2 shows the clinical parameters derived from retrospective studies, which indicate the low likelihood of clinical benefit from surgical management of MBO[3–7,20,26,28,29,33,35,37,38,40–42].

According to Krebs and Goplerud[4], the operative mortality rate was 44 per cent in the group of patients with ovarian carcinoma and two or more of factors numbered 3, 4, 5, 7; and it was significantly higher than the 13 per cent operative mortality among 32 patients who had no more than one risk factor. In the study of Jong *et al.*[27], successful palliation (defined as patient survival >60 days after surgery, ability to return home, and relief of obstruction postoperatively >60 days) was significantly associated with four prognostic factors, including absence of palpable abdominal or pelvic masses; volume of ascites less than 3l; unifocal obstruction; and preoperative weight loss less than 9 kg.

In the presence of favourable prognostic factors, the choice of the surgical approach should be based on individual clinical conditions, the aims of treatment, and expected survival (Table 10.2.4.3).

Proximal bowel decompression

Proximal bowel decompression may be achieved either by nasogastric suction or drainage or by venting gastrostomy. Short-term nasogastric tube (NGT) drainage is useful in achieving decompression of the stomach and/or intestine to break the vicious cycle of distension–secretion–distension before surgery or while a therapeutic decision is being made. This approach is generally not recommended for long-term drainage since a NGT is uncomfortable for the patient (Table 10.2.4.4). The distress caused by the tube could increase the volume of air swallowed and it may provoke many complications[43–45].

Prolonged nasogastric suction should only be considered for patients when pharmacological therapy for symptom control is ineffective; when gastrostomy cannot be carried out; as a temporary measure to reduce large volumes of secretions before starting pharmacological treatment; and during the first days of such treatment.

Gastrostomy is the procedure of choice for long-term decompression of unresolving bowel obstruction, as it is more acceptable than long-term use of a NGT and well-tolerated[46]. Intermittent venting of the gastrostomy provides patients the satisfaction of resuming oral intake of some foods, giving them significant psychological benefit, without the inconvenience of a nasal tube.

Table 10.2.4.3 Patients with a previous good performance status: surgical evaluation, indications, and problems.

	SNG	Gastrostomy	Stent	Surgery	Octreotide
Indications	Preparation for surgery (possibly avoided)	Long-term drainage in otherwise inoperable patients with prolonged expected survival	Postponing surgery	Benign cause	Preparation to surgery
	Contraindication for gastrostomy			Recent occurrence	
				Survival expectancy: >2 months	
				Good performance status	
				Exclusion of contraindication criteria	
Problems	Uncomfortable for long-term use	Hospitalization TPN (total parenteral nutrition)	Multiple levels of obstruction	Mortality–morbidity, hospitalization	

Gastrostomy can be inserted operatively or percutaneously either by an endoscopic or ultrasound-guided approach. Tube gastrostomy at the time of surgical exploration is the traditional method of long-term gastric decompression. It adds little time or morbidity to the surgical procedure, and should be done whenever the intra operative impression is that complete bowel obstruction may be prolonged, permanent, or imminent[47]. Previous surgery or

Table 10.2.4.4 Complications of prolonged nasogastric intubation.

Psychological distress

Pain

Epistaxis

Tube misplacement

Frequent spontaneous expulsions

Spontaneous migration of the tip of the tube

Nasal/pharyngeal irritation

Nasal cartilage erosion

Impairment of the function of the gastroesophageal sphincter causing or exacerbating oesophageal reflux

Oesophagitis

Oesophageal perforation, bleeding, strictures

Aspiration pneumonia

Pulmonary intubation

Interfere with coughing to clear pulmonary secretions

Otitis media

Tracheal-bronchial misplacement

Occlusions necessitating flushing or replacement

Source: Adapted from Pictus, D., Marx, M.V., and Weyman, P.J. (1988). Chronic intestinal obstruction: value of percutaneous gastrostomy tube placement. *American Journal of Radiology* **150**, 295–7. With permission. Adapted from Rees, R.G.P. *et al.* (1988). Spontaneous transpylorus passage and performance of fine bore polyurethane feeding under a controlled clinical trial. *Journal of Parenteral and Enteral Nutrition* **12**, 469–71. With permission. Adapted from Ripamonti, C. *et al.* (1996). Role of enteral nutrition in advanced cancer patients: indications and contraindications of the different techniques employed. *Tumori* **82**, 302–8. With permission.

massive carcinomatosis may make placement of the gastrostomy difficult or dangerous, but every effort should be made to place a gastrostomy tube at the time of surgical exploration if the clinical situation warrants it.

Percutaneous gastrostomy (PG) is the insertion of a tube into the stomach through the abdominal wall under fluoroscopic, ultrasound, or endoscopic guidance[48,49]. The addition of transcutaneous ultrasonography at the time of endoscopy permits accurate localization of the optimal site for PEG placement in patients with diffuse intra-abdominal disease and multiple prior surgeries [50,51]. The procedure may be performed under intravenous sedation and local anaesthesia[52]. Overall, this approach has been reported to control nausea and vomiting due to bowel obstruction in about 90 per cent of cases[53–58].

PG should be avoided in patients with portal hypertension, or large volume ascites, and in those predisposed to bleed, patients taking anticoagulants, and those with active gastric ulceration[46]. Other relative contraindications are multiple previous abdominal surgeries, carcinomatosis, colostomy, or open/infected abdominal wounds. In some patients with gastric outlet or proximal small bowel obstruction, some authors have described experience with the insertion of a draining gastrostomy with a concurrent feeding jejunostomy[59].

Self-expanding metallic stents (SEMS)

If palliative resections are not feasible, the implantation of SEMS is an alternative therapy option. In recent years, there has been growing experience in the use of expandable metallic stents in the management of obstruction in the gastric outlet, proximal small bowel, and colon. For manifest obstruction, placement of a SEMS is considered to be a suitable minimally invasive therapeutic option. Stent implantation presents lower morbidity (<25 per cent vs. <50 per cent) and mortality (<1 per cent vs. <10 per cent) in respect to surgical intervention[60–63]. Moreover, stent implantation provides a comparable prognosis and also avoids the need for a colostomy [64,65] thus keeping the quality for the remaining lifetime.

These stents may be useful in the management of patients with advanced metastatic disease, in patients who are poor surgical risks (ASA IV), or technically inoperable (revealed by imaging procedures), or as an interim procedure in patients presenting with large bowel obstruction in which a temporary decompression may allow treatment of coexisting medical complications to enable surgery to be carried out at a later date, after staging of the disease and thorough colonic preparation[66].

Among the contraindications are tumour stenosis of the lower third of the rectum (within 5 cm above the anocutaneous line) due to troublesome tenesmus and possible stent migration through the anal canal or anal incontinence[67].

Acute obstruction

The use of colorectal stents to alleviate acute MBO, followed by single-stage bowel resection and re-anastomosis is an application that is now well documented[68–71]. This technique can be palliative or can serve as an adjunct to curative resection. The goal is to convert an emergency procedure to a safer, elective operation and one that can be curative. In the report of Mainar et al.[72], in 83 per cent of the patients, the clinical and radiological findings of bowel obstruction resolved within 24 h after stent placement. Six days after complete resolution of the colonic obstruction, most patients underwent a single-stage surgical intervention. Soto et al.[70] describe a total of 63 self-expandable metallic stents implanted under endoscopic and fluoroscopic guidance. Clinical improvement and resolution of the obstruction were confirmed in 56 of the 58 patients within 48–72 h. Twelve patients had minor complications (pain, tenesmus or distal migration of the stent); whereas major complications occurred in 4 patients (colonic perforation in 3 patients and colovescical fistula in 1 patient 7 months after stent placement).

Preoperative stent placement (bridge to the elective surgery) is of additional value in patients with coexisting electrolyte imbalance, dehydration, or hyperglycaemia because the stent allows for time to get the patient into optimal condition before surgery.

Post-placement evaluation includes a water-soluble contrast-enhanced enema examination and abdominal radiographs to evaluate stent placement and patency and to exclude perforation.

Gastroduodenal stenosis

Gastric outlet obstruction is most commonly secondary to neoplastic invasion but more frequently due to extrinsic compression from carcinoma of the head of the pancreas or from compression by lymphadenopathy. Internal stenting of the lesion may be indicated in patients unfit for general anaesthesia and/or surgery or in patients unfit for a laparoscopic drainage procedure such as gastroenterostomy because of ascites and/or peritoneal metastases. Flexible, self-expanding metallic stents may be inserted using radiological or endoscopic techniques. The major limiting factor using the endoscopic technique is the inability to pass the endoscope through the stricture.

Several authors report relief of malignant gastric and/or duodenal obstruction in the majority of patients treated by per-oral endoscopic stent placement or via percutaneous insertion[63–70,73,74]. Most patients had immediate benefit and were able to eat small amounts of food without vomiting. No recurrence of gastric outlet obstruction was noted in the follow-up period of 1–5 months[75–77].

As with any procedure, complications are possible. The major complications reported are gastric ulceration, bowel perforation after balloon dilatation of the stent, biliary obstruction, stent dysfunction, and stent migration. Sometimes, subsequent endoscopic, radiologic, and surgical interventions were needed[73]. For these

reasons, this procedure should only be performed in experienced centres on selected patients.

According to some less recent reports, however, complications such as chest pain, blockage, gastro-oesophageal reflux, migration, perforation, and delayed massive bleeding occur in about 40–53 per cent of the patients[78–80].

Ross et al.[81] presented a case of malignant distal duodenal obstruction palliated by enteral stent placement using the double balloon enteroscope. This technique allows for endoscopic stent placement in patients with a single point of obstruction that is beyond the reach of conventional endoscopes.

Contraindications to stenting: Contraindications for the placement of a self-expanding stent are the presence of multiple stenoses and peritoneal carcinomatosis located distally in the small bowel that may not have been diagnosed at the pre-procedural radiological examination because of the severity of the duodenal stenosis. Failure to relieve the obstruction may be secondary to an inability to cross the stricture, incomplete opening of the stent, or stent malposition that fails to traverse the entire stricture. In this case, it is necessary to apply additional stents across the remaining obstruction.

Colon stenosis

The tumour site influences the decision regarding which patients are candidates for stent placement. Seventy per cent of colon and rectal cancers are left-sided and are considered accessible to stent placement[72].

In the study of Ptok et al.[67] carried out in 48 consecutive patients with malignant colorectal obstruction, 92 per cent of the patients had the obstruction resolved by means of stent placement. Four of the patients had stent dislocation. The median in situ time for the stents was 251 days, with 13 of the 44 patients treated with palliative therapy showing complications (29.5 per cent). Recurrent symptoms of a colorectal obstruction occurred 265 days after technically and clinically successful SEMS implantation.

Various authors have reported good results after insertion of colonic stents in colorectal obstruction[66,72,82–88].

Complications, which include perforation, bleeding, and stent migration, have been reported in fewer than 3 per cent of cases[79,80,82], and only in a few patients treated with self-expanding mesh stents was there a recurrent obstruction due to tumour growth. Temporary incontinence may be observed[88]. In the series of Canon et al.,[89] stent placement was successful in two out of four patients who needed a standard bowel cleansing before surgical resection with primary anastomosis and in five out of nine patients who had a stent as palliation of non-resectable tumours. Although colonic obstruction was relieved in 12 of 13 patients, seven (54 per cent) had some type of complication.

Mainar et al.[72] recommend self-expandable stents instead of balloon-expandable stents due to the risk of bowel perforation, secondary to the excessive manipulation of balloon dilation on the friable tumour. According to Feretis et al.[85], one of the possible disadvantages of the method may be the difficulty of treating tumour-bleeding, since laser and thermal methods of haemostasis cannot be safely applied to a tumour that is covered by an endoprosthesis.

Normal bowel contractions could cause stent migration, especially if the stent diameter is too small, if the stent length is too short, or if the stent is placed too distal in the lesion. The migration into the rectal ampulla can result in obstruction and in painful spasm. According to Wholey et al.[90], it is possible to retrieve stents from the rectum using fluoroscopic guidance.

According to Canon et al.[89], before a patient is selected as a candidate for having an expandable metal stent placed in the colon, three factors are determined: (1) the location of the lesion within the colon; (2) the length of the tumour; and (3) the presence or absence of a synchronous carcinoma.

Thus, meticulous evaluation of the digestive tract downstream is mandatory to avoid pointless stent placement.

In a recent cost-efficacy analysis[91], comparing stents and surgery showed that colonic stents reduced by 23 per cent operative procedures per patient and by 83 per cent the stoma requirement with a lower procedure-related mortality (7 per cent vs. 43 per cent) and a lower cost.

Further studies are necessary to identify those patients with advanced and terminal cancer and MBO who may have some benefit in terms of symptom control and quality of life after these procedures.

Pharmacological treatment in inoperable malignant bowel obstruction

The pharmacological management of MBO in inoperable patients focuses on the relief of nausea and vomiting, pain, and other possible distressing symptoms. It principally consists of a combination of antiemetics, antisecretory drugs, and analgesics. This approach has been found successful in both inpatients and outpatients. The drugs of choice vary to a certain extent between countries and centres, depending on personal clinical experience, drug availability, and costs, pending controlled studies, which would give clear therapeutic guidelines.

Vomiting may be controlled either symptomatically, using antiemetic drugs with specific central effects, or with anticholinergic drugs able to reduce gastrointestinal secretions. In recent years, steroids and somatostatin analogues have been successfully used as antisecretory–anti-inflammatory drugs, according to the most up-to-date views of the pathophysiology of bowel obstruction.

Clinical practice recommendations for the management of MBO in patients with end-stage cancer have recently been published by the Expert Working Group of the European Association for Palliative Care[20].

Route of administration

As oral administration is unreliable in most patients with nausea and/or vomiting, in the presence of bowel obstruction, an alternative route, mainly the parenteral one, is mandatory. A continuous subcutaneous infusion allows a constant drug infusion with minimal discomfort to the patient. In the presence of a pre-existing venous line, the intravenous route will be the route of choice. Although a continuous infusion is preferable, a nylon needle can be inserted to deliver drugs subcutaneously as boluses at fixed intervals, according to the characteristics of the drug chosen. Morphine, haloperidol, cyclizine, and octreotide appear to be compatible in different combinations and can be mixed in the same syringe[20,92–96] (Table 10.2.4.5). Rectal and sublingual administration can occasionally be used. Finally, some drugs, such as fentanyl and scopolamine, may be also administered by the transdermal route.

Drugs

Fig. 10.2.4.2 shows the drugs and their dosages used to control nausea and vomiting in bowel-obstructed patients according to the data of reference [20].

Antiemetics

Among the antiemetics, parenteral metoclopramide has been used successfully in patients with mainly functional or incomplete obstruction with no colicky pain rather than mechanical bowel obstruction. Metoclopramide (10 mg/4 h subcutaneously), used with dexamethasone, has been the drug of choice for patients with incomplete bowel obstruction [10]. However, its use is not recommended in complete mechanical bowel obstruction as it may increase colic and vomiting [8]. Other antiemetics include haloperidol and the phenothiazines. Their use, while effective in most circumstances, has only been reported in anecdotal experience in patients with inoperable bowel obstruction, and refers to clinical

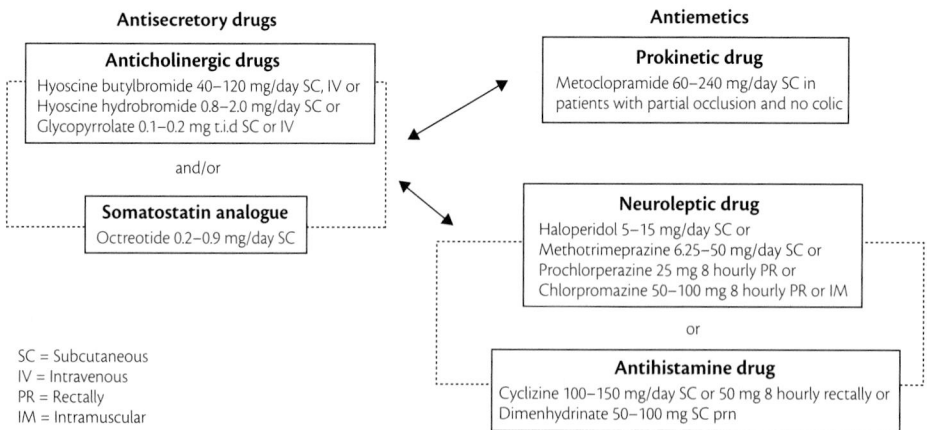

Figure 10.2.4.2 Drugs to control nausea and vomiting in bowel obstruction. The dosages of the different drugs have been reported in ref. [20]. (Reproduced with permission from Ripamonti et al. (2001). *Supportive Care in Cancer* **9**, 223–33.)

Table 10.2.4.5 Drug combinations in syringe drivers: compatibility and stability of opioids with antiemetics.

	Concentration	Antiemetics	Concentration (mg/ml)	Notes
Opioids tested in 5 per cent dextro				
Fentanyl citrate	25 mcg/ml	Atropine sulphate	0.4 undiluted	All the opioid solutions were compatible for at least 48 h with all the antiemetic tested[93]
Hydromorphone HCl	0.5 mg/ml	Diphenidramine HCl	2.0	
Methadone HCl	1.0 mg/ml	Haloperidol lactate	0.2	
Morphine sulphate	1.0 mg/ml	Hydroxyzine HCl	4.0	
		Methotrimeprazine	0.2	
		Metoclopramide HCl	5.0 undiluted	
		Scopolamine hydrobromide	0.05	
Opioids tested in distilled water				
Morphine sulphate	25 mg/ml	+Metoclopramide	25	Stable and compatible for 7 days
Hydromorphone HCl	10–20 mg/ml	+Metoclopramide	15	
Hydromorphone HCl	10 mg/ml	+Methotrimeprazine	10	
Morphine sulphate	20 mg/ml	+Haloperidol	2.0	Percipitable formulation[94]
Hydromorphone HCl	10–15 mg/ml	+Haloperidol	2.0	
Morphine sulphate	15 mg/ml	+Dexamethasone	0.02	No significant chemical degradation after 7 days at room temperature[92]
Morphine sulphate	15 mg/ml	+Metoclopramide	1.0	
Morphine sulphate	15 mg/ml	+Haloperidol	0.2	
Diamorphine	20–50–100 mg/ml	+Haloperidol	2.0	Stable and compatible after 7 days[95]
Diamorphine	20–50–100 mg/ml	+Haloperidol	3.0	
Diamorphine	20–50 mg/ml	+Haloperidol	4.0	
Diamorphine	50–100 mg/ml	+Cyclizine	4.0	Stable and compatible for 7 days[95]
Diamorphine	20 mg/ml	+Cyclizine	10.0	
Diamorphine	9 mg/ml	+Cyclizine	30.0	
Diamorphine	10 mg/ml	+Cyclizine	40.0	Stable and compatible for 48 h
Diamorphine	10 mg/ml	+Cyclizine	30.0	
Diamorphine	12 mg/ml	+Cyclizine	50.0	
Diamorphine	20 mg/ml	+Cyclizine	26.0	
Diamorphine	20 mg/ml	+Cyclizine	18.0	
Diamorphine	50 mg/ml	+Cyclizine	10.0	

Source: reproduced from Ripamonti, C. *et al.* (2001). Clinical-practice recommendations for the management of bowel obstruction in patients with end-stage cancer. *Supportive Care in Cancer* **9**, 223–33. With permission.

practice in different palliative care centres. Haloperidol, administered in varying doses, either intravenously or subcutaneously, titrated against effect, is a specific antidopaminergic drug, causing less sedation and having less anticholinergic effects compared with the phenothiazines. Among the phenothiazines, methotrimeprazine, chlorpromazine, and prochlorpromazine are commonly used. The two latter drugs may produce skin irritation when administered as a subcutaneous infusion [20,97].

Anticholinegic agents

Anticholinergic drugs, such as hyoscine butylbromide and glycopyrrolate, may reduce vomiting by virtue of their antisecretory effects. Their anticholinergic activity decreases the tone and peristalsis in smooth muscle and the secretory activity of mucosal cells by a competitive inhibition of muscarinic receptors and by impairment of ganglionic neural transmission. Many open studies have demonstrated that this class of drugs may be effective in controlling GI symptoms in inoperable MBO, in combination with other drugs[8,98–102]. In comparison with scopolamine hydrobromide, these drugs have poor central nervous system penetration, so they are unlikely to produce central adverse effects. However, this class of drugs acts on the myenteric cholinergic endings to reduce their activity, without influencing other intestinal processes, which have been found to have a relevant influence on the absorption and secretion of water and salts at the level of the intestinal lumen. Moreover, these agents also possess important haemodynamic and thermoregulatory effects.

Octreotide

This is a synthetic analogue of somatostatin, with a duration of action of 8–12 h and has been used in the management of the symptoms of bowel obstruction. In relation to somatostatin, octreotide has been shown to have the same biological effects, but greater specificity and potency in the inhibition of release of certain hormones, and to be longer acting (half-life 90–120 min) with a peak of action at 2 h and a duration of 12 h. Octreotide can be administered by continuous subcutaneous or intravenous infusion or by bolus parenteral injection. Octreotide inhibits the release of several GI hormones, thereby reducing gastric, pancreatic, biliary, and intestinal secretions, slowing down intestinal motility, and decreasing splanchnic blood flow, whilst at the same time increasing the absorption of water and electrolytes[103]. The rationale for using this drug can be explained by the mechanisms involved in the cascade of events presented in the section 'Pathophysiology'. Because the major morbidity of bowel obstruction relates to intestinal distension, electrolyte losses, and ischaemia, many experimental studies have been carried out to evaluate such features in animals treated with somatostatin or octreotide with respect to those treated with placebo[104-108].

Such experimental studies suggest that the principal mechanism of fluid secretion in bowel obstruction depends on VIP-induced inflammatory events[75,16]. VIP is released locally in the gut wall in the presence of ischaemia[107]. Octreotide has been shown to have a potent anti-VIP effect, resulting in the inhibition of intestinal secretion[14]. In an experimental preparation of rabbit ileum, the pro-absorptive effect of octreotide occurred without alterations in vascular resistance and was independent of systemic hormone interaction, thereby supporting a direct effect of octreotide on intestinal ionic transport[109].

Clinical studies have proven the benefits of octreotide in different clinical conditions. The preoperative use of octreotide administered at the dose of 0.3 mg/day for 2–5 days in cancer patients undergoing surgery for bowel obstruction, caused by extrinsic occlusion of the lumen, prevented the typical anatomical changes, such as oedema, vessel congestion, or necrosis of the bowel above the obstruction due to the accumulation of fluids in the lumen, commonly observed during surgery. Moreover, the study of some samples of the intestine above and below the obstruction showed a normal anatomical and biochemical pattern[108]. The prophylactic use of octreotide in cancer patients with recurrent episodes of obstruction was successful in maintaining or restoring the intestinal transit even for prolonged periods of time[110]. These preliminary results were confirmed in a randomized, double-blind clinical trial carried out on 54 consecutive patients with mechanical bowel obstruction. Patients who received somatostatin preoperatively required surgery less often than patients who did not receive the

drug. Moreover, severe dilatation and necrosis of the bowel proximal to the area of obstruction was significantly less frequent as compared with those patients who did not receive somatostatin preoperatively[111].

On the basis of these experiences, octreotide could be considered in an early phase, in the presence of intermittent states of obstruction, or preoperatively to improve the surgical conditions and prevent postoperative complications. Many uncontrolled studies report octreotide to be effective in relieving gastrointestinal symptoms in definitive MBO[112–116], even in patients in whom hyoscine butylbromide had failed. Randomized studies demonstrated that octreotide in doses of 0.3 mg daily was significantly more effective and had a shorter onset of action than hyoscine butylbromide in doses of 60 mg daily in reducing the intensity of nausea and the number of vomiting episodes[101], and the amount of gastrointestinal secretion, allowing for the removal of the nasogastric tube previously inserted[102]. On the other hand, the association of the two drugs may reduce GI secretions and vomiting in patients whenever one drug alone proves ineffective[117].

In a subsequent study performed in a larger sample of patients using higher doses of octreotide and scopolamine butylbromide (0.6–0.8 mg/day and 80 mg/day, respectively), and chlorpromazine 5–25 mg/day, nausea and vomiting significantly improved in patients treated with octreotide[118]. Long-acting octreotide, 20 mg every four weeks, could be a possible option[119]. Although octreotide is an expensive drug, its cost should be measured against the drug's ability to achieve rapid improvement of GI symptoms, which themselves affect admission to an inpatient unit and the length of hospitalization, in addition to the improved quality of life of the patient.

Steroids

The anti-inflammatory activity of steroids may reduce peri-tumoural oedema associated with a malignant lesion, thereby helping to resolve the obstruction and leading to consequent symptom relief. Steroids have been shown to increase water and salt absorption, thus reducing the net balance of water and electrolytes in the intestinal content. For this reason, this class of drugs can be considered as antisecretory agents. Steroids have been found to be effective in MBO in a series of studies[120,121].

A meta-analysis of these studies showed a trend towards resolution of bowel obstruction using the corticosteroid dexamethasone in doses ranging from 6 to 16 mg/day intravenously has been reported, with minimal morbidity, although this result did not achieve statistical significance[122]. These studies also were flawed by important methodological limitations[123].

Combination of drugs

A multimodal treatment, including different agents with relatively low toxicity and different mechanisms of action, may additively or sinergically improve gastrointestinal symptoms or partially resolve bowel obstruction. The treatment seems to be particularly effective if performed as early as possible with an aggressive treatment, before fecal impaction and oedema render obstruction irreversible. An early and intensive treatment may not only reduce gastrointestinal symptoms, but also reverse the bowel transit allowing a clear improvement in quality of life. The mixture includes metoclopramide 60 mg, octreotide 0.3 mg, dexamethasone 12 mg, daily, given intravenously and then maintained in the therapeutic

Table 10.2.4.6 Patients with a poor performance status with contraindications for surgical approach. Indications for the use of symptomatic drugs.

	Antiemetics	Metoclopramide	Steroids	Hyoscine	Octreotide	SNG
Indications	Symptom control	Functional subobstruction	Subobstructive states	Symptom control	Subobstructive states	Pts unresponsive to pharmacological treatment
		Symptom control			Symptom control	Temporary measure
Problems		Stop in definitive or complete obstruction				Uncomfortable for long-term use

regimen as an intravenous infusion, and an initial bolus of 50 ml of amidotrizoato orally[124].

Analgesics

Most patients presenting symptoms from bowel obstruction are on strong opioids, usually morphine, at the time of diagnosis. The dose of opioids should be titrated against effect, and must usually be administered parenterally, according to the WHO guidelines. In patients with subsequent episodes of subacute obstruction to which opioids may negatively contribute, it may be useful to choose the drug on the basis of presumed selectivity of distribution at the intestinal sites. Morphine tends to accumulate in intestinal tissues, interacting with local opioid receptors. It has been reported that more lipophilic drugs, like methadone and fentanyl, may limit their presence at the opioid intestinal receptors[125,126]. Experimental studies showed a more favourable constipation/analgesia ratio of fentanyl relative to morphine[127]. This is probably a reflection of the lipophilic properties of fentanyl. Some papers seem to indicate that transdermal fentanyl as well as methadone may have less constipating effects or may require lower laxative doses in comparison with morphine[128–130]. Moreover, switching from morphine to methadone improves GI tolerability[131] as well as switching the route of the opioid administration[132]. On the other hand, the use of NSAIDs may allow for a reduction of constipation induced by opioids[133] and may result in improvement in the opioid bowel syndrome[134].

The main recommendations for the use of symptomatic drugs or their combination, according to the aim of care and specific clinical conditions in patients with negative prognostic factors for surgery, are shown in Table 10.2.4.6.

Hydration and nutrition

The main goal of parenteral nutrition is to maintain or restore the patient's nutritional status and to correct or prevent malnutrition and its related symptoms[135]. The role of parenteral nutrition in the management of patients with inoperable bowel obstruction should be carefully considered on the basis of several factors. It rests on the ability to demonstrate genuine benefit for the patients[136]. The question is whether it improves quality of life and does not merely lengthen survival. Parenteral nutrition may prolong survival but can also lead to complications, add further suffering, and make prolonged hospitalization necessary[137].

In some circumstances in which bowel obstruction is temporary and can spontaneously resolve, rehydration is of value in maintaining an appropriate nutrient intake until the therapeutic intervention has had an effect. However, in most cases, this practice is unnecessary and may worsen the patient's burden. It is often employed as a psychological measure at the insistence of relatives. In most cases, parenteral nutrition is interrupted after an appropriate explanation about the short prognosis and the evidence of no benefit[138]. Therefore, routine use should be avoided when it is designed solely to prolong life. Parenteral nutrition should not be undertaken without a full discussion with the patient and family members. Only those patients who strongly support this decision after a clear explanation should be offered this approach. A home-care programme for such patients requires active participation of the patient's caregiver and the involvement of skilled nurses, pharmacists, and physicians.

Most patients with bowel obstruction are dehydrated, due to a steel fluid syndrome of water and electrolytes at the intestinal level and poor oral intake of fluids. The correction of this status does not have any effect on dry mouth and thirst, as the intensity of these symptoms seem to be independent of the amounts of fluids administered either by oral or parenteral route [20,139]. A high level of hydration may result in more bowel secretions. On the other hand, the intensity of nausea was significantly lower in patients treated with moderate amounts of water (>500 ml/day), probably due to the prevention of metabolic derangement associated with severe dehydration and reduction of stimulation of the chemoreceptor trigger zone [101,102]. Administration of 1–1.5 litre/day of solution containing electrolytes and glucose may be useful in preventing symptoms due to metabolic derangement.

Subcutaneous infusion is a valid alternative to intravenous administration of fluids for patients with poor vein availability or without a central venous catheter [140]. Providing sips of oral fluids, frequent attention to mouth care, and sucking ice cubes are of paramount importance in relieving dry mouth, commonly associated with the use of anticholinergics drugs[20].

Conclusions

MBO should be carefully evaluated by experienced physicians, considering individual and prognostic factors, as well as life expectancy. Different options may be chosen depending on the goals of intervention, and the modalities of occurrence of bowel obstruction, as well as the patient's conditions. Involvement of patients and family members in this therapeutic decision-making is mandatory, based on clear information about the clinical status and the possible evolution of the clinical course. Further controlled studies on large numbers of patients are needed, looking at the problems from an epidemiological and prognostic point of view. Comparative trials performed at different stages of bowel obstruction could make an important contribution to defining the best treatments in potentially reversible conditions as well as established MBO. Specifically, in inoperable MBO, the use of steroids or a combination of drugs, such as steroids with octreotide, or steroids with hyoscine butylbromide, should be investigated to improve gastrointestinal symptoms. The role and the level of hydration to administer to these patients should be assessed in studies with an appropriate design in a large number of patients.

References

1. Beattie, G.J., Leonard, R., and Smyth, J.F. (1989). Bowel obstruction in ovarian carcinoma: a retrospective study and review of the literature. *Palliative Medicine*, **3**, 275–80.

2. Lund, B. *et al.* (1989). Intestinal obstruction in patients with advanced carcinoma of the ovaries treated with combination chemotherapy. *Surgery, Gynecology and Obsterics*, **169**, 213–18.

3. Castaldo, T.W. *et al.* (1981). Intestinal operations in patients with ovarian carcinoma. *American Journal of Obstetrics and Gynecology*, **139**, 80–4.

4. Krebs, H.B. and Goplerud, D.R. (1983). Surgical management of bowel obstruction in advanced ovarian carcinoma. *Obstetrics and Gynecology*, **61**, 327–30.

5. Larson, J.E. *et al.* (1989). Bowel obstruction in patients with ovarian carcinoma: analysis of prognostic factors. *Gynecologic Oncology*, **35**, 61–5.

6. Fernandes, J.R., Seymour, R.J., and Suissa, S. (1988). Bowel obstruction in patients with ovarian cancer: a search for prognostic factors. *American Journal of Obstetrics and Gynecology*, **158**, 244–9.

7. Gallick, H.L. *et al.* (1986). Intestinal obstruction in cancer patients. An assessment of risk factors and outcome. *The American Surgeon*, **52**, 434–7.

8. Baines, M., Oliver, D.J., and Carter, R.L. (1985). Mechanical management of intestinal obstruction in patients with advanced malignant disease: a clinical and pathological study. *Lancet*, **II**, 990–3.

9. Mercadante, S. (1995). Bowel obstruction in home care cancer patients: four years of experience. *Supportive Care in Cancer*, **3**, 190–3.

10. Fainsinger, R.L. *et al.* (1994). Symptom control in terminally ill patients with malignant bowel obstruction. *Journal of Pain and Symptom Management*, **9**, 12–18.

11. Mercadante, S. (1997). Assessment and management of mechanical bowel obstruction. In *Topics in Palliative Care* Vol. 1 (ed. R.K. Portenoy and E. Bruera), pp. 113–30. New York: Oxford University Press.

12. Glare, P. and Lickiss, J.N. (1992). Unrecognized constipation in patients with advanced cancer. A review for therapeutic disaster. *Journal of Pain and Symptom Management*, **7**, 369–71.

13. Mercadante, S. (1995). Pain in inoperable bowel obstruction. *Pain Digest*, **5**, 9–13.

14. Nellgard, P., Bojo, L., and Cassuto, J. (1995). Importance of vasoactive intestinal peptide and somatostatin for fluid losses in small-bowel obstruction. *Scandinavian Journal of Gastroenterology*, **30**, 464–9.

15. Nellgard, P. and Cassuto, J. (1993). Inflammation as a major cause of fluid losses in small-bowel obstruction. *Scandinavian Journal of Gastroenterology*, **28**, 1035–41.

16. Basson, M.D. *et al.* (1989). Does vasoactive intestinal polypeptide mediate the pathophysiology of bowel obstruction? *American Journal of Surgery*, **157**, 109–15.

17. Neville, R. *et al.* (1991). Vascular responsiveness in obstructed gut. *Diseases of the Colon and Rectum*, **34**, 229–35.

18. Chan, A. and Woodruff, R.K. (1992). Intestinal obstruction in patients with widespread intra-abdominal malignancy. *Journal of Pain and Symptom Management*, **7**, 339–42.

19. Scott Jones, R. and Schirmer, B.D. (1989). Intestinal obstruction, pseudo-obstruction and ileus. In *Gastrointestinal Disease* (ed. M.H. Sleisinger and J.S. Fordtran), pp. 369–81. Philadelphia: JB Lippincott Co.

20. Ripamonti, C. *et al.* (2001). Clinical-practice recommendations for the management of bowel obstruction in patients with end-stage cancer. *Supportive Care in Cancer*, **9**, 223–33.

21. Welch, J.P. (1990). *Bowel Obstruction*. Philadelphia: WB Saunders.

22. Krebs, H.B. and Goplerud, D.R. (1984). The role of intestinal intubation in obstruction of the small intestine due to carcinoma of the ovary. *Surgery, Gynecology and Obstetrics*, **158**, 467–9.

23. Walsh, H.P.J. and Schofield, P.F. (1984). Is laparotomy for small bowel obstruction justified in patients with previously treated malignancy? *British Journal of Surgery*, **71**, 933–4.

24. Feuer, D.J. *et al.* (1999). Systematic review of surgery in malignant bowel obstruction in advanced gynaecological and gastrointestinal cancer. *Gynecologic Oncology*, **75**, 313–22.

25. Rubin, S.C. *et al.* (1989). Palliative surgery for intestinal obstruction in advanced ovarian cancer. *Gynecologic Oncology*, **34**, 16–19.

26. van Oojen, B. *et al.* (1993). Surgical treatment or gastric drainage only for intestinal obstruction in patients with carcinoma of the ovary or peritoneal carcinomatosis of other origin. *Surgery, Gynecology and Obstetrics*, **176**, 469–73.

27. Jong, P., Sturgeon, J., and Jamieson, C.G. (1995). Benefit of palliative surgery for bowel obstruction in advanced ovarian cancer. *Canadian Journal of Surgery*, **38** (5), 454–7.

28. Turnbull, A.D.M., Guerra, J., and Starners, H.F. (1989). Results of surgery for obstructing carcinomatosis of gastrointestinal, pancreatic, or biliary origin. *Journal of Clinical Oncology*, **7**, 381–6.

29. Butler, J.A. *et al.* (1991). Small bowel obstruction in patients with a prior history of cancer. *The American Journal of Surgery*, **162**, 624–8.

30. Lau, P.W. and Lorentz, T.G. (1993). Results of surgery for malignant bowel obstruction in advanced, unresectable, recurrent colorectal cancer. *Diseases of the Colon and Rectum*, **36** (1), 61–4.

31. Tang, E., Davis, J., and Silberman, H. (1995). Bowel obstruction in cancer patients. *Archives of Surgery*, **130**, 832–7.

32. Sun, X., Li, X., and Li, H. (1995). Management of intestinal obstruction in advanced ovarian cancer: an analysis of 57 cases. *Chung Hua Chung Liu Tsa Chih*, **17**, 39–42.

33. Yazdi, G.P., Miedema, B.W., and Humphrey, L.J. (1996). High mortality after abdominal operation in patients with large-volume malignant ascites. *Journal of Surgical Oncology*, **62**, 93–6.

34. Woolfson, R.G., Jennings, K., and Whalen, G.F. (1997). Management of bowel obstruction in patients with abdominal cancer. *Archives of Surgery*, **132**, 1093–7.

35. Tunca, J.C., Buchler, D.A., Mack, E.A. *et al.* (1981). The management of ovarian-cancer-caused bowel obstruction. *Gynecologic Oncology*, **12**, 186–92.

36. Piver, M.S. *et al.* (1982). Survival after ovarian cancer induced intestinal obstruction. *Gynecologic Oncology*, **13**, 44–9.

37. Aabo, K. *et al.* (1984). Surgical management of intestinal obstruction in the late course of malignant disease. *Acta Chirurgica Scandinavica*, **150**, 173–6.

38. Glass, R.L. and LeDuc, R.J. (1973). Small intestinal obstruction from peritoneal carcinomatosis. *American Journal of Surgery*, **125**, 316–17.

39. Rapin, Ch.H. *et al.* (1990). Pour une meilleure qualite' de vie en fin de vie: nutrition et hydratation. *Ageet nutrition*, **1**, 22–8.

40. Clarke-Pearson, D.L. *et al.* (1987). Surgical management of intestinal obstruction in ovarian cancer. I. Clinical features, postoperative complications, and survival. *Gynecologic Oncology*, **26**, 11–18.

41. Clarke-Pearson, D.L. *et al.* (1988). Surgical management of intestinal obstruction in ovarian cancer II. Analysis of factors associated with complications and survival. *Archives of Surgery*, **123**, 42–5.

42. Weiss, S.M., Skibber, J.M., and Rosato, F.E. (1984). Bowel obstruction in cancer patients: performance status as a predictor of survival. *Journal of Surgical Oncology*, **25**, 15–17.

43. Pictus, D., Marx, M.V., and Weyman, P.J. (1988). Chronic intestinal obstruction: value of percutaneous gastrostomy tube placement. *American Journal of Radiology*, **150**, 295–7.

44. Rees, R.G.P. *et al.* (1988). Spontaneous transpylorus passage and performance of fine bore polyurethane feeding under a controlled clinical trial. *Journal of Parenteral and Enteral Nutrition*, **12**, 469–71.

45. Ripamonti, C. *et al.* (1996). Role of enteral nutrition in advanced cancer patients: indications and contraindications of the different techniques employed. *Tumori*, **82**, 302–8.

46. Forgas, I., Macpherson, A., and Tibbs, C. (1992). Percutaneous endoscopic gastrostomy. The end of the line for nasogastric feeding? *British Medical Journal*, **304**, 1395–6.

47. Gleeson, N.C. *et al.* (1994). Gastrostomy tubes after gynecologic oncologic surgery. *Gynecologic Oncology*, **54**, 19–22.

48. Malone, J.M. *et al.* (1986). Palliation of small bowel obstructon by percutaneous gastrostomy in patients with progressive ovarian carcinoma. *Obstetrics and Gynecology*, **68**, 431–3.

49. George, J. *et al.* (1990). Percutaneous endoscopic gastrostomy: a two year experience. *Medical Journal of Australia*, **152**, 17–20.

50. Vargo, J.J. *et al.* (1993). Ultrasound-assisted percutaneous endoscopic gastrostomy in a patient with advanced ovarian carcinoma and recurrent intestinal obstruction. *American Journal of Gastroenterology*, **88**(11), 1946–8.

51. Cannizzaro, R. *et al.* (1995). Percutaneous endoscopic gastrostomy as a decompressive technique in bowel obstruction due to abdominal carcinomatosis. *Endoscopy*, **27**, 317–20.

52. Adelson, M.D. and Kazowits, M.H. (1993). Percutaneous endoscopic drainage gastrostomy in treatment of gastrointestinal obstruction from intraperitoneal malignancy. *Obstetrics and Gynecology*, **81**, 467–9.

53. Herman, L.L., Hoskins, W.J., and Shike, M. (1992). Percutaneous endoscopic gastrostomy for decompression of the stomach and small bowel. *Gastrointestinal Endoscopy*, **38**, 314–18.

54. Schwab, K.S. *et al.* (1993). Percutaneous endoscopic gastrostomy for decompression in patients with malignant carcinomatosis and radiation enteritis. *Gastrointestinal Endoscopy*, **39**, 288A.

55. Noyer, C. *et al.* (1993). Percutaneous endoscopic gastrostomy (PEG): gastric decompression in patients with carcinomatosis. *Gastrointestinal Endoscopy*, **39**, 282A.

56. Marks, W.H., Perkal, M.F., and Schwartz, P.E. (1993). Percutaneous endoscopic gastrostomy for gastric decompression in metastatic gynecologic malignancies. *Surgery, Gynecology and Obstetrics*, **177**, 573–6.

57. Cunningham, M.J. *et al.* (1995). Percutaneous gastrostomy for decompression in patients with advanced gynecologic malignancies. *Gynecologic Oncology*, **59**, 273–6.

58. Campagnutta, E. *et al.* (1996). Palliative treatment of upper intestinal obstruction by gynecological malignancy: the usefulness of percutaneous endoscopic gastrostomy. *Gynecologic Oncology*, **62**, 103–5.

59. Sriram, K., Sridhar, K., and Sridhar, R. (1996). Gastroduodenal decompression and simultaneous nasoenteral nutrition: 'extracorporeal gastrojejunostomy' (clinical conference) *Nutrition*, **12**, 440–1.

60. Rosen, S.A. *et al.* (2000). Initial presentation with stage IV colorectal cancer: how aggressive should we be? *Archives of Surgery*, **135**, 530–5.

61. Liu, S.K. *et al.* (1997). Operation in patients with incurable colon cancer: is it worthwhile? *Diseases of the Colon and Rectum*, **40**, 11–14.

62. Keymling, M. (2003). Colorectal stenting. *Endoscopy*, **35**, 234–8.

63. Lee, Y.M. *et al.* Emergency surgery for obstructing colorectal cancers: a comparison between right-sided and left-sided lesions. *Journal of the American College of Surgeons*, **192**, 19–25.

64. Johnson, R. *et al.* (2004). A comparison of two methods of palliation of large bowel obstruction due to irremovable colon cancer. *Annals of the Royal College of Surgeons of England*, **86**, 99–103.

65. Bhardwaj, R. and Parker, M.C. (2003). Palliative therapy of colorectal carcinoma: stent or surgery? *Colorectal Dos*, **5**, 518–21.

66. Wallis, F. *et al.* (1998). Self-expanding metal stents in the management of colorectal carcinoma—a preliminary report (see comments). *Clinical Radiology*, **53**, 251–4.

67. Ptok, H. *et al.* (2006). Palliative stent implantation in the treatment of malignant colorectal obstruction. *Surgical Endoscopy*, **20**, 909–14.

68. Lamah, M. *et al.* (1998). The use of rectosigmoid stents in the management of acute large bowel obstruction. *Journal of the Royal College of Surgeons, Edinburgh*, **43**, 318–21.

69. Pothuri, B. *et al.* (2004). The use of colorectal stents for palliation of large-bowel obstruction due to recurrent gynecologic cancer. *Gynecologic Oncology*, **95**, 513–7.

70. Soto, S. *et al.* (2006). Endoscopic treatment of acute colorectal obstruction with self-expandable metallic stents. *Surgical Endoscopy*, **20**, 1072–6.

71. Stefanidis, D. *et al.* (2005). Safety and efficacy of metallic stents in the management of colorectal obstruction. *Journal of the Society of Laparoendoscopic Surgeons*, **9**, 454–9.

72. Mainar, A. *et al.* (1996). Colorectal obstruction: treatment with metallic stents. *Radiology*, **198**, 761–4.

73. Mosler, P. *et al.* (2005). Palliation of gastric outlet obstruction and proximal small bowel obstruction with self-expandable metal stents (A single Center Series). *Journal of Clinical Gastroenterology*, **39**, 124–8.

74. Holt, A.P. *et al.* (2004), Palliation of patients with malignant gastroduodenal obstruction with self-expanding metallic stents: the treatment of choice? *Gastrointestinal Endoscopy*, **60**/6, 1010–7.

75. Park, H.S. *et al.* (1999). Upper gastrointestinal tract malignant obstruction: initial results of palliation with a flexible covered stent. *Radiology*, **210**, 865–70.

76. Keymling, M. *et al.* (1993). Relief of malignant duodenal obstruction by percutaneous insertion of a metal stent. *Gastrointestinal Endoscopy*, **39**(3), 439–41.

77. de Baere, T. *et al.* (1997). Self-expanding metallic stents as palliative treatment of malignant gastroduodenal stenosis. *American Journal of Roentgenology*, **169**, 1079–83.

78. Song, H.Y. *et al.* (1994). Covered, expandable esophageal metallic stent tubes: experiences in 119 patients. *Radiology*, **193**, 689–95.

79. Saxon, R.R. *et al.* (1995). Treatment of malignant esophageal obstructions with covered metallic Z stents: long-term results in 52 patients. *Journal of Vascular and Interventional Radiology*, **6**, 747–54.

80. Feins, R.H. *et al.* (1996). Palliation of inoperable esophageal carcinoma with the Wallstent endoprosthesis. *Annals of Thoracic Surgery*, **62**, 1603–7.

81. Ross, A.S. *et al.* (2006). Enteral stent placement by double balloon enteroscopy for palliation of malignant small bowel obstruction. *Gastrointestinal Endoscopy*, **64**/5, 835–7.

82. Arnell, T. *et al.* (1998). Colonic stents in colorectal obstruction. *American Surgery*, **64**, 986–8.

83. Tejero, E. *et al.* (1997). Initial results of a new procedure for treatment of malignant obstruction of the left colon. *Diseases of the Colon and Rectum*, **40**, 432–6.

84. Saida, Y. *et al.* (1996). Stent endoprosthesis for obstructing colorectal cancers. *Diseases of the Colon and Rectum*, **39**, 552–5.

85. Feretis, C. *et al.* (1996). Palliation of large-bowel obstruction due to recurrent rectosigmoid tumor using self-expandable endoprostheses. *Endoscopy*, **28**, 319–22.

86. Vandervoort, J. *et al.* (1996). Self-expanding metal stent for obstructing adenocarcinoma of the sigmoid. *Gastrointestinal Endoscopy*, **44**, 739–41.

87. Rey, J.F., Romanczyk, T., and Greff, M. (1995). Metal stents for palliation of rectal carcinoma: a preliminary report on 12 patients. *Endoscopy*, **27**, 501–4.

88. Dohomoto, M., Hunerbein, M., and Schlag, P.M. (1997). Application of rectal stents for palliation of obstructing rectosigmoid cancer. *Surgical Endoscopy*, **11**, 758–61.

89. Canon, C.L. *et al.* (1997). Treatment of colonic obstruction with expandable metal stents: radiologic features. *American Journal of Roentgenology*, **168**, 199–205.

90. Wholey, M.H. *et al.* (1997). Retrieval of migrated colonic stents from the rectum. *Cardiovascular and Interventional Radiology*, **20**, 477–80.

91. Targownick Le. *et al.* (2004). Colonic stent vs emergency surgery for management of acute left-sided malignant colonic obstruction: a decision analysis. *Gastrointestinal Endoscopy*, **60**/6, 865–74.

92. Swanson, G. *et al.* (1989). Patient-controlled analgesia for chronic cancer pain in the ambulatory setting. A report of 177 patients. *Journal of Clinical Oncology*, **7**, 1903–8.

93. Chandler, S.W., Trissel, L.A., and Weinstein, S.M. (1996). Combined administration of opioids with selected drugs to manage pain and other cancer symptoms: initial safety screening for compatibility. *Journal of Pain and Symptom Management*, **12**, 168–71.

94. Storey, P. *et al.* (1990). Subcutaneous infusions for control of cancer symptoms. *Journal of Pain and Symptom Management*, **5**, 33–41.

95. Grassby, P.F. and Hutchings, L. (1997). Drugs combinations in syringe drivers: the compatibility and stability of diamorphine with cyclizine and haloperidol. *Palliative Medicine*, **11**, 217–24.

96. Mercadante, S. (1995). Tolerability of continuous subcutaneous octreotide used in combination with other drugs. *Journal of Palliative Care*, **4**, 14–16.

97. Twycross, R. *et al.* (1998). Nausea and vomiting in advanced cancer. *European Journal of Palliative Care*, **5**, 39–45.

98. Ventafridda, V. *et al.* (1990). The management of inoperable gastrointestinal obstruction in terminal cancer patients. *Tumori.* 76, 389–93.

99. De Conno, F. *et al.* (1991). Continuous subcutaneous infusion of hyoscine butylbromide reduces secretions in patients with gastrointestinal obstruction. *Journal of Pain and Symptom Management*, **6**, 484–6.

100. Davis, M. and Furste, A. (1999). Glycopyrrolate: a useful drug in the palliation of mechanical bowel obstruction. *Journal of Pain and Symptom Management*, **18**, 153–4.

101. Ripamonti, C. *et al.* (2000). Role of octreotide, scopolamine butylbromide and hydration in symptom control of patients with inoperable bowel obstruction having a nasogastric tube. A prospective, randomized clinical trial. *Journal of Pain and Symptom Management*, **19**, 23–34.

102. Mercadante, S. *et al.* (2000). Comparison of octreotide and hyoscine butylbromide in controlling gastrointestinal symptoms due to malignant inoperable bowel obstruction. *Supportive Care in Cancer*, **8**, 188–91.

103. Mercadante, S. (1994). The role of octreotide in palliative care. *Journal of Pain and Symptom Management*, **9**, 406–11.

104. Guiro', F.F., Bertolini, G., and Salas, J.V. (1999). Improvement in the intestinal processes of hydroelectrolytic absorption and secretion in abdominal pathologies of surgical interest treated with SMS 201-995: experimental protocol. *Surgery Today*, **29**(5), 419–30.

105. Mulvihill, S.J. *et al.* (1988). The effect of somatostatin on experimental intestinal obstruction. *Annals of Surgery*, **207**(2), 169–73.

106. Yamaner, S., Bugra, D., Muslumanoglu, M. *et al.* (1995). Effects of octreotide on healing of intestinal anastomosis following small bowel obstruction in rats. *Diseases of the Colon and Rectum*, **38**(3), 308–12.

107. Modlin, I.M., Bloom, S.R., and Mitchell, S.C. (1978). Plasma vasoactive intestinal polypeptide (VIP) levels and intestinal ischemia. *Experientia*, **34**, 535–6.

108. Mercadante, S. *et al.* (1996). Octreotide prevents the pathological alterations of bowel obstruction in cancer patients. *Supportive Care in Cancer*, **4**, 393–4.

109. Anthone, G.J. *et al.* (1990). Direct proabsorptive effect of octreotide on ionic transport in the small intestine. *Surgery*, **108**(6), 1136–42.

110. Mercadante, S., Kargar, J., and Nicolosi, G. (1997). Octreotide may prevent definitive intestinal obstruction. *Journal of Pain and Symptom Management*, **13**, 352–5.

111. Bastounis, E. *et al.* (1989). Somatostatin as adjuvant therapy in the management of obstructive ileus. *Hepato-Gastroenterology* **36**(6), 538–9.

112. Mercadante, S. and Maddaloni, S. (1992). Octreotide in the management of inoperable bowel obstruction in terminal cancer patients. *Journal of Pain and Symptom Management*, **7**, 496–8.

113. Mercadante, S. *et al.* (1993). Octreotide in relieving gastrointestinal symptoms due to bowel obstruction. *Palliative Medicine*, **7**, 295–9.

114. Khoo, D., Riley J., and Waxman, J. (1992). Control of emesis in bowel obstruction in terminally ill patients. *Lancet*, **339**, 375–6.

115. Riley, J. and Fallon, M.T. (1994). Octreotide in terminal malignant obstruction of the gastrointestinal tract. *European Journal of Palliative Care*, **1**, 23–8.

116. Mangili, G. *et al.* (1996). Octreotide in the management of bowel obstruction in terminal ovarian cancer. *Gynecologic Oncology*, **61**, 345–8.

117. Mercadante, S. (1998). Scopolamine butylbromide plus octreotide in unresponsive bowel obstruction. *Journal of Pain and Symptom Management*, **16** (5), 278–9.

118. Mystakidou, K., Tsilika, E., Kalaidopoulou, O. *et al.* (2002). Comparison of octreotide administration vs conservative treatment in the management of inoperable bowel obstruction in patients with far advanced cancer: a randomized, double-blind, controlled clinical trial. *Anticancer Research*, **22**, 1187–92.

119. Matulonis, U.A. *et al.* (2005). Long-acting octreotide for the treatment and symptomatic relief of bowel obstruction in advanced ovarian cancer. **30**, 563–9.

120. Hardy, J. *et al.* (1988). Pitfalls in placebo-controlled trials in palliative care: dexamethasone for the palliation of malignant bowel obstruction. *Palliative Medicine*, **12**, 437–42.

121. Laval, G. *et al.* (2000). The use of steroids in the management of inoperable intestinal obstruction in terminal cancer patients: do they remove the obstruction? *Palliative Medicine*, **14**, 3–10.

122. Feuer, D.J. *et al.* (1999). Systematic review and meta-analysis of corticosteroids for the resolution of malignant bowel obstruction in advanced gynaecological and gastrointestinal cancers. *Annals of Oncology*, **10**, 1035–41.

123. Mercadante, S. Systematic review of etc.

124. Mercadante, S., Ferrera P., Villari P., Marrazzo A. (2004). Aggressive pharmacological treatment for reversing bowel obstruction. *Journal of Pain and Symptom Management*, **28**, 412–6.

125. Mercadante, S. (2001). What is the opioid of choice? *Progress in Palliative Care*, **9**, 190–3.

126. Mercadante, S., Sapio, M., and Serretta, R. (1997). Treatment of pain in chronic bowel subobstruction with self-administration of methadone. *Support Care in Cancer*, **5**, 327–9.

127. Hazen, L. *et al.* (1999) The constipation-inducing potential of morphine and transdermal fentanyl. *European Journal of Pain*, **3** (Suppl. A), 9–15.

128. Ahmedzai, S. and Brooks, D. (1997). Transdermal fentanyl versus sustained-release oral morphine in cancer pain: preference, efficacy, and quality of life. *Journal of Pain and Symptom Management*, **13**, 254–61.

129. Radbruck, L. *et al.* (2000). Constipation and the use of laxatives: a comparison between transdermal fentanyl and oral morphine. *Palliative Medicine*, **14**, 111–19.

130. Mancini, I.L. *et al.* (2000). Opioid type and other clinical predictors of laxatives dose in advanced cancer patients: a retrospective study. *Journal of Palliative Medicine*, **3**, 49–56.

131. Mercadante, S. *et al.* (2001). Switching from morphine to methadone to improve analgesia and tolerability in cancer patients: a prospective study. *Journal of Clinical Oncology*, **19**, 2898–904.

132. Cherny, N. *et al.* (2001). Strategies to manage the adverse effects of oral morphine: an evidence-based report. *Journal of Clinical Oncology*, **19**, 2542–54.

133. Mercadante, S. *et al.* (2002). A randomised controlled study on the use of anti-inflammatory drugs in patients with cancer pain on morphine therapy: effects on dose-escalation and pharmacoeconomical analysis. *European Journal of Cancer*, **38**, 1358–63.

134. Joishy, S.K. and Walsh, D. (1998). The opioid-sparing effects of intravenous ketorolac as an adjuvant analgesic in cancer pain: application in bone metastases and the opioid bowel syndrome. *Journal of Pain and Symptom Management*, **16**, 334–9.

135. Bozzetti, F. *et al.* (1996). Guidelines on artificial nutrition versus hydration in terminal cancer patients. *Nutrition*, **12**, 163–7.

136. Cozzaglio, L. *et al.* (1997). Outcome of cancer patients receiving home parenteral nutrition. *Journal of Parenteral and Enteral Nutrition*, **21**, 339–42.

137. Philip, J. and Depczynski, B. (1997). The role of total parenteral nutrition for patients with irreversible bowel obstruction secondary to gynecological malignancy. *Journal of Pain and Symptom Management*, **13**, 104–11.

138. Mercadante, S. (1995). Parenteral nutrition at home. *Journal of Pain and Symptom Management*, **10**, 476–80.

139. Burge, F.I. (1993). Dehydration symptoms of palliative care cancer patients. *Journal of Pain and Symptom Management*, **8**, 454–64.

140. Fainsinger, R.L. *et al.* (1994). The use of hypodermoclysis for rehydration in terminally ill cancer patients. *Journal of Pain and Symptom Management*, 9, 298–302.

10.2.5 Jaundice, ascites, and encephalopathy

Jeremy Keen

The development of jaundice or ascites is a clear signal to an individual and to those with whom he or she comes into contact that something is significantly amiss. For many, otherwise fit, individuals jaundice occurs as part of an episode of acute viral hepatitis, which in the case of infection with hepatitis A is likely to be self limiting.

However, in the context of chronic hepatic disease or malignancy, the onset of jaundice or ascites are usually indicators of advanced disease. In two series, 24 per cent and 42 per cent of patients with malignancy and admitted to hospital with jaundice died during their first admission.[1,2] Interestingly, one of the series also noted that 23 per cent of those with cirrhosis died during their first admission with jaundice.[1] In areas with specialist palliative care services, individuals with primary carcinoma or metastatic involvement of the liver will usually have the opportunity to have contact with such services but those with chronic liver disease are likely to have variable experiences. Advances in medical and surgical care of liver disease, particularly liver transplantation, whilst it is to be welcomed, has made patient care complex. Significant numbers of patients die on the transplant list and thus all patients should receive good palliative care. Tools such as the MELD[3] developed to predict prognosis as an aid to decisions about transplantation can also be an aid to prompting specialist input or ensuring a 'palliative approach' to care. Indeed some insurance companies in the United States now recognize the importance of input from specialist services and patients are allowed to benefit from hospice programmes whilst waiting for transplant and hospice cover revoked if surgery goes ahead.[4] Early input from palliative care services would also clearly smooth transition to increased input in the event of failed transplant.[5] The likely increase in numbers of patients with end stage liver disease (incidence correlates with age) and the associated poor quality of life will present increasing challenges for palliative care services.[6] Two recent studies from the UK[1] and Scandinavia[2] have analysed the cause of an elevated serum bilirubin level in consecutive samples received by biochemistry laboratories over a fixed period (neonatal samples excluded) (Table 10.2.5.1). Malignancy was found to be responsible in 33 per cent and 35 per cent of cases with primary pancreatic and cholangiocarcinoma being most frequent in the study from the UK and metastatic malignancy most frequently observed in the Scandinavian report. Clearly there will be geographical and cultural variation with, for example, primary hepatocellular carcinoma (HCC) being a very frequent cause of jaundice in South-East Asia (11.1 per cent of all admissions to a palliative care unit in Taiwan in a large reported series had HCC).[7] Carcinoma of the pancreas is relatively rarely seen in African countries, but has a very high rate in African Americans, indicating the likelihood of environmental contributors to the development of this particular malignancy. In areas with a high rate of HIV and hepatitis B and C infection, these will clearly be a significant contribution to those dying with cirrhosis or HCC.

Table 10.2.5.1 Causes of jaundice in a series of 121 patients in Wales[1] and 171 patients in Sweden[2].

Cause of jaundice	Wales (%)	Sweden (%)
Malignancy	35	33
Septicaemia	22	2.5
Cirrhosis	21	11
Gall stones	13	16
Drugs	6	1
Autoimmune hepatitis	1.5	2.5
Viral hepatitis	1.5	3.5

Table 10.2.5.2 A classification system for jaundice with examples.

Pre-hepatic	Hepatic	Post-hepatic
Gilbert's syndrome	Tumour infiltration	*Malignant*
Haemolysis	Viral hepatitis	Pancreas
Haematoma	Drug toxicity (including alcohol)	Ampulla
	Cholestasis	Cholangiocarcinoma
	Drugs	Lymphadenopathy
	Septicaemia	*Benign*
	Parenteral nutrition	Gall stones
	Graft versus host disease	Chronic pancreatitis
	Venous outflow block	Biliary stricture
	Severe heart failure	
	Budd–Chiari syndrome	

This chapter will cover three features of liver impairment that may be encountered in those for whom palliative care is appropriate but will concentrate the review of ascites on causes other than cirrhosis and portal hypertension.

Jaundice

The development of jaundice in a previously fit individual will usually prompt referral to hospital services for investigation and management. If the cause is found to be a malignancy or chronic progressive liver disease, then specialist palliative care input will often be appropriate given the associated poor prognosis. For individuals with known chronic progressive disease who develop jaundice, the responsibility for initiation of investigation and management may well rest on specialist palliative care services. The approach to the investigation and management of jaundice in palliative care should follow a logical progression, which aids the more difficult ethical decisions that often arise.

Classically, the disorders resulting in jaundice can be classified as in Table 10.2.5.2.

Prehepatic jaundice

Prehapatic causes of unconjugated hyperbilirubinaemia include Gilbert's syndrome, an inherited disorder characterized by mild chronic unconjugated hyperbilirubinaemia in the absence of liver disease or overt haemolysis. It has been estimated that 3–10 per cent of the general population may be affected by this syndrome,[8] who may demonstrate elevated bilirubin levels in response to stresses, including fasting and comorbidity. Therapeutic interventions for malignancy in individuals with Gilbert's may lead to hyperbilirubinaemia and mild jaundice[9–11] and there has been debate as to whether individuals with Gilbert's are more prone to toxic side effects with certain cytotoxic agents.[12] Prolonged parenteral nutrition has also been associated with hyperbilirubinaemia in individuals with Gilbert's syndrome.[13]

Hepatic jaundice

Hepatic causes of jaundice include any process that interferes with the excretion of conjugated bilirubin into the biliary system. Such processes either result in widespread necrosis of hepatocytes (hepatocellular jaundice) or impairment of bile excretory mechanisms (cholestatic jaundice). Worldwide, both chronic viral- and alcohol-related hepatitis with resultant cirrhosis are major causes of hepatic

jaundice. In England and Wales, the number of individuals with cirrhosis and HCC as a result of chronic hepatitis C infection more than doubled between 1995 and 2005 and may well double again by 2015.[14] The number of deaths almost tripled between 1997/8 and 2004/5, and chronic hepatitis C is now one of the most common indications for liver transplant. The existence and characteristics of chronic hepatitic viral infection is important information in those for whom immunosuppressive therapy for concomitant disorders is being considered. Fulminant liver failure is a well recognized complication of chemotherapy and other immunosuppressive therapy (immunosuppression allowing viral reactivation and proliferation) or, more frequently, its discontinuation (allowing an immune and inflammatory response).[15,16] Importantly, given their widespread use in palliative care, reactivation of hepatitis B infection has been related to the use of corticosteroids for comorbid conditions[17,18] and the inclusion of steroids in a cytotoxic regime.[19,20] The onset of jaundice, signs of portal hypertension, or the development of HCC are markers of decompensation in any patient with cirrhosis. In case series, jaundice has been the first indicator of decompensation in 30.1 per cent of patients with chronic hepatitis B and D with a consequent median survival of 26.1 months[21] and in 9 per cent with hepatitis C.[22] In these series, the most frequent first signs of decompensation were the development of ascites in hepatitis B and D (in 80 per cent of individuals) and HCC in hepatitis C-related cirrhosis (in 27 per cent). hepatitis C virus infection has been proposed as a factor in the rising incidence of intrahepatic cholangiocarcinoma in several disparate populations.[23,24]

Thankfully, the recent development of improved therapies appears to be changing the natural history of chronic liver disease secondary to the hepatitis viruses, but the likely benefit for those who already have cirrhosis is unclear.

Immunosuppression whether from drug therapy or comorbidity such as widespread metastatic carcinoma or AIDS can predispose to a number of infectious causes of hepatitis. End-stage chronic liver disease as result of infection with hepatitis B and C viruses is now a major cause of death for individuals infected with HIV.[25] The Data Collection on Adverse Events of Anti-HIV Drugs study, which followed over 23 000 HIV-infected persons from three continents reported that 14.5 per cent of deaths were from liver-related causes.[26] Of these, 16.9 per cent had active hepatitis B virus (HBV), 66.1 per cent had hepatitis C virus (HCV), and 7.1 per cent had dual viral hepatitis co-infections. In terms of absolute numbers, two post-mortem series from Nigeria and India noted the presence of tuberculous granulomata within the liver as the most frequent abnormal histological finding[27,28] and cholestatic, non-obstructive jaundice has been described as a consequence of hepatic involvement in tuberculosis.[29] Jaundice in individuals with AIDS, but without evidence of cirrhosis, may result from abnormalities within the biliary tract. Acalculous cholecystitis, secondary sclerosing cholangitis, and papillary stenosis have all been demonstrated and appear to be associated with cryptosporidia and cytomegaloviruis infection.[30] Where available, highly active anti-retroviral therapy (HAART) has dramatically improved the outlook for patients with AIDS-related cholangiopathy. However, a recent study determined that a massively raised (eight times normal value) level of alkaline phosphatase may be a marker of poor prognosis despite HAART. Cholecystectomy, papillotomy, and biliary stenting as determined by the form of cholangiopathy can significantly improve symptom control. Given the dramatic change in the natural history of HIV infection, liver transplantion should now be considered for individuals with end stage liver disease and early results suggest that results are as good as those in the population without HIV infection.[31]

Drug-induced liver disease

Hepatotoxicity from antimicrobial therapies is well recognized and these drugs make a major contribution to the global incidence of drug induced liver disease. Indeed, if paracetamol overdose is excluded, antiretroviral and antituberculous drugs are responsible for the vast majority of incidences of drug-induced hepatotoxicity.

Most drug effects simply lead to an increase in serum liver enzymes and do not result in jaundice (2–7 per cent of hospital admissions for non-obstructive jaundice[32]) but, in those that do so, there is a significant mortality. Drug-induced liver disease accounts for over 50 per cent of cases of acute liver failure in the United States of which approximately 70 per cent relate to paracetamol overdose and the remaining 30 per cent a result of idiosyncratic reaction to one of over 600 medicinal compounds that have been reported to cause hepatotoxicity of one form or another.[33] A recent Swedish audit reported that 77 of 1164 new referrals to a hepatology clinic were deemed to have drug-induced liver disease with 29 having clinical jaundice.[34] Flucloxacillin, diclofenac, and ciprofloxacin were the most frequently associated drugs with mean lengths of exposure of 10, 23, and 6 days, respectively. After discontinuation of each of the three drugs, the respective mean times to regain biochemical normality were 145, 35, and 54 days.

Jaundice in drug-induced liver disease can be both hepatocellular and cholestatic such that histological findings include acute hepatocyte necrosis, chronic hepatitis, vascular injury, and bile ductular injury. Drugs are thought to cause injury through a variety of mechanisms that often translate into differing clinical pictures. Predictable dose-dependent rapid-onset hepatotoxicity with paracetamol is well described. Drug-induced cholestasis resulting from disruption of bile secretion by the hepatocytes and cholangiocytes can occur as a result of immune-mediated hypersensitivity

but also possibly at receptor level through direct blocking of transporter polypeptides. Idiosyncratic cholestasis maybe explained by genetic variants in these transporters. Direct mitochondrial injury has been described, albeit rarely, with amiodarone, sodium valproate, and aspirin and produces a histological pattern resembling alcohol-induced liver disease. Sinusoidal cell injury and the development of veno-occlusive disease and hepatic necrosis is a recognized complication of high-dose myeloablative chemotherapy with such agents as cyclophosphamide, melphalan, and busulphan.

Immune-mediated drug-induced liver disease is usually accompanied by a latency period of 1–8 weeks and tends to be associated with fever, skin rash, arthralgia, and eosinophilia as well as jaundice and is characterized by a rapid recurrence on rechallenge. Hypersensitivity is thought to result from the creation of immunogens through the binding of the drug to proteins (as a result of its metabolism or bioactivation) and can result in acute hepatitic, cholestatic, or mixed reactions (Table 10.2.5.3). Raised serum hepatic enzyme levels will usually rapidly return to normal after withdrawal of the offending drug (a reduction of 50 per cent after 2 weeks and to baseline by 4 weeks is a general rule), but cholestatic reactions do have the potential of chronicity despite drug withdrawal. Amoxicillin/clavulanic acid is one of the most frequent causes of acute cholestasis and progression to chronic cholestasis has been associated with chlorpromazine and other phenothiazines.

When investigating possible drug-induced liver disease, it is important to enquire about non-prescription medications increasingly used by individuals receiving palliative care. Complementary medications may be responsible for up to 5 per cent of drug-induced liver disease and include preparations such as Germander and Mistletoe.[32,35,36]

Drug-induced liver disease can, rarely, become chronic either through direct injury as in the case of methotrexate or indirectly with the production of autoantibodies and a resultant autoimmune chronic hepatitis after an episode of acute drug-induced liver injury.

With an increasing incidence of chronic liver disease in the population, there is a need to be clear about the potential for exacerbation of liver disease by the prescription of certain drugs. In fact, whilst it is clear that patients with liver disease are at increased risk of drug toxicity secondary to slowed metabolism, there appears to be little evidence that there is an increased risk of drug-related hepatotoxicity. For example, individuals with cirrhosis tolerate therapeutic doses of paracetamol without deterioration in liver function.[37,38] Exceptions include the observation of an increased

Table 10.2.5.3 Drugs associated with immune-mediated liver disease.[2]

Hepatocellular reactions	Cholestatic/mixed reactions
Allopurinol	Amoxicillin/clavulanic acid
Germander	Chlorpromazine/levomepromazine
Other herbal medications	Erythromycin
Halothane	Tricyclic antidepressants
Minocycline	Fluoxetine
Phenytoin	Acetylcholinesterase inhibitors

rate of hepatotoxicity with the anti-androgens flutamide and cyproterone in those with chronic hepatitis B or C infection.[39]

Cholestatic, non-obstructive jaundice can clearly be seen in other chronic liver disorders such as primary biliary cirrhosis and sclerosing cholangitis but also as a result of sepsis or shock (21 per cent of cases of jaundice in one UK study).[1] Cholestasis secondary to sepsis may relate to hypotension and low hepatic blood flow but also to the direct inhibitory effects of endotoxin and inflammatory cytokines (interleukin-1, interleukin-6, and tumour necrosis factor-α) on bile secretion.[40]

Cardiac failure and the liver

Hypotension and low hepatic blood flow seen in sepsis is also partly responsible for the association between liver disease and heart failure. Eight patients out of 661 presenting with jaundice in a recent series were found to have cardiac failure as their main diagnosis.[41] Although clearly a rare presentation of heart failure, altered liver function is common in severe heart failure and is thought to be mainly a result of sinusoidal congestion, though significant hypotension (usually secondary to infarction or valvular disease) can lead to an ischaemic hepatitis signalled by a massive rise in aminotransferases and prolonged prothrombin time. Hepatic congestion produces a cholestatic derangement of liver enzymes thought to represent secondary damage to the bile canaliculae as a result of sinusoidal disruption.[42] Sinusoidal congestion is most marked in heart failure associated with tricuspid valve regurgitation and a clear correlation between severity of regurgitation and serum levels of alkaline phosphatase (ALP) and γ-glutamyl transferase (GGT) has been demonstrated.[43]

Graft versus host disease and venous occlusion

Jaundice resulting from sinusoidal congestion and obliteration or veno occlusive disease has been mentioned as a complication of myeloablative therapy prior to marrow transplantation. Cholestatic jaundice is, additionally, commonly seen after transplantation as a result of sepsis and acute graft versus host disease (GVHD).[44] Whilst jaundice and abnormal liver function usually respond to immunosuppressive therapy, occasionally cholestasis can progress as a manifestation of chronic GVHD to biliary cirrhosis. Ursodeoxycholic acid is widely used in cholestatic liver disease and is thought to work via several mechanisms including a change in the composition of bile salts within secreted bile and a consequent reduction in toxicity to damaged biliary epithelium.[45] In one study, the prophylactic administration of ursodeoxycholic acid has been studied in patients undergoing allogeneic stem cell transplantation with a resultant significant reduction in post-transplant hyperbilirubinaemia.[46] There are reports of successful liver transplantation in both acute and chronic GVHD. Reactivation of chronic viral hepatitis is not uncommonly seen during aggressive therapies requiring marrow transplantation and can lead to fulminant hepatic failure.

Patients with sinusoidal obliteration from myeloablative therapy can rapidly develop ascites and tender hepatomegaly along with jaundice. A similar rapid onset of symptoms can occur in the venous occlusion of the Budd–Chiari syndrome, although a chronic form of the syndrome resulting in the usual symptoms of chronic liver disease is more usual.[47] Chronic sinusoidal congestion leads on to chronic hepatitis and potentially cirrhosis. Venous obstruction can occur at any point from the hepatic venules to the right atrium and long lists of causative and associated disorders have

been described. The most commonly associated disorders are those that produce a hypercoagulable state such as the myeloproliferative disorders polycythaemia rubra vera and essential thrombocytosis. Malignancy is clearly associated with Budd–Chiari syndrome both through increased thrombogenicity, particularly if coupled with a genetic predisposition to hypercoagulability,[47] and local obstruction of the venous system by solid tumours. Clinically, progressive inferior vena caval obstruction maybe demonstrated by the development of increasing lower body oedema. Diagnosis relies on imaging by Doppler ultrasound in the first instance followed by CT or MR. Untreated acute Budd–Chiari syndrome is fatal in 80 per cent of cases and management therefore requires an urgent and aggressive approach (if appropriate given the individual's disease status) combining radiological and surgical interventions to relieve or bypass the venous obstruction. Inferior vena caval stenting and transjugular intrahepatic portosystemic shunt (TIPS) formation are relatively uninvasive procedures that can be of significant benefit in selected individuals. In those unsuitable for interventional procedures, a decision regarding anticoagulant therapy is required but the outlook with medical therapy alone is bleak with a mortality of over 80 per cent in one series.[48]

Malignant infiltration

Non-obstructive jaundice as a result of massive infiltration of the liver by primary or metastatic malignancy is rare, usually accompanied by signs of liver failure, and signals a very poor prognosis measured in days to weeks.[48] In the majority, this clinical picture develops during palliative care when anti-tumour therapies have been exhausted, although discussion with an oncologist may still be warranted.[49] Occasionally, liver failure will be the first presentation of malignancy and *if* the diagnosis is made pre-mortem, anti-tumour therapy can achieve a response sufficient to allow resolution of jaundice.

Obstructive jaundice

Obstruction of the biliary tract can occur at any point from within the liver to the ampulla of Vater. To give rise to jaundice this usually occurs at the confluence of the major ducts at the porta hepatis or more distally. In two recent studies of the causes of jaundice in consecutive, non-neonatal patients, obstructive jaundice caused by gall stones was diagnosed in 13 and 16 per cent.[1,2] The majority of cases of obstructive jaundice in these series were caused by malignancy, with carcinoma of the head of the pancreas, cholangiocarcinoma and metastatic disease (intrahepatic or porta hepatis lymphadenopathy) most frequently responsible. Obstruction at the porta hepatis is commonly secondary to cholangiocarcinoma but can be caused by benign strictures (57 per cent and 20 per cent of cases respectively in one series[50]), which, despite current imaging techniques, are difficult to distinguish from malignancy.

HCC, an increasingly common problem given the prevalence of chronic viral hepatitis and cirrhosis, can cause obstructive jaundice through a variety of mechanisms. Most frequently bile duct blockage is secondary to direct bile duct invasion and consequent haemobilia and thrombosis or obstruction by tumour debris. Less commonly, widespread diffuse tumour infiltration causes disruption of hepatic architecture and blockage of multiple small bile ducts. Occasionally, jaundice may also result from the external compression of the major bile ducts by direct tumour encasement or by metastatic lymphadenopathy at the porta hepatis.

Clinical presentation

Presenting symptoms of individuals with jaundice clearly, in part, relate to the underlying pathological process (Table 10.2.5.4). A large series of patients admitted to a palliative care unit with HCC, of whom 77 per cent had associated liver cirrhosis, has been reported.[7] The most common symptoms upon admission were pain, fatigue, weakness, anorexia, vomiting, peripheral oedema, cachexia, and ascites. Studies involving patients who have undergone procedures to relieve biliary obstruction give some indication of symptoms particularly related to hyperbilirubinaemia and malignant large biliary duct obstruction. In addition to the expected clearing of jaundice and relief of pruritus, significant improvements were noted in anorexia, indigestion, sleep pattern, and global health scores.[51,52] At an immunocytochemical level, studies have shown significant elevation of endotoxin, tumour necrosis factor-α, and interleukins 6 and 10 in malignant obstructive jaundice but reports vary with respect to the changes observed in levels of these factors after biliary drainage.[53–55] Biliary obstruction in an animal study reduced the activity of hepatic Kupffer cells, resulting in increased levels of systemic endotoxin but recovery of activity and reduction in endotoxin was noted after biliary drainage.[56] A Canadian study examined quality of life before and after biliary tract stenting in individuals with malignant obstruction. A significant association was demonstrated between the degree of reduction in bilirubin levels after stenting and an improvement in social function and mental health as assessed by the SF-36 Health Survey Questionnaire.[57] However, in a subgroup of individuals with baseline serum bilirubin levels above 13 mg/dl(222μmol/l), there was no improvement in social functioning after stent insertion. The authors propose, therefore, that careful assessment is carried prior to stent insertion in individuals with very high serum bilirubin levels.

Malignant obstructive jaundice is classically thought to be 'painless' and therefore distinguished from benign causes such as gallstones. However in a study of elderly patients with biliary duct obstruction, 32 per cent of those with a malignant cause alone (several patients in the study had both malignancy and gallstones casing obstruction) presented with abdominal pain.[58] Rarely individuals may present with malignant obstructive jaundice and symptoms of infective cholangitis. More commonly this is a complication of interventional manipulation of the biliary tract including stent placement.

Investigation

In a setting in which individuals are receiving palliative care, the onset of jaundice is likely to relate to a known underlying disease process. A careful history should elucidate the primary disease process and set the onset of jaundice in the context of other markers of disease status. A drug history from the patient including non-prescription items is clearly vital.

Physical examination may confirm signs of chronic liver disease, portal hypertension, or intra-abdominal malignancy and may give clues as to current liver function. It is important to assess cognitive function for signs of associated encephalopathy. In all cases, signs of infection must be looked for within the biliary tree or peritoneum (if ascites is present), particularly if the patient is immunosuppressed by chronic infection, including HIV, or drugs (including corticosteroids). Infective cholangitis is associated with a significant mortality rate.

Blood tests

A clinical diagnosis of jaundice is confirmed by serum hyperbilirubinaemia. Should there be no derangement of liver enzymes to suggest cholestasis or hepatocellular injury then relative levels of unconjugated and conjugated bilirubin can be measured to distinguish between prehepatic and hepatic causes of jaundice. Elevated levels of alkaline phosphatase and γ-glutamyl transferase with relatively normal, or only moderately increased, levels of aspartate transaminase and alanine transaminase would be a typical finding in cholestatic jaundice (Table 10.2.5.4). Isolated elevation of alkaline phosphatase is unusual in cholestasis and if present with normal γ-glutamyl transferase but elevated enzymes associated with hepatocellular injury may reflect bone disease. Isolated raised

Table 10.2.5.4 Clinical characteristics of jaundice of differing aetiologies.

	Type of jaundice			
Clinical factors	**Haemolytic**	**Hepatocellular**	**Intrahepatic/cholestatic**	**Posthepatic/cholestatic ('obstructive')**
Symptoms	Asymptomatic or back ache, arthralgia	Nausea, vomiting, anorexia, pyrexia	Deep jaundice, dark urine, light stools, Pruritus	Deep jaundice, dark urine, light stools, Pruritus, cholangitis, biliary colic
Physical	Splenomegaly	Tender hepatomegaly	Tender hepatomegaly	Hepatomegaly, palpable gallbladder
Liver function tests				
Bilirubin	<100 μmol/l	Variable	Variable may be >500 μmol/l	<500 μmol/l
ALT	Normal	>5-fold increase	2- to 5-fold increase	<2- to 3-fold increase but 3- to 5-fold increase with cholangitis
ALP	Normal	<2- to 3-fold increase	>3- to 5-fold increase	>3- to 5-fold increase
Prothrombin time	Normal	Prolonged	Prolonged	Prolonged
Corrected by Vitamin K?	—	No	Variable	Yes
Dilated bile ducts on ultrasound?	No	No	No	Yes

ALT, Alanine aminotransferase; ALP, Alkaline phosphatase.
Source: adapted with permission from Kamath *et al.*[59]

γ-glutamyl transferase may reflect a drug effect. Serum albumin levels and prothrombin time reflect, in part, the synthetic function of the liver and evidence of coagulopathy is vital information prior to performing invasive investigations and therapeutic procedures.

Imaging

It has been estimated that a thorough history, physical examination, and biochemical liver tests are sufficient for making an accurate diagnosis of the type of liver disease in at least 80 per cent of patients.[59] Imaging investigations in individuals with jaundice visualize the liver and biliary tree as an aid to confirming or identifying the underlying diagnosis, determining the location and extent of disease and the potential for treatment. Whilst ultrasound in combination with cholangiography either via the endoscopic or transcutaneous route have been the mainstay in imaging, improvements in CT and increasing availability of MRI has led to ongoing debates over the relative merits of each modality.

Ultrasound

Ultrasound remains the first imaging investigation of choice in the patient with jaundice. It can be used at the bedside, does not involve radiation, and is relatively cheap. In a patient with obstructive jaundice, ultrasound will detect bile duct dilatation with a sensitivity and specificity of between 95 and 99 per cent.[60,61] Ultrasound may also allow detection of primary or secondary malignant lesions within the liver, lymph nodes, or pancreas and visualization of the hepatic veins in the investigation of possible Budd–Chiari syndrome. Doppler can be used to demonstrate tumour vascularity and local invasion of major blood vessels such as the portal vein or, less accurately, the superior mesenteric artery. Contrast-enhanced power Doppler ultrasound is a promising method that can aid the differentiation of pancreatic malignancy from chronic pancreatitis.[62]

However, ultrasound is highly operator dependent and is problematic in obese patients and in situations where bowel gas overlies the region studied. Ducts may also be difficult to visualize in advanced cirrhosis and dilated ducts without obstruction may be seen after previous cholecystectomy. Indeed, a review of the use of standard transcutaneous ultrasound imaging to determine the level and aetiology of biliary obstruction reported respective sensitivities of only 71 per cent and 57 per cent.[63] However, the diagnostic accuracy of ultrasound in extrahepatic biliary obstruction has been considerably enhanced by the endoscopic placement of probes. Endoscopic ultrasonography not only allows the detection of very small lesions such as periampullary or intraductal carcinomas, often difficult to visualize even on CT or MR imaging, but also enables material to be obtained by needle aspiration, under imaging guidance, for histological diagnosis. This technique has significantly improved the rate of positive histological diagnoses of pancreatic masses and has also allowed cytological specimens to be obtained not only from the lower bile duct region but also from the hilum and even left lobe of the liver.[64] Endoscopic ultrasonography with fine needle injection has also been used to perform coeliac plexus neurolysis for pain control and even direct instillation of anti-tumour agents.[65,66]

Intraductal ultrasound can improve the visualization of longitudinal spread of cholangiocarcinoma and when used in conjunction with endoscopic retrograde cholangiopancreatography (ERCP) can significantly improve the differentiation between benign and malignant bile duct strictures.[67] The recent introduction of three-dimensional ultrasound scanning has improved the accuracy of localization of the site of obstruction and its aetiology in obstructive jaundice to levels comparable with magnetic resonance imaging (MRI) and direct cholangiography.[68]

Computed tomography (CT)

The role of CT scanning in the investigation of the individual with jaundice is dependent upon the local availability of other imaging hardware. CT imaging with intravenous contrast improves the imaging of liver parenchyma in hepatocellular causes of jaundice when compared with ultrasound. Localization and diagnosis of the cause of biliary obstruction may most frequently be obtained by a combination of ultrasound and cholangiography (either endoscopic or transcutaneous). The CT image used in conjunction with oral and intravenous contrast is, however, of use in determining the extent and stage of disease and hence treatment options. The introduction of spiral CT and, more recently, multi-detector CT has resulted in improved resolution for the detection and characterization of small lesions, and the enabled rapid accumulation of data with consequent reduced movement artefact has improved 3D imaging.[69] Multidetector CT if used in conjunction with biliary-specific contrast media can produce images as accurate as MR and direct cholangiography, but the presence of obstructive jaundice reduces the biliary excretion of contrast and which, in high levels of bilirubinaemia, is contra-indicated.[61]

Magnetic resonance cholangiopancreatography (MRCP)

MRCP is non-invasive, does not involve exposure to radiation, and does not require intra-venous injection of contrast medium. It is however, at present, an expensive procedure with relatively limited access. A large systematic review of the diagnostic ability of MRCP in biliary obstruction reported a pooled sensitivity of 95 per cent for the demonstration of the level of obstruction and an 88 per cent sensitivity in distinguishing between benign and malignant lesions.[70] Certainly in terms of demonstrating the level of obstruction, these results are similar to those achieved by direct cholangiography. ERCP can determine with greater accuracy the difference between benign and malignant lesions particularly at or near the ampulla because of the distortion caused to the MR image by duodenal gas. However, MRCP is more accurate than ERCP at distinguishing the nature and extent of perihilar cholangiocarcinoma (Klatskin tumours),[71] and determining the dominant ductal drainage to guide stent insertion.[72,73] Perhaps the most important advantage of MRCP over ERCP is that there are not the associated risks of cannulation of the biliary tract. MRCP allows a conventional MR image of the abdomen to be performed during the same session to determine the extent of disease and has therefore been proposed as the complete diagnostic study.[74] MR has been studied and found to be accurate in the demonstration of tumour thrombi as a cause of obstructive jaundice in HCC[75] but has been doubted in overall diagnostic accuracy in jaundice arising in those with HCC.[71] The use of new contrast agents with MR may well improve the visualization of liver parenchymal disorders.

At present, notwithstanding cost and access to scanners, many centres will use MRCP after initial ultrasound assessment as the definitive imaging technique with ERCP or PTC used only where therapeutic procedures are required. A recent review from the UK concluded that, overall, MRCP was more cost effective as a diagnostic imaging tool than ERCP, although in population analysis benefits were lost if the likelihood of choledocholithiasis was greater than 60 per cent.[76] The authors also admit theseconclusions are dependent on availability of scanners and waiting times. Developments in CT techniques will continue to challenge MR and relative cost effectiveness will need regular review.

Cholangiography

Given the advances in external imaging techniques and their relative safety, endoscopic and percutaneous cholangiography are now mainly used as part of a therapeutic procedure to manipulate the biliary tract in situations where definitive surgery is not contemplated. This, of course, may be simple choledocholithiasis, but in palliative care, obstructive jaundice is often related to extensive primary or metastatic malignancy. Access to the biliary tree via the percutaneous route is usually only attempted when the level of biliary obstruction is proximal to the common hepatic duct or when distorted anatomy often due to previous surgery or the presence of local tumour precludes ERCP (Fig. 10.2.5.1).

Both techniques allow cytological sampling, if needed, and palliative drainage of the biliary system via dilatation and stent insertion. The procedures are both associated with potentially fatal complications including bacterial cholangitis, bleeding, bile leakage, and pancreatitis after ERCP. The incidence of adverse events in both approaches is low, being reported in 0.5–5 per cent of patients and is, to an extent, operator dependent.[77,78] Various pharmacological agents have been trialled in attempts to reduce the incidence of post-ERCP pancreatitis.[79]

Positron emission tomography (PET)

PET is being used increasingly, where available, in staging of tumours where the accurate detection of the presence of metastatic disease is important in determining the potential for surgical resection of the primary lesion. PET has the potential to differentiate between benign and malignant lesions of the hepatobiliary tract.

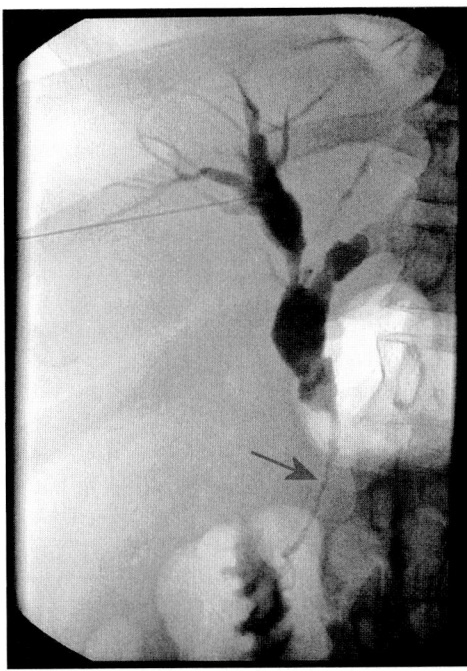

Figure 10.2.5.1 Transhepatic cholangiogram demonstrating long common bile duct stricture which could not be ccannulated via ERCP.

Unfortunately, PET has limited accuracy in detecting HCC arising in cirrhosis, a difficult but important diagnosis to make, because of low uptake of 18-F fluorodeoxyglucose, the labeled analogue of glucose used in the technique, in well-differentiated tumours.[80] The lack of ability to accurately display anatomical features and its expense mean that, at present, PET has little part to play in the investigation for palliative care of the individual with jaundice.

Management

The principles of management of jaundice in palliative care follow that of any condition arising in this phase of care. Treatment specific to the underlying cause should always, at least, be considered, with the approach to treatment always tailored to the individual's situation and after full and revisited discussion. Chemotherapy for sensitive malignancies, unless previously exhausted, may allow at least temporary relief of jaundice in those thought fit enough and for whom potential post-chemotherapy survival is deemed worthwhile. In individuals with certain chemosensitive tumours, chemotherapy can still be considered even in the presence of jaundice or signs of incipient hepatic failure resulting from widespread tumour infiltration. Careful drug selection and dose titration is required, but significant improvements in symptoms and survival can be achieved.[81,82] In obstructive jaundice, studies attest to the significant and rapid improvement in symptoms and overall quality of life after successful biliary drainage procedures.[51,52,57] If such procedures are combined with post-procedural anti-tumour therapy (systemic and intra-arterial local chemotherapy, hormone suppression,monoclonal antibodies, external radiotherapy, intra-luminal brachytherapy, and photodynamic therapy have all been described), then rapid predictable improvement in symptom control can be combined with potential prolonged survival and possible prolonged stent patency.[83,84]

Clearly, jaundice as a result of superinfection or malignancy in individuals with AIDS may well respond to specific treatment if adequate doses of antibacterial, antiviral, antifungal, or cytotoxic chemotherapy can be tolerated. Diagnosis is made serologically, by imaging sometimes accompanied by guided biopsy or, in the case of obstructive jaundice, at ERCP if AIDS-related cholangiopathy is suspected.

Biliary drainage procedures

Obstructive jaundice is present at the time of presentation in 70–80 per cent of individuals with pancreatic carcinoma and 85 per cent are deemed unsuitable for curative resection.[85] In one review of over 8000 patients with unresectable carcinoma of the pancreas those who underwent a surgical biliary bypass procedure, allowing biliary drainage, had a significant improvement in quality and length of survival.[86] Interestingly, one study of quality of life related to endoscopic biliary drainage demonstrated increased quality of life post-drainage but only in those individuals with pre-procedure serum bilirubin levels below 13 g/dl (222 μmol/l).[57] With improvement in endoscopic and percutaneous biliary cannulation and stent materials, there has been lengthy debate over the optimum approach to biliary drainage. A significant proportion of patients will be deemed unfit for surgery and if appropriate should be considered for biliary stenting via endoscopic or percutaneous routes. Five percent of individuals presenting with unresectable pancreatic carcinoma will have evidence of duodenal or gastric outlet obstruction and should therefore be considered for palliative duodenal and biliary bypass procedures. With ever-increasing interest in laparoscopic surgery, there are numerous reports of this approach being employed both for biliary and concomitant gastric drainage procedures.[87–89] If an individual prepared for tumour resection is found to have irresectable disease at the time of laparotomy, then a biliary bypass procedure is advised at the time of surgery.[85]

A recent, large, systematic review for the Cochrane Collaboration has confirmed the conclusions of earlier studies comparing endoscopic stenting and surgical bypass procedures for malignant biliary obstruction.[90] In the studies reviewed, there was no difference between the two interventions in terms of technical success, therapeutic success, survival, or quality of life. Endoscopic stenting with plastic stents is associated with fewer complications, a shorter total hospital stay, but a higher risk of recurrent biliary obstruction and consequent cholangitis than surgery. Only one published randomized trial was detected comparing percutaneous stents and surgery and reported no significant difference in outcome between both groups. Recurrent biliary obstruction is usually a result of stent blockage by debris or tumour overgrowth occurring, in the trials reviewed, after medians of 62–165 days for plastic stents. Occlusion is delayed to medians of 111–273 days by the use of relatively large bore self-expanding metal stents and is more often related to tumour in- or overgrowth. However, in the studies reviewed, the median length of survival ranged from 99 to 175 days, suggesting that many patients die before either stent occludes. Metal stents are expensive (approximately 20–30× that of plastic) and the plastic variety are, therefore, still preferred by many operators in situations where the prognosis is likely to be less than 6 months. A laparoscopic approach to surgical bypass is certainly to be favoured over laparotomy in terms of early complications, length of hospital stay, and postoperative recovery, but no trials comparing this technique to endoscopic stenting have been reported as yet. Additionally, access to local laparoscopic expertise remains limited.

It appears, therefore, that for the minority of individuals with pancreatic carcinoma having an estimated relatively long prognosis, of whom 13 per cent are likely to develop duodenal obstruction,[86] and a significant number would develop stent occlusion, consideration should be given to surgical biliary bypass with prophylactic gastric drainage. Individuals with malignant bile duct obstruction and evidence of hepatic or pulmonary metastases had a median survival of 2.5 months in one recent study whose authors therefore concluded that this particular population should undergo endoscopic placement of plastic stents as the primary drainage procedure.[91] Another group found that tumour size was the most powerful predictor of prognosis and concluded that biliary obstruction associated with tumours greater than 30mm should be managed by plastic stent insertion with metallic stents employed in tumours less than 30mm in diameter.[92]

Individuals with high bile duct obstruction or distorted duodenal anatomy may require a percutaneous approach either for stent placement or to allow external drainage of bile for symptomatic relief and to widen the choice, if appropriate, of systemic cytotoxic agents that maybe administered.[93] Chronic loss of bile through the drain can lead to nutritional deficiencies and if stents cannot be deployed then an attempt to pass an internal–external catheter via guidewire manipulation may be made. This catheter has side holes positioned proximal to the obstruction and the tip lies within the bowel to allow drainage of bile either externally or internally.[94]

Intraoperative pain management

Patients with obstructive jaundice secondary to pancreatic malignancy are highly likely to experience pain during their illness, which is not always easily controllable by opioids and adjuvants. Surgical bypass procedures offer an ideal opportunity to consider neurolytic procedures directed at either the coeliac plexus or the splachnic nerves. A prospective randomized controlled trial reported in 1993 compared intra operative coeliac plexus block with saline versus 50 per cent alcohol in patients with unresectable pancreatic carcinoma.[95] Individuals in whom neurolysis with alcohol was performed had significantly lower pain scores postoperatively and at all time points until death compared to the placebo group. Individuals in the alcohol group who experienced pain prior to operation had a significantly prolonged mean survival of 6 months in comparison to the placebo group who had a mean survival of 3 months. Individuals without pain prior to operation had a significantly prolonged period prior to the onset of pain (7.2 months) compared to the placebo group (3 months). There were no significant differences between the groups in terms of postoperative morbidity, mortality, or length of hospital stay. The authors understandably concluded that all individuals with unresectable pancreatic cancer should have an intraoperative neurolytic procedure. This recommendation is confirmed by recent UK national guidelines and is extended to include patients treated endoscopically.[96] Coeliac plexus block has been described with the aid of endoscopic ultrasound at the time of stenting procedures and has also been successfully performed laparoscopically at the time of bypass surgery.

Nutrition

Chronic cholestasis can lead to malabsorption of fat soluble vitamins such as vitamin K, which contributes to the prolonged clotting time that may be associated with jaundice.[97] The international normalized ratio (INR) should be regularly checked in jaundiced patients and vitamin K given either parenterally or orally (both routes, interestingly, seem as effective).[98] Even in patients with end-stage disease, this may reduce the likelihood of distressing haemorrhage.

Pruritus

Pruritus is likely to prove one of the most distressing symptoms in jaundiced individuals with diffuse liver disease or for whom biliary drainage procedures are inappropriate or have been unsuccessful. Given the significance of this symptom in chronic liver disease, it has been intensively investigated but the cause remains elusive and the optimal management is not clearly defined. Successful management is rare and the symptom so impacting on quality of life that severe pruritus can be an indication for liver transplant in chronic liver disease. Itch may be mild or severe, localized or generalized but a pattern in which itch typically starts on the palms of the hands and soles of the feet before becoming more generalized has been described.[100] Itching in cholestasis appears to be at its worst between 1200 and 1800 h.[101]

Theories as to the pathogenesis of pruritus in jaundice involve either the stimulation of peripheral itch receptors within the skin by an increased level of circulating bile acids and other pruritogens or alteration in neurotransmitters and generation of pruritus by central neural mechanisms. Histological evidence of mast cell activity within the skin in jaundiced individuals is conflicting and limited but clinical observation suggests that antihistamines are generally ineffective in relieving the itch associated with jaundice. Increasing interest has been reported in the central activity of endogenous opioids, in particular, but also serotonin, GABA, and cannibinoids.

Opioid systems

Pruritus, although a rare side effect of systemically administered opioids is experienced in 30 and 100 per cent of individuals after an epidural or intrathecal administration.[102] Opioid antagonists and the partial agonist buprenorphine have been shown to relieve pruritus in this situation. Opioid antagonists given to individuals with jaundice who are not taking opioid analgesics often produce an opioid withdrawal type reaction. Indeed, increased plasma levels of opioid peptides have been recorded in individuals with primary biliary cirrhosis,[103] and animal models suggest increased hepatic synthesis of enkephalins in cholestatic states. Furthermore, animals display naloxone-reversible scratching behaviour when given plasma extracts from humans with cholestasis and pruritus (but not from those without pruritus).[104]

Early reports described a significant improvement in cholestatic pruritus by both subjective and objective assessment after an intravenous infusion of naloxone.[101,105] Several studies including randomized controlled trials have shown similar effects with the oral opioid antagonists naltrexone and nalmefene.[106–109] All reports warn of a significant incidence of early and short-term opioid withdrawal-like side effects, principally nausea, hallucinations, and dysphoria. One small case series also warned of uncontrolled pain as complication requiring discontinuation of otherwise successful therapy with naltrexone.[110] Opioid withdrawal reactions tend to be more pronounced after initiation of therapy via the oral route than when given systemically.[111] At least one protocol has been advocated for avoidance of withdrawal by gradual upwards titration of opioid antagonist commencing with ultra-low doses of infusional naloxone before moving on to oral naltrexone for maintenance.[111,112] Clearly, the main difficulty in malignant biliary obstruction is the fact that the vast majority of individuals will be receiving opioid agonist analgesics and co-prescription of antagonists is likely to result in loss of pain control. However, recent trials in postoperative anaesthesia have demonstrated a reduction in opioid-induced side effects, including pruritus, without loss of pain control or increased opioid requirements, by the addition of low dose naloxone to morphine for intravenous infusion.[113,114] One case report of a lady with metastatic liver disease describes successful control of pain and pruritus with a combination of low dose tramadol and low dose naloxone followed by naltrexone.[111] Interestingly, one small trial reports a significant decrease in pruritus associated with perioperative intrathecal analgesia with morphine if low dose intravenous buprenorphine was co-administered.[115] A small case series found significant relief from cholestatic pruritus in two out of five patients treated with buprenorphine and intolerable side effects in three patients.[116] Interestingly, Cholestyramine, although thought principally to reduce pruritus by reducing circulating levels of bile acids through increased faecal excretion, has been shown to increase levels of cholecystokinin, which has anti-opioid actions.[117]

The apparent similarity between cholestatic pruritus and that induced by the spinal administration of opioids has fostered small trials of other potentially useful agents. Ondansetron,[118–120] droperidol,[121] propofol,[121,122] and intra-thecal bupivacaine[123] have all been shown to significantly reduce opioid-induced pruritus.

There are close links between the central opioidergic and seretonergic transmission systems. Early reports suggested substantial beneficial effects of seretonin type 3 (5-HT$_3$) receptor antagonists on cholestatic pruritus[124,125] but more recent controlled trials have suggested only modest or no benefit.[126,127] A case report suggested the beneficial effects of mirtazapine in a patient with pruritus and liver metastases may be related to its antagonist effects at certain seretonergic receptor sites[128] Interestingly there has been a case series attesting to the beneficial effects of the serotonin re-uptake inhibitor sertraline in cholestatic pruritus.[129]

Opioids antagonize the central inhibitory effects of GABA and several groups have shown recent interest in the use of propofol, a GABA agonist to reduce spinal opioid-induced pruritus. An early, small randomized trial showed benefit of subhypnotoc doses of propofol in cholestatic pruritus.[130] Phenobarbitone has been shown in two case series to improve itch in cholestasis associated with pregnancy and chronic liver disease.[131,132] This effect may be related to enzyme induction effects on the liver but Phenobarbitone is also a central GABA agonist. Another GABA enhancer, midazolam gave prolonged relief of cholestatic pruritus, without undue sedation, in one case report when given by continuous infusion.[133,117] One might postulate that the observation that pruritus tends to lessen in advancing liver failure may represent a decreased ability to synthesize pruritogens or may relate to increased levels of intrinsic GABA and GABAergic agonists noted in liver failure.[134]

A small study seemed to suggest a significant effect of the cannibinoid dronabinol in three patients who had found no benefit from multiple treatment including plasmapheresis.[135] The mechanism of action is unclear but probably relates to a close association with opiodergic neurotransmission.

One recent small randomized controlled study has shown prolonged relief of cholestatic pruritus after a 5-min intravenous infusion of 100 mg of lidocaine.[136] It is unclear whether any putative action of lidocaine is on the central or peripheral nervous system but maybe similar to the effect on opioid-induced pruritus seen with the addition of bupivacaine to epidural or intrathecal infusions.

Removal of pruritogens

Early studies of cholestatic pruritus centred on the use of anion exchange resins, most frequently cholestyramine, to chelate bile acids within the intestine with consequent reduction in reabsorption and lower plasma levels. Newer resins are available and colesevelam, at least, appears to be helpful in pruritus associated with chronic cholestasis.[137] The effectiveness of such chelating resins is dependent on a significant contribution to plasma bile acid levels by enterohepatic circulation and cholestyramine or other resins are unlikely to be helpful in complete bile obstruction. Stool colour may give an indication of the amount of bile reaching the intestine. Cholestyramine is not very palatable, can lead to bloating and constipation, and is usually poorly tolerated and potentially ineffective in a significant propoof individuals receiving palliative care.

Cholestyramine and other similar resins may bind other pruritogens that are in fact more influential in the generation of pruritus than bile acids. A recent study of extra corporeal plasma separation and anion adsorption demonstrated a significant reduction in cholestatic pruritus that did not correlate to plasma levels of bile acids and the authors suggested this as evidence for other unknown significant pruritogens in cholestasis.[138] Other extra-corporeal techniques for removing pruritogens have been suggested, including haemodialysis,[139] charcoal haemoperfusion,[140] plasmapheresis,[141] and albumin dialysis.[142]

Enzyme induction

Both rifampicin and phenobarbitone have been advocated in the management of cholestatic pruritis, although the mechanism of their action is unknown.[143,132] A trial in which both hepatic enzyme inducers were compared demonstrated that rifampicin was significantly more beneficial, and its effectiveness was suggested to relate to an additional inhibitory effect on bile acid uptake by the hepatocytes.[144] This in turn may minimize bile acid toxicity and release of other putative pruritogens. It has also been postulated that rifampicin may act as yet another opioid antagonist in situations of increased opioidergic tone.[145]

Antihistamines

There is no evidence in the pruritus of cholestasis, as opposed to allergic or other dermatological causes of pruritis that antihistamines are effective at relieving itch although their sedative actions may improve sleep.

Androgens

Reports from the 1950s and 1960s suggested the use of androgens in cholestatic pruritus, and their use has continued despite a lack of robust evidence of effectiveness. The method of action is unknown but a direct hepatotoxic effect has been postulated reducing production of endogenous opioids or other pruritogens.[100] One author, after a comprehensive review of the options for medical treatment of cholestatic pruritus, recommended androgens such as danozol or methyltestosterone as first-line therapy for patients on opioids.[100]

Non-pharmacological measures

The use of topical emollients on areas of pruritic dry skin and the maintenance of a cool and humid environment to lessen sweating may well be of help to many skin conditions that cause pruritus but their value in cholestatic pruritus is less clear. Most benefit may be obtained from keeping finger nails cut short and wearing cotton gloves at night to lessen damage to the skin through scratching.

One small pilot study, based on an observation of an apparent circadian rhythm to the scratching behaviour in cholestasis, has suggested a benefit of bright-light therapy directed towards the eyes.[99]

Summary

Cholestatic pruritus is a miserable symptom that intereferes significantly with the quality of life experienced particularly by those with chronic liver disease and end-stage malignancy. Despite over 50 years of research, the mechanism remains largely unknown. The most significant contributions rest with the finding of generalized increased opioidergic tone in animal models and clinical evidence of the benefit of opioid antagonists in symptom relief. Interest in the future lies in refining guidance for the use of low dose opioid antagonists or partial agonists and the optimum opioid analgesics to use alone or in combination with antagonists to minimize pruritus in cholestasis.

Ascites

The development of ascites as a complication of either chronic liver disease or malignancy not only heralds a poor prognosis in terms of survival but also can be associated with multiple distressing symptoms resulting from increased intra-abdominal pressure.

Cirrhosis is the precursor to ascites in approximately 75 per cent of individuals, malignancy is the main cause in 10 per cent, and cardiac failure and tuberculosis in 3 per cent and 2 per cent of individuals respectively.[146] Given the relatively high incidence of cirrhosis in the population, usually associated with either chronic alcoholic hepatitis or hepatitis C infection, there are several recently published and excellent reviews of the pathogenesis of associated ascites formation and its management to which the reader is directed.[147,148] The literature concerning malignant ascites is not as extensive or consensual and this form of ascites will become the focus for the ensuing section of the chapter.

Malignant ascites

A survey of Canadian physicians and their management of malignant ascites produced comments such as 'generally impossible to manage', 'it is a frustrating clinical situation', and 'a practical and effective solution is needed'.[149] The main frustrations in the management of ascites relate to questions such as the role of diuretic therapy, imaging, and the method of paracentesis, each of which remain poorly tested in formal trials. However, recent interest in the pathophysiology of ascites formation may lead to more individualized and novel methods of management.

Incidence/prevalence

Problems related to the presence of malignant ascites are present in 3.6–6 per cent of patients admitted to palliative care units.[150,151] Malignant ascites is most frequently associated with a primary diagnosis of ovarian carcinoma and less frequently with endometrial, breast, colonic, gastric, pancreatic, or unknown primary carcinoma.[152–154] The presence of ascites is usually an indicator of advanced disease and, unfortunately, is detectable at the time of initial diagnosis in over half of the patients in whom it develops.[155] Patients with ovarian cancer, however, do have a longer mean survival from the time of development of ascites compared with those with other malignancies.[154] This may relate to ascites being a complication of relatively early stage ovarian cancer and its relative sensitivity to cytotoxic chemotherapy. However, in one study of patients with stage III and IV disease receiving chemotherapy, the presence of ascites at the start of treatment reduced 5-year survival from 46 per cent to 5 per cent.[156] In another study of debulking surgery for patients with stage IV disease, the presence of ascites was the only independent predictive factor for early tumour progression.[157] Control of ascites often requires repeated inpatient episodes that, in one recent series of patients with ovarian cancer, showed a rapid increase in frequency over the last year of life to a median of seven admissions in the last 3 months.[158]

Symptoms

Symptoms requiring palliation relate to increased intra-abdominal pressure; discomfort of the abdominal wall, dyspnoea, anorexia, early satiety, nausea and vomiting, oesophageal reflux, poor mobility, insomnia related to general discomfort, pain in the groins and subcostal regions, and lower limb oedema. Abdominal Compartment

Syndrome with resultant multisystem failure has also been recently reported.[159] Easily overlooked can be the significant negative effect of abdominal distension on body image.

Pathophysiology

Ascites formation in cirrhosis occurs predominantly as a result of a cascade of events including portal hypertension and consequent splanchnic vasodilatation that results in both sodium and fluid retention and an increase in intestinal capillary pressure and permeability.[147] In contrast, it is tumour invasion of the visceral or parietal peritoneum that is the major cause of ascites in individuals with malignancy (50 per cent of cases). In 15 per cent of individuals with malignancy, ascites results from hepatic infiltration and portal venous compression, in 15 per cent it results from a combination of portal vein compression and peritoneal spread, and in 20 per cent ascites is chylous occurring after lymphatic invasion.[146]

The accumulation of ascites is a result of an imbalance in the normal state of influx and efflux of fluid from the peritoneal cavity. The absorption of radio-labelled serum albumin after intra-peritoneal injection has been measured in humans to be 4–5 ml/h.[160] Drainage of peritoneal fluid occurs via the lymphatic system with the open-ended diaphragmatic lymphatics probably providing the major pathway.

A decreased rate of fluid efflux may occur as a result of blockage of the lymphatic system by tumour and this has been shown histologically in association with malignant ascites in animal models.[161] In human subjects, one study demonstrated that 32 of 38 patients with malignant ascites showed no lymphatic absorption of radiolabelled sulphur colloid that had been injected into the peritoneum.[162] Conversely, 13 of 14 control subjects with either no ascites or non-malignant ascites did demonstrate lymphatic uptake of the colloid.

It is unlikely that a reduced rate of fluid efflux alone is sufficient to cause the accumulation of massive amounts of ascitic fluid. Indeed, the rate of efflux has been shown to increase as ascites accumulates and intra-abdominal pressure increases, possibly up to rates approaching 80 ml/h.[163]

The rate of fluid influx into the peritoneal space may be increased in malignancy as a result of two distinct mechanisms. Each mechanism will result in ascitic fluid of different biochemical properties and may respond to different modes of treatment.

1 Increased hepatic venous pressure, as an anatomical consequence of multiple hepatic metastases, or single large (sometimes benign) tumours causing a Budd–Chiari syndrome.[164] An increase in venous pressure results in both fluid leakage into the peritoneum from the sinusoids and, via an increase in plasma renin concentration, to the retention of salt and water by the kidneys. The ascitic fluid resulting from this mechanism is similar to that seen as a result of cirrhosis and has the properties of a transudate.

2 An exudate, of relatively high protein concentration, may be produced as a result of increased vascular permeability. Tumour neovasculature is thought to be intrinsically leaky, allowing extravasation of fluid, and from peritoneal tumour deposits would contribute to ascites formation. However, it has long been recognized that ascitic fluid also arises from areas of peritoneum unaffected by tumour.[163] Beecham and colleagues

observed marked neovascularization of the parietal peritoneum in patients with malignant ascites and ovarian carcinoma.[165]

In rats, there appears to be an increase in permeability of peritoneal capillaries after cell-free malignant ascitic fluid is infused intraperitoneally.[155] The permeability of normal microvessels, such as those that line the peritoneal cavity, can be increased by a variety of cytokines including transforming growth factors-α and -β, epidermal growth factor, and vascular endothelial growth factor (VEGF).[166] Cytokines may be secreted by tumour cells or inflammatory monocytes and macrophages.

VEGF is expressed by the normal ovary during phases of follicular development and copora lutea formation[167] and, in one series, the degree of tumour expression was related to patient survival.[168] VEGF not only increases capillary permeability but also stimulates angiogenesis, facilitating tumour growth and also, potentially, the observed neovascularization of normal peritoneum. Animal experiments have demonstrated a significant relationship between the degree of tumour cell expression of VEGF and observed levels of angiogenesis and ascites production.[169,170] VEGF has been detected in high concentrations in malignant as opposed to non-malignant ascites and associated with metastases from a variety of primary sites.[171–173] The exception has been the observation of high levels of VEGF in ovarian hyperstimulation syndrome, also associated with ascites formation.[174] The potential for therapeutic interventions that target the production or actions of VEGF will be discussed below.

In an individual patient, the relative contribution of the two principal mechanisms described of ascitic fluid production can be estimated from the calculation of the serum-ascites albumin gradient. The serum-ascites gradient is calculated by subtracting the albumin concentration of the ascitic fluid from that within a serum specimen obtained on the same day. The gradient correlates with the portal venous pressure and a value of ≥ 11 g/l is indicative of a transudate and the presence of portal hypertension.[175] This may be of importance in assessing the likelihood of response to diuretic therapy with an aldosterone antagonist.

The formation of chylous ascites is a complication of retroperitoneal tumour spread or its treatment and arises either from damage to lymphatic vessels or through obstruction of lymphatic flow through lymph nodes or the pancreas.

Diagnosis

The diagnosis of the presence of ascites in an individual is usually straight forward relying on relevant clinical history and examination.[176] Where there is doubt, usually with typical symptoms present in a patient with an obese abdomen or with potential bowel obstruction, ultrasound examination can detect as little as 100 ml of free fluid in the peritoneum.[177] CT is equally as accurate but not always as easily available as ultrasound. Plain abdominal X-rays may be helpful not only in excluding signs suggestive of bowel obstruction but also in demonstrating positive signs of ascites such as a 'ground glass' appearance, loss of psoas shadows and organ definition, and increased spacing of intestinal loops.

Clearly, the presence of ascites in a patient with known malignancy cannot always be assumed to be secondary to the presence of intra-abdominal tumour and other causes, such as cirrhosis, congestive heart failure, nephrotic syndrome, tuberculosis, and pancreatitis, which necessitate specific modalities of treatment, must be excluded.

Several tests have been proposed to differentiate malignant from other forms of ascites such as fluid levels of sialic acid,[178] telomerase,[179] β-HCG,[180] fibronectin,[181] or, in one study, a combination of total protein, lactate dehydrogenase, Tumour necrosis factor-α, C4, and haptoglobin.[182] Such diagnostic tests may, of course, be helpful in terms of prognosis and possibly decisions regarding anti-tumour therapy but not as an aid to decisions about other forms of palliative treatment.

Management

The palliation of all symptoms related to malignant disease follows the same broad principles of totally individualized care based on the best evidence available from larger populations. Guidelines and treatment algorithms for management of problems such as ascites have been developed and are helpful,[166,183,184] but the temptation is to manipulate every patient into particular protocols or guidelines and lose sight of the individual risk-benefit analyses for certain management plans. Furthermore, the evidence underlying common approaches is weak at best. A recent systematic review of the management of malignant ascites detected 32 studies, of which none were randomized trials and 26 were non-analytical studies such as case series.[185]

Anti-tumour therapy

For the relief of symptoms resulting from complications, such as ascites, which reflect tumour activity, specific anti-tumour therapy should always be considered particularly for patients with ovarian or breast carcinoma. The development of ascites often complicates ovarian carcinoma relatively early in the course of the disease and is, in fact, a presenting feature in a third of all cases.[186] Malik et al.[153] demonstrated complete clearance or significant reduction of ascites in 46 per cent of patients with ovarian cancer treated with systemic cytotoxic chemotherapy. Significant response in ovarian cancer can be observed with second and even third-line chemotherapy, and so should always be considered.

Cytotoxic agents have been given intraperitoneally from as early as the 1950s.[187] There has been a resurgence of interest with the development of a hyperthermic intraperitoneal technique that appears to allow greater tissue penetration and lowers levels of drug resistance.[188] This technique has been particularly used in combination with aggressive cytoreductive surgery.[189,190]

Chylous ascites, when associated with retroperitoneal lymphoma and a consequent disruption of normal lymphatic drainage pathways, may be expected to show some response to chemotherapy if it be first or second-line treatment. Radiotherapy may also have a role in the relief of symptoms of lymphoma.

The success of the intracavitary instillation of a variety of agents in the control of malignant pleural effusions has encouraged a similar approach to the treatment of malignant ascites. There have been numerous small trials and case series reporting the use of radioisotopes, cytotoxics, and more recently, biological agents and response modifiers to reduce ascitic fluid formation (Table 10.2.5.5). A recently reported phase II study found that intraperitoneal instillation of the corticosteroid triamcinolone hexacetonide resulted in a significant slowing of ascites accumulation.[191] The effect was noted particularly in patients with an albumin serum-ascites gradient of < 11g/l. The authors postulated the effect to have been mediated through a steroid-induced reduction of the secretion of VEGF.

Other approaches

Initial pre-clinical trials with anti-VEGF antibodies, anti-VEGF receptor antibodies, and an inhibitor of VEGF receptor tyrosine kinase activity[192] have been reported to show a reduction in ascites formation in animal models. Transfection of a mutated gene controlling production of VEGF has decreased ascites production in mice.[193] Tumour necrosis factor has been found to block reaccumulation of ascites in an animal model by inhibiting the expression of VEGF mRNA[194] and an early clinical study suggested benefit from the administration of recombinant TNFα.[195] Interestingly, a recent report of the use of the anti-TNF agent infliximab showed a reduction in levels of VEGF and angiogenesis in the synovia of patients with psoriatic arthritis.[196] VEGF expression and associated angiogenesis has also been shown to be reduced by ketoprofen,[197] green tea,[198] and angiotensin-converting enzyme inhibitors.[199]

Matrix metalloproteinases are a group of enzymes that, after loss of normal inhibitory control during tumour development, potentiate tumour invasion and metastases. Early clinical trials of metalloproteinase inhibitors have been reported to have benefit.[200]

Octreotide, the somatostatin analogue, has been suggested to have therapeutic potential for a myriad of different disorders and indeed, there has been a small case series demonstrating a reduction in malignant ascites in two of three patients treated.[201] The physiological mechanism remains unclear, although one other report does suggest a benefit to patients with hepatic cirrhosis and ascites.[202] A recent small case series reports the successful control of chylous ascites with the combination of octreotide and a fat-free diet.[203]

Diuretic therapy

Diuretic therapy remains the mainstay of the treatment of patients with ascites of non-malignant origin but the role of diuretics in the management of malignant ascites remains controversial. A recent Canadian survey of the management of malignant ascites reported that whilst 98 per cent of physicians used paracentesis only 61 per cent prescribed diuretics and of these one-quarter felt them to be ineffective.[149] The rates of response to diuretics in reported studies range from 38 per cent[204] to 86 per cent.[205] Theoretically, it would be expected that those patients who demonstrate raised plasma renin activity and hence increased sodium

Table 10.2.5.5 Agents reported to have been employed for intraperitoneal instillation in the management of peritoneal malignancy and ascites.

Thiotepa	^{198}Au
Fluorouracil	^{32}CrPO$_4$
Mustine	Interferon-α
Bleomycin	Interferon-β
Cisplatinum	Tumour necrosis factor
Carboplatin	Interleukin-2
Etoposide	Radiolabelled monoclonal antibodies
Mitomycin C	Metalloproteinase inhibitors
Adriamycin	Corticosteroids
Docetaxel	*Corynebacterium parvum*
Mitoxantrone	OK-432 (extract from *S. pyogene*)

and water retention would have a greater likelihood of response to diuretics. These patients are those who tend to demonstrate a serum-ascites albumin gradient of ≥11 g/l, where ascites is formed exclusively or principally as a result of intrahepatic metastases. A small study of the use of diuretics in patients with ascites and either massive hepatic metastases, 'peritoneal carcinomatosis' or chylous ascites only demonstrated a reduction in estimated ascitic volume in the group with hepatic metastases.[206] Each of the three patients in the group with hepatic metastases all had raised plasma renin levels, a high serum-ascites albumin gradient, and responded to the aldosterone antagonist, spironolactone. In another small series, 13 of 15 patients with malignant ascites responded to spironolactone therapy.[205] Plasma renin levels were measured in only five patients but were raised in each case. There is a significant body of evidence relating to the optimum use of diuretics in ascites secondary to cirrhosis, where 90 per cent of patients would be expected to respond to treatment.[175] The majority of trials report the use of spironolactone, but given the long half-life of the parent drug and its active metabolites, there is often a delay of up to 2 weeks before the onset of a significant diuresis. The alternative potassium-sparing diuretic, amiloride, has a much faster onset of action. Although amiloride is not a classical mineralocorticoid receptor antagonist, it appears to interfere with aldosterone effects in model systems.[207] Interestingly, both amiloride and spironolactone interfere with the effect of aldosterone on endothelial cells. Amiloride with a faster onset of action may be a more appropriate choice for patients with relatively short prognoses or in whom early prevention of reaccumulation of ascites after paracentesis is desired. The use of a loading dose of spironolactone has not been reported and the usual regime comprises a starting dose of 100 mg as a single daily dose increasing at 2–3 day intervals to 400 mg if needed and tolerated. Regular girth measurement may be a more appropriate method of monitoring response to treatment than daily weights and accurate fluid balance recordings. The response to diuretics is thought to occur, in part, as a result of a redistribution of fluid within body compartments rather than being wholly dependent on a diuresis.[208] The addition of a loop diuretic may improve the speed of response with one study reporting a rapid initial response to the use of an intravenous infusion of furosemide during the accumulation period of spironolactone therapy.[209]

The initiation of spironolactone therapy is not infrequently associated with nausea unrelated to electrolyte imbalance. The most debilitating side effects however relate to intravascular volume depletion and include postural hypotension, uraemia, and, in some cases, renal failure. A proportion of patients will have a concurrent paraneoplastic autonomic neuropathy and resultant postural hypotension[210] that will be augmented by aggressive diuretic therapy. Hepatic encephalopathy is an additional potential complication of aggressive diuresis in patients with limited residual hepatic function. It is important to monitor the response to diuretics and titrate the dose to a maintenance level to lessen the chance of side effects.

Paracentesis

Abdominal paracentesis remains the most commonly employed modality of treatment for malignant ascites.[149] It affords quick symptomatic relief in a population that often has a relatively short prognosis and for whom diuretic therapy, if effective, may include a significant lag period and be associated with postural hypotension.

The reported techniques and equipment used for the procedure are numerous and particularly amongst palliative care physicians appear to allow full expression of their creativity. The most significant differences in approach relate to the cannula or catheter used for puncturing the peritoneum, the rate of ascitic fluid drainage, and the necessity or not of maintenance of intravascular volume with albumin, colloid, or crystalloid infusions.

The large experience of the potential problems associated with paracentesis in patients with hepatic cirrhosis, particularly hypotension and renal impairment, has coloured the approach of many to the procedure in malignant ascites. It is likely that, in the absence of a serum-ascites gradient of of ≥11 g/l, these complications of paracentesis are rare in patients with malignant ascites and fluid maybe drained off relatively rapidly with no need to routinely administer intravenous colloid or albumin.[211] Indeed, the use of vacuum bottles allowing several litres to be removed in a matter of minutes, with apparently few complications, has been reported to be particularly useful in the outpatient clinic or even the patient's home.[212]

A study of 35 patients with ascites and ovarian cancer demonstrated a direct correlation between the measured value of intraperitoneal pressure and the severity of symptoms reported.[213] Another recent study helps to confirm that raised intra-abdominal pressure and related symptoms can be significantly relieved after drainage of just a 'few litres' over 2 h.[214] The group of patients reported had a mean of 5.3 l drained over 24 h but no significant improvement in symptom relief (of those assessed) after 24 h than that noted after only 2 h of drainage. Indeed only dyspnoea (and not discomfort, nausea, or vomiting) was improved significantly more at 72 h than at 2 h of ascitic drainage. It would be of interest if perception of body image had been factored into these studies.

Since symptoms can often be relieved by the removal of relatively small volumes of ascites over a short time period, this is to be recommended particularly in the very frail with a limited prognosis. One to two litres of fluid can be removed simply over 30 min via a plastic intra-venous cannula. The insertion of the cannula is simple and if used in conjunction with local infiltration of local anaesthetic is a relatively comfortable procedure. The removal of such a modest volume is unlikely to cause symptomatic hypovolaemia and the use of a small cannula for a short time is highly unlikely to cause local complications.

Clearly, however, ascites is likely to reaccumulate and should a prognosis be more than a few days, then frequent recurrent small volume paracenteses will be required. Two case series and two case reports suggest that this can be achieved by a permanent indwelling catheter that allows frequent small volume drainage without the risks of large volume fluid shifts and repeated peritoneal puncture.[215–218] However, most clinicians in this situation would give consideration to the less frequent drainage of larger volumes of ascites through some form of temporary catheter. Peritoneal dialysis, suprapubic urinary bladder, and self-retaining nephrostomy catheters have all been described as useful drainage devices.

Stephenson and Gilbert reported the successful introduction of guidelines for paracentesis into an oncology unit that resulted in reductions in the use of ultrasound to mark sites for drainage, the mean duration of drainage, and length of inpatient stay.[219] Catheters were left in for no more than 6 h with up to 5 l being drained and intravenous fluids only considered if patients were hypotensive, dehydrated, or known to have severe renal impairment. Patients without peripheral oedema may be particularly prone to hypovolaemia. It is prudent to monitor blood pressure during the procedure with intravascular volume replenished by intravenous infusion of either colloid or plasma protein solution should hypotension develop. A low threshold for the administration of intravenous fluid should be present for patients with high serum-ascitic albumin gradient who do not respond to diuretics and are treated by paracentesis.

After withdrawal of the drain, there is a tendency for a continued leakage of fluid from the drain site. This can be lessened by the use of a 'Z-technique' when introducing the catheter through the skin and then the peritoneal wall. Some operators tie a purse string suture around the site, others place a stoma bag over the site until leakage stops and one group have suggested the application of enbucrilate adhesive to seal the skin.[220]

Complications of paracentesis relate mainly to the potential for a relatively rapid shift of fluid between body compartments. One study reported two deaths from hypotension in a series of 109 consecutive paracenteses performed on 43 patients.[221] More likely, in malignant ascites, are procedural complications including bowel perforation, peritonitis, and localized cellulitis surrounding the drain site. One study reported two deaths from peritonitis in a series of 127 paracenteses in 100 patients.[160] Infection was a particular problem in a reported case series of patients with permanent implanted drains.[216] A recent series of 10 patients treated with tunnelled Pleurx® (Denver Biomedical, Denver, Colorado) catheters (soft 16F elastic catheter with a one-way valve originally developed for the drainage of pleural effusions see Fig. 10.2.5.2) recorded no catheter-related infections with a mean catheter survival of 70 days.[222] In this series, serial serum albumin measurements demonstrated a progressive decline. However, one

case report of the use of an implanted peritoneal dialysis catheter reported only one superficial infection in 17 months during which time the patient drained 1000–1500 ml of ascites twice a week and, interestingly, maintained serum albumin levels.[217] A similar recent report described a patient with a tunnelled Pleurx® catheter, who drained 2000 ml per day for 18 months.[203] However, anecdotal experience would suggest that many patients feel extremely tired for several days following paracentesis and both hyponatraemia and a progressive fall in plasma albumin concentration with repeated paracenteses has been recorded in some series. Patients with severely compromised hepatic function are at particular risk of hepatic failure and encephalopathy over the first 24 h after ascitic drainage.

Peritoneovenous shunting

Potential problems of repeated paracentesis such as intravascular hypovolaemia, hypoalbuminaemia, infection and visceral damage, and the expense, discomfort, and inconvenience of repeated hospital admissions have prompted the development of alternative drainage procedures. Peritoneovenous shunting was established in the mid-1970s[223] and remains the most common procedure performed. Shunting of ascitic fluid into the stomach[224] and urinary bladder[225] have also been reported but have presented too many technical difficulties to be useful at present. There have, however, been no randomized-controlled trials to date comparing peritoneovenous shunting with repeated abdominal paracentesis.

Two forms of shunt are commonly used, the original Le Veen and the Denver shunt. Both are designed to allow drainage of ascites into the central venous system, usually via the internal jugular or femoral veins. They may be placed surgically, laparoscopically, or percutaneously with a recent study reporting no difference in performance or complication rate on direct comparison of these methods.[226] The most common reason for shunt failure is lumen occlusion, which appears to occur more frequently during drainage of malignant ascites than cirrhotic ascites (for the control of which these shunts were first described). The Denver shunt has the theoretical advantage of a manual pumping mechanism to facilitate ascitic flow and clearance of debris. However, no statistical difference in the performance of the two shunts could be found in one comparative study.[227]

Successful resolution of ascites and symptom relief with the use of peritoneovenous shunts has been reported in between 62 and 87 per cent of patients.[204,228–231] One non-controlled study showed, in addition, a maintenace of serum albumin levels in comparison to a progressive decrease in patients treated with repeated paracentesis.[204] This same study measured 'quality of life' by a single question and VAS scale and found a non-significant trend to an improvement with either paracenteses or shunts and no difference between the two methods of drainage. In the previously quoted survey of physicians' practice, only 12 of 44 respondents had used peritoneovenous shunts and 7 found them to be useful.[149] The apparent reluctance to use this method is probably a result of the significant complication rate of both the operative procedure and the ongoing operation of the shunt. There is a significant operative mortality in patients with malignant ascites quoted as 13 per cent in one of the larger studies,[228] although this is less than that associated with the procedure for ascites associated with cirrhosis. Whilst this high mortality rate is in part to be expected in a frail population

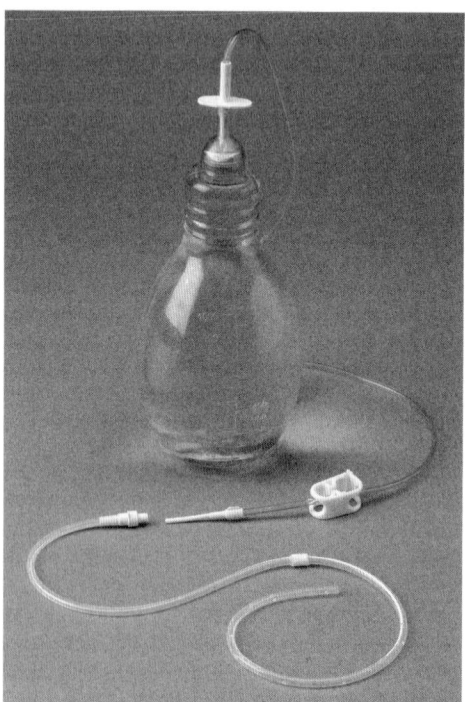

Figure 10.2.5.2 'Pleurx© ascitic drainage system of indwelling catheter and drainage bottle.'

undergoing a general anaesthetic or even local anaesthetic and sedation, specific procedure-related mortality is more commonly a result of pulmonary oedema. This complication of a sudden increase in fluid volume within the central venous system can be avoided, in part, by removing a proportion of the ascites (50–70 per cent quoted in one study[232]) at operation to reduce pressure and hence flow through the shunt. Many centres would still advocate 'intensive' monitoring with central venous pressure lines for the first 24 h after surgery.

Overall, complication rates of peritineovenous shunts of between 25 per cent and 50 per cent are reported.[204,228,229] The most common complication is shunt occlusion, either, more commonly, from thrombosis of the venous terminal or alternatively from debris in the peritoneal end. Two studies reported alterations in laboratory measurements of coagulation parameters (increased concentration of fibrinogen degradation products) consistent with subclinical disseminated intervascular coagulation (DIC) in all patients with patent shunts.[233,227] Indeed, while such findings may be used as surrogate evidence of shunt patency, frank DIC remains a rare complication. The incidence of DIC is greater in patients with shunts and cirrhotic ascites possibly as a result of a higher concentration of plasminogen-activator-inhibitor in malignant ascites with consequently less potential for fibrinolyitic activity.[234] The incidence of postoperative DIC can be reduced by removal of a significant proportion of the ascitic volume intra-operatively.[233] Other complications include thromboembolism, vena caval thrombosis, hepatic encephalopathy, peritonitis, and tumour seeding to the subcutaneous tissues of the anterior abdominal wall.

The potential effects of the introduction of tumour cells from the peritoneal cavity into the circulation via the shunt has been examined in a small series of post-mortem examinations.[235] The study reported a variety of observations but concluded that metastases, although occurring in some patients as a direct result of shunt placement, are not clinically significant and do not alter prognosis. This is likely to be related to the short prognosis of the majority of patients who develop malignant ascites.

Peritoneovenous shunts are clearly unsuitable for patients with loculated ascites and are not advised if the ascites is haemorrhagic or chylous or the patient has poor cardiac or renal function or a tendency to hepatic encephalopathy. Patients with elevated bilirubin levels have an increased risk of intravascular coagulation with shunting.[236] Portal hypertension, massive pleural effusion, and coagulation disorders are relative contraindications.[237,238] The presence of malignant cells in ascitic fluid, if no anti-tumour treatment is to be given, correlates with a poor prognosis (median survival of 26 days compared with 140 days if cytology is negative) and is thus also a relative contraindication.[239] A recently reported series of patients with ascites and non-gynaecological primary tumours showed the best outcomes of peritoneovenous shunts to occur in patients with normal renal function and tumours of non-gastrointestinal primary origin.[240] The relatively long survival of patients with ascites and gynaecological malignancies and the potential savings in terms of repeated hospitalizations for paracentesis makes peritoneovenous shunting an option to be considered in all cases.

Transjugular intrahepatic portosystemic shunts (TIPS)

The creation of an artificial porto-systemic shunt is a well established technique for the relief of complications of portal hypertension and

has been proposed as an option for the management of ascites refractory to diuretics and dietary sodium restriction. A recent Cochrane systematic review concluded that TIPS placement cleared ascites more effectively than repeat paracenteses with no difference in side effects between the approaches other than an increased risk of encephalopathy after TIPS.[241] If the resources are available then TIPS could be considered for the relatively few cases of ascites resulting from portal hypertension associated with malignancy.

Summary

The burden of ascites as a complication of malignancy remains highly significant particularly for the individual patient but also in terms of the health care resources consumed in clinical management. Despite numerous small studies of the intraperitoneal administration of various cytotoxic agents, radioisotopes, and immune/biological response modifiers, management continues to rely upon the use of diuretics, abdominal paracentesis, and peritoneovenous shunts. There is increasing interest in the use of 'long-term' indwelling drainage catheters including peritoneal dialysis and Pleurx® catheters. The use of these devices along with relatively large volume vacuum bottles is likely to become more widespread in the community to alleviate the need for repeated hospital attendance.

However, it is from recent studies into the pathophysiology of ascites production in intra-abdominal malignancy that new and specific ways to slow or halt ascitic fluid production are likely to emerge. In particular, the present interest in the role of VEGF in tumour angiogenesis along with the realization of the role of peritoneal neovascularization in ascites production has highlighted a possible new, specific target for therapy. One would hope, given the high frequency of occurrence of this complication of malignancy, that there would be good levels of recruitment to large, multi-centre trials. However, surprisingly, such trials have not been a feature of research into ascites management to date.

Hepatic encephalopathy

Hepatic encephalopathy manifests as a complex neuropsychiatric disturbance often developing as a consequence of progressive liver disease with cirrhosis. It may occur as an often fatal complication of acute liver failure associated with acute cerebral oedema or may also result from portosystemic bypass with no intrinsic hepatocellular disease. An international working party has recently proposed a nomenclature that defines hepatic encephalopathy with respect both to the underlying hepatic abnormality and the associated duration and characteristics of neurological signs and symptoms[242]. Encephalopathy can, relatively rarely, accompany liver failure occurring as a result of massive infiltration by metastatic tumour, but the prognosis in such cases is usually very bleak and measured in days.[243] Individuals with HCC in a recent study from Hong Kong had a median survival of one month following the first presentation with encephalopathy.[244]

Abnormal cognitive and motor function and psychiatric disorders are characteristic of hepatic encephalopathy with severity varying from mild abnormalities detected only by formal psychometric testing to deep coma. Encephalopathy is a sign of decompensation in cirrhosis, related to the development of significant portosystemic venous shunting, and the first episode is associated with a subsequent estimated 1-year survival of 42 per cent and a 3-year survival of 23 per cent.[245] Within this group, individuals with raised serum bilirubin, alkaline phosphatase, potassium, urea nitrogen, and reduced albumin and prothrombin activity have a significantly worse prognosis. The survival of all individuals with chronic liver disease after their first episode of acute encephalopathy is less than that associated with liver transplant and this procedure should therefore always be considered at this stage in the disease process.

Most authors would concur that raised blood ammonia levels are the most significant contributor to the development of encephalopathy and can be found in over 90 per cent of individuals with the clinical signs of the disorder. Two recent studies have demonstrated a correlation between blood levels (arterial and venous) of ammonia and severity of encephalopathy.[246,247] However, other studies have not demonstrated such a correlation and it is likely there are other variable factors and pathways involved in the pathogenesis of encephalopathy with hyperammonaemia as the principal predisposing factor. Ammonia is generated in the small intestine by the action of glutaminase on glutamine and in the colon by the activity of bacterial urease. Individuals with normal liver function will metabolize over 90 per cent of the ammonia in the portal system.[248] Raised ammonia levels in the systemic circulation are thought to come principally from portosystemic bypass of hepatic metabolic processing or from a reduction in processing capacity in liver failure. An intestinal protein load either from the diet or, for example, from oesophageal variceal haemorrhage will significantly increase ammonia levels and produce overt encephalopathy.

The importance of ammonia in the pathogenesis of encephalopathy has long been recognized but there is continuing debate as to the biochemical pathways involved. Ammonia readily passes through the blood–brain barrier and can be detoxified, in astrocytes, by scavenging processes producing glutamine from glutamate. Increased cerebral metabolism of ammonia has been demonstrated by PET in individuals with hepatic encephalopathy.[249] Interference with GABA-ergic and glutamatergic neurotransmission systems has been proposed as the most likely factor in the precipitation of encephalopathy by increased cerebral ammonia levels. Enhanced GABA-A receptor activity that is only, at best, partially reversed by a benzodiazepine antagonist such as flumazenil is emerging as a likely major pathway in the generation of hepatic encephalopathy. The increased production, or penetration through an altered blood brain-barrier, of GABA-A agonist ligands has been proposed. These ligands are distinct from endogenous benzodiazepine-like compounds and probably mainly comprising endogenous steroids such as pregnenolone and particularly its metabolite allopregnanolone.[250]

The cerebral effects of hyperammonaemia have been most studied but intestinal bacteria produce other potential central neurotoxins such as benzodiazepine-like compounds, mercaptans, phenols, and short- and medium-chain fatty acids, all of which have been found in relatively high levels in individuals with chronic liver disease.[251]

Elevated serum levels of manganese have also been detected in individuals with cirrhosis and encephalopathy and autopsy specimens have demonstrated increased deposition of manganese within the basal ganglia.[252] It has been postulated that the deposition of manganese, a known neurotoxin, may cause, either directly or via effects on dopamine receptors, the extra-pyramidal signs and symptoms noted in some individuals with encephalopathy.

Table 10.2.5.6 Common precipitating factors of hepatic encephalopathy.

- Infection
- Drugs (benzodiazepines, opioids, alcohol, and other sedatives)
- Gastrointestinal bleeding
- Excessive dietary protein
- Constipation
- Dehydration
- Uraemia
- Hypokalaemia
- Hypoglycaemia
- Anaemia
- Hypoxia

Manganese may also act synergistically with ammonia to increase the activity of GABA-ergic neurotransmission.[253]

Episodes of acute hepatic encephalopathy in chronic liver disease can be precipitated by a variety of factors most frequently infection, alcohol or other sedative drugs, gastrointestinal haemorrhage, electrolyte disturbance, dehydration, and constipation (Table 10.2.5.6). Infection can precipitate delirium in any individual but those with chronic liver disease seem particularly susceptible. It has been postulated that inflammatory cytokines produced in response to infection may affect the central nervous system at several different levels and working synergistically with pre-existing hyperammonaemia precipitate frank encephalopathy. Interleukins 1 and 6 and tumour necrosis factor-α have been particularly implicated.[254] Another theory suggests that the reduced cerebral blood flow associated with bacteraemia may augment the existing reduced cerebral flow associated with chronic liver disease.[254]

Diagnosis

The diagnosis of hepatic encephalopathy could be thought of as one of exclusion given the many possible causes of delirium associated with abnormal neurological signs. Other metabolic disorders, infection, cerebrovascular events, and intracranial space-occupying lesions may all present in a similar fashion. However, in individuals with known liver disease, the existence of a precipitating factor, or a prior history of hepatic encephalopathy, the diagnosis can usually be safely made. The presence of asterixis ('liver flap'), fetor hepaticus and extra pyramidal signs help strengthen the diagnosis but are not always present. Elevated blood ammonia levels may confirm the degree of underlying liver disease and susceptibility to encephalopathy.

Other objective diagnostic methods have been described including the measurement of visual and auditory evoked potentials,[255] electroencephalography, and more recently, actigraphy.[256] Whilst EEG recording has the most sensitivity, it is not specific and relatively inaccessible. An International Working Party of hepatologists has recommended the use of the West Haven criteria (see Table 10.2.5.7) and Glasgow Coma scales for grading and monitoring established encephalopathy.[242]

Table 10.2.5.7 West Haven Criteria of altered mental state in hepatic encephalopathy.

Stage 0	Lack of detectable changes in personality or behaviour
	Impairment noted only on formal psychomotor testing
	Asterixis absent
Stage 1	Mild lack of awareness
	Shortened attention span
	Altered sleep pattern
	Mild asterixis or tremor
Stage 2	Lethargy
	Disorientation
	Inappropriate behaviour
	Slurred speech
	Obvious asterixis
Stage 3	Somnolent but rousable
	Gross disorientation
	Bizarre behaviour
	Asterixis generally absent
	Increased muscle tone and hyperreflexia
Stage 4	Coma
	Decerebrate posturing

An estimated 50–80 per cent of individuals with cirrhosis will have subclinical or minimal encephalopathy, demonstrated only by altered formal psychometric testing, but who are at increased risk of acute episodes of frank encephalopathy.[242] Identification of individuals with this condition is important as the associated impaired daily functioning and disturbed sleep patterns, in addition to the potential progression to overt encephalopathy, are potentially reversible.[257,258] Whilst electroencephalography is the most accurate method of detecting encephalopathy, psychometric testing has been recommended by the International Working Party as a reliable method of detecting and monitoring minimal encephalopathy. The group recommended the use of at least two instruments of the following short list; the number connection tests-A or B, block design test, and digit symbol test.[242] The number connection tests are modified forms of the Trail Making Test, introduced in the 1950s and tests visual conceptual and visuo-motor tracking abilities. The tests involve drawing a line to link printed numbers (and letters in test B), in the correct order, as quickly as possible.[259] The block design test assesses visuo-spatial motor function and involves the assembly of small cubes to a given drawn design.[259] The digit symbol test is a subset of an adult intelligence test assessing motor speed and accuracy. Individuals have to correctly match numbers with shapes, as quickly as possible, on a test paper with the aid of a key.[260]

Treatment

The approach to the individual with encephalopathy will be similar to that taken with any individual with delirium. The environment and approach taken by care staff is particularly important for individuals likely to be disorientated and at risk of falls. The family and other lay carers are likely to need particular support and should be included in care procedures wherever possible.

Precipitating factors of encephalopathy in chronic liver disease have been well described (Table 10.2.5.7) and treatment must firstly be directed at such factors. A careful history should be taken with the checklist of possible precipitants in mind. Particular note should be made of symptoms suggestive of an infection or upper gastrointestinal haemorrhage and a review of recent psychotropic drug use, prescribed and otherwise.

It is generally agreed that bacterial production of ammonia and possibly other, as yet undefined, neurotoxins within the intestine is key to the pathogenesis of hepatic encephalopathy. Most proposed therapeutic options are therefore directed towards a reduction in ammonia production or increased clearance. Most interest has been shown in dietary factors, non-absorbable disaccharides, broad spectrum antibiotics, and central neurotransmitter manipulation.

Diet

A high protein diet can increase ammonia production and precipitate encephalopathy and in the acute stages restriction of dietary protein intake is usually suggested. However, one often-quoted study has shown no significant difference in outcome with individuals with cirrhosis presenting with acute encephalopathy randomized to receive either a normal or low protein diet.[260] Furthermore, in the longer term, protein restriction can aggravate encephalopathy, and in the setting of an increased catabolic rate often present in chronic liver disease lead to a reduced skeletal muscle mass with a consequent reduced ability to detoxify ammonia.[260] It has been suggested that a diet containing 1–1.5 g/kg/day of mainly vegetable protein is optimal.[261]

Disaccharides

The cornerstone of the medical management of encephalopathy has, for many years, been the use of non-absorbable disaccharides, such as lactulose. Lactulose is not broken down by intestinal enzymes and so reaches the colon where the sugar is metabolized by bacteria to acetic and lactic acid. Intestinal bacteria will preferentially take up carbohydrate over protein and lactulose or other carbohydrate in the diet will potentially, therefore, reduce ammonia production. Acidification of the intestinal contents converts ammonia to non-diffusable ammonium and helps catharsis and excretion of potential toxins.[203,262] Acidification of the intestinal contents may aid a change in microbial population away from urease-producing bacteria to acidophilic non-urese producing organisms. Protocols usually suggest titration of lactulose dosing to produce two or three soft stools per day. Lactulose can produce nausea, bloating, abdominal cramps, and in cases of excessive diarrhoea, dehydration and hypernatraemia, which can exacerbate encephalopathy. Despite the regular use of lactulose or other disaccharides in hepatic encephalopathy for many years, a recent Cochrane systematic review found only modest benefit overall and no significant benefit when only high quality trials were included in the analysis.[263] The authors concluded there was insufficient evidence to support or refute the use of disaccharides in encephalopathy. A secondary conclusion suggested that in head to head trials, antibiotics were superior to disaccharides in terms of improved symptoms and lowered ammonia levels.

Antibiotics

The use of antibiotics to reduce numbers of urease-producing bacteria in the intestine has also been employed for many years. The use of neomycin, metronidazole, ampicillin, and more recently, rifaximin have been described.[264] The evidence for the use of neomycin and metronidazole is modest and there is concern over the prolonged use of these agents because of the risks of renal and ototoxicity with neomycin and peripheral neuropathy and Antabuse-like reactions with metronidazole. Rifaximin is a broad spectrum, poorly absorbed antibiotic with a tolerability comparable to placebo.[265] Several trials have demonstrated its efficacy in relieving symptoms of encephalopathy, reducing blood ammonia levels and improving EEG abnormalities.[264] One recent study demonstrated lower serum levels of ammonia, benzodiazepine-like substances (thought to be bacterial products and potential cofactors in the pathogenesis of encephalopathy), and endotoxin in individuals treated with rifaximin.[266] Interestingly, this same study demonstrated that clinical improvement and low serum levels of potential toxins could be maintained by sequential administration of rifaximin followed by a probiotic mixture of lactobacilli and bifidobacter. Early studies of large quantities of orally administered lactobacilli to alter colonic flora in individuals with encephalopathy did not show a significant benefit. However, one later study with a non-urease-producing enterococcus did produce a reduction in blood ammonia and an improvement in performance in number connection tests to match that obtained with lactulose.[267]

Neurotransmitters

The use of the benzodiazepine antagonist flumazenil has been proposed in the management of encephalopathy. Although endogenous or bacterial benzodiazepine-like substances are thought to be involved in the pathogenesis of encephalopathy, studies of the use of flumazenil have produced a short-lived effect at best.[268] The use of this approach is probably limited to managing encephalopathy precipitated by the intake of benzodiazepine medications.

The presence of extra-pyramidal signs in some individuals with hepatic encephalopathy has generated a small number of studies into the use of the dopaminergic agonists such as L-dopa and bromocriptine. A recent Cochrane systematic review concluded that there was insufficient evidence to recommend their use.[269] Autopsy and imaging evidence suggesting manganese deposition in the basal ganglia has suggested this may relate to the development of extra-pyramidal signs. No studies to date have examined the role of manganese chelation in the management of encephalopathy.

Miscellaneous

The maintenance of circulating blood volume by correction of dehydration (often caused by overuse of diuretics) is important to maintain adequate renal excretion of ammonia.[270] Skeletal muscle reduces circulating ammonia through the synthesis of glutamine. L-ornithine L-aspartate provides intermediates that increase glutamate availability to muscle. Several studies suggest that administration of L-ornithine L-aspartate can improve the symptoms of encephalopathy.[270]

The role of external detoxification devices akin to dialysis in renal failure has been proposed for individuals with hepatic encephalopathy. Artificial support systems such as MARS (molecular adsorbents recirculating system) and bioartificial systems have been shown in a systematic review of a small number of trials to significantly improve symptoms of encephalopathy and are under continued investigation.[271] Interestingly, one trial showed significant improvement in encephalopathy with MARS without changes in blood levels of ammonia.[272]

Liver transplantation should always be considered with the development of hepatic encephalopathy in chronic liver disease but signs and symptoms do not always resolve, or do so only partially, indicating that permanent organic cerebral changes occur in chronic encephalopathy.[248]

There is a recent awakening of interest in the management of hepatic encephalopathy prompted by advances in molecular biology and imaging techniques. The role of anti-inflammatory agents, NMDA receptor antagonists, L-carnitine, sodium benzoate and phenylacetate, manganese chelators, and zinc supplementation are all under investigation.

Summary

At present, given the relative lack of evidence for any of the medical interventions described, it is imperative that any individual presenting with hepatic encephalopathy is, if appropriate given the stage of the associated disease process, intensively investigated for precipitating factors. If close attention is paid to treating infections, dehydration, acid–base and electrolyte disturbances, and constipation, this is likely to have the most significant impact on the clinical situation. If no precipitating factors are identified or symptoms are persistent, then antibiotics such as neomycin or particularly rifaximin, if available, should receive a trial of therapy. The management of minimal hepatic encephalopathy continues to be a worthy subject of debate.

References

1. Whitehead, M.W., Hainsworth, I., and Kingham, J.G. (2001). The causes of obvious jaundice in South West Wales: Perceptions versus reality. *Gut*, **48**, 409–13.

2. Bjornsson, E., Ismael, S., Nejdet, S. *et al.* (2003). Severe jaundice in Sweden in the new millennium: Causes, investigations, treatment and prognosis. *Scand J Gastroenterol*, **38**, 86–94.

3. Kamath, P.S., Wiesner, R.H., Malinchoc, M. *et al.* (2001). A model to predict survival in patients with end-stage liver disease. *Hepatology*, **33**, 464–70.

4. Rossaro, L., Troppmann, C., McVicar, J.P. *et al.* (2004). A strategy for the simultaneous provision of pre-operative palliative care for patients awaiting liver transplantation. *Transpl Int*, **17**, 473–5.

5. Adam, S.J. (2000). Palliative care for patients with a failed liver transplant. *Intensive Crit Care Nurs*, **16**, 396–402.

6. Sanchez, W. and Talwalkar, J.A. (2006). Palliative care for patients with end-stage liver disease ineligible for liver transplantation. *Gastroenterol Clin North Am*, **35**, 201–19.

7. Lin, M.H., Wu, P.Y., Tsai, S.T. *et al.* (2004). Hospice palliative care for patients with hepatocellular carcinoma in Taiwan. *Palliat Med*, **18**, 93–9.

8. Bosma, P.J., Chowdhury, J.R., Bakker, C. *et al* (1995). The genetic basis of the reduced expression of bilirubin UDP-glucuronosyltransferase 1 in Gilbert's syndrome. *N Engl J Med*, **333**, 1171–5.

9. Wasserman, E., Myara, A., Lokiec, F. *et al.* (1997). Severe CPT-11 toxicity in patients with Gilbert's syndrome: Two case reports. *Ann Oncol*, **8**, 1049–51.

10. Ruiz-Arguelles, G.J., Ruiz-Delgado, G.J., David Gomez-Rangel, J. *et al.* (2005). Gilbert's syndrome disclosed during the treatment of hematological malignancies. *Hematology*, **10**, 59–60.

11. Engin, H., Oksuzoglu, C.B., and Altundag, K. (2002). Interleukin-2-induced reversible hyperbilirubinemia and cholestasis in a patient with Gilbert's syndrome. *J Gastroenterol*, **37**, 145–6.

12. Mandala, M., Cremonesi, M., Cazzaniga, M. *et al.* (2004). Gilbert's syndrome and fluorouracil toxicity in colorectal cancer patients: Which correlation? *Colorectal Dis*, **6**, 129–30.

13. Au, W.Y., Cheung, W.C., and Tung, H.M. (2004). Gilbert's syndrome complicating long term parental nutrition. *J Hepatol*, **41**, 168–9.

14. Agarwal, K., Cross, T.J., and Gore, C. (2007). Chronic hepatitis C. *BMJ*, **334**, 54–5.

15. Xunrong, L., Yan, A.W., Liang, R. *et al.* (2001). Hepatitis B virus (HBV) reactivation after cytotoxic or immunosuppressive therapy—Pathogenesis and management. *Rev Med Virol*, **11**, 287–99.

16. Esteve, M., Saro, C., Gonzalez-Huix, F. *et al.* (2004). Chronic hepatitis B reactivation following infliximab therapy in Crohn's disease patients: Need for primary prophylaxis. *Gut*, **53**, 1363–5.

17. Koga, Y., Kumashiro, R., Yasumoto, K. *et al.* (1992). Two fatal cases of hepatitis B virus carriers after corticosteroid therapy for bronchial asthma. *Intern Med*, **31**, 208–13.

18. Hammond, A., Ramersdorfer, C., Palitzsch, K.D. *et al.* (1999). Fatal liver failure after corticosteroid treatment of a hepatitis B virus carrier. *Dtsch Med Wochenschr*, **124**, 687–90.

19. Yeo, W., Zee, B., Zhong, S. *et al.* (2004). Comprehensive analysis of risk factors associating with Hepatitis B virus (HBV) reactivation in cancer patients undergoing cytotoxic chemotherapy. *Br J Cancer*, **90**, 1306–11.

20. Cheng, A.L., Hsiung, C.A., Su, I.J. *et al.* (2003). Steroid-free chemotherapy decreases risk of hepatitis B virus (HBV) reactivation in HBV-carriers with lymphoma. *Hepatology*, **37**, 1320–8.

21. Gheorghe, L., Iacob, S., Simionov, I. *et al.* (2005). Natural history of compensated viral B and D cirrhosis. *Rom J Gastroenterol*, **14**, 329–35.

22. Sangiovanni, A., Prati, G.M., Fasani, P. *et al.* (2006). The natural history of compensated cirrhosis due to hepatitis C virus: A 17-year cohort study of 214 patients. *Hepatology*, **43**, 1303–10.

23. Shaib, Y.H., El Serag, H.B., Davila, J.A. *et al.* (2005). Risk factors of intrahepatic cholangiocarcinoma in the United States: A case-control study. *Gastroenterology*, **128**, 620–6.

24. Hai, S., Kubo, S., Yamamoto, S. *et al.* (2005). Clinicopathologic characteristics of hepatitis C virus-associated intrahepatic cholangiocarcinoma. *Dig Surg*, **22**, 432–9.

25. Williams, R. (2006). Global challenges in liver disease. *Hepatology*, **44**, 521–6.

26. Weber, R., Sabin, C.A., Friis-Moller, N. *et al.* (2006). Liver-related deaths in persons infected with the human immunodeficiency virus: The D:A:D study. *Arch Intern Med*, **166**, 1632–41.

27. Echejoh, G.O., Mandong, B.M., Tanko, M.N. *et al.* (2006). Hepatic histopathological findings in HIV patients at postmortem in Jos university teaching hospital, Nigeria. *Trop Doct*, **36**, 228–31.

28. Amarapurkar, A.D. and Sangle, N.A. (2005). Histological spectrum of liver in HIV—Autopsy study. *Ann Hepatol*, **4**, 47–51.

29. Ghoda, M.K. (2005). Hepatic tuberculosis presenting as cholestatic jaundice. A case report. *Trop Gastroenterol*, **26**, 203–4.

30. Yusuf, T.E. and Baron, T.H. (2004). AIDS Cholangiopathy. *Curr Treat Options Gastroenterol*, **7**, 111–17.

31. Roland, M.E. and Stock, P.G. (2006). Liver transplantation in HIV-infected recipients. *Semin Liver Dis*, **26**, 273–84.

32. Ryder, S.D. and Beckingham, I.J. (2001). ABC of diseases of liver, pancreas, and biliary system. Other causes of parenchymal liver disease. *BMJ*, **322**, 290–2.

33. Bissell, D.M., Gores, G.J., Laskin, D.L. *et al.* (2001). Drug-induced liver injury: Mechanisms and test systems. *Hepatology*, **33**, 1009–13.

34. De Valle, M.B., Av, K.V., Alem, N. *et al.* (2006). Drug-induced liver injury in a Swedish University hospital out-patient hepatology clinic. *Aliment Pharmacol Ther*, **24**, 1187–95.

35. Laliberte, L. and Villeneuve, J.P. (1996). Hepatitis after the use of germander, a herbal remedy. *CMAJ*, **154**, 1689–92.

36. Harvey, J. and Colin-Jones, D.G. (1981). Mistletoe hepatitis. *Br Med J (Clin Res Ed)*, **282**, 186–7.

37. Dart, R.C., Kuffner, E.K., and Rumack, B.H. (2000). Treatment of pain or fever with paracetamol (acetaminophen) in the alcoholic patient: A systematic review. *Am J Ther*, **7**, 123–34.

38. Ford-Dunn, S. (2005). Managing patients with cancer and advanced liver disease. *Palliat Med*, **19**, 563–5.

39. Pu, Y.S., Liu, C.M., Kao, J.H. *et al.* (1999). Antiandrogen hepatotoxicity in patients with chronic viral hepatitis. *Eur Urol*, **36**, 293–7.

40. Moseley, R.H. (2004). Sepsis and cholestasis. *Clin Liver Dis*, **8**, 83–94.

41. Van Lingen, R., Warshow, U., Dalton, H.R. *et al.* (2005). Jaundice as a presentation of heart failure. *J R Soc Med*, **98**, 357–9.

42. Cogger, V.C., Fraser, R., and Le Couteur, D.G. (2003). Liver dysfunction and heart failure. *Am J Cardiol*, **91**, 1399.

43. Lau, G.T., Tan, H.C., and Kritharides, L. (2002). Type of liver dysfunction in heart failure and its relation to the severity of tricuspid regurgitation. *Am J Cardiol*, **90**, 1405–9.

44. Hogan, W.J., Maris, M., Storer, B. *et al.* (2004). Hepatic injury after nonmyeloablative conditioning followed by allogeneic hematopoietic cell transplantation: A study of 193 patients. *Blood*, **103**, 78–84.

45. Paumgartner, G. and Beuers, U. (2004). Mechanisms of action and therapeutic efficacy of ursodeoxycholic acid in cholestatic liver disease. *Clin Liver Dis*, **8**, 67–81, vi.

46. Ruutu, T., Eriksson, B., Remes, K. *et al.* (2002). Ursodeoxycholic acid for the prevention of hepatic complications in allogeneic stem cell transplantation. *Blood*, **100**, 1977–83.

47. Zimmerman, M.A., Cameron, A.M., and Ghobrial, R.M. (2006). Budd-Chiari syndrome. *Clin Liver Dis*, **10**, 259–73, viii.

48. McCarthy, P.M., van Heerden, J.A., Adson, M.A. *et al.* (1985). The Budd-Chiari syndrome. Medical and surgical management of 30 patients. *Arch Surg*, **120**, 657–62.

49. Mano, M.S., Cassidy, J., and Canney, P. (2005). Liver metastases from breast cancer: Management of patients with significant liver dysfunction. *Cancer Treat Rev*, **31**, 35–48.

50. Koea, J., Holden, A., Chau, K. *et al.* (2004). Differential diagnosis of stenosing lesions at the hepatic hilus. *World J Surg*, **28**, 466–70.

51. Ballinger, A.B., McHugh, M., Catnach, S.M. *et al.* (1994). Symptom relief and quality of life after stenting for malignant bile duct obstruction. *Gut*, **35**, 467–70.

52. Luman, W., Cull, A., and Palmer, K.R. (1997). Quality of life in patients stented for malignant biliary obstructions. *Eur J Gastroenterol Hepatol*, **9**, 481–4.

53. Padillo, F.J., Andicoberry, B., Muntane, J. *et al.* (2001). Cytokines and acute-phase response markers derangements in patients with obstructive jaundice. *Hepatogastroenterology*, **48**, 378–81.

54. Kimmings, A.N., van Deventer, S.J., Obertop, H. *et al.* (2000). Endotoxin, cytokines, and endotoxin binding proteins in obstructive jaundice and after preoperative biliary drainage. *Gut*, **46**, 725–31.

55. Padillo, F.J., Muntane, J., Montero, J.L. *et al.* (2002). Effect of internal biliary drainage on plasma levels of endotoxin, cytokines, and C-reactive protein in patients with obstructive jaundice. *World J Surg*, **26**, 1328–32.

56. Clements, W.D., McCaigue, M., Erwin, P. *et al.* (1996). Biliary decompression promotes Kupffer cell recovery in obstructive jaundice. *Gut*, **38**, 925–31.

57. Abraham, N.S., Barkun, J.S., and Barkun, A.N. (2002). Palliation of malignant biliary obstruction: a prospective trial examining impact on quality of life. *Gastrointest Endosc*, **56**, 835–41.

58. Ashton, C.E., McNabb, W.R., Wilkinson, M.L. *et al.* (1998). Endoscopic retrograde cholangiopancreatography in elderly patients. *Age Ageing*, **27**, 683–8.

59. Kamath, P.S. (1996). Clinical approach to the patient with abnormal liver test results. *Mayo Clin Proc*, **71**, 1089–94.

60. Stott, M.A., Farrands, P.A., Guyer, P.B. *et al.* (1991). Ultrasound of the common bile duct in patients undergoing cholecystectomy. *J Clin Ultrasound*, **19**, 73–6.

61. Stroszczynski, C. and Hunerbein, M. (2005). Malignant biliary obstruction: Value of imaging findings. *Abdom Imaging*, **30**, 314–23.

62. Rickes, S., Unkrodt, K., Neye, H. *et al.* (2002). Differentiation of pancreatic tumours by conventional ultrasound, unenhanced and echo-enhanced power Doppler sonography. *Scand J Gastroenterol*, **37**, 1313–20.

63. Blackbourne, L.H., Earnhardt, R.C., Sistrom, C.L. *et al.* (1994). The sensitivity and role of ultrasound in the evaluation of biliary obstruction. *Am Surg*, **60**, 683–690.

64. Crowe, D.R., Eloubeidi, M.A., Chhieng, D.C. *et al.* (2006). Fine-needle aspiration biopsy of hepatic lesions: computerized tomographic-guided versus endoscopic ultrasound-guided FNA. *Cancer*, **108**, 180–5.

65. Gress, F., Schmitt, C., Sherman, S. *et al.* (1999). A prospective randomized comparison of endoscopic ultrasound- and computed tomography-guided celiac plexus block for managing chronic pancreatitis pain. *Am J Gastroenterol*, **94**, 900–5.

66. Chang, K.J. (2006). State of the art lecture: Endoscopic ultrasound (EUS) and FNA in pancreatico-biliary tumors. *Endoscopy*, **38**(Suppl 1), S56–60.

67. Domagk, D., Wessling, J., Reimer, P. *et al.* (2004). Endoscopic retrograde cholangiopancreatography, intraductal ultrasonography, and magnetic resonance cholangiopancreatography in bile duct strictures: A prospective comparison of imaging diagnostics with histopathological correlation. *Am J Gastroenterol*, **99**, 1684–9.

68. Hunerbein, M., Stroszczynski, C., Ulmer, C. *et al.* (2003). Prospective comparison of transcutaneous 3-dimensional US cholangiography, magnetic resonance cholangiography, and direct cholangiography in the evaluation of malignant biliary obstruction. *Gastrointest Endosc*, **58**, 853–8.

69. Mortele, K.J., McTavish, J., and Ros, P.R. (2002). Current techniques of computed tomography. Helical CT, multidetector CT, and 3D reconstruction. *Clin Liver Dis*, **6**, 29–52.

70. Romagnuolo, J., Bardou, M., Rahme, E. *et al.* (2003). Magnetic resonance cholangiopancreatography: a meta-analysis of test performance in suspected biliary disease. *Ann Intern Med*, **139**, 547–57.

71. Yeh, T.S., Jan, Y.Y., Tseng, J.H. *et al.* (2000). Malignant perihilar biliary obstruction: Magnetic resonance cholangiopancreatographic findings. *Am J Gastroenterol*, **95**, 432–40.

72. Hintze, R.E., Abou-Rebyeh, H., Adler, A. *et al.* (2001). Magnetic resonance cholangiopancreatography-guided unilateral endoscopic stent placement for Klatskin tumors. *Gastrointest Endosc*, **53**, 40–6.

73. Freeman, M.L. and Overby, C. (2003). Selective MRCP and CT-targeted drainage of malignant hilar biliary obstruction with self-expanding metallic stents. *Gastrointest Endosc*, **58**, 41–9.

74. Pavone, P., Laghi, A., and Passariello, R. (1999). MR cholangiopancreatography in malignant biliary obstruction. *Semin Ultrasound CT MR*, **20**, 317–23.

75. Gabata, T., Terayama, N., Kobayashi, S. *et al.* (2006). MR imaging of hepatocellular carcinomas with biliary tumor thrombi. *Abdom Imaging*, **32**, 470–4.

76. BravoVergel, Y., Chilcott, J., Kaltenthaler, E. *et al.* (2006). Economic evaluation of MR cholangiopancreatography compared to diagnostic ERCP for the investigation of biliary tree obstruction. *International Journal of Surgery*, **4**, 12–19.

77. Harbin, W.P., Mueller, P.R., and Ferrucci, J.T., Jr. (1980). Transhepatic cholangiography: complicatons and use patterns of the fine-needle technique: A multi-institutional survey. *Radiology*, **135**, 15–22.

78. Bilbao, M.K., Dotter, C.T., Lee, T.G. *et al.* (1976). Complications of endoscopic retrograde cholangiopancreatography (ERCP). A study of 10,000 cases. *Gastroenterology*, **70**, 314–20.

79. Testoni, P.A. (2006). Facts and fiction in the pharmacologic prevention of post-ERCP pancreatitis: A never-ending story. *Gastrointest Endosc*, **64**, 732–4.

80. Ros, P.R. and Mortele, K.J. (2002). Hepatic imaging. An overview. *Clin Liver Dis*, **6**, 1–16.

81. Gurevich, I. and Akerley, W. (2001). Treatment of the jaundiced patient with breast carcinoma: Case report and alternate therapeutic strategies. *Cancer,* **91**, 660–3.

82. Schull, B., Scheithauer, W., and Kornek, G.V. (2003). Capecitabine as salvage therapy for a breast cancer patient with extensive liver metastases and associated impairment of liver function. *Onkologie*, **26**, 578–80.

83. Van Laethem, J.L., De Broux, S., Eisendrath, P. *et al.* (2003). Clinical impact of biliary drainage and jaundice resolution in patients with obstructive metastases at the hilum. *Am J Gastroenterol*, **98**, 1271–7.

84. Qian, X.J., Zhai, R.Y., Dai, D.K. *et al.* (2006). Treatment of malignant biliary obstruction by combined percutaneous transhepatic biliary drainage with local tumor treatment. *World J Gastroenterol*, **12**, 331–5.

85. Andtbacka, R.H., Evans, D.B., and Pisters, P.W. (2004). Surgical and endoscopic palliation for pancreatic cancer. *Minerva Chir*, **59**, 123–36.

86. Sarr, M.G. and Cameron, J.L. (1982). Surgical management of unresectable carcinoma of the pancreas. *Surgery*, **91**, 123–33.

87. Ali, A.S. and Ammori, B.J. (2003). Concomitant laparoscopic gastric and biliary bypass and bilateral thoracoscopic splanchnotomy: The full package of minimally invasive palliation for pancreatic cancer. *Surg Endosc*, **17**, 2028–31.

88. Tang, C.N., Siu, W.T., Ha, J.P. *et al.* (2005). Endo-laparoscopic approach in the management of obstructive jaundice and malignant gastric outflow obstruction. *Hepatogastroenterology*, **52**, 128–34.

89. Ghanem, A.M., Hamade, A.M., Sheen, A.J. *et al.* (2006). Laparoscopic gastric and biliary bypass: A single-center cohort prospective study. *J Laparoendosc Adv Surg Tech A*, **16**, 21–6.

90. Moss, A.C., Morris, E., Leyden, J. *et al.* (2006). Malignant distal biliary obstruction: A systematic review and meta-analysis of endoscopic and surgical bypass results. *Cancer Treat Rev*, **33**, 213–21.

91. Soderlund, C. and Linder, S. (2006). Covered metal versus plastic stents for malignant common bile duct stenosis: A prospective, randomized, controlled trial. *Gastrointest Endosc*, **63**, 986–95.

92. Prat, F., Chapat, O., Ducot, B. *et al.* (1998). Predictive factors for survival of patients with inoperable malignant distal biliary strictures: A practical management guideline. *Gut*, **42**, 76–80.

93. Covey, A.M. and Brown, K.T. (2006). Palliative percutaneous drainage in malignant biliary obstruction. Part 1: Indications and preprocedure evaluation. *J Support Oncol*, **4**, 269–73.

94. Covey, A.M. and Brown, K.T. (2006). Palliative percutaneous drainage in malignant biliary obstruction. Part 2: Mechanisms and postprocedure management. *J Support Oncol*, **4**, 329–35.

95. Lillemoe, K.D., Cameron, J.L., Kaufman, H.S. *et al.* (1993). Chemical splanchnicectomy in patients with unresectable pancreatic cancer. A prospective randomized trial. *Ann Surg*, **217**, 447–55.

96. Pancreatic section of the British Society for Gastroenterology (2005). Guidelines for the management of patients with pancreatic cancer periampullary and ampullary carcinomas. *Gut*, **54**(Suppl 5), v1–16.

97. O'Brien, D.P., Shearer, M.J., Waldron, R.P. *et al.* (1994). The extent of vitamin K deficiency in patients with cholestatic jaundice: a preliminary communication. *J R Soc Med*, **87**, 320–2.

98. Green, B., Cairns, S., Harvey, R. *et al.* (2000). Phytomenadione or menadiol in the management of an elevated international normalized ratio (prothrombin time). *Aliment Pharmacol Ther*, **14**, 1685–9.

99. Bergasa, N.V., Link, M.J., Keogh, M. *et al.* (2001). Pilot study of bright-light therapy reflected toward the eyes for the pruritus of chronic liver disease. *Am J Gastroenterol*, **96**, 1563–70.

100. Twycross, R., Greaves, M.W., Handwerker, H. *et al.* (2003). Itch: Scratching more than the surface. *QJM*, **96**, 7–26.

101. Bergasa, N.V., Alling, D.W., Talbot, T.L. *et al.* (1995). Effects of naloxone infusions in patients with the pruritus of cholestasis. A double-blind, randomized, controlled trial. *Ann Intern Med*, **123**, 161–7.

102. Szarvas, S., Harmon, D., and Murphy, D. (2003). Neuraxial opioid-induced pruritus: A review. *J Clin Anesth*, **15**, 234–9.

103. Thornton, J.R. and Losowsky, M.S. (1988). Opioid peptides and primary biliary cirrhosis. *BMJ*, **297**, 1501–4.

104. Bergasa, N.V., Thomas, D.A., Vergalla, J. *et al.* (1993). Plasma from patients with the pruritus of cholestasis induces opioid receptor-mediated scratching in monkeys. *Life Sci*, **53**, 1253–7.

105. Bergasa, N.V., Talbot, T.L., Alling, D.W. *et al.* (1992). A controlled trial of naloxone infusions for the pruritus of chronic cholestasis. *Gastroenterology*, **102**, 544–9.

106. Carson, K.L., Tran, T.T., Cotton, P. *et al.* (1996). Pilot study of the use of naltrexone to treat the severe pruritus of cholestatic liver disease. *Am J Gastroenterol*, **91**, 1022–3.

107. Wolfhagen, F.H., Sternieri, E., Hop, W.C. *et al.* (1997). Oral naltrexone treatment for cholestatic pruritus: a double-blind, placebo-controlled study. *Gastroenterology*, **113**, 1264–9.

108. Bergasa, N.V., Schmitt, J.M., Talbot, T.L. *et al.* (1998). Open-label trial of oral nalmefene therapy for the pruritus of cholestasis. *Hepatology*, **27**, 679–84.

109. Terg, R., Coronel, E., Sorda, J. *et al.* (2002). Efficacy and safety of oral naltrexone treatment for pruritus of cholestasis, a crossover, double blind, placebo-controlled study. *J Hepatol*, **37**, 717–22.

110. McRae, C.A., Prince, M.I., Hudson, M. *et al.* (2003). Pain as a complication of use of opiate antagonists for symptom control in cholestasis. *Gastroenterology*, **125**, 591–6.

111. Jones, E.A. and Zylicz, Z. (2005). Treatment of pruritus caused by cholestasis with opioid antagonists. *J Palliat Med*, **8**, 1290–4.

112. Jones, E.A., Neuberger, J., and Bergasa, N.V. (2002). Opiate antagonist therapy for the pruritus of cholestasis: The avoidance of opioid withdrawal-like reactions. *QJM*, **95**, 547–52.

113. Cepeda, M.S., Alvarez, H., Morales, O. *et al.* (2004). Addition of ultralow dose naloxone to postoperative morphine PCA: Unchanged analgesia and opioid requirement but decreased incidence of opioid side effects. *Pain*, **107**, 41–6.

114. Maxwell, L.G., Kaufmann, S.C., Bitzer, S. *et al.* (2005). The effects of a small-dose naloxone infusion on opioid-induced side effects and analgesia in children and adolescents treated with intravenous patient-controlled analgesia: A double-blind, prospective, randomized, controlled study. *Anesth Analg*, **100**, 953–8.

115. Beltrutti, D., Niv, D., Ben Abraham, R. *et al.* (2002). Late antinociception and lower untoward effects of concomitant intrathecal morphine and intravenous buprenorphine in humans. *J Clin Anesth*, **14**, 441–6.

116. Juby, L.D., Wong, V.S., and Losowsky, M.S. (1994). Buprenorphine and hepatic pruritus. *Br J Clin Pract*, **48**, 331.

117. Prommer, E. (2005). Re: Pruritus in patients with advanced cancer. *J Pain Symptom Manage*, **30**, 201–2.

118. Borgeat, A. and Stirnemann, H.R. (1999). Ondansetron is effective to treat spinal or epidural morphine-induced pruritus. *Anesthesiology*, **90**, 432–6.

119. Pirat, A., Tuncay, S.F., Torgay, A. *et al.* (2005). Ondansetron, orally disintegrating tablets versus intravenous injection for prevention of intrathecal morphine-induced nausea, vomiting, and pruritus in young males. *Anesth Analg*, **101**, 1330–6.

120. Iatrou, C.A., Dragoumanis, C.K., Vogiatzaki, T.D. *et al.* (2005). Prophylactic intravenous ondansetron and dolasetron in intrathecal morphine-induced pruritus: A randomized, double-blinded, placebo-controlled study. *Anesth Analg*, **101**, 1516–20.

121. Horta, M.L., Morejon, L.C., da Cruz, A.W. *et al.* (2006). Study of the prophylactic effect of droperidol, alizapride, propofol and promethazine on spinal morphine-induced pruritus. *Br J Anaesth*, **96**, 796–800.

122. Torn, K., Tuominen, M., Tarkkila, P. *et al.* (1994). Effects of sub-hypnotic doses of propofol on the side effects of intrathecal morphine. *Br J Anaesth*, **73**, 411–12.

123. Asokumar, B., Newman, L.M., McCarthy, R.J. *et al.* (1998). Intrathecal bupivacaine reduces pruritus and prolongs duration of fentanyl analgesia during labor: A prospective, randomized controlled trial. *Anesth Analg*, **87**, 1309–15.

124. Raderer, M., Muller, C., and Scheithauer, W. (1994). Ondansetron for pruritus due to cholestasis. *N Engl J Med*, **330**, 1540.

125. Schworer, H., Hartmann, H., and Ramadori, G. (1995). Relief of cholestatic pruritus by a novel class of drugs: 5-Hydroxytryptamine type 3 (5-HT3) receptor antagonists: Effectiveness of ondansetron. *Pain*, **61**, 33–37.

126. Muller, C., Pongratz, S., Pidlich, J. *et al.* (1998). Treatment of pruritus in chronic liver disease with the 5-hydroxytryptamine receptor type 3 antagonist ondansetron: A randomized, placebo-controlled, double-blind cross-over trial. *Eur J Gastroenterol Hepatol*, **10**, 865–70.

127. O'Donohue, J.W., Pereira, S.P., Ashdown, A.C. *et al.* (2005). A controlled trial of ondansetron in the pruritus of cholestasis. *Aliment Pharmacol Ther*, **21**, 1041–5.

128. Davis, M.P., Frandsen, J.L., Walsh, D. *et al.* (2003). Mirtazapine for pruritus. *J Pain Symptom Manage*, **25**, 288–91.

129. Browning, J., Combes, B., and Mayo, M.J. (2003). Long-term efficacy of sertraline as a treatment for cholestatic pruritus in patients with primary biliary cirrhosis. *Am J Gastroenterol*, **98**, 2736–41.

130. Borgeat, A., Wilder-Smith, O.H., and Mentha, G. (1993). Subhypnotic doses of propofol relieve pruritus associated with liver disease. *Gastroenterology*, **104**, 244–7.

131. Heikkinen, J., Maentausta, O., Ylostalo, P. *et al.* (1982). Serum bile acid levels in intrahepatic cholestasis of pregnancy during treatment with phenobarbital or cholestyramine. *Eur J Obstet Gynecol Reprod Biol*, **14**, 153–62.

132. Bloomer, J.R. and Boyer, J.L. (1975). Phenobarbital effects in cholestatic liver diseases. *Ann Intern Med*, **82**, 310–17.

133. Prieto, L.N. (2004). The use of midazolam to treat itching in a terminally ill patient with biliary obstruction. *J Pain Symptom Manage*, **28**, 531–2.

134. Sargent, S. (2006). Management of patients with advanced liver cirrhosis. *Nurs Stand*, **21**, 48–56.

135. Neff, G.W., O'Brien, C.B., Reddy, K.R. *et al.* (2002). Preliminary observation with dronabinol in patients with intractable pruritus secondary to cholestatic liver disease. *Am J Gastroenterol*, **97**, 2117–19.

136. Villamil, A.G., Bandi, J.C., Galdame, O.A. *et al.* (2005). Efficacy of lidocaine in the treatment of pruritus in patients with chronic cholestatic liver diseases. *Am J Med*, **118**, 1160–3.

137. Bergasa, N.V. (2004). Pruritus in chronic liver disease: mechanisms and treatment. *Curr Gastroenterol Rep*, **6**, 10–16.

138. Pusl, T., Denk, G.U., Parhofer, K.G. *et al.* (2006). Plasma separation and anion adsorption transiently relieve intractable pruritus in primary biliary cirrhosis. *J Hepatol*, **45**, 887–91.

139. Hoek, F.J., Grijm, R., Sanders, G.T. *et al.* (1982). Removal of bile acids from the blood by hemodialysis with a polyacrylonitril membrane: Treatment of pruritus of cholestatic disease. *Digestion* **23**, 135–40.

140. Lauterburg, B.H., Taswell, H.F., Pineda, A.A. *et al.* (1980). Treatment of pruritus of cholestasis by plasma perfusion through USP-charcoal-coated glass beads. *Lancet*, **2**, 53–5.

141. Warren, J.E., Blaylock, R.C., and Silver, R.M. (2005). Plasmapheresis for the treatment of intrahepatic cholestasis of pregnancy refractory to medical treatment. *Am J Obstet Gynecol*, **192**, 2088–9.

142. Pares, A., Cisneros, L., Salmeron, J.M. *et al.* (2004). Extracorporeal albumin dialysis: A procedure for prolonged relief of intractable pruritus in patients with primary biliary cirrhosis. *Am J Gastroenterol*, **99**, 1105–10.

143. Ghent, C.N. and Carruthers, S.G. (1988). Treatment of pruritus in primary biliary cirrhosis with rifampin. Results of a double-blind, crossover, randomized trial. *Gastroenterology*, **94**, 488–93.

144. Bachs, L., Pares, A., Elena, M. *et al.* (1989). Comparison of rifampicin with phenobarbitone for treatment of pruritus in biliary cirrhosis. *Lancet*, **1**, 574–576.

145. Bergasa, N.V. (2004). An approach to the management of the pruritus of cholestasis. *Clin Liver Dis*, **8**, 55–66, vi.

146. Rosenberg, S.M. (2006). Palliation of malignant ascites. *Gastroenterol Clin North Am*, **35**, 189–99, xi.

147. Gines, P., Cardenas, A., Arroyo, V. *et al.* (2004). Management of cirrhosis and ascites. *N Engl J Med*, **350**, 1646–54.

148. Moore, K.P. and Aithal, G.P. (2006). Guidelines on the management of ascites in cirrhosis. *Gut*, **55** (Suppl 6), vi1–vi12.

149. Lee, C.W., Bociek, G., and Faught, W. (1998). A survey of practice in management of malignant ascites. *J Pain Symptom Manage*, **16**, 96–101.

150. Keen, J. and Fallon, M. (2002). Malignant ascites. In *Gastrointestinal symptoms in advanced cancer patients*(eds. C. Ripamonti and E. Bruera), pp 279–90. Oxford University Press, New York.

151. Preston, N. (1995). New strategies for the management of malignant ascites. *Eur J Cancer Care (Engl)*, **4**, 178–83.

152. Ringenberg, Q.S., Doll, D.C., Loy, T.S. *et al.* (1989). Malignant ascites of unknown origin. *Cancer*, **64**, 753–5.

153. Malik, I., Abubakar, S., Rizwana, I. *et al.* (1991). Clinical features and management of malignant ascites. *J Pak Med Assoc*, **41**, 38–40.

154. Parsons, S.L., Lang, M.W., and Steele, R.J. (1996). Malignant ascites: A 2-year review from a teaching hospital. *Eur J Surg Oncol*, **22**, 237–9.

155. Garrison, R.N., Kaelin, L.D., Galloway, R.H. *et al.* (1986). Malignant ascites. Clinical and experimental observations. *Ann Surg*, **203**, 644–51.

156. Puls, L.E., Duniho, T., Hunter, J.E. *et al.* (1996). The prognostic implication of ascites in advanced-stage ovarian cancer. *Gynecol Oncol*, **61**, 109–12.

157. Zang, R.Y., Zhang, Z.Y., Cai, S.M. *et al.* (1999). Cytoreductive surgery for stage IV epithelial ovarian cancer. *J Exp Clin Cancer Res*, 449–54.

158. von Gruenigen, V.E., Frasure, H.E., Reidy, A.M. *et al.* (2003). Clinical disease course during the last year in ovarian cancer. *Gynecol Oncol*, **90**, 619–24.

159. Etzion, Y., Barski, L., and Almog, Y. (2004). Malignant ascites presenting as abdominal compartment syndrome. *Am J Emerg Med*, **22**, 430–1.

160. Parsons, S.L., Watson, S.A., and Steele, R.J. (1996). Malignant ascites. *Br J Surg*, **83**, 6–14.

161. Feldman, G.B., Knapp, R.C., Order, S.E. *et al.* (1972). The role of lymphatic obstruction in the formation of ascites in a murine ovarian carcinoma. *Cancer Res*, **32**, 1663–6.

162. Coates, G., Bush, R.S., and Aspin, N. (1973). A study of ascites using lymphoscintography with 99m Tc-sulphur colloid. *Radiology*, **107**, 577–83.

163. Hirabayashi, K.I. and Graham, J. (1970). Genesis of ascites in ovarian cancer. *Am J Obstet Gynecol*, **106**, 492–7.

164. Sebastian, S., Tuite, D., Crotty, P. *et al.* (2004). Painful ascites. *Gut*, **53**, 1344–55.

165. Beecham, J.B., Kucera, P., Helmkamp, B.F. *et al.* (1983). Peritoneal angiogenesis in patients with ascites. *Gynecol Oncol*, **15**, 142.

166. De Simone, G.G. (1999). Treatment of malignant ascites. *Progress in Palliative Care*, **7**, 10–16.

167. Yamamoto, S., Konishi, I., Tsuruta, Y. *et al.* (1997). Expression of vascular endothelial growth factor (VEGF) during folliculogenesis and corpus luteum formation in the human ovary. *Gynecol Endocrinol*, **11**, 371–81.

168. Yamamoto, S., Konishi, I., Mandai, M. *et al.* (1997). Expression of vascular endothelial growth factor (VEGF) in epithelial ovarian neoplasms: Correlation with clinicopathology and patient survival, and analysis of serum VEGF levels. *Br J Cancer*, **76**, 1221–7.

169. Yoneda, J., Kuniyasu, H., Crispens, M.A. *et al.* (1998). Expression of angiogenesis-related genes and progression of human ovarian carcinomas in nude mice. *J Natl Cancer Inst*, **90**, 447–54.

170. Huang, S., Robinson, J.B., Deguzman, A. *et al.* (2000). Blockade of nuclear factor-kappaB signaling inhibits angiogenesis and tumorigenicity of human ovarian cancer cells by suppressing expression of vascular endothelial growth factor and interleukin 8. *Cancer Res*, **60**, 5334–9.

171. Zebrowski, B.K., Liu, W., Ramirez, K. *et al.* (1999). Markedly elevated levels of vascular endothelial growth factor in malignant ascites. *Ann Surg Oncol*, **6**, 373–8.

172. Verheul, H.M., Hoekman, K., Jorna, A.S. *et al.* (2000). Targeting vascular endothelial growth factor blockade: Ascites and pleural effusion formation. *Oncologist*, **5** (Suppl 1), 45–50.

173. Kraft, A., Weindel, K., Ochs, A. *et al.* (1999). Vascular endothelial growth factor in the sera and effusions of patients with malignant and nonmalignant disease. *Cancer*, **85**, 178–87.

174. Gomez, R., Simon, C., Remohi, J. *et al.* (2003). Administration of moderate and high doses of gonadotropins to female rats increases ovarian vascular endothelial growth factor (VEGF) and VEGF receptor-2 expression that is associated to vascular hyperpermeability. *Biol Reprod*, **68**, 2164–71.

175. Runyon, B.A. (1994). Care of patients with ascites. *N Engl J Med*, **330**, 337–42.

176. Williams, J.W., Jr. and Simel, D.L. (1992). The rational clinical examination. Does this patient have ascites? How to divine fluid in the abdomen. *JAMA*, **267**, 2645–8.

177. Goldberg, B.B., Goodman, G.A., and Clearfield, H.R. (1970). Evaluation of ascites by ultrasound. *Radiology*, **96**, 15–22.

178. Colli, A., Buccino, G., Cocciolo, M. *et al.* (1989). Diagnostic accuracy of sialic acid in the diagnosis of malignant ascites. *Cancer*, **63**, 912–16.

179. Tangkijvanich, P., Tresukosol, D., Sampatanukul, P. *et al.* (1999). Telomerase assay for differentiating between malignancy-related and nonmalignant ascites. *Clin Cancer Res*, **5**, 2470–5.

180. Gerbes, A.L., Hoermann, R., Mann, K. *et al.* (1996). Human chorionic gonadotropin-beta in the differentiation of malignancy-related and nonmalignant ascites. *Digestion*, **57**, 113–17.

181. Colli, A., Buccino, G., Cocciolo, M. et al. (1986). Diagnostic accuracy of fibronectin in the differential diagnosis of ascites. *Cancer*, **58**, 2489–93.

182. Alexandrakis, M.G., Moschandrea, J., Kyriakou, D.S. et al. (2001). Use of a variety of biological parameters in distinguishing cirrhotic from malignant ascites. *Int J Biol Markers*, **16**, 45–9.

183. Regnard, C. and Mannix, K. (1989). Management of ascites in advanced cancer—A flow diagram. *Palliat Med*, **4**, 45–7.

184. Stephenson, J. and Gilbert, J. (2002). The development of clinical guidelines on paracentesis for ascites related to malignancy. *Palliat Med*, **16**, 213–18.

185. Becker, G., Galandi, D., and Blum, H.E. (2006). Malignant ascites: systematic review and guideline for treatment. *Eur J Cancer*, **42**, 589–97.

186. Lifshitz, S. (1982). Ascites, pathophysiology and control measures. *Int J Radiat Oncol Biol Phys*, **8**, 1423–6.

187. Weisberger, A.S., Levine, B., and Storaasli, J.P. (1955). Use of nitrogen mustard in treatment of serous effusions of neoplastic origin. *JAMA*, **159**, 1704–7.

188. Witkamp, A.J., de Bree, E., Van Goethem, R. et al. (2001). Rationale and techniques of intra-operative hyperthermic intraperitoneal chemotherapy. *Cancer Treat Rev*, **27**, 365–74.

189. de Bree, E., Romanos, J., Michalakis, J. et al. (2003). Intraoperative hyperthermic intraperitoneal chemotherapy with docetaxel as second-line treatment for peritoneal carcinomatosis of gynaecological origin. *Anticancer Res*, **23**, 3019–27.

190. Loggie, B.W., Perini, M., Fleming, R.A. et al. (1997). Treatment and prevention of malignant ascites associated with disseminated intraperitoneal malignancies by aggressive combined-modality therapy. *Am Surg*, **63**, 137–43.

191. Mackey, J.R., Wood, L., Nabholtz, J. et al. (2000). A phase II trial of triamcinolone hexacetanide for symptomatic recurrent malignant ascites. *J Pain Symptom Manage*, **19**, 193–9.

192. Xu, L., Yoneda, J., Herrera, C. et al. (2000). Inhibition of malignant ascites and growth of human ovarian carcinoma by oral administration of a potent inhibitor of the vascular endothelial growth factor receptor tyrosine kinases. *Int J Oncol*, **16**, 445–54.

193. Huang, S., Robinson, J.B., Deguzman, A. et al. (2000). Blockade of nuclear factor-kappaB signaling inhibits angiogenesis and tumorigenicity of human ovarian cancer cells by suppressing expression of vascular endothelial growth factor and interleukin 8. *Cancer Res*, **60**, 5334–9.

194. Stoelcker, B., Echtenacher, B., Weich, H.A. et al. (2000). VEGF/Flk-1 interaction, a requirement for malignant ascites recurrence. *J Interferon Cytokine Res*, **20**, 511–17.

195. Rath, U., Kaufmann, M., Schmid, H. et al. (1991). Effect of intraperitoneal recombinant human tumour necrosis factor alpha on malignant ascites. *Eur J Cancer*, **27**, 121–5.

196. Canete, J.D., Pablos, J.L., Sanmarti, R. et al. (2004). Antiangiogenic effects of anti-tumor necrosis factor alpha therapy with infliximab in psoriatic arthritis. *Arthritis Rheum*, **50**, 1636–41.

197. Sakayama, K., Kidani, T., Miyazaki, T. et al. (2004). Effect of ketoprofen in topical formulation on vascular endothelial growth factor expression and tumor growth in nude mice with osteosarcoma. *J Orthop Res*, **22**, 1168–74.

198. Kojima-Yuasa, A., Hua, J.J., Kennedy, D.O. et al. (2003). Green tea extract inhibits angiogenesis of human umbilical vein endothelial cells through reduction of expression of VEGF receptors. *Life Sci*, **73**, 1299–313.

199. Yoshiji, H., Kuriyama, S., Noguchi, R. et al. (2004). Angiotensin-I converting enzyme inhibitors as potential anti-angiogenic agents for cancer therapy. *Curr Cancer Drug Targets*, **4**, 555–67.

200. Beattie, G.J. and Smyth, J.F. (1998). Phase I study of intraperitoneal metalloproteinase inhibitor BB94 in patients with malignant ascites. *Clin Cancer Res*, **4**, 1899–902.

201. Cairns, W. and Malone, R. (1999). Octreotide as an agent for the relief of malignant ascites in palliative care patients. *Palliat Med*, **13**, 429–30.

202. McCormick, P.A., Chin, J., Greenslade, L. et al. (1995). Cardiovascular effects of octreotide in patients with hepatic cirrhosis. *Hepatology*, **21**, 1255–60.

203. Brooks, R.A. and Herzog, T.J. (2006). Long-term semi-permanent catheter use for the palliation of malignant ascites. *Gynecol Oncol*, **101**, 360–2.

204. Gough, I.R. and Balderson, G.A. (1993). Malignant ascites. A comparison of peritoneovenous shunting and nonoperative management. *Cancer*, **71**, 2377–82.

205. Greenway, B., Johnson, P.J., and Williams, R. (1982). Control of malignant ascites with spironolactone. *Br J Surg*, **69**, 441–2.

206. Pockros, P.J., Esrason, K.T., Nguyen, C. et al. (1992). Mobilization of malignant ascites with diuretics is dependent on ascitic fluid characteristics. *Gastroenterology*, **103**, 1302–6.

207. Oberleithner, H., Ludwig, T., Riethmuller, C. et al. (2004). Human endothelium: Target for aldosterone. *Hypertension*, **43**, 952–6.

208. Twycross, R.G. and Lack, S.A. (1986). Ascites. 282–99.

209. Amiel, S.A., Blackburn, A.M., and Rubens, R.D. (1984). Intravenous infusion of frusemide as treatment for ascites in malignant disease. *Br Med J*, **288**, 1041.

210. Bruera, E., Chadwick, S., Fox, R. et al. (1986). Study of cardiovascular autonomic insufficiency in advanced cancer patients. *Cancer Treat Rep*, **70**, 1383–7.

211. Stephenson, J. and Gilbert, J. (2002). The development of clinical guidelines on paracentesis for ascites related to malignancy. *Palliat Med*, **16**, 213–18.

212. Moorsom, D. (2001). Paracentesis in a home care setting. *Palliat Med*, **15**, 169–70.

213. Gotleib, W.H., Feldman, B., Feldman-Moran, O. et al. (1998). Intraperitoneal pressures and clinical parameters of total paracentesis for palliation of symptomatic ascites in ovarian cancer. *Gynecol Oncol*, **71**, 381–5.

214. McNamara, P. (2000). Paracentesis—An effective method of symptom control in the palliative care setting? *Palliat Med*, **14**, 62–4.

215. Lee, A., Lau, T.N., and Yeong, K.Y. (2000). Indwelling catheters for the management of malignant ascites. *Support Care Cancer*, **8**, 493–9.

216. Belfort, M.A., Stevens, P.J., DeHaek, K. et al. (1990). A new approach to the management of malignant ascites; a permanently implanted abdominal drain. *Eur J Surg Oncol*, **16**, 47–53.

217. Bui, C.D.H., Martin, C.J., and Currow, D.C. (1999). Effective community palliation of intractable malignant ascites with a permanently implanted abdominal drain. *J Palliat Med*, **2**, 319–21.

218. Sabatelli, F.W., Glassman, M.L., Kerns, S.R. et al. (1994). Permanent indwelling peritoneal access device for the management of malignant ascites. *Cardiovasc Intervent Radiol*, **17**, 292–4.

219. Stephenson, J. and Gilbert, J. (2002). The development of clinical guidelines on paracentesis for ascites related to malignancy. *Palliat Med*, **16**, 213–18.

220. Blackwell, N. and Burrows, M. (1994). A sticky tip. *Palliat Med*, **8**, 256–7.

221. Ross, G.J., Kessler, H.B., Clair, M.R. et al. (1989). Sonographically guided paracentesis for palliation of symptomatic malignant ascites. *AJR Am J Roentgenol*, **153**, 1309–11.

222. Richard, H.M., III, Coldwell, D.M., Boyd-Kranis, R.L. et al. (2001). Pleurx tunneled catheter in the management of malignant ascites. *J Vasc Interv Radiol*, **12**, 373–5.

223. Le Veen, H.H., Christoudias, G., Moon, I.P. et al. (1974). Peritoneovenous shunting for ascites. *Ann Surg*, **180**, 580–90.

224. Lorentzen, T., Sengelov, L., Nolsoe, C.P. *et al.* (1995). Ultrasonically guided insertion of a peritoneo-gastric shunt in patients with malignant ascites. *Acta Radiol*, **36**, 481–4.

225. Stehman, F.B. and Ehrlich, C.E. (1984). Peritoneo-cystic shunt for malignant ascites. *Gynecol Oncol*, **18**, 402–7.

226. Clara, R., Righi, D., Bortolini, M. *et al.* (2004). Role of different techniques for the placement of Denver peritoneovenous shunt (PVS) in malignant ascites. *Surg Laparosc Endosc Percutan Tech*, **14**, 222–5.

227. Edney, J.A., Hill, A., and Armstrong, D. (1989). Peritoneovenous shunts palliate malignant ascites. *Am J Surg*, **158**, 598–601.

228. Schumacher, D.L., Saclarides, T.J., and Staren, E.D. (1994). Peritoneovenous shunts for palliation of the patient with malignant ascites. *Ann Surg Oncol*, **1**, 378–81.

229. Helzberg, J.H. and Greenberger, N.J. (1985). Peritoneovenous shunts in malignant ascites. *Dig Dis Sci*, **30**, 1104–7.

230. Adam, R.A. and Adam, Y.G. (2004). Malignant ascites: Past, present, and future. *J Am Coll Surg*, **198**, 999–1011.

231. Zanon, C., Grosso, M., Apra, F. *et al.* (2002). Palliative treatment of malignant refractory ascites by positioning of Denver peritoneovenous shunt. *Tumori*, **88**, 123–7.

232. Holm, A., Halpern, N.B., and Aldrete, J.S. (1989). Peritoneovenous shunt for intractable ascites of hepatic, nephrogenic, and malignant causes. *Am J Surg*, **158**, 162–6.

233. Reinhold, R.B., Lokich, J.J., Tomashefski, J. *et al.* (1983). Management of malignant ascites with peritoneovenous shunting. *Am J Surg*, **145**, 455–7.

234. Scott-Coombes, D.M., Whawell, S.A., Vipond, M.N. *et al.* (1993). Fibrinolytic activity of ascites caused by alcoholic cirrhosis and peritoneal malignancy. *Gut*, **34**, 1120–2.

235. Tarin, D., Price, J.E., Kettlewell, M.G. *et al.* (1984). Mechanisms of human tumor metastasis studied in patients with peritoneovenous shunts. *Cancer Res*, **44**, 3584–92.

236. Schwartz, M.L., Swaim, W.R., and Vogel, S.B. (1979). Coagulopathy following peritoneovenous shunting. *Surgery*, **85**, 671–6.

237. Markey, W., Payne, J.A., and Straus, A. (1979). Hemorrhage from esophageal varices after placement of the LeVeen shunt. *Gastroenterology*, **77**, 341–3.

238. Qazi, R. and Savlov, E.D. (1982). Peritoneovenous shunt for palliation of malignant ascites. *Cancer*, **49**, 600–2.

239. Cheung, D.K. and Raaf, J.H. (1982). Selection of patients with malignant ascites for a peritoneovenous shunt. *Cancer*, **50**, 1204–9.

240. Bieligk, S.C., Calvo, B.F., and Coit, D.G. (2001). Peritoneovenous shunting for nongynecologic malignant ascites. *Cancer*, **91**, 1247–55.

241. Saab, S., Nieto, J.M., Lewis, S.K. *et al.* (2006). TIPS versus paracentesis for cirrhotic patients with refractory ascites. *Cochrane Database Syst Rev*, CD004889.

242. Mullen, K.D. (2007). Review of the final report of the 1998 Working Party on definition, nomenclature and diagnosis of hepatic encephalopathy. *Aliment Pharmacol Ther*, **25** (Suppl 1), 11–16.

243. Alexopoulou, A., Koskinas, J., Deutsch, M. *et al.* (2006). Acute liver failure as the initial manifestation of hepatic infiltration by a solid tumor: Report of 5 cases and review of the literature. *Tumori*, **92**, 354–7.

244. Cheung, T.K., Lai, C.L., Wong, B.C. *et al.* (2006). Clinical features, biochemical parameters, and virological profiles of patients with hepatocellular carcinoma in Hong Kong. *Aliment Pharmacol Ther*, **24**, 573–83.

245. Bustamante, J., Rimola, A., Ventura, P.J. *et al.* (1999). Prognostic significance of hepatic encephalopathy in patients with cirrhosis. *J Hepatol*, **30**, 890–5.

246. Ong, J.P., Aggarwal, A., Krieger, D. *et al.* (2003). Correlation between ammonia levels and the severity of hepatic encephalopathy. *Am J Med*, **114**, 188–93.

247. Odeh, M., Sabo, E., Srugo, I. *et al.* (2005). Relationship between tumor necrosis factor-alpha and ammonia in patients with hepatic encephalopathy due to chronic liver failure. *Ann Med*, **37**, 603–12.

248. Mas, A. (2006). Hepatic encephalopathy: From pathophysiology to treatment. *Digestion*, **73** (Suppl 1), 86–93.

249. Lockwood, A.H. (2002). Positron emission tomography in the study of hepatic encephalopathy. *Metab Brain Dis*, **17**, 431–5.

250. Ahboucha, S., Pomier-Layrargues, G., Mamer, O. *et al.* (2006). Increased levels of pregnenolone and its neuroactive metabolite allopregnanolone in autopsied brain tissue from cirrhotic patients who died in hepatic coma. *Neurochem Int*, **49**, 372–8.

251. Williams, R. (2007). Review article: bacterial flora and pathogenesis in hepatic encephalopathy. *Aliment Pharmacol Ther*, **25** (Suppl 1), 17–22.

252. Rose, C., Butterworth, R.F., Zayed, J. *et al.* (1999). Manganese deposition in basal ganglia structures results from both portal-systemic shunting and liver dysfunction. *Gastroenterology*, **117**, 640–4.

253. Jones, E.A. and Basile, A.S. (1998). Does ammonia contribute to increased GABA-ergic neurotransmission in liver failure? *Metab Brain Dis*, **13**, 351–60.

254. Blei, A.T. (2004). Infection, inflammation and hepatic encephalopathy, synergism redefined. *J Hepatol*, **40**, 327–30.

255. Sandford, N.L. and Saul, R.E. (1988). Assessment of hepatic encephalopathy with visual evoked potentials compared with conventional methods. *Hepatology*, **8**, 1094–8.

256. Hourmand-Ollivier, I., Piquet, M.A., Toudic, J.P. *et al.* (2006). Actigraphy: A new diagnostic tool for hepatic encephalopathy. *World J Gastroenterol*, **12**, 2243–4.

257. Cordoba, J., Cabrera, J., Lataif, L. *et al.* (1998). High prevalence of sleep disturbance in cirrhosis. *Hepatology*, **27**, 339–45.

258. Groeneweg, M., Quero, J.C., De, B., I *et al.* (1998). Subclinical hepatic encephalopathy impairs daily functioning. *Hepatology*, **28**, 45–9.

259. Nolte, W., Wiltfang, J., Schindler, C. *et al.* (1998). Portosystemic hepatic encephalopathy after transjugular intrahepatic portosystemic shunt in patients with cirrhosis: Clinical, laboratory, psychometric, and electroencephalographic investigations. *Hepatology*, **28**, 1215–25.

260. Quero, J.C., Hartmann, I.J., Meulstee, J. *et al.* (1996). The diagnosis of subclinical hepatic encephalopathy in patients with cirrhosis using neuropsychological tests and automated electroencephalogram analysis. *Hepatology*, **24**, 556–60.

261. Blei, A.T. and Cordoba, J. (2001). Hepatic Encephalopathy. *Am J Gastroenterol*, **96**, 1968–76.

262. Bass, N.M. (2007). Review article: The current pharmacological therapies for hepatic encephalopathy. *Aliment Pharmacol Ther*, **25** (Suppl 1), 23–31.

263. Als-Nielsen, B., Gluud, L.L., and Gluud, C. (2004). Nonabsorbable disaccharides for hepatic encephalopathy. *Cochrane Database Syst Rev*, CD003044.

264. Festi, D., Vestito, A., Mazzella, G. *et al.* (2006). Management of hepatic encephalopathy: Focus on antibiotic therapy. *Digestion*, **73** (Suppl 1), 94–101.

265. Huang, D.B. and DuPont, H.L. (2005). Rifaximin—A novel antimicrobial for enteric infections. *J Infect*, **50**, 97–106.

266. Lighthouse, J., Naito, Y., Helmy, A. *et al.* (2004). Endotoxinemia and benzodiazepine-like substances in compensated cirrhotic patients: A randomized study comparing the effect of rifaximine alone and in association with a symbiotic preparation. *Hepatol Res*, **28**, 155–60.

267. Garcia-Tsao, G. and Wiest, R. (2004). Gut microflora in the pathogenesis of the complications of cirrhosis. *Best Pract Res Clin Gastroenterol*, **18**, 353–72.

268. Als-Nielsen, B., Gluud, L.L., and Gluud, C. (2004). Benzodiazepine receptor antagonists for hepatic encephalopathy. *Cochrane Database Syst Rev*, CD002798.

269. Als-Nielsen, B., Gluud, L.L., and Gluud, C. (2004). Dopaminergic agonists for hepatic encephalopathy. *Cochrane Database Syst Rev*, CD003047.

270. Shawcross, D. and Jalan, R. (2005). Dispelling myths in the treatment of hepatic encephalopathy. *Lancet*, **365**, 431–3.

271. Liu, J.P., Gluud, L.L., Als-Nielsen, B. *et al.* (2004). Artificial and bioartificial support systems for liver failure. *Cochrane Database Syst Rev*, CD003628.

272. Sen, S., Davies, N.A., Mookerjee, R.P. *et al.* (2004). Pathophysiological effects of albumin dialysis in acute-on-chronic liver failure: A randomized controlled study. *Liver Transpl*, **10**, 1109–19.

10.3

Weight loss in palliative medicine

Contents

10.3.1 Classification and pathophysiology of the anorexia–cachexia syndrome

Florian Strasser

Introduction

Most of the patients with advancing, incurable illness experience an involuntary loss of body weight and of most often appetite, accompanied by fatigue and muscle weakness and psychological distress, involving also their loved ones. This clinical condition can be summarized as cachexia syndrome (CS) or wasting disease. It is a very frequent, but poorly recognized clinical problem[1,2]. In cancer, prospective epidemiology data suggest that many patients suffering from cachexia are not recognized[3]. In contrast to this neglect, another clinical problem is the overtreatment of cachexia by artificial nutrition (lacking in advanced cancer illness often achievable meaningful treatment goals)[4] and probably also by pharmacological anti-cachexia interventions (narrow and short effect of progestins and corticosteroids)[5].

The strong meaning of eating (e.g. eating = life, expressing love by eating, my daily bread give me today)[6], at least in patients with certain cultures and religious backgrounds[7], may contribute to pressure of patients and families to preserve the normal and associated eating-related distress[8]. It remains challenging not only for patients, but also professionals, to understand 'what is happening with me', given the complex pathogenesis of cachexia. Also it's a hard piece of work and maturation to achieve a new meaning and hope with less physical function and food[9].

In order to improve the treatment of the cachexia, development of a consensus on how to define and perform staging of cachexia seems appropriate. The 'old' classification of anorexia–cachexia syndrome, applying only weight loss and loss of appetite is recognized as not sufficient to guide clinical practice and trials. New insight into the complexity of cachexia calls for more complex interventions.

This chapter will provide an update on the evolving understanding of anorexia–cachexia, with a focus on patients with advanced cancer. It reviews the current definition, diagnosis, and classification, the mechanism involved in primary cachexia, the causes of secondary/starvational anorexia and cachexia, implications on clinical decision-making, and finally provides an outlook to future therapeutic strategies and clinical trial design.

Current definition, diagnosis, and classification of cachexia

The classification of cachexia/wasting diseases was recently revised in a consensus meeting, and further discussed[12], the primary definition was involuntary weight loss and as additional diagnostic criteria (three out of five) decreased muscle strength, decreased muscle mass, fatigue, anorexia, and biochemical alterations (C-reactive protein; haemoglobin; albumin). This proposal may support collaborative work independent of primary diagnosis (cancer, COPD, chronic heart disease etc.). For cancer cachexia, the value of fatigue may require reconsideration[10]. Currently an international consensus process focus on cancer cachexia has been undertaken involving academic cancer cachexia experts, supported by systematic reviews of the literature, on factors to classify cancer cachexia and on secondary causes for decreased oral nutritional intake in cancer patients[11]. This work is supported by the European Palliative Care Research Collaborative (EPCRC), validation of these diagnostic criteria (including cut-off values) and classification are ongoing.

Definition of cachexia

Cachexia is considered by most experts to consist of an involuntary, ongoing, loss of body weight, accompanied by other factors which most often, but not always, occur, such as anorexia, muscle strength decline, or inflammation[12].

The term cachexia is used for cancer or cardiac cachexia patients, in contrast to the term HIV-wasting disease. Nevertheless, the pathogenesis and manifestations of cachexia within these diseases overlap, even though variable characteristics of the complex metabolic, neuroendocrine, or anabolic modifications in the context of a most-often-present inflammatory state occur (Table 10.3.1.3, Fig. 10.3.1.1). The cachexias are described in a variety of diseases, such as cancer[13,14], acquired immunodeficiency syndrome (AIDS)[15], chronic heart[16], liver[17], or renal failure[18], chronic obstructive pulmonary disease (COPD)[19], cystic fibrosis[20], and chronic infections[21]. The term failure to thrive refers mainly to children's malnutrition caused by dietary, organic, and social factors[22], whereas the term sarcopenia is used to describe the loss of muscle mass and strength (with age)[23].

In cancer, recently the old term anorexia–cachexia syndrome is replaced by the term cancer cachexia and a work definition has been elaborated by a group of clinical cancer cachexia experts[24]:

> Cancer cachexia is a multifactorial syndrome defined by a negative protein and energy balance driven by a variable combination of reduced food intake and abnormal metabolism. A key defining feature is ongoing loss of skeletal muscle mass, which cannot be fully reversed by conventional nutritional support, leading to progressive functional impairment.

Diagnosis of cachexia

Cancer cachexia is diagnosed by weight loss greater than 5 per cent over the last 6 months. Weight loss should be ongoing in the last 1–2 months.

In patients with significant fluid retention, large tumour mass or obesity (BMI >30 kg/m²) significant muscle wasting may occur in the absence of weight loss. In such patients, a direct measure of muscularity is recommended.

In advanced cancer patients, concurrent (secondary) causes for simple starvation (e.g. decreased oral nutritional intake or loss of nutrients) seem to occur frequently (e.g. stomatitis, constipation, pain, dyspnoea, nausea, vomiting, wrong (to healthy) diet, cognitive impairment, frequent paracentesis) and need to be diagnosed separately.

Classification of cachexia

Stages

Increasingly, it is recognized that cachexia is a process or spectrum, rather than a state, ranging from pre-clinical cachexia, to the clinically typical ACS syndrome, to finally the late (irreversible) cachexia[25]. Not all patients will progress down the spectrum.

Patients with pre-clinical cachexia (or early cachexia) include patients with cancer who manifest early clinical and metabolic—inflammatory signs of cachexia—without the presence of significant involuntary weight loss. This definition was proposed in late 2008, and merits prospective validation in clinical care.

Patients with late (irreversible) cancer cachexia have advanced muscle wasting (with or without loss of fat). Patients have a low performance status and short life expectancy (< 3months). It is evident that the burden of artificial nutritional support would outweigh any potential benefit. Therapeutic interventions focus typically on alleviating the consequences/complications of cachexia, e.g. symptom control (appetite stimulation, nausea), eating-related distress of patients and families.

Like pre-clinical cachexia is late (irreversible), cachexia is a relatively new concept, but of high clinical significance. Currently a consensus process is performed among cachexia experts to finalize these definitions, which will then be prospectively evaluated, whether they influence and change practice.

Severity

The severity of cachexia can be classified according to depleted energy/protein stores (cumulative deficit from the past) compounded by the sequelae of ongoing loss (current negative energy and protein balance). Also, whether a severity score will influence clinical practice and clinical trial evaluation merits prospective studies.

Domains

To further characterize cancer patients with cachexia, key components that contribute to cachexia may be used. Patients present with most but not necessarily all key components.

The following key components seem of high value for clinical assessment:

- Anorexia/loss of appetite and decreased oral food intake, accompanied by lack of central drive to eat, taste and smell abnormalities, and early satiety.
- Presence of a catabolic drive, caused by active, progressive tumour and inflammation, often accompanied by hypogonadism (in men) and insulin resistance.
- Decreased muscle mass and reduced strength of upper limb and lower limb muscles, and of the diaphragm.
- Reduced physical, psychosocial, and social function.

Symptoms

In palliative care, patient-perceived symptoms are almost a gold standard to express suffering; in cachexia, assessment symptoms are of variable value. They encompass 'a family of distinct characters'. Whereas group A are symptoms, for which a cause of cachexia can be associated with (e.g. early satiety as a symptom of decreased gastrointestinal motility), in group C, symptoms occur frequently in cachexia, since they are typical consequences, but they are too unspecific to reflect a cause (e.g., in advanced cancer patients many other causes than cachexia exist for fatigue).

A Symptoms mirroring the pathogenesis of cachexia (causes).

Early satiety, appetite loss, no desire to eat, muscle weakness/asthenia.

B Symptoms and syndromes causing simple starvation (co-morbidities).

Pain, vomiting, dyspnoea.

C Symptoms reflecting the impact of cachexia (consequences).

Fatigue, eating-related distress.

Mechanisms of primary–metabolic anorexia–cachexia

Based on the concepts of definition, diagnosis, and classification of cachexia, the pathogenesis of the 'metabolic syndrome' anorexia–cachexia, or so-called primary anorexia–cachexia is discussed following the three big groups of:

A   Anorexia—food intake caused by neuro-hormonal eating dysregulation (the gut–brain axis).

B   Catabolism—inflammation (the muscle–liver axis).

C   Anabolic dysbalance with muscle loss (the brain–muscle axis).

A key cause for primary anorexia–cachexia syndrome seems to be a catabolic drive mediated by immune alterations including (pro-inflammatory) cytokines and tumour-derived factors, however, the debate is ongoing[26], whether cachexia/wasting can occur without inflammation and—vice-versa—without alterations in the anabolic hormonal environment.

In the different diseases leading to primary anorexia–cachexia (Table 10.3.1.3) these mechanisms and causative factors might be observed, but with variable relative contribution. In patients with advanced cancer, for example, active cancer cells and their interactions with the host cause several overlapping syndromes of

Table 10.3.1.1 Secondary anorexia and secondary cachexia.

A) Starvation: secondary anorexia

Impaired oral intake

- Stomatitis, taste alterations, zinc deficiency
- Dry mouth (xerostomia), dehydration
- Dysphagia, odynophagia
- Gastro-oesophageal reflux, peptic disturbances
- Severe constipation, fear of faecal incontinence
- Bowel obstruction
- Autonomic failure
- Nausea, vomiting
- Severe symptoms such as pain, dyspnoea, or depression
- Cognitive impairment / delirium
- Social and financial obstacles
- Wrong diet ('too healthy')

Impaired gastrointestinal absorption

- Malabsorption
- Exocrine pancreatic insufficiency
- Chronic severe diarrhoea

B) Loss of muscle mass and of proteins: secondary cachexia

- Prolonged inactivity (bed rest, microgravity), deconditioning
- Hypogonadism, growth hormone deficiency
- Prolonged corticosteroid treatment
- Aging, sarcopenia
- Frequent drainage of ascites or pleural fluid punctions
- Nephrotic syndrome

C) Catabolic states and co-morbidities associated with cachexia

- Chronic and acute infections
- Treatment with pro-inflammatory cytokines
- Chronic heart failure (cardiac cachexia), severe lung disease, or renal failure
- Poorly controlled diabetes mellitus, liver cirrhosis
- Hyperthyroidism

anorexia–cachexia. Both hypermetabolism with metabolic alterations in the 'muscle–liver axis' (adapted term as proposed by Argiles, et al.[27] are present, as well as neuroendocrine alterations in the 'gut–brain axis' (term as proposed by Meguid, et al.[28]). However, research from other wasting conditions, such as cardiac cachexia or AIDS-wasting, has highlighted the role of the family of growth hormones and anabolic hormones. This 'endocrine-muscle/somatotropic axis' is of growing interest for cancer anorexia–cachexia syndrome. The immune alterations causing primary anorexia–cachexia syndrome are complex and involve systemic effects, which may be measurable in the blood, but in addition to predominantly local effects, including the brain and muscles (Fig. 10.3.1.3).

Anorexia—food intake caused by neuro-hormonal eating dysregulation (the gut–brain axis)

Food intake and consequently energy homeostasis is regulated by a highly complex process involving taste sensation, neural and humoral signals from the gastrointestinal tract, and neurotransmitters and peptides in the hypothalamus or other brain regions[29] (Fig. 10.3.1.2).

Satiety and adiposity signals from the periphery to the brain

Satiety signals from the upper gastrointestinal tract, the liver, and mediated by peptides, such as cholecystokinin (CCK), are transmitted through the vagus nerve and sympathetic fibres as well as the bloodstream to the autonomic centres of the hindbrain and possibly to the forebrain. The vagal nerve transmits meal-related signals (mechanical, chemical, hormonal) elicited by nutrient contact with the gastrointestinal tract to sites in the central nervous system that mediate ingestive behaviour[30]. The vagus nerve seems to be important as well to mediate anorexic effects of some[31], but not all[32], proinflammatory cytokines produced in the peritoneum.

Ghrelin is a recently discovered hormone produced predominantly by the stomach, and smaller amounts are formed in the bowel, pituitary, and hypothalamus[33]. Ghrelin has adipogenic and orexigenic effects, which are independent of its ability to stimulate growth hormone secretion[34]. Chronic administration of ghrelin was reported to improve left ventricular dysfunction and attenuates development of cardiac cachexia in rats with heart failure[35]. Ghrelin was found to have gastroprokinetic activity, as well as orexigenic activity through action on the hypothalamic neuropeptide Y receptor, which was lost after vagotomy[36]. Ghrelin expression in the stomach was found to be increased by fasting but decreased by administration of leptin, as well as by interleukin-1beta. Morning fasting levels of ghrelin in animals[37] or patients[38] with ACS are still poorly understood, both higher and lower ghrelin levels than controls are reported, differences in BMIs may explain the findings only partially. Ghrelin application (intravenous or subcutaneous) was reported to be safe and tolerable and preliminary data suggests its ability to stimulate orexigenic, prokinetic, and GH-releasing effects in patients with cachexia[39,40,41].

Peripheral adiposity signals are provided by leptin[42] (secreted by adipocytes) and insulin (secreted by the endocrine pancreas in proportion to adiposity). They are proposed to stimulate catabolic pathways (mediated by melanocortins) and inhibit anabolic pathways (neuropeptide-Y, agouti-related protein). They can act in the gastrointestinal tract[43] as well as centrally.

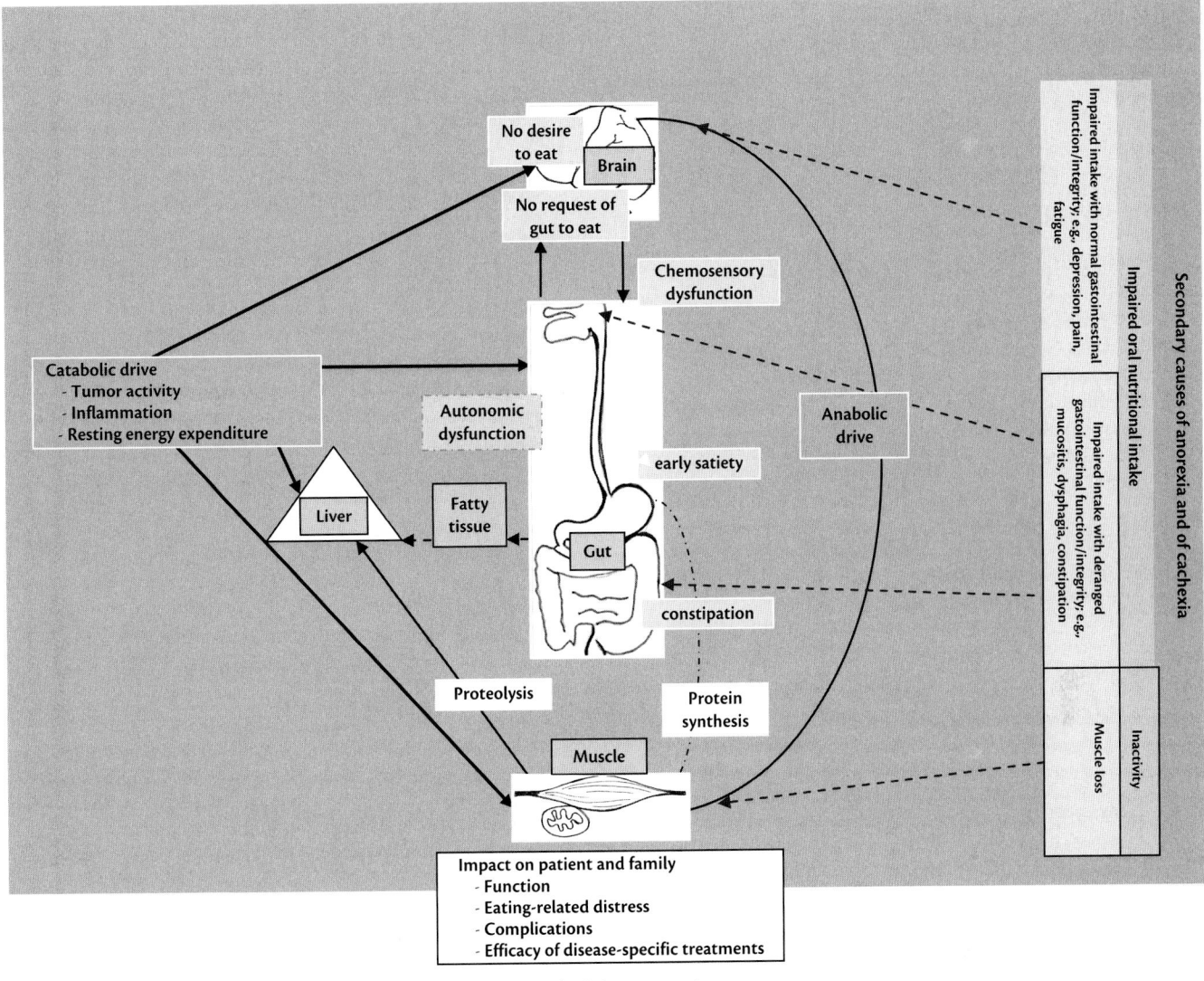

Figure 10.3.1.1 Main elements of the pathogenesis of primary anorexia–cachexia in cancer patients.

Hypothalamus and central nervous system control of food intake

In the hypothalamus, several neuropeptide-containing pathways mediating leptin and insulin action are under investigation[44].

Neuropeptide-Y (NPY) is an anabolic signalling molecule. NPY expression is stimulated by falls in circulating concentrations of insulin and leptin, both of which inhibit the hypothalamic NPY neurons[45]. NPY is expressed in a subset of hypothalamic neurons, which express leptin receptors (OB-Rb) too. Increased hypothalamic NPY expression is reported in underfed and insulin-deficient diabetic rats, suggesting a role in stimulating hunger and hyperphagia. However, mice lacking NPY have been found with intact feeding responses to leptin[46]. A recent study with cachectic (weight loss of 19 per cent compared to pair-fed controls) MAC16-tumour-bearing rats reported a normal regulation of leptin (decreased concentration in relation to loss of fat tissue, up-regulation of hypothalamic OB-Rb mRNA), insulin (reduction in both groups), and NPY (increase of hypothalamic NPY mRNA)[47]. These results suggest that in anorexia–cachexia related to cancer, a normal hypothalamic hyperphagic response to weight loss is overridden, maybe by mechanisms that interfere with NPY transport or release and/or neuronal targets downstream of NPY.

Several other neuropeptides promoting increased energy intake (orexigenic), such as Agouti-related protein (AGRP), melanin-concentrating hormone (MCH) or orexin A/B, and probably galanin and noradrenaline, are involved. The anorexigenic neuropeptides entail α-melanocyte-stimulating hormone (αMSH), corticotropin-releasing hormone (CRH), thyrotropin-releasing hormone (TRH), interleukin-1β (IL-1b), cocaine- or amphetamine-regulated transcript (CART), and probably serotonin, glucagon-like peptide 1, neurotensin, urocortin, and others[44]. Levels of free tryptophan, a precursor of serotonin, has been found to correlate with reduced food intake in cancer patients[48].

Leptin

Leptin has not been found to change the incorporation of amino acids in the skeletal muscle *in vitro* or increase skeletal muscle protein degradation[49]. Prolonged leptin treatment selectively reduces adipose tissue stores while the muscle mass remains unaffected[50]. It is possible, that a deficiency in leptin could contribute to immune dysfunction[51]. TNF-α has been shown to directly regulate leptin secretion of adipocytes in vitro, providing cytokine-induced hyperleptinaemia[52]. However, the opposite findings are reported too[53]. Leptin levels are increased in some

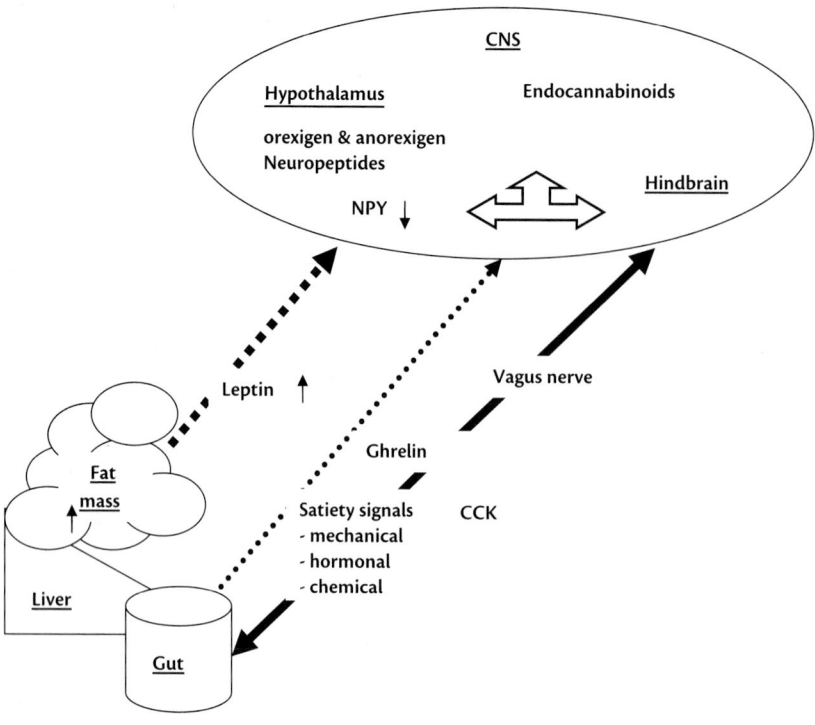

CNS—central nervous system; NPY—neuropeptide Y; CCK—cholecystokinine.

Figure 10.3.1.2 Aspects of neurohoromonal regulation of food intake.
CNS—central nervous system; NPY—neuropeptide Y; CCK—cholecystokinine.

models of inflammation[54,55]. In patients undergoing elective surgery, a positive correlation was reported for acute-phase response and plasma leptin[56]. However, in patients with cancer–related anorexia–cachexia, the leptin concentrations seem to be decreased, rather than increased, in comparison to healthy controls[57,58]. In 73 patients with 'incurable' cancer and more than 50 per cent decline in appetite during the last 2 months, lower values of NPY were found than from historic controls, but no difference in leptin or cholecystokinin-8 levels[59].

Endocannabinoid system

Cannabinoid receptor type 1 (CB1) receptor knockout mice eat less than their wild-type littermates, and the CB1 antagonist SR141716A reduces food intake in wild-type but not knockout mice. Defective leptin signalling is associated with elevated hypothalamic, but not cerebellar, levels of endocannabinoids (in obese db/db and ob/ob mice and Zucker rats) and acute leptin treatment of normal rats and ob/ob mice reduces anandamide and 2-arachidonoyl glycerol in the hypothalamus. These findings may indicate that endocannabinoids in the hypothalamus can tonically activate CB1 receptors to maintain food intake and form part of the neural circuitry regulated by leptin[60]. The endocannabinoid system was found to play a vital role in milk suckling, and hence in growth and development during the early stages of mouse life. The endocannabinoid 2-arachidonoyl glycerol is found in human milk. The administration of the CB1 antagonist SR141716A to newborn mice resulted in death within a week. This effect was reversed by feeding the mice Δ-9-THC, which binds to CB1 receptors, but not by cannabidinol, which binds to the CB2 receptor[61].

Melanocortin signalling system

The central melanocortin signalling system was found to remain active in cachectic tumour-bearing rats, despite marked loss of body weight. This system would be expected to be down-regulated to conserve energy stores. The intracerebroventricular injection of SHU9119, a melanocortin receptor antagonist, was found to increase food intake and promote weight gain in cachectic tumour-bearing rats, but not in their pair-fed controls. Interestingly, intracerebroventricular injection of both ghrelin and NPY did not improve oral intake or result in weight gain[62]. Various mixed and selective non-peptide antagonists (and inverse agonists) with high affinity and selectivity for melanocortin MC4 receptors achieved improved appetite and body mass in animals[63,64], clinical trials are currently considered.

Autonomic failure

Change in autonomic nerve function, called autonomic failure, may contribute to ACS. In 43 patients with advanced (locally recurrent or metastatic) breast cancer, 52 per cent of cardiovascular autonomic insufficiency tests were abnormal, in contrast to healthy controls (20 patients) with 7 per cent abnormal tests. In cancer patients, abnormal tests were correlated with decreased performance status, malnutrition, and increased basal heart rate[65]. In five patients with advanced breast, thyroid, and prostate cancer, complaining of unexplained chronic nausea and anorexia, an increased mean gastric emptying time in association with abnormal cardiovascular autonomic tests were reported[66]. These results of pathological ewing tests (valsalva, breathing, posture) in cancer patients were confirmed by two other studies[67,68].

Table 10.3.1.2 Alterations in primary anorexia–cachexia[a] compared to starvation.

	Primary anorexia–cachexia[a]	Starvation
Energy expenditure (per kg lean body mass)	⇑	⇓
Protein synthesis:		
◆ Overall	⇑	⇓
◆ Muscle proteins	⇓	⇓
◆ Acute-phase proteins	⇑	⇔
Proteolysis		
◆ Muscle proteins	⇑⇑	⇑
Lipogenesis	⇓	⇓
Lipolysis	⇑	⇑⇑
Glucose turnover	⇑	⇓
Ketone bodies	⇓	⇑
Hormones:		
◆ Leptin	⇔⇓	⇓
◆ Neuropeptide Y	⇔⇑	⇑
◆ Ghrelin	⇔⇑	⇑
◆ Testosterone	⇔⇓	⇓
◆ Growth hormone / IGF-1	⇔⇓	⇓
◆ Thyroxine (T4)	⇔	⇓
◆ Cortisol	⇑	⇓

Note: [a] Primary anorexia–cachexia refers mainly to cancer-related ACS.

Several of the symptoms of autonomic disorders, which are briefly discussed in the following paragraphs, are present in patients with advanced cancer: orthostatic abnormalities (postural hypotension), male sexual dysfunction, urinary incontinence, gastrointestinal symptoms (gastroparesis, pseudo-bowel obstruction, diarrhoea, constipation), and sleep dysfunction, suggesting a potential role of autonomic disorders in patients with advanced cancer.

The autonomic nervous system, through the sympathetic and parasympathetic pathways, supplies and influences every organ in the body. It closely integrates vital processes, such as blood pressure and body temperature[69]. Autonomic disorders are an increasingly recognized group of diseases, which may be localized (e.g., Horner's syndrome, Holmes–Adie pupil), or systemic. Three groups of systemic primary dysautonomia (pure autonomic failure, Parkinson's disease with autonomic failure, multiple-system atrophy [including Shy–Drager syndrome with pure orthostatic hypotension]) have been defined[70].

The symptoms of autonomic disorders have been proposed to be grouped in nine domains: (1) orthostatic; (2) secretomotor including sudomotor; (3) male sexual dysfunction; (4) urinary; (5) gastrointestinal including gastroparesis, diarrhoea, constipation; (6) pupillomotor, including visual symptoms; (7) vasomotor; (8) reflex syncope; and (9) sleep function[71].

Several gastrointestinal diseases may be linked to autonomic disorders. Primary enteric neuropathies may cause gastrointestinal motor dysfunction[72]. Idiopathic slow transit constipation has been hypothesized to be a consequence of pelvic autonomic dysfunction. Altered autonomic function has been involved as well in patients with gastro-oesophageal reflux disease, as well as functional disorders, such as irritable bowel syndrome or functional dyspepsia.

Secondary forms of autonomic disorders may include autonomic neuropathy secondary to neurotoxic treatments, or as a consequence of degenerative neuropathies associated with diabetes mellitus or amyloidosis[73]. Tumour-invasion of the sympathetic ganglia can result in pseudo-obstruction. Spinal cord pathology may also cause autonomic neuropathy. Gastrointestinal forms of a paraneoplastic neurological syndrome (such as polymyositis, Eaton–Lambert syndrome, etc.) may represent secondary autonomic failure. Paraneoplastic gastrointestinal motor dysfunction can precede diagnosis of the cancer by many months[74].

Significance of neuro-horomonal eating-dysregulation for clinical care and clinical research

Symptoms associated with the gut–brain axis are lack of hunger, taste and smell abnormalities, and profound early satiety. All of these symptoms should be considered as important indicators in the assessment and classification of cancer/cachexia. Therapeutic interventions currently focus on prokinetic agents have shown limited effectiveness: clinical research and currently explorative research on the effect of ghrelin (phase II clinical studies) and melanocortin-antagonists are ongoing (pre-clinical studies)[75].

Catabolism—inflammation (the muscle–liver axis)

In patients with primary ACS, an activation of the metabolism is observed, which evades normal regulatory mechanism. Simplified, it looks like that the muscles and other systems are obliged to provide all their energy to the liver[27] (Table 10.3.1.4).

Feeding, without modification of the complex metabolic alterations, was reported to increase only the synthesis of muscle protein without influencing proteolysis[76], and to accelerate the acute phase protein synthesis while not influencing albumin synthesis[77].

Energy balance and metabolism

The reports about increased energy expenditure (EE) in patients with ACS are heterogenous. Reasons for conflicting results may include: (1) differences of resting EE and total EE, influenced by physical activity; (2) variable methods of measuring EE (bicarbonate-urea, or whole-body indirect calorimetry); (3) unclear data about energy costs of feeding; (4) heterogeneous patient populations; and (5) calculating EE in relation to body weight rather than lean body mass. However, more precise approaches to measurement demonstrated that the energy expenditure [78] in relation to lean body mass is indeed increased in cancer anorexia–cachexia[79]. This hypermetabolic state is followed by a pre-terminal hypometabolism.

Carbohydrate metabolism

The glucose turnover is increased, including both the rates of hepatic gluconeogenesis[80] and the activity of futile cycles, such as recycling via lactate (Cori cycle)[81]. The insulin secretory response is delayed in ACS without a major difference in overall magnitude. This results in a delayed clearance of glucose. A relative glucose intolerance and insulin resistance is present with a decreased muscle insulin-stimulated glucose uptake. This is most likely

Table 10.3.1.3 Cachexia/wasting in different diseases.

	Clinical manifestation		Mechanism mediating the anorexia–cachexia syndrome			
	Weight loss	Anorexia	Metabolism	Neurohormonal	Anabolic hormones	Pro-inflamm. cytokines
Cancer (Cancer ACS)	+++	++	+++	++	+	+++
AIDS (HIV-wasting)	+++	+	++	++	+++	+++
Chronic heart failure (Cardiac cachexia)	++	+	+	++	++	++
Chronic renal failure (Renal cachexia)	++	+	+	+	++	++
Elderly patients (Sarcopoenia)	++	(+)	-	+	++	(+)

a result of impaired insulin responsiveness, rather than an abnormal insulin sensitivity, suggesting a post-receptor defect in insulin action[82–84]. The anabolic effects of insulin on skeletal muscle are abolished during inflammation[85] or infusion of TNF-α, indicating an insulin resistance regarding protein synthesis. A recent study in cancer patients suggests a role of insulin treatment in cachexia[86]. In addition, increases in counter-regulatory hormones, such as glucagon or glucocorticoids, seem to be involved too[81]. The concentration of ketone bodies, which seem to inhibit muscle proteolysis in starvation, is decreased through impaired ketogenesis and increased peripheral uptake. However, in patients with chronic heart failure, blood ketone bodies are elevated in proportion to the severity of cardiac dysfunction and neurohormonal activation (noradrenaline, growth hormone, interleukin-6)[87].

Lipid metabolism

In adipose tissue during primary ACS the glucose transport and *de novo* lipogenesis are inhibited and lipolysis activated[88]. In contrast, in the liver lipogenesis is increased, and hypertriglyceridaemia is present. Carnitine is involved in transporting long-chain fatty acids into the mitochondrial matrix. In tumour-bearing rats, the hepatic mitochondrial outer membrane carnitine palmitoyltransferase I (CPT I) was reported to be unaffected by the presence of the extra-hepatic tumour, whereas the mitochondrial inner-membrane carnitine palmitoyltransferase II (CPT II) activity was markedly decreased[89]. Preliminary reports suggest decreased carnitine levels[90] and beneficial effects of its replacement[91,92] in cancer cachexia; clinical trials are ongoing.

During cachectic states an increase in brown adipose tissue thermogenesis is reported. The uncoupling protein-1 (UCP-1) or thermogenin, uncouples oxidative phosphorylation in the mitochondrial compartment leading to energy released as heat rather than used for ATP-synthesis. The recently described UCP-2 and UCP-3 are elevated in skeletal muscle during tumour growth[93].

Protein metabolism

Whole-body protein turnover is increased in cachexia in association with progressive disease[94]. Protein synthesis shifts from normal muscle protein and other tissue protein synthesis to increased hepatic protein synthesis. The muscle fibrillar synthesis and the overall muscle amino acid uptake are reduced. A down-regulation of the MyoD mRNA[95] and of myosin, but not actin, synthesis[96]

were reported. DNA fragmentation is increased suggesting apoptosis[97]. The proteolysis of myofibrils is increased, provided mostly by the activated ATP-ubiquitine-proteasome system[98]. The two other proteolytic pathways (lysosomal cathepsins, calpains), are not up-regulated, rather than decreased[99]. The ATP-ubiquitine-proteasome system seems to be a common final pathway, with probably involvement of a lipoxygenase metabolite, both for muscle loss in starvation, aging, and cachexia[100,101]. The liver-protein synthesis is reprioritized with increased production of acute phase proteins (serum-amyloid A, C-reactive protein, haptoglobin, fibrinogen, among others), but decreased albumin synthesis[102]. The presence of acute phase protein reaction correlates with survival in cancer patients[103]. The circulating amino acid pattern changes in catabolic conditions[27]. The turnover of branched-chain amino acids (leucine, isoleucine, valine), which are normally poorly metabolized in the liver, but well in the muscle, is increased. The muscle increases the production of alanine and glutamine. Alanine is an alternative glycolytic end product to lactate for safe transport of 3C-ketoacids to the liver. The turnover of glutamine increases in order to provide a major source for energy as well as for nucleic acid synthesis, but for storage of nitrogen as an alternative to ammonia too[104].

Several of the described metabolic abnormalities in cancer patients such as increased energy expenditure[105] and insulin

Table 10.3.1.4 Inter-relationship between skeletal muscle and liver in ACS.

Muscle		Liver	
Proteolysis	⇑	Acute-phase protein synthesis	⇑
Glucagon: synthesis	⇑	Alanine and glucagon uptake	⇑
Alanine: synthesis	⇑	(liver unable to process BCAA)	
BCAA: uptake	⇑	Very-low densitiy lipoproteins	⇑
Muscle-protein synthesis	⇓		
Lactate: production	⇑		
Ketone bodies utilization	⇓		

Note: BCAA=branched-chained amino acids (leucine, isoleucine, valine).

resistance[106], are also reported in patients with AIDS and or cardiac desease.

Pro-inflammatory cytokines

Countless studies implicate cytokines in the pathogenesis of primary ACS in several diseases[107,108]. For example, in patients with lung cancer, a correlation of weight loss and height-adjusted lean body mass with sTNFR-p55 and sTNFR-p75 (soluble tumour necrosis factor receptors of molecular masses 55 and 75 kDa), but not with IL-6, was found[166]. In patients with non-small-cell lung cancer, a positive correlation between sTNF-55 and resting energy expenditure was shown[109]. A correlation between increased serum IL-6 and weight loss was found in patients with non-small-cell lung cancer[110]. Other examples are patients with chronic heart failure, in whom increased TNF-α levels were associated with exercise intolerance and neurohormonal (catecholamine) activation[111], as well as geriatric patients for which a correlation between the reduction of cytokine levels (TNFR-p55, TNFR-p75, sIL-2R, IL-6) after megestrol acetate treatment and fat-free mass was reported[112]. However, the relative role of pro-inflammatory cytokines in the pathogenesis of primary ACS may be different in the various diseases, with variable alterations of the three main mechanisms (axis).

Acute phase response as a physiological mechanism

Several of the clinical and metabolic features of the ACS may resemble a sustained, or protracted acute phase response. The acute phase response is a physiological reaction of adult mammals towards tissue damage or infection. It involves a variety of rapid systemic changes including a profound change in the synthesis of plasma proteins, hypermetabolism, fever, chills, somnolence, and anorexia. The acute phase response is mediated by pro-inflammatory cytokines, such as interleukin-6 (IL-6), interleukin-1 (IL-1), as well as tumour necrosis factor (TNF-α), interferon- γ (IFN-γ), or leukaemia inhibitory factor (LIF). The role of T-cell helper 1 and helper 2 subsets remains to be elucidated in primary ACS.

Pro-inflammatory cytokines mimic features of primary ACS

TNF-α administration can promote weight loss, increased energy expenditure, anorexia, acute phase protein response, increased thermogenesis, alterations in lipid metabolism and adipose tissue dissolution, insulin resistance, muscle wasting including activation of the ATP-dependent ubiquitin-proteasome pathway, inhibition of the myogenic differentiation, protein breakdown, and increased branched-chain amino acid metabolism. In tumour-bearing mice, a soluble pegylated 55-kDA TNF-α receptor construct improved food intake and led to weight gain compared to a vehicle treated control group[113]. In contrast, in rats bearing the Yoshida AH-130 acites hepatoma, treatment with goat anti-mTNF-α IgG did not affect weight loss but decreased protein degradation rates in heart, liver, and gastrocnemius muscle[114].

IL-6 is an inductor of the acute phase response, but seems to have few effects on TNF-α[115]. Whether IL-6 directly causes muscle catabolism or an induction of weight loss is controversial. Some groups found an involvement of IL-6 in experimental cachexia[116], whereas others found, that IL-6 did not cause weight loss in normal mice, but was associated with an increased acute phase protein production[117]. In mice bearing the colon-26 adenocarcinoma, serum IL-6 was associated with progression of cachexia, and administration of anti-IL-6 immunoglobulin reduced

the loss of gastrocnemius muscle[118]. The role of IL-6 may therefore be an epiphenomenon of the host cytokine cascade, mediating increased acute phase protein production, rather than being the key element in mediating muscle wasting and cachexia. However, blood levels of IL-6 [119] or of acute-phase proteins[103] in patients with anorexia–cachexia correlate with weight loss and survival.

IFN-γ and IL-1 were found to have procachectic activity, including the activation of muscle proteolysis[120]. In 64 patients with pancreatic adenocarcinoma and 101 healthy controls, it was observed that the possession of a genotype resulting in increased IL-1b production was associated with shortened survival and increased serum CRP level[121].

In vivo data from cytokine gene knockout mice showed that weight loss from implanted experimental tumours was not improved by knockout of the host cytokines TNF-α, IL-12 or IFN-γ, but that the host cytokine IL-6 could play a role in promoting an acute phase response. These data may suggest that these host cytokines could be less important in promoting primary ACS than tumour-derived factors[122].

Limitations of blood levels to assess cytokine effects

Systemic blood levels of cytokines only partially reflect their local effects. Paracrine–autocrine interactions within organs can sustain cytokine production independently of cytokine concentrations in the circulation. Besides, the systemic effects of pro-inflammatory cytokines during an acute phase response, their locally mediated effects are increasingly recognized, such as up-regulation of cytokine-receptors of muscle cells or central nervous system effects of cytokines, as discussed in the following paragraphs.

This may explain why the association of increased TNF-α levels in the blood of cancer patients with primary ACS is not consistent: some studies report a correlation of TNF-α with weight loss[123,124], while others do not[125,126]. Technical problems in measuring TNF-α and other cytokines may explain some of these inconsistent results, soluble TNF-α receptors (sTNF-R55&75) may be monitored instead[109,166]. The clinical value of measuring cytokines in patient's blood is questioned[127]. Instead, C-reactive protein seems a widely accepted marker of acute-phase response[24,107,128], also albumin might reflect more the acute phase response than nutritional status.

Local cytokine effects in the brain

The central-nervous effects of peripherally administered cytokines (IL-2, interferon-α, TNF-α) are well-known side effects of these treatments. Peripheral inflammatory responses, such as those caused by infections or cytokine administration, are associated with increased brain cytokine synthesis and release[129]. The phenomenon of anorexia, as observed during anorexia–cachexia, may be therefore directly related to peripheral cytokines acting in the brain. Besides systemic effects of cytokines on the brain, local cytokine effects have been shown in animal models. For example, athymic mice were injected intra-cerebrally with human A431 epidermoid carcinoma or OVCAR3 ovarian carcinoma and developed anorexia and weight loss within 7–10 days before a large tumour developed[130]. In contrast, mice injected intra-peritoneally or subcutaneously developed tumours without evidence of anorexia. Likewise, intra-cerebral injected GBLF glioma cells, used as a control, did not induce cachexia until day 20, when the tumour was large. Measurement of cytokines in the brain revealed that the carcinoma cells produced (human) cytokines, such as IL-1, IL-6, TNF-α, and LIF. Of the brain cytokines originating from the host (murine), only IL-6 was increased in the A431-bearing mice. The described effects occurred exclusively locally in the brain, since serum levels of both murine (host) and human (tumour) cytokines were not predictive of cancer cachexia development.

Cytokines and muscle

Diverse aspects of skeletal muscle function are regulated by pro-inflammatory cytokines. For example, it has been shown that TNF-α, which activates NF-κB: (1) prevented immature myoblasts from differentiating into major myotubes; (2) suppressed differentiated myotubes from synthesizing myosin; and (3) inhibited the synthesis of mRNA encoding the myogenenic transcription factor, myo-D, in muscle[95]. The muscle cytokine receptors mediating these functions have recently been characterized. Skeletal muscle of rats was found to express low levels of mRNAs encoding receptors for IL-1, IL-6, interferon, and TNF-α. These cytokine receptors were induced by intra-peritoneal administration of both endotoxin and TNF-α[131]. The capacity of the muscle for receptor induction provides, therefore. a mechanism for amplification of cytokine responses at the muscle level.

The recently discovered naturally occurring interleukin-15, which has 'IL-2-like' stimulatory activity on T cells, was reported to exert a preventative effect on muscle protein wasting in animal models[132], illuminating further the complexity of the cytokine–muscle interactions[27].

Corticosteroids

The role of cortisol in propagation of ACS is suspected, but not well documented. Elevated levels of cortisone and glucagon have been shown in patients with cancer[133]. However, in 20 patients with lung cancer, no association between loss of lean body mass and cortisol, but with systemic signs of inflammation or infection was reported[166]. Patients with COPD experience increased weight loss during corticosteroid treatment. Infusion of cortisol can cause protein loss, acute phase protein response, increased energy expenditure and glucose intolerance. Cytokines can trigger circulating cortisol levels and induce proteolysis. *In vivo* data from a mice model failed to show an improvement in weight loss after treatment with mifepristone/RU486, an anti-cortisol medication[134].

Tumour-derived catabolic factors

Effective antineoplastic treatments obviously not only shrink (or eliminate) the tumour, but as well improve tumour-related morbidity. Indeed, there is a growing body of literature documenting the symptomatic effect of antineoplastic treatments besides the 'classical' oncological outcome measurements (such as response rate, survival, time to progression), around the concepts of clinical benefit[135]. For several paraneoplastic phenomena tumour-derived products have been identified and their specific effects were demonstrated. A decade ago, tumour-derived products mediating anorexia–cachexia have been experimentally characterized[136], and many studies support the indeed important concept. However, until today, in humans, no clinical test is available for routine diagnosis of PIF-levels to monitor cachexia management[137], nor are clinical data applying experimental tests convincing[138].

Proteolysis-inducing factor (PIF)

PIF is a sulphated glyco-protein, which was associated with an accelerated rate of weight loss in patients with tumours of the pancreatic head, in comparison to patients, where PIF was not detectable in urine, who had less weight loss[139]. Another research group demonstrated the expression of PIF on tumour tissue from gastrointestinal cancers and has also found detectable PIF in urine associated with weight-loss[140]. Initially PIF, which is a 24-kD material, was believed to be a lipid-mobilizing factor[141], but this is now not thought to be the case[142].

PIF initiates directly muscle protein degradation, through activation of ATP-ubiquitin-dependent proteolysis[143], and decreases protein synthesis[144]. These direct effects of PIF inducing protein as well as muscle catabolism *in vitro* (rat model of cachexia) were found to follow a bell-shaped dose–response with a decrease of effect at higher doses of PIF and tumour burden, respectively. The rapid weight loss caused by PIF was found to be associated with a significant decrease in the weight of the spleen and soleus and gastrocnemius muscle, but with no effect on the weight of the heart or kidney[145]. The earlier described effects were found to be reversible by treatment with specific antibodies against PIF[146].

The exact site of PIF-induced protein degradation is under investigation. PIF induces an accumulation of ubiquitine protein conjugates in weight-losing mice[144]. PIF induces (*in vitro* data from C_2C_{12} myoblasts) an increased release of arachidonic acid as well with a dose–response curve parallel to that of protein degradation[144], and arachidonic acid was shown to be rapidly metabolized to prostaglandins E_2, $F_2\alpha$, and 15-HETE (hydroxyeicosatetraaenoic acid). The role of in mediating cachexia remains unclear. Indeed, it was suggested, that prostaglandins cause increased protein degradation of extremity muscles. In contrast, direct examination of prostaglandin E_2, both in normal and septic rats, revealed that PG_2 did not inhibit the proteolytic rate (which would lead also to protein degradation of muscles)[143]. Since 15-HETE produced *in vitro* a significant increase in protein degradation with the same bell-shaped dose curve as that produced by PIF, it has been suggested that the effect of PIF could be mediated by an increased synthesis of 15-HETE[144,145].

Substantial binding of PIF is reported only for skeletal muscle and liver, as cited by Cabal-Manzano R *et al.*[140]. In hepatocyte cultures, PIF was found to activate NF-κB resulting in increased IL-8 and IL-6 production, as well as the STAT3 pathway, which is involved in the acute phase protein response[147]. However, in clinical studies, PIF expression and the association with weight loss were found to be independent of the acute phase response[136].

Lipid-mobilizing factor (LMF)

LMF has been demonstrated in the serum and urine of cachetic cancer patients, which caused the immediate release of glycerol when intubated with epididymal adipodicytes. LMF was also found to correlate with the extent of weight loss as well as with the response to chemotherapy[139,141]. LMF, a 43-kD protein, is believed to counteract the two major mechanisms proposed to account for the decrease in body lipids in cancer cachexia, mainly the inhibition of the clearing enzyme lipoprotein lipase, which prevents adipocytes from extracting fatty acids from plasma lipoproteins for storage, as well as the direct stimulation of triglyceride hydrolysis in adipocytes by activation of triglyceride lipase. LMF was reported to induce lipolysis in white adipose tissue by stimulation of cAMP production, mediated possibly through a β-adrenergic receptor[148].

Parathyroid-hormone-related protein (PTHrP)

The plasma levels of TNF-α, IL-5, IL-8, IL-6 were higher in 24 patients with advanced cancer and elevated PTHrP compared to 26 cancer patients with normal PTHrP. PTHrP was found to correlate with blood levels of IL-6 and TNF-α. Anti-PTHrP monoclonal antibodies (Mabs) improved hypercalcemia and the author suggested, that in comparison to the effects of bisphosphonates and calcitonin, the Mab had an effect as well on symptoms (food intake, drinking, weight, behaviour) unrelated to hypercalcaemia[149]. PTHrP may therefore be seen as another tumour-derived procachectic factor.

Significance of catabolism: inflammation for clinical care and clinical research

From the biological markers discussed earlier, currently only C-reactive protein is considered to become part of a new classification system of cachexia. For all other biological markers associated with catabolism and inflammation, the clinical use remains to be determined and is considered experimental. Clinical trials of inflammatory-dominant cachexia applying a CRP-guided dose-escalation arm are currently considered.

For the muscle–liver axis, a typical phenomenon is the presence of inflammation, evident by clinical signs and/or laboratory markers, namely elevated C-reactive protein (in the absence of infection). For the understanding of the cachexia mechanisms, the metabolic–catabolic alterations are important, namely, to explain patients and family members 'what's happening'. The compassionate educational intervention emphasizing the 'broken fabric' to produce muscle proteins from food intake is based on the pathogenetic concepts discussed here, namely PIF and insulin resistance. However, after a decade of research, the proteolysis-inducing factor or LMF still did not enter diagnostic routine neither in clinical care nor clinical research, even though its mechanism is important for understanding and counseling. Likewise, the metabolic alterations have few implications in nutritional counselling (yet).

Therapeutic interventions currently focus on controlling the tumour and on exploring NSAIDs, but they are still lacking evidence from randomized clinical trials in various settings. Clinical trials investigate also anti-TNF interventions, but of unclear significance yet.

Anabolic–androgenic–hormones and the muscle: 'somatotropic axis'

The complex system of growth hormone (GH), insulin-like growth factors (IGFs), and anabolic (androgenic) hormones has been observed to be altered in patients with catabolic illnesses, contributing to wasting of lean body mass[150]. Among the diseases associated with primary ACS, these changes and their treatment have been best studied in patients with AIDS-wasting, to a far lesser extent in cancer patients. A possible reason might be that alterations of the somatotropic axis are a more prominent feature in AIDS compared to cancer, where metabolic and neuroendocrine alterations are more predominant. Alternatively, it might be argued that due to (outdated[151]) concerns about tumour growth stimulation by GH, the investigation of this axis is under-explored in cancer patients.

Growth hormone/IGFs

Growth hormone (GH) promotes nitrogen retention and improves the nitrogen balance. These anabolic effects on protein metabolism are mediated primarily through an increase in protein synthesis[152]. It is unclear, how GH acts directly on the skeletal muscle to stimulate its growth.

Circulating GH acts both on the liver to stimulate expression of the IGF-I and IGFBP3 genes, resulting in increased levels of these proteins in the circulation, as well as it stimulates expression of IGF-I genes in skeletal muscle. However, skeletal muscle IGF-I expression can be elevated in the absence of GH.

Insulin-like growth factors (IGFs) are mitogens, which play a pivotal role in regulation of cell proliferation, differentiation, and apoptosis. These effects are mediated through the IGF-1 receptor, at least six IGF-binding proteins (IGFBP), and IGFBP proteases[153].

IGF-I and IGF-II stimulate many anabolic responses in myoblasts, as they do in other cell types, and are critical factors in skeletal muscle development, regeneration, and hypertrophy. Since the skeletal muscle fibres are incapable of DNA synthesis, muscle growth and regeneration relies on proliferation and subsequent differentiation of undifferentiated skeletal muscle precursor cells, the myoblasts. IGF-I and IGF-II have the unusual property of stimulating both proliferation and differentiation of myoblasts[154].

The effects of IGFs are significantly modulated by IGFBPs secreted by myoblasts. Insulin-like growth factor-binding protein-1 (BP-1) is a multifunctional protein that binds IGF-I in solution and integrins on the cell surface. BP-1 was shown to both inhibit IGF-I-mediated protein synthesis by binding to IGF-I, and as well, acting independently of IGF-I, inhibit protein degradation[155].

Myoblasts express also sufficient amounts of autocrine IGF-II to stimulate myogenesis. Autocrine expression of IGFs is widely seen in cells responding to mitogenic stimuli, they may be seen as extracellular second messengers mediating many actions of agents that stimulate cell proliferation.

Interesting findings are reported from rats flying in space: in the microgravity environment, their muscle weight decreased 19–24 per cent, paralleled by increased myostatin/beta-actin mRNA ratios, increased myostatin protein levels, decreased IGF-II mRNA, unchanged IGF-1 mRNA, and unchanged proteolysis markers (3-methyl histidine, ubiquitin mRNA, proteasome 2C mRNA[156], suggesting a down-regulation of protein synthesis without activation of proteolysis.

Systemic inflammation (sepsis) and GH/IGFs

Catabolic illnesses induce a decrease in protein synthesis and an increase in proteolysis, as discussed earlier. These alterations in protein metabolism during catabolic diseases are found to be paralleled by an acquired resistance to GH, and GH-mediated induction of insulin-like growth factor I[157]. It is assumed that increased levels of inflammatory cytokines can inhibit the effects of GH on target tissues. Accordingly, GH has been found to have reduced effectiveness in retarding protein catabolism in septic patients, and to be associated with increased mortality in critically ill patients[158].

Likewise, IGF-1 was decreased in sepsis[159], whereas its binding protein (IGF-BP-1) is over-expressed and accumulates in skeletal muscle during catabolic illnesses. Muscle protein synthesis was reported decreased in association with endotoxins[160]. In muscle cells of burned rats, IGF-I treatment both *in vitro* and *in vivo* was shown to block the catabolic response[161]. However, this effect was not seen in muscles from septic rats incubated *in vitro* with IGF-1, even at high hormone concentrations, suggesting development of IGF-I resistance[162]. In contrast to the inability of IGF-1 to inhibit proteolysis, protein synthesis was found to be stimulated by intravenous IGF-1 even during sepsis[163]. Likewise, the administration of a binary complex of insulin-like growth factor I (IGF-I) complexed with IGF binding protein-3 (IGFBP-3) attenuated the sepsis-induced inhibition of protein synthesis[48]. Accordingly, *in vivo* experiments in septic rats revealed a reversal of the decreased muscle protein synthesis by IGF-1, but no effect on the increased myofibrillar muscle protein breakdown, even though a reduction of ubiquitin and $E2_{14k}$ mRNA levels was achieved[164].

GH/IGFs in primary ACS

In primary ACS, a decrease of IGF-1 is consistently reported in patients with cancer, cardiac cachexia, and AIDS, whereas few studies focused on GH alterations.

In 21 cachectic patients with chronic heart failure, an increase in total GH and immunologically intact GH, and a decrease in GH-binding protein, IGF-BP3, and IGF-I, was found, compared to 51 non-cachectic patients with chronic heart failure and 26 healthy control subjects[165].

In 20 patients with lung cancer and weight loss, an association between loss of BCM (body cell mass) and IGF-1 was found, as well as a correlation with inflammation[166]. From advanced breast cancer patients decreased IGF-1 levels are reported, which seem to increase during treatment with megestrol acetate. In those patients, an increased IGFBP-3 protease activity was found and may account for the decreased IGF-1 levels. The same group demonstrated in 128 patients with newly diagnosed breast cancer positive correlations

of an increased IGFBP-3 proteolysis associated with invasive cancer, compared with DCIS/benign conditions, with tumour mass, as well as with presence of metastases and stage, but a negative correlation with IGF-I and IGF-II[167]. In 16 patients with metastatic breast cancer treated with diethylstilboestrol (5 mg 3 times daily) a significant decrease of IGF-I, IGF-II, free IGF-I, IGFBP-2, IGFBP-3, and IGFBP-3 protease activity was found, but a significant increase of IGFBP-1, IGFBP-4[168].

Administration of GH was observed to increase lean body mass in patients with cardiac cachexia[169], aging[170], chronic obstructive pulmonary disease[171], or AIDS wasting[172]. Results from IGF-1 substitution are available only from studies in rats, where a reduction of weight loss is reported during starvation, diabetes, or during dexamethasone treatment. Only preliminary data are available from patients with cancer-related ACS, allowing no conclusion as to whether GH supplementation may reduce skeletal muscle loss.

Anabolic (androgenic) steroids

The effects of testosterone and its (mostly) less androgenic derivatives (e.g. nandrolone, oxandrolone, fluoxymesterone, oxymetholone, stanazolol, danazol, methandrostenolone) are mediated by the only one androgen receptor. Testosterone levels gradually decrease as a normal consequence of aging, and can lead to a decrease of bone mass, reduced bone marrow activity causing anaemia, reduced muscle strength, and diminished sexual function in men and women[173]. In addition, behavioural and cognitive deficits have been found to be associated with hypogonadism[174]. In women normal values of testosterone are not well defined, i.e. in postmenopausal states. In women, a syndrome of relative

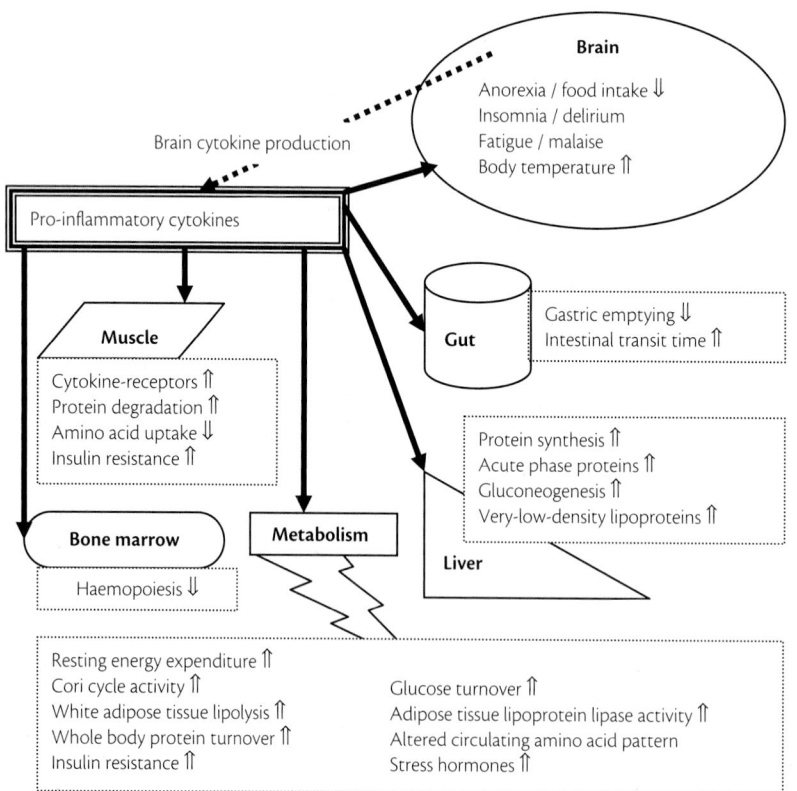

Figure 10.3.1.3 Cytokines effects on different organs.

androgen deficiency has been proposed. It has been suggested to be associated with alterations in mood, and energy, as well as sexual function[175].

Testosterone used in supraphysiologic doses was found to enhance muscle size and strength in eugonadal men[176]. Testosterone replacement in hypogonadal men, such as elderly patients, was reported to increase lean body mass[177], as well as in some, but not all studies, bone mineral density, haematocrit, prostate volume, self-reported sense of energy and sexual function, muscle size, and strength. The merits of hormone replacement in a normal aging population are presently debated.

Serum testosterone levels are decreased in primary ACS associated with HIV-infection, probably mostly due to hypogonadotropic hypogonadism[178]. In HIV-infected men, serum testo-sterone levels are lower in those with weight loss[143], correlate with deficits in muscle mass, low Karnofsky scores, and disease progression[179,180]. Likewise, low testosterone levels were found in female HIV patients[181]. Therapy with testosterone or its derivatives was found to be beneficial in HIV-infected patients, i.e. resulting in an increase of lean body mass and other improvements in some studies (muscle size and strength, haemaglobin), in both hypogonadal and eugonadal patients. Likewise, beneficial effects of testosterone therapy have been reported from HIV-infected women. Interestingly, exercise was found in one study to increase body weight, muscle mass, and strength in hypogonadal HIV-infected men to the same amount as testosterone replacement, and the combination of both did not increase the gain[182].

Hypogonadism is a frequent finding in patients with cancer[183,184], and associations with ACS are reported. For example, in 20 male patients with lung cancer, the patients with weight loss less than 10 per cent had higher serum testosterone values (21.5±5.6 nmol/litre), than those with weight loss greater than 10 per cent (13.2±7.5 nmol/litre), and a correlation between testosterone and loss of lean body mass was found[166]. Patients may have hypogonadism also due to impaired hypothalamic–pituitary axis function, antineoplastic treatments, or opioid therapy[183].

Chronic renal failure is associated with gonadal dysfunction, which is probably principally due to aberrant neuroendocrine regulation of GnRH secretion[185]. Therapy with anabolic androgenic steroids has been found to be beneficial in patients with chronic renal failure, for example, nandrolone was reported to improve lean body mass, function, and fatigue compared with placebo[186].

Likewise, in patients with chronic obstructive pulmonary disease, levels of free testosterone are reported decreased, both in patients without and concurrent with corticosteroid treatment[187]. Preliminary studies report that treatment with anabolic steroids increases fat-free mass in patients with ACS associated with chronic obstructive pulmonary disease[188], including male patients undergoing long-term glucocorticoid treatment[189].

Beta-2 adrenergic system

Alterations of the beta-2 adrenergic system have rarely been described in primary ACS, but animal and human data suggest a therapeutic role of beta-2-adrenergic agonists, which have anabolic effects[75]. They were found to promote muscle growth/hypertrophy and muscle strength, paralleled by a reduction of the body fat component, without requiring an increased food intake or exercise. In tumour-bearing animals, a normalization of protein breakdown rates was achieved by beta-2-agonists through a decrease in hyperactivation of the ATP-ubiquitin dependent proteolytic pathway. However, in heart-failure-related primary ACS, no effect of sustained-released salbutamol was found on muscle strength or fatigue in a small study.

Thyroid function

In critically-ill patients, thyroid function may be altered, manifest by the transient sick-euthyreot syndrome, where TSH, T3, as well as T4 are lowered. Administration of intra-arterial TNF-α was reported to cause the euthyreot sick syndrome[190]. However, in patients with cancer-related ACS, even though patients are often sick, preliminary data suggest a syndrome different from the euthyreot sick syndrome. No decrease of T3 and T4, despite an ongoing catabolic state, was observed in cancer ACS, whereas TSH levels seem not to be altered[191]. Likewise, in patients with HIV infection, unusual prolonged maintenance of normal T3 levels was reported[192].

Significance of anabolic–androgenic hormones and muscle for clinical care and research

The anabolic hormonal system seems important in cachexia care, practically hypogonadism can be detected, but the question of substitution remains the topic of ongoing research. Hypothyreosis seems to occur, rarely triggering substitution. Clinical trials with ghrelin aim also to influence GH, and other future trials will tackle the beta-adrenergic system, and directly the mitochondrial regulation in muscle tissues[5].

Causes for secondary anorexia and secondary cachexia

Many patients with advanced, incurable illness experience starvational complications of the disease (e.g. cancer)[193] or co-morbidities[194], which interfere with patients' appetite and ability to eat or digest food[2,195]. Patients' eating habits[196] and ability to cope with the complex eating problems[197] may also impact the response to dietary needs. The mechanism of this so-called starvational or secondary anorexia is different from the 'metabolic' anorexia–cachexia syndrome. Patients may also lose proteins from body fluids (e.g. frequent paracentesis)[198]and lose muscle mass from prolonged bed rest (inactivity) or from side effects of prolonged corticosteroid treatment[199]. These factors, also different from the metabolic anorexia–cachexia syndrome, are summarized as secondary cachexia.

Secondary anorexia–cachexia may be divided in three groups (Table 10.3.1.1).

Starvation/secondary anorexia

Secondary anorexia is a form of starvation, caused by impaired oral intake secondary to both altered function of the gastrointestinal tract and interfering symptoms. Typical causes are taste alterations[200,201], mucositis[202], nausea[203], constipation[204], pain[205], or shortness of breath[206]. The energy expenditure is reduced, proteins are conserved, and ketone bodies are utilized as an energy source. The result is weight loss, mostly at the expense of body fat. These features contrast to the alterations seen in primary ACS. Table 10.3.1.2 refers to the metabolic alterations in cancer-related primary ACS, compared to starvation. Starvation itself might impact the immune function or neuroendocrine regulation. Healthy adults die from starvation after a nitrogen loss of 35 per cent of the ideal weight, i.e. after 60–75 days, despite adequate adipose reserves, since the protein mass is the major determinant of starvation[207]. An estimate for dying from starvation equals about 15–30 days for patients with progressive, terminal cancer. If patients have, in addition, a systemically activated immune system caused by circulating cytokines, such as during infections (systemic inflammatory response syndrome) the number of days until death decreases further.

Even though countless authors mention the impact of starvational complications on patients, original research is scarce, as a systematic review of the literature of secondary causes for impaired oral nutritional intake found[208]. A reason for the paucity of research on the impact of secondary causes of impaired appetite is the lack of a quantitative screening instrument. The PG-SGA asks the patient about the presence of 'problems that have kept me from eating enough during the past two weeks', including no appetite, nausea, vomiting, constipation, diarrhoea, mouth sores, dry mouth, taste problems, bothering smell, swallow problems, early fullness, pain, and other reasons[209]. The PG-SGA has been proposed[210] and (effectively) used by many groups to screen for nutritional problems, namely malnutrition, in cancer patients having various tumours. Psychosocial and spiritual distress can also influence the sensation of hunger, appetite or satiety, culminating in expression of total suffering[211]. This cause of anorexia may be unrecognized, even when a careful assessment for causes of secondary anorexia–cachexia is performed. Currently, a new quantitative checklist for secondary anorexia is under development[2,24].

Deconditioning—secondary cachexia

Secondary cachexia can occur due to loss of muscle tissue in the absence of primary ACS, as a consequence of decreased muscle activity because of immobility (occurring, for example, during prolonged bed rest), or microgravity. This phenomenon has been called deconditioning. The failure to increase muscle mass in children (subgroup of failure to thrive), or the involuntary loss of muscle in elderly people (sarcopenia), despite adequate nutrition might be related to the phenomenon of deconditioning. In addition, patients can have a loss of proteins through body fluids.

Infections

Finally, concomitant acute or chronic infections can trigger a catabolic state[19]. In clinical reality, it is often difficult in patients presenting with clinical or laboratory signs of inflammation to sort out the contribution of infections and of cytokine-mediated primary ACS (see following paragraphs). The measurement of procalcitonin may assist in decisions.

Significance of secondary anorexia and secondary cachexia for clinical care and research

Secondary causes for impaired oral nutritional intake seem to occur frequently in the palliative care context, but are under-recognized. For clinical practice, a screening instrument or checklist should be applied (e.g. nutrition impact symptoms, PG-SGA, checklist for secondary anorexia, CNAQ). Prolonged bed rest and insufficient physical activity seems an under-recognized factor of muscle loss in ACS; current phase II trials encourage physical resistance training

also in the palliative care context; phase III trials currently explore its effectiveness.

Clinical implications of evolving pathogenetic concepts

An understanding of why patients with advanced incurable illnesses lose weight and appetite, and the implications for treatment are still evolving.

Recognition of a primary cachexia syndrome

Patients with advanced incurable illnesses, aware of their weight loss and decreased appetite, consequently express concerns about not eating enough. Fatigue and declining performance status is intuitively associated with insufficient nutritional intake. This belief about the cause of anorexia–cachexia triggers family members to insist on a sufficient amount of the right type of food for their loved one. Health-care professionals often base the concept of providing parenteral or enteral nutrition on the observation, that cancer patients who lose weight really have decreased calorie intake and that they lose fat tissue. Cachexia, at least in patients with cancer, was believed to be the result of a nutritional deficit caused by the combination of decreased energy intake due to tumour-related factors, which acted at the satiety centre in the central nervous system, as well as increased energy consumption by the tumour. However, attempts to increase (only) nutritional intake, including aggressive nutritional therapies, did not significantly improve clinical outcomes. The sometimes achieved weight gain by nutritional therapy was barely associated with an increase in lean body mass, but more with an increase in body water and fat[212]. Nutritional therapy remained controversial in patients with cancer, and was usually found not to be beneficial in patients with far advanced disease[213,214].

Pharmacological treatment of the primary anorexia–cachexia syndrome

Consequently, the nature of a primary cachexia was considered, and attempts were made to manipulate the metabolic, neuroendocrine, and anabolic alterations. Disease-modifying treatments, such as antineoplastic therapies for cancer or antiretroviral therapy for AIDS often improve primary ACS. In addition, pharmacological treatments of primary cachexia were established. For patients with cancer-related primary cachexia, three evidence-based therapies are now available (corticosteroids, progestins, and prokinetics), from other drugs, single positive trails await confirmation (thalidomide, ATP), while other initially promising drugs could not show in a placebo-controlled setting applying a one-size-fits-all cachexia definition a benefit over placebo (omega-3-fatty acids, cannabinoids)[215]. Other drugs, such as melatonin-receptor antagonists, ghrelin and analogues, anti-myostatin approaches, modern anabolic steroids, and anti-cytokine interventions are in the stage of clinical trials (from phase I to III) [75]. The options for patients with AIDS-related primary ACS include growth-hormone and 9-d-THC too. However, not all patients with primary ACS benefit from pharmacological treatments for several reasons. They may suffer from a relevant aggravating factor for anorexia–cachexia (Table 10.3.1.2, Fig. 10.3.1.1). Or they may belong to a subgroup of patients with a distinct primary ACS with variable importance of the pathogenetic mechanism (Fig. 10.3.1.1, Table 10.3.1.3). For example, a cancer patient suffering from a primary ACS involving mostly the somato-tropic axis may not profit from appetite-stimulation alone, but maybe from anabolic treatments. A third reason, for a limited benefit from pharmacological treatment for primary ACS, is the individual vulnerability to side effects, which requires a careful decision-making considering meaningful (symptomatic) outcomes (discussed in the next three chapters).

Identification of aggravating factors of anorexia–cachexia with a starvational component

There is an important subset of patients with anorexia–cachexia, which seem to benefit from nutritional interventions. These patients can be described as those having a relevant starvational component of anorexia–cachexia. Or in other words, they have relevant aggravating factors contributing to weight loss and anorexia, e.g. secondary anorexia–cachexia. Examples of patients with an important actual or predicted starvational component of anorexia–cachexia are patients: (1) with bowel obstruction (and slow-growing tumours and); (2) undergoing radiotherapy for head and neck cancers (often presenting with severe dysphagia); (3) with inadequate dietary intake because of interfering symptoms or psycho-social and financial factors; (4) undergoing surgery (i.e. upper gastrointestinal tract cancer); and (5) treated in high-dose chemo-therapy protocols.

Comprehensive nutritional approaches may therefore be bene-ficial for some patients with anorexia–cachexia. Clinicians may treat pharmacological the primary ACS ('fix the engine'), but pro-vide inadequate nutritional intake ('give fuel to the engine'). Likewise, social, psychological, economical, and neurological conditions contributing to impaired nutritional intake may be under-recognized.

However, for the diagnosis and assessment of the relative impor-tance of a starvational component of anorexia–cachexia, no cur-rent assessment instruments are available. Such instruments, which are under development, would facilitate the identification of patients with anorexia–cachexia, which have a higher likelihood of response to nutritional support.

Multi-dimensional treatment approaches

Current research aims on the one hand to better characterize the primary ACS, maybe allowing the targeting of interventions at multiple, different sites of action, resulting in either individualized therapies of subgroups or the development of combined treatment

Table 10.1.3.5 Pro-inflammatory and anti-inflammatory cytokines.

Pro-inflammatory cytokines	Anti-inflammatory cytokines
◆ Interleukin-1	◆ Interleukin-4
◆ Interleukin-6	◆ Interleukin-9
◆ Tumour necrosis factor-α	◆ Interleukin-10
◆ Interferon-γ	◆ Interleukin-12
	◆ Interleukin-15
	◆ Soluble TNF receptor

strategies[24]. On the other hand, efforts are made to improve the recognition and characterization of aggravating factors of anorexia–cachexia.

Conclusion

The pathophysiology of anorexia–cachexia is complex and multi-dimensional. Further characterization of the mechanism and causes of the primary ACS, involving metabolic, neurohormonal, and anabolic alterations, as well as inflammatory responses and specific pro-cachectic molecules, is required in the long term for the development of new therapies. Presently, an agreed-on defini-tion, diagnosis, classification, and assessment system carries a high potential to influence clinical routine decision-making and also clinical trial design. The active screening and assessment of aggravating and reversible factors of anorexia–cachexia, consid-ering multiple (physical, psychosocial, economical, and existen-tial) dimensions including an estimation of the starvational component of anorexia–cachexia, is also crucial for a balanced decision-making.

In late cachexia, the focus relies on relief of eating-related dis-tress, alleviating chronic nausea, counsel, and accompanying patients to cope with decreasing function. In contrast, for patients with anorexia–cachexia syndrome, the severity definition may be utilized to stratify patients in clinical trials, and cachexia domains may distinguish patient groups requiring variable interventions.

Interventions may be useful only for subgroups of patients (e.g. anti-inflammatory interventions for cachexia only for patients with elevated CRP, appetite-stimulants for patients with central loss of appetite, GI-motility enhancing agents for patients with severe early fullness despite good constipation control). It may become a new standard for clinical trials, that all patients receive basic nutritional support, physical activity interventions, and stan-dards of symptom control.

Further reading

Energy balance, metabolic alterations, and muscle wasting: 'muscle–liver axis'

Argiles, J.M., Busquets, S., and Lopez-Soriano, F. J. (2001). Metabolic interrelationships between liver and skeletal muscle in pathological states. *Life Science*, **69**(12), 1345–61.

Baracos, V.E. (2001). A deadly combination of anorexia and hypermetabolism. *Current Opinion in Clinical Nutrition and Metabolic Care*, **4**(3), 175–7.

Hasselgren, P.O. and Fischer, J.E. (2001). Muscle cachexia: current concepts of intracellular mechanisms and molecular regulation. *Annals of Surgery*, Jan, **233**(1), 9–17.

Tisdale, M.J.(2000). Biomedicine. Protein loss in cancer cachexia. *Science*, **289**(5488), 2293–4.

Neurohoromonal circuits and food intake: 'gut–brain axis'

Ahima, R.S. and Osei, S.Y. (2001). Molecular regulation of eating behavior: new insights and prospects for therapeutic strategies. *Trends in Molecular Medicine*, May, **7**(5), 205–13.

Meguid, M.M., Yang, Z.J., and Gleason, J.R. (1996). The gut-brain brain-gut axis in anorexia: toward an understanding of food intake regulation. *Nutrition*, **12**(1 Suppl), S57–62.

Schwartz, G.J. (2000). The role of gastrointestinal vagal afferents in the control of food intake: current prospects. *Nutrition*, **16**(10), 866–73.

Schwartz, M.W., Woods, S.C., Porte, D. Jr., *et al.* (2000). Central nervous system control of food intake. *Nature*, Apr 6, **404**(6778), 661–71.

Wren, A.M,, Seal, L.J., Cohen, M.A., Brynes, A.E., Frost, G.S., Murphy, K.G., *et al.* (2001). Ghrelin Enhances Appetite and Increases Food Intake in Humans. *Journal of Clinical Endocrinology and Metabolism*, **86**(12), 5992.

Growth hormone, IGFs, anabolic (androgenic) hormones: 'somatotropic axis'

Basaria, S., Wahlstrom, J.T., and Dobs, A.S. (2001). Anabolic-androgenic steroid therapy in the treatment of chronic diseases. *Journal of Clinical Endocrinology and Metabolism*, **86**(11), 5108–17.

Frost, R.A. and Lang, C.H. (1998). Growth factors in critical illness: regulation and therapeutic aspects. *Current Opinion in Clinical Nutrition and Metabolic Care*, **1**(2), 195–204.

Cytokines

Argiles, J.M. and Lopez-Soriano, F.J. (2000). New mediators in cancer cachexia. *Nestle Nutrition Workshop Series. Clinical and Performance Programme*, **4**, 147–62, discussion 163–5.

Plata-Salaman, C.R. (2000). Central nervous system mechanisms contributing to the cachexia-anorexia syndrome. *Nutrition*, **16**(10), 1009–12.

Tumour-derived cachectic factors

Tisdale, M.J. (2000). Catabolism of skeletal muscle proteins and its reversal in cancer cachexia. *Nestle Nutrition Workshop Series. Clinical and Performance Programme*, **4**,, 35–43, discussion 144–6.

References

1. Spiro, A., Baldwin, C., Patterson, A. *et al.* (2006). The views and practice of oncologists towards nutritional support in patients receiving chemotherapy. *British Journal of Cancer*, **95**, 431–4.

2. Omlin, A.G. and Strasser, F. (2007). Secondary causes of cancer-related anorexia: Recognition in daily practice by a novel checklist, a pilot study. *Journal of Clinical Oncology*, **25**, 18S (suppl abstract 9058).

3. Bozzetti, F. (2009). SCRINIO Working Group.Screening the nutritional status in oncology: a preliminary report on 1,000 outpatients. *Support Care Cancer*, **17**(3), 279–84.

4. Bozzetti, F. (2007). Total parenteral nutrition in cancer patients. *Current Opinion in Support Palliative Care*, **1**, 281–6.

5. Yavuzsen, T., Davis, M.P., Walsh, D. *et al.* (2005). Systematic review of the treatment of cancer-associated anorexia and weight loss. *Journal of Clinical Oncology*, **23**(33), 8500–11.

6. Mintz, S.W. *et al.* (2002). The Anthropology of food and eating.

7. Salomonsson, (1990). *Ethnologia Scandinavia*.

8. Strasser, F., Binswanger, J., Cerny, T. *et al.* (2007). Fighting a losing battle: eating-related distress of men with advanced cancer and their female partners. A mixed-methods study. *Palliative Medicine*, **21**, 129–37.

9. Calman, K.C. (1984). Quality of life in cancer patients-an hypothesis. *Journal of Medical Ethics*, **10**, 124–7.

10. Strasser, F. (2008). Diagnostic criteria of cachexia and their assessment: decreased muscle strength and fatigue. *Current Opinion in Clinical Nutrition and Metabolic Care*, **11**, 417–21.

11. Strasser, F., Omlin, A., Walker, J. *et al.* (2008). A novel Cachexia Classification for Palliative Cancer Care: Synthesis of systematic literature review and nominal experts' focus group. *Palliative Medicine*, **22**, 410 (Abstract 35).

12. Evans WJ, Morley JE, Argilés J. *et al.* (2008). Cachexia: a new definition. *Clin Nutr*, **27**(6), 793–9.

13. Walsh, D., Donnelly, S., and Rybicki, L. (2000). The symptoms of advanced cancer: relationship to age, gender, and performance status in 1,000 patients. *Supportive Care in Cancer*, **8**, 175–9.

14. Tishelman, C., Petersson, L.M., Degner, L.F. *et al.* (2007). Symptom prevalence, intensity, and distress in patients with inoperable lung cancer in relation to time of death. *Journal of Clinical Oncology*, **25**, 5381–9.

15. Mangili, A., Murman, D.H., Zampini, A.M. *et al.* (2006). Nutrition and HIV infection: review of weight loss and wasting in the era of highly active antiretroviral therapy from the nutrition for healthy living cohort. *Clinical Infectious Diseases*, **42**, 836–42.

16. on Haehling, S., Doehner, W., and Anker, S.D. (2007). Nutrition, metabolism, and the complex pathophysiology of cachexia in chronic heart failure. *Cardiovascular Research*, **73**, 298–309.

17. Roongpisuthipong, C., Sobhonslidsuk, A., Nantiruj, K. *et al.* (2001). Nutritional assessment in various stages of liver cirrhosis. *Nutrition*, **17**, 761–5.

18. Fouque, D., Kalantar-Zadeh, K., Kopple, J. *et al.* (2008). A proposed nomenclature and diagnostic criteria for protein-energy wasting in acute and chronic kidney disease. *Kidney International*, **73**, 391–8.

19. Remels, A.H., Gosker, H.R., van der Velden, J. *et al.* (2007). Systemic inflammation and skeletal muscle dysfunction in chronic obstructive pulmonary disease: state of the art and novel insights in regulation of muscle plasticity. *Clinics in Chest Medicine*, **28**, 537–52.

20. Marchand, V., Baker, S.S., Stark, T.J. *et al.* (2000). Randomized, double-blind, placebo-controlled pilot trial of megestrol acetate in malnourished children with cystic fibrosis. *Journal of Pediatric Gastroenterology and Nutrition*, **31**, 264–9.

21. Macallan, D.C., McNurlan, M.A., Kurpad, A.V. *et al.* (1998). Whole body protein metabolism in human pulmonary tuberculosis and undernutrition: evidence for anabolic block in tuberculosis. *Clinical Science (London)*, **94**, 321–31.

22. Altemeier, W.A., III, (2000). What is happening to children with failure to thrive? *Pediatric Annals*, **29**, 531, 534.

23. Thomas, D.R. (2007). Loss of skeletal muscle mass in aging: examining the relationship of starvation, sarcopenia and cachexia. *Clinical Nutrition*, **26**, 389–99.

24. Strasser F, Blum D, Omlin A. *et al.* (2008). A novel Cachexia Classification for Palliative Cancer Care: Synthesis of systematic literature review (SLR) and nominal experts' focus group. EAPC-Research Forum Trondheim. *Palliative Medicine*, **22**, 410 (Abstract 36).

25. Fearon, K.C. (2008). Cancer cachexia: Developing multimodal therapy for a multidimensional problem. *European Journal of Cancer*, **44**, 1124–32.

26. Cachexia conferences, www.cachexia.org (last accessed: September 2009).

27. Argiles, J.M., Busquets, S., and Lopez-Soriano, F.J. (2001). Metabolic interrelationships between liver and skeletal muscle in pathological states. *Life Science*, **69**, 1345–61.

28. Meguid, M.M., Yang, Z.J., and Gleason, J.R. (1996). The gut-brain brain-gut axis in anorexia: toward an understanding of food intake regulation. *Nutrition*, **12**, S57–62.

29. Schwartz, M.W., Woods, S.C., Porte, D. Jr. *et al.* (2000). Central nervous system control of food intake. *Nature*, **404**, 661–71.

30. Schwartz, G.J. (2000). The role of gastrointestinal vagal afferents in the control of food intake: current prospects. *Nutrition*, **16**, 866–73.

31. Konsman, J.P. and Dantzer, R. (2001). How the immune and nervous systems interact during disease-associated anorexia. *Nutrition*, **17**, 664–8.

32. Porter, M.H., Hrupka, B.J., Langhans, W. *et al.* (1998). Vagal and splanchnic afferents are not necessary for the anorexia produced by peripheral IL-1beta, LPS, and MDP. *The American Journal of Physiology*, **275**, R384–9.

33. Horvath, T.L., Diano, S., Sotonyi, P. *et al.* (2001). Minireview: ghrelin and the regulation of energy balance-a hypothalamic perspective. *Endocrinology*, **142**, 4163–9.

34. Nakazato, M., Murakami, N., Date, Y. *et al.* (2001). A role for ghrelin in the central regulation of feeding. *Nature*, **409**, 194–8.

35. Nagaya, N., Uematsu, M., Kojima, M. *et al.* (2001). Chronic administration of ghrelin improves left ventricular dysfunction and attenuates development of cardiac cachexia in rats with heart failure. *Circulation*, **104**,1430–5.

36. Asakawa, A., Inui, A., Kaga, T. *et al.* (2001). Ghrelin is an appetite-stimulatory signal from stomach with structural resemblance to motilin. *Gastroenterology*, **120**, 337–45.

37. Liu, Y.L., Malik, N.M., Sanger, G.J. *et al.* (2006). Ghrelin alleviates cancer chemotherapy-associated dyspepsia in rodents. *Cancer Chemotherapy and Pharmacology*, **58**, 326–33.

38. Wolf, I., Sadetzki, S., Kanety, H. *et al.* (2006). Adiponectin, ghrelin, and leptin in cancer cachexia in breast and colon cancer patients. *Cancer*, **106**, 966–73.

39. Neary, N.M., Small, C.J., Wren, A.M. *et al.* (2004). Ghrelin increases energy intake in cancer patients with impaired appetite: acute, randomized, placebo-controlled trial. *Journal of Clinical Endocrinology and Metabolism*, **89**, 2832–6.

40. Strasser, F., Lutz, T.A., Maeder, M.T. *et al.* (2008). Safety, tolerability and pharmacokinetics of intravenous ghrelin for cancer-related anorexia/cachexia: a randomised, placebo-controlled, double-blind, double-crossover study. *British Journal of Cancer*, **98**, 300–8.

41. Nagaya, N., Itoh, T., Murakami, S. *et al.* (2005). Treatment of cachexia with ghrelin in patients with COPD. *Chest*, **128**, 1187–93.

42. Friedman, J.M. and Halaas, J.L. (1998). Leptin and the regulation of body weight in mammals. *Nature*, **395**, 763–70.

43. Matson, C.A. and Ritter, R.C. (1999). Long-term CCK-leptin synergy suggests a role for CCK in the regulation of body weight. *The American Journal of Physiology*, **276**, R1038–45.

44. Wisse, B.E., Schwartz, M.W., and Cummings, D.E. (2003). Melanocortin signaling and anorexia in chronic disease states. *Annals of the New York Academy of Sciences*, **994**, 275–81.

45. Baskin, D.G., Figlewicz Lattemann, D., Seeley, R.J. *et al.* (1999). Insulin and leptin: dual adiposity signals to the brain for the regulation of food intake and body weight. *Brain Research*, **848**, 114–23.

46. Erickson, J.C., Clegg, K.E., and Palmiter, R.D. (1996). Sensitivity to leptin and susceptibility to seizures of mice lacking neuropeptide Y. *Nature*, **381**, 415–21.

47. Bing, C., Taylor, S., Tisdale, M.J. *et al.* (2001). Cachexia in MAC16 adenocarcinoma: suppression of hunger despite normal regulation of leptin, insulin and hypothalamic neuropeptide Y. *Journal of Neurochemistry*, **79**, 1004–12.

48. Cangiano, C., Testa, U., Muscaritoli, M. *et al.* (1994). Cytokines, tryptophan and anorexia in cancer patients before and after surgical tumor ablation. *Anticancer Research*, **14**, 1451–5.

49. Carbo, N., Ribas, V. V., Busquets, S. *et al.* (2000). Short-term effects of leptin on skeletal muscle protein metabolism in the rat. *The Journal of Nutritional Biochemistry*, **11**, 431–5.

50. Muzzin, P., Eisensmith, R.C., Copeland, K.C. *et al.* (1996). Correction of obesity and diabetes in genetically obese mice by leptin gene therapy. *Proceedings of the National Academy of Sciences of the United States of America*, **93**, 14804–8.

51. Lord, G.M., Matarese, G., Howard, J.K. *et al.* (1998). Leptin modulates the T-cell immune response and reverses starvation-induced immunosuppression. *Nature*, **394**, 897–901.

52. Finck, B.N. and Johnson, R.W. (2000). Tumor necrosis factor-alpha regulates secretion of the adipocyte-derived cytokine, leptin. *Microscopy Research and Technique*, **50**, 209–15.

53. Yamaguchi, M., Murakami, T., Tomimatsu, T. *et al.* (1998). Autocrine inhibition of leptin production by tumor necrosis factor-alpha (TNF-alpha) through TNF-alpha type-I receptor in vitro. *Biochemical and Biophysical Research Communications*, **244**, 30–4.

54. Mantzoros, C.S., Moschos, S., Avramopoulos, I. *et al.* (1997). Leptin concentrations in relation to body mass index and the tumor necrosis factor-alpha system in humans. *The Journal of Clinical Endocrinology and Metabolism*, **82**, 3408–13.

55. Sarraf, P., Frederich, R.C., Turner, E.M. *et al.* (1997). Multiple cytokines and acute inflammation raise mouse leptin levels: potential role in inflammatory anorexia. *The Journal of Experimental Medicine*, **185**, 171–5.

56. Moses, A.G., Dowidar, N., Holloway, B. *et al.* (2001). Leptin and its relation to weight loss, ob gene expression and the acute-phase response in surgical patients. *The British Journal of Surgery*, **88**, 588–93.

57. Wallace, A.M., Sattar, N., and McMillan, D.C. (1998). Effect of weight loss and the inflammatory response on leptin concentrations in gastrointestinal cancer patients. *Clinical Cancer Research*, **4**, 2977–9.

58. Simons, J.P., Schols, A.M., Campfield, L.A. *et al.* (1997). Plasma concentration of total leptin and human lung-cancer-associated cachexia. *Clinical Science (London)*, **93**, 273 –7.

59. Jatoi, A., Loprinzi, C.L., Sloan, J.A. *et al.* (2001). Neuropeptide Y, leptin, and cholecystokinin 8 in patients with advanced cancer and anorexia: a North Central Cancer Treatment Group exploratory investigation. *Cancer*, **92**, 629–33.

60. Di Marzo, V., Goparaju, S.K., Wang, L. *et al.* (2001). Leptin-regulated endocannabinoids are involved in maintaining food intake. *Nature*, **410**, 822–5.

61. Fride, E., Ginzburg, Y., Breuer, A. *et al.* (2001). Critical role of the endogenous cannabinoid system in mouse pup suckling and growth. *European Journal of Pharmacology*, **419**, 207–14.

62. Wisse, B.E., Frayo, R.S., Schwartz, M.W. *et al.* (2001). Reversal of cancer anorexia by blockade of central melanocortin receptors in rats. *Endocrinology*, **142**, 3292–301.

63. Joppa, M.A., Gogas, K.R., Foster, A.C. *et al.* (2007). Central infusion of the melanocortin receptor antagonist agouti-related peptide (AgRP(83-132)) prevents cachexia-related symptoms induced by radiation and colon-26 tumors in mice. *Peptides*, **28**, 636–42.

64. Nicholson, J.R., Kohler, G., Schaerer, F. *et al.* (2006). Peripheral administration of a melanocortin 4-receptor inverse agonist prevents loss of lean body mass in tumor-bearing mice. *Journal of Pharmacology and Experimental Therapeutics*, **317**, 771–7.

65. Bruera, E., Chadwick, S., Fox, R. *et al.* (1986). Study of cardiovascular autonomic insufficiency in advanced cancer patients. *Cancer Treatment Reports*, **70**, 1383–7.

66. Bruera, E., Catz, Z., Hooper, R. *et al.* (1987). Chronic nausea and anorexia in advanced cancer patients: a possible role for autonomic dysfunction. *Journal of Pain and Symptom Management*, **2**, 19–21.

67. Walsh, D. and Nelson, K.A. (2002). Autonomic nervous system dysfunction in advanced cancer. *Support Care Cancer*, **10**, 523–8.

68. Strasser, F., Palmer, J.L., Schover, L.R. *et al.* (2006). The impact of hypogonadism and autonomic dysfunction on fatigue, emotional function, and sexual desire in male patients with advanced cancer: a pilot study. *Cancer*, **107**, 2949–57.

69. Mathias, C.J. (1997). Autonomic disorders and their recognition. *The New England Journal of Medicine*, **336**, 721–4.

70. Consensus Committee of the American Autonomic Society and the American Academy of Neurology (1996). Consensus statement on the definition of orthostatic hypotension, pure autonomic failure, and multiple system atrophy. *Neurology*, **46**, 1470.

71. Suarez, G.A., Opfer-Gehrking, T.L., Offord, K.P. *et al.* (1999). The Autonomic Symptom Profile: a new instrument to assess autonomic symptoms. *Neurology*, **52**, 523–8.

72. De Giorgio, R., Stanghellini, V., Barbara, G. *et al.* (2000). Primary enteric neuropathies underlying gastrointestinal motor dysfunction. *Scandinavian Journal of Gastroenterology*, **35**, 114–22.

73. Corbo, M. and Balmaceda, C. (2001). Peripheral neuropathy in cancer patients. *Cancer Investigation*, **19**, 369–82.

74. Lee, H.R., Lennon, V.A., Camilleri, M. *et al.* (2001). Paraneoplastic gastrointestinal motor dysfunction: clinical and laboratory characteristics. *The American Journal of Gastroenterology*, **96**, 373–9.

75. Strasser, F. (2007). Appraisal of current and experimental approaches to the treatment of cachexia. *Current Opinion in Support in Palliative Care*, **1**, 312–6.

76. Bozzetti, F., Gavazzi, C., Ferrari, P. *et al.* (2000). Effect of total parenteral nutrition on the protein kinetics of patients with cancer cachexia. *Tumori*, **86**, 408–11.

77. Barber, M.D., Fearon, K.C., McMillan, D.C. *et al.* (2000). Liver export protein synthetic rates are increased by oral meal feeding in weight-losing cancer patients. *American Journal of Physiology, Endocrinology, and Metabolism*, **279**, E707–14.

78. Gibney, E., Elia, M., Jebb, S.A. *et al.* (1997). Total energy expenditure in patients with small-cell lung cancer: results of a validated study using the bicarbonate-urea method. *Metabolism*, **46**, 1412–7.

79. Falconer, J.S., Fearon, K.C., Plester, C.E. *et al.* (1994). Cytokines, the acute-phase response, and resting energy expenditure in cachectic patients with pancreatic cancer. *Annals of Surgery*, **219**, 325–31.

80. Leij-Halfwerk, S., van den Berg, J.W., Sijens, P.E. *et al.* (2000). Altered hepatic gluconeogenesis during L-alanine infusion in weight-losing lung cancer patients as observed by phosphorus magnetic resonance spectroscopy and turnover measurements. *Cancer Research*, **60**, 618–23.

81. Tayek, J.A. (1992). A review of cancer cachexia and abnormal glucose metabolism in humans with cancer. *Journal of the American College of Nutrition*, **11**, 445–56.

82. Barber, M.D., McMillan, D.C., Preston, T. *et al.* (2000). Metabolic response to feeding in weight-losing pancreatic cancer patients and its modulation by a fish-oil-enriched nutritional supplement. *Clinical Science (London)*, **98**, 389–99.

83. Yoshikawa, T., Noguchi, Y., Doi, C. *et al.* (2001). Insulin resistance in patients with cancer: relationships with tumor site, tumor stage, body-weight loss, acute-phase response, and energy expenditure. *Nutrition*, **17**, 590–3.

84. Kalaitzakis, E., Bosaeus, I., Ohman, L. *et al.* (2007). Altered postprandial glucose, insulin, leptin, and ghrelin in liver cirrhosis: correlations with energy intake and resting energy expenditure. *American Journal of Clinical Nutrition*, **85**, 808–15.

85. Jurasinski, C., Gray, K., Vary, T.C. (1995). Modulation of skeletal muscle protein synthesis by amino acids and insulin during sepsis. *Metabolism*, **44**, 1130–8.

86. Lundholm, K., Körner, U., Gunnebo, L. *et al.* (2007). Insulin treatment in cancer cachexia: effects on survival, metabolism, and physical functioning. *Clinical Cancer Research*, **13**, 2699–706.

87. Lommi, J., Kupari, M., Koskinen, P. *et al.* (1996). Blood ketone bodies in congestive heart failure. *Journal of the American College of Cardiology*, **28**, 665–72.

88. Vlassara, H., Spiegel, R.J., San Doval, D. *et al.* (1986). Reduced plasma lipoprotein lipase activity in patients with malignancy-associated weight loss. *Hormone and Metabolic Research*, **18**, 698–703.

89. Seelaender, M.C., Curi, R., Colquhoun, A. *et al.* (1998). Carnitine palmitoyltransferase II activity is decreased in liver mitochondria of cachectic rats bearing the Walker 256 carcinosarcoma: effect of indomethacin treatment. *Biochemistry and Molecular Biology International*, **44**, 185–93.

90. Malaguarnera, M., Risino, C., Gargante, M.P. *et al.* (2006). Decrease of serum carnitine levels in patients with or without gastrointestinal cancer cachexia. *World Journal of Gastroenterology*, **12**, 4541–5.

91. Gramignano, G., Lusso, M.R., Madeddu, C. *et al.* (2006). Efficacy of l-carnitine administration on fatigue, nutritional status, oxidative stress, and related quality of life in 12 advanced cancer patients undergoing anticancer therapy. *Nutrition*, **22**, 136–45.

92. Cruciani, R.A., Dvorkin, E., Homel, P. *et al.* (2006). Safety, tolerability and symptom outcomes associated with L-carnitine supplementation in patients with cancer, fatigue, and carnitine deficiency: a phase I/II study. *Journal of Pain and Symptom Management*, **32**, 551–9.

93. Busquets, S., Carbo, N., Almendro, V. *et al.* (2001). Hyperlipemia: a role in regulating UCP3 gene expression in skeletal muscle during cancer cachexia? *FEBS Letters*, **505**, 255–8.

94. Melville, S., McNurlan, M.A., Calder, A.G. *et al.* (1990). Increased protein turnover despite normal energy metabolism and responses to feeding in patients with lung cancer. *Cancer Research*, **50**, 1125–31.

95. Guttridge, D.C., Mayo, M.W., Madrid, L.V. *et al.* (2000). NF-kappaB-induced loss of MyoD messenger RNA: possible role in muscle decay and cachexia. *Science*, **289**, 2363–6.

96. Schmitt, T.L., Martignoni, M.E., Bachmann, J. *et al.* (2007). Activity of the Akt-dependent anabolic and catabolic pathways in muscle and liver samples in cancer-related cachexia. *Journal of Molecular Medicine*, **85**, 647–54.

97. van Royen, M., Carbo, N., Busquets, S. *et al.* (2000). DNA fragmentation occurs in skeletal muscle during tumor growth: A link with cancer cachexia? *Biochemical and Biophysical Research Communications*, **270**, 533–7.

98. Attaix, D., Ventadour, S., Codran, A. *et al.* (2005). The ubiquitin-proteasome system and skeletal muscle wasting. *Essays in Biochemistry*, **41**, 173–86.

99. Busquets, S., Garcia-Martinez, C., Alvarez, B., *et al.* (2000). Calpain-3 gene expression is decreased during experimental cancer cachexia. *Biochimica et Biophysica Acta*, **1475**, 5–9.

100. Whitehouse, A.S. and Tisdale, M.J. (2001). Downregulation of ubiquitin-dependent proteolysis by eicosapentaenoic acid in acute starvation. *Biochemical and Biophysical Research Communications*, **285**, 598–602.

101. Argilés, J.M., Busquets, S., Felipe, A. *et al.* (2006). Muscle wasting in cancer and ageing: cachexia versus sarcopenia. *Advances in Gerontology*, **18**, 39–54.

102. Fearon, K.C., Falconer, J.S., Slater, C. *et al.* (1998). Albumin synthesis rates are not decreased in hypoalbuminemic cachectic cancer patients with an ongoing acute-phase protein response. *Annals of Surgery*, **227**, 249–54.

103. Wigmore, S.J., McMahon, A.J., Sturgeon, C.M. *et al.* (2001). Acute-phase protein response, survival and tumour recurrence in patients with colorectal cancer. *The British Journal of Surgery*, **88**, 255–60.

104. De Blaauw, I., Heeneman, S., Deutz, N.E. *et al.* (1997). Increased whole-body protein and glutamine turnover in advanced cancer is not matched by an increased muscle protein and glutamine turnover. *The Journal of Surgical Research*, **68**, 44–55.

105. Toth, M.J., Gottlieb, S.S., Fisher, M.L. *et al.* (1997). Daily energy requirements in heart failure patients. *Metabolism*, **46**, 1294–8.

106. Swan, J.W., Anker, S.D., Walton, C. *et al.* (1997). Insulin resistance in chronic heart failure: relation to severity and etiology of heart failure. *Journal of the American College of Cardiology*, **30**, 527–32.

107. Fearon, K.C., Voss, A.C., Hustead, D.S. Cancer Cachexia Study Group (2006). Definition of cancer cachexia: effect of weight loss, reduced food intake, and systemic inflammation on functional status and prognosis. *American Journal of Clinical Nutrition*, **83**, 1345–50.

108. Fouladiun, M., Körner, U., Bosaeus, I. *et al.* (2005). Body composition and time course changes in regional distribution of fat and lean tissue in unselected cancer patients on palliative care--correlations with food intake, metabolism, exercise capacity, and hormones. *Cancer*, **103**, 2189–9.

109. Staal-van den Brekel, A.J., Schols, A.M., Dentener, M.A. *et al.* (1997). The effects of treatment with chemotherapy on energy metabolism and inflammatory mediators in small-cell lung carcinoma. *British Journal of Cancer*, **76**, 1630–5.

110. Scott, H.R., McMillan, D.C., Crilly, A. *et al.* (1996). The relationship between weight loss and interleukin 6 in non-small-cell lung cancer. *British Journal of Cancer*, **73**, 1560–2.

111. Cicoira, M., Bolger, A.P., Doehner, W. *et al.* (2001). High tumour necrosis factor-alpha levels are associated with exercise intolerance and neurohormonal activation in chronic heart failure patients. *Cytokine*, **15**, 80–6.

112. Yeh, S.S., Wu, S.Y., Levine, D.M. *et al.* (2001). The correlation of cytokine levels with body weight after megestrol acetate treatment in geriatric patients. *The Journals of Gerontology. Series A, Biological Sciences and Medical Sciences*, **56**, M48–54.

113. Torelli, G.F., Meguid, M.M., Moldawer, L.L. *et al.* (1999). Use of recombinant human soluble TNF receptor in anorectic tumor-bearing rats. *The American Journal of Physiology*, **277**, R850–5.

114. Costelli, P., Carbo, N., Tessitore, L. *et al.* (1993). Tumor necrosis factor-alpha mediates changes in tissue protein turnover in a rat cancer cachexia model. *The Journal of Clinical Investigation*, **92**, 2783–9.

115. Banks, R.E., Forbes, M.A., Patel, P.M. *et al.* (2000). Subcutaneous administration of recombinant glycosylated interleukin 6 in patients with cancer: pharmacokinetics, pharmacodynamics and immunomodulatory effects. *Cytokine*, **12**, 388–96.

116. Strassmann, G., Fong, M., Kenney, J.S. *et al.* (1992). Evidence for the involvement of interleukin 6 in experimental cancer cachexia. *The Journal of Clinical Investigation*, **89**, 1681–4.

117. Yasumoto, K., Mukaida, N., Harada, A. *et al.* (1995). Molecular analysis of the cytokine network involved in cachexia in colon 26 adenocarcinoma-bearing mice. *Cancer Research*, **55**, 921–7.

118. Fujita, J., Tsujinaka, T., Yano, M. *et al.* (1996). Anti-interleukin-6 receptor antibody prevents muscle atrophy in colon-26 adenocarcinoma-bearing mice with modulation of lysosomal and ATP-ubiquitin-dependent proteolytic pathways. *International Journal of Cancer*, **68**, 637–43.

119. Martin, F., Santolaria, F., Batista, N. *et al.* (1999). Cytokine levels (IL-6 and IFN-gamma), acute phase response and nutritional status as prognostic factors in lung cancer. *Cytokine*, **11**, 80–6.

120. Llovera, M., Carbo, N., Lopez-Soriano, J. *et al.* (1998). Different cytokines modulate ubiquitin gene expression in rat skeletal muscle. *Cancer Letters*, **133**, 83–7.

121. Barber, M.D., Powell, J.J., Lynch, S.F. *et al.* (2000). A polymorphism of the interleukin-1 beta gene influences survival in pancreatic cancer. *British Journal of Cancer*, **83**, 1443–7.

122. Cahlin, C., Korner, A., Axelsson, H. *et al.* (2000). Experimental cancer cachexia: the role of host-derived cytokines interleukin (IL)-6, IL-12, interferon-gamma, and tumor necrosis factor alpha evaluated in gene knockout, tumor-bearing mice on C57 Bl background and eicosanoid-dependent cachexia. *Cancer Research*, **60**, 5488–93.

123. Bossola, M., Muscaritoli, M., Bellantone, R. *et al.* (2000). Serum tumour necrosis factor-alpha levels in cancer patients are discontinuous and correlate with weight loss. *European Journal of Clinical Investigation*, **30**, 1107–12.

124. Karayiannakis, A.J., Syrigos, K.N., Polychronidis, A. *et al.* (2001). Serum levels of tumor necrosis factor-alpha and nutritional status in pancreatic cancer patients. *Anticancer Research*, **21**, 1355–8.

125. Socher, S.H., Martinez, D., Craig, J.B. *et al.* (1988). Tumor necrosis factor not detectable in patients with clinical cancer cachexia. *Journal of the National Cancer Institute*, **80**, 595–8.

126. Maltoni, M., Fabbri, L., Nanni, O. *et al.* (1997). Serum levels of tumour necrosis factor alpha and other cytokines do not correlate with weight loss and anorexia in cancer patients. *Supportive Care in Cancer*, **5**, 130–5.

127. Jatoi, A., Egner, J., Loprinzi, C.L. *et al.* (2004). Investigating the utility of serum cytokine measurements in a multi-institutional cancer anorexia/weight loss trial. *Support Care Cancer*, **12**, 640–4.

128. McMillan, D.C., Forrest, L.M., O'Gorman, P. *et al.* (2002). Performance status of male and female advanced cancer patients is independently predicted by mid-upper arm circumference measurement. *Nutrition and Cancer*, **42**, 191–3.

129. Plata-Salaman, C.R. (2000). Central nervous system mechanisms contributing to the cachexia-anorexia syndrome. *Nutrition*, **16**, 1009–12.

130. Negri, D.R., Mezzanzanica, D., Sacco, S. *et al.* (2001). Role of cytokines in cancer cachexia in a murine model of intracerebral injection of human tumours. *Cytokine*, **15**, 27–38.

131. Zhang, Y., Pilon, G., Marette, A. *et al.* (2000). Cytokines and endotoxin induce cytokine receptors in skeletal muscle. *American Journal of Physiology, Endocrinology and Metabolism*. **279**, E196–205.

132. Carbo, N., Lopez-Soriano, J., Costelli, P. *et al.* (2001). Interleukin-15 mediates reciprocal regulation of adipose and muscle mass: a potential role in body weight control. *Biochimica et Biophysica Acta*, **1526**, 17–24.

133. Knapp, M.L., al-Sheibani, S., Riches, P.G. *et al.* (1991). Hormonal factors associated with weight loss in patients with advanced breast cancer. *Annals of Clinical Biochemistry*, **28**, 480–6.

134. Llovera, M., Garcia-Martinez, C., Costelli, P. *et al.* (1996). Muscle hypercatabolism during cancer cachexia is not reversed by the glucocorticoid receptor antagonist RU38486. *Cancer Letters*, **99**, 7–14.

135. Koeberle D, Saletti P, Borner M. *et al.* (2008). Swiss Group for Clinical Cancer Research. Patient-reported outcomes of patients with advanced biliary tract cancers receiving gemcitabine plus capecitabine: a multicenter, phase II trial of the Swiss Group for Clinical Cancer Research. *J Clin Oncol*, **26**(22), 3702–8.

136. Todorov, P., Cariuk, P., McDevitt, T. *et al.* (1996). Characterization of a cancer cachectic factor. *Nature*, **379**, 739–42.

137. Wieland, B.M., Stewart, G.D., Skipworth, R.J. *et al.*(2007). Is there a human homologue to the murine proteolysis-inducing factor? *Clinical Cancer Research*, **13**, 4984–92.

138. Jatoi, A., Foster, N., Wieland, B. *et al.* (2006). The proteolysis-inducing factor: in search of its clinical relevance in patients with metastatic gastric/esophageal cancer. *Diseases of the Esophagus*, **19**, 241–7.

139. Wigmore, S.J., Todorov, P.T., Barber, M.D. *et al.* (2000). Characteristics of patients with pancreatic cancer expressing a novel cancer cachectic factor. *British Journal of Surgery*, **87**, 53–8.

140. Cabal-Manzano, R., Bhargava, P., Torres-Duarte, A. *et al.* (2001). Proteolysis-inducing factor is expressed in tumours of patients with gastrointestinal cancers and correlates with weight loss. *British Journal of Cancer*, **84**, 1599–601.

141. McDevitt, T.M., Todorov, P.T., Beck, S.A. *et al.* (1995). Purification and characterization of a lipid-mobilizing factor associated with cachexia-inducing tumors in mice and humans. *Cancer Research*, **55**, 1458–63.

142. Tisdale, M.J. (2000). Catabolism of skeletal muscle proteins and its reversal in cancer cachexia. *Nestle Nutrition Workshop Series. Clinical and Performance Programme*, **4**, 135–43.

143. Lorite, M.J., Smith, H.J., Arnold, J.A. *et al.* (2001). Activation of ATP-ubiquitin-dependent proteolysis in skeletal muscle in vivo and murine myoblasts in vitro by a proteolysis-inducing factor (PIF). *British Journal of Cancer*, **85**, 297–302.

144. Smith, H.J., Lorite, M.J., and Tisdale, M.J. (1999). Effect of a cancer cachectic factor on protein synthesis/degradation in murine C2C12 myoblasts: modulation by eicosapentaenoic acid. *Cancer Research*, **59**, 5507–13.

145. Lorite, M.J., Thompson, M.G., Drake, J.L. *et al.* (1998). Mechanism of muscle protein degradation induced by a cancer cachectic factor. *British Journal of Cancer*, **78**, 850–6.

146. Tisdale, M.J. (2000). Biomedicine. Protein loss in cancer cachexia. *Science*, **289**, 2293–4.

147. Watchorn, T.M., Waddell, I., Dowidar, N. *et al.* (2001). Proteolysis-inducing factor regulates hepatic gene expression via the transcription factors NF-(kappa)B and STAT3. *The FASEB Journal*, **15**, 562–4.

148. Islam-Ali, B., Khan, S., Price, S.A. *et al.* (2001). Modulation of adipocyte G-protein expression in cancer cachexia by a lipid-mobilizing factor (LMF). *British Journal of Cancer*, **85**, 758–63.

149. Ogata, E. (2000). Parathyroid hormone-related protein as a potential target of therapy for cancer-associated morbidity. *Cancer*, **88**, 2909–11.

150. Frost, R.A. and Lang, C.H. (1998). Growth factors in critical illness: regulation and therapeutic aspects. *Current Opinion in Clinical Nutrition and Metabolic Care*, **1**, 195–204.

151. Fiebig, H.H., Dengler, W., Hendriks, H.R. (2000). No evidence of tumor growth stimulation in human tumors in vitro following treatment with recombinant human growth hormone. *Anti-cancer Drugs*, **11**, 659–64.

152. Jenkins, R.C. and Ross, R.J. (1996). Growth hormone therapy for protein catabolism. *The Quarterly Journal of Medicine*, **89**, 813–9.

153. Yu, H. and Rohan, T. (2000). Role of the insulin-like growth factor family in cancer development and progression. *Journal of the National Cancer Institute*, **92**, 1472–89.

154. Florini, J.R., Ewton, D.Z., and Coolican, S.A. (1996). Growth hormone and the insulin-like growth factor system in myogenesis. *Endocrine Reviews*, **17**, 481–517.

155. Frost, R.A. and Lang, C.H. (1999). Differential effects of insulin-like growth factor I (IGF-I) and IGF-binding protein-1 on protein metabolism in human skeletal muscle cells. *Endocrinology*, **140**, 3962–70.

156. Lalani, R., Bhasin, S., Byhower, F. *et al.* (2000). Myostatin and insulin-like growth factor-I and -II expression in the muscle of rats exposed to the microgravity environment of the NeuroLab space shuttle flight. *The Journal of Endocrinology*, **167**, 417–28.

157. Jenkins, R.C. and Ross, R.J. (1996). Acquired growth hormone resistance in catabolic states. *Bailliere's Clinical Endocrinology and Metabolism*, **10**, 411–9.

158. Takala, J., Ruokonen, E., Webster, N.R. *et al.* (1999). Increased mortality associated with growth hormone treatment in critically ill adults. *The New England Journal of Medicine*, **341**, 785–92.

159. Svanberg, E., Frost, R.A., Lang, C.H. *et al.* (2000). IGF-I/IGFBP-3 binary complex modulates sepsis-induced inhibition of protein synthesis in skeletal muscle. *American Journal of Physiology, Endocrinology, and Metabolism*, **279**, E1145–58.

160. Lang, C.H., Frost, R.A., Jefferson, L.S. *et al.* (2000). Endotoxin-induced decrease in muscle protein synthesis is associated with changes in eIF2B, eIF4E, and IGF-I. *American Journal of Physiology, Endocrinology, and Metabolism*, **278**, E1133–43.

161. Fang, C.H., Li, B.G., Wang, J.J. *et al.* (1998). Treatment of burned rats with insulin-like growth factor I inhibits the catabolic response in skeletal muscle. *The American Journal of Physiology*, **275**, R1091–8.

162. Hobler, S.C., Williams, A.B., Fischer, J.E. *et al.* (1998). IGF-I stimulates protein synthesis but does not inhibit protein breakdown in muscle from septic rats. *The American Journal of Physiology*, **274**, R571–6.

163. Jurasinski, C.V. and Vary, T.C. (1995). Insulin-like growth factor I accelerates protein synthesis in skeletal muscle during sepsis. *The American Journal of Physiology*, **269**, E977–81.

164. Fang, C.H., Li, B.G., Sun, X. *et al.* (2000). Insulin-like growth factor I reduces ubiquitin and ubiquitin-conjugating enzyme gene expression but does not inhibit muscle proteolysis in septic rats. *Endocrinology*, **141**, 2743–51.

165. Anker, S.D., Volterrani, M., Pflaum, C.D. *et al.* (2001). Acquired growth hormone resistance in patients with chronic heart failure: implications for therapy with growth hormone. *Journal of the American College of Cardiology*, **38**, 443–52.

166. Simons, J.P., Schols, A.M., Buurman, W.A. *et al.* (1999). Weight loss and low body cell mass in males with lung cancer: relationship with systemic inflammation, acute-phase response, resting energy expenditure, and catabolic and anabolic hormones. *Clinical Science (London)*, **97**, 215–23.

167. Helle, S.I., Geisler, S., Aas, T. *et al.* (2001). Plasma insulin-like growth factor binding protein-3 proteolysis is increased in primary breast cancer. *British Journal of Cancer*, **85**, 74–7.

168. Helle, S.I., Geisler, J., Anker, G.B. *et al.* (2001). Alterations in the insulin-like growth factor system during treatment with diethylstilboestrol in patients with metastatic breast cancer. *British Journal of Cancer*, **85**, 147–51.

169. Osterziel, K.J., Strohm, O., Schuler, J. *et al.* (1998). Randomised, double-blind, placebo-controlled trial of human recombinant growth hormone in patients with chronic heart failure due to dilated cardiomyopathy. *Lancet*, **351**, 1233–7.

170. Papadakis, M.A., Grady, D., Black, D. *et al.* (1996). Growth hormone replacement in healthy older men improves body composition but not functional ability. *Annals of Internal Medicine*, **124**, 708–16.

171. Burdet, L., de Muralt, B., Schutz, Y. *et al.* (1997). Administration of growth hormone to underweight patients with chronic obstructive pulmonary disease. A prospective, randomized, controlled study. *American Journal of Respiratory and Critical Care Medicine*, **156**, 1800–6.

172. Schambelan, M., Mulligan, K., Grunfeld, C. *et al.* (1996). Recombinant human growth hormone in patients with HIV-associated wasting. A randomized, placebo-controlled trial. Serostim Study Group. *Annals of Internal Medicine*, **125**, 873–82.

173. Morley, J.E. (2001). Anorexia, body composition, and ageing. *Current Opinion in Clinical Nutrition and Metabolic Care*, **4**, 9–13.

174. Wang, C., Alexander, G., Berman, N. *et al.* (1996). Testosterone replacement therapy improves mood in hypogonadal men – a clinical research center study. *The Journal of Clinical Endocrinology and Metabolism*, **81**, 3578–83.

175. Lobo, R.A. (2001). Androgens in postmenopausal women: production, possible role, and replacement options. *Obstetrical and Gynecological Survey*, **56**, 361–76.

176. Bhasin, S., Storer, T.W., Berman, N. *et al.* (1996). The effects of supraphysiologic doses of testosterone on muscle size and strength in normal men. *The New England Journal of Medicine*, **335**, 1–7.

177. Snyder, P.J., Peachey, H., Berlin, J.A. *et al.* (2000). Effects of testosterone replacement in hypogonadal men. *The Journal of Clinical Endocrinology and Metabolism*, **85**, 2670–7.

178. Dobs, A.S., Few, W.L. 3rd,. Blackman, M.R. *et al.* (1996). Serum hormones in men with human immunodeficiency virus-associated wasting. *The Journal of Clinical Endocrinology and Metabolism*, **81**, 4108–12.

179. Grinspoon, S., Corcoran, C., Lee, K. *et al.* (1996). Loss of lean body and muscle mass correlates with androgen levels in hypogonadal men with acquired immunodeficiency syndrome and wasting. *The Journal of Clinical Endocrinology and Metabolism*, **81**, 4051–8.

180. Arver, S., Sinha-Hikim, I., Beall, G. *et al.* (1999). Serum dihydrotestosterone and testosterone concentrations in human immunodeficiency virus-infected men with and without weight loss. *Journal of Andrology*, **20**, 611–8.

181. Grinspoon, S., Corcoran, C., Miller, K. *et al.* (1997). Body composition and endocrine function in women with acquired immunodeficiency syndrome wasting. *The Journal of Clinical Endocrinology and Metabolism*, **82**, 1332–7.

182. Bhasin, S., Storer, T.W., Javanbakht, M. *et al.* (2000). Testosterone replacement and resistance exercise in HIV-infected men with weight loss and low testosterone levels. *Journal of the American Medical, Association*, **283**, 763–70.

183. Garcia, J.M., Li, H., Mann, D. *et al.* (2006). Hypogonadism in male patients with cancer. *Cancer*, **106**, 2583–91.

184. Abs, R., Verhelst, J., Maeyaert, J. et al. (2000). Endocrine consequences of long-term intrathecal administration of opioids. *The Journal of Clinical Endocrinology and Metabolism*, **85**, 2215–22.

185. Handelsman, D.J. and Dong, Q. (1993). Hypothalamo-pituitary gonadal axis in chronic renal failure. *Endocrinology and Metabolism Clinics of North America*, **22**, 145–61.

186. Johansen, K.L., Mulligan, K., and Schambelan, M. (1999). Anabolic effects of nandrolone decanoate in patients receiving dialysis: a randomized controlled trial. *Journal of the American Medical Association*, **281**, 1275–81.

187. Kamischke, A., Kemper, D.E., Castel, M.A. et al. (1998).Testosterone levels in men with chronic obstructive pulmonary disease with or without glucocorticoid therapy. *The European Respiratory Journal*, **11**, 41–5.

188. Schols, A.M., Soeters, P.B., Mostert, R. et al. (1995). Physiologic effects of nutritional support and anabolic steroids in patients with chronic obstructive pulmonary disease. A placebo-controlled randomized trial. *American Journal of Respiratory and Critical Care Medicine*, **152**,1268–74.

189. Reid, I.R., Wattie, D.J., Evans, M.C. et al. (1996). Testosterone therapy in glucocorticoid-treated men. *Archives of Internal Medicine*, **156**, 1173–7.

190. Feelders, R.A., Swaak, A.J., Romijn, J.A. et al. (1999). Characteristics of recovery from the euthyroid sick syndrome induced by tumor necrosis factor alpha in cancer patients. *Metabolism*, **48**, 324–9.

191. Knapp, M.L., al-Sheibani, S., Riches, P.G. et al. (1991). Hormonal factors associated with weight loss in patients with advanced breast cancer. *Annals of Clinical Biochemistry*, **28**, 480–6.

192. Lambert, M. (1994). Thyroid dysfunction in HIV infection. *Bailliere's Clinical Endocrinology and Metabolism*, **8**, 825–35.

193. Teunissen, S.C., Wesker, W., Kruitwagen, C. et al. (2007). Symptom prevalence in patients with incurable cancer: a systematic review. *Journal of Pain and Symptom Management*, **34**, 94–104.

194. Extermann, M. and Hurria, A. (2007). Comprehensive geriatric assessment for older patients with cancer. *Journal of Clinical Oncology*, **25**, 1824–31.

195. Del Fabbro, E., Dalal, S., Delgado, M. et al. (2007). Secondary vs primary cachexia in patients with advanced cancer. *Journal of Clinical Oncology*, **24**:49s (suppl; abstract 9128).

196. Hutton, J.L., Martin, L., Field, C.J. et al. (2006). Dietary patterns in patients with advanced cancer: implications for anorexia-cachexia therapy. *American Journal of Clinical Nutrition*, **84**, 1163–70.

197. Shragge, J.E., Wismer, W.V., Olson, K.L. et al. (2006). The management of anorexia by patients with advanced cancer: a critical review of the literature. *Palliative Medicine*, **20**, 623–9.

198. Zanon, C., Grosso, M., Aprà, F. et al. (2002). Palliative treatment of malignant refractory ascites by positioning of Denver peritoneovenous shunt. *Tumori*, **88**, 123–7.

199. Paddon-Jones, D., Sheffield-Moore, M., Cree, M.G. et al. (2006). Atrophy and impaired muscle protein synthesis during prolonged inactivity and stress. *Journal of Clinical Endocrinology and Metabolism*, **91**, 4836–41.

200. Hutton, J.L., Baracos, V.E., Wismer, W.V. (2007). Chemosensory dysfunction is a primary factor in the evolution of declining nutritional status and quality of life in patients with advanced cancer. *Journal of Pain and Symptom Management*, **33**, 156–65.

201. Bernhardson, B.M., Tishelman, C., Rutqvist, L.E. (2008). Self-reported taste and smell changes during cancer chemotherapy. *Support Care Cancer*, **16**, 275–83.

202. Rubenstein, E.B., Peterson, D.E., Schubert, M. et al. (2004). Mucositis Study Section of the Multinational Association for Supportive Care in Cancer; International Society for Oral Oncology. Clinical practice guidelines for the prevention and treatment of cancer therapy-induced oral and gastrointestinal mucositis. *Cancer*, **100**(9 Suppl), 2026–46.

203. Bruera, E., Moyano, J.R., Sala, R. et al. (2004). Dexamethasone in addition to metoclopramide for chronic nausea in patients with advanced cancer: a randomized controlled trial. *Journal of Pain and Symptom Management*, **28**, 381–8.

204. Qian, L., Orr, W.C., Chen, J.D. (2002). Inhibitory reflexive effect of rectal distension on postprandial gastric myoelectrical activity. *Digestive Diseases and Sciences*, **47**, 2473–9.

205. Mercadante, S., Villari, P., Ferrera, P. et al. (2006). Opioid-induced or pain relief-reduced symptoms in advanced cancer patients? *European Journal of Pain*, **10**, 153–9.

206. Chiu, T.Y., Hu, W.Y., Lue, B.H. et al. (2004). Dyspnea and its correlates in taiwanese patients with terminal cancer. *Journal of Pain and Symptom Management*, **28**, 123–32.

207. Cherel, Y., Robin, J.P., Heitz, A. et al. (1992). Relationships between lipid availability and protein utilization during prolonged fasting. *Journal of Comparative Physiology B. Biochemical, Systemic, and Environmental Physiology*, **162**, 305–13.

208. Omlin, A., Blum, D., Baumann, K. et al. (2008). The frequency, the relative role and reversibility of secondary causes of impaired oral nutritional intake in advanced cancer patients - a systematic literature review. *Palliative Medicine*, **22**, 451 (abstract 170).

209. Langer, C.J., Hoffman, J.P., Ottery, F.D. (2001). Clinical significance of weight loss in cancer patients: rationale for the use of anabolic agents in the treatment of cancer-related cachexia. *Nutrition*, **17**(Suppl 1):S1–20.

210. Barbosa-Silva, M.C. and Barros, A.J. (2006). Indications and limitations of the use of subjective global assessment in clinical practice: an update. *Current Opinion in Clinical Nutrition and Metabolic Care*, **9**, 263–9.

211. Clark D. 'Total pain', disciplinary power and the body in the work of Cicely Saunders, 1958–1967. *Social Science and Medicine*, **49**, 727–36.

212. Klein, S., Kinney, J., Jeejeebhoy, K. et al. (1997). Nutrition support in clinical practice: review of published data and recommendations for future research directions. Summary of a conference sponsored by the National Institutes of Health, American Society for Parenteral and Enteral Nutrition, and American Society for Clinical Nutrition. *The American Journal of Clinical Nutrition*, **66**, 683–706.

213. Bozzetti, F., Amadori, D., Bruera, E. et al. (1996). Guidelines on artificial nutrition versus hydration in terminal cancer patients. European Association for Palliative Care. *Nutrition*, **12**, 163–7.

214. Winter, S.M. (2000). Terminal nutrition: framing the debate for the withdrawal of nutritional support in terminally ill patients (Review). *The American Journal of Medicine*, **109**, 723–6.

10.3.2 Classification, clinical assessment, and treatment of the anorexia–cachexia syndrome

Kenneth C.H. Fearon, Vickie Baracos, and Sharon Watanabe

Introduction

The anorexia–cachexia syndrome is a complex multi-dimensional problem for which there has been no generally agreed classification system or treatment algorithm. This had led clinicians to feel that perhaps it is not worth trying to grapple with the difficult problem of assessment and treatment of patients with cachexia. The aim of this chapter is to resolve some of these issues and provide: (1) the reader with some background principles to classification; (2) a simple approach to patient assessment and a robust algorithm for basic multimodal treatment; and (3) an overview of the evidence base for different pharmacological interventions.

Cachexia affects a wide spectrum of patients with a variety of chronic diseases including cancer, chronic heart failure, end-stage renal failure, rheumatoid arthritis, and HIV. Whilst undoubtedly there are common mechanisms of wasting in each of these conditions, there are many unique aspects, which are too complex to explore in a single chapter. The present chapter focuses primarily on the patient with cancer. It is hoped that the principles outlined will provide a platform on which to build an approach for other groups of patients. To this end, comment is added on specific pharmacological interventions where the latter have been tested in large groups of cachectic patients with chronic diseases other than cancer.

Classification

A conceptual framework for classification

Cachexia is a syndrome of involuntary weight loss, progressing through various degrees of depletion and culminating in a cachectic (emaciated) state. The depletion pertains to body weight and its major elements, which constitute the physiological stores of energy and protein in the body (i.e. adipose tissue and skeletal muscle). Varying degrees of depletion are associated with quantifiable risks. The health risks that have been considered range from functional loss (e.g. physical function, immune function), morbidity (e.g. injuries from falls, infections), increased health service utilization and associated costs (e.g. hospital stay, emergency room visit) to mortality (Fig. 10.3.2.1). The timing of the emergence of and the magnitude of the clinical risks associated with body weight loss are affected by the patients' initial body weight (constituting the stores that may be mobilized) and the dynamic rate of loss of these constituents.

Weight and weight loss classification

It is important to be able to classify patients as overweight or underweight. The World Health Organization (WHO)[1] categories of body mass adjusted for stature [BMI: weight (kg)/height (m^2)] are widely used to classify clinically important deviations of body weight (Table 10.3.2.1). In addition to the risks from a variety of morbidities and mortality from secondary causes, depletion to a BMI in the vicinity of $10–11$ kg/m^2 is, of itself, fatal[2]. It should be noted that in patients over 65 years of age, a somewhat higher limit for underweight (20 kg/m^2) is generally accepted. During weight loss, individuals may pass through a zone conventionally referred to as 'normal', 'healthy', or 'ideal' body weight. However, depending on the intensity of weight loss, severe depletion will occur sooner or later; this situation is neither healthy nor ideal.

Various classification systems for grading weight loss show numerous inconsistencies. This is one possible explanation for the considerable confusion amongst oncologists as to what constitutes a clinically significant degree of weight loss[3]. The National Cancer Institute's Common Toxicity Criteria[4] are used widely to define cancer—and cancer therapy—associated toxicity and these define the total degree of loss relative to stable body weight as follows: Grade 0, <4.9 per cent loss; Grade 1, 5 –9.9 per cent; Grade 2, 10–19.9 per cent; and Grade 3, ≥20 per cent. Grade 4 (life-threatening) weight loss is not defined. Other weight loss grading systems in the clinical nutrition literature take into account rate of weight loss. The Scored Patient-Generated-Subjective Global Assessment (PG-SGA)[5] includes a useful grading system incorporating four weight loss grades that can be based on a 1-month or 6-month weight history, whichever is available (Table 10.3.2.2).

Measurement of tissue wasting

It is clear that the main constituents of body weight, adipose and lean tissues, merit separate consideration. This adds new orders of complexity to our understanding of wasting syndromes. Both muscle protein and adipose tissues can be considered as independent physiologic stores. The presence of a large adipose tissue reserve, at least up to a certain point, is a favourable prognostic factor in patients embarking on different types of wasting syndromes. By itself, depletion of muscle mass is associated with health risks, including frailty, functional problems in gait and balance, risk of falls, inability to complete tasks of daily living, extended hospital stay, and infectious and non-infectious complications in hospital, as well as overall mortality[6–10]. These health risks are seen to be independent of adiposity and are present in normal body weight ranges, as well as in obese persons.

The independent significance of muscle wasting requires some clinical capacity to determine muscle mass. Individuals within a population present with different degrees of muscularity, and this feature is variously expressed in the literature depending on the methods used for its determination. Whole-body muscle mass may be evaluated using image-based approaches, and is often expressed in the same units as BMI (kg skeletal muscle/m^2). Methods such as whole-body CT or MRI image analysis are required to determine this value. Dual energy X-ray absorptiometry may be used to quantify muscle in the arms and legs only, expressed as total appendicular skeletal muscle (kg/m^2). Anthropometrics constitute a simple tool to estimate skeletal muscle stores, as mid-arm muscle circumference. It should be noted that there are important methodological considerations. Ease of determination is often counterbalanced by low precision. Upper-arm measurements are prone to inter-observer variation. Scoring fatness and muscularity on physical examination has utility in the hands of a highly trained observer, but is otherwise difficult to standardize. Mid-arm muscle circumference is based on the assumption that the upper arm is perfectly cylindrical, which it is evidently not. The image-based methods enjoying high precision and the ability to discriminate muscle and adipose tissues require instrumentation, money, and time.

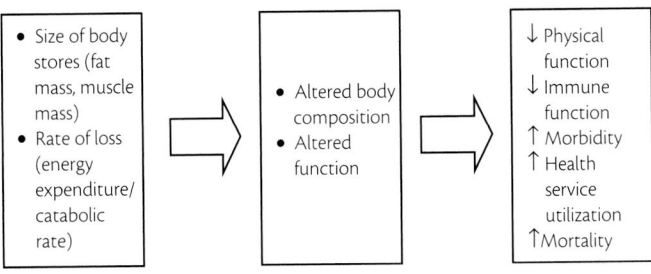

Figure 10.3.2.1 The timing and magnitude of the clinical risks associated with cachexia are determined, in part, by the size of the initial body stores and the rate at which they are lost.

Table 10.3.2.2 Weight loss score from the patient-generated-subjective global assessment.

Grade	1-month loss(%)	6-month loss (%)
0	0–1.9	0–1.9
1	2.0–2.9	2.0–5.9
2	3.0–4.9	6.0–9.9
3	5.0–9.9	10.0–19.9
4	≥ 10	≥ 20

Nevertheless, until image analysis becomes a routine facility, the CT- or MRI-based techniques will remain research techniques.

Cut-off points have been proposed for clinically important depletion of skeletal muscle (sarcopenia). Using dual-energy X-ray absorptiometry, low muscle mass has been defined as values > 2 standard deviations below the sex-specific mean for healthy, younger adults (<5.45 kg total appendicular skeletal muscle /m^2 for females and <7.26 kg /m^2 for males)[8,11]. Mid-arm muscle circumference below the 5th percentile is a related rule-of-thumb, and there are large data sets of reference values of this variable by sex and age.

Multiple-factor classification systems

Cachexia is a multi-dimensional problem and therefore it may not be possible to reflect the physiological change and clinical risks the patient sustains by a single measurement (e.g. loss of skeletal muscle mass). On the basis that risk derives from several key elements in the cachexia syndrome, a classification system based on weight loss (>10 per cent), reduced food intake (<1500 kcal/day) and systemic inflammation (serum C-reactive protein concentration >10mg/litre) has been proposed[12]. Patients with all three features have increased physiological impairment and reduced survival. Of key clinical importance is that patients with early stage of disease who demonstrate these features are at high risk of early demise and are therefore a key group to target for early and effective intervention.

Table 10.3.2.1 WHO classification of body mass adjusted for stature: body mass index (BMI).

	BMI (kg/m^2)
Severely underweight	<16
Moderately underweight	16–17
Mildly underweight	17–18.5[a]
Normal	18.5–25
Overweight	25–30
Class I obesity	30–35
Class II obesity	35–40
Morbid obesity	>40

Note: [a] Range extended 17–20 in elderly.

Clinical assessment and treatment strategy

When medical or nursing professionals who have not received specific training are confronted with a patient who requires nutritional assessment, the prospect can seem daunting. Moreover, the purpose of such assessment is often muddled since no clear link between assessment and treatment has been provided. The purpose of this section is to provide a clear, logical framework for patient assessment and to link this with a simple treatment algorithm.

Patients lose weight as a result of reduced food intake, abnormal metabolic activity, or most commonly, a combination of the two. Weight loss reflects that the patient has a negative energy balance (resulting in loss of fat mass: the main energy reserve) and a negative protein balance (resulting in loss of skeletal muscle: the main protein reserve). The purpose of nutritional assessment (Fig. 10.3.2.2) is to determine to what extent stores have been depleted, what contribution to this loss has been due to reduced food intake, what impact such changes are having on the patient's performance, and what potential there is for reversal of the situation? Each of these domains can be considered in relation to the patient's clinical journey (i.e. past, present, and future). The Scored PG-SGA[5] is a validated screening tool designed specifically for patients with cancer and is recommended by the Oncology Nutrition Dietetic Practice Group of the American Dietetic Association, and Oncology Nursing Society. Several elements of this instrument have practical utility for patient assessment, including the weight loss history (Table 10.3.2.2), the dietary intake component, checklist of 13 'nutrition impact' symptoms, and functional capacity component.

- *Stores*: the primary variables that are assessed readily are weight and weight loss history. Key questions include: height and current weight (kg), previous stable weight, duration of weight loss, and calculation of percentage weight loss. Weight loss Grade 3 or 4, Table 10.3.2.2) and/or a BMI <18.5 kg/m^2 are indicators of depletion of energy and/or protein reserves.

- *Intake*: routine clinical assessment with the PG-SGA includes such basic questions concerning type and amount of intake, loss of appetite, presence of early satiety, and other symptoms impeding dietary intake. This level of assessment is intended for non-specialists, and is useful for deciding when to refer patients to a nutrition health-care professional (dietitian or specialist in clinical nutrition). A detailed diet history or diet diary is a specialized assessment which is usually undertaken by a dietician. The information from such assessments can be used to estimate total energy and macronutrient intakes.

- *Performance*: every clinical, medical, or surgical oncologist is used to assessing the performance status of patients. The functional capacity component of the PG-SGA, is a version of the Eastern Cooperative Oncology Group (ECOG) performance status score; alternatively, either the WHO or Karnofsky scales may be used. Knowledge whether the patient is active and mobile is vital in determining not only how depletion of stores/intake is affecting quality of life but also what the nature of therapy should be. Bed-bound patients suffer from anabolic resistance and, in these circumstances, it is very difficult to improve muscle mass/function.

♦ *Potential*: knowledge of the patients' tumour type, stage of disease and purpose of current cancer therapy can give a ready impression of prognosis and the purpose of nutritional intervention. The presence or absence of systemic inflammation (serum C-reactive protein >10 mg/litre) may also identify the patient who requires early nutritional/metabolic support[12]. For the patient with relatively stable disease and with more than 2 months to live, it is reasonable to plan nutritional intervention. For the patient whose disease is progressing rapidly and has less than 2–3 months to live, symptomatic management (e.g. steroids) is perhaps more appropriate. It is also important to consider carefully the patients' expectations concerning the future benefits of any intervention. The burden of intervention (e.g. daily intake of oral nutritional supplements) has to match what the patient is willing to consider in the light of possible gains.

Intervention strategy

A simple treatment algorithm is outlined in Fig. 10.3.2.3. For those not at nutritional risk (e.g. weight stable, adequate macronutrient stores, normal appetite/intake, good performance status, and stable disease) it would be reasonable simply to review or ask the patients to seek further advice if they lose weight. For patients at nutritional risk (Grade 3 or 4 weight loss, BMI <18.5, evidence of depletion of lean body mass, reduced appetite/intake), it is vital to undertake a screen for reversible causes of anorexia/reduced food intake and to

ensure that their underlying primary disease and co-morbidities are being managed optimally. Key variables to consider in relation to secondary causes of reduced intake include oral ulceration, intestinal obstruction, constipation, diarrhoea, nausea, vomiting, uncontrolled pain, and side effects of drugs. Metabolism-related variables include the development of diabetes or malabsorption (e.g. both common associations with advanced pancreatic cancer) and, which, if not managed with insulin/pancreatic enzyme supplements, will result in continuing weight loss independent of any nutritional intervention.

The next stage in assessment involves consideration of the patients' performance status, prognosis and expectations. For patients reaching an end-of-life phase and whose main complaint is anorexia, it would be reasonable to consider the prescription of oral steroids or megestrol acetate. For patients with a better prognosis and who are not bed-bound, consideration should be given to four specific domains.

1 *Oral intake*: cancer patients are often anxious about whether their diet has contributed to the development of cancer or whether it may modify the course of established illness. In general, it is important to emphasize the need for a broad balanced diet and to explain the importance of maintaining a normal food intake in order to undergo cancer therapy or to optimize quality of life. It is vital to explore what patients consider to be a normal diet and to identify the principal daily source of protein in the diet. Two key basics in dietary advice are: (1) that the average daily calorie deficit in a weight-losing cancer patient is of the order of 250–400 kcal/day and (2) that it is vital to maintain protein intake at a high level in order to either stabilize or replete diminished skeletal muscle mass. Protein intake should generally be maintained between 1–1.5 g/kg/day[13]. In order to achieve this intake, patients will generally need to consume red or white meat or fish on a daily basis and supplement this with dairy products (e.g. milk or cheese). An alternative approach is to take an energy- and protein-dense oral nutritional supplement. A 250-ml carton with 1.5 kcal/ml should contain sufficient calories and protein to make up the average daily deficit. However, significant repletion of a patient with depleted stores will probably require consumption of two such supplements per day. Patients will often benefit from specialist dietary assessment and advice from a dietician especially if they continue to lose weight after initial management.

2 *Exercise*: the average physical activity levels of advanced cancer patients still attending the outpatient clinic is reduced by about 40–50 per cent[14]. Many patients with advanced cancer are elderly and may have significant co-morbidity. Thus, the idea of resistance exercise training to optimize muscle mass is beyond their capacity. However, it is vital to explain to patients the value of daily exercise to counteract muscle wasting. Simply maintaining mobility and going out for a regular daily walk are reasonable goals to set. Motivated patients may benefit from the advice of a physiotherapist.

3 *Anti-inflammatory*: there is growing evidence concerning the role of systemic inflammation in most forms of cachexia. Inflammatory mediators contribute to both reduced food intake and metabolic change. There is no ideal anti-inflammatory strategy that has been proven to be of benefit in cachexia. However, two common approaches are either non-steroidals

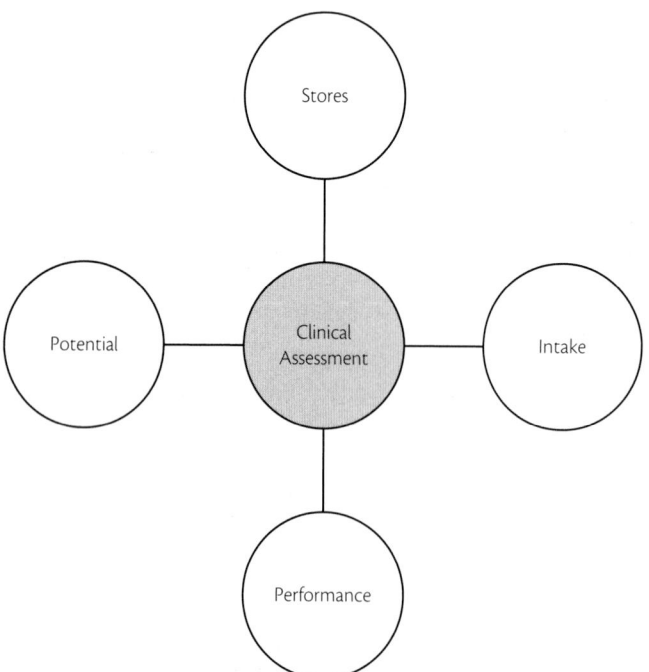

Figure 10.3.2.2 Components of clinical assessment.

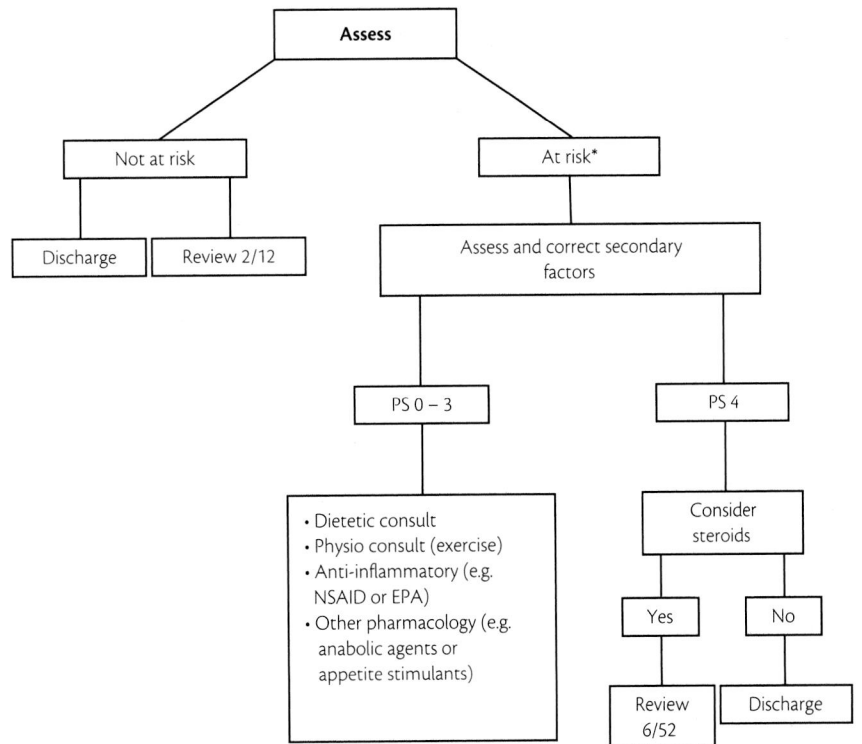

Figure 10.3.2.3 Cachexia intervention algorithm.
* At risk defined by the presence of persistent weight loss, reduced dietary intake,

(NSAIDs)[15] or fish oil (eicosapentaenoic acid). NSAIDs with a low incidence of GI side effects such as ibuprofen (400 mg x 3/day) can be taken long term with or without gastric mucosal protection. Fish oil represents a 'natural' alternative and may appeal more to some patients. A total dose of 1.5–2.0 g/day eicosapentaenoic acid is recommended and can be taken either as fish oil capsules[16] or as a fish-oil-enriched oral nutritional supplement[17,18].

4   *Other specific pharmacological agents*: see 'Pharmacological treatment'.

Pharmacological treatment

Pharmacological approaches to wasting syndromes have a number of specific treatment targets and have been evaluated in a variety of diseases, including cancer, AIDS, and chronic obstructive pulmonary disease. Such pharmacological treatments have been assessed in randomized clinical trials, and there are a number of high-quality systematic reviews (i.e. Cochrane Database) available, summarizing the evidence. The reader is referred to these reviews for full details; the results of the systematic reviews are summarized in the following paragraphs. Information from subsequently published trials has been added.

Cancer

In 2005, Yavuzsen and co-workers published a systematic review of pharmacological therapies for cancer-associated anorexia and weight loss in adult patients with non-hematological malignancies[19]. Databases searched were Ovid (MEDLINE, EMBASE), CINAHL, and Cochrane Control Trials Register. Only

randomized controlled trials published in English were considered. A total of 55 studies met inclusion criteria. Only two classes of drugs (progestins and corticosteroids) were found to have sufficient evidence to support their use in cancer patients. Studies with other agents had mixed outcomes, positive results in only a single trial, or were not adequately controlled. Note was made of heterogeneity amongst trials with respect to outcome measures, assessment tools, treatment duration, and timing of assessment.

Progestins

The largest number of studies involved progestins (29 trials were conducted in a total of 4139 patients). Twenty-three trials in 3436 patients involved megestrol acetate at doses of 160 mg to 1600 mg/day for 2 weeks to 2 years. Results for appetite and weight gain favored megestrol acetate over placebo. Five trials comparing different doses suggested that the optimal dose is between 480 and 800 mg/day. The influence of megestrol acetate on quality of life was minimal.

Five trials compared megestrol acetate with other drugs. Megestrol acetate was equivalent to corticosteroids and significantly better than dronabinol and fluoxymesterone for appetite stimulation. Compared with cisapride, megestrol acetate was associated with significantly less weight loss and better appetite. Ibuprofen plus megestrol acetate was better than megestrol acetate plus placebo at maintaining weight. A study comparing megestrol acetate with eicosapentaenoic acid will be discussed later.

Six trials in 703 patients involved medroxyprogesterone acetate at doses of 300 mg to 1200 mg/day for 6 to 12 weeks. Medroxyprogesterone acetate was associated with greater increase in weight and appetite versus placebo. Effects on quality of life were inconsistent.

In 2005, Berenstein and co-workers published a systematic review of megestrol acetate for the treatment of anorexia–cachexia syndrome in patients with cancer, AIDS or other underlying pathology[20]. Thirty randomized controlled trials involving 4123 patients were identified. Twenty-two were performed in cancer patients, while the remainder was in patients with AIDS, chronic obstructive lung disease, and cystic fibrosis, as well as in the elderly. Compared with placebo, relative risk for appetite improvement and weight gain in cancer patients was 3.09 (95 per cent confidence interval 1.68 to 5.69) and 2.14 (95 per cent confidence interval 1.41 to 3.24), respectively. Oedema of the lower limbs was the only side effect that occurred at a statistically significantly greater frequency with megestrol acetate compared with placebo (relative risk 1.74, 95 per cent confidence interval 1.29 to 2.35).

Corticosteroids

Corticosteroids was the subject of six studies conducted in a total of 637 patients. Three trials in 402 patients used methylprednisolone orally or methylprednisolone sodium succinate intravenously at doses of 32 mg to 125 mg/day for 1 to 8 weeks. Versus placebo, improvement was seen in appetite, pain, quality of life, vomiting, well-being, and performance status. Weight did not change significantly.

One trial in 61 patients involved prednisolone 10 mg/day for 6 weeks. Compared with placebo, appetite and well-being were improved. Two trials in 184 patients used dexamethasone 3 mg to 8 mg/day for 4 days or until time of death. A transient improvement in appetite compared to placebo was seen. Due to their well-known adverse effects, particularly with longer duration of use, corticosteroids may be more suitable for patients with a short life expectancy, especially if they have other symptoms that may be alleviated by this drug such as pain or nausea.

Eicosapentaenoic acid

A recent systematic review[21] last updated in 2006 included three trials in 689 patients, which examined the effects of eicosapentaenoic acid (EPA), given at a dosage of 1.2 to 2.2 g/day for 2 to 8 weeks. One study showed no differences in appetite, weight gain, well-being, or nutritional status compared with placebo. In a second study, the experimental group took a protein and energy-dense nutritional supplement enriched with n-3 fatty acids and antioxidants; no significant differences in outcomes were seen between the EPA and control groups by intent-to-treat analysis. A third study compared EPA plus placebo, megestrol acetate plus placebo, and EPA plus megestrol acetate; weight gain was greater with megestrol acetate compared with EPA, and improvement in appetite was similar between the two treatments; combining the treatments did not result in better outcomes compared to megestrol acetate alone. The review concluded that at present there was insufficient data to establish whether oral EPA was better than placebo. A different systematic review[22] concluded that administration of n-3 fatty acids in doses greater than or equal to 1.5 g/day for prolonged periods of time was associated with improvements in clinical, biological, and quality of life parameters. Neither review included the recent large randomized trial in 518 patients, which showed a non-significant, but clinically relevant treatment effect on lean body mass for 2 g EPA/day[23].

Cannabinoids

A systematic review[19] included one trial in 469 patients comparing dronabinol 5 mg/day versus megestrol acetate 800 mg/day versus the combination. Improvement in appetite was greater with megestrol acetate than with dronabinol alone. There was no additional benefit to combining the drugs[24].

In a multi-centre trial published in 2006, 243 patients were randomized in a double-blind manner to receive cannabis extract, dronabinol 2.5 mg, or placebo twice a day for 6 weeks. The study was terminated after the first interim analysis because of insufficient differences in the primary endpoint of appetite change between active treatment and placebo arms[25].

Androgenic steroids

Two trials[26,27] examining the effects of androgenic steroids have been conducted in 512 patients. The first compared chemotherapy plus nandrolone 200 mg intramuscularly weekly for 4 weeks versus chemotherapy alone. The nandrolone-treated patients demonstrated a trend towards less weight loss. The second trial, mentioned previously, compared fluoxymesterone with megestrol acetate or dexamethasone. Fluoxymesterone was inferior in terms of appetite and weight gain, and had greater toxicity.

Erythropoietin

Two trials[28,29] have examined the effects of erythropoietin in 417 patients using doses of 10 000 to 40 000 units per week for 8 weeks to 2.5 years. One study compared erythropoietin plus indomethacin with or without a specialized nutritional programme; since erythropoietin and indomethacin were given to all patients, no conclusions can be drawn about the specific effects of either drug. The other study compared indomethacin with or without erythropoietin, demonstrating greater weight loss in the group that received indomethacin alone.

Non-steroidal anti-inflammatory drugs

Two trials of indomethacin in combination with erythropoietin, and one trial of ibuprofen in combination with megestrol acetate, have been described in the relevant sections earlier. Gastrointestinal and renal toxicity are potential limitations to the use of non-steroidal anti-inflammatory drugs in advanced cancer patients.

Melatonin

Two trials[30,31] have examined the effects of melatonin in 186 patients, using doses of 20 mg/day for 1 to 16 weeks. Patients on melatonin lost less weight than control patients. No improvement was seen in nutritional intake and appetite.

Pentoxifylline

One trial[32] examined the effects of pentoxifylline 1200 mg/day compared with placebo in 70 patients. No benefit was found with the active drug.

Adenosine 5′-triphosphate

In a single-centre trial, 58 stage IIIB or IV non-small cell lung cancer patients were randomized in an open manner to receive adenosine 5′-triphophate and supportive care, or supportive care alone. ATP was administered by 30-h intravenous infusion every two weeks for 7 weeks, and then every 4 weeks for 3 doses. Treatment was given on an inpatient basis. Compared with placebo, ATP was associated with significantly less weight loss, improved upper and lower extremity strength, and better quality of life. Loss of fat mass, fat-free mass and mid-upper arm muscle area was attenuated with ATP. Energy intake and appetite were greater with ATP. Survival was not different between the two groups. The need for intravenous infusion is a potential limitation of this drug[33].

Thalidomide

In a randomized double-blind single-centre trial, 50 weight-losing patients with inoperable pancreatic cancer were treated with thalidomide 200 mg or placebo orally daily for 6 months. At 4 and 8 weeks, patients who received thalidomide demonstrated a significant increase in weight and bone-free muscle area, compared with controls. There were no differences in muscle strength, quality of life, or survival[34].

HIV

Anabolic steroids

In 2005, Johns *et al.* published a systematic review of anabolic steroids for the treatment of weight loss in HIV-infected individuals[35]. The review included randomized controlled trials of anabolic steroids in HIV-infected adults who had lost any amount of weight. Databases searched included CENTRAL, MEDLINE, AIDSLINE, CINAHL, Current Contents, EMBASE, AIDSearch, and NLM until 2005. Thirteen randomized controlled trials met inclusion criteria. Meta-analysis of change from baseline in lean body mass revealed a weighted mean difference of 1.3 kg (95 per cent confidence interval 0.6 to 2.0). Meta-analysis of change from baseline in body weight showed a weighted mean difference of 1.1 kg (95 per cent confidence interval 0.3 to 2.0). The trials involved different anabolic steroid analogues, routes of delivery, doses, duration of therapy, and methodology of reporting adverse events. Adverse events were usually reported as mild and reversible. The magnitude of increase in lean body mass and body weight was not large and may not be clinically relevant. Also, sample sizes were small and significant heterogeneity was found. It is unknown if changes in lean body mass and body weight correlate with survival, muscle strength, physical functioning, or quality of life.

Subsequent to the systematic review, a multi-centre trial[36] was published in which 262 weight-losing HIV-infected men were randomized in a double-blind manner to receive oxandrolone 20, 40 or 80 mg/day or placebo for 12 weeks. All patients then received oxandrolone 20 mg/day in an open label fashion. At 12 weeks or the last measurement, weight gain was greater in the oxandrolone 40 mg/day group than the placebo group. Increase in body cell mass was greater in the oxandrolone 40 mg and 80 mg/day groups than the placebo group. There were no differences in quality of life and total work output. By 24 weeks, weight gain was not different between groups. Oxandrolone treatment was accompanied by significant increases in transaminases and low-density lipoprotein and decreases in high-density lipoprotein.

Recombinant human growth hormone

In a randomized, double-blind, multi-centre trial, 60 patients with AIDS-associated wasting received subcutaneous injections of recombinant human growth hormone (rhGH) 1.4 mg/day plus placebo, recombinant insulin-like growth factor 1 (rhIGF-1) 5 mg bid plus placebo, the combination of the two drugs, or placebo only for 12 weeks. Weight increased in the rhGH and combination groups by 6 weeks, but there were no significant differences between groups by 12 weeks. Lean body mass increased in the rhGH, rhIGF-1 and combination groups by 6 weeks, but only in the combination group by 12 weeks. No differences were seen between groups in muscle function or quality of life[37].

In another randomized, double-blind, multi-centre trial 178 patients received rhGH 0.1 mg/kg or placebo subcutaneously daily for 12 weeks. Weight, lean body mass, and work output increased significantly, and fat mass decreased significantly, in the rhGH group but not in the placebo group. There were no differences between groups in quality of life[38].

In a 12-week trial, HIV-infected men with weight loss were randomized to receive nandrolone 10 mg or placebo intramuscularly in a double-blind manner, or rhGH 6 mg subcutaneously daily in an open label manner. Increases in lean body mass and fat-free mass were greater with nandrolone compared with placebo, but equivalent to rhGH. Fat mass decreased to a greater degree with rhGH than nandrolone or placebo. There were no significant differences between groups in measures of muscle performance, physical function, and endurance. Side effects (peripheral oedema, arthralgia, carpal tunnel syndrome) and rate of discontinuation were greater with rhGH[39].

Megestrol acetate

In a multi-centre trial, 271 patients with AIDS-related cachexia were randomized in a double-blind manner to receive megestrol acetate 100 mg, 400 mg, or 800 mg, or placebo daily for 12 weeks. Maximum weight change, percentage of patients gaining at least 5 lb, and mean change in lean body mass were greater in the group that received megestrol acetate 800 mg daily, compared with the group that received placebo. Also, perception of well-being, change in caloric intake, and improvement in appetite were greater in this group[40].

In another multi-centre trial, 100 patients with AIDS-related cachexia were randomized in a double-blind manner to receive megestrol acetate 800 mg or placebo daily for 12 weeks. Changes in caloric intake, protein intake, weight, body mass index, fat mass, anthropometric measurements, and well-being scores favoured megestrol acetate. There were no differences between groups in body water, lean body mass, performance status, and survival[41].

Forty patients with HIV-related weight loss were randomized in a multi-centre study to receive megestrol acetate 800 mg daily or oxandrolone 10 mg twice daily for 2 months in an open manner. In both groups, weight, body mass index, fat, and lean body mass increased significantly with no differences between groups[42].

Chronic obstructive pulmonary disease

Anabolic steroids

In a single-centre trial, 230 patients with moderate to severe COPD who were admitted to an inpatient pulmonary rehabilitation programme were randomized to receive placebo intramuscularly every 2 weeks for 4 doses, placebo injections plus nutritional supplementation, or nandrolone decanoate (50 mg for men and 25 mg for women) intramuscularly every 2 weeks for 4 doses plus nutritional supplementation. The injections were given in a double-blind manner. Patients in both groups that received nutritional supplementation gained weight. However, patients who did not receive nandrolone gained fat mass, whereas those who also received nandrolone gained fat-free mass. Maximal inspiratory pressure improved in both treatment groups at 4 weeks, but was sustained only in combination group at 8 weeks[43].

Megestrol acetate

In a multi-centre trial, 145 underweight COPD patients were randomized to receive megestrol acetate 800 mg or placebo daily for 8 weeks in a double-blind manner. The group that received megestrol acetate gained more weight compared to the placebo group. The weight gain was determined to be fat mass. $PaCO_2$ decreased and PaO$_2$ increased in the megestrol acetate group, consistent with stimulation of ventilation. There were no significant differences between groups in respiratory muscle strength. Distance walked in 6 min and dyspnoea score were worse in the megestrol acetate group compared to placebo, but body image and appetite scores were better[44].

Summary and future perspectives

At the present time there is a basis to adopt a proactive approach to screening, assessment, and early intervention for involuntary weight loss in cancer cachexia. There are clinically useful evaluations and the efficacy of a number of treatments have been established in randomized clinical trials. A future goal will be to further improve surveillance, especially the development of more clinically practical ways of assessing body composition so that losses of lean body mass and skeletal muscle may be detected early. A number of investigational new drugs are appearing in phase I/II clinical trials and these are targeted at stimulation of appetite in the hypothalamus as well as skeletal muscle anabolism. These agents provide further promise of slowing down or reversing weight loss and functional loss. Investigations of nutrient requirements are required to define the unique needs of patients with cachexia syndromes and underpin the development of nutritional recommendations or nutritional support products.

References

1. World Health Organ Tech Rep Ser. (2000). Obesity: Preventing and Managing the Global Epidemic. Report of a WHO consultation. **894**, i–xii, 1–253.

2. Rigaud, D., Hassid, J., Meulemans, A. *et al.* (2000). A paradoxical increase in resting energy expenditure in malnourished patients near death: the king penguin syndrome. *American Journal of Clinical Nutrition*, **72**, 355–60.

3. Spiro, A., Baldwin, C., Patterson, A. *et al.* (2006). The views and practice of oncologists towards nutritional support in patients receiving chemotherapy. *British Journal of Cancer*, **95**, 431–4.

4. Cancer Therapy Evaluation Program, Common Terminology Criteria for Adverse Events, Version 3.0, DCTD, NCI, NIH, DHHS March 31, 2003. (http://ctep.cancer.gov), Published Date: August 9, 2006.

5. Ottery, F.D. (1996). Definition of standardized nutritional assessment and interventional pathways in oncology. *Nutrition*, **12**, S15–9.

6. Morley, J.E., Baumgartner, R.N., Roubenoff, R. *et al.* (2001). Sarcopenia. *Journal of Laboratory and Clinical Medicine*, **137**, 231–43.

7. Cosqueric, G., Sebag, A., Ducolombier, C. *et al.* (2006). Sarcopenia is predictive of nosocomial infection in care of the elderly. *British Journal of Nutrition*, **96**, 895–901.

8. Baumgartner, R.N., Koehler, K.M., Gallagher, D. *et al.* (1998). Epidemiology of sarcopenia among the elderly in New Mexico. *American Journal of Epidemiology*, **147**, 755–63.

9. Roubenoff, R. (2003). Sarcopenia: effects on body composition and function. *Journal of Gerontology. Series A, Biological Sciences and Medical Sciences*, **58**, 1012–7.

10. Kyle, U.G., Pirlich, M., Lochs, H. *et al.* (2005). Increased length of hospital stay in underweight and overweight patients at hospital admission: a controlled population study. *Clinical Nutrition*, **24**, 133–42.

11. Janssen, I., Baumgartner, R.N., Ross, R. *et al.* (2004). Skeletal muscle cutpoints associated with elevated physical disability risk in older men and women. *American Journal of Epidemiology*, 159, 413–21.

12. Fearon, K.C.H., Voss, A.C., Hustead, D.S. on behalf of the Cancer Cachexia Study Group (2006). Definition of cancer cachexia: effect of weight loss, reduced food intake and systemic inflammation on functional status and prognosis. *American Journal of Clinial Nutrition*, **83**, 1345–50.

13. Wolfe, R.R. (2006). The underappreciated role of muscle in health and disease. *American Journal of Clinical Nutrition*, **84**, 475–82.

14. Dahele, M., Skipworth, R., Wall, L. *et al.* (2007). Objective physical activity and self-reported quality of life in patients receiving palliative chemotherapy. *Journal of Pain and Symptom Management*, **33**, 676–85.

15. Preston, T., Fearon, K.C.H., McMillan, D.C. *et al.* (1995). Effect of Ibuprofen on the acute phase response and protein metabolism in weight-losing cancer patients. *British Journal of Surgery*, **82**, 229–34.

16. Wigmore, S.J., Ross, J.A., Falconer, J.S. *et al.* (1996). The effect of polyunsaturated fatty acids on the progress of cachexia in patients with pancreatic cancer. *Nutrition*, **12**, S27–S30.

17. Fearon, K.C.H., von Meyenfeldt, M., Moses, A.G.W. *et al.* (2003). An energy and protein dense, high n-3 fatty acid oral supplement promotes weight gain in cancer cachexia. *Gut*, **52**, 1479–86.

18. Moses, A.W.G., Slater, C., Preston, T. *et al.* (2004). Reduced total energy expenditure and physical activity in cachectic patients with pancreatic cancer can be modulated by an energy and protein dense oral supplement enriched with n-3 fatty acids. *British Journal of Cancer*, **90**, 996–1002.

19. Yavuzsen, T., Davis, M.P., Walsh, D. *et al.* (2005). Systematic review of the treatment of cancer-associated anorexia and weight loss. *Journal of Clinical Oncology*, **23**, 8500–11.

20. Berenstein, E.G. and Ortiz, Z. (2005). Megestrol acetate for the treatment of anorexia-cachexia syndrome. *Cochrane Database of Systematic Reviews*, **2**, CD004310.

21. Dewey, A., Baughan, C., Dean, T. *et al.* (2007). Eicosapentaenoic acid (EPA, an omega-3 fatty acid from fish oils) for the treatment of cancer cachexia. *Cochrane Database of Systematic Reviews*, **1**: CD004597.

22. Colomer, R., Moreno-Nogueira, J.M., Garcia-Luna, P.P. *et al.* (2007). n-3 Fatty acids, cancer and cachexia: a systematic review of the literature. *British Journal of Nutrition*, **97**, 823–31.

23. Fearon, K.C.H., Barber, M.D., Moses, A.G. *et al.* (2006). Double-blind, placebo-controlled, randomized study of eicosapentaenoic acid diester in patients with cancer cachexia. *Journal of Clinical Oncology*, **24**, 3401–7.

24. Jatoi, A., Windschitl, H.E., Loprinzi, C.L. *et al.* (2002). Dronabinol versus megestrol acetate versus comgination therapy for cancer associated anorexia: A North Central Cancer Treatment Group study. *Journal of Clinical Oncology*, **20**, 567–73.

25. Strasser, F., Luftner, D., Possinger, K. *et al.* (2006). Comparison of orally administered cannabis extract and delta-9-tetrahydrocannabinol in treating patients with cancer-related anorexia-cachexia syndrome: a multicenter, Phase III, randomized, double-blind, placebo-controlled clinical trial from the Cannabis-In-Cachexia-Study-Group. *Journal of Clinical Oncology*, **24**, 3394–00.

26. Chlebowski, R.T., Herrold, J., Ali, I. *et al.* (1986). Influence of nandrolonte decanoate on weight loss in non-small cell lung cancer. *Cancer*, **58**, 183–6.

27. Loprinzi, C.L., Kugler, J.W., Sloan, J.A. *et al.* Randomized comparison of megestrol acetate versus fluoxymesterone for the treatment of cancer anorexia cachexia (1999). *Journal of Clinical Oncology*, **17**, 3299–306.

28. Lundholm, K., Daneryd, P., Bosaeus, I. *et al.* (2004). Palliative nutritional intervention in addition to cyclooxygenase and EPO treatment for patients with malignant disease: Effects on survival, metabolism, and function. *Cancer*, **100**, 1967–77.

29. Daneryd, P., Svanberg, E., Korner, U. *et al.* (1998). Protection of metabolic and exercise capacity in unselected weight losing cancer patients following treatment with recombinant erythropoietin: A randomized prospective study. *Cancer Research*, **58**, 5374–9.

30. Lissoni, P., Paolorossi, F., Tancini, G. *et al.* (2006). Is there a role for melatonin in the treatment of neoplastic cachexia? *European Journal of Cancer*, **32A**, 1340–3.

31. Lissoni, P., Chielelli, M., Villa, S. *et al.* (2003). Five years survival in metastatic nonsmall cell lung cancer patients treatment with chemotherapy alone or chemotherapy and melatonin: A randomized trial. *Journal of Pineal Research*, **35**, 12–5.

32. Goldberg, R.M., Loprinzi, C.L., Mailliard, J.A. *et al.* (1995). Pentoxifylline for treatment of cancer anorexia and cachexia? A randomized double blind placebo trial. *Journal of Clinical Oncology*, **13**, 2856–9.

33. Argteresch, H.J., Dagnelie, P.C., van der Gaast, A. *et al.* (2000). Randomized clinical trial of adenosine 5'-triphosphate in patients with advanced non-small-cell lung cancer. *Journal of the National Cancer Institute*, **92**, 321–28.

34. Gordon, J.N., Trebble, T.M., Ellis, R.D. *et al.* (2005). Thalidomide in the treatment of cancer cachexia: a randomized placebo controlled trial. *Gut*, **54**, 540–5.

35. Johns, K., Beddall, M.J., Corrin, R.C. (2005). Anabolic steroids for the treatment of weight loss in HIV-infected individuals. *Cochrane Database of Systematic Reviews*, **4**, CD005483.

36. Grunfeld, C., Kotler, D.P., Dobs, A., Glesby, M., Bhasin, S. (2006). Oxandrolone in the treatment of HIV-associated weight loss in men. *Journal of Acquired Immune Deficiency Syndrome*, **41**, 304–14.

37. Waters, D.W., Danska, J., Hardy, K. *et al.* (1996). Recombinant human growth hormone, insulin-like growth factor 1, and combination therapy in AIDS-associated wasting. A randomized, double-blind, placebo-controlled trial. *Annals of Internal Medicine*, **125**, 865–72.

38. Schambelan, M., Mulligan, K., Grunfeld, C. *et al.* (1996). Recombinant human growth hormone in patients with HIV-associated wasting. A randomized, placebo-controlled trial. *Annals of Internal Medicine*, **125**, 874–82.

39. Storer, T.W., Woodhouse, L.J., Sattler, F. *et al.* (2005). A randomized, placebo-controlled trial of nandrolone decanoate in human immunodeficiency virus-infected men with mild to moderate weight loss with recombinant human growth hormone as active reference treatment. *Journal of Clinical Endocrinology and Metabolism*, **90**, 4474–82.

40. Von Roenn, J.H., Armstrong, D., Kotler, D.P. *et al.* (1994). Megestrol acetate in patients with AIDS-related cachexia. *Annals of Internal Medicine*, **121**, 393–99.

41. Oster, M.H., Enders, S.R., Samuels, S.J. *et al.* (1994). Megestrol acetate in patients with AIDS and cachexia. *Annals of Internal Medicine*, **121**, 400–8.

42. Mwamburi, D.M., Gerrior, J., Wilson, I.B. *et al.* (2004). Comparing megestrol acetate therapy with oxandrolone therapy for HIV related weight loss: similar results in 2 months. *Clinical Infectious Diseases*, **38**, 895–902.

43. Schols, A.M.W.J., Soeters, P.B., Mostert, R. *et al.* (1995). Physiologic effects of nutritional support and anabolic steroids in patients with chronic obstructive pulmonary disease: a placebo-controlled randomized trial. *American Journal of Respiratory and Critical Care Medicine*, **152**, 1268–74.

44. Weisberg, J., Wanger, J., Olson, J. *et al.* (2002). Megestrol acetate stimulates weight gain and ventilation in underweight COPD patients. *Chest*, **121**, 1070–78.

10.4

Fatigue and asthenia

Sriram Yennurajalingam and
Eduardo Bruera

Introduction

Fatigue is the most frequent symptom in patients with advanced cancer and has a prevalence of 60–90 per cent in various studies[1–5]. In the palliative care setting, the prevalence ranges from 48 per cent to 78 per cent[6].

In the past, the term 'asthenia' was used to describe a subjective sensation of tiredness and the term 'fatigue' was used to describe a symptom of tiredness precipitated by effort. However, the terms are currently often used in the same context. In this chapter, we consider the two terms synonymous, and by convention, 'fatigue' is generally used.

Fatigue may include three major features:

1 Easy tiring and reduced capacity to maintain performance.

2 Generalized weakness, defined as the anticipatory sensation of difficulty in initiating a certain activity; and

3 Mental fatigue, defined as the presence of impaired mental concetration, loss of memory, and emotional lability[7,8].

Fatigue occurs as a result of both cancer and its treatment. The onset of fatigue may precede the diagnosis of cancer or it may occur at any stage in the course of the illness. It may first occur after or be exacerbated by chemotherapy, radiotherapy, or surgery, and may be present for prolonged periods after these treatments[9]. In patients with advanced cancer, fatigue usually coexists with a number of other symptoms, among them pain, anorexia, nausea, vomiting, dyspnoea, sleep disturbance, anxiety, and depression.

Fatigue can interfere with a patient's ability to perform physical and social activities. It may influence patients' decision-making regarding future treatment and lead to refusal of potentially curative treatment. In recent years, as the management of other symptoms (such as pain, dyspnoea, and nausea) has improved, there has been an increased awareness of the importance of fatigue as symptom deserving of attention. The purpose of this chapter is to highlight the importance of fatigue in palliative care; to discuss this symptom's pathophysiology, assessment, and management in palliative care patients; and to stimulate an interest in research into this prevalent and troublesome symptom. Most of the evidence presented in this chapter relates to studies in cancer patients. However, similar principles can be applied to fatigue in patients with other diseases such as HIV infection and cardiac conditions.

Pathophysiology

In the majority of patients with advanced cancer, the aetiology of fatigue is unclear. The basic mechanisms by which fatigue is caused are not well understood, and in addition, several possible underlying causes of fatigue exist in most patients. Occasionally one predominant abnormality is present and appears to be the main contributor to the symptom; however, in most cases several abnormalities and other symptoms are present that may contribute to the genesis of fatigue.

In patients with cancer, complex interactions occur between tumour and host. These interactions, which are not well understood, can result in fatigue in several ways. Table 10.4.1 outlines mechanisms by which tumours have the potential to directly or indirectly produce fatigue in patients with advanced cancer. Fig. 10.4.1 summarizes contributors to fatigue in cancer patients.

Tumour, host-derived factors, and cytokines

Tumours can produce various byproducts, including lipolytic and proteolytic factors capable of interfering with host metabolism. These factors are believed to play a role in the development of cancer cachexia[10–12]. The relationship between cachexia and fatigue is

Table 10.4.1 Mechanism by which tumours may directly or indirectly cause fatigue.

Direct effects	Induced host factors	Accompanying factors
Lipolytic factors	Interleukin-6	Psychological issues
Proteolytic factors	Interleukin-1	Anaemia
Tumour degradation products	Tumour necrosis factor	Cancer-related symptoms: pain, sleep disturbance, dyspnoea, drowsiness
Invasion of brain or pituitary gland by tumour or metastases		Cachexia, hypoxia, and infection; metabolic disorders; dehydration; neurological disorders; endocrine disorders; paraneoplastic syndromes

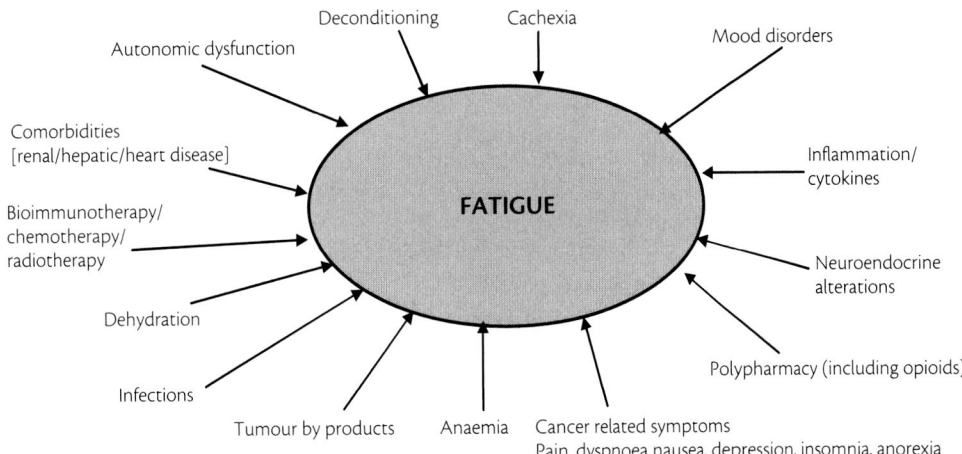

Figure 10.4.1 Contributors to fatigue.

discussed below. The presence of a tumour and cancer-related treatment can also induce the production of such inflammatory cytokines as tumour necrosis factor-alpha (TNF-α), interleukin (IL)-1, and IL-6. These cytokines have been implicated in the pathophysiology of fatigue by acting at multiple levels, including mood, muscle mass, strength, and metabolic status[13–15]. Rats and mice showed increased signs of fatigue when infection and other conditions associated with an increase in pro-inflammatory cytokines were present[16]. Drugs such as interferon-alpha (IFN-α), IL-2, and TNF-α have been associated with symptoms of fatigue, mood swings, sleep disturbance, and cognitive changes[17]. Cytokine-associated symptoms such as anorexia or cachexia, chronic nausea, fever, depression, pain, and sleep disorders may also contribute to fatigue[18].

Muscle abnormalities

Impaired muscle function may be one of the main underlying mechanisms in fatigue. The cause of these muscular abnormalities may relate in part to known abnormalities in cytokine production, but the production of other fatigue-inducing substances by the tumour or the host has been postulated. Muscle alterations in tumour-bearing patients are well known. Cachexia leads to a loss of muscle and fat, which may partially explain the relationship between cachexia and fatigue. However, tumour-bearing patients can have muscle abnormalities even in the presence of normal caloric intake and a constant body weight and lean body mass. Tumour-free muscle tissue of cancer patients has been found to contain excessive amounts of lactate[19]. It is unclear whether lactate is part of the pathogenic mechanism of weakness or a consequence of it. Atrophy of type II muscle fibres has been suggested to be a systemic effect of cancer, even in early or non-metastatic stages[20]. Tumour-free muscle from tumour-bearing animals shows alterations in the activity of various enzymes, the distribution of isoenzymes, and the synthesis and breakdown of myofibrillar and sarcoplasmic proteins[11]. Our group found impaired maximal strength, decreased relaxation velocity, and increased fatigue after electrical stimulation of the abductor pollicis muscle via the ulnar nerve in patients with breast cancer as compared to normal controls[21].

Myopathies can also be caused by medications used in cancer patients. Corticosteroids can cause loss of muscle mass, and

cyclosporine has been implicated as a cause of mitochondrial myopathy[22].

Deconditioning

Prolonged bed rest and immobility lead to loss of muscle mass and reduced cardiac output. This deconditioning results in reduced endurance for exercise and activities of daily living and may be compounded by other muscle abnormalities in patients with cancer[23,24]. Recent studies have found that endurance exercise training can reduce fatigue and improve physical performance in cancer patients undergoing chemotherapy[25] and in patients who have undergone bone marrow or autologous stem-cell transplantation[26,27]. Exercise may have a beneficial effect on muscle mass and cardiovascular fitness. In a randomized controlled trial of patients who underwent high-dose chemotherapy and peripheral blood stem-cell transplantation, significantly higher haemoglobin concentrations were found in the exercise group than in the control group. Improved physical performance can also result in improved mood, higher self-esteem, and less anxiety[28].

Overexertion

Overexertion is frequent cause of fatigue in non-cancer patients[29]. It should also be considered in young cancer patients who are receiving aggressive antineoplastic treatment, such as radiotherapy and chemotherapy, and who are trying to maintain their social and professional activities. Research in sports medicine has shown that for prolonged endurance, it is important to provide muscles with adequate substrate (carbohydrate loading). Unfortunately, cancer patients frequently present with abnormalities in muscle metabolism that may not allow adequate utilization of this substrate[30].

Central nervous system abnormalities

The mechanisms by which fatigue is perceived or induced in the central nervous system (CNS) are poorly understood. It has been suggested that the reticular activating system is responsible for controlling the experience of fatigue. The reticular activating system receives descending stimuli from the cortex on a feedback system based on ascending information from a number of sensory organs[31]. Chronic stimuli, such as pain, may generate fatigue through unremitting reticular stimulation. It has also been suggested that physiological fatigue might have an important protective function against overexertion. Cancer fatigue could be due to a breakdown of this particular mediated mechanism by environmental and cortical stimuli, humoural factors, or both.

Primary or secondary tumours involving the CNS and leading to invasion of brain tissue (particularly the pituitary gland, with resulting endocrine abnormalities) appear to be possible causes of fatigue in cancer patients. Disturbed cognitive functioning may be caused by fatigue but may also contribute to fatigue. Brain tumours can cause cognitive dysfunction, and other tumours, such as small cell lung cancers, can affect brain function by producing hormones or neurotransmitters[32]. Antineoplastic treatments, such as chemotherapy and radiotherapy, and drugs used to treat complications of cancer, such as opioids and corticosteroids, can also affect the CNS[33–35]. It has been observed that more than 70 per cent of patients receiving cranial radiotherapy for acute lymphoblastic leukaemia experience fatigue, depression, and some somnolence[33]. Recent research findings suggest that inflammatory cytokines play a role in mental fatigue[36]. However, much more research is needed to improve our understanding of the mechanisms by which fatigue is induced at the CNS level.

Relationship between fatigue and cachexia

Fatigue and cachexia coexist in the great majority of patients with advanced cancer, and it is likely that malnutrition is a major contributor to fatigue. The loss of muscle mass resulting from progressive cachexia provides a reason for profound weakness and fatigue. As previously discussed, even in the presence of normal protein and caloric intake and normal body weight, structural and biochemical muscle abnormalities are frequently found in cancer patients[19,37,38]. Similar abnormalities often are used to explain fatigue associated with chronic cardiac and respiratory disease. Some metabolic abnormalities related to cachexia are specifically responsible for muscle breakdown, including an increased concentration of cathepsin-D (a lysosomal enzyme involved in the intracellular degradation of macromolecules)[39].

It is important to recognize, however, that profound fatigue can exist in the absence of significant weight loss. Fatigue is common in patients with breast cancer and lymphomas, in which the prevalence of cachexia is low. In non-malignant conditions, such as chronic fatigue syndrome and depression, profound fatigue is generally not associated with malnutrition. Our group found no correlation between fatigue and nutritional status or weight in a population of breast cancer patients[40]. On the other hand, severe malnutrition without fatigue can be observed in patients with anorexia nervosa and in some patient populations with solid tumours. Fig. 10.4.2 illustrates the model to show the potential relationship between cachexia and fatigue.

It has been proposed that anorexia and fatigue may be part of an expression of the major metabolic abnormalities that occur in cancer patients, rather than simply an expression of malnutrition per se[41]. This situation would be similar to that experienced when a catabolic state occurs, such as a viral infection or in the early postoperative period. In these conditions, patients experience anorexia and fatigue that are secondary to the metabolic abnormalities rather than being causes of those abnormalities. Some interventions used to treat cancer cachexia, such as corticosteroids and progestational agents, have been found to be effective in the management of fatigue. The mechanisms by which these agents

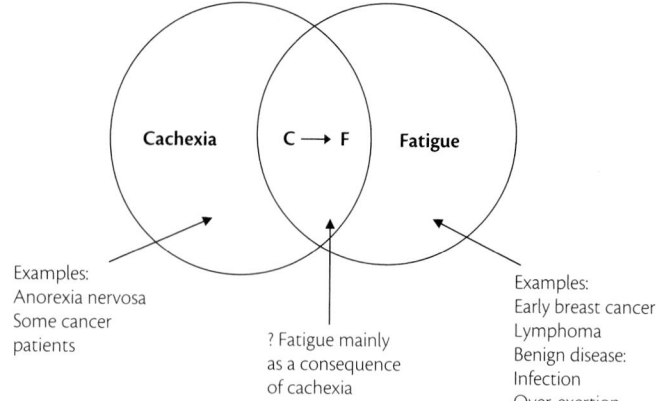

Figure 10.4.2 Possible relationship between cachexia and fatigue.

ameliorate cachexia and fatigue, however, are not well understood. Current pharmacological interventions for cachexia are discussed elsewhere in this book.

Infection

Fatigue is frequently associated with infections, particularly those that are recurrent or protracted. It may occur as a prodromal symptom, and it may outlast the infection by weeks or even months[42,43]. In patients with cancer, immunosuppression due to the cancer itself or cancer treatment increases the risk of infection and its complications. Chronic infection and cancer induce the same mediators for cachexia, including inflammatory cytokines[13]. It can be hypothesized that they share similar mediators for fatigue as well.

Anaemia

Anaemia is prevalent in cancer patients. Common causes of anaemia in cancer patients are myelosuppression by chemotherapeutic agents, iron deficiency, bleeding, haemolysis, nutritional deficiencies, and anaemia of chronic disease. Severe anaemia (haemoglobin <8 g/dl) is known to be a cause of profound fatigue. In patients receiving chemotherapy, treating less severe anaemia has been shown to improve energy levels, activity levels, and quality of life. In a prospective, open-label study of epoetin-alpha in 2342 anaemic patients receiving chemotherapy, mean energy levels, activity levels, and quality of life were found to improve with increases in mean haemoglobin levels from approximately 9–11 g/dl[44]. The improvements were independent of tumour response and correlated with the increases in haemoglobin levels. Similar findings were reported in a study of 2289 patients receiving chemotherapy; increased haemoglobin was correlated with improvements in energy, activity, and quality of life[45]. Although these data suggest an association between anaemia and fatigue, there are limited studies that specifically assess this relationship in populations with advanced illness.

Autonomic dysfunction

Autonomic dysfunction is a common complication of advanced cancer[46]. This syndrome includes malnutrition, delayed gastric emptying, chronic nausea, anorexia, and poor performance status[46,47].

Postural hypotension has been documented in patients with a specific type of severe chronic fatigue syndrome[48]. Autonomic dysfunction may contribute to fatigue as well as to orthostatic hypotension. The association between fatigue and autonomic dysfunction has not been established in cancer patients and should be investigated in future research[49].

Psychological issues

Anxiety, depression, and psychological distress can all contribute to fatigue. However, the nature of these relationships is unclear. In almost 75 per cent of non-cancer patients who present with fatigue, the final diagnosis is psychological (depression, anxiety, or another psychological disorder)[50]. While some depressive symptoms are frequent in cancer patients, only a minority of patients develop adjustment disorders and only a small percentage present with major depressive or anxiety disorders[51,52]. The diagnosis of a major depressive episode in patients with advanced cancer is difficult because they frequently present with neurovegetative and somatic symptoms that are part of the disease itself. The diagnosis of major depression thus should rely more on the presence of psychological and cognitive signs and symptoms in these patients than in those without advanced cancer[53], as discussed elsewhere in this book. Nevertheless, cancer patients presenting with an adjustment disorder or a major depressive disorder can have fatigue as one of the prevalent symptoms. Some authors who found an association between fatigue and mood changes in patients with breast cancer attributed the relationship to a combination of the disease and its therapy[54]. One prospective cohort study of elderly patients with cancer found a significant association between the intensity of fatigue and psychological symptoms, such as anxiety and depression[55]. In a double-blind clinical trial of 94 women with breast cancer, depression was significantly reduced in the 44 patients receiving paroxetine compared to the 50 patients receiving placebo, indicating that a biologically active dose was used; however, the groups did not differ in regard to any measures of fatigue[56]. Thus, the role of psychological factors, including anxiety and depression, in the development of fatigue among cancer patients needs further research.

Metabolic and endocrine disorders

Endocrine disorders, such as diabetes mellitus, Addison's disease, and hypothyroidism, and electrolyte disorders, such as hyponatraemia, hypokalaemia, and hypercalcaemia, are possible causes of fatigue and in many instances have relatively simple and effective treatments.

Interest in hypogonadism as a cause of fatigue and loss of muscle mass has increased in recent years as a result of the prevalence of these symptoms in HIV-infected men. Testosterone deficiency results in loss of muscle mass, fatigue, reduced libido, and reduced haemoglobin[57]. Androgen insufficiency in cancer patients can result from the anorexia–cachexia syndrome[58]. In addition, chemotherapy and radiotherapy can cause hypogonadism. Hormonal ablative therapy has been found to double the incidence of fatigue in patients with prostate cancer[59]. In patients with testosterone insufficiency due to HIV disease and other causes, treatment with androgenic anabolic steroids, including testosterone and its derivatives, has been found to increase muscle mass[60–63], improve energy and libido[60], and increase haemoglobin levels[60,64]. Androgenic anabolic steroids are regularly used for the

treatment of hypogonadism in HIV-infected men. A randomized, single-blind, placebo-controlled trial of testosterone replacement in 35 men with mild Leydig cell insufficiency after chemotherapy found that physical fatigue significantly improved in the testosterone-treated group and was associated a borderline increase in physical activity[65]. Other variables such as bone mineral density and body composition, were not significantly altered. The effects of treating hypogonadism in cancer patients should be researched further.

Abnormalities of the hypothalamic–pituitary–adrenal (HPA) axis concerning corticotrophin-releasing factor have been postulated as another possible endocrine-related cause of fatigue. Corticotrophin-releasing factor levels increase in situations of during physical or emotional stress and thus may cause fatigue[66]. In addition, HPA axis is activated by stress; while hyperactivity in this system can lead to depression[67], reduced HPA activity also has been postulated as a possible cause of chronic fatigue syndrome[68]. Proinflammatory cytokines IL-1, IL-6, and TNF-α are central mediators of the inflammatory process that can result in the activation of the HPA axis and the secretion of mediators that induce such symptoms as pain, fatigue, anxiety, and depression, leading to an impaired quality of life[13]. Further research is needed to clarify the role of abnormalities of the HPA axis in the genesis of fatigue.

Paraneoplastic neurological syndromes

Paraneoplastic neurological syndromes are rare but are important to recognize since many of these syndromes can precede the clinical presentation of a malignancy. They may be partially reversible with primary treatment of the tumour. Table 10.4.2 summarizes some of the paraneoplastic neurological syndromes associated with fatigue[69].

Other cancer-related symptoms

Various correlative studies have shown that fatigue is associated with pain, such psychological symptoms as anxiety and depression, dyspnoea, sleep disturbances, anorexia, and constipation. However, the intensity of the individual symptoms in a given patient may determine their ultimate contribution to causing fatigue[55].

Side effects of cancer treatment

Treatments for both cancer and the symptoms and conditions caused by cancer can cause or aggravate fatigue. Worsening of fatigue is common during chemotherapy and radiotherapy[70–73]. The mechanisms by which these treatment modalities cause fatigue are not fully understood. Radiotherapy can result in anaemia, diarrhoea, anorexia, and weight loss, and chemotherapy commonly causes anorexia, nausea, vomiting, and anaemia; all these events may contribute to fatigue. In addition, the two types of treatment have secondary effects that may cause or exacerbate fatigue; for instance, fatigue may be a consequence of chronic pain resulting from radiotherapy or chemotherapy-induced immunosuppression that predisposes patients to infection. Such effects may persist long-term. One study found that breast cancer patients who had undergone adjuvant chemotherapy or autologous bone marrow transplantation appeared to experience fatigue for months to years after the completion of treatment[74].

Biological response-modifying agents have also been implicated in fatigue; for instance, IFN-α was shown to cause fatigue in

Table 10.4.2 Paraneoplastic neurological syndromes associated with fatigue.

Syndrome	Comment
Progressive multifocal leucoencephalopathy	Leukaemia and lymphoma are the cancers in which this syndrome is most often found
Paraneoplastic encephalomyelitis	70% of cases occur in patients with lung cancers and 30% in others
Amyotrophic lateral sclerosis	
Subacute motor neuropathy	Proximal or distal, often asymmetric (e.g. after radiotherapy for lymphoma)
Subacute necrotic myelopathy	Mainly lung cancer
Peripheral paraneoplastic neurological syndrome	Often precedes diagnosis of the primary tumour, similar to Guillain–Barré syndrome
Ascending acute polyneuropathy (Guillain–Barré syndrome)	Lymphoma
Neuromuscular paraneoplastic syndromes	
Dermatomyositis, polymyositis	Associated with malignancy in about 50% of cases (onset within 1 year)
Eaton–Lambert syndrome	Strongly associated with small cell lung cancer. Can precede detection of tumour by months. Improves with successful treatment
Myasthenia gravis	30% of cases occur in patients with thymoma, while most of the rest occur in those with lymphoma

70 per cent of patients[75]. In fact, fatigue is the most frequent dose-limiting side effect in patients receiving biological response-modifying treatments for cancer.

Opioids such as morphine have significant effects on the reticular system and are capable of inducing sedation, cognitive changes, and fatigue in some patients. In addition, anxiolytics, hypnotics, and other drugs may cause sedation and fatigue. Table 10.4.3 outlines cancer therapies and drugs that frequently contribute to fatigue in patients with cancer.

In summary, evidence clearly shows that fatigue is a complex, subjective multidimensional syndrome that can be attributed to multiple contributing causes. It is particularly important to note that not only cancer but also cancer treatments, cancer related symptoms (including anorexia–cachexia, pain, sleep disturbances, drowsiness, anxiety depression, cognitive dysfunction and dysnoea), metabolic causes, endocrine (including HPA-axis dysfunction, inflammatory(including cytokine dysregulation), and neuromuscular dysfunction may be among those causes, making careful assessment of paramount importance.

Assessment

The assessment of fatigue should involve evaluation of the severity of the fatigue; its onset, duration, and level of interference with everyday life; associated psychological or social problems; and possible underlying causes.

Fatigue is a subjective sensation and at present no 'gold standard' tool exists for its assessment. Its multidimensional nature adds to the complexity of assessment. Table 10.4.4 outlines some assessment tools for fatigue; several others also exist.

Functional capacity tests attempt to objectively determine a patient's ability to perform a standard task, such as walking on a treadmill, riding a bicycle, or driving for a prolonged period (in a simulator). However, these tests are of very limited value in cancer care and research, as they are very difficult for patients with advanced cancer to perform. A suitable alternative is measuring daily physical activity by means of actigraphy[76]. An actigraph can also be used to record and evaluate sleep quantity and quality, daytime activity levels, and napping. Roscoe et al.[77] found that actigraph measurements significantly correlated with fatigue in patients with breast cancer. Conversely, Dimsdale and colleagues found no correlation between fatigue expression and actigraph measurements in healthy controls[78]. Task-related fatigue tests attempt to assess the fatigue induced by standard tasks. The six-minute walk test, for example, is commonly used to assess physical function[79].

Assessment of performance status is the most commonly used measure of a patient's physical condition in oncology. Two popular

Table 10.4.3 Cancer therapies and medications that commonly contribute to fatigue.

♦ Cytotoxic therapeutic agents
♦ Radiotherapy
♦ Biological response modifiers (e.g. interferon)
♦ Opioids
♦ Polypharmacy: hypnotics/anxiolytics, anticholinergics, antiepileptics, neuroleptics, opioids, alpha adrenergic blocking agents, diuretics, selective serotonin reuptake inhibitors and tricyclic antidepressants, and benzodiazepines

Table 10.4.4 Assessment approaches for fatigue.

Functional capacity	Task-related fatigue
♦ Treadmill performance (speed, duration)	♦ Visual analogue/numerical rating scale
	♦ Pearson and Byars Fatigue Feeling Checklist
♦ Number of errors (pilot, driver)	
♦ Six-minute walk[79]	
Performance status	**Subjective assessment tools**
♦ Karnofsky Performance Status[80]	♦ Visual analogue/numerical rating scale
♦ European Cooperative Oncology Group criteria[81]	♦ Functional Assessment of Cancer Therapy-Fatigue[83]
♦ Edmonton Functional Assessment Tool[82]	♦ Piper Fatigue Scale[84]
	♦ Brief Fatigue Inventory[85]

tools, the Karnofsky Performance Status score[80] and the European Cooperative Oncology Group score[81], rely on a physician's rating of the patient's functional capabilities after a regular medical consult. Another tool used in oncology, the Edmonton Functional Assessment Test (EFAT)[82], is administered by a physiotherapist and attempts to determine a patient's functional status in addition to identifying obstacles to clinical performance.

Subjective measures of fatigue are generally considered to be the most relevant in clinical practice and in clinical trials. Visual analogue scales, numerical scales, the Functional Assessment of Cancer Therapy–Fatigue (FACIT–F)[83], the Piper Fatigue Scale (PFS)[84], and the Brief Fatigue Inventory (BFI)[85] have all been validated and can be used in both pharmacological and non-pharmacological studies. In addition to these tools, there are validated functional assessments of fatigue in most frequently applied quality-of-life questionnaires, such as the EORTC QLQ-C30 and FACT-G. However, there are studies indicating that the short scales within these instruments have certain limitations[86]. For more details see chapter on quality of life assessment in this textbook.

Tools that are multidimensional are generally preferred to those that are not because they give a broader picture of the problem and can highlight both general and specific management approaches that may benefit a specific patient. Examples of multidimensional tools used to assess fatigue include PFS[84], Fatigue Questionnaire[87], and Multidimensional Assessment of Fatigue[88].

Assessment of fatigue also involves assessment of possible underlying causes, including those factors shown in Fig. 10.4.1. A full assessment therefore involves a careful systems review and psychological assessment, a detailed physical examination, and blood tests that would detect anaemia and electrolyte or endocrine abnormalities. Multiple causes should be suspected in all patients, and the possible impact of various factors should be weighed according to their severity.

Screening for fatigue

Patients may not report fatigue spontaneously, as they may believe it is 'normal' and untreatable. That may delay or prevent cancer treatment. Furthermore, physicians may fail to screen for fatigue, as they may be unsure that they can treat it effectively[4,89–91]. The recently published guidelines of the National Comprehensive Cancer Network Fatigue Practice Guidelines Panel recommend that patients be screened for the presence and severity of fatigue at the time of their initial contact with a doctor and that ongoing assessments be made. The guidelines suggest that the screening data be used to designate the fatigue as mild, moderate, or severe (on a 0–10 numerical rating scale, with 1–3 considered mild, 4–6 moderate, and 7–10 severe). Mild fatigue would be re-evaluated on an ongoing basis, while moderate or severe fatigue would undergo more focused assessment and intervention.

Management

Since fatigue is a complex multidimensional symptom, it is crucial that an adequate therapeutic approach be used to identify and prioritize the different underlying factors. Alterations in fatigue over time may demonstrate a relationship with a particular factor (for example, fatigue may increase following an increase in tumour size, a change of medication, or a reduction in the haemoglobin concentration). This temporal pattern underlines the importance of continuous assessment and monitoring of symptoms and signs even in palliative medicine. In planning the therapeutic approach, it is also important to answer the following questions:

1 Is fatigue a symptom of primary concern to this patient?

2 What are the major probable causes?

3 Are there therapeutic measures available that have a reasonable cost/benefit ratio?

An intervention may have the purpose of decreasing the intensity of fatigue, allowing the patient to express a maximal level of functioning with a stable level of fatigue, or both. In palliative care, the satisfactory treatment of a symptom such as fatigue does not mean that the symptom must be eliminated completely. Even minor improvements can be enough to shift fatigue downward on the patient's list of priorities.

In a given patient, it is often impossible to determine with certainty whether or not an identified problem is a major contributor to fatigue or simply coexists with the fatigue. Therefore, it is of great importance to measure the intensity of fatigue and the patient's performance status before and after treating any suspected contributing factor. For example, fatigue should be measured before and after correcting hypercalcaemia or treating anaemia. This can be done in a number of ways, including using a simple numerical scale (e.g. 0 = best, 10 = worst) or a visual analogue scale (e.g. 0 = best, 100 = worst imaginable). If the level of fatigue does not improve after correction of an underlying abnormality, then it is clear that further treatment of that abnormality will not improve the fatigue in the future.

Fig. 10.4.3 outlines some general and specific measures that may be useful in the management of fatigue in cancer patients. In many patients, no reversible causes will be identified. Several pharmacological and non-pharmacological approaches may be effective in these patients, however, including those that reduce energy expenditure or levels of fatigue. Specific treatments may also be used to address underlying abnormalities believed to contribute the fatigue in an individual patient.

Non-specific measures

Non-pharmacological approaches

Counselling can be very useful for both patients and families. Patients frequently underestimate the side effect burden at the beginning of chemotherapy. In one study, only 8 per cent of patients expected tiredness but 86 per cent experienced it[90]. This result suggests that many patients undergo treatment without sufficient information to develop realistic expectations about what that treatment entails. Counselling and informing the patient of the possible causes of fatigue and the types of therapeutic options available may allow the patient the opportunity to develop realistic expectations. As the disease progresses, the patient will be required to adapt to further limitations in physical functioning and activity; likewise, the family will need to have realistic expectations for the patient.

If patients are empowered by receiving correct and full information and by undergoing counselling, they may combat fatigue by

1 Adapting their activities of daily living by reducing the amount of housework they do or by enlisting the help of others to perform physical duties;

2 Spending more time in bed or, alternatively, exercising more (the latter if deconditioning is considered to be a contributor to the fatigue);

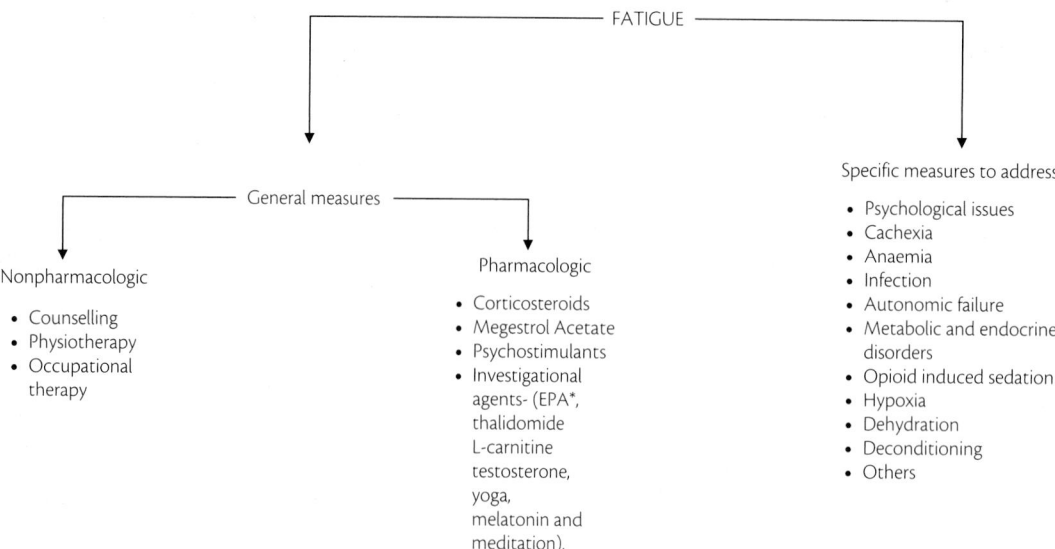

Figure 10.4.3 Therapeutic approach to managing fatigue.
* Eicosapentanoic acid.

3 Rearranging their schedules within the day, depending on their fatigue patterns;

4 Requesting changes in medications perceived to be causing a loss of energy; and

5 Avoiding expending energy on unnecessary activities.

Deconditioning due to inactivity should be treated if appropriate. A physiotherapist can suggest suitable exercises and encourage increased activity, which may have beneficial effects from both physical and psychosocial perspectives. In addition, if the patient is immobile, a physiotherapist can perform passive movements that will help the patient maintain flexibility and decrease painful tendon retraction. Occupational therapists can allow patients to remain safe and increase their activity at home by providing such resources as ramps, wheelchairs and walkers, elevated toilets, safety devices for bathrooms, and hospital beds. In addition, these therapists can give patients and families useful tips that enhance mobility and help prevent further muscle atrophy, tendon retraction, and pressure ulcers. A recent preliminary study showed that physical exercise is a feasible intervention and improves fatigue in patients with advanced cancer[92].

Pharmacological treatments

In patients with fatigue of unknown origin and those in who specific treatment is not available, several non-specific pharmacological interventions have been proposed, chief among them corticosteroids, megestrol acetate and other anti-cachexia agents, and psychostimulant drugs.

Corticosteroids

Studies have suggested that corticosteroids decrease fatigue in cancer patients. In a randomized, controlled, double-blind cross-over trial, both patients and investigators identified methylprednisolone administered at a dose of 32 mg/day as more effective than placebo in reducing levels of fatigue[93]. Two multicentre European trials have confirmed that corticosteroids can reduce fatigue[94,95]. Corticosteroids can also have beneficial effects on several other symptoms that are common in patients with advanced cancer, such as nausea, impaired appetite, and pain.

The mechanism of action by which corticosteroids combat fatigue is unknown. The inhibition of tumour or tumour-induced substances, as well as central euphoriant effects, are potential mechanisms[96]. The effects of these drugs are probably not due to their demonstrated appetite stimulation since corticosteroids do not result in significant improvements in nutritional status.

Corticosteroid effects usually last only 2–4 weeks. In addition, corticosteroids can cause metabolic abnormalities and serious long-term toxic effects, including osteoporosis, myopathies, and increased risk of infections. Therefore, long-term treatment should generally be avoided. In addition, the best type and dose of corticosteroids as a treatment for fatigue have not been established. Most studies have used doses equivalent to approximately 40 mg/day of prednisone.

Megestrol acetate

Studies involving terminally ill patients have demonstrated rapid (within 10 days) improvement in fatigue and general well-being in patients treated with megestrol acetate at a dose of 160–480 mg/day as compared to placebo, without any significant change in nutritional status[97,98]. The mechanism of action by which progestational agents confer these benefits is unclear, although it is believed to be related to glucocorticoid or anabolic activity, as well as effects on cytokine release.

Other agents of potential benefit in the management of cachexia

Other pharmacological agents that are of potential benefit in the management of cachexia, such as thalidomide and omega-3 fatty acids, may also have a beneficial effect on fatigue. Thalidomide was found to preserve performance status in a randomized, double-blind, placebo-controlled study of 28 patients with advanced HIV disease and cachexia[99]. A pilot study of thalidomide (100 mg/day) in 37 evaluable cancer patients with cachexia found that the patients' sense of well-being had improved after 10 days of treatment[100]. In a study looking at the effect of an oral nutritional supplement enriched with eicosapentanoic acid (EPA; an omega-3 fatty acid found in fish oil) in weight-losing cancer patients, performance status was significantly improved after 3 weeks of treatment[101]. Further research is needed to study the potential beneficial effects of these agents on fatigue in cancer patients.

Treating malnutrition as a cause of fatigue in cancer patients remains controversial. In general, malnourished patients are known to have significant levels of fatigue. However, it has not been clearly demonstrated that attempts to reverse the level of malnutrition result in significant improvement in the level of fatigue[102,103].

Psychostimulants

Clinical experience with cancer patients indicates that psychostimulants promote a sense of well-being, decrease fatigue, and alleviate depression. Psychostimulants are also effective in treating fatigue related to opioid-induced sedation. Randomized controlled trials have shown that methylphenidate and dextroamphetamine can antagonize the sedating effect of opioids as compared to placebo[103–105]. Preliminary reports have suggested that methylphenidate has efficacy in treating fatigue in cancer patients, as well as in patients with other chronic illnesses[105–107] and ambulatory patients with HIV infection[106]. Methylphenidate has been used to manage opioid-induced sedation and depression in the palliative care setting[109–111]. Sarhill and colleagues reported that this agent caused a rapid reduction of fatigue in 9 of 11 consecutively treated patients in an open-label study[112]. A pilot study of 14 evaluable patients with advanced cancer found that methylphenidate at a dose of 5–10 mg/day significantly improved fatigue after 7 days[113].

Modafinil is a novel psychostimulant that appears to have a mode of action different to that of the amphetamine derivatives[112]. A recent study in DSP-4-treated mice showed that non-noradrenergic, dopamine-dependent adrenergic signalling was associated with activation of the wake-promoting mechanism of modafinil[113]. Modafinil is indicated in the treatment of excessive daytime sleepiness (EDS) in patients with narcolepsy and such conditions as Parkinson's disease and obstructive sleep apnoea[114–117]. It appears to have less potential for abuse than amphetamines[118,119]. This agent also reduces fatigue in healthy individuals during sustained mental work and may have fewer side effects than d-amphetamine[118,119]. In a 9-week study of 72 patients with multiple sclerosis who received either 200 mg/day modafinil or placebo for 2 weeks, the patients in the treatment arm had a significant improvement in fatigue ($P < 0.001$)[119]. Modafinil's role in patients with advanced cancer, however, has not been established, and in general, more research is needed to define the role of psychostimulants in the management of fatigue in patients with advanced cancer.

Specific measures

As previously discussed, fatigue is often multicausal and may appear as a consequence of other conditions, such as cachexia, infection, or anaemia. Any intervention capable of reversing an underlying contributor should alleviate fatigue. Thus, it is useful to consider all factors that may be contributing to fatigue in any given patient, with the aim of identifying reversible causes. It is also important to remember that reversible causes, such as dehydration, metabolic disorders, or severe anaemia, may coexist with nonreversible causes.

Infections should be treated appropriately. Factors leading to recurrent infections should be addressed where possible.

In patients with anaemia, determining the underlying cause is important, as it may influence the choice of treatment. Treatment may also be influenced by the acuity with which anaemia develops. Severe anaemia (haemoglobin <8 g/dl) is usually treated with blood transfusion. As noted earlier, there is evidence that patients with less severe anaemia also benefit from increases in haemoglobin levels when receiving chemotherapy[44,45].

Epoetin-alpha at a dose of 10 000 units 3 times weekly and then increasing to as much as 20 000 units 3 times weekly (depending on response) has been found to effectively combat anaemia in patients receiving chemotherapy[44]. Gabrilove et al. found that weekly dosing with 40 000 units of epoetin-alpha (increasing to 60 000 units after 4 weeks, depending on response) produced clinical benefits similar to treatment with a three-times-weekly regimen[120]. A recent systematic review of controlled clinical trials of epoetin treatment of anaemia associated with cancer therapy found that only studies in which patients had mean baseline haemoglobin concentrations of 10 g/dl or less reported significant benefits of treatment on quality of life[121]. The main disadvantages of epoetin-alpha include its cost, recent evidence that it may cause increased thrombotic events, suggestions that it may reduce survival times[122], and the delay of 4–8 weeks until an increase of 1–2 g/dl in haemoglobin concentration, with resulting symptomatic improvement, can be observed. These disadvantages are particularly relevant in palliative care patients who have short life expectancy.

Although treatment of anaemia has been shown to decrease fatigue in patients receiving chemotherapy, the correction of anaemia in advanced cancer patients at the end of life was found to have limited impact on the intensity of fatigue[123,124]. This is probably due to the fact that multiple factors contribute to fatigue in these patients, including cachexia, depression, pain, and deconditioning.

Autonomic failure in patients with diabetes and neurological disorders has been effectively managed by midodrine, a specific alpha 1-sympathomimetic agent[125,126]. Other measures that could be considered include (1) adjusting the dose medications that contribute to fatigue or ceasing polypharmacy so as to reduce drug interactions; (2) having the patient exercise; (3) increasing the patient's salt intake or considering mineralocorticoid (fludrocortisone), if indicated; and (4) having the patient avoid triggers of autonomic insufficiency, such as large morning meals, heat (including showers), alcohol intake, and motionless standing.

Counselling should be considered for patients with adjustment disorders, depression, anxiety, and coping difficulties. Various randomized clinical trials have shown that supportive interventions (group and individual), such as education and stress management groups, coping strategies training, and behavioural interventions, can help cancer patients manage their fatigue. Patients with major depression should be treated with antidepressant medication. As in the general population, the choice of antidepressant in a patient with advanced cancer will depend on other patient factors. Selective serotonin reuptake inhibitors are commonly used and have fewer side effects than tricyclic antidepressants. An alternative is to consider using a psychostimulant, such as methylphenidate, modafinil, or dextroamphetamine, to treat the depression. Psychostimulants have been found to be effective antidepressants and are also useful in the treatment of opioid-induced sedation[107]. An advantage of psychostimulants is their rapid antidepressant effect, which is usually apparent within a few days. Disadvantages include their neurotoxic side effects and the risk that patients will develop tolerance or dependency.

Metabolic disorders, such as hypercalcaemia, hyponatraemia, and hypokalaemia, should be corrected where possible. Endocrine deficiencies, such as hypothyroidism and Addison's disease, require treatment with hormones. Testosterone replacement therapy can be considered for patients with hypogonadism. Future studies are needed to look at the effects of testosterone replacement in cancer patients with fa tigue and to determine which of these patients are most likely to benefit from treatment.

Other possible contributors to fatigue should also be considered and treated. The list of prescribed drugs should be monitored regularly to ensure that the fatigue is not an iatrogenic effect. Dehydration and hypoxia should be managed as appropriate, and the treatment of underlying cardiac or respiratory conditions should be optimized.

Studies have found that the micronutrient carnitine is frequently deficient in patients with advanced cancer, and preliminary studies using escalating doses (250–3000 mg/day) of carnitine supplementation have shown improvements in fatigue. Randomized controlled studies are now under way to test the effects of carnitine supplementation in patients with cancer and AIDS.

Conclusion

Fatigue in cancer patients is now accepted as a symptom that should be studied in its own right. Unfortunately, few studies have addressed fatigue in palliative cancer populations. Consequently, most of the insight into the complexity of fatigue need to be based upon extrapolation from studies performed in the patients earlier in the disease trajectory. To improve treatment, we must gain a better understanding of the many aspects of fatigue. Thus, identifying tumour or tumour-induced factors that cause fatigue is important. Assessment and staging tools that are valid and reliable are needed to assist in clinical practice and research. Clinical syndromes of fatigue (cognitive, affective, and physical) also must be characterized better. The role of nutritional interventions and the roles of commonly used agents, such as megestrol acetate and corticosteroids, also need to be more thoroughly investigated. The potential of such agents as EPA, thalidomide, L-carnitine, and anabolic steroids must be explored in studies where fatigue is a primary endpoint. Finally, the role of psychostimulants such as modafinil should be further researched, and the importance of counselling, rest, and exercise in cancer patients receiving palliative care should be clarified.

References

1. Bruera, E. (1998). Research into symptoms other than pain. In *Oxford Textbook of Palliative Medicine* (eds. D. Doyle, G. Hanks, and N. MacDonald), pp. 179–85. Oxford University Press, Oxford.
2. Coyle, N., Adelhardt, J., Foley, K.M. *et al.* (1990). Character of terminal illness in the advanced cancer patient: Pain and other symptoms during the last four weeks of life. *Journal of Pain & Symptom Management*, 5, 83–93.
3. Cella, D.F. *et al.* (1993). The Functional Assessment of Cancer Therapy scale: development and validation of the general measure. *Journal of Clinical Oncology*, 11, 570–9.
4. Vogelzang, N.J. *et al.* (1997). Patient, caregiver, and oncologist perceptions of cancer-related fatigue: Results of a tripart assessment survey. The Fatigue Coalition. *Seminars in Hematology*, 34, 4–12.
5. Portenoy, R.K. *et al.* (1994). Symptom prevalence, characteristics and distress in a cancer population. *Quality of Life Research*, 3, 183–9.
6. Smets, E.M., Garssen, B., Schuster-Uitterhoeve, A.L. *et al.* (1993). Fatigue in cancer patients. *British Journal of Cancer*, 68(2), 220–4.
7. Theologides, A. (1982). Asthenia in cancer. *American Journal of Medicine*, 73, 1–3.
8. Bruera, E. and MacDonald, R.N. (1988). Asthenia in patients with advanced cancer. Issues in symptom control. Part 1. *Journal of Pain & Symptom Management*, 3, 9–14.
9. Berglund, G., Bolund, C., Fornander, T. *et al.* (1991) Late effects of adjuvant chemotherapy and postoperative radiotherapy on quality of life among breast cancer patients. *European Journal of Cancer*, 27, 1075–81.
10. Tisdale, M.J. (1998). New cachexic factors. *Current Opinion in Clinical Nutrition and Metabolic Care*, 1, 253–6.
11. Theologides, A. (1986). Anorexins, asthenins, and cachectins in cancer. *American Journal of Medicine*, 81, 696–8.
12. Beutler, B. and Cerami, A. (1987). Cachectin: More than a tumor necrosis factor. *New England Journal of Medicine*, 316, 379–85.
13. Lee, B.N., Dantzer, R., Langley, K. *et al.* (2004). A cytokine-based neuroimmunologic mechanism of cancer-related symptom. *Neuroimmnomodulation*, 11, 279–92.
14. Michalaki, V., Syrigos, K., Charles, P. *et al.* (2004). Serum levels of IL-6 and TNF-α correlate with clinicopathological features and patient survival in patients with prostate cancer. *British Journal of Cancer*, 90, 2312–6.
15. Adler, H.L., McCurdy, M.A., Kattan, M.W. *et al.* (1999). Elevated levels of circulating interleukin-6 and transforming growth factor-β1 in patients with metastatic prostatic carcinoma. *Journal of Urology*, 161, 182–7.
16. Gupta, S., Aggarwal, S., See, D. *et al.* (1997). Cytokine production by adherent and non-adherent mononuclear cells in chronic fatigue syndrome. *Journal of Psychiatric Research*, 31(1), 149–56.
17. Cheney, P.R., Dorman, S.E., and Bell, D.S. (1989). Letters and corrections: Interleukins-2 and the chronic fatigue syndrome. *Annals of Internal Medicine*, 110(4), 321.
18. Moss, R.B., Mercandetti, A., and Vojdani, A. (1999). TNF-α and chronic fatigue syndrome. *Journal of Clinical Immunology*, 19(5), 314–6.
19. Holroyde, C.P., Axelrod, R.S., Skutches, C.L. *et al.* (1979). Lactate metabolism in patients with metastatic colorectal cancer. *Cancer Research*, 39, 4900–4.
20. Warmolts, J.R. (1975). Type II muscle fibre atrophy (II-atrophy): An early systemic effect of cancer. *Neurology*, 2, 374.
21. Bruera, E., Brenneis, C., Michaud, M. *et al.* (1988). Muscle electrophysiology in patients with advanced breast cancer. *Journal of the National Cancer Institute*, 80, 282–5.
22. Tirdel, G.B., Girgis, R., Fishman, R.S. *et al.* (1998). Metabolic myopathy as a cause of the exercise limitation in lung transplant recipients. *Journal of Heart and Lung Transplantation*, 17, 1231–7.
23. Germain, P., Guell, A., and Marini, J.F. (1995). Muscle strength during bedrest with and without muscle exercise as a countermeasure. *European Journal of Applied Physiology and Occupational Physiology*, 71, 342–8.
24. Levine, B.D., Zuckerman, J.H., and Pawelczyk, J.A. (1997). Cardiac atrophy after bed-rest deconditioning: A nonneural mechanism for orthostatic intolerance. *Circulation*, 96, 517–25.
25. Schmitz, K.H., Holtzman, J., Courneya, K.S. *et al.* (2005). Controlled physical activity trials in cancer survivors: a systematic review and meta-analysis. *Cancer Epidemiology, Biomarkers and Prevention*, 14, 1588–95.
26. Dimeo, F., Fetscher, S., Lange, W. *et al.* (1997). Effects of aerobic exercise on the physical performance and incidence of treatment-related complications after high-dose chemotherapy. *Blood*, 90, 3390–4.

27. Dimeo, F., Bertz, H., Finke, J. *et al.* (1996). An aerobic exercise program for patients with haematological malignancies after bone marrow transplantation. *Bone Marrow Transplant*, **18**, 1157–60.

28. Dimeo, F.C. (2001). Effects of exercise on cancer-related fatigue. *Cancer*, **92**, 1689–93.

29. Plum, F. (1988). Asthenia, weakness and fatigue. In *Cecil Textbook of Medicine* (eds. J. Wyngaarden and L. Smith), pp. 2044. WB Saunders Company, Philadelphia.

30. Burnfoot, A. (1994). The brain connection. *Runners World*, **29**, 70–5.

31. Grandjean, E.P. (1970). Fatigue. *American Industrial Hygiène Association Journal*, **31**, 401–11.

32. Valentine, A.D. and Meyers, C.A. (2001). Cognitive and mood disturbance as causes and symptoms of fatigue in cancer patients. *Cancer*, **92**, 1694–8.

33. Proctor, S.J., Kernaham, J., and Taylor, P. (1981). Depression as component of post-cranial irradiation somnolence syndrome. *Lancet*, **1**, 1215–6.

34. Schagen, S.B., van Dam, F.S., Muller, M.J. *et al.* (1999) Cognitive deficits after postoperative adjuvant chemotherapy for breast carcinoma. *Cancer*, **85**, 640–50.

35. Schagen, S.B., Hamburger, H.L., Muller, M.J. *et al.* (2001). Neurophysiological evaluation of late effects of adjuvant high-dose chemotherapy on cognitive function. *Journal of Neurooncology*, **51**, 159–65.

36. Ronnback, L. and Hansson, E. (2004). On the potential role of glutamate transport in mental fatigue. *Journal of Neuroinflammation*, **1**(1), 22.

37. Beck, S.A., Mulligan, H.D., and Tisdale, M.J. (1990). Lipolytic factors associated with murine and human cancer cachexia. *Journal of the National Cancer Institute*, **82**, 1922–6.

38. Smith, K.L. and Tisdale, M.J. (1993). Mechanism of muscle protein degradation in cancer cachexia. *British Journal of Cancer*, **68**, 314–8.

39. Beck, S.A. and Tisdale, M.J. (1987). Production of lipolytic and proteolytic factors by a murine tumor-producing cachexia in the host. *Cancer Research*, **47**, 5919–23.

40. Bruera, E., Brenneis, C., Michaud, M. *et al.* (1989). Association between asthenia and nutritional status, lean body mass, anemia, psychological status, and tumor mass in patients with advanced breast cancer. *Journal of Pain & Symptom Management*, **4**, 59–63.

41. Bruera, E. (1992). Current pharmacological management of anorexia in cancer patients. *Oncology (Huntington)*, **6**, 125–30.

42. Jones, J.F., Ray, C.G., Minnich, L.L. *et al.* (1985). Evidence for active Epstein-Barr virus infection in patients with persistent, unexplained illnesses: Elevated anti-early antigen antibodies. *Annals of Internal Medicine*, **102**, 1–7.

43. Straus, S.E., Tosato, G., Armstrong, G. *et al.* (1985). Persisting illness and fatigue in adults with evidence of Epstein-Barr virus infection. *Annals of Internal Medicine*, **102**, 7–16.

44. Glaspy, J., Bukowski, R., Steinberg, D. *et al.* (1997). Impact of therapy with epoetin alfa on clinical outcomes in patients with nonmyeloid malignancies during cancer chemotherapy in community oncology practice. Procrit Study Group. *Journal of Clinical Oncology*, **15**, 1218–34.

45. Demetri, G.D., Kris, M., Wade, J. *et al.* (1998). Quality-of-life benefit in chemotherapy patients treated with epoetin alfa is independent of disease response or tumor type: Results from a prospective community oncology study. Procrit Study Group. *Journal of Clinical Oncology*, **16**, 3412–25.

46. Bruera, E., Chadwick, S., Fox, R. *et al.* (1986). Study of cardiovascular autonomic insufficiency in advanced cancer patients. *Cancer Treatment Reports*, **70**, 1383–7.

47. Henrich, W.L. (1982). Autonomic insufficiency. *Archives of Internal Medicine*, **142**, 339–44.

48. Calkins, H. and Rowe, P.C. (1998). Relationship between chronic fatigue syndrome and neurally mediated hypotension. *Cardiology Reviews*, **6**, 125–34.

49. Strasser, F., Palmer, J.L., Schover, L.R. *et al.* (2006). The impact of hypogonadism and autonomic dysfunction on fatigue, emotional function, and sexual desire in male patients with advanced cancer: A pilot study. *Cancer*, **107**(12), 2949–57.

50. Adams, R. (1993). Anxiety, depression, asthenia and personality disorders. In *Harrison's Principles of Internal Medicine* (eds. R. Petersdorf, R. Adams, and E. Brawnnald), pp. 68–75. McGraw-Hill, New York.

51. Derogatis, L.R. (1993). The prevalence of psychiatric disorders among cancer patients. *Journal of the American Medical Association*, **249**, 751–7.

52. Hayes, J.R. (1991). Depression and chronic fatigue in cancer patients. *Primary Care*, **18**, 327–39.

53. Breitbart, W., Chochinov, H., and Passik, S. (1998). Psychiatric aspects of palliative care. In *Oxford Textbook of Palliative Medicine* (eds. D. Doyle and G.W. Hanks), pp. 933–54. Oxford University Press, Oxford.

54. Piper, B.F. (1993). Fatigue. In *Pathophysiological Phenomena in Nursing: Human Responses to Illness* (eds. V. Carrieri, A. Lindsey, and C. West), pp. 279–302. Saunders, Philadelphia.

55. Respini, D., Jacobsen, P.B., Thors, C. *et al.* (2003). The prevalence and correlates of fatigue in older cancer patients. *Critical Reviews of Oncology and Hematology*, **47**, 273–9.

56. Roscoe, J.A., Morrow, G.R. *et al.* (2005). Effect of paroxetine hydrochloride (Paxil®) on fatigue and depression in breast cancer patients receiving chemotherapy. *Breast Cancer Research and Treatment*, **89**, 243–9.

57. Basaria, S., Wahlstrom, J.T., and Dobs, A.S. (2001). Clinical review 138: Anabolic-androgenic steroid therapy in the treatment of chronic diseases. *Journal of Clinical Endocrinology and Metabolism*, **86**, 5108–17.

58. Todd, B.D. (1988). Pancreatic carcinoma and low serum testosterone: A correlation secondary to cancer cachexia? *European Journal of Surgical Oncology*, **14**, 199–202.

59. Stone, P., Hardy, J., Huddart, R. *et al.* (2000). Fatigue in patients with prostate cancer receiving hormone therapy. *European Journal of Cancer*, **36**, 1134–41.

60. Snyder, P.J., Peachey, H., Berlin, J.A. *et al.* (2000). Effects of testosterone replacement in hypogonadal men. *Journal of Clinical Endocrinology and Metabolism*, **85**, 2670–7.

61. Bhasin, S., Storer, T.W., Berman, N. *et al.* (1997). Testosterone replacement increases fat-free mass and muscle size in hypogonadal men. *Journal of Clinical Endocrinology and Metabolism*, **82**, 407–13.

62. Bhasin, S., Storer, T.W., Asbel-Sethi, N. *et al.* (1998). Effects of testosterone replacement with a nongenital, transdermal system, Androderm, in human immunodeficiency virus-infected men with low testosterone levels. *Journal of Clinical Endocrinology and Metabolism*, **83**, 3155–62.

63. Grinspoon, S., Corcoran, C., Stanley, T. *et al* (1998). Effects of androgen administration in men with the AIDS wasting syndrome. A randomized, double-blind, placebo-controlled trial. *Annals of Internal Medicine*, **129**, 18–26.

64. Wang, C., Cunningham, G., Dobs, A. *et al.* (2000). Long-term testosterone gel (AndroGel) treatment maintains beneficial effects on sexual function and mood, lean and fat mass, and bone mineral density in hypogonadal men. *Journal of Clinical Endocrinology and Metabolism*, **89**(5), 2085–98.

65. Howell, S.J., Radford, J.A., Adams, J.E. *et al.* (2001). Randomized placebo-controlled trial of testosterone replacement in men with mild Leydig cell insufficiency following cytotoxic chemotherapy. *Clinical Endocrinology*, **55**, 315–24.

66. Gutstein, H.B. (2001). The biologic basis of fatigue. *Cancer*, **92**, 1678–83.

67. Checkley, S. (1996). The neuroendocrinology of depression and chronic stress. *British Medical Bulletin*, **52**, 597–617.

68. Scott, L.V. and Dinan, T.G. (1999). The neuroendocrinology of chronic fatigue syndrome: Focus on the hypothalamic-pituitary-adrenal axis. *Functional Neurology*, **14**, 3–11.

69. Warenius, H.M. (1989). Paraneoplastic neurological syndromes. In *The Clinical Neurology of Old Age* (ed. R. Tallis), pp. 323–34. John Wiley and Sons Ltd, New York.

70. Greene, D., Nail, L.M., Fieler, V.K. *et al.* (1994). A comparison of patient-reported side effects among three chemotherapy regimens for breast cancer. *Cancer Practice*, **2**, 57–62.

71. Stone, P., Richards, M., A'Hern, R. *et al.* (2001). Fatigue in patients with cancers of the breast or prostate undergoing radical radiotherapy. *Journal of Pain and Symptom Management*, **22**, 1007–15.

72. Irvine, D., Vincent, L., Graydon, J.E. *et al.* (1994). The prevalence and correlates of fatigue in patients receiving treatment with chemotherapy and radiotherapy. A comparison with the fatigue experienced by healthy individuals. *Cancer Nursing*, **17**, 367–78.

73. Blesch, K.S., Paice, J.A., Wickham, R. *et al.* (1991). Correlates of fatigue in people with breast or lung cancer. *Oncology Nursing Forum*, **18**, 81–7.

74. Jacobsen, P.B. and Stein, K. (1999). Is fatigue a long-term side effect of breast cancer treatment? *Cancer Control*, **6**, 256–63.

75. Jones, T.H., Wadler, S., and Hupart, K.H. (1998). Endocrine-mediated mechanisms of fatigue during treatment with interferon-alpha. *Seminars in Oncology*, **25**, 54–63.

76. Sugimoto, A., Hara, Y., Findley, T.W. *et al.* (1997). A useful method for measuring daily physical activity by a three-direction monitor. *Scandinavian Journal of Rehabilitation Medicine*, **29**, 37–42.

77. Roscoe, J.A., Morrow, G.R., and Hickok, J.T. (2002). Temporal interrelationships among fatigue, circadian rhythm and depression in breast cancer patients undergoing chemotherapy treatment. *Support Care Cancer*, **10**, 329–36.

78. Dimsdale, J.E., Ancoli-Israel, S., Elsmore, T.F. *et al.* (2003). Taking fatigue seriously: I. Variations in fatigue sampled repeatedly in healthy controls. *Journal of Medical Engineering & Technology*, **27**, 218–22.

79. American Thoracic Society. (2002). ATS Statement: Guidelines for the Six-Minute Walk Test. *American Journal of Respiratory and Critical Care Medicine*, **166**, 111–17.

80. Karnofsky, D.A. and Burchenal, J.H. (1949). The clinical evaluation of chemotherapeutic agents in cancer. In *Evaluation of Chemotherapeutic Agents* (ed. C.M. Macleod), pp. 191–205. Columbia University Press, New York.

81. Zubrod, C.G. (1960). Appraisal of methods for the study of chemotherapy of cancer in man: Comparative therapeutic trial of nitrogen mustard and triethylene thiophosphoramide. *Journal of Chronic Disease*, **11**, 7–33.

82. Kaasa, T., Loomis, J., Gillis, K. *et al.* (1997). The Edmonton Functional Assessment Tool: Preliminary development and evaluation for use in palliative care. *Journal of Pain & Symptom Management*, **13**, 10–19.

83. Cella, D. (1997). Manual of the Functional Assessment of Chronic illness Therapy (FACIT) Measurement System. Center on Outcomes, Research and Education (CORE), Evanston Northwestern Healthcare and Northwestern University. Version 4.

84. Piper, B.F., Dibble, S.L., Dodd, M.J. *et al.* (1998). The revised Piper Fatigue Scale: Psychometric evaluation in women with breast cancer. *Oncology Nursing Forum*, **25**, 677–84.

85. Mendoza, T.R., Wang, X.S., Cleeland, C.S. *et al.* (1999). The rapid assessment of fatigue severity in cancer patients: Use of the Brief Fatigue Inventory. *Cancer*, **85**, 1186–96.

86. Knobel, H., Loge, J.H., Brenne, E. *et al.* (2003). The validity of EORTC QLQ-C30 fatigue scale in advanced cancer patients and cancer survivors. *Palliative Medicine*, **17**(8), 664–72.

87. Chalder, T., Berelowitz, G., Pawlikowska, T. *et al.* (1993). Development of a fatigue scale. *Journal of Psychosomatic Research*, **37**, 147–153.

88. Smets, E.M.A., Garssen, B., Bonke, B. *et al.* (1995). The Multidimensional Fatigue Inventory. *Journal of Psychosomatic Research*, **39**, 315–25.

89. Belza, B., Steele, B.G., Hunziker, J. *et al* (2001). Correlates of physical activity in chronic obstructive pulmonary disease. *Nursing Research*, 50, 195–202.

90. Kirsh, K.L., Passik, S., Holtsclaw, E. *et al.* (2001). I get tired for no reason: A single item screening for cancer-related fatigue. *Journal of Pain & Symptom Management*, **22**, 931–7.

91. Mock, V. (2001). Fatigue management: evidence and guidelines for practice. *Cancer*, **92**, 1699–707.

92. Oldervoll, L.M., Loge, J.H., Paltiel, H. *et al.* (2006). The effect of a physical exercise program in palliative care. *Journal of Pain Symptom and Management*, **31**, 421–430.

93. Bruera, E., Roca, E., Cedaro, L. *et al.* (1985). Action of oral methylprednisolone in terminal cancer patients: a prospective randomized double-blind study. *Cancer Treatment Reports*, **69**, 751–4.

94. Della Cuna, G.R., Pellegrini, A., and Piazzi, M. (1989). Effect of methylprednisolone sodium succinate on quality of life in preterminal cancer patients: A placebo-controlled, multicenter study. The Methylprednisolone Preterminal Cancer Study Group. *European Journal of Cancer and Clinical Oncology*, **25**, 1817–21.

95. Popiela, T., Lucchi, R., and Giongo, F. (1989). Methylprednisolone as palliative therapy for female terminal cancer patients. The Methylprednisolone Female Preterminal Cancer Study Group. *European Journal of Cancer and Clinical Oncology*, **25**, 1823–9.

96. Love, R.R., Leventhal, H., Easterling, D.V. *et al.* (1989). Side effects and emotional distress during cancer chemotherapy. *Cancer*, **63**, 604–12.

97. Bruera, E., Ernst, S., Hagen, N. *et al.* (1998). Effectiveness of megestrol acetate in patients with advanced cancer: a randomized, double-blind, crossover study. *Cancer Prevention and Control*, **2**, 74–8.

98. De Conno, F., Martini, C., Zecca, E. *et al.* (1998). Megestrol acetate for anorexia in patients with far-advanced cancer: A double-blind controlled clinical trial. *European Journal of Cancer*, **34**, 1705–9.

99. Reyes-Terán, G., Sierra-Madero, J.G., Martínez del Cerro, V. *et al.* (1996). Effects of thalidomide on HIV-associated wasting syndrome: A randomized, double-blind, placebo-controlled clinical trial. *AIDS*, **10**, 1501–7.

100. Bruera, E., Neumann, C.M., Pituskin, E. *et al.* (1999). Thalidomide in patients with cachexia due to terminal cancer: Preliminary report. *Annals of Oncology*, **10**, 857–9.

101. Barber, M.D., Ross, J.A., Voss, A.C. *et al.* (1999). The effect of an oral nutritional supplement enriched with fish oil on weight-loss in patients with pancreatic cancer. *British Journal of Cancer*, **81**, 80–6.

102. Koretz, R.L. (1984). Parental nutrition: Is it oncologically logical? *Journal of Clinical Oncology*, **2**, 534–8.

103. Evans, W., Macmillan, K., and Daly, J. (1986). A randomized study of standard or augmented oral nutritional support versus ad lib nutrition intake in patients with advanced cancer. *Clinical and Investigative Medicine*, **9**, 127 (Abstract).

104. Olin, J. and Masand, P. (1996). Psychostimulants for depression in hospitalized cancer patients. *Psychosomatics*, **37**, 57–62.

105. Masand, P.S. and Tesar, G.E. (1996). Use of stimulants in the medically ill. *Psychiatric Clinics of North America*, **19**, 515–47.

106. Schwartz, A.L., Thompson, J.A., and Masood, N. ((2002). Interferon-induced fatigue in patients with melanoma: A pilot study of exercise and methylphenidate. *Oncology Nursing Forum*, **29**, E85–90.

107. Breitbart, W., Rosenfeld, B., Kaim, M. *et al.* (2001). A randomized, double-blind, placebo-controlled trial of psychostimulants for the treatment of fatigue in ambulatory patients with human immunodeficiency virus disease. *Archives of Internal Medicine*, **161**, 411–20.

108. Breitbart, W., Rosenfeld, B., Kaim, M. *et al.* (2001). A randomized, double-blind, placebo-controlled trial of psychostimulants for the treatment of fatigue in ambulatory patients with human immunodeficiency virus disease. *Archives of Internal Medicine*, **161**, 411–420.

109. Bruera, E., Brenneis, C., Chadwick, S. *et al.* (1987). Methylphenidate associated with narcotics for the treatment of cancer pain. *Cancer Treatments Report*, **71**, 67–70.

110. Homsi, J., Nelson, K.A., Sarhill, N. *et al.* (2001). A phase II study of methylphenidate for depression in advanced cancer. *American Journal of Hospice and Palliative Care*, **18**, 403–7.

111. Fernandez, F., Adams, F., Holmes, V.F. *et al.* (1987). Methylphenidate for depressive disorders in cancer patients. An alternative to standard antidepressants. *Psychosomatics*, **28**, 455–61.

112. Sarhill, N., Walsh, D., Nelson, K.A. *et al.* (2001). Methylphenidate for fatigue in advance cancer: A prospective open-label pilot study. *American Journal of Hospice and Palliative Care*, **18**(3), 187–92.

113. Sugawara, Y., Akechi, T., Shima, Y. *et al.* (2002). Efficacy of methylphenidate for fatigue in advanced cancer patients: A preliminary study. *Palliative Medicine*, **16**(3), 261–3.

114. Anonymous (2000). Randomized trial of modafinil as a treatment for the excessive daytime somnolence of narcolepsy: US Modafinil in Narcolepsy Multicenter Study Group. *Neurology*, **54**, 1166–75.

115. Wisor, J.P. and Eriksson, K.S. (2005). Dopaminergic–adrenergic interactions in the wake promoting mechanism of modafinil. *Neuroscience*, **132**(4), 1027–34.

116. Broughton, R.J., Fleming, J.A., George, C.F. *et al.* (1997). Randomized, double-blind, placebo-controlled crossover trial of modafinil in the treatment of excessive daytime sleepiness in narcolepsy. *Neurology*, **49**, 444–51.

117. Beusterien, K.M., Rogers, A.E., Walsleben, J.A. *et al.* (1999). Health-related quality of life effects of modafinil for treatment of narcolepsy. *Sleep*, **22**, 757–65.

118. Schwartz, J.R., Feldman, N.T., Fry, J.M. *et al.* (2003). Efficacy and safety of modafinil for improving daytime wakefulness in patients treated previously with psychostimulants. *Sleep Medicine*, **4**(1), 43–9.

119. Rammohan, K.W., Rosenberg, J.H., Lynn, D.J. *et al.* (2002) Efficacy and safety of modafinil (Provigil) for the treatment of fatigue in multiple sclerosis: a two centre phase 2 study. *Journal of Neurology, Neurosurgery, and Psychiatry*, **72**(2), 179–83.

120. Gabrilove, J.L., Cleeland, C.S., Livingston, R.B. *et al.* (2001). Clinical evaluation of once-weekly dosing of epoetin alfa in chemotherapy patients: Improvements in hemoglobin and quality of life are similar to three-times-weekly dosing. *Journal of Clinical Oncology*, **19**, 2875–82.

121. Seidenfeld, J., Piper, M., Flamm, C. *et al.* (2001). Epoetin treatment of anemia associated with cancer therapy: A systematic review and meta-analysis of controlled clinical trials. *Journal of the National Cancer Institute*, **93**, 1204–14.

122. FDA. (April 2007). Alert: New safety information about the erythropoiesis-stimulating agents increased risk thrombosis and reduced survival.

123. Stone, P., Richards, M., A'Hern, R. *et al.* (2000). A study to investigate the prevalence, severity and correlates of fatigue among patients with cancer in comparison with a control group of volunteers without cancer. *Annals of Oncology*, **11**, 561–7.

124. Munch, T.N., Zhang, T., Willey, J. *et al.* (2005). The association between anemia and fatigue in patients with advanced cancer receiving palliative care. *Journal of Palliative Medicine*, **8**, 1144–1149.

125. Fouad-Tarazi, F.M., Okabe, M.,and Goren, H. (1995). Alpha sympathomimetic treatment of autonomic insufficiency with orthostatic hypotension. *American Journal of Medicine*, **99**, 604–10.

126. Wright, R.A., Kaufmann, H.C., Perera, R. *et al.* (1998). A double-blind, dose-response study of midodrine in neurogenic orthostatic hypotension. *Neurology*, **51**, 120–4.

10.5

Clinical management of anaemia, cytopenias, and thrombosis in palliative medicine

A. Robert Turner

Introduction

The illnesses, malignant or benign, that bring patients to a palliative care setting are often complicated by haematological problems such as anaemia, marrow failure, or thrombosis. Supportive therapy for these problems can provide gratifying relief of symptoms and improvement in overall quality of life, permitting resumption of pleasurable activities. This chapter emphasizes a practical approach to assessment and therapy intended to maximize quality of life.

Anaemia

Anaemia is present in over 50 per cent of patients in palliative care[1]. It is associated with symptomatology, which includes[2]

- easy fatigability;
- reduced mental acuity;
- dyspnoea;
- anorexia;
- oedema;
- exacerbation of angina;
- postural hypotension.

Determining the cause of anaemia in the palliative care setting can be challenging, since the aetiology of anaemia is often multifactorial.

The differential diagnosis of the cause of anaemia in a patient seen in a palliative care setting is different from the differential diagnosis in a general medical context. The major entities that should be considered are[3]

- anaemia of chronic disorders (ACD);
- marrow suppression;
- acute and chronic haemorrhage;
- haemolysis;
- malnutrition;
- underlying chronic or congenital anaemia.

Anaemia of chronic disorders[4] (ACD)

This is a hypoproliferative anaemia that is unresponsive to haematinic therapy. Severe anaemia is unusual but transfusions are sometimes required to maintain the patient's activity levels. The anaemia of chronic disorders is caused by an immunological reaction to the presence of a malignancy or inflammation. Several cytokines are released in this reaction. Interleukin 1 (IL1β) is one of a large family of glycoprotein hormones that carry signals from various types of leucocytes to other types of white cells. IL-1β, previously known as endogenous pyrogen, is released by macrophages. It interacts with other cytokines, such as tumour necrosis factor (TNFα) and gamma interferon (IFγ), to mediate an immune response. IL-1β affects the haematologic system in many ways. One of these is to impede the transfer of iron molecules from storage sites in the reticuloendothelial system to red cell precursors. This results in the paradoxical situation of iron deficient erythropoiesis occurring in a marrow replete with iron. IL-1β also causes stimulation of splenic macrophages, which leads to hypersplenism and a shortened red cell survival. TNFα and IFγ both impair red cell precursor proliferation. Interleukin 6 (IL-6), another pro-inflammatory cytokine, is up-regulated in malignant disorders causing a low-grade anaemia as well as decreased serum albumin. Hepcidin is a protein made in the liver. It controls iron absorption from the gastrointestinal tract as well as suppressing iron uptake by marrow cells. Inflammatory cytokines stimulate hepcidin release from the liver.

The diagnosis of ACD is often based on the exclusion of other forms of anaemia. However, ACD should always be considered in the palliative care setting. The anaemia will be slightly microcytic or near the lower limits of the mean corpuscular volume. The reticulocyte count will be low, reflecting a reduced marrow output. Serum iron studies should be interpreted carefully. The serum iron may be low but the total iron binding capacity (transferrin) is also low and the iron saturation is >15 percent. (In iron deficiency, the total iron binding capacity would be elevated resulting in a very low iron saturation index.) Hepcidin is the cause of the low serum iron. The transferring levels are low because of normal or elevated tissue iron stores. Serum ferritin gives the best estimate of 'true' iron levels, but it can be influenced by an acute phase reaction.

If the ferritin is <100 ng/ml, iron supplementation can be prescribed (orally or parenterally). Erythropoietin (Epo) stimulates proliferation and differentiation of red cell precursors. It counteracts the antiproliferative effects of the cytokines, which are causing the anaemia of chronic disorders. Epo treatment is discussed below.

Marrow suppression[5]

Low blood counts are frequent in patients presenting for palliative care. Patients who have had extensive treatments with myelotoxic chemotherapy or radiation, or whose marrow has been infiltrated with metastatic cancer, myelodysplasia, or fibrosis will not be able to produce blood cells on demand. Thrombocytopenia may lead to purpura and haemorrhage. If the neutrophil count is $<0.5 \times 10^9/l$, bacterial sepsis is a risk.

The presence of a leucoerythroblastic blood reaction (the presence of immature red and white blood cells in the peripheral blood) as well as the presence of tear drop-shaped red cells points to the presence of metastasis or fibrosis within the bone marrow. A bone marrow aspirate and biopsy can document the metastasis or fibrosis but a bone marrow examination is rarely done in a palliative care setting, since the test is uncomfortable and there are few therapies that would benefit the patient beyond transfusion support.

Myelodysplasia (refractory anaemia, pre-leukaemia) is a marrow failure state that may be primary or may be a complication of chemotherapy. It is very frustrating to manage. No evidence-based therapy exists other than red cell transfusion support.

If neutropenic sepsis is a problem, filgrastim (G-CSF) 300–480 mg SC q.d. will raise the neutrophil count and may be an effective preventative[6].

Acute and chronic haemorrhage[7] (see also Chapter 10.14)

Haemorrhage can occur in palliative care patients due to bleeding from neoplastic lesions within the gastrointestinal tract, the upper and lower respiratory tract, or the genitourinary system. Less commonly, haemorrhage can occur within tumour masses or around a pathologic fracture. This bleeding can be acute and massive, resulting in a rapid depletion of intravascular volume and consequent shock. More commonly, the bleeding is of a chronic nature with a loss of a few millilitres of blood daily. Chronic loss of blood can lead to iron deficiency. In most cases, the chronic blood loss is obvious from the presence of blood in bodily fluids but, occasionally, tests for occult blood or endoscopic examinations are necessary to determine the presence and site of the bleeding.

The first priority is to control the bleeding lesion if practical. This may be accomplished surgically, endoscopically, or by radiation of the bleeding lesion. Medical therapy is helpful for some patients with chronic haemorrhage who are bleeding from non-neoplastic lesions within the gastrointestinal tract. H_2 antagonists, such as ranitidine, are of use in treating chronic gastrointestinal bleeding. Other agents that have been utilized are omeprazole, misoprostol, and sucralfate. Patients whose chronic bleeding has led to iron deficiency can be treated with an orally administered simple iron salt such as ferrous sulphate or ferrous gluconate (300 mg, two to three times daily). Intravenous administration of 1–2 g of iron dextran is a very useful way to provide a reserve of iron dextran when oral iron preparations cannot be tolerated or are poorly absorbed. Transfusion therapy will be discussed in a separate section below.

Chronic haemorrhage can also be seen in patients with thrombocytopenia secondary to marrow failure or coagulation factor deficiencies due to liver failure or disseminated intramuscular coagulation (DIC) (see below). Extensive ecchymoses are often evident in patients whose platelet count is less than $50 \times 10^9/l$ or whose prothrombin time or activated partial thromboplastin time is prolonged. These patients tend to have a gradual drop in their haemoglobin levels without gross evidence of blood in the stool or other body fluids.

An important cause of anaemia in patients in any type of institutional setting is chronic bloodletting for laboratory testing purposes. Each vial of blood that is drawn represents 7–10 ml of whole blood. Routine, repetitive laboratory testing should be limited.

Malnutrition

Most patients in a palliative care setting have protein or calorie malnutrition. Along with protein/calorie malnutrition, there will be deficiencies in the dietary intake of haematologically important nutrients such as iron or folic acid. Iron deficiency usually results from chronic or acute haemorrhage and not from malnutrition alone, but patients can readily become deficient in folic acid if they have not had it in their diet for 4–6 weeks. Patients with chronic anaemias, rapidly growing tumours and prior treatment with folic antagonists such as methotrexate are at especially high risk for this easily correctable deficiency. Folic acid, 5 mg. daily, can be administered orally or subcutaneously.

Deficiencies of iron should be suspected when the mean corpuscular volume (MCV) is reduced. A serum ferritin test should be done to establish the diagnosis as ACD often causes a very similar microcytic picture. Megaloblastic effects of the chemotherapy should be suspected in a patient who has a macrocytic anaemia. Other important causes of a macrocytic anaemia in a patient in palliative care include liver disease, folate deficiency, and B_{12} deficiency.

Chronic protein malnutrition can lead to a generalized hypoproteinemia that is often accompanied by a normocytic anaemia and marrow failure. The anaemia in these patients may respond to improvement in overall nutrition if the anorexia–cachexia syndrome is not present.

Chronic haemolysis[8,9]

Haemolysis is rarely a major contributor to anaemia in the palliative care setting. Some neoplasms are associated with haemolysis such as chronic lymphocytic leukaemia, non-Hodgkin's lymphomas, thymomas, and adenocarcinomas of diverse origins. Haemolysis should be suspected in the patient who has a progressive anaemia and in whom chronic haemorrhage cannot be documented. The laboratory evaluation of these patients may show an elevation lactate dehydrogenase (LDH), indirect bilirubin, and a reduction in serum haptoglobin. Because of the effects of ACD or marrow failure, a reticulocytosis may not be seen despite active haemolysis.

Three general types of haemolysis can be seen in these patients. They are

- immune haemolysis (Coombs positive or cold agglutinin);

- microangiopathic haemolytic anaemia; and

- hypersplenism.

Immune haemolysis is due to the presence of an immunoglobulin or complement on the surface of red cells causing red cell lysis or macrophage engulfment in the reticulo-endothelial system. The Coombs test (direct antiglobulin test) or the cold agglutinin screen detects the immunoglobulin or complement. If active haemolysis is occurring, there will be evidence of red cell breakdown (including elevation of red cell derived LDH) and evidence of increased haemoglobin release (that is, increased indirect bilirubin and decreased haptoglobin). An examination of peripheral blood may show spherocytes or agglutinated red cells.

Immune haemolysis not due to cold agglutinin may be treated with corticosteroids (prednisolone, 0.5–1.0 mg/kg). Other forms of treatment include splenectomy or the use of immunosuppressive drugs such as cyclophosphamide or azathioprine but they are not often utilized in the palliative care setting. Cold agglutinin haemolysis does not respond to corticosteroids or splenectomy. Transfusions are the mainstay of therapy.

Microangiopathic haemolytic anaemia may be seen when there is destruction of the red cell membrane as it passes through abnormal vasculature within a tumour or in a disorder sometimes associated with vascular neoplasms or chemotherapy agents such as mitomycin C. There are striking changes noted in the peripheral blood of these patients, prominent red cell fragmentation is seen. The therapy of these disorders has been unrewarding.

Hypersplenism is a disorder in which an enlarged or overactive spleen causes an increased rate of destruction of red blood cells and other blood elements. This disorder can be treated with splenectomy or by radiation to the spleen. The latter approach may be attractive in palliative care when the general condition of the patient would make surgery difficult. Surgical advances have made laparoscopic splenectomy much less traumatic than removing a spleen through a laparotomy incision.

Chronic or congenital haematological disorders[3]

Patients receiving palliative care bring with them a variety of medical disorders. Some of these can be associated with anaemia and should not be disregarded in the differential diagnosis of the cause of anaemia in the palliative care patient. Examples of chronic disorders include rheumatological diseases, inflammatory bowel disorders, or chronic infections. Perhaps the most common cause of chronic anaemia in the world is the presence of α- or β-thalassemia trait. Thalassemia trait will cause a chronic anaemia marked by the presence of severe microcytosis and target cells in the peripheral blood. It can be confused with iron deficiency or ACD. Many patients with thalassemia trait will have a positive family history. β-thalassemia trait can be diagnosed by demonstrating an elevation in the proportion of haemoglobin A_2 on haemoglobin electrophoresis.

General approach to the diagnosis of anaemia[3]

In the palliative care setting, anaemia is very common and is almost always multifactorial in aetiology (Table 10.5.1). Any patient who has a neoplasm or chronic infection will have some degree of anaemia of chronic disorders. Many of these patients will also have chronic haemorrhage and marrow failure. Haemolysis and malnutrition occur in a minority of patients but need to be recognized,

Table 10.5.1 Approach to the diagnosis of anaemia in a palliative care setting.

Anaemias	Diagnosis	Therapy
ACD	Exclude other causes	Transfuse
		Erythropoietin
Haemorrhage	Determine site	Control haemorrhage
		Proton pump inhibitor
Marrow failure	Marrow examination	Transfuse
Malnutrition	Iron, albumin	Increase calories
		Iron or folate
Haemolysis	Coombs test, cold agglutinin, haptoglobin, LDH, indirect bilirubin, blood smear	Prednisolone
		Splenectomy
		Transfuse

since the therapeutic options will be influenced. Laboratory investigation needs to be individualized to each patient depending upon their prognosis and the likelihood of remediable causes of the anaemia. The peripheral blood smear often gives very valuable clues as to the diagnosis and the cause of anaemia. Estimates of iron stores using a serum ferritin level and the demonstration of immune haemolysis with the direct antiglobulin test (Coombs) are commonly used. A bone marrow examination is done infrequently.

Transfusions in the palliative care setting

In the past, for many patients, transfusion therapy represented the extent of palliation. Transfusion of packed red cells remains a very important part of the comprehensive care of palliative care patients. In addition to red cells, platelets and plasma components can also be administered. Advances in the delivery of transfusions in the home setting have expanded greatly the number of patients whose quality of life is improved. Guidelines for transfusion are given in Table 10.5.2.

Indications for transfusion of red blood cells[10–15]

Red blood cells provide two important factors to patients. Oxygen transport to tissues from the lung is augmented and intravascular volume expansion is provided. Other blood products provide superior means to produce plasma volume expansion and will be discussed later. Red cell concentrates can only provide oxygen carrying capacity.

This discussion will deal exclusively with the provision of red cell concentrates in the chronically anaemic patient. The management of acute haemorrhage will not be dealt with here.

The most important factor in determining the need for red cell transfusion in the patient with chronic anaemia is the presence or absence of symptoms attributable to the anaemia. Patients who have developed their anaemia chronically will tolerate levels of haemoglobin much lower than that tolerated by patients suffering an acute haemorrhage. Therefore, no specific guidelines can be given as to the degree of anaemia, which necessitates transfusion. If the

Table 10.5.2 Transfusion guidelines.

Product	Transfusion trigger	Comments
Red blood cells	Symptoms Hb < 80 g/l	Watch for fluid overload
Platelet concentrate	Symptoms (no critical no.)	Tranexamic acid may help
Albumin	If diuresis needed	
Frozen plasma	Prothrombin time (PT)	Vitamin K helpful
Cryoprecipitate	International normalized ratio (INR) > 5 Fibrinogen < 1.0 g/l	1-Deamino-8-d-arginine vasopressin (DDAVP) if von Willebrand's

patient is symptomatic from dyspneoa, angina, postural hypotension, headache, or peripheral oedema and there are no other medical explanations for these symptoms, the patient should be transfused.

One can anticipate the progression of anaemia in many patients in the palliative care setting. Patients who have marrow failure develop anaemia at the rate of approximately 10 g/l per week. It is common to transfuse these patients at a rate of 3–4 units of red cells every 3–4 weeks.

In estimating the number of units required, it is convenient to aim for a post-transfusion haemoglobin of 110–120 g/l. Each unit of packed red cells administered to an adult will result in a rise in haemoglobin concentration of 10 g/l. In a patient with a haemoglobin of 80 g, a transfusion of 3–4 units will raise the haemoglobin concentration to 110–120 g/l.

There are three types of complications that can be seen with red blood cell transfusion in the palliative care setting. They are

- volume overloading;
- febrile/urticarial reactions;
- iron overloading.

Many patients in a palliative care setting have a compromised cardiovascular system that will not tolerate the rapid addition of several hundred millilitres of fluid. Each red cell unit provides the equivalent of approximately 450 ml of fluid. Three units therefore have in excess of 1200 ml and this cannot be tolerated over a short period by many palliative care patients. Volume overload problems can be avoided by administering a small amount of frusemide (furosemide) (20 mg) with alternate units and by administering the blood slowly. Each unit can be administered over a period of 3–4 h. It is advisable to administer no more than 2 units per day.

Febrile and urticarial reactions used to occur frequently in patients receiving blood products because of the presence of white blood cells in the transfused product carrying HLA antigens to which the patient has become immunized. Most transfusion services are now providing red cell (and platelet) concentrates that have been subjected to leucodepletion. These leucodepleted products are a significant improvement in transfusion therapy. Most patients do not require premedication with antihistamines or paracetamol (acetaminophen). Occasional patients continue to have febrile reactions to blood products. These patients are likely

sensitized to proteins in the plasma. These reactions can be attenuated with an antihistamine such as diphenhydramine (50 mg) or by the use of washed red cells or platelets.

Iron overload is not often a concern in the palliative care setting since it does not become evident until between 50 and 75 units of red cells have been transfused to the patient. Each unit of blood adds 250 mg of iron to the patient's iron stores. Patients with more than 20 g of iron in their stores are at risk for haemosiderosis. Haemosiderosis can cause heart, liver dysfunction, or failure of pancreatic endocrine function. The best way to avoid the problem of haemosiderosis is to transfuse red blood cells only when the patient's symptoms demand it. Iron chelation therapy (desferrioxamine) can remove iron from patient stores but is very rarely indicated in the palliative care setting.

Infectious complications of blood transfusion have been minimized by recent improvements in the screening of blood donations. AIDS, hepatitis B, hepatitis C, HTLV-1/2, West Nile Fever, and syphilis can be screened for and the risk of these infections arising from a blood transfusion, prepared in a blood bank with these procedures in place, are minimal. In most situations, the benefit of improved quality of life with the transfusion of red blood cells would outweigh the potential risk from infectious complications. Although there is some experimental evidence that transfusion might induce immunosuppression and enhance the growth of neoplasms, this complication of transfusion is not of practical importance in the palliative care setting. The removal of white cells in the leucodepletion process would also reduce the risk of immunosuppression.

Erythropoietin and other pharmacological agents[16]

Erythropoietin (Epo), a hormone made in the kidney, stimulates red cell production in the marrow. Its use during chemotherapy treatments has been shown to reduce the need for red cell transfusions and to improve patients' quality of life, in particular to counteract fatigue. There have been intriguing suggestions from the data of the quality of life studies that Epo can counteract deleterious effects of cytokines causing ACD and anorexia–cachexia syndrome.

If Epo were not so expensive, there would be little disagreement over its use during active cancer chemotherapy or radiotherapy, but it is only 'cost-effective' compared to transfusions when large transfusion liability litigation costs are factored in.

In the palliative care setting, reduction of fatigue and anaemia symptoms and the avoidance of transfusions is unlikely to shift the cost equation in favour of routine use of Epo.

The Hg should be kept <120 g/l to minimize risk of cardiovascular and thromboembolic risks. Other pharmacological agents[16] sometimes used to control these symptoms include androgens such as danazol or halotestin and modest doses of prednisone[10]. Little or no scientific data supports their use and hormone related exacerbation of thrombosis or tumour growth must always be considered.

Transfusion of other blood products
Platelets

Thrombocytopenia may be seen in the palliative care setting when the patient has extensive marrow involvement by their neoplasm, has an immune reaction resulting in thrombocytopenia, has a disseminated coagulopathy (DIC), has an enlarged spleen, or has received extensive myelotoxic therapy. Platelet counts of less than $50 \times 10^9/l$ can be associated with bleeding problems. If the patient has a platelet count of less than $50 \times 10^9/l$ and is bleeding, transfusion of 5 units of platelet concentrate may be helpful in curtailing the bleeding for a short period of time. In most patients in the palliative care setting, thrombocytopenia is a chronic problem. Some patients with chronic purpura will have less bleeding with the use of an anti-fibrinolytic medication such as tranexamic acid (1000 mg, 3 times daily).

Albumin[17]

Many patients in a palliative care setting are hypoalbuminemic. This is not an indication for the transfusion of albumin. Albumin should be administered only when there is a need for an acute expansion of plasma volume such as when acute diuresis is necessary. There is no point in transfusing albumin to the patient with chronic hypoalbuminemia for 'nutritional' purposes. In most cases, hypoalbuminemia is a feature of the anorexia–cachexia syndrome.

Other plasma components

Fresh plasma and cryoprecipitate should be used only when specific and documented bleeding diathesis remediable by plasma or cryoprecipitate are present. Examples of this would be the correction of a prolonged prothrombin time due to liver failure or warfarin anticoagulation by frozen plasma or the correction of an abnormal bleeding time due to a deficiency of von Willebrand's factor (vWf) by cryoprecipitate. DDAVP (desmopressin), 20 mcg intravenously, is a useful way to raise vWf activity, if required. DDAVP is helpful in reducing the bleeding diathesis, due to diminished vWf, seen in chronic renal failure.

Thrombosis[18,19]

There is a well-known association between cancer and hypercoagulability. Thrombophlebitis is quite common is cancer patients. Hypercoagulability may have preceded the diagnosis of cancer and patients who have cancer-related hypercoagulability have a worse prognosis than those patients whose cancer is not associated with hypercoagulability. There are some types of cancers that appear to have a particular predilection to induce hypercoagu-lability: prostate, pancreas, breast, and ovary. It is thought that cancer-related thrombosis results from activation of the coagulation cascade as well as an inhibition of anticoagulant proteins and fibrinolysis.

Another issue related to cancer-related hypercoagulability is whether anticoagulation would prolong survival by 'treating' the underlying malignant disease. Warfarin, heparin, fibrinolytics, and anti-platelet agents disrupt the growth of cancer cells *in vitro* and also impair the metastatic process. Patients treated with chemotherapy and warfarin or low molecular weight heparin seem to have a survival benefit. A practical question for palliative medicine research to resolve is whether anticoagulation extends the lives of patients not receiving chemotherapy or radiation therapy.

Acute deep venous thrombosis

Acute deep venous thrombosis can produce painful swelling of a lower limb, or less commonly, an upper limb. Extension and embolization of these clots can occur if the clotting is present above the popliteal fossae. An important complication is pulmonary embolization. This may contribute to the cause of death in the majority of patients with end-stage cancer. Other patients will have a very painful swelling of the entire limb (phlegmasia cerulea dolens).

The diagnostic and therapeutic approach has to be individualized to each patient's circumstances. If the decision to treat has been made, the deep venous thrombosis should be documented by venography, plethmysography or Doppler studies. The presence or absence of pulmonary embolism can be difficult to establish with certainty and routine diagnostic imaging tests available for this condition (such as ventilation perfusion scans) are not very specific. A high resolution CT scan of the chest is the most specific.

The therapy of acute deep venous thrombosis usually involves the administration of a low-molecular-weight heparin (LMWH) such as dalteparin at 100 U/kg. Oral warfarin should be started at a dose of 5–10 mg and continued daily until the PT INR is between 2 and 3. Once a therapeutic PT INR is achieved, the LMWH can be discontinued and the warfarin continued indefinitely. Recurrent thrombosis should be managed by intensive LMWH.

The decision to use heparin in the patient in the palliative care setting is often a complex one. Many of these patients have major or minor contraindications to the use of heparin. Major contraindications include active gastrointestinal haemorrhage, active bleeding from any other site, an intracranial neoplasm, and uncontrolled hypertension. Minor contraindications include a past history of gastrointestinal haemorrhage, retinopathy, and the presence of bleeding disorders. It is the author's approach to recommend full anticoagulation in most patients without major contraindications whose prognosis exceeds a few days and who are having significant symptoms from the deep venous thrombosis.

LMWH, such as dalteparin or enoxaparin, has the dual advantage of requiring much less monitoring than warfarin or unfractionated heparin and being administered by once daily SC injections. These expensive agents may be useful in the palliative setting where blood letting should be minimized for patient comfort. LMWH also has advantages over warfarin in patients with abnormal liver function.

Venocaval filters may prevent pulmonary embolization in patients with recurrent deep venous thrombosis on therapy, or in patients with major contraindications to anticoagulation but are associated with painful engorgement of both lower limbs.

Chronic venous thrombosis

Patients with neoplastic lesions obstructing veins or with a hypercoagulability related to disseminated malignancy can have chronic venous thrombosis. Two therapeutic approaches are suggested for these patients: chronic warfarin and subcutaneous whole heparin or LMWH.

Chronic warfarin therapy can be administered quite safely if the prothrombin time is monitored closely. The PT INR should be checked every 1–2 weeks after establishment of the initial therapeutic dose. The INR should be kept within 2 to 3. Some patients will have continued thrombosis despite maintenance therapy with coumarins and an INR between 2 and 3. In some of those patients, increasing the warfarin dose so that the INR is between 3 and 4 will

Table 10.5.3 Anticoagulation guidelines.

Thrombosis issue	Strategy
Acute DVT/PE	Full dose IV heparin
	Warfarin → PT INR 2-3
Chronic DVT	Warfarin → PT INR 2-3
	LMWH once daily SC
Contraindication to anticoagulation	IVC filter
Cancer hypercoagulability	Warfarin → PT INR 2-3
	LMWH (prophylactic dose)
Superficial thrombophlebitis	ASA, indomethacin

be successful in controlling the thrombotic tendency but many of those patients will have bleeding complications. If warfarin therapy has to be reversed rapidly, the administrations of 3–4 units of fresh plasma and 10 mg of vitamin K will bring the PT INR back to baseline rapidly.

In those patients who continue to have thrombotic problems despite warfarin therapy, subcutaneous whole heparin or LMWH should be considered. This approach involves subcutaneous injection of whole heparin thrice daily or LMWH once daily. Many patients can self-administer heparin and it does not necessarily involve increased use of medical personnel. For whole heparin, a starting dose of 5000 units is given every 8 h. If the patient has been receiving intravenous heparin therapy, the total dose administered over a 24-h period can be used as a guide to selecting the initial subcutaneous dose. Half of the total 24-h dose is administered each 12 h. Standard prophylactic and therapeutic doses for each LMWH are listed in prescribing information sheets.

Trousseau's syndrome is a migratory polyphlebitis affecting superficial veins primarily but also causing venous and arterial clotting. It can be very bothersome and may not be adequately treated with either warfarin or subcutaneous heparin. Indomethacin at a dose of 25 mg, 3–4 times daily, is a useful adjunct in these patients, but gastrointestinal side effects must be monitored.

Guidelines for anticoagulation are given in Table 10.5.3. Chronic DIC may be seen in patients with metastatic prostatic carcinoma as well as some other solid tumours and haematological neoplasms. Chronic DIC is produced by an activation of the clotting process but the result is the consumption of the components of the clotting system. Thrombocytopenia, hypofibrinogenanaemia, and prolongation of the PT INR and PTT are commonly present. Chronic DIC can lead to troublesome bleeding. Effective therapy is difficult when the underlying neoplasm cannot be eradicated or suppressed in the case of hormone sensitive prostate cancer. If therapeutic measures are to be utilized, emphasis should be placed upon augmenting the fibrinogen levels with cryoprecipitate and transfusing platelets when there is thrombocytopenic bleeding. Heparin is rarely used now.

References

1. Mercadante, S., Gebbia, V., Marrazzo, A. *et al.* (2000). Anaemia in cancer: Pathophysiology and treatment. *Cancer Treat Rev*, **26(4)**, 303–11.
2. Ludwig, H. and Strasser, K. (2001). Symptomatology of anemia. *Semin Onocl*, **28(2 Suppl 8)**, 7–14.
3. Turner, A.R. and Turner, E.H. (2006). Anemias in the Elderly. *Can J Cont Med Edu*, **18(9)**, 75–9.
4. Weiss, G. and Goodnough, L.T. (2005). Anemia of chronic disease. *N Eng J Med*, **352(10)**, 1011–23.
5. Prachal, J.T. (2006). Anemia associated with marrow infiltration. In *Williams Hematology*, (eds. M.A. Lichtman, E. Beutler, T.J. Kipps, U. Seligsohn, K. Kaushansky, J.T. Prchal), 7th edition, pp. 561–3. McGraw-Hill, New York.
6. Mughal, T.I. (2004). Current and future use of hematopoietic growth factors in cancer medicine. *Hemat Oncol*, **22**, 121–34.
7. Hillman, R.S. and Hershko, C. (2006). Acute blood loss anaemia. In *Williams Hematology*, (eds. M.A. Lichtman, E. Beutler, T.J. Kipps, U. Seligsohn, K. Kaushansky, J.T. Prchal), 7th edition, pp. 767–72. McGraw-Hill, New York.
8. Rytting, M., Worth, L., and Joffe, N. (1996). Hemolytic disorders associated with cancer. *Hematol Oncol Clin North Am*, **10**, 365–76.
9. Ruggenenti, P. and Remuzzi, G. (1991). Thrombotic microangiopathies. *Crit Rev Onc/Hem*, **11**, 243–65.
10. Menitove, J.E. (1999). Red cell transfusion therapy in chronic anaemia. In *Transfusion therapy: Clinical principles and practice*, (ed. P.D. Muntz), 1–12. AABB Press, Bethesda, MD.
11. Vanvakas, E.C. and Blajchman, M.A. (2001). Universal WBC reduction: The case for and against. *Transfusion*, **41**, 691–712.
12. Girot, R., Hagege, I., Deux, J.F. *et al.* (2006). Treatment of iron overload in haematological diseases (heredity hemochromatosis excluded). *Hematologie*, **12(3)**, 181–93.
13. Jinger, Y. and Shvartzman, P. (1998). The feasibility and advisability of administering home blood transfusions to the terminally ill patient. *J Palliat Care*, **14**, 46–8.
14. Cella, D. (1998). Factors influencing quality of life in cancer patients: Anaemia and fatigue. *Semin Oncol*, **25**, 43–6.
15. Turner, A.R., Anglin, P., Burkes, R. *et al.* (2001). Erythropoietin alfa in cancer patients: Evidence-based guidelines. *J Pain Symptom Management*, **22(5)**, 954–65.
16. Singh, A.K., Szczech, L., Tan, K.L. *et al.* (2006). Correctioin of anemia with epoetin alfa in chronic kidney disease. *N Engl J Med*, **355(20)**, 2085–98.
17. Lee, A.Y.Y. (2004). Management of thrombosis in cancer: Primary prevention and secondary prophylaxis. *Br J Haematol*, **128**, 291–302.
18. Kirkova, J., Oneschuk, D., and Hanson, J. (2005). Deep vein thrombosis (DVT) in advanced cancer patients with lower extremity edema referred for assessment. *Am J Hospice Palliat Med*, **22(2)**, 145–9.
19. Rosovsky, R.P. and Kuter, D.J. (2005). Catheter-related thrombosis in cancer patients: Pathophysiology, diagnosis, and management. *Hematol Oncol Clin N Am*, **19**, 183–202.

10.6

Pruritus and sweating in palliative medicine

Mark R. Pittelkow and Charles L. Loprinzi

Introduction

Itching (pruritus) and sweating (perspiration, diaphoresis) are physiological functions of the skin that normally serve human existence well. Itching is the sensory input arising from the skin and mucous membranes that alerts man to potentially harmful insults from physical, chemical, and biological sources. The reflex of scratching is closely linked to the perception of itch, and in most situations functions effectively as an aversive motor response to relieve the sensation and protect the skin. Similarly, sweating is a well-developed and finely coordinated sudomotor response designed to regulate body temperature and prevent hyperthermia.

However, both pruritus and sweating have the potential to function aberrantly and develop into pathological conditions that create significant suffering and morbidity. Since these skin responses encompass both normal and abnormal functions, effective treatments to alleviate or eliminate the pathological component are challenging. In this chapter, we provide a practical overview of the normal function and pathophysiology of pruritus and sweating, and offer a variety of therapeutic options and general comforting measures for patients experiencing these maladies.

Pruritus

Terminology

Itch and pruritus are terms used to describe both physiological and pathological sensory perception. Itch is a distinctive and common cutaneous sensation that arises from the superficial layers of the skin and mucous membranes. It is often fleeting, and the sensation may pass relatively unnoticed since the reflex action of scratching is largely involuntary and typically relieves the temporary discomfort.

Itch (itching, itchy, or itchiness) and pruritus (from the Latin *prurire*, to itch) are generally considered to have equivalent meanings. Itch and related descriptions such as 'terrible itching' are terms commonly used by the patient to convey this distinctive symptom. However, subtle differences in the terminology of itch and pruritus have evolved in the medical literature. In this respect, the terms itch and pruritus have been used to characterize the spectrum of unique cutaneous sensations ranging from the physiological response to severe pathological symptoms[1–5]. Physiological itch is the short-lived cutaneous response to the usual events of living, while pruritus is more closely associated with pathological itch[1,2]. Use of the term pruritus represents the symptomatic level or quality of itch that is defined as an intense cutaneous discomfort occurring with pathological change in the skin or body and eliciting vigorous scratching.

The definition of pruritus or itch is subjective and not entirely precise. Although the general sensation is well known and implicitly understood, many patients with more severe symptoms assimilate itch with various other discomforting or unpleasant sensation. The term itch frequently encompasses a range of descriptive or qualifying terms such as tickle, prickle, pins and needles, burning, stinging, chafed, raw, aching, and even 'painful' sensations[2].

To avoid confusion and to focus on the palliative medicine perspective, the terms itch and pruritus are used interchangeably to describe this pathological symptom. Patients experiencing pruritus may develop this symptom only mildly and transiently, or itching may be so severe and unrelenting that it preoccupies and completely disrupts their daily existence. It must be recognized that itch or pruritus is variable in its perceived quality and intensity. As with pain, the perception and tolerance of pruritus and the response to this sensation depends significantly on the individual's physical and emotional states, the functional level of activity, adaptive coping mechanisms, and the overall outlook. Attempts to develop questionnaires that assess severity of pruritus have been developed based on modified pain questionnaires[6]. These quantitative measuring tools will be useful to better standardize symptoms and treatment responses.

Anatomy and physiology

Pruritus is a discrete sensation and a primary sensory modality arising from the activation and integration of cutaneous sensory neural receptors, afferent pathways, and central nervous system processing centres[7] (Fig. 10.6.1). In the past, itch was considered to be a low-threshold form or submodality of pain based on various clinical and experimental observations. Both pain and itch are induced by noxious stimuli and therefore are designated 'nociceptive'.

A prevailing theory was that itch and pain were related sensations that differed only in the strength of the stimulus, with itch being a response to a weak stimulus and pain being elicited by a stronger stimulus. Further investigation of pain and pruritus not only revealed similarities but also clearly demonstrated the distinctive differences between these two sensations. Recent research has conclusively demonstrated that itch and pain are represented by distinct nerve fibres. Itch neurons are specific type C fibres in skin,

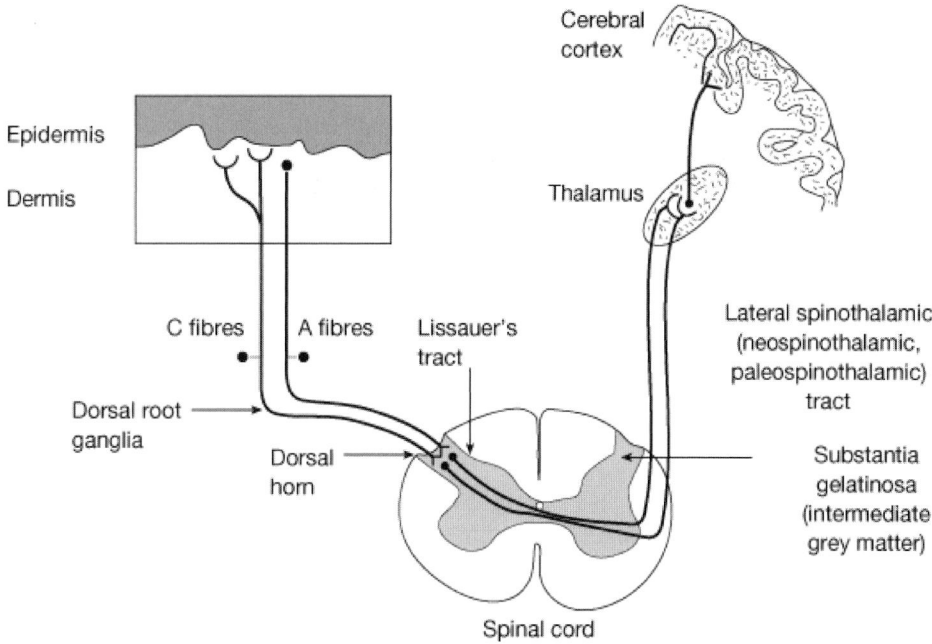

Figure 10.6.1 Pathway for transmission of itch sensation. The C fibres terminate in substantia gelatinosa. Spinothalamic relay axons cross and ascend contralaterally at the spinal level of entering sensory neurons. Larger-diameter A fibres and other interneuronal and central pathways may modulate signalling information. (Modified with permission[2,10].)

each having a wide innervation territory, thin axon, and very low conduction velocity[8]. The central neural pathway for itch has also been recently localized to spinothalamic lamina I neurons that are selectively sensitive to histamine[9].

Many definitions of pruritus specifically include the reflex action of scratching. Scratching illustrates the distinctive sensation of pruritus, and the scratching reflex is routinely elicited and intimately coupled to itch. Scratching is regarded as a protective reflex, much as withdrawal (flexion) and guarding are comparable reflexes in response to painful stimuli.

Pruritogenic stimuli

Pruritus is induced in skin by various stimuli. Both exogenous and endogenous factors have the capacity to elicit itch[10,11]. Most experimental and spontaneous triggering factors are mediated via the exogenous or external route. Cutaneous sensory nerves that convey the pruritic signal become activated through the application of either physical or chemical stimuli to the skin (Fig. 10.6.2). Many physical stimuli induce pruritus, including pressure, thermal stimulation, low-intensity electrical stimulation, formation of suction blisters, and epicutaneous application of caustic substances.

Chemical stimuli include histamine, proteases, prostaglandins, and neuropeptides[7]. Delivery of histamine to the upper layers of skin by injection or iontophoresis has been a quantitative and reproducible method of examining pruritus experimentally. Histamine is also secreted in skin by mast cells. It acts directly on free nerve endings in skin.

Proteases such as trypsin, chymotrypsin, papain, and kallikrein have the ability to induce pruritus when injected into skin. For example, the spicules of the plant cowhage (*Mucuna pruriens*) contain an endopeptidase. These fine spicules are an active ingredient of itching powder and induce an itching sensation when they penetrate

into the epidermal layers or dermoepidermal junction of skin. Other natural proteases produced in cells and tissues of the body or by microorganisms such as bacterial or fungal microflora of the skin also have the potential to induce pruritus.

Mediators of pruritus

The nerve fibres that conduct signals representing itch are located predominantly at the epidermal–dermal junction and have free endings extending into the epidermis[10]. Many of these nerve fibres contain neuropeptides such as substance P, neurokinin A, and calcitonin gene-related peptide (CGRP) (Fig. 10.6.2). Other neuropeptides contained in nerves deeper in the dermis and located around blood vessels include vasoactive intestinal peptide (VIP) and neuropeptide Y. Substance P, which is the best-characterized pruritogenic neuropeptide, is a sensory transmitter of nociception. It is localized to sensory nerve endings in the skin and is abundant in the prevertebral ganglia, the dorsal roots of the spinal cord, and the brain. Administration of substance P intrathecally causes intense scratching that can be blocked by an antagonist. Nerve fibres containing substance P appear to transmit direct synaptic sensory impulses for the itch sensation.

Capsaicin, an alkaloid derived from the common pepper plant, is a well-known stimulant of erythema and pain when applied to mucous membrane or skin. It depletes substance P from the sensory nerves and excites the type C polymodal nerve fibres conveying pain. However, after initial stimulation, capsaicin blocks C fibre conduction and mediates neuronal toxicity which eventually decreases fibre density. These activities of capsaicin have stimulated the use of this agent for the treatment of pruritus[12].

Neuromediators directly influence vascular permeability and erythema (Fig. 10.6.2). They also activate release of other mediators such as interleukins, prostaglandins, bradykinin, serotonin, and

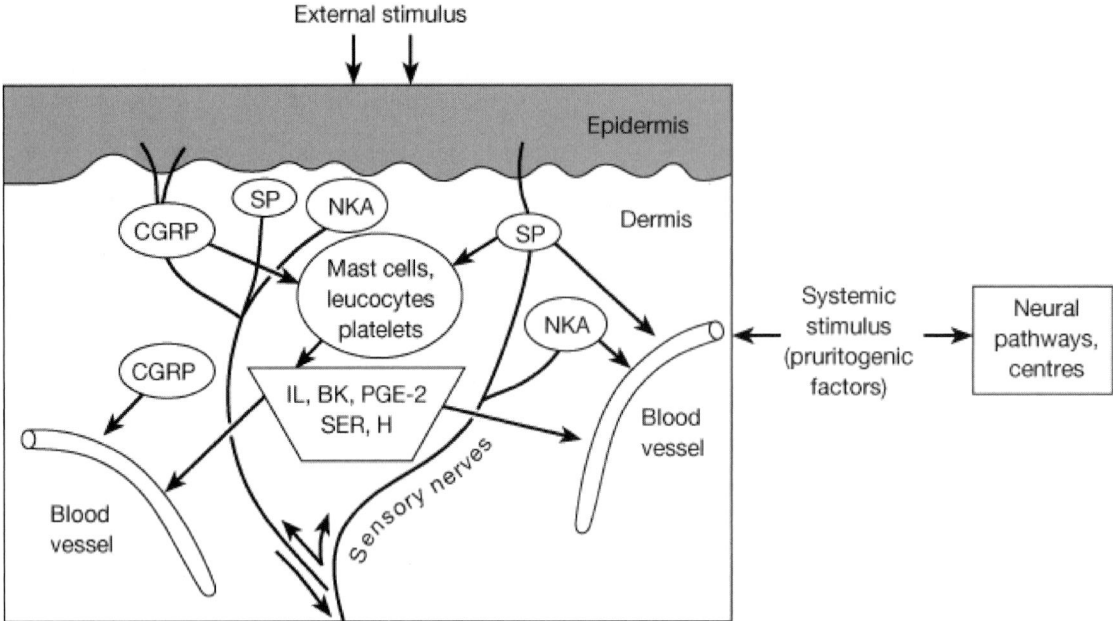

Figure 10.6.2 Stimuli of itch in skin or at peripheral and central neural sites. External or endogenous (systemic) routes of activation trigger nerve fibre stimulation in the skin and the release of neuropeptides including substance P (SP), neurokinin A (NKA), and calcitonin gene-related peptide (CGRP). These mediators trigger inflammatory cells in the skin to release histamine (H), bradykinins (BK), serotonin (S), interleukins (IL), and prostaglandin E2 (PGE-2). Vascular permeability, inflammatory cell infiltration, and nerve stimulation are evoked by stimuli. (Modified with permission[10].)

histamine from infiltrating leucocytes and tissue-localized mast cells. Together, these neural and cellular mediators induce the sensation of itch, augment local activation of inflammatory responses that often accompany itch, and create areas of hyper-responsiveness around the primary stimulus zone for itch. For example, the phenomenon of 'itchy skin' (alloknesis) may be due to regional hyper-responsiveness as well as a lowering of the threshold to itch stimuli at the level of the spinal cord. Additionally, neuro-mediator release is probably augmented through antidromic nerve stimulation.

Cutaneous neural input

Human skin is supplied principally by nerve fibre networks composed of A and D myelinated fibres and thin type C unmyelinated fibres. Afferent type C fibres include C mechanoreceptors, cold thermoreceptors, C polymodal, and C itch nociceptors. Itch is primarily conveyed by the C itch fibres that represent approximately 15–20 per cent of unmyelinated nerve fibres in skin. The remaining polymodal C fibres constitute about 80 per cent of all afferent C fibres (Fig. 10.6.1). The exact location and unique identity of the itch receptor is unknown, but it is likely resides in free nerve endings.

Itch, therefore, is separate from the slow, aching, dull, or burning pain that is conducted by type C polymodal fibres[13,14]. Myelinated A delta nociceptors conveying sharp pain also have been identified. Physiological and pharmacological studies have shown that separate independent sensory channels conduct itch and pain stimuli. The latency between stimulation and onset of the sensation of pain coincides with the relatively low rates of conduction (2 m/s) by the neurons that serve these sensory functions. Itch fibres have very slow velocities of 0.5–0.7 m/s[8,9]. Some investigators have suggested separating 'itch' into the 'pricking' sensation carried by myelinated

fibres and the 'burning' sensation conveyed by unmyelinated fibres. This classification of sensations correlates with the two different systems of sensation described by Head[15] in 1905 as the epicritic or specific well-defined sensation that mediates spontaneous itch and the protopathic or diffuse poorly localized sensation that conveys the perception of itchy skin. On the basis of current scientific knowledge, pain and itch are largely separable cutaneous sensations. However, there is evidence of secondary neuron interactions with 'itch-specific' fibres being suppressed by coactivation of pain nociceptors using agents such as capsaicin.

In addition to the external or exogenous pathway for initiation of the itch sensation, there is considerable clinical evidence for the endogenous activation of pruritus[1–5] (Fig. 10.6.2). The endogenous route for stimulation of pruritus represents a major and clinically relevant pathway; however, it is poorly understood. The potential sites of stimulation (the peripheral nervous system, the spinal cord, and the central nervous system), the inciting agents and mediators, and the relative overlap of exogenous versus endogenous activation pathways remain to be clearly delineated and applied effectively in the clinical setting. The systemic or endogenous stimuli for itch have been only partially characterized, and the biochemical causes for pruritus associated with a spectrum of systemic illnesses, including metabolic disease, organ failure, and various malignancies, continue to be ill-defined and vexing problems.

Several substances have been shown to mediate different or opposing effects on itch when tested experimentally. Their activities depend on the route of administration and their specific responses at the peripheral, spinal cord, and central nervous system levels. These observations support the concept of itch as a neural message that is interpreted in the context of signal reception, transmission, and modulation at each level of the nervous system.

Opioid and serotonergic mediators

Opioids are one example of substances that exert separate and potentially disparate responses in modulating the transmission and perception of itch and pain at different levels of the nervous system[2,16]. Uncovering the existence of central opioid receptors led to the discovery of encephalins, endogenous pentapeptides that bind to these receptors. Opioids are powerful analgesics that mimic the effects of encephalins. However, opioids mediate both excitatory and modulatory effects on pruritus at several levels. At the spinal level, encephalins released from short spinal interneurons and opioids stimulate an inhibitory presynaptic signal transmitted to primary afferents that modulates secondary transmission of itch. However, within some regions of the central nervous system, opioids directly trigger itch. Clinically, intrathecal or epideral morphine has been known to induce localized or generalized itching. At the peripheral level within skin, opioids stimulate mast cell degranulation and release of histamine which produces itch. Furthermore, based on the recent identification and characterization of itch-specific primary nerve fibres, opioids may induce itching by blocking the painful stimuli that suppress activity of central itch neurons.

Central activation of itch by opioids appears to play a dominant role in some diseases, since opioid antagonists have been shown to exert significant antipruritic effects[16,17]. The parenterally administered opioid antagonist naloxone inhibits induction of itch following histamine injection of skin. Pruritus of cholestatic liver disease (primary or secondary biliary cirrhosis) can be dramatically reduced with naloxone or the oral antagonist nalmephene[7,18].

Serotonergic compounds are another group of agents that modulate effects on pruritus primarily at the peripheral level, although receptors for serotonin are present in the peripheral and central nervous systems. Cutaneous injection but not intravenous infusion of a serotonergic agonist increases the scratching reflex in animals. Peripheral serotonin receptors in humans are presumed to play a role in the mediation of pruritus. Temperature-dependent pruritus experienced by patients with polycythaemia vera may be stimulated by serotonin. Serotonin reuptake inhibitors, specifically paroxetine, have recently been reported to be useful for treatment of polycythemia vera-related pruritus[19]. Of potential clinical significance, generalized pruritus of hepatic cholestatic disease and chronic renal insufficiency have been relieved dramatically with intravenous administration of the type 3 serotonin (5-HT$_3$) receptor antagonist ondansetron[20,21]. However, other recent placebo-controlled studies have refuted this finding in uraemic pruritus[22]. Nonetheless, opioid and serotonin receptor antagonists have revealed the complex mechanisms involved in transmitting signals for pruritus at the peripheral and central nervous system levels.

Pathogenic correlates in management of pruritus

The similarity of the symptoms of exogenous and endogenous forms of pruritus has prompted empirical use of similar treatment measures for both types of conditions. Frequently, however, effective therapy for pruritus caused by one condition is not particularly beneficial for pruritis of another cause. Also, treatments that ameliorate or relieve pruritus induced by exogenous agents have limited or minimal effects on alleviating pruritus of endogenous cause. This is probably related to the site and mode of activity of these treatments and their limitations in targeting the receptors, mediators, or central neural pathways that control expression of endogenous versus exogenous pruritus.

The nuclei of the afferent C itch and polymodal nerves reside in the dorsal root ganglia and axon extensions that synapse in the dorsal horn of the substantia gelatinosa (Fig. 10.6.1). Secondary neurons cross the spinal cord to the contralateral spinothalamic tract of the venterolateral quadrant before ascending to the thalamus. Lamina I of the spinothalamic tract contains type C itch fibres[9]. There is also evidence in animals that pathways in addition to the anterolateral system can transmit pruritogenic stimuli. Both the ventral posterior inferior nucleus and the ventral periphery of the ventral posterior lateral nucleus of the thalamus contain itch fibres projecting from lamina I[9]. The synaptic neurons within the thalamus project to the somatosensory cortex of the postcentral gyrus. Scratching is the spinal reflex in response to itching but also has input from higher neural centres.

Perception of itch has the potential to be modulated at the level of the spinal cord and, probably at other levels, by additional neural input as described for pain by Melzak and Wall[23]. The description of 'a gate control system that modulates sensory input from the skin before it evokes pain perception' can also be applied to the perception of itch.

A fibre impulse conduction is self-regulated by a negative feedback pathway that tends to dampen continued firing. It also interrupts summation of sensations of itch and pain conveyed by the C itch and polymodal fibres. The 'gate' has the ability to control neural transmission. Gate closure is envisaged to produce inhibition at the spinal cord level such that stimulation of A fibres by scratching would induce or enhance inhibition of conduction. Although the gate-control theory has been intensively evaluated and revised over the past three decades and its operational functionality has been challenged, practical application based on this theory appears to have been made in the control of pain and itch using transcutaneous electrical nerve stimulation[24,25].

Clinical evaluation and treatment of pruritus

The clinical approach to pruritus can present a considerable diagnostic as well as therapeutic challenge. To formulate a simple clinical strategy for diagnosis and treatment of pruritus, pathological itch can be classified as primary or secondary (Table 10.6.1). Secondary pruritus is caused by either dermatological or systemic disease[1–4]. Pruritus can be further separated into localized and generalized forms based on the location and extent of body surface involvement.

Table 10.6.1 Pruritus: causes and distribution.

Aetiology	Distribution
Primary:	Localized
Idiopathic	Generalized, diffuse
Essential	
Secondary:	
Dermatological	
Systemic	

In most cases, localized pruritus is due to cutaneous infections or other regionalized expressions of dermatological disease.

Generalized or diffuse pruritus typically presents more troublesome symptoms for the patient and a greater challenge for the physician. Diffuse pruritus is usually related to a dermatological or systemic disorder affecting the entire skin surface. However, even pruritus which is generalized or diffuse exhibits symptoms that may be accentuated and localized to certain regions of the body, and these symptoms may fluctuate, migrate, or extend over time.

Primary pruritus

Primary or idiopathic pruritus is identified in the majority (more than 70 per cent) of patients where dermatological disease (secondary pruritus) has been excluded as a cause for itching.[26] Idiopathic pruritus may be fairly limited in extent and intensity. Symptoms can be reasonably controlled by conscientious skin care and topical soothing measures. However, other cases of primary pruritus prove to be quite extensive, severe, and chronic. The diagnosis of primary pruritus is established following a thorough medical and dermatological evaluation to exclude secondary causes of itching.

Evaluation and management of idiopathic pruritus is frequently a frustrating experience for the patient and physician as possible causes and beneficial treatments are sought. When no clear aetiology is delineated, both the patient and physician may experience disappointment. With severe idiopathic pruritus, there is also lingering uncertainty whether an occult disease, particularly malignancy, may eventually be uncovered. However, several clinical studies have shown that only a small percentage of patients referred to dermatologists for generalized pruritus will develop a malignancy during follow-up evaluation[26,27]. The majority manifest haematological malignancies, particularly lymphomas, and therefore periodic clinical surveillance is warranted. However, the duration and severity of chronic primary pruritus may be sufficiently debilitating for palliative intervention and the identification of effective therapies to become the principal goals.

Secondary pruritus—dermatological

Secondary pruritus is associated with a variety of disorders including both dermatological and systemic diseases (Tables 10.6.2 and 10.6.3). For example, contact dermatitis is a common characteristic skin disease that has itching and scratching as its hallmarks. Table 10.6.2 lists the major dermatological entities that are accompanied by pruritus. Some disorders, such as scabies, insect bites, folliculitis, and allergic contact dermatitis, are caused by exogenous agents that elicit pruritus. Other conditions, including atopic dermatitis, bullous pemphigoid, lichen planus, psoriasis, and urticaria, are endogenously mediated inflammatory skin conditions that exhibit variably intense symptoms of pruritus.

The mechanisms that induce itching have been partially characterized for some of these disorders. Specific inflammatory cell types, such as mast cells, lymphocytes, and eosinophils, play important roles in the pathogenesis of specific diseases and the development of pruritus. Neuropeptides, cytokines, and proteases, among other mediators, are the main cellular products initiating pruritus (Fig. 10.6.3). These mediators probably act in addition to specific neurotransmitters that directly convey a pruritogenic signal to the itch receptor. Treatment of the specific skin condition and elimination of any offending exogenous agent(s) typically alleviate the

Table 10.6.2 Skin diseases associated with pruritus.

Aquagenic pruritus
Atopic dermatitis (eczema)
Bullous pemphigoid
Contact dermatitis
Cutaneous T-cell lymphoma (mycosis fungoides, Sézarys syndrome)
Dermatitis herpetiformis
Drugs (dermatitis medicamentosa)
Folliculitis
Grover's disease
Insect bites
Lichen planus
Lichen simplex chronicus
Mastocytosis
Miliaria
Pediculosis
Pityriasis rosea
Prurigo
Prurigo nodularis
Pruritus ani and vulvae
Psoriasis
Scabies
Sunburn
Systemic parasitic infection (onchocerciasis, trichinosis, echinococcosis)
Urticaria, dermographism
Xerosis

symptoms of pruritus. When dealing with pruritus, which may be skin related, it is crucial to identify and classify any primary skin lesions and obtain appropriate skin sample specimens or skin biopsies. This information is often very helpful in establishing a diagnosis. The correct diagnosis and appropriate therapy for dermatological disorders should be sought through specialist consultation and is well described in standard dermatology textbooks.

Cutaneous diseases that cause pruritus should not be overlooked. For example, unrelenting pruritus caused by scabies infestation, sometimes lasting for months to years, has been mistakenly attributed to concurrent malignancy (Fig. 10.6.4). Other cutaneous infections, irritant or allergic contact dermatitis (Fig. 10.6.5), or autoimmune blistering diseases such as bullous pemphigoid (Fig. 10.6.6) have been repeatedly observed to develop during the course of malignancies or other systemic illnesses. By recognizing that pruritus is due to a supervening dermatological condition, prompt and appropriate treatment can be instituted and the skin disease and pruritus both resolve. Therefore, the periodic evaluation and re-evaluation of the causes of idiopathic or poorly controlled pruritus may uncover new information that will significantly benefit total patient care and improve overall comfort.

Some dermatological conditions provide instructive lessons on the aetiology and limitations of managing pruritus. For example,

Table 10.6.3 Systemic disorders associated with pruritus.

Biliary and hepatic disease
Biliary atresia
Primary biliary cirrhosis
Sclerosing cholangitis
Extrahepatic biliary obstruction
Cholestasis of pregnancy
Drug-induced cholestasis
Chronic renal failure—uraemia
Drugs
Opioids
Amphetamines
Cocaine
Acetylsalicylic acid
Quinidine
Niacinamide
Etretinate-acitretin
Other medications
Subclinical drug sensitivity
Endocrine diseases
Diabetes insipidus
Diabetes mellitus
Parathyroid disease
Thyroid disease (hypothyroidism, thyrotoxicosis)
Haematopoietic diseases
Hodgkin's and non-Hodgkin's lymphoma
Cutaneous T-cell lymphoma (mycosis fungoides, Sézary's syndrome)
Systemic mastocytosis
Multiple myeloma
Polycythaemia vera
Iron-deficiency anaemia
Infectious diseases
Syphilis
Parasitic
HIV
Fungal
Malignancy
Breast, stomach, lung, etc.
Carcinoid syndrome
Neurological disorders
Distal small-fibre neuropathy
Stroke
Multiple sclerosis
Tabes dorsalis
Brain abscess/tumours
Psychosis, psychogenic causes
Delusions of parasitosis

prurigo nodularis is a distinctive pruritic dermatosis that can be chronic and is often recalcitrant to therapy[28]. The symptom of pruritus appears to play a more central role in the pathogenesis and propagation of this disease. The pruritus of prurigo nodularis largely localizes to the nodular lesions that appear to develop and become more prominent as a result of scratching (Fig. 10.6.7). Cutaneous nerve elements are accentuated within the lesions and are often difficult to block effectively or eliminate. These factors probably account for the refractory nature of the condition to various treatments. Clinical and therapeutic observations on prurigo nodularis potentially have aetiological and practical relevance to non-dermatological disorders that are associated with pruritus, since some of these conditions may also be quite refractory to many therapeutic measures directed at alleviating the itch.

Secondary pruritus—systemic

Pruritus is a feature of a broad range of systemic diseases (Table 10.6.3). For some diseases, specific medical or surgical treatment provides cure of the illness and pruritus. However, with many of the chronic systemic diseases, patients may survive for long periods with adequate control of the illness. Unfortunately, pruritus often continues to be a major symptom and may cause considerable morbidity.

Topical antipruritic agents

A variety of topical medications have been developed through the years to provide symptomatic relief of itching[29,30]. Many of the active ingredients have long been known to ease the symptoms of itch. A list of the common therapeutic antipruritic lotions, creams, and gels, together with their active ingredients, is given in Table 10.6.4. Topical medications are not convenient to apply to the entire body surface on a routine basis, but even patients with more generalized pruritus often have localized areas of accentuated itching that are more troublesome to control. Therefore, topical agents have a role in treating both regionalized accentuation of generalized pruritus and localized itching.

Phenol in dilute solution (0.5–2 per cent) alleviates pruritus by anaesthetizing cutaneous nerve endings. Phenol is potentially neurotoxic and hepatotoxic, and should be avoided in pregnancy and in infants less than 1 year of age. Menthol and camphor relieve itching by counter-irritant and anaesthetic properties. Menthol (typically 0.25–2 per cent, but can be as high as 16 per cent) produces a cool sensation, and camphor (typically 1–3 per cent, but can be as high as 9 per cent) exerts similar effects. Zinc oxide, coal tars, calamine, glycerine, and salicylates also have been used in many preparations with reported benefit, although their specific modes of action have not been elucidated.

Pramoxine hydrochloride is a topical anaesthetic similar to dyclonine that has been used as the sole ingredient or has been compounded with hydrocortisone or menthol and is available as an aerosol, foam, cream, gel, or lotion. Newer anaesthetic prescription medications include EMLA® cream, a combination of the caine drugs lignocaine (lidocaine) and prilocaine that are absorbed transcutaneously and produce anaesthesia as well as abolish itch. Lignocaine patches (Lidoderm®) are also available that can be applied to problematic pruritic areas[31]. Doxepin has been demonstrated to be effective in relieving the itch of skin disease and may be useful for pruritus of various aetiologies. Capsaicin has been reported to be effective in localized neurogenic pruritus of

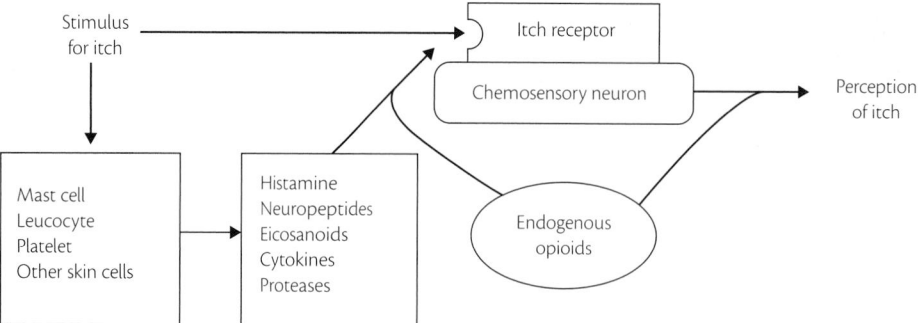

Figure 10.6.3 Factors mediating itch: direct or indirect activation of itch receptor by specific pruritogens. The itch signal is transmitted to a chemosensory neuron, which is activated and conveys perception centrally in the nervous sytem. Endogenous opioids, among other factors, modulate pruritogenic signals. (Modified with permission[2]).

various causes and has demonstrated benefit in other conditions accompanied by itch. Initial applications of the medication produce burning sensations and other discomfort. The patient must be alerted to these sensations and coaxed to continue if sustained use is planned and benefit is to be obtained.

Systemic therapies and other treatments

A plethora of systemic medications and various other modalities have been used in the treatment of pruritus[1,4,5,30,32,33]. These agents are organized and listed in Table 10.6.5 according to their standard pharmacological activities. On examining this list, it becomes apparent that no drug has ever been successfully developed, tested, and produced exclusively or even primarily for pruritus. This fact alone reveals the potential difficulties that are encountered in the pharmacological treatment of chronic and severe cases of pruritus. All too frequently, patients requiring palliative relief from intractable itching are subjected to trials of various medicines in an attempt to discover which one 'works best' for them. With persistence and luck, a particular drug or modality can be identified that offers benefit and has tolerable side effects. Combinations of systemic and topical agents often seem to provide the best relief. Clinical experience has also shown that certain medications or treatment modalities seem to provide more consistent benefit for specific types of secondary pruritus, as is the case for ultraviolet B (UVB) phototherapy and the pruritus of chronic renal

failure. Unfortunately, few controlled clinical studies have ever been conducted on the palliative management of pruritus, and a well-developed and simple clinical management strategy does not exist. Therefore, as outlined above, the practical aspects of establishing the probable cause(s), selecting a treatment, and assessing its benefit, side effects, and potential risks must all be addressed routinely as part of the process of providing palliative care for the patient with pruritus. In addition, several simple measures can be adopted to give patients and their skin some relief from the anguish of itching and the injury of scratching.

Pruritus of malignancy

Itching associated with malignancy presents special challenges and dilemmas. It can be among the most severe and recalcitrant forms of secondary pruritus. Patients with malignancy-associated pruritus represent a significant percentage of those requiring palliation, and many may manifest this symptom at some time during their illness. However, the frequency, chronicity, and severity of pruritus associated with malignancy and its response to treatment are difficult parameters to determine, and they have not been examined systematically and reported in the literature. For example, the percentage of patients for whom the symptoms of itching have been relieved by primary treatment of the malignancy versus those

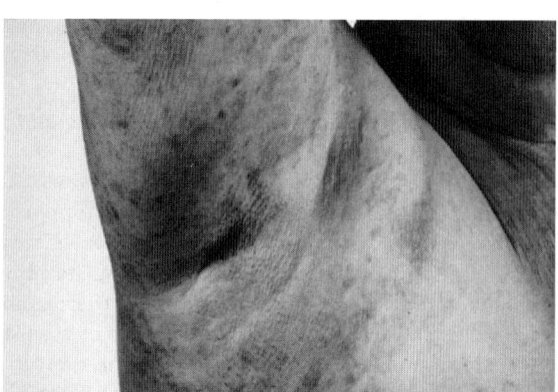

Figure 10.6.4 Scabies: erythematous papules, crusts, and excoriations. Mite burrows can be identified under magnification.

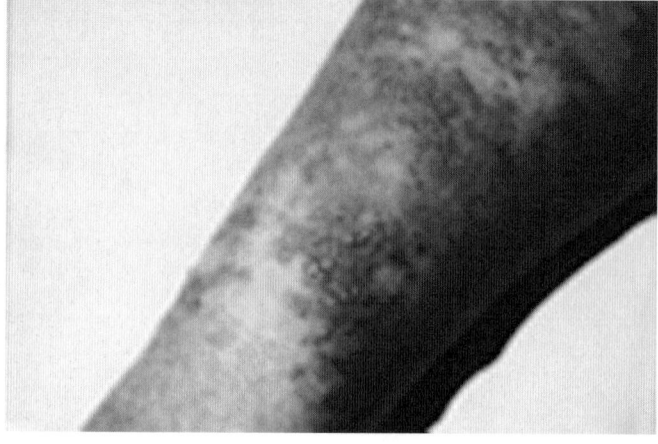

Figure 10.6.5 Acute dermatitis: erythema, scaling, and blister formation due to allergy after application of triple antibiotic ointment containing neomycin.

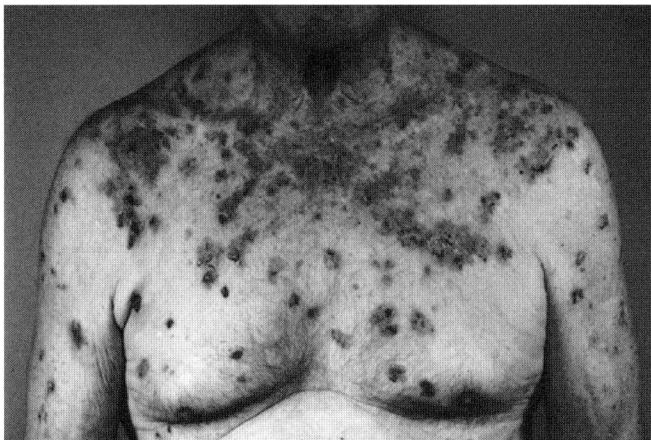

Figure 10.6.6 Bullous pemphigoid: tense blisters on an erythematous and urticarial base with rupture of secondary blisters, erosions, and crust formation.

Table 10.6.4 Topical antipruritic agents.

Preparation	Active ingredient
Dodd's lotion	Phenol, glycerine, zinc oxide
Lerner's lotion	Ethyl alcohol, glycerine, zinc oxide
Pamscol	Phenol, acetylsalicylic acid
Sarna	Menthol, camphor, phenol
Schamberg's lotion	Menthol, phenol, zinc oxide
Topic gel	Benzl alcohol, ethyl alcohol, methol, phenol
Wibi lotion	Menthol
Crude coal tar 3%–10% solution	Crude coal tar
Caladryl	Diphenhydramine, calamine, camphor
Pramosone, Prax	Pramoxine
Quotane	Dimethisoquin
EMLA	Lignocaine, prilocaine
Lignocaine patch	Lignocaine
Zonalon	Doxepin
Zostrix	Capsaicin

Modified from Ref. 30.

who have benefited from symptomatic therapies has not been defined in this population of patients. As a result, a single, specific, and effective treatment plan for pruritus of malignancy is not available.

Symptomatic skin care

Patients with itching of malignancy may manifest different types of pruritic skin lesions that warrant individualized therapies. Many patients will demonstrate excoriations due to scratching and injury of the skin from fingernails or other implements (brushes, etc.) (Fig. 10.6.8). Other patients show discrete papular, crusted, or excoriated lesions more characteristic of prurigo (Fig. 10.6.9). As a routine, close trimming and filing of sharp edges of fingernails as well as wearing cotton gloves, if necessary, are initial steps to minimize further skin injury. Tepid (not too warm or too hot) baths are usually soothing and temporarily relieve the itch. Patients often relate that a hot bath or shower feels more relaxing and offers symptom relief, but the itch is worse afterwards due in part to vasodilation and the accentuated neural response of cutaneous heating. Immediately following the bath and a light towelling, the patient or caregiver should lubricate the skin with a fragrance-free

cream-base emollient containing phenol or menthol if this is found to be beneficial. Applying a cream results in better maintenance of skin hydration and lessens the chance of further aggravation of pruritus from xerosis. Wearing clothing that is loose fitting, less irritating (e.g. avoid wools), and minimizes heat retention and sweating (e.g. avoid synthetics) can also be helpful in lessening the frequency and intensity of itch. Cotton fabric clothing usually meets these requirements.

For patients with numerous excoriations and crusting due to scratching, application of tap water wet dressings (or cotton long underwear soaked in water) to the affected areas several times daily for 1–2 h provides temporary relief and hastens healing of injured skin. A low- to medium-potency corticosteroid cream containing 1–2.5 per cent hydrocortisone can be applied to the skin prior to the wet dressings for topical anti-inflammatory action. A more potent corticosteroid such as triamcinolone 0.05–0.1 per cent in a cream base can be used for 7–10 days as needed on an intermittent basis, but prolonged use should be avoided to prevent atrophy and bruising of the skin, secondary skin infections, or hypothalamic–pituitary–adrenal suppression.

Oral corticosteroids

Various systemic anti-inflammatory agents are useful in the management of pruritus. Oral corticosteroids often improve the symptoms of itching for patients with primary or secondary pruritus. In many patients, the specific activity is unknown. The corticosteroid may inhibit release of pruritogens, inflammatory factors, or neuromediators, or it may block pruritogen activity or alter its metabolism. As with topical steroids, prolonged use has significant adverse side effects. However, in cases where the duration of treatment is limited, an oral corticosteroid can provide much sought relief of itching.

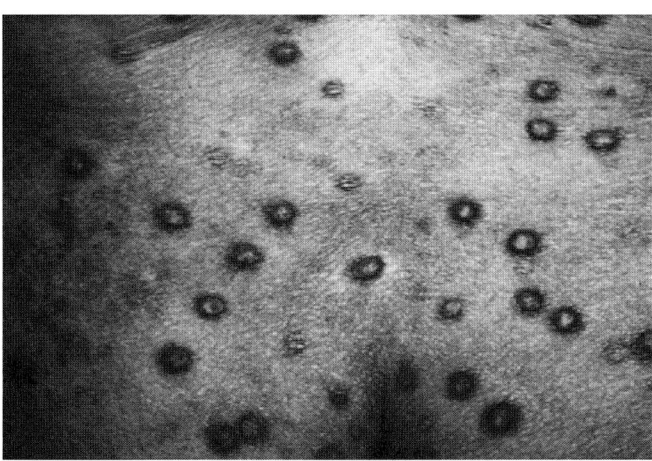

Figure 10.6.7 Prurigo nodularis: discrete firm pruritic globular nodules over the sacral area that often have a verrucous crust and an excoriated surface.

Table 10.6.5 Pruritus therapies.

Anti-inflammatory agents
Corticosteroids
H_1, H_2, H_3 blocking agents
Salicylates
Cromolyn
Thalidomide
Vasoactive drugs
α-Blockers
β-Blockers (e.g. propranolol)
Central and peripheral nervous system agents
Anaesthetic agents
Lignocaine etc.
Propofol
Antidepressant agents (tricyclic, SSRI[34])
Neuroleptic agents
Tranquillizing agents
Sedatives
Opioid antagonists (naloxone, naltrexone, nalmephene)
Serotonin antagonists (ondestranon)
Analgesic (non-conventional, voltage-gated calcium channel)
Gabapentin
Pregabalin
Sequestrants
Cholestyramine
Charcoal
Heparin (IV)
Miscellaneous
Disease-specific drugs and therapies
Cholestatic disease[35]: rifampicin, methyltestosterone ursodeoxycholic acid, partial external biliary diversion[30,36–38]
Uraemia: erythropoietin, parathyroidectomy, ultraviolet B phototherapy[39–41]
Polycythaemia vera: α-interferon,[42] paroxetine[19]
Neurofibromatosis (neurofibroma): ketotifen[43]
Phototherapy: ultraviolet A, ultraviolet B, photochemotherapy (PUVA)[30,41]
Transcutaneous nerve stimulation[24,25]
Plasma exchange, apheresis[30]
Acupuncture[30]
Psychotherapy, biofeedback, relaxation techniques[30]

Antihistamines

Antihistamines are another class of agent that offers benefit in treatment of itching. More than 30 different antihistaminic compounds of at least six different classes are available over the counter or by prescription. Although antihistamines provide minimal benefit for some patients with problematic itching such as that associated with Hodgkin's disease, obstructive jaundice, or uraemic pruritus, they have a good safety profile and should be used at full dose to attempt amelioration of pruritus. For example, pruritis is an early manifestation of HIV infection, and antihistamines, sometimes at high dosages, are used to control symptoms. Studies have shown superior efficacy of sedating over low-sedating antihistamines for relieving itch. Low-sedating antihistamines (e.g. fexofenadine, cetirizine, loratadine) should be reserved for the histamine-mediated whealing disorders that are accompanied by pruritus. Longer-acting antihistamines with central nervous system sedation are preferred for control of itch. These include chlorpheniramine, diphenhydramine, clemastine, hydroxyzine, and cyproheptadine. Agents of different classes should be tried if an antihistamine of one class is not effective. Sometimes, combination of agents from different classes is efficacious when a single agent is ineffective.

Other drug therapies

Cromones and thalidomide are anti-inflammatory agents that have been reported to be useful in pruritus associated with several different types of chronic or malignant disease. Disodium chromoglycate improves the flushing and pruritus of systemic mast cell disease[44]. It also has been reported to improve the pruritus of Hodgkin's disease when other therapies have failed[45]. Thalidomide has been found to relieve the intractable pruritus and development of skin lesions in prurigo nodularis[46]. More recently, thalidomide (100 mg/day) was found to produce significant relief of uraemic pruritus[47]. This drug is used primarily in the treatment of leprosy reactions and graft-versus-host disease. Because of its neuropathic and teratogenic side-effects, thalidomide is not routinely available for prescription.

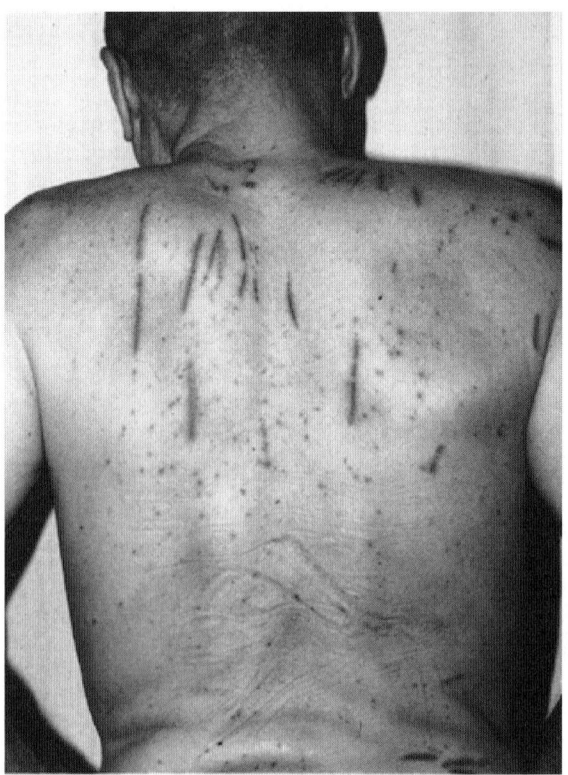

Figure 10.6.8 Linear excoriations, erosions, and crusts resulting from unrelenting pruritus and scratching by a patient with small-cell carcinoma of the lung.

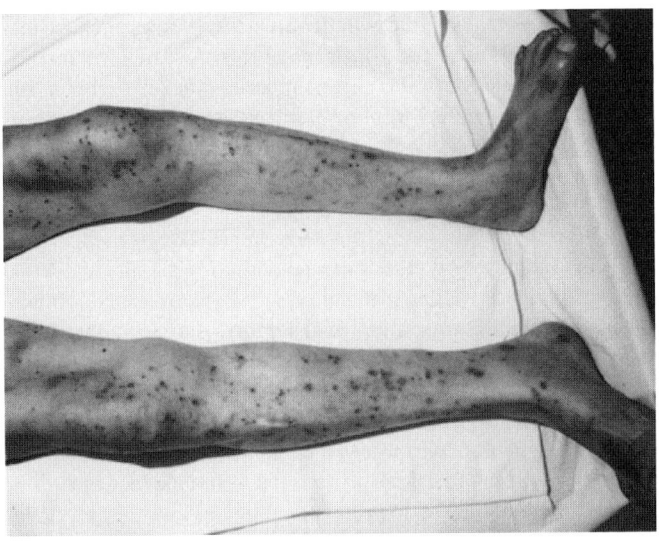

Figure 10.6.9 Discrete, crusted, and haemorrhagic prurigo-like lesions accompanying generalized pruritus of chronic renal failure and diabetes mellitus.

However, selected patients who require only a limited course of therapy and can be monitored regularly may be candidates for thalidomide when an alternative medication is sought.

Many drugs have effects on the peripheral or central nervous system, and some of these agents have been found to be very useful in the treatment of itching from many causes. Anaesthetic agents administered by the intradermal, intravenous, or intra-arterial routes have effects similar to topical anaesthetics in blocking sensory input and transmission, including the sensation of pruritus. Parenteral lignocaine (200 mg in 100 ml saline by an intra-arterial line) alleviates refractory pruritus in hepatic cholestasis and chronic renal failure[48,49]. Hypotension, cardiovascular effects, seizures, and psychosis are possible side effects. Recently, the anaesthetic sedative propofol, used at subhypnotic doses (15 mg) daily when itch was most severe or by continuous infusion at 1–1.5 mg/kg/h, produced significant reduction in pruritus due to cholestatic disease of pancreatic neoplasia, hepatic and bile duct metastasis, cholangitis, and primary biliary cirrhosis[50,51]. A rapid onset of action within 5–10 min was observed. Propofol also relieves pruritus from spinal morphine administration, and it is postulated that propofol blocks effects of opioid-like pruritogens at the spinal level[52]. Parenterally administered agents such as lignocaine, propofol, and naloxone are of relatively limited use in chronic pruritus. However, if acute severe episodes of pruritus become incapacitating, these agents can often provide much sought relief and re-establish some measure of symptom control.

Antidepressant drugs, including doxepin, amitriptyline, nortriptyline, and imipramine, have antihistaminic effects as well as psychoactive and analgesic properties that make them useful in the management of various pain and itch states. Serotonin reuptake inhibitors such as paroxetine have demonstrated significant actitvity in controlling recalcitrant types of pruritus, especially secondary to polycythemia vera[19], as well as various other advanced cancers[34]. Neuropathic pain with protopathic features of diffuse burning itch as well as the sensation of pain is improved by chronic anti-depressant treatment[53]. These medications may also benefit patients with pruritus where depression appears to be playing a role in the prominence or severity of symptoms.[54] Neuroleptic medications, including pimozide and haloperidol as well as risperidone, drugs useful in the management of delusions of parasitosis, may play a therapeutic role in some clinical situations. Although not indicated for the primary treatment of organic pruritus, these agents may be useful when patients exhibit delusional ideation in conjunction with their disease process. Treatment improves the symptoms of psychosis and diminishes the mental fixation on pruritus[54].

Sedative medications such as diazepam have been shown to be ineffective in reducing experimental itch, although mechanically induced pruritus was eliminated with this agent[33,55]. Sedatives in conjunction with other antipruritic agents appear to offer greater relief if the patient is experiencing anxiety as part of the chronic pruritic reaction. In addition to the sedative effects of antihistamines such as hydroxyzine, doxepin, and diphenhydramine, specific anxiolytic agents, including buspirone, clomipramine, and benzodiazepines such as alprazolam, can be used when anxiety appears to be playing a role in magnifying the symptoms of pruritus. Long-term treatment with benzodiazapines should be avoided as there is a risk of habituation[54].

The opioid and serotonin antagonists, as reviewed earlier, have been found to be very effective in selected types of chronic pruritus. The opioid antagonists have been evaluated most extensively in the clinical setting of pruritus of cholestasis where they show significant benefit in symptom relief[17,56]. Naloxone must be administered parenterally. Naltrexone and nalmephene are orally active agents that may be useful as longer-term therapeutic agents for chronic pruritus. Some studies have clearly demonstrated benefit for cholestatic pruritus[35], though randomized, blinded, and placebo-controlled studies in uraemic pruritus seem to indicate no significant improvement in symptoms[57]. Serotonin (5-HT) antagonists are few in number and less well evaluated in pruritus. However, the 5-HT$_3$ receptor antagonist ondestranon shows promise as the first in a new class of agents to alleviate the symptoms of generalized pruritus in patients with cholestasis and chronic renal failure[20,21], although recent studies have refuted its efficacy in uraemic pruritus[22].

Gabapentin and the newer analogue pregabalin are anticonvulsant drugs with analgesic activity but with no appreciable anti-inflammatory activities. These novel agents have recently been shown to bind to the alpha 2-delta-1 subunit of the voltage-dependent calcium channel and mediate analgesic properties in the brain and spinal cord levels. Both agents have activity in neuropathic pain, and recent clinical evidence indicates effectiveness in pruritus due to uraemic states as well as other types of primary and secondary pruritus, including pruritus following burn injury.

Sequestrants such as cholestyramine or charcoal administered orally or heparin administered by intravenous infusion have been reported to be helpful in the treatment of obstructive biliary pruritus[30]. Cholestyramine was also observed to improve itching in polycythaemia vera and uraemia. These treatments may be useful as adjuvant or alternative therapies during the management of chronic pruritus due to these diseases.

A variety of miscellaneous therapies are listed in Table 10.6.5, which also includes additional disease-specific medications reported to benefit chronic pruritus and other treatment modalities such as phototherapy, transcutaneous nerve stimulation, plasma exchange, and acupuncture. Pertinent references reporting the benefit of specific therapies are cited for each modality. For example, several medications and physical modalities have been found to relieve the pruritus of chronic renal failure. Despite our lack of knowledge regarding specific pruritogenic factors and their expression and activity in chronic renal failure, UVB phototherapy often provides symptomatic relief. UVB phototherapy is well tolerated, has few side effects, and can be administered at many dermatological practices or regional clinical phototherapy centres. A combination of a arrow band UVB and crotamiton has been reported to alleviate pruritus of metastatic breast carcinoma to the skin[58]. Erythropoietin and thalidomide have been reported to improve uraemic pruritus. Interferon-α and rifampicin have been found to be effective for polycythemia vera and malignant cholestatic pruritus, respectively[59,60]. Parenteral lignocaine is typically reserved for severe recalcitrant episodes of pruritus in uraemic patients unresponsive to other measures.

The multitude and variety of medications and sundry other therapeutic modalities reviewed in this chapter attest to the magnitude, severity, and chronicity of pruritus. All these drugs and therapies have been successful, to some extent, in ameliorating or abolishing this troublesome symptom. In managing the symptom of pruritus as well as the disease, it behoves the physician to make the best possible assessment of the specific physical and emotional factors that may be contributing to the intensity and character of a patient's problem of itch. With reassurance, flexibility, creativity, persistence, and a demonstrated concern by the physician, most patients will find relief and comfort.

Sweating

Anatomy and physiology

Sweating is a physiological sudomotor response of skin that has pathological counterparts. Abnormalities of sweating can be classified in terms of quantitative or qualitative dysfunction. From the perspective of palliative care, the most troublesome sudomotor symptoms relate to inappropriate or excessive sweating that occurs as part of malignant disease or its treatment. To understand the aetiological factors contributing to abnormal sweating and its palliative management, the anatomy and physiology of the peripheral and central thermoregulatory systems of the human are presented and reviewed.

Sweating or perspiration is a unique function of the skin of humans and apes that allows evaporative heat loss and regulation of body temperature in a hot environment or during physical exertion. Other mammals must pant, seek a cooler location, rest, or splash the skin with water to lower body temperature thermally. The crucial function and efficiency of sweat production is witnessed in individuals with the inherited disorder anhidrotic ectodermal hypoplasia who are unable to rely on evaporative heat loss through sweating. Physical inactivity, a cool ambient environment, or wetting the clothing or skin with water substitutes for sweating in order to achieve thermoregulation. Another group of persons particularly susceptible to the adverse consequences of thermal stress are young infants and the sedentary elderly who fail to sweat sufficiently and are also more likely to develop and succumb to hyperthermia.

Temperature regulation

Sweating is an important component of the elaborate thermoregulatory system of humans that is shown diagrammatically in Fig. 10.6.10[61]. The hypothalamus integrates inputs from central and peripheral thermoreceptors with the efferent response mechanisms, particularly sweating. The two types of thermosensitive neurons, warm-sensitive and cold-sensitive, are located in the preoptic and anterior hypothalamus (POAH). Warm-sensitive neurons respond to a rise in peripheral body temperature and are more abundant than cold-sensitive neurons that are activated by a decrease in peripheral temperature.

Body temperature is sensed at several crucial sites within the body, including specific thermoreceptors in the skin, spinal cord, and brainstem as well as thermal responses from the abdominal viscera. The POAH integrates thermal information from these sites and others in the body. Body temperature appears to be regulated to match a set-point. An abnormal upward shift of the set-point is believed to be the mechanism for production of fever. Additional control of the central thermoregulatory centre is mediated at several other sites in the brain with projections to the POAH, including the midbrain reticular formation, the raphe nucleus, the amygdala, the hippocampal formation, the sulcal prefrontal cortex, and the medial forebrain bundle. Thermoregulatory control of the hypothalamus can be modified by higher brain activity such as sleep, mental stress, and emotional excitement.

Hypercapnia, plasma osmolality, intravascular volume changes, and dehydration also alter the body temperature and set-point. Chemical mediators, including neurotransmitters such as catecholamines and acetylcholine and the eicosanoid prostaglandin E, play central roles in the control of normal thermoregulation as well as in the expression of fever. Hypothalamic peptides, including thyrotropin-releasing hormone, bombesin, neurotensin, ACTH, and vasopressin, are also important in the modulation of central thermoregulation.

Autonomic control

The afferent input and efferent responses of thermoregulation are complex but are intimately coupled and controlled by both peripheral and central mechanisms (Fig. 10.6.11). The main thermoregulatory response affecting vasomotion and sweating is mediated through the autonomic system. The cutaneous vasculature is innervated mainly by adrenergic vasoconstrictor nerve fibres. Vasodilation and constriction are coordinated with sweating responses and interact to control blood flow and dissipate or preserve body heat. Sympathetic efferent pathways descend from the hypothalamus through the brainstem to the spinal cord and the preganglionic neurons. From here the fibres exit the cord and enter the sympathetic chain. Postganglionic sympathetic axons innervate sweat glands, blood vessels, and pilomotor muscles in skin. Eccrine glands are innervated by cholinergic fibres. Sweating is produced by both thermal and mental stimulation of eccrine glands, but the distribution and inciting factors causing the sudomotor response are different. Thermal sweating results from excess temperature that is perceived by the body. A local thermal stimulus will generate a uniform sweat response over the body surface while sparing the palms and soles.

The palms and soles show a baseline sweat pattern in the waking state, and mental excitement and stress will increase the rate. This response is called mental sweating. Mental sweating is controlled by the cerebral neocortex limbic system as well as by the hypothalamus. Thermal and mental sweating have some overlap in their central control but are also coordinated independently. General body surface sweating can be affected by various mental stresses.

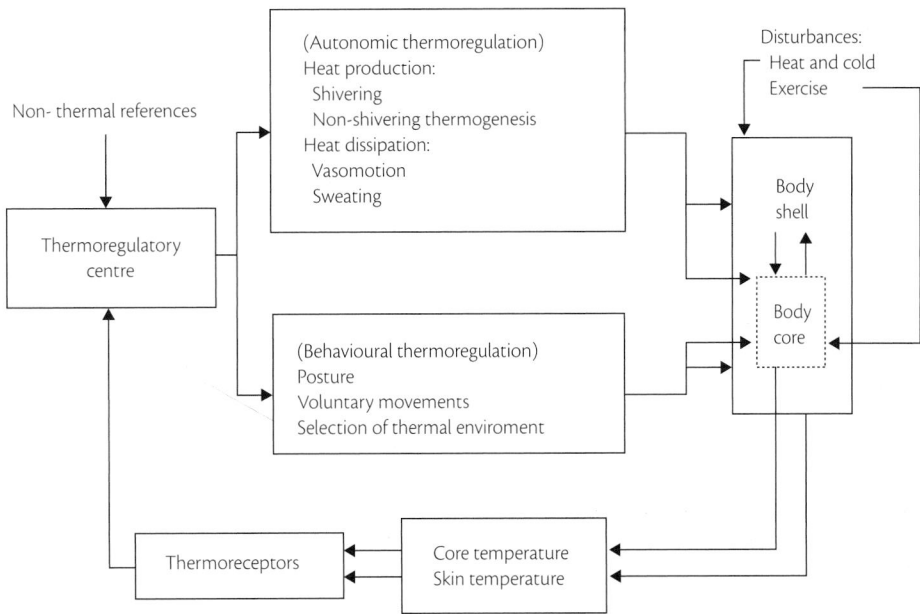

Figure 10.6.10 The human thermoregulatory system. (Reproduced with permission[61].)

Mental sweating may augment or depress the thermal response of sweating over the body surface, but always increases sweating of the palms and soles. Axillary and, in some individuals, forehead sweating have a lower threshold to stimulation and are often active when there is no thermal sweating elsewhere.

Thermal sweating normally occurs uniformly over the body. Various factors, including body position, exercise, dehydration, sweat gland blood flow, ambient humidity, gender, and age, have also been shown to exert significant effects on the distribution, rate of production, activation thresholds, and other functional aspects of sweating. These factors must be taken into consideration in determining whether sweating responses are physiological or pathological.

Hyperhidrosis

In considering the palliative aspects of sweat dysfunction, most patients are typically bothered by hyperhidrosis (excessive sweating) or the distinctive symptom of nocturnal diaphoresis (night sweats).[63] A variety of underlying disorders contribute to localized or generalized hyperhidrosis (Table 10.6.6). Hyperhidrosis can be further classified as primary or secondary. It also should be appreciated that it may be a compensatory response to anhidrosis at other body sites (Fig. 10.6.12). Therefore, the cause of hyperhidrosis should be determined if possible, and attempts should be made to alleviate underlying abnormalities that may induce pathological states of excessive or insufficient sweat production.

Clinical evaluation

Determination of sweating abnormalities can be based on the clinical history and examination, or on more comprehensive evaluations such as thermoregulatory sweat testing or specific measurements such as quantitative sudomotor axon reflex tests (QSART).[62] QSART measures the pattern of sweat response and discriminates whether abnormalities in sweat production are pre- or postganglionic. Postganglionic abnormalities demonstrate alterations in the QSART, while disturbances at the preganglionic level typically spare QSART function.

Thermoregulatory sweat testing assesses the integrity of the peripheral and central sympathetic sudomotor pathways[62]. Thermal stimulation is achieved by raising the skin temperature and the central or core body temperature. An environmentally controlled cabinet that warms the ambient air temperature to 45–50°C and also heats the skin with infrared lamps is used to raise central (oral or tympanic membrane) temperature and skin temperature to levels that stimulate sweating. Sweating on the skin surface is visualized with a special indicator powder containing iodinated corn starch, iodine solution, or alizarin-red-containing corn starch and sodium carbonate. Reduced or absent sweating can be delineated clearly (Fig. 10.6.12), and the distribution and extent of sweat loss is useful in further characterizing potential pathological abnormalities of the pre- or postganglionic pathways (Fig. 10.6.13) or the end organ, that is, the sweat glands (Fig. 10.6.14).

Disruption of the sympathetic chain or white rami produces localized loss of sweating as can be seen with a Pancoast tumour involving the apical lung (Fig. 10.6.13). In contrast, irritation of the sympathetic chain by encroachment of a neoplasm such as bronchial carcinoma, mesothelioma, or osteoma may also produce ipsilateral hyperhidrosis[64]. Stroke rarely causes contralateral hyperhidrosis if large infarcts affect both the superficial and deep cerebral structures. Basilar artery strokes have been known to produce focal symmetrical sweating.

Generalized or regionalized hyperhidrosis

Generalized hyperhidrosis occurs with various systemic diseases, including endocrine disorders, menopause, infections, lymphomas and other cancers, carcinoid syndrome, and drug withdrawal[65]. Endocrine disturbances observed to cause excessive sweating include acromegaly, diabetes mellitus, diabetes insipidus, hypopituitarism, hypoglycaemia thyrotoxicosis, and phaeochromocytoma.

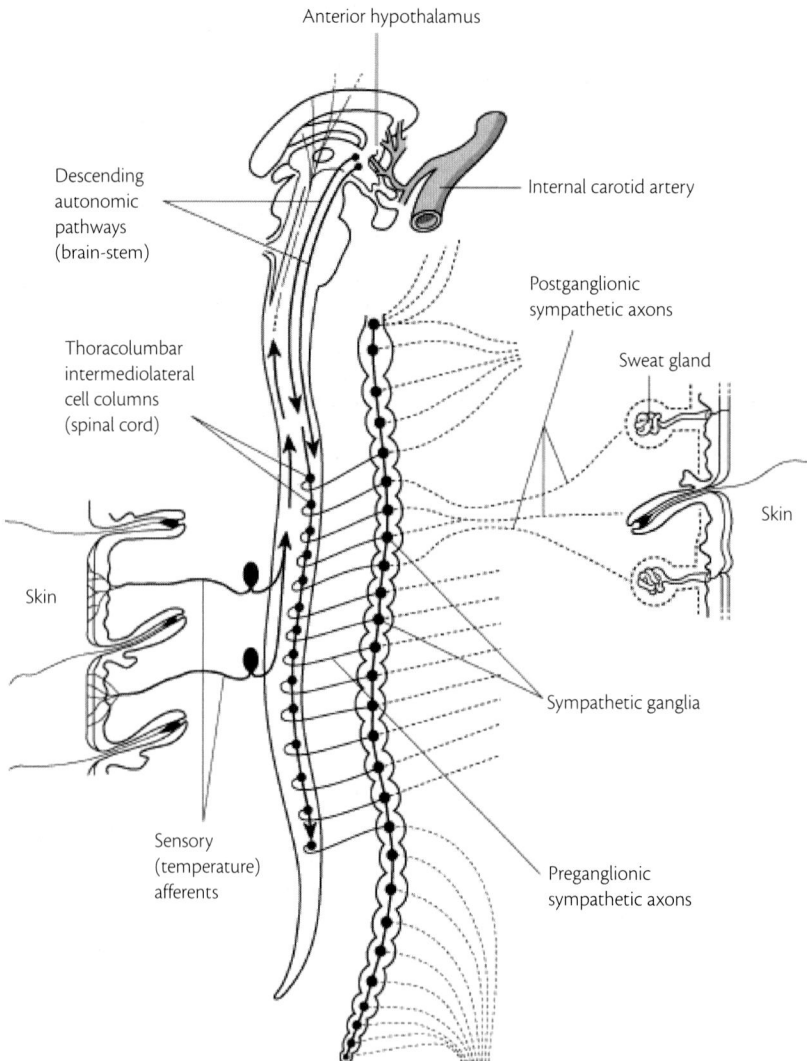

Figure 10.6.11 Autonomic thermoregulatory sweat pathways: afferent and efferent limbs integrating temperature sensation and sudomotor response. (Reproduced with permission[62].)

Drugs reported to cause hyperhidrosis include opioid analgesics such as morphine, diamorphine, methadone, butorphanol, and pentazocine, antidepressants such as fluoxetine, acyclovir, and naproxen. If patients experience significant symptoms of sweat excess as a result of a particular medication, switching to an alternative drug may provide significant relief. Although the mechanism producing hyperhidrosis is not clearly understood and may be different for each of these causes, a downward shift of the set-point of the POAH could stimulate inappropriate sweating.

The patient may confuse excessive regionalized sweating with generalized hyperhidrosis. Compensatory hyperhidrosis may occur within normal sweat-producing areas of the skin in response to anhidrosis that involves other areas of the skin. The patient may not notice the loss of sweating, but, rather, experiences discomfort from the exaggerated sweating response. In this case, detection of the underlying cause of the loss of sweating would guide further treatment and appropriate management for symptomatic hyperhidrosis.

Treatment of sweating

The management of hyperhidrosis is based on identifying the primary cause underlying the abnormal sweat response as well as eliminating any potential aggravating factors that may further augment sweating. Primary hyperhidrosis will not be considered in the discussion of the palliative management of sweating. A variety of therapies offer benefit in treatment of primary hyperhidrosis but are not usually applicable to management of secondary hyperhidrosis[66]. For primary localized hyperhidrosis, endoscopic thoracic sympathectomy or botulinum toxin injections into the affected skin regions are the most popular therapies[67,68].

Hot flushes

Hot flushes are a prominent cause of excessive sweating in patients with cancer. A detailed discussion of the proposed pathophysiological mechanisms for this problem is outside the scope of this chapter but can be found elsewhere[69–71]. Hot flushes classically occur in

Table 10.6.6 Hyperhidrosis.

Localized hyperhidrosis	Generalized hyperhidrosis
Essential (primary)	Systemic illness
Neurogenic	Phaeochromocytoma
Spinal cord disease	Thyrotoxicosis
Peripheral neuropathy	Hypopituitarism
Cerebrovascular disease (stroke)	Diabetes insipidus
Intrathoracic neoplasms or masses	Diabetes mellitus
Unilateral circumscribed	Acromegaly
Cold-induced	Hypoglycaemia
Associated with cutaneous lesions	Carcinoid syndrome
Gustatory	Menopause
	Tuberculosis
	Lymphoma
	Endocarditis
	Angina
	Malignancy
	Nocturnal
	Episodic
	Medication-induced

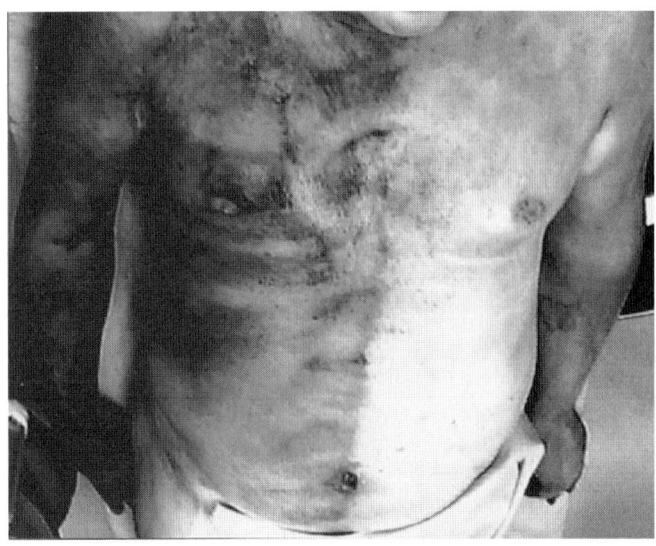

Figure 10.6.12 Compensatory hyperhidrosis resulting from hemitruncal anhidrosis measured by thermoregulatory sweat testing (sweat indicated by dark areas). (Courtesy of Dr R. Fealey, Mayo Clinic.)

menopausal women and are associated with oestrogen depletion. Breast cancer survivors are not exempt from this clinical problem; in fact, they are more at risk for several reasons. First, adjuvant chemotherapy given to premenopausal women can frequently result in premature ovarian failure with all the sequelae of oestrogen-depletion problems; second, the commonly used anti-oestrogen, tamoxifen, causes hot flushes as its most common toxicity; third, commonly used aromatase inhibitors also cause hot flushes; and fourth, general clinical practice has been to deny hormone replacement therapy to these women because of theoretical concerns that oestrogen replacement might harm them.

Given that breast cancer is a commonly diagnosed cancer whose incidence is rising, particularly among younger women, and that hot flushes are a very common clinical problem, what therapeutic options are available? Potential options can be grouped into two classes: hormonal and non-hormonal. Non-hormonal options will be considered first.

Non-hormonal treatment options for women

Twenty years ago, the most common non-hormonal treatment option for treating hot flushes was Bellergal. This is a mixture of phenobarbital and belladonna alkaloids. Review of studies, however, show minimal suggestions of efficacy for hot flushes[72].

Clonidine is the next non-hormonal agent that was studied and utilized for hot flushes. Well-conducted, placebo-controlled trials demonstrated that it reduces hot flushes more than does a placebo[73,74]. However, it only reduces hot flushes by about one hot flush per person per day, on average. It is also associated with toxicities such as dry mouth, constipation, and sleeping troubles. Thus, it is not very useful for most women.

In the 1990s data became available looking at the newer antidepressants as agents to decrease hot flushes. A placebo-controlled clinical trial looked at venlafaxine in a dose-finding study[75]. This demonstrated that venlafaxine, at a target dose of 75 mg per day (with an initiation dose of 37.5 mg per day), decreased hot flushes by about 60 per cent from baseline, compared to a 27 per cent reduction with a placebo arm. This agent does cause some toxicities, with nausea and vomiting being the biggest problem. In 5–10 per cent of patients, this is severe enough to prevent continuation

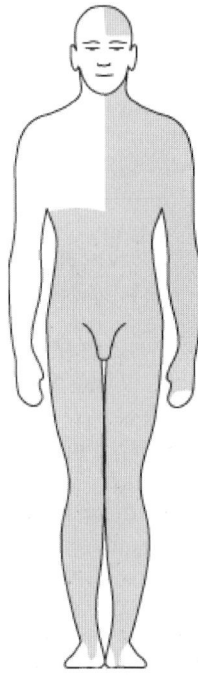

Figure 10.6.13 Anhidrosis (light-coloured areas) of the right head, upper trunk, and upper extremity due to a right-sided Pancoast tumour. Distal sweat loss is due to peripheral neuropathy. (Reproduced with permission[62].)

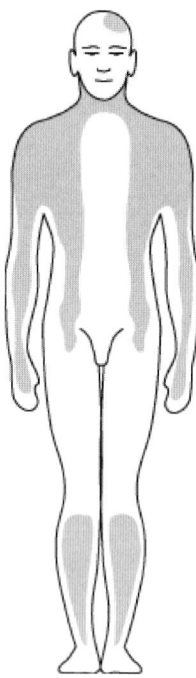

Figure 10.6.14 Loss of sweating in the distribution of the truncal radiation port. Anhidrosis is caused by damage to the dermis and loss of sweat gland function. (Reproduced with permission[62].)

of medication. In the rest of them, however, the nausea generally abates with continuation of the drug for longer than 1 week.

Paroxetine has also been studied and appears to decrease hot flushes to a similar degree as what is seen with venlafaxine[76–78]. However, this drug should not be used with tamoxifen as it interferes with an enzyme (CYP 2D6), which is utilized to convert tamoxifen to its active metabolite, endoxifen[79].

Fluoxetine and sertraline appear to also reduce hot flashes, but to a less substantial degree than is seen with venlafaxine and paroxetine[80–82]. There are other antidepressants, such as citalopram, which are currently being investigated[83,81].

Subsequent to information regarding antidepressant use, data became available demonstrating that gabapentin also reduces hot flushes. At a target dose of 900 mg per day, it reduces hot flashes by about 50 per cent[84,85]. A recent trial looked at target doses of 2400 mg per day. In a single trial, with small patient numbers, this appeared to be as effective as was Premarin®[86]. This needs to be confirmed in further trials.

There are other non-hormonal agents, such as black cohosh and vitamin E, that do not appear to be very efficacious[87,88].

Hormonal agents

Soy products have been examined in multiple placebo-controlled clinical trials. The bulk of the information available suggests that soy is not very helpful for reducing hot flushes[89]. There have been some studies that have reported positive results and eventually further investigation might define some soy product that does help hot flushes. Nonetheless, until this has been done, soy phyto-oestrogens should not be recommended as therapy for hot flushes.

Progestational agents, however, do clearly decrease hot flushes. A placebo-controlled trial examined megestrol acetate vs. a placebo[90]. This demonstrated approximately an 85 per cent reduction of hot

flushes, with low doses of megestrol acetate, results similar to what would be expected with oestrogen therapy. A subsequent clinical trial compared oral megestrol acetate to intramuscular medroxy-progesterone acetate (MPA)[91]. Both of these agents appeared similarly advantageous, with a suggestion that the MPA was slightly better. A subsequent trial compared a single intramuscular dose of MPA to continuous oral venlafaxine. MPA did reduce hot flushes more substantially then did venlafaxine[92].

There are hypothetical concerns with regards to the use of low doses of progestational agents in women with breast cancer[92]. There are some data to suggest that it might promote breast cancer growth, while there are other data suggesting that it might actually have antitumor activity. Many oncologists are currently concerned about giving this therapy to women with a history of breast cancer, especially hormonal receptor positive breast cancer.

Oestrogen also decreases hot flushes by approximately 80–90 per cent[93]. New concerns were raised with combined hormonal therapy (oestrogen plus progesterone) in a relatively recent publication of the Women's Health Initiative[94]. This therapy increased the risk of breast cancer and increased the risk of cardiovascular trouble, including thromboembolic problems. This has raised concern for the use of this therapy, both in women with breast cancer and women without a history of breast cancer. A subsequent Women's Health Initiative trial reported on the use of oestrogen therapy alone (without a progestational agent) in women who had had a hysterectomy[95]. In this situation there was no increased risk of breast cancer, with a suggestion that there was actually a decreased incidence of breast cancer in women receiving Premarin®, vs. the placebo group. There are mixed reports with regards to the safety of oestrogen use in women with a history of breast cancer[96–100]. All-in-all, oestrogen is frequently not utilized in patients with a history of breast cancer because of the concerns noted above.

Another group of cancer patients who suffer from hot flushes are men who have had androgen ablation therapy for prostate cancer. Hot flushes affect approximately 75 per cent of such men and can be a very substantial problem[70,71]. A placebo-controlled trial demonstrated that clonidine does not appear to decrease hot flushes in men[101]. However, low-dose megestrol acetate alleviates hot flushes in men as well as it does in women[90]. It should be noted that megestrol acetate has occasionally been associated with rising PSA concentrations, however[102,103]. Lastly, venlafaxine, paroxetine, and gabapentin all appear to help hot flushes in men as well as they do in women[104–107], and so it is reasonable to try one of these agents first, saving progestational agents for patients who do not get relief from venlafaxine. A randomized, placebo-controlled, dose-finding, double-blinded clinical trial evaluating gabapentin for treating hot flushes in men has recently completed accrual of 220 patients. Results from this trial reveal that gabapentin appears to decrease hot flashes in men to a similar degree to what it does in women[108].

Treatment of other causes of sweating

Another cause of sweating is related to fever. Sweating is a physiological response to fever, and documented fevers that elicit diaphoresis either during or following the episodes need to be investigated and treated appropriately. Sweating can be a prominent clinical problem in patients with advanced cancer who have tumour fever. Antipyretic agents such as aspirin and paracetamol (acetaminophen) appear to reduce fever by resetting the POAH set-point, and these agents improve symptoms, including sweating, that are associated with fever. At times, however, patients with tumour fever are relatively asymptomatic while they are febrile, but they may perspire and chill during defervescence. A simple solution to this problem is to discontinue antipyretic medications. Asymptomatic fever may continue but symptomatic periods of defervescence decrease. Another method of treating tumour fever is to use non-aspirin-containing non-steroidal anti-inflammatory drugs (NSAIDs) such as naproxen. These drugs can be remarkably successful in alleviating tumour fevers and associated sweating[109–111]. While the efficacy may cease after a period of weeks or months, switching to another NSAID may again induce defervescence[109].

Sweating may be a chronic and prominent concern for many patients who do not have any malignancy or infectious aetiology. Even in patients with malignancy, where antipyretic therapies have either been instituted or discontinued to attempt symptom relief, diaphoresis may continue to be a major symptom. Various medications, including H_2-antagonists, have been tried empirically in attempts to provide relief. Although a specific mechanism of action is not well defined and documented clinical trials are lacking, clinical experience has indicated marked benefit from cimetidine (400–800 mg twice daily) in both idiopathic and malignancy-associated sweating. Whether other newer H_2-blockers exhibit a better or worse clinical response is not known.

Thalidomide is another medication that may exert significant benefit in reducing sweating as well as improving other symptoms and syndromes of advanced cancer, such as cachexia, nausea, and insomnia[112]. Both low-dose (100 mg orally every night) and high-dose (300 mg twice daily) thalidomide have been reported to improve sweating in the majority of affected patients.[113,114] Thalidomide has been shown to reduce tumour necrosis factor-α production as well as modulate other interleukins and cytokines. Besides peripheral neuropathy, severe constipation, headache, cutaneous eruptions-skin sloughing, and oedema have been reported. However, the relative safety of the drug in advanced cancer favours judicious use. It is hoped that improved therapies will follow as the peripheral and central neural controls of sweating become better understood.

References

1. Winkelmann, R.K. and Muller, S.A. (1964). Pruritus. *Annual Reviews of Medicine*, **15**, 53–64.
2. Bernhard, J.D. (1994). *Itch: Mechanisms and management of pruritus.* McGraw-Hill, New York.
3. Winkelmann, R.K. (1961). Dermatological clinics. 1. Comments on pruritus related to systemic disease. *Mayo Clinic Proceedings*, **36**, 187–96.
4. Gilchrest, B.A. (1982). Pruritus: Pathogenesis, therapy, and significance in systemic disease states. *Archives of Internal Medicine*, **142**, 101–5.
5. Denman, S.T. (1986). A review of pruritus. *Journal of the American Academy of Dermatology*, **14**, 375–92.
6. Yosipovitch, G. *et al.* (2001). A questionnaire for the assessment of pruritus: Validation in uremic patients. *Acta Dermatologica Venereologia*, **81**, 108–11.
7. Paus, R. *et al.* (2006). Frontiers in pruritus research: Scratching the brain for more effective itch therapy. *Journal of Clinical Investigation*, **116**, 1174–86.
8. Schmelz, M. *et al.* (1997). Specific C-receptors for itch in human skin. *Journal of Neuroscience*, **17**, 8003–8.
9. Andrew, D. and Craig, A.D. (2001). Spinothalamic lamina I neurons selectively sensitive to histamine: A central neural pathway for itch. *Nature Neuroscience*, **4**, 72–7.
10. Wallengren, J. (1993). The pathophysiology of itch. *European Journal of Dermatology*, **3**, 643–7.
11. Hägermark, O. (1992). Peripheral and central mediators of itch. *Skin Pharmacology*, **5**, 1–8.
12. Bernstein, J.E. (1992). Capsaicin and substance P. *Clinics in Dermatology*, **9**, 497–503.
13. Winkelmann, R.K. (1988). Cutaneous sensory nerves. *Seminars in Dermatology*, **7**, 236–68.
14. Handwerker, H.O., Forster, C., and Kirchhoff, C. (1991). Discharge patterns of human C-fibres induced by itching and burning stimuli. *Journal of Neurophysiology*, **66**, 307–15.
15. Head, H. (1905). The afferent nervous system from a new aspect. *Brain*, **28**, 99–115.
16. Lowitt, M.H. and Bernhard, J.D. (1992). Pruritus. *Seminars in Neurology*, **12**, 374–84.
17. Bergasa, N.V. *et al.* (1995). Effects of naloxone infusions in patients with the pruritus of cholestasis. *Annals of Internal Medicine*, **123**, 161–7.
18. Khandelwal, M. and Malet, P.F. (1994). Pruritus associated with cholestasis: A review of pathogenesis and management. *Digestive Diseases Sciences*, **39**, 1–7.
19. Diehn, F. and Tefferi, A. (2001). Pruritus in polycythaemia vera: Prevalence, laboratory correlates and management. *British Journal of Haematology*, **115**, 619–21.
20. Schworer, H. and Ramadori, G. (1993). Treatment of pruritus: A new indication for serotonin type 3 receptor antagonists. *Clinical Investigation*, **71**, 659–62.
21. Raderer, M., Muller, C., and Scheithauer, W. (1994). Ondansetron for pruritus due to cholestasis. *New England Journal of Medicine*, **330**, 1540.
22. Ashmore, S.D. *et al.* (2000). Ondansetron therapy for uremic pruritus in hemodialysis patients. *American Journal of Kidney Disease*, **35**, 827–31.
23. Melzack, R. and Wall, P.D. (1965). Pain mechanisms: A new theory. *Science*, **150**, 971–9.
24. Carlsson, C.-A. *et al.* (1975). Electrical transcutaneous nerve stimulation for relief of itch. *Experientia*, **31**, 191.
25. Monk, B.E. (1993). Transcutaneous electronic nerve stimulation in the treatment of generalized pruritus. *Clinical and Experimental Dermatology*, **18**, 67–8.
26. Paul, R., Paul, R., and Jansen, C.T. (1987). Itch and malignancy prognosis in generalized pruritus: A 6-year-follow-up of 125 patients. *Journal of the American Academy of Dermatology*, **16**, 1179–82.
27. Kantor, G.R. and Lookingbill, D.P. (1983). Generalized pruritus and systemic disease. *Journal of the American Academy of Dermatology*, **9**, 375–8.
28. Doyle, J.A. *et al.* (1979). Prurigo nodularis: A reappraisal of the clinical and histological features. *Journal of Cutaneous Pathology*, **6**, 392–403.
29. Arndt, K.A., Bowers, K.E., and Chuttani, A.R. (1995). *Manual of Dermatological Therapeutics: With Essentials of Diagnosis*, 5th edtion, pp. 145–8, 317–22. Little Brown, New York.
30. Fransway, A.F. and Winkelmann, R.K. (1988). Treatment of pruritus. *Seminars in Dermatology*, **7**, 310–25.
31. Devers, A. and Galer, B.S. (2000). Topical lidocaine patch relieves a variety of neuropathic pain conditions: An open-label study. *Clinical Journal of Pain*, **16**, 205–8.
32. Winkelmann, R.K. (1982). Pharmacologic control of pruritus. *Medical Clinics of North America*, **66**, 1119–33.
33. Lorette, G. and Vaillant, L. (1990). Pruritus: Current concepts in pathogenesis and treatment. *Drugs*, **39**, 218–23.
34. Zylicz, Z., Smits, C., and Krajnik, M. (1998). Paroxetine for pruritus in advanced cancer. *Journal of Pain and Symptom Management*, **16**, 121–4.

35. Jones, E.A. and Bergasa, N.V. (2000). Evolving concepts of the pathogenesis and treatment of the pruritus of cholestasis. *Cancer Journal of Gastroenterology*, **14**, 33–40.

36. Ghent, C.N. and Carruthers, S.G. (1988). Treatment of pruritus in primary biliary cirrhosis with rifampin. *Gastroenterology*, **94**, 488–93.

37. Gregorio, G.V. *et al.* (1993). Effect of rifampicin in the treatment of pruritus in hepatic cholestasis. *Archives of Disease in Childhood*, **69**, 141–3.

38. Whitington, P.F. and Whitington, G.L. (1988). Partial external diversion of bile for the treatment of intractable pruritus associated with intrahepatic cholestasis. *Gastroenterology*, **95**, 130–6.

39. Marchi, S. *et al.* (1992). Relief of pruritus and decreases in plasma histamine concentrations during erythropoietin therapy in patients with uremia. *New England Journal of Medicine*, **326**, 969–74.

40. Hampers, C. *et al.* (1986). Disappearance of uraemic itching after subtotal parathyroidectomy. *New England Journal of Medicine*, **279**, 695–700.

41. Gilchrist, B. *et al.* (1977). Relief of uraemic pruritus with ultraviolet phototherapy. *New England Journal of Medicine*, **297**, 136–8.

42. Finelli, C. *et al.* (1993). Relief of intractable pruritus in polycythemia vera with recombinant interferon alfa. *American Journal of Hematology*, **43**, 316–18.

43. Riccardi, V.M. (1993). A controlled multiphase trial of ketotifen to minimize neurofibroma-associated pain and itching. *Archives of Dermatology*, **129**, 577–81.

44. Soter, N.A., Austin, K.F., and Wasserman, S.I. (1979). Oral disodium cromoglycate in the treatment of systemic mastocytosis. *New England Journal of Medicine*, **301**, 465–9.

45. Leven, A. *et al.* (1979). Sodium cromoglycate and Hodgkin's pruritus. *British Medical Journal*, **2**, 896.

46. Winkelmann, R.K. *et al.* (1984). Thalidomide treatment of prurigo nodularis. *Acta Dermatologica Venereologica*, **64**, 412–17.

47. Silva, S.R.B. *et al.* (1994). Thalidomide for the treatment of uraemic pruritus: A crossover randomized double-blind trial. *Nephrology*, **67**, 270–3.

48. Levy, M. and Catalano, R. (1985). Control of common physical symptoms other than pain in patients with terminal disease. *Seminars in Oncology*, **12**, 411–30.

49. Tapia, L. *et al.* (1977). Pruritus in dialysis patients treated with parenteral lidocaine. *New England Journal of Medicine*, **296**, 261–2.

50. Borgeat, A., Wilder-Smith, O.H.G., and Mentha, G. (1993). Subhypnotic doses of propofol relieve pruritus associated with liver disease. *Gastroenterology*, **104**, 244–7.

51. Borgeat, A. *et al.* (1994). Intractable cholestatic pruritus after liver transplantation—Management with propofol. *Transplantation*, **58**, 727–30.

52. Borgeat, A. *et al.* (1992). Subhypnotic doses of propofol relieve pruritus induced by epidural and intrathecal morphine. *Anesthiology*, **76**, 510–12.

53. Willner, C. and Low, P.A. (1993). Pharmacologic approaches to neuropathic pain. In *Peripheral Neuropathy*, 3rd edition. (ed. P. Dyck *et al.*), pp. 1700–20. Saunders, Philadelphia, PA.

54. Fried, R.G. (1994). Evaluation and treatment of 'psychogenic' pruritus and self-excoriation. *Journal of the American Academy of Dermatology*, **30**, 993–9.

55. Hagermark, K.O. (1973). Influence of antihistamines, sedatives and aspirin on experimental itch. *Acta Dermatologica Venereologia*, **53**, 363–8.

56. Jones, E.A. and Bergasa, N.V. (1990). The pruritus of cholestasis: From bile acids to opiate agonists. *Hepatology*, **11**, 884–7.

57. Pauli-Magnus, C. *et al.* (2000). Naltrexone does not relieve uremic pruritus: Results of a randomized, double-blind, placebo-controlled crossover study. *Journal of the American Society of Nephrology*, **11**, 514–19.

58. Holme, S.A. and Mills, C.M. (2001). Crotamiton and narrow-band UVB phototherapy: Novel approaches to alleviate pruritus of breast carcinoma skin infiltration. *Journal of Pain and Symptom Management*, **22**, 803–5.

59. Lengfelder, E., Berger, U., and Hehlmann, R. (2000). Interferon alpha in the treatment of polycythemia vera. *Annals of Hematology*, **79**, 103–9.

60. Price, T.J., Patterson, W.K., and Olver, I.N. (1998). Rifampicin as treatment for pruritus in malignant cholestasis. *Support Care Cancer*, **6**, 533–5.

61. Ogawa, T. and Low, P. (1992). Autonomic regulation of temperature and sweating. In *Clinical Autonomic Disorders: Evaluation and Management* (ed. P.A. Low), pp. 79–91. Little Brown, Boston, MA.

62. Fealey, R.D. (1992). The thermoregulatory sweat test. In *Clinical Autonomic Disorders: Evaluation and Management* (ed. P.A. Low), pp. 217–29. Little Brown, Boston, MA.

63. Lea, M.J. and Aber, R.C. (1985). Descriptive epidemiology of night sweats upon admission to a university hospital. *Southern Medical Journal*, **78**, 1065–7.

64. Walsh, J.C., Low, P.A., and Allsop, J.L. (1976). Localized sympathetic overactivity: An uncommon complication of lung cancer. *Journal of Neurology, Neurosurgery and Psychiatry*, **39**, 93–5.

65. Freeman, R., Waldorf, H.A., and Dover, J.S. (1992). Autonomic neurodermatology (Part II): Disorders of sweating and flushing. *Seminars in Neurology*, **12**, 394–407.

66. White, J.W. (1986). Treatment of primary hyperhidrosis. *Mayo Clinic Proceedings*, **61**, 951–6.

67. Vallieres, E. (2001). Endoscopic upper thoracic sympathectomy. *Neurosurgery Clinics of North America*, **12**, 321–7.

68. Heckmann, M., Ceballos-Baumann, A.O., and Plewig, G. (2001). Botulinum toxin A for axillary hyperhidrosis (excessive sweating). *New England Journal of Medicine*, **344**, 488–93.

69. Casper, R.F. and Yen S.S. (1985). Neuroendocrinology of menopausal flushes: An hypothesis of flush mechanism. *Clin Endocrinol (Oxf)*, **22**(3), 293–312.

70. Charig, C.R. and Rundle, J.S. (1989). Flushing. Long-term side effect of orchiectomy in treatment of prostatic carcinoma. *Urology*, **33**(3), 175–8.

71. Quella, S., Loprinzi, C.L. *et al.* (1994). A qualitative approach to defining "hot flashes" in men. *Urology and Nursing*, **14**(4), 155–8.

72. Bergmans, M.G., Merkus, J.M. *et al.* (1987). Effect of Bellergal Retard on climacteric complaints: A double-blind, placebo-controlled study. *Maturitas*, **9**(3), 227–34.

73. Goldberg, R.M., Loprinzi, C.L. *et al.* (1994). Transdermal clonidine for ameliorating tamoxifen-induced hot flashes. *Journal of Clinical Oncology*, **12**(1), 155–8.

74. Pandya, K.J., Raubertas, R.F. *et al.* (2000). Oral clonidine in postmenopausal patients with breast cancer experiencing tamoxifen-induced hot flashes: A University of Rochester Cancer Center Community Clinical Oncology Program study. *Annals of Internal Medicine*, **132**(10), 788–93.

75. Loprinzi, C.L., Kugler, J.W. *et al.* (2000). Venlafaxine in management of hot flashes in survivors of breast cancer: A randomised controlled trial. *Lancet*, **356**(9247), 2059–63.

76. Stearns, V., Isaacs, C. *et al.* (2000). A pilot trial assessing the efficacy of paroxetine hydrochloride (Paxil) in controlling hot flashes in breast cancer survivors. *Annals of Oncology*, **11**(1), 17–22.

77. Stearns, V., Beebe, K.L. *et al.* (2003). Paroxetine controlled release in the treatment of menopausal hot flashes: A randomized controlled trial. *JAMA*, **289**(21), 2827–34.

78. Stearns, V., Slack, R. *et al.* (2005). Paroxetine is an effective treatment for hot flashes: Results from a prospective randomized clinical trial. *Journal of Clinical Oncology*, **23**(28), 6919–30.

79. Stearns, V., Johnson, M. *et al.* (2003). Active tamoxifen metabolite plasma concentrations after coadministration of tamoxifen and the selective serotonin reuptake inhibitor paroxetine. *Journal of National Cancer Institute*, **95**, 1758–64.

80. Loprinzi, C.L., Sloan, J.A. *et al.* (2002). Phase III evaluation of fluoxetine for treatment of hot flashes. *Journal of Clinical Oncology*, **20**(6), 1578–83.

81. Suvanto-Luukkonen, E., Koivunen, R. *et al.* (2005). Citalopram and fluoxetine in the treatment of postmenopausal symptoms: A prospective, randomized, 9-month, placebo-controlled, double-blind study. *Menopause*, **12**(1), 18–26.

82. Kimmick, G. G., Lovato, J. *et al.* (2006). Randomized, double-blind, placebo-controlled, crossover study of sertraline (Zoloft) for the treatment of hot flashes in women with early stage breast cancer taking tamoxifen. *Breast Journal*, **12**(2), 114–22.

83. Loprinzi, C.L., Flynn, P.J. *et al.* (2005). Pilot evaluation of citalopram for the treatment of hot flashes in women with inadequate benefit from venlafaxine. *Journal of Palliative Medicine*, **8**(5), 924–30.

84. Guttuso, T., Jr., Kurlan, R. *et al.* (2003). Gabapentin's effects on hot flashes in postmenopausal women: A randomized controlled trial. *Obstetrics and Gynecology*, **101**(2), 337–45.

85. Pandya, K.J., Morrow, G.R. *et al.* (2005). Gabapentin for hot flashes in 420 women with breast cancer: A randomised double-blind placebo-controlled trial. *Lancet*, **366**(9488), 818–24.

86. Reddy, S.Y., Warner, H. *et al.* (2006). Gabapentin, estrogen, and placebo for treating hot flushes: A randomized controlled trial. *Obstetrics and Gynecology*, **108**(1), 41–48.

87. Barton, D.L., Loprinzi, C.L. *et al.* (1998). Prospective evaluation of vitamin E for hot flashes in breast cancer survivors. *Journal of Clinical Oncology*, **16**(2), 495–500.

88. Pockaj, B.A., Gallagher, J.G. *et al.* (2006). Phase III double-blind, randomized, placebo-controlled crossover trial of black cohosh in the management of hot flashes: NCCTG Trial N01CC1. *Journal of Clinical Oncology*, **24**(18), 2836–41.

89. Quella, S.K., Loprinzi, C.L. *et al.* (2000). Evaluation of soy phytoestrogens for the treatment of hot flashes in breast cancer survivors: A North Central Cancer Treatment Group Trial. *Journal of Clinical Oncology*, **18**(5), 1068–74.

90. Loprinzi, C.L., Michalak, J.C. *et al.* (1994). Megestrol acetate for the prevention of hot flashes. *New England Journal of Medicine*, **331**(6), 347–52.

91. Bertelli, G., Venturini, M. *et al.* (2002). Intramuscular depot medroxyprogesterone versus oral megestrol for the control of postmenopausal hot flashes in breast cancer patients: A randomized study. *Annals of Oncology*, **13**(6), 883–8.

92. Loprinzi, C.L., Levitt, R. *et al.* (2006). Phase III comparison of depomedroxyprogesterone acetate to venlafaxine for managing hot flashes: North Central Cancer Treatment Group Trial N99C7. *Journal of Clinical Oncology*, **24**(9), 1409–14.

93. Society, N.A.M. (2004). Recommendations for estrogen and progestogen use in peri- and post-menopausal women: October 2004 position statements of The North American Menopause Society. *Menopause*, **11**, 589–600.

94. Rossouw, J.E., Anderson, G.L. *et al.* (2002). Risks and benefits of estrogen plus progestin in healthy postmenopausal women: Principal results From the Women's Health Initiative randomized controlled trial. *JAMA*, **288**(3), 321–33.

95. Anderson, G.L., Limacher, M. *et al.* (2004). Effects of conjugated equine estrogen in postmenopausal women with hysterectomy: The Women's Health Initiative randomized controlled trial. *JAMA*, **291**(14), 1701–12.

96. Vassilopoulou-Sellin, R., Theriault, R. *et al.* (1997). Estrogen replacement therapy in women with prior diagnosis and treatment for breast cancer. *Gynecologic Oncology*, **65**(1), 89–93.

97. Dew, J., Eden, J. *et al.* (1998). A cohort study of hormone replacement therapy given to women previously treated for breast cancer. *Climacteric*, **1**(2), 137–42.

98. Vassilopoulou-Sellin, R., Asmar, L. *et al.* (1999). Estrogen replacement therapy after localized breast cancer: clinical outcome of 319 women followed prospectively. *Journal of Clinical Oncology*, **17**(5), 1482–7.

99. Col, N.F., Hirota, L.K. *et al.* (2001). Hormone replacement therapy after breast cancer: A systematic review and quantitative assessment of risk. *Journal of Clinical Oncology*, **19**(8), 2357–63.

100. Vassilopoulou-Sellin, R., Cohen, D.S. *et al.* (2002). Estrogen replacement therapy for menopausal women with a history of breast carcinoma: Results of a 5-year, prospective study. *Cancer*, **95**(9), 1817–26.

101. Loprinzi, C.L., Goldberg, R.M. *et al.* (1994). Transdermal clonidine for ameliorating post-orchiectomy hot flashes. *Journal of Urology*, **151**(3), 634–6.

102. Burch, P.A. and Loprinzi, C.L. (1999). Prostate-specific antigen decline after withdrawal of low-dose megestrol acetate. *Journal of Clinical Oncology*, **17**(3), 1087–8.

103. Sartor, O. and Eastham, J.A. (1999). Progressive prostate cancer associated with use of megestrol acetate administered for control of hot flashes. *Southern Medical Journal*, **92**(4), 415–6.

104. Roth, A.J. and Scher, H.I. (1998). Sertraline relieves hot flashes secondary to medical castration as treatment of advanced prostate cancer. *Psychooncology*, **7**(2), 129–32.

105. Quella, S.K., Loprinzi, C.L. *et al.* (1999). Pilot evaluation of venlafaxine for the treatment of hot flashes in men undergoing androgen ablation therapy for prostate cancer. *Journal of Urology*, **162**(1), 98–102.

106. Guttuso, T.J., Jr. (2000). Gabapentin's effects on hot flashes and hypothermia. *Neurology*, **54**(11), 2161–3.

107. Loprinzi, C.L., Barton, D.L. *et al.* (2004). Pilot evaluation of paroxetine for treating hot flashes in men. *Mayo Clinic Proceedings*, **79**(10), 1247–51.

108. Loprinzi, C.L., Khoyratty, B.S., Dueck, A. *et al.* (2007). Gabapentin for hot flashes in men: NCCTG trial N00CB. JCO 2007 ASCO Annual Meeting Proceedings Part I, **25**(18S), abstract 9005.

109. Tsavaris, N. *et al.* (1990). A randomized trial of the effect of three non-steroid anti-inflammatory agents in ameliorating cancer-induced fever. *Journal of Internal Medicine*, **228**, 451–5.

110. Chang, J.C. and Gross, H.M. (1984). Utility of naproxen in the differential diagnosis of fever of undetermined origin in patients with cancer. *American Journal of Medicine*, **76**, 597–603.

111. Chang, J.C. and Hawley, H.B. (1995). Neutropenic fever of undetermined origin (N-FUO): Why not use the naproxen test? *Cancer Investigation*, **13**, 448–50.

112. Peuckmann, V., Fisch, M., and Bruera, E. (2000). Potential novel uses of thalidomide: Focus on palliative care. *Drugs*, **60**, 273–92.

113. Deaner, P.B. (2000). The use of thalidomide in the management of severe sweating in patients with advanced malignancy: Trial report. *Palliative Medicine*, **14**, 429–31.

114. Eisen, T.G. (2000). Thalidomide in solid tumors: The London experience. *Oncology*, **14**, 17–20.

Skin problems in palliative medicine

Contents

10.7.1 Skin problems in palliative medicine

Michal Lotem

Introduction: skin in disease

Perception of reality is based on visual inputs, and part of living experience is a reflection of what meets the eye. The skin is the largest and most visible organ of the body. It can be a passive participant in states of disease or be directly involved by disease or by its treatment. The skin may manifest the disease or subtly hint at its existence. For the physician, the skin may be a diagnostic aid, though often enigmatic.

For the patient, the skin is part of what their sense of illness derives from. Cancer progression is often more of an abstract notion. In contrast, skin manifestations are easily perceived, measured, and followed. They focus attention and cause distress that often outsize their real risk, being a constant reminder of the harboured disease. The most alarming aspect of skin involvement in cancer is the threat of disfigurement. When a distressing skin symptom is addressed and treated successfully, the patient may derive relief and hope that reflect on their motivation and active partnership in their therapy.

Skin structure and function

The basic function of the skin is to serve as a barrier, separating the human body from the external environment. The skin is made up of three distinct layers.

Epidermis

The epidermis is comprised mainly of keratinocytes. Intercalated among them are the immigrant cells: melanocytes that produce melanin, Langerhans cells, which serve as antigen presenting cells, and Merkel cells, cells of neuroendocrine features, which take part in mechanoreception.

The base of the epidemis is the germinative layer of the skin, the basal layer, composed of columnar keratinocytes that undergo a process of differentiation while they move upwards towards the surface[1]. Differentiating keratinocytes produce and contain keratin filaments arranged in bundles that anchor each keratinocyte to adjacent cells and produce adherent forces that resist external traction. Cellular adhesion is lost at the surface of the skin, where keratinocytes detach as flakes and scales, which are usually unnoticeable. Pathological states of the skin associated with inflammation result in an increased turn-over of keratinocytes. A small proportion of keratinocytes are constantly dividing to replace cells that are injured and removed. The regenerative potential of the skin is harboured in colony-forming cells that reside in the hair follicles[2]. In states of damage to the skin, these cells will generate a new epidermal covering.

The epidermis is anchored to the dermis through a basement membrane complex. This highly specialized basal lamina acts as a highly selective pathway for the migration of cells and transport of macromolecules. The basal cells are anchored to the basal lamina through an array of tonofilaments and hemidesmosomes. Epidermal integrity may be disrupted by any pathology that weakens keratinocyte adhesion or damages the basal lamina. Deposition of antibodies against proteins or collagen sub types that build these structures can split the epidermis and lead to the formation of blisters. Excessive accumulation of fluids in the dermis can generate similar forces and damage skin integrity by distending the intercellular matrix, causing cells to detach from each other.

The skin appendages are specialized differentiated subunits with unique functions. They include the hair follicle, sebaceous gland,

and the eccrine and apocrine sweat glands. The hair sebaceous unit in humans mainly serves a social function. The sweat glands are part of the thermoregulatory mechanism of the body.

Dermis

The dermis is a network of collagen and elastin fibres embedded in an amorphic extracellular matrix of mucopolysaccharides, which nests below the epidermis. The fibres and extracellular matrix of the dermis are synthesized by fibroblasts, cells that are dispersed throughout the dermis. The dermis also contains the blood supply for the non-vascularized epidermis tissue. Two webs of capillary blood vessels, deep and superficial, stretch along the dermis to oxygenate and nourish both layers. Parallel lymphatic vessels remove fluids from the skin back into the intravascular compartment. Trafficking immune cells traverse the lymphatic channels to and from regional lymph nodes as part of a screening and defence process against invasion. Inflammation of the skin—dermatitis—results in oedema of the dermis, vasodilatation, and accumulation of leucocytes and lymphocytes in the dermis.

Subcutaneous fat

This adipose tissue serves as a layer of padding and thermal isolation. In states of starvation and cachexia, the subcutaneous fat is severely depleted and the skin is exposed to pressure without the protective effect of fat.

Skin manifestations of neoplastic disease

Skin involvement in the patient with advanced cancer is unique compared to other organs of the body. While the sequels of metastatic spread to internal organs would generally be replacement of normal tissue and resultant organ failure—widespread replacement of skin with a neoplasm is uncommon. Yet, even a local disruption of skin integrity can cause deterioration in the quality of life, debilitation, and even mortality. Other aspects of neoplastic disorders affecting the skin include accumulation of abnormally produced metabolites, adverse effects to treatment, and paraneoplastic syndromes.

Direct invasion of skin by tumour

Metastases to the skin are not an infrequent occurrence in cancer patients. In a retrospective series of 4020 metastatic cancer patients, 10 per cent had skin involvement[3]. The skin may be involved with the primary tumour or may be the target of systemic metastatic spread[4].

Direct invasion of the skin results from an uncontrolled local-regional disease, as in melanoma and breast cancer, where the tumour invades the superficial lymphatic vessels and infiltrates the skin (Fig. 10.7.1.1). This commonly appears as discrete nodules, but can also form a diffuse pattern similar to oedema, or an inflammatory plaque may occur, often mistaken for erysipelas until diagnosed correctly. Any aggressive tumour that arises in an adjacent organ may directly extend to the overlying skin. The pressure of a tumour mass interferes with cutaneous blood supply and may lead to ulcerating wounds that discharge foul smelling necrotic material. Local discomfort can be alleviated by daily washing and the use of hydrocolloids or absorbant dressings. 'Sister Mary Joseph nodules' have long been recognized as clinical manifestations of intra-abdominal tumours extending via the umbilical vessels into the peri-umbilical skin. Incisional metastases are also a common cause of abdominal skin involvement[3].

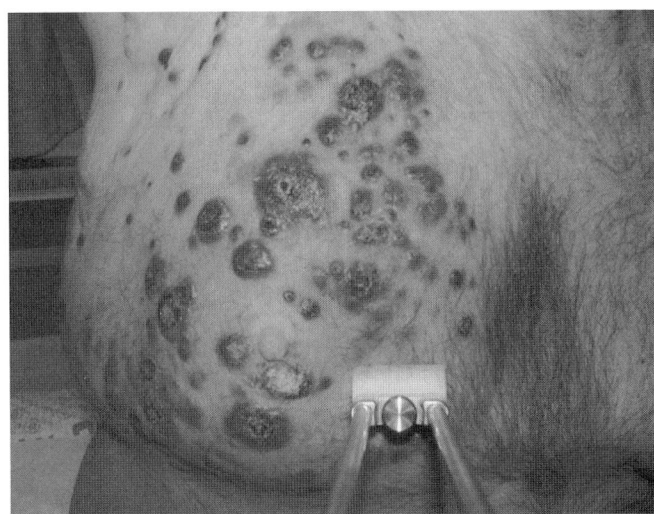

Figure 10.7.1.1 Dermal spread of melanoma nodules originating in local lymphatic invasion.

Hematogenic spread to the skin may also occur with dermotropic distant metastases. Breast cancer, lung cancer, melanoma, and colon cancer are common neoplasms that tend to involve the skin[5]. Common locations of skin metastases are the scalp, chest, and abdominal wall and less frequently to the limbs[6]. Dermal metastases are more likely to cause pain and ulceration than metastases to the subcutaneous fat. Diagnosis of skin metastases is simple in the context of a patient already diagnosed with metastatic cancer.

Discolouration

The colour of the skin is based on the reflection of chromophores, which are normal constituents of skin, that may form abnormal deposits as part of disease. Brown discolouration is intuitively attributed to melanin. Generalized melanosis, darkening of the skin because of shower of single melanoma cell dissemination, may occur with advanced melanin-producing metastatic malignant melanoma[7]. Dark urine often accompanies this condition.

Mild darkening of the skin may be seen with adrenal insufficiency, with ACTH-producing tumours such as primary tumours of the pituitary gland, or with other malignant tumours metastatic to the pituitary gland. Increased melanization of the basal layer leading to hyperpigmentation may be a side effect of chemotherapeutic agents[8]. It may occur in skin overlying a vein used for chemotherapy administered with no apparent extravasation injury; this is typical for 5-fluorouracil. Bleomycin (Fig. 10.7.1.2), busulphan, capecitabin, and hydroxyurea can cause generalized persistent hyperpigmentation[9]. Drug-induced hyperpigmentation may be limited to mucosae, nails, palms, and soles.

Brown discolouration may also result from hemosiderin sedimentation. Widespread inflammation of the skin from any cause results in post inflammatory hyperpigmentation and persistent brown tint. Yellowish orange discolouration is associated with states of hyperbilirubinemia.

Pruritus

One of the most distressing skin symptoms of advanced cancer is pruritus. In severe cases, it can lead to sleep deprivation and contribute to significant psychological distress. Cancer per se can

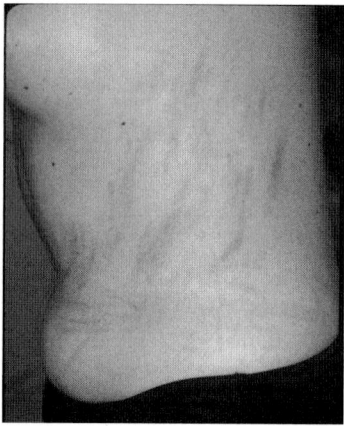

Figure 10.7.1.2 Typical linear hyperpigmentation following bleomycin administration.

cause pruritus with an unknown mechanism possibly related to serotonin. Long-term use of systemic or intrathecal opioids or intractable pain can cause pruritus[10]. However, biliary obstruction and cholestasis are the most common causes of pruritus in advanced disease. Topical therapies for immediate itch relief include 1 per cent menthol in cream base or lotion, but systemic therapy is usually required.

In the mamagement of choleststic itch, first line therapies such as antihistamines have limited effectiveness. Other types of therapies are available, which have shown some effectiveness. Anticholestatic agents have proven effectual in certain cases. Cholestyramine is effective for cholestatic pruritus but is of limited use in total biliary obstruction[11]. It chelates intestinal bile acids, thereby reducing the enterohepatic circulation of bile salts. Treatment consists of 4 g administered before meals; however, patients may find the preparation nauseating. Ursodeoxycholic acid (UDCA) exerts anticholestatic effects in various cholestatic disorders. Several potential mechanisms could explain its beneficial effects, including protection of injured cholangiocytes against the toxic effects of bile acids and stimulation of impaired hepatocellular secretion[12].

Paroxetine, a selective serotonin reuptake inhibitor, may show some effect in cancer related pruritus. Rifampicin, acting as a hepatic enzyme inducer, has been reported to relieve itching[13]. Oral opioid μ-receptor blockers (naltrexone, nalmefene) and continuous infusion with granisetron, a 5HT3 antagonist, were also reported to relieve cancer-related pruritus[14].

Topical application of the opioid antagonist naltrexone was recently reported as having the advantage of avoiding opiate withdrawal-like symptoms, and has been documented as providing relief from itching[15]. For patients with good performance status, phototherapy using ultraviolet B spectrum is a good option[16], but takes several weeks to exert its beneficial effect.

Dryness and erythroderma

General dryness, xerosis, is a common skin condition in cancer patients. Xerosis may follow chemotherapy administration, a period of decreased food intake and hypoproteinemia. Gentle flakes or larger scales generate an ichtyosiform appearance. Lack of elasticity of the drying skin creates cracking lines over the trunk and lower limbs, resulting in itching and soreness (Fig. 10.7.1.3). Daily use of emollient is effective and should be encouraged.

The term 'erythroderma' refers to general redness of the skin often associated with exfoliation. Essentially, erythroderma is an end stage of many skin diseases, including psoriasis and papulosquamous disorders. Sezary syndrome is a rare variant of cutaneous T-cell lymphoma with erythroderma featuring as a clinical hallmark. In the wider oncological context, erythroderma may accompany leukaemia and lymphoma[17] and, less commonly, solid tumours. The mechanism of this eruption is unknown. Use of emollients and systemic steroids may relieve symptoms.

Radiation-induced toxicities

Radiation effects on the skin are usually divided into acute and chronic effects. Early effects occur during the course of radiation and in the weeks thereafter, and late effects occur months and years later. The acute effects are thought to result from germinative cell failure to reproduce and replenish epidermal keratinocytes[18]. Radiotherapy destroys a section of the basal keratinocytes; non-cycling basal cells are then stimulated into a cycling phase; however, the continued destruction of basal cells from ongoing radiation treatment causes extensive injury. Damage to dermal vasculature leads to capillary disruption, extravasation, extracapillary cell damage, and inflammatory responses. Histamine and serotonin induce vasodilation and hence erythema, oedema, and a burning sensation. Hair growth is interrupted as hair follicles revert to a resting phase and new hairs are shed. Complete hair loss depends on the total dose and fractionation of the radiation. Sweat and sebaceous glands can be permanently destroyed after approximately 30 Gy in fractions of 2 Gy per day.

Acute radiodermatitis varies in severity and is dependent on radiation energy, total dose, and fractionation, the use of bolus material that reduces the skin-sparing effect of megavoltage units, and on the individual's sensitivity[19]. Addition of an electron beam boost to enhance the dose to the tumour is often associated with severe local skin reactions. Erythema and oedema are the first to occur, appearing after 1 to 2 weeks of treatment, peaking around week 3–4. Dry desquamation and moist desquamation then ensue, and in severe cases erosions and even ulcers may develop and be associated with severe pain. Areas of skin folding are at particular risk of developing severe reactions. Co-morbidities, older age, and previous sun damage to the irradiated skin are aggravating factors[20].

There is no effective prophylaxis for radiodermatitis. The basic care for radiodermatitis consists of the use of ointments, creams and lotions to moisten the skin, ease the burning sensation, restore

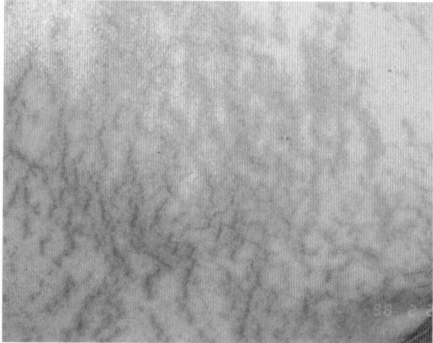

Figure 10.7.1.3 Extreme skin dryness and crackling of the trunk in a child with carcinoma of the nasopharynx treated with 5-fluorouracil.

elasticity, and prevent breakage and erosions. Practices such as daily washing with mild soaps, avoiding the use of deodorants, and electric razors may also be helpful.

It is important to note that the vehicle of the beneficial preparation may be as influential in its effectiveness as the active component in it. Gels are soothing but increase drying. Fatty ointments protect well from moisture loss, but may increase itching. Corticosteroid creams and ointments may reduce vasodilation and inflammation, but have no preventative effect and their advantage over non steroidal preparations is doubtful. Oil-in-water emulsions are a good option (Biafine®, aqueous creams)[21]. Calendula oil, sucralfate, and barrier films were tried with favourable effects.

Ulcers and erosions are treated with silver sulfadiazine (silverol) and hydrophylic dressings such as Tegaderm® and Vaseline® gauze.

Chronic radiodermatitis: delayed damage to the skin is primarily a function of radiation effects on the vasculature; an initial wave of dermal atrophy is seen within 4–6 months. A second phase of dermal thinning tends to develop after more than 52 weeks, often accompanied by the appearance of telangiectasia[18]. The skin is seen to appear thin and tight, hyperpigmented, and dry. Marked fibrosis may limit flexibility or movement. Radiation-induced skin necrosis and chronic ulcers may develop and persist indefinitely (Fig. 10.7.1.4), especially over the scalp and leg. Trauma, chronic friction, and pressure contribute to the development of radiation ulcers. Keratoses and squamous cell carcinoma (SCC) may develop. Histopathology is often required to differentiate SCC from non neoplastic radionecrosis.

Basic treatment for intact skin consists of oil-in-water emollients and prevention of trauma. Radiation ulcers are resistant to treatment and a realistic goal would be to prevent secondary infection, pain, and fetid smell. This can be achieved with the use of hydrocolloids, but the prospects of healing are limited.

Radiation recall refers to inflammatory reactions triggered by cytotoxic agents that develop in previously irradiated areas, mainly in the skin. Typically, a well-circumscribed erythema arises that perfectly fits the radiation field of past treatment. The treatment could have been delivered days to years ago.

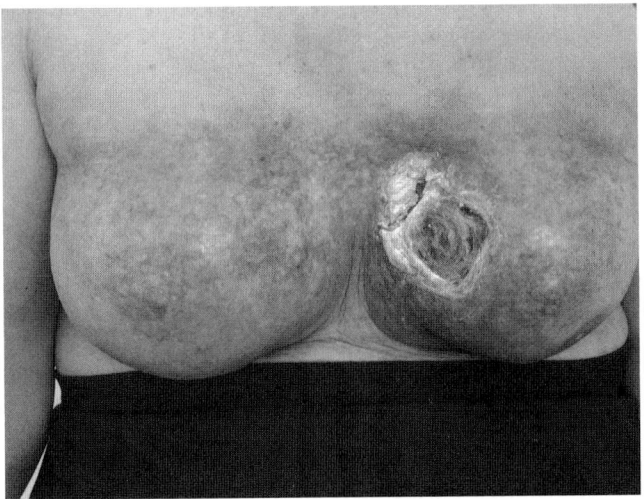

Figure 10.7.1.4 Skin fibrosis and non-healing ulcers of chronic radiodermatitis of the chest wall.

The most common chemotherapeutic agents implicated are anthracyclines and taxanes. Gemcitabine, a nucleotide analog, was implicated recently in several cases[22]. Histopathology of affected skin reveals mixed non-specific inflammatory infiltrate. The condition may not necessarily require any special treatment. Withdrawal of the offending agent produces prompt improvement. Alternatively, corticosteroids or the use of non-steroidal anti-inflammatory agents may help[23].

Paraneoplastic syndromes with skin manifestations

Paraneoplastic syndrome refers to a pathological state generated by cancer in an unrelated organ or system. The syndromes may be due to tumour production of substances that directly or indirectly cause distant symptoms, depletion of normal substances or host response to the tumour that results in the syndrome. There is a variety of paraneoplastic syndromes involving the skin. In the palliative patient, however, the discomfort caused by skin manifestations is often overshadowed by the neoplastic disease itself. Skin manifestations can precede or succeed the diagnosis of cancer, indicate a recurrence of disease, or have no correlation with the course of the neoplastic disease. Some of the more common paraneoplastic syndromes are detailed here:

Dermatomyositis

Dermatomyositis (DM) is associated with solid tumours, often melanoma and lymphoma in 15–50 per cent of adults over the age of 40 years[24]. Carcinoma may involve almost any organ, affecting patients with ovarian cancer, lung, pancreatic, stomach, or colorectal cancer[25]. In 1992, Sigurgeirsson *et al.* established the connection between DM and cancer. The relative risk of cancer in their series of 392 patients was 2.4 in male and 3.4 in female patients. In another series, the two independent predictive factors for malignancy ($P < 0.05$) in patients with DM were an older age at onset (>45 years) and male gender[26]. As for polymyositis, which is often mentioned together with DM, although patients with polymyositis had a slight increase in cancer frequency, it was not highly significant and could be explained by a more aggressive cancer search.

The characteristic and possibly pathognomonic cutaneous features of DM are the heliotrope rash and Gottron's papules (Fig. 10.7.1.5). The heliotrope is a violaceous rash with or without oedema involving periorbital skin. Gottron's papules are mainly found over the finger joints. They may also be found overlying the elbows, knees, and feet. The lesions consist of slightly elevated, violaceous papules and plaques. There may be a slight scale and, on some occasions, there is a thick psoriasiform scale. Telangiectasia often accompanies the lesions. Erythematous eruption in a photosensitive distribution and periungual changes are characteristic features of DM.

The diagnosis of DM is based on the clinical presentation, elevations of creatine kinase, aldolase, lactic dehydrogenase, or alanine aminotransferase. An evaluation of malignancy should be considered in all adult patients with DM[27]. Corticosteroids are the mainstay of DM therapy. In resistant cases immunosuppressive agents, such as methotrexate, azathioprine, cyclophosphamide, mycophenolate mofetil, chlorambucil, or cyclosporin, may be helpful in inducing remission. Skin lesions may persist even when systemic effect prevails, and are controlled by topical steroids

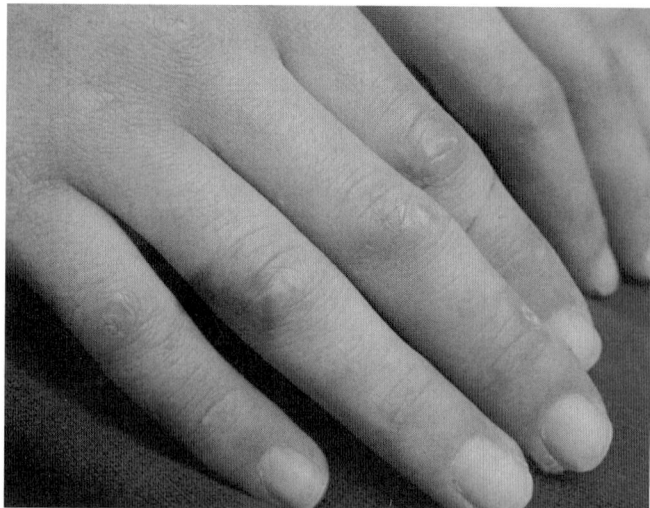

Figure 10.7.1.5 Erythematous papules over finger joints in a patient with dermatomyositis (Gothron's sign).

or topical immunosupressants, such as 0.1 per cent tacrolimus ointment.

Bazex syndrome

Bazex syndrome, also known as acrokeratosis paraneoplastica, was first described in 1965 in a man with carcinoma of the pyriform fossa and scaly erythematous lesions of the extremities. The eruption in Bazex syndrome consists of scaly papules and plaques over the nose, ears, nails, knees, and elbows. Thickening of the skin of the palms is a frequent occurrence. Squamous cell carcinoma of the oropharynx, larynx, oesophagus, and lung are the most common associated tumours[28].

Acanthosis nigricans

The majority of cases of acanthosis nigricans in the clinics are associated with obesity and diabetes mellitus. When associated with internal malignancy, most tumours are intra-abdominal, mainly gastric carcinoma. This syndrome is characterized by dark velvety plaques of skinfolds: axillae, neck, behind elbows, and knees and sometimes it may show as papillomatous lesions in mucosal membranes. Sudden appearance in the absence of known causative disorders should prompt the search for an underlying cancer. About 20 per cent of cases precede malignancy.

Sign of Leser-Trélat

Abrupt appearance of numerous seborrhoeic keratoses is traditionally mentioned among paraneoplastic signs, although its association with this group is sometimes doubted. The Leser-Trélat sign was reported with the same cancer association as acanthosis nigricans and thus can represent a variant with a same initiating mechanism.

Paraneoplastic pemphigus

The autoimmune bullous dermatoses are a group of diseases characterized by the formation of slits within the epidermis or between the epidermis and the dermis. In pemphigus, intra-epidermal tears occur by loss of cell–cell adhesion (acantholysis) due to autoantibodies to epithelial cell surface protein desmoglein 3. The classical variant, pemphugus vulgaris, consists of loose vesicles and erosions involving skin and mucosal membranes. Treatment consists of systemic corticosteroids and steroid sparing agents.

It has long been noted that pemphigus vulgaris appears in combination with neoplastic disease[29]. Non-Hodgkin's lymphoma, chronic lymphatic leukaemia, and thymoma were the most commonly reported diseases. It was not until 1990, however, that Anhalt *et al.* defined paraneoplastic pemphigus as a clinically and immunologically distinct disease and suggested five criteria for its diagnosis[30]. The mechanisms underlying this condition are not completely clear. Interferon alpha treatment was associated with the disease, suggesting that other immunomodulators may act similarly. Anti-tumour responses against tumour antigens may cross react with epidermal components, thus creating the skin pathology. A variety of antigens were described with paraneoplastic pemphigus, to desmosomal and hemidesmosomal proteins. Clinically, the disease manifests itself not only as flaccid or tense blisters and erosions, but also as lichenoid and erythema multiforme-like lesions. Confluent erythema was often seen.

As in pemphigus vulgaris, treatment consists of a combination of prednisone and cyclosporine[31]. In resistant cases, cyclophosphamide, azathioprine, mycophenolate mofetil, plasmapheresis, and intravenous gammaglobulins may be required.

Skin toxicities of chemotherapeutic agents

The skin is a natural target for toxicities and adverse effects of anti-cancer drugs. Since the skin, hair, nails, and mucous membranes are composed of rapidly dividing cells, they would be targeted by these agents. Cancer therapy has widened extensively during recent years. New molecular targeting therapies and monoclonal antibodies now comprise a larger part in the arsenal of anti-neoplastic drugs. Alongside new indications and combinations of these drugs, novel toxicities also appeared, including skin toxicity. Common skin toxicities of chemotherapy will be detailed first followed by those of the widely used EGFR inhibitors.

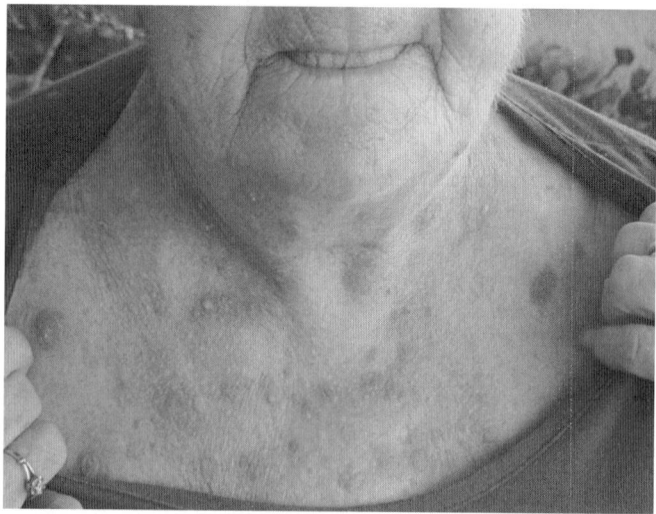

Figure 10.7.1.6 Paraneoplastic pemphigus.

Common cutaneous adverse effects of chemotherapeutic agents

Alopecia is one of the most common and most distressing side effects of chemotherapeutic agents. Since these drugs act on rapidly dividing and proliferating cells, the hair follicle is a natural target. Paclitaxel and doxorubicin are major causes of alopecia in the oncology clinic. Scalp hair is affected to a larger extent than the slowly growing eyelashes, eyebrows, and body hair.

Mucositis: this term includes damage to mucosal membranes—most frequently of the oral cavity—and is characterized by redness, swelling, white exudates, and in severe cases can lead to ulceration. Difficulty in chewing, swallowing, and speech may arise. Patients avoid food intake, oral medications, and in severe cases water due to distressing pain. Severity of chemotherapy-related mucositis is drug and patient dependent. Almost all anti-neoplastic agents are associated with mucositis. Drugs that are administered continuously by slow release mechanisms are likely to produce mucositis, such as continuous 5-FU, daily capecitabine, and liposomal doxorubicin. Other drugs with high rates of mucositis include methotrexate, cytarabine, and taxanes. Myeloablative conditioning may cause severe stomatitis worsened by mucosal candidiasis secondary to reduced immunity. Superimposed herpes simplex infection may severely complicate chemotherapy induced stomatitis. Extensive erosive components and circumscribed ulcers should raise the suspicion of HSV infection. Damaged mucosal barriers give rise to a higher rate of septicaemia.

Patient susceptibility to mucositis may be genetically determined, perhaps related to the expression levels of proapoptotic and anti-apoptotic genes[32].

Prevention of chemotherapy-related oral complications is difficult. Good dental and oral hygiene are helpful. Daily chlorhexidine mouthwash is often recommended for preventing chemotherapy-induced oral mucositis, but its efficacy is doubtful. Povidone-iodine, NaCl 0.9 per cent, water salt soda solution, and chamomile mouthwash are recommended and are not associated with dental staining typically produced by chlorhexidine[33]. Mucosal protectants such as sucralfate yield inconsistent results[34, 35]. Systemic administration of GM-CSF apparently reduces the development of radiation- and chemotherapy-related mucositis[36]. Palifermin (recombinant human keratinocyte growth factor) was recently shown to decrease severity and duration of oral mucosal injury induced by intensive chemotherapy for hematological malignancies[37]. Data on Palifermin in patients with solid tumours are limited and its use is not advocated as there is a theoretical risk of stimulating tumour growth. Topical non-steroidal anti-inflammatory agents and corticosteroids have been used with varying success. In some cases, pain may be so excruciating as to require opioid analgesics.

Nail changes and paronychia

Although less commonly encountered than alopecia and mucositis, nail changes can significantly interfere with manual activities and locomotion, due to their sensitive location. Taxans, especially docetaxel, are the main drugs causing nail abnormalities in 30–40 per cent of patients[38]. Recently, paronychia was reported to occur with the new EGF receptor inhibitors (HU). Discolouration, nail bed bleeding, and detachment of the corny material from the nail plate (onychlysis) occur[39]. Purulent exudates may accumulate beneath the nail and soft tissue swelling of the nail bed ensues. Development of onycholysis seems to be unrelated to the drug dose or frequency of administration. There is a tendency for nail changes to resolve gradually over weeks, despite continued treatment[40]. Nail changes may be partly reduced by soaking the tips of the fingers in ice water. Topical disinfectants like povidone iodine and 6 per cent peroxide and topical antibiotics can reduce secondary bacterial infection.

Hand and foot syndrome

Also known as toxic acral erythema and palmar-plantar erythrodysesthesia syndrome, HF syndrome is a common skin reaction. The earliest sign is painful erythema of the palms, soles, and fingers that later becomes oedematous, changes colour to violet, then dries off, and desquamates. In severe cases, blisters develop, later leaving erosive surfaces, with considerable impairment in function. Hand–foot syndrome is often the dose-limiting toxic effect, especially for liposomal doxorubicin.

Pharmacologic agents that have been evaluated for hand–foot syndrome include pyridoxine or vitamin B6, dexamethasone, amifostine, and COX-2 inhibitors.

Chronic graft versus host disease

Allogeneic haematopoietic stem cell transplantation (SCT) remains the major therapy that can consistently eradicate all evidence of chronic myeloid leukaemia, which is the most common indication of this treatment. The success of allogeneic SCT depends on the degree of HLA matching. The therapeutic success is offset by a large percentage of patients who develop clinical graft versus host disease (GVHD) that is part of the graft versus tumour responses. Early withdrawal of post-transplant immunosuppression and use of donor lymphocyte infusions to incite a graft-versus-malignancy effect in patients with residual or progressive disease enhance acute and chronic GVHD. GVHD is initiated when immunocompetent T cells from the graft react against the immunocompromised host via recognition of alloantigens displayed by host antigen-presenting cells. Th1 cytokines secreted by activated donor T cells are responsible in part for the acute phase changes, while Th2 cytokines, including IL-4 and IL-5 generate some of the chronic phase pathology[41,42]. The skin is only one organ involved, others being the GI tract, liver, respiratory tract, musculoskeletal, and hematopoietic system.

The majority of patients with chronic GVHD have had prior acute GVHD. In HLA-matched marrow grafting with primarily methotrexate-based prophylaxis, skin (65–80 per cent), mouth (48–72 per cent), liver (40–73 per cent), and eye (18–47 per cent) involvement are most commonly reported[43].

The cutaneous hallmark of chronic GVHD is a lichenoid eruption, an erythematous, papular rash that resembles lichen planus and

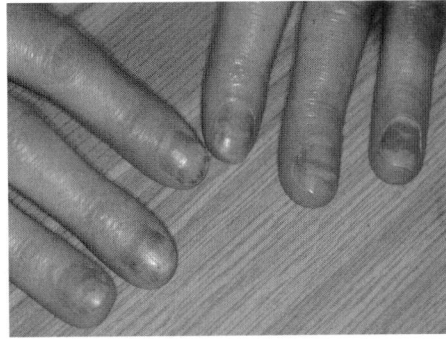

Figure 10.7.1.7 Nail discolouration and paronychia caused by docetaxel.

leaves hyperpigmented spots when resolved. In sclerodermatous GVHD, the skin is thickened, tight, and fragile[44]. Atrophic patches of lichen sclerosus are often described. Poor wound-healing and ulcerations occur on areas subjected to tension or trauma. Hair loss and reduced sweating occur as a result of dermal fibrosis. Brittle hair, fingernails, and toenails develop and premature graying of hair may occur. Ocular GVHD presents with irritation, burning, dry eyes, or photophobia from irreversible destruction of the lacrimal glands[44]. Salivary gland dysfunction leads to xerostomia. Mucosal involvement by lichenoid eruption causes food sensitivity and in severe cases can develop to ulceration especially at the biting line.

Basic skin lubrication to maintain flexibility and eye and mouth wetting preparations are required. Antimicrobial agents against complicating herpes simplex infection may be required. Extracorporeal photopheresis was reported to improve refractory GVHD. This may be due to an increase in regulatory T cells that suppress autoreactivity[45].

Skin toxicity of epidermal growth factor receptor (EGFR) inhibitors

This group is comprised of: (1) monoclonal antibodies that target the extracellular ligand-binding domain of the molecule, thereby preventing binding of the ligand to the same receptor, such is cetuximab; and (2) small molecules that target the intercellular tyrosine kynase domain of the receptor. These agents include erlotinib (Tarceva®; OSI Pharmaceuticals, Melville, NY) and gefitinib

(Iressa®; AstraZeneca, Wilmington, DE) and act by competing with adenosine triphosphate (ATP) binding at the TK site.

Skin eruptions are the most common and sometimes distressing side effect of this category of drugs affecting 45–100 per cent of users[46,47]. The characteristic rash is composed of acneiform pustules on a background of seborrhoeic dermatitis-like erythematous plaques with oily scales (Fig. 10.7.1.9). The rash begins during the first week of treatment and may vary in severity with repeated treatments, tending to increase initially and then partially decrease. A correlation between the clinical response to the drug and the presence of skin rash has been observed[48,49]. Typical distribution of the rash is on the face, upper chest, and back and less often the scalp. Unlike acne, closed and open comedones will not appear, and in contrast to steroid-induced acne, the EGFR inhibitors may induce oily scales and dried pus crusts with severe dermatitis rather than small pustular lesions that are prominent on normal skin.

Microscopically, infiltration with T lymphocytes around the follicular infundibulum is seen, which can be followed by superficial lymphocytic perifolliculitis, leading to follicular rupture and suppurative superficial folliculitis. The basic pathology is directly related to the inhibition of the EGF receptors on epidermal cells and is non-infectious. Secondary bacterial infection can occur.

Treatment is based on acne drugs and therapies. Mild soaps and emulsions can be used for skin wash. Oil-free moisturizing creams are used to relive dryness and itching. In severe cases, anti-histamines can alleviate pruritus. Treatment with topical agents consists of hydrocortisone (2.5 per cent cream) and clindamycin (1 per cent gel). In more severe cases, pimecrolimus (Elidel®; Novartis) (1 per cent cream) is recommended. Addition of systemic treatment with doxycycline (100 mg, PO twice a day) or minocycline (100 mg, PO bid) can expedite recovery. Dose reduction should be considered in non remitting, severe skin symptoms[50].

Skin problems of bedridden patients

Prolonged incapacitation and loss of mobility lead to increasing dependency on bed rest. The recumbent patient suffers debilitating effects on many systems including the skin. Immobilization, decreased

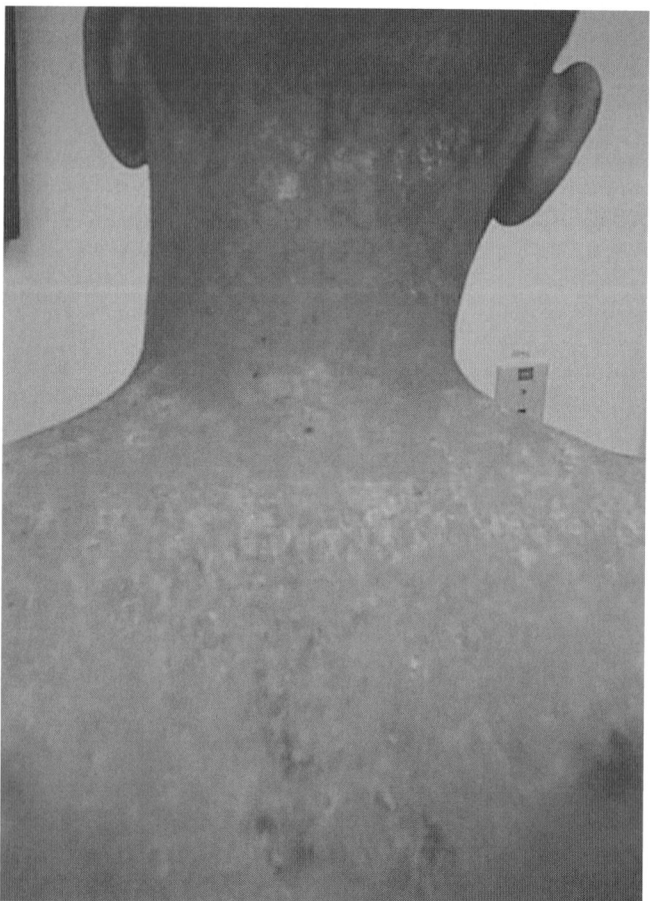

Figure 10.7.1.8 Chronic graft versus host disease.

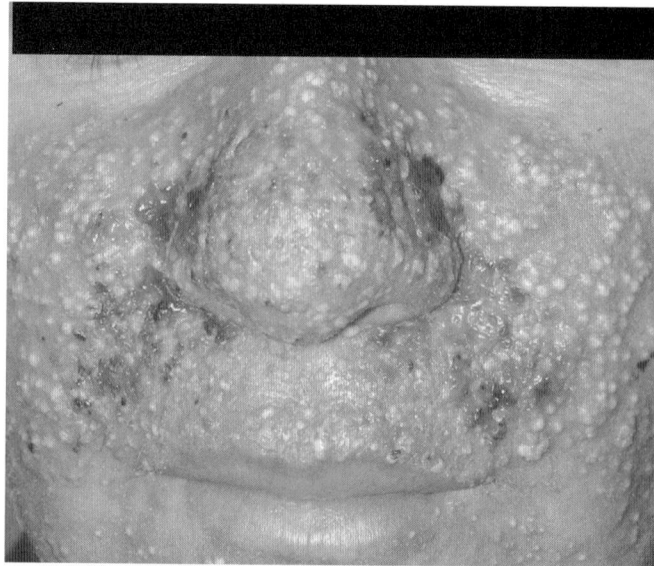

Figure 10.7.1.9 Cetuximab-induced acneiform erruption.

body hygiene, urinary incontinence, and spilled body fluids expose the patient to the development of decubitus ulcers, hair follicle and sweat gland occlusion, irritant contact dermatitis, and skin infections caused by yeasts and dermatophytes.

Fungal skin infections

Tinea corporis and cruris: the typical presentation is of large, confluent polycyclic or psoriasiform plaques extending over the buttocks, lower back, inguinal region, inner aspects of the thigh, pubic region, genitalia, and peri anal skin. A common causative agent is the dermatophyte trichophyton rubrum. Although the clinical picture is useful for diagnosis, KOH skin scraping may reveal hyphea. Tinea corporis may resemble psoriasis, seborrhoeic dermatitis, and nummular eczema.

Topical agents such as the allylamines, imidazoles, tolnaftate, butenafine, or ciclopirox are effective. In resistant cases, fluconazole 150 mg weekly for 4–6 weeks or terbinafine 250 mg daily for 2 weeks can be effective.

Mucocutaneous candidiasis

Candida albicans is an opportunistic human pathogen that produces skin infection under debilitating conditions and immune suppression. The non-albicans *Candida* species have been detected more frequently in clinical isolates in recent years, particularly from oropharyngeal cultures in patients who are HIV-positive. White patches over buccal mucosa and a yellow velvety membrane over the tongue typically appear in oral candidiasis also called 'oral thrush' and 'black hairy tongue'[51]. Once sloughing, the tongue may appear red and atrophic. Angular cheilitis—fissuring of the angles of the mouth may accompany the oral infection.

Nystatin suspension, amphotericin B, and clotrimazole oral preparations are helpful[52]. However, immune compromised hosts often do not respond to topical treatment. A short course of systemic fluconazole 100–200 mg daily for 5–10 days may expedite relief.

Vaginal candidiasis

The clinical picture of candida vulvovaginitis is quite similar to that of oral infection. The symptoms include irritation and discomfort associated with a creamy discharge[53]. Skin lesions may spread from the vulva to the groin area. Small 'satellite' pustules overlie intertriginous patches of the outer labial skin and groin region. Topically applied Nystatin or miconazole is usually successful. Alternatively, oral treatment with single-dose fluconazole or itraconzole for 3–5 days is effective.

Other forms of skin infection with pathogenic candida species include nail involvement and peri-ungual inflammation and intertriginous eczema.

Diaper dermatitis

Urinary incontinence leads to prolonged periods of wetness and soaking of the skin. Maceration of the skin and barrier damage enhances the irritant effect of urine and faeces. Inflamed patches evolve over affected regions, usually the buttocks and genitalia, and cause a burning sensation. Erosions may aggravate the pain. Preventive use of 5 per cent dexpanthenol and zinc oxide ointments restore the barrier and protect skin from the irritant effect of stool, urine, and sweat[54]. Topical corticosteroids are advocated when painful and disturbing dermatitis has already occurred, but should be combined with the barrier restoring agents and totally replaced once improvement is detected.

Pressure ulcers

Immobilization puts the cancer patient at an immediate risk of developing pressure ulcers. Other factors such as old age, malnutrition, dehydration, immune suppression, cancer-related coagulopathy and hypoperfusion, and increased susceptibility to skin infections contribute to a significantly increased level of morbidity and deterioration[55]. In the hospice population, 14–28 per cent develop ulcers, similar to the prevalence of this disorder in long-term care settings (2.3–28 per cent)[56]. Areas subjected to pressure in the supine patients will be prone to develop sores, the most common being the sacrum region. Pressure ulcers often become a major source of distress for the patient and for the caregiver because of unsightliness, pain, odour, exudates, bleeding, and the potential of infection.

The exact aetiology of pressure ulcers is unclear. Prolonged pressure obstructs capillaries, which cannot re-perfuse, leading to dermal hypoxia. The ischaemia results in necrosis that progresses from superficial discolouration to full thickness skin loss.

The key to good wound care is prevention, if possible. Frequent repositioning and weight support for better distribution of pressure on body parts is necessary. Alternating pressure mattresses and absorbing overlays aid in achieving this goal. Careful assessment for early evolving pressure wounds must be done on a daily basis.

Local wound care consists of absorbent dressing (activated charcoal, cellulose, or soft alginate) local and systemic infection control (metronidazole and antibiotics), and surgical debridement.

Conclusion

While there is a lot that cannot be changed in the course of incurable cancer, many dermatological aspects can be solved successfully. It is important to give dermatological aspects of disease their appropriate attention, because these can be the ones that may be dealt with efficiently, using simple and effective treatments. The dermatologist is an important participant of the multi-disciplinary team. An ambitious approach to seemingly minor aspects of disease improve the patient's quality of life and provides a message of care, attention, and respect.

References

1. Chu, D., Haake, A., Holbrook, K. *et al.* (2003). The structure and development of skin. In *Fitzpatrick's Dermatology in General Medicine*, (ed. I. Freedberg), 6th edition. McGraw-Hill, New York.
2. Oshima, H., Rochat, A., Kedzia, C. *et al.* (2001). Morphogenesis and renewal of hair follicles from adult multipotent stem cells. *Cell*, **104**(2), 233–45.
3. Lookingbill, D.P., Spangler, N., and Helm, K.F. (1993). Cutaneous metastases in patients with metastatic carcinoma: A retrospective study of 4020 patients. *J Am Acad Dermatol*, **29**(2 Pt 1), 228–36.
4. Brenner, S., Tamir, E., Maharshak, N. *et al.* (2001). Cutaneous manifestations of internal malignancies. *Clin Dermatol*, **19**(3), 290–7.
5. Brownstein, M.H. and Helwig, E.B. (1972). Metastatic tumours of the skin. *Cancer*, **29**(5), 1298–307.
6. Brownstein, M.H. and Helwig, E.B. (1972). Patterns of cutaneous metastasis. *Arch Dermatol*, **105**(6), 862–8.
7. Schuler, G., Honigsmann, H., and Wolff, K. (1980). Diffuse melanosis in metastatic melanoma. Further evidence for disseminated single cell metastases in the skin. *J Am Acad Dermatol*, **3**(4), 363–9.
8. Alley, E., Green, R., and Schuchter, L. (2002). Cutaneous toxicities of cancer therapy. *Curr Opin Oncol*, **14**(2), 212–16.

9. Singal, R., Tunnessen, W.W., Jr., Wiley, J.M. *et al.* (1991). Discrete pigmentation after chemotherapy. *Pediatr Dermatol*, **8**(3), 231–5.

10. Ruan, X. (2007). Drug-related side effects of long-term intrathecal morphine therapy. *Pain Physician*, **10**(2), 357–66.

11. Bosonnet, L. (2003). Pruritis: Scratching the surface. *Eur J Cancer Care (Engl)*, **12**(2), 162–5.

12. Paumgartner, G. and Beuers, U. (2002). Ursodeoxycholic acid in cholestatic liver disease: Mechanisms of action and therapeutic use revisited. *Hepatology*, **36**(3), 525–31.

13. Tandon, P., Rowe, B.H., Vandermeer, B. *et al.* (2007). The efficacy and safety of bile Acid binding agents, opioid antagonists, or rifampin in the treatment of cholestasis-associated pruritus. *Am J Gastroenterol*, **102**(7), 1528–36.

14. Porzio, G., Aielli, F., Narducci, F. *et al.* (2004). Pruritus in a patient with advanced cancer successfully treated with continuous infusion of granisetron. *Support Care Cancer*, **12**(3), 208–9.

15. Bigliardi, P.L., Stammer, H., Jost, G. *et al.* (2007). Treatment of pruritus with topically applied opiate receptor antagonist. *J Am Acad Dermatol*, **56**(6), 979–88.

16. Seckin, D., Demircay, Z., and Akin, O. (2007). Generalized pruritus treated with narrowband UVB. *Int J Dermatol*, **46**(4), 367–70.

17. Robak, E. and Robak, T. (2007). Skin lesions in chronic lymphocytic leukemia. *Leuk Lymphoma*, **48**(5), 855–65.

18. Hopewell, J.W. (1990). The skin: Its structure and response to ionizing radiation. *Int J Radiat Biol*, **57**(4), 751–73.

19. Denham, J.W., Hamilton, C.S., Simpson, S.A. *et al.* (1995). Factors influencing the degree of erythematous skin reactions in humans. *Radiother Oncol*, **36**(2), 107–20.

20. Porock, D. (2002). Factors influencing the severity of radiation skin and oral mucosal reactions: Development of a conceptual framework. *Eur J Cancer Care (Engl)*, **11**(1), 33–43.

21. McQuestion, M. (2006). Evidence-based skin care management in radiation therapy. *Semin Oncol Nurs*, **22**(3), 163–73.

22. Friedlander, P.A., Bansal, R., Schwartz, L. *et al.* (2004). Gemcitabine-related radiation recall preferentially involves internal tissue and organs. *Cancer*, **100**(9), 1793–9.

23. Azria, D., Magne, N., Zouhair, A. *et al.* (2005). Radiation recall: A well recognized but neglected phenomenon. *Cancer Treat Rev*, **31**(7), 555–70.

24. Braverman, I.M. (2002). Skin manifestations of internal malignancy. *Clin Geriatr Med*, **18**(1), 1–19, v.

25. Hill, C.L., Zhang, Y., Sigurgeirsson, B. *et al.* (2001). Frequency of specific cancer types in dermatomyositis and polymyositis: A population-based study. *Lancet*, **357**(9250), 96–100.

26. Chen, Y.J., Wu, C.Y., and Shen, J.L. (2001). Predicting factors of malignancy in dermatomyositis and polymyositis: a case-control study. *Br J Dermatol*, **144**(4), 825–31.

27. Callen, J.P. (1982). The value of malignancy evaluation in patients with dermatomyositis. *J Am Acad Dermatol*, **6**(2), 253–9.

28. Bolognia, J.L., Brewer, Y.P., and Cooper, D.L. (1991). Bazex syndrome (acrokeratosis paraneoplastica). An analytic review. *Medicine (Baltimore)*, **70**(4), 269–80.

29. Krain, L.S. and Bierman, S.M. (1974). Pemphigus vulgaris and internal malignancy. *Cancer*, **33**(4), 1091–9.

30. Anhalt, G.J., Kim, S.C., Stanley, J.R. *et al.* (1990). Paraneoplastic pemphigus. An autoimmune mucocutaneous disease associated with neoplasia. *N Engl J Med*, **323**(25), 1729–35.

31. Anhalt, G.J. (1997). Paraneoplastic pemphigus. *Adv Dermatol*, **12**, 77–96, discussion 97.

32. Sonis, S.T., Elting, L.S., Keefe, D. *et al.* (2004). Perspectives on cancer therapy-induced mucosal injury: pathogenesis, measurement, epidemiology, and consequences for patients. *Cancer*, **100**(9 Suppl), 1995–2025.

33. Potting, C.M., Uitterhoeve, R., Op Reimer, W.S. *et al.* (2006). The effectiveness of commonly used mouthwashes for the prevention of chemotherapy-induced oral mucositis: A systematic review. *Eur J Cancer Care (Engl)*, **15**(5), 431–9.

34. Nottage, M., McLachlan, S.A., Brittain, M.A. *et al.* (2003). Sucralfate mouthwash for prevention and treatment of 5-fluorouracil-induced mucositis: A randomized, placebo-controlled trial. *Support Care Cancer*, **11**(1), 41–7.

35. Pfeiffer, P., Madsen, E.L., Hansen, O. *et al.* (1990). Effect of prophylactic sucralfate suspension on stomatitis induced by cancer chemotherapy. A randomized, double-blind cross-over study. *Acta Oncol*, **29**(2), 171–3.

36. Stokman, M.A., Spijkervet, F.K., Boezen, H.M. *et al.* (2006). Preventive intervention possibilities in radiotherapy- and chemotherapy-induced oral mucositis: Results of meta-analyses. *J Dent Res*, **85**(8), 690–700.

37. Spielberger, R., Stiff, P., Bensinger, W. *et al.* (2004). Palifermin for oral mucositis after intensive therapy for hematologic cancers. *N Engl J Med*, **351**(25), 2590–8.

38. Hussain, S., Anderson, D.N., Salvatti, M.E. *et al.* (2000). Onycholysis as a complication of systemic chemotherapy: Report of five cases associated with prolonged weekly paclitaxel therapy and review of the literature. *Cancer*, **88**(10), 2367–71.

39. Nicolopoulos, J. and Howard, A. (2002). Docetaxel-induced nail dystrophy. *Australas J Dermatol*, **43**(4), 293–6.

40. Flory, S.M., Solimando, D.A., Jr., Webster, G.F. *et al.* (1999). Onycholysis associated with weekly administration of paclitaxel. *Ann Pharmacother*, **33**(5), 584–6.

41. Hofmeister, C.C., Quinn, A., Cooke, K.R. *et al.* (2004). Graft-versus-host disease of the skin: Life and death on the epidermal edge. *Biol Blood Marrow Transplant*, **10**(6), 366–72.

42. Okamoto, I., Kohno, K., Tanimoto, T. *et al.* (2000). IL-18 prevents the development of chronic graft-versus-host disease in mice. *J Immunol*, **164**(11), 6067–74.

43. Sullivan, K.M., Agura, E., Anasetti, C. *et al.* (1991). Chronic graft-versus-host disease and other late complications of bone marrow transplantation. *Semin Hematol*, **28**(3), 250–59.

44. Higman, M.A. and Vogelsang, G.B. (2004). Chronic graft versus host disease. *Br J Haematol*, **125**(4), 435–54.

45. Biagi, E., Di Biaso, I., Leoni, V. *et al.* (2007). Extracorporeal photochemotherapy is accompanied by increasing levels of circulating CD4+CD25+GITR+Foxp3+CD62L+ functional regulatory T-cells in patients with graft-versus-host disease. *Transplantation*, **84**(1), 31–9.

46. Shepherd, F.A., Rodrigues Pereira, J., Ciuleanu, T. *et al.* (2005). Erlotinib in previously treated non-small-cell lung cancer. *N Engl J Med*, **353**(2), 123–32.

47. Perez-Soler, R. and Saltz, L. (2005). Cutaneous adverse effects with HER1/EGFR-targeted agents: Is there a silver lining? *J Clin Oncol*, **23**(22), 5235–46.

48. Clark, C., Perez-Soler, R., and Siu, L. (2003). Rash severity is predictive of increased survival with erlotinib HCL [abstract]. *Proc Am Soc Clin Oncol*, **22**, 196.

49. Saltz, L.B., Meropol, N.J., Loehrer, P.J., Sr. *et al.* (2004). Phase II trial of cetuximab in patients with refractory colorectal cancer that expresses the epidermal growth factor receptor. *J Clin Oncol*, **22**(7), 1201–8.

50. Lynch, T.J., Jr., Kim, E.S., Eaby, B. *et al.* (2007). Epidermal growth factor receptor inhibitor-associated cutaneous toxicities: An evolving paradigm in clinical management. *Oncologist*, **12**(5), 610–21.

51. Samaranayake, L. and Yaacob, H. (1990). Classification of oral candidiasis. In *Oral candidiasis*, (ed. T.W. Slam), pp. 82–101. Wright, London.

52. Hay, R.J. (1999). The management of superficial candidiasis. *J Am Acad Dermatol*, **40**(6 Pt 2), S35–42.

53. Sobel, J.D. (1984). Vulvovaginal candidiasis—What we do and do not know. *Ann Intern Med*, **101**(3), 390–2.

54. Wananukul, S., Limpongsanuruk, W., Singalavanija, S. *et al.* (2006). Comparison of dexpanthenol and zinc oxide ointment with ointment base in the treatment of irritant diaper dermatitis from diarrhea: A multicenter study. *J Med Assoc Thai*, **89**(10), 1654–8.

55. McDonald, A. and Lesage, P. (2006). Palliative management of pressure ulcers and malignant wounds in patients with advanced illness. *J Palliat Med*, **9**(2), 285–95.

56. Cuddigan, J., Berlowitz, D. and Ayello, E. (2001). Pressure ulcers in America: Prevalence, incidence and implications for the Future. An executive summary of the National Pressure Ulcer Advisory Panel Monograph. *Adv Skin Wound Care*, **14**, 208–15.

10.7.2 Skin problems in palliative care—nursing aspects

Patricia Grocott and Vicky Robinson

Introduction

The purpose of this chapter is to apply principles of palliative care to wound care for patients with advanced disease. Skin problems are almost inevitable in patients receiving palliative care. Wound management in palliative care is dedicated to achieving a myriad of goals related to symptom relief, patient comfort, and dignity, thereby enhancing the quality of life of patients and families. Wound management in palliative care encompasses the nursing care of patients, of all ages, with a weakened skin barrier together with the management of wounds caused by advanced and intractable diseases and conditions.

The incidence and prevalence of wounds in palliative care patients is unknown, nor has this population been clearly defined. The aim of wound care normally is to achieve healing with a preference for evidence-based treatments evaluated in randomized controlled trials. Healing is the main outcome measure. The problem with this is that patients with longstanding 'hard to heal' wounds, such as fungating malignant wounds, are substantively excluded from clinical trials of new treatments for wounds and perceived to be a marginal group. However, patients with intractable wounds are heavy users of health-care services and dressing products. As such they may be the outliers of a bell-shaped population curve, but they command a significant proportion of wound care resources.

Because wound management in palliative care is under research, it has not been fully formalized into rational standards of care supported by appropriate protocols and products. In this chapter, the authors have drawn on their clinical experience and research outputs to describe components of good skin care and three core principles of wound management in palliative care. These are linked with clinical decision-making and outcome measurement tools, which illustrate how the core principles relate to clinical care, and how they can be validated by the collection of outcome data.

Palliative care patients requiring wound care

As with other aspects of palliative care, careful assessment is required in order to determine the most appropriate treatment[1]. That said the principles of wound management in palliative care that we propose are essentially components of appropriate patient care, which could complement curative wound care protocols. The management emphasis for patients who are dying, and for patients at an earlier stage of their disease will be different. However, the difference between 'curative' and 'palliative' wound care, in our view, has more to do with goal setting and outcome measures than radically different clinical interventions. For example goals include the management of odour, exudate, bleeding, pain, and the maintenance of an intact dressing system, which are interim goals towards wound healing by secondary intention[2]. Fig. 10.7.2.1 illustrates the patient groups that might benefit from palliative care measures, including people with intractable diseases for whom skin breakdown is a significant and challenging aspect of daily life.

Principles of wound management in palliative care

Wound care can be organized around three core principles within a framework of supportive care to patients, families, and friends:

- Treatment of the underlying problem, if possible.
- Local wound management.
- Symptom control.

These principles will be illustrated in this chapter in relation to good skin care, and the management of pressure ulcers and fungating malignant wounds. Symptom control and local wound management are themes that cut across all wound groups, for example exudate and odour feature in a range of wounds of different aetiologies. The interventions overlap, and, as with all palliative care practice, must be taken into account in care planning, at each intervention, and in methods of evaluation.

Clinical assessment, decision-making, and evaluation

Clinical assessment, documentation, and evaluation are particularly important in wound management in palliative care where the theory and evidence base is not established.

Decision-making algorithms have been developed by the Skin and Wound Care Group at St Christopher's Hospice, London. They highlight in particular the interrelationships between wound management problems and interventions. A clinical note-making tool, based on the TELER® system of treatment evaluation, has been developed for wound care[3]. During the course of this

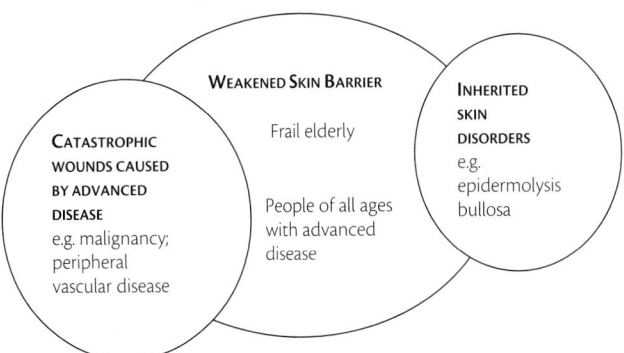

Figure 10.7.2.1 Overview of patient groups that may benefit from palliative wound care.

chapter examples will be given of the decision-making algorithms linked to the note-making tool.

TELER is a system of note-making with clinical indicators, which assess interventions and outcomes in a numerical format. The indicators measure dressing performance, optimal wound management, and symptom control on an ordinal scale with 5 being the management goal and 0 the problem to be resolved, or avoided. The indicators therefore define patient-centred goals of care in relation to a wound and measure the outcomes numerically.

Three forms of data are generated from the system: factual information about disease aetiology and treatment, numerical TELER codes, and minimal written observations by clinicians. Data analysis is conducted in two steps. The first comprises a qualitative narrative analysis of the treatment and observational data. The second involves the calculation of two indices of the treatment and care given: a Patient Outcome Index and a Quality of Care Outcome Index[4].

Together the algorithms and the note-making system offer the following:

- A link between theory and practice.
- Systematic decision-making.
- Measuring outcomes:
  - Longitudinal observational evaluation.
  - Patient-centred experiential outcomes.

- Training and skills development in clinical care and product use.
- Clinical and cost-effectiveness evidence of wound care.
- Knowledge transfer for needs-driven products and industrial innovation.

Patients with a weakened skin barrier: good skin care

Skin problems in advanced disease are largely attributable to skin that is weakened by general effects of chronic disease, such as malnutrition, dehydration, and immobility[5]. There are many factors that predispose palliative care patients to skin problems: if they are taken into account when taking a history and assessing the patient, it may be possible to mitigate their effects. Nursing care is clearly not able to prevent and resolve all the problems of advanced disease, for example immobility and anorexia. However, dedicated interventions to prevent morbidity resulting from these problems, for example pressure ulcers and dry skin conditions, may be possible.

Good skin care has three cornerstones: avoiding pressure damage, cleansing and protection, and continuous assessment. It is not a highly technical activity. It requires practical knowledge and skill, and above all, dedicated attention to detail if the patient's skin is to remain intact and the patient free of distressing symptoms. An algorithm has been developed to guide clinical assessment and care planning (Fig. 10.7.2.2).

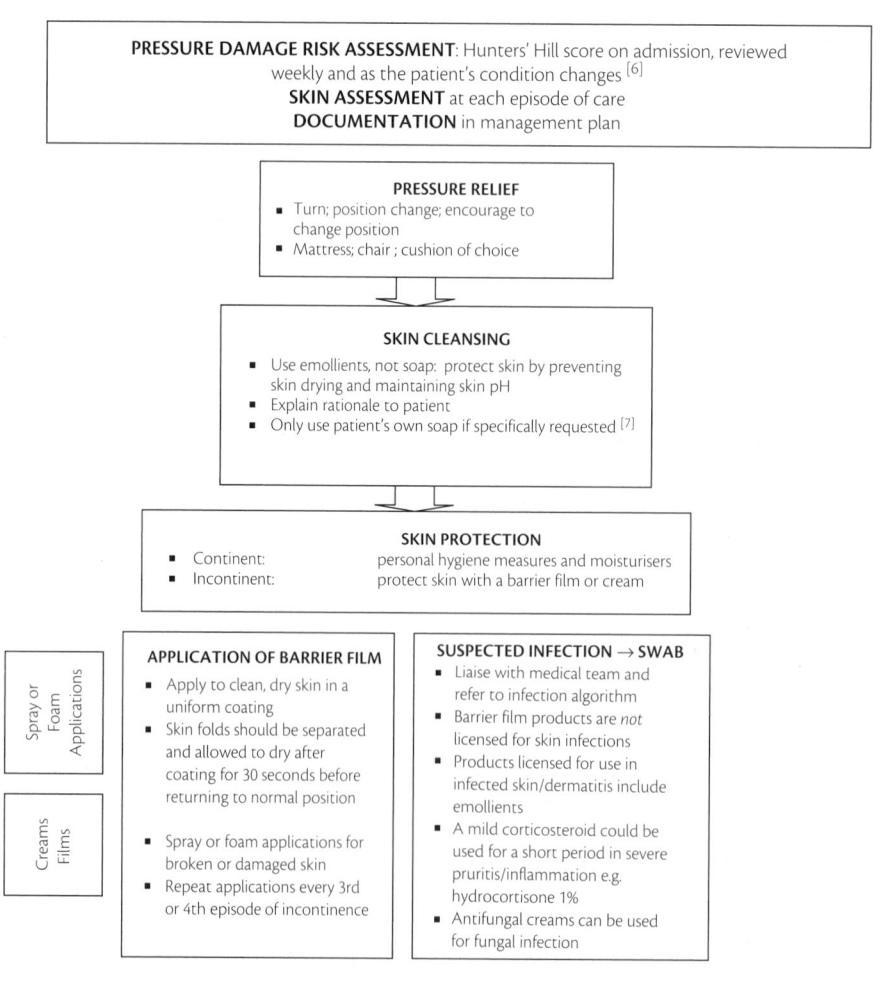

Figure 10.7.2.2 St. Christopher's Hospice good skin care algorithm.

Code 5	Skin appears intact
4	Skin has pale pink patches (or pale discoloured patches)
3	Skin has patchy reddening (or patchy discolouration)
2	Skin has fiery red patches (or dense discoloured patches)
1	Skin is diffuse fiery red (or diffusely discoloured)
0	Skin is diffuse fiery red and shiny (or diffusely discoloured and shiny e.g. in dark skin)

Figure 10.7.2.3 Clinical indicator: Irritant dermatitis.

Figure 10.7.2.3 shows an example of a clinical indicator. It is used to monitor skin condition relative to irritant dermatitis from body fluids, for example urine and exudate.

Principle I: treatment of the underlying cause

Pressure ulcers

There is an extensive literature on the management of pressure ulcers, including clinical guidelines, which can be drawn on to guide pressure relieving strategies and local wound management[8]. The focus in this section is to put general principles of pressure relief and ulcer management into the context of wound management in palliative care.

Treatment of pressure ulcers is inextricably linked with prevention. As and when pressure damage occurs, interventions that relieve pressure are maintained. Prevention of skin damage from pressure, friction, and shear forces is fundamental to good skin care in vulnerable patients. The Hunter's Hill risk assessment tool has been developed specifically for palliative care patients who are, in the main, at considerable risk of developing pressure sores[6]. In our experience, patients will require regular repositioning on pressure relieving devices (mattresses, seating), regardless of the quality of the device. Repositioning is also essential to maintain movement in joints, to prevent contractures, and for psycho-social reasons. The frequency of position change will be based on assessment of risk, the general condition of the patient, and the equipment being used[9].

Skin condition is the best indicator of how often position changes need to occur. This is assessed by lightly pressing an area of skin on which the patient was lying prior to turning. The skin should go white (blanche) and then return to its normal colour. The time taken to return to normal should be no longer than twice the length of time for which the finger pressure was applied. A fixed red mark that does not fade within 20 min after pressure has been relieved is indicative of pressure damage, loss of tissue viability, and varying degrees of skin breakdown and ulceration[10].

Patients with no evidence of pressure damage simply require good skin care and ongoing monitoring. Those with evidence of minor damage can benefit from the application of a transparent film dressing to protect the vulnerable skin and reduce friction. Pressure ulcers can still occur in spite of rigorous assessment and monitoring and the use of first class pressure relieving devices for beds and chairs.

The development of a pressure ulcer is understandably distressing for patients, families, and clinicians. Once an ulcer is established, care and management revolve around pressure relief, local wound management, and symptom management.

The nature and stage of the damage dictates treatment interventions together with curative or palliative goals. Several pressure ulcer grading tools exist. St. Christopher's has adopted the Stirling system[11]. Once there is evidence of a pressure ulcer, characterized by devitalized tissue following interruption of the blood supply, the management plan will be guided by whether the aim is to heal the wound or to palliate. Local wound management and symptom control strategies will be discussed further using the conceptual framework of wound bed preparation (WBP).

Fungating malignant wounds

Fungating malignant wounds are caused by tumour infiltration of the skin and its supporting blood and lymph vessels. The tumours may be locally advanced, metastatic, or recurrent. Unless they can be treated by single or combination anti-cancer treatments, there is the potential for massive skin damage. This occurs through a combination of tumour growth, loss of local blood supply, and consequent loss of tissue viability[5]. The dead tissue is colonized by anaerobic and aerobic bacteria, which are associated with malodour and exudate[12,13].

Fungating tumours present with proliferative tissue growth, progressing to ulceration as and when the blood supply to the area is interrupted. The wounds can be full thickness, also extending into organs, or superficial and extensive[14]. Fig. 10.7.2.4 illustrates a full thickness, ulcerating, and fungating breast tumour. Fig. 10.7.2.5 is an example of 'en cuirasse' fungation of the chest wall from primary breast cancer.

Diagnosis is based on histological assessment and the treatment aim is to control tumour growth, arrest surface haemorrhage, and promote healing whenever possible. Mainstream treatment protocols may involve one or more of the following: surgery, radiotherapy, hormone manipulation, or chemotherapy. The adoption of strict lines of demarcation between curative and palliative approaches is considered inappropriate as disease-modifying treatments can be used palliatively to make the day-to-day management of a wound easier, enhancing quality of life[5,15]. Treatment selection is based on balancing effects that will cause minimal harm and maximum benefit to the patient.

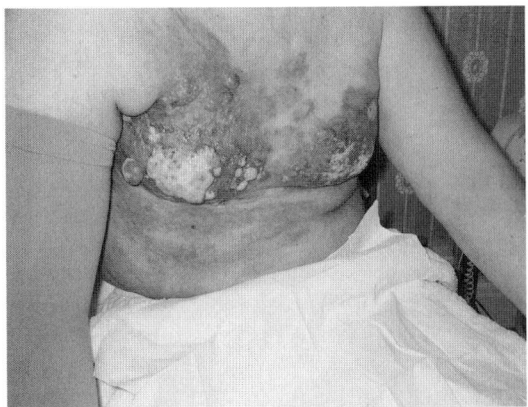

Figure 10.7.2.4 Ulcerating and fungating breast tumour.

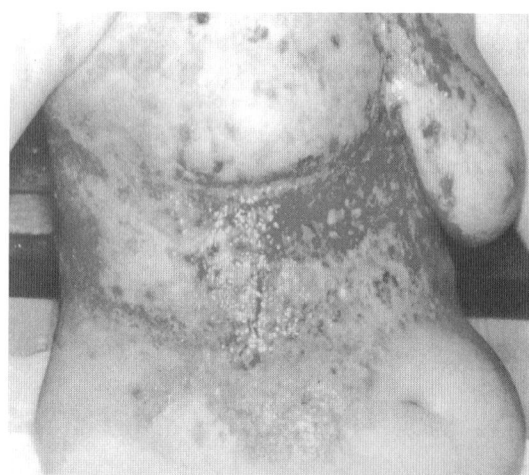

Figure 10.7.2.5 'En cuirasse' fungating breast cancer.

Fungating tumours that are sensitive to conventional anti-cancer treatments can be resolved to the point of healing. Unfortunately, tumour recurrence with fungation is not uncommon. Without treatment, fungation can extend catastrophically and is associated with significant co-morbidity.

Management requires a team approach with the patient and their family central to planning and decision-making. The psychological, social, and spiritual impact of advancing disease is covered in other chapters. The nursing care of patients with these wounds is complex, requiring skills in a range of specialisms, for example stoma care, continence care, lymphoedema management, nutrition and parenteral feeding, symptom control, and tissue viability.

Fungating wounds have a significant impact on the individual, the family and health service resources, over a potentially lengthy period. Crucially, these wounds can be a source of revulsion for all concerned. The individual with the wound may lose their sense of self with gradual separation from family and friends in the face of disfigurement, uncontrolled body fluid, and malodour[16]. Clinicians can share such revulsion whilst also hiding their feelings to minimize distress[17]. Conversely, as we will illustrate in the following case study, a patient with an advancing fungating wound (Fig. 10.7.2.6) can experience positive care outcomes[18].

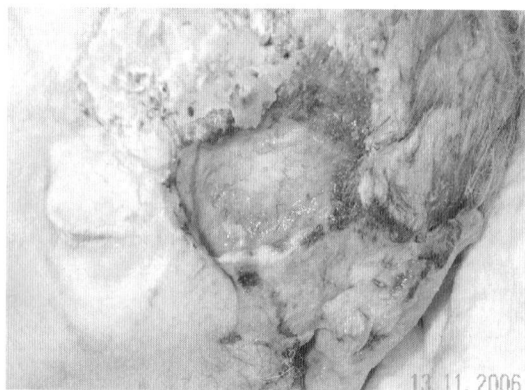

Figure 10.7.2.6 Advanced fungating facial wound across the left side of the face.

Case study

Overview

Joe was a 78-year-old man with a squamous cell carcinoma of the left temple. In March 2004, the carcinoma was excised. Skin was grafted on to the site and he received postoperative radiotherapy. The grafted area became chronically infected and the graft failed to take.

In May 2005, there was local disease recurrence and he was diagnosed with a second primary in the lung (non-small-cell lung cancer). He was given palliative radiotherapy and chemotherapy.

His medical notes indicated ongoing problems with infections and the need for regular dressings. Joe lived with his wife, his daughter, and grandchildren. In June 2006, Joe was referred to his local community palliative care team by his general practitioner (GP). He had been for an oncology appointment and he had been told that there were no more options available to treat either of his two cancers. His GP wanted assistance with pain and symptom management.

It was clear at first assessment that one of Joe's biggest problems was his wound management. A different nurse was arriving each day to do the dressings, which meant there was no continuity for Joe. Most days, the outer dressing fell off soon after the nurse's visit. Joe's distress was profound. His young grandson now refused to go near his grandfather due to the smell and appearance of the wound—'grandad looked scary'.

In addition to the dressing problems, there were personal hygiene problems. Joe had not had a shower or hair wash for 6 months: he and his family were anxious about causing trauma and pain to the wound. He was admitted to the hospice just over 2 weeks before his death for wound care and symptom management.

Fig. 10.7.2.6 shows the wound on admission. In the centre of the image is a crater about the size of a golf ball and in front of the crater there is a collection of dead skin. The tumour had eroded through the left side of his face and into the temporal bone. His hair and his beard were matted with dried exudate. On the right of the image you can see the ear. The tumour had advanced into his ear—he was now deaf in that ear. Just below the ear a small sinus had developed—this was discharging small amounts. This was the only painful area of the wound. He was also blind in the left eye and had a VIIth nerve palsy. His speech was quite badly affected and it was at times difficult to understand what Joe was saying.

Wound condition: advancing fungating wound with sinus formation, discharging progressively purulent exudate, malodorous.

Local wound management: dry, scaly scalp surrounding wound, immediate wound margins macerated by exudate; exudate, malodour; dressing fixation and stability between dressing changes.

Guided by the skin care algorithm (Fig. 10.7.2.2), interventions included attention to personal hygiene including the use of emollients to dry skin and scalp. Guided by the exudate management algorithm (Fig. 10.7.2.12), fibrous absorbent cavity dressings were applied, covered by a non-adherent silicone mesh dressing, with an additional large dressing pad secured with a tubular bandage. A complete dressing change was effected on alternate days with additional changes of the dressing pad if strikethrough (exudate breeches the surface of the pad) occurred. Figures 10.7.2.7–10.7.2.9 illustrate the dressing system.

Symptom management: the fungating tumour was advancing with increasing impact on vital structures and function of the left

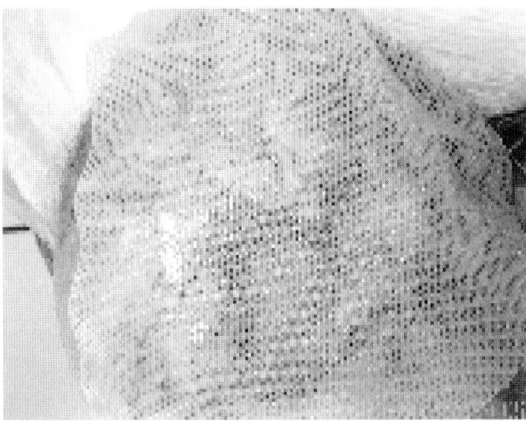

Figure 10.7.2.7 Silicone mesh dressing.

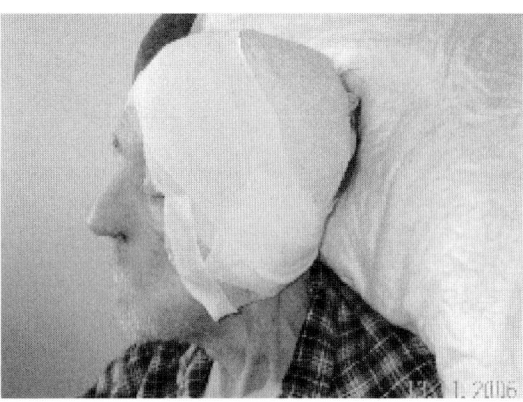

Figure 10.7.2.9 Modified tubular bandage.

side of Joe's face, including loss of sight and hearing. Localized pain at wound site exacerbated at dressing changes. The risk of a serious bleed was high because of the location and inward tumour invasion. The intervention for symptom management included an oral opioid spray at dressing changes.

Fig. 10.7.2.10 is a graphical representation of the outcomes of local wound and symptom management over 12 days. According to the TELER system, the scale is 5 to 0, where 5 is the optimal management goal[3]. Joe's view of the wound was that it was *better* following the interventions, even though it was advancing rapidly. Fig. 10.7.2.10 illustrates how palliative interventions can improve a patient's quality of life whilst the disease process (in this case, a fungating lesion) rapidly advances.

Joe's grandson came to visit him in the hospice a number of days before his death. He was able to crawl up on to Joe's knee and give him a cuddle. He then visited each day until Joe's death.

Principle II: local wound management

As illustrated in the above case study, wound dressings in conjunction with symptom management can significantly relieve the physical and psychosocial problems, and the overall impact of the wound[18]. There are however limitations in the performance of dressing systems currently available for the extensive wounds that fall within the remit of palliative care.

Local wound management is determined by the location, size, and shape of the wounds together with presenting problems.

Current practice in wound care, including the manufacturing focus for wound dressings, is substantially based on Winter's theory of moist wound healing. It explains the profound influence on epithelialization of restricting the evaporation of water from the wound surface[19]. It does not explain the management of advanced wounds[20].

Tissue hypoxia in pressure ulcers and fungating wounds is a significant factor in local wound management because of the consequential loss of tissue viability, necrosis, and odour. The activity of anaerobic bacteria, which proliferate in these hypoxic conditions, combined with facultative aerobic species is attributed to the characteristic symptoms of malodour and another distressing symptom, profuse exudate. Exudate represents a further consequence of loss of vascularity and necrosis. Exudate production is also attributed to bacterial enzymes (proteases) and their assistance in the autolytic processes of tissue breakdown and liquefaction[21].

Wound bed preparation (WBP) is a framework for chronic wound care that is increasingly adopted in clinical care[22]. Fig. 10.7.2.11 illustrates the components of wound bed preparation applied to wound management in palliative care.

Essentially WBP is a framework for managing the local wound environment, including clinical signs of bacterial overload, infection, the state of wound tissue, exudate, and the peri-wound skin. The rationale underpinning WBP is that if healing is the goal, the wound bed needs to be free of bacteria and harmful enzymes that may delay healing. If palliation is the goal, clearance of dead tissue and management of bacterial overload, for example, can reduce odour and exudate, and damage to the peri-wound skin. Correction of cellular dysfunction and cellular imbalance refers to a number of factors that include cell senescence and the over expression of

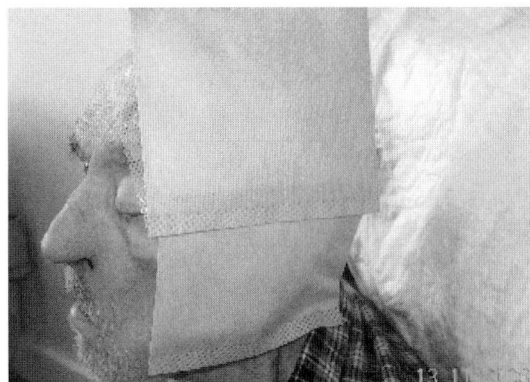

Figure 10.7.2.8 Super absorbent pads.

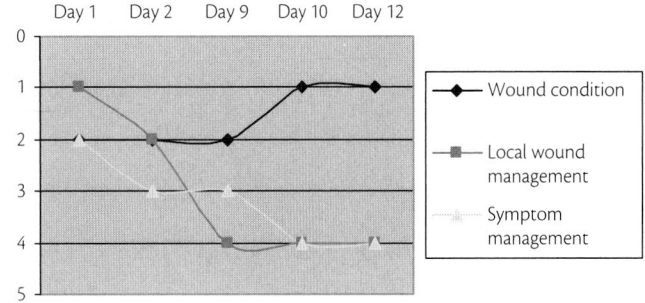

Figure 10.7.2.10 Graph illustrating the case study outcomes.

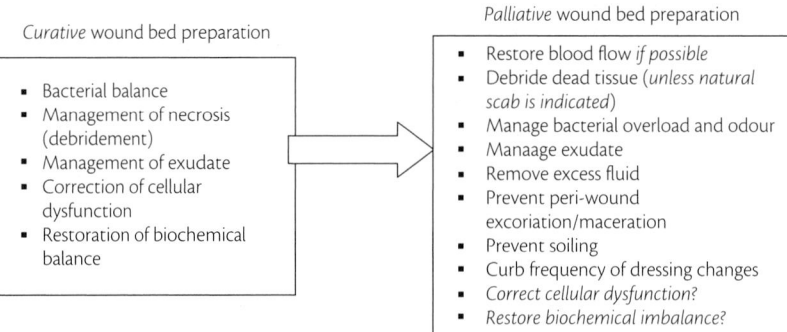

Figure 10.7.2.11 Components of wound bed preparation applied to palliative wound care.

proteolytic enzymes. Enzyme imbalance can apparently be corrected with advanced wound products such as topical protein-ase modulating agents. However, dysfunction at the cellular level is challenging to address in practical and measurable ways, and the evidence base for the effectiveness of these agents, which are costly, remains weak. The approach we are proposing emphasises the removal of dead tissue (unless preservation of natural scab is indicated) and the control of symptoms such as exudate and odour (see Figs. 10.7.2.12 and 10.7.2.16 in the section below).

Debridement of dead tissue

Dead tissue is unsightly and a focus for bacteria. Bacteria metabolize dead tissue and the by-products of this metabolism are malodorous[13]. This is a natural autolytic process of dead tissue removal. A number of methods have been advanced to speed the removal of dead tissue. These include surgical, sharp, larval, enzymatic, and mechanical methods[22]. Debridement in long term wounds

will need to be repeated. Therefore, careful attention needs to be paid to the choice of method, so that it minimizes side effects and is acceptable to the patient. In addition, the clinical gains to the individual patient need to be assessed critically. For example, patients with extensive wounds covered with scab may not benefit from debridement if life expectancy is short and the consequent exudate profuse. In these circumstances, the aim will be to maintain a dry wound environment.

The use of honey dressings to debride and deodorize a range of extensive, complex wounds, including fungating lesions, has been reported[23]. For some patients, the introduction of honey into a wound can be painful, attributed to the osmotic pull exerted by the honey on fluid and tissues within the wound. The pain may be transient as the honey liquefies. However, for some patients, this symptom is intolerable and alternative debriding agents such as hydrogels or iodine preparations will be indicated. Because honey promotes autolysis, the devitalized tissue is liquefied and separated

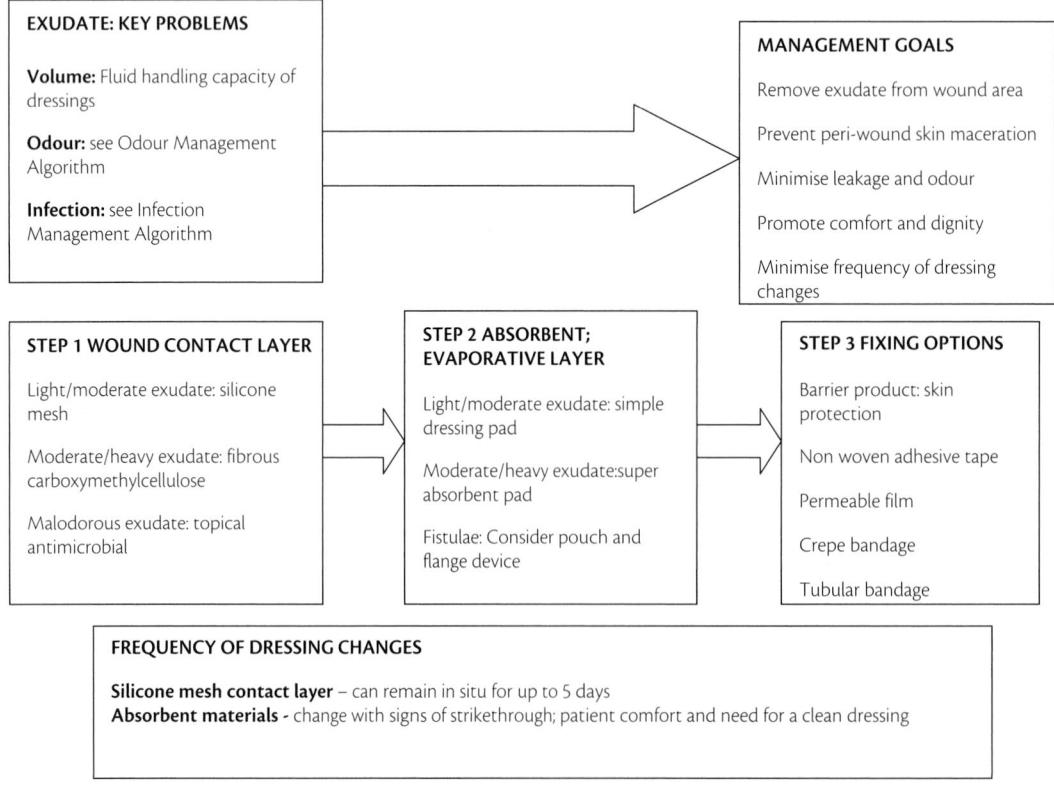

Figure 10.7.2.12 St Christopher's Hospice Exudate Management Algorithm©.

Code 5	No exudate leakage* between routine/planned dressing change
4	Exudate leakage within 24 hours of next dressing change
3	Exudate leakage within 18 hours of next dressing change
2	Exudate leakage within 12 hours of dressing change
1	Exudate leakage within 8 hours of dressing change
0	Exudate leakage within 2 hours of dressing change

* exudate leakage = strike through

Figure 10.7.2.13 Exudate leakage (daily dressings).

from the wound bed. This exudate has to be contained with wound dressings otherwise the patients experience a further unpleasant problem or the aggravation of an existing problem. The management of exudate is discussed further in the following section.

Exudate

Without control of exudate, the physical and psychosocial impact of a wound is compounded by leakage, soiling, frequent dressing changes or re-padding, peri-wound maceration, and odour. Effective control of exudate substantially resolves the wound management problems, and patients can regain a degree of independence and control over their daily lives[4]. The algorithm at Fig. 10.7.2.12 sets out core activities relative to exudate management.

Currently, absorption is the main method of managing exudate. Reliance on absorption into moisture conserving dressing materials is not adequate, particularly when there is a lot of exudate and problems fitting dressings too extensive, or with eccentrically shaped wounds and curved body surfaces. Grocott's (2000) study indicates that breathable, high moisture loss materials manage exudate in a thin conformable system. The system is built up of membranes with the following three functions:

1 Conservation of surface humidity and moisture to prevent adherence and trauma.

2 Reservoir capacity for exudate that is excess to the purpose of (1).

3 High moisture vapour loss (HVML) through the back surface of the dressing to evaporate the water content of exudate.

To be effective, the system depends crucially on the fit of the dressing to the size and site of the wound, fast uptake of exudate, and fluid venting capacity. The choice of adhesives and the configuration of the adhesive on films and tapes are also critical to prevent skin stripping.[20]

The majority of dressings have moisture vapour loss (MVL) values that are considerably lower than 15 000 $g/m^2/24$ h and designed to conserve moisture, for example Opsite® (Smith and Nephew Limited) has a MVL of around 700 $g/m^2/24$ h.

The fluid handling systems included in the algorithm (Fig. 10.7.2.12) are based on the functions described above but are limited by the bulk of dressing pads. A recent addition to the portfolio of dressings available in the UK is indicative of a promising shift towards fluid handling via moisture loss systems. The new products need to be evaluated clinically in relation to their fluid handling properties. The pre-sized, pre-shaped presentations of the products may limit their applicability to eccentrically shaped and extensive wounds. However, in principle, they appear to constitute an advance on existing absorbent and moisture conserving dressings with respect to fluid handling properties.

As previously mentioned, there are circumstances when a dry wound environment is the kindest option for the patient. At the time of writing, research is in progress in the UK to evaluate *dry* wound management, actively promoting scab formation.

Fistula management

The management of fluid from fistulae is particularly challenging with immense variation in presentation between patients. A fistula is an abnormal track that communicates between two hollow organs. An enterocutaneous fistula is a connection between a hollow organ and the skin. There are multiple causes of fistulae, for example they may develop as a complication of surgery, infection, radiotherapy, and progressive malignant disease.

The nursing care of patients with fistulae follows substantially the principles of stoma care. These principles are listed below and the reader is referred to the relevant chapter on stoma management in this textbook and the following reference[24].

Summary of the principles of fistula management

- Prevention of skin excoriation with barrier products.
- Collection of effluent in closed stoma devices or wound manager devices.
- Management of odour in a closed device; the use of odour-neutralizing sprays when bags are emptied and changed.
- Nutrition and fluids to maintain a balance between intake and loss, which may require enteral or parenteral feeding.
- Supportive care to protect the patient's sense of self, autonomy and ability to socialize.

The location and advancement of the fistula may however preclude the application of a stoma device. Clinicians are challenged in these circumstances to find novel approaches to manage the lesions. Custom built solutions need to be found using stomahesive pastes to which a drainage bag(s) can be attached. Alternatively, it may be possible to fit silicone mesh dressings over a fistula. The dressing, which can be left *in situ* for 3–4 days, unless clogged with debris, can assist in directing the flow of fluid, whilst preserving the integrity of the skin, into a super absorbent pad with a waterproof backing. The pads will need to be fixed with an adhesive, waterproof tape or film to avoid leakage. Given that the pads will need to be changed several times a day, when heavily soiled, but not saturated, the skin under the adhesive needs to be protected with a barrier product.

Principle III: symptom management

Symptom management measures are both systemic and local. The measures focused on in this chapter are predominantly linked to local wound management. The key issue here is that the management of advanced wounds is complex and requires an interdisciplinary approach. The patients need to be referred to palliative care teams who have specialist knowledge and expertise in the art and science of symptom control. In addition to textbooks such as this, there are a number of useful resources, including web-based ones, which share current best practice in both the management of wounds, and symptom management, for example the SIGN and PRODIGY guidelines and the Palliative Care Formulary[25–27].

Symptoms specifically related to the wound include: pain, soreness, and irritation from excoriated skin, pruritis, odour, spontaneous bleeding, and haemorrhage. Frequently, more than one problem needs to be managed at a given time. For example it is

The pain experienced by a patient in relation to a chronic wound may have a number of causes. Before deciding if the pain is opioid sensitive, and therefore suitable for management with topical opioids, a number of factors need to be considered. Please consider the following questions and circle your responses. This process should help you to clarify and justify your decision whether to use or not use topical opioids for the management of the patient's wound pain.

1. Does the patient experience the wound pain only when the dressing is removed?

YES   NO

If you answered YES, the dressing is probably sticking to the wound, causing pain on removal. The dressing needs to be changed to a non adherent dressing, then re-evaluate the pain problem before you proceed to topical opioids.

2. Does the patient experience the wound pain when they move?

YES   NO

If you answered YES, the dressing may be tugging or causing friction. Revise your dressing plan, and re-evaluate the pain problem before getting topical opioids prescribed.
The pain may also be caused by unrelieved pressure, in which case you need to devise a re-positioning regime and provide pressure relief.

3. Is the wound heavily exuding?

YES   NO

If you answered YES the surrounding skin may be becoming damaged, irritated, sore/stinging and macerated by the exudate. You need to apply an alcohol free barrier product. You need to repeat the applications at <u>every dressing change,</u> covering all the skin that may be affected by the exudate. Review the pain problem once you have established this routine for at least 3 days before topical opioids are used.

4. Are you using adhesive dressings and tapes?

YES   NO

If you answered YES the pain may be due to the removal of the dressings and tapes. Consider using a tapeless garment or tubular bandage. If this is not possible, apply a barrier product to the skin to which you are applying the adhesive product. Review the pain problem once you and your colleagues have established this routine, before proceeding to topical opioids.

5. Are you using gauze products?

YES   NO

If you answered YES the wound may be drying out. When this happens, the nerve endings can be stimulated and cause pain. If you apply a moisture-conserving dressing the wound will become moist and the pain may be relieved.

6. Are there signs of clinical infection of the surrounding tissues with irregular redness radiating from the wound, stabbing pain, skin that is hot to the touch, increased odour and exudate, and where the patient is febrile and less well? *

YES   NO

If you answered YES, the pain may be caused by cellulitis, which is bacterial invasion of the surrounding skin. Do a wound swab and commence the appropriate antibiotic treatment and the pain should subside as the infection subsides.

7. Is the wound a full thickness cavity wound?

YES   NO

If you answered YES, the pain may not be due to the wound itself because the nerve supply to the wound may be lost. Review the above possible causes to determine the source of the pain.

AFTER YOU HAVE REVIEWED THE ABOVE, TAKEN THE PROPOSED ACTIONS THAT WERE APPROPRIATE FOR THE PATIENT CONCERNED AND THE PAIN PERSISTS, CONSIDER THE FOLLOWING:

8. Is the pain from the wound constant and unrelieved?

YES   NO

If you answered YES, a topical opioid is probably indicated.
If the patient has cellulitis and cannot take antibiotics, consider topical metronidazole gel, and consider prescribing topical opioids. The opioid can be safely incorporated into metronidazole gel.

If you are applying topical opioids, follow the hospice protocol and consider the following system to apply over the wound. The reason for suggesting this is to avoid absorbing the opioid gel into the dressing. The silicone mesh has a water repellent silicone layer, which may help to leave the opioid in the wound, where it is needed:

• Non adherent silicone mesh and a simple gauze pad. The mesh should not be changed at every dressing change. As long as the tiny holes are not clogged with debris, the dressing can be peeled back, the wound cleaned, the topical opioids applied, the dressing arranged back and the pad applied.

You may have to use super absorbent pads, or alginates and foams because of heavy exudate. In this case you may need to titrate the amount of opioid required and the frequency of the applications to reach a therapeutic effect for the individual patient. It is important to remember that a dressing change disturbs the wound and may aggravate the pain, or cause the wound and surrounding skin to deteriorate further by the dressing/tape removal. Conversely, leaving wet dressings on a wound may aggravate the pain problem. All of this means that you need to observe what is happening to the dressings, and listen to the patients' accounts of their pain carefully.

Figure 10.7.2.14 Decision-making for the selection of topical opioids for the management of painful wounds ©King's College London. * see Fig. 10.7.2.17.

well known that wounds can bleed, can be malodorous and painful. If the wounds become infected, problems of pain, odour and bleeding are exacerbated, the wound extends, and the frequency of dressing changes increases, including the amount of product required[28]. Accurate diagnosis and treatment can reduce the severity of the problems.

Pain

The causes of pain may be multiple, and include emotional factors. Pain associated with pressure ulcers and fungating wounds is generally of a mixed aetiology. Patients can experience stinging, burning, aching and sharp pain, depending on the size, position, and nature of the wound. Some will have no pain at all, others just at dressing changes, whilst some will have constant pain.

Pain management requires careful assessment, administration of combinations of drugs, monitoring of pain levels and emotional support[25,29]. Analgesia can be given systemically or locally. For pain at dressing changes, a short acting analgesic can be administered and repeated if the dressing change is lengthy.

Topical opioids are useful for pain and stinging from damaged and ulcerated skin[30]. Opioids were considered to act systemically until receptors were identified in inflamed peripheral tissues[31]. Krajnik and Zylicz observed that the analgesic effect of topical morphine is achieved at low doses. They concluded that it is unlikely that the effect is mediated systemically[32,33]. In a single case study, local pain management was similarly achieved at low doses[34]. This needs further research before recommendations can be made. Fig. 10.7.2.14 offers a decision-making tool for identifying the circumstances where topical opioids may be indicated. Fig. 10.7.2.15 is a clinical indicator for monitoring and evaluating the outcomes of interventions for local pain management.

Soreness and irritation from macerated and excoriated skin conditions

As already indicated in relation to a weakened skin barrier, exudate and body fluids cause predictable and inevitable damage to the skin in the form of inflammation, pruritis, and progressive damage to the tissues. The interventions indicated earlier are applicable to the prevention and treatment of maceration and excoriation from exudate in relation to pressure ulcers and fungating wounds. To maintain skin integrity, interventions need to cover the area of skin that is vulnerable, repeating the process at dressing and pad changes.

Cutaneous, pruritic irritation (see Chapter 10.6)

This form of irritation is quite distinct from the irritation caused by maceration. It is a creeping, intense itching sensation attributed to a number of diseases and disorders, for example tumours and liver disease. Inflammatory breast disease with cutaneous infiltration is a particular example. Pruritis can be extremely disabling and difficult to treat[35] and is discussed in detail in Chapter 10.6. It is worth considering non-pharmacological interventions, for example

significant relief from the intensity of pruritis was achieved with the use of TENS (transcutaneous electrical nerve stimulation)[34]. The application of TENS involves a degree of trial and error. It is therefore important to involve experts in the administration of this treatment[36] (see Chapter 10.1.11).

Odour

A number of approaches are adopted for the management of odour, including systemic antibiotics, topical antimicrobials, and charcoal dressings. In addition, debridement of the dead tissue harbouring the bacteria can improve the performance of antimicrobials, or render them unnecessary. The algorithm at Fig. 10.7.2.16 aids decision-making and gives additional measures that can assist when odour is difficult to bring under control. A key issue here is that there are limitations to absolute control of odour, which may be attributable to the size and eccentric shape of the wounds, the liquefaction of dead tissue, and the management of consequent exudate. Therefore, additional, creative measures may be required to minimize odour for patients and families, and to support front line clinical staff.

Systemic antibiotics

These are used to reduce bacterial colonization and control the offensive odour from volatile metabolic end-products. One of the limitations of systemic antibiotics is the increasing incidence of antibiotic resistance[38]. A further limitation is their side effects, though these may be avoided at low doses without losing the therapeutic effect on the odour[27].

Topical antimicrobials

Topical agents, such as metronidazole gels and silver impregnated dressings, are alternatives to systemic antibiotics, though they tend to be more expensive[13,39]. There are practical issues around the application of topical agents and dressings to extensive wounds to achieve sufficient inhibitory concentration of the active ingredients of the agents to deodorize. The issues include the size of the wounds and a lack of tissue penetration to bacteria located below the surface. In addition the site of the wound, for example the perineum, may limit the efficacy of topical gels, which are absorbed into dressings and pads.

Debridement of dead tissue

The rationale for removal of dead tissue has been covered in the section on local wound management.

Adsorption of volatile malodorous chemicals by charcoal cloth

Activated charcoal dressings act as filters to absorb the volatile malodorous chemicals from the wound, before they pass into the air[40]. They must therefore be fitted as a sealed unit or these chemicals simply escape into the air. Air tight charcoal garments may overcome this limitation when the wounds are extensive or sited in body curves that are difficult to dress[41]. In addition, charcoal is

Code 5	Pain controlled by the medicine
4	Aware of pain about 30 minutes before the next dose
3	For about an hour I was waiting for the next dose because of pain
2	Relief for about 2 hours after taking/applying the medicine, then the pain returned
1	Some relief after taking/applying the medicine, but it did not last long (less than 1½ hours)
0	Pain not controlled by the medicine

Figure 10.7.2.15 Clinical indicator: wound pain due to underlying disease—effectiveness of medications.

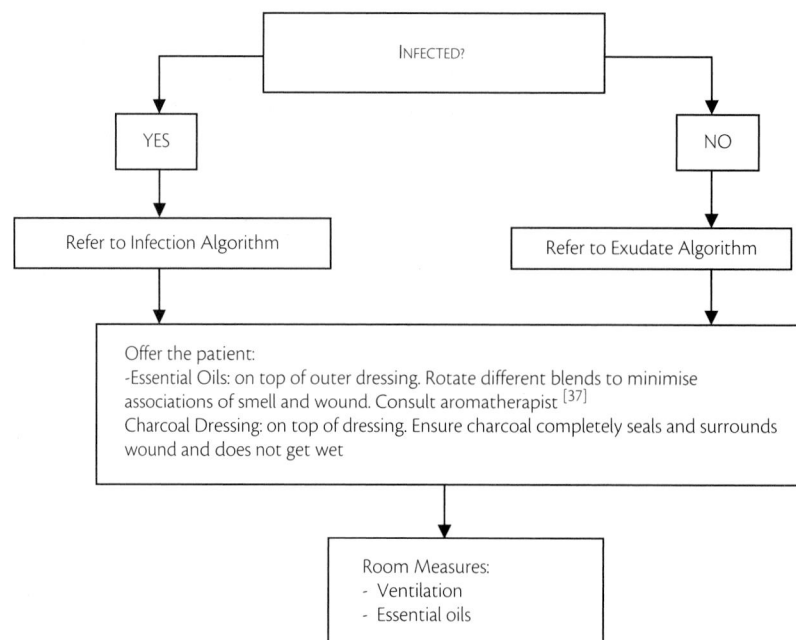

Figure 10.7.2.16 St Christopher's Hospice Odour Management Algorithm©.

inactivated if it becomes wet; therefore, the dressings need to be applied as the outer dressing, and changed if wet.

Infection

As with other interventions in wound care, the aim is to provide maximum comfort and minimum distress to the patient. If a wound is showing no signs of improvement, and the patient's condition is sufficiently good to allow for wound healing, heavy bacterial colonization and infection may be root causes. The algo-rithm at Fig. 10.7.2.17 guides decision-making when wound infec-tion is suspected. Signs of local infection, advancing redness of the skin with heat for example, are sufficient to consider the wound infected, and to initiate topical anti-microbial dressing products. It may not be necessary or indicated to take a wound swab if the patient's prognosis is short, particularly if they are unable to take oral antibiotics.

Systemic medication of proven sensitivity to the culture from the wound swab is otherwise indicated for the management of infection

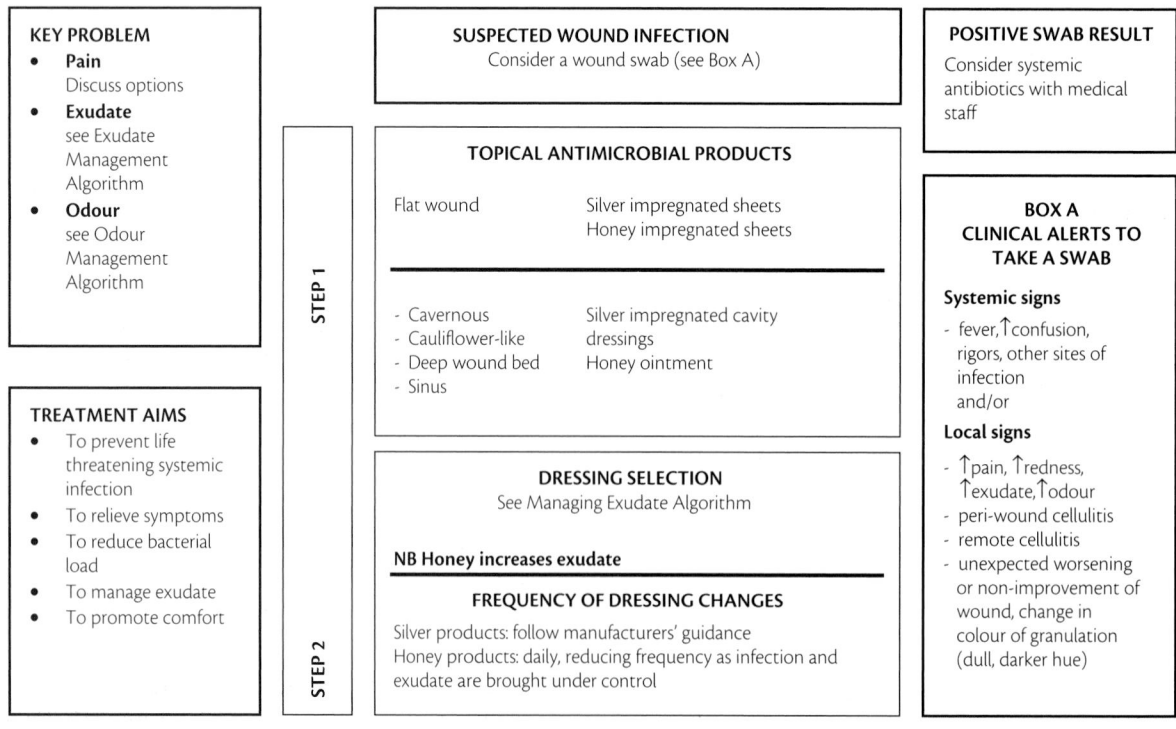

Figure 10.7.2.17 St Christopher's Hospice Wound Infection Management Algorithm©.

as bacteria have invaded local tissues. Topical agents can additionally help to reduce the microbial load on the wound, and assist the management of exudate and odour (see Fig. 10.7.2.17).

The role of wound dressing in infected wounds is threefold: to contain the infection and prevent contamination to and from the wound, to keep anti-microbial agents in contact with the wound, and to contain exudate and odour.

Some of the advanced dressings, for example silver impregnated products can be left *in situ* for several days as they are designed to release the active antimicrobial agent over a specified time period. The manufacturers' guidance assists decisions around frequency of changes when using these products. Exudate levels will however dictate the frequency of changes required on an individual basis.

Bleeding

On rare occasions, tumours will erode a major vessel, causing a fatal bleed. These situations are extremely distressing to witness and manage. Death will normally occur within a few minutes and the patient will lose consciousness some time before that.

Attention to the following can reduce the incidence of more minor bleeding at the dressing changes: dressing application and removal techniques, maintenance of humidity at the wound/dressing interface, and cleaning techniques.

Particularly for fungating wounds, when capillaries are visible on the surface of fungating wounds, mechanical damage and bleeding can occur with fibrous materials such as alginates[42]. Alternative non-fibrous systems include silicone wound contact dressings with dressing pads, or gel sheets. In addition, radiotherapy is used to control spontaneous bleeding from eroding blood vessels. It is therefore important to have contacts with oncology centres for rapid patient referrals for emergency control of bleeding. Topical measures such as adrenaline 1:1000 may be useful. Surgical haemostatic sponges (e.g. Spongostan®: Johnson & Johnson Ltd.) are alternative, practical emergency measures for controlling fast capillary bleeding, though they are expensive on a unit cost basis. Sucralfate suspension is advocated by some palliative care specialists as a cost-effective alternative[43].

Conclusions

Wound management in palliative care can be complex and is an interdisciplinary responsibility drawing on colleagues who can contribute specific knowledge, skills, and experience to problem-solve for the patients. Effective management is based on treatment of the underlying cause wherever possible, local wound care and control of associated symptoms. These are crucial to the physical and psychological well-being of the patients and families. There remain significant limitations in the design and presentation of dressings for extensive wounds, particularly in relation to exudate management, which need further research and development.

Further reading

Grocott, P., Browne, N., and Richardson, A. (2003). Palliative wound care: Optimising the use of classification systems. *Polish Palliative Medicine*, **2**, 222–32.

Le Roux, A.A. (1993). TELER: The Concept. *Physiotherapy*, **79**,11, 755–59.

Naylor, W. (2001). Assessment and management of pain in fungating wounds. *BJN (Supplement)*, **10**, S33–58.

Naylor, W., Laverty, D., and Mallet, J. (eds.). (2001). *The Royal Marsden Handbook of Wound Management in Cancer Care*. Blackwell Science, London.

White, R.J., Cooper, R.A., and Molan, P. (eds.). (2005). *Honey: A Modern Wound Management Product*. Wounds UK, Glasgow. (Sponsored by Avancis Medical Limited).

References

1. Ennis, W.J. and Meneses, P. (2005). Palliative care and Wound care: 2 emerging fields, with similar needs for outcomes data. *Wounds*, **19**, 99–104.
2. Dealey, C. (2005). Managing wounds. In *Care of Wounds A Guide for Nurses*, 3rd edition. pp. 72–6. Blackwell Publishing. Oxford.
3. Browne, N., Grocott, P., and Cowley, S. *et al.* (2004). Woundcare research for appropriate products (WRAP): Validation of the TELER method involving users. *IJNS*, **41**, 559–71.
4. Grocott, P., Browne, N., and Cowley, S. (2005). Quality of life: Assessing the impact and benefits of care to patients with fungating wounds. *WOUNDS: A compendium of clinical research and practice*, **17**, 8–15.
5. Pearson, I.C. and Mortimer, P. (2004). Skin problems in palliative medicine: Medical aspects. In *The Oxford Textbook of Palliative Medicine*, (eds. D. Doyle, G. Hanks, N. Cherny, and K. Calman), 3rd edition. pp. 618–28. Oxford University Press, Oxford.
6. Chaplin, J. (2000). Pressure sore risk assessment in palliative care. *Journal of Tissue Viability*, **10**, 27–31.
7. Lafferty, A.M. (2003). *An exploration of nurses views on the use of soap and water to cleanse patients' skin after episodes of incontinence in a palliative care inpatient setting - a research proposal*. Unpublished BSc Dissertation. University of London.
8. Grocott, P. and Dealey, C. (2004). Skin problems in palliative medicine: Nursing aspects. In *The Oxford Textbook of Palliative Medicine*, (eds. D. Doyle, G. Hanks, N. Cherny, and K. Calman), 3rd edition. pp. 628–39. Oxford University Press, Oxford.
9. NICE (2001). *Pressure Ulcer Risk Assessment and Prevention*. London, National Institute of Health and Clinical Excellence,
10. Salisbury Health Care. (2004). Policy and guidelines for the prevention and management of pressure sores.
11. Reid, J. and Morrison, M. (1994). Towards a consensus: Classification of pressure sores. *JWC*, **3**, 157–60.
12. Rotimi, V. and Durosinmietti, O. (1984). The bacteriology of infected malignant ulcers. *Journal of Clinical Pathology*, **37**, 592–95.
13. Thomas, S. and Hay, N.P. (1991). The anti microbial properties of two metronidazole medicated dressings to treat malodorous wounds. *The Pharmaceutical Journal*, **246**, 261–66.
14. Haisfield-Wolfe, M.E. and Baxendale-Cox, L.M. (1999). Staging of malignant cutaneous wounds: A pilot study. *Oncology Nurse Forum*, **26**, 1055–64.
15. Hoskin P.J. (2004). Radiotherapy in symptom management. In *The Oxford Textbook of Palliative Medicine*, (eds. D. Doyle, G. Hanks, N. Cherny, and K. Calman), 3rd edition. pp. 239–55. Oxford University Press, Oxford.
16. Lawton, J. (2000). *The Dying Process: Patients' experiences of palliative care*. Routledge, London.
17. Wilkes, L.M., Boxer, E., and White, K. (2003).The hidden side of nursing: Why caring for patients with, malignant malodorous wounds is so difficult. *JWC*, **12**, 76–80
18. Lund-Nielsen, B., Muller, K., and Adamsen, L. (2005). Qualitative and quantitative evaluation of a new regimen for malignant wounds in women with advanced breast cancer. *JWC*, **14**, 69–73.
19. Winter, G.D. (1962). Formation of the scab and the rate of epithelialisation of superficial wounds in the skin of the young domestic pig. *Nature*, **193**, 293–4.

20. Grocott, P. (2000). The palliative management of fungating malignant wounds. *JWC*, **9**, 4–9.

21. Cutting, K.F. and Harding, K. (1994). Criteria for identifying wound infection. *JWC*, **3**, 198–201.

22. Vowden, K. and Vowden, P. (2002). Wound bed preparation. *World Wide Wounds*, URL at http://www.worldwidewounds.co.uk. Last accessed 13 September 2006.

23. Molan, P. (2006). The Evidence Supporting the Use of Honey as a Wound Dressing. *The International Journal of Lower Extremity Wounds*, **5**, 40–54.

24. Pringle, W. (1995). The management of patients with enterocutaneous fistulas. *JWC*, **4**, 211–13.

25. Scottish Intercollegiate Guidelines Network (SIGN). Guidelines. URL at: http://www.sign.ac.uk/guidelines/fulltext/44/section5.html. Last accessed 22 November 2006.

26. PRODIGY Guidance. URL: http://www.prodigy.nhs.uk/patient_information/pils/malignant_skin_ulcers.htm. Last accessed 22 November 2006.

27. Twycross, R., Wilcock, A., Charlesworth, S. *et al.* (2002). *Palliative Care Formulary PCF1*, 2nd edition. Radcliffe Medical Press, Oxford.

28. Cooper, R. and Molan, P. (1999). The use of honey as an antiseptic in managing Pseudomonas infection. *JWC*, **8**, 161–9.

29. Wiles, J., Rutter, D., Exton, L. *et al.* (2004). Management of pain. In *Management of Advanced Disease*, (eds. N. Sykes, P. Edmonds, and J. Wiles), 4th edition. pp. 175–205. Arnold, London.

30. Flock, P. (2002). Pilot study to determine the effectiveness of diamorphine gel to control pressure ulcer pain. *Journal of pain and symptom management*, **25**, 547–54.

31. Stein, C. (1994). Interaction of Immune-Competent Cells and Nociceptors. In *7th World Congress on Pain*, (eds. G. Gebhardt, D.L. Hammond, and T.S. Jensen), pp. 285–97. IASP Press, Seattle, USA.

32. Krajnik, M. and Zylicz, A. (1999). Potential use of topical opioids in palliative care—Report of six cases. *Pain*, **80**, 121–25.

33. Krajnik, M. and Zylicz, Z. (1997). Topical morphine for cutaneous cancer pain. *Palliative Medicine*, **11**, 326.

34. Grocott, P. (2000). Palliative management of fungating malignant wounds. *Journal of Community Nursing*, **14**, 31–40.

35. Thorns, A. and Edmonds, P. (2004). Pruritis. In *Management of Advanced Disease*, (eds. N. Sykes, P. Edmonds, and J. Wiles), 4th Edition. pp. 207–13. Arnold, London.

36. Bercovitch, M. and Waller, J.W. (2004). Transcutaneous Nerve Stimulation (TENS). In *The Oxford Textbook of Palliative Medicine*, (eds. D. Doyle, G. Hanks, N. Cherny, and K. Calman), 3rd edition. pp. 405–10. Oxford University Press, Oxford.

37. Mercier, D. and Knevitt, A. (2005). Using topical aromatherapy for the management of fungating wounds in a palliative care unit. *JWC*, **14**, 497–501.

38. Dunford, C., Cooper, R., Molan, P. *et al.* (2000). The use of honey in wound management. *Nursing Standard*, **15**, 63–8.

39. Thomas, S., Fisher, B., Fram, P.J. *et al.* (1998). Odour-absorbing dressings. *JWC*, **7**, 246–50.

40. Sibbald, G.R., Meaume, S., Kirsner, R.S. *et al.* (2005). Review of the clinical RCT evidence and cost effectiveness data of a sustained-release silver foam dressing in the healing of critically colonised wounds. *World Wide Wounds*, URL at: http://www.worldwidewounds.com. Last accessed 12 September 2006.

41. Suarez, F.L., Springfield, J., and Levitt, M.D. (1998). Identification of gases responsible for the odour of human flatus and evaluation of a device purported to reduce this odour. *Gut*, **43**, 100–4.

42. Grocott, P. (2004). Malignant Wounds. In *Management of Advanced Disease*, (eds. N. Sykes, P. Edmonds, and J. Wiles), 4th edition. pp. 295–305. Arnold, London.

43. Regnard, C. and Hockley, J. (2003). *A Guide to Symptom Relief in Palliative Care*, 5th edition. Radcliffe Medical Press. Oxford.

10.7.3 **Lymphoedema**

Vaughan Keeley

Introduction

Lymphoedema is a chronic oedema developing as a result of failure of the lymphatic system to drain fluid and other substances from the tissues. It typically affects the limbs but can involve any part of the body. It can result from damage to the lymphatic system by injury, surgery, radiotherapy, cancer, and infections ('secondary lymphoedema'), or can occur because of maldevelopment of the lymphatics ('primary lymphoedema').

The management of all types of lymphoedema is largely palliative in nature in that there are no surgical or other treatments that offer a cure for the problem in the vast majority of cases. In the UK, most lymphoedema services are provided by palliative care services and hospices[1]. Some of these treat only cancer-related lymphoedema (either treatment-related or due to active disease), whereas others treat all types of lymphoedema and other chronic oedemas, e.g. those related to venous disease.

In light of this, this chapter will consider all types of lymphoedema but will focus on cancer treatment-related lymphoedema and oedema associated with advanced cancer and chronic diseases.

Classification

Pure lymphoedema arises as a result of failure of the lymphatic system draining a particular area. This may be the situation in many primary lymphoedemas, e.g. Milroy's disease (see below). However, in many other situations, the oedema often occurs as a result of a number of coexisting factors, e.g. a mixture of lymphatic and venous disease such as in the chronic dependency oedema seen in people with immobility who spend much of their time sitting in a chair. Even in situations once thought to be pure lymphoedemas such as that resulting from the treatment of breast cancer, there is evidence that these are multifactorial in origin with changes in both arterial and venous flow contributing to the development of swelling as well as damage to the lymphatic system[2]. Equally, in oedemas once thought to be entirely venous in origin, e.g. that associated with venous leg ulcers, there is evidence of a lymphatic component[3].

Thus in clinical practice pure lymphoedema is probably quite rare. To take this into account, the term 'chronic oedema' has been used in a recent epidemiological study of the prevalence of 'lymphoedema'[4]. 'Chronic oedema' is 'a broad term used to describe oedema which has been present for more than 3 months and involves one or more of the following areas: limb/s, hands/feet, upper body (breast, chest, shoulder, back), lower body (buttocks, abdomen), genital (scrotum, penis, vulva), head, neck, or face. Oedema which develops as a result of failure of the lymphatic system is referred to as lymphoedema but chronic oedema may have a more complex underlying aetiology'[4].

From a practical clinical viewpoint, it is still useful to classify chronic oedemas according to the predominant abnormality, e.g.:

♦ Lymphoedema (primary and secondary).

♦ Venous oedema.

- Lymphovenous oedema.
- Oedema of advanced cancer.

In the oedema of advanced cancer, the swelling can have particularly complex aetiology, which may include:

- Lymphatic damage due to treatment or malignant lymphadenopathy.
- Venous obstruction due to extrinsic venous compression by tumour or by intrinsic obstruction by thrombosis or tumour, including that of large veins such as the superior vena cava or inferior vena cava.
- Hypoalbuminaemia.
- Lymphovenous malfunction due to immobility (dependency oedema).
- General fluid retention due to drugs, e.g. corticosteroids.

Primary lymphoedemas

Although the focus of this chapter is on lymphoedema associated with cancer or its treatment, primary lymphoedema will be considered briefly. There are many types of primary lymphoedema and comparatively little is known about most of them. What they have in common is that they are believed to be due an intrinsic developmental abnormality of part or occasionally all of the lymphatic system. Overt oedema may be present at birth or may develop around puberty or even later in life, depending upon the type. At first sight, it may seem difficult to consider a condition that presents in later life to be due to a developmental abnormality. However, it is postulated that in this situation, there may be a relatively minor developmental abnormality of the lymphatics, which in itself is insufficient to cause clinical oedema in early life. With aging, injury, or infection, relatively minor damage may mean that the transport capacity of the system is further reduced and overt swelling develops. Alternatively, some of what we, at present, consider to be primary lymphoedemas may in fact be 'secondary', but the extrinsic cause is not yet known.

Some primary lymphoedemas are inherited and in recent years there has been a growth in the knowledge of the genetics of these. Milroy's disease is one such condition. It is due to a mutation in the gene for VEGFR3 (vascular endothelial growth factor receptor 3)[5]. This receptor binds with VEGF (vascular endothelial growth factors) C and D, which are believed to be involved in the development of the lymphatic system. People with this mutation develop lower limb lymphoedema at or shortly after birth. The abnormality of the lymphatics is distal hypoplasia. There do not seem to be any associated abnormalities of other systems, although there is a high incidence of hydrocoeles in males with Milroy's disease.

Milroy's disease is inherited as an autosomal dominant condition with incomplete penetrance. However, some patients present with what seems to be Milroy's disease clinically but without a family history. It is likely that these patients may have new mutations. The term 'Milroy's disease' is sometimes used inaccurately to describe a wide variety of primary lymphoedemas. Therefore, current estimates of its prevalence are likely to be inaccurate.

Lymphoedema distichiasis is a rarer autosomal dominantly inherited lymphoedema. It is due to mutation of the FOXC2 gene. This codes for a transcription factor. Patients tend to develop lymphoedema around puberty but have distichiasis (the presence of a second aberrant row of eyelashes that tend to ingrow and irritate the eye) from earlier on. They also may have other problems reflecting the nature of the gene abnormality including cleft palate, varicose veins, and cardiac abnormalities[6]. It has been suggested that the lymphatic abnormality is maldevelopment of the valves that leads to incompetence and reflux (as with varicose veins).

Meige's syndrome is probably the most common type of inherited primary lymphoedema but the gene abnormality causing it has not yet been identified. It presents with leg oedema after puberty and may be associated with other abnormalities. However, it is possible that what we currently call Meige's syndrome may represent a number of separate conditions with different genetic abnormalities that have yet to be elucidated.

Chronic oedema: incidence and prevalence

In the past, in the UK, lymphoedema has been considered to be an uncommon problem about which little can be done to help. There has been little research carried out and little investment in the development of services to treat the problem. To date there has been no national strategy or framework for service development. A national project, 'the Lymphoedema Framework Project', is currently in progress to define the extent of the problem, assess the needs of patients, and develop models of service provision.

As an initial stage of this project, an epidemiological study of the prevalence of chronic oedema, as defined above, using a case ascertainment method was carried out[4]. This found a crude prevalence of 1.33/1000 in a population in south-west London. The prevalence increased with age, being 5.4/1000 in those over 65 years of age and 10.3/1000 in those over 85 years and was higher in women (2.15/1000) than in men (0.47/1000).

Although this technique did not differentiate between the various types of chronic oedema, it suggests that chronic oedema is more common than previously thought and is about as common as venous leg ulcers. Furthermore, the results provide a valuable basis upon which to calculate the likely health care needs of a population and plan services accordingly.

Incidence after cancer treatments

The incidence of lymphoedema following the treatment of cancer, particularly breast cancer, has been the subject of much research[7]. However, it is often difficult to compare the results of one series with another as there is no internationally agreed definition of what constitutes lymphoedema. For example, some studies of the incidence of arm oedema after the treatment of breast cancer define lymphoedema as a measurable difference in arm circumference or volume in the treated size compared with the untreated (e.g. >5 per cent or >10 per cent difference), whereas others compare the circumference or volume of the arm pre- and post-treatment (e.g. >100 ml or >200 ml increase). Furthermore, it is well recognized that arm oedema may take many years to develop after the treatment of breast cancer, particularly following radiotherapy, and so the length of follow-up of patients in different studies is likely to affect the incidence found. In addition, patients may develop oedema as a result of disease recurrence and so it is important to take these into account in studies of purely treatment-related oedema. Finally, in recent years, modifications to surgical and radiotherapy techniques have been introduced to reduce the

Table 10.7.3.1 Incidence of oedema following treatment for different cancers.*

Site of cancer	Site of oedema	Incidence reported (range)
Breast cancer	Arm	1–54%
Malignant melanoma (of leg)	Leg	6–80%
Genitourinary cancers	Leg/genital	10–100%
Gynaecological cancers	Leg	1–48%

*Derived from Ref. (7) (NB: breast cancer studies from 1995)

risks of developing post-treatment oedema whilst retaining an effective anti-cancer result, e.g. sentinel node biopsy in breast cancer treatment. Therefore, older studies may yield different results from newer ones.

Table 10.7.3.1 summarizes the incidence of post-cancer treatment oedema from a number of studies[7]. The wide ranges reflect the factors described above and make it difficult to use these figures in service planning.

Pathophysiology of chronic oedema

To understand the clinical features of and ways of treating different types of chronic oedema, it is helpful to consider the underlying pathophysiology. In the initial stages of oedema formation, there may be no clear distinguishing appearances, but as the oedema persists, skin and tissue changes occur.

Tissue fluid formation

The amount of fluid in the tissues depends upon the balance between fluid entering by capillary filtration and that leaving by lymphatic drainage. Under normal circumstances, the two are balanced and there is no build-up of fluid (oedema). If capillary filtration exceeds lymphatic drainage, then oedema develops[8].

Capillary filtration and lymphatic drainage

The amount of capillary filtration depends upon the so-called 'Starling forces' across the capillary wall.

♦ The hydrostatic pressure gradient across the capillary wall that tends to push fluid out of the capillary.

♦ Colloid osmotic (oncotic) pressure due to plasma proteins that tends to draw fluid into the capillary.

The net effect of these opposing forces, together with the permeability of the capillary wall, will determine the rate of flow out of the capillary. Fluid within the tissue (interstitial) space then drains away via the lymphatics. The flow into the lymphatics will depend upon similar forces.

The flow along the lymphatics is dependant upon a number of factors:

♦ An intrinsic 'pumping' effect of smooth muscle within the walls of larger lymph vessels, the direction of flow being determined by valves.

♦ Extrinsic compression of the lymphatics by skeletal muscle activity, similar to that which enhances venous flow.

Oedema formation

Oedema occurs when capillary filtration exceeds lymphatic drainage. This can occur in a number of circumstances:

♦ Failure of lymphatic drainage (lymphoedema). This can result from:
  • Maldevelopment of the lymphatics (primary lymphoedema).
  • Damage to the lymphatics from surgery, radiotherapy, infection, trauma, and cancer (secondary lymphoedema).
  • Malfunction of the lymphatics due to reduced extrinsic compression by skeletal muscles in conditions resulting in immobility, e.g. paraparesis (this causes a lymphovenous oedema as there will also be reduced venous drainage).

♦ Increased venous pressure (causing increased capillary hydrostatic pressure and capillary filtration rate) e.g. in:
  • Deep vein thrombosis and post-thrombotic syndrome.
  • Chronic venous hypertension secondary to varicose veins.
  • Heart failure.
  • Chronic immobility (see above).

♦ Hypoalbuminaemia (resulting in increased capillary filtration as the plasma colloid osmotic pressure is reduced) e.g. in:
  • Advanced cancer.
  • Nephrotic syndrome.

In some situations, e.g. in oedema in advanced cancer, several factors coexist and virtually all chronic oedemas have a lymphatic component. For example, in chronic venous hypertension, the increased capillary filtration results in increased flow in the lymphatic system, which clears more fluid from the tissues. It is only when the demand exceeds the maximum transport capacity of the lymphatic system that oedema develops (high output failure of the lymphatics). If the high flow in the lymphatics continues for a prolonged period, the lymphatics become damaged, resulting in a low output lymphoedema.

Tissue changes in chronic oedema

The above disturbances to the normal balance between capillary filtration and lymphatic drainage explain the immediate cause of fluid accumulation in the different types of oedema. However, in chronic oedema, changes occur in the tissues and skin, which give the characteristic clinical features of the different aetiologies.

In lymphoedema, the oedema that is soft and pitting initially becomes firmer and pits less easily. This is due to the accumulation of adipose tissue and fibrosis, which arises from a chronic inflammatory process[9,10].

In chronic venous oedema, chronic lipodermatosclerosis is a common finding along with ulceration. There is a loss of subcutaneous tissue with fibrosis, which typically distorts the shape of the leg causing the 'inverted champagne bottle' appearance[11].

In conditions with mixed aetiology, the skin and subcutaneous changes can also be mixed.

Clinical features

General features of lymphoedema

Lymphoedema can occur in any part of the body but is most commonly seen in the limbs. When it first develops, it is a soft pitting oedema but over time the swelling typically becomes firmer and it is more difficult to pit.

Skin changes

At first the skin appears normal or a little stretched but again with time various changes occur (Table 10.7.3.2). These skin changes are usually more obvious in leg lymphoedema than in the arm but can occur anywhere (see Fig. 10.7.3.1).

Pain

The limb often feels heavy and the skin stretched or tight. Patients may experience pain, which is often described as an ache, tightness, or heaviness rather than a severe sharp pain[12]. Typically the pain is worse when the swelling is worse, e.g. towards the evening in active patients with leg lymphoedema. In addition, the weight of the limb can cause pain at its root, e.g. shoulder pain in patients with arm oedema.

Impaired mobility/use of limb

Lymphoedema can impair the use of a limb by the weight of the swelling making it more difficult to move or by causing stiffness due to firm swelling around the joints. This is particularly problematic in the leg with stiffness of the ankle joint resulting in restricted contraction of the calf muscles and thus impairment of the muscle pump, which would normally aid lymphatic and venous flow. This in turn exacerbates the swelling.

Psychological aspects

Many patients experience significant distress as a result of their lymphoedema[13]. This may include alteration of body image, loss of independence, loss/change of employment, and difficulty in finding suitable clothes and shoes to wear.

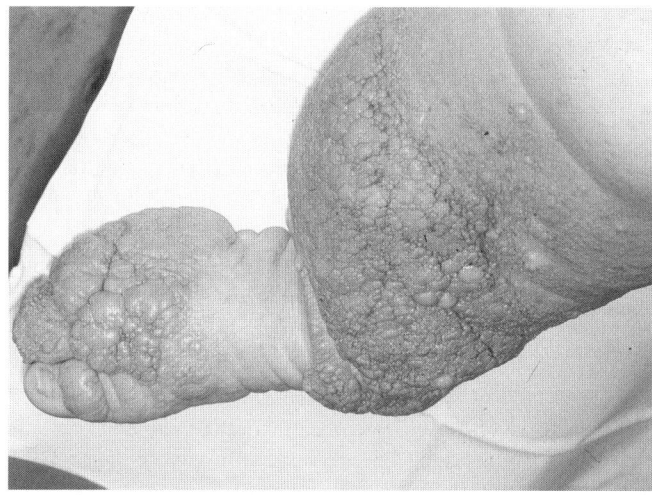

Figure 10.7.3.1 Severe skin changes in a lymphoedematous leg.

It can be particularly difficult for patients who have undergone treatment for cancer, e.g. mastectomy, hair loss from chemotherapy, to face another disfigurement in the form of post-treatment oedema.

Specific situations

Breast cancer treatment-related oedema

Following surgical and radiotherapy treatment for breast cancer, arm oedema can develop almost immediately or following many years[14]. Initially, women often notice a change in how the arm feels and this may occur before overt pitting oedema is present. Sometimes precipitating factors are reported, e.g. an infection or strenuous exercise such as gardening or decorating.

Understandably the woman may be concerned that the appearance of swelling may represent recurrence of the cancer. Indeed, sometimes this is the case and assessment of a woman who develops arm oedema following breast cancer treatment should include examination and, if necessary, appropriate investigations, e.g. ultrasound examination of the axilla to exclude or confirm suspected recurrence.

The part of the arm affected by oedema is variable. Sometimes it is the hand only, sometimes the forearm and upper arm with the hand spared, sometimes mainly around the elbow and sometimes the whole arm including the hand and fingers.

In women who have had a mastectomy, the chest wall can become oedematous. This can be remarkably painful. Women who have had a wide local excision of the cancer and post-operative radiotherapy may develop breast oedema.

Advanced breast cancer

Oedema in advanced breast cancer can be particularly distressing. It can occur as a result of recurrent disease in the axilla, when it may be associated with a brachial plexopathy, which, by causing paralysis of the arm, can exacerbate the swelling.

In addition, metastatic cancer can develop in the skin of the chest wall (cancer en cuirasse) and upper arm. This tends to obstruct the skin lymphatics and may cause gross oedema of the arm with the skin becoming tense, stretched, and fragile. In these circumstances, the limb can become useless, very heavy, and painful. The fingers and hand can become very deformed and may look like a 'boxing glove'.

Table 10.7.3.2 Typical skin changes in lymphoedema.

Skin change	Description
Skin thickening	
Hyperkeratosis	Build up of the horny layer of the skin
Lymphangiectasia	Dilated lymph vessels that appear on the skin surface like small blisters, which if damaged can leak lymph (lymphorrhoea)
Papillomata	These skin lesions are similar to lymphangiectasia but also contain fibrous tissue, giving them a firmer consistency; they often occur in groups producing a cobblestone-like appearance to the skin
Increased skin creases particularly around the joints	These can become very deep in severe swelling causing deformity of the limb
Chronic inflammation	This leads to erythema of the skin and can be similar to the chronic lipodermatosclerosis seen in venous disease
Stemmer's sign (usually positive)	This is the inability to pick up a fold of skin at the base of the second toe in lymphoedema of the leg and reflects the skin and subcutaneous tissue changes described above. In normal toes Stemmer's sign is negative i.e. one can pickup a fold of skin at the toe base

The skin can break, leading to profuse lymphorrhoea and predisposing to infection and ulceration (Fig. 10.7.3.2).

The extreme nature of the oedema in this situation is probably explained by the combination of damage to the deeper lymphatics by surgery, radiotherapy, and possibly tumour and damage to the superficial skin lymphatics by tumour. It is believed that the superficial lymphatics act as collateral system of drainage when the deeper system is damaged, a process exploited by the compression and massage techniques used in the treatment of lymphoedema. When these are blocked by tumour, the collateral route is no longer available and so severe oedema develops. There may be additional factors such as extrinsic compression of the axillary vein that can contribute to the swelling.

Advanced pelvic and abdominal cancer

Gross oedema of the legs, genitalia and abdomen can occur in patients with advanced pelvic and abdominal cancers. The clinical features may include

◆ soft, pitting, or firm oedema of the legs;

◆ stretched, shiny, fragile skin;

◆ lymphorrhoea;

◆ ulceration;

◆ genital oedema—scrotal, penile, and vulval;

◆ pitting oedema of the abdominal wall;

◆ ascites;

◆ dilated veins on the abdominal wall in inferior vena caval obstruction (IVCO);

◆ Stemmer's sign may be negative.

There may be no skin changes typical of chronic lymphoedema, unless there has been a preceding treatment-related oedema.

Gross oedema can severely restrict mobility. Patients may be unable to walk, climb stairs, get up from a chair, or lift their own legs on to their bed. This may exacerbate existing problems resulting from the muscle weakness of advanced cancer. Patients may find the appearance of their limbs and genitalia difficult to cope with. Furthermore, in men, penile oedema may lead to problems with micturition and sexual function. It may be difficult to insert a catheter per urethram, if needed, and so sometimes a suprapubic catheter is necessary.

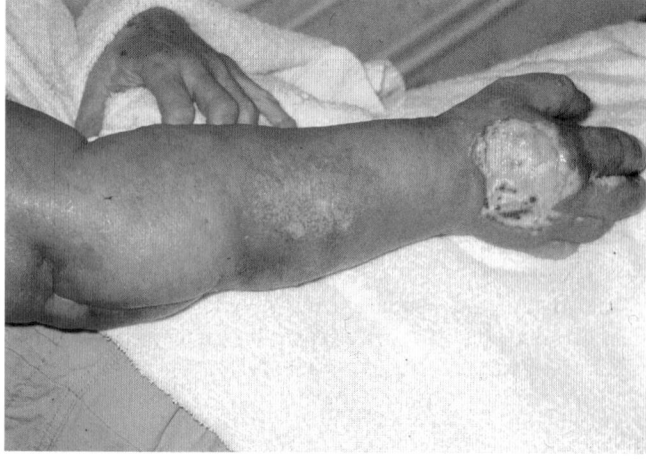

Figure 10.7.3.2 Arm oedema in locally advanced breast cancer.

Differential diagnosis and investigations

Differential diagnosis

Making a diagnosis in chronic oedema relies on the conventional method of a history, examination, and appropriate investigations. The causes of chronic oedema are summarized in Table 10.7.3.3. This is not an exhaustive list and reference to general medical texts is suggested for a more detailed discussion of the causes of oedema. In many patients, there may be multiple factors contributing to the overall picture of oedema. Some common clinical scenarios are

◆ Fluid retaining drugs e.g. NSAIDs in an elderly patient with chronic lymphovenous oedema secondary to immobility due to an inflammatory arthritis.

◆ An element of chronic heart failure in an immobile patient with chronic leg oedema.

◆ Cyclical oedema in a woman with primary lymphoedema.

One type of non-oedematous limb enlargement is worthy of further more detailed discussion here, as it is quite commonly seen in lymphoedema clinics, probably because it presents as a non-pitting swelling. This is lipoedema.

Lipoedema

Lipoedema is a type of lipodystrophy, a lipohypertrophy. There is a bilateral, symmetrical enlargement of the legs and lower half of the body usually from the hips down to the ankles due to an abnormal

Table 10.7.3.3 Causes of chronic oedema.

General causes
Heart failure
Hepatic disease, e.g. cirrhosis
Renal disease, e.g. nephrotic syndrome
Drugs, e.g. corticosteroids, calcium channel blockers, non-steroidal anti-inflammatory drugs (NSAIDs)
Endocrine conditions, e.g. hypothyroidism, cyclical oedema in women

Local causes:
I. Lymphatic: primary and secondary lymphoedema
II. Venous disease:
a. Post-thrombotic syndrome
b. Chronic venous disease
III. Mixed aetiology:
a. Lymphovenous disease e.g. secondary to chronic immobility e.g. due to paraplegia, chronic respiratory disease
b. Oedema of advanced cancer

Non-oedematous limb enlargement*
I. Lipoedema
II. Limb hypertrophies:
a. In congenital vascular malformations such as Klippel–Trenaunay syndrome
b. Hemihypertrophy
III. Tumours e.g. lymphangiomas, lipomas, neurofibromas

* May be associated with superadded oedema

deposition of fat[15] (Fig. 10.7.3). The feet are not involved. It tends to develop around the time of puberty and seems to almost exclusively affect women. There may be a family history in some patients.

There is usually no oedema but some women do develop pitting oedema of the feet and ankles (sometimes known as lipolymphoedema). Stemmer's sign is negative. Patients commonly experience pain in the lower leg, with tenderness of the shins and a tendency for easy bruising of the legs. Characteristically, when the patient tries to lose weight, she often reports that fat may go from the top part of the body (trunk and arms) but remains unchanged in the legs.

Investigations

In many patients, the history and examination will give the diagnosis and further investigation is unlikely to be necessary. However, even in apparently straightforward cases, e.g. in a woman with arm oedema following treatment for breast cancer, contributing factors such as deep venous thrombosis or even disease recurrence need to be considered and investigated if necessary.

Investigations that may be helpful in the assessment of chronic oedema are shown in Table 10.7.3.4. The choice of investigations, if any, will depend upon the initial clinical assessment. Other investigations may be necessary to confirm that it is safe to carry out planned compression treatments, e.g. arterial brachial pressure index (ABPI) or arterial ultrasound studies to investigate possible peripheral vascular disease.

In the early stages of the development of chronic oedema, the characteristic skin and subcutaneous tissue changes may not be present, and so the clinical features may not be diagnostic. The combination of lymphoscintigraphy and colour Doppler ultrasound in the assessment of leg oedema of unknown cause has been

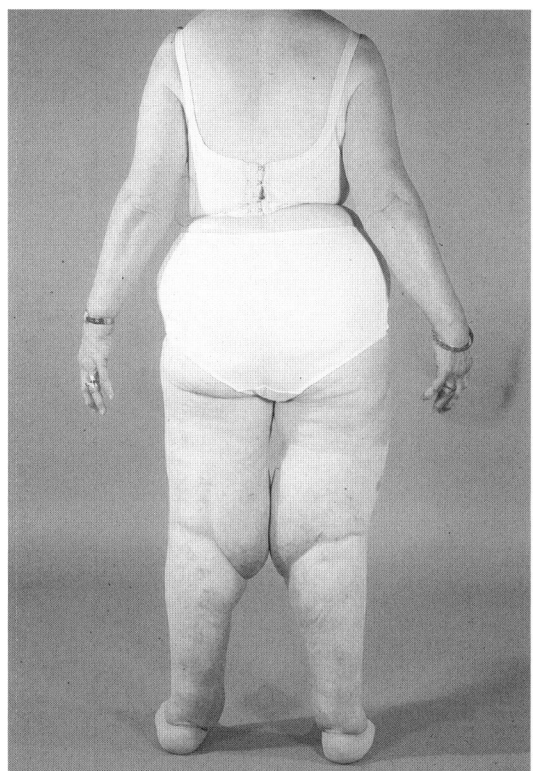

Figure 10.7.3.3 A patient with lipoedema.

Table 10.7.3.4 Investigations that may be used in the assessment of chronic oedema.

Investigation	To assess
Blood tests	
Full blood count	Anaemia
Urea and electrolytes	Renal function
Liver function tests	Hepatic disease
Plasma proteins	Hypoalbuminaemia
Brain natriuretic peptide (BNP)	Heart failure
Ultrasound examinations	
Venous system	Venous disease, incompetence, thrombosis
Abdomen	Intra-abdominal disease e.g. malignancy
Axilla/breast	Breast cancer recurrence
Lymphoscintigraphy	Lymphatic function
CT/MR scans	Underlying malignancy

shown to establish the diagnosis in >80 per cent of patients[16]. Lymphoscintigraphy can be particularly useful in the assessment of patients with probable primary lymphoedema[17]. A detailed discussion of the technique of isotope lymphoscintigraphy is beyond the scope of this chapter but can be found in Ref. 17.

Treatment

General principles

The current management of lymphoedema and other chronic oedemas, e.g. lymphovenous oedema, is largely based upon a combination of physical techniques:

◆ compression;

◆ massage;

◆ exercise;

◆ skin care.

This approach is known by various terms, e.g. decongestive lymphatic therapy (DLT), combined decongestive therapy (CDT).

Although there is evidence that the combination of these techniques is effective in reducing the volume of limb oedema and the incidence of cellulitis in chronic lymphoedema[18], there are few reports on the effectiveness of each component[19]. As a consequence, an international consensus approach has recently been taken to produce a guidance document, 'Best practice for the management of lymphoedema'[20].

Compression

Compression is a key component of management. It is provided in a number of ways: bandaging, elastic compression garments, and intermittent pneumatic compression pumps, although the last is not frequently used in routine management.

Multi-layer lymphoedema bandaging (MLLB)

This technique comprises a series of layers of bandage applied to a swollen limb, which creates a graduated compression with the pressure reducing from the distal to proximal part of the limb. The layers consist of:

◆ Finger or toe bandaging.

◆ A tubular bandage which provides a protective layer to the skin.

◆ A soft synthetic wool or foam which protects the skin, 'normalizes' the shape of the limb and facilitates the distribution of pressure provided by the other layers.

◆ Inelastic bandages that produce relatively low pressures at rest but which increase on exercise.

Compression bandages need to be applied by skilled trained practitioners as, if incorrectly used, they may cause damage to the skin and subcutaneous tissues.

They are particularly useful for the initial management of lymphoedema to reduce swelling and improve limb shape before applying an elastic compression garment. They are also used if there is broken, ulcerated, or fragile skin and for the control of lymphorrhoea. Skin changes, e.g. hyperkeratosis and papillomatosis, can be improved with MLLB.

Contraindications to MLLB are shown in Table 10.7.3.5. In some circumstances, MLLB can be applied with a lower pressure and careful monitoring to minimize the risks, e.g. in peripheral vascular disease (ABPI <0.5), in controlled heart failure (where, in addition, one limb may be bandaged at a time), in diabetic peripheral neuropathy, and following cellulitis.

In patients with oedema of advanced cancer and lymphorrhoea, a modified lower pressure 'palliative bandage' can help control symptoms of heaviness and leakage.

Elastic compression garments

Graduated elastic compression garments are used in the long-term management of lymphoedema and other chronic oedemas. They are available 'off the shelf' or 'made to measure' and in a number of different strengths of compression. The classification of compression strength is different in different countries and so it preferable to describe compression strength in terms of mmHg rather than Class 1, 2, 3, etc. The choice between the different compression strengths depends upon the cause of the oedema and what can be tolerated by the patient. High compression i.e. 50-60 mmHg may be needed for a primary lymphoedema of the legs but inevitably higher compression garments are more difficult to put on and take off. Therefore, sometimes a lower compression garment may need to be used at the expense of less good control of the oedema. This is particularly true for elderly or frail patients who usually need help to apply the garments and so the availability of carers to do this becomes an additional consideration.

Contraindications to using compression garments are shown in Table 10.7.3.6. Successful use of compression garments requires skilled measurement, fitting, monitoring of effectiveness, and timely replacement as the garments lose elasticity with regular use.

Intermittent pneumatic compression (IPC) pumps

The use of intermittent compression pumps has largely 'gone out of fashion' in the management of lymphoedema in the UK. They are believed to reduce capillary filtration rather than improve lymph drainage. Multichamber devices that inflate in a sequential fashion provide a massage effect from the distal part of the limb to the proximal. They are said to be more effective in oedemas associated with immobility, and venous disease. However, there is little evidence to guide their most appropriate use. It is important to use compression garments/bandaging as part of the management plan, as any improvement in swelling following a treatment session can rapidly reverse if not. Contraindications include acute DVT, thrombophlebitis, acute cellulitis, uncontrolled heart failure, pulmonary oedema, and peripheral vascular disease. IPC can exacerbate swelling at the root of the limb or in the trunk.

Massage techniques

Manual lymphatic drainage (MLD)

This is a technique of light superficial massage that improves lymphatic drainage. It is carried out by trained professionals as part of a programme of management, usually combined with other modes of treatment particularly compression. The concept behind the technique is that it encourages collateral flow around damaged/absent lymphatics by stimulating superficial lymphatic drainage away from congested areas. There is little research evidence to support its use but it is valued by patients and therapists. It seems to be particularly useful in the management of midline oedemas such as breast, trunk, genital, and head and neck oedema and where there is swelling at the root of an oedematous limb. These are all areas where it is difficult to create effective compression garments.

MLD is said to be contraindicated in acute cellulitis, severe heart failure, renal failure, hypertension, ascites, superior vena caval obstruction, around primary tumours, and metastases[19]. In the latter, it is felt theoretically possible that MLD facilitates metastatic spread. However, in the oedema of advanced cancer, MLD may be helpful in providing symptomatic relief. In this situation, it seems reasonable to use MLD if the benefit is likely to outweigh the risks and the patient gives informed consent.

Table 10.7.3.6 Contraindications to the use of compression garments.

Contraindication	Reason
Arterial insufficiency	Exacerbation of problem
Acute heart failure	
A distorted limb shape with deep skin creases	Damage to skin increasing the risk of infection
Ulceration	
Lymphorrhoea	
Numbness, e.g. peripheral neuropathy	

Table 10.7.3.5 Contraindications to MLLB.

Contraindication	Reason
Severe arterial insufficiency	Exacerbation of problem
Uncontrolled heart failure	
Numbness of skin, e.g. due to peripheral neuropathy	Damage to skin and risk of infection
Acute cellulitis	Painful

There are various 'schools' of MLD techniques but a typical procedure would involve the following:

♦ Diaphragmatic breathing (to improve thoracic duct flow).

♦ Gentle massage to unaffected areas of the body first (to improve drainage here).

♦ Gentle massage from proximal to distal in the affected limb with the massage strokes being in a proximal direction (to clear fluid from the proximal parts so that they can receive the fluid moved subsequently from the distal areas).

Simple lymphatic drainage

This is a technique based upon MLD but which patients and carers can be taught to apply themselves. Again there is little research base for this but many patients seem to find it helpful. It is usually carried out daily and the patient or carer needs to be motivated to do it regularly. Contraindications to SLD are the same as for MLD.

Skin care

The aim of skin care is to maintain the integrity of the skin and minimize the risk of infection. The routine use of moisturisers such as Aqueous cream is recommended for all patients. Other conditions such as eczema and Athlete's foot should be treated appropriately.

Exercise

Muscular activity is known to improve lymphatic and venous drainage. However, there is little evidence to guide the best exercise for individual patients with lymphoedema. It is usually suggested that patients carry out normal activity whilst wearing compression garments. Specific exercises for patients with joint stiffness may be recommended following a physiotherapy assessment. It is commonly recommended that some activity such as heavy lifting is avoided as it is believed this may exacerbate the oedema.

Phasing of treatments

Patients with moderate to severe oedema are usually managed by an initial 'intensive phase' of treatment of approximately 2 weeks duration consisting of

♦ MLLB;

♦ ± MLD;

♦ skin care;

♦ exercises as appropriate.

This is followed by a 'maintenance phase' of

♦ elastic compression garment;

♦ ± SLD;

♦ skin care;

♦ exercises as appropriate.

It has been shown that MLLB as an initial phase of treatment for moderate to severe unilateral lymphoedema followed by hosiery achieves a greater and more sustained reduction in limb volume than hosiery alone[21]. The place of MLD and SLD is less clear. Studies have shown that the addition of MLD to MLLB may give an added reduction in volume (mean = 27 ml)[22] and MLD may also produce a greater volume reduction when compared to SLD

(mean = 39 ml)[23]. It is not known whether these small differences are of clinical significance.

Patients with mild oedema and no distortion of limb shape may go straight to the 'maintenance phase'. Mid-line oedemas are mainly managed with MLD and SLD.

Outcome measures

The conventional outcome measure for the treatment of lymphoedema of the limbs used in the UK is an improvement in limb volume. Limb volumes may be measured by a tape measure method or an opto-electronic device (e.g. Perometer). In the former, a series of circumferences is measured along the limb and these are converted into an estimated volume.

However, it is recognized that this approach is limited and the introduction of other measures, such as an improvement in the skin condition, a reduction in the firmness of subcutaneous tissues, a reduction in the incidence of cellulitis, and the use of a condition-specific quality of life measure, should give a better indication of the effectiveness of treatments[24].

In patients with oedema in advanced cancer, the aims of treatment are usually different and therefore other measures of symptom improvement such as the relief of pain may be more relevant.

Other treatments

Surgical treatments for lymphoedema are rarely carried out in the UK. Genital oedema as part of a primary lymphoedema in men is sometimes treated by reduction surgery. One group in Sweden has pioneered the use of liposuction in the management of breast cancer treatment-related arm oedema where physical treatments have failed[25]. Limb volume reduction is good but patients need to continue to wear compression garments to prevent the accumulation of fluid.

Drug treatments also have little place in management. Diuretics, e.g. furosemide, seem to be ineffective in lymphoedema, although they may have a place where there is also fluid retention, e.g. due to drugs. Benzopyrones have been advocated by some but the evidence for their effectiveness is mixed[26] and the risk of side effects, e.g. hepatic toxicity, is such they are not generally used in the UK.

Management of oedema in advanced cancer

The general principles of symptom management in palliative care can be applied to oedema in advanced cancer:

♦ Determining the underlying cause(s).

♦ Considering potentially reversible factors including psychosocial issues.

♦ Deriving treatment options, taking into account likely prognosis.

♦ Ensuring the burdens of treatment do not outweigh the benefits.

♦ Enabling patients and their carers to make an informed decision.

Potentially reversible factors and their treatment are summarized in Table 10.7.3.7.[27] Details of a number of these approaches can be found elsewhere in this book or in a textbook of general medicine. Some factors, e.g. hypoalbuminaemia, are difficult to reverse.

Corticosteroids can sometimes be helpful in relieving lymphatic and extrinsic venous obstruction. It is usual to give a trial of high dose steroids, e.g. dexamethasone 6 mg twice daily for 1 week to assess effectiveness. After this, the drug can either be discontinued

Table 10.7.3.7 Potentially reversible factors in oedema of advanced cancer and their management.

Factor	Possible management
Anaemia	Blood transfusion
DVT	Anticoagulation
Ascites	Paracentesis, diuretics
Fluid retaining drugs	Discontinue if possible, diuretics
SVCO	Metal stent[28], corticosteroids + radiotherapy, chemotherapy
IVCO	Corticosteroids, stent
Heart failure	Diuretics, digoxin, ACE inhibitors, etc.
Lymphadenopathy	Corticosteroids, anticancer treatment

if ineffective or 'down-titrated' to the minimum effective dose, balancing benefit against unwanted effects.

If there are no reversible factors or the unwanted effects of treatment outweigh the benefits, then a purely symptomatic approach may be necessary. This may include:

♦ Analgesia.

♦ Skin care.

♦ Modified, supportive bandaging for comfort, or controlling lymphorrhoea.

♦ Shaped tubular bandage, e.g. Tubigrip if unable to tolerate an elastic compression garment.

♦ Support and positioning, e.g. the use of a Lancaster sling to support a paralysed swollen arm with a brachial plexopathy.

♦ Passive movements to help reduce stiffness.

♦ Gentle massage techniques (MLD, SLD).

♦ Aids to mobility and function.

The skin is often very fragile in patients with advanced disease and the oedema can be very extensive and so the physical management techniques described above need to be modified accordingly. The aim of treatment is comfort rather than limb volume reduction.

Some patients, e.g. those with advanced breast cancer, may have associated fungating lesions. If bandaging is applied to an oedematous arm with an ipsilateral fungating breast lesion, there may be an increase in any discharge from the lesion. This can be distressing for patients and it is important to warn them about this possibility.

Needle drainage of oedema

There has recently been renewed interest in the physical drainage of oedema fluid in patients with advanced cancer. A good symptomatic response has been reported in eight patients with severe oedema using subcutaneous needles draining into a closed bag system[29]. No patients developed an infection but the median survival was only 2 weeks. There would normally be concerns about introducing needles into a lymphoedematous limb because of the risk of infection and worsened swelling. However, this technique may have a place in selected patients with advanced cancer, a short prognosis, and severe symptomatic oedema that has been unresponsive to other conventional approaches.

Complications of lymphoedema and their treatment

Cellulitis

Clinical features

Patients with lymphoedema are more prone to developing skin infections in the affected limb (cellulitis)[30]. The typical clinical presentation is the onset of 'flu-like symptoms that may include malaise, fever, myalgia, nausea, vomiting, and headaches. This usually precedes symptoms in the affected limb, which can include pain, redness, and increased swelling. On examination, the patient may have a red, warm, tender swollen limb, or part of the limb. There may be lymphangitis, lymphadenitis, and in severe cases the skin may blister and desquamate in places. In very severe cases, this may progress to necrotising fasciitis.

This classical presentation is, however, not seen in many patients who may have a variety of different rashes in the affected limb and variable systemic symptoms.

There may be evidence of a likely portal of entry of infection, e.g., a scratch or cut, insect bite, skin cracking due to Tinea pedis (Athlete's foot), an ingrowing toenail, dermatitis, etc. However, in many cases, there is no obvious source. It has been postulated that in some cases the infection arises at a distant site, e.g. tonsillitis.

The cause of most of these infections is believed to be the Group A Streptococcus but it is not easy to prove this with swabs or blood cultures. Indeed, the degree of uncertainty as to the aetiology of these episodes has led to them also being known as 'acute inflammatory episodes' (AIEs). Some episodes may be inflammatory rather than infective but because of the often rapid progression of symptoms that can result in hospital admission for i.v. antibiotics, it is usual practice at present to treat them all as infective.

The differential diagnosis includes acute deep vein thrombosis (DVT), acute inflammatory skin conditions such as eczema and acute lipodermatosclerosis arising from acutely increased venous pressure. The propensity to develop these infections is believed to be related to a local immune paresis in lymphoedematous limbs, as normally functioning lymphatics are an essential part of the local immune response to infection[31].

Management

Treatment is aimed at the Group A beta-haemolytic Streptococcus. Many patients who present early can be managed with oral antibiotics and rest at home but some with severe cellulitis may need to be admitted to hospital for IV antibiotics, either at presentation or if their condition progresses despite appropriate oral antibiotics.

There is no research evidence at present as to the best antibiotic regimen but recently a group of UK clinicians has produced a 'consensus' guideline[32]. The recommended antibiotics are shown in Table 10.7.3.8. It is worth taking swabs from any area of broken skin but the results may be unhelpful. Blood tests (white cell count, erythrocyte sedimentation rate [ESR], and C-reactive protein [CRP]) may be helpful in monitoring progress as is marking and dating the edge of the rash/erythema.

Bed rest seems to improve the rate of recovery. Compression garments used to treat the lymphoedema may need to be removed temporarily because of discomfort but, ideally, this should be for as short a time as possible. The use of lower strength compression or bandages should be considered. Massage should be avoided in the acute episode.

Table 10.7.3.8 Antibiotic treatment for cellulitis in lymphoedema.

1. *Management at home*
a. Amoxicillin 500 mg 8 hourly
b. Clindamycin 300 mg 6 hourly, if allergic to penicillin or if not responding satisfactorily to amoxicillin after 48 h
c. Flucloxacillin 500 mg 6 hourly may be added if there is a suspicion of a staphylococcal infection e.g. folliculitis, crusted dermatitis
Antibiotics should be continued for at least 14 days or until signs of inflammation have resolved.
2. *Management in hospital*
a. Amoxicillin 2 g 8 hourly IV or benzylpenicillin 1200–2400 mg 6 hourly IV
b. Clindamycin 600 mg 6 hourly—if penicillin allergic or if poor response to amoxicillin after 48 h
Antibiotics can be changed to the oral route when temperature is normal for 48 hrs. and the inflammation is much resolved.

NB Local hospital antibiotic guidelines may determine the choice of regimen

Recurrent cellulitis

Some patients may suffer from repeated bouts of cellulitis. There may be an underlying reason, e.g. recurrent Tinea pedis, ingrowing toenail, eczema, and any such cause should be treated vigorously. However, there is often no obvious predisposing factor other than the lymphoedema itself. It has been shown that controlling the degree of swelling with combined physical treatments reduces the likelihood of developing cellulitis[18]. Good skin care is also felt to be important in preventing cellulitis.

Nevertheless, despite these approaches, some patients continue to have recurrent episodes of cellulitis and antibiotic prophylaxis should be considered in those who have 2 or more episodes of cellulitis per year[17]. Table 10.7.3.9 shows the recommended regimens.

Lymphorrhoea

Lymphorrhoea is the leakage of lymph from an oedematous limb through defects in the skin. It can result from direct trauma, e.g. cuts and abrasions, or from rupture of cutaneous lymphangiectasia or papillomata. The leakage can be quite profuse and distressing for patients. Any damage to the skin is also likely to increase the risk of infection and therefore, lymphorrhoea should be treated promptly.

Lymphorrhoea is best treated by the application of a compression bandage with absorbent padding but the compression applied may need to be modified in patients with fragile skin, e.g. in advanced cancer[33] (see below). The bandage may need to be changed several times per day to begin with because of 'strike through' but often the leakage can be sealed within a few days. However, in some situations

Table 10.7.3.9 Antibiotic prophylaxis for recurrent cellulitis in lymphoedema.

1. Phenoxymethylpenicillin 500 mg per day (1 g per day if weight >75 kg)
2. Erythromycin 250 mg per day if allergic to penicillin
3. Clindamycin 150 mg per day or clarithromycin 250 mg per day if above not effective

NB: after 1 year it may be possible to reduce the penicillin dose to 250 mg per day (500 mg per day if weight >75 kg)

particularly with severe oedema and skin breakdown, the leakage may be persistent and require prolonged bandaging.

Malignancy

Patients with lymphoedema are at risk of developing malignancies in the affected area. There are a number of reports in the literature of different skin cancers in lymphoedematous limbs but a direct causal link is not established for many. The most established link is the development on lymphangiosarcomas in women with arm oedema following the treatment of breast cancer (Stewart-Treves syndrome)[34]. Fortunately, these are rare (incidence <0.45 per cent). The mean time of onset in this situation is about 10 years. Lymphangiosarcomas present as bluish/red nodules in the skin or subcutaneous tissues, which spread rapidly and tend to form satellite lesions. Early metastasis to the lungs is common. Unfortunately, prognosis is poor with a median survival of <3 years.

Conclusions

The management of all chronic oedemas requires an accurate diagnosis and consideration of appropriate treatment options. In patients with oedema of advanced cancer, it is particularly important to ensure that the benefits of treatment should outweigh the burdens.

Much of the assessment and management requires specialist input from appropriately trained health care professionals. However, the maintenance treatment of patients with stable uncomplicated oedema can be carried out by trained generalists[20]. Unfortunately, in the UK, specialist services are not available in all areas. It is clear that chronic oedemas are more common than previously thought and that effective ways of management are now available, although there are as yet no simple curative procedures.

Further reading

Browse, N., Burnand, K., and Mortimer, P. (2003). *Diseases of the Lymphatics*. Arnold, London.

Twycross, R., Jenns, K., Todd, J. (eds.) (2000). *Lymphoedema*. Radcliffe Medical Press, Oxon, UK. (New edition due to be published)

References

1. British Lymphology Society Directory of Services. Available at http://www.lymphoedema.org/bls.

2. Mortimer, P.S. (2003). Management of the upper limb. In *Diseases of the Lymphatics* (eds. N. Browse, K.G. Burnand, and P.S. Mortimer), pp. 231–42, Arnold, London.

3. Bull, R.H., Gane, J.N., Evans, J.E.C. *et al.* (1993). Abnormal lymph drainage in patients with chronic venous leg ulcers. *Journal of the American Academy of Dermatology*, **28**, 585–90.

4. Moffatt, C.J., Franks, P.J., Doherty, D.C. *et al.* (2003). Lymphoedema: An underestimated health problem. *Quarterly Journal of Medicine*, **96**, 731–8.

5. Karkkainen, M.J., Ferrell, R.E., Lawrence, E.C. *et al.* (2000). Missense mutations interfere with VEGFR-3 signalling in primary lymphoedema. *Nature Genetics*, **25**, 153–9.

6. Brice, G., Mansour, S., Bell, R. *et al.* (2002). Analysis of the phenotypic abnormalities in lymphoedema-distichiasis syndrome in 74 patients with FOXC2 mutations or linkage to 16q.24. *Journal of Medical Genetics*, **39**, 472–83

7. Williams, A.F., Franks, P.J., and Moffatt, C.J. (2005). Lymphoedema: Estimating the size of the problem. *Palliative Medicine*, 19, 300–13.

8. Levick, J. and McHale, N. (2003). The physiology of lymph production and propulsion. In *Diseases of the Lymphatics* (eds. N. Browse, K. Burnand, and P. Mortimer), pp. 44–64. Arnold, London.

9. Daroczy, J., Wolfe, J., and Mentzel, T. (2003). Pathology. In *Diseases of the Lymphatics* (eds. N. Browse, K. Burnand, and P. Mortimer), pp. 65–101. Arnold, London.

10. Brorson, H., Aberg, M., and Svensson, H. (1999). High content of adipose tissue in chronic arm lymphoedema—An important factor limiting treatment outcome. *Lymphology*, **32**(suppl), 52–54.

11. Mortimer, P.S. and Burnand, K.S. (2004). Diseases of the veins and arteries: Leg ulcers. In *Rook's Textbook of Dermatology* (T. Burns *et.al.*), 7th edition. Ch. 50, pp. 25–6. Blackwell Publishing, Oxford UK.

12. Badger, C.M., Mortimer, P.S., Regnard, C.F.B. *et al.* (1998). Pain in the chronically swollen limb. *Progress in Lymphology*, **11**, 243–6.

13. Woods, M. (2000). Psychosocial aspects of lymphoedema. In *Lymphoedema* (eds. R. Twycross, K. Jenns, and J. Todd), pp. 89–96. Radcliffe Medical Press, Oxon, UK.

14. Franks, P., Williams, A., and Moffatt, C. (2006). A review of the epidemiology of BCRL. *Journal of lymphoedema*, **1**, 66–71.

15. Wold, L.E., Hines, E.A., and Allen, E.V. (1951). Lipoedema of the legs: A syndrome characterised by fat legs and oedema. *Annals of Internal Medicine*, **34**, 1243–50.

16. Wheatley, D.C., Wastie, M.L., Whitaker, S.C. *et al.* (1996). Lymphoscintigraphy and colour Doppler sonography in the assessment of leg oedema of unknown cause. *British Journal of Radiology*, **69**, 1117–24.

17. Keeley, V.L. (2006). The use of lymphoscintigraphy in the management of chronic oedema. *Journal of Lymphoedema*, **1**, 42–57.

18. Ko, D.S.C., Lerner, R., Klose, G. *et al.* (1998). Effective treatment of lymphoedema of the extremities. *Archives of Surgery*, **133**, 452–8.

19. Badger, C., Preston, N., Seers, K. *et al.* (2004). Physical therapies for reducing and controlling lymphoedema of the limbs. *Cochrane Database of Systemic Reviews*, **4**, CD003141.

20. Lymphoedema Framework. (2006). *Best practice for the management of lymphoedema*. International consensus, MEP Ltd., London.

21. Badger, C.M.A., Peacock, J.L., and Mortimer, P.S. (2000). A randomised controlled parallel group clinical trial comparing multilayer bandaging followed by hosiery versus hosiery alone in the treatment of patients with lymphoedema of the limb. Cancer, **88**, 283–7.

22. Johansson, K., Albertsson, M., Ingvar, C. *et al.* (1999). Effects of compression bandaging with or without manual lymphatic drainage treatment in patients with postoperative arm lymphoedema. *Lymphology*, **32**, 103–10

23. Williams, A.F., Vadgama, A., Franks, P. *et al.* (2002). A randomised controlled cross-over study of manual lymphatic drainage therapy in women with breast cancer-related lymphoedema. *European Journal of Cancer Care*, **11**, 254–61.

24. Morgan, P.A., Franks, P.J., and Moffatt, C.J. (2005). Health-related quality of life with lymphoedema: A review of the literature. *International Wounds Journal*, **2**, 47–62.

25. Brorson, H. and Svensson, H. (1998). Liposuction combined with controlled compression therapy reduces arm lymphoedema more effectively than controlled compression therapy alone. *Plastic and Reconstructive Surgery*, **102**, 1058–67.

26. Badger, C., Preston, N., Seers, K. *et al.* (2004). Benzo-pyrones for reducing and controlling lymphoedema of the limbs. *Cochrane Database of Systemic Reviews*, **2**, CD003140.

27. Keeley, V.L. (2000). Oedema of advanced cancer. In *Lymphodema* (eds. R Twycross, K Jenns and J Todd), pp. 338–358. Radcliffe Medical Press, Oxon, UK

28. National Institute for Clinical Excellence (2004). Stent placement for vena caval obstruction. *Interventional Procedure Guidance*, **79**, NICE, UK.

29. Clein, L.J. and Pugachev, E. (2004). Reduction of oedema of lower extremities by subcutaneous controlled drainage: Eight cases. *American Journal of Hospice and Palliative Medicine*, **21**(3), 228–32.

30. Mortimer, P. and O'Donnell. (2003). Principles of medical and physical treatment. In *Diseases of the Lymphatics* (eds. N. Browse, K. Burnand, and P. Mortimer), pp.167–78, Arnold, London.

31. Mallon, E., Powell, S., Mortimer, P. *et al.* (1997). Evidence for altered cell-mediated immunity in postmastectomy lymphoedema. *British Journal of Dermatology*, **137**, 928–33.

32. British Lymphology Society and Lymphoedema Support Network. (2005). Guidelines on the management of cellulitis in lymphoedema. Available at: http://www.thebls.com.

33. Anderson, I. (2003). The management of fluid leakage in grossly oedematous legs. *Nursing Times*, **99**, 54–6.

34. Janse, A.J., van Coevorden, F., Hans, P. *et al.* (1995). Lymphoedema-induced lymphangiosarcoma. *European Journal of Surgical Oncology*, **21**, 155–8.

10.8

Genitourinary problems in palliative medicine

Richard W. Norman and Greg G. Bailly

Introduction

The genitourinary system may produce a variety of disturbing symptoms or life-threatening conditions in patients receiving palliative care. Unilateral or bilateral ureteral obstructions occur commonly in association with primary or secondary malignancies involving the retroperitoneum and pelvis. This can lead to pain and impaired renal function. Lower-tract obstruction may be associated with benign or malignant conditions involving the bladder neck, prostate, or urethra. Anticholinergic drugs, frequently prescribed for patients receiving palliative care, may be responsible for voiding dysfunction and may need modification of type or dosage. Interaction between the bladder and other pelvic organs may be significant and can lead to fistula formation. Haematuria requires investigation to determine whether it is of upper- or lower-tract origin and, if severe, will need intervention.

This chapter is concerned with the practical aspects of symptom control in patients receiving palliative care and suffering from urinary tract dysfunction; arguably the most difficult management decision is choosing the right option in the context of the patient's total situation. Factors to consider include the patient's pre-morbid health and performance status, adequacy of symptom control, disease progression, and the burden versus the benefit balance of investigation and intervention. Emphasis is placed on less aggressive, non-invasive therapies, in keeping with the general condition of these patients. Decisions to recommend more complex, invasive procedures may be appropriate but should always be based on the quality of life anticipated, stage of the disease, and reasonable likelihood of symptomatic improvement.

Pathophysiology and factors governing voiding

The bladder wall is composed of a mesh of smooth muscle fibres that become organized in layers at the bladder neck (detrusor muscle). The outer layer extends throughout the length of the female urethra (Fig. 10.8.1)[1] and to the distal aspect of the prostate in the male, where its arrangement (circular/spiral) is responsible for the major involuntary sphincter (Fig. 10.8.2)[2]. The middle circular layer ends at the bladder neck and contributes to sphincteric function. Internal fibres remain longitudinal and extend to the distal end of the urethra in the female and the prostate in the male. Converging, they form the muscle of the vesical neck, which contributes to urinary continence.

The bladder receives its principal nerve supply from one paired somatic and two paired autonomic nerves. The hypogastric nerves, arising from lumbar spinal segments, mediate sympathetic activity, while the pelvic nerves, derived from S2–S4, contain parasympathetic fibres. The pudendal nerves (S2–S4) primarily serve as a conduit for non-autonomic fibres. With distension of the bladder wall, stretch receptors trigger pelvic nerve fibres, which, unless inhibited by higher centres, will lead to a parasympathetic motor response and bladder contraction (Fig. 10.8.3).

The voluntary external sphincter is made up of striated muscle, which is located between the layers of the urogenital diaphragm. In the male, these fibres are concentrated at the distal aspect of the prostate; in the female, they are found mainly in relation to the middle third of the urethra. Smooth muscle investing the vesical neck and posterior urethra is under sympathetic control, mediated through the hypogastric nerve with thoracolumbar origin (T11–L2). Norepinephrine is the neurotransmitter in this sympathetic release. The external sphincter is under pudendal nerve control (S2–S4) and influenced by autonomic as well as somatic innervation from the pelvic floor. All are coordinated by higher centres to initiate or inhibit bladder emptying.

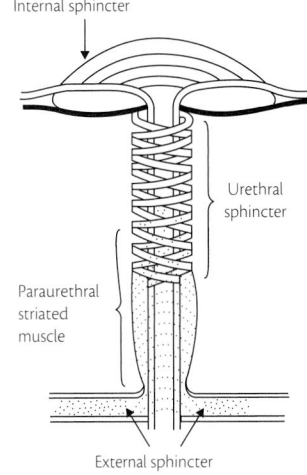

Figure 10.8.1 Sphincter arrangement in the female.

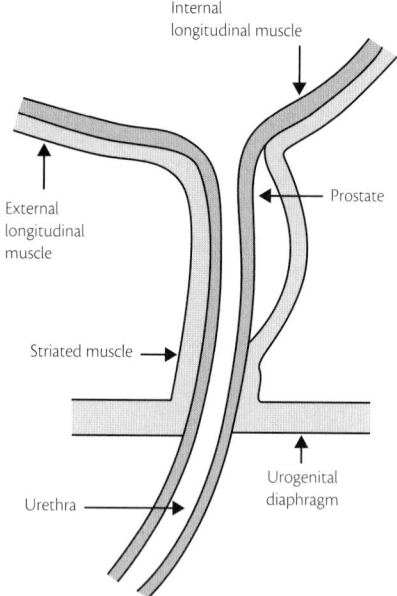

Figure 10.8.2 Sagittal section of the male urethra.

Satisfactory voiding requires an unobstructed passage from the bladder to the urethral meatus, in addition to a functioning detrusor muscle, an intact bladder wall, and integrity of the nerves initiating and coordinating detrusor and sphincteric activities. Stimulation of the parasympathetic bladder nerves causes contraction of the detrusor muscle and relaxation of the bladder neck sphincter. Stimulation of the sympathetic system (T10–T12, L1) has the reverse effect.

Neurological damage associated with metastases to the spine and epidural space causing spinal cord compression or nerve root injury secondary to tumour infiltration may interfere with voiding. Drugs required for control of pain and other symptoms in patients

with advanced cancer also have an important impact on bladder function. Anticholinergic drugs can interfere by causing contraction of the bladder neck sphincter and relaxation of the detrusor muscle. Drugs with such effects that are frequently used in patients with advanced cancer include phenothiazines, haloperidol, antihistamines, and tricyclic antidepressants. Opioid drugs have little impact on bladder function unless combined with other problems, for example, faecal impaction, which, when significant, adds an obstructive component by pressure on the urethra. Particular caution is indicated in the use of these drugs in the elderly and in patients who have pre-existing early bladder outlet obstruction and coexisting immobility.

Bladder outlet obstruction with distension produces great physical distress, which may be masked in the elderly and in patients taking opioid drugs and neuroleptic agents. Confusion is a common presentation, particularly in the elderly. This may result from the physical discomfort or as a result of metabolic disturbances from impaired renal function. In the evaluation of dysfunction, the anatomical and functional integrities of the bladder and urethra should be considered. Spinal cord or nerve root damage should be ruled out. The patient's drug profile must be reviewed. If possible, drugs with anticholinergic effects should be eliminated or their dosages reduced. Constipation should be considered. Biochemical abnormalities that may increase urinary flow must be remembered—hypercalcaemia, hyperglycaemia, and diabetes insipidus should be excluded.

Urinary incontinence

Involuntary loss of urine or urinary incontinence is described as total, overflow, urgency, or stress. In patients with advanced malignant disease, total urethral incontinence or extraurethral loss from urinary fistulae are the most common and significant. Proper management is very important as incontinence predisposes to perineal rashes, pressure ulcers, urinary tract infections, urosepsis, falls, and fractures.

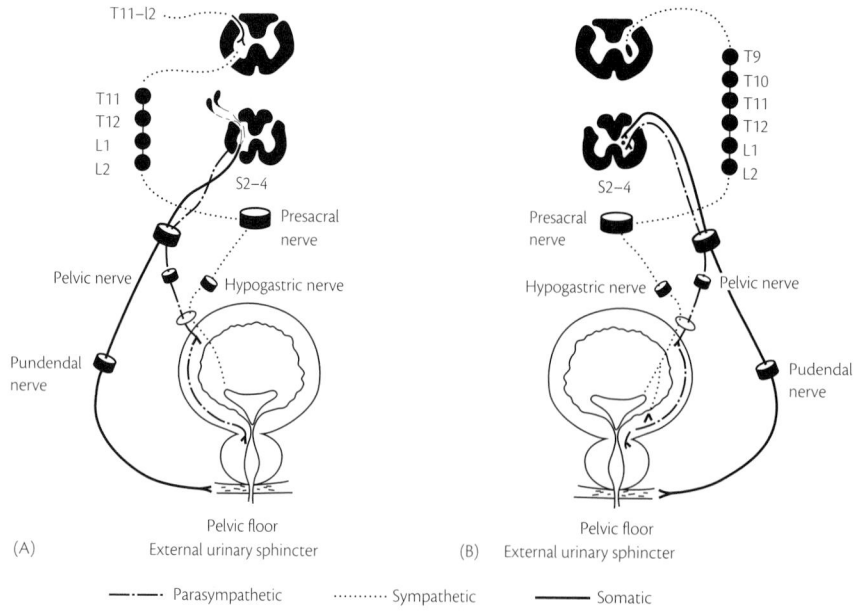

Figure 10.8.3 Innervation of bladder and sites of drug activity.

Total urethral incontinence

This is associated with sphincteric incompetence. Direct tumour invasion, surgical intervention, or loss of innervation from spinal cord or nerve root damage represents the usual responsible factors in patients in palliative care. Direct visualization confirms the urethral nature of the loss. Endoscopic examination and urodynamic evaluation may be necessary to establish a diagnosis. The presence of other motor or sensory abnormalities suggesting spinal cord or nerve root damage may provide the necessary evidence to implicate a neurological deficit. Management usually entails use of an indwelling Foley catheter in women and condom drainage or a penile clamp in men. If the condom or penile clamp is not well tolerated, a Foley catheter would be the next choice. Although artificial sphincters are being used with increasing frequency, their use in patients with active and advanced malignant disease is ordinarily inappropriate.

Overflow incontinence

This type of urinary incontinence is associated with bladder outlet or urethral obstruction. Initially associated with the acute distress of acute retention, voiding occurs in small amounts and without control. The bladder is distended and usually palpable except in the very obese or in patients with pelvic masses or extensive lymphoedema involving the lower abdominal wall.

Catheterization is indicated. Definitive treatment must be individualized and may include surgical or other interventional techniques to correct the obstruction, long-term dependence on an indwelling catheter, intermittent catheterization, or an intraurethral stent.

Urgency incontinence

Detrusor overactivity is associated with increased spontaneous activity of detrusor smooth muscle, leading to excessive detrusor force in relation to urethral sphincter tone. The urge is sudden and urinary loss may be severe. The impaired mobility of patients in a palliative care setting may be an aggravating factor in preventing them from reaching the toilet in time. Causes include intrinsic and extrinsic tumours, which produce irritation of the bladder wall, particularly in the region of the trigone and vesical neck. It may also be associated with inflammatory changes from physical agents (e.g. previous radiation), drugs (e.g. cyclophosphamide), or bacteria. An irritable bladder producing urgency incontinence may be of non-specific type or related to lack of inhibition from neural deficiency, as seen in association with cerebrovascular insufficiency. It usually responds to anticholinergic therapy, such as oxybutynin 2.5 mg orally two to three times per day. In the elderly, a single low dose daily is recommended and 'as necessary' dosing considered. If this is not tolerated other drugs can be considered to reduce detrusor overactivity (Fig. 10.8.3, Table 10.8.1).

Stress incontinence

Stress incontinence consists of involuntary urethral loss of urine associated with increased intra-abdominal pressure from coughing, sneezing, jumping, laughing, or, in severe cases, even walking. It is associated with faulty urethral support, wherein the increased intravesical pressure cannot be resisted. This does not usually represent a major problem in patients in palliative care. Surgery is the usual treatment but it is unlikely to be appropriate in patients with advanced cancer. If not contraindicated by other conditions, treatment with an alpha agonist such as phenylpropandamine (50–100 mg/day in divided doses)[3], or a tricyclic antidepressant, such as imipramine, may be appropriate (Fig. 10.8.3, Table 10.8.1). Long-term catheterization may be necessary in severe cases. Minimally invasive procedures such as cystoscopic injection of intraurethral bulking agents such as collagen or small solid particles of specially treated silicone in a water-based carrier gel may be appropriate for some patients.

Extraurethral incontinence

Urinary fistulae are covered elsewhere in the chapter.

Investigation and management of sudden urinary stoppage

Sudden and marked decrease in urinary output can be both a distressing and potentially lethal problem for patients if it persists and is associated with the metabolic abnormalities characteristic of acute renal failure. Complete cessation of urinary output usually implies obstruction of either the lower urinary tract at the level of the bladder neck, prostate, or urethra or upper-tract obstruction of both ureters or obstruction of a single functioning kidney.

Lower-tract obstruction as a cause of sudden urinary stoppage

Most patients who develop urinary retention will have had some milder, usually progressive, symptoms of obstruction, including hesitancy, decreased urinary stream, and inability to empty the bladder satisfactorily. Symptoms of urinary frequency, nocturia, incontinence, and urinary tract infection may also be apparent. Past history of urethral instrumentation, injury, or infection may point towards the development of a urethral stricture. The use of anticholinergic or α-adrenergic drug may be a contributing factor. On physical examination, these patients are usually restless and uncomfortable due to a painfully overfilled bladder—usually one is able to see, palpate, and percuss the distended organ. Attention should be paid to the urethral meatus, to rule out significant meatal stenosis, and to the entire length of the urethra, to identify areas of scarring or induration, which could imply stricture or tumour formation. Rectal examination is imperative in order to assess the size and consistency of the prostate gland. Firm irregularities may be indicative of cancer of the prostate.

The most appropriate treatment at this time is passage of a urethral catheter to drain the bladder. If this is impossible, insertion of a suprapubic catheter will permit satisfactory bladder drainage and allow relief of symptoms until further definitive endoscopic assessment of the lower urinary tract can be arranged. It is important that the subsequent urinary output of these patients be measured on an hourly basis for several hours to ensure that they do not develop a significant post-obstructive diuresis. Although most of these patients with prostatic enlargement will benefit from a limited transurethral prostatectomy, sometimes referred to as a 'channel TURP', careful case selection is advised because this population of patients often have increased risk of bleeding,

Table 10.8.1 Characteristics of drugs commonly used to control detrusor overactivity.

Action	Dosage	Comments
Flavoxate hydrochloride is a papaverine-like antispasmodic with some anticholinergic and anaesthetic properties	200 mg by mouth three or four times daily up to a maximum of 1200 mg/day may be used	Low incidence of side effects. Recommended for elderly patients and patients who have trouble tolerating other drugs
Dicyclomine chlorhydrate has both musculotropic and anticholinergic effects on smooth muscles	Some formulations provide continuous-release. Up to 80 mg by mouth per day in three or four doses	Recommended for elderly patients and patients who have trouble tolerating other drugs
Oxybutynin chloride has anticholinergic, antispasmodic, and anaesthetic properties	2.5 mg by mouth once daily to 5mg four times a day. For elderly patients try 2.5 mg once or twice a day	Often associated with dry mouth and eyes. May be taken on a necessary basis
Oxybutynin chloride ER has similar actions as its predecessor, oxybutinin, but slow release delivery system	5–15 mg by mouth once daily	Relatively constant plasma concentrations throughout 24 h. Better tolerated than oxybutynin
Oxybutynin chloride transdermal system, slow release through the skin	36 mg skin patch twice weekly	Low incidence of side effects
Tolterodine is a muscarinic receptor antagonist	2–4 mg by mouth twice daily	Because of greater bladder selectivity, less anticholinergic side effects than oxybutinin
Tolterodine LA is a long-acting form of its precessor, tolterodine	2–4 mg by mouth once daily	Better tolerated than tolterodine
Solifenacin succinate is a competitive muscurinic receptor antagonist	5–10 mg by mouth once daily	Because of greater bladder selectivity, less anticholinergic side effects than oxybutinin
Darifenacin is a competitive muscurinic receptor antagonist	7.5–15 mg by mouth once daily	Because of greater bladder selectivity, less anticholinergic side effects than oxybutinin
Trospium chloride is an antispasmodic, antimuscurinic agent	20 mg by mouth once daily	Does not cross blood–brain barrier, possible lower incidence of confusion in elderly
Propantheline bromide is a cholinergic receptor competitor	From 7.5 mg by mouth once daily to 15 mg by mouth four times a day. Where absorption in the digestive tract is incomplete up to 30 mg by mouth four times a day may be necessary	Frequent dosing usually required
Imipramine chlorhydrate is a tricyclic antidepressant with anxiolytic, anticholinergic, direct musculotropic, and adrenergic properties. It also has mild anaesthetic and antihistamine effects. Inhibits the noredrenaline reuptake at presynaptic nerve terminals lesions	Increase gradually to about 25 mg twice daily, but up to a maximum of 200 mg/day can be used if necessary	Imipramine should not be given along with MAO inhibitors
Belladonna/opium suppositories have analgesic, anticholinergic, and antispasmodic properties. Because of their potential addictiveness, they should only used over the short term, e.g., to control pain and bladder spasm after bladder or prostate surgery	One suppository every 3–4 h as required	Useful in management of bladder spasms in those who can not tolerate medication orally

clot retention, infection, and persistent failure to void. Alternatives to prostatectomy include intraurethral stent[4], transurethral microwave therapy, transurethral needle ablation, and holmium laser enucleation. Medical therapy, such as the use of α-blockers and 5α-reductase inhibitors, has gained in popularity for the management of men with symptomatic benign prostatic hyperplasia but is not indicated in men with refractory urinary retention.

Case study

A 79-year-old man presented with mild obstructive voiding symptoms and lower back discomfort. He underwent a digital rectal examination and cystoscopy, which confirmed the presence of a large necrotic nodular prostatic tumour mass with invasion into the right side of the trigone. Biopsies confirmed poorly differentiated adenocarcinoma of the prostate. Renal ultrasound was consistent with right-sided hydronephrosis and a bone scan showed diffuse metastases. Serum prostate specific antigen measured 987 ng/ml. He was treated with total androgen blockade with some improvement in his voiding symptoms and back discomfort. Three months later, he suffered a myocardial infarction. Two weeks following discharge he went into urinary retention and, despite attempts at catheter removal, was unable to void spontaneously. He found the catheter very uncomfortable, but because of his recent cardiovascular problem, he was not felt to be a suitable candidate for a transurethral resection of the prostate. He was treated by placement of an intraurethral stent (Fig. 10.8.4) under local anaesthesia and subsequently voided normally.

There are an increasing number of alternatives for the management of bladder outlet obstruction and it is important to individualize therapy for a specific patient. In this particular case, it was

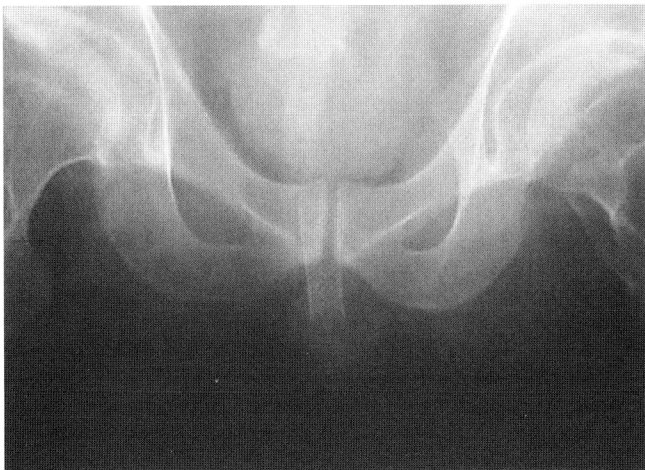

Figure 10.8.4 Urethral stent bridging prostatic urethra.

possible to treat this man's problem in a palliative fashion and improve his quality of life without the catheter, despite his serious underlying malignant and cardiovascular diseases.

Bilateral ureteric obstruction as a cause of sudden urinary stoppage

Acute renal failure secondary to bilateral ureteric obstruction is a common problem in palliative care. Obstruction in the cancer patient may be secondary to tumour invasion, compression of the ureter by retroperitoneal tumour, encasement of the ureter by retroperitoneal or pelvic lymph nodes involved with metastatic disease, or, rarely, by direct metastases to the ureter. In 75 per cent of patients within this group, an underlying malignant disorder will be diagnosed[5]. In almost one-half, the development of bilateral ureteric obstruction is the initial manifestation of the underlying cancer. About three-quarters of the tumours are pelvic in origin; the most common in women is carcinoma of the cervix, and in men, carcinoma of the prostate. The most frequent benign diagnosis is retroperitoneal fibrosis[6].

Common symptoms are a lack of urinary output and abdominal pain. Acute ureteral obstruction usually causes flank pain and colic typical of urolithiasis. Chronic renal obstruction is usually a silent event that is often detected as hydronephrosis with atrophy of the renal cortex on upper abdominal imaging. Physical examination may reveal evidence of flank masses or tenderness. The bladder will not be distended and the urethra should be unremarkable. The importance of an adequate rectal and pelvic examination is emphasized in view of the anticipated causes of obstruction.

Because the obstruction may have been progressing over several days prior to causing complete urinary stoppage, most of these patients will reveal laboratory evidence of acute renal failure with elevated levels of serum creatinine and potassium, metabolic acidosis, and fluid overload, and as a result, investigation and treatment become urgent. Intravenous pyelography is contraindicated in acute renal failure, but renal ultrasono-graphy can be extremely useful in identifying both kidneys and the degree of obstruction. Occasionally, it may show obstructing stones in the upper ureter or renal pelvis. More recently, unenhanced spiral computed tomography (CT) has become an effective and safe initial imaging tool

in the evaluation of renal obstruction, providing more useful information than ultrasonography[7].

Regardless of the method used to acutely relieve bilateral renal obstruction, these patients must be observed closely for changes in their potassium and creatinine levels, as well as the volume of urinary output, following relief of obstruction, which often is followed by a diuresis. If fluid and electrolyte abnormalities are severe, it may be necessary to arrange early temporary haemodialysis to correct life-threatening problems.

In the presence of bilateral ureteric obstruction, cystoscopy and bilateral retrograde pyelograms are usually done next. These studies can reveal abnormalities within the urinary bladder, such as a primary or secondary tumour involving the trigone, and will outline the ureters to define the level, and often the cause, of the ureteric obstruction. Once this has been accomplished, an indwelling ureteric stent can be passed, under cystoscopic control, up the ureter such that one end lies within the renal pelvis and the other within the bladder[8]. This would usually be attempted on both sides if feasible and both kidneys appear to have reasonable potential for regaining function (Fig. 10.8.5). When single stents have failed, placement of two parallel stents simultaneously in extrinsically obstructed ureters may improve drainage of the kidney [9]. Others have described the placement of self-expandable metallic mesh stents as an alternative to traditional ureteric stents, although experience is limited[10–12].

In circumstances in which it is impossible to endoscopically position ureteric stents, one would proceed to percutaneous placement of a nephrostomy tube under ultrasound guidance. Antegrade nephrostograms can then be performed to localize the site and extent of obstruction (Fig. 10.8.6). Nephrostomy tubes can sometimes be replaced by antegrade insertion of ureteric stents and eliminate the need for an external drainage device. If indwelling stents are not successful, long-term management of obstruction can be provided by several means. Percutaneous nephrostomy tubes are often difficult to manage for many patients because the posterior exit site increases the risk of displacement, infection, and blockage. Subcutaneous tunnelling of nephrostomy tubes obviates these problems[13]. The procedure may be done with local

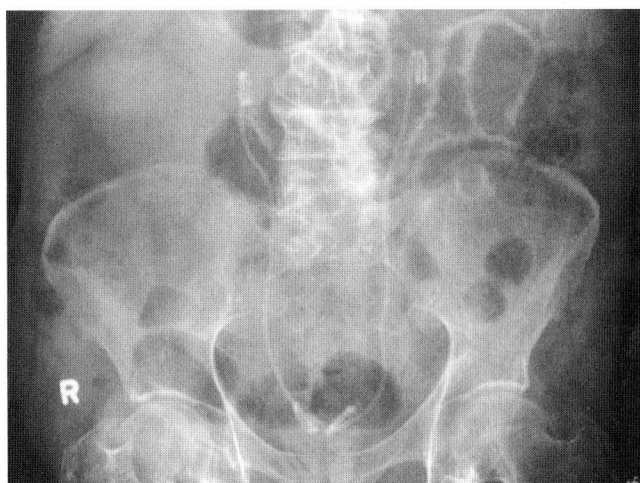

Figure 10.8.5 Bilateral ureteric stents draining obstructed ureters secondary to bladder cancer.

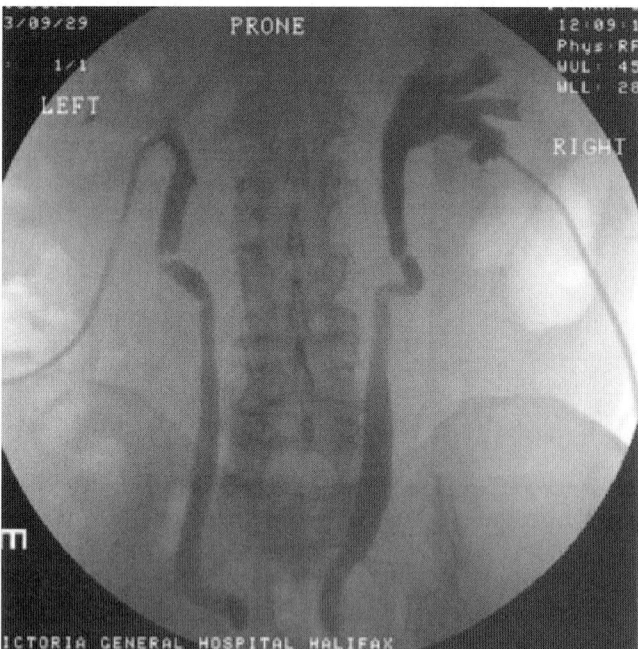

Figure 10.8.6 Bilateral nephrostograms demonstrate complete obstruction of both ureters by prostate cancer.

anaesthesia and conscious sedation, as conventional 8F tubes are replaced by larger 12F tubes under fluoroscopic guidance. Each tube is tunnelled subcutaneously anteriorly where it exits through a common opening in the skin in the right lower quadrant (Fig. 10.8.7(A–D)). The patient can manage the urinary drainage with an external ostomy appliance and drainage bag. Tube exchange is performed every 3 months on an outpatient basis.

Once a ureteral stent or nephrostomy tube is placed, subsequent management requires close follow-up, including periodic monitoring of renal function and periodic stent or tube replacement (every 4–6 months). Permanent indwelling metallic ureteric stents are starting to become available and may avoid the necessity of regular stent changes[14]. If a specific treatment, for example, radiation or chemotherapy, eliminates the lesion responsible for the obstruction, then removal of the nephrostomy tubes or stents can be done, provided imaging studies confirm that the kidneys are draining freely. In advanced prostate cancer patients, androgen blockade is an important palliative treatment that may reduce tumour volume and induce ureteric patency, eliminating the need for long-term stents or tubes.

In situations where this scenario is the result of long-term progression of an underlying malignancy, active intervention at this stage may not be warranted. Posed with a difficult ethical question, the physician and patient must consider the benefits of facilitating treatment and palliation of symptoms versus merely prolonging the patient's suffering. This option should be discussed with the patient and family. In cases where this is the initial manifestation of underlying cancer, therapy is usually tailored towards the underlying malignancy in the hope of relieving the obstruction. Ordinarily, definitive surgical intervention would be entertained only in this situation.

Case study

A 79-year-old man with advanced metastatic prostate cancer treated with total androgen blockade, presented to hospital with a 1-month history of increasing fatigue, anorexia, nausea, vomiting, and decreased urine output. On examination he was tachypnoeic, and had an elevated JVP, bilateral pulmonary rales, and significant paedal oedema. Digital rectal exam revealed a large, hard, nodular prostate. Investigations showed a creatinine of 988 mmol/l, potassium of 7.2 meq/l, and bicarbonate of 9 meq/l. Renal ultrasound revealed severe bilateral hydronephrosis and normal parenchymal thickness. Electrolyte disturbances were treated medically and the patient had urgent insertion of percutaneous nephrostomy tubes bilaterally (Fig. 10.8.6). Over the next 5 days, electrolytes and creatinine returned to normal. Cystoscopy was performed and showed infiltration of the trigone by tumour with obliteration of the ureteric orifices making it impossible to insert ureteric stents in a retrograde fashion. Attempted antegrade placement was also unsuccessful. After discussion with the patient, the nephrostomy tubes were tunnelled subcutaneously and urine drainage was managed with an ostomy appliance (Fig. 10.8.7(d)). The patient managed well for 16 months before succumbing to his disease from diffuse metastatic disease.

Most patients who have advanced inoperable pelvic malignancy with significant bilateral ureteric obstruction should be managed initially with ureteric stents. With recurrent obstruction or failure of stent insertion, appropriate management may include subcutaneously tunnelled nephrostomy tubes if the obstruction is anticipated to be indefinite.

Unilateral ureteric involvement by underlying malignancy

Because of their long length through either side of the retroperitoneum, the ureters are susceptible to involvement by a wide variety of primary and secondary malignancies. In many cases, this can be insidious and asymptomatic; in other instances, the effect can be sudden and associated with significant discomfort. In either case, the presence of ureteric obstruction is usually established by intravenous pyelography, renal ultrasonography, or CT of the abdomen. These studies may also give further clues to the possible underlying cause of obstruction.

Physical examination of the abdomen, pelvis, and rectum is critical and may provide important information that will assist in determining the underlying problem. Because of the presence of obstruction and the associated decrease in renal function, intravenous pyelography may fail to demonstrate the site of blockage. Many patients, therefore, will require cystourethroscopy and a retrograde study. This will provide important information in terms of the site, degree, and cause of obstruction.

If the involved side is symptomatic, or if the contralateral side is absent or non-functioning, cystoscopic placement of an indwelling ureteric stent is useful in providing temporary relief of the obstruction while further investigation and treatment can be established. When this is impossible, percutaneous placement of an indwelling nephrostomy tube can be a useful means of drainage and can permit injection of contrast medium into the upper tract further to define the site and degree of obstruction. Antegrade stenting or subcutaneous tunnelling may be considered for patient comfort. In general, the ultimate outcome in these circumstances will be dictated by the underlying disease. Open surgical therapy to divert the urine or to lyse the ureters is not usually indicated in the face of advanced underlying malignancy. Assuming the contralateral

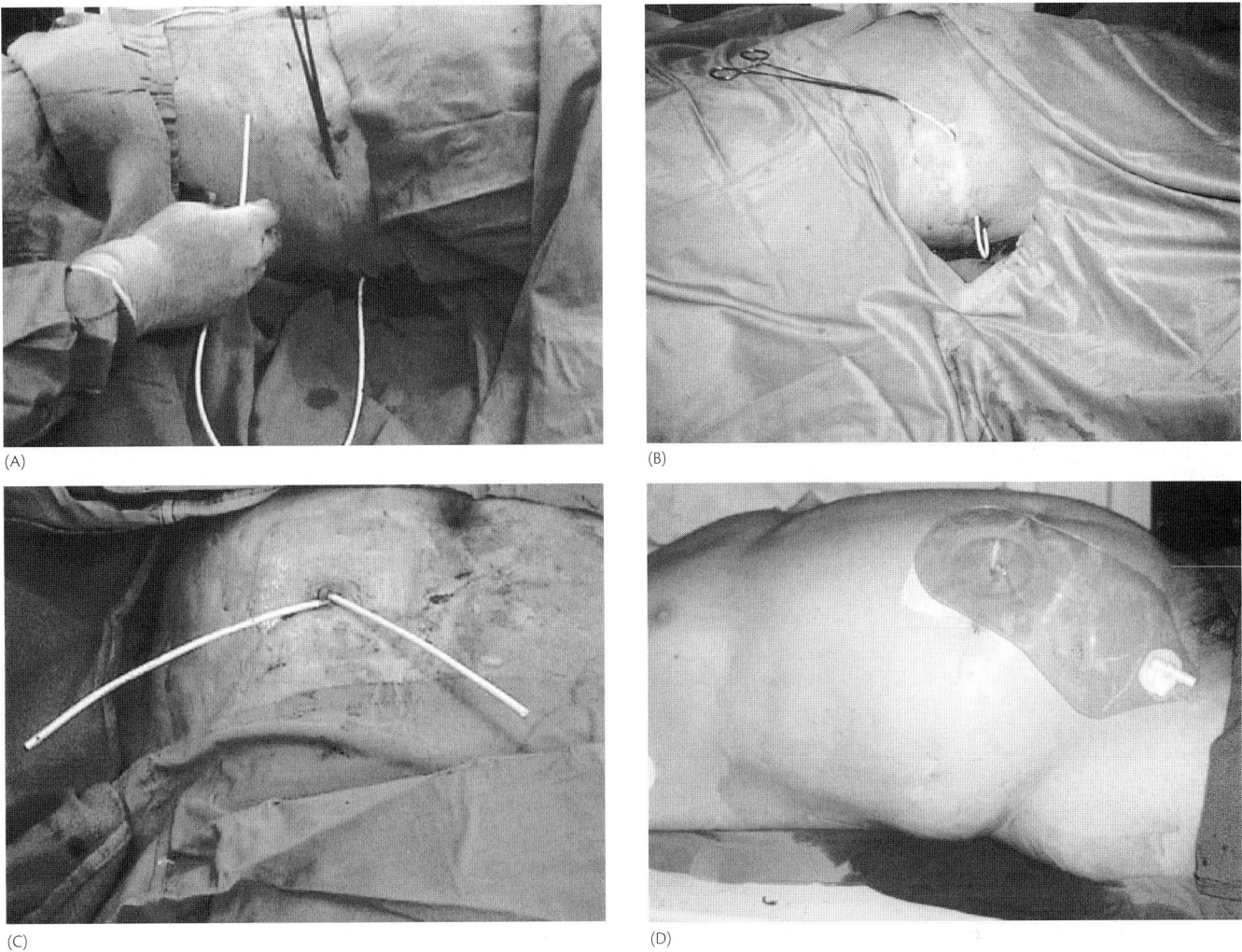

Figure 10.8.7 Operative steps in placement of subcutaneously tunnelled nephrostomy tubes. (A) Instrument is passed subcutaneously into a 1-cm stab wound in the left anterior flank and will be brought out through another stab wound posteriorly beside the nephrostomy tube. (B) Left nephrostomy tube is being pulled out through the anterior incision. This will be repeated until the left and right tubes are brought out through a single site in the right lower quadrant. (C) Both nephrostomy tubes have been tunnelled subcutaneously and are exiting through a single stab wound in the right lower quadrant. (D) The nephrostomy tubes have been cut so that 2 cm protrude from the skin and they can easily be inserted into and covered by an appliance.

kidney to be functioning reasonably well, it is sometimes necessary to remove the involved, obstructed kidney if it continues to be symptomatic, despite satisfactory internal or external drainage. This is often better tolerated than a heroic attempt at reconstruction. In circumstances where the obstructed kidney is completely asymptomatic and the contralateral kidney is functioning well, intervention is usually not required.

Case study

A 57-year-old man complained of some mild fullness and discomfort in the right flank for 6 weeks. Past history revealed that he had undergone an abdominoperineal resection for carcinoma of the rectum 2 years previously. At that time, the surgical margins were clear and the lymph nodes were negative. Current investigations included a renal ultrasound, which showed high-grade ureteric obstruction on the right side with a normal left kidney. Cystoscopy and a right retrograde pyelogram confirmed the presence of marked obstruction of the lower end of the right ureter, secondary to an extrinsic mass. An abdominal and pelvic CT scan were consistent with liver metastases, right hydroureteronephrosis, and a large right pelvic mass encasing the lower end of the ureter (Fig. 10.8.8(A) and (B)). Attempts at insertion of a ureteric stent were unsuccessful and in view of the fact that the patient was coping well, it was decided to perform no further interventions to the right kidney or ureter.

There are a number of endoscopic and percutaneous approaches to the obstructed ureter, but when a patient has a variety of other underlying problems, it is not always appropriate to intervene unless there are significant symptoms. In this situation, the patient was reasonably comfortable and it was decided not to get involved in any more complicated interventional procedures.

Haematuria

Haematuria is a frequent symptom and sign of underlying urological disease, but the degree of bleeding does not always correlate with the seriousness of the underlying condition[15]. Although a specific cause for asymptomatic microscopic haematuria can often not be determined, it may signal the presence of an underlying malignancy.

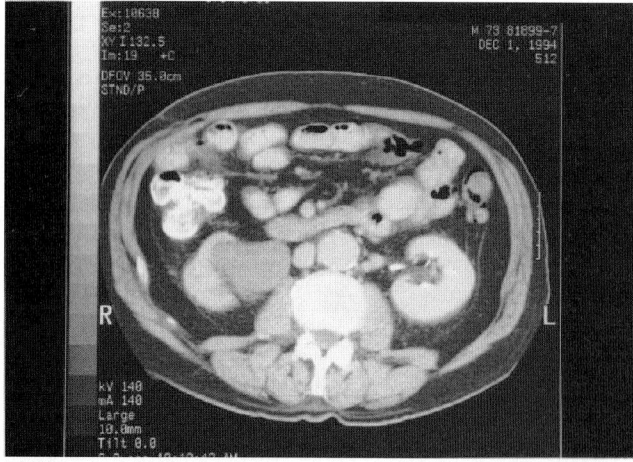

(A)

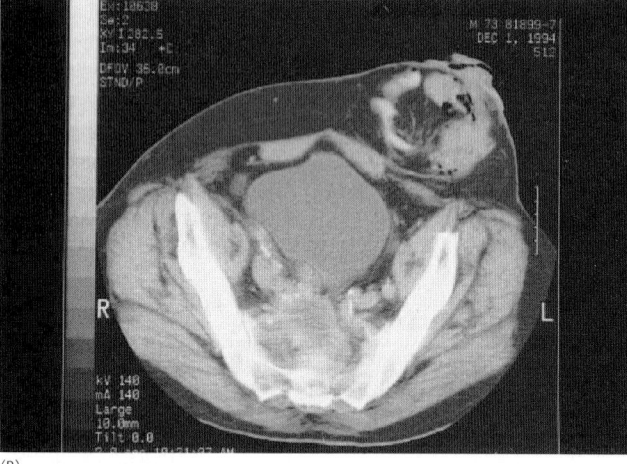

(B)

Figure 10.8.8 CT scan showing (A) obstructed and dilated right renal pelvis and (B) large tumour mass behind the bladder and obstructing the right ureter.

It is important, therefore, that all degrees of newly diagnosed haematuria be assessed. A key feature in the history relates to whether the urine has been previously examined and whether the presence of blood is a new and persistent finding. Other associated symptoms, such as dysuria and urinary frequency and urgency, may point towards a urinary tract infection, which can be diagnosed with an adequate urinalysis and urine culture, or less commonly malignant invasion of the bladder diagnosed endoscopically. Use of non-steroidal anti-inflammatory drugs and aspirin has been associated with microhaematuria. Danthron, a common component of laxatives used in palliative care, may tint alkaline urine a harmless pink or orange and cause confusion. Lower abdominal or flank discomfort may point towards abnormalities in the bladder, ureter, or kidney as the cause. Unfortunately, physical examination often fails to provide satisfactory clues. In these patients, an intravenous pyelogram will allow assessment of the upper tracts in terms of presence, function, and drainage. Renal ultrasonography and CT may be required to accurately characterize renal masses. Although the bladder is also seen, small lesions within it can be missed radiographically and complete cystourethroscopy is indicated when upper-tract radiological procedures do not establish a diagnosis. Specific therapy will be directed towards individual abnormalities.

One of the most frightening symptoms is the sudden onset of gross haematuria. This may simply mean the passage of brown-, black-, or red-coloured urine, or it could involve the passage of large clots or the development of clot retention or colic. Either will require prompt urological consultation. In the palliative care setting, knowledge of the site of an underlying malignancy, possibility of a major coagulation disorder, history of cyclophosphamide use, or prior pelvic irradiation may be significant. In less urgent cases, investigations as described above would be necessary.

Lower tract

Patients with clot retention require immediate intervention and management prior to the initiation of specific studies. Most of these patients will be frightened and uncomfortable due to bladder distension from blood clots and urine. Usually they are extremely restless and unable to remain still because of discomfort, but in rare cases bleeding may have been sufficient to cause hypotension and shock. On physical examination, the distended bladder can be seen, palpated, and percussed. Tenderness or a mass in either flank may hint at an upper-tract cause for the bleeding. Rectal examination is important in men to assess the size and consistency of the prostate and pelvic and rectal examinations are important in women to try to identify a pelvic abnormality.

Adequate initial management requires complete evacuation of clots from the bladder. This is best achieved with urethral placement of a 24F or 26F multieyed Robinson catheter. Percutaneous insertion of a suprapubic catheter is contraindicated in the presence of clot retention because of the inability to place a catheter of satisfactory size to provide adequate irrigation and the potential for seeding of the percutaneous tract by an unsuspected bladder carcinoma. Once the urethral catheter has been passed into the bladder, vigorous irrigation with water or saline, using a Toomey syringe, will usually permit removal of all clots. Bladder irrigation can be very uncomfortable and may require additional analgesia. Manual irrigation should be continued until no further clots are obtained and the backflow is clear. At this stage the Robinson catheter should be replaced with a 22F or 24F three-way indwelling catheter and continuous bladder irrigation should be established using cold water or saline.

Unsuccessful attempts at initial placement of a satisfactory urethral catheter, or continued bleeding and recurrent obstruction of the irrigating catheter, are specific indications for early endoscopic evaluation. Recurrent obstruction of the urethral catheter is usually related either to the persistence of clots or to significant continuous bleeding. Cystourethroscopy permits complete evaluation of the entire penile and prostatic urethra as well as the bladder. In these circumstances, it is important to rule out causes of obstruction and to identify sites of bleeding. The larger and more rigid cystoscope or resectoscope sheath (compared with the urethral catheter) allows improved evacuation of bladder clots. In the majority of instances, this type of bleeding will be caused by local disease involving either the bladder or the prostate. Depending upon the specific circumstances, small and isolated bleeding sites can be cauterized or fulgurated at this time, but usually there is a requirement for transurethral resection of specific lesions to stop the bleeding and to obtain tissue for histological diagnosis. When these procedures have been completed, continuous bladder irrigation is established using an indwelling three-way Foley catheter.

Significant or recurrent haematuria may be the result of a condition known as haemorrhagic cystitis, defined as an acute or insidious diffuse bladder inflammation with haemorrhage. In cancer patients, metabolites of chemotherapeutic agents (e.g. cyclophosphamide), bladder injury secondary to radiation therapy, and viral infections account for the vast majority of cases. If the bleeding is refractory to these conservative measures, bladder instillations with formalin under general anaesthesia and direction of a urologist[16,17], silver nitrate (100 cc of 0.5–1.0 per cent in sterile water instilled for 10–20 min followed by saline irrigation and repeated as necessary)[17], alum (1 per cent solution of the ammonium salt of aluminium in sterile water administered by continuous bladder irrigation over 12–24 h)[17], or epsilon aminocaproic acid[18] may be tried. Haemorrhagic cystitis secondary to cyclophosphamide responds to oral pentosan polysulphate[19] or intravesical instillation of carboprost tromethane, an F2-α prostaglandin in more than 50 per cent of cases[20]. Bleeding from established radiation cystitis may respond to hyperbaric oxygen and chronic or recurrent episodes may benefit from oral pentosan polysulphate[21,22]. On the other hand, local irradiation of the bladder can be palliative in the presence of unresectable cancer and oral tranexamic acid may be helpful, but can cause clot formation and retention. Rarely, it is necessary to resort to surgical intervention, such as hypogastric artery ligation or embolization, or proximal urinary diversion with or without cystectomy.

Upper tract

Occasionally gross haematuria is not due to local bladder pathology but due to upper-tract bleeding. Cystoscopy under these circumstances is again useful in confirming the side from which the blood is coming, and in permitting removal of bladder clots. Retrograde pyelography is occasionally useful under these circumstances, but it should be remembered that many apparent filling defects within the ureter or renal pelvis at these times often represent blood clots.

The next investigation would be an intravenous pyelogram, if renal function is satisfactory, or a renal ultrasound/CT if not. The most likely causes of upper-tract bleeding, under these circumstances, would be the presence of renal tumour, such as a renal cell carcinoma or transitional cell carcinoma of the renal pelvis or ureter, or a stone. Rarely, a specific cause will not be identified with these studies and it may be necessary to progress to renal arteriography. Selective injections permit optimal visualization of the intrarenal vasculature and can identify small arteriovenous malformations, small neoplasms, or renal vein varices. Occasionally, even the renal arteriogram will be normal, despite continued gross haematuria, and in these circumstances, flexible ureteroscopy can be helpful to identify the specific site of haemorrhage, which can be biopsied or cauterized.

In the event that a renal tumour is identified, appropriate management requires metastatic work-up and, if this is negative, a radical nephrectomy is performed. Radical nephroureterectomy with removal of a bladder cuff is usually indicated if it is a transitional cell lesion of the upper tract.

Occasionally the chest radiograph, abdominal computed tomography scan, or bone scan will confirm the presence of metastases, which would obviate the need for radical surgery. In these circumstances, therapeutic arteriography with the injection of pharmacodynamic agents and clot or gelfoam can be used to control bleeding.

If bleeding persists, palliative nephrectomy may be required despite the presence of metastases[23].

Urinary fistulae

A fistula (from the Latin word *pipe*) is a non-anatomic connection between two epithelial-lined organs and is commonly related to inflammation, both benign and malignant in nature. In patients with underlying malignancy, the symptoms associated with urinary tract fistulae can be devastating. The psychological distress and physical afflictions associated with these problems can make patients, their families, and their care givers distraught and give them a sense of hopelessness. The four most common urinary fistulae are vesicoenteric, vesicovaginal, urethrocutaneous, and rectourethral.

Vesicoenteric fistulae

Fistulization between the bladder and the alimentary tract can involve any segment of bowel. Usually the problem is secondary to colonic malignancy or diverticulitis or small bowel inflammatory disease. Rarely, the primary problem originates from the bladder. The most common complaint associated with vesicoenteric fistulae is dysuria (73 per cent), which almost always precedes the development of pneumaturia, that is, the passage of gas or froth in the urine (65 per cent)[24]. Because of a connection between the bowel and urinary tract, many patients will suffer from persistent urinary tract infections, particularly when the colon is involved. The urine usually has a foul odour. In circumstances where the connection is large, patients may be aware of passing particulate faecal matter in the urine. Physical examination may reveal the presence of an associated bowel-related mass from underlying disease, but it is often non-contributory. Diagnostic confirmation of a fistula may be difficult. Cystoscopy has been repeatedly reported as the most accurate diagnostic modality and is considered the first line investigation[25]. One usually observes a localized area of erythema and bullous inflammation at the fistulous site, which is frequently high on the posterior wall. Small amounts of stool may be seen extruding from the involved area. The remainder of the bladder may or may not appear inflamed. Occasionally, the fistulous site may be so small that it cannot be appreciated at the time of endoscopy, and in these circumstances, a variety of other tests, including cystography (sensitivity 32–56 per cent), intestinal barium studies from above or below, visible contrast media, oral ^{51}Cr-labelled sodium chromate[26], and oral or rectal charcoal[25] or indocyanine green solution[27] may be required to identify the abnormal communication. CT scan and MRI are the most sensitive methods used to detect enterovesical fistulae. Overall, CT scanning with oral and rectal contrast, together with cystoscopy, should be adequate to demonstrate an enterovesical fistula in most cases[28].

Management of enterovesical fistulae is usually dictated by the underlying bowel disease, and patient comorbidity. Ideally, the segment of bowel and bladder are removed together and remaining healthy bowel and bladder integrity are re-established. If this is not technically feasible, intestinal diversion may redirect enough of the faecal stream to reduce the urinary symptoms to a tolerable level. In rare circumstances, when massive bladder involvement is present, a total cystectomy, with or without complete pelvic exenteration, and ileal conduit urinary diversion may be necessary.

Placement of bilateral percutaneous nephrostomy tubes, with subsequent tunnelling, is sometimes performed to divert the urine.

Case study

An 83-year-old woman with severe, chronic obstructive lung disease was admitted to hospital with pneumonia. She deteriorated rapidly and required endotracheal intubation and ventilation. She was treated with anti-biotics, bronchodilators, and steroids and eventually required a tracheostomy. Although she remained alert and was able to communicate with sign language, mouthing of words, and writing, it was impossible to wean her from the respirator. As a result she had difficulty mobilizing. Three weeks later, her urine developed a foul smell and was noted to contain large particles of faeces. Cystoscopic evaluation revealed a large fistula arising from the posterior aspect of the bladder in the midline, above the trigone. Barium enema confirmed a large colovesical fistula (Fig. 10.8.9). She was not felt to be a candidate for a major surgical procedure because of her underlying respiratory difficulties and she was therefore treated with a defunctioning colostomy.

Comment

In a healthy patient, an enterovesical fistula would be treated with bowel resection and closure of the bladder. In the palliative care setting, the optimal therapy is often not possible because of underlying restrictions on choices because of the idiosyncrasies of the patients. In this case, it was felt that the patient would not tolerate any further insult to her tenuous respiratory status and the minimal procedure of faecal diversion was carried out to eliminate the faecaluria and associated symptomatology.

Vesicovaginal urinary fistulae

Most vesicovaginal fistulae are the result of gynaecological surgery or local trauma[29]. The characteristic symptom is leakage of urine

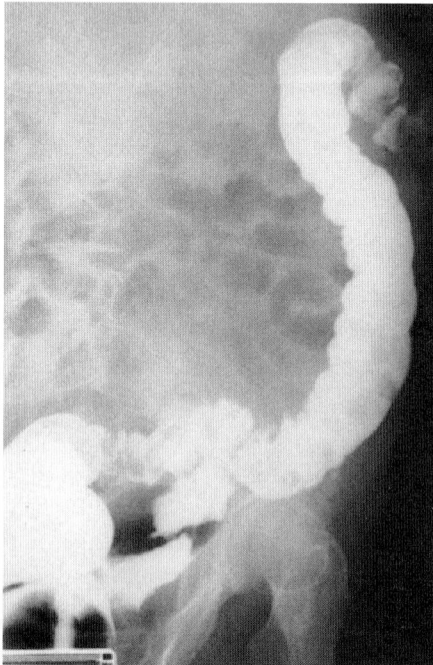

Figure 10.8.9 Barium enema showing large vesicoenteric fistula originating in sigmoid colon.

from the bladder into the vagina. Routine physical examination is usually unrewarding, although occasionally one may be able to identify a large fistulous site on pelvic examination. Intravenous pyelography, or more recently computed tomography intravenous urography (CT-IVU) is necessary to exclude the presence of ureteric involvement in the fistula. The latter is usually heralded by evidence of associated obstruction or significant displacement of the ureter. Cystoscopy will allow characterization of the vesicovaginal fistula in terms of size, site, and multiplicity. It is usually present low on the posterior wall, but the demonstration of proximity to a ureteric orifice is crucial to planning corrective surgery. Escape of irrigating fluid from the vagina while filling the bladder confirms the diagnosis. Vaginoscopy may be confirmatory. When the fistula is small it is occasionally helpful to place a vaginal pack and then fill the bladder with methylene blue to demonstrate the connection. In circumstances where the cause of the fistula is not obvious, a biopsy of the involved area at the time of cystoscopy is imperative to establish a specific diagnosis.

In the absence of underlying malignancy or other significant pathology, small fistulae occasionally close spontaneously following 4–6 weeks of urethral or suprapubic catheter drainage. Usually, it will be necessary to proceed with a surgical repair and this can be accomplished vaginally or transabdominally, with interposition of an omental pedicle graft. Success of surgical management is dependent upon gentle and selective tissue handling, layered closure, lack of tension along suture lines, use of absorbable sutures, use of suprapubic catheter drainage of the bladder post-operatively, and administration of appropriate antibiotics peri-operatively[30].

In circumstances where there is extensive pelvic disease, which is not manageable by surgical reconstruction or requiring anterior or pelvic exenteration, urinary diversion may be required.

When the patient has diffuse metastases or is unable to tolerate major surgery, placement of bilateral percutaneous nephrostomy tubes, with or without subcutaneous tunnelling, may be indicated as a means of diverting the urine and restoring continence. Indwelling urethral or suprapubic catheterization may be appropriate to reduce, but not eliminate urine leakage in some patients with chronic disease states.

Urethrocutaneous fistulae

Urethrocutaneous urinary fistulae are most frequently a complication of hypospadias repair, but may be the result of primary or secondary urethral or penile malignancies. Patients complain of a localized penile mass and drainage of urine through the fistulous site. Ultimate management usually requires a proximal, total, or partial penectomy with subsequent adjuvant surgical or pharmacological therapy as necessary. In those patients who are not candidates for definitive therapy, a percutaneous suprapubic cystostomy would be the ideal form of urinary diversion.

Rectourethral fistulae

Rectourethral fistulae occur most often as a complication of radical prostatectomy, but they are seen occasionally in association with locally invasive prostatic or rectal cancer. Most patients will complain of the passage of urine *per rectum* or pneumaturia and the passage of faecal material *per urethram*. The diagnosis is usually confirmed at the time of cystourethroscopy or proctoscopy. If the fistulous site is small, it may occasionally close spontaneously following a temporary diverting colostomy and bladder catheterization. If this is unsuccessful and there is no obvious persisting local malignancy, surgical repair is indicated. If persistent malignancy is present, the optimal treatment for the underlying malignancy should be determined and urinary or faecal diversion may be necessary.

Urethral catheters

The indwelling urethral catheter remains one of the most useful and commonly used urological instruments. Its primary uses are to provide continuous drainage of urine from the bladder in patients who are unable to void spontaneously or who suffer from marked urinary incontinence not amenable to condom drainage. Occasionally, urethral catheters are used as a means of assessing the degree of bladder emptying, irrigating blood clots from the bladder, and measuring hourly urine output.

The most frequently used urethral catheters are made from latex rubber and are blunt-tipped. These have one channel for draining the urine and another smaller channel for inflating the balloon which prevents displacement of the catheter. Because of a tendency towards encrustation, irritation, and infection, a variety of new hydrophilic polymers have been developed to improve catheter biocompatibility. These lubricious coatings provide protection against irritation of urethral mucosa, help to minimize encrustation, and enhance patient comfort. Their effectiveness has reduced the need for more expensive silicone catheters. Silver-impregnated catheters, antibiotic-coated catheters, and electrified catheters may diminish bacteriuria for a few days, but are costly and have no role in long-term catheterization[31].

A critical factor to be considered when choosing the catheter is the size. Most are labelled with respect to the measurement of the outer circumference of the catheter. The most frequently used system is the F-scale and conversion to the diameter of the catheter is possible by remembering that each number of the F-scale equals 0.33 mm. In the usual situation of using an indwelling urethral catheter, one would use a 16F or a 18F. Catheters smaller than this are less useful because of their tendency to coil up in the urethra during passage and to obstruct with bladder debris. It is best to minimize bladder irritation by using 5 or 10 ml balloons.

In patients for whom urethral catheterization is difficult, it is useful to fill the urethra with 10 ml of 2 per cent lignocaine (lidocaine) jelly; one should allow 5 min for this to take effect. This lubricates the urethra, allows the external sphincter to relax, and decreases some of the discomfort. Occasionally, a curved or Coudé catheter can be used to simplify passage through the external sphincter and prostatic urethra or bladder neck.

When it is impossible to pass a urethral catheter to drain a distended bladder, a suprapubic drainage system can be used. There are many kits to permit placement of a suprapubic catheter, but the principles of the technique involve placing the patient in a slight Trendelenburg position, treating the suprapubic area with an appropriate antiseptic, infiltrating a small area of skin 5 cm above the pubis in the midline with a local anaesthetic, and using a syringe and needle to aspirate urine through this area to confirm the position of the distended bladder. Once this had been accomplished, a plastic trocar and sheath can be passed through the same tract into the bladder. The trocar is then removed and the indwelling catheter passed through the sheath, which is then withdrawn or peeled away. The catheter is sutured in place and left indwelling. This can be an extremely important technique in patients with extensive urethral stricture disease.

The incidence of urinary tract infections in patients with indwelling urinary catheters is related to the duration of catheterization[32]. This acquired bacteriuria occurs at a rate of about 5–10 per cent per day of catheterization, with 50 per cent of patients bacteriuric within 10–14 days, and virtually all by 6 weeks[33]. Since it is impossible to eliminate catheter-associated infections, and the bacterial flora changes rapidly in patients with chronic indwelling urethral catheters, treatment of asymptomatic bladder bacteriuria or funguria is not recommended[34]. Antibiotic prophylaxis simply promotes the emergence of antibiotic-resistant microbes. Because of the risk of blockage and encrustation and formation of stones on the catheter, it is recommended that it be changed every 4–6 weeks, although the ideal frequency is not known. Patients whose catheter's block are metabolically different from patients without blocked catheters and should receive fresh catheters at 7–10 days to avoid obstruction[35]. It would be appropriate to use a short course of antibiotics around the time of manipulation; the authors use an oral fluoroquinolone for 24 h when changing a catheter has been difficult or traumatic. In some instances, if patients are physically able to or if they have assistance, it can be beneficial to initiate a programme of regular intermittent clean catheterization to maintain low urinary residuals. This technique is useful in both males and females[36]. The frequency may be individualized, depending on bladder capacity. This type of protocol is associated with fewer urinary tract infections and obviates the problems of a long-term indwelling catheter.

Having an intravesical balloon inflated with 5 cc of water as the mechanism of preventing displacement, these urethral catheters may produce considerable bladder irritation and discomfort in some patients, and occasionally, loss of urine around the catheter. Bladder spasms are described as intermittent episodes of excruciating suprapubic discomfort, often associated with leakage of small amounts of urine through the urethra alongside the catheter when the bladder contracts. These can often be reduced by using a catheter with a smaller balloon or evacuating some of the fluid within the balloon. This tip is especially useful if a 30-cc balloon was used initially. In patients in whom this does not provide symptomatic improvement, the use of belladonna and opium (B and O) suppositories *per rectum* every 4 h or low-dose oxybutynin 2.5 mg orally two times per day can be helpful. There is a tendency to treat urine leakage secondary to bladder spasms by increasing the size of the catheter and balloon; this is counterproductive and tends to aggravate the underlying problem.

Failure of the catheter balloon to deflate after aspiration of its contents has been attempted, is not uncommon, and can make removal of the catheter difficult or impossible. Gentle passage of a ureteric wire stylet along the inflation channel will puncture the balloon and correct the problem[37].

Pain

Renal colic

Pain associated with urinary dysfunction represents one of the most distressing types of acute pain. In the absence of personal experience as sufferer or observer, it is unlikely that the distress of severe ureteric colic can be appreciated fully. Induced by acute ureteric obstruction, usually a stone or blood clot, pain in renal distribution is thought to be due to capsular distension. The severe colicky-type pain, which is probably due to ureteric muscle spasm, extends from the costovertebral angle, along the course of the ureter, and radiates to the ipsilateral testis or labium. The associated autonomic outpouring is reflected in a characteristic response associated with severe restlessness, pallor, and diaphoresis. An intravenous opioid, such as morphine, or an intramuscular injection of a non-steroidal anti-inflammatory drug such as ketorolac or diclofenac are effective in relieving this discomfort[38]. Under-dosing is a common error and should be avoided, but keep in mind that non-steroidal anti-inflammatory drugs may be associated with numerous side effects, including renal failure, gastrointestinal bleeding, and platelet dysfunction, and they must be used with care in the palliative care population, especially those with underlying urinary tract obstruction.

Bladder pain

This may be identified as obstructive or irritative.

Obstructive

Chronic distension of the bladder, developing over a period of weeks or months, is usually associated with little more than a sense of fullness in addition to the symptoms of chronic urinary retention. Overflow incontinence may occur. On the other hand, acute retention of sudden onset will produce agonizing lower abdominal pain, severe restlessness, and a constant and compelling urge to void. If the obstruction is not relieved spontaneously or by passage of a catheter, the acute urge will gradually subside but bladder distension will persist. Symptoms, particularly in the elderly and those on opioid drugs, may be masked. Confusion may be the major presenting symptom.

Irritative symptoms

Inflammation of the bladder is most often due to infection and symptoms consist of excessive urinary frequency, dysuria, and urgency incontinence. Dysuria at the end of voiding suggests prostatic origin in the male and trigone in the female.

Irritative bladder symptoms are frequently associated with external radiation and with certain chemotherapeutic agents, such as cyclophosphamide. Idiopathic detrusor instability and central neurological disease may also be responsible. Metabolic abnormalities producing polyuria should be excluded. Intravesical or extravesical tumours may produce irritative bladder symptoms and, along with other agents, may be responsible for the development of bladder spasms, which comprise an exquisitely painful sensation felt mainly in the bladder region. These spasms are due to severe contraction of the detrusor muscle responding to some irritation, usually on the trigone. In addition to tumour, infection, radiation, and calculi may be responsible—irritation is often associated with an indwelling catheter, particularly with encrustation. Treatment of this condition is covered under the section on 'Catheters'.

References

1. Hutch, J.A. (1967). A new theory of the anatomy of the internal urinary sphincter and the physiology of micturition. IV. The urinary sphincteric mechanism. *Journal of Urology*, **97**, 705–12.

2. Hutch, J.A. and Rambo, O.A. (1967). A new theory of the anatomy of the internal urinary sphincter and the physiology of micturition. III. Anatomy of the urethra. *Journal of Urology*, **97**, 696–704.

3. Urinary Incontinence Guideline Panel. *Urinary Incontinence in Adults: Clinical Practice Guidelines, AHCPR Pub. No. 92-0038.* Agency for Health Care Policy and Research, Public Health Service, US Department of Health and Human Services, Rockville MD, March, 1992.

4. Chiou, R.K. *et al.* (1996). Long-term outcome of prostatic stent treatment for benign prostatic hyperplasia. *Urology*, **48**, 589–93.

5. Feng, M.I., Bellman, G.C., and Shapiro, C.E. (1999). Management of ureteral obstruction secondary to pelvic malignancies. *Journal of Endourology*, **13**, 521–4.

6. Norman, R.W. *et al.* (1982). Acute renal failure secondary to bilateral ureteric obstruction: Review of 50 cases. *Canadian Medical Association Journal*, **127**, 601–4.

7. Koelliker, S.L. and Cronan, J.J. (1997). Acute urinary tract obstruction: imaging update. *Urology Clinics of North America*, **24**, 571–82.

8. Andriole, G.L. *et al.* (1984). Indwelling double-J ureteral stents for temporary and permanent urinary drainage: Experience with 87 patients. *Journal of Urology*, **131**, 239–41.

9. Lui, J.S. and Hrebinko, R.L. (1998). The use of two ipsilateral ureteric stents for relief of ureteral obstruction from extrinsic compression. *Journal of Urology*, **159**, 179–81.

10. Ahmed, M. *et al.* (1999). Metal mesh stents for ureteral obstruction caused by hormone resistant carcinoma of prostate. *Journal of Endourology*, **13**, 221–4.

11. VanSonnenberg, E. *et al.* (1994). Malignant ureteral obstruction: treatment with metal stents—Technique, results, and observations with percutaneous untraluminal US. *Radiology,* **191**, 765–8.

12. Pauer, W. and Lugmayr, H. (1992). Metallic wallstents: A new therapy for extrinsic ureteral obstruction. *Journal of Urology*, **148**, 281–4.

13. Wilcox, D.T., De Bruyn, R., and Mouriquand, P.D. (1999). The tunnelled nephrosotmy tube. *BJU International*, **83**, 506–7.

14. Borin, J.F., Melamud, O., and Clayman, R.V. (2006). Initial experience with full-length metal stent to relieve malignant ureteral obstruction. *J Endourology*, **20**, 300–4.

15. Mariani, A.J. *et al.* (1989). The significance of adult hematuria: 1000 hematuria evaluations including a risk-benefit and cost-effectiveness analysis. *Journal of Urology*, **141**, 350–5.

16. Donahue, L.A. and Frank, I.N. (1989). Intravesical formalin for hemorrhagic cystitis: Analysis of therapy. *Journal of Urology*, **141**, 809–12.

17. DeVries, C.R. and Freiha, F.S. (1990). Hemorrhagic cystitis: A review. *Journal of Urology*, **143**, 1–9.

18. Singh, I. and Laungani, G.B. (1992). Intravesical epsilon aminocaproic acid in management of intractable bladder hemorrhage. *Urology*, **40**, 227–9.

19. Toren, P.J. and Norman, R.W. (2005). Cyclophosphamide induced hemorrhagic cystitis successfully treated with pentosanpolysulphate. *Journal of Urology*, **173**, 103.

20. Levine, L.A. and Jarrard, D.F. (1993). Treatment of cyclophosphamide-induced hemorrhagic cystitis with intravesical carboprost tromehamine. *Journal of Urology*, **149**, 719–23.

21. Norkool, D.M. *et al.* (1993). Hyperbaric oxygen therapy for radiation-induced hemorrhagic cystitis. *Journal of Urology*, **150**, 332–4.

22. Mathews, R. *et al.* (1999). Hyperbaric oxygen for radiation induced hemorrhagic cystitis. *Journal of Urology*, **161**, 435–7.

23. Flanigan, R.C. (1987). The failure of infarction and/or nephrectomy in stage IV renal cell cancer to influence survival or metastatic regression. *Urology Clinics of North America*, **14**, 757–62.

24. McNamara, M.J. *et al.* (1990). Surgical treament of enterovesical fistulas in Crohn's disease. *Diseases of the Colon and Rectum*, **33**, 271–6.

25. Kavanagh, D. *et al.* (2005). Diagnosis and treatment of enterovesical fistulae. *Colorectal Disease*, **7**(3), 286–291.

26. Lippert, M.C., Teates, C.D., and Howards, S.S. (1984). Detection of enteric-urinary fistulas with a non-invasive quantitative method. *Journal of Urology*, **132**, 1134–6.

27. Sou, S. *et al.* (1999). Preoperative detection of occult enterovesical fistulas in patients with Crohn's disease: Efficacy of oral or rectal administration of indocyanine green solution. *Diseases of the Colon and Rectum*, **42**, 266–70.

28. Manganiotis, A.N., Banner, M.P., and Malkowicz, S.B. (2001). Urologic complications of Crohn's Disease. *Surgery Clinics of North America*, **81**, 197–215.

29. Domochowski, R. (2002). Surgery for vesicovaginal fistula, urethrovaginal fistula and urethral diverticulum. In *Campbell's Urology*, 8th edition, (eds. P.C. Walsh, *et al.*), pp. 1195–217. WB Saunders, Philadelphia, PA.

30. Turner-Warwick, R. (1986). Urinary fistulae in the female. In *Campbell's Urology*, 5th edition, (eds. P.C. Walsh *et al.*), pp. 2718–38. WB Saunders, Philadelphia, PA.

31. Cravens, D.D. and Zweig, S. (2000). Urinary catheter management. *American Family Physician*, **61**, 369–76.

32. Platt, R. *et al.* (1986). Risk factors for nosocomial urinary tract infection. *American Journal of Epidemiology*, **124**, 977–85.

33. Sedor, J. and Mulholland, S.G. (1999). Hospital-acquired urinary tract infection associated with the indwelling catheter. *Urology Clinics of North America*, **26**, 821–8.

34. Yoshikawa, T.T., Nicolle, L.E., and Norman, D.C. (1996). Management of complicated urinary tract infection in older patients. *Journal of the American Geriatric Society*, **44**, 1235–41.

35. Kunin, C.M., Chin, Q.F., and Chambers, S. (1987). Indwelling urinary catheters in the elderly: Relation of 'catheter life' to formation of encrustations in patients with and without blocked catheters. *American Journal of Medicine*, **82**, 405–11.

36. Wyndaele, J.J. and Maes, D. (1990). Clean intermittent self catheterization: A 12 year follow-up. *Journal of Urology*, **143**, 906–8.

37. Browning, G.G., Barr, L., and Horsburgh, A.G. (1984). Management of obstructed balloon catheters. *British Medical Journal*, **289**, 89–91.

38. Oosterlinck, W. *et al.* (1990). A double-blind single dose comparison of intramuscular ketorolac tromethamine and pethidine in the treatment of renal colic. *Journal of Clinical Pharmacology*, **30**, 336–41.

10.9

Mouth care

Franco De Conno, Cinzia Martini,
Alberto Sbanotto, Carla Ripamonti,
and Vittorio Ventafridda

Introduction

Lesions of the oral cavity may have a great impact on quality of life, compromising both physical and psychological functions, often affecting body image, communication, and nutrition. In patients with cancer, lesions, and/or dysfunctions of the oral cavity may be due to progression of oral cancer and/or to the consequences of antineoplastic therapies. Oral complications of chemotherapy and/ or radiotherapy include stomatitis, xerostomia, oral infection, dental caries, loss of taste, and osteoradionecrosis.

Oral care protocols

The oral cavity consists of the lip, floor of the mouth, oral tongue (the anterior two-thirds of the tongue), buccal mucosa, upper and lower gingivae, hard palate, and retromolar trigone.

The assessment and monitoring of the oral cavity, assessment of oral symptoms, and patient education on oral hygiene and in oncology is necessary to limit problems due to progression of head and neck cancer and to preserve the integrity of oral cavity during antineoplastic treatments, are all needed in all patients with advanced illness.

Good oral hygiene is fundamental to prevent oral infection, decay, periodontal disease, and oral symptoms especially halitosis; to prevent further damage to the oral mucosa in patients undergoing antineoplastic and pharmacological treatments; to relieve oral pain and discomfort and increase or maintain oral intake; to minimize psychological distress and social isolation and increase family involvement; and to maintain the patient's dignity even as death is approaching. The aim of oral hygiene is to keep lips and oral mucosa clean, soft, and intact, as far as possible; and remove plaque and debris. The first step is the oral cavity examination (Table 10.9.1). It should be carried out routinely wherever the patient is being cared for. Daily brushing with a soft-bristle toothbrush, use of unwaxed dental floss, and rinsing with a mild solution of sodium bicarbonate (one teaspoonful per large cup of water) form the basis of good oral hygiene. A thick paste of sodium bicarbonate and a few drops of warm water can be applied by the patient with a soft toothbrush in a 'pat and push' manner into the gingival sulcus and around the teeth. This technique is an effective complementary regimen to mechanical plaque debridement for reducing sulcus/pocket organisms and improving periodontal health. Commercial mouthwashes

Table 10.9.1 Oral cavity: routine examination.

Equipment: examination gloves, light, tongue depressor, hand mirror
1. External examination of the lips, degree of mouth opening
2. Remove dentures (if present)
3. Assess oral hygiene
4. Assess dental disease
5. Observe the state of all the structures of oral cavity
6. Observe the presence of cancer lesions, infections, ulceration, haemorrhages
7. Evaluate the presence of symptoms (pain, xerostomia, sialorrhoea, dysphagia, taste alteration, halitosis)
8. Note systemic factors such as medications and nutritional status

may be helpful, but patients with stomatitis may have to avoid products containing alcohol, lemon, and glycerine as well as hard toothbrushes.

Many patients wear partial or complete dentures. Cachectic patients may find that their dentures are loose and ill-fitting, with consequent abrasions and ulcerations of soft tissue, associated with pain. Some principles for the care of dentures are presented in Table 10.9.2.

Nurses should teach oral hygiene techniques and reinforce oral hygiene practices continuously.

Oral symptoms

Xerostomia

Xerostomia is the subjective feeling of dryness of the mouth, not always accompanied by a detectable decrease in saliva flow[1]. Prevalence in palliative care is between 30 and 90 per cent[2]. Probably all patients suffer from a dry mouth at some point during the terminal stage of many diseases. In one series of patients with advanced cancer receiving care in the community or in hospice, 88 per cent reported dry mouth of a mean intensity of 6.2 (SD 2.21) on a 0–10 scale[3]. In a study of 529 adults in a primary-care setting, the prevalence of xerostomia was 29 per cent[1]. Women were more frequently affected and there was a positive correlation with age. Despite the high prevalence of this symptom in palliative care and the great impact on quality of life, xerostomia has received little attention.

Table 10.9.2 Care of dentures.

Realign dentures if they are loose
Brush and clean well after meals
Remove dentures overnight and leave them (non-metal) in an antiseptic solution (1% sodium hypochlorite)
Brush metal dentures with povidone–iodine solution
If dentures are stained, soak in warm water with a commercial denture cleaner (brushing and rinsing before reinserting)
If oropharyngeal candidiasis is present, leave dentures in nystatin suspension

Note: [a] Many disinfectant solutions can also promote certain microbial growth if left to stagnate for more than 24 h.

The assessment and the study of patients with xerostomia could be improved by the use of a specific questionnaire. One such tool to evaluate xerostomia is the Xerostomia Index, an 11-item instrument that measures dry-mouth symptoms. Responses are recorded using a 5-point likert scale (1 = never, 2 = hardly ever, 3 = occasionally, 4 = fairly often, 5 = very often). A summary score is computed by adding scores for the responses to the 11 statements. Scores range from 11 to 55, with a higher score indicating more severe dry mouth symptoms[4].

Saliva is very important for oral integrity. The primary constituents are water, proteins, and electrolytes. They have a protective effect on the mucous membranes in the oral cavity and in the upper digestive tract and provide antimicrobial and buffering activities that protect the teeth from dental caries. In the absence or reduction of saliva, both the hard and soft tissues of the oral cavity may be severely damaged, with an increase in ulceration, oral infection, dental decay, and taste alteration. Swallowing and chewing become difficult and painful and there is usually an effect on speech. Patients report the need to do something to keep the mouth moist, the need to get up at night to drink water, burning and tingling sensations on the tongue, and the presence of cracks or fissures at the corners of the lips. Dental prostheses will frequently traumatize the vulnerable mucosa. These symptoms can contribute to anorexia, loss of weight, and cachexia.

Normally, about 1000–1500 ml of saliva are produced daily by the parotid, submaxillary, and sublingual glands and by hundreds of minor salivary glands of the oral cavity. Salivary pH is about 6–7, favouring the digestive action of a salivary enzyme, α-amylase. Its production is reduced by gland damage, as occurs following radiotherapy[5]. Saliva is composed of a serous part (α-amylase), devoted to starch digestion, and a mucous component, which acts as a lubricant. The bicarbonate content of saliva enables it to buffer and produces the conditions necessary for the digestion of plaque, which holds acid in contact with the teeth. In addition, saliva helps with bolus formation and lubricates the throat for the easy passage of food. The organic and inorganic components of the salivary secretions have a protective potential. They act as a barrier to irritants and as a means of removing cellular and bacterial debris. Saliva contains various components involved in defence against bacterial and viral invasions, including mucins, lipids, secretory immunoglobulin, lysozymes, lactoferrin, salivary peroxidase, and myeloperoxidase. The release of lysozyme, lactoferrin, and myeloperoxidase from the polymorphonuclear leucocytes is increased following oral inflammation[6]. Although the minor glands only produce approximately 10 per cent of the total salivary output, they account for 70 per cent of the total mucin in saliva[7]. This substance protects the oral tissues from chemical and mechanical trauma and infections, and lubricates the oral membranes[8]. Salivary flow is categorized as unstimulated, or resting, and stimulated, as it occurs when an exogenous factor is acting on the secretory mechanisms. Both the parasympathetic and sympathetic nervous systems innervate the salivary glands. Parasympathetic stimulation induces more watery secretions, whereas the sympathetic system produces a sparser and more viscous flow. In general, unstimulated whole salivary flow rates of less than 0.1 ml/min are considered low and indicative of xerostomia[9].

Causes of xerostomia are listed in Table 10.9.3.

Xerostomia due to radiotherapy

Patients treated with radiotherapy for oral or head and neck cancer often suffer from xerostomia from the beginning of treatment. Radiation can affect one or both parotid glands and the submandibular salivary glands, resulting in a marked diminution in the normal salivary flow, as a consequence of inflammation and degeneration of the acini and ducts, connective tissue, and vascular components of the salivary glands[5,10–13]. The most important factor affecting salivary flow after a curative dose of radiotherapy seems to be the volume of the major salivary glands irradiated[14], particularly the parotid as it is more radiosensitive than the other major salivary glands[15–17]. The flow rate of an irradiated parotid gland is almost negligible after only two treatments of 2.25 Gy each[18]. When 100 per cent of the parotid gland is irradiated, no saliva is produced; however, exclusion of 10–20 per cent of the gland from the radiation field allows the continued production of saliva[15]. A sharp decrease in salivary flow usually occurs after the first week of radiotherapy with a dose of about 10 Gy. The decrease in the flow rate continues throughout the treatment, which may lead to persistent xerostomia[12,16]. While one study noted a partial return of salivary flow 8 months after the end of radiotherapy[11], others found minimal, if any, improvement some years after radiotherapy[19,20].

Table 10.9.3 Causes of xerostomia.

1. Medications
◆ Anticholinergics
◆ Antidepressants and antipsychotics
◆ Diuretics
◆ Antihypertensives
◆ Sedative and anxiolytics
◆ Muscle relaxants
◆ Analgesics
◆ Antihistamines
◆ Anticonvulsants
2. Radiotherapy and/or chemotherapy of the head and neck regions
3. Progression of oral cancer
4. Oral infections
5. Dehydration
6. Depression, anxiety
7. Connective tissue or immunological disorders

Irradiation of the salivary glands causes saliva to become more viscous, and more acidic, with a loss of organic and inorganic components. Production of the aqueous component of whole saliva is much more sharply depressed than that of the protein component during xerostomia. Therefore, the capacity of saliva to act as a barrier against irritating substances or to remove bacterial and cellular debris is reduced. The bicarbonate content also diminishes, further impairing the cleansing action of saliva, and there is an increase in the salivary content of Na^+, Cl^-, Mg^{++}, and protein[10,13,17]. The reduction in salivary flow, together with these qualitative changes, can alter the oral microbial flora and result in increased growth of *Streptococcus, Lactobacillus,* and *Candida*. These often irreversible changes can damage dental structures rapidly and increase tooth decay[21]. In patients undergoing radiotherapy, tooth decay can be rapid and lesions can be manifest within 3–6 months[10]. The process of decay may cause pain in the oral cavity, adding to the suffering of the patient. Loss of already-decaying teeth causes further difficulty in mastication, which, when added to xerostomia, may cause difficulty in swallowing and digestion. Saving the minor oral glands may play an important role in protection against new colonization by micro-organisms or against tooth decay. Apart from flow rate measurements, the level of α-amylase seems to be the best indicator of salivary gland function during radiotherapy, whereas albumin and lactoferrin are good indicators of the inflammatory reactions often related to irradiation[5].

Drug-induced xerostomia

A large number of drugs cause dryness of the mouth, including anticholinergic drugs, tricyclic antidepressants, antihistamines, anticonvulsants, antipsychotics, hypnotics, β-blockers, and diuretics[22]. They may reduce the flow of saliva directly or indirectly and some have a parasympatholytic effect. In the study of Sreebny et al.[23], almost 60 per cent of those patients with a dry mouth were taking drugs known to cause this symptom. The intake of xerostomia-inducing medications is positively correlated with age and with the total number of drugs taken daily and it is highest among institutionalized patients[23,24]. Reduced salivation in the elderly may be related to drug use rather than to age. Xerostomia was not generally recognized as a side effect of morphine but clinical experience suggested that it was a common problem in cancer patients treated with morphine[25]. Ventafridda et al.[26] observed a significantly higher incidence of dry mouth following treatment with oral aqueous morphine than with methadone or controlled-release morphine tablets[27]. Another study, carried out for a two-month period after initial treatment, noted that dry mouth was present 35 per cent of the time during treatment with an anti-inflammatory and/or adjuvant drugs, 36 per cent of the time during treatment with weak opioids and/or adjuvants, and 51 per cent of the time during treatment with strong opioids and/or adjuvants[28].

Other factors, which may contribute to xerostomia
Dehydration

Patients with advanced cancer are often dehydrated, with consequent thirst and dry mouth. There have been no controlled clinical trials which have demonstrated any relief of xerostomia following hydration, and the use of parenteral hydration in the palliative care setting remains controversial but generally should be based on individual needs. One study did not show any association between the severity of thirst and fluid intake in palliative care patients[29]. Symptoms related to dehydration are often manageable with simple measures, such as oral fluids or ice cubes and lubrication of the lips.

Decreased mastication

Mastication plays an important role in the regulation of salivary secretion, its effects being mediated through somatic afferent nerves of the oral mucosa and in the periodontal tissues. Patients taking a liquid diet or with immobilized jaws following oral surgery show a significant decrease in salivary flow. No data are available concerning decreased salivation in enterally fed patients or those with a gastrostomy or affected by trismus.

Psychological factors

Psychological factors, including anxiety, are known to reduce salivary flow. Hyposalivation and xerostomia may be observed in patients suffering from depression[30,31].

Prevention and treatment of xerostomia

The regimen currently used by the authors involves good oral hygiene, the prevention and treatment of infections such as candidiasis by administration of clotrimazole or fluconazole (especially in high-risk patients such as those undergoing high-dose corticosteroid therapy or radiotherapy for head and neck cancer), and a review of the drug regimen to avoid the use of drugs that may induce xerostomia.

Xerostomia after radiation therapy may be the most difficult to treat because of irreversible damage to the salivary glands.

It is a serious complication after conventional radiotherapy for nasopharyngeal carcinoma that severely impairs quality of life. Intensity-modulated radiotherapy is an advanced form of conformal radiotherapy that conforms to a high dose to the target volume while conforming a low dose to normal tissues. For nasopharyngeal carcinoma it may spare the parotid glands from excessive radiation and in other head and neck cancers it has been shown to preserve salivary function without compromising the local control[32].

The submandibular glands contribute up to 90 per cent of the unstimulated salivary output. Seikaly and colleagues[33] in a prospective non-randomized study of patients with head and neck cancer, transferred one submandibular gland from the side of the neck with the least risk of metastases to the submental area during neck dissection. This technique successfully prevented radiation-induced xerostomia. More recently, a study attempted to preserve submandibular gland function using intensity-modulated radiotherapy in the treatment of head and neck cancer[34].

A randomized controlled trial of standard fractionated radiation with or without amifostine (200 mg/m²) before each fraction of radiation, was conducted in 315 patients with head and neck cancer. Amifostine administration was associated with a reduced incidence of grade 2 or higher xerostomia over two years of follow-up ($p = 0.002$), an increase in the proportion of patients with meaningful (>0.1 g) unstimulated saliva production at 24 months ($p = 0.011$) and reduced mouth dryness scores on a patient benefit questionnaire at 24 months ($p < 0.001$)[35].

Currently available therapies for xerostomia are listed in Table 10.9.4.

Current therapy for chronic xerostomia includes the use of saliva substitutes or salivary stimulants. Water, glycerine preparations, and artificial saliva are used as substitutes for saliva, while sialogogues, sugarless sweets, and chewing gum stimulate the production of saliva[36]. An open, crossover, randomized trial compared artificial saliva with sugar-free chewing gum for xerostomia in 43 advanced

Table 10.9.4 Treatments for xerostomia.

Oral hygiene every 2 h
Humidified air
Suck: ice cubes, vitamin C tablets, frozen tonic water
Chew: sugarless chewing gum, lemon sugar candy, acid substances, pieces of pineapple
Artifical saliva and oral lubricants
Dentures which include a reservoir for the release of artificial saliva
Avoid alcohol and mouth rinses containing alcohol
Pilocarpine
Cevimeline
Xerostomia caused by drugs
Reduce the dosage and/or change the drug if possible
Application of fluoride gel to avoid dental damage
Xerostomia caused by systemic dehydration
Correct the cause
Increase liquid intake by mouth
Hypodermoclysis
Intravenous hydration in selected patients

cancer patients. Chewing gum produces an increase in salivary flow, and both treatments were effective, but 61 per cent of the patients preferred the chewing gum[37].

Many commercial products are formulated as solutions, sprays, or gels. Formulations have multiple contents including carboxymethyl- or hydroxymethylcellulose, electrolytes, and flavouring. Most salivary substitutes provide relief for only a limited time. They are most useful when used immediately before bedtime or speaking. There are few data to indicate superiority of any of the products. Artificial preparations of saliva that contain mucin provide substantially more symptomatic relief to patients with xerostomia than do conventional, non-mucin substitutes[38–40].

A comparison was made of Oral Balance gel delivered by slow release via a novel intra-oral device versus an oral bolus of gel on the oral health condition and oral-health-related quality of life in patients who had received standard head and neck irradiation for nasopharyngeal carcinoma. Slow release of gel via intra-oral device did not appear to improve quality of life, whereas gel alone reduced the severity of xerostomia symptoms and was the treatment of choice[41].

Pilocarpine, an alkaloid, functions primarily as a muscarinic–cholinergic agonist and has potent effects on both smooth muscle and exocrine tissues. It has been shown to be effective in patients treated with radiotherapy or who have had bone marrow transplantation and in those with Sjögren's syndrome. The peak secretory effects of pilocarpine are assumed to occur within one hour of its intake. Controlled studies have been carried out on the use of oral pilocarpine for radiation-induced xerostomia[42–44]. All these studies show that pilocarpine produces clinically significant benefits with acceptable side effects. Best results are obtained with continuous treatment for more than 8 weeks with doses of 5 mg, three times a day, when both efficacy and side effects are considered. Higher doses (10 mg three times a day) can increase clinical

benefits; however, an increase in side effects (mainly sweating) may occur. Caution is important in patients subject to bronchospasm or who have pre-existing bradycardia. Pilocarpine-treated patients require lesser amounts of artificial saliva; furthermore, patients treated with pilocarpine report that improvements in xerostomia, comfort, and speaking occur immediately. A French study evaluated the action of pilocarpine hydrochloride against xerostomia and the relationship of the response to dose/volume radiotherapy parameters[45]. The response to pilocarpine was independent of the dose of radiotherapy, suggesting that pilocarpine acts primarily by stimulating minor salivary glands and may be of benefit to patients with severe xerostomia, regardless of the radiotherapy dose. A controlled trial showed contrasting results: pilocarpine at a dose of 5 mg five times a day did not improve the production of saliva[46].

Another cholinergic agent, cevimeline hydrochloride, recently was approved for use in patients with Sjögren's syndrome.

Anethole-trithione (Sialor®, Sulfarlem®) seems to act directly on the secretory cells of the salivary glands. Some studies have found it to improve salivary flow, while others have not. Epstein and Schubert reported a phase I–II trial of the combined use of pilocarpine and anethole-trithione in patients who had not responded with increased saliva production to either agent alone[47]. A statistically significant increase in salivary volume and improved symptoms were reported. Apparently, the anethole-trithione prepared the salivary glands' cells for the stimulation provided by pilocarpine. Acupuncture has been shown to be effective in patients with pilocarpine-resistant xerostomia after radiotherapy[48, 49].

Dietary advice includes the ingestion of foods with high moisture content and the drinking of plenty of liquids with meals to facilitate mastication.

Sialorrhoea

Sialorrhoea (excessive salivation) is uncommon in advanced cancer patients but can cause discomfort, inconvenience, and social embarrassment; it can impair masticatory function, interfere with speech, favour perioral infection (particularly by *Candida albicans*) and result in irritation of lips, commissure, and chin. The most frequent causes are: radical mandibular resection procedures, recurrent oral cancer, which suspends the mouth in an open position, oral pain (apthous ulcers), local irritants (ill-fitting dentures), drugs (lithium, cholinesterase inhibitors, cholinergic agonists), psychosis, and epilepsy.

Salivation is mainly mediated through parasympathetic stimulation. Acetylcholine is the active neurotransmitter, binding to muscarinic receptors in the salivary glands. Cholinergic antagonists such as atropine, scopolamine (hyoscine), or glycopyrronium bromide can be used to treat sialorrhoea. These drugs are contraindicated when there are cardiac problems, closed-angle glaucoma, prostate hypertrophy, paralytic ileus, pyloric obstruction, cognitive impairment, and dementia. The clinical response is often incomplete but high doses cause significant side effects such as dry mouth, constipation, urinary retention, blurred vision, irritability, and confusion.

Atropine administered sublingually is readily available[50].

Scopoderm transdermal therapeutic system (TTS) is a dermal patch delivering scopolamine, usually applied to prevent nausea associated with motion sickness. Dryness of the mouth is its most common side effect. The lesser peak-concentration side effects are a specific advantage. It was reported to be used successfully for sialorrhoea in one cancer patient[51].

In a controlled clinical trial, a single dose of 0.02 mg/kg of hyoscine (scopolamine) hydrobromide solution, rinsed in the mouth for 5 min before swallowing, reduced non-stimulated and paraffin-stimulated salivation at 60 min, by 81 and 80 per cent, respectively. The heart rate of these patients increased significantly when compared with those given placebo and subjective sedation and relaxation were experienced by most of the volunteers[52]. Zeppetella successfully used scopolamine via nebulization in three patients, two of whom had not improved with the transdermal form. With nebulized delivery, scopolamine is absorbed faster and can be used on an 'as required' basis[53].

No data are available about the long-term use of anticholinergic drugs in patients suffering from sialorrhoea. Mier et al. in a placebo-controlled double-blind cross-over dose-ranging study demonstrated that glycopyrrolate is effective in the control of excessive sialorrhoea in children with developmental disabilities[54].

Glycopyrrolate is a quaternary ammonium antimuscarinic and does not cross the blood–brain barrier, so it is relatively free of central effects. It can be used orally, 0.4 mg three times a day[55] or subcutaneously but the use of nebulized glycopyrrolate is also described to treat sialorrhoea in motor neuron disease[56].

Andersen et al. treated the severe drooling with radiotherapy in 18 patients with amyotrophic lateral sclerosis and a life expectancy of fewer than two years. Irradiation of the larger part of the parotid glands and the posterior part of the submandibular glands with 7.0–7.5 Gy in a single fraction reduced drooling without producing permanent xerostomia, except in one patient[57].

There are also surgical methods for treating drooling problems such as bilateral parotid duct relocation, bilateral duct ligation of the parotid glands, combined with submandibular gland removal or relocation. The latter is performed alone or in combination, but is a common procedure usually reserved for patients with mental impairment.

There are several studies on botulinum toxin serotype A and serotype B in the treatment of sialorrhoea. When injected in the salivary gland, botulinum toxin inhibits acetylcholine release in the cholinergic nerve endings, mainly at neurosecretory junctions. The injection is made percutaneously, and ultrasound guidance improves efficacy and safety. The duration of action varies from 6 weeks to 6 months[58].

Taste alteration

Taste alterations are common in patients with cancer and can be the result of the disease itself and /or its treatment[59]. It occurs as a reduction in taste sensitivity (hypogeusia), an absence of taste sensation (ageusia), or a distortion of normal taste (dysgeusia). The incidence of these symptoms is unknown, but according to Twycross, between 25 and 50 per cent of cancer patients have a diminished taste sensation[60]. Specifically, chemotherapy and radiotherapy to the head and neck area have been shown to induce significant taste changes. Taste alterations can lead to food aversions, a reduction in food intake, and nutritional deficits. Many patients typically report that 'the food is tasteless' or 'the food is bitter' or 'the presence of a metallic aftertaste'. The sensation of taste is mediated through specific chemoreceptors (taste buds) each of which contains about 50 cells, which are renewed continuously. Their number decreases with age. They are found in the tongue, between the hard and soft palates, in the pharynx, larynx, epiglottis and uvula, lips and cheeks, and in the upper third of the oesophagus.

The tongue is most sensitive to sweetness on the anterior surface and tip, to salt and sour tastes on the two lateral sides and to bitter tastes on the circumvillate papillae on the posterior surface. Sour and bitter tastes are perceived most acutely on the palate; salt and sweet are most sensitive on the tongue. The pharynx has decreased sensitivity to all four tastes. Because smell and taste are closely linked, and both are required for the full sensation of flavour, changes to a patient's sense of smell can affect how foods taste. The chemical components of food stimulate the hair-like protrusions of taste receptors, which are bathed in saliva and, as a result, nerve impulses are sent by way of the fifth, seventh, ninth, and tenth cranial nerves to the medulla (nucleus of the tractus solitarius) and from there through pons and thalamus to the cortical area subserving taste. Information in this pathway is also projected to the lateral hypothalamus. A lesion in any one of these areas can alter taste perception.

Taste changes partly result from the influence of amino-acid-like substances secreted by tumour cells and such alterations are associated with disease progression. Taste loss and alteration can also occur as a consequence of cancer treatment. The average lifespan of a taste receptor is 10 days and of an olfactory receptor is 30 days. This fast proliferation is susceptible to inhibition by chemotherapeutic drugs, in keeping with the impact of chemotherapy on all rapidly dividing cells. Taste changes may also be related to surgery, radiation therapy, and non-chemotherapy drugs such as opioids or antibiotics.

The effect of cancer on taste is unknown. Potential causes of taste alteration are listed in Table 10.9.5. Taste abnormalities in cancer patients may be correlated with the site or extent of the tumour, independent of the histological type. A positive correlation exists between weight loss and the presence of abnormal taste sensation[61]. Disturbances in taste can also alter digestion because stimulation of taste organs can increase salivary and pancreatic flow, gastric

Table 10.9.5 Causes of taste alteration.

Local disease of the mouth and tongue caused by cancer
Partial glossectomy
Tobacco usage
Elimination of the olfactory component of taste after laryngectomy
Surgical removal of the palate
Damage to the nervous system following surgery or cerebral lesions
Alteration of the cell renewing, or cell regenerating cycle: ◆ Malnutrition   ◆ Radiotherapy   ◆ Drugs   ◆ Metabolic disturbances   ◆ Xerostomia   ◆ Stomatitis and oral infections   ◆ Endocrine factors (thyroidectomy, hypophysectomy, adrenalectomy)
Modification in the receptor cells due to alteration of saliva by metabolic agents, drugs, radiation
Dental pathology
Bad dental hygiene

contractions, and bowel motility[62]. There is also an association between advanced disease and an abnormality in the recognition of sugar and urea. A higher concentration of sweetness is needed for the solution to be recognized[61].

Williams and Cohen demonstrated elevated thresholds for recognition of sour (HCl), but not bitter (urea), sweet (sucrose), or salt (NaCl) in a group of patients with lung cancer who were tested before receiving chemotherapy or radiotherapy[61]. An elevated threshold of detection for all four basic tastes was reported in a group of patients with laryngeal cancer who were examined before laryngectomy.

Chemotherapy

Between 36 and 75 per cent of patients receiving chemotherapy report distressing changes in taste[59]. Patients undergoing haemotopoietic stem cell transplantation, where patients receive high-dose chemotherapy, often experience a complete loss of taste prior to replacement of their own stem cell. Taste disturbances have also been reported in patients receiving stem cells from donors, possibly related to the use of methotrexate to prevent graft-versus-host disease in the high-risk period immediately after transplantation[59].

The chemotherapeutic agents most commonly associated with taste changes include carboplatin, cisplatin, cyclophosphamide, doxorubicin, 5-fluorouracil, levamisole, methotrexate, and paclitaxel. Of these, cisplatin and doxorubicin were the most often reported as being associated with severe taste changes. Taste changes may occur during chemotherapy administration and can last from a few hours to several days, weeks or even months[59]. In a study of 284 patients with cancer receiving chemotherapy, 193 patients (68 per cent) reported taste changes; of these, the most common changes reported were loss of taste acuity or a metallic taste[63].

Taste alterations are a direct consequence of radiotherapy for tumours in the head and neck regions. This may be due to the direct toxic effect of radiation on the cells of the tongue, microvilli, and taste buds and their innervating nerve fibres. Furthermore, saliva production may be irreversibly reduced or impaired by radiation therapy, resulting in altered taste sensation and altered perception of food texture, plus difficulty in physically chewing foods due to lack of saliva. Patients report becoming more or less sensitive to sweetness. Perception of bitterness may be the most affected, with loss of the ability to taste sweetness occurring if the tip of the tongue is included in the field of irradiation. Taste loss is not observed until radiation doses of 20 Gy have been administered[64,65]. At doses of 20–40 Gy taste loss increases rapidly, and a dose of 60 Gy causes a relative taste loss of over 90 per cent[64]. Mossman et al.[20] demonstrated that curative courses of radiotherapy for tumours of the head and neck resulted in long-term changes in taste and salivary function; the maximum tolerated doses resulting in a 50 per cent complication rate, five years after treatment, were estimated to be 40–65 Gy for xerostomia and 50–65 Gy for taste loss.

Taste changes caused by irradiation usually begin to improve between three and eight weeks post-treatment and are fully restored within two to four months. When the total radiation dose to the head and neck region exceeds 60 Gy, taste may be permanently impaired.

Zinc deficiency has been noted as a potential cause of anorexia, dysgeusia, or hypogeusia. Plasma zinc levels have been found to be reduced in patients with bronchial carcinoma compared to the healthy population, and the zinc level in leukaemic cells appears to be lower than that in normal white blood cells[66]. The administration of zinc has been reported to correct abnormalities of taste in some patients[67,68], and copper and nickel have also been used with good result in clinical trials. Patients treated prophylactically with 25 mg of oral zinc four times a day prior to radiotherapy developed less severe hypogeusia than those given radiotherapy without zinc treatment[68]. Zinc must be administered in the middle of a meal to reduce potential gastrointestinal symptoms. Ripamonti et al., in a randomized, double-blind, placebo-controlled trial, described the beneficial effects of oral zinc sulphate tablets (45 mg three times a day) in 18 patients with cancer, receiving external beam radiotherapy to the head and neck region. One month after radiotherapy was terminated, the patients receiving zinc sulphate had a quicker recovery of taste acuity than those receiving placebo[69].

Patients suffering from taste alterations need good oral hygiene, treatment to increase salivation, the withdrawal of drugs that can induce or increase the symptoms, and dietary advice. Patients can sometimes take food with a strong smell; the addition of lemon, pineapple, or vinegar being useful if stomatitis or mouth ulcers are not present.

Halitosis

Halitosis (unpleasant or bad breath), occurs when exhaled air is combined with foul-smelling substances coming from various sections of the respiratory tract or from the upper digestive tract[70]. No epidemiological data are available about the incidence and prevalence of this symptom in cancer patients. Table 10.9.6 shows the most important causes of halitosis.

Between 56 and 85 per cent of the cases of halitosis are a consequence of diseases of the oral cavity[71,72]. The most likely cause of oral malodour is the accumulation of food debris and dental bacterial plaque on the teeth and tongue, resulting from poor oral hygiene, and resultant gingival and periodontal inflammation or sometimes nasopharyngeal disease. A careful history and examination of the oral cavity, sinuses, and the upper respiratory tract must be carried out to exclude inflammatory, infective, or neoplastic conditions[73,74]. Xerostomia and sometimes wearing dentures can cause or enhance malodour.

In people with nasal obstruction or sleeping in a hot, dry atmosphere, halitosis arises after sleep.

Some substances, such as garlic, leeks, onions, and alcohol contain volatile products which are absorbed by the intestinal wall and then excreted through the lungs. Alcohol also causes a decrease in salivary flow. The sulphur-containing amino acids in meat and fish can cause halitosis. A decreased intake of food can deplete body fat stores, with acidosis and ketosis giving an acetone odour. The role of smoking is controversial, but may modify the oral environment, exerting a local effect upon the oral mucosa.

When the sensation of halitosis is subjective, without objective evidence, it is necessary to investigate neurological or psychiatric illness (a form of delusion or monosymptomatic hypochondriasis). Sometimes, dysgeusia or dysosmia can cause these disturbances.

The treatment of halitosis is summarized in Table 10.9.7.

Hygiene measures, mainly use of a toothbrush and dental floss, are extremely important. Oral rinses, such as 0.2 per cent aqueous chlorhexidine gluconate, are helpful[75]. It is necessary to individualize

Table 10.9.6 Causes of halitosis.

Diseases of the oral cavity
Poor oral hygiene
Dental plaque, decay, cancer, bleeding gums
Tongue coating
Xerostomia
Acute necrotizing ulcerative gingivitis
Gingivostomatitis, periodontitis, pericoronitis
Inflammatory–suppurative phenomena
Oral malignancy
Diseases of the respiratory tract
Infection of the nose, tongue, nasal sinuses, pharynx, lungs
Tonsillar abscess, necrotic ulcers
Chronic rhinitis and rhinopharyngitis
Pharyngeal–laryngeal cancer with superinfection
Bronchiectasis, lung abscess
Abscess-forming lung cancer
Diseases of the digestive tract
Oesophageal diverticula, hiatus hernia, gastric stasis
Gastro-oesophageal reflux disease
Pyloric stenosis or duodenal obstruction
Altered secretion or bile-composition, colon stasis
Metabolic failure
Diabetic ketoacidosis (sweet acetone breath)
Renal failure (ammoniacal smell)
Hepatic failure (foetor hepaticus)
Drugs
Causing xerostomia and/or taste alteration
Cytotoxic drugs causing oral complications
Dimethylsulfoxide, antibiotics
Nitrites and nitrates, chloral hydrate, or iodine-based drugs
Foods
Garlic, onions, leeks, radishes
Alcohol, tobacco

Table 10.9.7 Treatment of halitosis.

General measures
Oral hygiene: toothbrushing, tongue scraping, and dental flossing
Regular use of antimicrobial toothpastes and mouthwashes (e.g. povidone–iodine mouthwash, chlorhexidine 0.2%, hydrogen peroxide 1%)
Denture care
Dietary advice: reduce alcohol intake and smoking
Specific measures
Treatment of possible non-oral causes
Drugs: discontinue use of drugs causing the symptom, if possible

drug treatment according to the likely cause and the general condition of the patient.

Infections of oral cavity

In normal subjects, most infections of the oral cavity are odontogenic infections with dental caries, gingivitis, and periodontitis being the most common. In comparison to normal subjects, the oral flora of patients with advanced cancer more often includes yeasts (83 per cent), coliforms (49 per cent), and coagulase-positive staphylococci (28 per cent)[76]. Such data indicate a loss of resistance to colonization of the oral mucosa in terminal cancer patients.

Many predisposing factors for candidiasis may be present, including antibiotics and immunosuppressive agents, nutritional factors, and low salivary rates[77, 78]. Increased oral coliforms have been reported in several groups of compromised patients, including those on cytotoxic therapy for malignant disease[79], patients who have received radiotherapy for oral and laryngeal cancer[80] and those with acute leukaemia[81]. Perhaps the release of endotoxin by Gram-negative bacilli may be responsible for oral soreness and clinical inflammation of the oral mucosa[82]. Microbial factors, such as adhesion and interbacterial interference, exogenous factors, including antimicrobial therapy, and miscellaneous host factors, such as xerostomia, seem to play an important part in the loss of resistance to bacterial colonization.

Fungal infections

Many patients receiving palliative care for advanced cancer are treated with repeated courses of antifungal medication for recurrent fungal infections. These drugs are often prescribed without confirmation of the diagnosis of an oral fungal infection by culture. In routine clinical practice, therefore, the identities and antifungal susceptibility profiles of the species involved in the infections are frequently unknown.

Candidiasis is the most common fungal infection seen in cancer patients[83]. *Candida* species are reported to be present in the normal oral flora of 40–60 per cent of the population[84]. Clinically evident candidiasis developed in up to 27 per cent of patients admitted to an oncology ward[85]. Oropharyngeal candidiasis can be the source of regional and systemic dissemination, particularly in granulocytopenic and immunosuppressed patients.

The primary pathogen is candida albicans, but other candida species and other fungi, including *Aspergillus*, may be involved. More recently, the oral mycological flora in hospice patients has been shown in several studies to host a significant proportion of non-*Candida albicans* yeasts. In 120 patients with advanced cancer, oral yeast carriage was present in 66 per cent of cases, and the frequency of isolation of individual species was: *Candida albicans*, 46 per cent; *Candida glabrata*, 18 per cent; *Candida dubliniensis*, 5 per cent; others, less than 5 per cent[86]. In a multi-centre study, the oral mycological flora of 207 patients receiving palliative care for advanced malignant disease was examined. In total, 194 yeasts were isolated, of which 95 (49 per cent) were *Candida albicans*. There was a high prevalence of *Candida glabrata* isolates[47] of which 72 per cent were resistant to both fluconazole and itraconazole[87].

Table 10.9.8 Main factors involved in fungal infections of oral cavity.

Local factors	Systemic factors
Wearing dentures	Diabetes
Xerostomia	Immunosuppression
Saliva composition alterations[a]	Medical therapies (e.g. steroids)
Oral mucosa disruption[b]	Nutritional status alterations
Microbial alterations	
Reduced mechanical debridement[c]	
Previous infections	
Poor oral hygiene	

[a] Mainly proteins and electrolytes.

[b] Radiotherapy, chemotherapy, surgery, cancer.

[c] Comatose patients, enterally/parenterally fed patients, trismus, etc.

The development of clinically evident oral candidiasis depends on local and/or systemic factors commonly involved in other oral infections and symptoms (Table 10.9.8). The role of xerostomia and drugs (such as steroids) should be emphasized; about 40 per cent of patients receiving adrenal corticosteroid therapy and about 30 per cent of those receiving antibiotics, develop oropharyngeal candidiasis[88]. Oral candida infection usually presents as acute pseudo-membranous candidiasis (thrush), acute atrophic candidiasis (or acute erythematous candidiasis), chronic atrophic (or chronic erythematous) candidiasis, chronic hyperplastic candidiasis, or candidal cheilosis (Table 10.9.9).

The thrush presentation appears as a white–yellowish plaque, which is easily wiped off, leaving a bleeding, painful surface. The acute atrophic form is often related to broad-spectrum antibiotics; white plaques are minimal, and painful lesions of the oral mucosa and depapillation of the dorsum of the tongue are present. Chronic atrophic candidiasis is characterized by erythema and oedema, usually localized to the part of the palatal mucosa in contact with dentures. This particular form of candidiasis occurs in up to 65 per cent of elderly individuals who wear complete maxillary dentures and is more common in women. Individuals with denture-related chronic atrophic candidiasis often also have angular cheilitis, characterized by soreness, redness, and cracks at the corners of the mouth. It can be either erosive or granular in type; habitual licking of the corners of the mouth and a reduction in the vertical dimensions of the lower third of the face, due to edentia, play a major role

Table 10.9.9 Common clinical pictures of oral candidiasis.

Type	Signs/symptoms (see text for more details)
Thrush (acute pseudomembranous form)	Typical white–yellowish plaques; usually accompanied by tenderness, burning, dysphagia, dysgeusia
Acute atrophic	More generalized red lesions, tongue depapillation; dysgeusia usually present
Chronic atrophic	Bright red surface (denture print); dysgeusia usually present
Chronic hyperplastic	Usually resembles leukoplakia; symptoms are usually absent
Angular cheilitis	it can be moderately painful and bleeding

in this clinical form. Chronic candidal infections are also capable of producing a hyperplastic clinical picture which can resemble leucoplakia, especially when occurring in the retrocommissural area; its role as a precancerous lesion remains open to debate[89].

Both topical and systemic treatments are available and they can be used together in more severe cases. Nystatin suspension (100 000 U/ml, 4–6 ml every 6 h) is the classic, topical treatment of oral candidiasis, but results can sometimes be disappointing. (Its action is limited to the time of contact with the mucosal surface; consequently, ice lollies made of nystatin diluted with water are a soothing and effective alternative). Any combination with chlorhexidine reduces its activity[90]. Clotrimazole lozenges (10 mg five times a day) have good antimycotic activity, even in nystatin-resistant patients, and are well tolerated and seem to be an effective drug for the prevention of oropharyngeal candidiasis[91]. Miconazole, an imidazole derivative, is another suggested topical treatment and is very effective in the form of lozenges (250 mg four times daily) or gel (two to four times daily), although the taste of lozenges may be found to be unpleasant. Amphotericin B lozenges can also be used for oral candidiasis, but are not as effective as clotrimazole and miconazole[92]. Intravenous amphotericin is not indicated in the treatment of oral candidal infection due to the low concentrations that are achieved in saliva.

Among systemic treatments, ketoconazole (200 mg once daily) has largely been replaced by more recent triazole derivatives, such as fluconazole (50–150 mg once daily) and itraconazole (100–200 mg once daily), which have fewer side effects. These are well absorbed by the gastrointestinal tract and have a long half-life, allowing once-daily administration. Their spectrum of action is wide; they are active against many different fungi and hence are useful in the treatment of oropharyngeal candidiasis and systemic and deep fungal infections[93–95]. Fluconazole treatment of oropharyngeal candidiasis (50 g once daily for 7–14 days) is possibly more effective than traditional treatments such as nystatin and ketoconazole and its once-a-day schedule makes it an attractive alternative for patients with advanced cancer.

The prolonged or repeated exposure to fluconazole may be associated with emergence of fluconazole resistence among strains of candida albicans and the potential selection of non-albicans species of yeast such as *Candida glabrata* and *Candida krusei* that are less responsive to fluconazole.

There is a need to assess new antifungal drugs for both the prevention and management of fungal infections in patients with advanced cancer because of the increasing incidence of colonization and infection with non-albicans yeasts with reduced susceptibility to the first-generation azoles. Voriconazole, a second-generation azole antifungal, may be a useful additional agent for the management of oral fungal infections caused by strains resistant to fluconazole and itraconazole, but susceptibility cannot be assumed and evaluation is recommended[96].

Caspofungin belongs to a new class of antifungal agents that have a different mode of action to azoles and polyenes. It is the first inhibitor of fungal glucan synthesis to receive approval for the treatment of mucosal and invasive candidiasis and invasive aspergillosis. It is well-tolerated and represents an option for patients with azole-resistant candida infection or who cannot tolerate amphotericin B[97].

Posaconazolo is a new triazole antifungal agent, it is active against candida, cryptococcus, and other yeast species, including those resistant to fluconazole and itraconazole. It is administered as an oral suspension. In a comparative, multi-centre, phase III study in patients with advanced HIV infection who had azole-refractory oropharyngeal and/or oesophageal candidiasis, posaconazole 400 or 800 mg/day resulted in a clinical response in 132 of 176 patients (75 per cent) with good tolerance[98].

The activity of voriconazole, caspofungin, and posaconazole is very potent *in vitro* against the majority of the isolates tested. Posaconazole is a useful therapeutic option for treating infections due to rare emerging species or for those mycoses caused by resistant isolates[99].

In conclusion, 75 per cent of the oral isolates were susceptible to fluconazole and this drug is likely to continue as the mainstay of treatment for oral fungal infections in the terminally ill, but a significant proportion of yeasts showed reduced susceptibility to fluconazole and itraconazole.

When using opioids in combination with antifungal the possibility of metabolic interactions should be considered. Opioids which are mainly metabolized by isoenzymes of the cytochrome P450 chain (methadone and fentanyl) can cause unexpected toxicity due to inhibition of their metabolism by azolic antifungal drugs[100,101].

Bacterial infections

Few data are available concerning oral bacterial infections in patients with advanced or terminal cancer[102].

A compromised mucosal barrier can contribute to local invasion by colonizing microorganisms and, subsequently, to systemic infection. Historically, Gram-negative bacteraemia has been the most problematic bacterial infection in neutropenic patients, but its incidence has reduced over time because of the use of prophylactic antibiotics. There has been a shift in the type of infecting organisms responsible for bacteraemia in these patients, from predominantly Gram-negative organisms to Gram-positive cocci. Oral colonizers such as *Streptococcus mitis*, *Streptococcus oralis*, and *Streptococcus sangulis* are the most frequently identified pathogens[103].

Periodontal disease is very common in the healthy population: about 70–80 per cent of adults are affected by minor periodontitis. About 15 per cent of those between the ages of 60 and 64 are affected by more severe levels of periodontal destruction[104]. Studies in patients with acute leukaemia suggest that periodontal disease may be an important cause of death during myelosuppression[105,106]. While the common oral flora is characterized by a prevalence of Gram-positive bacteria, a shift of oral flora towards Gram-negative colonization can be caused by: xerostomia, chemotherapy, radiotherapy, and immunosuppression cause[107]. The presence of heterogeneous flora, including candida and other species, makes bacterial cultures difficult to interpret, and interactions between bacteria and fungi contribute to the adherence and colonization of host tissues by micro-organisms[108]. Small haemorrhages, pain localized to the peridontium, and fever can be present, especially during chemotherapy. Secondary infection can be present in nearby structures, and radiographic signs of periapical abscess may exist[105,106].

The treatment of bacterial infections depends first on adequate hygiene (Table 10.9.10). Periodontal probing and scaling could possibly reduce postchemotherapy oral complications: the exact role of these treatments in advanced cancer patients has to be

Table 10.9.10 Causes of poor oral hygiene and treatment.

Pain
If possible, treat the basic cause
Good titration of systemic analgesic drugs
Analgesic gargles with:
◆ Benzydamine hydrochloride 0.15%, 15 ml every 2 h
◆ Xylocaine viscous 2%, 5–15 ml every 4 h
◆ Xylocaine spray 10%, every 4 h
◆ Diphenhydramine hydrochloride elixir 12.5 mg/5 ml and aluminum hydroxide in equal parts up to 30 ml every 2 h
◆ Choline salicylate dental paste 8.7%, every 3–4 h on the oral and perioral lesions
◆ Aluminum hydroxide and lignocaine 2% in equal parts
◆ Dyclonine hydrochloride
◆ Cetacaine (benzocaine) 20% solution
◆ Systemic analgesics
◆ Avoid alcohol and lemon-containing mouthwashes
Haemorrhage
Treat the basic cause (e.g. thrombocytopaenia)
Avoid using toothbrush and dental floss
Use a low-pressure dental jet and/or a gauze pad wrapped around a finger or a disposable sponge (toothette) moistened in a mild solution of baking soda and water
Gargles with:
◆ Saline solution
◆ Hexetidine 0.1%
◆ Sodium perborate
◆ Chlorhexidine 0.2%
◆ Povidone–iodine 1%
◆ Bicarbonate of soda
◆ Cetylpyridinium
◆ H_2O_2 3–6% in water 1:4
Gargles or soaked gauzes with antihaemorrhagic drugs:
◆ Thrombin 1–2 g/day
◆ Tranexamic acid 2–4 g/day
Debility or unconsciousness
Assisted oral hygiene by using a brush, gargles, spray, dental jet, cotton swabs moistened with mouthwash, gauze
Lips cracking prevention (petroleum jelly)
Room humidifier

evaluated. In acute periodontal infection, broad-spectrum antibiotic therapy is usually initiated, followed by more specific therapy based on the bacterial cultures, if possible and if indicated. Amoxicillin/clavulanic acid is one of the antibiotics recommended for the treatment of odontogenic infections due to its wide spectrum, low incidence of resistance, pharmacokinetic profile, tolerance, and dosage[109]. Teeth debridement with 2 per cent hydrogen peroxide and frequent rinsing are helpful. Povidone iodine and chlorhexidine 0.2-per cent mouthwashes can be added to the oral hygiene schedule, especially in the presence of fungating cancer lesions. In a palliative care setting pain treatment, usually non-steroidal anti-inflammatory drugs and topical treatments may play an important role.

Viral infections

Herpes simplex, cytomegalovirus, varicella zoster, and Epstein–Barr virus are the main causes of viral infections of the oral cavity[110]. Herpes simplex virus type 1 is the most common in patients receiving cancer chemotherapy; the reported incidence ranges from about 11 to 65 per cent[111,112], and different studies suggest a strong correlation of oral mucositis with isolation of herpes simplex virus[113–115]. Oral lesions due to herpes simplex appear to represent recurrent rather than primary infection. There are no data on the incidence of this infection in patients with advanced disease.

Herpetic infections appear as yellowish lesions, which are easily removed from the mucosa and are extremely painful; vesicles can also appear on the lips (cold sores) and fever, anorexia, and malaise may coexist. In severe infections, pain can be so intense as to produce complete dysphagia. The diagnosis of herpes simplex virus infection is mainly clinical: some difficulties can arise from the presence of other oral infections. When needed, exfoliative cytology permits an accurate diagnosis (95 per cent) in a short time[116]. The infection should be differentiated from aphthous ulcers: a history of vesicles preceding ulcers, a location on hard gingiva and hard palate, and crops of lesions are indicative of herpetic infection rather than aphthous ulcers.

Specific treatment of the herpes infection is provided by acyclovir, which can be administered orally or intravenously, with few side-effects, although patients must be hydrated and creatinine clearance monitored[117,118]. Venous extravasation must be avoided. Acyclovir can be employed also for prophylaxis in patients undergoing antineoplastic chemotherapy: screening for anti-HSV antibodies might be useful in order to identify patients at high risk for herpes simplex virus infection[119]. In patients with advanced cancer, the oral and topical routes (5 per cent acyclovir ointment) are better employed. Control of associated infections and oral hygiene are necessary. Chlorhexidine (0. 2 per cent twice daily rinsing) may be beneficial with herpes simplex virus type 1 infection[120]. Extraoral lesions may become secondarily infected; topical antibiotics are then indicated.

Oral lesions due to cytomegalovirus are not frequent in cancer patients, while they are the most common causes of oral diseases associated with AIDS patients. Active viral replication in the oral tissue produces ulcerations, aphthous stomatitis, necrotizing gingivitis, and acute periodontal infection. There are three systemic drugs approved for cytomegalovirus treatment: ganciclovir, or its prodrug valganciclovir, foscarnet, and cidofovir[121].

Radiotherapy- and chemotherapy-induced stomatitis

Oral mucositis represents a major non-haematological complication of chemotherapy, radiotherapy, and chemoradiation and in the conditioning before bone marrow transplantation–hemopoietic stem cell transplantation. It significantly affects the quality of life with significant morbidity, pain, ability to talk, eat, swallow, and subsequent dehydration and malnutrition. Indeed, symptoms are often of such severity as to require an interruption or curtailment of therapy or lead to dose reduction of the cancer therapy or treatment delay, to require the placement of feeding tubes and hospitalization.

In a recent meta-analysis of studies of radiation therapy, with or without chemotherapy in patients with head and neck cancer, the incidence of mucositis was of 80 per cent[122]. Factors that were found to be significantly associated with an increased risk of oral mucositis were nasopharyngeal or oropharyngeal tumour location, a cumulative radiation dose greater than or equal to 5000 cGy, and concomitant chemotherapy[123]. Anywere in randomized controlled trials comparing conventional versus different fractionations of radiation therapy or combined radiation and chemotherapy, severe oral mucositis has been reported in up to 60 per cent of patients receiving standard therapy and as many as 100 per cent of those receiving either hyperfractionation or accelerated hyperfractionation regimens[123].

Mucositis is a dose- and rate-limiting toxicity of therapy for cancer, and severe oral toxicities can compromise the delivery of optimal cancer therapy protocols. Mucositis has significant clinical implications, including severe pain requiring opioid analgesics and affects the quality of life. This dysfunction interferes with important functions such as swallowing and speech, leading to serious consequences such as weight loss[124–127].

Radiation-induced oral mucositis is due to the direct cytotoxic effect of radiation. The epithelial cells of the oral mucosa undergo rapid turnover, usually every seven to 14 days, which makes these cells susceptible to the effects of cytotoxic therapy. Mucosal erythema occurs in the first week in patients treated with standard 200 cGy of daily fractionated radiotherapy programmes. Patchy or confluent mucositis peaks during the fourth to fifth weeks of treatment with the same dose of radiation. It is characterized clinically by diffuse erythema, pseudomembrane formation and ulceration, xerostomia, taste alterations, pain, and oral intake can be markedly reduced. Mucositis caused by interstitial radioactive implants usually appears in seven to 10 days and peaks after 2 weeks. Stomatitis is self-limiting and heals within two to three weeks of the end of radiation treatment. The severity of stomatitis may be increased by environmental factors, including poor oral hygiene, tobacco use, xerostomia, low neutrophil count, blood urea, creatinine, older age, chronic periodontal disease and combined chemotherapy and radiation therapy[126–128].

A wide variety of agents may produce direct toxicity: antimetabolites (5-fluorouracil, methotrexate), anthracyclines (doxorubicin, epirubicin), alkylating agents, taxanes, and vinca alkaloids. It is estimated that there is an increased risk of mucositis development with bolus and continuous infusions, compared to prolonged or repetitive administration of lower doses of cytotoxic agents. Mucositis is a form of mucosal barrier injury and can be complicated by the infection of Gram-negative bacteria and fungal species. Patients are at increased risk of oral infections when they are neutropenic. The onset of mucositis secondary to myelosuppression varies, depending upon the timing of the neutrophil nadir associated with the chemotherapy agent administered, but typically develops anywhere from 10 to 21 days after chemotherapy administration. Patients with poor oral health have a higher risk of oral infections following chemotherapy. In the presence of neutropenia, mucositis predisposes to septicaemia, bacteraemia, and fungaemia.

Stomatotoxicity involves four phases, proposed by Sonis in 1998[129], in which the reduction of the renewal rate of the mucosa results in atrophic changes and ulceration. It most often affects the non-keratinized oral mucosa, including the cheek, soft palate, lips, ventral surface of the tongue, and the floor of the mouth. The first inflammatory phase includes the release of mediators (free radicals, cytokines, prostaglandins, and tumour necrosis factor) that cause damage by increasing vascular permeability, thereby enhancing cytotoxic drug uptake into the oral mucosa. In the second epithelial phase, chemotherapy reduces epithelial turnover and renewal, resulting in epithelial breakdown. This results in erythema from increased vascularity and epithelial atrophy, so microtrauma from speech, swallowing, and mastication leads to ulceration. In the third phase, the loss of epithelium and exudation leads to the formation of pseudomembranes and ulcers. Ulcerative mucositis can then provide a portal for microbial entry and can thus lead to local and sometimes systemic infections, which may even be life-threatening. Microbial colonization of damaged mucosal surfaces by Gram-negative organisms and yeast occurs and this may be exacerbated by concomitant neutropenia. Not only does mucositis open the way to adherence and invasion by oral commensals, but the floral changes seen in such patients lead to the appearance of, or increase in, potential pathogens such as α-haemolytic streptococci, which can lead to bacteraemia. The prevalence of an oral focus in febrile neutropenia has been reported in up to 30 per cent of cases. Bacteria, *Candida* species, or herpes viruses may be responsible, and xerostomia after cancer treatment further predisposes to infection. *Streptococcus oralis* and *mitis* are among the most common bacterial isolates from blood. Mucositis may also be a site of origin of mycoses, typically infection with *Candida albicans*, but also with *Candida krusei*, *Candida tropicalis*, *Candida parapsilosis*, *Candida glabrata*, and *Aspergillus* and *Mucor*[126].

The fourth healing phase usually lasts from 12 to 16 days. Sonis has recently proposed a five-phase biological model of stomatitis that includes dynamic interactions that promote initiation, message generation, signaling and amplification, ulceration and healing[127].

Assessment of oral pathology is essential to minimize acute and chronic oral and systemic sequelae of antineoplastic and radiation therapy[130].

To describe the toxicities associated with chemotherapeutic drugs, WHO (1979)[131] and the National Cancer Institute Common Terminology Criteria for Adverse Events v.3.0 (2003)[132], which incorporate both objective and subjective signs of oral mucositis, are widely used. There are also specific tools:

- The Oral Assessment Guide evaluates oral cavity changes related to cancer therapy, using eight categories (voice, swallow, lips, tongue, saliva, mucous membranes, gingival, and teeth/dentures), each rated on three levels of descriptors: normal findings, mild alterations, definitely compromised. An overall oral assessment score is the summation of the sub-scale scores, giving a possible range of 8 to 24[133].

- The Oral Mucositis Rating Scale was developed to assess stomatitis after bone marrow transplantation. It is a research tool consisting of 91 items for 13 areas of the mouth that are assessed for several types of changes. The total possible score is the sum of all item scores, with a possible range of 0 to 273[134].

- The Oral Mucositis Assessment Scale was developed by a group including dentists, oncologists, and oncology nurses from the United States, Canada, and Europe, as a scoring system for evaluating the anatomical extent and severity of stomatitis in research studies[135].

Validity and reliability have been demonstrated for the tools mentioned.

Treatment of the oral lesions induced by chemo- or radiotherapy can be problematic; therefore, prophylaxis is emphasized.

Oral hygiene should be stressed: mouth care protocols, including toothbrushing, flossing, mouth rinsing and fluoride applications, can significantly decrease the frequency of oral complications (Table 10.9.10). Patient education on routine mouth care is stressed. They should be counselled to rinse the mouth thoroughly after every meal so that the food particles do not remain in the mouth. Routine oral care includes removal of dentures, debridement of necrotic tissues, and regular oral rinse with saline. Hydrogen peroxide rinsing seems to be helpful for removing debris and mucus from the teeth [136a,136b].

Antibiotic rinses such as chlorhexidine may also be used; however, there is insufficient evidence to support or refute that chlorhexidine is better than placebo.

Few have an evidence base in the prophylaxis of mucositis, and there are no universally accepted treatment protocols. Two systematic reviews have focused on the prevention of oral mucositis in patients with cancer. One published in 1998 concluded that for most strategies reviewed there is insufficient evidence to draw any conclusions regarding their effectiveness[137]. The other review focused on patients with head and neck cancer only and found a beneficial effect of prophylactic interventions[138]. The most significant development has been the publication of the evidence-based guidelines of the Multinational Association of Supportive Care in Cancer and International Society for Oral Oncology for |the prevention and treatment of oral mucositis[139,140]. These guidelines were based on the consensus of 36 panelists after an exhaustive review of literature published between 1996 and 2002. They only recommend a few effective strategies, but highlight a variety of strategies to be avoided in clinical practice.

A recent Cochrane review[141] was conducted to evaluate the effectiveness of prophylactic agents for oral mucositis in patients with cancer, receiving treatment, compared with other potentially active interventions, placebo, or no treatment. It included 5217 randomized patients and evaluated the following treatments: acyclovir, allopurinol mouth rinse, aloe vera, amifostine, antibiotic pastille or paste, benzydamine, beta carotene, calcium phosphate, camomile, chlorhexidine, clarithromycin, folinic acid, glutamine, GM-CSF, honey, hydrolytic enzymes, ice cubes, iseganan, keratinocyte GF, misonidazole, oral care, pentoxifylline, povidone, prednisone, propantheline, prostaglandin, sucralfate, traumeel, and zinc sulphate. Of the 29 interventions included in trials, 10 showed some evidence of a benefit, sometimes weak, for either preventing or reducing the severity of mucositis. Only in the following treatments did more than one trial in the meta-analysis find a significant difference when compared with a placebo or no treatment: amifostine, antibiotic paste or pastille, hydrolytic enzymes, and ice cubes; the first three for patients with head and neck cancer and the last one for patients undergoing chemotherapy with 5-FU. Other interventions, each showing some benefit in only one study were: benzydamine, calcium phosphate, honey, oral care protocols, povidone, and zinc sulphate[141].

The strategy of therapy is based on pain control, improving healing and preventing infective complications. Minimizing mucosal trauma and controlling oral pain are the main principles of the palliative treatment of mucositis. Severe oral pain may require systemically administered medications. Systemic analgesics with non-steroidal agents and other non-opioids are used first and combined with opioids when pain is severe. Morphine and other opioids can be administered orally or parenterally. In bone-marrow transplant recipients, where severe mucositis is often present, continuous intravenous infusion of morphine is used routinely with good results[142]. Patient-controlled analgesia provides the most effective pain control, with lower total doses of opioid and less sedation and difficulty in concentrating[143].

The potential analgesic effect on mucositis-related pain of topically applied opioids has been explored in two studies. In one study, two different strengths of transmucosal fentanyl were not superior to placebo for radiation-induced oral mucositis[144]. In another study, mouth rinses with morphine were superior to topical lidocaine in treating pain due to chemotherapy-associated mucositis[145].

Anaesthetic rinses containing lignocaine hydrochloride may allow simple oral intake.

Patients should be told to avoid foods that irritate the mouth or throat, to cook solid foods until tender, use moist sauces, and choose soft, bland, low-salt foods. Patients should be informed of lifestyle changes, such as avoiding alcohol, tobacco, and spices to minimize oral complications.

Some benefits can be obtained with:

Cryotherapy: cooling of oral mucosa using ice chips will reduce the blood flow to reducing the availability of chemotherapeutic agents to the oral mucosa. Controlled clinical trial data demonstrate that ice chips placed in the mouth for 5 min before bolus administration of 5-FU, and then for a further 25 min have been shown to reduce stomatitis by approximately 50 per cent. Cryotherapy to induce vasoconstriction should be considered for patients receiving 5-FU or melphalan administered over short infusion times[146,147].

Antimicrobial: concurrent oral infections should be energetically treated. These approaches include the use of antibiotics, antivirals (acyclovir, valacyclovir, ganciclovir) and the antifungal agent, fluconazole. The oral mucosa of cancer patients is colonized by a variety of potentially pathogenic microorganisms such as Gram-positive and Gram-negative opportunistic bacteria and fungi. Antibiotic lozenges containing polymyxin E, tobramycin, and amphotericin B have shown contrasting results in preventing severe forms of oral mucositis, compared to controls in patients with radiation treatment in head and neck cancers. Although fungi are not primarily involved in the development of oral mucositis, they account for the most frequent infections of the damaged mucosa in the immunosuppressed patients. Viruses, particularly herpes simplex virus type I and varicella zoster, represent the most common pathogens aggravating stomatitis in the course of antineoplastic therapy. For seropositive and myelosuppressed patients, topical and systemic acyclovir treatment is effective in the management of oral herpetic infections[148].

The role of infections in the pathophysiology of mucositis has been reviewed by Donnelly [149], but no firm conclusion could be drawn due to the lack of a clear pattern of patient type, cancer treatment, type of antimicrobial agent used, and of consistent stomatitis assessment.

Benzydamine, a non-steroidal agent with anti-inflammatory and topical analgesic properties, has been found to be efficacious for stomatitis in patients receiving radiation therapy. In a controlled study, benzydamine hydrochloride mouth rinse produced significant pain relief and a reduction in the area of ulceration in radiation-induced stomatitis[150].

Chlorhexidine is a broad-spetrum topical antiseptic, but the results in controlling chemotherapy-associated oral mucositis are inconclusive. No studies have shown any benefit of chlorhexidine on radiation-induced mucositis. Results of studies on the efficacy of chlorhexidine as an adjunct to oral hygiene measures, suggest that its value is no more than sterile saline[128].

Although initial pilot studies showed beneficial effects of allopurinol mouthwash[151,152], results from controlled clinical studies have been controversial[153,154].

The oral mucosal defence mechanism is enhanced by local accumulation of activated neutrophils subsequent to subcutaneous administration of granulocyte colony-stimulating factor (G-CSF) and granulocyte-macrophage colony-stimulating factor (GM-CSF)[124]. Results of clinical trials are conflicting; the efficacy seems only partially dependent on the marrow-stimulating effect. GM-CSF mouthwashes have been shown to cause marked reduction of oral mucositis, but in contrast to these findings, prophylaxis with GM-CSF mouthwash in a randomized trial of 90 patients, undergoing high-dose chemotherapy and autologous peripheral blood stem cell transplantation, did not reduce frequency and duration of severe stomatitis[155]. The use of colony-stimulating factors in the treatment of stomatitis remains investigational[156].

Suspension of glutamine has been tried in different trials with inconclusive results. Huang and colleagues observed a reduction in the severity of radiation-induced mucositis[157]. Some studies have shown a positive result on mucositis due to chemotherapy[158]. In another study, Jebb *et al.* evaluated 5-FU-induced and folinic acid-induced mucositis and concluded that there is no effect of oral glutamine supplementation. No benefit was found from IV glutamine in haemopoietic stem cell transplantation[159].

Results of prostaglandin E2, which is a naturally occurring cytoprotective agent, administration for stomatitis are controversial[160]. It has been reported to be beneficial in healing gastric ulcers and chronic leg ulcers and work suggests a potential use as preventive treatment to chemotherapy-induced and radiation-induced mucositis. In a randomized double-blind placebo-controlled study, 60 patients undergoing bone marrow transplantation, treated with prostaglandin E2 prophylactically had no significant benefit in comparison with placebo administration. Importantly, the incidence of herpes simplex virus infection was significantly higher in patients receiving prostaglandin E2[161].

Amifostine is an inorganic thiophosphate that has been demonstrated to protect normal tissues against the toxic effects of some chemotherapy drugs and radiotherapy. This drug was approved by the Food and Drug Administration to reduce nephrotoxicity from chemotherapy containing cisplatin and to diminish xerostomia secondary to radiation therapy. A recent meta-analysis of 14 randomized controlled studies, comprising 1451 patients, compared the use of radiotherapy versus radiotherapy plus amifostine for cancer treatment. It has shown that amifostine significantly reduces the side effects of radiation therapy and that the efficacy of radiotherapy was not itself affected by the use of this drug. Furthermore, the patients receiving amifostine were able to achieve higher rates of complete response. Possible side effects are nausea, vomiting, hypotension, and cutaneous rash[162]. A randomized, double-blind, placebo-controlled, phase III study to evaluate the efficacy and safety of intravenous amifostine during radiochemotherapy for head and neck cancer was published recently. The results did not show any mucosal or salivary protection. A higher dose of amifostine may possibly be necessary, however, for protection of normal tissues when radiotherapy is combined with chemotherapy[163].

The camomile plant has anti-inflammatory, antibacterial, and antifungal properties. Preliminary uncontrolled studies suggested that it has shown good results in reducing the severity and duration of mucositis in a smaller group of patients[127]. Phase III trials have failed to conclude that camomile given in mouthwash formulation is effective in patients with chemotherapy-induced mucositis[164].

Traumeel S, a homeopathic medication in the form of mouth rinse, has been tried on patients undergoing allogeneic or autologous stem cell transplantation. The severity and duration of chemotherapy-induced stomatitis were reduced significantly; however, the limited number of patients was not sufficient to prove its efficacy[165].

Sucralfate, an oral, non-absorbable aluminium salt of sucrose octasulfate, with both local and systemic mucosal protective effects, has been investigated for possible prophylactic use in patients receiving radiotherapy to the head and neck and/or chemotherapy[166]. When it is used as a rinse, it is only 3 to 5 per cent systemically absorbed. Different controlled studies have failed to confirm any efficacy in the prevention of mucositis; however, oral pain has been reported to improve[167]. Other topical coating agents, such as magnesium hydroxide and hydroxypropyl cellulose, may be useful in treating established stomatitis[127].

Gelclair is a concentrated, bioadherent gel indicated for the management of stomatitis-related oral pain. It creates a protective barrier for susceptible tissues and sensitized nociceptors[124].

One approach to minimizing mucositis is to decrease the total dose of radiation and/or the volume of mucosa treated. Some of the risk factors for mucositis have been minimized by today's improved oral hygiene and dental care. Initially, the focus was on using single-agent antimicrobial agents to minimize and ameliorate mucositis, but this has been largely unsuccessful. Prophylaxis of herpes simplex virus in intensive chemotherapy and hematopoietic cell transplantation has been successful. More recently, some evidence suggests that severe mucositis can be decreased using a combination of antibiotics for Gram-negative infections and antifungal compounds[124]. More research is needed for conclusive data.

Graft-versus-host disease oral lesions

Chronic GVHD oral lesions present as tissue atrophy and erythema, lichenoid changes, and pseudomembranous ulcerations occurring typically on buccal and labial mucosa and the lateral tongue, angular stomatitis, and xerostomia. Oral pain, decreased oral intake, and risk of infection are serious problems in these patients. Oral symptoms benefit from topical steroids such as dexamethasone elixir, fluocinonide, and the high-potency steroid clobetasol 0.05 per cent. These treatments, however, need proper evaluation[168].

Osteonecrosis of the jaw

Patients with multiple myeloma and cancer metastatic to bone who are receiving intravenous, nitrogen-containing bisphosphonates are at greatest risk of osteonecrosis of the jaw[169]. A recent review on 368 cases showed that 94 per cent of patients were treated with pamidronate or zoledronic acid or both; 85 per cent of affected patients had cancer and 4 per cent osteoporosis. The prevalence of osteonecrosis in patients with cancer is 6 to 10 per cent. Osteonecrosis seems to be time- and dose-dependent because of the long half-life of aminobisphosphonates. The mandible is more commonly affected than the maxilla, and 60 per cent of cases are preceded by a dental surgical procedure, the remaining 40 per cent are probably related to infection, denture, or other physical trauma[170]. Oversuppression of bone turnover is probably the primary mechanism for the development of this condition, but there are factors that can contribute to this toxicity. Local oral factors include oral-health status, infection, and previous radiation therapy. All sites of potential infection should be eliminated before bisphosphonate therapy is initiated to reduce the necessity of subsequent dentoalveolar surgery. Exacerbating factors include diabetes mellitus, immunosuppression, the use of other drugs such as chemotherapeutic agents, corticosteroids, and antiangiogenic agents (thalidomide and bortezomib).

The oral lesions associated with bisphosphonates are similar in appearance to those of radiation-induced osteonecrosis. Clinically, they appear as ragged oral mucosal ulcerations that expose underlying bone and are often extremely painful. The clinical characteristics of necrosis of bone are a growing, painful, and unilateral swelling with jaw pain and difficulty chewing and brushing teeth.

The risk of developing this complication appears to increase with duration of use of the drug. A study in 252 patients with advanced cancer evaluated the incidence, characteristics, and risk factors for the development of osteonecrosis of the jaw. In patients treated for 4–12 months, the incidence was 1.5 per cent and in patients treated for 37–48 months it was 7.7 per cent. The cumulative risk was significantly higher with zoledronic acid compared with pamidronate alone or pamidronate and zoledronic acid sequentially ($P < 0.001$)[171].

A survey, conducted by the International Myeloma Foundation, in 1203 patients (904 with myeloma and 299 with breast cancer) receiving intravenous bisphosphonate therapy, showed that 81 per cent of the patients with myeloma and 69 per cent of the patients with breast cancer, who developed osteonecrosis, had a dental infection or had had a dental extraction[172].

Prevention of osteonecrosis is the best approach to management of this complication with removal of all foci of dental infection before starting bisphosphonate therapy. Conservative debridement of necrotic bone, pain control, infection management, use of antimicrobial oral rinses, and withdrawal of bisphosphonates are preferable to aggressive surgical measures for treating this condition. Hyperbaric oxygen therapy showed poor efficacy[173, 170] in some studies, however, some evidence exists for its use (see Chapter 11.2).

Local complications of oral tumours

Facial trismus

Facial trismus is the consequence of tumour invasion of the muscles of mastication, usually the pterygoid. It is common in retromolar trigone lesions, in very advanced anterior tonsillar pillar and tonsillar fossa tumours, and in soft palate lesions[124]. It is often accompanied by local pain or by pain felt in the external ear, in the pre-auricular or in the temporal area. Occasionally, the cranial nerves may be involved. Rarely a neoplasm originating in the pharygotympanic tube region can present with sharp, neuralgic pain in the distribution of the third division of the trigeminal nerve, associated with trismus (sinus of Morgagni syndrome).

Radiotherapy, when appropriate, can produce good results in alleviating facial trismus, and chemotherapy may also be helpful. Systemic analgesics, steroids, anticonvulsants (such as carbamazepine), muscle relaxants, such as diazepam, and local anaesthetic infiltration may help when trismus develops in response to a painful stimulus. Oral hygiene presents many problems due to reduced access to the oral cavity. Cotton swabs soaked with antiseptics, sprays, and dental jet can help. Liquid or semisolid feeding is not always possible: whenever indicated, a nasogastric or a gastrostomy tube should be inserted (see Chapter 11.2).

Abscesses, fistulas

Infections are very common in head and neck cancer patients, reported to contribute to 44–46 per cent of causes of death in this population.

Cellulitis, tumour infections, and orocutaneous fistulas make up about 22 per cent of febrile episodes in patients with head and neck cancers. Such patients are very often malnourished, with a previous history of alcoholism and of chronic lung disease and with decreased salivary flow and secretory IgA levels. In addition, surgery, radiotherapy, and chemotherapy often seriously damage head and neck structures in this patient group.

Shifting of oral flora, towards a Gram-negative population, including aerobic enterobacteria and *Pseudomonas aeruginosa*, is particularly important. Anaerobic Gram-negative bacteria also play an important role in head and neck infection. All of these aspects must be considered when approaching the management of abscesses and orocutaneous fistulas. A simple povidone-iodine solution is a sufficient preventive measure in patients at risk of developing secondary bacterial infections. The same antiseptics can be used as oral medication when an abscess is already present. In the presence of signs of sepsis or of local pain or discharge, broad-spectrum antibiotics, including metronidazole, should be administered. Carers will usually need careful education about management and mediation. In addition, information about what

Table 10.9.12 Family education programme.

The importance of oral hygiene in advanced and terminal cancer
Family-oriented oral cavity examination
The correct use of toothbrushes, dental floss, gauzes, toothette, gloves
Different mouthwashes: preparation, indication, and uses
The main oral complications of patients with advanced cancer
General
Specific to their relative
Personalized oral care programme (centred on the patient and their family)
Dietary and behavioural advice (e.g. if mucositis, dysgeusia, xerostomia)
Oral care in the unconscious patient

to do in any emergency, including the unlikely event of a massive haemorrhage is important (Table 10.9.10).

Tumour discharge

Many oral cavity tumours discharge, causing problems in swallowing and dysphagia and creating a chronic bad taste in the mouth. Radiotherapy may help this symptom, reducing the tumour mass and its secretions, but if this is not possible, local measures must be applied. Frequent rinsing with hydrogen peroxide can help by removing tumour debris. Benzydamine hydrochloride rinse can reduce the colonization of the oral cavity and help patients with

Table 10.9.13 Future research.

Perform epidemiological studies, evaluating the incidence and prevalence of oral-cavity problem in patients with advanced cancer, including the role of pre-existing infections (e.g. HSV)
Define the impact of oral complications on the quality of life of patients with advanced and terminal cancer
Develop quantifiable and reproducible criteria for assessing and classifying oral cavity pathologies in patients with advanced and terminal cancer
Define the importance of long-term oral side effects of anticancer therapies and their optimal planning, according to these aspects (e.g. radio therapy-fractionation schedules, different kinds of destructive and/or reconstructive surgery)
Study the interactions between oral-cavity problems and different systemic conditions present in advanced cancer (e.g. cachexia, anorexia, malnutrition)
Develop controlled studies in patients with advanced cancer, completely integrated with antineoplastic therapies
Develop appropriate evaluation methods for xerostomia and its treatment
Define and develop appropriate diagnostic tools for oral care in patients with advanced cancer
Develop and determine the role of oral care protocols in the palliative care setting
Develop adequate education tools to get the family involved in their relative's oral care
Determine the preventive and therapeutic role of the different antifungal drugs according to their administration schedules, to their compliance, their side effects, and costs
Perform clinical studies evaluting the oral complications of drugs currently used in palliative care (e.g. steroids, morphine, anticholinergic drugs)
Evaluate the role of biological response modifiers in preventing oral complications due to antineoplastic treatment performed in patients with advanced cancer
Evaluate the topical and systemic treatments for the prevention and management of taste alterations
Evaluate the role of systemic hydration in the management of xerostomia
Conduct appropriate studies to define and select topical and systemic analgesics for mucositis
Evaluate the different treatments for the management of fistulas, abscesses, and fungating tumours, in head and neck cancers
Develop prevention and treatment strategies for oral problems, which are feasible in developing countries
Develop new treatments specifically for oral-cavity problems

oral cleansing. Prevention and treatment of other oral problems such as candidiasis is very important (Table 10.9.10).

Conclusions

Health professionals involved in cancer management should be trained in the prevention, assessment, and treatment of oral problems[174]. Patients and family education, counselling, and motivation are needed to promote successful preventive strategies. An oral-disease prevention programme for patients receiving radiation and chemotherapy should be available at every institution involved in cancer care. Carers/family should be involved in the patient's oral care, especially in a palliative care setting, when patients are often unable to take care of themselves. The palliative care team should have a teaching programme for oral care: this can be applied during hospice and/or hospital admissions and continued during home care (Table 10.9.12).

Many aspects of oral care need improved evidence. The main areas of research should include the epidemiology of oral complications, their impact on quality of life, evaluation tools, and appropriately designed clinical studies. Table 10.9.13 indicates the main directions for future research.

References

1. Sreebny, L.M. and Valdini, A. (1988). Xerostomia. Part I: Relationship to other oral symptoms and salivary gland hypofunction. *Oral Surgery, Oral Medicine, Oral Pathology*, 66, 451–8.
2. Sweeney, M.P., Bagg, J., Baxter W.P. *et al.* (1998). Oral disease in terminally ill cancer patients with xerostomia. *Oral Oncology*, 34,123–6.
3. Oneschuk, D., Hanson, J., and Bruera, E. (2000). A survey of mouth pain and dryness in patients with advanced cancer. *Support Care Cancer*, 8, 372–6.
4. Thomson, W.M., Chalmers, J.M., Spencer, A.J. *et al.* (1999). The xerostomia inventory: a multi-item approach to measuring dry mouth. *Community Dental Health*, 16,12–7.
5. Makkonen, T.A., Tenovuo, J., Vilja, P. *et al.* (1986). Changes in the protein composition of whole saliva during radiotherapy in patients with oral or pharyngeal cancer. *Oral Surgery*, 62, 270–5.
6. Mandel, I.D. (1980). Sialochemistry in diseases and clinical situations affecting salivary glands. *CRC Critical Reviews in Clinical and Laboratory Science*, 11, 321–66.
7. Milne, R.W. and Dawes, C. (1973). The relative contributions of different salivary glands to the blood group activity of whole saliva in humans. *Vox Sanguinis*, 25, 298–307.
8. Tabak, L.A., Levine, M.J., Mandel, I.D. *et al.* (1982). Role of salivary mucins in the protection of the oral cavity. *Journal of Oral Pathology*, 11, 1–17.
9. Sreebny, L.M. and Valdini, A. (1987). Xerostomia. A neglected symptom. *Archives of Internal Medicine*, 147, 1333–7.
10. Brown, L.R., Dreizen, S. and Rider, I. (1976). The effect of radiation-induced xerostomia on saliva and serum lysozyme and immunoglobulin levels. *Oral Surgery*, 41, 83–92.
11. Eneroth, C.M., Henrikson, C.O. and Jakobsson, P.A. (1972). Effect of fractionated radiotherapy on salivary gland function. *Cancer*, 30, 1147–53.
12. Wescott, W.B., Mira, J.G., Starcke, E.N. *et al.* (1978). Alterations in whole saliva flow rate induced by fractionated radiotherapy. *American Journal of Roentgenology*, 130, 145–9.
13. Dreizen, S., Brown, L.R., Handler, S. *et al.* (1976). Radiation-induced xerostomia in cancer patients. Effect on salivary and serum electrolytes. *Cancer*, 38, 273–8.
14. Makkonen, T.A. and Nordman, E. (1987). Estimation of long-term salivary gland damage induced by radiotherapy. *Acta Oncologica*, 26, 307–12.
15. Cheng, V.S.T., Downs, J., Herbert, D. *et al.* (1981). The function of the parotid gland following radiation therapy for head and neck cancer. *International Journal of Radiation Oncology, Biology, Physics*, 7, 253–8.
16. Wescott, W.B., Starcke, E.N., and Shannon, I.L. (1981). Some factors influencing salivary function when treating with radiotherapy. *International Journal of Radiation Oncology, Biology, Physics*, 7, 535–41.
17. Kuten, A., Ben Aryeh, H., Berdicevsky, I. *et al.* (1986). Oral side-effects of head and neck irradiation: correlation between clinical manifestations and laboratory data. *International Journal of Radiation Oncology, Biology, Physics*, 12, 401–5.
18. Shannon, I.L., Trodhal, J.N., and Starcke, E.N. (1978). Radiosensitivity of the human parotid gland. *Proceedings of the Society of Experimental Biology and Medicine*, 157, 50–3.
19. Liu, R.P., Fleming, T.J., Toth, B.B. *et al.* (1990). Salivary flow rates in patients with head and neck cancer 0.5 to 25 years after radiotherapy. *Oral Surgery, Oral Medicine, Oral Pathology*, 70, 724–9.
20. Mossman, K., Shatzman, A. and Checharick, J. (1982). Long term effects of radiotherapy on taste and salivary function in man. *International Journal of Radiation Oncology, Biology, Physics*, 8, 991–7.
21. Carl, W. (1980). Dental management of head and neck cancer patients. *Journal of Surgical Oncology*, 15, 265–81.
22. Sreebny, L.M. and Schwartz, S.S. (1986). Reference guide to drugs and dry mouth. *Gerodontology*, 5, 75–99.
23. Sreebny, L.M., Valdini, A., and Yu, A. (1989). Xerostomia. Part II. Relationship to nonoral symptoms, drugs, and diseases. *Oral Surgery, Oral Medicine, Oral Pathology*, 68, 419–27.
24. Handelman, S.L., Baric, J.M., Espeland, M.A. *et al.* (1986). Prevalence of drugs causing hyposalivation in an institutionalized geriatric population. *Oral Surgery, Oral Medicine, Oral Pathology*, 62, 26–31.
25. White, I.D., Hoskin, P.J., Hanks, G.W. *et al.* (1989). Morphine and dryness of the mouth. *British Medical Journal*, 298,1222–3.
26. Ventafridda, V., Ripamonti, C., Bianchi, M. *et al.* (1986). A randomized study on oral morphine and methadone in the treatment of cancer pain. *Journal of Pain and Symptom Management*, 1, 203–7.
27. Ventafridda, V., Saita, L., Barletta, L. *et al.* (1989). Clinical observations on controlled-release morphine in cancer pain. *Journal of Pain and Symptom Management*, 4, 124–9.
28. Ventafridda, V., Tamburini, M., Caraceni, A. *et al.* (1987). A validation study of the WHO method for cancer pain relief. *Cancer*, 59, 850–6.
29. Burge, F.I. (1993). Dehydration symptoms of palliative care cancer patients. *Journal of Pain and Symptom Management*, 8, 454–64.
30. Mathew, R.J., Weinman, M., and Claghorn, J.L. (1979). Xerostomia and sialorrhea in depression. *American Journal of Psychiatry*, 136, 1476–7.
31. Anttila, S.S., Knuuttila, M.L. and Sakki, T.K. (1998). Depressive symptoms as an underlying factor of the sensation of dry mouth. *Psychosomatic Medicine*, 60, 215–8.
32. McMillan, A.S., Pow, E.H., Kwong, D.L. *et al.* (2006). Preservation of quality of life after intensity-modulated radiotherapy for early-stage nasopharyngeal carcinoma: results of a prospective longitudinal study. *Head and Neck*, 28, 712–22.
33. Seikaly, H., Jha, N., McGaw, T. *et al.* (2001). Submandibular gland transfer: a new method of preventing radiation-induced xerostomia. *Laryngoscope*, 111(2), 347–52.
34. Saarilahti, K., Kouri, M., Collan, J. *et al.* (2006). Sparing of the submandibular glands by intensity modulated radiotherapy in the treatment of head and neck cancer. *Radiotherapy and Oncology*, 78, 270–5.
35. Wasserman, T.H., Brizel, D.M., Henke, M. *et al.* (2005). Influence of intravenous amifostine on xerostomia, tumour control, and survival after radiotherapy for head-and-neck cancer: 2-year follow up of a prospective, randomised, phase III trial. International Journal of Radiation Oncology, Biology, Physics, 63, 985–90.
36. Levine, M.J., Aguirre, A., Hatton, M.N. *et al.* (1987). Artificial salivas: present and future. *Journal of Dental Research*, 66, 693–8.

37. Davies, A.N. (2000). A comparison of artificial saliva and chewing gum in the management of xerostomia in patients with advanced cancer. *Palliative Medicine*, **14**, 197–203.

38. Duxbury, A.J., Thakker, N.S., and Wastell, D.G. (1989). A double-blind cross-over trial of a mucin-containing artificial saliva. *British Dental Journal*, **166**, 115–20.

39. Vissink, A., Schaub, R.M., van Rijn, L.J. *et al.* (1987). The efficacy of mucin-containing artificial saliva in alleviating symptoms of xerostomia. *Gerodontology*, **6**, 95–101.

40. Visch, L.L., Gravenmade, E.J., Schaub, R.M. *et al.* (1986). A double-blind crossover trial of CMC- and mucin-containing saliva substitutes. *International Journal of Oral and Maxillofacial Surgery*, **15**, 395–400.

41. McMillan, A.S., Tsang, P.C.S. Wong, M.C.M. *et al.* (2006). Efficacy of a novel lubricating system in the management of radiotherapy-related xerostomia. *Oral Oncology*, **42**, 842–8.

42. LeVeque, F.G., Montgomery, M., Potter, D. *et al.* (1993). A multicenter, randomized, double-blind, placebo-controlled, dose-titration study of oral pilocarpine for treatment of radiation-induced xerostomia in head and neck cancer patients. *Journal of Clinical Oncology*, **11**, 1124–31.

43. Johnson, J.T., Ferretti, G.A., Nethery, W.J. *et al.* (1993). Oral pilocarpine for post-irradiation xerostomia in patients with head and neck cancer. *New England Journal of Medicine*, **329**, 390–5.

44. Rieke, J.W., Hafermann, M.D., and Johnson, J.T. *et al.* (1995). Oral pilocarpine for radiation-induced xerostomia: integrated efficacy and safety results from two prospective randomized clinical trials. *International Journal of Radiation Oncology, Biology, Physics*, **31**, 661–9.

45. Horiot, J.C., Lipinski, F., Schraub, S. (2000). Post-radiation severe xerostomia relieved by pilocarpine: a prospective French cooperative study. *Radiotherapy in Oncology*, **55**(3), 233–9.

46. Gornitsky, M., Shenouda, G., Sultanem, K. *et al.* (2004). Double-blind randomized, placebo-controlled study of pilocarpine to salvage salivary gland function during radiotherapy of patients with head and neck cancer. *Oral Surgery Oral Medicine, Oral Pathology, Oral Radiology and Endodontics*, **98**, 45–52.

47. Epstein, J.B. and Schubert, M.M. (1987). Synergistic effect of sialagogues in management of xerostomia after radiation therapy. *Oral Surgery, Oral Medicine, Oral Pathology*, **64**, 179–82.

48. Rydholm, M. and Strang, P. (1999). Acupuncture for patients in hospital-based home care suffering from xerostomia. *Journal of Palliative Care*, **15**, 20–3.

49. Johnstone, P.A.S., Peng, Y.P., May, B.C. *et al.* (2001). Acupuncture for pilocarpine-resistant xerostomia following radiotherapy for head and neck malignancies. *International Journal of Radiation Oncology, Biology, Physics*, **50**, 353–7.

50. Hyson, H.C., Johnson, A.M., and Jog, M.S. (2002). Sublingual atropine for sialorrhea secondary to parkinsonism: a pilot study. *Movement Disorders*, **17**, 1318–20.

51. Tassinari, D., Poggi, B., Fantini, M. *et al.* (2005). Treating sialorrhea with transdermal scopolamine. Exploiting a side effect to treat an uncommon symptom in cancer patients. *Support Care Cancer*, **13**, 559–61.

52. Lieblich, S. (1989). Episodic supersalivation (idiopathic paroxysmal sialorrhea): description of a new clinical syndrome. *Oral Surgery, Oral Medicine, Oral Pathology*, **68**, 159–61.

53. Zeppetella, G. (1999). Nebulized scopolamine in the management od oral dribbling: three case reports. *Journal of Pain and Symptom Management*, **17**, 293–5.

54. Mier, R.J., Bachrach, S.J., Lakin R.C. *et al.* (2000). Treatment of sialorrhea with glycopyrrolate. *Archives of Pediatric Adolescent Medicine*, **154**, 1214–8.

55. Olsen, A.K. and Sjogren, P. (1999). Oral glycopyrrolate alleviates drooling in a patient with tongue cancer. *Journal of Pain and Symptom Management*, **18**, 300–2.

56. Strutt, R., Fardell, B., and Chye, R. (2002). Nebulized glycopyrrolate for drooling in a motor neuron patient. *Journal of Pain and Symptom Management*, **23**, 2–3.

57. Andersen, P.M., Gronberg, H. *et al.* (2001). External radiation of the parotid glands significantly reduces drooling in patients with motor neurone disease with bulbar paresis. *Journal of Neurological Science*, **191**, 111–4.

58. Meningaud, J.P., Pitak-Arnnop, P., Chikhani, L. *et al.* (2006). Drooling of saliva: a review of the etiology and management options. *Oral Surgery, Oral Medicine, Oral Pathology, Oral Radiology in Endodontics*, **101**, 48–57.

59. Ravasco, P. (2005). Aspects of taste and compliance in patients with cancer. *European Journal of Oncology Nursing*, **9**, S84–S91.

60. Twycross, R.G. and Lack, S.A., comps. (1986). Taste change. *Control of Alimentary Symptoms in Far Advanced Cancer*, vol. 4, pp. 57–65. Edinburgh: Churchill Livingstone.

61. Williams, L.R. and Cohen, M.H. (1978). Altered taste thresholds in lung cancer. *American Journal of Clinical Nutrition*, **31**, 122–5.

62. DeWys, W.D. and Walters, K. (1975). Abnormalities of taste sensation in cancer patients. *Cancer*, **36**, 1888–96.

63. Wickham, R.S., Rehwaldt, M., and Kefer, C. (1999). Taste changes experienced by patients receiving chemotherapy. *Oncology Nursing Forum*, **26**, 697–706.

64. Herrmann, T., Adamski, K., and Stefan, M. (1984). Storungen von Speichelproduktion und Geschmacksempfindung nach Bestrahlung intramuscular oropharyngeal Bereich. *Radiobiology Radiotherapy*, **25**, 621–9.

65. Mossman, K.L. and Henkin, R.I. (1978). Radiation-induced changes in taste acuity in cancer patients. *International Journal of Radiation Oncology, Biology, Physics*, **4**, 663–70.

66. Henkin, R.I. and Brandley, D.F. (1970). Hypogeusia corrected by Ni++ and Zn++. *Life Science*, **9**, 701–9.

67. Henkin, R.I., Schechter, P.J., Hoye, R.C. *et al.* (1971). Idiopathic hypogeusia with dysgeusia, hyposmia and dysosmia: a new syndrome. *Journal of the American Medical Association*, **217**, 434–40.

68. Henkin, R.I. (1972). Prevention and treatment of hypogeusia due to head and neck irradiation. *Journal of the American Medical Association*, **220**, 870–1.

69. Ripamonti, C., Zecca, E., Brunelli, C. *et al.* (1998). A randomized, controlled clinical trial to evaluate the effects of zinc sulphate on cancer patients with taste alterations caused by head and neck irradiation. *Cancer*, **82**, 1938–45.

70. Porter, S.R. and Scully, C. (2006). Oral malodour (halitosis). *British Medical Journal*, **333**, 632–5.

71. Attia, E.L. and Marshall, G.L. (1982). Halitosis. *Canadian Medical Assocation Journal*, **126**, 1281.

72. Scully, C., Porter, S., and Greenman, J. (1994). What to do about halitosis. *British Medical Journal*, **308**, 217–8.

73. Richardson, H.C. and Prichard, A.J.N. (1994). Managing halitosis (letter). *British Medical Journal*, **308**, 652.

74. Parmar, S.C. and Naik, P.C. (1994). Remember the tongue (letter). *British Medical Journal*, **308**, 652.

75. Rosenberg, M. (1992). Halitosis—the need for further research and education. *Journal of Dental Research*, **71**, 424.

76. Jobbins, J., Bagg, J., Parsons, K. *et al.* (1992). Oral carriage of yeasts, coliforms and staphylococci in patients with advanced malignant disease. *Journal of Oral Pathology and Medicine*, **21**, 305–8.

77. Aldred, M.J., Addy, M., Bagg, J. *et al.* (1991). Oral health in the terminally ill: a cross sectional pilot survey. *Specialist Care in Dentistry*, **11**, 59–62.

78. Finlay, I.G. (1986). Oral symptoms and candida in the terminally ill. *British Medical Journal*, **292**, 592–3.

79. Samaranayake, L.P., Calman, K.C., Ferguson, M.M. *et al.* (1984). The oral carriage of yeasts and coliforms in patients on cytotoxic therapy. *Journal of Oral Pathology*, **13**, 390–3.

80. Martin, M.V., Al-Tikriti, U., and Bramley, P. (1981). Yeasts flora of the mouth and skin during and after irradiation for oral and laryngeal cancer. *Journal of Medical Microbiology*, **14**, 457–61.

81. Wahlin, Y.B. and Holm, A.K. (1988). Changes in the oral microflora in patients with acute leukaemia and related disorders during the period of induction therapy. *Oral Surgery, Oral Medcine, Oral Pathology*, **65**, 411–17.

82. Spijkervet, F.K.L., van-Saene, H.K., van-Saene, J.J. (1990). Mucositis prevention by selective elimination of oral flora in irradiated head and neck cancer patients. *Journal of Oral Pathology and Medicine*, **19**, 486–9.

83. Bodey, G.P. (1984). Candidiasis in cancer patients. *American Journal of Medicine*, **77D**, 13–19.

84. Epstein, J.B., Truelove, E.L., and Izutzu, K.T. (1984). Oral candidiasis: pathogenesis and host defense. *Reviews of the Infectious Diseases*, **6**, 96–106.

85. Yeo, E., Alvarado, T., Fainstein, V. *et al.* (1985). Prophylaxis of oropharyngeal candidiasis with clotrimazole. *Journal of Clinical Oncology*, **3**, 1668–71.

86. Davies, A.N., Brailsford, S., Broadley, K. *et al.* (2002). Oral yeast carriage in patients with advanced cancer. *Oral Microbiology and Immunology*, **17**, 79–84.

87. Bagg, J., Sweeney, M.P., Lewis, M.A.O. *et al.* (2003). High prevalence of non-albicans yeasts and detection of anti-fungal resistance in the oral flora of patients with advanced cancer. *Palliative Medicine*, **17**, 477–81.

88. Bodey, G.P., Samonis, G., and Rolston, K. (1990). Prophylaxis of candidiasis in cancer patients. *Seminars in Oncology*, **17**, 24–8.

89. Regezi, J.A. and Sciubba, J.J., ed. (1989). White lesions. In *Oral pathology: Clinical-Pathologic Correlations*, 3rd edition, pp. 84–124. Philadelphia PA: WB Saunders.

90. Barkvoll, P. and Attramadal, A. (1989). Effect of nystatin and chlorexidine digluconate on Candida Albicans. *Oral Surgery, Oral Medicine, Oral Pathology*, **67**, 279–81.

91. Meunier, F., Paesmans, M., and Autier, P. (1994). Value of antifungal prophylaxis with antifungal drugs against oropharyngeal candidiasis in cancer patients. *Oral Oncology, European Journal of Cancer*, **30B**, 196–9.

92. de Vries-Hospers, G.H. and van der Waaij, D. (1980). Salivary concentrations of amphotericin B following its use as an oral lozenges. *Infection*, **8**, 63–5.

93. Saag, M.S. and Dismukes, W.E. (1988). Azole antifungal agents: emphasis on new triazoles. *Antimicrobial Agents and Chemotherapy*, **32**, 1–8.

94. Cauwenbergh, G., Doncker, P.D., Stoops, K. *et al.* (1987). Itraconazole in the treatment of human mycoses: Review of three years of clinical experience. *Reviews of the Infectious Diseases*, **9**, S146–52.

95. Dupont, B. and Drouhet, E. (1988). Fluconazole for the treatment of fungal diseases in immunosuppressed patients. *Annals of the New York Academy of Sciences*, **544**, 564–70.

96. Bagg, J., Sweeney, M P., Davies, A.N. *et al.* (2005). Voriconazole susceptibility of yeasts isolated from the mouths of patients with advanced cancer. *Journal of Medical Microbiology*, **54**, 959–64.

97. Garbino, J. (2004). Caspofungin-a new therapeutic option for oropharyngeal candidiasis. *Clinical Microbiology Infections*, **10**, 187–9.

98. Keating, G.M. (2005). Posaconazole. *Drugs*, **65**, 1553–67.

99. Sabatelli, F., Patel, R., Mann, P.A. *et al.* (2006). In vitro activities of posaconazole, fluconazole, itraconazole, voriconazole, and amphotericin B against a large collectioof clinically important molds and yeasts. *Antimicrobial Agents and Chemotherapy*, **50**, 2009–15.

100. Tarumi, Y., Pereira, J., and Watanabe, S. (2002). Methadone and fluconazole: respiratory depression by drug interaction. *Journal of Pain and Symptom Management*, **23**, 148–53.

101. Mercadante, S., Villari, P., and Ferrera, P. (2002). Itraconazole-fentanyl interaction in a cancer patient. *Journal of Pain and Symptom Management*, **24**, 284–6.

102. Poland, J.M. (1987). Stomatitis and specific oral infections of the oncologic patients. *American Journal of Hospice Care*, Sep/Oct, 30–2.

103. Khan, S.A. and Wingard, J.R. (2001). Infection and mucosal injury in cancer treatment. *Journal of the National Cancer Institute, Monographs*, **29**, 31–6.

104. Epidemiology and Oral Disease Prevention Program, National Institute of Dental Research. (1987). Oral Health of United States Adults: the National Survey of Oral Health in US Employed Adults and Seniors, 1985–86: National Findings. Bethesda, MD: Department of Health and Human Services, Public Health Service, National Institutes of Health (NIH publication no. 87–2868).

105. Overholser, C.D., Peterson, D.E., Williams, L.T. *et al.* (1982). Periodontal infections in patients with acute non lymphocytic leukemia: prevalence of acute exacerbations. *Archives of Internal Medicine*, **142**, 551–4.

106. Peterson, D.E. and Overholser, C.D. (1981). Increased morbidity associated with oral infections in patients with non acute lymphocytic leukemia. *Oral Surgery, Oral Medicine, Oral Pathology*, **51**, 390–3.

107. Minah, G.E., Rednor, J.L., Peterson, D.E. *et al.* (1986). Oral succession of gram-negative bacilli in myelosuppressed cancer patients. *Journal of Clinical Microbiology*, **24**, 210–13.

108. Peterson, D.E., Minah, G.E., Reynolds, M.A. *et al.* (1990). Effect of granulocytopenia on oral microbial relationships in patients with acute leukemia. *Oral Surgery, Oral Medicine, Oral Pathology*, **70**, 720–3.

109. Maestre-Vera, J.R. (2004). Treatment options in odontogenic infection. *Med Oral Patol Oral Cir Bucal*, **9**, 25–31.

110. Barret, A.P. (1986). A long term prospective clinical study of orofacial herpes simplex virus infection in acute leukemia. *Oral Surgery, Oral Medicine, Oral Pathology*, **61**, 149–52.

111. Rand, H.R., Kramer, B., and Johnson, A.C. Cancer chemotherapy and associated symptomatic stomatitis and the role of herpes simplex virus. *Cancer*, **50**, 1262.

112. Barret, A.P. (1987). A long term prospective clinical study of oral complications during conventional chemotherapy for acute leukemia. *Oral Surgery, Oral Medicine, Oral Pathology*, **63**, 313–16.

113. Montgomery, R.T., Redding, S.W., and Le Maistre, C.F. (1986). The incidence of oral herpes simplex virus infection in patients undergoing cancer chemotherapy. *Oral Surgery, Oral Medicine, Oral Pathology*, **61**, 238–42.

114. Beattie, G., Whelan, J., Cassidy, J. *et al.* (1989). Herpes simplex virus, Candida Albicans and mouth ulcers in neutropenic patients with non-haematological malignancy. *Cancer Chemotherapy and Pharmacology*, **25**, 75–6.

115. Bergmann, O.J., Mogensen, S.C., and Ellegard, J. (1990). Herpes simplex virus and intraoral ulcers in immunocompromised patients with haematological malignancies. *European Journal of Clinical Microbiology and Infectious Disease*, **9**, 184–90.

116. Barret, A.P., Buckley, D.J., and Greenberg, M.L. (1986). The value of exfoliative cytology in diagnosing of oral herpes infection in immunosuppressed patients. *Oral Surgery, Oral Medicine, Oral Pathology*, **62**, 175–8.

117. Hann, J.M., Prentice, H.G., Blacklock, H.A. *et al.* (1983). Acyclovir prophylaxis against herpes virus infections in severely immunocompromised patients: a randomised double blind study. *British Medical Journal*, **287**, 384–8.

118. Leflore, S., Anderson, P.L., and Fletcher, C.V. (2000). A risk-benefit evaluation of acyclovir for the treatment and prophylaxis of herpes simplex virus infections. *Drug Safety*, **23**(2), 131–42.

119. Carrega, G., Castagnola, E., Canessa, A. *et al.* (1994). Herpes simplex virus and oral mucositis in children with cancer. *Support Care-Cancer*, **2**, 266–9.

120. Park, J.B. and Park, N.H. (1989). Effect of chlorexidine on the *in vitro* and *in vivo* herpes simplex virus infection. *Oral Surgery, Oral Medicine, Oral Pathology*, **67**, 149–53.

121. Biron, K.K. (2006). Antiviral drugs for citomegalovirus diseases. *Antiviral Research*, **71**, 154–63.

122. Trotti, A., Bellm, L.A., Epstein, J.B. *et al.* (2003). Mucositis incidence, severity and associated outcomes in patients with head and neck

cancer receiving radiotherapy with or without chemotherapy: a systematic literature review. *Radiotherapy and Oncology, 66*, 253–62.

123. Vera-Llonch, M., Oster, G., Hagiwara, M. *et al.* (2005). Oral mucositis in patients undergoing radiation treatment for head and neck carcinoma. Risk factors and clinical consequences. *Cancer, 106*, 329–36.

124. Berger, A.M. and Fall-Dickson, J.M. (2005). Oral complications. In *Cancer: principles and practice of oncology* (eds. T.D. DeVita, S. Hellman, and S.A. Rosemberg), 7th edition. pp. 2523–5. Lippincott Williams and Wilkins, Philadelphia.

125. Raber-Durlacher, J.E., Weijl, N.I., Abu Saris. M. *et al.* (2000). Oral mucositis in patients treated with chemotherapy for solid tumours: a retrospective analysis of 150 cases. *Support Care Cancer, 8*(5), 366–71.

126. Scully, C., Epstein, J., and Sonis, S. (2003). Oral mucositis: a challenging complication of radiotherapy, chemotherapy, and radiochemotheraphy: part 1, pathogenesis and prophylaxis of mucositis. *Head and Neck, 25*,1057–70.

127. Naidu, M.U., Ramana, G.V., Rani, P.U. *et al.* (2004). Chemotherapy-induced and/or radiation therapy-induced oral mucositis— Complicating the treatment of cancer. *Neoplasia, 6*, 423–31.

128. Scully, C., Epstein, J., and Sonis, S. (2004). Oral mucositis: a challenging complication of radiotherapy, chemotherapy, and radiochemotheraphy: part 2, diagnosis and management of mucositis. *Head and Neck, 26*, 77–84.

129. Sonis, S.T. (1998). Mucositis as a biological process- a new hypothesis for the development of chemotherapy induced stomatotoxicity. *Oral Oncology. 34*, 39–43.

130. Stone, R., Fliedner, M.C., and Smiet, A.C.M. (2005). Management of oral mucositis in patients with cancer. *European Journal of Oncology Nursing, 9*, S24-S32.

131. World Health Organization, (1979). *Handbook for reporting results of cancer treatment*, pp. 15–22. World Health Organization, Geneva, Switzerland.

132. Cancer Therapy Evaluation Program. (2003). Common terminology criteria for adverse events, version 3.0. DCTD, NCI, NIH, DHHS, June 10.

133. Eilers, J., Berger, A.M., and Petersen, M.C. (1988). Development, testing, and application of the oral assessment guide. *Oncology Nursing Forum, 15*, 325.

134. Schubert, M.M., Williams, B.E., Lloid, M.E. *et al.* (1992). Clinical scale for the rating of oral mucosal changes associated with bone marrow transplantation. Development of an oral mucositis index. *Cancer, 69*, 2469.

135. Sonis, S.T., Eilers, J.P., Epstein, J.B., for the Mucositis Study Group (1999). Validation of a new scoring system for the assessment of clinical trial research of oral mucositis induced by radiation or chemotherapy. *Cancer, 85*, 2103–13.

136a. Daeffler, R. (1980). Oral hygiene measures for patients with cancer I. *Cancer Nursing* Oct, 347–56.

136b. Daeffler, R. (1980). Oral hygiene measures for patients with cancer II. *Cancer Nursing*, Dec, 427–32.

137. Kovanko, I. (1998). The effectiveness of strategies for preventing and treating chemotherapy and radiation induced oral mucositis in patients with cancer, pp. 1–84. Joanna Briggs Institute for evidence based nursing and midwifery, Adelaide, S. Australia,

138. Sutherland, S.E. and Browman, G.P. (2001). Prophylaxis of oral mucositis in irradiated head-and-neck cancer patients: a proposed classification scheme of interventions and meta-analysis of randomized controlled trials. *International Journal of Radiation Oncology, Biology and Physics, 49*, 917–30.

139. Rubenstein, E.B., Peterson, D.E., Schubert, M. *et al.* (2004). Clinical practice guidelines for the prevention and treatment of cancer therapy-induced oral and gastrointestinal mucositis. *Cancer Supplement, 100*, 2026–46.

140. Sonis, S.T., Elting, L.S., Keefe, D. *et al.* (2004). Perspectives on cancer therapy-induced mucosal injury. *Cancer Supplement, 100*, 1995–2025.

141. Worthington, H.V., Clarkson, J.E., and Eden, O.B. (2006). Interventions for preventing oral mucositis for patients with cancer receiving treatment. *Cochrane Database of Systematic Reviews, 2*, CD000978.

142. Hill, H.F., Chapman, C.R., Kornell J.A. *et al.* (1990). Self-administration of morphine in bone-marrow transplant patients reduces drug requirements. *Pain, 40*, 121–9.

143. Mackie, A.M., Coda, B.C., and Hill, H.F. (1991). Adolescents use patient-controlled analgesia effectively for relief from prolonged oropharyngeal mucositis pain. *Pain, 46*, 265–9.

144. Shaiova, L., Lapin, J., Manco, L.S. *et al.* (2004). Tolerability and effects of two formulations of oral transmucosal fentanyl citrate (OTFC; ACTIQ) in patients with radiation-induced oral mucositis. *Support Care Cancer, 12*, 268–73.

145. Cerchietti, L., Navigante, A.H., and Bonomi, M.R. (2002). Effect of topical morphine for mucositis-associated pain following concomitant chemoradiotherapy for head and neck carcinoma. *Cancer, 95*, 2230–6.

146. Mahood, D.J., Dose, A.M., Loprinzi, C.L. *et al.* (1991). Inhibition of fluouracil-induced stomatitis by oral cryotherapy. *Journal of Clinical Oncology, 9*, 449–52.

147. Cascinu, S., Fedeli, A., Fedeli, S.L. *et al.* (1994). Oral cooling (cryotherapy), aneffective treatment for the prevention of 5-fluorouracil-induced stomatitis. *European Journal of Cancer B Oral Oncology, 30B*, 234–6.

148. Arduino, P.G. and Porter, S.R. (2006). Oral and perioral herpes simplex virus type I (HSV-1) infection: review of its management. *Oral Diseases, 12*, 254–70.

149. Donnelly, J.P. *et al.* (2003). Antimicrobial therapy to prevent or treat oral mucositis. *Lancet Infectious Diseases, 3*, 405.

150. Epstein, J.B., Stevenson-Moore, P., Jackson, S.M. *et al.* (1989). Prevention of oral mucositis in radiation therapy: a controlled study with benzydamine hydrochloride rinse. *International Journal of Radiation Oncology, Biology, Physics, 16*, 1571–5.

151. Clark, P.I. and Slevin, M.L. (1985). Allopurinol mouthwash and 5-fluoruracil-induced oral toxicity. *European Journal of Surgical Oncology, 11*, 267–8.

152. Bleyer, J.P. (1990). A controlled evaluation of an allopurinol mouth-washes as prophylaxis against 5 FU induced stomatitis. *Cancer*, 1879.

153. Dose, A.M. (1989). A controlled evaluation of an allopurinol mouthwash as prophylaxis against 5-fluoruracil (5-FU)-induced stomatitis: a North Central Treatment Group and Mayo Clinic Study. *Proceedings of the American Society of Clinical Oncology, 8*, 341.

154. Porta, C., Moroni, M., and Nastasi, G. (1994). Allopurinol mouthwashes in the treatment of 5-Fluorouracil-induced stomatitis. *American Journal of Clinical Oncology 17*, 246–7.

155. Dazzi, C., Cariello, A., Giovanis, P. *et al.* (2003). Prophylaxis with GM-CSF mouthwashes does not reduce frequency and duration of severe oral mucositis in patients with solid tumours undergoing high-dose chemotherapy with autologous peripheral blood stem cell transplantation rescue: a double blind, randomized, placebo-controlled study. *Annals of Oncology, 14*, 559.

156. Makkonen, T.A., Minn, H., and Jekunen, A. (2000). Granulocyte macrophage-colony stimulating factor (GM-CSF) and sucralfate in prevention of radiation-induced mucositis: a prospective randomized study. *International Journal of Radiation Oncology, Biology, Physics, 46*, 525–34.

157. Huang, E.Y., Leung, S.W., and Wang, C.J. (2000). Oral glutamine to alleviate radiation-induced oral mucositis: a pilot randomized trial. *International Journal of Radiation Oncology, Biology, Physics, 46*(3), 535–9.

158. Anderson, P.M., Schroeder, G., and Skubitz, K.M. (1998). Oral glutamine reduces the duration and severity of stomatitis after cytotoxic cancer chemotherapy. *Cancer*, **83**, 1433–9.

159. Schloerb, P.R. and Skikne, B.S. (1999). Oral and parenteral glutamine in one marrow transplantation: a randomized, double-blind study. *Journal of Parenteral and Enteral Nutrition*, **23**,117–22.

160. Kuhrer, I., Kuzmits, R., Linkesch, W. *et al.* (1986). Topical PGE2 enhances healing of chemotherapy-associated mucosal lesions. *Lancet*, **1**, 623.

161. Labar, B., Mrsic, M., Pavletic, Z. *et al.* (1993). Prostaglandin E2 for prophylaxis of oral mucositis following BMT. *Bone Marrow Transplant*, **11**, 379–82.

162. Sasse, A.D. and Clark, O.A.C. (2006). Amifostine reduces side effects and improves complete response rate during radiotherapy: results of a meta-analysis. *International Journal of Radiation Oncology, Biology, Physics*, **64**, 784–91.

163. Buentzel, J., Micke, O., and Adamietz, I.A. (2006). Intravenous amifostine during chemotherapy for head and neck cancer: a randomized placebo-controlled phase III study. *International Journal of Radiation Oncology, Biology, Physics*, **64**, 684–91.

164. Fidler, P., Loprinzi, C.L., O'Fallon, J.R. *et al.* (1996). Prospective evaluation of chamomile mouthwash for prevention of 5FU-induced oral mucositis. *Cancer*, **77**, 522–5.

165. Menachem, O. (2001). A randomized controlled clinical trial of the homeopathic medication Traumeel Sr in the treatment of chemotherapy induced stomatitis in chidren undergoing stem cell transplantation. *Cancer*, **92**, 684–90.

166. Etiz, D., Erkal, H.S., Serin, M. *et al.* (2000). Clinical and histopathological evaluation of sucralfate in prevention of oral mucositis induced by radiation therapy in patients with head and neck malignancies. *Oral Oncology*, **36**, 116–20.

167. Epstein, J.B. and Wong, F.L. (1994). The efficacy of sucralfate suspension in the prevention of oral mucositis due to radiation therapy. *International Journal of Radiation Oncology, Biology, Physics*, **28**, 693–8.

168. Vogelsang, G.B. (2001). How I treat chronic graft-versus-host-disease. *Blood*, **97**, 1196.

169. Ruggiero, S.L., Mehrotra, B., Rosenberg, T.J. (2004). Osteonecrosis of the jaws associated with the use of bisphosphonates: a review of 63 cases. *Journal of Oral Maxillofacial Surgery*, **62**, 527–34.

170. Woo, S.B., Hellstein, J.W., and Kalmar, J.R. (2006). Systematic review: bisphosphonates and osteonecrosis of the jaws. *Annals of Internal Medicine*, **144**, 753–61.

171. Bamias, A., Kastritis, E., Bamia, C. (2005). Osteonecrosis of the jaw in cancer after treatment with bisphosphonates: incidence and risk factors. *Journal of Clinical Oncology*, **23**, 8580–7.

172. Durie, B.G.M., Kats, M., and Crowley, J. (2005). Osteonecrosis of the jaw and bisphosphonates. *New England Journal of Medicine*, **353**, 99–100.

173. Migliorati, C.A., Casiglia, J., Epstein, J. *et al.* (2005). Managing the care of patients with bisphosphonates-associated osteonecrosis. An American Academy of Oral Medicine position paper. *Journal of the American Dental Association*, **136**, 1658–68.

174. Regnard, C. and Fitton, S. (1989). Mouth care: a flow diagram. *Palliative Medicine*, **3**, 67–9.

10.10

Endocrine and metabolic complications of advanced cancer

Mark Bower and Sarah Cox

Introduction

Cancer produces endocrine and metabolic complications in two ways. First, the primary tumour or its metastases may interfere with the function of endocrine glands, kidneys, or liver by invasion or obstruction. Second, tumours may give rise to remote effects without local spread. Generally, these paraneoplastic syndromes arise from secretion by tumours of hormones, cytokines, and growth factors, but also occur when normal cells secrete products in response to the presence of tumour. For example, antibodies produced in this fashion are responsible for many paraneoplastic neurological syndromes including cerebellar degeneration, Lambert–Eaton myaesthenic syndrome, and paraneoplastic retinopathy.

This chapter reviews the pathogenesis, epidemiology, and management of the commonest paraneoplastic endocrinopathies and concludes with a brief discussion of the management of diabetes mellitus, renal failure, and liver failure in the context of advanced malignancy.

Paraneoplastic syndromes

Hypercalcaemia

Hypercalcaemia is the commonest life-threatening metabolic disorder associated with cancer. It usually occurs in patients with advanced disseminated malignancy and produces a number of distressing symptoms. The treatment of hypercalcaemia of malignancy frequently ameliorates these symptoms and for this reason the diagnosis should always be sought.

Pathogenesis

Three related mechanisms contribute to hypercalcaemia:

1 Increased osteoclastic bone resorption.

2 Decreased renal clearance of calcium.

3 Enhanced calcium absorption from the gut.

All three processes occur in malignancy and in different circumstances each contributes to a greater or lesser extent. Bone resorption in malignant hypercalcaemia is universal and may be related to both local factors produced in response to metastases and humoral factors produced by tumours. It is mediated by osteoclasts, which are multinucleated giant cells derived from the fusion of macrophages and reside in Howship's lacunae in bone. Osteoclasts resorb bone at their ruffled border where cellular proton pumps secrete hydrogen and chloride ions that dissolve hydroxyapatite and liberate bicarbonate and calcium phosphate into the blood stream. In addition, osteoclasts produce lytic proteases including lysosomal proteases, metalloproteinases, and cystine proteases that dissolve bone matrix. Decreased renal calcium excretion occurs with low glomerular filtration rates and increased tubular reabsorption of calcium in response to parathyroid hormone or its relatives. Haematological neoplasms rarely produce 1,25-dihydroxycholecalciferol ($1,25(OH)_2D_3$, calcitriol) causing increased gastrointestinal absorption of calcium.

RANKL/RANK/OPG

The final common pathway of osteolysis has recently been elucidated at the molecular level and involves a triad of OPG (osteoprotegerin), RANK (receptor activator of NF kappa B), and RANKL (receptor activator of NF kappa B Ligand). Bone destruction in the presence of osteolytic skeletal metastases is not caused directly by tumour cells but by osteoclasts. The tumour cells either produce RANKL (as in the case of myeloma cells) directly or produce growth factors that stimulate bone stromal cells to produce RANKL. RANKL is an osteoclast activating factor belonging to the TNF (tumour necrosis factor) gene family that stimulates the RANK membrane receptor on osteoclast precursors. In conjunction with M-CSF (macrophage colony stimulating factor), RANKL causes the differentiation of these precursors into osteoclasts and the fusion and activation of osteoclasts into functional multinucleated osteoclasts that are responsible for bone resorption. OPG (also known as OCIF: osteoclastogenesis inhibitory factor) is a soluble decoy receptor for RANKL that acts as an inhibitor of RANK by competing for RANKL binding. The production of OPG may be diminished in myeloma and metastatic prostate cancer. This RANKL/RANK/OPG equilibrium is disrupted by cytokines, chemokines, and prostaglandins, uncoupling the usual homeostatic balance between osteoclastic bone resorption and osteoblastic bone formation. In addition, osteotropic factors such as 1,25 dihydroxy vitamin D3 and PTHrP as well as interleukins 1 and 6 enhance RANKL expression and diminish OPG expression. Germ line mutation of OPG causes juvenile Paget's disease whilst mutation of RANK causes familial expansile osteolysis.

Parathyroid hormone

In most cases of malignancy-associated-hypercalcaemia cytokine-mediated osteoclastic bone resorption appears to be the dominant factor; however, in up to 20 per cent of cases no bone metastases are present, so called humoral hypercalcaemia of malignancy. In these patients, ectopic secretion of factors by the tumour accounts for the disturbance of calcium homeostasis. Humoral hypercalcaemia of malignancy resembles primary hyperparathyroidism biochemically with hypercalcaemia, hypophosphataemia, renal phosphate wasting, increased tubular resorption of calcium, and enhanced osteoclastic bone resorption. However, the ratio of deoxypyridinoline to osteocalcin, which is normal in primary hyperparathyroidism, is markedly raised in malignancy-associated-hypercalcaemia[1]. Early suggestions of ectopic parathyroid hormone (PTH) secretion by tumours have not been supported by radioimmunoassay and gene expression studies, although very occasionally true ectopic secretion of PTH has been described in nonparathyroid tumours.

Parathyroid hormone-related protein

Parathyroid hormone related protein (PTHrP) is a 16 kDa peptide that resembles PTH in bioactivity but has different immunoreactivity. Competitive binding assays show that PTHrP (1-141) and PTH act via the same receptor. The PTH receptor 1 is a large, heptahelical G-protein coupled, membrane spanning receptor that binds PTH and PTHrP with equal affinity. In addition to the actions on calcium metabolism, PTHrP is a mitogen in rat carcinoma models[2] and PTHrP expression is upregulated by H-ras and v-src oncogenes[3]. Whilst PTH is only expressed in parathyroid glands, PTHrP gene expression is found in several tissues including keratinocytes, placenta, breast tissue, parathyroid glands, fetal liver, and brain. Knock-out mice experiments demonstrated that PTHrP appears to play a central role in endochondrial bone formation promoting chondrocyte proliferation. The PTHrP driven chondrocyte proliferation is in equilibrium with cartilage differentiation that is stimulated by the Indian hedgehog protein, the human homologue of a secreted patterning protein of Drosophila fruit flies[4,5]. In addition, PTHrP has been implicated in breast morphogenesis and transplacental calcium flux[6].

Early studies demonstrated that PTHrP immunoperoxidase staining is strongly positive in human squamous cell carcinomas from various sites[7]. Moreover, PTHrP mRNA expression was detected in all tumours obtained from patients with humoral hypercalcaemia of malignancy, but not in any of those from normocalcaemic control patients with cancer[8]. Furthermore, cancer patients with hypercalcaemia have elevated serum levels of PTHrP measured by immunoassay (>2.5 pg/ml)[9]. Thus PTHrP assays may facilitate the diagnosis of the cause of hypercalcaemia[10]. PTHrP may also have a limited role as a prognostic tumour marker, predicting the development of bone metastases in women with breast cancer[11].

At least 80 per cent of patients with solid tumours and hypercalcaemia have elevated serum levels of PTHrP[12] including over 60 per cent of patients with bone metastases[13]. Antibodies to PTHrP alleviate hypercalcaemia in animal models of humoral hypercalcaemia of malignancy[14,15] and it has been reported that serum levels of PTHrP fell in parallel with serum calcium in three patients with humoral hypercalcaemia of malignancy who had successful curative surgery[16]. Nevertheless, PTHrP cannot explain all the biochemical findings in humoral hypercalcaemia of malignancy. In contrast to primary hyperparathyoidism, there is impaired intestinal calcium absorption, low 1,25 $(OH)_2D_3$ levels, and osteoclastic bone resorption is far more prominent. These features suggest that other factors (probably cytokines) have an important role in humoral hypercalcaemia of malignancy even in the absence of bone metastases.

Vitamin D

Gut absorption of calcium and levels of vitamin D are generally suppressed in patients with humoral hypercalcaemia of malignancy. However, a number of cases of Hodgkin's disease, non-Hodgkin's lymphoma, and human T-cell lymphotrophic virus type 1 (HTLV-1)-associated adult T-cell leukaemia/lymphoma (ATLL) have been reported in which ectopic production of 1,25 $(OH)_2D_3$ resulted in hypercalcaemia[17]. The mechanism is thought to involve extra-renal hydroxylation of 25(OH)D_3 by 1 alpha-hydroxylase to 1,25 $(OH)_2D_3$[18]. Tumour-related vitamin D excess causing increased gut absorption of calcium has implications for therapy. Hypercalcaemia of malignancy is usually associated with low absorption and dietary calcium restriction is unnecessary; however, with elevated 1,25 $(OH)_2D_3$ levels, a low calcium diet is needed to control hypercalcaemia.

Epidemiology

Ten per cent of cancer patients develop hypercalcaemia and malignancy accounts for about half the cases of hypercalcaemia amongst hospital inpatients. Hypercalcaemia occurs most frequently with myeloma (up to 50 per cent of patients), breast, lung, and renal cancers, and up to 20 per cent of cases occur in the absence of bone metastases. Most patients with hypercalcaemia of malignancy have disseminated disease and 80 per cent die within 1 year. The prognosis is grave with a median survival of 3–4 months. Thus hypercalcaemia is usually a complication of advanced disease and its treatment should be directed at symptom palliation. Occasionally patients with myeloma or metastatic breast cancer present with hypercalcaemia.

Clinical features

The clinical manifestations of hypercalcaemia are myriad and many symptoms that may have been attributed to the underlying malignancy may resolve on correction of the hypercalcaemia. Although the severity of symptoms is not correlated with degree of elevation of serum calcium, most patients initially develop malaise and lethargy followed by thirst, nausea, and constipation before neurological (drowsiness and confusion) and cardiological features appear. A diagnosis of hypercalcaemia can only be made by biochemical investigation and so all symptomatic patients with malignancy should have their serum calcium measured if treatment is likely to be appropriate.

Treatment

In parallel with the advances in the understanding of the pathogenesis of hypercalcaemia in the late 1980s and early 1990s came improvements in therapy. These new therapies are more effective, less toxic, and easier to administer. They represent a major

Table 10.10.1 Clinical features of hypercalcaemia of malignancy.

General	Gastrointestinal	Neurological	Cardiological
Dehydration	Anorexia	Fatigue	Bradycardia
Polydipsia	Weight loss	Lethargy	Atrial arrhythmias
Polyuria	Nausea	Confusion	Ventricular arrhythmias
Pruritis	Vomiting Constipation Ileus	Myopathy Hyporeflexia Seizures Psychosis Coma	Prolonged P-R interval Reduced Q-T interval Wide T waves

improvement in palliative therapy for cancer patients. The treatment of hypercalcaemia should be determined on the basis of attributable symptoms and the corrected serum calcium calculated from the formula:

$$\text{Corrected calcium} = \text{measured calcium} + [(40 - \text{serum albumin (g/l)}) \times 0.02]$$

Rehydration followed by the administration of calcium-lowering agents is the mainstay of therapy. Low calcium diets are unpalatable, impractical, and exacerbate malnutrition and have no place in palliative therapy. Drugs promoting hypercalcaemia (thiazide diuretics, vitamins A and D) should be withdrawn.

Intravenous fluids

Dehydration due to polyuria and vomiting is a prominent feature of hypercalcaemia and intravenous rehydration is an essential component of acute therapy for severe or symptomatic hypercalcaemia. Although large volumes of fluid will lower serum calcium, patients rarely achieve normocalcaemia and careful monitoring to avoid fluid overload is necessary. In view of this, 2–3 l/day of fluid is now the accepted practice with daily serum electrolyte measurement to prevent hypokalaemia and hyponatraemia. Loop diuretics are often prescribed as an adjunct to intravenous fluids and cause calciuresis. However, there is little evidence of any benefit and they may exacerbate hypovolaemia, hypokalaemia, and hypomagnesaemia and are best avoided.

Corticosteroids

Glucocorticoids have been widely used in cancer-related hypercalcaemia and rapidly inhibit osteoclastic bone resorption *in vitro* as well as reducing calcium absorption from the gut. However, their limited clinical benefit is chiefly confined to tumours that respond to the cytostatic effects of steroids, such as myeloma, lymphoma, leukaemia, and occasionally breast cancer when hypercalcaemia occurs as a flare effect caused by endocrine therapy. Thus their role in severe hypercalcaemia is limited to haematological malignancies and oral prednisolone 40–100 mg/day is usually effective in these circumstances although they may take 4–10 days to lower the serum calcium.

Bisphosphonates

Bisphosphonates are synthetic pyrophosphate analogues characterized by a phosphorus–carbon–phosphorus bond, making them resistant to enzymatic hydrolysis. They reduce bone resorption by inhibiting directly osteoclast function, leading to disappearance of the ruffled border, decreased acid production, and altered enzyme activity[19,20] Bisphosphonates bind hydroxyapatite crystals with a high affinity and affect osteoclast recruitment and activation. They are highly effective in controlling hypercalcaemia of malignancy causing a gradual fall in serum calcium over a few days. Etidronate is a first generation bisphosphonate that has weak activity and requires repeated infusions over three days[21]. Clodronate has been shown to be more effective than placebo (in the only randomized controlled study) and may be administered as a single 1.5 g infusion over 4 h[22]. However, the most commonly prescribed bisphosphonate is pamidronate, which may be administered as a single infusion of 90 mg administered at 1 mg/min, irrespective of the serum calcium level and repeated every 3–4 weeks[23]. A randomized trial has shown that pamidronate is superior to clodronate in terms of the duration of normocalcaemia achieved[24,25]. Maintenance therapy with oral bisphosphonates has been reported for both etidronate and clodronate; however, the low bioavailability and considerable gastrointestinal toxicity limit their value in this context. Bisphosphonates do not alter PTHrP levels, renal calcium reabsorption, RANKL, or osteoprotegerin levels and so they may fail to control humoral hypercalcaemia of malignancy without bone metastases[26,27]. Indeed, there is a correlation between the responsiveness to pamidronate in humoral hypercalcaemia and the plasma PTHrP level. Non-responders have levels above 75 pg/ml and so PTHrP measurement may allow the identification of patients requiring higher doses of bisphosphonates and increased dose frequency[28].

A number of third generation bisphosphonates have been developed in an attempt to enhance oral bioavailability and reduce gastrointestinal toxicity. Of the new bisphosphonates, only ibandronate (4 mg intravenous infusion over 2 h)[29,30] and zoledronate[31,32] have been shown to be effective in studies in humoral hypercalcaemia of malignancy. Recently, zoledronate has been found to achieve a normal corrected serum calcium in more patients, faster and for longer than pamidronate, as well as only requiring a 5-min infusion[32]. The differences between the two agents were not great however and the choice is based largely on cost and convenience. In our unit, intravenous pamidronate is used for inpatients, whilst outpatients are treated with the briefer zoledronate infusions. A randomized study comparing ibandronate and pamidronate suggested similar efficacy but longer duration of normocalcaemia with ibandronate, although the study used stratified dosing based on serum calcium levels[30]. In addition to these actions, intravenous bisphosphonates have valuable analgesic activity in patients with metastatic bone pain and reduce skeletal morbidity in patients with breast cancer and myeloma. Osteonecrosis of the jaw is a recognized complication of bisphosphonate therapy associated with prolonged use, old age in patients with multiple myeloma, and a history of recent dental extraction. Symptoms can mimic dental problems and the patient may develop severe pain. The usual management is with antibiotics and surgical debridement[33].

Calcitonin

Calcitonin is secreted by the parafollicular cells of the thyroid gland, although its physiological role in calcium homeostasis remains undefined. In the much higher pharmacological doses, calcitonin reduces osteoclastic bone resorption and increases calciuresis, thereby reducing serum calcium. It is effective in around a third of patients and usually causes a fall in calcium within 4 h (compared to 48 h for bispohosphonates) but normocalcaemia is rare and the effect is short-lived, usually requiring daily repeat dosing. Doses of up to 8 IU/kg salmon calcitonin may be injected subcutaneously or intramuscularly every 6–12 h and this therapy has minimal toxicity (nausea is the most frequent side effect and occasional hypersensitivity reactions are seen).

Calcitonin and calcitonin gene-related peptide (CGRP) are produced by alternate exon splicing from the same gene on chromosome 11p15.5 close to the PTH gene. Calcitonin expression is regulated by serum calcium via the same calcium sensing receptor (CASR) that controls PTH secretion. CASR is a plasma membrane G protein-coupled receptor that is expressed in the parathyroid hormone-producing chief cells of the parathyroid gland and the cells lining the kidney tubule and acts by modulating PTH secretion and renal cation handling to achieve calcium homeostasis. Calcitonin acts via a heptahelical G protein-coupled receptor expressed by osteoclasts and osteoblasts, whilst CGRP also acts through a separate receptor as a neurotransmitter and vasodilator. Both may be produced by tumours but no clinical syndrome has been attributed to their production and conversely athymic patients who produce no calcitonin have no disturbance of calcium metabolism. Although production of calcitonin and CGRP is common in many tumours, its main value to the oncologist is as a tumour marker for medullary cell carcinoma of the thyroid and multiple endocrine neoplasia type II.

Plicamycin

Plicamycin (formerly mithramycin), a cytotoxic antibiotic, is toxic to osteoclasts by blocking RNA synthesis and hence reduces bone resorption, producing prompt and effective lowering of serum calcium. It is administered as an intravenous bolus or 2 h infusion at a dosage of 25 mcg/kg. It produces normocalcaemia within 3 days in 80 per cent of patients and is usually repeated weekly. The disadvantage of this highly effective treatment is its toxicity; cumulative nephrotoxicity, and hepatotoxicity occur and thrombocytopenia is common; nausea is frequent and may be reduced when plicamycin is given as an infusion. Plicamycin is now very rarely used.

Phosphates

Oral phosphates may be effective in mild hypercalcaemia by a combination of effects on calcium metabolism. The usual recommended dose is 0.5–3 g/day phosphate (as sodium cellulose phosphate powder) and this frequently causes nausea and diarrhoea. Intravenous phosphate is a highly effective therapy for acute life-threatening hypercalcaemia and the onset of hypocalcaemic action is more rapid than with any other agent. However, the severe toxicity of parenteral phosphate includes extensive extraskeletal calcification and hence it has been abandoned in all but exceptional cases. Recommended dosing is 1.5 g (50 mmol) elemental phosphate diluted in 1 l of saline over 6–8 h and should preferably be given in intensive care where the patient's cardiac and renal function can be monitored closely.

Gallium nitrate

Gallium nitrate is incorporated into bone, rendering hydroxyapatite less soluble[34]. It inhibits bone resorption directly without killing osteoclasts and is not associated with the nausea or myelosuppression caused by plicamycin. Gallium is highly effective, producing normocalcaemia in 80 per cent of patients with hypercalcaemia of malignancy. Two randomized double-blind trials have demonstrated the superiority of gallium compared to calcitonin[35] and etidronate[36]. The main drawback of gallium is that it requires continuous intravenous infusion (100–200 mg/m² per day) for 5 days and it causes nephrotoxicity. Gallium nitrate is not licensed in the United Kingdom.

Future approaches

Passive immunization with monoclonal antibodies against PTHrP reduces serum calcium in nude mice bearing human tumour xenografts secreting PTHrP[37], suppresses osteolytic bone metastasis of human breast cancer cells injected into mice[38], and lowers calcium levels of hypercalcemic mice bearing human pancreatic or lung cancer xenografts that secrete PTHrP[39]. These data suggest a potential role in the clinical management of humoral hypercalcaemia of malignancy. Osteoprotegerin, the decoy receptor for RANKL, reduces serum calcium levels faster and further than pamidronate in murine models of malignancy-associated-hypercalcaemia[40] and has been trialed in patients with myeloma and breast cancer[41]. Similarly, denosumab, a fully human monoclonal antibody to RANKL has been studied in postmenopausal women with osteoporosis[42] and patients with myeloma and breast cancer[43]. A final novel approach that is again based on the molecular basis of calcium homeostasis uses calcimimetics. Circulating levels of ionized calcium ion are sensed and hence regulated via a cell-surface calcium sensing receptor (CASR) that belongs to the superfamily of G protein-coupled receptors. Calcium sensor mimetics or calcimimetics are small organic molecules that potentiate the effect of calcium on the CASR and suppress PTH secretion. Calcimimetics have been used successfully in primary and secondary hyperparathyroidism[44], although not in hypercalcaemia of malignancy. All these and other approaches may yield clinical advances in the management of hypercalcaemia.

Treatment summary

Symptomatic or severe hypercalcaemia requires intravenous rehydration with 2–3 l/day followed by a single infusion of pamidronate at 1 mg/minute according to the corrected serum calcium. This combination will control hypercalcaemia in most patients simply, promptly, and with minimal toxicity. The majority of patients will remain normocalcaemic for 2–4 weeks with encouragement of oral hydration. In the absence of effective treatment of the malignancy; however, hypercalcaemia will recur and the serum calcium should be rechecked every 3–4 weeks. Maintenance pamidronate infusions over 2 h or zoledronate over 5 min can be managed on an outpatient basis. Second-line therapy for humoral hypercalcaemia of malignancy resistant to bisphosphonates should probably be with gallium nitrate, although this is rarely available.

Cushing's syndrome

Ectopic secretion of adrenocorticotrophic hormone (ACTH) by non-endocrine-derived tumours rarely causes clinically overt Cushing's syndrome. However, the production of pro-opiomelanocortin (POMC) derived peptides by tumours is not uncommon and the infrequency of clinical signs and symptoms reflects the

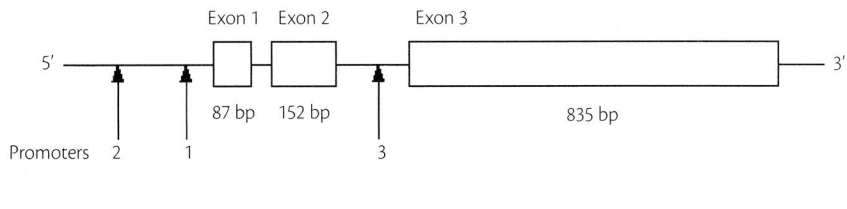

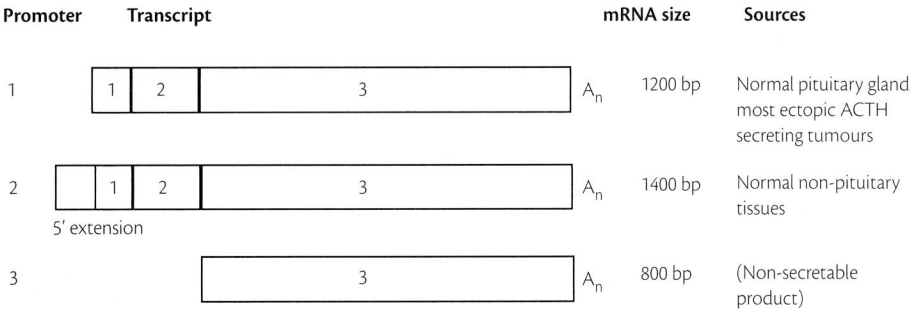

Figure 10.10.1 The molecular biology of pro-opiomelanocortin gene expression.

subtle and complex control of hormone production from this gene. Symptoms usually arise as a consequence of excessive ACTH production by tumours through uncontrolled POMC gene expression following promoter switches or transcription activation. The mRNA transcripts may be of altered lengths and give rise to different POMC peptides by variation in protein cleavage and glycosylation.

Pathogenesis

The POMC gene is located on the short arm of chromosome 2 at p23 and includes three exons and three putative promoter sites, which are active to varying degrees in different tissues . The expression of the POMC gene is influenced by glucocorticoids, which suppress transcription, and corticotrophin, which stimulates transcription. Glucocorticoids bind to steroid hormone receptors, which in turn bind to a glucocorticoid inhibitory element sequence of POMC gene. In this way, steroids downregulate POMC transcription only when it is driven by promoter 1, yielding the 1200 base transcript, and this may account for the failure of high dose dexamethasone to suppress ectopic ACTH production when alternative promoters are active.

Post-translational processing of POMC peptide gives rise to a large number of different peptides, many of which have been detected in tumour extracts and cell lines. Some of these peptides have also been identified in patients' plasma and are active biologically Following the development of monoclonal antibodies to these peptides, high specificity two-site immunoradiometric assays (IRMA) have been introduced. IRMA is able to discriminate between ACTH and its larger precursors (pro-ACTH and POMC). This methodology has been used to demonstrate that most patients with ectopic ACTH secrete pro-ACTH, which has only 5 per cent of the steroidogenic activity of ACTH 1-39, whilst patients with pituitary adenomas produce normal 1200 base POMC transcripts and the peptide product undergoes normal proteolysis and glycosylation culminating in the secretion of ACTH 1-39. Thus, two-site directed IRMA may help in the differential diagnosis of Cushing's disease and ectopic ACTH. However, occasionally large aggressive pituitary adenomas secrete pro-ACTH and these patients

often have a biochemical profile more indicative of ectopic ACTH rather than Cushing's disease[45,46].

Elevated plasma levels and tumour extract concentrations of various other POMC-derived peptides have been described. Although melanocyte-stimulating hormone (MSH) production is not light-sensitive (unlike melatonin), it regulates skin pigmentation by affecting directly dermal melanocyte growth and melanin production. Hence ectopic secretion of MSH containing peptides (α-MSH, ACTH, pro-ACTH, β-MSH, γ-MSH, β-LPH), γ-LPH, N-POC, pro-γ-MSH) may lead to generalized hyperpigmentation, but this symptom is rarely distressing. Leptin, the adipocyte derived regulator of food balance and energy homeostasis enhances expression of α-MSH[47] and mouse models of obesity produced by deleting the POMC gene can be rescued by α-MSH[48]. The Agouti-related protein (AGRP) is a natural neuropeptide antagonist of the action of alpha-melanocyte stimulating hormone (alpha-MSH) at the melanocortin receptors (MCR)[49,50]. Transgenic mice overexpressing AGRP are also hyperphagic and eventually become obese, whilst humans with common single nucleotide polymorphisms (SNPs) in the promoter or the coding region are leaner and resistant to late-onset obesity than wild-type individuals[51]. Thus MSH and AGRP may be critical components in a complex regulatory system that exists to maintain energy balance. Whilst other physiological roles for α-, β- and γ-MSH have been described, no other clinical correlates in the setting of ectopic MSH secretion have been reported.

The secretion of endorphins and enkephalins derived from the POMC gene occurs frequently in conjunction with ectopic ACTH secretion[52,53]. Numerous clinical effects within the central nervous system have been postulated for these endogenous opioids that bind G-protein-coupled receptors, inhibiting net cAMP synthesis by antagonizing adenyl cyclase and activating phosphodiesterase. However, these opioid molecules cross the blood–brain barrier with difficulty and although one-third of patients with Cushing's syndrome have psychiatric disturbances, the proportion is lower in Nelson's syndrome, which suggests that these symptoms are related to excess steroids rather than opioids[54].

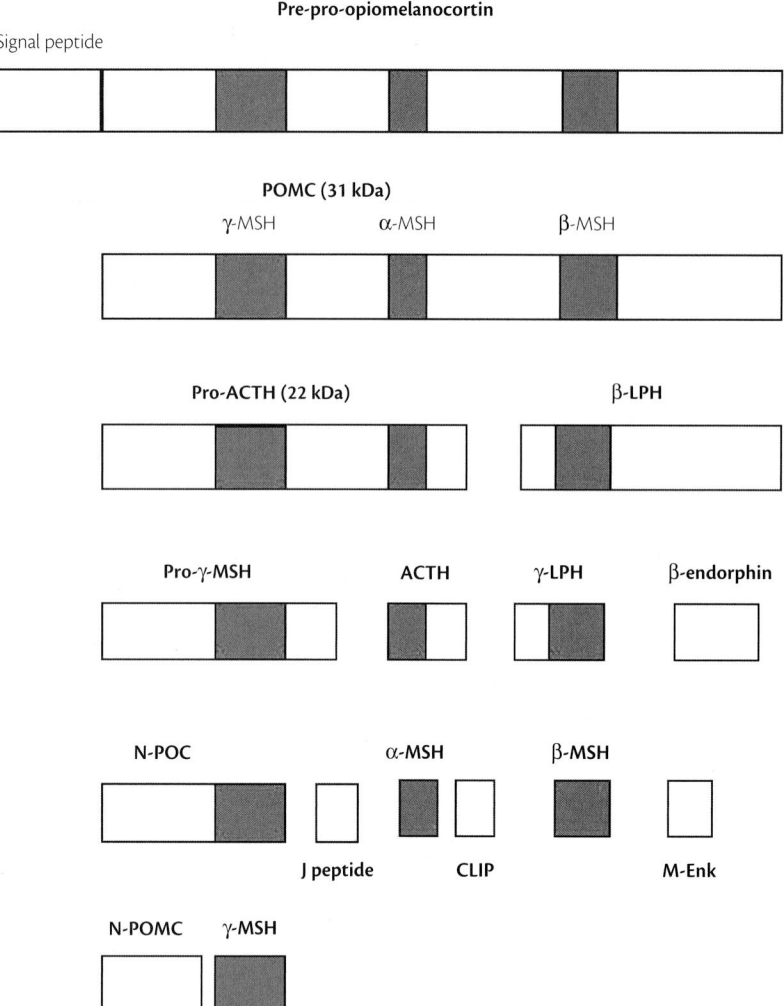

Figure 10.10.2 Pro-opiomelanocortin (POMC) derived peptides. POMC, Pro-opiomelanocortin; MSH, melanocyte stimulating hormone; LPH, lipotropin; POC, pro-opiocortin; CLIP, corticotropin-like intermediate lobe peptide; Enk, enkephalin.

Epidemiology

Ectopic ACTH secretion by a tumour accounts for 12 per cent of cases of Cushing's syndrome and the cancer is frequently occult at presentation[55]. For this reason, the differential diagnosis between an ACTH secreting pituitary adenoma and ectopic ACTH production is important clinically but biochemical overlap often makes this difficult. Half the cases of ectopic ACTH syndrome are due to lung cancer divided evenly between small-cell lung cancer and bronchial carcinoids[56]. Islet cell tumour of the pancreas (16 per cent) and thymic carcinoids (10 per cent) make up most of the remaining cases[57]. In small-cell lung cancer, ectopic secretion of ACTH is generally thought not to be correlated with either stage or survival, although one retrospective analysis suggested an association with poor outcome and a high incidence of infectious complications[58]. The levels of ACTH may decline in response to chemotherapy or radiotherapy[59], but any correlation between declining ACTH levels and tumour response is anecdotal only and elevation of ACTH may persist in long-term survivors following chemotherapy[60].

Clinical features

The typical presentation is of a middle-aged male smoker with features of severe hypercortisolism and hypokalaemic metabolic alkalosis. Patients have muscle weakness or atrophy, oedema, hypertension, mental changes, glucose intolerance, and weight loss. When ectopic ACTH production arises from a slower growing tumour (e.g. bronchial carcinoid or thymoma), the other classical features of Cushing's syndrome may be present, including truncal obesity, moon facies, and cutaneous striae often making the clinical distinction from pituitary-dependant Cushing's disease impossible. Furthermore, biochemical tests do not always differentiate reliably a pituitary from an ectopic tumour as the source of ACTH.

Diagnosis

In addition to the clinical features, the diagnosis of Cushing's syndrome may be confirmed by elevated urinary free cortisol, loss of diurnal variation of plasma cortisol, and failure of cortisol suppression in the low-dose dexamethasone (2 mg) test. After establishing the diagnosis, an elevated plasma ACTH supports the

Table 10.10.2 Diagnosis of syndrome of inappropriate diuresis (SIAD).

Essential criteria to establish this diagnosis are:

1. Plasma hypo-osmolality (plasma osmolality <275 mosm/kg H_2O and plasma sodium <135 mmol/l)

2. Concentrated urine (urine osmolality >100 mosm/kg H_2O)

3. Normal plasma/extracellular fluid volume

4. High urinary sodium (urine sodium>20 mEq/l) on a normal salt and water intake

5. Exclude (i) hypothyroidism, (ii) hypoadrenalism, and (iii) diuretics

Supportive criteria for this diagnosis are:

1. Abnormal water load test (unable to excrete >90 per cent of a 20 ml/kg water load in 4h, and/or failure to dilute urine to osmolality <100 mosmol/kg H_2O)

2. Elevated plasma AVP

diagnosis of pituitary adenoma or ectopic ACTH syndrome. Failure of cortisol to suppress following high dose dexamethasone (2 mg four times daily for two days, or 8 mg overnight) and very high levels of ACTH (>200 pg/ml) suggest an ectopic source of ACTH. However, half of the cases of ectopic ACTH from carcinoid tumours suppress with dexamethasone and have ACTH levels in the lower range; circadian rhythms of secretion may even be maintained. In difficult cases, a corticotrophin-releasing hormone stimulation test, selective venous catheterization of inferior petrosal sinus with ACTH estimations and two-site directed IRMA for pro-ACTH and ACTH measurements may be necessary to determine the source of ACTH[46,55]. Recently, both somatostatin analogue scintigraphy[61] and [99]technetium methoxyisobutylisonitrile (MIBI) imaging[62] have been used for localization of ectopic ACTH-producing tumours.

Further difficulties in differential diagnosis have arisen with the description of ectopic corticotrophin-releasing hormone secretion by tumours giving rise to Cushing's syndrome[63]. In these circumstances, ectopically secreted corticotrophin-releasing-hormone stimulates the normal pituitary to secrete excess ACTH resulting in Cushing's syndrome. A patient with medullary carcinoma of the thyroid developed Cushing's syndrome due to ectopic production of a bombesin-like peptide that is thought to stimulate ACTH secretion by pituitary corticotrophs. This provides a further diagnostic complication.

Treatment

The mainstay of palliative therapy for Cushing's syndrome due to ectopic ACTH production is inhibition of steroid synthesis, although inhibition of ACTH release and blocking glucocorticoid receptors have also been attempted. Several steroid synthesis inhibitors are available and successful use in these circumstances has been reported with aminoglutethamide, metyrapone, mitotane, ketoconazole, and octreotide. On rare occasions, laparoscopic bilateral adrenalectomy or adrenal artery embolization may be necessary to control symptoms[55].

Aminoglutethamide inhibits 20, 22-desmolase enzyme which catalyses the cholesterol side chain cleavage which gives rise to Δ5-pregnenolone. In this way the production of glucocorticoids, mineralocorticoids and androgens is inhibited at higher doses

(1.5–3 g/day), whilst at lower doses (125 mg twice daily) aminoglutethamide inhibits aromatase, which converts androgens to oestrogens. The latter is responsible for the efficacy of aminoglutethamide in post-menopausal breast cancer. The high doses used to treat Cushing's syndrome are associated with considerable toxicity, in particular sedation, ataxia, and rashes.

Metyrapone inhibits 11-β-hydroxylase, the final step in cortisol and corticosterone synthesis and has been shown to be effective in ectopic ACTH syndrome at doses of 250–750 mg four times a day. The short half-life of metyrapone and gastrointestinal toxicity (chiefly nausea) are drawbacks and very high levels of ACTH may over-ride the effects of metyrapone. For these reasons, it has been suggested that metyrapone should be used in conjunction with low dose aminoglutethamide (250 mg twice daily) to reduce the toxicities of both compounds[63].

Mitotane is an adrenal cytotoxic, structurally related to the insecticide DDT, which irreversibly inhibits 11-β-hydroxylase and 18-hydroxylase, thus reducing glucocorticoid, mineralocorticoid, and androgen production. It produces focal atrophy and necrosis of the zona fasiculata and zona reticularis. Doses of 1–12 g/day in four divided doses have been used and it is also active against primary adrenal tumours. Mitotane is a toxic drug with gastrointestinal side effects (anorexia, nausea, vomiting, diarrhoea) reported in 80 per cent of patients and lethargy and somnolence in 40 per cent[64].

The imidazole antifungal ketoconazole inhibits cytochrome P450-dependent steroid hydroxylases and case reports document its successful use in Cushing's syndrome due to ectopic ACTH secretion[65,66]. The potential side effects include nausea, headaches, pruritic rashes, and liver failure. Bromocriptine has also been advocated for use in these circumstances. Bromocriptine acts on dopamine-2 receptors, inhibiting cAMP production and decreasing POMC expression *in vitro*, but it is rarely successful *in vivo*[67].

The suppression of ectopic ACTH secretion by the administration of octreotide, a long acting somatostatin analogue, has been documented and may be supplemented by dopamine agonists.[68] The mechanism of this action is unknown but may reflect the wide distribution of somatostatin receptors on tumours and the diverse endocrine effects of somatostatin[69]. However, somatostatin analogues occasionally cause a paradoxical rise in plasma ACTH and cortisol levels in patients with ectopic ACTH production and therefore a preliminary evaluation of their therapeutic efficacy is suggested[70].

Mifepristone (RU-486) is a progesterone partial agonist that inhibits the separation of heat shock protein (hsp90) from the progesterone receptor. Case reports describe symptomatic improvement in patients with Cushing's syndrome, although it has yet to be used in ectopic ACTH secretion[46]. Antisense oligonucleotide complementary to a region of β-endorphin reduced the synthesis of POMC derived peptides *in vitro* and this approach may prove fruitful in the future[71].

Treatment summary

The first-line therapy for paraneoplastic Cushing's syndrome should be aminoglutethamide 250 mg twice daily and metyrapone 250 mg four times daily used together. The efficacy of treatment should be monitored and this is most easily achieved by measuring 24 h urinary cortisol excretion. As levels return to normal in these patients, hormone replacement therapy is frequently necessary.

Regimens similar to those used in Addison's disease should be used (e.g. hydrocortisone 20 mg at 0800 h and 10 mg at 1800 h, fludrocortisone 0.05–0.15 mg daily). Mitotane is second-line therapy, although it should be used as first-line therapy in patients with primary adrenal tumours. Mitotane is currently not licensed in Europe but may be obtained from the USA.

Syndrome of inappropriate antidiuresis

Hyponatraemia, usually defined as serum Na^+ <136 mmol/l, is a common finding in association with advanced malignancy and many factors may contribute including cardiac and hepatic failure, hyperglycaemia, diuretics, and the sick-cell syndrome. However, the detection of concentrated urine in conjunction with hypo-osmolar plasma suggests abnormal renal free water excretion and the presence of the syndrome of inappropriate antidiuresis (SIAD). This acronym is more suitable than 'SIADH', since there is no vasopressin secretion in approximately 15 per cent of cases[72].

Pathogenesis

The vasopressin gene on human chromosome 20 comprises three exons encoding a transcript of 700 base pairs. The peptide product includes the nine amino acid arginine vasopressin (AVP) and a 90 amino acid peptide, vasopressin-specific neurophysin II (NP II). This peptide complex is flanked by an N-terminal signal peptide and a C-terminal glycoprotein (absent in the oxytocin-NP I peptide). The AVP-NP II polypeptide is transported by axonal streaming from its site of synthesis in the supraoptic and paraventricular nuclei of the hypothalamus to the posterior pituitary gland. The peptide is cleaved and secreted by the posterior pituitary to produce a nonapeptide (AVP) and the 10 kDa transport peptide (NP II). This molecular mechanism is mimicked by oxytocin-neurophysin I whose gene is adjacent on chromosome 20p13 but in mirror image orientation. Three AVP receptors have been identified (V_{1A}, V_{1B}, and V_2); V2 receptors are located on renal collecting duct cells and mediate the antidiuretic actions of AVP. Following ligand binding, V_2 receptor activation acts via cAMP to result in the insertion of aquaporin-2 (AQP2) water channels into the apical plasma membrane of collecting duct cells. Aquaporins are a group of membrane channels that allow the passage of free water but not ions across cell membranes. Thus, enhanced AQP2 expression in the collecting ducts increases water reabsorption and leads to reduced free water excretion.

Epidemiology

Stimulation of hypothalamic-pituitary secretion of AVP or a direct effect on distal nephrons accounts for most cases of SIAD. However, in paraneoplastic SIAD, tumours secrete ectopic AVP, or vasopressin-like peptides[73]. SIAD is most frequently associated with small-cell lung cancer or carcinoid tumours but has also been described in pancreatic, oesophageal, prostatic, and haematological malignancies. In one series of 523 patients with small cell lung cancer, 9 per cent had clinically evident SIAD, 32–44 per cent elevated AVP detectable by radioimmunoassay and 53–68 per cent had abnormal renal handling of water loads[74,75]. In another study 58 per cent of small-cell lung cancer patients had raised plasma neurophysins (NP I, 14 per cent; NP II, 44 per cent)[76], although the high incidence of vasopressin/oxytocin gene expression in lung cancer is confined to neuroendocrine tumours[77] and both normal and abnormal gene products are found[78]. Prognosis, stage

at diagnosis and response to chemotherapy are similar in small cell lung cancer patients with and without SIAD[79]. Furthermore, although correction of hyponatraemia may correlate with tumour response to chemotherapy[80,81] complete restoration of normal renal water handling is rare even when complete remissions are achieved[82].

Clinical features

Significant symptoms of hyponatraemia appear at plasma sodium levels below 120 mmol/l with confusion progressing to stupor, coma, and seizures as levels fall. Nausea, vomiting, and focal neurological deficits may also occur. The clinical features depend on both the levels of plasma sodium and the rate of decline; with gradual falls in sodium the brain cells are able to compensate against cerebral oedema by secreting potassium and other intracellular solutes. Asymptomatic hyponatraemia therefore suggests chronic SIAD rather than acute SIAD. The division into chronic and acute SIAD is of therapeutic importance as their management differs[83].

Diagnosis

The diagnosis of SIAD requires the demonstration of plasma hyponatraemia and hypo-osmolality in the presence of concentrated urine and normal extracellular fluid volume There are a number of causes of SIAD, including ectopic AVP production by tumours and several may play a role in hyponatraemia in patients with advanced malignancy. Pulmonary, meningeal, and cerebral infections are common causes and drug-induced SIAD may also present in patients with cancer. Most drugs cause SIAD by stimulating hypophyseal secretion of AVP, although prostaglandin synthesis inhibitors inhibit directly renal tubular excretion of free water. The list of drugs implicated is long and includes morphine, phenothiazines, tricyclic antidepressants, and non-steroidal anti-inflammatory drugs, all frequently used in palliative care, as well as the cytotoxic drugs vincristine and cyclophosphamide and nicotine. The possibility of drug-related SIAD should always be considered before invoking ectopic AVP secretion by tumours and in most cases the hyponatraemia resolves when the drug is stopped. When SIAD presents with no identifiable cause, a thorough search for occult malignancy (especially small cell lung cancer) should be undertaken, as SIAD may be the presenting symptom and may precede radiological evidence by up to 1 year[84].

Treatment

The management of SIAD depends upon the rate of onset of hyponatraemia and the presence of neurological complications. Acute SIAD with an onset over 2–3 days and falls in serum sodium in excess of 0.5 mmol/l per day is associated with neurological sequelae and require prompt correction by intravenous hypertonic saline. In contrast, the mainstay of therapy for chronic asymptomatic SIAD is fluid restriction and inhibition of tubular reabsorption of water with drugs including demeclocycline.

Acute hyponatraemia with neurological symptoms has a mortality of 5–8 per cent, partly reflecting the underlying pathology. Rapid correction of hyponatraemia by intravenous hypertonic saline causes osmotic demyelination, leading to central pontine and extrapontine myelinosis. Central pontine myelinosis usually presents 1–2 days after correcting hyponatraemia with quadriparesis and bulbar palsy and is related to the rapidity of correction of sodium. A safe balance between overzealous correction causing irreversible myelinosis and the considerable mortality of uncorrected SIAD is required[85,86]. Hypertonic saline infusions should correct serum sodium at a rate of 0.5 mmol/l per hour[87], although a correction rate of up to 2 mmol/l per hour is said to be safe[88]. The total rise in serum sodium should not exceed 25 mmol/l and correction should stop once the serum sodium exceeds 120 mmol/l and symptoms have resolved. To achieve a correction rate of 0.5 mmol/l per hour requires 0.3 × body weight in kg (mmol Na$^+$/h). Hypertonic (twice normal) saline solution of 1.8 per cent contains 0.3 mmol/l Na$^+$. So the correct rate of infusion is 1 ml/kg body weight per hour of 1.8 per cent sodium chloride[89]; although more complex formulae may prove more accurate, they tend to be more difficult to calculate[90].

The mainstay of treatment of chronic asymptomatic SIAD is fluid restriction. It is suggested that intake is limited to 500 ml/day and the daily urine output should be less than 500 ml/day. This should include all fluids and takes several days to influence the hyponatraemia. In the context of palliative care, fluid restriction is frequently undesirable as it is unpleasant for patients and onerous for their carers. Alternative strategies for chronic SIAD include the use of distal nephron inhibitors preventing water reabsorption and osmotic diuretics.

The tetracycline analogue demeclocycline (desmethylchlortetracycline) causes nephrogenic diabetes insipidus by inhibiting vasopressin-induced cAMP formation in distal tubules and is used in the treatment of chronic SAD. Demeclocycline administered orally in two divided doses equivalent to 900–1200 mg/day will reverse chronic SIAD gradually over three to four days and should be followed by a maintenance dosage of 600–900 mg/day. The main side-effects of demeclocycline are gastrointestinal disturbances and hypersensitivity reactions, although reversible nephrotoxicity may occur with prolonged use, especially when hepatic function is impaired. Lithium carbonate, which has a similar effect on tubular water reabsorption, has also been used in the treatment of SIAD, but is not recommended as its efficacy is less consistent and its toxicity is greater.

Urea acts as an osmotic diuretic increasing free water excretion and in addition reduces natriuresis by increasing intramedullary urea levels. It is effective in controlling SIAD when given both intravenously and orally. Oral urea should be given once daily at a dose of 30 g dissolved in orange juice to mask the taste. There is no need to restrict fluid intake of patients treated with oral urea because of its diuretic properties[91].

The development of vasopressin analogues that may act as specific antagonists is underway and these may hold the key to the control of SIAD in the future. A series of oral nonpeptide antagonists of vasopressin receptor subtypes have been synthesized, including selective V_2 receptor antagonists (lixivaptan and tolvaptan) and V_{1A}/V_2 receptor antagonists (conivaptan). Lixivaptan has shown promise in trials in heart failure[92], whilst Tolvaptan reverses hyponatraemia more effectively than fluid restriction[93] and conivaptan was effective in a randomized placebo-controlled trial of patients with hyponatraemia[94]. This class of drugs has been christened aquaretics in recognition of their different mechanism of diuresis compared to the saliuretic actions of more familiar diuretics such as frusemide and most of the research has focused on their role in the treatment of heart failure and cirrhosis rather than SIAD[95].

Atrial natriuretic peptide

Atrial natriuretic peptide (ANP) is secreted by atrial monocytes and acts to regulate natriuresis and diuresis via the kidney and adrenals. A role for ectopic or inappropriate ANP secretion had been proposed to account for cases of SIAD when vasopressin is undetectable[96]. Ectopic production of ANP has been identified by radioimmunoassay in various neuroendocrine tumours[97] and elevated serum levels of ANP have been found in small-cell lung cancer patients with SIAD who had normal levels of AVP[98].

The natriuretic peptide family is now known to include four peptides: atrial natriuretic peptide, brain natriuretic peptide (BNP), C-type natriuretic peptide (CNP), and urodilatin, which share a similar cysteine bridge structure and function. ANP and BNP are secreted by cardiac myocytes, CNP is produced by endothelial cells, while urodilatin is secreted by renal tubular cells. ANP and BNP act via two gyuanylyl cyclase receptors and a third peptide clearance receptor[99]. The exact role of natriuretic peptides in SIAD remains to be established and ANP inhibitors may in the future have a place in treating SIAD[100].

Non-islet cell tumour hypoglycaemia

Tumour-related hypoglycaemia is a frequent complication of beta islet cell tumours of the pancreas, which secrete insulin, but occurs uncommonly with non-islet cell tumours. Although ectopic insulin secretion has been documented in a woman with cervical cancer[101], most non-islet cell tumours produce hypoglycaemia by increased glucose use by tumours, secretion of insulin-like factors, and failure of the normal compensatory mechanisms[102].

Pathogenesis

Increased glucose utilization by tumours has been documented in association with anaerobic metabolism by measuring arteriovenous differences in glucose concentrations. Daily glucose consumption by tumours may reach 200 g/kg per day. In addition, hepatic glucose production falls despite normal glycogen stores, producing an acquired glycogen storage disease, which may contribute to hypoglycaemia. Finally, suppression of other compensatory mechanisms, including growth hormone and glucagon secretion is believed to play a role.

Insulin-like growth factors (formerly named somatomedins) are a family of peptides involved in cellular growth, differentiation, and metabolism. They cross-react with insulin in both bioassay and radioreceptor assay but may be differentiated from insulin by radioimmunoassay. Two insulin-like growth factors (IGFs) have been characterized and both have sequence homology with insulin. In many cases, non-islet cell tumours associated with hypoglycaemia secrete an abnormal precursor of IGF-2 (formerly known as somatomedin A). This pro-IGF-2 has not undergone processing to remove the E domain that is normally cleaved from it during intracellular peptide processing. This is analogous to the conversion of pro-insulin to insulin and it is worth recalling that pro-insulin rather than insulin dominates in the plasma of patients with insulinomas. IGF-2 binds at least two receptors: An insulin-receptor-like tyrosine kinase for which IGF-1 is also a ligand and the mannose-6-phosphate receptor. IGF-2 expression is induced by human placental lactogen, especially during fetal life where the expression of IGF-2 and its type 2 receptor are reciprocally modulated by genomic imprinting. Unlike insulin, the IGFs are bound to at least six plasma IGF-binding proteins. At high levels of IGF-2, there is a specificity spill-over so that lower affinity binding to the insulin receptor occurs and this may mediate hypoglycaemia. In addition, suppression of counter-regulatory hormones including growth hormone and glucagon is a feature of non-islet cell hypoglycaemia. IGF-2 suppresses growth hormone secretion and thus reduces the production of IGF binding proteins by the liver[103]. Decreased IGF binding protein levels permit free IGF-2 levels to rise, leading to the inhibition of hepatic glucose release and stimulation of peripheral glucose uptake. The role of IGFs, their binding proteins, and their receptors in the pathogenesis of cell transformation remains under close scrutiny[104,105]. Rarely, other mechanisms contribute to non-islet cell hypoglycaemia, including the development of autoantibodies to the insulin receptor in Hodgkin's disease[106,107], as well as overwhelming hepatic destruction.

Epidemiology

Non-islet cell tumours associated with hypoglycaemia are usually large (average 2.4 kg), retroperitoneal, or intrathoracic, often with liver invasion and follow a protracted time-course over several years. Histologically half these tumours are mesenchymal (mesothelioma, neurofibroma, fibrosarcoma, leiomyosarcoma, rhabdomyosarcoma, neurofibrosarcoma, haemangiopericytoma, and spindle cell carcinoma), 20 per cent hepatoma, 5–10 per cent adrenal carcinoma (chiefly androgen-secreting), and 5–10 per cent gastrointestinal tumours. Unlike other endocrine complications of malignancy, hypoglycaemia is very rarely associated with lung cancer.

Clinical features

Hypoglycaemia may be a presenting symptom but more commonly occurs in the terminal stages of the disease. The clinical manifestations are associated with cerebral hypoglycaemia and secondary secretion of catecholamines. Neurological findings include agitation, stupor, coma, and seizures, which usually follow exercise or fasting and occur most often in the early morning and late afternoon. Focal neurological deficits may be present especially when cerebral circulation is poor.

Tumour-related hypoglycaemia should be differentiated from other causes of hypoglycaemia including drugs (e.g. sulphonylureas), hypoadrenalism, hypopituitarism, and liver failure. In advanced malignancy, the most common cause of hypoglycaemia is continued oral hypoglycaemic medication in long-standing diabetics.

Treatment

The reversal of life-threatening or symptomatic hypoglycaemia initially requires intravenous glucose infusion. Hyperosmolar glucose solutions in excess of 10 per cent should be administered via central lines; serum glucose levels require frequent monitoring to ensure optimal correction of hypoglycaemia. Up to 2000 g/day may be required to control tumour-related hypoglycaemia. Debulking surgery and effective chemotherapy frequently improve paraneoplastic hypoglycaemia and should therefore be considered even in a palliative context. Dietary supplementation with frequent feeding, including during the night, may control symptoms of mild paraneoplastic hypoglycaemia. Corticosteroids in high doses, parenteral glucagon, and human growth hormone have all been of benefit in some patients, whilst diazoxide, which inhibits insulin secretion, and somatostatin have been ineffective[105].

Arterial embolization of tumours may also be used to palliate paraneoplastic hypoglycaemia.

Future approaches

The discovery of the role of IGFs in the pathogenesis of non-islet cell tumour hypoglycaemia suggests that antagonists of these peptides may become useful as therapy and may reduce the dependence on continuous glucose infusions to control hypoglycaemia in these circumstances.

Enteropancreatic hormone syndromes

Enteropancreatic hormone production is relatively uncommon in malignant disease; however, there are a variety of clinical syndromes associated with hormone secretion by endocrine tumours of the pancreas and, less frequently, tumours arising in other organs. The majority of pancreatic islet cell tumours are malignant (with the exception of most insulinomas) and metastases are frequently present at diagnosis. Surgical excision of small localized tumours is optimal treatment and unresectable malignant secretory tumours may respond to chemotherapy. However, in many patients, the distressing clinical manifestations arising from excessive secretion of gastrointestinal peptides require palliation and this may be difficult to achieve. These tumours often secrete more than one polypeptide hormone and may switch their hormone production during follow-up. Furthermore, many molecular species of the hormones, including precursor peptides with varying bioactivity, may be found in the circulation.

Treatment

The clinical manifestations listed according to the major hormone product of secretory endocrine tumours are shown in along with the palliative endocrine manoeuvres that may control them. The control of insulinoma-related hypoglycaemia is similar to the management of paraneoplastic hypoglycaemia (see above), except that diazoxide may be a valuable additional agent in insulinoma. Diazoxide inhibits insulin release from beta islet cells but may cause salt and water retention and so is usually prescribed with chlorothiazide. Palliation of acid hypersecretion in Zollinger–Ellison syndrome is most effectively achieved by proton pump inhibitors, although other drugs including high dose histamine H2 receptor antagonists may be useful. The symptomatic control of other secretory tumours has been revolutionized by the introduction of long acting somatostatin analogues.

Somatostatin is a widely distributed 14-amino acid cyclic neuroendocrine peptide, which plays an inhibitory role in homeostatic mechanisms of the nervous system, gastrointestinal tract, and both endocrine and exocrine pancreas. A single gene on chromosome 3 encodes somatostatin, which is translated as the 116 amino acid pre-pro-somatostatin that includes a signal peptide. Extensive post-translational processing yields SOM-14, the biologically active form. SOM-14 acts via five somatostatin receptors (sstr1-5) that activate G proteins, which in turn reduce adenyl cyclase activity, decrease conductance of voltage-sensitive calcium channels, activate potassium channels, and stimulate tyrosine kinase activity[108]. Somatostatin has a short duration of action, requires intravenous administration, and rebound hypersecretion of hormones may occur following the infusion. These shortcomings have been overcome by the use of the synthetic analogue octreotide, an eight-amino acid analogue that is given by subcutaneous injection. Octreotide acts on three of the somatostatin receptor subtypes and appears to exert

Table 10.10.3 Clinical manifestations of secretory endocrine tumours.

Tumour	Major feature	Minor feature	Common sites	Malignant	MEN associated	Palliative therapies
Insulinoma	Neuroglycopenia (confusion, fits)	Permanent neurological deficits	Pancreas (β cells) >99%	10%	4–5%	Frequent feeding, glucose, glucagon, diazoxide and chlorothiazide; Octreotide (if scan +ve)
Gastrinoma (Zollinger–Ellison syndrome)	Peptic ulceration	Diarrhoea, weight loss, malabsorption, dumping	Pancreas (D cells) 25%, duodenum 70%	>50%	20–25%	Gastrectomy, proton pump inhibitors, H2 receptor antagonists, Octreotide
VIPoma (WDHA or Werner–Morrison syndrome)	Watery diarrhoea, hypokalaemia, achlorhydria	Hypercalcaemia, hyperglycaemia, hypomagnesaemia	Pancreas (A–D cells) 90%, neuroblastoma, SCLC, phaeochromocytoma	>50%	6%	Octreotide, glucocorticoids, potassium and bicarbonate during attacks
Glucagonoma	Migratory necrolytic erythema, mild diabetes mellitus, muscle wasting, anaemia	Diarrhoea, thromboembolism, stomatitis, hypoaminoacidaemia, encephalitis	Pancreas (α cells) 99%	>70 %	1–20%	Octreotide, oral hypoglycaemics, prophylactic anticoagulation
Somatostatinoma	Diabetes mellitus, cholelithiasis, steatorrhoea, malabsorption	Anaemia, diarrhoea, weight loss, hypoglycaemia	Pancreas (β cells) 55%, duodenum and jejunum 45%	>60%	45%	Pancreatic enzyme supplements, Insulin for diabetes
PPoma	None	Diarrhoea, hypokalaemia, achlorhydria, weight loss	Pancreas (interacinar F cells) 99%	>60%	18–44%	

Abbreviations: MEN, multiple endocrine neoplasia; SCLC, small cell lung cancer; VIP, vasoactive intestinal polypeptide; PP, pancreatic polypeptide; H2, histamine type 2; WDHA, watery diarrhoea, hypokalaemic achlorhydria.

its clinical effect via binding to receptor subtype 2[108]. A similar octapeptide, lanreotide is also now available and is formulated for prolonged action over one to four weeks.

The control of clinical symptoms associated with enteropancreatic hormone hypersecretion including profuse diarrhoea, hypokalaemia, hypoglycaemia, peptic ulceration, necrolytic skin lesions, and even Cushing's syndrome can be achieved by 100–600 mcg octreotide subcutaneously daily in many patients with endocrine pancreatic tumours. Once adequate symptom control has been achieved, patients may be switched to a slow-release depot formulation such as octreotide depot (Sandostatin LAR®) or lanreotide (Somatuline LA®). The response to octreotide seems to depend upon the presence of somatostatin receptors on the tumours and this has been exploited for tumour localization using *in vivo* scintigraphy with labelled octreotide.[109] Somatostatin receptor scintigraphy has a sensitivity of 90 per cent and specificity of 80 per cent for enteropancreatic neuroendocrine tumours except insulinomas, which often do not express these receptors and are less responsive to somatostatin analogue therapy[110]. Somatostatin analogues provide valuable symptom palliation in insulinomas, glucagonomas, gastrinomas, and VIPomas but there is little evidence to suggest that they control tumour growth. Resistance may develop with chronic use of octreotide and this is thought to occur due to the emergence of tumour cells lacking somatostatin receptors. Octreotide therapy is well tolerated; although initially abdominal cramps and diarrhoea may occur; significant steatorrhoea and malabsorption have not been observed. Amongst the more recent advances in the management of these tumours is the use of radiolabelled somatostatin analogues[111].

Carcinoid syndrome

Carcinoid tumours arise from serotonin-producing enterochromaffin cells principally in the gastrointestinal tract, pancreas, and lungs but occasionally in the thymus and gonads. The incidence of these uncommon neoplasms is 1.5 per 100 000. The carcinoid syndrome develops in 6–18 per cent of patients with these tumours and these patients almost invariably have hepatic metastases[108,112,113]. The features of carcinoid tumours vary by their sites of origin and are shown in Table 10.10.4.

The cardinal feature of the carcinoid syndrome is the combination of diarrhoea and flushing, which occurs in at least 75 per cent of patients, and may be associated with endomyocardial fibrosis, asthma, and pellagra. One-third of patients develop cardiac manifestations, which are late complications, typically involving the right side of the heart and leading to pulmonary valve stenosis and tricuspid valve regurgitation. Asthma and pellagra are less common. The pellagroid rash is thought to arise secondary to the diversion of tryptophan for 5-hydroxytryptamine (5HT) synthesis rather than nicotinamide production[114]. The clinical features are mediated by several potentially active substances secreted by these tumours including 5HT, 5-hydroxytryptophan, kallikrein, tachykinins (substance P, neuropeptide K), prostaglandins, catecholamines, and histamine. The diagnosis is usually established by measuring the urinary excretion of 5-hydroxyindoloacetic acid formed by the action of monoamine oxidase on 5HT. However, platelet 5HT levels are a more sensitive diagnostic test and are unaffected by diet[115]. Tumour localization may be achieved using somatostatin receptor scintigraphy or by positron emission tomography (PET) scanning after injecting ^{11}C-labelled 5-hydroxytryptophan[116].

Table 10.10.4 Comparison of carcinoid tumours by site of origin.

	Foregut (2–33% carcinoid tumours)	Midgut (75–87% carcinoid tumours)	Hindgut (1–8% carcinoid tumours)
Site	Respiratory tract, pancreas, stomach, proximal duodenum	Jejunum, ileum, appendix, Meckle's diverticulum, ascending colon	Transverse and descending colon, rectum
Tumour products	Low 5HTP, multihormones*	High 5HTP, multihormones*	Rarely 5HTP, multihormones*
Blood	5HTP, histamine, multihormones,* occasionally ACTH	5HT, multihormones,* rarely ACTH	Rarely 5HT or ACTH
Urine	5HTP, 5HT, 5HIAA, histamine	5HT, 5HIAA	Negative
Carcinoid syndrome	Occurs but is atypical	Occurs frequently with metastases	Rarely occurs
Metastases to bone	Common	Rare	Common

*Multihormones include tachykinins (substance P, substance K, neuropeptide K), neurotensin, PYY, enkephalin, insulin, glucagon, glicentin, VIP, somatostatin, pancreatic polypeptide, ACTH, α-subunit of human chorionic gonadotrophin.

Abbreviations: 5HT, 5-hydroxytryptamine (serotonin), 5HTP, 5-hydroxytryptophan,; 5HIAA, 5-hydroxyindole acetic acid.

The pharmacological control of carcinoid syndrome is primarily directed at inhibiting the synthesis, release, and peripheral action of circulating tumour products, principally 5HT. The choice of drugs remains empirical in view of the varied profiles of active substances released by different tumours. Parachlorophenylalanine and methyldopa block 5HT synthesis but are poorly tolerated and, therefore, rarely used. At least 16 5HT receptors have been cloned and most have been found to be G-protein coupled, although the $5HT_3$ receptor is a ligand-gated ion channel. The development of selective 5HT receptor ligands and antagonists will allow the investigation of the physiological roles of each receptor. However, the relevance of the different receptors in the clinical manifestations of carcinoid syndrome remains uncertain and is obscured by the secretion of multiple products by these tumours. Of the drugs which block $5HT_2$ receptors, cyproheptadine (4–7 mg three times daily) improves diarrhoea in 60 per cent of patients and flushing in 47 per cent with a mean duration of response of 8 months. In contrast, ketanserin (40-160mg once daily) ameliorates flushing in 50 per cent but only 20 per cent derive relief from diarrhoea. Selective $5HT_3$ receptor inhibitors have been shown to reduce diarrhoea in carcinoid syndrome. Metoclopramide and cisapride are believed to stimulate gastric motility via the $5HT_4$ receptor and antagonists of this receptor, which are in development, may prove useful in the palliation of carcinoid syndrome.

Somatostatin analogues are considered by most physicians to be the first-line treatment of choice for patients with carcinoid syndrome. Octreotide in doses of 50–150 mcg two or three times daily subcutaneously, reduces 5HT secretion and its peripheral action and is valuable in controlling both flushing and diarrhoea in the carcinoid syndrome. It produces initial relief of symptoms in 80 per cent of patients[117]. Sandostatin LAR® and lanreotide, a related peptide, are long acting analogues that have been found to be efficacious[118–120]. A reuction in tumour rarely occurs, however, and the effects of treatment diminish with time.

Palliative debulking surgery may be offered to selected patients with metastatic disease as it can delay the development of the carcinoid syndrome. Hepatic artery embolization similarly can be employed and may produce good symptom palliation. Chemotherapy and alpha interferon have also been used successfully to palliate symptoms in carcinoid syndrome[116]. Interferon alpha is of benefit for carcinoid tumours that are somatostatin receptor negative[121] but the addition of interferon α to somatostatin analogues does not improve the outcome overall for carcinoid tumours[122]. Finally, ^{131}I-met-iodobenzylguanidine has been used in patients with disabling symptoms in whom other therapeutic options have failed[123].

Palliation of the clinical manifestations of carcinoid syndrome includes symptomatic therapy of diarrhoea (codeine phosphate, loperamide, or diphenoxylate), $β_2$ adrenergic agonists for wheezing, and avoidance of precipitating factors to reduce flushing (including alcohol and some foods).

Phaeochromocytoma

Catecholamine-secreting tumours may arise from the adrenal medulla (phaeochromocytomas) or from other neural crest derived tissues. Phaeochromocytomas arise from the chromaffin cells of the sympathetic nervous system most frequently in the adrenal medulla but occasionally from sympathetic ganglia (paragangiomas). Phaeochromocytomas commonly secrete norepinephrine and epinephrine but in some cases, significant quantities of dopamine are also produced. The catecholamines cause intermittent, episodic, or sustained hypertension and other clinical manifestations including anxiety, tremor, palpitations, sweating, flushing, headaches, gastrointestinal disturbances, and polyuria. These symptoms are all attributable to excessive adrenergic stimulation and when surgery and chemotherapy are unable to control the disease, palliative treatment is usually achieved by α and β adrenergic receptor blockade. However, these tumours may elaborate and secrete other peptide hormones that may cause symptoms refractory to adrenergic inhibition, but this is rare. Initial treatment should be α blockade to control hypertension (e.g phenoxybenzamine 10 mg twice daily and gradually increasing the dosage until symptoms are palliated) followed by β blockade to control tachycardia (e.g propranolol 20–80 mg three times daily). This combination will control symptoms in most patients with malignant phaeochromocytoma. If palliation is not achieved despite full adrenergic receptor blockade, α-methylparatyrosine (metirosine 250 mg twice daily increasing up to 4 g/day) may be used but is not widely available (metirosine is only available on a named patient basis in the UK). Metirosine is a competitive inhibitor of tyrosine hydroxylase, the rate limiting enzyme in catecholamine synthesis, and reduces catecholamine production by up to 75 per cent but it is poorly tolerated due to sedation, extrapyramidal effects, and diarrhoea. The norepinephrine analogue metiodobenzylguanidine (MIBG) is taken up by catecholamine synthesizing tissues and ^{131}I-MIBG is useful for imaging phaeochromocytomas. At higher doses, ^{131}I-MIBG may be used as therapy for phaeochromocytoma and neuroblastoma and it reduces catecholamine synthesis in patients with malignant phaeochromocytoma[124].

Gonadotrophin secretion

Follicle stimulating hormone, luteinizing hormone, and human chorionic gonadotrophin (hCG) may be secreted by pituitary, trophoblastic, or germ cell tumours and ectopically by tumours arising in other organs. All three gonadotrophins are dimeric glycoproteins sharing the same β subunit with thyroid stimulating hormone but each has a unique α subunit that confers biological activity. The overproduction by tumours of gonadotrophins may result in precocious puberty in children, secondary amenorrhoea in women, gynaecomastia in men, and rarely, hyperthyroidism. HCG is a valuable tumour marker for detecting and monitoring therapy in trophoblastic and germ cell tumours.

Precocious puberty

Central precocious puberty occurs with central nervous system tumours secreting gonadotrophins that activate the hypothalamic-pituitary axis. Incomplete or peripheral precocious puberty may result from hCG secretion by germinomas, teratomas, chorioepitheliomas, and hepatomas and oestrogen or testosterone production by adrenal, testicular (Leydig cell), and ovarian (granulosa thecal cell) tumours. The treatment of precocious puberty includes psychological counselling for boys with increased aggression and excessive masturbation. Medical therapy is required to control both the psychosocial aspects and sustained effects on skeletal maturation. Central precocious puberty is amenable to gonadorelin analogues that, following an initial phase of stimulation, lead to pituitary gonadotrophin receptor desensitization, resulting in suppressed luteinizing hormone and follicle-stimulating-hormone secretion. The management of incomplete precocious puberty is more difficult and requires the use of antiandrogens (e.g. flutamide, bicalutamide, cyproterone acetate, and spironolactone) and inhibitors of androgen synthesis (e.g. ketoconazole, dutasteride, and finasteride).

Amenorrhoea

Secondary amenorrhoea in women with cancer may occasionally be a consequence of gonadotrophin, prolactin, oestrogen, or androgen-secreting tumours, although iatrogenic causes are far more common. The vasomotor symptoms associated with menopause may be palliated by hormone replacement therapy if appropriate and dyspareunia caused by vaginal atrophy may be alleviated by topical oestrogen preparations.

Gynaecomastia

Gynaecomastia results from elevation in the oestrogen:androgen ratio that may be either a consequence of decreased androgen production or activity or increased oestrogen formation (usually by peripheral aromatization of circulating androgens to oestrogens). In men with advanced cancer, gynaecomastia is most often a consequence of drug therapy, either chemotherapy (alkylating agents, vinca alkaloids, nitrosoureas), antiemetics (metoclopramide and phenothiazines), antiandrogens (cyproterone acetate, flutamide, bicalutamide), or gonadorelin analogues (goserelin, leuprorelin, buserelin, and triptorelin). Occasionally other drugs are implicated or tumour secretion of oestrogens or gonadotrophins may be responsible.

Testicular Leydig-cell tumours and feminizing adrenocortical tumours may secrete oestrogens, whilst peripheral aromatization is a feature of Sertoli cell tumours, trophoblastic germ cell tumours, and sex cord tumours of the testes and hepatocellular cancers. The elevated, circulating oestrogen levels induce ductal, lobular, and alveolar growth of the breast leading to gynaecomastia. HCG-secreting tumours (including testicular tumours, trophoblastic tumours, non-small cell lung cancers, hepatoma, and islet cell tumours of the pancreas) stimulate oestradiol production by interstitial and Sertoli cells of the testes resulting in gynaecomastia. Symptomatic therapy for gynaecomastia should include discontinuation of any incriminated drugs and treatment of the primary tumour. Tamoxifen, clomiphene, topical dihydrotestosterone, and danazol have all been used with some success, as have liposuction, subcutaneous mastectomy, and low dosage radiotherapy for palliation of painful gynaecomastia[125,126].

Hyperthyroidism

On account of the structural similarities to thyroid stimulating hormone, hCG has intrinsic thyrotropic action via a thyroid stimulating hormone receptor spill-over effect[127]. Clinically overt hyperthyroidism caused in this way only occurs with tumours secreting very large quantities of hCG, usually trophoblastic tumours[128]. The hyperthyroidism resolves after surgical removal of the tumour and therefore palliation of the hyperthyroidism should be with drugs (e.g carbimazole) rather than radioactive iodine or thyroidectomy.

Prolactin

Ectopic prolactin secretion from non-pituitary tumours is very rare and uncommonly causes galactorrhoea. Small-cell lung cancer and renal cell cancer have been associated with elevated prolactin levels, although the mechanism remains uncertain. Elevated serum prolactin is a poor prognostic indicator in women with breast cancer[129] and prolactin promotes the growth *in vitro* of human breast cancer cells. Galactorrhoea due to ectopic prolactin production may be treated by the dopaminergic agonist bromocriptine.

Oxytocin

The molecular biology of oxytocin resembles that of AVP with similar genes, precursor proteins, and transport by axonal streaming. Furthermore, ectopic secretion of both oxytocin and its carrier protein neurophysin I have demonstrated in small-cell lung cancer, usually in conjunction with ectopic AVP production. Although water intoxication and hyponatraemia may follow oxytocin infusions in women with obstetric problems, ectopic oxytocin secretion is not thought to contribute to SIAD nor any other clinical symptoms.

Pyrexia

Pyrexia is a common feature of terminal cancer and is usually attributable to infection or drugs. In one study of fever of unknown origin, 15 per cent of cases were attributed to malignancy,[130] although amongst patients with cancer infection, chemotherapy, or other treatments account for most cases of pyrexia. Paraneoplastic pyrexia is a diagnosis of exclusion established after other causes of fever have been ruled out. Hodgkin's disease, renal cell adenocarcinoma, lymphoma, leukaemia, hepatoma, myxoma, and osteogenic sarcoma account for most cases of paraneoplastic fever.[131] Although neither CRP nor ESR levels are valuable in differentiating paraneoplastic pyrexia from infection[132], resolution of fever with naproxen 250 mg bd has been found to be diagnostic of paraneoplastic pyrexia in some[133] but not all studies[134].

Pathogenesis

Pyrexia is a consequence of endogenous pyrogenic cytokines (including TNF, IL-1, IL-6, and interferons), stimulating the organum vasculosum of the lamina terminalis, which lacks a blood–brain barrier. This results in the synthesis and release of prostaglandin E_2 from the preoptic anterior hypothalamus that mediates thermal homeostasis. Indeed, microsomal prostaglandin E synthase-1 appears to be the central switch determining fever at least in mice[135]. Resetting the thermostatic set point by one to four degrees centigrade enhances macrophage killing of bacteria and also impairs replication of micro-organisms[136–138]. Tumour related pyrexia is thought to be a consequence of cytokine production by neoplastic cells or by normal cells in response to tumour presence. Evidence for the former includes TNF-α production in Hodgkin's disease, which may be localized by *in vitro* hybridization to the Reed Sternberg cell[139]. Furthermore, the abnormal lymphocytes in Castleman's disease (an angiofollicular lymph node hyperplasia related to lymphoma and associated with fever) produce IL-6. After complete surgical excision of these tumours circulating plasma IL-6 is no longer detectable and symptoms resolve. In addition, anti-interleukin-6 receptor antibody therapy has been shown to be a useful therapy for multicentric Castleman's disease[140]. A similar mechanism has been elucidated in phaeo-chromocytoma where tumour cells produce IL-6, resulting in paraneoplastic pyrexia that resolves with tumour resection[141]. In addition, raised serum levels of TNF-α, IL-1, and IL-6 are found in patients with renal cell carcinoma and serum IL-6 may be used as a tumour marker in these patients[142].

Therapy

Definitive therapy of the tumour will resolve paraneoplastic pyrexias in most cases of Hodgkin's disease and many lymphomas. Sponging, ice-packs, and fans may often relieve discomfort. Pharmacological agents such as paracetamol, aspirin, non-steroidal anti-inflammatory drugs, and steroids are effective antipyretics. Advances in the understanding of the pathogenesis of paraneoplastic pyrexia propose a role for cytokine antagonists in therapy. The development of IL-1 false receptors is an attractive approach to cytokine induced pyrexia that has already been usurped in nature by vaccinia virus. Vaccinia secretes virally encoded IL-1 receptors that compete with endogenous IL-1 receptors on T-lymphocytes, thus attenuating the host response to infection including pyrexia[143]. Similar strategies based upon IL-1 receptor antagonists including IL-1RA, which is structurally related to IL-1, have been explored in paraneoplastic pyrexia along with strategies aimed at blocking IL-6 signalling[144,145].

Non-paraneoplastic complications

Hyperglycaemia

The prevalence of hyperglycaemia in cancer patients is higher than in the general population. Diabetes mellitus has been proposed repeatedly as a risk factor for the development of pancreatic cancer. However, a multicentre study involving 720 patients failed to confirm this[146]. Several mechanisms may contribute to hyperglycaemia in advanced cancers including increased gluconeogenesis and Cori cycle activity (conversion of muscle derived lactate to glucose), diminished glucose tolerance and turnover along with insulin resistance[147,148]. These changes may arise as a consequence of hepatic dysfunction, altered glucose metabolism by tumour cells, and the secretion of insulin antagonists. Furthermore, the frequent use of corticosteroids in palliative medicine may contribute, since one in five patients on high-dose steroids will develop steroid-induced diabetes mellitus.

The conventional treatment of diabetes advocates tight control of blood sugar to delay the onset of both macrovascular and microvascular complications. In contrast the aims of therapy in palliative care are to minimize symptoms associated with hypoglycaemia or marked hyperglycaemia. For this reason, a wider range of blood sugar is acceptable and close blood glucose monitoring is unnecessary.

Weight loss and anorexia reduce the need for hypoglycaemic agents as cancer progresses and strict dietary restrictions are unnecessary and burdensome. Oral hypoglycaemic drugs can usually be reduced or stopped in non-insulin-dependent diabetics without symptomatic hyperglycaemia ensuing. Similarly, the insulin requirements of insulin-dependent diabetics with advanced malignancy fall and insulin regimens can usually be simplified to once daily, long-acting insulin such as human mixed insulin zinc suspensions (e.g. Human monotard, Humulin lente) or human crystalline insulin zinc suspensions (e.g. human Ultratard, Humulin Zn). Alternatively, twice a day regimens using biphasic isophane insulin preparations such as Mixtard can be used and may reduce the chance of hypoglycaemia. Blood sugars may be allowed to stay on the high side (e.g. 8–15) to prevent the distressing symptoms of hypoglycaemia. Where possible, monitoring should be performed by urinalysis rather than blood sampling. Steroid-induced diabetes, which occurs frequently in advanced cancer, is usually asymptomatic and requires no therapy; however, if polyuria and polydipsia develop a short acting sulphonylurea may be useful (e.g. gliclazide 40–80 mg once daily). Biguanides (e.g. metformin) and alpha-glucosidase inhibitors (e.g. acarbose) are best avoided in view of their unpleasant gastrointestinal side effects, whilst thiazolidinediones (e.g. rosiglitazone, pioglitazone) require monitoring of liver function[149].

Renal failure

Renal failure is a common feature of advanced malignancy and many aetiological factors play a role in its pathogenesis. In the context of incurable malignant disease, reversible causes may be addressed but aggressive treatment such as renal replacement therapy is usually not appropriate. Conversely, there is increasing awareness of palliative measures and end of life care amongst nephrologists treating patients with end stage renal failure[150].

Potentially reversible metabolic causes of renal failure include urate nephropathy, hypercalcaemia, and tumour lysis syndrome.

Table 10.10.5 Causes of renal failure in malignancy.

1.	Infiltration by tumour
2.	Fluid depletion
3.	Electrolyte imbalance
	Uric acid (tumour lysis syndrome)
	Hypercalcaemia
	Paraprotein (e.g. myeloma)
	Amyloid (e.g. myeloma)
	Lysozyme (e.g. acute myelomonocytic leukaemia)
	Mucoprotein (e.g. pancreatic adenocarcinoma)
	Nephrogenic diabetes insipidus (e.g.leiomyosarcoma)
4.	Urinary tract obstruction
5.	Iatrogenic
	Chemotherapy
	Radiotherapy
6.	Paraneoplastic
	Membranous glomerulonephritis (e.g. carcinomas)
	Minimal change glomerulonephritis (e.g. Hodgkin's disease)
	Membranoproliferative glomerulonephritis (e.g. non-Hodgkin's lymphoma)
7.	Pre-existing chronic renal failure

Prerenal and obstructive renal failure may be reversible, although treatment may not be appropriate if the patient is very frail and antitumour options have been exhausted[151]. Tumour infiltration can sometimes be improved if effective anticancer therapy is available as in newly diagnosed lymphoma.

Symptomatic management of renal failure is important. Patients may experience nausea, vomiting, drowsiness, and confusion as the kidneys fail. Dry mouth and anorexia are frequent symptoms of advanced cancer and may be exacerbated by renal impairment. Appropriate and sensitive explanation to the patient and family should be accompanied by medication to relieve any unpleasant symptoms. In the context of renal failure doses or dose frequency of some medications, including opioid analgesics, may need to be reduced or stopped to avoid drug accumulation or deterioration of renal function (see Chapter 12.6). Patients already receiving renal dialysis for pre-existing chronic renal failure usually choose to continue this until it becomes impractical.

Obstructive nephropathy may cause colicky or constant pain in addition to the non-specific symptoms of renal failure. Although analgesics and antispasmodics may ameliorate the pain, longer lasting relief of symptoms can be achieved with percutaneous nephrostomy. This procedure, performed under sedation, can be followed by antegrade catheterization of the ureters. Nephrostomy tube insertion is an invasive procedure and is appropriate in selected cases where prognosis may be longer or antitumour treatment is planned[152,153].

Liver failure

Liver failure in cancer patients is usually a consequence of biliary obstruction, very extensive hepatic metastases, or drug therapy, although paraneoplastic hepatopathy has been described in Hodgkin's lymphoma[154] and renal cancer[155]. After excluding drug causes, it is important to differentiate obstructive and parenchymal causes as the approach to palliation differs.

Obstructive jaundice may be differentiated from other causes by the detection of urinary bilirubin in the absence of urinary urobilinogen using dipstick testing. Biliary obstruction may be confirmed by ultrasonography and drainage may be undertaken to relieve jaundice and associated symptoms (anorexia, nausea, pruritus) (see Chapter 10.2.5). Biliary drainage may be obtained by percutaneous transhepatic biliary drainage or endoscopic retrograde biliary drainage and both techniques provide good palliation.

Hepatic failure due to massive metastases may produce jaundice, pruritis, anorexia, liver capsule pain, ascites, disturbances of haemostasis, malabsorption, and electrolyte disturbances, culminating in hepatic encephalopathy. The palliative treatment of liver failure needs to be tailored to the particular symptoms of each patient. Liver capsule pain may be helped by non-steroidal anti-inflammatory drugs or corticosteroids together with conventional analgesics. Symptoms of functional gastric outlet obstruction may be relieved by metoclopramide before meals. Nausea secondary to liver failure may require centrally acting antiemetics such as haloperidol. Pruritus may be reduced by using emollients and night sedation. Naltrexone and stanozolol have also been found to be effective in pruritis from intrahepatic cholestasis and obstructive jaundice respectively (see Chapter 10.2.5). If the cause is obstructive, then stenting provides the most effective palliation[156].

Hepatic encephalopathy is thought to be due to an excess of γ-aminobutyric acid (GABA) activity, ammonia, and other toxins in the central nervous system. Conventional therapies for hepatic encephalopathy include restriction of dietary protein and sodium, bowel clearance with magnesium sulphate enemas and lactulose, as well as bowel sterilization with neomycin in an attempt to reduce ammonia production by gut microflora. Since hepatic encephalopathy is a terminal event in the context of advanced malignancy, these unpleasant treatments are rarely appropriate. The main symptom of encephalopathy is confusion and after establishing the cause of confusion, familiar company, a light and quiet environment and a regular routine should be provided together with explanation, reassurance and reorientation. Sedation may be necessary if the patient is agitated. Under these circumstances, haloperidol (1.5–5 mg) or levomepromazine (6.25–150 mg) may be given orally or subcutaneously and will also have an antiemetic action (see Chapter 19.2). The combination of portal hypertension and abnormal coagulation in liver failure predisposes to gastrointestinal haemorrhage. Major haemorrhage should usually be managed symptomatically (see Chapter 10.14).

Lactic acidosis

Lactic acidosis in cancer patients is most frequently type A lactic acidosis due to impaired tissue oxygenation secondary to hypoperfusion as a consequence of septicaemia shock. Less commonly type B lactic acidosis occurs with large tumour burdens and where the underlying malignancy is haematological. Increased lactate production by tumour cells owing to uncoupled oxidative phosphorylation and glycolysis and reduced lactate clearance due to liver dysfunction have both been implicated in the pathogenesis of malignancy-associated lactic acidosis. Lactic acidosis presents clinically with hyperventilation and hypotension and the diagnosis is established biochemically by the combination of wide anion gap acidosis and raised plasma lactate (>2 mEq/l). High volume haemofiltration and intravenous sodium bicarbonate may be used to correct the metabolic acidosis but should obviously only be used if effective anticancer therapy is available and appropriate[157].

References

1. Nakayama, K., Fukumoto, S., Takeda, S. *et al.* (1996). Differences in bone and vitamin D metabolism between primary hyperparathyroidism and malignancy-associated hypercalcemia. *J Clin Endocrinol Metab*, **81**, 607–11.

2. Benitez-Verguizas, J. and Esbrit, P. (1994). Proliferative effect of parathyroid hormone-related protein on the hypercalcemic Walker 256 carcinoma cell line. *Biochem Biophys Res Commun*, **198**(3), 1281–9.

3. Li, X. and Drucker, D.J. (1994). Parathyroid hormone-related peptide is a downstream target for ras and src activation. *J Biol Chem*, **269**(9), 6263–6.

4. Vortkamp, A., Lee, K., Lanske, B. *et al.* (1996). Regulation of rate of cartilage differentiation by Indian hedgehog and PTH-related peptide. *Science*, **273**, 613–22.

5. Lanske, B., Karaplis, A.C., Lee, K. *et al.* (1996). PTH/PTHrP receptor in early development and Indian hedgehog-regulated bone growth. *Science*, **273**, 663–6.

6. Strewler, G.J. (2000). The physiology of parathyroid hormone-related protein. *N Engl J Med*, **342**(3), 177–85.

7. Danks, J.A., Ebeling, P.R., Hayman, J. *et al.* (1989). Parathyroid hormone-related protein of cancer: Immunohistochemical localisation in cancers and in normal skin. *J Bone Miner Res*, **4**, 273–8.

8. Honda, S., Yamaguchi, K., Suzuki, M. *et al.* (1988). Expression of parathyroid hormone-related protein mRNA in tumours obtained from patients with humoral hypercalcaemia of malignancy. *Jpn J Cancer Res*, **79**, 677–83.

9. Budayr, A.A., Nissenson, R.A., Klein, R.F. *et al.* (1989). Increased serum levels of a parathyroid hormone-like protein in malignancy-associated hypercalcaemia. *Ann Intern Med*, **111**, 807–12.

10. Hutchesson, A.C., Dunne, F., Bundred, N.J. *et al.* (1993). Parathyroid hormone-related protein as a tumour marker in humoral hypercalcaemia associated with occult malignancy. *Postgrad Med J*, **69**(814), 640–2.

11. Bouizar, Z., Spyratos, F., Deytieux, S. *et al.* (1993). Polymerase chain reaction analysis of parathyroid hormone-related protein gene expression in breast cancer patients and occurrence of bone metastases. *Cancer Res*, **53**(21), 5076–8.

12. Wysolmerski, J.J. and Broadus, A.E. (1994). Hypercalcemia of malignancy: The central role of parathyroid hormone-related protein. *Annu Rev Med*, **45**, 189–200.

13. Grill, V., Ho, P., Body, J.J. *et al.* (1991). Parathyroid hormone-related protein: Elevated levels in both humoral hypercalcemia of malignancy and hypercalcemia complicating metastatic breast cancer. *J Clin Endocrinol Metab*, **73**, 1309–15.

14. Kukreja, S.C., Shevrin, D.H., Wimbiscus, S.A. *et al.* (1988). Antibodies to parathyroid hormone-related protein lower serum calcium in athymic mouse models of malignancy associated hypercalcemia of cancer. *J Clin Invest*, **82**, 1798–802.

15. Henderson, J., Bernier, S., D'Amour, P. *et al.* (1990). Effects of passive immunization against parathyroid hormone (PTH)-like peptide and PTH in hypercalcaemic tumour-bearing rats and normocalcaemic controls. *Endocrinology*, **127**, 1310–18.

16. Burtis, W.J., Brady, T.G., Orloff, J.J. *et al.* (1990). Immunocytochemical characterisation of circulating parathyroid hormone-related protein in patients with humoral hypercalcaemia of malignancy. *N Engl J Med*, **322**, 1106–12.

17. Seymour, J.F. and Gagel, R.F. (1993). Calcitriol: The major humoral mediator of hypercalcemia in Hodgkin's disease and non-Hodgkin's lymphomas. *Blood*, **82**(5), 1383–94.

18. Davies, M., Hayes, M., Yin, J. *et al.* (1994). Abnormal synthesis of 1,25-dihydroxyvitamin D in patients with malignant lymphoma. *J Clin Endocrinol Metab*, **78**, 1202–7.

19. Sato, M., Grasser, W., Endo, N. *et al.* (1991). Bisphosphonate action. Aldendronate localization in rat bone and effects on osteoclast ultrastructure. *J Clin Invest*, **88**, 2095–105.

20. Zimolo, Z., Wesolowski, G., and Rodan, G. (1995). Acid extrusion is induced by osteoclast attachment to bone. Inhibition by aledronate and calcitonin. *J Clin Invest*, **96**, 2324–33.

21. Gucalp, R., Ritch, P., Wiernik, P.H. *et al.* (1992). Comparative study of pamidronate disodium and etidronate disodium in the treatment of cancer-related hypercalcaemia. *J Clin Oncol*, **10**, 134–42.

22. O'Rourke, N.P., McCloskey, E.V., Vasikaran, S. *et al.* (1993). Effective treatment of malignant hypercalcaemia with a single intravenous infusion of clodronate. *Br J Cancer*, **67**, 560–563.

23. Hillner, B.E., Ingle, J.N., Chlebowski, R.T. *et al.* (2003). American Society of Clinical Oncology 2003 update on the role of bisphosphonates and bone health issues in women with breast cancer. *J Clin Oncol*, **21**(21), 4042–57. Epub 2003 Sep 8.

24. Purohit, O.P., Radstone, C.R., Anthony, C. *et al.* (1995). A randomised double-blind comparison of intravenous pamidronate and clodronate in the hypercalcaemia of malignancy. *Br J Cancer*, **72**, 1289–93.

25. Vinholes, J., Guo, C.-Y., Purohit, O. *et al.* (1997). Evaluation of new bone resorption markers in a randomized comparison of pamidronate or clodronate for hypercalcemia of malignany. *J Clin Oncol*, **15**, 131–8.

26. Walls, J., Ratcliffe, W., Howell, A. *et al.* (1994). Response to intravenous bisphosphonate therapy in hypercalcaemic patietns with and without bone metastases: The role of parathyroid hormone-related protein. *Br J Cancer*, **58**, 556–7.

27. Zojer, N., Brenner, K., Beke, D. *et al.* (2005). Bisphosphonate treatment does not affect serum levels of osteoprotegerin and RANKL in hypercalcemic cancer patients. *Anticancer Res*, **25**(5), 3607–12.

28. Wimalwansa, S. (1994). Significance of plasma PTH-rp in patients with hypercalcaemia of malignancy treated with bisphosphonate. *Cancer*, **73**, 2223–30.

29. Ralston, S.H., Thiebaud, D., Herrmann, Z. *et al.* (1997). Dose-response study of ibandronate in the treatment of cancer-associated hypercalcaemia. *Br J Cancer*, **75**, 295–300.

30. Pecherstorfer, M., Steinhauer, E.U., Rizzoli, R. *et al.* (2003). Efficacy and safety of ibandronate in the treatment of hypercalcemia of malignancy: A randomized multicentric comparison to pamidronate. *Support Care Cancer*, **11**(8), 539–47. Epub 2003 Jun 3.

31. Body, J., Lortholary, A., Romieu, G. *et al.* (1999). A dose-finding study of zoledronate in hypercalcemic cancer patients. *J Bone Mineral Res*, **14**, 1557–61.

32. Major, P., Lortholary, A., Hon, J. *et al.* (2001). Zoledronic acid is superior to pamidronate in the treatment of hypercalcemia of malignancy: A pooled analysis of two randomized, controlled clinical trials. *J Clin Oncol*, **19**(2), 558–67.

33. Migliorati, C.A., Siegel, M.A., and Elting, L.S. (2006). Bisphosphonate-associated osteonecrosis: A long-term complication of bisphosphonate treatment. *Lancet Oncol*, **7**(6), 508–14.

34. Bockman, R.S., Repo, M.A., Warrell, R.P., Jr. *et al.* (1990). Distribution of trace levels of therapeutic gallium in bone as mapped by synchrotron x-ray microscopy. *Proc Natl Acad Sci USA*, **87**(11), 4149–53.

35. Warrell, R., Israel, R., Frisone, M. *et al.* A randomised double-blind study of gallium nitrate versus calcitonin for acute treatment of cancer-related hypercalcaemia. *Ann Int Med*, **108**, 669–674.

36. Warrell, R., Heller, G., W. M, Schulman P, O'Dwyer P. (1991). A randomised double-blind study of gallium nitrate compared to etidronate for acute control of cancer related hypercalcemia. *J Clin Oncol*, **9**, 1467–75.

37. Sato, K., Yamakawa, Y., Shizume, K. *et al.* (1993). Passive immunization with anti-parathyroid hormone-related protein monoclonal antibody markedly prolongs survival time of hypercalcemic nude mice bearing transplanted human PTHrP-producing tumors. *J Bone Miner Res*, **8**(7), 849–60.

38. Saito, H., Tsunenari, T., Onuma, E. *et al.* (2005). Humanized monoclonal antibody against parathyroid hormone-related protein suppresses osteolytic bone metastasis of human breast cancer cells derived from MDA-MB-231. *Anticancer Res*, **25**(6B), 3817–23.

39. Onuma, E., Sato, K., Saito, H. *et al.* (2004). Generation of a humanized monoclonal antibody against human parathyroid hormone-related protein and its efficacy against humoral hypercalcemia of malignancy. *Anticancer Res*, **24**(5A), 2665–73.

40. Capparelli, C., Kostenuik, P.J., Morony, S. *et al.* (2000). Osteoprotegerin prevents and reverses hypercalcemia in a murine model of humoral hypercalcemia of malignancy. *Cancer Res*, **60**(4), 783–7.

41. Body, J.J., Greipp, P., Coleman, R.E. *et al.* (2003). A phase I study of AMGN-0007, a recombinant osteoprotegerin construct, in patients with multiple myeloma or breast carcinoma related bone metastases. *Cancer*, **97**(3 Suppl), 887–92.

42. McClung, M.R., Lewiecki, E.M., Cohen, S.B. *et al.* (2006). Denosumab in postmenopausal women with low bone mineral density. *N Engl J Med*, **354**(8), 821–31.

43. Body, J.J., Facon, T., Coleman, R.E. *et al.* (2006). A study of the biological receptor activator of nuclear factor-kappaB ligand inhibitor, denosumab, in patients with multiple myeloma or bone metastases from breast cancer. *Clin Cancer Res*, **12**(4), 1221–8.

44. Block, G.A., Martin, K.J., de Francisco, A.L. *et al.* (2004). Cinacalcet for secondary hyperparathyroidism in patients receiving hemodialysis. *N Engl J Med*, **350**(15), 1516–25.

45. Hale, A.C., Millar, J.B., Ratter, S.J. *et al.* (1985). A case of pituitary dependent Cushing's disease with clinical and biochemical features of the ectopic ACTH syndrome. *Clin Endocrinol (Oxf)*, **22**(4), 479–88.

46. Orth, D. (1995). Cushing's Syndrome. *N Engl J Med*, **332**, 791–803.

47. Friedman, J. and Halaas, J. (1998). Leptin and the regulation of body weight in mammals. *Nature*, **395**, 763–770.

48. Yaswen, L., Diehl, N., Brennan, M. *et al.* (1999). Obesity in the mouse model of pro-opiomelanocortin deficiency responds to peripheral melanocortin. *Nature Medicine*, **5**, 1066–70.

49. Lu, D., Willard, D., Patel, I.R., *et al.* (1994). Agouti protein is an antagonist of the melanocyte-stimulating-hormone receptor. *Nature*, **371**(6500), 799–802.

50. Ollmann, M.M., Wilson, B.D., Yang, Y.K. *et al.* (1997). Antagonism of central melanocortin receptors in vitro and in vivo by agouti-related protein. *Science*, **278**(5335), 135–8.

51. Stutz, A.M., Morrison, C.D., and Argyropoulos, G. (2005). The Agouti-related protein and its role in energy homeostasis. *Peptides*, **26**(10), 1771–81.

52. Pullan, P.T., Clement-Jones, V., Corder, R. *et al.* (1980). Ectopic production of methionine enkephalin and beta-endorphin. *Br Med J*, **280**(6216), 758–9.

53. Chatikhine, V.A., Chevrier, A., Chauzy, C. *et al.* (1994). Expression of opioid peptides in cells and stroma of human breast cancer and adenofibromas. *Cancer Lett*, **77**(1), 51–6.

54. Jeffcoate, W., Silverstone, J., Edwards, C. *et al.* (1979). Psychiatric manifestations of Cushing's syndrome: response to lowering plasma cortisol. *Quart J Med*, **48**, 465–72.

55. Boscaro, M., Barzon, L., Fallo, F. *et al.* (2001). Cushing's syndrome. *Lancet*, **357**(9258), 783–91.

56. Isidori, A.M., Kaltsas, G.A., Pozza, C. *et al.* (2006). The ectopic adrenocorticotropin syndrome: Clinical features, diagnosis, management, and long-term follow-up. *J Clin Endocrinol Metab*, **91**(2), 371–7. Epub 2005 Nov 22.

57. Beuschlein, F. and Hammer, G.D. (2002). Ectopic pro-opiomelanocortin syndrome. *Endocrinol Metab Clin North Am*, **31**(1), 191–234.

58. Delisle, L., Boyer, M.J., Warr, D. *et al.* (1993). Ectopic corticotropin syndrome and small-cell carcinoma of the lung. Clinical features, outcome, and complications. *Arch Intern Med*, **153**(6), 746–52.

59. Abeloff, M., Trump, D., and Baylin, S. (1981). Ectopic adrenocorticotrophin (ACTH). syndrome and small cell carcinoma of the lung: Assessment of clinical implications in patients on combination chemotherapy. *Cancer*, **48**, 1082–1087.

60. Hansen, M., Hammer, M., and Hammer, L. (1980). ACTH, ADH and calcitonin concentrations as markers of response and relapse in small cell carcinoma of the lung. *Cancer*, **46**, 2062–7.

61. de Herder, W.W., Krenning, E.P., Malchoff, C.D. *et al.* (1994). Somatostatin receptor scintigraphy: Its value in tumor localization in patients with Cushing's syndrome caused by ectopic corticotropin or corticotropin-releasing hormone secretion. *Am J Med*, **96**(4), 305–12.

62. Jacobsson, H., Wallin, G., Werner, S. *et al.* (1994). Techetium-99 methoxyisobutylisonitrile localizes an ectopic ACTH-producing tumour: Case report and review of the literature. *Eur J Nucl Med*, **21**, 582–6.

63. Carey, R.M., Varma, S.K., Drake, C.R., Jr. *et al.* (1984). Ectopic secretion of corticotropin-releasing factor as a cause of Cushing's syndrome. A clinical, morphologic, and biochemical study. *N Engl J Med*, **311**(1), 13–20.

64. Wajchenberg, B.L., Albergaria Pereira, M.A., Medonca, B.B. *et al.* (2000). Adrenocortical carcinoma: Clinical and laboratory observations. *Cancer*, **88**(4), 711–36.

65. Hoffman, D. and Boigham, B. (1991). The use of ketoconazole in ectopic adrenocorticotropic hormone syndrome. *Cancer*, **67**, 1447–1449.

66. Winquist, E.W., Laskey, J., Crump, M. *et al.* (1995). Ketoconazole in the managemtn of paraneoplastic Cushing's syndrome secondary to ectopic adrenal corticotropin production. *J Clin Oncol*, **13**, 157–64.

67. Farrell, W., Clark, A., Stewart, M. *et al.* (1992). Bromocriptine inhibits pro-opiomelanocortin mRNA and ACTH precursor secretion in small cell lung cancer cell lines. *J Clin Invest*, **90**, 705–710.

68. Pivonello, R., Ferone, D., Lamberts, S.W. *et al.* (2005)Cabergoline plus lanreotide for ectopic Cushing's syndrome. *N Engl J Med*, **352**(23), 2457–8.

69. Woodhouse, N.J., Dagogo-Jack, S., Ahmed, M. *et al.* (1993). Acute and long-term effects of octreotide in patients with ACTH-dependent Cushing's syndrome. *Am J Med*, **95**, 305–308.

70. Rieu, M., Rosilio, M., Richard, A. *et al.* (1993). Paradoxical effect of somatostatin analogues on the ectopic secretion of corticotropin in two cases of small cell lung carcinoma. *Horm Res*, **39**(5–6), 207–12.

71. Spampinato, S., Canossa, M., Carboni, L. *et al.* (1994). Inhibition of proopiomelanocortin expression by an oligonucleotide complementary to beta-endorphin mRNA. *Proc Nat Acad Sci USA*, **91**, 8072–6.

72. Verbalis, J. (1989). Hyponatraemia. *Balliere's Clin Endocrinol Metab*, **3**, 499–530.

73. Smitz, S., Legros, J., Franchimont, P. *et al.* (1988). Identification of vasopressin-like peptides in the plasma of a patient with the syndrome of inappropriate secretion of antidiuretic hormone and an oat cell carcinoma. *Acta Endocinol (Copenhagen)*, **119**, 567–574.

74. Hansen, M., Hammer, M., and Hummer, L. (1980). Diagnostic and therapeutic implications of ectopic hormone production in small cell lung cancer. *Thorax*, **35**, 101–106.

75. Comis, R., Miller, M., and Ginsberg, S. (1980). Abnormalities in water homeostasis in small cell anaplastic lung cancer. *Cancer*, **45**, 2414–21.

76. North, W., Ware, J., Maurer, L. *et al.* (1988). Neurophysins as tumour markers for small cell carcinoma of the lung. A cancer and leukemia group B evaluation. *Cancer*, **62**, 1343–7.

77. Friedmann, A., Memoli, V., and North, W. (1993). Vasopressin and oxytocin production by non-neuroendocrine lung carcinomas: An apparent low incidence of gene expression. *Cancer Lett*, **75**, 79–85.

78. Friedmann, A., Malott, K., Memoli, V. *et al.* (1994). Products of vasopressin gene expression in small cell carcinoma of the lung. *Br J Cancer*, **69**, 260–263.

79. List, A.F., Hainsworth, J.D., Davis, B.W. *et al.* (1986). The syndrome of inappropriate secretion of antidiuretic hormone (SIADH). in small-cell lung cancer. *J Clin Oncol*, **4**(8), 1191–8.

80. Cohen, M.H., Bunn, P.A., Jr., Ihde, D.C. *et al.* (1978). Chemotherapy rather than demeclocycline for inappropriate secretion of antidiuretic hormone. *N Engl J Med*, **298**(25), 1423–4.

81. Vanhees, S., Paridaens, R., and Vansteenkiste, J. (2000). Syndrome of inappropriate antidiuretic hormone associated with chemotherapy-induced tumour lysis in small cell lung cancer: Case report and review of the litterature. *Ann Oncol*, **11**, 1061–5.

82. Srensen, J., Kristjansen, P., Osterlind, K. *et al.* (1987). Syndrome of inappropriate antidiuresis in small cell lung cancer. Classification and effect of tumour regression. *Acta Medica Scandanavica*, **222**, 155–61.

83. Hojer, J. (1994). Management of symptomatic hyponataemia: Dependence on the duration of development. *J Intern Med*, **235**, 497–501.

84. Cohen, I., Warren, S., and Skowsky, W. (1984). Occult pulmonary malignancy in syndrome of inappropriate ADH secretion with normal ADH levels. *Chest*, **86**, 929–31.

85. Chitmans, F. and Meinders, A. (1990). Management of severe hyponatremia: Rapid or slow correction. *Am J Med*, **88**, 161–6.

86. Sterns, R. (1990). The treatment of hyponatremia: First do no harm. *Am J Med*, **88**, 557–60.

87. Sterns, R. (1987). Severe symtomatic hyponatremia: Treatment and outcome. *Ann Intern Med*, **107**, 656–64.

88. Ayus, J., Olivero, J., and Frommer, J. (1982). Rapid correction of severe hyponatremia with intravenous hypertonic saline solution. *Am J Med*, **72**, 43–8.

89. Adrogue, H. and Madias, N. (2000). Hyponatremia. *N Eng J Med*, **342**, 1581–9.

90. Nguyen, M.K. and Kurtz, I. (2005). An analysis of current quantitative approaches to the treatment of severe symptomatic SIADH with intravenous saline therapy. *Clin Exp Nephrol*, **9**(1), 1–4.

91. Decaux, G., Prospert, F., Pennincks, R. *et al.* (1993). 5-year treatment of the chronic syndrome of inappropriate secretion of ADH with oral urea. *Nephron*, **63**, 468–70.

92. Abraham, W.T., Shamshirsaz, A.A., McFann, K. *et al.* (2006). Aquaretic effect of Lixivaptan, an oral, non-peptide, selective v2 receptor vasopressin antagonist, in New York Heart Association functional class II and III chronic heart failure patients. *J Am Coll Cardiol*, **47**(8), 1615–21. Epub 2006 Mar 29.

93. Gheorghiade, M., Gottlieb, S.S., Udelson, J.E. *et al.* (2006). Vasopressin v(2). receptor blockade with tolvaptan versus fluid restriction in the treatment of hyponatremia. *Am J Cardiol*, **97**(7), 1064–7. Epub 2006 Feb 17.

94. Ghali, J.K., Koren, M.J., Taylor, J.R. *et al.* (2006). Efficacy and safety of oral conivaptan: A V1A/V2 vasopressin-receptor antagonist, assessed in a randomized, placebo-controlled trial in patients with euvolemic or hypervolemic hyponatremia. *J Clin Endocrinol Metab*, **7**, 7.

95. Rabinstein, A.A. (2006). Vasopressin antagonism: potential impact on neurologic disease. *Clin Neuropharmacol*, **29**(2), 87–93.

96. Cogan, E., Debieve, M.F., Philipart, I. *et al.* (1986). High plasma levels of atrial natriuretic factor in SIADH. *N Engl J Med*, **314**(19), 1258–9.

97. Yoshinaga, K., Yamaguchi, K., Abe, K. *et al.* (1994). Production of immunoreactive atrial natriuretic polypeptide in neuroendocrine tumors. *Cancer*, **73**, 1292–6.

98. Chute, J.P., Taylor, E., Williams, J. *et al.* (2006). A metabolic study of patients with lung cancer and hyponatremia of malignancy. *Clin Cancer Res*, **12**(3 Pt 1), 888–96.

99. Levin, E., Gardner, D., andSamson W. (1998). Natriuretic peptides. *N Engl J Med*, **339**, 321–8.

100. Morishita, Y., Sano, T., Kase, H. *et al.* (1992). HS-142-1, a novel nonpeptide atrial natriuretic peptide (ANP) antagonist, blocks ANP-induced renal responses through a specific interaction with guanylyl cyclase-linked receptors. *Eur J Pharmacol*, **225**, 203–7.

101. Kiang, D., Baner, G., and Kennedy, B. (1973). Immunoassayable insulin in carcinoma of the cervix. *Cancer*, **31**, 801–5.

102. Gorden, P., Hendricks, C.M., Kahn, C.R. *et al.* (1981). Hypoglycemia associated with non-islet-cell tumor and insulin-like growth factors. *N Engl J Med*, **305**(24), 1452–5.

103. Marks, V. and Teale, J. (1998). Tumours producing hypoglycaemia. *Endocrine-related Cancer*, **5**, 111–29.

104. Yu, H. and Rohan, T. (2000). Roel of the insulin-like growth factor family in cancer development and progression. *J Natl Cancer Inst*, **92**, 1472–89.

105. Teale, J.D. and Wark, G. (2004). The effectiveness of different treatment options for non-islet cell tumour hypoglycaemia. *Clin Endocrinol*, **60**(4), 457–60.

106. Braund, W., Naylor, B., Williamson, D. *et al.* (1987). Autoimmunity to insulin receptor and hypoglycaemia in patients with Hodgkin's disease. *Lancet*, **i**, 237–240.

107. Walters, E., Tavare, J., Denton, R. *et al.* (1987). Hypoglycaemia due to an insulin-receptor antibody in Hodgkin's disease. *Lancet*, **i**, 241–243.

108. Kulke, M.H. and Mayer, R.J. (1999). Carcinoid tumors. *N Engl J Med*, **340**(11), 858–68.

109. Ricke, J., Klose, K.J., Mignon, M. *et al.* (2001). Standardisation of imaging in neuroendocrine tumours: Results of a European delphi process. *Eur J Radiol*, **37**(1), 8–17.

110. Barakat, M.T., Meeran, K., and Bloom, S.R. (2004). Neuroendocrine tumours. *Endocr Relat Cancer*, **11**(1), 1–18.

111. Kaltsas, G.A., Papadogias, D., Makras, P. *et al.* (2005). Treatment of advanced neuroendocrine tumours with radiolabelled somatostatin analogues. *Endocr Relat Cancer*, **12**(4), 683–99.

112. Feldman, J. (1987). Carcinoid tumours and syndrome. *Sem Oncol*, **14**, 237–46.

113. Modlin, I. and Sandor, A. (1997). An analysis of 8305 cases of carcinoid tumors. *Cancer*, **79**, 813–29.

114. Vinik, A.I., McLeod, M.K., Fig, L.M. *et al.* (1989). Clinical features, diagnosis, and localization of carcinoid tumors and their management. *Gastroenterol Clin North Am*, **18**(4), 865–96.

115. Kema, I.P., Schellings, A.M., Meiborg, G. *et al.* (1992). Influence of a serotonin- and dopamine-rich diet on platelet serotonin content and urinary excretion of biogenic amines and their metabolites. *Clin Chem*, **38**(9), 1730–6.

116. Jensen, R.T. (2000). Carcinoid and pancreatic endocrine tumors: Recent advances in molecular pathogenesis, localization, and treatment. *Curr Opin Oncol*, **12**(4), 368–77.

117. Kvols, L.K. and Reubi, J.C. (1993). Metastatic carcinoid tumors and the malignant carcinoid syndrome. *Acta Oncol*, **32**(2), 197–201.

118. di Bartolomeo, M., Bajetta, E., Buzzoni, R. *et al.* (1996). Clinical efficacy of octreotide in the treatment of metastatic neuroendocrine tumors. A study by the Italian Trials in Medical Oncology Group. *Cancer*, **77**(2), 402–8.

119. O'Toole, D., Ducreux, M., Bommelaer, G. *et al.* (2000). Treatment of carcinoid syndrome: A prospective crossover evaluation of lanreotide versus octreotide in terms of efficacy, patient acceptability, and tolerance. *Cancer*, **88**(4), 770–6.

120. Rubin, J., Ajani, J., Schirmer, W. *et al.* (1999). Octreotide acetate long-acting formulation versus open-label subcutaneous octreotide acetate in malignant carcinoid syndrome. *J Clin Oncol*, **17**(2), 600–6.

121. Oberg, K. (2000). Interferon in the management of neuroendocrine GEP-tumors: A review. *Digestion*, **62**(Suppl 1), 92–7.

122. Faiss, S., Pape, U.F., Bohmig, M. *et al.* (2003). Prospective, randomized, multicenter trial on the antiproliferative effect of lanreotide, interferon alfa, and their combination for therapy of metastatic neuroendocrine gastroenteropancreatic tumors—The International Lanreotide and Interferon Alfa Study Group. *J Clin Oncol*, **21**(14), 2689–96.

123. Taal, B.G., Hoefnagel, C.A., Valdes Olmos, R.A. *et al.* (1996). Palliative effect of metaiodobenzylguanidine in metastatic carcinoid tumors. *J Clin Oncol*, **14**(6), 1829–38.

124. Lenders, J.W., Eisenhofer, G., Mannelli, M. *et al.* (2005). Phaeochromocytoma. *Lancet*, **366**(9486), 665–75.

125. Braunstein, G. (1993). Current concepts: Gynaecomastia. *N Engl J Med*, **328**, 490–5.

126. Di Lorenzo, G., Autorino, R., Perdona, S. *et al.* (2005). Management of gynaecomastia in patients with prostate cancer: A systematic review. *Lancet Oncol*, **6**(12), 972–9.

127. Fradkin, J., Eastman, R., Lesniak, M., *et al.* (1989). Specificity spillover at the hormone receptor—Exploring its role in human disease. *N Engl J Med*, **320**, 640–5.

128. Giralt, S., Dexeus, F., Amato, R. *et al.* (1992). Hyperthyroidism in men with germ cell tumors and high levels of beta-human chorionic gonadotrophin. *Cancer*, **69**, 1286–90.

129. Dowsett, M., McGarrick, G., Harris, A. *et al.* (1983). Prognostic significance of serum prolactin levels in advanced breast cancer. *Br J Cancer*, **47**, 763–769.

130. Vanderschueren, S., Knockaert, D., Adriaenssens, T. *et al.* (2003). From prolonged febrile illness to fever of unknown origin: the challenge continues. *Arch Intern Med*, **163**(9), 1033–41.

131. Zell, J.A. and Chang, J.C. (2005). Neoplastic fever: A neglected paraneoplastic syndrome. *Support Care Cancer*, **13**(11), 870–7. Epub 2005 Apr 29.

132. Kallio, R., Bloigu, A., Surcel, H.M. *et al.* (2001). C-reactive protein and erythrocyte sedimentation rate in differential diagnosis between infections and neoplastic fever in patients with solid tumours and lymphomas. *Support Care Cancer*, **9**(2), 124–8.

133. Chang, J.C. (1987). How to differentiate neoplastic fever from infectious fever in patients with cancer: usefulness of the naproxen test. *Heart Lung*, **16**(2), 122–7.

134. Vanderschueren, S., Knockaert, D.C., Peetermans, W.E. *et al.* (1987). Lack of value of the naproxen test in the differential diagnosis of prolonged febrile illnesses. *Am J Med*, **115**(7), 572–5.

135. Engblom, D., Saha, S., Engstrom, L. *et al.* (2003). Microsomal prostaglandin E synthase-1 is the central switch during immune-induced pyresis. *Nat Neurosci*, **6**(11), 1137–8. Epub 2003 Oct 19.

136. Saper, C. and Breder, CD. (1994). Seminars in Medicine of the Beth Israel Hospital, Boston: The neurologic basis of fever. *N Engl J Med*, **330**, 1880–6.

137. Netea, M., Kullberg, B., and Van der Meer, J. (2000). Circulating cytokines as mediators of fever. *Clin Infect Dis*, **31**, S178–84.

138. Blatteis, C., Sehic, E., Li, S. (2000). Pyrogens sensing and signalling: Old views and new concepts. *Clin Infect Dis*, **31**, S168–177.

139. Kretschmer C, *et al.* (1990). Tumor necrosis factor alpha and lymphotoxin production in Hodgkin's disease. *Am J Pathol*, **137**, 341–51.

140. Nishimoto, N., Sasai, M., Nakagawa, M. *et al.* (2000). Improvement in Castleman's disease by humanized anti-interleukin-6 receptor antibody therapy. *Blood*, **95**, 56–61.

141. Fukumoto, S., Matsumo, T., Harada, S. *et al.* (1991). Phaeochromocytoma with pyrexia and marked inflammatory signs: A paraneoplastic syndrome with possible relation to interleukin 6 production. *J Clin Endocrinol Metab*, **73**, 871–81.

142. Dosquet, C., Schaetz, A., Faucher, C. *et al.* (1994). Tumour necrosis factor-alpha, interleukin-1 beta and interleukin-6 in patients with renal cell carcinoma. *Eur J Cancer*, **30A**(2), 162–7.

143. Alcami, A. and Smith, G.L. (1996). A mechanism for the inhibition of fever by a virus. *Proc Natl Acad Sci USA*, **93**(20), 11029–34.

144. Eisenberg, S.P., Brewer, M.T., Verderber, E. *et al.* (1991). Interleukin 1 receptor antagonist is a member of the interleukin 1 gene family: Evolution of a cytokine control mechanism. *Proc Natl Acad Sci USA*, **88**(12), 5232–6.

145. Dalal, S. and Zhukovsky, D.S. (2006). Pathophysiology and management of fever. *J Support Oncol*, **4**(1), 9–16.

146. Gullo, L., Pezzilli, R., and Morselli-Labate, A.M. (1994). Diabetes and the risk of pancreatic cancer. Italian Pancreatic Cancer Study Group. *N Engl J Med*, **331**(2), 81–4.

147. Nelson, K.A., Walsh, D., and Sheehan, F.A. (1994). The cancer anorexia-cachexia syndrome. *J Clin Oncol*, **12**(1), 213–25.

148. Poulson, J. (1997). The management of diabetes in patients with advanced cancer. *J Pain Symptom Manage*, **13**(6), 339–46.

149. McCoubrie, R., Jeffrey, D., Paton, C. *et al.* (2005). Managing diabetes mellitus in patients with advanced cancer: a case note audit and guidelines. *Eur J Cancer Care (Engl)*, **14**(3), 244–8.

150. Poppel, D.M., Cohen, L.M., and Germain, M.J. (2003). The renal palliative care initiative. *J Palliat Med*, **6**(2), 321–6.

151. Garnick, M.B. and Mayer, R.J. (1978). Acute renal failure associated with neoplastic disease and its treatment. *Semin Oncol*, **5**(2), 155–65.

152. Harrington, K.J., Pandha, H.S., Kelly, S.A. *et al.* (1995). Palliation of obstructive nephropathy due to malignancy. *Br J Urol*, **76**(1), 101–7.

153. Little, B., Ho, K.J., Gawley, S. *et al.* (2003). Use of nephrostomy tubes in ureteric obstruction from incurable malignancy. *Int J Clin Pract*, **57**(3), 180–1.

154. Dourakis, S.P., Tzemanakis, E., Deutsch, M. *et al.* (1999). Fulminant hepatic failure as a presenting paraneoplastic manifestation of Hodgkin's disease. *Eur J Gastroenterol Hepatol*, **11**(9), 1055–8.

155. Fang, J.W., Lau, J.Y., Wu, P.C. *et al.* (1992). Fulminant hepatic failure in nonmetastatic renal cell carcinoma. *Dig Dis Sci*, **37**(3), 474–7.

156. Bergasa, N.V. (2005). The pruritus of cholestasis. *J Hepatol*, **43**(6), 1078–88. Epub 2005 Oct 6.

157. Fall, P.J. and Szerlip, H.M. (2005). Lactic acidosis: From sour milk to septic shock. *J Intensive Care Med*, **20**(5), 255–71.

10.11

Neurological problems in advanced cancer

Augusto Caraceni, Cinzia Martini, and Fabio Simonetti

Introduction

Neurological complications are frequent in populations with advanced cancer. An adequate neurological assessment must always be part of patient evaluation. In some cases, this assessment will be symptom-focused. Pain, for example, is highly prevalent and must be evaluated from the neurological perspective to adequately clarify the pathophysiology and cause. Characterization of the pain in terms of pathophysiology, aetiology, and syndrome is necessary to achieve successful treatment and anticipate complications.

In other situations, the neurological assessment is necessary to evaluate the possibility of specific neurological syndromes, such as intracranial hypertension, seizures, or delirium. All these disorders occur frequently in advanced cancer.

Intracranial hypertension

General aspects

Intracranial content includes brain, 80 per cent (in adults 1400 g); blood, 10 per cent (32–58 ml); and cerebrospinal fluid 10 per cent (in adult 140 ml, including 23 ml in the cerebral ventricles, 37 ml in the subarachnoid space, and 80 ml in the spine). Cerebrospinal fluid (CSF) is produced at a rate of about 0.35 ml/min (which accounts for a three-times-a-day turnover) by the choroidal plexus, which is located in the walls of the lateral ventricles and in the roof of the third and fourth ventricles. CSF flows from the fourth ventricle through the foramina of Lushka and Magendie and into the cisternae, spaces where pia and arachnoid are widely separated. There, it is actively reabsorbed by the arachnoid villi, microscopic excrescences of arachnoid membrane, which are aggregated to form granulations (of Pacchioni) and protrude through the meningeal layer of the dura mainly into the superior sagittal and other dural sinuses.

Intracranial pressure (ICP) is a function of the volumes occupied by brain, blood, and CSF. ICP is not constant but depends on systemic blood pressure, and on venous and intrathoracic pressure. The values of ICP range in adults from 5 to 15 mmHg (1 mmHg = 1.36 cm H_2O), and usually is less than 20 mmHg; the pressure is 2.4–4.2 mmHg in neonates; 5–10 mmHg in infants; and 10–15 mmHg in older children. Minor increases in ICP occur with Valsalva manoeuvers and periodically during the cardiac cycle. More significant increases occur occasionally, such as during sneezing or coughing. The normal brain can tolerate these variations without clinical consequences.

The interrelationship between changes in the volume of intracranial contents and changes in ICP characterize the *intracranial compliance*, which is defined as the ability to accommodate increases in intracranial volume without change in ICP. This concept was developed by Alexander Monro in 1783 and his former pupil George Kellie in 1824: George Burrows introduced CSF volume into the 'Monro–Kellie hypothesis' in 1846. Others demonstred that the sum of the volume of brain parenchyma, blood, and CSF is, in an intact skull, constant; an increase in one element either is accompanied by a reduction in another, or in an increase of ICP.

Pathological processes, such as tumours, abscesses, or haematomas, increase intracranial contents that compress brain parenchyma. They also disrupt the blood–brain barrier, which may lead to increased intracranial blood volume. If this occurs slowly, there may be no increase in ICP, at least temporarily. This is due to compensatory mechanisms, such as enhanced CSF reabsorption, reduced intracranial blood volume, and increased drainage through the lymphatic and circulatory system. When these mechanisms are insufficient or if the process is acute, ICP rises rapidly and may cause death, with or without brain distortion or herniation (see below).

Clinical findings

The clinical picture of increased ICP is characterized by an altered state of consciousness, headache, nausea and vomiting, papilloedema, and, at times, focal signs. An altered state of consciousness is the most frequent sign, starting with psychomotor retardation, and slowing of verbal and motor responses. This can progress stupor and then coma.

Headache progresses and can be severe. It usually is diffuse, more intense in the supine position, and worse in the morning immediately after awakening. It can awaken the patient from sleep, and also is worsened by head movements, cough, and the Valsalva manoeuvre. Nausea and vomiting frequently accompany the headache. Vomiting may be projectile in children with posterior fossa lesions, which can directly stimulate the trigger zone in the fourth ventricle.

Papilloedema is a specific sign of increased ICP. It may, however, be absent, even in severe cases. The development of increased ICP associated with typical symptoms and signs, but no papilloedema, is more likely in the elderly who develop intracranial lesions.

Among the focal signs that occur frequently in those with increased ICP, the most frequent is diplopia due to paralysis of the abducens nerve. This nerve has a long intracranial course and is particularly sensitive to traction. Other signs may occur in either the sensory or motor systems. Seizures also may occur in the setting of increased ICP.

In children, increased ICP often is accompanied by nonspecific findings or may manifest as irritability, labile mood, negativism, or aggressive or hostile behaviours. A focal sign relatively more common in children is the 'sunset' sign (or Collier's sign). This phenomenon includes eyelid retraction and eyes rotation downward, and is due to compression of the quadrigeminal plate, with damage to prenuclear structure for eyelid control and to fibres for conjugate upward gaze.

Acute pressure symptoms

In the setting of intracranial hypertension, the physiologic fluctuation in ICP pressure can be suddenly interrupted by a abnormal pressure waves (Table 10.11.1), including waves of very high pressure, or plateau waves, as described originally by by Lundberg[1]. These pressure waves, which usually last seconds to minutes, may be accompanied by acute pressure symptoms (Table 10.11.2).

Herniation

Dural reflections of the falx cerebri and tentorium cerebelli divide cranial box into compartments, and raised ICP can result in pressure gradients between compartments. These pressure gradients can, in turn, lead to shifts of brain parenchyma. When severe, herniation of brain structures from one compartment to another can occur, with life-threatening consequences. These phenomena are usually described by topographic and anatomical criteria as central, subfalcial, uncal, and cerebellar tonsil herniation.

Central herniation syndrome

In central herniation syndrome, clinical findings are due to the development of a pressure cone originating in upper brain structures, which force a shift in intracranial contents in an up–down direction and leads to progressive compression of the cerebral structure of the diencephalon and brainstem. In the diencephalic

Table 10.11.1 Three types of ICP waves.

A waves—recurrent plateau waves, reaching 50–100 mmHg, duration 5–20 min, associated with deterioration and clinical signs. A waves are indicative of a greatly reduced intracranial compliance
B waves—shorter duration, rhythmical, 0.5–2 per min, of variable amplitude, lower than 50 mmHg. They are related to respiratory movements, associated with clinical signs, and are also indicative of reduced compliance
C waves—small oscillations, rhythmical at about 6 per min, with amplitude of only 20 mmHg, and related to intracranial transmission of the arterial pulse, usually do not have clinical consequences

Table 10.11.2 Signs and symptoms of ICP waves.

Altered state of consciousness, agitation, delirium
Headache, neck pain
Focal or generalized seizures
Cerebellar fits (opisthotonus)
Decerebration (hypertonus, extension, and internal rotation of four limbs)
Amaurosis, midriasis
II, IV, VI nerve paralysis, conjugated eye deviation
Ocular microtremor (seen only with ophthalmoscophe, personal observation)
Nystagmus, tinnitus
Myoclonus of face and limb muscles
Dysarthria, dysphagia
Pyramidal signs, paresthesias
Cardiovascular or respiratory disturbances, yawning
Hyperthermia, face cyanosis, flushing, pallor, sweating
Nausea, vomiting, hiccup, sialorrhoea, diarrhoea, incontinence

stage of compression, consciousness starts to deteriorate, there is Cheyne–Stokes respiration, pupils are miotic but reactive to light, and the 'doll's eyes' phenomenon is present. Paratonic rigidity (as opposed to forced extension of limbs, which is called gegenhalten) and pyramidal signs are present. Painful stimuli may induce decorticate rigidity (upper arm flexion and lower limb extension), which can begin contralaterally to the lesion, and then become bilateral. With worsening of the pressure cone, this diencephalic stage progresses through a mesencephalic, pontine, and bulbar stages, with changing neurological signs. Ultimately, coma, respiratory rhythm alteration, fixed pupils, oculovestibular abnormalities, and decerebrate rigidity occur. Flaccidity of the limbs and loss of brainstem reflexes may occur before death.

Uncal herniation

Uncal herniation is the displacement of part of the temporal lobe underneath the cerebellar tentorium. Neurological signs are first due to compression of the structures to the side of the lesion, including the oculomotor nerve. The pupil ipsilateral to the lesion typically becomes mydriatic and then nonreactive to light; occasionally, brainstem displacement toward opposite tentorial edge occurs, trapping the contralateral oculomotor nerve and producing initial pupillary changes on the contralateral side. These pupillary changes (which are followed by paresis of the extraocular muscles innervated by the oculomotor nerve) may be accompanied by visual field defects, which are caused by compression of the ipsilateral posterior cerebral artery. Subsequently, consciousness deteriorates, hyperventilation may occur and be followed by Cheyne–Stokes breathing, complete paralysis of the oculomotor nerve occurs, 'doll's eyes' become abnormal, and painful stimulation evokes may evoke decorticate responses ipsilateral to the lesion and decerebrate responses contralaterally.

Cerebellar herniation

Cerebellar herniation is due to the descent of cerebellar structures through the occipital foramen by a so-called 'cerebellar pressure cone'. The syndrome is characterized by occipital or frontal headache, hiccup and vomiting, followed by deterioration of consciousness, abnormality of breathing, and 'cerebellar fits', which are characterized by opisthotonus and episodes of decerebration.

Brain oedema and treatment of increased ICP

Brain oedema

In both primary and secondary brain tumours, oedema is a important cause of increased ICP. The underlying pathogenic mechanism of oedema is the loss of osmotically active substances such as albumin from the circulatory system into the brain interstitial tissue, which is caused by disruption of the blood–brain barrier within the tumour and in the surrounding cerebral parenchima. According to the classic classification of Klatzo[2], there are four broad types of brain oedema:

Vasogenic oedema is caused by an increase of the extracellular space. It results from increased capillary permeability and can be produced by any lesion that damages the blood–brain barrier.

Cytotoxic oedema is caused by an increase of intracellular volume. It results from ischaemic or hypoxic cellular damage. Cellular dysfunction of the ion pump system produces intracellular accumulation of sodium followed by influx of extracellular fluid. It is now referred to as cellular swelling.

Interstitial oedema is caused by an increase of the extracellular space due to blockade of CSF reabsorption at any level.

Osmotic oedema is caused by an increase of the water content of the brain parenchyma due to plasma hypo-osmolarity. This may occur, for example, in water intoxication or in SIADH.

Tumour-induced brain oedema is mainly sustained, at least initially, by vasogenic mechanisms. Interstitial and osmotic oedema are rare and do not apply to the perturbations produced by a tumour.

Treatment of increased ICP

Conservative management of cerebral oedema has two main goals: maintenance of cerebral perfusion pressure (CPP) and reduction of vasogenic oedema[3]. CPP is defined as mean arterial pressure minus ICP. Intracranial processes can impair CPP by increasing ICP and disrupting cerebrovascular autoregulation. The consequences of reduced CPP are cerebral ischaemia, compensatory, and dilatation of cerebral vessels, with further increase of ICP. Since hypovolemia reduces arterial pressure and therefore CPP, the patient with elevated ICP does not require fluid restriction, but should be kept euvolemic with adequate fluid intake.

Interventions that assist in maintaining CPP and reducing vasogenic oedema are varied. Consideration of these interventions depends on the goals of care. Aggressive management strategies, such as assisted ventilation to lower the P_{CO_2} may not be considered when the goals are purely palliative.

Positioning: a neutral head position should be adopted, with the head at least 30° above the heart to facilitate venous drainage from the head.

Hyperventilation: by reducing P_{CO_2} and causing vasoconstriction, intracranial blood volume may be reduced. In the past, P_{CO_2} was routinely kept at 20–25 mmHg. This intervention has become more controversial because of concern that reduced blood flow associated with vasoconstriction actually may reduce CPP. Hyperventilation usually is tried when ICP appears to be rising, and in the relatively stable patient, may be used intermittently to

deal with pressure waves. When patients become clinically stable, P_{CO_2} is allowed to return to normal levels.

Infusion of hypertonic solutions: rapid reduction of ICP and cerebral oedema with hypertonic solutions has been utilized since 1925[4]. Nowadays, hyperosmolar solutions include mannitol, glycerol, and hypertonic saline solutions. Mannitol is the most commonly used agent[5]. Its activity is based primarily on an increase in blood flow, leading to improved CPP. It later creates an osmolar gradient between blood and brain and can extract water from the cerebral compartment. Usually more water than sodium is eliminated, resulting in hypovolemia and hyponatremia. There is no interaction between mannitol and glucose metabolism. There are a number of other actions associated with the therapeutic effect of mannitol, including a diuretic effect, an increase in red cell deformability, and a rapid reduction of the diameter of arterioles and small veins of the brain surface. Mannitol is not metabolized and is excreted by the kidneys; with moderate reduction of glomerular filtration, it can accumulate in the central compartment.

Although it can be administered orally, bioavailability is very poor and the usual approach is IV infusion, aiming to achieve concentrations higher than 5 mmol/l, which is osmotically active and persists for 4–6 h.

Mannitol 18 or 20 per cent solutions are used and the suggested dose regimen for both adults and children is 0.25–1 g/kg delivered over 15–60 min every 6 or 12 h. The regimen can vary according to the severity of symptoms. If symptoms are severe and a rapid onset is needed, 1 g/kg can be given in 15–20 min. For a less urgent intervention and to have a more long-lasting effect, 0.5–1 g/kg can be given in 60 min. Daily doses vary from 1 to 4 g/kg and should never be higher than 150–200 g/day. Renal disease, congestive heart failure, and intracerebral haemorrhage contraindicate the use of mannitol. Mannitol therapy should never extend for more than 3–4 days. Salt and water balance should be carefully monitored to avoid dehydration and hypotension. Hyperosmolality should also be prevented by cessation of therapy at values of 320 mosmol/kg.

When mannitol or another hyperosmolar solution is used for a longer period than a few days, a risk for a mannitol rebound effect exists. This rebound effect is in part a consequence of the osmotic agents entering the intracranial compartment, with inversion of the osmotic gradient between blood, extracellular fluid, and brain. The manifestation is increased ICP.

Corticosteroids: after the early observation by Galicich and French of the anti-peritumoral oedema effect of dexamethasone[6], corticosteroids gained wide application in neuro-oncology. The mechanism of action is fundamentally based on their ability to block the outflow of blood components from the capillary bed into the brain tissue at the site of blood–brain barrier damage. Dexamethasone does not reduce the water content of the swelling brain tissue (as mannitol does), and reduction of ICP does not occur before 48–72 h. Nonetheless, it is common to observe a clinical improvement before this and within the first 24 h.

Doses and administration schedules of corticosteroids have never been established by specific guidelines. It is therefore worthwhile considering the relative potency of the different drugs and their pharmacological characteristic[7] (Table 10.11.3).

Dexamethasone is found in higher concentrations within the CSF compared with prednisolone because it is less bound to plasma proteins. This should be taken into account when switching from one to another steroid, in addition to the data shown in Table 10.11.3.

Table 10.11.3 Relative potency of different drugs.

	Anti-inflammatory activity	Duration of action, hours	Equivalent dose, mg
Cortisone	0.8	8–12	25
Prednisone	4	12–36	5
6 α-Methylprednisolone	5	12–36	4
Dexamethasone	25	36–54	0.75
Bethamethasone	30	36–54	0.75
Cortisol	1	8–12	20

Sodium retention activity is 1 for cortisol, 0.8 for hydrocortisone, 0.8 for prednisone and methylprednisolone, and 0 for bethamethasone and dexamethasone.

The dose of dexamethasone used in metastatic or primary brain tumours varies according to the clinical findings and degree of oedema from 4 mg every 6 h to 96 mg/day in patients with more severe symptoms or impending herniation. Once the patient is clinically stabilized, the total dose can be given in one or two daily doses, as suggested by the drug's pharmacokinetic profile. In children, the suggested initial dose of dexamethasone is 1 mg/kg followed by doses of 0.4–1 mg/kg in one or more daily doses. Clinical experience suggests that higher doses can be administered safely, if needed.

In some centres, immunocompetent patients with brain tumours who are receiving long-term treatment with a steroid also receive prophylactic therapy for *Pneumocystis carinii* pneumonia. A common regimen is one double strength tablet of trimethoprim–sulphamethoxazole on three consecutive days each week.[8]

Although it is common for steroids to be continued indefinitely, continuation of steroid therapy must always be under constant review. Steroids should not be continued if there is no clear medical indication for therapy or the clinical benefit is exceeded by side effects. Steroid side effects are significant and some may add to the disability of patients (e.g. weakness due to myopathy). Table 10.11.4 lists the side effects of corticosteroids. Although not all are relevant to short-term management of symptoms in palliative care, many can seriously impact on the quality of life of patients and require careful balancing with therapeutic effects. If a steroid is no longer indicated, it should be tapered and discontinued.

Seizures in patients with advanced illness

A seizure is a transient occurrence of signs or symptoms due to abnormal excessive or synchronous neuronal activity in the brain[21]. A distinction must be made between seizures, which is the clinical event, and epilepsy, which refers to a set of diseases associated with recurrent seizures and usually other clinical signs.

Seizures are not infrequently encountered in palliative medicine. They may be caused by structural disease of the brain, nonstructural causes, or both. Structural problems include metastatic cerebral lesions and infectious causes. The most common nonstructural causes include metabolic derangement and drug toxicity[22].

Seizure definition and classification[23]

Seizures are classified according to their electroencephalographic (EEG) features as partial or focal, which applies to any seizure related to an initiating focus that can be identified in a specific brain area, and generalized, which refers to seizures that appear to begin bilaterally. Seizures that originate as truly generalized electrical discarges are defined as primary generalized seizures; those that begin locally and evolve into generalized tonic–clonic seizures are termed secondary generalized seizures.

Depending on the level of consciousness during attacks, partial or focal seizures are classified as follows:

Simple partial seizures are associated with a normal level of consciousness. Only a selective area of the cortex participates in the seizure activity, causing symptoms that depend on the function of that part of the cortex. Therefore, partial motor, sensory, autonomic, and affective seizures are possible. At times when symptoms of this kind precede the onset of a generalized seizure they are called an 'aura'.

Complex partial seizures combine focal symptoms with an altered state of consciousness. These are the most common type of seizures in adults and probably the most common encountered in palliative care. The patient seems awake but is not meaningfully engaged with the environment. If there is verbal output, questions are not answered appropriately and the patient may repeat words or sentences. Eyes can be fixed or rolling purposelessly. The patient may be immobile or engaged in repetitive behaviours (motor automatisms), such as grimacing, snapping fingers, chewing, running, or undressing. If physically restrained, behaviours can become hostile or aggressive. The seizure lasts on average 3 min and is followed by a post-ictal phase, which can include somnolence, delirium, and headache, and can last for several hours. After complete recovery, the patient has no recall of the event, but sometimes may remember the aura. The partial complex seizure can itself be preceded by an aura, which may be equivalent to a simple partial seizures.

Generalized seizures can be non-convulsive, which also are called absence or *petit mal*, or convulsive, which are known as tonic-clonic or *grand mal* seizures:

Absence (petit mal) seizures rarely begin before the fourth year of age or after puberty. They can last for 5–10 s and can occur ten to hundreds of times a day. The patient stops whatever he/she is doing and is unresponsive; the eyes usually are fixed. If the seizure lasts for more than 10 s, the patient may blink or smack lips repetitively. Atypical absences can be of longer duration and can be associated with flaccidity or muscle rigidity.

Generalized tonic–clonic (grand mal) seizures start with a sudden loss of consciousness, at times accompanied by shouting (due to forced air expiration by sudden contraction of the diaphragm). Diffuse muscle rigidity follows, which is accompanied by cyanosis. After a short time, myoclonus and muscle fasciculations occur and the patient can bite his or her tongue. The latter clonic phase typically lasts two minutes or less, but more prolonged episodes can occur. At the end, post-ictal phase presents with deep sleep and slow deep breathing. Later the patient gradually awakens, often complaining of headache.

Absence and tonic–clonic seizures are the most typical clinical presentation of generalized seizures. This category also includes *clonic seizures* (characterized by rhythmic contractions of upper limb, neck, and face muscles); *myoclonic seizures* (brief segmental contractions of the limbs, occurring alone or in clusters without loss of consciousness); *tonic seizures* (sudden generalized muscle rigidity associated with loss of consciousness and falls); and *atonic seizures* (sudden loss of muscle tone).

Table 10.11.4 Side effects of corticosteroids.

Infections (especially relevant if associated with chemotherapy): reactivation of TB, candida, pneumocystis pneumonia
Metabolic disturbances: hyperglycaemia, electrolyte imbalances, fluid retention, hyperlipidaemia
Dystrophic reaction: delay in wound healing, purpura, dermal atrophy, acne
Myopathy:[9] weakness affects mainly the pelvic girdle muscles, but also head flexor and shoulder muscles are affected. Muscle enzymes and EMG are normal. On the contrary, cretinuria is elevated. Myopathy occurs as early as 2 weeks of starting dexamethasone, manifesting with difficulties in climbing stairs and standing from a sitting position. Some authors suggest that substitution with non-fluorinated steroids (methylprednisolone or prednisone) is effective in reducing myopathic effects
Bone: osteoporosis probably due to the reduced intestinal absorption of calcium and reduced tubular reuptake with increased calciuria. These mechanisms cause hypocalcaemia, which reflects on parathyroid activation and subsequent increased bone re-absorption. Phenobarbital causes osteopathy and so it is preferable to use different anticonvulsants in combined therapies
Aseptic bone necrosis (usually of the femoral head). Two hypotheses have been proposed to explain this complication. Fat embolism due to altered lipid metabolism and osteomedullary ischaemia. Bone necrosis has been seen after relatively short-term treatment with dexamethasone (cumulative doses of 220 mg)[10]
GI side effects: peptic ulcer disease: the use of steroids alone in patients in good general condition is not associated with damage to the GI tract. There are, however, specific risk factors that are associated with peptic ulceration and bleeding, such as, very high doses, systemic neoplasm, previous peptic ulcer, and combined use of NSAIDs. It is also well known that patients with intracranial lesions are at risk of GI bleeding.[11] Prophylaxis with proton pump inhibitors is therefore suggested in patients at increased risk
Hiccup: chronic hiccup has been observed in association with the use of dexamethasone or high-dose methylprednisolone. The physiopathology of this effect is unknown[12]
Psychiatric:[13] euphoria with mild insomnia. Hyperalert reaction: anxiety can be associated with confusion. Steroid psychosis: can have hypomanic, depressive, and psychotic features with high inter- and intraindividual variability. This reaction is usually seen within 2 weeks of therapy at doses above 40 mg of prednisone per day. The steroid dose should be tapered and symptoms usually subside spontaneously in about 3 weeks
Anaphylaxis: has been observed after IV methylprednisolone[14]
Ocular toxicity: glaucoma,[15] cataract
Perineal burning sensation[16]
Endocrine effects: adrenal suppression is seen after 10 days of therapy with doses in excess of 7.5 mg prednisone per day. It is therefore useful to follow some practical suggestions to minimize this effect:[17] Morning administration matches the physiological zenith of ACTH secretion while evening administration favours the inhibition of ACTH secretion. Single administration should be preferred and when possible on alternate days. Before withholding therapy, it is important to check adrenal function (morning cortisol and response to ACTH stimulation)
Steroid withdrawal syndrome: this syndrome can occur with sudden discontinuation of therapy and includes, pseudo-rheumatism, headache, lethargy, nausea, vomiting, postural hypotension, papilloedema[18]
Epidural lipomatosis: this complication can cause slowly developing spinal cord compression[19]
Pseudo-tumour cerebri: papilloedema and headache can occur without focal neurological signs and normal CSF. It has been described in patients with Addison's disease and after steroid withdrawal and it has also been reported after chronic steroid use[20]

Treatment[24]

All anticonvulsants have potentially serious side effects and most interact with other drugs, are sedative, and produce cognitive impairment. For these reasons, prophylactic therapy of seizures in palliative medicine usually should not be undertaken if the patient has never had seizures. Although prophylactic anticonvulsant treatment in patients with primary brain tumours or metastases may be considered in selected cases, very few studies have addressed the efficacy of this approach and one randomized clinical trial confirmed that prophylactic treatment did not prevent seizures in patients with brain metastases who had never had seizures[25]. Metastases from melanoma, choriocarcinoma, and cancer of the testis are more often associated with seizures, possibly because these lesions are often haemorrhagic and, in the case of melanoma, tend to invade the grey matter. Many clinicians do consider prophylaxis for patients with these tumour types, particularly those with melanoma. In patients with primary brain tumours without seizures, it is suggested that anticonvulsant therapy be withdrawn 1 week after surgery[26].

Seizures worsen brain oedema and oedema can, in turn, cause seizures[27]. Therefore, it is advisable to optimize antioedema therapies before modifying anticonvulsant regimen in patients who develop new seizures in spite of anticonvulsant therapy.

Pharmacological therapy

The general characteristics of commonly-used anticonvulsants are summarized in Table 10.11.5 together with the recommended dosage. The ideal drug for palliative care is not easy to establish as the classic anticonvulsants cause a variety of metabolic interactions and significant side effects. The newer anti-epileptic drugs may be easier to use and better tolerated, but these often lack parenteral formulations and require slow titration schedules, which limit their usefulness in palliative medicine. Blood levels of some anticonvulsants should be monitored because of the unpredictability of metabolic changes and drug interactions, but it must be remembered that clinical response and not blood levels should guide dosage.

Table 10.11.5 Main indications and therapeutic dosing schedules of some anticonvulsivants used in palliative medicine.

Drug	Indication	Therapeutic daily dose	Schedule
Phenobarbital	Broad spectrum	1–5 mg/kg in adults; 3–8 mg/kg in children	qhs
Phenyoin	Broad spectrum	200–400 mg in adults; 4–8 mg/kg children	q8–12h
Sodium valproate	Broad spectrum	1000–3000 mg in adults; 30–60 mg/kg in children	q12h
Carbamazepine	Broad spectrum	400–1800 mg in adults; 12–20 mg/kg in children	q8–12h
Oxcarbazepine	Focal	900–2400 mg in adults; 20–40 mg/kg in children	q12h
Clonazepam	Focal	1–6 mg in adults; 0.2 mg/kg in children	q8–12h
Clobazam	Broad spectrum as second line	10–30mg	q12h
Gabapentin	Broad spectrum	1800–3600 mg in adults; 30–45 mg/kg in children	q8h
topiramate	Broad spectrum	75–200 mg in adults; 5–10 mg/kg in children	q12h
Lamotrigine	Broad spectrum	100–400 mg in adults; 5–10 mg/kg in children; if association with valproate 1–5 mg/kg	q12h
Levetiracetam	Broad spectrum	750–3000 mg in adults; 20–45 mg/kg in children	q12h
Zonisamide	Broad spectrum	200–600 mg; 4–12 mg/kg in children	q12–24h

Phenobarbital is available in oral and parenteral formulations. It is effective in both partial and generalized tonic–clonic seizures. It is metabolized by liver cytochrome P450 and has a very slow plasma clearance (4–5 days), which can be prolonged by liver disease. It has a wide therapeutic index but can cause drowsiness, ataxia, and severe rash (Stevens–Johnson syndrome and the more extensive toxic epidermal necrolysis, Lyell syndrome). It can interfere with the metabolism of several chemotherapy agents and in chronic use is associated with pseudo-rheumatism, which can worsen the symptoms of a concurrent steroid-induced osteoporosis.

Phenytoin is the first line drug in simple and complex partial seizures, and in generalized tonic–clonic seizures. Dosing can vary from 4 to 8 mg/kg/day in two to three daily administrations, preferably after eating. The intravenous formulation of phenytoin, or fosphenytoin, can be systemically loaded and provide rapid control of seizures. The advantages of phenytoin are the relative lack of sedative effects, and good tolerability at higher than recommended doses. Side effects due to chronic use include ataxia, GI disturbances, gingival hypertrophy, hirsutism, osteoporosis, and megaloblastic anaemia. The use of phenytoin also may be problematic due to variation in blood levels produced by the administration of many other drugs that interfere with liver metabolism, absorption, or protein binding. Interactions have been demonstrated with cyclosporin, cis-platinum, and paclitaxel. Significant pharmacokinetic interaction is found with concurrent dexamethasone, which can reduce phenytoin plasma levels by 50 per cent. Severe allergic reactions involving rash, hypersensitivity reactions, liver toxicity, and myelo-suppression have been reported, but are rare.

Sodium valproate is active in most types of generalized seizures (tonic, myoclonic, absence, tonic–clonic), including secondary generalized partial seizures. Doses start at 250–500 mg/day and are increased by 250 mg/week up to 1000–3000 mg/day. In children, the initial dose is 10–15 mg/kg/day, increased by the same incremental doses. Dose escalation can occur more quickly if needed and an intravenous formulation is available in some countries, which can allow tolerable loading doses. Common side effects of sodium valproate are tremors, sedation, ataxia, GI symptoms, and thrombocytopenia. Liver enzymes and blood ammonia can be increased. Although severe liver toxicity can occur (usually in the first 6 months of therapy), all reported cases occurred in children under the age of three years who also were receiving other anticonvulsants.

Carbamazepine is only available in oral formulations. It is effective in the treatment of simple and complex partial seizures, and in tonic–clonic generalized seizures. Doses should start low at 200 mg/day, increasing by 200 mg per week (Table 10.11.5). Acute intoxication can cause stupor and coma, convulsions, and respiratory depression. After chronic administration, sedation, vertigo, ataxia, diplopia, and myelo-suppression can occur. Myelotoxicity can occur, and aplastic anaemia has been reported rarely (one case per 200 000 patients).

Oxcarbazepine is chemically related to carbamazepine, but has less pharmacological interaction liability because of a relatively lower propensity to induce liver enzymes. Like carbamazepine, its mechanism of action appears to involve sodium channel modulation. It is approved for partial and generalized tonic-clonic seizures, both as mono- and add-on therapy. It is equivalent to carbamazepine in efficacy but usually is better tolerated. Initial dose ranges from 300–600 mg in two to three daily administration and it is usually titrated up to 600–1800 mg/day.

Clonazepam is approved for the prophylaxis of absence, atypical absence, and myoclonic epilepsy. It can also be used as a temporary treatment to control and prevent seizures not controlled by ongoing therapy. In children, initial doses start with 0.01–0.03 mg/kg/day. Doses usually are increased by 0.25–0.5 mg every 3 days. The most relevant side effect is sedation. Paradoxical excitation is rare.

Clobazam is considered a second-line drug for all seizure types. It usually is well tolered but has been associated with a rare idiosyncratic rash. The usual starting dose in adults is 10 mg, and the dailly maintenance dose is 10–30 mg.

Gabapentin is effective in monotherapy for partial seizures with or without secondary generalization. Its use is facilitated by the lack of binding to plasma proteins and lack of hepatic metabolism. Elimination is renal and influenced only by renal function. Usual daily doses are given in Table 10.11.5 but doses 2–3 times higher than recommended in children and doses as high as 3600–6000 mg/day in adults have been used without severe side effects. Side effects include ataxia, weight gain, and dizziness.

Topiramate is indicated in partial and generalized seizures in children and adults. Initial doses should be low (25 mg) and increased by 25–50 mg/week. The usually effective dose in adults ranges from 200 to 400 mg. In children, the initial dose is 0.5–1 mg/kg/day; this is increased weekly by the same amount, up to 5–9 mg/kg. The usual side effects include sedation, unsteadiness, memory disturbances, and concentration problems.

Lamotrigine has been approved for absence seizures, but is used as monotherapy for partial and secondary generalized seizures in adults. It is metabolized by the liver and has significant interactions with all the classic anticonvulsants (phenobarbitone, phenytoin, carbamazepine). Cases of severe rashes, including Stevens–Johnson syndrome have been observed and are related to a rapid titration of the drug dose. With slow initiation of therapy, the risk of skin rash is comparable with that seen with phenytoin. It is therefore important to titrate the dose slowly with weekly increments of 25 or 50 mg up to 300–500 mg/day. The risk also is increased in patients younger than 16 years of age and when the drug is combined with sodium valproate. In patients who are already taking liver enzyme-inducing antiepileptic drugs (with the exception of sodium valproate), the starting dose should be 50 mg/day for 2 weeks, then increased by 100 mg/day (in two divided doses) to a maintenance dose of 300–500 mg/day. If added to a sodium valproate containing regimen, lamotrigine should be started at 25 mg every other day for 2 weeks and titrated even more carefully.

Levetiracetam is used for partial and secondary generalized tonic–clonic seizures. The drug is well tolerated, and the most frequent side effects are somnolence, asthenia, and dizziness. The starting dose may be the same as the minimally effective dose of 750–1000 mg/daily.

Zonisamide is well absorbed after oral administration. Its efficacy in addition to other anticonvulsants has been demonstred for partial and secondary generalized tonic–clonic seizures. It is usually well tolerated. Somnolence, dizziness, and anorexia as most common side effects; it also is associated with renal calculi in approximately 1 per cent of patients. This drug has urinary excretion

Status epilepticus

Mechanistically, status epilepticus represents the failure of the natural homeostatic seizure-suppressing mechanisms responsible for seizure termination[28]. As defined for adults and children older than age five, status epilepticus is a seizure that lasts 30 min or more, or two or more seizures that occur without complete recovery of consciousness in between. Although the definition requires a continuous seizure for 30 min, it should be recognized that the mean behavioural and electroecephalographical duration of generalized convulsive seizures in adults is exceeded after 1 min and the likelihood of spontaneous resolution becomes small after 5 min. For this reason, the treatment used for status epilepticus should be considered whenever a seizure lasts 5 min or more.

Clinical characteristics of status epilepticus

Status epilepticus may be classified by the type of seizure[28]. The broadest classification distinguishes non-convulsive status epilepticus from convulsive status epilepticus. Non-convulsive status epilepticus can manifest as an absence type and as a partial complex type. The most common convulsive status epilepticus in populations with advanced illness presents as continuous or repeated tonic–clonic seizures. There are numerous other subtypes, however, including epilepsia partialis continua, supplementary motor area (SMA) status eoilepticus, aura continua, tonic status epilepticus, absence status epilepticus, myoclonic status epilepticus, and subtle status epilepticus.

Non-convulsive status epilepticus is characterized by EEG seizure activity without convulsive activity. It is a significant cause of impaired consciousness in patients with complex toxic–metabolic encephalopathies, occurring in 8 per cent of comatose patients according to recent data[29]. According to some authors, most patients with altered state of consciousness and mild motor signs have EEG findings compatible with seizures.

Partial complex non-convulsive status epilepticus may be particularly challenging to diagnose and treat. Seizure activity may fluctuate and often originates from a temporal cortical area that may not be evident on routine EEG. The syndrome may present as a confusional state with variable clinical findings. It may be continuous or frequently recurrent, or discontinuous, with recurrent partial complex seizures and recovery of consciousness between episodes. The duration of a status episode is highly variable and can be as long as weeks. In 40 per cent of cases, the episode is shorter than 24 h; in another 40 per cent, the episode lasts from 1 to 10 days. The clinical manifestations may take the form of a prolonged delirium, with or without psychotic behaviours and automatisms, or have a more baffling presentation. Some patients have minimal difficulty answering questions but demonstrate affective changes, such as fear, or paranoid ideation.

In a patient without brain metastases, the treatment of non-convulsive status epilepticus can be delayed, or introduced gradually. Although, the drugs selected for the treatment of this condition mirrors the treatment of convulsive status epilepticus in most cases, the syndrome rarely causes significative cerebral injury and the potential risk of emergent administration of antiepileptic drugs outweighs the risk involved in a more gradual introduction of medications.

Convulsive status epilepticus takes the form of continuous or frequently recurrent abnormal motor movements and loss of consciousness. The risk of cerebral damage and serious complications, including acidosis and rhabdomyolysis, usually mandates an emergent approach to management[30]. Treatment has a high rate of success if initiated early, before neuronal injury and time-dependent pharmacoresistence develop. A suggested algorithm for the management of status epilepticus is given in Table 10.11.6.

Lorazepam[31] often is considered the drug of choice for the emergent management of convulsive status epilepticus. The mean time to clinical effect is 3 min. The half-life is 10–15 h, but effective brain levels are maintained for 8–24 h. It has no active metabolites. It should be infused IV not faster than 2 mg/min, to reduce the risk of respiratory depression. It is well absorbed also after intramuscular (IM) administration.

Diazepam enters the brain in a few seconds but because of its high lipid solubility, redistribution to all body tissues is rapid, with a consequent fall in brain concentration. Its anticonvulsant effect is therefore very brief and a second dose may be necessary after only 20–30 min. Rectal formulations are available. Recommended doses are 10 mg in adults and 5 mg (0.5 mg/kg) in children. Rectal administration at these doses does not cause respiratory depression.

Table 10.11.6 Algorithm for the management of status epilepticus.

Minutes	Treatment
0	Stabilize the patient: ABC, protect airway—ensure breathing—maintain the circulation.
>5	*Lorazepam* IV, 0.1–0.15 mg/kg in children and 4–8 mg in adult (regarding the body weight), at rate of 2 mg/min; may repeat once after 20,
	or
	midazolam IV 0.2 mg/kg as bolus, continuous venous infusion of 0.1–0.6 mg/kg/h. Midazolam is well absorbed also IM and SC, and can be given at the same doses when venous access in not feasible;
	midazolam against buccal or nasal mucosa is also an alternative, at dose of 0.5 mg/kg, 2.5 mg for children, 6–12 months old; 5 mg 1–4 years; 7.5 mg 5–9 years; 10 mg for children 10 years or older,
	or
	intravenous *diazepam* 0.15–0.25 mg/kg, at rate of 5 mg/min, until a total of 20 mg in adults; may repeat once after 5min; *rectal diazepam*, 0.5 mg/kg or 2.5 mg for children 6–12 months old; 5 mg for 1–4 years; 7.5 mg 5–9 years; 10 mg for children 10 years, or more, older;
Additional drug therapy may be not required if seizure stops and the cause of SE is treated	then
	intravenous *valproic acid* 15 mg/kg over in 3 min, but higher doses, up to 25–60 mg/kg, at 3 mg/kg/min, have been used without serious side effects. This bolus must be followed by continous infusione of 1–2 mg/kg/h*,
	or
	intravenous *phenytoin* 15(in the elderly)–20 mg/kg, at infusion rate no more that 50 mg/min in adults or 1 mg/kg/min in children (monitor for hypotension and electrocardigraphic QT prolongation), in *normal saline*, followed by a dose of 4–8 mg/kg/daily oral or IV.
	If ineffective, give supplemental intravenous **phenytoin** 5 mg/kg, which can be repeated until a total dose of 30 mg/kg.
	* in some guidelines, phenytoin is suggested before valproic acid, but a number of papers have documented the successful use of intravenous valproate in SE, without serious cardiovascular side effects; fosfenytoin is better tolerated than phenytoin, but is not available in all countries.
	If seizure continues:
	phenobarbital IV, 20 mg/kg, infusion rate of 60 mg/min; caution to respiratory depression, mostly in patients treated before with benzodiazepines;
	if ineffective,
	supplemental intravenous *phenobarbital* 5-10 mg/kg.
>60	*Refractory status epilepticus*: to be treated in intensive care unit, where the patient can be treated with general anaesthesia, for example:
	propofol 1–2 mg/kg over in 5–10 min, followed by infusion of 2–10 mg/kg/h;
	pentobarbital loading up to 10 mg/kg at no more than 25 mg/min, followed by infusion of 0.25–2.0 mg/kg/h or higher, until burst-suppression EEG pattern is evident

After IM administration, absorption is very variable and unpredictable and this route should generally be avoided.

Midazolam is water soluble, has a very short half-life, and has no active metabolites. Its onset of action is 3 min after IV administration, and 5 min and 15 min, respectively, after IM and oral administration. The good IM and SC absorption are an important advantage in cases of difficult venous access. In refractory SE, the initial dose is 0.2 mg/kg, followed by 0.05–0.5 mg/kg/h IV infusion. Higher dose may be used in refractory status epilepticus without significant morbidity[32].

Sodium valproate is available as a parenteral formulation and provides an alternative to phenytoin. Studies confirm the efficacy and safety of valproate infusion, including infusion at high doses in patients with repetitive seizures, and its superiority to phenytoin.[33] Valproate is relatively contraindicated in cirrhosis or hepatic failure, and liver function should be monitored during therapy. However, fatalities have been reported only in children under 2 years who were concurrently treated with other anticonvulsant drugs.

Phenytoin,[34] when given intravenously, has an relatively rapid onset of action (10–20 min). It has no sedative effects, does not cause respiratory depression, and has a long duration of action. It may be used to abort the seizure in benzodiazepine-refractory status epilepticus. In the latter situation, it may be given IV infusion at a rate that should not exceed 50 mg/min. After diluting phenytoin in saline, the solution should be infused within 1 h. The loading dose usually is 20 mg/kg but should be less, and 15 mg/kg in elderly patients. A loading dose of 15–20 mg/kg can be also administered orally but poor gastric tolerability limits the use of this route in some patients. Side effects may be related to excessively fast infusion rates, as may occur in emergency situations, and include cardiac arrhythmias, hypotension, and CNS depression. The 'purple glove syndrome' is due to the high pH of the drug (−13), which manifests as blue discolouration and distal oedema near the site of infusion about 2 h after administration. After the loading dose, the duration of the therapeutic effect is about 24 h. Blood levels can be checked 120 min after the end of the infusion.

Phenobarbital is an option if benzodiazepines, valproic acid, or phenytoin fail. The peak clinical effect is delayed for 20–60 min after administration.

Propofol[35] has an effect on GABA receptors similar to that of benzodiazepines and barbiturates. Its use requires intensive care support and is reserved for cases of status epilepticus, which are refractory to standard treatment. Hypotensive effects should be carefully managed.

Pentobarbital is highly lipid soluble and for this reason undergoes rapid redistribution, resulting in a shorter elimination half-life than phenobarbital, which result in faster recovery of consciousness after withdrawal. It is associated with hypotension and respiratory depression, and in some cases, awakening may be complicated by decrebrate posturing or flaccid paralysis, which may persist for weeks.

Differential diagnosis of status epilepticus

It is important to keep in mind that acute conditions with an altered state of consciousness, at times associated with motor or behavioural abnormalities, are often erroneously considered seizures. The most frequent of these conditions is listed in Table 10.11.7[36].

Delirium

Definition

Delirium has been defined as a transient organic brain syndrome characterized by the acute onset of disordered attention and cognition, accompanied by disturbances of cognition, psychomotor behaviour, and perception[37]. Delirium is considered to be a single taxonomic entity, and the DSM-IV proposes specific diagnostic criteria for its diagnosis (Table 10.11.8)[38].

Delirium may be considered to be a stereotyped response of the brain to a spectrum of insults and as a distinctive state on the continuum between normal wakefulness and stupor and coma. Other terms for this condition include 'encephalopathy' and 'acute confusional state'. The latter descriptions are used commonly by neurologists to describe acute changes in mental status, and as a result, there are semantic differences between the psychiatric and neurologic literature. Delirium also has been described by Engels and Romano as a syndrome of cerebral insufficiency, but this term is not generally used[39].

The EEG of patients with delirium, regardless of aetiology, demonstrates generalized symmetric slowing with reduction of the alpha rhythm and an increase in delta and theta frequencies[39]. These

Table 10.11.7 Conditions associated with motor and behavioural abnormalities.

Psychiatric disturbances: somatoform reactions, panic attacks, psychotic dissociative episodes, Munchausen syndrome
Cardiovascular disorders: syncope, arrhythmia, transient ischaemic attacks (TIA)
Headache: hemicrania complicata, hemicrania basilare
Movement disorders: tremor, dyskinesia, tic, myoclonus
Parasomnias and sleep disturbances: nightmares, somnambulism, narcolepsy, cataplexy, nocturnal paroxysmal dystonia
Gastrointestinal symptom: nausea or colic
Delirium

Table 10.11.8 DSM IV criteria for diagnosing delirium due to a general medical condition.[38]

A.	Disturbance of consciousness with reduced ability to focus, sustain, and shift attention
B.	Change in cognition (such as memory deficit, disorientation, language disturbances, or perception disturbances not better explained by a pre-existing stabilized or evolving dementia)
C.	The disturbance develops over a short period of time and tends to fluctuate during the course of the day
D.	There is evidence from the history, physical examination, or laboratory findings that the disturbance is caused by the direct physiological consequences of a general medical condition

changes are not dissimilar to those found in stages of the sleep pattern. In general, the degree of EEG slowing correlates with a decrease in arousal. In some conditions, EEG fast wave activity, beta activity, is also present. This activity is more prevalent in delirium characterized by hyperactive phenomena, such as delirium tremens.

Clinical diagnosis

The diagnosis of delirium requires that consciousness and attention are assessed together with cognitive function and performance. This is best done by instruments that are sensitive to the derangement of these areas of brain function. The Mini Mental State Examination (MMSE) is the most widely used method and can be applied to bedside patient assessment. It assesses cognitive function but is not a diagnostic tool. It screens for cognitive failure and can be abnormal in dementia or delirium, or in other disorders that affect cognitive performance.

In contrast to the MMSE, the Confusion Assessment Method is a diagnostic system that can be used to apply the DSM criteria for the diagnosis of delirium. It is very sensitive and specific when applied by trained personnel[40,41].

The Delirium Rating Scale (DRS)[42] and the Memorial Delirium Assessment Scale (MDAS)[43] are instruments specifically designed to assess delirium and its severity. These tools can be used to evaluate a range of symptoms that occur in patients with delirium.

Whether or not the clinical evaluation of a possible delirium includes the application of a validated assessment instrument, symptoms and signs fluctuate and the diagnosis may be overlooked if careful attention is not paid to the changes in mental status over time. Additionally, subtle changes frequently precede the onset of delirium. These minor symptoms and behavioural changes may go unnoticed, only to be recalled later in family or staff interviews. A patient who becomes restless, anxious, depressed, irritable, angry, or emotionally labile may be manifesting these premonitory symptoms of delirium. The differential diagnosis is complex, however, and includes adjustment disorder and any of a large number of neurological conditions, including dementia.

The variation in symptoms and signs also creates a diagnostic challenge. In the early stages of delirium, or while recovering from an episode, there may be isolated disturbances that do not themselves fulfil the criteria for a diagnosis of delirium. These findings may include daytime somnolence with night-time insomnia, subtle mood and personality changes, or hallucinations.

The first of the DSM diagnostic criteria for delirium relates to disturbance of consciousness and impaired attention. This disturbance can be highly variable, characterized by increased or decreased arousal, or merely by distractibility and reduced responsiveness. Three clinical variants of delirium have been described based on the type of arousal disturbance: hypoalert–hypoactive, hyperalert–hyperactive, and mixed type (with fluctuations from hypoalert to hyperalert)[37,44].

Attention is affected not only by the level of arousal but also by changes in the patient's ability to concentrate, which can be subtle. Attention disturbances may be evidenced by an inability to maintain a conversation or to attend to its flow, language abnormalities, and difficulties in writing[45].

The second DSM criterion for delirium relates to the presence of changed cognition. This may take the form of disorientation, memory deficits, or disturbances of language, reasoning, or perception. It is important to recognize that a diagnosis of delirium may be established in the presence of any one of these cognitive abnormalities. The use of the MMSE or another tool provides a method to globally assess these potential disturbances.

Language abnormalities are frequent in delirium and are often compounded by the presence of incoherent reasoning. Language may lack fluency and spontaneity, and conversation may be prolonged and interrupted by long pauses or repetitions. The language may reflect an inability to find the correct word or to name objects (anomia) or may be characterized by 'passepartout' words (nonspecific phrases that substitute for specific language, for example, 'you know what I mean'), perseveration, stereotypes, and cliches. Writing abilities are affected early and more severely than other language-related skills[46,47]. Delirium affects reasoning and patients frequently demonstrate irrelevant or rambling thinking, abnormal conceptualization, and altered insight with anosognosia.

Perceptual abnormalities and delusions are not considered by the MMSE, but also may be typical of delirium, especially in some subtypes such as delirium tremens or other types of hyperactive delirium. These disturbances in perception are systematically assessed in the DRS and the MDAS.

Delusions may be associated with hallucinations. These delusions are frequently poorly organized and characterized by paranoid features, which may incorporate themes that relate, for example, to homicide, imprisonment, or jealousy. Occupational delusions are among the most common, with the patient locating himself or herself in a familiar time and space, and attending to usual activities. Lipowski describes 'the law of the unfamiliar mistaken for the familiar'[48] and suggests that perceptions are influenced by the emotional colour of the situation and the patient's personality characteristics[49].

Delirium can significantly interfere with family and staff understanding of patient's suffering. A recent small study of 14 patients with cancer pain and severe cognitive failure found that during episodes of agitated cognitive failure, pain intensity as assessed by a nurse was significantly higher than the patient's assessment had been before and after the episode[50]. Upon complete recovery, none of these patients recalled having had any discomfort during the episode.

The third and fourth criteria for diagnosis of delirium relates to the time course and organic aetiology of the disturbance. For diagnosis, there must be evidence confirming that the disturbance has developed over a short period of time and tends to fluctuate during the course of the day. Fluctuation in the clinical manifestations of delirium is usually apparent in disturbance of the sleep–wake cycle.

Patients usually experience insomnia and may be agitated at night and somnolent during the day. As noted previously, this change in sleep pattern is often found to be among the prodromal symptoms of the syndrome. The phenomenon known as 'sundowning' refers to the worsening of symptoms toward evening and probably has to do with sleep–wake abnormalities that are aggravated by environmental factors.

In addition to mental status changes, neurological examination of the patient with delirium may identify findings associated with diffuse brain dysfunction, such as multifocal myoclonus and asterixis. Some findings may be relatively specific for one or more aetiologies. For example, tremulousness is typical of alcohol withdrawal states; miosis and mydriasis suggest opioid toxicity and anticholinergic toxicity, respectively; and tachypnoea may be a manifestation of a central process, or of sepsis or hypoxaemia.

Frequency

A study performed in the early 1980s found that the prevalence of organic brain syndromes was 4 per cent among hospitalized cancer patients[51]. No prevalence data based on a specific definition of delirium are available for the general cancer population. More recently, delirium prevalence has been studied in the elderly, patients in the postoperative period, and patients presenting to the emergency room[52,53]. Altered mental state is the second most common reason for neurological consultation at a tertiary cancer centre[54]. In patients admitted to inpatient hospice or to home palliative care programmes, prevalence of delirium is about 30 per cent[55].

In a study by Gagnon et al., 18 of 89 cancer patients (20 per cent) consecutively hospitalized for terminal care were delirious on admission and, among the 71 who were free of delirium at admission, the incidence of confirmed delirium was 32 per cent[56]. In a sample of 104 patients admitted to an acute palliative care unit in a university-affiliated teaching hospital, Lawlor et al. diagnosed delirium in 44 patients (42 per cent), and of the remaining 60, delirium developed in 27 (45 per cent)[57]. Reversal of delirium occurred in 46 (49 per cent) of 94 episodes in 71 patients and terminal delirium occurred in 46 (88 per cent) of the 52 deaths[57].

These prevalence figures may under-represent the problem. In the emergency room setting, for example, one study demonstrated that only 6 per cent of delirium diagnoses were detected by the emergency room physician[58]. In a series of elderly medical patients, the physicians' diagnoses correctly identified only eight of 47 patients as being delirious or acutely confused[59].

Aetiologic factors in delirium and multifactorial risk model

Risk factors

The socio-demographic and disease-related factors that may predispose to delirium or predict its occurrence have not been documented in cancer patients. The studies that have investigated delirium in the oncology setting have generally sought to address the spectrum and prevalence of a range of psychiatric diagnoses rather than to address factors involved in specific diagnoses, such as delirium. As a consequence, the number of delirious cancer patients that has been studied has not been large enough to allow investigators to draw conclusions that relate to predictive factors. In one recent study, dyspnoea, anorexia, presence of brain metastases, performance status, and physician estimate prediction of survival were associated with the diagnosis of delirium but only univariate statistics were applied[55].

Inouye and Charpentier have proposed a multifactorial model for delirium in the hospitalized elderly that may be relevant in the cancer population[60]. The model involves the interaction between 'baseline vulnerability' and 'precipitating factors or insults'. In this model, baseline vulnerability is defined by the predisposing factors present at the time of admission to hospital, and the precipitating factors are the noxious insults that occurred during hospitalization. Patients who have high baseline vulnerability may develop delirium with any precipitating factor, whereas those with low baseline vulnerability will be more resistant to the development of delirium, even with noxious insults. The factors that Inouye et al. specifically demonstrated to be contributory to baseline vulnerability in the elderly include visual impairment, severity of illness, cognitive impairment, and an elevated serum urea nitrogen/creatinine ratio of 18 or greater (dehydration)[60]. Other studies have implicated risk factors, including each of the aforementioned factors, age, dementia, depression, alcohol abuse, the preoperative use of anticholinergic drugs, poor functional status, and markedly abnormal preoperative serum sodium, potassium, or glucose levels[61,62]. Certain medications have also been implicated as risk factors for delirium, including neuroleptics, opioids, and anticholinergic drugs[52,61,37].

Aetiology

In cancer patients, the potential aetiologies of delirium, as distinct from 'risk factors', may be divided into direct effects related to tumour involvement and indirect effects. The latter category includes drugs, electrolyte imbalance, cranial irradiation, organ failure, nutritional deficiencies, vascular complications, paraneoplastic syndromes, and many other factors (Table 10.11.9).

A survey of 140 confused cancer patients referred initially for a neurology consultation demonstrated a single cause of the altered mental status in 31 per cent and multiple causes in 69 per cent; the median number of probable contributing factors in each patient was 3[63]. Drugs, especially opioids, were associated with altered mental status in 64 per cent of patients, metabolic abnormalities in 53 per cent, infection in 46 per cent, and recent surgery in 32 per cent. A structural brain lesion was the sole cause of encephalopathy in 15 per cent of patients. Lateralizing neurological signs were found in 41 per cent of patients, and of those with lateralizing findings, 42 per cent had cerebral metastases. Importantly, however, it was noted that 25 per cent of patients without lateralizing signs who had neuro-imaging had a focal cerebral lesion defined as a cause or a contributory factor to the delirium. Two-thirds of the patients in this survey recovered cognitive function when the cause of the delirium was treated.

In the study by Lawlor et al., of 104 patients with advanced cancer admitted to a palliative care unit[57], the median number of precipitating factors was 3, and 49 per cent of patients had delirium that was reversible. Although the use of psychoactive medications, predominantly opioids, was the precipitating factor that was independently associated with reversibility of the delirium, the authors concluded that more than one factor (e.g. opioid medication and dehydration) usually requires attention if the delirium is to be reversed[57]. Other studies have demonstrated that drug interactions with opioid metabolism and metabolic failure (especially renal impairment) can produce unexpected toxicities, especially in the patient with advanced disease[37,64,65].

Table 10.11.9 Aetiological factors implicated in the onset of delirium in patients with cancer.

Primary CNS tumour
Secondary CNS tumour
Brain metastases
Meningeal metastases
Non-metastatic complications of cancer
Metabolic encephalopathy due to hepatic, renal, or pulmonary failure
Electrolyte abnormalities
Glucose abnormalities
Infections
Haematological abnormalities
Nutritional deficiency (thiamine, folic acid, vitamin B12 deficiency)
Vasculitis
Paraneoplastic neurological syndromes
Toxicity of antineoplastic therapies
Chemotherapy: methotrexate, cisplatin, vincristine, procarbazine, asparaginase, citosina arabinoside, 5-fluorouracil, ifosfamide, tamoxifene (rare), etoposide (high doses), nitrosurea (high doses or arterial route)
Radiation to brain
Acute and delayed encephalopathy
Toxicity of other drugs
Anticholinergics: belladonna alkaloids, scopolamine, atropine, hyoscine
Drugs with established anticholinergic activity: tricyclic antidepressants, diphenhydramine, promethazine, triesifenidile, chlorpromazine, and other neuroleptics: hyoscine butylbromide
Anxiolytics, hypnotics
Steroids, opioids, digitalis, cyprofloxacine, acyclovir, gancyclovir, NSAIDs, anticonvulsants, H2 blockers, omeprazole, interferons, interleukins, cyclosporin, levodopa, lithium
Other diseases not related to neoplasms
CNS diseases or trauma
Cardiac disease
Lung disease
Endocrinopathy
Alcohol or drug abuse or withdrawal

Cognitive compromise is likely one of the most common presenting symptoms or signs of brain[8] and leptomeningeal metastases.[66] Paraneoplastic encephalitis, which can be associated with anti-Hu and other antineuronal antibodies, also should be considered a potential rare cause of delirium[8].

Non-convulsive epileptic status, which can occur in association with complex metabolic problems and also with ifosfamide encephalopathy, is a condition that also can result in altered consciousness manifesting with delirium[67]. EEG can be used to confirm this diagnosis, which is likely to be more frequent than suspected[29].

In reviewing the many causes of delirium, it is important to recognize that many are common and potentially reversible in the population with advance illness. These factors include, among others, dehydration, borderline renal function, infections, metabolic disturbances, drug withdrawal, and the use of psycho-active medications such as opioids[37].

General assessment recommendations

Given the high prevalence of delirium in populations with advanced illness, clinicians must be prepared to offer a routine assessment whenever the syndrome is suspected. Clinical assessment should include careful physical and neurological examination. Specific mental status assessment can follow the above-mentioned recommendations and can be helped by the systematic use of the MMSE, DRS, or MDAS, and also by screening with the CAM. Aetiological screening should involve a rational and stepwise implementation of procedures, noting that any specific procedure may be appropriate or inappropriate depending on the patient's condition, wishes, prognosis, and goals of care (Table 10.11.10). The completeness of the list is not inconsistent with a policy of avoiding procedures that are determined to be inappropriate in the individual case.

EEG may be useful in assessing delirium, clarifying the differential diagnosis and severity, and providing a better method for serial monitoring[68]. EEG findings, specifically decreased alpha and increased delta and theta frequencies, have been demonstrated to correlate with low MMSE scores in delirious patients. The utility of EEG in the differential diagnosis of delirium has also been demonstrated in the differentiation of non-convulsive status epilepticus from delirium and several specific diagnostic entities. For example, the EEG associated with delirium produced by high-dose ifosfamide shows rhythmic complexes typical of seizure-like activity, in contrast to generalized symmetric slowing of the EEG considered to be typical of other types of delirium[67].

Treatment

Aetiological interventions are aimed at correcting infectious and toxic-metabolic causes or risk factors, as reviewed in Table 10.11.10. Symptomatic management often is required both in reversible and irreversible cases, and is based on non-pharmacological and pharmacological therapies.

Environmental interventions

In a classic study by Inouye et al., systematic reorientation and a risk-modifying protocol reduced the incidence of delirium among elderly hospitalized patients[60]. A calm, quiet environment, with good light, is important to allow for potential recovery and to help the patient to reorient to time and space. The process may be further assisted by placing a clock or calendar where the patient can see them, and by permitting the patient to see or touch a well-known object from the patient's house. Presence in the room of family members can be very important.

Communication with patient and family

In managing the delirious patient, a close collaboration between staff and family is fundamental. Special attention needs to be focused on communication. Family members may be particularly stressed by observing the change of the patient's usual behaviour and by a new barrier to communication. The family must be informed about the characteristics of delirium, including fluctuation of cognitive function, its relationship with the disease conditions, potential for reversibility, role of therapies, and short-term prognosis.

Table 10.11.10 Screening process for delirium aetiology in advanced cancer.

Toxic factors	Bedside screen of medication profile
	Urine or blood drug screening
Sepsis	Temperature
	Blood/urine and other cultures for infection screen
	Leucocyte count
	Urinalysis
	Red cell count
Glucose-oxidative brain deficiency	Pulse oximetry
	Blood gases and acid–base balance
	Blood glucose
Electrolyte imbalances	Serum electrolytes (Na, K, Cl, Mg, Ca)
Renal failure	Urea, creatinine, creatinine clearance
Liver failure	Liver function tests
	Ammonia
CNS vascular, infectious or structural lesion	DIC screening and coagulation profile
	CSF examination: blood, glucose, proteins, lymphocytes, leucocytes, malignant cells, culture
	Brain CT or MRI
Paraneoplastic disease	Autoantibodies Anti-Hu, Yo, Ma, etc.
Cofactor deficiency malnutrition	B12 levels—administer B1 1 g/day[a]
Endocrine dysfunction	Thyroid hormone and TSH
	Adrenal function

[a] Because the determination of B1 levels is problematic, it is reasonable to supplement B1 in every patient with poor nutritional status.

In the care of patients with advanced illness, the goals of care must be clarified and discussed, and the level of patient suffering assessed and explained to family members. Family members may require special care as they react to what they interpret as the patient suffering, or pain. The behaviour of families, particularly those strained by the burden of caregiving, can swing from requests to withdraw medication to advocating sedation; caregiver distress may be compounded by personal problems in facing suffering and death[37].

It is very important to clarify the potential aetiologic role of existing therapies. For example, it is customary to blame opioid medications for mental changes that are actually caused by the complex interaction of several factors. This idea may be reinforced by previous experience, or by the erroneous statements of healthcare professionals, and can result in the caregiver guilt for administering drugs that they believe caused the change of mental status. If the aetiology cannot be established, this should be explained to the family and decisions about using drugs that may contribute to the delirium should be based on the priority of providing symptom control and comfort care.

In communicating with the patient, the clinician should show empathy and to ask simple questions ('Do you feel confused?'). The patient may be fearful and should be reassured. As needed, logic and rational communication should be supplanted by more direct nonverbal communication. The patient should be encouraged to communicate with well-known family members, and this communication should focus more on affective aspects than on discussions that could confuse or frighten the delirious patient.

Pharmacological therapy

Agitated delirium often requires pharmacological treatment to control behaviours that could result in harm for the patient and others, and to treat hallucinations or delusions that may be contributing to patient suffering. The treatment of hypoactive deliria is more debatable and will depend on individual clinical judgement.

The usual first choice drug for agitated delirium is haloperidol[69,70], since it has relatively low sedating potency and less anticholinergic and cardiovascular effects than other neuroleptics. Table 10.11.11 gives guidelines for the use of haloperidol and alternative drugs.

Haloperidol has been used via IV infusion, although it is not licensed for this route of administration[70]. Very high IV doses, up to 1200 mg per day, have been safely administered. Therapeutic effects in hyperactive delirium typically are seen at doses of 6–12 mg/day; difficult cases may require higher doses or sedation with other drugs. Careful titration of the dose at the bedside is the most important recommendation to improve outcome. ECG monitoring should be considered during haloperidol therapy to monitor possible prolongation of the Q–T interval that can occasionally occur with most neuroleptics; torsade de pointe has been described as a rare complication of haloperidol administration via the IV and oral routes[71].

Alternative neuroleptics can be used if greater sedation is desired or haloperidol is contraindicated. Droperidol and chlorpromazine are relatively sedating, and recently, risperidone, clozapine, quetiapine, zipasidone and olanzapine have been used[37].

Benzodiazepines are first choice agents in the treatment of delirium related to alchohol or other sedative-hypnotic withdrawal. They also can be added in cases of delirium when anxiolytic and sedative effects are considered particularly desirable or in cases unresponsive to neuroleptic medications. They should be used cautiously, however, because they can worsen delirium, especially in the elderly[69], they should not be used in hepatic encephalopathy.

In the management of delirium in the setting of advanced illness, more than a single drug may be needed. In one case series of 39 patients, only 20 per cent could be managed by haloperidol alone[72]. When sedation is the goal of therapy, and especially when delirium occurs with other severe complications such as pain, haemorrhage, or dyspnoea, the combination of an opioid with a neuroleptic and an antihistamine such as promethazine can be particularly effective.

Other neurological complications of cancer

Although intracranial hypertension, seizures, and delirium are the most common challenging neurological complications of advanced cancer, there are numerous others that may be encountered, particularly in populations with advanced illness. Indeed, neurological complications are estimated to occur in up to 20 per cent of patients

Table 10.11.11 Pharmacological therapy of delirium (regimens suggested for general guidance; each case will need specific dose adjustment).

Haloperidol; oral	0.5–5 mg every 8–12 h; a dose of 2 mg/day can be efficacious in mild cases
Haloperidol; SC, IM, or IV	0.5–2 mg per dose titrating dose to clinical effect hourly IV infusion 0.2–1 mg/h with careful titration to clinical effect can be used in difficult cases. ECG monitoring is recommended
Chlorpromazine; oral, IM, or IV	12.5–50 mg every 8–12 h. More sedating, anticholinergic, and hypotensive effects
Clozapine; oral	12.5–50 mg at night (monitoring of blood cell count is needed) very sedative, has less extrapyramidal effects than other neuroleptics
Risperidone; oral	From 0.5–1 mg/day up to 2–4 mg/day. In the elderly, has less extrapyramidal effects
Olanzapine; OS IM	5 mg qhs to be titrated up to clinical effect
Lorazepam; oral, SL, or IV	0.5–2 mg every 6–8 h if sedating anxiolytic effects required
Midazolam; SC or IV	20–100 mg 24 h IV or SC continuous infusion for sedation in refractory cases. 3–5 mg IV priming dose if rapid sedation is required. Start IV infusion with 1 mg/h, dose should be frequently titrated to effect
Promethazine; IM or IV	50 mg every 8–12 h; antihistamine very sedative; useful if sedation desired

with cancer[73]. In a large consultation survey conducted at a comprehensive cancer centre, the most frequent complaints were pain and altered mental status (Table 10.11.12)[54].

Brain metastases

Pathology

Intracranial metastases are found at autopsy in about 25 per cent of patients who died of cancer[8]. Other common intracranial lesions involve the skull and meninges. The choroid plexus and the pituitary are less commonly affected. There is evidence that the incidence of brain metastases and leptomeningeal metastases is increasing, because of better control of systemic disease and longer survival, which allow 'sanctuary' cells in the central nervous system to evolve into clinically significant lesions. Lung cancer, melanoma, and breast cancer are the primary tumours most frequently associated with metastatic spread to the brain parenchyma. Tumours such as melanoma usually cause multiple lesions, while breast cancer more often causes single lesions (some 50 per cent of breast cancer patients have a single lesion and 20 per cent two lesions). It is important to bear this in mind when planning surgery or focal radiation treatment.

Brain metastases usually originate from neoplastic emboli. Tumour emboli lodge in the white matter at the grey/white matter junction, usually involving the watershed territories at the end of the arterial supply. Once implanted, they grow as spherical masses that displace, rather than infiltrate, the brain. Their geographic distribution of metastases in the brain relates to blood flow. Thus, the

Table 10.11.12 Cancer-related and treatment related neurological diagnoses in 851 patients with cancer[a].

Diagnosis	Percentage
Brain metastasis	15.9
Metabolic or drug related encephalopathy	10.2
Pain associated with bone metastasis	9.9
Epidural tumour	8.5
Tumour plexopathy	5.8
Leptomeningeal metastasis	5.1
Chemotherapy peripheral neuropathy	3.2
Radiculopathy	2.7
Base-of-skull metastasis	2.7
Seizures due to metastasis	2.7
Seizures not due to metastasis	1.8
Paraneoplastic syndromes	1.2
Intracranial haemorrhage related to thrombocytopenia	1.3
Radiation myelopathy	1.2
Radiation plexopathy	1.1
Intracranial haemorrhage from tumour	0.6

[a] Modified from Clouston et al., 1992.[54] A total of 1042 diagnoses were given with up to three per patient. Among the non-cancer-related diagnoses, cerebro-vascular disease, headache, and degenerative spine disease were the most common diagnoses.

supratentorial regions are more often affected (85 per cent of all central nervous system metastases). However, vasculature is not the only factor to influence the metastatic process. For example, some pelvic tumours tend to metastasize to the posterior fossa and the cerebellum (53 per cent of central nervous system metastases from pelvic tumours, excluding gastrointestinal tumours).

Brain metastases can cause symptoms by compression, local destruction, irritation of brain tissue, brain oedema, and bleeding. The most common effect of a metastatic lesion is brain oedema and increased ICP. Focal symptoms can be due to oedema or bleeding. As discussed previously, typical presentations include cognitive failure, seizures, and the syndrome of intracranial hypertension.

Clinical course

After clinical presentation of a brain metastasis, the median survival is about 2 months if no treatment is given, depending on tumour type[8]. Patients who have access to brain radiotherapy and respond favourably to this modality usually die of their systemic disease. Patients who do not receive radiotherapy or do not respond often die of direct effects related to the brain metastasis[74].

The signs and symptoms of brain metastases are highly variable (Table 10.11.13). Symptoms can present progressively and deceptively, or alternatively, can be sudden, and 'stroke-like'. It should be remembered that in many patients formal neurological tests of strength and mental function will reveal signs of changes in the central nervous system that are not otherwise apparent[8].

Headache is an important symptom of brain metastasis. The headache usually is aching in quality and moderate in intensity. It is caused by compression or traction of intracranial pain-sensitive structures. With supratentorial lesions, it is often bifrontal, although it can occur on one side—always that of the tumour. Headache occurs more frequently and is more severe with infratentorial lesions, and in this case, is referred to the nuchal region and the neck[8].

ICP is not always elevated with brain metastases. When it occurs, the clinical features can be distinctive, as explained previously.

Treatment

The treatment of a brain metastasis requires a careful assessment of the the type of cancer and its sensitivity to radiation and chemotherapy, the neurological status of the patient, the extent of systemic disease, symptoms and other complications and comorbidities, expectations concerning quality of life with and without treatment, and both the goals of care expressed at the time of diagnosis and the broader values of the patient. It should be understood that the provision of supportive treatment only is among the therapeutic options available.

Surgery is indicated only for single metastases with limited or no systemic disease, especially with radioresistant tumours[75]. Whole brain irradiation (WBRT) produces neurological improvement in the majority of patients but survival after treatment is only 4–6 months. Metastases from breast and lung cancers usually have a relatively good response to radiotherapy, showing both clinical and radiological improvement. Treatment should never be withheld solely on the basis of histology, however, because, on occasion, lesions from radioresistant tumours do respond. Clinical improvement in the absence of radiological improvement is relatively common during treatment of metastases from melanoma, colon cancer, or renal cancer.

Newer techniques for focal radiation may be of benefit. Focal brain irradiation or 'radiosurgery' can have a role in treating single, or occasionally two, brain metastases, sometimes in combination with whole brain irradiation. The aim of this strategy is eradication of disease from the brain[75] and radiosurgery is used as a substitute for surgery in this context[75]. Radiosurgery also may be considered for palliation of single or double lesions in the brain when the disease is advanced and a shorter course of treatment (and a shorter expected latency for symptomatic improvement) would be greatly preferred. It can also be used in cases where there is recurrence in the brain after whole brain irradiation. The role of focal brain irradiation in combination or not with WBRT remain to be clearly defined and should follow rational guidelines[75].

Corticosteroids

Treatment with steroids is recommended for all symptomatic patients with brain metastases or primary brain tumour. The main therapeutic effect is probably related to a reduction in peri-tumoral

Table 10.11.13 Symptoms and signs due to cerebral metastases.

Symptoms more frequent	Symptoms less frequent	Signs more frequent	Signs less frequent
Headache	Ataxia	Impaired cognition	Unilateral sensory loss
Focal weakness	Aphasia	Hemiparesis	Papilloedema
Mental change			Ataxia
Seizures			Aphasia

oedema from partial restoration of the blood–brain barrier. Steroids are also recommended for all patients undergoing brain irradiation. Treatment should start 48 h before radiation. A traditional regimen is dexamethasone 16 mg/day in four divided doses, which is tapered beginning the second week of radiation. Tapering should be gradual (2–4 mg every fifth day).

Higher steroid doses can be given acutely if symptoms recur (e.g. restarting 16 mg/day) or if there are signs of increased ICP or cerebral herniation (e.g. 16–100 mg IV once, followed again by tapering). If a steroid cannot be discontinued, the dose should be tapered to the minimum required for symptom control. Dexamethasone taper and discontinuation should always be attempted after completion of radiation treatment, since in most patients steroids are not necessary to preserve neurological function.

Spinal cord compression

Pathology

Most cases of epidural spinal cord compression in populations with cancer are caused by a vertebral body metastasis invading the epidural space posteriorly and compressing the spinal cord or cauda equina. Invasion of the epidural space through the intervertebral foramina by a paraspinal lesion also can occur, and is relatively more likely in lymphoma and neuroblastoma; the absence of a bony lesion on radiography in these cases can lead to misdiagnosis. Very rarely, spinal cord syndromes are due to epidural or cord metastases. Metastases from breast, lung, and prostate cancers more often affect the thoracic spine, whereas the lumbar spine is more often affected by metastases from colorectal and other pelvic tumours.

Other causes of epidural compression include epidural abscess or haemorrhage, herniated disc, and other rare epidural masses (such as epidural lipomatosis and extramedullary haematopoiesis). Spinal cord, including conus medullaris, and cauda equina lesions have similar aetiologies, mechanisms, and clinical implications, and are therefore usually considered together.

Clinical course

Spinal cord compression occurs in 5–10 per cent of cases of cancer.[8] It is a neurological emergency, as functional outcome is dependent on the degree of neurological impairment at diagnosis and the initial response to therapy. Other factors important in prognosis are tumour histology and rate of progression of the neurological symptoms. The importance of early diagnosis cannot be over-emphasized; symptoms are usually present for some weeks before the neurological emergency occurs. Pain precedes other neurological symptoms in almost every case, but diagnosis is often delayed until the onset of neurological symptoms and signs.

Pain of long duration, which suddenly changes its characteristics, should prompt re-evaluation and spinal imaging. Pain in a crescendo pattern is particularly worrisome, as is pain aggravated by recumbency, pain associated with the Valsalva manoeuvre, and radicular pain (pain occurring or radiating in a dermatomal distribution).

The occurrence of a Lhermitte's sign also should raise concern about the possibility of tumour compression of the spinal cord. A Lhermitte's sign, also described as 'barber's chair sign' in the British literature, is a shock-like sensation passing down the trunk and one or more extremities when the neck is flexed. It also may occur

spontaneously or be precipitated by sudden limb movements, or by coughing or sneezing. It is due to demyelination or compression of the posterior column of the spinal cord in the cervical or upper thoracic regions. Lhermitte's sign is frequent in multiple sclerosis, but it is not uncommon in cancer-related spinal cord dysfunction. In the cancer population, the differential diagnosis ranges from relatively benign conditions such as transient radiation myelopathy and cisplatin injury, to severe complications such as cord compression and progressive radiation myelopathy[76].

Diagnosis

The neurological signs associated with epidural disease depend on the location of the compressive lesion. If the spinal cord is involved (typically with lesions at or above, the T12–L1 spinal level), signs are consistent with myelopathy and usually begin with paraesthesiae or sensory loss in the feet, which ascends as the compression worsens. Weakness of hip flexors, and then other lower extremity muscles, also occurs. The sensory signs may be helpful in defining the level of the compression (Table 10.11.14). If the lesion is at the T12–L1 level, a conus medullaris syndrome may be the presenting phenomenology, with early loss of sphincter control and 'saddle' sensory symptoms or signs. A more caudal lesion causes a cauda equine syndrome, which may mimic myelopathy or be prominently asymmetric, with weakness or sensory changes affecting one leg more than another.

Emergency imaging of the spinal cord and canal should be carried out in patients with cancer and back pain who have symptoms of myelopathy (including conus medullaris) or cauda equine syndrome. Ideally, this should be done when the characteristic back pain is noted and before significant neurological signs ensue[77].

Other clinical and radiological characteristics are often associated with epidural invasion. In patients with back pain and bone changes on spine radiograph, epidural invasion has occurred in 60–70 per cent of cases, and in 80 per cent of cases where there is vertebral collapse of more than 50 per cent. In patients with radiculopathy, there is epidural invasion in 60 per cent of cases. Ninety per cent of patients with radiculopathy and bone changes on radiograph have epidural invasion. However, in cases of lymphoma, radiographs that show no bony changes may be misleading (because tumour grows in through the intervertebral foramina from the paraspinal gutter without injuring bone) and false-negative results can be as high as 70 per cent[8]. A positive bone scan without radiological changes is associated with epidural invasion in only 17 per cent of patients[78].

Fig. 10.11.1 summarizes the clinical and radiological findings that should prompt either immediate treatment or spinal cord imaging with magnetic resonance imaging (MRI), the results of which will dictate the treatment modality[77]. Although MRI is the best imaging procedure in these patients, myelography or computed tomography (CT) still has a place when MRI is unavailable. There may be multiple lesions and the whole spine should be evaluated.

Treatment (see also Chapter 9.2)

If the goals of care support aggressive treatment of epidural spinal cord or cauda equine compression, steroids and radiation should be offered[79,80]. Steroids can reduce pain, preserve neurological function, and improve functional outcome after definitive treatment[81]. Dexamethasone in high doses is recommended for high-degree lesions, as shown by severe or rapidly progressing neurologcal

Table 10.11.14 Localizing signs with spinal cord lesions.

Sign	Clinical level		
	Cord	Conus and epiconus medullaris	Cauda equina
Motor	Paraparesis usually flaccid	If epiconus involved L5–S3 weakness	Never pyramidal signs
	Pyramidal signs can be present	If conus S2–S3 weakness	Often asymmetrical weakness
Reflex	Absent or hyperactive	Patellar hyperactive	Hypoactive
		Ankle hypoactive	Asymmetrical
Babinski sign	Usually present	Present only if lesion of epiconus	Never present
Sensory	Symmetrical level of dermatomal level sensory loss (locates compression within two dermatomes above the sensory level)	If conus S2–S5 'saddle' sensory loss	Asymmetrical findings in the lower extremities and perineum
		If epiconus L4–S5	
Sphincter control	Can be initially preserved	Early involved sometimes selectively	Can be preserved

abnormalities, or by MRI evidence of a severe lesion or myelographic block (80 per cent or more). A low-dose regimen should be used for low-degree lesions, as suggested by stable or slowly progressing neurological findings, or by MRI or myelography. The high-dose regimen includes an initial intravenous bolus of 100 mg followed by a tapering schedule of 96 mg orally for 3 days and subsequent halving of the dose every third day until the end of radiation treatment[8,80]. The use of high doses for epidural spinal cord compression has been questioned[82], but experimental data favour this method.

In the past, posterior laminectomy and radiation were the most used treatment modalities. Review of the literature and one randomized trial showed no advantage for posterior laminectomy plus radiation over the use of radiation alone[83], and indeed posterior laminectomy can aggravate spine instability and neurological compromise.[83] A more rational surgical approach for anteriorly compressing lesions is vertebral body resection[84], but the procedure requires intact vertebral elements above and below the affected level to stabilize the spine after surgery. Surgery is the first choice where the site of the primary tumour is unknown, where there is relapse after radiation treatment, and in cases of spinal instability or vertebral displacement. It should also be considered when neurological symptoms progress during radiotherapy, in plegia of rapid onset, and when the tumours is not likely to be radiosensitive.

An evaluation of overall results of radiation and posterior laminectomy showed that ambulatory patients retained ambulation, and about half of paraparetic patients regained ambulation; paraplegic patients rarely recovered[83]. Some series showed impressive results with vertebral resection. In one series, 13 of 36 paraplegic patients regained ambulation[84]. One controlled clinical trial suggests that surgery can be the efirst choice for selected patients with better prognosis[85]. However, the numbers of patients are still too small to assess the benefits of this type of surgery. Prognosis and expected quality of life should influence the decision; it seems certainly worthwhile in some cases.

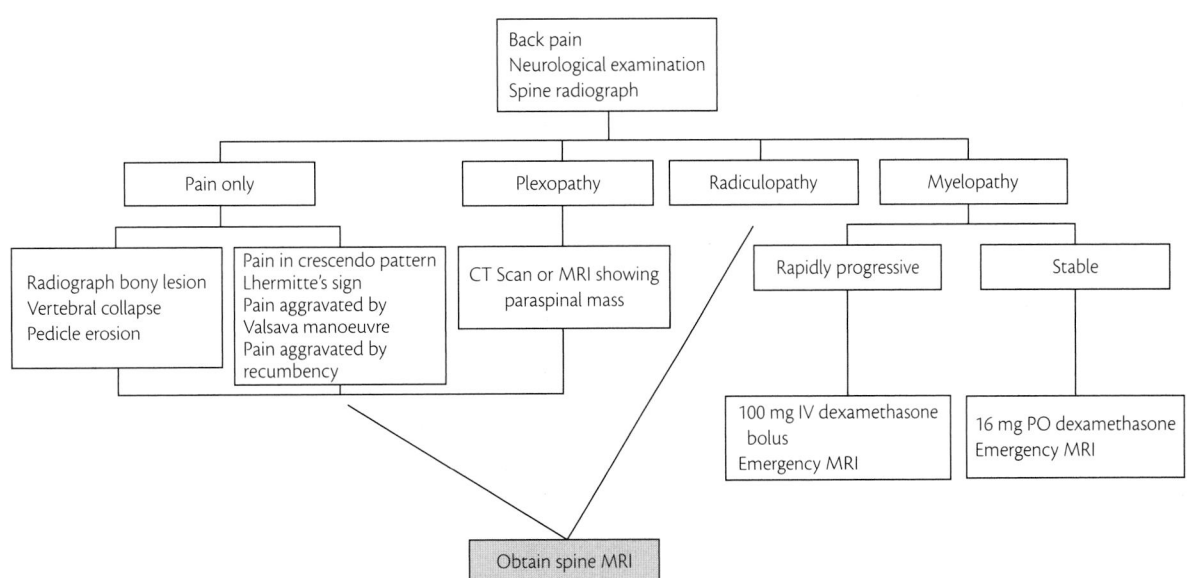

Figure 10.11.1 Algorithm for the evaluation of back pain in the patient with cancer.

Leptomeningeal metastases

Pathology

Leptomeningeal metastases (also known as carcinomatous meningitis or meningeal carcinomatosis) are caused by the dissemination of cancerous cells throughout the subarachnoid space. These cells can reach the meninges through the general circulation or the perineural spaces along nerve roots, by direct invasion from epidural lesions, or by direct seeding from existing brain tumours[160]. Meningeal involvement can be multifocal or diffuse, and either visible on imaging as discrete masses or not visible on imaging because of microscopic infiltration.

Clinical course

Leptomeningeal metastases were once considered an unusual complication of systemic cancer (1–8 per cent of cases at autopsy)[8] but these are increasingly seen nowadays, usually as a result of breast or lung cancer, lymphoma, leukaemia, or melanoma. Life expectancy is usually short, ranging from 3 to 6 months in patients who have received intensive treatment. Many patients are not offered treatment and their survival is shorter[8,86].

The clinical findings associated with leptomeningeal disease may relate to central nervous system or peripheral nervous system dysfunction, or some combination. The clinical syndromes are highly variable. The pathophysiology includes abnormality in the flow and absorption of cerebrospinal fluid (which can result in hydrocephalus)[164], direct involvement of the cranial and peripheral nerve meningeal sheets, competition with brain metabolism, invasion of the brain parenchyma or nerve roots, and areas of focal ischaemia.

The most common symptoms are headache, change in mental status, and radicular-type pain[8,86,87], but cranial nerve involvement, seizures, polyradiculopathy, and cauda equina syndrome also occur in varying combinations. Meningismus is uncommon, unlike infectious meningitis. Multiple symptoms, from involvement of different levels of the neuraxis, are often seen.

Diagnosis

Diagnosis is usually confirmed from examination of the cerebrospinal fluid (CSF)[86]. While malignant cells may not be apparent in the first sample of CSF, other abnormalities are usually found, such as high opening pressure, high protein content, increased white cell count, or low glucose content. In one series, only 3 per cent of the first samples were completely normal[86]. Other markers and immunocytochemical techniques have not been found to have clinical value[86]. Repeated lumbar punctures often are needed to establish the diagnosis. Contrast-enhanced MRI also can be useful[87] (Fig. 10.11.2), as the only sign of leptomeningeal metastases may be slight enhancement of the meninges due to blood–brain barrier disruption or focal enlargement of roots.

Therapy

Traditionally, treatment modalities have been based on a combination of corticosteroids, radiotherapy, and intrathecal or intraventricular chemotherapy. Systemic chemotherapy may also be helpful in some cases with appropriate tumour histology. In one series, only 23 per cent of treated patients could be regarded as long-term survivors. Intrathecal chemotherapy did not achieve better results than systemic chemotherapy (median survival 23 months)[86,88],

and caused a treatment-related leucoencephalopathy in 58 per cent of cases. The role of intrathecal chemotherapy therefore requires prospective study.

Base of the skull and cranial nerve syndromes

Lesions at the base of the skull are commonly caused by metastasis from breast, prostate, and other tumours[89] or from local invasion by advanced head and neck tumours[90]. Symptoms secondary to bone lesions are commonly associated with alterations of cranial nerve function. Headache at the site of the lesion or referred to the vertex or to the entire affected side of the head is also frequent[8,89]. The best imaging procedure for all these syndromes is CT scan with bone window studies. Treatment with radiation is indicated, to control pain and neurological dysfunction.

Orbital syndrome

Progressive retro-orbital and supraorbital pain characterizes this syndrome, which may also be associated with blurred vision and diplopia. Chemosis, proptosis, external ophthalmoplegia, ipsilateral papilloedema, and sensory loss (in a trigeminal distribution) are common.

Parasellar and cavernous sinus syndrome

In this syndrome, unilateral supraorbital and frontal headache is associated with ocular palsies, diplopia, and unilateral papilloedema. There may be hemianopsia or quadrantanopsia, secondary to optic chiasm compression.

Middle cranial fossa syndrome

The common symptom is facial pain associated with numbness along the distribution of the second or third trigeminal nerves. The pain can be continuous and dull, be referred to the affected side of the head, and be associated with paroxysmal episodes of lancinating pain in a trigeminal distribution. There may be ocular palsies, caused by contiguous extension to the cavernous sinus.

Jugular foramen syndrome

This syndrome usually presents with hoarseness and dysphagia. Pain is referred to the mastoid region, the neck, or the shoulder,

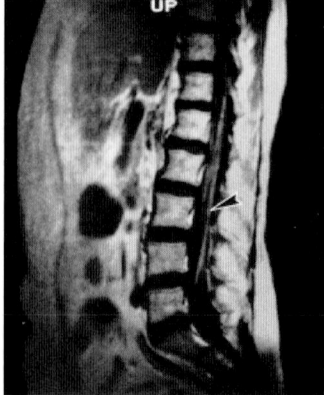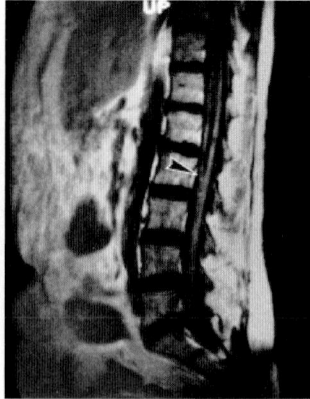

Figure 10.11.2 MRI, gadolium enhanced. The white enhancement of the meningeal sheath around the cauda equina (left side, arrow) and the thecal sac (right side arrow) due to meningeal infiltration.

with an associated diffuse, unilateral headache. Horner's syndrome and IX, X, XI, and sometimes XII nerve palsy can occur.

Occipital condyle syndrome

Unilateral nuchal pain, aggravated by neck flexion, with neck stiffness and a characteristic tilt of the head, occur in this syndrome. There is limited movement of the head and tenderness over the occipitocervical junction. The XI and XII nerves are often affected.

Clivus syndrome

While vertex headache may occur, the pain can often be referred behind the eye, radiating posteriorly to the occiput. XI and XII nerve dysfunction is the most common finding, but other lower cranial nerves (VI–IX) can be affected. Symptoms can occur on one or both sides.

Sphenoid and ethmoid sinus syndromes

These usually present with bilateral frontal headaches, nasal congestion and discharge, and diplopia secondary to VI nerve involvement.

Other cranial neuropathy syndromes

Glossopharyngeal nerve

The typical patient has throat and neck pain, which radiates to the ear and is aggravated by swallowing. Pharyngeal and other carcinomas of the neck can present with odynophagia with reflex otalgia. Severe pain may be associated with syncope[92]. Although it has been described with leptomeningeal disease, it commonly results from local nerve infiltration in the neck or base of the skull.

Trigeminal nerve

The most common presentation is a constant dull, well-localized pain related to the underlying disease of bone and other somatic structures. This pain may be associated with paroxysmal episodes of lancinating or throbbing pain. The quality of the pain sometimes can mimic classical trigeminal neuralgia, but an atypical facial pain is more common[93]. Atypical trigeminal pain and sensory abnormalities in the peripheral distribution of the V nerve, occasionally associated with incomplete lesions of the VII nerve, have been reported with different facial neoplasms[93].

Involvement of the mental nerve does not usually produce pain but can cause the 'numb chin syndrome'. This is a sign of bony disease of jaw or foramen ovale, but can also be found with tumours of the base of the skull or leptomeninges and local perineural spread of lip carcinoma. The symptom can occur months before the discovery of a bony lesion[94].

Radiculopathy

Radiculopathy is usually caused by the compression of nerve roots by vertebral or paraspinal lesions, or by leptomeningeal metastases. The pain of a root lesion is usually focal and radiates in the distribution of the affected root. It is sometimes difficult to distinguish a polyradiculopathy from a plexus lesion; in these cases, the neurological assessment can be supplemented by electrodiagnostic studies of the paraspinal muscles, thus identifying the level of the lesion. CT and MRI are useful for imaging non-bony paraspinal lesions. MRI is necessary for imaging the epidural space.

Herpes zoster and post-herpetic neuralgia are common in patients with cancer and should always be considered in the differential diagnosis of painful radiculopathies.

Cervical plexopathy

Infiltration of the cervical plexus by tumour can be a result of compression by head and neck neoplasms or metastases to cervical nodes. Symptoms usually include local lancinating or dysaesthetic pain referred to the retro-auricular and nuchal areas, the shoulder, and the jaw. Sensory abnormalities define the affected (greater auricular and greater occipital) nerves[90]. The differential diagnosis should include post-radical neck dissection syndrome. The diagnosis in patients with head and neck cancer may be difficult because of the postoperative and postradiation changes often found in these patients.

CT or MRI scan is appropriate, and imaging of the cervical spine and paraspinal structures is very important in distinguishing between bony lesions, cervical radiculopathy, and epidural spinal cord compression.

Brachial plexopathy

Five per cent of the neurological consultations at a comprehensive cancer centre were found to be initiated by brachial plexopathy[54]. It occurs most often with breast and lung carcinoma, and with lymphoma. The plexus can be compressed or infiltrated by tumour lying in contiguous structures, such as axillary or supraclavicular nodes, or the apex of the lung. Pain is the first symptom in 85 per cent of patients[95], preceding other neurological symptoms or signs by weeks or months.

Breast and lung malignancies typically affect the lower plexus (C7–T1) (Fig. 10.11.3) and cause pain in the shoulder, elbow, hand, and the fourth and fifth finger. Lung tumours can affect the intercostobrachial nerve, giving rise to a pain syndrome and associated sensory disturbances in the axilla (C8–T1–T2). The upper brachial plexus (C5–C6) can also be affected, especially by breast cancer, when pain is usually referred to the paraspinal region, shoulder, biceps region, elbow, and hand; burning dysaesthesia in the index finger or thumb is common. The hallmark of the syndrome is the neuropathic nature of the pain with numbness, paraesthesia, allodynia, and hyperaesthesia.

CT scan with narrow sections and contrast enhancement is effective in imaging soft tissue and bony structures in the plexus area. All patients with symptoms of brachial plexopathy should have a scan of the contiguous paravertebral region before radiation therapy, since extension of disease in this region is common (13/41 cases in one series). MRI is particularly useful in imaging the contiguous epidural space. While use of both techniques can give helpful complementary information in doubtful cases, sometimes neither is helpful even in cases of proven metastatic plexopathy[96]. Comparative data on specificity and sensitivity of the two techniques is lacking.

Epidural invasion eventually will occur in some patients with brachial plexopathy (Fig. 10.11.4). Imaging of the epidural space is essential when patients develop Horner's syndrome, panplexopathy, vertebral body erosion, or a paraspinal mass detected on CT scan. These are often hallmark symptoms of tumour progression into the epidural space.

Radiation fibrosis is important in the differential diagnosis of brachial plexopathy in cancer (Table 10.11.15), particularly in

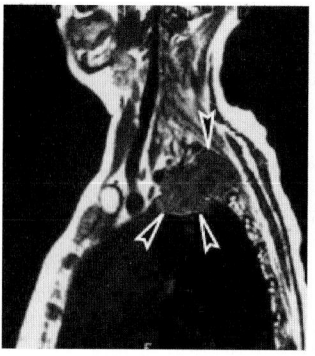
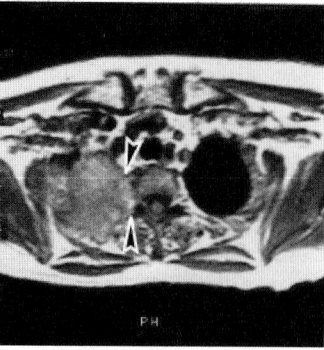

Figure 10.11.3 MRI image. Lung tumour in the upper lobe compressing the lower trunk of the brachial plexus. Pain was reported in the inner aspect of the arm and paraesthesiae in the 5th and 4th finger. Left side: the arrows show the tumour mass invading the tissue planes in the area of the brachial plexus. Right side: the tumour is invading the left upper lobe, the arrows show the tumour invading one thoracic vertebral body. Reproduced with permission from Caraceni, A. (1996). Clinicopathologic correlates of common cancer pain syndromes. *Hematology and Oncology Clinics of North America,* **10**, 57–78.

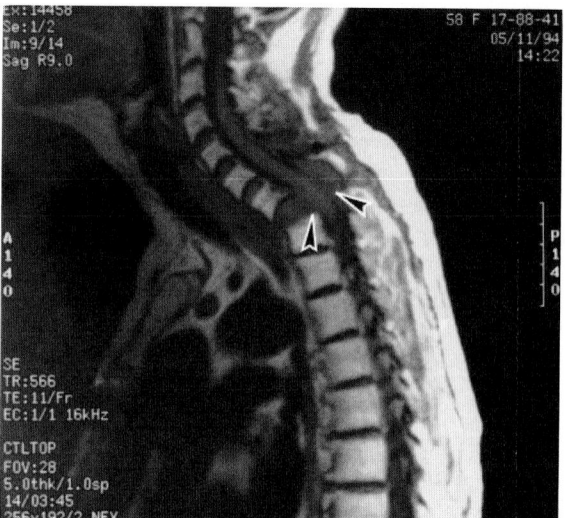

Figure 10.11.4 MRI image in the same case as shown in Fig. 10.11.3. The tumour is invading the epidural canal and compressing the spinal cord. Reproduced with permission from Caraceni, A. (1996). Clinicopathologic correlates of common cancer pain syndromes. *Hematology and Oncology Clinics of North America,* **10**, 57–78.

patients who have had radiotherapy and who present with upper plexus signs. Pain is often less prominent in patients with radiation-induced plexopathy.

Although electrodiagnostic studies and imaging may distinguish radiation-induced plexopathy from malignant invasion[97], this differential diagnosis sometimes is difficult. In these cases, PET scan can be very useful but, at times, surgical exploration of the plexus is necessary to rule out fibrosis, a new primary tumour, a radiation-induced tumour, or recurrent cancer.

Lumbosacral plexopathy

Lumbosacral plexopathy is one of the most disabling complications of cancer. Although it is commonly associated with colorectal, cervical, and other pelvic malignancies (bladder, uterus, prostate, sarcoma, lymphoma), it can also be caused by breast or lung cancer or melanoma. Retroperitoneal tumours (e.g. sarcoma, metastatic nodal tumours) may affect the lumbosacral plexus or its roots more proximally.

The presenting symptom in almost all cases (93 per cent)[98] is pain in the buttocks or the legs. Pain often precedes other symptoms by weeks or months. It is usually followed by numbness, paraesthesia, weakness, and, later, leg oedema. The pain is usually aching or pressure-like in quality, and is rarely burning or dysaesthetic. In one series[98], an upper plexopathy (L1–L4) was found in about one-third of cases, a lower plexopathy (L4–S1) in one-half of cases, and panplexopathy (L1–S3) in about 20 per cent (Table 10.11.16).

Other structures can be involved. These include nerve roots from proximal extension of the tumour, or contiguous structures, such as the sympathetic chain or the psoas muscle. Selective involvement of the L1, iliohypogastric, ilioinguinal, or genitofemoral nerves can produce pain and paraesthesia in the inguinal and scrotal region.

A sacral plexopathy, often overlapping a sacral polyradiculopathy, can be produced from direct extension of a presacral mass invading the sacrum, as sometimes occurs with rectosigmoid and bladder carcinomas. The coccygeal plexus is usually affected in patients with sphincter dysfunction and perineal 'saddle' sensory loss.

Tumour is often found in the lumbar vertebrae, sacrum, or pelvis of patients with lumbosacral plexopathy (45/76 patients) and

epidural extension is also common, especially with retroperitoneal tumours. Hydroureter or hydronephrosis is extremely common at diagnosis[98,99].

Lumbosacral plexopathy can occur after pelvic irradiation. Thomas et al.[99] reported that radiation-induced lumbosacral plexopathy very rarely presents with pain and has a median latency of 5 years from radiotherapy. Motor involvement is bilateral in 80 per cent of cases and electromyography can be a useful diagnostic tool. Other differential diagnoses include leptomeningeal carcinomatosis, cauda equina compression, and non-cancer-related causes of lumbar plexopathy, such as iliopsoas muscle haemorrhage or abscess, aortic aneurysm, idiopathic acute lumbosacral neuritis, or post-surgical compressive lesions.

MRI and CT scanning both image the lumbosacral plexus effectively. CT gives more information on the bony structures, while MRI is more accurate for soft tissues. The assessment should extend from L1 through the true pelvis[98], and should include the spine and adjacent pelvic soft tissues.

Mononeuropathy

Mononeuropathy is less common than plexopathy or radicular lesions[100]. It is caused by compression or infiltration of a nerve by bony lesions or by soft tissue masses in the limbs. Intercostal nerve neuropathy from invasion of the chest wall is the most common of the mononeuropathies caused by cancer. Obturator, femoral, and sciatic neuropathies are seen when tumour involves the soft tissue along the nerve distribution in the pelvis and thigh. Peroneal mononeuropathy can occur with bony lesions of the head of the fibula and sarcoma of the popliteal fossa. Ulnar and radial neuropathies result from bony lesions in the elbow or humerus. These mononeuropathies must be distinguished from traumatic or compressive lesions, and from nutritional–metabolic lesions of nerves.

Palliative treatment of peripheral nerve compression

Radiation is the first-line therapy for plexopathy, mononeuropathy, and radiculopathy caused by tumour compression. However,

Table 10.11.15 Differential diagnosis of brachial plexopathy.

	Tumour infiltration	Radiation fibrosis
Incidence of pain	89%	18%
Severity of pain	Severe in 98%	Mild to moderate
Dose of radiotherapy	—	>6000 cGy large fractions (>1900 cGy/day)
Latency	Not indicative	>6 months <5 years
Course	Progressive neurological dysfunction	Progressive weakness
	Pain progression with dysaesthetic quality	Pain stabilizing with onset of weakness
	C7–T1 distribution[a]	C5–C6 distribution
Horner	Can be present	Absent
CT scan findings[b]	Mass with tissue infiltration	Diffuse infiltration of tissue planes
MRI scan findings[b]	High signal intensity mass on T2-weighted images	Low signal intensity lesion on T_2-weighted images
Electromyography findings	Denervation no myokymia	Myokymia

[a] The distribution of the neurological findings can be helpful in some cases but it is not always indicative (see text for more details).

[b] The use of both techniques may provide complementary information. No method is totally credible in differentiating fibrosis from tumour. PET scan nowadays can be an important diagnostic tool.

the results of radiotherapy in brachial plexopathy have been disappointing, with only 46 per cent of patients reporting relief from pain in a retrospective series.[95] Lesions caused by radio-resistant tumours, such as sarcomas, are particularly unlikely to respond.

Management of pain is often difficult in these syndromes; opioids are indicated and adjuvants for neuropathic pain should be used for specific indications. Clinical experience suggests that dexamethasone can be particularly effective for pain due to compression and oedema of peripheral nerves.

Interventional strategies may be considered in selected cases. Non-neurolytic approaches include peripheral nerve stimulation and dorsal column stimulation, and neuraxial analgesia delivered via external or implanted pump also is a possibility. Peripheral neurolytic blocks, with alcohol or phenol, can be considered for severe arm and leg pain in patients with advanced plexus lesions. These blocks are sometimes associated with significant side effects, such as paresis and incontinence. Sacral root blockade with phenol for perineal pain caused by root invasion is more acceptable when patients already have established urinary and rectal sphincter dysfunction. Late onset dysaesthesia may occur in long-term survivors.

Percutaneous cordotomy also is feasible for the pain of lumbosacral plexopathy. Brachial plexopathy is more difficult to treat

Table 10.11.16 Clinical findings in lumbosacral plexopathy due to cancer.

	Upper plexopathy	Lower plexopathy	Panplexopathy
Local pain	Lower abdomen	Buttock, perineum	Lumbosacral
Referred pain	Flank, iliac crest	Hip and ankle	Variable
Radicular pain	Anterolateral thigh	Posterolateral thigh, leg	Variable
Paraesthesiae	Anterior thigh	Perineum, thigh, sole	Anterior thigh, leg, foot
Motor and reflex changes	L2–L4	L5–S1	L2–S2
	Proximal leg weakness	Distal leg weakness	Weakness can affect different muscle groups and reflexes
	Patella reflex	Ankle reflex	
Sensory loss	Anterolateral thigh	Posterior thigh, sole	Anterior thigh, leg
Tenderness	Lumbar	Sciatic notch, sacrum	Lumbosacral
Positive SLRT			
Direct	50%	50%	83%
Reverse	15%	50%	83%
Leg oedema	41%	37%	83%
Rectal mass	25%	43%	15%
Anal sphincter weakness	0	50%	0

SLRT, straight leg raising test or Lasegue manoeuvre.

Source: modified from Jaeckle *et al.* (1985),[98] with permission.

with cordotomy because the cervical dermatomes up to C4 must be included. This is technically difficult and increases the risk of respiratory depression and neurological sequelae. A short prognosis (6 months to 1 year) is required to avoid long-term post-cordotomy dysaesthetic pain.

Peripheral polyneuropathy

Polyneuropathy in cancer patients can be caused by chemotherapy, metabolic disturbance or nutritional deficiency, or paraneoplastic syndromes (Table 10.11.17)[100]. Subclinical dysfunction of small and large sensory fibres can be demonstrated with quantitative sensory testing in 30–40 per cent of cancer patients[101].

Peripheral neuropathy is characterized by a stocking–glove distribution of negative sensory and positive sensory symptoms. Loss of sensation may predominate, or there may be painless paraesthesia or distressing burning dysaesthesia, allodynia, and hyperalgesia. Early sensory loss and later motor signs (weakness) are characteristic of some drug-induced sensorimotor neuropathies (vincristine, paclitaxel). Sensory involvement can be selective in neuropathies associated with cisplatin or paraneoplastic syndromes. Often the only early sign of polyneuropathy is reduction or loss of the ankle reflex. Muscle cramps may be associated with neuropathy and can sometimes be prominent symptoms in vincristine neuropathy.

Table 10.11.17 Polyneuropathies and peripheral neuropathies.

Related to cancer
Myeloma associated neuropathies
Paraneoplastic sensory neuronopathy (Denny–Brown)
Sensory–motor peripheral neuropathy
Nutritional factors (cachexia-associated neuromyopathy[a])
Cancer related metabolic dysfunction: hepatic, renal
Infiltration of peripheral nerves (lymphomas, leukaemias)[b]
Vascular (haemorrhagic or ischaemic) peripheral nervelesion[b]
Related to chemotherapy and radiation
Vincristine
Vinblastine
Vinorelbine
Cisplatin
Oxaliplatin
Paclitaxel
Suramin
Epothilones
Thalidomide
Bortezomid
Radiation to limbs with worsening of vincristine neuropathy
Non-cancer related
Metabolic dysfunction: diabetes

[a] Very frequent.

[b] Mononeuritis multiplex.

Muscle cramps are relatively frequent in cancer (see Table 10.11.18 for different aetiologies).

Paraneoplastic sensory neuropathy and sensory neuropathy caused by vincristine or paclitaxel is often more painful than that caused by cisplatin. Cisplatin induces a sensory neuronopathy mainly affecting the cells of the dorsal root ganglia. There is predominant involvement of the large fibre functions (proprioception), which causes sensory ataxia rather than pain. Vinca alkaloids and paclitaxel produce a mostly sensory axonopathy with some motor component. New antineoplastic drugs that interfere with specific metabolic pathways, such as bortezomid, also have distinct toxic effects on the peripheral nervous system[100].

Clinical examination is usually sufficient for diagnosis of a polyneuropathy, although nerve conduction studies and electromyography may provide additional information[201]. Treatment is palliative, with analgesics and adjuvants.

Cerebrovascular disorders in patients with cancer

Cerebrovascular disease in patients with cancer is not uncommon. It is often tumour-related, either as a direct effect of the tumour or its treatment or as an indirect effect of coagulation changes. Coronary and cerebral arteriosclerosis is less common in patients dying of cancer than in the general population. In one study, cerebrovascular lesions were found at autopsy in 15 per cent of cases[102] and half of these patients had clinical symptoms related to the pathological findings. There were 500 cerebrovascular lesions, of which 244 were haemorrhagic and 256 ischaemic. Only 72 of the ischaemic lesions were related to atherosclerosis and nine haemorrhages were hypertensive; the remaining lesions were related to tumour-associated conditions. Haemorrhagic diatheses (thrombocytopenia, disseminated intravascular coagulation) or hypercoagulability states are common causes.

Cerebral haematoma is more common than subarachnoid haemorrhage and is the complication most frequently seen in leukaemia. Ischaemic complications caused by thrombotic emboli due to nonbacterial thrombotic endocarditis are a frequent finding at autopsy in patients with advanced cancer but are difficult to demonstrate during life since transoesophageal echocardiography is required[103]. If the diagnosis is made, treatment with heparin is recommended[103].

Multiple microinfarcts can produce a global encephalopathy associated with mild disseminated intravascular coagulation, but with no laboratory abnormalities, in patients with leukaemia, lymphoma, or breast cancer[104]. Other syndromes are listed in Table 10.11.19.

Table 10.11.18 Muscle cramps in cancer.

Aetiology	Number of patients
Peripheral neuropathy	22
Root and plexus pathology	17
Polymyositis	2
Hypomagnesaemia	1
Unknown	9

Source: modified from Steiner, I. and Siegal, T. (1989). Muscle cramps in cancer patients. *Cancer*, **63**, 574–7, with permission.

Table 10.11.19 Cerebrovascular complications of cancer.

Central nervous system complication	Mechanism
Cerebral haemorrhage	Intratumoural bleeding[a]
	Disseminated intravascular coagulation[b]
	Coagulopathy[b]
	Leucostasis[c]
Subdural haematoma	Dural metastases[d]
	Coagulopathy[d]
Embolic infarct	Non-bacterial thrombotic endocarditis[d]
	Tumour embolism[d]
	Fungal embolism[b]
Sinus thrombosis	Dural, bony tumour[d]
	Coagulopathy[d]
	L-asparaginase[b]
Thrombotic microinfarcts	Disseminated intravascular coagulation[b,d]

[a]Associated with cerebral and leptomeningeal tumour.

[b]Associated with leukaemia/lymphoma.

[c]Only found with leucocytes ≥ 100 000.

[d]Associated with solid tumours.

Paraneoplastic syndromes

The pathogenesis of remote effects of systemic cancer on the nervous system is unknown, although autoimmune processes are seen in many syndromes and autoantibody determinations are sometimes helpful in diagnosis. Paraneoplastic syndromes are rare, probably affecting less than 1 per cent of patients with cancer (see also Table 10.11.1)[8,105,106]. Some classic paraneoplastic syndromes can be recognized and diagnosed with confidence (Table 10.11.20). Cerebellar degeneration associated with ovarian and lung cancer, or peripheral neuronopathy and limbic encephalitis associated with small-cell tumours of the lung are relatively stereotyped clinico-pathological entities associated with the presence of specific autoantibodies (anti-Yo for cerebellar degeneration and anti-Hu for neuronopathy with encephalomyelitis). Opsoclonus–myoclonus and Lambert–Eaton myasthenic syndrome occurring in children with neuroblastomas and in small-cell lung cancer, respectively, are also classic in their presentation. However, many syndromes present with varying symptoms, affecting the brain and cranial nerves, spinal cord and dorsal root ganglia, or peripheral nerves

Table 10.11.20 Paraneoplastic neurological syndromes.

Lambert–Eaton myasthenic syndrome
Sub-acute cerebellar degeneration
Sub-acute sensory neuronopathy
Opsoclonus–myoclonus
Motor neuronopathy (with lymphoma)
Limbic encephalitis

and muscles, and pose difficult diagnostic problems[8,105–107]. There is little in the literature on these syndromes, although the term encephalomyelitis is reserved by some authors for those patients with evidence of widespread neurological dysfunction without findings predominantly in one particular area[105].

In general, neurological symptoms and signs related to paraneoplastic phenomena develop acutely and are severe. Subtle, long-lasting symptoms are not usually caused by paraneoplastic syndromes. Examination of CSF and immunofluorescence techniques for testing circulating autoantibodies can aid diagnosis. MRI scans are usually normal[107].

The clinical course is independent of that of the original tumour, which in 50 per cent of cases is found after the onset of neurological symptoms. The associated tumour often is small and slow growing, and may have a relatively benign course. Remission of the neurological symptoms only occasionally follows treatment of the tumour. Spontaneous remissions have been seen, but the syndrome is usually irreversible. The results of treatment are poor; steroids and plasmapheresis are not effective except in the Lambert–Eaton syndrome, where plasmapheresis is indicated. The administration of immunoglobulin preparation can be worthwhile in peripheral syndromes[106].

The Lambert–Eaton syndrome is the only paraneoplastic syndrome for which an autoimmune pathogenesis has been proved with animal models. The syndrome is caused by a reduced release of acetylcholine from presynaptic membranes. It presents with muscle weakness and fatiguability. Proximal muscles are affected and bulbar musculature usually are spared. Strength initially improves with exercise and examination can therefore be ambiguous since power can improve during testing, although weakness recurs after continuous effort. Fifty per cent of patients have dry mouth and impotence. The diagnosis is made by electromyography, with a classic finding of small compound action potentials that increase with exercise. Repetitive stimulation at a low and high rate produces a decrease and increase in the compound action potential, respectively. Most patients have autoantibodies that react with the calcium channels at the cholinergic synapse level. It often responds to immunosuppression and plasmapheresis.

Adverse neurological effects of anticancer therapy

Surgery, chemotherapy, or radiation can cause neurological syndromes. They are discussed in greater detail elsewhere in this textbook (see Section 9). In particular, irradiation of the brain can produce multiple acute and chronic adverse effects; acute effects include worsening of neurological symptoms, somnolence, and Lhermitte's sign, and the main chronic effect is dementia caused by radiation necrosis and leucoencephalopathy.

References

1. Lundberg, N. (1960). Continuous recording and control of ventricular fluid pressure in neurosurgical practice. *Acta Psychiatrica et Neurologica Scandinavica*, **36** (Suppl 149).
2. Klatzo, I. (1967). Neuropathological aspects of brain edema. *Journal of Neuropathology and Experimental Neurology*, **26**, 1–14.
3. Rosner, M., Rosner, S., and Johnson, A. (1995). Cerebral perfusion pressure: management protocol and clinical results. *Journal of Neurosurgery*, **83**, 949–62.

4. Howe, H. (1925). Reduction of normal cerebrospinal fluid pressure by intravenous administration of hypertonic solutions. *Archives of Neurology and Psychiatry*, **14**, 315–26.

5. Nau, R. (2000). Osmotherapy for elevated intracranial pressure. A critical reappraisal. *Clinical Pharmacokinetics*, **38**, 23–40.

6. Galicich, J.H. and French, L.A. (1961). Use of dexamethasone in the treatment of cerebral edema resulting from brain tumors and surgery. *American Practitioner and Digest of Treatment*, **12**, 169–74.

7. Schimmer, B. and Parker, K. (2006). Adrenocorticotropic hormone: Adrenocortical steroids and their synthetic analogs; inhibitors of the synthesis and actions of adrenocortical hormones. In *Goodman & Gilman's The Pharmacological Basis of Therapeutics* (eds L.B. Brunton, J.S. Lazo, and K.L. Parker), pp. 1587–612. McGraw-Hill, New York.

8. Posner, J.B. (1995). Neurologic complications of cancer. *Contemporary Neurology Series, Vol. 45*. F.A. Davis, Philadelphia.

9. Batchelor, T., Taylor, L., Thaler, H. *et al.* (1997). Steroid myopathy in cancer patients. *Neurology*, **48**, 1234–8.

10. McCluskey, J. and Gutteridge, D. (1982). Avascular necrosis of bone after high doses of dexamethasone during neurosurgery. *British Medical Journal*, **284**, 333–4.

11. Cushing, H. (1932). Peptic ulcers and the interbrain. *Surgery, Gynecology and Obstetrics*, **55**, 1–35.

12. LeWitt, P., Barton, N., and Posner, J. (1982). Hiccup with dexamethasone therapy. *Annals of Neurology*, **12**, 405–6.

13. Vanelle, J.-M., Aubin, F., and Michel, F. (1990). Les complications psychiatriques de la corticotherapie. *La Revue du Praticien*, **40**, 556–8.

14. Freedmann, M., Schocket, A., Chapel, N. *et al.* (1981). Anaphylaxis after intravenous methylprednisolone administration. *Journal of the American Medical Association*, **245**, 607–8.

15. Garbe, E., LeLorier, J., Boivin, J.-F. *et al.* (1997). Risk of ocular hypertension or open-angle glaucoma in elderly patients on oral glucocorticoids. *Lancet*, **350**, 979–82.

16. Baharav, E., Harpaz, D., Mittelman, M. *et al.* (1986). Dexamethasone-induced perineal irritation. *New England Journal of Medicine*, **314**, 315–16.

17. Helfer, E. and Rose, L. (1989). Corticosteroids and adrenal suppression. Characterising and avoiding the problem. *Drugs*, **38**, 838–45.

18. Dixon, R.A. and Christy, N.P. (1980). On the various forms of corticosteroid withdrawal syndrome. *American Journal of Medicine*, **68**, 224–30.

19. Jalladeau, E., Carpentier, A., Napolitano, M. *et al.* (2000). Lipomatosi epidurale cortico-induite. *Revue Neurologique*, **156**, 517–19.

20. Walker, A. and Adamkiewicz, J. (1964). Pseudotumor cerebri associated with prolonged corticosteroid therapy. *Journal of the American Medical Association*, **188**, 779–84.

21. Fisher, R.S., van Emde Boas, W., Blume, W. *et al.* (2005). Epileptic seizures and epilepsy. Definition proposed by the International League against Epilepsy (ILAE) and the International Bureau for Epilepsy (IBE). *Epilepsia*, **46**, 470–2.

22. Delanty, N., Vaughan, C., and French, J. (1998). Medical causes of seizures. *Lancet*, **352**, 383–90.

23. Ropper, A.H. and Brown, R.H. (2005). *Adams and Victor's principles of neurology*, 8th edition. McGraw-Hill, New York.

24. Duncan, J.S., Sander, J.W., Sisodiya, S.M. *et al.* (2006). Adult epilepsy. *Lancet*, **367**, 1087–100

25. Glantz, M. *et al.* (1994). Double blind randomized, placebo-controlled trial of anticonvulsants prophylaxis in adults with newly diagnosed brain metastases. *Proceedings of the American Society of Clinical Oncologists*, **13**, 176.

26. Glantz, M. *et al.* (2000). Practice parameter: Anticonvulsant prophylaxis in patients with newly diagnosed brain tumors. *Neurology*, **54**, 1886–93.

27. Gabor, A., Brooks, A., Scobey, R. *et al.* (1984). Intracranial pressure during epileptic seizures. *Electroencephalography and Clinical Neurophysiology*, **57**, 497–506.

28. Engel, J., Jr. (2006). Report of the ILAE Classification Core Group. *Epilepsia*, **47**, 1558–8.

29. Towne, A. *et al.* (2000). Prevelence of nonconvulsive status epilepticus in comatose patients. *Neurology*, **54**, 340–5.

30. Chen, J.W.Y. and Wasterlain, C.G. (2006). Status epilepticus: Pathophysiology and management in adults. *Lancet Neurol*, **5**, 246–56.

31. Prasad, K., Al-Roomi, K., Krishnan, P.R. *et al* (2005). Anticonvulsivant therapy for status epilepticus. *The Cochrane Database of Systematic Reviews*, **4**, CD003723.

32. Morrison, G., Gibbons, E., and Whitehouse, W.P. (2006). High-dose midazolam therapy for refractory status epilepticus in children. *Intensive Care Med*, september 15, Epub ahead print.

33. Misra, U.K., Kalita, J., and Patel, R. (2006). Sodium valproate vs phenytoin in status epilepticus: A pilot study. *Neurology*, **67**, 340–2

34. Wheless, J. (1998). Pediatric use of intravenous and intramuscular phenytoin: Lesson learned. *Journal of Child Neurology*, **13**, s11–14.

35. van gestel, J.P.J., van Oud, B., Malingré, M. *et al.*(2005). Propofol and thiopental for refractory status epilepticus in children. *Neurology*, **65**, 591–2.

36. Krumholz, A. (1999). Nonepileptic seizures: Diagnosis and management. *Neurology*, **52**, s76–83.

37. Caraceni, A. and Grassi, L. (2003). Delirium acute confusional states in palliative medicine. Oxford, Oxford University Press.

38. American Psychiatric Association. (2000). *Diagnostic and statistical manual of mental disorders*, 4th edn. Text revision. DSM IV-TR. American Psychiatric Press, Washington DC.

39. Engel, G.L. and Romano, J. (1959). Delirium: A syndrome of cerebral insufficiency. *Journal of Chronic Diseases*, **9**, 260–77.

40. Inouye, S.K., van Dyck, C.H., Alessi, C.A. *et al.* (1990). Clarifying confusion: The confusion assessment method. A new method for detection of delirium. *Annals of Internal Medicine*, **113**, 941–8.

41. Inouye, S.K., Foreman, M.D., Mion, L.C. *et al.* (2001). Nurses' recognition of delirium and its symptoms: Comparison of nurse and researcher ratings. *Archives of Internal Medicine*, **161**, 2467–73.

42. Trzepacz, P.T., Mittal, D., Torres, R. *et al.* (2001). Validation of the delirium rating scale-revised-98: Comparison with the delirium rating scale and the cognitive test for delirium. *Journal of Neuropsychiatry and Clinical Neurosciences*, **13**, 229–42.

43. Breitbart, W., Rosenfeld, B., Roth, A. *et al.* (1997). The memorial delirium assessment scale. *Journal of Pain and Symptom Management*, **13**, 128–37.

44. Liptzin, B. and Levkoff, S.E. (1992). An empirical study of delirium subtypes. *British Journal of Psychiatry*, **161**, 843–5.

45. Wallesch, C.W. and Hundsaltz, A. (1994). Language function in delirium: A comparison of single word processing in acute confusional state and probable Alzheimer's disease. *Brain & Language*, **46**, 592–606.

46. Macleod, A.D. and Whitehead, L.E. (1997). Dysgraphia in terminal delirium. *Palliative Medicine*, **11**, 127–32.

47. Chedru, F. and Geschwind, N. (1972). Disorders of higher cortical functions in acute confusional states. *Cortex*, **8**, 395–411.

48. Lipowski, Z.J. (1990).*Delirium: Acute confusional states*. Oxford University Press, New York, p. 490.

49. Wolf, H.G. and Curran, D. (1935). Nature of delirium and allied states. The disergastic reaction. *Archives of Neurology and Psychiatry*, **33**, 1175–215.

50. Bruera, E., Fainsinger, R.L., Miller, M.J. *et al.* (1992). The assessment of pain intensity in patients with cognitive failure: A preliminary report. *Journal of Pain and Symptom Management*, **7**, 267–70.

51. Derogatis, L.R., Morrow, G.R., Fetting, J. *et al.* (1983). The prevalence of psychiatric disorders among cancer patients. *Journal of the American Medical Association*, **249**, 751–7.

52. Francis, J., Martin, D., and Kapoor, W.N. (1990). A prospective study of delirium in hospitalized elderly. *Journal of the American Medical Association*, **263**, 1097–101.

53. Levkoff, S.E. *et al.* (1992). Delirium. The occurence and persistence of symptoms among elderly hospitalized patients. *Archives of Internal Medicine*, **152**, 334–40.

54. Clouston, P.D., De Angelis, L., and Posner, J.B. (1992). The spectrum of neurological disease in patients with systemic cancer. *Annals of Neurology*, **31**, 268–73.

55. Caraceni, A. *et al.* (2000). The impact of delirium on the short-term prognosis of advanced cancer patients. *Cancer*, **89**, 1145–8.

56. Gagnon, P., Allard, P., Masse, B. *et al.* (2000). Delirium in terminal cancer: A prospective study using daily screening, early diagnosis and continuous monitoring. *Journal of Pain and Symptom Management*, **19**, 412–26.

57. Lawlor, P.G. *et al.* (2000). Occurrence, causes and outcome of delirium in patients with advanced cancer. *Archives of Internal Medicine*, **160**, 786–94.

58. Lewis, L.M., Miller, D.K., Morley, J.E. *et al.* (1995). Unrecognized delirium in ED geriatric patients. *American Journal of Emergency Medicine*, **13**, 142–5.

59. Johnson, J.C., Kerse, N.M., Gottlieb, G. *et al.* (1992). Prospective versus retrospective methods of identifying patients with delirium. *Journal of the American Geriatrics Society*, **40**, 316–19.

60. Inouye, S.K. *et al.* (1999). A multicomponent intervention to prevent delirium in hospitalized older patients. *New England Journal of Medicine*, **340**, 669–76.

61. Schor, J.D. *et al.* (1992). Risk factors for delirium in hospitalized elderly. *Journal of the American Medical Association*, **267**, 827–31.

62. Marcantonio, E.R. *et al.* (1994). A clinical prediction rule for delirium after elective noncardiac surgery. *Journal of the American Medical Association*, **271**, 134–9.

63. Tuma, R. and DeAngelis, L.M. (2000). Altered mental status in patients with cancer. *Archives of Neurology*, **57**, 1727–31.

64. Fainsinger, R., Schoeller, T., Boiskin, M. *et al.* (1993). Palliative care round: cognitive failure (CF) and coma after renal failure in a patient receiving captopril and hydromorphone. *Journal of Palliative Care*, **9**, 53–5.

65. Bortolussi, R. *et al.* (1994). Acute morphine intoxication during high-dose recombinant Interleukin-2 treatment for metastatic renal cell cancer. *European Journal of Cancer*, **30A**, 1905–7.

66. Weitzener, M.A., Olofson, S.M., and Forman, A.D. (1995). Patients with malignant meningitis presenting with neuropsychiatric manifestations. *Cancer*, **76**, 1804–8.

67. Wengs, W.J., Talwar, D., and Bernard, J. (1993). Ifosfamide-induced nonconvulsive status epilepticus. *Archives of Neurology*, **50**, 1104–5.

68. Jacobson, S. and Jerrier, H. (2000). EEG in delirium. *Seminars in Clinical Neuropsychiatry*, **5**, 86–92.

69. Breitbart, W., Marotta, R., Platt, M.M. *et al.* (1996). A double-blind trial of haloperidol, chlorpromazine and lorazepam in the treatment of delirium in hospitalized AIDS patients. *American Journal of Psychiatry*, **153**, 231–7.

70. American Psychiatric Association. (1999). Practice guideline for the treatment of patients with delirium. *American Journal of Psychiatry*, **156**, 1–20.

71. Jackson, T., Ditmanson, L., and Phibbs, B. (1997). Torsade de pointes and low-dose oral haloperidol. *Archives of Internal Medicine*, **157**, 2013–15.

72. Stiefel, F., Fainsinger, R., and Bruera, E. (1992). Acute confusional states in patients with advanced cancer. *Journal of Pain and Symptom Management*, **7**, 94–8.

73. Gilbert, M.R. and Grossman, S.A. (1986). Incidence and nature of neurologic problems in patients with solid tumor. *American Journal of Medicine*, **81**, 951–4.

74. Boogerd, W., Vos, V.W., Hart, A.A.M. *et al.* (1993). Brain metastases in breast cancer; Natural history, prognostic factors and outcome. *Journal of Neuro-oncology*, **15**, 165–74.

75. Kaal, C.A., Niel, C.G.J.H., and Vecht, C.J. (2005). Therapeutic management of brain metastasis. *Lancet Neurology*, **4**, 289–98.

76. Ventafridda, V., Caraceni, A., Martini, C. *et al.* (1991). On the significance of Lhermitte's sign in oncology. *Journal of Neuro-oncology*, **10**, 133–7.

77. Portenoy, R.K., Lipton, R.B., and Foley, K.M. (1987). Back pain in the cancer patient: An algorithm for evaluation and management. *Neurology*, **37**, 134–8.

78. Portenoy, R.K. *et al.* (1989). Identification of epidural neoplasm. Radiography and bone scintigraphy in the symptomatic and asymptomatic spine. *Cancer*, **64**, 2207–13.

79. Ingham, J., Beveridge, A., and Cooney, N.J. (1993). The management of spinal cord compression in patients with advanced malignancy. *Journal of Pain and Symptom Management*, **8**, 1–6.

80. Spinazzé, S., Caraceni, A., and Schrijvers, D. (2005). Epidural spinal cord compression. *Crit Rev Oncol Hematol*, **56**, 397–406.

81. Sorensen, P.S. *et al.* (1994). Effect of high-dose dexamethasone in carcinomatous metastatic spinal cord compression treated with radiotherapy. A randomized trial. *European Journal of Cancer*, **30A**, 22–7.

82. Vecht, C.J., Haaxma-Reiche, H., van Putten, W.L.J. *et al.* (1989). Initial bolus of conventional versus high-dose dexamethasone in metastatic spinal cord compression. *Neurology*, **39**, 1255–7.

83. Findlay, G.F. (1984). Adverse effects of the management of malignant spinal cord compression. *Journal of Neurology, Neurosurgery, and Psychiatry*, **47**, 761–8.

84. Harrington, K.D. (1988). Anterior decompression and stabilization of the spine as treatment for vertebral collapse and spinal cord compression from metastatic cancer. *Clinical Orthopaedics*, **233**, 177–97.

85. Patchell, R., Tibbs, P., Regine, W. *et al.* (2005). Direct decompressive surgical resection in the treatment of spinal cord compression caused by metastatic cancer: A randomized trial. *Lancet*, **366**, 643–8.

86. Chamberlain, M.C. (2006) Neoplastic meningitis. *The Neurologist*, **12**, 179–87.

87. Formaglio, F. and Caraceni, A. (1998). Meningeal metastases clinical aspects and diagnosis. *Italian Journal of Neurological Sciences*, **19**, 133–49.

88. Siegal, T., Lossos, A., and Pfeffer, M.R. (1994). Leptomeningeal metastases. Analysis of 31 patients with sustained off-therapy response following combined-modality therapy. *Neurology*, **44**, 1463–9.

89. Greenberg, H.S. *et al.* (1981). Metastasis to the base of the skull: Clinical findings in 43 patients. *Neurology*, **31**, 530–7.

90. Vecht, C.J., Hoff, A.M., Kansen, P.J. *et al.* (1992). Types and causes of pain in cancer of the head and neck. *Cancer*, **70**, 178–84.

91. Foley, K.M. (1979). Pain syndromes in patients with cancer. In *Advances in Pain Research and Therapy*, Vol. 2 (eds J.J. Bonica and V. Ventafridda), pp. 59–75. Raven Press, New York.

92. Weinstein, R.E., Herec, D., and Friedman, J.H. (1986). Hypotension due to glossopharyngeal neuralgia. *Archives of Neurology*, **40**, 90–2.

93. Cheng, T.M., Cascino, T.L., and Onofrio, B.M. (1993). Comprehensive study of diagnosis and treatment of trigeminal neuralgia secondary to tumors. *Neurology*, **43**, 2298–302.

94. Burt, R.K., Sharfam, W.H., Karp, B.I. *et al.* (1992). Mental neuropathy (Numb chin syndrome). A harbinger of tumor progression or relapse. *Cancer*, **70**, 877–81.

95. Kori, S.H. *et al.* (1981). Brachial plexus lesions in patients with cancer 100 cases. *Neurology*, **31**, 45–50.

96. Krol, G. (1993). Evaluation of neoplastic involvement of brachial and lumbar plexus: Imaging aspects. *Journal of Back and Musculoskeletal Rehabilitation*, **3**, 35–43.

97. Harper, C.M., Thomas, J.E., Cascino, T.L. *et al.* (1989). Distinction between neoplastic and radiation-induced brachial plexopathy, with emphasis on EMG. *Neurology*, **39**, 502–6.

98. Jaeckle, K.A., Young, D.F., and Foley, K.M. (1985). The natural history of lumbosacral plexopathy in cancer. *Neurology*, **35**, 8–15.

99. Thomas, J.E., Cascino, T.L., and Earl, J.D. (1985). Differential diagnosis between radiation and tumor plexopathy of the pelvis. *Neurology*, **35**, 1–7.

100. Anoine, J.C. and Camdessanché, J.P. (2007). Peripheral nervous systeminvolvement in patients with cancer *Lancet Neurology*, **6**, 75–86.

101. Lipton, R.B. *et al.* (1991). Large and small fibre type sensory dysfunction in patients with cancer. *Journal of Neurology, Neurosurgery, and Psychiatry*, **54**, 706–9.

102. Rogers, L.H., Cho, E.S., Kempin, S. *et al.* (1987). Cerebral infarction from non-bacterial thrombotic endocarditis. A clinical and pathological study including the effects of anticoagulation. *American Journal of Medicine*, **83**, 746.

103. Rogers, L.R. (2004). Cerebrovascular complications in patients with cancer. *Seminars in Neurology*, **24**, 453–60.

104. Collins, R.C., Al-Mondhiry, H., Chernik, N.L. *et al.* (1975). Neurologic manifestations of intravascular coagulation in patients with cancer. A clinicopathological analysis of 12 cases. *Neurology*, **25**, 795.

105. Voltz, R. (2002). Paraneoplastic neurological syndromes: An update on diagnosis, pathogenesis and therapy. *Lancet Neurology*, **1**, 294–305.

106. Vedeler, C.A. *et al.* (2006) Mangement of paraneoplastic neurological syndromes: Report of an EFNS task force. *European Journal of Neurology*, **13**, 682–90.

107. Glantz, M.J., Biran, H., Myers, M.E. *et al.* (1994). The radiographic diagnosis and treatment of paraneoplastic central nervous system disease. *Cancer*, **73**, 168–75.

Sleep in palliative care

Michael J. Sateia and Ira R. Byock

Introduction

Sleep disorders have been recognized for centuries as a frequent complication of medical illness. The last several decades have produced an explosive growth in our knowledge and understanding of sleep physiology and pathophysiology. Unfortunately, the practical application of this knowledge has been slow in reaching the majority of health-care providers, including those in palliative medicine. However, examination of the literature on this subject does suggest a growing recognition on the part of clinicians that attention to patients' sleep is a necessary and an important aspect of care in this population. Problems related to sleep are among the most commonly reported complaints of patients with advanced illness who are hospitalized or who reside in hospice settings. A good night's sleep can provide a seriously ill person valuable respite from the physical discomforts, worries, and sorrows of the day, and may allow the person to meet the next day with enhanced energy and motivation. Therefore, it is important that palliative care clinicians routinely ask their patients how they are sleeping at night, and whether they are bothered by daytime sleepiness or other sleep–wake-related disturbances. In this chapter, we review basic aspects of sleep and sleep disorders, particularly as they apply to palliative care, and discuss strategies for the evaluation and treatment of these conditions.

Sleep physiology

Human sleep is a complex and dynamic physiologic function, the nature of which we have only begun to unravel. Contrary to the historical view of sleep as a passive state of little medical interest or relevance, it has become increasingly clear that sleep is an active condition that is affected by waking physiological and psychological states and which, in turn, has significant effects on those waking conditions. This is particularly true in the case of serious medical illnesses in which marked perturbations in somatic and psychological functions may result in severe disruption of sleep and concomitant waking complications.

Normal sleep consists of two distinct states. Non-rapid eye movement (NREM) sleep accounts for approximately 75 per cent of the night; the remainder consists of rapid eye movement (REM) sleep. Recent changes in sleep stage scoring now classify NREM sleep as N1 (stage 1), N2 (stage 2), N3 (stages 3/4), and R (REM)[1]. In the NREM sleep of the healthy young adult, N1 (light sleep) normally represents only 5–10 per cent of total sleep, N2 represents approximately 50 per cent, and N3 (slow wave, or delta, sleep)

represents about 20 per cent. These stages, along with REM sleep, repeat themselves in cyclical fashion through the night. The deepest stages of NREM sleep occur predominantly during the first half of sleep, while REM periods are significantly longer and more intense during the second half of the night. NREM sleep is a period of relative physiological and cognitive quiescence, quite distinct from REM sleep, which is characterized by cortical activation and regionally increased cerebral blood flow, muscle atonia, dreaming, and autonomic variability. Autonomic changes include periodic increases in pulse and blood pressure, decreased temperature regulation, and erection activity in males. Ventilatory response to hypercapnoea and hypoxemia are diminished, resulting in greater likelihood of hypoventilation in susceptible individuals. The sleep–wake cycle is a component of the body's overall circadian rhythm. As such, its timing is synchronized with other biological rhythms, including temperature oscillation, melatonin release, and cortisol and growth hormone secretion. Onset and maintenance of normal sleep patterns are dependent on a number of conditions, including appropriate timing of sleep within the 24-h circadian rhythm, adequate homeostatic sleep drive (a function of time since last sleep), an adequate level of physical comfort, an acceptable sleeping environment, an intact central nervous system function, and relative absence of psychological distress and psychophysiologic arousal.

The restorative functions of sleep are dependent on a well-organized and reasonably uninterrupted structure or 'sleep architecture'. In many medical conditions, as well as with advancing age, there is a tendency towards lighter sleep, with an increase in N1 and decrease in N3. The percentage of REM sleep remains relatively constant in a healthy elderly population, but is typically decreased when cognitive impairment or certain other medical conditions are present. Sleep often becomes more fragmented, with increased awakenings through the night, resulting in complaints of poor sleep and associated daytime consequences.

Sleep impacts numerous other physiologic functions. Sleep as a mediating factor in pain regulation is discussed in later sections. Of particular interest in cancer or AIDS patients is the observation that sleep deprivation results in alterations of immune system function[2–4]. Immune activation has a stimulating effect on slow-wave sleep (mediated, at least in part, by cytokine production) and, conversely, slow-wave sleep enhances immune function[5]. Thus, it seems likely that sleep is an important factor in recuperative processes, including recovery from infection. More recent studies have demonstrated alterations in natural killer cell activity associated with sleep deprivation[6,7]. Savard et al., assessing women at risk for cervical cancer, demonstrated that satisfaction with sleep quality was positively associated with levels of helper T cells and cytotoxic/suppressor T cells[8]. This same group reported increase in interferon-gamma and IL-1 beta following cognitive behavioural therapy for insomnia in cancer patients[9]. Sleep loss has also been associated with elevated levels of interleukin-6 and tumour necrosis factor[10].

Classification of sleep disorders

Sleep disorders are classified according to the International Classification of Sleep Disorders, 2nd edition, of the American Academy of Sleep Medicine[11]. The major categories and representative diagnoses within these categories are listed in Table 10.12.1. It is important to note that specific symptoms, such as insomnia, may be observed within any number of these broad categories. The categories are comprised of specific diagnoses that most closely fit the category from a phenomenological perspective.

Clinical approach to insomnia

In clinical practice, insomnia can be defined as a subjective complaint by the patient of sleep disturbance despite adequate opportunity to sleep. These disturbances encompass complaints of difficulty initiating or maintaining sleep, interrupted sleep, or poor quality ('non-restorative') sleep. The term 'insomnia' denotes a symptom or general condition, but is not a sufficient diagnosis in its own right. It is incumbent upon the clinician to clarify the nature of the complaint and to consider potential aetiologies in developing a differential diagnosis of this disorder. In the case of insomnia that occurs in the context of medical conditions, there are often numerous contributing physiological, psychological, and environmental factors that contribute to a patient's sleep disturbance. Among the most common physiological determinants are pain, toxic and metabolic disturbance, medications, sleep-related breathing disorder (e.g. obstructive and central sleep apnoea, nocturnal asthma), movement disorders, and diseases of the central

nervous system. Depression and anxiety are leading psychological contributors to insomnia in medically ill patients. Environmental circumstances such as unfamiliar surroundings, frequent interruptions, lack of privacy, or noise are particularly important problems for patients in hospital. The most frequent factors contributing to insomnia among patients with advanced illness are outlined in Table 10.12.2.

Insomnia by definition must be associated with daytime consequences. These may include progressive fatigue, subjective complaints of sleepiness, impairment of concentration, depressed mood and irritability, and a variety of non-specific physical complaints[12,13]. Although insomnia is often triggered by identifiable factors such as psychological stress or medical illness, the current understanding of the condition suggests that conditioned psychological and behavioural factors such as arousal in response to efforts to sleep and negative expectations are key in the perpetuation of the condition. Recent investigations of the biology of insomnia suggest psychophysiologic 'hyperarousal' as a common final pathway. Psychophysiologic changes include increased

Table 10.12.1 Major categories of sleep disorders.

Diagnostic category	Common diagnoses
Insomnia	Primary insomnia; insomnia due to medical or mental disorder
Sleep related breathing disorders	Obstructive and central sleep apnoea; hypoventilation/hypoxemia syndromes
Hypersomnolence not due to other sleep disorders	Narcolepsy; idiopathic hypersomnolence
Circadian rhythm disorders	Delayed or advanced sleep phase; shift work; irregular sleep–wake rhythm
Movement disorders	Restless legs syndrome; periodic limb movement
Parasomnias	Night terrors; sleepwalking; REM sleep behaviour disorder; nightmares
Isolated symptoms and normal variants	Primary snoring; sleep talking; long/short sleepers
Other sleep disorders	Environmental sleep disorder

Table 10.12.2 Common contributing factors to insomnia in seriously ill patients.

Depression	Major depressive illness related to loss, chronic pain, effects of tumour on central nervous system, metabolic/endocrine disturbance
Anxiety	Adjustment disorder or generalized anxiety related to fears of illness, procedures, pain or death; medication; direct effects on central nervous system
Cognitive impairment disorder	Delirium secondary to medication, metabolic derangement, direct involvement of central nervous system, or non-specific delirium-inducing factors
Fever	With or without sweats, chills
Pain	Related to direct tumour effects, diagnostic or treatment interventions, non-specific causes
Nausea and vomiting	Associated with chemotherapy, medications, or primary gastrointestinal disturbance
Respiratory distress	Dyspnoea due to hypoxia and/or anxiety, obstructive sleep apnoea, pleuritic pain
Medications	Stimulants, bronchodilators, steroids, some antihypertensives, activating antidepressants; withdrawal or rebound from sedative hypnotics or analgesics
Psychophysiologic insomnia	Caused by conditional arousal response, negative expectations and poor sleep habits
Sleep–wake schedule disorder	Associated with disruption of normal schedule, excessive time in bed or napping, disturbed nocturnal sleep
Environmental factors	Light, noise (including device alarms, overhead paging, and snoring, moaning, crying of other patients), frequent interruptions (e.g. for vital signs, glucose monitoring or adjustment of infusions), lack of privacy
Periodic limb movement/restless legs syndrome	Secondary to peripheral neuropathy, Parkinson's disease, iron deficiency, antidepressant medication, caffeinism, sedative hypnotic withdrawal, anaemia, uraemia, leukaemia

24-h metabolic rate, activation of the hypothalamic–pituitary–adrenal axis, autonomic hyperactivity, increased sleep EEG frequencies, alteration of cytokine production, regionally increased CBF, and cognitive hyperactivity[14–18].

Clinical approach to excessive daytime sleepiness

Excessive sleepiness is a common and frequently overlooked symptom, particularly among patients with serious medical illness. Despite its frequency, there is little formal data on the prevalence of sleepiness as a symptom in patients with terminal malignancies or other end-stage disease. Because sleepiness renders many individuals more quiet and 'compliant', care providers may dismiss sleepiness as a problem. As Kubler-Ross[19] pointed out, health professionals may actually encourage daytime sedation as a means of dealing with their own discomfort with the dying patient. While some degree of daytime sedation can be desirable in certain cases, this is by no means uniformly the case. Excessive somnolence is potentially disabling symptom that may further compromise a seriously ill patient's already tenuous functional capacity. Patients who are sleepy tend to be inactive, weakly motivated, and less capable of participating in treatment. Inactivity heightens the risk of deep vein thrombosis, pulmonary embolism, and decubitus ulcers. Sleepy patients' ability to pay attention, learn, and retain information is compromised. They may become irritable, depressed, and withdrawn. Sleepiness can impair social interactions and rob people who have only weeks or days to live of important opportunities to attend to their affairs, visit and communicate with friends and family, and engage in activities of life review, and life completion. Depression, irritability, and emotional or social withdrawal are also potential complications of pathological sleepiness.

Sleepiness must be distinguished from more general and vague complaints of 'tiredness' and 'fatigue', which are very common among patients receiving palliative care. Specifically, it must be determined to what extent an individual experiences drowsiness or episodes of irresistible sleepiness, especially under circumstances of physical inactivity, or takes naps during normal waking hours. The most widely employed scale for assessment of subjective sleepiness is the Epworth Sleepiness Scale, an eight-item measure of sleep tendency in various settings[20]. When appropriate, an objective measure of pathological sleepiness, the Multiple Sleep Latency Test[21], is utilized. Diagnostic blurring may arise in the final stages of disease when the distinction between excessive somnolence and alteration of consciousness associated with delirium becomes blurred.

There are many potential causes of excessive sleepiness in this population. They include insufficient or disturbed night-time sleep, medication (analgesic, sedative-hypnotic, antidepressant, anticholinergic, and chemotherapeutic), metabolic disorders, and disruption of the sleep–wake schedule. Repetitive sleep disruption due to breathing or movement disorders in sleep is a common cause of sleepiness. In some cases, subjective sleepiness may occur as a form of psychological and social withdrawal or as an atypical symptom of depressive illness. For many patients, the aetiology is multifactorial. A careful review of potential causes must be conducted in order to identify the source(s) of the complaint. Most importantly, it is essential that clinicians not dismiss excessive sleepiness as an inevitable part of illness, but rather approach it as an important and treatable symptom.

Disorders of the sleep–wake schedule

Maintenance of a normal sleep pattern is dependent on adherence to a well-established schedule of sleep and wakefulness. Because of frequent disruptions of night-time sleep, an absence of usual daytime schedule demands, and relative inactivity during normal waking hours, individuals with advanced illness are particularly prone to disturbances of the sleep–wake schedule. When night sleep has been poor, there is an inclination to delay the hour of rising and/or to engage in lengthy daytime naps. While these practices are understandable, they pose a problem in that the onset of sleep may be significantly delayed on the subsequent night. This, in turn, can result in further delays in morning rising times and increased daytime napping. Ultimately, the consequence can be pronounced difficulty falling asleep until early morning hours, with subsequent sleep often stretching into the early afternoon. This disturbance is referred to as delayed sleep phase disorder. In other cases, the fatigue and sedation so often associated with major medical illness may give rise to advancement of the normal sleep–wake schedule, resulting in early morning awakening, coupled with evening sleepiness and/or earlier bedtimes (advanced sleep phase disorder). For some, a normal sleep–wake rhythm disappears altogether and is replaced by a pattern of multiple shorter sleep periods that are interspersed with wakefulness throughout the 24-h cycle (irregular sleep–wake schedule).

While such sleep–wake patterns may be acceptable to some patients, it is poorly tolerated by many, resulting in complaints of insomnia, excessive sleepiness, or both, depending on the specific nature of the schedule disturbance and a variety of patient-specific factors. In addition to the dysfunction and frustration that these disorders engender for the patient, the burden imposed on caregivers can be substantial in that they are required to respond to the needs of a patient who is awake at all hours.

Sleep–wake schedule disorders of the type described may respond to straightforward efforts at regularization of the circadian rhythm and maintenance of proper sleep hygiene, as described later in this chapter. Short-term treatment with hypnotic medications may be helpful in re-establishing a normal sleep–wake cycle in some patients. Bright light therapy and melatonin can be administered at specific times to advance or delay sleep phase[22–24]. For some patients, the more formal behavioural approach of 'chronotherapy' (e.g. progressive delay of sleep phase) is required to correct the rhythm disturbance[25].

Sleep disturbances in cancer

People living with advanced cancer comprise an important population for palliative care and for many, sleep disturbance is an important and troubling symptom. Women with metastatic breast cancer rated sleep in the highest quartile of quality of life items[26], while patients undergoing radiation therapy ranked sleep disturbance as one of the 10 most troubling difficulties associated with their illness[27]. Current data suggests that sleep is disturbed in 50 per cent or more of those with advanced cancer, particularly when pain is a complicating factor[28–32]. The prevalence of sleep disturbance in cancer patients has been reviewed by Savard and Morin[33]. They note that comparisons of insomnia or sleep disturbance data across these studies are difficult in light of the variability in definitions and measurement devices. They add that, in their own analysis of 300 women with breast cancer (non-metastatic),

51 per cent reported insomnia symptoms but only 19 per cent met specific criteria for the full 'insomnia syndrome'. Of these, about one in three described the onset of sleep problems as occurring after the cancer diagnosis. Recent studies confirm that sleep-related complaints are among the most common and most severe symptoms in cancer patients[34–38].

Insomnia in cancer patients

Despite the fact that insomnia occurs on an almost nightly basis for many patients, many do not report the problem to their physicians, perhaps assuming that it is an inevitable aspect of their illness or that there is little that can be done to help. Engstrom and colleagues found that 85 per cent of cancer patients with sleep disturbance did not discuss the problem with a health-care provider[39]. The same population reported that physicians and other health-care providers generally did not ask about sleep-related problems. However, more recent data suggest that reporting may be a function of degree of concern rather than symptom severity, in that 92 per cent of palliative cancer patients with elevated levels of concern about sleep difficulties did discuss the condition with a health-care provider[40].

Patients with cancer sleep less at night and are more likely to sit, lie down, and sleep during the day than healthy people[41]. In an early report, Beszterczey and Lipowski found that 45 per cent of a mixed group of cancer patients referred for radiotherapy had a total sleep time of less than 50 h week, while 23 per cent slept for less than 40 h per week[42]. A comparison of sleep in these patients with that in an independent group of mixed medical and surgical patients revealed less sleep in the patients with neoplastic disease. Other comparisons between cancer patients and those with non-malignant disease or normal controls have yielded mixed results. Lamb found no difference between the sleep of newly diagnosed cancer patients and a group with non-malignant medical illness[43]. Another survey that compared patients with cancer with cardiac patients and normal controls indicated that the cancer group had no less difficulty falling asleep than cardiac patients, but they reported significantly more problems in maintaining sleep than either of the two comparison groups[44]. Approximately 30 per cent of the cancer patients with sleep maintenance complaints described pain as a cause of awakening. Interpretation of this study is complicated by the use of hypnotics or analgesics in a higher percentage (33 per cent) of the cancer group. Engstrom also reported that about half of the patients with sleep problems experienced the disturbance on an almost nightly basis[39]. Midcycle awakening was the most common symptom, followed by insufficient sleep and difficulty getting back to sleep. Reports of sleep problems correlated with a pre-morbid history of sleep disturbance. These nocturnal disturbances may be associated with any of the factors listed in Table 10.12.2, although pain is of particular importance in cancer patients.

Objective evaluation of sleep in cancer patients is limited. Silberfarb et al.[45] reported on a group of 14 patients with unresectable lung cancer. Nine patients were self-described 'good sleepers' and five were 'poor sleepers'. All patients were studied for three consecutive nights in a sleep laboratory. The groups did not differ with respect to sleep efficiency, sleep latency, or distribution of sleep stages, with the exception that good sleepers spent a significantly greater amount of time in stages 3/4 (delta) sleep. The authors suggest that, for cancer patients, the subjective appraisal of quality of sleep may relate to the amount of time spent in delta sleep, although both groups spent so little time in deep sleep that this explanation should be considered preliminary. In a continuation of this study[46], the sleep architecture of 17 patients with unresectable lung cancer and 15 with breast cancer (in various stages of their disease) was compared to that of 32 insomnia patients without medical illness and an equal number of normal controls. All cancer patients were ambulatory and, for the most part, only mildly impaired by their illness, with mean Karnofsky functional scale ratings of 85.4 and 92.8 for the lung and breast cancer groups, respectively. Overall, cancer patients slept as long as the controls and significantly longer than the insomniacs. Patients with breast cancer were not distinguishable from controls on polysomnographic variables. Lung cancer patients achieved total sleep times that were comparable with those of the controls by spending significantly more time in bed. However, their sleep was clearly more disturbed, with prolonged latency to stage 2 sleep, lower sleep efficiency, increased stage 1, and increased awakenings through the night. Curiously, and in contradistinction to the usual reports of insomniacs, the lung cancer group under-reported the sleep disturbance, denying the presence of sleep problems despite polysomnographic evidence to the contrary. Psychological questionnaires and interviews suggested that the differences observed were not a function of psychological disturbance which was, in fact, not evident in this group of cancer patients. Others have reported polysomnographic data in groups of cancer patients, but these studies have focused primarily on evaluation of obstructive sleep apnoea[47,48] or assessment of insomnia treatment response (see below)[9].

Actigraphic study of women with breast cancer prior to chemotherapy demonstrated an average of approximately 6 h of sleep per night with reduced efficiency and increased awakenings[49]. Similarly, an investigation of actigraphically recorded sleep in a population of women with various cancers, compared to a control group, showed lower sleep efficiency, more waking after sleep onset, and less activity during normal waking hours in the patient group[36]. In contrast to other studies, however, there was little evidence of correlation between poor nocturnal sleep and fatigue scales in this group.

Daytime fatigue and sleepiness in cancer patients

Daytime fatigue and sleepiness may occur as a result of tumour effects (e.g. mediated by cytokines), treatment, or disturbance of quantity, quality, or timing of nocturnal sleep. One survey found that about 40 per cent of cancer patients described sleeping at unusual times (mid-morning/afternoon). Munro et al.[27] noted 'sleeping more than usual' as one of the most troublesome symptoms of patients undergoing radiation therapy, although others found no increase in subjective sleepiness, as measured by the Epworth Sleepiness Scale during radiation therapy for prostate cancer[50,51]. Sixty per cent of a large cohort of cancer patients undergoing radiation therapy reported subjective problems with drowsiness prior to initiation of treatment, with substantial worsening of the problem during treatment[35]. Epworth scores in various other cancer groups have ranged from means of 6.0 to 18 (range 0–24; normal <10 with model score ~6; 10–13 = mild sleepiness; 14–17 = moderate sleepiness; 18–24 = severe sleepiness)[52]. Excessive sedation is described in association with opioid analgesics[53,54] and some forms of chemotherapy[55,56].

Other aetiologies of sleepiness in cancer patients, including breathing disturbance, movement disorder, and sleep–wake schedule disturbances are discussed elsewhere. To date, there has been no systematic analysis of the risk factors and relative contributions to sleepiness in cancer patients or others with serious illness.

There is limited, and largely anecdotal, information relating specific cancers to sleep disorders. Symptoms of narcolepsy/cataplexy have been described in association with midbrain or brainstem tumours, including those in the region of the third ventricle[57,58]. Centrally mediated respiratory disorders that disrupt sleep have been described in patients with brainstem tumours[59]. It seems certain that other primary malignancies or metastases of the central nervous system may affect sleep indirectly, through cerebral oedema, or directly through structures subserving sleep. An understanding of such effects awaits further investigation.

Fatigue in cancer patients accounts for a significant degree of functional disability. It is important to note that fatigue is not synonymous with sleepiness, the latter being associated with a somewhat more circumscribed set of aetiologies. Sleepiness is typically accompanied by fatigue, although fatigue is not necessarily accompanied by sleepiness. Available evidence suggests that sleep–wake disturbances account for a portion of the fatigue experienced by cancer patients, although correlations are variable[36–38,60]. Significant associations between sleep disturbance and severe fatigue have been noted in two samples of breast cancer survivors[61,62]. Berger and Farr also reported a strong association between night-time awakenings and cancer-related fatigue[63]. Investigation of patients undergoing radiation treatments revealed substantial increases in fatigue during therapy, apparently unrelated to depression or sleepiness[51]. Fernandes found no correlation between sleep disturbance and fatigue severity in cancer inpatients[36]. Other data underscore the potential importance of sleep disturbance as an intermediate variable between pain and cancer-related fatigue[60]. The United States National Comprehensive Cancer Network Guidelines include sleep disturbance as a primary factor associated with fatigue, along with pain, anaemia, emotional distress, and hypothyroidism[64]. Clearly, fatigue in this population is a multifactorial problem that requires careful assessment and a multifaceted therapeutic approach. Causes, correlates, and management of fatigue in cancer patients have been reviewed by Groopman[65].

Sleep disturbances in HIV/AIDS (see also Chapter 12.2)

Insomnia, fatigue, and daytime sleepiness have been commonly reported in HIV/AIDS patients[66,67]. As in all epidemiological studies of insomnia, prevalence data vary with the stringency of criteria for the diagnosis. Sixty per cent of HIV-infected patients reported 'dissatisfaction with the quality of sleep', while about one in four described sleep as 'poor' or 'very poor'[68]. In another investigation, nearly three-quarters of outpatients with HIV/AIDS were defined as having an insomnia problem by the Pittsburgh Sleep Quality Index (PSQI)[69]. Occurrence of insomnia correlated with depression, anxiety, cognitive impairment, night sweats, chills, and headaches. Nokes and Kendrew described sleep impairment in HIV patients, and examined correlates of sleep quality as measured by PSQI, but did not report prevalence of insomnia, per se[70]. This area has been reviewed in detail by Reid and Dwyer who point out

that these studies all lack adequate comparison groups of healthy individuals or those with other chronic medical illness[71]. Thus, it remains to be seen to what extent HIV/AIDS is associated with rates of insomnia that are actually higher than the general population or others with chronic illness. In this regard, it is noteworthy that one study comparing insomnia subscales of Hamilton Anxiety and Depression ratings found no difference in frequency of insomnia between HIV-positive patients and a control group of non-infected gay men[72].

Patients with moderate or advanced stages of HIV infection are more likely to experience sleep-related problems. St Kubicki et al.[73] described disturbance of sleep, including diminished slow-wave sleep, in patients with diagnosed cerebral disease. Cognitive impairment in patients with AIDS-related CNS involvement is highly predictive of insomnia[69].

As with cancer patients, sleep problems in HIV/AIDS patients are often unrecognized by health-care providers. No consistent relationship between stage of disease and insomnia has been described except in late stage patients with AIDS-defining illnesses[72]. Sleep disorders and their consequences are one of numerous factors that contribute to fatigue in persons with HIV/AIDS. Darko et al.[74] postulated that the debilitating fatigue of these patients may be related to elevated levels of somnogenic humoral factors such as interferon, tumour necrosis factor, and interleukin-1.

Sleep architecture and sleep-related problems have been studied in a number of HIV-infected patients, including some with clinical manifestations of AIDS. In a series of early reports, Norman et al.[75–77] reported alterations in the sleep of asymptomatic HIV-infected males. These patients demonstrated an increase in total slow-wave sleep, particularly as a result of increased slow-wave sleep in the second half of the night, when compared with normal controls. These investigators speculated that the alterations in sleep might represent early changes in the central nervous system associated with the infection or an adaptation to bolster immune response. Similar findings were reported by White et al. who noted correlation between CD4 T cell counts and increase in delta sleep during the last half of the night[78]. They found no evidence of pathological daytime sleepiness. More recent investigations have failed to confirm evidence of increased slow-wave activity[79,80].

Cytokine production has been identified as a potential source of enhanced nocturnal slow-wave activity as well as daytime sleepiness in HIV patients. This theory is supported by the findings of Darko et al. who noted that, in 6/10 HIV patients, fluctuations in the levels of tumour necrosis factor-alpha (TNF-alpha) were coupled to peak periods of slow-wave activity (SWA) in sleep[74]. The strength of this association was proportional to the CD4 cell count, suggesting that, as patients became more ill and cell counts dropped, this physiological coupling of TNK-alpha and SWA declines and, with it, slow-wave sleep. However, evaluation of correlation between CD4 counts and other PSG variables or insomnia complaints have yielded mixed results.

Sleep disturbance has also been described in association with treatment for HIV/AIDS. Early reports suggested that insomnia is a side effect of AZT[81,82], although this association has been questioned by others[80,83]. Severe sleepiness when receiving a combination of AZT and acyclovir[84] has also been described. One polysomnographic investigation of sleep in HIV patients taking zidovudine found no significant alterations in sleep physiology compared to that of unmedicated HIV patients[83]. Larger, more recent investigations have found significant correlation between plasma efavirenz levels and odds ratios for insomnia[85] as well as a significantly higher rate of insomnia among efavirenz users versus those taking protease inhibitor regimens[86]. Of note, increased insomnia did not appear to translate to poorer quality of life in that population.

Co-morbidities and complications also affect the sleep of HIV-infected individuals. The sleep of asymptomatic infected persons is predictably quite different from that in late-stage AIDS with concomitant cancer or opportunistic infections. Although specific effects of depression, anxiety, and dementia, particularly AIDS dementia complex, have not been clearly elucidated, they each can have major impact on sleep of HIV-infected patients. Hintz *et al.* reported the response to antidepressant medications in 90 adult male outpatients with depression, 45 of whom were HIV-positive. Decreased sleep was a particularly prominent finding among the HIV-positive sample. Patients with asymptomatic infection responded better to antidepressant medication[87]. CNS involvement in late stage illness has been associated with high rates of insomnia complaint[69].

Sleep disturbances in cardiorespiratory diseases

Cheyne–Stokes pattern of periodic respirations is common in congestive heart failure patients, occurring in nearly 50 per cent of patients with low ejection fractions[88,89]. A 30 per cent incidence of nocturnal periodic breathing was found in a cohort of 20 German patients being evaluated for pharmacologic treatment of advanced pulmonary hypertension[90]. The disturbance was largely ameliorated by night-time nasal oxygen. In patients with Cheyne–Stokes respirations and congestive heart failure with left-bundle branch block, cardiac resynchronization therapy was associated with significant decrease in apnoeic episodes, reported sleep disturbances, and improved oxygen saturation[91]. A single dose of acetazolamide before bedtime can decrease episodes of sleep apnoea and oxygen desaturation in patients with CHF and may improve daytime symptoms[92]. A case study of a patient with end-stage primary pulmonary hypertension who underwent lung transplantation showed resolution of periodic breathing at night[93]. Disordered breathing during sleep in advanced congestive heart failure has been associated with a higher risk of nocturnal onset ischaemic stroke[94].

Sleep disturbances are recognized to be common in patients with chronic respiratory disease with greater than 50 per cent of patients reporting difficulty falling asleep, staying asleep, or general insomnia. Sleep disturbances tend to worsen as respiratory function deteriorates[95,96]. Theophylline treatment exacerbates sleep disturbances[97]. Anticholinergic inhalers, such as ipratropium bromide, may improve breathing at night without stimulating side-effects of beta adrenergic agonists[96]. Some patients with respiratory insufficiency may benefit greatly from non-invasive nocturnal ventilation. Hypnotic medications must be used cautiously due to their potential to decrease the normal central nervous system respiratory response to hypoxia and hypercapnoea and diminish muscle tone in the upper airway. Short-acting benzodiazepine receptor blockers, such as triazolam, zolpidem, and zaleplon, may be used in selected patients with COPD[95]. Sedating antidepressant medications may improve sleep without respiratory compromise.

Sleep disturbances in end-stage renal failure

Sleep disorders are common in patients with chronic kidney disease[98], including restless leg syndrome, periodic limb movements, and sleep apnoea. In a study of pre-dialysis patients, 53 per cent of subjects reported poor sleep[99]. Disorders of sleep are particularly frequent in patients treated with haemodialysis[98,100]. In one study[101], 77 per cent of dialysis patients had either subclinical or clinical sleep disorders, as assessed by the Sleep Disorders Questionnaire. Most physiologic parameters were not predictive of sleep disturbances, including body weight, body mass index, plasma creatinine, urea, albumin, PTH, or haemoglobin. Those without sleep disorders had significantly fewer co-morbidities. Age, dialytic age, dialysis shift, and antihypertensive prescriptions also were associated with sleep disturbances.

Restless leg syndrome (RLS) is frequent in dialysis patients. In a large Italian study that applied strict diagnostic criteria, Gigli *et al.* found a prevalence of 21 per cent of RLS in a dialysis population[102]. Affected patients had a very high incidence of reported sleep disturbances. Among an array of physiologic and behavioural variables, only the period of dialysis dependence was significantly associated with RLS. RLS patients were taking lower doses of anti-hypertensives and phosphorus binders.

Transplantation is associated with improved quality of life, lower incidences of depression, and sleep disturbances. In a large Hungarian population study, the incidence of insomnia among patients who underwent kidney transplantation was comparable to the general population and far lower than that of transplant wait-list patients. However, the incidence of depression was significantly associated with insomnia and being wait-listed, making it impossible to distinguish an independent impact of transplantation on sleep disturbances[103]. In a study of 100 renal transplant recipients, the incidence of poor sleep (by PSQI) was 30 per cent, slightly above the general population, and was highly associated with depression assessed by the Beck Depression Inventory[104].

Factors contributing to sleep disorder
Depression (see also Chapter 15.5)

Sleep disturbance is a hallmark of major depression. It is generally reported that 90 per cent or more of depressed patients exhibit abnormalities of their sleep patterns. Although early morning awakening is most commonly associated with depression, difficulty initiating sleep and repeated awakenings are common, particularly when depression is associated with medical illness and its attendant complications. Specific disturbances in the continuity of sleep, decreased latency to the first REM sleep period, and diminished slow-wave sleep (N3) can be identified in the sleep EEG of many patients with major depression[105]. The extent to which these findings are pertinent to depression in the context of palliative care patients has not been determined. What is certain is that the sleep disturbance experienced by depressed, seriously ill, and dying patients is a major source of concern, frustration, and added disability.

Depression is common among cancer patients. That much is certain; however, the manner in which the cancer patients were screened and the criteria for assigning a diagnosis of 'depression' have varied widely from one investigator to another, making comparisons of prevalence data difficult and definitive statements of incidence and prevalence impossible. Depressive illness accounts for approximately 50 per cent of psychiatric consultations in cancer patients[106]. Investigation of psychiatric disorders in Japanese cancer patients found that sleep disorders were the second most common reason for initiation of a psychiatric consultation, and that these patients showed high rates of depression, anxiety, and cognitive disturbance[107]. Current estimates, based on investigations utilizing various assessment techniques, place the prevalence of depression in cancer patients at about 25 per cent[108–110]. In those with advanced disease, rates have been estimated at 23–58 per cent[111]. The variation in these numbers reflects differences in patient populations, sampling methods, and inconsistency in diagnostic criteria used to identify depression, as well as the difficulties inherent in diagnosing mood disorder in patients with medical illnesses (see below).

Available prevalence statistics suggest that depression is a significant cause of sleep pathology among people with advanced illness. In light of this, it is surprising to find that antidepressant medication is administered to a relatively small percentage of cancer patients. A 1970s multicentre study of psychotropic drug utilization by the Psychosocial Collaborative Oncology Group (PSYCOG) found that antidepressant medications accounted for only 1 per cent of all psychotropic prescriptions[112]. In the study of Bukberg and colleagues[113] in which 42 per cent of patients met criteria for depression, only 6 per cent were receiving an antidepressant. Jaeger et al.[114] found that 10 per cent of patients with advanced cancer (life expectancy less than 3 months) received antidepressants. This higher rate of administration may reflect a greater degree of overt psychological distress among people who are approaching death. More recent data suggests that this situation may not have improved greatly. Review of antidepressant prescriptions in over 1000 patients receiving palliative care for cancer demonstrated that only 10 per cent received antidepressant medications from the palliative care team and that the majority of these were administered this medication only in the last 2 weeks of life, when it was unlikely to have much effect[115]. This apparently low rate of treatment intervention for depression is, at least in part, a function of the low rate of recognition of the disorder[110].

Under-recognition and under-treatment of mood disorder may in part be a function of the complexity of establishing a diagnosis of depression in this context. The boundaries between adjustment to illness, grief, and clinical depression are not well-defined. In addition, uncertainty exists regarding the use of somatic symptoms (including sleep) in establishing the diagnosis of depression, inasmuch as such symptoms (fatigue, loss of appetite/weight loss, and sleep disturbance) are often a function of the medical disorder. Some evidence suggests that sleep-related symptoms may be of particular importance in identifying depressive illness in cancer patients. One analysis of the association between insomnia and depression, anxiety, and pain revealed that insomnia was closely correlated with depression and anxiety[42]. A study designed to address the specificity of somatic symptoms in the diagnosis of depression in cancer patients found that, with the exception of insomnia, somatic symptoms did not distinguish the patients with depression from the non-depressed cancer population[113]. Although no statistical analysis is offered, the data strongly suggest that early, middle, and late insomnia were more diagnostic of depression. In contrast, Plumb and Holland[116] reported that

depressed patients with malignant disease did not manifest significantly greater insomnia than their next of kin, and reported less insomnia than a comparison psychiatric group with depression and suicide attempt. Unfortunately, the researchers do not make clear whether their findings indicate little insomnia among the cancer patients or a relatively high degree of insomnia in the next-of-kin[116]. Recent analysis of the association between physical symptoms, including sleep disturbance, and depression in palliative care patients revealed that, while increased ratings of physical symptoms were closely associated with presence of depression, a semi-structured DSM-based diagnostic approach outperformed physical symptom ratings coupled with verbal mood rating in identifying depression[117]. Numerous studies have assessed methodologies for evaluation of mood disorders. For the most part, these suggest that depression rating scales or semi-structured interview are superior to single item assessment ('Are you depressed') in detecting significant mood disorder[118,119].

There is no specific evidence regarding the efficacy of antidepressant medications in the treatment of insomnia associated with depression in the terminally ill. First generation antidepressant medications, particularly the more sedating compounds such as amitriptyline, doxepin, and trazodone, have been effective in the treatment of chronic pain syndromes that are frequently accompanied by depression and insomnia[120–122]. Patients with combined pain, depression, and insomnia may benefit not only from sedative and antidepressant effects of tricyclic medication, but also from the analgesic activity of these compounds[123,124]. However, troubling side effects often limit the use and dosages of these agents. More recent generation antidepressants may offer some advantages in terms of fewer side effects and higher compliance rates. For those patients with insomnia complaints, a more sedating compound such as mirtazapine (which can also stimulate appetite) may be appropriate. In patients who are already sedated from opioid or other sources, less sedating/more stimulating medications such as fluoxetine or buproprion may be better choices. There is no clear consensus with regard to greater efficacy for a particular antidepressant or group of antidepressants in cancer patients. Various studies have suggested efficacy of tricyclics[125], possible superiority of fluoxetine versus tricyclics in advanced cancer[126], and lack of significant improvement with fluoxetine[127]. A review of antidepressant efficacy for depression in medical illnesses, including cancer, suggested efficacy for both tricyclics and SSRIs, with a trend towards greater effectiveness, but also higher dropout rates with tricyclics[128].

There are a number of potential reasons for the low rate of antidepressant prescribing, including a wish to avoid polypharmacy, drug interactions, and side effects of antidepressants including sedation or delirium. In some patients the palliative care team may choose a psychostimulant that has a rapid onset of action, rather than tricyclic, SSRI or newer antidepressants. In other patients, the team may use corticosteroids as co-analgesics while exploiting the mood-elevating side effects that often occur. However, use of psychostimulants or steroids requires close attention to the potential disruptive effects that these agents may have on sleep. Lastly, in some patients, supportive counselling that includes problem-solving and anticipatory guidance is quite effective, obviating the need for additional medications.

The available literature makes it clear that depression is a common cause of insomnia among patients with advanced malignancies and that this aspect of their condition frequently goes unrecognized or untreated. Insomnia is an important diagnostic marker for depressive illness that must not be overlooked, particularly in light of the fact that effective treatment is available.

Anxiety

Although there has been little specific investigation of the relationship between advanced illness, specifically cancer, and anxiety symptoms, the available literature supports the common-sense conclusion that anxiety is frequent among these patients[43,129,130]. Anxiety symptoms may be directly related to aspects of the patient's medical condition or treatment. Pain is frequently associated with increased anxiety. Early delirium, withdrawal from analgesics or sedative-hypnotics, and shortness of breath can frequently result in anxiety symptoms. Among patients with significant anxiety, sleep disturbance is common. Battelli et al.[131] reported that 63 per cent of cancer patients with anxiety had insomnia. A survey of 100 oncology clinic patients found a significant correlation between difficulty falling asleep (reported by 40 per cent of the population surveyed) and anxiety symptoms.

Fears that are masked by activities and distractions during daylight hours may come rapidly to the fore in the stillness of night. Anxieties regarding the illness itself, concerns about forthcoming procedures, worries regarding family, work-related responsibilities, or financial matters are but a few of the tensions that can disrupt the onset or maintenance of sleep. Pain may escalate during the night (owing to inadequate medication and lack of distraction), exacerbating anxiety about the meaning of the pain as a possible sign of advancing disease and impending death. For patients in the final stages of their illness, the prospect of sleep may provoke anxieties about the possibility that they will never awaken.

As sleeplessness ensues, the inability to fall asleep may give rise to additional anxiety, setting in motion a vicious cycle in which an ill person with an initially transient sleep disturbance develops a self-fulfilling dread of another tension- and frustration-laden night in bed. For such patients, bed or the coming of night become powerful conditioned stimuli for anxiety and arousal that prevent the onset of sleep. This dilemma may be particularly difficult for patients who are not ambulatory and, thus, unable to assert control over their environment. This combination of heightened internal arousal and conditioned anxiety resulting in chronic, self-propagating sleep disturbance is referred to as psychophysiologic insomnia. This condition may include an increase in muscle tension, sympathetic arousal, and unrelenting cognitive activity. As sleep steadily worsens, daytime anxiety and rumination regarding the inability to obtain a restful night may further erode the ill person's quality of life.

Limited research regarding sleep of patients with diagnosed anxiety disorders has been conducted. Laboratory studies have demonstrated prolonged sleep latency, decreased sleep efficiency (the percentage of time in bed which is spent asleep), increased awake time during the night, decreased deep sleep, and higher percentages of light sleep[40,132,133]. In addition to these alterations of sleep architecture, specific anxiety-related disturbances, such as nocturnal anxiety attacks or nightmares, may occur[134]. Nightmares are dream anxiety episodes that ordinarily arise from REM sleep. They are accompanied by awakening from sleep with a sense of dread or terror and a moderate level of autonomic arousal. The frightening dream content is recalled in detail upon awakening.

Nightmares may occur as a complication of severe anxiety or other psychiatric illness, prior physical or psychological trauma, use of drugs, or administration of certain medications, such as some antidepressants, β-blockers, L-dopa, amantadine, or reserpine.

Psychological and behavioural therapeutic measures including support, reassurance, healthy sleep practices and behavioural techniques, such as relaxation training, counselling involving problem-solving, normalization, and affirmation of self-worth may help to ameliorate the sleep disturbance associated with anxiety. Benzodiazepines have been effective in treating anxiety-related insomnia. Battelli et al. found that 80 per cent of patients with insomnia were sleeping normally after 2 weeks of treatment with lorazepam[131]. Diazepam has also been used with similar beneficial effects, although many patients experienced daytime sedation. Psychotherapy, benzodiazepines, tricyclic, SSRI and antipsychotic medications, and more recently prazosin, have been employed with some success in the treatment of recurrent nightmares[135,136]. Imagery rehearsal, a therapeutic approach designed to teach nightmare sufferers to replace distressing dream images with neutral or pleasant imagery through cognitive rehearsal techniques, has also proven quite helpful[137]. Psychological and behavioural therapies for insomnia and related anxiety are discussed in greater detail in the treatment section.

Cognitive impairment disorders

Numerous investigations have revealed that cognitive dysfunction, particularly delirium, is common among cancer patients[106,138]. The incidence of delirium is particularly high among those in the terminal stages of illness[139] (see Chapter 19.1). Disturbance of the sleep–wake schedule is an intrinsic component of delirium. As described by Lipowski[140], wakefulness during the daytime hours is typically reduced, while night-time often brings increased alertness and agitation. The normal circadian rhythm may be reversed or severely disrupted in this population. The multiple aetiologies of delirium in patients with terminal malignancies have been reviewed elsewhere[141,142]. Sleep deprivation itself may predispose to the development of delirium[143]. Polysomnographic studies of delirium have been limited to withdrawal states[144], and the applicability of these findings to the sleep of patients with delirium due to other causes is uncertain.

Dementia may be encountered in seriously ill patients seen by palliative care teams[130], particularly in the geriatric population. This disorder is often associated with nocturnal delirium (sundowning). Sleep studies of dementia patients reveal increased sleep latencies, lighter sleep, reduced REM sleep, and increased awakening after sleep onset[145–147]. A characteristic finding in dementia patients is loss of the normal sleep–wake rhythm, with increased periods of daytime sleep and diminished nocturnal sleep. This pattern often poses a particularly difficult challenge for care providers who may be stressed beyond their endurance by having to provide not only daytime care and supervision but night-time attendance as well.

Sleep disturbances associated with cognitive impairment disorders can be exceedingly difficult to manage. Accurate diagnosis is the first step. Delirium often goes unrecognized, particularly in its early stages, and may be mistaken for depression or anxiety in some patients. Attempts to treat or control the specific causes of delirium constitute the primary approach. This may include treatments to correct metabolic abnormalities such as elevated serum ammonia levels, hyponatraemia, and hypercalcaemia. Medication lists must be carefully scrutinized and potentially offending medications withdrawn or diminished whenever possible. Alcohol withdrawal has been noted as an overlooked cause of delirium in patients with advanced malignancy[148]. The list of medications that can cause or worsen delirium is long, but common agents include H-1 antihistamines, anticholinergics, anti-parkinsonian medications, analgesics, corticosteroids, hypnotics, and antidepressants. Efforts to prevent excessive sleep and encourage activity during the daytime are advisable. Patients with cognitive dysfunction may sleep better in a lit room, where disorientation and agitation are minimized. Conventional hypnotic medications have typically been avoided, because of concerns regarding side effects such as falls or aggravation of delirium. However, newer generation short-acting hypnotics in lower dosages may prove helpful to some. The traditional pharmacological treatment for patients with non-drug-related delirium and disruptive behaviour is low-dose neuroleptic medication such as haloperidol 0.5–2.0 mg or risperidone 0.5–1.0 mg. Atypical anti-psychotic medications do not consistently have therapeutic advantages over older agents in this setting, are more expensive, and have their own side effects (e.g. sedation and metabolic effects), which may be problematic in a palliative care population[149–151]. In patients whose agitation is largely limited to the night-time, it is often helpful to begin administration of the medication in the late afternoon before agitation begins to escalate. Subcutaneous midazolam has been used effectively in patients with terminal delirium or agitation when other agents were not helpful[152,153].

Pain

A number of issues must be taken into consideration in assessing the relationship between pain and sleep in ill patients. What are the effects of pain on sleep? How does sleep deprivation affect pain threshold and perception? To what extent does pain lower the threshold of waking from sleep? What concomitant variables, such as psychiatric disorders, influence the relationship between pain and sleep?

Pain undoubtedly plays an important role in sleep disturbance in advanced illness with most research having been conducted with cancer patients. Up to 50 per cent of all cancer patients and 60–90 per cent of those with advanced disease experience pain[154–156]. Of 200 patients referred to a cancer pain clinic, 124 (61 per cent) reported that pain interrupted sleep[157]. Dorrepaal and colleagues evaluated pain experience and management in a group of 240 cancer patients in hospital[158]. They found that upon admission, 37 per cent of patients with pain reported that it interfered with sleep onset, while 65 per cent complained of difficulty in maintaining sleep through the night because of pain. Similarly, 56 per cent of 91 lung and colon cancer patients stated that pain interfered 'moderately' or 'greatly' with sleep[159]. A study investigating the influence of cancer-related pain on various quality of life indicators revealed that 58 per cent of cancer patients woke during the night because of pain[160]. Pain intensity has also been demonstrated to correlate inversely with total hours of sleep in patients with advanced cancer[161]. The contribution of pain to fatigue is explained, in part, by its impact on sleep quality[60]. Psychological distress, particularly depression and anxiety, secondary to chronic pain may also contribute to insomnia and fatigue[162].

Donovan et al. examined the issue of pain in hospitalized patients and the effects of inadequate analgesia[163]. In this mixed group, which consisted of predominantly non-cancer patients with acute or chronic pain, 61 per cent reported that they were awakened by pain. The patients were receiving an average of less than 25 per cent of the total analgesic dosage ordered. Of note, the incidence and severity of pain in this population did not differ between those with and without cancer.

Pain models and related variables

Understanding the effects of pain on sleep provides further insight into this problem. In assessing peak pain-related symptoms, Kinsman et al.[164] reported that 60 per cent of the group complained of frequent sleep disturbance. In a population of patients attending a pain clinic, sleep was characterized as 'poor' by 70 per cent of the group[165]. The poor sleepers reported greater pain intensity, less total sleep time, and a tendency towards greater disability. Pain intensity and depression were the only significant predictors of sleep disturbance, leading the investigators to speculate that degree of insomnia may serve as a useful marker for pain intensity. Closs found that pain was the most common factor resulting in sleep disturbance in postoperative patients. Pain relief was the most effective intervention for improving sleep maintenance[166].

Animal models of chronic pain demonstrate an increase in wakefulness, a shift to lighter stages of NREM sleep, reduction in paradoxical (REM) sleep, and fragmentation of sleep[167,168]. There was a concomitant loss of the normal diurnal variation of sleep–wake cycles. Similar polysomnographic findings have been described in humans with rheumatic and other pain conditions[169,170].

It is well established that people in pain often do not sleep well, but the impact of pain on sleep is not a simple cause and effect relationship. Associated factors, particularly psychological distress (including, as discussed, depression, and anxiety) contribute to disrupting normal sleep. For example, the incidence of pain among cancer patients with a psychiatric disorder is twice that of those without a psychiatric diagnosis[169]. This may reflect the fact that patients with pain are also likely to have more advanced illness and therefore to be more susceptible to depression or cognitive impairment disorders. Nevertheless, it is apparent that psychiatric comorbidity may account for sleep disturbance as much as the pain per se. Beszterczey and Lipowski[42] described decreased total sleep time in a group of cancer patients referred for radiation therapy. In their analysis, insomnia correlated far better with the degree of depression and anxiety than with pain. A study of chronic pain patients found that presleep cognitive arousal was more predictive of poor sleep than pain severity. Thus, while pain may be an important determinant of sleep disturbance, a range of other factors, some of which co-vary with pain, may be of equal importance.

Sleep deprivation and pain

Analysis of the relationship between sleep and pain, must take into account how sleep disturbances can affect pain perception and, conversely, to what extent improving sleep can produce a beneficial effect on pain. Several investigations have reported that pain threshold in rats is decreased in response to deprivation of REM sleep[171,172], and that the effect persisted for up to 96 h following the deprivation[171]. This may be related to the fact that opioid receptor binding decreases after sleep deprivation[173]. It has been shown that sleep deprivation, and specifically REM deprivation, lowers pain threshold in human controls[172,174]. Likewise, reversal of sleep deprivation produces significant increases in threshold[172]. Burn patients reported higher levels of background pain during the night-time and this correlated strongly with poor sleep quality[175]. In addition, poor sleep quality predicted higher levels of pain on the following day. Repeated interruptions of sleep induced experimentally result in a pain syndrome, which is akin to fibromyalgia[176]. The work of Moldofsky and others related to fibromyalgia syndrome suggests that sleep may play an important role in pain modulation and that disturbance of sleep might predispose to the development of rheumatic pain disorder. The relationship of these findings to pain of other origins is uncertain.

Clinical experience suggests that patients whose coping skills are enhanced by improved sleep are in a far better position to maintain optimal function despite their pain and, perhaps, to perceive the pain as less severe. This notion is supported by reports from hospital patients with acute and chronic pain that sleep helped to reduce their pain[160]. Moreover, administration of delta-sleep-inducing peptide to chronic pain patients resulted in reduction of pain and associated symptoms of depression[177].

In summary, pain is a frequent symptom of cancer and other advanced illnesses and often contributes to the development and persistence of sleep disturbances. Sleep deprivation, in turn, may exacerbate pain problems and erode the often tenuous function and quality of life of seriously ill patients. Common associated problems, including co-varying conditions, such as depression and anxiety, play a contributory role. The interrelationship of factors suggests that by controlling pain, clinicians may foster a therapeutic cascade of improved sleep, diminished psychological distress, and better cognitive function, resulting in improved overall quality of life.

Medication

Medications in common use can disturb sleep in a variety of ways. Attention is warranted to medications that can interfere with normal sleep, as well as those that can cause excessive or undesirable sedation. The effects of specific hypnotic medication are discussed in the treatment section of this chapter.

Clinical experience suggests that corticosteroids can disturb sleep in some patients, although this has not been well documented. Steroids do appear to decrease REM sleep[178], but the clinical implications of this are uncertain. Although use of other anti-inflammatory alternatives or minimization of steroid dosage may reduce the potential risk of sleep disturbance, this is not a realistic possibility in many cases. In such circumstances, use of otherpharmacological and non-pharmacological strategies to minimize the impact on sleep is necessary. Methylxanthine derivatives (bronchodilators) have theoretical potential for disturbing sleep, although the extent to which this occurs clinically is not known. Central nervous system stimulants, increasingly employed to counteract opioid-induced sedation, have clear potential for disrupting sleep when given too close to bedtime, as do certain types of antidepressants (e.g. monoamine oxidase inhibitors, fluoxetine, or bupropion). Withdrawal from certain short-acting sedative-hypnotic medication or SSRI antidepressants is also a potentially important cause of insomnia. Certain antihypertensives, such as methyldopa and propranolol,

have been reported to cause insomnia; the latter also associated with nightmare activity in some patients. Medications used for Parkinson's disease, including L-dopa, selegiline, pramipexole, and amantadine, can interfere with sleep and cause nightmares. Dopamine agonists have also been associated with excessive sleepiness in Parkinson's disease patients.

Relatively little attention has been given to the effects of cancer chemotherapy agents on sleep. Some studies demonstrate an association between chemotherapy, poor sleep, and increased fatigue in cancer patients, either prior to or during treatment[38,179–181]. Some chemotherapeutic agents may produce insomnia as a result of their potential for inducing nausea or cognitive dysfunction.

Psychotropic agents

Excessive sleepiness and associated daytime impairment induced by medication can severely compromise function of patients already impaired by other aspects of their disease. The most common offending agents are psychotropics prescribed for anxiety, sleep, and depression, or employed as antiemetics. Older patients with medical illness are susceptible to sedating effects of generally safe medications, such as antihistamines, and are particularly vulnerable to excess sedation due to drug accumulation as a result of delayed metabolism and excretion. Sedating antidepressants, such as amitriptyline, doxepin, or trazodone, may result in daytime sleepiness, even when given at bedtime. Phenothiazines and other dopamine antagonists used in the treatment of nausea due to chemotherapy can be very sedating. This is especially true for aliphatic and piperidine compounds, but less so for piperazine derivatives and butyrophenones. H_1 antagonist antihistamines are routinely administered before chemotherapy and transfusions, are commonly prescribed for pruritis, and are sometimes used as hypnotics. As noted above, they are a common cause of daytime sleepiness especially in elderly and ill patients. H_2 antagonists have less effect on the central nervous system.

Opioids and other analgesics

The effects of opioids on sleep and wakefulness are complex and appear to include both stimulant and sedative properties[182]. The effects of opioids on sleep structure vary with duration of usage. Acute administration in healthy adults produces diminished slow wave and REM sleep[183]. With long-term use, there is diminished difficulty falling asleep, but more time awake during the night. Similarly, drowsiness is common after morphine administration for acute pain, but tends to abate with chronic use. The prominent initial effect of REM suppression is less evident with longer-term administration. The effects on NREM sleep vary according to type of drug, length of usage, and specific sleep stage. There is some evidence to suggest that daytime psychomotor performance is slowed as a result of opioid administration[184] but other data show minimal or no effects of opioids. The adverse effects of opioids on breathing in sleep are discussed in the following section.

Although these data are helpful in understanding the effects of opioid analgesics on sleep, most are derived from small studies, often with subjects who were not seriously ill or not in pain. As discussed, effective analgesia typically results in improved sleep for pain patients, and any alterations of 'normal' sleep that may be induced by medication are outweighed by the benefits attributable to relief of pain. A notable advance in this area has been the use of controlled-release opioids for pain control. Hanks *et al.* describe improved sleep in a group of advanced cancer patients in response to crossover from aqueous morphine sulfate administered 4-hourly to controlled-release morphine[53]. Ventafridda *et al.* reported that mean total sleep time was doubled in patients with cancer pain treated according to the WHO guidelines[185]. Similar observations have been described by other investigators[54,186]. Comparisons of controlled-release morphine and transdermal fentanyl have demonstrated improved sleep with both medications[187–189]. One study suggested that the transdermal fentanyl may be associated with somewhat less daytime sedation and poorer sleep quality than controlled-release morphine[187]. While opioids can produce some degree of daytime drowsiness, particularly in the earlier phases of administration, this is not always the case and, in some, may be considered a potentially unavoidable sequela of adequate pain relief. While a clinician, in careful discussion with a patient, should attempt to strike an appropriate balance between pain relief and sedation, sufficient analgesia usually takes precedence. Effective strategies for control of daytime sedation with stimulant medications have been described[190,191].

Significant improvements in sleep have also been reported with the use of non-steroidal anti-inflammatory drugs (NSAIDs) in advanced cancer pain[192]. Carrol *et al.*[193] demonstrated that a combined regimen of methadone, NSAID, tricyclics, and hydroxyzine produced marked improvement in pain and sleep in patients not responsive to single drug therapy. For patients refractory to all other routes of opioid administration, combined, long-term intrathecal morphine and bupivacaine have produced prolonged improvement in sleep and pain[194]. A multi-disciplinary approach that included various combinations of oral and epidural opioids, non-opioid analgesics, antidepressants, benzodiazepines, anticonvulsants, and nerve blocks produced an almost 80 per cent reduction in the number of cancer patients whose sleep was interrupted by pain[157]. In appropriate circumstances, continuous infusion *and* or patient-controlled analgesia will be superior to immediate release oral opioids in fostering sustained sleep. A comparison of the effects of a mild sedative with those of a mild analgesic on sleep in non-cancer patients demonstrated that the analgesic was most important in improving sleep for those with pain[195]. The pharmacological effects of opioids on sleep physiology and wakefulness are discussed below.

Respiratory disorders

Respiratory disturbance during sleep is a common cause of sleep disorder. Obstructive sleep apnoea is associated primarily with heavy snoring and excessive daytime sleepiness, although some patients report frequent nocturnal awakening. The syndrome is observed more commonly in older patients and those who are obese. There is no clear connection between obstructive sleep apnoea and malignancy in general, although it should be noted that patients whose upper airway structure or function is compromised directly as a result of tumour mass or indirectly through treatment may be predisposed to the development of obstruction during sleep. This has been described in patients with parapharyngeal tumour mass[196,197], medulloblastoma[198], other head and neck cancers, both pre- and post-treatment[47,48], and in those who have undergone mandibulectomy without reconstruction[199]. In patients with AIDS, daytime sleepiness has been described in association with sleep apnoea due to tonsillar hypertrophy[200].

Others have reported OSA associated with obesity and lipodystrophy in HIV-infected patients[201].

Perhaps of greater importance for the majority of patients with advanced disease being seen by palliative care teams is the fact that respiratory depressant medications, particularly opioid analgesics, but also benzodiazepines, can exacerbate this condition. Etches described severe respiratory depression associated with patient-controlled opioid analgesia[202]. Pre-existing sleep apnoea and concomitant use of sedative-hypnotics were associated with the development of respiratory compromise. Opioid analgesics have been associated with worsening of obstructive sleep apnoea, particularly in the acute postoperative period. Central sleep apnoea has been linked to chronic opioid usage, especially methadone, as well as to certain malignancies[203,204]. Sleep apnoea frequently goes unrecognized and may be a source of major compromise of function (due to sleepiness and attendant neuropsychological factors) in patients with advanced illness. Positive airway pressure (PAP) remains the recommended treatment for moderate to severe OSA, although its application in a palliative care population will depend on assessment of the particular advantages and disadvantages for a given patient. Bilevel PAP may also be used effectively for non-invasive ventilation in patients with significant hypoventilation due to lower airway obstructive disease, neuromuscular weakness, or restrictive disease, including obesity.

Dyspnoea is a disturbing symptom for many palliative care patients, particularly those with far advanced respiratory failure from intrinsic pulmonary diseases or from intractable congestive heart failure, as well as those with primary lung cancer, pulmonary metastases, and lymphangitic spread of tumour. Pulmonary involvement may give rise to complaints of insomnia through two primary mechanisms. Patients describe the sensation of breathlessness as psychologically disturbing and have difficulty initiating or maintaining sleep as a result of heightened arousal associated with this anxiety. Studies of patients with chronic obstructive pulmonary disease also suggest that severe hypoxia and/or hypercapnoea, and especially chronic cough, may play a role in determining sleep disturbance. Decreased total sleep time, increased light sleep, multiple arousals, and decreased REM sleep have been reported in such patients[205]. Non-pharmacological treatment (e.g. relaxation training) for heightened arousal associated with breathlessness may aid sleep in patients with dyspnoea. Nocturnal oxygen supplementation is indicated for hypoxic patients. Pharmacological treatment with benzodiazepines may be used cautiously in patients without major blood gas alterations, but is contraindicated in more severely hypoxic or hypercapnoeic patients.

Gastrointestinal disorders

Nausea and vomiting following certain forms of chemotherapy can disrupt sleep and impair quality of life[206]. Some patients with advanced illness report nocturnal diarrhoea or discomfort associated with chronic constipation as a cause of repeated sleep disruption. These complications may occur as a result of autonomic dysfunction, medication, or other forms of treatment. Gastro-oesophageal reflux is commonly aggravated during sleep, giving rise to epigastric pain, heartburn, and cough, with repeated disruption of sleep. Patients with nasogastric tubes commonly report irritation in their nose or hypopharynx that interferes with sleep. Patients receiving nocturnally administered nutrition via gastrostomy or jejunostomy tubes may experience intestinal bloating or cramping that interrupts sleep.

Hospital admission

It is well known that admission to hospital can be associated with marked disruption of sleep[207,208]. Although this issue has been examined primarily in patients in surgical and intensive care units, it stands to reason that other seriously ill patients also experience frequent interruptions of sleep as a direct result of the hospital environment. Potential interruptions include intrusions by staff to monitor vital signs, check lines, infusion pumps and other equipment, or administer medications, excessive noise or light, difficulties experienced by other patients occupying the same room, or conversations among staff in the hallway or nursing station. Under these circumstances sleep may become highly fragmented and total sleep time markedly reduced, giving rise to increased napping and disturbance of the sleep–wake cycle. Efforts by staff to minimize such disrupting factors are likely to result in improved sleep[209].

Other conditions affecting sleep and wakefulness

Numerous other disorders may predispose to poor sleep in the terminally ill. Nocturia is a common source of repetitive awakening in patients receiving diuretics. Similarly, patients may suffer from frequent nocturnal headaches that disrupt sleep. Endocrine disturbance can give rise to sleep disorder. A specific endocrine issue that has been identified as a significant cause of sleep disturbance is that of hot flushes. Carpenter *et al.* reported that 65 per cent of post-menopausal breast cancer patients experienced hot flushes[210]. Among those with hot flushes, 86 per cent had some form of nocturnal hot flushes. Studies of post-menopausal women have demonstrated that hot flushes are associated with sleep disruption and that treatment with hormone replacement therapy (HRT) improves sleep[211]. Unfortunately, HRT may be contraindicated in the population of breast cancer patients, who are most susceptible to this problem. SSRI and serotonin-norepinephrine reuptake inhibitors represent alternative approaches for managing hot flushes though their reported efficacy is somewhat less than HRT[193,212].

Other primary sleep disorders may occur in seriously ill patients. The most notable of those not mentioned elsewhere in this chapter are restless legs syndrome (RLS) and periodic limb movement in sleep (PLMS). RLS is a waking dysaesthesia, most often localized to the calves, which occurs primarily in evening hours with inactivity. The major manifestation of this dysaesthesia is an irresistible urge to move the legs. RLS may interfere with sleep onset or maintenance, as well as cause the sufferer great torment while waking. PLMS, often observed in patients with RLS, consists of repetitive, stereotyped leg or arm movements that occur at intervals of 20–40 sec during sleep, typically in clusters throughout the night. The repetitive movements may result in frequent arousals during sleep, leading to complaints of light or non-restorative sleep, sleep maintenance disturbance, or daytime sleepiness. Potential aetiologies of the disorders are noted in Table 10.12.2, although they are frequently idiopathic. These conditions may respond to correction of the underlying causative factor, when one can be identified. In most cases, dopamine agonists are the treatment of choice. Clonazepam, opioids, and gabapentin have also been employed with good results in some cases. Low iron stores have also been associated with RLS. Current recommendations suggest that ferritin levels less than 40 ng/ml. should be treated with iron supplementation in RLS patients.

Evaluation

The most serious and fundamental problem in the identification and treatment of sleep disorders is that patients are frequently never asked about their sleep. When complaints are offered by the patient, they are too often dismissed by clinicians as insignificant or because they assume little can be done. It is essential that healthcare practitioners recognize the importance of adequate sleep and alertness to the psychological, social, and physical well-being of their patients. Two basic questions should be asked of all patients as a component of the general systems review: How are you sleeping at night? Are you excessively sleepy during the day? When sleep-related complaints are elicited, a more detailed history is required. As previously emphasized, insomnia and hypersomnolence are not diagnoses in their own right. Further assessment is required to determine the significance of these complaints to the patient, as well as to define the potential causes of these complaints. The basic principles of evaluation are outlined in Table 10.12.3.

A complaint of 'insomnia' may arise as a result of several different types of sleep-related disturbance. Although insomnia is most often associated with, reports of difficulty in initiating or maintaining sleep, other factors such as the perceived quality of sleep, timing of the sleep–wake cycle, or total duration of sleep may also give rise to sleep complaints. Since these varied presentations may suggest different causative factors, an effort must be made to clarify these components of the disorder. It is helpful to identify the context in which the sleep disturbance began, with consideration of possible precipitating factors. Elaboration of the influence of intervening variables, including treatment efforts, may also yield useful information regarding aetiology. The patient's 24-h schedule must be determined. Sleep medicine clinicians frequently employ sleep logs for this purpose. An example of a typical

Table 10.12.3 Evaluation of sleep disorders.

Identify the primary complaint: insomnia, excessive sleepiness, parasomnia, (abnormal event), sleep–wake schedule disturbance
Characterize the complaint: difficulty initiating sleep, recurrent nocturnal awakening, insufficient total sleep, non-restorative sleep, advanced or delayed sleep onset, excessively long sleep, chronic drowsiness, sleep attacks
Document the sleep–wake cycle: sleep logs including night-time sleep schedule, naps, activities, medications (see below)
Identify possible precipitants of disturbance: information from patient and spouse or family members (see Table 10.12.2)
Consider the particular sleep requirements of the patients: short/average/long sleepers, variation in sleep habits with age and situation
Medical and neuropsychiatric history
Substance use: medication, alcohol, drugs, caffeine, nicotine
Physical examination and laboratory data
Polysomnography, particularly in elderly medically ill patients with excessive sleepiness or those with histories suggesting underlying physiological disturbance (breathing or movement disorder)
Multiple Sleep Latency Test; evaluation of otherwise unexplained excessive daytime sleepiness

Table 10.12.4 Sample sleep log.

How tired were you at bedtime? 1–5 (1=most tired; 5=not tired at all)	
What time did you get into bed last night?	
What time did you turn out the lights?	
How long did it take you to fall asleep?	
How many times did you awaken during the night?	
What was the total time of these awakenings?	
What time did you awaken for the day?	
What time did you wish to awaken?	
What time did you get out of bed?	
Estimate your total sleep time for last night	
How rested were you when you awoke? 1–5 (1= very rested; 5= not rested at all)	
What was the quality of your sleep last night? (1–5; 1= most refreshing; 5= least refreshing)	
Did you nap during the day? When? For how long?	
How many alcoholic beverages did you consume?	
How many caffeine beverages did you consume? At what time?	
List your medications for each day:	
Please describe, by day, any unusual stresses or events that might have affected your sleep:	

sleep log is seen in Table 10.12.4. Such logs are completed for a period of 1–2 weeks. Some patients report that the mere process of completing such a log helps them to identify conditions unfavourable to sleep.

Difficulty falling asleep is often associated with negative expectations regarding sleep, specific anxieties, ruminations, and, in some cases, heightened physiologic arousal (increased heart rate, respiratory rate, or muscle tension). In a medically ill population, physical factors, most notably pain, may interfere with the onset of sleep. To gain an understanding of associated patterns of cognition, affect, and behaviour that may further contribute to delayed sleep onset or prolonged nocturnal awakenings, it is necessary to determine what the patient thinks, feels, and does during the time in bed awake. Identification of anxieties regarding the course of illness, upcoming procedures, family matters, and death is of particular importance in terminally ill patients.

When patients have difficulty maintaining sleep, an effort must be made to identify possible precipitants for the awakenings. Although psychological factors, particularly depression, may contribute to awakening and difficulty in returning to sleep, midcycle awakening, especially repeated brief awakenings, should increase the clinician's suspicion of an underlying physiological cause. Failure to provide analgesia of sufficient dosage and duration often results in awakening due to pain. Other readily identifiable causes must be sought, such as nocturia, respiratory disturbance (sleep apnoea, congestive heart failure, primary, or metastatic pulmonary disease), headache, or non-specific musculoskeletal discomfort. Repeated awakenings may be associated with specific sleep-related conditions such as periodic movements in sleep, sleep apnoea, or nightmares. Disease of the central nervous system can result in

severe disruption of the normal sleep–wake architecture and inability to maintain sound sleep for any length of time.

In evaluating complaints of insomnia, the clinician must keep in mind that the duration of normal sleep varies significantly from person to person. The 'normal' amount of sleep for a given individual is best defined as that amount which is required to achieve sustained daytime alertness, concentration, and energy. This may be difficult to assess in seriously ill patients and, for this reason, it is necessary to rely on the patient's pre-morbid sleep history to determine how many hours of sleep that individual can reasonably expect. The severity of the impact of sleep disturbance on the patient's quality of life must be gauged. A complaint of insomnia should include evidence of impairment of daytime function that is attributable to insufficient or poor quality sleep. There are some individuals who may complain of fatigue and sleepiness in spite of obtaining what the clinician assumes to be a normal amount of sleep. These patients may be 'long-sleepers' who are essentially sleep-deprived with 'average' total sleep times. Although no systematic investigation has been conducted, it seems plausible that a need for extra sleep may arise in conditions of systemic illness.

For some patients, the complaint of insomnia may be more related to the timing of sleep in the 24-h cycle. Specifically, patients may complain of difficulty in falling asleep although, once asleep, they are capable of achieving an appropriate amount of sleep. This and other sleep–wake rhythm disorders have been discussed earlier in this chapter.

A careful review of medication, drugs, and alcohol usage is a crucial component in assessing complaints of insomnia and excessive sleepiness. The role of medication has been discussed. Patients who are experiencing difficulty sleeping often resort to alcohol in an effort to alleviate their symptoms. Although sufficient amounts of alcohol will ultimately induce sleep onset, sleep during later stages of the night is often light and marked by frequent awakenings and increased autonomic arousal. Alcohol may also aggravate sleep-related breathing disorders. Caffeine is an obvious, but surprisingly overlooked, cause of sleep disturbance. In assessing its role, one must be aware of the fact that some individuals experience marked and prolonged arousal in response to even small quantities of caffeine. Nicotine has also been demonstrated to have similar disruptive effects on sleep in normal subjects although nicotine may improve mood and sleep in depressed patients. The impact of nicotine transdermal patches on patients trying to quite smoking is complex and remains under study[213]. Stimulant medications have been used increasingly in the management of daytime sedation due to opioids. In such usages, caution must be exercised to avoid adverse effects on nocturnal sleep due to excessive or late dosages of the stimulant.

The physical examination and laboratory data must also be considered an essential part of the evaluation of patients with sleep disorder. Particular attention must be paid to the evaluation of pain and to the neurological, endocrine, and cardiopulmonary examinations. General laboratory screening may include a full blood count and biochemistry as well as screening for nutritional deficiency, endocrine disturbance, and medication levels, as indicated. Serum ferritin levels may be helpful in identifying low iron stores as a cause of restless legs syndrome.

Overnight sleep study (polysomnography) is an important element in the assessment of sleep disorders. However, such studies should clearly be used in a judicious manner for patients receiving palliative care. Nevertheless, when proper indications exist, the information gained from such studies may allow dramatic improvements in the quality of life. Standard polysomnography typically includes monitoring of sleep EEG, submental EMG, eye movement, airflow, respiratory effort, oxygen saturation, ECG, and leg movements, with additional parameters as indicated. An adequate diagnostic study can usually be accomplished in one night, with minimum discomfort or inconvenience for the patient. Such studies are most useful when an underlying physiological disturbance, such as periodic limb movement or sleep-related breathing disorder, is suspected. Further characterization of abnormal events (parasomnias) or medical conditions in sleep may also be productive. Polysomnography is not indicated in the routine assessment of primary insomnia or insomnia due to mental disorders such as depression or anxiety[214]. When complaints of unexplained daytime fatigue or sleepiness are present, daytime nap studies (Multiple Sleep Latency Test) that follow overnight sleep study can provide an objective determination of the degree of sleepiness, as well as shedding light on certain specific diagnoses, such as narcolepsy.

Treatment

The treatment of sleep disorders must be carefully tailored to the aetiology of the condition and the particular needs and specific situation of the patient. Just as there are usually a number of contributing factors in the genesis and maintenance of a sleep disorder, treatment must correspondingly be multifaceted. When insomnia or excessive sleepiness is secondary to a serious medical or psychiatric condition, ideally the primary condition would be identified and effectively treated as a means of effecting significant improvement in sleep. However, in the context of palliative care, a patient's underlying condition is typically advanced and even with optimal treatment, continued medical and psychological complications, as well as perpetuating psychophysiologic factors may complicate insomnia and excessive sleepiness. By definition, it is not possible to abolish the primary disease process for palliative care patients, but it is usually feasible to control aspects of the process in a manner that will have a positive impact on sleep.

Sleep hygiene

Most people are aware of the common-sense guidelines and advice for promoting good sleep. Nevertheless, failure to adhere to these practical steps is an almost ubiquitous component of many sleep disorders. The problems in this area are so common that the International Classification of Sleep Disorders nosology designates a diagnosis for 'Inadequate Sleep Hygiene'. Adequate sleep is dependent on the proper internal (psychophysiologic) and external (environmental) circumstances; the recognized components of good sleep hygiene can be seen as an effort optimize the individual's internal and external milieu. Suggestions for sleep hygiene in palliative care patients are summarized in Table 10.12.5.

Excessive arousal in bed is a frequent cause and effect of insomnia. A patient with serious, progressive illness may carry multiple concerns to bed and their level of arousal may be pronounced. Lying in bed, mind racing, agitated and tense, despite fatigue, there may be little possibility of falling asleep soon. Remaining in bed may be distinctly frustrating and counterproductive. However, this is often what patients with insomnia do, either by choice or, in the

Table 10.12.5 Sleep hygiene for palliative care patients.

Maintain as regular a sleep–wake schedule as possible, particularly with respect to the hour of morning awakening
Avoid unnecessary time in bed during the day; for bedridden patients, provide as much cognitive and physical stimulation during daytime hours as conditions permit
Nap only as necessary and avoid napping in the late afternoon and evening, whenever possible
Keep as active a daytime schedule as possible: this should include social contacts and, when able, light exercise
Minimize night-time sleep interruptions due to medication, noise, or other environmental conditions
Avoid lying in bed for prolonged periods at night in an alert and frustrated or tense state; read or engage in other relaxing activity (out of bed, when appropriate) including relaxation exercises, meditation, or prayer until drowsiness ensues
Remove unpleasant conditioned stimuli, such as clocks, from sight and sound
Identify problems and concerns of the day before trying to sleep, and address these issues with an active problem-solving approach
Avoid stimulating medication and other substances (e.g. caffeine, nicotine), particularly in the hours before bedtime
Maintain adequate pain relief through the night, preferably with long-acting analgesics
Use sleep medication as indicated after proper evaluation of the sleep problem and avoid overusage

case of non-ambulatory patients, because they have no option. Under the mistaken impression that they are 'resting', or because getting out of bed is a sign of defeat, they remain in bed, sometimes for hours, fully awake. When this occurs on a regular basis for weeks or months, the bed becomes associated not with relaxation and sleep but, rather, with frustration and tension. In time, the mere sight of the bed evokes increased arousal.

When an individual is unable to fall asleep within a reasonable period (typically within 20–30 min), he should get out of bed and engage in some relaxing activity until he feels ready to sleep. For patients who require assistance to get out of bed, this presents a problem. In such cases, some provision should be made to allow for some relaxing activity (e.g. reading, music, or hand-work) in bed. It is most important that the focus be turned away from a pressure to fall asleep. This is a situation in which patients may benefit from being taught simple relaxation exercises or meditation that involves an affirming focus or content. Patients who are comfortable with prayer can be encouraged to use wakeful periods at night as an opportunity to deepen their spiritual practice.

Other stimuli may also come to evoke a response of wakefulness. One of the most common is the clock. When unable to fall asleep, or following an awakening, patients often stare at the clock. In time, the clock becomes a very powerful reminder of their inability to fall asleep. If this occurs, clocks and similar conditioned stimuli must be identified and removed from sight or sound.

Palliative care patients are especially susceptible to alterations of their normal schedules. Because of fatigue, immobility, discomfort, or lack of motivation, the daytime level of activity is often severely curtailed. When this occurs, the division between day and night becomes blurred. This is particularly true if napping and time in bed are a significant part of the daily routine. Lacking many of the usual environmental cues (zeitgebers) that serve to strengthen basic circadian rhythms, the affected individual is no longer well entrained to an organized sleep–wake rhythm. As a result, the sleep pattern may become chaotic and unpredictable. The therapeutic approach to this problem involves taking steps to reinforce the basic rest/activity–sleep/wake cycle. A regular hour of bedtime and arising is the most essential part of this. Complete avoidance of daytime napping and recumbent rest is not realistic for very sick patients, but such time should be limited and scheduled as early in the day as possible, to foster a prolonged period of wakeful activity prior to bedtime. A programme of physical activity and cognitive and social stimulation will underscore day–night differences and strengthen biological rhythms. Although vigorous physical exercise is not usually possible in this population, even mild exercise in a sitting or recumbent position may be helpful. However, excessive physical stimulation should be avoided in the pre-bedtime hours as this may interfere with sleep onset.

It is frequently the case that patients manage to avoid anxieties during the day by means of distraction, only to be inundated with worries as they lie in bed in the quiet privacy of their thoughts. There may, therefore, be therapeutic benefit in addressing anxieties, concerns, and disappointments in a direct fashion during waking hours. Helping patients to identify their concerns and problem-solve and encouraging them to take an active role in resolving problems and completing their affairs, supporting people both in asking for forgiveness and in granting forgiveness to others can all be part of supportive counselling in the context of palliative care.

Finally, patients often benefit from help in accepting those aspects of their situation that cannot be changed.

Particularly for patients who reside in an institutional setting, the sleeping environment must not be overlooked as a potential source of sleep disturbance. Patients in a hospital or nursing facility often experience frequent interruptions of sleep as a result of staff activities, background noise, lighting, or other factors. It is necessary to identify environmental circumstances of this nature and seek solutions in conjunction with the patient. For example, some patients prefer a darker sleeping environment while others, particularly those with some degree of cognitive disturbance, find a partially lit room to be orienting and reassuring. Hospital beds may assist some patients in attaining comfortable positions that are not possible in standard beds. For individuals who are not ambulatory and require special assistance in meeting minimal needs, it will be reassuring to have access to necessary articles at the bedside as well as a reliable means of calling for assistance. One advantage to transition to a home environment can be the ability to sleep with a spouse or with a beloved pet on the patient's bed.

Substances such as caffeine, nicotine, and alcohol, which may interfere with sleep, should be avoided well before bedtime. The effects of food intake on sleep are not clear. Some patients find a snack at bedtime comforting, while others insist that food before bedtime promotes wakefulness. l-Tryptophan, found in higher concentrations in certain foodstuffs, has been promoted as a potential sleep aid, although laboratory studies indicate only modest effect.[215]

Psychological and behavioural treatment of insomnia

Cognitive behavioural approaches have emerged as mainstays in the treatment of chronic insomnia. Reviews and meta-analyses of this subject are available[94]. There is no single most effective behavioural approach and mulitcomponent strategies are frequently employed. For many palliative care patients, behavioural interventions may require some adaptation but can nevertheless be effective.

Successful applications of behavioural techniques for control of sleep disturbance in cancer patients have been reported. Cannici et al.[216] described the first use of muscle relaxation training in 15 patients with insomnia 'secondary to cancer'. They reported a significant reduction in sleep latency and increase in total sleep time for the treatment group following 3 days of relaxation training. Anecdotal reports indicate that other behavioural approaches, including hypnosis[217] and somatic focus/imagery training[218] have been effective for insomnia in cancer patients. In a related vein, behavioural interventions are frequently employed for patients with cancer pain and chronic pain syndromes[219,220]. Currie and others demonstrated effectiveness of a multicomponent cognitive behavioural approach to insomnia in chronic pain patients, with maintenance of gains after 3 months[221]. This aspect of treatment, which is highly relevant to sleep disturbance, is reviewed in Chapter 10.1.13. Savard and colleagues conducted the first larger scale, controlled outcome assessment of CBT administered to breast cancer patients. They demonstrated that a multicomponent CBT intervention resulted in improved sleep, less medication usage, and improved mood and quality of life ratings in comparison to waiting list controls. The effects were sustained over a 12-month follow-up period[9]. Moreover, multiple measures of immune function suggested improved function following treatment[33].

Numerous specific techniques are included in the cognitive behavioural approach. These approaches are summarized in Table 10.12.6. Some have proven more effective than others in the management of insomnia. Progressive muscle relaxation therapy has been used widely in the treatment of insomnia, and is effective when used alone or as a part of multicomponent treatment. This approach is designed to reduce not only muscle tension but also other elements of physiological and cognitive hyperarousal that interfere with sleep onset or maintenance. Relaxation training can be practised by means of a bedside tape-recorded training session, although patients with more severe or chronic insomnia may require the intervention of a skilled behavioural therapist.

It has previously been noted that many patients with insomnia spend excessive time in bed in a waking and aroused state. Two commonly employed and effective strategies that address this important aspect of insomnia are stimulus control and sleep restriction[222,223]. Both of these approaches can be quite stressful on patients in their early phases and may result in some initial sleep deprivation, rendering them of limited practicality for very sick patients. Other behavioural approaches such as biofeedback, hypnosis, autogenic training, systematic desensitization, or meditation may be helpful for some patients.

In addition to the specific behavioural strategies described, identification and restructuring of cognitive distortions related to the insomnia is often a useful component. Common maladaptive cognitions include such things as 'I can't sleep without medication' or 'If I can't sleep I should stay in bed and try harder to fall asleep'. 'Catastrophization' regarding the consequences of poor sleep is also a common distortion that should be addressed.

Finally, supportive brief psychotherapy contacts that allow the patient to ventilate hopes and fears may yield indirect benefit for sleep problems. Although some of the therapeutic time may be spent in discussion of the sleep problem per se, it is advisable for the therapist to turn the patient's attention towards anxieties, conflicts, or disappointments that commonly arise in life-threatening conditions. A practical, problem-solving approach to these matters is particularly appropriate in later stages of illness.

Pharmacological treatment

The conventional wisdom regarding the use of hypnotic medications for the treatment of insomnia is that they should be largely limited to short-term use. This traditional approach is predicated on concerns regarding tolerance, dosage escalation, psychological addiction, and physical dependency. While such concerns are legitimate, they are of less importance in the population of palliative care patients for whom life expectancy is limited and alleviation of symptoms and suffering are primary goals. Moreover, some newer generation sleep medications do not carry the same limitations to short-term usage and have been shown to maintain efficacy without dosage escalation or significant safety issues for periods as long as 24 months.

It is clear from data previously cited that hypnotic medications are used frequently in cancer patients. Unfortunately, these data do not provide information about the specific medications used, their effectiveness, appropriateness, or their side effects. Depending on which medications are prescribed, their dosage, and their indications, hypnotics may greatly enhance the quality of remaining life in the terminally ill, or may further complicate an already difficult period.

Benzodiazepine receptor agonists

Benzodiazepine (BZD), imidazopyridine (zolpidem), pyrazolopyrimidine (zaleplon), and cyclopyrrolone (zopiclone/eszopiclone)

Table 10.12.6 Psychological and behavioural therapies.

Treatment	Description
Stimulus control	Go to bed only when sleepy; maintain a regular schedule; avoid naps; use the bed only for sleep; if unable to fall asleep (or back to sleep) within 20 min, remove yourself from bed—engage in relaxing activity until drowsy then return to bed—repeat this as necessary
Progressive muscle relaxation	Methodical tensing and relaxing different muscle groups throughout patient's body; useful in patients displaying high levels of arousal both at night and in the daytime
Cognitive therapy (coupled with behavioural treatments)	Altering patient's faulty beliefs and attitudes about sleep using multiple patient-specific techniques to replace identified dysfunctional concepts about sleep with more appropriate ones; increasingly used as part of multicomponent strategies
Sleep restriction	Maintain a sleep log; determine mean total sleep time (TST) for baseline period; initiate total time in bed (TIB)=baseline mean TST (not <4.5 h); for sleep efficiency (TST/TIB) >90% over 5–7 days, increase TIB by 15 min; for SE < 80%, decrease TIB by 15 min; repeat TIB adjustment q. 5–7 days
Paradoxical intention	Training patient to confront most feared behaviour, deliberately trying to remain awake when sleep desired; eliminates performance anxiety that inhibits sleep onset
Multicomponent CBT-I	Varying combinations of psychological (aimed at changing patient's beliefs and attitudes about insomnia) and behavioural (e.g. stimulus control, progressive muscle relaxation, sleep restriction) interventions
Biofeedback	Providing visual and auditory feedback to assist patient in controlling some physiologic parameters (e.g. muscle tension) to seek reduction in somatic arousal
Sleep hygiene	Maintain a regular sleep–wake schedule; do not nap, especially close to bedtime; avoid 'sleeping in' after a poor night; avoid watching the clock; do not lie in bed for prolonged periods awake (see stimulus control); avoid excessive liquids or heavy evening meals; exercise regularly, but not within 3–4 h of bedtime; minimize/avoid caffeine (none after noon), alcohol, tobacco, stimulants

hypnotics are the standard medications of choice in the treatment of transient or short-term insomnia. Before such drugs are prescribed, however, the clinician must carefully consider the differential diagnosis in an effort to identify treatable comorbidities that contribute to the sleep disturbance. Having done so, it is then reasonable to consider use of a hypnotic as a component of a comprehensive treatment approach to insomnia. The patient's stated preferences regarding use of sleep medications and the care provider's assessment of consequences of the insomnia and potential adverse effects of the medication play important roles in deciding whether or not to use a hypnotic. When pharmacological treatment is employed in the acute or chronic insomnia setting, education and other non-pharmacological approaches remain key components of the overall therapeutic approach.

There have been no systematic studies of efficacy of various hypnotic medications in palliative care[224]. Several factors must be considered in prescribing hypnotic medication. These include the short- and long-term effectiveness of the drug, its rate of absorption and metabolism, and the potential risks or side effects. Characteristics of selected hypnotics, and other benzodiazepines often employed as hypnotics, are summarized in Table 10.12.7.

These medications, as a group, have a reasonably well-established record of effectiveness in the short-term treatment of insomnia. Studies report reductions in sleep latency and wake time after sleep onset[225,226]. There has been substantial historical controversy over the issue of long-term effectiveness of these medications. At present, most are recommended primarily for short-term usage. However, some newer benzodiazepine receptor agonists do not carry short-term usage restrictions and have been used chronically in primary insomnia patients without apparent adverse effect.

Most benzodiazepines, as well as the non-benzodiazepine hypnotics, are absorbed quickly, reaching peak concentrations within approximately 1 h or less. Triazolam, temazepam, and flurazepam were the most widely used in the past but they have been supplanted to a great extent by newer benzodiazepine receptor agonists in the past 10–15 years. Lorazepam and oxazepam have not been extensively studied or marketed as hypnotic medications, but are frequently used as such. The half-life of flurazepam's major active metabolite (*n*-desalkyl flurazepam) is in excess of 50 h, resulting in significant accumulation when the compound is used on a nightly basis. For this reason, the use of flurazepam has declined markedly since the introduction of shorter-acting agents.

Table 10.12.7 Characteristics of hypnotic medications.

Medication	Dosage[a]	Elimination half-life[b]	T_{max}[b]	Active metabolites	Comments[c]
Benzodiazepines					
Triazolam[d]	0.125	2–4	1.0	No	Promotes rapid sleep onset with minimal accumulation of drug over time; may be less effective for sleep maintenance problems; rebound insomnia, anterograde amnesia, untoward drug reactions described with triazolam
Temazepam	7.5–15	8–13	1.0	No	Promote sleep onset/maintenance with minimal accumulation; lorazepam not approved/marketed as a hypnotic but widely used as such
Lorazepam	0.5 mg	12–15	2.0	No	
Flurazepam	15 mg	47–100[f]	1.0	Yes	Effective for sleep onset and maintenance; but extended half-life and accumulation increases risk for daytime sedation; performance decrements; drug accumulation; especially in elderly or those with delayed metabolism
Quazepam	7.5[e]	29–73[f]	2.0	Yes	
Other benzodiazepine receptor agonists					
Zolpidem/Zolpidem CR	5	1.5–4.0	1.0–1.5	No	
Zaleplon	5	1.0	0.5–1.0	No	Manufacturer suggests zaleplon may be taken for middle of the night insomnia but not less than 4 hours before morning awakening
Zopiclone	3.7	5–7	0.5–2.0	Minimal	
Eszopiclone	2				
Melatonin agonists					
Ramelteon	8	1.0–2.0	0.5–1.0	No	Not a controlled substance

[a] Recommended starting dosage in elderly and medically ill patients.

[b] Elimination half-life and T_{max} represent estimated averages for healthy adults.

[c] All benzodiazepines carry potential for dosage escalation and for psychological and physical dependence.

[d] Not available in numerous EU and other countries.

[e] Manufacturer recommends initial dosage of 15 mg with reduction to 7.5 mg after 1–2 nights.

[f] *n*-desalky-flurazepam metabolite

The non-benzodiazepine hypnotics zolpidem and zaleplon as well as the benzodiazepine triazolam (triazolam has been removed from the market in numerous countries) are rapidly metabolized to inactive compounds. Zaleplon's ultra-short elimination half-life of about 1 h makes it potentially suitable for middle of the night usage, provided that there are at least 4 h before time of arising. Zopiclone and eszopiclone (the s-isomer of zopiclone marketed in the US) are also rapidly absorbed and have durations of clinical action that make them suitable for sleep onset and maintenance problems. In normal subjects eszopiclone does not accumulate with once daily dosing and does not carry a short-term usage restriction in the US. Temazepam, lorazepam, and oxazepam have intermediate half-lives ranging from about 8 to 15 h. These figures have been established for healthy adults. It is essential to recognize that rate of metabolism may be substantially slower in medically ill and elderly patients, predisposing to greater accumulation of the drug and daytime carry-over effects.

The benefits that may be achieved through the use of hypnotic medication in palliative care patients must be weighed against the potential for complications and side effects associated with their use. Perhaps the most common undesirable effect is that of daytime sedation and performance decrement. In populations of otherwise healthy insomnia patients, there is clear evidence that longer-acting benzodiazepines, such as flurazepam, are associated with significant deficits in daytime performance. However, some question exists as to the relevance of the psychomotor tasks on which these findings are based to the population of palliative care patients. Long-acting hypnotics can have daytime carry-over anxiolytic effects that may be beneficial for some patients. Performance decrement and daytime sedation are not prominent characteristics of shorter-acting hypnotics. Benzodiazepines and similar drugs may also predispose to nocturnal confusion and behavioural disturbance, particularly in individuals with baseline cognitive dysfunction. Likewise, respiratory disturbance in sleep, most prominent in geriatric patients, may be exacerbated by benzodiazepine hypnotic medication, although comparable findings have not been reported for the non-benzodiazepines.

In prescribing hypnotic medication, the clinician must consider the complication of rebound insomnia. Evidence suggests that the shortest-acting benzodiazepines (e.g. triazolam) predispose to transient insomnia following abrupt withdrawal of the medication, even after short-term use[227]. It has also been suggested that these medications may result in increased daytime anxiety and morning insomnia. These phenomena do not appear to be present with long-acting benzodiazepines and have not been clearly demonstrated with the non-benzodiazepine hypnotics. The clinical safety of these agents has been well established. Their lethality in the absence of other central nervous system depressants is very low. When any of these medications are discontinued after regular usage, clinicians must be mindful of the possibility of withdrawal symptoms and taper medications appropriately.

Other sleep medications

A number of medications other than standard hypnotics have been employed in the treatment of insomnia. Barbiturates, although effective in short-term treatment, result in rapid development of tolerance and are more dangerous and potentially lethal in overdose situations. These medications, and similar barbiturate-like compounds, are not recommended in the treatment of sleep disturbance. Chloral hydrate appears to have moderate short-term efficacy, but is more toxic than benzodiazepines. Sedating antidepressant drugs have assumed a more important role in the treatment of various forms of insomnia and non-restorative sleep in the past decade. These medications can be administered over long periods of time without concerns regarding physiological addiction. However, despite their widespread usage, evidence for their efficacy in the treatment of insomnia is quite limited. Of this class, trazodone has been most extensively studied as a sleep aid, but these investigations are limited to comparatively small numbers of patients with insomnia associated with major depression. The data do suggest that low-dose trazodone (25–100 mg) may improve sleep when used as an adjunct with other antidepressant medication. Trazodone has milder anticholinergic effects and a somewhat shorter half-life than most tricyclics. Likewise, sedating tricyclics, such as amitriptyline or doxepin, may be helpful adjuncts when administered in lower dosages (10–50 mg) than are typically required for treatment of major depression. Anticholinergic side-effects and daytime sedation can be problematic, especially in frail elderly or medically ill individuals. Delirium, due to central anticholinergic activity, is a potential complicating factor, as is lethality in overdose situations. Secondary amine tricyclics, such as desipramine or nortriptyline, may be beneficial while producing fewer anticholinergic complications. Newer-generation sedating antidepressants, such as mirtazapine, may be effective sleep aids, but are used primarily in treatment of depressed persons with insomnia. Nefazodone, another newer generation sedating antidepressant has been withdrawn in Europe, Canada, and several other countries due to concerns regarding hepatotoxicity, but continues to be marketed (with warning) in the US at the current time.

The melatonin agonist, ramelteon, is the first such agent to be marketed for treatment of insomnia. It has a favorable safety profile and carries no significant risk for dependency. However, it is very short-acting and suitable primarily for use in sleep initiation problems.

Melatonin has received widespread attention as a treatment for insomnia and other sleep disorders. The popularity of melatonin in recent years has far exceeded the scientific basis for its use as a treatment for all types of insomnia. Melatonin has been effectively used in the treatment of sleep–wake schedule disorders and has documented phase-shifting capability[228,229]. There is also mixed evidence that suggests possible benefit from melatonin treatment of insomnia among elderly patients, who may exhibit decreased melatonin secretion as a result of aging[230,231]. No large-scale controlled trials have yet demonstrated effectiveness of melatonin for the symptomatic treatment of insomnia. It should also be recognized that 'off the shelf' preparations for insomnia are not regulated as a drug in many countries and, as a result, the contents and source of the material may not be identifiable by the consumer. Finally, users should be aware that melatonin is a potent hormone with a variety of physiological effects, including reproductive and cardiovascular. While the ultimate clinical effects of exogenous melatonin are not known, and millions have apparently used it without major adverse effect, some degree of caution still seems advisable. Herbal preparations have also been used widely but with the possible exception of valerian extract (for which there is limited evidence of some short-term efficacy); these compounds have not been shown to be efficacious in the treatment of insomnia. Likewise, over-the-counter preparations, which are typically an antihistamine such as diphenhydramine, have very limited evidence to support their efficacy as hypnotic medications and are not recommended for long-term use.

The choice of a particular pharmacological treatment for insomnia must be based on the particular situation in which it will be used. Considerations include the nature of the insomnia complaint, the expected duration of treatment, potential side effects, including daytime sedation and performance decrement, and patient tolerance. Non-benzodiazepine drugs are generally considered first-line treatment base on efficacy and safety considerations, although benzodiazepines may be a less expensive and preferred choice for some patients. Once pharmacotherapy is initiated, it is most important to determine efficacy and complications and adjust dosage or type of medication accordingly.

It is noteworthy that at least one group of investigators has reported improvement of cognition in a population of cancer patients following rapid withdrawal of hypnotic medication (predominantly BZDs). The withdrawal was accomplished without significant worsening of insomnia, but numerous confounding variables leave some doubt as to whether improvements in cognition were a direct result of elimination of BZDs[232].

Choice of hypnotics in the elderly and infirm

The choice of a hypnotic medication in the elderly or the infirm must be predicated on achieving a careful balance between therapeutic efficacy and adverse consequences, for which this population is particularly at risk. A number of studies suggest that the use of sedative-hypnotics in the elderly, especially longer-acting drugs, is associated with increased risk of falls, hip fracture, and cognitive impairment[233–235].

Alterations in drug sensitivity and pharmacokinetics among the elderly and sick must be taken into account in prescribing. Older patients may have heightened sensitivity to hypnotic medications compared to younger persons, even at comparable plasma levels. In addition, drug clearance of at least some benzodiazepines is decreased in the elderly.

Benzodiazepines and their active metabolites, which undergo oxidative metabolism in the liver (e.g. diazepam, quazepam-flurazepam/desalkylflurazepam, alprazolam, and triazolam,) are cleared more slowly in the elderly. In contrast, drugs that are directly metabolized to inactive substances (e.g. zolpidem, zaleplon, temazepam, oxazepam, lorazepam) show little change in rate of clearance in older compared with younger age groups[236]. Furthermore, epidemiological evidence suggests a relationship between longer-acting benzodiazepine hypnotics and risk of injury[234]. These data would seem to suggest that the optimal choice of hypnotic in the elderly and debilitated would be a shorter-acting drug, typically a non-benzodiazepine, which undergoes direct inactivation (e.g. zolpidem or zopiclone), or, in the case of sleep-onset insomnia, ramelteon.

Concerns about sensitivity and drug accumulation have prompted manufacturers and clinicians to recommend lower dosages of these medications in elderly patients and those with severe medical illness. Recommended starting dosages for these populations are included in Table 10.12.6. Although nightly use of benzodiazepine or other hypnotics may be appropriate for patients in the terminal phase of illness, short-term, intermittent use may suffice and will minimize the possibility of drug accumulation. Aggravation of existing cognitive impairment, risk of fall and injury, worsening of nocturnal respiratory disturbance, and unwanted daytime sedation with its attendant impact on mood and behaviour are particular concerns in the elderly and infirm.

The metabolism of heterocyclic antidepressants may be substantially slowed in medically ill and older patients. Low starting dosages should be utilized and the potential for accumulation must be recognized. Development of excessive sedation, orthostatic hypotension, cardiotoxicity, and anticholinergic side effects are the major risks associated with elevated plasma levels of several of these agents.

Sleep in family and care providers (see Chapter 15.3)

Palliative care includes attention to the needs and difficulties of the patient's family and other care providers. This is certainly true with respect to sleep disturbances, which are common in this group. Focus on these problems for family care givers is especially important because sleep disruption and fatigue may contribute to loss of hope[237]. Grief, anxiety, and depression are frequently cited psychological disturbances that may cause insomnia among relatives[238]. Carter and Chang noted that 95 per cent of cancer care givers reported severe sleep problems, as measured by the Pittsburgh Sleep Quality Index[239]. These problems affected all aspects of sleep and were associated with evidence of clinical depression in over half of the group. For those providing direct care, frequent night-time interruptions to attend to the patient fragment sleep and, in time, can result in psychophysiologic insomnia. Care providers may feel compelled to 'keep one eye open' through the night so as not to miss a call for assistance.

Inquiries about the sleep patterns of family should be a component in assessing how well the palliative care system is succeeding. Discussion of sleep hygiene issues and practical problem-solving approaches to reducing night-time interruptions may be helpful. A multicomponent approach of stimulus control therapy, relaxation, cognitive therapy, and sleep hygiene education was successful in improving sleep in a group of caregivers for patients with cancer[240]. For some, short-term use of a benzodiazepine hypnotic or an anti-depressant medication may be indicated and can appropriately be addressed by their own health-care professionals. While it is clearly not advisable to employ sedating medication or antidepressants as a means of inhibiting normal grief, it must also be recognized that sleep deprivation and its sequelae may significantly interfere with the quality of relationships in the palliative care period and complicate bereavement following the patient's death.

References

1. Iber, C.A.S., Chesson, A, and Quan, S.F. for the American Academy, Medicine. (2007). *The AASM manual for the scoring of sleep and associated events: Rules, terminology and technical specifications*, 1st edition American Academy of Sleep Medicine, Westchester, Illinois.

2. Bryant, P.A., Trinder, J., and Curtis, N. (2004). Sick and tired: Does sleep have a vital role in the immune system? *Nat Rev Immunol*, **4**(6), 457–67.

3. Irwin, M. (2002). Effects of sleep and sleep loss on immunity and cytokines. *Brain Behav Immun*, **16**(5), 503–12.

4. Majde, J.A. and Krueger, J.M. (2005). Links between the innate immune system and sleep. *J Allergy Clin Immunol*, **116**(6), 1188–98.

5. Morley, J.E., Kay, N.E., Solomon, G.F. *et al.* (1987). Neuropeptides: Conductors of the immune orchestra. *Life Sci*, **41**(5), 527–44.

6. Heiser, P., Dickhaus, B., Schreiber, W. *et al.* (2000). White blood cells and cortisol after sleep deprivation and recovery sleep in humans. *Eur Arch Psychiatry Clin Neurosci*, **250**(1), 16–23.

7. Irwin, M., Mascovich, A., Gillin, J.C. *et al.* (1994). Partial sleep deprivation reduces natural killer cell activity in humans. *Psychosom Med*, **56**(6), 493–8.

8. Savard, J., Miller, S.M., Mills, M. *et al.* (1999). Association between subjective sleep quality and depression on immunocompetence in low-income women at risk for cervical cancer. *Psychosom Med*, **61**(4), 496–507.

9. Savard, J., Simard, S., Ivers, H. *et al.* (2005). Randomized study on the efficacy of cognitive-behavioral therapy for insomnia secondary to breast cancer, part I: Sleep and psychological effects. *J Clin Oncol*, **23**(25), 6083–96.

10. Irwin, M.R., Wang, M., Campomayor, C.O. *et al.* (2006). Sleep deprivation and activation of morning levels of cellular and genomic markers of inflammation. *Arch Intern Med*, **166**(16), 1756–62.

11. American Academy of Sleep Medicine. (2005). *International classification of sleep disorders: Diagnostic and coding manual*, 2nd edition. American Academy of Sleep Medicine, Westchester, IL.

12. Roth, T. and Ancoli-Israel, S. (1999). Daytime consequences and correlates of insomnia in the United States: Results of the 1991 National Sleep Foundation Survey. II. *Sleep*, **22**(Suppl 2), S354–8.

13. Zammit, G.K., Weiner, J., Damato, N. *et al.* (1999). Quality of life in people with insomnia. *Sleep*, **22**(Suppl 2), S379–85.

14. Bonnet, M.H. and Arand, D.L. (2003). Situational insomnia: Consistency, predictors, and outcomes. *Sleep*, **26**(8), 1029–36.

15. Bonnet, M.H. and Arand, D.L. (2000). Activity, arousal, and the MSLT in patients with insomnia. *Sleep*, **23**(2), 205–12.

16. Nofzinger, E.A., Buysse, D.J., Germain, A. *et al.* (2004). Functional neuroimaging evidence for hyperarousal in insomnia. *Am J Psychiatry*, **161**(11), 2126–8.

17. Pavlova, M., Berg, O., Gleason, R. *et al.* (2001). Self-reported hyperarousal traits among insomnia patients. *J Psychosom Res*, **51**(2), 435–41.

18. Smith, M.T., Perlis, M.L., and Haythornthwaite, J.A. (2004). Suicidal ideation in outpatients with chronic musculoskeletal pain: An exploratory study of the role of sleep onset insomnia and pain intensity. *Clin J Pain*, **20**(2), 111–8.

19. Kubler-Ross, E. (1973). In *On the use of psychopharmacologic agents for the dying patient and the bereaved. In Psycho-pharmacological Agents for the Terminally Ill and Bereaved* (eds. I.K. Goldberg, S. Malitz, and A.H. Kutscher), pp. 3–6. Columbia University Press, New York.

20. Johns, M.W. (1991). A new method for measuring daytime sleepiness: The Epworth sleepiness scale. *Sleep*, **14**(6), 540–5.

21. Carskadon, M.A., Dement, W.C., Mitler, M.M. *et al.* (1986). Guidelines for the multiple sleep latency test (MSLT): A standard measure of sleepiness. *Sleep*, **9**(4), 519–24.

22. Chesson, A.L., Jr., Littner, M., Davila, D. *et al.* (1999). Practice parameters for the use of light therapy in the treatment of sleep disorders. Standards of Practice Committee, American Academy of Sleep Medicine. *Sleep*, **22**(5), 641–60.

23. Kamei, Y., Hayakawa, T., Urata, J. *et al.* (2000). Melatonin treatment for circadian rhythm sleep disorders. *Psychiatry Clin Neurosci*, **54**(3), 381–2.

24. Okawa, M., Uchiyama, M., Ozaki, S. *et al.* (1998). Melatonin treatment for circadian rhythm sleep disorders. *Psychiatry Clin Neurosci*, **52**(2), 259–60.

25. Czeisler, C.A., Richardson, G.S., Coleman, R.M. *et al.* (1981). Chronotherapy: Resetting the circadian clocks of patients with delayed sleep phase insomnia. *Sleep*, **4**(1), 1–21.

26. Sutherland, H.J., Lockwood, G.A., and Boyd, N.F. (1990). Ratings of the importance of quality of life variables: Therapeutic implications for patients with metastatic breast cancer. *J Clin Epidemiol*, **43**(7), 661–6.

27. Munro, A.J., Biruls, R., Griffin, A.V. *et al.* (1989). Distress associated with radiotherapy for malignant disease: A quantitative analysis based on patients perceptions. *Br J Cancer*, **60**(3), 370–4.

28. Ginsburg, M.L., Quirt, C., Ginsburg, A.D. *et al.* (1995). Psychiatric illness and psychosocial concerns of patients with newly diagnosed lung cancer.[see comment]. *CMAJ Can Med Associat J*, **152**(5), 701–8.

29. Grond, S., Zech, D., Diefenbach, C. *et al.* (1994). Prevalence and pattern of symptoms in patients with cancer pain: A prospective evaluation of 1635 cancer patients referred to a pain clinic. *J Pain Symptom Manage*, **9**(6), 372–82.

30. Krech, R.L. and Walsh, D. (1991). Symptoms of pancreatic cancer. *J Pain Symptom Manage*, **6**(6), 360–7.

31. Portenoy, R.K., Thaler, H.T., Kornblith, A.B. *et al.* (1994). Symptom prevalence, characteristics and distress in a cancer population. *Qual Life Res*, **3**(3), 183–9.

32. Walsh, D., Donnelly, S., and Rybicki, L. (2000). The symptoms of advanced cancer: Relationship to age, gender, and performance status in 1,000 patients. *Support Care Cancer*, **8**(3), 175–9.

33. Savard, J. and Morin, C.M. (2001). Insomnia in the context of cancer: a review of a neglected problem. *J Clin Oncol*, **19**(3), 895–908.

34. Vena, C., Parker, K., Allen, R. *et al.* (2006). Sleep–wake disturbances and quality of life in patients with advanced lung cancer. *Oncology Nursing Forum Online*, **33**(4), 761–9.

35. Hickok, J.T., Morrow, G.R., Roscoe, J.A. *et al.* (2005). Occurrence, severity, and longitudinal course of twelve common symptoms in 1129 consecutive patients during radiotherapy for cancer. *J Pain Symptom Manage*, **30**(5), 433–42.

36. Fernandes, R., Stone, P., Andrews, P. *et al.* (2006). Comparison between fatigue, sleep disturbance, and circadian rhythm in cancer inpatients and healthy volunteers: Evaluation of diagnostic criteria for cancer-related fatigue. *J Pain Symptom Manage*, **32**(3), 245–54.

37. Byar, K.L., Berger, A.M., Bakken, S.L. *et al.* (2006). Impact of adjuvant breast cancer chemotherapy on fatigue, other symptoms, and quality of life. *Oncology Nursing Forum Online*, **33**(1), E18–26.

38. Ancoli-Israel, S., Liu, L., Marler, M.R. *et al.* (2006). Fatigue, sleep, and circadian rhythms prior to chemotherapy for breast cancer. *Support Care Cancer*, **14**(3), 201–9.

39. Engstrom, C.A., Strohl, R.A., Rose, L. *et al.* (1999). Sleep alterations in cancer patients. *Cancer Nurs*, **22**(2), 143–8.

40. Sela, R.A., Watanabe, S., and Nekolaichuk, C.L. (2005). Sleep disturbances in palliative cancer patients attending a pain and symptom control clinic. *Palliative & Supportive Care*, **3**(1), 23–31.

41. Malone, M., Harris, A.L., and Luscombe, D.K. (1994). Assessment of the impact of cancer on work, recreation, home management and sleep using a general health status measure. *J R Soc Med*, **87**(7), 386–9.

42. Beszterczey, A. and Lipowski, Z.J. (1977). Insomnia in cancer patients. *Can Med Assoc J*, **116**(4), 355.

43. Lamb, M.A. (1982). The sleeping patterns of patients with malignant and nonmalignant diseases. *Cancer Nurs*, **5**(5), 389–96.

44. Kaye, J., Kaye, K., and Madow, L. (1983). Sleep patterns in patients with cancer and patients with cardiac disease. *J Psychol*, **114**(1st Half), 107–13.

45. Silberfarb, P.M., Hauri, P.J., Oxman, T.E. *et al.* (1985). Insomnia in cancer patients. *Soc Sci Med*, **20**(8), 849–50.

46. Silberfarb, P.M., Hauri, P.J., Oxman, T.E. *et al.* (1993). Assessment of sleep in patients with lung cancer and breast cancer. *J Clin Oncol*, **11**(5), 997–1004.

47. Payne, R.J., Hier, M.P., Kost, K.M. *et al.* (2005). High prevalence of obstructive sleep apnea among patients with head and neck cancer. *J Otolaryngol*, **34**(5), 304–11.

48. Nesse, W., Hoekema, A., Stegenga, B. *et al.* (2006). Prevalence of obstructive sleep apnoea following head and neck cancer treatment: A cross-sectional study. *Oral Oncol*, **42**(1), 108–14.

49. Ancoli-Israel, S. (2006). The impact and prevalence of chronic insomnia and other sleep disturbances associated with chronic illness. *Am J Manag Care*, **12**(8 Suppl), S221–9.

50. Monga, U., Kerrigan, A.J., Thornby, J. *et al.* (2005). Longitudinal study of quality of life in patients with localized prostate cancer undergoing radiotherapy. *J Rehabil Res Development*, **42**(3), 391–9.

51. Monga, U., Kerrigan, A.J., Thornby, J. *et al.* (1999). Prospective study of fatigue in localized prostate cancer patients undergoing radiotherapy. *Radiat Oncol Investig*, **7**(3), 178–85.

52. Slatkin, N.E. and Rhiner, M. (2003). Treatment of opiate-related sedation: Utility of the cholinesterase inhibitors. *J Supportive Oncol*, **1**(1), 53–63.

53. Hanks, G.W., Twycross, R.G., and Bliss, J.M. (1987). Controlled release morphine tablets: A double-blind trial in patients with advanced cancer. *Anaesthesia*, **42**(8), 840–4.

54. Lapin, J., Portenoy, R.K., Coyle, N. *et al.* (1989). Guidelines for use of controlled-release oral morphine in cancer pain management. Correlation with clinical experience. *Cancer Nurs*, **12**(4), 202–8.

55. Harris, A.L., Powles, T.J., and Smith, I.E. (1982). Aminoglutethimide in the treatment of advanced postmenopausal breast cancer. *Cancer Res*, **42**(8 Suppl), 3405s–8s.

56. Smedley, H., Katrak, M., Sikora, K. *et al.* (1983). Neurological effects of recombinant human interferon. *Br Med J Clin Res Ed*, **286**(6361), 262–4.

57. Anderson, M. and Salmon, M.V. (1977). Symptomatic cataplexy. *J Neurol Neurosurg Psychiatry*, **40**(2), 186–91.

58. Stahl, S.M., Layzer, R.B., Aminoff, M.J. *et al.* (1980). Continuous cataplexy in a patient with a midbrain tumor: The limp man syndrome. *Neurology*, **30**(10), 1115–8.

59. Jaeckle, K.A., Digre, K.B., Jones, C.R. *et al.* (1990). Central neurogenic hyperventilation: Pharmacologic intervention with morphine sulfate and correlative analysis of respiratory, sleep, and ocular motor dysfunction. *Neurology*, **40**(11), 1715–20.

60. Beck, S.L., Dudley, W.N., and Barsevick, A. (2005). Pain, sleep disturbance, and fatigue in patients with cancer: Using a mediation model to test a symptom cluster. *Oncology Nursing Forum Online*, **32**(3), 542.

61. Bower, J.E., Ganz, P.A., Desmond, K.A. *et al.* (2000). Fatigue in breast cancer survivors: Occurrence, correlates, and impact on quality of life. *J Clin Oncol*, **18**(4), 743–53.

62. Okuyama, T., Akechi, T., Kugaya, A. *et al.* (2000). Factors correlated with fatigue in disease-free breast cancer patients: Application of the Cancer Fatigue Scale. *Support Care Cancer*, **8**(3), 215–22.

63. Berger, A.M. and Farr, L. (1999). The influence of daytime inactivity and nighttime restlessness on cancer-related fatigue. *Oncol Nurs Forum*, **26**(10), 1663–71.

64. Mock, V., Atkinson, A., Barsevick, A. *et al.* (2000). NCCN practice guidelines for cancer-related fatigue. *Oncology (Huntington)*, **14**(11A), 151–61.

65. Groopman, J.E. (1998). Fatigue in cancer and HIV/AIDS. *Oncology (Huntington)*, **12**(3), 335–44; discussion 45–6.

66. Darko, D.F., McCutchan, J.A., Kripke, D.F. *et al.* (1992). Fatigue sleep disturbance, disability, and indices of progression of HIV infection. *Am J Psychiatry*, **149**(4), 514–20.

67. Moeller, A.A., Oechsner, M., Backmund, H.C. *et al.* (1991). Self-reported sleep quality in HIV infection: correlation to the stage of infection and zidovudine therapy. *J Acquir Immune Defic Syndr*, **4**(10), 1000–3.

68. Cohen, F.L., Ferrans, C.E., Vizgirda, V. *et al.* (1996). Sleep in men and women infected with human immunodeficiency virus. *Holist Nurs Pract*, **10**(4), 33–43.

69. Rubinstein, M.L. and Selwyn, P.A. (1998). High prevalence of insomnia in an outpatient population with HIV infection. *J Acquir Immune Defic Syndr Hum Retrovirol*, **19**(3), 260–5.

70. Nokes, K.M. and Kendrew, J. (2001). Correlates of sleep quality in persons with HIV disease. *J Assoc Nurses AIDS Care*, **12**(1), 17–22.

71. Reid, S. and Dwyer, J. (2005). Insomnia in HIV infection: A systematic review of prevalence, correlates, and management. *Psychosom Med*, **67**(2), 260–9.

72. Perkins, D.O., Leserman, J., Stern, R.A. *et al.* (1995). Somatic symptoms and HIV infection: Relationship to depressive symptoms and indicators of HIV disease. *Am J Psychiatry*, **152**(12), 1776–81.

73. St Kubicki Hea. (1988). AIDS-related sleep disturbances-a preliminary report. In *HIV and Nervous System* (eds. St. H. Kubicki HH, H. Bienzle, and H.D. Pokle), pp. 97–105. Gustar Fischer; Stuttgart.

74. Darko, D.F., Miller, J.C., Gallen, C. *et al.* (1995). Sleep electroencephalogram delta-frequency amplitude, night plasma levels of tumor necrosis factor alpha, and human immunodeficiency virus infection. *Proc Natl Acad Sci USA*, **92**(26), 12080–4.

75. Norman, S.E., Chediak, A.D., Freeman, C. *et al.* (1992). Sleep disturbances in men with asymptomatic human immunodeficiency (HIV) infection. *Sleep*, **15**(2), 150–5.

76. Norman, S.E., Chediak, A.D., Kiel, M. *et al.* (1990). Sleep disturbances in HIV-infected homosexual men. *AIDS*, **4**(8), 775–81.

77. Norman, S.E., Resnick, L., Cohn, M.A. *et al.* (1988). Sleep disturbances in HIV-seropositive patients. *JAMA*, **260**(7), 922.

78. White, J.L., Darko, D.F., Brown, S.J. *et al.* (1995). Early central nervous system response to HIV infection: sleep distortion and cognitive-motor decrements. *AIDS*, **9**(9), 1043–50.

79. Smirne, S. and Ferini-Strambi, L. (1999). Clinical applications of cyclic alternating pattern. *Electroencephalography & Clinical Neurophysiology (Supplement)*, **50**, 109–12.

80. Wiegand, M., Moller, A.A., Schreiber, W. *et al.* (1991). Alterations of nocturnal sleep in patients with HIV infection. *Acta Neurol Scand*, **83**(2), 141–2.

81. Richman, D.D., Fischl, M.A., Grieco, M.H. *et al.* (1987). The toxicity of azidothymidine (AZT) in the treatment of patients with AIDS and AIDS-related complex. A double-blind, placebo-controlled trial. *N Engl J Med*, **317**(4), 192–7.

82. (1988). Azidothymidine in the treatment of AIDS. *N Engl J Med*. **318**(4), 250–1.

83. Moeller, A.A., Wiegand, M., Oechsner, M. *et al.* (1992). Effects of zidovudine on EEG sleep in HIV-infected men. *J Acquir Immune Defic Syndr*, **5**(6), 636–7.

84. Bach, M.C. (1987). Possible drug interaction during therapy with azidothymidine and acyclovir for AIDS. *N Engl J Med*, **316**(9), 547.

85. Nunez, M., Gonzalez de Requena, D., Gallego, L. *et al.* (2001). Higher efavirenz plasma levels correlate with development of insomnia. *J Acquir Immune Defic Syndr*, **28**(4), 399–400.

86. Fumaz, C.R., Munoz-Moreno, J.A., Molto, J. *et al.* (2005). Long-term neuropsychiatric disorders on efavirenz-based approaches: Quality of life, psychologic issues, and adherence. *J Acquir Immune Defic Syndr*, **38**(5), 560–5.

87. Hintz, S., Kuck, J., Peterkin, J.J. *et al.* (1990). Depression in the context of human immunodeficiency virus infection: Implications for treatment. *J Clin Psychiatry*, **51**(12), 497–501.

88. Javaheri, S., Parker, T.J., Liming, J.D. *et al.* (1998). Sleep apnea in 81 ambulatory male patients with stable heart failure. Types and their prevalences, consequences, and presentations. *Circulation*, **97**(21), 2154–9.

89. Javaheri, S., Parker, T.J., Wexler, L. *et al.* (1995). Occult sleep-disordered breathing in stable congestive heart failure. *Ann Intern Med*, **122**(7), 487–92.

90. Davidson, J.R., MacLean, A.W., Brundage, M.D. *et al.* (2002). Sleep disturbance in cancer patients. *Soc Sci Med*, **54**(9), 1309–21.

91. Sinha, A.M., Skobel, E.C., Breithardt, O.A. *et al.* (2004). Cardiac resynchronization therapy improves central sleep apnea and Cheyne-Stokes respiration in patients with chronic heart failure. *J Am Coll Cardiol*, **44**(1), 68–71.

92. Javaheri, S. (2006). Acetazolamide improves central sleep apnea in heart failure: A double-blind, prospective study. *Am J Respir Crit Care Med*, **173**(2), 234–7.

93. Schulz, R., Fegbeutel, C., Olschewski, H. *et al.* (2004). Reversal of nocturnal periodic breathing in primary pulmonary hypertension after lung transplantation. *Chest*, **125**(1), 344–7.

94. Kario, K., Morinari, M., Murata, M. *et al.* (2004). Nocturnal onset ischemic stroke provoked by sleep-disordered breathing advanced with congestive heart failure. *Am J Hypertens*, **17**(7), 636–7.

95. George, C.F. (2000). Perspectives on the management of insomnia in patients with chronic respiratory disorders. *Sleep*, **23**(Suppl 1), S31–5; discussion S6–8.

96. George, C.F. and Bayliff, C.D. (2003). Management of insomnia in patients with chronic obstructive pulmonary disease. *Drugs*, **63**(4), 379–87.

97. Sacco, C., Braghiroli, A., Grossi, E. *et al.* (1995). The effects of doxofylline versus theophylline on sleep architecture in COPD patients. *Monaldi Arch Chest Dis*, **50**(2), 98–103.

98. Novak, M., Shapiro, C.M., Mendelssohn, D. *et al.* (2006). Diagnosis and management of insomnia in dialysis patients. *Semin Dial*, **19**(1), 25–31.

99. Iliescu, E.A., Yeates, K.E., and Holland, D.C. (2004). Quality of sleep in patients with chronic kidney disease. *Nephrol Dial Transplant*, **19**(1), 95–9.

100. Molnar, M.Z., Novak, M., and Mucsi, I. (2006). Management of restless legs syndrome in patients on dialysis. *Drugs*, **66**(5), 607–24.

101. De Santo, R.M., Lucidi, F., Violani, C. *et al.* (2005). Sleep disorders in hemodialyzed patients—The role of comorbidities. *Int J Artif Organs*, **28**(6), 557–65.

102. Merlino, G., Piani, A., Dolso, P. *et al.* (2006). Sleep disorders in patients with end-stage renal disease undergoing dialysis therapy. *Nephrol Dial Transplant*, **21**(1), 184–90.

103. Novak, M., Molnar, M.Z., Ambrus, C. *et al.* (2006). Chronic insomnia in kidney transplant recipients. *Am J Kidney Dis*, **47**(4), 655–65.

104. Eryilmaz, M.M., Ozdemir, C., Yurtman, F. *et al.* (2005). Quality of sleep and quality of life in renal transplantation patients. *Transplant Proc*, **37**(5), 2072–6.

105. Benca, R.M. (2000). Mood disorders. In *Principles and Practice of Sleep Medicine*, 3rd edition. pp. 1140–57. WB Saunders, Philadelphia. PA.

106. Levine, P.M., Silberfarb, P.M., and Lipowski, Z.J. (1978). Mental disorders in cancer patients: A study of 100 psychiatric referrals. *Cancer*, **42**(3), 1385–91.

107. Akechi, T., Nakano, T., Okamura, H. *et al.* (2001). Psychiatric disorders in cancer patients: Descriptive analysis of 1721 psychiatric referrals at two Japanese cancer center hospitals. *Jpn J Clin Oncol*, **31**(5), 188–94.

108. Lloyd-Williams, M. (2001). Screening for depression in palliative care patients: A review. *Eur J Cancer Care*, **10**(1), 31–5.

109. Grabsch, B., Clarke, D.M., Love, A. *et al.* (2006). Psychological morbidity and quality of life in women with advanced breast cancer: A cross-sectional survey. *Palliat Supportive Care*, **4**(1), 47–56.

110. Fulton, C. (1998). The prevalence and detection of psychiatric morbidity in patients with metastatic breast cancer. *Eur J Cancer Care*, **7**(4), 232–9.

111. Breitbart, W., Bruera, E., Chochinov, H. *et al.* (1995). Neuropsychiatric syndromes and psychological symptoms in patients with advanced cancer. *J Pain Symptom Manage*, **10**(2), 131–41.

112. Derogatis, L.R., Feldstein, M., Morrow, G. *et al.* (1979). A survey of psychotropic drug prescriptions in an oncology population. *Cancer*, **44**(5), 1919–29.

113. Bukberg, J., Penman, D., and Holland, J.C. (1984). Depression in hospitalized cancer patients. *Psychosom Med*, **46**(3), 199–212.

114. Jaeger, H., Morrow, G.R., Carpenter, P.J. *et al.* (1985). A survey of psychotropic drug utilization by patients with advanced neoplastic disease. *Gen Hosp Psychiatry*, **7**(4), 353–60.

115. Lloyd–Williams, M. and Friedman, T. (1999). Depression in terminally ill patients. *Am J Hosp Palliat Care*, **16**(6), 704–5.

116. Plumb, M.M. and Holland, J. (1977). Comparative studies of psychological function in patients with advanced cancer. I. Self-reported depressive symptoms. *Psychosom Med*, **39**(4), 264–76.

117. Lloyd-Williams, M., Dennis, M., and Taylor, F. (2004). A prospective study to compare three depression screening tools in patients who are terminally ill. *Gen Hosp Psychiatry*, **26**(5), 384–9.

118. Lawrie, I., Lloyd-Williams, M., and Taylor, F. (2004). How do palliative medicine physicians assess and manage depression. *Palliat Med*, **18**(3), 234–8.

119. Akechi, T., Okuyama, T., Sugawara, Y. *et al.* (2006). Screening for depression in terminally ill cancer patients in Japan. *J Pain Symptom Manage*, **31**(1), 5–12.

120. Hameroff, S.R., Cork, R.C., Scherer, K. *et al.* (1982). Doxepin effects on chronic pain, depression and plasma opioids. *J Clin Psychiatry*, **43**(8 Pt 2), 22–7.

121. Hameroff, S.R., Weiss, J.L., Lerman, J.C. *et al.* (1984). Doxepin's effects on chronic pain and depression, a controlled study. *J Clin Psychiatry*, **45**(3 Pt 2), 47–53.

122. Walsh, T.D. (1983). Antidepressants in chronic pain. *Clin Neuropharmacol*, **6**(4), 271–95.

123. Spiegel, K., Kalb, R., and Pasternak, G.W. (1983). Analgesic activity of tricyclic antidepressants. *Ann Neurol*, **13**(4), 462–5.

124. Miller, K.E., Adams, S.M., and Miller, M.M. (2006). Antidepressant medication use in palliative care. *Am J Hosp Palliat Care*, **23**(2), 127–33.

125. Kugaya, A., Akechi, T., Nakano, T. *et al.* (1999). Successful antidepressant treatment for five terminally ill cancer patients with major depression, suicidal ideation and a desire for death. *Support Care Cancer*, **7**(6), 432–6.

126. Holland, J.C., Romano, S.J., Heiligenstein, J.H. *et al.* (1998). A controlled trial of fluoxetine and desipramine in depressed women with advanced cancer. *Psychooncology*, **7**(4), 291–300.

127. Cheer, S.M. and Goa, K.L. (2001). Fluoxetine: a review of its therapeutic potential in the treatment of depression associated with physical illness. *Drugs*, **61**(1), 81–110.

128. Gill, D. and Hatcher, S. (2000). Antidepressants for depression in medical illness.[update of Cochrane Database Syst Rev 2000; 2, CD001312; PMID, 10796770]. *Cochrane Database Syst Rev*, **4**, CD001312.

129. Craig, T.J. and Abeloff, M.D. (1974). Psychiatric symptomatology among hospitalized cancer patients. *Am J Psychiatry*, **131**(12), 1323–7.

130. Derogatis, L.R., Morrow, G.R., Fetting, J. *et al.* (1983). The prevalence of psychiatric disorders among cancer patients. *JAMA*, **249**(6), 751–7.

131. Battelli, T., Bonsignori, M., Manocchi, P. *et al.* (1976). Anxiety therapy in the neoplastic patient. *Curr Med Res Opin*, **4**(3), 185–8.

132. Reynolds, C.F., 3rd, Shaw, D.H., Newton, T.F. *et al.* (1983). EEG sleep in outpatients with generalized anxiety: A preliminary comparison with depressed outpatients. *Psychiatry Res*, **8**(2), 81–9.

133. Rosa, R.R., Bonnet, M.H., and Kramer, M. (1983). The relationship of sleep and anxiety in anxious subjects. *Biol Psychol*, **16**(1–2), 119–26.

134. Neuhaus, W., Lanij, B., Ahr, A. *et al.* (1994). [Psychological disease adjustment in breast cancer patients]. *Geburtshilfe Frauenheilkd*, **54**(10), 564–8.

135. David, D., De Faria, L., and Mellman, T.A. (2006). Adjunctive risperidone treatment and sleep symptoms in combat veterans with chronic PTSD. *Depress Anxiety*, **23**(8), 489–91.

136. Peskind, E.R., Bonner, L.T., Hoff, D.J. *et al.* (2003). Prazosin reduces trauma-related nightmares in older men with chronic posttraumatic stress disorder. *J Geriatr Psychiatry Neurol*, **16**(3), 165–71.

137. Germain, A. and Nielsen, T. (2003). Impact of imagery rehearsal treatment on distressing dreams, psychological distress, and sleep parameters in nightmare patients. *Behavioral Sleep Medicine*, **1**(3), 140–54.

138. Massie, M.J., Holland, J., and Glass, E. (1983). Delirium in terminally ill cancer patients. *Am J Psychiatry*, **140**(8), 1048–50.

139. Fainsinger, R., Miller, M.J., Bruera, E. *et al.* (1991). Symptom control during the last week of life on a palliative care unit. *J Palliat Care*, **7**(1), 5–11.

140. Lipowski, Z.J. (1987). Delirium (acute confusional states). *JAMA*, **258**(13), 1789–92.

141. Posner, J.B. (1979). Neurological complications of systemic cancer. *Med Clin North Am*, **63**(4), 783–800.

142. Silberfarb, P.M. (1988). Psychiatric treatment of the patient during cancer therapy. *CA Cancer J Clin*, **38**(3), 133–7.

143. Safer, D.J. (1970). The concomitant effects of mild sleep loss and an anticholinergic drug. *Psychopharmacologia*, **17**(5), 425–33.

144. Evans, J.I. and Lewis, S.A. (1968). Sleep studies in early delirium and during drug withdrawal in normal subjects and the effect of phenothiazines on such states. *Electroencephalogr Clin Neurophysiol*, **25**(5), 508–9.

145. Dein, S. and George, R. (2002). The use of psychostimulants by palliative care consultants in the UK: A retrospective telephone survey. *Palliat Med*, **16**(2), 167–8.

146. Prinz, P.N., Vitaliano, P.P., Vitiello, M.V. *et al.* (1982). Sleep, EEG and mental function changes in senile dementia of the Alzheimer's type. *Neurobiol Aging*, **3**(4), 361–70.

147. Reynolds, C.F., 3rd, Kupfer, D.J., Taska, L.S. *et al.* (1985). EEG sleep in elderly depressed, demented, and healthy subjects. *Biol Psychiatry*, **20**(4), 431–42.

148. Irwin, P., Murray, S., Bilinski, A. *et al.* (2005). Alcohol withdrawal as an underrated cause of agitated delirium and terminal restlessness in patients with advanced malignancy. *J Pain Symptom Manage*, **29**(1), 104–8.

149. Lieberman, J.A. (2007). Effectiveness of antipsychotic drugs in patients with chronic schizophrenia: efficacy, safety and cost outcomes of CATIE and other trials. *J Clin Psychiatry*, **68**(2), e04.

150. Meltzer, H.Y. and Bobo, W.V. (2006). Interpreting the efficacy findings in the CATIE study: What clinicians should know. *Cns Spectrums*, **11**(7 Suppl 7), 14–24.

151. McEvoy, J.P. (2006). An overview of the clinical antipsychotic trials of intervention effectiveness (CATIE) study. *Cns Spectrums*, **11**(7 Suppl 7), 4–8.

152. Burke, A.L., Diamond, P.L., Hulbert, J. *et al.* (1991). Terminal restlessness—Its management and the role of midazolam.[see comment]. *Med J Aust*, **155**(7), 485–7.

153. Stiefel, F., Fainsinger, R., Bruera, E. (1992). Acute confusional states in patients with advanced cancer. *J Pain Symptom Manage*, **7**(2), 94–8.

154. Bonica, J.J. (1979). Importance of the problem. In *Advances in Pain Research and Therapy, Vol. 2* (eds. J.J. Bonica and V. Ventafridda), pp. 1–12. Raven Press, New York.

155. Panutti, Fea. (1979). The role of endocrine therapy for the relief of pain due to cancer. In *Advances in Pain Research and Therapy Vol. 2*, (eds. J.J. Bonica and V. Ventafridda), pp. 59–77. Raven Press, New York.

156. Twycross, R.G. and Fairfield, S. (1982). Pain in far-advanced cancer. *Pain*, **14**(3), 303–10.

157. Banning, A., Sjogren, P., and Henriksen, H. (1991). Treatment outcome in a multidisciplinary cancer pain clinic.[see comment]. *Pain*, **47**(2), 129–34; discussion 7–8.

158. Dorrepaal, K.L., Aaronson, N.K., and van Dam, F.S. (1989). Pain experience and pain management among hospitalized cancer patients. A clinical study. *Cancer*, **63**(3), 593–8.

159. Portenoy, R.K., Miransky, J., Thaler, H.T. *et al.* (1992). Pain in ambulatory patients with lung or colon cancer. Prevalence, characteristics, and effect. *Cancer*, **70**(6), 1616–24.

160. Strang, P. and Qvarner, H. (1990). Cancer-related pain and its influence on quality of life. *Anticancer Res*, **10**(1), 109–12.

161. Tamburini, M., Selmi, S., De Conno, F. *et al.* (1987). Semantic descriptors of pain. *Pain*, **29**(2), 187–93.

162. Mystakidou, K., Tsilika, E., Parpa, E. *et al.* (2006). Psychological distress of patients with advanced cancer: Influence and contribution of pain severity and pain interference. *Cancer Nurs*, **29**(5), 400–5.

163. Donovan, M.I. and Dillon, P. (1987). Incidence and characteristics of pain in a sample of hospitalized cancer patients. *Cancer Nurs*, **10**(2), 85–92.

164. Kinsman, R., Dirks, J.F., Wunder, J. *et al.* (1989). Multidimensional analysis of peak pain symptoms and experiences. *Psychother Psychosom*, **51**(2), 101–12.

165. Pilowsky, I., Crettenden, I., and Townley, M. (1985). Sleep disturbance in pain clinic patients. *Pain*, **23**(1), 27–33.

166. Closs, S.J. (1992). Patients' night-time pain, analgesic provision and sleep after surgery. *Int J Nurs Stud*, **29**(4), 381–92.

167. Carli, G., Montesano, A., Rapezzi, S. *et al.* (1987). Differential effects of persistent nociceptive stimulation on sleep stages. *Behav Brain Res*, **26**(2–3), 89–98.

168. Landis, C.A., Levine, J.D., and Robinson, C.R. (1989). Decreased slow-wave and paradoxical sleep in a rat chronic pain model. *Sleep*, **12**(2), 167–77.

169. Breitbart, W. (1989). Psychiatric management of cancer pain. *Cancer*, **63**(11 Suppl), 2336–42.

170. Moldofsky, H., Lue, F.A., and Smythe HA (1983). Alpha EEG sleep and morning symptoms in rheumatoid arthritis. *J Rheumatol*, **10**(3), 373–9.

171. Hicks, R.A., Coleman, D.D., Ferrante, F. *et al.* (1979). Pain thresholds in rats during recovery from REM sleep deprivation. *Percept Mot Skills*, **48**(3 Pt 1), 687–90.

172. Onen, S.H., Alloui, A., Gross, A. *et al.* (2001). The effects of total sleep deprivation, selective sleep interruption and sleep recovery on pain tolerance thresholds in healthy subjects. *J Sleep Res*, **10**(1), 35–42.

173. Fadda, P., Tortorella, A., and Fratta, W. (1991). Sleep deprivation decreases mu and delta opioid receptor binding in the rat limbic system. *Neurosci Lett*, **129**(2), 315–7.

174. Roehrs, T., Hyde, M., Blaisdell, B. *et al.* (2006). Sleep loss and REM sleep loss are hyperalgesic.[see comment]. *Sleep*, **29**(2), 145–51.

175. Raymond, I., Nielsen, T.A., Lavigne, G. *et al.* (2001). Quality of sleep and its daily relationship to pain intensity in hospitalized adult burn patients. *Pain*, **92**(3), 381–8.

176. Moldofsky, H. and Scarisbrick, P. (1976). Induction of neurasthenic musculoskeletal pain syndrome by selective sleep stage deprivation. *Psychosom Med*, **38**(1), 35–44.

177. Larbig, W., Gerber, W.D., Kluck, M. *et al.* (1984). Therapeutic effects of delta-sleep-inducing peptide (DSIP) in patients with chronic, pronounced pain episodes. A clinical pilot study. *Eur Neurol*, **23**(5), 372–85.

178. Gillin, J.C., Jacobs, L.S., Fram, D.H. *et al.* (1972). Acute effect of a glucocorticoid on normal human sleep. *Nature*, **237**(5355), 398–9.

179. Kuo, H.-H., Chiu, M.-J., Liao, W.-C. *et al.* (2006). Quality of sleep and related factors during chemotherapy in patients with stage I/II breast cancer. *J Formos Med Assoc*, **105**(1), 64–9.

180. Berger, A.M. and Higginbotham, P. (2000). Correlates of fatigue during and following adjuvant breast cancer chemotherapy: A pilot study. *Oncol Nurs Forum*, **27**(9), 1443–8.

181. Broeckel, J.A., Jacobsen, P.B., Horton, J. *et al.* (1998). Characteristics and correlates of fatigue after adjuvant chemotherapy for breast cancer. *J Clin Oncol*, **16**(5), 1689–96.

182. Kay, D.C. and Samiuddin, Z. (1988). Sleep disorders associated with drug abuse and drugs of abuse. In *Sleep Disorders: Diagnosis and Treatment* (eds. R.L. Williams, I. Karacan, and C.A. Moore), pp. 315–71. Wiley, New York.

183. Shaw, I.R., Lavigne, G., Mayer, P. *et al.* (2005). Acute intravenous administration of morphine perturbs sleep architecture in healthy pain-free young adults: A preliminary study.[erratum appears in

Sleep, 2006 Feb 1, **29**(2), 136 Note: dosage error in text]. *Sleep*, **28**(6), 677–82.

184. Nicholson, A.N., Bradley, C.M., and Pascoe, P.A. (1989). Medications: Effect on sleep and wakefulness. In *Principles and Practice of Sleep Medicine* (eds. M.H. Kryger T. Roth, and W.C. Dement), pp. 228–36. WB Saunders, Philadelphia, PA.

185. Ventafridda, V., Tamburini, M., Caraceni, A. *et al.* (1987). A validation study of the WHO method for cancer pain relief. *Cancer*, **59**(4), 850–6.

186. Goughnour, B.R., Arkinstall, W.W., and Stewart, J.H. (1989). Analgesic response to single and multiple doses of controlled-release morphine tablets and morphine oral solution in cancer patients. *Cancer*, **63**(11 Suppl), 2294–7.

187. Ahmedzai, S. and Brooks, D. (1997). Transdermal fentanyl versus sustained-release oral morphine in cancer pain: preference, efficacy, and quality of life. The TTS-Fentanyl Comparative Trial Group.[see comment]. *J Pain Symptom Manage*, **13**(5), 254–61.

188. Payne, R., Mathias, S.D., Pasta, D.J. *et al.* (1998). Quality of life and cancer pain: satisfaction and side effects with transdermal fentanyl versus oral morphine. *J Clin Oncol*, **16**(4), 1588–93.

189. Wong, J.O., Chiu, G.L., Tsao, C.J. *et al.* (1997). Comparison of oral controlled-release morphine with transdermal fentanyl in terminal cancer pain.[erratum appears in *Acta Anaesthesiol Sin* 1007 Sep, **35**(3), 191]. *Acta Anaesthesiol Sin*, **35**(1), 25–32.

190. Bruera, E., Fainsinger, R., MacEachern, T. *et al.* (1992). The use of methylphenidate in patients with incident cancer pain receiving regular opiates. A preliminary report. *Pain*, **50**(1), 75–7.

191. Wilwerding, M.B., Loprinzi, C.L., Mailliard, J.A. *et al.* (1995). A randomized, crossover evaluation of methylphenidate in cancer patients receiving strong narcotics. *Support Care Cancer*, **3**(2), 135–8.

192. Corli, O., Cozzolino, A., and Scaricabarozzi, I. (1993). Nimesulide and diclofenac in the control of cancer-related pain. Comparison between oral and rectal administration. *Drugs*. **46**(Suppl 1), 152–5.

193. Carrol, E.N., Fine, E., Ruff, R.L. *et al.* (1994). A four-drug pain regimen for head and neck cancers. *Laryngoscope*, **104**(6 Pt 1), 694–700.

194. Sjoberg, M., Appelgren, L., Einarsson, S. *et al.* (1991). Long-term intrathecal morphine and bupivacaine in "refractory" cancer pain. I. Results from the first series of 52 patients. *Acta Anaesthesiol Scand*, **35**(1), 30–43.

195. Smith, G.M. and Smith, P.H. (1985). Effects of doxylamine and acetaminophen on postoperative sleep. *Clin Pharmacol Ther*, **37**(5), 549–57.

196. Veitch, D., Rogers, M., and Blanshard, J. (1989). Parapharyngeal mass presenting with sleep apnoea. *J Laryngol Otol*, **103**(10), 961–3.

197. Zorick, F., Roth, T., Kramer, M. *et al.* (1980). Exacerbation of upper-airway sleep apnea by lymphocytic lymphoma. *Chest*, **77**(5), 689–90.

198. Greenough, G., Sateia, M., and Fadul, C.E. (1999). Obstructive sleep apnea syndrome in a patient with medulloblastoma. *Neuro-Oncology*, **1**(4), 289–91.

199. Panje, W.R. and Holmes, D.K. (1984). Mandibulectomy without reconstruction can cause sleep apnea. *Laryngoscope*, **94**(12 Pt 1), 1591–4.

200. Epstein, L.J., Strollo, P.J., Jr., Donegan, R.B. *et al.* (1995). Obstructive sleep apnea in patients with human immunodeficiency virus (HIV) disease. *Sleep*, **18**(5), 368–76.

201. Lo Re, V., 3rd, Schutte-Rodin, S., and Kostman, J.R. (2006). Obstructive sleep apnoea among HIV patients. *Int J STD AIDS*, **17**(9), 614–20.

202. Etches, R.C. (1994). Respiratory depression associated with patient-controlled analgesia: A review of eight cases.[see comment]. *Can J Anaesth*, **41**(2), 125–32.

203. Wang, D., Teichtahl, H., Drummer, O. *et al.* (2005). Central sleep apnea in stable methadone maintenance treatment patients. *Chest*, **128**(3), 1348–56.

204. Thomas, M., von Eiff, M., and van de Loo, J. (1993). [Central sleep apnea syndrome as a cause of impaired wakefulness in multiple myeloma]. *Dtsch Med Wochenschr*, **118**(51–52), 1884–8.

205. Flenley, D.C. (1989). Chronic obstructive pulmonary disease. In *Principles and Practice of Sleep Medicine* (eds. M.H. Kryger TR, and W.C. Dement), pp. 601–10. WB Saunders, Philadelphia, PA.

206. Osoba, D., Zee, B., Warr, D. *et al.* (1997). Effect of postchemotherapy nausea and vomiting on health-related quality of life. The Quality of Life and Symptom Control Committees of the National Cancer Institute of Canada Clinical Trials Group. *Support Care Cancer*, **5**(4), 307–13.

207. Dlin, B.M., Rosen, H., Dickstein, K. *et al.* (1971). The problems of sleep and rest in the intensive care unit. *Psychosomatics*, **12**(3), 155–63.

208. Topf, M. and Thompson, S. (2001). Interactive relationships between hospital patients' noise-induced stress and other stress with sleep. *Heart Lung*, **30**(4), 237–43.

209. Fabijan, L. and Gosselin, M.D. (1982). [How to recognize sleep deprivation in your ICU patient and what to do about it.]. *Can Nurse*, **78**(4), 20–3.

210. Carpenter, J.S., Gautam, S., Freedman, R.R. *et al.* (2001). Circadian rhythm of objectively recorded hot flashes in postmenopausal breast cancer survivors. *Menopause*, **8**(3), 181–8.

211. Polo-Kantola, P., Erkkola, R., Helenius, H. *et al.* (1998). When does estrogen replacement therapy improve sleep quality? *Am J Obstet Gynecol*, **178**(5), 1002–9.

212. Loprinzi, C.L., Levitt, R., Barton, D. *et al.* (2006). Phase III comparison of depomedroxyprogesterone acetate to venlafaxine for managing hot flashes: North Central Cancer Treatment Group Trial N99C7. *J Clin Oncol*, **24**(9), 1409–14.

213. Salin-Pascual, R.J. (2006). Effects of nicotine replacement therapies on sleep.[comment]. *Sleep Medicine*, **7**(2), 105–6.

214. Chesson, A.L., Jr., Ferber, R.A., Fry, J.M. *et al.* (1997). The indications for polysomnography and related procedures. *Sleep*, **20**(6), 423–87.

215. Hartmann, E. (1977). L-tryptophan: A rational hypnotic with clinical potential. *Am J Psychiatry*, **134**(4), 366–70.

216. Cannici, J., Malcolm, R., and Peek, L.A. (1983). Treatment of insomnia in cancer patients using muscle relaxation training. *J Behav Ther Exp Psychiatry*, **14**(3), 251–6.

217. LaClave, L.J. and Blix, S. (1989). Hypnosis in the management of symptoms in a young girl with malignant astrocytoma: A challenge to the therapist. *Int J Clin Exp Hypn*, **37**(1), 6–14.

218. Stam, H.J. and Bultz, B.D. (1986). The treatment of severe insomnia in a cancer patient. *J Behav Ther Exp Psychiatry*, **17**(1), 33–7.

219. Fishman, B. and Loscalzo, M. (1987). Cognitive-behavioral interventions in management of cancer pain: Principles and applications. *Med Clin North Am*, **71**(2), 271–87.

220. Morin, C.M., Kowatch, R.A., and Wade, J.B. (1989). Behavioral management of sleep disturbances secondary to chronic pain. *J Behav Ther Exp Psychiatry*, **20**(4), 295–302.

221. Currie, S.R., Wilson, K.G., Pontefract, A.J. *et al.* (2000). Cognitive-behavioral treatment of insomnia secondary to chronic pain. *J Consult Clin Psychol*, **68**(3), 407–16.

222. Bootzin, R. and Nicassio, P. (1978). Behavioral treatments of insomnia. In *Progress in Behavior Modification* (eds. M. Hersen, R. Eissler, and P. Miller), pp. 1–45. Academic Press, New York.

223. Spielman, A.J., Saskin, P., and Thorpy, M.J. (1983). Sleep restriction: A new treatment of insomnia. *Sleep Res*, **12**, 286.

224. Hirst, A. and Sloan, R. (2002). Benzodiazepines and related drugs for insomnia in palliative care. *Cochrane Database Syst Rev*, (4), CD003346.

225. Spinweber, C.L. and Johnson, L.C. (1982). Effects of triazolam (0.5 mg) on sleep, performance, memory, and arousal threshold. *Psychopharmacology (Berl)*, **76**(1), 5–12.

226. Nowell, P.D., Mazumdar, S., Buysse, D.J. *et al.* (1997). Benzodiazepines and zolpidem for chronic insomnia: a meta-analysis of treatment efficacy. *JAMA*, **278**(24), 2170–7.

227. Vogel, G., Thurmond, A., Gibbons, P. *et al.* (1975). The effect of triazolam on the sleep of insomniacs. *Psychopharmacologia*, **41**(1), 65–9.

228. Attenburrow, M.E., Dowling, B.A., Sargent, P.A. *et al.* (1995). Melatonin phase advances circadian rhythm. *Psychopharmacology (Berl)*, **121**(4), 503–5.

229. Lewy, A.J., Sack, R.L., Blood, M.L. *et al.* (1995). Melatonin marks circadian phase position and resets the endogenous circadian pacemaker in humans. *Ciba Found Symp*, **183**, 303–17; discussion 17–21.

230. Garfinkel, D., Laudon, M., Nof, D. *et al.* (1995). Improvement of sleep quality in elderly people by controlled-release melatonin. [see comment]. *Lancet*, **346**(8974), 541–4.

231. Haimov, I., Lavie, P., Laudon, M. *et al.* (1995). Melatonin replacement therapy of elderly insomniacs. *Sleep*, **18**(7), 598–603.

232. Bruera, E., Fainsinger, R.L., Schoeller, T. *et al.* (1996). Rapid discontinuation of hypnotics in terminal cancer patients: A prospective study. *Ann Oncol*, **7**(8), 855–6.

233. Larson, E.B., Kukull, W.A., Buchner, D. *et al.* (1987). Adverse drug reactions associated with global cognitive impairment in elderly persons. *Ann Intern Med*, **107**(2), 169–73.

234. Ray, W.A., Griffin, M.R., and Downey, W. (1989). Benzodiazepines of long and short elimination half-life and the risk of hip fracture. [see comment]. *JAMA*, **262**(23), 3303–7.

235. Robbins, A.S., Rubenstein, L.Z., Josephson, K.R. *et al.* (1989). Predictors of falls among elderly people. Results of two population-based studies. *Arch Intern Med*, **149**(7), 1628–33.

236. Greenblatt, D.J., Harmatz, J.S., and Shader, R.I. (1991). Clinical pharmacokinetics of anxiolytics and hypnotics in the elderly. Therapeutic considerations (Part I). *Clin Pharmacokinet*, **21**(3), 165–77.

237. Herth, K. (1993). Hope in the family caregiver of terminally ill people. *J Adv Nurs*, **18**(4), 538–48.

238. Sawyer, M.G., Antoniou, G., Toogood, I. *et al.* (1993). A prospective study of the psychological adjustment of parents and families of children with cancer. *J Paediatr Child Health*, **29**(5), 352–6.

239. Carter, P.A. and Chang, B.L. (2000). Sleep and depression in cancer caregivers. *Cancer Nurs*, **23**(6), 410–5.

240. Carter, P.A. (2006). A brief behavioral sleep intervention for family caregivers of persons with cancer. *Cancer Nurs*, **29**(2), 95–103.

10.13

Withdrawing life support: clinical advice for challenging scenarios

Gordon D. Rubenfeld

Death in or after care in an intensive care unit (ICU) occurs in 22 per cent of all deaths in the United States and most of these deaths occur after decisions to limit or withdraw life-support[1,2]. The ethical principles guiding decision-making in these cases and many of the issues around pharmacologic symptom control are addressed in other chapters in this text (Chapters 5.6 and 12.7). Many practical questions about withdrawal of life-support in specific types of cases are perplexing and controversial: should the endotracheal tube be left in place? Should the ventilator be weaned slowly or quickly? When and how should sedation be increased? How can the concerns about relieving suffering be reconciled with fears of killing the patient? Should neuromuscular blockade be discontinued? These questions are important because clinicians face them frequently and are still confused by the goals and process of withdrawing life-support and because patients who die after withdrawal of life-support may receive inadequate pain and symptom management[3,4].

Principles of withdrawing life-sustaining treatment

In this era of evidence-based medicine, there is a lack of data to direct clinicians in the optimal management of the dying critically ill patient. Despite the lack of data on optimal management of some aspects of withdrawing life-sustaining treatment, a general consensus exists on the ethical and clinical principles that should guide this care. These six principles are listed in Table 10.13.1[5,6,7].

Understanding that the goal of withdrawing life-sustaining treatments is to remove unwanted treatments rather than to hasten death is essential in clarifying the distinction between active euthanasia (providing drugs or toxins that hasten death) and death that accompanies the withdrawal of life support in the ICU. Ethicists draw a line between withdrawing life-sustaining treatments when the expected but unintended effect is to hasten death and providing a treatment with the sole intent of hastening death. Despite the well-established principle that 'withholding and withdrawing are equivalent' some clinicians find it difficult to stop treatments that are currently being provided and choose to withhold future

treatments while continuing current levels of support. Frequently, clinicians are faced with multiple decisions about a variety of current or potential life-sustaining treatments. For example, consider a patient with respiratory failure, shock, and worsening acidosis with anuria. A family conference is held and a decision, based on the surrogate decision-maker's judgement of the patient's values, is made to withhold dialysis. In this case, clinicians should strongly consider whether continuing vasopressors and mechanical ventilation while withholding dialysis makes clinical sense. There is no distinction from an ethical or medical standpoint between withdrawing mechanical ventilation, vasopressors, dialysis, antibiotics, blood products, intravenous fluids, or nutrition. All medical treatments, even nutrition and fluids, can be legally, ethically, and compassionately stopped in the appropriate setting. The withdrawal of mechanical ventilation is special in several ways. It is one of the few life-sustaining treatments whose withdrawal can cause discomfort. Mechanical ventilation has profound symbolic significance for clinicians and families. In patients not receiving intensive cardiovascular support, the withdrawal of mechanical ventilation is usually the event that most proximally precedes death[8,9]. The recommendations in this chapter are based on the premise that the withdrawal of life-sustaining treatments is a clinical procedure, and, as such, merits the same meticulous preparation and expectation of quality that clinicians provide when they perform other procedures to initiate life support. Therefore, the steps clinicians take when they withdraw life-support should parallel the steps they take when they perform intubation, cardiopulmonary resuscitation, an appendectomy or bronchoscopy (Table 10.13.2).

The decision to withdraw life-sustaining treatments

Ethical and legal guidelines for decisions to withdraw life-sustaining treatments are well established and have been presented elsewhere[10,6]. Competent, informed patients may refuse any life-sustaining treatment. For incompetent patients, appropriate surrogates may refuse life-sustaining treatments based on written advance directives or, in almost all states, the patient's previously

Table 10.13.1 Principles of withdrawing life support.

1 The goal of withdrawing life-sustaining treatments is to remove treatments that are no longer desired or do not provide comfort to the patient
2 Withholding life-sustaining treatments is morally and legally equivalent to withdrawing them
3 Actions whose sole goal is to hasten death are morally and legally problematic
4 Any treatment can be withheld or withdrawn
5 Withdrawal of life-sustaining treatment is a medical procedure
6 Corollary to 1 and 2: when circumstances justify withholding one indicated life-sustaining treatment, strong consideration should be given to withdrawing all current life-sustaining treatments

stated wishes, values, or best interests. In some circumstances, it is ethically appropriate for physicians to limit treatment in the absence of a surrogate or advance directive[11].

There should be consensus among the health-care team about the decision to withdraw life-support. Frequently, members of the critical care team will reach the conclusion to limit life-sustaining treatment at different times. While the attending physician must take ultimate responsibility for the decision, it would be imprudent to insist on a plan in the face of persistent, thoughtful disagreement by members of the health-care team. Withdrawing life-support is seldom an emergency decision and time should be taken to resolve disagreements among the staff and with family members. Strategies to improve consensus include allaying fears of legal liability, encouraging face-to-face discussions between health-care professionals who disagree on the prognosis, eliciting the views of clinicians who are providing bedside care, and consulting with a senior clinician or ethics committee. When engaging in these discussions, clinicians should temper the certainty of their convictions about the utility of life-sustaining treatment with the knowledge that a large body of data shows that clinicians apply personal values and biases rather than ethical principles and outcome data when making clinical decisions[12–14]. All team members, particularly those in direct patient care roles, should feel that they have had meaningful input into the final plan.

Informed consent

Like other medical procedures, withdrawal of life-support should be accompanied by informed consent, or at least assent,

Table 10.13.2 Routine steps in performing a procedure.

1 Decision is made to perform the procedure
2 Informed consent is obtained
3 An explicit plan for performing the procedure and handling complications is formed
4 The patient is moved to an appropriate setting
5 Adequate sedation and analgesia are begun
6 The plan is carried out
7 The process is documented in the medical record
8 The outcomes are evaluated in an attempt to improve the procedure

and documentation of this process in the medical record. Informed consent for the procedure of withdrawing life-sustaining treatment does not refer to the process of signing a consent form. It refers to a process of communication between caregivers and families that focuses on the burdens and benefits of life-sustaining treatment and the options for alternate care. Competent patients or the surrogates of incompetent patients should understand and agree with the decision to withdraw life-support. In many cases, patients or families will initiate the request that life-support be withdrawn. In rare cases, patients or surrogates may insist on interventions that the health-care team regards as futile. While there is no ethical obligation to provide futile care, there is considerable controversy over what interventions are futile and can be withdrawn over the objections of the patient or surrogate[15]. Fortunately, almost all patients or surrogates eventually agree with physicians' recommendations to withdraw or withhold interventions[16]. Even in the few extraordinary cases where consensus cannot be achieved and life-sustaining treatment are withdrawn over the determined requests of a family member, the ethical principles of truth-telling and respect for persons dictate that they should be informed of the decision or clinicians should determine that the decision-makers do not wish to be informed. These discussions can be uncomfortable for clinicians and family members but this is not a justification for covert clinical activity like 'slow codes' or replacing vasopressor drips with normal saline.

Physicians must provide clear recommendations while respecting the right of patients or their surrogates to make decisions about the process. It is important to explain to the family members how interventions will be withdrawn, to solicit their feedback and to respect strong preferences regarding how interventions will be withdrawn. Some patients or their families may assign particular symbolic significance to certain aspects of care. For example, there may be strong wishes to remove the endotracheal tube while mechanical ventilation is being withdrawn or to continue feeding and hydration when dialysis and vasopressors are stopped. These wishes should be respected as long as they do not interfere with the primary goal of enhancing patient comfort and removing technology that does not fulfil the shared goals. Although it is important for patients and families to have some control over the dying process, it is confusing and inhumane to ask family members to give specific consent for each step of the withdrawal process. Clinicians should specifically avoid providing patients with an entire menu of life-sustaining treatment options to choose from. Families who are not medically sophisticated may have unrealistic expectations and understanding of life-sustaining technology[17]. Generally, once families set the goals of care, for example, to maximize comfort and forego attempts to prolong survival, it is up to clinicians to decide how to meet these goals. With rare exceptions, when discussions with families about withdrawing life-sustaining treatments occur, personnel within the appropriate organ procurement agency should be notified to screen the patient for consideration of organ donation.

Appropriate setting and monitoring

Transforming the ICU into a suitable place to fulfil the new goals of terminal care is not a simple task. The ICU and its staff are poised to respond to minor physiologic changes. Comfort, dignity, family access, and quiet may not always receive the highest priority.

Particularly when family members and friends will be in attendance, the goal should be to have the patient clean and comfortable in a quiet room devoid of technology and alarms that affords the patient and family privacy. The following are suggestions for creating a humane and private environment for the dying patient and family or surrogate:

◆ Separate the patient from the commotion of the ICU by moving the patient to a separate area or an isolated room. In open units, curtains should be closed.

◆ Turn off monitors and, if possible, remove them from the room. Remove electrocardiographic leads, pulse oximeter, and haemodynamic monitoring catheters. There is no point to monitoring physiologic parameters when the data generated will not alter care. Families attending the dying patient can become preoccupied with irrelevant numbers and waveforms instead of focusing their attention on the patient. Removing monitors also eliminates the alarms that will sound as patients die. Intensive nursing care supplemented by physical examination of the patient for blood pressure, pulse, and respiratory rate is sufficient to identify manifestations of suffering and to determine when death occurs. Removing patients from electronic monitoring is an essential step in the transition from curative to comfort care. Unfortunately, it is extremely difficult for clinicians to give up this technologic tether precisely because this step symbolizes the break from the physiologic monitoring that identifies the ICU.

◆ Remove all tubes, lines and drains if this can be done without significant discomfort. Catheters whose removal would lead to painful obstruction, for example, Foley catheters or biliary drains, may be left in place. Intravenous access should be maintained to administer analgesic medication. Remove unused intravenous pumps, resuscitation carts, and other mobile technology from the room.

◆ Liberalize visitation to the extent that it does not interfere with the delivery of care to other patients. Children should be allowed to visit if their parents approve.

◆ Do not obtain further laboratory or imaging studies.

Sedation and analgesia

Prior to performing uncomfortable procedures, clinicians provide patients with adequate medication to prevent anxiety and suffering. Critically ill, haemodynamically unstable patients may not receive optimal sedation when drug related hypotension or respiratory suppression compromises the goals of maintaining life or liberation from mechanical ventilation. However, when the goal of care is changed to assuring patient comfort, any dosage of medication that is required to meet this goal is justified, even if it hastens death. The sole purpose of administering sedatives to dying patients is to relieve symptoms associated with this process. Although rare in the modern ICU, patients capable of communicating their wishes during the withdrawal of life-sustaining treatments should determine how much sedation they receive. Before patients are removed from life-support, they should be completely comfortable as judged by the cessation of tachypnoea, grimacing, agitated behaviour, and autonomic hyperactivity. This is accomplished by titrating medication until objective signs of discomfort have been eliminated. In many cases this will require medication sufficient to induce unconsciousness. Doses should not be increased in the absence of demonstrable signs of discomfort or for behaviour that cannot plausibly be interpreted as distress. Distinguishing signs of true discomfort from autonomic responses that are purely physiologic is challenging[18]. When these goals are achieved, further increases in sedation are unnecessary and ethically problematic.

Although variations in clinical practice are expected, some regimens are unacceptable. Large boluses of medication similar to those used for the induction of general anaesthesia are excessive unless smaller doses have failed to provide adequate sedation. There is an important ethical difference between escalating sedative doses in order to achieve rapid relief of symptoms and administering a large initial bolus intended to induce apnoea or hypotension. There is no role for paralytic agents in the withdrawal of life-sustaining treatments. In fact, these drugs are contraindicated since they will hide manifestations of discomfort like grimacing and tachypnoea.

Given the variability in individual responses and drug tolerance, it is impossible to outline a single pharmacologic regimen to apply in every case. Current guidelines on the management of pain and anxiety in critical care and palliative sedation recommend a combination of morphine or similar narcotic with a benzodiazepine[19,20]. These medications, dosed appropriately, will provide adequate analgesia and sedation in virtually all cases when life-support is withdrawn. The individual clinician's experience or the failure of the opiate/benzodiazepine combination may justify the use of barbiturates, haloperidol, or propofol[21].

The following principles can guide dosing decisions:

◆ Specific doses of medication are less important goals than titration to achieve the desired effect. In patients with painful surgical wounds, high ventilatory drives, or prior exposure to narcotics, large doses of narcotics may be necessary to relieve discomfort. Perhaps, the most important concept is that no ceiling should be placed on dosage if the goal of relieving patient distress has not been achieved. There is no substitute for close bedside evaluation in assessing the efficacy of the sedative medication.

◆ Because of its flexibility and reliability, continuous infusion is the route of choice for drug delivery. Increases in dosage should be preceded by a bolus so that steady state levels are achieved rapidly.

◆ Critical care nurses, who have extensive experience in evaluating suffering in patients who cannot communicate, should be afforded wide latitude in drug dosing, with clear indications for changing the dose. For example, the order might read: '*Titrate morphine drip to keep respiratory rate < 30, heart rate < 100, and eliminate grimacing and agitation*'.

◆ It is essential that nurses be trained to document the objective rationale for escalating doses of palliative medication. For example, charting *Morphine drip increased to 15 mg/h after 15 mg IV bolus administered for grimacing and agitation* is preferable to simply documenting the dose increase. This allows chart auditing for quality of care and provides a factual response in the unlikely event that the nurse is accused of over-dosing medication at the end-of-life.

A plan for withdrawal

Before physicians perform procedures like intubation or central venous catheterization, they have a clear plan of action as well as contingency plans for complications. A similar plan should be developed for withdrawing mechanical ventilation. Physicians need to consider which life-support measures will be discontinued, in what order, and by whom.

Once a decision has been made to orient the patient's care to comfort, the only criterion to use to judge whether a treatment should be initiated, withheld, or withdrawn is whether it contributes to the patient's comfort. All treatments can be withdrawn including vasopressors, drugs, antibiotics, blood transfusions, and nutritional support. Many health-care workers feel more comfortable withholding treatments rather than withdrawing them after they have been initiated[22]. Unfortunately, this leads many clinicians to a strategy that withdraws life support in a series of steps over several days[8]. The decision to provide 'partial' life support, that is, to provide some forms of life-sustaining treatments while withholding or withdrawing others, should be carefully scrutinized. In some cases, these decisions are justifiable. Rarely, patients may have strong reservations about specific medical treatments based on personal experience with the treatment, strongly held religious beliefs, or an assessment of the treatment's burdens and benefits. However, the decision to provide 'stuttering withholding and withdrawal', for example, orders such as 'no second vasopressors drug' or 'no further increases in PEEP', is likely to reflect *clinicians*' values rather than patients' or surrogates'[23,24]. Rarely, such measures are indicated as negotiating techniques with family members or to fulfil specific goals such as trying to sustain life until a relative can arrive while still minimizing burdensome treatments. Clinicians may engage in this stepped withdrawal because a gradual series of steps minimizes the psychological linkage between their actions and the patient's death[25]. Although potentially psychologically reassuring, a gradual approach to withdrawing life-sustaining treatments over several days is not ethically or legally necessary and runs the risk of exposing the patient to pain and suffering without a significant chance of benefit and prolongs the grief experience for the family. Generally, circumstances that justify withholding one indicated life-sustaining treatment also justify the withdrawal of current life-sustaining treatments[26]. When partial treatment strategies are entertained, clinicians should be clear about the goals of care and the rationale for their decision and to ensure that this rationale is based on a specific family request rather than their own discomfort with withdrawal of a particular life-sustaining treatment.

Withdrawing life-sustaining treatments

The time course over which a life-sustaining treatment should be withdrawn is determined by the potential for discomfort as the life-sustaining treatment is stopped. The only rationale for weaning or slowly tapering any life-sustaining treatment is to allow time to meet the patient's needs for pain relief. Mechanical ventilation is one of the few life-support devices whose abrupt termination is likely to lead to profound discomfort due to dyspnoea and therefore deserves specific attention to the timecourse of its withdrawal. There is little justification for 'weaning' other interventions. After adequate sedation has been achieved, vasopressors, pacemakers, intra-aortic balloon pumps, and other therapy not oriented toward meeting the comfort goals of care should be turned off. Tapering these treatments serves no role other than delaying death and prolonging the patient's potential discomfort. Since the withdrawal of mechanical ventilation poses the greatest problems with ensuring comfort, all other life-support devices should be withdrawn before the ventilator. Patients requiring high levels of haemodynamic support may sustain a rapid cardiac death just by withdrawing haemodynamic support before any attention can be devoted to withdrawing the ventilator. Physically turning these devices off can be an emotional task, and the attending physician should be prepared to perform this task or be present when it occurs. Physicians-in-training do not perform other medical procedures independently prior to demonstrating their competence in a supervised setting, and the same rules should apply to the withdrawal of life-support.

Withdrawing mechanical ventilation

Unless the patient specifically requests otherwise, sedation and analgesia sufficient to prevent grimacing or response to painful stimuli should be provided before withdrawing mechanical ventilatory support. After adequate sedation is achieved, reduce the inspired oxygen concentration to 0.21, remove positive end expiratory pressure, and set the ventilator at an intermittent mandatory ventilation (IMV) rate equal to the spontaneous respiratory rate or a level of pressure support (PS) sufficient to fully meet ventilatory requirements. These ventilator settings give the patient a fully supported ventilator breath with every inspiratory attempt and allow clinicians time to modify the sedation before completely removing ventilator assistance. Air hunger, as manifested by tachypnoea or agitation, should be treated with a bolus of the chosen medication followed by an increase in the continuous infusion. After the patient is comfortable, ventilatory support is weaned rapidly in either IMV or PS mode until the patient is comfortable with an IMV rate of zero or a PS of zero cm H_2O at which point the patient can be placed on a T-piece on humidified air. Unless extraordinary levels of dyspnoea are encountered or in the unusual case of an awake patient where clinicians are trying to withdraw ventilatory support and maintain some level of consciousness, there is no reason for the transition from full ventilatory support to T-piece or extubation to take more than 15–30 min. Families may wish to be present for this process or not—If they choose to attend, they should be prepared for the possibility of some transient increases in agitation or respiratory rate as sedation is being titrated. It is extremely important to disable ventilator alarms during this period as patients' terminal hypoventilation may trigger them. Some ventilator's alarms can not be disabled and this should direct clinicians to use a T-piece or to extubate rather than to leave the patient attached to the ventilator. An experienced physician should attend this early phase of withdrawal from the bedside to reassure the patient and family and observe for complications like intractable discomfort that would require immediate intervention.

There are no specific data to guide the decision about managing the endotracheal tube after withdrawal of mechanical ventilation. It may be appropriate to extubate the patient, particularly when the patient may be able to communicate or when prolonged survival off of life-support is possible. Some families or providers may feel strongly about whether to remove the endotracheal tube. These wishes should be respected. If the endotracheal tube is removed, specific plans should be formulated to anticipate secretion problems and agonal airway obstruction and the family should be prepared for these possibilities. If other aspects of the withdrawal of life-sustaining treatments are managed well, including communication with the family and adequate sedation, the decision to remove or leave the endotracheal tube may not be of paramount importance.

The time course leading to death will vary according to the clinical situation and cannot be predicted accurately in every case[27]. However, care givers should inform the patient and family of the probable course of events once life-support is withdrawn. The critically ill patient on several vasopressor agents who is pacemaker-dependent will survive for only a few minutes when these are discontinued. A neurologically devastated teenager with a closed head injury whose only life-support is an endotracheal tube, antibiotics, and enteral nutrition will have a more prolonged course. Plans should be made for alternative care sites if death is delayed. When patients are transferred out of the ICU, the ICU team should communicate the goals and plan communicated to the new team and introduce the new team to the patient and family, so that continuity of care is maintained.

Pastoral, nursing, and emotional support

Before interventions are withdrawn, the family should be asked if a priest, pastor, rabbi, or other religious advisor should be called. Caring for patients after life-sustaining technology is withdrawn can require the same level of vigilance and time that aggressive life-support requires. Nursing attention should be directed to hygiene, skin care, interacting with family members, and maintaining a quiet environment within the busy ICU. Treatments that may alleviate or prevent uncomfortable complications should be instituted or continued. For example, cooling blankets, antipyretics, and anticonvulsants fulfil the goals of patient comfort and usually should be continued. Suggestions and feedback from the family members should be regularly solicited. Members of the health-care team should ask the family in an open-ended manner how they feel things are going and whether they have any questions or suggestions for supportive care. Our approach is to invite the family to play an active role in the care, without making them feel responsible for how interventions are withdrawn.

Just as potential medical complications should be anticipated, the health-care team needs to plan how to respond to the family's emotional reactions and needs. Family members, as well as some members of the health-care team, often believe that they are causing the patient's death by withdrawing interventions. The physician should address these issues directly: 'Many family members ask themselves whether they are causing the patient's death by agreeing to withdraw the ventilator. Do you feel that way?' Generally, people feel more comfortable with withdrawing interventions after these feelings are acknowledged, legitimized as common reactions, and discussed openly. Until these issues are addressed on an emotional level, it is unproductive to discuss the lack of philosophical and legal distinctions between withdrawing and withholding interventions.

If the patient survives longer than expected, family members and health-care workers may feel impatient, frustrated, or angry. Again, the best course is to address the issue directly. A simple comment may broach the topic: 'It's hard to have to wait like this, isn't it?'

Our approach emphasizes that the exact time of death is out of the hands of the physicians and nurses. Some health-care workers may feel comfortable saying, 'It is now in God's hands.' Death is traditionally marked by ceremonies and rituals that extend support and sympathy to the survivors. Health-care workers can ask open ended questions such as, 'Tell me about his life as a young man.' After the patient dies, the attending physician can observe a moment of silence, say a few words of remembrance, and console the family. Empathetic comments such as 'It must be hard to accept'; 'This must be very painful for you'; and questions such as 'How can I be of help' are better received than identification with the family, such as 'I know how you feel' or reassurance, such as 'Time makes it easier'; or 'God had a purpose'. Physicians and nurses need not hide tears they shed. Physical acts of sympathy, from a handshake to a hug, are appropriate, but will vary with the cultural and personal backgrounds of the health-care workers and families.

Documentation

Progress notes in the medical record should document the meetings leading up to the decision to withdraw support, the specific plans for withdrawal, and the pharmacologic plan for sedation. This is particularly important because nurses or covering physicians who implement the plan may not have been involved in the original decision or discussions. Although meetings with surrogates need not address specific decisions regarding every piece of life-support technology, communication with other health-care providers must be detailed. This is particularly important when clinicians choose to withhold some life-sustaining treatments while continuing others. In these cases, the rationale, proscribed treatments, and plan should be clearly documented in the progress notes and orders.

Specific orders for withdrawing interventions and for sedation should be written in the medical record. Orders that simply say 'no heroic measures' or 'comfort care only' can be confusing to a covering physician who must make decisions about antibiotics or blood transfusions. Institutions should develop guidelines, pathways, pre-printed orders, and nursing and respiratory care documentation standards for the withdrawal of life-support, as they currently do for other common clinical situations. Examples from the literature exist and have been shown to increase physician and nurse satisfaction with care[28]. Implementation of this order form was associated with increased use of narcotics and benzodiazepines during the process of withdrawing life support, but was not associated with any change in the time for ventilator withdrawal to death suggesting that medications were used to increase patient comfort without hastening death.

Evaluation

Quality improvement procedures are important for evaluating the withdrawal of life-support and the process of dying, just as they are for other hospital procedures. Members of the hospital critical care committee should review the circumstances of these deaths to evaluate the care. Those involved in the withdrawal of care, including family members, should have the opportunity to evaluate the quality of dying and suggest improvements for the future. These suggestions should be incorporated into the processes in this document and made a part of the local ICU guidelines.

Special cases

Brain death

Although there are cultures that do not accept the diagnosis, brain dead patients are not considered alive according to current ethical and legal guidelines. The decision to withdraw life-sustaining treatments should not be presented as an option in brain-dead patients. Discussions should focus on the timing of withdrawal of life-sustaining treatments and the needs of the family. Appropriate personnel to address potential organ donation should be notified. Sedation and analgesia is not necessary in the management of brain-dead patients and, if organ donation is not being considered, life-sustaining treatments should simply be turned off.

Coma

Many of the patients from whom life-sustaining treatments are withdrawn are neurologically devastated[2]. In these cases, the decision to use sedation during withdrawal of life support is complicated by concerns that unconscious patients, by definition, cannot perceive pain and therefore may not require sedation or analgesia. Studies indicate that physicians do use sedation when withdrawing life-support from patients with catastrophic neurologic injury[29]. While facial electromyography and augmented electroencephalographic techniques may be helpful in determining level of arousal, they have not been validated in this setting. In selected cases, clinicians may rely on the neurologic exam and imaging studies to try to assess whether a patient's injury is compatible with the ability to experience pain. Because these assessments can rarely be made with absolute certainty and there is no gold standard test for perception of discomfort, clinicians will face two possible concerns in the palliative care of comatose patients. By not sedating comatose patients there is, at least, the possibility that some patients will experience discomfort that might be prevented with medication. Alternatively, sedating comatose patients during the withdrawal of life-sustaining treatments may lead clinicians to believe that they are shortening comatose patients' lives without offering them any benefit if they are unconscious. This concern is probably misplaced as higher levels of opioids and sedatives are not associated with reduced time until death[20].

One approach to resolving this dilemma is to select the average adult dosage of medication used in a large series of patients receiving withdrawal of life support (diazepam 10 mg/h and morphine sulfate 10 mg/h or equivalent) that is not adjusted unless objective signs of breakthrough suffering are detected[30]. If patients had been placed on sedatives earlier in the course of their critical illness and show no signs of discomfort, it is not necessary to reduce these medications to withdraw life-sustaining treatment. Obviously, if patients show signs of clinical distress during the withdrawal of life support, then this dose should be increased.

Non-invasive mechanical ventilation

The increasing availability of non-invasive mechanical ventilation provides another option for managing ventilatory support. At least some patients with respiratory failure who were expected to die without intubation and mechanical ventilation can be managed with non-invasive mechanical ventilation[31]. To determine whether this is appropriate, it is essential that clinicians clarify what a patient is refusing when they request not to be 'intubated'.

Clinicians should view non-invasive mechanical ventilation in these cases as either (1) a form of life-sustaining mechanical ventilation that does not use an endotracheal tube for patients who are specifically refusing intubation but not mechanical ventilation or (2) a palliative modality where the goal is relief of discomfort. If a patient is specifically refusing an endotracheal tube because of the lack of ability to communicate with family or concerns over discomfort, then non-invasive mechanical ventilation may be an option. In this situation, clinicians would offer all other forms of life-sustaining treatment except an endotracheal tube. In these cases, if the patient's condition worsens and a trial of non-invasive mechanical ventilation fails, the goals of care would shift to palliation. Non-invasive mechanical ventilation in the patient who refuses ventilatory support because they no longer wish the burdens of aggressive life-sustaining treatment is purely palliative. The sole rationale for using non-invasive mechanical ventilation in these cases is that it objectively improves the patient's symptoms. Although improvements in gas exchange and other physiologic measures are reassuring for intensivists, the primary goal of palliative non-invasive mechanical ventilation in the patient who has refused life-sustaining treatment is palliation of symptoms. Under these circumstances, if the patient does not receive symptomatic benefit from non-invasive ventilation, it should be stopped.

Although the term 'non-invasive' is used to describe mechanical ventilation provided by mask, it is somewhat of a misnomer when applied to option (1) above. Remember that most of these patients will be managed in an ICU, require arterial blood gas and other blood draws, and may receive less than optimal sedation or require restraints to guarantee a more secure airway. Therefore, it is essential, particularly when using non-invasive mechanical ventilation, that the goals and limits of care be established.

Withdrawal of mechanical ventilation with potential survival

Some patients and families, particularly in cases of severe pulmonary or neuromuscular disease, request that ventilatory support be withdrawn when survival off the ventilator is unlikely but possible. Such requests pose a dilemma for clinicians because the goals of care are mixed. It is difficult to simultaneously provide palliative sedation and maximize respiratory function to provide the best chance at survival without a ventilator. In cases when survival is possible and families hope to maximize this goal, sedation should be held to a minimum, respiratory function optimized with bronchodilator therapy, antibiotics, diuresis, and pulmonary toilet; and the patient should be extubated to supplemental oxygen. If it is consistent with the patient's goals, non-invasive ventilatory support can be used as a bridge to unassisted breathing. Prior to and just after extubation, the medical team and patient must formulate specific plans regarding recurrent respiratory failure. Clinicians have two options in this situation: to reinitiate mechanical ventilation (either using an endotracheal tube or mask) or to initiate aggressive symptom management of dyspnoea without ventilatory support. Waiting until the patient develops respiratory failure to formulate a plan leads to chaotic decision-making in the middle of the night with an acutely ill and dyspnoeic patient. If the patient and family choose not to reinitiate mechanical ventilation, then sedation and other treatment as outlined elsewhere are begun acknowledging that the goal of unassisted breathing is no longer attainable. Clinicians may be tempted to 'make sure' the patient still refuses intubation at the time of respiratory compromise; however, intubation need not be specifically offered if the patient has already participated in a decision to withhold it.

Despite clinicians' best efforts to clarify the choices and formulate a prospective plan for patients who develop respiratory failure after extubation, some patients or their families who initially refuse reintubation change their minds. These situations can be harrowing for providers because of the urgency of the decision to choose between reintubation and palliative sedation; and the difficulty in ascertaining which request represents the patient's true wishes. Because mechanical ventilation can be ethically, legally, and humanely withdrawn later, an informed request by the patient for intubation should be fulfilled even when it violates prior requests. Complex and subtle discussions regarding end-of-life treatment choices should never occur at the bedside of a dyspnoeic acutely ill patient in imminent danger of cardiopulmonary arrest.

Prolonged survival despite withdrawal of life-sustaining treatment

The available data suggest that prolonged survival after a decision to withdraw life support is uncommon[30]. Patients who survive the withdrawal of life-sustaining treatments present clinicians with several challenges. Families and clinicians can become frustrated and hope for some means to expedite death. These requests should be dealt with honestly and compassionately. Treatments solely intended to hasten death or increases in sedation that are not necessary to relieve discomfort are not justified under current ethical and legal guidelines[6]. Families should be reassured that their loved one is comfortable and that the timing of death is out of the control of the clinical team. It is appropriate to transfer these patients out of the ICU to an area in the hospital with more privacy as long as the family has been prepared for the move. Prolonged survival may cause those involved to question their decision to withdraw life-sustaining treatments. Because so little is known about the timing of death after withdrawal of life support, clinicians should be wary of revising their plans and prognosis based on a perceived delay in the expected timing of death. These changes in plans can have a devastating effect on loved ones and staff.

Pharmacologic paralysis

Despite the fact that most intensivists are using pharmacologic paralysis less frequently because of the long-term neuromuscular sequelae attributed to the drugs, patients who have received these medications present unique challenges during the withdrawal of mechanical ventilation[32,33]. Agents like pancuronium and vecuronium are used in critically ill patients to improve ventilator synchrony and reduce oxygen consumption; however, they serve no purpose in fulfilling the comfort goals during the withdrawal of life-support. Although the argument has been made that paralytic drugs ease the family's distress by making the dying patient appear comfortable, they actually prevent clinicians from adequately assessing patients' discomfort and therefore may contribute to the patient's suffering. Paralytic drugs are also ethically problematic because they may hasten death by preventing respiration without offering any beneficial effects to the patient.

The primary concern about withdrawing ventilation in the face of pharmacologic paralysis is its masking effect on patient discomfort.

For this reason, paralytic drugs should be stopped as soon as the withdrawal of life-sustaining treatments is considered. Some clinicians may choose to try to reverse pharmacologic paralysis in an effort to restore some of the patient's ability to manifest discomfort to help guide sedation requirements. Unfortunately, after an extended course of these drugs, some critically ill patients will not regain normal neuromuscular function for days or weeks[34]. Some physicians may regard withdrawing mechanical ventilation in a partially paralysed patient as euthanasia and wish to delay until neuromuscular function returns to normal. This delay is not justified. Neuromuscular weakness after pharmacologic paralysis initiated to treat critical illness is a complication of treatment of the patient's illness. Withdrawing life-support in the face of treatment complications is justified because the complications, even if iatrogenic, are part of the patient's illness, may not resolve, and continued therapy of the complication imposes an unwanted burden on the patient. Patients who are receiving pharmacologic paralysis should have it stopped prior to the withdrawal of life-sustaining treatments. Clinicians should wait for the return of sufficient neuromuscular function to detect spontaneous movements and attempts at respiration so that sedation needs can be monitored. Therefore, physicians should stop neuromuscular blocking drugs as soon as the withdrawal of life-support is anticipated, but need not wait for the effects of these drugs to disappear completely before withdrawing life-sustaining treatments. Obviously, caregivers should be aware, as they are in all patients who have received pharmacologic paralysis, that physical manifestations of discomfort may be blunted by muscle weakness. A similar argument can be made for patients receiving high doses of barbiturates or propofol to induce coma for intractable intracranial hypertension.

Request to reduce sedation to allow communication with family

Families sometimes request that sedation be stopped in critically ill patients either to try to elicit the patient's decisions about ongoing intensive care or to allow family members to reach some closure with the patient. This is a reasonable request; however, families and ethics committees should be prepared for the realistic outcomes of this procedure. It is routine in most ICUs to implement a daily 'sedation vacation' and stop sedating medications until patients are awake enough to follow instructions or until they become uncomfortable or agitated[35]. Given the prevalence of agitated delirium in critically ill patients who are sick enough to be considering withdrawal of life-sustaining treatment, most patients become agitated and uncomfortable without regaining meaningful levels of consciousness[36]. Even those who are able to follow commands are likely to be sufficiently impaired by delirium and an endotracheal tube to impede their participation in subtle decisions about limiting life support.

Non-heart beating donors

Organ procurement after declaration of cardiopulmonary death rather than brain death is increasingly common[37]. In these cases, life support is withdrawn in a controlled fashion, frequently in the operating room after placement of cannulae to preserve organ perfusion. Patients who are expected to survive for longer than 30–45 min without life-sustaining treatment are poor candidates for this procedure due to concerns about organ viability. After death is declared, the organs are removed for transplantation. In some programmes, families are permitted to accompany their loved one to the operating room until death is declared. As a general rule, care of the patient before and after organ donation is provided by completely separate teams to avoid even the appearance of a conflict. Care of the non-heart beating donor can present challenges to the clinical team. For example, how long must a patient be asystolic before organ procurement can begin? Once a decision has been made for the patient to be a non-heart beating donor and the surgical team is assembling, how should haemodynamic and respiratory complications in the potential donor be handled? If cardiopulmonary death is imminent, should it be forestalled to protect organ viability? Clinicians should look to local policies governing this evolving area of clinical practice.

Conclusion

The clinician's responsibility to the patient does not end with a decision to limit medical treatment, but continues through the dying process. Every effort should be made to ensure that withdrawing life-support occurs with the same quality and attention to detail as is routinely provided when life-support is initiated. Approaching the withdrawal of life-support as a medical procedure provides clinicians with a recognizable framework for their actions. Key steps in this process are identifying and communicating explicit shared goals for the process, approaching withdrawal of life-sustaining treatments as a medical procedure, and preparing protocols and materials to assure consistent care. Our hope is that adopting a more formal approach to this common procedure will improve the care of patients dying in ICUs.

References

1. Vincent, J.L., Parquier, J.N., Preiser, J.C. *et al.* (1989). Terminal events in the intensive care unit: Review of 258 fatal cases in one year. *Crit Care Med*, **17**(6), 530–3.
2. Prendergast, T.J. and Luce, J.M. (1997). Increasing incidence of withholding and withdrawal of life support from the critically ill. *Am J Respir Crit Care Med*, **155**(1), 15–20.
3. Asch, D.A. (1996). The role of critical care nurses in euthanasia and assisted suicide. *N Engl J Med*, **334**(21), 1374–9.
4. 1995. A controlled trial to improve care for seriously ill hospitalized patients. The study to understand prognoses and preferences for outcomes and risks of treatments (SUPPORT). The SUPPORT Principal Investigators. *JAMA*, **274**(20), 1591–8.
5. 1991. Withholding and withdrawing life-sustaining therapy. This Official Statement of the American Thoracic Society was adopted by the ATS Board of Directors, March 1991. *Am Rev Respir Dis*, **144**(3 Pt 1), 726–31.
6. Lo, B. (1995). *Resolving ethical dilemmas: A guide for clinicians*. Williams & Wilkins, Baltimore.
7. Jonsen, A.R., Siegler, M., and Winslade, W.J. (1998). *Clinical ethics: A practical approach to ethical decisions in clinical medicine*, 4th edition. McGraw Hill, New York.
8. Faber-Langendoen, K. (1996). A multi-institutional study of care given to patients dying in hospitals. Ethical and practice implications. *Arch Intern Med*, **156**(18), 2130–6.
9. Faber-Langendoen, K. and Bartels, D.M. (1992). Process of forgoing life-sustaining treatment in a university hospital: An empirical study. *Crit Care Med*, **20**(5), 570–7.
10. Beauchamp, T.L. and Childress, J.F. (1994). *Principles of biomedical ethics*, 4th edition. Oxford University Press, New York.
11. Asch, D.A., Hansen, F.-J., and Lanken, P.N. (1995). Decisions to limit or continue life-sustaining treatment by critical care physicians in the United States: Conflicts between physicians' practices and patients' wishes. *Am J Resp Crit Care Med*, **151**(2 Pt 1), 288–92.
12. Wachter, R.M., Luce, J.M., Hearst, N. *et al.* (1989). Decisions about resuscitation: Inequities among patients with different diseases but similar prognoses *Ann Intern Med*, **111**(6), 525–32.
13. Cook, D.J., Guyatt, G.H., Jaeschke, R. *et al.* (1995). Determinants in Canadian health care workers of the decision to withdraw life support from the critically ill. *JAMA*, **273**(9), 703–8.
14. Hanson, L.C., Danis, M., Garrett, J.M. *et al.* (1996). Who decides? Physicians' willingness to use life-sustaining treatment. *Arch Intern Med*, **156**(7), 785–9.
15. Truog, R.D., Brett, A.S., and Frader, J. (1992). The problem with futility. *N Engl J Med*, **326**(23), 1560–4.
16. Prendergast, T.J., Claessens, M.T., and Luce, J.M. (1998). A national survey of end-of-life care for critically ill patients. *Am J Respir Crit Care Med*, **158**(4), 1163–7.
17. Diem, S.J., Lantos, J.D., and Tulsky, J.A. (1996). Cardiopulmonary resuscitation on television. Miracles and misinformation. *N Engl J Med*, **334**(24), 1578–82.
18. Campbell, M.L., Bizek, K.S., and Thill, M. (1999). Patient responses during rapid terminal weaning from mechanical ventilation: A prospective study. *Crit Care Med*, **27**(1), 73–7.
19. Shapiro, B.A., Warren, J., Egol, A.B. *et al.* (1995). Practice parameters for intravenous analgesia and sedation for adult patients in the intensive-care unit—An Executive Summary. *Crit Care Med*, **23**(9), 1596–600.
20. Lo, B. and Rubenfeld, G. (2005). Palliative sedation in dying patients: 'We turn to it when everything else hasn't worked'. *JAMA*, **12294**(14), 1810–16.
21. Truog, R.D., Berde, C.B., Mitchell, C. *et al.* (1992). Barbiturates in the care of the terminally ill. *N Engl J Med*, **3327**(23), 1678–82.
22. Solomon, M.Z., O'Donnell, L., Jennings, B. *et al.* (1993). Decisions near the end of life: Professional views on life-sustaining treatments. *Am J Public Health*, **83**(1), 14–23.
23. Christakis, N.A. and Asch, D.A. (1993). Biases in how physicians choose to withdraw life support. *Lancet*, **342**(8872), 642–6.
24. Christakis, N.A. and Asch, D.A. (1995). Medical specialists prefer to withdraw familiar technologies when discontinuing life support. *J Gen Intern Med*, **10**(9), 491–4.
25. Gianakos, D. (1995). Terminal Weaning. *Chest*, **108**(5), 1405–6.
26. 1983. *President's Commission for the Study of Ethical Problems in Medicine and Biomedical and Behavioral Research. Deciding to Forego Life-sustaining Treatment*. U.S. Government Printing Office, Washington.
27. Campbell, M.L. (1993). Case studies in terminal weaning from mechanical ventilation. *Am J Crit Care*, **2**(5), 354–8.
28. Treece, P.D., Engelberg, R.A., Crowley, L. *et al.* (2004). Evaluation of a standardized order form for the withdrawal of life support in the intensive care unit. *Crit Care Med*. **32**(5), 1141–8
29. Mayer, S.A. and Kossoff, S.B. (1999). Withdrawal of life support in the neurological intensive care unit. *Neurology*, **52**(8), 1602–9.
30. Wilson, W.C., Smedira, N.G., Fink, C. *et al.* (1992). Ordering and administration of sedatives and analgesics during the withholding and withdrawal of life support from critically ill patients. *JAMA*, **267**(7), 949–53.
31. Benditt, J.O. (2000). Noninvasive ventilation at the end of life. *Respir Care*, **45**(11), 1376–81, discussion 1381–4.
32. Kirkland, L. (1994). Neuromuscular paralysis and withdrawal of mechanical ventilation. *J Clin Ethics*, **5**(1), 38–9, discussion 39–42.
33. Truog, R.D., Burns, J.P., Mitchell, C. *et al.* (2000). Pharmacologic paralysis and withdrawal of mechanical ventilation at the end of life. *N Engl J Med*, **342**(7), 508–11.

34. Segredo, V., Caldwell, J.E., Matthay, M.A. *et al.* (1992). Persistent paralysis in critically ill patients after long-term administration of vecuronium. *N Engl J Med*, **327**(8), 524–8.

35. Kress, J.P., Pohlman, A.S., O'Connor, M.F. *et al.* (2000). Daily interruption of sedative infusions in critically ill patients undergoing mechanical ventilation. *N Engl J Med*, **342**(20), 1471–7.

36. Ely, E.W., Inouye, S.K., Bernard, G.R. *et al.* (2001). Delirium in mechanically ventilated patients: Validity and reliability of the confusion assessment method for the intensive care unit (CAM- ICU). *JAMA*, **286**(21), 2703–10.

37. Zawistowski, C. and DeVita, M. (2003). Non-heartbeating organ donation: a review. *J Intensive Care Med*, **18**, 189–97.

Clinical management of bleeding complications

Jose Pereira and Sophie Pautex

Haemorrhaging is amongst the most distressing complications for palliative patients and their caregivers[1]. It can provoke pronounced anxiety and fear in patients. A major catastrophic haemorrhage from a ruptured carotid artery due to invasive cancer is one of the most alarming events to experience and witness in palliative care. Often patients and families are ill-prepared to deal with these situations when they arise. This section provides a review of causes and treatment options for these complications. The focus is on visible haemorrhaging.

Causes

Although bleeding may be associated with non-cancer palliative situations such as life-threatening Goodpasture's syndrome, it is more common in cancer[2]. Approximately 6–10 per cent of patients with advanced cancer experience some form of haemorrhaging during their illness[2]. In some types of cancers, the incidence can be higher. In lung cancer, for example, up to 50 per cent of patients may experience haemoptysis some time in their illness.

The causes and mechanisms of bleeding in palliative patients are varied and include perforation of blood vessels by cancer, tissue destruction and inflammation, and systemic abnormalities such as blood clotting dysfunction resulting from complications such as liver failure, disseminated intravascular coagulopathy (DIC), and thrombocytopenia[2]. In cancer patients, bleeding may be related to primary or metastatic disease. Haematuria, for example, may arise from primary cancer in the genitourinary tract, local infiltration of an advanced cervical or rectal cancer, or from metastases in the kidneys. Cancer treatments may cause bleeding. The chemotherapy agents cyclophosphamide and ifosfamide, for example, may cause a chemical cystitis with bleeding. A late complication of high dose radiotherapy to the bladder is telangiectasia, which can result in severe bleeding. Non-steroidal anti-inflammatory drugs (NSAIDs) used in the management of pain are associated with a well-recognized risk of gastrointestinal bleeds. Excessive anticoagulation therapy, either by over-dosing or drug interactions, is not uncommon in patients with advanced cancer on anticoagulation treatment[3]. Bleeding may also result from causes not associated with the cancer or other terminal illness. These include pre-existing duodenal ulcer disease or auto-immune platelet diseases.

Clinical presentation

Haemorrhaging manifests clinically in a variety of ways. In terms of site, it may present as haematemesis, haematochezia, haemoptysis, haematuria, epistaxis, or vaginal bleeding. It can also appear from an ulcerated surface wound or as ecchymoses, petechiae, or bruising. In systemic causes of bleeding it is not uncommon for haemorrhaging to present simultaneously at multiple sites. Sometimes its presentation is more insidious, as in the case of melaena. In terms of duration and volume, bleeding can be a one-time event, recur intermittently or be continuous. Small intermittent bleeds may herald larger future bleeds. Large ulcerating chest lesions from advanced breast cancer, for example, may present as continuous low-grade oozing from the underlying vascular bed, losing several millilitres of blood per day. In rare cases, haemorrhaging can be massive and catastrophic, causing hypovolaemia and death within minutes.

Management: general measures

Treatment, as with any palliative intervention, needs to be individualized. Several factors need to be considered. These include goals of care and a patient's wishes, life expectancy, likelihood of reversing or controlling the underlying cause of the bleeding, and the availability of treatment options. An interventional approach, using radiotherapy or endoscopic laser cautery, may be warranted in a patient with haemoptysis from lung cancer whose life expectancy is still in the order of many months and whose quality of life is acceptable, while a more conservative approach, focusing largely on comfort measures, may be more appropriate for patients in the terminal phases of their lives. Clearly, the goals of care need to be established. When it is unclear as to whether or not a local or systemic measure will be of benefit, a time-limited trial may be warranted.

Management generally focuses on identifying and treating, where possible and appropriate, the underlying cause and controlling the bleeding. Depending on the origin of the bleeding and the goals of care, a variety of options may be available, including non-pharmacological, pharmacological, endoscopic, radiation, and surgical interventions. An appropriate history and focused physical examination is required. A review of concurrent medications and other concurrent illnesses is essential. The burden versus risks of continuing prophylactic anti-coagulation need to be reviewed in patients bleeding from excessive anti-coagulation treatment[3]. Investigations may be helpful in select cases. Full blood counts and clotting profiles may reveal systemic problems while angiography or endoscopic studies may identify the site of bleeding.

Patients at a high risk of bleeding should be identified and preventative measures taken before a crisis occurs. Patients at increased risk include patients with severe thrombocytopenia (particularly platelet counts below 5000–10 000/mm^3), large head and neck carcinomas, large centrally located lung cancers, severe liver disease, refractory acute and chronic leukaemias, and patients with advanced cancer on oral anticoagulants. Episodic, low-volume haemoptysis may herald larger, catastrophic haemorrhages and pre-emptive treatment such as irradiation should be considered. Caregivers of patients at risk for major bleeds ought to be informed and prepared for such an event.

The treatment options available depending on the site of bleeding are listed in Tables 10.14.1 and 10.14.2 and are discussed in more detail below.

Management: local interventions

Compression dressings and packing

Compression dressing is the simplest modality to stem bleeding from a surface wound. However, it requires that the site be accessible to circular bandaging. If circular bandaging is not possible, applying a pressure bandage by using adhesive bandaging to the surrounding skin may work as a temporary solution but may become uncomfortable and damage skin that is already friable. Haemostatic or vasoconstrictive agents may be added to the dressings.

Packing with dry or saline-soaked dressings or surgical swabs can be used to achieve haemostasis in bleeding from the nose, vagina, or rectum. If possible, the frequency of dressings should be reduced and non-adherent dressings used. Haemostatic or vasoconstrictive agents may also be added to the dressings. Vaginal bleeding, for example, has been controlled with packs soaked with formalin or acetone[4,5]. Vasoconstrictors such as cocaine, epinephrine, or astringents such as silver nitrate have been used for controlling epistaxis[6].

Specially designed catheters with inflatable balloons may be used to control severe epistaxis from posterior nasal bleeding. In emergency cases, urinary catheters have been used. Such measures are temporary since prolonged pressure may cause ischaemia and tissue necrosis.

Vasoconstrictive and cauterizing agents

These are particularly useful for managing localized, capillary bleeding. The type of agent varies depending on the site of bleeding.

Astringent agents

These agents induce chemical cauterization and are more appropriately used to control relatively small bleeds. The two most commonly used astringents are silver nitrate and aluminium-based astringents. Silver nitrate acts as a strong oxidizing agent, causing tissue coagulation[7]. Silver nitrate has been used to control bladder haemorrhages and epistaxis[8]. Thin wooden applicators with tips containing the silver nitrate fused with potassium nitrate are then applied to the bleeding focus. It is relatively inexpensive and application requires minimal technical skill. Alum (either aluminium

Table 10.14.1 Local measures for controlling local bleeding in palliative care.

- ◆ Compression dressings
- ◆ Packing
- ◆ Vasoconstrictive agents
  - • Astringents
    - ◦ Silver nitrate
    - ◦ Aluminum astringents
  - • Epinephrine
  - • Topical cocaine
  - • Sucralfate
  - • Prostaglandins E$_2$ & F$_2$
  - • Acetone
  - • Formalin
- ◆ Other haemostatic agents
  - • Alginates
- ◆ Absorbable haemostatic agents
  - • Gelatin (porcine or bovine)
  - • Microfibrillar collagen (bovine)
  - • Regenerated oxidized cellulose
  - • Thrombin (bovine)
  - • Combination
  - • Flowable bovine collagen and bovine platelets
  - • Flowable bovine gelatin matrix and bovine thrombin
- ◆ Non-absorbable haemostatic materials
  - • Fibrin sealants
  - • Microporus polysaccharide or zeolite particles
- ◆ Radiotherapy
- ◆ Surgery
  - • Vessel ligation
  - • Tissue resection
- ◆ Endoscopy
- ◆ Interventional radiology
  - • Transcutaneous arterial embolization
  - • Transcutaneous arterial balloons
- ◆ Inhaled ornopressin

ammonium sulphate or aluminium potassium sulphate) causes the precipitation of protein in the interstitial tissue spaces, resulting in decreased capillary permeability, vasoconstriction, constriction of the interstitial spaces and hardening of the capillary endothelium. One percent alum has been administered via irrigation in intractable tumour- or irradiation-related haematuria originating from the bladder[9]. Patients with a damaged bladder wall or renal impairment are at increased risk of developing aluminum toxicity, which may manifest in lethargy, confusion, seizures, anorexia, vomiting, abdominal pain, or dysarthria. Treatment involves haemodialysis and desferrioxamine.

Sucralfate

Sucralfate has been used most often for the treatment of radiation proctitis and cutaneous oozing. Its cytoprotective action seems to

Table 10.14.2 Systemic measures to control bleeding in palliative care.

- Vitamin K (phytonadione)
- Vasopressin/desmopressin
- Somatostatin analogues (octreotide)
- Antifibrinolytic agents
  - Tranexamic acid
  - Aminocaproic acid
  - Aprotinin
- Plasma/blood products
  - Platelets
  - Fresh frozen plasma
  - Packed red blood cells
  - Cryoprecipitate
  - Recombinant F VIIa

originate from the production of prostaglandins and promotion of epithelial cell proliferation. Application of 20 ml of 10 per cent rectal sucralfate suspension enemas twice a day until rectal bleeding stops has been used to control bleeding from radiation proctitis[10]. It can be mixed with a water soluble gel such as KY® jelly to form a paste for direct application[11]. A preparation made up of a 1-g tablet of sucralfate, crushed and mixed into 5 ml of water soluble gel for twice daily application, has been reported[12].

Formalin
Formalin 2–5 per cent, a safe and inexpensive option, acts as a chemical cautery and has been used successfully to control haemorrhaging from radiation proctitis, bladder lesions, vaginal/cervix tumours, and cutaneous ulcers[13–17]. In the case of rectal bleeds, formalin solution is either used to irrigate the rectum or soaked in a gauze and applied through a rectoscope. In one case series, topical formalin controlled bleeding in 49 of 55 patients (89 per cent)[18]. Endoscopically aided insertion of cotton pledgets soaked in 5 per cent formalin has been used to control bleeding from specific foci in the bladder[19,20]. However, bladder instillations of formalin may result in bladder spasms. These can be controlled with antispasmodic medications such as hyoscine butylbromide.

Acetone
Acetone-soaked packs have been used to control vaginal bleeding[5]. It is particularly useful when embolic techniques are neither immediately available nor practical, or in patients who have previously been irradiated and who cannot safely be treated with additional radiotherapy.

Others
Cancer-related vaginal bleeding has been treated with formaldehyde[21]. Cocaine can be applied to cotton pledgets and packed into the nasopharynx[22]. Four ml of a 4 per cent solution may be used to minimize cardiovascular adverse effects. Prostaglandins E_2 and F_2 have been used to control intractable haemorrhagic cystitis but bladder spasms may limit their utility[23]. Epinephrine can also be used but liberal use is discouraged[24]. Local application of antifibrinolytic agents has been reported. This includes tranexamic acid 500 mg tablets crushed and dissolved in 5 ml of normal saline, soaked in gauze and applied to skin wounds for 10 min[25]; local instillation to control haemothoraces and rectal bleeding (5 ml diluted in 50–100 ml of water and applied once or twice a day); and as a mouthwash (1 g diluted in 20–50 ml of water given three to four times a day) for oral lesions[26,27].

Absorbable haemostatic agents
Haemostatic agents stop bleeding mechanically or by augmenting the coagulation cascade. Tissue sealants on the other hand bind to and close defects in tissue. They are primarily used in surgery to stem low-volume bleeding from surgical sites (particularly capillary oozing during surgery involving the liver, spleen, and nervous tissues) when more conventional methods such as suturing, ligature, and cauterization are ineffective or impractical. They may be considered in the palliative setting to control continuous oozing of blood from malignant fungating surface lesions where simpler strategies, such as pressure dressings or radiotherapy, are ineffective or not possible. Typically, these agents are not administered according to standardized dosing regimens. Their high costs, particularly the absorbable haemostatic agents, may be prohibitive for long-term treatment.

Absorbable haemostatic agents usually dissolve spontaneously after a few weeks (usually 4–8 weeks). In some cases, they leave behind radiographic traces that could be misinterpreted as abscesses or necrotic processes. They are particularly useful for controlling capillary bleeding and usually exert their pharmacologic effects by mimicking the final phases of the coagulation cascade. The agents largely contain porcine or bovine gelatin, bovine collagen, or regenerated oxidized cellulose[28]. They have also been used to control bleeding from fistula-puncture sites and closure of fistulae[29,30]. They may be considered for off-label use to control refractory capillary bleeding from chest or skin ulcerating tumours.

In general, adverse effects are not common with these products. These include minor burning and stinging sensations, allergic reactions, and local fibrosis. Because of the propensity of these agents to increase in size, it is generally not indicated for use in neurosurgical, ophthalmic, and urological procedures when compression of sensitive tissues such as nerve tissues can cause paralysis or blindness.

Gelatin (porcine or bovine)
Porcine gelatin, usually moulded into a sponge, applied to an area of bleeding causes fibrin to be deposited in the interstices of the gelatine foam and platelets to be activated. This results in swelling of the sponge and creation of a synthetic clot[31–33]. It is also available in powder form. Since it activates the intrinsic clotting pathway, clotting factors and co-factors need to be present and functional to achieve optimal haemostasis. It can be applied dry directly to the surface or after being soaked with saline and squeezed to remove the air bubbles. Gelatin sponge is usually absorbed approximately 4–6 weeks following application, but in the nasal mucosa it liquefies within 2–5 days.

Microfibrillar or sponge-based collagen (bovine)
Collagen, available as a bovine-derived microfibrillar mesh or sponge, creates a clot when it comes into contact with blood by provoking the clotting cascade[34,35]. The mesh form may be cut to size. The collagen sponge preparations can be stored at room temperature and are basically ready to use out of the box.

Regenerated oxidized cellulose

Regenerated oxidized cellulose is derived from α-cellulose that is plant-based and activates the intrinsic clotting pathway. Its use has been reported in palliative care[36].

Thrombin (bovine)

Thromboplastin (also known as factor III) is a protein present in subendothelial tissue, platelets, and leucocytes necessary for the initiation of thrombin formation and coagulation of blood. Thrombin is usually obtained from bovine plasma. It is generally available as a sterile freeze-dried powder that can either be sprinkled over the exposed capillary bed or reconstituted in 0.9 per cent sodium chloride and mixed with the gelatin matrix in the operating room just before use[37]. It may be used in combination with the other absorbable haemostatic agents, particularly absorbable gelatin sponge. Because thrombin preparations are of bovine origin, patients may develop antibodies to bovine coagulation factors that may cross-react with endogenous human clotting proteins. Allergic reactions, usually presenting as rashes, have been reported but are scarce. Three deaths have been reported following intravenous and naso-gastric administration.

Combination agents

Combinations products made up of fluid bovine collagen and bovine platelets are available, as are products of fluid bovine gelatin matrix and bovine thrombin. The two components work independently to promote clot formation at the bleeding site. In the latter, a preparatory time of 1–3 min is required. Once mixed, it is usable for about 2 h.

Other absorbable agents

A number of other absorbable haemostatic agents, including cyanoacrylates, bovine serum/albumin/glutaraldehyde, and polyethylene glycol hydrogels may become more widely available in the future.

Other haemostatic agents

Alginates

Alginates are dressings derived from seaweed and cause clotting by activating the intrinsic clotting pathway[38,39]. Calcium ions in the dressings catalyse coagulation, drawing in water and fluids that cause the alginate fibres to swell and form a gel. These act as a tamponade. The degree of swelling is determined principally by the chemical composition of the alginate[40]. Alginates containing zinc ions appear to have a superior effect. Bupivicaine hydrochloride (0.5 per cent) soaked in calcium alginate may reduce pain.

Alginates are available for topical use only and maintain a physiologically moist microenvironment that promotes healing and the formation of granulation tissue. They can be rinsed away with saline irrigation and so removal of the dressing does not interfere with granulation tissue. They absorb drainage from wounds with moderate to heavy drainage and often swell to many times their own weight. Because these dressings are highly adsorbent and require moisture to function correctly, they are best used in wounds with moderate to heavy drainage and not indicated for dry wounds.

Alginate dressings are usually packed into the wound bed as the primary dressing. They should not be moistened prior to application. A secondary dressing is then added to hold the alginate in place and maintain the moist healing environment. Choosing an appropriate secondary dressing is important. Petrolatum gauzes or foams will secure the alginate and keep it from drying out. If the wound is infected, the secondary dressing should be non-occlusive. Alginate fibres left *in situ* for long periods of time may elicit an allergic reaction[41]. The value of alginates has been challenged in a randomized clinical trial related to tooth extractions in young children[42].

Fibrin sealants

Fibrin sealants (also known as fibrin glues) are a type of surgical tissue adhesive derived from human and bovine blood products. They are used in a wide range of surgeries (including cardiovascular, hepatic, and splenic surgery) primarily as haemostatic agents, but also to assist in tissue sealing and wound healing[43,44]. While all fibrin sealants contain fibrinogen (a protein) and thrombin (an enzyme), they differ in their final composition. These ingredients interact during application to form a stable clot composed of fibrin. Many sealants have two additional ingredients, human blood factor XIII and a substance called aprotinin, which is derived from cows' lungs. Factor XIII is a compound that strengthens blood clots by forming cross-links between strands of fibrin, while aprotinin inhibits the enzymes that break down blood clots.

These products are usually supplied in syringes with long tubes. Fibrin sealants with a fibrinogen component of low viscosity are easier to apply than highly viscous solutions. Most products consist of a two-vial system and require preparation of about 5–15 min. Once these elements are mixed, the product has to be used within a few hours. Fibrin sealants generally need to be kept in cold storage and thawed prior to usage. Bovine thrombin can cause an IgE-mediated allergic reaction. Antibodies formed against bovine factor V or thrombin can cross react with human factor V, causing haemorrhage. Thromboembolic events can result if the sealant is introduced into large blood vessels. Although fibrin sealants have been used in a variety of settings, the evidence in their support is largely based on animal models, case reports, and small series.

Microporus polysaccharide or zeolite particles

New haemostatic agents consisting of zeolite granules and microporus polysaccharide particles that are directly poured onto a bleeding wound have recently been reported in the management of significant haemorrhaging resulting from trauma, on and off the battlefield. The granules, which are non-allergenic and resemble granular sand, are poured onto the bleeding site. The particles absorb water from blood and plasma, resulting in concentration of clotting factors and platelets. Concerns have been expressed about local hyperthermia from an exothermic process. There have been no reports of use of these materials in the palliative setting but they may hold potential. The granules are non-allergenic.

Radiotherapy

Radiotherapy is one of the more useful modalities for controlling bleeding caused by malignant conditions, including cancers of the lung[45,46], skin, soft-tissues, vagina and cervix[47], rectum, and bladder[48].

Haemoptysis caused by lung cancer is amenable to external beam radiotherapy and control rates of up to 80 per cent have been reported with palliative doses of external beam radiotherapy[45,46]. Single or dual fractions appear as effective and safe as multiple fractions. Palliative endobronchial brachytherapy has also been reported. Patients with good performance status and stage III lung cancer may benefit from higher radiotherapy doses. Radiotherapy should be considered in patients with small-cell lung cancer if chemotherapy has failed or is not possible. Where haemoptysis is associated with extensive pulmonary metastases, treatment with radiotherapy may be more difficult unless a specific site of haemorrhaging can be identified through bronchoscopy. Low-dose whole lung radiotherapy delivered in 20 fractions over several weeks has been reported but should be reserved for very exceptional cases where the functional status is good and the cancer is radio-sensitive, such as Ewing's sarcoma. Large asymptomatic lung cancers (10 cm or greater in size) may be considered for prophylactic radiotherapy since they may be at greater risk of haemorrhaging.

External beam irradiation is an option in treating haematuria from bladder cancer particularly in patients whose cancer is inoperable and where other local or conservative measures have failed or are not possible[49]. Radiotherapy improves haematuria in up to 63 per cent of these patients. In most cases, results are noted within several days but in some cases the maximal benefit may only manifest up to 3 months after treatment. Shorter fraction protocols appear to be as effective and safe as protocols relying on multiple fractions. In the case of bladder tumours, the site of bleeding needs to be localized using a cystogram or CT scan. In a patient who has a poor performance status, a single dose of radiotherapy should be considered. Although nephrectomy is often preferred in cases of haematuria from renal cell carcinoma, inoperable renal carcinoma may also be treated with radiotherapy. However, renal damage is a real danger and radiotherapy should not be attempted in a patient whose other kidney is impaired. Radiotherapy to the bladder or kidney may result in diarrhoea and nausea.

Uterine and vaginal bleeding can be treated with either external beam or intra-cavitary irradiation[47]. Intra-cavitary irradiation is usually considered in cases where bleeding is from superficial small volume disease.

Radiotherapy has been used successfully to control bleeding from lower gastrointestinal tract lesions, particularly in the rectum or recto-sigmoid colon. Response has been noted in up to 85 per cent of cases, with up to three-quarters of these patients experiencing complete cessation of bleeding[50]. Low doses may be considered in patients who have previously been irradiated. Tumours in the lower sigmoid colon, rectum, and anal canal can be irradiated using intra-luminal brachytherapy in select cases.

Radiotherapy is a good option for controlling bleeding from large fungating ulcerated skin or anterior chest wall. Radiotherapy may also be considered with bleeding related to advanced head and neck cancers, but further radiotherapy is often difficult because these patients have often been irradiated previously with large doses.

Endoscopy

Endoscopic interventions have proven useful for managing cancer-related haemorrhaging of the upper gastrointestinal tract,[51,52] lungs[53,54], and bladder[55]. The vessel needs to be visualized, which can be difficult if there is massive active bleeding. It is then surgically ligated or sclerozed using agents such as ethanol[56,57], hyperosmotic saline epinephrine, gelatin solutions[58], and sodium tetradecyl sulfate[59]. Alternatively, the site of bleeding may be cauterized with heat, usually by polar, laser, or argon plasma coagulation[60–62]. Laser-beam coagulation has been reported to control bleeding from the upper gastrointestinal tract and from rectal cancers[63]. Symptoms of tenesmus may also respond, although evidence in support of this is less well established. Argon plasma coagulation

(APC) has replaced laser therapy in many gastrointestinal endoscopy units because of its lower cost and ease of use[64]. Small pilot studies have examined the use of photodynamic therapy for the palliation of rectal cancer[65]. However, patients must avoid significant sun exposure for up to 6 weeks following treatment.

One of the most common indications for endoscopic interventions in controlling bleeding is in the management of bleeding from upper gastrointestinal varices. Endoscopy can be considered as a first-line treatment strategy or second-line when systemic therapies such as vasopressin or somatostatin analogues have failed. Endoscopic techniques, which achieve control of bleeding in about 70–95 per cent of cases, have been reported to be superior to balloon tamponade[66]. Complications occur in 5–15 per cent of cases. This included worsening of the bleeding and perforation of the tract.

Endoscopic procedures have been used to control bleeding from gastrointestinal cancers, including the oesophagus, stomach, duodenum, and lower gastrointestinal tract[51,59,67,68].

Cystoscopic-assisted cautery by either heat or laser has been used in the treatment of haematuria in patients with bladder cancer[69]. Its role is mainly in patients where continuous bladder irrigation and lavage have failed. Under direct vision, the urologist identifies the source of bleeding and fulgurates the vessel or tumour[70].

In the case of haemoptysis, several endoscopic options are available if the site of bleeding is from a visible proximal source. The site can be coagulated with laser phototherapy, compressed by balloon tamponade[71], or have thrombin or fibrinogen applied topically[54]. However, when bleeding is coming from peripheral lesions that cannot be visualized, bronchoscopic options are fewer. Instillation of cold saline, epinephrine solution, or anti-diuretic hormone derivates such as ornipressin or terlipressin can be attempted[72]. When an invasive intervention is appropriate and justified, the goal may be to prevent hypoxia when the blood floods the other lung. Endoscopically-assisted tamponade may be attempted of the large bronchus that the bleeding is coming from with glue, balloon, or embolization with a silicone spigot[73,74]. Unlike endobronchial glue injection, the spigot is a reversible treatment and can be followed up with a more definitive treatment of the bleeding such as arterial embolization.

Interventional radiology

Transcutaneous arterial embolization (TAE) may be considered in well-selected patients, particularly where bleeding continues despite attempts at controlling it with other measures[75]. The procedure is usually performed via a femoral or axillary approach under local anaesthetic and is generally well tolerated, requiring only mild sedation. The blood vessel supplying the affected site is first identified by arteriography, followed by the insertion of a haemostatic agent, often in the form of a micro-coil. Limiting factors include the presence of a bleeding disorder and the availability of the appropriate expertise. Embolization is restricted to areas where the blood vessels are accessible by the catheter and where embolization of the blood vessel does not result in ischaemia of key organs. Benefits have been reported in patients with cancers involving the head and neck[76–78], bladder[79], pelvis[80–83], lung[75,84], liver[8586], and gastrointestinal tract embolization[87].

Nabi et al. reported a small case series of bilateral internal iliac artery embolization with permanent coils to control intractable haemorrhage from advanced pelvic urological cancers[80]. Bleeding was controlled in 5 of 6 patients at the first attempt. The person that did not respond in the initial attempts responded when retreated. Complications were minor and included temporary nausea, vomiting, and fever.

TAE has been used to manage carotid artery rupture in cancer patients. Bates and Shamsham report a patient whose episodes of profuse carotid haemorrhage were successfully controlled by an endovascular technique that combined placement of a flexible self-expanding stent-graft to protect the common and internal carotid artery with selective coil embolization of the affected external carotid artery branches[88]. Sakakibara and colleagues used an endoluminal balloon to staunch bleeding in three patients prior to undergoing surgical ligation of the arteries[89].

TAE was used to control bleeding in 5 patients with bleeding from oesophageal varices or direct invasion of the duodenum, transverse colon or stomach from inoperable hepatocellular cancer[86], and four patients with spontaneous rupture of hepatocellular carcinoma[90]. Wu and colleagues reported that upper gastrointestinal bleeding is a potential complication following TAE in patients with hepatocellular cancer, but the bleeding in these isolated cases was probably due to concurrent gastric and duodenal ulcers and oesophageal varices[91].

Surgery

Surgery may be appropriate for a small group of well-selected patients who have failed conservative measures and who are deemed fit for surgery. Surgery consists of ligation of larger vessels[92] or the removal of bleeding tissue[93]. Two surgical approaches have been described for the management of carotid artery rupture: resection with reconstruction or ligation of the artery. Witz et al. reported three patients with head and neck cancers whose carotid arteries were successfully ligated following acute or imminent carotid artery rupture[92]. Ligation of a vessel was successful in some patients who presented with bleeding from radiation proctitis[94].

Management: systemic interventions

Vitamin K (phytonadione)

Vitamin K is necessary for the hepatic production of a number of clotting factors, including factors II, VII, IX, and X. Liver disease, decreased intake of green vegetables, small bowel disease or resection, and intrahepatic and extrahepatic biliary obstruction can lead to deficiencies in the clotting factors. Coagulation screening studies usually reveal a prolonged prothrombin time or international normalized ratio (INR) and partial thromboplastin time with normal thrombin time, fibrinogen, and serum fibrin-fibrinogen degradation products.

Vitamin K treatment is indicated in the control of bleeding resulting from a lack of these clotting factors or excessive warfarin therapy. Doses of between 2.5 mg and 10 mg are recommended, depending on the severity of the bleeding. It can be administered via a number of routes, including the oral, subcutaneous, and intravenous routes. Oral administration of vitamin K appears to be more reliable than the subcutaneous route, although the onset of action is slower than the intravenous route[95]. A dose range of 1.0–2.5 mg is effective when the INR is between 5.0 and 9.0, but larger doses (5mg or more) are required to correct INRs greater than 9.0[96]. Anaphylactic reactions have been reported more frequently with intravenous administration. In a retrospective study of 105

patients, two (1.9 per cent) patients experienced serious systemic allergic reactions following intravenous administration[97]. When intravenous administration is considered unavoidable, the drug should be injected slowly, probably not exceeding 1 mg per minute. In a serious situation where over-anticoagulation needs to be reversed rapidly, a repeated parenteral dose may be considered 6–8 h after initial treatment if the INR is not satisfactorily lowered. However, in serious cases requiring rapid anti-coagulation reversal, an infusion of fresh frozen plasma may be more appropriate in select cases.

Whitling et al. evaluated four different routes of vitamin K administration for reversing excessive anticoagulation: high-dose intravenous (1–10 mg), low-dose intravenous (≤0.5 mg), subcutaneous (1–10 mg), and oral (2.5–5 mg)[98]. Satisfactory anticoagulation was achieved in all four groups. The high-dose intravenous method was the most effective in lowering INR levels to less than 5 but was also more often associated with overcorrection. Byrd and colleagues reported effective and safe reversal of excess warfarin anticoagulation using subcutaneous phytonadione at doses of 1 mg for INR levels between 8 and 14 and 2 mg for levels greater than 14[99]. The mean INR reductions were between 49 per cent and 67 per cent, respectively, and INR levels were below 4.5 after 48 h. No haemorrhagic or thrombotic complications were reported. Subcutaneous phytonadione did not correct the INR as rapidly or as effectively as when administered intravenously in a randomized trial[100]. However, higher doses of subcutaneous phytonadione may be required for full anticoagulation reversal[101].

A randomized, double-blind, placebo-controlled study comparing oral vitamin K (2.5 mg) versus omission alone in 30 asymptomatic patients with INR levels of 6–10 found that treatment with oral phytonadione (accompanied by holding further warfarin dosing) reduced the time to achieve a normal INR by a day[102]. Adverse effects did not differ between the two groups. Fondevilla et al., on the other hand, found no advantage of adding a small oral dose of vitamin K (1 mg) to a regimen of simply discontinuing the warfarin in patients with excessive oral anticoagulation[103]. Oral menadiol (vitamin K) (20 mg daily for 3 days) was found to be as effective as intravenous phytomenadione (1 mg daily) in normalizing INR levels in 26 patients with cholestasis[104].

The role of prophylactic vitamin K administration to asymptomatic patients with significantly increased INR levels because of end-stage liver involvement with the goal of preventing symptomatic bleeding is unclear in the palliative care setting and warrants further investigation.

Vasoactive drugs

Vasopressin/desmopressin

Vasopressin is a posterior pituitary hormone that causes splanchnic arteriolar constriction and reduction in portal pressure when injected intravenously or intra-arterially[105]. The vasopressin analogue 1-desamino-8-D-arginine vasopressin (desmopressin, DDAVP) is usually used and is the treatment of choice for patients with von Willebrand's disease and mild haemophilia A. The compound has also proved useful for the treatment of patients with other inherited or acquired haemostasis disorders. It has been used extensively in the management of variceal bleeding related to portal hypertension[106,107].

In cancer care, a pilot study evaluated the use of vasopressin in 15 patients with various haematologic malignancies and thrombocytopenia for the treatment or prevention of bleeding episodes.

Desmopressin (0.4 mcg/kg), diluted in 100 ml of isotonic saline, was infused over 30 min to 15 patients with various haematological malignancies and thrombocytopenia. All the patients responded to a single infusion without toxicities. Desmopressin may minimize the need for transfusions in patients with treatment-related thrombocytopenia or thrombocytopenia due to haematologic malignancy[108]. Vasopressin therapy, given in doses of 0.1–0.4 mg by continuous infusion, appears to stop bleeding in about half of patients with active bleeding from stomach cancer[109]. Vasoconstrictor effects on the myocardial, mesenteric, and cerebral circulations may cause problems but are relatively uncommon.

Inhaled ornipressin

Five units (1 ml) of ornithine-8-vasopressin diluted in 1 or 2 mL of physiological saline solution and administered in aerosol as needed halted haemoptysis a few hours after beginning of the inhaled treatment in 3 patients with mild to moderate haemoptysis who received it[110].

Somatostatin analogues

Octreotide, an analogue of somatostatin, has been used to manage upper gastrointestinal bleeds, particularly from peptic ulcers[111] and peptic ulcer disease. It has also been reported perioperatively to prevent perioperative bleeding in pancreatic cancer resections postoperatively[112]. Somatostatin reduces splanchnic flow and pressure by causing venous dilatation, thereby reducing portal pressure and portal venous flow. A starting dose of 50–100 mcg twice daily subcutaneously or intravenously is recommended[113]. The dose may be titrated, up to 600 mcg per day if needed. An alternative regimen consists of a bolus of 50 mcg given intravenously or subcutaneously, followed by a continuous subcutaneous or intravenous infusion of 50 mcg/h for 48 h.[114] Few side effects are reported at low doses but nausea, abdominal discomfort, and diarrhoea may occur at higher doses (greater than 100 mcg/h.)

D'Amico et al., in a meta-analysis, concluded that in variceal bleeding, vasoactive drugs (octreotide, somatostatin, vasopressin, and terlipresin) should be used before trying sclerotherapy[107]. The vasoactive drugs were effective in approximately 83 per cent of cases. A more recent meta-analysis reported that ligation appears to be the most effective treatment for bleeding varices[106]. It was effective in 91 per cent of cases compared to 69 per cent of cases treated with vasoconstrictive treatment (vasopressin/terlipressin) and 76 per cent of cases each with vasoactive treatments (octreotide) and sclerotherapy. The difference between ligation and sclerotherapy was not significant.

Antifibrinolytic agents

Antifibrinolytic agents or fibrinolytic inhibitors are synthetic agents that block the binding sites of plasminogen, thereby inhibiting the conversion of plasminogen into plasmin by tissue plasminogen activator. This results in decreased lysis of fibrin clots. Tranexamic acid (TA) and aminocaproic acid (EACA) are the two most commonly used antifibrinolytic agents and TA is more potent than EACA in vitro. Fibrinolytic inhibitors have been used successfully in a variety of oncological and non-oncological settings, including to assist in controlling bleeding in patients with thrombocytopenia[115], disseminated intravascular coagulation[116], lung cancer[117], mesothelioma[118], and leukaemia[119,120].

Non-oncological uses have included control of bleeding following dental extractions[121], subarachnoid haemorrhages[122], and gastrointestinal bleeds[123].

In the palliative care setting, Dean and Tuffin found that cessation of bleeding occurred in 14 out of 16 cancer patients treated with tranexamic acid for a variety of bleeding problems, including haematuria, haemoptysis, and bleeding from fungating tumours and the rectum[124]. The average time until significant improvement in bleeding was just 2 days and the average time for complete cessation was 4 days. TA and EACA have been administered orally and intravenously. Doses of tranexamic acid were 1.5 g followed by 1 g three times a day. Aminocaproic acid was dosed at a 5-g load followed by 1 g four times a day. Treatment was continued for another 7 days after the bleeding stopped. The suggested intravenous dose of TA is 10 mg/kg three to four times a day, infused over about 1 h, while that of EACA is 4–5 g in 250 ml over the first hour, then 1 g per hour in 50 ml administered continuously for 8 h or until the bleeding is controlled[125]. The most common adverse effects are gastrointestinal in nature (nausea, vomiting and diarrhoea) and occur in 25 per cent of cases[126]. Adverse effects appear to be dose dependent and thromboembolism is uncommon[127].

A systematic review of randomized trials to evaluate the effectiveness of haemostatic medications (TA, EACA, desmopressin, and aprotinin) for reducing surgery-related bleeding found that there is generally limited or contradictory evidence of efficacy[128].

Plasma/blood products

In palliative care, the most likely situations for which these modalities will be considered are in the symptomatic treatment of patients with bleeding secondary to end-stage liver disease or coumarin (warfarin) therapy. Occasionally, it may also be considered in the management of disseminated intravascular coagulopathy. The options include platelets, fresh frozen plasma (FFP), cryoprecipitate, and recombinant Factor VIIa. Clearly these, in the palliative care setting, are indicated only in a small select group of patients.

Platelet transfusions

The frequency and severity of haemorrhages increases as the platelet count declines below 20 000/ul[129]. A single unit of platelets should increase the platelet count in an average adult by approximately 6000–10 000/ul, assuming normal splenic pooling. Four to six units are usually required to control bleeding. There is no strong scientific basis for establishing a 'cut-off' level of 20 000/mm³" below which an infusion should be initiated[130,131]. However, the risk of spontaneous bleeding appears to rise when count is below 5–10 000/mm³. Patients with chronic autoimmune thrombocytopenia can tolerate platelet counts in the range of 5–10 000/mm³ for long periods of time.

Platelet transfusion in the setting of advanced cancer should be on a case-by-case basis with the aim of controlling symptoms. The short half-life of platelets limits the usefulness of platelet transfusions in patients with end-stage disease. Moreover, the half life decreases further as the platelet count drops. Indications for platelet transfusions in patients with advanced haematologic malignancies have been suggested[132]. These include: (1) continuous bleeding of the mouth and gums; (2) overt haemorrhage (gastrointestinal, gynaecological, and urinary); (3) extensive and painful haematoma; (4) recent disturbed vision (in the setting of thrombocytopenia); (5) severe and recent headache (in the setting of thrombocytopenia); and (6) severe anaemia (and thrombocytopenia).

The issue of whether or not to continue platelet transfusions in thrombocytopenic patients with end-stage disease may pose an ethical dilemma. While ongoing transfusions may be helpful in some select patients in the terminal phases, they are more often futile and patients and families often perceive the cessation of transfusions as withdrawal of life-sustaining therapy. Sensitive and empathic discussions between patients, their families and the attending health team are essential to explore their expectations, fears, and concerns and to reassure them of ongoing support and commitment to providing optimal comfort care.

Fresh frozen plasma (FFP)

FFP contains plasma clotting factors. It is reserved for a very select group of patients with life expectancies greater than days to weeks. These include: (1) patients with specific deficiencies in certain coagulation factors; (2) patients in whom the effects of warfarin need to be reversed urgently; (3) patients who require urgent invasive interventions such as thoracentesis or surgery; and (4) when

appropriate, in the treatment of DIC. Similarly, packed red cell transfusions are indicated when anaemia resulting from blood loss causes or aggravates symptoms such as fatigue and dyspnoea.

Packed red blood cells

Guidelines for red blood transfusions in palliative patients are described elsewhere[133,134]. They may be considered in a select group of patients with symptomatic anaemia from recurrent bleeding. Transfusions are generally not felt to be useful in patients who are in the terminal phases.

Cryoprecipitate and recombinant factor VIIa

Cryoprecipitate is prepared from plasma and contains, in each 15-ml unit, about 100 units of factor VIII, 350 mg of fibrinogen, von Willebrand factor, and factor XIII. Its indications therefore include haemophilia, von Willebrand's disease, hypofibrinogenaemia, and bleeding from excessive anticoagulation. Recombinant FVIIa was developed for the treatment of bleeding in haemophiliac patients but has also been used successfully in non-haemophiliac patients who have acquired antibodies against factor VIII[135]. It has been used to reduce bleeding in advanced gynaecological malignancies. These products are generally costly.

Table 10.14.3 General first and second-line treatment options in specific clinical palliative situations[a].

	First-line options	Second-line options	Third-line options
Skin and chest wall lesions	◆ Pressure ◆ Pressure bandaging ◆ Radiotherapy	◆ Absorbable haemostatic agents ◆ Non-absorbable haemostatic agents ◆ Alginates	◆ Microporus polysaccharide or zeolite particles (large bleeds from large open wounds) ◆ Vasocontrictive and cauterizing agents
Haemoptysis	◆ Radiotherapy ◆ Chemotherapy for chemotherapy-sensitive tumours	◆ Bronchoscopic procedures	◆ Transcutaneous arterial embolization in select cases ◆ Vasoactive drugs
Haematuria	◆ Continuous bladder irrigation and lavage ◆ Instillation of vasocontrictive and cauterizing agents, including with astringents	◆ Radiotherapy ◆ Cystoscopic-assisted cautery	◆ Transcutaneous arterial embolization in select cases
Vaginal bleeding	◆ Gelatin dressings or packs soaked with acetone or formalin	◆ Radiotherapy	◆ Vasocontrictive and cauterizing agents ◆ Transcutaneous arterial embolization in select cases
Rectal bleeding	◆ Radiotherapy	◆ Packing ◆ Gelatin dressings	◆ Transcutaneous arterial embolization in select cases
Haematemesis	◆ Endoscopic procedures	◆ Endoscopic procedures ◆ Vasoconstrictive and cauterizing agents ◆ Radiotherapy	◆ Transcutaneous arterial embolization in select cases
Melaena	◆ Endoscopic procedures		◆ Transcutaneous arterial embolization in select cases ◆ Vasoactive drugs
Epistaxis	◆ Packing with cocaine, epinephrine or silver nitrate	◆ Balloon catheter ◆ Gelatin dressings	
Massive external haemorrhaging	◆ Pressure and pressure bandaging or packing plus dark towels plus sedation	◆ Microporus polysaccharide or zeolite particles	
Haemorrhaging from thrombocytopenia or other blood clotting abnormalities	◆ Local measures if bleeding is local (e.g. epistaxis)	◆ Systemic treatment with Vit K or transfusion of plasma products, depending on the underlying cause	

[a] Refer to the text for details of each of these options. Whether or not a treatment is 1st, 2nd, or 3rd line depends on the individual circumstances of a patient.

Management of specific problems

A summary of the options available in various clinical situations is listed in Table 10.14.3. They include suggested first-, second-, and third-line treatments. Clearly these need to be individualized and in some cases, a third-line option may be used as a first-line strategy.

Massive bleeds

One of the most distressing events in palliative care, for patients and caregivers alike, is a massive haemorrhage in which over a short period of time, large volumes of blood are lost leading to hypovolaemia and death. These gruesome events may prompt families and caregivers to panic and call on emergency services, potentially resulting in inappropriate attempts at resuscitation in patients whose goals of care are comfort. It is therefore important where possible, to prepare families and caregivers for such as event. Planning may minimize unnecessary calls to emergency response centres. Planning for such a possible event includes[136]: (1) identifying patients at risk; (2) having dark towels available to apply on the site of bleeding or place at the side of the mouth or nose if the bleeding is from those sites; (3) instructing family and caregivers how to apply pressure if there is a specific bleeding site and positioning patients with massive haemoptysis or haematemesis; and (4) providing sedatives for treatment of anxiety. Risk factors include large fungating, ulcerating lesions in the areas of carotid arteries and veins or in proximity of other large vessels, recurrent haemoptysis or haematemesis, and extremely low platelet counts. Midazolam, a quick-acting sedative, should be available for sedation. Midazolam 2.5 mg or 5 mg may be given intravenously, intramuscularly, or subcutaneously. If necessary, it can be repeated after 5–10 min. It can be stored in a dark place at room temperature. Families and caregivers should be instructed how to administer the medication subcutaneously. The presence of a subcutaneous butterfly will facilitate this.

Conclusion

Bleeding in the palliative setting can be caused by a variety of underlying processes and can present clinically in different ways. These include continuous low-volume oozing to massive haemorrhages that could lead to death. They are the source of considerable distress for patients and caregivers. Several strategies, either local or systemic or combinations of the two, exist for the patient experiencing bleeding. The majority of these treatments are supported only by case reports and series in the palliative care setting and controlled or comparative trials are lacking.

Treatment options will vary according to the goals of care of individual patients, their life expectancies, functional status, setting of care, and availability of treatment options. Patients at risk of major haemorrhages should be identified and their families and caregivers prepared for these events.

References

1. Gagnon, B., Mancini, I., and Pereira, J. (1998). Palliative management of bleeding events in advanced cancer patients. *J Pall Care*, **14**, 50–4.
2. Dutcher, J.P. (1987). Hematologic abnormalities in patients with nonhematologic malignancies. *Hematol Oncol Clin North Am*, **1**(2), 281–9.
3. Johnson, M.J. (1997). Problems of anticoagulation within a palliative care setting: An audit of hospice patients taking warfarin. *Palliat Med*, **11**(4), 306–12.
4. Fletcher, H., Wharfe, G., Mitchell, S. *et al.* (2002). Treatment of intractable vaginal bleeding with formaldehyde soaked packs. *J Obstet Gynaecol*, **22**, 570–1.
5. Patsner, B. (1993). Topical acetone for control of life-threatening vaginal hemorrhage from recurrent gynecologic cancer. *Eur J Gynaecol Oncol*, **14**, 33–5.
6. Shinkwin, C.A., Beasley, N., Simo, R. *et al.* (1996). Evaluation of Surgicel Nu-knit, Merocel and Vasolene gauze nasal packs: A randomized trial. *Rhinology*, **34**(1), 413.
7. Hanif, J., Tasca, R.A., Frosh, A. *et al.* (2003). Silver nitrate: Histological effects of cautery on epithelial surfaces with varying contact times. *Clin Otolaryngol*, **28**, 368–70.
8. Vijan, S.R., Keating, M.A., and Althausen, A.F. (1988). Ureteral stenosis after silver nitrate instillation in the treatment of essential hematuria. *J Urology*, **139**(5), 1015–16.
9. Russo, P. (1993). Urologic emergencies. In *Cancer, principles & practice of oncology* (eds. Vincent T. Devita, Jr., Samuel Hellman, and Steven A. Rosenberg), pp. 2159–60. JB Lippincott Co., Philadelphia, PA.
10. Cotti, G., Seid, V., Araujo, S. *et al.* (2003). Conservative therapies for hemorrhagic radiation proctitis: A review. *Rev Hosp Clin Fac Med Sao Paulo*, **58**, 284–92.
11. Regnard, C.F. (1991). Control of bleeding in advanced cancer. *Lancet*, **337**, 974.
12. Woodruff, R. (1993). Haematological problems. In *Palliative medicine: Symptomatic and supportive care for patients with advanced cancer and AIDS* (ed. R. Woodruff) pp. 228–52. Aperula Pty Ltd., Melbourne.
13. Roche, B., Chautems, R., and Marti, M.C. (1996). Application of formaldehyde for treatment of hemorrhagic radiation-induced proctitis. *World J of Surg*, **20**(8), 1092–4.
14. Biswal, B.M., Lal, P., Rath, G.K. *et al.* (1995). Intrarectal formalin application, an effective treatment for grade III haemorrhagic radiation proctitis. *Radiotherapy & Oncology*, **35**(3), 212–15.
15. Russo, P. (1993). Urologic emergencies. In *Cancer, principles & practice of oncology* (eds. Vincent T. Devita, Jr., Samuel Hellman, Steven A. Rosenberg), pp. 2159–60. JB Lippincott Co., Philadelphia, PA.
16. Yegappan, M., Ho, Y.H., Nyam, D. *et al.* (1998). The surgical management of colorectal complications from irradiation for carcinoma of the cervix. *Ann Acad Med Singapore*, **27**(5), 627–30.
17. Adebamowo, C.A. (2000). Topical formalin for management of bleeding malignant ulcers. *World J Surg*, **24**, 518–20.
18. Cotti, G., Seid, V., Araujo, S. *et al.* (2003). Conservative therapies for hemorrhagic radiation proctitis: A review. *Rev Hosp Clin Fac Med Sao Paulo*, **58**, 284–92.
19. Lowe, B.A. and Stamey, T.A. (1997). Endoscopic topical placement of formalin soaked pledgets to control localized hemorrhage due to radiation cystitis. *J Urol*, **158**, 528–9.
20. Choong, S.K., Walkden, M., and Kirby, R. (2000). The management of intractable haematuria. *BJU Int*, **86**, 951–9.
21. Fletcher, H., Wharfe, G., Mitchell, S. *et al.* (2002). Treatment of intractable vaginal bleeding with formaldehyde soaked packs. *J Obstet Gynaecol*, **22**, 570–1.
22. Kothari, P., Patel, S.K., and O'Malley, S. (2001). Application of cocaine to the nasal mucosa: A novel method. *J Laryngol Otol*, **115**, 650–1.
23. Russo, P. (1993). Urologic emergencies. In *Cancer, principles & practice of oncology* (eds. Vincent T. Devita, Jr., Samuel Hellman, and Steven A. Rosenberg) pp. 2159–60, JB Lippincott Co, Philadelphia, PA.
24. Atkinson, L.J. and Fortunato, N.H. (1996). Hemostasis and blood loss replacement. In *Operating room technique* (eds. L.J. Atkinson and N.H. Fortunato) pp. 469–89, 8th Edition. Mosby, St. Louis.
25. Twycross, R. and Wilcock, A. (2001). *Symptom management in advanced cancer*, 3rd edition. Radcliffe Medical Press, Oxford, UK.
26. de Boer, W. (1991). Tranexamic acid treatment of haemothorax in two patients with malignant mesothelioma. *Chest*, **100**, 847–8.
27. McElligott, E. (1991). Tranexamic acid and rectal bleeding. *Lancet*, **337**, 431.

28. Schonauer, C., Tessitore, E., Barbagallo, G. *et al.* (2004). The use of local agents: Bone wax, gelatin, collagen, oxidized cellulose. *Eur Spine J*, **13** (suppl 1), S89–96.

29. Gabay, M. (2006). Absorbable hemostatic agents. *Am J Health-Syst Pharm*, **63**(13), 1244–53.

30. Kanaoka, Y., Hirai, K., Ishiko, O. *et al.* (2001). Vesicovaginal fistula treated with fibrin glue. *Int J Gynaecol Obstet*, **73**, 147–9.

31. Gall, R.M., Witterick, I.J., Shargill, N.S. *et al.* (2002). Control of bleeding in endoscopic sinus surgery: use of a novel gelatin-based hemostatic agent. *J Otolaryngol*, **31**(5), 2714.

32. Weaver, F.A., Hood, D.B., Zatina, M. *et al.* (2002). Gelatin-thrombin-based hemostatic sealant for intraoperative bleeding in vascular surgery. *Ann Vasc Surg*, **16**(3), 28693.

33. Harris, W.H., Crothers, O.D., Moyen, B.J. *et al.* (1978). Topical hemostatic agents for bone bleeding in humans. A quantitative comparison of gelatin paste, gelatin sponge plus bovine thrombin, and microfibrillar collagen. *J Bone Joint Surg Am*, **60**(4), 454–6.

34. Sirlak, M., Eryilmaz, S., Yazicioglu, L. *et al.* (2003). Comparative study of microfibrillar collagen hemostat (Colgel) and oxidized cellulose (Surgicel) in high transfusion-risk cardiac surgery. *J Thorac Cardiovasc Surg*, **126**(3), 666–70.

35. Schenk, W.G., 3rd, Burks, S.G., Gagne, P.J. *et al.* (2003). Fibrin sealant improves hemostasis in peripheral vascular surgery: A randomized prospective trial. *Ann Surg*, **237**(6), 871–6.

36. Lagman, R., Walsh, D., and Day, K. (2002). Oxidized cellulose dressings for persistent bleeding from a superficial malignant tumor. *Am J Hosp Palliat Care*, **19**, 417–18.

37. Thrombostat. (1997). Compendium of pharmaceuticals and specialties. *Canadian Pharmacists Association. Ottawa*, **32**, 1587.

38. Motta, G.J. (1989). Calcium alginate topical wound dressings: a new dimension in the cost-effective treatment for exudating dermal wounds and pressure sores. *Ostomy Wound Manage*, **25**, 52–6.

39. Thomas, S. (2000). Alginate dressings in surgery and wound management: Part 2. *Journal of Wound Care*, **9**(3), 115–19

40. Segal, H.C., Hunt, B.J., and Gilding, K. (1998). The effects of alginate and non-alginate wound dressings on blood coagulation and platelet activation. *J Biomater Appl*, **12**, 249–57.

41. Odell, E.W., Oades, P., and Lombardi, T. (1994). Symptomatic foreign body reaction to haemostatic alginate. *Br J Oral Maxillofac Surg*, **32**(3), 178–9.

42. Henderson, N.J., Crawford, P.J., and Reeves, B.C. (1998). A randomised trial of calcium alginate swabs to control blood loss in 3–5-year-old children. *Br Dent J*, **28**, 184(4), 187–90.

43. Kanaoka, Y., Hirai, K., Ishiko, O. *et al.* (2001). Vesicovaginal fistula treated with fibrin glue. *Int J Gynaecol Obstet*, **73**, 147–49.

44. Mankad, P.S. and Codispoti, M. (2001). The role of fibrin sealants in hemostasis. *American Journal of Surgery*, **82**(2 Suppl), 21S–8.

45. Brundage, M.D., Bezjak, A., Dixon, P. *et al.* (1996). The role of palliative thoracic radiotherapy in non-small cell lung cancer. *Canadian J of Oncol*, **6**(1), 25–32.

46. Medical Research Council Lung Cancer Working Party. (1992). A Medical Research Council (MRC) randomised trial of palliative radiotherapy with two fractions or a single fraction in patients with inoperable non-small cell lung cancer (NSCLC) and poor performance status. *Br J Cancer*, **65**, 934–41.

47. Biswall, B.M., Lal, P., Rath, G.K. *et al.* (1995). Hemostatic radiotherapy in carcinoma of the uterine cervix. *Int'l J of Gynaecology & Obstetrics*, **50**(3), 281–5.

48. Srinivasan, V., Brown, C.H., and Turner, A.G. (1994). A comparison of two radiotherapy regimens for the treatment of symptoms from advanced bladder cancer. *Clin Oncol*, **6**, 11–13.

49. Duchesne, G.M. *et al.* (2000). A randomized trial of hypofractionated schedules of palliative radiotherapy in the management of bladder carcinoma: Results of the Medical Research Council Trial BA09. *Int J Radiation Oncol Biol Physics*, **47**, 379–88.

50. Taylor, R.E., Kerr, G.R., and Arnott, S.J. (1987). External beam radiotherapy for rectal adenocarcinoma. *British Journal of Surgery*, **74**, 455–9.

51. Akhtar, K., Byrne, J.P., Bancewicz, J. *et al.* (2000). Argon beam plasma coagulation in the management of cancers of the esophagus and stomach. *Surg Endosc*, **14**(12), 1127–30.

52. Loftus, E.V., Alexander, G.L., Ahlquist, D.A. *et al.* (1994). Endoscopic treatment of major bleeding from advanced gastroduodenal malignant lesions. *Mayo Clin Proc*, **69**, 736–40.

53. Knott-Craig, C.J., Oostuizen, J.G., and Rossouw, G. (1993). Management and prognosis of massive hemoptysis. *J Thoracic Cardio Surg*, **105**(3), 394–7.

54. Patel, U., Pattison, C.W., and Raphael, M. (1994). Management of massive haemoptysis. *Brit J of Hosp Med*, **52**(2–3), 74, 76–8.

55. MacKinnon, K.J. and Norman, R.W. (1993). Genitourinary disorders in palliative medicine. In *Oxford textbook of palliative medicine* (eds. D. Doyle and G.W.C. Hanks), pp. 415–22. Oxford.

56. Loscos, J.M., Calvo, E., and Alvarez-Sala, J.L. (1993). Treatment of dysphagia and massive hemorrhage in esophageal carcinoma by ethanol injection. *Endoscopy*, **25**(8), 544.

57. Gupta, P.K. and Fleischer, D.E. (1993). Nonvariceal upper gastrointestinal bleeding. *Med Clinics N Amer*, **77**(5), 973–91.

58. Tajika, M., Kato, T., and Magaki, M. (1996). Endoscopic injection of gelatin solution for server. *Gastrointestinal Endoscopy*, **43**(3), 247–50.

59. Loftus, E.V., Alexander, G.L., Ahlquist, D.A. *et al.* (1994). Endoscopic treatment of major bleeding from advanced gastroduodenal malignant lesions. *Mayo Clin Proc*, **69**, 736–40.

60. Savides, T.J., Jensen, D.M, and Cohen, J. (1996). Severe upper gastrointestinal tumor bleeding: Endoscopic findings, treatment, and outcome. *Endoscopy*, **28**, 244–8.

61. Suzuki, H., Miho, O., Watanabe, Y. *et al.* (1989). Endoscopic laser therapy in the curative and palliative treatment of upper gastrointestinal cancer. *World J Surg*, **13**, 158–64.

62. Mathus-Vliegen, E.M.H. and Tytgat, G.N.J. (1990). Analysis of Failures and Complications of Neodymium-YAG Laser Photocogulation in Gastrointestinal Tract Tumors. *Endoscopy*, **22**, 17–23

63. von Ditfurth, B., Buhl, K., and Friedl, P. (1990). Palliative endoscopic therapy for rectal cancer with neodymium. *YAG laser Eur J Surg Oncol*, **16**, 376–9.

64. Birnbaum, P.L. and Mercer, C.D. (1990). Laser fulguration for palliation of rectal tumours. *Can J Surg*, **33**, 299–301.

65. Kimmey, M.B. (2004). Endoscopic methods (other than stents) for palliation of rectal carcinoma. *J Gastrointest Surg*, **8**, 270–273.

66. Burnett, D.A. and Rikkers, L.F. (1990). Nonoperative emergency treatment of variceal hemorrhage. *Surg Clin North Amer*, **70**(2), 291–306.

67. Schulze, S. and Lyng, K.M. (1994). Palliation of Rectosigmoid Neoplasms with Nd:YAG I. *Dis Colon Rectum*, **37**(9), 882–4.

68. Schrock, T.R. (1989). Colonoscopic diagnosis and treatment of lower gastrointestinal bleeding. *Surg Clin North Amer*, **69**(6), 1309–25.

69. MacKinnon, K.J. and Norman, R.W. (1993). Genitourinary disorders in palliative medicine. In *Oxford textbook of palliative medicine* (eds. D. Doyle, G.W.C. Hanks), pp. 415–22. Oxford.

70. Russo, P. (1993). Urologic emergencies. In *Cancer, principles & practice of oncology* (eds. Vincent T. Devita, Jr., Samuel Hellman, and Steven A. Rosenberg), pp. 2159–60. JB Lippincott Co., Philadelphia, PA.

71. Kato, R., Sawafuji, M., Kawamura, M. *et al.* (1996). Massive hemoptysis successfully treated by modified bronchoscopic balloon tamponade technique. *Chest*, **109**(3), 842–3.

72. Tüller, C., Tüller, D., Tamm, M. *et al.* (2004). Hemodynamic effects of endobronchial application of ornipressin versus terlipressin. *Respiration*, **71**, 397–401.

73. de Gracia, J., de la Rosa, D., Catalan, E. *et al.* (2003). Use of endoscopic fibrinogen-thrombin in the treatment of severe hemoptysis. *Respir Med*, **97**, 790–5.

74. Freitag, L. (1993). Development of a new balloon catheter for management of hemoptysis with bronchofiberscope. *Chest*, **103**, 593.

75. Broadley, K.E., Kurowska, A., Dick, R. *et al.* (1995). The role of embolization in palliative care. *Palliative Med*, **9**, 331–5.

76. Bates, M.C. and Shamsham, F.M. (2003). Endovascular management of impending carotid rupture in a patient with advanced head and neck cancer. *J Endovasc Ther*, **10**(1), 547.

77. Sakakibara, Y., Kuramoto, K., and Jikuya, T. (1998). An approach for acute disruption of large arteries in patients with advanced cervical cancer: Endoluminal balloon occlusion technique. *Ann Surg*, **227**(1), 134–7.

78. Morrissey, D.D., Andersen, P.E., Nesbit, G.M. *et al.* (1997). Endovascular management of hemorrhage in patients with head and neck cancer. *Arch Otolaryngol*, **123**(1), 15–19.

79. Hays, M.C., Wilson, N.M., Page, A. *et al.* (1996). Selective embolization of bladder tumors. *Brit J Urology*, **78**(2), 311–12.

80. Nabi, G., Sheikh, N., Greene, D. *et al.* (2003). Therapeutic transcatheter haemorrhage from pelvic urological malignancies: preliminary experience and long-term follow-up. *BJU Int*, **92** (3), 245–7.

81. Wells, I. (1996). Internal iliac artery embolization in the management of pelvic bleeding. *Clin Rad*, **51**(12), 825–7.

82. Yamashita, Y., Harada, M., Yamamoto, H. *et al.* (1994). Transcatheter arterial embolization of obstetric and gynaecological bleeding: Efficacy and clinical outcome. *Brit J Rad*, **67**(798), 530–4.

83. Jenkins, C.N. and McIvor, J. (1996). Survival after embolization of the internal iliac arteries in ten patients with severe haematuria due to recurrent pelvic carcinoma. *Clin Rad*, **51**(12), 865–8.

84. Canellos, G.P., Cohen, G., and Posner, M. (1981). Pulmonary emergencies in neoplastic disease. *Oncol Emerg*, 301–22.

85. Recordare, A., Bonarial, L., Caratozzolo, E. *et al.* (2002). Management of spontaneous bleeding due to hepatocellular carcinoma. *Minerva Chir*, **57**(3), 347–56.

86. Srivastava, D.N., Gandhi, D., Julka, P.K. *et al.* (2000). Gastrointestinal hemorrhage in hepatocellular carcinoma management with transhepatic arterioembolization. *Abdom Imaging*, **25**(4), 380–4.

87. Mal, H., Rullon, I., Mellot, F. *et al.* (1999). Immediate and long-term results of bronchial artery embolization for life-threatening hemoptysis. *Chest*, **115**, 996–1001.

88. Bates, M.C. and Shamsham, F.M. (2003). Endovascular management of impending carotid rupture in a patient with advanced head and neck cancer. *J Endovasc Ther*, **10**(1), 547.

89. Sakakibara, Y., Kuramoto, K., Jikuya, T. *et al.* (1998). An approach for acute disruption of large arteries in patients with advanced cervical cancer: Endoluminal balloon occlusion technique. *Ann Surg*, **227**(1), 134–7.

90. Recordare, A., Bonarial, L., and Caratozzolo, E. (2002). Management of spontaneous bleeding due to hepatocellular carcinoma. *Minerva Chir*, **57**(3), 347–56.

91. Wu, J.X., Huang, J.F., Yu, Z.J. *et al.* (2002). Factors related to acute upper gastrointestinal bleeding after transcatheter arterial chemoembolization in patients with hepatocellular carcinoma. *Ai Zheng*, **21**(8), 881–4.

92. Witz, M., Korzets, Z., and Shnaker, A. (2002). Delayed carotid artery rupture in advanced cervical cancer: A dilemma in emergency management. *Eur Arch Otorhinolaryngol*, **259**(1), 37–9.

93. Baum, M., Breach, N.M., and Shepherd, J.H. (1993). Surgical palliation. In: *Oxford textbook of palliative medicine* (eds. D. Doyle and G.W.C. Hanks), pp. 129–40. Oxford.

94. Yegappan, M., Ho, Y.H., Nyam, D. *et al.* (1998). The surgical management of colorectal complications from irradiation for carcinoma of the cervix. *Ann Acad Med Singapore*, **27**(5), 627–30.

95. Ansell, J., Hirsh, J., Poller, L. *et al.* (2004). The pharmacology and management of the vitamin K antagonists: The seventh ACCP conference on antithrombotic and thrombolytic therapy. *Chest*, **126**(suppl 3), 204S–33.

96. Jenkins, C.N. and McIvor, J. (1996). Survival after embolization of the internal iliac arteries in ten patients with severe haematuria due to recurrent pelvic carcinoma. *Clin Rad*, **51**(12), 865–8.

97. Shields, R.C., McBance, R.D., Kuiper, J.D. *et al.* (2001). Efficacy and safety of intravenous phytonadione (vitamin K1) in patients on long-term oral anticoagulant therapy. *Mayo Clinic Proceedings*, **76**(3), 260–6.

98. Whitling, A.M., Bussey, H.I., and Lyons, R.M. (1998). Comparing different routes and doses of phytonadione for reversing excessive anticoagulation. *Arch Intern Med*, **158**(19), 2136–40.

99. Byrd, D.C., Stephens, M.A., Hammann, G.L. *et al.* (1999). Subcutaneous phytonadione for reversal of warfarin-induced elevation of the International Ratio. *Am J Health System Pharmacy*, **56**(22), 2312–15.

100. Raj, G., Kumar, R., and McKinney, W.P. (1999). Time course of reversal of anticoagulant effect of warfarin by intravenous and subcutaneous phytonadione. *Arch Intern Med*, **159**(22), 2721–4.

101. Nee, R., Doppenschmidt, D., Donovan, D.J. *et al.* (1999). Intravenous versus subcutaneous vitamin K1 I reversing excessive oral anticoagulation. *Am J Cardiology*, **83**(2), 286–8.

102. Patel, R.J., Saseen, J.J., Tillman, D.J. *et al.* (2000). Randomized, placebo-controlled trial of oral phytonadione for excessive anticoagulation. *Pharmacotherapy*, **20**(10), 1159–66.

103. Fondevila, C.G., Grosso, S.H., Santarelli, M.T. *et al.* (2001). Reversal of excessive oral anticoagulation with a low dose of vitamin K1 compared with acenocoumarine discontinuation. A prospective, randomized, open study. *Blood Coagul Fibrinolysis*, (**1**), 9–16.

104. Green, B., Carinis, S., Harvey, R. *et al.* (2000). Phytomenadione or menadiol in the management of elevated international normalized ration (prothrombin time). *Aliment Pharmacol Ther*, **14**(12), 1685–9.

105. Stein, C. and Korula, J. (1995). Variceal bleeding. *Postgrad Med*, **98**(6), 143–52.

106. Gross, M., Schiemann, U., Muhlofer, A. *et al.* (2001). Meta-analysis: Efficacy of therapeutic regimens in ongoing variceal bleeding. *Endoscopy*, **33**(9), 737–46.

107. D'Amico, G., Peitrosic, G., Tarantino, I. *et al.* (2003). Emergency sclerotherapy versus vasoactive drugs for variceal bleeding in cirrhosis: A Cochrane meta-analysis. *Gastroenterology*, **124**(5), 1277–91.

108. Castaman, G., Bona, E.D., Schiavotto, C. *et al.* (1997). Pilot study on the safety and efficacy of desmopressin for the treatment or prevention of bleeding in patients with hematologic malignancies. *Haematologica*, **82**, 584–7.

109. Allurn, W.H., Brearley, S., Wheatley, K.E. *et al.* (1990). Acute haemorrhage from gastric malignancy. *Brit J Surgery*, **77**(1), 19–20.

110. Anwar, D., Schaad, N., and Mazzocato, C. (2005). Aerolized vasopressin is a safe and effective treatment for mild to moderate recurrent hemoptysis in palliative care patients. *J Pain Symptom Manage*, **29**, 427–9.

111. Lin, H.J., Perng, C.L., Wang, K. *et al.* (1995). Octreotide for arrest of peptic ulcer hemorrhage: A prospective, randomized controlled trial. *Hepto-Gastroenterology*, **42**(6), 856–60.

112. Halloran, C.M., Ghaneh, P., Bosonnet, L. *et al.* (2002). Complications of pancreatic cancer resection. *Digestive Surgery*, **19**(2), 130–46.

113. Lamberts, S.W.J., Van Der Lely, A.J., De Herder, *et al.* (1996). Octreotide. *New Eng J Med*, 246–54.

114. Burroughs, A.K., McCormick, P.A., Hughes, M.D. *et al.* (1990). Randomized, double-blind, placebo-controlled trial of somatostatin for variceal bleeding: Emergency control and prevention of early variceal rebleeding. *Gastroenterology*, **99**, 1388–95.

115. Garewal, H.S. and Durie, B.G. (1985). Anti-fibrinolytic therapy with aminocaproic acid for the control of bleeding in thrombocytopenic patients. *Scand J Haematol*, **35**, 497–500.

116. Cooper, D.L., Sandler, A.B., Wilson, L.D. *et al.* (1992). Disseminated intravascular coagulation and excessive fibrinolysis in a patient with metastic prostate cancer: Response to epsilon-aminocaproic acid. *Cancer*, **70**, 656–8.

117. Kaufman, B. and Wise, A. (1993). Antifibrinolytic therapy for haemoptysis related to bronchial carcinoma. *Postgrad Med J*, **69**, 80–1.

118. De Boer, W.A., Koolen, M.G.J., Roos, C.M. *et al.* (1991). Tranexamic acid treatment of haemothorax in two patients with malignant mesothelioma. *Chest*, **100**, 847–8.

119. Shpilberg, O., Blumenthal, R., Sofer, O. *et al.* (1995). A controlled trial of tranexamic acid therapy for the reduction of bleeding during treatment of acute myeloid leukemia. *Leukemia Lymphoma*, **19**(1–2), 141–4.

120. Avvisat, G., Buller, H.R., Cate, J.W.T. *et al.* (1989). Tranexamic acid for control of haemorrhage in acute promyelocytic leukaemia. *Lancet*, **2**(8655), 122–4.

121. Ramstrom, G., Sindet-Pedersen, S., Hall, G. *et al.* (1993). Prevention of post-surgical bleeding in oral surgery using tranexamicacid without dose modification or oral anticogulants. *J Oral Maxillofac Surg*, **51**, 1211–16.

122. Chandra, B. (1978). Treatment of subarachnoid haemorrhage from ruptured intracranial aneurysm with tranexamic acid: A double blind clinical trial. *Ann Neurol*, **3**, 502–4.

123. Biggs, J.C., Hugh, T.B., and Dodds, A.J. (1976). Tranexamic acid and uppergastrointestinal haemorrhage: A double blind trial. *Gut*, **17**, 729–34.

124. Dean, A. and Tuffin, P. (1997). Fibrinolytic inhibitors for cancer-associated bleeding problems. *J Pain Symptom Manage*, **13**(1), 20–4.

125. Herfindal, E.T., Gourley, and D.R. (eds.) (1996). *Textbook of therapeutics: Drug and disease management*, 6th edition. Willians and Wilkins, Baltimore.

126. Cada, D.J. (ed.) (1997). *Drug facts and comparisons*, p. 91. St Louis.

127. Hashimoto, S., Koike, T., Tatewaki, W. *et al.* (1994). Fatal thromboembolism in acute promyelocytic leukemia during all-trans retinoic acid therapy combined with antifibrinolytic therapy for prophylaxis of hemorrhage. *Leukemia*, **8**(6), 1113–15.

128. Erstad, B.L. (2001). Systemic hemostatic medications for reducing surgical blood loss. *Ann Pharmacother*, **35**(7–8), 925–34.

129. Aderka, D., Praff, G., Santo, M. *et al.* (1986). Bleeding due to thrombocytopenia in acute leukemias and reevaluation of the prophylactic platelet tranfusion policy. *Am J Med Sci*, **291**, 147.

130. Pisciotto, P.T., Benson, K., Hume, A.B. *et al.* (1995). Prophylactic versus therapeutic platelet transfusion practices in hematology and/or oncology patients. *Tranfusion*, **35**(6), 498–502.

131. Beutler, E. (1993). Platelet transfusions: The 20,000/µL trigger. *Blood*, **81**, 1411–13.

132. Lassauniere, J.M., Bertolino, M., Hunault, M. *et al.* (1996). Platelet transfusions in advanced hematological malignancies: A position paper. *J Palliat Care*, **12**, 38–41.

133. Gleeson, C. and Spencer, D. (1995). Blood transfusion and its benefits in palliative care. *Palliat Med*, **9**, 307–13.

134. Monti, M., Castellani, L., Berlusconi, A. *et al.* (1996). Use of red blood cell transfusions in terminally ill cancer patients admitted to a palliative care unit. *J Pain Symptom Manage*, **12**(1), 18–22.

135. Sajdak, S., Moszynski, R., and Opala, T. (2002). Bleeding from endometrial and vaginal malignant tumors treated with activated recombinant factor VII. *Eur J Gynaecol Oncol*, **23**, 325–6.

136. Gagnon, B., Mancini, I., Pereira, J. *et al.* (1998). Palliative management of bleeding events in advanced cancer patients. *J Pall Care*, **14**, 50–4.

SECTION 11

Issues in specific neoplastic disease

Palliative medicine in malignant respiratory diseases

Kin-Sang Chan, Doris M.W. Tse,
Michael M.K. Sham, and Anne Berit Thorsen

Introduction

The Lord God formed man from the dust of the ground and breathed into his nostrils the breath of life, and man became a living creature. *(Genesis)*

A breath is a vital sign of a living creature. When one dies, one expires. A breath, however, serves more than physiological purposes. A sigh often carries unspeakable messages from the inner being. Hence a breath is filled with physiological, psychological, and spiritual signals.

Every day, millions of people throughout the world are distressed by breathlessness and other respiratory symptoms. Besides, millions are sighing from their suffering.

Breathing, an automatic activity which one undergoes hundreds of millions of cycles throughout one's life, is mostly effortless. However, when the respiratory system is compromized by diseases, every breath becomes laborious. Control of respiratory symptoms remains challenging towards the end of life[1]. Upon longitudinal follow up, dyspnoea in advanced cancer patients followed the 'decrease-increase' pattern as patients approaching end of life[1] Another study also identified factors that predict the will to live, including depression, anxiety, shortness of breath and sense of well-being; and dyspnoea became a critical factor affecting the will to live while approaching death[2].

Care for patients at the end of life aim at maximizing quality of remaining lives, sustaining the will to live, and finally achieving a peaceful death. For patients with respiratory malignancy, these goals can only be achieved when distresses related to respiratory symptoms are addressed. The suboptimal outcome of dyspnoea control calls for a persistent search to unravel its underlying pathophysiological mechanisms and the development of new drugs for specific treatment of dyspnoea. Cough, which was previously under-addressed, is an area with rapid growth in new findings and insights. With the emergence of new chemotherapeutic agents and novel molecular targeted therapy; patient with lung cancers will be put on more options of anti-cancer treatment till the later phases of their disease, even when goal of treatment is of palliative intent.

While hopefully witnessing the recent advances in this area, it is just as important, if not more, for the palliative care team to accompany our patients, to provide appropriate psychological, social, and spiritual support, so that the last journey will be filled with peace.

Lung cancer

Changing scenario of managing advanced lung cancer

Lung cancer is the most common cancer and the leading cause of cancer death in the world, accounting for 1.3 million deaths per year (17 per cent of all cancer deaths). The 5-year survival has been relatively static at about 15 per cent in the past decades in developed countries[3]. Seventy per cent of patients with lung cancer are presented late. In the past, many of them were offered best supportive care or palliative care. Currently, many patients with late stage lung cancer with performance status WHO 0 or 1 may be offered chemotherapy, with potential improvement in symptom relief, disease control, quality of life, and survival. Meta-analysis showed a modest survival benefit for platinum-based chemotherapy by approximately 9 weeks. The second-generation chemotherapeutic agents (ifofasmide, vinblastine, vindescine, mitomycin C, and carboplatin) are less toxic and the third-generation chemotherapeutic agents (gemcitabine, paclitaxol, vinorelbine, and docetaxel) have been shown to have significant activity against non-small-cell lung cancer[4].

Molecular-targeted therapies with different mechanisms of action from chemotherapy are recently discovered, these include epidermal growth factor receptor (EGFR), tyrosine kinase inhibitors (TKIs), and antibody against vascular endothelial growth factor (VEGF) that plays a critical role in tumour angiogenesis. Bevacizumab, a humanized monoclonal antibody which binds to and inhibits VEGF, when used in combination with standard chemotherapy, was found to prolong survival of patients with advanced lung cancer[5]. EGFR is a transmembrane receptor tyrosine kinase which binds to ligands and causes a host of downstream interactions that lead to cell growth, proliferation and survival. Both gefitinib and erlotinib are reversible inhibitors of EGFR that compete with adenosine triphosphate (ATP) at its binding site.

For patients with advanced non-small-cell lung cancer who fail to respond to chemotherapy, TKIs have been shown to prolong survival; especially for patients with adenocarcinoma cell type and who are non-smokers, women, and Asian in ethnic origin. Other than survival benefits, patients put on erlotinib had significantly longer median time to deterioration for cough, dyspnoea, and pain as compared with placebo. About one-third of patients receiving erlotinib had improvement in these symptoms, accompanied by an improvement in the physical function and global quality of life[6]. These oral agents are better tolerated than the usual chemotherapeutic drugs, except for the most common adverse effects of skin rashes and diarrhoea. With these new options, decisions on chemotherapy in the palliative phase have to take into consideration these new balancing factors.

Distress and burden of lung cancer

Lung cancer is associated with considerable burden in physical, psychological, and social aspects of care[7,8]. Lung cancer patients were found to have the highest prevalence of psychological distress[9], and the greatest number of symptoms and existential concerns than patients with other malignancies[10].

In a study on 100 lung cancer patients referred to palliative care, patients had a median number of nine symptoms, among which pain, dyspnoea, and anorexia were most common and most severe[11]. In another study on 650 lung cancer patients on presentation to treatment, multiple symptoms were identified, including tiredness, lack of energy, worry, anxiety, cough, dyspnoea, lack of appetite, and difficulty sleeping[12]. Even for ambulatory lung cancer patients in the community, 55 per cent of the 157 patients studied experienced dyspnoea that interfered with daily activities including physical activities (52 per cent) and psychological domain (23 per cent)[13].

Longitudinal studies showed that intial symptom distress was a predictor for distress at the later stage. In one study on lung cancer patients who underwent tumour treatment, fatigue and pain were the most distressing symptoms in all treatment groups and at 0, 3, and 6 months[14]. Moreover, symptom distress at entry to study was a strong predictor of nine distressing symptoms at 3 months and six distressing symptoms at 6 months[14]. Similarly, in a study on 400 inoperable lung cancer patients who were followed up for a maximum of 1 year, symptoms of breathlessness, pain, and fatigue remained most distressing at all time points and in all subgroups of treatment[15].

Results from these longitudinal studies also illustrated the emerging concept of symptom cluster[14,15]. Symptom cluster can be defined as three or more concurrent symptoms that are related to each other that may or may not have a common mechanism or aetiology[16]. Gift et al.[17] reported seven symptoms as a cluster in lung cancer patients, including fatigue, weakness, nausea, vomiting, loss of appetite, weight loss, and altered taste, which remained present and related at 3 months and 6 months; with the symptom cluster was an independent predictor of death. Newer findings in this area may guide us on the symptom assessment and intervention strategy in lung cancer.

Psychological distress of lung cancer

On average, one out of four patients with lung cancer experienced periods of depression or other psychosocial problems during their illness[8]. In a large scale study of 4496 patients with 14 cancer diagnosis, lung cancer patients had the highest prevalence rate of psychological distress (43.4 per cent versus 35.1 per cent in overall group)[9]. In another recent study on 1721 cancer patients who were referred to psychiatrists, lung cancer patients were the most common, constituting 19 per cent of the total referrals[18].

Studies also suggested that psychological distress persisted along the course of disease. Hopwood and Stephens evaluated 987 inoperable lung cancer patients who underwent palliative treatment trials[19]. Upon self-rating, 33 per cent of patients reported depression, which persisted in more than half of them. In one longitudinal study on 85 newly diagnosed advanced NSCLC, most forms of psychological distress including anger – hostility, vigour, fatigue, and confusion as experienced by patients persisted till 6 months after diagnosis[20]. The initial psychological distress after cancer diagnosis was the most important predictor of subsequent psychological distress[20].

Lung cancer also has its own special feature of being associated with smoking. Because of this casual relationship, lung cancer patients reported experience of shame and stigma; fear of lack of access to medical care and a dreadful death while 'gasping for air'[21].

Unmet needs of lung cancer

In one recent study on the needs of various cancers, lung cancer patients had the highest mean number of unmet needs at 15.6 (95 per cent CI 12.1–19.1) compared with 10.9 (95 per cent CI 10.0–11.8) in other cancers, mainly accounted by unmet psychological needs and unmet needs in physical and in daily activities[22]. Having a lung cancer diagnosis was an independent predictor of high level of psychological need (RR 2.00, 95 per cent CI 1.13–3.56) and daily living need (RR 2.81, 95 per cent CI 1.60–4.95)[22]. A national questionnaire survey in UK had identified that unmet need was most apparent during periods away from acute service sectors[23]. Only 40 per cent of the patients participated in the survey received as much help as they needed from community services[23].

Results from this survey also revealed the unmet need of the informal caregivers, who reported considerable psychological distress as they felt fearful, sad, low, anxious or angry. However, their needs were largely overlooked by hospital staff. Even among the patients, only 29 per cent of patients identified their caregivers to be in need[23]. Relationship distress or conflicts between the patient and caregiver is an issue of concern. Continued smoking after diagnosis of lung cancer has been shown to be a major source of conflict between spouses[24].

Overall, lung cancer is a disease with significant volume among cancers, causing significant symptom and psychological distress. Early intervention to patients' distress may help to prevent or reduce subsequent distress in patients and families as disease progresses, also narrowing gaps in unmet needs.

Dyspnoea

Definition of dyspnoea

Dyspnoea is the term generally applied to unpleasant or uncomfortable respiratory sensations experienced by individuals. The American Thoracic Society defines dyspnoea as 'a subjective experience of breathing discomfort that consists of qualitatively distinct sensations that vary in intensity'[25]. The experience is derived from interaction among physiological, psychological, social, and environmental factors, and may induce secondary physiological and behavioural responses[25].

It is emphasized that dyspnoea is subjective, and can only be described and interpreted by the patient; therefore most accurate when reported by patient[25]. Dyspnoea is a term we use for a symptom that patients often describe as breathlessness. In the following text, the two terms are used interchangeably.

Pathophysiology of dyspnoea

Control of breathing

The respiratory rhythm is under the automatic control of the respiratory centre in the medulla which integrates afferent inputs from the chemoreceptors and mechanoreceptors from the airway, lung, chest wall, and respiratory muscle. The motor outputs of the brainstem can also be influenced by voluntary control from the cerebral cortex, which modifies the breathing pattern of the individual.

Neuroimaging of voluntary breathing

The recent advances in neuroimaging enable us to localize the sites of cerebral activations during breathing. McKay et al. investigated the functional neuroanatomy of voluntary respiratory control by using blood O_2 level-dependent functional magnetic resonance imaging (MRI) in six healthy right-handed individuals during voluntary hyperpnoea[26]. Functional images of the brain were acquired during 30-s periods of spontaneous breathing alternated with 30-s periods of isocapnic hyperpnoea. Voluntary hyperpnoea was found to be associated with significant neural activity bilaterally in the primary sensory and motor cortices, supplementary motor area, cerebellum, thalamus, caudate nucleus, and globus pallidum. Significant increase in activity was also identified in the medulla in a superior dorsal position. Activity within the medulla suggests that the brain stem respiratory centres may have a role in mediating the voluntary control of breathing in humans[26].

Mechanisms of dyspnoea

The possible mechanisms of dyspnoea include: (1) increase afferent input from chemoreceptors and mechanoreceptors from upper airway, chest wall, and lung; (2) increase sense of respiratory effort; and (3) afferent mismatch. For a patient who feels breathless from a disease, the dyspnoea may mediate through multiple mechanisms (Fig. 11.1.1).

Chemoreceptors

The central chemoreceptors, postulated to be within the raphé and retrotrapezoid nucleus of medulla, are sensitive to small changes in pH of cerebral spinal fluid resulting from diffusion of carbon dioxide (CO_2) from the blood[27]. The peripheral chemoreceptors are situated in the carotid body and aortic body that respond primarily to changes in PO_2 in the blood, and to a lesser degree, the PCO_2.

Hypoxia and hypercapnia are postulated to be associated with 'air hunger' (an urge to breath) via central or peripheral chemoreceptors. Anecdotal observation suggested that hypoxia does not elicit dyspnoea. An opposing view is that any stimulus to medullary respiratory centres generates dyspnoea via 'corollary discharge' to higher centres, absence of dyspnoea during low-inspired PO_2 may result from increased ventilation and hypocapnia. In the recent study performed by Moosavi et al., steady state levels of hypoxic normocapnia (end-tidal PO_2 = 60–40 Torr), and hypercapnic hyperoxia (end-tidal PCO_2 = 40–50 Torr) were induced in naïve subjects when there were free breathing and during fixed mechanical ventilation[28]. In a separate experiment, normocapnic hypoxia and normoxic hypercapnia, matched by ventilation free-breathing trials, were presented to experienced subjects breathing with constrained rate and tidal volume and 'air hunger' was rated. Air hunger-$PETO_2$ curves rose sharply at $PETO_2$ <50 Torr. Hypercapnia was perceptually indistinguishable from hypoxia. The authors concluded hypoxia and hypercapnia had equal potency for air hunger when matched by ventilatory drive[28].

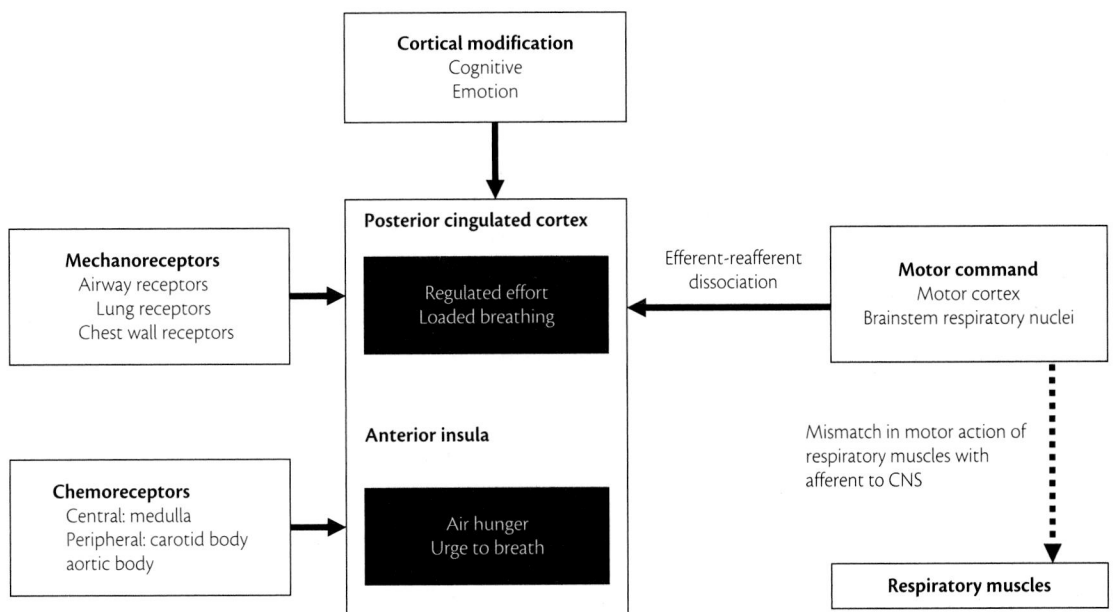

Figure 11.1.1 Mechanism and pathophysiology of dyspnoea.

For the role of PCO_2, earlier studies showed that hypercapnia did not produce air hunger in the absence of respiratory muscle activity. However, later studies on quadriplegic subjects[29] or in volunteers paralysed by neuromuscular blocker[30], hypercapnia induced the sense of 'air hunger'. This suggests that air hunger induced by hypercapnia occurs independently of any associated increase in respiratory activity. The sensation of air hunger induced by hypercapnia can be modulated by changes in tidal volume in the absence of afferent information from the lung, as similar magnitude of reduction in air hunger occurred in heart lung transplant subjects and control subjects[31].

For chronic hypercapnia, a study was performed involving four ventilator-dependent subjects participated in a 2-week study during which they were ventilated with air or air rich in CO_2. It was found that subjects' sensation of 'air hunger' fully adapted to the chronic hypercapnia[32]. The threshold for triggering air hunger sensation to hypercapnia can be increased by inhaling hyperoxia gas mixture and decreased by inhaling hypoxia gas mixture[33].

Mechanoreceptors in upper airway, lung, and chest wall

Mechanoreceptors that reside in the airway, lung, and chest wall may contribute to the control of breathing. There are three types of vagal mediated receptors in the lung: (1) the slowly adapting stretch receptors in the airways respond to lung inflation and participate in the termination of inspiration; (2) the rapidly adapting or irritant receptors in airway epithelium respond to a variety of mechanical and chemical stimuli and mediate bronchoconstriction; and (3) the C fibres (juxta-pulmonary or J) receptors located in the alveolar wall and blood vessels respond to interstitial congestion. Stimulation of different receptors may occur in different diseases. For example, stimulation of irritant receptors occurs in asthma, stimulation of J receptors occurs in pulmonary oedema, lymphangitis carcinomatosis, pneumonia, and pulmonary embolism (PE).

In a study performed by Binks et al. in patients with asthma, bronchoconstriction was induced by inhaled methacholine in 15 subjects with mild asthma[34]. Subjects were mechanically ventilated so as to relieve the work of breathing, and thereby minimise activation of respiratory muscle afferents and motor command. During bronchoconstriction, ratings of 'effort' were greater during spontaneous breathing than during mechanical ventilation. Ratings of 'tightness' were unchanged by the absence of respiratory muscle activity. The authors concluded that 'tightness' was not related to the increase in respiratory work during bronchoconstriction, and postulated that changes within the airway itself and the associated activity of pulmonary receptors generated tightness and the persistent respiratory discomfort[34].

Moreover, clinical observation suggests that upper airway and facial receptors modify the sensation of dyspnoea. Patients sometimes notice a decrease in dyspnoea when sitting by a fan or open window[35]. Mechanoreceptors in the joints, tendons, and muscle of the chest wall may affect the sensation of dyspnoea.

Sense of respiratory effort

Respiratory muscles play an important role in the mechanism of dyspnoea. When the outgoing motor command is sent to the respiratory muscles, a corollary discharge is sent from the motor cortex or possibly brainstem respiratory centre to the sensory cortex, producing a sense of effort. The sense of effort is related to the ratio of the pressure generated by respiratory muscles to the maximum pressure-generating capacity of the muscles[36]. The sense of respiratory effort increases whenever the central motor command to the respiratory muscles is increased. This occurs when the muscle load is increased, or the muscles are weakened by fatigue, paralysis, or an increase in lung volume. Dyspnoea that can possibly be explained by increased sense of effort include that experienced by patients with obstructive airway diseases (e.g. COPD and asthma) and restrictive lung diseases (e.g. interstitial lung disease and respiratory muscle weakness).

It was hypothesized that different afferent sources produce two qualitatively different sensations of 'respiratory work and effort' and 'air hunger'. In a study performed by Lansing et al. in five normal subjects, 'work or effort' ratings changed more steeply when ventilation was altered and PCO_2 was constant; 'air hunger' ratings changed more steeply when PCO_2 was altered and ventilation was constant[37].

Afferent mismatch

In response to afferent information the central nervous system sends efferent impulses to the respiratory muscles in order to increase respiration. This concept of 'neuromechanical dissociation' reflects a 'mismatch' between afferent information to the central nervous system and the outgoing motor command to the respiratory muscles. Based on this concept, the brain anticipates a certain ventilatory response according to the associated afferent information. It is believed that instead of being directly related to muscular activities, dyspnoea is experienced when there is a mismatch between the outgoing motor command to the respiratory muscles and the incoming afferent information[36]. In an early study performed by Schwartzstein et al., 10 naïve normal subjects breathed at various levels of ventilation while end-tidal PCO_2 was held at 55 mmHg[38]. Subjects used a visual target to adjust ventilation to five different levels ranging from 50 per cent below to 50 per cent above the chemically driven ventilation. The intensity of breathlessness was correlated with ventilation and not with measures of respiratory effort. It was speculated that the dissociation between chemical drive and afferent signals produced by motion of the lung and chest wall is important in modulating the sensation of breathlessness[37]. Subsequent studies involving constraining of thoracic displacement during hypercapnia[39] reduced tidal volume at fixed PCO_2 in ventilated quadriplegics[40] and chest wall restriction during exercise[41]; all supported this hypothesis. Banzett et al. termed this process 'efferent-reafferent dissociation'[30].

Dyspnoea generated from multiple mechanisms

There is accumulating evidence that in many patients, dyspnoea is multi-factorial in aetiology. For example, the mechanisms of dyspnoea in patients with asthma are caused by sense of effort, irritant receptor C-fibre, afferent mismatch, with or without the effects from hypoxia or hypercapnia[42]. In a recent study performed by Nishino et al., the sensation of dyspnoea was induced by hypercapnia alone and a combination of hypercapnia and flow-resistive loading in 23 healthy subjects. Dyspnoea was assessed by the use of visual analogue scale (VAS) and the use of 13 listed descriptors[43]. Hypercapnia alone caused a modest degree of dyspnoea characterized by both air hunger and work/effort sensations. An addition of inspiratory flow-resistive loading (IRL) caused an increase in inspiratory difficulty and some attenuation of 'work/effort.' The addition of expiratory flow-resistive loading (ERL) caused an increase in expiratory difficulty and attenuation of 'air hunger.' The addition of both IRL and ERL caused a marked increase in dyspnoea, the amount of which was close to the sum of the increases obtained individually by IRL and by ERL, while the quality of dyspnoea was characterized predominantly by work/effort. These results suggest that despite the difference in quality of sensations, the intensity of dyspnoea would sum linearly when the two kinds of loads are presented at the same time[43].

Breathlessness descriptors

It is postulated that different mechanisms of dyspnoea produce distinct sensory experiences. The sense of air hunger appears to arise out of an increased brain stem drive to breathe as a result of stimulation from chemoreceptors, the sense of tightness arises from stimulation of lung receptors and the increased sense of effort arises from an increased mechanical load. For a patient who feels breathless from a disease, the dyspnoea may mediate through multiple mechanisms, so one will use different combination of descriptors to describe their breathlessness. In the study performed by Simon et al. in 1990, 15 descriptors used by breathless patients were grouped under eight clusters (rapid, exhalation, shallow, work, suffocating, hunger, tight, and heavy); and there was an association between certain groups of descriptors and specific conditions producing dyspnoea[44]. These breathlessness descriptors were applied to patients with cancer and other cardiopulmonary diseases by Wilcock et al.[45]. It was found that all patient groups were characterized by more than one cluster and several clusters were shared between groups; but the relationship does not appear to be sufficient robust for the questionnaire to aid differential diagnosis.

Neuroimaging of cerebral activations during air hunger and loaded breathing

In an experimental model, Evans et al. employed blood oxygen level dependent functional MRI to examine activation during air hunger[46]. Six healthy men and women were mechanically ventilated at 12–14 breaths/min. The primary experiment was conducted at mean end-tidal PCO_2 of 41 Torr. Moderate to severe 'air hunger' was evoked during 42-s epochs of lower tidal volume (mean = 0.75 l). Subjects described the sensation as 'like breathhold,' 'urge to breathe,' and 'starved for air.' Limbic and paralimbic loci activated were within anterior insula, anterior cingulate, operculum, cerebellum, amygdala, thalamus, and basal ganglia. Elements of frontoparietal attentional networks were also identified. The activation of anterior insular activation had been a consistent finding in previous studies, suggesting that the insula is essential to dyspnoea perception, probably acts in concert with a larger neural network[46].

In another experimental model performed by Peiffer et al., regional blood flow measured by functional brain imaging positron emission tomography (PET) was performed in eight healthy subjects during loaded breathing[47]. High-loaded breathing (as reflected by the amplitude of mouth pressure) was associated with neural activation in three distinct brain regions, the right anterior insula, the cerebellar vermis, and the medial pons. There was an area in the right posterior cingulated cortex where neural activation was specifically associated with perceived intensity of respiratory discomfort that is not related to the amplitude of mouth pressure. It was hypothesized this area of brain may be involved in the integration of the effect on perception of the various factors such as menthol, chest wall vibration, and other cognitive/affective factors. Respiratory discomfort related to loaded breathing may be

subserved by two distinct neural networks, the first being involved in the concomitant processing of the genesis and perception of respiratory discomfort and the second in the modulation of perceived intensity of the sensation by various factors[47].

In summary, breathing is automatically regulated by the medulla which integrates afferent inputs from the central and peripheral chemoreceptors and mechanoreceptors from the airway, lung, chest wall, and respiratory muscle. Chemoreceptors are triggered by hypoxia, hypercapnoea, and changes in pH of cerebrospinal fluid; whereas mechanoreceptors are triggered by mechanical or stretch signals as caused by different lung pathologies. Cortical activities such as cognition and emotion modify breathing. Dyspnoea, as a complex sensation, is likely to be mediated through multiple mechanisms. The sensation of 'air hunger' or 'urge to breathe' is differentiated from 'respiratory effort' or 'loaded breathing' in quality, underlying mechanism, and sites of cerebral activiation. Air hunger is related to increased afferent from chemoreceptors while respiratory effort is related to increased afferent from mechanoreceptors and the sensation of increased motor command to respiratory muscles. A mismatch in the afferent and the efferent to the respiratory muscles is also an important mechanism of dyspnoea. Advances in neuroimaging provide data on sites of cerebral activation, for example, the involvement of anterior insula in air hunger and the posterior cingular cortex in respiratory effort (see Fig. 11.1.1). Further evidences are required to elucidate the complexity of the sensation of dyspnoea, the underlying mechanisms, and the neural network involved.

Dyspnoea in cancer patients—magnitude and burden

Prevalence of dyspnoea in advanced cancer

The prevalence of dyspnoea varies with the site of primary cancers and the stage of illness. Dyspnoea is common in the general cancer population, ranging from 46 to 59 per cent in recent studies, and often of moderate to severe intensity[48–53]. In patients with primary lung cancers, the prevalence and intensity of dyspnoea reported were even higher, ranging from 75 to 87 per cent[54–56].

Towards the end of life, or as the functional status of the patient decreases, there is a tendency for dyspnoea to become more prevalent and more severe. Early in the National Hospice Study[57], the prevalence of dyspnoea increased from 49 to 64 per cent during the last 6 weeks of life. The progressive trend in dyspnoea intensity towards end of life has also been reported in more recent studies[1,53,58]. Dyspnoea intensity at end of life was found to increase progressively as Karnofsky Performance Scale (KPS) fell below 60 and peaked at KPS 30 and 20[58]. Chiu et al.[53] reported that 60 per cent of the terminal cancer patients had dyspnoea at two days before death, of which two-thirds were of moderate to severe intensity. Tsai et al., in studying symptom patterns of advanced cancer, found that dyspnoea progression was that of decrease–increase pattern, one which initially improved, but deteriorated again at two days before death[1].

Dyspnoea as a multi-dimensional symptom with significant impact

As a multi-dimensional symptom, dyspnoea should be assessed not only by its occurrence, namely the intensity, frequency, and duration, but also by the distress as experienced by the patient. Dyspnoea can cause significant impact to cancer patients in multiple aspects, including physical, emotional, social, and functional[59].

Dyspnoea can cause significant limitations to the daily activities of cancer patients, and with implications on personal life and self[59]. A study on 171 advanced lung cancer patients had shown that dyspnoea interfered with at least one daily life activity in more than half of the patients. Dyspnoea rated as low severity (1–3 on a 0–10 numerical scale) were severe enough to interfere with at least one daily activity[60].

Dyspnoea can be chronic or intermittent, or with episodic exacerbations[59]. Sudden episodes of severe dyspnoea may mean differently to patient as compared with a constant level of dyspnoea but of lower intensity. The unpredictability and the uncertainty of the occurrence of dyspnoea are difficult to bear with, and increasing breathlessness is perceived as worsening of illness. Emotions associated with their description of dyspnoea included anxiety, fear, panic, feeling of impending death, helplessness, loneliness and guilt[59].

Under recognition of dyspnoea by health-care workers add more to patients' helplessness. Patients with dyspnoea feel that health-care workers do not understand them or cannot help them, and they have to develop their own coping strategies. Patients try to cope by limiting their activity or stay quiet, so that the impact of dyspnoea on activity may not be noticed by staff[59]. In one recent study on 100 cancer patients, significant discrepancies were observed between the patient and the doctor reporting presence of dyspnoea, as well as intensity and distress[61].

Dyspnoea and its correlates

Various factors have been reported to be correlated with dyspnoea in cancer, including smoking, lung disease such as asthma or COPD, lung involvement by cancer, and lung irradiation, exposure to asbestos, coal dust, cotton dust, or grain.[51,52] Anxiety was reported to be related to presence or intensity of dyspnoea in various studies[51,53,62].

The correlation of lung function parameters with dyspnoea intensity has not been well established. Spirometry readings have poor correlation with intensity of dyspnoea[63]. It has also been shown that dyspnoea in the terminally ill does not correlate with the degree of hypoxaemia, as in other respiratory conditions[51]. The maximum inspiratory pressure (MIP), a measure of the inspiratory muscle strength through the mouth, was associated with dyspnoea severity in one study[51] but not in another[62].

Dyspnoea as a prognostic indicator

Dyspnoea is one of the clinical variables reported to correlate significantly with survival in cancer[64–68]. In a study on 1574 advanced cancer patients who were followed up till death, clinical variables, including dyspnoea, were found to be strongly associated with survival (HR, 2.16; 95 per cent CI, 1.55–3.00)[68]. In another recent study of 248 advanced cancer patients, the hazards of dying increased by 28 per cent in the presence of dyspnoea[67].

In one other study, respiratory rate above 28/min was identified as a risk factor for imminent death in cancer patients presented with acute dyspnoea, and predicted a survival of <2 weeks[69]. Sanchez *et al.* recently reported three independent variables for prediction of survival for home-care patients as assessed by the home-care support team; (1) Palliative Performance Score of 50 or under; (2) heart rate of 100 per minute or more; and (3) respiratory rate of 24 per minute or more[70].

Dyspnoea is also incorporated in various prognostic models. Pirovano *et al.* reported a palliative prognostic score including six variables, inclusive of dyspnoea, for prediction of survival at 30 days[71]. Morita *et al.* reported a prognostic model including performance status, oedema, delirium, and dyspnoea at rest for predicting survival at 3 and 6 weeks[72].

Current consensus among palliative care experts is that cancer symptoms, such as anorexia–cachexic syndrome, dyspnoea, delirium, together with performance status are useful for predicting prognosis[73]. Future studies will help to further define the role of using dyspnoea as a prognostic indicator, and hence facilitating care planning.

Underlying causes of dyspnoea in advanced cancer

In any cancer patient presented with dyspnoea, multiple underlying causes can be responsible. Elucidation of all the underlying causes of dyspnoea guides its treatment and maximises the potential for good control. Causes of dyspnoea can be classified according to: (1) local cardiopulmonary causes versus systemic causes; and (2) malignant versus paramalignant, non-malignant causes. However, this serves only as a guide in evaluation and each classification is supplementary to each other (Table 11.1.1).

Local cardiopulmonary causes versus systemic causes

Cardiopulmonary causes are the main causes of dyspnoea. It is useful to identify specific causes of dyspnoea among the cardiopulmonary causes, or specific dyspnoea syndromes as defined in this chapter. Each dyspnoea syndrome has its own distinct clinical features and specific treatment approach. Major dyspnoea syndromes in cancer, as illustrated in the latter part of the text, include: (1) pleural effusion; (2) pleural tumour; (3) pericardial effusion; (4) superior vena cava obstruction (SVCO); (5) major airway obstruction (MAO); (6) PE; (7) pulmonary lymphangitis carcinomatosis; (8) respiratory muscle weakness; (9) chest infection; and (10) other miscellaneous syndromes.

Systemic causes may occur concomitantly. They should be looked for when there is no apparent cardiopulmonary cause for the dyspnoea, or the degree of dyspnoea is disproportionate to the extent of cardiopulmonary embarrassment. Examples include anaemia, ascites, hepatomegaly, and respiratory muscle weakness.

Malignant versus paramalignant, non-malignant causes

Causes of dyspnoea can also be classified as malignant, para-malignant, or non-malignant causes. With smoking as a common casual factor, coexistence of other illnesses such as COPD or heart disease should be considered. In one study on 294 patients with lung cancer, lung function tests were reviewed to look for airflow obstruction. Patients with FEV_1/FVC ratio of <70 per cent was considered to have COPD. With this criterion, COPD was present in 72.8 per cent of male patients and 52.5 per cent of female patients[74]. In another study on lung cancer patients, 49 per cent patients were found to have airflow obstruction, but only 14.4 per cent of patients received bronchodilator therapy[75].

Para-malignant causes include the para-neoplastic syndromes and causes related to cancer treatment. Surgical resection of lung segments reduces pulmonary reserve, especially in presence of co-existing cardiopulmonary morbidities. Chemotherapy and radiotherapy can give rise to pulmonary toxicity, and its development during and after therapy often poses significant diagnostic problems. Radiotherapy can cause lung injury in the form of acute respiratory distress syndrome, acute pneumonitis, and subsequent fibrosis. Symptoms of acute pneumonitis develop one to 6 months after radiotherapy, and its symptomatic form occurs in 5 per cent to 15 per cent of lung cancer patients. Chemotherapy-induced lung

Table 11.1.1 Underlying causes of dyspnoea in advanced cancer.

	Local cardiopulmonary causes		Systemic causes
Malignant causes (directly due to cancer) and Paramalignant causes (indirectly due to cancer)	Lung parenchymal involvement: ◆ Lung cancer ◆ Pulmonary metastasis Pleural involvement: ◆ Pleural tumour, mesothelioma ◆ Pleural effusion Pericardial: ◆ Effusion Major airway obstruction: ◆ Tracheal obstruction Blood vessels: ◆ Superior vena cava obstruction ◆ Pulmonary artery: tumour embolism tumour encasement ◆ Pulmonary veno-occlusion Lymphatics: ◆ Lymphangitis carcinomatosis Phrenic nerve paralysis Chest wall infiltration	Pneumothorax Pneumonia: ◆ Aspiration ◆ Tracheo-oesophageal fistula ◆ Opportunistic infection Pulmonary embolism *Treatment related* Surgery: ◆ Pneumonectomy ◆ Lobectomy Chemotherapy: ◆ Pulmonary toxicity ◆ Cardiac toxicity Radiotherapy: ◆ ARDS ◆ Acute pneumonitis ◆ Pulmonary fibrosis ◆ Post-irradiation pericarditis	Respiratory muscle weakness: ◆ Cancer cachexia ◆ Paraneoplastic syndrome ◆ Steroid myopathy ◆ Electrolyte and metabolic abnormality Blood: ◆ Anaemia ◆ Hyperviscosity syndrome Elevated diaphragm: ◆ Diaphragmatic paralysis ◆ Ascites ◆ Hepatomegaly Metabolic acidosis: ◆ Renal failure
Non-malignant causes	Obstructive pulmonary disease: ◆ COPD ◆ Asthma Restrictive lung disease Interstitial lung disease Chest wall deformity Pulmonary vascular disease: ◆ Pulmonary AV malformation Cardiac disease: ◆ Congestive heart failure ◆ Ischaemic heart disease ◆ Cardiac arrhythmia		Retrosternal goitre Neuromuscular disorder Hepatopulmonary syndrome Respiratory panic attack Hyperventilation Obesity

injury is associated with a wide range of agents, especially that associated with cyclophosphamide, bleomycin, and gemcitabine. Gemcitabine can cause dyspnoea within a few hours of treatment and is thought to be related to bronchospasm, but it is also related to many reports of gemcitabine induced severe pulmonary toxicity (GISPT). The newer agent, the EGFR inhibitor gefitinib, is also reported to have association with life-threatening diffuse alveolar damage during the first 3 months of treatment. The incidence of gefitinib-related lung injury ranges from 0.34 to 1.9 per cent, with higher percentages reported in Japan. Diagnosis requires exclusion of other causes of dyspnoea, and in some indicated patients, bronchoscopy and high resolution computed tomography (CT) may be required[76].

Assessment of dyspnoea in advanced cancer: clinical approach

In clinical palliative care practice, the objectives of dyspnoea assessment is to identify all underlying causes of dyspnoea and to understand the impact and distress as experienced by patient. The vehicles for assessment included a detailed history and physical examination, carefully selected investigations, and use of measuring tools appropriate to the clinical context.

Good history taking in dyspnoeic cancer patients

No objective test can replace patient's own description of the symptom and related features. A good history on dyspnoea is extremely helpful in elucidating the underlying causes of dyspnoea; exploring the symptom profile, experience, and distress; and assessing the impact on patients in various aspects of life (Table 11.1.2).

Detailed physical examination

Physical examination can yield useful clues to the underlying causes of dyspnoea. In patients who are too dyspnoeic to talk, or too distressed to undergo more investigations, physical examination will be heavily relied on as a source of clinical information (Table 11.1.3).

Carefully selected investigations

The choice of investigations depends on the invasiveness, availability, costing, potential gain, and patient's preference. Investigations should be carefully selected to guide specific treatment. First-line

Table 11.1.2 History findings in cancer patients with dyspnoea.

Elucidating underlying causes	
Smoking	
Occupational exposure	Asbestos, cotton wool
Drug history	Beta blocker, non-steroidal anti-inflammatory drugs (NSAIDs) precipitating heart failure
	Long-term steroid causing respiratory muscle weakness
Past anti-cancer treatment	Chemotherapy agents with cardiopulmonary toxicity
	Radiation to lung and mediastinum
Concomitant medical illness	COPD, asthma, heart disease, anxiety
Associated respiratory symptoms	Cough, sputum, haemoptysis, wheeze, stridor
	Pleuritic chest pain e.g. pleural effusion, pneumothorax, pulmonary embolism
	Severe chest wall pain e.g. tumour invasion, mesothelioma
Special patterns of dyspnoea	Nocturnal or early morning dyspnoea e.g. asthma
	Orthopnoea e.g. congestive heart failure, superior vena cava syndrome, gross ascites, diaphragmatic paralysis and respiratory muscle weakness
	Platyspnoea i.e. worsening of dyspnoea on sitting up e.g. pulmonary arteriovenous malformation, hepatopulmonary syndrome
Exploring the symptom experience	
Description of breathlessness	The sensation is most accurate when self-described by the patient
Severity of dyspnoea	As verbalized by patient
	Simple or unidimensional scale e.g. VAS or NRS is helpful in clinical practice
	Choice of other tools depends on context
Precipitating factors	Physical activities or posture
	Mechanical factors e.g. crying and laughing
	Environmental factors e.g. bad weather, pollens, smoke
	Emotional factors e.g. anxiety, frustration, excitement, and fear
Trajectory of dyspnoea	Chronic or intermittent
	Duration and frequency of attack, interval between attacks
Concurrent symptoms	Fatigue, loss of concentration, loss of appetite, pain, insomnia, sweating
Past dyspnoea experience	Experience of dyspnoea after the diagnosis of cancer
	History of frightening experience of dyspnoea
Assessing the impact and coping strategies[59]	
Emotional disturbance	Anxiety, depressive mood, anger, helplessness, nervousness, fear, loneliness
Functional impairment	Note the indoor and outdoor activities that have to stopped, slow down, modified, or transferred to others
Social restriction	Impact on sexual life, social roles, recreational activities and the degree of isolation
Coping strategies	Immediate coping strategies e.g. positioning, moving more slowly, posture, use of medications, pursed-lip breathing
	Long-term adaptive strategies e.g. decrease, slow down, modification, or advanced planning of activities; home modification, breathing strategy, avoidance of precipitants, improving ventilation, relaxation techniques, diversional activities
	Emotional coping by acceptance, stay calm, avoid being alone, avoid thinking about it, seek support from family

investigations include haemoglobin level, oxygen saturation by oximetry, and chest radiograph. Oximetry is non-invasive and can detect hypoxia. Chest radiograph is informative in defining specific dyspnoea syndromes (Table 11.1.4). Bedside lung function tests including spirometry, MIP, or nasal sniff inspiratory pressure (NSIP) can help to detect concomitant obstructive airway disease and inspiratory muscle weakness.

Second-line investigations are non-invasive but are more expensive and less readily available in palliative care setting. Echocardiogram and Doppler ultrasound may be diagnostic in some cardiopulmonary conditions, or helpful in guiding procedures such as pleural or pericardial tapping. Lung function test of a flow volume loop is a simple, fast, and non-invasive investigation to look for upper airway obstruction.

Table 11.1.3 Physical examination findings in cancer patients with dyspnoea.

General examination	Pallor, plethora, cyanosis, engorged neck and upper chest wall veins, leg oedema, cachexia, muscle wasting
	Retrosternal goitre, tense ascites, hepatomegaly
Respiratory system	
Abnormal chest wall expansion	Localized decreased expansion
	Wasted accessory respiratory muscle and insucking intercostal muscle e.g. respiratory muscle weakness
Abnormal breathing pattern	Prolonged expiration e.g. COPD
	Rapid shallow breathing e.g. restrictive lung disease
	Paradoxical breathing e.g. upper airway obstruction, respiratory muscle weakness
	Hyperventilation e.g. panic attack
	Kussmaul breathing in acidosis
Breath sounds	Stridor or inspiratory noise in major airway obstruction
	Expiratory wheeze in COPD
	Silent chest in the presence of severe dyspnoea e.g. in critical airway stenosis, severe asthma, respiratory muscle weakness
Cardiovascular system	
Pulse	Paradoxical pulse (defined by an inspiratory fall of systolic pressure of 10 mmHg or more) in pericardial effusion
Jugular venous pressure	Raised in heart failure, cardiac tamponade, pulmonary embolism, and cor pulmonale
Heart sounds	Gallop rhythm in heart failure
	Muffled in massive pericardial effusion

The third-line investigations should be considered in highly selected cases, and subject to availability of resource and benefit versus burden analysis. CT may be valuable in diagnosing conditions that cannot be confirmed on the chest radiograph, for example, PE, MAO, SVCO, and lymphangitis carcinomatosis.

Dyspnoea measurement tools

Dyspnoea can be assessed in various dimensions. A comprehensive approach for assessing dyspnoea in advanced cancer patients in palliative care setting is well illustrated by the Breathlessness Assessment Guide, which covers the characteristics and the dimensions of dyspnoea in cancer as elaborated in this chapter[77]. However, this tool has not been tested formally on its psychometric properties. Many other measuring tools are being validated for assessment of dyspnoea, though most were developed for COPD patients initially. At present, there is no ideal or universally accepted tool for measuring the complex symptom of dyspnoea[78,79]. A simplistic and yet practical way of grouping these dyspnoea measurement tools is based on: (1) the dimension specificity; (2) the symptom specificity; and (3) the disease specificity (Table 11.1.5).

Dyspnoea can be assessed in various dimensions, though when only a single dimension is being assessed by tools, it is usually the intensity. Tools commonly used include the VAS, the numerical rating scale (NRS), and the Modified Borg Scale[78,79]. Application is relatively easy, even in cancer patients who have lost their mobility. NRS has been shown to be more repeatable than VAS in assessing dyspnoea, and requires a smaller sample size than VAS for evidence of intervention effectiveness[80,79]. VAS and NRS are useful for comparison within patient but not so satisfactory between groups[78]. At present, there is no sufficient evidence to conclude on the level of change in VAS or NRS score in order for it to be meaningful in clinical setting. In a recent meeting among the experts, the consensus regarded the change of 10 per cent (1 cm) in VAS from baseline, or a 1-point change in the BORG scale as a reasonable minimum for current use[81].

Dyspnoea can also be assessed by its burden, in terms of its distress experienced by the patient and its limitation on function. The Cancer Dyspnoea Scale (CDS)[82] is one evaluated in lung cancer patients for assessing dyspnoea in terms of sense of effort, anxiety, and discomfort; but requires further assessment of construct validity and responsiveness[79]. The Lung Cancer Symptom Scale (LCSS) is also validated in lung cancer patients, items on other respiratory symptoms and the gobal quality of life are also included[83]. Apart from these more specific tools, dyspnoea is also among the symptoms measured in various multi-dimensional general cancer symptom scales. Some examples of these scales include the Memorial Symptom Assessment Scale (MSAS)[84], the Rotterdam Symptom Checklist (RSCL)[85], the Edmonton Symptom Assessment System (ESAS)[86], the MD Anderson Symptom Inventory (MDASI)[87], and the Symptom Distress Scale (SDS)[88].

Tools mainly for assessing the limitation of dyspnoea on functional, daily activities, or exercise tolerance are mostly validated for non-cancer disease, mainly the chronic respiratory disease. Examples include the Baseline Dyspnoea Index (BDI)[89], the Transitional Dyspnoea Index (TDI)[89], the Modified Dyspnoea Index (MDI)[90], and the Medical Research Council (MRC) dyspnoea scale[91]. However, they may not be applicable for advanced cancer patients with poor performance status, or sensitive enough to detect the effect of intervention. The Chronic Respiratory Questionnaire dyspnoea subscale (CRQ-D) has been evaluated in chronic lung diseases and heart failure. With its face and construct validity, test-retest reliability, and responsiveness, CRQ-D may show promise for use in palliative care[79]. The shuttle walking test (SWT) had been applied to cancer patients with reproducible results[92]. Tools such as the Reading Numbers Aloud Test[93], or the upper limbs exercise test[94] are developed for cancer patients, and applicable for those who cannot walk.

Overall, dyspnoea is closely related to patient satisfaction with quality of life and has been incorporated in quality of life assessment tools. A notable example is the EORTC Quality of Life Questionnaire which is used widely in cancer research[95]. Dyspnoea is an item assessed in both the generic questionnaire, the EORTC QLQ C-30, and in the modular questionnaire developed for lung cancer patients (EORTC QLQ-LC13)[96]. An independent shortened questionnaire has been developed for cancer patients in palliative care setting (EORTC QLQ-C15-PAL), a 15-item questionnaire including the symptom of dyspnoea[97]. In a recent study on 954 advanced cancer patients, the intensity of dyspnoea as measured

Table 11.1.4 Chest radiograph interpretation in dyspnoeic cancer patient.

Anatomical site	X-ray findings	Possible causes of dyspnoea
Parenchymal	Lung masses	Primary or secondary lung tumours
	Infiltration	Pneumonia
	Collapse consolidation	Major airway obstruction
		Pulmonary embolism
	Reticular shadow	Lymphangitis carcinomatosis
		Radiation related lung injury
		Chemotherapy related lung injury
Pleural	Blurring of costophrenic angle	Pleural effusion
	Subpulmonary effusion mimic raised diaphragm	
	Pseudotumour	
	Opacification of whole lung field	
	Pleural base opacity	Pleural tumour
	Pleural calcification	
	Visible pleural line	Pneumothorax
Trachea and major airway	Deviation	Massive pleural effusion
		Lung collapse
	Narrowing	Endobronchial tumour
		Mediastinal mass
		Retrosternal goitre
Mediastinum	Mediastinal shift	Massive pleural effusion
		Lung collapse
	Mediastinal widening	Mediastinal mass including mediastinal lymphadenopathy
		SVCO
Diaphragm	Elevation	Diaphragmatic paralysis
		Diaphragmatic muscle weakness
		Phrenic nerve paralysis
		Gross hepatomegaly
		Tense ascites
		Subpulmonary effusion
Cardiac shadow	Cardiomegaly	Pericardial effusion
		Congestive heart failure
		Cor pulmonale
Pulmonary vessels	Enlarged pulmonary conus	Pulmonary hypertension
Normal chest radiograph	Pulmonary causes	Major airway obstruction
		SVCO
		Pulmonary embolism
		Lymphangitis carcinomatosis
		Pneumonia
	General causes	Respiratory muscle weakness
		Anaemia
		Ascites
		Metabolic acidosis
		Hyperventilation
		Obesity

Table 11.1.5 Dyspnoea assessment tools.

		VAS/NRS	Modified Borg	CDS	LCSS	MSAS ESAS RSCL MDASI SDS	CRQ-D BDI TDI MRC MDI SWT	Reading numbers Aloud test upper limbs exercise test
Dimension specificity	Symptom intensity	✓	✓		✓	✓	✓	
	Symptom distress			✓		✓		
	Functional limitation				✓	✓	✓	✓
Symptom specificity	Specific for dyspnoea		✓	✓			✓	✓
	General cancer symptom	✓						
	Defined group of symptoms				✓	✓		
Disease specificity	Cancer specific			✓	✓	✓		✓
	Other disease specific		✓				✓	✓

by the EORTC dyspnoea subscale was strongly correlated with patient satisfaction with QOL[98].

The choice of the measuring tool depends on the objectives of measurement, the clinical condition of the patient, and the availability of manpower and time. The burden of the test on both the patient and the staff is always an important consideration especially when a battery of scales is employed. Currently, it has been recommended that a simple scale such as VAS, NRS, or Modified Borg Scale can be used for general clinical questions such as evaluating effectiveness of intervention[78,79]. Additional information, if desired, can be supplemented by more sophisticated scales or qualitative interviews[78].

With the evolving concept of symptom cluster, it may be possible to reduce assessment burden by narrowing the symptoms to those which are likely to occur in clusters[16]. This concept also embraces the notion that the overall burden is not necessary a summation of all symptoms, as some may carry a weight heavier than the other. Moreover, the temporal relationships between different symptoms in a cluster can be revealed[16].

There are still more to be explored in searching for newer ways of assessing this complex symptom of dyspnoea. The clinical application of dyspnoea descriptors and the use of changes in physiological parameters in assessing the sensation of dyspnoea await further studies.

Management of dyspnoea

Management of dyspnoea in cancer patients involves the following stepwise approach:

1 assessment of dyspnoea;

2 management of specific dyspnoea syndrome;

3 non-pharmacological management;

4 oxygen;

5 pharmacological treatment;

6 other potential drugs; and

7 palliative sedation.

Management of dyspnoea syndromes

Malignant pleural effusion (MPE)

The presence of malignant cells in pleural fluid and/or parietal pleura signifies disseminated or advanced disease. The median survival following diagnosis of MPE ranges from 3 to 12 months, depending on the stage and the type of the underlying malignancy. The shortest survival time is observed in MPE secondary to lung cancer and the longest in ovarian cancer. Combining the data of five series, the most common metastatic tumour to the pleura was lung cancer in men and breast cancer in women. These two cancers account for approximately 50–65 per cent of all malignant effusions, with lymphomas, tumours of the genitourinary tract and gastrointestinal tract as a group account for a further 25 per cent[99]. The pathogenesis of MPE involves the following cascade: (1) loss of adherence of malignant cell from primary tumour, (2) adherence and penetration of blood vessel wall, (3) migration through the pleura, (4) constitutive production of autocrine growth factors, and (5) induction of angiogenesis[100]. The expression of VEGFs in tumours is considered to be associated with tumour development via capillary and lymph vessel neogenesis[101].

Clinical approach to MPE

Dyspnoea, cough, and chest discomfort are common symptoms. Symptom severity is usually related to the rate of accumulation, size of effusion, baseline lung function, and the underlying cause of the effusion.

The cause of the pleural effusion in patient with malignancy should be first identified. Pleural effusion in patient with known malignancy is most commonly caused by pleural metastases. Other causes include the para-malignant conditions such as local effect of tumour (e.g. bronchial obstruction with atelectasis, lymphatic obstruction, and venous obstruction as in superior vena cava syndrome), or systemic effects of malignancy such as PE and hypoalbuminaemia. Non-malignant causes including congestive heart failure, liver cirrhosis, nephrotic syndrome, and infection should be looked for and treated accordingly. In 5–15 per cent of MPE, it has features of transudation that can be caused by concomitant heart failure, hypoalbuminaemia, or atelectasis of lung.

The chest radiograph is helpful for evaluation of MPE. In massive MPE, contralateral mediastinal shift is expected. An ipsilateral mediastinal shift may indicate bronchial obstruction with atelectasis or a trapped lung resulting from pleural encasement. Trapped lung should be suspected clinically when a negative suction pressure is encountered during thoracocentesis and pleural effusion recurs rapidly. Massive effusion with no mediastinal shift may signify mediastinal tumour infiltration. Massive lung consolidation can be differentiated from pleural effusion radiologically by a decubitus radiograph or ultrasound of chest. Coexisting pericardial effusion has to be ruled out in the presence of cardiomegaly.

Treatment options for MPEs are determined by several factors: symptoms and performance status of the patient, the primary tumour and its response to systemic therapy, and lung re-expansion following pleural fluid evacuation[999]. Tumour-targeted treatment is an option to consider in selected cases. Small-cell lung cancer, lymphoma, and breast cancer usually respond to chemotherapy, and some advanced NSCLC may respond to new chemotherapeutic agents and molecular-targeted therapy. However, evidences on the degree of symptom relief with these tumour treatments have to be carefully interpreted when patient outcome is otherwise defined.

The treatment options for symptomatic MPE include:

♦ therapeutic thoracocentesis;

♦ chemical pleurodesis: either via chest tube or thoracoscopy;

♦ chronic indwelling pleural catheter;

♦ pleuroperitoneal shunt; and

♦ pleural abrasion and pleurectomy.

Therapeutic thoracocentesis

Thoracocentesis should be considered when MPE is symptomatic. Needle thoracocentesis is usually performed in the hospital setting where supportive facilities are readily available for managing complications including pneumothorax. The advisable site of thoracocentesis is anterior to the mid-axillary line to avoid pain on lying flat in case local deposits occur. An early aspiration may prevent sudden deterioration in patient with massive effusion or contralateral mediastinal shift on chest radiograph. The amount of fluid evacuated is guided by clinical symptoms and should be limited to 1–1.5 l each time. Large pleural effusion should be drained in a controlled manner to avoid re-expansion pulmonary oedema[99] In the case of ipsilateral mediastinal shift towards the side of the pleural effusion, which may suggest atelectasis or trapped lung, a therapeutic tapping of <300 ml can be attempted. Aspiration should be abandoned if there is increasing dyspnoea, chest discomfort, and persistent cough during the procedure. Alternatively, monitoring and keeping the pleural pressure at not <−20 cm H_2O will minimise the risk of re-expansion pulmonary oedema[102]. Ultrasound guidance is helpful in guiding tapping of loculated or organized effusion. Routine chest radiograghs for detecting pneumothorax after needle thoracocentesis may not be necessary if the procedure is smooth and the patient has no deterioration of symptoms during or after the procedure. The risk of pneumothorax will be minimised if aspiration is performed with a small needle and guided by ultrasound. If pleurodesis is not considered after

aspiration, tube thoracostomy should be avoided because of high recurrence rate[99]. Repeating pleural aspiration instead of pleurodesis is recommended for the palliation of breathlessness in patients with a very short life expectancy and poor performance status[99]. Needle thoracocentesis can relieve dyspnoea in the terminally ill if effusion is the major casual factor for the dyspnoea.

Chemical pleurodesis

Chemical pleurodesis involves the introduction of sclerosing agents into the pleural space either by tube thoracostomy or thoracoscopy. By inducing an exuberant fibrotic response on the surface of the visceral and parietal pleura, it serves to achieve symphysis between the visceral and parietal pleural layers, hence preventing accumulation of fluid in the pleural space. The fibrotic response involves a large number of fibroblasts, and fibroblast growth is dependent on the presence of growth factors such as fibroblast growth factor (FGF) and platelet-derived growth factor (PDGF). Sclersoing agent such as talc can induce release of basic fibroblast growth factor (bFGF) from mesothelial cell, an important mediator of early pleural response to sclerosants. Patients with extensive tumour involvement of the pleural mesothelium have a significantly lower pleural fluid bFGF response to talc compared with those who have limited involvement. Patients with limited pleural disease and higher bFGF responses are factors favouring successful pleurodesis[103]. Increased pleural fibrinolytic activity as measured by pleural D-dimer is associated with failure of pleurodesis. A study showed that pleural neutrophilic and fibrinolytic response to talc can predict outcome of pleurodesis[104].

Chemical pleurodesis should be considered in recurrent MPE if relief of dyspnoea is evident after thoracocentesis in the presence of satisfactory performance status. Many workers would only consider pleurodesis if the estimated survival is longer than one month. Before inserting an intercostal tube, features suggesting of trapped lung should be looked for as the chance of full lung expansion is low.

Historically, more than 30 sclerosing agents have been used achieving different rates of success, including antibiotics, antineoplastics, pro-inflammatory drugs and biological response modifiers. The sclerosants commonly used are talc, tetracycline hydrochloride, doxycycline, minocycline, bleomycin, and *Corynebacterium parvum*. The choice of agent depends on its accessibility, efficacy, safety, ease of administration and cost. Optimal dosage of different intrapleural agents and side effects are listed in Table 11.1.6.

In a web-based survey involving 859 pulmonologists in five English speaking countries, preferred sclerosants agent chosen by respondents were: 56 per cent for talc slurry, 12 per cent for talc poudrage, 26 per cent for tetracycline derivatives, and 7 per cent for bleomycin[105]. The efficacy of different pleurodesis agents was compared in two meta-analysis. A systematic review in 2004 reported that the use of sclerosants compared with control was associated with an increased efficacy of pleurodesis. Based on ten studies comprising 308 subjects comparing different sclerosants, talc was found to be the most efficacious. The RR of effusion non-recurrence was 1.34 (95 per cent CI, 1.16–1.55) in favour of talc compared with bleomycin, tetracycline, mustine, or tube drainage alone. This was not associated with increased mortality post-pleurodesis[106]. In another systematic review, talc was compared with other agents in nine studies that included 341 patients. Talc tended to be associated with fewer recurrences when compared with bleomycin (RR, 0.64; 95 per cent CI, 0.34–1.20) and, with

Table 11.1.6 Sclerosing agents for pleurodesis: dosage, success rate, and adverse effects.

Agent	Optimal intrapleural dosage[99]	Reported success rate[99]	Reported adverse effects and concerns
Tetracycline	1.0 to 1.5 g or 20 mg/kg	50–92 per cent; mean 65 per cent	Transient fever and pleuritic chest pain
Doxycyline	500 mg	65–100 per cent; mean 76 per cent	Fever and mild to moderate pleuritic chest pain
Bleomycin	60 units	58–85 per cent; mean 61 per cent	Fever, chest pain, and nausea 45 per cent of the drug is absorbed systemically Cost
Talc (graded talc)	2–5 g	88–100 per cent; mean 90 per cent	Fever, chest pain Acute pneumonitis, adult respiratory distress syndrome, acute respiratory failure when small particle size of talc was used

more uncertainty, to tetracycline (RR, 0.50; 95 per cent CI, 0.06–4.42). Tetracycline (or doxycycline) was not superior to bleomycin (RR, 0.92; 95 per cent CI, 0.61–1.38)[107].

Based on the above evidences, talc should be the sclerosant of choice. Talc ($Mg_3Si_4O_{10}(OH)_2$) is a trilayered magnesium silicate sheet that is inert. Talc used for intrapleural administration is asbestos-free and sterilized effectively by dry heat exposure, ethylene oxide, and gamma radiation. There is marked variation in the diameter of the talc particles produced from different countries, with the median diameter varied from 7.8 to 31.3 µm.

In the comparison of thoracoscopic versus medical pleurodesis, thoracoscopic pleurodesis was found to be more effective in a systematic review[106]. A larger prospective randomized trial compared thoracoscopy with talc insufflation (TTI) (n = 242) to thoracostomy and talc slurry (TS) (n = 240) for patients with documented MPE. Overall, there was no difference between both groups for successful 30-day outcomes (TTI, 78 per cent; TS, 71 per cent). However, the subgroup of patients with primary lung or breast cancer had higher success with TTI than with TS (82 per cent vs 67 per cent)[108].

The risk of developing acute respiratory distress syndrome (ARDS) after receiving talc pleurodesis has raised lingering concern, especially in association with high doses of talc. In animal study, pulmonary injury and dissemination to other organs are related to a talc particle size of <10 µm[109]. Another report had shown that talc pleurodesis with a mean particle size of <15 µm ('mixed' talc) produces more lung and systemic inflammation than tetracycline or 'graded' talc (most particles < 10 µm were removed). Therefore the routine use of 'graded' talc for pleurodesis should be recommended for reducing the morbidity of this procedure[110]. Other safety precautions include avoiding simultaneous bilateral procedures, concomitant pulmonary biopsies and use of more than 5 g of talc[109].

Inexpensive agents for pleurodesis are alternatives when common agents are unavailable. These include: 20 ml of 0.5 per cent silver nitrate, quinacrine 500 mg in 200 ml normal saline, and 20 ml 10 per cent iodopovidone in 80 ml normal saline, but experience are much less with these agents[111].

Technical aspect of pleurodesis

A systematic review had evaluated the role of patient rotation after instillation of sclerosant, the duration of chest drain affecting outcome and the size of chest tube affecting outcome of pleurodesis[107]. Two RCTs using tetracycline or talc showed no difference in recurrence conferred by rotation. Two RCTs found

no difference in recurrence when comparing the standard protocol of draining to dryness before tube removal to the shorter protocol of removing the tube after 24 h. No RCT compared large versus small chest tubes using the same method of tube insertion. One RCT of 18 patients compared large chest tube placed during thoracoscopy with small catheters which were percutaneously inserted[51]. The recurrence rates were similar, but the larger tubes caused more discomfort.

Full lung expansion is often considered a prerequisite for successful pleurodesis, but successful pleurodesis with partial lung re-expansion was reported in a small series[112]. Where patient is not suitable for surgical intervention, pleurodesis should still be attempted even in incomplete lung re-expansion or pleural apposition[99]. Pleural analgesia with lignocaine (3 mg/kg, maximum 250 mg) as pre-medication was recommended[99]. Based on above evidences, the procedures of pleurodesis are summarized as follow:

1 Similar efficacy for medical pleurodesis by tube thoracostomy or thoracoscopic pleurodesis.

2 For tube thoracostomy, a small bore intercostal tube (10–14 F) gives similar efficacy.

3 Controlled evacuation of pleural fluid in massive effusion to avoid re-expansion pulmonary oedema.

4 Confirm full lung re-expansion by chest radiograph.

5 Administer premedication intrapleurally prior to pleurodesis (lignocaine solution 3 mg/kg maximum up to 250 mg).

6 Install sclerosant of choice and clamp tube for 1 h.

7 Patient rotation following pleurodesis is not necessary.

8 Remove intercostal tube within 12–72 h if lung remains fully re-expanded.

Other interventions

When pleurodesis fails due to trap lung, an indwelling pleural drainage may be considered[113]. Pleuroperitoneal shunt had been performed safely in a large series of 160 patients with trapped lung and recurrent effusion with a median survival of 7.7 months[114]. Tunnelled pleural catheter (TPC) has been studied as a first line treatment for MPE. In a large series of 250 cases with TPC placement, no further ipsilateral pleural procedures were required in 90.1 per cent of cases. Complication rate was low and the overall median survival time following TPC insertion was 144 days[115].

Pleural tumour-malignant mesothelioma (MM)

Despite new evidence in the basic science, diagnostic tools, and new chemotherapy in the past few years, malignant mesothelioma (MM) remains a challenge in medicine. Diagnosis is often delayed at 2 or 3 months after the onset of the symptoms. Only a small proportion of patients (1–5 per cent) are suitable for surgical management. Radiotherapy and chemotherapy remain palliative, and patients have a median survival of 9–12 months. Projections suggest that the incidence is expected to rise by at least 50 per cent over the next 20 years in Western Europe and Australia. In the UK, mortality from MM is expected to peak between 2012 and 2015, and MM is predicted to account for 65 000 deaths between 2001 and 2050. However, the incidence is falling in the USA[116].

The response of MM to chemotherapy has been poor. In the UK, a large multi-centre Phase III randomized trial of the most widely used treatments, mitomycin, vinblastine, and cisplatin against vinorelbine and compared with active symptom control is under way[117]. In the large single-blind control study of 448 patients comparing pemetrexed and cisplatin with cisplatin alone, Pemetrexed with folic acid and vitamin B_{12} supplementation has been shown to be an effective agent in the treatment of MM with a significant gain in survival of 2.8 months when used in combination with cisplatin compared with single agent cisplatin in good performance status patients (ECOG performance status 0 and 1 patients)[118]. Response rates were 41.3 per cent in the pemetrexed/cisplatin arm, versus 16.6 per cent in the control arm ($p < 0.0001$). Median survival time was 12.1 months in the pemetrexed/cisplatin arm, versus 9.3 months in the control arm ($p = 0.020$). This study has been criticized for adopting the single agent cisplatin in the control arm which was not universally accepted as the standard of care for the management of advanced disease; and for the lack of a clearly defined number of treatment cycles in the protocol. The combination arm patients received a median of six cycles of chemotherapy compared with a median of four cycles in the platinum alone arm, which may be a contributing factor to the difference in survival rates[116]. Moreover, there are reservations in the use of this regimen based on economic evaluation[119].

Radiotherapy has never been evaluated in prospective randomized trials in comparison to chemotherapy or surgery or to best supportive care (as part of combination therapy)[120]. Prophylactic radiotherapy may have a role in prevention of local chest wall deposits after needle aspiration or biopsy.

Management of dyspnoea in MM

Most patients with MM require symptom palliation from the time of diagnosis onwards. The most common symptoms are dyspnoea, chest pain, and cough. Possible causes of dyspnoea in MM include:

- pleural effusion which occurs in 95 per cent of patients and at an earlier stage of disease;

- pleural encasement which causes restrictive lung or trapped lung in severe cases; and

- mediastinal structure invasion, for example, superior vena cava, pulmonary vessels encroachment at later stage of disease.

Pleural effusion is a key management issue in MM. Pleurodesis by medical or surgical approach is effective in preventing fluid accumulation and should be considered as early as possible. With disease progression, presence of trapped lung may preclude pleurodesis.

Various chemical agents have been used for pleurodesis. When using talc poudrage by thoracoscopy, the response rate of 78.8 per cent at 1 month was reported in 88 patients[121]. Another study of 117 patients showed a response rate of 76.2 per cent for oxytetracycline and 76.3 per cent for *Corynebacterium parvum* at 90 days[122]. In a systematic review of chemical pleurodesis for MPE, talc was found to be most efficacious among other sclerosants. Thoracoscopic pleurodesis was also found to be more efficacious compare with tube pleurodesis[106]. However, a randomized control study performed by the Cooperative Group Cancer and Leukaemia Group B showed that both methods of talc delivery are similar in efficacy[123]. A recent study reported a long survival of 26 MM patients who had undergone talc poudrage as a primary therapy. The mean survival was 23.8 ± 16.3 months[124]. This survival benefit of talc pleurodesis awaits confirmation by larger series.

It is interesting to find that in an *in vitro* model, talc induced significant apoptosis in MM cells at a therapeutically achievable concentration (6 mg/cm^2), while talc did not induce apoptosis in pleural mesothelial cells[125].

Pleuroperitoneal shunt has been performed for cases with trapped lung. In the largest series, 36 cases of mesothelioma with trapped lung had undergone this procedure with a median survival of 10.1 months[114]. TPC has been inserted for recurrent symptomatic MPE. In the largest series of 250 cases reported, 29 patients were inserted for pleural effusion of MM. The median survival was 203 days (95 per cent CI, 162–244 days)[126].

Malignant cardiac disease and pericardial effusion

The heart is more often involved by tumour metastasis than as a primary site. Malignant cardiac involvement may also occur as the first presentation of cancer[127,128]. Other causes of cardiac involvement in cancer are related to cancer treatment, including irradiation to mediastinum or to the thyroid, chemotherapy with anthracycline drugs, and immunosuppression predisposing to infective pericarditis. As the gross appearance and biochemistry of the pericardial fluid are not diagnostic, malignancy cannot be excluded by a negative biopsy and cytology.

The reported incidence of cardiac metastases ranged from 2.3 per cent to 18.3 per cent[127]. The heart can be invaded through various routes, namely direct invasion, lymphatic spread, blood dissemination, and intracavitary diffusion through inferior vena cava or pulmonary veins. Retrograde lymphatic spread through tracheal or mediastinal lymph nodes is an important route of spread especially to pericardium. In a large autopsy series of 7289 cancer deaths, cardiac metastases occurred in 9.1 per cent. Among them, pericardium was involved in 69.4 per cent, epicardium in 34.2 per cent, myocardium in 31.8 per cent, and endocardium in only 5 per cent[127]. Lung cancer is often the most common primary reported, accounting for one-third or more of the cases[128,129]. Breast cancer is the second commonest, other common primaries are leukaemia and lymphoma. Melanoma also has a high propensity for metastases to the heart. Adenocarcinoma is the most common cell type, followed by squamous cell carcinoma[127,129].

Pericardial effusion can present with subtle features or as an emergency in case of cardiac tamponade. Cardiac tamponade occurs when the pericardial effusion accumulation compromises the ventricular function causing hypotension and low cardiac output. The enlarged cardiac silhouette can be obscured by concomitant pleural effusion in chest radiograph.

Echocardiogram is an important tool for diagnosis of pericardial effusion, assessment of cardiac function, and guidance of pericardial drainage by catheter insertion with a high success rate[130]. After initial relief of symptoms, prevention of recurrence of pericardial effusion should be contemplated unless a very short life span is anticipated. Recurrence of pericardial fluid after intial tapping was reported to be 21.5 per cent in one series. Independent predictors for recurrence included absence of pericardial catheter for extended drainage, large effusion size, and emergency procedures[130].

Intrapericardial sclerotherapy is a strategy to prevent recurrence. Various sclerosing or cytotoxic agents have been instilled into the pericardial cavity, including doxycycline, minocycline, bleomycin, thiotepa, or radionuclides[131]. When outcome is defined as absence of pericardial effusions at 30 days after drainage, success is observed in 70–90 per cent of all treated patients[131].

Other surgical procedures have been reported to be successful. Subxiphoid pericardiotomy and percutaneous balloon pericardiotomy can be performed under local anaesthesia. Other more invasive surgical procedures, such as rigid pericardioscopy, video-assisted thoracoscopy, pleuropericardiotomy, or pericardectomy require the patient to be haemodynamically stable, and therefore not suitable for rapid relief.

In general, survival of cancer patients after manifestation of pericardial effusion is guarded. The median survival of a cohort of 275 cancer patients with pericardial effusion was 135 days[130]. The underlying disease appears to be a significant factor in determining the prognosis. Patients who had haemodynamic collapse on presentation were reported to perform poorer[130].

There is no consensus on the best modality of treatment for malignant pericardial effusion as there is a lack of randomized controlled trials comparing different approaches. Provision of rapid symptom relief by percutaneous drainage under echocardiographic guidance should always be considered as an initial treatment. Consideration for sclerotherapy to prevent recurrence and for more invasive interventions will depend on the choice and prognosis of patients and the accessibility to various expertise and facilities.

Superior vena cava obstruction

SVCO is a condition in which venous return of blood from the head, upper limb, and thorax to the right atrium is interrupted by obstruction of the SVC, which is situated in a confined space in the superior mediastinum. The incidence of SVCO at the diagnosis of small-cell lung cancer is 10 per cent and for non-small-cell lung cancer 1.7 per cent[132]. The compressing or obstructive lesion can be a tumour arising from the right main or upper lobe bronchus or the bulky mediastinal lymph nodes typically arising from the right paratracheal or pre-carinal stations as in lung cancer, lymphoma or other metastases. Other causes of SVCO include fibrosis, or thrombosis (e.g. due to partial obstruction by tumour, presence of venous catheter, pacemaker wire).

SVCO is usually diagnosed clinically. The severity of clinical features depends on the speed of obstruction. Four patterns of collaterals were described in SVCO, with the azygos-hemiazygos system being the main collateral pathway. Greater degrees of collateral development occur with greater extent of obstruction and concomitant occlusion of the azygos system[133]. The clinical signs and symptoms are the net effect of the venous hypertension, the impairment of venous circulation, the development of venous collaterals, and the underlying pathology[133]. The patient may complain of dyspnoea, cough, orthopnoea, facial oedema, headache, and dizziness. A florid picture may include facial and arm swelling, neck vein distension, upper body plethora, glossal oedema, and cerebral oedema. The features may be alarming and distressing to the patient, but the syndrome itself is usually not life-threatening.

The survival of SVCO is closely related to that of the underlying cancer. Patients with lymphoma and breast cancer survive longer than those with lung cancer[134]. However, in the presence of concomitant compression of trachea, there is a potential threat of MAO[133,134] and could be fatal[135].

Investigations

Chest radiography may show widening of the superior mediastinum and associated pulmonary lesions, and pleural effusion in one-quarter of SVCO. Contrast-enhanced CT especially multi-slice CT[136] and MRI can provide information on the location and extent of occlusion, the mechanism of obstruction, the collateral development; serving as guidance for radiotherapy planning or as baseline for assessment of response to chemotherapy[132]. Venography, mostly carried out as a prelude of stenting, will detect SVC stenosis or occlusion and the extent of thrombus formation.

Treatment

The objective of treatment of SVCO is to relieve the symptoms by reducing the obstruction, which may be mediated or accompanied by reduction in tumour mass. Propping up the patient and an empirical trial of steroid therapy can be considered before other interventions. Radiotherapy or chemotherapy, depending upon the chemo/radiosensitivity, is most commonly used and stent insertion has also emerged as an effective intervention for rapid relief of symptoms.

A systematic review of SVCO in lung cancer identified two randomized trails and 44 non-randomized trials on the treatment of SVCO by steroids, radiotherapy, chemotherapy, and endovascular stent[132]. Among 22 studies, the median survival of patients in chemotherapy/ radiotherapy studies ranged from 2 to 9.5 months. The review reported that chemotherapy and/or radiotherapy relieved SVCO in 77 per cent with SCLC. Of those treated, 17 per cent had a recurrence of SVCO, giving a relapse free rate of 60 per cent. In NSCLC, chemotherapy and/or radiotherapy relieved SVCO in 60 per cent; with 19 per cent of those treated had a recurrence, giving a relapse free rate of 41 per cent. The rates of relief of SVCO were very similar for chemotherapy and for radiotherapy in both cell types; 77 per cent and 78 per cent, respectively, in SCLC and 59 per cent and 63 per cent, respectively, in NSCLC. Effectiveness was not clearly related to any particular radiotherapy fractionation schedule or chemotherapy regimen. Response time reported ranged from 1 to 3 weeks.

For endovascular stenting for treating SVCO in lung cancer, no randomized controlled study was conducted, but 23 small non-randomized studies were identified in a systematic review[132]. The median survival of patients in stent studies ranged from 1.5 to 6.5 months. Insertion of SVC stent relieved SVCO in 95 per cent with 11 per cent of patients developing recurrent SVCO ranging from 3 days to 8 months, with a median of 1–2 months. Relapse in stented patients was often due to stent thrombus but tumour ingrowth was also found. Stent patency was restored by thrombolysis or further stent insertion. This gave a primary patency rate of 84.3 per cent and secondary patency rate of 92.5 per cent. There were variations in the practice of anti-coagulation. Heparin was used during placement in some studies, while warfarin was commenced after placement in others. Higher morbidity rate was associated with administration of thrombolytics. The response to stenting was reported to be immediate for headache, within 24 h for facial oedema, and up to 72 h for oedema of arm or trunk. Stent insertion appears to provide relief in more patients more rapidly.

Outcome of stenting for 40 studies were summarized by another paper[137], these include a technical success rate of 99 per cent (range 95–100 per cent), a clinical success rate of 96 per cent (range 80–95 per cent), a recurrence rate of 13 per cent (range 0–40 per cent), and a complication rate of 5.8 per cent (range 0–19 per cent). Periprocedural or post-procedural complications include SVC rupture, haemorrhage, haemoptysis, epistaxis, pericardial tamponade, cardiac failure, recurrent laryngeal palsy, stent migration, pulmonary embolism, and groin haematoma.

Stenting may evolve as a primary treatment for SVCO, or as secondary treatment for those who fail to respond to chemotherapy or radiotherapy, or who develop recurrence following an initial response to treatment. The application of stenting for SVCO in the terminally ill awaits further study among this group of patients.

Corticosteroids are often given in high doses and in short courses to treat SVCO along with radiotherapy or chemotherapy before their effect takes place. However, systematic review identified no report on its treatment effectiveness[132]. Dexamethasone at a daily dose of 16 mg can be tried empirically, and then gradually tapered.

For patients with SVCO who are too ill for chemotherapy, radiotherapy or stenting, a trial of high dose corticosteroid may be warranted. Cautious use of diuretics may be tried for relieving the symptoms.

Major airway obstruction

MAO is defined here as airway obstruction from the level of the larynx to the level of the lobar bronchi. In advanced cancer, MAO often results from occlusion by endoluminal tumours or extrinsic compression by tumours or mediastinal masses. Other causes include bilateral vocal cord paralysis, stricture as a complication of endobronchial intubation, brachytherapy, or tracheostomy, displacement of tracheostomy tube or stent, retention of sputum, or foreign body.

Dyspnoea, cough, sputum, and haemoptysis are common presenting symptoms. The clinical picture depends on the level of obstruction; it can be that of life threatening respiratory distress with risk of suffocation in case of tracheal obstruction, or masquerading as asthma or COPD in case of lower airway obstruction.

MAO can be distressing and yet potentially reversible. Clinical acuity is crucial in identifying patients at risk. Clinical clues include inspiratory stridor, paradoxical breathing, wheeze poorly responded to bronchodilators, lung collapse or persistent cough with normal chest radiograph. The choice of non-invasive tests include a high kV chest radiograph lung function test (a truncated inspiratory or expiratory flow volume loop in case of upper airway obstruction) and CT of the thorax. Emergency diagnostic or interventional bronchoscopic examination may be life-saving in some situations.

Management

Sputum retention, blockade of airway stent, or kinking of a tracheostomy tube should be looked for. For tumour obstructing airway, the treatment choice depends on its clinical urgency and the performance status of the patient.

In acute situations, endobronchial lesions can be treated by rigid bronchoscopic debulking, laser therapy, and electrocautery; and extrinsic compression by stenting. In sub-acute cases, other endoluminal therapies such as cryotherapy, brachytherapy, and photodynamic therapy, can be considered; but they require longer time to take effect. For extrinsic compression, external irradiation or brachytherapy are alternatives to stenting.

Interventional bronchoscopic procedures

Laser is commonly employed to relieve obstruction due to endoluminal lesion. It provides rapid relief, and can be repeated if indicated. The neodynium–yttrium aluminium garnet (Nd-YAG) laser is most commonly used for tracheobronchial lesions. Contraindications include extrinsic obstruction, coagulation disorders, tumour invading or close to a major vessel. A systematic review reporting four case series (with a total of more than 2500 patients) achieving palliation of dyspnoea in 80 per cent of patients. Success rate was higher in central lesions (70–95 per cent) compared with those with lobal lesions (40–60 per cent), or patients with complete occlusion (57 per cent). The mortality rate was 0.4 to 3 per cent, with a complication rate of 3 per cent. Between 50 and 60 per cent of patients were retreated 3–4 months later, with a median survival of 6 months[138]. For long-standing bronchial obstruction of more than 4–6 weeks, re-expansion of the involved lung is unlikely.

Cryotherapy in advanced cancer is used for relief of obstruction due to endoluminal tumours. A systematic review of three case series (with a total of 411 patients) found that palliation was achieved in 65–68 per cent of patients, with a higher rate of palliation in patients with central lesions (60 per cent) compared with peripheral lesions (35 per cent)[138]. Cryotherapy may be safer than laser for distal lesions in terms of lower risk of perforation and better patient tolerance. However, its effect is not immediate and repeated treatments are often needed.

Endobronchial stents are commonly used in patients with endobronchial obstruction and extrinsic compression. There are two main types of endobronchial stents: the tube silicone stent and the expandable metallic stent. A systematic review of three case series (with a total of 413 patients) found that endobronchial stent provided relief in 90 per cent of patients, of whom the majority were patients with severe airway obstruction from central tumour. Stent migration and mucus retention occurred in 10–20 per cent of patients[138].

Radiotherapy

Radiotherapy is another modality commonly employed for relieving symptoms caused by major airway tumours. A systematic review examined 14 randomized controlled trials (with 3576 evaluable patients) comparing different external palliative radiotherapy regimens for non-small-cell lung cancer[139]. It was found that symptoms improved under all regimens, with no clear additional benefit in giving higher doses. There was strong evidence for a modest increase in survival (5 per cent at 1 year and 3 per cent at 2 years) in patients with localized disease and better performance status. However, regimens with higher doses give more toxicity, especially radiation oesophagitis. It was recommended that patients with locally advanced non-small-cell lung cancer and thoracic symptoms, especially those with poor performance status, should be treated with short courses of palliative radiotherapy (such as 10 Gy in one fraction or 17 Gy in two fractions). Care should be taken to avoid irradiating, or to reduce the dose to the spinal cord if giving 17 Gy in two fractions. Selected patients with good performance status should be considered for treatment with higher dose palliative regimens (such as 36 Gy in 12 fractions), if the chance of a modest increase in survival outweighs the increased treatment burden and toxicity.

Brachytherapy, as given via a fibreoptic bronchoscope, has the advantage of limiting the radiation to the tumour tissue, and may be repeated in case of tumour recurrence or initiated after failure of conventional therapy. Palliation was reported as 69–00 per cent for haemoptysis, 24–89 per cent for dyspnoea, and 24–88 per cent for cough. Brachytherapy can be given alone or in combination with external irradiation, laser therapy, or cryotherapy[140].

A systematic review on the role of high-dose-rate brachytherapy (HDREB) in the palliation of symptoms in patients with non-small-cell lung cancer had included 29 eligible trials[140]. Six randomized trials involved HDREB alone or with external beam radiation therapy (EBR) or laser therapy. EBR alone is more effective than HDREB for symptom palliation in previously untreated patients with endobronchial non-small-cell lung cancer. HDREB with EBR seems to provide better symptom relief than EBR alone. HDREB is recommended for symptomatic patients with recurrent endobronchial obstruction previously treated by EBR, providing it is technically feasible. Median and 1-year survival ranged from 4 to 10 months and from 11 to 38 per cent, respectively. Fatal haemoptysis occurred in 7–22 per cent.

Pulmonary embolism (PE) in cancer patients

Venous thromboembolic disease (VTE) has long been recognized in its association with cancer. Hospitalized cancer patients have four to sevenfold higher incidence of VTE than those without cancer[141]. In a large study in USA on the incidence of VTE in patients hospitalized with cancer between 1979 and 1999, 0.6 per cent of all hospitalizations (40 787 000 discharges) had diagnosis of PE, twice the rates in non-cancer patients[142]. The presence of advanced malignancies and distant metastases increase the risk of VTE[143]. In palliative care setting, thromboembolism was found in 52 per cent of patients[144].

Diagnosis and risk stratification of PE

The goal is to achieve early diagnosis of PE and risk stratification so that appropriate treatment options can be identified. A past history of VTE should raise the alertness. Presenting symptoms may be non-specific, including breathlessness, chest pain, cough, syncope, and haemoptysis; and can be attributed to cancer or concomitant illness[145]. Blood gases, electrocardiogram, and chest radiography are more helpful in excluding other diagnosis than in diagnosing PE. A near normal chest radiograph in the presence of respiratory distress can be suggestive of PE. Clinical prediction scores such as the Wells' clinical prediction score and the revised Geneva score have been developed to assist in clinical assessment of the likelihood of PE. The usefulness and accuracy of these scores as compared with implicit clinical judgement in cancer patients await further evidence.

Helical-computed tomography (hCT) has become the main imaging modality for diagnosis of PE. Single detector hCT was reported to have an accuracy of only 70 per cent, and had been supplemented by compression ultrasonography (CUS) for detection of DVT to increase the yield. The new generation of multi-detector hCT allows thinner collimation of 1–2 mm thickness and detection of emboli in subsegmental pulmonary arteries. In the recent study PIOPED II study on diagnosis of PE in 824 patients, multi-detector hCT gave a sensitivity of 83 per cent and a specificity of 96 per cent. Positive predictive value was up to 95 per cent in the presence of concordant clinical judgement; and sensitivity was increased to 90 per cent when combined with venous phase of hCT in detecting DVT[146].

Risk stratification helps to guide treatment in PE, and echocardiogram is an important non-invasive tool. Dysfunction and dilatation of right ventricle (RV) is a predictor of adverse outcome in PE, and was shown to be associated with higher inpatient mortality as compared with those without RV dysfunction[147]. Cardiac troponins and natriuretic peptides released in proportion to RV dysfunction have emerged as biomarkers[148].

D-dimer lacks its specificity as it is usually elevated in cancer. Pulmonary angiogram is seldom done except for anticipation of catheter-related intervention. Pulmonary radionuclide perfusion scintigraphy is surpassed by hCT as the main imaging tool, but has its role in patients with renal insufficiency or contrast allergy[141].

Management of PE in cancer

1   Prophylaxis of VTE.

2   Detection and risk stratification.

3   Anticoagulation if not contraindicated:
    a   initial heparin and then oral anticoagulation; and
    b   initial heparin and maintained on heparin.

4   In carefully selected cases:
    a   thrombolysis;
    b   embolectomy; and
    c   inferior vena caval (IVC) filter.

Given the propensity of cancer patients to develop VTE, its management in cancer patients should begin with prevention or prophylaxis. The expert panel of National Comprehensive Cancer Network of USA recommended prophylactic anticoagulation for all inpatients with a diagnosis of cancer if not contradindicated[141].

The mainstay of specific treatment of PE is to prevent death and recurrent PE. Most cancer patients will not survive long enough to develop post-thrombotic sequelae. However, in cancer patients with shorter life expectancy, treatment selection may be difficult and limited.

For patients with massive PE, as manifested by right ventricular dysfunction, hypotension or cardiogenic shock, thrombolysis, and embolectomy may provide survival benefit[148]. Patients with PE but with normal haemodynamic status and right ventricular function have good prognosis when treated with anticoagulation alone. For patients with submassive PE, who are normotensive but with evidence of right ventricular dysfunction, the role of thrombolysis is debatable[148].

Anticoagulation

Anticoagulation should be commenced as soon as PE is diagnosed. This will not dissolve the clot, but will prevent propagation. Heparin, either in the form of unfractionated heparin (UFH) or low-molecular-weight heparin (LMWH), is given in the acute stage. LMWH gives a stable and sustainable anticoagulant effect without laboratory monitoring when given once or twice daily. Short acting UFH is the choice if catheter or surgical procedure is contemplated. UFH can be given as body weight adjustment monograms (80 units/kg load, then 18 units/kg/h, target aPTT to 2.0–2.9 of control). LMWH approved by FDA for treatment of PE include: enoxaparin 1 mg/kg twice daily or 1.5 mg/kg once daily (reduce to 1.0 mg/kg once daily if CrCl<30 ml/min); tinzaparin 175 units/kg once daily (dose adjustment for impaired renal function); and fondaparinux 5 mg for patients <50 kg, 7.5 mg for >50 kg but <75 kg, 10 mg for >100 kg (contraindicated in CrCl<30 ml/min and body weight < 50 kg). Dalteparin, as given in 100 mg/kg twice daily or 200 unit/kg daily, has not yet been approved by FDA for treatment of PE.

Switching from heparin to maintenance with oral anticoagulant can be problematic in cancer. Cancer patients, as compared with non-cancer patients, have a threefold higher incidence of recurrent VTE, a 2.5–6 times higher chance of major bleeding even at a similar therapeutic range of anticoagulation. Anticoagulation in cancer also requires more burdensome monitoring as the therapeutic international normalized ratios (INRs) are difficult to achieve[149,150] Concomitant chemotherapy, invasive provedures, hormonal treatment, long-term catheter, poor nutrition infection, impaired liver function are factors complicating the situation.

Maintenance on LMWH instead of switching to oral anticoagulant has its potential merits in advanced cancer patients. It does not require frequent blood monitoring and is not affected by nutrition problems or liver impairment. Several studies have shown therapeutic advantage and safer profile of LMWH over warfarin in cancer patients. The CLOT study found that dalteparin was more effective than oral anticoagulant in reducing the risk of recurrent VTE without increasing the risk of bleeding[151]. Enoxaparin was also found to cause less bleeding than warfarin when used for 3 months in secondary prevention of VTE in cancer patients in another randomized controlled study[152]. LMWH also emerges as an option for abbreviated hospital stay or home treatment of VTE or PE[153].

In view of the continual presence of malignancy as risk factor for VTE in palliative care patients, treatment is often life long if not contraindicated. A quality study reported that LMWH is acceptable to inpatients with advanced cancer receiving palliative care and has a positive impact on overall quality of life[154].

Thrombolysis and embolectomy

Thrombolytic agents, such as urokinase, streptokinase, and tissue-type plasminogen activator (t-PA) may restore patency of pulmonary arteries, and potentially life saving in massive PE with shock or haemodynamic instability. However, its use in unselected PE patients is more debatable[145,155]. Bleeding, which could be intracranial or life threatening, is a risk of concern. In one recent study, the respective bleeding rates were 19.2 and 5 per cent, with cancer as one of the independent predictors of major haemorrhage[156]. Contrary results were, however, reported by the MAPPET-3 study. When comparing t-PA plus UFH with UFH alone in patients with submassive PE, as defined as those who had normal blood pressure but had RV dysfunction, the t-PA plus UFH group had a better outcome with no fatal or intracerebral bleeding. Further evidence is required to support the routine consideration of use of thrombolytics in palliative cancer patients.

Inferior vena caval (IVC) filters

IVC filters are increasingly used in patients with advanced-stage cancer for prophylaxis of PE[157]. The indications of IVC filter include: contraindication to anticoagulation therapy; recurrent VTE despite oral anticoagulation therapy; patient's non-compliance with prescribed anticoagulation; and patients with documented multiple PE[141]. The IVC filter can prevent further migration of thrombus to pulmonary arteries, but cannot prevent further thrombosis. In the 8-year follow up of patients in the PREPIC study, results showed that IVC filters reduced the risk for symptomatic PE, but increased the risk of DVT, and had no effect on survival[158].

Overall, PE poses a diagnostic challenge and a complicated decision-making process in palliative care. Patency of arteries and restoration of haemodynamic status may not necessarily represent a meaningful survival in individual cancer patients, but chances of good survival should not be ignored. Indeed changes in attitude among palliative care workers towards treatment of VTE have been noted. When comparing survey conducted in palliative care units in 2000 and 2005, thromboprophylaxis guidelines were being developed in 19 per cent of units (versus 2 per cent) and only 18 per cent of units surveyed would stop LMWH in a patient already receiving thromboprophylaxis (versus 75 per cent)[159].

Pulmonary lymphangitis carcinomatosis

Pulmonary lymphangitis carcinomatosis is caused by tumour spread through the pulmonary interstitium and lymphatics, often resulting in respiratory failure and cor pulmonale. Spreading can be through the haematogenous route, with microtumour emboli to the lung that subsequently infiltrate through the lung interstitium; or by retrograde spread from tumour-laden hilar lymph nodes; or by local spread from the primary lung tumour. A study of 222 autopsies showed that lymphangitis carcinomatosis was morphologically distinct from arterial tumour embolism, but similar in signs and symptoms, though death from respiratory distress was significantly more frequent in arterial tumour emboli[160]. Lymphangitic carcinomatosis is most commonly seen with adenocarcinoma originating from the lung, breast, gastrointestinal tract, or prostate. Distribution may be bilateral; but it can be presented locally related to a primary lung tumour[54].

Clinical features

Patients can present with non-specifc features of exertional dyspnoea, cough, chest pain, haemoptysis, severe pulmonary hypertension and respiratory failure. Diagnosis is supported by imaging.

Chest radiographic changes are variable, though typically described as widespread linear, micronodular (<3 mm), or reticulonodular interstitial infiltrates. Larger nodules (up to 1 cm) may also be present. Other features reported include Kerley A and B lines, hilar lymphadenopathy, thickening of fissures, perihilar haze, consolidation, reduced lung volume, or a miliary pattern.

High-resolution CT is helpful in differentiating lymphangitis carcinomatosis from other interstitial lung diseases. The characteristic features are smooth or nodular thickening of the interlobular septa and peribronchovascular and subpleural interstitium, with preservation of the normal lung and lobular architecture. Discrete small nodules may also coexist[161]. In a small series,[161] F-FDG PET scan was performed in patients with lung cancer identified as pulmonary lymphangitic carcinomatosis on CT scan, which showed the intensity of uptake in diseased lung is significantly greater than in corresponding normal contralateral lung or in the lungs of normal controls[162].

Treatment

Specific oncological treatment with chemotherapy has been tried with success in patients with sensitive tumours. In a recent report from Japan, patients with advanced adenocarcinoma of lung were treated with tyrosine kinase inhibitor gefitinib, the group presented with lymphangitic carcinomatosis has a high response rate of 50 per cent, with the highest adjusted odd ratios among four factors (lymphangitic carcinomatosis, performance status, female, and never smoker[163]. Survival need to be re-examined in the era of new chemotherapy.

Steroid is commonly prescribed anecdotally for symptomatic treatment of dyspnoea[164]. Dexamethasone can be started empirically in the range of 4–12 mg/day.

Respiratory muscle weakness

Respiratory muscle weakness has been described as the cause of dyspnoea in advanced cancer patients. The National Hospice Study reported 24 per cent of the patients with dyspnoea among 1754 terminal cancer patients, had no identifiable underlying parenchymal, pleural, or other cardiopulmonary disease[57]. It was postulated that dyspnoea in this group might be due to 'debility of terminal cancer' which included general muscle weakness and associated medical complications. Study showing the positive correlation between dyspnoea and poor performance status also suggested that general causes other than local lung or cardiac, might contribute to dyspnoea[58].

In a prospective study on 100 dyspnoeic cancer patients reported by Dudgeon, the median maximal inspiratory pressure (MIP) of −16 cm H_2O was grossly lower than the quoted normal value of −50 cm H_2O[165]. In another prospective study on 144 ambulatory terminally ill cancer patients reported by Bruera, 40 per cent of patients who reported moderate dyspnoea (defined by VAS > 30/100) had normal chest radiography. Multi-variate analysis in patients with moderate to severe dyspnoea demonstrated that anxiety and MIP were independent correlates of the intensity of dyspnoea[51]. The finding suggested the possible contributory role of respiratory muscle weakness in causing dyspnoea.

Respiratory muscle weakness can be assessed by sniff nasal inspiratory pressure (SNIP), as an alternative test to MIP. SNIP was performed in 40 breathless cancer patients with ECOG performance status of 0–2[166]. Patients found SNIP easy to perform. Adjusted for age and sex, the mean maximum SNIP was 51 per cent of predicted. SNIP was weakly but significantly correlated with hand-grip strength, but not with Dyspnoea Exertion Scale, FEV_1, or FVC.

Causes of respiratory muscle weakness

Respiratory muscle weakness can be due to direct effect of cancer cachexia, metabolic and electrolytes inbalance, anaemia, sepsis, and drugs. In a study that explored factors affecting low MIP, it was found that diaphragmatic excursion, haemoglobin, serum phosphate, oxygen saturation, total lung capacity, forced vital capacity, and the predicted vital capacity percentage explained 58 per cent of variance in MIP in the multi-variate model[62]. Anorexia–cachexia syndrome is common in advanced cancer patients with loss of muscle and fat. Steroid myopathy present

acutely after a high dose of steroid, or chronically after prolonged treatment with moderate dosage[167]. In a prospective study of steroid myopathy in cancer patients, nine out of 15 patients developed peripheral muscle weakness. Of these nine patients, eight experienced a significant decline in respiratory function, with symptomatic dyspnoea developing in four. Respiratory muscle weakness could occur when proximal limb muscle remained strong and it could be reversed with the reduction or discontinuation of steroid[168].

Treatment

Evidence of treating respiratory muscle weakness related to cancer process is largely lacking. Potentially reversible causes should be treated, including correction of metabolic and electrolyte imbalance and withdrawal of steroid. Theophylline has been demonstrated to improve respiratory muscle function in patients with COPD but its effect in cancer is unknown. Respiratory support in the form of non-invasive positive pressure ventilation (NIPPV) is an established treatment in neuromuscular conditions.

Infection of the chest

Infection is common among advanced cancer patients. In one study with 1598 hospice patients, 38.9 per cent of patients developed clinical infections[169]. Apart from infection of the urinary tract, the chest is also commonly affected. In one review, 60–72 per cent of patients with infection were treated by antibiotics[170]. However, in another study on palliative car patients largely of Karnofsky Performance Score of ≤ 60, 31 per cent of patients would choose no antimicrobial, and 48.2 per cent would choose antimicrobial for symptomatic use only[171]. Studies have also shown that survival of advanced cancer patients was not affected by the presence of infection or the use of antibiotics[169,171]. Therefore, use of antibiotic for symptom control may become the major indication for the use of antimicrobial for the treatment of infections. Antimicrobial for controlling respiratory symptom in chest infection appears less promising than urinary tract infection, often with less than half of patients with symptoms responded[172]. In specific circumstances, a beneficial role exists for the use of parental antibiotics in palliative care setting[172].

Choice of antibiotic is guided by the predicted organisms and the local antibiotic sensitivity pattern. The most common infected organisms for patients with COPD are *Haemophilus influenzae* and *Streptococcus pneumoniae*, which have an increasing trend of resistance to penicillin. Residents of long-term care facility are commonly colonised by Gram-negative organisms or methicillin-resistant *Staphylococcus aureus*. A study conducted in a palliative care setting of USA, out of 221 episodes of respiratory tract infections, the most common organisms isolated were *Staphylococcus aureus*, *Klebsiella pneumoniae*, and *Pseudomonas aeruginosa*[169].

First-line antibiotics include oral preparations of amoxicillin/clavulanate potassium and quinolones. In case of Gram-negative organisms, fluroquinolone with anti-*pseudomonas* activity, or parental antibiotics like anti-pseudomonal penicillin, third-generation cephalosporin, or aminoglycosides may be considered in special circumstances.

Pulmonary tuberculosis

Presentation of pulmonary tuberculosis may be atypical in patients with advanced cancer. The single most useful test is sputum smear examination for acid-fast bacilli and palliative care units should have access to this test. In situation where multi-resistant tuberculosis is suspected, drug sensitivity testing should be considered for public health purpose.

Anti-tuberculosis treatment is often considered not for the patient's long-term benefit as treatment duration may exceed patient's survival, but for prevention of cross infection. Respiratory isolation for the terminally ill will give extra barrier for end-of-life care. In general, the infectious status will be minimised if the AFB smear is converted to negative status, which often occur with 2–3 weeks of treatment. Treatment regimen should consist of at least three standard antituberculosis drugs, namely isoniazid, rifampicin, and pyrazinamide. In areas where multi-resistant tuberculosis is common, medications should be modified according to the resistance pattern.

Aspiration

Many factors predispose advanced cancer patients to aspiration. These include general factors including old age, impaired conscious level, impaired cough or gag reflex, near-supine position during feeding, and local factors including cranial nerve palsy, structural diseases of larynx and pharynx, for example, head and neck tumour, vocal cord palsy, problems of major airways such as tracheostomy tube, tracheo-oesophageal fistula, and oesophageal or gastric obstruction. Aspiration can give rise to chemical pneumonitis when gastric content is aspirated, pneumonia when colonised oropharyngeal secretion is aspirated or asphyxiation if the airway is obstructed.

Bedside clinical assessment is important. Choking after feeding is a clue, but cough may be absent in those with silent aspiration. Noisy breathing, cough, or dyspnoea at night may be due to accumulation of oropharyngeal secretions due to suppressed cough reflex by sedatives, hypnotics, or opioids. A comprehensive swallowing assessment depends on the asessibility to speech therapist. The golden test of videofluoroscopy is uncommonly performed in palliative care settings.

The following precautions should be taken during oral feeding: adopt an upright position, feed slowly in small bolus, ask patient to tuck the chin to the chest and swallow repeatedly. The food can be prepared in the best consistency as defined by the swallowing assessment. Family members should be educated on the correct method feeding. Failing all these measures, one may have to consider feeding through nasogastric or gastrostomy tube. However, both may not reduce the incidence of aspiration. Aspiration from colonized oral secretions may still occur, so vigorous oral care should be continued. When saliva accumulates in the oropharynx due to a swallowing problem, anticholinergic medications may be given to reduce the secretion.

Preferred antibiotics for aspiration pneumonia involving anaerobic, organisms include β-lactam/β-lactamase inhibitor or clindamycin. For patients who are frail or with a history of repeated hospitalization, coverage for Gram-negative organisms by anti-*Pseudomonas* penicillins and second- or third-generation cephalosporins is recommended.

Miscellaneous syndromes

Other medical causes can also contribute to dyspnoea in cancer patients, including chronic airflow obstruction, arrhythmia, heart failure, anaemia, ascites and metabolic acidosis. Smoking is a common cause for both lung cancer and COPD. A study on newly diagnosed lung cancer patients showed that COPD was present in 72.8 per cent of men and in 52.5 per cent of women[74]. COPD can be diagnosed clinically or aided by a spirometry test in subclinical cases. A value of FEV_1/FVC of <70 per cent indicates airway obstruction. Medications in treating dyspnoea in COPD include short acting inhaled bronchodilators like $β_2$-agonists or anticholinergic ipratropium; long acting bronchodilators like formoterol or salmeterol; and long acting anti-cholinergic tiotropium, and inhalation steroids. Oral theophylline can be effective in relieving dysonoea, with a potential role of enhancing diaphragmatic strength and endurance. However, cautions should be taken for its narrow therapeutic margin, drug interactions, and potential toxicities.

Anaemia from various causes is commonly found in advanced cancer patients. In one study, anaemia of chronic disease was present in 76.7 per cent of women and 46.8 per cent of men; while occult folate deficiency was suggested in 28.6 per cent of patients[173].

Hyperventilation is physiologically defined as breathing in excess of the metabolic needs of the body. It is characterized by tachypnoea with low blood CO_2 level and a normal alveolar–arterial (A-a) oxygen gradient. Central neurogenic hyperventilation has been described in cerebral tumour, especially cerebral lymphoma. Panicky attacks can occur in dyspnoiec patients. Hyperventilation provocation test was positive in 20.9 per cent of cancer patients in one study, indicating the contributory role of hyperventilation in cancer patients with dyspnoea[174].

Symptomatic management of dyspnoea

Non-pharmacological management of dyspnoea

The core concept of non-pharmacological intervention consists of an integrative model in which the psychological experience of breathlessness is considered inseparable from the physical aspects of the symptom. This model of care is based on biopsychosocial care and 'patient-empowerment'. The key intervention strategies consist of detail assessment, psychosocial support, breathing control, and problem-focused, and emotional-focused coping delivered by a multi-disciplinary approach. The success of this model depends on the patent's ability to learn, to cope, and ultimately feel self-empowered to deal with the dyspnoeic episodes.

Non-pharmacological interventions have been proven to be effective by two randomized controlled studies. One was performed in 20 NSCLC patients, and interventions were rovided by a nurse research practitioner over 3–6 weeks, including weekly sessions of counselling, breathing retraining, relaxation, and coping and adaptation strategies[175]. Another study was conducted in 119 patients with lung cancer and mesothelioma[176]. Patients in the intervention group attended a weekly nursing clinic for up to 8 weeks. Interventions provided included: (1) detailed assessment; (2) advice and support provided to patients and families on management of dyspnoea; (3) exploration of the meaning of breathlessness; (4) training in breathing control techniques; (5) goal setting to complement breathing and relaxation techniques and management of functional and social activities; and (6) early recognition of problems warranting pharmacological and medical intervention. The intervention group improved significantly at 8 weeks in 5 of the 11 items assessed: breathlessness at rest, WHO performance status, level of depression, and two Rotterdam Symptom Checklist measures (physical symptom distress and breathlessness).

The experiences of these research works have been translated into practices with the setting up of breathlessness clinic, which is either led by physiotherapist or nurse–physiotherapist collaboration[177,178].

Strategy of non-pharmacological intervention

The clinical framework for assessment of dyspnoea is important as illustrated earlier in this chapter. It is important to document the triggers for breathlessness, including the physical activities, environmental, or emotional factors. The overall strategy of non-pharmacological approach is outlined in Table 11.1.7[179,180].

Psychosocial support and empowerment

Qualitative results from the report of breathlessness clinic showed that several aspects of patient's psychology need to be addressed: (1) trauma of diagnosis; (2) difficulty in adjusting, both to diagnosis and the limitation imposed by breathlessness; and (3) issues related to death[177].

Information giving and education to the disease and underlying causes of breathlessness may alleviate anxieties. Education on medications, equipment and respiratory care will empower the patients and families for self-management. The availability of a home-care team or a 'hot line' service will support the patient when the symptom is at its worst.

Control breathlessness techniques

Controlled breathing techniques include positioning, pursed-lip breathing (PLB), breathing exercises, and coordinated breathing training. Positioning is the simplest and most common adopted strategy to relieve dyspnoea. Classically, the patient is instructed to lean forward with arms bracing, a chair or knees with the upper body supported.

A study on newly diagnosed lung cancer patients showed that COPD was present in 72.8 per cent of men and in 52.5 per cent of women[74]. PLB has frequently been practised by patients with COPD. Patients inhale through their nose for several seconds with their mouths closed; they then exhale slowly for 4–6 s through pursed lips held in a whistling or kissing position. PLB should be performed during exercise and whenever dyspnoea is triggered. PLB can potentially relieve perception of dyspnoea, increase tidal volume, decrease respiratory rate, and improve gas parameters in patients with chronic chest ailments.

Activities or emotions can often precipitate dyspnoeic episodes. A severe dyspnoeic attack can evoke fear and precipitate a respiratory panic attack, as uncoordinated breathing can further worsen ventilation. Training in coordinated breathing during dyspnoeic attacks may be effective in aborting the respiratory panic attack.

Various problem-focused and emotional-focused coping techniques are summarized in Table 11.1.7. Support for respiratory home-care equipments can help patient to cope more effectively at home.

Other non-drug modalities

Cold facial stimulation by a flow of cold air onto the face or using a fan is simple and can be effective[35]. Further, airflow over the face and nasal mucosa during oxygen administration may improve dyspnoea. The use of external nasal dilator strips (ENDS) may improve breathlessness in some cancer patients[181]. Acupuncture was not

Table 11.1.7 Non-pharmacological intervention for dyspnoea in advanced cancer patients.

Intervention goals	Intervention strategy and modalities
Detailed assessment of breathlessness	◆ History, physical examination, and selected investigations
Support for patients and their families on ways of managing breathlessness	◆ Provide information ◆ Psychological support ◆ Home-care support, e.g. respiratory equipment ◆ Breathlessness clinic
Exploring perception of patient and family on breathlessness and their disease	◆ Explore trauma of diagnosis ◆ Explore effects of breathlessness on daily living and social role ◆ Explore anxiety, fear and panic attack associated with breathlessness attack ◆ Work on losses related to disease deterioration and issue related to death
Control breathlessness technique[179]	◆ Posture and positioning ◆ Breathing retraining: pursed-lip breathing, coordinated breathing
Emotional coping during dyspnoea episode	◆ Relaxation technique ◆ Desensitization and guided mastery technique [180]
Problem-focused coping	◆ Exercise training ◆ Training in activities of daily living ◆ Energy conservation techniques ◆ Home environment modification ◆ Arrangement for home respiratory equipment and adaptive device, e.g. oxygen concentrator, portable oxygen, wheelchair ◆ Planning of daily activities
Early recognition of attacks requiring drug or medical intervention	◆ Support from home-care team ◆ Self-management plan

shown to be more effective than placebo in relieving breathlessness in cancer in a randomized controlled trial[182]. Non-invasive ventilation has been used as a palliation treatment of acute respiratory failure in patients with end-stage solid cancer. The causes of acute respiratory failure include COPD exacerbation, pneumonia, heart failure, PE and acute lung injury. At 1 h, NIV significantly improved PaO_2/FiO_2 and Borg dyspnoea score[183]. The role of NIV as a means for dyspnoea palliation remains to be explored.

Oxygen therapy

Hypoxia triggers the sense of air hunger via stimulation of peripheral chemoreceptor. In experimental model, the threshold for triggering air hunger sensation to hypercapnia can be increased by inhaling hyperoxia gas mixture and decreased by inhaling hypoxia gas mixture[33].

Oxygen therapy has been widely used in acute hypoxaemic conditions. Long-term oxygen therapy is derived from studies in patients of COPD who suffered chronic hypoxaemia with the aim to improve long-term survival. Other forms of oxygen therapy are suggested with the aim to decrease dyspnoea or improve exercise capacity. These include: ambulatory oxygen therapy, which is defined as oxygen therapy during exercise; and short-burst oxygen therapy, which is defined as intermittent use of oxygen for relief of breathlessness, before or after exercise. Ambulatory oxygen has been shown to improve dyspnoea and exercise capacity in some COPD patients who presented with significant exercise-induced hypoxaemia[184]. Recent studies on short-burst oxygen therapy in patients with COPD had not confirmed its benefits in the relief of dyspnoea following exercise[185], and improved quality of life and health-care utilization[186].

The goal of oxygen therapy in palliative care setting is mainly for the relief of dyspnoea, and it is often delivered intermittently for this purpose. The other physiological benefits of oxygen such as improvement in neuropsychological function or survival are uncertain in advanced cancer patients. In a study of 100 dyspnoeic cancer patients[165], 40 per cent had hypoxia. It has been shown that dyspnoea in the terminally ill does not correlate with the degree of hypoxaemia[51]. This can be explained by the multiple causes and pathophysiologies of dyspnoea in cancer.

Five randomized controlled studies have been performed to compare the effect of oxygen and air on dyspnoea in advanced cancer patients. Four trials were conducted with patients at rest, and one conducted during exercise. Oxygen therapy had been shown to be effective in a single hypoxaemia advanced cancer patients at rest by the N of 1 randomized controlled trial[187]. Bruera et al. reported a double-blind study on 12 hypoxaemic cancer patients comparing air and oxygen at 5 l/min at rest[188]. Oxygen is significantly better than air in terms of oxygen saturation, respiratory effort, respiratory rate, and the dyspnoea VAS score. Both patients and investigators consistently preferred oxygen to air.

In another single-blind study on 38 patients, Booth et al. reported that air was just as effective as oxygen at 4 l/min in relieving dyspnoea at rest, with significant reduction of baseline dyspnoea VAS score $(p < 0.001)$[189]. However, the improvement with oxygen was quantitatively greater and its effect appeared to carry over into the air phase. The improvement in dyspnoea with oxygen could not be predicted from the baseline hypoxic level. It is noteworthy that only six patients in this study had oxygen saturation below 90 per cent. The authors concluded that air, as well as oxygen, could have a

significant effect in reducing dyspnoea at rest in patients with advanced cancer. Possible mechanisms in play include the airflow produced by nasal prong stimulates nasal receptors or the placebo effect of nasal prong.

Another double–blind, crossover, randomized, controlled study compared the effects of 5 l/min of oxygen versus air in dyspnoeic cancer patients with no hypoxaemia (oxygen saturation >90 per cent at rest)[190]. In 33 evaluable patients, no significant differences were observed between treatment groups in dyspnoea, fatigue, and 6-minute walk test. The authors did not recommend the routine use of oxygen for exercise-induced dyspnoea in cancer patients without hypoxia. However this study had not examined those with borderline saturation at rest who might desaturate with exercise.

A recently conducted randomized, double-blind, crossover trial examined the effect of oxygen versus air on the relief of dyspnoea in 51 advanced cancer patients[191]. Symptoms improved with air and oxygen to similar degree. The subgroup of 17 hypoxic patients did not demonstrate a significant difference in symptom improvement between air and oxygen, though oxygen did improve the oxygen saturation. However, the causes of dyspnoea for patients in this study group were heterogeneous. Cancer was deemed to be solely responsible for the symptom in 29 patients out of 51. The remaining patients had other causes of dyspnoea related either to complications of cancer, such as pneumonia, or to the treatment of cancer, such as radiation pneumonitis. Fifteen patients (29 per cent) had unrelated causes contributing to dyspnoea, including 11 patients with COPD. Further studies are required to explore the efficacy of oxygen in relieving dyspnoea directly related to cancer in hypoxic patients.

Falling short of a unified recommendation on oxygen therapy for dyspnoeic patients with cancer, there are great variations of physicians' practices of prescribing oxygen in palliative care setting[192]. As a practice guideline, dyspnoeic cancer patients with resting oxygen saturation <90 per cent, oxygen therapy can be prescribed as intermittent basis for symptom relief and its effect monitored. Oximeter monitoring may guide the initial titration of the amount of oxygen delivered. However, subsequent routine regular monitoring of oxygen saturation by oximeter is often not warranted, as this may add undue burden to patient, family or staff. In hypoxaemic cancer patients who suffer little dyspnoea, the goal of oxygen therapy has to be clarified, balancing benefit, and burden of treatment. For any dyspnoeic cancer individual who is not hypoxic, oxygen therapy should not be routinely recommended. As oxygen therapy is not without risk, a trial of oxygen or air by the method of N of 1 trial can be considered to document its effect[187]. The patient can put on either air or oxygen sequentially to evaluate its effect in relieving dyspnoea.

Oxygen delivery

Oxygen therapy carries potential risk, burden, cost, and possible psychological dependence to the patient. The patient's abstinence from smoking is a prerequisite for oxygen therapy to avoid fire hazard. Over prescription of oxygen in chronic hypoxaemic patient can suppress hypoxic ventilatory drive resulting in hypercapnia and CO_2 narcosis, especially in COPD patients. When patient develops progressive somnolence despite good oxygenation, oxygen flow should be lowered to maintain the oxygen saturation at around 90 per cent.

Oxygen mask will impede functional activities including speech, communication, or eating. Nasal oxygen cannulae are generally more comfortable and convenient than the oxygen masks. In the case of refractory hypoxia despite high oxygen flow, the effectiveness of oxygen delivery can be enhanced by high flow oxygen bag, or a reservoir cannula (oximizer or oximizer pendant).

The oxygen concentrator is a convenient way of delivering oxygen at home. The flow is usually limited to a maximum of 51/min for most models. An oxygen cylinder is an alternative when the oxygen concentrator is not readily available. A portable cylinder enables patient to continue with some outdoor activities.

Opioids for symptomatic management of dyspnoea

Mechanisms of opioids on dyspnoea

The presence of opioid terminals and neuronal bodies in the respiratory nuclei strongly suggests that endogenous opioid has a modulatory role in the function of the nuclei. Opioid receptors are found in high densities in the brain stem. The mu receptor clearly has an inhibitory influence on respiration, the delta receptor has a modest effect, the kappa has little, and the sigma receptor may stimulate respiration[193]. Opioid receptors, the conventional (μ, κ, δ) and the non-conventional ones, are also found widely distributed in the lung.

Exogenous opioids have been used for reducing dyspnoea, but the exact site of action is unknown. A central site of action is likely. Administration of exogenous opioid leads to a dose-dependent reduction in minute ventilation leading to increase in PCO_2 and a depression of the ventilatory response to CO_2 demonstrated by displacement of the CO_2 response curve to the right, or reduction in slope, or both[193]. In animal study of newborn rat brainstem-spinal cord preparations, Mu- and kappa-opioid receptor agonists caused reduction of final motor outputs by mainly inhibiting medullary inspiratory neuron network[194]. This inhibition of inspiratory neurons seems to be a result of both a presynaptic and post-synaptic inhibition. The central respiratory rhythm as reflected by the preinspiratory neuron burst rate was essentially unaltered by the agonists. Opioid induced breathing depression is caused by direct inhibition of rhythm-generating respiratory neurons in the Pre-Böetzinger complex (PBC) of the brainstem. It was found that serotonin 4(a) [5-HT$_4$(a)] receptors are strongly expressed in respiratory PBC neurons and that their selective activation protects spontaneous respiratory activity. Treatment of rats with a 5-HT$_4$ receptor-specific agonist overcame fentanyl-induced respiratory depression and reestablished stable respiratory rhythm without loss of fentanyl's analgesic effect[195].

In another clinical trial involving nine advanced emphysema patients, epidural methadone perfusion at thoracic level had effectively palliated dyspnoea, improved exercise capacity, and quality of life[196]. $PaCO_2$ also decreased after 1 week of treatment. There was no demonstrated effect on ventilatory control and respiratory perception. The overall pattern of response to epidural methadone is compatible with a change in the operating lung volumes in these hyperinflated COPD patients. It was speculated that reduction in the reflex activation of the intercostal muscles due to an interruption in the local spinal reflexes that are mediated at the level of the posterior horn cells, which could have increased the compliance of the chest wall muscles and allowed the end-expiratory lung volume to fall. Alternatively, the fall in respiratory frequency may promote better lung emptying and a fall in operating lung volume.

Opioid receptors are located throughout the respiratory tract, in most abundance within the alveolar walls, and less lining the

smooth muscle within the trachea and main bronchi. In addition to μ, δ, and κ opioid receptors, 'non-conventional' opioid binding sites have been suggested, although the function of opioid receptors in the pulmonary tract is not known[197]. Recent studies on peripheral acting mu-selective opioid receptor agonist frakefamide may help in exploring the role of peripheral opioid receptors. In a double-blind, randomized, double dummy four-way crossover study in 12 healthy male subjects, the effects on resting ventilation of frakefamide and two dose levels of morphine were compared with placebo[198]. During resting ventilation, frakefamide, unlike morphine, did not cause central respiratory depression. In another similar trial, a double-blind, randomized, double-dummy, four-way, crossover study was conducted to investigate the effects of frakefamide comparing with morphine and placebo on hypercarbic and hypoxic ventilation[199]. There were no ventilatory effects caused by frakefamide or placebo, whereas large doses of morphine influenced both hypercarbic and hypoxic ventilatory responses. Earlier study on inhaled morphine bioavailability varied from 9 to 35 per cent, with a mean of 17 per cent[200]. However, recent conducted studies via advanced pulmonary delivery system designed to deliver bolus aerosols of drug to the peripheral lung efficiently, have shown new understanding on the pharmacokinetics of inhaled opioid[201]. These studies showed that the time courses of plasma concentration after pulmonary delivery and by intravenous infusion were similar. The absolute bioavailability of aerosol-delivered morphine was approximately 100 per cent with similar inter-subject variability in area-under-curve for both routes of administration. Therefore in studies conducted on nebulized opioid, data on systemic bioavailability of the nebulized route or different pulmonary delivery system is required for interpretation. For the study of the role of peripheral opioid receptors in controlling dyspnoea, a pure peripheral opioid receptor agonist may be the drug of choice.

Clinical studies on opioids for relieving dyspnoea

There were two placebo, randomized, controlled studies conducted in cancer patients with dyspnoea and both showed improvement of dyspnoea to subcutaneous injection of morphine[202,203]. One study used 50 per cent higher than the regularly scheduled dose[202] and the other used 5 mg in opioid-naïve patients or 50 per cent on top of the regularly scheduled dose[203]. A systematic review was conducted on the use of opioids in the management of dyspnoea[204]. It included nine placebo-controlled studies of oral or parenteral opioids; with one study performed in patients with cancer, one performed in patients with heart failure, and seven performed in patients with COPD. All included small samples, with the largest consisting of only 19 patients, and the total number of patients included in the oral or parental studies was 116. There were three studies on the use of nebulized opioids, with one study performed in cancer, two studies performed in patients with chronic lung diseases. The studies were again small in size, with the largest consisting of only 79 patients, and the total number of patients was 106. Meta-analysis of the nine non-nebulized studies showed a highly significant result in reducing dyspnoea ($p = 0.0006$) with a standardized mean difference of −0.40 (the standardized mean difference can be converted to units of visual analogue scale or Borg scale by multiplying the standard deviation for a particular study) (95 per cent CI: −0.63 to −0.71). However, the clinical effect of oral and parental opioids appears to be small. Possible reasons to account for this finding include: the opioid doses were relatively small in some of the studies; the doses were not titrated in any of the studies; the dosing intervals were probably too long in some of the studies; and the opioids would not have reached steady state in the single dose studies. The review found no significant effect of nebulized opioids in relieving dyspnoea ($p = 0.31$), with a standardized mean difference of −0.11 (95 per cent CI: −0.32 to 0.10). There was no evidence to indicate that the use of opioids was associated with a deleterious effect on arterial blood gases or oxygen saturation in the patient populations studied. Suggested possible mechanisms of action of opioids include reduction in the central perception of dyspnoea, reduction in anxiety associated with dyspnoea, reduction in sensitivity to hypercapnia, reduction in oxygen consumption, and improved cardiovascular function[204].

Subsequent to this review, another randomized, double-blind, placebo-controlled, crossover study of oral morphine on 38 patients with predominantly COPD was reported[205]. Patients were randomized to 4 days of 20 mg oral morphine with sustained release followed by four days of identically formulated placebo, or vice versa. The results showed that sustained release morphine was superior to placebo in diminishing dyspnoea. This confirms the result of the systematic review, and is the first adequately powered randomized controlled trial showing the efficacy of oral morphine for relieving dyspnoea.

Another double-blind, randomized cross-over controlled trial was conducted comparing the effects of nebulized versus subcutaneous morphine for patients with cancer dyspnoea[206]. Patients were recruited if they had dyspnoea related to advanced cancer with predominantly restrictive ventilation and a resting dyspnoea intensity of at least 3 on a 0–10 scale. In addition to patients' regularly scheduled opioid dose, eligible patients were randomly assigned to receive half of their scheduled equivalent opioid dose, either in the form of subcutaneous injection or nebulization. Eleven patients completed the study. Dyspnoea decreased from a median of 5 (range, 3–8) to 3 (range, 0–7) after SC morphine ($p = 0.025$) and from 4 (range, 3–9) to 2 (range, 0–9) after nebulized morphine ($p = 0.007$). There was no significant difference in dyspnoea intensity between nebulized and subcutaneous morphine at 60 min. However, there was insufficient power to rule out a significant difference between both routes of administration. Results showed that nebulized morphine offered dyspnoea relief similar to that of subcutaneous morphine. However, these results may not be generalizable to patients with more severe respiratory distress. This study differed from previous studies with nebulized opioids studies in that a larger opioid dose was used. The exact role of nebulized opioids in dyspnoea control warrants further research.

Ethical issues involving safety of taking opioids and acceptance by patient, family or health-care staff, are issues of concern. A study performed in Taiwan showed that using morphine for dyspnoea, both on admission and in the 48 h before death, did not significantly influence the patients' survival. Positive ethical acceptability and satisfaction with using morphine for dyspnoea control were found in both medical staff and family[207].

Clinical use of opioids

The best available evidences support the use of systemic opioids in the form of oral or subcutaneous morphine injection for relieving dyspnoea in cancer patients[204,205]. Use of nebulized opioid is not supported by the systematic review[204]. However, with a recent

randomized controlled study showing a similar efficacy of nebulized morphine to subcutaneous morphine[206], it is recommended that nebulized opioid should be used in trial setting.

Case reports and randomized controlled studies have reported the usefulness of 25–50 per cent of the 4-hourly opioid dose for dyspnoea control. In a dosage comparison study comparing 25–50 per cent of the 4-hourly opioid dose for dyspnoea in terminally ill cancer patients, patients showed similar preference to either 25 or 50 per cent of regular morphine dose[208]. Therefore for patients who are on regular morphine for pain control, a dosage of 25–50 per cent on top of the regularly 4-hourly analgesic dose is recommended for relieving dyspnoea. The dosage can be titrated up according to clinical response. For opioid-naïve patient, a small dose of 2.5–5 mg oral morphine prn is recommended as a trial, with the efficacy and side effects carefully monitored. A monitoring chart which records the respiratory rate and level of consciousness regularly is helpful. If more than 2–3 prn doses of morphine are required for dyspnoea control within 24 h, regular morphine can be considered. The choice of regimen (i.e. intermittent or regular) depends on the profile of the dyspnoeic episodes of individual patients. Other than morphine, there is no randomized controlled study documenting the efficacy of other opioids for controlling dyspnoea in cancer patients. The use of oral transmucosal fentanyl citrate was reported to be helpful in the management of dyspnoea crisis in anecdotal report[209].

Other drugs for symptomatic management of dyspnoea

Anxiolytics and tranquillizers

Anxiety and panic disorder appear to be more common in patients with respiratory diseases[210]. Hyperventilation syndrome was reported to be common in advanced cancer patients[174]. However, the role of anxiolytics and tranquillizers in dyspnoea relief in relation to these findings is not certain. Use of sedatives in palliative sedation is discussed in a separate section, as palliative sedation has its own clinical and ethical consideration. Several small-scale controlled studies performed in COPD and in healthy volunteers gave inconsistent results and anxiolytics were generally poorly tolerated[25]. The report on the use of chlorpromazine in controlling dyspnoea and restlessness in the advanced cancer patients was anecdotal[211]. One recent study reported the effective use of subcutaneous midazolam as adjunct therapy to morphine in the alleviation of severe dyspnoea in cancer patients. These patients had anxiety level correlated with their degree of dyspnoea. However, patients were recruited when life expectancy is limited to <1 week[212]. More research is needed to establish the role of tranquillizers in the control of dyspnoea.

Other potential drugs

Stimulation of cold receptor of the upper airway with nasal inhalation of l-menthol was shown to reduce sensation of respiratory discomfort associated with loaded breathing in normal subjects[213]. There are anecdotal reports on the successful use of inhaled furosemide in relieving dyspnoea in cancer patients[214,215]. In a randomized, double-blind, crossover, placebo-controlled study, Inhaled aerosolized furosemide (40 mg) reduced air hunger in normal subjects[216]. In another double-blind, randomized, crossover study, inhaled furosemide reduced dyspnoea induced by constant-load exercise in stable COPD[217].

In a phase II double-blind, randomized, crossover, controlled study comparing Heliox28 (72 per cent He/28 per cent O_2) with oxygen-enriched air (72 per cent N_2/28 per cent O_2) on dyspnoea in lung cancer. Heliox 28 was shown to be more effective than oxygen-enriched air in improving oxygen saturation, exercise capacity and dyspnoea scores[218].

Cough in cancer patients

Prevalence of cough

Cough is the forceful expiration of air with a partially closed glottis that produces a noise. Cough has a prevalence of 47–86 per cent in lung cancer and 23–37 per cent in general cancer patients. Cough of moderate to severe intensity occurred in 13 per cent of general cancer patients[49,84] and in up to 48 per cent of lung cancer patients[54,55]. Cough was also the most frequent symptom in very young and very old patients with non-small-cell lung cancer[219].

Neurophysiology of the cough reflex

Our current understanding of the afferent neuronal pathways regulating the cough reflex is derived almost entirely from animal studies. Afferent pathways that innervate respective sites (airway and pleural, external auditory canal, pharynx, larynx, stomach, heart, and oesophagus) are transmitted mainly via the vagus nerve, and the afferent signals are integrated at the brainstem in the nucleus tractus solitarius. Input from the higher cortex is likely as cough can be voluntarily suppressed or initiated. The motor efferent then goes from the ventral respiratory group/Bötzinger complex neurons to the inspiratory and expiratory muscles through the phrenic and other spinal motor nerves, and to the larynx and bronchial tree through the recurrent laryngeal branches of the vagi.

There are two types of vagal-mediated afferent nerve innervating the airway: low threshold mechanosensors and chemosensors. Two classic types of low threshold mechanosensors have been described in the mammalian intrapulmonary airways, namely the rapidly adapting receptors (RARs) and slowly adapting receptors (SARs). Airway chemosensors are the C-fibre and Aδ-fibre, both resided at intrapulmonary and extrapulmonary airways[220]. The capsaicin receptor, the transient receptor potential vanilloid (TRPV-1) was recently cloned[221]. Recent studies in guinea pigs also support the notion of 'cough receptors', which are found primarily in the extrapulmonary airways (i.e. larynx, trachea, and mainstem bronchi) where cough is most readily initiated. The putative cough receptors, unlike RARs, are unresponsive to a wide variety of spasmogens that induce airway smooth muscle contraction. Unlike C-fibres, it is myelinated, unresponsive to capsaicin, bradykinin, or hypertonic saline solution, and do not express TRPV-1[222].

It is postulated that the basic primary defensive cough pathway (i.e., uncontrollable cough in response to an acute stimulus such as aspiration) is likely mediated primarily by extrapulmonary low threshold mechanosensors (cough receptors). However, cough associated with airways obstruction or more chronic airway irritation may involve the recruitment of other afferent (RAR and/ or chemosensor) pathways[221].

RARs can be defined as dynamic receptors that respond to changes in airway mechanical properties. RARs are insensitive to many 'direct' chemical stimuli, however, activated by stimuli that evoke bronchospasm or obstruction resulting from mucus secretion or oedema. Substances such as histamine, capsaicin, substance P, and bradykinin activate RARs can be markedly inhibited by preventing the local end-organ effects that these stimuli produce (e.g. bronchospasm and mucus secretion)[222]. The majority of afferent nerves innervating the airways and lungs are unmyelinated C-fibres. Airway C-fibres are relatively insensitive to mechanical stimulation. C-fibres are further distinguished from RARs by their direct activation by bradykinin and capsaicin, not indirectly through effects on smooth muscle or the airway vasculature[222].

Cough can be triggered indirectly by C-fibre via interacting with RARs. C-fibre can interact peripherally via axon reflex-dependent activation of RARs, or interact centrally by acting synergistically with RARs at nucleus tractus solitarius at the level of brainstem[222].

Physiology of cough

Cough efficiency relies on the adequate tidal volume, high expiratory pressure, and airflow velocity generated to expel mucus and droplets, which in turn depends on the optimal function of the respiratory muscles, closure of the glottis, dynamic compression of the major airways, the mucus properties, and mucociliary clearance. However, in cancer patients, cough can be ineffective for various reasons (Table 11.1.8).

Causes of cough in cancer patients

Chronic cough in the general population is due to multiple causes in up to 93 per cent. In cancer, it is likely that multiple causes and hence multiple mechanisms are responsible[223] (Table 11.1.9).

Assessment of cough in cancer patients

History, physical examination, and chest radiograph are important in identification of the cause of the cough. A diagnostic protocol based on the anatomical distribution of cough receptor afferent nerves may be helpful. The history should include assessment of frequency, severity, provocative factors, associated chest symptoms like appearance of sputum, and impact of daily activities. Cough is a distress to patient by causing exhaustion, sleep disturbances, and social inconveniences.

However, few studies have quantitatively examined the distress caused by cough in cancer patients. Lack of standardized assessment tool is an issue. Currently, there are three cough-specific health-related quality-of-life questionnaires developed: cough-specific quality of life questionnaire (developed in USA), the Leicester cough questionnaire (developed in UK), and the chronic cough impact questionnaire (developed in Italy). Recently, a disease specific 'Lung Cancer Cough Questionnaire' was validated for self evaluation of cough occurrence, frequency and severity and its impact[224].

Management of cough in cancer

Cough as a defence mechanism to prevent entry of noxious materials into the respiratory system and clears foreign materials and excess secretions from the respiratory tract and should generally be encouraged. It is pathological when it is ineffective and causing distresses. Clinically it is important to differentiate the wet cough serving to clear up airway secretions from a dry cough resulting from irritations. The following approach to the management of cough is suggested: (1) identify and treat the underlying cause of the distressing cough (Table 11.1.10), although the search for a specific cause in advanced cancer patients may be limited by the burden of investigations; (2) enhance expectoration of sputum or secretions if present (see section on airway secretion); (3) suppress cough if

Table 11.1.8 Factors leading to ineffective cough in cancer patients.

Muscle factor	General debility	Anaemia, weakness, impaired conscious level
	Weakness of respiratory muscles	Cachexia syndrome, steroid myopathy
	Neurological problem	Brain metastasis, spinal cord compression
	Ineffective use of respiratory muscles	Weakness of abdominal muscles, gross ascites, hepatomegaly
Airway factor	Vocal cord problem	Paralysis
	Non-compressible airway	Tumour, stent insertion
Mucus factor	Reduction of water content of mucus	Reduced fluid intake, effect of drugs
Mucociliary factor	Impaired mucociliary function	Airway diseases

there is little airway secretion, the above manoeuvres fail, or the symptom is too distressing. Specific oncological treatments include radiotherapy and endobronchial treatment for tumours causing cough (see section on MAO). Single new chemotherapeutic agent like gemcitabine alone with relatively lower toxicity profile has been shown to decrease cough in patients with non-small-cell lung cancer[225].

Agents used for suppressing cough in cancer

Two classes of antitussive drugs are available: (1) centrally acting, opioid and non-opioid (2) peripheral acting, directly and indirectly.

Availability of antitussive varies in different places of the world. Many antitussives, such as codeine, hydrocodone, and dextromethorphan, have been extensively studied in the acute and chronic cough settings for their efficacy and safety profiles. The drugs that have been specifically studied in cancer are hydrocodone, dihydrocodeine, levodropropizine, benzonatate, and sodium cromoglycate.

Centrally acting drugs

Opioids Opioids have been long advocated for the suppression of cough. Its cough suppression action has been shown to be mediated

Table 11.1.9 Causes of cough in cancer.

Cancer unrelated	Cancer related
Heart failure	Major airway or endobronchial lesions
Asthma	Lung parenchymal infiltration
Chronic bronchitis	Pleural disease—effusion, mesothelioma
Bronchiectasis	Pericardial effusion
Post-nasal drip syndrome (PNDS)	Mediastinal involvement
Gastro-oesophageal reflux (GERD)	Lymphangitis carcinomatosis
Post-infectious	Aspiration (e.g. head and neck tumour, tracheo-oesophageal fistula, vocal cord paralysis)
Drugs: angiotensin-converting enzyme inhibitor (ACEI),	
Eosinophilic bronchitis	Radiation-induced fibrosis
	Chemotherapy-induced fibrosis
	Pneumonia
	Microembolism

through mu, kappa, delta, and sigma receptors[226]. Codeine is widely perceived as the 'gold standard' cough suppressant drug due to its efficacy in animal models and in several older studies in humans. Dextromethorphan, the most common over-the-counter antitussive in the USA, has also been shown to be effective in patients with chronic bronchitis in a placebo-controlled study[227]. Contradictory to earlier reports and the wide spread perception, recent double-blind, placebo-controlled studies showed that codeine was no more effective than placebo in reducing cough in healthy subjects[228], patients with upper respiratory tract infection[229], and COPD[230]. Similarly, the effectiveness of dextromethorphan was also not confirmed by study[231]. The causes of these discrepancies are not entirely known. Workers have postulated the existence of a complex hierarchical control system that regulates the expression of coughing. This system, known as a holarchy, is composed of regulatory elements known as 'holons' that interact with one another to regulate cough. Based on work in animal models, codeine is proposed to act on an intermediate order holon that may not be critical for coughing under some situations in humans[232].

Codeine and derivatives Experience of codeine on cough suppression is based on its use in non-cancer patients. Codeine has an antitussive action lasting for 4 h following oral administration. The elimination half-life is 2.5–4 h. Codeine is a prodrug that is metabolized by liver to morphine, norcodeine, normorphine, and hydrocodone. The usual adult antitussive dosage is 10–20 mg every 4–6 h administered orally, with a daily dose no higher than 120 mg[223]. Codeine can also be administered as intramuscular and subcutaneous injections.

Hydrocodone is a codeine derivative, with a molecular structure similar to hydromorphone and naloxone. The antitussive duration of action is 4–6 h following oral administration. The elimination half-life is 3.8 h, with hydromoprhone as one of the metabolites. The usual adult antitussive dose is 5–0 mg every 4–6 h administered orally, with a daily dose no higher than 60 mg[223]. In a phase II dose-titration study of 25 patients with advanced cancer who had cough, 5 mg of hydrocodone was administered twice daily[233].

Table 11.1.10 Specific treatment of cough.

Lung parenchymal tumour	Radiotherapy, chemotherapy, steroid
Endobronchial tumour	Endobronchial therapy: brachytherapy, laser, cryotherapy
Tracheo-oesophageal fistula	Stent insertion
Lymphangitis carcinomatosis	Steroid
Post-irradiation lung damage	Steroid
Pleural and pericardial effusion	Fluid aspiration
Aspiration pneumonia	Prevention of aspiration, antibiotics
Congestive heart failure	Diuretics
Asthma	Bronchodilators, steroid
Post-nasal drip syndrome (PNDS)	Antihistamine
Gastro-oesophageal reflux (GERD)	H2 blocker, proton pump inhibitor, diet modification
Eosinophilic bronchitis	Steroid

The dose was increased daily until there was an improvement of ≥50 per cent in the frequency of cough and then was maintained for 3 consecutive days. The median best response was 70 per cent in cough frequency, which was achieved with a median hydrocodone dose of 10 mg/day (range 5–30 mg/day).[223] Cough severity, frequency, associated symptoms and complications, and activities of daily living improved significantly. Side effects of hydrocodone (dry mouth, nausea, and drowsiness) were tolerable and rated as mild.

Dextromethorphan Experience of dextromethorphan is based on its use in non-cancer patients. Dextromethorphan is the methyl ether of the dextrorotatory form of levorphanol. It has been shown to be an effective antitussive in randomized controlled trials, but tends to cause fewer side effects on the gastrointestinal tract and the central nervous system[234]. Dextromethorphan acts on sigma opioid receptor and is a non-competitive antagonist of the NMDA receptors in animal models. The antitussive action is via central or peripheral sigma receptors as shown in guinea pig experiment[235]. Its antitussive action can be reverted by haloperidol, a non-selective sigma antagonist[236]. Dextromethorphan is not associated with addiction potential. The antitussive duration of action is 3–6 h following oral administration. It is metabolized in the liver by the cytochrome P450 isoform CYP2D6. It is administered orally as 10–20 mg every 4–6 h, with the total daily dose not to exceed 120 mg[223]. Drug interaction is an issue, and serotonergic syndrome was reported when dextromethorphan was combined with paroxetine.

Morphine In a recent double-blind, placebo-controlled study in patients with chronic persistent cough of more than 3 months' duration who failed to respond to specific measures, morphine sulfate has shown to be an effective antitussive in intractable chronic cough at the doses of 5–10 mg twice daily. Results showed that there was significant improvement of 3.2 points over baseline on the Leicester Cough Questionnaire, and a rapid and highly significant reduction by 40 per cent in daily cough scores among patients who have taken slow-release morphine[237].

Other opioids It is often said all opioids have antitussive activity, but none has been studied specifically in cancer-related cough. Clinical experiences show that heroin, hydromorphone, levopropoxyphene, methadone, oxycodone, and pholcodine, all have an antitussive action.

Use of opioids in cough The recommendation of clinical use of opioid in cough is based on empirical experience. If the patient is opioid naïve, start with a weak opioid such as codeine. If codeine is ineffective, consider a shift to morphine. The starting dose of morphine in opioid naïve patient is 2.5 mg 4 hourly and as required. If morphine has been prescribed for pain control, do not use codeine for cough. Morphine can be given as required dosage for controlling cough, and the total dose given over 24 h can be calculated and add to the regular 4 hourly morphine dose. Repeat this process every 1–2 days until the cough is controlled.

Non-opioids centrally acting drugs There are more than 10 non-opioids centrally acting drugs available mainly in European countries. Clobutinol is one of the drugs that commonly used as antitussive. Its experience for controlling cough in cancer patients is uncertain.

Peripheral acting drugs

Benzonatate This is a peripheral acting drug related to the local anaesthetic group of procaine, which dampens the activity of the stretch receptors. Benzonatate acts in 15–20 min and its effect can last for 3–8 h. Doses of 100–200 mg tid have been used as for cough when hydrocodone failed[238]. The patient should be instructed not to chew the capsule to avoid local anaesthetic effect in the oropharynx.

Levodropropizine Levodropropizine, like benzonatate, acts on the periphery by modulation of C fibre activity. In one multi-centre, parallel group, randomized, double-blind controlled study comparing levodropropizine (75 mg tid) and dihydrocodeine (10 mg tid) for treatment of cough in lung cancer, both were equally effective in controlling cough, but somnolence was significantly less in the levodropropizine group (8 versus 22 per cent)[239].

Sodium cromoglycate Sodium cromoglycate is believed to have an inhibitory action on C fibres. In a double-blind, randomized controlled trial, sodium cromoglycate given at 2 puffs bid (total 40 mg/day) significantly reduced cough in lung cancer patients without significant side effects[240].

Lignocaine (lidocaine) Lignocaine has been reported to be useful in preventing cough during bronchoscopy and other surgical procedures. Inhaled lignocaine in the dose of 20 mg and 40 mg were reported to suppress capsaicin-induced cough in healthy volunteers[241,242]. The action of inhaled lignocaine is often transient, with side effects of oropharyngeal numbness, possible lead to bronchospasm and risk of systemic toxicity if patient is given a too high dosage. This should only be given with caution when other treatment failed. Some workers would use 5 ml of 2 per cent lignocaine up to 6-hourly, or 5 ml 0.25 per cent (12.5 mg) bupivacaine up to 8-hourly. Before giving nebulized lignocaine, it is recommended to pretreat with salbutamol because of the risk of bronchospasm. Patients should be advised to stop oral intake, preferably 4 h before, and for a minimum of 2 h afterwards, or till the local anaesthetic effect wears off.

Other agents

Menthol which stimulates the cold receptor is a commonly used ingredient in many over the counter cough remedies. Its efficacy in cough suppression had been demonstrated in citric acid induced cough in normal subjects[243] and guinea pigs[244]. There are anecdotal reports on the usage of gabapentin and paroxetine in opioid resistant chronic cough[245,246]. There is a growing interest in the development of new group of drugs for cough, with more exploration of underlying neurophysiology of cough. These include new opioids, neurokinin receptor anagonists, bradykinin receptor anagonists, transient receptor potential vanilloid (TRPV-1) blockers, and potassium channel openers.

Airway secretion in cancer patients

Airway secretions are produced from two sources, salivary gland and bronchial mucosa. In cancer patients, airway secretion can be classified as: (1) airway secretions that occur during the terminal phase of cancer that commonly called 'death rattle', (2) airway secretions that are generated from underlying airway or pulmonary pathology that occur during any phase of the disease. The first type is labelled by some workers as 'real' death rattle or 'type I' rattle, whereas the second type as 'pseudo' death rattle or 'type II' rattle[247,248,249].

It is hypothesized that the 'type I' rattle is caused by the combined syndromes of aspiration of predominately saliva due to dysphagia and the inability to expectorate; whereas the 'type II' rattle is caused by predominately bronchial secretions that caused by airway or pulmonary pathology and the inability to expectorate[248]. These can be due to non-malignant causes like chronic bronchitis, bronchiectasis and pulmonary oedema, or malignancy-related causes like tumour in the lung, infection, tracheo-oesophageal fistulae, and bleeding. In a prospective study of 310 terminally ill cancer patients, bronchial secretions were observed in 41 per cent in the final 3 weeks of life, with 4.5 per cent classified as severe (clearly audible at about 6 m, or at the door of the room)[248]. Multiple logistic regression analyses showed that the determinants of the development of bronchial secretion were primary lung cancer, pneumonia, and dysphagia; there were no significant effects of severity of oedema and pleural effusion[248]. 'Real' death rattle is a strong predictor of death, with 76 per cent died within 48 h of onset reported in one study[249].

Excessive airway secretion affects cancer patients by interfering normal sleep, inducing cough, predisposing to infection, and increasing dyspnoea by further compromising the airway. The embarrassment on the airway depends on the physical properties of the secretion, including volume and tenacity. These vary from the tenacious or inspissated sputum in the dehydrated and debilitated terminally ill, to the very watery voluminous secretion in bronchorrhoea.

Death rattle is often perceived as a distress to relatives. However, recent studies showed that at least half of the relatives interviewed were not distressed by the sound; some even found it helpful, as a warning sign of impending death[250,251]. Moreover, the interpretation of the sound by relatives was influenced by the patient's appearance, being less concerned if the patient was not obviously disturbed. Relatives were distressed when they thought that when the sound of death rattle indicated the patient might be drowning or choking. Skilful communication should enable health professionals to check out relatives' interpretation and fantasies when they hear the sound of death rattle.

Management of death rattle

Positioning of patient in comforting position and gentle suction of secretion may be helpful. Low dose of anti-muscarinics will readily inhibit salivary secretion. As non-muscarinic mechanisms play an important role in regulating baseline bronchial secretions, the clinical effects of anti-muscarinics drugs on bronchial secretion will be less than on salivary secretions. Bronchial secretions that occur in response to vagal stimulation are only inhibited by high dose anti-muscarinics.

A systematic review showed that about three quarters of patients with death rattle received anti-muscarinic drugs and beneficial responses were observed in 80 per cent. About 20 per cent of patients who do not benefit from anti-muscarinics are possibly due to bronchial secretions resulting from pulmonary pathology like infection or pulmonary oedema[252]. Experiences on anti-muscarinic drugs are mostly based on single dose studies. In volunteers, both parental hyoscine butylbromide and hyoscine hydrobromide gave a rapid onset of action [about 30 min after intramuscular (IM)

injection] but with short duration of effect (<1 h for hyoscine butylbromide and 2–3 h for hyoscine hydrobromide). The peak effects of IM or SC glycopyrronium occurred after 1–2 h and were dose dependent, with 50 per cent decrease in salivary secretions still apparent at 6 h post-injection. In one study, SC hyoscine hydrobromide 400 mcg was demonstrated to be more effective in symptom control at 30 min than glycopyrronium 200 mcg, but no significant difference in improvement at 1 h, or at the last record before death[253]. Another study comparing glycopyrronium with historical case matched control of hyoscine hydrobromide suggests that glycopyrronium may be at least as effective as hyoscine hydrobromide in controlling respiratory tract secretion in dying patients[254]. The side effects of hyoscine hydrobromide include bradycardia and mental confusion as it crosses blood–brain barrier. The following anti-muscarinics are recommended for the treatment of death rattle[252]:

- Hyoscine hydrobromide 400 mcg SC injection. To gauge response after 30 min; if effective, consider 1.2–2.0 mg continuous SC infusion over 24 h. (assuming a single dose of 400 mcg would produce effects lasting between 5 and 8 h).

- Glycopyrronium 200 mcg SC injection. To gauge response after 1 h. Doses of 400 mcg are likely to produce faster results at 30 minutes; if effective, further injection or to consider 1.2–2.0 mg continuous SC infusion over 24 h (assuming a single dose of 400 mcg would produce effects lasting between 5 and 8 h).

- Hyoscine butylbromide 20 mg SC injection. To gauge response after 30 minutes. May need dosage higher than 400 mg continuous SC infusion over 24 h (assuming a single dose of 20 mg would produce effects lasting for 1 h).

Management of bronchial and mucus secretion

The elucidation of the underlying causes of bronchial secretion may help to guide aetiological-based therapy (e.g. steroid for tumour secretion, antibiotics for infection, diuretics for pulmonary oedema, physical therapy for aspiration, mucoactive medications for airway diseases).

Airway mucociliary clearance depends on the properties and volume of secreted mucus, ciliary function, and mucociliary interactions. In chronic airway diseases, mucus viscoelasticity is higher than the optimal values for mucociliary clearance. The mucous glycoproteins (MGs) are produced by goblet and submucosal gland cells and are the most important determinants of the viscoelasticity of normal respiratory mucus, although with chronic infection and inflammation neutrophil-derived DNA and F-actin assume an important role. The quantities and structures of MGs mainly determine the rheological properties of mucus. Mucoactive medications serve either to increase the ability to expectorate sputum or to decrease mucus hypersecretion. Mucoactive agents include[255]:

- Expectorants: iodinated compounds, guaifenesin, and simple hydration have not been shown to be as effective as expectorants. However, long-term use of inhaled hyperosmolar saline has been shown to be beneficial to patients with cystic fibrosis and bronchiectasis from other causes.

- Mucolytics: these include classical mycolytics that depolymerise the mucin network like N-acetylcysteine severs disulfide bond linking mucin oligomers, peptide mucolytics that depolymerise

DNA-actin polymer network like dornase alfa that hydrolyses DNA polymer with reduction in DNA length.

- Mucoregulatory medications: these include anticholinergic agents, corticosteroids, aerosolized indomethacin, and the macrolide antibiotics.

- Cough clearance promoters: these include bronchodilators which improve cough clearance by increasing expiratory flow, aerosolize surfactant that decrease sputum adhesiveness.

Non-pharmacological airway therapy

A formal systematic review of non-pharmacologic protussive therapies was performed in non-malignant chest conditions[256]. Some principles in non-cancer conditions may also be applicable to cancer patients:

- Manually assisted cough should be considered to reduce respiratory complications in patients with expiratory muscle weakness.

- Huffing should be taught as an adjunct to other methods of sputum clearance in patients with COPD and cystic fibrosis.

- Expiratory muscle training is recommended to improve peak expiratory pressure, which may have a beneficial effect on cough in patients with neuromuscular weakness and impaired cough.

- Mechanical cough assist devices are recommended to prevent respiratory complications in patients with neuromuscular disease with impaired cough.

Bronchorrhoea

Bronchorrhoea is a condition in which voluminous sputum is produced. It is arbitrarily defined as watery sputum production of more than 100 ml/day[257]. It occurs in mucinous bronchioloalveolar carcinoma of the lung, or occasionally in pulmonary metastasis from other tumours. Non-malignant conditions include chronic bronchitis, asthma, and endobronchial tuberculosis. The volume of sputum production reported ranged from a few hundred millilitres to massive bronchorrhoea of several litres, up to the maximum of 91/day[258]. Due to the large volume of secretion involved, patient has to bend forward constantly to expectorate the sputum[257]. It can cause cough, disturbance to sleep, dehydration, electrolyte disturbance[259], dyspnoea, and even respiratory failure.

Management

Management of bronchorrhoea includes general supportive measures to promote comfort, to maintain fluid and electrolyte balance, and to decrease sputum production.

Radiotherapy and chemotherapy has been used to alleviate bronchorrhoea with variable effect. Prompt control of bronchorrhoea by EGFR tyrosine kinase inhibitor gefitinib in patients with bronchioloalveolar carcinoma have been demonstrated recently in several reports, with resolution of lung infiltrations, dyspnoea, and oxygen requirement within hours, days, to weeks[260,261]. Epidermal growth factor has its role in regulating mucin secretion in normal goblet cells of the respiratory tract, such as the major mucin MUC5AC. In lung cancer cell lines, gefitinib has been shown to suppress MUC5AC mRNA levels subsequent to a decrease in intracellular and secreted MUC5AC protein, and this inhibitory effect may be mediated through mitogen activating kinase (MAPK) and Akt

pathways downstream of the EGFR[262]. As bronchorrhoea was improved too rapid to be explained by cell apoptosis, gefitinib may inhibit mucin production in bronchioloalveolar carcinoma apart from its anti-proliferative effects[262].

There are anecdotal reports on other agents. Anticholinergic drugs given in various routes often fail to improve bronchorrhoea[258,259]. Erythromycin inhibits the synthesis and secretion of a mucus secretagogue from pulmonary macrophages, and has been used to treat bronchorrhoea with variable outcome[263]. Octreotide up to a dosage of 500 mcg over 24 h was reported to be effective in decreasing bronchorrhoea[264]. Cyclooxygenase-2 has been implicated in the pathogenesis of bronchorrhoea, and inhaled indomethacin had been reported to improve bronchorrhoea, dyspnoea, and hypoxaemia[265] Pulse steroid in the dosage of methylprednisolone 1000 mg per day for 3 days had been shown to be effective in a patient of bronchioloalevolar carcinoma producing CA 19-9[266].

Haemoptysis

Haemoptysis is often alarming to patients and their families. The degree of haemoptysis varies from a mild to a massive episode that cause asphyxiation. The definition of massive haemoptysis, as defined as expectoration of at least 100–600 ml of blood within 24 h, covers a broad range[267]. However, some workers preferred a definition of massive haemoptysis as the volume that is life threatening by virtue of airway obstruction or blood loss, with the anatomical dead space of the major airway of 100–200 ml as a reference[268].

Causes of haemoptysis in cancer

The causes of haemoptysis in cancer patient are listed in Table 11.1.11 Bronchogenic carcinoma is the most common primary cancer responsible. In a large retrospective autopsy analysis of 877 cases of lung cancer, the overall incidence of haemoptysis was 19.3 per cent[269]. Twenty-nine patients (3.3 per cent) had massive terminal haemoptysis, which was strongly associated with squamous cell type, cavitation, and major airway involvement. Of non-small-cell lung cancer patients with poor performance status referred for palliative radiotherapy, up to 75 per cent were referred for haemoptysis[270].

Clinical approach

One has to assess if the bleeding is a recent or old, the severity of bleeding, the risk of recurrent haemoptysis, and the cause of bleeding.

Table 11.1.11 Causes of haemoptysis in cancer.

Malignant	Paramalignant	Non-malignant
Lung cancer	Thrombocytopenia	Pneumonia
Tracheal tumour	Platelet dysfunction	Tuberculosis
Endobronchial tumour: carcinoid,	Tumour-related coagulopathy	Fungal pneumonia
Endobronchial metastasis: breast, colon, renal cell carcinoma	Disseminated intravascular coagulopathy (DIC)	Bronchiectasis
		Liver disease
Haematological malignancy	Pulmonary embolism	Medications:
Tumour-vessel fistula		- Anticoagulation (warfarin, LMWH)
		- NSAID

Systemic causes of bleeding tendency should be looked for, and the site of bleeding should be located as far as possible.

The severity of haemoptysis will guide the prognosis and further therapy. Prognostic features associated with death in massive haemoptysis include: (1) bleeding exceeding 1000 ml in 24 h; (2) radiographic evidence of aspiration; (3) haemodynamic instability; and (4) massive haemoptysis caused by a neoplasm. Other features associated with high mortality include factors that exclude patients from surgical intervention, namely inadequate pulmonary function, debilitated states, bilateral pulmonary bleeding sources, inability to localize source of bleeding, and metastatic cancer[271].

Localization of the site and source of bleeding may define the best treatment for stopping the bleeding. Bleeding can come from bronchial or pulmonary circulation. For major haemoptysis, the bleeding often comes from bronchial arteries and collaterals from systemic circulation.

Baseline investigations include complete blood count, renal and liver function tests, prothrombin time, and activated partial thromboplastin time. Chest radiography and CT will identify lung pathology and may help to localize the bleeding site. Multi-detector CT is recently used as a non-invasive investigation in localising the vascular source of haemoptysis from bronchial or systemic artery[272]. In the case of significant haemoptysis, localization of bleeding site by bronchoscopy may guide specific bronchoscopic therapy. Treatment options of haemoptysis include: (1) general resuscitation and management; (2) pharmacological therapy; (3) invasive interventions: bronchoscopic procedure, endobronchial therapies, and bronchial artery embolization; (4) oncological treatment (radiotherapy); and (5) palliative management of fatal haemoptysis.

General management

Haemoptysis will more often cause respiratory distress than haemodynamic disturbance. Fluid can be given in haemodynamic disturbance and airway should be cleared by suction and oxygen delivered to correct hypoxaemia. The patient should be put in the lateral decubitus position towards the site of bleeding to avoid drowning of the other lung segments. Underlying coagulopathy or thrombocytopenia should be corrected by fresh frozen plasma or platelet transfusion respectively. Drugs such as non-steroidal anti-inflammatory agent or anticoagulant should be withheld.

Pharmacological treatment

In case of bleeding caused by prolonged clotting resulting from oral anticoagulant, liver disease and disseminated intravascular coagulopathy (DIC); vitamin K should be administered either intravenously or orally. A dose of 1.0–2.5 mg is effective while the INR is between 5.0 and 9.0, but larger doses like 5 mg are required to correct INRs >9.0[273]. Antifibrinolytic agents such as tranexamic acid or aminocaproic acid are frequently used empirically but their beneficial effects were only reported anecdotally[274]. Doses of tranexamic acid were 1.5 g followed by 1 g thrice a day. Aminocaproic acid was dosed at 5 g load followed by 1 g four times a day. Aerosolized vasopressin in the dosage of 5 units of orthnithine-8-vasopressin was reported to be effective for mild to moderate recurrent haemoptysis[275]. Recombinant factor VIIa have been found to enhance thrombin generation and helpful in providing haemostasis in situations with profuse bleeding. It has shown to be effective in stopping massive haemoptysis resulting from invasive aspergillosis in a patient with leukaemia[276].

Invasive intervention for massive haemoptysis

The prognosis of massive haemoptysis is poor without specific treatment. If the episode occurs at the terminal stage of the disease, promoting comfort with minimal aggressive treatment is the goal. If invasive intervention is contemplated, maintainence of adequate airway is the priority. This usually requires endotracheal intubation, and a single-lumen endotracheal tube is generally more beneficial than a double-lumen endotracheal tube[267]. Bronchoscopy is usually needed to locate the source of bleeding. When only the location of bleeding is identified but no direct source is found, the bleeding segment can be tamponaded by balloon endobronchially with balloon remains in place for 24–48 h[277]. Vasoactive drugs such as 1:10 000 epinephrine solution, iced saline solution lavage[278], and fibrinogen-thrombin[279] have also been reported anecdotally with success. A recent study on massive haemoptysis as defined as bleeding rate more than 150 ml/h or on one occasion, together with impaired respiratory function (PaO$_2$ < 8 kPa); bronchoscopy-guided topical haemostatic tamponade therapy (THT) with oxidized regenerated cellulose was successfully performed on 56 of 57 patients (98 per cent) with immediate arrest of massive haemoptysis. Recurrence of haemoptysis developed in 10.5 per cent. For visible lesions in the trachea and proximal bronchi; laser, cryotherapy, or electrocautery treatment is useful (see under 'MAO'). Massive bleeding is more likely to come from the high-pressure bronchial arteries, which may be stopped by embolization with the aid of bronchoscopy and angiography. The immediate and long-term success rate is high in the range of 60–100 per cent in non-cancer patients[268]. The procedure has been performed in cancer-related haemoptysis[280].

Oncological treatment: radiotherapy

Haemoptysis is an indication for radiotherapy. A systematic review examined 14 randomized controlled trials (with 3576 evaluable patients) comparing different external palliative radiotherapy regimens for non-small-cell lung cancer[281]. Symptoms improved under all regimens with no additional advantage in giving a higher dosage. It was recommended that patients with poor performance status should be treated with short courses of palliative radiotherapy (such as 10 Gy in one fraction or 17 Gy in two fractions). Brachytherapy, as given via a fibreoptic bronchoscope, has the advantage of limiting the radiation to the tumour tissue, and may be repeated in case of tumour recurrence or initiated after failure of conventional therapy. Palliation was reported as 69–100 per cent for haemoptysis[282].

Management of fatal haemoptysis

If a patient is at risk of massive haemoptysis, it is essential to establish a plan of action. The family needs to be informed, psychologically prepared, with possible treatment options discussed. If a massive life-threatening haemoptysis occurs, sedation to relieve the distress should be given as soon as possible. Midazolam 2.5–5.0 mg can be given intravenously or via the subcutaneous route. Diazepam given per rectal is an alternative. Morphine can also lessen the dyspnoea and distress. A dark towel to cover the patient and dark basin for collecting blood helps to reduce the visual impact. Keeping an 'emergency box' with the necessary drugs and towels in the ward facilitates timely intervention of such crisis. The psychological impact of a patient dying from massive haemoptysis is enormous. Support and attention should be given to the family and persons who witness the event. It is important that support will also be given to the staff after the incident.

Palliative sedation for refractory respiratory symptom

Palliative sedation is defined as the use of specific sedative medications to relieve intolerable suffering from refractory symptoms by a reduction in patient consciousness, using appropriate drugs carefully titrated to the cessation of symptoms[283]. It is often considered a last option for relieving suffering that arises from refractory symptoms. Towards death, a significant proportion of patients are still facing uncontrolled or refractory dyspnoea, requiring sedation. In a recent retrospective review on sedation of 548 cancer patients at 48 h before death, about 35 per cent were sedated for dyspnoea[284]. In a survey on 105 representative physicians in Japan, dyspnoea was the most common indication for continuous deep sedation in terms of the perceived appropriateness, where 87 per cent of physicians thought dyspnoea was an indicator, or a strong indicator[285].

Considerations for palliative sedation

Palliative sedation for refractory symptom and its distress, including dyspnoea, is a complex ethical and clinical decision. Recommendations from experts in palliative care help in guiding the practice in the clinical setting[283]. 'Refractoriness' of symptom, being not an absolute phenomenon, should be carefully explored for the condition or symptom concerned. A symptom is generally considered refractory, as suggested by Cherny and Portenoy[286], when further interventions: (1) will not bring adequate relief; (2) will be associated with intolerable morbidity; and (3) are unlikely to bring relief within a reasonable time frame. Systematic and careful elucidation of all underlying causes of dyspnoea, team discussion, and assessment by palliative care specialists help to define the refractoriness, and distinguishing a 'refractory' symptom from a 'difficult' symptom.

Without the indication and the intention of sedation being clearly defined, there is always a concern that liberal use of palliative sedation represents a kind of 'slow euthanasia'. Palliative sedation is an option of palliation ethically provided the intention and the goal of sedation is to relieve distress from intractable dyspnoea. Sedation is a proportionate intervention, and that death of the patient is not a criterion of success or the mean to relieve the suffering of dyspnoea. Although sedation in patients with respiratory problem can evoke the concern of excessive respiratory suppression, studies have shown that use of sedatives in the last days of life for various indications are not associated with a shortened survival[207,287]. A clear understanding of the ethical and clinical background and established guidelines can facilitate the discussion of the care plan, and to address the concerns of patient, family and staff concerned.

Before sedation, the following steps should be undertaken. The decision should be based on the conditions that the symptom is refractory. Patients and their families have to be involved in the discussion, and informed consent should be obtained. The unbearable suffering is most accurate when expressed by patient, but when patient is unable to communicate freely, a surrogate decision maker shall be involved. The goal of sedation should be clearly communicated. They have to be reassured that as sedation is only a means of treatment, it will be under constant review, and both

continuation and reversal of sedation can be considered if deemed appropriate. The medication used and the details of the regimen should be explained. The level of sedation and the possible loss of ability to communicate with each other should be carefully considered. Adverse effects, sedation level, and degree of relief will be assessed regularly and documented.

Drugs used for palliative sedation in various studies include: (1) anxiolytics, e.g. midazolam, lorazepam; (2) antipsychotics, e.g. haloperidol, methotrimeprazine, chlorpromazine; (3) barbiturates, e.g. phenobarbital; and (4) anaesthetics, e.g. propofol. Midazolam given subcutaneously or intravenously is the most commonly used drugs for sedation for refractory symptoms[288,283]. Midazolam is short and fast acting, has minimal cardiovascular effects, facilitating titration against clinical response. It has properties of an anxiolytic, a sedative, a muscle relaxant and an anti-epileptic. This should be considered a first line drug for palliative sedation. Recent systematic review showed that the mean dosages of midazolam used for palliative sedation ranged from 20 to 70 mg per 24 h, and median dosages range from 30 to 45 mg per 24 h[283]. Alternative drugs have been used as listed above, especially when midazolam fails[289]. The depth of sedation can vary from mild (somnolence) to intermediate (stupor) to deep coma; while the administration of sedatives can be intermittent or continuous[283]. When time and the situation allows, reversal of sedation for reviewing the symptoms is an option. When sedation is given near the end of life, it may be reasonable to continue the sedation till death to avoid recurrence of distressing symptoms. Continuous deep sedation is generally recommended for patients with limited life expectancy of hours or days[283]. The issue of provision of fluid and nutrition while patient is sedated is a more controversial issue. Although a separate ethical issue by itself, the plan to continue, to discontinue or to initiate parenteral fluid and nutrition is often affected by the life expectancy when sedation is initiated.

The frequency and the practice of sedation for refractory dyspnoea were variably reported by palliative care workers in different places. This may be due to the differences in the condition of patients, prescription habit, culture, social values, and hospice policies. Sedation should be tailored to the individual need and expectation of the patient with intractable suffering from dyspnoea. For patients who choose relieving dyspnoea while trading off consciousness, palliative sedation remains an option. For those patients who decline sedation despite overwhelming discomforts, it remains of the palliative care workers to hold, to accompany, and to walk with the patients in their last journey.

References

1. Tsai, J.S., Wu, C.H., Chiu, T.Y. et al. (2006). Symptom patterns of advanced cancer patients in a palliative care unit. *Palliative Medicine*, **20**, 617–22.
2. Chochinov, H.M., Tataryn, D., Clinch, J.J. et al. (1999). Will to live in the Terminally ill. *Lancet*, **354**, 816–9.
3. Jemal, A., Murray, T., Ward, E. et al. (2005). Cancer statistics, 2005. *CA: A Cancer Journal For Clinicians*, **55**, 10–30.
4. The Diagnosis and Treatment of Lung Cancer. (2005). *National Institute for Clinical Excellence.*
5. Sandler, A., Gray, R., Perry, M.C. et al. (2006). Paclitaxel-carboplatin alone or with bevacizumab for non-small-cell lung cancer. *New England Journal of Medicine*, **355**, 2542–50.
6. Bezjak, A., Tu, D., Seymour, L. et al. (2006). Symptom improvement in lung cancer patients treated with erlotinib: quality of life analysis of the

National Cancer Institute of Canada Clinical Trials Group Study BR.21. *Journal of Clinical Oncology*, **24**, 3831–7.

7. Cooley, M.E. (2000). Symptoms in adults with lung cancer. A systematic research review. *Journal of Pain and Symptom Management*, **19**, 137–53.

8. Carlsen, K., Jensen, A.B, Jacobsen, E. *et al.* (2005). Psychosocial aspects of lung cancer. *Lung Cancer*, **47**, 293–300.

9. Zabora, J., BrintzenhofeSzoc, K., Curbow, B. *et al.* (2001). The prevalence of psychological distress by cancer site. *Psychooncology*, **10**, 19–28.

10. Degner, L.F., and Sloan, J.A. (1995). Symptom distress in newly diagnosed ambulatory cancer patients and as a predictor of survival in lung cancer. *Journal of Pain and Symptom Management*, **10**, 423–31.

11. Krech, R., Davis, J., Walsh, D. *et al.* (1992). Symptom of lung cancer. *Palliative Medicine*, **6**, 309–305.

12. Hopwood, P., and Stephens, R.J. (1995). Symptoms at presentation for treatment in patients with lung cancer: implications for the evaluation of palliative treatment. The Medical Research Council (MRC) Lung Cancer Working Party. *British Journal of Cancer*, **71**, 633–6.

13. Tanaka, K., Akechi, T., Okuyama, T. *et al.* (2002). Prevalence and screening of dyspnea interfering with daily life activities in ambulatory patients with advanced lung cancer. *Journal of Pain and Symptom Management*, **23**, 484–9.

14. Cooley, M.E., Short, T.H., and Moriarty, H.J. (2003). Symptom prevalence, distress, and change over time in adults receiving treatment for lung cancer. *Psychooncology*, **12**, 694–708.

15. Tishelman C, Degner, L.F., Rudman, A. *et al.* (2005). Symptoms in patients with lung carcinoma: distinguishing distress from intensity. *Cancer*, **104**, 2013–21.

16. Dodd, M. J., Miaskowski, C. Paul, S. M. (2001). Symptom clusters and their effect on the functional status of patients with cancer. *Oncology Nursing Forum*, **28**, 465–70.

17. Gift, A.G., Stommel, M., Jablonski, A. *et al.* (2003). A cluster of symptoms over time in patients with lung cancer. *Nursing Research*, **52**, 393–400.

18. Akechi, T., Nakano, T., Okamura, H. *et al.* (2001). Psychiatric disorders in cancer patients: descriptive analysis of 1721 psychiatric referrals at two Japanese cancer center hospitals. *Japan Journal of Clinical Oncology*, **31**, 188–94.

19. Hopwood, P., Stephens, R.J. (2000). Depression in patients with lung cancer: prevalence and risk factors derived from quality-of-life data. *Journal of Clinical Oncology*, **18**, 893–903.

20. Akechi, T., Okuyama, T., Akizuki, N. *et al.* (2006). Course of psychological distress and its predictors in advanced non-small cell lung cancer patients. *Psychooncology*, **15**, 463–73.

21. Chapple, A., Ziebland, S., and McPherson, A. (2004). Stigma, shame, and blame experienced by patients with lung cancer: qualitative study. *British Medical Journal*, **328**, 1470.

22. Li, J. and Girgis, A. (2006). Supportive care needs: are patients with lung cancer a neglected population? *Psychooncology*, **15**, 509–16.

23. Krishnasamy, M., Wilkie, E., and Haviland, J. (2001). Lung cancer health care needs assessment: patients' and informal carers' responses to a national mail questionnaire survey. *Palliative Medicine*, **15**, 213–27.

24. Badr, H., and Taylor, C.L. (2006). Social constraints and spousal communication in lung cancer. *Psychooncology*, **15**, 673–83.

25. Dyspnea. Mechanisms, assessment, and management: a consensus statement. (1999). American Thoracic Society. *American Journal of Respiratory and Critical Care Medicine*, **159**, 321–40.

26. McKay, L.C., Evans K.C., Frackowiak, R.S. *et al.* (2003). Neural correlates of voluntary breathing in humans. *Journal of Applied Physiology*, **95**, 1170–8.

27. Richerson, G.B., Wang, W., Hodges, M.R. *et al.* (2005). Homing in on the specific phenotype(s) of central respiratory chemoreceptors. *Experimental Physiology*, **90**: 259–66; discussion 266–9.

28. Moosavi, S.H., Golestanian, E., Binks, A.P. *et al.* (2003). Hypoxic and hypercapnic drives to breathe generate equivalent levels of air hunger in humans. *Journal of Applied Physiology*, **94**, 141–54.

29. Banzett, R.B., Lansing, R.W. Reid, M.B. *et al.* (1989). 'Air hunger' arising from increased PCO_2 in mechanically ventilated quadriplegics. *Respiration Physiology*, **76**, 53–67.

30. Banzett, R.B., Lansing, R.W., Brown, R. *et al.* (1990). 'Air hunger' from increased PCO_2 persists after complete neuromuscular block in humans. *Respiration Physiology*, **81**, 1–17.

31. Harty, H.R., Mummery, C.J., Adams, L. *et al.* (1996). Ventilatory relief of the sensation of the urge to breathe in humans: are pulmonary receptors important? *Journal of Physiology*, **490** (Pt 3), 805–15.

32. Bloch-Salisbury, E., Shea, S.A., Brown, R. *et al.* (1996). Air hunger induced by acute increase in PCO_2 adapts to chronic elevation of PCO_2 in ventilated humans. *Journal of Applied Physiology*, **81**, 949–56.

33. Banzett, R.B., Lansing, R.W., Evans, K.C. *et al.* (1996). Stimulus-response characteristics of CO_2-induced air hunger in normal subjects. *Respiration Physiology*, **103**, 19–31.

34. Binks, A.P., Moosavi, S.H., Banzett, R.B. *et al.* (2002). "Tightness" sensation of asthma does not arise from the work of breathing. *American Journal of Respiratory and Critical Care Medicine*, **165**, 78–82.

35. Schwartzstein, R.M., Lahive, K., Pope, A. *et al.* (1987). Cold facial stimulation reduces breathlessness induced in normal subjects. *American Review of Respiratory Disease*, **136**, 58–61.

36. Manning, H., and Schwartzstein, R.M. (1999). Dyspnea and the control of breathing. In control of breathing in Health and Disease (Ed. M.D. Altose and T. Kamakami). *Marcel Dekker, New York*.

37. Lansing, R.W., Im, B.S., Thwing, J. I. *et al.* (2000). The perception of respiratory work and effort can be independent of the perception of air hunger. *American Journal of Respiratory and Critical Care Medicine*, **162**, 1690–6.

38. Schwartzstein, R.M., Simon, P.M., Weiss, J.W. *et al.* (1989). Breathlessness induced by dissociation between ventilation and chemical drive. *American Review of Respiratory Disease*, **139**, 1231–7.

39. Chonan, T., Mulholland, M.B., Cherniack, N.S. *et al.* (1987). Effects of voluntary constraining of thoracic displacement during hypercapnia. *Journal of Applied Physiology*, **63**, 1822–8.

40. Manning, H.L., Shea, S.A., Schwartzstein, R.M. *et al.* (1992). Reduced tidal volume increases 'air hunger' at fixed PCO_2 in ventilated quadriplegics. *Respiration Physiology*, **90**, 19–30.

41. O'Donnell, D.E., Hong, H.H., Webb, K.A. (2000). Respiratory sensation during chest wall restriction and dead space loading in exercising men. *Journal of Applied Physiology*, **88**, 1859–69.

42. Manning, H.L., Mahler, D.A. (2001). Pathophysiology of dyspnea. *Monaldi Archives for Chest Disorder*, **56**, 325–30.

43. Nishino, T., Isono, S., Ishikawa, T. *et al.* (2007). An additive interaction between different qualities of dyspnea produced in normal human subjects. *Respiration Physiology and Neurobiology*, **155**, 14–21.

44. Simon, P.M., Schwartzstein, R.M., Weiss, J. W. *et al.* (1990). Distinguishable types of dyspnea in patients with shortness of breath. *American Review of Respiratory Disease*, **142**, 1009–14.

45. Wilcock, A., Crosby, V., Hughes, A. *et al.* (2002). Descriptors of breathlessness in patients with cancer and other cardiorespiratory diseases. *Journal of Pain and Symptom Management*, **23**, 182–9.

46. Evans, K.C., Banzett, R.B., Adams, L. *et al.* (2002). fMRI identifies limbic, paralimbic, and cerebellar activation during air hunger. *Journal of Neurophysiology*, **88**, 1500–11.

47. Peiffer, C., Poline, J.B., Thivard, L. *et al.* (2001). Neural substrates for the perception of acutely induced dyspnea. *American Journal of Respiratory and Critical Care Medicine*, **163**, 951–7.

48. Walsh, D., Donnelly, S., Rybicki, L. (2000). The symptoms of advanced cancer: relationship to age, gender, and performance status in 1,000 patients. *Supportive Care in Cancer*, **8**, 175–9.

49. Chang, V.T., Hwang, S.S., Feuerman, M. *et al.* (2000). Symptom and quality of life survey of medical oncology patients at a veterans affairs medical center: a role for symptom assessment. *Cancer*, **88**, 1175–83.

50. Chiu, T.Y., Hu, W.Y., Chen, C.Y. (2000). Prevalence and severity of symptoms in terminal cancer patients: a study in Taiwan. *Supportive Care in Cancer*, **8**, 311–3.

51. Bruera, E., Schmitz, B., Pither, J. *et al.* (2000). The frequency and correlates of dyspnea in patients with advanced cancer. *Journal of Pain and Symptom Management*, **19**, 357–62.

52. Dudgeon, D.J., Kristjanson, L., Sloan, J.A. *et al.* (2001). Dyspnea in cancer patients: prevalence and associated factors. *Journal of Pain and Symptom Management*, **21**, 95–102.

53. Chiu, T.Y., Hu, W.Y., Lue, B.H. *et al.* (2004). Dyspnea and its correlates in taiwanese patients with terminal cancer. *Journal of Pain and Symptom Management*, **28**, 123–32.

54. Muers, M.F., and Round, C.E. (1993). Palliation of symptoms in non-small cell lung cancer: a study by the Yorkshire Regional Cancer Organisation Thoracic Group. *Thorax*, **48**, 339–43.

55. Hopwood, P., and Stephens, R.J. (1995). Symptoms at presentation for treatment in patients with lung cancer: implications for the evaluation of palliative treatment. The Medical Research Council (MRC) Lung Cancer Working Party. *British Journal of Cancer*, **71**, 633–6.

56. Smith, E.L., Hann, D.M., Ahles, T.A. *et al* (2001). Dyspnea, anxiety, body consciousness, and quality of life in patients with lung cancer. *Journal of Pain and Symptom Management*, **21**, 323–9.

57. Reuben, D.B., and Mor, V. (1986). Dyspnea in terminally ill cancer patients. *Chest*, **89**, 234–6.

58. Mercadante, S., Casuccio, A., and Fulfaro, F. (2000). The course of symptom frequency and intensity in advanced cancer patients followed at home. *Journal of Pain and Symptom Management*, **20**, 104–12.

59. O'Driscoll, M., Corner, J., and Bailey, C. (1999). The experience of breathlessness in lung cancer. *European Journal of Cancer Care (England)*, **8**, 37–43.

60. Tanaka, K., Akechi, T., Okuyama, T. *et al.* (2002). Prevalence and screening of dyspnea interfering with daily life activities in ambulatory patients with advanced lung cancer. *Journal of Pain and Symptom Management*, **23**, 484–9.

61. Hayes, A.W., Philip, J., Spruyt, O.W. (2006). Patient reporting and doctor recognition of dyspnoea in a comprehensive cancer centre. *Internal Medicine Journal*, **36**, 381–4.

62. Dudgeon, D.J., Lertzman, M., and Askew, G.R. (2001). Physiological changes and clinical correlations of dyspnea in cancer outpatients. *Journal of Pain and Symptom Management*, **21**, 373–9.

63. Heyse-Moore, L., Beynon, T., and Ross, V. (2000). Does spirometry predict dyspnoea in advanced cancer? *Palliative Medicine*, **14**, 189–95.

64. Maltoni, M., Pirovano, M., and Scarpi, E. *et al.* (1995). Prediction of survival of patients terminally ill with cancer. Results of an Italian prospective multicenter study. *Cancer*, **75**, 2613–22.

65. Vitetta, L., Kenner, D., Kissane, D. *et al.* (2001). Clinical outcomes in terminally ill patients admitted to hospice care: diagnostic and therapeutic interventions. *Journal of Palliative Care*, **17**, 69–77.

66. Morita, T., Tsunoda, J., Inoue, S. *et al.* (1999). Survival prediction of terminally ill cancer patients by clinical symptoms: development of a simple indicator. *Japanese Journal of Clinical Oncology*, **29**, 156–9.

67. Vigano, A., Donaldson, N., Higginson, I.J. *et al.* (2004). Quality of life and survival prediction in terminal cancer patients: a multicenter study. *Cancer*, **101**, 1090–8.

68. Toscani, P., Brunelli, C., Miccinesi, G. *et al.* (2005). Predicting survival in terminal cancer patients: clinical observation or quality-of-life evaluation? *Palliative Medicine*, **19**, 220–7.

69. Escalante, C.P., Martin, C.G., Elting, L.S. *et al.* (2000). Identifying risk factors for imminent death in cancer patients with acute dyspnea. *Journal of Pain and Symptom Management*, **20**, 318–25.

70. De Miguel Sanchez, C., Elustondo, S.G., Estirado, A. *et al.* (2006). Palliative performance status, heart rate and respiratory rate as predictive factors of survival time in terminally ill cancer patients. *Journal of Pain and Symptom Management*, **31**, 485–92.

71. Pirovano, M., Maltoni, M., Nanni, O. *et al.* (1999). A new palliative prognostic score: a first step for the staging of terminally ill cancer patients. Italian Multicenter and Study Group on Palliative Care. *Journal of Pain and Symptom Management*, **17**, 231–9.

72. Morita, T., Tsunoda, J., Inoue, S. *et al.* (1999). Survival prediction of terminally ill cancer patients by clinical symptoms: development of a simple indicator. *Japanese Journal of Clinical Oncology*, **29**, 156–9.

73. Maltoni, M., Caraceni, A., Brunelli, C. *et al.* (2005). Prognostic factors in advanced cancer patients: evidence-based clinical recommendations—a study by the Steering Committee of the European Association for Palliative Care. *Journal of Clinical Oncology*, **23**, 6240–8.

74. Loganathan, R.S., Stover, D.E., Shi, W. *et al.* (2006). Prevalence of COPD in women compared to men around the time of diagnosis of primary lung cancer. *Chest*, **129**, 1305–12.

75. Congleton, J., and Muers, M.F. (1995). The incidence of airflow obstruction in bronchial carcinoma, its relation to breathlessness, and response to bronchodilator therapy. *Respiratory Medicine*, **89**, 291–6.

76. Danson, S., Blackhall, F., Hulse, P. *et al.* (2005). Interstitial lung disease in lung cancer: separating disease progression from treatment effects. *Drug Safety*, **28**, 103–13.

77. Corner, J., and O'Driscoll, M. (1999). Development of a breathlessness assessment guide for use in palliative care. *Palliative Medicine*, **13**, 375–84.

78. Bausewein, C., Farquhar, M., Booth, S. *et al.* (2007). Measurement of breathlessness in advanced disease: A systematic review. *Respiratory Medicine*, **101**, 399–410.

79. Dorman, S., Byrne, A., Edwards, A. (2007). Which measurement scales should we use to measure breathlessness in palliative care? A systematic review. *Palliative Medicine*, **21**, 177–91.

80. Wilcock, A., Crosby, V., Clarke, D. *et al.* (1999). Repeatability of breathlessness measurements in cancer patients. *Thorax*, **54**, 375.

81. Booth, S. (2006). Reporting of 'Improving research methology in breathlessness' meeting held by MRC Clinical Trials Unit and Cicely Saunders Foundation. *Palliative Medicine*, **20**, 219–20.

82. Tanaka, K., Akechi, T., Okuyama, T. *et al.* (2000). Development and validation of the Cancer Dyspnoea Scale: a multidimensional, brief, self-rating scale. *British Journal of Cancer*, **82**, 800–5.

83. Hollen, P.J., Gralla, R. J., Kris, M.G. *et al.* (1993). Quality of life assessment in individuals with lung cancer: testing the Lung Cancer Symptom Scale (LCSS). *European Journal of Cancer*, **29A** (Suppl 1), S51–8.

84. Portenoy, R.K., Thaler, H.T., Kornblith, A.B. *et al.* (1994). The Memorial Symptom Assessment Scale: an instrument for the evaluation of symptom prevalence, characteristics and distress. *European Journal of Cancer*, **30A**, 1326–36.

85. de Haes, J.C., van Knippenberg, F.C., Neijt, J.P. (1990). Measuring psychological and physical distress in cancer patients: structure and application of the Rotterdam Symptom Checklist. *British Journal of Cancer*, **62**, 1034–8.

86. Bruera, E., Kuehn, N., Miller, M.J. *et al.* (1991). The Edmonton Symptom Assessment System (ESAS): a simple method for the assessment of palliative care patients. *Journal of Palliative Care*, **7**, 6–9.

87. Cleeland, C.S., Mendoza, T.R., Wang, X.S. *et al.* (2000). Assessing symptom distress in cancer patients: the M.D. Anderson Symptom Inventory. *Cancer*, **89**, 1634–46.

88. McCorkle, R. and Young, K. (1978). Development of a symptom distress scale. *Cancer Nursing*, **1**, 373–8.

89. Mahler, D.A., Weinberg, D.H., Wells, C.K. *et al.* (1984). The measurement of dyspnea. Contents, interobserver agreement, and physiologic correlates of two new clinical indexes. *Chest*, **85**, 751–8.

90. Stoller, J.K., Ferranti, R., and Feinstein, A.R. (1986). Further specification and evaluation of a new clinical index for dyspnea. *American Review of Respiratory Disease*, **134**, 1129–34.

91. Mahler, D.A., and Wells, C.K. (1988). Evaluation of clinical methods for rating dyspnea. *Chest*, **93**, 580-6.

92. Booth, S., and Adams, L. (2001). The shuttle walking test: a reproducible method for evaluating the impact of shortness of breath on functional capacity in patients with advanced cancer. *Thorax*, **56**, 146–50.

93. Wilcock, A., Crosby, V., Clarke, D. *et al.* (1999). Reading numbers aloud: a measure of the limiting effect of breathlessness in patients with cancer. *Thorax*, **54**, 1099–103.

94. Wilcock, A., Walker, G., Manderson, C. *et al.* (2005). Use of upper limb exercise to assess breathlessness in patients with cancer: tolerability, repeatability, and sensitivity. *Journal of Pain and Symptom Management*, **29**, 559–64.

95. Aaronson, N.K., Ahmedzai, S., Bergman, B. *et al.* (1993). The European Organization for Research and Treatment of Cancer QLQ-C30: a quality-of-life instrument for use in international clinical trials in oncology. *Journal of National Cancer Institute*, **85**, 365–376.

96. Bergman, B., Aaronson, N.K., Ahmedzai, S. *et al.* (1994) The EORTC QLQ-LC13: a modular supplement to the EORTC Core Quality of Life Questionnaire (QLQ-C30) for use in lung cancer clinical trials. EORTC Study Group on Quality of Life. *European Journal of Cancer*, **30A**, 635–642.

97. Groenvold, M., Petersen, M.A., Aaronson, N.K. *et al.* (2006). The development of the EORTC QLQ-C15-PAL: a shortened questionnaire for cancer patients in palliative care. *European Journal of Cancer*, **42**, 55–64.

98. Gupta, D., Lis, C.G. and Grutsch, J.F. (2007). The relationship between dyspnea and patient satisfaction with quality of life in advanced cancer. *Supportive Care in Cancer*, **15**, 533–8.

99. Antunes, G., Neville, E., Duffy, J. *et al.* (2003). BTS guidelines for the management of malignant pleural effusions. *Thorax*, **58** (Suppl 2), ii29–38.

100. Antony, V.B. (1999). Pathogenesis of malignant pleural effusions and talc pleurodesis. *Pneumologie*, **53**, 493–8.

101. Ishii, H., Yazawa, T., Sato, H. *et al.* (2004). Enhancement of pleural dissemination and lymph node metastasis of intrathoracic lung cancer cells by vascular endothelial growth factors (VEGFs). *Lung Cancer*, **45**, 325–37.

102. Management of malignant pleural effusions. (2000). *American Journal of Respiratory and Critical Care Medicine*, **162**, 1987–2001.

103. Antony, V.B., Nasreen, N., Mohammed, K.A. *et al.* (2004). Talc pleurodesis: basic fibroblast growth factor mediates pleural fibrosis. *Chest*, **126**, 1522–8.

104. Psathakis, K., Calderon-Osuna, E., Romero-Romero, B. *et al.* (2006). The neutrophilic and fibrinolytic response to talc can predict the outcome of pleurodesis. *European Respiratory Journal*, **27**, 817–21.

105. Lee, Y.C., Baumann, M.H., Maskell, N.A. *et al.* (2003). Pleurodesis practice for malignant pleural effusions in five English-speaking countries: survey of pulmonologists. *Chest*, **124**, 2229–38.

106. Shaw, P. and Agarwal, R. (2004). Pleurodesis for malignant pleural effusions. *Cochrane Database System Review*, CD002916.

107. Tan, C., Sedrakyan, A., Browne, J. *et al.* (2006). The evidence on the effectiveness of management for malignant pleural effusion: a systematic review. *European Journal Cardiothoracic Surgery*, **29**, 829–38.

108. Dresler, C.M., Olak, J., Herndon, J.E., 2nd, *et al.* (2005). Phase III intergroup study of talc poudrage vs talc slurry sclerosis for malignant pleural effusion. *Chest*, **127**, 909–15.

109. Janssen, J. P. (2004). Is thoracoscopic talc pleurodesis really safe? *Monaldi Archives for Chest Disorder*, **61**, 35–8.

110. Maskell, N.A., Lee, Y.C., Gleeson, F.V. *et al.* (2004). Randomized trials describing lung inflammation after pleurodesis with talc of varying particle size. *American Journal of Respiratory and Critical Care Medicine*, **170**, 377–82.

111. Dikensoy, O. and Light, R.W. (2005). Alternative widely available, inexpensive agents for pleurodesis. *Current Opinion in Pulmonary Medicine*, **11**, 340–4.

112. Robinson, L.A., Fleming, W. and H.Galbraith, T.A. (1993). Intrapleural doxycycline control of malignant pleural effusions. *Annals of Thoracic Surgery*, **55**, 1115–21; discussion 1121–2.

113. Ohm, C., Park, D., Vogen, M. *et al.* (2003). Use of an indwelling pleural catheter compared with thorascopic talc pleurodesis in the management of malignant pleural effusions. *American Journal of Surgery*, **69**, 198–202; discussion 202.

114. Genc, O., Petrou, M., Ladas, G. *et al.* (2000). The long-term morbidity of pleuroperitoneal shunts in the management of recurrent malignant effusions. *European Journal of Cardiothoracic Surgery*, **18**, 143–6.

115. Tremblay, A.Michaud, G. (2006). Single-center experience with 250 tunnelled pleural catheter insertions for malignant pleural effusion. *Chest*, **129**, 362–8.

116. Green, J., Dundar, Y., Dodd, S. *et al.* (2007). Pemetrexed disodium in combination with cisplatin versus other cytotoxic agents or supportive care for the treatment of malignant pleural mesothelioma. *Cochrane Database System Review*, CD005574.

117. Muers, M.F., Rudd,R.M., O'Brien, M.E. *et al.* (2004). BTS randomised feasibility study of active symptom control with or without chemotherapy in malignant pleural mesothelioma: ISRCTN 54469112. *Thorax*, **59**, 144–8.

118. Vogelzang, N.J., Rusthoven, J.J., Symanowski, J. *et al.* (2003). Phase III study of pemetrexed in combination with cisplatin versus cisplatin alone in patients with malignant pleural mesothelioma. *Journal of Clinical Oncology*, **21**, 2636–44.

119. Dundar, Y., Bagust, A., Dickson, R. *et al.* (2007). Pemetrexed disodium for the treatment of malignant pleural mesothelioma: a systematic review and economic evaluation. *Health Technology Assessment*, **11**, 1–90.

120. Chapman, E., Berenstein, E.G., Dieguez, M. *et al.* (2006). Radiotherapy for malignant pleural mesothelioma. *Cochrane Database System Review*, **3**, CD003880.

121. Viallat, J. R., Rey, F., Astoul, P. *et al.* (1996). Thoracoscopic talc poudrage pleurodesis for malignant effusions. A review of 360 cases. *Chest*, **110**, 1387–93.

122. Senyigit, A., Bayram, H., Babayigit, C. *et al.* (2000). Comparison of the effectiveness of some pleural sclerosing agents used for control of effusions in malignant pleural mesothelioma: a review of 117 cases. *Respiration*, **67**, 623–9.

123. Dresler, C.M., Olak, J., Herndon, J.E., 2nd, *et al.* (2005). Phase III intergroup study of talc poudrage vs talc slurry sclerosis for malignant pleural effusion. *Chest*, **127**, 909–15.

124. Aelony, Y., and Yao, J.F. (2005). Prolonged survival after talc poudrage for malignant pleural mesothelioma: case series. *Respirology*, **10**, 649–55.

125. Nasreen N., Mohammed, K.A., Dowling, P.A. *et al.* (2000). Talc induces apoptosis in human malignant mesothelioma cells in vitro. *American Journal of Respiratory and Critical Care Medicine*, **161**, 595–600.

126. Tremblay, A., and Michaud, G. (2006). Single-center experience with 250 tunnelled pleural catheter insertions for malignant pleural effusion. *Chest*, **129**, 362–8.

127. Bussani, R., De-Giorgio, F., Abbate, A. *et al.* (2007). Cardiac metastases. *Journal of Clinical Pathology*, **60**, 27–34.

128. Garcia-Riego, A., Cuinas, C., and Vilanova, J.J. (2001). Malignant pericardial effusion. *Acta Cytologica*, **45**, 561–6.

129. Klatt, E.C. and Heitz, D.R. (1990). Cardiac metastases. *Cancer*, **65**, 1456–9.

130. Tsang, T.S., Seward, J.B., Barnes, M.E. *et al.* (2000). Outcomes of primary and secondary treatment of pericardial effusion in patients with malignancy. *Mayo Clinic Proceedings*, **75**, 248–53.

131. Martinoni, A., Cipolla, C.M., Civelli, M. *et al.* (2000). Intrapericardial treatment of neoplastic pericardial effusions. *Herz*, **25**, 787–93.

132. Rowell, N.P. and Gleeson, F.V. (2001). Steroids, radiotherapy, chemotherapy and stents for superior vena caval obstruction in carcinoma of the bronchus. *Cochrane Database System Review*, CD001316.

133. Baker, G.L. and Barnes, H.J. (1992). Superior vena cava syndrome: aetiology, diagnosis, and treatment. *American Journal of Critical Care*, **1**, 54–64.

134. Ahmann, F.R. (1984). A reassessment of the clinical implications of the superior vena caval syndrome. *Journal of Clinical Oncology*, **2**, 961–9.

135. Hon, K.L., Leung, A., Chik, K.W. *et al.* (2005). Critical airway obstruction, superior vena cava syndrome, and spontaneous cardiac arrest in a child with acute leukemia. *Pediatric Emergency Care*, **21**, 844–6.

136. Eren, S., Karaman, A., and Okur, A. (2006). The superior vena cava syndrome caused by malignant disease. Imaging with multi-detector row CT. *European Journal of Radiology*, **59**, 93–103.

137. Uberoi, R. (2006). Quality assurance guidelines for superior vena cava stenting in malignant disease. *Cardiovascular and Interventional Radiology*, **29**, 319–22.

138. Detterbeck, F., Jones, D., and Morris, D. (2001). Palliative treatment of lung cancer. In *Diagnosis and treatment of lung cancer. An evidence guideline for the practising clinician* (eds. Detterbeck FC, Rivera, MP Socinski, MC, Roseman, JD), pp. 419–36, WB Saunders, Philadelphia.

139. Lester, J.F., Macbeth, F.R., Toy, E. *et al.* (2006). Palliative radiotherapy regimens for non-small cell lung cancer. *Cochrane Database System Review*, CD002143.

140. Ung, Y.C., Yu, E., Falkson, C. *et al.* and Lung Cancer Disease Site Group Of Cancer Care Ontario's Program In Evidence-Based, C. (2006). The role of high-dose-rate brachytherapy in the palliation of symptoms in patients with non-small-cell lung cancer: a systematic review. *Brachytherapy*, **5**, 189–202.

141. Streiff, M.B. (2007). The NCCN Guidelines on Venous Thromboembolism. *Clinical Advancement in Hematology and Oncology*, **5**, 117–9.

142. Stein, P.D., Beemath, A., Meyers, F.A. *et al.* (2006). Pulmonary embolism as a cause of death in patients who died with cancer. *American Journal of Medicine*, **119**, 163–5.

143. Blom, J.W., Doggen, C.J., Osanto, S. *et al.* (2005). Malignancies, prothrombotic mutations, and the risk of venous thrombosis. *JAMA*, **293**, 715–22.

144. Johnson, M.J., Sproule, M.W. and Paul, J. (1999). The prevalence and associated variables of deep venous thrombosis in patients with advanced cancer. *Clinical Oncology (Royal College of Radiologists)*, **11**, 105–10.

145. Goldhaber, S.Z., Haire, W.D., Feldstein, M.L. *et al.* (1993). Alteplase versus heparin in acute pulmonary embolism: randomised trial assessing right-ventricular function and pulmonary perfusion. *Lancet*, **341**, 507–11.

146. Stein, P.D., Fowler, S.E., Goodman, L.R. *et al.* (2006). Multidetector computed tomography for acute pulmonary embolism. *New England Journal of Medicine*, **354**, 2317–27.

147. Kasper, W., Konstantinides, S., Geibel, A. *et al.* (1997). Prognostic significance of right ventricular afterload stress detected by echocardiography in patients with clinically suspected pulmonary embolism. *Heart*, **77**, 346–9.

148. Giannitsis, E. and Katus, H.A. (2005). Risk stratification in pulmonary embolism based on biomarkers and echocardiography. *Circulation*, **112**, 1520–1.

149. Hutten, B.A., Prins, M.H., Gent, M. *et al.* (2000). Incidence of recurrent thromboembolic and bleeding complications among patients with venous thromboembolism in relation to both malignancy and achieved international normalized ratio: a retrospective analysis. *Journal of Clinical Oncology*, **18**, 3078–83.

150. Palareti, G., Legnani, C., Lee, A. *et al.* (2000). A comparison of the safety and efficacy of oral anticoagulation for the treatment of venous thromboembolic disease in patients with or without malignancy. *Thrombosis and Haemostasis*, **84**, 805–10.

151. Lee, A.Y., Levine, M.N., Baker, R.I. *et al.* (2003). Low-molecular-weight heparin versus a coumarin for the prevention of recurrent venous thromboembolism in patients with cancer. *New England Journal of Medicine*, **349**, 146–53.

152. Meyer, G., Marjanovic, Z., Valcke, J. *et al.* (2002). Comparison of low-molecular-weight heparin and warfarin for the secondary prevention of venous thromboembolism in patients with cancer: a randomized controlled study. *Archives Internal Medicine*, **162**, 1729–35.

153. Siragusa, S., Arcara, C., Malato, A. *et al.* (2005). Home therapy for deep vein thrombosis and pulmonary embolism in cancer patients. *Annals of Oncology*, **16**, iv136–iv139.

154. Noble, S.I., Nelson, A., Turner, C.F. *et al.* (2006). Acceptability of low molecular weight heparin thromboprophylaxis for inpatients receiving palliative care: qualitative study. *British Medical Journal*, **332**, 577–80.

155. Wan, S., Quinlan, D.J., Agnelli, G. *et al.* (2004). Thrombolysis compared with heparin for the initial treatment of pulmonary embolism: a meta-analysis of the randomized controlled trials. *Circulation*, **110**, 744–9.

156. Fiumara, K., Kucher, N., Fanikos, J. *et al.* (2006). Predictors of major hemorrhage following fibrinolysis for acute pulmonary embolism. *American Journal of Cardiology*, **97**, 127–9.

157. Stein, P.D., Kayali, F. and Olson, R.E. (2004). Twenty-one-year trends in the use of inferior vena cava filters. *Archives Internal Medicine*, **164**, 1541–5.

158. Eight-year follow-up of patients with permanent vena cava filters in the prevention of pulmonary embolism: the PREPIC (Prevention du Risque d'Embolie Pulmonaire par Interruption Cave) randomized study. (2005) *Circulation*, **112**, 416–22.

159. Noble, S.I. and Finlay, I.G. (2006). Have palliative care teams' attitudes toward venous thromboembolism changed? A survey of thromboprophylaxis practice across British specialist palliative care units in the years 2000 and 2005. *Journal of Pain and Symptom Management*, **32**, 38–43.

160. Soares, F.A., Pinto, A.P., Landell, G.A. *et al.* (1993). Pulmonary tumor embolism to arterial vessels and carcinomatous lymphangitis. A comparative clinicopathological study. *Archives of Pathology and Laboratory Medcine*, **117**, 827–31.

161. Stein, M.G., Mayo, J., Muller, N. *et al.* (1987). Pulmonary lymphangitic spread of carcinoma: appearance on CT scans. *Radiology*, **162**, 371–5.

162. Digumarthy, S.R., Fischman, A.J., Kwek, B.H. *et al.* (2005). Fluorodeoxyglucose positron emission tomography pattern of pulmonary lymphangitic carcinomatosis. *Journal of Computer Assisted Tomography*, **29**, 346–9.

163. Naito, T., Hasegawa, H., Asada, K. *et al.* (2006). Lymphangitis carcinomatosis as a potential predictor for a response to gefitinib. *Clinical Oncology (Royal College of Radiologists)*, **18**, 573–4.

164. Bruce, D.M., Heys, S.D., Eremin, O. (1996). Lymphangitis carcinomatosa: a literature review. *Journals of Royal College of Surgeons of Edinburgh*, **41**, 7–13.

165. Dudgeon, D.J., Lertzman, M. (1998). Dyspnea in the advanced cancer patient. *Journal of Pain and Symptom Management*, **16**, 212–9.

166. Feathers, L.S., Wilcock, A., Manderson, C. *et al.* (2003). Measuring inspiratory muscle weakness in patients with cancer and breathlessness. *Journal of Pain and Symptom Management*, **25**, 305–306.

167. Dekhuijzen, P.N., and Decramer, M. (1992). Steroid-induced myopathy and its significance to respiratory disease: a known disease rediscovered. *European Respiratory Journal*, **5**, 997–1003.

168. Batchelor, T.T., Taylor, L.P., Thaler, H.T. *et al.* (1997.) Steroid myopathy in cancer patients. *Neurology*, **48**, 1234–8.

169. Reinbolt, R.E., Shenk, A.M., White, P.H. *et al.* (2005). Symptomatic treatment of infections in patients with advanced cancer receiving hospice care. *Journal of Pain and Symptom Management*, **30**, 175–82.

170. Nagy-Agren, S. and Haley, H. (2002). Management of infections in palliative care patients with advanced cancer. *Journal of Pain and Symptom Management*, **24**, 64–70.

171. White, P.H., Kuhlenschmidt, H.L., Vancura, B.G. *et al.* (2003). Antimicrobial use in patients with advanced cancer receiving hospice care. *Journal of Pain and Symptom Management*, **25**, 438–43.

172. Clayton, J., Fardell, B., Hutton-Potts, J. *et al.* (2003). Parenteral antibiotics in a palliative care unit: prospective analysis of current practice. *Palliative Medicine*, **17**, 44–8.

173. Dunn, A., Carter, J.Carter, H. (2003). Anemia at the end of life: prevalence, significance, and causes in patients receiving palliative care. *Journal of Pain and Symptom Management*, **26**, 1132–9.

174. Heyse-Moore, L.H. (1993). On dyspnoea in advanced cancer. University of Southampton.

175. Corner, J., Plant, H., A'Hern, R. *et al.* (1996). Non-pharmacological intervention for breathlessness in lung cancer. *Palliative Medicine*, **10**, 299–305.

176. Bredin, M., Corner, J., Krishnasamy, M. *et al.* (1999). Multicentre randomised controlled trial of nursing intervention for breathlessness in patients with lung cancer. *BMJ*, **318**, 901–4.

177. Hately, J., Laurence, V., Scott, A. *et al.* (2003). Breathlessness clinics within specialist palliative care settings can improve the quality of life and functional capacity of patients with lung cancer. *Palliative Medicine*, **17**, 410–7.

178. Syrett, E. and Taylor, J. (2003). Non-pharmacological management of breathlessness: a collaborative nurse–physiotherapist approach. *International Journal of Palliative Nursing*, **9**, 150–6.

179. Gallo-Silver, L. and Pollack, B. (2000). Behavioral interventions for lung cancer-related breathlessness. *Cancer Practice*, **8**, 268–73.

180. Carrieri-Kohlman, V., Douglas, M.K., Gormley, J.M. *et al.* (1993). Desensitization and guided mastery: treatment approaches for the management of dyspnea. *Heart and Lung*, **22**, 226–34.

181. Neuenschwander, H., Molto, A., and Bianchi, M. (2006). External nasal dilator strips (ENDS) may improve breathlessness in cancer patients. *Supportive Care in Cancer*, **14**, 386–388.

182. Vickers, A.J., Feinstein, M.B., Deng, G.E. *et al.* (2005). Acupuncture for dyspnea in advanced cancer: a randomized, placebo-controlled pilot trial [ISRCTN89462491]. *BMC Palliative Care*, **4**, 5.

183. Cuomo, A., Delmastro, M., Ceriana, P. *et al.* (2004). Noninvasive mechanical ventilation as a palliative treatment of acute respiratory failure in patients with end-stage solid cancer. *Palliative Medicine*, **18**, 602–610.

184. Eaton, T., Garrett, J. E., Young, P. *et al.* (2002). Ambulatory oxygen improves quality of life of COPD patients: a randomised controlled study. *European Respiratory Journal*, **20**, 306–12.

185. Stevenson, N.J., Calverley, P.M. (2004). Effect of oxygen on recovery from maximal exercise in patients with chronic obstructive pulmonary disease. *Thorax*, **59**, 668–72.

186. Eaton, T., Fergusson, W., Kolbe, J. *et al.* (2006). Short-burst oxygen therapy for COPD patients: a 6-month randomised, controlled study. *European Respiratory Journal*, **27**, 697–704.

187. Bruera, E., Schoeller, T., and MacEachern, T. (1992). Symptomatic benefit of supplemental oxygen in hypoxemic patients with terminal cancer: the use of the N of 1 randomized controlled trial. *Journal of Pain and Symptom Management*, **7**, 365–8.

188. Bruera, E., de Stoutz, N., Velasco-Leiva, A. *et al.* (1993). Effects of oxygen on dyspnoea in hypoxaemic terminal-cancer patients. *Lancet*, **342**, 13–4.

189. Booth, S., Kelly, M.J., Cox, N.P. *et al.* (1996). Does oxygen help dyspnea in patients with cancer? *American Journal of Respiratory and Critical Care Medicine*, **153**, 1515–8.

190. Bruera, E., Sweeney, C., Willey, J. *et al.* (2003). A randomized controlled trial of supplemental oxygen versus air in cancer patients with dyspnea. *Palliative Medicine*, **17**, 659–63.

191. Philip, J., Gold, M., Milner, A. *et al.* (2006). A randomized, double-blind, crossover trial of the effect of oxygen on dyspnea in patients with advanced cancer. *Journal of Pain and Symptom Management*, **32**, 541–50.

192. Stringer, E., McParland, C., Hernandez, P. (2004). Physician practices for prescribing supplemental oxygen in the palliative care setting. *Journal of Palliative Care*, **20**, 303–7.

193. Florez, J. (1993). *Opioid, respiration and vomiting*. Springer, Berlin.

194. Takeda, S., Eriksson, L.I., Yamamoto, Y. *et al.* (2001). Opioid action on respiratory neuron activity of the isolated respiratory network in newborn rats. *Anesthesiology*, **95**, 740–9.

195. Manzke, T., Guenther, U., Ponimaskin, E.G. *et al.* (2003). 5-HT4(a) receptors avert opioid-induced breathing depression without loss of analgesia. *Science*, **301**, 226–9.

196. Juan, G., Ramon, M., Valia, J.C. *et al.* (2005). Palliative treatment of dyspnea with epidural methadone in advanced emphysema. *Chest*, **128**, 3322–8.

197. Zebraski, S.E., Kochenash, S.M., and Raffa, R.B. (2000). Lung opioid receptors: pharmacology and possible target for nebulized morphine in dyspnea. *Life Science*, **66**, 2221–31.

198. Modalen, A.O., Quiding, H., Frey, J. *et al.* (2005). A novel molecule (frakefamide) with peripheral opioid properties: the effects on resting ventilation compared with morphine and placebo. *Anesthesia and Analgesia*, **100** 713–7.

199. Modalen, A.O., Quiding, H., Frey, J. *et al.* (2006). A novel molecule with peripheral opioid properties: the effects on hypercarbic and hypoxic ventilation at steady-state compared with morphine and placebo. *Anesthesia and Analgesia*, **102**, 104–9.

200. Chrubasik, J., Wust, H., Friedrich, G. *et al.* (1988). Absorption and bioavailability of nebulized morphine. *British Journal of Anaesthesia*, **61**, 228–30.

201. Farr, S.J. and Otulana, B.A. (2006). Pulmonary delivery of opioids as pain therapeutics. *Advanced Drug Delivery Review*, **58**, 1076–88.

202. Bruera, E., MacEachern, T., Ripamonti, C. *et al.* (1993). Subcutaneous morphine for dyspnea in cancer patients. *Annals Internal Medicine*, **119**, 906–7.

203. Mazzocato, C., Buclin, T., and Rapin, C.H. (1999). The effects of morphine on dyspnea and ventilatory function in elderly patients with advanced cancer: a randomized double-blind controlled trial. *Annals of Oncology*, **10**, 1511–4.

204. Jennings, A.L., Davies, A.N., Higgins, J.P. *et al.* (2002). A systematic review of the use of opioids in the management of dyspnoea. *Thorax*, **57**, 939–44.

205. Abernethy, A.P., Currow, D.C., Frith, P. *et al.* (2003.) Randomised, double blind, placebo controlled crossover trial of sustained release morphine for the management of refractory dyspnoea. *British Medical Journal*, **327**, 523–8.

206. Bruera, E., Sala, R., Spruyt, O. *et al.* (2005). Nebulized versus subcutaneous morphine for patients with cancer dyspnea: a preliminary study. *Journal of Pain and Symptom Management*, **29**, 613–8.

207. Chiu, T.Y., Hu, W.Y., Lue, B.H. *et al.* (2001). Sedation for refractory symptoms of terminal cancer patients in Taiwan. *Journal of Pain and Symptom Management*, **21**, 467–72.

208. Allard. P., Lamontagne, C., Bernard, P. *et al.* (1999). How effective are supplementary doses of opioids for dyspnea in terminally ill cancer patients? A randomized continuous sequential clinical trial. *Journal of Pain and Symptom Management*, **17**, 256–65.

209. Benitez-Rosario, M.A., Martin, A.S., Feria, M. *et al.* (2005). Oral transmucosal fentanyl citrate in the management of dyspnea crises in cancer patients. *Journal of Pain and Symptom Management*, **30**, 395–7.

210. Smoller, J.W., Pollack, M.H., Otto, M.W. *et al.* (1996). Panic anxiety, dyspnea, and respiratory disease. Theoretical and clinical considerations. *American Journal of Respiratory and Critical Care Medicine*, **154**, 6–17.

211. McIver, B., Walsh, D.Nelson, K. (1994). The use of chlorpromazine for symptom control in dying cancer patients. *Journal of Pain and Symptom Management*, **9**, 341–5.

212. Navigante, A.H., Cerchietti, L.C., Castro, M.A. *et al.* (2006). Midazolam as adjunct therapy to morphine in the alleviation of severe dyspnea perception in patients with advanced cancer. *Journal of Pain and Symptom Management*, **31**, 38–47.

213. Nishino, T., Tagaito, Y., Sakurai, Y. (1997). Nasal inhalation of l-menthol reduces respiratory discomfort associated with loaded breathing. *American Journal of Respiratory and Critical Care Medicine*, **156**, 309–13.

214. Kohara, H., Ueoka, H., Aoe, K. *et al.* (2003). Effect of nebulized furosemide in terminally ill cancer patients with dyspnea. *Journal of Pain and Symptom Management*, **26**, 962–7.

215. Shimoyama, N. and Shimoyama, M. (2002). Nebulized furosemide as a novel treatment for dyspnea in terminal cancer patients. *Journal of Pain and Symptom Management*, **23**, 73–6.

216. Moosavi, S.H., Binks, A.P., Lansing, R.W. *et al.* (2007). Effect of inhaled furosemide on air hunger induced in healthy humans. *Respiration Physiology and Neurobiology*, **156**, 1–8.

217. Ong, K.C., Kor, A.C., Chong, W.F. *et al.* (2004). Effects of inhaled furosemide on exertional dyspnea in chronic obstructive pulmonary disease. *American Journal of Respiratory and Critical Care Medicine*, **169**, 1028–33.

218. Ahmedzai, S.H., Laude, E., Robertson, A. *et al.* (2004). A double-blind, randomised, controlled Phase II trial of Heliox28 gas mixture in lung cancer patients with dyspnoea on exertion. *British Journal of Cancer*, **90**, 366–71.

219. Kuo, C.W., Chen, Y.M., Chao, J.Y. *et al.* (2000). Non-small cell lung cancer in very young and very old patients. *Chest*, **117**, 354–7.

220. Mazzone, S.B. (2005). An overview of the sensory receptors regulating cough. *Cough*, **1**, 2.

221. Caterina, M.J., Schumacher, M.A., Tominaga, M. *et al.* (1997). The capsaicin receptor: a heat-activated ion channel in the pain pathway. *Nature*, **389**, 816–824.

222. Canning, B.J. (2006). Anatomy and neurophysiology of the cough reflex: ACCP evidence-based clinical practice guidelines. *Chest*, **129**, 33S–47S.

223. Homsi, J., Walsh, D., and Nelson, K.A. (2001). Important drugs for cough in advanced cancer. *Supportive Care in Cancer*, **9**, 565–74.

224. Chernecky, C., Sarna, L., Waller, J.L. *et al.* (2004.) Assessing coughing and wheezing in lung cancer: a pilot study. *Oncology Nursing Forum*, **31**, 1095–101.

225. Thatcher, N., Jayson, G., Bradley, B. *et al.* (1997). Gemcitabine: symptomatic benefit in advanced non-small cell lung cancer. *Seminars in Oncology*, **24**, S8-6–S8-12.

226. Kotzer, C.J., Hay, D.W., Dondio, G. *et al.* (2000). The antitussive activity of delta-opioid receptor stimulation in guinea pigs. *Journal of Pharmacology and Experimental Therapeutics*, **292**, 803–9.

227. Aylward, M., Maddock, J., Davies, D.E. *et al.* (1984). Dextromethorphan and codeine: comparison of plasma kinetics and antitussive effects. *European Journal of Respiratory Disease*, **65**, 283–91.

228. Hutchings, H.A., and Eccles, R. (1994). The opioid agonist codeine and antagonist naltrexone do not affect voluntary suppression of capsaicin induced cough in healthy subjects. *European Respiratory Journal*, **7**, 715–9.

229. Freestone, C., and Eccles, R. (1997). Assessment of the antitussive efficacy of codeine in cough associated with common cold. *Journal of Pharmacy and Pharmacology*, **49**, 1045–9.

230. Smith, J., Owen, E., Earis, J. *et al.* (2006). Effect of codeine on objective measurement of cough in chronic obstructive pulmonary disease. *Journal of Allergy and Clinical Immunology*, **117**, 831–5.

231. Lee, P.C.L., Jawad, M.S., and Eccles, R. (2000). Antitussive efficacy of dextromethorphan in cough associated with acute upper respiratory tract infection. *Journal of Pharmacy and Pharmacology*, **52**, 1137–42.

232. Bolser, D.C., and Davenport, P.W. (2007). Codeine and cough: an ineffective gold standard. *Current Opinion in Allergy and Clinical Immunology*, **7**, 32–6.

233. Homsi, J., Walsh, D., Nelson, K.A. *et al.* (2002). A phase II study of hydrocodone for cough in advanced cancer. *The American Journal of Hospice & Palliative Care*, **19**, 49–56.

234. Hagen, N.A. (1991). An approach to cough in cancer patients. *Journal of Pain and Symptom Management*, **6**, 257–62.

235. Brown, C., Fezoui, M., Selig, W.M. *et al.* (2004). Antitussive activity of sigma-1 receptor agonists in the guinea-pig. *British Journal of Pharmacology*, **141**, 233–40.

236. Kamei, J., Iwamoto, Y., Kawashima, N. *et al.* (1992). Involvement of haloperidol-sensitive sigma-sites in antitussive effects. *European Journal of Pharmacology*, **224**, 39–43.

237. Morice, A.H., Menon.,M.S, Mulrennan,S.A. *et al.* (2007). Opiate therapy in chronic cough. *American Journal of Respiratory and Critical Care Medicine*, **175**, 312–5.

238. Doona, M., Walsh, D. (1998). Benzonatate for opioid-resistant cough in advanced cancer. *Palliativie Medicine*, **12**, 55–8.

239. Luporini, G., Barni, S., Marchi, E. *et al.* (1998). Efficacy and safety of levodropropizine and dihydrocodeine on nonproductive cough in primary and metastatic lung cancer. *European Respiratory Journal*, **12**, 97–101.

240. Moroni, M., Porta, C., Gualtier, G. *et al.* (1996). Inhaled sodium cromoglycate to treat cough in advanced lung cancer patients. *British Journal of Cancer*, **74**, 309–11.

241. Hansson, L., Midgren, B., Karlsson, J.A. (1994). Effects of inhaled lignocaine and adrenaline on capsaicin-induced cough in humans. *Thorax*, **49**, 1166–8.

242. Choudry, N.B., Fuller, R.W., Anderson, N. *et al.* (1990). Separation of cough and reflex bronchoconstriction by inhaled local anaesthetics. *European Respiratory Journal*, **3**, 579–83.

243. Morice, A.H., Marshall, A.E., Higgins, K.S. *et al.* (1994). Effect of inhaled menthol on citric acid induced cough in normal subjects. *Thorax*, **49**, 1024–6.

244. Laude, E.A., Morice, A.H., Grattan, T.J. (1994). The antitussive effects of menthol, camphor and cineole in conscious guinea-pigs. *Pulmonary Pharmacology*, **7**, 179–84.

245. Mintz, S., and Lee, J.K. (2006). Gabapentin in the treatment of intractable idiopathic chronic cough: case reports. *American Journal of Medicine*, **119**, e13–15.

246. Zylicz, Z. and Krajnik, M. (2004). What has dry cough in common with pruritus? Treatment of dry cough with paroxetine. *Journal of Pain and Symptom Management*, **27**, 180–4.

247. Bennett, M. I. (1996). Death rattle: an audit of hyoscine (scopolamine) use and review of management. *Journal of Pain and Symptom Management*, **12**, 229–33.

248. Morita, T., Hyodo, I., Yoshimi, T. *et al.* (2004). Incidence and underlying etiologies of bronchial secretion in terminally ill cancer patients: a multicentre, prospective, observational study. *Journal of Pain and Symptom Management*, **27**, 533–9.

249. Wildiers, H., and Menten, J. (2002). Death rattle: prevalence, prevention and treatment. *Journal of Pain and Symptom Management*, **23**, 310–7.

250. Wee, B.L., Coleman, P.G., Hillier, R. *et al.* (2006). The sound of death rattle I: are relatives distressed by hearing this sound? *Palliative Medicine*, **20**, 171–5.

251. Wee, B.L., Coleman, P.G., Hillier, R. *et al.* (2006). The sound of death rattle II: how do relatives interpret the sound? *Palliative Medicine*, **20**, 177–81.

252. Bennett, M., Lucas, V., Brennan, M. *et al.* (2002). Using anti-muscarinic drugs in the management of death rattle: evidence-based guidelines for palliative care. *Palliative Medicine*, **16**, 369–74.

253. Back, I.N., Jenkins, K., Blower, A. *et al.* (2001). A study comparing hyoscine hydrobromide and glycopyrrolate in the treatment of death rattle. *Palliative Medicine*, **15**, 329–36.

254. Hugel, H., Ellershaw, J., Gambles, M. (2006). Respiratory tract secretions in the dying patient: a comparison between glycopyrronium and hyoscine hydrobromide. *Journal of Palliative*, **9**, 279–84.

255. Rubin, B.K. (2006). The pharmacologic approach to airway clearance: mucoactive agents. *Paediatric Respiratory Reviews*, **7** (Suppl 1), S215–9.

256. McCool, F.D., and Rosen, M.J. (2006). Nonpharmacologic airway clearance therapies: ACCP evidence-based clinical practice guidelines. *Chest*, **129**, 250S–259S.

257. Shimura, S., Sasaki, T., Sasaki, H. *et al.* (1988). Viscoelastic properties of bronchorrhoea sputum in bronchial asthmatics. *Biorheology*, **25**, 173–9.

258. Hidaka, N., and Nagao, K. (1996). Bronchioloalveolar carcinoma accompanied by severe bronchorrhea. *Chest*, **110**, 281–2.

259. Lembo, T., and Donnelly, T.J. (1995). A case of pancreatic carcinoma causing massive bronchial fluid production and electrolyte abnormalities. *Chest*, **108**, 1161–3.

260. Milton, D.T., Kris, M.G., Gomez, J.E. *et al.* (2005). Prompt control of bronchorrhea in patients with bronchioloalveolar carcinoma treated with gefitinib (Iressa). *Supportive Care in Cancer*, **13**, 70–2.

261. Takao, M., Inoue, K., Watanabe, F. *et al.* (2003). Successful treatment of persistent bronchorrhea by gefitinib in a case with Recurrent Bronchioloalveolar Carcinoma: a case report. *World Journal of Surgical Oncology*, **1**, 8.

262. Kitazaki, T., Soda, H., Doi, S. *et al.* (2005). Gefitinib inhibits MUC5AC synthesis in mucin-secreting non-small cell lung cancer cells. *Lung and Cancer*, **50**, 19–24.

263. Marom, Z.M., and Goswami, S.K. (1991). Respiratory mucus hypersecretion (bronchorrhea): a case discussion—possible mechanisms(s) and treatment. *Journal of Allergy and Clinical Immunology*, **87**, 1050–1055.

264. Hudson, E., Lester, J.F., Attanoos, R.L. *et al.* (2006). Successful treatment of bronchorrhea with octreotide in a patient with adenocarcinoma of the lung. *Journal of Pain and Symptom Management*, **32**, 200–2.

265. Tamaoki, J., Kohri, K., Isono, K. *et al.* (2000). Inhaled indomethacin in bronchorrhea in bronchioloalveolar carcinoma: role of cyclooxygenase. *Chest*, **117**, 1213–4.

266. Nakajima, T., Terashima, T., Nishida, J. *et al.* (2002). Treatment of bronchorrhea by corticosteroids in a case of bronchioloalveolar carcinoma producing CA19-9. *Internal Medicine*, **41**, 225–8.

267. Kvale, P.A., Simoff, M., Prakash, U.B. (2003). Lung cancer. Palliative care. *Chest*, **123**, 284S–311S.

268. Lordan, J. L., Gascoigne, A., Corris, P. A. (2003). The pulmonary physician in critical care * Illustrative case 7: Assessment and management of massive haemoptysis. *Thorax*, **58**, 814–9.

269. Miller, R. R., McGregor, D. H. (1980). Hemorrhage from carcinoma of the lung. *Cancer*, **46**, 200–5.

270. A Medical Research Council (MRC) randomised trial of palliative radiotherapy with two fractions or a single fraction in patients with inoperable non-small-cell lung cancer (NSCLC) and poor performance status. Medical Research Council Lung Cancer Working Party. (1992). *British Journal of Cancer*, **65**, 934–41.

271. Kavuru, M.S., Dweik, R.A., Thomassen, M.J. *et al.* (1999). Role of bronchoscopy in asthma research. *Clinics in Chest Medicine*, **20**, 153–89.

272. Bruzzi, J.F., Remy-Jardin, M., Delhaye, D. *et al.* (2006). Multi-detector row CT of hemoptysis. *Radiographics*, **26**, 3–22.

273. Ansell, J., Hirsh, J., Poller, L. *et al.* (2004). The pharmacology and management of the vitamin K antagonists: the Seventh ACCP Conference on Antithrombotic and Thrombolytic Therapy. *Chest*, **126**, 204S–233S.

274. Dean, A., Tuffin, P. (1997). Fibrinolytic inhibitors for cancer-associated bleeding problems. *Journal of Pain and Symptom Management*, **13**, 20–4.

275. Anwar, D., Schaad, N., Mazzocato, C. (2005). Aerosolized vasopressin is a safe and effective treatment for mild to moderate recurrent hemoptysis in palliative care patients. *Journal of Pain and Symptom Management*, **29**, 427–9.

276. Meijer, K., de Graaff, W. E., Daenen, S.M. *et al.* (2000). Successful treatment of massive hemoptysis in acute leukemia with recombinant factor VIIa. *Archives Internal Medicine*, **160**, 2216–7.

277. Freitag, L., Tekolf, E., Stamatis, G. *et al.* (1994). Three years experience with a new balloon catheter for the management of haemoptysis. *European Respiratory Journal*, **7**, 2033–7.

278. Conlan, A.A., Hurwitz, S.S., Krige, L. *et al.* (1983). Massive hemoptysis. Review of 123 cases. *Journal of Thoracic Cardiovascular Surgery*, **85**, 120–4.

279. Tsukamoto, T., Sasaki, H., Nakamura, H. (1989). Treatment of hemoptysis patients by thrombin and fibrinogen-thrombin infusion therapy using a fiberoptic bronchoscope. *Chest*, **96**, 473–6.

280. Fernando, H.C., Stein, M., Benfield, J. R. *et al.* (1998). Role of bronchial artery embolization in the management of hemoptysis. *Archives of Surgery*, **133**, 862–6.

281. Lester, J.F., Macbeth, F.R., Toy, E. *et al.* (2006). Palliative radiotherapy regimens for non-small cell lung cancer. *Cochrane Database System Review*, CD002143.

282. Ung, Y.C., Yu, E., Falkson, C. *et al.* and Lung Cancer Disease Site Group Of Cancer Care Ontario's Program In Evidence-Based, C. (2006). The role of high-dose-rate brachytherapy in the palliation of symptoms in patients with non-small-cell lung cancer: a systematic review. *Brachytherapy*, **5**, 189–202.

283. Graeff, A.D., and Dean, M. (2007). Palliative sedation therapy in the last weeks of life: a literature review and recommendations for standards. *Journal of Palliative Medicine*, **10**, 67–85.

284. Muller-Busch, H.C., Andres, I., Jehser, T. (2003). Sedation in palliative care – a critical analysis of 7 years experience. *BMC Palliative Care*, **2**.

285. Morita, T. (2004). Differences in physician-reported practice in palliative sedation therapy. *Supportive Care in Cancer*, **12**, 584–92.

286. Cherny, N.I., Portenoy, R.K. (1994). Sedation in the management of refractory symptoms: guidelines for evaluation and treatment. *Journal of Palliative Care*, **10**, 31–8.

287. Morita, T., Tsunoda, J., Inoue, S. *et al.* (2001). Effects of high dose opioids and sedatives on survival in terminally ill cancer patients. *Journal of Pain and Symptom Management*, **21**, 282–9.

288. Cowan, J.D., and Walsh, D. (2001). Terminal sedation in palliative medicine—definition and review of the literature. *Supportive Care in Cancer,* **9**, 403–7.

289. Cheng, C, Roemer-Becuwe, C., and Pereira, J. (2002). When midazolam fails. *Journal of Pain and Symptom Management*, **23**, 256–65.

11.2

Palliative issues in the care of patients with cancer of the head and neck

Barbara A. Murphy, Anthony Cmelak,
Stephen Bayles, Ellie Dowling, MS, CCC-SLP
Cheryl R. Billante, Sheila H. Ridner,
Kirsten Haman, Stewart M. Bond,
Ann Marie Flores, and
Panarut Wisawatapnimit

Introduction

By convention, head and neck cancer (HNC) refers to tumours arising from the epithelial lining of the upper aero-digestive tract. This includes patients with tumours of the oral cavity, larynx, pharynx, paranasal sinuses, and salivary glands. There are approximately 50 000 cases of HNC diagnosed annually within the USA[1]. The vast majority of tumours (>90 per cent) are squamous cell carcinomas. Due to the higher rate of smoking and heavy drinking in males, this type of cancer affects men disproportionately. Patients with HNC experience a wide array of palliative problems. Symptoms may be related to the tumour, acute toxicities of treatment, or the long-term sequelae of therapy. Although some symptoms are common to all cancers, HNC patients experience a host of unique problems which require special consideration. In addition, palliation is a major issue throughout the disease trajectory. Symptoms are usually present at the time of diagnosis and remain problematic through the terminal phase. For those patients who are cured, long-term biopsychosocial sequellae may persist for years. Thus, assessment and treatment of palliative issues is an intrinsic and vital component of care for the HNC patient. This chapter will address the palliative issues unique to this cohort of patients. It has been divided into four sections: (1) a review of presenting symptoms, initial evaluation, and contemporary treatment; (2) quality of life (QOL) and psychosocial issues; (3) functional deficits (speech and voice); and (4) symptom-control issues specific to HNC. The reader is referred to other chapters in this text to address general symptom-control problems.

Presenting symptoms, initial evaluation, and treatment

Presenting symptoms

As with all patients being evaluated for malignancy, patients with carcinoma arising in the head and neck region demand a comprehensive history and physical examination. A complete history should be obtained with particular attention to type and duration of symptoms. Patients with a known head and neck primary carcinoma additionally carry a 5–15 per cent risk of a synchronous primary elsewhere in the aero-digestive tract, thus, appropriate assessment includes questions directed at symptoms that may relate to a second primary aero-digestive tumour[2].

Presenting symptoms are often the result of encroachment of normal structures within the upper aero-digestive system and may be predictive of the primary tumour's location. Symptoms of hoarseness, for example, would implicate laryngeal involvement, whereas dysphagia may be more indicative of hypopharyngeal or oropharyngeal involvement. Early in the disease process symptoms may mimic routine complaints seen by a primary care physician, such as sore throat, nasal congestion, hoarseness, swollen glands, and earache. Symptoms not resolving or improving spontaneously within 3 weeks with conservative measures warrant additional attention and specialty evaluation, particularly in patients with risk factors of smoking and alcohol use. Attention should be given to more subtle symptoms such as otalgia with no evidence of ear disease, for this may represent referred pain from a lesion of the upper

Table 11.2.1 Head and neck staging.

Stage grouping*			
Stage 0	Tis	N0	M0
Stage I	T1	N0	M0
Stage II	T2	N0	M0
Stage III	T3	N0	M0
	T1	N1	M0
	T2	N1	M0
	T3	N1	M0
Stage IVA	T4	N0	M0
	T4	N1	M0
	Any T	N2	M0
Stage IVB	Any T	N3	M0
Stage IVC	Any T	Any N	M1

Regional lymph nodes (N)

NX Regional lymph nodes cannot be assessed

N0 No regional lymph node metastasis

N1 Metastasis in a single ipsilateral lymph node, 3 cm or less in greatest dimension

N2 Metastasis in a single ipsilateral lymph node, more than 3 cm but not more than 6 cm in greatest dimension; or in multiple ipsilateral lymph nodes, none more than 6 cm in greatest dimension; or in bilateral or contralateral lymph nodes, none more than 6 cm in greatest dimension

  N2a Metastasis in single ipsilateral lymph node more than 3 cm but not more than 6 cm in greatest dimension

  N2b Metastasis in multiple ipsilateral lymph nodes, none more than 6 cm in greatest dimension

  N2c Metastasis in bilateral or contralateral lymph nodes, none more than 6 cm in greatest dimension

N3 Metastasis in a lymph node more than 6 cm in greatest dimension

Distant metastasis (M)

MX Distant metastasis cannot be assessed

M0 No distant metastasis

M1 Distant metastasis

*T stage is dependent on the primary site

aero-digestive tract. Conductive hearing loss with a unilateral serous otitis media is highly suggestive of a nasopharyngeal mass obstructing the Eustachian tube. More ominous symptoms of airway obstruction, oral bleeding, and haemoptysis deserve emergent assessment.

Physical examination

A thorough examination involves inspection and palpation of each region of the head and neck. Initial assessment of the skin and scalp area may identify cutaneous malignancies. A complete cranial nerve exam is necessary as patients with advanced carcinomas may display signs of perineural spread or extension into the skull base. Otoscopy is performed to assess for the possibility of serous effusion, which may herald a mass in the nasopharynx obstructing the eustachian tube. Unilateral serous otitis media in an adult demands

direct visualization of the nasopharynx. Nasal exam begins with anterior rhinoscopy to assess the vestibule, turbinates, and septum. The oral cavity is then inspected for mucosal abnormalities. Ulceration and leukoplakia are suspicious for malignancy. Bimanual palpation of the oral cavity and the oropharynx is essential to identify submucosal masses that are not visualized by surface change to the mucosa and to assess for contiguous extension of visible primaries. Tumours of the base of tongue and tonsil are often missed because they are not immediately evident on simple oral visualization but can often be identified by palpation of a firm mass within the region. Fixation of tumour to the mandible and loose dentition are indicative of bony involvement. Trismus may be the result of extension of tumour into the deep pterygomaxillary space. Visualization of the larynx is either accomplished with a mirror examination or more commonly with a fibre-optic scope. The use of a fibre-optic scope through a transnasal route also allows for additional inspection of the nasopharynx and posterior soft palate as well as the larynx and hypopharyngeal inlet. Attention should be given to subsites of laryngeal involvement and the impact that any tumour has on vocal cord mobility, for this ultimately will impact on overall tumour stage. The neck is then palpated with attention to nodal basins. The parotids, suboccipital, submental, jugulodigastric, and paratracheal nodes are bimanually palpated and any mass is characterized by its size, location, consistency and mobility. Fixation of nodal metastasis often suggests extra-capsular extension with potential involvement of the carotid artery or deep neck musculature, which may be unresectable.

Radiographic and laboratory assessment

CT scans and MRIs are routinely used in the assessment of head and neck carcinoma. MRI imaging can be valuable in assessing skull-base involvement and perineural spread of tumour, while CT scans are more useful for bone evaluation and nodal assessment. Workup must include an evaluation for potential distant metastatic disease. Chest radiographs or CT of the chest are used to rule out metastatic disease or a second primary tumour. Increasingly, PET scans are used as a part of the staging work-up. Of note, they may be particularly useful in the setting of an unknown primary[3]. PET scans are used for follow-up where they may be helpful in distinguishing post-treatment scar tissue from recurrent disease[4] Blood counts and complete metabolic profile should be obtained to screen for organ system dysfunction. Elevations in liver enzymes may indicate potential hepatic metastasis. Elevations of alkaline phosphatase may herald bony metastasis and warrant bone scanning.

Endoscopy

Operative endoscopy is performed commonly to assess completely extension of tumour not easily viewed in the clinic setting. Additionally, due to the complexity and overlap of mucosal folds within the oral cavity, oropharynx, pharynx, and hypopharynx, standard images often fail to delineate the exact location of a tumour. For example, a tumour arising on the post-cricoid aspect of the larynx on CT scan cannot be differentiated from a tumour arising on the posterior pharyngeal wall behind the larynx because these two surfaces are in contact with one another. Operative endoscopy offers the opportunity to manipulate the region, lift the larynx off the posterior pharyngeal wall, and define the site of origin and extent of the tumour. Mapping of the tumour becomes critical in assessing the ability to resect the tumour and defining the

Table 11.2.2 Common toxicity and adverse event criteria 3.0 (CTCAE) grading for select toxicities of head and neck therapy.

Adverse event	1	2	3	4	5
Induration/fibrosis (skin and subcutaneous tissue)	Increased density on palpation	Moderate impairment of function not interfering with ADL; marked increase in density and firmness on palpation with or without minimal retraction	Dysfunction interfering with ADL; very marked density, retraction or fixation	C	C
Dermatitis associated with radiation	Faint erythema or dry desquamation	Moderate to brisk erythema; patchy moist desquamation, mostly confined to skin folds and creases; moderate oedema	Moist desquamation other than skin folds and creases; bleeding induced by minor trauma or abrasion	Skin necrosis or ulceration of full thickness dermis; spontaneous bleeding from involved site	Death
Dry mouth/ salivary gland (xerostomia)	Symptomatic (dry or thick saliva) without significant dietary alteration; unstimulated saliva flow >0.2 ml/min	Symptomatic and significant oral intake alteration (e.g. copious water, other lubricants, diet limited to purees and/or soft, moist foods); unstimulated saliva 0.1–0.2 ml/min	Symptoms leading to inability to adequately aliment orally; IV fluids, tube feedings, or TPN indicated; unstimulated saliva <0.1 ml/min	C	C
Dysphagia (difficulty swallowing)	Symptomatic, able to eat regular diet	Symptomatic and altered eating/ swallowing (e.g. altered dietary habits, oral supplements); IV fluids indicated <24 h	Symptomatic and severely altered eating/ swallowing (e.g. inadequate oral calorific or fluid intake); IV fluids, tube feedings, or TPN indicated ≥24 h	Life-threatening consequences (e.g. obstruction, perforation)	Death
Mucositis/stomatitis (clinical exam)	Erythema of the mucosa	Patchy ulcerations or pseudomembranes	Confluent ulcerations or pseudomembranes; bleeding with minor trauma	Tissue necrosis; significant spontaneous bleeding; life-threatening consequences	Death
Mucositis/stomatitis (functional/ symptomatic)	Upper aero-digestive tract sites: Minimal symptoms, normal diet; minimal respiratory symptoms but not interfering with function Lower GI sites: minimal discomfort, intervention not indicated	Upper aero-digestive tract sites: symptomatic but can eat and swallow modified diet; respiratory symptoms interfering with function but not interfering with ADL Lower GI sites: symptomatic, medical intervention indicated but not interfering with ADL	Upper aero-digestive tract sites: symptomatic and unable to adequately aliment or hydrate orally; respiratory symptoms interfering with ADL Lower GI sites: stool incontinence or other symptoms interfering with ADL	Symptoms associated with life-threatening consequences	Death
Stricture/stenosis (including anastomotic), GI	Asymptomatic radiographic findings only	Symptomatic; altered GI function (e.g. altered dietary habits, vomiting, bleeding, diarrhoea); IV fluids indicated <24 h	Symptomatic and severely altered GI function (e.g. altered dietary habits, diarrhoea, or GI fluid loss); IV fluids, tube feedings, or TPN indicated ≥24 h: operative intervention indicated	Life-threatening consequences; operative intervention requiring complete organ resection (e.g. total colectomy)	Death

potential defect that would be created so a reconstructive effort may be planned.

Treatment and outcome

Upon completion of the initial evaluation, the tumour is characterized based on stage and the site of origin. The staging process must be carried out in a thorough and deliberate fashion as both treatment and outcome are heavily dependent on the extent of disease and the site of primary. Patients with early stage tumours $(T_{1-2}N_0M_0)$ have a cure rate of between 70 and 90 per cent with either radiation or surgery[5]. Unfortunately, the majority of patients present with locally advanced disease $(T_{3-4}$ or N+). Patients with locally advanced disease are usually treated with combined modality therapy. Patients with resectable disease are treated with surgery followed by radiation therapy (plus or minus concurrent chemotherapy) which is added in order to eliminate microscopic residual disease. In some patients, surgical-based treatment may be found to lead to severe functional compromise. Patients at particular risk of poor functional outcome with a surgical approach included those patients with laryngeal, hypopharyngeal, and base-of-tongue primaries. In this cohort of patients, a radiation-based treatment approach may be undertaken in order to avoid the morbidity of surgery[6]. Depending on the stage and the site of primary, 3-year survival for patients with resectable locally advanced disease was 30–70 per cent[5]. Patients with unresectable disease are treated with a combination of chemotherapy and radiation. Survival for unresectable patients using aggressive chemoradiation is approximately 20–30 per cent[7]. Of note, combined modality therapy for locally advanced disease is associated with increase in both acute and long-term toxicities. The clinician is, therefore, challenged to provide sufficient symptom control to ensure completion of this aggressive therapy. In addition, attempts to minimize long-term sequellae of treatment through rehabilitation, nutritional counselling, and general support services are mandatory.

Quality of life and psychosocial issues

Quality of life and symptom burden

QOL is a global construct that reflects a patient's general sense of well-being. It is influenced by numerous factors including: beliefs, expectations, and personal experience[8,9]. There are four core domains included in health-related QOL: functional, emotional, social and, physical well-being. It is important that QOL be distinguished from symptom assessment. Symptom assessment is directed at a specific problem or a related group of problems. Symptoms are a component of QOL assessment, but the emphasis of QOL assessment is on the overall sense of well-being, not specific contributing factors. The relationship between symptom burden and QOL is complex and may change over time as patients adapt to symptom-control issues.

Historically, QOL research in HNC patients has been limited by: (1) lack of adequate tools; (2) lack of prospective data collection with appropriate baseline and long-term follow-up; (3) inadequate power due to small sample size; and (4) heterogeneous patient selection and lack of treatment uniformity. Over the past decade, numerous tools have been developed to assess QOL in patients with cancer. The two most commonly used are the Functional Assessment of Cancer Therapy (FACT/FACIT)[10,11] and the European Organization for Research into the Treatment of Cancer

Quality of Life Questionnaire for HNC (EORTC QLQ-30)[12]. Both of these instruments have head and neck subscales which address disease specific symptoms. The sensitivity, reliability, validity, and responsiveness to change of these tools have been well summarized in a recent review of QOL instruments for HNC[13]. Prospective QOL assessments using these and other validated tools are now being reported. The reader is referred to a recent review for a detailed discussion of QOL in the HNC population[14].

Worth noting is the general trajectory of QOL in patients undergoing therapy for locally advanced disease. Regardless of the treatment approach used, patients with HNC experience an initial drop in QOL post-treatment. The QOL then rises slowly towards baseline levels as acute symptoms abate, function improves, and as patients adapt to new physical limitations. Weymuller evaluated QOL in 210 consecutive patients treated with either primary surgery or radiation. Composite QOL scores were *not* affected by treatment method (surgery versus chemoradiation) with the exception of 12 patients with advanced laryngeal cancer[15]. Using the University of Washington QOL tool (UW-QOL), Rogers *et al.* assessed pre-treatment QOL in 48 patients undergoing surgical resection for oral cavity tumours[16]. QOL was reassessed at 3 and 12 months. Twenty-five of 29 surviving patients completed the 1-year post-treatment assessment. The results demonstrate a drop in overall QOL 3 months after primary surgery with a return to pre-treatment levels at 12 months. Investigators were able to identify prognostic indicators for poor outcome which included: more advanced stage, the need for adjuvant radiation and anterior oral cavity lesions. Similarly, Murry reported the QOL outcome of 58 patients treated with intra-arterial chemoradiation for organ preservation. Overall QOL and physical/functional parameters worsened with therapy. At 6 months, overall QOL had improved above baseline. The degree of QOL improvement was site specific with laryngeal and hypopharyngeal cancer patients showing improved QOL, while QOL was unchanged for patients with oral cavity tumours. This study was limited by the relatively low number of patients who completed the 6 month assessment (n = 27)[17].

Co-morbid disease

Primary risk factors for HNC include smoking and drinking, both of which may lead to the development of co-morbid disease[18]. While some co-morbid diseases are mild and do not affect outcome, others may be severe enough to affect treatment tolerance, disease specific and overall survival. As combined modality treatment regimens are being used with increased frequency, it has become recognized that aggressive regimens may not be appropriate for all patients. Thus, there is a heightened awareness that we must understand the relationship between co-morbid disease and treatment outcome.

Piccirillo developed the Washington University Head and Neck Co-morbidity Index (WUHNCI) in order to relate co-morbid disease to treatment outcome in the HNC population[19]. In a chart review of 1153 HNC patients, the most common co-morbidities were pulmonary disease (17.9 per cent), other controlled cancers (8.6 per cent), diabetes mellitus (7.9 per cent), myocardial infarction (6.7 per cent), peptic ulcer disease (5.2 per cent), and cerebrovascular disease (4.6 per cent). Seven conditions (congestive heart failure, cardiac arrhythmia, peripheral vascular disease, pulmonary disease, renal disease, controlled cancer, and uncontrolled cancer) were related to survival and thus deemed 'predictive co-morbidities'.

The WUHNCI score is the sum of the weights of each of these seven conditions. Results demonstrated that the WUHNCI co-morbidity score was strongly associated with survival (log rank = 0.7717, $p < 0.001$). An added issue in the HNC population is the high prevalence of alcohol abuse. Investigators have identified alcoholism as an independent risk factor for survival in HNC[20].

Thus, an extensive medical evaluation is mandatory for all patients prior to initiating therapy. In particular, clinicians should assess carefully those co-morbidities that have been identified as 'prognostic for survival'. Patients with a number of poor prognostic co-morbidities may be suitable for less aggressive therapy. Interestingly, Hollenbeak conducted a separate analysis of 1780 Medicare patients with HNC to determine whether co-morbidity predicted cost of treatment. No difference in 1-year cost was noted based on the WUHNC score, however, the 5-year cost of therapy was higher for those patients with predictive co-morbidities[21].

Socio-economic status

In addition to complex medical problems, patients with HNC have significant psychosocial issues. After treatment, patients often experience prolonged treatment side effects and increasing social isolation. Using QOL questionnaires, Epstein *et al.* reported on the psychosocial effect of HNC on a cohort of patients who had completed therapy. Moderate or severe adverse effects were reported on family interactions (16.9 per cent), social interactions (30.8 per cent), and finances (30.8 per cent)[22].

Family issues

HNC patients identify the family as their primary social support, followed by friends, health-care providers, and self help groups[23–24]. Families play an important role in helping patients to control side effects of HNC and its treatment as well as providing psychological support. Sherman[25] found that HNC patients who do not have family support have worse adaptation and increased distress. De Leeuw also found that available appraisal support, emotional support, and the number of informal social networks were associated with decreased depression[26].

From a family systems perspective, dysfunction or illness in one family member affects other family members, because a family unit functions as an interconnected whole[27]. Research has documented that HNC affects the patient's family, including psychological problems, family relationships, and general concerns. Based on secondary analysis of studies, a research team at the Vanderbilt University School of Nursing and the Vanderbilt-Ingram Cancer Center found that of 61 HNC patient-family caregiver dyads, 69 per cent of patients, and 17.8 per cent of caregivers had depressed mood, based on the Center for Epidemiologic Studies Depression Scale[28]. Caregiver burden was significantly related to psychological vulnerability, confrontive coping, distraction, wishful thinking, self-castigation, self-isolation, general disengagement, and depressed mood in the patients and their family caregivers[30]. Vickery studied the impact of HNC and side effects of treatment (in particular, facial disfigurement) on the QOL of patients and their partners[30]. They found that HNC patients' partners reported higher levels of HNC-related anxiety than the patients themselves. Thus it is clear that HNC causes psychological problems for both patients and their families.

Wisawatapnimit[29] also analyzed secondary qualitative data in 11 HNC patients after treatment and six family caregivers and found that patients and their family caregivers had closer family relationships than before they had cancer, but they were faced with role transition challenges. Most patients reported that they had closer or better relationship with their families than before they had cancer, and appreciated how important the family was to them to cope with cancer. However, some patients who had side effects and stayed at home felt helpless and frustrated because they did not want to be a burden on their family. Family caregivers reported that it was difficult for them to adjust to their new role. Further, if the patient could not work, it affected their financial status, which in turn led to additional problems for them and their families.

Both patients and their families reported similar concerns about fear of cancer recurrence[31–34]. However, there were some differences in concerns between HNC patients and their family members that highlight the importance of assessing family members. Patients' concerns focused on their physical, functional, and social problems. On the other hand, family caregivers were concerned about their caregiver roles and about taking care of themselves. Thus, individuals' concerns varied depending on their roles, and differences appear to increase with time after the surgery[33,34].

Social issues

The disfigurement and dysfunction resulting from HNC and its treatment strongly affects the social domain, with the major social problems of HNC patients being social interaction and communication. HNC patients with visible scars and distorted features often feel stigmatized and reluctant to participate in public activities such as eating and speaking[36]. This is especially true in larynx cancer patients who have lost the ability to speak.

In general, HNC patients have to cope with social interaction challenges more than patients with other types of cancer, because the features of HNC and its treatment, especially surgery, can be clearly visible to other people. Because of the changes in their perceived or actual body image, HNC patients often do not want to go outside or to participate in social activities. Thus, social interaction problems are often reported by these patients. For example, Epstein found that 60 per cent of HNC patients reported moderate or severe effects of their cancer on social activities[22]. In particular, laryngectomized patients frequently report troubles with their friends and acquaintances and decreased participation in social events away from home[36]. Unfortunately, patients' social lives and functioning do not improve over time from treatment[37], which suggests that HNC patients may face these problems permanently. Further, social withdrawal and decreased social activities are themselves associated with patients' impaired psychosocial adjustment, as higher levels of social activity are associated with better psychosocial adjustment[38].

Communication problems are particularly prevalent among HNC patients and are particularly problematic because of cancer patients' need to associate with and relate to families and significant others to obtain social support[39]. Wisawatapnimit[30] analyzed secondary qualitative data and found that HNC patients identified that communication problems are 'devastating' for patients, because it affects their work, relationships with others, and emotions. Although some patients reported better communicative functioning 2 years post-treatment[40], other patients had this problem permanently or indefinitely, depending on the type of treatment they received.

Financial issues

Unfortunately, HNC patients frequently have few resources to cope with the complex array of medical and psychological problems. In a study of the long-term psychosocial implications of surgery for HNC patients, over half of patients were unable to return to work after treatment[41]. The financial implications for the patient and the patient's family may be significant. Inadequate resources may impact on both QOL and survival. In a recent report from Canada, patients with a lower socio-economic status had worse treatment outcomes than patients with a higher socio-economic status. The cause-specific 5-year survival was from 65.4 per cent in the highest quintile compared with 51.7 per cent in the lowest quintile (CI 11.1–16.3)[42]. Providing adequate medical and psychosocial support for HNC patients can challenge the treatment team. Aggressive social work involvement is needed from the time of diagnosis and throughout treatment to aid the patient and the treatment team and optimize therapeutic outcome.

Functional deficits: swallowing and voice

HNC may affect profoundly two vital life functions: swallowing and vocalization. Abnormalities in swallowing and voice may be the result of either progressive tumour or treatment-related sequelae[43,44]. Functional damage due to tumour may be irreparable; however, investigators have attempted to identify therapies which optimize outcome. 'Function preservation' or 'tissue sparing' treatment is directed at providing patients with a curative treatment that limits function loss. Techniques which have been investigated as potential function sparing approaches include: function sparing surgery, altered fractionation radiation therapy, and chemoradiation. Equally important for maximizing function is to ensure adequate access to rehabilitation services. The speech-language pathologist (SLP) should be considered an integral member of the multi-disciplinary team which carries out the comprehensive care and complex rehabilitation of these patients.

For early stage diseases, both surgery and radiation-based function preservation approaches have become standard treatment options[45]. Radiation therapy as a single modality has long been utilized as a treatment for patients with stage I, stage II, and good risk stage III squamous carcinomas of the larynx. Over the past two decades, surgical function sparing therapies have been also become popular. Such techniques include: microflap resection of carcinoma *in situ*, partial cordotomy, total cordotomy, supraglottic laryngectomies, and hemilaryngectomies. As with single modality radiation therapy, the majority of function-sparing surgical approaches have demonstrated feasibility in patients with early

Table 11.2.3 Survival and economic status in head and neck cancer patients.[42]

Income group	Percentage of survival
Quintile 1	65.4
Quintile 2	60.1
Quintile 3	60.6
Quintile 4	60.3
Quintile 5	51.7

stage disease. While surgery and radiation have long been accepted as function sparing approaches for early stage disease (stage I and II), it is only within the past two decades that function-preserving approaches using chemoradiation have been utilized in locally advanced HNC (stage III and IV). As data have accumulated, concern has been expressed that tissue-preserving therapy may not result in good functional outcome, particularly in patients treated with aggressive regimens[46]. Thus, there is tremendous interest in the evaluation and comparison of functional outcome for patients treated with various approaches. The outcome parameters of the most vital interest are swallowing and voice.

When addressing functional issues in patients with HNC, one must frame the discussion in a meaningful manner. It is often helpful to distinguish functional impairment from disability and handicap. Most HNC patients have an amazing ability to adapt to functional deficits. However, functional deficits may lead to disability (effect of dysfunction on self) or handicap (effect of dysfunction in relationship to others). More often than not, physicians are unaware of the extent and severity of functional deficits, disabilities, and handicaps experienced by their patients[47]. Rehabilitation services can identify more effectively the type and extent of functional deficits. Therapy can be undertaken to improve function and minimize the disability and handicap resulting from function loss.

Swallow function and dysfunction

Swallowing is a complex series of mechanical processes that allows for nutritional intake. It can be broken down into several phases: oral, pharyngeal, and oesophageal. The oral phase can be described as having two separate components: the oral preparation phase and the oral transport phase[48]. During the oral phase, the lips and tongue play a vital role in oral bolus preparation and bolus propulsion to the oropharynx. During the subsequent pharyngeal phase, the tongue acts as the driving force for the food bolus while a complex sequence of physiologic processes propels the bolus towards the oesophagus. These physiologic processes include: (1) closure of the velopharyngeal port; (2) elevation and anterior movement of the larynx and hyoid; (3) closure of the larynx at the level of the true and false vocal cords and epiglottis; and (4) opening of the upper oesophageal sphincter allowing for bolus passage into the oesophagus[49]. The pharyngeal phase takes about 800 ms from entry of the pharynx to exit into the oesophagus [50]. The oesophageal phase, which typically lasts 8–20 s, begins at the cricopharyngeal juncture or upper oesophageal sphincter and ends at the gastrooesophageal juncture or lower oesophageal sphincter. Oesophageal peristalsis carries the bolus to the stomach.

Deficits in any one of these phases can result in significant levels of disability. Swallowing dysfunction may require patients to alter substantially the consistencies and type of foods they ingest[51]. These dietary changes may lead to nutritional deficits and the numerous complications of malnutrition. Furthermore, functional deficits may lead to handicaps such as inability to eat in public or at social gatherings. The most severe complication of swallowing dysfunction is aspiration. Patients who aspirate are at risk of pneumonia. In the stroke population, aspiration results in 40 000 deaths per year[52]. The number of deaths due to aspiration in the HNC population is unknown. Lundy reported on 166 consecutive patients referred for swallowing evaluation with various underlying medical problems[53]. Eighty patients had neurological problems, 38 medical problems, and 33 HNC. HNC patients had the highest rate of aspiration with a total of 76 per cent versus 49 per cent for patients with a neurological diagnosis and 43 per cent of patients who had a medical diagnosis. Nyguyn conducted a retrospective chart review of 114 HNC patients treated with concurrent chemoradiation for locally advanced disease in order to assess the incidence of aspiration during therapy[54]. Aspiration was defined as: (1) chest X-ray consistent with pneumonia or (2) aspiration on the modified barium swallow (MBS) during their treatment. Fifteen patients (13 per cent) developed aspiration during chemoradiation (12 identified on chest X-ray, three on MBS alone, and three both). All 15 patients had severe mucositis at the time of the aspiration. Six patients (5 per cent) died. Thus, it is likely that aspiration is a significant and frequently unrecognized problem in the HNC population. It is imperative that physicians are aware of the possibility of aspiration in this patient population and that appropriate evaluation and therapy be undertaken when indicated.

Assessment of swallowing dysfunction

Various instrumental techniques have been used to study swallowing, including electromyography, manometry, scintigraphy, ultrasound, endoscopy and videofluoroscopy[55]. The most commonly used technique in the clinical setting and what is considered 'the gold standard' for swallowing assessment is the videofluoroscopy, also referred to as the modified barium swallow study (MBSS). The MBSS provides information on oral and pharyngeal transit deficits as well as the presence and, most importantly, aetiology of aspiration. The MBSS also provides information to the clinician regarding the effectiveness of diet modification and compensatory strategies that may be utilized to improve swallowing safety and function. Flexible endoscopic evaluation of swallowing (FEES) is an endoscopic procedure for the assessment of sensory and motor swallowing function. It may be used to evaluate airway protection as well as bolus transport[56]. Scintigraphy may be used to assess bolus flow; however, anatomic structures are not well defined. In addition, patient report tools have been developed to assess swallowing. Examples include the MD Anderson Dysphagia Specific Quality-of-Life tool[57], the SWAL-QOL[58] and the Vanderbilt Head and Neck Symptom Survey[59].

Pre-treatment swallowing abnormalities

To understand clearly the effect of therapy on swallowing abnormalities in HNC patients, prospective longitudinal studies are needed. Unfortunately, few studies have been conducted in this manner. The majority of studies are cross-sectional evaluations of swallowing function after therapy has been completed. Thus, baseline data are missing. Stenson undertook an analysis of HNC patients prior to treatment in order to provide insight into the baseline swallowing abnormalities [60]. The tools selected for assessment were the MBSS and the Swallowing Performance Status Scale (SPSS). The SPSS is a global assessment tool for reporting the results of a MBSS. It is rated on a scale of 1 (normal) to 7 (severe impairment—requires PEG tube). As expected, the type of impairment was site specific with oral cavity, and oropharynx tumours manifesting oral impairment; larynx and hypopharynx tumours manifesting pharyngeal impairment; and hypopharyngeal tumours manifesting oesophageal impairment. The degree of impairment was site specific with hypopharyngeal and laryngeal patients experiencing the most impaired swallowing with a SPSS score of 4.1 and 3.7, respectively. Similarly, patients with hypopharyngeal and

laryngeal carcinomas were the most likely to experience aspiration (80 per cent and 67 per cent, respectively). Interestingly, there was no association between T-stage or overall stage and swallowing dysfunction. The high rate of baseline swallowing dysfunction underscores the need for prospective trials in order to ascertain clearly the long-term effects of treatment.

Post-treatment swallowing abnormalities

Patients who undergo surgery of an organ involved in swallowing may expect some alteration in function. The degree of functional deficit is largely dependent on the extent of surgery. McConnel evaluated 30 patients who underwent resection of oral cavity cancers. The percentage of oral and tongue base resected were the only parameters prognostic for swallowing outcome[61]. This has been confirmed by other investigators[62]. In addition to extent of resection, Logemann demonstrated that the degree of swallowing dysfunction was also related to the site of resection. Patients undergoing floor of mouth or tongue base resections had more swallowing difficulty than those undergoing supraglottic laryngectomies[63]. Adjuvant radiation may worsen postoperative swallowing by increasing oedema, fibrosis, and xerostomia[64]. Finally, the method of reconstruction may also affect functional outcome. Borggreven conducted a prospective study of 80 patients who underwent microvascular soft tissue reconstruction for primary tumours of the oral cavity and oropharynx[65]. Patients underwent MBS and scintigraphy at baseline, 6 and 12 months post-treatment. Abnormalities in oral and oropharyngeal swallow were noted in more than half of patients at 6 months post-treatment. No significant improvement was noted between 6 and 12 months. Factors predictive for poor swallow outcome include: co-morbid condition, T3 or T4 tumours, and combined resection of the base of tongue and soft palate.

Swallowing abnormalities have also been noted in patients who undergo primary radiation therapy. These deficits can be divided into abnormalities related to acute toxicities and those associated with long-term effects. Acutely during therapy, patients develop severe mucosal ulcers and soft tissue oedema. These result in painful swallowing and dysphagia. Acute toxicities resolve slowly within 4–12 weeks of completing therapy. Late effects may begin to appear simultaneously with the resolution of acute toxicities. Persistent oedema and the development of fibrosis result in mechanical alterations in swallow function. Swallowing abnormalities can be seen in the oral preparation, oral, pharyngeal, and oesophageal phases. The most commonly identified swallowing abnormalities include: decreased tongue base retraction, decreased laryngeal elevation, decreased epiglottic inversion, decreased pharyngeal wall motion and aspiration.

In an attempt to study the late effects of chemoradiation on HNC patients, investigators undertook a correlative study to assess functional outcome[66] in patients enrolled on ECOG 2399, a phase II organ preservation study using induction chemotherapy followed by concomitant chemoradiation (CCR) in patients with squamous cancer of the larynx or oropharynx[67]. Swallow evaluations were done at baseline, 3, 12, and 24 months post-treatment. Measures included: (1) the MBS score using the Dysphagia Outcome Severity Scale and the Functional Communication Measure; and (2) self-report measures consisted of the PSS-HN and FACT-HN. Results are noted in Table 11.2.4. The majority of patients presented with mild objective abnormalities on MBS. Few patients had moderate or severe swallowing abnormalities at baseline. At 3 months

Table 11.2.4 Results of modified barium swallow studies on E 2399.

Score (per cent)	Normal (7)		Mild (5–6)		Moderate (3–4)		Severe (1–2)	
Scale	D	F	D	F	D	F	D	F
Baseline	20	73	68	16	9	7	4	4
3 month	0	23	63	36	20	21	18	24
12 month	3	44	83	37	11	12	5	7
24 month	4	46	84	43	12	4	0	8

D = Dysphagia Outcome Severity Scale, F = Functional Communication Measure.

post-treatment, swallowing had deteriorated markedly. Eighteen and 24 per cent of patients had severe swallowing deficits on the DOSS and FCM, respectively, while 20 and 21 per cent of patients had moderate swallowing deficits. At 12 months, swallowing function had improved for the majority of patients with <10 per cent of patients having severe swallowing effects. Conversely, some investigators have reported high rates of PEG feeding tubes 1–2 years post-treatment[68].

Recently, considerable effort has been directed at attempts to identify patients who are at risk of poor swallowing function after radiation-based therapy. Kendall conducted a study of swallowing function in patients 12 months after primary radiation therapy[69]. Although flawed by the lack of baseline measurements, he demonstrated abnormal swallowing in all patients. Of significance, the tongue base tumours were found to have a high incidence of aspiration. This has been confirmed by other investigators. Using the Head and Neck Radiotherapy Questionnaire and a swallowing questionnaire, Murry et al. identified disease site as a predictor for swallowing outcome after aggressive treatment with intra-arterial chemoradiation for organ preservation[17]. In addition to site specificity as potential predictors for swallowing outcome, retrospective studies of primary radiation therapy demonstrate a worse functional outcome for patients with a higher T-stage. Risk factors for poor functional outcome may also include a patient's characteristics which reflect general health and psychosocial support.

Of interest, patients often attribute difficulty swallowing to xerostomia. Logemann evaluated the effect of xerostomia on bolus transport in patients treated with chemoradiation. Although patients with xerostomia perceived swallowing deficits, bolus transport was unaffected[70]. Hamlet demonstrated that xerostomia does affect mastication and oral manipulation of dry food[71].

Various techniques are available for swallowing therapy and rehabilitation; however, the role of swallowing therapy in HNC patients remains to be clarified. Issues that require further study include: (1) the optimal techniques for specific deficits; (2) timing of therapy; (3) duration of therapy; and (4) identification of those most likely to benefit. Dejonckere reported the results of a retrospective analysis of swallowing function in patients who have completed therapy: 87 per cent were treated with surgery with or without postoperative radiation and 13 per cent were treated with radiation. Post-treatment, all patients underwent evaluation of swallowing function followed by rehabilitation. Rehabilitation lasted fewer than 12 weeks for 45 per cent of patients and fewer than 24 weeks for 78 per cent of patients. Patients underwent reassessment post-treatment. There was a marked improvement in swallowing

function ($p = 0.0001$) post-treatment. Nine of 82 patients had significant swallowing abnormalities post-rehabilitation. While this study does not have a control arm and some degree of improvement over time should be expected, the results support the efficacy of speech language pathology therapy.

Voice

The ability to communicate is a critical human function and vocalization is our most important communication method. Without an intact voice, patients often become isolated and experience a marked decrease in their social interactions. Furthermore, conducting activities of daily living may be difficult without vocal ability. Treatment of HNC often necessitates resection of structures critical to the production of normal speech, resonance, and voice. Further, resection of a malignancy may require sacrifice of the nerve supply which innervates these structures, leaving the patient with paralysis of the tongue, pharynx, palate, or larynx. In general, the greater the extent of resection, the more severe the resultant communication disorder. Primary or adjuvant radiation may also affect vocalization. Listed below are brief descriptions of the voice abnormalities noted in HNC patients. For further information on evaluation and treatment, please see Chapter 4.9.

Disordered speech

Lip Most early lip lesions can be treated effectively with resection or radiation therapy. Small local wedge-shaped defects can be closed primarily. More serious tissue deficits can be reconstructed with pedicle flaps[72]. This may result in altered articulation of bilabial sounds /b, p, m/, and labiodental sounds /f, v/. Injury to the second and third branches of the trigeminal nerve disrupts sensation to the lips, while motor function is supplied by a branch of the facial nerve (upper lip) or marginal mandibular nerve (lower lip). Labial paralysis prevents normal articulation of related sounds.

Tongue Reconstruction of lingual tissue defects are usually achieved with primary closure or local, regional or distant flaps. In the case of minor deficits, speech and swallowing can be largely preserved. However, in the case of advanced disease, total glossectomy severely alters articulation. In such cases, the focus of speech therapy is to maximize remaining function through range of motion and flexibility drills, and to devise alternative articulatory placements for affected speech sounds. In cases where disability is extreme, an augmentative system of communication, such as computerized speech is indicated. A prosthesis may be helpful in rehabilitating the communication of the glossectomy patient. Involvement or sacrifice of the hypoglossal nerve creates a unilateral lingual paralysis. Dysarthria, weak and imprecise articulation, is the resulting speech disability.

Teeth Loss of or extraction of teeth associated with tumour involvement or radiation therapy, or mandibular osteoradionecrosis (ORN), can impact negatively on articulation and overall intelligibility. Lingual and labiodental placements may be modified and speech therapy may provide compensatory articulatory postures.

Hard palate Hard palate defects resulting from maxillary involvement of tumour potentially affect the production of lingua-alveolar sounds [t, d, n, l] and lingual-palatal sounds [sh, zh, ch, j]. Often a flap is used to close the defect. Alternatively, the team prosthodontist can design an obturator to cover and seal the defect to normalize articulation of these sounds[72].

Disordered resonance

During speech production, the soft palate makes contact with the posterior pharyngeal wall to separate the nasal and oral cavities and allow for normal articulation of 'plosive' consonants such as /p, b, k, g, t, d, ch, sh/. In the patient with unilateral palatal paralysis, the inability of the soft palate to contact the posterior pharyngeal wall creates a constant air leak in the vocal tract. The abnormal leak of air through the nose during speech production results in a hypernasal quality to the voice. When severe, the patient's speech may be distorted to the point of being unintelligible[73]. Vocal volume is abnormally soft, because as much as 10 dB of sound is lost through the nose[74]. When a malignancy requires surgical resection of the soft palate, the resulting tissue deficit creates velopharyngeal insufficiency. Similarly, when tumour involvement or its removal necessitates disruption of cranial nerves IX or X, the resulting unilateral palatal paralysis creates a velopharyngeal gap.

There are several options to restore velopharyngeal closure if the neurological input to these structures is intact. When the velopharyngeal gap is minimal, behavioural therapy may facilitate over articulation of speech sounds sufficient to reduce nasality and optimize intelligibility[75]. However, in the case of a moderately-sized or large gap, a surgical solution for velopharyngeal incompetence is indicated. Gaps of small to moderate size have been managed with a pharyngeal wall implant, which moves the posterior pharyngeal wall into range of contact with soft palate elevation. Silicone, Teflon, and collagen have been used, but migration of these substances has been a concern[76,77]. The most popular surgical solution traditionally has been a pharyngeal flap. In this procedure, a superiorly-based flap from the posterior pharyngeal wall is sutured to the velum to bridge the space and obturate the gap.

In the case of palatal paralysis following involvement or sacrifice of the vagus nerve for skull base tumours, a palatal adhesion effectively eliminates hyper nasality and nasal regurgitation. In this procedure, the paralysed side of the soft palate is sutured to the posterior pharyngeal wall to close the gap between the oral and nasal cavities[78]. Alternatively, a palatal lift prosthesis can be fashioned to place the soft palate in a position favourable to assist velopharyngeal contact. In the most severe cases of velopharyngeal incompetence, where a lack of tissue prevents a flap procedure, a speech bulb/obturator can be fitted by the prosthodontist. The appliance fills the velopharyngeal space as the lateral pharyngeal walls move to surround the bulb snugly[79].

Disordered voice

Neurological abnormalities

The voice disorder resulting from laryngeal paralysis is extremely debilitating. Most patients present with a very soft, breathy voice quality or even a whisper[80]. Attempts to force enough vocal volume to be heard results in rapid fatigue of laryngeal and respiratory muscles and patients may avoid communication because of the effort required. The lack of volume is very problematic or potentially dangerous for patients who work in a noisy environment or who must communicate with hard-of-hearing family members. Professional voice users, such as teachers or salespeople may be unable to fulfil the vocal demands of their work and may find their career in jeopardy.

In patients with unilateral vocal fold paralysis, medialization laryngoplasty is performed to reposition the immobile vocal fold into a more favourable midline position to allow contact with its contra lateral, mobile partner[81]. A small silastic implant is placed lateral to the paralysed vocal fold, which pushes the muscle towards the laryngeal midline. Improved vocal fold contact restores voice and prevents aspiration. Studies have documented that voice quality is normal or better following phonosurgery[82,83]. Injection of collagen has been recommended for vocal fold immobility[84]. Numerous other materials have been evaluated for vocal fold immobility. New concern over potential bioreaction has prompted testing of autologous materials. Injection of fat tissue has been found to improve glottal closure in case of laryngeal paresis[85,86]; however, its abbreviated life span of <12 months has been corroborated histologically.

Surgical organ preservation procedures

Operative procedures which spare some glottic structures and mobility yield varying voice results. Vocal cordectomy or cordotomy remove a portion of the sound source of phonation and create a breathy dysphonia. When a malignancy involves one vocal fold and surrounding structures, a vertical hemilaryngectomy may provide a mechanism for voicing; the uninvolved vocal fold vibrates against the tissue of the neolarynx, preserving a functional voice. In the case of supraglottic tumour, the entire laryngeal vestibule may be excised, with the membranous vocal folds left intact to provide for phonation[87]. When laryngeal cancer requires a supracricoid laryngectomy, all laryngeal structures above the level of the glottis are removed as well as the membranous vocal folds. In general, one or both mobile arytenoid cartilages are spared[88]. The arytenoids approximate on adduction and make contact with the base of tongue to produce a vibratory source and generate 'voice'. In general, the voice quality is very breathy and low-pitched. Finally, the near total-laryngectomy requires removal of an entire hemilarynx and the anterior two-thirds of the contra lateral hemilarynx. The laryngeal remnant is not sufficient to allow normal air exchange, so a permanent tracheostoma is constructed[89]. A tracheopharyngeal tract is created to form a vibratory source for sound production. Voice quality is very similar to that achieved with a tracheooesophageal voice prosthesis.

Total laryngectomy

There are several options for rehabilitation of communication in the patient who undergoes total laryngectomy. An artificial larynx (electrolarynx) is a device which provides an external sound source. The most common type of electrolarynx is a small, handheld machine which is placed against the neck or into the mouth with a tubular adapter. The patient's articulation of speech sounds is superimposed over the robotic sound source to produce a mechanical-sounding voice. The greatest advantage of the electrolarynx is that it provides immediacy of communication. With minimal training on placement and over-articulation, the patient can begin to 'speak' in the perioperative period[90]. A second type of speech method is the use of oesophageal speech. This requires a long commitment to therapy but allows for greatest communicative independence. In this method, air is pumped via swallow or inhaled into the cervical oesophagus and immediately exhaled. The pharyngooesophageal segment is vibrated by the expelled air and sound is produced, similar to a controlled belch[91]. Generally, the patient can produce a few syllables per air change. Some patients become quite proficient at this, and do not have to rely on a mechanical or prosthetic device to communicate. Creation of a tracheooesophageal tract allows insertion of a one-way valve. With the stoma occluded, air from the lungs is shunted through the prosthesis and into the oesophagus. The air vibrates tissue in the superior aspect of the oesophagus to produce sound[92]. The patient uses the sound to articulate audible voice. The advantage of prosthetic speech over oesophageal speech is that the patient removes the device periodically for cleaning. More recently, the development of an indwelling prosthesis allows a patient to wear the device for several months without removal.

Specific symptom-control issues

Airway control

Advanced HNC patients may experience a number of problems that may lead to progressive airway compromise. Airway compromise is one of the most distressing symptoms of progressive disease. The airway must be divided into multiple levels—the nasal cavity, nasopharynx, oral cavity oropharynx, larynx, extra-thoracic and intra-thoracic trachea, and lungs. Obstruction can occur in any area along the airway and the symptoms and treatment differ depending on the level of obstruction. Initial assessment of the airway begins with an observation of breathing pattern to determine grossly the level of airway obstruction. Mouth breathing with normal inspiratory and expiratory duration and without noise may be indicative of purely nasal obstruction; whereas, sonorous mouth breathing without stridor would suggest obstruction at the level of base of tongue or oral cavity that could be palliated immediately with a nasal trumpet and upright positioning until more definitive procedure could be performed. Inspiratory or biphasic stridor is more indicative of a fixed laryngotracheal obstruction, which will probably require bypass, most often in the form of a tracheostomy. Anxiety, agitation, confusion, and claustrophobia are all signs of progressive hypercarbia and air hunger resulting from obstruction and immediate intervention is warranted. Flexible fibre-optic laryngoscopy can be performed further to assess the mass effect of the tumour and its overall degree of obstruction. Laryngoscopy also permits a determination as to whether a patient may be amenable to intubation in the event of complete airway loss. Additional factors such as trismus and neck immobility from prior radiation or direct tumour involvement may, however, complicate intubation, and a tracheostomy under local anaesthetic may be simpler than an attempted intubation which may result in loss of the airway due to inability to expose the larynx. If the tumour is extremely friable, then a tracheostomy under local anaesthetic may be more prudent to avoid manipulation of the tumour. Ultimately for patients with known incurable disease, an honest discussion with the patient about the potential future need for tracheostomy and early placement may avoid emergent intervention under duress.

The most common and definitive procedure that can be offered is a tracheostomy. This can be performed under local or general anaesthesia. An incision is made approximately 1–2 cm below the cricoid cartilage, either vertically or horizontally. The strap muscles of the neck are reflected laterally to provide access to the trachea. If the thyroid isthmus is encountered, it may be ligated or reflected superiorly or inferiorly for exposure of the trachea. The trachea is generally entered between tracheal rings 2 and 3, however, may be entered lower if necessary to bypass any subglottic extension of tumour. Tracheostomy tubes come in a variety of sizes and shapes depending on the individual vendor, however, most generally have three components—an outer cannula, an inner cannula, and an obturator. The obturator is placed through the outer cannula to provide a smooth tip to allow for easy insertion. Once the tracheostomy has been inserted, the obturator is removed and an inner cannula is inserted into the outer cannula. The inner cannula can be

removed frequently to facilitate cleaning and prevent plugging of the tracheostomy. The initial tracheostomy change should be performed by the surgeon, but after a mature tract has formed, usually within 1–2 weeks, the tracheostomy can be changed with ease by the patient or care provider. The tracheostomy is maintained patent by encouraging patients to cough. Additional saline lavage and deep suctioning can also clear secretions and should be done routinely initially every 4 hours and as needed. Patients often need supplemental humidification to thin secretions when they have a tracheostomy, for the natural humidification provided by airflow through the mouth and nose is lost when the upper airway is bypassed. A bedside humidifier, humidified trach collar and frequent instillation of saline drops through the tracheostomy can provide the necessary humidification. The addition of mucolytics such as guaifenesin or nebulized Mucomyst® may be of added benefit to patients with thick secretions, which are difficult to clear. Added modifications to tracheostomy tubes include high volume low-pressure cuffs. A cuffed tube is initially placed at the time of surgery to prevent any blood from passing distally into the airway. Cuffed tracheostomy tubes, however, are usually only necessary for patients requiring positive pressure ventilation, which requires a seal of the trachea to achieve the necessary pressure. A common misconception is that patients need a cuffed tube to prevent aspiration of secretions around the tracheostomy tube from above. Inflation of a cuff places pressure on the posterior common wall between the trachea and oesophagus, and this added obstruction to the oesophagus can actually induce greater secretion pooling and potentiate aspiration to a degree. In general, after a mature tract has formed, a cuffless tracheostomy tube can be used in the cancer patient, which will permit enough collateral flow around the tube, if appropriately sized, to allow a patient to occlude the lumen with a finger or a passy-muir valve and still speak. Another modification to the tracheostomy tube is the addition of a fenestrated opening in the canula to permit added airflow past the trach with occlusion of the lumen. This design is meant to enhance glottal airflow with occlusion and improve speech. However, fenestrations in the tracheostomy tube often create a rough surface, which incite granulation tissue formation in the airway that can be problematic. The added benefit of a fenestrated tube is often minimal and should be used only with reservation.

Auditory function

HNC patients may experience a decrease in hearing as a result of therapy. Sensorineural hearing loss may result from therapy with either radiation or systemic chemotherapy agents such as cisplatin. In a longitudinal study of hearing loss in 294 patients treated with radiation or radiochemotherapy for nasopharyngeal carcinoma[93], 31 per cent of patients had a measurable sensorineural hearing deficit 3 months after completing therapy. Hearing deficits improved over time in only 40 per cent of patients. Older patients (>50 years of age) and patients with pre-treatment hearing deficits were more likely to develop measurable sensorineural hearing loss. Concomitant chemotherapy did not worsen hearing outcome. In a separate analysis, Bhandare[94] assessed 325 patients who received either radiation or chemoradiation for HNC. Sensorineural hearing loss was noted in 15.1 per cent of patients. Predictive factors included age, dose to cochlea, and concurrent chemotherapy. Freedom from sensorineural hearing loss after 5 and 10 years was 70 per cent for patients treated with chemoradiation and 82 per cent for patients treated with radiation only ($p = 0.0281$). Rarely, destruction of the inner ear apparatus by infiltrative tumours results in sensorineural hearing loss. Patients with a clinically significant sensorineural hearing loss should be referred for hearing aids. Middle ear effusions are a common cause of non-sensorineural hearing loss and should be identified and treated appropriately.

Dermatitis

Similar to oral mucositis, patients receiving treatment with external beam radiation can develop severe dermal and soft tissue reactions. Acute radiation dermatitis usually begins 2–3 weeks after therapy is initiated. The first manifestation of radiation dermatitis is erythema with mild oedema. As treatment progresses, the skin may begin to blister, ulcerate, and slough. As with mucositis, radiation dermatitis can be graded according to a variety of toxicity scales. The severity of radiation-induced dermal damage may increase if chemotherapy is given concomitantly. In addition, patients with tracheostomy tubes in place may have increased irritation and ulceration. Acute radiation-induced dermal damage begins to heal within 2–4 weeks after radiation is completed. Treatment for radiation dermatitis is largely supportive. Important principles of care include: cleansing with mild agents, avoiding topical irritants such as clothing that rubs against affected skin, avoiding aluminium- or magnesium-based salts which may increase radiation dermatitis and the use of emollients to maintain moisture[95]. Techniques for treatment of wet desquamation and ulceration are similar to those used in general wound care[96]. General guidelines for assessment and treatment of radiation dermatitis have recently been published and provide a good framework for treatment[96].

Laboratory abnormalities

Hypothyroidism

After primary surgery, neck dissection or radiation therapies, patients frequently develop hypothyroidism. In a study by Tell, thyroid function was measured in 264 consecutive patients who received radiation to at least part of the thyroid gland. The risk for developing clinical or chemical hypothyroidism 3 years post-treatment was 15 and 40 per cent, respectively[97]. Routine follow-up should include a careful history and physical exam directed towards signs or symptoms of hypothyroidism. Periodic monitoring with a serum TSH is appropriate for any patient who has received radiation to the low neck. For recommendations regarding treatment of hypothyroidism, please reference the American Thyroid Association Standards of Care Committee guidelines[98].

Hypercalcaemia

Hypercalcaemia is common in patients with squamous carcinoma of the head and neck. The majority of patients' tumours express parathyroid-hormone-related protein (PTHrP) which causes release of calcium from the skeleton[99]. Although an occasional patient with curable locally advanced squamous carcinoma of the head and neck will present with hypercalcaemia, the majority of patients have metastatic disease. Treatment of the underlying disease should be attempted where possible. Intravenous hydration, bisphosphonates and other pharmacologic agents should be used as indicated by the clinical setting.

Anaemia

Anaemia is a common presenting haematological abnormality in patients with HNC and may worsen throughout the course of radiation or chemoradiation. Compelling data in a number of tumour sites, including HNC, demonstrate that anaemia is a strong predictor for outcome with radiation-based treatment regimens[100]. It is hypothesized that low numbers of circulating red blood cells may increase the fraction of cancer cells that are hypoxic. Hypoxic tumour cells are resistant to radiation therapy. Thus anaemia may lead to increased radiation resistance. In a recent analysis of RTOG 8527, patients were assigned randomly to radiation alone or radiation plus etanidazole (a radiation sensitizing agent). Primary analysis demonstrated no survival advantage to concomitant therapy with etanidazole[101]. A secondary analysis was conducted to evaluate the association between pre-treatment anaemia and overall survival, local regional control and radiation therapy complications. Results of this study indicated that patients with a normal haemoglobin (>14. g/ml in men and >13 g/ml in women) had a statistically significant improvement in overall survival and local regional control. The survival advantage for normal haemoglobin level persisted at 5 years. In addition to the survival and local regional control advantage, late toxicity was diminished in patients with a normal haemoglobin level at initiation of therapy. Additional studies confirm the predictive value of haemoglobin level on treatment outcome. Fien et al. reported on pre-treatment haemoglobin level with patients undergoing radiation therapy for $T_{1/2}$ squamous carcinoma of the glottic larynx[102]. The 2 year local control in patients with a haemoglobin of <13 g/dl was 66 per cent ($p = 0.018$). For patients with haemoglobin of > 13 g/dl, the 2 year local control was 95 per cent. For normal and abnormal haemoglobin levels, similarly 2 year survival was 46 per cent and 88 per cent, respectively ($p < 0.001$). Overgard et al. reported on predictive factors for outcome of radiation therapy for laryngeal and pharyngeal carcinoma[103]. Nine hundred and fifty patients received primary irradiation in doses ranging from 60 to 68 Gy in 6–7 weeks. Pre-treatment haemoglobin was associated with tumour control and survival in patients with pharyngeal and supraglottic tumours.

Based on the above data, studies were undertaken within the USA and Europe to determine whether erythropoetic agents could ameliorate radiation-induced haematological toxicity and enhance treatment efficacy. Several studies have been reported recently that raise concern about the potential adverse effect of erythropoietin on treatment outcome. Henke reported the results of a clinical trial investigating the role of epoietin beta in HNC patients receiving radiation therapy[104]. Epoietin beta was initiated at a haemoglobin level of 12 g/dl in women and 13 g/dl in men. The haemoglobin was driven to levels above those currently recommended for erythropoietin agents. Results demonstrated reduced loco-regional control in patients treated with epoietin beta when compared with placebo. Based on a recent re-review of the available data, it has been recommended that erythropoetic agents be used only as specified by regulatory agencies.

Lymphoedema

Lymphoedema is a condition in which excessive fluid and protein accumulate in the extra-vascular and interstitial space[105]. This accumulation of fluid and protein occurs when the lymphatic system can no longer transport the normal fluid and protein load from the blood capillary-interstitial interface into the lymphatic vessels or when there is reduced lymphatic transport capacity coupled with increased lymph[106–108]. Cancer treatment is the most common cause of lymphoedema in developed countries[109].

HNC patients are believed to experience lymphoedema more than any other cancer group. European literature suggests that 30–56 per cent of all HNC patients develop lymphoedema, a larger percentage than lymphoedema associated with breast cancer[110,111]. The high rate of lymphoedema in HNC patients is due to the fact that surgery, radiation and cancer alter structures vital to fluid exchange at the blood capillary-interstitial-lymphatic-interface[106,109]. Lymphoedema may occur acutely after surgery and during radiation treatment[112] or months after treatment is completed[112,113].

The incidence of lymphoedema and its manifestations in HNC patients are largely unknown. Methadological issues plague the study of lymphoedema in this cohort of patients. Unlike limb lymphoedema where multiple valid and reliable measurement methods are available to draw from, such methods do not exist for the head and neck area. In addition, distinguishing between the progression of lymphoedema and oedema related to direct tumour spread and/or other systemic diseases may be difficult[114]. Finally, lymphoedema may involve tissues of the oral cavity, paranasal sinuses, pharynx, larynx, face, neck, and shoulders. Thus, the clinical manifestations are varied and often unrecognized.

Presenting symptoms vary depending on the site of involvement. Subtle or overt swelling of the soft tissues of the neck and face are often the first indicator of lymphoedema[115]. Soft tissue swelling may progress over time resulting in fibrosis and impaired range of motion. Lymphoedema of the larynx may result in airway compromise or altered voice quality while pharyngeal oedema may impair swallowing. If swelling appears suddenly or if pre-existing lymphoedema worsens[115] other medical conditions such as renal failure, liver failure, myxoedema, cancer recurrence, or infectious complications should be considered. Thus, a thorough history coupled with a physical assessment is needed to ascertain causative factors and better plan treatment. The history should include: onset of swelling (new or pre-existing), location of swelling, type of symptoms being experienced, and exacerbation and remission patterns of symptoms. The physical assessment should include: (1) laryngoscopic evaluation to assess oedema of the pharynx, larynx and paranasal sinuses, and (2) careful examination of skin and soft tissues of the face, neck and shoulders with attention to range of motion and signs of infection or inflammation.

If infection is noted during the physical assessment it must be treated and resolved prior to initiating other lymphoedema treatment. Olsezewski suggests treatment with antibiotics such as penicillin or erythromycin which are known to be effective in most cases of lymphoedema-related infections[116]. If there is no infection or the infection has resolved, therapy is recommended to achieve maximum symptomatic relief. Although controlled trials of lymphoedema therapy are lacking, clinical experience would indicate that appropriate treatment may result in improved patient comfort, increased neck and shoulder range of motion, decrease respiratory compromise, improved swallowing function, and decreased risk of infection and skin breakdown. Treatment of lymphoedema includes Manual lymphatic drainage (MLD), the use of compression garments, and education. MLD should only be undertaken by lymphoedema therapists trained in head and neck drainage techniques. Compression garments should be fitted appropriately for maximal effectiveness and tolerability. Education should include postural techniques to minimize symptoms, identification and prevention of infections and exercises to maintain neck and shoulder mobility.

One of the greatest challenges for lymphoedema therapists is caring for HNC patients with advanced disease and/or those at end of life who have symptomatic lymphoedema[114]. Standard MLD approaches to lymphoedema management may need to be modified substantially as massage and garments may be poorly tolerated. Family members and other care-givers may need to be enlisted to help with the self-care components of MLD. Patient tolerance of treatment must be assessed constantly and managed carefully. If the patient can tolerate some degree of treatment, then it is warranted; however, if the treatment causes more discomfort than the end-of-life patient can tolerate, then no treatment may be the best option.

Mood disorders in the head and neck cancer patient

Clinical experience would indicate that mental health issues are frequent in the HNC population. Unfortunately, there are few well-designed studies addressing this issue in the literature. Many studies focus on 'psychological distress', which describes the psychological turmoil surrounding the cancer diagnosis and its treatment. However, distress is not synonymous with depression or anxiety[117,118]. Additionally, most studies of depression and anxiety in cancer patients rely on self-report tools which provide insufficient information to determine a diagnosis per standard psychiatric criteria. Haman et al. conducted a cross sectional study to clarify the prevalence of anxiety and depression disorders in the HNC population. Using the structured clinical interview (SCID) for DSM-IV, Haman determined the prevalence of a continuum of psychological syndromes for both current and lifetime periods. Thirteen per cent of patients had a pre-cancer history of an anxiety or depression disorder. Post-treatment, the prevalence of new onset depression and anxiety was 24 per cent and 4 per cent, respectively. Both anxiety and depression had a significant negative impact on QOL measures[119,120].

In order to address this issue effectively, the aetiology of the prevalence of mood disorders in this patient population must be understood. Certainly, several well-recognized risk factors may play a role. For example, therapy can result in the inability to communicate or impair the ability to eat, leading to social avoidance, depression and anxiety. A close relationship exists between substance abuse and psychopathology. HNC patients have a high rate of substance abuse (past and ongoing), pointing to maladaptive coping strategies which can increase the likelihood of depression and anxiety[121–123]. Interestingly, as cytokines may have a role in depression, the biology of the tumour or the treatment and resultant inflammation may also play a role in the biological basis of mood disorders in this population[124–127].

Despite the unanswered questions, the fact remains that mood disorders represent a significant problem in the HNC patient and can impact negatively on QOL. Additionally, mood disorders and associated ongoing substance abuse can undermine the ability of the patient to change positively modifiable risk factors (tobacco and alcohol) which can affect disease free survival. Males with HNC demonstrate some of the highest suicide rates of all cancer patients. In fact, characteristics common to this population such as male gender, advanced disease, little social or cultural support, and limited treatment options all contribute to this high rate[128]. Physicians who treat HNC must be sensitive to both the physical and psychological sequelae of the diagnosis and treatment. In order to maximize the quality of survivorship, a mental health professional should be included in the multi-disciplinary team of HNC providers.

Mucositis

Oral and pharyngeal mucositis is the most devastating acute complication of radiotherapy for HNC. Over the past decade our understanding of the pathophysiology of mucositis has progressed dramatically. Sonis has developed a 'multiple mechanism model' describing the numerous events that contribute to the development and manifestations of mucositis[129]. Clinically, oral mucositis usually begins after 10–14 days after radiation therapy is initiated. The initial observation is a transient, patchy white discolouration of the mucosa followed by a confluent deep erythema and pseudomembrane formation. The most severe manifestation is frank ulceration of the mucosa. Risk factors for the development of mucositis include: total dose of radiation, fractionation, the extent of the involved field and the use of concurrent chemotherapy[130]. In addition to causing pain, mucositis impairs eating, swallowing, and speech[131]. When severe, mucositis may lead to hospitalization for malnutrition or dehydration, and may result in interruptions in treatment[130]. Overwhelming data indicate that breaks in treatment decrease local control and overall survival, thus treatment breaks due to mucositis must be avoided[132]. A plethora of traditional treatments for oropharyngeal mucositis have been reported. Currently, the only FDA approved agent available for the treatment of oral mucositis in HNC patients is Caphosol®. The Multi-national Association for Supportive Care in Cancer has reviewed the literature on prevention and treatment of oral mucositis and generated guidelines to aid clinicians. Guidelines are available for review at http://www.mascc.org. It is clear that new agents are needed for the prevention and treatment of this acute toxicity[133]. For further information on treatment of mucositis and other oral cavity lesions, please see Chapter 10.9.

Neurocognitive impairment

Neurocognitive impairment is a clinically significant problem in the HNC population. Patients may present with baseline neurocognitive impairment, or they may develop impairment acutely during therapy or as a late effect of treatment. The ramifications of neurocognitive impairment are protean. Patients with baseline neurocognitive impairment may be at increased risk for delirium and worsened neurocognitive impairment during the post-treatment period. Patients with neurocognitive impairment may have difficulty learning new information and understanding the scope of their disease and treatment. Furthermore, pre-treatment neurocognitive impairment may also affect negatively treatment tolerance and compliance, follow-up, and rehabilitation[134,135].

Baseline neurocognitive impairment

The prevalence of neurocognitive impairment in the HNC population at baseline is underappreciated and understudied. McCaffery[135] assessed preoperative HNC patients and found that alcohol abuse, depression, and neurocognitive impairment are common. Risk factors for baseline neurocognitive impairment include alcohol abuse and co-morbid medical and psychological conditions. Of note, McCaffery found that alcohol-dependent patients were at increased risk of greater preoperative neurocognitive impairment demonstrating difficulties in three of five cognitive subsets including initiation and perseveration (frontal lobe function), conceptualization (reasoning ability, frontal lobe function), and construction (visual–spatial ability).

Acute neurocognitive impairment

Acute neurocognitive impairment in HNC patients has been studied primarily in the context of postoperative delirium. The incidence of postoperative delirium in HNC patients ranges from 13 to 26 per cent[136–138]. The incidence of postoperative delirium in these studies is probably underestimated because delirium identification was based on psychiatric referrals for delirium symptoms, clinical documentation of confusion and documentation of agitated behaviours that interfered with postoperative recovery. These approaches to measuring delirium may miss or undercount episodes of hypoactive or quiet delirium. Preoperative risk factors for delirium include the following: older age[136], hypertension[136], living alone[137], the American Society of Anesthesiologists (ASA) classification[137] and preoperative white blood cell count[137]. An operative time of more than 10 h was the only intraoperative factor associated independently with postoperative delirium[138]. The length of surgery of more than 10 h suggests that more extensive surgery is a risk factor for postoperative delirium. Postoperative factors associated with delirium were: low oxygen saturation[136], decreased haemoglobin level[136], and lack of use of minor tranquilizers for sleep[138].

Weed[137] used a previously identified predictive model for postoperative delirium[139] to stratify patients into three cohorts with an increasing risk of postoperative delirium. Delirium risk was determined by assigning one point for each of the following factors: age ≥ 70 years; alcohol abuse; poor cognitive status; poor functional status; markedly abnormal serum sodium, potassium, or glucose level; and high-risk surgery. The total number of points determined the risk category: 1 point = low risk; 2 points = moderate risk; and ≥ 3 points = high risk. Postoperative delirium increased progressively as risk factors multiplied. The percentage of patients with delirium among those with one risk factor was 9 per cent; two risk factors, 19 per cent; and three or more factors, 25 per cent.

Long-term neurocognitive impairment

Long-term neurocognitive impairment has been studied predominantly in the setting of inpatients with nasopharyngeal carcinoma (NPC) and paranasal sinus cancers who were treated with radiation, as incidental brain irradiation is most common in these disease sites. Early studies indicated that NPC patients treated with primary radiation were at risk for significant neurocognitive impairment. Lee[140] found that patients (n = 16) treated with radiation a median of 5.5 years earlier exhibited lower overall IQ, impaired non-verbal memory recall, and increased self-reports of memory complaints compared with control subjects. In another study, Woo[141] described the development of combined neurocognitive impairment and endocrine dysfunction in 11 patients following radiation therapy for NPC.

Although improvements in treatment techniques have evolved, more recent studies also have demonstrated similar problems in neurocognitive functioning following radiation therapy for HNC. Meyers[142] identified problems with learning and memory in 19 patients who received paranasal sinus radiation; 50 per cent had difficulty learning new information and 80 per cent forgot the information over time. Additionally, a third of the patients had difficulty with visual motor speed, executive functioning, and fine motor coordination. Cheung[143] found that patients with no temporal lobe necrosis following radiation for NPC performed similar to controls, but that patients with post-radiation necrosis had significant impairments in multiple domains including verbal and visual memory, language, motor ability, planning, overall cognitive ability, and abstract thinking. In contrast, Lam[144] found that NPC patients treated with radiation more than 2 years before, exhibited greater memory impairment when compared with controls, regardless of evidence of radiation-induced temporal lobe injury.

The pathogenesis of neurocognitive impairment following radiation therapy for HNC is multi-factorial. In a review, Abayomi[145] identified multiple contributing factors including radiation-induced vascular injury and inflammation, radionecrosis, radiation-injury to subcortical white matter, pituitary and hypothalamic dysfunction, cerebral atrophy, and co-morbid conditions such as hypertension, diabetes, hyperlipidaemia, obesity, and smoking. In studies of NPC patients, neurocognitive impairment was associated with the extent of radiation necrosis[146] the total RT dose[142], and time since treatment[142]. In the study by Cheung[146], patients who were older at the time of radiation therapy had more extensive radiation necrosis. The location of radionecrosis lesions also affected the pattern of neurocognitive impairment. For example, left hemisphere lesions were associated with language deficits and impaired verbal memory, whereas right hemisphere lesions were strongly associated with visual memory impairments.

Additional studies examining the development of symptomatic temporal lobe necrosis following radiation therapy for NPC[147–149] identified the following risk factors: fractional dose, overall treatment time, administration techniques and treatment schedule. Accelerated-hyperfractionated treatment regimens with twice-daily dosing resulted in an increased incidence of symptomatic temporal lobe necrosis[147,148]. In addition, Teo[149] noted that accelerated-hyperfractionated radiation therapy resulted in radiation-induced damage to other central nervous system structures and functions.

Nutrition

Nutritional deficits are present in a high percentage of patients with newly diagnosed or recurrent HNC. Malnutrition is often multi-factorial in nature. Careful assessment and treatment of weight loss and the institution of preventive measures during therapy are mandatory to optimize therapeutic outcome. Clinical trials have demonstrated that weight loss at the time of diagnosis is prognostic for survival and ability to tolerate treatment[150,151]. Further studies have demonstrated that aggressive nutritional intervention can minimize weight loss and decrease treatment-related toxicity[152]. Thus, aggressive nutritional intervention is an important component of care for HNC patients. In addition, the presence of cytokines known to be associated with cancer cachexia (tumour necrosis factor and Interleukin-6) may carry prognostic value[152].

Prior to instituting therapy, the causes of weight loss should be identified and treatable causes must be attended to quickly. Decreased oral intake may be caused by a wide array of functional problems including oral pain, difficulty swallowing, or mechanical obstruction caused by the tumour[153]. Patients with oral pain due to cancer should be given adequate pain medications. If functional abnormalities are present, a swallowing evaluation and swallowing therapy may prove beneficial. In patients with mild to moderate swallowing deficits, soft, puréed foods and liquid supplements can stabilize weight loss. Patients with severe swallowing difficulty require more aggressive therapy such as placement of a PEG feeding tube.

Weight loss secondary to treatment is almost universal with the exception of patients with small lesions amenable to surgical resection or lesions requiring a small radiation port. Patients who have extensive surgical procedures and are expected to have difficulty swallowing usually have a PEG tube or NG tube placed. In this setting, PEG tubes have demonstrated a decrease in length of hospital stay and diminished complication rate when compared with nasogastric tubes[154]. Patients undergoing primary radiation therapy or combined chemoradiation may develop severe mucositis which results in a profoundly diminished oral intake. In a report by Newman, patients undergoing aggressive chemoradiotherapy lost an average of 10 per cent body weight during therapy[246]. The aggressive use of PEG feeding tubes can minimize weight loss during therapy and improve QOL. In a study reported by Tyldesley, patients who received an elective PEG tube prior to radiation therapy had a 3 per cent weight loss at week 6 of therapy versus 9 per cent in the control group. The difference was maintained at 3 months (3 per cent versus 12 per cent)[247]. It should be noted, however, that concern has been expressed that prophylactic feeding tube placement may lead to increased rates of long-term feeding tube dependence. Several potential contributing factors have been hypothesized including; disuse atrophy, loss of normal swallowing reflex, and psychological dependence. Thus, patients with a feeding tube should be seen by a licensed Speech and Language Pathologist so that they may be given appropriate swallowing exercises to maintain swallow function. In addition, patients should be encouraged to return to oral intake as soon as it is feasible. The use of a nasogastric tube should be avoided since patients receiving radiation therapy usually require prolonged nutritional support and NG tubes may exacerbate radiation-induced mucositis.

The placement of a feeding tube does not guarantee adequate calorific or fluid intake. Feeding tubes require considerable time and effort to manage. Elderly or debilitated patients who undergo feeding tube placement may require assistance from caregivers. The time required to manage feeding tubes should not be underappreciated. One study reported that in elderly HNC patients between 1 and 3 months post-feeding tube placement, caregivers reported an average of 62 h of direct patient care per week[248].

Post-treatment, nutrition remains an issue of concern for many patients. There are numerous late effects of therapy that contribute to the dietary alterations noted in post-treatment HNC patients: (1) swallowing abnormalities due to tumour or treatment; (2) xerostomia from salivary gland radiation inhibits food bolus formation; (3) dental extractions alter the ability to chew solid foods; (4) alterations in taste cause food aversions; and (5) pain due to mucosal sensitivity. These factors lead to decreased food intake with or without restriction in the consistencies and type of foods ingested. Adaptations may result in micronutrient deficits that have heretofore been unrecognized. In a pilot study to assess dietary adaptations in HNC patients, investigators found that 12 months post-treatment, 20 per cent of patients required ongoing use of nutritional supplements. Patients reported decreased intake of dry foods (such as bread and rice) and fruits (due to acidity). Due to dietary alterations, a high percentage of patients were deficient in key micronutrients[51]. Similar results were reported by Beeker et al[154]. Twenty-four patients who completed therapy for HNC at least 1 year prior to study entry (average 3 years, range 1.6–7 years) were evaluated. Seventy-two per cent of patients reported dietary modifications: 12 patients ate no dry foods and five ate only soft food consistencies. Of note, increasing dietary modifications were associated with decreased energy and protein intake. Non-treatment-related factors which must be considered in the nutritional assessment include co-morbid diseases, the adequacy of socio-economic support and the presence of alcohol abuse. It is important to identify all factors contributing to malnutrition in order to establish an effective treatment plan. Periodic dietary assessment is critical to minimize the late effects of treatment on nutritional quality.

In addition to the functional causes of weight loss, patients with locally advanced, metastatic, or recurrent disease may also have cancer cachexia[155,156,157]. Cancers are able to affect profoundly the normal metabolic pathways resulting in weight loss, loss of lean muscle mass[158] and adipose tissue[159]. Similar wasting syndromes have been noted in a number of disease states including: burn victims, advanced congestive heart failure, advanced COPD and HIV. These phenomena are at least partially mediated by pro-inflammatory cytokines[160]. Of note, patients undergoing aggressive therapy with chemoradiation may develop a similar clinical syndrome which is characterized by anorexia, rapid weight loss, muscle mass loss, loss of subcutaneous fat, fatigue, and generalized weakness. It may be hypothesized that treatment results in local and systemic tissue damage. The body responds in a stereotypic fashion, activating biological pathways intended to aid in healing and repair[161]. Unfortunately, when the biological response to tissue damage is over-exuberant or protracted, repair mechanisms may actually adversely affect the host. Investigators conducted a pilot study to assess weight loss in HNC patients undergoing chemoradiation[162]. Seventeen patients with locally advanced disease underwent the following assessment pre- and post-treatment: (1) weight; (2) oral intake via 24-h diet recall using a telephone survey; (3) lean body mass via DEXA; (4) cytokine levels; (5) measures of oxidative stress; (6) C-reactive protein; (7) physical performance and activity level; and (8) resting energy expenditure. Results demonstrated the following: average weight loss of 10.1 kg, average lean muscle mass loss of 6.8 kg, no difference in resting energy expenditure, and no significant difference in calorific intake between the two time points. Thus, decreased calorific intake could not explain the either significant loss of weight nor lean muscle mass. The decrease in lean muscle mass was associated with decreased physical function and an increase in pro-inflammatory cytokines. In addition, levels of F2-isoprostanes were elevated post-treatment and were also associated with loss of fat and fat free mass. Further studies of the metabolic effects of chemoradiation are under way.

Osteoradionecrosis

ORN is one of the most serious complications from head and neck irradiation. The incidence of this varies depending upon total radiation dose, fractionation, volume irradiated, follow-up time, the status of dentition and reporting institution[171–174]. It is more common in edentulous patients; however, ORN is often reported as occurring after dental extractions following irradiation. The pathogenesis of ORN include a decrease in cellularity, suppressed osteoblastic activity, disorganization of the bone remodelling apparatus, avascularity and fibrosis that leads to poor wound healing after dental trauma and an increased risk of secondary infection from bacterial flora [175]. Ultimately, ORN can result in exposure of bone, fistula formation, or pathological fracture. Radiographic

signs include crestal bone irregularity, density changes, osteolysis, obvious sequestration, and frank pathological fracture. As tissue changes induced by radiation are long-term and the risk of dental trauma is lifelong, careful attention must be paid to the dentition and gingiva before, during and after radiation treatment.

Prevention

Before initiation of treatment, all patients scheduled to receive high dose (>50 Gy) radiation to one or both jaws should be evaluated by a skilled dentist familiar with radiation side effects. Panoramic radiographs are essential for the evaluation. All grossly diseased maxillary and mandibular teeth should be extracted immediately, and alveolar tori trimmed and carefully smoothed so that primary closure of the mucosa can be performed under little or no tension. Antibiotic prophylaxis should be used and a minimum of 14 days (preferably 21 days) should be allowed for healing prior to onset of radiation.

Following treatment, prevention of ORN has evolved naturally around minimizing trauma or local irritants that have been shown to precipitate the process[249]. Periodontal disease has been shown to be a major predisposing factor, particularly when dental extractions are performed in a portion of the previously irradiated jaw. Although a certain number of cases will arise spontaneously in spite of conscientious care, the patient can be instructed on ways to decrease overall risk. A correlation between higher ORN and continued tobacco and alcohol use has been reported. Improvement of salivary function with sialogogues such as pilocarpine hydrochloride, and bromhexine can decrease bacterial decay. Daily use of fluoride via sprays or liquids before bedtime are effective in minimizing dental caries. Diseased teeth should be maintained, if possible, through meticulous endodontic therapy with or without coronal recontouring (crown amputation). It has been shown that endodontic management of teeth in previously irradiated cancer patients does not increase the risk of ORN[178]. For periodontally involved or cariously unrestorable teeth, the retention of roots (with or without endodontic therapy), and the use of overdentures are preferable to extractions.

Treatment of established ORN

Treatment of ORN via the *non-surgical* route prior to the use of hyperbaric oxygen (HBO) therapy consists of improving oral hygiene and removing local irritants like alcohol and tobacco. Irrigation, packing, and systemic antibiotics may also be useful. Pentoxifylline, a methylxanthine derivative introduced in 1984 for the treatment of intermittent claudication and venous stasis ulcers, has been shown to improve erythrocyte flexibility and increase tissue oxygen levels. It has been helpful in promoting healing of radiation soft tissue necrosis, fibrosis and atrophy due to head and neck irradiation[250]. Unfortunately, a randomized trial in the USA comparing pentoxifylline (400 mg every 8 hours) to best supportive care for patients with ORN closed before completion due to poor accrual. HBO therapy was shown to be an effective treatment for ORN in 1975[251]. Early ORN (stage I) without fractures of fistulae may be cured by HBO alone. A suggested regimen is 30 dives of 90 min at 2.5 atmospheres[252].

If conservative measures fail or in advanced cases (stage II or III), then HBO in combination with surgical management is necessary. In stage III ORN, Marx reported good results using 30 dives HBO followed by transoral alveolar sequestrectomy with a primary mucosal closure[253]. Adjunctive HBO is recommended, varying from 10 to 30 dives. Others have reported good results using 5–10 preoperative dives of 2.5–2.8 atmospheres for 90 to 120 min, followed by 5–7 dives postoperatively. In severe cases (stage III), 30 dives have been recommended followed by resection, using tetracycline fluorescence under ultraviolet light or the presence of bleeding bone to determine margins. Stabilization of the mandible with either an extra-skeletal pin or maxillofacial fixation is usually necessary. HBO is then performed until a healthy mucosal closure is seen (usually 20–30 dives). It has been advocated that reconstruction can be accomplished 10 weeks later, using HBO preoperatively for 20 dives, then operating strictly from a transcutaneous approach to avoid oral contamination. Ten additional dives are recommended postoperatively.

Pain

Pain in the patient with HNC is a multi-dimensional symptom complex with physical, emotional, and cultural factors contributing to the overall pain experience. All of these factors must be addressed in order to provide adequate palliation. It is beyond the scope of this chapter to review the basics of cancer pain management. The reader is referred to the chapters on pain assessment and management elsewhere in this text. There are, however, specific problems that confront HNC patients that merit special attention.

Grond *et al.* reported on the type of pain experienced by HNC patients prior to, during and after treatment[179]. Of 167 patients studied, 138 (83 per cent) patients had pain due to tumour. Of 138 patients with tumour-related pain, 80 per cent had soft tissue pain, 20 per cent had bone pain, and 35 per cent had neuropathic pain. Clearly some patients had mixed pain. Head and neck tumours are often deeply ulcerative causing severe somatic pain. Irritation of an ulcerative tumour by movement from speech or swallowing can diminish function and make pain control a challenge. Tumour invasion into nerves either peripherally or at the level of the base of skull can lead to refractory pain syndromes as well as debilitating neurological deficits. Tumours such as adenoid cystic carcinoma may track along peripheral nerves (perineural invasion) and into nerve roots resulting in painful peripheral neuropathies[180]. Finally, maxillofacial pain thought to be due to benign processes such as sinusitis, temporomandibular joint dysfunction, or maxillofacial neuralgias can be the first manifestation of carcinomas[181–187]. Determining the aetiology of pain in the head and neck patient requires familiarity with anatomy and often calls for consultation with the treating otolaryngologist and neuroradiologist.

Patients undergoing surgical resection will experience postoperative pain which can be treated per recommendations in the Agency for Health Care Policy and Research Clinical Practice Guidelines for Acute Pain Management[188]. Adequate treatment of postoperative pain in HNC patients can present specific challenges. Tracheostomy tube placement, loss of speech function, or severe oral pain may make it difficult for patients to communicate effectively with caregivers, thus interfering with pain assessment. As patients recuperate, postoperative pain subsides. However, it is important to emphasize that chronic postoperative pain is common in the head and neck population. In a report by Chaplin *et al.*, 26 per cent of patients had pain 2 years after completing therapy[189]. Pain was described as moderate or severe in 14 per cent of patients. Predictors for chronic pain included pain at 3 months post-treatment and neck dissection. Peripheral nerves may be damaged during resection resulting in the development of neuropathic pain. Less commonly, patients may have associated syncopal episodes[190]. Patients may also develop contractures and tissue scarring in the neck and shoulders. This can lead to severe and debilitating musculoskeletal dysfunction with resultant pain. The degree of musculoskeletal pain may be determined by the extent of surgery or amount of adjuvant radiation therapy used for treatment. For example, Short demonstrated that sparing of the spinal accessory nerve during neck dissection resulted in diminished postoperative shoulder pain[191]. The utilization of non-pharmacological interventions to prevent and treat this sequela is extremely important. Physical therapy consultation can help guide patients in exercises which can decrease contractures and preserve function and range of motion[192].

Radiation therapy may be used as primary treatment or as adjuvant therapy in the postoperative setting. In general, the dose of radiation therapy used for the treatment of HNC is high (70 Gy for primary treatment and 50–60 Gy for adjuvant therapy). These doses are expected to result in significant damage to the mucous membranes, soft tissue and skin. The severity of symptoms is usually related to the size of the radiation field and the area involved. Patients with large fields and those receiving radiation to the oral cavity experience severe debilitating mucositis and radiation dermatitis.

Mucositis-related pain is often severe and may impact dramatically on function. Investigators conducted a secondary analysis of data from a prospective, longitudinal, multi-centre study of mucositis in patients receiving radiation with or without chemotherapy for HNC[131]. Seventy-five patients were enrolled from six centres (67 per cent of patients received concurrent chemoradiation). Outcome measures included mouth/throat pain and function loss due to mouth/throat pain. Over the first 6 weeks of therapy, 57 (76 per cent) patients experienced severe mouth and throat pain. Sixty-four (85 per cent) patients were prescribed opioid analgesics. Pain and impaired function secondary to pain increased dramatically during therapy, despite the use of opioids. Severe swallowing difficulty was noted in 38 per cent of patients during weeks 1–2 of therapy. This increased to 59 per cent during weeks 5–6 of therapy. A similar decrease in function was noted for difficulty eating, drinking, talking, and sleeping.

The treatment of mucositis-induced pain requires close and frequent monitoring. It is imperative that pain treatment be aggressive. A small study reported from the Medical College of Wisconsin demonstrated that daily nursing assessment with aggressive treatment of mucositis resulted in decreased pain, improved sleep and eating and a better energy level when compared with historical controls[193]. During the first 2–3 weeks of RT oral discomfort is usually mild. The use of topical lidocaine solution and combined opioid/non-opioid medication is usually adequate. By week 4–5, oral and dermal pain begins to increase substantially. At the same time, patients' ability to swallow decreases substantially[194]. Fentanyl patches are a very convenient method for administering long acting opioids in this patient population, although care has to be taken to titrate the opioid dose downwards as pain is resolving. Short-acting liquid opioids should be used for breakthrough pain. Pain due to radiation mucositis takes weeks to months to resolve. Although detailed epidemiological data regarding chronic post-radiation pain is lacking, there is a significant cohort of patients with persistent pain months to years after completion of therapy[189].

Pain due to local recurrence is a major palliative issue in terminal HNC patients. More importantly, it may be the first symptom indicating recurrent disease. In a recent report by Smit, pain was the first symptom indicative of recurrence in 70 per cent of patients, with a median lag time of 4 months between the onset of pain and the diagnosis of recurrent disease[195]. Thus, new onset pain in a previously treated HNC patient should be investigated carefully.

Physical therapy examination and treatment for the patient with head and neck cancer

Surgical or radiation-based treatment approaches may result in head and neck specific and generalized alterations of physical performance. Examples of head and neck specific functional loss include decrease range of motion in the jaw, neck and shoulders. Generalized physical functional abnormalities include weakness and deconditioning secondary to therapy. Thus, the majority of HNC patients with locally advanced disease would potentially benefit from physiotherapy (PT).

PT of HNC patients ideally begins prior to cancer treatment and is continued throughout the illness trajectory. The goals of PT are to optimize the patient's physical function, fitness, physical activity and improve health-related QOL, while also providing education about the physical and biomechanical changes related to their cancer treatment. Physiotherapists will individualize, modify and update a home exercise programme targeting the involved areas, fatigue and cardiovascular fitness throughout the entire illness trajectory. The recovery of a 'new normal' for physical function is a critical role that PT can fulfil and is arguably an important link for smooth transition to cancer survivorship after treatment[196,197]. The majority of the literature on physical function and exercise in HNC concerns temperomandibular joint hypomobility, trismus and spinal accessory nerve resection (also known as 'shoulder syndrome')[198]. In addition to these specific problems, PT can also address problems further up and down the 'chain' of movement that involves the anterior and posterior neck, bilateral shoulder and upper back musculature. Such additional problems include disuse atrophy and associated weakness, postural malalignment, chemotherapy-induced fatigue, radiation therapy-induced tissue fibrosis and lymphoedema. These are all aspects of physical recovery amenable to PT interventions throughout the illness trajectory.

Phase I: prior to cancer treatment

Prior to treatment, a baseline PT evaluation will determine physical function and provide pre-treatment exercise programming and education to the patient and caregivers. At this time, the physiotherapist can take advantage of a 'teachable moment' and discuss physical recovery milestones as well as expected physical and biomechanical changes and the importance of exercise to cancer survivorship[199,200]. Assessment should include active and passive range of motion, muscle strength and length (flexibility), endurance and extent of physical performance, especially as they concern the temperomandibular joint, shoulder joint complex, cervical and upper thoracic vertebrae, postural alignment, facial symmetry, and tongue mobility[7–10,201–203]. Skin integrity, skin sensation, and, if indicated, a systems-based evaluation of balance and coordination (somatosensory organization of visual, proprioceptive, vestibular systems) may also be included as part of the baseline evaluation[204–206].

An individualized home exercise programme targeting postural alignment, active and passive range of motion for muscle lengthening, resistive exercises for muscle strengthening, and balance/coordination activities are recommended. The home exercise programme prior to treatment optimizes strength, length, posture, and physical function thereby lessening the effects of disuse and tissue shortening due to surgery, chemotherapy and radiation therapy. Additionally, aerobic activity such as walking or bicycling for cardiovascular fitness should be recommended, to optimize the physical condition of the patient prior to treatment. After considering the patient's cardiac status, a target heart rate should be calculated[207].

Phase II: acute phase—after cancer surgery

For those undergoing neck dissection involving sacrifice of motor nerves (e.g. facial and/or spinal accessory nerves), removal of muscle tissue and/or reconstruction, the patient should be informed about expected biomechanical changes and sensory changes of the involved tissues at the time of the baseline evaluation. Part of the patient's preparation for the acute phase is an understanding of postoperative precautions, general exercise precautions for the patient with cancer and specific impairments commonly encountered after active treatment.

Postoperative precautions and general exercise precautions During the acute phase, the home exercise programme should be modified to account for postoperative movement and activity precautions. After surgery, active range of motion as tolerated is generally indicated. However, in the case of reconstruction, active range of motion and flexibility exercises of the involved area should be restricted to preserve tissue integrity and promote healing. Depending on the extent of reconstruction (e.g. bone, microvascular flaps, alloderm) movement may be restricted up to 6–8 weeks after surgery. During this time, isometric exercises of the cervical and associated shoulder muscles can help prevent muscle atrophy, excessive oedema, and decrease pain. The individualized aerobic fitness (walking or bicycling) programme can be maintained after surgery provided that adherence to postoperative precautions continue. Postural alignment exercises may also be performed while supine on a firm but supported surface or standing against a wall. The patient will also need to be instructed on positioning to remain comfortable and best protect the affected area. For example, moving from sitting to supine will require support of the head and/or neck throughout the movement and, once supine, the patient may feel more comfortable with several pillows supporting the head and neck.

Special considerations for surgeries involving sternocleidomastioid resection and spinal accessory nerve damage Unilateral removal of the sternocleidomastoid will result in cervical rotation with the chin pointing towards the involved side. In severe cases, this may also result in cervical flexion, rotation and lateral flexion towards the uninvolved side mimicking torticollis. This dysfunctional movement pattern can be exacerbated with radiation-induced tissue fibrosis shortening the remaining ipsilateral tissue and, in some cases, the contralateral tissue. Left untreated, the cervical vertebrae lose mobility and abnormal biomechanics are translated up and down the involved vertebral segments and, in some cases, the shoulder to accommodate for these abnormalities. Pain, muscle length and strength imbalances, adhesive capsulitis and inadequate muscular timing for postural control and efficient movement stem from these biomechanical changes.

Similarly, a lack of preservation of the spinal accessory nerve will result in 'shoulder syndrome' in which both the sternocleidomastoid and trapezius are affected[198]. Together this results in the appearance of a lower shoulder on the involved side with visible atrophy of the trapezius[198]. The patient presents typically with the same appearance as the person who has had removal of the sternocleidomastoid, but the involved scapula will drift upward and downwardly rotate with visible winging of the scapula[203]. Furthermore, while the patient may have full passive range of motion of the shoulder, active range will be limited due to the lack of muscle innervation[198]. To compensate for the loss of the trapezius, the smaller scapular stabilizers (rhomboids, teres minor, levator scapula) are overused and can contribute to pain[208,198]. Taken together, these biomechanical changes alter scapular stabilization and scapulothoracic rhythm[209]. Left untreated, this can lead to shoulder impairment such as adhesive capsulitis[210]. The physiotherapist will use therapeutic exercise, postural re-education and manual therapy techniques (including passive range of motion) to normalize altered cervical and shoulder biomechanics.

Trismus Trismus (limited mouth closing/TMJ hypomobility) may be caused by a variety of mechanisms including the tumour occupying muscle tissue, radiation-induced tissue fibrosis, or muscle spasm of the masseters, pterygoids, and/or temporalis muscles. Trismus is the most problematic of physical function impairments because it directly affects nutritional intake and will result in weight loss and energy imbalances. Trismus has been treated effectively with physical rehabilitation methods such as sustained stretch devices (e.g. Therabite®[211]), application of electrical stimulation and exercise[212,213]. Sustained stretch devices are cited as the single most effective method[211] to improve trismus with some evidence that early use may be helpful[214]. Nevertheless, co-morbid factors that affect the integrity of the mandible and temperomandibular joint may contraindicate the use of a sustained stretch device (e.g. bone occupying tumour, loss of dentition, mucositis, mouth reconstruction, tongue resection). These co-morbid factors may make it difficult for the patient to adhere to the physiotherapy programme[215].

Phase III: sub-acute, phases—during and after treatment and return to fitness

Therapeutic exercise During active treatment, it is critical to monitor the individualized home exercise programme. PT coordinated with chemotherapy and radiation treatment sessions will enable effective monitoring and modification of the home exercise and fitness programme while continuing to target cervical and shoulder range of motion, strength, flexibility, balance, coordination, cardiovascular fitness, and postural alignment. The importance of postural alignment cannot be overemphasized as poor postural alignment of the head and neck is commonly observed (see Fig. 11.2.1). Exercises targeting postural alignment that accommodate the stage of recovery (e.g. performing exercises in supine or against a wall during phases I and II or in advanced positions as in phases III and IV) can provide dramatic results (see Fig. 11.2.1).

During this time, special precautions must be taken to ensure that exercise is not causing or contributing to ataxia, cachexia, dehydration, dyspnea, fatigue, hypoxia, infection, nausea, lymphoedema, and pathological fracture[216,217]. Low haemoglobin (<8 g/dl) and oxygen saturation (<90 per cent) indicate poor oxygen exchange and can contribute to fatigue, underlining the need to reduce exercise intensity. A low platelet count places the patient at a higher risk of haemorrhage or ecchymosis thus high intensity exercises, especially those performed with high levels of resistance, are also contraindicated. A low neutrophil count and/or fever may be the first signs of infection and as such exercise intensity and frequency should also be reduced until the infection is resolved. Bone metastases preclude resistive exercise due to the risk of pathological fracture. In cases where the patient reports dizziness, vertigo, loss of balance, or peripheral sensation, the physiotherapist should reduce the intensity and frequency of exercise or stop exercise until these neurological signs are reduced. Changing the mode of exercise and modifying frequency and intensity may be helpful to combat any or all of these special considerations[216, 217]. In cases of balance and coordination impairments, retraining for reliance on other aspects of sensory input (visual, vestibular and somatosensory) may also be effective to reduce the impact of these physiological responses to exercise[204,206,218,219].

Scar management

After active treatment and successful scar closure, scar massage and mobility may be initiated with the goals of softening, flattening and reducing the size of the scar, improving mobility over underlying tissues and the cosmetic appearance of the scar (see Figs. 11.2.3 and 11.2.4)[220,221]. Special care must be taken to not blister the skin with over-aggressive scar mobility[220,221]. The scar should also be monitored for any changes such as infection, tumour recurrence, and lymphoedema.

Radiation-induced tissue fibrosis

As described earlier, radiation-induced tissue fibrosis presents as hardened and inflexible tissue that may also be accompanied by lymphoedema (see lymphoedema section). Physiotherapists use a variety of modalities and techniques to combat radiation tissue fibrosis such as myofascial release, sustained stretching, scar tissue mobility, manual lymph drainage, compression bandaging or garments, and electrical stimulation. While these approaches continue to be used, a promising study on the use of microcurrent electrical stimulation to soften tissue fibrosis was reported by Lennox et al.[7]. Using a 5-day, twice daily microcurrent protocol (using alternating microampere current with frequencies between 0.5 and 100 Hz and with a maximum of 600 µA) cervical range of motion was improved for between 81 per cent and 92 per cent of their 29 participants. Three months later, 91 per cent either maintained

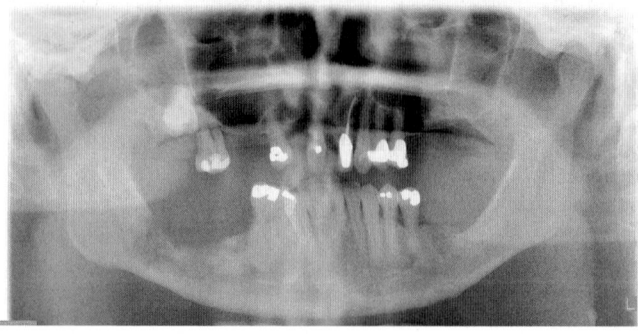

Figure 11.2.1 Osteoradionecrosis of the right mandible after a dental extraction.

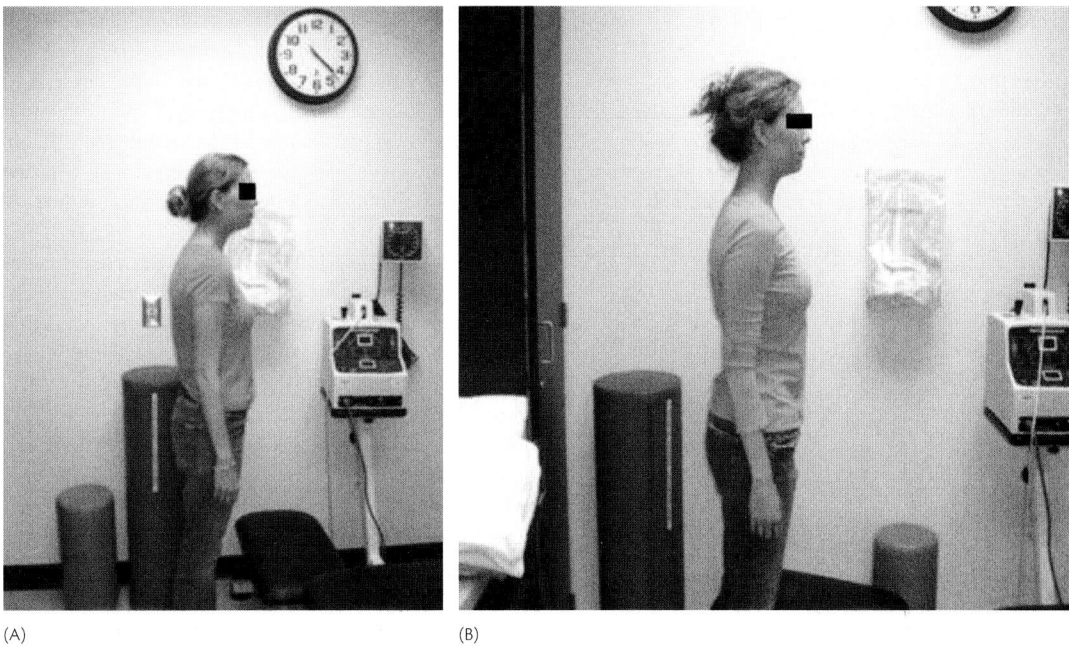

(A)   (B)

Figure 11.2.2 Right sagittal postural alignment. (a) 6th post-operative week (b) 10th post-operative week

or improved their range of motion. Improvements were also noted for tongue mobility, facial symmetry, xerostomia, muscle spasm, trismus, and tenderness. Unfortunately, this study did not include controls for comparison and, to date, no randomized clinical trials have been attempted to test the efficacy of this protocol.

The goals of PT after active cancer treatment are to maximize muscle strength, soft tissue length, postural alignment, endurance, balance/coordination along with scar and tissue mobility. Likewise, PT aims to minimize pain, fatigue, lymphoedema, and improve overall physical function and return the patient to fitness.

Taste alteration

The majority of taste buds are located on the tongue. They may also be found scattered throughout the upper aero-digestive system. Taste buds are composed of 50–100 receptor cells with associated support cells. Receptor cells transmit signals to the trigeminal nerve fibres which carry information to the brain. Loss of taste may be caused by a wide variety of medical illnesses and pharmaceutical agents including many chemotherapy drugs[170]. Radiation therapy, which is an integral part of treatment for all patients with locally advanced disease, may result in severe and permanent alteration in taste sensation. The exact mechanism of radiation-induced taste alteration remains to be elucidated. Taste alteration may begin 2–3 days after initiating therapy and taste bud degeneration may be seen 6–7 days after starting radiation therapy. Accumulated doses over 6000 cGy may be associated with permanent damage.

Loss of taste may have a profound effect on nutritional status and QOL. Patients may describe an inability to take nutrition orally due to severe loss of taste or altered taste sensation. The taste of food may become noxious resulting in nausea and vomiting. Taste slowly returns for the majority of patients weeks to months after the completion of therapy. However, some patients have a permanent alteration in taste sensation. To date, there are no

known preventative or treatment measures for taste alterations. Although small studies have reported that zinc improves taste alterations, a randomized trial of zinc in HNC patients failed to demonstrate efficacy for the prevention of radiation-induced taste alterations[223].

Xerostomia

Xerostomia can be a severe and permanent complication of external beam radiation therapy[224,225]. It results from damage to the acinar cells and stromal matrix of the major and minor salivary glands. The degree of xerostomia is related to the amount of salivary gland tissues within the radiation port and the radiation dose delivered. The sparing of at least one salivary gland can reduce significantly

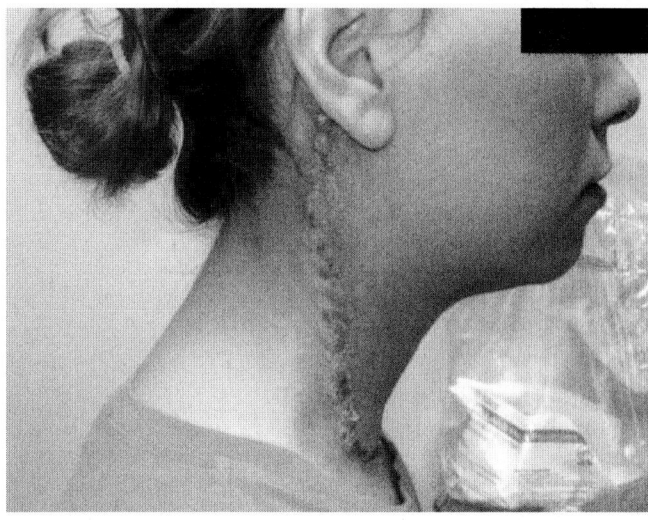

Figure 11.2.3 Right sagittal view of thyroidectomy scar – 6th post-operative week

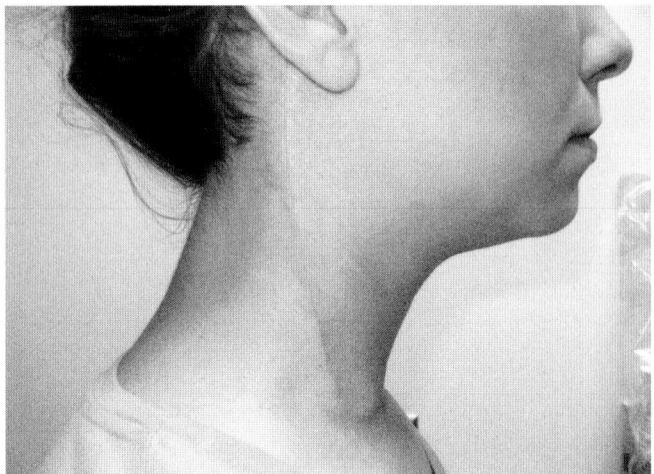

Figure 11.2.4 Right sagittal view of thyroidectomy scar – 10th post-operative week and after 4 weeks of physical therapy.

sequellae of radiation therapy to the oral cavity. Damage to the acinar cells is evident at low doses of radiation therapy. Salivary gland function, both stimulated and unstimulated, drops rapidly to 5–30 per cent of normal within the first 2–3 weeks of therapy and remains low (<10 per cent of normal) following completion of radiation for a prolonged period of time[163–166]. In general, recovery of function is slow and partial.

Saliva is vital for normal oral function[224,225] Symptoms due to hyposalivation are numerous and can profoundly decrease QOL. Saliva plays an important role in moistening food to allow bolus formation. Even mild xerostomia can result in a significant decrease in the variety and types of food that patients can eat. Difficulty forming a food bolus makes deglutition difficult. Saliva maintains oral flora, thus preventing the development of dental caries. It lubricates mucosal membranes allowing normal speech and swallowing[226,227]. Finally, xerostomia results in mucosal irritation which can be extremely severe at night and in dry conditions. A number of palliative and therapeutic interventions can be attempted to improve symptoms of xerostomia and its associated complications.

Patients with severe xerostomia usually carry water with them to swish and swallow on a frequent basis. The soothing effect is short lived. Patients with severe xerostomia may drink litres of fluid daily merely for comfort purposes. The use of a sodium bicarbonate rinse can help maintain dental hygiene as well as sooth the mucosal surface. Caphosol®, a concentrated calcium and phosphate solution, has recently been FDA approved for palliation of xerostomia of all causes. Caphosol® is administered as a 'swish and spit' agent four to ten times per day as indicated clinically. A number of commercial salivary gland substitutes are available. Although some patients find these products useful, the majority of patients fail to find significant benefit. For an extensive listing of palliative agents, please visit Oral Health in Cancer Therapy at http://www.doep.org.

With increasing use of primary radiation therapy plus or minus chemotherapy for treatment of squamous carcinomas of the head and neck, attention has turned to methods for ameliorating treatment-related toxicity. Prevention of xerostomia has been an area of active clinical research. Several agents merit mention because

they are now approved for and commonly used in the treatment of xerostomia.

Pilocarpine is a parasympathomimetic that acts as a muscarinic agonist. It has a time to peak effect of 1 h (unstimulated salivation) and a duration of effect of between 3 and 5 h. Pilot trials demonstrated promising results with pilocarpine for the treatment of xerostomia[167]. Subsequently, two double-blind controlled trials were undertaken to confirm the efficacy of pilocarpine in the treatment of radiation-induced xerostomia. Johnson *et al.* reported on 207 patients who received ~4000 cGy with at least one parotid gland within the radiation port. Patients were assigned randomly to placebo or pilocarpine at one of two doses (5 mg and 10 mg tabs tid). Results demonstrated an improvement in xerostomia-related symptoms for both the 5 and 10 mg tablet[168]. The results of the objective saliva production were less clear. In a study conducted by LeVeque in 162 patients with radiation-induced xerostomia, similar results were reported[169]. In both trials, the most common side effects include sweating, nausea, rhinitis, chills, flushing, urinary frequency, dizziness, and asthenia. Thus, pilocarpine at a dose of 5 mg PO three to four times per day may produce a modest but significant subjective improvement in oral symptoms related to xerostomia with generally mild side effects. Symptom relief was maximal at 4 months and a prolonged drug trial may be required to determine efficacy in a given patient. Pilocarpine has been investigated as a prophylactic treatment during radiation therapy. A small phase II trial has demonstrated a reduction in radiation-induced xerostomia when patients received pilocarpine during radiation therapy[229]. A subsequent randomized phase III trial conducted through the RTOG demonstrated an improvement in unstimulated salivary flow with the concomitant use of oral pilocarpine; however, patient reported outcomes were not improved[230].

Cevimeline, a cholinergic agent with muscarinic agonist activity, has been used for the treatment of xerostomia in collagen vascular disorders[231]. Investigators recently reported the results of a combined data analysis of two randomized trials evaluating the efficacy of cevimeline in HNC patients with radiation-induced xerostomia[232,233]. Five hundred and seventy subjects were entered into the study. Both studies demonstrated a significant increase in unstimulated salivary flow with cevimeline when compared with placebo. No differences in stimulated salivary flow were noted. Select patient reported outcomes were improved in one study. Thus, cevimeline administration of 30–45 mg of cevimeline three times daily increased unstimulated salivary flow. The potential benefit of increased unstimulated salivary flow of oral function and oral health was not investigated.

Amifostine (WR-2721) is a free radical scavenger that has been investigated for its potential to protect cells from chemotherapy and radiation-induced DNA damage. Amifostine has been FDA approved for reduction in xerostomia in patients undergoing postoperative radiation treatment for HNC when the radiation port includes a large segment of salivary gland tissue (>75 per cent of both salivary glands included in the radiation port). In a randomized trial of 315 patients receiving postoperative radiation therapy, patients receiving amifostine 200 mg/m² 15 to 30 min prior to each fractionation of radiation had a significantly decreased rate of grade 2 or greater xerostomia. The rate of acute xerostomia dropped from 78 per cent to 51 per cent ($p <0.0001$) and late xerostomia dropped from 57 per cent to 35 per cent ($p = 0.0016$). Side-effects to amifostine are significant with hypotension reported in

15 per cent of patients. A number of subsequent trials have been conducted to delineate more clearly the role of amifostine in the HNC population, however, the results were mixed. Therefore, a meta-analysis was performed which demonstrated that amifostine decreased acute (OR, 0.24; CI 0.15–0.36; $p < 0.00001$) and late xerostomia (OR 0.33; CI, 0.21–0.51; $p < 0.00001$). Subcutaneous amifostine was compared with IV dosing and was found to be equally effective with an improved toxicity profile[234].

Non-pharmacological techniques have also been evaluated to prevent xerostomia. Surgical transfer of the contralateral submandibular gland to the submental triangle before radiation has demonstrated efficacy in preventing xerostomia[235]. Intensity-modulated radiation therapy (IMRT) technology is available in more centres, allowing improved sparing (mean dose ≤ 26Gy) of the parotids without compromising tumour control. Measurements of salivary flow after IMRT show considerable decreases in xerostomia and improved QOL compared with patients treated with standard 3-dimension conformal irradiation techniques[236–240].

Wound care, fistulas, and carotid rupture

With the advancement in reconstructive techniques in the past two decades, our ability to handle larger and more complex wounds in the head and neck has improved. Regional and distant tissue transfer techniques have expanded the ability to cover vital organs such as the carotid artery and bring well-vascularized tissue into a contaminated operative field that can resist infection and postoperative radiation therapy. In general, if distant tissue is used to reconstruct a wound created by resection of a tumour, the blood supply to that tissue is preserved by isolating the tissue on a pedicle artery and vein. If the tissue is simply rotated on its pedicle to reach the defect, it is called a pedicled flap, such as a pectoralis muscle or the latissimus muscle flap. If the vascular pedicle has to be divided to allow movement of the flap from a remote site, such as the fibula, then the arterial and venous blood supply must be re-established through a microvascular anastamosis in the neck and this is referred to as a free flap. In all cases, the reconstruction, particularly in the immediate postoperative period, is solely dependent on its blood supply and careful attention must be given to placing any dressings around the neck, which may compress the pedicle vessels. Tracheostomies are typically sewn in place to avoid a circumferential dressing around the neck until the wound appears to be sealed.

Despite newer reconstructive techniques, patients who have undergone prior radiation therapy or combined chemo-radiation therapy are at greater risk for wound breakdown as a result of the small vessel arteritis that reduces oxygen tissue exchange in the area. Additionally, patients' preoperative nutritional status and smoking history complicate their wound healing capacity. Pharyngocutaneous fistulas may result from wound breakdown if a watertight seal of the pharynx cannot be maintained. Patients who have had a breech of the pharynx during their resection are often maintained with nasogastric feedings to limit the contamination of the suture lines for 1–2 weeks. Fistula formation is usually heralded by erythema of the neck, tenderness and low-grade fevers. The saliva in the neck must be drained and the path of drainage directed away from the carotid artery. Saliva, with its digestive enzymes, has the ability to necrose the great vessels resulting in life threatening haemorrhage. Additionally, exposure of the vessels to the external environment leads to desiccation and potential carotid rupture.

Exposure of the neck vessels as a result of loss of overlying skin or fistula formation represents a surgical emergency. The vessels should be covered with saline soaked gauze until vascularized tissue can be placed over the vessels. Any continuous bleeding from an exposed area must be taken seriously for it may herald an early leak from the carotid artery and surgical exploration to repair the vessel may be necessary.

If a fistula does form, and the great vessels are not exposed, the wound can often be managed conservatively until secondary healing occurs. The patient should continue to be fed through a non-oral route to minimize contamination. The wound should be packed with wet to dry gauze dressings twice a day or more frequently if contamination is excessive.

In patients who have unresectable disease in the neck, ulceration of the tumour with necrotic debris may become problematic. Tumour hygiene can be achieved through gentle debridement with hydrogen peroxide. Desiccating powders may be applied if wound remains moist. Intermittent use of antibiotics to cover anaerobic floral contaminants will often assist with sterilizing the field and assist with odour control. Oral hygiene can be maintained with use of the Water Pik made by Teledyne, Inc. set on low settings to debride tissue. Use of frequent mouth rinses with saline and soda or similar proprietary preparations can also assist in cleansing as well.

A carotid rupture is an uncommon but catastrophic complication of HNC and its therapy. Carotid rupture may occur in patients undergoing extensive resection, external beam radiation therapy, brachytherapy, or those with recurrent/advanced cancers of the neck. Although initial retrospective reviews in the 1950s and 1960s demonstrated rates of carotid rupture as high as 14 per cent[241] the numbers are much lower with contemporary treatment methods[242]. The investigators at MSKCC reviewed the data of 2346 patients undergoing head and neck surgical procedures between 1994 and 1995. Only one case of carotid rupture was identified[243]. When possible, patients with carotid rupture should undergo evaluation with angiography. In patients with controlled tumour (i.e. the postoperative setting), aggressive intervention with surgery or invasive radiological procedures are indicated. Unfortunately data on the success of radiological procedures (i.e. balloon occlusion and embolization) are scant[244]. In one series reported by Citardi, 12 patients with carotid rupture were treated with endovascular occlusion[245]. All 12 patients survived without neurologic sequelae. In patients will terminal disease, palliative measures are usually undertaken.

Conclusions

Patients with HNC suffer from a variety of cancer and treatment-related symptom-control problems. Some of the palliative issues are unique to the head and neck population. Optimal palliation requires a multi-modality team of physicians, nurses, social workers, dentists, physiotherapists and speech/swallowing therapists in order to address the multitude of needs. As many of these patients have poor social support systems, the treatment team may need to spend substantially more time with the patient to ensure adequate symptom palliation. The added effort and attention can result in improved cure rates, diminished long-term side effects and decreased existential distress for the patient and family. For those patients who are destined to die of their disease, adequate medical support can mean the difference between an agonizing death and one that is both physically and emotionally comfortable.

Fruther reading

Lennox, Wong, R.K., Jones, G.W. *et al.* (2002), A phase I–II study of acupunctur-like trancutaneous merve stimulating in the treatment of radiation-induced Xerostemice in head & meck cancer patients treated with radical radiotherapy. *Int J Rasiat Oncol Biol Plays*, 2003 oct1: **57**(2), 472–80.

Dejonckere, P.H., Hordijk, G.J. (1998). Prognostic factors for swallowing after head & med clini Otolaryngol allied sci, **23**(3), 218–23.

Brizel, D.M., Waserman, T.H., Henke, M. *et al.* (2000). Phase III Randomized in Head & Neck cancer, *J Clin oncol*, **18**(19), 3339–45.

Sasse, A.D. *et al.* Cemifostine reduces side effects and improves complete response rate during radiotherapy results of a meta-analysis. *Int J Radiation Biol Phy*, **64**(1), 784–91

Reuther, T. *et al.*, Osteoradionecrosis of the jaws as a side effect of radiotherapy of head and neck tumour patients–a report of a thirty year retrospective review. *Int J Oral Maxillofac Surg*, **32**(3), 289–295.

References

1. Jemal, A., Siegal, R., Ward, E. *et al.* (2007). Cancer statistics, *CA: A Cancer Journal for Clinicians*, **57**(1), 43–66.

2. Braakhuis, B.J.M., Brackenhoff, R.H., and Leemans, C.R. (2005). Second field tumors: a new opportunity for cancer prevention? *Oncologist*, **10**(7), 493–500.

3. Donta, T.S., and Smoker, R. (2007). Head and neck cancer: carcinoma of unknown primary. *Topics In Magnetic Resonance Imaging*, **18**(4), 281–92.

4. Nayak, J.V., Walvekar, R.R., Andrade, R.S. *et al.* (2007). Deferring Planned Neck Dissection Following Chemoradiation for Stage IV Head and Neck Cancer: The Utility of PET-CT. *Laryngoscope*, **117**, pp2129–2134.

5. Shah, J.P., and Lydiatt, W. (1995). Treatment of cancer of the head and neck. *CA: A Cancer Journal for Clinicians*, **45**(6), 352–368.

6. Forastiere, A.A., Goepfert, H., Maor, M. *et al.* (2003). Concurrent chemotherapy and radiotherapy for organ preservation in advanced laryngeal cancer. *New England Journal of Medicine*, **349**(22), 2091–8.

7. Adelstein, D., Adams, G.L., Wagner, H. *et al.* (2000). A phase III comparison of standard radiation therapy (RT) versus RT plus concurrent cisplatin (DDP) versus split-course RT plus CCP and F-flurouracil (5FU) in patients with unresectable squamous cell head and neck cancer (SCHNC): an Intergroup study. *Proceedings of American Society of Clinical Oncology*, **19**, 411A Abstract 1624.

8. Berzon, R. (2000). Understanding and using health-related quality of life instruments within clinical research studies, In *Quality of life assessment in clinical trials, methods and practice* (Staquet, M.J., ed.), pp. 3–5, Maurice J Staguet, Ron, D. Hayes and Peter M Fayaers Oxford: Oxford.

9. Osoba, D. (2000). Guidelines for measuring health-related quality of life clinical trials, In *Quality of life assessment in clinical trials, methods and practice* (Staquet, M.J., ed.), pp. 19–35, Maurice, J. Staguet, Ron, D. Hayes, and Peter, M. Fayaers Oxford: Oxford.

10. Cella, D.F., Tulsky, D.S., Gray, G. *et al.* (1993). The functional assessment of cancer therapy (FACT) scale: Development and validation of a general measure. *Journal of Clinical Oncology*, **11**, 570–579.

11. Cella, D. (1994). Manual for the Functional Assessment of Therapy (FACT) Measurement System (Version 3). Rush Medical Center, Chicago IL.

12. Sherman, A.C., Simonton, S., Adams, D.C. *et al.* (2000). Assessing Quality of Life in Patients with Head and Neck Cancer: Cross-Validation of the European Organization for Research and Treatment of Cancer (EORTC) Quality of Life Head and Neck Module (QLQ-H&N35). *Archives of Otolaryngology—Head and Neck Surgery*, **126**(4), 459–467.

13. Ringash, J., and Bezjak, A. (2001). A stuctured review of quality of life instruments for head and neck cancer patients. *Head and Neck*, **23**, 201–213.

14. Murphy, B.A., Wells, N., Ridner, S. *et al.* (2007). Quality of life research in head and neck cancer: a review of the current state of the science. *Critical Reviews in Oncology/Hematology*, **62**, 251–267.

15. Weymuller, E., Yueh, B., Deleyiannis, F.W. *et al.* (2000). Quality of life in patients with head and neck cancer. *Archives of Otolaryngology—Head and Neck Surgery*, **126**, 329–335.

16. Rogers, S., Lowe, D., Brown, J.S. *et al.* (1999). The University of Washington Head and Neck Cancer Measure as a predictor of outcome following primary surgery for oral cancer. *Head and Neck*, **21**, 394–401.

17. Murry, T., Madasu, R., Martin, A. *et al.* (1998). Acute and chronic changes in swallowing and quality of life following intraarterial chemoradiation for organ preservation in patients with advanced head and neck cancer. *Head and Neck*, **20**, 31–37.

18. Blot, W.J., McLaughlin, J.K., Winn, D.M. *et al.* (1988). Smoking and drinking in relation to oral and pharyngeal cancer. *Cancer Research*, **48**(11), 3282–3287.

19. Piccirillo, J.F., Lacy, P.D., Basu, A. *et al.* (2002). Development of a new head and neck cancer-specific comorbidity index. *Archives of Otolaryngology—Head and Neck Surgery*, **128**(10), 1172–9.

20. Deleyiannis, F., Thomas, D.B., Vaughan, T.L. *et al.* (1996) Alcoholism: independent predictor of survival in patients with head and neck cancer. *J Natl Cancer Inst*, **88**, 542–9.

21. Hollenbeak, C.S., Stack, B.C. Jr, Daley, S.M. *et al.* (2007). Using comorbidity indexes to predict costs for head and neck cancer. *Archives of Otolaryngology—Head and Neck Surgery*, **133**(1), 24–7.

22. Epstein, J.B. *et al.* (1999). Quality of life and oral function following radiotherapy for head and neck cancer. *Head and Neck*, **21**, 1–11.

23. Hutton, J.M. and Williams, M. (2001). An investigation of psychological distress in patients who have been treated for head and neck cancer. *British Journal of Oral and Maxillofacial Surgery*, **39**, 333–9.

24. Relic, A., Mazemda, P., Arens, C. *et al.* (2001). Investigating quality of life and coping resources after laryngectomy. *European Archives of Oto-Rhino-Laryngology*, **258**(10), 514–7.

25. Sherman, A.C., Simonton, S., Adams, D.C. *et al.* (2000). Coping with head and neck cancer during different phases of treatment. *Head and Neck*, **22**(8), 787–93.

26. de Leeuw, J.R., de Graeff, A., Ros, W.J. *et al.* (2001). Prediction of depression 6 months to 3 years after treatment of head and neck cancer. *Head & Neck*, **23**(10), 892–8.

27. Friedman Marilyn, M., Bowden Vicky, R., Jones, E. (2002). *Family nursing: research, theory, and practice*, 5th edition, Prentice Hall, Upper Saddle River, NJ, pp. 151–69.

28. Wisawatapnimit, P., Dwyer, K.A., and Murphy, B. (2005). Predicting depressed mood in head and neck cancer patients, Poster session presented at the 19th Annual Conference of the Southern Nursing Research Society, Atlanta, Georgia.

29. Wisawatapnimit, P., Dwyer, K., Murphy, B. (2006). Life experience of head and neck cancer patients and their caregivers after treatment. In *Southern Nursing Research Society Meeting*. Memphis TN.

30. Vickery, L.E., Latchford, G., Hewison, J. *et al.* (2003). The impact of head and neck cancer and facial disfigurement on the quality of life of patients and their partners. *Head Neck*, **25**(4), 289–96.

31. Watt-Watson, J. and Graydon, J. (1995). Impact of surgery on head and neck cancer patients and their caregivers. *Nursing Clinics of North America*, **30**(4), 659–71.

32. Deschler, D.G., Walsh, K.A., Friedman, S. *et al.* (1999). Quality of life assessment in patients undergoing head and neck surgery as evaluated by lay caregivers. *Laryngoscope*, **109**(1), 42–6.

33. Deschler, D.G., Walsh K.A., and Hayden, R.E. (2004). Follow-up quality of life assessment in patients after head and neck surgery as evaluated by lay caregivers. *ORL Head and Neck Nursing*, **22**(1), 26–32.

34. Mood, D. (1997). Cancers of the head and neck. In *A cancer source book for nurses* (Eds. Varricchio, M.P.C., Walker, C.L., and Ades, T.B), pp. 271–83, *American Cancer Society*, Atlanta.

36. Nalbadian, M., Nikolaidis, V., Petridis, D. *et al.* (2001). Factors influencing quality of life in laryngectomized patients. *European Archives of Oto-Rhino-Laryngology*, **258**(7), 336–40.

37. De Graeff, A., de.Leeeuw.R., Ros, W.J.G. *et al.* (1999). A prospective study of quality of life of laryngeal cancer patients treated with radiotherapy. *Head and Neck*, **21**, 291–6.

38. Ramirez, M.J., Ferriol, E.E., Domenech, F.G. *et al.* (2003). Psychosocial adjustment in patients surgically treated for laryngeal cancer. *Otolaryngology—Head and Neck Surgery*, **129**(1), 92–7.

39. Taylor, E.J. (2003). Spiritual needs of patients with cancer and family caregivers. *Cancer Nursing*, **26**(4), 260–6.

40. Deleyiannis, F.W.B., Weymuller EA Jr, Coltrera, M.D. *et al.* (1999). Quality of life after laryngectomy: are functional disabilities important?. *Head and Neck*, **21**, 319–24.

41. David, D.J. and Barritt, J.A. (1982). Psychosocial implications of surgery for head and neck cancer. *Symposium on Social and Psychological Considerations in Plastic Surgery*, **9**(3), 327–36.

42. Boyd, C., Zhang-Salomons, J.Y., Groome, P.A. *et al.* (1999). Associations between community income and cancer survival in Ontario, Canada and the United States. *Journal of Clinical Oncology*, **17**, 2244–55.

43. Simpson, C.B., Postma, G.N., Stone, R.E. Jr. *et al.* (1997). Speech outcomes after laryngeal cancer management. *Otolaryngologic Clinics of North America*, **30**(2), 189–206.

44. Blaylock, D. (1997). Speech rehabilitation after treatment of laryngeal carcinoma. *Otolaryngologic Clinics of North America*, **30**(2), 179–88.

45. National Comprehensive Cancer Network (2005) www.nccn.org/ professionals/physician_gls/f_guidelines.asp.

46. Epstein, J.B., Robertson, M., Emerton, S. *et al.* (2001). Quality of life and oral function in patients treated with radiation therapy for head and neck cancer. *Head and Neck*, **23**(5), 389–98.

47. Perry, A. and Shaw, M. (2000). Evaluation of functional outcomes (speech, swallowing and voice) in patients attending speech pathology after head and neck cancer treatment(s), development of a multi-centre database. **114**, 605–15.

48. Perlman, A. (1994). Disordered Swallowing, In *Diagnosis in speech-language pathology* (eds. Morris, H., and Spriestersback, D.), pp. 361–82, Singular Publishing Group, San Diego.

49. Logemann, J. (1998). Evaluation and treatment of swallowing disorders. Pro-ed., Austin, TX.

50. McConnel, F., Cerenko, D., Jackson, R. *et al.* (1988). Timing of major events of pharyngeal swallowing. *Archives of Otolaryngology—Head and Neck Surgery*, **114**, 1413–8.

51. Murphy, B.A., F.J., Dowling, E., Cheatham, R., Cmela, A. (2002). Dietary intake and adapations in head and neck cancer patients treated with chemoradiation. *Proceedings of American Society Clinical Oncology*, **21**, abstract 932.

52. Aviv, J., Martin, J.H., Sacco, R.L. *et al.* (1996). Supraglottic and pharyngeal sensory abnormalities in stroke patients with dysphagia. *Ann Otol Rhinol Laryngeal*, **105**, 92–7.

53. Lundy, D., Smith, C., Colangelo, L. *et al.* (1999). Aspiration: Cause and implications. *Otolaryngology—Head and Neck Surgery*, **120**, 474–8.

54. Nguyen, N.P., S.H., Duttan, S. *et al.* (2007). Aspiration occurence during chemoradiation for head and neck cancer. *Anticancer Drugs*, **3B**, 1669–72.

55. Sonies, B.C. and Baum, B.J. (1988). Evaluation of swallowing pathophysiology. *Otolaryngologic Clinics of North America*, **21**(4), 637–48.

56. Hiss, S.G., P.G., (2003). Fiberoptic endoscopic evaluation of swallowing. *The Laryngoscope*, **113**(8), 1386–1383.

57. Chen, A.Y., Frankowski, R., Bishop-Leone, J., Hebert, T. *et al.* (2001). The development and validation of a dysphagia-specific quality-of-life questionnaire for patients with head and neck cancer: The MD Anderson Dysphyagia Inventory. *Archives of Otolaryngology—Head and Neck Surgery*, **127**, 870–6.

58. McHorney, C.A., Martin-Harris, B., Robbins, J. *et al.* (2006). Clinical validity of the SWAL-QOL and SWAL-CARE outcome tools with respect to bolus flow measures. *Dysphagia*, **21**(3), 141–8.

59. Murphy, B.A., Wells, N., Cmelak, A. *et al.* (2004). Reliability and validity for the Vanderbilt Head and Neck Symptom Survey (VHNSS): A new tool to assess symptom burden in patients undergoing chemoradiation. *Proceedings of American Society Clinical Oncology*, **23**, abstract 5569.

60. Stenson, K., MacCracken, E., List, M. *et al.* (2000). Swallowing function in patients with head and neck cancer prior to treatment. *Archives of Otolaryngology—Head and Neck Surgery*, **126**, 371–7.

61. McConnel, F., L.J., Rademaker, A.W. *et al.* (1994). Surgical variagles affecting postoperative swallowing efficiency in oral cancer patients: a Pilot Study *Laryngoscope*, **104**, 87–90.

62. Hirano, M., Kuroiwa, Y., Tanaka, S. *et al.* (1992). Dysphagia following various degrees of surgical resection for oral cancer. *Ann Otol Rhinol Laryngeal*, **101**, 138–41.

63. Logemann, J. and Bytell, D. (1979). Swallowing disorders in three types of head and neck surgical patients. *Cancer*, **44**, 1095–105.

64. Pauloski, B., Rademaker, A.W., Logemann, J.A. *et al.* (1998). Speech and swallowing in irradiated and nonirradiated postsurgical oral cancer patients. *Otolaryngology—Head and Neck Surgery*, **118**, 616–24.

65. Borggreven, P.A., Leeuw, I.V., Rinkel, R.N. *et al.* (2007). Swallowing after major surgery of the oral cavity or oropharynx: a prospective and longitudinal assessment of patients treated by microvascular soft tissue reconstruction. *Head and Neck*, **29**(7), 638–47.

66. Murphy, B.A., S.K., Dowling, E. *et al.* (2006). Swallowing function for patients treated on E2399: A phase II trial of function preservation with induction paclitaxel/carboplatin followed by radiation plus weekly paclitxel. *Proceedings of American Society Clinical Oncology*, **24**, abstract 5524, 286.

67. Cmelak, A.J., Li, S., Meredith, A. *et al.* (2007). Phase II trial of chemoradiation for organ preservation in resectable stage III or IV squamous cell carcinomas of the larynx or oropharynx: results of Eastern Cooperative Oncology Group Study E2399. *Journal of Clinical Oncology*, **25**(25), 3971–7.

68. Rosenthal, D.I., Lewin, J.S., and Eisbruch, A. (2006). Prevention and treatment of dysphagia and aspiration after chemoradiation for head and neck cancer. *Journal of Clinical Oncology*, **24**, 2636–43.

69. Kendall, K.A., McKenzie, S.W., Leonard, R.J. *et al.* (1998). Structural mobility in deglutition after single modality treatment of head and neck carcinomas with radiotherapy. *Head and Neck*, **20**, 720–5.

70. Logemann, J., Smith, C.H., Pauloski, B.R. *et al.* (2001). Effects of xerostomia on perception and performance of swallow function. *Head and Neck*, **23**, 317–21.

71. Hamlet, S., Faull, J., Klein, B. *et al.* (1997). Mastication and swallowing in patients with postirradiation xerostomia. *International Journal of Radiation Oncology, Biology, Physics*, **37**, 789–96.

72. Baker, S. (1990). Current management of cancer of the lip. *Oncology*, **4**, 107–20[Karnell, 2000 253].

73. Hardin, M., Van Demark, D., and Morris, H. (1990). Long-term speech results of cleft palate speakers with marginal velopharyngeal competence. *Journal of Communication Disorders*, **23**, 401–16.

74. McWIlliams, B., Morris, H., and Shelton, R. (1994). *Cleft palate speech*. C.V. Mosby Company, St Louia.

75. Nylen, B. (1961). Cleft palate speech. *Acta Radiologica Supplementum*, **203**.

76. Blocksma, R. (1963). Correction of velopharyngeal insufficiency by silastic pharyngeal implant. *Plastic and Reconstructive Surgery*, **31**, 268.

77. Lewy, R., Cole, R., and Wepman (1965). Teflon injection in the correction of velopharyngeal insufficiency. *Ann Otol Rhinol Laryngeal*, **74**, 874.

78. Netterville, J. and Vrabed, J. (1994). Unilateral palatal adhesions for paralysis after high vagal injury. *Archives of Otolaryngology—Head and Neck Surgery*, **120**, 218–21.

79. Johnson, J., Aramany, M., and Myers, E. (1983). Palatal Neoplasms: reconstruction considerations. *Otolaryngologic Clinics in North America*, **16**, 441.

80. Colton, R. and Casper, J. (1996). *Understanding voice problems*. Williams & Williams, Baltimore, Maryland.

81. Issihiki, N. *et al.* (1974). Thyroplasty as anew phonosurgical technique. *Acta Oto-Laryngologica*, **78**, 451–7.

82. Netterville, J. *et al.* (1993). Silastic medializaton and arytenoid adduction: the Vanderbilt experience. A review of 116 phonosurgical procedures. *Ann Otol Rhinol Laryngeal*, **102**(6), 413–24.

83. Wanamaker, J., Netterville, J., and Ossoff, R. (1993). Phonosurgery: silastic medialization for unilateral vocal fold paralysis. *Oper Tech Otolaryngol Head Neck Surg*, **4**(3), 207–17.

84. Ford, C., Bless, D., and Loftus, J. (1992). Role of injectable collagen in the treatment of glottic insufficiency: a study of 119 patients. *Ann Otol Rhinol Laryngeal*, **101**(3), 237–47.

85. Shindo, M., Saretsky, L., and Rice, D. (1996). Autologous fat injection for unilateral vocal fold paralysis. *Ann Otol Rhinol Laryngeal*, **105**(8), 602–6.

86. Mikaelian, D., Lowry, L., and Sataloff, R. (1991). Lipoinjection for unilateral vocal cord paralysis. *Laryngoscope*, **101**, 465–8.

87. Bocca, E., Pignataro, O., and Oldini, C. (1983). Supraglottic laryngectomy: 30 years of experience. *Ann Otol Rhinol Laryngeal*, **92**, 14–9.

88. Levine, P. *et al.* (1997). Management of advanced-stage cancer. *Otolaryngologic Clinics in North America*, **30**(1), 101–12.

89. DeSanto, L., Pearson, B., and Olsen, K. (1989). Utility of near-total laryngectomy for supraglottic, pharyngeal, base-of-tongue, and other cancers. *Ann Otol Rhinol Laryngeal*, **98**(1), 2–7.

90. Keith, R., and Thomas, J. (1986). *A handbook for the laryngectomy*, 4th edition, Pro-ed, Austin, Texas.

91. Case, J. (1984). *Clinical management of voice disorders*. Aspen Publishers, Inc., Rockville, Maryland, 237–84.

92. Singer, M., and Blom, E. (1980). Tracheostoma valve for postlaryngectomy voice rehabilitation. *Ann Otol Rhinol Laryngol*, **91**, 576–8.

93. Ho, W-K., Wei, W.I., Kwong, D.L.W. *et al.* (1999). Long-term sensorineural hearing deficit following radiotherapy in patients suffering from nasopharyngeal carcinoma: a prospective study. *Head and Neck*, **21**, 547–53.

94. Bhandare, N., Antonelli, P.J., Morris, C.G. *et al.* (2007). Ototoxicity after radiotherapy for head and neck tumors. *International Journal of Radiation Oncology, Biology, Physics*, **67**(2), 469–79.

95. Hymes, S.R., Strom, E.A., and Fife, C. (2006). Radiation dermatitis: clinical presentation, pathophysiology, and treatment 2006. *Journal of American Academy of Dermatology*, **54**(1), 28–46.

96. Bernier, J., Bonner, J., Vermorken, J.B. *et al.* (2007). Consensus guidelines for the management of radiation dermatitis and coexisting acne-like rash in patients receiving radiotherapy plus EGFR inhibitors for the treatment of squamous cell carcinoma of the head and neck. *Annals of Oncology*, **19**(1), 142–9.

97. Tell, R., Sjodin, H., Lundell, G. *et al.* (1997). Hypothyroidism after external radiotherapy for head and neck cancer. *International Journal of Radiation Oncology, Biology, Physics*, **39**(2), 303–8.

98. Singer, P. *et al.* (1995). Treatment guidelines for patients with hyperthyroidism and hypothyroidism. Standards of Care Committee. American Thyroid Association. *JAMA*, **173**, 80–812.

99. Wysolmerski, J. and Broadus, A. (1994). Hypercalcemia of malignancy: the central role of parathyroid hormone-related proteins. *Annual Review of Medicine*, **45**, 189–200.

100. Dische, S., Saunders, I., and Warburton, M. (1986). Hemoglobin, radiation, morbidity and survival. *International Journal of Radiation Oncology, Biology, Physics*, **12**, 1335–7.

101. Lee, D-J., Cosmatos, D., Marcial, V.A. *et al.* (1995). Results of an RTOG phase III trial (RTOG-85-27) comparing radiotherapy plus etanidazole with radiotherapy alone for locally advanced head and neck carcinomas. *International Journal of Radiation Oncology, Biology, Physics*, **32**(3), 567–76.

102. Fein, D.A., Lee, W.R., Hanlon, A.L. *et al.* (1995). Pretreatment hemoglobin level influences local control and survival of T1-T2 squamous cell carcinomas of the glottic larynx. *Journal of Clinical Oncology*, **13**, 2077–83.

103. Overgaard, J., Hansen H,S., Jsrgensen, K. *et al.* (1986). Primary radiotherapy of larynx and pharynx carcinoma-an analysis of some factors influencing local control and survival. *International Journal of Radiation Oncology, Biology, Physics*, **12**, 515–21.

104. Henke, M., Laszig, R., Rube, C. *et al.* (2003). Erythropoietin to treat head and neck cancer patients with anaemia undergoing radiotherapy: Randomised, double-blind, placebo-controlled trial. *Lancet*, **362**, 1255–60.

105. Rockson, S. (2001). Lymphedema. *The American Journal of Medicine*, **110**, 288–95.

106. Browse, N., Burnand, B.K., Mortimer, P.S. (2003). *Diseases of the lymphatics*, Arnold, London, 45–101.

107. Guyton, A.C. and Hall, J. (2000). *Textbook of medical physiology*, 10th edition, Saunders, Philadelphia, 162–4.

108. Ridner, S.H. (2002). Breast cancer lymphedema: Pathophysiology and risk reduction guidelines. *Oncology Nursing Forum*, **29**, 1285–93.

109. Foldi, M., Foldi, E., and Kubik, S. (2003). *Textbook of lymphology for physicians and lymphedema therapists*. Urban & Fischer, Muchen, Germany, 231–319.

110. Bruns, F., Micke, O., and Bremer, M. (2003). Current status of selenium and other treatments for secondary lymphedema. *Journal of Supportive Oncology*, **1**(2), 121–30.

111. Micke, O., Bruns, F., Mucke, R. *et al.* (2003). Selenium in the treatment of radiation-associated secondary lymphedema. *International Journal of Radiation Oncology, Biology, Physics*, **56**(1), 40–9.

112. Fajardo, L.F. (1994). Effects of ionizing radiation on lymph nodes. *Frontiers of Radiation Therapy and Oncology*, **28**, 37–45.

113. Weissleder, H., Schuchhardt C (eds). (2001). *Lymphedema diagnosis and therapy*. Viavital Verlag GmbH, Koln, Germany, 222–6

114. Cheville, A. (2002). Lymphedema and palliative care. National Lymphedema Network, LymphLink, **14**, 1–4 (reprint).

115. Armer, J. and Ridner, S.H. (2005). *Lymphedema, in Palliative and End-of-Life Care: Clinical practice guidelines* (eds. K.K. Kuebler, D.E. Heidrich, P. Espers). Saunders Elsevier: St. Louis, 417–30.

116. Olszewski, W. (1996). Inflammatory changes of skin in lymphedema of extremities and efficacy of benzathine penicillin administration. *National Lymphedema Network LymphLink*, **8**, 1–2.

117. Pandey, M. *et al.* (2007). Distress overlaps with anxiety and depression in patients with head and neck cancer. *Psychooncology*, **16**(6), 582–6.

118. Zabora, J., BrintzenhofeSzoc, K., Curbow, B. *et al.* (2001). The prevalence of psychological distress by cancer site. *Psychooncology*, **10**, 19–28.

119. Haman, K., Murphy, B., and Compas, B. (2005). Social anxiety in head and neck cancer patients. *In American Psychological Oncology Society Annual Meeting*. Pheonix, AZ.

120. Haman, K., S.B., Murphy, B. *et al.* (2006). Predictors of quality of life in head and neck cancer patients, *In American Psychological Oncological Society Annual Meeting*, Amelia Island, FL.

121. Raison, C.L., Capuron, L., and Miller, A.H. (2006). Cytokines sing the blues: inflammation and the pathogenesis of depression. *Trends in Immunology*, **27**, 24–31.

122. Schiepers, O.J.G., W.M., and Maes, M. (2005). Cytokines and major depression. *Progress in Neuro-Psychopharmacology and Biological Psychiatry*, **29**, 201–17.

123. Pitsavos, C. et al. (2006). Anxiety in relation to inflammation and coagulation markers, among healthy adults: the ATTICA study. *Atherosclerosis*, **185**(2), 320–6.

124. Druzgal, C.H., C.Z., Yeh, N.T. et al. (2005). A pilot study of longitudinal serum cytokine and angiogenesis factor levels as markers of therapeutic response and survival in patients with head and neck squamous cell carcinoma. *Head & Neck*, **27**, 771–84.

125. Linkov, F., Lisovich, A., Yurkovetsky, Z. et al. (2007). Early detection of head and neck cancer: development of a novel screening tool using multiplexed immunobead-based biomarker profiling. *Cancer Epidemiology, Biomarkers and Prevention*, **16**(1), 102–7.

126. Gridley, D.S., Bush, D.A., Bonnet, R.B. et al. (2004). Time course of serum cytokines in patients receiving proton or combined photon/proton beam radiation for resectable but medically inoperable non-small-cell lung cancer. *International Journal of Radiation Oncology, Biology, Physics*, **60**(3), 759–66.

127. Pusztai, L., Mendoza, T., Reuben, J.M. et al. (2004). Changes in plasma levels of inflammatory cytokines in response to paclitaxel chemotherapy. *Cytokine*, **25**, 94–102.

128. Kendel, W. (2007). Suicide and cancer: a gender-comparative study. *Annals of Oncology*, **18**(2), 381–7.

129. Sonis, S., Pathobiology of Oral Mucositis: Novel Insights and Opportunities. *Supportive Oncology*, **5**(9), 3–11.

130. Murphy, B. (2007). Clinical and economic consequences of mucositis indiced by chemotherapy and/or radiation therapy. *Supportive Oncology*, **5**(9), 13–21.

131. Isitt, J., Murphy, B., Beaumont, J.L. et al. (2006). Oral mucositis (OM) related morbidity and resource utilization is a prospective study of head and neck cancer (HNC) patients. *Proceedings of American Society for Clinical Oncology*, **24**, abstract 5539, 289.

132. Rosenthal, D. (2007). Consequences of mucositis-induced treatment breaks and dose reductions on head and neck cancer treatment outcomes. *Supportive Oncology*, **5**(9), 23–31.

133. Posner, M., H.R., (2007). Novel agents for the treatment of mucositis. *Supportive Oncology*, **5**(9), 33–9.

134. Bjordal, K. and Kaasa, S. (1995). Psychological distress in head and neck cancer patients 7–11 years after curative treatment. *British Journal of Cancer*, **71**(3), 592–7.

135. McCaffery, M. and Ferrell, B. (1997). Nurses' knowledge of pain assessment and management: How much progress have we made? *Journal of Pain and Symptom Management*, **13**(3), 175–88.

136. Wang, S.G., Lee, U.J., Goh, E.K. et al. (2004). Factors associated with postoperative delirium after major head and neck surgery. *Ann Otol Rhinol Laryngol*, **113**(1), 48–51.

137. Weed, H., Lutman, C.V., Young, D.C. et al. (1995). Preoperative identification of patients at risk for delirium after major head and neck cancer surgery. *Laryngoscope*, **105**, 1066–8.

138. Yamagata, K., Onizawa, K., Yusa, H. et al. (2005). Risk factors for postoperative delirium in patients undergoing head and neck surgery. *International Journal of Oral and Maxillofacial Surgery*, **34**, 33–6.

139. Marcantoni, E.R., Goldman, L., Mangione, C.M. et al. (1994). A clinical prediction rule for delirium after elective noncardiac surgery. *JAMA*, **271**(2), 134–9.

140. Lee, P.W., Hung, B.K.M., Choy, D. et al. (1989). Effects of radiation therapy on neuropsychological functioning in patients with nasopharyngeal carcinoma. *Journal of Neurology, Neurosurgery and Psychiatry*, **52**(4), 488–92.

141. Woo, E., Lam, K., Yu, Y.L. et al. (1988). Temporal lobe and hypothalamic-pituitary dysfunctions after radiotheraphy for nasopharyngeal carcinoma: a distinct clinical syndrome. *Journal of Neurology, Neurosurgery and Psychiatry*, **51**, 1302–7.

142. Meyers, C.A., Geara, F., Wong, P.F. et al. (2000). Neurocognitive effects of therapeutic irradiation for base of skull tumors. *International Journal of Radiation Oncology and Biological Physics*, **46**(1), 51–5.

143. Cheung, M.C., Chan, A.S., Law, S.C. et al. (2000). Cognitive function of patients with nasopharyngeal carcinoma with and without temporal lobe radionecrosis. *Archives of Neurology*, **57**, 1347–52.

144. Lam, L.C.W., Leung, S.F., and Chan, Y.L. (2003). Progress of memory function after radiation therapy in patients with nasopharyngeal carcinoma. *Journal of Neuropsychiatry and Clinical Neurosciences*, **15**(1), 90–7.

145. Abayomi, O. (2002). Pathogenesis of cognitive decline following therapeutic irradiation for head and neck tumors. *Acta Oncologica*, **41**, 346–51.

146. Cheung, M.C., Chan, A.S., Law S.C. et al. (2003). Impact of radionecrosis on cognitive dysfunction in patients after radiotherapy for nasopharyngeal carcinoma. *Cancer*, **97**(8), 2019–26.

147. Jen, Y.M., Hsu, W.L., Chen, C.Y. et al. (2001). Different risks of symptomatic brain necrosis in NPC patients treated with different altered fractionated radiotherapy techniques. *International Journal of Radiation Oncology and Biological Physics*, **51**(2), 344–8.

148. Lee, A.W.M., Kwong, D.L.W., Leung, S.F. et al. (2002). Factors affecting risk of symptomatic temporal lobe necrosis: significance of fractional dose and treatment time. *International Journal of Radiation Oncology and Biological Physics*, **53**(1), 75–85.

149. Teo, P.M., Leung, S.F., Chan, A.T.C. et al. (2000). Final report of a randomized trial on altered-fractionated radiotherapy in nasopharyngeal carcinoma prematurely terminated by significant increase in neurologic complications. *International Journal of Radiation Oncology and Biological Physics*, **48**(5), 1311–22.

150. Dewys, W., Begg, C., Lavin PT. et al.(1980). Prognostic effect of weight loss prior to chemotherapy in cancer patients. *American Journal of Medicine*, **69**, 491–7.

151. Hammerlid, E., Wirblad, B., Sandin, C. et al. (1998). Malnutrition and food in take in relation to quality of life in head and neck cancer patients. *Head and Neck*, **20**, 540–8.

152. Brookes, GB. (1985). Nutritional status—a prognostic indicator in head and neck cancer. *Otolaryngology—Head and Neck Surgery*, **93**, 69–74.

153. Silver, H.J., Wells, N., Arnold, D.J. et al. (2004). Older adults on home enteral nutrition: enteral regimen, provider involvement, and health care outcomes. *Journal of Parenteral and Enteral Nutrition*, (28), 92–8.

154. Beecken, L. and Calaman, F. (1994). A return to "normal eating" after curative treatment for oral cancer. *Eur J Cancer B Oral Oncol*, **30B**, 387–92.

155. Lopez, M.J. et al. (1994). Nutritional support and prognosis in patients with head and neck cancer. *Journal of Surgical Oncology*, **55**, 33–6.

156. van Bokhorst-devan der Schueren, M.A.E., von Blombergi-van der Flier, M.E., Kuik, D.J., et al. (2000). Survival of malnourished head and neck cancer patients can be predicted by human leukocyte antigen-DR expression and interleukin-6/tumor necrosis factor-alpha response of the monocyte. *Journal of Parenteral and Enteral Nutrition*, **24**, 329–36.

157. Tisdale, M. (2000). Metabolic Alterations in Cachexia and Anorexia. *Nutrition*, **16**, 1013–4.

158. Baracos, V. (2000). Regulation of skeletal-muscle-protein turnover in cancer-associated cachexia. *Nutrition*, **16**, 1015–8.

159. Innui, A. (2002). Cancer anorexia-cachexia syndrome: current issues in research and management. *CA: A Cancer Journal for Clinicians*, **52**, 72–91.

160. Plata-Salaman, C. (2000). Central nervous system mechanisms contributing to the cachexia-anorexia syndrome. *Nutrition*, **16**, 1009–12.

161. Selye, H. (1936) A syndrome produced by diverse nocuous agents. *Nature*, **138**, 32.

162. Silver, H.J., D.M., and Murphy BA. (2007). Loss of lean body mass and associated physical function decline in the context of increased energy expenditure and inflammatory state in head and neck cancer patients undergoing concurrent chemo-radiation therapy *Head and Neck*. On Line-Early View.

163. Frazen, L., Funegard, U., Ericson, T. *et al.* (1992). Parotid gland function during and following radiotherapy of malignancies in the head and neck. *British Journal of Cancer*, **28**, 457–62.

164. Cheng, V.S., Downs, J., Herbert, D. *et al.* (1989). The function of the parotid gland following radiation therphy for head and neck cancer. *International Journal of Radiation Oncology and Biological Physics*, **7**(2), 253–8.

165. Mandel, I.D. (1989). The role of saliva in maintaining oral homeostasis. *Journal of American Dental Association*, **119**(2), 298–304.

166. Wolff, A. *et al.* (1990) Pretherapy interventions to modify salivary dysfunction. *NCI Monograph*, **9**, 87–90.

167. Vladez, I.H. *et al.* (1992). Use of pilocarpine during head and neck radiation therapy to reduce xerostomia and salivary dysfunction. *Cancer*, **1993**, 848–51.

168. Johnson, J.T., Ferretti G,A., Nethery, W.J. *et al.* (1993). Oral pilocarpine for post-irradiation xerostomia in patients with head and neck cancer. *New England Journal of Medicine*, **329**, 390–5.

169. LeVequ, F. *et al.* (1996). Salivary gland sheltering using concurrent pilocarpine (PC) in irradiated head and neck cancer patients. *Proc Amer Soc Clin Oncol*, **15**, 1665.

170. Nelson, G.M. (1998). Biology of taste buds and the clinical problem of taste loss. *Anatomical Record* (New Anat), **253**, 70–8.

171. Fujita, M., Hirokawa, Y., and Kashiwado, K. (1996). An analysis of mandibular bone complications in radiotherapy for T1 and T2 carcinoma of the oral tongue. *International Journal of Radiation Oncology and Biological Physics*, **34**(2), 333–9.

172. Beumer, J., Curtis, T., and Morrish, R. (1976). Radiation Complications in edentulous patients. *Journal of Prosthetic Dentistry*, **36**, 193–302.

173. Wang, C. (1972). Management and prognosis of squamous cell carcinoma of the tonsillar region. *Radiology*, **104**, 667–71.

174. Murray, C., Herson, J., and Daly, T. (1980). Radiation necrosis of the mandible: a 10-year study, part 1. Factors influencing the onset of necrosis. *International Journal of Radiation Oncology and Biological Physics*, **6**, 543–8.

175. Larson, D., Lindberg, R., and Lane, E. (1983). Major complications of radiotherapy in cancer of the oral cavity and oropharynx. *American Journal of Surgery*, **146**, 531–6.

176. Emami, B., Bignardi, M., Spector, G.J. *et al.* (1987). Reirradiation of recurrent head and neck cancers. *Laryngoscope*. 85–8.

177. Withers, H. Peter, L., and Taylor, J. (1995). Late normal tissue sequelae from radiation therapy for carcinoma of the tonsil: patterns of fractionation study of radiobiology. *International Journal of Radiation Oncology and Biological Physics*, **33**, 563–8.

178. Silverman, S.J. (1999). Current concepts in the management of oral/dental adverse sequelae of head and neck radiotherapy. Radition Injury—advances in management and prevention, In (eds. J. Meyers, and J. Vaeth) Vol. 32, Karger.

179. Grond, S. (1993). Validation of world health organization guidelines for pain relief in head and neck cancer. *Ann Otto Rhino Laryngol*, **102**, 342–8.

180. Boerman,R. *et al.* (1999). Trigeminal neuropathy secondary to perineural invasion of head and neck carcinomas. *Neurology*, **53**, 213–6.

181. Trumpy, I.G., and Lyberg, T. (1993). Temporomandibular joint dysfunction and facial pain caused by neoplasms. *Oral Surgery, Oral Medicine, Oral Pathology, Oral Radiology and Endodontics*, **76**, 149–52.

182. Cohen, S.G. and Quinn, P.D. (1988). Facila trismus and myofacial pain associated with infections and malignant disease. *Oral Surg Oral Med Oral Path*, **65**, 538–44.

183. Bullitt, E., Tew, J., and Boyd, J. (1986). Intracranial tumors in patients with facial pain. *Journal of Neurosurgery*, **64**, 865–71.

184. Huntley, T. and Wiesenfeld, D. (1994). Delayed diagnosis of the cause of facial pain in patients with neoplastic disease: a report of eight cases. *Journal of Oral and Maxillofacial Surgery*, **52**, 81–5.

185. Gouda, J.J. and Brown, J.A. (1997). Atypical facial pain and other pain syndromes. *Neurosurgery Clinics of North America*, **8**(1), 87–100.

186. Donlon, W.C. and Jacobson, A.L. (1984). Maxillofacial Pain. *AFP*, **30**, 151–63.

187. Thaller, S. and Thaller, J. (1990). Head and Neck Symptoms Is the problem in the ears, face, neck, or oral cavity? *Postgraduate Medical Journal*, **87**, 75–86.

188. Carr, D., Jacox, A., and Chapman, C. (1992). Acute pain management: Operative or medical procedures and trauma. Clinical Practice Guideline No. 1. Agency for Health Care Policy and Research Pub. No. 92-0032. Rockville, MD, Agency for Health Care Policy and Research, Public Health Service, US Department of Health and Human Services.

189. Chaplin, J.M. and Morton, R.P. (1999). A prospective, longitudinal study of pain in head and neck cancer patients. *Head and Neck*, **21**, 531–7.

190. Butler, J.D. and Miles, J. (1998). Dysaesthetic neck pain with syncope. *Pain*, **75**, p. 395–7.

191. Short, S.O., Kaplan, J.N., Laramore, G.E. *et al.* (1984). Shoulder Pain and function after neck dissection with or without preservation of the spinal accessory nerve. *American Journal of Surgery*, **148**, 478–82.

192. Barrett, N.V.J., Martin, J.W., Jacob, R.F. *et al.* (1988). Physical therapy techniques in the treatment of the head and neck patient. *Journal of Prosthetic Dentistry*, **59**, 343–6.

193. Jannjan, N., Weissman, D., and Pahule, A. (1992). Improved pain management with daily nursing intervention during radiation therapy for head and neck carcinoma. *International Journal of Radiation Oncology and Biological Physics*, **23**, 647–52.

194. Epstein, J.B. and Stewart, K.H. (1993). Radiation therapy and pain in patients with head and neck cancer. *European Journal of Cancer. Part B, Oral Oncology*, **29b**, 191–3.

195. Smit, M. *et al.* (2001). Pain as sign of recurrent disease in head and neck squamous cell carcinoma. *Head and Neck*, **23**, 372–5.

196. Mutrie, N., Campbell, A.M., Whyte, F. *et al.* (2007). Benefits of supervised group exercise programme for women being treated for early stage breast cancer: pragmatic randomised controlled trial. *BMJ*, **334**(7592), 517.

197. Institute of Medicine Report: From Cancer patient to cancer survivor: lost in translation. (2006). National Academies Press, Washington, DC.

198. Nahum, A.M., Mullally, W., and Marmor, L. (1961). A syndrome resulting from radical neck dissection. *Archives of Otolaryngology*, **74**, 424–8.

199. Demark-Wahnefried, W. *et al.* (2005). Riding the crest of the teachable moment: promoting long-term health after the diagnosis of cancer. *Journal of Clinical Oncology*, **23**(24), 5814–30.

200. Courneya, K., Mackey, J.R., and McKenzie, D.C. (2002). Exercise for breast cancer survivors: Research evidence and clinical guidelines. *Phys Sports med*, **30**, 33–42.

201. Guldiken, Y., Onizawa, K., Demirel, T. *et al.* (2005). Assessment of shoulder impairment after functional neck dissection: Long term results. *Auris Nasus larynx*, **32**, 387–91.

202. Choy, N.L., Johnson, N., Treleaven, J. *et al.* (2006). Balance, mobility and gaze stability deficits remain following surgical

removal of vestibular schwannoma (acoustic neuroma): an observational study. *Australian Journal of Physiotherapy*, **52**(3), 211–6.

203. Cappiello, J., Piazza, C., Giudice, M. *et al.* (2005). Shoulder disability after different selective neck dissections (level II–IV versus levels II–V): A Comparative Study. *The Laryngoscope*, **115**, 259–63.

204. Herdman, S.J., Clendaniel, R., Mattox, D.E. *et al.* (1995). Vestibular adaptation exercises and recovery: acute stage after acoustic neuroma resection. *Otolaryngol Head Neck Surg*, **113**(1), 77–87.

205. Enticott, J.C., O'Leary, S., and Briggs, R.J. (2005). Effects of vestibulo-ocular reflex exercises on vestibular compensation after vestibular schwannoma surgery. *Otol Neurotol*, **26**(2), 265–9.

206. Patten, C., H.F., and Krebs DE. (2003). Head and body center of gravity control strategies: adaptations following vestibular rehabilitation. *Acta Otolaryngol*, **123**(1), 32–40.

207. Neiman, D.C. and C.K. (2005). Immunological conditions. In *ACSM resource manual for guidelines for exercise testing and prescription* (eds. B.K. Kaminsky, L.A., Garber, C.E, Glass *et al.*), pp. 528–42, ACSM.

208. Piazza, C., Cappiello, J., and Nicolai, P. (2002). Sternoclavicular joint hypertrophy following neck dissection and upper trapezius myocutaneous flap transposition. *Otolaryngology—Head And Neck Surgery*, **126**, 193–4.

209. McQuade, K.J., Dawson, J., and Smidt, G.L. (1998). Scapulothoracic muscle fatigue associated with alterations in scapulohumeral rhythm kinematics during maximum resistive shoulder elevation. *Journal of Orthopaedic And Sports Physical Therapy*, **28**(2), 74–80.

210. Patten, C. and Hillel, A. (1993). The 11th nerve syndrome. Accessory nerve palsy or adhesive capsulitis? *Archives of Otolaryngology—Head and Neck Surgery*, **119**(2), 215–20.

211. Dijkstra, P.U., Kalk, W., and Roodenburg, J.L.N. (2004). Trismus in head and neck oncology: a systematic review. *Oral Oncology*, **40**, 879–89.

212. Wong, R.K., Jones, G., Sagar, S.M. *et al.* (2003). A Phase I–II study in the use of acupuncture-like transcutaneous nerve stimulation in the treatment of radiation-induced xerostomia in head-and-neck cancer patients treated with radical radiotherapy. *International Journal of Radiation Oncology and Biological Physics*, **57**(2), 472–80.

213. Dijkstra, P.U., Sterken, M., Pater, R. *et al.* (2007). Exercise therapy for trismus in head and neck cancer. *Oral Oncology*, **43**, 389–94.

214. Cohen, E.G., Deschler, D., Walsh, K. *et al.* (2005). Early use of a mechanical stretching device to improve mandibular mobility after composite resection: a pilot study. *Archives of Physical Medicine and Rehabilitation*, **86**(7), 1416–9.

215. Grandi, G., S.M., Steit, C., and Wagner, J.C.B. (2007). A mobilization regimen to prevent mandibular hypomobility in irradiated patients: an analysis and comparison of two techniques. *Medicina Oral, Patología Oral y Cirugía Bucal*, **12**, E105–E109.

216. Doyle, C., K.L., Byers, T., Courtneya, K.S. *et al.* (2006). Nutrition and physical activity during and after cancer treatment: an American Cancer Society guide for informed choices. *Cancer J. Clin*, **56**(6), 323–53.

217. Courneya, K.S., Mackey, J., and Jones, L.W. (2000). Coping with cancer: Can exercises help? *Phys Sports med*, **28**, 49–73.

218. Dozza, M., C.L., and Horak FB. (1995). Audio-feedback improves balance in patients with bilateral vestibular loss. *Archives of Physical Medicine and Rehabilitation*, **86**(7), 1401–3.

219. Endicott, J.C., O.L.S., and Briggs, R.J. (2005). Effects of vestibulo-ocular reflex exercises on vestibular compensation after vestibular schwannoma surgery. *Otology & Neurotology*, **26**(2), 265–9.

220. Mustoe, T.A., Cooter, R.D., Gold, M.H. *et al.* (2002). International Advisory Panel on Scar Management. International clinical recommendations on scar management. *Plastic and Reconstructive Surgery*, **110**(2), 560–71.

221. Edwards, J. (2003). Scar management. *Nursing Standard*, **17**(520), 39–42.

222. Marunick, M., Seyedsadr, M., Ahmad, K. *et al.* (1991). The effect of head and neck cancer treatment on whole salivary flow. *Journal of Surgical Oncology*, **48**, 81–6.

223. Halyard, M.Y., J.A., Sloan, J.A. *et al.* (2007). Does zinc sulfate prevent radiation-induced taste alterations ("Dysgeusia") in head and neck cancer patients? A North Central Cancer Treatment Group (NCCTG) placebo-controlled trial (N01C4). *Proceedings Multidisciplinary Head and Neck Cancer Symposium*, **111**, abstract 32.

224. Brosky, M.E. (2007). The role of saliva in oral health: strategies for prevention and management of xerostomia. *Journal of Supportive Oncology*, **5**(5), 215–25.

225. Chambers, M.S., G.A., Kies, M.S., and Martin, J.W. (2007). Radiation-induced xerostomia in patients with head and neck cancer: pathogenesis, impact on quality of life, and management. *Head and Neck*, **26**, 796–2004.

226. Rhodus, N.L., Moller, K., Colby, S. *et al.* (1995). Articulatory speech performance in patients with salivary galnd dysfunction: a pilot study. *Quintessence International*, **26**, 805–810.

227. Roh, J.L., K.A., and Cho MJ. (2005). Xerostomia following radiotherapy of the head and neck affects vocal function. *Journal of Clinical Oncology*, **13**, 3016–23.

229. Wong, W.W., Mick, R., Haraf, D.J., *et al.* (1994). Time-dose relationship for local tumor control following alternate week concomitant radiation and chemotherapy of advanced head and neck cancer. *International Journal of Radiation Oncology and Biological Physics*, **29**, 153–62.

230. Scarantino, C., LeVeque, F., Swann, R.S. *et al.* (2006). Effect of pilocarpine during radiation therapy: results of RTOG 97-09, a phase III randomized study in head and neck cancer patients. *Journal of Supportive Oncology*, **4**(5), 252–8.

231. Fife, R.S., Chase, W., Dore, R.K. *et al.* (2002). Cevimeline for the treatment of xerostomia in patients with Sjorgren syndrome: a randomized trial. *Achieves Internal Medicine*, **162**(11), 45–52.

232. Chambers, M.S., Jones, C.U., Biel, M.A. *et al.* (2007). Open-label, long-term safety study of cevimeline in the treatment of postirradiation xerostomia. *International Journal of Radiation Oncology and Biological Physics*, **69**, 1369–76.

233. Chambers, M., Posner, M., Jones, C.U. *et al.* (2007). Cevimeline for the treatment of postirradiation xerostomia in patients with head and neck cancer. *International Journal of Radiation Oncology and Biological Physics*, **68**(4), 1102–9.

234. Bardet, E., Martin, L., Calais, G. *et al.* (2005). Subcutaneous versus intravenous administration of amifostine for head and neck cancer patients receiving radiotherapy: preliminary results of the GORTEC 2000-02 randomized trial. *International Journal of Radiation Oncology and Biological Physics*, **63**(2), S127.

235. Seikaly, H., Jha, N., Harris, J.R. *et al.* (2004). Long-term outcomes of submandibular gland transfer for prevention of postradiation xerostomia. *Archives of Otolaryngology*, **130**(8), 956–61.

236. Henson, B.S., Inglehart, M., Eisbruch, A. *et al.* (2001). Preserved salivary output and xerostomia-related quality-of-life in head and neck cancer patients receiving parotid-sparing radiotherapy. *Oral Oncology*, **1**, 84–93.

237. Lin, A., Kim, H., Terrell, J.E. *et al.* (2003). Quality of life after parotid-sparing IMRT for head and neck cancer: A prospective longitudinal study. *International Journal of Radiation Oncology and Biological Physics*, **57**(12), 61–70.

238. Saarilahti, K., Kouri, M., Collan, J. *et al.* (2006). Sparing of the submandibular glands by intensity modulated radiotherapy in the treatment of head and neck cancer. *Radiotherapy and Oncology*, **78**(3), 270–5.

239. Pacholke, H.D., Amdur, R.J., Morris, C.G. *et al.* (2005). Late xerostomia after intensity-modulated radiation therapy versus

conventional radiotherapy. *American Journal of Clinical Oncology*, **28**(4), 351–8.

240. Chao, K.S., Majhail, N., Huang, C.J. *et al.* (2001). Intensity-modulated radiation therapy reduces late salivary toxicity without compromising tumor control in patients with oropharyngeal carcinoma: a comparison with conventional techniques. *Radiotherapy and Oncology*, **61**(3), 275–80.

241. Marks, J.E., Freeman, R.B., Lee, F. *et al.* (1978). Pharyngeal wall cancer: an analysis of treatment results complications and patterns of failure. *International Journal of Radiation Oncology and Biological Physics*, **4**(7–8), 587–93.

242. Gall, A.M., Sessions, D.G., Ogura, J.H. (1977). Complications following surgery for cancer of the larynx and hypopharynx. *Cancer*, **39**(2),624–31.

243. Downey, R.J., Friedlander, P., Groeger, J. *et al.* (1999). Criitcal care for the severely ill head and neck patient. *Critical Care Medicine*, **27**(1), 95–7.

244. Lam, H.C., Abdullah, V.J., Wormald, P.J. *et al.* (2001). Internal carotid artery hemorrhage after irradiation and osteoradionecrosis of the skull base. *Otolaryngology—Head and Neck Surgery*, **125**(5), 522–7.

245. Citardi, M.J., Chaloupka, J.C., Son, Y.H. *et al.* (1995). Management of carotid artery rupture by monitored endovascular therapeutic occlusion (1988–1994). *Laryngoscope*, **105**(10), 1086–92

246. Newman, L.A. *et al.,* (1998). Eating and weight changes following chemoradiation therapy for advanced head and neck cancer. *Arch Otolaryngol Head Neck Surg,* **124**, 589–592.

247. Tyldesley, S. et al., (1996). The use of radiologically placed gastrostomy tubes in head and neck cancer patients receiving radiotherapy. *Int J Radiation Onolocy Biol Phys*, **36**(5), 1205–1209.

248. Silver, H.J., Wellman, N.S., Arnold, D.J., Livingstone, A.S., Byers, P.M, (2004). Older adults on home enteral nutrition: enteral regimen, provider involvement, and health care outcomes. *J Parenter Enteral Nutr*, (28), 92–98.

249. Freidman, R., (1990). Osteoradionecrosis: causes and preention. *NCI Monogr*, **9**, 145–149.

250. Futran, N.D., A. Trotti, and C. Gwede, (1997). Pentoxifylline in the treatment of radiation-related soft tissue injury: preliminary observations. *Laryngoscope*, **107**(3), 391–5.

251. Mainous, E. and G. Hart, (1975). Osteoradionecrosis of the mandible. *Arch Otolaryngol Head Neck Surg*, **101**, 173–177.

252. Aitasalo, K. *et al.*, (1983). A modified protocol for early treatment of osteomyelitis and osteoradionecrosis of the mandible. *Head Neck*, **20**, 411–417.

253. Marx, R.E. Johnson, R.P., Kline, S.N, (1985). Prevention of osteoradionecrosis: a randomized prospective clinical trial of hyperbaric oxygen versus penicillin. *J Am Dent Assoc*, **111**(1), 49–54.

11.3

Primary brain tumours

Claudia Bausewein, Gian Domenico Borasio, and Raymond Voltz

Introduction

Patients with primary brain tumours comprise about 2 per cent of all new cases of cancer[1]. The age-adjusted incidence rate is currently about 6–11 new cases/100.000 population per year in men and 4–11 new cases in women[2]. Primary brain tumours comprise several histological entities, from more benign forms such as ependymomas to very malignant tumours with a poor prognosis such as glioblastoma multi-forme (GBM) (Table 11.3.1)[3]. Some tumours, e.g. astrocytomas, may progress over time from less to more malignant forms.

Depending on the histology of the brain tumour, different disease-modifying therapeutic options exist: most patients undergo surgery, radiotherapy, chemotherapy, or a combination of these treatments, but the chances of cure are very low[4,5]. The average life expectancy of a patient with GBM lies between several weeks and several months after postoperative radiotherapy[4]. Only few patients survive 2 years. Most supposed long-term survivors of GBM had a wrong histological diagnosis[6].

In most countries, patients with malignant brain tumours are usually seen by neurologists and neurosurgeons who are not familiar with basic medical, legal, and ethical issues in palliative care[7]. Given the lack of curative treatments and the short life expectancy of most patients, good palliative care is essential starting from the time of diagnosis.

Communication

Patients and families should be informed early in the course of the disease that the tumour—depending on its localization—will most probably lead to cognitive impairment, with the consequence of limitations in decision-making and legal capacity. Information about prognosis should be tailored to coping styles of individual patients and their relatives[8]. In most patients, communication becomes progressively difficult during the course of the disease because of dysphasia, confusion, or somnolence. Therefore, anticipation regarding end-of-life issues such as tube feedings, life-sustaining treatments, resuscitation or discontinuation of steroids is essential, and the patients should be encouraged to formulate an advance directive and name a health-care proxy[9–11].

Caring for patients and relatives

Psychosocial issues play a major role in care of patients with brain tumour. The patients not only have to face their life-threatening disease but also the possibility of future change in personality, cognitive impairment, and functional decline. Emotional reactions of patients with brain tumours comprise a variety of feelings, including shock, anxiety, despair, anger, fear, and sadness[12]. At the time of diagnosis, most patients with malignant glioma seem unaware or only partly aware of their poor prognosis, while their relatives appear more aware and more distressed[8,13]. Patients with brain tumour seldom seem to reach a state of acceptance of the disease, possibly due to progressive cognitive dysfunction[12].

The psychological burden for relatives becomes higher during the course of the disease. The relatives feel progressively estranged from the patient and often experience the social death of the patient long before the actual death. Therefore, the family members need special attention, counselling, and care from the interdisciplinary team, and they should be involved in medical decisions and care from the beginning.

Organization of care

Patients with primary brain tumours are diagnosed in most cases by a neurologist, and then handed over to neurosurgeons and radiotherapists for tumour-specific treatment. As the disease progresses, however, these specialities may be withdrawn and the patient may be returned to the care of a neurologist, sometimes to receive chemotherapy. In areas where palliative care is available, there is a frequent misconception that patients with brain tumour have no treatable symptoms and that their life expectancy is too long for a hospice or palliative care unit[14]. This perspective is unfortunate. Patients with brain tumours and their families have multi-dimensional problems, which may benefit from early involvement of a multi-professional and interdisciplinary team, including physiotherapy, occupational therapy, and speech therapy. This effort may be coordinated by the general practitioner, with the support of the neurologist or the palliative care specialist[15].

Symptom control

The disease-related symptoms experienced by patients with brain tumours usually are caused either by raised intracranial pressure or by direct impingement of the tumour on brain structures. Concurrent and interrelated causes of raised intracranial pressure include the expanding tumour mass, cerebral oedema, and impaired absorption of cerebrospinal fluid.

Headache

About 60 per cent of the patients with brain tumour experience headaches during the course of their disease, 20 per cent in the

Table 11.3.1 Histological types and prognosis of primary brain tumours.

		Incidence	Relative survival rates (per cent)		
			1 year	**2 years**	**5 years**
Astrocytic tumours	Pilocytic astrocytoma WHO I	10 per cent of cerebral astrocytomas most common in children	95.7	94.3	91.3
	Diffuse astrocytomas WHO II	10–15 per cent of astrocytic tumours	73.9	61.8	46.9
	Anaplastic astrocytomas WHO III		60.3	44.0	29.4
	Glioblastoma multi-forme WHO IV	50–60 per cent of astrocytomas 12–15 per cent of all intracranial neoplasms	29.3	8.7	3.3
Oligodendroglial tumours	Oligodendroglioma WHO II		89.7	83.4	70.5
Ependymal tumours	Ependymoma/anaplastic ependymoma		87.6	81.4	70.6

Source: Modified from CBTRUS, 2005[3].

initial stages. Only a small group experiences the 'classic' brain tumour headache, which is more severe on awakening, eases off after arising, and may be associated with nausea and vomiting. Most patients complain of a dull generalized headache similar to tension headache, while a small group describes their headache like a migraine. Headaches are caused by traction on pain-sensitive structures, such as meninges, cranial nerves, and venous sinuses due to raised intracranial pressure. They often correlate with the degree of raised intracranial pressure, cerebral oedema, or shift of midline structures, but not with the size of the tumour mass itself[16]. A strong pain with acute onset might indicate a quick raise of intracranial pressure, e.g. due to tumour haemorrhage.

Steroids are very important drugs in symptom management of patients with brain tumours. They reduce the raised intracranial pressure by reducing vasogenic peritumoural oedema. The effect of steroids on headache, reduced consciousness, nausea and vomiting, and neurological deficits is often dramatic, occurring within days. Depending on the extent and tempo of the disease, these benefits may not be long lasting. This needs to be explained in advance to patients and relatives, together with the fact that steroids have no influence on tumour progression. There are no clear guidelines regarding dose, type of steroid, or duration of treatment. In a randomized controlled trial in patients with brain tumours, doses of 4 mg dexamethasone per day were as effective as 16 mg/day, but caused fewer side effects[17]. Prescription and dosage of steroids should be reviewed regularly. Many patients are given doses of steroids that are unnecessarily high, predisposing them to severe side effects, including Cushing's syndrome, psychosis, and myopathy. In the case of acutely raised intracranial pressure, treatment may be started with relatively high doses (dexamethasone 16–24 mg/day), given in the morning as a single dose—the biological half-life of dexamethasone is 36–72 h—and not in the evening to reduce the risk of sleep disturbances. The dosage should be tapered after symptom control has been achieved to the lowest effective dose, which is often as low as 2 mg/day. Alternatively, extract from *Boswellia serrata* (H15, 1200–3600 mg/day) can be used or combined with steroids to reduce oedema. Based on clinical observation, about half of the patients report a positive effect and the main side effects observed are nausea and vomiting[18].

In addition to the usual and well-recognized side effects from steroid drugs, the risk of drug–drug interactions must be noted. For example, the concomitant use of anti-convulsants, such as phenytoin, may decrease the blood levels of dexamethasone by as much as two-thirds[19].

If headache worsens with progression of the disease, titration of the steroid dose can be tried as an analgesic strategy. Daily doses can become quite high at the end of life, as repeated dose increments are undertaken with each episode of worsening headache. If steroids alone are not sufficient, analgesic therapy also should be employed. Opioids are the mainstay and typically are administered as recommended in the World Health Organization's 'analgesic ladder' approach. There is no reason to withhold opioids in patients with brain tumours. Cognitive impairment in more advanced stages makes pain assessment difficult. Physical signs such as rubbing of the head or moaning may be taken as indication for headache[9].

Dysphagia

Patients with primary brain tumours may develop dysphagia as a consequence of cranial nerve or bulbar palsy. In contrast to dysphagia due to obstruction, it is easier for patients with neurogenic dysphagia to swallow solids than fluids. Aspiration and malnutrition are the main complications of dysphagia. If appropriate given the status of disease, and the patient's wishes, placement of a feeding tube via percutaneous endoscopic gastrostomy may address these complications.

Cognitive and behavioural dysfunction

Patients with brain tumours develop cognitive dysfunction much earlier than other patients with terminal illness. Fluctuation of these symptoms is common. The patients present with a variety of symptoms, ranging from attention deficit to personality changes and psychiatric problems. The most common types of cognitive dysfunction are summarized in Table 11.3.2. Brain imaging and laboratory tests may be necessary to differentiate among the varied causes and assess the potential for reversibility with treatment. Anti-epileptic drugs should be considered as a common cause of cognitive changes[9]. Risperidone, a new class neuroleptic with serotonin ($5 HT_2$) and dopamine (D_2) antagonist properties, seems to be more effective than haloperidol when the patient is aggressive, agitated, or confused[20].

Table 11.3.2 Types and causes of cognitive and behavioural dysfunction in patients with brain tumour.

Type	Description	Anatomical localization	Treatment
Anosognosia	Inability to accept the reality of one's illness	Posterior parietal non-dominant hemisphere	Acceptance and explanation to the relatives
Aphasia	Difficulty in speaking and/or understanding (see Table 11.3.3)	Dominant (usually left) parieto-temporal hemisphere	Logopaedic therapy (if slow course)
Apraxia	Inability to plan and perform complex movements	Parietal lobes	Occupational therapy to improve activities of daily living
Neglect	Loss of interest in one side of the body	Non-dominant (usually right) parietal hemisphere	Occupational therapy, neuropsychological training (of limited value if rapid progression)
Memory loss	Short-term memory is usually affected first	Hippocampus, temporal lobes	As above
Attention deficit	Insidious onset, fluctuations	Fronto-parietal lobes	As above
Apathy	May be so severe as to simulate unconsciousness	Frontal lobes	As above
Affective disinhibition	Loss of distance, inadequate emotional expression	Frontal lobes	Psychosocial adjustment, explanation to the family
Personality change	May range from apathy to aggression; very troublesome for relatives; often presenting symptom	Variable	Psychosocial adjustment, explanation to the family
Psychosis	May present with hallucinations and/or paranoid ideas	Variable; consider steroid-induced psychosis	Neuroleptics; beware of lowered seizure threshold!
Depression	May mimic cognitive dysfunction (pseudodementia)	N/A	Psychotherapy (consider family therapy), antidepressants
Delirium	May be hypo- or hyperactive	Generalized, often metabolic or drug-induced	Causal treatment if possible (see Chapter 10.11)

Speech and language problems

Disturbed speech and language are important symptoms in patients with brain tumours. About one-third of patients with high-grade gliomas have speech deficits at first presentation, requiring early access to speech therapy[21]. One must distinguish between dysphasia (Table 11.3.3), a loss of production or comprehension of spoken and/or written language (cortical dysfunction), and dysarthria (Table 11.3.4), a disturbance in articulation (dysfunction of brainstem, cranial nerves, or muscles). Comprehension of dysphasic patients is normally worse than anticipated. Questions should be asked slowly and clearly. It is important to develop a yes/no code or to find alternative strategies like pointing, writing, or painting. Patients with fluent dysphasia should be taught to slow their speech and those with hesitant speaking should be encouraged to speak nonetheless. Patience, time, and empathy are necessary to maintain communication. In patients with severe dysarthria, communication boards or electronic aids might be helpful.

Seizures

Seizures are a frequent problem in patients with brain tumours. In about 20 per cent of supratentorial brain tumours, a presenting seizure leads to the diagnosis, and about 70 per cent of the patients will experience seizures during the course of their illness[22]. Seizures must be differentiated from other forms of involuntary movements, such as myoclonus (e.g. with opioid therapy), drug-induced hyperkinesias (e.g. with haloperidol), or movement patterns related to terminal elevation of intracranial pressure.

Seizure phenomenology should be described in detail, as this approach localizes the epileptogenic regions of the cortex best. During the seizure, care must be taken that the patient does not get hurt. A single generalized tonic–clonic seizure, which usually lasts around 3–5 min, requires no acute anti-convulsant therapy. However, status epilepticus, a seizure that persists more than 5 min or repeated seizures without return of consciousness between, warrants aggressive therapy because of its high mortality rate.

Prophylactic anti-convulsant therapy is not recommended in newly diagnosed brain tumours as it does not provide substantial benefit and is associated with a higher incidence of side effects[23]. However, long-term prophylaxis is necessary after a first seizure has occurred. Choosing the right drug depends on several considerations:

- *Time factor:* if a rapid onset of effect is needed, clobazam or diazepam (also available as rectal formulation) may be best. Therapeutic valproate or phenytoin levels are reached within a short time, as both are available as intravenous preparations and can be administered in a regimen that includes a loading dose. With drugs which are available only orally, loading regimens usually are not tolerated and it may take several days before therapeutic levels are reached.

- *Drug interactions:* anti-convulsants such as phenytoin and carbamazepine may lower serum levels of other medications, such as steroids or chemotherapy, and vice versa. This may be counteracted by increasing the doses of the medication. However, the danger of reaching toxic levels exists, especially with phenytoin, as this drug has non-linear pharmacokinetics. Drug toxicity from anti-convulsants may mimic tumour symptoms such as ataxia,

Table 11.3.3 Dysphasia.

	Comprehension	Speaking	Reading/writing
Global dysphasia	Disturbed	Repetition of syllables instead of words	Totally disturbed
Wernicke's dysphasia	Disturbed	Non-sensical but fluent disfigurement of words	Similar to comprehension and speaking
Broca's dysphasia	Good	Hesitant, telegraphic style, grammar disturbed	Similar to comprehension and speaking
Amnestic dysphasia	Hardly disturbed	Difficulty in wording, correct construction of sentences	Hardly disturbed

double vision, or gait disturbance. Valproate and the newer anti-convulsants, such as levetiracetam, do not interact with other medications to the same extent as phenytoin[24,25]; these drugs may be preferred for this reason.

- *Efficacy and side effects:* anti-convulsant drug doses should be increased until no more seizures occur, or side effects appear. Here, the upper limit of drug levels is of less clinical value than commonly believed. Sometimes, patients have side effects long before this 'upper limit' is reached; others have no side effects even above it. The patient's response, and not the serum level, should guide treatment. Carbamazepine may be switched to oxcarbazepine on a milligram to milligram basis if side effects occur with carbamazepine treatment; oxcarbazepine may be increased as this generally is less toxic[24,25]. Carbamazepine may have an adverse effect on late radiation toxicity[26]. Another severe side effect, especially relevant for patients with brain tumour, is the so-called Stevens–Johnson syndrome (potentially lethal multi-form exudating erythema) in patients receiving phenytoin, and sometimes carbamazepine, who have received cranial irradiation and are on decreasing doses of steroids[27,28].

- *Route of administration:* once patients are no longer able to swallow, a parenteral route of application must be considered. Pheny-toin, valproate, and levetiracetam are available as IV preparations. Alternatively, lorazepam can be given sublingually (0.5–1.0 mg thrice per day) or clonazepam can be given subcutaneously (e.g. 0.5 mg thrice per day or by continuous subcutaneous infusion).

Venous thromboembolism

Compared with other malignancies patients with brain tumours have a higher risk for venous thromboembolism, such as deep

Table 11.3.4 Dysarthria.

Type of dysarthria	Localization	Clinical feature
Cortical	Motor cortex, descending motor pathway	Reduced articulation, often combined with dysphasia
Suprabulbar corticobulbar	Descending motor pathways	'Staccato'-speech
Extrapyramidal system	Basal ganglia	Low voice, stuttering
Cerebellar	Cerebellum	Scanning speech (abnormal separation of syllables)
Bulbar	Brainstem	Hollow, unarticulated

venous thrombosis or pulmonary embolism[29]. Anti-coagulation is recommended in these patients, both prophylactically (when mobility is reduced) and when patients are symptomatic[30]. Both for primary and secondary prevention, low molecular weight heparin seems to be effective and safe[31].

Mobility problems

In patients with brain tumours, mobility may be impaired due to hemiplegia, increasing weakness or obesity after long-term treatment with steroids. Problems with coordination may evolve from ataxia. Steroid myopathy affecting proximal muscles of legs and arms occurs often, and may develop after short-term treatment. Patients then find it difficult to get up from a chair or climb steps.

Any little gain in mobility decreases the need for care and increases the independence of the patient. If mobility can be improved, the patient might be able to stay longer at home and the burden for the relatives can be reduced. Physiotherapy and occupational therapy should be organized early on and adapted to the patient's actual situation, abilities, and skills.

Specific issues in the terminal phase

Little is known about the terminal phase of patients with brain tumours. In a retrospective study, the main symptoms during the last 72 h of life were somnolence (84 per cent), pain (33 per cent), death rattle (18 per cent), seizures (9 per cent), and restlessness (9 per cent)[32]. In this series, a peaceful death was observed in 85 per cent of the patients. Reasons for a non-peaceful death were uncontrolled symptoms, such as pain or dyspnoea, or seizures.

With increasing weakness, dysphagia, or deteriorating consciousness, the patient will be unable to take medication orally. Therefore, alternative routes of drug administration, such as transdermal, rectal or subcutaneous, are necessary for symptom control and should be planned in advance of the terminal phase.

Most patients with brain tumour receive long-term steroid therapy. When their condition deteriorates, it has to be decided whether to increase the dose or to discontinue the treatment. A raise in steroid dose should be limited to 5–7 days if possible. If no effect is seen within that time, they should be reduced again. In dying patients who cannot take oral medication, continuation of steroids might prolong the dying phase, while discontinuation might lead to exacerbation of cerebral oedema (unlikely if the fluid intake is reduced) and to adrenal insufficiency (unlikely to result in significant suffering). Thus, parenteral continuation of steroids in the dying phase is rarely appropriate or necessary. If steroids are discontinued, intensified symptom monitoring is required, as increasing analgesic, anti-emetic and anti-convulsant medication may be necessary.

References

1. Prados, M.D. and Levin, V. (2000). Biology and treatment of malignant glioma, *Seminars in Oncology*, **27**(3), Suppl **6**, 1–10.

2. Ohgaki, H. and Kleihues, P. (2005). Epidemiology and etiology of gliomas. *Acta Neuropathologica*, **109**, 93–108.

3. CBTRUS (2005). *Statistical Report: Primary Brain Tumors in the United States, 1998-2002*. Published by the Central Brain Tumor Registry of the United States. www.cbtrus.org

4. Davis, F.G., Freels, S., Grutsch, J. *et al.* (1998). Survival rates in patients with primary malignant brain tumours stratified by patients age and tumour histological type: an analysis based on Surveillance, Epidemiology and End Results (SEER) data, 1973–1991. *Journal of Neurosurgery*, **88**(1), 1–10.

5. Blomgren, H. Brain tumours (1996), *Acta Oncologica*, **35**(Suppl 7), 16–21.

6. Stupp, R., Mason, W.P., van den Bent, M.J. *et al.* (2005). European Organisation for Research and Treatment of Cancer Brain Tumor and Radiotherapy Groups; National Cancer Institute of Canada Clinical Trials Group. Radiotherapy plus concomitant and adjuvant temozolomide for glioblastoma. *New England Journal of Medicine*, **352**(10), 987–96.

7. Morita, M., Rosenblum, M.K., Bilsky, M.H. *et al.* (1996). Long-term survivors of glioblastoma multiforme: clinical and molecular characteristics. *Journal of Neuro-Oncology*, **27**(3), 259–66.

8. Carver, A.C., Vickrey, B.G., and Bernat, J.L. (1999). End-of-life-care: A survey of US neurologists' attitudes, behaviour and knowledge. *Neurology*, **53**, 284–93.

9. Davies, E. and Higginson, I.J. (2003). Communication, information and support for adults with malignant cerebral glioma: a systematic literature review. *Support Cancer Care*, **11**, 21–9.

10. Peterson, K. (2001). Brain tumours, In *Neurologic Clinics: Palliative Care* (Eds. A. Carver, and K.M. Foley), Vol. 19, No. 4, pp. 887–902, WB Saunders Philadelphia.

11. Taillibert, S., Laigle-Donadey, F., and Sanson, M. (2004). Palliative care in patients with primary brain tumours. *Current Opinion in Oncology*, **16**, 587–92.

12. Voltz, R., Akabayashi, A., Reese, C. *et al.* (1998). End-of-life decisions and advance directives in palliative care: A crosscultural survey of patients and health care professionals. *Journal of Pain and Symptom Management*, **16**, 153–62.

13. Adelbratt, S. and Strang, P. (2000). Death anxiety in brain tumour patients and their spouses. *Palliative Medicine*, **14**, 499–507.

14. Davies, E., Clarke, C., and Hopkins, A. (1996). Malignant cerebral glioma II: Perspectives of patients and relatives on the value of radiotherapy. *BMJ*, **313**, 1512–6.

15. Behar, R. and Abu Rkih, R. (2001). Does the patient with a primary brain tumour need hospice? *Eur J Pall Care* Abstracts of the 7th Congress of EAPC. p. 1200.

16. Faithfull, S., Cook, K., and Lucas, C. (2005). Palliative care of patients with a primary malignant brain tumour: case review of service use and support provided. *Palliative Medicine*, **19**(7), 545–50.

17. Forsyth, P.A. and Posner, J.B. (1993). Headaches in patients with brain tumours. *Neuorology*, **43**, 1678–83.

18. Vecht, C.J., Hovestadt, A., Verbiest, H.B. *et al.* (1994). Dose–effect relationship of dexamethasone on Karnofsky performance in metastatic brain tumours: a randomized study of doses of 4, 8 and 16 mg per day. *Neurology*, **44**(4), 675–80.

19. Winking, M., Böker, D.K., and Simmet, T. (1996). Boswellic acid as an inhibitor of the perifocal edema in malignant glioma in man. *Journal of Neuro-Oncology*, **30**, 104.

20. Chalk, J.B., Ridgeway, K., Brophy, T. *et al.* (1984). Phenytoin impairs the bioavailability of dexamethasone in neurological and neurosurgical patients. *Journal of Neurology, Neurosurgery and Psychiatry*, **47**(10), 1087–90.

21. Lee, M.A., Leng, M.E.F., and Tiernan, E.J.J. (2001). Risperidone: a useful adjunct for behavioural disturbance in primary cerebral tumours. *Palliative Medicine*, **15**, 255–6.

22. Thomas, R., O'Connor, A.M., and Ashley, S. (1995). Speech and language disorders in patients with high grade glioma and its influence on prognosis, *Journal of Neuro-Oncology*, **23**(3), 265–70.

23. Cloughesy, T., Selch, M.T., Liau, L.M.(2001). Brain. In *Cancer treatment* (ed. Haskell CM), 5th edn, pp. 1106–42, WB Saunders Co, Philadelphia.

24. Glantz, M.J., Cole, B.F., Forsyth, P.A. *et al.* (2000). Practice parameter: anticonvulsant prophylaxis in patients with newly diagnosed brain tumours. Report of the Quality Standards Subcommittee of the American Academy of Neurology. *Neurology*, **54**(10), 1886–93.

25. McAuley, J.W., Biederman, T.S., Smith, J.C. *et al.* (2002). Newer therapies in the drug treatment of epilepsy. *Annals of Pharmacotherapy*, **36**(1), 119–29.

26. Thompson, D., Takeshita, J., Thompson, T. *et al.* (2006). Selecting antiepileptic drugs for symptomatic patients with brain tumors. *The Journal of Supportive Oncology*, **4**(8), 411–6.

27. Nieder, C., Leicht, A., Motaref, B. *et al.* (1999). Late radiation toxicity after whole brain radiotherapy: the influence of antiepileptic drugs. *American Journal of Clinical Oncology*, **22**(6), 573–9.

28. Delattre, J.Y., Safai, B., and Posner, J.B. (1998). Erythema multiforme and Stevens-Johnson syndrome in patients receiving cranial irradiation and phenytoin. *Neurology*, **38**(2), 194–8.

29. Eralp, Y., Aydiner, A., Tas, F. *et al.* (2001). Stevens-Johnson syndrome in a patient receiving anticonvulsant therapy during cranial irradiation. *American Journal of Clinical Oncology*, **24**(4), 347–50.

30. Marras, L.C., Geerts, W.H., and Perry, J.R. (2000). The risk of venous thromboembolism is increased throughout the course of malignant glioma: an evidence-based review. *Cancer*, **89**, 640–6.

31. Batchelor, T. and Byrne, T. (2006). Supportive care of brain tumor patients. *Hematology/Oncology Clinics of North America*, **20**, 1337–61

32. van Dongen, C.J. and van den Belt, A.G. (2004). Fixed dose subcutaneous low molecular weight heparins versus adjusted dose unfractionated heparin for venous thromboembolism. *Cochrane Database System Review*, **4**, CD001100.

33. Bausewein, C., Hau, P., Voltz, R. *et al.* (2003). How do patients with brain tumours die? *Palliative Medicine*, **17**, 558–9.

SECTION 12

Palliative medicine in non-malignant disease

12.1

Palliative medicine in non-malignant disease

Marie Fallon and Norma O'Leary

Introduction

The needs of patients with progressive, incurable, non-malignant disease and the needs of their families are similar to those of patients with advanced cancer. However, 40 years after the founding of the modern hospice movement, only a small minority of non-cancer patients access specialist palliative care services. There is, however, a significant difference in the degree of coverage between the United Kingdom and the United States of America.

The ingredients of specialist palliative care

The modern hospice movement was established, nurtured, and developed through a complex mixture of compassion, imagination, knowledge, conviction, creativity, and determination. The ability to listen, observe, learn, experiment, adapt, and listen again were essential qualities. Clearly, charismatic personalities were a fundamental part of this process. We can see that no ready-made formula existed for specialist cancer palliative care, as indeed no formula exists for non-cancer palliative care, and we know that the growth of cancer palliative care has been marked by its diversity. Palliative care provision for non-cancer patients will also take diverse forms and already does so according to disease, patient, and family wishes, the health-care system, and, importantly, those who provide continuing care for such patients at present. With the call for improved palliative care for all, including non-cancer patients, it is important to stand back and examine the following:

♦ The range of non-cancer diagnoses and problems that most commonly require palliative care.

♦ The professionals caring for the patients with advanced non-malignant disease at present.

♦ Voluntary groups.

♦ Current practice and problems.

♦ Research evidence for the management of specific problems and models of care.

♦ Evolving natural history of non-cancer chronic illness (e.g. HIV disease with the advent of new life-prolonging treatments and, potentially, multiple sclerosis and amyotrophic lateral sclerosis—ALS).

♦ Research from palliative cancer care into physical symptom control, psychosocial care, and models of care to avoid the extension of management based purely on anecdotal experience into other areas of patient care[1].

♦ Problems in current cancer palliative care that may inform developments in palliative care of non-malignant disease.

♦ The background and characteristics of current practice of palliative care professionals, which clearly will influence the type of approach the profession will take to developing non-cancer palliative care.

Increasingly, more people in the developed world die from chronic rather than acute diseases. The percentage of the population over 65 has increased and will continue to increase. The main causes of mortality are: heart disease, cerebrovascular disorders, chronic respiratory disease, and cancer.

The above points will help to inform the fundamental question: should specialists provide palliative care for non-malignant disease, or should the principles of palliative care be promoted and adopted for all non-cancer patients with chronic, progressive disease? From this question flow other questions—if palliative care specialists, both doctors and nurses, should be the ones providing the palliative care, is the time coming when we shall have to have sub-specialties for the many non-malignant conditions within palliative care? This would have important and far-reaching implications for recruitment and training, and raise the possibility of de-skilling the specialists who usually care for such patients. Of course, as described elsewhere in this textbook, there are few countries where palliative medicine or palliative care nursing are recognized as specialties—most countries electing to promote and facilitate the teaching of the principles of palliative care throughout their caring professions. In this case, it must be questioned whether there are sufficient people with experience of providing palliative care for non-malignant conditions to be able to teach it and, if the answer is no, how is the necessary experience to be gained? Are fundamental changes needed in current palliative medicine training courses?

A number of key factors will influence the response to these questions. Not only will the education, skills, and attitudes of palliative care professionals play a large part but the knowledge and attitudes of the professionals currently looking after patients with non-cancer chronic progressive disease will need to be addressed if they, too, are to be better informed and trained in this care and know how to access and take full advantage of the skills of their specialist palliative medicine colleagues. The knowledge and attitudes of

Theory	Modelling	Exploratory	Definitive RCT	Long-term implementation
Explore relevant theory to ensure best choice of intervention and hypothesis and to predict major confounders and strategic design issues	Identify the components of the intervention, and the underlying mechanisms by which they will influence outcomes to provide evidence allowing prediction of their relation to and interaction with each phase	Describe the constant and variable components of a replicable intervention and a feasible protocol for comparison of the intervention with an appropriate alternative	Compare a fully defined intervention to an appropriate alternative using a protocol that is theoretically-defensible, reproducible and adequately controlled, in a study with appropriate statistical power	Determine whether others can reliably replicate the intervention and results in uncontrolled settings over the long-term
Pre-clinical	Phase 1	Phase 2	Phase 3	Phase 4

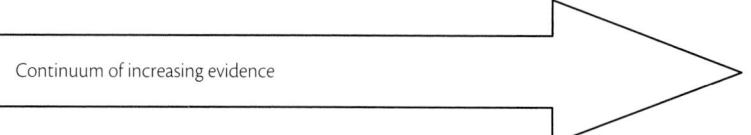

Continuum of increasing evidence

Figure 12.1.1 Framework for trials of complex interventions. Reproduced with permission from the Medical Research Council (2000)[2].

patients and family is important and, of course, last but not least, the issue that often drives the development of most services—financial support and the informed understanding of politicians and health-care planners, are all important. For some reason, people have come to believe that cancer is the principal 'killer' in the world and the one associated with the worst pain and suffering. It will take considerable public education to change this perception. It is likely to take some time before many doctors, whether generalist or specialist, are as sensitive to the palliative care needs of their non-malignant patients as are currently to their cancer patients.

It is the unequivocal view of the editors of this textbook that in terms of needs, care provision, and quality of care, there can be no distinction between the care of patients with malignant and non-malignant disease, hence the many chapters devoted to this in the book.

Since the last edition of the *Oxford Textbook of Palliative Medicine*, a significant amount has been written about the concept and reality of palliative care in chronic non-malignant disease, and we have seen the emergence of more research. While the vast majority of palliative care is provided for patients with cancer, there has been a definite positive shift in interest and knowledge of chronic non-malignant disease and palliative care.

Palliative care is a complex intervention comprising a number of components, which may act both independently and inter-dependently. It is difficult to determine the core or active ingredient of a palliative care intervention. The Medical Research Council (MRC) published a framework for the development and evaluation of complex interventions, such as palliative care, to improve health. It describes a series of stages of investigation in the process[2]. Theoretical and early modelling research will identify,

in preliminary form, the kind of intervention needed to meet the palliative care needs of non-cancer patients. This informs the next stage of research, which evaluates the effectiveness of active components of care and their inter-relationships, which will further inform the development of effective models of service and delivery. (Fig. 12.1.1). The MRC framework is currently under review. It is expected that modification will take into account the iterative nature of the process on each stage.

Modifications based on practical research experience in palliative care have already been proposed (Fig. 12.1.2)[3].

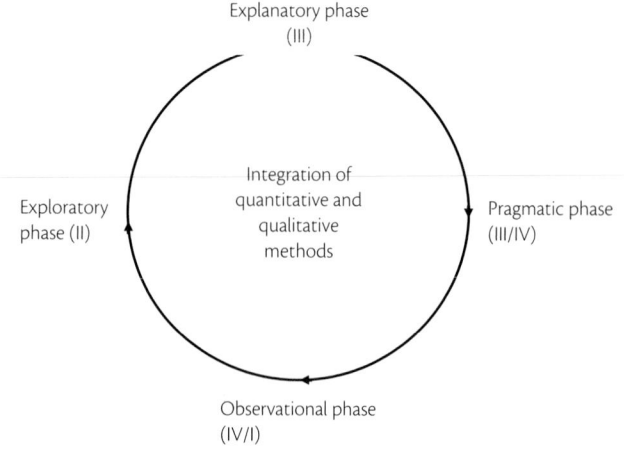

Figure 12.1.2 Modifications based on practical research experience.

Dame Cicely Saunders envisaged that hospice care would be available to all patients regardless of diagnosis. This decision was informed, in part, by the evidence from Hinton's work published in 1963[4]. He found that patients dying from non-malignant diseases were just as likely to experience distressing symptoms as cancer patients, but were less likely to have these symptoms relieved. Cicely Saunders made it clear that her original 'vision' included the care of people with conditions other than cancer: 'terminal care should not be a facet of oncology, but of geriatric medicine, neurology, general practice and throughout medicine'[5].

Early experiences in hospices exposed the problems of indeterminate prognosis. Although some palliative care literature addresses specific needs of patients with non-malignant diseases, it was not until the emergence of AIDS in the mid-1980s that the hospice movement was widely confronted by the challenge of non-malignant conditions[5]. Several recent studies have maintained this challenge by emphasizing the unmet needs of patients with advanced disease with conditions other than cancer[6–10].

Despite its initial aspirations, the early hospice movement became synonymous with terminal care. It focused on diseases with a predictable terminal phase. Cancer was the dominant diagnostic group, with a small number of patients with motor neuron disease also receiving care. Palliative care for cancer patients has evolved since the early days. It is no longer confined to the terminal phase of the cancer disease trajectory. Indeed, the concepts of continuity and totality of care, which are inherent to palliative care, are applicable at any stage along the cancer disease journey, depending on patient need.

Hospice care has a long tradition of service development, relying heavily on emotive appeals and reflecting the enthusiasms and energies of local lobbyists and advocates. The modern hospice movement expanded quickly on the strength of these pioneering individuals. However, in the current era of tight budgets and evidence-based practice, determination of need is required to make a case for service expansion.

Patients living with potentially life-limiting diseases experience losses. These losses are experienced on many different levels such as loss of physical functioning, loss of financial income, loss of hope for the future. These can be experienced over a long period of time and can be exaggerated in patients having multiple co-morbid illnesses.

The challenge for specialist palliative care service planners and policy makers is to determine which of these multiple needs fall within the specialist palliative care domain and which could or should be addressed more effectively by other health- and social-care professionals.

Need is defined as 'the ability to benefit from health care'[6]. The ability of the population to benefit from healthcare depends on two things: the number of individuals affected, that is, the incidence and prevalence of the condition under question, and the effectiveness of the services available to deal with it[7].

Need is different from demand. Demand is defined as 'what people ask for'[7]. Demand is changeable and is influenced by, among other things, social and educational backgrounds, the media, and the medical profession. Demands may be made for the extension of specialist palliative care services for non-cancer patients on the grounds of equity and justice. However, it could also be argued that it is unjust to offer specialist palliative care if a more effective service or intervention exists. For the expansion of specialist palliative care services, there is a need to provide evidence that specialist palliative care is the most appropriate health-care response.

A recently published report of the Scottish Partnership for Palliative Care, entitled *Joined Up Thinking Joined Up Care*, outlined six areas of unmet palliative care need in patients with ten specific progressive life-threatening conditions: cystic fibrosis, dementia, heart failure, HIV/AIDS, motor neuron disease, multiple sclerosis, muscular dystrophy, Parkinson's disease, renal failure, and respiratory failure[8]. The palliative care needs identified were classified as follows: information, practical help, symptom management, joint working, psychosocial education and training. It may be tempting for specialist palliative care services to give immediate attention to those needs. However, when examined more closely, specialist palliative care professionals may not have the most appropriate skills. For example, regarding information needs, groups identified the need for knowledge about their entitlement to financial help and when it is appropriate to apply for benefits. They wanted information about using public transport, accessible facilities, how to get holiday insurance, and how to get help when on holiday. They wanted information on how their informal carers could get time off work. They wanted information on local facilities such as day centres, respite care and buddy schemes, and how to access them. It may be argued that information needs fall within the general palliative care domain. General palliative care needs are not specific to specialist palliative care but are no less important to the patient. Even though specialist palliative care services may not take direct responsibility for addressing these needs, they have a responsibility to ensure that generalists have the skills to address them.

Predicted causes of death

Technological advances in medicine and improvements in public health have enabled people in developed countries to live longer and to survive potentially life-threatening events such as childbirth, infectious disease, and injury. A result of these advances has been the emergence of serious chronic diseases as a major pathway towards death.

In line with the ageing of the population, the pattern of diseases that people suffer and die from is also changing. The top five predicted causes of death for 2020 are listed in Table 12.1.1[9].

The predicted increase in the number of old and frail people with chronic cardio-respiratory disease is a very real challenge for health services generally and palliative care services specifically. Among these chronic cardio-respiratory diseases, congestive cardiac failure (CCF) and chronic obstructive pulmonary disease (COPD) have been identified as being especially suited to specialist palliative care services, for three reasons; first, there are usually symptoms to control; second, the prevalence is high and increasing; and third, the prognosis is poor. Of patients with heart failure, 20 per cent are dead within a year of diagnosis, 50 per cent within 5 years[10].

Table 12.1.1 Top five predicted causes of death in 2020.

Ischaemic heart disease
Cerebrovascular disease
Chronic obstructive pulmonary disease
Respiratory infection
Lung cancer

Patients hospitalized with an acute exacerbation of COPD have a median survival of 2 years and 50 per cent of patients are readmitted to the hospital within 6 months[11].

With the exception of patients with motor neuron disease, most publications on non-cancer palliative care have been concerned with patients with CCF and COPD, with most written about patients with CCF. COPD has received less attention as it is frequently diagnosed late within the disease process, as the symptoms are not apparent until the lung function is significantly affected, often less than 50 per cent of normal[12]. Often, individuals with advanced COPD experience episodes of severe illness, followed by a significant recovery. This can lead to a deceptive picture for all concerned and conceals the true pathway of the disease process. Many patients are never formally diagnosed with the condition or are managed at primary care level without tertiary referral. As a result, they are not entered onto registers and it is harder to identify them for inclusion in research studies. Mortality data are known to underestimate COPD as a cause of death, because it is more likely to be cited as a contributory rather than an underlying cause of death[13]. COPD patients may not seek medical attention if they feel little can be done for them. They may think that the medical profession is disinterested in their plight, as their condition is self-inflicted.

The following sections summarize existing knowledge of the palliative care needs of the different patient groups and the gaps in current research are also outlined. To clarify further the role of palliative care, let us look at some of the issues that arise in the chronic, progressive diseases.

Progressive neurological illness

In the United Kingdom, at least 75 per cent of inpatient palliative care units in a 1998 survey were involved in the care of amyotrophic lateral sclerosis (ALS, also known as motor neuron disease) patients and while only 15 per cent of patients were referred for symptom control, many were found to have uncontrolled symptoms on assessment[14]. Research and experience has gone some way to inform the important role of specialist palliative care services in the provision of care to patients with neurodegenerative diseases and their families[15]. The causes of the neurodegenerative disorders, including ALS, are as yet unidentified and in general there are no known cures. Much research is concerned with gaining a greater understanding of the precise aetiologies and in developing disease-modifying drugs. Treatments such as riluzol for ALS are developed to slow the progression of the disease process and, in the future, it is not impossible that treatments may be developed to reverse or even cure such illnesses as ALS. However, while research for disease-modifying agents continues, patients must be offered an optimal level of palliation to ensure that they have the best possible quality of life. ALS has a prevalence of 4–6 per 100 000. While the peak incidence occurs between 60 and 70 years, it can affect patients aged from their late teens to the tenth decade. While part of the basic definition of palliative care is that it does not aim either to hasten death or prolong life, there is no doubt that the process of good palliation will not infrequently involve a prolongation of life and this also applies to chronic, progressive, non-cancer illness as well as cancer. Issues in ALS such as gastrostomy feeding or ventilatory support can clearly affect prognosis and survival of the patient as well as some aspects of quality of life. The range of issues affecting a patient with ALS and most other progressive neurological disorders

very much mirror the issues affecting a patient with cancer. The issue of communicating the diagnosis in the broadest sense, along with symptom control, including pain, dysphagia, nutritional problems, salivary dribbling, breathlessness, and upper-respiratory problems, dysarthria, anarthria, communication difficulties, sometimes bladder dysfunction, and, of course, depression and/or anxiety, are all commonly encountered. The care of the family and the need for interdisciplinary team work remain vital. All these issues are addressed in Sections 4, 6, and 15.

Congestive cardiac failure

Most cardiovascular diseases which affect the heart, such as hypertension, coronary artery disease, significant heart valve stenosis or regurgitation, and primary myocardial diseases, cause myocardial damage resulting in CCF. The clinical definition of CCF is a syndrome associated with symptoms, signs, and objective evidence of left ventricular dysfunction[16]. It is the only cardiovascular disease with increasing prevalence, incidence, and mortality. It accounts for more hospitalizations than any other condition and is mainly a disease of old age[16]. The estimated prevalence (per 1000 population) is between 3.8 and 29.4 rising to 80.4 for people over the age of 65 years and up to 190 for those over the age of 75[18]. Mortality rates are high; 40 per cent in the first year following diagnosis and 45–75 per cent at five years, with a high risk of sudden death[19].

The Regional Study of the Care for the Dying (RSCD) and the Study to Understand Prognosis and Preferences for Outcomes and Risks of Treatment (SUPPORT) were among the first studies to outline the palliative care needs of CCF patients[20,21].

The RSCD was a population-based retrospective survey of a random sample of people dying in 20 English health districts, including 683 deaths from heart disease. People who died from heart disease experienced a wide range of symptoms, which were often distressing and lasted for more than 6 months[22]. Breathlessness, pain, nausea, constipation, and low mood were common, and poorly controlled. In a secondary analysis, a comparison was made between heart disease and cancer patients, with regard to pain characteristics. Pain was less common in the last year of life in patients with heart disease than cancer (77 per cent vs. 88 per cent), but it was more likely to last longer than 6 months (75 per cent vs. 58 per cent). A similar pattern was found for mood; the majority of either heart disease or cancer patients reported to have felt low at some point in the last year (59 per cent and 69 per cent) and this was more likely to have lasted 6 months or more in heart disease (82 per cent vs. 54 per cent). This was a landmark study. For the first time evidence was provided showing that patients with heart disease have palliative care needs. However, this important study did not describe the cardiac diseases it included, so information specific to heart failure could not be extracted. The information gathered was reliant on proxy accounts. Studies that have examined the concordance of preferences for end-of-life care between patients and their family caregivers have found poor to moderate consistency in preferences[23]. Furthermore, this can often change over time for a variety of obvious reasons.

While the RSCD was a retrospective study, the SUPPORT was a prospective US national multi-centre study of outcomes, preferences, and decision-making among seriously ill, hospitalized adults. It provided further evidence of the unmet needs of heart patients. The study defined the conditions considered. It included 263 patients with acute exacerbation of CCF. Patients and their identified surrogates were interviewed prospectively from the index hospitalization up until 4–10 weeks after the patient's death. This showed severe symptoms in the last 3 days of life; 65 per cent were breathless and 42 per cent had severe pain. Of these patients, 40 per cent received a major treatment intervention in the last 3 days of life, suggesting the doctors had not recognized the closeness of death. Family members, however, believed that patients would have preferred comfort to life-sustaining treatments[24].

These two studies are important as they highlight the plight of patients dying from heart disease. More recently, studies reporting direct heart failure patient accounts of their physical, psychosocial, emotional, and information needs have been published.

Fatigue and breathlessness are the two most prevalent symptoms experienced by heart failure patients[25–27]. Symptoms such as breathlessness and fatigue can limit the extent of daily physical activities, requiring careful planning to allow for slow performance and frequent stops[28]. In addition to breathlessness and fatigue, Nordgren found that patients experienced a wide range of other symptoms, such as limb swelling, pain, nausea, sleeplessness, palpitations, and loss of appetite[27]. In fact, up to 21 symptoms were noted, and patients had an average of seven symptoms. However, this study was a retrospective review of medical records, nursing records, and medication charts, and, as such, provided an indirect approach to the patients, being more of a reflection of the perception of symptoms of the medical staff. The reliability of proxy symptom ratings is quite variable[29]. A more robust study that directly evaluated heart failure patients attending a specialist heart failure clinic using a validated symptom assessment tool (Memorial Symptom Assessment Scale-Heart Failure) found that they experienced a mean of 15.1 symptoms[30].

The prevalence of pain in patients with heart failure is variable. In a group of heart failure patients requiring admission to a hospice, 75 per cent of patients reported no pain, whereas 3 per cent reported chest pain and 20 per cent reported other pains. The other primary symptoms documented in the last week of life included oedema, incontinence of bowel or bladder, and some confusion[31]. A systematic review of symptoms experienced by patients with one of five progressive conditions (cancer, AIDS, heart disease, COPD, renal disease) found that pain, fatigue, and breathlessness were universal and frequent—with prevalence often well above 50 per cent[31]. There may be a common pathway towards the end of life in terms of symptomatology in patients with advanced disease. The common pathway is a useful concept as it means that pain, breathlessness, and fatigue should be at the top of the palliative care research agenda. The effectiveness of palliative care interventions for these three symptoms needs to be evaluated. This information will help to determine which symptoms would benefit from specialist palliative care intervention and therefore, guide referral of patients. One of the current barriers to the extension of specialist palliative care to heart failure patients is the lack of proven effectiveness of specialist palliative care interventions.

Physical symptoms that remain poorly controlled have emotional and social consequences. In the community, heart failure patients with a high symptom burden had feelings of uselessness and confusion. Loss of independence and increased reliance on others for activities of daily living was thought to pose the most worry for patients. Many self-reported symptoms of depression[26]. In another qualitative, community-based study, patients experienced significant losses in their lives relating to the inability to carry out many activities they had previously done with ease. Difficulties in performing simple tasks changed patients' roles in the family and society, which caused them to be housebound and leading to isolation and loneliness[32]. Social isolation can lead to an increased risk of fatal and non-fatal cardiovascular events[33]. Willems examined the patient 'work' in living with advanced heart failure[34]. Four categories of work were described and were considered all-consuming for patients:

♦ Managing the illness—the work done in organizing medications and care, following regimens, and obtaining the care needed.

♦ Everyday work to keep life going—organizing daily life, including the pacing of rest and activity.

♦ Biographical work—dealing with the threat of increasing loss, while maintaining a coherent biography.

♦ Arrangement work—organizing mobility and infrastructure, obtaining devices and adaptations for the home.

Heart failure impacts significantly on the lives of informal carers. Patients experience increased reliance on carers as they lose their independence[26]. Levenson analysed data from the SUPPORT study and found that the patients' heart failure had marked financial impact on their families, with 23 per cent of patients' families reporting the loss of most or all of family savings at the time of the patient's death[24]. Carers for a group of heart failure patients based in London identified feelings of dread, frustration, guilt, and anxiety. They reported fearing the patient's deterioration or death[19].

Anxiety and depression

In addition to having a high physical symptom burden, CCF patients have also been shown to have significant psychological morbidity. Carers in particular have reported that patients often experience anger, frustration, anxiety, and depression[19]. The prevalence of depression in outpatient heart failure patients has been found to be as high as 42 per cent. In a hospitalized cohort, 20 per cent of the patients met the DSM4 criteria for a major depressive episode, 16 per cent for a minor depressive episode, and 51 per cent scored above the cut-off for depression on the Beck Depression Inventory[35]. Depression has a negative impact on both CCF patients and their spouses[36]. In a recent study, over 90 per cent of depressed patients did not receive drug treatment for their depression[37].

The studies described thus far have highlighted high symptoms burdens and emotional distress in heart failure patients. However, the documentation of need does not imply that it is specialist palliative care need. One attempt to determine which needs fall within the specialist palliative care domain, uses cancer patients as a reference point. Murray compared the illness trajectories, needs, and service use of patients with heart failure and cancer[38].

The conclusions of the study were that patients with advanced heart failure may benefit from specific models of care with strategic planning across primary and secondary care, involvement of health- and social-care services, and specialist palliative care providers. Models of care that focus on quality of life, symptom control, and psychosocial support for patients and their families, while continuing active treatment, were recommended[39]. However, a significant limitation with these studies was that the study samples were poorly described in relation to, for example, the extent of disease, aetiological factors, and presence of co-morbidities. The heart failure patients had not been entered onto chronic illness management programmes, which is the current reference standard of care[40]. Nonetheless, these studies have been useful for highlighting the relative neglect of heart failure patients. They are widely cited as evidence supporting the need for specialist palliative care services. It would, however, be more accurate to say that they provide evidence for the need for better coordinated health-care, incorporating the principles of general palliative care.

CCF patients have been shown to have unmet information and communication needs. Rogers carried out a qualitative analysis of in-depth interviews with heart failure patients[41]. Participants sought information from the research interviewer about their heart failure, their prognosis, and likely manner of death. Many patients felt that their symptoms were a result of growing older and, at least before diagnosis, something for which nothing could be done. Some patients were apparently unaware of their likely prognosis, with two reporting that 'heart failure' sounded too terminal. Some patients' narratives suggested that they were aware of, but had not (or did not wish to) openly acknowledged their prognosis. This illustrated their ambivalent attitude towards gaining greater knowledge of their condition. Patients also described several factors that could inhibit successful communication with their doctors. These included difficulties in getting to hospital appointments, confusion, short-term memory loss, and the belief that doctors did not want to provide patients with too much information.

In a qualitative study by Gillian Horne, community-based patients expressed need for better communication from their physicians in the form of explanation, education, and information[32]. Typical comments were 'nobody ever tells you anything' and the 'doctor didn't explain'. Selman found that the silence around end-of-life issues was a source of fear and anxiety for both patients and carers, and yet most participants were willing to discuss their end-of-life preferences[19]. Even though this study contrasts somewhat with the findings of Rogers, it highlights the feasibility of raising these issues which, in turn, may reduce the fear and anxiety experienced by patients and carers[41]. Willems found that patients with heart failure only thought about death during exacerbations[42]. Patients described aspects of dying that they felt were important to them: a degree of usefulness, prognostic knowledge, appropriate duration, and mental awareness. Few respondents were in favour of euthanasia or suicide, but all wanted life-prolonging treatment to be withheld or withdrawn when appropriate.

The end of life for heart failure patients has been revolutionized by implantable cardioverter defibrillators (ICD). These devices improve survival by reducing the likelihood of arrhythmic death. (This is discussed in Chapter 12.4.) However, at the end of life, these devices may subject patients to a prolonged, more uncomfortable process of dying. Since ICD discharges can cause pain and anxiety and avoiding an arrhythmic death may become undesirable in light of other modes of dying that the patient faces, some patients may prefer to deactivate their ICD near end of life. Goldstein found that next of kin reported that clinicians discussed deactivating the ICD in only 27 of 100 cases[43]. Most discussions occurred in the last days of life. Family members reported that eight patients received a shock from their ICD in the minutes before death.

A Spanish study examined preferences concerning cardiopulmonary resuscitation and end-of-life care in 80 elderly patients hospitalized for heart failure. Of these, 40 per cent expressed a wish not to have CPR. Only two had previously discussed their preferences

with their physicians. While recovery from the illness was considered unlikely, 40 (50 per cent) participants preferred to receive treatment at home, 32 (40 per cent) preferred in-hospital management, and eight were unsure. Of the participants, 33 (41 per cent) expressed a desire for spiritual support, 38 (48 per cent) said not, and the remainder were indifferent. The authors concluded that advance planning of end-of-life procedures and doctor–patient communication regarding these issues remains poor and must be improved[44]. These findings are not culturally specific, as studies from the US and elsewhere have found that when given the choice, patients with life-limiting illnesses would choose treatments that improve quality of life at the expense of life-prolonging treatments and most patients would prefer to die at home[45].

These studies highlight the challenge of communicating with heart-failure patients regarding end-of-life issues. Patients differ in their needs. Some want frank and open conversations other avoid such conversations. This is further complicated by the unpredictable disease trajectory. Formiga found that decision-making at the end of life, in patients with heart failure, was hindered by their lack of awareness of the proximity of death[44]. How can doctors be expected to give accurate prognoses to patients with unpredictable disease trajectories? Patients should, at least, be given the opportunity to address their information needs. These studies have highlighted two points in time when health-care professionals should consider initiating such discussions: at the time of ICD insertion and following recovery from an acute exacerbation. Which healthcare professional should address information needs? Do they fall solely within the specialist palliative care domain or are they the responsibility of cardiology professionals? Who is likely to be more accurate in their prognostications?

Many studies have documented the unmet palliative care needs of patients with CCF. Fatigue and breathlessness are the most prevalent symptoms. The chronic condition impacts negatively on functional status and quality of life. Carers experience emotional and psychosocial distress. However, there are limitations to these studies. The original studies were based on proxy accounts or were retrospective. In studies that reported direct patient accounts, the study samples were poorly described. No study examined the palliative care needs of patients receiving the current reference standard of care for heart failure patients, which is coordinated and multi-disciplinary. Even though many palliative care needs were documented, no attempt was made to differentiate between general and specialist palliative care needs. Despite a significant body of literature, a question still remains unanswered: do heart failure patients receiving the current reference standard of care have unmet specialist palliative care needs?

Chronic obstructive pulmonary disease

Chronic obstructive pulmonary disease (COPD) is a syndrome defined by breathing-related symptoms and signs: chronic cough, expectoration, varying degrees of exertional dyspnoea, and a significant and progressive reduction in expiratory airflow. It is a progressive illness with no cure. For those with severe COPD, prognosis can be very poor, with one hospital-based study identifying 50 per cent mortality at 2 years after admission for an acute exacerbation of severe COPD[46]. Since the publication of the landmark RSCD and SUPPORT studies, a palliative care approach has been advocated in the management of end-stage COPD.

The SUPPORT study enrolled seriously ill, hospitalized patients with one of nine illnesses, including COPD. SUPPORT found that, compared to patients with lung cancer, patients with COPD were much more likely to die with dyspnoea, in the intensive care unit on mechanical ventilation. These differences in care occurred despite the fact that most patients with COPD preferred treatment focused on comfort rather than on prolonging life. In fact, the SUPPORT investigators found that patients with lung cancer and COPD were equally likely to prefer not to be intubated[47,48]. Data from the RSCD study conducted in 1990 was analysed. No differences were found in the mean number of symptoms reported by the groups (lung cancer and COPD) in the final year or week of life, although the COPD patients were more likely to have experienced these symptoms over a longer period. Significantly, more patients with COPD experienced breathlessness in the final year and final week of life[49].

Physical needs

As with heart failure patients, many studies have highlighted the unmet palliative care needs of patients with COPD. The nature of the physical needs differs between the two groups. Dyspnoea is undisputedly the most common and distressing symptom experienced by people with COPD. It is a frightening, disabling, and restricting symptom resulting in enormous losses in working and personal lives[50]. Seamark describes loss of personal liberty and dignity, and of expectations of the future[51]. In turn, these losses can lead to increased feelings of frustration, tension, and anxiety that, in themselves, can trigger episodes of breathlessness[52]. Bailey describes this eloquently as the 'dyspnoea–anxiety–dyspnoea cycle'[53]. As COPD is generally smoking-related, patients can experience feelings of self-blame. They feel undeserving of medical attention, which further fuels anxiety[50].

Breathlessness restricts patients' freedom by impairing their mobility and their ability to leave their home. The treatments also impose lifestyle restrictions. Oxygen dependence means patients feel unable to leave home[54]. Extreme breathlessness leads to social isolation[55]. Fatigue, weakness, disturbed sleeping patterns, and low mood are also frequently experienced[56,57].

Patients generally rate their quality of life as poor. Lynn et al. looked at the experiences of COPD patients who died within 1 year of an index hospitalization[58]. They found that in the last 6 months of life, 75 per cent described their quality of life as fair or poor and that they spent about 20 per cent of their time in hospital. Skilbeck interviewed 63 individuals with advanced COPD[56]. Poor quality of life was evident, relating to a high degree of social isolation and emotional distress, associated with a high symptom load, low physical functioning, and disability. She describes these patients as invisible to medical and social supports until they require symptom management in an acute phase of the illness. This emphasis on acute care led to fragmented services with obvious gaps in community care. On the whole, services were delivered on an ad hoc basis and what emerged was reactive crisis intervention, rather than supportive preventative services. Family members and carers felt helpless, powerless, and anxious when watching their loved one gasp for breath. Booth describes them as 'the invisible victims'[50].

Comparison with cancer patients

As in Murray's work, Gore attempted further to define the needs of COPD patients by comparing them with the needs of cancer patients[59]. This frequently cited study highlights the inequity of care for patients with COPD compared with cancer. This was a prospective comparative study between patients with end-stage COPD and lung cancer. The COPD patients had worse activities of daily living scores, physical, social, and emotional functioning in comparison to the cancer cohort. They had a lack of information regarding their diagnosis, prognosis, and social supports. Some 26 per cent of the COPD patients implied that they did not know that they would die of their disease. They were less likely to die at home and much less likely to receive palliative care services. Of these patients, 90 per cent had clinically relevant anxiety or depression, but did not receive specific treatment for emotional problems. The study population in this paper is not unusual and not comparable as lung cancer patients were long-term survivors, whereas COPD patients were end stage.

Anxiety and depression

Patients with advanced COPD and their partners or family members often report significant mood disturbance and sometimes even suicidal thoughts[60]. Both anxiety and depression are common (affecting 40–50 per cent of patients) and much more prevalent than in the general population[61]. Unfortunately, both symptoms often go untreated in the COPD population[62]. Depression is an independent predictor of mortality in advanced COPD and depression is linked to how patients make choices about potentially life-sustaining treatments[63,64]. A higher burden of depressive symptoms was significantly associated with a preference against CPR[65]. Treatment of depression can have beneficial effects on many aspects of living with COPD, including a positive effect on dyspnoea and, in fact, appears to have more beneficial effects on dyspnoea than the use of anxiolytics[66,67]. Recognition of the psychosocial needs of patients and care providers with COPD has come relatively late but should be recognized as a key facet to the provision of quality of care in advanced stages of COPD[50].

Information and communication needs

Studies from three continents have shown that physicians, though they may recognize the need, often do not discuss prognosis with their COPD patients[68,65]. Only a minority of patients with moderate to severe COPD have discussed treatment preferences and end-of-life care issues with their physicians[69]. Further, the majority of these patients believe that their physicians do not know their preferences for end-of-life care[70]. Only a third of patients with oxygen dependent COPD discussed end-of-life care with their physicians and fewer than 25 per cent of physicians had discussed some particularly important aspects of end-of-life care with their patients[65]. These infrequently discussed aspects include talking about how long the patient might live, talking about what dying might be like, talking with family about what dying might be like, and asking patients about their spiritual or religious beliefs. Going back to the concept of need, is it a need that can be met? Is the apparent side-stepping of end-of-life issues a reflection of the difficulty of prognosticating in COPD?

Jones found that most patients interviewed wanted more information about their disease and prognosis[71]. However, this study also reported that some patients did not want this type of information. These findings highlight an important challenge for physicians: how to distinguish patients who desire prognostic information from those who do not. A study that examined 115 patients with oxygen-dependent COPD, and the difficulties in communication about end of life, found the barriers to be diverse and patient specific[72]. Of the 15 barriers identified, only two were endorsed by more than 50 per cent of patients:

- I'd rather concentrate on staying alive than talk about death.

- I'm not sure which physician will be taking care of me if I get sick.

Sudden life-threatening exacerbations of COPD or episodes of acute respiratory failure often demand immediate answers from patients and families about the implementation of life supportive care. There is evidence that little discussion about treatment preferences of people with COPD occurs before such a crisis. Canadian respiratory physicians revealed that many respondents initiated discussions about mechanical ventilation late in the progression of advanced lung disease, if at all[73]. While understandable, this approach is counter to patient expectations. Virtually all of the study participants, in a survey of pulmonary rehabilitation, expressed interest in discussing end-of-life decisions with their physicians[70]. Reluctance to discuss prognosis inhibits terminally ill patients from speaking openly about their hopes and fears and from planning actively for death. Patients' end-of-life preferences are highly individualized and influenced largely by personal beliefs that cannot be assumed or predicted[74]. This underlines the importance of proactively addressing end-of-life issues with patients. The approach requires skill and must be sensitive to the individual needs to the patient.

Political/policy recognition

From the mid-1990s onwards, due to the increasing body of evidence of their unmet palliative care needs, non-cancer patients have taken centre stage on palliative care policy agendas. Internationally, in 2004, the WHO released a booklet entitled *The Solid Facts*[75]. It recommended that policy makers should plan to meet the care needs of ageing populations towards the end of life. It proposed that health-care systems must place much greater emphasis on the care of people of all ages who are living with and dying from a range of serious chronic diseases. The recommendation of the EU Committee of Ministers to member states on the organization of palliative care, suggested that it was the responsibility of health-care planners in each country to assess their specific needs and to plan accordingly[76].

The impetus to extend palliative care services beyond cancer has come from within palliative care circles rather than from external sources. In recent years, the care for chronically ill people has improved significantly with the development of coordinated multi-disciplinary approaches that incorporate the principles of self-management[77]. End-of-life care is now increasingly recognized as an integral part of the care package for patients. The American College of Chest Physicians strongly supports the position that palliative and end–of-life care of patients with an acute devastating or chronically progressive pulmonary or cardiac disease and their families, would be an integral part of cardiopulmonary medicine[78]. The new National Institute for Health and Clinical Excellence (NICE) guidelines for the management of COPD acknowledge that a full range of palliative care services should be offered to those with advanced COPD, for example, the use of opioids, access to multi-disciplinary palliative care teams, and so forth[79]. The NICE guidelines for heart failure also recommend palliative care as an intrinsic part of patient care[80].

However, palliative care for non-malignant diseases has not been universally endorsed outside specialist palliative care circles.

For example, the British Thoracic Society guidelines for the management of COPD suggest that there should be provision for terminal and respite care for patients with the most severe COPD[81]. However, this is not mentioned in the main body of the document and only appears in an appendix listing the provisions a district hospital should have[81]. The Global Initiative for Chronic Obstructive Lung Disease (GOLD) is an organization that aims to improve the prevention and management of COPD worldwide, with similar goals to the BTS, and works in collaboration with the US National Heart, Lung and Blood Institute and the WHO. GOLD published a management plan for COPD in 2003, which does not include palliative care[82]. Even though there is increasing recognition that palliative care should be incorporated into the care provided to all patients, there is not universal recognition at policy level.

Many reasons have been postulated as to why palliative care has not become mainstream for non-cancer conditions.

For those who endorse the extension of palliative care to non-cancer patients, these factors are viewed as barriers that need to be broken down. Those who feel that palliative care is irrelevant to non-cancer patients view these factors as valid reasons to interrupt the non-cancer palliative care movement. The factors can be categorized into patient/carer issues, professional concerns, funding issues, variable non-cancer disease trajectory, service structure issues, and lack of referral criteria.

Patient/carer issues

Patients with non-cancer conditions may be focused on cure and may be unwilling to forego futile curative attempts even for the sake of relieving suffering. They may not wish to entertain discussion of treatment with palliative intent. Carers may feel that talk of palliative care could result in their loved ones giving up hope. Patients and carers may view palliative care as synonymous with cancer or as having connotations with death. They may be fearful of it[83,84].

Professional concerns

Although palliative care interventions are effective for cancer patients, they cannot be assumed to be effective for the non-cancer population[85]. Acute care specialists, as well as specialist palliative care providers, may have concerns about the lack of disease-specific expertise within the specialty of palliative medicine[86]. The wide breadth of non-cancer conditions that could be referred is another concern for specialist palliative care providers. Due to the lack of proven effectiveness of specialist palliative care interventions for non-cancer conditions, specialist palliative care providers may be unsure as to what they can offer. There may be blurring of boundaries between professional groups: which needs can be classified as general palliative care and which are specialist? Professionals may feel that they are already doing an adequate job at caring for their own dying patients and that specialist palliative care services are try to 'steal patients'. They may believe that, if they relinquish the care of their own dying patients to others, they will become deskilled in caring for the dying[87].

Funding issues

Who will fund the expansion of palliative care services to non-cancer conditions? Will fundraising initiatives or statutory funding for cancer patients be adversely affected[80]? Some groups may have vested interests in maintaining the present health service arrangements.

For example, a survey of volunteers in the United Kingdom, who are often largely responsible for fundraising initiatives, found that they were slow to endorse hospice care for non-cancer patients[88].

Non-cancer disease trajectory

The variable non-cancer disease trajectory is, arguably, the most significant barrier. The delivery of specialist palliative care in most developed countries has traditionally been predicated on the cancer trajectory, whereby intervention is confined predominantly to the 'terminal phase'[89]. This is recognizable by a marked decline in weight and function. Three other dying trajectories have been described, which are more commonly associated with non-cancer conditions. These are:

- Sudden death with little prior warning and minimal interaction with health services before death. Up to 50 per cent of heart failure patients die suddenly and unexpectedly.

- Death from organ failure (including heart failure and COPD), where a gradual decline in functional status occurs, interspersed with acute periods of deterioration, which could cause death.

- Death following progressive deterioration accompanying frailty, stroke, or dementia[90].

Theoretical models of dying can provide a framework for service planning (Fig. 12.1.2). When Glaser and Strauss introduced the idea of dying trajectories, they were referring not only to the physiological unfolding of a patient's disease, but to the total organization of work done over the course of illness that impacts on those involved with that work and its organization[91]. Attempts have been made to describe variables that can be used to identify the end of life for non-cancer patients and help to plan and provide relevant services.

A recent study by Gott has challenged the idea of planning and delivering services on the basis of theorized trajectory[89]. In this prospective, longitudinal study of physical function in heart failure patients prior to death, no typical dying trajectory was identified.

Service structure issues

There are many questions about the best service configuration to meet non-cancer patients' needs. Developing models of care that are responsible to the fluctuating needs of non-cancer patients is a challenge.

Lack of referral criteria

Referral criteria for cancer patients have traditionally been based on prognosis. Prognostication is difficult in non-cancer conditions due to the variable disease trajectory. Referral criteria should be developed that identify patients most in need and not simply those who are closest to death. The current lack of policies is a barrier.

Renal disease

Renal failure results from various diseases irreversibly damaging both kidneys resulting in uraemic symptoms. These are commonly nausea and vomiting, anorexia, tiredness, itching, weakness, decreased sexual function and libido. Without dialysis or transplantation, the patient would become comatose and die. In developed countries, there is nearly universal access to dialysis treatment. Consequently, the population of patients receiving dialysis support has steadily grown and aged over the last decade. The acceptance of sicker patients whose renal disease results from, or is associated

with, more severe, co-morbid conditions, has also increased. These factors affect both the quality and length of patients' lives. The annual mortality rate of patients on dialysis in the United States is approximately 25 per cent, which is clearly higher than that of AIDS or of most cancers[92]. Cardiovascular complications account for at least half of the deaths. It is easy to see that including all the physical symptom control issues to be managed, there are, of course, significant psychosocial family and communication issues and the difficulties associated with end-of-life decision-making, particularly withdrawal of dialysis (see Chapter 12.6).

Liver disease

The profile of terminal chronic liver disease has been modified greatly in countries with active liver transplant programmes, and many patients do not develop the range of complications considered here. However, in the United Kingdom, at least four people die from chronic liver disease for every one transplanted. In addition, those parts of the world with the highest incidence of liver disease have limited access to transplantation. Patients with end-stage liver disease have a number of symptoms and signs, and a few

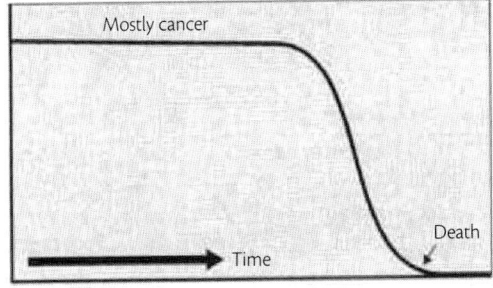

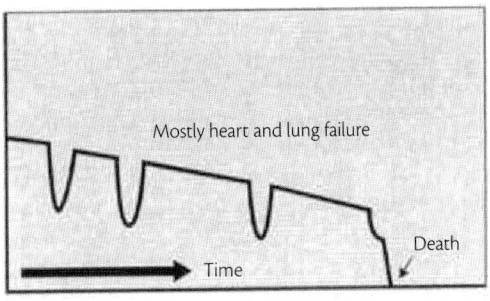

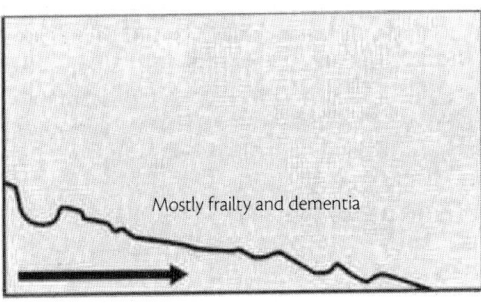

Figure 12.1.3 Typical trajectories upon which services are developed.

patients may develop hepatocellular carcinoma. All patients will have ascites, jaundice, or encephalopathy as elements of their disease, with the majority of patients having all three during the last days of life. In the terminal stages, good symptomatic management is essential. Bleeding from varices in the oesophagus or stomach is the final cause of death in about one-third of those to die. There is a general consensus that optimal management plans for such patients and their families have not been adequately worked out by the staff looking after them, but a willingness to discuss this with palliative care colleagues is growing.

Dementia

Dementia is among the commonest conditions experienced by patients in nursing homes where care is given by a mix of registered nurses and nursing care assistants. The focus of care is the resident and little provision is made for support of relatives or for bereavement care. The culture in which patients are looked after in the nursing home is one of encouraging 'normalization' and this is clearly not always appropriate for every patient and in particular for those who are actively dying. It would seem that a great deal of work is required to be done in nursing homes before adequate palliative care for patients with dementia becomes the norm. It is likely that palliative care expertise in this important and challenging area will only be developed through collaboration between specialist services and with an initial focus in a specialist unit. This was certainly the only way cancer palliative care succeeded (see Chapter 14.1).

Stroke

Estimates of the number of people suffering from stroke and fatality rates vary significantly because of difficulties with recording the data. However, it is estimated that a typical health authority in England of 250 000 may expect 500 new strokes and 1000 recurrent strokes each year. In such an area, it would be expected that 1500 survivors of stroke would be living in the community, half of whom will have significant disability. Twelve per cent of stroke survivors will be admitted to institutional care within a year[93]. While it is difficult to get accurate figures of the numbers of people with strokes for whom palliative care may be appropriate (not least because of the lack of clarity about the role of palliative care in stroke), it can be concluded that approximately one-third of people having a stroke will have died within 2 years. Studies of prognostic indicators suggest people living with stroke but with poor prospects of functional recovery will have major medical, health-related, and social needs[94]. Patients with poor prognosis stroke will have a range of problems including communication difficulties, feeding, terminal care, and bereavement support. Stroke survivors living in the community, but functionally dependent on others, are likely to be concerned with coping with ongoing uncertainty and disability, incontinence, post-stroke pain, and depression. Their informal carers may need respite care. Clearly, patients with stroke raise difficult end-of-life dilemmas as well as other problems and there is no doubt that these are areas in which specialist palliative care has expertise. Research, however, into the needs of patients with stroke is surprisingly lacking.

HIV disease

Therapeutic advances have had enormous impact on the clinical course of HIV infection. When HIV/AIDS first emerged, it was a disease characterized by peaks and troughs. As immunity gradually faded, patients repeatedly faced life-threatening crises from successive, variably treatable opportunistic infections and malignancies, as part of a fairly rapid terminal phase. Initially, HIV was regarded as an infection and, therefore, curable, until with time it became obvious that all patients eventually died and palliation was, in fact, necessary. Control of symptoms and complications evolved and then with the introduction of anti-retroviral treatments, the possibility of disease control was seen. However, it was not until the latter part of the 1990s, when combination therapies of reverse transcriptase and protease inhibitors and improved prophylactics were introduced, that we saw the most dramatic change in HIV management. It was then that survival increased dramatically and inpatient bed use declined[95]. Clinicians and patients are now able to expect a longer term of survival with some centres now seeing HIV as a predominantly outpatient problem. Sadly, however, drug resistance will become more of a problem and as treatment fails, the need for greater palliative care input may change once again. In general, however, those who currently are in need of palliation are the late presenters who are usually those with the most complex social circumstances involving not just themselves but other family members. HIV/AIDS is a good example of how a disease process can fluctuate with time, how palliative care physicians need to work with HIV specialists, and how adaptability of the service must be in-built to cope with fluctuation.

Clearly, the situation in the developing world with HIV/AIDS—in particular Central and Southern Africa—is very different, with the only treatment being care, and palliation is obviously a pressing need. As in other chronic progressive diseases, maintaining quality of life with the minimum symptomatic load is essential for patients living with uncertainty and any symptom issues highlighted in studies are around pain[96,97]. Other symptoms include breathlessness, nausea, gastrointestinal disturbance, fatigue, and weight loss. However, there are some major differences between HIV/AIDS and other chronic progressive diseases, particularly the need for vigilance around reversible or treatable conditions.

Chronic non-malignant painful conditions such as sickle cell disease

It is estimated that the number of patients in the United Kingdom with sickle cell disease is more than 10 000[98]. The median life expectancy for men and women with homozygous sickle cell anaemia in the United States is 42 and 48 years, respectively[99]. The most common causes of death from sickle cell disease are pulmonary complications, cerebrovascular accidents, causes related to infection, acute splenic sequestration, and chronic organ damage and failure[99,100]. In patients over 20 years old, more frequent (more than three per year) episodes of painful crisis are associated with an increased mortality[101]. In the cooperative study of sickle cell disease, only 18 per cent of deaths were in patients with chronically obvious organ failure such as renal failure, congestive heart failure, or chronic stroke. Thirty-three per cent of patients died acutely during a sickle crisis, most commonly a pain crisis, acute chest syndrome, or acute stroke[99]. A cooperative study of sickle cell disease also reported that only 5.2 per cent of patients with sickle cell disease experienced 3–10 episodes of pain each year. From these data we could say that, while specialist palliative care based on symptom control would be required for a relatively small number of patients, many more patients would benefit from a palliative care approach to a varying extent at different points in their illness. The use of opioid analgesia in the management of pain due to sickle cell disease is worth a special mention. There is an incorrect perception that significant numbers of patients with sickle cell disease and pain are addicted to drugs such as pethidine and morphine. It has been reported that 9 per cent of American haematologists and 22 per cent of Emergency Department physicians thought that more than 50 per cent of adult sickle cell patients were addicted to strong opioids[102]. There are numerous other studies that agree with such findings. While the palliative care needs of sickle cell patients have not been clearly defined, there is undoubtedly a subgroup with a poor prognosis and frequent pain crises who would benefit from specialist palliative care involvement. Well-conducted research with this group of patients would be very beneficial.

Chronic non-malignant gastrointestinal pathologies

There is a group of patients who not uncommonly come to the attention of specialist palliative care services when it is felt that nothing else can be done. This includes patients with a history of inflammatory bowel disease, which is not necessarily currently active, motility disorders either inherited or acquired, patients with chronic complications of surgery, and rare diseases such as porphyria. They are not uncommonly labelled as difficult personalities with opioid dependence and often have a background of chronic pathology that has been perceived as being cured or quiescent. This group of patients suffers from great physical and non-physical morbidity, spends much time in hospital, or in their general practitioner's surgery/office, and is often incapacitated from the point of view of working and leading any sort of normal life. They are traditionally not well-dealt with by any of the usual services available. They constitute a group of patients who may benefit from specialist palliative care involvement in parallel with their standard medical care for a limited period of time. Further exploration of this area is needed.

Other patient groups and care settings

It has long been recognized that care of the elderly and palliative care have many features in common. As demonstrated in Chapter 14.2, though relatively few patients in a care-of-the-elderly unit have malignant disease many need palliative care, which can usually be provided by the staff of the unit, though occasionally, a palliative medicine specialist may be needed.

Though few would normally speak of palliative care and intensive care in the same breath, there is a place for the principles of palliative care in an intensive care unit as Cohen and Prendergast explain in Chapter 12.7.

Summary

The myriad palliative care needs of non-cancer patients have been outlined with a particular focus on patients with CCF and COPD. Barriers to the extension of specialist palliative care services to non-cancer patients exist. The challenge for palliative care services is to overcome these barriers and develop flexible and integrated models of care that are responsive to the unmet needs of these patients. Specialist palliative care services no longer have the monopoly on multi-disciplinary holistic care. Increasingly, specialist providers are providing coordinated holistic care. Despite such holistic care,

there is evidence that acute specialists are reluctant to address end-of-life issues. How can specialist palliative care services blend with existing services to ensure quality of end–of-life care? Recognition by all involved of a transition point where the focus of care should be palliative is important. A collaborative research programme between specialist palliative care providers and specific care input or general input (e.g. cardiologists and general practitioners) continues to be necessary to improve understanding of what are the main areas of care which need specialist palliative care input or general input. In addition, models of care clearly need evaluation.

Conclusions

Some of the strong messages from the spectrum of non-cancer/chronic disease categories discussed in this chapter are:

◆ The spectrum of problems presented by chronic progressive, non-malignant disease is wide, with the intensity of physical, psychosocial, and spiritual suffering often as intense as in malignant disease.

◆ Clinicians already involved in the care of these patients are all highly trained and skilled in the diagnosis and various aspects of the management of these diseases. They recognize the need for high-quality palliative care, many already working with Clinical Nurse Specialists and other professionals with specialist expertise in these areas.

◆ No palliative care professional can have knowledge to a specialist level in even one of these areas, let alone several. They can, however, help to make more widely known, and encourage the adoption of, the principles of palliative care.

◆ There appears to be a lack of evidence of systematic communication between palliative medicine as a specialty and the different specialties managing the diseases above. Palliative care needs assessments should be conducted jointly with various specialties.

◆ Not surprisingly, there is a lack of research evidence into specific areas of symptom control in the various progressive non-malignant diseases and research into potential best models for looking after such patients in a compassionate and knowledgeable way.

◆ The key areas that will benefit from specialist palliative care input, along with those which need general palliative care input need to be identified in the same way that they have been identified for patients with cancer.

It is evident that to avoid mistakes and to do our best for patients and families with a range of chronic, non-malignant disease, each with a very different disease trajectory, we need to go back to communication. We have useful glimpses of patient needs and more experience in some areas, for example, ALS. We need to set up a dialogue with the various specialties about how we can best explore a partnership to help with the optimization of patient care at every point during their illness and care for some patients as required at certain points in their illness. Clearly combined research is fundamental to taking this important area forward. For that, as for any research, funding will be needed and for that to be made available there will need to be a greater appreciation and agreement of the need for the principles of palliative care to be applied to non-malignant disease.

References

1. Hinton, J. (1963). The physical and mental distress of the dying. *Quarterly Journal of Medicine*, **32**, 1–21.

2. Medical Research Council. (2000). *A Framework for Development and Evaluation of RCTs for Complex Interventions to Improve Health.* London: MRC.

3. Booth, S. (2008). Abstract COMPASS Scientific Meeting, Edinburgh.

4. Hinton, J.M. (1963). The physical and mental distress of the dying. *Quarterly Journal of Medicine NS*, **32**, 1–20.

5. Saunders, C. and Baines, M. (1996). *Living with dying: the management of terminal disease.* Oxford: Oxford University Press.

6. Stevens, A. and Gillam, S. (1998). Needs Assessment: from theory to practice. *British Medical Journal*, **316**, 1448–52.

7. Stevens, A. and Gabbay, J. (1991). Need assessments needs assessment. *Health Trends*, **23**, 1, 20–3.

8. Scottish Partnership for Palliative Care. (2006). *Joined Up Thinking Joined Up Care.* Increasing access to palliative care for people with life-threatening conditions other than cancer.

9. Murray, C.J.L. and Lopez, A.D. (1997). Alternative projections of mortality and disability by causes 1990-2020: Global burden of disease study. *Lancet*, **349**, 1498–1504.

10. Ward, C. (2002). The need for palliative care in the management of heart failure. *Heart*, **87**, 294–8.

11. Connors, A.F. Jr., Dawson, N.V., Thomas, C. *et al.* (1996). Outcomes following acute exacerbation of severe chronic obstructive lung disease. The SUPPORT investigators (Study to Understand Prognoses and Preferences for Outcomes and Risks of Treatments). *American Journal Respiratory and Critical Care Medicine*, **154**, 959–67.

12. Engstrom, C.P., Persson, L.O., Larsson, S. *et al.* (2001). Health related quality of life in COPD: why both disease-specific and generic measures should be used. *European Respiratory Journal*, **18**, 69–76.

13. Pauwel, R. (2001). Global initiative for chronic obstructive lung disease (GOLD): time to ace. *European Respiratory Journal*, **18**(6), 901–2.

14. Oliver, D. and Webb, S. (2000). The involvement of specialist palliative care in the care of people with motor neuron disease. *Palliative Medicine*, **14**(5), 427–8.

15. O'Brien, T., Kelly, M., and Saunders, C. (1992). Motor neuron disease: a hospice perspective. *British Medical Journal*, **304**, 471–3.

16. Task force of the working group on heart failure of the European Society of Cardiology. (1997). The treatment of heart failure. *European Heart Journal*, **18**, 736–53.

17. Rich, M.W. (1997). Epidemiology, pathophysiology and aetiology of CHF in older adults. *Journal of the American Geriatric Society*, **45**, 968–74.

18. Cowie, M.R., Mostard, A., Wood, D.A. *et al.* (1997). The epidemiology of heart failure. *European Heart Journal*, **18**(2), 208–25.

19. Selman, L., Harding, R., Beynon, T. *et al.* (2007). Improving end of life care for chronic heart failure patients. *British Medical Journal.*

20. Addington-Hall, J.M. and McCarthy, M. (1995). The regional study of care for the dying: methods and sample characteristics. *Palliative Medicine*, **9**, 27–35.

21. Lynn, J., Harrell, F., Cohn, F. *et al.* (1997). Prognoses of seriously ill hospitalized patients on the days before death: implications for patient care and public policy. *New Horizon*, **5**, 56–61.

22. McCarthy, M., Lay, M., Addington–Hall, J. (1996). Dying from heart disease. *Journal of the Royal College of Physicians, London*, **30**, 325–8.

23. Tang, S.T., Liu, T.W., Lai, L.N. *et al.* (2005). Concordance of preferences for end of life care between terminally ill cancer patients and their family caregivers in Taiwan. *Journal of Pain and Symptom Management*, **30**(6), 510–8.

24. Levenson, J.W., McCarthy, E.P., Lynn, J. *et al.* (2000). The Last Six Months of Life for Patients with Congestive Heart Failure. *Journal of the American Geriatric Society*, **48**(5), S101–09.

25. Walke, L., Byers, A.L., McCorkle, R. *et al.* (2006). Symptom Assessment in Community-Dwelling Older Adults with Advanced Chronic Disease. *Journal of Pain and Symptom Management*, **31**(1), 31–7.

26. Barnes, S., Gott, M., Payne, S. *et al.* (2006). Prevalence of symptoms in a community based sample of heart failure patients. *Journal of Pain and Symptom Management*, **32**(3), 208–16.

27. Nodgren, L. and Sorensen, S. (2003). Symptoms experienced in the last six months of life in patients with end stage heart failure. *European Journal of Cardiovascular Nursing*, **2**, 213–7.

28. Mayou, R.J., Blackwood, R., Bryant, B. *et al.* (1991). Cardiac failure: symptoms and functional status. *Psychosomatic Research*, **35**(4/5), 399–407.

29. Nekolaichuk, C.L., Bruera, E., Spachynski, K. *et al.* (1999). A comparison of patient and proxy symptom assessments in advanced cancer patients. *Palliative Medicine*, **4**, 311–23.

30. Zambroski, C.H., Moser, D.K., Bhat, G. *et al.* (2005). Impact of symptom prevalence and symptom burden on quality of life in patients with heart failure. *European Journal of Cardiovascular Nursing*, **4**, 198–206.

31. Solan, J.P., Gomes, B., Higginson, I.J. (2006). A comparison of symptom prevalence in far advanced cancer, AIDS, heart disease, chronic obstructive pulmonary disease and renal disease. *Journal of Pain and Symptom Management*, **1**, 58–69.

32. Horne, G. and Payne, S. (2004). Removing the boundaries: palliative care for patients with heart failure. *Palliative Medicine*, **18**, 291–6.

33. Krumholz, H.M., Phillips, R.S., Hamel, M.B. *et al.* (1998). Resuscitation preferences among patients with severe congestive heart failure: results from the SUPPORT project. Study to Understand Prognoses and Preferences for Outcomes and Risks of Treatments. *Circulation*, **98**(7), 648–55.

34. Willems, D.L., Hak, A., Visser, F. *et al.* (2006). Patient work in end stage heart failure: a prospective longitudinal multiple care study. *Palliative Medicine*, **1**, 25–33.

35. Freedland, K.E., Rich, M.W., Skala, J.A. *et al.* (2003). Prevalence of depression in hospitalised patients with congestive heart failure. *Psychosomatic Medicine*, **1**, 119–28.

36. Martensson, J., Dracup, K., Canary, C. *et al.* (2003). Living with heart failure: depression and quality of life in patients and spouses. *Journal of Heart and Lung Transplantation*, **4**, 460–7.

37. Gottlieb, S.S., Khatta, M., Friedmann, E. *et al.* (2004). The influence of age, gender and race on the prevalence of depression in heart failure patients. *Journal of the American College of Cardiologists*, **43**(9), 1542–9.

38. Murray, S.A., Boyd, K., Kendall, M. *et al.* (2002). Dying from lung cancer or cardiac failure: prospective qualitative interview study of patients and their carers in the community. *British Medical Journal*, **325**, 929–32.

39. Boyd, K.J., Murray, S.A., Kendall, M. *et al.* (2004). Living with advanced heart failure: a prospective, community based study of patients and their carers. *European Journal of Heart Failure*, **5**, 585–91.

40. Holland, R., Battersby, J., Harvey, I. *et al.* (2005). Systematic review of multi-disciplinary intervention in heart failure. *Heart*, **91**, 899–906.

41. Rogers, A.E., Addington-Hall, J.M., Abery, A.J. *et al.* (2000). Knowledge and communication difficulties for patients with chronic heart failure: qualitative study. *British Medical Journal*, **321**, 605–7.

42. Willems, D.L., Hak, A., Visser, F. *et al.* (2004). Thoughts of patients with advanced heart failure in dying. *Palliative Medicine*, **18**, 564–72.

43. Goldstein, N.E., Lampert, R., Bradley, E. *et al.* (2004). Management of implantable cardioverter defibrillators in end of life care. *Annals of Internal Medicine*, **141**, 835–8.

44. Formiga, F., Chivite, D., Ortega, C. *et al.* (2004). End of life preferences in elderly patients admitted for heart failure. *Quarterly Journal of Medicine*, **97**, 8803–8.

45. Lynn, J., Teno, J.M., Phillips, R.S. *et al.* (1997). Perceptions by family members of the dying experience of older and seriously ill patients. *Annals of Internal Medicine*, **126**, 97–106.

46. Connors, A.F. Jr, Dawson, N.V., Thomas, C. *et al.* (1996). Outcomes following acute exacerbation of severe chronic obstructive lung disease. The SUPPORT investigators (Study to Understand Prognoses and Preferences for Outcomes and Risks of Treatments). *American Journal of Respiratory Care Medicine*, **154**, 959–67.

47. SUPPORT principal investigators. (1995). A controlled trial to improve care for seriously ill hospitalized patients. (Study to Understand Prognoses and Preferences for Outcomes and Risks of Treatments) *Journal of the American Medical Association*, **274**, 1591–8.

48. Claessens, M.T., Lynn, J., Zhong, Z. *et al.* (2000). Dying with lung cancer or chronic obstructive pulmonary disease, insights from SUPPORT. *Journal of the American Geriatric Society*, **48**, S146–S153.

49. Edmonds, P., Karlsen, S., Addington-Hall, J. (2001). Palliative care needs of hospital inpatients. *Palliative Medicine*, **14**, 227–8.

50. Booth, S., Silvester, S., and Todd, C. (2003). Breathlessness in cancer and chronic obstructive pulmonary disease: Using a qualitative approach to describe the experience of patients and carers. *Palliative Support Care*, **1**, 337–44.

51. Seamark, D.A., Blake, S.D., Seamark, C.J. *et al.* (2004). Living with severe chronic obstructive pulmonary disease (COPD): perceptions of patients and their carers. An interpretative phenomenological analysis. *Palliative Medicine*, **18**, 619–25.

52. Bredin, M., Corner, J. *et al.* (1999). Multi-centre randomised controlled trial of nursing intervention for breathlessness in patients with lung cancer. *British Medical Journal*, **318**, 901–4.

53. Bailey, P.H. (2004). The dyspnoea-anxiety-dyspnoea cycle. COPD patients' stories of breathlessness: It's scary when you can't breathe. *Quality Health Research*, **14**(6), 760–8.

54. Elkington, H., White, P., Addington-Hall, J.M. *et al.* (2004). The last year of life of COPD; a qualitative study of symptoms and services. *Respiratory Medicine*, **98**, 439–45.

55. Shee, C.D. (1995). Palliation in chronic respiratory disease. *Palliative Medicine*, **9**, 3–12.

56. Skilbeck, J., Mott, L., Page, H. *et al.* (1998). Palliative care in chronic obstructive airways disease: a needs assessment. *Palliative Medicine*, **12**, 245–54.

57. Elkington, H., White, P., Addington-Hall, J.M. *et al.* (2005). The healthcare needs of chronic obstructive pulmonary disease patients in the last year of life. *Palliative Medicine*, **19**, 485–91.

58. Lynn, J., Ely, E.W., Zhong, Z. *et al.* (2000). Living and dying with chronic obstructive pulmonary disease. *Journal of the American Geriatric Society*, **48**, S91–S100.

59. Gore, J.M., Brophy, C.J., and Greenstone, M.A. (2000). How well do we care for patients with end stage chronic obstructive pulmonary disease (COPD)? A comparision of palliative care and quality of life in COPD and lung cancer. *Thorax*, **55**, 1000–6.

60. Guthrie, S.J., Hill, K.M., Muers, M.F. (2001). Living with severe COPD. A qualitative exploration of the experience of patients in Leeds. *Respiratory Medicine*, **95**, 196–204.

61. van Ede, L., Yzermans, C.J., and Brouwer, H.J. (1999), Prevalence of depression in patients with chronic obstructive pulmonary disease: a systematic review. *Thorax*, **54**, 688–92.

62. Kim, H.F., Kunik, M.E., Molinari, *et al.* (2000). Functional impairment in COPD patients: the impact of anxiety and depression. *Psychosomatics*, **41**(6), 465–71.

63. Stage, K.B., Middelboe, T., and Pisinger, C. (2005). Depression and chronic obstructive pulmonary disease (COPD). Impact on survival. *Acta Psychiatrica Scandinavica*, **111**(4), 320–3.

64. Stapleton, R.D., Nielson, E.l., Engelberg, R.A. *et al.* (2005). Association of depression and life sustaining treatment preferences in patients with COPD. *Chest*, **127**, 328–34.

65. Curtis, J.R., Engelberg, R.A., Nielsen, E.L. *et al.* (2004). Patient-physician communication about end of life care for patients with severe COPD. *European Respiratory Journal*, **24**, 200–5.

66. Borson, S., McDonald, G.J., Gayle, T. *et al.* (1992). Improvement in mood, physical symptoms and function with nortriptyline for depression in patients with chronic obstructive pulmonary disease. *Psychosomatics*, **33**(2), 190–201.

67. Manning, H.L. (2000). Dyspnoea treatment. *Respiratory Care*, **45**, 1342–50; discussion 1350–54.

68. Mulcahy, P., Buetow, S., Osman, L. *et al.* (2005). GPs' attitudes to discussing prognosis in severe COPD: an Auckland (NZ) to London(UK) comparison. *Family Practice*, **22**, 538–40.

69. Heffner, J.E., Fahry, B., Hilling, L. *et al.* (1997). Attitudes regarding advance directives among patients in pulmonary rehabilitation. *American Journal of Respiratory and Critical Care Medicine*, **155**, 1735–40.

70. Heffner, J.E., Fahry, B., Hilling, L. *et al.* (1996). Attitudes regarding advance directives among patients in pulmonary rehabilitation *American Journal of Respiratory and Critical Care Medicine*, **154**, 1735–40.

71. Jones, I., Kirby, A., Ormiston, P. *et al.* (2004). The needs of patients dying of chronic obstructive pulmonary disease in the community. *Family Practice*, **21**, 310–3.

72. Knauft, E., Nielsen, E., Engelberg, R.A. *et al.* Barriers and facilitators to end of life care communication for patients with COPD. *Chest*, **127**, 2188–96.

73. Sullivan, K.E., Hebert, P.C., Logan, J. *et al.* (1996). What do physicians tell patients with end stage COPD about intubation and mechanical ventilation? *Chest*, **109**(1), 258–64.

74. Danis, M., Patrick, D.L., Southerland, L.I. *et al.* (1988). Patients' and families' preferences for medical intensive care. *Journal of the American Medical Association*, **260**(6), 797–802.

75. World Health Organization. (2004). *The Solid Facts Palliative Care.* Eds E. Davies and I.J. Higginson.

76. Recommendation Rec. (2003). 24 of the Committee of Ministers to member states on the organisation of palliative care. Council of Europe.

77. Wagner, E.H. (2001). Meeting the needs of chronically ill people. *British Medical Journal*, **323**, 945–6.

78. Selecky, P.A., Eliasson, C.A., Hall, R.I. *et al.* (2005). Palliative and end of life care for patients with cardiopulmonary diseases: American College of Chest Physicians position statement. *Chest*, **128**, 3599–610.

79. NICE. (2004). www.nice.org.uk/CG12.

80. NICE. (2003). www.nice.org.uk/CG5.

81. British Thoracic Society. (1997). www.britthoracic.org.uk/guidelines_since_1997.html.

82. GOLD. (2003). GOLD Workshop Report, Global strategy for diagnosis, management and prevention of COPD. www.goldcopd.com.

83. Addington-Hall, J.M., Fakhoury, W., and McCarthy, M. (1998). Specialist palliative care in non-malignant disease. *Palliative Medicine*, **12**, 417–27.

84. Field, D. and Addington-Hall, J.M. (1999). Extending specialist palliative care to all? *Social Science and Medicine*, **48**, 1271–80.

85. Addington-Hall, J.M. (1998). Reaching Out: Specialist Palliative Care for Adults with Non-malignant Disease. The National Council for Palliative Care.

86. Hanratty, B., Hibbert, D., and Mair, F. (2002). Doctors' perceptions of palliative care for heart failure: focus group study. *British Medical Journal*, **325**, 581–5.

87. Addington-Hall, J.M. and Higginson, I.J. (2001). *Palliative Care for Non-Cancer Patients.* OUP.

88. Addington-Hall, J.M. and Karlsen, S. (2005). A national survey of health professionals and volunteers working in voluntary hospice services in the UK. 1. Attitudes to current issues affecting hospices and palliative care. *Palliative Medicine*, **19**(1), 40–8.

89. Gott, M., Barnes, S., Parker, C. *et al.* (2007). Dying trajectories in heart failure. *Palliative Medicine*, **21**, 95–9.

90. Lunney, J.R., Lynn, J., and Hogan, C. (2002). Profiles of older Medicare decedents. *Journal of the American Geriatric Society*, **50**(6), 1108–12.

91. Glaser, B.G. and Strauss, A.L. (1981). Time for Dying Aldine 1968. Sentimental work in the technologised hospital. *Sov Health Illn*, **4**, 254–78.

92. United States Renal Data System 1998 Annual Report. (1998). The Excerpts. *American Journal of Kidney Diseases*, **32**(2), 51–213.

93. Effective Health Care Bulletin. (1992). *Stroke Rehabilitation*. Leeds: University of Leeds,.

94. Kwakkel, G. *et al.* (1996). Predicting disability in stroke—a critical review of the literature. *Age and Ageing*, **25**, 479–89.

95. Aalen, O. *et al.* (1999). New therapy explains the fall in AIDS incidence with a substantial rise in number of persons on treatment expected. *AIDS*, **13**, 103–8.

96. Breitbart, W. (1996). Pain management and psychosocial issues in HIV and AIDS. *The American Journal of Hospice and Palliative Care*, January/February, 21–9.

97. Hewitt, D. *et al.* (1997). Pain syndromes and aetiologies in ambulatory AIDS patients. *Pain*, **70**, 117–23.

98. Streetly, A., Maxwell, K., and Mejia, A. (1997). Sickle Cell Disorders in Greater London: A Needs Assessment of Screening and Care Services. London: Bexley and Greenwich Health Authority.

99. Platt, O.S. *et al.* (1994). Mortality in sickle cell disease. Life expectancy and risk factors for early death. *New England Journal of Medicine*, **330**, 1639–44.

100. Gray, A. *et al.* (1991). Patterns of mortality in sickle cell disease in the UK. *Journal of Clinical Pathology*, **44**, 459–63.

101. Platt, O.S. *et al.* (1991). Pain in sickle cell disease: rates and risk factors. *New England Journal of Medicine*, **325**, 11–16.

102. Shapiro, B.S. *et al.* (1997). Sickle cell related pain: perceptions of medical practitioners. *Journal of Pain and Symptom Management*, **14**(3), 168–74.

HIV/AIDS in adults

Roger Woodruff and David Cameron

The natural history of infection with the human immunodeficiency virus (HIV) is that it evolves over a period of years into the acquired immune deficiency syndrome (AIDS)[1]. More than 25 million people have died of HIV/AIDS in the 25 years since the syndrome was first described in 1981[2]. The estimates made by the Joint United Nations Programme on HIV/AIDS[3] demonstrate the enormity of the HIV/AIDS pandemic, reflecting mortality and morbidity of catastrophic proportions (Table 12.2.1)[3].

In developed countries, the introduction of effective anti-retroviral therapy during the 1990s led to a reduction in both the incidence and mortality of AIDS[4]. But in less developed countries, where 95% of the world's HIV-infected people live, the epidemic is having devastating effects. Anti-retroviral therapy has recently become available although it is estimated that only one-fifth of the people who need it have access to it[5]. The life expectancy of patients in these countries is less than those in developed countries and there are noticeable effects on national life expectancies and economic productivity[3].

The first part of this chapter describes the clinical features of HIV infection and AIDS, and the opportunistic infections and malignancies with which they are associated, followed by a section outlining the treatment of pain and common symptoms. The final section deals with the role of palliative care in the management of HIV/AIDS, including the differences in delivering palliative care to patients with HIV/AIDS compared with diseases like cancer, the evolving interface between HIV medicine and palliative care, and the provision of appropriate palliative care for patients with advanced disease. The specifics of the treatments for HIV infection, the opportunistic infections and the AIDS-related cancers are not detailed here as it is assumed a palliative care specialist would be working in collaboration with specialists in HIV medicine, infectious diseases and oncology.

HIV infection and AIDS

Epidemiology

HIV infection is transmitted by sexual contact, by exposure to infected blood or blood products, body fluids or tissue, and by perinatal transmission from mother to child[1]. HIV infection was first reported in 1981 in male homosexuals, but it soon became apparent that the disease was also occurring in injecting drug users (IDUs), in haemophiliacs, and other patients who had received infected blood or blood products, and in children born to women with the disease.

In developed countries, the majority of patients with HIV infection have been either male homosexuals or IDUs and these groups represent the majority of the people living with HIV infection. There has been a gradual increase in the incidence of HIV infection attributed to heterosexual activity and data from the UK showed that heterosexual contact was the most frequent probable route of infection in 2000, although it was noted that the majority of these infections were contracted outside the UK, mainly in Africa.

The incidence of new cases of AIDS in developed countries began to fall in the early 1990s as a result of previously instituted public health policies and public education. The introduction of effective anti-retroviral therapy in the mid-1990s led to a dramatic fall in both the incidence and mortality of AIDS (Fig. 12.2.1). However, data from the UK show an increasing incidence of new HIV infection over the last few years, which has been attributed to an increase in unsafe behaviours in the high-risk groups (male homosexuals and IDUs) and to increasing spread to the heterosexual population[6].

It is in less-developed countries that the HIV/AIDS epidemic has reached alarming proportions. In sub-Saharan Africa, the Caribbean and areas of South America, the disease is now transmitted primarily by heterosexual contact and there are increasing signs of similar changes in Asia. The situation is worst in some African countries where tuberculosis is endemic and there are high rates of co-infection[3]. In an attempt to provide care for the large numbers of patients in resource-poor settings, WHO have proposed a public-health approach to the management of HIV/AIDS[7].

Pathogenesis

HIV is a retrovirus, with a genome made up exclusively of RNA[1]. Following introduction into the body, the virus binds to the CD4 surface receptors on CD4-positive T-lymphocytes and to a lesser extent on monocytes and macrophages. After gaining access to the cell, the enzyme reverse transcriptase produces a double-stranded

Table 12.2.1 UNAIDS estimates of the HIV/AIDS epidemic *(in millions)*.

	1995	2000	2005
People newly infected with HIV in previous year	4.7	5.3	4.9
Total number of people living with HIV	15	36.1	40.3
Deaths from HIV/AIDS in previous year	1.0	2.1	3.1

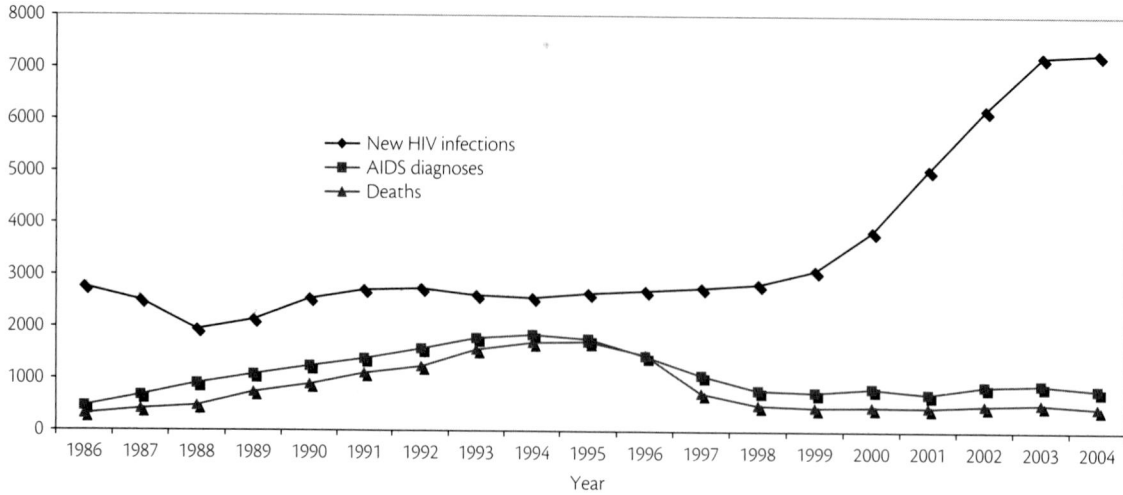

Figure 12.2.1 New HIV and AIDS diagnoses and deaths (UK data [6]).

DNA replica of the original RNA genome, which is then incorporated in the host cell genome. Activation of this material leads to production by the cell of large amounts of viral RNA, which is then processed to produce complete virus particles; HIV-derived protease is an important enzyme in this assembly process. Virions produced bud from the surface of the host cell and repeat the retroviral life cycle by infecting other CD4-positive cells.

CD4-positive T-lymphocytes serve as both essential regulators and effectors of the normal immune response. HIV infection leads to a progressive depletion of these cells, resulting in the progressive immunodeficiency that characterizes the disease.

Natural history

The natural history of HIV infection, without anti-retroviral therapy, is that it progresses to AIDS and death over a period of about 10 years. However, there is considerable individual variation with a few individuals dying of AIDS within months of the initial infection, whilst a few remain alive and well with only mild immunodeficiency more than 10 years after the initial infection. There are no significant differences in the rate of disease progression or survival associated with sex, race, injection drug use, or other exposure category. The differences in survival between developed and less-developed countries relate to other factors including nutrition, the availability of antibiotics to treat and prevent opportunistic infections, co-infection with tuberculosis, and the availability of anti-retroviral therapy[3].

Phases of HIV infection

There is no universally accepted clinical staging system for HIV/AIDS. The different phases of the disease were originally shown to parallel the degree of immunodeficiency as measured by the numbers of CD4-positive T-lymphocytes (CD4) in the blood (Fig. 12.2.2). However, there are no sharp dividing lines and the different phases form part of a clinical continuum. The more recently introduced measurements of plasma HIV RNA or viral load have been shown to provide a more accurate assessment of disease progression and response to therapy. In general, plasma HIV RNA levels increase as the CD4 counts decrease, and the prognosis is most accurately defined using both the plasma HIV RNA and the CD4 count together. High RNA titres predict rapid disease progression, whatever the CD4 count. The plasma HIV RNA levels are reported to be lower in women and perhaps in other groups,

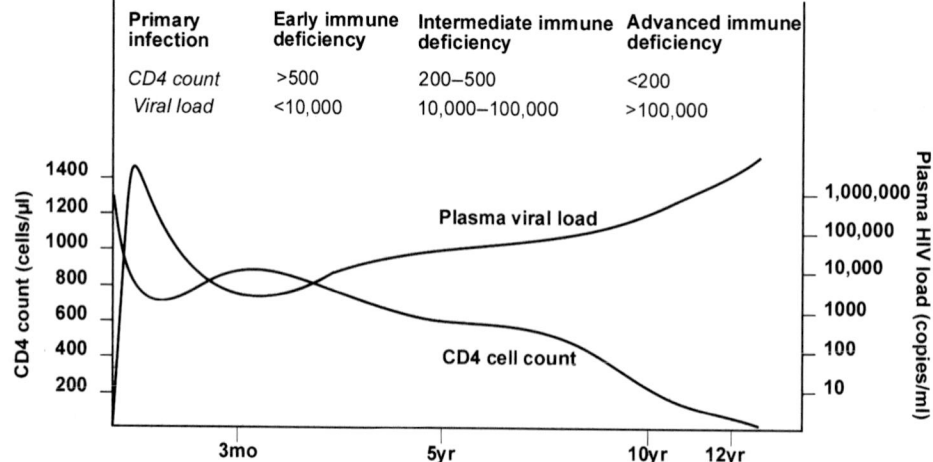

Figure 12.2.2 Schematic representation of the natural history of HIV infection.

Table 12.2.2 AIDS-defining conditions.

Candidiasis (oesophageal, tracheobronchial or pulmonary)

Cervical cancer, invasive

Coccidioidomycosis (disseminated or extrapulmonary)

Cryptococcosis (extrapulmonary)

Cryptosporidiosis (>1 month)

Cytomegalovirus (retinitis, or other than liver, spleen, nodes)

Encephalopathy, HIV-related

Herpes simplex (ulceration >1 month, or oesophageal, pulmonary)

Histoplasmosis (disseminated or extrapulmonary)

Isosporiasis (>1 month)

Kaposi's sarcoma

Lymphoma (systemic or primary cerebral)

Mycobacterium tuberculosis, any site

Mycobacteria, other species (disseminated or extrapulmonary)

Pneumocystis carinii pneumonia

Salmonella septicaemia, recurrent

Toxoplasmosis, cerebral

Wasting syndrome due to AIDS

but this is not associated with differences in the rate of progression to AIDS or survival.

Primary infection

Acute infection is characterized by a glandular fever-like illness, which typically occurs 2–4 weeks after infection. Common manifestations include fever, fatigue, skin rash, myalgia, headache, pharyngitis, and lymphadenopathy. The illness usually lasts 10–14 days, following which there is return to normal clinical health.

Diagnosis is made by the detection of specific HIV proteins, serum antibodies to the proteins, or both. The development of assays to detect HIV-specific RNA in plasma, which is often detectable before the appearance of antibodies, has greatly facilitated the diagnostic process.

Early immune deficiency

The second phase lasts an average of 4–5 years and is often asymptomatic. Some patients will develop autoimmune-type illnesses such as immune thrombocytopenic purpura (ITP) or the Guillain–Barré syndrome and others develop persistent lymphadenopathy. Serial measurements during this phase show a gradual fall in CD4 lymphocyte count and a gradual rise in the HIV RNA titre.

Intermediate immune deficiency

The third or chronic symptomatic phase lasts an average of 4–5 years. During the first few years, the CD4 counts decline slowly and the HIV RNA titre continues to rise. The patients usually remain clinically well except for minor infections. Towards the end of this period, the CD4 lymphocyte counts decline more quickly and there is a parallel increase in the HIV RNA titres. More patients develop persistent lymphadenopathy and some develop AIDS-related malignancies. Anti-retroviral therapy is usually started during this period.

Advanced immune deficiency (AIDS)

The last phase or clinical AIDS may be defined by a CD4 lymphocyte count <200/μl or by the occurrence of AIDS-defining conditions as set out by the Centers for Disease Control and Prevention (CDC) in 1992[8] (Table 12.2.2). In a population of HIV-positive people, the CD4 count falls below 200/μl 1–2 years before AIDS-defining conditions develop, which has an obvious effect on the measurement of the survival of patients with AIDS. Prior to the use of anti-retroviral therapy, survival from the time the CD4 lymphocyte count was <200/μl was 2–3 years, but only 1 year after the first AIDS-defining condition.

Clinical course of AIDS

The clinical course of AIDS is characterized by the occurrence of opportunistic infections and AIDS-related constitutional symptoms (weight loss, fever, and diarrhoea). Some patients will develop AIDS-related malignancy or AIDS-related neurological disease. Anti-retroviral therapy is continued and prophylaxis against other infections started. Patients suffer increasingly frequent infections that may become less responsive to therapy and from which they recover progressively less well. Serial measurements will show a continuing decline in the CD4 lymphocyte count and a corresponding rise in the HIV RNA titre.

The clinical course of AIDS follows a fluctuating course, punctuated by opportunistic infections requiring acute therapy, and there is considerable individual variation. The clinical course of AIDS has also been changed since the introduction of effective combination anti-retroviral therapy. These factors complicate the timing and delivery of palliative care to these patients and underline the need for palliative care involvement long before the terminal phase, complementary to other medical care and not sequential to it. For patients who have failed anti-retroviral therapy, or never had the opportunity to have it, the clinical course of AIDS can be broadly grouped into four phases that show the gradual shift in the goals of treatment with progression of the disease[9] (Table 12.2.3).

Anti-retroviral therapy

Anti-retroviral therapy has had a profound impact on the clinical course of HIV infection and AIDS. Following the introduction of

Table 12.2.3 Clinical course of AIDS.

Early stage	Recent diagnosis of AIDS
	Good response to antiretroviral therapy and treatment of infections
	Normal activities, work
Progressive stage	Increasing number and frequency of infections
	Progressive weight loss, increasing fatigue
	Capable of partial activity, work
Advanced stage	Increasing or constant infections, with poor response to treatment
	Fatigue and debility seriously affect daily function
	Active treatment should be stopped and the goal of treatment shifted to comfort
Terminal stage	Totally dependent
	Death can be anticipated within days to a few months
	Care is entirely comfort orientated

zidovudine in the 1980s, a number of new drugs, of differing classes and mechanisms of action, have been developed (Table 12.2. 4)[1]. The major changes occurred in the mid-1990s when the very potent protease inhibitors and a growing list of reverse transcriptase inhibitors enabled the development of combination therapy with three or four drugs aimed at durable suppression of viral replication. These combinations are collectively known as highly active anti-retroviral therapy (HAART). The optimal use of these drugs—when they should be started and in what combination—remains the subject of on-going clinical research, and regularly updated expert recommendations are available on the internet[10]. Enfuvirtide, the first of a new class of fusion inhibitors that prevent viral attachment and entry into cells, has recently been introduced into clinical practice and the search for more effective drugs is on-going.

Effects

The introduction of HAART has transformed AIDS from an inevitably fatal condition to a chronic, manageable disease in some settings. Patients responding to HAART showed marked reduction in HIV RNA levels, often to undetectable levels, associated with increases in the CD4 count, often by several hundred cells/µl. This was associated with symptomatic improvement with increased appetite with weight gain as well as improved energy and well-being. This has translated into a prolongation of the time to the development of AIDS, and improved survival both after a diagnosis of AIDS and overall. The magnitude of the effect parallels the intensity of the anti-retroviral treatment, combination therapy being superior to monotherapy, and combination therapy that includes a protease inhibitor confers additional benefit.

There is a dramatic reduction in the incidence of opportunistic infections in patients taking HAART and patients with low or undetectable HIV RNA levels and significant and sustained increases in CD4 counts are able to safely stop prophylaxis for these infections.

Treatment with HAART produces noticeable effects on the neurological disease of AIDS. Successful therapy leads to a reduction in the incidence of AIDS dementia and there may be improvement in cognitive and neurological function, AIDS dementia and progressive multi-focal leucoencephalopathy (PML).

The pattern of AIDS-related malignancies has changed since the introduction of HAART[11]. There has been a marked decrease in the incidence of Kaposi's sarcoma and cerebral lymphoma, but not in the incidence of systemic non-Hodgkin's lymphoma, Hodgkin's disease, or cervical cancer.

The recovery of immune function following HAART may cause immune reconstitutions syndromes, caused by increased tissue inflammation directed against opportunistic infections or AIDS-related malignancies[12].

HAART has changed the pattern of HIV disease. Patients responding to HAART are less likely to have an opportunistic infection as the AIDS-defining illness and are more likely to have malignant lymphoma. Similarly, the cause of death is more likely to relate to malignancy or chronic organ failure rather than opportunistic infections[13]. However, a more recently published collaborative study of more than 20 000 patients treated with HAART showed that despite improved early virological response (plasma HIV load), there was no significant improvements in early immunological response (CD4 counts), and no significant reduction in AIDS and all-cause mortality; these apparently anomalous results may be attributable to the changing demographics of the population being treated or to co-morbidities such as tuberculosis[14].

Side effects

The side effects of HAART are considerable, and the majority of patients will suffer some adverse reaction[15]. The principal toxicities include mitochondrial toxicity, drug hypersensitivity, and lipodystrophy; numerous other side effects are recorded for individual drugs.

◆ Mitochondrial toxicity due to reverse transcriptase inhibitors includes myopathy, neuropathy, hepatic steatosis with lactic acidaemia, and pancreatitis.

◆ Drug hypersensitivity occurs much more frequently in patients with HIV/AIDS than the general population, and 10–20% of patients treated with amprenavir or a non-nucleoside reverse transcriptase inhibitor will develop a reaction. This is usually manifest as a morbilliform or maculopapular rash with fever, fatigue, myalgia, and mucosal ulceration.

The lipodystrophy syndrome consists of peripheral lipoatrophy from the face and limbs with central fat accumulation in the abdomen and over the lower cervical spine (the so-called 'buffalo hump'), associated with hypertriglyceridaemia, hypercholesterolaemia, insulin resistance, and type II diabetes mellitus.

There are a large number of potential drug interactions both between different anti-retroviral drugs and between anti-retroviral drugs and other medications and recreational drugs[16,17].

Small but significant numbers of patients fail to complete trials of HAART because of adverse events; others have difficulty with the complicated treatment regimens and adherence to HAART is often suboptimal[18]. Interventions to improve compliance have been reviewed[19].

Limitations

HAART is not curative and is not effective for all patients[1]. A small proportion of patients will show no virological (reduced plasma HIV RNA levels) or immunological (increased CD4 counts) response and their disease will progress to AIDS and death. There is evidence of drug resistance in a significant proportion of people newly infected with HIV, who are unlikely to benefit from currently available HAART. Other patients, particularly those with advanced disease at the time of starting drug therapy, may show a partial or transient response only, following which their disease

Table 12.2.4 Anti-retroviral therapy.

Reverse transcriptase inhibitors		Protease inhibitors
Nucleoside analogues	Non-nucleoside analogues	
Abacavir	Delavirdine	Amprenavir
Didanosine	Efavirenz	Atazanavir
Emtricitabine	Nevirapine	Darunavir
Lamivudine		Indinavir
Stavudine		Lopinavir
Tenofovir		Nelfinavir
Zalcitabine		Ritonavir
Zidovudine		Saquinavir
		Tipranavir

will progress. Even for patients who show an optimal response, viral rebound with increasing HIV RNA levels can occur within a year. Reservoirs of HIV can be detected in peripheral blood mononuclear cells and in lymphoid tissue of patients with undetectable plasma HIV RNA levels and discontinuation of HAART can lead to rebound of the plasma HIV RNA levels within weeks.

The other limitations of HAART are that it is expensive and that it is not available to the majority of people afflicted with HIV infection. Major clinical improvements have occurred in the 10 years since HAART was first introduced and it is to be hoped that continued research and development will result in therapy that is more effective and less toxic and, most importantly, affordable in developing countries where the great majority of people with HIV infection live.

HIV-associated infections

AIDS is characterized by the occurrence of multiple opportunist infections caused by a host of different pathogens. Expert recommendations, regularly updated and comprehensively referenced, regarding diagnosis, prophylaxis, and treatment are available on the internet[10,20].

Fungal infections

Pneumocystis carinii

Pneumocystis carinii pneumonia (PCP, but officially renamed Pneumocystis jiroveci pneumonia) occurred in about 85% of patients with AIDS before PCP prophylaxis became standard. PCP usually presents with fever, dry cough, and progressive dyspnoea occurring over several weeks. Examination may be unremarkable or show tachypnoea and dry rales. Chest X-ray usually shows bilateral, symmetrical perihilar interstitial infiltrates. Diagnosis is by demonstration of the organism in an induced sputum specimen or bronchial washings.

Treatment

Treatment is with trimethoprim/sulfamethoxazole (TMP-SMX), given orally for mild and intravenously for moderate or severe infection. This is effective in the majority of patients although side-effects are frequent. Some patients with severe infection will develop respiratory failure requiring mechanical ventilation and PCP still carries a significant mortality. Patients unable to take TMP-SMX or whose disease is unresponsive can be treated with trimethoprim/dapsone or pentamidine. Patients with PCP who are hypoxic should be treated with corticosteroids, started at the same time as anti-fungal therapy. This ameliorates or prevents the progressive hypoxia often seen 2–3 days after starting treatment and has been shown to significantly reduce both morbidity and mortality[21].

Prophylaxis

Primary prophylaxis against PCP is recommended for any patient with a CD4 count <200/µl. Standard therapy is with oral TMP-SMX. Patients unable to take this can be treated with dapsone or atovaquone. Aerosolized pentamidine is less effective than systemic therapy in preventing PCP and does not protect against extrapulmonary pneumocystis infections that may occur in patients with severe immunodeficiency. Indefinite secondary prophylaxis or maintenance therapy is required after infection with PCP, using the same medications as for primary prophylaxis. Patients treated with HAART with sustained CD4 counts >200/µl can safely discontinue primary or secondary PCP prophylaxis; patients relapsing from HAART should restart prophylaxis when the CD4 count is 200/µl.

Candidiasis

Candida frequently causes oropharyngeal, oesophageal, and vaginal infection, but dissemination may occur with advanced immunodeficiency. Oropharyngeal candidiasis produces characteristic white plaques or may appear as smooth erythematous patches on the palate and tongue; it may also cause angular cheilosis with fissuring and cracking at the corners of the mouth. Diagnosis of oropharyngeal and vaginal candidiasis is made on clinical grounds and microbiological studies. Oesophageal candidiasis causes odynophagia, dysphagia and substernal chest pain. The diagnosis is frequently made on clinical grounds, especially if there is oropharyngeal candidiasis; radiological studies and endoscopy are reserved for patients not responding to empiric therapy.

Treatment

Oropharyngeal infection is treated with topical therapy such as nystatin, amphotericin, or miconazole. Severe oral infection and oesophagitis are treated with fluconazole; itraconazole, and ketoconazole are alternatives[22]. Caspofungin may be an effective alternative for patients with refractory disease[23]. Uncomplicated vulvovaginal infection usually responds well to topical nystatin or miconazole; oral fluconazole, or itraconazole can be used for prolonged or repeated infections[24].

Prophylaxis

Prophylactic therapy for mucosal candidiasis is not usually recommended because of the effectiveness of treatment for acute disease. Daily or weekly fluconazole maintenance can be considered for patients with oesophageal candidiasis or recurrent mucosal infections not controlled with topical therapy.

Cryptococcosis

Infection with Cryptococcus neoformans characteristically causes meningitis; pneumonia, and skin infiltrates are the common extraneural lesions. Meningitis presents with fever and mild headache and meningeal signs are often absent. There may be focal neurological signs and seizures. The diagnosis is established by the demonstration of cryptococci or cryptococcal antigen in the CSF.

Treatment

Treatment is with amphotericin, with or without flucytosine, for 2 weeks, followed by fluconazole for 8–10 weeks.

Prophylaxis

Life-long secondary prophylaxis or maintenance therapy with fluconazole is required. Although not proven in prospective studies, it would seem reasonable to suspend prophylactic therapy in patients with sustained response (CD4 counts >200/µl) to HAART[25].

Other fungal infections

Histoplasmosis

Infection with Histoplasma capsulatum occurs frequently in areas where the infection is endemic, particularly the central USA, Central and South America. The clinical features are non-specific and include fever, weight loss and pneumonia. Diagnosis is made on bone marrow, liver, or lymph node biopsy or by culture of the organism from the blood, bone marrow, or sputum. Treatment is with itraconazole, which needs to be continued indefinitely. Patients presenting with a septicaemic or meningitic illness should initially be treated with amphotericin.

Coccidioidomycosis

Infection with *Coccidioides immitis* occurs in the endemic areas of Latin America and the south western USA. In AIDS patients, coccidioidomycosis presents with malaise, fever, weight loss and pneumonia. The diagnosis is established by demonstration of the organism in sputum or bronchial washings. Treatment is with amphotericin followed by indefinite maintenance therapy with itraconazole.

Penicilliosis

Infection with *Penicillium marneffei* is common in HIV-infected patients in Southeast Asia. It presents with fever, anaemia and weight loss; skin lesions resembling *Molluscum contagiosum* are common. The diagnosis is made by isolation of the organism from blood, skin lesions, or bone marrow. Treatment is with amphotericin followed by itraconazole, which needs to be continued indefinitely.

Aspergillosis

Infection with *Aspergillus* species usually occurs in patients with advanced disease and severe immunodeficiency. Pulmonary infection causes focal or bilateral infiltrates and there may be cavitation. Treatment is with amphotericin but the mortality is high.

Nocardiosis

Infection with *Nocardi* species may produce pneumonia, cerebral abscesses, or disseminated disease. It is treated with high doses of TMP-SMX similar to PCP, and continued TMP-SMX prophylaxis is required. The widespread use of TMP-SMX prophylaxis for Pneumocystis may explain the relative infrequency of Nocardia infections in patients with AIDS.

Protozoal infections

Toxoplasmosis

Infection with *Toxoplasma gondii* is common and in normal individuals causes either no symptoms or a mild illness with fever and lymphadenopathy. Reactivation and dissemination of infection in patients with AIDS usually causes encephalitis. Cerebral toxoplasmosis presents with fever, headache and focal neurological signs. Hemiparesis is the most common focal neurological sign and seizures are common. There may be an altered mental state with confusion and cognitive impairment, delusional behaviour, or psychosis; some patients present in coma. The clinical diagnosis is made on the basis of positive serology for toxoplasma and the characteristic CT scan appearance of multiple, bilateral hypodense lesions that show ring enhancement with contrast. The definitive diagnosis can only be made on brain biopsy, which is usually reserved for patients not responding to appropriate therapy and those with a solitary lesion.

Treatment

Active treatment is with pyrimethamine and either sulfadiazine or clindamycin[26].

Prophylaxis

Primary prophylaxis with TMP-SMX is recommended for patients with CD4 lymphocytes <100/µl who are seropositive for toxoplasma. Seronegative patients are advised to avoid undercooked or raw meat,

to ensure that all food is thoroughly washed and to avoid any direct contact with animal or human faeces. Indefinite secondary prophylaxis or maintenance therapy is required and the combination of pyrimethamine and sulfadiazine is probably superior to other regimens and also provides adequate prophylaxis against *Pneumocystis* infection. Patients having a sustained response to HAART with CD4 counts >200/µl can safely discontinue prophylaxis.

Cryptosporidiosis

Infection with *Cryptosporidium* species causes a self-limited diarrhoeal illness in persons with normal immunity. In patients with AIDS it causes severe enteritis with voluminous watery diarrhoea associated with colic, pain, anorexia, malaise, and weight loss. The infection may resolve spontaneously in patients with higher CD4 lymphocyte counts but patients with counts <100/µl can experience severe unremitting diarrhoea. The diagnosis is established by identification of the organism in the faeces.

Treatment

There is no consistently effective anti-microbial therapy. Azithromycin and paromomycin may reduce stool volume and lessen symptoms for some patients but do not eradicate the infection. Successful treatment with HAART leads to resolution of the infection, although it is likely to recur if the CD4 count falls.

Prophylaxis

Patients with CD4 lymphocyte <200/µl should be advised to use only boiled water, as cryptosporidial infection is primarily waterborne and infective oocysts are destroyed by boiling. Rifabutin or clarithromycin taken for prophylaxis of *M. avium* infection may prevent cryptosporidiosis.

Other protozoal infections

Microsporidiosis

Infection with microsporidia causes a diarrhoeal illness similar to cryptosporidia. Diagnosis is made by identification of the organism in the stool or small bowel biopsy. Some patients respond to albendazole or fumagillin, but there is no consistently effective anti-microbial therapy. Successful treatment with HAART leads to resolution of the infection.

Isosporiasis and cyclosporiasis

Infection with *Isospora belli* or *Cyclospora cayetanensis* causes a diarrhoeal illness similar to cryptosporidia. Diagnosis is made by identification of the organism in the stool or small bowel biopsy. Treatment is with TMP-SMX and continued maintenance therapy at a lower dose is recommended. Patients intolerant of TMP-SMX can be treated with ciprafloxacin or metronidazole.

Giardiasis

Infection with *Giardia lamblia*, a frequent cause of the 'gay bowel syndrome' in homosexual men, may cause diarrhoea in patients with AIDS. Diagnosis is made by identification of the organism in the stool or small bowel biopsy. Treatment is with oral metronidazole.

Leishmaniasis

Infection with *Leishmania* species causes visceral leishmaniasis or kala-azar, probably as the result of recrudescence of previous asymptomatic infection. Co-infection with HIV and *Leishmania* has been reported in southern Europe and is likely to occur elsewhere as the HIV epidemic spreads. The clinical features include fever, hepatosplenomegaly and anaemia. Diagnosis is made by identification of the parasite in the bone marrow or blood. Treatment is with a pentavalent anti-monial compound, pentamidine, or amphotericin and continued suppressive therapy is necessary.

Trypanosomiasis

American trypanosomiasis (*T. cruzi*; Chagas' disease) may be reactivated by co-infection with HIV, causing meningoencephalitis and cardiac disease. Coinfection with HIV does not appear to exacerbate African trypanosomiasis (*T. brucei*; sleeping sickness).

Bacterial infections

Mycobacterium tuberculosis

There is a markedly increased risk of tuberculosis (TB) in HIV-infected people. Because of impaired cellular immunity, HIV-positive individuals are at increased risk of primary infection, reactivation of prior infection, or a second infection from exogenous sources. Whilst many cases of TB were thought to be reactivation of previous infections, it has now been demonstrated that new infection is responsible for up to half the cases in HIV-positive individuals. TB has a detrimental affect on HIV infection and may accelerate the course of the disease. In developing countries where TB is endemic, high rates of HIV co-infection are frustrating TB control programmes and the mortality from TB may be increasing.

Clinical features

The clinical features are more likely to be atypical in patients with advanced immunodeficiency. Patients with mild immunodeficiency (CD4 count >200/µl) usually present with typical features with upper lobe consolidation and cavitation and the tuberculin skin test is often positive. Since the introduction of HAART, more HIV-positive patients have presented with 'typical' features. Patients with more severe immunodeficiency may present with non-specific symptoms of fever, weight loss and fatigue, and are more likely to have atypical pulmonary disease with diffuse or lower zone infiltrates without cavitation; extra pulmonary disease occurs frequently and common sites of infection include lymph nodes, liver, bone marrow and the central nervous system. The chest X-ray is usually abnormal, but 5% of HIV-positive patients with positive sputum have a normal chest X-ray. The diagnosis is made by identification of the organism in smears and cultures of sputum or other affected tissue.

Treatment

Specific recommendations regarding treatment of active infection vary in different countries. Some recommend quadruple therapy (isoniazid, rifampicin, pyrazinamide, and ethambutol) for at least 2 months followed by isoniazid and rifampicin for another 4 months, whilst others recommend that quadruple therapy be continued for longer periods. HIV-positive patients are likely to respond more slowly, and treatment should be continued until at least 4 months after cultures become negative.

There are complex interactions between anti-retroviral drugs and the medications used for the treatment of TB. Patients being treated for TB who are commenced on anti-retroviral therapy may suffer a paradoxical worsening of their disease, due to intensification of the immune response to the infection; it is usually self-limited.

Highly drug-resistant strains of TB have been isolated from patients with AIDS. Outbreaks of nosocomial multi-drug-resistant (MDR) TB occurred in New York and Miami in the early 1990s with a mortality rate of up to 80% in HIV-infected patients. Stringent infection-control measures are required to control these outbreaks and prevent similar incidents. These organisms constitute a risk to others, including health care workers and particularly other patients with HIV/AIDS. Co-infection with HIV and extensively drug-resistant (XDR) TB in South Africa carries a very high mortality and threatens the success of the treatment programmes for both diseases[27].

Prophylaxis

Primary prophylaxis is recommended for HIV-positive patients if they have a positive tuberculin test, have had TB in the past, or have had recent contact with an infectious person. Treatment with rifampicin/pyrazinamide for 2 months or isoniazid for 6–12 months is recommended; the incidence of overt tuberculosis in HIV-positive patients given isoniazid prophylaxis is less after longer treatment. Indefinite secondary prophylaxis or maintenance therapy with isoniazid should be given after the completion of acute therapy[28].

Mycobacterium avium

Mycobacterium avium is an atypical mycobacterium that rarely causes disease in HIV-negative individuals, but between one-third and one-half of patients with AIDS and advanced immunodeficiency will develop disseminated *M. avium* complex (MAC) infection. Infection is usually manifest as a constitutional illness (with fever, malaise, anaemia and weight loss) or gastrointestinal disease with chronic diarrhoea and abdominal pain sometimes associated with malabsorption and obstructive jaundice. The diagnosis is made by isolation of the organism from blood, bone marrow or other tissue.

Treatment

Treatment is with ethambutol and either clarithromycin or azithromycin, which will lead to clinical and bacteriological improvement in half of the patients. Patients commenced on HAART may present with high fevers and increased lymphadenopathy caused by an increased inflammatory response to previously asymptomatic MAC infection.

Prophylaxis

Primary prophylaxis with either clarithromycin or azithromycin is recommended for patients with a CD4 count <50/µl. Adding other drugs increases the risks of side effects and the potential for drug interactions without significantly improving efficacy. Patients treated for MAC require continuing therapy (secondary prophylaxis) with ethambutol and either clarithromycin or azithromycin. Patients showing a sustained response to HAART with CD4 counts >100/µl can have their prophylaxis withdrawn safely.

Bacillary angiomatosis

Infection with the small gram negative bacilli, *Bartonella henselae*, and quintana, occurs more frequently in patients with advanced immunodeficiency. It presents as a few to many purple or red papules and nodules that may resemble Kaposi's sarcoma. The skin lesions may be the predominant manifestation of the infection or part of a systemic illness with fever, hepatitis, lymphadenopathy, and bone lesions. The diagnosis is made on biopsy. Treatment is with erythromycin or doxycycline and should be continued for 8 weeks for cutaneous disease, longer for visceral infection.

Response may be dramatic but recurrence is common and maintenance therapy is often required.

Pyomyositis

Muscle abscesses, usually caused by *Staphylococcus aureus*, cause local pain and tenderness. The creatine phosphokinase is normal. Diagnosis is made on microbiological studies and treatment is with appropriate antibiotics, initially given parentally, for a number of weeks.

Other bacterial infections

Bacterial infections are common in patients with AIDS because of HIV-related immunodeficiency, which may be compounded by neutropenia caused by anti-retroviral therapy or chemotherapy. Infections are likely to be more severe than in immunocompetent individuals and there is a high incidence of bacteraemia. Recurrent infections are common because protective levels of antibodies fail to develop. Diagnosis is made on microbiological studies. Treatment is with appropriate antibiotics and, compared with patients without HIV infection, initial therapy may need to be given for a longer period. For some infections, notably salmonella, long-term suppressive therapy is required to prevent recurrence.

Viral infections

Cytomegalovirus (CMV)

Approximately half of the general population has serological evidence of previous infection with CMV. In patients with AIDS, the infection can reactivate and disseminate causing a variety of clinical problems including retinitis, colitis, encephalitis and myelitis, pneumonitis, and hepatitis. CMV retinitis occurs in about 20% of patients with AIDS. It presents as diminished visual acuity that leads to blindness if untreated. The diagnosis is made on the characteristic fungal appearance of large yellowish-white granular areas with perivascular exudates and haemorrhages in a patient with HIV infection and antibodies to CMV. The diagnosis of CMV infection at other sites is made by demonstration of the characteristic viral inclusions on biopsy or the detection of CMV antigen or nucleic acid.

Treatment

Treatment of systemic infection is with parenteral ganciclovir, foscarnet, or cidofovir. Ganciclovir causes myelosuppression, foscarnet can be nephrotoxic, and cidofovir can cause uveitis and nephrotoxicity. Treatment of retinitis is usually effective in preventing progression, but visual field defects present at the time of starting therapy do not improve. Ganciclovir can be given by intravitreal injection and ganciclovir implants have been developed for continuing intravitreal therapy. Systemic therapy is required in addition to the ganciclovir implant to provide protection for the other eye and other tissues. Treatment with ganciclovir implant and oral ganciclovir produces equivalent results to parenteral cidofovir, although the two treatments have different side-effect profiles. Patients started on HAART may suffer severe intraocular inflammation or 'immune reconstitution uveitis' caused by increased immune response to CMV and which can lead to further loss of vision.

Prophylaxis

Primary prophylaxis with oral ganciclovir can be considered for patients with CD4 counts <50/μl who have antibodies to CMV.

Life-long secondary prophylaxis or chronic maintenance therapy is required. Patients treated with HAART who achieve sustained elevation of the CD4 count to >100–150/μl can safely have prophylaxis withdrawn.

Herpes simplex virus (HSV)

Herpes simplex viruses types 1 and 2 (HSV-1, HSV-2) cause recurrent herpetic lesions in the orolabial and anogenital regions. More than 95% of patients with AIDS have serological evidence of previous infection with HSV and recurrent infections occur frequently. Recurrent HSV infections in patients with AIDS are likely to be more severe, with prolonged new lesion formation and delayed healing, associated with persistent local pain lasting several weeks. The frequency and the severity of the attacks increase with increasing immunodeficiency. Orofacial infection may commence with painful vesicles along the lips and spread to involve the oropharyngeal mucosa as well as adjacent areas of the face. Genital herpes causes proctitis (with pain, tenesmus, and mucosal ulceration), perianal infection (vesicle formation, pain, and ulceration), and may be associated with neurological symptoms in the distribution of the sacral plexus. HSV infection can also cause oesophagitis and encephalitis. The diagnosis is made on the basis of the clinical features and confirmed by direct microscopy and culture or by the detection of viral antigen or nucleic acid in the affected tissue.

Treatment

Treatment is with aciclovir, which can usually be given orally. Therapy should be continued until all mucocutaneous lesions have crusted or re-epithelialized. Intravenous therapy is reserved for patients with severe infection or visceral involvement and those unable to take oral medication. Famciclovir and valaciclovir are also effective in the treatment of HSV infection; foscarnet or cidofovir are used for aciclovir-resistant HSV infection. Successful topical treatment has been reported with cidofovir, imiquimod, and foscarnet. Patients suffering frequent attacks and those with severe immunodeficiency can be considered for continued maintenance therapy with oral aciclovir.

Varicella zoster virus (VZV)

Herpes zoster occurs in approximately 20% of HIV-infected patients and 20–30% of these will have multiple attacks. Herpes zoster in patients with AIDS is more likely to involve multiple dermatomes and cutaneous lesions outside the affected dermatome(s) occur more frequently; healing times may be prolonged and bacterial superinfection is common. Herpes zoster is occasionally complicated by cutaneous dissemination (producing a disease indistinguishable from primary varicella or chicken pox), and less commonly by visceral dissemination that can cause pneumonitis, hepatitis, transverse myelitis, or encephalitis. The diagnosis is made on the clinical features and confirmed by microscopy and culture or the detection of viral antigen.

Treatment

Treatment is with aciclovir, famciclovir, or valaciclovir. Therapy is continued for at least 7 days or until all external lesions are crusted. Intravenous therapy is used if there is evidence of dissemination. Foscarnet can be used for aciclovir-resistant VZV. Topical treatment of the rash is symptomatic and includes saline-soaked gauze pads or Burow's solution (aluminium acetate) for early, weeping lesions and calamine lotion for pruritic, healing lesions. Secondary infection should be treated appropriately.

Other viral infections

Molluscum contagiosum

This poxvirus infection causes multiple umbilicated papules with a predilection for the face (especially the eyelids) and the anogenital region. Diagnosis should be made by biopsy as a number of other benign and infective conditions may have a similar appearance. Treatment is with cryotherapy, electrocautery, curettage, or application of topical caustics. Repeated treatments are necessary as it is difficult or impossible to eradicate the infection. Successful topical treatment has been reported with cidofovir and imiquimod. The lesions may regress when anti-retroviral therapy is given[29].

Human papilloma virus (HPV)

HPV infection causes squamous papillomas or warts. Warts occur in greater numbers and in a wider distribution in patients with HIV infection, and this trend increases with progressive immunodeficiency. Treatment of warts is similar to molluscum with cryotherapy and the application of topical caustics. Successful topical treatment has been reported with cidofovir and imiquimod. In HIV-infected people, HPV infection in the anogenital region is associated with the increased incidence of anal cancer in men and cervical cancer in women.

JC virus

This papova virus infection causes progressive multi-focal PML. It is discussed in the section on neurological disease.

HIV-related cancer

There is a greatly increased incidence of cancer in patients with HIV-AIDS. A quarter of patients with AIDS develop cancer and it is a major contributory cause of death in about 15% of patients. The cancers that occur with increased frequency can be broadly grouped by whether or not there is an increasing risk with increasing immunodeficiency. Kaposi's sarcoma (KS), cerebral non-Hodgkin's lymphoma (NHL), and Hodgkin's disease (HD) occur with increasing frequency as the disease progresses, possibly related to the fact that they are believed to be caused by viral infection (human herpes virus type 8 (HH8) in KS, Epstein–Barr virus (EBV) in lymphoma). The human papilloma virus (HPV)-associated anal and cervical cancers occur with increased frequency in patients with HIV/AIDS but there is no increasing incidence with increasing immunodeficiency, suggesting the excess results from sexually acquired HPV infection and not because of immunodeficiency. This grouping of AIDS-associated cancers is supported by observations following HAART therapy and from Africa. In developed countries, introduction of HAART has greatly reduced the incidence of KS and some lymphomas, but the incidence of cervical and anal cancers is unchanged; in Africa, the incidence of KS and NHL are increasing rapidly but not cervical or anal cancer[11].

Kaposi's sarcoma (KS)

KS was a rarely reported malignancy before the AIDS epidemic but it is the most common cancer in HIV-infected persons. In developed countries, the incidence of KS has fallen dramatically since the introduction of HAART. KS is caused by infection with the human herpes virus type 8 (HHV8). It was originally thought that transmission was primarily via anal intercourse amongst homosexual men, but it is more likely that the transmission is via the salivary route to susceptible individuals. In developed countries, KS is rare in HIV-infected women but in Africa it is seen in the two sexes almost equally and also in children and adolescents.

AIDS-related KS is characterized by widespread lesions in the skin and mucous membranes and frequent visceral involvement. The skin lesions appear as red or purplish macules or nodules that usually increase in size and number with time. The lesions are usually multiple and may coalesce to form plaques of tumour. AIDS-related KS has a variable clinical course, depending primarily on the patient's immune status, ranging from a few indolent skin nodules to rapidly progressive systemic disease. Extra-cutaneous KS may involve any tissue but the common sites are the mucous membranes of the mouth and pharynx, the gastrointestinal tract, lymph nodes and the lung. Gastrointestinal KS is usually asymptomatic but may cause obstruction and bleeding. Lymphatic involvement leads to local oedema. Pulmonary KS causes progressive dyspnoea and cough with a diffuse interstitial infiltrate on chest X-ray. Pulmonary KS may respond less well to treatment than other visceral sites of involvement. The diagnosis is made by biopsy of the skin lesion or other involved tissue.

Treatment

Indications for treatment include cosmetic concerns for unsightly lesions, the palliation of symptoms for painful or bulky lesions and those causing oedema, and progressive systemic disease[30].

Local therapy

Local forms of therapy are of most use for non-bulky local disease. Local therapies employed include excision, cryotherapy, laser treatment, photodynamic therapy, intralesional vinblastine, and radiotherapy. Radiotherapy is effective but is associated with more mucositis and soft tissue damage than would be expected in patients without AIDS. Topical treatment with alitretinoin and docosanol is reported.

Systemic therapy

Systemic therapy is indicated for widespread, bulky or rapidly progressive disease. The best responses are seen with liposomal doxorubicin and paclitaxel. Interferon, vinorelbine, and docetaxel may also have a role.

Non-Hodgkin's lymphoma (NHL)

There is a greatly increased incidence of NHL in patients with HIV infection that affects all risk groups. NHL may manifest as either systemic lymphoma or as a primary cerebral lymphoma. Epstein–Barr virus (EBV) DNA has been isolated from most cerebral and some systemic NHL in patients with HIV infection. Since the advent of HAART, there has been a significant fall in the incidence of primary cerebral lymphomas and possibly systemic NHL of the immunoblastic type, but there has been no significant change in the incidence of other types of systemic NHL[11].

Primary cerebral lymphoma

Primary cerebral lymphomas are usually immunoblastic in type and occur in patients with advanced immunodeficiency (CD4<100/μl, usually <50/μl). Patients present with headache in association with confusion, lethargy, and memory loss or there may be hemiparesis, cranial nerve abnormalities, and seizures. Meningeal and ocular involvement is common. Scanning demonstrates one or more mass lesions that may be difficult to distinguish from toxoplasmosis: toxoplasmosis presents as a solitary lesion in 20% of cases and 50% of cerebral lymphomas present with multiple lesions. Detection of

EBV DNA in the cerebrospinal fluid is strongly indicative of cerebral lymphoma. Definitive diagnosis is made on biopsy.

Treatment

Dexamethasone or other corticosteroid is given to reduce intracranial pressure. If there is significant neurological improvement and the patient is not too debilitated from other complications of AIDS, treatment with radiotherapy can be considered. However, despite apparently good clinical response rates with radiotherapy, the average life expectancy is only 1–4 months. For patients who are comatose, those who do not improve with dexamethasone, and those severely debilitated from other effects of AIDS, radiotherapy is inappropriate. For the uncommon patient presenting with a good performance status and a CD4 count >200/μl, better results have been reported with combination chemotherapy and radiotherapy.

Systemic NHL

Systemic NHL can occur at any time during HIV infection although the incidence rises as immunodeficiency increases. The majority of these tumours occur in patients with lower CD4 counts and are high-grade tumours associated with poor prognostic features. The disease is usually widespread at the time of diagnosis with a high incidence of involvement of extranodal sites including the gastrointestinal tract, central nervous system, bone marrow and liver. Severe constitutional symptoms including fevers, night sweats and weight loss are common. Diagnosis is established on biopsy.

Treatment

Combination chemotherapy will alleviate pain and distressing systemic symptoms and stop weight loss in many patients, although only about half will achieve remission. Few of the remissions are durable and the overall median survival is less than a year. Patients in whom HAART improves the underlying HIV infection (and reduces the risk of opportunistic infections) fare best. The use of granulocyte-colony stimulating factor (G-CSF) reduces the incidence of severe neutropenia and sepsis associated with treatment. The role of rituximab is controversial, as it may temporarily aggravate the degree of immunosuppression[31]. Patients presenting at an earlier stage with better performance status, higher CD4 counts and less aggressive histology may do well with aggressive therapy. Radiotherapy is used for localized disease and to treat areas of residual or bulky disease in patients responding to chemotherapy.

Hodgkin's disease

The incidence of Hodgkin's disease is increased two-to-five fold in patients with HIV infection. Compared with patients without HIV infection, EBV DNA is detected more frequently in the tumour cells. In patients with HIV infection, biopsy usually shows a more aggressive (mixed cellularity or lymphocyte depleted) histological type. The disease is usually disseminated (Stage III or IV) at diagnosis and extra nodal involvement is frequent. Nearly all patients have constitutional 'B' symptoms.

Treatment

Treatment is with combination chemotherapy, given with G-CSF to reduce myelotoxicity. However, whilst the majority of patients may respond, the responses are not durable and the median survival is of the order of 16 months. Patients responding to HAART fare better. Radiotherapy is used for local complications of the disease.

Cervical cancer

Women with HIV infection have an increased incidence of cervical intraepithelial neoplasia (CIN) and invasive carcinoma of the cervix (ICC), attributed to HPV infection. HIV-infected women are more likely to have persistent HPV infection that is more likely to include HPV subtypes known to be oncogenic, and the incidence increases with increasing immunodeficiency. The incidence of CIN is increased compared with HIV-negative women, is more advanced at presentation, and the frequency increases with increasing immunodeficiency. There is an increased incidence of ICC but the frequency is not related to progressive immunodeficiency and has not decreased since the introduction of HAART. Following standard treatment for ICC, the majority of HIV-infected women relapse and the median survival is less than a year.

Anal cancer

Homosexual men have an increased incidence of anal HPV infection, anal intraepithelial neoplasia (AIN) and anal cancer. Patients who are HIV-positive are more likely to have heavy and persistent HPV infection and AIN and the incidence of both increase with increasing immunodeficiency. AIN lesions do not regress after commencement of HAART and the incidence of invasive anal cancer has not decreased[32]. AIN is more advanced at the time of presentation than in non-AIDS patients. AIN is treated by cryotherapy or electrocautery and regular follow up. Invasive cancer is treated by combination chemoradiotherapy. However, invasive anal cancer in patients with HIV/AIDS presents in a more advanced state and has a higher recurrence rate and a poorer prognosis.

Symptom control

Patients with AIDS present a spectrum of distressing physical and psychological symptoms that involves every body system and which may have a significant effect on the quality of life (QOL)[33,34]. The prevalence of symptoms in a series of South African patients with AIDS is shown in Table 12.2.5[34]. Some symptoms are similar to those seen with cancer, some quite different. There are reports that despite the availability of efficacious therapies, many patients with AIDS continue to experience significant symptoms[35].

This section deals with the diagnosis and management of some of the common syndromes seen with AIDS, and the reader is

Table 12.2.5 Symptom prevalence in AIDS.

Symptom	Prevalence (per cent)
Pain	98
Weight loss	81
Loss of appetite	71
Low mood	70
Weakness	66
Dry skin	56
Diarrhoea	53
Nausea and vomiting	45
Cough	45
Fatigue	43

referred to other sections of this book for more detailed discussion of symptoms that occur frequently in other diseases.

As with most medical problems in palliative care, symptoms are best managed by identifying and treating the underlying pathology, where this is possible and clinically appropriate. All palliative treatment should be appropriate to the stage of the patient's disease and the prognosis. Over-enthusiastic therapy and patient neglect are equally deplorable. The prescription of appropriate therapy is particularly important in palliative care because of the additional unnecessary suffering that may be caused by inappropriately active therapy or by lack of treatment. The fluctuating course of AIDS, punctuated by episodes requiring acute interventions, can make decisions about appropriate therapy quite difficult.

Many symptoms in AIDS can be ameliorated by treatment with corticosteroids, but they have traditionally been withheld for fear of compromising immunity and predisposing to infection. For patients on HAART, a controlled study of prednisolone therapy (0.5 mg/kg/day for 8 weeks) showed the treatment was safe and had no deleterious effect on CD4 counts or HIV RNA levels[36].

Pain

AIDS-related pain and cancer pain: similarities and differences

Pain is a common problem in patients with HIV infection, particularly when it progresses to AIDS. AIDS-related pain has many similarities with cancer pain, particularly the increasing incidence with advancing disease and the impact on the QOL (Table 12.2.6).

There are also significant differences that make AIDS-related pain more difficult to assess and treat (Table 12.2.7)[37]. The pain syndromes that are common in HIV/AIDS are considered difficult pain problems when they occur in patients with cancer. The assessment and treatment of pain may be complicated by psychosocial issues related to alternative lifestyles or intravenous drug use and the high incidence of psychiatric problems and dementia. There is less evidence for the efficacy of pharmacological therapies for AIDS-related pain than for cancer pain, and whilst there is substantial clinical experience in using strong opioids for AIDS-related pain, the level of evidence is only modest at the present time.

Incidence

Pain occurs frequently in patients with HIV/AIDS, the incidence increasing as the disease progresses. Pain is reported by about 25% of patients in the 'asymptomatic' phase, 40–50% of ambulatory patients with AIDS, and over 80% of hospitalized patients with advanced disease[33,38–40]. The number of pains reported per patient also increases through the course of AIDS. Many patients with AIDS had pain rated to be moderate or severe, with significant

Table 12.2.6 Similarities between AIDS-related pain and cancer pain.

Increasing incidence with disease progression

Moderate/severe in intensity

Profound effect on the quality of life

Usefully classified into pain due to (a) disease, (b) treatment, (c) debility, or (d) unrelated to disease or treatment

Multiple concurrent pains, the number increasing with disease progression

Under-treatment is problematic

Table 12.2.7 Management of AIDS-related pain: differences compared with cancer pain.

Higher incidence of 'difficult to manage' pain syndromes e.g. neuropathic pain, abdominal pain, headache

Disease-specific therapy often appropriate even in advanced stages

More problems with polypharmacy, drug side effects and interactions

Higher incidence of IDUs

Higher incidence of psychiatric disorders and dementia

Psychosocial problems associated with alternative lifestyles and other marginalized social groups

Lack of access to specialist pain clinics

Limited evidence for efficacy of analgesics

impairment of activities of daily living[41,39]. A number of studies have documented the strong relationship between pain and psychological function, with pain being associated with increased levels of psychosocial distress, depression, hopelessness, and poorer QOL[40].

Pain in patients with AIDS may be acute or chronic. The types of pains were described in one series as 45% somatic, 15% visceral, 19% neuropathic and 4% not defined (in addition to 17% who reported headache)[42]. The prevalence of pain at different anatomic sites in another series was lower limb pain (66%), mouth pain (50.5%), headache (42.3%), throat pain (39.8%), and chest pain (17.5%)[34].

Cause

Pain may be caused by the HIV infection itself, the treatment, general debility or an unrelated cause. Some examples are given in Table 12.2.8.

Assessment

The assessment of pain in HIV/AIDS is similar to the approach in patients with cancer. It requires a multi-disciplinary approach to

Table 12.2.8 Examples of causes of pain in AIDS.

Pain due to HIV infection	HIV infection: neuropathy, arthropathy, aseptic meningitis
	HIV-related infection: fungal, protozoal, viral, bacterial
	HIV-related cancer: Kaposi's sarcoma, non-Hodgkin's lymphoma
Pain associated with treatment	Diagnostic procedures
	Anti-retrovirals: painful neuropathy, myopathy
	Radiotherapy: mucositis
Pain related to debilitating disease	Pressure sores
	Musculoskeletal pain secondary to inactivity, wasting
	Constipation
Pain unrelated to HIV infection or treatment	Haemophiliac arthropathy

determine both the underlying cause of the pain and the psychosocial factors affecting the pain experience.

Patients with AIDS and pain have high levels of psychosocial and emotional distress and assessment for anxiety, depression and other psychosocial problems is particularly important as these may greatly influence the severity or persistence of pain.

Treatment

Multi-modality therapy

As with cancer, the treatment of pain in patients with AIDS involves a number of different modalities, including analgesics and adjuvant analgesics, disease-specific therapy, invasive treatments, physical therapies, and psychosocial interventions (Table 12.2.9).

If an underlying cause can be defined, then it should be treated where possible and clinically appropriate. The best way to relieve pain caused by an opportunistic infection or malignancy is to treat the underlying pathology and such disease-specific therapy is often appropriate until the terminal stages.

Treatment of pain in patients with AIDS includes management of any associated psychosocial problems. This may involve medications for anxiety or depression as well as non-pharmacological treatments directed at pain control such as relaxation exercises, supportive psychotherapy and physical therapies.

Treatment with HAART lessens the number of patients progressing to AIDS but it does not reduce the incidence or severity of pain in patients with AIDS[43].

Analgesics

The choice of analgesic depends on the type and severity of pain, and the WHO analgesic ladder, designed originally for the treatment of cancer pain, applies equally well to pain in AIDS. Patients with chronic pain should receive regular analgesics to both relieve the pain and prevent its recurrence.

Table 12.2.9 Examples of different modalities for the treatment of AIDS-related pain.

Disease-specific therapies:

* Treatment of opportunistic infections: antibiotics, anti-fungals, etc
* Anticancer therapy for HIV-related cancer: radiotherapy, chemotherapy
* HAART

Analgesics:

* Non-opioids
* Opioids
* Adjuvant analgesics
* Spinal analgesia

Invasive therapies e.g.nerve blocks

Physical therapies e.g. exercise, TENS

Psychosocial interventions:

* Management of anxiety, depression: medications, supportive psychotherapy
* Supportive counselling
* Group therapy
* Non-pharmacological therapies e.g. relaxation, meditation

The neuropathic pain that occurs frequently in AIDS, for which adjuvant analgesics should be used, has been the subject of a number of treatment trials. Acupuncture, amitriptyline, and mexilitene have not been shown to be more effective than placebo[44]. Lamotrigine has been shown to be effective for the treatment of painful peripheral neuropathy[45] and gabapentin is also reported to be effective[46].

Patients requiring opioid analgesics should be treated by the oral route whenever possible, although patients with severe gastrointestinal disease may not absorb the medication. Oral slow-release morphine preparations are effective in AIDS patients[47]. Patients unable to take oral medication will require parenteral treatment or transdermal fentanyl[48].

A number of important drug interactions may occur between opioid analgesics and some of the antibiotics and anti-retroviral agents taken by patients with AIDS[16,17], and consultation with the HIV and infectious diseases specialists is required.

Barriers to treatment

Pain associated with AIDS is poorly treated. In a study from New York, 85% of patients received inadequate analgesia as classified by the Pain Management Index (PMI) and only 8% of patients with severe pain received a strong opioid analgesic. Women, IDUs and less-educated patients were most likely to be inadequately treated[41]. In another study, 57% of patients who reported pain received no analgesia and only 22% got an opioid drug[38]. The reason for this seems to lie with both patient and physician. A study of clinicians identified an admitted lack of knowledge about the treatment of pain and concerns about substance abuse as the most likely reasons for under treatment of pain in patients with AIDS[49]. In another study, the doctor underestimated the pain severity in 52% of cases and this was more likely to occur when patients reported moderate or severe pain[38]. A study of patients showed they were apprehensive about taking analgesics because of fears about addiction and side effects. These barriers were most noticeable amongst the non-Caucasians, the less educated and those with higher levels of psychosocial distress[50].

Patients with a history of substance abuse

The principles of management of pain in IDUs and other patients with a history of substance abuse are no different from other patients although in practice treatment may be complicated by considerable tolerance to opioids and by the psychosocial problems that accompany substance abuse.

The incidence of pain in patients with a history of drug use is reported to be the same or a bit higher compared with those without such a history[51]. Reports of pain intensity and pain-related functional impairment were similar in the two groups[51]. However, the patients with a history of drug use were significantly more likely to receive inadequate analgesia, reported lower levels of pain relief and suffered greater psychological distress[51].

Pain in a patient with a history of substance abuse is carefully assessed as for any other patient. If opioid therapy is appropriate, the required dose is likely to be much higher than for other patients and needs to 'cover' what they were injecting or receiving on a maintenance programme. Morphine is effective for the treatment of pain in patients with a history of drug use[52]. Oral medication such as methadone and slow-release morphine or transdermal fentanyl are preferred as they have a lower abuse potential. Patients on maintenance programmes receive methadone once a day to prevent withdrawal; this needs to be increased to 6- or 8-hourly for analgesia. Reports of increased pain and requests for increased doses need to be carefully assessed, as some patients with a history of substance abuse are habitually manipulative. Some will require increased doses because of progressive physical disease and, as with patients without a history of substance abuse, some complaints of pain are really a manifestation of underlying psychosocial distress that requires skilled and sensitive management. For others, it may relate to psychological dependence and these patients are more likely to report 'loss' of prescribed drugs or prescriptions, make unsanctioned dose escalations or be found to be obtaining opioids from multiple sources; boundaries may need to be set and specialists in the management of drug dependence should be involved.

Constitutional symptoms

Anorexia

There are many possible causes for anorexia, or a reduced desire to eat, in patients with AIDS (Table 12.2.10) and it may be a significant contributing factor to weight loss in some.

Treatment

The treatment of anorexia is that of the cause and many of those listed in Table 12.2.10 are amenable to some degree of palliation. The assistance of a dietitian may be invaluable.

Appetite stimulants

A number of appetite stimulants have been recommended. Corticosteroids will produce subjective improvement in appetite in the majority of patients, although the effect may last only a few weeks and the possibility that corticosteroids may further compromise immunity or predispose to infection has to be considered. Treatment with the progestogen, megestrol acetate, given in higher

Table 12.2.10 Causes of anorexia.

Systemic infection	
Medications	Drugs for opportunistic infections
	Anti-retrovirals
	Drugs for symptom palliation
Intracranial disease	Infection, malignancy, radiotherapy
Abnormal taste, smell	Stomatitis, xerostomia
	Radiotherapy, chemotherapy Medications
Gastrointestinal	Stomatitis, oesophagitis, enterocolitis Malignancy
	Opioid-related constipation, delayed gastric emptying
	Chemotherapy, abdominal radiotherapy Liver disease
	Medication-related nausea
Metabolic	Abnormalities of sodium, calcium, sugar
	Organ failure: liver, kidney, adrenal
Psychological	Anxiety, depression, confusion, dementia Fear of making diarrhoea worse
Organizational Advanced cancer pain	Poor food preparation, presentation

dosage (800 mg/day) has been shown in placebo-controlled studies to improve appetite and weight, although the weight gained is predominately fat[53]; lower doses may stimulate the appetite without leading to weight gain. Side effects are not insignificant and include fluid retention, oedema, and thrombosis. The cannabis derivative, dronabinol, stimulates appetite but weight gain is minimal and troublesome side effects may occur, including dysphoria, dizziness, and sedation[53].

Weight loss and wasting

Weight loss and wasting, defined as the involuntary loss of 10% or more of the baseline body weight, occurs frequently in patients with AIDS. This may relate to reduced intake (related to anorexia, a functional blockage, or vomiting), malabsorption (caused by opportunistic infections, HIV enteropathy or medications), increased energy expenditure, or hypogonadism[54]. There is evidence of increased energy expenditure in patients with HIV/AIDS during periods when the clinical condition is stable, exacerbated by the occurrence of opportunistic infections[53]. Patients with AIDS and advanced cancer can develop a cachexia syndrome in which weight loss is primarily due to metabolic alterations induced by the tumour.

Significant weight loss in patients with AIDS is an ominous prognostic sign and has important psychological connotations. In the pre-HAART era, weight loss during the course of opportunistic infections was seldom completely regained. Progressive weight loss is associated with other clinical signs of progression of the HIV infection, and changes in the serum HIV RNA have been shown to correlate with weight loss[55]. Weight loss has also been shown to correlate with depression and QOL scores[56].

The introduction of HAART has lessened the tendency to weight loss in patients with advanced HIV infection and has allowed some to regain lost weight. However, some patients continue to loose weight despite HAART therapy[53].

Treatment

Treatment is directed at the underlying cause, where possible, and at the maintenance of weight. Patients with hypogonadism should receive physiological androgen replacement[54]. Optimal nutrition is crucial and the assistance of a dietitian is important. Progressive resistance training and other exercise programmes have been advocated.

Testosterone has been shown to improve weight and muscle mass in both hypogonadal and eugonadal men[53] and a meta-analysis of randomized placebo-controlled trials shows a positive effect on lean body mass[57]. Physiological replacement in women with weight loss and low testosterone levels produced a non-significant increase in lean body mass[58,59].

Anabolic steroids are effective in increasing lean body mass and are generally well tolerated[57,60], although there is a lack of information about long-term benefits and adverse effects. A small trial of nandrolone for women with weight loss reported a significant improvement in lean body mass[57]; virilization was not reported as a troublesome side effect.

Recombinant human growth hormone (rhGH) is also reported to increase lean body mass. However, while its effectiveness is similar to nandrolone, it is less well tolerated and much more expensive[57].

Megestrol acetate, 800 mg/day, will increase body weight more than nandrolone, although the weight gained is primarily fat[61]. In addition, there is concern that megestrol may cause adrenal and testosterone deficiencies.

The use of total parenteral nutrition (TPN) has been shown to be effective in preventing weight loss and regaining weight lost in patients with continuing diarrhoea or evidence of malabsorption. The use of TPN in patients without malabsorption is ineffective[53].

Many dietary and nutritional supplements have been advocated but few have shown significant benefit. A placebo-controlled study of the combination of β-hydroxy-β-methylbutyrate (a metabolite of leucine), L-glutamine, and L-arginine was shown to significantly increase weight and lean body mass[62].

Asthenia: weakness and fatigue

Asthenia is generalized weakness associated with fatigue and lassitude. Fatigue may be under-reported by patients and poorly acknowledged by health-care professionals[63]. There are many possible causes in patients with AIDS (Table 12.2.11).

Treatment is directed at the underlying cause, where possible. Assessment for anxiety and depression are important, given the study correlating fatigue with psychological concerns and not with the stage of the HIV infection[64]. The management of the AIDS-related conditions that lead to asthenia are discussed elsewhere in this chapter. Patients responding to HAART may experience considerable improvement. Psychostimulants have also been shown to improve fatigue and QOL in patients with AIDS[65,66].

Neurological disease in AIDS

Progressive neurological disease is one of the most debilitating features of AIDS. At least 40% of patients have clinically significant CNS dysfunction and autopsies have shown CNS damage in up to 90% of cases. The common causes are listed in Table 12.2.12[67].

Encephalopathy: disease involving the brain
Infection
The diagnosis and treatment of opportunistic infections involving the CNS are discussed in the section on infections. The clinical

Table 12.2.11 Causes of generalized weakness and asthenia.

Weight loss with muscle wasting systemic infections	
Medications	Anti-retrovirals
	Interferon
	Sedatives
	Other medications
Neuromuscular	Intracranial infection, malignancy
	Acute confusion or delirium
	Myelopathy, neuropathy, myopathy
	Overactivity, prolonged immobility
Metabolic	Hypogonadism
	Electrolyte imbalance, dehydration
	Renal, hepatic, adrenal failure
	Anaemia
Malnutrition	Inanition, malabsorption
Cancer	Chemotherapy, radiotherapy
	Cancer cachexia
Psychological	Anxiety, depression
	Dependency, boredom, insomnia

picture frequently includes altered mental state and diminished alertness. Diseases caused by HIV and JC virus infection are discussed below.

Primary cerebral lymphoma

The diagnosis and treatment of primary cerebral lymphoma, which may also cause alterations in mental state and consciousness, are discussed in Section 9.

Acute confusion or delirium

The investigation and management of acute confusion or delirium are discussed elsewhere. In patients with AIDS there are a considerable number of potential causes and in many cases it is due to more than one cause. The most frequent causes relate to systemic infection and intracranial pathology. Metabolic encephalopathy also occurs frequently in patients with advanced disease due to hypoxia, electrolyte imbalance, and multi-organ failure. Drug toxicity, which includes illicit or recreational drugs as well as prescribed medications, is a frequent and reversible cause of confusion and is more likely in debilitated patients.

Neuroleptic drugs with anti-dopaminergic action should be used with care in patients with AIDS, who are particularly susceptible to the extrapyramidal side effects[68].

HIV encephalopathy (AIDS dementia complex)

HIV encephalopathy or AIDS dementia complex is a syndrome of subcortical dementia characterized by the triad of cognitive impairment, motor slowing, and behavioural dysfunction. An alternative name is the HIV-associated cognitive-motor complex. It is attributed to HIV infection of the CNS. The AIDS dementia complex is clinically evident in 25% of patients with AIDS, although autopsy studies show changes in 80–90% of patients. The incidence of AIDS dementia complex rises with increasing immunodeficiency. A clinical staging system for AIDS dementia complex is shown in Table 12.2.13[67].

The clinical picture is one of progressive decline in cognitive ability and motor function. Initially there may be difficulties with concentration or memory, reading or performing complex tasks. It may cause the patient to be socially withdrawn and lead to an inappropriate diagnosis of depression. Progression leads to complete intellectual disability. The initial signs of motor dysfunction include an unsteady gait or poor balance, tremor and difficulty with rapid alternating movements. Progression leads to increasing weakness and an ataxic spastic paraparesis; urinary and faecal incontinence are common in the late stages. Some of these features are due to vacuolar degeneration in the spinal cord that is part of the AIDS dementia complex. Behavioural dysfunction manifests initially as apathy and lack of initiative; occasionally patients show agitation and mild mania. Progression leads to a vegetative state.

The diagnosis of HIV encephalopathy is made on clinical grounds and by exclusion of CNS infections and tumours and other potential causes (Table 12.2.14). The CT or MRI scan characteristically shows cerebral atrophy and the CSF findings are non-specific. The diagnosis requires mental state and neuropsychological examination; the HIV Dementia Scale (HDS) and the Executive Interview (EXIT) have been validated for the assessment of dementia in HIV/AIDS[69].

The introduction of HAART has reduced the incidence of HIV encephalopathy and dementia and leads to stabilization or improvement in neurological and cognitive function for a proportion of patients[70,71].

Table 12.2.12 Neurological disease in AIDS.

	Common	Uncommon
Brain: encephalopathy		
Focal brain disease	Toxoplasmosis	Tuberculosis
	Primary cerebral lymphoma	Cryptococcosis
	JC virus (PML)	VZV encephalitis
		Vascular disease
Diffuse brain disease	AIDS dementia complex (HIV)	HSV encephalitis
	Metabolic encephalopathy	
	CMV encephalopathy	
	Toxoplasmosis	
Spinal cord: myelopathy		
	Vacuolar myelopathy (HIV)	VZV myelitis
		Lymphoma
Meninges		
	Cryptococcal meningitis	Lymphomatous meningitis
	Aseptic meningitis (HIV)	Tuberculous meningitis
		Syphilitic meningitis
Peripheral nerve: neuropathy		
	Sensory polyneuropathy	Mononeuritis multiplex
	Herpes zoster (VZV)	CMV polyradiculopathy
	Demyelinating neuropathies	
	Toxic neuropathy	
Muscle: myopathy		
	Polymyositis	
	Toxic myopathy (zidovudine)	
	Corticosteroid myopathy	

For patients who have failed to respond to HAART, or never had access to it, treatment is by symptomatic and supportive care. Patients with mild dementia may require no specific treatment unless a secondary acute confusional state develops. Patients with dementia will fare better in familiar surroundings, which should be simplified as much as possible to reduce demands on them. They are not kept in hospital unless necessary and their neuropsychiatric condition may improve after discharge home. In contrast to dementia occurring in patients without HIV infection, patients with AIDS dementia become progressively physically incapacitated as well as cognitively impaired and require increasing levels of support and assistance.

Progressive multi-focal PML

PML is an opportunistic infection caused by the JC virus, a ubiquitous human papova virus. It is reported to occur in 5% of patients with AIDS and the untreated median survival is <6 months[72].

Patients present with multiple and progressive focal neurological deficits without change in the level of consciousness. Focal neurological signs include hemiparesis, hemianopia, aphasia, and ataxia. The condition is progressive although spontaneous remissions are reported. Dementia, encephalopathy, and coma can occur in the later stages. The MRI scan shows subcortical white matter lesions corresponding with the clinical abnormalities. Routine CSF examination usually shows non-specific changes, but the detection of JC virus DNA in the CSF is diagnostic in the appropriate clinical setting.

HAART is reported to reduce JC virus levels in the CSF, which can be associated with neurological improvement or stabilization and improved survival[73,74]. There is conflicting evidence whether HAART given in conjunction with cidofovir is more effective[75,76].

Aseptic meningitis (HIV meningoencephalitis)

Patients with AIDS may present with several weeks or months of generalized headache, with or without meningismus and photophobia, for which no cause other than HIV infection can be found. Aseptic meningitis may occur at the time of initial seroconversion but is more frequent as immunodeficiency progresses. Cerebral and meningeal diseases have to be excluded, as do other common causes of headache (Table 12.2.15). CSF examination is usually inconclusive. Treatment of aseptic meningitis or 'HIV headache' is symptomatic. Some patients are reported to respond to amitriptyline.

Table 12.2.13 Clinical staging of AIDS dementia complex.

Stage	Characteristics
Stage 0 (normal)	Normal mental and motor function
Stage 0.5 (equivocal)	Minimal or equivocal symptoms of cognitive or motor function
	Normal capacity for work and activities of daily living (ADL)
	Normal gait and strength
Stage 1 (mild)	Unequivocal intellectual or motor impairment
	Able to do all but the more demanding work and ADL
	Can walk without assistance
Stage 2 (moderate)	Cannot work or perform demanding ADL
	Capable of basic self care
	Ambulatory but may need a single support
Stage 3 (severe)	Major intellectual disability
	Cannot walk unassisted
Stage 4 (end-stage)	Nearly vegetative; mute or almost mute
	Rudimentary intellectual and social comprehension and Response
	Paraparetic or paraplegic with urinary and faecal incontinence

Seizures

Seizures are a relatively frequent complication of HIV infection and are reported to occur in up to 50% of patients with AIDS dementia complex, 40% of patients with cerebral toxoplasmosis, and 30% of patients with primary cerebral lymphoma. Causes of seizures in AIDS patients are listed in Table 12.2.16, although no definite cause may be found in 20% of patients.

The clinical features and investigation of seizures are discussed elsewhere (see Chapter 10.11). Seizures recur in up to 70% of patients with AIDS, so anti-convulsant treatment should be instituted after the first episode. Patients with AIDS have an increased incidence of hypersensitivity reactions to phenytoin and carbamazepine may cause leucopenia; sodium valproate or clonazepam are better first line drugs in this population. Careful observation is

Table 12.2.14 Causes of dementia.

Related to HIV infection or treatment	AIDS dementia complex
	CNS infection: JC virus, toxoplasmosis, tuberculosis, syphilis
	Primary cerebral lymphoma
	Obstructive hydrocephalus: infection, lymphoma
	Radiotherapy
Unrelated to HIV infection or treatment	Alzheimer's disease
	Alcoholic dementia
	Cerebrovascular disease
	Other: hydrocephalus, thyroid dysfunction, thiamine deficiency

Table 12.2.15 Causes of headache.

Aseptic meningitis (HIV)

Cerebral disease (including toxoplasmosis, lymphoma)

Meningeal disease (including cryptococcosis, tuberculosis, lymphoma)

Sinusitis

Migraine

Other causes of headache

needed to ensure anti-convulsant therapy does not exacerbate liver disease. Protease inhibitors may markedly alter metabolism of some medications and anti-convulsant drug levels should be carefully monitored.

Spinal cord disease: myelopathy

Acute myelopathies

The causes of acute myelopathies include spinal cord compression by lymphoma, infection with VZV or other viruses, and bacterial or mycobacterial infections. If spinal cord compression is suspected, assessment and investigations must be carried out promptly, as the prognosis for recovery depends on the neurological function at the time of initiation of treatment. A MRI scan or CT myelogram is the investigation of choice. The CSF should be examined for evidence of infection or malignancy. The ability to detect viral and mycobacterial nucleic acids in CSF greatly facilitates the diagnostic process. Treatment of lymphoma and opportunistic infections are dealt with in the relevant sections.

HIV myelopathy

About 20% of patients with AIDS develop spinal cord disease. Vacuolar degeneration, thought to be due to HIV infection, may occur as part of the AIDS dementia complex. It presents initially as ataxia and progresses to cause spastic paraparesis with urinary and faecal incontinence. Other patients may develop a dorsal column syndrome with pure sensory ataxia or sensory myelopathy with paraesthesiae and dysaesthesiae in the lower limbs. Abnormalities are demonstrable on MRI scanning. In contrast to the cerebral features of the AIDS dementia complex, spinal cord disease does not appear to respond to anti-retroviral therapy and treatment is supportive.

Peripheral neuropathy

Peripheral neuropathy occurs frequently in patients with HIV/AIDS[77]. The treatment of painful neuropathy with adjuvant analgesics is discussed in the section on pain in this chapter and elsewhere (see Chapter 10.11).

Table 12.2.16 Causes of seizures.

Infection	HIV, toxoplasmosis, cryptococcus, tuberculosis, JC virus (PML)
Tumour	Primary cerebral lymphoma
Metabolic	Hepatic encephalopathy, uraemia
Drug toxicity	Pethidine (meperidine)
Drug withdrawal	Opioids, barbiturates, alcohol, benzodiazepines

Distal sensory polyneuropathy

This produces a symmetrical tingling, numbness and burning pain in the feet and may spread up the lower limbs with time. It is thought to be due to HIV infection. It is clinically manifest in one-third of AIDS patients and tests are abnormal in a further one-third. Anti-retroviral therapy is not of benefit.

Toxic neuropathy

Didanosine, zalcitabine, and stavudine can produce painful peripheral neuropathy, usually when used in higher doses. The neuropathy will resolve a few weeks after discontinuation of the drugs. There are no tests available to determine whether a patient's neuropathy is drug related. Thalidomide also causes peripheral neuropathy.

Demyelinating polyneuropathy

This syndrome is characterized by progressive weakness, loss of reflexes and mild sensory disturbances. It may be acute or chronic. The acute form resembles the Guillain–Barré syndrome and may occur at the time of seroconversion or during the phase of intermediate immune deficiency. Therapy, if required, is with plasmapheresis, intravenous immunoglobulin, or corticosteroids.

Mononeuritis multiplex

The acute onset of multiple nerve palsies that may be widespread and progressive is described in patients with AIDS. It is often due to CMV infection and may respond to therapy with ganciclovir or foscarnet.

CMV polyradiculopathy

This is a painful sensorimotor neuropathy that starts in the lumbosacral roots and progresses proximally. Autonomic involvement with bowel and bladder dysfunction can occur. It is usually caused by CMV and may respond to therapy with ganciclovir or foscarnet.

Myopathy

HIV myopathy

Polymyositis with proximal muscle weakness and myalgia may occur in AIDS. It ranges in severity from a mild complaint to a severe illness with progressive weakness and pain. The creatine phosphokinase level is increased and the EMG abnormal. Muscle biopsy may show inflammatory changes. Treatment, if required, is with corticosteroids or intravenous immunoglobulin and physiotherapy.

Zidovudine myopathy

Patients treated with zidovudine for longer periods (usually more than a year) may develop proximal muscle weakness that is usually more marked in the lower limbs with wasting of the gluteal and thigh muscles. It may be difficult to distinguish from HIV polymyositis and inflammatory changes can be seen on biopsy. If zidovudine is suspected of causing myopathy, alternative anti-retroviral therapy should be substituted. The myopathy usually resolves within 6–12 weeks of stopping zidovudine.

Corticosteroid myopathy

Patients treated with corticosteroids for more than a few weeks are at risk of developing proximal muscle weakness. The myopathy will improve within a few weeks of stopping the drug.

Eye disease

Conjunctivitis

Conjunctivitis is common in patients with AIDS and is usually due to infection (Table 12.2.17). Culture negative conjunctivitis occurs in about 10% of patients with AIDS, which probably relate to allergy or systemic medications. Another 10% of AIDS patients develop a dry eye syndrome, possibly related to autoimmunity or systemic medications. Conjunctivitis causes mild discomfort associated with watering, itching, and a gritty feeling in the eye. Vision is well preserved. Examination shows diffuse inflammation of the conjunctiva; a suppurative discharge suggests infection.

The treatment of conjunctivitis is with regular saline washes and appropriate anti-microbial therapy for specific infections. Aseptic conjunctivitis is treated with saline washes, cool compresses and topical antibiotics to prevent bacterial infection. Dry eyes are treated with lubricant drops or artificial tears.

Keratitis

Keratitis or corneal inflammation is usually due to infection, the common causes being HSV, VZV, bacteria, fungi, and microsporidia. It is characterized by conjunctivitis, pain, photophobia, watering of the eye, and there is usually some blurring of vision. Infection with HSV is usually associated with signs of nasolabial infection and dendritic ulceration is seen on ophthalmologic examination. Infection with VZV occurs in association with herpes zoster of the ophthalmic nerves and corneal ulceration is seen on examination. Herpetic infection is treated with topical aciclovir and corticosteroid. Other infections are treated appropriately.

Anterior uveitis

Anterior uveitis and iritis present as a painful red eye associated with photophobia. Formal ophthalmologic assessment should be arranged. Causes include CMV, VZV, HSV, or other opportunistic infection, usually in conjunction with retinal involvement. Anterior uveitis occurs in a significant proportion of patients treated with rifabutin or cidofovir. If present, infection is treated appropriately. Drug-related uveitis is treated with topical corticosteroids and, if necessary, reducing the dose of the drug.

Retinal disease

Patients with AIDS who complain of visual disturbances should be assessed by an ophthalmologist, so that CMV retinitis can be diagnosed and treated before it causes blindness. CMV retinitis is seen most frequently in patients with a CD4 count <50/μl, and it is recommended that these patients have regular ophthalmologic assessment.

Retinal abnormalities occur frequently in AIDS[78]. Cotton wool spots, seen in 50% of patients, appear as hard white spots with irregular edges and are areas of retinal ischaemia caused by

Table 12.2.17 Conjunctival disease.

Conjunctivitis:	
Infective	HSV, VZV, bacterial
Non-infective	Allergy, medication side effects, radiotherapy (acute)
Dry eyes	Autoimmune, medication side effects, radiotherapy (late)
Tumour	Kaposi's sarcoma, squamous cell carcinoma

microvascular disease. CMV retinitis produces perivascular haemorrhage and exudates. Pneumocystis carinii causes raised yellow white plaques. Toxoplasma retinitis may look similar to CMV but usually occurs with cerebral toxoplasmosis. Herpetic infections cause multiple pale grey patches in the retina. CMV retinitis occurs in 25% of patients with AIDS, the other infections less frequently.

Cotton wool spots do not compromise vision and do not require therapy. Appropriate anti-microbial therapy is given for the various infections as described in the section on infections.

Psychiatric disorders

Many patients with HIV/AIDS will experience psychiatric problems at some stage during the course of their illness[79,80]. However, because of the high incidence of organic brain disease in patients with HIV/AIDS, all new psychiatric disorders should be considered to have an organic basis until proven otherwise.

Depression

A number of studies have reported that there is no increased risk of depression in HIV-positive people, although re-examination of this data by meta-analysis suggests the incidence of depression may be twice as high in HIV-infected people[81]. It has also been reported that depression and other psychological symptoms predict progression of the underlying HIV infection[82,83].

The difficulties encountered in the diagnosis of depression in medically ill patients is discussed elsewhere see Chapter 15.5. This is even more difficult in patients with HIV/AIDS because of the high incidence of organic brain disease. The symptoms upon which a diagnosis of depression is made in physically health individuals are shown in Table 12.2.18. These are not easily applicable to patients with HIV/AIDS, as both the cognitive and somatic symptoms may have an organic cause. For example, apathy has been ascribed as primarily related to neuropathology by some, and to psychopathology by others.

A number of different measures or scales have been validated for the diagnosis of depression in patients with HIV/AIDS[84], although it has been suggested that deletion of the somatic symptoms increases the sensitivity of the ratings[85], and that the use of self-report measures may significantly overestimate the true incidence of psychological illness[86].

Most patients with HIV/AIDS will experience symptoms of depression at some time during their illness (Table 12.2.19). Depressive symptoms and anxiety occur as part of the normal psychological stress response at times of crisis such as treatment failure or disease progression. These reactions last 1–2 weeks and resolve spontaneously with time and appropriate support.

Table 12.2.18 Symptoms of depression.

Psychological	Depressed mood
	Diminished interests or pleasure in activities
	Psychomotor agitation or retardation
	Diminished self esteem, feelings of guilt
	Lack of concentration or indecision
	Thoughts of death or suicide
Somatic	Significant change in appetite and/or weight
	Insomnia or hypersomnia
	Fatigue and/or loss of energy

Table 12.2.19 Causes of depressive symptoms in patients with HIV/AIDS.

Normal	Part of transient normal response to crises, stress
Adjustment disorder	Reactive depression ± reactive anxiety
Major depressive illness	
Organic brain syndromes	Acute confusion (delirium)
	Dementia
	Side effects of drugs

Reactive depression or an adjustment disorder differs from the normal self-limited stress response in either degree or duration. Symptoms last longer than expected (more than 2 weeks) and may be more severe or intense, causing more disruption and interference with daily functioning, social activities, and relationships with others. Major or endogenous depression occurs in a small proportion of patients with HIV/AIDS. The symptoms are usually more severe than in reactive depression and the mood is incongruent with the disease outlook and does not respond to support, understanding or distraction. Patients with acute confusional states (delirium) or dementia may exhibit features of depression. A number of drugs can also cause depressive symptoms, including corticosteroids, barbiturates, amphotericin, and interferon. In the case of delirium, dementia and drug side effects, mental state examination will reveal evidence of organic brain dysfunction.

Treatment

If an organic brain syndrome is present, it is treated appropriately. Other problems causing or aggravating depression, particularly pain, should be treated. Patients with transient depressive symptoms occurring in response to acute crises usually require only good general supportive care. Psychotherapy is not usually required although relaxation training may be helpful if anxiety is pronounced.

A variety of different forms of psychotherapy have been reported for patients with HIV/AIDS. Cognitive behavioural therapy has been reported to be of benefit[87,88]. Anti-depressants are effective although side effects and drug interactions may be problematical; tricyclic anti-depressants may be effective but less well tolerated than newer SSRIs[89,90].

Three other forms of treatment have been used in patients with HIV/AIDS and depressive symptoms, the success of which suggests the possibility that a significant proportion of psychological symptomatology relates to neuropathology. First, treatment with psychostimulants (dextroamphetamine, methylphenidate, and pemoline) has been shown in placebo-controlled trials to significantly reduce levels of depression and psychological distress[65,66]. Second, a proportion of males with HIV/AIDS have hypogonadism and treatment with testosterone in blinded, placebo-controlled studies showed significant improvements in depression ratings[91,92]. Third, treatment with HAART, known to be of benefit to neuropsychological function, leads to significant improvement in depression scores[93,94].

Demoralization syndrome

Demoralization is a prominent form of existential distress in which meaninglessness, hopelessness and helplessness predominate and

Table 12.2.20 Diagnosis of the demoralization syndrome.

Symptoms of existential distress: meaninglessness, pointlessness, hopelessness
Sense of pessimism, helplessness, loss of motivation to cope differently, desire to die
Associated social isolation, alienation or lack of support
Phenomena persist over more than 2 weeks

which may lead to a desire to die[95,96]. The diagnostic criteria are listed in Table 12.2.20 and it can be distinguished from depression in that demoralized patients can enjoy the present, their lack of hope being confined to the future. In the past, the features of this syndrome have probably been regarded as sub-clinical depression.

Demoralization can be actively treated with cognitive behavioural therapy to counter the sense of pessimism and promote the setting of goals, meaning-based therapy that explores continued role and purpose, and supportive therapies to reduce feelings of isolation and dependence.

Anxiety

The assessment and management of anxiety is discussed in detail elsewhere (see Chapter 15.5). Anxiety occurs frequently in patients with HIV/AIDS[97]. Cognitive behavioural stress management is reported to be effective.

Psychosis

Mania and psychoses in patients with HIV/AIDS are usually attributable to organic brain disease or the effects of drugs (both medicinal and recreational). Presentation with psychosis occurs more frequently in patients with AIDS than in the earlier phases of HIV infection, and patients may show signs of cognitive impairment and have abnormalities on CT scanning of the brain[98]. Follow-up of these patients shows an increased incidence of cognitive impairment and AIDS dementia[98].

Mania

The typical features of mania are listed in Table 12.2.21. In addition, there may be cognitive defects that may persist after resolution of the manic episode. In hypomania, the symptoms are not severe enough to cause serious impairment of social or occupational functioning and there are no psychotic features. In mania, there is functional impairment and there may be psychotic features, including delusions, hallucinations, disorganized speech and grossly disorganized or catatonic behaviour.

Table 12.2.21 Typical features of mania.

Persistently elevated, expansive or irritable mood
Unrealistically inflated self-esteem or grandiosity
Decreased need for sleep
Increased talkativeness
Flight of ideas or subjective experience that thoughts are racing
Easily distracted
Hyperactivity
Involvement in activities without regard to probable adverse consequences

Initial therapy is with a potent neuroleptic. Any causative or precipitating factors related or organic brain disease or drugs are sought and treated appropriately. Continued therapy is with a lower potency neuroleptic or one of the mood altering drugs such carbamazepine or sodium valproate. Lithium therapy can be very difficult to manage in patients with advanced HIV infection and is not recommended.

Respiratory symptoms

The investigation and management of respiratory symptoms are dealt with elsewhere in this book, including dyspnoea, cough, haemoptysis, pleural effusion, hoarseness, and terminal respiratory congestion.

Pneumonia

Treatment of pneumonia in patients with HIV infection and AIDS is with the appropriate specific anti-microbial therapy[99]. Treatment must be appropriate to the stage of the disease and the prognosis. Intensive therapy is only appropriate if it is felt that successful treatment of the infection will allow the patient to survive a significant period of time with reasonable QOL. Treatment of *Pneumocystis carinii* and mycobacterial pneumonia is outlined in the section on opportunistic infections.

Gastrointestinal disease

Stomatitis

Stomatitis occurs frequently in AIDS, due to a variety of causes (Table 12.2.22).

The common symptoms are pain, altered taste, and halitosis. Severe stomatitis may prevent eating or drinking and cause difficulty taking medications. Infective stomatitis can be caused by a wide range or organisms, and as the clinical features are often atypical, appropriate microbiological studies and biopsies should be performed.

Candida usually presents in the pseudomembranous form (removable, creamy white plaques) but may manifest in an

Table 12.2.22 Stomatitis: causative and predisposing factors.

Causes	
Infection:	
Fungal	*Candida*, other fungi
Bacterial	Gingivitis, periodontitis, other bacteria
Viral	HSV, CMV, HPV, hairy leucoplakia
Aphthous ulcers	
Radiotherapy	Direct mucosal damage, xerostomia
Chemotherapy	Direct mucosal damage, neutropenic sepsis
Predisposing factors	
Xerostomia	Diminished amount of less alkaline saliva
Poor oral hygiene	
Poor nutrition	Thin atrophic mucous membranes
Drugs	Steroids, antibiotics predispose to fungal infection
Cancer	Kaposi's sarcoma, non-Hodgkin's lymphoma

erythematous form (flat red patches) or cause angular cheilosis. HSV causes clusters of painful small vesicles that rupture and ulcerate, usually on keratinized mucosa (the hard palate or gingiva). VZV infection causes vesicles that coalesce to form large ulcers and always occurs in association with skin lesions involving the maxillary or mandibular branches of the trigeminal nerve. HPV infection can cause solitary or multiple nodules, which may be sessile or pedunculated and usually require biopsy for diagnosis. Oral CMV infection that occurs as part of systemic CMV disease causes ulcers that look necrotic with a white halo. Hairy leucoplakia is a white thickening of the oral mucosa that has a corrugated surface or 'hairy' appearance, typically occurring along the lateral margin of the tongue. It is an EBV-induced benign hyperplasia. Linear gingival erythema is a bacterial gingivitis that presents with a bright red band of erythema at the gingival margin, even in clean mouths. It may progress to a necrotizing ulcerative gingivitis and periodontitis in which there is rapid loss of gingival and periodontal tissues with destruction of supporting bone and loss of teeth; it is usually associated with severe pain. Bacillary angiomatosis causes vascular papular lesions in the mucosa that can mimic Kaposi's sarcoma. Aphthous ulcers are common and may be single or multiple, small or large, and are frequently recurrent. They occur on non-keratinized mucosa and have an erythematous margin. Kaposi's sarcoma presents as purplish lesions in the mucosa that may be raised or flat, single or multiple. Non-Hodgkin's lymphoma may present as a painless swelling that may ulcerate.

Treatment

Preventive. All patients with advanced HIV infection and AIDS, particularly those receiving chemotherapy or radiotherapy, require a programme of preventive mouth care including regular mouth washing, attention to dental hygiene and avoidance of very hot or very hard food. Prophylactic topical anti-fungal therapy should be considered for all patients with CD4 lymphocytes <200/µl. Addition of an antiseptic such as chlorhexidine reduces the incidence of bacterial stomatitis in myelosuppressed patients.

Treatment of pain

Mild to moderate pain can usually be managed using mouthwashes containing anaesthetic or analgesic agents, with or without oral analgesics. Severe pain is treated with opioid analgesics.

Specific therapy

Specific treatments for different causes of stomatitis are listed in Table 12.2.23. Candidal infection not responding to topical antifungal agents is treated with oral fluconazole. Aciclovir may improve the rate of healing of HSV lesions, and in higher dose VZV lesions. Hairy leucoplakia is not routinely treated and the response to oral aciclovir is usually short-lived. Linear gingival erythema is treated with regular mouth washing with either chlorhexidine or povidone-iodine. Necrotizing gingivitis requires plaque removal and local debridement, mouth washing with chlorhexidine or povidone-iodine and oral antibiotic therapy with metronidazole or clindamycin. Aphthous ulcers are treated with topical steroid in orabase or a steroid mouthwash. Systemic steroids may be considered for severe aphthous ulcers or if there are also oesophageal lesions. Thalidomide (200 mg/day) is effective in the short-term treatment of aphthous ulcers but may cause somnolence, rash, and peripheral neuropathy. Thalidomide taken intermittently at lower dose does not protect against recurrent aphthous ulcers.

Table 12.2.23 Treatment of stomatitis.

Candida	Topical antifungal therapy, oral fluconazole
HSV, VZV	Oral aciclovir
CMV	Ganciclovir
HPV	Excision, cryotherapy, cautery or laser therapy
Leucoplakia	High dose oral aciclovir
Other fungi	Antifungal therapy
Gingivitis	Chlorhexidine or povidone-iodine mouthwash
Periodontitis	Removal of necrotic tissue
	Chlorhexidine or povidone-iodine mouthwash
	Oral metronidazole or clindamycin
Other bacteria	Antibiotics selected on basis of culture results
Aphthous ulcers	Topical corticosteroid or corticosteroid mouthwash
	Thalidomide

Topical application of granulocyte macrophage colony stimulating factor (GM-CSF) is reported to be effective for recalcitrant aphthous ulcers[100].

Nausea and vomiting

The causes and management of nausea and vomiting are discussed elsewhere. In patients with AIDS, additional causes might include the side effects of medications (anti-retrovirals and anti-microbials), opportunistic infections, malignancy or infection affecting the central nervous system, and psychological factors. Management includes the identification and palliation of the cause, where possible, and anti-emetics. There is an increased incidence of extrapyramidal side effects in patients with AIDS and the doses of anti-dopaminergic drugs should be kept as low as possible[68]. If a prokinetic drug is required, domperidone should be used in preference to metoclopramide as the former does not cross the blood–brain barrier.

Oesophagitis

The common causes of oesophagitis in AIDS are listed in Table 12.2.24. Oesophagitis causes pain on swallowing (odynophagia), some degree of difficulty with swallowing (dysphagia) and may produce anterior chest pain. Reflux oesophagitis causes characteristic burning retrosternal discomfort or 'heartburn'.

Table 12.2.24 Causes of oesophagitis.

Infection	*Candida*, CMV, HSV
Idiopathic ulcers	
Radiation	Mucosal damage, predisposition to infection
Chemotherapy	Mucosal damage, predisposition to infection
Reflux oesophagitis	Raised intra-abdominal pressure (any cause)
	Prolonged recumbent posture
	Persistent vomiting
	Anticholinergic drugs, anti-cholinergic side effects of drugs

Barium examination will show mucosal irregularity or ulceration. Endoscopy to obtain biopsies and specimens for microbiological examination is frequently required. *Candida* infection produces white or yellow-white plaques, which may become confluent and cause oesophageal narrowing in severe cases; oropharyngeal infection is usually present. CMV infection produces either diffuse oesophagitis or multiple shallow ulcers; giant ulcers (>1cm) are sometimes seen. Idiopathic ulcers, in which no pathogen can be identified, are typically large and shallow.

Treatment

Therapy includes treatment of infection, pain relief, measures to aid healing of ulceration and avoidance of reflux (Table 12.2.25). In milder cases thought to be due to *Candida* because of the presence of oropharyngeal infection, radiological, and endoscopic assessment may be delayed a few days to see if there is response to fluconazole. Idiopathic ulcers do not respond to the treatments used for infective oesophagitis but frequently respond to corticosteroids; thalidomide is also reported to be beneficial.

Diarrhoea

Diarrhoea affects up to 90% of patients with HIV infection and AIDS. The incidence increases with progressive immunodeficiency and there has been a marked reduction in the incidence in patients treated with HAART. In most cases it is due to an opportunistic infection (Table 12.2.26) and infection with more than one organism may occur at any given time. Non-infective causes (Table 12.2.27) also occur and both infection and infection-induced malabsorption may occur at the same time[101].

Infective causes of diarrhoea can be broadly grouped by whether they cause enteritis or colitis (Table 12.2.26) although the distinction is not always clear and some organisms can affect all parts of

Table 12.2.26 Infective causes of diarrhoea.

Enteritis—predominantly small bowel	
Bacteria	*Mycobacterium avium*, *Salmonella* spp.
Protozoa	Cryptosporidia, microsporidia, *Cyclospora* spp. *Isospora* spp. *Giardia lamblia*
Viruses	Enteroviruses, HIV

Colitis—predominantly colon	
Bacteria	*Campylobacter* spp. *Shigella* spp. *Yersinia* spp. *Aeromonas* spp. *Cl. difficile*
Protozoa	*Entamoeba histolytica*
Viruses	CMV, adenovirus, HSV

the bowel. Small bowel disease is characterized by large volumes of watery diarrhoea associated with bloating and central abdominal pain. Colitis is associated with lower abdominal pain and cramping, urgency, and the frequent passage of small volumes of stool that often contains blood, mucous and pus. The bacterial pathogens usually cause an acute diarrhoeal illness whilst infection with protozoa, viruses and mycobacteria characteristically causes chronic diarrhoea.

Initial assessment includes microscopy and culture of three stool specimens. Tests for *Cl. difficile* toxin should be performed if there is a history of antibiotic use or pseudomembranous colitis is suspected. Blood cultures should be taken. If no pathogen is identified, endoscopy for biopsies and cultures should be considered: upper gastrointestinal endoscopy and small bowel biopsy are performed if the clinical features suggest enteritis, and sigmoidoscopy or colonoscopy is done for colitis-type diarrhoea. In a proportion of patients, no pathogen will be identified despite rigorous investigation. It has been suggested that some of these cases are due to HIV infection ('HIV enteropathy') but a causal association is unproven.

Treatment

Treatment of infection. After collection of stool specimens, patients should be given ciprofloxacin to which most enteric bacteria in HIV-positive patients are sensitive. Pseudomembranous colitis is treated with oral vancomycin. If a pathogen is identified, specific treatment is instituted, as described earlier in the section on infection. Maintenance therapy is necessary for some infections, particularly

Table 12.2.25 Management of oesophagitis.

Infection-specific antimicrobial therapy	*Candida*	fluconazole
	CMV	ganciclovir, foscarnet
	HSV	aciclovir
Idiopathic ulcers	Corticosteroids, thalidomide	
Pain relief	Topical local anaesthetics: oxethazaine, lignocaine, cocaine	
	Oral analgesics (mild pain), parenteral opioids (severe pain)	
	Antacids	
	Dietary advice: liquid or semisolid diet, avoid very hot or cold foods	
Prevention and healing of ulceration	Antacids combined with coating agent alginate	
	Sucralfate	
	Reduce gastric acid production: H$_2$-receptor antagonist, proton pump inhibitor	
Avoidance of reflux	Reduce increased intra-abdominal pressure	
	Dietary: avoid large meals, carbonated drinks, alcohol	
	Posture: avoid stooping, lying flat	
	Increase lower oesophageal sphincter tone: metoclopramide, cisapride	

Table 12.2.27 Non-infective causes of diarrhoea.

Dietary	Excess roughage, fibre; enteric supplements
Drugs	Laxatives, antibiotics, anti-retrovirals, others
Haemorrhage	
Inflammation	Radiation, drugs
Cancer	Kaposi's sarcoma, non-Hodgkin's lymphoma
Lactose intolerance	
Steatorrhoea	Pancreatic insufficiency
	Biliary obstruction
	Bacterial overgrowth
Psychological	Anxiety

those more likely to occur when the CD4 count is <100/µl: CMV, MAC, cryptosporidia, microsporidia, and cyclospora.

General measures

Maintenance of hydration is important except in the terminally ill. Commercially available soft drinks or oral rehydration solutions can be used. Intravenous rehydration may be necessary if diarrhoea is severe or if there is vomiting. Dietary modifications to both reduce diarrhoea and ensure adequate nutrition are important and the assistance of a dietician is useful. Patients with severe or prolonged diarrhoea may require consideration for enteral nutrition, either by nasogastric tube or percutaneous gastrostomy; patients with continuing diarrhoea and malabsorption benefit from TPN[53]. Drugs that may be causing or aggravating diarrhoea should be stopped, if possible.

Anti-diarrhoeal agents

The opioid drugs such as loperamide, diphenoxylate, and codeine reduce diarrhoea by inhibiting peristalsis. Unless morphine or codeine is being given for analgesia, loperamide is the agent of choice. The hydrophilic bulking agents such as methylcellulose and ispaghula may reduce diarrhoea by absorbing excess fluid. Adsorbent agents such as the kaolin preparations are of questionable value and may interfere with absorption of other drugs. The somatostatin analogue, octreotide, reduces intestinal secretion and motility and is of benefit in a proportion of AIDS patients with diarrhoea[102]. It is more likely to help patients without a defined pathogen and recent studies suggest it may be more effective at higher doses. Acetorphan, an orally active encephalinase inhibitor benefits some patients[103].

Anorectal disease

Anorectal disease is common in patients with AIDS, particularly male homosexuals (Table 12.2.28). Anorectal ulceration is most frequently caused by HSV, less often by CMV. Warts due to HPV infection are common. Proctitis is most frequently caused by chlamydia or gonorrhoea and less often by other bacterial infections, including syphilis. Kaposi's sarcoma, non-Hodgkin's lymphoma and anal cancer can present as either mass lesions or ulceration. Idiopathic ulcers occur for which no pathogen can be identified, similar to idiopathic oesophageal ulcers. Fistulas, fissures and haemorrhoids are common and may be caused or aggravated by local infections or severe diarrhoea. Assessment is by proctoscopy to view lesions and to obtain biopsies and specimens for microbiological studies. Examination should be thorough, including biopsy of any suspicious areas, given the high incidence of intraepithelial neoplasia in patients referred for benign conditions[104].

Treatment is directed at the cause. Gonorrhoea is treated with a third generation cephalosporin or ciprofloxacin, chlamydia with tetracycline and HSV with oral aciclovir. Symptomatic measures including analgesia and stool softening (if appropriate) are instituted. Preparations for rectal use containing a local anaesthetic and

Table 12.2.28 Anorectal disease.

Infection	Chlamydia, gonorrhoea, HSV, CMV, HPV, other bacteria
Cancer	Kaposi's sarcoma, non-Hodgkin's lymphoma, anal cancer
Other	Idiopathic ulcers, fissures, fistulas, haemorrhoids

Table 12.2.29 Causes of liver disease.

Pre-existing liver disease	Cancer:
Biliary disease	Kaposi's sarcoma
Infection:	Non-Hodgkin's lymphoma
M. avium	Drugs:
CMV	Anti-retroviral e.g. didanosine
M. tuberculosis	Anti-viral e.g. foscarnet
Cryptococcosis	Anti-fungal e.g. ketoconazole
Histoplasmosis	Anti-mycobacterial e.g. isoniazid
P. carinii	Anti-protozoal e.g. pentamidine
Rochalimaea henselae	Complementary medications
Viral hepatitis B, C	Recreational drugs
	Alcohol

corticosteroid can be of significant symptomatic benefit. Idiopathic ulcers respond to local or systemic corticosteroid and may respond to thalidomide.

Liver disease

Liver disease or abnormalities of liver function occur commonly and relate to pre-existing liver disease, infection, drug toxicity or malignancy (Table 12.2.29). The infections that most commonly involve the liver are due to mycobacteria and CMV and occur as part of a systemic illness with fever and constitutional symptoms. Drug toxicity usually produces a diffuse hepatitic picture and ranges in severity from asymptomatic biochemical abnormalities to hepatic failure.

The history, other clinical features and liver function tests may provide clues to the diagnosis. Imaging may show evidence of diffuse or focal liver disease or biliary pathology. Opportunistic infections can often be diagnosed by non-invasive means such as blood cultures. Liver biopsy may be necessary if the diagnosis cannot be made by other means.

Treatment

Treatment is directed at the underlying cause. Drugs causing toxicity are withdrawn or the dose modified. Infections are treated appropriately.

Co-infection with hepatitis viruses

In patients with AIDS, progressive immunodeficiency may lead to activation of hepatitis B (HBV) and hepatitis C (HCV) infections, and previously asymptomatic carriers may develop clinical hepatitis. Patients with HBV or HCV co-infection are less likely to tolerate treatment with protease inhibitors and HCV patients respond less well to HAART. HBV co-infection does not accelerate progression to AIDS, although there may be increased mortality related to liver disease[105]. HCV co-infection is associated with increased mortality from liver disease and more rapid progression to AIDS, although some report no effect on the HIV infection[106,107]. Patients earlier in the course of their HIV infection and those who have responded to HAART should be considered for treatment of HBV and HCV, and control of HCV infection may facilitate the delivery of HAART. However, in patients with AIDS who have either failed HAART or never had access to it, the HIV infection is

Table 12.2.30 Biliary disease.

Sclerosing cholangitis ± papillary stenosis	CMV, cryptosporidia
Acalculous cholangitis	CMV, cryptosporidia, microsporidia
Biliary strictures	Infection, Kaposi's sarcoma, lymphoma, cholangiocarcinoma

Table 12.2.31 Causes of anaemia.

Decreased red cell production	HIV infection
	Opportunistic marrow infection
	Marrow infiltration
	Marrow suppression:
	Drugs: anti-retrovirals, drugs for opportunistic infections
	Chemotherapy
	Radiation
	Iron deficiency
	Vitamin B12, folate deficiency
Red blood cell loss	Bleeding
Increased red cell destruction (haemolysis)	Infection
	Drugs
	Autoimmune

regarded as the major determinate of their life expectancy and treatment of the hepatitis virus infection with interferon (with all its attendant toxicity) is not usually recommended.

Biliary disease

Sclerosing cholangitis and acalculous cholecystitis occur with increased frequency in patients with HIV/AIDS. They are related to an opportunistic infection in most cases; occasionally, strictures are due to malignant infiltration (Table 12.2.30).

Patients present with biliary-type abdominal pain that may be severe. Examination reveals fever and local tenderness. Liver function tests show progressive cholestasis. Imaging will usually show some dilatation of the biliary tree. In sclerosing cholangitis, endoscopic retrograde cholangiopancreatography (ERCP) may show multiple focal strictures and dilatations of both the intrahepatic and extrahepatic bile ducts, often associated with papillary stenosis at the ampulla. Large or solitary strictures suggest the possibility of malignancy.

Treatment

Sclerosing cholangitis is treated by endoscopic sphincterotomy and therapy directed at the underlying infection. This frequently provides good pain relief although the liver function tests may not improve significantly if there is continuing intrahepatic cholangitis. If severe or recurrent, acalculous cholecystitis is treated by cholecystectomy.

Haematological disorders

Anaemia

Up to 80% of patients develop symptomatic anaemia during the course of HIV infection and AIDS, the incidence and severity increasing with progressive immunodeficiency[108].

Cause

The anaemia is frequently multi-factorial (Table 12.2.31). For most patients with AIDS, anaemia is attributed to direct infection of the marrow by HIV. It is usually a diagnosis of exclusion, no other cause for anaemia being found. It has the features of an anaemia of chronic disease with normochromic, normocytic anaemia, a low reticulocyte count and inappropriately low erythropoietin levels. More recently, patients have been reported with elevated erythropoietin levels associated with low testosterone levels[109]. Mycobacterial (*M. tuberculosis*, *M. avium*) and fungal (cryptococcosis, histoplasmosis, coccidioidomycosis) infections frequently involve the marrow. Infection with parvovirus B19, associated with transient aplasia in immunocompetent individuals, can cause severe and chronic anaemia in AIDS patients. Bone marrow infiltration occurs frequently with non-Hodgkin's lymphoma and Hodgkin's disease and the blood film may show a leucoerythroblastic picture. Cancer chemotherapy routinely causes a transient pancytopenia and a number of the drugs used in the treatment of

HIV and opportunistic infections may also cause bone marrow suppression. Iron deficiency due to inadequate intake or bleeding produces a hypochromic, microcytic anaemia. Vitamin B12 or folate deficiency may occur secondary to intestinal malabsorption caused by infection and produce a macrocytic anaemia with megaloblastic changes in the marrow.

Iron deficiency anaemia will occur with significant bleeding at any site. The most frequent is bleeding from the gastrointestinal tract due to malignant infiltration or severe infection. Patients with haemophilia or severe thrombocytopenia are also at increased risk of haemorrhage.

Some degree of haemolysis (shortened red cell survival) occurs with many of the infections complicating AIDS. More severe haemolysis occurs when patients with G6PD deficiency are given sulfonamides or dapsone.

Treatment

Treatment of specific causes. Anaemia in patients with AIDS is frequently multi-factorial and treatment is initially directed at specific causes, where possible. Bone marrow infection is treated with specific anti-microbial therapy; parvovirus B19 infection is treated with intravenous immunoglobulin. Malignant lymphoma is treated with chemotherapy. Drug-induced bone marrow suppression requires consideration of dose reduction or use of different drugs. Iron, vitamin B12 and folate deficiencies are treated with replacement therapy. The underlying cause of bleeding is treated appropriately. The haemolysis associated with infections responds to treatment of the infection. Drug-induced haemolytic anaemia requires the offending drugs be withheld. Patients with low testosterone levels should receive androgen replacement.

Transfusion

Decisions regarding blood transfusion depend on the speed of onset and the severity of the symptoms of anaemia. Acute anaemia due to blood loss or serious infection usually requires transfusion. Recommendations regarding transfusion for patients with chronic anaemia are summarized in Table 12.2.32. Patients without antibodies to CMV should receive CMV-negative blood. There is no benefit in using leucocyte-reduced red cell transfusions[110].

Table 12.2.32 Indications for blood transfusion for chronic anaemia.

Hb < 80–90 g/l	and	Symptomatic
Hb 80–90 g/l	and	Continued or likely haemorrhage
		Planned surgery
		Planned radiotherapy
		Planned chemotherapy
		Serious infection
		Doubt about symptomatic benefit
		Unexplained weakness, fatigue, or dyspnoea
Hb > 90–100 g/l	and	Symptomatic (cardiac or respiratory insufficiency)

Erythropoietin

Treatment of patients with AIDS and anaemia with recombinant human erythropoietin (EPO) leads to a significant rise in haemoglobin and improvement in the QOL[111]. It is effective in patients with low endogenous erythropoietin levels (<500 IU/l) but may not produce improvement in patients with opportunistic infections or taking zidovudine. It is administered by subcutaneous injection (100 µg/kg) three times weekly and is well tolerated. EPO therapy is very expensive.

Lymphopenia

Progressive lymphopenia is the hallmark of HIV infection. Lymphopenia also occurs with chemotherapy, radiotherapy, and treatment with corticosteroids.

Neutropenia

HIV infection results in impaired neutrophil production, an effect that increases with progressive immunodeficiency. Neutropenia may also occur with marrow involvement by opportunistic infections or malignant infiltration. A considerable number of drugs used in the treatment of AIDS patients may cause neutropenia. Neutropenia predisposes to bacterial infection and also causes mucositis, particularly involving the gastrointestinal tract.

Treatment

Treatment of specific causes. Where possible, the specific cause is treated appropriately. Drug-related neutropenia requires consideration of dose reduction or the substitution of a different agent.

Growth factors

The neutrophil growth factors, G-CSF (granulocyte colony stimulating factor) and GM-CSF (granulocyte-macrophage colony stimulating factor), are effective in patients with persistent neutropenia and may allow other essential but myelotoxic medications to be continued. The CSFs are administered by daily subcutaneous injection. Side effects are few although the treatment is expensive. GM-CSF has been shown to augment HIV replication *in vitro* and, whilst there is no evidence that it has deleterious effect *in vivo*, it is customary for patients receiving GM-CSF to be also on anti-retroviral therapy.

Thrombocytopenia

Immune thrombocytopenia (ITP) may occur at any stage of HIV infection. Thrombocytopenia may also occur with various marrow disorders (Table 12.2.33). Thrombocytopenia related to HIV infection of the marrow increases in frequency and severity with progressive immunodeficiency.

Table 12.2.33 Causes of thrombocytopenia.

Diminished platelet production:
HIV infection
Opportunistic infection of marrow
Malignant infiltration of marrow
Vitamin B12 or folate deficiency
Cancer treatment: chemotherapy, radiotherapy
Drugs
Increased platelet destruction:
Immune thrombocytopenia (ITP)

Most patients with AIDS have mild thrombocytopenia and are asymptomatic. Bone marrow examination should be considered for patients with a platelet count $<50 \times 10^9$/l for which the cause is not apparent. This will distinguish impaired production from increased peripheral destruction and will demonstrate any marrow pathology.

Treatment

Specific causes of diminished platelet production are treated, where possible. Anti-retroviral therapy frequently produces improvement in the platelet count.

Treatment of more severe ITP in patients with HIV infection and AIDS is with corticosteroids, intravenous immunoglobulin and splenectomy. Corticosteroids produce improvement in 50–75% of patients but thrombocytopenia frequently recurs when the dose is tapered. Intravenous immunoglobulin produces a response in 75–90% of patients; the response is transient but is useful in patients who are bleeding or are scheduled for surgery. Splenectomy is reported to benefit 80% of patients.

Thrombotic thrombocytopenic purpura

Thrombotic thrombocytopenic purpura (TTP) is a rare condition characterized by severe thrombocytopenia, microangiopathic haemolytic anaemia, neurological signs, renal impairment, and fever. TTP occurs in patients with advanced HIV infection and AIDS, usually in association with opportunistic infections. Untreated, the condition is often rapidly fatal. Treatment is by plasma exchange with fresh frozen plasma[112].

Skin disease

Skin disorders are extremely common in patients with HIV infection and AIDS. The frequency increases with progressive immunodeficiency and the lesions may be clinically more severe and respond less well to therapy. Atypical clinical presentations are common and skin biopsies are often necessary to establish the diagnosis.

Skin infections

Bacterial infections

Staphylococcal infection may present as folliculitis with pustules affecting the trunk, inguinal regions and face, sometimes associated with severe pruritus. Other presentations include cellulitis, bullous impetigo, and ecthyma (punched-out ulcers, most frequently on the lower leg). Diagnosis is made on the clinical features and the results of cultures. Treatment is with appropriate antibiotics, and benzoyl peroxide washes or anti-bacterial soaps can be helpful.

Patients with recurrent infections can be given a short course of rifampicin.

Bacillary angiomatosis presents as a few to many purple or red papules and nodules, which may resemble Kaposi's sarcoma or pyogenic infection. The diagnosis is made by biopsy. Treatment is with erythromycin or doxycycline.

Other bacterial infections, including syphilis and systemic mycobacterial infections, can produce unusual or atypical skin lesions. Biopsies and cultures are essential for diagnosis.

Viral infections

Infections with herpes simplex (HSV), varicella zoster (VZV), molluscum contagiosum, and human papilloma virus (HPV) are discussed above in the section on infections.

Fungal infection

Infections with dermatophytes (fungi that infect the skin, hair, and nails) occur more frequently in patients with HIV infection and become more widespread and less responsive to treatment with progressive immunodeficiency. Tinea infections may be severe and widespread with prominent nail involvement. Trichophyton rubrum is a common cause of nail infection in patients with severe immunodeficiency and produces the characteristic proximal white subungual onychomycosis. Diagnosis is made by microscopy and culture.

Treatment is with topical anti-fungal agents including ketoconazole, clotrimazole, and terbinafine. More severe infections require systemic therapy using griseofulvin, an imidazole or terbinafine. Oral therapy is more effective but more likely to cause side effects and drug interactions.

Candida usually affects the mouth and oesophagus but may also cause vulvovaginitis, balanitis, angular cheilosis, paronychia, and onychomycosis. Diagnosis is made on microscopy and culture.

Skin lesions are common in patients with other systemic fungal infections. The lesions can resemble molluscum, making biopsy essential.

Parasitic infection

The mite that causes scabies, *Sarcoptes scabiei*, proliferates unchecked in patients with severe immunodeficiency, leading to heavy infestation that may involve much of the body surface. Diagnosis is by identification of mites or biopsy. Treatment is with topical benzyl benzoate, lindane, or permethrin, with or without oral ivermectin[113]. Close contacts of the patient must also be treated.

Skin disorders

Xerosis and ichthyosis

Xerosis or dry, fine scaling of the skin is common in AIDS. Treatment is symptomatic with topical moisturizing applications. Ichthyosis, predominantly affecting the lower limbs, occurs in a quarter of patients with HIV infection. The skin is dry with a 'fish-scale' appearance. Treatment is with emollients to keep the skin as moist as possible; if scaling is severe, a keratolytic such as 2% salicylic acid can be added to the emollient.

Seborrhoeic dermatitis

Seborrhoeic dermatitis is reported to occur in up to 90% of patients with HIV infection, the incidence and severity increasing with progressive immunodeficiency. Erythematous patches covered with greasy scales characteristically occur on the face and scalp and may also involve the central chest, axillae, and groins. Treatment is with a topical corticosteroid preparation and anti-dandruff shampoos are useful for the scalp. The role of *Pitysporum orbiculare* in the causation of seborrhoeic dermatitis is controversial but the rash often responds well to ketoconazole cream in HIV-infected patients.

Psoriasis

Psoriasis typically presents as erythematous-rounded plaques covered by silvery micaceous scale, predominantly affecting the elbows, knees, and scalp. In HIV-infected patients, the disease can be more severe and widespread and prove resistant to therapy; psoriatic arthritis is also more frequent. Treatment includes conventional topical tar products and topical corticosteroids, which may be ineffective in severe cases. Ultraviolet light therapy (either UV-A with psoralen (PUVA) or UV-B) is usually effective for patients with widespread disease. A high-energy excimer laser produces more rapid responses. Other therapies include topical calcipotriol (a vitamin D analogue) and oral retinoid therapy with acitretin or etretinate. Methotrexate may compromise immune function and is not used.

Eosinophilic folliculitis

Eosinophilic folliculitis is an uncommon skin condition that occurs much more frequently in patients with HIV infection. It presents with follicular and perifollicular urticarial papules and plaques scattered on the upper trunk, head and neck, and the upper arms, often associated with severe pruritus. Diagnosis is made on biopsy, which shows eosinophilic infiltration of the hair follicle. Treatment with anti-histamines, topical corticosteroids, and ultraviolet light may be helpful. Some improve with itraconazole, suggesting an infective aetiology.

Hypersensitivity reactions

Photosensitivity

Patients with HIV infection are often very photosensitive and can suffer burns as a result of exposure to sunlight or radiation therapy. Treatment is with topical corticosteroids and discontinuance of any medications that may act as a photosensitiser. Advice should be given regarding the use of sunscreens and protective clothing.

Insect bite reactions

Mosquito and other insect bites can produce florid reactions in patients with HIV infection. Treatment is with anti-histamines and topical corticosteroids and the avoidance of further bites by the use of insecticides, insect repellents, and protective clothing.

Drug reactions

Drug reactions are common in patients with AIDS and are usually due to sulfonamides or other antibiotics. The most common reaction is a widespread maculopapular rash; other patterns include urticaria, erythema multi-forme and, less often, the Stevens–Johnson syndrome, and toxic epidermal necrolysis. Mild reactions should be observed and may resolve. Symptomatic treatment is with anti-histamines and topical corticosteroids. More severe reactions require withdrawal of the offending agent.

Other disorders

Arthropathy

Arthralgia occurs in about one-third of patients with HIV/AIDS for a variety of reasons. Treatment of TB with pyrazinamide can cause arthropathy.

HIV polyarthritis

A transient widespread mild polyarthralgia may occur at the time of seroconversion or during the 'asymptomatic' phase of HIV infection. Less frequently, a persistent symmetrical polyarthritis may develop in patients with advanced HIV infection or AIDS. If warranted, treatment is with NSAIDs.

HIV arthropathy

This is oligoarticular arthritis which involves large joints, predominantly the knees and ankles. It is non-erosive with few inflammatory changes in the synovial fluid. The onset is subacute, developing over 1–6 weeks, and it lasts 6 weeks to 6 months. Treatment with NSAIDs is often unhelpful but the condition usually responds to intra-articular corticosteroids.

Septic arthritis

Septic arthritis occurs relatively infrequently in patients with AIDS, given the high incidence of septicaemic illness. It can be caused by bacteria (e.g. *S. aureus*), mycobacteria or fungi. Gonococcal infection may produce a widespread polyarthritis with mild joint swelling which is thought to be an immune reaction, or typical gonococcal arthritis with severe pain and swelling of a single joint and from which the organism can be cultured.

Reiter's syndrome

This is the triad of urethritis, arthritis and conjunctivitis and may be triggered by sexually transmitted chlamydial infection. Persistent, painful, lower extremity oligoarthritis develops and may persist for months. Treatment is with NSAIDs and physiotherapy. Doxycycline is given if there is evidence of active chlamydial infection.

Psoriatic arthritis

Up to one-third of patients with HIV infection and psoriasis will develop psoriatic arthritis. It usually causes chronic, painful oligoarthritis involving the large joints in the lower limbs; sacroileitis; Achilles tendonitis; and plantar fasciitis may occur. Treatment is with NSAIDs and physiotherapy. Systemic steroids are avoided, if possible, because of the increased risk of infection. Methotrexate should be avoided because it may cause both myelosuppression and immunosuppression.

Renal failure

Renal impairment is most frequently caused by pre-renal factors and nephrotoxic drugs (Table 12.2.34). Drugs may cause renal damage by direct effects on renal cells, by precipitation in tubules or as part of a hypersensitive reaction causing interstitial nephritis. Nephrotoxicity is more likely in dehydrated or debilitated patients, those with pre-existing renal impairment, or if two or more of the drugs are used at the same time.

Two forms of glomerulonephritis are associated with HIV infection. A proliferative glomerulonephritis associated with immune complex deposition occurs and is thought to be due to HIV infection. It usually follows an indolent course with stable renal function over months or years. Focal and sclerosing glomerulosclerosis or HIV nephropathy presents as a nephrotic syndrome progressing to renal failure in months.

The treatment of renal failure depends on the cause, the degree of impairment and the stage of the patient's HIV illness. Pre-renal factors are corrected where possible. Care in prescribing potentially nephrotoxic drugs will reduce the incidence of reactions. If acute

Table 12.2.34 Causes of renal impairment in patients with HIV/AIDS.

Pre-renal	
Dehydration	
Sepsis	
NSAIDs	
Renal	
Glomerulonephritis	Immune complex proliferative Glomerulonephritis
	Focal and sclerosing glomerulosclerosis
Interstitial nephritis	Infections
	Drug hypersensitivity
Nephrotoxic drugs	Antibiotics, anti-virals, anti-protozoals, anti-fungals
	Chemotherapy
	Radiological contrast media
Radiation	
Pyelonephritis	
Post-renal	
Ureteric obstruction by retroperitoneal lymphadenopathy	

renal failure does occur, dialysis may be considered if this is appropriate to the stage of the patient's disease and general condition. Proliferative glomerulonephritis may require no therapy; dialysis may be considered if renal failure develops. Glomerulosclerosis responds to corticosteroid therapy.

Gynaecological infections

Vaginal candidiasis

The incidence and severity of vaginal candidiasis increase with progressive immunodeficiency. Diagnosis is made on the clinical features and culture. Treatment is with topical nystatin or clotrimazole. Oral fluconazole is reserved for severe infections not responding to topical therapy. Maintenance therapy, either topical or systemic, can be considered for women with frequent infections.

Herpes simplex virus (HSV)

The frequency and severity of ulcerative genital herpes increase with progressive immunodeficiency. Treatment is with aciclovir, followed by maintenance therapy for women with severe or frequent recurrences.

Aphthous ulceration

Giant idiopathic genital ulcers are uncommon but can be very painful. Diagnosis is by exclusion of all possible infective causes and malignancy. The pathogenesis may be similar to oesophageal aphthous ulcers, but the efficacy of steroids or thalidomide for genital ulceration is not documented.

Pelvic inflammatory disease

Pelvic inflammatory disease may be more severe in women with advanced immunodeficiency. Treatment is with standard antibiotic regimes incorporating anaerobic cover.

Human papilloma virus (HPV)

Warts may become extensive and florid with advanced immunodeficiency. Treatment is with topical trichloroacetic acid or podophyllin or by cryotherapy, but the recurrence rate is high. Successful topical treatment has been reported with cidofovir and imiquimod[114].

Pregnancy

The majority of HIV-positive women are of childbearing age and much research has been conducted to reduce the risk of transmission from mother to child[115]. The risk of infection in utero is probably dependent on the stage of the mother's infection, reflected by the CD4 count and plasma HIV RNA load. Risk factors during the perinatal period include the mother's CD4 count and a viral load, duration of ruptured membranes, maternal genital ulceration and HIV shedding, and the mode of delivery. Breastfeeding is a well-documented mode of transmission.

In developed countries, the risk of mother-to-child transmission can be reduced from about 30% in untreated mother–child pairs to about 2% with anti-retroviral therapy given during the antenatal and neonatal periods, elective Caesarean delivery, and avoidance of breastfeeding[116,117]. However, what constitutes optimal anti-retroviral therapy in this situation, including minimizing adverse effects on the child, is uncertain.

In developing countries, short courses of antenatal anti-retroviral therapy have been shown to significantly reduce perinatal transmission[118]. In breastfeeding populations, 30–50% of transmission is attributable to breastfeeding. However, in resource-poor situations in developing countries, avoidance of breastfeeding may jeopardise the health of the child; safe replacement feeding may not be available, affordable, or culturally acceptable. Anti-retroviral therapy during breastfeeding reduces the risk of transmission, but continued therapy for the duration of breastfeeding is presently not possible in most resource-poor settings.

Palliative care and HIV/AIDS

HIV/AIDS has provided many challenges for palliative care and will continue to do so as the epidemic evolves. In developed countries, the role of palliative care in the management of patients with HIV/AIDS has at times been controversial and is again being questioned following the introduction of HAART.

During the early years of the epidemic, the concept of palliative care was resisted and equated with giving up hope. The patient population was young and there was a natural tendency for both patients and clinicians to pursue aggressive investigation and therapy right up until they died. Conventional palliative care, originally developed to cater for the diverse and multi-disciplinary needs of the dying, with its emphasis on symptom control and psychological care, together with minimization of investigations and treatment, was not acceptable. Concerns were also expressed that palliative care services would discriminate against male homosexuals and IDUs.

By the early 1990s, before the advent of HAART, increasing numbers of patients and clinicians came to accept the value of palliative care, acknowledging that there comes a point when continuing to pursue active therapy is counterproductive to a patient concluding their life in a dignified, orderly and meaningful way. Many patients with advanced AIDS were managed by palliative care services and a number of AIDS hospices were established.

The major textbooks on HIV/AIDS even included a chapter dealing with palliative care and matters related to death and dying.

HAART has had a dramatic effect on HIV/AIDS in developed countries. Progression of HIV infection to AIDS has been slowed, as has the rate of progression of patients with AIDS, and the numbers dying of AIDS has fallen sharply (see Fig. 12.2.1). It has been argued that HIV/AIDS is now a chronic, stable problem—even possibly curable—with no need for palliative care and that talk of death and dying is unduly negative. Textbooks on HIV/AIDS no longer have chapters relating to palliative and terminal care. However, the long-term outlook for patients currently responding to HAART is unknown: there is increasing evidence of emerging drug resistance to HAART, and improved survival may be associated with an increased incidence of AIDS-related malignancies. In addition, not all patients will respond to HAART, others are unable to tolerate it, and some present late in the course of the disease and have a poorer prognosis even with HAART. It therefore seems likely that there will continue to be patients with advanced AIDS who will benefit from palliative care.

Palliative care has also evolved during the 25 years of the AIDS epidemic. In the past, palliative care has been regarded as primarily the care of the dying, to be employed when all avenues of treating the underlying disease are exhausted and further active medical treatment is considered inappropriate (Fig. 12.2.3).

More recently, the advantages of integrating palliative care with acute care have been explored in specialties such as oncology and HIV/AIDS. Even though HIV infection is incurable and ultimately fatal, its various manifestations are eminently treatable, and it is appropriate to provide pain relief, symptom control and psychosocial support to patients with far-advanced disease while they continue to pursue disease-controlling therapies. Comprehensive symptomatic and supportive care, addressing all aspects of a patient's suffering and provided by an interdisciplinary team, should be made available for all patients with cancer or AIDS, long before the terminal phase of the illness. This treatment is complementary to (and not in competition with) all the active medical aspects of treatment, and should be integrated in a seamless manner with other aspects of the patient's care (Fig. 12.2.4); this has been termed the 'mixed management model' of end-of-life care[119]. However, one recent survey of oncologists and HIV specialists indicated they felt strongly that palliative care was only appropriate for dying patients, only when all avenues of treatment for the disease had been exhausted, and that there should be restrained prescriptive power for physicians providing palliative care[120].

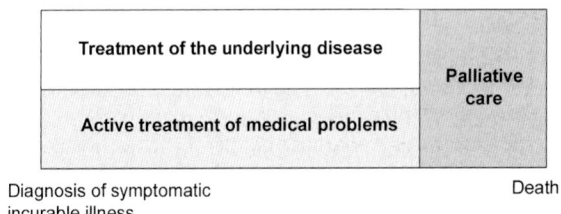

Figure 12.2.3 A traditional view of palliative care. (Reproduced with permission from Woodruff, R. (2004) *Palliative Medicine. Evidence-based symptomatic and supportive care for patients with advanced cancer* 4th edition, Oxford University Press.)

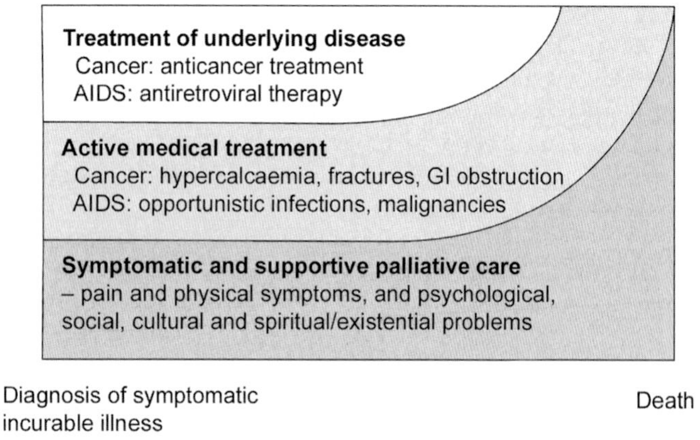

Treatment of underlying disease
Cancer: anticancer treatment
AIDS: antiretroviral therapy

Active medical treatment
Cancer: hypercalcaemia, fractures, GI obstruction
AIDS: opportunistic infections, malignancies

Symptomatic and supportive palliative care
– pain and physical symptoms, and psychological,
social, cultural and spiritual/existential problems

Diagnosis of symptomatic   Death
incurable illness

Figure 12.2.4 Modern palliative care. Symptomatic and supportive palliative care is complementary to, and seamlessly integrated with, active treatment of the underlying disease. (Reproduced with permission from Woodruff, R. (2004) *Palliative Medicine. Evidence-based symptomatic and supportive care for patients with advanced cancer* 4th edition, Oxford University Press.)

As well as expertise in pain and symptom control, palliative care brings to this partnership an interdisciplinary and holistic approach to care that is so important for the management of psychosocial problems but which is often lacking in modern disease-orientated medicine.

The evolution of palliative care to provide services that are complementary to acute medical care earlier in the course of the disease, together with the observation that a proportion of patients with HIV infection will continue to progress to the advanced stages of AIDS, suggests that the need for palliative care in the management of patients with HIV/AIDS will continue for the foreseeable future[121,122].

The population of patients with HIV/AIDS in developed countries is also changing, with an increasing incidence in women, in minority and migrant populations, and in the socially disadvantaged. Palliative care stands to make a positive contribution to meeting the needs of this increasingly heterogeneous patient population.

Palliative care in resource-poor countries

The management of the HIV/AIDS epidemic in resource-poor countries of the developing world presents unparalleled challenges[3,123].

In resource-poor countries, disease progression is more rapid and survival is shorter[3]. Poverty, malnutrition and social inequalities are major co-factors in the epidemic in poorer countries. Gender inequality, in particular, has been singled out as the main reason that, globally, HIV infection is now more frequent in women than men[3,124].

In resource-poor countries, basic health care services may not be available, or cannot be accessed or afforded. Medications for opportunistic infections may be unavailable or unaffordable. The risk of transmission of HIV by blood transfusion remains high. High rates of co-infection with TB complicate both epidemics in southern Africa[125].

How resource-poor countries should address the problems of HIV/AIDS is much debated. Prevention must remain a priority, requiring education of the population at large. Voluntary testing and counselling is reported to be cost-effective. There is increasing debate that instead of having to opt-in, people have to opt-out of being tested.

Treating HIV infection in resource-poor countries provides many challenges. It requires not only drugs but also the creation of a sustainable primary care system, as well as programmes for identifying HIV-infected people before the terminal stage of the disease. Drug costs can be reduced and will lead to more widespread use. To maximize the benefits and minimize the risks of drug-resistant disease, programmes will then be required to oversee optimal use and adherence, perhaps similar to the successful directly observed therapy (DOTS) programmes for tuberculosis. Good adherence and response rates to anti-retroviral therapy are reported from home-based programmes in rural Africa[126], but the cost of such programmes may deprive many others of access to treatment[127].

Even in the absence of antibiotic and anti-retroviral therapy, there is much that palliative care can do to improve the QOL of patients with AIDS[128]. Palliative care can promote basic medical care and symptom control, such as the use of opioids for pain control. Social supports can be strengthened and services accessed. Patients can be counselled and allowed to talk about how they feel, what to expect, and how they can help themselves. Families can be shown how to care for someone with AIDS, how to give emotional and spiritual support, and about safe waste disposal. Palliative care can help dispel fear and ignorance in carers and in the community, reducing the stigmatization that is often associated with AIDS.

Palliative care for advanced aids

Palliative care for patients with advanced or terminal AIDS is about QOL and is directed at the alleviation of pain and physical symptoms as well as the assessment and management of psychological, social and spiritual/existential problems. It also involves care and support of family members or partners, including bereavement follow-up. It requires a holistic approach to care and is best provided by a well-coordinated interdisciplinary team. It must be provided in a manner that shows respect for the individual patient—their dignity, their culture, their choices or wishes regarding treatment, and their goals and unfinished business. Continuity of care through the terminal illness is also very important.

Surveys of what patients believe constitutes quality end-of-life care report simpler, more specific concerns, focused on outcomes[129]. One study identified five domains: receiving adequate pain and symptom management, avoiding inappropriate prolongation of dying, achieving a sense of control, relieving burden, and strengthening relationships with loved ones[130].

Palliative care for AIDS can be delivered in the patient's home or in a hospice or hospital—the principles and practices are the same. It is important that a palliative care consultation service be available in acute hospitals treating patients with AIDS.

Palliative care for AIDS must accommodate the social and cultural background of the patients and provide service that is non-discriminatory and culturally sensitive[131]. In the UK, many new cases are occurring in immigrants who are socially disadvantaged, isolated, less aware of the health care to which they are entitled, and more likely to present only when symptomatic[132]. In the USA, the patients are disproportionately male, black, and poor[133]. There is lack of equitable access to palliative care services in both the UK and the USA[134].

Patients with AIDS can place an enormous burden on their caregivers. High levels of stress can lead to depression[135] and, in some societies, the caregivers themselves face stigma and prejudice[136].

Medical care

The medical management of patients with AIDS is complicated by a number of factors related to the underlying disease. The population is younger, making the transition to palliative care and advance care planning more difficult. There may be uncertainties about the trajectory of the illness and the prognosis[134]. Patients may present with multiple and complex medical problems: as well as underlying AIDS, they may be suffering from one or more opportunistic infections, hepatitis B or C, side effects of HAART such as diabetes, and other unrelated medical conditions. There may also be a history of drug or alcohol abuse.

The palliative care of patients with AIDS also involves difficult decisions about such matters as aggressive investigation and treatment of complications, or the withdrawal of anti-retroviral or infection prophylaxis therapies. These decisions have to be made with each individual patient and must be concordant with their goals, priorities and expectations, albeit that these can change frequently.

Advance care planning

Advance care planning is the process of planning future medical care, particularly for the situation where patients may no longer be able to make their own decisions[137]. Such planning would be particularly appropriate to AIDS, given the high incidence of organic brain dysfunction in the later stages. However, only about 50% of patients with HIV/AIDS have discussions about end-of-life care; the proportion is lower in those with a lower educational level and IDUs. A study of barriers preventing such discussions suggests it may relate more to the clinicians than the patients[138]. Advance care planning in patients with advanced cancer has been said to foster feelings of personal resolution, but in patients with HIV/AIDS the response rate was low and it led to lessening of patients' overall satisfaction with care[139].

Goals of care and appropriate treatment

Many difficult clinical and ethical problems can arise in the advanced and terminal stages of AIDS. These arise because on the one hand the underlying retroviral infection is incurable, progressive and ultimately fatal, but on the other hand many of its manifestations, which are responsible for much of the morbidity and mortality of AIDS, are eminently treatable. However, as patients become increasingly weak and debilitated, whether some investigations and therapies are appropriate has to be questioned. Patients with advanced disease are less able to tolerate invasive procedures and are more likely to suffer side effects of medication. Whether or not there has been advance care planning, there needs to be an ongoing partnership of care between the patient and the treatment team, with honest and open communication, to define the goals of care. The physician must be able to convey prognosis, even with its uncertainties, and what it is reasonable for the patient to hope for. This allows patients to make informed decisions about their own care and treatment, and ensures that all decisions about therapy are individualized.

What constitutes medical futility is rarely unequivocal and can lead to disagreement. This may occur if there are misunderstandings about prognosis or if the physician or the patient is pursuing unrealistic goals, matters that can usually be resolved by discussion. One survey showed that the majority of patients accepted that the doctor was not obliged to talk about treatments considered futile[140].

Decisions should be made according to what is in the patient's best interest and directed at the QOL. Investigations and therapies should only be pursued if they will provide benefit to the patient in terms of QOL or in the context of their goals and unfinished business.

Polypharmacy

Patients with AIDS are frequently taking multiple medications. These may include anti-retroviral drugs, multiple medications for the treatment and prevention of opportunistic infections, medications for symptom control, as well as drugs for unrelated medical conditions. There is a high incidence of drug side effects and a significant risk of drug interactions[17]. Medications should be continually reviewed and those that are not essential or worthwhile discontinued.

Stopping anti-retroviral therapy

Anti-retroviral therapy given during the earlier phases of AIDS may be of great clinical benefit to the patient. However, in the advanced stages, it is possibly of no benefit and, as it is usually associated with significant clinical toxicity, a decision may have to be made about continuing treatment. This may constitute a major psychological and emotional step for the patient to take and requires careful and compassionate discussion. Many patients have a considerable psychological investment in continuing anti-retroviral medication and a decision to discontinue it requires an acknowledgement of the state of their disease and prognosis.

Stopping infection prophylaxis

Patients with AIDS are frequently taking large numbers of tablets, many with significant side effects, as prophylaxis against various infections. As the disease progresses, the question arises as to when these treatments can be withdrawn. The decision is finally up to the patients and depends on their appreciation of the state of their disease, which in turn depends upon the adequacy of medical communication. A decision to discontinue prophylactic therapy should be based on the inconvenience and toxicity of the treatment, the likelihood that recurrent infection will occur within the patient's expected time of survival, and whether or not the symptoms of such infection can be adequately palliated.

Prophylactic therapy for candidiasis and HSV infection should be continued indefinitely or until the patient is unable to swallow. These medications are not associated with significant toxicity and painful or distressing infection may occur within days or a week or two of stopping the treatment. Prophylaxis for pneumocystis and toxoplasmosis with cotrimoxazole is relatively free of side effects and can be continued as long as the patient is taking oral medications. Prophylaxis for MAC infection usually involves multiple drugs with significant side effects; for patients with advanced or terminal AIDS the symptoms of *M. avium* infection may be better controlled with NSAIDs or corticosteroids than by the use of multiple antibiotics. Ganciclovir maintenance therapy for CMV retinitis is the most difficult for patients to discontinue, as half will develop significant deterioration of vision or blindness within a few weeks.

Treatment of infections

Whether or not to actively treat opportunistic infections can pose problems and, given uncertainty about the prognosis of the underlying disease, the decision is often made to proceed with treatment. However, the patient's wishes, their tolerance of the side effects of treatment, and their general condition (including signs of advanced disease or dementia) have all to be considered and the decisions individualized.

Parenteral nutrition

Whether or not patients with advanced disease and severe or chronic diarrhoea should receive parenteral hydration and nutrition can be problematic. Decisions need to be individualized and based both on the wishes of the patients and their general condition (excluding the effects of the diarrhoea). Parenteral nutrition is expensive and not without side effects and its use can lead to difficult decisions about discontinuation at a later stage.

Corticosteroids

The use of corticosteroids can be of major symptomatic benefit in patients with advanced AIDS. It may lead to significant improvement in neuropathic and musculoskeletal pain, headache, dyspnoea, nausea and anorexia, lethargy and weakness, fevers and sweats. Many patients experience a feeling of improved well-being. However, corticosteroids may further compromise immune function and predispose to infection. The decision to use corticosteroids usually requires that the patient has accepted a shift from disease control to symptom control and depends on whether the patient believes that the short-term benefits outweigh the possible risk of additional infection.

Terminal care

The final pathway of terminal AIDS is not very different to that of cancer. Although the duration of the terminal phase may be more variable, the last few days of life of AIDS involve debility and dependency, semi-consciousness, poor oral intake, and may feature generalized pain, restlessness, and rattling respiration. These symptoms respond to the usual measures, including subcutaneous analgesia, anxiolytics, and anti-cholinergics.

Infection control

In managing patients with AIDS, all blood and body substances should be regarded as infectious and standard precautions should be followed. This will protect caregivers from infection with HIV, hepatitis and enteric pathogens. Gloves are worn if there is, or may be, exposure to blood, mucous membranes, non-intact skin or any other body fluid or material. Cuts or abrasions on worker's hands should be covered with an occlusive waterproof dressing. Masks, including eye protection, are used if there is risk of splashing of blood or other body fluid; this includes the management of patients with chest infection who are coughing. Procedures should be established for the disposal of contaminated linen, equipment and waste, and for the management of spillages of blood or body fluids. Care is required when implementing these procedures as excessive or unreasonable safety precautions can accentuate a patient's feelings of isolation and discrimination.

The estimated risk of contracting HIV infection from a percutaneous injury (such as a needle stick) is 0.3%[141]. The risk of mucous membrane exposure (splashes) is much smaller and there are only two anecdotal reports of such infection and none were observed in prospective studies. There is no evidence for infection resulting from cutaneous exposure, such as spilling blood on intact skin. Workers who are immunosuppressed or have exfoliative dermatitis should seek advice before working with AIDS patients.

AIDS patients with pulmonary tuberculosis can pose a risk to health-care workers, especially if the infection is drug-resistant[142]. The management of patients with TB should be in conjunction with respiratory and infectious disease specialists, and good quality face masks that effectively filter the inspired air are required.

Infection control precautions must be continued after the patient's death. Tissue and fluid from the body remain infectious for days. There should be minimal handling of the body, which is placed in a special sealed plastic bag. Embalming is not performed. Further viewing of the body may not be possible and the bereaved should be made aware of this before the body is sealed away.

Psychosocial and spiritual/existential problems

Psychological problems

The psychological impact of AIDS on patients and their caregivers is enormous and the possible sources of psychological distress are legion (Table 12.2.35). The importance of assessing and treating

Table 12.2.35 Sources of psychological distress.

Disease	Progressive disease, uncertain life expectancy
	Unrelieved pain and physical symptoms
	Disfigurement, disabilities
	Long illness leading to psychological exhaustion
Patient	Fear of pain, paralysis, dementia, death
	Loss (or fear of loss) of control, independence, dignity
	Loss (or fear of loss) of job, social position
	Helplessness, hopelessness
	Unfinished business: personal, interpersonal, financial
	Anxious personality: neuroticism, hypochondriasis
Treatment team	Poor communication, lack of information
	Lack of involvement in decisions regarding care
	Exclusion of care givers, partners
Treatment	Side effects
	Multiple failed treatments
	Diagnostic delays
	Bureaucratic red-tape
Social	Stigmatization within family, communities, society
	Discrimination, alienation
	Need for confidentiality, secrecy
	Lack or failure of social supports, resources
	Multiple previous bereavements
	Financial hardship
	Disassociation of biological and social family
	Accessing appropriate care

Table 12.2.36 Some clinical features of psychological distress.

Anxiety	Sadness, misery, remorse
Depression	Regression
Anger, frustration, irritability	Withdrawal
Hopelessness, despair	Passivity
Helplessness	Avoidance
Denial	Inappropriate compensation (joyful)
Guilt	Lack of co-operation with carers
Fear	Unresponsive pain or physical symptoms
Grief	

psychological distress is that it may have a profound effect on QOL and it is reported that high levels of stress and coping by denial are associated with disease progression[82,83,143].

Psychological distress is often described simply in terms of anxiety and depression, but in practice a wide range of psychological reactions and physical symptoms may be manifest (Table 12.2.36)[144]. Most importantly, it should be remembered that unresolved psychosocial and spiritual/existential problems may manifest clinically as pain and physical symptoms unresponsive to treatment. Depression, anxiety, and demoralization have been discussed in the section on psychiatric disorders.

Patients from the male homosexual community, IDUs, and immigrants from areas where HIV is heterosexually endemic may have experienced multiple previous bereavements as friends and family died of AIDS. This may serve to heighten their distress as their own health deteriorates.

Male homosexuals may be distressed by the visible deterioration in their physical appearance that occurs with AIDS. Their sexual orientation may not have been disclosed to their biological family and the boundaries established between their biological and social families are often breached in the face of a life-threatening illness. A life-threatening illness often exposes the conflicts and guilt relating to the homosexual lifestyle, but dealing with these conflicts is usually left until late in the disease and non-resolution may aggravate both physical symptoms and psychological distress. There is often great concern about the maintenance of confidentiality regarding the diagnosis, for fear of the repercussions it might have for them, their families or friends. Many homosexual communities have developed good support networks, but the fact that many have suffered multiple previous bereavements and that the carer may also be infected complicates their effectiveness. Male homosexual couples may need special legal advice to ensure the rights and financial security of the surviving partner.

Intravenous drug users (IDUs) often have poor social networks and have problems with poor nutrition and poor housing. Chaotic lifestyles and the continued use of mind-altering drugs, together with a negative perception of health institutions, often lead to problems with compliance.

The increasing incidence of AIDS in minority and immigrant groups has highlighted problems related to accessing care and patients from these groups tend to take up services late in the course of their illness. These groups usually have low socio-economic status, poor housing, and financial problems. Migrant groups may bring with them different perceptions of health and language barriers may complicate care.

Treatment includes support and counselling and the provision of appropriate services. A trial designed to enable patients to identify sources of stress and develop adapting coping responses led to improved emotional health[145]. Cognitive behavioural and other therapies incorporating stress management may be useful[146,147]. Whether the patients are from the male homosexual or IDU communities, immigrants or other minority groups, support and counselling need to be done in a culturally appropriate and sensitive manner.

Social problems

Social problems encountered in the management of patients with AIDS may relate to alternative life styles with disassociation of biological and social family or to the socio-economic problems experienced by marginalized and minority groups. The high incidence of dementia in the terminal stage makes it important that matters of guardianship and wills are dealt with at a relatively early stage. Because of the discrimination that exists in society, the patient's privacy and confidentiality need to be protected. Patients with AIDS can have difficulty obtaining or keeping accommodation and some are homeless. Housing is a particular problem for otherwise well, younger patients with moderate to severe dementia; if alternative accommodation cannot be provided, long-term residential care for these individuals often falls on palliative care units. Social discrimination may lead to problems with employment

The adequacy of, and satisfaction with, social supports can have significant effect on QOL[148,149]. Interventions to improve social supports and services may be of great benefit.

Spiritual and existential problems

Questions pertaining to spiritual and existential issues, questions about meaning and purpose, may arise as the result of any life event, but occur most frequently in response to a life-threatening illness. Spiritual or existential distress may manifest clinically as a need to discuss issues or as pain and physical symptoms that respond poorly to appropriate therapy. The management of existential distress is discussed elsewhere (see Chapter 15.1). For patients with HIV/AIDS, therapy must be in a culturally appropriate manner.

Quality of life

A number of different tools have been developed to measure QOL in patients with HIV/AIDS[148,150,151].

Multiple bereavements

Multiple losses result in significant psychological, social and spiritual problems, and facilitating grief work can reduce abnormal grieving reactions and promote effective coping skills[152]. A trial of a brief group intervention significantly reduced distress and assisted resolution of the grieving process[153].

Euthanasia and physician assisted suicide

It is reported that more than half of patients with HIV/AIDS in developed countries consider physician-assisted suicide (PAS) or euthanasia[154,155].

In the Netherlands, one-third of patients dying with AIDS receive euthanasia or PAS[156,157]; given the paucity of palliative care services in that country, it is unlikely these patients received any significant palliative care. In the San Francisco Bay area, a significant proportion of doctors looking after patients with HIV/AIDS admit to performing PAS[158]; these were mostly general practitioners who are likely to have had little or no training in palliative care. Another study from the USA reported that 12% of patients dying with AIDS were given increased doses of medications by their partner with the intention of hastening death[159].

In contrast, a report from the Mildmay Mission Hospice, a specialist palliative care service caring for patients with AIDS in London, recorded only one request for euthanasia amongst 1800 admissions over a 3-year period[160]. In the state of Oregon, where PAS is legalized, only one patient with HIV/AIDS is reported to have used the programme[161].

Requests for assisted death from patients with HIV/AIDS have been linked to psychological and psychosocial distress, and to poor control of pain and symptoms. It is documented that people with HIV/AIDS have a higher rate of psychiatric symptoms such as depression and a higher risk of suicide[162], and pre-morbid and co-morbid psychiatric syndromes, as distinct from the physical and psychological consequences of the disease itself, have been advanced as a possible explanation of the high rate of suicide in men with HIV/AIDS[163]. Patients with HIV/AIDS may be susceptible to the demoralization syndrome[95,96].

The strongest predictors of interest in PAS are reported to be depression, hopelessness, experience with terminal illness in a family member or friend, and lack of social supports[154]. Cognitive impairment may also play a role[164]. A study to validate the Schedule of Attitudes Toward Hastened Death in patients with HIV/AIDS showed good correlation with ratings of depression and psychological distress and also with pain intensity and physical symptom distress[165].

A study of the origins of the desire for assisted death in people with HIV/AIDS suggests it is a way of limiting the loss of self due to personal disintegration. Such disintegration results from symptoms and loss of function, and from loss of community that is in turn due to the individual's inability to initiate and maintain personal relationships[162].

These studies underline the importance of comprehensive palliative care in the treatment of patients with HIV/AIDS. All patients should have access to quality palliative care services, practised by interdisciplinary teams experienced in palliative care, and with attention to both the physical and psychosocial aspects of care. A request for euthanasia should be handled like any other distressing symptom occurring in the palliative care setting; it requires careful assessment, identification and treatment of the cause or causes where possible, and provision of comprehensive multidisciplinary symptomatic and supportive care.

References

1. Simon, V., Ho, D.D., and Abdool Karim, Q. (2006). HIV/AIDS epidemiology, pathogenesis, prevention, and treatment. *Lancet*, **368**, 489–504.

2. Merson, M.H. (2006). The HIV-AIDS pandemic at 25–the global response. *New England Journal of Medicine*, **354**, 2414–7.

3. UNAIDS. (2005). AIDS epidemic update, December. http://www.unaids.org/

4. Sepkowitz, K.A. (2006). One disease, two epidemics--AIDS at 25. *New England Journal of Medicine*, **354**, 2411–4.

5. Schwartlander, B., Grubb, I., and Perriens, J. (2006). The 10-year struggle to provide antiretroviral treatment to people with HIV in the developing world. *Lancet*, **368**, 541–6.

6. The UK Collaborative Group for HIV and STI Surveillance (2005). HIV and other Sexually Transmitted Infections in the United Kingdom:http://www.hpa.org.uk/publications/2005/hiv_sti_2005/

7. Gilks, C.F. *et al.* (2006). The WHO public-health approach to antiretroviral treatment against HIV in resource-limited settings. *Lancet*, **368**, 505–10.

8. Centers for Disease Control and Prevention (1992). 1993 revised classification system for HIV infection and expanded surveillance case definition for AIDS among adolescents and adults. Morbidty and Mortality Weekly Report (MMWR). *Recommendations and Reports*, **41**, 1–19.

9. Expert Working Group on Integrated Palliative Care for Persons with AIDS (1988). Summary of a report submitted to Health and Welfare, Canada. *Journal of Palliative Care*, **4**, 76–86.

10. U.S. Department of Health and Human Services (2006). AIDSinfo, the HIV/AIDS Treatment Information Service (HIVATIS). http://aidsinfo.nih.gov/

11. Appleby, P. *et al.* (2000). Highly Active Antiretroviral Therapy and Incidence of Cancer in Human Immunodeficiency Virus-Infected Adults. *Journal of National Cancer Institute*, **92**, 1823–30.

12. DeSimone, J.A., Pomerantz, R.J., and Babinchak, T.J. (2000). Inflammatory Reactions in HIV-1-Infected Persons after Initiation of Highly Active Antiretroviral Therapy. *Annals of Internal Medicine*, **133**, 447–54.

13. Sansone, G.R. and Frengley, J.D. (2000). Impact of HAART on causes of death of persons with late-stage AIDS. *Journal of Urban Health*, **77**, 166–75.

14. May, M.T. *et al.* (2006). HIV treatment response and prognosis in Europe and North America in the first decade of highly active antiretroviral therapy: a collaborative analysis. *Lancet*, **368**, 451–8.

15. Carr, A. and Cooper, D.A. (2000). Adverse effects of antiretroviral therapy. *Lancet*, **356**, 1423–30.

16. Piscitelli, S.C. and Gallicano, K.D. (2001). Interactions among drugs for HIV and opportunistic infections. *New England Journal of Medicine*, **344**, 984–96.

17. Back, D.J. (2006). Drug-drug interactions that matter. Top HIV Med, **14**, 88–92. Also available on line at http://www.iasusa.org/pub/topics/2006/issue2/88.pdf

18. Brook, M.G. *et al.* (2001). Adherence to highly active antiretroviral therapy in the real world: experience of twelve English HIV units. *AIDS Patient Care STDS*, **15**, 491–4.

19. Rueda, S. *et al.* (2006). Patient support and education for promoting adherence to highly active antiretroviral therapy for HIV/AIDS. *Cochrane Database System Review*, **3**, CD001442.

20. Centers for Disease Control and Prevention, National Institutes of Health, and the HIV Medicine Association/Infectious Diseases Society of America (2004). Treating Opportunistic Infections Among HIV-Infected Adults and Adolescents. http://www.cdc.gov/mmwr/preview/mmwrhtml/rr5315a1.htm

21. Briel, M. *et al.* (2006). Adjunctive corticosteroids for Pneumocystis jiroveci pneumonia in patients with HIV-infection. *Cochrane Database System Review*, **3**, CD006150.

22. Pienaar, E.D., Young, T., and Holmes, H. (2006). Interventions for the prevention and management of oropharyngeal candidiasis associated with HIV infection in adults and children. *Cochrane Database System Review*, **3**, CD003940.

23. Dinubile, M.J. *et al.* (2002). Response and relapse rates of candidal esophagitis in HIV-infected patients treated with caspofungin. *AIDS Research and Human Retroviruses*, **18**, 903–8.

24. Watson, M.C. *et al.* (2001). Oral versus intra-vaginal imidazole and triazole anti-fungal treatment of uncomplicated vulvovaginal candidiasis (thrush). *Cochrane Database System Review*, CD002845.

25. Chang, L.W. *et al.* (2005). Antifungal interventions for the primary prevention of cryptococcal disease in adults with HIV. *Cochrane Database System Review*, CD004773.

26. Dedicoat, M. and Livesley, N. (2006). Management of toxoplasmic encephalitis in HIV-infected adults (with an emphasis on resource-poor settings). *Cochrane Database System Review*, CD005420.

27. Gandhi, N.R. *et al.* (2006). Extensively drug-resistant tuberculosis as a cause of death in patients co-infected with tuberculosis and HIV in a rural area of South Africa. *Lancet*, **368**, 1575–80.

28. Woldehanna, S. and Volmink, J. (2004). Treatment of latent tuberculosis infection in HIV infected persons. *Cochrane Database System Review*, CD000171.

29. van der Wouden, J.C. *et al.* (2006). Interventions for cutaneous molluscum contagiosum. *Cochrane Database System Review*, CD004767.

30. Dedicoat, M., Vaithilingum, M., and Newton, R. (2003). Treatment of Kaposi's sarcoma in HIV-1 infected individuals with emphasis on resource poor settings. *Cochrane Database System Review*, CD003256.

31. Kaplan, L.D. *et al.* (2005). Rituximab does not improve clinical outcome in a randomized phase 3 trial of CHOP with or without rituximab in patients with HIV-associated non-Hodgkin lymphoma: AIDS-Malignancies Consortium Trial 010. *Blood,* **106**, 1538–43.

32. Bower, M. *et al.* (2004). HIV-associated anal cancer: has highly active antiretroviral therapy reduced the incidence or improved the outcome? *Journal of Acquired Immune Deficiency Syndrome*, **37**, 1563–5.

33. Shawn, E.R. *et al.* (2005). The spectrum of symptoms among rural South Africans with HIV infection. *Journal of the Association of Nurses in Aids Care*, **16**, 12–23.

34. Norval, D.A. (2004). Symptoms and sites of pain experienced by AIDS patients. *South African Medical Journal*, **94**, 450–4.

35. Karus, D. *et al.* (2005). Patient reports of symptoms and their treatment at three palliative care projects servicing individuals with HIV/AIDS. *Journal of Pain and Symptom Management*, **30**, 408–17.

36. McComsey, G.A. *et al.* (2001). Placebo-controlled trial of prednisone in advanced HIV-1 infection. *Aids*, **15**, 321–7.

37. Glare, P.A. and Cooney, N.J. (1996). Managing HIV. Part 5: Treating secondary outcomes. 5.19 HIV and palliative care. *Medical Journal of Australia*, **164**, 612–5.

38. Larue, F., Fontaine, A., and Colleau, S.M. (1997). Underestimation and undertreatment of pain in HIV disease: multicentre study. *BMJ*, **314**, 23–8.

39. Frich, L.M. and Borgbjerg, F.M. (2000). Pain and pain treatment in AIDS patients: a longitudinal study. *Journal of Pain and Symptom Management*, **19**, 339–47.

40. Rotheram-Borus, M.J. (2000). Variations in perceived pain associated with emotional distress and social identity in AIDS. *AIDS Patient Care STDS*, **14**, 659–65.

41. Breitbart, W. *et al.* (1996). Pain in ambulatory AIDS patients. I: Pain characteristics and medical correlates. *Pain*, **68**, 315–21.

42. Hewitt, D.J. *et al.* (1997). Pain syndromes and etiologies in ambulatory AIDS patients. *Pain*, **70**, 117–23.

43. Brechtl, J.R. *et al.* (2001). The use of highly active antiretroviral therapy (haart) in patients with advanced HIV infection. impact on medical, palliative care, and quality of life outcomes. *Journal of Pain and Symptom Management*, **21**, 41–51.

44. Shlay, J.C. *et al.* (1998). Acupuncture and amitriptyline for pain due to HIV-related peripheral neuropathy: a randomized controlled trial. Terry Beirn Community Programs for Clinical Research on AIDS. *JAMA*, **280**, 1590–5.

45. Simpson, D.M. *et al.* (2000). A placebo-controlled trial of lamotrigine for painful HIV-associated neuropathy. *Neurology*, **54**, 2115–9.

46. La Spina, I. *et al.* (2001). Gabapentin in painful HIV-related neuropathy: a report of 19 patients, preliminary observations. *European Journal of Neurology*, **8**, 71–5.

47. Kaplan, R. *et al.* (1996). Sustained-release morphine sulfate in the management of pain associated with acquired immune deficiency syndrome. *Journal of Pain and Symptom Management*, **12**, 150–60.

48. Newshan, G. and Lefkowitz, M. (2001). Transdermal fentanyl for chronic pain in AIDS: a pilot study. *Journal of Pain and Symptom Management*, **21**, 69–77.

49. Breitbart, W., Kaim, M., and Rosenfeld, B. (1999). Clinicians' perceptions of barriers to pain management in AIDS. *Journal of Pain and Symptom Management*, **18**, 203–12.

50. Breitbart, W. *et al.* (1998). Patient-related barriers to pain management in ambulatory AIDS patients. *Pain*, **76**, 9–16.

51. Breitbart, W. *et al.* (1997). A comparison of pain report and adequacy of analgesic therapy in ambulatory AIDS patients with and without a history of substance abuse. *Pain*, **72**, 235–43.

52. Kaplan, R. *et al.* (2000). A titrated morphine analgesic regimen comparing substance users and non- users with AIDS-related pain. *Journal of Pain and Symptom Management*, **19**, 265–73.

53. Corcoran, C., and Grinspoon, S. (1999). Treatments for wasting in patients with the acquired immunodeficiency syndrome. *New England Journal Medicine*, **340**, 1740–50.

54. Rietschel, P. *et al.* (2000). Prevalence of hypogonadism among men with weight loss related to human immunodeficiency virus infection who were receiving highly active antiretroviral therapy. *Clinical Infect Disaster*, **31**, 1240–4.

55. Lyles, R.H. *et al.* (1999). Virologic, immunologic, and immune activation markers as predictors of HIV-associated weight loss prior to AIDS. Multicenter AIDS Cohort Study. *Journal of Acquired Immune Deficiency Syndrome*, **22**, 386–94.

56. Wagner, G.J. and Rabkin, J.G. (1999). Development of the Impact of Weight Loss Scale (IWLS): a psychometric study in a sample of men with HIV/AIDS. *AIDS Care*, **11**, 453–7.

57. Mulligan, K. *et al.* (2005). Effect of nandrolone decanoate therapy on weight and lean body mass in HIV-infected women with weight loss: a randomized, double-blind, placebo-controlled, multicenter trial. A randomized, placebo-controlled trial of nandrolone decanoate in human immunodeficiency virus-infected men with mild to moderate weight loss with recombinant human growth hormone as active reference treatment. Testosterone therapy in HIV wasting syndrome: systematic review and meta-analysis. Anabolic steroids for the treatment of weight loss in HIV-infected individuals. *Archives of Internal Medicine*, **165**, 578–85.

58. Dolan, S. *et al.* (2004). Effects of testosterone administration in human immunodeficiency virus-infected women with low weight: a randomized placebo-controlled study. *Achieves of Internal Medicine*, **164**, 897–904.

59. Choi, H.H. *et al.* (2005). Effects of testosterone replacement in human immunodeficiency virus-infected women with weight loss. *Journal of Clinical Endocrinology Metabolism*, **90**, 1531–41.

60. Johns, K., Beddall, M.J., and Corrin, R.C. (2005). Anabolic steroids for the treatment of weight loss in HIV-infected individuals. *Cochrane Database System Review*, CD005483.

61. Batterham, M.J. and Garsia, R. (2001). A comparison of megestrol acetate, nandrolone decanoate and dietary counselling for HIV associated weight loss. *International Journal of Andrology*, **24**, 232–40.

62. Clark, R.H. *et al.* (2000). Nutritional treatment for acquired immunodeficiency virus-associated wasting using beta-hydroxy beta-methylbutyrate, glutamine, and arginine: a randomized, double-blind, placebo-controlled study. *JPEN Journal of Parenteral and Enteral Nutrition*, **24**, 133–9.

63. Jenkin, P., Koch, T., and Kralik, D. (2006). The experience of fatigue for adults living with HIV. *Journal of Clinical Nursing*, **15**, 1123–31.

64. Henderson, M. *et al.* (2005). Fatigue among HIV-infected patients in the era of highly active antiretroviral therapy. *HIV Med 6*, 347–52.

65. Wagner, G.J., and Rabkin, R. (2000). Effects of dextroamphetamine on depression and fatigue in men with HIV: a double-blind, placebo-controlled trial. *Journal of Clinical Psychiatry*, **61**, 436–40.

66. Breitbart, W. *et al.* (2001). A randomized, double-blind, placebo-controlled trial of psychostimulants for the treatment of fatigue in ambulatory patients with human immunodeficiency virus disease. *Achieves of Internal Medicine*, **161**, 411–20.

67. Price, R.W. (1999). Management of the neurological complications of HIV-1 infection and AIDS. In *The medical management of AIDS*

(eds. M.A. Sande and P. Volberding), pp. 217–40, Philadelphia, W. B. Saunders.

68. Hriso, E. *et al.* (1991). Extrapyramidal symptoms due to dopamine-blocking agents in patients with AIDS encephalopathy. *American Journal of Psychiatry*, **148**, 1558–61.

69. Berghuis, J.P., Uldall, K.K., and Lalonde, B. (1999). Validity of two scales in identifying HIV-associated dementia. *Journal of Acquired Immune Deficiency Syndromes*, **21**, 134–40.

70. Price, R.W. *et al.* (1999). Neurological outcomes in late HIV infection: adverse impact of neurological impairment on survival and protective effect of antiviral therapy. AIDS Clinical Trial Group and Neurological AIDS Research Consortium study team. *AIDS*, **13**, 1677–85.

71. Sacktor, N. *et al.* (2001). HIV-associated neurologic disease incidence changes: Multicenter AIDS Cohort Study, 1990-1998. *Neurology*, **56**, 257–60.

72. Berger, J.R. and Major, E.O. (1999). Progressive multifocal leukoencephalopathy. *Seminars in Neurology*, **19**, 193–200.

73. Giudici, B. *et al.* (2000). Highly active antiretroviral therapy and progressive multifocal leukoencephalopathy: effects on cerebrospinal fluid markers of JC virus replication and immune response. *Clinical Infectious Disorder*, **30**, 95–9.

74. Dworkin, M.S. *et al.* (1999). Progressive multifocal leukoencephalopathy: improved survival of human immunodeficiency virus-infected patients in the protease inhibitor era. *Journal of Infectious Disorder*, **180**, 621–5.

75. De Luca, A. *et al.* (2000). Cidofovir added to HAART improves virological and clinical outcome in AIDS-associated progressive multifocal leukoencephalopathy. *AIDS*, **14**, F117–F121.

76. Wyen, C. *et al.* (2004). Progressive multifocal leukencephalopathy in patients on highly active antiretroviral therapy: survival and risk factors of death. *Journal of Acquired Immune Deficiency Syndromes*, **37**, 1263–8.

77. Wulff, E.A., Wang, A.K., and Simpson, D.M. (2000). HIV-associated peripheral neuropathy: epidemiology, pathophysiology and treatment. *Drugs*, **59**, 1251–60.

78. Cunningham, E.T., Jr. and Margolis, T.P. (1998). Ocular manifestations of HIV infection. *New England Journal of Medicine*, **339**, 236–44.

79. Karus, D. *et al.* (2004). Mental health status of clients from three HIV/AIDS palliative care projects. *Palliat Support Care*, **2**, 125–38.

80. Pence, B.W. *et al.* (2006). Prevalence of DSM-IV-defined mood, anxiety, and substance use disorders in an HIV clinic in the Southeastern United States. *Journal of Acquired Immune Deficiency Syndromes*, **42**, 298–306.

81. Ciesla, J.A. and Roberts, J.E. (2001). Meta-analysis of the relationship between hiv infection and risk for depressive disorders. *American Journal of Psychiatry*, **158**, 725–30.

82. Leserman, J. *et al.* (2000). Impact of stressful life events, depression, social support, coping, and cortisol on progression to AIDS. *American Journal of Psychiatry*, **157**, 1221–8.

83. Ironson, G. *et al.* (2005). Psychosocial factors predict CD4 and viral load change in men and women with human immunodeficiency virus in the era of highly active antiretroviral treatment. *Psychosomatic Medicine*, **67**, 1013–21.

84. Cockram, A. *et al.* (1999). The evaluation of depression in inpatients with HIV disease. *Australian and New Zealand Journal of Psychiatry*, **33**, 344–52.

85. Kalichman, S.C., Rompa, D., and Cage, M. (2000). Distinguishing between overlapping somatic symptoms of depression and HIV disease in people living with HIV-AIDS. *Journal of Nervous and Mental Disorder*, **188**, 662–70.

86. Richardson, M.A. *et al.* (1999). Effects of depressed mood versus clinical depression on neuropsychological test performance among African American men impacted by HIV/AIDS. *Journal of Clinical and Experimental Neuropsychology*, **21**, 769–83.

87. Carrico, A.W. *et al.* (2006). Reductions in depressed mood and denial coping during cognitive behavioural stress management with HIV-Positive gay men treated with HAART. *Annals of Behavioral Medicine*, **31**, 155–64.

88. Laperriere, A. *et al.* (2005). Decreased depression up to one year following CBSM+ intervention in depressed women with AIDS: the smart/EST women's project. *Journal of Health and Psychology*, **10**, 223–31.

89. Himelhoch, S. and Medoff, D.R. (2005). Efficacy of antidepressant medication among HIV-positive individuals with depression: a systematic review and meta-analysis. *AIDS Patient Care STDS*, **19**, 813–22.

90. Caballero, J. and Nahata, M.C. (2005). Use of selective serotonin-reuptake inhibitors in the treatment of depression in adults with HIV. *Annals of Pharmacotherapy*, **39**, 141–5.

91. Grinspoon, S. *et al.* (2000). Effects of hypogonadism and testosterone administration on depression indices in HIV-infected men. *Journal of Clinical Endocrinology and Metabolism*, **85**, 60–5.

92. Rabkin, J.G., Wagner, G.J., and Rabkin, R. (2000). A double-blind, placebo-controlled trial of testosterone therapy for HIV-positive men with hypogonadal symptoms. *Archives General Psychiatry*, **57**, 141–7; discussion 155–6.

93. Judd, F.K. *et al.* (2000). Depressive symptoms reduced in individuals with HIV/AIDS treated with highly active antiretroviral therapy: a longitudinal study. *Australian and New Zealand Journal of Psychiatry*, **34**, 1015–21.

94. Low-Beer, S. *et al.* (2000). Depressive symptoms decline among persons on HIV protease inhibitors. *Journal of Acquired Immune Deficiency Syndromes*, **23**, 295–301.

95. Chochinov, H.M. *et al.* (1999). Will to live in the terminally ill. *Lancet*, **354**, 816–9.

96. Kissane, D.W. (2001). Demoralisation: its impact on informed consent and medical care. *Medical Journal of Australia*, **175**, 537–9.

97. Sewell, M.C. *et al.* (2000). Anxiety syndromes and symptoms among men with AIDS: a longitudinal controlled study. *Psychosomatics*, **41**, 294–300.

98. Ellen, S.R. *et al.* (1999). Secondary mania in patients with HIV infection. *Australian and New Zealand Journal of Psychiatry*, **33**, 353–60.

99. Afessa, B. and Green, B. (2000). Bacterial pneumonia in hospitalized patients with HIV infection: the Pulmonary Complications, ICU Support, and Prognostic Factors of Hospitalized Patients with HIV (PIP) Study. *Chest*, **117**, 1017–22.

100. Herranz, P. *et al.* (2000). Successful treatment of aphthous ulcerations in AIDS patients using topical granulocyte-macrophage colony-stimulating factor. *British Journal of Dermatology*, **142**, 171–6.

101. Knox, T.A. *et al.* (2000). Diarrhea and abnormalities of gastrointestinal function in a cohort of men and women with HIV infection. *American Journal of Gastroenterology*, **95**, 3482–9.

102. Lamberts, S.W. *et al.* (1996). Octreotide. *New England Journal of Medicine*, **334**, 246–54.

103. Beaugerie, L. *et al.* (1996). Treatment of refractory diarrhoea in AIDS with acetorphan and octreotide: a randomized crossover study. *European Journal of Gastroenterology and Hepatology*, **8**, 485–9.

104. Goldstone, S.E. *et al.* (2001). High Prevalence of Anal Squamous Intraepithelial Lesions and Squamous- Cell Carcinoma in Men Who Have Sex With Men as Seen in a Surgical Practice. *Diseases of The Colon and Rectum*, **44**, 690–8.

105. Konopnicki, D. *et al.* (2005). Hepatitis B and HIV: prevalence, AIDS progression, response to highly active antiretroviral therapy and increased mortality in the EuroSIDA cohort. *AIDS*, **19**, 593–601.

106. Law, W.P. *et al.* (2004). Impact of viral hepatitis co-infection on response to antiretroviral therapy and HIV disease progression in the HIV-NAT cohort. *AIDS*, **18**, 1169–77.

107. Weis, N. *et al.* (2006). Impact of hepatitis C virus coinfection on response to highly active antiretroviral therapy and outcome in HIV-infected individuals: a nationwide cohort study. *Clinical Infectious Disease*, **42**, 1481–7.

108. Volberding, P. (2000). Consensus statement: anemia in HIV infection--current trends, treatment options, and practice strategies. Anemia in HIV Working Group. *Clinical Therapy*, **22**, 1004–20; discussion 1003.

109. Behler, C. *et al.* (2005). Anemia and HIV in the antiretroviral era: potential significance of testosterone. *AIDS Research and Human Retroviruses*, **21**, 200–6.

110. Collier, A.C. *et al.* (2001). Leukocyte-reduced red blood cell transfusions in patients with anemia and human immunodeficiency virus infection: the Viral Activation Transfusion Study: a randomized controlled trial. *JAMA*, **285**, 1592–601.

111. Abrams, D.I., Steinhart, C., and Frascino, R. (2000). Epoetin alfa therapy for anaemia in HIV-infected patients: impact on quality of life. *International Journal of STD and AIDS*, **11**, 659–65.

112. Tamkus, D. *et al.* (2006). Thrombotic microangiopathy syndrome as an AIDS-defining illness: the experience of J. Stroger Hospital of Cook County. *Clinical Advances in Hematology and Oncology*, **4**, 145–9.

113. Obasanjo, O.O. *et al.* (2001). An outbreak of scabies in a teaching hospital: lessons learned. *Infection Control and Hospital Epidemiology*, **22**, 13–8.

114. Hengge, U.R. *et al.* (2000). Self-administered topical 5% imiquimod for the treatment of common warts and molluscum contagiosum. *British Journal of Dermatology*, **143**, 1026–31.

115. Peckham, C. and Newell, M.L. (2000). Preventing vertical transmission of HIV infection. *New England Journal of Medicine*, **343**, 1036–7.

116. Brocklehurst, P. (2002). Interventions for reducing the risk of mother-to-child transmission of HIV infection. *Cochrane Database Systematic Review*, CD000102.

117. Read, J.S. and Newell, M.K. (2005). Efficacy and safety of cesarean delivery for prevention of mother-to-child transmission of HIV-1. *Cochrane Database Systematic Review* CD005479.

118. Brocklehurst, P. and Volmink, J. (2002). Antiretrovirals for reducing the risk of mother-to-child transmission of HIV infection. *Cochrane Database Systematic Review*, CD003510.

119. Glare, P.A. and Virik, K. (2001). Can we do better in end-of-life care? The mixed management model and palliative care. *Medical Journal of Australia*, **175**, 530–3.

120. Peretti-Watel, P. *et al.* (2004). Opinions toward pain management and palliative care: comparison between HIV specialists and oncologists. *AIDS Care*, **16**, 619–27.

121. Easterbrook, P. and Meadway, J. (2001). The changing epidemiology of HIV infection: new challenges for HIV palliative care. *Journal of Royal Society of Medicine*, **94**, 442–8.

122. Matheny, S.C. (2001). Clinical dilemmas in palliative care for HIV infection. *Journal of Royal Society of Medicine*, **94**, 449–51.

123. Grant, A.D. and De Cock, K.M. (2001). ABC of AIDS. HIV infection and AIDS in the developing world. *BMJ*, **322**, 1475–8.

124. Rankin, W. and Wilson, C. (2000). African women with HIV. *BMJ*, **321**, 1543–4.

125. Harries, A.D. *et al.* (2001). Deaths from tuberculosis in sub-Saharan African countries with a high prevalence of HIV-1. *Lancet*, **357**, 1519–23.

126. Weidle, P.J. *et al.* (2006). Adherence to antiretroviral therapy in a home-based AIDS care programme in rural Uganda. *Lancet*, **368**, 1587–94.

127. Gill, C.J. (2006). Antiretroviral programme in rural Uganda. *Lancet*, **368**, 1556–7.

128. Merriman, A. (1999). Hospice Uganda: 1993-1998. *Journal of Palliative Care*, **15**, 50–2.

129. Steinhauser, K.E. *et al.* (2000). Factors considered important at the end of life by patients, family, physicians, and other care providers. *JAMA*, **284**, 2476–82.

130. Singer, P.A., Martin, D.K., and Kelner, M. (1999). Quality end-of-life care: patients' perspectives. *JAMA*, **281**, 163–8.

131. Armes, P.J. and Higginson, I.J. (1999). What constitutes high-quality HIV/AIDS palliative care? *Journal of Palliative Care*, **15**, 5–12.

132. James, J.H. (2001). Healthcare financing for the under-served: UK. *Journal of Royal Society of Medicine*, **94**, 462–5; discussion 466–7.

133. Bozzette, S.A. *et al.* (1998). The care of HIV-infected adults in the United States. HIV Cost and Services Utilization Study Consortium. *New England Journal of Medicine*, **339**, 1897–904.

134. Higginson, I.J. and O'Neill, J. (2001). Palliative care in the age of HIV/AIDS. Conclusions from the meeting. *Journal of Royal Society of Medicine*, **94**, 496–8.

135. Pirraglia, P.A. *et al.* (2005). Caregiver burden and depression among informal caregivers of HIV-infected individuals. *Journal of General Internal Medicine*, **20**, 510–4.

136. Orner, P. (2006). Psychosocial impacts on caregivers of people living with AIDS. *AIDS Care*, **18**, 236–40.

137. Martin, D.K., Emanuel, L.L., and Singer, P.A. (2000). Planning for the end of life. *Lancet*, **356**, 1672–6.

138. Curtis, J.R. *et al.* (2000). Why don't patients and physicians talk about end-of-life care? Barriers to communication for patients with acquired immunodeficiency syndrome and their primary care clinicians. *Archives of Internal Medicine*, **160**, 1690–6.

139. Ho, V.W. *et al.* (2000). The effect of advance care planning on completion of advance directives and patient satisfaction in people with HIV/AIDS. *AIDS Care*, **12**, 97–108.

140. Curtis, J.R. *et al.* (2000). The attitudes of patients with advanced AIDS toward use of the medical futility rationale in decisions to forego mechanical ventilation. *Archives of Internal Medicine*, **160**, 1597–601.

141. Evans, B. *et al.* (2001). Exposure of healthcare workers in England, Wales, and Northern Ireland to bloodborne viruses between July 1997 and June 2000: analysis of surveillance data. *BMJ*, **322**, 397–8.

142. Hannan, M.M. *et al.* (2001). Investigation and control of a large outbreak of multi-drug resistant tuberculosis at a central Lisbon hospital. *Journal of Hospital Infection*, **47**, 91–7.

143. Moskowitz, J.T. (2003). Positive affect predicts lower risk of AIDS mortality. *Psychosomatic Medicine*, **65**, 620–6.

144. Kelly, B. *et al.* (2000). Measuring psychological adjustment to HIV infection. *International Journal of Psychiatry Medicine*, **30**, 41–59.

145. Heckman, T.G. *et al.* (2001). A pilot coping improvement intervention for late middle-aged and older adults living with HIV/AIDS in the USA. *AIDS Care*, **13**, 129–39.

146. Ozsoy, M. and Ernst, E. (1999). How effective are complementary therapies for HIV and AIDs?--A systematic review. *International Journal of STD and AIDS*, **10**, 629–35.

147. Lechner, S.C. *et al.* (2003). Cognitive-behavioural interventions improve quality of life in women with AIDS. *Journal of Psychosomatic Research*, **54**, 253–61.

148. Holmes, W.C. and Shea, J.A. (1999). Two approaches to measuring quality of life in the HIV/AIDS population: HAT-QoL and MOS-HIV. *Quality of Life Research*, **8**, 515–27.

149. Swindells, S. *et al.* (1999). Quality of life in patients with human immunodeficiency virus infection: impact of social support, coping style and hopelessness. *International Journal of STD and AIDS*, **10**, 383–91.

150. McDonnell, K.A. *et al.* (2000). Measuring health related quality of life among women living with HIV. *Quality of Life Research*, **9**, 931–40.

151. Kemppainen, J.K. (2001). Predictors of quality of life in AIDS patients. *Journal of the Association of Nurses in AIDS Care*, **12**, 61–70.

152. Mallinson, R.K. (1999). Grief work of HIV positive persons and their survivors. *Nursing Clinics in North America*, **34**, 163–77.

153. Goodkin, K. *et al.* (1999). A randomized controlled clinical trial of a bereavement support group intervention in human immunodeficiency virus type 1-seropositive and - seronegative homosexual men. *Archives of General Psychiatry*, **56**, 52–9.

154. Breitbart, W., Rosenfeld, B.D., and Passik, S.D. (1996). Interest in physician-assisted suicide among ambulatory HIV-infected patients. *American Journal of Psychiatry*, **153**, 238–42.

155. Starace, F. and Sherr, L. (1998). Suicidal behaviours, euthanasia and AIDS. *AIDS*, **12**, 339–47.

156. Bindels, P.J. *et al.* (1996). Euthanasia and physician-assisted suicide in homosexual men with AIDS. *Lancet*, **347**, 499–504.

157. Onwuteaka-Philipsen, B.D. and van der Wal, G. (1998). Cases of euthanasia and physician assisted suicide among AIDS patients reported to the Public Prosecutor in North Holland. *Public Health*, **112**, 53–6.

158. Slome, L.R. *et al.* (1997). Physician-assisted suicide and patients with human immunodeficiency virus disease. *New England Journal of Medicine*, **336**, 417–21.

159. Cooke, M. *et al.* (1998). Informal caregivers and the intention to hasten AIDS-related death. *Archives of Internal Medicine*, **158**, 69–75.

160. McKeogh, M. (1997). Physician-assisted suicide and patients with AIDS. *New England Journal of Medicine*, **337**, 56.

161. Hedberg, K., Hopkins, D., and Kohn, M. (2003). Five years of legal physician-assisted suicide in Oregon. *New England Journal of Medicine*, **348**, 961–4.

162. Lavery, J.V. *et al.* (2001). Origins of the desire for euthanasia and assisted suicide in people with HIV-1 or AIDS: a qualitative study. *Lancet*, **358**, 362–7.

163. Mishara, B.L. (1998). Suicide, euthanasia and AIDS. *Crisis*, **19**, 87–96.

164. Pessin, H. *et al.* (2003). The role of cognitive impairment in desire for hastened death: a study of patients with advanced AIDS. *General Hospital Psychiatry*, **25**, 194–9.

165. Rosenfeld, B. *et al.* (1999). Measuring desire for death among patients with HIV/AIDS: the schedule of attitudes toward hastened death. *American Journal of Psychiatry*, **156**, 94–100.

12.3

Palliative care in non-malignant, end-stage respiratory disease

Richard M. Leach

Introduction

There is an increasing awareness that non-malignant, end-stage respiratory disease requires 'palliative' and compassionate end-of-life management and this is increasingly reflected in management guidelines, department of health directives, and published research. Unlike malignant disease, the course of chronic respiratory disease is often one of slow inexorable decline with relapsing but increasing periods of disabling dyspnoea and reduced exercise tolerance, recurrent hospital admissions, and premature death. In many patients, loss of dignity, self respect, social isolation, and psychological problems are often present during and well before the terminal phase of the disease. Good prognostic data demonstrate convincingly that the variability and unpredictability of survival even in advanced end-stage respiratory disease makes accurate prognosis impossible, except when the patient is actually dying. This prolonged and arbitrary deterioration places family members, carers, and medical teams under considerable pressure which may manifest in many ways including denial, hostility, and communication difficulties within families and in relation to medical carers.

Despite recent interest, these long-suffering incurable patients have not fully benefited from the holistic approach to the management of the physical, psychological, social, and spiritual needs developed and provided by specialist palliative care medicine. Recognition of these unmet needs is not new. When John Hinton first reported the requirements of dying patients in 1963, he recognized that cancer patients were not alone in suffering uncontrolled symptoms in the last days of life. Indeed, he reported that patients with non-malignant disease often suffered the greatest physical distress[1]. Since this seminal article, the considerable success of the hospice movement in the management of cancer patients has further highlighted the plight of terminally-ill, non-cancer patients and the widening gap in their access to adequate palliative care[2]. In recent years, there has been a growing awareness of the need for palliative and hospice care of patients dying of non-malignant disease. Nevertheless, there is still surprisingly little research or data examining the needs of patients with non-malignant, end-stage respiratory disease, which is a substantial and increasing cause of disability and mortality in the developed world. In some countries like the USA, a high proportion of patients with non-malignant disease are already admitted to hospice inpatient units (30 per cent in 1994–1995)[3]. In contrast, such facilities are limited in the UK accounting for <4 per cent of hospice inpatient admissions in 1994–1995 and are only available to small numbers of specific groups of end-stage neurological and HIV disease (Table 12.3.1)[4].

Recent studies have recognized the similarity between symptoms in patients dying with malignant and non-malignant disease[5,6]. Although pain is often reported to be a greater problem in cancer patients[7], recent reports suggest that moderate and severe pain can occur as often in non-cancer patients[8,9]. The SUPPORT study, a major American investigation of decision-making in the last days of life, reported severe pain in 40 per cent of patients, and moderate or severe dyspnoea in 25 per cent irrespective of the disease[10]. Similar findings in end-stage patients with renal failure[11], motor neuron disease[12], heart disease[13], stroke[14], and chronic obstructive pulmonary disease (COPD)[15–17] demonstrated the considerable physical and psychological needs of the non-malignant dying patient.

These deficiencies have been recognized by a number of Government Committee's in the UK who have recommended that all non-malignant dying patients who require palliative care services should have access to them[2,18,19]. The National Council for Hospice and Specialist Palliative Care Services and Scottish Partnership Agency for Palliative and Cancer Care Diseases assessed the need, potential demand, and resource implications of these directives in their 1998 publication entitled 'Reaching out: Specialist palliative care for adults with non-malignant diseases'[2]. There are, without doubt, considerable difficulties to be overcome if adequate palliative care facilities are to be provided to sufferers of non-malignant disease[2] and many of these are particularly applicable

Table 12.3.1 Adult patients who received care from hospices/palliative care services in 1994–1995.

	Malignancy (per cent)	Neurological (per cent)	HIV/AIDS (per cent)	Other (per cent)
New inpatients	96.7	1.3	0.5	1.6
Home care patients	96.3	0.6	0.6	2.5
Day care patients	96.3	0.2	0.2	1.2

to the management of end-stage respiratory disease. Not least is the potential size and resource implications of this requirement and the fear, expressed by many palliative care physicians, that this demand may be detrimental to the delivery of care to cancer patients and may reduce charitable donations. Determining when chronic disease becomes terminal is another major issue. Unlike cancer many non-malignant diseases, particularly end-stage respiratory disease, have long periods of stability interrupted by major life-threatening exacerbations which make end-of-life management decisions difficult. Finally, concern has also been raised as to whether specialists in palliative care have the necessary skills to manage a wide variety of terminal disease processes.

The potential requirement for palliative care in end-stage pulmonary disease

In most developed countries, lung cancer and chronic lung diseases are a significant and increasing cause of morbidity and mortality. Respiratory diseases accounted for 117 456 of 587 808 deaths in the UK in 2004[20,22,23], more than ischaemic heart disease (106 081 cases) and just less than non-respiratory cancer (122 512 cases). Of the respiratory deaths, acute infectious diseases including pneumonia and influenza accounted for 33 986, respiratory cancer for 34 721, and pulmonary circulatory disease 3926 cases. Progressive, non-malignant diseases, in particular COPD (27 478 cases), but also including less common chronic lung diseases such as pneumoconiosis (3024 cases), pulmonary fibrosis and cystic fibrosis account for about 22 per cent of all respiratory deaths (Table 12.3.2).

Chronic obstructive pulmonary disease is recognized as a major although neglected medical and social problem. In the UK, chronic respiratory disability causes about 9–13 per cent of adult disability and COPD is the major cause[20,23]. Exact figures for the prevalence of COPD are difficult to determine due to problems of definition. In the UK, 9–11 per cent of patients over the age of 45 years old have non-reversible chronic airflow obstruction and will account for 1000 inpatient admissions and 25 000 primary care consultations annually in an average health district[20,24,25]. However, it should be recognized that respiratory disease and in particular COPD is twice as frequent in the UK (age standardized death rate: 105 per 100 000 population) compared with other European Union countries (57 per 100 000 population)[20,26]. In the

USA about 2 million people have emphysema and about 50 per cent of these have reduced exercise tolerance[27]. Although smoking appears to be decreasing in developed countries, and eventually the incidence of COPD will fall, it appears to be increasing in developing countries and current low levels of COPD in these countries is likely to rise in the future[28].

The cause of end-stage respiratory disease requiring palliative care varies geographically in relation to socio-economic factors. HIV-related respiratory diseases and post-tuberculous bronchiectasis are common problems in developing countries. In contrast, COPD, cystic fibrosis, restrictive chest wall diseases (e.g. scoliosis, thoracoplasty), and neuro-muscular disorders (e.g. motor neuron disease, muscular dystrophies, old poliomyelitis) are more common in the USA and Europe. In developed countries, diseases which affect younger patients including cystic fibrosis and the muscular dystrophies, are better resourced and the terminal needs of these patients are often well managed. In comparison, COPD and the less common fibrotic lung diseases have the same palliative care requirements but there is inadequate resource to meet these needs.

From the data in Table 12.3.2, it is apparent that equal numbers of patients with non-malignant, end-stage respiratory disease (mainly COPD), and lung cancer are experiencing pre-terminal disease and are likely to require similar medical and social services. Both conditions are managed by the same health-care professionals and intuition and a number of recent UK studies suggest that patients with end-stage respiratory disease do not receive the care appropriate to their needs[2,15,16]. However, in comparison with malignant disease, there has been remarkably little research into the symptomatology, survival, appropriate care, and service utilization of patients with chronic lung disease. This information is vital if appropriate and manageable solutions to the current weaknesses in care delivery are to be addressed.

Terminal symptoms, quality of life, and survival of patients with end-stage pulmonary disease

Quality of life in patients with chronic lung disease is often poor and survival statistics may be worse than for many malignant conditions. Prognosis is inversely related to age and directly to FEV_1 and hypoxaemia. Unfortunately, in the individual case, these measurements are of little help in predicting survival as the patient may struggle from one crisis to another for many years before sudden deterioration and death over a few days. In the Medical Research Council trial of domiciliary oxygen in patients with COPD and stable hypoxaemia, survival of men and women in the control arm was only 42 per cent and 28 per cent, respectively, at 3 years[29]. There is further evidence from the SUPPORT study that judging time to death is difficult in non-malignant disease. On the day before death, hospitalized lung cancer patients were predicted to have <20 per cent chance of living for 2 months, compared with a 60 per cent predicted chance of doing so in patients with heart failure[9].

In patients with COPD there have been several recent studies demonstrating the difficulty of accurate prognostication[30–32]. In a study of 110 COPD patients who survived severe acute hypercapnic respiratory failure after non-invasive ventilation, 80 per cent were readmitted within a year, 63 per cent experienced a further life threatening event but only 50 per cent had died that year and it was

Table 12.3.2 Respiratory disease deaths 2004.

All respiratory disease	117 456 cases (100 per cent)
Pneumonia and TB	34 345 cases (29.2 per cent)
Cancer	34 721 cases (29.6 per cent)
Progressive non-malignant causes	35 979 cases (30.6 per cent)
COPD	27 478 cases (23.3 per cent)
Pulmonary circulatory disease	3926 cases (3.3 per cent)
Pneumoconiosis	3024 cases (2.6 per cent)
Asthma	1381 cases (1.2 per cent)
Cystic fibrosis	139 cases (0.1 per cent)
Sarcoidosis	31 cases (0.07 per cent)
Others (congenital, foreign body, etc)	12 411 cases (10.6 per cent)

Table 12.3.3 Factors associated with poor prognosis in COPD.

Low BMI/low fat-free body mass
Low FEV$_1$/dyspnoea
Low SaO$_2$/long-term oxygen treatment
Low 6-min walking distance (6MWD)
Two or more hospital admissions in the previous year
Maintenance treatment with oral steroids
Concomitant congestive cardiac failure
Low serum albumin
Cor pulmonale

Table 12.3.4 Symptoms reported in the final year of life.

Symptom	Chronic lung disease		Lung cancer	
	All (per cent)	Very distressing (per cent)	All (per cent)	Very distressing (per cent)
Pain	77	56	85	56
Breathlessness	94	76	78	60
Cough	59	46	56	40
Anorexia	67	15	76	19
Constipation	44	25	59	55
Insomnia	65	42	60	35
Low mood	71	57	68	51

impossible to differentiate those who survived from those who died[31]. In a further small study of 19 patients who elected to decline further mechanical ventilation in the event of deterioration, the mean length of subsequent survival was 210 days and more than 50 per cent were still alive after1 year[32]. Further attempts to quantify prognosis and construct a prognostic index for COPD have confirmed the importance of key elements of the patient's condition (Table 12.3.3). The BODE index used the body–mass index, airflow obstruction, dyspnoea, and exercise capacity index but the correlation between these elements and survival was not good enough to enable an accurate assessment in the individual[33]. As a result it is difficult to make end-of-life decisions and the inability to predict disease trajectory has led to some concern that hospice facilities will be blocked by non-malignant cases who are gravely ill at admission but recover to their previous state of chronic ill-health[2]. However, it must be recognized that only half of hospice admissions in cancer patients in 1994/1995 ended in death, with many patients returning home following resolution of the immediate problem[4].

The poor quality of life experienced by patients with end-stage COPD was recognized and reported in the Nocturnal Oxygen Therapy Trial in 1980 as disturbances in both emotional and social functioning and marked impairment in activities in daily living[34]. Recent studies have documented the symptoms (Table 12.3.4), quality of life, palliative care needs and service utilization of patients dying of chronic respiratory disease during the final weeks and months of life[15–17]. Breathlessness and pain were reported as 'very distressing' in 76 per cent and 56 per cent of patients during the final year[16]. In this study, the overall burden of symptoms both in the last week and year of life was similar to those experienced by lung cancer patients. In chronic lung disease, symptoms had been present for longer and the severity and frequency of breathlessness was greater. In contrast, constipation and anorexia were more frequent in lung cancer patients.

When compared with patients dying with unresectable, non-small cell lung cancer patients, end-stage COPD patients have a significantly worse quality of life[15]. However, assessing quality of life is complex, being both individual and multi-dimensional[35]. Many quantitative instruments are available to measure 'generic' health-related quality of life (HRQoL). In the medical context these grade physical symptoms, psychological well-being and limitations in physical and social activity (e.g. Medical Outcomes Study Short Form 36 (SF-36)). They can be compared with data from normal populations but have limitations in relation to chronic disease[36].

Disease-specific instruments examine features specific to the disease studied. The St George's Respiratory Questionnaire (SGRQ) and the Chronic Respiratory Disease Questionnaire (CRDQ) are often used to measure HRQoL in respiratory patients[37,38]. In cancer patients the European Organisation for the Research and Treatment of Cancer Core questionnaire (EORTC QLQ-C30) and the site-specific module LC-17 for lung cancer are well validated as an outcome measure[39]. In the study comparing quality of life in patients with COPD and lung cancer, both 'generic' and 'disease-specific' measures demonstrated a worse quality of life in COPD patients[15]. Physical, social, and emotional functioning, as well as activities of daily living, were worse in COPD patients. Clinical depression measured with the Hospital Anxiety and Depression Scale (HADS) also affected 90 per cent of COPD compared with 52 per cent of lung cancer patients. However, some care should be exercised in interpreting the results of this study[35], as previous studies reported greater levels of depression using HADS scores in patients with inoperable cancer[40] and lower EORTC scores for emotional function in lung cancer[41].

Current service provision and utilization by patients with end-stage pulmonary disease

In the UK, few (<5 per cent) of the 75 per cent of patients who die from non-malignant disease, die in a hospice or under the care of a domiciliary palliative care team (Table 12.3.5) although a larger proportion receive such care outside the UK[3]. A recent UK study reported that non-cancer patients accounted for between 0 per cent and 12 per cent (median 5 per cent) of the palliative care team's workload[2]. In contrast, at least 20 per cent of cancer patients die in a hospice and a further 40 per cent die whilst under the care of a specialist domiciliary care team[4]. These figures may be an underestimate as many cancer patients receive domiciliary care from, or attended, a hospice day unit and die elsewhere. In comparison, the vast majority of patients with end-stage non-malignant respiratory disease are admitted to, and die, on hospital wards or high dependency units in order to receive adequate palliation of their pre-terminal respiratory symptoms, as they have little access to either hospice or home support.

There is little data on the value of palliative care in non-malignant disease except in motor neuron disease and dementia[2,11,14]. It is also recognized that the majority of patients

Table 12.3.5 Place of death in a random sample in 20 UK health districts in 1990.

Place of death	Cancer (per cent n = 2063)	Chronic lung disease (per cent; n = 87)	Heart disease (per cent; n = 683)	Stroke (per cent; n = 229)
Home	29	12	29	9
Hospital	50	72	55	67
Hospice	14	0	0	0
Other	7	16	16	24

Source: adapted from references (2) and (13).

with heart disease and stroke die in hospital or residential/nursing homes and that there are deficits in their end-of-life care[5,6,42]. Likewise, most respiratory health workers would accept the assumption that patients with end-stage respiratory disease are less well provided for than cancer patients in the UK[15], although the British Thoracic Society survey in 1997 reported that <30 per cent of lung cancer units had access to a specialist cancer nurse[43]. Despite this, there is little doubt that more palliative care services are available to cancer patients[2].

There have been two direct comparisons of end-of-life care in lung cancer and chronic respiratory disease[15,16]. Patients with chronic respiratory disease were more likely to die in hospital and lung cancer patients at home or in a hospice. Chronic lung disease patients were often admitted as emergencies, and as a result lung cancer patients were observed to spend longer in their place of death[16]. Access to primary medical care was good for both groups[15,16] although only a small percentage received treatment for anxiety and depression despite high levels of these symptoms[15]. Financial support (mobility allowance or income support) and aids (including wheelchairs, bed aid, bath aids) were available to both groups but more frequent in COPD patients due to the longer course of the illness and because most of these patients were housebound and 30 per cent wheelchair bound. In both studies, access to palliative care services for patients with chronic respiratory disease was poor[15,16]. Thirty per cent of cancer patients received help from a Marie- Curie nurse, Macmillan nurse, or hospice centre, and a further 56 per cent had been offered or were aware of the availability of these services[15]. In contrast none of the COPD patients received or were offered access to these services or any equivalent service. However, a respiratory nurse visited about 25 per cent of COPD patients, although her primary responsibility was for tuberculosis-contact tracing. A concern in both studies was the lack of information relating to treatment, management, and prognosis. Lung cancer patients were more likely to be told that they would die of the disease by the hospital doctor than patients with COPD. Most COPD patients determined their prognosis by talking to other health personnel (e.g. district nurse) and during acute admissions.

There is currently little evidence as to the effectiveness or feasibility of specialist palliative care services in end-stage, non-malignant respiratory disease. As early as 1981 the Royal College of Physicians (UK) recommended the creation of respiratory health worker posts to help with the management of patients with chronic respiratory diseases[44]. Home visits to advise on both psychosocial and respiratory problems and to improve compliance with treatment were envisaged[45]. The 1997 British Thoracic Society guidelines for the management of COPD conclude that there are

no data to show how end-stage COPD should be managed to achieve the best combination of clinical and cost effectiveness[24]. Currently, there are about 140 respiratory nurses in the UK[46]. Patients under the care of these nurses may live longer but their impact on improving quality of life has been questioned in some studies[45,47]. However, chest clinics employing specialist respiratory nurses recognize their role in symptom control and compliance with therapy. In addition, despite the lack of evidence of objective improvement, patients valued these visits and wanted them to continue[45]. Recent studies in acute exacerbations of COPD suggest that early discharge and 'care at home programmes' run by respiratory outreach nurses are both safe and cost effective[48,49]. In addition, both patients and carer's reported that home care was their preferred option[50].

Symptom pathophysiology and assessment

Chronic end stage lung disease is associated with the symptoms of breathlessness, cough (± sputum production), fever (± sweats), infection (± halitosis), haemoptysis, stridor, and chest wall pain. The pathophysiology and assessment of most of these symptoms has been examined in the chapter relating to malignant respiratory conditions. This brief review will concentrate on the relationship to non-malignant disease. The treatment of each symptom and therapeutic modalities will be discussed in the management of individual disease process.

Dyspnoea

Dyspnoea is derived from the Greek *dys*: meaning painful or difficult and *pneuma* meaning breath and is used to describe a variety of sensations experienced when breathing is difficult, uncomfortable or laboured or when the subject feels a need for more air[51]. This sensation of breathlessness is experienced by healthy individuals under stress (e.g. altitude, exercise) and patients with a wide spectrum of respiratory, cardiac, neurological, renal, and other diseases. It is multi-factorial and influenced by many modifying factors (e.g. physiological, psychological, and social) and is distinct from other symptoms like tachypnoea, hyperinflation, or cyanosis. The American Thoracic Society in its 1999 consensus conference defined dyspnoea as: '*a term used to characterize a subjective experience of breathing discomfort that is comprised of qualitatively distinct sensations that vary in intensity. The experience derives from interactions among multiple physiological, psychological, social and environmental factors, and may induce secondary physiological and behavioural responses*' and remains the current definition but, depending on future developments, is likely to be subject to modification[52].

Like pain, breathlessness has specific descriptors and refers to a number of different sensations including chest tightness, the need for deep inspiration, frequency, and depth of ventilation[53,54]. Both normal subjects and COPD patients were able to distinguish the intensity of breathlessness from the distress it causes[55]. Unfortunately, the 'language of dyspnoea' is not specific and individual descriptions are dependent on physiological context, personality, social, and ethnic factors[56]. Thus, as with pain, a good history is invaluable in the assessment of dyspnoea.

Prevalence of dyspnoea

Breathlessness is the most frequent symptom experienced in end-stage respiratory disease. In the SUPPORT trial, dyspnoea was the major complaint of 416 patients dying with COPD, and was twice as common as pain or confusion throughout the 6 months of their dying[10]. In chronic lung disease breathlessness was reported in 94 per cent during the last year and 91 per cent during the last week of life, compared with 78 per cent and 69 per cent respectively in lung cancer patients[16].

Mechanisms of dyspnoea

The mechanism of dyspnoea is extensively reviewed in the chapter on malignant respiratory disease. Fig. 12.3.1 is a simplified representation of the complex and poorly understood mechanism of dyspnoea. At its simplest level the mechanism of dyspnoea may be expressed as:

◆ A central drive or 'urge to breath' that functions to satisfy the metabolic requirements of the body by maintaining blood-gas and acid–base homeostasis by modulating ventilatory activity. This drive to breath incorporates all the sensory afferent input from chemosensors (e.g. medulla, carotid, and aortic bodies), mechanoreceptors (e.g. chest wall, lung and pulmonary vessel receptors, peripheral muscle receptors) and higher cerebral cortex activity (e.g. anxiety, personality).

◆ *The 'sense of respiratory effort' or work of breathing associated with ventilation.* When the efferent motor command to the respiratory muscles is discharged, a corollary message is sent to higher brain centres and results in a conscious awareness of the outgoing motor command. The resulting *'sense of effort'* is the ratio of the pressure actually generated by the respiratory muscles to the maximum that could be generated[52].

An attractive unifying theory is that dyspnoea results from a dissociation or mismatch between central motor activity and incoming afferent information from chemo- and mechanoreceptors[52]. The sensation of dyspnoea depends on the degree to which the respiratory neurons and neurotransmittor agents in the diffuse brainstem 'respiratory complex' are stimulated[57,58] by factors like hypoxia, hypercapnia, exercise, and metabolic acidosis. In addition, most studies demonstrate that stimulation of ventilation is necessary for breathlessness to occur[57]. However, the relationship between ventilatory response to stimuli and dyspnoea is not maintained in all circumstances and the sensation of dyspnoea may be directly affected by inputs from chemoreceptors. Thus, relief of exercise-induced hypoxaemia by administration of oxygen in COPD patients results in a reduction of dyspnoea out of proportion to the reduction in ventilation[59]. Similarly, ventilator-dependent quadriplegics with high cervical spinal cord transections experience breathlessness when PCO_2 is increased when there should be no change in afferent feedback from the chest wall[60].

Prolonged severe hypoxia and hypercapnia may also occur in the complete absence of dyspnoea suggesting that in some patients the medullary respiratory centre adapts to prolonged stimulation. There is further evidence that stimulation of lung (e.g. mechano, juxta-pulmonary, irritant) and peripheral (e.g. chest wall, skeletal muscle, facial skin) afferent receptors modulates dyspnoea[52,61]. Thus, blowing cold air on the face may decrease dyspnoea[62].

The 'sense of effort' in peripheral muscles has been demonstrated to be separate from the 'urge or drive' to breath in hyperventilating normal subjects in whom the addition of CO_2 resulted in an increased urge to breath but reduced awareness of the effort of breathing[63]. Similarly patients with lung disease and normal subjects with constraints to breathing (e.g. external respiratory loads) also report increased effort during breathing[52]. An individual's emotional state, personality, experience and cognitive function may also influence the perception of dyspnoea[64]. Dyspnoea is worse when it occurs suddenly, unexpectedly, in inappropriate situations or is perceived to be life threatening. The intensity of the dyspnoea is often also influenced by previous experience of the sensation[65].

Assessment of dyspnoea

Evaluation of dyspnoea should first attempt to establish the underlying pathophysiology (Table 12.3.6). A good history and examination is essential and will often establish the causal system and probable cause (e.g. heart, lung, neuromuscular). Diagnostic testing commonly follows to confirm the underlying pathology (Table 12.3.7). As the underlying disease progresses assessment of severity of dyspnoea aids decision-making and may indicate the success of a particular therapy. In general, the simpler the measurement technique the more likely it is to be used in end-stage lung disease. Severity may be assessed by:

◆ *Verbally reported intensity:* a number of instruments are available that allow reasonably reproducible ratings of dyspnoea intensity on linear or numerical scales. Clinicians often rely on a simple verbal numerical rating scale from 0 to 10[66]. The visual analogue scale (VAS) is a horizontal or vertical line,

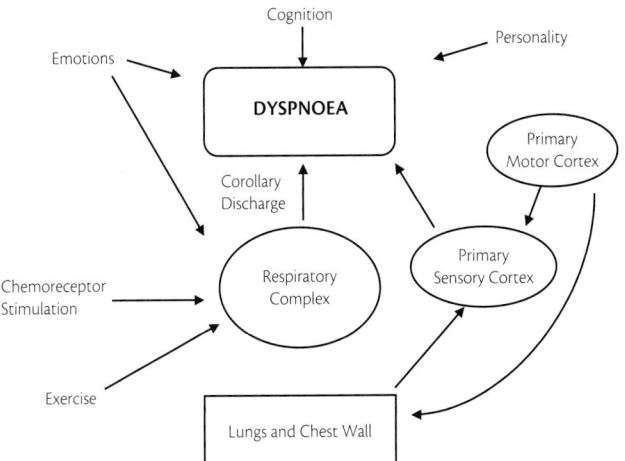

Figure 12.3.1 Control of ventilation; involving the brainstem respiratory complex, higher cortical functions and afferent input from the lungs, chest wall and chemoreceptors.

Table 12.3.6 The pathophysiological causes of dyspnoea.

Pathophysiological mechanism	Typical causes
Increased respiratory drive	
Hypoxaemia	Many respiratory and cardiac diseases
Metabolic acidosis	Renal failure, cardiac failure
Intrapulmonary receptor stimulation	Infiltrative disease, pulmonary oedema
Mechanical impedance	
Airflow obstruction	Asthma, COPD, tumour, stenosis
Mechanical chest wall restriction	Kyphoscoliosis, obesity, pregnancy
Reduced compliance ('stiff lungs')	Interstitial fibrosis, lymphangitis carcinomatosis
Respiratory muscle failure	
Muscle disease / paralysis	Poliomyelitis, muscular dystrophy
Mechanical disadvantage	Hyperinflation, pneumothorax, pleural effusion
Wasted ventilation	
Large vessel obstruction	Pulmonary emboli, pulmonary vasculitis
Capillary damage	Interstitial lung disease, emphysema
Psychological	
Anxiety, depression	Hyperventilation syndrome

Table 12.3.7 Diagnostic tests for the evaluation of dyspnoea.

Pulmonary function tests	Arterial blood gases
	Exercise testing
	Lung volumes and flow rates
	Gas transfer/diffusing capacity (D_{LCO})
	Bronchial challenge
Imaging techniques	Ventilation-perfusion scanning
	High resolution CT scanning
	Angiography
	Diaphragmatic fluoroscopy
	Positron emission tomography (PET)
Cardiac evaluation	Echocardiography
	Cardiac angiography
	Myocardial perfusion scan
	ECG monitoring
Other techniques	Sleep studies
	Oesophageal pH monitoring
	Otolaryngoscopy

usually 10 cm long, with no breathlessness and maximum breathlessness at the two ends. In response to the question 'how breathless are you?' the patient marks a point along the line so that the length reflects the intensity of the dyspnoea[66]. The Borg Scale (Table 12.3.8) is a 12-point category scale with extremes of no breathlessness and maximal breathlessness with verbal descriptors like 'slight' and 'severe' to assist the subject to rate the symptom[67]. Many other dyspnoea scales are available[52].

♦ *Quality of life (QOL) measurements:* are designed to measure how patients function physically, emotionally, and socially in response to their symptoms and disease[52]. Improvements in these measures may be independent of changes in the severity of the disease. Several questionnaires have been specifically developed to assess the impact of respiratory disease on QOL but are most likely to be of value in research projects rather than the clinical setting. The most commonly used are (a) The Chronic Respiratory Disease Questionnaire which evaluates dyspnoea, fatigue, emotional function, and mastery in a 20-item questionnaire. Dyspnoea is assessed by determining the five most bothersome activities and grading these on a 7-point scale[52]. (b) The Saint George's Respiratory Questionnaire is a 76-item questionnaire which assesses symptoms, activity and impact of disease on daily life[68]. (c) The Pulmonary Functional Status Scale measures mental, physical, and social functioning in COPD patients to assess the effect of respiratory distress on functional activity[52]. Development of new and better validation of pre-existing, QOL scales is ongoing particularly in relation to COPD and non-malignant respiratory disease[69].

♦ *Physiological techniques:* simple spirometry and saturation monitoring are relatively easy to perform even in severe lung disease. Unfortunately, a patient's FEV_1 is a poor predictor of the degree of dyspnoea[52]. Similarly, improvements in dyspnoea after bronchodilators do not match changes in FEV_1[70]. In 34 COPD patients observed over time, loss of FEV_1 did not correlate with changes in dyspnoea[71]. Despite these limitations, spirometry has a role in the assessment of reversibility in airways obstruction. Exercise tolerance (e.g. endurance, 6 min or shuttle walking) may also be used to assess the response to therapy even in patients with limited mobility[72]. Many other investigations assist evaluation of dyspnoea (Table 12.3.7) but are less reliable and increasingly difficult to perform in end-stage respiratory disease.

Table 12.3.8 Modified Borg dyspnoea scale.

Intensity of sensation	Rating
Nothing at all	0
Very, very slight	0.5
Very slight	1
Slight	2
Moderate	3
Somewhat severe	4
Severe	5
	6
Very severe	7
	8
Very, very severe	9
Maximal	10

Treatment of dyspnoea

Nearly every end-stage respiratory disease will be associated with breathlessness but the focus of treatment will vary depending on the underlying mechanism and the specific disease process[52].

Treatment aims are:

- Reduction of ventilatory demand by:
  - Exercise training and supplemental oxygen to reduce metabolic demand.
  - Decreasing central drive using pharmacological therapy (oxygen, opiates, anxiolytics), altering afferent input to the medulla (inhaled pharmacological therapy, facial fans), and improving CO_2 elimination by breathing therapy.

- Reduction of work of breathing (i.e. to reduce ventilatory impedance):
  - Bronchodilation (β_2 agonists, muscurinic receptor antagonists, steroids).
  - Reduce or counterbalance lung hyperinflation by continuous airways pressure to match auto-PEEP or surgical volume reduction.

- Improve inspiratory muscle function:
  - nutrition;
  - inspiratory muscle training including rehabilitation programmes;
  - positioning;
  - partial ventilatory support (BIPAP, CPAP, NIPPV); and
  - avoiding oral steroids.

- Alter perception:
  - education, desensitization and behavioural approaches; and
  - pharmacological therapy.

Dyspnoea is most effectively alleviated by treatment of the underlying condition and its complications (Table 12.3.6). As the terminal phase approaches and dyspnoea persists despite optimal treatment of the underlying disease, therapy should focus on symptom relief (Table 12.3.9) and the mechanisms contributing to an individual's dyspnoea (e.g. anxiety, hypoxaemia, respiratory muscle weakness). Determining the point at which active treatment of the underlying disease should give way to symptomatic relief of symptoms and palliative care can be extremely difficult.

Cough

Cough is not a common occurrence in normal subjects but it may become a distressing symptom in many pulmonary diseases (Table 12.3.10). Mucociliary transport is responsible for the majority of airways clearance but is impaired in lung disease. In chronic bronchitis mucociliary clearance is 50 per cent of that in healthy subjects. Cough is normally a reserve mechanism but in chronic bronchitis contributes 20 per cent to sputum clearance compared with 2.5 per cent in healthy individuals[73]. In end-stage respiratory disease there are few data relating to the frequency, severity, and management of cough. However, in one of the few studies examining cough in the final year of life, 59 per cent of these patients complained of cough and this was very distressing in 46 per cent[16]. In the last week of life cough was reported

in 52 per cent of patients. These figures were very similar to the incidence of cough in lung cancer patients.

Mechanism of cough (see Chapter 11.1)

Involuntary cough is initiated by rapidly adapting 'irritant' receptors (RARs) that transmit through fast-velocity myelinated vagal fibres. The most sensitive sites for cough induction are the larynx, main carina, and branching points in the tracheobronchial tree. Stimulation of smaller airways and alveoli does not cause cough. RARs respond to a wide variety of chemical (e.g. smoke), inflammatory (e.g. histamine), and mechanical (e.g. foreign body) stimuli and also cause bronchoconstriction and mucous hypersecretion[74]. C-fibres lying in close proximity to RARs respond to the same stimuli but do not cause cough although they may stimulate RARs to initiate cough[75].

Table 12.3.9 Symptomatic relief of dyspnoea.

Treatment	
Reduce work of breathing (e.g. sense of effort / improve muscle function)	Breathing strategies (e.g. purse-lip breathing)
	Position (e.g. upright posture / lean forward)
	Rest respiratory muscles (NIPPV, cuirass)
	Medication (e.g. theophylline)
	Correct nutrition / obesity
Exercise training / rehabilitation	Optimize muscle strength
	Dyspnoea desensitization
	Improve movement efficiency
Decrease respiratory drive	Oxygen
	Sedatives and opiates
	Vagal nerve / carotid body resection
Psychological strategies	Education
	Coping strategies, psychotherapy
	Anxiolytics

Table 12.3.10 Non-malignant causes of cough.

Cause of cough	Typical examples
Acute infection	Viral, bronchopneumonia
Chronic infection	Bronchiectasis, cystic fibrosis
Airways disease	Asthma, COPD
Cardiovascular	Left ventricular failure
Parenchymal disease	Interstitial fibrosis
Irritant	Oesophageal reflux, foreign body
Recurrent aspiration	Motor neuron disease, stroke
Drug induced	ACE inhibitors, inhaled drugs
Pleural disease	Pneumothorax, pleural effusion
Vocal cord disease	Paralysis or nodules

Cough is integrated in the medulla. Afferent fibres are relayed through the nucleus of the tractus solitarius and motor output dispatched via the nucleus ambigualis to the larynx and bronchial tree and via the nucleus retroambigualis to the respiratory muscles. The central nervous receptors for cough include serotonin, opiods, GABA, and dopamine which may have potential therapeutic implications[76]. Voluntary cough, initiated by the cerebral cortex, can bypass these integrative centres as patients with brainstem damage and no spontaneous cough reflex can consciously induce cough to clear the airways. It is also possible for most patients to suppress involuntary cough for 5–20 min.

Cough has two functions; to prevent foreign material entering the lower respiratory tract and to clear secretions from the lungs and bronchial tree. The mechanics of cough rely on the generation of high expiratory pressures (e.g. intrapleural pressures up to 40 kPa) and rapid airflow velocity (500 mile/h). Glottic closure is not essential as the expiratory muscles are able to generate effective cough even with an endotracheal tube in place. Failure to generate an adequate airflow causes ineffective cough and subsequent atelectasis, infection and eventually bronchiectasis. Conditions that interfere with the ability to maintain a clear airway include:

- Extrapulmonary disorders—rib fractures, costochondritis, acute abdomen, recent surgery, respiratory muscle weakness; upper airway obstruction, and central cough depression.

- Intrathoracic conditions—COPD, pulmonary fibrosis, and bronchiectasis.

Excessive cough may impair quality of life by preventing sleep, interrupting communication, and causing social embarrassment. In addition, the high pressures, rapid airflow and energy associated with effective cough can cause haemodynamic changes (e.g. arrhythmias), ruptured vessels (e.g. eyes, nasal, bronchial), urinary incontinence, hernia, neurological problems (e.g. syncope, headache), lung barotrauma (e.g. pneumothorax), and rib fractures[77].

Assessment of cough and cough effectiveness

Cough assessment must determine the cause, effectiveness, and impact on quality of life[78]. Many causes are amenable to therapy including excessive secretions, recurrent infections, bronchoconstriction, aspiration, postnasal drips, and gastric reflux. If cough is excessive and distressing (e.g. preventing sleep), and a reversible component cannot be established, suppressive therapy may be indicated. Inadequate cough is a common problem and determining when there is a significant risk of atelectasis, pneumonia, or hypoventilation is important. However, the only studies assessing cough effectiveness have been performed in patients with myasthenia gravis[79] and muscular dystrophy[80]. These demonstrated that maximal expiratory mouth pressures <4 kPa were associated with difficulty expectorating secretions[79] and suggested the need for enhancement of cough and secretion clearance.

Cough therapy

Cough therapy is usually successful if the cause is established[77,78,81].

Treatment of the cause: therapy aimed at treating the underlying cause is essential[81]. Exacerbating factors should be identified and simple measures like change of posture can be very effective. Drainage of a pleural effusion or dilation of an oesophageal stricture to prevent recurrent aspiration may be necessary. Stopping smoking abolished cough in 50 per cent of COPD cases[81] and treatment

of underlying lung disease (e.g. bronchodilators, steroids) is essential. Diuretics relieve cough in heart failure, nasal anticongestants in post-nasal drip and H_2 antagonists in gastrooesophageal reflux[81]. Antibiotics may be required in bronchiectasis and other chronic infective conditions.

Protussive therapy: makes cough more effective: Inability to clear airways secretions due to excessive production, ineffective cough, or reduced mucociliary clearance in diseases like chronic bronchitis and bronchiectasis leads to recurrent infection, dyspnoea, cough, and airways obstruction with atelectasis. Measures to improve cough and secretion clearance are described in relation to individual diseases but include:

- Adequate hydration, steam inhalations, and nebulized saline to loosen tenacious secretions and aid expectoration.

- Physiotherapy with forced exhalation, airways vibration, postural drainage, and assisted cough techniques[77] but improvement in morbidity or mortality have not been established[82].

- Pharyngeal suctioning.

- Occasionally a mini-tracheostomy inserted through the cricothyroid membrane is required to clear tracheal secretions that cannot be coughed past the vocal cords.

- Bronchorrhoea (watery sputum >100 ml but occasionally several litres/day) can occur in non-malignant conditions (e.g. asthma, tuberculosis) and may respond to steroids, erythromycin, or inhaled indomethacin[83].

- Pharmacological protussive therapies including aerosolized hypertonic saline which induces cough and fluid influx from the mucosa, cysteine derivatives (e.g. N-acetylcysteine, rhDNase) which liquefy lung secretions and beta agonists (e.g. salbutamol) have been demonstrated to increase secretion clearance in randomized controlled trials[78,81,84].

Antitussive therapy: prevents or eliminates cough: Non-specific antitussive therapy is indicated when the cause of the cough is not reversible or cannot be controlled by specific therapy. Usually they are used for dry rather than productive coughs. Medications demonstrated to be effective in randomized, placebo-controlled trials include:

- *Opiods:* are the most effective antitussive agents. Strong opiods like morphine have the most pronounced effects. All act on the central cough centre. Methadone is useful at night but because of its long half-life can accumulate[85]. Hydrocodeine (5–10 mg every 4–6 h) is often preferred to codeine (15–30 mg every 4–6 h) as it causes less constipation and neuropsychological side-effects. Dextromethorphan also causes fewer gastrointestinal and neurological side effects.

- *Oral local anaesthetics:* benzonate (100–200 mg every 8 h) is related to procaine and inhibits the effects of stretch receptors[86]. Levodroproizine modulates C-fibre activity and has been demonstrated to be as effective as dihydrocodeine in cough suppression but is less sedative[87]. Benzociane and lignocaine lozenges may be useful for laryngeal, pharyngeal, or tracheal irritation but the risk of aspiration must be considered.

- *Nebulized local anaesthetics:* lignocaine (5 ml of 2 per cent solution every 6 h) and bupivicaine (5 ml 0.25 per cent solution every 6 h) have been recommended for intractable cough but can cause bronchospasm requiring bronchodilators. Efficacy has not been established and in view of the largyngeal anaesthesia all fluid and food intake should be stopped for at least 1–2 h after use to avoid inadvertent aspiration[77,88].

◆ *Other antitussive agents:* theophyllines and β_2 agonists stimulate mucociliary clearance and may be beneficial in chronic bronchitis and bronchiectasis[81]. Sodium cromoglycate inhibits C fibres and may reduce cough related to allergy and cancer[77,89]. Steroids are effective in many obstructive (e.g. asthma, endobronchial tumour) and pulmonary infiltratitive disorders (e.g. sarcoidosis, lymphangitis carcinomatosis). A wide variety of over the counter antitussive medications including antihistamine-decongestant (e.g. pseudoephedrine, dexbrompheniramine) and expectorant (e.g. guaifenesin) preparations are available with varying and unproven efficacy[78,90].

◆ *Antimuscarinics:* antimuscarinic bronchodilators e.g. inhaled ipratropium bromide, tiotropium bromide) are useful in chronic bronchitis and may reduce secretion without increasing mucous viscosity or impairing mucociliary clearance. Hyoscine hydrobromide (0.2–0.4 mg SC prn) or glycopyrronium bromide (0.2–0.4 mg IM prn) may be essential for the control of the distressing 'chest rattle' due to loose secretions in the terminal phase of chronic lung disease. Both cause sedation and dysphoria and occasionally, in the elderly, central anticholinergic syndrome with excitement, ataxia, and hallucinations.

Chest pain

Chest pain is a component of many chronic lung diseases and may exacerbate breathlessness, inhibit secretion clearance, and impair quality of life. Management depends on identifying and treating the cause. Despite the proximity of various organs and the visceral nature of the pain it is usually possible to clinically differentiate most types of pain although simple investigations (e.g. chest radiography) may be helpful.

Musculoskeletal disorders

Chest wall pain is usually associated with localized tenderness. Rib fractures due to cough, tumour, or trauma may limit chest wall movement with the risk of hypoventilation and atelectasis. Adequate analgesia will often involve combinations of oral opiate analgesia and intercostals nerve blocks. Local nerve blocks with subcostal bupivicaine 0.25 per cent (+ adrenaline 1:200 000) are useful but, if feasible, a thoracic epidural may be more effective[91]. External chest wall stabilization (e.g. taping, sandbagging, fixation) is ineffective and by limiting chest wall movement encourages atelectasis. Costochondritis (*Tietze's syndrome*), fibrositis, and subcostal pain due to diaphragmatic and intercostal muscle fatigue are all recognized[92]. Intercostal radiculitis from cervical and thoracic spine osteoarthritis may cause significant chest wall pain, hyperalgesia, and skin anaesthesia in immobile or bedridden end-stage respiratory disease patients. Other neuropathic pains should be considered including herpes zoster infection which may be associated with immune suppression and brachial plexus invasion by a Pancoast's tumour.

Pleuropulmonary disorders

Inflammation of parietal pleura causes pleuritic pain with its typical relationship to breathing movements. The character of the pain can vary but there is usually no localized tenderness. The speed of development provides a clue to the cause. Sudden onset suggests a pneumothorax, pulmonary embolism, or rib fracture. Development over days may herald pneumonia particularly if associated with fever and rigors. Slow onset with weight loss and lethargy may indicate malignancy or tuberculosis. The pain of tracheobronchitis is characteristically substernal. It is a sharp, raw, or burning pain worse with coughing. Pulmonary hypertension (PHT) is also frequently associated with acute crushing central chest pain which may radiate into the neck and arms and is difficult to differentiate from myocardial ischaemia. It has been reported in acute PHT (e.g. massive pulmonary embolus) and chronic PHT (e.g. primary PHT, mitral stenosis)[93].

Visceral disorders

A variety of cardiovascular (e.g. ischaemic heart disease, pericarditis), gastrointestinal (e.g. oesophagitis, cholecystitis) and psychological disorders (e.g. anxiety/panic disorders, hyperventilation syndrome) may present with chest pain. Missed diagnosis and delayed treatment may result in unnecessary discomfort.

If pain is refractory to treatment of the underlying cause then symptomatic therapy may be necessary. The World Health Organization's guidelines for the use of analgesic drugs have been discussed in previous chapters and the principles are identical in end-stage respiratory disease[94].

Haemoptysis

Haemoptysis is a dramatic, and sometimes life-threatening development in end-stage lung disease[95,96]. The majority of episodes are mild to moderate, and massive haemoptysis (defined as 500–1000 ml blood/day or any life-threatening haemoptysis) accounts for less than 20 per cent of episodes of haemoptysis[95]. Most cases are due to infective causes (~80 per cent) including tuberculosis, lung abscess and bronchiectasis. Only a minority are due to malignancy (~20 per cent)[95,96]. Death results from asphyxia, due to alveolar flooding, rather than circulatory collapse and mortality is directly related to the rate and volume of blood loss and underlying pathology. Haemoptysis of >600 ml within a 4-h period is associated with 71 per cent mortality, compared with 45 per cent in patients expectorating the same quantity over 4–16 h and 5 per cent during 16–48 h[97].

Initial assessment

A good history and examination are essential and the characteristic clinical picture of diseases like pulmonary embolism and bronchiectasis may direct subsequent investigation and management. Examination of expectorated blood may provide clues. Food particles suggest the possibility of haematemesis whereas purulent material in the sputum may indicate bronchiectasis or a lung abscess. Microbiology may isolate tubercle bacilli and associated haematuria raises the possibility of alveolar haemorrhage syndrome. Important diagnostic information includes evidence of a mass or abscess on chest radiography, although diffuse alveolar shadowing, caused by widespread distribution of blood during coughing may obscure the site and cause of bleeding[98].

Management

Active management may be inappropriate in many patients with end-stage respiratory disease. However, dying with haemoptysis is distressing for both the patient and relatives. If massive haemoptysis is a potential risk (i.e. previous haemoptysis), careful planning (e.g. warning relatives and immediate access to drugs) improves management of the terminal event. Simple measures like the use of green bed linen and towels to mask the evidence of blood, nursing the patient with the affected chest side down and the calming influence of a controlled situation are invaluable. Palliative treatment should aim to reduce awareness and fear. Both opiod and anxiolytic therapy may be required[85].

If resuscitation is appropriate the key aspects of management are[95–98]:

- Maintain a patent airway and ensure adequate oxygenation with supplemental oxygen as asphyxia is the immediate risk. Endotracheal intubation and mechanical ventilation may be required.

- Promote drainage and prevent alveolar 'soiling' of the unaffected lung, by positioning the patient slightly head down in the lateral decubitus position with the 'presumed' bleeding side down.

- Determine the cause, site, and severity of the bleeding (see below): haematemesis and upper airways bleeding (e.g. nose, pharynx) may be confused with haemoptysis.

- Avoid excessive chest manipulation (e.g. physiotherapy, spirometry) as this may increase or restart bleeding. Cough suppression with codeine 30–60 mg every 6 h may be helpful.

- Institute appropriate therapeutic measures depending on the underlying pathology and clinical circumstances (e.g. antibiotics in bronchiectasis, anticoagulation in pulmonary embolism).

Determining the site and cause of haemoptysis

Once the patient has been stabilized, the site and cause of bleeding must be established.

- Early bronchoscopy is essential and is superior to other diagnostic techniques including bronchial arteriograms and computer tomography (CT) scans[96,98].

- If bronchoscopy is unsuccessful, CT scans with contrast may detect the bleeding site, tumours, and other structural abnormalities. Combination of bronchoscopy and CT scanning has the highest diagnostic yield[95–98]. Occasionally, radionucleotide scans may be useful.

- Bronchial or pulmonary angiography is occasionally required.

Control of haemoptysis

Control of bleeding is usually required during ongoing investigation and includes immediate temporising measures or bronchial embolization. When the patient's condition has stabilized definitive surgery may be necessary.

Immediate: control of bleeding is achieved in 95 per cent of cases with bronchoscope directed iced saline and adrenaline (10 ml; 1:10000 dilution) lavage[99]. Occasionally, topical thrombin application[100], balloon catheter tamponade[95], tranexamic acis or intravenous vasoconstrictors (e.g. terlipressin) may be useful.

Bronchial angiography and embolization: bronchial artery embolization is the established therapeutic technique for immediate control of haemoptysis and is successful in 70–100 per cent of cases[101]. The best results occur in patients with dilated bronchial arteries (e.g. bronchiectasis). Early rebleeding is common but long-term control

(>3 months) is reported in 45 per cent of cases[102]. Infarction of the anterior spinal artery and paraplegia occurs in about 5 per cent. Rare complications include ischaemic necrosis of the bronchus and arterial dissection[101].

Medical versus surgical treatment: medical management may be mandatory due to end-stage lung disease (FEV_1<40 per cent predicted), poor cardiac reserve or severe bleeding diathesis. In other patients, lesions may be multi-focal or not amenable to surgical resection. However, if appropriate, surgical therapy has the best long-term outcome with control of bleeding in 82 to 92 per cent of isolated lesions[95–98]. In conservative studies, when surgery would have been feasible, success rates were between 46 and 68 per cent[103].

Stridor

Laryngeal or major airway obstruction results in a hoarse inspiratory wheeze termed stridor. Airways infection (e.g. epiglottitis, diphtheria), tumours, anaphylaxis, aspirated foreign bodies (e.g. food), blood clots, sputum plugs, and dislodged tumour can obstruct the upper airways. Management requires immediate removal of the cause of the obstruction. Postural manipulation and physiotherapy may relieve obstruction but occasionally laryngoscopy, bronchoscopy, or surgical intervention are required to assess the cause and determine appropriate management. Corticosteroid therapy can provide rapid relief when oedema or inflammatory changes are a significant cause of obstruction. Heliox inhalation (helium and oxygen in a ratio of 4:1) may provide short-term relief by reducing airflow resistance. Endoscopically placed stents (bronchial or tracheal) or tracheostomy to bypass laryngeal obstruction may be appropriate in some cases.

Recurrent aspiration

Recurrent aspiration occurs in the terminal phase of many diseases and is an important factor in the development of respiratory failure[104]. Bulbar involvement in neuromuscular (e.g. multiple sclerosis) and cerebrovascular disease is associated with recurrent aspiration due to impairment of complex swallowing reflexes. Repeated micro-aspiration causes infection, bronchiectasis, and lung scarring. The right main bronchus is the most direct path for aspirated material and consequently the right lower lobe is most involved. Posture affects susceptibility to aspiration and nursing in the semi-recumbent position may reduce the risk[105]. Recurrent aspiration is often missed but coughing after drinking or eating and crepitations in the right lower lobe are characteristic clues. Recurrent pneumonia and chest radiographic changes of atelectasis or inflammation in the right lower lobe should raise suspicion and detection of dyes (e.g. methylene blue) added to drinks in tracheal aspirates suggests the diagnosis. Barium swallow confirms aspiration when barium enters the bronchial tree. It may occasionally demonstrate an oesophageal-tracheal fistula that requires stenting or surgical intervention.

If aspiration is suspected, swallowing must be assessed by a speech therapist and strategies for prevention tested, including posture manipulation and thickening of food[104]. If these fail, fine bore nasogastric feeding, or gastric pegs should be considered although this will depend on the stage of the illness. The pneumonia and atelectasis associated with aspiration are treated with physiotherapy and broad spectrum antibiotics that cover nasopharyngeal organisms (e.g. anaerobes).

Management of end-stage respiratory disease

In respiratory disease there is often no clear event that signifies the onset of the end-stage after many years of gradual deterioration. Carers must be alert to the subtle change in symptoms and psycho-social status that indicate declining health and the beginning of this terminal phase including:

- persistent breathlessness despite optimization of medical therapy;
- inability to mobilize and get out of the house despite pulmonary rehabilitation;
- increasing numbers of hospital admissions;
- limited improvement following admission;
- expressions of fear or anxiety and panic attacks; and
- patient awareness of a change and expressions of concern about dying.

At present end-stage management, and particularly the last 48 h, of respiratory disease is mainly in hospital following an acute exacerbation of the chronic lung disease. About 72 per cent of patients die in hospital, 12 per cent at home and none in hospice[16]. Recently, there has been a trend toward the management of acute exacerbations of COPD at home. This 'hospital at home' (HaH) management has been demonstrated to be safe and cost effective[46–48] and 95 per cent of 184 patients in a recent study of acute exacerbations of COPD, reported satisfaction with HaH care[47]. However, the 32 COPD patient cohort of another randomized control study expressed a preference for inpatient care[106]. Many respiratory nurses already provide domicillary care for some patients with end-stage respiratory disease, including emotional/psychological support and assistance with oxygen and nebulizer therapy[107]. There is some early data suggesting that HaH is cost effective in COPD patients. A recent Spanish trial examining the health-care costs of HaH management of COPD exacerbations demonstrated an average cost saving of € 810 (CI 418–1169) per episode in HaH patients compared with conventionally treated hospital patients[108].

Important factors in the management of chronic lung disease are respiratory failure (including hypoventilation, V/Q mismatching, airflow obstruction), chronic infection (± sputum retention), pneumothorax, pleural effusions, and thromboembolic disease. The emphasis of treatment will vary according to which components predominate in individual diseases.

Respiratory failure

Respiratory failure is defined as the inability of the respiratory system to supply adequate oxygen for tissue metabolic requirements and/or failure of carbon dioxide clearance. Most end-stage respiratory diseases are associated with respiratory failure, although the underlying mechanisms differ. In neuromuscular disease treatment focuses on secretion clearance and support of respiratory muscle function (e.g. non-invasive ventilation) to prevent hypoventilation and CO_2 retention whereas in fibrotic lung disease correction of hypoxaemia with oxygen therapy may be paramount. Overall, the majority of patients (~75 per cent) with end-stage respiratory disease and respiratory failure will have COPD.

Chronic obstructive pulmonary disease (COPD)

Extensive guidelines for the clinical management of COPD have recently been published[25,109,110]. End-stage management of COPD with respiratory failure[111] includes: (1) *pharmacological therapies:* to reduce airways obstruction, correct hypoxaemia and relieve dyspnoea; and (2) *non-pharmacological therapies:* to improve respiratory muscle function/ventilation and enhance gas exchange.

Pharmacological therapies

Bronchodilators: inhaled β₂-agonists are well-established bronchodilators for the treatment of dyspnoea. In COPD, they reduce resting and exercise-induced dyspnoea and dynamic hyperinflation without necessarily increasing FEV_1 or FVC[109,110]. Anticholinergic agents, including ipratropium and oxitropium bromide, also reduce dyspnoea, improve exercise tolerance and increase FEV_1[112]. Tiotropium bromide, a once daily therapy is superior to ipratropium bromide as it acts specifically on the M3 bronchodilator muscurinic receptor whereas ipratropium bromide acts on three muscurinic receptors M1, M2, and M3 where M1 and M3 receptors are bronchodilator and M2 bronchoconstrictor. Recent studies have confirmed that tiotropium reduces exacerbations and related hospital admissions, improves quality of life, increases exercise tolerance, reduces functional residual capacity (i.e. hyperinflation) and may slow decline in FEV_1 compared with ipratropium[113,114]. Anticholinergics can aggravate prostatism and glaucoma and should be used with care in patients with these conditions. Inhaler technique must be examined as incorrect use is a frequent cause of lack of effect. Dry powder inhalers may improve delivery in patients with poor co-ordination using metered dose aerosol inhalers.

Current evidence suggests that the clinical and bronchodilator effects of anticholinergics are greater than those of β₂-agonists in COPD. Analysis from seven trials comparing ipratropium with β₂-agonists given for at least 90 days reported a greater increase in FEV_1 with ipratropium bromide and this bronchodilation was sustained whereas the β₂-agonist effect waned with prolonged use[115]. Combinations of β₂-agonists and anticholinergic agents are additive with greater effect than either agent alone and fewer side effects. In a randomized, controlled trial of 534 COPD patients, combining ipratropium with a β₂-agonist improved the FEV_1 beyond that with either agent alone[116].

There is contradictory evidence for the use of nebulizer therapy in COPD[117] but study comparisons are difficult because nebulizer devices differ and patient groups are small. In general, nebulizers deliver more drug to the lungs but in a less efficient manner than metered dose inhalers. Nebulizers also cause more side effects, have increased administration times and higher costs. Comparisons between nebulizers and inhalers (± spacer) have not shown significant benefits on dyspnoea, bronchodilation, exercise tolerance, or reduced rescue therapy in patients with stable COPD. Nevertheless, many patients prefer nebulized bronchodilators despite this lack of objective response. Benefit in acute exacerbations and during end-of-life management is reported. Current recommendations suggest the initial use of metered dose inhalers provided that inhaler technique is adequate. Near the end of life, or during acute exacerbations, patients may be too weak to use metered dose inhalers effectively and nebulizer therapy both at home and in hospital becomes the better option.

Inhaled and oral steroids: inhaled corticosteroids do not reduce long-term decline in FEV_1 in patients with COPD[25,108,109]. In mild and moderate COPD long-term treatment with inhaled corticosteroids is only recommended if a previous trial of inhaled or oral steroids has shown a beneficial spirometric response. However, the combination of an inhaled corticosteroid with a long-acting β_2-agonist is recommended in patients with an FEV_1<50 per cent predicted who have had two or more exacerbations requiring oral steroids ($\pm$ antibiotics) over the previous 12 months, as this has been demonstrated to decrease the frequency of further exacerbations. Long-term treatment with oral corticosteroids is not recommended in COPD and benefits <25 per cent of patients. Steroid-induced myopathy and other systemic side effects of oral steroids may contribute to muscle weakness and early respiratory failure. In acute exacerbations of COPD high-dose oral steroids may be beneficial but should be rapidly reduced after 10 days and either stopped or replaced by inhaled steroids as appropriate[25].

Methylxanthines: theophylline and aminophylline are usually prescribed as slow-release oral preparations and improve exercise tolerance and blood gases at serum concentrations between 10 and 20 mcg/ml but have negligible effects on spirometry[25]. In addition to their bronchodilator effects they may improve respiratory drive, diaphragmatic strength and mucociliary clearance[118]. Withdrawal results in deterioration[118]. However, recent use has declined due to potential toxicity and the need for monitoring of plasma levels at higher doses. If used judiciously, theophylline continues to have a useful role and should be prescribed once or twice daily to achieve levels between 10 and 12 mcg/ml.

Oxygen therapy: patients with severe COPD often commence oxygen therapy at home several years before the disease reaches the terminal phase. Depending on the circumstances it will be provided from cylinders, an oxygen concentrator or as liquid oxygen. It is commonly delivered by a face mask or nasal prongs, with or without humidification. At the onset of treatment, oxygen space is usually provided overnight, intermittently during the day and on exercise if a portable supply is available (i.e. liquid oxygen in the USA). As a patient becomes increasingly unwell their dependence on oxygen will increase. Continuous use is not uncommon towards the end-stage of the disease and panic may result if it is removed[85]. Oxygen saturations should be monitored. The development of headache, drowsiness, or confusion may indicate CO_2 retention and the need to check an arterial blood gas although routine blood gases are not necessary. Many patients find that the flow of air or oxygen over the face reduces breathlessness and the use of venturi masks to entrain air and increase flow may be beneficial[62].

Long-term oxygen therapy (LTOT): extends life expectancy in hypoxaemic COPD patients if administered for at least 12–15 h a day and benefit increases with continuous use[29,119]. In the MRC trial, mortality at 3 years was 45 per cent in patients treated with oxygen (2 l/min) for 15 h/day compared with 67 per cent in controls[29]. In the Nocturnal Oxygen Therapy Trial in the USA mortality was 22 per cent in patients treated with continuous oxygen (~18 h/day) and 41 per cent in patients receiving nocturnal therapy[119]. Reductions in dyspnoea, haemocrit, and improved pulmonary haemodynamic performance were also reported. Quality of life was not changed significantly although there were some modest neuropsychiatric improvements[119]. In contrast to these studies, the 2001 Cochrane review identified a number of recent trials that had not shown benefit with nocturnal oxygen therapy[120].

Table 12.3.11 UK department of health guidelines for LTOT prescription.

Indications for LTOT
COPD (+ cystic fibrosis):
• PaO_2 <7.3 kPa (55 mmHg) when breathing air
• $PaCO_2$ may be normal or >6.0 kPa
• Two measurement separated by 4 weeks when clinically stable
• Clinical stability = No exacerbations or peripheral oedema for 4 weeks
• FEV_1 <1.5 L and FVC <2.0 L
• Non-smokers
Or
• PaO_2 between 7.3–8.0 kPa (56–59 mmHg) together with
• Secondary polycythaemia, peripheral oedema or PHT
• Nocturnal hypoxaemia (SaO_2 below 90 per cent for >30 per cent of the night)
Interstitial lung disease or PHT (without parenchymal involvement):
• PaO_2 <8 kPa
Other indications:
• Palliation of dyspnoea due to terminal disease
• Obstructive sleep apnoea with persistant nocturnal hypoxaemia despite CPAP
• Neuromuscular and skeletal disorders
• Heart failure with PaO_2 <7.3 kPa (55 mmHg) or nocturnal hypoxaemia

PHT = pulmonary hypertension.

The criteria for LTOT prescription vary in different countries[25,108] but current guidelines in the UK are listed in Table 12.3.11. In practice, compliance with these guidelines is poor[121]. In the UK, an oxygen concentrator is recommended for LTOT delivery as it is cheaper than cylinder oxygen. Liquid oxygen systems are preferred in the USA as they allow mobility outside the home. Nasal cannulae are a comfortable mode of administration and a flow rate of 1–3 l/min is usually adequate to achieve a saturation >90 per cent. The baseline flow rate is often increased by 1 l/min at night and during exercise to prevent desaturation. The low concentrations of oxygen administered with LTOT cause only small increases in $PaCO_2$ in patients with hypercapnoea. Unfortunately, a proportion of LTOT patients continue to smoke!

Oxygen during exercise: in patients with resting or exercise-induced hypoxaemia supplemental oxygen augments exercise capacity and reduces dyspnoea[122]. This benefit is greater with higher flow rates[72]. A diffusing capacity below 55 per cent predicted, accurately predicts exercise-induced desaturation[123]. Portable cylinder or liquid oxygen systems may improve mobility and quality of life in patients who benefit in controlled exercise assessments. They are widely available in the USA but less so in Europe[72].

Palliative oxygen therapy: a significant proportion of patients with end-stage lung disease including COPD will have resting hypoxaemia, although the degree of hypoxaemia does not necessarily correlate with the level of dyspnoea[124]. Both dyspnoea and exercise tolerance are substantially improved with supplemental oxygen[72,124]. In patients with refractory hypoxaemia despite high flow oxygen, a nasal reservoir (e.g. oximizer), which stores oxygen during expiration and delivers a larger bolus at the onset of inspiration may be useful. However, at high flow rates, oxygen therapy can cause CO_2 narcosis. Progressive somnolence in a patient with a good saturation on oximetry should raise suspicion. A blood gas should be measured or end tidal CO_2 checked to confirm hypercapnia and the oxygen flow rate reduced whilst monitoring CO_2 and mental function.

Palliative oxygen in the absence of hypoxaemia: even in the absence of resting hypoxaemia or with minimal exercise-induced desaturation, supplemental oxygen may relieve dyspnoea in some COPD patients[124]. A 'blinded' comparison of air and oxygen may confirm this benefit[72]. The likely mechanism for dyspnoea relief is that oxygen reduces carotid body afferent output, altering carbon dioxide sensitivity and thereby reducing minute ventilation and work of breathing. In these patients intermittent 'palliative' oxygen therapy is usually adequate, as few will require continuous therapy[124]. Oxygen is usually delivered from cylinders, although an oxygen concentrator may be supplied if life expectancy is >3 months and oxygen usage high.

Drug treatment for the relief of dyspnoea

Drug treatment of dyspnoea is controversial, with differing opinions and conflicting evidence. In general, the therapeutic benefit has been small and the side effects considerable[124].

Anxiolytic agents and promethazine: anxiety aggravates breathlessness and some patients experience severe panic attacks. Patients must be advised how to stay calm by purse-lip breathing, slow expiration and shoulder and chest wall muscle relaxation. Early work with anxiolytic therapy reported that oral diazepam reduced dyspnoea in 'pink puffer' type COPD patients but subsequent studies failed to show improvement in dyspnoea, exercise tolerance or sense of well-being with either diazepam or alprazolam[125,126]. Indeed, diazepam caused drowsiness, decreased exercise tolerance and dyspnoea was unchanged[126]. Promethazine use is equally controversial as initial reports suggested increased exercise tolerance and decreased dyspnoea with no notable side effects[126] whereas a later study found no significant changes from baseline after use for 1 month[127]. Equally conflicting reports have been published in small studies examining the use of buspirone hydrochloride, a non-sedating, non-addictive anxiolytic agent. Anxiety scores, exercise performance and dyspnoea all improved on 20 mg a day for 15 days but in a second study no effect was demonstrated with at least 30 mg/day for 6 weeks[128]. Despite these inconclusive results, clinical experience suggests that low dose anxiolytics have a beneficial effect in the management of breathlessness as a consequence of their anxiolytic, muscle relaxant, and sedative effects and not only in those prone to anxiety or panic attacks. Concerns about respiratory depression are largely unfounded.

Antidepressant drugs: a high proportion of COPD patients have psychiatric illness. Studies examining the effect of tricyclic antidepressants, serotonin reuptake inhibitors, and phenothiazines have been reported to be beneficial for anxiety but effects on dyspnoea are inconclusive[124]. However, chlorpromazine was effective for the control of dyspnoea and restlessness in advanced cancer[129].

Oral opiods: the site of action may be central, affecting the opiate receptors in the brainstem and reducing ventilation, by decreasing anxiety or by affecting peripheral receptors in the lung. Exogenous opiates cause dose-dependent reduction in ventilation with increased $PaCO_2$ and a depression of the ventilatory response to CO_2[130]. However, oral dihydrocodeine reduced breathlessness in COPD without an increase in CO_2[131]. Oral morphine has also been demonstrated to reduce breathlessness and increase exercise tolerance but with drowsiness, a fall in PaO_2 and an increase in $PaCO_2$ as significant side effects[132]. In contrast, sustained release morphine given for 6 weeks at a mean dose of 25 mg daily had no effect on quality of life, exercise tolerance, or dyspnoea[133]. Further studies examining diamorphine, dextromethorphan, and codeine have failed to demonstrate useful benefit and codeine caused significant $PaCO_2$ increases[127,134]. Given that opiods may cause serious side effects including CO_2 retention, nausea and drowsiness, and that clinical benefit is unproven, their routine prescription for COPD cannot be recommended. However in severely dyspnoeic, end-stage COPD patients without carbon dioxide retention, a trial of dihydrocodeine or opiate with close monitoring is appropriate. The dose of opiod is titrated in the same way as for pain, but lower doses and smaller increments should be given. As little as 2.5 mg of morphine elixir every 4 h may be sufficient[85]. For patients unable to swallow, subcutaneous diamorphine is recommended. In the terminal phase opiate therapy is justified for the relief of breathlessness and restlessness even with coexisting hypoxaemia and carbon dioxide retention. Similarly, apprehension about respiratory depression must be tempered to avoid unnecessary patient suffering. Laxatives and stool softeners should be started at the onset of opiod therapy

Nebulized opiods: act on peripheral lung receptors. An early study reported increased exercise tolerance with nebulized morphine but a series of subsequent investigations has shown no reduction in dyspnoea in patients with COPD or interstitial lung disease[135,136]. There is currently no good evidence to support the use of nebulized opiods in chronic lung disease.

Mucolytics: viscid or copious mucous production, impaired mucociliary clearance and cough often complicate chronic lung disease. Sputum expectoration may vary from a few millilitres daily to bronchorrhoea with more than 100 ml/day. Avoiding irritants, especially cigarette smoke can reduce secretion dramatically although cough and expectoration may temporarily increase for several weeks after stopping smoking. In COPD, N-acyetylcysteine can be used as a mucolytic agent and is associated with symptom improvement and reduced exacerbations[137]. Recombinant human DNAse although useful in cystic fibrosis has not been beneficial in COPD. Thick secretions may be better expectorated after steam inhalations or nebulized normal (0.9 per cent) or hypertonic (3–7 per cent) saline but specific expectorants like glycerol guaiacolate are of limited value[123]. Bronchorrhoea may be controlled by oral steroid, inhaled atropine or indomethacin[138]. B_2-agonists and theophyllines also aid mucociliary clearance.

Other drugs: nebulized lignocaine to anaesthetize airways receptors and reduce dyspnoea was not beneficial in interstitial lung disease[139]. No improvement in dyspnoea was reported with alcohol, caffeine, indomethacin, or carbimazole[124].

Non-pharmacological therapies

General factors:

◆ *Vaccinations:* influenza and pneumococcal vaccinations should be given to severe COPD patients.

◆ *General nursing:* a fan to blow cool air over the face[62] or being near an open window may help relieve breathlessness. Good nursing care and regular repositioning prevent pressure sores and alleviate the musculoskeletal pain that may be associated with immobility. Relief of constipation and assistance with personal hygiene are essential.

◆ *Nutrition:* patients with end-stage emphysema may lose weight and become frankly cachexic. The main consequence is reduced muscle strength with weakness of both inspiratory and expiratory muscles[25,109]. Weight loss is attributed to a 15–25 per cent increase in resting energy expenditure, due to increased work of breathing, increased metabolic requirement for daily activities, reduced calorie intake and increased inflammatory cytokines[140]. Improved nutrition improves respiratory muscle strength but this only occurs after weight gain which can be difficult to achieve as patients tolerate concentrated nutritional supplements poorly[141]. In contrast, patients with hypercapnic COPD may be overweight. In these patients weight loss may improve breathlessness and exercise tolerance.

◆ *Physiotherapy:* an effective cough is the most efficient means of expelling airways secretions. Forced expiratory techniques and controlled coughing are also helpful. The cleansing action of cough occurs during the first one or two coughs in a sequence. With controlled cough the patient takes a deep breath and coughs 2–3 times with the mouth open without taking another breath. Forced expiratory techniques involve forced exhalation without glottic closure starting at mid-lung volume ('huffing'). This is followed by force expectoration (or controlled cough) at full lung volume to clear central airways. In patients with large volumes of secretion, chest percussion/vibration or postural drainage in the 25 degree head down position for 20 min is safe and effective. Patients with small quantities of secretion derive no benefit from these techniques. In the terminal phase of chronic lung disease physiotherapy may be inappropriate and the right to decline or accept physiotherapy in a modified form should be accepted[107].

◆ *Psychosocial support and counselling:* the level of advice and support offered depends on the patient's level of understanding. The aim is to help them cope, provide strategies to relieve symptoms and improve quality of life. Many patients will want to be involved with their terminal care, providing a 'living will' with instructions on levels of care and use of mechanical ventilation. Many will simply want to 'leave their house in order' or say 'goodbye to loved ones'. Relatives as well as patients will need support and counselling. They must also be involved in discussing the issues associated with death and helped through the grieving process[107].

Pulmonary rehabilitation: pulmonary rehabilitation attempts to return patients to their highest possible level of functional capacity and has become an essential component in the comprehensive care of patients with end-stage lung disease. Numerous studies have confirmed the value of these programmes to reduce dyspnoea, improve quality of life, increase independence, extend exercise capacity, and decrease time in hospital for COPD patients[142,143]. Exercise conditioning is the single most important aspect of rehabilitation. Patients should undertake both general exercises (e.g. stair climbing, stationary cycling) and specific muscle training, particularly the upper limbs and shoulder girdle which act as accessory muscles of respiration. The value of respiratory muscle training with an inspiratory resistance breathing device is controversial and

recent studies have reported no benefit over general exercise reconditioning alone[142,145]. Training should be continued at home, using supplemental oxygen if there is exercise-desaturation. The addition of domiciliary non-invasive positive pressure ventilation (see below) to an exercise training programme has been shown to further improve exercise tolerance and quality of life[145].

Controlled breathing techniques: these include purse-lip breathing, slow expiration, manual upper abdominal compression, and the standing bent forward position with the arms supporting the body. Purse-lip breathing helps improve alveolar ventilation and gas exchange by stenting the airways, preventing dynamic airways collapse and thus decreasing gas trapping[146]. The associated slow expiratory phase is an important component in overcoming the panic attacks that often develop in the severely breathless patient[107]. The bending forwards posture improves diaphragmatic function by increasing abdominal pressure and helps relieve dyspnoea[147]. Nursing positions that facilitate breathing and reduce respiratory distress are illustrated in Fig. 12.3.2.

Non-invasive mechanical ventilation: treatment of hypercapnic COPD exacerbations with non-invasive positive pressure ventilation (NIPPV) is associated with quicker improvement in pH, $PaCO_2$, respiratory rate and breathlessness, as compared with standard treatment alone, and is associated with a reduction in endotracheal intubation rates (~25–30 per cent), decreased mortality (~10 per cent), and shorter hospital stays (~4–6 days)[148,149]. Most studies have included highly selected COPD cases with moderately severe respiratory failure (pH <7.35; $PaCO_2$ 6–8 kPa, respiratory rate >25 breaths/min) and demonstrated failure rates of 20–30 per cent as judged by death or the requirement for endotracheal intubation. Most studies report that the response to the first 2 h of NIPPV (as measured by improvement in pH and $PaCO_2$) is predictive of success or failure. Higher failure rates (35–49 per cent) have been reported in series of less carefully selected patients[149].

NIPPV is usually applied through a nasal or full facemask and dramatically reduces respiratory distress in some patients although others are unable to tolerate the tight fitting mask despite careful explanation and slow introduction of respiratory support.

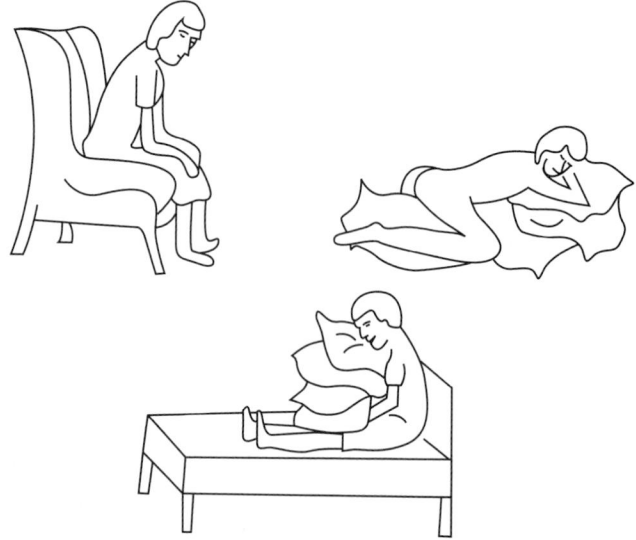

Figure 12.3.2 Patient positioning to alleviate breathlessness.

Non-invasive ventilation in an acute exacerabation often provides time to assess potential reversibility and discuss the patient, carer, and physician's views on full mechanical ventilation.

The value of domiciliary non-invasive ventilation to 'rest' respiratory muscles in stable COPD with chronic respiratory failure has not been established. Failure to improve respiratory muscle function, exercise endurance or sleep and poor tolerance has been reported. A more positive view has been presented by other investigators who demonstrated reduced dyspnoea, improved ventilatory drive, reduced gas trapping, and better sleep[150,151].

Lung reduction surgery and lung transplantation: in a small number of suitable patients with severe emphysema, lung reduction surgery (LRS) produces improvement in both walking distance and quality of life at 6 months[25,152]. The FEV_1 increased by 25–58 per cent (range 16–96 per cent) and FVC between 12 and 40 per cent, 3–6 months after bilateral sur-gery[152]. However improvements were short-lived due to an increase in the annual decline in FEV^1 from ~40 ml/year to 93–163 ml/year in post-surgical patients and overall mortality benefit was small[153,154]. Results from the National Emphysema Treatment Trial has reported that patients with an FEV_1 or gas transfer <20 per cent predicted and lower-lobe emphysema had a high mortality and were unlikely to benefit from LRS[155]. Recent work has examined the possibility of bronchoscopic volume reduction[156].

Lung transplantation (LT) is a therapeutic option for patients with end-stage COPD (FEV_1<25 per cent, PaO_2 <7.3 kPa, elevated pulmonary artery pressure) but mortality is significantly higher in older patients (>65 years old). COPD accounted for 47 per cent of 7204 single and 20 per cent of 5420 bilateral LT reported to the International Transplant Registry[25,157]. In a case series of LT for emphysema, hospital mortality was 3.9 per cent with an overall 5-year survival of 58.6 per cent (with no difference in α_1-antitrypsin deficient patients) although 5-year survival was better in bilateral compared with single LT (67 per cent versus 45 per cent respectively)[158]. FEV_1, exercise capacity and quality of life were improved by LT[159].

However, the availability of lung transplantation has greatly complicated the management of end-stage respiratory disease, especially for those with cystic fibrosis. Due to limited organ availability only a small percentage of patients assessed will be successful recipients. Patients and their families undergo considerable stress waiting for transplants. Acknowledgement that the end-stage has been reached and provision of appropriate palliative care is often delayed, with unnecessary pain and suffering, in the hope of a 'last minute transplant'[107].

Interstitial/fibrotic lung disease

Table 12.3.12 lists the extensive spectrum of diseases that cause progressive fibrotic lung damage, pulmonary hypertension, and hypoxaemic respiratory failure. However, these conditions are relative rare; the commonest group, the pneumoconioses account for about 3024 deaths/year and sarcoidosis for 31 deaths/year compared with over 27 478 deaths/year from COPD[20]. Idiopathic pulmonary fibrosis (previously cryptogenic fibrosing alveolitis) has an incidence of about 3–5/10 0000. The overall mortality is high at ~50 per cent at 5 years but the course is very variable and dependent on the clinico-pathological classification. Acute interstitial pneumonitis leads to death in a few months whereas desquamative interstitial pneumonitis is associated with a 70 per cent 10-year survival[160]. Sarcoidosis follows a relapsing course with two-thirds of cases resolving spontaneously. In a small minority, pulmonary fibrosis progresses relentlessly over many years to respiratory failure. Connective tissue diseases are often associated with pulmonary fibrosis and hypertension. In systemic sclerosis, lung disease and recurrent aspiration (as a result of the oesophageal strictures) accounts for 21 per cent of all deaths[161]. Minor pulmonary fibrosis may occur in up to 60 per cent of patients with rheumatoid arthritis but severe progressive disease is rare and has a 5-year survival of <50 per cent. Bronchiectasis, organizing pneumonia and obliterative bronchiolitis occasionally lead to end-stage lung disease in rheumatoid arthritis.

Immunosuppressive therapies including oral steroids, cyclophosphamide, azothioprine, and penicillamine are used to treat fibrotic lung diseases with variable success[160]. Increasing pulmonary damage is associated with dyspnoea, decreased exercise tolerance, hypoxaemia, pulmonary hypertension, and cor pulmonale. It is rare for CO_2 retention to occur and it is safe to use high inspired concentrations of oxygen. Although benefit with oxygen therapy is poorly documented, it is widely prescribed to relieve breathlessness and improve exercise tolerance[160]. Drug therapy for relief of dyspnoea may be required as the disease progresses. Guidelines for the selection of patients with progressive pulmonary fibrosis for lung transplantation have been published but shortage of organs limits the value of this therapeutic option[160].

Table 12.3.12 Classification of interstitial lung diseases.

Classification	Examples
Idiopathic fibrotic disorders	Idiopathic interstitial pneumonitis, cyptogenic organizing pneumonitis, desquamative interstital pneumonitis, non-specific interstitial pneumonitis, acute interstitial pneumonitis etc
Connective tissue diseases	Systemic lupus erythematosis, rheumatoid arthritis, scleraderma, ankylosing spondylitis etc
Drug induced diseases	Antibiotics (furantoin), antiarrhythmics (amiodarone), anti-inflammatory (gold, penacillamine), chemotherapeutic agents (bleomycin), paraquat, therapeutic radiation etc
Occupational	*Inorganic:* silicosis, asbestosis, coal workers pneumoconiosis, berylliosis, stanosis *Organic:* farmers lung, pigeon fanciers lung etc
Primary unclassified	Sarcoidosis, amyloidosis, pulmonary vasculitis, lymphangitis carcinomatosis, gauchers disease, AIDS, ARDS, eosinophilic granulomatosis etc

AIDS = acquired immunodeficiency syndrome, ARDS = acute respiratory distress syndrome.

Neuromuscular, restrictive, and chest wall disease

Neuromuscular and chest wall disease cause restrictive defects in ventilatory function due to either respiratory muscle weakness or loss of compliance in the thoracic cage[162]. Rapid, shallow breathing, atelectasis, and aspiration due to loss of cough result in ventilatory failure and pneumonia. Neuromuscular diseases affect the respiratory muscles at multiple sites from the spinal cord (e.g. trauma, motor neuron disease) to the muscles themselves (e.g. myopathies, dystrophies). A number of other factors influence respiratory function:

- Ventilatory drive is increased in most of these conditions but with inadequate ventilatory response. However, patients with quadriplegia, congenital myopathies and myotonic dystrophy may also have reduced ventilatory drive. Hypercapnia and sleep abnormalities are the main features in these patients.

- Sleep disorders commonly affect neuromuscular (~42 per cent) and quadreplegic patients (~28 per cent), with respiratory disturbance indicators >15/h[163].

- Unbalanced weakness of spinal and thoracic muscle leads to kyphoscoliosis in poliomyelitis and the muscular dystrophies, causing loss of compliance and increased work of breathing.

- Bulbar incoordination (e.g. multiple sclerosis) may cause upper airways obstruction from aspirated food or foreign bodies. Micro-aspiration results in recurrent pneumonia.

- Diaphragmatic paralysis is a feature of many neuromuscular diseases and may occur after trauma or thoracic surgery. Unilateral paralysis has a good outcome but bilateral paralysis is associated with severe symptoms, ventilatory failure, and pneumonia. The manifestations of bilateral paralysis are much worse in the supine position.

- Pulmonary embolism is a constant threat to immobilized patients but prophylactic anticoagulation reduces mortality.

General supportive measures including oxygen therapy, antibiotics and physiotherapy are required. Clearing secretions is of particular importance and techniques to improve cough capacity have been developed. Coughing can be augmented by synchronizing cough with manual abdominal compressions[164]. An insufflator/exsufflator, 'cough machine' provides a deep insufflation by mask followed by rapid decompression[165]. High cervical injury patients often learn the technique of glossopharyngeal breathing. This involves using the tongue, cheek, pharyngeal and laryngeal muscles in a coordinated way to 'gulp/inject' small boluses of air into the trachea augmenting VC by up to a litre. The larger inspiration, is associated with better passive recoil and cough[164].

Inspiratory muscle training with a daily regime of forced inspiration and expiration through resistances has been advocated in neuromuscular diseases to reduce dependence on mechanical ventilation but not all studies have reported benefit[166]. Occasionally phrenic or abdominal nerve stimulation may be useful[167] for those patients with failure of central drive (e.g. high cervical paralysis) but in anterior horn cell diseases, neuropathies or myopathies the muscles are no more likely to respond to electrical stimulation than to voluntary or automatic effort. Beta-adrenergic agonists can improve mucociliary clearance in the absence of airways obstruction and mucolytics like nebulized acetylcholine may help loosen thick tenacious secretions.

Nasotracheal suctioning, postural drainage and bronchoscopy may be required to clear thick secretions.

When neuromuscular and chest wall diseases are advanced and hypercapnic respiratory failure is developing, ventilatory support is required if patients are to survive. Improved respiratory care and specialist respiratory facilities have made it possible for patients to live for long periods with an acceptable quality of life on mechanical ventilation with or without tracheostomy[168]. However, many patients choose not to accept either tracheostomy or ventilatory support. There are several categories of non-invasive mechanical ventilation many of which are suitable for domiciliary use:

- *Rocking beds:* utilize gravity to assist diaphragmatic movement and are useful for patients with diaphragmatic paralysis who have reasonable respiratory function when upright but not supine.

- *Abdominal pneumatic belts*: assist upward diaphragmatic movement by intermittent compression of the abdomen, with passive recoil during the non-compressive phase. It is most efficient when the patient is sitting upright.

- *Negative pressure body ventilators*: have been extensively used for many neuromuscular diseases and have the advantage of allowing unimpeded speech. The early iron lungs were too cumbersome for practical use but the smaller cuirass and body wrap ventilators are more acceptable to most patients but require considerable skill for successful operation.

- *Non-invasive positive pressure ventilation*: has been used with great success in neuromuscular and chest wall diseases and may prevent the need for tracheostomy[164,168]. It is usually delivered through a nasal mask using a portable volume or pressure cycled ventilator. Full-facemasks and mouthpieces can be used. The tidal volume is adjusted for mouth and mask leaks which can be troublesome and occasionally a chin strap is required to hold the mouth closed particularly during sleep. It is generally well tolerated but skin breakdown at sites in contact with the mask and sinusitis or nasal congestion can be problems[168].

- *Nasal continuous positive airways pressure*: prevents atelectasis, upper airways collapse, and upper airways obstruction in patients with neuromuscular and chest wall diseases. However CPAP has the potential to worsen inspiratory muscle weakness by increasing FRC and is probably best suited to patients with upper airway obstruction due to paresis of upper airways musculature or in diaphragmatic paralysis. It should be used with caution and close monitoring in most neuromuscular diseases.

Specialist respiratory centres with domiciliary nursing facilities are required to provide home ventilation for patients with neuromuscular and chest wall diseases. In most countries these facilities are poorly financed and coordinated although there are exceptions (e.g. France). In these centres staff are proficient in the management of end-stage respiratory disease, providing high quality palliative care for patients that they may have treated and nursed for many years.

Chronic infection

Many respiratory diseases result in chronic or recurrent infection due to structural abnormalities, ineffective cough, or inadequate immune function. Parenchymal damage due to ongoing infection results in ventilation/perfusion mismatching and progressive hypoxaemic respiratory failure. Chronic infection also results in excessive pulmonary secretions with severe cough and atelectasis, weight loss, recurrent fever, and halitosis.

Bronchiectasis and cystic fibrosis

The prognosis for patients with bronchiectasis in the pre-antibiotic era was dismal with only 15 per cent of patients living for more than 20 years. Their lives were characterized by progressive decline in health punctuated by episodes of acute infection and haemoptysis. This picture has been transformed by the advent of antibiotics and survival is much improved[169]. Table 12.3.13 reports conditions associated with bronchiectasis. Diagnosis was previously made with bronchography which is now obsolete and has been replaced by high-resolution, thin-section CT scan of the chest which has a specificity of more than 90 per cent to detect bronchiectasis at the segmental level[170]. Detection should promote a search for the underlying cause including protein electrophoresis for α_1-antitrypsin deficiency, hypogammaglobulinaemia, pilocarpine ionophoresis (sweat test) for cystic fibrosis, *Aspergillus* precipitins for aspergillosis, and electron microscopy for primary ciliary dyskinesia. Regular determination of bacterial colonization in sputum aids management[171].

Treatment requires management of infection, secretions, haemoptysis, and obstructive airways disease and includes:

◆ *Antimicrobial drugs*: which are the mainstay of therapy and are directed by sputum culture. Combinations of broad spectrum antibiotics that have good lung penetration and cover anaerobic and gram negative organisms including *Pseudomonas* are required including metronidozole, augmentin, and ciprofloxcin. They often have to be administered intravenously. Most physician only treat acute infective exacerbations but some patients may require continuous or intermittent cycles of antibiotic therapy to maintain good health. Treatment has to be given for longer periods, often 3–4 weeks, continuously or in cycles of therapy to minimize the risk of resistance. Higher doses are required to achieve therapeutic antibiotic levels in the infection filled endobronchial spaces[172]. Nebulized antibiotics including gentamycin and tobramycin have been administered successfully in cystic fibrosis to control airways inflammation and secretion[173].

◆ *Bronchodilator therapy*: including β_2-agonists (metered dose and nebulized), antimuscurinic agents and oral theophyllines are all used to relieve airways bronchoconstriction (see COPD)

Table 12.3.13 Conditions associated with bronchiectasis.

Cystic fibrosis
HIV infection
Rheumatoid arthritis
Infection, inflammation
Bronchopulmonary sequestration
Allergic bronchopulmonary aspergillosis
Alpha₁-antitrypsin deficiency
Congenital cartilage deficiency
Immunodeficiency
Yellow nail syndrome
Bronchial obstruction
Unilateral hyperlucent lung

◆ *Chest physical therapy*: with postural drainage, chest clapping, humidification and the use of mucolytics increase sputum clearance[174]. Chest clapping can be administered by family members with considerable psychological benefit. Mucociliary clearance is increased by β_2-agonists and nebulized amiloride or hypertonic saline (with cough) in cystic fibrosis[175].

◆ *Nebulized recombinant human deoxyribonuclease (DNAse)*: facilitates secretion clearance by hydrolysing the extracellular deoxyribonucleic acid that accumulates with other neutrophil degradation products in infected airways but does not reduce acute infective exacerbations[176,177].

◆ *Anti-inflammatory therapy*: inhaled indomethacin improves sputum viscosity and relieves symptoms in patients with chronic bronchitis and bronchiectasis[138]. Oral ibuprofen twice daily reduced decline in lung function, radiographic deterioration and loss of weight in patients with cystic fibrosis[178]. Oral steroids are associated with side effects with little additional benefit except in allergic bronchopulmonary aspergillosis.

◆ *Supplemental oxygen and mechanical ventilation*: are required in hypoxaemic respiratory failure complicating bronchiectasis and cystic fibrosis, as for COPD.

◆ *Other pharmacotherapies*: include immunoglobulin administration in hypogammaglobulinaemia and enzyme replacement in α_1-antitrypsin deficiency. Gene replacement therapy is currently being studied in cystic fibrosis. Good nutrition with a high caloric intake is required and pancreatic supplements may be required in cystic fibrosis.

◆ *Surgery*: segmental resection may be considered in localized bronchiectasis with recurrent severe haemoptysis but otherwise the benefits of surgery are limited. Double lung and heart lung transplantation has been most successful in the end-stage management of cystic fibrosis but is also an option in severe bronchiectasis (see COPD).

◆ *Haemoptysis*: is a common problem in bronchiectasis. For the majority it is relatively minor with only flecks of blood in sputum. However, because the disease affects the high pressure bronchial circulation it can be massive and life-threatening. Its management has been discussed above.

◆ *Halatosis*: is an often neglected problem in bronchiectasis. It can be severe, causing social embarrassment and difficulty managing patients both at home and in hospital. Although chronic lung infection is the most likely cause, oral hygiene including dentistry and gum disease must be addressed. The causative anaerobic or gram negative lung infections are managed with high dose, prolonged, antibiotic therapy (± nebulized antibiotics) as determined by sputum culture and sensitivity (see above). Aggressive physiotherapy and postural drainage are required to clear the foul smelling respiratory secretions. Simple measures including mouth scents, good ventilation, and air fresheners will help, particularly in the terminal phase of the disease when physiotherapy and postural drainage become more difficult.

Cystic fibrosis affects 1 in 2500 children and the gene responsible has been identified. The defect alters ion and water transport across epithelial cells causing recurrent pulmonary infection, bronchiectasis, lung fibrosis, and pancreatic insufficiency. Survival has improved progressively over the last 20 years and median survival is now about

12 per cent of cases in the PIOPED study[191] and the features were often non-specific particularly in patients with concurrent respiratory disease (e.g. atelectasis, hilar enlargement, oligaemia). Doppler ultrasonography and contrast venography are standard techniques for establishing the presence of DVT. Investigations to establish a diagnosis of PE include ventilation/perfusion scans, angiography, and contrast spiral CT scans. At present V/Q scanning remains the first-line investigation. A normal V/Q scan excludes and a high probability scan confirms PE. An indeterminate scan or low probability scan with high clinical probability suggest the need for angiography or CT scan[191,193]. Angiography remains the 'gold' standard test but is relatively invasive[191]. CT scanning is sensitive, specific, and non-invasive and is its role as the first-line investigation is currently being assessed[191].

The importance of prevention in the immobile, cardiorespiratory patient cannot be overstressed. Simple factors like hydration, mobility, and reduction of venous obstruction by uncrossing legs should not be overlooked. The use of compression 'anti-embolism' stockings in end-stage disease is questionable and the associated discomfort must be balanced against likely benefit. Low-molecular-weight heparin offers substantial advantages over unfractionated heparin in the prevention of DVT and PE in terminally ill patients[194]. It is equally effective, has better bioavailability, predictable anticoagulant response and less complications (e.g. bleeding, thrombocytopaenia). Once daily dosing with some preparations is feasible because of the longer duration of action. Except in renal failure and marked obesity monitoring is not required reducing the need for repeated blood tests. These properties make it valuable in hospice and domiciliary therapy if carers are taught to administer the daily injection. In patients with proven DVT or PE, maintenance therapy with warfarin is standard procedure after initial heparinization. The aim is to maintain the INR between 2 and 3[195]. However, the use of warfarin in patients with terminal disease can cause problems because of the need for repeated monitoring of the INR which may fluctuate according to drug therapy, liver function and diet. As a result continuation of low-molecular-weight heparin is becoming increasingly popular[194].

The decision to use more aggressive therapies in the management of DVT and PE in end-stage lung disease is difficult. In general, the use of thrombolytic therapy (e.g. recombinant tissue plasminogen activator) in PE, with the associated risks of haemorrhage, should probably be reserved for those with acute, severe, haemodynamic instability and even in this situation survival benefit over heparinization alone is unproven[195]. Where risk of PE is very high but anticoagulation contraindicated vena caval filters may be considered although lower limb oedema may be a significant problem. Catheter or surgical embolectomy must be carefully considered in patients with end-stage disease.

Pneumothorax and pleural disease

In end-stage lung disease even a small collection of air or fluid in the pleural space may have serious implications because respiratory reserve to compensate for the loss of ventilatory capacity (due to lung compression) is reduced in these patients[196]. The incidence of 'spontaneous' pneumothorax increases with age and severity of the underlying lung disease. It is most commonly associated with COPD but may affect a wide variety of other lung diseases that damage lung architecture or the pleura. Iatrogenic damage during aspiration of a pleural effusion may also result in a pneumothorax.

Early recognition and wide-bore, intercostal tube drainage with an underwater seal is necessary in most patients and is often life-saving[196]. However, in the terminally ill patient the decision may be taken to treat the patient symptomatically with oxygen, analgesics and opiods to avoid the distress of moving them to a unit with the appropriate facilities to insert and manage a chest drain.

Pleural effusions and empyema also result in exaggerated respiratory embarrassment in chronic lung diseases due to lung compression. Intermittent aspiration or tube drainage provides valuable symptomatic relief of breathlessness in most patients. There are a wide variety of potential causes including infection, cardiac failure, low albumin, and renal impairment, and the underlying cause must be addressed. However, if the cause is irreversible the possibility of chemical pleurodesis may have to be considered. Pleurodesis is discussed in Chapter 11.1. Localized pleural pain due to rib fractures, infection or pneumothorax may respond to normal analgesic regimes. However, local anaesthetic intercostals nerve blocks or intrapleural instillation of bupivicaine may also be useful.

Patient–physician communication about end-of-life care

Patients with end-stage respiratory disease are less likely to discuss end-of-life care and their treatment preferences with their physician than patients with respiratory or other forms of cancer[197]. Thus despite the poor prognosis of hospitalized COPD patients (median 2-year survival) and a 50 per cent probability of readmission within 2 months, these patients are more likely to die with aggressive technological care directed at preserving life rather than with home nursing and palliative care than patients with lung cancer, despite having similar preferences for palliative care[198]. The reasons for this are complex but the lack of data to guide physicians on how best to achieve patient-physician end-of-life communication in end-stage respiratory disease has been highlighted in recent COPD guidelines[118].

In a recent study of patient-physician communication undertaken in end-stage COPD the patients reported that most physicians do not discuss prognosis (i.e. how long the patient has to live), what dying might be like or the patients spirituality[197]. Common barriers to communication endorsed by patients when asked about end-of life care were 'I would rather concentrate on staying alive than talk about death' (75 per cent) and 'I don't know what kind of care I would want if I get very sick' (37 per cent). The physician endorsed barriers were 'There is too little time during our appointments to discuss everything we should' (64 per cent) and 'I worry that discussing end-of-life care will take away hope' (23 per cent). Some of the patient facilitators to these discussions were 'I trust my doctor' (87 per cent) and 'I have family or friends who have died' (88 per cent) and for physicians 'I have cared for many patients with lung disease' (80 per cent) and 'The patient has been very sick in the past' (71 per cent)[199]. Improving patient-physician communication is essential to ensure that patients receive the care they desire. Those practising clinicians who do address prognosis and future management in the outpatient setting often report that patients rarely encourage or welcome these discussions which, in many cases are counterproductive and unrealistic. Whether this difficulty in addressing prognosis in the stable patients stems from a lack of training is not established but it is clear that excessive pulmonary secretions with severe cough and atelectasis, weight loss, recurrent fever, and halitosis.

Bronchiectasis and cystic fibrosis

The prognosis for patients with bronchiectasis in the pre-antibiotic era was dismal with only 15 per cent of patients living for more than 20 years. Their lives were characterized by progressive decline in health punctuated by episodes of acute infection and haemoptysis. This picture has been transformed by the advent of antibiotics and survival is much improved[169]. Table 12.3.13 reports conditions associated with bronchiectasis. Diagnosis was previously made with bronchography which is now obsolete and has been replaced by high-resolution, thin-section CT scan of the chest which has a specificity of more than 90 per cent to detect bronchiectasis at the segmental level[170]. Detection should promote a search for the underlying cause including protein electrophoresis for α_1-antitrypsin deficiency, hypogammaglobulinaemia, pilocarpine ionophoresis (sweat test) for cystic fibrosis, *Aspergillus* precipitins for aspergillosis, and electron microscopy for primary ciliary dyskinesia. Regular determination of bacterial colonization in sputum aids management[171].

Treatment requires management of infection, secretions, haemoptysis, and obstructive airways disease and includes:

♦ *Antimicrobial drugs*: which are the mainstay of therapy and are directed by sputum culture. Combinations of broad spectrum antibiotics that have good lung penetration and cover anaerobic and gram negative organisms including *Pseudomonas* are required including metronidozole, augmentin, and ciprofloxcin. They often have to be administered intravenously. Most physician only treat acute infective exacerbations but some patients may require continuous or intermittent cycles of antibiotic therapy to maintain good health. Treatment has to be given for longer periods, often 3–4 weeks, continuously or in cycles of therapy to minimize the risk of resistance. Higher doses are required to achieve therapeutic antibiotic levels in the infection filled endobronchial spaces[172]. Nebulized antibiotics including gentamycin and tobramycin have been administered successfully in cystic fibrosis to control airways inflammation and secretion[173].

♦ *Bronchodilator therapy*: including β_2-agonists (metered dose and nebulized), antimuscurinic agents and oral theophyllines are all used to relieve airways bronchoconstriction (see COPD)

Table 12.3.13 Conditions associated with bronchiectasis.

Cystic fibrosis
HIV infection
Rheumatoid arthritis
Infection, inflammation
Bronchopulmonary sequestration
Allergic bronchopulmonary aspergillosis
Alpha$_1$-antitrypsin deficiency
Congenital cartilage deficiency
Immunodeficiency
Yellow nail syndrome
Bronchial obstruction
Unilateral hyperlucent lung

♦ *Chest physical therapy*: with postural drainage, chest clapping, humidification and the use of mucolytics increase sputum clearance[174]. Chest clapping can be administered by family members with considerable psychological benefit. Mucociliary clearance is increased by β_2-agonists and nebulized amiloride or hypertonic saline (with cough) in cystic fibrosis[175].

♦ *Nebulized recombinant human deoxyribonuclease (DNAse)*: facilitates secretion clearance by hydrolysing the extracellular deoxyribonucleic acid that accumulates with other neutrophil degradation products in infected airways but does not reduce acute infective exacerbations[176,177].

♦ *Anti-inflammatory therapy*: inhaled indomethacin improves sputum viscosity and relieves symptoms in patients with chronic bronchitis and bronchiectasis[138]. Oral ibuprofen twice daily reduced decline in lung function, radiographic deterioration and loss of weight in patients with cystic fibrosis[178]. Oral steroids are associated with side effects with little additional benefit except in allergic bronchopulmonary aspergillosis.

♦ *Supplemental oxygen and mechanical ventilation*: are required in hypoxaemic respiratory failure complicating bronchiectasis and cystic fibrosis, as for COPD.

♦ *Other pharmacotherapies*: include immunoglobulin administration in hypogammaglobulinaemia and enzyme replacement in α_1-antitrypsin deficiency. Gene replacement therapy is currently being studied in cystic fibrosis. Good nutrition with a high caloric intake is required and pancreatic supplements may be required in cystic fibrosis.

♦ *Surgery*: segmental resection may be considered in localized bronchiectasis with recurrent severe haemoptysis but otherwise the benefits of surgery are limited. Double lung and heart lung transplantation has been most successful in the end-stage management of cystic fibrosis but is also an option in severe bronchiectasis (see COPD).

♦ *Haemoptysis*: is a common problem in bronchiectasis. For the majority it is relatively minor with only flecks of blood in sputum. However, because the disease affects the high pressure bronchial circulation it can be massive and life-threatening. Its management has been discussed above.

♦ *Halatosis*: is an often neglected problem in bronchiectasis. It can be severe, causing social embarrassment and difficulty managing patients both at home and in hospital. Although chronic lung infection is the most likely cause, oral hygiene including dentistry and gum disease must be addressed. The causative anaerobic or gram negative lung infections are managed with high dose, prolonged, antibiotic therapy (± nebulized antibiotics) as determined by sputum culture and sensitivity (see above). Aggressive physiotherapy and postural drainage are required to clear the foul smelling respiratory secretions. Simple measures including mouth scents, good ventilation, and air fresheners will help, particularly in the terminal phase of the disease when physiotherapy and postural drainage become more difficult.

Cystic fibrosis affects 1 in 2500 children and the gene responsible has been identified. The defect alters ion and water transport across epithelial cells causing recurrent pulmonary infection, bronchiectasis, lung fibrosis, and pancreatic insufficiency. Survival has improved progressively over the last 20 years and median survival is now about

Table 12.3.14 Infective and non-infective pulmonary complications of HIV disease.

Pulmonary complications	Examples
Infection:	
Bacterial	*Streptococcus pneumoniae, Haemophilus* spp. *Pseudomonas aeruginosa*
Mycobacterial	*M. tuberculosis, M. avian complex, M. kanasii*
Fungi	*Pneumocystis carinii (jirovecii), Cryptococcus neoformans, Histoplasma capsulatum, Aspergillus* species, *Blastomyces dermatitidis, Penicillium marneffei*
Viruses	Cytomegalovirus
Parasites	*Toxoplasma gondii*
Malignancies	Kaposi's sarcoma, non-Hodgkin's lymphoma, bronchogenic carcinoma
Interstitial pneumonitides	Lymphocytic and non-specific interstitial pneumonitis
Other	COPD, PHT, diffuse alveolar damage, bronchiolitis obliterans organizing pneumonia, alveolar proteinosis

COPD = chronic obstructive pulmonary disease, PHT = pulmonary hypertension.

30 years. Most patients with cystic fibrosis will be cared for in specialized units, with home support teams and staff trained in the principles of palliative care. They are encouraged to manage their own disease and most will be familiar with the course of the disease. Psychosocial support from family and well established carers is usually excellent and many will have discussed their end-of-life management, often at the time when a peer dies. In general, these young patients manage remarkably well although psychological problems are common. The option of lung transplantation has complicated 'end-of-life' decision-making. Delay in acknowledging that the end-stage has been reached, and that lung transplantation is no longer a realistic option, should not be allowed to delay effective palliative care. In comparison terminal care in older adults with end-stage bronchiectasis is often poor.

HIV-associated chronic infection

Pulmonary involvement in HIV disease is a major source of morbidity and mortality[179]. The Pulmonary Complications of HIV Infection Study (PCHIS) has demonstrated that the prevalence of HIV-associated pulmonary diseases depends on geographical factors and appears to be changing with time[179,180]. Although there is a wide range of pulmonary manifestations both infectious and non-infectious (Table 12.3.14), respiratory disease is often a small component in a complex scenario including fever, wasting, skin disease, gastrointestinal, eye, and neurological complications. Good palliative care is a major challenge. In developed countries most patients are managed in specialized units which provide optimal medical and nursing management. The palliative management of end-stage HIV infection and its respiratory complications is reviewed in Chapter 12.2.

Tuberculosis

Poorly treated tuberculosis may result in pulmonary scarring, cavitation, and secondary *Aspergillus* infection. Respiratory failure and massive haemoptysis may develop. In active tuberculosis infection patients must be isolated in a negative pressure room but otherwise treatment of the respiratory failure and chronic infection does not differ from that previously described. Considerable care must be taken to avoid transmission to other patients and self-infection. Tuberculosis must be actively treated with appropriate antibiotics depending on sensitivities determined from culture. Surgical and antimicrobial therapy of secondary *Aspergillus* infection is often required.

Pulmonary vascular disease

Pulmonary hypertension[181] and thromboembolic disease may be the cause or secondary problems of end-stage respiratory disease. The breathlessness, fatigue (due to poor cardiac output), and fluid retention (cor pulmonale) that accompany these conditions are significant clinical challenges. Primary pulmonary hypertension, emphysema due to α_1-antitrypsin deficiency and thromboembolic disease (e.g. antiphospholipid syndrome) often affect young adults whereas COPD and fibrotic lung disease usually involve older age groups. Prevention of thromboembolism is essential in all terminally ill-patients. Failure to prevent deep venous thrombosis or pulmonary embolism leads to unnecessary discomfort and complicates care. The degree of investigation, intervention and treatment undertaken is adjusted according to the needs of the individual patient and the level of terminal care.

Pulmonary hypertension and cor pulmonale

Most respiratory disease can result in pulmonary hypertension (PHT) which eventually leads to right ventricular hypertrophy, dilation and cor pulmonale. Many mechanisms contribute to the development of PHT (Table 12.3.15) including hypoxaemic pulmonary vasoconstriction (HPV), multiple obstructive lesions, and primary pulmonary hypertension.

Chronic bronchitis and emphysema: cause PHT due to progressive hypoxic pulmonary vasoconstriction and associated vascular

Table 12.3.15 Classification of pulmonary hypertension.

Mechanisms of pulmonary hypertension
Idiopathic (e.g. primary pulmonary hypertension)
Hypoxic (e.g. hypoxic pulmonary vasoconstriction)
Passive (e.g. LVF / mitral stenosis / elevated LAP)
Hyperkinetic
Obliterative (e.g. chronic thromboembolic disease)
Dietary/drug induced
Vasoconstrictive

LVF = left ventricular failure, LAP = left atrial pressure.

remodelling but is usually relatively mild. Management aims to improve the underlying lung disorder. Oxygen therapy reverses hypoxic pulmonary artery vasoconstriction and reduces right ventricular afterload, although reductions in PHT were small with LTOT[118]. Diuretics are the mainstay of the management of fluid retention and ankle oedema in the acute phase of cor pulmonale. Pulmonary vasodilators including calcium channel (e.g. nifedipine), angiotensin-converting enzyme and angiotensin II inhibitors, and endothelin antagonsists reduce pulmonary artery pressure but cause systemic hypotension, increase ventilation/perfusion mismatch, and impair gas exchange with no clinically useful amelioration of PHT or cor pulmonale in chronic stable COPD.

Obstructive pulmonary hypertension: is often caused by repetitive, silent, pulmonary emboli arising from deep vein thromboses over prolonged periods of time[182]. Other causes of obstructive PHT include vasculitis, sickle cell anaemia or infective endocarditis. World wide schistosomiasis is one of the commonest causes of PHT due to the obstructive effect of the parasitic organism itself and the acute inflammatory response it evokes. Chronic thromboembolic disease is a risk in many terminal diseases including chronic lung disease due to immobility and the increased tendency to coagulation[183]. It highlights the importance of prophylactic anticoagulation, compression stockings and maintained mobility (see below). Chronic thromboembolic PHT as a consequence of repeated small emboli that have not previously been recognized requires careful assessment to determine whether pulmonary thromboendarterectomy is an option. Occasionally, if accumulated clot can be successfully removed the improvement in the PHT can be dramatic[184]. If surgery is not justified, management is focused on preventing further embolism by adequate anticoagulation, the occasional use of thrombolytic agents and inferior vena cava filters. Pulmonary blood flow is also optimized by correcting hypoxaemia and maximising pulmonary vasodilation.

Idiopathic pulmonary hypertension (IPH): is a disease of unknown aetiology causing progressive PHT[181]. The prognosis is poor with a median survival in the US registry of 2.8 years[181]. Although, a rare condition it has a relatively high profile because it often affects young women of child bearing age (mean age 36 years) and as an end-stage condition presents all the problems of terminal care in young adults. The primary clinical symptoms are progressive dyspnoea, reduced exercise tolerance, central chest pain, syncope, and occasional haemoptysis. In the terminal phase it is often associated with fluid accumulation and ankle oedema. Sudden death occurs in severe PHT due to acute right ventricular decompensation, arrhythmias or thromboembolic events. In end-stage disease oxygen therapy provides symptomatic relief and may be beneficial in the management of the cor pulmonale. Most patients are anticoagulated because it is difficult to exclude the possibility of recurrent embolism and *in situ* thrombosis is perceived as part of the pathogenesis of the condition. Previous studies have reported improved survival in anticoagulated patients[181].

There have been rapid advances in the treatment IPH with associated improved survival[181]. Calcium channel blockers (e.g. nifedipine) are beneficial in the 10 per cent of patients who respond to acute vasodilators (e.g. adenosine) but only about 50 per cent have sustained vasodilation. Sildenafil, a potent, orally active, cGMP-phosphodiesterase type 5 inhibitor which increases cGMP, has been demonstrated to improve exercise capacity, functional class and haemodynamics in IPH (NYHA class II and III)[185].

Likewise, bosentan, a dual endothelin receptor (ET_A and ET_B) antagonist, improved exercise tolerance, symptoms, haemodynamics, and functional class in recent trials[186]. Prostacyclin, an intravenously administered vasodilator produces substantial haemodynamic and symptomatic improvement when given by continuous infusion with reductions in pulmonary artery pressure and vascular resistance and improved survival[181,187]. Prostacyclin (iloprost) inhalation 6–9 times daily has also been reported to improve exercise tolerance, haemodynamics and functional class[187]. IPH patients are often listed for lung transplantation which may increase survival but lack of donor organs limits the application of this technique and complicates end-stage palliative care.

Pulmonary embolism (PE)

In the USA, approximately 5 million episodes of deep venous thrombosis (DVT) occur, 10 per cent embolize and 10 per cent of those who have an embolic event (~50 000) die[188]. The majority are not due to therapeutic failure but prophylactic oversight or diagnostic error. The incidence is increasing particularly in the dependent, hospitalized patients in the terminal phase of chronic cardiopulmonary disease who are relatively immobile, with an increased thrombotic tendency and often longstanding peripheral vascular disease[189]. About 90 per cent of clinically significant PE arise from the deep veins in the lower extremities. Calf vein thrombi are rarely associated with PE whereas over 50 per cent of thrombi in the popliteal or ileofemoral systems will embolize[189]. Acute cardiovascular collapse and rapid death may occur with a large embolus and is the cause of death in many end-stage terminally ill patients who expire suddenly during an apparently unremarkable exertion.

Clinical diagnosis of PE is imprecise although acute dyspnoea is the most frequent presenting symptom in most studies[190]. The PIOPED study (Prospective Investigation of Pulmonary Embolism Diagnosis) trial examined the clinical probability of PE on the basis of history, examination, CXR, ECG, and blood gases[191]. In 90 patients estimated to have a >80 per cent clinical probability of PE, 32 per cent did not have confirmatory angiographic evidence. In 228 patients estimated to have a probability of <19 per cent, 9 per cent had positive angiograms. In patients without prior cardiopulmonary disease in the PIOPED study the combination of pleuritic pain or haemoptysis was the most common mode of presentation of pulmonary embolism in 65 per cent of cases, isolated dyspnoea in 22 per cent and circulatory collapse in 8 per cent. Dyspnoea was not present in 27 per cent of patients with confirmed PE. In addition, prospective studies demonstrate that asymptomatic PE occurs in 40 per cent of high risk patients with proximal deep vein thrombosis[189]. It is apparent that the 'typical' picture of PE is relatively rare and that presentation is often atypical or subtle. However, recent meta-analysis of clinical prediction strategies for DVT and PE provides strong evidence to support the use of a clinical prediction rule for establishing the pre-test probability of disease in a patient before more definitive testing. In addition, use of a D-dimer assay with a clinical prediction rule has a very high negative predictive value[192].

The extent and type of investigations for PE in end-stage lung disease is to a large extent determined by life expectancy and the level of potential discomfort that may be inflicted. Basic investigations should include blood gases, ECG, and chest radiography but these are generally non-specific. Chest radiography was normal in

12 per cent of cases in the PIOPED study[191] and the features were often non-specific particularly in patients with concurrent respiratory disease (e.g. atelectasis, hilar enlargement, oligaemia). Doppler ultrasonography and contrast venography are standard techniques for establishing the presence of DVT. Investigations to establish a diagnosis of PE include ventilation/perfusion scans, angiography, and contrast spiral CT scans. At present V/Q scanning remains the first-line investigation. A normal V/Q scan excludes and a high probability scan confirms PE. An indeterminate scan or low probability scan with high clinical probability suggest the need for angiography or CT scan[191,193]. Angiography remains the 'gold' standard test but is relatively invasive[191]. CT scanning is sensitive, specific, and non-invasive and is its role as the first-line investigation is currently being assessed[191].

The importance of prevention in the immobile, cardiorespiratory patient cannot be overstressed. Simple factors like hydration, mobility, and reduction of venous obstruction by uncrossing legs should not be overlooked. The use of compression 'anti-embolism' stockings in end-stage disease is questionable and the associated discomfort must be balanced against likely benefit. Low-molecular-weight heparin offers substantial advantages over unfractionated heparin in the prevention of DVT and PE in terminally ill patients[194]. It is equally effective, has better bioavailability, predictable anticoagulant response and less complications (e.g. bleeding, thrombocytopaenia). Once daily dosing with some preparations is feasible because of the longer duration of action. Except in renal failure and marked obesity monitoring is not required reducing the need for repeated blood tests. These properties make it valuable in hospice and domiciliary therapy if carers are taught to administer the daily injection. In patients with proven DVT or PE, maintenance therapy with warfarin is standard procedure after initial heparinization. The aim is to maintain the INR between 2 and 3[195]. However, the use of warfarin in patients with terminal disease can cause problems because of the need for repeated monitoring of the INR which may fluctuate according to drug therapy, liver function and diet. As a result continuation of low-molecular-weight heparin is becoming increasingly popular[194].

The decision to use more aggressive therapies in the management of DVT and PE in end-stage lung disease is difficult. In general, the use of thrombolytic therapy (e.g. recombinant tissue plasminogen activator) in PE, with the associated risks of haemorrhage, should probably be reserved for those with acute, severe, haemodynamic instability and even in this situation survival benefit over heparinization alone is unproven[195]. Where risk of PE is very high but anticoagulation contraindicated vena caval filters may be considered although lower limb oedema may be a significant problem. Catheter or surgical embolectomy must be carefully considered in patients with end-stage disease.

Pneumothorax and pleural disease

In end-stage lung disease even a small collection of air or fluid in the pleural space may have serious implications because respiratory reserve to compensate for the loss of ventilatory capacity (due to lung compression) is reduced in these patients[196]. The incidence of 'spontaneous' pneumothorax increases with age and severity of the underlying lung disease. It is most commonly associated with COPD but may affect a wide variety of other lung diseases that damage lung architecture or the pleura. Iatrogenic damage during aspiration of a pleural effusion may also result in a pneumothorax.

Early recognition and wide-bore, intercostal tube drainage with an underwater seal is necessary in most patients and is often life-saving[196]. However, in the terminally ill patient the decision may be taken to treat the patient symptomatically with oxygen, analgesics and opiods to avoid the distress of moving them to a unit with the appropriate facilities to insert and manage a chest drain.

Pleural effusions and empyema also result in exaggerated respiratory embarrassment in chronic lung diseases due to lung compression. Intermittent aspiration or tube drainage provides valuable symptomatic relief of breathlessness in most patients. There are a wide variety of potential causes including infection, cardiac failure, low albumin, and renal impairment, and the underlying cause must be addressed. However, if the cause is irreversible the possibility of chemical pleurodesis may have to be considered. Pleurodesis is discussed in Chapter 11.1. Localized pleural pain due to rib fractures, infection or pneumothorax may respond to normal analgesic regimes. However, local anaesthetic intercostals nerve blocks or intrapleural instillation of bupivicaine may also be useful.

Patient–physician communication about end-of-life care

Patients with end-stage respiratory disease are less likely to discuss end-of-life care and their treatment preferences with their physician than patients with respiratory or other forms of cancer[197]. Thus despite the poor prognosis of hospitalized COPD patients (median 2-year survival) and a 50 per cent probability of readmission within 2 months, these patients are more likely to die with aggressive technological care directed at preserving life rather than with home nursing and palliative care than patients with lung cancer, despite having similar preferences for palliative care[198]. The reasons for this are complex but the lack of data to guide physicians on how best to achieve patient-physician end-of-life communication in end-stage respiratory disease has been highlighted in recent COPD guidelines[118].

In a recent study of patient-physician communication undertaken in end-stage COPD the patients reported that most physicians do not discuss prognosis (i.e. how long the patient has to live), what dying might be like or the patients spirituality[197]. Common barriers to communication endorsed by patients when asked about end-of life care were 'I would rather concentrate on staying alive than talk about death' (75 per cent) and 'I don't know what kind of care I would want if I get very sick' (37 per cent). The physician endorsed barriers were 'There is too little time during our appointments to discuss everything we should' (64 per cent) and 'I worry that discussing end-of-life care will take away hope' (23 per cent). Some of the patient facilitators to these discussions were 'I trust my doctor' (87 per cent) and 'I have family or friends who have died' (88 per cent) and for physicians 'I have cared for many patients with lung disease' (80 per cent) and 'The patient has been very sick in the past' (71 per cent)[199]. Improving patient-physician communication is essential to ensure that patients receive the care they desire. Those practising clinicians who do address prognosis and future management in the outpatient setting often report that patients rarely encourage or welcome these discussions which, in many cases are counterproductive and unrealistic. Whether this difficulty in addressing prognosis in the stable patients stems from a lack of training is not established but it is clear that neither postgraduate training nor textbooks in internal medicine devote adequate resource to this aspect of medical care.

Respiratory terminal care and palliative sedation

During the terminal phase of end-stage respiratory disease simple nursing measures including a constant draught from an open window or fan, regular sips of water to moisten the mouth (particularly when using oxygen), and sitting upright may be beneficial. If confined to bed the patient may be propped up with pillows as there is a significant loss of diaphragmatic function, increased risk of pulmonary oedema associated with cardiac failure, and lower lobe atelectasis when lying flat. In addition, recurrent micro-aspiration is more likely in the recumbent position.

At this stage, the emphasis of management changes from active interventions to purely supportive and symptomatic measures. Non-invasive ventilatory support and active physiotherapy may be withdrawn to facilitate greater comfort for the patient but drug treatments aimed at palliating symptoms of pain, breathlessness, constipation, and haemoptysis are often unavoidable. If possible drugs should be given orally using sustained release preparations but subcutaneous infusions or intermittent, intramuscular injections may be necessary. Often these patients will have been on oxygen therapy for long-periods and may become distressed if this is removed. Use of nasal prongs facilitates communication with relatives and carers. Similarly, nebulizers should be continued as long as practically possible to provide bronchodilators, local anaesthetics, and opioids to alleviate breathlessness and cough. The 'rattle' associated with loose respiratory secretions in the short period before death may be distressing to relatives although most patients will be unaware of the noise at this stage. Hyoscine should be administered to reduce respiratory secretions, although repositioning or gentle suctioning may also be required[200].

The use of palliative sedation for the relief of refractory dyspnoea is particularly difficult because of the perceived risk of respiratory depression. A recent multi-centre study reported that the use of sedation varied considerably between different hospice units although this was primarily in cancer patients rather than those with end-stage respiratory disease[200]. However, several studies examining the use of sedation for refractory symptoms during the terminal phase have not shown a difference in survival between sedated and non-sedated patients with respiratory distress[201–203]. As many patients approaching death with end-stage respiratory disease will have uncontrolled breathlessness, sedation and opioid use should not be withheld because of an inappropriate fear of respiratory depression. When the risk of respiratory depression is considerable, the risks and benefits must be carefully considered and the justification for sedation clearly defined. Such decisions are usually made by teams rather than individuals and it is appropriate that patients and families are fully involved in decision-making and should understand that sedation is a means of relieving distressing symptoms. Before starting sedation it should be clear that other interventions to relieve refractory dyspnoea have not provided relief, or will not do so in an appropriate time period.

The degree of sedation may be varied throughout the course of the terminal stage by periods of discontinuation or titrating drug effect to the desired level. However, as death approaches and if breathlessness becomes intolerable, sedation to unconsciousness may be the last resort to alleviate suffering. For those patients and their families who do not wish to accept sedation during the dying period, it is the duty of the carer to relieve suffering as best possible and to support the patient through to death.

Summary: the future for palliative care in end-stage respiratory disease

In the UK, the number of specialist respiratory nurses is increasing but remains relatively small[49]. They are based in hospital but many make domiciliary visits. Patients cared for by these nurses live longer but quality of life is not necessarily improved[45,50]. Nevertheless patients valued these visits and wanted them to continue. Despite the efforts of respiratory physicians and nurses, support for patients with terminal lung disease is less well developed than that available for patients with malignant disease. A number of exceptions include care for patients with cystic fibrosis and HIV related respiratory disease. Nevertheless, there is a major unmet need in the care of the patient with end-stage respiratory disease.

In response to recommendations that all patients should have access to palliative care[2,15,16], the need, potential demand and, resource implications of this directive have been assessed[2]. There are clearly problems that will have to be overcome if the goal of 'palliative care for all' is to be achieved[2]. These include lack of current service provision, difficulty projecting disease trajectory in chronic lung disease, the need for specialist respiratory skills and inadequate resources. Overcoming these problems will be difficult. Education in palliative care will be essential at all levels of doctor and nurse training and it is clear that respiratory physicians and specialist nurses will need to adopt the palliative care approach. A potential solution to the current lack of palliative care provision in the management of chronic lung disease may be to expand the limited specialist respiratory nurse service following further training in the principles of palliative care. In the short-term specialists in palliative care medicine may be able to provide consultancy services and advice on training. In addition, there may be scope for short term involvement of the palliative care team in the management of individual patient problems[2]. In the longer term, the need for increased funding of specialist respiratory nurses with palliative skills and the possibility of specialist units for the management of end-stage respiratory disease must be explored.

References

1. Hinton, J.M. (1963). The physical and mental distress of the dying. *Quarterly Medical Journal*, **32**, 1–21.
2. Addington-Hall, J. (1998). For The National Council for Hospice and Specialist Palliative Care Services and Scottish Partnership Agency for Palliative and Cancer Care. Reaching Out: *Specialist Palliative Care for Adults with Non-Malignant Diseases*. Land & Unwin (Data Sciences) Ltd, Northamptonshire, UK.
3. Lupu, D. (1996). Hospice inpatient care: an overview of NHO's 1995 inpatient survey results. *Hospice Journal*, **11**, 2–39.
4. Eve, A., Smith, A.M., and Tebbit, P. (1997). Hospice and palliative care in the UK 1994–5, including a summary of trends 1990–5. *Palliative Medicine*, **11**, 31–43.
5. Wilkes, E. (1984). Dying now. *Lancet*, **i**, 950–952.
6. Mills, M., Davies, T.O., and Macrae, W.A. (1994). Care of dying patients in hospital. *British Medical Journal*, **309**, 583–586.
7. Seale, C. (1991). Death from cancer and death from other causes: the relevance of the hospice approach. *Palliative Medicine*, **5**, 13–20.
8. Hockley, J.M., Dunlop, R., and Davies, R.J. (1988). Survey of distressing symptoms in dying patients and their families in hospital and the

response to a symptom control team. *British Medical Journal*, **296**, 1715–17.

9. Lynn, J. *et al.* (1997). Perceptions by family members of the dying experience of older and seriously ill patients. *Annals Internal Medicine*, **126**, 97–106.

10. The SUPPORT Principal Investigators (1995). A Controlled trial to improve care for seriously ill hospitalised patients. The Study to Understand Prognoses and Preferences for Outcomes and Risks of Treatment (SUPPORT). *Journal of the American Medical Association*, **274**, 1591–8.

11. Cohen, L.M. *et al.* (1995). Dialysis discontinuation. A 'good' death? *Archives Internal Medicine*, **155**, 42–7.

12. Barby, T., Leigh, P.N. (1995). Palliative care in motor neuron disease. *International Journal Palliative Nursing*, **1**, 183–8.

13. McCarthy, M., Lay, M., and Addington Hall, J.M. (1996). Dying from heart disease. *Journal of the Royal College of Physicians*, **30**, 325–8.

14. Addington Hall, J.M. *et al.* (1995). Symptom control, communication with health professionals and hospital care of stroke patients in the last year of life, as reported by surviving family, friends and carers. *Stroke*, **26**, 2242–8.

15. Gore, J.M., Brophy, C.J., and Greenstone, M.A. (2000). How well do we care for patients with end stage chronic obstructive pulmonary disease (COPD)? A comparison of palliative care and quality of life in COPD and lung cancer. *Thorax*, **55**, 1000–6.

16. Edmonds, P. *et al.* (2001). A comparison of the palliative care needs of patients dying from chronic respiratory diseases and lung cancer. *Palliative Medicine*, **15**, 287–95.

17. Skilbeck, J. *et al.* (1998). Palliative care in chronic obstructive airways disease: a needs assessment. *Palliative Medicine*, **12**, 245–54.

18. Standing Medical Advisory Committee, Standing Nursing and Midwifery Advisory Committee (1992). *The Principles and Provision of Palliative Care*. Standing Medical Advisory Committee and Standing Nurse and Midwifery Advisory Committee, London.

19. The Scottish Office NHS in Scotland Management Executive. *Contracting for Specialist Palliative Care Services*.

20. The British Thoracic Society (2006). *The Burden of Lung Disease, 2nd edition*. www.brit-thoracic.org.uk.

21. Office for National Statistics (2000). *Mortality Statistics by Cause*. Series DH2 no. 26. The Stationary Office: London.

22. Royal College of Physicians (1986). Physical disability in 1986 and beyond. *Journal of the Royal College of Physicians London*, **3**, 160–94.

23. Cox, B.D. (1987). Blood pressure and respiratory function. In *The health and lifestyle survey. Preliminary report of a nationwide survey of the physical and mental health attitudes and lifestyle of a random survey of 9003 British adults*, pp 17–33, London Health Promotion Research Trust.

24. COPD Guidelines Group of the Standards of Care Committee of the BTS (1997). BTS guidelines for the management of chronic obstructive pulmonary disease. *Thorax*, **52**(Suppl 5), S1–S28.

25. (2004). National clinical guideline on management of chronic obstructive pulmonary disease in adults in primary and secondary care (NICE guidelines). *Thorax*; **59**(Suppl 1), 1–232.

26. Thorn, T.J. (1989). International comparisons in COPD mortality. *American Review of Respiratory Disease*, **140**, S27–S34.

27. Higgins, M. (1993). Epidemiology of obstructive pulmonary disease. In *Principles and practice of pulmonary rehabilitation* (eds. Casaburi, R., Pett, T.L.), pp 10–17.Philadelphia: Saunders.

28. Gustafsson, P.M. (2001). A world galloping into breathlessness. *Respiration*, **68**, 2–3.

29. Medical Research Council Working Party (1981). Long term domicillary oxygen therapy in chronic hypoxic cor pulmonale complicating chronic bronchitis and emphysema. *Lancet*, **i**, 681–6.

30. Almagro, P., Calbo, E., Ochoa de, E.A. *et al.* (2002). Mortality after hospitalisation for COPD. *Chest*, **121**(5), 1441–8.

31. Chu, C.M., Chan, V.L., Lin, A.W. *et al.* (2004). Readmission rates and life threatening events in COPD survivors treated with non-invasive ventilation for acute hypercapnnic respiratory failure. *Thorax*, **59**(12), 1020–5.

32. Pang, S.M., Tse, C.Y., Chan, K.S. *et al.* (2004). An empirical analysis of the decision-making of limiting life sustaining treatment for patients with advanced chronic obstructive pulmonary disease in Hong Kong, China. *J Critical Care*, **19**(3), 135–44.

33. Celli, B.R., Cote, C.G., Marin, J.M. *et al.* (2004). The body-mass index, airflow obstruction, dyspnoea, and exercise capacity index in chronic obstructive pulmonary disease. *New England Journal of Medicine*, **350**(10), 1005–12.

34. Nocturnal Oxygen Therapy Trial Group (1980). Continuous or nocturnal oxygen therapy in hypoxaemic chronic obstructive lung disease: a clinical trial. *Annals Internal Medicine*, **93**, 391–8.

35. Hill, K.M. and Muers, M.F. (2000). Palliative care for patients with non-malignant end stage respiratory disease. *Thorax*, **55**, 978–81.

36. McHorney, C.A., Ware, J.E. Jr, and Raczek, A.E. (1993). The MOS 36-Item Short-Form Health Survey (SF-36). II Psychometric and clinical tests of validity in measuring physical and mental health constructs. *Medical Care*, **31**, 247–63.

37. Jones, P.W., Quirk, F.H., and Baveystock, C.M. (1992). A self-complete measure of health status for chronic airflow limitation. *American Review of Respiratory Disease*, **144**, 1321–7.

38. Guyatt, G.H. *et al.* (1987). A measure of quality of life for clinical trials in chronic lung disease. *Thorax*, **42**, 773–8.

39. Bergman, B. *et al.* (1994). For the European Organisation for Research and Treatment of Cancer (EORTC) Study Group on Quality of Life. The EORTC QLQ LC-13: a modular supplement to the EORTC Core Quality of Life Questionaire (QLQ-C30) for use in lung cancer clinical trials. *European Journal of Cancer*, **30**, 635–42.

40. Aass, N. *et al.* (1997). Prevalence of anxiety and depression in cancer patients seen at the Norwegian Radium Hospital. *European Journal of Cancer*, **33**, 1597–604.

41. Langendijk, J.A. *et al.* (2000). Quality of life after palliative radiotherapy in non-small cell lung cancer: a prospective study. *International Journal of Radiation Oncology, Biology, Physics*, **47**, 149–55.

42. Gibbs, G. (1995). Nurses in private nursing homes: a study of their knowledge and attitudes to pain management in palliative care. *Palliative Medicine*, **9**, 245–53.

43. British Thoracic Society (BTS) Standards of Care Committee (1997). *Survey of resources used by respiratory physicians for the diagnosis and management of lung cancer*. BTS, London.

44. Royal College of Physicians (1981). Disabling Chest Disease: Prevention and Care. *Journal of the Royal College Physicians London*, **15**, 69–87.

45. Cockroft, A. *et al.* (1987). Controlled trial of respiratory health worker visiting patients with chronic respiratory disability. *British Medical Journal*, **294**, 225–8.

46. Cotton, M.M. *et al.* (2000). Early discharge for patients with exacerbations of chronic obstructive pulmonary disease: A randomised controlled trial. *Thorax*, **55**, 902–6.

47. Skwarska, E. *et al.* (2000). Randomised controlled trial of supported discharge in patients with exacerbations of chronic obstructive pulmonary disease. *Thorax*, **55**, 907–12.

48. Ojoo, J.C. *et al.* (2002). Patients' and carers' preferences in two models of care for acute exacerbations of COPD: results of a randomised controlled trial. *Thorax*, **57**, 167–9.

49. Heslop, A. (1993). Role of the respiratory nurse specialist. *British Journal of Hospital Medicine*, **50**, 88–90.

50. Littlejohns, P. *et al.* (1991). Randomised controlled trial of the effectiveness of a respiratory health worker in reducing impairment, disability and handicap due to chronic airflow limitation. *Thorax*, **46**, 559–64.

51. Tobin, M.J. (1990). Dyspnea: pathophysiologic basis, clinical presentation, and management. *Archives of Internal Medicine*, **150**, 1604–13.

52. Dyspnea Mechanisms, assessment and management (1999). A consensus statement. American Thoracic Society. *American Journal of Respiratory & Critical Care Medicine*, **159**, 321–40.

53. Elliott, M.W. *et al.* (1991). The language of breathlessness: use of verbal descriptors by patients with cardiorespiratory disease. *American Review of Respiratory Disease*, **144**, 826–32.

54. O'Donnell, D.E., Chau, L., and Webb, K.A. (1998). Qualitative aspects of exertional dyspnoea in patients with interstitial disease. *Journal of Applied Physiology*, **84**, 2000–9.

55. Wilson, R.C. and Jones, P.W. (1991). Differentiation between intensity of breathlessness and the distress it evokes in normal subjects during exercise. *Clinical Science*, **80**, 65–70.

56. Mahler, D.A. (2000). Do you speak the Language of dyspnoea? *Chest*, **117**, 928–9.

57. Freedman, S., Lane, R., and Guz, A. (1987). Breathlessness and respiratory mechanics during reflex or voluntary hyperventilation in patients with chronic airflow limitation. *Clinical Science*, **73**, 311–8.

58. Lindsey, B.G. *et al.* (2000). Respiratory neuronal assemblies. *Respiration Physiology*, **122**, 183–96.

59. Lane, R. *et al.* (1987). Arterial oxygen saturation and breathlessness in patients with chronic obstructive airways disease. *Clinical Science*, **72**, 693–8.

60. Banzett, R.B., Lansing, R.W., and Brown, R. (1990). 'Air hunger' from increased P_{CO_2} persists after complete neuromuscular block in humans. *Respiration Physiology*, **81**, 1–17.

61. Cristiano, L.M. and Schwartzstein, R.M. (1997). Effect of chest wall vibration on dyspnoea during hypercapnia and exercise in chronic obstructive pulmonary disease. *American Journal of Respiratory & Critical Care Medicine*, **155**, 1552–9.

62. Schwartzstein, R.M. *et al.* (1987). Cold facial stimulation reduces breathlessness induced in normal subjects. *American Review of Respiratory Disease*, **136**, 58–61.

63. Demediuk, B.H. *et al.* (1992). Dissociation between dyspnoea and respiratory effort. *American Review of Respiratory Disease*, **146**, 1222–5.

64. Chetta, A. *et al.* (1998). Personality profiles and breathlessness perception in outpatients with different gradings of asthma. *American Journal of Respiratory & Critical Care Medicine*, **157**, 116–22.

65. Smoller, J.W. *et al.* (1996). Panic anxiety, dyspnoea, respiratory disease: Theoretical and clinical considerations. *American Journal of Respiratory & Critical Care Medicine*, **154**, 6–17.

66. Gift, A.G. and Narsavage, G. (1998). Validity of the numeric rating scale as a measure of dyspnoea. *American Journal Critical Care 1998*; **7**, 200–4.

67. Borg, G. (1978). Subjective effort and physical activities. *Scandinavian Journal Rehabilitation Medicine*, **6**, 108–13.

68. Jones, P.W. *et al.* (1992). A self-complete measure of health status for chronic airflow limitation. *American Review of Respiratory Disease*, **145**, 1321–7.

69. Hu, J. and Meek, P. (2005) Health related quality of life in individuals with chronic obstructive pulmonary disease. *Heart Lung*, **34**(6), 415–22.

70. Wolkove, N., Dajczman, E., Colacone, A. *et al.* (1989). The relationship between pulmonary function and dyspnoea in obstructive lung disease. *Chest*, **96**, 1247–51.

71. Lareau, S.C. *et al.* (1999). Dyspnea in patients with chronic obstructive pulmonary disease: does dyspnoea worsen longitudinally in the presence of declining lung function? *Heart & Lung*, **28**, 65–73.

72. Leach, R.M. *et al.* (1992). Portable liquid oxygen and exercise ability in severe respiratory disability. *Thorax*, **47**, 781–9.

73. Puchelle, E. *et al.* (1980). Mucociliary transport in vivo and in vitro: Relations to sputum properties in chronic bronchitis. *European Journal of Respiratory Disease*, **61**, 254–64.

74. Sant'Ambrogio, G. and Widdicombe, J.G. (2001). Reflexes from airway rapidly adapting receptors. *Respiration Physiology*, **125**, 33–45.

75. Tatar, M., Webber, S.E., and Widdicombe, J.G. (1988): Lung C-fibre receptor activation and defensive reflexes in anaesthetised cats. *Journal of Physiology*, **402**, 411–20.

76. Kamai, J. (1996). Role of opioidergic and serotonergic mechanisms in cough and antitussives. *Pulmonary Pharmacology*, **9**, 349–56.

77. Irwin, R.S. *et al.* (1998). Managing cough as a defence mechanism and as a symptom: A consensus panel report of the American College of Chest Physicians. Managing cough as a defence mechanism and as a symptom. *Chest*, **114**, 133S–81S.

78. Morice, A.H., McGarvey, L., Pavord, I. on behalf of the British Thoracic Society Cough Guideline Group (2006). Recommendations for the management of cough in adults. *Thorax*, **61**(Suppl 1), 1–24.

79. Gracey, D.R., Divertie, M.B., and Howard, F.M. Jr. (1983). Mechanical ventilation for respiratory failure in myasthenia gravis: Two year experience with 22 patients. *Mayo Clinic Proceedings*, **58**, 597–602.

80. Szienberg, A. *et al.* (1988). Cough capacity in patients with muscular dystrophy. *Chest*, **94**, 1232–5.

81. Irwin, R.S., Curley, F.J., and French, C.L. (1990). Chronic cough: The spectrum and frequency of causes, key components of the diagnostic evaluation, and outcome of specific therapy. *American Review of Respiratory Disease*, **141**, 640–7.

82. Jones, A.P., Rowe, B.H. Bronchopulmonary hygiene physical therapy for chronic obstructive pulmonary disease and bronchiectasis. *The Cochrane Library* **2**.

83. Tamaoki, J. *et al.* (2000). Inhaled indomethacin in bronchorrhoea in bronchoalveolar carcinoma: role of cyclooxygenase. *Chest*, **117**, 1213–4.

84. Wills, P., Greenstone, M. Inhaled hyperosmolar agents for bronchiectasis. *The Cochrane Library*, **2**.

85. Davies, C.L. (1997). ABC of Palliative care: Breathlessness, cough, and other respiratory problems. *British Medical Journal*, **315**, 931–4.

86. Doona, M. and Walsh, D. (1998). Benzoate for opiod-resistant cough in advanced cancer. *Palliative Medicine*, **12**, 55–8.

87. Luporini, G. *et al.* (1998). Efficacy and safety of levodropropizine and dihydrocodeine on non-productive cough in primary and metastatic lung cancer. *European Respiratory Journal*, **12**, 97–101.

88. Louie, K., Bertolino, M., and Fainsinger, R. (1992). Management of intractable cough. *Journal of Palliative Care*, **8**, 46–8.

89. Moroni, M. *et al.* (1996). Inhaled sodium cromoglycate to treat cough in advanced lung cancer patients. *British Journal of Cancer*, **74**, 309–11.

90. Schroeder, K. and Fahey, T. (2002). Systematic review of randomised controlled trials of over the counter cough medicines for acute cough in adults. *British Medical Journal*, **324**, 1–6.

91. Luchette, F. *et al.* (1994). Prospective evaluation of epidural versus intrapleural catheters for analgesis in chest wall trauma. *Journal of Trauma*, **36**, 865–70.

92. Wise, C.M. (1994). Chest wall syndromes. *Current Opinion in Rheumatology*, **6**, 197–202.

93. Viar, W.N. and Harrison, T.R. (1952). Chest pain in association with pulmonary hypertension: Its similarity to the pain of coronary disease. *Circulation*, **5**, 1–11.

94. Adam, J. (1997). ABC of palliative care: The last 48 hours. *British Medical Journal*, **315**, 1600–3.

95. Hirshberg, B., Biran, I., Glazer, M. *et al.* (1997). Hemoptysis; aetiology, evaluation, and outcome in a tertiary referral hospital. *Chest*, **112**, 440–4.

96. Patel, U., Pattison, C.W., and Raphael, M. (1994). Management of massive haemoptysis. *British Journal of Hospital Medicine*, **74**, 76–8.

97. Crocco, J.A. *et al.* (1968). Massive haemoptysis. *Archives of Internal Medicine*, **121**, 495–8.

98. Gong, H. and Salvatierra, C. (1981). Clinical efficacy of early and delayed fibreoptic bronchoscopy in patients with hemoptysis. *American Review of Respiratory Disease*, **124**, 221–5.

99. Conlan, A.A. and Hurwitz, S.S. (1980). Management of massive haemoptysis with the rigid broncoscope and iced saline lavage. *Thorax*, **35**, 901–7.

100. Bense, L. (1990). Intrabronchial selective coagulative treatment of hemoptysis. *Chest*, **97**, 990–6.

101. Tan, R.T., McGahan, J.P., Link, D.P. *et al.* (1991). Bronchial artery embolisation in management of haemoptysis. *Journal of Interventional Radiology*, **6**, 67–76.

102. Mal, H. *et al.* (1999). Immediate and long-term results of bronchial artery embolisation for life-threatening hemoptysis. *Chest*, **115**, 996–1001.

103. Jones, K.D. and Davies, R.J. (1990). Massive haemoptysis. *British Medical Journal*, **300**, 889–900.

104. Lomotan, J.R., George, S.S., and Brandsetter, R.D. (1997). Aspiration pneumonia. Strategies for early recognition and prevention. *Postgraduate Medicine*, **102**, 229–31.

105. Drakulovic, M.B. *et al.* (1999). Supine body position as a risk factor for nosocomial pneumonia in mechanically ventilated patients; a randomised trial. *Lancet*, **354**, 1851–8.

106. Shepperd, S. *et al.* (1998). Randomised controlled trial comparing hospital at home care with inpatient hospital care. I; Three month follow-up of health outcomes. *British Medical Journal*, **316**, 1786–91.

107. Madge, S. and Esmond G (2001). End-stage management of respiratory disease. In *Respiratory Nursing* (ed G. Esmond), pp 229–40. Bailliere Tindall, London.

108. Puig-Junoy, J., Font-Planells, J., Escarrabill, J. *et al.* (2007). The impact of home hospitalization on healthcare costs of exacerbations in COPD patients. *Eur J Health Econ*, **8**, 325–32.

109. Pauwels, R.A. *et al.* (2001). Global strategy for the diagnosis, management, and prevention of chronic obstructive pulmonary disease. NHLBI/WHO Global Initiative For Chronic Obstructive Lung Disease (GOLD) workshop summary. *American Journal of Respiratory & Critical Care Medicine*, **163**, 1256–76.

110. Celli, B.R., MacNee, W. and the ATS/ERS Task Force. (2004). Standards for the diagnosis and treatment of patients with COPD: a summary of the ATS/ERS position paper. *European Respiratory Journal*, **23**, 932–46.

111. Shee, C.D. (1995). Palliation in chronic respiratory disease. *Palliative Medicine*, **9**, 312.

112. Teramoto, S., Fukuchi, Y., and Orimo, H. (1993). Effects of inhaled anticholinergic drug on dyspnoea and gas exchange during exercise in patients with chronic obstructive airways disease. *Chest*, **103**, 1774–82.

113. Barr, R.G., Bourbeau, J., Camargo, C.A. *et al.* (2006). Tiotropium for stable chronic obstructive pulmonary disease: a meta-analysis. *Thorax* **61**, 854–62.

114. O'Donnell, D.E., Fluge, T., Gerken, F. *et al.* (2004). Effects of tiotropium on lung hyperinflation, dyspnoea, and exercise tolerance in COPD. *European Respiratory Journal*, **23**, 832–40.

115. Rennard, S.I. *et al.* (1996). Extended therapy with ipratropium is associated with improved lung function in patients with COPD: a retrospective analysis of data from seven clinical trials. *Chest*, **110**, 62–70.

116. Combivent Inhalation Aerosol Study Group (1994). In chronic obstructive pulmonary disease, a combination of ipratropium and albuterol is more effective than either agent alone: an 85-day multicenter trial. *Chest*, **105**, 1411–9.

117. The Nebuliser Project Group of the British Thoracic Society Standards of Care Committee (1997). Current Best Practice for Nebuliser Treatment. *Thorax*, **52**, S1–S106.

118. Kirsten, D.K., Wegner, R.E., Jorres, R.A. *et al.* (1993). Effects of theophylline withdrawal in severe chronic obstructive pulmonary disease. *Chest*, **104**, 1101–7.

119. Nocturnal Oxygen Therapy Trial Group (1980). Continuous or nocturnal oxygen therapy in hypoxaemic chronic obstructive lung disease: a clinical trial. *Annals Internal Medicine*, **93**, 391–398.

120. Crockett, A.J., Cranston, J.M., Moss, J.R. *et al.* (2001). Domiciliary oxygen for chronic obstructive pulmonary disease (Cochrane Review). In: the Cochrane Library, Issue 4. Oxford:Update Software.

121. Ringbaek, T., Lange, P., and Viskum, K. (1999). Compliance with LTOT and consumption of mobile oxygen. *Respiratory Medicine*, **93**, 333–7.

122. Woodcock, A.A., Gross, E.R., and Geddes, D.M. (1981). Oxygen relieves breathlessness in "pink puffers". *Lancet*, **i**, 907–09.

123. Kelley, M.A., Panettieri, R.A., and Krupinski, A.V. (1986). Resting single-breath diffusing capacity as a screening test for exercise-induced hypoxemia. *American Journal of Medicine*, **80**, 807–12.

124. Luce, J.M. and Luce, J.A. (2001). Management of dyspnoea in patients with far-advanced lung disease. *Journal of the American Medical Association*, **285**, 1331–7.

125. Man, G.C., Hsu, K., and Sproule, B.J. (1986). Effect of alprazolam on exercise and dyspnoea in patients with chronic obstructive pulmonary disease. *Chest*, **90**, 832–6.

126. Woodcock, A.A., Gross, E.R., and Geddes, D.M. (1981). Drug treatment of breathlessness: contrasting effects of diazepam and promethazine in pink puffers. *British Medical Journal*, **283**, 343–5.

127. Rice, K.L. *et al.* (1987). Effects of chronic administration of codeine and promethazine on breathlessness and exercise tolerance in patients with chronic airflow obstruction. *British Journal Diseases of the Chest*, **81**, 287–91.

128. Singh, N.P. *et al.* (1993). Effects of buspirone on anxiety levels and exercise tolerance in patients with chronic airflow obstruction and mild anxiety. *Chest*, **103**, 800–4.

129. McIver, B., Walsh, D., and Nelson, K. (1994). The use of chlorpromazine for symptom control in dying cancer patients. *Journal of Pain and Symptom Management*, **9**, 341–5.

130. Zebraski, S.E., Kochenash, S.M., and Raffa, R.B. (2000). Lung opiod receptors: pharmacology and possible target for nebulized morphine in dyspnoea. *Life Sciences*, **66**, 2221–31.

131. Johnson, M.A., Woodcock, A.A., and Geddes, D.M. (1983). Dihydrocodeine for breathlessness in "pink puffers". *British Medical Journal*, **286**, 675–77.

132. Light, R.W. *et al.* (1989). Effects of oral morphine on breathlessness and exercise tolerance in patients with chronic obstructive pulmonary disease. *American Review of Respiratory Disease*, **139**, 126–33.

133. Poole, P.J., Veale, A.G., and Black, P.N. (1998). The effect of sustained-release morphine on breathlessness and quality of life in severe chronic obstructive pulmonary disease. *American Journal of Respiratory & Critical Care Medicine*, **157**, 1877–80.

134. Eiser, N., Denman, W.T., West, C. *et al.* (1991). Oral diamorphine: lack of effect on dyspnoea and exercise tolerance in the "pink puffer" syndrome. *European Respiratory Journal*, **4**, 926–31.

135. Leung, R., Hill, P., and Burdon, J. (1996). Effect of inhaled morphine on the development of breathlessness during exercise in patients with chronic lung disease. *Thorax*, **51**, 596–600.

136. Harris-Eze, A.O. *et al.* (1995). Low dose nebulized morphine does not improve exercise in interstitial lung disease. *American Journal of Respiratory & Critical Care Medicine*, **152**, 1940–5.

137. Multicentre Study Group (1980). Long-term oral acetylcysteine in chronic bronchitis, a double blind controlled study. *European Journal Respiratory Disease*, **61**, 93–108.

138. Tamaoki, J. *et al.* (1992). Effect of indomethacin on bronchorrhea in patients with chronic bronchitis, diffuse panbronchitis, or bronchiectasis. *American Review of Respiratory Disease*, **145**, 548–52.

139. Winning, A.J., Hamilton, R.D., and Guz, A. (1988). Ventilation and breathlessness on maximal exercise in patients with interstitial lung disease after local anaesthetic aerosol inhalation. *Clinical Science*, **74**, 275–81.

140. de Godoy, I. *et al.* (1996). Elevated TNF-alpha production by peripheral blood monocytes of weight-losing COPD patients. *American Journal of Respiratory & Critical Care Medicine*, **153**, 633–7.

141. Whittaker, J.S. *et al.* (1990). The effects of refeeding on peripheral and respiratory muscle function in malnourished chronic obstructive pulmonary disease patients. *American Review of Respiratory Disease*, **142**, 283–8.

142. American Association of Cardiovascular and Pulmonary Rehabilitation (1997). Pulmonary rehabilitation: Joint ACCP/AACVPR evidence-based guidelines. ACCP/AACVPR Pulmonary Rehabilitation Guidelines Panel. American College of Chest Physicians. *Chest*, **112**, 1363–96.

143. Guell, R. *et al.* (2000). Longterm effects of outpatient rehabilitation of COPD: a randomised trial. *Chest*, **117**, 976–83.

144. Weiner, P. *et al.* (2000). The cumulative effect of long-acting bronchodilators, exercise, and inspiratory muscle training on the perception of dyspnoea in patients with advanced COPD. *Chest*, **118**, 672–8.

145. Garrod, R., Mikelsons, C., Paul, E.A. *et al.* (2000). Randomised controlled trial of domiciliary non-invasive positive pressure ventilation and physical training in severe chronic obstructive pulmonary disease. *American Journal of Respiratory & Critical Care Medicine*, **162**, 1335–41.

146. Tiep, B.L. *et al.* (1986). Pursed lips breathing training using ear oximetry. *Chest*, **90**, 218–21.

147. Sharp, J.T. *et al.* (1980). Postural relief of dyspnoea in severe chronic obstructive pulmonary disease. *American Review of Respiratory Disease*, **122**, 201–11.

148. Hillberg, R.E. and Johnson, D.C. (1997). Noninvasive ventilation. *New England Journal of Medicine*, **337**, 1746–52.

149. Ram, F., Picot, J., Lightowler, J. *et al.* (2004). Non-invasive positive pressure ventilation for the treatment of respiratory failure due to exacerbations of chronic obstructive pulmonary disease. *Cochrane Database of Systematic Reviews*, **1**, CD004104.

150. Elliott, M.W. *et al.* (1991). Domicilliary nocturnal nasal intermittent positive pressure ventilation in COPD: Mechanisms underlying changes in arterial blood gas tensions. *European Respiratory Journal*, **4**, 1044–52.

151. Krachman, S.L. *et al.* (1997). Effects of non-invasive positive pressure ventilation on gas exchange and sleep in COPD patients. *Chest*, **112**, 623–8.

152. Toma, T.P., Goldstraw, P., and Geddes, D.M. (2002). Lung volume reduction surgery. *Thorax*, **57**, 5–6.

153. Brenner, M. *et al.* (1998). Rate of FEV change following lung volume reduction surgery. *Chest*, **113**, 652–9.

154. Ingenito, E.P. *et al.* (1998). Relation between preoperative inspiratory lung resistance and outcome of lung-volume-reduction surgery for emphysema. *New England Journal of Medicine*, **338**, 1181–5.

155. National Emphysema Treatment Trial Research Group (2003). A randomised trial comparing lung-volume-reduction surgery with medical therapy for severe emphysema. *New England Journal of Medicine*, **348**, 2059–73.

156. Ingenito, E.P. *et al.* (2001). Bronchoscopic volume reduction. A safe and effective alternative to surgical therapy for emphysema. *American Journal of Respiratory & Critical Care Medicine*, **164**, 295–301.

157. Hosenpud, J.D. *et al.* (1997). The Registry of the International Society for Heart and Lung Transplantation: Fourteenth official report 1997. *Journal of Heart Lung Transplantion*, **16**, 691–712.

158. Cassivi, S.D., Meyers, B.F., Battafarano, R.J. *et al.* (2002) Thirteen-year experience in lung transplantation for emphysema. *Ann Thoracic Surg* 2002;74, 1663–9.

159. Trulock, E.P. (1998). Lung Transplantation for COPD. *Chest*, **113**(4), 269S–276S.

160. Joint statement of the American Thoracic Society (ATS) and the European Respiratory Society (ERS). (2000). Idiopathic pulmonary fibrosis: diagnosis and treatment. International Consensus Statement 1999. *American Journal of Respiratory and Critical Care Medicine*, **161**, 646–64.

161. Silman, A.J. (1997). Scleroderma—demographics and survival. *Journal of Rheumatology*, **48**, 58–61.

162. Frankel, H.L. *et al.* (1998). Long-term survival in spinal cord injury: a fifty year investigation. *Spinal Cord*, **36**, 266–74.

163. Labanowski, J., Schmidt-Nowara, W., and Guilleminault, C. (1996). Sleep and neuromuscular disease: Frequency of sleep disordered breathing in a neuromuscular disease clinic population. *Neurology*, **47**, 1173–80.

164. Bach, J.R. and Alba, A.S. (1990). Non-invasive options for ventilatory support of the traumatic high level quadriplegic patient. *Chest*, **98**, 613–9.

165. Bach, J.R. *et al.* (1993). Airways secretion clearance by mechanical exsufflation for post-poliomyelitis ventilator-assisted individuals. *Archives Physical Medical Rehabilitation*, **74**, 170–7.

166. Uijl, S.G., Houtman, S., Folgering, H.T. *et al.* (1999). Training of the respiratory muscles in individuals with tetraplegia. *Spinal Cord*, **37**, 575–9.

167. Lin, V.W. *et al.* (1998). Functional magnetic stimulation for restoring cough in patients with tetraplegia. *Archives Physical Medicine Rehabilitation*, **79**, 517–22.

168. Bach, J.R. *et al.* (1998). Neuromuscular ventilatory insufficiency: Effect of home mechanical ventilator use v oxygen therapy on pneumonia and hospitalisation rates. *American Journal Physical Medicine Rehabilitation*, **77**, 8–19.

169. Ellis, D.A. *et al.* (1981). Present outlook in bronchiectasis: Clinical and social study and review of factors influencing prognosis. *Thorax*, **36**, 659–64.

170. Grenier, P. *et al.* (1986). Bronchiectasis: Assessment by thin-section CT. *Radiology*, **161**, 95–9.

171. Angrill, J. *et al.* (2002). Bacterial colonisation in patients with bronchiectasis: microbiological pattern and risk factors. *Thorax*, **57**, 15–7.

172. Ramsey, B.W. (1996). Management of pulmonary disease in patients with cystic fibrosis. *New England Journal of Medicine*, **335**, 179–88.

173. Lin, H-C. *et al.* (1997). Inhaled gentamicin reduces airway neutrophil activity and mucous secretion in bronchiectasis. *American Journal of Respiratory & Critical Care Medicine*, **155**, 2024–9.

174. Thomas, J., Cook, D.J., and Brooks, D. (1995). Chest physical therapy management of patients with cystic fibrosis. *American Journal of Respiratory & Critical Care Medicine*, **151**, 846–50.

175. Robinson, M. *et al.* (1996). Effect of hypertonic saline, amiloride, and cough on mucociliary clearance in patients with cystic fibrosis. *American Journal of Respiratory & Critical Care Medicine*, **153**, 1503–9.

176. Fuchs, H.J. *et al.* (1994). Effect of aerosolised recombinant human DNAse on exacerbations of respiratory symptoms and on pulmonary function in patients with cystic fibrosis. *New England Journal of Medicine*, **331**, 637–42.

177. O'Donnell, A.E. *et al.* (1998). Treatment of idiopathic bronchiectasis with aeroslozed recombinant human DNAse. *Chest*, **113**, 1329–34.

178. Konstan, M.W. *et al.* (1995). Effect of high-dose ibuprofen in patients with cystic fibrosis. *New England Journal of Medicine*, **332**, 848–54.

179. Wallace, J.M. *et al.* (1997). Respiratory disease trends in the Pulmonary Complications of HIV Infection Study cohort. Pulmonary Complications of HIV Infection Study Group. *American Journal of Respiratory & Critical Care Medicine*, **155**, 72–80.

180. UNAIDS and WHO (1997). *Report on the Global HIV/AIDS Epidemic.* Geneva: WHO, December 1997 pp 1–26.

181. The task force on diagnosis and treatment of pulmonary arterial hypertension of the European Society of Cardiology (2004). Guidelines on the diagnosis and treatment of pulmonary arterial hypertension. *European Heart Journal*, **25**, 2243–78.

182. Fedullo, P.F. *et al.* (1995). Chronic thromboembolic pulmonary hypertension. *Clinical Chest Medicine*, **16**, 353–74.

183. Hyers, T.M. (1999). Venous thromboembolism. *American Journal of Respiratory & Critical Care Medicine*, **159**, 1–14.

184. Archibald, C.J. *et al.* (1999). Long-term outcome after pulmonary thromboendarterectomy. *American Journal of Respiratory & Critical Care Medicine,* **160,** 523–8.

185. Galie, N., Ghofrani, H., Torbicki, A. *et al.* (2005). Sildenafil citrate therapy for pulmonary hypertension. *New England Journal of Medicine,* **353,** 2148–57.

186. Rubin, L.J., Badesch, D.B., Barst, R.J. *et al.* (2002). Bosentan therapy for pulmonary arterial hypertension. *New England Journal of Medicine,* **346,** 896–903.

187. Galie, N., Seeger, W., Naeije, Simonneau, G. *et al.* (2004). Comparative analysis of clinical trials and evidence based treatment algorithm in pulmonary arterial hypertension. *Journal of the American College of Cardiology.* **43,** 81S–88S.

188. Siverstein, M.D. *et al.* (1998). Trends in the incidence of deep vein thrombosis and pulmonary embolism. *Archives Internal Medicine,* **158,** 585–93.

189. Ryu, J.H., Olson, E.J., and Pellikka, P.A. (1998). Clinical recognition of pulmonary embolism: Problem of unrecognised and asymptomatic cases. *Mayo Clinic Proceedings,* **73,** 873–9.

190. Wells, P.S. *et al.* (1995). Accuracy of clinical assessment of deep-vein thrombosis. *Lancet,* **345,** 1326–30.

191. The PIOPED Investigators (1990). Value of the ventilation/perfusion scan in acute pulmonary embolism. Results of the Prospective Investigation Of Pulmonary Embolism Diagnosis (PIOPED). *Journal of the American Medical Association,* **263,** 2753–9.

192. Segal, J.B., Eng, J., Tamariz, L.J. *et al.* (2007) Review of the evidence on diagnosis of deep venous thrombosis and pulmonary embolism. *Annals of Family Medicine,* **5,** 63–73.

193. Miniati, M. *et al.* (1996). Value of perfusion lung scan in the diagnosis of pulmonary embolism. Results of the Prospective Investigative Study of Acute Pulmonary Embolism Diagnosis (PISA-PED). *American Journal of Respiratory & Critical Care Medicine,* **154,** 1387–93.

194. Simonneau, G. *et al.* (1997). A comparison of low-molecular weight heparin and unfractionated heparin for acute pulmonary embolism. *New England Journal of Medicine,* **337,** 663–9.

195. Martin, R. (2001). Acute pulmonary embolism 2: treatment. *Heart,* **85,** 351-60.

196. Millar, A.C. and Harvey, J.E. (1993). On behalf of Standards of Care Committee, British Thoracic Society. Guidelines for the management of spontaneous pneumothorax. *British Medical Journal,* **307,** 114–6.

197. Curtis, J.R., Engelberg, R.A., Nielsen, E.L. *et al.* (2004). Patient-physician communication about end-of-life care for patients with severe COPD. *European Respiratory Journal,* **24,** 200–5.

198. Claessens, M.T., Lynn, J., Zhong, Z. *et al.* (2000). Dying with lung cancer or chronic obstructive pulmonary disease: insights from SUPPORT. *Journal of the American Geriatrics Society,* **48,** S146–S153.

199. Knauft, E., Nielsen, E.L., Engelberg, R.A. *et al.* (2005). Barriers and facilitators to end-of-life care communication for patients with COPD. *Chest,* **127,** 2188–96.

200. Doyle, D. (1987). *Domiciliary Terminal Care.* Edinburgh: Churchill Livingstone.

201. Fainsinger, R.L. *et al.* (2000). A multicentre international study of sedation for uncontrolled symptoms in terminally ill patients. *Palliative Medicine,* **14,** 257–65.

202. Thorns, A. and Sykes, N. (2000). Opiod use in the last week of life and the implications for end-of-life decision-making. *Lancet,* **356,** 398–9.

203. Chater, S. *et al.* (1998). Sedation for intractable distress in the dying—a survey of experts. *Palliative Medicine,* **12,** 255–69.

12.4

Palliative care for patients with end-stage heart disease

Andrew D. McGavigan, Carolyn L. Datta, and Francis G. Dunn

Introduction

It is perhaps surprising that it has taken so long for the principles of palliative care to be applied to patients with end-stage cardiac disease, given that the term cardiac cachexia has been in use for many decades, and there are some striking clinical similarities to patients with advanced cancer. Patients with end-stage cardiac disease have a greatly reduced quality of life, inadequate support in terms of counselling and communication, and an infrastructure that is not yet widely in place for home management. It has to be acknowledged, however, that there are challenges in applying palliative care principles to patients with end-stage cardiac disease as illustrated by these two short clinical scenarios.

1 A 72-year-old retired teacher initially presented in 1993 with progressive breathlessness and was found to have severe left ventricular dysfunction. So poor was his left ventricular function that it was felt at that time that survival beyond 1 year was considered most unlikely and his family was informed of this probable outcome. He responded well to medical management and some 14 years later he continues to be stable with an excellent quality of life.

2 A 76-year-old patient with a previous history of myocardial infarction was admitted with severe dyspnoea caused by cardiac failure. Echo assessment of left ventricular function revealed it to be substantially impaired. He made good progress with medication and was discharged 5 days later essentially symptom free. Following discharge from hospital he joined a supervised cardiac rehabilitation exercise programme, which he found helpful. Two weeks later he died suddenly during the night.

Definitions and natural history

For the purposes of this article, end-stage cardiac disease is defined as patients with heart disease who have a predicted life expectancy of 6 months or less. Such patients usually have grade-4 breathlessness (New York Heart Association Classification—NYHA), hypotension, clinical features of cardiac failure, and an ejection fraction of less than 20 per cent[1]. In addition, the extent of the disease will also be manifest by recurrent hospital admissions. The patients who fall within this definition will usually have had a past history of cardiac failure, but there are also cohorts who develop intractable heart failure or cardiogenic shock with renal failure following acute myocardial infarction and in whom palliative care is particularly appropriate.

Heart failure is an extremely common disorder affecting 1–3 per cent of the general population. There is a marked age-related increase with up to 10 per cent of elderly patients being affected. With the rising number of elderly patients in the population, the burden of heart failure is likely to further increase and the magnitude of this rise between 2000 and 2020 is expected to be in excess of 20 per cent[2]. The incidence of heart failure ranges from one to five cases per 1000 of the population per year[3]. Although the main cause of cardiac failure in the United Kingdom is coronary artery disease, other causes include hypertension, alcohol excess, viral infections, metabolic disorders, and the cardiomyopathies[3]. Coronary artery disease also accounts for over 300 000 myocardial infarctions every year in the United Kingdom, and over 2 million patients have angina[4]. A significant percentage of these patients will have continuing symptoms despite optimum medical management and appropriate revascularization.

The overall prognosis in patients with congestive heart failure (CHF) is equivalent to many types of advanced cancer, with an estimated 1-year survival of less than 50 per cent[5]. The mortality even in the milder forms of heart failure approaches 50 per cent within 5 years, a prognosis, which is worse than many forms of cancer[6]. Heart failure also has the greatest negative effect on quality of life compared to other major chronic illnesses such as diabetes, arthritis, and hypertension[7]. The devastating impact of CHF on quality of life is demonstrated by a study conducted in 99 patients with advanced heart failure (NYHA functional class III/IV)[8]. Nearly half of those patients felt that they had such poor quality of life that they would be willing to trade at least half their remaining life expectancy in order to feel better. The high morbidity of heart failure is reflected by the number of hospital admissions. In the United Kingdom that number currently exceeds 120 000 cases per year with a cost to the NHS in excess of £500 million[9]. The total cost of treating heart failure, including long-term nursing home care, is predicted at 4 per cent of the total NHS expenditure in the United Kingdom.

Mechanisms

Heart failure is a clinical syndrome characterized by the inability of the heart to maintain a cardiac output adequate for the requirements of metabolizing tissues. This is usually due to left ventricular (LV) systolic dysfunction, but heart failure with preserved LV systolic function is increasingly being recognized as a clinical entity[10].

In addition to the mechanical problems associated with pump failure, the heart failure syndrome is associated with complex inflammatory and neurohumoral abnormalities. The initial response of myocardial injury and incipient failure is cellular and structural remodelling due to activation of adaptive neurohumoral mechanisms[11], producing a shift to the right along the Frank–Starling curve. This is protective in the short term and is achieved via a number of mechanisms including activation of the renin–angiotensin–aldosterone system (RAAS), which increases vascular tone through increased circulating levels of angiotensin II. The endothelin and adrenergic nervous systems contribute to the maintenance of adequate blood pressure and perfusion of vital organs. Adrenergic activation also has positive inotropic effects.

These responses improve haemodynamics in the short term, but continued activation soon becomes maladaptive, and a vicious cycle ensues. Increased levels of circulating adrenaline, endothelin, and effectors of the RAAS cause endothelial dysfunction, cardiac and vascular fibrosis, sodium and water retention, promote arrhythmogenesis, and facilitate ventricular and vascular remodelling[11]. These are all improved by drugs which antagonize these systems[12].

Heart failure is also an inflammatory syndrome with increased circulating levels of the interleukin family and tumour necrosis factor[13]. The exact role of these mediators in the pathophysiology of heart failure is an area of considerable research. They may be responsible for reduced skeletal muscle mass and function[14] and may contribute to the low-grade pyrexia found in heart failure, although hyperstimulation of the adrenergic system may also play a role in this.

Clinical features

The symptoms associated with end-stage cardiac disease are diverse, ranging from the well recognized triad of breathlessness, fatigue, and ankle swelling to less specific ones of anorexia, muscle wasting, and pain. Symptoms are often severe and have many parallels with malignancy, although there are some key differences (Table 12.4.1).

Similarities to malignancy

Cachexia is a frequent complication of both advanced cardiac disease and malignancy, occurring in up to 50 per cent of patients with the former[15], although this is sometimes masked by oedema (Fig. 12.4.1). The loss of muscle mass compounds exercise intolerance and is an independent predictor of reduced survival[16]. Reduced energy reserve, muscle pain, and easy fatigability occur due to lactic acidosis caused by poor perfusion of skeletal muscle. Increased basal metabolic rate and reduced energy intake due to anorexia contribute to the problem. Anorexia and nausea may either be due to heart failure itself or as a consequence of therapy. Reduced perfusion of the gastrointestinal tract, gut or liver congestion, activation of the sympathetic nervous system, and uraemia, all play a role. Marked lethargy is a characteristic of both illnesses and in cardiac failure is due in part to relative hypoxia, anaemia,

Table 12.4.1 Comparison of clinical characteristics between heart disease and cancer.

Similarities to malignancy
- Breathlessness
- Weight loss (reduced muscle mass countered by fluid retention)
- Cachexia
- Lethargy
- Pain
- Anxiety and depression
- Poor mobility
- Insomnia and confusion
- Postural hypotension
- Jaundice with abnormalities of liver function tests
- Increased infection risk
- Anaemia
- Polypharmacy
- Fear of the future

Differences from malignancy
- Prediction of life expectancy more difficult
- Mistaken belief that condition is more benign than cancer
- Oedema more prominent in heart failure
- Lack of local pressure effects

Source: adapted with permission from O'Brien, T., Welsh, J., and Dunn, F.G. (1998). ABC of palliative care. Non-malignant conditions. *British Medical Journal*, **316**, 286–9.

and biochemical abnormalities. Paroxysmal nocturnal dyspnoea, nocturia, anxiety or depression may contribute to daytime fatigue and somnolence, as may sleep apnoea, which is known to be highly prevalent in patients with heart failure[17].

Anaemia, common in patients with malignancy (~67 per cent with Hb <10 g/dL)[18], is now increasingly recognized in cardiac disease. The aetiology is undoubtedly multifactorial, including gastrointestinal blood loss secondary to antiplatelet or anticoagulant therapy, bone marrow suppression, intestinal congestion producing malnutrition, leading to iron or folate deficiency, and haemolysis as a consequence of a damaged native or prosthetic heart valve. In addition, chronic renal impairment or increased cytokine production leads to reduced erythropoietin production in up to half of heart failure patients[19]. Anaemia is a poor prognostic indicator in cardiac failure[19]. The level of haemoglobin at which blood transfusion is indicated has not been clarified. A therapeutic trial of transfusion should be considered in all symptomatic patients with anaemia, with care to avoid circulatory volume overload. Subcutaneous erythropoietin and intravenous iron have been shown to improve symptoms, cardiac, and renal function and exercise capability.

Traditionally, pain has not been thought to be a major symptom in heart failure, although problems with concomitant angina have long been recognized. However, the SUPPORT study showed an incidence of pain of 43 per cent in patients with advanced heart failure, with 90 per cent of patients unhappy with the level of pain control received[1]. A number of studies have looked at pain in the terminal phase, although none at the aetiology, which is probably multi-factorial—angina, pain from co-morbidities such as diabetic neuropathy, osteoarthritis, musculoskeletal pain or abdominal discomfort from intestinal oedema or ascites. Perhaps increased recognition of pain as a symptom of end-stage cardiac disease may allow us to offer better analgesic regimens.

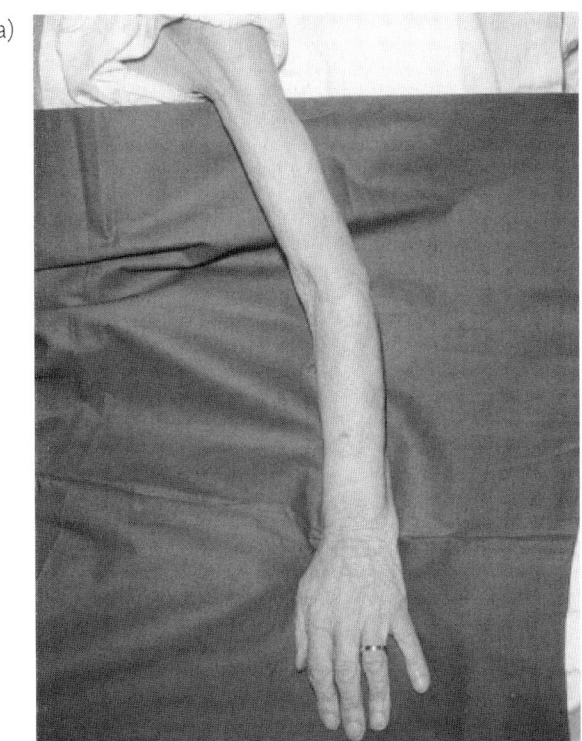

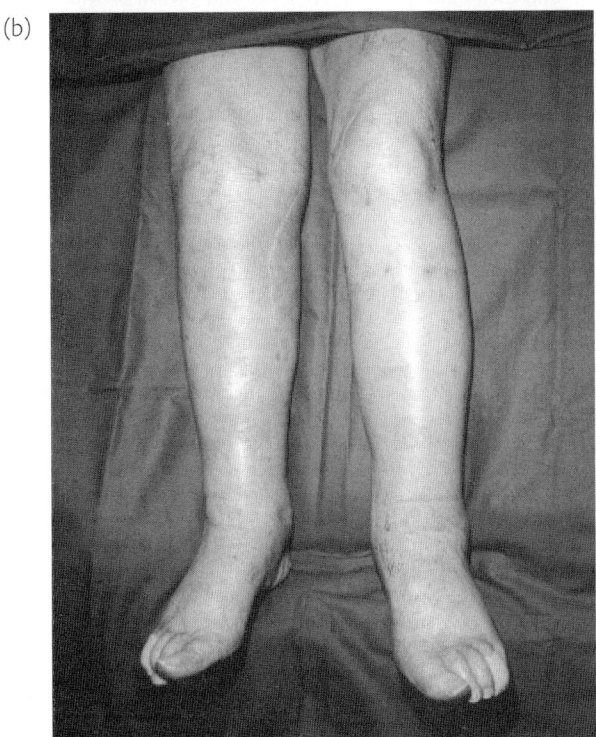

Figure 12.4.1 Photographs of a patient with advanced cardiac failure. Note the marked oedema of the legs but marked muscle wasting of the arms. Reproduced with permission from O'Brien, T., Welsh, J., and Dunn, F.G. (1998). ABC of palliative care. Non-malignant conditions. *British Medical Journal*, **316**, 286–9.

Breathlessness and oedema are not unique to heart failure and are often found in patients with advanced malignancy. In cardiac failure, the aetiology of the oedema is predominately circulatory overload, sometimes combined with malnutrition causing hypoalbuminaemia. In cancer patients, however, hypoalbuminaemia and lymphoedema are the key factors. These symptoms can be very debilitating, contributing to anxiety and insomnia.

Cognitive impairment may occur in both subtypes of patients. Those with cardiac failure may suffer from cerebrovascular disease or cerebral hypoperfusion and have been shown to demonstrate attention and memory deficits[20]. Patients with malignancy may have cerebral metastases, opioid side effects, or hypercalcaemia. Both groups may have biochemical abnormalities resulting from malnutrition, poor renal function, or diuretics.

As with all patients with chronic and potentially life-threatening conditions, depression and anxiety are frequent symptoms, although often under-diagnosed. Quality-of-life scores are markedly reduced in heart failure, and with advancing symptoms comes an increased incidence of depression[7]. Anxiety and fear of the future can be provoked by severe episodes of breathlessness and many patients report apprehension regarding attacks, especially at night. Feelings of social isolation and increasing dependency are common. It is imperative to actively seek out the signs and symptoms in order that they may be treated accordingly and not add to patient-suffering. Moderately and severely depressed patients with heart failure have a significantly higher mortality, being four times more likely to die within 2 years compared with those classified as not depressed[21]. Drug and non-drug approaches are both equally important and the role of clinical psychology and cognitive behavioural therapy should be considered. Selective serotonin reuptake inhibitors (SSRIs), such as citalopram and sertraline are generally safe, but tricyclic antidepressants should be avoided due to the risk of arrhythmias. Small doses of benzodiazepines are useful in the management of anxiety.

Differences from malignancy

With increasing severity of heart disease, symptoms become more specific (Table 12.4.1) with oedema and breathlessness becoming much more pronounced. The patient with end-stage cardiac disease will often experience debilitating orthopnoea and paroxysmal nocturnal dyspnoea with signs of pulmonary congestion and gross oedema often being present. However, there are two key differences between advanced heart disease and malignancy, neither of which are a function of symptoms or signs.

Firstly, predicting mortality on an individual basis in heart failure is difficult. Heart failure patients have episodes of decompensation interspersed with periods of stability[2], unlike the classical progressive decline seen in many malignancies. The unpredictable response to therapy and the spectre of sudden cardiac death make the prediction of proximity to death particularly difficult in end-stage cardiac disease. In the vasodilator in heart failure (V-HEFT) trials, 64 per cent of cardiac deaths occurred suddenly and only 30 per cent were preceded by any reported worsening of cardiac symptoms[22]. These patients also have a lower inpatient mortality than those with other chronic diseases, further emphasizing the difficulty in predicting life expectancy. Patients even within 2–3 days of death may have a prognosis predicted by their physicians of 2–3 months[1]. Secondly, most patients and health-care professionals do not view heart failure as a terminal disease, despite the appalling mortality seen in the condition. These two factors hinder the palliative care of advanced heart failure. Improved identification of patients who are likely to be in the end stages of heart failure and a change in attitude to their treatment and prognosis are required from health-care workers, the patient and their families. Despite these differences, lessons can be drawn from experience of palliative care in other disease processes and applied to the patient with advanced heart disease.

General palliative care issues

Location of management

Many patients with end-stage cardiac disease state a preference for home over hospital management[23]. This has not been achieved uniformly in the United Kingdom and the reasons for this are complex and include concerns about the patient's stability, a bias towards hospital care among health professionals and lack of resources and suitable infrastructure. The outstanding success of Community Palliative Care Nurse Specialists has led to an exploration of home management in patients with advanced cardiac failure using a similar model. In Glasgow, a programme has been developed using Specialist Heart Failure Liaison Nurses who provide a link between hospital consultants and the community. Clear protocols have been drawn up identifying patients who can be managed in this shared way and when they require hospital admission. This system has already been shown to reduce hospital admission and improve the patient's quality of life[24].

Pain control

Adequate pain control is essential in advanced heart disease. Standard anti-anginal therapy to control symptoms arising from myocardial ischaemia can be used. Opioids may be necessary to achieve adequate pain control and are useful for associated breathlessness and anxiety. The need for short- and long-acting opioids should be assessed regularly. These may be given orally, transdermally, nebulized, subcutaneously, or intravenously. Non-steroidal anti-inflammatory drugs should be avoided due to their adverse effect on renal function and their propensity to increase fluid retention.

Resuscitation issues

There is a common misconception amongst patients and healthcare staff that cardiac disease is a more benign condition than cancer. Often patients' expectations are such that their physician is expected to actively treat them under any circumstance and, indeed, cardiologists may focus on what can be done rather than what should be done. This, coupled with the difficulty in predicting life expectancy, leaves many physicians feeling uncomfortable discussing resuscitation issues with their patients. In addition, even in endstage cardiac disease there are many correctable causes of cardiac arrest. This is clearly a complex issue, but it is imperative that it is faced and approached with delicacy and understanding and in the knowledge that patients with end-stage cardiac disease may change their views from time to time regarding resuscitation preferences.

The SUPPORT study provided important information on resuscitation preferences of patients with end-stage cardiac failure[25]. In hospital it was found that 'do not resuscitate' (DNR) orders were less common in heart failure. They were written for only 5 per cent of patients admitted with cardiac failure in comparison to 47 per cent of those with malignancy and 52 per cent of patients with AIDS. Twenty-three per cent of patients stated that they did not wish resuscitation and 40 per cent of these patients subsequently changed their mind in favour of resuscitation. The number of patients wishing cardiopulmonary resuscitation has been shown to decrease, however once they have been provided with information regarding estimated probability of survival[26].

Many hospitals have or are currently in the process of creating DNR policies. The importance of such policies cannot be over emphasized. There are three key situations in which a DNR order is appropriate. Firstly, when CPR is unlikely to be effective; secondly, when it is known that the patient does not wish to receive CPR; and thirdly, where successful CPR would not prolong, or more importantly, improve quality of life.

The patient may not always be able to participate in the decisionmaking regarding DNR decisions. In this situation, a previous request by the patient should be adhered to and discussion with the family is also helpful. Such discussions, however, must be approached with sensitivity and understanding, and a full explanation is extremely important for all members of staff to know what the patient's resuscitation status is, which should always be clearly documented in the case notes. It is crucial to highlight that the DNR order only applies to cardiopulmonary resuscitation and does not in any way limit other medical or nursing care the patient is receiving. A DNR order should be reviewed on a regular basis as there are situations when it may have to be reversed.

There has been some debate in the past about whether all patients presenting to hospital should be asked about their resuscitation preferences. At the moment, this is done on a selective basis, but in the future, living wills or advance directives may well become the norm. These are important in setting goals of care, including preferences and limitations and discussing end-of-life issues.

Polypharmacy and withdrawing treatment

Treatment of traditional risk factors for cardiovascular disease such as hypertension and hyperlipidaemia becomes less important in the severe heart disease population due to the high mortality. However, the risk of death on an individual basis is difficult to predict and standard therapy should be maintained provided it is well tolerated.

Patients with terminal illnesses are often on a variety of medications and patients with cardiac failure take an average of 6.3 ± 2.3 drugs[27]. These may be to treat the underlying condition, but also to alleviate associated symptoms. As symptoms become more intractable, the number of medicines can multiply greatly. This is important for several reasons. Firstly, the potential for drug interactions increases as the number of medicines grows and secondly it may be progressively more difficult for patients to swallow tablets. It is therefore important to critically review a patient's medication regularly, discontinuing medication that confers no symptomatic benefit, particularly in the pre-terminal and terminal stages of their illness. In fact, in the last few days of life, patients may be able to be managed without the need for medicines. The withdrawal of regular cardiac medicines for some patients may send a strong signal that death is imminent and many may feel that their cardiology team is 'giving up' on them. It can help if this is done gradually, with a palliative-minded approach being adopted from early on in their management.

Diet, bed rest, and exercise

Cardiac cachexia is known to be a poor prognostic marker regardless of the severity of LV dysfunction. Nutrition, therefore, has an important role in the management of cardiac disease, and a dietician should be involved as part of the multi-disciplinary team. The diet should be palatable and tailored to the patient's individual needs. Restriction of sodium intake and fluid may be employed if the patient is symptomatic from fluid accumulation. With the introduction of powerful diuretics in recent years, sodium can be restricted simply to 'no added salt' and fluid intake may be restricted to 1.5–2 l. Frequent light meals are often better tolerated than heavy meals, and vitamin supplementation may be required since the absorption of these is reduced in patients with cardiac failure. It is worth considering the use of thiamine, both because it may be a contributing factor in patients with alcohol-related cardiomyopathy and also because diuretic use may cause reduced thiamine levels[28]. Studies have shown micronutrients to be beneficial in improving LV function and quality of life in theory by reducing oxidative stress[29].

Until the last 10 years, exercise was actively discouraged in patients with end-stage cardiac disease because of concern about metabolic abnormalities and hypoperfusion of skeletal muscle giving rise to fatigue. The ability to remain mobile is obviously related to the degree of oedema present; however, inactivity can contribute to muscle atrophy and deconditioning, setting up a vicious circle. Furthermore, controlled trials in recent years have revealed an improvement in exercise capacity and symptomatic well-being with tailored exercise programmes[30]. There is also some evidence that exercise programmes are associated with a reduced incidence of arrhythmias and increased survival[31]. Clearly, these programmes become less appropriate in the latter stages of the disease process, but if possible, activity should still be encouraged with appropriate physiotherapy. Bed rest should be reserved for periods of decompensation as it enhances response to diuretic therapy[32].

Complementary and alternative medicine

Throughout the Western world there is increasing interest in the use of complementary and alternative medicines (CAM). There are roughly 200 different modalities under the broad heading of CAM, including many herbs and supplements. There is little data on potential herb or nutrient– drug interactions, although it is recognized that a number of these supplements have an interaction with anticoagulants and antiplatelets[33]. Patients may use CAM for associated symptoms including anxiety and depression. Therapies such as aromatherapy, reiki, reflexology, acupuncture, and hypnotherapy are now practised in a wide variety of palliative care settings. Acupuncture stimulates release of endogenous opioids in animal models, inhibiting sympathetic nervous activity, which may help explain its reported benefit in heart failure patients[34]. The popularity of these therapies is undoubtedly increasing and they may become a significant aspect of the management of some patients in conjunction with mainstream therapies.

Thromboprophylaxis

Cardiac thromboembolism is a common problem, with severe LV systolic dysfunction increasing the risk of stroke by up to five times, even in patients with normal sinus rhythm. It is generally accepted that anticoagulation is warranted for those with LV dysfunction, coupled with atrial fibrillation or LV thrombus[35]. However, the decision to anticoagulate should not be made lightly as it brings its own attendant risks, and monitoring can be burdensome for both the patient and physician. There is probably only a limited role for warfarin in a truly palliative care arena. There is ongoing debate as to whether or not patients with terminal illnesses should receive prophylaxis against venous thromboembolism and there are many arguments for and against. Ultimately, each case should be examined carefully on individual merit, taking into account such details as life expectancy, patient choice, and assessing the risks and benefits.

Hypotension

Hypotension may arise as a result of an inadequate circulating volume due to pump failure or as a consequence of arrhythmias, over-diuresis, anti-hypertensive medication, sedative drugs, autonomic failure, or loss of body mass. Withdrawal of hypotensive drugs and careful monitoring of fluid status may help alleviate associated symptoms.

Communication

There is evidence showing that symptom relief is inadequate in 60–75 per cent of patients with advanced heart disease, and management plans did not take into account the wishes of the patient in approximately one-third of cases[36]. Patients often have a poor understanding of their illness and many questions go unanswered[37]. The importance of good communication with patients and their families at every step in their illness cannot be over-emphasized and is the key to quality care. It is also important to recognize the burden that cardiac disease places on carers and to be empathetic to their needs. Discussing goals of care should be done openly in order for patients to be able to express their wishes and avoid misunderstanding at a later date. In addition, they should be given the opportunity to understand the difficulties in prognosticating given the higher risk of sudden cardiac death. Many patients would appreciate a timely and frank discussion about these issues to help them to prepare for the end of life, including expressing their preferred place of care and death.

There is a well-developed support network for patients with cancer. This is not yet in place for patients with end-stage cardiac disease, and there are a number of studies indicating a lack of appropriate communication between physician and patients with end-stage cardiac disease[36]. However, increased recognition of this has produced improvements in communication between hospital staff, GPs, and patients with end-stage cardiac disease in recent years. This has been facilitated by cardiac rehabilitation programmes throughout the country, which provide a platform for education with regard to drugs, diet, and psychological aspects of cardiac failure in addition to structured exercise programmes. This multi-disciplinary approach is reaping benefits in terms of helping patients and their families to cope with advanced cardiac failure and other forms of end-stage cardiac disease.

Issues specific to the cardiac patient

Although many of the general tenets of palliative care can be applied in the treatment of those with end-stage cardiac disease, there are several issues unique to the cardiac patient. The most obvious of these is cardio-active drug therapy for the treatment of heart failure, but other treatment issues encompass the treatment of refractory angina, control of symptomatic arrhythmias, the use of pacemakers, and other device therapies and cardiac transplantation.

Pharmacological treatment of heart failure

The pharmacological treatment of heart failure is rapidly developing, partly due to our increasing understanding of the pathophysiology of the syndrome. The last decade or so has brought a clear evidence base for drug prescribing in heart failure of all classes to reduce mortality and hospital admissions, improve symptoms and functional status, and to delay progression of adverse remodelling. Although all these aspects are important, the severity of heart failure determines the relative importance of each one.

Heart failure is characterized by symptoms of congestion and diuretics are the mainstay of treatment. They are more effective at reducing breathlessness and oedema and improving exercise tolerance than any other treatment[38]. Diuretic requirements change, and the dose should be tailored to the patient's symptoms, fluctuation in weight, and renal function. Episodes of decompensation should be treated with intravenous diuretics to circumvent poor oral absorption caused by intestinal oedema. Although loop diuretics, such as furosemide, are the most commonly prescribed diuretic, it may be necessary to add a thiazide diuretic or metolazone which act on the distal convoluted tubule. Often, only a few days of treatment are required in the acute setting, but a combined diuretic regime may also be given in the stable phase to patients resistant to loop diuretics alone. The addition of a potassium-sparing diuretic (spironolactone) also increases diuresis. The need for monitoring blood chemistry is increased when using combinations of diuretics.

Current drug therapy: the evidence base

There is now a strong evidence base for a number of agents in reducing hospital admissions and mortality and improving NYHA class and functional status (Table 12.4.2). Tolerability is generally good, and side-effect profiles are at an acceptable level.

Neurohumoral modulation is effected by angiotensin-converting enzyme (ACE) inhibitors, which inhibit the production of angiotensin II and, as a by-product, increase bradykinin concentration. In addition to vasodilatation, inhibition of the RAAS by ACE inhibitors causes improvements in remodelling, improving LV geometry and function[39]. They improve survival and symptoms in all classes of heart failure. Dose-limiting factors include hypotension, hyperkalaemia, and cough[39,40]. However, two points are important to remember. Firstly, cough is a common symptom of heart failure itself, occurring in up to 31 per cent of patients. The incidence is only 6 per cent higher with ACE inhibitors[40]. Secondly, there is a common misconception that ACE inhibitors are highly nephrotoxic and contraindicated in patients with renal impairment. They cause reduced glomerular blood flow with an associated rise in serum creatinine, which reflects a functional change that is reversible on discontinuation of the drug[5]. Creatinine values up to 200 µg/litre should not be regarded as a contraindication to starting an ACE inhibitor, but regular monitoring of renal function is mandatory. Angiotensin II receptor blockers (ARBs) deliver similar benefits to ACE inhibitors, both in the post myocardial infarction setting[41] and in chronic heart failure[42]. Thus in patients with a troublesome cough

or angioneurotic oedema, the ACE inhibitor should be replaced by an ARB[43]. There is evidence from the CHARM study that in chronic heart failure the combination of ACEI/ARB provides additional benefit to the patient[44].

Inhibition of the RAAS can also be achieved by spironolactone. In addition to its diuretic effects, there seems to be a reduction in fibrosis and improvement in myocyte function with antagonism of aldosterone. Clinically, its use improves NYHA class and reduces hospital admissions and mortality[45]. Small doses are used, and the risk of hyperkalaemia seems small, although must be borne in mind. Breast tenderness and troublesome gynaecomastia can occur, which may necessitate discontinuation of the drug. Future studies may reveal that the newer aldosterone antagonist eplerenone can replace spironolactone but its role is yet to be determined.

Inhibition of the sympathetic nervous system by beta-blockers, traditionally thought to be contraindicated, is an effective form of treatment for heart failure. In the last decade, trials have demonstrated improved symptoms and reduction in NYHA class in addition to mortality benefit. However, only carvedilol to date has demonstrated safety, tolerability, and efficacy in class IV heart failure[46]. Beta-blockade should be initiated when the patient is stable and not during an episode of acute decompensation. The dose should be up-titrated as symptomatic status, heart rate, and blood pressure allow.

Although digoxin is the archetypal treatment for heart failure, its use was not supported by evidence until the 1990s. It does not confer a survival benefit, but reduces hospital admissions and improves symptoms[47]. It is therefore a useful adjunct in the treatment of severe heart failure and as a rate control agent in atrial fibrillation.

Treatment of refractory angina

Refractory angina is distressing and limiting. Multiple drug classes, including beta-blockers, calcium channel blockers, nitrates, and nicorandil are useful in reducing the ischaemic burden, thereby reducing symptoms. However, in addition to standard anti-ischaemic therapy and use of opioids, several additional strategies can be considered.

Surgical or percutaneous revascularization should be considered for those with anginal symptoms in an attempt to achieve symptomatic relief. However, it is known that up to 40 per cent of patients referred for cardiac transplantation may be suitable for surgical revascularization with reasonable survival rates[48], and there is now considerable interest in revascularization as a treatment for heart failure, with two large clinical trials ongoing. Currently, one

Table 12.4.2 Drug groups and their use in the four classes of heart failure as assessed by clinical trials with their effects on survival, hospital admission and functional status.

Drug	NYHA I	NYHA II	NYHA III	NYHA IV	Improved survival	Reduced hospital admissions and improved functional status
Diuretic	No	Yes	Yes	Yes	No	Yes
ACEI/ARB	Yes/Not studied	Yes	Yes	Yes	Yes	Yes
Spironolactone	Not studied	No	Yes	Yes	Yes	Yes
Beta-blocker	Not studied	Yes	Yes	Yes	Yes	Yes
Digoxin	Not studied	Yes	Yes	Yes	No	Yes
Combined ACEI/ARB	Not studied	Yes	Yes	Yes	Yes	Yes

Note: NYHA = New York Heart Association class.

would only consider this outside a trial setting if a significant area of ischaemia can be identified through non-invasive assessment with suitable surgical targets apparent at angiography.

Other therapies include enhanced external pneumatic counter-pulsation, consisting of inflatable bands for the limbs that inflate in diastole improving blood flow to the coronary arteries and improving haemodynamics. Although experimental, recent evidence suggests it may be useful in the palliation of severe anginal symptoms[49]. Another useful device for symptom palliation is the implantable spinal cord stimulator. Its use is based on the gate theory of pain and the device is inserted into the epidural space, providing paraesthetic stimuli over the area where anginal symptoms are present (typically T2 to T5 dermatomes). The patient controls how much stimulus is given.

Arrhythmia control and implantable defibrillators

Myocardial infarction, hypertensive heart disease, and LV dysfunction produce areas of scarring and adverse cardiac remodelling, providing a substrate for arrhythmogenesis. This, coupled with adverse cardiac haemodynamics, altered biochemistry associated with chronic diuretic use, super-activation of the renin–angiotensin and sympathetic nervous systems and the potential for pro-arrhythmia with many cardio-active drugs, means that disturbances of cardiac rhythm are common in those with advanced heart disease[50]. These range from symptomatically important supraventricular arrhythmias including atrial fibrillation (AF), the incidence of which rises sharply with advancing heart disease[51], to the life-threatening arrhythmias of ventricular tachycardia and fibrillation. Careful attention to risk factors and potential pro-arrhythmic therapy is required, but more specific therapy may ultimately be needed.

Simple pharmacological measures, such as rate control with beta-blockers or digoxin may improve symptoms and functional status in AF and much of the increased survival seen with beta-blocker, ACE inhibitor, and spironolactone use in the heart failure setting is driven by a reduction in sudden arrhythmic death. Most anti-arrhythmic drugs have a cardio-depressant effect, and the use of some agents is associated with an increase in mortality. The drugs of choice are digoxin or beta-blockers for atrial arrhythmias and amiodarone for life-threatening ventricular arrhythmias. Restoration to sinus rhythm may improve symptoms in those who develop AF.

Increased understanding of the pathophysiology of arrhythmogenesis and improvements in electrophysiological techniques has widened the therapeutic options for the treatment of arrhythmias. Some of these are suitable in patients with advanced heart failure if symptoms cannot be effectively controlled by pharmacological means or side effects of antiarrhythmic therapy occur. Radiofrequency ablation is a percutaneous trans-catheter means of arrhythmia control. The application of radiofrequency energy produces interruption of an arrhythmia circuit or modifies the substrate for arrhythmogenesis and is curative in some arrhythmias. However, with regard to ventricular arrhythmias, a discrete arrhythmogenic focus is seldom found in this group of patients and catheter ablation is of limited use, although may be considered for intractable VT.

Implantable cardioverter defibrillators (ICD) are advanced pacemaker systems allowing recognition of broad complex tachycardias and ventricular fibrillation. They are able to terminate the arrhythmia with anti-tachycardia pacing or the delivery of a small internal electrical shock provided by a capacitor. Improvements in technology mean these devices are now not much bigger than a standard pacemaker and can be inserted percutaneously, obviating the need for major surgery. Up to 60 per cent of deaths in patients with severe heart failure are due to sudden cardiac death[22], and several large trials have demonstrated a reduction in sudden cardiac death in heart failure patients, both in those who have survived a ventricular arrhythmic event[52] and as primary prevention in the wider heart failure population[53]. Although the insertion of a defibrillator would be contraindicated in those with a life expectancy of less than 6 months, the decision to implant may have been taken at an earlier stage in the patient's disease. It is therefore to be expected that patients with ICDs will increasingly be encountered in palliative care settings, and this raises major end-of-life and other ethical issues. A recent study of terminally ill patients with ICDs showed only one-third had shock therapy withdrawn as part of a palliative care comfort strategy[54]. This scenario is likely to become more common in the future, and an active decision on whether to continue shock capability of the ICD should be made following full and frank discussion with the patient, carers, and health professionals involved in their care.

Pacemakers and cardiac resynchronization

Pacemakers have long been used for the treatment of bradyarrhythmias and should be considered in patients with advanced heart disease and symptomatic heart block. However, pacing to improve haemodynamics and symptoms in advanced heart failure in the absence of a bradyarrhythmia has increased over the last decade. Many patients with severe LV systolic dysfunction will have inter- and intra-ventricular conduction delay, manifest by widening of the QRS complex on the ECG and causing dys-synchronous activation and contraction of the left ventricle. Synchronous pacing of both ventricles, unlike traditional single RV pacing, improves haemodynamics, ejection fraction, and cardiac index and reduces mortality[55]. More importantly, it is associated with improved functional status and reduced hospital admissions[55].

Transplantation and LV assist devices

The place of orthoptic cardiac transplantation in the treatment of end-stage heart disease is constantly changing and is the subject of considerable debate[56]. Improved survival post-transplant has become a reality with advances in immunosuppressive therapy[57]. However, advances in the treatment of chronic heart failure, coupled with the difficulty in determining those who are truly 'end-stage' makes it difficult to determine who will actually benefit. The key lies in careful patient selection. Transplantation requires great commitment from the patient and their families. Psychological evaluation and continued support are essential. Patients should be considered only if they have severe symptoms from cardiac disease refractory to all other forms of conventional treatment, including other surgical options, and have 1-year mortality in excess of 20 per cent. However, transplantation may be considered on a purely symptomatic basis, if no other treatment options are available.

The limiting factor is usually the availability of donor organs and this has fuelled interest in mechanical devices to support the circulation. These range from short-term support with intra-aortic balloon pumps to left ventricular assist devices (LVAD) as a bridge to transplantation, or as a stand-alone therapy[58]. The widespread adoption of LVADs has been hindered by high complication rates, but improvements in device technology may overcome this in the future.

Integrated strategy for end-stage cardiac disease

In palliative cardiac care, treatment strategies often combine many of the pharmacological and non-pharmacological treatments outlined previously. Not all these options will be relevant, and it is vital that treatment is appropriate and tailored to the individual. Table 12.4.3 gives an overview of the management of symptoms.

Dedicated heart failure clinics and community nurse specialists have a key role in continually assessing the suitability, efficacy, and potential detrimental effects of treatment, and to institute change where required in response to monitoring of weight. At times, it may be difficult to tease out side effects of therapy from symptoms of heart failure.

Despite the large number of advances in the management of cardiac disease in recent times, ultimately, patients die from their disease. When is the right time to involve palliative medicine teams in their management? Although there is no 'right time', it could be argued that it is when the answer to the question, 'Would you be surprised if your patient died within the next 6 months?' is 'no'. Others would argue that it is when patients have opted for a non-interventional/non-aggressive approach to treatment or when a further admission to hospital would not be in their best interests or indeed, their wish. Input from palliative care should be a gradual, seamless transition overlapping with active interventional treatment (Fig. 12.4.2). Regardless of the stage of their illness, patients benefit from a holistic approach, and the involvement of a multi-professional team in order to ensure all their needs, including social, psychological, and financial are met. Ultimately, bereavement support for family or carers is also essential.

Decompensation and hospital admission

Periods of hospitalization will inevitably be required to allow more intensive therapy. It is often difficult to judge when hospital admission is necessary, as one has to balance the risks in inappropriately delaying hospitalization against the psychological and other benefits of care at home. The decision to hospitalize will depend on many factors. Table 12.4.4 offers a guide to those who should be considered for admission. Some centres adopt a 'hospital at home' approach for episodes of decompensation, allowing infusions of diuretics and even inotropes to be given at home. It is important that a cause of deterioration is sought and reversed if possible. In hospital, intravenous loop diuretics are usually given, and inotropic agents such as dobutamine and low-dose dopamine may be required. Strategies to reduce afterload, such as intravenous nitrates, can also be employed. Some centres advocate the use of phosphodiesterase inhibitors such as milrinone as a positive inotropic agent, but there is little evidence to support this. The role of invasive haemodynamic monitoring is questionable.

What often appears to be the final admission may not be and the patient and their family should be made aware of the uncertainty in predicting the terminal phase. The input of the cardiac liaison nursing staff that care for the patient in the community is very important at this stage.

Future developments
Home management

Considerable further changes are needed to take the end-of-life care of patients with cardiac failure to a level where home management equivalent to that in hospital or hospice can be provided

Table 12.4.3 Integrated management for the treatment of advanced heart disease.

Breathlessness
- Oxygen
- Drugs: diuretics, digoxin, ACE inhibitors, beta-blockers, vasodilators, sublingual GTN for acute breathlessness
- Opioids: regular quick release oral morphine, intravenous diamorphine if acutely distressed
- Non-drug measures: fan, positioning in bed/chair, easier access to toilet, consider CPAP etc
- Assess need for admission to hospital

Oedema
- Early detection important
- Monitor weight regularly
- Aim for weight loss 0.5–1 kg/day
- Diuretics: furosemide remains first line, consider addition of bendrofluazide 5 mg od or metolazone 2.5 mg od in resistant oedema
- Fluid restriction: 1.5–2 l/day
- Mild salt restriction: no adding salt at table
- Decrease lower limb dependency: bed-rest in early stages, raise lower limbs by footstool or recliner when sitting
- Assess need for admission to hospital

Lightheadedness
- Check for postural hypotension
- Reassess need for drugs: vasodilator, beta-blocker, diuretic
- Exclude arrhythmia as a cause
- Reassure and educate patient

Muscle wasting and fatigue
- Physiotherapy
- Exercise: if possible
- Assess diet and energy intake: consider supplements
- Consider anticytokine therapy
- Review medications: consider stopping beta-blocker

Nausea, taste disturbance, anorexia
- Check biochemistry: uraemia and liver function tests
- Review medications
- Assess diet and energy intake: encourage frequent small meals and consider supplements
- Consider supplementation of fat soluble vitamins
- Consider appetite stimulants: small amounts of alcohol, megestrol acetate
- Consider pro-motility agents: metoclopramide/domperidone

Depression and anxiety
- Regularly assess mental state
- Morphine or temazepam at night may help reduce nocturnal anxiety
- Exercise programme
- Relaxation exercises
- Antidepressant therapy: avoid tricyclics
- Reassure and educate the patient

Pain
- Analgesics: avoid NSAIDs, consider opioids
- Consider increasing anti-ischaemic medication
- Non-drug measures: relaxation exercises, TENS, hot packs, device therapy
- Review need for admission to hospital

Source: Adapted with permission from O'Brien, T., Welsh, J., and Dunn, F.G. (1998). ABC of palliative care. Non-malignant conditions. *British Medical Journal*, **316**, 286–9.

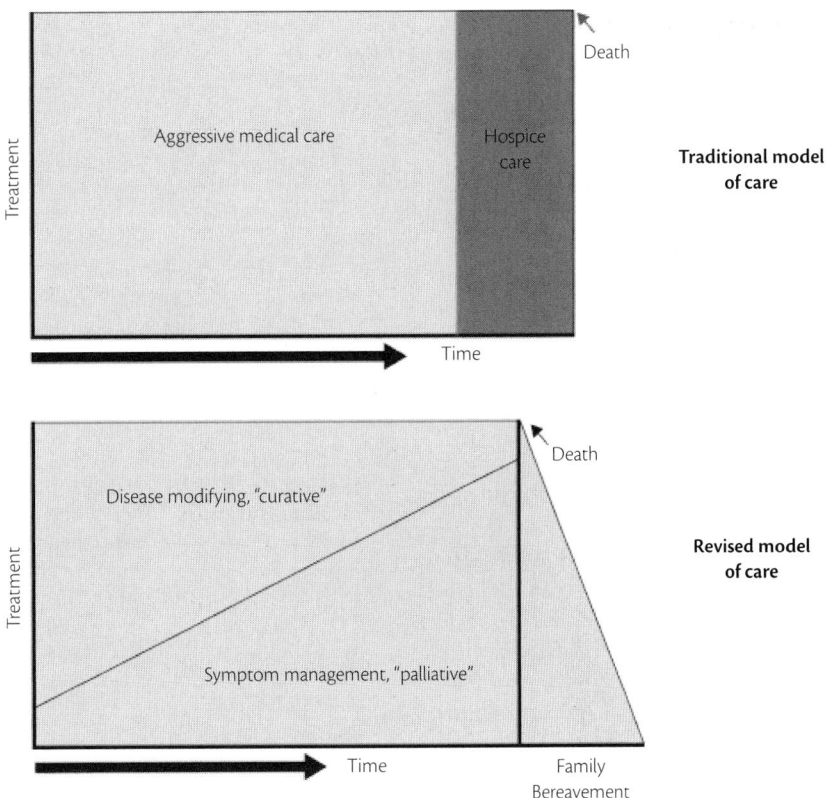

Figure 12.4.2 Traditional model for heart disease management vs. revised model. Aim should be seamless transition from a primarily disease modification approach to increasing focus on symptomatic management as disease progresses. Reproduced from Lynn, J. and Adamson, D. Living Well At The End Of Life: Adapting Health Care To Serious Chronic Illnesses In Old Age. RAND document WP-137. Copyright RAND Corporation. Used with permission.

right up until the time of death. The infrastructure has to be in place to meet patients' needs, if they choose to remain at home. The provision of the Heart Failure Liaison Service is inconsistent presently, and it is important that this service be deployed evenly and completely throughout the country. Thereafter, the service has to be taken to a level where in addition to all necessary appliances in the home; there are facilities for infusions of opioids and other agents along with round the clock nursing and medical support if required. How the care of these patients is coordinated between cardiology teams, palliative care teams, and GPs is a matter for discussion at a local level.

Hospice management

Hospices also have a role to play in the management of patients with cardiac disease, although it would be naïve to think that they could provide care to all patients with end-stage cardiac disease

Table 12.4.4 Guide for the need for hospital admission.

- ◆ Need for intravenous therapy
- ◆ Persistent paroxysmal nocturnal breathlessness or orthopnoea
- ◆ Refractory dependent oedema despite high dose oral therapy
- ◆ Fluid leakage from lower limbs
- ◆ Symptomatic postural hypotension
- ◆ Development of arrhythmias
- ◆ Refractory pain: ischaemic pain or otherwise
- ◆ Anaemia requiring blood transfusion

without being overwhelmed[59]. Patients may be visited by Community Palliative Care Nurse Specialists who can facilitate admission to the hospice for symptom management, respite for carers or end-of-life care. Furthermore, attending Day Hospices may provide some support.

Psychological support

This is an important element of palliative care, which has not been adequately dealt with in the past. Both patients and carers will at some stage suffer symptoms of anxiety and depression, and patients, in particular, will often experience emotions which they do not clearly recognize as being due to their disease. Additionally, when such issues as resuscitation preference are discussed, considerable support from carers is required. Good psychological support and counselling skills are likely to make a significant impact on the patient's quality of life.

Physician education and research

Cardiologists may be unfamiliar with the principles of palliative care and how they can be applied to patients with end-stage cardiac disease. There may be ignorance and misunderstanding on the part of both cardiologists and palliative care physicians when it comes to looking after patients with cardiac disease. Cardiologists are thoroughly competent in the specific aspects of the management of heart failure, but may be less familiar with the optimal management of pain, constipation, or anxiety and depression, plus the other clinical features that arise towards the end of life. Education about the principles of palliative care can be most easily attained by collaborating closely with the local palliative care team, and by recognizing the similar problems that patients experience towards the end of their life regardless of the underlying disease.

There are currently large gaps in knowledge, practice, and research related to the supportive care of patients with advanced cardiac disease. Barriers to research need to be overcome in order that we may provide our patients and their families with the best evidenced based care.

Conclusion

The unmet needs of patients living with end-stage cardiac disease and their families or carers affect every facet of life, and there is little doubt that the traditional view that palliative care be directed only towards the patient with advanced cancer is changing. It is now recognized that end-stage cardiac disease has many characteristics that lend themselves to the principles of palliative care, and the management of cardiac disease at all stages has a substantial palliative component. Much still needs to be achieved in this area. It may be regarded as a paradox that despite the considerable reduction in mortality and morbidity from cardiac failure because of new treatments, the number of patients with end-stage cardiac disease is likely to rise. In anticipation of this, it is important to establish a multi-disciplinary approach to the management of end-stage cardiac disease with enhanced integration of cardiology and palliative medicine services. This will greatly improve the quality of life for these patients in the final days and hours of their lives and will also ease the burden on patients' families and friends in the same way that palliative care with cancer has done so impressively over the past 40 years.

References

1. Levenson, J.W., McCarthy, E.P., Lynn, J. *et al.* (2000). The last six months of life for patients with congestive heart failure. *Journal of the American Geriatric Society*, **48**(5 Suppl), S101–S109.
2. Stewart, S., MacIntyre, K., Capewell, S. *et al.* (2003). Heart failure and the ageing population: an increasing burden in the 21st Century? *Heart* **89**, 49–53.
3. Cowie, M.R., Wood, D.A., Coats, A.J.S. *et al.* (1999). Incidence and aetiology of heart failure. A population-based study. *European Heart Journal*, **20**(421), 428.
4. Tunstall-Pedoe, H., Kuulasmaa, K., Malhonen, M. *et al.* for the WHO MONICA Project. (1999). Contribution of trends in survival and coronary event rates to changes in coronary heart disease mortality: 10 year results form the 37 WHO Monica Project populations. *Lancet*, **353**, 1547–57.
5. The Consensus Trial Study Group. (1987). Effects of enalapril on mortality in severe congestive heart failure. Results of the Cooperative North Scandinavian Enalapril Survival Study (CONSENSUS). *New England Journal of Medicine*, **316**, 1429–35.
6. McKee, P.A., Castelli, W.P., McNamara, P.M. *et al.* (1971). The natural history of congestive heart failure: the Framingham study. *New England Journal of Medicine*, **285**, 1441–46.
7. Stewart, A.L., Greenfield, S., Hays, R.D. *et al.* (1989). Functional status and well-being of patients with chronic conditions. Results from the Medical Outcomes Study. *Journal of the American Medical Association*, **262**, 907–13.
8. Lewis, E.F., Johnson, P.A., Johnson, W. *et al.* (2001). Preferences for quality of life or survival expressed by patients with heart failure. *Journal of Heart and Lung Transplantation*, **20**, 1016–24.
9. Stewart, S., Jenkins, Q., Buchan, S. *et al.* (2002). The current cost of heart failure to the National health service in the UK. *European Heart Journal*, **4**(361), 371.
10. Feld, Y., Dubi, S., Reisner, Y. *et al.* (2006). Future strategies for the treatment of diastolic heart failure. *Acute Cardiac Care*, **8**, 13–20.
11. Francis, G.S. (2001). Pathophysiology of chronic heart failure. *American Journal of Medicine*, **110**(Suppl 7A), 37S–46S.
12. Lombardi, W. and Gilbert, E. (2000). The effects of neurohormonal antagonism on pathologic left ventricular remodeling in heart failure. *Current Cardiology Reports*, **2**, 90–8.
13. Matsumori, A. and Sasayama, S. (2001). The role of inflammatory mediators in the failing heart: immunomodulation of cytokines in experimental models of heart failure. *Heart Failure Reviews*, **6**, 129–36.
14. Herrera-Garza, E., Stetson, S.J., Cubillos-Garzon, A. *et al.* (1999). Tumour necrosis factor-alpha: a mediator of disease progression in the failing human heart. *Chest*, **115**, 1170–4.
15. Carr, J.G., Stevenson, L.W., Walden, J.A. *et al.* (1989). Prevalence and hemodynamic correlates of malnutrition in severe congestive heart failure secondary to ischemic or idiopathic dilated cardiomyopathy. *American Journal of Cardiology*, **63**, 709–13.
16. Anker, S.D., Ponikowski, P., Varney, S. *et al.* (1997). Wasting as independent risk factor for mortality in chronic heart failure. *Lancet*, **349**, 1050–3.
17. Ferrier, K., Campbell, A., Yee, B. *et al.* (2005). Sleep-disordered breathing occurs frequently in stable outpatients with congestive heart failure. *Chest*, **128**, 2116–22.
18. Ludwig, B.S., Van Belle, S., Barrett-Lee, P. *et al.* (2004). The European Cancer Anaemia Survey (ECAS): a large, multinational, prospective survey defining the prevalence, incidence, and treatment of anaemia in cancer patients. *European Journal of Cancer*, **40**, 2293–306.
19. Silverberg, D.S., Wexler, D.B., Iaina, A. (2004). The role of anemia in the progression of congestive heart failure. Is there a place for erythropoietin and intravenous iron? *Journal of Nephrology*, **17**, 749–61.
20. Almeida, O.P. and Flicker, L. (2001). The mind of a failing heart: a systematic review of the association between congestive heart failure and cognitive functioning. *Internal Medicine Journal*, **31**, 290–5.
21. Murberg, T.A., Bru, E., Svebak, R. *et al.* (1999). Depressed mood and subjective health symptoms as predictors of mortality in patients with congestive heart failure: a two-years follow-up study. *International Journal of Psychiatry in Medicine*, **29**, 311–26.
22. Cohn, J.N., Archibald, D., Ziesche, S. *et al.* (1986). Effect of vasodilator therapy on mortality in chronic congestive heart failure. Results of a Veterans Administration Cooperative Study. *New England Journal of Medicine*, **314**, 1547–52.
23. Fried, T.R., van Doorn, C., O'Leary, J.R. *et al.* (1999). Older persons' preferences for site of terminal care [published erratum appears in Ann Intern Med 2000 Mar 7;132(5):419]. *Annals of Internal Medicine*, **131**(2), 109–12.
24. Blue, L., Lang, E., McMurray, J.J.V. *et al.* (2001). Randomised controlled trial of specialist nurse intervention in heart failure. *British Medical Journal*, **323**, 715–8.
25. Krumholz, H.M., Phillips, R.S., Hamel, M.B. *et al.* (1998). Resuscitation preferences among patients with severe congestive heart failure: results from the SUPPORT project. Study to Understand Prognoses and Preferences for Outcomes and Risks of Treatments. *Circulation*, **98**, 648–55.
26. Murphy, D.J., Burrows, D., Santilli, S. *et al.* (1994). The influence of the probability of survival on patients' preferences regarding cardiopulmonary resuscitation. *New England Journal of Medicine*, **330**, 545–9.
27. Lainscak, M. and Keber, I. (2003). Patient's view of heart failure: from the understanding to the quality of life. *European Journal Cardiovascular Nursing*, **2**, 275–81.

28. Seligmann, H., Halkin, H., Rauchfleisch, S. *et al.* (1991). Thiamine deficiency in patients with congestive heart failure receiving long-term furosemide therapy: a pilot study. *American Journal of Medicine*, **91**, 151–5.

29. Witte, K.A.A., Nikitin, N.P., Parker, A.C. *et al.* (2005). The effect of micronutrient supplementation on quality-of-life and left ventricular function in elderly patients with chronic heart failure. *European Heart Journal*, **26**, 2238–44.

30. Meyer, K., Samek, L., and Schwalbold, M. (1996). Physical responses to different modes of interval exercise in patients with chronic heart failure: application to exercise training. *European Heart Journal*, **17**, 1040–7.

31. Meta-analysis finds that exercise training improves survival in people with heart failure. (2004). *Evidence-Based Cardiovascular Medicine*, **177**, 178–9.

32. Abildgaard, U., Aldershvile, J., Ring-Larsen, H. *et al.* (1985). Bed rest and increased diuretic treatment in chronic congestive heart failure. *European Heart Journal*, **6**, 1040–6.

33. Miller, K.L., Liebowitz, R.S., and Newby, L.K. (2004). Complementary and alternative medicine in cardiovascular disease: a review of biologically based approaches. *American Heart Journal*, **147**, 401–11.

34. Middlekauff, H.R. (2004). Acupuncture in the treatment of heart failure. *Cardiology in Review*, **12**, 171–3.

35. Diet, F. and Erdmann, E. (2000). Thromboembolism in heart failure: who should be treated? *European Journal of Heart Failure*, **2**, 355–63.

36. McCarthy, M., Hall, J.A., and Ley, M. (1997).Communication and choice in dying from heart disease. *Journal of the Royal Society of Medicine*, **90**(3), 128–31.

37. Murray, S.A., Boyd, K., Kendall, M. *et al.* (2002). Dying of lung cancer or cardiac failure: prospective qualitative interview study of patients and their carers in the community. *British Medical Journal*, **325**, 929.

38. Mujais, S.K., Nora, N.A., and Levin, M.L. (1992). Principles and clinical uses of diuretic therapy. *Progressive Cardiovascular Diseases*, **35**, 221–45.

39. Pfeffer, M.A., Lamas, G.A., Vaughan, D.E. *et al.* (1988). Effect of captopril on progressive ventricular dilatation after anterior myocardial infarction. *New England Journal of Medicine*, **319**, 80–6.

40. SOLVD investigators. (1988). Effect of enalapril on survival in patients with reduced left ventricular ejection fractions and congestive heart failure. *New England Journal of Medicine*, **325**, 293–302.

41. Pfeffer, M.A., McMurray, J.J.V., and Velazquez, E. (2003). Valsartan, captopril or both in myocardial Infarction cmplicated by heart Failure, left ventricular dysfunction or both. *New England Journal of Medicine*, **249**, 1893–1906.

42. Pfeffer, M.A., Swedberg, K., Granger, C.B. *et al.* (2003). Effects of candesartan on mortality and morbidity in patients with chronic heart failure: the CHARM-Overall programme. *Lancet*, **362**, 759–66.

43. Granger, C.B., McMurray, J.J.V., Yusuf, S. *et al.* (2003). Effects of candesartan in patients with chronic heart failure and reduced left-ventricular systolic function intolerant to angiotensin-converting-enzyme inhibitors: the CHARM-Alternative trial. *Lancet*, **362**, 772–6.

44. McMurray, J.J.V., Ostergren, J., Swedberg, K. *et al.* (2003). Effects of candesartan in patients with chronic heart failure and reduced left-ventricular systolic function taking angiotensin-converting-enzyme inhibitors: the CHARM-Added trial. *Lancet*, **362**, 767–71.

45. Pitt, B., Zannad, F., Remme, W.J. *et al.* (1999). The effect of spironolactone on morbidity and mortality in patients with severe heart failure. Randomized Aldactone Evaluation Study Investigators. *New England Journal of Medicine*, **341**, 709–17.

46. Tendera, M. and Ochala, A. (2001). Overview of the results from the recent beta-blocker trials. *Current Opinion in Cardiology*, **16**, 180–5.

47. The Digitalis Investigation Group. (1997). The effect of digoxin on mortality and morbidity in patients with heart failure. *New England Journal of Medicine*, **336**(525), 533.

48. Elefteriades, J.A., Tolis, G., Levi, E. *et al.* (1993). Coronary artery bypass grafting in severe left ventricular dysfunction: excellent survival with improved ejection fraction and functional state. *Journal of the American College of Cardiology*, **22**, 1411–7.

49. Loh, P., Louis, A., Windram, J. *et al.* (2006). The immediate and long-term outcome of enhanced external counterpulsation in treatment of chronic stable refractory angina. *Journal of Internal Medicine*, **259**, 276–84.

50. Cleland, J.G., Chattopadhyay, S., Khand, A. *et al.* (2002). Prevalence and incidence of arrhythmias and sudden death in heart failure. *Heart Failure Reviews*, **7**, 229–42.

51. Heist, E.K. and Ruskin, J.N. (2006). Atrial fibrillation and congestive heart failure: risk factors, mechanisms, and treatment. *Progressive Cardiovascular Diseases*, **48**, 256–69.

52. Connolly, S.J., Hallstrom, A., Cappato, R. *et al.* (2000). Meta-analysis of the implantable cardioverter defibrillator secondary prevention trials. AVID, CASH and CIDS studies. Antiarrhythmics vs Implantable Defibrillator study. Cardiac Arrest Study Hamburg. Canadian Implantable Defibrillator Study. *European Heart Journal*, **21**, 2071–8.

53. Duray, G., Israel, C.W., Hohnloser, S.H. Recent primary prevention implantable cardioverter defibrillator trials. *Current Opinion in Cardiology*, **21**, 15–9.

54. Lewis, W.R., Leubke, D.L., Johnson, N.J. *et al.* (2006). Withdrawing implantable defibrillator shock therapy in terminally ill patients. *American Journal of Medicine*, **119**, 892–6.

55. Abraham, W.T., Fisher, W.G., Smith, A.L. *et al.* (2002). Cardiac resynchronization in chronic heart failure.[see comment]. *New England Journal of Medicine*, **346**(24), 1845–53.

56. Gardner, R.G., McDonagh, T.A., McDonald, M. *et al.* (2006). Who needs a heart transplant? *European Heart Journal*, **27**, 770–2.

57. Trulock, E.P., Edwards, L.B., Taylor, D.O. *et al.* (2005). Registry of the International Society for Heart and Lung Transplantation: twenty-second official adult lung and heart-lung transplant report--2005. *Journal of Heart and Lung Transplantation*, **24**, 956–67.

58. Mancini, D. and Burkhoff, D. (2005). Mechanical device-based methods of managing and treating heart failure. *Circulation*, **112**, 438–48.

59. Gannon, C. (1995). Palliative care in terminal cardiac failure. Hospices cannot fulfil such a vast and diverse role. *British Medical Journal*, **310**, 1410–11.

12.5

Palliative care in non-malignant neurological disorders

Gian Domenico Borasio, Stefan Lorenzl, Angela Rogers, and Raymond Voltz

Neurological disorders are among the leading causes of death in the Western world. Stroke alone accounts for around 60 deaths/100 000 population/year in Europe. Other disorders such as multiple sclerosis and Parkinson's disease are highly prevalent, and ultimately lead to premature death, although death is usually ascribed to terminal complications such as pneumonia. In addition, there are a plethora of rare neurological disorders with progressive course (amyotrophic lateral sclerosis, Huntington's disease, progressive supranuclear palsy, central nervous system infections, muscle disorders, etc.) which nonetheless, when summed together, constitute an epidemiologically relevant group. Primary brain tumours and dementias are dealt with elsewhere in this textbook.

The differences in approach to palliative care between neurology and oncology stem primarily from the different time courses of neurological disorders, which are outlined in Table 12.5.1. In addition, the distribution and prevalence of symptoms is quite different from oncology. Generally speaking, pain is less prominent, while impairment in mobility as well as behavioural and cognitive changes are more prevalent The following section outlines principles of palliative care for some of the most important neurological disorders.

Amyotrophic lateral sclerosis/motor neuron disease

Amyotrophic lateral sclerosis (ALS, aka motor neuron disease in the UK and Lou Gehrig's disease in the USA) is the most common degenerative disorder of the motoneuronal system in adults. The incidence of ALS is 1.5–2/100 000/year and the prevalence is around 6–8/100 000. Most cases begin after age 40, with a mean age at onset of 58 years and an average disease duration of 3–4 years. 10 per cent of patients survive >10 years. There is no satisfactory treatment; the only approved drug (riluzole) prolongs life by about 3 months.

Patients present with fasciculations and slowly progressing pareses of voluntary muscles, coupled with hyperreflexia and spasticity due to concomitant involvement of upper and lower motor neurons. Bulbar onset with slurred speech (dysarthria) and/or difficulty in swallowing (dysphagia) occurs in 20–30 per cent of all cases, particularly in older females. Extraocular movements, sphincter continence, and cognitive functions are usually spared, and sensation is normal. The main symptoms of ALS are shown in Table 12.5.2.

Palliative care in ALS starts with the communication of the diagnosis and goes all the way to bereavement counselling

Table 12.5.1 Different time courses of neurological disorders.

(Sub)-acute progressive (days–weeks)	Progressive stroke, meningitis/encephalitis, Creutzfeldt–Jakob disease
Chronic progressive (months–years)	Amyotrophic lateral sclerosis, brain tumours, Huntington's disease, muscular dystrophies, multiple sclerosis (some), Alzheimer's disease
Chronic disability (± fluctuations)	Stroke, persistent vegetative state, multiple sclerosis (some), Parkinson's disease

Table 12.5.2 Symptoms due to ALS (either as a direct consequence of motoneuronal degeneration or indirectly as a consequence of the primary symptoms).

Directly	Indirectly
Weakness and atrophy	Psychological disturbances
Fasciculations and muscle cramps	Sleep disturbances
Spasticity	Constipation
Dysarthria	Drooling
Dysphagia	Thick mucous secretions
Dyspnoea	Symptoms of chronic hypoventilation
Pathological laughing/crying	Pain

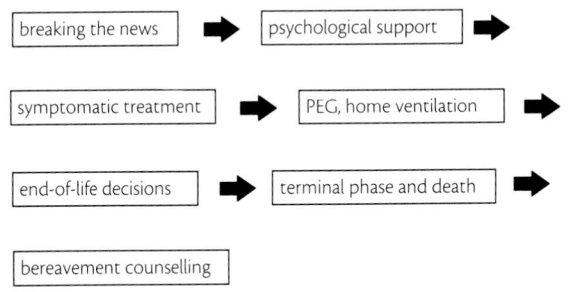

Figure. 12.5.1 The course of palliative care in ALS.

Table 12.5.4 Symptoms of chronic hypoventilation.

Daytime fatigue and sleepiness, concentration problems
Difficulty falling asleep, disturbed sleep, nightmares
Morning headache
Nervousness, tremor, increased sweating, tachycardia
Depression, anxiety
Tachypnoea, dyspnoea, phonation difficulties
Visible efforts of auxiliary respiratory muscles
Reduced appetite, weight loss, recurrent gastritis
Recurrent or chronic upper respiratory tract infections
Cyanosis, oedema
Vision disturbances, dizziness, syncope
Diffuse pain in head, neck, and extremities

(Fig. 12.5.1). Despite first attempts at establishing evidence-based guidelines, standards of palliative treatment in ALS are still largely based on expert opinion and differ between countries[1–3].

Palliative care in ALS involves a large number of different professionals (Table 12.5.3). In the UK, at least 75 per cent of inpatient palliative care/hospice units are involved in the care of patients with ALS[3]. This figure is lower (between 25 and 50 per cent) for the rest of Europe, no US data are currently available. Early and close cooperation between the neurologist and the local palliative care/hospice team can be of invaluable help for patients and family. Ideally, all members of the palliative care team should be trained and receive ongoing support and education in this area. A comprehensive volume on this subject has been published[4].

Breaking the news

This is a crucial step and the start of palliative care. The patient should dictate the pace and depth of the information flow, while the doctor retains the difficult task of responding appropriately to the patient's cues[5]. As many patients with ALS turn to alternative treatments[6], this topic should be discussed proactively in order to protect the patient from serious financial and/or medical risks, while preserving hope and maintaining trust in the patient–physician relationship.

At the onset of dyspnoea, symptoms of chronic nocturnal hypoventilation (see Table 12.5.4), or when the forced vital capacity (FVC) drops below 50 per cent, the patient should be offered information about the terminal phase, as most patients at this point fear that they will 'choke to death'. Describing the mechanism of terminal hypercapnic coma and the resulting peaceful death during sleep will relieve this fear in most patients[5].

At the same time, patients should be asked whether they would wish to be intubated and ventilated in the event of a terminal

respiratory failure. Patients who have been informed about the possible subsequent clinical course, which may end up in a 'locked-in' syndrome on an intensive care unit, will usually deny permission for such a procedure. This denial must be documented in writing by the physician and should be incorporated into an advance directive[7]. The consequences of such a decision must be discussed with the patient, family, and the primary physician. Advance directives should be reviewed at regular intervals, as ALS patients' preferences for life-sustaining treatments have been shown to change over time.

Symptom control

Muscle weakness should be managed by regular exercise, never to the point of fatigue, and by the use of appropriate aids (cane, ankle-foot-orthosis, wheelchair, aids for clothing and eating, etc.), in order to maintain as high as possible a degree of independence and mobility. Occasionally, a short-term (few weeks) increase of muscle strength may be achieved with pyridostigmine 40–60 mg tid. Because of its cholinergic side effects (e.g. diarrhoea), the medication should be stopped after a week if there is no subjective benefit.

Dysphagia should first be treated by an adjustment in diet consistency (recipe books for ALS patients are available from several lay associations, see below). Specific swallowing techniques (such as supraglottic swallowing) can help to prevent aspiration. When oral food intake becomes intolerable due to choking, or the calorie intake is insufficient (weight loss >10 per cent), it is best to perform a percutaneous endoscopic gastrostomy (PEG), which is usually very well tolerated, provided the vital capacity is >50 per cent at the time of introduction. As the mortality of the procedure increases with worsening of the pulmonary function, patient and family should be encouraged to make an early decision regarding PEG placement. It is important to remember that a PEG does not prevent aspiration pneumonia, which indeed is frequent if overfeeding by PEG occurs. A radiologically inserted gastrostomy may be an alternative in advanced disease[8].

Dysarthria can lead to a complete loss of oral communication abilities. Speech therapy is helpful at the beginning. In advanced cases, modern computer technology offers several options that enable even patients with almost total paresis of voluntary muscles

Table 12.5.3 Palliative care in ALS: who is involved?

Chaplain	Physical therapist
Counsellor	Physician
Dietitian	Psychologist
Hospice volunteers	Relatives
Lay associations	Social worker
Nurse	Speech therapist
Occupational therapist	Swallowing therapist

to communicate, e.g. via myoelectrically controlled switches. First attempts at directly exploiting brain electric currents to control computers have shown encouraging results[9].

Dyspnoea is the most severe symptom in ALS. At the onset of dyspnoea, chest physiotherapy is helpful. Dyspnoeic attacks usually have a pronounced anxiety component and are best managed by short-acting benzodiazepines (lorazepam SL 0.5–1 mg). In acute and chronic dyspnoea, the subjective feeling of shortness of breath is reduced by the administration of morphine (2.5–5 mg PO or 1–2 mg SC/IV q4h). Titration of the morphine dose against the clinical effect will almost never lead to a life-threatening respiratory depression[10].

Months to years before terminal respiratory failure symptoms of chronic nocturnal hypoventilation ensue, which may considerably hamper the patient's quality of life (Table 12.5.4). Non-invasive intermittent ventilation via mask (NIV) is an efficient and cost-effective means of alleviating these symptoms[11,12]. Patients and families should be informed about the temporary nature of the measure, which is primarily directed at improving quality of life, rather than prolonging life (as opposed to tracheostomy). The problems with mechanical ventilation are usually not related to cost or technical difficulties, but to the increasing care needs of the ventilated patients. A slow progression, good communication skills, mild bulbar involvement, a strong motivation on the patient's part, and a supportive family environment argue in favour of the initiation of NIV. To be effective, NIV needs to be administered for at least 4 h/day, most preferably at night[13]. It is very important to reassure the patients that, whenever they may decide to stop NIV, all necessary care and appropriate medication will be available to ensure a peaceful death. If a patient requests discontinuation of NIV, the physician has a legal and ethical duty to honour it and to provide appropriate medication to ensure a peaceful death[14].

Psychological symptoms. Most if not all patients with ALS undergo a phase of reactive depression after being told the diagnosis. Counselling is of paramount importance at this stage. Although full-fledged major depression according to DSM-IV criteria is infrequent (around 10 per cent), self-reported depressive symptoms have been described in 22–75 per cent of ALS patients[15]. Clinically significant depression should be looked for and treated at all disease stages. SSRIs are most frequently used; however, the old-fashioned amitriptyline has its advantages in ALS, as it may exert favourable effects on other symptoms such as drooling, emotional lability, and sleep disturbance. As the concordance of depression and distress levels between patients and caregivers is high, attention to the mental health of the caregiver may alleviate the patient's distress as well[16].

Sleep disorders are usually a consequence of the inability to change position during sleep. Psychological problems, muscle cramps, fasciculations, dysphagia, and dyspnoea can also impair sleep. Sedatives should be used sparingly, as they may impair residual muscle force.

Thick mucous secretions: this symptom, which results from a combination of diminished fluid intake and reduced coughing pressure, is difficult to treat. N-acetylcysteine is helpful only in a minority of cases. Suction is usually not fully effective unless performed via a tracheostomy. Physical therapy with vibration massage may be helpful in the initial stages. Both manually assisted coughing techniques and mechanical insufflation–exsufflation can assist in extracting excess mucus from the airway[17].

Pathological laughing/crying: this symptom is also referred to as 'pseudobulbar affect' and occurs in up to 50 per cent of patients. It is not a mood disorder, but rather an abnormal display of affect, which can be very disturbing for the patients in social situations. As this symptom is seldom volunteered, physicians should ask for it and point out that it responds well to medication (Table 12.5.5). A combination of dextromethorphan and quinidine has been recently shown to be effective in a randomized study, but further experience on the long-term side effects and tolerability is needed[18].

Other symptoms of ALS which can be relieved by appropriate medication include *muscle cramps*, *fasciculations*, *spasticity*, and *drooling*. Treatment options for these symptoms are shown in Table 12.5.5. For anti-spasticity drugs, the patient has to titrate the dose against the clinical effect, as a moderate degree of spasticity is usually better for mobility than a fully flaccid paresis. Dantrolene should not be used as first-line medication in ALS, because it enhances weakness; however, we have witnessed a case of extreme spasticity in the terminal phase, which could only be relieved by

Table 12.5.5 Symptomatic medication in ALS (in order of recommendation).

	Dosage*
Fasciculations and muscle cramps	
If mild:	
Magnesium	5 mmol qd–tid
Vitamin E	400 IU bid
If severe:	
Quinine sulphate	200 mg bid
Carbamazepine	200 mg bid
Phenytoin	100 mg qd–tid
Spasticity	
Baclofen	10–80 mg
Tizanidine	6–24 mg
Memantine	10–60 mg
Tetrazepam	100–200 mg
Drooling	
Glycopyrrolate	0.1–0.2 mg SC/IM tid
Transdermal hyoscine patches	1–2 patches
Amitriptyline	10–150 mg
Atropine/benztropine	0.25–0.75 mg/1–2 mg
Clonidine	0.15–0.3 mg
Pathologic laughing/crying	
Amitriptyline	10–150 mg
Fluvoxamine	100–200 mg
Lithium carbonate	400–800 mg
L-dopa	500–600 mg

* Usual range of adult daily dosage; some patients may require higher dosages, e.g. of antispastic medication.

high doses of IV dantrolene. If severe spasticity is a problem earlier in the disease, intrathecal baclofen may be an option. For patients with therapy-refractory drooling, botulinum toxin injections[19], or irradiation of the salivary glands[20] may be considered.

Constipation. Lack of exercise can promote the development of constipation in patients with ALS. The first step is dietary measures (foods with high fibre content such as 'power pudding'—equal measure of prunes, prune juice, bran, and apple sauce). Care should be taken to ensure adequate fluid intake, as dysphagia-induced dehydration may worsen constipation. The medication should be reviewed, as muscle relaxants, sedatives, and anti-cholinergics reduce bowel mobility. Mild laxative therapy should be prophylactically initiated in bed-ridden patients and in those receiving opioids.

Pain. Up to 73 per cent of ALS patients complain of pain. Although ALS itself does not usually involve sensory fibres, musculoskeletal pain often arises in the later stages of the disease as a result of stress on the bones and joints which have lost their protective muscular ensheathment due to atrophy. In addition, muscle contractures and joint stiffness (e.g. frozen shoulder) may be painful. These symptoms are usually best treated with non-steroidal anti-inflammatory drugs (NSAIDs) and physiotherapy. Another cause of pain in ALS is skin pressure pain, due to immobility. Special attention must be given to the nursing care, which requires frequent changes in the patient's position, both at night and during daytime. If NSAIDs are insufficient, opioid analgesics should be started.

Gastro-oesophageal reflux disease may occur in ALS due to diaphragmatic weakness involving the lower oesophageal sphincter. Particular care is needed when starting a patient on PEG because of possible overfeeding which may lead to gastro-oesophageal reflux and even aspiration. Treatment includes peristaltic agents (e.g. metoclopramide) and antacids.

Dependent oedema of the hands and feet occurs in weak limbs because of reduced muscle pump activity. Limb elevation, physiotherapy, and compression hose are helpful. If pain develops or swelling persists despite prolonged elevation, a deep venous thrombosis should be ruled out.

Urinary urgency and frequency in the absence of urinary tract infections can be due to spasticity of the bladder and respond favourably to oxybutinin (2.5–5 mg qd–tid).

Jaw quivering or clenching may develop in patients with pseudobulbar involvement in response to noxious stimuli such as cold, anxiety, or pain, and is relieved by benzodiazepines (e.g. lorazepam SL or clonazepam).

Laryngospasm (a sudden reflex closure of the vocal chords) can cause panic due to a sensation of choking. Several types of stimuli (e.g. emotions, strong flavours or smells, cold air, fluid aspiration, sinus drainage, or gastro-oesophageal reflux) may provoke this symptom, which usually resolves spontaneously within a few seconds. Repeated swallowing while breathing through the nose can accelerate resolution. Patients also benefit from reassurance and education about this distressing symptom. H_1 or H_2 blocking agents (anti-histamines or antacids) may also be helpful.

Nasal congestion in bulbar patients with a weakening of the nasopharyngeal muscles can be helped by elevating the nasal bridge with nasal tape and application of topical decongestants.

Psychosocial care

According to data from the USA, a large proportion of patients with ALS show an interest in physician-assisted suicide, which in our experience is often the result of the fear of becoming a burden to their families, or of a sense of hopelessness and loss of meaning in life. Although suicidal actions are relatively rare in ALS[21], 20 per cent of ALS patients in the Netherlands have been reported to die through active euthanasia or physician-assisted suicide[22]. When asked about the most important aspects of their quality of life (QOL), 100 per cent of the patients mentioned their family, while health-related items were nominated in about half of the cases[23]. Correspondingly, several studies indicate that QOL in ALS depends on factors other than strength and physical function[24]. In ALS, the burden of the relatives often exceeds that of the patients and deserves particular attention. The physician must be particularly sensitive to the needs and fears of the patients' children, and the importance of helping patients in their role as parents. Assessing for hopelessness and instituting early non-pharmacological interventions aimed at maintaining hope and a sense of meaning in life is likely to be the best way of preventing wishes for hastened death in ALS. Patients' associations (see note below) may provide invaluable help and assistance, and should be involved in patient care from the very beginning.

Spiritual care and bereavement

The role of spiritual care is often underestimated. Available data indicate that spirituality or religiousness may affect the use of PEG and NIV in ALS, and may be a source of comfort to the patients[25]. Cases of patients whose spiritual practice greatly enhanced their ability to cope with ALS have been reported[26]. Spiritual care is not limited to patients, but should encompass the whole family as a means of preventing complicated bereavement, which may be particularly severe in ALS families. It is important to acknowledge that the process of bereavement in ALS actually starts immediately after the diagnosis is communicated, in the form of so-called 'anticipatory grief', and that callous delivery of the diagnosis may affect the psychological adjustment to bereavement.

Terminal phase

A retrospective survey of 171 patients with ALS showed that around 90 per cent of the patients died peacefully, mostly in their sleep, and none of the patients choked to death[21]. If patients with ALS are not mechanically ventilated, the death process usually begins with the patients slipping from sleep into coma due to increasing hypercapnia. If restlessness or signs of dyspnoea develop, morphine should be administered beginning with 2.5–5 mg PO, SC, or IV every 4 h (if necessary in combination with an anti-emetic). As morphine is not an anxiolytic drug, if anxiety is present, it should be treated with lorazepam SL (beginning with 1–2.5 mg) or midazolam PO/SC (beginning with 1–2 mg). The dosage of morphine and anxiolytics should be increased until satisfactory symptom control is achieved. According to a recent meta-analysis, there is virtually no risk of shortening life through these measures[10].

Most patients with ALS wish to die at home. This can often best be achieved through enrolment of the patient in a hospice or other palliative care programme. It is advisable for the physician to initiate contact with the hospice institution, where available, well in advance of the terminal phase.

Note: A list of ALS patients' associations worldwide can be found under www.alsmndalliance.org; a list of ALS centres worldwide is at www.wfnals.org

Stroke

Stroke is a heterogeneous group of diseases including brain infarction (84 per cent), intracerebral bleeding (7 per cent), subarachnoid haemorrhage (7 per cent), and various rare entities like vasculitis, dissections, and sinus thrombosis (1.4 per cent). Typical symptoms include paresis (mostly as hemiparesis), hypoesthesia, hemianopia, diplopia, visual loss, headache, acute vomiting, aphasia, and loss of consciousness. The aetiology of brain infarction includes emboli originating from the heart, aorta or major brain supplying vessels, haemodynamic changes from severe stenosis or occlusions, *in situ* thrombosis of intracranial arteries and microangiopathy caused by diabetes or hypertension. The long-term prognosis following a stroke is rather poor: 20 per cent of patients die within 1 month, a further 10 per cent within a year, and another 5 per cent within 2 years. In addition, up to 25 per cent of patients develop post-stroke dementia, and only about 25 per cent survive without disability. At least 12 per cent of stroke survivors will be admitted to institutional care within a year.

Prevalence and incidence of stroke varies between different populations and age is the major determinant. The incidence in 45–54-year-olds is about 0.8/1000 rising to 9.4/1000 in 75- to 84-year-olds. The lowest death rates are found in USA, Canada, Australia, and Switzerland (30/100 000/year). Western European countries show rates around 60/100 000, while eastern European countries have extremely high death rates from stroke (up to 250/100 000).

About 30–50 per cent of all stroke victims present with a so-called stroke-in-evolution with progression after arrival at the hospital. In the setting of an acute stroke unit about 7–11 per cent develop a severe clinical worsening with the urgent need to transfer them to an ICU. In acute stroke treated with thrombolysis, clinical deterioration is often related to secondary haemorrhagic transformation or the development of brain swelling with an increase in intracranial pressure.

Predictors of functional recovery following stroke include age, previous stroke, urinary continence, consciousness at onset, disorientation in time and place, admission activities of daily living score, and level of social support[27]. Many of these factors (e.g. unconsciousness and hemiplegia or incontinence) are interdependent and are by themselves good indicators of death. Severe strokes appear to be more common among older patients, in which significant co-morbidity is likely to be present.

Two different epidemiological trends exist: the growing ageing population with a rise in stroke incidence and severity, and the decline in stroke incidence and death rate caused by lifestyle factors and healthier behaviour. On the whole, more strokes and more severe strokes are to be expected in the coming decades, which will increase the demand for palliative care in these patients.

The most common types of stroke with a fatal outcome include[28]: *malignant middle cerebral artery infarction*, which may be amenable to decompressive neurosurgery; *basilar artery thrombosis/severe brain stem infarction*, where local intraarterial thrombolysis can reduce mortality to 50 per cent or less; and *severe intracerebral or subarachnoid haemorrhage*, with a mortality around 50 per cent.

The *locked-in-syndrome* is a severe form of brainstem infarction where the patients are tetraplegic but fully awake. The prognosis is bad for recovery, but survival may be as long as 2–18 years. The key issues for long-term survivors are means of communication and the emotional and physical stress for the patient's caregivers. Promising results have been obtained using EEG-recorded potentials to operate communicating devices[29].

Symptom control

Currently, there is very limited data on the palliative care needs in stroke and little is known about the extent to which hospice, hospital- or community-based specialist palliative care units are involved in the care of these patients. However, the UK National Clinical Guidelines for Stroke recommends that all stroke patients should have access to specialist palliative care expertise when needed.

A population-based survey involving 237 patients who died from stroke showed that 65 per cent were reported to experience pain, 57 per cent low mood, 56 per cent urinary incontinence, and 51 per cent confusion. Pain control was judged to be inadequate in 37 per cent and in 25 per cent there was a feeling of insufficient choice about treatments and interventions[30]. A recently published international review of the literature found only seven papers that look directly at the palliative care needs of stroke patients[31].

Loss of consciousness

A variety of stroke syndromes result in reduced levels of consciousness or alertness, which may progress into coma. This should not, however, lead to an assumption that these patients are not suffering. Non-verbal and physiological clues, such as grimacing, blushing, stiff neck, or increased respiratory rate, blood pressure, or pulse frequency may be indicators of distress. Adequate nursing care and analgesic medication are required, especially in situations where a cause for pain is evident, for example large intracranial haemorrhage.

Communication

Communication is often hampered by aphasia and/or dysarthria in patients who suffer strokes involving the dominant (usually the left) temporo-parietal hemisphere. Aphasia may significantly impact on palliative care. Kehayia *et al.* found that aphasic stroke patients received less pain medication than those without aphasia[32]. The patients' communication deficits may be further compromised due to accompanying neuropsychological deficits such as apraxia, agnosia, neglect, and impaired visuo-spatial orientation. However, it is important always to work on the assumption that the patients understand everything that is being said to and around them.

Stroke patients and their families are eager for information about their illness and its prognosis, while studies indicate that health professionals tend to avoid these subjects. Open and ongoing dialogue with patients' relatives in severe stroke is essential, as health-care professionals will be reliant on their knowledge of the patient's previous functional status and probable wishes for care.

Incontinence and constipation

Urinary and faecal incontinence are common in stroke patient and are associated with high mortality and morbidity. Impaired communication and reduced mobility may contribute to the development of incontinence, which can reduce morale and thus influence recovery. The management of urinary incontinence with catheter facilitates nursing care, but carries a risk of infection and should be restricted to severely impaired patients. Faecal incontinence is a very distressing symptom for patients and relatives. Poor management of faecal incontinence may lead to skin damage and thus to pain and discomfort. Constipation should be expected and anticipated after stroke, due to immobility and decreased oral intake. Anti-cholinergic and opioid medication may worsen constipation. Prophylaxis includes increased fluid intake, high-fibre diet, and laxatives.

Nutrition

In the acute and sub-acute phases of stroke, dysphagia occurs in about half of all patients; about two-thirds of aspirations are 'silent'. About half of dysphagic stroke patients die or recover spontaneously within 2 weeks of stroke. A recently published London-based study of first stroke patients found that dysphagia was associated with both more severe stroke and poorer long-term outcome[33].

Predominant dysphagic symptoms after stroke are delayed pharyngeal swallow, disturbed lingual movements, and reduced tongue base reaction. In addition, stroke patients may eat less due to facial weakness, poor arm function, and fatigue. Functional swallowing therapy includes specific exercises and techniques such as supraglottic swallowing, which however require intact cognition and good co-operation. Malnutrition is present in up to 40 per cent of stroke patients and can result in reduced muscle strength, lower resistance to infection, and impaired wound healing. A naso-gastric tube (NG) for feeding is uncomfortable and often dislodges. The alternative is a PEG tube, inserted directly into the stomach. A controlled trial of PEG and NG feeding found greater mortality and decreased nutritional intake among NG patients[34]. However, PEG feeding has also been associated with high mortality rates and does not prevent aspirations, thought to be a common cause of pneumonia in stroke patients. Results from a large international multi-centre randomized trial of feeding policies for patients admitted to hospital following stroke suggests that supplemented diets are probably of no benefit following stroke in previously well-nourished patients who are able to swallow[35].

Early tube feeding may substantially reduce the risk of dying in stroke patients with dysphagia; however, improved survival rates may mean that more people survive their stroke with poor outcome. The question of whether to feed poor prognosis stroke patients can be a crucial issue with a strong emotional impact on the family. Every effort should be made to determine what the patient's own wishes would be in the current situation. Involvement of a palliative care specialist may be helpful at this time, especially if there are disagreements between health professionals and family members or within the health care team.

Pain

Pain in stroke patients may be directly due to the brain lesion, the result of pressure sores or contractures or stem from unrelated chronic conditions such as diabetic neuropathy or arthritis. Between 18 and 23 per cent of stroke patients suffer post-stroke headaches, while shoulder hand–syndrome occurs in up to 30 per cent. The latter begins with pain and oedema of the shoulder, wrist and hand and progresses to trophic skin changes, muscular atrophy, and contractures. Treatment with a rapidly tapering short course of oral steroids was effective in 86 per cent of patients in a controlled study and prevention of shoulder trauma in the acute phase reduced the frequency of shoulder–hand syndrome from 27 to 8 per cent[36].

Eight per cent of patients suffer from 'central post-stroke pain', a neuropathic pain syndrome which is thought to arise from the vascular lesion and is characterized by pain the corresponding body part. This pain is particularly resistant to opioids and difficult to treat; amitriptyline and lamotrigine have shown benefit in controlled trials.

Depression, anxiety, and confusion

A Scandinavian study of 486 stroke patients found major depression in 26 per cent of and minor depression in 14 per cent. The only predictors of post-stroke depression were dependency in daily life and pre-stroke depression[37]. Post-stroke depression has both organic and psychological causes, is generally under-diagnosed but may be relieved with appropriate psychological and medical therapies. Serotonin uptake inhibitors are usually preferable to tricyclics for these patients. Anxiety disorders have been detected in 28 per cent of stroke patients in the acute phases. They correlate with depression and may worsen its prognosis. Disorientation and confusion are common after stroke and agitation may be severe enough to warrant sedation.

Caregivers

Most informal care of people following stroke is provided by spouses. The level of care needed is predicted by the severity of stroke and the patient's ability to undertake activities of daily living. The 'burden' experienced by informal carers is also associated with the carers' personal characteristics. Stroke survivors living in the community are generally under-served by both health and social services and may have unmet psychosocial and health-care needs, both of which increase the load for informal carers[38]. Relatives who are involved in end-of-life decision-making may experience considerable distress and anxiety, and may benefit from counselling and bereavement support.

Care in the last days of life

Good supportive nursing care of patients dying from stroke is essential. The Liverpool Care Pathway has been successfully used in managing the care of dying stroke patients over a longer period of time[39]. However, its use did not impact on next of kin's awareness that the patient had entered a dying phase. This may be crucial as timely transfer from the acute care unit to a more peaceful environment or home setting should ideally be considered and discussed with the family to help ensure the patient dies in their preferred place of care or failing this in the most appropriate place of care.

Multiple sclerosis

Multiple sclerosis (MS) is the most frequent inflammatory demyelinating disorder of the central nervous system. The exact cause and pathogenesis are still unknown. Several factors are discussed such as genetic influence, environmental factors, and most importantly autoimmune mechanisms. There are at least four pathological entities with different pathomechanisms which clinically are subsumed under the term MS. Not only demyelination but also clear axonal damages in the grey matter are now recognized features of MS. New diagnostic criteria set up by an international consensus group now allow the diagnosis of MS even after a single clinical episode[40].

The last 15 years have been dominated by the advent of effective immunomodulatory treatment options such as interferon beta, copolymer-1, mitoxantrone, or most recently natalizumab[41]. The beneficial effect of these drugs, however, is still relatively modest, e.g. reduction of relapse rate by one-third, or delaying the necessity of a wheel-chair by 6–9 months. These advances—after decades without useful treatment options—have in some respect overshadowed the aspect of symptomatic and palliative care for patients with MS. Although MS is not a progressive lethal disorder in the strict palliative care definition, several aspects of palliative care are important for MS and should be respected from the initial telling of the diagnosis until the patient's death.

When communicating the diagnosis, the fact that MS—in general—does not reduce life expectancy, will be important to the patient. However, it should be known to the treating physician that patients with MS are at increased risk for suicide, especially within the first 5 years of diagnosis. Therefore, care must be taken to detect and treat reactive depression in the initial stages. Importantly, treatment with interferon-beta may exacerbate depressive symptoms. The wish for active euthanasia is frequent in patients with MS. In the Netherlands, euthanasia is the cause of death in one out of 20 MS patients. Risk factors for suicide or the wish for euthanasia are not so much physical symptoms, but rather loneliness, unemployment, and lack of psychosocial support or spiritual background. Therefore, from the beginning, introducing any form of help—for instance via the national MS societies (e.g. www.ifmss.org.uk)—is an essential part of palliative care.

It is a frequent experience of nurses caring for MS patients in nursing homes that many of the patients tend to overestimate their abilities which may lead to tensions between the patient and the team. On the other hand, many patients with MS perceive a reduced quality of life which is dependent on the effect of their disease in the physical, cognitive, and psychosocial domains (see Table 12.5.6)[42]. Symptoms perceived by the professionals are not necessarily the most disabling to the patients. The physician and MS sufferer J.K. Wolf considers depressive symptoms to be the most disabling, spasticity to be the most frequent, bladder symptoms to be the most confusing, and bowel symptoms to be the most humiliating[43].

Table 12.5.6 Three domains of multiple sclerosis care.

Physical	Cognitive	Psychosocial
Motor function	Memory	Mood
Coordination	Thought processing	Partnership
Sensory function	Attention	Family
Vision	Judgement	Stress
Gaze	Decision-making	Friendships
Speech	Concentration	Work
Swallowing	Abstract reasoning	Money
Bladder	Orientation (person, time, space, situation)	Spiritual
Bowel		
Sexual		

More than 50 per cent of patients severely affected by MS suffer from six symptoms or more at the same time[44] For optimal symptom control, a multi-disciplinary team is necessary which includes general practitioner, neurologist, urologist, psychiatrist, pain physician, neuroradiologist, nurse, physiotherapist, social worker, occupational therapist, psychologist, speech therapist, clergy, and lay organizations. MS neurologists perceive a lack of professional help for their patients, with main shortages in psychology, occupational therapy, speech therapy, and palliative care[45]. Loss and change is the most prevalent emotional experience in MS patients[46]. This combination suggests that offering a complementary palliative care service may be of great value for these patients and their families[47].

Once advanced neurological deficits have accumulated, mortality is increased four times. Causes of death are complications of chronic illness in about half of the patients, i.e. pneumonia, pulmonary embolism, renal insufficiency, or urinary tract infections. Other causes of death are tumours (16 per cent), suicide (15 per cent), heart attack (11 per cent), or stroke (5 per cent).[48] In patients with advanced disease who repeatedly develop potentially lethal complications, a shift in the goals of care may be appropriate. To this aim, DNR orders must be discussed early with the patient and relatives. Decisions should be recorded in the medical notes, and if possible a disease-specific advance directive should be set up[49].

Symptom control

Symptoms in MS may arise as a direct (primary) or indirect (secondary) consequence of the loss of myelin and axons (see Table 12.5.7). Tertiary symptoms depend on the progression of the disease. A multitude of therapy options are available to MS patients, even in the later stages of their disease when immunomodulatory treatment options are no longer indicated[50].

Oculomotor disturbances: an acquired nystagmus may be ameliorated using either the GABA-B-agonist baclofen

Table 12.5.7 Symptoms in multiple sclerosis.

Primary	Secondary	Tertiary
Weakness	Disuse weakness	Psychological issues
Numbness	Bladder infections	Reactive depression
Paresthesias	Pressure sores	Social isolation
Dysbalance	Demineralization of bone	Unemployment
Visual loss	Fractures	Role changes
Incontinence	Contractures	Financial issues
Sexual problems	Falls	Divorce
Cognitive impairment	Injuries	Decreased independence
Dysarthria	Aspiration pneumonia decreased activities of daily living	Denial
Dysphasia		Bereavement
Dysphagia		
Epileptic seizures		
Pain		

(orally, 5–10 mg thrice daily), the GABA-A agonist clonazepam (3×0.5 mg/day) or—especially in acquired fixation pendular nystagmus—the NMDA antagonist memantine (40–60 mg/day), or alternatively gabapentin (600–1500 mg/day)[51].

Tremor: in some patients with MS-related tremor, wrist weights may be helpful. Despite early reports of the beneficial effect of the 5-HT$_3$-antagonist ondansetron, a further small study has found no effect in MS patients with cerebellar tremor[52]. Propranolol (3–4×10–20 mg/day), isoniazid (800–1200 mg/day distributed over 3–4 doses), or clonazepam (2–4 mg/day, starting at 0.5 mg/day) may be tried. In very severe cases, tremor may be ameliorated using deep brain stimulation which can be performed at specialized centres.

Spasticity: the mainstay of treatment is regular and intensive physiotherapy. In a Cochrane review, no specific anti-spastic drug could be identified as being superior over the others due to insufficient data[53]. Therefore, one should use the drug which one is familiar with. To avoid side effects, it is important to start any anti-spastic medication at low doses, slowly titrating against the clinical effect. If overdosed, patients will complain of increasing weakness. Drug options include baclofen (orally, 3–4×5–25 mg; in severe cases, intrathecal application may be necessary), tizanidine (3×2–8 mg), gabapentin (3×600–900 mg), dantrolene (2×25–200 mg), memantine (2–3×10–20 mg), tetrazepam (1×50–4×100 mg), and other benzodiazepines. Cannabinoids may be helpful in some patients, as may be local botulinum toxin injections in cases with focal spasticity; both should only be used in specialized centres[50].

Urinary symptoms: patients may develop a hyperreflexia of the detrusor muscle, if the lesion is above the sacral micturition centre. A pragmatic approach includes counselling for adequate fluid intake (more in the morning, less in the afternoon) and if possible passing water every 2–4 h. Medication is based on anti-cholinergics such as oxybutinin (2–3×5 mg), propiverin (3×10 mg/day), or imipramine (3×10–25 mg/day). If nocturnal incontinence is still present, desmopressin (spray) at night might be very helpful. If the lesion lies between the sacral and pontine micturition centre, a dyssynergia of detrusor and sphincter muscles may result. Urge incontinence and incomplete emptying of the bladder are the clinical hallmarks. In most patients—especially if the residual urine volume lies above 100 ml—intermittent catheter use will be necessary. Alpha-blockers (phenoxybenzamine, 2×10–3×20 mg/day), anti-spasticity drugs (see above) or botulinum toxin injection into the external sphincter may be helpful[50].

Pain occurs in 50–60 per cent of MS patients, with increasing prevalence over time. Pains may be directly MS-related, an indirect sequel of other MS symptoms such as spasticity, they may follow drug treatment (interferons), or may be MS-independent. Causes of acute pain include trigeminal neuralgia, paroxysmal dysaesthetic pain, and painful tonic spasms. Trigeminal neuralgia may be the first manifestation of MS and is clinically indistinguishable from the idiopathic form. Lhermitte's sign, the most common form of paroxysmal dysaesthetic pain, may occur spontaneously or in response to triggers such as movement (particularly neck flexion) or tactile stimuli. In painful tonic spasms (sometimes referred to as 'brainstem seizures'), paroxysmal activation of the pyramidal tract leads to sudden bursts of spasticity in the upper or lower extremities, or the whole body, without loss of consciousness but with severe pain. Paroxysmal manifestations probably arise through the loss of the insulating myelin sheath which renders axons susceptible to uncontrolled spreading of potentials across the whole pathway ('ephaptic activation'). They respond well to anti-convulsant treatment (carbamazepine and gabapentin)[50]. For painful tonic spasms, benzodiazepines, and acetazolamide may also be effective.

Headache is frequent in MS and any headache type may be encountered. Optic neuritis may produce retro-orbital pain aggravated by eye movement. A case of cluster headache attributed to MS-induced demyelination has been reported[54].

Chronic pain in MS occurs as dysaesthetic central pain, low back pain, and painful leg spasms due to spasticity. Central dysaesthetic pain arises through lesions of the spinothalamic tract and is associated with sensory abnormalities. It is usually described as a burning pain in the legs, but may affect trunk and arms as well. It may also be aching, stabbing, or squeezing, and is best treated with anti-convulsants and analgesics for neuropathic pain. For therapy-refractory cases, intrathecal analgesia (e.g. bupivacaine)[55] can be considered. Low back pain is related to degenerative changes and scoliosis of the lumbosacral spine, and is aggravated by prolonged sitting. It may overlap with spasticity-related pain. Visceral pain in MS can be due to constipation, bladder spasms, or bladder distension.

Fatigue: a very common symptom in MS, it probably is also one of the most under-treated ones. If the fatigue is part of a depressive syndrome, this must be treated first. Cooling of the body or of extremities may be helpful[50]. For fatigue, the indirect dopaminergic agonist and NMDA antagonist amantadine (e.g. 2×100 mg) has been in use for some time with good effect. Alternatively, the potassium channel blockers 4-aminopyridine[56] or the anti-narcoleptic drug modafinil[57] have been shown to have some efficacy in this regard.

Psychobehavioural and cognitive symptoms: adjustment to the disease progression can be difficult and require psychotherapeutic intervention. Denial is very frequent in late stage MS. It is predominantly organically determined leading to reduced compliance and problems with the caregivers. Depression is frequent in MS (40–50 per cent) and is related to the amount of cerebral pathology and steroid treatment, but not to disease duration or disability. It is often under-recognized and under-treated, SSRI's are the drugs of choice because of their good tolerability. Disorders of emotional expression (pathological laughing and crying, emotional incontinence) occur in 10–25 per cent of patients and may respond to amitriptyline or SSRIs. Cognitive deficits can be detected in 40–60 per cent of patients and are severe in 21–33 per cent. Management includes education of patient and relatives, as well as cognitive retraining and learning of compensatory strategies. Personality changes may manifest as irritability, apathy, or disinhibition. They are often cause of great distress to the family and require careful psychosocial intervention[58].

Parkinson's disease and progressive supranuclear palsy

Parkinson's disease and progressive supranuclear palsy (PSP) are examples of degenerative neurological diseases with a long chronic course, which not necessarily lies within the strict definition of palliative care. However, no curative approaches are currently available, and during the course of these diseases a multitude of symptoms occur which affect the quality of life of the patients and their relatives. Care requires an expert multi-professional and interdisciplinary approach. At some point, the shift of goals of care will also be relevant to patients with these disorders. This may be the case once the patient, despite optimal therapy, becomes more and more disabled and persistent neuropsychiatric problems arise. Whether under the current organization of care this is recognized in time and handled according to the established palliative care principles may be doubted[59]. Mortality is about twice the normal. Usually the patients die in nursing homes or in general hospitals. There is little published information about the way these patients die. In most cases, this will probably be due to complications of the longstanding chronic disease such as bronchopneumonia or aspiration pneumonia (especially in PSP) or complications from falls. Currently, many palliative care programmes decline to take care of these patients as it is difficult to predict prognosis. The onset of dysphagia has been shown to predict a survival time of 15–24 months in several movement disorders including Parkinson's disease and PSP[60]. Evidence from a recent study indicates that palliative care may be very beneficial for these patients and their families[61].

Parkinson's disease

Parkinson's syndrome is a clinical diagnosis consisting of the classical triad of tremor, akinesia, and rigidity. 'Idiopathic' Parkinson's disease is highly likely if there are no obvious causes (such as drug-induced Parkinson's syndrome) and there is a good response to L-dopa therapy. L-dopa mainly improves akinesia but does not have a positive effect on many other symptoms (Table 12.5.8). The long-term use of L-dopa also leads to problems such as drug-induced fluctuations (on–off phenomenon), dyskinesias, or neuropsychological problems. Therefore, in the early stages of the disease, an L-dopa sparing approach should be taken and treatment should be started with dopaminergic agonists, especially in younger patients. Patients with long off time during the day or with severe dyskinesias should be evaluated for deep brain stimulation.

Symptom control

An essential part of palliative care in Parkinson's disease is good nursing care. Skin care (complicated by the typical seborrhoic dermatitis), positioning, constipation, and oral hygiene are only a few examples of the nursing needs of these patients.

Motor symptoms: balance, gait and 'freezing' attacks may be ameliorated by ergonomic advice and physiotherapy (educating about cueing tricks, use of external or internal pacing). Acute episodes of hypokinesia usually respond to sc administration of apomorphine. Hyperkinesias—which generally are better tolerated—may still be very burdensome to some patients. In hyperkinetic crises potent neuroleptic drugs (e.g. risperidone) may be necessary. Contractures may be difficult to prevent. Recently, the use of botulinum toxin has been a very helpful addition to the therapeutic spectrum. Severe cases may require surgical tenotomies.

Pain: although not intuitively obvious, pain is a very common problem in the end-stages of Parkinson's disease[62]. It may arise from stiffness, rigidity, or dystonic spasms. Uncomfortable posture as well as constipation may contribute to pain. If these

Table 12.5.8 Symptoms of Parkinson's disease.

Parkinsonian triad	Akinesia
	Rigor
	Tremor
Other symptoms	Anxiety
	Confusion
	Constipation
	Dementia
	Depression
	Drooling
	Dysarthria
	Dyskinesia
	Dysphagia
	Dystonia
	Falls
	Freezing attacks
	Fixed stooped posture
	Hallucinations
	Immobility
	Incontinence
	Orthostatic hypotension
	Pain
	Postural imbalance
	Seborrhoea
	Sleep attacks
	Weakness

cannot be alleviated by treating the underlying cause (e.g. with L-dopa, laxatives, nursing care), analgesics according to the WHO ladder should be used. When treating opioid-induced nausea and vomiting, the possible Parkinson-aggravating side-effects of some neuroleptics (haloperidol and prochlorperazine) should be kept in mind. Anti-emetics such as domperidone, which does not block cerebral dopamine receptors, may be preferable.

Neuropsychiatric symptoms: depression is a frequent symptom in Parkinson's disease and is often overlooked. Confusion and hallucinations may occur as part of the disease process or may be induced by dopaminergic drugs. The drugs used must be reviewed and dopaminergic or anti-cholinergic drugs reduced where possible. If required, atypical neuroleptics such as quetiapine should be used instead of haloperidol. Development of dementia is frequent in late stages, and usually causes severe psychosocial problems. The ensuing reduction in competence should be anticipated by the early introduction of advance directives.

Progressive supranuclear palsy

Progressive supranuclear palsy (PSP) is a rare and fatal neurodegenerative disorder, which is frequently under-recognized.

PSP is referred to as Parkinson-Plus syndrome because of the associated clinical features but exhibits distinctive pathological characteristics, poor response to Parkinson's medication and a poorer prognosis. The course of PSP is usually rapidly progressive with a median survival time of 9 years. Patients typically present with loss of balance and unexplained falls. An abnormality of the extraocular eye movements, known as supranuclear gaze palsy, is the classical symptom. Many patients report dizziness. The facial expression has been described as the appearance of sustained surprise or stone face, due to contracted facial muscles. The patient and the family should be educated about the progression of PSP early in its course. Advance directives and living will are important issues, but often not discussed with the patients.

Symptom control

As PSP is more rapidly progressive than Parkinson's disease with not only motor symptoms but also neuropsychiatric symptoms like slow informational processing, angry outbursts and dementia, multi-disciplinary treatment approaches are needed. Nursing care and home support groups play an important role.

Motor symptoms: dopaminergic medication may offer some relief at the onset of the disease. The most common drugs used in PSP are carbidopa/levodopa, amantadine, imipramine, and selegiline. Zolpidem has been reported to improve eye movements, but benefit is brief and sedation is likely[63]. With the progression of the disease the effect of these drugs is reduced and they may be withdrawn. Rigidity of the neck muscles and the extremities is often present. Some patients develop blepharospasm or eyelid apraxia and botulinum toxin injections may be necessary. The frequent falls can cause serious injury and therefore gait training is important. Additionally, a helmet for the head may be necessary, as well as and preventive measures aimed at avoiding or buffering falls (e.g. transfer belt, grab bars).

Pain: although systematic research is lacking, pain is a common problem in PSP patients. Most common are neck and back pain. Compared with Parkinson's disease, it arises from stiffness, rigidity or dystonic spasms. If local treatment of dystonic muscles with botulinum toxin fails, analgesics should be prescribed according to the WHO ladder.

Dysphagia and dysarthria are linked to severe neuronal damage within the brainstem and its connection to higher brain centres. A combination of slowed reflexes and dystonia places the patient at risk of choking and aspiration[64]. As in ALS, when oral food intake becomes burdensome, it is best to perform a PEG.

Neuropsychiatric symptoms: personality and mood changes are common in PSP patients. Emotional incontinence with sudden bouts of crying or laughing may occur. With progressive disease patients develop subcortical dementia characterized by mental slowing, language difficulties, impaired memory, apathy, and irritability. Although cholinergic deficits are thought to underlie the postural instability and cognitive impairment of PSP, trials of cholinergic agonists and cholinesterase inhibitors have failed to show improvement[65].

Note: More information on the disease can be found at: www.pspeur.org

References

1. Andersen, P.M., Borasio, G.D., Dengler, R. *et al.* (2005). EFNS task force on Management of Amyotrophic Lateral Sclerosis: Guidelines for diagnosing and clinical care of patients and relatives. An evidence-based review with Good Practice Points. *European Journal of Neurology*, **12**, 921–8.

2. Simmons, Z. (2005). Management strategies for patients with amyotrophic lateral sclerosis from diagnosis through death. *Neurologist*, **11**, 257–70.

3. Borasio, G.D., Shaw, P.J., Hardiman, O. *et al.* (2001). Standards of palliative care for patients with amyotrophic lateral sclerosis: results of a European survey. *Amyotrophic Lateral Sclerosis & Other Motor Neuron Disorders*, **2**, 159–64.

4. Oliver, D., Borasio, G.D., and Walsh, D. (eds.) (2006). *Palliative care in amyotrophic lateral sclerosis – from diagnosis to bereavement*, 2nd edition. Oxford University Press, Oxford.

5. Borasio, G.D., Sloan, R., Pongratz, D.E. (1998). Breaking the news in amyotrophic lateral sclerosis. *Journal of Neurological Science*, **160**, 127–33.

6. Wasner, M., Klier, H., and Borasio, G.D. (2001). The use of alternative medicine by patients with amyotrophic lateral sclerosis. *Journal of Neurological Science*, **191**, 151–4.

7. Borasio, G.D., Voltz, R. (2006). Advance directives. In *Palliative care in amyotrophic lateral sclerosis* (eds. D. Oliver, G.D. Borasio, and D. Walsh), pp. 55–61. Oxford University Press, Oxford.

8. Chio, A., Galletti, R., Finocchiaro, C. *et al.* (2004). Percutaneous radiological gastrostomy: a safe and effective method of nutritional tube placement in advanced ALS. *Journal of Neurology, Neurosurgery Psychiatry*, **75**, 645–7.

9. Kubler, A., Nijboer, F., Mellinger, J. *et al.* (2005). Patients with ALS can use sensorimotor rhythms to operate a brain-computer interface. *Neurology*, **64**, 1775–7.

10. Sykes, N. and Thorns, A. (2003). The use of opioids and sedatives at the end of life. *Lancet Oncology*, **4**, 312–8.

11. Bourke, S., Tomlinson, T., Williams, T. *et al.* (2006). Effects of non-invasive ventilation on survival and quality of life in patients with amyotrophic lateral sclerosis, a randomised controlled trial. *Lancet Neurol*, **5**, 140–7.

12. Mustfa, N., Walsh, E., Bryant, V. *et al.* (2006). The effect of non-invasive ventilation on ALS patients and their caregivers. *Neurology*, **66**, 1211–7.

13. Kleopa, K.A., Sherman, M., Neal, B. *et al.* (1999). Bipap improves survival and rate of pulmonary function decline in patients with ALS. *Journal of Neurological Science*, **164**, 82–8.

14. Borasio, G.D. and Voltz, R. (1998). Discontinuation of life support in patients with amyotrophic lateral sclerosis. *Journal of Neurology*, **245**, 717–22.

15. Rabkin, J.G., Albert, S.M., Del Bene, M.L. *et al.* (2005). Prevalence of depressive disorders and change over time in late-stage ALS. *Neurology*, **65**, 62–7.

16. Rabkin, J.G., Wagner, G.J., and Del Bene, M. (2000). Resilience and distress among amyotrophic lateral sclerosis patients and caregivers. *Psychosomatic Medicine*, **62**, 271–9.

17. Sancho, J., Servera, E., Diaz, J. *et al.* (2004). Efficacy of mechanical insufflation-exsufflation in medically stable patients with amyotrophic lateral sclerosis. *Chest*, **125**, 1400–5.

18. Brooks, B.R., Thisted, R.A., Appel, S.H. *et al.* (2004). Treatment of pseudobulbar affect in ALS with dextromethorphan/quinidine: A randomized trial. *Neurology*, **63**, 1364–70.

19. Giess, R., Naumann, M., Werner, E. *et al.* (2000). Injections of botulinum toxin A into the salivary glands improve sialorrhoea in amyotrophic lateral sclerosis. *Journal of Neurology, Neurosurgery Psychiatry*, **69**, 121–3.

20. Stalpers, L.J. and Moser, E.C. (2002). Results of radiotherapy for drooling in amyotrophic lateral sclerosis. *Neurology, 58*, 1308.

21. Neudert, C., Oliver, D., Wasner, M. *et al.* (2001). The course of the terminal phase in patients with amyotrophic lateral sclerosis. *Journal of Neurology, 248*, 612–6.

22. Veldink, J.H., Wokke, J.H., van der Wal, G. *et al.* (2002). Euthanasia and physician-assisted suicide among patients with amyotrophic lateral sclerosis in the Netherlands. *New England Journal of Medicine, 346*, 1638–44.

23. Neudert, C., Wasner, M., and Borasio, G.D. (2001). Patients' assessment of quality of life instruments: a randomised study of SIP, SF-36 and SEIQoL-DW in patients with amyotrophic lateral sclerosis. *Journal of Neurological Science, 191*, 103–9.

24. Neudert, C., Wasner, M., and Borasio, G.D. (2004). Individual quality of life is not correlated with health-related quality of life or physical function in patients with amyotrophic lateral sclerosis. *Journal of Palliative Medicine, 7*, 551–7.

25. Murphy, P.L., Albert, S.M., Weber, C. *et al.* (2000). Impact of spirituality and religiousness on outcomes in patients with ALS. *Neurology, 55*, 1581–4.

26. Borasio, G.D. (2001). Meditation and ALS. In *Amyotrophic lateral sclerosis: a comprehensive guide to management* (eds. H. Mitsumoto and T. Munsat), pp. 271–6. Demos Medical Publ., New York.

27. Kwakkel, G., Wagenaar, R.C., Kollen, B.J. *et al.* (1996). Predicting disability in stroke – a critical review of the literature. *Age Ageing, 25*, 479–89.

28. Hamann, G.F., Rogers, A., and Addington-Hall, J. (2004). Palliative care in stroke. In *Palliative care in neurology* (eds. R. Voltz, J. Bernat, G.D. Borasio, I. Maddocks, D. Oliver, R. Portenoy), pp. 13–26. Oxford University Press, Oxford.

29. Hinterberger, T., Kubler, A., Kaiser, J. *et al.* (2003). A brain–computer interface (BCI) for the locked-in: comparison of different EEG classifications for the thought translation device. *Clinical Neurophysiology, 114*, 416–25.

30. Addington-Hall, J.M., Lay, M., Altmann, D. *et al.* (1995). Symptom control, communication with health professionals, and hospital care of stroke patients in the last year of life as reported by surviving family, friends, and officials. *Stroke, 26*, 2242–8.

31. Stevens, T., Payne, S.A., Burton, C. *et al.* (2007). Palliative Care in Stroke: a critical review of the literature. *Palliative Medicine, 21*, 323–31.

32. Kehayia, E., Korner-Bitensky, N., Singer, F. *et al.* (1997). Differences in pain medication use in stroke patients with aphasia and without aphasia. *Stroke, 28*, 1867–70.

33. Smithard, D.G., Smeeton, N.C., and Wolfe, C.D.A. (2007). Long-term outcome after stroke: does dysphagia matter? *Age and Ageing, 36*, 90–4.

34. Norton, B., Homer-Ward, M., Donnelly, M.T. *et al.* (1996). A randomised prospective comparison of percutaneous endoscopic gastrostomy and nasogastric tube feeding after acute dysphagic stroke. *British Medical Journal, 312*, 13–6.

35. Dennis, M., Lewis, S., Cranswick, G. *et al.* on behalf of the FOOD Trial Collaboration (2006). FOOD: a multicentre randomised trial evaluating feeding policies in patients admitted to hospital with a recent stroke. *Health Technology Assessment, 10*, 1–120.

36. Barus, D.F., Krauss, J.K., and Strobel, J. (1994). The shoulder hand syndrome after stroke: a prospective clinical trial. *Annals of Neurology, 36*, 728–33.

37. Gainotti, G., and Marra, C. (2002). Determinants and consequences of post-stroke depression. *Current Opinion in Neurology, 15*, 85–9.

38. Scholte op Reimer, W.J., de Haan, R.J., Rijnders, P.T. *et al.* (1998). The burden of caregiving in partners of long-term stroke survivors. *Stroke, 29*, 1605–11.

39. Jack, C., Jones, L., Jack, B.A. *et al.* (2004). Towards a good death: the impact of the care of the dying pathway in an acute stroke unit. *Age Ageing, 33*, 625–6.

40. Metz, L.M., McFarland, H.F., O'Connor, P.W. *et al.* (2005). Diagnostic criteria for multiple sclerosis: 2005 revisions to the "McDonald Criteria". *Annals of Neurology, 58*, 840–6.

41. Polman, C.H., O'Connor, P.W., Havrdova, E. *et al.* (2006). A randomized, placebo-controlled trial of natalizumab for relapsing multiple sclerosis. *New England Journal of Medicine, 354*, 899–910.

42. Gruenewald, D.A., Higginson, I.J., Vivat, B. *et al.* (2004). Quality of life measures for the palliative care of people severely affected by multiple sclerosis: a systematic review. *Multiple Sclerosis, 10*, 690–704.

43. Wolf, J.K. (1996). *Mastering MS: handbook of management.* Academy Books, Rutland, Vermont.

44. Higginson, I.J., Hart, S., Silber, E. *et al.* (2006). Symptom prevalence and severity in people severely affected by multiple sclerosis. *Journal of Palliative Care, 22*, 158–65.

45. Kümpfel, T., Hoffmann, L.A., Pollmann, W. *et al.* (2007). Palliative care in patients with severe multiple sclerosis: two case reports and a survey among German MS neurologists. *Palliative Medicine, 21*, 109–14.

46. Edmonds, P., Vivat, B., Burman, R. *et al.* (2007). Loss and change: experiences of people severely affected by multiple sclerosis. *Palliative Medicine, 21*, 101–7.

47. Higginson, I.J., Vivat, B., Silber, E. *et al.* (2006). Study protocol: delayed intervention randomised controlled trial within the Medical Research Council (MRC) Framework to assess the effectiveness of a new palliative care service. *BMC Palliative Care, 5*(7).

48. Sadovnick, A.D., Eisen, K., Ebers, G.C. *et al.* (1991). Cause of death in patients attending multiple sclerosis clinics. *Neurology 41*, 1193–6.

49. Voltz, R., Akabayashi, A., Reese, C. *et al.* (1998). End-of-life decisions and advance directives in palliative care: a cross-cultural survey of patients and health-care professionals. *Journal of Pain and Symptom Management, 16*, 153–62.

50. Henze, T., Rieckmann, P., Toyka, K.V., Multiple Sclerosis Therapy Consensus Group of the German Multiple Sclerosis Society (2006). Symptomatic treatment of multiple sclerosis. *European Neurology, 56*, 78–105.

51. Dieterich, M., Straube, A., Brandt, T. *et al.* (1991). The effects of baclofen and cholinergic drugs on upbeat and downbeat nystagmus. *Journal of Neurology, Neurosurgery and Psychiatry, 54*, 627–32.

52. Gbadamosi, J., Buhmann, C., Moench, A. *et al.* (2001). Failure of ondansetron in treating cerebellar tremor in MS patients—an open label pilot study, *Acta Neurologica Scandinavica, 104*, 308–11.

53. Shakespeare, D.T., Boggild, M., and Young, C. (2001). Anti-spasticity agents in multiple sclerosis (Cochrane Review). Cochrane Library, 4, Oxford.

54. Leandri, M., Cruccu, G., and Gottlieb, A. (1999). Cluster headache-like pain in multiple sclerosis. *Cephalalgia, 19*, 732–4.

55. Dahm, P.O., Nitescu, P.V., Appelgren, L.K. *et al.* (1998). Long-term intrathecal (i.t.) infusion of bupivacaine relieved intractable pain and spasticity in a patient with multiple sclerosis. *European Journal of Pain, 2*, 81–5.

56. Solari, A., Uitdehaag, B., Giuliani, G. *et al.* (2001). Aminopyridines for symptomatic treatment in multiple sclerosis (Cochrane Review), The Cochrane Library, 4, Oxford.

57. Rammohan, K.W., Rosenberg, J.H., Lynn, D.J. *et al.* (2002). Efficacy and safety of modafinil (Provigil(R)) for the treatment of fatigue in multiple sclerosis: a two centre phase 2 study. *Journal of Neurology, Neurosurgery and Psychiatry, 72*, 179–83.

58. MacLeod, A.D., and Formaglio, F., (2004). Demyelinating disease. In Palliative care in neurology (R. Voltz, J. Bernat, G.D. Borasio, I. Maddocks, D. Oliver, R. Portenoy), Oxford University Press, Oxford, pp. 27–36.

59. Clough, C.G., and Blockley, A. (2004). Parkinson's Disease and related disorders. In *Palliative care in neurology* (R. Voltz, J. Bernat, G.D. Borasio, I. Maddocks, D. Oliver, R. Portenoy), pp. 48–58, Oxford University Press, Oxford.

60. Müller, J., Wenning, K.G., Verny, M. *et al.* (2001). Progression of dysarthria and dysphagia in postmortem-confirmed parkinsonian disorders. *Archives of Neurology*, **58**, 259–64.

61. Hudson, P.L., Toye, C., and Kristjanson, L.J. (2006). Would people with Parkinson's disease benefit from palliative care? *Palliative Medicine*, **20**, 87–94.

62. Quinn, N.P., Lang, A.E., Koller, W.C. *et al.* (1986). Painful Parkinson's disease. *Lancet* **1**, 1366–9.

63. Daniele, A., Moro, E., and Bentivoglio, A.R. (1999). Zolpidem in progressive supranuclear palsy. *New England Journal of Medicine*, **341**, 543–4.

64. Nath, U., Ben-Shlomo, Y., Thomson, R.G. *et al.* (2003). Clinical features and natural history of progressive supranuclear palsy: a clinical cohort study. *Neurology*, **60**, 910–6.

65. Warren, N.M., Pigott, M.A., Perry, E.K. *et al.* (2005). Cholinergic systems in progressive supranuclear palsy. *Brain*, **128**, 239–49.

12.6

Palliative medicine in end-stage renal failure

E. Joanna Chambers

SM was 66 when he died; he received a renal transplant at age 55 after 15 years of dialysis for end-stage renal disease (ESRD) from diabetic nephropathy. He first met the palliative care team for help with the management of severe pain from an acute arthritis of his left foot 6 months before his death. Three months earlier he had a right below-knee amputation for peripheral vascular disease; rehabilitation at home with enormous support from his wife was ongoing. At the time of referral his renal function was deteriorating. Pain relief was established and he was able to go home on regular analgesia and to continue rehabilitation. From this time onward, increasing symptoms, progressive physical decline, and multiple hospital admissions followed leading to a rapid deterioration in his quality of life. He was a man who loved his home, his family, and to follow football with his sons. Time in hospital was time wasted.

Each admission, first with polyarthritis, then a series of infections weakened him markedly with concomitant deterioration in renal function. Finally, he needed dialysis through an emergency line. Throughout this he did not appear to consider that things might not return to how they had been. Clinical improvement with dialysis enabled him to return home with outpatient dialysis. Within days, however, he was readmitted with further infection, physical deterioration, and the development of calciphylaxis in multiple areas. He remained in hospital and was bed bound for the last weeks of life, pain was controlled with fentanyl, but intense anguish and acute anxiety predominated until, with the support and care of his wife and the teams caring for them, he came to accept the irreversibility of his condition. When he was semi-conscious it was agreed that dialysis should stop, he rallied for a few days leading to further anguish, the deterioration in his physical state, however, was relentless with calciphylaxis and skin breakdown in many areas progressing. He demonstrated his acceptance finally by asking his sons to care for his wife and gradually he achieved peace of mind.

Main palliative care issues:

- Initial severe pain in the presence of renal impairment.

- Deteriorating functional status because of amputation and increasing weakness.

- All previous severe illness had been reversible and therefore difficulty for him, his family, and the team caring for him to see that this might be different.

- It was always still possible to dialyse though this would not reverse the physical complications of renal disease and co-morbid conditions.

- Acknowledgement of difficulty of reversing complications which were occurring and reduced life expectancy.

- The role of an advisory team in taking forward the communication about entering a terminal phase while active investigation and management continue.

- Personal anguish about the situation, which was difficult to express—previous problems had always been put right.

Definitions

The internationally accepted definition of chronic kidney disease (CKD) is:

- Kidney damage for 3 or 4 months, as defined by structural or functional abnormalities, with or without decreased glomerular filtration rate (GFR), manifested by pathological abnormalities or markers of kidney damage, including abnormalities in the composition of the blood or urine or abnormalities in imaging tests. It is divided into stages according to GFR. See Table 12.6.1.

- Or a GFR <60 ml/min/1.73 m^2 for 3 months, with or without signs of kidney damage as described above.

This definition is irrespective of cause. The treatment necessary will depend on the disease stage. Patients with stage 4–5 disease are likely to be symptomatic with increased mortality rates; most patients

Table 12.6.1 Stages of chronic kidney disease.

Stage of CKD	Percentage of population	GFR ml/min/1.73/m²	Comments
All stages	10	-	
Stage 1		Normal >90	Plus persistent albuminuria
Stage 2		60–90	Plus persistent albuminuria
Stage 3		30–59	Evaluation and management renal disease and co-morbidity
Stage 4	0.2	15–29	Patients experience many of the complications of renal failure; increased mortality particularly from cardiovascular disease. Preparation for renal replacement therapy (RRT)
Stage 5	0.2	<15	= ESRD, majority require RRT

on reaching stage 5 require renal replacement therapy (RRT) in the form of dialysis or a renal transplant unless a decision is taken not to dialyse. For this, latter group ongoing management of kidney disease will continue in order to optimize renal function and quality of life. This is now a recognized management option described as conservative management or optimal medical management.

Extent of the problem from chronic kidney disease

CKD affects about 10 per cent of the population with an estimated prevalence of renal RRT in the UK at the end of 2004 of 638 persons per million population (pmp)[1]. The numbers with stages 1–4 have not changed greatly between the early and late 1990s however there has been a doubling of those with stage 5 disease in that time; these patients still represent the minority though they require the majority of services. The incidence of stage 5 CKD in the Afro-Caribbean and South Asian population is 3–4 times higher than the general population.

The changed demography of renal patients

Age

In the late 1960s and early 1970s when dialysis techniques were developing, treatment was confined to the fit young breadwinner. As techniques have improved, greater numbers of people are entering dialysis programmes. This has resulted in a change in the characteristics of patients on dialysis with a marked increase in the elderly (Fig. 12.6.1) and those with significant co-morbidity. By 2004, one-quarter of patients starting dialysis was over 75 years in the UK[1].

Co-morbidity in prevalent patients

Hypertension and cardiovascular disease are the commonest causes of renal failure requiring RRT; however, diabetes is increasingly present in patients who dialyse and is now the index cause in 20 per cent of new dialysis patients in the UK[1] (>40 per cent in the USA). Fig. 12.6.2 illustrates the considerable extent of co-morbidity in UK patients accepted onto RRT programme in 2003; Nearly one-third of patients over 65 have cardiovascular disease including one-forth with a history of angina, and in this age group peripheral vascular disease, cerebrovascular disease, malignancy, recent

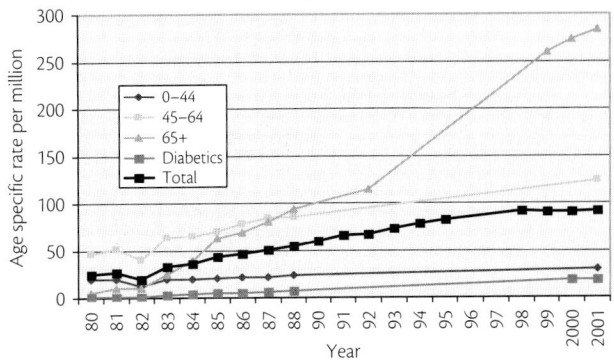

Figure 12.6.1 Age specific rate/million of patients accepted for RRT in UK. UK Renal Registry 2002.

myocardial infarction, diabetes, and a history of smoking are present in 15 per cent or more of patients starting RRT. The presence of co-morbidity affects both the quality of life of dialysis patients and mortality adversely[2].

Primary renal causes of renal failure such as glomerular nephritis and familial cause such as adult polycystic kidney disease (APKD) are more common in younger patients. There is no change in the incidence of these as cause for ESRD.

Prognosis

The prognosis for ESRD is equivalent to or worse than that for many malignancies with a 5 year survival of incident patients on RRT in the UK in 2004 of 43 per cent[1]; this survival varies from 64 per cent for the under 65 to 14 per cent for those older. There is also a large variation with co-morbidity[2]. Figs. 12.6.3 and 12.6.4 demonstrate this and show an increase in mortality compared with the general population of about 18 times for the 45–54 age group and four times for the over 75 age group.

Renal replacement therapy

Renal transplant

Patients who are transplanted have the best overall prognosis, with a 1-year survival in the UK of over 90 per cent[1]; however, if the

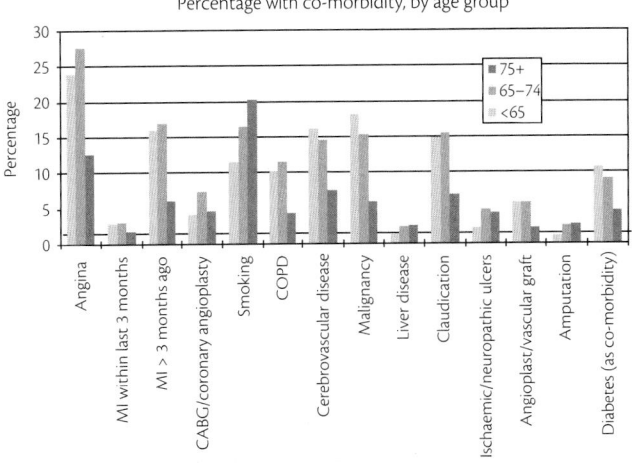

Figure 12.6.2 Chart to show percentage with co-morbidity, by age group. UK Renal Registry report 2004.

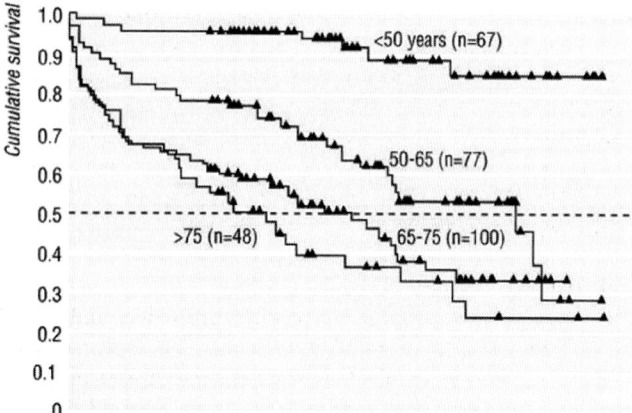

Figure 12.6.3 Kaplan–Meier survival curve to show effect of age on survival. Reproduced with permission from Chandna *et al.* (1999)[2].

patient has co-morbid conditions, progression of these diseases will not be delayed; and any complications of renal failure already present such as renal osteodystrophy may continue to cause symptoms. The patient has to remain on immunosuppression for life with the consequent increase in risk of malignancy and infection, added to which these drugs may have unpleasant side effects and can accelerate vascular disease with risk of stroke and myocardial infarction increased compared with age-matched controls. There is a gradual attrition rate for transplanted kidneys due to chronic rejection so some patients receive second or third grafts, or have to return to dialysis.

Dialysis

Dialysis is the artificial removal of waste products from the body by diffusion across a thin membrane. The membrane is either within a machine through which the patient's blood passes known as haemodialysis or within the patients themselves in the peritoneum known as peritoneal dialysis. Dialysis does not correct for the normal hormones produced by the kidney, namely 1,25-dihydroxycholecalciferol (vitamin D) and erythropoietin so these may need replacing for life.

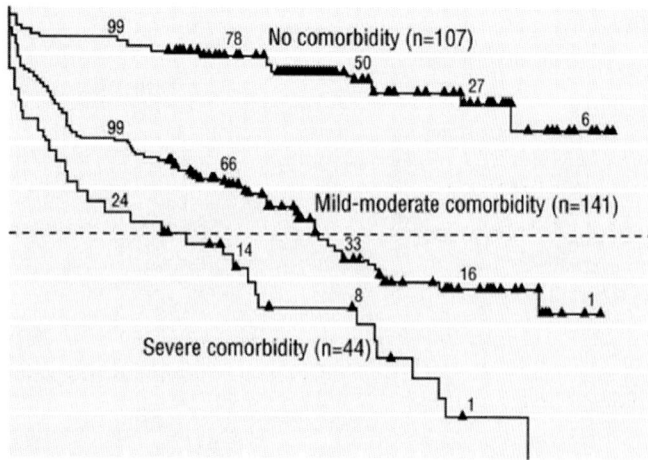

Figure 12.6.4 Kaplan–Meier survival curve to show effect of co-morbidity on survival. Reproduced with permission from Chandna *et al.* (1999)[2].

Haemodialysis (HD)

Permanent access to the circulation is required; for the patient who is being prepared for dialysis this is via a fistula usually in the forearm and it takes many months to 'ripen' ready for regular access; for the patient who is unprepared, or in whom fistula formation has failed, access is through temporary or tunnelled lines. These can be a source of infection and at end of life may become gradually more difficult to achieve. Sessions of 4 h are most commonly conducted three times a week at a dialysis centre or for a small proportion of patients at home.

Peritoneal dialysis (PD)

Fluid is introduced into the peritoneal cavity either for several hours or for 30–40 min several times a day and then withdrawn. The patient usually carries out his or her own dialysis in their own home. A permanent peritoneal catheter is needed and meticulous sterile technique is imperative.

Problems, advantages, and disadvantages for patients of dialysis

As will be seen below the symptom burden for dialysis patients is high; added to which are concerns peculiar to the mode of dialysis: for HD patients these include disfiguration from the fistula appearance, thrice weekly commitment to the dialysis machine which prevents holidays away from dialysis centres, and for those dialysing in HD units, transport delays and difficulty negotiating flexibility in treatment times to fit in with social circumstances. Those peculiar to PD patients include feeling bloated, fear of infection, negative body image from permanent catheter, and social isolation. As a group all patients have to contend with dietary and fluid restrictions which impinge on many social activities and a high medication burden to maintain optimal cardiovascular function, calcium phosphate balance and correction of deficiencies of erythropoietin and iron. From this, it can readily be seen that the treatment of this illness impacts hugely on quality of life.

Symptoms in the patient with ESRD and their management

Patients with stage 4 and 5 CKD are as symptomatic as patients with metastatic malignancy, indeed studies suggest that the number and severity of symptoms they experience may be greater. Symptoms are caused by the patients' co-morbid conditions, renal disease, particularly uraemia, the consequences of management of their renal failure, and some relate to the dialysis procedure itself. The incidence, severity and impact on quality of life of these symptoms has only recently been recognized[3–5]. Management is complicated by the patients co-morbid conditions, the multiple drug regimens most need to take and the altered handling of drugs by the body in renal failure. Patients considered in this chapter can be divided into four groups: patients with stage 4 disease who are likely to progress to renal RRT, those on dialysis, those who are transplanted, and those who choose not to dialyse or for whom it is not recommended and who are therefore managed on a conservative pathway. End-of-life care for those stopping dialysis will be considered separately. Transplanted patients are likely to have fewer symptoms as uraemia resolves; however, pain from co-morbid conditions particular arthritis and diabetic neuropathy will continue and there may be residual symptoms from long-standing renal impairment. The other three groups have similar symptoms and will be discussed together with any important differences highlighted.

Pain

Incidence and causes and severity

Significant pain is experienced by more than 50 per cent of haemodialysis patients, and is moderate to severe in at least half[6,7]. The commonest group of pains are musculoskeletal; the precise cause of pain may not be clear as osteoarthritis may not be distinguished from renal osteodystrophy, for example, and osteoporosis is common in the age group represented but more common in ESRD. Studies suggest this pain is as severe as the pain from peripheral vascular disease[6]. The different groups of causes are listed in Table 12.6.2. Significant pain during dialysis affects over a quarter of patients; occurring more than once a week for those who report it and lasting >2 h per session present for a median of 2 years. Non-dialysis pains had a similar intensity and median duration occurring on at least 4 days a week[7].

Impact of pain

Pain in a population of haemodialysis patients has been shown to correlate significantly with depression, reduced physical and mental quality of life, and insomnia[3,8]; unrelieved pain may contribute to a patient's decision to discontinue dialysis[8]. Patients with moderate to severe pain had an incidence of depression of 34 per cent and insomnia of 75 per cent compared with 18 per cent and 35 per cent, respectively for those with none or mild pain. A separate study[7] showed that pain interfered with many aspects of everyday living in particular general activity, enjoyment of life and normal work as measured by the brief pain inventory interference score. In the few studies of symptoms at end of life, pain is a significant symptom in around 50 per cent and may continue or be severe in last 24 h for up to 25 per cent[9,10].

Types of pain

ESRD patients experience nociceptive, neuropathic, and mixed pains in about equal proportions as would be expected from the common causes described earlier. Ischaemia and neuropathy are major contributors to the overall pain burden. In addition, the high incidence of musculoskeletal pains means that many are movement related with the recognized difficulty associated with its management.

Obstacles to pain management in ESRD

Factors which contribute to the difficulty of managing pain in ESRD include: elderly patients with multiple co-morbidity and complex drug regimens who may not report their pain; a lack of recognition of the problem until recently by physicians combined with a paucity of research and evidence from which to obtain the skills to manage it. Complicated drug handling in ESRD together with the similarity between opioid side effects and symptoms of uraemia contribute to a well-documented failure to relieve pain in this group of patients[7,11,12]. In addition, a fear of the use of opioids by the

Table 12.6.2 Causes of pain in ESRD.

Causes	Examples	Comments
Concurrent co morbidity	Diabetic neuropathy	Incidence DM depends on age and country but incidence in ESRD 25–50 per cent
	Peripheral vascular disease	Critical limb ischaemia, phantom limb pain, ischaemic leg ulcers
	Arthritis osteoporosis	
Primary renal disease	Adult polycystic kidney disease (APCK)	Pain from liver or kidney distension, infected cysts
	Renal calculi	
Complications of renal failure	Renal osteodystrophy	
	Gout	
	Other crystal arthropathies	
	Dialysis amyloid arthropathy	Carpal tunnel
	Calciphylaxis	Skin ischaemia and ulceration
	Peripheral polyneuropathy	Feature of long standing dialysis
Dialysis related	Cramps	Occur during and between dialysis
	Headaches	
	Fistula pain (HD)	Ischaemia from diversion of blood flow
	Abdominal pain (PD)	Distension, peritonitis
	Pain of fistula needling (HD)	
Infection	Discitis	Associated with needing catheters for HD
	Septic arthritis	
	Peritonitis (PD)	
Miscellaneous	Malignancy	Increased incidence in both dialysis and transplanted patients

clinician, the patients, and their relatives and it is not surprising that there is inadequate prescribing of analgesia. One recent study suggested that using the WHO analgesic ladder, with appropriate modifications can help relieve pain,[13] though long-term studies are lacking.

Drug handling in renal failure

The major cause of increased drug sensitivity and hence toxicity in patients with reduced renal function is the accumulation of the drug or its active metabolites. Other factors listed in Table 12.6.3 are of lesser importance, some effects are inconsistent and therefore difficult to predict. In addition, most studies of pharmacokinetics are single-dose studies and therefore difficult to extrapolate to chronic dosing. Tables which suggest dose modification in renal failure are not consistent in their advice[14].

Management

Assessment

The assessment of pain will be as for any comparable situation in palliative medicine, with special reference to the underlying co-morbid conditions and complications of renal disease suffered by the patient. Current medication and previous experience of analgesics need considering. Establishing pain relief may take time, so it is important to build a relationship with the patient through an explanation of the plan of action and the nature of individualizing treatment through titration to give them a realistic expectation. As most pain has been present for some time it is better to titrate slowly with the aim of minimizing toxicity than to lose the patient and renal team's confidence through rapid escalation and risk early toxicity.

Table 12.6.3 Factors which influence the clinical effect of drugs in severe renal impairment in addition to renal excretion.

- ◆ Bioavailability:
  - Varies more in uraemia than normal renal function; may be both increased or decreased
- ◆ Distribution:
  - Increased in oedematous states
  - Decreased in dehydration
- ◆ Plasma albumin:
  - Reduced plasma protein binding may lead to increased toxicity
  - E.g. phenytoin
- ◆ Metabolism:
  - Reduction in uraemia particularly hydrolysis
  - Glucuronidation not usually effected
- ◆ Pharmacokinetics:
  - Usually calculated from single dose studies and mathematical models may not be relevant to repeated dosing seen in palliative care
- ◆ Drug removal by extracorporeal techniques:
  - Many factors involved include:
    - ○ Molecular weight
    - ○ Lipid solubility
    - ○ Dialysis membrane (pore size, biocompatibility)
    - ○ Blood and dialysate flow rates
    - ○ Protein binding

WHO analgesic ladder

The WHO analgesic ladder, which was developed for the management of cancer pain, can be applied here with modification to recommended regimens[15–18]. Non-opioids and adjuvants, particularly for neuropathic pain are indicated as for cancer pain management. Table 12.6.4 shows analgesics and other drugs commonly used in palliative care with suggested modifications for renal disease. NSAIDs are not recommended for patients with impaired renal function or those who dialyse and have significant residual renal function because of the risk of further decline. Where NSAIDS are clinically indicated for those who dialyse an individual decision should be made; non-renal side effects are increased in ESRD; if used the lowest effective dose should be used for as short a time as possible.

Step 1: non-opioid ± adjuvants
Paracetamol can be given at normal doses with adjuvants as clinically indicated.

Step 2: opioids for mild to moderate pain ± non-opioid ± adjuvants
Codeine is metabolized to codeine-6-glucuronide and morphine; this metabolite and those of morphine accumulate. There are well-documented cases of narcosis with codeine in ESRD patients though the incidence appears to be idiosyncratic. If used, the dose should be titrated from a low base with careful monitoring; this is easier to achieve if it is prescribed in a separate tablet from paracetamol.

There are reports of CNS depression with dihydrocodeine and very little data regarding its use in ESRD; it is should therefore be avoided. Dextropropoxyphene is contraindicated due to the accumulation of toxic metabolites.

Tramadol is mainly excreted by the kidney, 30 per cent unchanged; dose reductions are recommended in renal failure and when these are adhered to the incidence of side effects is likely to be similar to that for people without renal disease. For patients on the conservative management pathway, 50 mg twice a day and for those on dialysis 50 mg four times a day can provide useful analgesia for mild to moderate pain for some patients.

Step 3: opioids for severe pain ± non-opioid ± adjuvants
Morphine

The metabolites of morphine, morphine-3-glucuronide and morphine-6-glucuronide (M6G) are retained in renal failure, M6G is a potent analgesic and probably the cause of morphine toxicity in patients with renal impairment and ESRD[19]; causing, sedation, cognitive impairment, and myoclonus. Morphine is not recommended for chronic dosing in this group of patients.

Hydromorphone

Hydromorphone is metabolized mainly to hydromorphone-3-glucuronide (H3G), an active metabolite. In the only study[20] looking at the pharmacodynamics and pharmacokinetics of hydromorphone in ESRD, it was shown in 12 dialysis patients taking multiple doses of hydromorphone that hydromorphone neither accumulate in renal failure nor is it removed by dialysis; however, H3G was retained and shown to be removed by dialysis. Hydromorphone was shown to be an effective analgesic without serious adverse effects though there was the suggestion that analgesia became less effective between dialysis treatments with the proposal that this was caused by an antagonistic effect of H3G.

Table 12.6.4 Modification of drugs commonly used for symptom control in patients with ESRD either on dialysis, being managed without dialysis (conservative pathway) or following withdrawal of dialysis.

Symptom group	Drug	Modifications	Suggested doses	Comments
Analgesia				
Step 1	Paracetamol	None	1 g qds	
Step 2	Codeine	Titrate carefully	15–30mg qds	Profound narcosis reported (idiosyncratic)
	Tramadol	HD 50 per cent	50 mg qds	Side effects common in the elderly
		No D 25 per cent	50 mg bd –tds	
Step 3	**All step 3 drugs have doses individually titrated. (See also text and Table 12.6.5)**			
	Alfentanil			1. Use for procedural pain
				2. SC in syringe driver where mod-high-dose opioid indicated
	Buprenorphine			Possible role; insufficient evidence for recommendation
	Fentanyl			Parenteral drug of choice
				Titrate with alternative opioid prior to TD fentanyl
	Hydromorphone			Low dose; careful monitoring prior to TD fentanyl
	Methadone			Use only by those familiar with methadone
	Morphine			Avoid chronic dosing
	Oxycodone			Insufficient evidence for recommendation
Neuropathic pain				
	Amitriptyline	None		Side effects may limit dose achievable
	Gabapentin	Depends on eGFR till ESRD	HD loading dose 300 mg then 200–300mg after each dialysis	Excreted unchanged in urine, accumulates in renal failure
			No D individual titration, max 300 mg alt days	
	Clonazepam	50 per cent dose	500 mcg on–2 mg/24 h	Max 2 mg/24 h
				Useful for rapid onset of action and at end of life for ease of administration
Nausea and vomiting				
	Cyclizine	None	25–50 mg 8 hourly	Avoid if possible because of dry mouth
	Haloperidol	Reduce dose		
	Levomepromazine	Low dose only	6 mg PO od to bd	May cause sedation in moderate doses
	Metoclopramide	Max 50 per cent dose	10 mg tds	Max 30 mg/24 h
Anxiolytics and sedatives				
	Diazepam	None	2–10 mg od	Active metabolites accumulate (with normal renal function) reduce dose after a number of days
	Midazolam	Use at approx 50 per cent	Stat 2.5–5 mg and prn hrly	Active metabolite accumulate
			SC 24 h infusion 10–15 mg	
Antisecretory drugs				
	Hyoscine butylbromide	None	Stat 20 mg and prn 2 hourly	Does not cause sedation
			SC 24 h infusion 160–240 mg	
	Glycopyrronium	Minor dose reduction	Stat 200 mcg and prn 4 hourly	Excreted renally
			SC 24 h infusion 800–1200 mcg	Caution drug interactions
				Does not cause sedation
Restless legs				
	Clonazepam	50 per cent dose	Stat 500 mcg on	Useful once daily dosing
			PO or SC 2 mg/24 h	

HD = haemodialysis, No D = no dialysis.

Case reports of neurotoxicity in two patients who went into *acute renal failure* while taking very high doses of hydromorphone suggest neurotoxicity; however, one report which demonstrated a high H3G to hydromorphone ratio in a patient with severe renal impairment also reported the patient to have normal cognitive function[21]. This data, personal experience and a retrospective review[22], suggest that hydromorphone can be used in patients who dialyse but great caution should be exercised in those on the conservative pathway or who stop dialysis in view of the accumulation of H3G. Personal practice is to use immediate release preparations at low dose for titration with careful monitoring followed by the introduction of transdermal fentanyl instead of the regular hydromorphone when the dose reaches 12 mg per 24 h if a dialysis patient requires continuous analgesia.

Oxycodone

There is prolongation of elimination of the main metabolites of oxycodone; noroxycodone, and oxymorphone in patients with renal failure as evidenced by a single-dose study of 13 patients prior to transplant[23]; both metabolites are active though their significance in pain management is uncertain. A single case study showed that oxycodone and its metabolites were removed by dialysis; however, a further case report detailed respiratory depression in a patient with ESRD who received regular doses of oxycodone 5 mg/paracetamol 325 mg over 8 days for pain relief following removal of an infected AV graft, the patient continued to dialyse but more than 4 days naloxone infusion was required to reverse the opioid toxicity[24]. Short-term low-dose oxycodone was used in some patients in the study which looked at the use of the WHO analgesic ladder in ESRD[13]. There are no studies of chronic use in renal failure; there is therefore insufficient evidence currently for a recommendation.

Fentanyl and alfentanil

Both fentanyl and alfentanil are metabolized to inactive, non-toxic metabolites; <10 per cent of fentanyl and 1 per cent alfentanil are excreted in the urine; it is not thought that fentanyl is removed by dialysis. For these reasons, this group of drugs have characteristics which are favourable for their use in renal failure, however, as there is no oral formulation titration will either need an alternative strong opioid for oral use initially or subcutaneous fentanyl can be used where parenteral drugs are indicated. Personal practice is to use hydromorphone to titrate prior to the use of transdermal fentanyl where pain is continuous. Subcutaneous fentanyl is widely used as the parenteral drug of choice for titration for end-of-life care; if doses greater than 600 mcg/24 h are needed in a syringe driver a change to alfentanil can be made as it is more soluble and can therefore be given in a smaller volume despite being one quarter as potent. See also 'End-of-life care' and Table 12.6.5[15,16].

Great care must be taken with all strong opioids in renal patients as toxicity can be precipitated following a period of stability if pain intensity reduces or sepsis intervenes. The depot of fentanyl remaining on removal of TD fentanyl means that if naloxone is required an infusion may be necessary.

Buprenorphine

Buprenorphine is extensively metabolized to buprenorphine-3-glucuronide (B3G) and norbuprenorphine (NorB); the majority of buprenorphine is eliminated through the faeces though the

Table 12.6.5 Suggested drugs to be available at end of life in ESRD—see also text.

Symptom	Anticipatory prescribing	
	Drug	Initial (range) syringe driver doses/24 h
Pain	Fentanyl 12.5–25 mcg prn hourly	100 (100–300) mcg
Dyspnoea	Fentanyl 12.5–25 mcg prn hourly	
Agitation	Midazolam 2.5–5 mg prn hourly	5 (5–20) mg
	Haloperidol 0.5 – 1.5 mg prn 8-hourly	1.5 (1.5–5) mg
Fits/myoclonus	Midazolam 2.5–5mg prn hourly	5 (5–20) mg
Nausea and vomiting	Levomepromazine 5 mg prn 8-hourly	5 (5–15) mg
Retained respiratory secretions	Hyoscine butylbromide 20 mg prn 2-hourly	40 (40–240) mg

metabolites are excreted renally. B3G and NorB were increased 15- and fourfold respectively in eight renal failure patients receiving a continuous IV infusion in ITU with ventilation[25]. B3G is inactive. Norbuprenorphine is a less potent analgesic in humans but more potent respiratory depressant than buprenorphine rats[26] an effect that can be reversed with naloxone. One week of low dose (median 52.5 mcg/h) TD buprenorphine given to 10 haemodialysis patients did not cause an increase in NorB. An unknown number of patients who could not tolerate it were excluded from the study[27]. Doses of buprenorphine in patients with renal failure *may* not need to be adjusted; however, further studies of long-term use with clear selection criteria are needed in this group of patients before recommendations can be given.

Methadone

Methadone has inactive metabolites both the parent drug and its metabolites are excreted in the faeces and the urine; though excretion is almost exclusively faecal in the anuric patient and <1 per cent is removed by dialysis. It has a well recognized role in pain management within palliative care in the hands of those familiar with it use. Its pharmacokinetic characteristics suggest it may be a safe drug for those familiar with its use in ESRD but recommendations for dose adjustments vary and it should not be used by those unfamiliar

Specific renal conditions which are painful

Adult polycystic kidney disease (APKD)

Both renal and liver cysts can cause pain through size, infection, or rupture. Nephrectomy is sometimes necessary to relieve pain; the liver too can reach an enormous size causing back pain from lumbar lordosis, and mechanical problems from its size; rarely liver transplantation has been done to relieve this.

Calciphylaxis

Calciphylaxis is a condition where calcification of small vessels leads to tissue ischaemia with the development of extremely painful skin lesions. Skin discolouration or nodules may progress rapidly to ischaemic ulceration on the thighs, buttocks, lower abdomen as well as the lower limbs. Pain is characteristically severe and neuropathic in nature often with extreme allodynia. Skilled and meticulous nursing care with adequate pain relief is essential. Psychological care of the patient and family are also needed as this condition is associated with a very poor prognosis and often heralds the terminal phase of the patient's illness.

Non-pain symptoms

Recent studies[3,4] and a systematic review of studies[5] demonstrate not only the high prevalence of symptoms that ESRD patients experience but also their severity and impact on quality of life. The mean number of symptoms experienced in outpatient haemodialysis patients is nine[3,4]. Three-quarters experience dry skin, 69 per cent lethargy, and 54 per cent itch and bone or joint pain. The most severe symptoms have been demonstrated in a group of patients with high co-morbidity these include: constipation, pain, difficulty sleeping, itching, and dry mouth. Dry skin, itch, restless legs, cramps, and symptoms from diabetic neuropathy occur more commonly than in cancer patients. Patients on the conservative pathway are a less-studied group; an ongoing study suggests they experience a similar spectrum of symptoms with pain and dyspnoea more common than dialysis patients.

Both depression and anxiety occur in up to one quarter of dialysis patients. Depression is associated with pain and reduced quality of life. Levels of anxiety will fluctuate according to the stage of disease with increasing incidence at diagnosis and with the development of significant toxicity or life limiting or life threatening complications. The disruption to life style is well recognized as is the burden of loss as dialysis and the symptoms described above impinge on functioning leading to loss of job and status both at work and in the family.

Management

The management of individual symptoms will depend on their severity, the adverse effects of the treatment, the stage of disease and the time to response to treatment. Only symptoms that are particularly prevalent in renal disease will be discussed here. **Nearly all non-pain symptoms can be helped by an optimal dialysis prescription, effective anaemia management, and the optimal use of phosphate binders; these should be addressed prior to consideration of drug or non-drug measures.** Other symptoms are managed using the same principles as for cancer patients but with particular reference to drug interactions and toxicity from drugs which have active metabolites and are excreted through the kidney.

Pruritus

Pruritus occurs in about half ESRD patients[28] and is severe in half of those. It may be localized or generalized, has different aetiological factors of which uraemia is important but it may also relate to secondary hyperparathyroidism and release of dermal histamine and cytokines. The pathophysiology and management described in Section 10 applies also to those with renal disease.

Topical treatments such as capsaicin cream and tacrolimus ointment have been shown in double-blind and prospective studies, respectively, to reduce the severity of uraemic itch. Systemic treatments such as ultraviolet B phototherapy show consistent benefit whereas there is little evidence for antihistamines, though they are widely used. Small studies, including a randomized placebo-controlled study of gabapentin and observation study of thalidomide report significant reduction in itch while similar small studies of ondansetron are conflicting with the most recent randomized controlled trial reporting no benefit.

For the individual patient with a relatively short prognosis, consideration of time to response, other symptoms that might benefit, and potential for toxicity will be important when choosing an agent.

Restless leg syndrome (RLS)

RLS is the symptom complex of persistent and extremely uncomfortable crawling sensation in the lower limbs which is present in 10–15 per cent of the general population[29] but affects 20–30 per cent patients with ESRD. It is a form of neuropathy involving dopaminergic dysfunction. Factors in dialysis patients which may contribute include: anaemia from iron deficiency (present in one-quarter of sufferers), low ferritin (inversely related to severity), inadequate dialysis, low parathyroid hormone, age, diabetes, pruritus, and medication. It causes significant sleep disturbance and therefore contributes to day time lethargy and tiredness. Reversible and contributory factors, such as caffeine and drugs, should be excluded or minimized. Specific treatments include dopamine receptor agonists, considered first line treatment; benzodiazepines, particularly clonazepam, and gabapentin (with appropriate dose adjustment).

Psychological symptoms

Education and information programmes run by renal units provide an important source of non-pharmacological support to the renal patient which contributes to the management of psychological ill health. In addition patients need access to trained counsellors or psychologists for the more severe and complex symptoms and situations. Drug treatment is often necessary for defined episodes of severe disability or long-term treatment where symptoms are chronic and refractory to non-drug measures. The majority of antidepressants can be used without dose adjustment in renal failure because they are fat soluble, metabolized in the liver, secreted in the bile and are not dialysable. However, their side effect profile, particularly sedation and dry mouth from the tricyclic anti-depressants may limit doses that can be achieved. Of the SSRIs, citalopram, fluoxetene, and sertraline can be used without dose adjustment

Dialysis-related symptoms

These are common and affect up to 40 per cent of patients. One-quarter experience cramps; a smaller number headache, symptomatic hypotension, nausea, and pruritus during dialysis. In addition, patients may feel washed out for 24 h post-dialysis. Key to management is the optimization of dialysis and target dry weight; if this is insufficient to relieve the symptom; drug measures such as quinine and carnitine have been shown to be effective in reducing cramps and the latter may improve cardiovascular symptoms as well.

Conservative management of ESRD

Patients with significant co-morbidity and those in the older age group are known to have a poorer prognosis on dialysis (Figs. 12.6.3 and 12.6.4). Longitudinal studies have looked at the option of optimal medical management, which includes anaemia management with erythropoietin, but without dialysis[30], though no studies are randomized to determine if there are differences in survival. These studies suggest that quality of life may not be reduced with conservative management, and as a surrogate for better end-of-life care, it was noted that more died at home in this study. Survival comparison is complicated because of the difficulty of identifying a starting point for those who don't dialyse. Preliminary data using a regression analysis of renal function in a dialysed group of patients who were compared with a conservatively managed group with the same eGFR suggests a reduction in median survival for those who do not dialyse.

This highly symptomatic group of patients, with survival measured in months, should receive supportive care in the primary care setting in a similar fashion to someone with metastatic malignancy. The expertise of the renal team is needed to optimize renal and cardiac function and to manage the complications of renal failure; in addition, the patient and family should have recourse to specialist palliative care if symptoms are difficult to manage or patient in need of specialist psychosocial support[31,32].

Withdrawal from dialysis

The percentage of dialysis patients who choose to withdraw from dialysis varies with age from about 10 per cent of those under 65 to 25 per cent of those over 75. The median survival from withdrawal is 8–10 days; a few patients with some residual renal function may live several weeks or occasionally months.

Reasons for withdrawal include: increasing dependence on others for every day functioning, progressive peripheral vascular disease, stroke and the development of an untreated or incurable malignancy or other irreversible organ failure, particularly heart failure. Up to 18 per cent patients stop dialysis within 90 days of starting, when it is recognized that the suffering the patient is experiencing is not reversed or improved by dialysis.

There are a number of important areas for consideration prior to cessation of dialysis. Reversible medical and social conditions that may have led to the decision must be considered and acted upon where possible. The clinician must ensure the patient has decision-making capacity and understands the consequences of his or her choice. Ideally discussion regarding withdrawal from dialysis should have been initiated earlier through advance care planning. Many renal units provide patients with written information about withdrawal of dialysis so patients are aware of the possibility, though the timing of such introduction will need to be sensitive. Some patients who are experiencing poor quality of life through ongoing disease burden are however unaware of the possibility. It is important to reassure patients that cessation of dialysis is neither suicide nor euthanasia.

Communication is crucial. Within the team, communication before the decision enables all members of the team to contribute to a better understanding of the patient and his or her situation and after the decision it is imperative that all team members are aware and support it. Family members also need sensitive communication,

with permission of the patient if they have capacity. Sometimes they are not privy to discussions that have been held between patient and nephrologist and so the decision to stop dialysis causes anger and distress. Where the patient loses capacity and has not made his or her wishes clear prior to this loss, decisions are made in the patient's best interest by the consultant. This will take into account the views of the renal team and those close to the patient who may be able to help the renal team discern what the patient's views are likely to have been.

Patients with another life limiting condition such as cancer may choose to stop dialysis as a means of controlling time of death or prefer to continue to dialyse and let nature take its course.

Causes of death

The commonest cause of death in ESRD is cardiac disease accounting for nearly one-third of deaths; infection, cessation of dialysis, and malignancy account for 14 per cent, 11 per cent, and 8 per cent, respectively. In addition, up to 15 per cent of patients with stage 5 disease, some of whom die from other causes and some from renal failure, do not enter a renal replacement programme; a significant but unknown number are never referred to a nephrologist so do not appear in renal statistics.

Recognizing the need for palliative care and the terminal phase

Recognizing that someone is reaching the end of their life can be difficult where there remains the ability to replace the kidney's function. It is important; however, to recognize that someone is in the last months of life and has supportive care needs which are social, psychological, physical, and spiritual.

Physical indicators include a change in performance status with increasing dependence, weight loss >0 per cent without explanation, an increase in episodes of hospitalization for recurrent infections or with complications of RRT, underlying disease progression particularly peripheral or cerebrovascular disease, intractable fluid overload or the development of calciphylaxis.

It is equally important to recognize the terminal phase in those who continue to dialyse. Withdrawal of interest in their surroundings, perhaps declining food and medications while still accepting dialysis should be seen as a possible indication that someone is approaching the end of their life. It is an opportunity to open discussion and explore their concerns and fears. Sensitivity to a patient's wishes and feelings at this time should enable staff to clarify their wishes and act on verbal and non-verbal clues.

End-of-life care

For those who choose to stop dialysis there is a clear and usually well-defined period of 7–10 days between cessation and death. Ideally, discussions regarding the person's preferred place of care at end of life would take place prior to this time, though frequently the clinical deterioration that leads to the decision creeps up on both patient and medical team and decisions have to be made rapidly. The emphasis of care changes from one of prolongation of life and prevention of morbidity to relief of symptoms, maintenance of comfort, and attention to psychological, social, and spiritual concerns. Those symptoms already present will continue; a worsening of the symptoms from uraemia can develop particularly increasing sedation, cognitive impairment, pruritus, pericarditis, and fits. In addition, symptoms from fluid overload can be extremely distressing for a few. Pain is not a feature of renal failure per se; however, pains already present are likely to remain and may already be severe. In addition, the joint and skin pain of decreased mobility mean that many who had no pain at the time dialysis stopped will need low doses of analgesia to maintain comfort until death. The few studies of the symptoms experienced by those who withdraw from dialysis are retrospective. One of 35 patients[10] suggests that two-thirds of patients are confused, and about a half experience pain and shortness of breath. More than one-fifth suffer nausea, twitching, psychological distress, pulmonary congestion, pruritus, and oedema. Only a half of patient were mentally competent at the time of withdrawal; this illustrates the difficulties faced by patients, families, and clinicians around the decision to withdraw from dialysis and argues for earlier discussion about end-of-life care options and the provision of advance care planning.

The principles of end-of-life care are those for any person who is dying, with special consideration of the drug modifications necessary when dying with renal failure and when prescribing in anticipation of likely symptoms[32,33]. Where end-of-life care pathways are in use, these can start at cessation of dialysis and contain the appropriate drug modifications. Table 12.6.5 contains a suggested list of drugs.

End-of-life symptom control

Drugs from the fentanyl/alfentanil group are the parenteral analgesics of choice for pain. Fentanyl is chosen for prn use as it has a longer duration of action than alfentanil and titration is therefore easier; however, alfentanil may be substituted for fentanyl where 24 h subcutaneous doses of fentanyl exceed 600 mcg because of the volume of diluent needed for such doses. Subcutaneous alfentanil is about one quarter as potent as fentanyl and ten times as potent as subcutaneous diamorphine; the doses required can usually be calculated from this, with the usual opioid switch precautions. For patients not previously on a strong opioid, pain relief is frequently achievable with low 24 h fentanyl doses between 100 and 300 mcg without sedation or confusion. The short duration of action of alfentanil can, however, be used to advantage for incident pain such as dressing change and a buccal or intranasal preparation can be useful here.

Nausea may be severe and drugs acting at the chemoreceptor trigger zone such as haloperidol or the broader spectrum levomepromazine are suggested for control. Doses are kept to the lowest possible to relieve symptoms. If the patient is already on metoclopramide and it is effective this can be given parenterally at doses up to 50 per cent that used for those with normal renal function. Cyclizine is best avoided as these patients usually already suffer from a dry mouth. Where a benzodiazepine is indicated midazolam can be used; doses should be kept low as there is accumulation of an active metabolite. Clonazepam is indicated for twitching, myoclonus, restless legs, agitation and can be substituted for neuropathic pain where the patient's oral medication can no longer be taken. It is generally recommended that a maximum of 2 mg/24 h is used in renal impairment; it can be given orally or subcutaneously by single daily dose or in a syringe driver starting at 500 mcg.

Fluid overload occurs less frequently than might be expected, however. it is extremely distressing when it does. In the imminently dying, symptom relief through management of dyspnoea with opioids (fentanyl) and reduction in retained secretions with hyoscine butylbromide or glycopyrronium with sedation if needed will be used along with non-drug measures of positioning, fan, and oxygen. Occasionally, ultra filtration is used with good relief of symptoms where appropriate for the stage of disease and is in accordance with the patient wishes.

Rarer symptoms such as uraemic pericarditis or pain from a kidney being acutely rejected need steroids for symptom relief and empiric doses of dexamethasone can be used.

The renal team and the place of palliative care

The supportive care for the renal patient is delivered largely by the renal multi-disciplinary team. Renal physicians look after the majority of their patient from diagnosis to death. Some patients particularly those who have severe symptoms, complex communication, and support needs or where there is profound distress as end of life approaches are likely to benefit from a palliative care referral. Patients who are on a conservative management pathway will principally be cared for by primary care, with renal specialist advice, until they die, many at home. The trigger for referral to a community palliative care service or hospice should be based on need not diagnosis. Many patients choose to die in hospital in the care of those they trust and have known for many years; a few ask for hospice care for the last days. Some, when the decision to stop dialysis is made in hospital will wish to return to their own homes. Joint working between primary care, the renal and palliative care teams will be crucial in addition as each has an educational role with the others[34].

References

1. Ansell, D., Feest, T., Williams, A.J. et al. (2005). *The eighth annual report of the UK Renal Registry*. Bristol: UK Renal Registry.

2. Chandna, S.M., Schulz, J., Lawrence, C. et al. (1999). Is there a rationale for rationing chronic dialysis? A hospital based cohort study of factors affecting survival and morbidity. *British Medical Journal*, 318, 217–23.

3. Weisbord, S.D., Fried, L.F., Arnold, R.M. et al. (2005). Prevalence, severity, and importance of physical and emotional symptoms in chronic hemodialysis patients. *Journal of American Society of Nephrology*, 16(8), 2487–94.

4. Davison, S.N., Jhangri, G.S., and Johnson, J.A. (2006). Cross-sectional validity of a modified Edmonton symptom assessment system in dialysis patients: A simple assessment of symptom burden. *Kidney International*, 69(9), 1621–5.

5. Murtagh, F.E.M., Addington-Hall, J., Higginson, I.J. (in press). The prevalence of symptoms in end-stage renal disease: a systematic review. *Advances in Chronic Kidney Disease*.

6. Davison, S.N. (2003). Pain in Hemodialysis Patients: Prevalence, Cause, Severity, and Management. *American Journal of Kidney Diseases*, 42, 1239–47.

7. Cornish, C. (2005). A survey of pain in haemodialysis patients: prevalence, characteristics, management and impact. MSc dissertation.

8. Davison, S.N., and Jhangri, G.S. (2005). The impact of chronic pain on depression, sleep, and the desire to withdraw from dialysis in hemodialysis patients. *Journal of Pain and Symptom Management*, 30, 465–73.

9. Cohen, L.M., Germain, M., Poppel, D.M. *et al.* (2000). Dialysis Discontinuation and Palliative Care. *American Journal of Kidney Diseases,* **36**, 140–14.

10. Chater, S., Davison, S.N., Germain, M.J. *et al.* (2006). Withdrawal from dialysis: a palliative care perspective. *Clinical Nephrology,* **66**, 364–72.

11. Bailie, G.R., Mason, N.A., Bragg-Gresham, J.L. *et al.* (2004). Analgesic prescription patterns among hemodialysis patients in the DOPPS: Potential for underprescription, *Kidney International,* **65**, 2419–25.

12. Davison, S.N. (2002). Pain in haemodialysis patients: prevalence, aetiology, severity and analgesic use. *Journal of American Society of Nephrology,* **42**(6), 1239–47.

13. Barakzoy, A., and Moss, A.H. (2006). Efficacy of the world health organization analgesic ladder to treat pain in end-stage renal disease. *Journal of American Society of Nephrology,* **17**, 3198–203.

14. Vidal, L., Shavit, M., Fraser, A. *et al.* (2005). Systematic comparison of four sources of drug information regarding adjustments of dose for renal function. *British Medical Journal,* **331**, 263–6.

15. Murtagh, F.E.M., Chai, M.O., Donohoe, P. *et al.* (2007). The Use of Opioid Analgesia in End-Stage Renal Disease Patients Managed without Dialysis: Recommendations for Practice. Accepted for publication. *Journal of Pain and Palliative Care Pharmacotherapy,* **21**(2).

16. Ferro, C.J., Chambers, E.J., and Davison, S. (2004). Management of Pain in renal failure. In *Supportive care for the renal patient* (eds. E.J. Chambers, M. Germain, and E. Brown), pp 105–53. Oxford University Press: Oxford.

17. Kurella, M., Bennett, W.M., and Chertow, G.M. (2003). Analgesia in Patients With ESRD: A Review of the Available Evidence. *American Journal of Kidney Diseases,* **42**, 217–28.

18. Dean, M. (2004). Opioids in renal failure and dialysis patients. *Journal of Pain and Symptom Management,* **28**(5), 497–504.

19. Osborne, R., Joel, S., Slevin, M. (1986). Morphine intoxication in renal failure; the role of morphine-6-glucuronide. *British Medical Journal,* **292**, 1548–9.

20. Davison, S.N. (2006). The Pharmacokinetics and Pharmaocdynamics of Hydromorphone in Hemodialysis Patients. ASN Abstract.

21. Babul, N., Darke, A.C., and Hagen, N.. Hydromorphone metabolite accumulation in renal failure. (1995). *Journal of Pain and Symptom Management,* **10**, 184–6.

22. Lee, M.A., Leng, M.E., and Tiernan, E.J. (2001). Retrospective study of the use of hydromorphone in palliative care patients with normal and abnormal urea and creatinine. *Palliative Medicine,* **15**, 26–34.

23. Kirvela, M., Lindgren, L., Seppala, T. *et al.* (1996). The pharmacokinetics of Oxycodone in Uremic patients Undergoing Renal Transplantation. *Journl of Clinical Anesthesia,* **8**, 13–8.

24. Foral, P.A., Ineck, J.R., and Nystrom, K.K. (2007). Oxycodone Accumulation in a Hemodialysis Patient. *Southern Medical Journal* **100**(2), 212–4.

25. Hand, C.W., Sear, J.W., Uppington, J. *et al.* (1990). Buprenorphine disposition in patients with renal impairment: single and continuous dosing, with special reference to metabolites. *British Journal of Anaesthesia,* **64**, 276–82.

26. Ohtani, M., Kotaki, H., Nishitateno, K. *et al.* (1997). Kinetics of respiratory depression in rats induced by Buprenorphine and its metabolite norbuprenorphine. *Journal of Pharmacology and Experimental Therapeutics,* **281**, 428–33.

27. Filitz, J., Griessinger, N., Sittl, R. *et al.* (2006). Effects of intermittent hemodialysis on buprenorphine and norbubrenorphine plasma concentrations in chronic pain patients treated with transdermal buprenorphine. *European Journal of Pain,* **10**, 743–8.

28. Lugon, J.R. (2005). Uraemic Pruritus; A review. *Hemodialysis International,* **9**, 180–8.

29. Medcalf, P., and Bhatia, K.P. (2006). Restless legs syndrome is treatable but under-recognised. *British Medical Journal,* **333**, 457–8.

30. Smith, C., Da Silva-Gane, M., Chandna, S. *et al.* (2003). choosing Not to Dialyse: Evaluation of Planned Non-Dialytic management in a Cohort of Patients with End-Stage Renal Failure. *Nephron. Clinical practice,* **95**, c40–c46.

31. Murtagh, F.E., Addington-Hall, J.M., Donohoe, P. *et al.* (2006). Symptom management in patients with established renal failure managed without dialysis. *EDTNA/ERCA Journal,* **32**(2), 93–8.

32. Murtagh, F.E., Murphy, E., Shepherd, K.A. *et al.* (2006). End-of-life Care in end-stage renal disease: renal and palliative care. *British Journal of Nursing,* **15**, 8–11.

33. Chambers, E.J. (2004). End of Life Care, the terminal phase *In Supportive care for the renal patient,* (eds. E.J. Chambers, M. Germain, and E. Brown), pp. 255–65, Oxford University Press, Oxford.

34. Levy, J.B., Chambers, E.J., and Brown, E.A. (2004). Supportive Care for the renal patient. *Nephrology, Dialysis, Transplantation,* **19**, 1357–60.

12.7

Palliative medicine in intensive care

S.L. Cohen and T.J. Prendergast

Introduction

At first glance, it may seem contradictory to assert that palliative medicine has a place in intensive care. Intensive care units (ICUs) are hospital locations where the prime aim is to prevent patients from dying, principally by stabilizing and reversing organ system failure, often through invasive and highly technology-dependent interventions. Palliative care directs its efforts towards control of suffering, emphasizing quality of life over prolonging life in patients whose illnesses are known to be unresponsive to curative treatment. Palliative medicine specialists typically focus on the period near the end of life, when the complexity of the medical, psychosocial, and spiritual issues often require the input of a team with special competencies in the care of the dying. The seemingly disparate approaches of palliative care and intensive care meet in the ICU for two main reasons: A significant percentage of patients entering ICUs die, and their deaths must be actively managed by physicians who specialize in intensive care (intensivists).

ICU mortality rates vary depending on selection criteria and on the type of patients treated, from <5 per cent to upwards of 40 per cent[1]. Dying in an ICU has evolved over the past two decades in Europe and North America so that death now occurs most often following a considered decision to withhold or withdraw treatment modalities[2]. The high mortality rate in ICUs, and the prevalence of death following decisions to limit therapy, together highlight the importance of integrating the rescue and palliation functions of intensive care.

Despite this common focus on patients at high risk of dying, there are many reasons why physicians and nurses find it difficult to be simultaneous advocates of rescue and palliative medicine. Most importantly, there is a mindset that is common among clinicians in all disciplines that limits palliative care to symptom relief of the dying patient, and sees acknowledgement of dying as inimical to intensive care practice[3]. This mindset can compromise the quality of care. One of the central goals of palliative care, to facilitate communication and promote careful decision-making that maintains focus on patient preferences, can improve the ICU experience for patients and clinicians. Other difficulties pertinent to the ICU that may impede efforts to integrate a palliative care perspective include pervasive uncertainty about prognosis, which makes it difficult to predict which individual patient is going to die[4]; pressure from families to persist in what appears to be ineffective treatment; pressure from colleagues to continue intrusive efforts to save patients recognized as dying by the dispassionate observer; and necessity in many cases to make abrupt transitions from saving life at all costs to allowing the patient to die with dignity, which may confuse relatives and allow them no time to adjust to impending loss.

Palliative and intensive care may seem unlikely partners but, over the past decade, multiple researchers with interest and expertize in both disciplines have begun to develop an evidence-based rationale for their integration. We now understand more clearly the limitations of pain and symptom management in ICUs[5-6]; how families of ICU patients may fail to understand basic information about diagnosis, prognosis, and treatment[7], or experience depression and anxiety[8]; how medical decision-making may not accord with patient preferences[9]; how conflict[10] and burnout[11] are common among clinicians; and how organizational structures may promote or mitigate negative interactions[12,13,14]. There are increasingly sophisticated tools for assessing the quality of palliative care practice within intensive care[15,16] and a growing literature to guide practice[17,18,19] and support-specific interventions[20]. As a result of this deeper understanding of intensive care practice, the intensive care community in Europe and North America increasingly accepts palliative care as integral to the care of critically ill patients, including those who wish to pursue every reasonable measure to prolong life[21,22,23].

Communication: vital for palliative care in intensive care

Several structural factors inherent in intensive care contribute to problems of communication. Most ICU admissions are acute emergencies in patients who did not begin the day anticipating critical illness or contemplating their imminent mortality. Nearly all ICU patients are too ill to take part in discussions about their treatment and very few have established relationships with the intensivists now charged with their care. The intensivist therefore must discuss preferences for care and decision-making with surrogates who may or may not have specific knowledge of the patient's wishes in the particular situation. Family members seek guidance through medical information and inevitably ask about prognosis, but it is genuinely difficult to predict outcomes for individual patients[24].

ICUs contain a large team of clinicians from various disciplines, including nurses, respiratory therapists, physiotherapists, dieticians, and others. Interactions between the family and multiple clinical services create the possibility for conflicting messages and confusion. It is very important to effective communications that there is a shared understanding about patient-care planning, particularly in end-of-life decisions. Physicians must take the initiative to keep all other members of the multi-disciplinary team aware of changing goals of care.

Physicians' own feelings of grief and inadequacy in dealing with dying patients may affect family interactions[25]. Physicians' subspecialty training[13], religious and cultural background[26], and practice location[27,28] profoundly affect attitudes towards withdrawal of life support. Many ICUs, particularly in urban areas, serve multi-ethnic and multi-cultural communities, whose diverse values must be respected. For example, African-Americans in the USA are more likely to want full and prolonged life support than European-Americans[29].

In this complicated environment, one consistent research finding is the importance that surrogates place on communication. In a meta-analysis addressing needs of family members with relatives in intensive care, 8 of the 10 needs identified related to communication with clinicians[30]. As physicians usually have little training in communication about dying or medical decision-making, it is not surprising that the quality of communication remains poor[31,32].

Studies indicate that some strategies to improve communication with families are surprisingly straightforward. Family satisfaction improves when physicians spent more time listening and less time talking[21,33] and when communication aides are provided. In one French study[34], for example, investigators gave families at their first meeting with the intensivist a specially designed leaflet containing general information on the ICU and hospital, the name of the intensivist caring for the patient, a diagram of a typical ICU room with the names of all the devices, and a glossary of 12 terms commonly used in ICUs. The leaflet improved comprehension of family members, and was associated with improved family satisfaction.

In order to improve the quality of communication, physicians should plan and prepare the discussion, as they would any other procedure in intensive care. The clinician should ensure that the discussion can occur in a quiet, private place, without disturbance from mobile telephones or beepers. Various members of the multi-disciplinary team who are involved in the care of the patient should be present. The family should be asked whom they would like to be present at the discussion; it is important to ensure that the most significant relatives and friends are present, if possible. Planning should include reviewing the details of the patient's illness and any knowledge of the patient's attitudes and aspirations. Finally, the clinician planning to discuss life-and-death issues with a patient or family should try to examine his or her own personal feelings, ttitudes, biases, and grief, to understand how these emotions may affect clinical judgement or the ability to communicate with the family.

As discussion with the patient or family begins, the clinician should try to put all participants at ease. It is often best to begin by trying to determine what the patient or family understands, and how much the patient or family wants to know. Although most patients in developed countries, when given the option, want to know the truth about their illness, there are broad individual and cultural differences in this desire. Some patients or families will not want to discuss end-of-life care, and some patients will defer to their families.

Whoever receives the information, it is important to try to discuss the medical issues and the prognosis frankly and openly, and in a way that the family understands. Too often, families are blinded by technical jargon or misinformed by being given uninterpretable information, such as 'the platelet count has risen today and the patient's multi-organ system failure persists'. One must not support unrealistic expectations for survival or improvement, but it is important not to quash all hope. The crucial insight is to redirect hope towards the possible, to focus on alleviating suffering and on healing or cementing relationships. If withdrawal of life-sustaining treatment is suggested, it should be made abundantly clear that a shift in the emphasis of care from cure to comfort does not imply withdrawal of care. The patient is not being abandoned. The patient and family should be reassured that the patient's comfort will be a high priority.

These discussions cannot be rushed. It is useful to allow for periods of silence and to give the family opportunities to ask questions. The aim should be to achieve a common understanding of the disease and the treatment plan. One should make it clear that the patient is continuing to undergo reassessment and that staff will be available for further discussions.

Effective communication also depends on the clinician being able to recognize that a problematic situation exists and then to address it promptly and appropriately. If there is miscommunication, and a corrective discussion takes place too late, ends abruptly, or is inadequate to meet the family's needs, families may feel betrayed or abandoned, leading to conflict between families and physicians[14].

In contrast to intensive care clinicians, for whom death becomes part of their routine, the family often experiences the death of a loved one as an unexpected tragedy. It is commonplace for families to have feelings of guilt, and one should never leave a family feeling that they are responsible for a patient's death. A recommendation to withdraw treatment is a medical decision based on the patient's clinical condition in the setting of his or her wishes for care. To the extent that the family may be involved in decisions to limit therapy, their role is to represent and support the patient. It should be stressed that the withdrawal of treatment modalities does not hasten death so much as it stops the fruitless prolongation of dying.

Some families require time to come to terms with the death of a loved one. If conflict arises, it may be necessary to repeat conversations at frequent intervals. Families should be encouraged to bring whatever support they find meaningful to help them resolve the situation, including outside opinions, spiritual advisors, and others. In many hospitals, ethics committees help to defuse conflict situations.

Symptom control in the intensive care unit

ICUs have a higher concentration of physicians, nurses, and professional staff than other departments of the hospital. Higher staffing ratios should mean that palliation of symptoms is more readily achievable in the ICU than elsewhere. Palliative care is already an essential part of ICU nursing, and applies equally to patients who will survive as it does to those who are going to die. ICU nurses should have the training and experience to assess the needs of the patients and families, speak meaningfully about every planned manoeuvre, and provide support even to patients who are deeply unconscious. Good ICU nursing care is good palliative care.

Many intensive care patients are unconscious on admission or rendered so shortly thereafter. As a consequence, all aspects of pain—physical, psychological, emotional, and spiritual—are difficult to assess. Nonetheless, a surprising percentage of patients can report their symptom burden. In one study, hunger, thirst, and disruption of sleep were reported as moderate or severe by more than 50 per cent of ICU patients[5]. In those ICU patients who cannot report their subjective experience, it is important to look for potential sources of pain, such as pressure sores, infection, poor mouth hygiene, oesophageal candidiasis, and a host of other potential sources. Many procedures regarded as routine in intensive care, such as insertion of lines, intubation, and mechanical ventilation, may cause pain, in addition to distress and anxiety[35].

There is evidence that intensivists systematically under treat pain. In the SUPPORT study, a large US survey of patients with life-threatening illness, 22 per cent of those interviewed in the second week of the study said that they had moderate or severe pain all, most, or half the time[36].

Intensivists also may rely excessively on sedation. Kress et al[37], reported that daily interruption of sedative infusions in critically ill patients undergoing mechanical ventilation resulted in a shorter duration of mechanical ventilation and shorter ICU stay than in a comparable group in whom sedation was not interrupted. Unnecessary sedation may occur, particularly when local practice encourages continuous infusion rather than intermittent dosing.

Delirium is increasingly recognized among ICU patients[38]. It is more common among the elderly, particularly those with underlying dementia, and appears to carry an independent risk for both prolonged hospitalization and increased mortality. The memory impairment and confusion may be very upsetting to families of affected patients, as is the tendency for patients' agitation not to improve or to worsen with well-intentioned, simple reassurance. Haloperidol is the drug of choice.

Clinicians may not become fully aware of patients' symptoms until they are beginning to recover from the insult that led to the ICU admission. After mechanical ventilation has been discontinued and patients are better able to communicate, a frequent request is to be moved into a darkened side room so that the patient may sleep. A need for privacy and an appropriate environment is another common request in recovering patients. Open visiting by family members and, on occasion, by beloved pets, may be of great value in this situation.

Competent symptom management depends on understanding the specific needs of different types of patient. For instance, patients with cirrhosis of the liver or renal impairment may handle drugs very differently than patients with uncomplicated respiratory failure. It is important to understand the pharmacology of a small number of drug families in order to achieve good symptom control. Opioids are of great value and may improve tolerance of an endotracheal tube, suppress coughing, or reduce struggling against a ventilator. However, opioids are only mildly sedative and do not have any specific anxiolytic effects apart from those consequent upon pain reduction. Occasionally, active metabolites of morphine may accumulate in patients with renal failure and contribute to excessive sedation or other adverse effects.

Benzodiazepines and neuroleptics are generally safe and inexpensive drugs to manage the need for sedation, anxiolysis, or other symptoms in ICU patients. Benzodiazepines have potent anxiolytic and amnestic properties, and are mild hypnotics. They have no intrinsic analgesic effects but may be synergistic with opioids in causing central respiratory depression. Haloperidol is the usual neuroleptic of choice for the management of delirium and psychosis; chlorpromazine is a more sedating agent with similar clinical effects.

When a decision to withdraw treatment has been made, it is commonplace to administer both analgesics and sedatives. The amount of opioid necessary to control acute pain or dyspnoea varies widely, and large doses can be necessary. The dose is not fixed, but rather, should be matched to the patient's needs[35]. Administration of neuromuscular blocking agents should be discontinued following a decision to withdraw mechanical ventilation. Neuromuscular blockade is not desirable because it renders clinical assessment of pain difficult or impossible[39].

Many families find the experience of a family member being treated in the ICU to be distressing and even traumatic[40,41]. It is part of the ICU team's remit to try to address the problems of the family as well as the patient[42]. A proactive communication strategy, combined with written informational materials, has been shown to lessen the burden of bereavement[21]. Counsellors and spiritual advisors should be available for patients and relatives as part of the ICU service.

Withholding and withdrawing intensive care treatment

The shared understanding that it is generally inappropriate to use intensive care to prolong dying represents a recent and difficult consensus[43]. A high proportion of hospital deaths occurs in ICUs, now most often following a considered decision to withhold or withdraw life-sustaining treatment[2,44]. Medical treatment, founded on beneficence and compassion for the patient, is no different in an era when death in the ICU has become a managed process. Good communication based on collaboration and consensus among doctors, patients, and families is essential, especially when treatment limitation is proposed[45].

There are many factors involved in decisions to limit life-sustaining therapy. How this decision is made, and who is ultimately responsible, varies from institution to institution and from country to country. From the medical point of view, the first requirement is that there is at least acceptance and at best consensus agreement among all the members of the medical team, to limit therapy when hope for recovery is outweighed by burden of the treatment. This decision should be supported by the senior physician responsible for the patient. The patient's wishes for continued treatment are of paramount importance; unfortunately, in the ICU, these views are usually not known directly from the patient, but are represented by the family. It is very important, therefore, that the views of the family be taken into consideration and attempts made to avoid conflict at this sensitive time. For clinicians working in intensive care, it must always be remembered that the passing of a loved one may be a potent source of grief and guilt for family members, so the maximum sensitivity in handling the situation is essential.

Meeting the needs of a dying patient's family may be particularly challenging given ongoing changes in the relationship between the medical profession and the general public. Sjokvist reported in 1999 that patients and families wanted to be involved in decisions to limit treatment, and only 5 per cent of the Swedish public supported a physician-only approach[46]. Along with diminishing trust in the medical profession, medical information is increasingly available from a variety of sources of highly variable reliability. Very fine information and gross misinformation are available side-by-side on the Internet, and families who search for information may be unable to weigh the quality of what they read. Many popular television shows[47] maximize recovery from critical illness in a way that also fuels unrealistic expectations that families may bring to the bedside. At the same time, intensivists recognize that prognosis in critical illness is often uncertain. Morbidity and mortality are high despite their best efforts, and clinicians may be challenged to respond patiently to the naïve optimism expressed by family members. Physicians, nurses, and families often disagree about how to value a small chance of improvement or how to weigh the continuing burdens of treatment[48]. In this complex environment, different perspectives complicate communication with patients and families, and communication among members of the multidisciplinary team. These complications may be magnified in a discussion of withdrawal of life supporting therapies.

In the current climate, decision-making must be open and accountable to the patient, family, and all concerned. All discussions and decisions should be detailed in the patient's record. The role and legal position of surrogate decision makers depend on the particular country, and may not be clearly defined. The UK law, for example, allows the senior physician to make a decision to withdraw life support but, at the very least, this should be done with the assent of the family. In the USA, both the medical community and the public accuse each other of over-treatment, but the evidence suggests that physicians and families are roughly equally responsible[49]. Many physicians, unhappy with patient and family decisions that they regard as medically inappropriate, attempt to apply the concept of medical futility in order to reassert their prerogative to make the decision they favour at the end of life[50]. Such use of the concept of medical futility is seriously flawed and may lead to complete breakdown of communications.

Guidelines for limitation of intensive care treatment

Decision-making concerning the withdrawal of life-sustaining therapy, and the implementation of a plan of care once such decisions are made, are both exceedingly complex processes. It is possible, nonetheless, to develop guidelines that emphasize best practices, in order to reduce variation and to counter perceptions that life-and-death decisions are ever pursued in an ad hoc or capricious way. The guidelines that follow are founded on ethical principles and reflect a high level of professional competency.

Ethics

Almost all ethical authorities agree that there is no moral difference between withholding and withdrawing treatments. In practice, however, many clinicians feel more comfortable withholding treatments, particularly in the first instance, rather than withdrawing treatment.

Any life-sustaining therapy may be withdrawn or withheld, including blood products, haemofiltration, vasopressors, parenteral nutrition, antibiotics, mechanical ventilation, and artificial nutrition and hydration. Artificial nutrition and hydration have a privileged legal status in some countries, and often need special care because of their association with feeding and nurturing, the perceived withdrawal of which may give rise to dissent.

Medical treatment should only be withdrawn on clinical grounds. Every withdrawal decision should be made upon its own merits and must not be made on the basis of either cost or medical convenience (e.g. to avoid the cancellation of a surgical/medical procedure, or to transfer out of an ICU bed). Limitation of treatment should be regarded as a formal ICU procedure subject to the same preparation, thought, care, and consent as any other procedure.

In a physiologically fragile and dying patient, the administration of opioids or sedatives in doses adequate to ensure comfort may hasten death. Therefore, the management of treatment withdrawal may uncover a conflict between two primary duties of the clinician: to provide comfort always, and to do no harm. There is broad consensus among physicians, bioethicists, legal scholars, and the public, that attention to symptom control is not only permissible but also essential, provided that the intention of the clinician is to relieve suffering, and that dosing is carefully titrated toward that end. The intellectual and legal justification for this practice is the so-called principle of 'double-effect'[51].

Some physicians and nurses may have conscientious objection to treatment withdrawal. Their view should be respected and they should be allowed not to involve themselves with procedures that violate their principles. If necessary, the patient should be transferred to another physician.

When patients are admitted to the ICU there must be a clear plan for management, including identification of surrogate decision makers, clarification of the goals of care, and definition of any limits on invasive interventions, including resuscitation status. It is good practice for the physician in charge of the patient to meet with the family within 24 h of the time of admission.

If the patient is competent, then the patient's wishes and preferences for treatment are of the greatest importance and must be ascertained. It is essential that all discussions and decisions be clearly recorded in the patient's notes. This may be invaluable if decisions are challenged at a later date. In the case of patients who are incompetent or who lack the decisional capacity to guide specific actions, laws that vary across and within countries help to define the specific right of the family. If the patient has legally designated an individual to be his or her health-care agent, then this person can make decisions for the patient which reflect the patient's previously expressed wishes or best interests. If the patient who is unable to make decisions lacks a family or other surrogate decision makers, the physician has to determine what is in the best interest of the patient, consistent with local custom, and statute[52]. Assistance by an Ethics Committee experienced in such matters may be invaluable.

It is the responsibility and duty of the intensivist to recognize a dying patient and to know when the burdens of aggressive, disease-modifying therapies outweigh the potential benefits. In this setting, palliative care becomes the overriding approach. All members of the multi-disciplinary team should recognize that families frequently need time to come to terms with their impending loss. Intensivists also need to understand death and bereavement, and how to support the family in their time of grief and despair.

Training

There is a paramount need for improved training for all ICU personnel in all the relevant domains of palliative care, including communication, comprehensive assessment, pain and symptom control, care of the needs of the actively dying, and others. In all discussions with surrogates, sufficient time must be given for the family to speak; the doctor conducting the meeting should not monopolize conversation, and should invite the perspective of the family and allow for silences. Clinicians should avoid referring to the patient by their disease; the statement, 'This is the case of alcoholic liver failure', is an extremely insensitive way to address the patient or their family. It is important to try to build a picture of the patient as a person in their pre-morbid state by asking about their occupation, activities, and interests. This approach may enhance trust between physicians and the family.

Withdrawal of treatment

Patients and families should be given the maximum possible access and privacy during withdrawal of life support. If possible, the patient should be in a private room; otherwise, the curtains should be drawn. All unnecessary alarms and monitors should be removed from the patient. Although treatment may be withdrawn, the patient's care should continue to be compassionate and attentive at the highest level. To this end, it is important to relieve the patient's pain and distress by judicious administration of suitable drugs (such as opioids and benzodiazepines) in appropriate doses by intravenous bolus or infusion. The dosage needs to be adjusted to relieve the patient's suffering but not to hasten death. At the time of withdrawal of life support, however, the comfort of the patient is paramount. If comfort can only be achieved with doses of medications that may hasten death, such administration is appropriate if the intention of the clinician is the relief of suffering.

Treatments aimed at maintaining organ function that prolong death but do not contribute to palliation of symptoms should be withdrawn. Examples include vasoactive drugs, antibiotics, and intravenous fluids. The practice of withdrawal of respiratory support is variable. In the sickest patients, positive end expiratory pressure is eliminated and the inspired oxygen concentration is reduced to ambient air (21 per cent). Where appropriate the patient may be extubated. Adequate analgesia and sedation are of paramount importance. Neuromuscular blocking agents should be avoided at this time as they render impossible assessment of the patient's awareness and degree of suffering.

The issue sometimes arises whether the patient should be transferred to a different floor or facility that may be more conducive to dying in peace. Although this approach may be appropriate in some institutions, it eliminates the potential benefit that can be derived by the continuing involvement of a multi-disciplinary ICU team that has established relationships with the patients and their families. In many cases, transfer out of the ICU can be disruptive, diminish the quality of care, and potentially give rise to a feeling of abandonment.

The way forward

The ICU has an important role as a palliative care facility. Brett describes the problems of admitting patients to the ICU who have little or no hope of survival[53]. There are a variety of reasons for this practice, including the inability to identify the dying with certainty, disagreement among the clinicians involved over diagnosis and prognosis, overwhelming pressure from the patient, family or referring physicians, and the need to preserve working relationships within an institution. Patients who have suffered an iatrogenic injury may be preferentially admitted. It is important to transfer a very sick patient from a ward environment where they cannot receive proper nursing care to the ICU, particularly if the atmosphere on the ward has become highly charged.

Palliative care is important for patients and their relatives who make requests for a better death. That is not to say that patients should ever be deprived of curative therapy, just that the physicians in the ICU need to be sensitive to these sorts of request[54]

In some settings, the single most important step in implementing palliative care in the ICU is to institute mandatory family meetings with the senior physician in charge. The purpose of such meetings is to inform the family about the patient and his illness from the perspective of the treating physicians, to allow clinicians to orient the family to the ICU, to establish a strategy for future communication, and to reassure the family of their involvement in the process while permitting the clinician to gain insight into the attitudes of the family. Family meetings also enable the clinician to see the patient as a person rather than a disease in a bed. Sequential meetings over time convey the extraordinary efforts of the ICU team to care for patients, engender trust with the family, and reduce the frequency of conflict by helping family to feel well informed.

Additional key measures in ensuring that good palliative care is performed in the ICU include identifying surrogate decision makers; clarifying the patient's goals of care, including wishes for resuscitation (particularly if there is a completed advance directive); providing family and friends with written information about the ICU and ICU policies; instituting regular pain and symptom assessment; and developing a multi-disciplinary approach that provides for counselling and spiritual support for those families in need.[17]

Good communication skills must be part of the training and reassessment of all intensive care clinicians. Such skills will help clinicians and families to cope with uncertainty, unstable and changing situations, intense personal relationships, and emotions on both sides of the clinician/family divide. Techniques such as videotaping clinicians when they are conducting interviews may be of great value. It is important that trainees be involved in these discussions, but family meetings should generally be led by the clinician in charge.

References

1. Prendergast, T.J., Claessens, M.T., and Luce, J.M. (1998). A national survey of end-of-life care for critically ill patients. *Amercian Journal of Respiratory and Critical Care Medicine*, **158**, 1163–7.
2. Luce, J.M. and Prendergast, T.J. (2001). The changing nature of death in the ICU. In: *Managing death in the intensive care unit*. (eds. J.R. Curtis and G.D. Rubenfeld), pp 19–29, Oxford University Press, New York.
3. Nelson, J.E. (2006). Identifying and overcoming the barriers to high-quality palliative care in the intensive care unit. *Critical Care Medicine*, **34** (Suppl 11), S324–S331.
4. Teres, D. and Lemeshaw, S. (1994). Why severity models should be used with caution. *Critical Care Clinics*, **10**, 93–110, discussion 111–5.
5. Nelson, J.E., Meier, D.E., Oei, E.J. *et al.* (2001). Self reported symptom experience of critically ill cancer patients receiving intensive care. *Critical Care Medicine*, **29**, 277–82.

6. Somogyi-Zalud, E., Zhong, Z., Lynn, J. et al. (2000). Dying with acute respiratory failure or multiple organ system failure with sepsis. J Am Geriatr Soc, **48**, S140–S145.

6. Desbiens, N.A., Wu, A.W., Broste, S.K. et al. (1996). Pain and satisfaction with pain control in seriously ill hospitalized adults: findings from the SUPPORT research investigations. Critical Care Medicine, **24**, 1953–61.

7. Azoulay, E., Chevret, S., Leleu, G. et al. (2000). Half the families of intensive care unit patients experience inadequate communication with physicians. Critical Care Medicine, **28**, 3044–9.

8. Pochard, F., Azoulay, E., Chevret, S. et al. for the French FAMIREA Study Group (2001). Symptoms of anxiety and depression in family members of intensive care unit patients: ethical hypothesis regarding decision-making capacity. Critical Care Medicine, **29**, 1893–7.

9. Cook, D.J., Guyatt, G., Rocker, G.M. et al. (2001). Cardiopulmonary resuscitation directives on admission to intensive-care unit: n international observational study. Lancet, **358**, 1941–5.

10. Studdert, D.M., Mello, M.M., Burns, J.P. et al. (2003). Conflict in the care of patients with prolonged stay in the ICU: types, sources, and predictors. Intensive Care Medicine, **29**, 1489–97.

11. Embriaco, N., Azoulay, E., Barrau, K. et al. (2007). High level of burnout in intensivists: prevalence and associated factors. American Journal of Respiratory Critical Care Medicine, **175**, 686–92.

12. Cassell, J., Buchman, T.G., Streat, S. et al. (2003). Surgeons, intensivists, and the covenant of care: administrative models and values affecting care at the end of life—Updated. Critical Care Medicine, **31**, 1551–7, discussion 1557–9.

13. Fins, J.J. and Solomon, M.Z. (2001). Communication in intensive care settings: the challenge of futility disputes. Critical Care Medicine, **29** (Suppl 2), N10–N15.

14. Nelson, J.E., Angus, D.C., Weissfeld, L. et al., for the Critical Care Peer Workgroup of the Promoting Excellence in End-of-Life Care Project. (2006). End-of-life care for the critically ill: A national intensive care unit survey. Critical Care Medicine, **34**, 2547–53.

15. Mularski, R.A., Curtis, J.R., Billings, J.A. et al. (2006). Proposed quality measures for palliative care in the critically ill: a consensus from the Robert Wood Johnson Foundation Critical Care Workgroup. Critical Care Medicine, **34** (Suppl 11), S404–S411.

16. Nelson, J.E., Mulkerin, C.M., Adams, L.L. et al. (2006). Improving comfort and communication in the ICU: a practical new tool for palliative care performance measurement and feedback. Quality and Safety in Health Care, **15**, 264–71.

17. Prendergast, T.J. and Puntillo, K.A. (2002). Withdrawal of life support: intensive caring at the end of life. JAMA, **288**, 2732–40.

18. Azoulay, E. and Sprung, C.L. (2004). Family-physician interactions in the intensive care unit. Critical Care Medcine, **32**, 2323–8.

19. Fassier, T., Lautrette, A., Ciroldi, M. et al. (2005). Care at the end of life in critically ill patients: the European perspective. Current Opinion in Critical Care, **11**, 616–23.

20. Lautrette, A., Darmon, M., Megarbane, B. et al. (2007). A communication strategy and brochure for relatives of patients dying in the ICU. New England Journal of Medicine, **356**, 469–78.

21. Carlet, J., Thijs, L.G., Antonelli, M. et al. (2004). Challenges in end-of-life care in the ICU. Statement of the 5th International Consensus Conference in Critical Care: Brussels, Belgium, April 2003. Intensive Care Medicine, **30**, 770–84.

22. Truog, R.D., Cist, A.F., Brackett, S.E. et al. (2001). Recommendations for end-of-life care in the intensive care unit: The Ethics Committee of the Society of Critical Care Medicine. Critical Care Medicine, **29**, 2332–48.

23. Selecky, P.A., Eliasson, C.A., Hall, R.I. et al. (2005). Palliative and end-of-life care for patients with cardiopulmonary diseases: American College of Chest Physicians position statement. Chest, **128**, 3599–610.

24. Barnato, A.E. and Angus, D.C. (2004). Value and role of intensive care unit outcome prediction models in end-of-life decision-making. Critical Care Clinics, **20**, 345–62.

25. Curtis, J.R. and Patrick, D.L. (2001) How to discuss dying and death in the ICU. In Managing death in the intensive care unit. (eds. J.R. Curtis and G.D. Rubenfeld), pp 85–102, Oxford University Press, New York.

26. Yaguchi, A., Truog, R.D., Curtis, J.R. et al. (2005). International differences in end-of-life attitudes in the intensive care unit: results of a survey. Archives of Internal Medicine, **165**, 1970–5.

27. Vincent, J.L. (1999). Forgoing life support in Western European ICUs. The results of an ethical questionnaire. Critical Care Medicine, **27**, 1626–33.

28. Sprung, C.L., Cohen, S.L., Sjokvist, P. et al. for the Ethicus Study Group. (2003). End-of-life practices in European intensive care units: the Ethicus Study. JAMA, **290**, 790–7.

29. Blackhall, L.J., Frank, G., Murphy, S.T. et al. (1999). Ethinicity and attitudes towards life sustaining technology. Social Science and Medicine, **48**, 1779–89.

30. Hickey, M. (1990). What are the needs of families of critically ill patients? A review of the literature since 1975. Heart Lung, **19**, 401–15.

31. White, D.B., Braddock, C.H. 3rd, Bereknyei, S. et al. (2007). Toward shared decision-making at the end of life in intensive care units: opportunities for improvement. Archives of Internal Medicine, **167**, 461–7.

32. Curtis, J.R., Engelberg, R.A., Wenrich, M.D. et al. (2005). Missed opportunities during family conferences about end-of-life care in the intensive care unit. American Journal of Respiratory and Critical Care Medicine, **171**, 844–9.

33. McDonagh, J.R., Elliott, T.B., Engelberg, R.A. et al. (2004). Family satisfaction with family conferences about end-of-life care in the intensive care unit: increased proportion of family speech is associated with increased satisfaction. Critical Care Medicine, **32**, 1484–8.

34. Azoulay, E., Pochard, F., Chevret, S. et al. (2002). Impact of a family information leaflet on effectiveness of information provided to family members of intensive care unit patients: a multicenter, prospective, randomized, controlled trial. American Journal of Respiratory. Critical Care Medicine, **165**, 438–42.

35. Prendergast, T.J. (2007). Palliative Care in the Intensive Care Unit Setting. In Principles and practice of supportive oncology, 3rd edition., Chapter 76 (eds. A.M.Berger, J.L. Shuster, Jr., and J.H. VonRoenn), pp. 849–65. Lippincott, Williams and Wilkins, Philadelphia.

36. The SUPPORT Investigators (1995). A controlled trial to improve care for seriously ill hospitalised patients. The study to understand prognosis and preferences for outcomes and types of treatments. JAMA, **274**, 1591–8.

37. Kress, J.P., Pohlman, A.S., O'Connor, M.F. et al. (2000). Daily interruption of sedative infusions in critically ill patients undergoing mechanical ventilation. New England Journal of Medicine, **342**, 1471–7.

38. Ely, E.W., Shintani, A., Truman, B. et al. (2004). Delirium as a predictor of mortality in mechanically ventilated patients in the intensive care unit. JAMA, **291**, 1753–62.

39. Truog, R.D., Burns, J.P., Mitchell, C. et al. (2000). Pharmacologic paralysis and withdrawal of mechanical ventilation at the end of life. New England Journal of Medicine, **342**, 508–11.

40. Heyland, D.K., Rocker, G.M., O'Callaghan, C.J. et al. (2003). Dying in the ICU: perspectives of family members. Chest, **124**, 392–7.

41. Azoulay, E., Pochard, F., Kentish-Barnes, N. et al. for the FAMIREA Study Group (2005). Risk of post-traumatic stress symptoms in family members of intensive care unit patients. American Journal of Respiratory and Critical Care Medicine, **171**, 987–94.

42. Davidson, J.E., Powers, K., Hedayat, K.M. et al. (2007). Clinical practice guidelines for support of the family in the patient-centered intensive care unit: American College of Critical Care Medicine Task Force 2004-2005, Society of Critical Care Medicine. Critical Care Medicine, **35**, 605–22.

43. Luce, J.M. and Alpers, A. (2000). Legal aspects of withholding and withdrawing life support from critically ill patients in the United States and providing palliative care to them. *American Journal of Respiratory and Critical Care Medicine*, **162**, 2029–32.

44. Angus, D.C., Barnato, A.E., Linde-Zwirble, W.T. *et al.* for the Robert Wood Johnson Foundation ICU End-Of-Life Peer Group (2004). Use of intensive care at the end of life in the United States: an epidemiologic study. *Critical Care Medicine*, **32**, 638–43.

45. Cohen, S.L., Ridley, S., and Goldhill, D. (2002). Guidelines for limitation of intensive care treatment in adults. UK Intensive Care Society, http://www.ics.ac.uk/icmprof/downloads/LimitTreatGuidelines2003.pdf

46. Sjokvist, P., Nilstun, T., Svantesson, M. *et al.* (1999). Withdrawal of life support – who should decide? Differences in attitudes among the general public, nurses and physicians. *Intensive Care Medicine*, **25**, 949–54.

47. Diem, S.J., Lantos, J.D., and Tulsky, J.A. (1996). Cardiopulmonary resuscitation on television. Miracles and misinformation. *New England Journal of Medicine*, **334**, 1578–82.

48. Asch, D.A. (1996). The role of critical care nurses in euthanasia nd assisted suicide. *New England Journal of Medicine*, **334**, 1374–9.

49. Prendergast, T.J. (1997). Resolving conflicts surrounding end of life care. *New Horizons*, **5**, 62–71.

50. Prendergast, T.J. (1995). Futility and the common cold. How requests for antibiotics can illuminate care at the end of life. *Chest*, **107**, 836–44.

51. Sulmasy, D.P. and Pellegrino, E.D. (1999). The rule of double effect: clearing up the double talk. *Archives of Internal Medicine*, **159**, 545–50.

52. White, D.B., Curtis, J.R., Wolf, L.E. *et al.* (2007). Life Support for Patients without a Surrogate Decision Maker: Who Decides? *Annals of Internal Medicine*, **147**, 34–40.

53. Brett, S. (2001). Ethical questions for the new millennium. *Proceedings of the Brussels Intensive Care Symposium*, 708–715.

54. Back, A.L. and Pearlman, R.A. (2001). Desire for physician assisted suicide requests for a better death. *Lancet*, **358**, 362–3.

SECTION 13

Paediatric palliative medicine

Children in palliative medicine: an overview

Betty Davies and Harold Siden

Differences between palliative care for adults and children

The concept of *paediatric* palliative care is an extension of palliative care philosophy, but with specific differences that distinguish it from adult palliative care. Taken broadly, the phrase paediatric palliative care designates a programme or approach to care that seeks to maximize present quality of life by adapting principles of palliative care to children themselves, including newborn infants and adolescents, or their family members, and to other concerned persons who are coping with any of the following as they relate to a child: living with serious or life-threatening illness, the imminent likelihood of dying, or the aftermath of death[1].

Several consensus groups and committees have developed formalized statements elucidating these concepts[2–5]. Care is provided to *children and their families* who live with progressive life-threatening diseases. Various alternative terms include 'life-limiting' instead of 'life-threatening' and 'condition' instead of 'disease'. Nevertheless, at the core they all describe a population of children with severely impaired health who have a high risk of dying before they reach adulthood.

Since the late 1960s, the adult palliative care movement increased in size and sophistication as a result of a growing awareness of the needs of terminally ill people and their families. Palliative care for adults has evolved to a stage where it is understood and is perceived as a reasonable option of care for individuals who may be suffering from an incurable illness. Palliative care for children, however, is in much earlier stages of acceptance and only beginning to receive its place in the spectrum of health-care services. The strongly held belief that 'children are not supposed to die' creates societal barriers to facing this reality.

It has been said sometimes regarding adult and paediatric palliative care that the fields 'share the same words but mean different things'. For example, using aggressive, curative interventions up until death is quite common in paediatrics. There is far less acceptance of the inevitability of death and therefore an emphasis on cure, or at least intervention, throughout the trajectory. Since palliative care can be introduced early in the course of illness, for example soon after diagnosis of an incurable life-threatening disease, children may be in a paediatric palliative programme for many years. The term 'length of stay' therefore means something quite different to paediatric and adult clinicians. Children require specialized approaches and services to meet their unique needs and they require a combination of specialized caregivers in addition to their family. Additionally, family members, especially siblings, have special unique needs and concerns. Their needs and how they are met will vary greatly according to the characteristics and age of each child, the family, and caregivers involved.

Background
Diagnoses

Children who could benefit from palliative care have different diagnoses than do most adults receiving palliative care. Life-threatening diseases in paediatrics are those diseases that are likely to end in death sometime between diagnosis and full adulthood, generally accepted to be in the third decade of life. The common perception is that children's programmes are just for children dying of cancer, as is still the case for the majority of adult palliative care patients. With children however, only about 20 per cent of those admitted to palliative care programmes have cancer. The majority of children needing palliative care have a wide range of diagnoses including pulmonary disease, congenital anomalies, and progressive neurological and metabolic diseases, many with a range of associated mental and physical impairments. These diagnoses mean that a major focus of paediatric palliative care must be on the need for respite services due to the extended experience of illness. Most adult programmes admit patients who are within weeks to days of death. In contrast, children's programmes seek to admit children and their families as they progress through the various phases of the illness trajectory and into bereavement. Accordingly, the length of stay may be considerably longer than is typical in adult programmes. In paediatrics, the emphasis is often on continuing life-prolonging interventions, 'buying time' and preserving hope. In the end, the quality of life for the child can be vastly improved, even if the quantity of life cannot be dramatically changed, through the support and expertise of the palliative care team.

The 1997 ACT/Royal College of Paediatrics and Child Health report[4], revised in 2003, provided a very helpful categorization of the kinds of children accessing palliative care. Children in the first category have diseases that are often curable, but the cure has not been successful. Cancer is a paradigm illness for this category; however, there are many diseases in this group, especially in industrialized countries where advanced medical technology is readily available. The second category constitutes diseases where cure, i.e. elimination of the underlying, pathophysiological disturbance, is not available, but where therapies alter significantly the natural course and prolong life. Cystic fibrosis is a classic example—until now, gene therapy has not been able to cure the disease, but a number of advances in disease management have prolonged life expectancy significantly, in fact into young adulthood[6]. Many other diseases are now in this second category, for example Duchenne's muscular dystrophy can now be considered a Category 2 disease. Category 3 diseases are those without cure or even a directed or disease-modified treatment; symptom management is the core approach. The classical metabolic diseases are amongst the many diseases in this group.

The fourth category comprises a challenging group. In these conditions, the inherent disease itself is not progressive, but is static, and the sequelae constitute the life-limiting aspect. Secondary effects to the disease compromise the child's health and become life-threatening. The paradigmatic situation is the child with an encephalopathy due to an anoxic brain injury (e.g. near-drowning). Subsequently, the injury does not continue; however, the disruptions in function can be massive. In the most severely affected, problems include poorly controlled seizures, repeated aspiration pneumonias, worsening scoliosis with cardio-respiratory dysfunction, compromised nutrition, and skin breakdown. All of these problems may compound and lead to an earlier-than-expected death. Unlike the first three categories, the 'disease' here is entirely functional, and therefore harder to prognosticate.

Another and complementary formulation of the diagnostic categories seen in paediatric palliative care uses the concept of Complex Chronic Conditions (CCC)[7]. On the basis of ICD-9 coding, categories of disease are described, including cardiac, malignancy, neuromuscular, respiratory, renal, gastrointestinal, immunodeficiency, and metabolic, genetic, and other congenital anomalies. Information is available on the CCCs from large databases. The CCC approach is another way of describing the conditions of the children and families frequently receiving paediatric palliative care. It has the advantage of enabling a detailed examination of different diagnostic groups. The ACT/RCPCH formulation speaks directly to the Life-Threatening Diseases and may be useful in addressing the types of care that children and families require.

Prognoses

The key reason that it is so important to understand the range of diagnoses in children with life-threatening disease is how diagnosis interacts with prognosis. As is known from adult research studies, making even somewhat accurate prognostications for patients with advanced diseases is difficult[8]. In children, prognostication becomes even more difficult for several reasons. Most of the Life-Threatening Diseases/Complex Chronic Conditions are highly rare. For example in the United Kingdom, 1500 new cases of cancer are diagnosed each year. In the US, the data are 9746 new cases diagnosed in children aged 0–14, in the years 2000–2003[9].

Arguably, cancer is the most closely studied of the childhood life-threatening diseases in the industrialized countries because of an extensive network that collects data for therapy trials, in parallel to the adult system. When one begins to examine the other significant diagnostic groups of life-threatening diseases, such as genetic-cellular, metabolic, neurodegenerative, and severe neurological

impairments due to prematurity, abnormalities of nervous system genesis, and anoxic injury, no similar databases exist.

Yet it is the latter diagnoses that make up the majority of life-threatening diseases as followed by paediatric palliative care teams. For example, among the number of children followed by the paediatric palliative care team at Canuck Place Children's Hospice in Vancouver, Canada, at a single point in time, cancer makes up 5 per cent of the cases, whereas the combined diagnoses of central nervous system (CNS) disease, metabolic-genetic diseases, or multi-organ chromosomal conditions comprise 49 per cent. Receiving paediatric palliative care means access to respite/family care, acute symptom management, and end-of-life care. In contrast, from the same organization, when looking at 'deaths on programme' as incidence over several years, cancer makes up 41 per cent of those cases, with the aforementioned conditions at 43 per cent.

Second, what is known about these most unusual conditions is based on early studies, some published even before the advent of modern care for these children. Older textbooks contain out-dated information on mean and median survival based on small numbers or even case reports. For many of these diseases, the emphasis of biomedical research has been in uncovering the underlying genetic-cellular pathways leading to the disturbed pathophysiology. For those diseases not amenable to cure or significant life-prolonging therapy, there has been no attention paid to improving the understanding of the epidemiology and natural trajectory of the diseases.

A third factor that alters the prognostic profile of the disease conditions is simple improvements in care. Attention to hygiene, artificial routes of nutrition, improved seizure management, powerful but easily delivered antibiotics (including oral), significant changes in seating, and mobility systems to minimize musculoskeletal complications have all combined to change the outcome for even the most affected children. Because there are only limited registries and databases following children with these conditions, and those registries were not designed to distinguish children by functional health status, there is little opportunity to examine how the prognoses have changed over the years.

The fourth factor affecting prognosis is the tremendous underlying 'resiliency' of children. This is really a reflection of the fact that most of a child's cellular and organ systems are oriented towards rapid growth and repair. It is uncommon for children to have the multi-organ disease adults often have. For example, it is likely that a child with severe neurological impairment still has healthy cardiac, renal, and immunologic systems. These systems will continue to function well until very near the end of life.

The end result is that parents, clinicians, and health-care planners are often faced with outdated and very limited data regarding longevity and trajectory.

Epidemiology

Specific epidemiologic data on children receiving paediatric palliative services is difficult to come by in the United States, Canada, or the United Kingdom. In part, this has to do with the lack of universal agreement as to which diseases constitute the life-threatening group as described. Furthermore, for many diagnoses, such as the cellular, classical metabolic, and neurological diseases, diagnosis alone can be a poor predictor of prognosis—close attention to clinical course, function, and progression is more important. Therefore, categorization of diseases in large population databases may not add much information.

Nevertheless, there are some rough numbers describing the population for western industrialized nations. A series of studies in the United Kingdom[4] all suggest that somewhere between 1 in 700 and 1 in 1500 children have conditions that would be addressed by paediatric palliative care services. Studies in the United States describing the population of children with Complex Chronic Conditions suggest that 15 000 children die each year and that 5000 are within their last 6 months of life[7]. The data are not readily comparable to the studies informing the ACT/RCPCH report as the US data looks at children assumed to be within their last 6 months of life. Nevertheless, these studies begin to develop the basis for planning; it is within the CCC population that those with progressive, life-threatening disease will be found.

The situation is entirely different in the developing world. Much attention has been focused on HIV-AIDS in Africa and there is a body of literature regarding methods of providing palliative care to children. Only a small fraction of people living with HIV/AIDS are children, but the numbers are rising and have devastating implications for the future. Children, defined by UNAIDS as persons under age 15, comprised 7.6 per cent of the infected population, 1.6 per cent of new infections and 1.9 per cent of AIDS deaths in 2002. Infections in the womb are still common. Out of global total of 14 million AIDS orphans, 11 million live in sub-Saharan Africa[10]. Palliative care is highly contextual and thus, while HIV can be controlled in industrialized countries, it must be considered a life-threatening disease in the context of developing world counties where treatment is not reliably available. Nevertheless, similar principles of care, including delineating the critical distinctions between adults and children, still apply.

The child

Developmental considerations in child health

The major obvious difference that strikes observers is the 'developmental nature' of child health. Not only are the diagnoses and overall epidemiology different between adults and children but the significance of the developmental trajectory is a critical factor. Moreover, what makes this issue even more complex is that paediatric clinicians must deal with both children experiencing illness alongside normal healthy development and children whose illness is linked to severely disrupted development. Within each of these two groups, there are various levels of developmental stage and sequence and the patient must be approached at the appropriate level, whilst keeping in mind the possibility of transformation into the next level. This is a complex dynamic, as the following examples may illustrate:

A 15-year-old young man had a diagnosis of osteosarcoma. He was referred to the paediatric hospice palliative care team for symptom management, discussion of advanced directives, and family support. He was a healthy, intelligent, and athletic child when he was initially diagnosed at age 11. After a relapse at age 13, he underwent limb amputation and acquired a prosthetic leg; chemotherapy was re-introduced leading to alopecia. Numerous metastatic lesions appeared. He underwent two surgical procedures for palliative purposes to remove tumours impinging on his heart and on spine. Subsequently, he developed paraplegia and was required to use a wheelchair for mobility. Transfers for daily care including bathing became a challenge. All of the alterations in body image, ability, and function occurred in the setting of a young teen experiencing and attempting to fulfil normal adolescent development and transition.

He tried to stay in school as much as possible, socialize with friends, and find athletic outlets such as wheelchair basketball. His variable health status compromised all of this. Some of his friends, although not all, found it awkward to be around him but his social life was very compromised. He could be moody and not always communicative about symptoms such as pain and constipation. The anger and frustration were sometimes attributed to emotional response to disease, sometimes to healthy adolescent expression and sometimes to mood modifying drugs such as steroids. It was noted that some members of the clinical team treated him as the happy but essentially dependent 11-year-old they had first met, while others saw him as a young man with clear ideas regarding his own needs and wishes.

This case illustrates the complexity of dealing with the rapidly transforming individual within a matrix whose elements include the transition from childhood to adolescence, burdens of disease, and a progressive life-altering and life-threatening condition.

The second case illustrates the other commonly encountered developmental challenge—the child with severely compromised development:

An 8-year-old girl was referred to the paediatric hospice palliative care team by her General Practitioner (GP). She was the product of a 36 week uncomplicated pregnancy with a birth weight of 1.9 kg and microcephaly. After hospital discharge she had difficulty with sucking and swallowing, requiring naso-gastric feeding. At age four months, she experienced the onset of generalized seizures. An extensive genetic-metabolic workup did not reveal a specific gene or cellular condition; CNS imaging showed a poorly developing brain with large ventricles and periventricular leucomalacia. At age 5, she was physically small with weight and estimated length less than the 10th percentile. She was wheelchair dependent with marked hypertonicity, spasticity, and rigidity. She had cortical visual impairment. Seizures occurred typically one to two times per month but when she was ill they would be daily. Feeding was exclusively by gastrostomy; she had moderate reflux controlled with medications. She did not have language but did vocalize; her parents and school caregiver used some combinations of vocalization and gesture as simple communication, consistent with yes/no, happy/sad. These adults also consistently interpreted her feelings and moods through more subtle signs that they were not able to describe easily. For her first 6 years of life, she was seldom ill. In the prior 2 years, she had undergone hospitalization multiple times for worsening reflux disease, repeated aspiration pneumonia and influenza, and more frequent seizures. There were episodes of unexplained crying and arching. She had been admitted to the Intensive Care unit once for respiratory distress, but had not received ventilator support.

This second case illustrates two points. First, paediatric palliative care involves working with children whose development is severely compromised. This is not simply arrest along the spectrum of normal child development—instead it takes on its own trajectory. Non-verbal children require a new approach to detecting, assessing, and managing symptoms. Tools are being developed for pain assessment in these children and this is an emerging field[11-12]. Second, even the child with multi-handicaps due to severe neurological impairment is never static—there are subtle developmental dynamics that must be taken into account. The child described above has developed some basic communication patterns through vocalizations and movements, which caregivers experienced *with that individual child* can interpret. This form of communication may not develop for many years, if at all, but when it does it can be one more reliable source to assist in care.

One can argue that there is actually a third category of children we meet in paediatric palliative care: pre-verbal children.

These children are expected to experience normal development progression but at the time they are experiencing a life-threatening illness, they are too young to talk or are just acquiring language. Examples include the premature neonate with severe lung disease or the two-year-old with cancer. They represent a mix of the first and second types of cases described above.

Childhood development progresses through an orderly sequence of increasing comprehension, interpretation, and independence (see Chapter 13.4, Table 13.4.1). The ill child may be delayed in reaching his/her milestones, and with prolonged or serious illness, will probably regress. This does not mean, however, that strategies to facilitate the ill child's developmental progress can be ignored, since most children with serious illness seem to mature beyond their years in their perception of death and ability to cope.

Many adults assume that children are less affected than adults by serious illness, death, and grief because they are 'too young to understand', or because they 'will forget as time passes by'. Children may be less verbal and communicate their thoughts and feelings in different ways than adults, but it is not at all true that children are not affected by such events. Children are often not asked or approached appropriately to obtain their insights and perspectives; professional caregivers and parents often find greater comfort in talking with each other than with the children about sensitive topics, making assumptive decisions regarding care based on this exchange of information and sideline support. An approach that recognizes these patients are children *first* and seriously ill *second* helps to focus individualized priorities appropriately with the child and family.

Overall developmental considerations are a complex, core issue in the provision of paediatric palliative care services. They have implications for the front-line clinicians in medicine, nursing and counselling, for support staff, and for managers and programme planners. Articles and texts often use shorthand and simply say refer to 'development' as one important aspect of providing paediatric palliative care. As can be seen, it is not a simple issue at all, and the full scope of the complexity cannot be captured in a single term.

Children as dependents within family

As the typically or 'normally' developing child progresses from birth through adolescence to adulthood, the degree of his/her dependency is in constant flux, moving steadily towards the capability to be totally independent. This dependent status creates a significant challenge for the health-care team. The team must understand the child as a unique individual with needs and wants, rights, and opportunities. As well, the team must understand the child as a member of a family with parents who are, to a greater or lesser extent, responsible spokespersons and even proxies. The family element is described in a subsequent section, as family is not always a set of married parents, but can involve numerous combinations of extended family and often the courts or community organizations. The challenges of dealing with children along the developmental trajectory refer to more than the cognitive/language/function stream described previously; challenges also exist in negotiating decision-making within a dependent context.

A child's innate drive to independence never proceeds along a smooth course even in healthy children; when impeded by serious illness, it compounds stress and confusion for the child. Parents, overwhelmed by their fear of the impending loss of their child, may cling more protectively and seek to be all things to the child as a means of gaining some sense of control over their destiny. Younger children, dependent for all things, usually adjust accordingly, but older children and adolescents may chafe under such restrictions. These circumstances create opportunities for the palliative care team to foster alternate perspectives and approaches to children's experience of illness, treatment, and family responses. Providing avenues for even limited decision-making can be helpful. Children of all ages respond to consistency and sameness and an emphasis on the 'ordinariness' (even when it is not ordinary) of daily life with its attendant responsibilities and rights. Consequently, many children's hospice and palliative care programmes offer a school programme—it is a child's 'job' to go to school each day, regardless of their disease, disability, or prognosis[13].

Legal and ethical status of children

In adult palliative care programmes, patient wishes are paramount and receive attention and protection. When caring for children, it is somewhat more difficult to determine whose wishes and goals are being followed or are directing the plan of care. Parents sometimes see the child's needs and options quite differently to the child. Parents' and various staff caregivers' views may also differ. Professionals must consider the age, cognitive level, and illness experience of the child; they are challenged to find ways to seek the input, perspectives, and personal experience of the ill child as a guide for care giving decisions[14]. Traditionally, most professionals have had little training or experience in assuring the child's understanding of the disease process, treatment and therapies, identifying the child's personal goals, or exploring quality of life as defined by the patient's/family's experience.

In addition, the child's legal status must be considered. As minors in the eyes of the law, children are subservient to the will of their parents in day-to-day circumstances. In some countries, the law has changed a great deal in the last decade. Where there were once clear legal concepts (and laws) regarding the age of majority especially regarding health care, some jurisdictions have done away with all of these. Rather than trying arbitrarily to establish an age of consent at 12, 15, or 18, these jurisdictions have determined that there is no lower limit on the age of consent for medical procedures. In part, this approach enables governments to avoid charges of ageism for both the elderly and youth equally. Seen in a somewhat better light, it is a move to acknowledge the uniqueness and essential claim on the rights of all individuals. Practically it has put health-care providers at a significant disadvantage in their ability to identify with those with whom they need to communicate. Some jurisdictions acknowledge that children are not always capable of giving consent, but at least they must be asked to express assent, and an attempt at attaining that assent must be carried out to a reasonable degree.

Because of the changing nature of the law regarding the issue of child/youth consent, and the differences that exist from one jurisdiction to another, practitioners must seek advice locally and continue to be up-to-date with changes in the local governing law. It is helpful to have a connection to local experts in law and ethics.

Despite the legislative moves away from an age of majority, the courts are still willing to intervene and protect a child's interests, especially when the wishes of the parents and a perceived but vague societal norm conflict. If children are unable to speak for themselves, an ombudsman may intercede on their behalf to assure that the children's best interests are met.

Standard ethical approaches recognize the child as an individual deserving of a voice in his/her own destiny[15]. Ethics supports the concept of individual autonomy as a fundamental basis of all ethical decision-making. When an individual is not capable of manifesting an autonomous stance, then the default is for society to act in accordance with the individual's best interests. The challenge becomes one of determining that best interest, by whom and based upon what standard. When possible, children themselves may be able to express a desire or decision. Often, even for older children and adolescents, these desires may not be expressed in spoken or written directions—other modalities such as art and play analysis can help children express their feelings, even regarding how they might perceive the inevitability (or not) of their dying and preference for comfort or curative/sustaining treatments. Their overt and covert communication must be noted to reveal their level of acceptance of the inevitability of their demise, their desire for more interventions or their ambivalence about the continuation of therapies, discouragement with how their life is impacted, and their quality of life as seen through their own eyes. A hospice palliative team comprised of trained, skilled, and experienced child-health clinicians from multiple disciplines can assist in ascertaining a child's beliefs, values, and concerns and can facilitate a discussion with parents and the health-care team to unify perceptions.

In the situation of prenatal hospice, parents may decide on a palliative care approach during pregnancy, making incremental decisions about interventions, both medical and non-medical, at time of birth. Other challenging situations requiring legal or ethical considerations are children in foster care, withdrawal of ventilator support, hydration, or nutrition. For further discussion of related ethical issues, see Chapter 5.4.

The family

Family constellation

Families of young children tend to be more inclusive and extensive and, therefore, life-threatening disease creates a broad scope of impact. Parents and grandparents are still living, siblings are often present, and school/neighbourhood friends are part of the affected group, all requiring attention from the palliative team. Moreover, most family members will not have faced the death of a child before and so the task of meeting family needs requires special attention, skills, and considerable time. Siblings of the seriously ill child require focused attention and ongoing evaluation of support for their own needs, fears, concerns, and struggles both at home and at school. For school children and especially adolescents, friends are crucial partners and are sometimes seen to be as close as or closer than some siblings.

Another factor to consider is the myriad forms that family structures take. With divorce rates and second marriage rates at 40–50 per cent in many countries, children are highly likely to have single parents, step-parents, and step-siblings. Step-parents and biological parents may share aspects of legal custody and emotional allegiance with the child. It is not uncommon for grandparents to be the primary caregivers for grandchildren. In industrialized countries, this is often due to teenage pregnancy—in the developing countries it is now an unfortunate result of the HIV-AIDS epidemic.

Ramifications of diverse family structures have a clear impact on family dynamics and on the interactions of the child–family and health-care team. It is important that an up-to-date, extended family genogram be in every child's health record. This should show not only the specifics of structure, but also dynamics, for example who actually lives in the home. Similarly, accurate information recorded from relevant legal documents, such as divorce decrees specifying guardianship and custody, needs to be noted in the record. All too often clinicians assume that because they are talking to a parent, that person actually has a legal decision-making role. A child's illness changes the life of everyone in the family constellation.

Siblings, friends, and pets

For most children, parents are the most important people in the world; but for many, siblings and friends run a close second. Complete provision of paediatric palliative care must take this fact into account. Care for healthy siblings is rated by families as one of their highest concerns in paediatric palliative care and in paediatric chronic illness care in general[16–17]. Parents often feel guilt and conflict over spending all their time with their ill child while neglecting their other children. Siblings' comments indicate that they too carry a sense of conflict over the needs of their ill sibling and their own desires for parent attention and for family normality.

Paediatric hospice palliative care programmes can provide valuable support to siblings. Trained volunteers can provide recreational and therapeutic outlets for siblings, leaving time for parents to be with their ill child or to find support and rest for themselves. Healthy siblings benefit from the services of professionals in dealing with their own worries, vulnerabilities, and losses. A number of modalities can enable a communicative and therapeutic relationship to develop, including art, music, and play, conducted individually or in groups[18–19].

A second, related question often asked by parents is how to talk to their healthy children about what is happening to the ill youngster. Families need guidance and support around finding helpful language and opportunities in discussing difficult issues. They sometimes need advice about child development, what words to use and what reactions are normal or indications of trouble. Similarly, a child's closest friends, especially teenagers, will be affected by their experience of being close to someone with a life-threatening illness. They too benefit from receiving information and support and, in turn, they will be able to be present for their friend rather than withdrawing out of fear or anxiety. Many children's hospices have adopted policies and approaches that support a friend staying with an ill child.

Lastly, professionals must remember the importance of animals in a child's life, particularly as a source of support and solace for many children. A last request of many children has been to see their favourite pet one more time. For some children, just the presence of a non-judgemental animal, perhaps one not known to them previously, is supportive; thus many programmes have adopted regular visits by a therapy-trained pet, usually a dog. Again, paediatric hospice palliative programmes need to create policy to accommodate these desires.

Provision of care by the family

Parents expect to be the ones providing complete care for their children. Under ordinary circumstances care begins with food, clothing, and shelter and then extends to health, education, opportunity, and a secure future. This normal pattern of expectations is disrupted when a child has a life-threatening condition. Moreover, some grief-filled parents seeking to assuage the anguish and pain of the possibility of death may compensate by trying to be all things at all times to their sick child and tend to resist help from outsiders. In addition, parents are often coping with pre-existing psychosocial and emotional issues and conflicts within the family. The health-care system, with its wide variety of caregivers, often puts parents in an ambiguous position of appreciating the expert care while resenting the control exerted over their child and themselves by authoritative professionals. Some parents, when inadvertently displaced from the bedside by well-meaning staff, have been electing to reclaim their autonomy by caring for their dying children at home, reluctantly turning to home care support where available. More importantly, this choice may also indicate that parents identify home as the most appropriate setting to achieve any sense of normality as a family. Parents' need to 'be everything' and maintaining control of their child's life helps dissipate their anguish and grief. Assisting the sick child, parents and siblings alike gain control over the aspects of care and their own lives and experiencing choice contributes to a lessening of their intense feelings of powerlessness. There are many subtle yet significant decisions regarding care that can enhance or impact negatively on the child's experience as a passive recipient or an active participant. Caregivers value and respect the child's experience by addressing such questions as: Does the child routinely get offered pre-medication for any painful procedure along with relaxation strategies to reduce fear and anxiety? Is care at home routinely offered or discussed as an option instead of deciding for the child/family that home care is not appropriate? Does the child want to master a particular aspect of care himself? Does the medical team 'talk over' the child as they discuss needs and changes? Has there been a discussion with the child regarding his/her desired place for the dying process and death to occur? Has there been discussion regarding the desired intensity of care related to specific symptoms and changes anticipated and their benefit/burden on the child? Are there friends who can be encouraged to visit? Are there simple changes in routines that might reduce anxiety or stress for the child? At all times, the care must fit the child, whether at home or in hospital, rather than fitting the child into the rigid structure of a particular setting.

It is essential that professional caregivers do not violate the relationship between parent and child; professionals must continuously reflect on their answer to the question, 'Whose need is this meeting: the parents or my own?' Professionals must create opportunities to strengthen parents' responsibility and authority in decisions and discussions related to their child's care and needs. Paediatric palliative care programmes need to provide skilled, accessible, and coordinated assistance in a sensitive and responsive manner in accordance with the parents' desires and child/family-directed goals.

Provision of care for the family

If one of the core philosophical tenets of paediatric palliative care is a family-centred approach, then programmes must both accommodate care *by* family, but also provide care *for* the family. Creating supportive responsive programmes that respect the parents' primary role, as described above, is only one aspect of paediatric palliative care. Another critical aspect is recognizing that the stress

and work of caring for a child with a life-threatening disease is an extraordinary circumstance and requires extraordinary support.

Depending upon the duration and intensity of the child's illness, parents must either prepare for a sprint requiring courage and intense focus or a marathon, running the distance on an uphill and downhill course with unexpected turns that require strength and endurance of body, spirit, and will. Parents tackle the situation without prior training or life experience to guide them. Thus, respite should be a core service of paediatric palliative care programmes. Respite takes place in many settings—children's hospices, children's hospitals, long-term care homes, and, of course, within the family home. Respite can take many forms, with many types of caregivers and arrangements. The presence of trained caregivers who can provide care for the sick child is key. If families have confidence in a caregiver they can obtain much-needed rest, spend time with their other children, and meet personal needs. Respite needs to be provided by trained, though not necessarily professional, caregivers. It needs to be reliable and of sufficient frequency and duration to provide a real break for parents.

Providing home care to a seriously ill child often becomes impossible for families without the support of home care services and some form of respite care. With periodic respite from their caregiving burden and associated responsibilities, families gain a much-needed period of rest and revitalization and are better able to resume care, refreshed. Even a short period of respite helps maintain parents' endurance and resiliency. Ill children themselves have reported that respite for their parents provides them with a welcome break from their parents. Respite care may be needed under other circumstances as well; for example, when a sibling or parent is ill, particularly if someone is ill with a contagious disease, which could spread to the already debilitated child[18].

Few resources exist in most countries to meet this ongoing and significant demand. Insurers do not cover it and there are rarely the financial resources available for families to pay for this, and so they go without, patching together some occasional relief through the kindness of friends or relatives. Through hospices, home visits of the home health aid can be of some relief for parents. In countries, such as the United Kingdom, where children's hospices provide respite care, families report the vital role of this service. Volunteers can also play a vital role in palliative care service, as companions for siblings, a listening ear for the child, or practical assistance for parents.

Other aspects of care for the family include financial support. Some jurisdictions have systems of financial support for health-care expenses incurred for the sick children—schemes however vary greatly from one location to another and financial burden is also identified as one of the greatest stressors affecting families. A related support issue is 'administrative support'. In many countries, families find themselves in the position of 'case manager' for their child's care, negotiating a myriad of health, education, and insurance systems. A skilled social worker, ombudsman, or advocate can be an important source of support for families experiencing this burden of care.

For many fortunate children, life can be full of treats, special events, and extraordinary adventures. The opportunity to experience these is often denied to families living with a childhood life-threatening disease. Barriers can be of several kinds—not just financial, but also logistical in relationship to moving children who require wheelchairs, medical equipment including ventilators, and even one-to-one nursing care. Programmes have met these challenges successfully as highlighted by the efforts of a number of charities, such as Make-A-Wish®, to accommodate children's special wishes. Many similar programmes exist in North America and Europe to address these requests. Not only do these charities meet a child's requests for a 'special' time, but they support parents' desire to have these opportunities for their family—for both the vulnerable child and siblings.

Bereavement needs

As a rule, families suffer the death of a child more intensely than the death of an adult. And, because of the composition of the family group and the differences in age of its members, potential exists for more disruption for a prolonged time. Bereavement care is a required programme component, with family-oriented support provided more frequently, to a more diverse group of bereaved family members and for a longer time than in typical adult hospice programmes. Such care must be malleable enough to meet the needs of survivors of various cultures whose children had a range of conditions.

The families of children who die outside of the typical palliative care model, such as in prenatal or infant death, consistently do not receive bereavement care, or do not have access to such care. The support available may vary by programme but 'after care' is not routinely offered or available in many institutional settings or by traditional home care agencies. This is largely because of limited resources—human and financial, and the absence of reimbursement for such programmes. The practical limits of unit or field staff keeping up with the cumulative bereaved families, over time, along with current clients is finite. Institutions may have a protocol for use at the time of death and provide families with a packet of community and grief resources but the actual *mechanism* to ensure automatic and routine connections for follow-up does not usually exist. Parents who have a baby die receive keepsake items and often a memory box, but this same practice often does not exist in other paediatric settings, such as in emergency or intensive care units, although there are useful recommendations for these settings[20]. Essential for optimal well-being and healing of family survivors is a seamless continuum of care (across settings and caregivers) that begins at diagnosis and continues through the illness experience where many losses are grieved and on into bereavement care after the child dies.

Caregivers

Knowledge base

Successful palliation permits the child and family to share each day to the fullest degree possible, defining appropriate care plans with their caregivers. Since emphasizing quality of daily life is the desired outcome, a specific knowledge base is needed for caregivers. The historical emphasis on adult palliative care has resulted in little available research, experience, and knowledge pertaining to the principles and details of care for paediatric patients and their families[21]. This is particularly apparent in the lack of accessible expertise and skills in strategies for pain and symptom management for the diverse ages and conditions of childhood, and for settings where children are cared for. Adapting existing knowledge to the care of children and seeking new approaches to the prevention and management of problems (physical, psychosocial, spiritual)

and coordination of care should be major programme goals of any children's palliative care programme. Therefore, a significant need exists for teaching both parents and health-care professionals appropriate end of life care skills and about potential resources. As well, the scarcity of expertise and mentors in the evolving field of paediatric palliative care must be addressed. Health-care professionals often lack paediatric specific knowledge of pain and other complex symptom management strategies as the disease condition advances, knowledge about the actual disease trajectory for the wide range of paediatric diagnoses that are life-threatening, and how to meet needs across the paediatric spectrum: newborn through older adolescence and young adults.

Caregivers require extensive developmental and baseline knowledge of children and their perceptions of illness, death, and dying. Caregivers knowledgeable and experienced in childhood development assess and respond appropriately to children's changing and evolving status and design care plans according to children's functional rather than chronological stage. Such caregivers facilitate a match between children's desires and waning capabilities and their parents' expectations, as well as the directives of the medical team. They communicate with ill children in accordance with their developmental level, encouraging them to express their feelings, needs, wishes, and fears more freely. Understanding children's functional level permits professional caregivers to provide children with as much control over their life and circumstances, as they are willing and able to handle. Sharing the developmental evaluation with the parents enlightens them as they seek to cope with their child's behaviour and will reassure them that the regressive patterns are the expected norm.

Understanding of best practices regarding communication and coordination is also key knowledge for all caregivers involved with children with life-threatening conditions. The palliative care team assists children and families to identify their goals and then works to help facilitate accomplishing them through ongoing communication among family and professionals and collaboration among all providers—both inpatient and home providers. The palliative care team, child/family, medical specialists, and primary care team all have contributions and perspectives to offer; a continuous feedback process must be organized for optimal communication to occur about such questions as: Do the parents (and child when appropriate) have the same understanding as the medical teams of the intent and purpose of the therapies/interventions? Have their mutual goals been evaluated for compatibility to achieve the desired outcome? Families may place very different values on interventions and treatments than do professionals. Centralized coordination of care of all providers keep patient/family wishes uniformly centre stage, well understood, and actively pursued. Patient/family wishes should be driving the care planning process with input from the interdisciplinary health-care team in order to create one voice for the family and relieve them of the burden of what seems to be 'running a business' of health care for their seriously ill child.

A basic understanding of the many forms of childhood disease encountered in paediatric palliative care, the myriad trajectories and the complex interactions of symptoms, disease trajectories, emotional needs, family-social aspects, and spiritual challenge is required for all members of the palliative team, including ancillary support staff and volunteers. Recognition of how paediatric palliative care differs from adult care, as described in this and other chapters, is necessary. Not all providers or caregivers will be directly involved in symptom management, but all should be aware that for some children the palliative trajectory only lasts days to weeks, while for others it is months to years, even bridging into young adulthood. This understanding sets the context for the flexible approach required in the provision of paediatric palliative care. Fortunately, knowledge dissemination and translation are now occurring more rapidly than when the field first began—there are a number of workshops and training courses, handbooks, and texts and on-line resources available for providers to increase their knowledge regarding paediatric palliative care.

Teamwork

Special services for children require a highly skilled team that attends to the needs of each member of the family, not only the patient[22–23]. Experienced caregivers must be closely attuned to the emotional, mental, spiritual and physical stamina, and resilience of children's parents as well as siblings' responses to the illness and family changes. Paediatric personnel must acquire a thorough understanding of the family's lifestyle, personalities, spirituality and religion, cultural mores, and parent–child–sibling relationships. Ill children usually want all care to be rendered by their parents, with whom they feel safest, but most children will respond to sensitive caregivers if the parents take the lead in accepting assistance from and demonstrating trust in the staff. Parents' ability to function well and remain in charge will benefit from consistent support and guidance by an empathetic staff that incorporate the needs of all family members into the care plan and help the entire family to cope. The team then must function as a coach— always guiding and supporting but never 'taking over' the course. Working parents require an approach from the palliative care team that fosters a sense of inclusiveness for both parents even when both are not available at the same time. Having the social worker/ counsellor or chaplain meet regularly with the working parent later in the day, or at lunchtime, helps him/her feel connected to and perceived as part of the palliative care team. Such attention provides opportunity to clarify concerns and ask questions regarding the child's needs and their own. This can validate and reinforce their role as a parent when the burden of work, marriage, family, and a sick child become very heavy and isolating. Many families are challenged additionally with poverty, drug abuse, single parent households, or grandparent caregivers—each of which has a different set of complexities.

Effective teamwork guides parents in reinvesting *some* of the energy singularly focused on a cure to a few short-term, realistic goals that can revitalize the spirit of the family. Hope is an intangible force that fuels families through the unspeakable field of trials, sorrows, and fears. As one parent said 'It is hope that allows me to put one foot in front of the other each day, to keep me going at least for today, for this hour, this moment. Without hope, the weight of all this would paralyse me completely'. Hope allows families to raise their sights above the immediacy of their burdens and their fears of the present to the possibilities and opportunities that do exist, and to weave some small measure of 'normality' into their lives.

The pioneer efforts of Martinson in 1978, and later Lauer *et al.*, demonstrated the value of the team concept in providing support to families[24–29]. This support permitted parents, even those living at a distance from the patient's hospital base, to be involved fully in the care of their child in the home, even choosing the place for

death to occur. An important element in facilitating such involvement is careful forward planning so that priorities are established and needless suffering is avoided. The resolution of a crisis or sudden change can serve as an opportunity for the team to help the family view it as a rehearsal of sorts for subsequent changes. Team members can encourage family members to discuss what they might do differently, what worked, and what can be prevented or anticipated for next time something similar happens. It might be as simple as improving communication between regular and after-hours staff, leaving more detailed, up-to-date information in the home or having a particular medication at hand. Using the 'teachable moments' as they arise gradually helps to mitigate the fears associated with parental anxiety of 'What will I do if something terrible happens?'

Bonds of trust, communication, and support with caregivers develop from the time of diagnosis and are essential to sustaining children and families—for children, particularly when ill, do not adapt well to changes in caregivers, unless such changes are handled with great sensitivity and preparation. Continuity of care must be established and maintained so that families do not experience fragmented services or feelings of abandonment resulting from disruptive shifting of care among home and hospital and hospice. This same level of disruption can occur when communication is poor among the multiple specialists involved, various residents, and other staff who change over the length of illness. The goals of care, regardless of setting, diagnosis, or length of illness are to normalize living to the degree possible, to optimize quality of life, and to create opportunities for living fully. To meet these goals, inpatient care must always be an option. Families may need assistance with symptom control or they may become increasingly anxious and need the reassurance of the familiar hospital or the quiet support of the hospice environment. Services offered among various locations must be coordinated, with children and families always supported to achieve their goals. The palliative care programme should ensure a seamless continuum of care—across settings, across caregivers, and over time.

Recruitment and retention of competent and sensitive caregivers is often difficult because of the personal pain and sadness associated with the impending death of a child (see Chapter 13.5). Staff need to be protected from emotional exhaustion and depletion, as they must sustain the entire family in their supportive caregiving role as well as each other within the team. Adaptation to this specialty takes time, mentoring, and clinical supervision. In addition to the learning/coping needs of staff, managers have considerable responsibility to facilitate opportunities for thriving in this unique environment of care.

People who have had previous experience with sick infants, children, and adolescents and their anxious parents best meet the many needs of the dying child. This is not to exclude those who wish to learn to relate to children who are seriously or terminally ill, but, since time is of the essence for these children, the dying child deserves access to skilled paediatric caregivers. The learning curve for becoming such a caregiver is slow for persons starting from no experience, as the process of integrating child development, child psychology, cultural and religious influences, pathophysiology of the range of disease processes, therapeutic treatment modalities, pain control, and other symptom management is long and difficult. The care of a child receiving palliation demands the same commitment to excellence and the same level of monitoring and skilled intervention as does acute care. Currently, there are few resources and research-based clinical competencies for interdisciplinary team members in paediatric palliative care. The model required is one of mentoring over time based on best practice and current trends in clinical care. Most communities do not have this depth of local expertise and thereby rely on scattered, fragmented approaches. Unfortunately, some try to approach the care of these children as small adults and the results can be very negative from the family's point of view.

Nurses

In palliative care, the nurse emerges as a key caregiver and in some programmes is the natural coordinator of the plan of care. Time spent with the children and the ability to read their body language and incorporate pertinent pieces of scientific knowledge into effective care plans equips the nurse with the ability to coordinate collaborative team efforts, which may influence significantly the emotional burden and stress and ease the coming events. The nurse must be mindful not to displace the parents in their need to care for their child and simultaneously not demand more of them than they can handle. In addition, the nurse serves as the 'control tower navigator', recognizing when to call in the strengths, services, and consultation of others. In times of limited resources or in areas less well endowed, the nurse may need to fill multiple roles as well as train volunteers to assist. Besides knowledge and skill in physical palliative care, the nurse must also weave the psychosocial and spiritual dimensions of the child's experience into his/her care as they are all closely intertwined and interconnected. The nurse has far more responsibility than simply 'body care'. It is equally important for the nurse keenly to be aware of his/her own limitations, to reflect on his/her own practice, and to take the time for self-care in order to provide ongoing optimal care.

Physicians

The physician has a vital role in adapting treatment through the ongoing changes in a child's physical condition and in anticipating what to expect as a result. Since the realm of palliative care extends from pre-natal diagnoses through adolescent medicine, a wide range of providers may participate in the direction of medical care. For example, the obstetrician/perinatologist or the geneticist may be involved at various stages. In other situations, the paediatrician may provide coordination of care during high acuity in hospital. The family physician may be in a unique position to be the thread of continuity before and after the child's illness and death. Each is in a unique position to evaluate the coping and need for support. Provision of the core of paediatric palliative medicine requires knowledge of paediatrics because of the nature of the complex chronic diseases children face, and knowledge of palliative medicine because of the need to provide advanced symptom management, especially at end-of-life. There are only a few training programmes in the United Kingdom, Australia, Canada, and the United States that provide paediatricians and palliative physicians with the relevant training. In most situations, clinicians develop their own self-learning programme to acquire the necessary skills.

Most seriously ill and dying children are treated by multiple physician specialists. To optimize communication and facilitate supportive services, specialists need to work in close collaboration with the child's primary physician. With the transitioning of goals over time from curative to palliative care, parents need to know which one person will serve as their primary physician. Close collaboration between the physician and nurse is needed to achieve optimal symptom control and to provide continuity of care for patients and reassurance to families. Constancy of caregivers is essential, for, as children weaken, they (and the family) want to interact with fewer and fewer people.

Many parents find comfort in a follow-up visit with the physician to review the cause of death, what happened, and what implications there might be for future pregnancies or the other siblings. Families often find a meeting with the physician to discuss autopsy results particularly beneficial.

Psychologists/psychiatrists

Mental health professionals may be more likely to be involved early in a child's illness and are probably under-utilized later in the illness, but should have an ongoing role with children and their families. Given that mental-health professionals vary in type and extent of preparation and areas of expertise, it is important to match the individuals available in local settings with the needs of children and families. Psychologists are trained in a variety of techniques to help children explore their emotional issues. Adolescents, often filled with anger, ambivalence, conflict and resentment as well as fear, may benefit from the psychologist's role as a sounding board and may be most amenable to supportive therapies or cognitive behavioural approaches depending on the issues. 'Talking therapy' is only one modality and younger children will more readily find support through therapies structured around art, music, or play. All of these modalities require specific training, usually quite extensive, backed-up by appropriate fundamental grounding in psychological theory. Another role for mental health therapists is to contend with symptoms. Hypnosis, which goes by various names such as relaxation-imagery, mind–body therapy, and imagination medicine, can be immensely helpful to children in contending with pain, other symptoms, and anxiety. Clinical consultation on anxiety, escalating anger, behaviour problems and assessment for clinical depression, and substance abuse issues are also all appropriate indicators for mental health clinicians' involvement in the child's care. Psychologists will also have expertise in testing and assessment as part of their training; this is not typically required in paediatric palliative care, but there are times when this service is important in clarifying skills, abilities, and challenges for children living with life-threatening disease.

Psychiatrists represent the medical arm of the mental health professions. In addition to skill in supportive and therapeutic counselling, they bring an understanding of severe psychopathology and skill in the use of medications to treat them. They are familiar with medications such as neuroleptics that play important roles in symptom management and should be accessed as resources in these situations.

Social workers

As an experienced listener, the social worker prioritizes the problems and concerns of all involved parties and seeks to expedite solutions for them. Resources and pertinent information are provided, as is expert negotiation of management crises and bureaucratic obstacles. The social worker's contributions to and support of the family include facilitation of family conflict and communication. Social workers also can address sibling issues during the illness, assist and guide the family in memory-making activities and rituals and facilitate expression of feelings and concerns. Social work services do not end with the death, but may, in some programmes, continue throughout the bereavement period. The social worker fulfils a valuable liaison role—parents, nurse, physician, psychologist, clergy, and others are well served by an experienced social worker. Social workers should also be available to families who are not receiving hospital-based care.

Play and recreation therapists

Play and recreation therapies are recognized modalities of care for all children. Play is the work of all children; meaningful play is the ideal way to help the young patient express his feelings and reduce anxiety, anger, depression, and fears. Child life specialists are often especially trained to assist with such techniques, but such professionals are currently not a standard component of hospice and palliative care. They may be accessed through paediatric clinical settings and, in some areas, are actually being integrated into adult hospital settings to meet better the emotional needs of children whose parents are ill.

Clergy

The goal of spiritual care is to provide non-judgemental love and the promise of non-abandonment. Spiritual care is not only appropriate but is an innate need of all persons, religious or not. In offering spiritual care, the caregiver goes the extra mile to seek out the inner person of the patient or family member, share their anguish, provide solace, and perhaps help them find meaning in their experience[30]. Clergy provide formal rites, hear concerns, fears and confessions, offer counselling, serve as non-judgemental companions on the journey, facilitate personalized rituals, and support families to find meaning in their experience and, most importantly, symbolize a link to an uncertain future. Even when families do not identify a religious affiliation (and perhaps especially) a supportive clergyman can help the family identify issues and concerns regarding the meaning of their experience and how to approach an unknown future. Whenever possible, a clergy person of the family's religious background should be recruited to collaborate with the team, in addition to the clergy usually associated with the palliative care team. The palliative care chaplain often is the bridge between the palliative team and the family's religious support base.

The palliative care chaplain also has a role in supporting the inherent spiritual work of the other clinicians on the team. Care directed to the physical body without concern for the mind and spirit is incomplete and frequently ineffective. Providing spiritual care transcends the empathetic communication used to meet the family's daily psychosocial needs and invokes a sharing of self through listening and presence when needed. Caregivers are challenged to reach beyond their personal religious belief system to help each family probe, access, and utilize its own religious ties and nurture them. The clergy member of the palliative team can have an important role, not only in connecting directly with the child and family but also in supporting clinical members of the team as they provide spiritual support.

Location of care for children

In the provision of palliative care for children with life-limiting conditions, location of care is a major issue. At the time of onset, diagnosis, and initial workup for a disease, children may be hospitalized for lengthy periods of time as well as intermittently returning to hospital for exacerbations or additional treatments or procedures. Parents report this early phase as highly traumatic and stressful, requiring a depth of resources to be mobilized. Ideally, the palliative care team should be involved in the early phase of treatment to ensure adequate attention to quality of life for children and families and to model an interdisciplinary holistic approach. Later, when options are limited or exhausted, children facing the possibility of death and their parents reserve the right to select where the child's final days or weeks should be spent, and deserve the full endorsement and help of the caregiving staff to plan accordingly to accomplish this.

Hospital

Hospitals, the most important site of care over the past four decades, have become less essential since parents have become more knowledgeable and assertive in their active involvement in care, as pain control, and other symptom management strategies and support systems for the patient are now available in the home. However, hospital admission should always be readily available for those families with acute clinical needs, episodes of exacerbation of illness or symptoms, fear of being a burden, for the sense of security and availability of sophisticated personnel[29], or for individual cultural needs and wishes of the family. Most paediatric deaths occur as a result of trauma; consequently, most children who die do so in hospitals; they and their families deserve to receive palliative care[31]. These children and families can benefit from brief yet intensive involvement of the palliative care team. Deliberate attention to the details of the child's and family's experience can shape the survivors' perceptions for years to come. Staff need to allow parents and even siblings the opportunity to be alone with the child, before death if possible, and then after the death in a private setting and for the time they feel is needed before letting the child's body be taken away. Important rituals, memories, and keepsakes can be created at this very sorrowful time.

Children themselves rarely prefer the hospital; when they sense their parents' inability to cope at home and to protect them, some children will subjugate their own wishes to those of their parents. Or, if children perceive no alternative or recognize the hospital as the desired site for higher acuity needs, or prefer care from trusted caregivers, they may select the hospital for care. However, children's dependent relationship within the family makes the isolation of the hospital, with separation from the familiar, undesirable for most children under any circumstance. In the final stages of a terminal illness, the emotional tensions of the despairing family and the potential subtle withdrawal of discomfited hospital staff, including physicians, can confuse and disturb children who may already be anxious. Ill children and their families often perceive such changes as rejection and abandonment; the clinician's role is still essential even if cure is not attainable. This sense of abandonment can trigger deeply hostile responses leading to intense conflicts and even legal actions. Failure to maintain relationships with the family all the way through the experience can have dire consequences.

Hospice

Thirty-five years ago, Martinson's[24,32] home care programme for children with cancer was one of the first models for developing hospice programmes in the United States. It was followed by a community-based hospice home care programme (Edmarc) in Virginia in 1979 and Helen House, the first free-standing hospice for children that provided respite care, opened in Oxford, England, in 1982. Since that time, numerous similar facilities have opened in the United Kingdom, Canada, Australia, Western Europe, and most recently, the United States.

Paediatric hospices focus on maximizing quality of life for children with life-limiting conditions by providing a holistic programme of services that meet the combined physical, social, emotional, and spiritual needs of the child and family members. The type and scope of services provided are based on initial and ongoing assessments of the needs of the child and family. The exact combination of services and level of care (such as frequency of visits, number of hours of care by various team members) is unique to each child and family and changes as the child's and family's needs evolve. After the child has died, the emotional support must continue as families learn to face life without their child.

A free-standing children's hospice is one approach to offering the type of care that acute care hospitals or home-care programmes are often unable to provide to children and families at the end of life. A hospice can provide a safe haven for families when their child is dying, and may be a source of information and respite that allows families to continue caring for their child at home for as long as possible. As hospices have developed over the past decade, there has also been increasing activity in the area of developing standards for paediatric hospice care. Evaluations of existing programmes also provide direction for future development[18,19,33–37].

Overall, families themselves are strongly positive in their assessment of children's hospice services. They report that the hospice filled a major gap and provided services not available anywhere else. However, upon first hearing about the hospice programme, many parents did not believe the programme would be suitable for them, often because it was extremely difficult for them to accept the inevitability of their child's death. Once they visit the hospice, however, parents change their minds, recognizing the value of a place for respite where their child is cared for by experienced, competent, and compassionate staff and where their needs for rest and nurture are also met. With increasing trends towards home care of children with even the most complex conditions and care requirements, respite becomes critical in improving the quality of life for terminally ill children and their families[18]. Parents were particularly satisfied with the focus on each member of the family. Family-centred care is a central principle of paediatric palliative care; despite this emphasis, however, traditionally, the focus is on the ill child with little attention on the other members of the family. Parents were also satisfied with their role in making decisions about their child's care and felt included as part of the team, attributing these feelings to open, honest, and respectful communication. Parents also appreciated the sense of freedom that came from knowing that emergency services were available, learning from other parents about how to manage various aspects of the children's care, and knowing they would be supported when their child died. Despite the fact that some parents found the exposure to death difficult, most parents felt this experience helped prepare them for what lay ahead[36–37].

Both ill children and their siblings rated the hospice positively[19]. They particularly liked the informal, comfortable and home-like environment that typically characterizes children's hospices. They enjoyed interacting with other ill children and siblings where they were not seen 'as different from other kids'. The ill children valued the rare opportunity of being independent from their parents, and the siblings liked being involved in their brother or sister's care. They too valued time spent with staff who understood and listened to their concerns about the future.

The emotional support offered by staff plays a central role in assisting families to deal with the devastating effect of their child's impending death. Providing such support requires that staff understand the family's predicament and is not reluctant to talk about death with families. Thus, staffing levels for hospice care may need to incorporate a higher nurse/patient ratio than might be usual in a hospital setting. Models of care may need to allow for the increased costs associated with this approach, although cost analysis research continues to be needed in this area.

Home

Home-based palliative care programmes, as an adjunct to hospital care, are needed to provide skilled, accessible, and coordinated assistance in a sensitive and responsive manner in accordance with the parents' desires and child/family-directed goals. Many parents identify home as the most appropriate setting to achieve any sense of normality as a family.

Although home would be the natural place for children to want to spend their final days, this decision must be reached within the context of individual families, with awareness of the impact that the impending death will have on all family members and with consideration given to the family's cultural mores. Children's physical condition and possible emergency needs, available resources and physical care-giving responsibilities must be anticipated, with plans in place, so that parents are prepared to cope with a sudden or unexpected change of status. Without the security of appropriate physical care in the home, children's sense of safety and protection can be lost. Anxiety can easily escalate and exacerbate the physical symptoms. The decision regarding location of care is weighty and should be made with serious attention to all aspects of family life and the ability of the chosen location to meet the quality of life expectations of the child and the parents[33]. Examination of the specific fears of the child and parents regarding care at home—or in the inpatient setting near death—can be discussed at a discharge planning conference. Typically, these are areas where parents will not want to feel out of control nor see their child suffer needlessly. For example, if parents' greatest and worst fear is sudden onset severe pain or acute shortness of breath, a plan can be made with the home-care team to have a quick-acting medication available as a 'first responder' in the home. If severe bleeding is the fear and it is a distinct possibility, family members need to know what to look for and what to do in case of bleeding of a severe nature. Despite the emphasis on home care, relatively few children in the industrialized world die at home. This may be due, in part, to certain conditions not being met; such conditions are requisite to paediatric home care.

Four conditions are requisite for paediatric home care. First, parent or other responsible person must be available, able, and willing to care for the child with some outside help and support. In today's economy, most parents must work outside the home. Various insurance programmes may relieve some of the burden and fears of job loss. But in all countries, including those with government insurance programmes, many smaller companies cannot afford to hold jobs open for extended periods of time. The palliative care team may, at times, need to advocate for parents with employers, or keep employers informed as to the challenges families face. Second, primary health-care teams in local communities may rarely encounter dying children and often feel ill equipped to deal with the medical, emotional, or spiritual needs of the child and family. Moreover, since most health-care professionals' education occurs in hospital settings, most health-care workers are neither comfortable with nor skilled at providing care in the home. Responding to changes in the home requires a very different approach for which caregivers must be educated. A third condition necessary for paediatric palliative homecare has been put forward by those pioneers who implemented and evaluated such programmes[32,34,38]. These researchers concluded that the effectiveness of a programme depended upon a nurse being available 24 h a day, seven days a week for professional consultation, support, and visits when necessary. It is also important that nurses' are able to access medical consultation and pharmacy and ancillary team member support services as needed, to provide optimal care to children and families. This single component of consultation availability can become a most effective safety net in home care. It is also important to have an available means of immediate response in the home for sudden changes that may occur, in order to prevent unnecessary suffering or unwanted hospitalization. For example, having an emergency kit of medications for anticipated/feared symptoms enables many parents to manage calmly at home until the nurse arrives rather than waiting in panic, calling an ambulance, or rushing to the emergency room. Finally, care across settings must be coordinated. Families are greatly reassured by the knowledge that an alternative exists if they find themselves unable to care for their child at home and when no guilt is attached to their choice for location of care. There is often an idealized notion that the 'best death' takes place at home, that everyone should die at home to have a 'good death'. Anyone who does not follow this path may be judged as failing in 'doing it right'. Coordination of services is also needed for children and families who do not change settings—the multitude of physicians and other professional caregivers who enter the child's life must be coordinated and organized so that families are not overwhelmed by sheer numbers of helpers and are clear as to who does what for the child. The suggestion of a 'cornerstone carer' or a care coordinator is a worthy one—where one key individual is identified as the family's primary contact person who ensures consistency of care while assisting them through the maze of other helpers[39]. Unfortunately, for children with non-traditional life-threatening illness—of which there are many—there are few, if any, centralized providers or organizations locally to advocate for the child's needs and to assist families to navigate the system.

Other supportive environments for children

School

For many children, school is their second 'family' community that includes classmates, teachers, counsellors, school nurses, other parents, and team mates. Consequently, children with life-threatening conditions who experience many weeks to months of ups and downs and slow decline must be assisted to attend school as a source of satisfaction and even pleasure through participation in normal activities with peers and through striving for personal

goals. Schools are required to meet the needs of special needs children and yet they may not be equipped to meet the additional needs and issues surrounding a dying child in their midst. For children who cannot attend school, home school assistance is another option that helps the child maintain connections with the classroom and fulfil a sense of accomplishment. School conferences with representatives of the palliative care team can facilitate children's ongoing desires to attend school and, at the same time, integrate the health-care team into the existing supports available at school. The nurse can speak to the child's classmates, be a resource to the teacher and suggest ways to establish an emotionally and clinically safe environment for children in the school. The school can also facilitate connection with the homebound child through the assistance of classmates and teachers with the palliative care team.

Day care

Day care programmes for daytime activities and companionship, increasingly utilized for adult patients with cancer and Alzheimer's disease, have not yet found widespread use in paediatrics, although such programmes are able to offer respite to parents and an opportunity for some freedom from surveillance and physical care for the significant number of children whose illness and terminal course is prolonged. For the pre-school child, day care provides the peer companionship, stimulation, and sense of belonging that school provides for the older child. St Mary's Hospital for Children in Bayside, New York, provides a stimulating day-care programme for their special needs children and has extended enrollment to some of the terminally ill children from the hospice unit no longer able to attend school[40]. Personal communication from several other hospital-based programmes indicates that a variety of day programmes for family respite are being explored but are still experimental.

Other supportive resources

Parent/peer group support

When available, supportive family members are invaluable in rallying round stricken families. However, not all parents have extended family members present; moreover, many parents find themselves socially and emotionally isolated as friends and family also struggle with their difficult situation. Parent/peer support groups become important to such parents and become increasingly effective as parents adjust to their changed lives and identify with others who share similar challenges. Parent groups can be most beneficial if they provide participants with freedom to move in and out of the group until they find their own level of comfort and choose to participate with the group. Encouragement by caregivers, and sensitivity on their part to introduce parents likely to be compatible, smoothes the adjustment for parents and children and helps create a supportive ambience for all concerned. Consideration of confidentiality is important before the contact is made. Some families are fortunate to connect with other parents through a disease-specific organization but those whose children have rare or less familiar diseases, are more isolated. One alternative has been the explosion of Web-based supports where parents can often find others in a similar situation. However, caution is advisable since the information shared and the presented facts can sometimes be largely unsubstantiated and even harmful. However, the Internet has helped many families of children with progressive, life-limiting conditions.

Volunteers and community figures

To attain the goal of meeting the needs of the ill children and their families, the team needs to include, on an ad hoc basis, whoever is most capable of accomplishing each given task, or helping children and families reach their goals. Classmates, teachers, coaches, scout leaders, or others may contribute to the ill children's sense of still belonging to a peer group and may encourage children to participate in accord with their wishes, emotional state, and physical reserves.

Volunteers have proven to be a valuable asset in staffing home, hospice, and inpatient care programmes. Volunteers should be well trained so that they augment the staff, benefit families, and in no way antagonize or inadvertently do harm to patients or families. Volunteers often bring a fresh outlook to the scene, provide beneficial services to children and families and relieve parents and staff, providing them with respite from stress. In paediatric situations, volunteers are especially beneficial in providing attention and companionship to siblings. Volunteers require training by skilled professionals in how to work with families, and ongoing supervision and support around working with children and families.

Ombudsmen are invaluable in ascertaining that children's points of view are heard and that decisions are made in their best interests. The parent–child relationship is of such magnitude that bringing in a third party is not common, but utilizing an ombudsman as a 'neutral observer' may provide excellent service in prevention of miscommunication, particularly in acute care hospital settings where the environment may predispose to a focus on curative efforts.

Cost of paediatric palliative care

Palliative care must be quality care—efficient and yet cost-effective. In the field of paediatrics, particularly in life-threatening illnesses, families tend not to let cost deprive their children of life-saving care. Many exhaust all financial resources in the pursuit of additional treatments or possibility of a cure. As technology has increased in sophistication, with its resultant escalation in costs, families are facing unbearable financial burdens, which impact on all the members. In some countries, families can become impoverished as a result.

The growth and success of the palliative care movement since the 1960s has been described as a social movement provoked by rising health-care costs[41,42]. Certainly, the survival of the hospice philosophy of home care in a highly competitive hospital-dominated environment can be attributed, in part, to the need to control rising costs recognized by both provider and consumer. It would be inappropriate, however, if the intent of pioneer Sister Francis Dominica and her associates—to relieve pain, alleviate symptoms, and provide comfort to children who suffer from life-threatening conditions—and the contributions of countless numbers of volunteers committed to paediatric palliative care were perceived to be driven primarily by money.

The outstanding advances in pain control made through research in pharmacology and neurology have been welcomed, but the price of these gains is to increase the cost of care that will need further evaluation to demonstrate if the benefits gained are truly cost-effective. Analysis of the elements of cost, the rightful assignment of charges, and the measurement of out-of-pocket costs must also include the savings in hospital costs, in-kind contributions of family and volunteers and reduction in physical and mental health costs in survivors[41,43]. Work by Birenbaum[44], comparing hospital care and home care costs for children, indicates the importance of a breakdown of sub-categories of cost in order to identify the burden of cost to families using home care who must bear the higher out-of-pocket social costs and direct non-health costs. The literature reports a variety of conflicting observations, but in general seems to favour the position that home care in toto is less costly than hospital admission[45]. More definitive studies are needed to analyse actual costs in a prospective manner, since retrospective studies, even with diaries, are limited in their ability to capture many of the important details. In the United States, financial assistance for non-medical expenses is sorely needed as, increasingly, the financial burden can break an already emotionally strained marriage and leave the family with an insurmountable debt as well as an irreparable marital relationship. Definitive cost analyses will be essential to move the policy-makers to provide the additional financing needed for the current unacknowledged expenditures.

Children present a particularly poignant problem, especially in the United States where there is no national system of universal health insurance. Most young parents are poorly insured, if at all. Federal and state programmes for hospital therapeutic care may sustain the most impoverished, but little is available for comprehensive services. Both Bloom et al.[46] and Lansky et al.[47] have provided data suggesting that, although the family portions of the total costs may be only 5 per cent, on a per family basis this will consume approximately 38 per cent of the gross annual family income. Of note is the initiative by American-based Children's Hospital International in concert with the Center for Medicare and Medicaid Services to allow demonstration projects that will do away with the barriers to paediatric palliative and end-of-life care—primarily the need for a prognosis of 6 months or less and the requirement to forego life-prolonging and life-sustaining treatments most importantly[48]. In California alone, it is estimated that 16 000 children with life-threatening conditions would benefit from concurrent hospice and palliative care[49]. To that end, California's Children's Hospice and Palliative Care Coalition passed legislation requiring the state to submit a federal paediatric hospice eligibility waiver by January 2008[50]. Under the waiver, pilot projects have been established to demonstrate the efficacy and benefit of offering children hospice and palliative care concurrent with curative or life-prolonging treatment. The State of Florida acquired a similar waiver in 2005. Such initiatives provide hope for paediatric palliative care.

Paediatric palliative care costs more than adult care, primarily because of the large number of specialized personnel needed to provide definitive paediatric care and support services to entire families and the need for care over an indeterminate length of time. Further studies on cost-effectiveness and cost–benefit of palliative care will be critical to its continued existence as an integral part of the health-care system. Survival of palliative care may hinge on cost wise management and hard evidence that the cost-benefit ratio is favourable[51].

Research and evaluation of palliative care

The opportunities for research in paediatric palliative care are unlimited, since well-controlled studies with significant data are minimal in most areas of the field. To date, very few paediatric centres or programmes have been able to conduct large-scale controlled evaluations on either the physical or behavioural aspects of palliative therapy or to provide validated outcome measures. Most hospice programmes are service oriented and lack the skill and resources for research. There is rarely a well-established relationship between the academic settings and the care provider systems for hospice or palliative care, which grossly limits the advancement of research in the care setting. Indeed, the most common phrases about paediatric palliative care research in the report by the American Institute of Medicine are that 'research is limited' and 'systematic data are not available'[31]. As a result, clinical decision-making in paediatric palliative care is often made with little guidance from clinical or health services research.

Despite these limitations, however, research in paediatric palliative care has begun to grow during the past several years. Various national or federal initiatives have contributed to this development. For example, since 1997, the National Institute for Nursing Research, under the auspices of the US National Institutes of Health, identified a specific priority for end-of-life research which encompasses research in paediatric palliative care. The Center for Medicare and Medicaid Services is funding several demonstration projects that are intended to provide information about the development, operation, effectiveness, and costs of comprehensive programmes of palliative care for children and families from the time of diagnosis through to bereavement. Private foundations have also provided funding for various programmes in the United States. In 2003, the Canadian Institute for Health Research announced a strategic initiative to build research capacity, enhance research resources, and fund research in palliative and end of life care. One programme funded by this new initiative is New Emerging Teams (NETs), designed to address the long-term issue of capacity building within the field of palliative and end-of-life care by creating new interdisciplinary research teams or expanding small existing teams. One successfully funded NET 'Transitions in Pediatric Palliative and End-of-Life Care' has as its goal to establish multi-centre research in three main but overlapping themes. These themes are: (1) biomedical and clinical indicators to generate evidence based instruments to guide in diagnosis, prognosis, and management of childhood life-limiting conditions; (2) families studies to uncover and document experiences of child, family members, friends, and caregivers as they move through illness trajectory (transitioning); and (3) health services research to support and optimize quality, coordination, and continuity of care with a focus on identifying, refining, and describing development, operations, and impact of paediatric palliative care programmes to serve as prototype for an expanding network of these programmes[52].

Advances in paediatric palliative care research are summarized in several comprehensive publications[31,53,54]. Despite some progress, however, challenges remain. Research in paediatric palliative care is inherently difficult to undertake. Paediatric patients present a demanding challenge to investigators in questions of design, measurement, analysis, and ethics[55,56]. The problems of conducting randomized controlled studies of paediatric palliative care procedures and services seem overwhelming. For children,

most evaluation tools lack validation. The behaviour of a developing infant or child is in constant flux, with continuously changing norms. Children frequently present barriers to communication-limited comprehension, unpredictable behaviour, and capricious cooperation, which may frustrate efforts to evaluate even the simplest actions. In the adolescent age group, the natural rebelliousness and need for control are heightened by the teenager's anger at the injustice of a foreshortened life. The more tenuous the child's hold on life, the less inclined will the patient or family be to participate in any but the most necessary activities, and even the most cooperative will become resistant to measurements and evaluations that impinge on their remaining time. The researcher, in turn, feels guilty about adding to the burden of a family under such agonizing stress.

Research questions should be addressed to infants, children, and youth across each age and developmental category, with the data analysed accordingly rather than amassed under the single euphemism of 'children'. Although there may be similar responses to research questions, regardless of age, the variations at each developmental milestone are of such a magnitude as to cloud the outcome if not segregated carefully before the fact. Additionally, cultural variations in child-rearing practices and subsequent child behaviour may be so different across countries that data will not be compatible, but will have to be viewed and interpreted culturally.

For example, in palliative care, the quality of remaining life, regardless of its length, for the child is primary and is a product of optimal relief of suffering and excellent symptom control[57,58]. Evaluation of quality of life is both complex and multi-factorial; one major difficulty has been separation of the child's statements and values from those of the parents. Very few paediatric programmes have evaluated critical issues such as staff attitudes towards children dying in a 'do not resuscitate' status, patient-controlled opioid administration, acceptance of the parent as a co-caregiver, or, most basically, how, when and by whom decisions should be made along the trajectory of care. The coping mechanisms most useful to parents to handle the stress, the influence of various types of support services, the role reversal between parent and clinical caregivers and the grief work necessary for each member of the family, as well as the patient, the benefit of extending hospice care principles into pregnancy with a potentially fatal prenatal diagnosis are just a few of the issues requiring well-controlled studies.

Studies need to be done regarding settings of care. Many of the same questions need to be addressed to the child and his/her family in each of the different locations where a child might receive palliative care. If indeed, as earlier studies have shown[26,27], the child with terminal illness wants to be in his/her own home, further definitive research is needed to identify the ideal characteristics of successful home care. In many countries, there has recently been a groundswell of renewed interest in the integration of paediatric palliative and end-of-life care into the overall management of children in intensive and acute care settings, from the time of diagnosis, through treatment and ultimately into the bereavement period. More opportunities are needed for collaboration between clinical and non-clinical researchers from different paediatric disciplines. Regardless of location, research is needed on the components and provisions of quality care during a child's final weeks.

Financial support from health agencies and foundations will continue only if there is hard evidence of the values to be realized by high-calibre palliative care. Regulatory and reviewing bodies do not seem to take note of the lack of paediatric specific standards for hospice and home care. With children, clinical judgement, clouded by emotional overlay, may influence the evaluation and interfere with the orderly collection of comparative data needed for improved quantitative systems of review. Within the National Health Service of the United Kingdom, efforts to evaluate care have focused increasingly on cost. Audit tools, particularly performance indicators, used in the National Health Service compare one hospital with another rather than with best-practice standards. For many hospitals, these indicators serve the same purpose as the diagnosis-related groups in the United States, to encourage early discharge of patients who are incurable, with little concern for the patient's wishes or quality of care.

The need for 'hospice' or specialist palliative care facilities for paediatric patients, an ongoing debate in the United Kingdom, deserves study in the light of criticisms regarding the use of limited resources for such highly specialized low-census centres[59,60]. Demographic research of regions or districts could better define the extent of the need for facilities offered in respite care to children with chronic disease and their parents. The marked difference in geography and population distribution in countries such as Canada, the United States, and Australia, compared with the United Kingdom, will require multi-site studies of the similarities and disparities of styles, services, and staffing to render the findings applicable across countries. Moreover, as technology advances, society will continue to struggle with ethical and legal issues around 'appropriate' utilization of health-care resources and quality of care issues toward and at the end of life. Only through rigorous scientific research can sound, evidence-based decisions be made by clinical practitioners and policy makers. Such research should focus on the values, experiences, processes of care, and outcomes of all seriously ill patients, and basic investigations into the mechanisms producing and alleviating distressing symptoms experienced at the end of life. Legal and ethical research on end-of-life issues will also influence policy decisions and clinical practice in this field.

A further barrier to access to palliative and end-of-life care is one of attitude, in that patients, families, and many health professionals tend to avoid the issue because they associate it with lack of hope. If palliative care is to succeed, we must not only understand better how to improve people's views towards it but also study strategies to optimize access to paediatric palliative and end-of-life care that go beyond the availability of services. Current models of paediatric palliative and end-of-life care will need to adapt to meet the needs of different patient groups.

The future of paediatric palliative care

The last half of the 20th century saw a dramatic fall in morbidity and mortality in children, with improved survival rates for many diseases. Most families have never experienced the death of a child, and even the demise of elderly parents or relatives may only have occurred at a distance, in hospital, or a nursing home. However, in contrast, many families over many generations have experienced a birth tragedy of one type or another and yet this type of death is still barely recognized as a valid reason for mourning in modern society. At a time when families have become less confident in their competence to care for their severely ill children, the hospitals, beset with burgeoning costs to sustain the new technology, cannot assign expensive paediatric beds to patients needing in some health-care systems, such as the US, non-reimbursable, symptom-directed palliation. The disincentive exists for pursuit of palliative care when higher reimbursement ends because 'comfort care only' appears in the medical record. Children in need of palliative care may be discharged prematurely to an unprepared community environment or into the hands of their overwhelmed parents and other family members.

The community has responded to the needs of such patients with significant improvements in broader services, increased availability of home care nursing, and the development of hospice programmes and facilities[22,61]. Collaborations between hospices and hospitals can extend the limited resources of both and extend the support further into the community. Community-based partnerships that seek to avoid duplication and identify unmet needs may actually reduce costs and the burden of responsibility. These previously mentioned limits may prevent those who are not curable from being discharged, but only if financing of their care can be procured and guaranteed. The equally difficult challenge of educating health professionals to recognize that medicine was designed to serve the patient, not the disease, and to perfect the skills necessary to provide compassionate care until death and into bereavement will be much harder to influence.

For parents, the decision to move their child from a course of further therapeutic care—the unfortunate interpretation from early hospice days that palliation replaces *all* treatment modalities—has been a serious drawback to timely and effective symptom control. It permeates the language of medicine through this 'all or none' mentality. Successful palliative care often requires full utilization of chemotherapy, radiation, antibiotics and even surgical intervention on occasion. The goal of palliative care—to affect the best quality of life for the patient—will be met best by utilizing every means appropriate to alleviate children's symptoms. In fact, only the goals and the type of treatment changes, never a cessation of care. Asking parents to choose between continuing treatments or giving up is all too common in attempts to discuss transition to hospice care with parents. Even the most realistic parents cling to the hope that some event will transpire to prevent the death of their child.

Palliative care has served an even larger and more diverse group of patients as the public and professional acceptance of home care for irreversible and chronic illness has increased. The paediatric conditions previously excluded from most palliative care services by nature of the unpredictability of the date of death and the long terminal trajectory, namely cystic fibrosis, congenital anomalies and abnormalities, genetic disorders, neurodegenerative disorders, severe CNS impairment, metabolic disorders, cardiac disease, an array of rare and fatal disorders, and, most recently, AIDS, are pressing for much needed support. The nature of each of these conditions will require special services and collaboration amongst the many disciplines and policy decision makers involved in children's care to ensure for them the optimal quality of life, throughout their lifetime. 'All living things have lifetimes. And lifetimes are really all the same, they have beginnings and endings ... and there is living in between'. We must set our sights on the living and focus our collective energy to make the necessary improvements in service.

References

1. Corr, C.A. and Corr, D.M. (1988). In our opinion ... What is paediatric hospice care? *Children's Health Care*, **17**, 4–11.

2. American Academy of Pediatrics, Committee on Palliative Care for Children. (2000). Palliative care for children. *Pediatrics*, **106**(2), 351–7.

3. CHIPPS (Children's International Project on Palliative/Hospice Services). (2001). *A call for change: Recommendations to improve the care of children living with life-threatening conditions.* National Hospice and Palliative Care Organization, Alexandria, VA.

4. ACT (Association for Children with Life-threatening and Terminal Conditions and their Families) and the RCPCH (Royal College of Paediatrics and Child Health). (1997). *A guide to the development of children's palliative care services.* RCPCH, London.

5. Canadian Network of Palliative Care for Children. http://cnpcc.ca/. Accessed on 1 March 2007.

6. Elborn, J.S., Shale, D.J., and Britton, J.R. (1991). Cystic fibrosis: Current survival and population estimates to the year 2000. *Thorax*, **46**, 881–5.

7. Feudtner, C., Hays, R.M., Haynes, G. *et al.* (2001). Deaths attributed to paediatric complex chronic conditions: National trends and implications for supportive care services. *Pediatrics*, **107**(6), e99.

8. Christakis, N.A. and Lamont, E.B. (2000). Extent and determination of error in doctors' prognoses in terminally ill patients: Prospective cohort study. *British Medical Journal*, **320**(7233), 469–72.

9. Ries, L.A.G., Harkins, D., Krapcho, M. *et al.* (eds). SEER Cancer Statistics Review, 1975–2003, National Cancer Institute. Bethesda, MD, http://seer.cancer.gov/csr/1975_2003/, based on November 2005 SEER data submission, posted to the SEER web site, 2006.

10. http://www.prcdc.org/ summaries/ aidsworldwide/ aidsworldwide. Html

11. Hunt, A.M. (1990). A survey of signs, symptoms, and symptom control in 30 terminally ill children. *Developmental Medicine and Child Neurology*, **32**(4), 341–346.

12. Hunt, A., Goldman, A., Seers, K. *et al.* (2004). Clinical validation of the paediatric pain profile. *Developmental Medicine and Child Neurology*, **46**(1), 9–18.

13. Wood, I. (2006). School. In *Oxford Textbook of Palliative Care for Children.* (eds. A. Goldman, R. Hain, and S. Liben,), pp. 128–42. Oxford University Press, Oxford.

14. American Academy of Pediatrics, Committee on Bioethics. (1996). Ethics and the care of critically ill infants and children. *Pediatrics*, **98**, 149–52.

15. American Academy of Pediatrics, Committee on Bioethics. (1995). Informed consent, parental permission, and assent in paediatric practice. *Pediatrics*, **95**, 314–17.

16. Davies, B. (1999). *Shadows in the sun: Experiences of sibling bereavement.* Brunner/Mazel, Philadelphia, PA.

17. Silverman, P. (2000). *Never too young to know: Death in children's lives.* OUP, New York.

18. Davies, B., Steele, R., Collins, J.B. *et al.* (2004). The impact on families of respite care in a children's hospice program. *Journal of Palliative Care*, **20**(4), 277–86.

19. Davies, B., Collins, J.B., Steele, R. *et al.* (2005). Children's perspectives of a paediatric hospice program. *Journal of Palliative Care*, **21**(4), 252–61.

20. Charles, G. (2003). Stack Bereavement in paediatric intensive care. *Pediatric Anesthesia*, **13**(8), 651–4.

21. Cooley, C., Adeodu, S., Aldred, H. *et al.* (2000). Paediatric palliative care: A lack of research-based evidence. *International Journal of Palliative Nursing*, **6**(7), 346–51.

22. Wallace, A. and Jackson, D. (1995). Establishing a district palliative care team for children. *Child: Care, Health and Development*, **21**(6), 383–5.

23. Sumner, L. (2001). *Staff support in paediatric hospice care. Hospice Care for Children*, pp. 190–212. Oxford University Press, New York.

24. Martinson, I.M., Armstrong, G.D., and Geis, D.P. (1978). Home care for children dying of cancer. *Pediatrics*, **62**, 106–13.

25. Lauer, M.E. (1983). A comparison study of parental adaptation following a child's death at home or in the hospital. *Pediatrics*, **71**, 107–11.

26. Mulhern, R.K., Lauer, M.E., and Hoffman, R.G. (1983). Death of a child at home or in the hospital: Subsequent psychological adjustment of the family. *Pediatrics*, **71**, 743–7.

27. Lauer, M.E., Mulhern, R.K., Hoffman, R.G. *et al.* (1986). Utilization of hospice/home care in paediatric oncology: a national survey. *Cancer Nursing*, **9**, 102–7.

28. Lauer, M.E., Mulhern, R.K., Schell, M.J. *et al.* (1989). Long term follow-up of parental adjustment following a child's death at home or hospital. *Cancer*, **63**, 988–94.

29. Lauer, M.E. and Mulhern, R.K. (1984). Home-care referral: Parental self selection versus psychosocial predictors of capacity. *American Journal of Hospice Care*, **1**, 35–8.

30. Davies, B., Brenner, P., Orloff, S. *et al.* (2002). Addressing spirituality in paediatric hospice and palliative care. *Journal of Palliative Care*, **1**, 59–67.

31. Field, M.J. and Behrman, R.E. (2003). *When children die: Improving palliative and end-of-life care for children and their families.* Report of the Institute of Medicine Task Force. National Academy Press, Washington, DC.

32. Martinson, I.M. and Enos, M. (1985). The dying child: At home. In *Hospice Approaches to Pediatric Care*, pp. 31–42. Springer Publishing Company, New York.

33. Singleton, R. (1992). Palliative home care program for terminally ill children. *Leadership in Health Services*, **1**(1), 21–7.

34. Duffy, C. *et al.* (1990). Home based palliative care for children. Part 2: The benefits of an established program. *Journal of Palliative Care*, **6**(2), 8–14

35. Dangel, T., Fowler-Kerry, S., Karwack, M. *et al.* (2000). An evaluation of a home palliative care programme for children. *Ambulatory Child Health*, **6**(2), 101–14.

36. Davies, B., Steele, R., Collins, J. *et al.* (2003). The impact on families of a children's hospice program. *Journal of Palliative Care*, **19**(1), 15–26.

37. Steele, R., Davies, B., Collins, J.B. *et al.* (2005). End-of-life care in a children's hospice program. *Journal of Palliative Care*, **21**(1), 5–11.

38. Martin, B.B. (1985). *Home care for terminally ill children and their families. Hospice Approaches to Pediatric Care*, pp. 65–86. Springer Publishing Company, New York.

39. Stein, A., Forrest, G.G., Woolley, H. *et al.* (1989). Life threatening illness and hospice care. *Archives of Disease in Childhood*, **64**, 114–18.

40. Grebin, B. (2001). Palliative care in an inpatient hospital setting. *Hospice Care for Children*, pp. 313–22. Oxford University Press, New York.

41. Mor, V. and Kidder, D. (1985). Cost savings in hospice: Final results of the National Hospice Study. *Health Services Research*, **20**, 407–22.

42. Paradis, L.F. (1988). An assessment of sociology's contributions to hospice: priorities for future research. *Hospice Journal*, **4**, 57–71.

43. Houts, P.S., Lipton, A., Harvey, H.A. *et al.* (1984). Non-medical costs to patients and their families associated with outpatient chemotherapy. *Cancer*, **53**, 2388–92.

44. Birenbaum, L.K. (1990). Cost of terminal care for families of children with cancer. Phyllis F. Verhonick Nursing Research Conference, Delivering Nursing Care in the 90s: Growing Needs, Shrinking Resources. Charlottesville, VA, 6 April 1990.

45. Bloom, B.S. (1987). Is hospice care least expensive for the terminally ill? *Hospice Journal*, **3**, 67–76.

46. Bloom, B.S., Knorr, R., and Evans, A. (1985). The epidemiology of disease expenses. *Journal of the American Medical Association*, **253**, 2393–9.

47. Lansky, S.B., Black, J.L., and Cairns, N.U. (1983). Childhood cancer: medical costs. *Cancer*, **52**, 762–6.

48. CHI (Children's Hospice International). Implementation manual: Program for all-inclusive care for children and their families (PACC)

49. Dalsey M, M.D., MPH, Chief, California Medical Services Branch; Published Minutes from the Pediatric Palliative Care Stakeholders Meeting, Sacramento, November 29, 2006. http://www.dhs.ca.gov/pcfh/cms/ppc/meetings.htm).

50. Nick Snow Bill (Legislation - AB1745 Nick Snow Children's Hospice & Palliative Care Act of 2006, Authored by Assemblywoman Wilma Chan, Principal Co-Author SenatorDon Perata. www.childrenshospice.org).

51. Hill, F. and Oliver, C. (1989). Hospice—an update on the cost of patient care. *Palliative Medicine*, **3**, 119–24.

52. NET pedspallcare. website http://www.pallpedsnet.ca, accessed on 1 March 2006.

53. Toce, S.S. and Andresen, E. (2002). Roles of data collection, evaluation and research in paediatric palliative care. *Supportive Voice*, **8**, 5–6.

54. Himelstein, B.P., Hilden, J.M., Boldt, A.M. *et al.* (2004). Pediatric palliative care. *New England Journal of Medicine*, **350**(17), 1752–62.

55. Davies, B. and Steele, R. (1996). Challenges of identifying children for palliative care. *Journal of Palliative Care*, **12**(30), 5–8.

56. Moore, I.M. and Ruccione, K. (1989). Challenges to conducting research with children with cancer. *Oncology Nursing Forum*, **16**, 587–932.

57. Robbins, M. (2001). *Evaluating palliative care: Establishing the evidence base*. Oxford University Press, Oxford.

58. Scriven, M. (1993). Hard-won lessons in program evaluation. *New Directions for Program Evaluation*, **58**, 1–101.

59. Chambers, T.L. (1987). Hospices for children. *British Medical Journal*, **295**, 1309–10.

60. Wilkinson, J.M. *et al.* (1987). Hospices for children? *British Medical Journal*, **295**, 210–11 (Correspondence).

61. Davies, B. (1996). Assessment of need for a children's hospice program. *Death Studies*, **20**, 247–68.

13.2

Pain control

Stephen C. Brown and Patricia A. McGrath

Introduction

Pain control is an integral component of paediatric palliative care. Children may experience many different types of pain from invasive procedures, the cumulative effects of toxic therapies, progressive disease, or psychological factors. The pain is often complex with multiple sources, comprised of nociceptive and neuropathic components. In addition, several situational factors usually contribute to children's pain, distress, and disability. Thus, to treat pain adequately in children receiving palliative care, we must evaluate the primary pain sources and ascertain which situational factors are relevant for which children and families. Treatment emphasis should shift accordingly from an exclusive disease-centred framework to a more child-centred focus.

In this chapter, we describe a child-centred framework for understanding and controlling pain for children receiving palliative care. Pain control should include regular pain assessments, appropriate analgesics administered at regular dosing intervals, adjunctive drug therapy for symptom and side-effects control and non-drug interventions to modify the situational factors that can exacerbate pain and suffering. Basic information on pathophysiology, pharmacology, and physical interventions is not repeated in this chapter, but presented elsewhere in this textbook. This chapter provides a complementary focus to the other authors' contributions by describing the unique nature of children's pain including the primary factors that affect their pain and quality of life, presenting guidelines for selecting and administering drug therapy in accordance with the nociceptive and neuropathic components, and recommending practical non-drug therapies for integration within a hospital, home, or hospice setting.

The nature of children's pain

Throughout the last decade, we have gained an increasing appreciation for the plasticity and complexity of children's pain. As with adults, children's pain is often initiated by tissue damage caused by noxious stimulation, but the consequent pain is neither simply nor directly related to the amount of tissue damage. Perhaps even more than in adults, differing pain responses to the same tissue damage are noted. The eventual pain evoked by a relatively constant noxious stimulus can be different depending on children's expectations, perceived control, or the significance that they attach to the pain [1]. Children do not sustain tissue damage in an isolated manner, devoid of a particular context, but actively interpret the strength and quality of any pain sensations, determine the relevance of any hurting, and learn how to interpret the pain by observing the general environment, especially the behaviour of other people. Children's perceptions of pain is defined by their age and cognitive level; their previous pain experiences, against which they evaluate each new pain; the relevance of the pain or disease causing pain; their expectations for obtaining eventual recovery and pain relief; and their ability to control the pain themselves. While plasticity and complexity are critical features for all pain perception, plasticity seems an even more important feature for controlling children's pain.

Much research has been conducted to identify the critical factors responsible for the plasticity of pain perception [2]. Animal behaviour studies, in which the physiological responses activated by a noxious stimulus are directly recorded, have demonstrated that certain factors, such as the primate's attention, the predictability of a painful stimulus, and the relevance of the stimulus can directly modify the intensity of the physiological responses evoked by a constant noxious stimulus. Parallel psychophysical studies, in which adults rate the painfulness of constant noxious stimuli in different contexts, have demonstrated that these same factors can modify the perceived intensity and unpleasantness of the consequent pain sensations. Psychologically mediated modulation of pain can occur at the earliest levels of pain processing, but also at the highest levels. Both PET and functional MRI studies have demonstrated that painful stimulation activates different cortical regions—depending on an individual's expectations and attention [3]. Human studies evaluating the impact of environmental and psychological factors on the perception of experimentally induced pain have been conducted primarily in adults. However, results from laboratory studies conducted with children are consistent with those from adult studies [4,5]. In addition, much compelling evidence about the powerful mediating role of psychological factors in children's pain derives from clinical studies of acute, recurrent, and chronic pain. These studies highlight the need to recognize and evaluate the mediating impact of these factors in order to control children's pain optimally.

The model illustrated in Fig. 13.2.1 provides a framework for assessing these factors, based on our knowledge of the plasticity and complexity of children's pain. Some factors are relatively stable for a child, such as gender, temperament, and cultural background, while other factors change progressively, such as age, cognitive level, previous pain experience, and family learning (listed in the open box in the figure). These child characteristics shape how children generally interpret and experience the various sensations caused by tissue damage. In contrast, the cognitive, behavioural, and emotional factors (listed in the shaded boxes) are not stable.

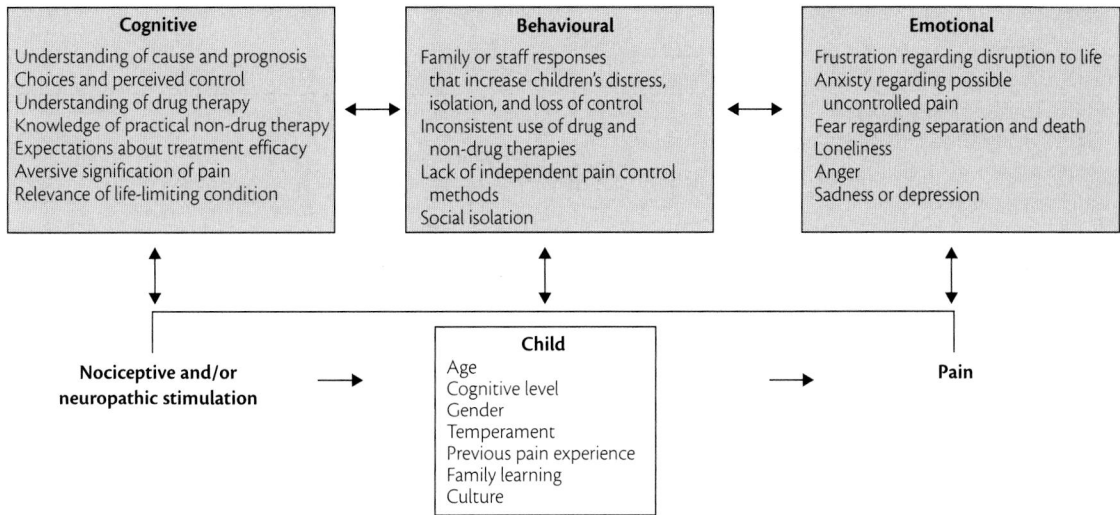

Figure 13.2.1 A model depicting the situational factors that modify children's pain perception.

They represent a unique interaction between the child and the situation in which the pain is experienced[1,6]. These situational factors can vary dynamically throughout the course of a child's illness, depending on the specific circumstances in which children experience pain. For example, a child receiving treatment for cancer will have repeated injections, portacatheter access, and lumbar punctures—all of which may cause some pain (depending on the analgesics, anaesthetics, or sedatives used). Even though the tissue damage from these procedures is the same each time, the particular set of situational factors for each treatment is unique for a child—depending on a child's (and parent's) expectations, a child's (and parent's *and* staff's) behaviours, and on a child's (and family's) emotional state. Although the causal relationship between an injury and a consequent pain seems direct and obvious, what children understand, what they do, and how they feel all affect their pain. Certain factors can intensify pain, exacerbate suffering, or affect adversely a child's quality of life[4]. While parents and health-care providers may be unable to change the more stable child characteristics, they can modify situational factors and dramatically improve children's pain and lives.

The impact of situational factors on children's pain

Cognitive factors include children's understanding about the pain source, their ability to control what will happen, their expectations regarding the quality and strength of pain sensations that they will experience, their primary focus of attention (that is distracted away from or focused primarily on the pain), and their knowledge of pain control strategies. In general, children's pain can be lessened by providing accurate age-appropriate information about pain, for example emphasizing the specific sensations that children will experience (such as the stinging quality of an injection, rather than the general hurting aspects), by increasing their control and choices, by explaining the rationale for what can be done to reduce pain, and by teaching them some independent pain reducing strategies[1,7,8]. For children receiving palliative care, key cognitive factors also include the relevance or meaning of their illness—particularly its

life-threatening potential, their beliefs about death, and their understanding of the significance of their lives.

Behavioural factors refer to the specific behaviours of children, parents, and staff when children experience pain and also encompass parents' and children's wider behaviours in response to a chronic pain problem or progressive illness. Common behavioural factors include children's distress or coping reactions (e.g. crying, using a pain control strategy, withdrawing from life) and parent's and health staff's subsequent reactions to them (e.g. displaying frustration, calmly providing encouragement for children to use pain control strategies, engaging them in conversation and activities)[4]. They also include the extent to which children are physically restrained during invasive or aversive treatments and the broader physical and social restrictions on children's and family's lives as children become sicker. Distress behaviours and some altered behavioural patterns may initiate, exacerbate, or maintain children's pain. In general, as children's mental or physical activity increases, as children use coping and pain control methods, as their distress and disability behaviours decrease and as staff and parental responses become more consistent in encouraging them to use pain control methods, their pain should lessen. Children receiving palliative care seem to report less pain, feel less distressed by pain and have a higher quality of life when families and staff encourage them to remain engaged in life and live as fully as possible.

Emotional factors include parents' and children's feelings in response to pain, to the daily effects of the underlying illness or condition, and to the subsequent impact of the children's deaths on the family. Children's emotions affect their ability to understand what is happening, their ability to cope positively, their behaviours, and ultimately their pain. Children's immediate emotional reactions to pain may vary from a relatively neutral acceptance to annoyance, anxiety, fear, frustration, anger, or sadness. The specific emotions depend on the nature of the pain—type, cause, intensity, and duration—and its impact on their lives. In general, the more emotionally distressed children are, the stronger or more unpleasant their pain. When children do not understand what is happening, when they lack control and do not know independent pain control strategies, their emotional distress increases and their pain intensifies. Similarly, when children's behaviours are restricted, when they are physically restrained during medical procedures, or when their usual daily activities and social interactions are disrupted, their emotional distress and pain can intensify. Children with life-threatening conditions may not understand what they are feeling or may be unable to articulate their fears and anxieties. Yet, almost all children will become aware of differences in how their parents and families respond to them as they progress from receiving active curative treatments to receiving only palliative therapies. Even very subtle behavioural cues can still evoke fear, uncertainty, apprehension, or depression depending on children's ages and what they understand about death and separation. Thus, an essential component of pain control should be evaluating whether these emotions are exacerbating children's pain and distress and impairing the quality of their lives.

Situational factors in paediatric palliative care

Cognitive and emotional factors are the most salient situational factors that affect pain for children receiving palliative care. Children probably have already endured a prolonged period of intermittent pain, physical disability, and multiple aversive treatments. Children who were receiving curative therapies become more focused on the future consequences of their disease. Their thoughts, behaviours, and feelings change as they begin to understand that they are dying. Naturally, the type of support, information, and guidance children require also changes. While the impact is profound for all children and families, each child and family is unique with respect to their specific psychological, medical, social, and spiritual needs. All families experience anguish and grief, but they may also experience denial, anxiety, anger, guilt, frustration, and depression. It is essential that health professionals listen attentively and observe carefully, not only to ensure that all the needs of both the child and family are met, but also to resolve the myriad factors that can exacerbate children's pain and suffering. The primary situational factors in paediatric palliative care are listed in Table 13.2.1. This summary has evolved from our treatment of children referred to our pain clinic. Child and family factors are listed in italics; the factors that are relevant for health staff, as well as families, are listed in roman print.

The shift in care from curative to palliative therapies may signify to some children and families that health professionals are giving up on the child. Children and families must understand that stopping ineffective therapies is not giving up, but represents a rational decision based on children's best interests. Pain control is an essential component of palliative care[9–15]. Children and parents should not fear that health professionals have given up on controlling pain and aversive symptoms. Pain and all symptoms must be treated aggressively from the dual perspective of targeting the primary source of tissue damage and modifying the secondary contributing factors. Although most families receive accurate information about their disease and required treatments, few children or their parents receive concrete information about their pain, the factors that can attenuate or exacerbate it, a rationale for the interventions they receive and training in effective non-drug pain control methods. The latter may be particularly important for children in palliative care, who have diminishing control in their lives. Children and their parents often do not understand that pain control therapies may vary in efficacy due to changing disease, the effects of other

Table 13.2.1 Situational factors in paediatric palliative care.

Cognitive factors
Meaning of death
Inaccurate understanding:
Impact of situational factors on pain and quality of life
Course of disease
Palliative versus curative therapy
Little independent control over pain
Limited choices
Expectation for continuing pain and suffering
Misunderstanding of drug therapy:
Opioids
Dosing and administration
Criteria for evaluating effectiveness
Behavioural factors
Social withdrawal
Physical inactivity
Passive approach to pain control
Secondary gains:
Stress reduction
Emotional denial
Parent or staff attention
Inappropriate drug management:
Choice or mode of drug administration
Failure to treat aggressively opioid-related side effects
Failure to evaluate pain sources and document pain level
Failure to use effective non-drug therapies
Emotional factors
Anxiety about:
Dying and death
Suffering
Meaning of life
Fear of:
Separation
Inadequate pain control
Increasing adverse symptoms
Impact on family
Anger
Sadness or depression
Distancing by staff and friends

drugs and situational factors. Thus, their confidence in certain pain control therapies can decrease, even though these therapies would effectively alleviate pain at another time. The fear of inadequate pain control places an enormous emotional burden on an already distressed child and family and can create a situation in which children's pain and disability intensifies.

Generally, children's physical activity has been progressively restricted due to the disability caused by their condition. Parents who encourage children to adopt passive patient roles, to behave differently to other children, and to depend primarily on others for pain control will undoubtedly create a situation wherein children's pain is maximized. Even when children are somnolent, it is possible to create some 'normal environment' in which children can participate and actively involve themselves during their alert periods. Children should live as fully as possible, even though they are also dying.

Children who experienced adverse physical effects from medication, such as hair loss and weight gain, may have become acutely self-conscious about their appearance. As a result, these children may have progressively withdrawn from social interactions with their peers because they anticipated negative reactions. Children become more distant from the people and activities that they had enjoyed. Moreover, many children may lose the opportunity to be regarded as unique individuals by the friends and classmates they value; instead, they are regarded increasingly as sick, different, or even dying. Their peers and their daily accomplishments (whether social, academic, or athletic) had provided special meaning about children's unique value in the world. While families emphasize children's value to them and to the world, children often lose the objective feedback they routinely received. The increased withdrawal and social isolation can exacerbate their pain and emotional distress. Their withdrawal may increase when treatment emphasis shifts from cure and palliation to palliation alone. Parents may 'close-in', spending even more exclusive time with the dying child as a closed family unit. While important for children and families, the exclusive focus on the family increases a child's social isolation and may cause more anxiety for some children—particularly when the family does not openly address the child's concerns about death and dying. Inadvertently, the family may prevent children from interacting both with peers who can lessen their anxiety through play and conversation and also with health professionals who can help them to resolve their anxiety and fears about dying. Children seem to know intuitively, even when dying has not been discussed directly with them. They fear separation and abandonment; some children may fear that their illness is a punishment. Dying children may feel frightened, isolated, and guilty unless they are able to express and resolve their concerns openly. Many observers have noted that children who are dying have a level of maturity 'far beyond their years'. It is essential to acknowledge and resolve their fears. Children should receive accurate information, consistent with their spiritual beliefs, presented in a calm reassuring manner. They may need concrete reassurance that they will not suffer when they die, that they will not be alone, and that their families will remember them. Unresolved emotions add anguish and may intensify their pain. (For the comprehensive care of the dying child, please see references[13,16–21].)

Optimal pain control for children

Pain control is an intrinsic component of paediatric palliative care. Since children may experience complex pains due to myriad physical and psychological factors, pain control must be child-centred rather than disease-centred. Health-care providers must evaluate carefully the varied causes and contributing factors to select the most effective therapies for each child's pain.

Table 13.2.2 Primary components of pain assessment.

Sensory characteristics
Onset
Location
Intensity
Quality
Duration
Spread to other sites (consistent with neurological pattern)
Radiation
Temporal pattern
Accompanying symptoms
Medical/surgical
Investigations conducted
Radiological and laboratory results
Consult results
Analgesic and adjuvant medications (type, dose, frequency, route, length of medication trial)
Clinical factors
Environmental features
Roles of medical and associated health professionals
Nature of interventions
Complementary and alternative therapy
Documentation of pain
Criteria for determining analgesic effectiveness
Cognitive factors
Understanding of pain source
Understanding of diagnosis, treatment, and prognosis
Expectations
Perceived control
Relevance of disease or painful treatments
Knowledge of pain control
Behavioural factors
General coping style
Learned pain behaviours
Overt distress level
Parents' behaviours
Physical activities and limitations
Social activities and limitations
Emotional factors
Frustration
Anxiety
Fear
Denial
Sadness
Anger
Depression

Onset, location, intensity, quality, duration (or frequency, if recurring), spatial extent, temporal pattern, and accompanying physical symptoms are the key pain characteristics for assessment, as listed in Table 13.2.2. All these characteristics should be evaluated as part of the initial clinical examination, with pain intensity and any other characteristics that are clinically relevant for children monitored regularly. Children's descriptions about the nature of their pain (when self-report is available) complete the information obtained through radiological and laboratory investigations. Since several situational factors usually contribute to children's pain, distress, and disability, health-care providers should evaluate the extent to which these may be relevant for a child—building on their knowledge of the child and family's previous experiences throughout the child's illness and their observations of the current situation.

In palliative care, the differential diagnosis of a child's pain is a dynamic process that guides our clinical management. We should select specific therapies to target the responsible central and peripheral mechanisms and to mitigate the pain-exacerbating impact of situational factors, recognizing that the multiple causes and contributing factors will vary over time. Drug therapies—analgesics, analgesic-adjuvants, and anaesthetics are essential for pain control, but non-drug therapies—cognitive, physical, and behavioural are also essential. As we monitor the child's improvement in response to the therapies initiated, we refine our pain diagnosis and treatment plan accordingly. Pain control is achieved practically by adjusting both drug and non-drug therapies in a rational child-centred manner based on the assessment process, as outlined by the treatment algorithm in Fig. 13.2.2. (The different therapies are described later in the chapter.) Controlling children's pain requires an integrated approach because many factors are responsible, no matter how seemingly clear cut the aetiology. Adequate analgesic prescriptions, administered at regular dosing intervals, must be

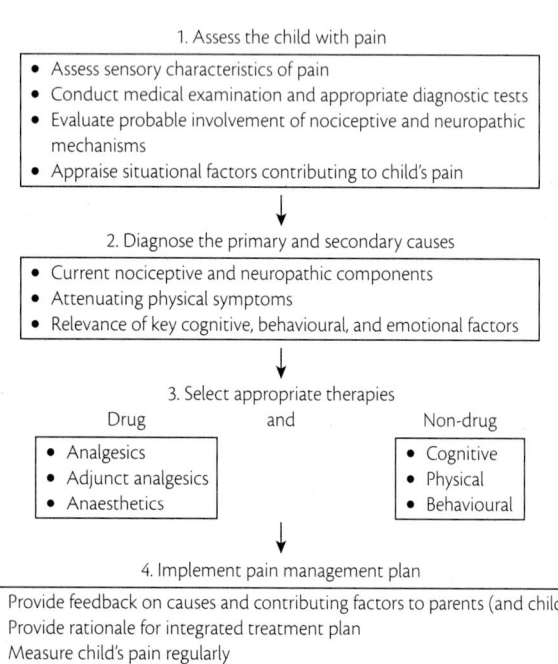

Figure 13.2.2 A treatment algorithm for controlling children's pain.

complemented by a practical cognitive behavioural approach to ensure optimal pain relief.

Misconceptions regarding pain control in children

Several misconceptions have led to inadequate pain control in children as described in the following (revised from reference[1]).

Misconceptions about children's pain systems

Many health-care providers continue to treat children's pain from an erroneous disease model perspective wherein pain is always proportional to the extent and severity of tissue damage. As a result of misconceptions about the plasticity and complexity of children's nociceptive systems, they focus on the primary source of noxious stimulation but not on all the causative and contributing factors that affect nociceptive processing. As a result of misconceptions about nociceptive and neuropathic components of pain, they fail to use the wide range of analgesic and analgesic-adjuvants available to control pain.

Misconceptions about the pharmacodynamics and pharmacokinetics of opioid analgesics

As a result of misconceptions about the pharmacodynamics and pharmacokinetics of opioid analgesics, health professionals do not always select the most appropriate drugs, doses, dosing intervals, or administration routes.

Misconceptions about the risk of addiction

Some health-care providers and parents believe that opioid analgesics should be administered only as a last resort, to avoid drug addiction. They have not understood that Tolerance + Physical Dependence ≠ Addiction. As a result, children have not always received the potent analgesics required to relieve severe pain. Moreover, they may not understand that opioid-related side-effects should be treated aggressively so that the potential efficacy of these drugs for controlling pain is not compromised by adverse side effects.

Misconceptions about the efficacy of non-drug therapies

Many health professionals do not realize that relatively simple non-drug strategies can lessen children's pain. As a result, they have not taught children or their parents how to use practical cognitive, physical, and behavioural strategies that are effective for reducing pain, distress, and pain-related disability. Similarly, they have not taught parents the importance of evaluating and modifying situational and familial factors to lessen children's pain.

Misconceptions about comprehensive pain control

Many health-care providers believe that drug therapies are both necessary and sufficient to control children's pain. They have not prescribed non-drug therapies to supplement or complement analgesics, even when situational factors are impeding analgesic efficacy.

Misconceptions about pain assessment

Many health-care providers do not know how to assess children's pain levels routinely or the factors that intensify their pain and distress. As a result, it may be difficult to evaluate the effectiveness of changes in drug therapy, complementary therapies, and situational factors.

Misconceptions about who is in charge of pain control

One individual should assume primary responsibility for ensuring that a child's pain is controlled adequately. Diffusion of responsibility among various health-care providers leads to gaps in recognizing a child's pain and treating pain appropriately.

Misconceptions about the importance of consistent pain control

The medical specialties, which provide care to children throughout their illness, do not always adopt a consistent approach to pain assessment and pain control, similar to their consistent approach to disease diagnosis and medical treatment. The failure to regard pain control as important throughout a child's treatment can lead to difficulties for children in palliative care, whose previous experiences with inadequate pain management can create undue stress and anxiety for them and their parents.

Guidelines for assessment, analgesic selection and administration, and non-pharmacological interventions

The principles of analgesic therapy, the guidelines for drug administration, and the guidelines for a supportive cognitive behavioural approach are those that should be followed in all paediatric palliative care, including the care of children with cancer, neurodegenerative diseases, and acquired human immunodeficiency virus (HIV) infection.

Evaluating children's pain

Pain assessment is an integral component of diagnosis and treatment for children. A thorough medical history, physical examination and assessment of pain characteristics, and contributing factors are necessary to establish a correct clinical diagnosis. Subsequent assessments of pain intensity enable us to determine when treatments are effective and to identify those children for whom they are most effective. Health-care providers need pain measures that are convenient to administer and whose resulting pain scores provide meaningful information about children's pain experiences. An extensive array of pain measures have been developed and validated for use with infants, children, and adolescents[22–24].

Like adult pain measures, children's pain measures are classified as physiological, behavioural, and psychological, depending on what is monitored—physical parameters (e.g. heart rate, sweat index, blood pressure, cortisol level), distress behaviours (e.g. grimaces, cries, protective guarding gestures), or children's own descriptions of what they are experiencing (e.g. words, drawings, numerical ratings). Physiological and behavioural measures provide indirect estimates of pain because health-care providers must infer the location and strength of a child's pain solely from his or her responses. In contrast, psychological measures can provide direct information about the location, strength, quality, affect, and duration.

The criteria for an accurate pain measure are similar to those required for any measuring instrument. A pain measure must be valid, in that it measures a specific aspect of pain so that changes in pain ratings reflect meaningful differences in a child's pain experience. The measure must be reliable, in that it provides consistent and trustworthy pain ratings regardless of the time of testing, the clinical setting, or who is administering the measure. The measure must be relatively free from bias, in that children should be able to use it similarly, regardless of differences in how they may wish to please adults. The pain measure should be practical and versatile for assessing different types of pain (e.g. disease-related, procedural pain) in many different children (according to age, cognitive level, cultural background) and for use in diverse clinical and home settings.

Physiological and behavioural pain scales

Although physiological parameters can provide valuable information about a child's distress state, more research is required to develop a sensitive system for interpreting how these parameters reflect pain strength. At present, there are no valid physiological pain scales for children.

Most behavioural pain scales are checklists of the different distress behaviours that children exhibit when they experience a certain type of pain[22,25,26]. To develop these scales, trained health-care providers carefully observe children when they are in pain (e.g. after surgery) and document any behaviours that seem caused by the pain. They then list these 'presumed pain' behaviours (e.g. crying, facial expression, limb rigidity) on an itemized checklist. Parents complete the pain scale by checking which of the listed behaviours they see when children are ill. On many scales, parents also rate the intensity of the behaviours. The intensity scores for each of the observed behaviours are summed to produce a composite pain score. Although most behavioural scales measure acute pain, there remains a need to develop sensitive measures for children who are cognitively or physically impaired[27]. The current behavioural scales may not be adequate for children receiving palliative care. The complexity of a child's disease or health condition, concomitant drug therapy and the other distress sources in the health-care environment, may limit children's ability to behave so that the pain score is not meaningful. Their pain behaviours may be very different from those of the children studied to develop the original scales. Moreover, the most salient pain behaviour might be very child-dependent and vary widely among different children or change throughout the course of their illness. At present, health-care providers must use their content expertise and consult with parents to consider carefully which behaviour or behaviours are the most relevant indices of pain for a particular child. They can chart the presence and intensity of these behaviours (it is likely that these will be more subtle indices than on current standardized scales) and interpret them as an indirect measure of pain.

Psychological pain scales

Psychological or self-report pain scales directly capture an individual's subjective experience of pain. Interviews, questionnaires, adjective checklists, and numerous pain intensity scales are available for children, each with some evidence of validity and reliability[22,28]. Clinical interviews are ideally suited for learning about the sensory characteristics of pain, the aversive component, and contributing cognitive, behavioural, and emotional factors. Interviews should also include a simple rating scale to document pain strength. Children choose a level on the scale that best matches the strength of their own pain (i.e. a level on a number or thermometer scale, a number of objects, a mark on a visual analogue scale, a face from a series of faces varying in emotional expression, or a particular word from adjective lists). Pain intensity scales are easy to administer, requiring only a few seconds once children understand how to use them. Many of these scales yield pain scores on a 0–10 scale. Visual and coloured analogue scales are versatile for use with acute, recurrent, and chronic pain and provide a convenient and flexible pain measure for use in hospital and at home.

Health-care providers must consider the age and cognitive ability of a child when selecting a pain scale. Most toddlers (approximately 2 years of age) can communicate the presence of pain, using words learned from their parents to describe the sensations they feel when they hurt themselves. They use concrete analogies to describe their perceptions. Gradually children learn to differentiate and describe three levels of pain intensity—'a little', 'some or medium', and 'a lot'. By the age of 5, most children can differentiate a wider range of pain intensities and many can use simple pain intensity scales.

Children's understanding and descriptions of pain naturally depend on their age, cognitive level, and previous pain experience. Children begin to understand pain through their own hurting experiences; they learn to describe the different characteristics of their pains (intensity, quality, duration, and location) in the same way that they learn specific words to describe different sounds, tastes, smells, and colours. Most children can communicate meaningful information about their pain. Gradually they develop an increasing ability to describe specific pain features—the quality (aching, burning, pounding, sharp), intensity (mild to severe), duration and frequency (a few seconds to years), location (from a diffuse location on their skin to more precise internal localization), and unpleasantness (mild annoyance to an intolerable discomfort). Children's understanding of pain and the language that they use to describe pain comes from the words and expressions used by their families and peers and from characters depicted in books, videos, and movies. (For a more extensive review of developmental factors in children's pain, see references[1,6,29–33].) Physicians should always ask children directly about their pain. Pain onset, location, frequency (if recurring), quality, intensity, accompanying physical symptoms, and pain-related disability should be assessed as part of children's clinical examination. Health-care providers should also assess relevant situational factors in order to modify their pain-exacerbating impact, especially the factors listed in Table 13.2.1.

Analgesic selection and administration

Pain control should include regular pain assessments, appropriate analgesics and adjuvant analgesics administered at regular dosing intervals, adjunctive drug therapy for symptom and side effects control, and non-drug therapies to modify the situational factors that can exacerbate pain and suffering. Analgesics include acetaminophen, non-steroidal anti-inflammatory drugs (NSAIDs), and opioids. Adjuvant analgesics include a variety of drugs with analgesic properties that were initially developed to treat other health problems, such as anticonvulsants and antidepressants. The use of adjuvant analgesics has become a cornerstone of pain control in paediatric palliative care. They are especially crucial when pain has a neuropathic component.

The guiding principles of analgesic administration are 'by the ladder', 'by the clock', 'by the child', and 'by the mouth'. 'By the ladder' refers to a three-step approach for selecting drugs according to their analgesic potency based on the child's pain level—acetaminophen to control mild pain, codeine to control moderate pain and morphine for strong pain[34]. The ladder approach was based on our scientific understanding of how analgesics affect pain of nociceptive origins. If pain persists despite starting with the appropriate drug, recommended doses and dosing schedule, move up the ladder and administer the next more potent analgesic. Even when children require opioid analgesics, they should continue to receive acetaminophen (and NSAIDs, if appropriate) as supplemental analgesics. The analgesic ladder approach is based on the premise that acetaminophen, codeine, and morphine should be available in all countries and that doctors and health-care providers can relieve pain in the majority of children with a few drugs. The WHO model of: (1) appropriate policies; (2) adequate drug availability; (3) education of the health-care workers, policymakers, and the public; and (4) implementation has been shown to provide an effective strategy to establish palliative care[35,36]. Oral morphine remains, in either immediate release or sustained release form, the analgesic of choice for moderate or severe cancer pain[37,38]. The higher use of opioids and sedatives (when required) takes place when end-of-life care (EOLC) discussions are an integral component of palliative care, as discussed elsewhere in this textbook[39].

However, increasing attention is focusing on 'thinking beyond the ladder' in accordance with our improved understanding of pain of neuropathic origins[40,41]. Children should receive adjuvant analgesics to target neuropathic mechanisms more specifically. Regrettably, two of the main classes of adjuvant analgesics, antidepressants and anticonvulsants, have unfortunate names. Proper education of health-care providers, parents, and children should lead to a wider acceptance and use of these medications for pain management. For example, amitriptyline may require 4–6 weeks to affect depression, but often requires only 1–2 weeks to affect pain. The newer classes of antidepressants, the selective serotonin reuptake inhibitors (SSRIs), may be beneficial to treat depression for a child with pain but have not been shown to be beneficial for pain management. The other main class of adjuvant analgesics is the anticonvulsants. The two principal medications used for this purpose in paediatrics are carbamazepine and gabapentin. With gabapentin, the main dose-limiting side effect is sedation so that a slow titration to maximal dose is required. Because of its greater number of significant side effects, the use of carbamazepine has decreased and the use of gabapentin has increased. While some reports support the use of gabapentin in children[42–44], we still await published studies to support this wider use in children generally and specifically in palliative care[45].

NSAIDs are similar in potency to aspirin. NSAIDs are used primarily to treat inflammatory disorders and to lessen mild to moderate acute pain. They should be used with caution in patients with hepatic or renal impairment, compromised cardiac function, hypertension (since they may cause fluid retention, oedema), and a history of GI bleeding or ulcers. NSAIDs may also inhibit platelet aggregation and thus must be monitored closely in patients with prolonged bleeding times. Indications for NSAIDs are much narrower for children with cancer (due to the concern for bleeding problems) than for children with other painful conditions. Although acetaminophen should be considered the routine non-opioid analgesic for children with cancer, NSAIDs are effective for patients with bony metastases, who have adequate platelets.

Tramadol was launched in the area of pain practice over 30 years ago in Germany. It has recently been released in North America in a long-acting oral preparation and as a combination drug with acetaminophen. Its release has been welcomed as an additional analgesic in our drug armamentarium with a potency compatible with step two of the WHO analgesic ladder.

Tramadol is a synthetic 4-phenyl-piperidine analog of codeine, which is marketed as a racemic mixture of (+) and (−) enantiomers. The opioid activity of tramadol results from low affinity binding of the (+) enantiomer to mu opioid receptors. The (+) enantiomer inhibits serotonin uptake and has a direct serotonin-releasing action, while the (−) enantiomer is a more effective inhibitor of norepinephrine uptake[46]. The analgesic potency of tramadol is considered to be medium, having one-tenth the potency of morphine. Its advantages over opioids are mainly the lower incidence of side effects such as respiratory depression, nausea, vomiting, constipation, sedation, and a low potential for dependence or abuse.

Rose reported that in 113 children aged 7–16 years, the use of oral tramadol (50 mg) at 1 mg/kg every 4–6 h for various conditions was well tolerated[47]. Tramadol may prove particularly useful in patients with poor cardiopulmonary, renal, or hepatic function and in those for whom non-steroidal anti-inflammatory drugs are not recommended or need to be used with caution[48].

A growing number of studies and case reports[49,50] show the safety and efficacy of tramadol. Because of insufficient studies in this population, while it continues to be prescribed in Europe and North America for paediatric patients, it is not recommended for patients under 18 years of age in Canada.

Although the specific drugs and doses are determined by the needs of each child, general guidelines for drug therapies to control pain for children in palliative care have been developed through a Consensus Conference on the Management of Pain in Childhood Cancer, published as a supplement to *Pediatrics*[51], in a monograph, *Cancer Pain Relief and Palliative Care for Children*[15], and in clinical practice guidelines[52–54]. The drugs listed in this chapter are based on these sources and guidelines from our institution[55]. Recommended starting doses for analgesic medications to control children's disease-related pain are listed in Tables 13.2.3 and 13.2.4; starting doses for adjuvant analgesic medications to control pain, drug related side effects, and other symptoms are listed in Table 13.2.5. (For further review of analgesics and adjuvant analgesics in children, see references[41, 56–63].)

Children should receive analgesics at regular times, 'by the clock', to provide consistent pain relief and prevent breakthrough pain. The specific drug schedule (e.g. every 4 or 6 h) is based on the drug's duration of action and the child's pain severity. Although breakthrough pain episodes have been recognized as a problem in adult pain control, they may represent an even more serious problem for children. Unlike adults, who generally realize that they can demand more potent analgesic medications or demand more frequent dosing intervals, children have little control, little awareness of alternatives, and fear that their pain cannot be controlled. They may become progressively frightened, upset, and preoccupied with their symptoms. Thus, it is essential to establish and maintain a therapeutic window of pain relief for children.

Analgesic doses should be adjusted 'by the child'. There is no one dose that will be appropriate for all children with pain. The goal is to select a dose that prevents children from experiencing pain before they receive the next dose. It is essential to monitor the child's pain regularly and adjust analgesic doses as necessary to control the pain. The effective opioid dose to relieve pain varies widely among different children or in the same child at different times. Some children require massive opioid doses at frequent

Table 13.2.3 Non-opioid drugs for relieving cancer pain in children.

Drug	Dosage	Comments
Acetaminophen	10–15 mg/kg PO, every 4–6 h	Lacks GI and haematological side effects; lacks anti-inflammatory effects (may mask infection-associated fever)
		Dose limit of 65 mg/kg/day or 4 g/day, whichever is less
Ibuprofen	5–10 mg/kg PO, every 6–8 h	Anti-inflammatory activity
		Use with caution in patients with hepatic or renal impairment, compromised cardiac function or hypertension (may cause fluid retention, oedema), history of GI bleeding or ulcers, may inhibit platelet aggregation
		Dose limit of 40 mg/kg/day; max. dose of 2400 mg/day
Naproxen	10–20 mg/kg/day PO, divided every 12 h	Anti-inflammatory activity. Use with caution and monitor closely in patients with impaired renal function. Avoid in patients with severe renal impairment
		Dose limit of 1 g/day
Diclofenac	1 mg/kg PO, every 8–12 h	Anti-inflammatory activity. Similar GI, renal and hepatic precautions as noted above for ibuprofen and naproxen
		Dose limit of 50 mg/dose

Note: Increasing the dose of non-opioids beyond the recommended therapeutic level produces a 'ceiling effect', in that there is no additional analgesia but there are major increases in toxicity and side effects.

PO, by mouth; GI, gastrointestinal.

Table 13.2.4 Opioid analgesics: usual starting doses.

Drug	Equianalgesic dose (parenteral)	Starting dose IV	IV:PO ratio	Starting dose PO/transdermal	Duration of action
Morphine	10 mg	Bolus dose = 0.05–0.1 mg/kg every 2–4 h Continuous infusion = 0.01–0.04 mg/kg/h	1:3	0.15–0.3 mg/kg/dose every 4 h	3–4 h
Hydromorphone	1.5 mg	0.015–0.02 mg/kg every 4 h	1:5	0.06 mg/kg every 3–4 h	2–4 h
Codeine	120 mg	Not recommended		1.0 mg/kg every 4 h	3–4 h (dose limit 1.5 mg/kg/dose)
Oxycodone	5–10 mg	Not recommended		0.1–0.2 mg/kg every 3–4 h	3–4 h
Meperidine[a]	75 mg	0.5–1.0 mg/kg every 3–4 h	1:4	1.0–2.0 mg/kg every 3–4 h (dose limit 150 mg)	1–3 h
Fentanyl[b]	100 mcg	1–2 mcg/kg/h as continuous infusion		25 mcg patch	72 h (patch)
Controlled-release morphine[c,d]				0.6 mg/kg every 8 h or 0.9 mg/kg every 12 h	
Controlled-release hydromorphone[d]				0.18 mg/kg every 12 h	
Controlled-release codeine[d]				3 mg/kg every 12 h	
Controlled-release oxycodone[d]				0.6 mg/kg every 12 h	
Methadone	10 mg	0.1 mg/kg every 4–8 h	1:2	0.2 mg/kg every 4–8 h	12–50 h
Tramadol	100 mg	2.0 mg/kg every 4–6 h		1 mg/kg every 4–6 h (dose limit 400 mg/day)	4–6 h

Doses are for opioid naïve patients. For infants under 6 months, start at one-quarter to one-third the suggested dose and titrate to effect.

PO, by mouth; IV, intravenous.

Principles of opioid administration:

1. If inadequate pain relief and no toxicity at peak onset of opioid action, increase dose in 50% increments.

2. Avoid IM administration.

3. Whenever using continuous infusion, plan for hourly rescue doses with short onset opioids if needed. Rescue dose is usually 50–200% of continuous hourly dose. If greater than six rescues are necessary in 24-h period, increase daily infusion total by the total amount of rescues for previous 24 h. An alternative is to increase infusion by 50%.

4. To change opioids—because of incomplete cross-tolerance: if changing between opioids with short duration of action, start new opioid at 50% of equianalgesic dose. Titrate to effect. If changing between opioids from short to long duration of action (i.e. morphine to methadone), start at 25% of equianalgesic dose and titrate to effect.

5. To taper opioids—anyone on opioids over 1 week must be tapered to avoid withdrawal: taper by 50% for 2 days, and then decrease by 25% every 2 days. When dose is equianalgesic to an oral morphine dose of 0.6 mg/kg/day; opioid may be stopped. Some patients on opioids for prolonged periods may require much slower weaning.

[a] Avoid use in renal impairment. Metabolite may cause seizures.

[b] Potentially highly toxic. Not for use in acute pain control.

[c] Use may be hampered by child's difficulty in swallowing large tablets.

[d] The widely-used equianalgesic doses in adults are used as guidelines in paediatric practice but have not been substantiated in children.

intervals to control their pain. If such large doses are necessary for effective pain control, and the side effects can be managed by adjunctive medication so that children are comfortable, then the doses are appropriate. Children receiving opioids may develop altered sleep patterns so that they are awake at night, fearful and complaining about pain and they sleep intermittently throughout the day. They should receive adequate analgesics at night with antidepressants or hypnotics as necessary to enable them to sleep throughout the night. To relieve severe ongoing pain, opioid doses should be increased steadily until comfort is achieved, unless the child experiences unacceptable side effects such as somnolence or respiratory depression (Table 13.2.6).

'By the mouth' refers to the oral route of drug administration. Medication should be administered to children by the simplest and most effective route, usually by mouth. Since children are afraid of painful injections they may deny that they have pain or they may not request medication. When possible, children should receive medications through routes that do not cause additional pain. Although optimal analgesic administration for children requires flexibility in selecting routes according to children's needs,

Table 13.2.5 Adjuvant analgesic drugs.

Drug category	Drug, dosage	Indications	Comments
Antidepressants	Amitryptyline, 0.2–0.5 mg/kg PO. Titrate upward by 0.25 mg/kg every 2–3 days Maintenance: 0.2–3.0 mg/kg	Neuropathic pain (i.e. vincristine-induced, radiation plexopathy, tumour invasion, CRPS-1)	Usually improved sleep and pain relief within 3–5 days
	Alternatives: nortriptyline, doxepin, imipramine, venlafaxine	Insomnia	Anticholinergic side effects are dose-limiting. Use with caution for children with increased risk for cardiac dysfunction
Anticonvulsants	Carbamazepine, initial dosing: 10 mg/kg/day PO divided OD or BID. Maintenance: up to 20–30 mg/kg/day PO divided every 8 h Increase dose gradually over 2–4 weeks	Neuropathic pain, especially shooting, stabbing pain	Monitor for haematological, hepatic and allergic reactions
	Alternatives: phenytoin, clonazepam		Side effects: gastrointestinal upset, ataxia, dizziness, disorientation, somnolence
	Gabapentin, 5 mg/kg/day PO. Titrate upward over 3–7 days. Maintenance: 15–50 mg/kg/day PO divided TID		
Sedatives, hypnotics, anxiolytics	Diazepam, 0.025–0.2 mg/kg PO every 6 h	Acute anxiety, muscle spasm	Sedative effect may limit opioid use. Other side effects include depression and dependence with prolonged use
	Lorazepam, 0.05 mg/kg/dose SL	Premedication for painful procedures	
	Midazolam, 0.5 mg/kg/dose PO administered 15–30 min prior to procedure; 0.05 mg/kg/dose IV for sedation		
Antihistamines	Hydroxyzine, 0.5 mg/kg PO every 6 h	Opioid-induced pruritus, anxiety, nausea	Sedative side effects may be helpful
	Diphenhydramine, 0.5–1.0 mg/kg PO/IV every 6 h		
Psychostimulants	Dextroamphetamine, methylphenidate, 0.1–0.2 mg/kg BID. Escalate to 0.3–0.5 mg/kg as needed	Opioid-induced somnolence Potentiation of opioid analgesia	Side effects include agitation, sleep disturbance and anorexia. Administer second dose in afternoon to avoid sleep disturbances
Corticosteroids	Prednisone, prednisolone, and dexamethasone dosage depends on clinical situation (i.e. dexamethasone initial dosing: 0.2 mg/kg IV. Dose limit 10 mg. Subsequent dose 0.3 mg/kg/day IV divided every 6 h)	Headache from increased intracranial pressure, spinal, or nerve compression; widespread metastases	Side effects include oedema, dyspeptic symptoms and occasional gastrointestinal bleeding

CRPS-1, complex regional pain syndrome, Type 1; PO, by mouth; IV, intravenous; SL, sublingual.

parenteral administration is often the most efficient route for providing direct and rapid pain relief. Since intravenous, intramuscular, and subcutaneous routes cause additional pain for children, serious efforts have been expended on developing more pain-free modes of administration that still provide relatively direct and rapid analgesia. Attention has focused on improving the effectiveness of oral routes. As an example, oral transmucosal fentanyl citrate (OTFC) provides rapid onset analgesia via a pleasant route for children with cancer receiving painful medical procedures. OTFC produces significant serum concentrations after 15–20 minutes[64]. Children aged 2–14 years have shown good cooperation and sedation when given OTFC as a premedication[65,66]. OTFC produced safe and effective analgesia for outpatient wound care in children and the taste was preferred to oral oxycodone[67].

Many hospitals have restricted the use of intramuscular injections because they are painful and drug absorption is not reliable;

they advocate the use of intravenous lines into which drugs can be administered directly without causing further pain. Topical anaesthetic creams should also be applied prior to the insertion of intravenous lines in children. The use of portacatheters has become the gold standard in paediatrics, particularly for children with cancer who require administration of multiple drugs at weekly intervals.

Continuous infusion has several advantages over intermittent subcutaneous, intramuscular, or intravenous routes. This method circumvents repetitive injections, prevents delays in analgesic drug administration and provides continuous levels of pain control without children experiencing increased side effects at peak level and pain breakthroughs at trough level. Continuous infusion should be considered when children have pain for which oral and intermittent parenteral opioids do not provide satisfactory pain control, when intractable vomiting prevents oral medications, when intravenous lines are not desirable, and when children would

Table 13.2.6 Opioid side effects.

Side effect	Management
Respiratory depression	Reduction in opioid dose by 50%, titrate to maintain pain relief without respiratory depression
Respiratory arrest	Naloxone, titrate to effect with 0.01 mg/kg/dose IV/ETT increments or 0.1 mg/kg/dose IV/ETT, repeat PRN. Small frequent doses of diluted naloxone or naloxone drip preferable for patients on chronic opioid therapy to avoid severe, painful withdrawal syndrome. Repeated doses often required until opioid side effect subsides
Drowsiness/sedation	Frequently subsides after a few days without dosage reduction; methylphenidate or dextroamphetamine (0.1 mg/kg administered twice daily, in the morning and mid-day so as not to interfere with night-time sleep). The dose can be escalated in increments of 0.05–0.1 mg/kg to a maximum of 10 mg/dose for dextroamphetamine and 20 mg/dose for methylphenidate
Constipation	Increased fluids and bulk, prophylactic laxatives as indicated
Nausea/vomiting	Administer an antiemetic (e.g. ondansetron, 0.1 mg/kg IV/PO every 8 h)
	Antihistamines (e.g. dimenhydrinate 0.5 mg/kg/dose every 4–6 h IV/PO) may be used. Pre-chemotherapy, nabilone 0.5–1.0 mg PO and then every 12 h may also be used
Confusion, nightmares, hallucinations	Reassurance only, if symptoms mild. A reduced dosage of opioid or a change to a different opioid or add neuroleptic (e.g. haloperidol 0.1 mg/kg PO/IV every 8 h to a maximum of 30 mg/day)
Multifocal myoclonus; seizures	Generally occur only during extremely high dose therapy; reduction in opioid dose indicated if possible. Add a benzodiazepine (e.g. clonazepam 0.05 mg/kg/day divided bid or tid increasing by 0.05 mg/kg/day every 3 days PRN up to 0.2 mg/kg/day. Dose limit of 20 mg/day)
Urinary retention	Rule out bladder outlet obstruction, neurogenic bladder, and other precipitating drug factors (e.g. tricyclic antidepressant). Particularly common with epidural opioids. Change of opioid, route of administration, and dose may relieve symptom. Bethanechol or catheter may be required

IV, intravenous; PO, by mouth; ETT, endotracheal tube; PRN, as needed.

like to remain at home despite severe pain. Children receiving a continuous infusion should continue to receive 'rescue doses' to control breakthrough pain, as necessary. As outlined in Table 13.2.4, the rescue doses should be 50–200 per cent of the continuous infusion hourly dose. If children experience repeated breakthrough pain, the basal rate can be increased by 50 per cent or by the total amount of morphine administered through the rescue doses over a 24-h period (divided by 24 h).

Patient-controlled analgesia (PCA) enables children to administer analgesic doses according to their pain level. PCA provides children with a continuum of analgesia that is prompt, economical, not nurse dependent and a lower overall opioid use[68–73]. It has a high degree of safety, allows for wide variability between patients and there is no delay in analgesic administration (for review, see ref. 49). It can now be regarded as a standard for the delivery of analgesia in children aged more than 5 years[74]. However, there are opposing views about the use of background infusions with PCA. Although they may improve efficacy, they may increase the occurrence of adverse effects such as nausea and respiratory depression. In a comparison of PCA with and without a background infusion for children having lower extremity surgery, the total morphine requirements were reduced in the PCA only group and the background infusion offered no advantage[75]. In another study comparing background infusion and PCA, children between 9 and 15 achieved better pain relief with PCA while children between 5 and 8 showed no difference[76]. Although data on the use of background infusions in combination with PCA for the paediatric palliative care patient is limited, our current standard is to add a background infusion to the PCA if the pain is not controlled adequately with PCA alone. The selection of opioid used in PCA is perhaps less critical than the appropriate selection of parameters such as bolus dose, lockout, and background infusion rate.

The opioid choice may be based on adverse effect profile rather than efficacy. Clearly, patient controlled analgesia offers special advantages to children who have little control and who are extremely frightened about uncontrolled pain. PCA is as it states, patient controlled analgesia. When special circumstances require that alternate people administer the medication, we do allow both nurse and parent controlled analgesia. Under these circumstances, parents require our nurse educators to educate them fully on the use of PCA.

Fentanyl is a potent synthetic opioid, which like morphine binds to mu receptors. However, fentanyl is 75–100 times more potent than morphine. The intravenous preparation of fentanyl has been used extensively in children. A transdermal preparation of fentanyl was introduced in 1991 for use with chronic pain. This route provides a noninvasive but continuously controlled delivery system. Although limited data is available on transdermal fentanyl (TF) in children, its use is increasing for children with stable and chronic cancer pain. In one study, TF was well tolerated with effective pain relief in 11 of 13 children and provided an ideal approach for children, where compliance with oral analgesics was problematic[77]. Children in palliative care were converted from oral morphine doses to TF; the investigators noted diminished side effects and improved convenience with TF[78]. The majority of parents and investigators considered TF to be better than previous treatment. No serious adverse events were attributed to fentanyl, suggesting that TF was both effective and acceptable for children and their families. Similarly, no adverse effects were noted in a study of TF for children with pain due to sickle-cell crisis[79]. This study showed a significant relationship between TF dose and fentanyl concentration; pain control with the use of TF was improved in 7 of 10 patients in comparison to PCA alone. In a multicentre crossover study in adults, TF caused significantly less constipation and less daytime drowsiness in comparison to morphine, but greater sleep disturbance and shorter sleep duration[80]. Of those patients able to express a preference, significantly more preferred fentanyl patches. As with all opioids, fatal adult complications have been noted with the use of multiple transdermal patches[81].

The use of regional techniques (epidural and spinal) for the administration of local anaesthetics and analgesics for children continues to be an integral part of pain control in children[82]. Experience from many centres suggests that these techniques can be extremely useful for children with advanced cancer with resulting pain that may be difficult to control by more conventional means. It is also feasible for children to receive epidural and spinal infusions at home on an extended basis.

When one undertakes the administration of potent analgesics and anaesthetics, whether by intravenous or a regional anaesthetic technique, such as an epidural or spinal approach, appropriate monitoring must be paramount for the safety of our patients. This involves the education and training of staff; immediate availability of resuscitative drugs and equipment; and an accurate and timely pain record consisting of vital signs, pain, and sedation scores. A complete set of intravenous and epidural monitoring guidelines have been included in Table 13.2.7.

Dosing considerations for neonates and infants

Research on controlling pain in neonates has led to improved rational therapeutic regimens that provide safe and effective analgesia with a minimum of side effects[83–90]. Neonates and infants require the same three categories of analgesic drugs as older children. However, the differences in pharmacokinetics and pharmacodynamics among neonates, pre-term infants, and full-term infants, warrant special dosing considerations for infants and close monitoring when they receive opioids. Acetaminophen can be safely administered to neonates and infants without concern for hepatotoxicity, when given for short courses at the recommended dose (10–15 mg/kg PO). The rate of absorption is slower in neonates and its plasma half-life prolonged, and so peak serum concentrations are reached at approximately 60 min after an oral dose, and subsequent doses may be required after 6 h rather than 4 h. Acetaminophen does not cause respiratory depression and does not produce tolerance.

Opioid analgesics are the mainstay of treatment for controlling severe pain in neonates. When compared to Table 13.2.4, the starting doses for opioid analgesics in infants under 6 months of age are one-quarter to one-third the suggested doses. As for children, the dosage and mode of administration of opioids needs to be titrated between the degree of analgesia required and a reasonable level of sedation. (Note: theoretically postulated long-term effects of opioid administration include the alteration of endogenous opioid receptor development but these effects are irrelevant in neonatal palliative care.) The drug clearance and the analgesic effects of morphine, fentanyl, sufentanil, and methadone for infants above the age of six months and children resemble those for young adults. Thus, the general clinical impression is that morphine and other opioids have a reasonable margin of safety and excellent efficacy for most children over 6 months of age with cancer pain. However, premature and term newborns show reduced clearance of most opioids. The widely observed sensitivity of new-borns to morphine is probably due to kinetic factors, including smaller volume of distribution, diminished clearance, immaturity of the blood–brain barrier, and increased sensitivity on a pharmacodynamic basis associated with the immaturity of ventilatory responses to hypoxaemia and hypercarbia. Therefore, opioids must be used more cautiously with infants under the age of 6 months and appropriate monitoring must be instituted. Proper dosing and careful monitoring will help minimize side-effects. Tolerance has significance only as a signal of receptor function or as a potential indicator of withdrawal when therapy is discontinued.

Table 13.2.7 Analgesia monitoring guidelines.

Baseline assessment
Obtain RR, HR, BP, O_2 saturation, sedation score, and pain score before administering a single or intermittent dose or initiating continuous infusion
Intermittent intravenous administration
RR, HR, BP, and sedation score every 5 min × 4, then every 30 min × 2 and then as per child's condition/pre-existing orders
Pain score every 20–30 min
Continuously monitor O_2 saturation only for children whose underlying condition predisposes them to respiratory depression
Intravenous additive (to run over 15–20 min)
RR, HR, BP, and sedation score every 10 min × 2, then every 30 min × 2 and then as per child's condition
Pain score at completion of the flush, then every 30 min × 2 and then as per child's condition/pre-existing orders
Continuously monitor O_2 saturation only for children whose underlying condition predisposes them to respiratory depression
Continuous IV infusion/PCA
RR, HR, BP, pain score, and sedation score every 1 h × 4, then RR and sedation score every 1 h and then HR, BP, and pain score every 4 h
Continuously monitor O_2 saturation and document reading every 1 h
Intermittent epidural administration
RR, HR, and BP every 5 min for the first 20 min following a bolus dose, and then RR and sedation score every 1 h
HR, BP, pain score, and motor block score every 4 h
Continuously monitor only for children whose underlying condition predisposes them to respiratory depression
Continuous epidural infusion[a,b]
RR, HR, BP, sedation score, pain score, and motor block score every 1 h × 4 h, then RR and sedation score every 1 h and HR, BP, pain score, and motor block score every 4 h
Continuously monitor O_2 saturation and document reading every 1 h

[a] Opioids used with bupivacaine.

[b] After any change in drug dose, infusion rate or if transferred between patient care areas, return to assessments every 1 h for 4 h. Continuous respiratory rate/apnoea monitoring may provide additional benefits for certain children who are receiving continuous opioid infusions by alerting the nurse to a decreasing respiratory rate. Respiratory rate monitoring is not, however, a substitute for frequent patient observation and vital sign monitoring. ECG monitoring is not routinely required, but may be ordered if the child's underlying condition predisposes them to ECG abnormalities. *Source*: adapted from 2001–2002 Drug Formulary, The Hospital for Sick Children, Toronto, Ontario.

Neonates who have pain severe enough to require opioids usually have an intravenous line in place. If a limited number of doses is needed and if intravenous access is not available, intramuscular or subcutaneous routes may be used occasionally in full-term neonates. However, these routes are painful and not suitable for preterm neonates because of their sparse muscle mass and delicate skin. They are also not suitable for long-term pain management in term neonates because plasma levels and clinical effects are less controlled and difficult to titrate from intramuscular administrations. Similarly, intravenous doses may produce peak levels resulting in coma and respiratory depression with rapid decline in plasma levels, causing alternate periods of pain and analgesia. Thus, continuous intravenous infusion of opioids, producing constant blood levels and minimal fluctuations in analgesia, is the most effective route. The use of peripherally inserted central catheters (PICCs) has become standard practice for the neonate with difficult venous access or for the patient that may require access for a prolonged period. Anand *et al.* recommend a loading dose of 50 mcg/kg followed by a continuous infusion of morphine at 10–20 mcg/kg/h[84]. Further increases in the infusion rate may be required to titrate to clinical effect or with the development of tolerance. However, infants must be monitored carefully because most opioids have prolonged duration of action in neonates, so that continuous infusions can result in slow accumulation of the drug over time with high blood levels that may not be detected immediately.

The principal and potentially life-threatening side effect of all opioid drugs is the dose-dependent respiratory depression leading to apnoea, which may be observed in infants and neonates at relatively low doses. This is advantageous in ventilated patients, but poses considerable challenges when using opioids for spontaneously breathing newborns. Opioid-induced respiratory depression can be reversed with naloxone, but the effect of the drug diminishes within 30 min so that repeated naloxone dosing may be required. If apnoea does occur, stimulation of the baby will usually elicit some respiratory effort temporarily while emergency arrangements are made to inject naloxone and provide respiratory support. Naloxone should be titrated to effect in increments of 10 mcg/kg until a desired effect is obtained, or up to a total dose of 100 mcg/kg. High doses of naloxone may produce a massive stress response from sudden nociception and withdrawal, or may result in undesirable fluid shifts. Following an effective dose of naloxone, the neonate should be monitored closely for at least 24 h. In fact, because plasma concentrations of morphine can increase in some neonates, even after an opioid infusion is discontinued, neonates require close monitoring for at least 24 h after morphine administration is discontinued.

Young infants, especially premature babies or those who have neurological abnormalities or pulmonary disease, are more susceptible to apnoea and respiratory depression when systemic opioids are used. The infants' metabolism is altered so that the elimination half-life is longer and there may be possible increased entry into the brain, due to immaturity of the blood–brain barrier. Both factors result in young infants having higher concentrations of opioids in the brain for a given dose than mature infants or adults. Thus, non-ventilated infants who are less than 1 year of age should be monitored closely when they receive opioids because extreme sedation and decreased respiratory effort may be difficult to assess. Institutions where neonates and infants are treated for cancer should train personnel in the safe and effective administration of

analgesia and provide appropriate technologies for monitoring. Monitoring should include respiratory rate, heart rate, blood pressure, sedation score and pain score, as shown in Table 13.2.7.

Epidural analgesia is now widely used for infants with postoperative pain. The haemodynamic effects of major regional analgesia in infants with postoperative pain appear minimal. For paediatric epidural infusions, the standard local anaesthetic we use is bupivacaine in an infusion rate of 0.2–0.4 mg/kg/h. Epidural infusions that exceed the recommended rate may lead to convulsions. Epidural opioids such as morphine and fentanyl have been used successfully, even for very young infants with cancer. The proper use of infusions or intermittent doses of epidural opioids or local anaesthetics requires expertise and appropriate monitoring, as shown in Table 13.2.7.

Physical dependence, tolerance, and addiction

Physical dependence is defined as a state of adaptation that often includes tolerance and is manifested by a drug class specific withdrawal syndrome that can be produced by abrupt cessation, rapid dose reduction, decrease in the blood level of drug and administration of an antagonist. Tolerance is a state of adaptation in which exposure to a drug induces changes that result in a diminution of one or more of the drug's effects over time. Addiction is a primary, chronic, neurobiological disease, with genetic, psychosocial, and environmental factors influencing its development and manifestations. It is characterized by behaviours that include one or more of the following four 'C's: impaired Control over drug use, Compulsive use, continued use despite harm (Consequences), and Craving[91].

The fear of opioid addiction in children has been greatly exaggerated. While physical dependence is common, gradual tapering protocols can control the withdrawal syndromes caused by an abrupt cessation of the medication. Physical dependence may develop in as short a period as 7–10 days. Tolerance is also an expected change to be seen and anticipated in children. There is no empirical evidence that children receiving opioid analgesics for pain control are at risk of addiction. In contrast, children who do not receive appropriate analgesic medications are probably more at risk of 'pseudoaddiction' by becoming excessively concerned about receiving their next medication dose in the hope that it might eventually relieve their suffering.

Parents, and occasionally staff, may have misconceptions about the use of potent opioids. Although the sensory characteristics of children's pain should be consistent with the known pattern from the presumed source of tissue injury, the source is not easily identified for all children. This is particularly true for children who have cancer, since there may be multiple sources of noxious stimulation due to disease and the effects of curative therapies. Yet, children's pain must be controlled, even when the specific aetiology is not yet determined. Otherwise, children become increasingly anxious, fearful, and distressed—beginning a cycle of increasing pain that will be more difficult to alleviate.

Parents are often anxious about opioids for their children, particularly when children require increased dose increments. Staff must educate parents that physical dependence and tolerance are very different from addiction. Parents will then understand that physical dependence and tolerance are normal drug effects and these do not mean that their children with pain have become addicted. Physical drug dependence is well recognized. When opioids are withdrawn suddenly, children may suffer from irritability, anxiety, insomnia, diaphoresis, rhinorrhoea, nausea, vomiting, abdominal cramps, and diarrhoea. These withdrawal symptoms can be prevented by the gradual tapering of an opioid. Even though children with severe pain require progressively higher and more frequent opioid doses due to drug tolerance, they should receive the doses they need to relieve their pain. However, children who require increased opioids to relieve previously controlled pain should be assessed carefully to determine whether the disease has progressed, since pain may be the first sign of advancing disease.

Therapists can use familiar analogies to explain dependence, tolerance, and addiction. For example parents are often accustomed to drinking coffee in the morning. They know that they will experience some noticeable effects without their usual caffeine intake, but they also know that they can withdraw from coffee by gradually lowering their daily consumption. The fact that their body is used to a certain amount of caffeine at certain times of the day means that they are dependent. Similarly, many people become accustomed to a certain level of salt for a food to taste 'salty'. After a while they may need to increase their salt intake if they want foods to taste the same, because their bodies have adjusted to or now tolerate the previous amount of salt so that it no longer has the same effect. In the same way, their children can become tolerant to a morphine dose so that they require a slightly higher dose to achieve the same pain reduction. These benign examples of a body's normal responses to substances often help parents understand that when opioids are prescribed for their children, the effects of those drugs are well known, well understood, and will not lead to adverse effects, including addiction.

Opioid-related side effects

The safe, rational use of opioid analgesics requires an understanding of their clinical pharmacology. The potent opioids that we use to treat children for palliative pain control have no fixed upper dosage limit. The dose can be increased as necessary to maximize pain control, as long as children do not experience dose-limiting side effects (i.e. vomiting, respiratory depression). The goal should be titration of medication either up or down for maximum clinical effect. Side effects must be anticipated and treated aggressively. Since opioids produce physical dependence and tolerance, doses must be increased over time to control pain. Doses must be adjusted according to the child's need, depending on pain severity, prior analgesic medication use, and the bioavailability and drug distribution of the medication.

All opioids have a similar spectrum of side effects. These well-known problems should be anticipated and treated whenever opioids are administered, so that children can receive pain control without suffering untoward effects. Children may not report all side effects (i.e. constipation, dysphoria) voluntarily, and so they should be asked specifically about these problems. Some side effects may resolve within the first 1 or 2 weeks of initiating therapy as the child develops tolerance to them (e.g. nausea, vomiting, and drowsiness). The clinician must educate the patient about these problems and encourage them to give the medication an adequate trial. Slow titration may minimize this problem. Other side-effects may require aggressive treatment. If they persist despite appropriate

interventions, conversion to an alternate opioid may be indicated. There is generally incomplete cross-tolerance between opioids, so that the guidelines for converting from one opioid to another is to begin at the lower dosing range, considering the presence or absence of central nervous system side effects, and titrate upward. When used in therapeutic doses, opioids have not been demonstrated to cause long-term permanent organ toxicity. This makes them a safe choice for use in children. There is evidence that untreated severe chronic pain may cause cognitive impairment, which is improved with opioid therapy. The treatment of opioid side effects is summarized in Table 13.2.6.

Non-drug therapies
Cognitive and behavioural approaches

An extensive array of non-drug therapies is available to treat children's pain, including counselling, guided imagery, hypnosis, biofeedback, behavioural management, acupuncture, massage, homeopathic remedies, naturopathic approaches, and herbal medicines. Non-drug therapies are generally regarded as safe, with few contra-indications for their use in otherwise healthy children. However, little is known about the safety and effectiveness of certain therapies for children in palliative care. In particular, almost no paediatric research has been conducted on many of the therapies regarded as complementary to traditional medical approaches. Thus, the efficacy of complementary therapies for treating children's pain is unknown, even though children are increasingly using complementary therapies[92]. In contrast, the evidence base supporting the efficacy of cognitive and behavioural approaches is strong[4,5,15,93–104]. These methods can mitigate some of the factors that intensify pain, distress, and disability for children in palliative care.

The primary cognitive and behavioural therapies are listed in Table 13.2.8. Cognitive therapies are directed at a child's beliefs, expectations, and coping abilities. They encompass a wide range of approaches from basic patient education to formal psychotherapy. Most children and families benefit from supportive counselling. Accurate information about what will happen and what children may feel should improve children's understanding, increase their control, lessen their distress, and reduce their pain.

In addition, health-care providers can teach children how to use a few pain control methods to lessen pain and guide families to recognize the particular circumstances that exacerbate pain and

Table 13.2.8 Cognitive and behavioural therapies.

Cognitive	Behavioural
Information	Simple exercise
Choices and control	Participation in activities
Supportive counselling	Desensitization training
Counselling	Relaxation training
Stress management	Biofeedback
Attention and distraction	Behavioural modification
Guided imagery	
Hypnosis	

distress. These methods provide children with some independent strategies—either to relieve mild pain or to complement the medication needed to relieve strong pain. Children should begin by learning a few basic methods. As they acquire confidence in using these methods, they seem to adapt them naturally to fit their personality or invent new equally effective methods. A therapist guides them throughout this process. Children should be interested and motivated in learning some independent pain control methods. They seem more adept than adults at using non-drug therapies, presumably because they are usually less biased than adults about their potential efficacy.

Distraction is a simple and effective pain control method. When children attend intently to something other than their pain, they can lessen its intensity and unpleasantness. Distraction is often incorrectly perceived as a simple diversionary tactic; the implication is that the pain is still there but the child is momentarily focused elsewhere. However, when children's attention is fully absorbed in some engaging topic or activity, distraction is a very active process that can reduce the neuronal responses to a noxious stimulus. Children do not simply ignore their pain, but are actually reducing it. The essential feature for achieving pain relief is a child's ability to attend fully to and concentrate on something else besides the pain. Therefore, the choice of a distraction is crucial and varies according to children's ages and interests. Young children usually need to be actively involved with their parents or peers, while older children and adolescents can distract themselves more independently. Children should work with their parents or a therapist to choose distracting activities that children can incorporate practically into their lives. Guided imagery is a specific method of distraction and attention. A health-care provider guides children to concentrate fully on the image of an experience or situation. Children recall and vividly describe what they experienced—the colours, sounds, tastes, and feel of the situation. Children are guided to become as immersed in their image as if it were occurring in the present situation.

There is considerable overlap among the interventions of attention/distraction, guided imagery, and hypnosis. Hypnosis usually begins with an induction procedure in which a child's full attention is focused gradually on the therapist and his/her suggestions. The therapist guides the child into a very relaxed physical and mental state, an altered level of consciousness—distinct from an alert or sleep state. The induction procedure typically includes guided imagery for children and progressive muscle relaxation for adolescents. The induction can be very simple for young children. They can be guided into a hypnotic state as they imagine vividly their favourite television shows, movies, books, or cartoon characters[105–107]. As they imagine an activity, scene, or character, they gradually receive suggestions for relaxation, reduced anxiety, increased control, and pain reduction. The therapist provides consistent positive suggestions, rather than authoritative commands. The emphasis is on the child's own natural abilities, as in 'Notice that your back, legs (painful body areas) feels lighter, the heaviness, and pain are starting to lessen. It seems as if your back doesn't hurt as much as before. You are doing well at turning down the pain switch'.

During a hypnotic state, individuals become extremely susceptible to suggestions, including suggestions for pain relief. Children become so involved in thoughts or ideas that they dissociate from a 'reality orientation'[106]. Hypnosis enables children to re-direct attention from the painful sensation or to reinterpret the sensation

as something more pleasant/less aversive and less bothersome[107]. Like adults, children differ in their ability to be hypnotized. Children's ability to use their imagination is the key component in determining their hypnotic susceptibility.

Behaviour therapy is often used in combination with cognitive therapy. The goals are to lessen the specific behaviours (i.e. child, family, and staff) that may increase pain, distress, or disability, while concomitantly increasing healthy behaviours that engage children in living as fully as possible. Relaxation training is a common method used for children with chronic pain. Therapists train children how to achieve a state of mental and physical relaxation so that children can eventually relax independently when they experience pain or feel stressed and fearful about their condition. Therapists may use guided imagery, hypnosis, deep breathing, or progressive relaxation exercises to train children. Biofeedback is a useful tool for teaching children to recognize when their bodies are relaxed. Surface electrodes, attached to the skin or specific muscle groups, transform the electrical activity of the body into easily observable signals.

Pain control methods

Health professionals and parents can relieve children's pain, not only by administering analgesic drugs, but also by increasing their understanding and control, decreasing their emotional distress and teaching them some simple methods to reduce their pain and anxiety. In addition to providing support and reassurance, parents can help children to understand what will happen, make choices, gain whatever control is possible within the setting, and independently use pain reducing methods. Thus, the family, as well as health professionals, shares a fundamental role in managing their children's cancer pain. The key concept underlying the use of all analgesic and non-analgesic therapies for children is 'by the child', as described above.

Specific pain control methods that require the child to concentrate and focus attention should always be used for children with cancer pain. Beales noted critical differences between adults and children in their perceptions of pain, especially cancer pain[108]. Children's cancer pain seemed even less positively correlated with pathology than adults' cancer pain. Beales suggested that some of the psychological mechanisms involved in pain perception may be manipulated more easily in children than in adults, consistent with our clinical observations that children's cancer pain is more plastic than that of adults[1,101]. Children seem to possess an enhanced ability to absorb themselves completely in a task, game, or imagined event and thus, might be more able than adults to trigger endogenous pain-inhibitory mechanisms. Even very young children can learn easily to use a variety of practical pain control methods. The goals of therapy are to enable children to understand what is happening and to have something that they can actively do to lessen their anxiety, distress, and pain.

The specific methods selected depend on the age of the child, the type of pain experienced, and the resources available. Simple methods such as deep breathing, blowing bubbles, alternately tightening and relaxing their fists, squeezing their mother's hand, listening to stories or music, and imagining that they are in a pleasant setting can be very effective for reducing procedural-related pain, when used with appropriate analgesics. When possible, children should learn a few basic methods to reduce their pain and distress. They should not be encouraged to develop a false reliance on the magical benefits of any one method. Instead, they should understand that these practical methods relieve pain because they change the factors that usually increase pain and they help to restore normal sensory input.

All children should learn that pain from some procedures is generally less when they are able to choose the site and rub the area before and after the injection or finger prick. They should learn that pain is less when they are very relaxed. Progressive muscle relaxation with simple exercises in which they tense and relax their body limbs, and biofeedback can help to show them that any type of pain can be intensified if the muscles are always tightened. Children should learn that fear and anxiety can make them tense and increase pain. Then, they need practical tools to alleviate their fear about the cancer or their anxiety towards necessary treatments. Children and families must learn that what they think, how they behave and how they feel affects their children's pain. Then they can begin to work independently and with staff to create additional non-drug pain control methods based on the child's interest, the cultural setting, and the availability of resources. Specific interventions should be selected and administered to children as part of a comprehensive pain programme, in the same manner as the most appropriate analgesics are selected and administered in adequate doses, at regular dosing intervals, through the most efficient routes.

Summary

Optimal pain control for children in palliative care requires an integrated treatment plan with both drug and non-drug therapies. However, the specific interventions must be selected after determination of the primary and secondary sources of noxious stimulation and after a thorough assessment of the unique situational, behavioural, emotional, and familial factors that affect a child's pain. It is impossible to relieve children's pain adequately from a unidimensional perspective, in which pain is considered as synonymous with the nature and extent of tissue damage. Childhood pain must be viewed from a multidimensional perspective because multiple sensory, environmental, and emotional factors are responsible for the pain—no matter how apparently clear cut an aetiology. Treatment begins with a thorough assessment of these multiple factors, using structured interviews and standardized measures. Pharmacological, physical, and psychological strategies must be incorporated into a flexible intervention programme for children, in which parents and siblings form an essential component of treatment.

All analgesics should be selected 'by the ladder' and administered 'by the clock', 'by the child', and in an effective and painless route. Dosing intervals should be frequent enough to control pain adequately, so that children do not experience an alternating cycle of pain, drowsy analgesia, pain, etc. Children should also learn some simple pain control strategies so that they can reduce acute pain caused by invasive treatments and disease or therapy related pain. Adjuvant medications should be administered to control aversive symptoms and side-effects. Non-drug therapies should also be used to control pain.

Special problems in pain control may arise when children die at home, unless parents and medical and nursing teams communicate openly about the availability of potent analgesics and the flexibility of dosing routes and regimens. Parents may be unduly anxious because even small children, like adults with cancer, may require larger opioid doses at more frequent intervals. Parents' fears can lead them to deny the extent to which their children are in pain or children may fail to report pain because they do not want to distress parents further or because they fear injections.

Multiple sources of noxious stimulation are usually responsible for pain in dying children, as the disease progressively affects many systems. Increased disability, toxic side effects of medication, physical impairment, and the emotional adjustment of children and their families can intensify pain and suffering. Like adults, children's pain affects the entire family and must be viewed within a broader context. Effective pain control is possible when the goals are to reduce or block nociceptive activity by attenuating responses in peripheral afferents and central pathways, activate endogenous pain inhibitory systems and modify situational factors that exacerbate pain. Thus, the choice for pain control is not merely 'drug versus non-drug therapy', but rather a therapy that mitigates both the causative and contributing factors for pain. Pain management is a continuous dynamic process, since the disease state and factors that influence pain are not static. Different combinations of drug and non-drug therapies will be required at different times. Thus, health professionals continually must assume as much responsibility for monitoring and relieving children's pain as for managing their diseases medically. Children should not suffer. We have the knowledge to ensure that children receive adequate pain control, from the time they are diagnosed to their death. Parents' memories of their children should not be marred by memories that they experienced unrelieved pain.

References

1. McGrath, P.A. (1990). *Pain in children: Nature, assessment and treatment.* Guilford Publications, New York.
2. Price, D.D. (1999). *Psychological mechanisms of pain and analgesia.* IASP Press, Seattle.
3. Casey, K. and Bushnell, M.C. (eds.)(2000). *Pain imaging.* IASP Press, Seattle.
4. McGrath, P.A. and Hillier, L.M. (2003). Modifying the psychological factors that intensify children's pain and prolong disability. In *Pain in infants, children, and adolescents*, 2nd edition, (eds. N.L. Schechter, C.B. Berde, and M. Yaster), pp. 85–104. Lippincott Williams & Wilkins, Philadelphia.
5. Schechter, N., Berde, C.B., and Yaster, M. (eds.)(2003). *Pain in infants, children, and adolescents*, 2nd edition. Lippincott Williams & Wilkins, Philadelphia.
6. Ross, D.M. and Ross, S.A. (1988). *Childhood pain: Current issues, research, and management.* Urban & Schwarzenberg, Baltimore.
7. McGrath, P.A. and de Veber, L.L. (1986). The management of acute pain evoked by medical procedures in children with cancer. *J Pain Symptom Manage*, **1**(3), 145–50.
8. Poltorak, D.Y. and Benore, E. (2006). Cognitive–behavioral interventions for physical symptom management in paediatric palliative medicine. *Child Adolesc Psychiatr Clin N Am*, **15**(3), 683–91.
9. Goldman, A. (eds) (1994). *Care of the dying child.* Oxford University Press, New York.
10. Goldman, A., Frager, G., and Pomietto, M. (2003). Pain and palliative care. In *Pain in infants, children, and adolescents*, 2nd edition (eds. N.L. Schechter, C.B. Berde, and M. Yaster), pp. 539–600. Lippincott Williams & Wilkins, Philadelphia.
11. Chaffee, S. (2001). Pediatric palliative care. *Prim Care*, **28**(2), 365–90.
12. American Academy of Pediatrics. Committee on Bioethics and Committee on Hospital Care. (2000). Palliative care for children. *Pediatrics*, **106**(2 Pt 1), 351–7.

13. Goldman, A. (1998). ABC of palliative care. Special problems of children. *BMJ*, **316**(7124), 49–52.

14. Frager, G. (1997). Palliative care and terminal care of children. *Child and Adolescent Psychiatric Clinics of North America*, **6**, 889–900.

15. World Health Organization (1998). *Cancer pain relief and palliative care in children*. World Health Organization, Geneva.

16. Stevens, M. (2004). Care of the dying child and adolescent: Family adjustment and support. In *Oxford textbook of palliative medicine*, 3rd edition (eds. D. Doyle, G. Hanks, and N. MacDonald), pp. 806–22. Oxford University Press, Oxford.

17. Stevens, M. (2004). Psychological adaptation of the dying child. In *Oxford textbook of palliative medicine*, 3rd edition (eds. D. Doyle, G. Hanks, and N. MacDonald), pp. 798–806. Oxford University Press, Oxford.

18. Howell, D. and Martinson, I. (1993). Management of the dying child. In *Principles and practice of paediatric oncology* (eds. P. Pizzo and D. Poplack), pp. 1115–24. Lippincott, Philadelphia.

19. Davies, B. and Howell, D. (1998). Special services for children. In *Oxford textbook of palliative medicine*, 2nd edition (eds. D. Doyle, G. Hanks, and N. MacDonald), pp. 1078–84. Oxford University Press, Oxford.

20. Sourkes, B.M. (1996). The broken heart: Anticipatory grief in the child facing death. *J Palliat Care*, **12**(3), 56–9.

21. Collins, J.J. (2002). Palliative care and the child with cancer. *Hematol Oncol Clin North Am*, **16**(3), 657–70.

22. McGrath, P.A. and Gillespie, J. (2001). Pain assessment in children and adolescents. In *Handbook of pain assessment*, 2nd edition (eds. D. Turk and R. Melzack), pp. 97–118. Guilford Press, New York.

23. Finley, G.A. and McGrath, P.J. (eds.) (1998). *Measurement of pain in infants and children. Progress in pain research and management*, IASP Press, Seattle.

24. Royal College of Nursing Institute (1999). *Clinical guideline for the recognition and assessment of acute pain in children: Recommendations*. Royal College of Nursing Institute, London.

25. McGrath, P.J. (1998). Behavioral measures of pain. In *Measurement of pain in infants and children* (eds. G.A. Finley and P.J. McGrath), pp. 83–102. IASP Press, Seattle, WA.

26. Sweet, S.D. and McGrath, P.J. (1998). Physiological Measures of pain, In *Measurement of pain in infants and children* (eds. G.A. Finley and P.J. McGrath), pp. 59–81. IASP Press, Seattle, WA.

27. Hunt, A.M. Goldman, A., Mastroyannopoulou, K. *et al.* (1999). Identification of pain cues of children with severe neurological impairment. In Proceedings of the 9th World Congress on Pain. Abstract 84, IASP Press, Seattle, WA.

28. Champion, G.D. Goodenough, B., von Baeyer, C.L. *et al.* (1998). Measurement of pain by self-report. In *Measurement of pain in infants and children* (eds. G.A. Finley and P.J. McGrath), pp. 123–60. IASP Press, Seattle, WA.

29. Bush, J.P. and Harkins, S.W. (eds.) (1991). *Children in pain: Clinical and research issues from a developmental perspective.* Springer-Verlag, New York.

30. Gaffney, A., McGrath, P.J., and Dick, B. (2003). Measuring pain in children: Developmental and instrumental issues In *Pain in infants, children and adolescents*, 2nd edition (eds. N.L. Schechter, C.B. Berde, and M. Yaster), pp. 128–41. Lippincott Williams and Wilkins, Philadelphia.

31. McGrath, P.J. and Unruh, A.M. (1987). *Pain in children and adolescents. Pain research and clinical management*, Elsevier, Amsterdam.

32. Peterson, L. Harbeck, C., Farmer, J. *et al.* (1991). Developmental contributions to the assessment of children's pain: Conceptual and methodological implications In *Children in pain: Clinical and research issues from a developmental perspective* (eds. J.P. Bush and S.W. Harkins), pp. 33–58. Springer-Verlag, New York.

33. Pichard-Leandri, E. and Gauvain-Piquard, A. (eds.) (1989). *La Douleur Chez l'Enfant*. Medsi/McGraw-Hill, Paris.

34. World Health Organization (1990). *Cancer pain relief and palliative care*. World Health Organization, Geneva.

35. Stjernsward, J. (2007). Palliative care: The public health strategy. *J Public Health Policy*, **28**(1), 42–55.

36. Monteiro Caran, E.M. Dias, C.G., Serber, A. *et al.* (2005). Clinical aspects and treatment of pain in children and adolescents with cancer. *Pediatr Blood Cancer*, **45**(7), 925–32.

37. Wiffen, P.J. Edwards, J.E., Barden, J. *et al.* (2003). Oral morphine for cancer pain. *Cochrane Database Syst Rev*, (4), CD003868.

38. Hain, R.D. Miser, A., Devins, M. *et al.* (2005). Strong opioids in paediatric palliative medicine. *Paediatr Drugs*, **7**(1), 1–9.

39. Tan, G.H. Totapally, B.R., Torbati, D. *et al.* (2006). End-of-life decisions and palliative care in a children's hospital. *J Palliat Med*, **9**(2), 332–42.

40. Staats, P.S. (1998). Cancer pain: Beyond the ladder. *Journal of Back and Musculoskeletal Rehabilitation*, **10**, 67–80.

41. Galloway, K.S. and Yaster, M. (2000). Pain and symptom control in terminally ill children. *Pediatr Clin North Am*, **47**(3), 711–46.

42. Hauer, J.M., Wical, B.S., and Charnas, L. (2007). Gabapentin successfully manages chronic unexplained irritability in children with severe neurologic impairment. *Pediatrics*, **119**(2), e519–22.

43. Butkovic, D., Toljan, S., and Mihovilovic-Novak, B. (2006). Experience with gabapentin for neuropathic pain in adolescents: Report of five cases. *Paediatr Anaesth*, **16**(3), 325–9.

44. Lauder, G.R. and White, M.C. (2005). Neuropathic pain following multilevel surgery in children with cerebral palsy: A case series and review. *Paediatr Anaesth*, **15**(5), 412–20.

45. Klepstad, Kaasa, S. Cherry, N.P. *et al.* (2005). Pain and pain treatments in European palliative care units. A cross sectional survey from the European Association for Palliative Care Research Network. *Palliat Med*, **19**(6), 477–84.

46. Bozkurt, P. (2005). Use of tramadol in children. *Paediatr Anaesth*, **15**(12), 1041–7.

47. Rose, J.B. Finkel, J.C., Arqueda-Mohns, A. *et al.* (2003). Oral tramadol for the treatment of pain of 7–30 days' duration in children. *Anesth Analg*, **96**(1), 78–81, table of contents.

48. Scott, L.J. and Perry, C.M. (2000). Tramadol: A review of its use in perioperative pain. *Drugs*, **60**(1), 139–76.

49. Hullett, B.J. Chambers, N.A., Pascoe, E.M. *et al.* (2006). Tramadol vs morphine during adenotonsillectomy for obstructive sleep apnea in children. *Paediatr Anaesth*, **16**(6), 648–53.

50. Brown, S.C. and Stinson, J.(2004). Treatment of paediatric chronic pain with tramadol hydrochloride: Siblings with Ehlers-Danlos syndrome—Hypermobility type. *Pain Res Mana*, **9**(4), 209–11.

51. Schechter, N., Altman, A., and Weisman, S. (1990). Report of the consensus conference on the management of pain in childhood cancer. *Pediatrics*, **86**(Suppl 5).

52. Acute Pain Management Guideline Panel (1992). In *Clinical practice guideline: Acute pain management in infants, children and adolescents: Operative and medical procedures*. Agency for Health Care Policy and Research, Rockville.

53. Consensus Panel (1999). *Pediatric pain and symptom algorithms for palliative care*. Children's Hospital, Seattle.

54. Jacox, A., Payne, R. Carr, D.B. *et al.* (1994). *Management of cancer pain, clinical practice guideline*. Agency for Health Care Policy and Research, U.S. Department of Health and Human Services, Service PH (ed.) Rockville, MD.

55. The Hospital for Sick Children. *Drug Handbook and Formulary 2007–2008*. The Hospital for Sick Children, Toronto, ON.

56. Houlahan, K.E. Branowicki, P.A., Mack, J.W. *et al.* (2006). Can end of life care for the paediatric patient suffering with escalating and intractable symptoms be improved? *J Pediatr Oncol Nurs*, **23**(1), 45–51.

57. Collins, J.J. and Weisman, S.J. (2003). Management of pain in childhood cancer. In *Pain in infants, children, and adolescents*, 2nd

Edition (eds. N.L. Schechter, C.B. Berde, and M. Yaster) pp. 517–38. Lippincott Williams and Wilkins, Baltimore.

58. Krane, E.J. Leong, M.S., Golianu, B. *et al.* (2003). Treatment of paediatric pain with nonconventional analgesics. In *Pain in infants, children, and adolescents*, 2nd edition (eds. N.L. Schechter, C.B. Berde, and M. Yaster), pp. 225–40. Lippincott Williams and Wilkins, Philadelphia.

59. Maunuksela, E.L. and Olkkola, K.T. (2003). Nonsteroidal anti–inflammatory drugs in paediatric pain management. In *Pain in infants, children, and adolescents*, 2nd edition (eds. N.L. Schechter, C.B. Berde, and M. Yaster), pp. 171–81. Lippincott Williams and Wilkins, Philadelphia.

60. Yaster, M., Kost-Byerly, S. and Maxwell, L.G. (2003). Opioid agonists and antagonists. In *Pain in infants, children, and adolescents*, 2nd edition (eds. N.L. Schechter, C.B. Berde, and M. Yaster), pp. 181–224. Lippincott Williams and Wilkins, Philadelphia.

61. Yaster, M., J.R. Tobin, and S. Kost-Byerly. (2003). Local anesthetics. In *Pain in infants, children, and adolescents*, 2nd edition (eds. N.L. Schechter, C.B. Berde, and M. Yaster), pp. 241–64. Lippincott Williams and Wilkins, Philadelphia.

62. Mercadante, S. (2004). Cancer pain management in children. *Palliat Med*, **18**(7), 654–62.

63. Gregoire, M.C. and Frager, G. (2006). Ensuring pain relief for children at the end of life. *Pain Res Manag*, **11**(3), 163–71.

64. Schutzman, S.A. Liabelt, E., Wisk, M. *et al.* (1996). Comparison of oral transmucosal fentanyl citrate and intramuscular meperidine, promethazine, and chlorpromazine for conscious sedation of children undergoing laceration repair. *Ann Emerg Med*, **28**(4), 385–90.

65. Dsida, R.M. Wheeler, M., Birmingham, P.K. *et al.* (1998). Premedication of paediatric tonsillectomy patients with oral transmucosal fentanyl citrate. *Anesth Analg*, **86**(1), 66–70.

66. Malviya, S. Voepel-Lewis, T., Huntington, J. *et al.* (1997). Effects of anesthetic technique on side effects associated with fentanyl Oralet premedication. *J Clin Anesth*, **9**(5), 374–8.

67. Sharar, S.R. Carrougher, C.R. *et al.* (2002). A comparison of oral transmucosal fentanyl citrate and oral oxycodone for paediatric outpatient wound care. *J Burn Care Rehabil*, **23**(1), 27–31.

68. Gaukroger, P. (1993). Patient-controlled analgesia in children. In *Pain in infants, children, and adolescents* (eds. N.L. Schechter, C.B. Berde, and M. Yaster), pp. 203–12. Lippincott Williams & Wilkins, Baltimore.

69. Hill, H.F. Chapman, C.R., Kornell, J.A. *et al.* (1990). Self-administration of morphine in bone marrow transplant patients reduces drug requirement. *Pain*, **40**(2), 121–9.

70. Rodgers, B.M. Webb, C.J., Stergios, D. *et al.* (1988). Patient-controlled analgesia in paediatric surgery. *J Pediatr Surg*, **23**(3), 259–62.

71. Shapiro, B.C., Cohen, D.E., and Howe, C.J., (1991). Patient-controlled analgesia for patients with sickle cell related disease. *J Pain Symptom Manage*, **8**(1), 22–80

72. Tahmooressi, J., Schmalzle, S., and Tobin, J. (1991). Patient-controlled analgesia in the adolescent undergoing Cotrel-Dubosset Rod. *J Pain Symptom Manage*, **6**, 160.

73. Webb,C., Paarlberg, J., and Sussman, M. (1991).The use of a PCA device by parents or nurses for postoperative pain in children with cerebral palsy. *J Pain Symptom Manage*, **6**, 160.

74. McDonald, A.J. and Cooper, M.G. (2001). Patient-controlled analgesia: an appropriate method of pain control in children. *Paediatric Drugs*, **3**(4), 273–84.

75. McNeely, J.K. and Trentadue, N.C. (1997). Comparison of patient-controlled analgesia with and without nighttime morphine infusion following lower extremity surgery in children. *J Pain Symptom Manag*, **13**(5), 268–73.

76. Bray, R. Woodhams, A.M., Vallis, C.J. *et al.* (1996). A double-blind comparison of morphine infusion and patient controlled analgesia in children. *Paediatr Anaesth*, **6**(2), 121–7.

77. Noyes, M. and Irving, H. (2001). The use of transdermal fentanyl in paediatric oncology palliative care. *Am J Hosp Palliat Care*, **18**(6), 411–6.

78. Hunt, A. Goldman, A., Devine, T. *et al.* (2001). Transdermal fentanyl for pain relief in a paediatric palliative care population. *Palliat Med*, **15**(5), 405–12.

79. Christensen, M.L. Wang, W.C., Harris S. *et al.* (1996). Transdermal fentanyl administration in children and adolescents with sickle cell pain crisis. *J Pediatr Hematol Oncol*, **18**(4), 372–6.

80. Ahmedzai, S. and Brooks, D. (1997). Transdermal fentanyl versus sustained-release oral morphine in cancer pain: preference, efficacy, and quality of life. The TTS-Fentanyl Comparative Trial Group. *J Pain Symptom Manage*, **13**(5), 254–61.

81. Edinboro, L.E. Poklis, A., Trautman, D. *et al.* (1997). Fatal fentanyl intoxication following excessive transdermal application. *J Forensic Sci*, **42**(4), 741–3.

82. Wilder, R.T. (2003). Regional anesthetic techniques for chronic pain management in children. In *Pain in infants, children, and adolescents*, 2nd edition (eds. N.L. Schechter, C.B. Berde, and M. Yaster), pp. 396–416. Lippincott Williams and Wilkins, Philadelphia.

83. Anand, K., Stevens, B.J., and McGrath, P. (eds.) (2007). *Pain in neonates*. 3rd edition Elsevier, New York.

84. Anand, K., Shapiro, B., and Berde, C. (2007). Pharmacotherapy with systemic analgesics. In *Pain in neonates* (eds. K. Anand and P. McGrath), pp. 155–98. Elsevier, New York.

85. Fitzgerald, M. and Howard, R. (2003). The neurological basis of paediatric pain. In *Pain in infants, children, and adolescents*, 2nd edition (eds. N.L. Schechter, C.B. Berde, and M. Yaster) pp.19–43. Lippincott Williams and Wilkins, Baltimore.

86. Franck L and Gregory G. (1993). Clinical evaluation and treatment of infant pain in the neonatal intensive care unit. In *Pain in infants, children, and adolescents* (eds. N.L. Schechter, C.B. Berde, and M. Yaster), pp. 519–36. Lippincott Williams & Wilkins, Baltimore.

87. Greeley, W., Boyd, J., and Kern, F. (1993). Pharmacokinetics of analgesic drugs. In *Pain in neonates* (eds. K. Anand and P. McGrath), pp. 107–54. Elsevier, New York.

88. Koren, G. Butt, W., Chinyanga, H. *et al.* (1985). Postoperative morphine infusion in newborn infants: Assessment of disposition characteristics and safety. *J Pediatr*, **107**(6), 963–7.

89. Collins, C. Koren, G., Crean, P. *et al.* (1985). Fentanyl pharmacokinetics and hemodynamic effects in preterm infants during ligation of patent ductus arteriosus. *Anesth Analg*, **64**(11), 1078–80.

90. Lynn, S. and Slattery, J. (1987). Morphine pharmacokinetics in early infancy. *Anesthesiology*, **66**, 136–139.

91. oney, R.D. (2002). *Managing pain: The Canadian Health Care Professional's Reference*, pp. 64–66. Healthcare and Financial Publishing, Rogers Media.

92. Spigelblatt, L. Laine-Ammara, G., Pless, I.B. *et al.* (1994). The use of alternative medicine by children. *Pediatrics*, **94**(6 Pt 1), 811–4.

93. Dahlquist, L.M. Gil, K.M., Armstrong, F.D. *et al.* (1985). Behavioral management of children's distress during chemotherapy. *J Behav Ther Exp Psychiatry*, **16**(4), 325–9.

94. Dash, J. (1980). Hypnosis for symptom amelioration. In *Psychologic aspects of childhood cancer* (ed. J. Kellerman), pp. 215–30. C.C. Thomas, Springfield, IL.

95. Hartman, G.A. (1981). Hypnosis as an adjuvant in the treatment of childhood cancer. In *Living with childhood cancer* (ed. P. Deasy-Spinetta), pp. 143–52. Mosby, St. Louis.

96. Hilgard, R. and LeBaron, S. (1982). Relief of anxiety and pain in children and adolescents with cancer: Quantitative measures and clinical observations. *Int J Clin Exp Hypn*, **30**(4), 417–42.

97. Hilgard, J.R. and LeBaron, S. (1984). *Hypnotherapy of pain in children with cancer*, p. 250. Kaufmann, Los Altos, CA.

98. Jay, S.M. Elliot, C.H., Ozolins, M. *et al.* (1985). Behavioral management of children's distress during painful medical procedures. *Behav Res Ther*, **23**(5), 513–20.

99. Katz, E., Kellerman, J., and Ellenberg, L. (1987). Hypnosis in the reduction of acute pain and distress in children with cancer. *J Pediatr Psychol*, **12**(3), 379–94.

100. LaBaw, W. Holton, C., Tewell, K. *et al.* (1975). The use of self-hypnosis by children with cancer. *Am J Clin Hypn*, **17**(4), 233–8.

101. McGrath, P.A. and Hillier, L.M. *et al.* (2002). A practical cognitive–behavioral approach for controlling children's pain. In *Psychological approaches to pain manangement*. 2nd edition, (ed. D.C. Turk), pp. 534–52. Guilford Press, New York.

102. Olness, K. (1981). Imagery (self-hypnosis) as adjunct therapy in childhood cancer: Clinical experience with 25 patients. *Am J Pediatr Hematol Oncol*, **3**(3), 313–21.

103. Olness, K. (1981). Hypnosis in paediatric practice. *Curr Probl Pediatr*, **12**(2), 1–47.

104. Zeltzer, L. and LeBaron, S. (1982). Hypnosis and nonhypnotic techniques for reduction of pain and anxiety during painful procedures in children and adolescents with cancer. *J Pediatr*, **101**(6), 1032–5.

105. Hall, H. (1999). Hypnosis and paediatrics. In *Medical hypnosis: An introduction and clinical guide* (ed. R. Tennes), pp. 79–93.Churchill Livingstone, New York.

106. LeBaron, S. and Zeltzer, L. (1996). Children in pain. In *Hypnosis and suggestion in the treatment of pain: A clinical guide* (ed. J. Barber), pp. 305–40. W.W. Norton, New York.

107. Olness, K. and Kohen, D.P. (1996). *Hypnosis and hypnotherapy with children*, 3rd edition. Guilford Press, New York.

108. Beales, J. (1979). Pain in children with cancer. In *Advances in pain research and therapy* (ed. J. Bonica and V. Ventafridda), pp. 89–98. Raven Press, New York.

13.3

Symptom control in life-threatening illness in children

John J. Collins

Introduction

Palliative care may begin at diagnosis and, for children with slowly progressive illnesses, palliative care may last for years. A common misconception, based on an older, traditional model, erroneously equates palliative care with terminal care. This chapter focuses primarily on the end-of-life component within the broader context of palliative care. Dying children are often highly symptomatic and their symptom burden may increase with time, especially when the terminal phase is reached. This symptom burden consists of physical, psychological, spiritual, and other factors. Although the entire matrix needs to be considered in the symptom assessment of the dying child, the reader is referred to the other sections that cover the psychological and cognitive, social, spiritual, and existential domains of caring for a dying child.

Physical symptoms may be caused by either the underlying illness, side effects related to medical interventions and treatment, or to causes unrelated to either the primary disease or its treatment. The assessment and diagnosis of symptoms is fundamental to the clinical care of dying children. Palliative therapeutics should generally only be implemented once the underlying causative mechanisms have been established, since therapies directed at the primary cause may ultimately have a more effective outcome for symptom management.

Clinical assessment of symptoms is complemented by symptom measurement. Measurement refers to the application of a metric to a specific dimension of symptom experience. The measurement of symptoms in children often utilizes formal scales that assess symptom intensity or frequency. Intensity is the most frequently measured dimension of pain, for example, and is often the dimension measured clinically to monitor success or otherwise of analgesic prescription.

Symptoms, symptom burden, and quality of life in children

It is frequently assumed that a child's quality of life is directly related to their degree of symptom burden. This is not necessarily true as quality of life is a complex, multi-factorial, and dynamic process. This complexity is compounded in paediatrics by quality of life measurement. Quality of life measures frequently assess functional status rather than involve a comprehensive evaluation of the health-related quality of the child's physical, emotional, and social domains of life. Even with measures tailored appropriately to the child's capacity, a variety of barriers to the inclusion of QOL endpoints in clinical trials have been identified[1]. Attitudinal bias against self-reported health questionnaire data, lack of validated measures, and the absence of a QOL 'gold standard' are some of the difficulties faced when incorporating these measures into clinical research and practice[1].

Current status of symptom measurement and symptom management drug trials in children with life-threatening illness

The progress in symptom control for adults receiving palliative care does not have a parallel experience in children. The Cochrane Library has few systematic reviews of symptom management trials in children[2]. This is due, in part, to the paucity of symptom control research in children and explains the reliance of best practice in paediatric palliative care on the best evidence in adult palliative care. In addition, most of the validated symptom assessment tools in paediatrics have focused on two common symptoms, pain and nausea. In contrast to instruments measuring nausea and vomiting, instruments measuring pain in children have largely been validated in predominantly the non-cancer setting. Few multi-dimensional symptom assessment scales exist for children. Systematic symptom assessment may be useful in assessing symptom burden as part of decision-making towards palliative care and in future epidemiological studies of symptoms in dying children.

There are general and specific problems peculiar to conducting symptom management studies in children. Although many of the difficulties encountered in performing these trials in children can be overcome, few studies have been performed in children receiving palliative care. For example, the ethical issue of performing novel drug trials in paediatrics is somewhat mitigated by delaying such studies until the safety, efficacy, and tolerability data are available from adult studies. Similarly, obtaining the assent of a child for a drug trial, using age-appropriate explanations, mitigates the issue of only obtaining an informed consent from a proxy (usually a parent). The compromise to the problem of repeated venipuncture in children for drug assays is utilizing intravenous cannulae inserted at the time of anaesthesia or blood collection from a central venous line.

Another major difficulty in performing symptom management studies in dying children pertains to the heterogeneous nature of symptoms in this population. If cancer were to be the disease model, for example, one difficulty relates to the treatment of childhood cancer. Children tend to receive therapies directed at control of their tumours until very late in the course of their illnesses and are frequently very ill and highly symptomatic. These epidemiological and treatment variables make it less likely that a sub-population of children receiving palliative care exists who have a stable, chronic pattern of symptoms amenable to evaluation in a trial. The lack of an appropriate analgesic study design to account for small numbers of subjects is a further impediment to progress in symptom management for these children.

Instruments for the assessment of pain

Unidimensional self-report measures: self-report measures of pain in children have largely focused on the assessment of pain severity. Generally, the data support the use of visual analogue scales or numerical rating scales for children over the age of 5. Visual analogue scales have been used in the assessment of paediatric cancer pain[3,4]. To use such scales, children must understand the concept of proportionality, be able to conceptualize their pain experience along a continuum and be able to translate that understanding to the visual representations of the line and the anchors.

Similar strategies, such as Likert scales with anchor points of 1 ('no pain') and 5 ('extreme pain'), have been used to assess pain in children with cancer[5]. However, research on the use of verbal rating scales with children (9 years and older) has not established clearly the utility of this approach over visual analogue scales[6]. In the context of childhood cancer, other investigators have used visual cues, such as different pictures of a child's face, which are graded from neutral or happy expressions (no pain) to sad/distressed expressions (extreme pain)[7–10].

Behavioural observation measures: the subjective distress of acute pain, particularly after traumatic medical procedures, often manifests itself in certain facial expressions, verbal, and motor responses. Behavioural methods for assessing pain in children require independent observers to record the physical behaviours of children in pain, as well as the frequency of their occurrence[5,11,12]. Observation methods have generally been used to obtain data on specific, treatment-related pain-distress reactions in children with cancer (e.g. bone marrow aspiration (BMA), lumbar puncture (LP), postoperative pain, etc.).

The *Gauvain-Piquard rating scale*[13] is an observation scale designed for the assessment of chronic pain in paediatric oncology patients aged 2–6 years. The scale consists of 17 items, seven of which are related to pain assessment (antalgic rest position, spontaneous protection of painful areas, somatic complaints, the child points out painful areas, antalgic behaviour during movement, control exerted by child when moved, emotional reactions to medical examination of painful regions), 6 are related to depression (child retires 'into his shell', lack of expressiveness, lack of interest in surroundings, slowness and rarity of movements, signs of regression, social withdrawal), and 4 assess anxiety

(nervousness/anxiety, ability to protest, moodiness/irritability, tendency to cry). Kappa statistics analysing the correlation between observers were low, ranging from 0.24 to 0.60.

Pain measurement in children with neuro-cognitive impairment

Many neurodegenerative diseases impact profoundly on a child's ability to communicate verbally and children with neuro-cognitive impairment require specific measures to ensure pain is adequately evaluated and treated. Physical aspects of certain illnesses, such as grimacing or muscles spasms, can mimic features or behaviours commonly attributed to pain.

In one study, 24 children with cognitive impairment were rated by their care-givers and researchers as to the perceived intensity of the child's pain pre- and post-surgery[14]. One outcome was that familiarity with the individual child was not necessary for observers to have congruent pain measurement assessments[14]. Another study generated a checklist of typical pain behaviours of children with cognitive impairment. Seven observational items were predictive of numerical pain ratings with 85 per cent sensitivity and 89 per cent specificity. Pain cues reported by 29 caregivers of non-communicative children with life-limiting conditions were compared against a checklist of 203 items. This study yielded a common 'core' set of six pain cues. These included screaming/yelling, crying, distressed facial expression, tense body, difficult to comfort, and flinching when touched[15].

Instruments for the assessment of nausea in children

A comparison of child and parental ratings of children's nausea and emesis symptoms was assessed among 33 children (aged 1.7–17.5 years, median 4.7 years) with acute lymphoblastic leukaemia receiving identical chemotherapy[16]. The measures utilized nausea and vomiting vignettes designed to assess the frequency and severity of nausea and emesis symptoms as reported by children and their parents based on the previous chemotherapy experience of the child. The vignettes, based on the work of Zeltzer[17], consisted of 12 questions assessing separately nausea and emesis at three time intervals: prior to, during, and after chemotherapy. A five-point Likert-type rating scale ranging from 'not at all' to 'all the time' for the frequency items and from 'not bad' to 'real bad' on the severity items were employed. A composite nausea/vomiting score was determined by calculating the mean of the 12 frequency and severity items.

This study demonstrated a significant correlation between child and parent ratings of nausea. Significant inter-rater correlations for nausea frequency and severity but not for emesis frequency or severity were found. Lastly, a rating scale for nausea and vomiting utilizing verbal descriptors was used in a series of assessment studies in children with cancer aged 5–18[18–21]. There was 80 per cent agreement between parent and child rating when they were assessed independently.

The measurement of fatigue in children

Previous surveys of children with cancer have indicated that fatigue is highly prevalent and distressing[22,23]. Three instruments to measure fatigue from the perspectives of the child, parents, and staff were developed and tested in a recent study[24]. The study consisted of three phases: instrument development, content validation, and estimations of psychometric properties of the three fatigue instruments. One hundred and forty-nine children between the ages of 7–12 years receiving chemotherapy for cancer, 147 parents, and 124 staff participated in this study. The instruments demonstrated strong initial validity and reliability estimates.

A new Children's Fatigue Scale (CFS), was tested in 7–12-year-old oncology patients (*n* = 149), just over half of whom were within 6 months of diagnosis[62]. The most frequently endorsed items included not being able to play, being tired in the morning, sleeping more at night, not being able to run, and lying around. Children and adolescents noted distressing fatigue at the time of their cancer diagnosis, throughout treatment, and for several years following successful treatment[6,63,64]. Associated factors in cancer-related fatigue include altered sleep, sadness or depression, anaemia, hospitalization, inadequate nutrition, and lack of enjoyment for social encounters[6,62,65].

Multidimensional symptom assessment tools for children

The Memorial Symptom Assessment Scale is a 30-item patient-rated instrument adapted from a previously validated adult version to provide multidimensional information about the symptoms experienced by children aged 10–18 with cancer[22]. The analyses supported the reliability and validity of the MSAS 10–18 subscale scores as measures of physical, psychological, and global symptom distress, respectively. The majority of patients could easily complete the scale in a mean of 11 minutes.

A revised Memorial Symptom Assessment Scale (MSAS) was created as an instrument for the assessment of symptoms in children aged 7–12 years with cancer[23]. Validity was evaluated by comparison with the medical record, parental report, and concurrent assessment on visual analogue scales for selected symptoms. The data provide evidence of the reliability and validity of MSAS (7–12) and demonstrated that children as young as seven years with cancer could report clinically relevant and consistent information about their symptom experience. The completion rate for MSAS 7–12 was high and the majority of children completed the instrument in a short period of time and with little difficulty. The instrument appeared to be age appropriate and may be helpful to older children unable to complete MSAS 10–18 independently.

Symptom epidemiology in children with life-limiting illness

The child dying in hospital

Following the publication of recent data from the United States[25], there has been an increasing awareness of the need for better symptom management of dying children. Wolfe[25] found that 89 per cent of 103 parents whose children died of cancer in a hospital setting reported retrospectively that their children experienced 'a lot' or 'a great deal' from at least one symptom in their last month of life. In the children who were treated for specific symptoms, treatment was thought to be successful in only 27 per cent of those with pain and in only 16 per cent of those with dyspnoea. Apart from the humanitarian perspective, another driving force towards a better standard of symptom management in dying children is the

insight that perceived, unrelieved pain, and suffering will be carried for many years in the memories of their parents[25].

A retrospective survey to describe the course of terminal care provided to 77 dying hospitalized children in terms of symptom assessment and management, and communication and decision-making, at the end of life was performed in Edmonton, Canada[26]. Eighty-three per cent of children died in intensive care settings (64/77), and 78 per cent (60/77) were intubated prior to their death. Opioid analgesia was provided in 84 per cent of all cases (65/77), 6 (8 per cent) patients had do not resuscitate (DNR) orders preceding final hospital admission, and 56/71 (79 per cent) patients had documented discussion resulting in a DNR decision during final hospital admission. Median time from DNR to death was <1 day. Decision-making regarding end-of-life issues in this paediatric population was deferred very close to the time of death and only after no remaining curative therapy was available. Acuity of care was very high prior to death for most children. Children in this survey were rarely told that they were dying.

Another retrospective study examined symptom prevalence, characteristics, and distress of 30 children dying at the Children's Hospital, Westmead, Australia[27]. Symptoms and their characteristics during the last day of life were determined from an interview of a nurse who cared for that child during the last day of life using a symptom assessment instrument. The dominant disease process was cancer, while the most likely location of death was intensive care. The mean duration of the 'active phase of dying' was 25.2 h and the major physiological disturbances at this time were respiratory failure and encephalopathy. The mean (± SD) number of symptoms per patient was 11.1 ± 5.6 with significantly more (<0.02) symptoms for children dying on the ward (14.3 ± 6.1) compared to children dying in intensive care (9.5 ± 4.7). Six symptoms (lack of energy, drowsiness, skin changes, irritability, pain, and oedema of the extremities) occurred with a high prevalence (affecting 50 per cent or more of the children) in the last week of life. Symptoms in the last day of life, even if they occurred with a high prevalence, frequency ('a lot' to 'almost always') or severity ('moderate' to 'very severe') were, in general, not associated with a high level of distress ('quite a lot' to 'almost always'). Lack of energy was the only symptom where over 30 per cent of children with the symptom had a high level of distress ('quite a bit' to 'very much'). The level of patient comfort, as perceived from the medical notes, indicated that the majority of children were 'always comfortable' to 'usually comfortable' in the last week (64 per cent), day (76.6 per cent), and hour (93.4 per cent) of life[27].

In summary, the symptom burden of children dying in hospital is high. Ironically, in Drake's survey[27], the symptom burden was significantly reduced in the intensive care unit where the most aggressive interventions were undertaken.

The child dying in an inpatient hospice

There are few epidemiological data on the symptoms experienced by children with life-limiting and life-threatening illness dying in a children's inpatient hospice unit. A retrospective survey of 30 children at a children's hospice indicated pain, secretions, dyspnoea, oral symptoms, and cough to be common problems for children in the last week of life[28]. This survey was dependent upon the report of carers, since many of the children were cognitively impaired. As such, this survey may be under-reporting the frequency with which these symptoms occurred.

Table 13.3.1   Prevalence and characteristics of symptoms determined by the memorial symptom assessment scale in 159 children with cancer[22].

Symptom	Degree when symptom was present			
	Overall prevalence (%)	Intensity, Mod–VSev (%)[a]	Frequency, A lot–AA (%)[b]	Distress, QB–VM (%)[c]
Lack of energy	49.7	61.6	40.9	21.4
Pain	49.1	80.8	35.9	39.1
Feeling drowsy	48.4	64.0	34.6	18.6
Nausea	44.7	65.9	23.0	36.6
Cough	40.9	47.7	23.0	16.3
Lack of appetite	39.6	66.3	39.7	35.8
Feeling sad	35.8	59.6	17.5	39.5
Feeling nervous	35.8	56.1	28.1	23.7
Worrying	35.4	66.1	28.6	27.2
Feeling irritable	34.6	63.6	30.9	34.7
Itching	32.7	63.4	26.9	30.0
Insomnia	30.8	66.7	38.8	58.7
Dry mouth	30.8	50.2	28.6	23.5
Hair loss	28.3	66.6	NE	48.0
Vomiting	27.7	67.5	32.3	45.2
Weight loss	26.6	51.2	NE	25.0
Dizziness	24.5	55.2	15.4	21.9
Numbness/tingling in hands/feet	22.0	36.0	28.6	22.7
Sweating	20.3	54.7	25.0	10.8
Lack of concentration	20.1	54.5	21.9	30.3
Diarrhoea	20.1	61.6	28.1	33.4
Skin changes	20.1	68.8	NE	46.1
Dyspnoea	16.5	69.1	22.9	29.1
Change in the way food tastes	16.5	77.0	NE	30.4
'I don't look like myself'	15.8	76.0	NE	49.5
Mouth sores	13.9	59.2	NE	56.9
Difficulty swallowing	12.6	83.8	56.3	76.1
Constipation	13.8	81.8	NE	25.9
Swelling of arms/legs	12.0	52.8	NE	8.0
Problems with urination	6.3	90.0	70	45.0

[a] Percentage moderate to very severe.

[b] Percentage a lot to almost always.

[c] Percentage quite a bit to very much. NE, not evaluated.

[*Source*: Collins, J.J., Byrnes, M.E., Dunkel, I. *et al.* (2000). The Memorial Symptom Assessment Scale (MSAS): Validation study in children aged 10–18. *Journal of Pain and Symptom Management*, **19**(5), 363–77.]

The symptoms of children with cancer

Children aged 10–18 with cancer were surveyed at Memorial Sloan-Kettering, New York, for symptom prevalence and distress[22]. Symptom prevalence ranged from 49.7 per cent for lack of energy to 6.3 per cent for problems with urination (Table 13.3.1). The mean (±SD) number of symptoms per inpatient was 12.7 ± 4.9 (range, 4–26), significantly more than the mean 6.5 ± 5.7 (range, 0–28) symptoms per outpatient. Patients who had recently received chemotherapy had significantly more symptoms than patients who had not received chemotherapy for more than four months (11.6 ± 6.0 vs. 5.2 ± 5.1), and those patients with solid tumours had significantly more symptoms than patients

Table 13.3.2   Symptom prevalence (%) in four tumour types (n = 131)[22].

Symptom	Prevalence (%)			
	Leukaemia (*n* = 33)	Lymphoma (*n* = 26)	Solid tumour (*n* = 54)	CNS tumour (*n* = 18)
Lack of energy	43.8	50.0	53.7	66.7
Pain	43.8	26.9	63.0	50.0
Feeling drowsy	50.0	38.5	57.4	33.3
Nausea	43.8	34.6	53.7	50.0
Cough	34.4	38.5	48.1	22.2
Lack of appetite	28.1	30.8	51.9	33.3
Feeling sad	34.4	26.9	37.0	38.9
Feeling nervous	28.1	23.1	42.6	22.2
Worrying	31.3	36.0	37.0	22.2
Feeling irritable	34.4	34.6	38.9	27.8
Itching	40.6	15.4	35.2	38.9
Insomnia	28.1	30.8	29.6	27.8
Dry mouth	21.9	11.5	40.7	55.6
Hair loss	9.4	50.0	38.9	22.2
Vomiting	12.5	15.4	38.9	33.3
Weight loss	15.6	19.2	29.6	47.1
Dizziness	21.9	15.4	31.5	22.2
Numbness/tingling in hands/feet	25.0	34.6	16.7	22.2
Sweating	12.9	26.9	24.1	16.7
Lack of concentration	21.9	15.4	20.4	27.8
Diarrhoea	21.9	11.5	24.1	16.7
Skin changes	15.6	15.4	20.4	22.2
Dyspnoea	21.9	11.5	18.5	5.6
Change in the way food tastes	9.4	7.7	27.8	11.8
'I don't look like myself'	—	23.1	24.1	11.1
Mouth sores	9.4	15.4	20.4	5.9
Difficulty swallowing	3.1	3.8	18.5	11.1
Constipation	6.3	—	24.1	16.7
Swelling of arms/legs	6.3	15.4	14.8	11.8
Problems with urination	—	3.8	9.3	11.1

[*Source*: Collins, J.J., Byrnes, M.E., Dunkel, I. *et al.* (2000). The Memorial Symptom Assessment Scale (MSAS): Validation study in children aged 10–18. *Journal of Pain and Symptom Management*, **19**(5), 363–77.]

with either leukaemia, lymphoma, or central nervous system malignancies (9.9 ± 7.0 vs. 6.8 ± 5.5 vs. 6.8 ± 5.0 vs. 8.0 ± 6.1) (Table 13.3.2). The most common symptoms (prevalence >35 per cent) were lack of energy, pain, drowsiness, nausea, cough, lack of appetite, and psychological symptoms (feeling sad, feeling nervous, worrying, feeling irritable). Of the symptoms with prevalence rates >35 per cent, those that caused high distress in more than one-third of patients were feeling sad, pain, nausea, lack of appetite, and feeling irritable. These data confirm a high prevalence of symptoms overall and the existence of subgroups with high distress

associated with one or multiple symptoms. Systematic symptom assessment may be useful in future epidemiological studies of symptoms and in clinical chemotherapeutic trials. Symptom epidemiology may also provide a focus for future clinical trials related to symptom management in children with cancer.

A survey of symptom prevalence and distress was performed in younger children aged 7–12 with cancer[23]. Of the eight symptoms surveyed, the mean number of symptoms experienced by younger children was 1.9 (±1.6). Symptom prevalence during the 48 h prior to the completion of the questionnaire included: tiredness (35.6 per cent),

Table 13.3.3   Prevalence and characteristics of symptoms determined by the memorial symptom assessment scale (7–12) in children with cancer aged 7–12[23].

Symptom	Degree when symptom was present			
	Overall prevalence (%)	Intensity, medium amount—a lot (%)	Frequency, medium amount— almost all the time (%)	Distress, medium amount—very much (%)
Lethargy	53 (35.6)	51	64	5
Pain	48 (32.4)	56	54	37
Insomnia	46 (31.1)	—	—	39
Itch	37 (25.0)	56	54	38
Lack of appetite	33 (22.3)	—	52	12
Worry	30 (20.1)	43	43	30
Nausea	20 (13.4)	—	45	65
Sadness	15 (10.1)	60	53	50

[*Source*: Collins, J.J., Devine, T.B., Dick, G. *et al.* (2002). The measurement of symptoms in young children with cancer: The validation of the Memorial Symptom Assessment Scale in children aged 7–12. *Journal of Pain and Symptom Management*, **23**(1), 10–6.]

pain (32.4 per cent), insomnia (31.1 per cent), itch (25.0 per cent), lack of appetite (22.3 per cent), worry (20.1 per cent), nausea (13.4 per cent), and sadness (10.1 per cent) (Table 13.3.3). More than half the children who endorsed pain as a symptom rated their pain as a 'medium amount' to 'a lot'. Although sadness was the least prevalent symptom, more than half of the patients who experienced it rated it as severe, frequent, and distressing. Tiredness and lack of appetite were less likely to be causes of high distress than pain, insomnia, itch, nausea, or worry[23]. These data confirm the ability of young children to quantify their symptomatology in terms of severity, frequency, and distress.

Pain in children with cystic fibrosis at the end of life

A retrospective chart review at a tertiary care hospital was conducted summarizing the end-of-life care of US patients more than 5 years of age and dying from cystic fibrosis[29]. Twenty-five per cent of these patients had been receiving opioids for the treatment of chronic headache or chest pain for more than their last 3 months of life. When opioids were used for the treatment of breathlessness or chest pain, the proportion increased to 86 per cent. When pain was present, it was described as 'serious' pain with chest, head, extremity, abdomen, and back being the more common locations. Increasing pain for this patient population may signal advanced, progressive disease[30].

Pain and other symptoms in children with neurodegenerative illnesses

Pain, breathlessness, and oral symptoms (i.e. secretions) were highlighted as the most common symptoms by caregiver's proxy report for children in the last month of life at an inpatient hospice[28]. Half of the children reported on in the study were non-communicative, indicating the potential for under-reporting in this patient population.

The epidemiology of intractable pain in children

Pain that cannot be relieved using conventional treatment is intractable. Intractable pain that does not respond to therapies

beyond conventional practice is refractory. The relief of refractory pain may require a therapy that compromises consciousness. Intractable pain in childhood is rare and is usually seen in the setting of cancer pain. Intractable childhood cancer pain is usually associated with disease-related syndromes. It is rare, however, for a paediatric patient to have persistent tumour-related pain from diagnosis[31]. Disease-related pain often recurs at the time of tumour recurrence and when the cancer becomes unresponsive to treatment.

The opioid requirements of 199 children with terminal malignancy were examined in a retrospective study[32]. Twelve (6 per cent) of the patients in this study required therapies beyond conventional opioid pharmacotherapy. The majority of the patients had neuropathic pain as the basis of their intractability. Eleven of the patients had spinal cord compression, solid tumour metastatic to the spinal nerve roots, nerve plexus, or large peripheral nerve. Half of the patients had adequate analgesia with either regional anaesthesia or with opioid infusion alone. The remaining patients required the addition of sedation to control refractory pain.

Since the publication of the above report, practice has become more sophisticated with a greater understanding of the management of the paediatric pain crisis, the calculation of opioid 'rescue' dosing and dose escalation, opioid switching, greater understanding of the management of opioid side effects to permit greater opioid dose escalation, the *N*-methyl-D-aspartate (NMDA) antagonists as new therapeutic options, and a better understanding of invasive approaches to pain management in children (see discussion of these therapeutic options later in the text). Given the advances in therapeutics, it may be that fewer children need to be sedated to reduce conscious awareness of intractable symptoms.

Symptom management in children with life-threatening illness

The adequate, proficient, and timely management of symptoms in the dying child is of critical importance. Not only is it important from an humanitarian viewpoint, but also it is apparent that the memory of unrelieved symptoms in dying children may be retained in the memory of parents many years after their child has died[25]. It will be impossible for children and their families to negotiate the domains of psychological and spiritual care if physical symptomatology has not been adequately treated. The following outlines the management of the major symptoms experienced by children receiving palliative care. As few controlled studies of symptom management have been performed in childhood, many of the therapies used in children have been devised utilizing best practice for adults. The reader is referred to the adult section of this volume for the principles of management of unusual symptoms. An emphasis has been given in this chapter to the palliative care emergencies of childhood. Less urgent symptoms have been discussed in alphabetical order.

The palliative care emergencies of childhood

Intractable pain

The modalities of pain control for the management of intractable cancer pain in paediatric patients include opioid dose titration, opioid side-effect management, opioid rotation, NMDA receptor antagonists, adjuvant analgesics (covered in a previous section), regional anaesthesia, and sedation. Non-pharmacologic methods of pain control have a secondary role in the setting of intractable pain.

The paediatric pain crisis

The pain crisis in a child is an emergency and requires treatment beyond conventional means. A specific diagnosis must be made, as therapies directed at the primary cause may be more effective in the longer term. The management of intractable pain requires the clinician to be at the patient's bedside, to titrate incremental intravenous doses every 10–15 min until effective analgesia has been achieved. The analgesic effects of opioids increase in a log-linear function, with incremental opioid dosing required until either analgesia is achieved or somnolence occurs[33]. The total amount of opioid administered to achieve this reduction in pain intensity is considered the opioid loading dose. A continuous infusion of opioid may need to be commenced to maintain this level of analgesia and the infusion rate is often based on the opioid administered as a loading dose[33]. An alternative to a continuous infusion of opioid is intermittent parenteral opioid, especially in the setting of an unpredictable pain syndrome.

Breakthrough doses or 'rescues'

Breakthrough doses or 'rescues' are additional doses of opioid incorporated into the analgesic regimen to allow for additional analgesia if required by the patient. Rescue doses of opioid may be calculated as approximately 5–10 per cent of the total daily opioid requirement and may be administered orally every hour[33].

A prospective study was performed to determine the prevalence, characteristics, and impact of breakthrough pain in children with cancer[34]. Twenty-seven paediatric in- and outpatients with cancer (age 7–18 years) who had severe pain requiring treatment with opioids and who received care at the Oncology Unit at the Children's Hospital at Westmead, Sydney, Australia, participated in this study. The children responded to a structured interview (Breakthrough Pain Questionnaire for Children [BPQC]), designed to characterize breakthrough pain in children. Measures of pain, anxiety, and depressed mood were completed. Fifty-seven per cent of the children experienced one or more episodes of breakthrough pain during the preceding 24 h, each episode lasting seconds to minutes, occurring three to four times/day, and most commonly characterized by the children as sharp and shooting. Younger children (7–12 years) had a significantly higher risk of experiencing breakthrough pain compared to teenagers. Although no statistical difference could be shown between children with and without breakthrough pain in regard to anxiety and depression, children with breakthrough pain reported significantly more interpersonal problems on a Child Depression Inventory subtest. The most effective treatment of an episode of breakthrough pain was a patient controlled analgesia (PCA) opioid bolus dose. Postoperative data suggest that 7-year-old children of normal intelligence can use PCA effectively to provide analgesia[35].

Opioid dose escalation

If pain can be controlled by the opioid loading technique (above), then the subsequent opioid dose escalation may be calculated as follows:

1 If greater than approximately six rescue doses of opioid are required in a 24 h period, then the hourly average of this total daily rescue opioid should be added to the baseline opioid infusion. An alternative would be to increase the baseline infusion by 50 per cent[33].

2 Rescue doses are kept as a proportion of the baseline opioid infusion rate and are re-calculated as between 50 per cent and 200 per cent of the hourly basal infusion rate[33].

Opioid side effects

Children do not necessarily report opioid side effects voluntarily (e.g. constipation, pruritus, dreams, etc.) and should be asked specifically about these problems. An assessment of opioid side effects is included in an assessment of analgesic effectiveness. All opioids can potentially cause the same constellation of side effects. If opioid side effects limit opioid dose escalation, then consideration should be given to an opioid switch. Tolerance to some opioid side effects (e.g. sedation, nausea and vomiting, pruritus) often develops within the first week of starting opioids. Children do not develop tolerance to constipation and concurrent treatment with laxatives should be provided.

There is a tendency to attribute new symptoms to the adverse side effects of opioid therapy. Other potential causes should always be considered. In comparison to adults, children are far less accepting of a slightly adverse opioid analgesic/side effect ratio[36]. Any potential side effect must be anticipated and actively managed.

At the end of life, confusion can be one of the more distressing adverse effects, sometimes much more so for those close to the child than for the child themselves. To lose aspects of the child's personality through medications rather than, or in addition to, illness or death, is profoundly tragic[36]. It is also frequently ossible to prevent or ameliorate through judicious analgesic titration, opioid switching, the use of adjuvant analgesics to minimize drug-related toxicities while ensuring adequate pain relief.

When confusion is attributed to opioid toxicity, it is appropriate to switch to an alternative opioid. The decision to change analgesic therapy should be based on several factors, including the expected proximity to the child's death, what the anticipated time course would be for effective pain relief with the analgesic alternative and the attendant possible side-effect profile[36].

Opioid switching

The usual indication for switching to an alternative opioid is dose-limiting opioid toxicity. In the setting of intractability, opioid dose escalation may be limited by opioid-related side effects. An observation is that a switch from one opioid to another is often accompanied by change in the balance between analgesia and side effects[37]. A favourable change in opioid analgesia to side-effect profile will be experienced if there is less cross-tolerance at the opioid receptors mediating analgesia, than at those mediating adverse effects[38].

A retrospective study examined the therapeutic value of opioid switching in children attending a large paediatric oncology centre for treatment[39]. The details for opioid prescriptions, over the course of a year, were obtained from the medical records of children with cancer who had a rotation of opioid during their admission. Twenty-two children (14 per cent) had 30 opioid switches. Mucositis was the cause of pain in 19 (70 per cent) children, bone pain in 3 (11 per cent) children, and postoperative, visceral, or neuropathic pain in the remainder. The opioid was switched either for excessive side effects with adequate analgesia (70 per cent), excessive side effects with inadequate analgesia (16.7 per cent), or tolerance (6.7 per cent). Five (23 per cent) children required two switches, three during the same admission. The favoured switches were morphine to fentanyl in 20 (67 per cent) children and fentanyl to hydromorphone in six (20 per cent). Adverse opioid effects were resolved in 90 per cent of cases; all failures occurred when morphine was rotated to fentanyl. There was no significant loss of pain control or increase in mean morphine equivalent dose requirements. Opioid switching had a positive impact on managing dose-limiting side effects of, or tolerance to, opioid therapy during cancer pain treatment in children. This was accomplished without loss of pain control or having to increase the dose of opioid therapy significantly[39].

Following a prolonged period of regular dosing with one opioid, equivalent analgesia may be attained with a dose of a second opioid that is smaller than that calculated from an equianalgesic table (see previous sections). An opioid switch is usually accompanied by a reduction in the equianalgesic dose (approximately 50 per cent for short half-life opioids).

In contrast to short half-life opioids, the doses of methadone required for equivalent analgesia after switching may be of the order of 10–20 per cent of the equianalgesic dose of the previously used short half-life opioid. A protocol for methadone dose conversion and titration has been documented for adults[40].

NMDA receptor antagonists

NMDA-receptor antagonists depress central sensitization in animal experiments and in humans[41–44]. Among others, dextromethorphan, dextrorphan, ketamine, memantine, and amantadine have been shown to have NMDA-receptor antagonist activities. The clinical usefulness of some of these medications is compromised by a high adverse side effect to analgesic ratio. There are no data of their utility in paediatrics, other than procedural pain management. Clinical usage is increasing, particularly in the setting

of severe neuropathic pain and rapid opioid dose escalation and perceived tolerance.

Invasive approaches to intractable paediatric cancer pain

Anaesthetic approaches

In contrast to the adult population, the experience of using regional anaesthesia for children with intractable pain is limited. A retrospective study of children with terminal cancer[45] showed that regional anaesthesia is appropriate in a highly select subset of children. The indications for regional anaesthesia in this group were largely related to either dose-limiting side effects of opioids or opioid unresponsiveness in patients where pain was confined to one region of the body. Rapid intravenous opioid dose reduction was required in some cases. Technique modifications appropriate to children have been recommended[46]. The recommendations included the use of sedation and imaging for epidural insertion.

Neurosurgical approaches

Experience with neurodestructive procedures in children is limited. Matson described his experience with cordotomy in children[47] with intractable pain. It is unclear whether these cases may have been effectively managed by current pharmacologic techniques. In selected cases neurosurgical approaches to pain management may be appropriate.

Sedation as a therapeutic modality for intractable pain

The use of sedation in the setting of refractory pain generally assumes that therapies beyond the conventional have been utilized and that there is no acceptable means of providing analgesia without compromising consciousness. This trade-off between sedation and inadequate pain relief requires the consideration of the wishes of the child and his or her family. The ethical issues surrounding prolonged sedation in paediatrics, including the principle of double effect have been previously discussed[48–50]. The continuation of high-dose opioid infusions in these circumstances is recommended to avoid situations in which a patient may have unrelieved pain but inadequate clarity to express pain perception. A variety of drugs have been used in this setting, including barbiturates, benzodiazepines, and phenothiazines[49].

Seizure control

Seizures in palliative care patients may be either recent in onset or part of a long-standing underlying seizure disorder. In the former situation, the onset will usually be frightening to patients and families and may be due to many possible causes (e.g. cerebral metastases, infection, metabolic disorder, hypoxia, etc.), which must be excluded as treatment directed at the primary causes may be appropriate whilst anti-convulsant therapy is implemented. In the latter situation, worsening seizure control in a patient with an underlying seizure disorder may indicate either disease progression or factors related to anti-convulsant dose, class, or administration which should be reviewed.

Refractory seizure control has been the subject of two reviews[51,52]. Initial treatment of status epilepticus in children typically consists of either diazepam or lorazepam, immediately followed by phenytoin or phenobarbitone[51]. Buccal midazolam has been shown to be at least as effective as rectal diazepam in the acute treatment of seizures[52]. Administration via the mouth is more socially acceptable and convenient and may become the preferred treatment for long seizures that occur outside hospital[52]. The buccal dose is the same as the oral dose of midazolam used for sedation (0.3 mg/kg per dose, maximum dose 15 mg) and should be used as a single dose only.

Traditionally, refractory status epilepticus is treated with barbiturate coma or general anaesthetics, both of which require invasive cardiorespiratory and haemodynamic monitoring and are associated with significant complications. Midazolam has been effective in terminating seizures refractory to diazepam, lorazepam, phenytoin, and phenobarbitone in paediatric patients[51].

Spinal cord compression

Spinal cord compression is an unusual complication of childhood cancer and occurs most often late in a child's illness. Back pain, more often than abnormal neurologic signs or symptoms, is the usual initial presenting sign of spinal cord compression in children[53]. Spinal cord compression is an emergency, since adult data show that if treated whilst a patient is ambulatory, the probability of retaining ambulant status is 89 per cent to 94 per cent[54]. The mainstays of management are firstly radiological diagnosis and treatment with radiotherapy for radiosensitive tumour and corticosteroids[55].

Bleeding

Although the fear of external bleeding is paramount in the minds of families and caregivers of children dying of either haematological malignancy or children dying of liver failure, massive external bleeding as a mode of death in childhood is uncommon. While some children with malignancy receive blood products indefinitely, this is not always feasible or appropriate. Many families negotiate the use of blood products only if minor bleeding or anaemia becomes problematic. If the fear of external bleeding is overwhelming for families, this may influence their choice of location of the child's death and attitude towards blood product transfusion.

Terminal dyspnoea

Dyspnoea is an uncomfortable awareness of breathing[56]. In the terminal phase, it is often highly distressing to patients and for families to watch. Terminal dyspnoea may be due to a variety, and perhaps combination, of causes. These include pulmonary metastases, intrinsic lung disease or infection, cardiac failure, acidosis,

Table 13.3.4 Indicators of end-stage respiratory disease in children.

Persistent dyspnoea despite optimization of medical management
Decreased mobility because of above
Resistant respiratory pathogens
Limited improvement following hospital admission
Increasing number of hospitalizations for chest infection or respiratory decompensation
Oxygen dependence
Pulmonary hypertension

muscle weakness, etc. Again, diagnosis is important as this may influence choice of therapies. Non-invasive ventilation may be a viable choice for symptom management of dyspnoea related to muscle weakness, for example, and bronchospasm could be easily reversed with bronchodilators. Table 13.3.4 shows indicators of end-stage respiratory disease in children.

Most of the data on the management of terminal dyspnoea are from studies of adults with terminal malignancy. There are no data on the appropriate management of dyspnoea related to muscle weakness or complications of cystic fibrosis, for example. The goal of palliative therapies for terminal dyspnoea is to improve the patient's subjective sensation. A double blind, cross-over trial studied the effects of supplemental oxygen on dyspnoea in adult patients with terminal cancer[57]. The subjective sensation of dyspnoea was improved in patients receiving supplemental oxygen. In addition, systemic opioid therapy[56,58] and cognitive–behavioural strategies[59] have been shown to be of benefit to patients with dyspnoea related to terminal malignancy. As anxiety is often a component of terminal dyspnoea, judicious prescription of a benzodiazepine may be warranted.

Secretions

The management of noisy secretions in an unconscious patient is aimed at reducing the distress of family, other patients, and staff. The sound of noisy secretions can be haunting to all concerned and should be given some priority by the attending clinician. While there is no standard of care for the management of noisy secretions, accepted management includes explanation to relatives, positioning, suction, and anticholinergics (e.g. hyoscine hydrobromide or glycopyrolate)[60].

Terminal delirium

Delirium during the final phase of dying is one of the most distressing symptoms for care-givers to watch, especially if the delirium is agitated. The interpretation of the latter may be that the delirium is a manifestation of an internal existential angst. This latter interpretation is unlikely, since the aetiology of delirium in the setting of an actively dying patient is usually multifactorial with a physical rather psychological basis (eg. hypoxia, metabolic derangement, central nervous system disease, infection, fever, etc). Simple causes that can be corrected, hypoxia for example, should be excluded. As terminal delirium cannot be predicted, a therapeutic plan for its management should be considered in every dying child. The usual therapies consist of haloperidol for delirium per se with consideration of adding a benzodiazepine if there is agitation as well.

The palliation of other symptoms in childhood

Constipation

Although constipation is a relatively common symptom in children, it is more likely to be distressing to the child's caregivers than to the child. The aetiology of constipation is often multifactorial and may include reduced physical activity, mechanical obstruction, metabolic derangement, poor diet and low fluid intake, bowel atony due to opioids, etc. Although unusual, bowel

Table 13.3.5 Guidelines for the management of opioid induced constipation in children.

Non-drug measures
Dietary change
Increase fluids
Increase physical activity

Principles of laxative prescription
By a pleasant route of administration (i.e. avoid per rectum administration)
Individualize to avoid side effects
Around the clock dosing
Simple dosing regimen

Laxative prescription[68]
1 Try a stimulant laxative first (e.g. senna 7.5 mg once or twice daily)
2 If this is ineffective, increase the dose
3 If this is ineffective add lactulose (1 ml/kg/dose once or twice daily). This dose frequency may need to be increased
4 Bisacodyl suppository +/− an enema may be required if the above fails to produce a response
5 Consider Movicol-half® for older children instead of the above regimens

obstruction and faecal impaction must be excluded and treated urgently in any child presenting with constipation.

Generally, dietary changes are recommended in the first instance (increased vegetables and fruity, bulk, prune juice, etc.). In addition, attention should be given to hydration, mobility, and other activities of daily living. Chronic opioid therapy necessitates the prescription of a regular laxative. There is little evidence to guide the prescription of laxatives in children. Whilst there are emerging adult data to suggest oral naloxone may be appropriate for the management of opioid induced constipation[61], a senna and lactulose combination is often prescribed in the adult population[62]. It is not clear if a senna/lactulose combination is appropriate for children. Table 13.3.5 gives some guidelines for the management of opioid induced constipation in children. The osmotic laxative, Movicol-half® is being used increasingly to treat constipation in children. There are, however, no data on its use for children aged 2–11 years.

Fatigue

Fatigue is a common symptom of children with cancer[22,23,25,63] and one that is often highly distressing. The aetiology of fatigue in children dying of cancer may be due to a combination of factors including anaemia, poor nutrition, insomnia,

Table 13.3.6 Nausea and vomiting: paediatric palliative care.

Cause	Putative mechanism (-S)[68]	Treatment
Gastrointestinal causes:		
Poor mouth care	Cerebral cortex, vagus	Regular mouth care
Gastric irritation	Vagus	Exclude drug related causes, consider prescription of H1 antagonists
Intestinal obstruction	Vagus	May require surgical opinion
Constipation	Vagus	Laxatives (see below)
Hepatic distension	Vagus	Depends on aetiology (e.g. frusemide for cardiac failure, dexamethasone for tumour related causes)
Metabolic causes:		
Renal failure	Chemoreceptor trigger zone (CTZ)	Consider anti-emetics if more invasive therapies not appropriate
Hypercalcaemia	CTZ	If appropriate, consider hydration, diuretic (osteoclast inhibitors may also be appropriate)
NS causes:		
Raised intracranial	Vomiting centre	Dexamethasone
Pressure	Vestibular apparatus	Anti-histamine
Vestibulitis		
Treatment related causes:		
Medications (chemotherapy, opioids, etc.)	Chemoreceptor trigger zone, vagus	Consider an opioid switch for dose limiting side effects
Psychological trigger:		
Anxiety	Cerebral cortex	Consider cognitive behavioural therapy
Emotional distress	Cerebral cortex	
Other causes:		
Pain	Vagus	Treat the primary cause
Infection	Chemoreceptor trigger zone	Treat the primary cause
Migraine headache	Vomiting centre	Anti-migraine therapies
Situational triggers (unpalatable food, etc.)	Vagus	Alter situation
	Cerebral cortex	

metabolic derangement, the increased work of breathing in patients with dyspnoea, side effects of medication, and psychological factors.

In the assessment of fatigue in a child and the matrix of its potential causes, it is important to establish if this symptom is distressing to the child or his family. If so, the potential remediable causes should be considered. Therapies directed at the primary cause should be instituted only if these therapies are not of substantial burden to the patient or his/her family. There are adult and limited paediatric data on the use of stimulant medication for the treatment of opioid induced somnolence[64–66]. In children it has become more common practice to switch opioids (see above) for somnolence as a dose-limiting side effect of opioid therapy.

Insomnia

Sleep disturbance is common in children with life-threatening illness[67]. In the context of cancer, insomnia is both prevalent and distressing to children and, by inference, distressing to caregivers (Table 13.3.1). The aetiology of insomnia is multi-factorial and is often a combination of physical, psychological, and perhaps environmental factors. When depression is a factor, consideration should be given to psychotherapy and pharmacologic treatment. Fatigue often coexists with sleep disturbance. Lifestyle changes, including improved sleep hygiene, exposure to sunlight and exercise may be helpful to improved sleep. Low dose amitriptyline,

if not contraindicted, is often a helpful pharmacologic agent for the management of insomnia in terminally ill children, particularly if pain is a symptom management issue.

Mouth care and hydration

Routine mouth care promotes patient comfort and ability to eat and drink, prevents halitosis and helps identify problems such as dry mouth, candidiasis, and ulceration[68]. Lip emolients and mouthwashes are important therapies for mouth care. The sensation of a dry mouth may be due to local (e.g. mouth breathing, candidiasis, radiotherapy to salivary glands, etc.) and systemic causes (e.g. dehydration, anticholinergic drugs, uraemia, etc.) and is often distressing. The issue of hydration in dying patients is a contentious issue. Small but frequent volumes of fluid to maintain insensible losses may be appropriate via the oral route. However, this may be impossible in some instances unless other routes of administration are considered. As with all therapies, the benefits, and deficits of any intervention must be discussed with the patient and family before any therapeutic intervention is implemented.

Nausea and vomiting

Nausea and vomiting are not uncommon in children receiving palliative care. Nausea and vomiting occur when the vomiting centre in the brain is activated by any of the following: cerebral cortex (e.g. anxiety), vestibular apparatus, chemoreceptor trigger zone

Table 13.3.7 Anti-emetic drug therapy in paediatric palliative care.

Drug category	Putative mechanism of action[68]	Drugs	Dosing regimen	Route of administration	Side effects/caution
Prokinetic drugs	Promote gastric emptying via a cholinergic mechanism All act on the CTZ	Metoclopramide	0.15 mg/kg/dose 6–8 hourly prn	O/IV/IM/SC	Extrapyramidal side effects more common in children
5HT$_3$ antagonists	Central action on CTZ and vomiting centre. Block serotonin receptors on vagal efferents in the bowel	Ondansetron	0.15 mg/kg/dose 8–12 hourly prn OR 5 mg/m^2/dose 8–12 hourly prn	O/IV	Dose limit 8 mg/dose
Corticosteroids	Probably act via peripheral mechanisms. Useful for chemotherapy related emesis	Dexamethasone	0.1–1.0 mg/kg/day 6–8 hourly prn	O/IV/SC* *Incompatible in combination with many other drugs via SC route	Cushingoid effects with long-term use Gastric irritation Mood instability Poor contol of blood sugar levels
Antihistamines	Act on the vomiting centre	Cyclizine	0.8 mg/kg/dose 6 hourly prn	O/IV/SC	Anticholinergic side effects, drowsiness Max. dose 50 mg
Neuroleptic drugs	Act on the CTZ	Haloperidol	10–50 mcg/kg/day 8–12 hourly prn	O/SC	Extrapyramidal side-effects Drowsiness
Anticholinergic drugs	Act on the vomiting centre	Hyoscine hydrobromide (Scopolamine)	6–10 mcg/kg/dose 6 hourly prn	O/IV/IM/SC	Maximum dose = 400 mcg/dose
Benzodiazepines	Act on the cerebral cortex	Lorazepam	25–50 mcg/kg/dose 6–8 hourly prn	O/IV	Drowsiness Max. dose 1 mg

Abbreviations: O, oral; SC, subcutaneous; IM, intramuscular; prn, when required; IV, intravenous.

Table 13.3.8   Resources to assist with assessment and management of symptoms in children with life-limiting illnesses.

Web site	List serv
www.act.org.uk	A list-serv accessible world-wide through e-mail/internet for issues relating to paediatric palliative care is accessible by sending an e-mail to paedpalcare@act.org.uk with subscribe as the subject line
www.nhpco.org	A list-serv accessible world-wide through e-mail/internet for issues relating to paediatric pain is accessible by sending an e-mail to LISTSERV@is.dal.ca with the message SUB PEDIATRIC-PAIN and your first then last name
www.ippcweb.org	
www.childendoflifecare.org	
www.cnpcc.ca	
www.ich.ucl.ac.uk/cpap	

(CTZ), vagus nerve, or by direct action on the vomiting centre. A clear diagnosis must be sought as to aetiology, as the list of potential causes is great and therapies different, depending on the putative mechanism (see Table 13.3.6).

Antiemetic drug trials in children

Apart from pain, the only other symptom control therapy for which clinical trials have been undertaken in children are the antiemetics. Antiemetic drug trials have been conducted with an increasing degree of sophistication in this population, ranging from open label studies[69] to randomized double blind cross over studies[70] (Table 13.3.7). Unfortunately, these studies are few in number, have a small number of recruited subjects and may be flawed by virtue of the measures used. In addition, the context for most of these nausea and emesis drugs trials is related to cancer chemotherapy. Table 13.3.8 outlines one approach to antiemetic prescription in children receiving palliative care. There are no data on the use of 5HT3 for non-chemotherapy/non-postoperative induced nausea and vomiting in children.

Summary

Symptom management is one of many domains of care of the dying child. A recent report[25] indicates that the memory of a dying child's symptomatology lingers for a long time in the memory of parents and care-givers. This same report and others indicate that the dying child is often highly symptomatic and these symptoms need to be prioritized and treated meticulously.

References

1. Bradlyn, A., Harris, C., and Speith, L. (1995). Quality of life assessment in paediatric oncology: A retrospective review of Phase III reports. *Soc Sci Med*, **41**(10), 1463–5.
2. Cochrane. (2007). Internet Communication.
3. Jay, S.M., Elliott, C., Katz, E. *et al.* (1987). Cogitive, behavioral, and pharmacologic interventions for children's distress during painful medical procedures. *Journal of Consult Clinical Psychology*, **55**, 860–5.
4. Elliott, C., Jay, S.M., and Woody, P. (1987). An observational scale for measuring children's distress during medical procedures. *J Pediatr Psychol*, **12**, 543–51.
5. LeBaron, S. and Zeltzer, L. (1984). Assessment of acute pain and anxiety in children and adolescents by self-reports, observer reports and a behavior checklist. *J Cons Clin Psych*, **52**, 729–38.
6. Savedra, M., Gibbons, P., Tesler, M. *et al.* (1982). How do children describe pain? A tentative assessment. *Pain*, **14**, 95–104.
7. Kuttner, L., Bowman, M., and Teasdale, M. (1988). Psychological treatment of distress, pain and anxiety for children with cancer. *Dev Behav Pediatr*, **9**, 374–81.
8. Manne, S.L., Bakeman, R., Jacobsen, P. *et al.* (1992). Adult and child interaction during invasive medical procedures: sequential analysis. *Health Psychol*, **11**, 241–9.
9. Champion, G.D., Goodenough, B., von Baeyer, C.L. *et al.* (1998). Measurement of pain by self-report. In *Measurement of pain in infants and children* (eds. G.A. Finlay and P.J. McGrath), pp. 123–60. IASP Press, Seattle.
10. Hicks, C.L., von Baeyer, C.L., Spafford, P. *et al.* (2001). The faces pain scale-revised: Toward a common metric in paediatric pain measurement. *Pain*, **93**, 173–83.
11. Jay SM, Elliott C, Ozolins M, *et al.* (1985). Behavioral management of children's distress during painful medical procedures. *Behav Res Ther*, **5**, 513–20.
12. Jay, S.M., Ozolins, M., Elliott, C. *et al.* (1983). Assessment of children's distress during painful medical procedures. *J Health Psych*, **2**, 133–47.
13. Gauvain-Piquard, A., Rodary, C., Rezvani, A. *et al.* (1987). Pain in children aged 2–6 years: A new observational rating scale elaborated in a paediatric oncology unit: A preliminary report. *Pain*, **31**, 177–88.
14. Breau, L.M., Finley, G.A., McGrath, P.J. *et al.* (2002). Validation of the non-communicating children's pain checklist-postoperative version. *Anesthesiology*, **96**(3), 523–6.
15. Stallard, P., Williams, A., Velleman, R. *et al.* (2002). Brief report: Behaviors identified by caegivers to detect pain in noncommunicating children. *Pediatr Psychology*, **27**, 209–14.
16. Tyc, V.L., Mulhearn, R.K., FAirclough, D. *et al.* (1993). Chemotherapy induced nausea and emesis in paediatric cancer patients: External validity of child and parent ratings. *Dev Behav Pediatr*, **14**(4), 236–41.
17. Zeltzer, L., LeBaron, S., Richie, D.M. *et al.* (1988). Can children understand and use a rating scale to quantify somatic symptoms? Assessment of nausea and vomiting as a model. *Journal of Consult Clinical Psychology*, **56**(4), 567–72.
18. Zeltzer, L., Kellerman, J., Ellenberg, L. *et al.* (1983). Hypnosis for reduction of vomiting associated with chemotherapy and disease in adolescents with cancer. *Journal of Adolescent Health Care*, **4**(77), 84.
19. Zeltzer, L., LeBaron, S., and Zeltzer, P.M. (1984). The effectiveness of behavioral intervention for reducing nausea and vomiting in children and adolescents receiving chemotherapy. *Journal of Clinical Oncology*, **2**, 683–90.
20. Zeltzer, L., LeBaron, S., and Zeltzer, P.M. (1984). A prospective assessment of chemotherapy related nausea and vomiting in children with cancer. *American Journal of Pediatric Hematology/Oncology*, **6**, 5–16.

21. LeBaron, S. and Zeltzer, L. (1984). Behavioral intervention for reducing chemotherapy-related nausea and vomiting in adolescents with cancer. *Journal of Adolescent Health Care*, **5**(178), 182.

22. Collins, J.J., Byrnes, M.E., Dunkel, I. *et al.* (2000). The memorial symptom assessment scale (MSAS): Validation study in children aged 10–18. *Journal of Pain and Symptom Management*, **19**(5), 363–7.

23. Collins, J.J., Devine, T.B., Dick, G. *et al.* (2002). The measurement of symptoms in young children with cancer: The validation of the Memorial Symptom Assessment Scale in children aged 7–12. *Journal of Pain and Symptom Management*, **23**(1), 10–6.

24. Hockenberry, M., Hinds, P., Barrera, P. *et al.* (2003). Three instruments to assess fatigue in children with cancer: The child, parent and staff perspectives. *Journal of Pain & Symptom Management*, **25**(4), 319–28.

25. Wolfe J, Grier H.E., Klar N. *et al.* (2000). Symptoms and suffering at the end of life in children with cancer. *New England Journal of Medicine*, **342**(5), 326–33.

26. McCallum DE, Byrne P, Bruera E. (2000). How children die in hospital. *Journal of Pain & Symptom Management*, **20**(6), 417–23.

27. Drake R, Frost J, Collins JJ. (2003). The symptoms of dying children. *Journal of Pain & Symptom Management*, **27**(7), 6–10.

28. Hunt AM. (1990). A survey of signs, symptoms and symptom control in 30 terminally ill children. *Dev Med Child Neurol*, **32**, 347–55.

29. Robinson, W.M., Ravilly, S., Berde, C.B. *et al.* (1997). End-of-life care in cystic fibrosis. *Pediatrics*, **100**, 205–9.

30. Ravilly, S., Robinson, W., Suresh, S. *et al.* (1996). Chronic pain in cystic fibrosis. *Pediatrics*, **98**, 741–7.

31. Miser, A.W., Dothage, P., Wesley, R.A. *et al.* (1987). The prevalence of pain in a paediatric and young adult population. *Pain*, **29**, 265–6.

32. Collins, J.J., Grier, H.E., Kinney, H.C. *et al.* (1995). Control of severe pain in terminal paediatric malignancy. *Journal of Pediatrics*, **126**(4), 653–7.

33. Cherny, N.I. and Foley, K.M. (1996). Nonopioid and opioid analgesic pharmacotherapy of cancer pain. *Hematol Oncol Clin North Amer*, **10**, 79–102.

34. Friedrichsdorf, S., Finney, D., Bergin, M. *et al.* (2007). Breakthrough pain in children with cancer. *Journal of Pain & Symptom Management*, **34**, 209–16.

35. Berde, C.B., Lehn, B.M., Yee, J.D. *et al.* (1991). Patient controlled analgesia in children and adolescents: A randomized, prospective comparison with intramuscular morphine for postoperative analgesia. *Journal of Pediatrics*, **118**, 460–6.

36. Frager, G. and Collins, J.J. (2005). Symptoms in life-limiting conditions. In *Textbook of paediatric palliative care* (eds. R. Hain, A. Goldman, and S. Liben). Oxford University Press.

37. Galer, B.S., Coyle, N., Pasternak, G.W. *et al.* (1992). Individual variability in the response to different opioids: Report of five cases. *Pain*, **49**, 87–91.

38. Portenoy, R.K. (1994). Opioid tolerance and responsiveness: research findings and clinical observations. In *Progress in pain research and management* (eds. G.F. Gebhart, D.I. Hammond, and T.S. Jensen), pp. 615–9. IASP Press, Seattle.

39. Drake, R., Longworth, J., and Collins, J.J. (2004). Opioid rotation in children with cancer. *Journal of Palliative Medicine*, **7**(3), 419–22.

40. Inturrisi, C.E., Portenoy, R.K., Max, M. *et al.* (1990). Pharmacokinetic-pharmacodynamic relationships of methadone infusions in patients with cancer pain. *Clin Pharmacol Ther*, **47**, 565–77.

41. Eide, P.K., Jorum, E., Stubhaug, A. *et al.* (1994). Relief of post-herpetic neuralgia with the *N*-methyl-D-aspartic acid receptor antagonist ketamine: A double-blind cross-over comparison with morphine and placebo. *Pain*, **58**, 347–54.

42. Persson, J., Axelsson, G., Hallin, R.G. *et al.* (1995). Beneficial effects of ketamine in a chronic pain state with allodynia. *Pain*, **60**, 217–22.

43. Nelson, K.A., Park, K.M., Robinovitz, E. *et al.* (1997). High dose dextromethorphan versus placebo in painful diabetic neuropathy and postherpetic neuralgia. *Neurology*, **48**, 1212–8.

44. Eisenberg, E. and Pud, D. (1994). Can patients with chronic neuropathic pain be cured by acute administration of the NMDA-receptor antagonist amantadine? *Pain*, **74**, 37–9.

45. Collins, J.J., Grier, H.E., Sethna, N.F. *et al.* (1996). Regional anesthesia for pain associated with terminal malignancy. *Pain*, **65**, 63–9.

46. Berde, C.B. (1989). Regional analgesia in the management of chronic pain in childhood. *Journal of Pain & Symptom Management*, **4**(4), 232–7.

47. Matson, D.D. (1969). Neurosurgery of Infancy and Childhood. Charles C. Thomas, Springfield.

48. Truog, R.D., Berde, C.B., Mitchell, C. *et al.* (1992). Barbiturates in the care of the terminally ill. *New England Journal of Medicine*, **327**, 1678–82.

49. Kenny, N.P. and Frager, G. (1996). Refractory symptoms and terminal sedation in children: Ethical issues and practical management. *J Palliat Care*, **12**, 40–5.

50. Truog, R.D., Burns, J.P., Shurin, S.B. *et al.* (2002). Ethical considerations in paediatric oncology. In *Principles and practice of paediatric oncology*, 4th edition (eds. P.A. Pizzo and D.G. Poplack), pp. 1411–30. Lippincott Williams & Wilkins, Philadelphia.

51. Pellock, J.M. (1998). Use of midazolam for refractory status epilepticus in paediatric patients. *Journal of Child Neurology*, **13**(12), 581–7.

52. Scott, R.C., Besag, F.M., and Neville, B.G. (2002). Buccal midazolam and rectal diazepam for treatment of prolonged seizures in childhood and adolescence: A randomised trial. *Lancet*, **353**, 623–6.

53. Lewis, D., Packer, R., and Raney, B. (1986). Incidence, presentation, and outcome of spinal cord disease in children with systemic cancer. *Pediatrics*, **78**, 438–43.

54. Loblaw, D.A. and Laperriere, N.J. (1998). Emergency treatment of malignant extradural spinal cord compression: An evidence-based guideline. *J Clin Oncol*, **16**(4), 1613–24.

55. Abrahm, J.L. (1999). Management of pain and spinal cord compression in patients with advanced cancer. *Ann Intern Med*, **131**(1), 37–46.

56. Bruera, E., MacEachern, T., Ripamonti, C. *et al.* (1993). Subcutaneous morphine for dyspnoea in cancer patients. *Annals of Internal Medicine*, **119**(9), 906–7.

57. Bruera, E., de Stoutz, N., Velasco-Leiva, A. *et al.* (1993). Effects of oxygen on dyspnoea in hypoxemic terminal cancer patients. *Lancet*, **342**(8862), 13–4.

58. Boyd, K.J. and Kelly, M. (1997). Oral morphine as symptomatic treatment of dyspnoea in patients with advanced cancer. *Palliative Medicine*, **11**, 277–81.

59. Corner, J., Planth, H., Hern, R. *et al.* (1996). Non-pharmacological interventions for breathlessness in ling cancer. *Palliative Medicine*, **10**(4), 299–305.

60. Hughes, A.C., Wilcock, A., and Corcoran R. (1996). Management of "Death Rattle". *Lancet*, **12**(6), 271–2.

61. Culpepper-Morgan, J.A., Adelhardt, J. *et al.* (1992). Treatment of opioid-induced constipation with oral naloxone: A pilot study. *Clinical Pharmacological Therapy*, **52**, 90–5.

62. Abu-Saad, H.H. and Courtens A. (2001). *Pain and Symptom Management*. 63–87.

63. Hockenberry-Eaton, M., Hinds, P.S., Alcoss, P. *et al.* (1998). Fatigue in children and adolescents with cancer. *J Pediatr Oncol Nurs*, **15**, 172–82.

64. Bruera, E., Faisinger, R., MacEachern, T. *et al.* (1992). The use of methylphenidate in patients with incident pain receiving regular opiates: A preliminary report. *Pain*, **50**, 75–7.

65. Bruera, E., Miller, M.J., Macmillan, K. *et al.* (1992). Neuropsychological effects of methylphenidate in patients receiving a continuous infusion of narcotics for cancer pain. *Pain*, **48**, 163–6.

66. Yee, J.D. and Berde, C.B. (1994). Dextroamphetamine or methylphenidate as adjuvants to opioid analgesia for adolescents with cancer. *Journal of Pain and Symptom Management*, **9**, 122–5.

67. Herbert, A. Sleeping patterns in children with life limiting conditions—A survey of hospitalised children with and without life limiting conditions. 2-11-2007. Personal Communication.

68. *Symptom Relief in Terminal Illness*. (1998). World Health Organization, Geneva.

69. Pinkerton, C.R., Williams, D., Wooton, C. *et al.* (1990). 5-HT3 antagonist ondansetron—An effective outpatient antiemetic in cancer treatment. *Arch Dis Child*, **65**, 822–5.

70. Alvarez, O., Freeman, A., and Bedros, A. (1995). Randomized double-blind cross-over ondansetron-dexamethasone versus ondansetron-placebo study for treatment of chemotherapy induced nausea and vomiting in paediatric patients with malignancies. *Journal of Pediatric Hematology and Oncology*, **17**(2), 145–50.

Psychological adaptation of the dying child

Michael M. Stevens

What do children think and fear about death—particularly their own death? Do children who are dying develop insight to adjust and cope? These questions are clearly relevant to paediatric palliative medicine and are discussed in this chapter.

Psychological development of the normal child

An understanding of what sick children think and fear about death and how they adjust requires a brief discussion of how healthy children begin to think and form concepts including a concept of death.

Jean Piaget (1896–1980) is regarded as one of the most significant psychologists of the 20th century. His stage theory of child development[1,2] describes the development of the child's intellect (thoughts, perceptions, judgement, reasoning) as an orderly hierarchical sequence of three major periods, each integrating and extending the previous one. This theory is widely used as a model in experimental child psychology (Table 13.4.1).

In the first period (sensorimotor intelligence, birth to 2 years), intellectual development begins with motor and sensory actions, which, by being repeated, become behavioural sequences. These form the basis for later intellectual structure. Piaget believed infants in this period are still unable to think or form concepts.

The second period (preparation and organization of concrete operations, early childhood to adolescence) consists of two stages, referred to as pre-operational thought and concrete operations. During the stage of pre-operational thought (age 2–7 years), the child is still unable to differentiate between the internal and external worlds (egocentricity), and has thoughts that do not follow logical rules. The child will attribute life and consciousness to inanimate objects (animistic thinking) and believes that inanimate objects can be commanded to obey actions or thoughts (magical thinking). This assists the child in making order out of the world and ascribing causes to events. The child will ascribe magical prelogical explanations in discovering what differentiates life from death. The child will also believe that all objects and events in the world are manufactured to serve people (artificialism).

During the stage of concrete operations (age 7–12 years), the child gradually becomes less egocentrically orientated. Animistic, magical, and artificialistic thinking decrease and gradually disappear and the child comes to realize the personal nature of his or her views. Language and communication skills increase dramatically and the child acquires the concepts of conservation, space, time, and rate. The child's thinking becomes logical and influenced by the rules of disciplines such as arithmetic and mechanics. The child is concerned with the actual, rather than the hypothetical and his or her reasoning will be connected as much as possible to beliefs based on direct observation. The child confronted by death will now know that animals and people do not die because a magic spell was put upon them that can be lifted, and will seek to discover what differentiates life from death.

During formal operations (adolescence to adulthood), previous cognitive structures and functions are integrated to achieve full intellectual capacities, including the ability to deal effectively with the world of abstract ideas.

The sequence of these periods will be orderly in all children, but children may differ widely in the ages at which they move through the sequence. Occasional reversions to a less-developed mode of thought will occur.

The well child's concept of death and its development

The development of an understanding of death in the well child parallels Piaget's sequence of periods of cognitive development.

Specific cognitive achievements suggested as essential for understanding the various components of a concept of death include classification abilities (ability to categorize in hierarchies and to attend to multiple classifications simultaneously, e.g. a banana is yellow and long and belongs to the fruit family), the ability to focus on transformations as well as states, a linear notion of time, the ability to perform reversible operations (ability to follow a process from beginning to end and retrace steps back to the starting point), reciprocity skills (recognition that others may feel and/or think differently to oneself) that enable children to learn from the experience of others, increased objectivity, decreased egocentrism, and the universal application of rules. A child's concept of death will vary according to his or her level of cognitive development.

Maria Nagy conducted 484 assessments on 378 Hungarian children aged between three and 10 years in Budapest and its environs, using compositions written by those aged 7–10 years on the subject of death, drawings by those aged 6–10 years, and discussions with those aged 3–10 years. Her results were published in English in

Table 13.4.1 The child's cognitive development and development of death concepts: recommendations for caregivers.

Period/stage of cognitive development (Piaget)[a]	Life period[b]	Some major characteristics	Predominant death concepts	Recommendations for caregivers[c]
I. Period of sensori-motor intelligence	Infancy (0–2)	'Intelligence' consists of sensory and motor actions. No conscious thinking. Limited language,[d] no concept of reality	No concept of death	Provide maximum physical relief and comfort
II. Period of preparation and organization of concrete operations				
1. Stage of pre-operational thought	Early childhood (2–7)	Egocentric orientation. Magical, animistic, and artificialistic thinking. Thinking is irreversible. Reality is subjective	Death is reversible: a temporary restriction, departure, or sleep	Minimize child's separation from parents. If parents unavailable, provide reliable and consistent substitute. Correct misperception of illness as punishment for bad thoughts or actions. Evaluate for feelings of guilt, rejection, anger, resentment of self or others
2. Stage of concrete operations	Middle childhood/ pre-adolescence (7–11/12)	Orientation ego-decentred. Thinking is limited to actual (although possibly absent) features of a situation rather than exploring abstract relationships and hypotheses. More adaptive thinking but confined to objects No abstract reasoning. Understands conservation, reversibility. Multiple classification ability	Death is irreversible but capricious: external-internal physiological explanations	Evaluate for fears of abandonment, destruction, or body mutilation. Be truthful and open. Provide details about treatments. Reassure treatments are not punishments. Maintain access to peers. Foster child's sense of control, mastery
III. Period of formal operations	Adolescence and adulthood (12+)	Propositional and hypodeductive thinking. Generality of thinking. Reality is objective	Death is irreversible, universal, personal, but distant: natural, physiological, and theological explanations	Reinforce comfortable body image, self-esteem. Allow ventilation of anger. Provide privacy. Support reasonable measures for independence. Be clear, honest, and direct. Maintain access to peers. Consider mutual support groups

[a] Each stage includes an initial period of preparation and a final period of attainment; thus, whatever characterizes a stage is in the process of formation.

[b] There are individual differences in chronological ages.

[c] Adapted from Rando, T. A. (1984). *Grief, dying and death: Clinical interventions for caregivers*, pp. 385–91. Research Press, Champaign, IL.

[d] By the end of their second year children, on the average, have attained a vocabulary of approximately 250–300 words. Adapted from ref.. 4 with permission of Routledge/Taylor & Francis Group, LLC.

1948[5], although much of the work was done as early as 1936. Nagy found three stages of development of a concept of death:

1 Age 3–5 years: death seen as temporary and reversible and not distinguished completely from life.

2 Age 5–9 years: death is personified and imagined as a separate person.

3 Age 9 years and upwards: death is seen as the cessation of corporal activities, and is universal and inevitable.

Sylvia Anthony studied definitions of the word 'dead' by 128 children[6]. Their responses fell into five categories:

1 Apparent ignorance of the meaning of the word 'dead'.

2 Limited or erroneous concept.

3 No evidence of non-comprehension of the meaning of 'dead' but definition by reference to (a) associated phenomena that were not biologically or logically essential or (b) humans specifically but not other living things.

4 Correct, essential, but limited reference.

5 General, logical, or biological definition or description.

As the child grew older, his or her concept of 'dead' changed in the order of the classification from (1) to (5). Anthony noted that immature death concepts take the form of oral fantasy. She also observed that fairy tales are full of such oral fantasy about death of a kind which is not death: Red Riding Hood's grandmother is eaten by the wolf and is later recovered from the beast's belly; Hansel and Gretel eat part of the witch's house, and she welcomes them inside but plans to cook and eat them.

Components of the child's concept of death: the current view

Although earlier studies have been valuable, it now appears that the child's concept of death is virtually complete by the age of 8 years. Studies have confirmed that different components of the child's concept of death are acquired at differing ages. In one study, 3-year-olds were found often to have some realization of death, but only at the age of 12 years would a child be likely to have an accurate idea of what a dead body would look like[7].

In a review of three key components of a death concept[8], it was concluded that, under at least some circumstances, young children think that death is reversible, attribute various life-defining functions to dead things, and think that certain individuals (often including themselves) will not die. Irreversibility, non-functionality, and universality are understood at roughly the same time (for most children between 5–7 years). In a second study[9] of the age of acquisition of seven of Kane's[7] components of the concept (separation, universality, causality, irrevocability, appearance of the body, insensitivity, and cessation of body function) in well children, about 60 per cent of the 5-year-olds, 70 per cent of the 6-year-olds, and 66 per cent of the 7-year-olds had complete or almost complete concepts. By the age of 8 and 9 years the figures were almost 100 per cent.

Some caution is required in comparing various studies of age of acquisition.

1 Differing statistical criteria are used by various investigators (e.g. a varying percentage of positive responses are defined to consider a concept acquired).

2 There are variations in the socioeconomic and educational standards of the children tested.

3 There are other influences related to the date of the particular study (e.g. the opportunity for the child to encounter death more commonly in the modern media).

The currently accepted components of the concept of death as summarized by Schonfeld[10] are presented in Table 13.4.2, with examples of incomplete understanding and implications of incomplete understanding for adjustment to loss.

Development in well children of fears and anxieties concerning death

There are at least three views on how children acquire fears and anxieties about death[12].

1 The psychoanalytic view suggests that death anxieties and fears in children and adults are derivatives of other anxieties and fears that develop in early life, principally separation anxiety, fear of object loss, fear of castration, fear of abandonment, and fears of physical immobility and the dark. Anthony[13] suggests that risk-taking behaviour such as 'dares' is one type of defence against such anxieties.

2 The cognitive view relates children's fears and anxieties about death to the stage of development of their concept of death. The young child may fear waking up after death and being trapped in the grave. After the child develops the concept of irreversibility of death, there will be a fear of its permanence.

3 The social learning view puts forward the idea that children's ideas and feelings are influenced by their experiences and by the observations of others. Thus, death fears and anxieties in children will be influenced by their parents, as well as by siblings, peers, teachers, and relatives. Siblings and peers can provide 'information' about death that can be truly frightening. The media (particularly television), children's books and fairy tales have also been noted to be significant influences.

Death education

Educating children about death is advocated on the basis that it is desirable to promote conceptual development related to death and that death should be introduced as a general concept prior to the child's exposure to personal loss in order to lessen anxiety about death and assist more successful adjustment to loss[11,14].

The sick child's perception of death

Although the survival rates for a variety of chronic illnesses have dramatically improved over the last 30 years, many children still do not survive. Thus, the issue of their concept of death is still pertinent. Anxiety about death is an issue for all chronically ill children, particularly those with leukaemia and other malignancies, whether or not they eventually survive.

Prior to 1970, most caregivers believed that unless a child was aged over 10 years, he or she was incapable of understanding death

Table 13.4.2 Concepts of death and implications of incomplete understanding for adjustment to loss.

Component of death concept	Definition	Example of incomplete understanding	Implication of incomplete understanding
Irreversibility	The understanding that once a living thing dies, its physical body cannot be made alive again. Death as final, as irrevocable, as permanent	The child expects the deceased to return, as if from a trip	Failure to comprehend this concept prevents the child from detaching personal ties to the deceased, a necessary first step in mourning
Finality: (non-functionality, dysfunctionality, cessation)	The understanding that all life-defining functions cease completely at death	The child worries about a buried relative being cold or in pain; the child wishes to bury food with the deceased	May lead to preoccupation with the physical suffering of the deceased and impair adjustment
Universality (inevitability)	The understanding that all living things die. Death as a natural phenomenon that no living being can escape indefinitely	The child views significant individuals (i.e. self, parents) as immortal	If the child does not view death as inevitable, he or she is likely to view death as punishment (either for actions or thoughts of the deceased, or the child) leading to excessive guilt and shame
Causality	A realistic understanding of the causes of death	Child who relies on magical thinking is apt to assume responsibility for death of a loved one by assuming that bad thoughts or unrelated actions were causative	Tends to lead to excessive guilt that is difficult for the child to resolve

Reproduced from ref. 10 with permission Sage Publications Inc; additional data taken from refs. 8 and 11.

and therefore did not experience anxiety about it. It was felt that children did not need information about their disease and that they would be incapable of coping with the distress and anxiety of knowing that they were dying. A closed protective approach was advocated[15–18].

Revised concepts of illness and death in children with leukaemia

In the late 1960s and early 1970s, pioneering work by Vernick and Karon[19,20], Waechter[21], and Bluebond-Langner[22] prompted a complete revision of this perspective.

The views of those advocating a closed protective approach were challenged bluntly for the first time in 1971 by the late Eugenia Waechter. In a key article[21] published in mid-1971, which was prepared from research on anxiety about death in terminally ill children conducted for her doctoral dissertation, Waechter reported on 64 children between the ages of 6 and 10 divided into four groups of equal size: those with a fatal disorder, those with a chronic non-fatal disease, those with a brief illness, and a group of well elementary school children who were not in hospital. A General Anxiety Scale for Children[23], measuring concerns in

many areas of living, was administered to each child. A set of eight pictures was also shown individually to each child and stories were requested in order to elicit fantasy expression of the child's concern regarding present and future body integrity and functioning. Four pictures were selected from the Thermatic Apperception Test[24]. Four others that were designed specifically for the study are reproduced in Fig. 13.4.1.

Parents of children in the first three groups were interviewed to assess how the quality and quantity of the fatally ill children's concerns about death were influenced by their previous experience with death, the religious devoutness within the family, the quality of maternal warmth towards them and the opportunities that they had to discuss their concerns or the nature of their illness with their parents, professional personnel, or other meaningful adults.

Although only two of the 16 fatally ill children had been told their prognoses, the generalized anxiety was extremely high in all 16 cases, almost double that of the two comparison groups of children in hospital and three times that of healthy children. The children threatened with death discussed loneliness, separation, and death much more frequently in their fantasy stories. Waechter's most striking finding was the dichotomy between the children's degree of

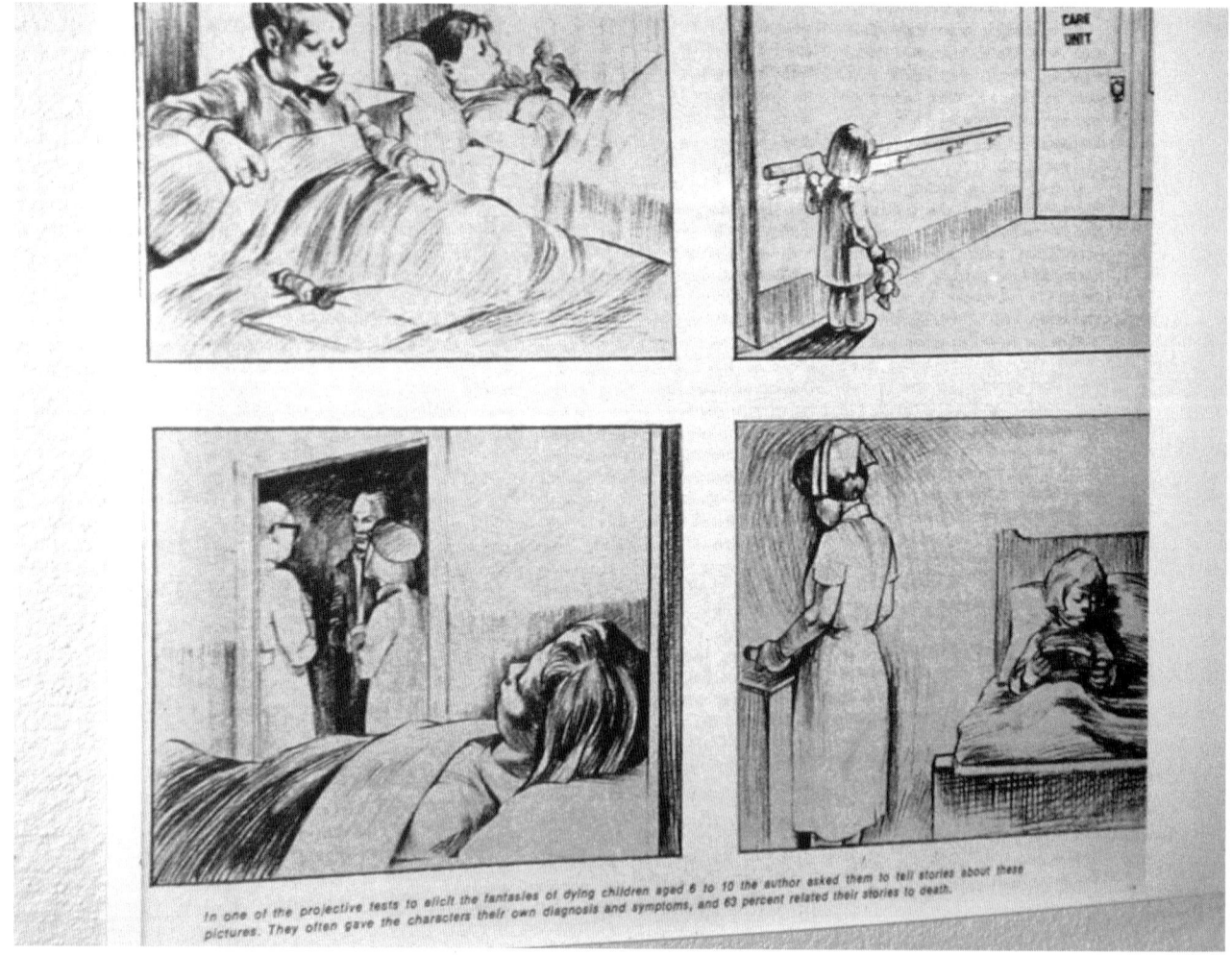

Figure 13.4.1 Four specifically designed pictures used by Waechter to elicit fantasy expressions of concerns related to present and future body integrity from dying children aged 6–10 years. The children were asked to tell stories about the pictures. They often gave the characters their own diagnosis and symptoms and 63 per cent related their stories to death. (Reproduced with permission of the *American Journal of Nursing Company*, Lippincott Williams & Wilkins).

Table 13.4.3 Stages in a sick child's acquisition of information about illness, and critical experiences required for passage through stages.

Stage of acquisition of information	Child's information	Experience required for passage to this stage	Child's self-concept at this stage
First stage	'It' is a serious illness (not all know the name of the disease)	Parents being informed of diagnosis	I was previously well but am now seriously ill
Second stage	The names of the drugs used in treatment, how they are given, and their side effects	Parents being informed that child is in remission, child speaking to other children at clinic	I am seriously ill and will get better
Third stage	Purposes of special procedures and additional treatments consequent to the side effects of therapy, and the relationship between particular symptoms and procedures	The first relapse	I am always ill and will get better
Fourth stage	A larger perspective of the disease as an endless series of relapses and remissions	Several further relapses and remissions	I am always ill and will never get better
Fifth stage	The disease as a series of relapses and remissions, ending in death	Child learns of the death of an ill peer	I am dying

Adapted from ref. 22.

awareness of their prognosis, as inferred from their imaginative stories, and the parents' beliefs about their child's awareness. Only two of the 16 fatally ill children had discussed their concerns about death with their parents, yet 63 per cent of stories told by these children related to death. The children often gave the characters in the stories their own diagnoses and symptoms; they frequently depicted death in their drawings and occasionally they would express awareness of their prognoses to persons outside their immediate family. Waechter concluded that denial and protectiveness by adults may not be entirely effective in preventing these children from experiencing anxiety or in keeping their diagnosis and probable prognosis from them. She recommended that the child's questions and concerns should be dealt with in a way that did not further alienate and isolate the child from the parents and other meaningful adults.

In the early 1970s, Myra Bluebond-Langner, an anthropologist, confirmed and extended Waechter's research by conducting detailed, long-term observations of leukaemic children, their parents, and the various health professionals caring for them in the haematology/oncology clinic and ward of an American hospital. Her observations and conclusions, published in 1978[22], together with those of Waechter, have been pivotal in changing the establishment's views on how to work most effectively with dying children.

Stages of acquisition of factual information about the disease (Bluebond-Langner)

Although parents and staff provided little or no information to the child about any aspect of the illness in the hope of lessening his or her anxiety, it was found that over time such children acquired information about their disease in five stages and that particular experiences were critical to passage through these stages. As the children passed through these stages, they also passed through five different definitions of themselves (Table 13.4.3).

The children's personal experiences were a much more significant determinant than age or intellectual ability in determining concepts of their sickness. Thus a 3- or 4-year-old child might know more about his or her prognosis than a very intelligent 9-year-old child.

Mutual pretence

Bluebond-Langner's research confirmed that not only did terminally ill children know they were dying before death became imminent, but they also kept such knowledge a secret, mainly to avoid upsetting their parents and to lessen the probability of being abandoned by loved ones or caregivers because of the anxieties that such disclosures might cause in the latter. Instead, the children, together with their parents and the caregivers, practised an elaborate ritual of mutual pretence, in which all parties defined the patient as dying but acted as if the patient was going to live (Table 13.4.4).

Interestingly, in the children studied by Bluebond-Langner, breaches in these rules did not lead to open awareness. Mutual pretence remained the dominant mode of interaction in all children studied, who practised it to the end.

Many patients practise mutual pretence because they find it the most comfortable way to relate to many staff members in the treatment team. The important thing is to be aware that it exists and that it is not a suitable medium for honest communication.

Table 13.4.4 Rules for practice of mutual pretence[a].

1. All parties to the interaction should avoid dangerous topics
2. Talk about dangerous topics is permissible as long as neither party breaks down
3. All parties to the interaction should focus on safe topics and activities
4. Props should be used to sustain the 'crucial illusion'
5. When something happens, or is said which tends to expose the fiction that both parties are attempting to sustain, then each must pretend that nothing has gone awry
6. All parties to the interaction must strive to keep the interaction normal
7. All parties must strive to keep the interaction brief
8. When the rules become impossible to follow and the breakdown of mutual pretence appears imminent, avoid or terminate the interaction

[a] Dying children, their parents, and caregivers are observed to adhere to these rules when practising mutual pretence.

Data from refs. 22 and 25.

Other research on sick children's concepts of death, illness, and isolation

An evaluation of anxiety and withdrawal in children aged between 6 and 10 years who were terminally ill with leukaemia was conducted in 1974[26,27]. It was found that they appeared to be aware of the seriousness of their illness (even though they might not be yet capable of talking about this awareness in adult terms), expressed more anxiety than controls and, of greater concern, perceived a growing psychological distance from those around them.

A later study[28] of concepts of death, illness, and isolation in 21 children with leukaemia aged between 4 and 9 years, conducted in 1988 in the United Kingdom, found no indications that the sick children interviewed had radically different concepts of death than have been shown by healthy children. Some of the perceptions of the sick children about themselves in hospital were worrying. The children's feelings of being alone, even with ample company, suggested deprivation of another sort. There was a large variation in the concept of death among individual children, particularly in those younger than eight years.

The family's culture and environment and the child's concept of death

Little information is yet available to indicate how a child's concept of death will be affected by the family's culture and environment. However, there is a recurrent theme in the death literature that the way in which parents and others discuss death within the family will have a significant effect on the child's developing concept. Virtually all the literature encourages openness, honesty, and opportunity for the child to talk about the subject. Some cultures, for example that of the Lebanese, are rich in mourning rituals but have a closed attitude to discussion of death. It is not yet known how Lebanese children who attend a relative's funeral or who are seriously ill themselves deal with the sudden massive displays of emotion that they witness without the benefit of discussion with other members of the family.

Guidelines for working with the dying child

Clearly, seriously ill and dying children are much more aware of their illness and prognosis than it is comfortable to acknowledge. They are known to harbour anxiety about their situation and are helped by the provision of age-appropriate information. Equipped with this knowledge, the caregiver certainly can be more attentive to the child's verbal and non-verbal communications and seek, where possible, to lessen the child's anxiety.

The emotional needs of the dying child are as follows:

- Those of all children regardless of health.
- Those arising from the child's reaction to illness and admission to hospital.
- Those arising from the child's concept of death.

The following guidelines[29] can be used to help seriously ill children communicate the inner experiences related to their illness:

1   Before proceeding with communication, ascertain the child's own perception of the situation, taking into account his or her developmental level and experience.

2   Understand the child's symbolic language. Children often experience emotions without being able to put them into concepts or words and young children can use symbolic language to communicate their worries.

3   Clarify reality and dispel fantasy. Children often have difficulty distinguishing between reality and fantasy and between actions and thoughts. A common fantasy of sick children is that of being responsible for the illness. Thus, admission to hospital and medical procedures are interpreted as punishment.

4   Encourage the expression of feelings. When children are allowed to express their anger, sadness, and anxiety, they are able to examine these feelings, place them in perspective and gain control over them.

5   Promote self-esteem through mastery. The self-esteem of the child with cancer is threatened by pain, frustration, deprivation, changes in body image, and the possibility of death. As a result, his or her school attendance and peer relationships may both suffer. School is the ideal setting in which to encourage the child to communicate about his or her illness in a way that will promote self-esteem through mastery.

6   When approaching the child with cancer, make no assumptions about what the situation will entail. Be open to what each encounter can teach. Do not underestimate the child's ability to master life's challenges creatively and with humour and dignity.

A child who asks 'Am I going to die?' has already picked the person to ask. The wisest and best response is to be honest and confirm that such is the case. How one replies and the words one uses will vary greatly because the details of each child's situation and management and the relationship with the caregiver asked the question, make every case unique. The important thing is to be honest, confirm that the answer to the question is 'yes' and stay with the child to deal with whatever specific concerns he or she may mention next. Like adults, children are concerned that they will be comfortable, safe, and not alone.

Recommendations for caregivers working with a terminally ill child are referred to in Table 13.4.1.

Methods of assessing children's psychological adaptation

Art therapy and music therapy are both forms of expressive therapy that can be used for effective communication by the child. Both can also be used as effective measures of the child's psychological adaptation.

Art therapy

Children are natural artists and can express themselves with few inhibitions. The child's art may communicate what words cannot. While the therapist needs to understand the images produced by children, interpretations of their work are most reliable when provided by the children themselves.

Art therapy can be used to rechannel acting-out behaviour and aggression, provide periods of normality in the midst of frequent examinations, tests and treatments, and provide opportunity for the children's expressions of creativity. Group art therapy provides opportunities for socializing and communication with peers and for countering feelings of withdrawal or isolation.

The art work of terminally ill children has been found to share common features and to follow particular trends. Objects and forms tend to move towards the upper left quadrant of a page as death approaches. An unusual treatment of a body area has corresponded to new areas of disease unsuspected by the medical staff. Pictures depicting extreme weather conditions have been noted frequently in the art work of terminally ill children: clouds, heavy rain, or snow (often with a brightly shining sun nearby) are said to indicate feelings of anxiety or of being overwhelmed. There may also be a decreased selection of bright colours as the disease progresses, reflecting decreased physical stamina and emotional energy. The interested reader is referred to a report[30] for a more detailed account of this useful medium for communication and assessment.

Music therapy

Music therapy is also effective in uncovering and working through fears and anxieties related to death and mourning, and it offers the opportunity for creative acts. As illustrated by the case histories of one therapist working with children terminally ill with cancer[31], music therapy may energize or relax, promote thought or distract, and provide an opportunity for expression. A variety of music therapy techniques, including song writing and selection, lyric substitution, improvization, and guided imagery, can all be used to encourage the child to release his or her fears through a creative act. Music may facilitate a therapeutic relationship, which in turn may supply the security and trust that enables the child to let go of his or her fears. Concerns that are too threatening to be talked about openly can be expressed indirectly during music-therapy activities.

Fortunately, the use of music therapy in paediatric settings, previously confined largely to the United States, is finding application and acceptance more recently in numerous countries.

Books about death for adults and children

There is a wide variety of books dealing with death in both fiction and non-fiction for children and parents, including such well-known works as *Little Women* by L.M. Alcott and *Charlotte's Web* by E.B. White. There is some difference of opinion about the usefulness of such material for working with children[32–35]. Such books are useful when they assist parents or health professionals in explaining aspects of death to a questioning child, particularly when they allow a dialogue on the subject to develop between parent and child. Lists of recommended titles for adults and children appear in Tables 13.4.5 and 13.4.6.

The terminally ill child at school

As a result of their illness, children with cancer will have acquired concepts and experiences of pain, loss, and grief, which will have changed them and will distinguish them from their peers. Children who receive treatment for cancer encounter a loss of self-esteem. Their unusual situation requires them to deal with new and significant issues, occasionally with some anxiety, so that they may have less attention and energy for the day-to-day matters of school. They will be less assertive. They will be more reluctant than their healthy peers to attempt new concepts in which failure is possible because of the risk of losing more self-esteem through failure. Schooling for these children should always start out from areas and levels of competence in which they feel absolutely comfortable.

Table 13.4.5 Books for adults about death.

Adams, D.W. (1979). *Childhood malignancy: The psychosocial care of the child and his family*. Charles C. Thomas, Springfield, IL

Adams, D.W. and Deveau, E.J. (1993). *Coping with childhood cancer—Where do we go from here?* 3rd edition.: Kinbridge Publications, Hamilton, Ontario

Deitrick, R. and Armstrong-Dailey, A. *Approaching grief* (pamphlet), Children's Hospice International, Washington, DC

Grollman, E.A. (1976). *Talking about death: A dialogue between parent and child*. Beacon Press, Boston, MA

Martinson, I.M. (1976). *Home care for the dying child: Professional and family perspectives*. Appleton-Century-Crofts, New York

Miles, M.S. *The grief of parents*. Privately printed 1978. Available from Compassionate Friends Inc., IL

Schiff, H.S. (1977). *The bereaved parent*. Crown Publishers, New York

Schulman, J.L. (1976). *Coping with tragedy: Successfully facing the problem of a seriously ill child*. Follett Publishing, Chicago

Sherman, M. (1976). *The leukemic child*. US Department of Health, Education & Welfare, Washington, DC, Publication No. (NIH) 76–863

Stephens, S. (1973). *Death comes home*. Morehouse-Barlow, New York

Wass, H. and Corr, C.A. (ed.). (1984). *Helping children cope with death: Guidelines and resources*, 2nd edition. Hemisphere, Washington, DC

Wells, R. *Helping children cope with grief—Facing a death in the family*. Sheldon Press, London

Zagdanski, D. (1990). *Something I've never felt before—How teenagers cope with grief*. Hill of Content Press, Melbourne

Children who are terminally ill with cancer may continue to receive treatment and in many cases will remain well enough to attend school for many months. Even though they may be in an advanced stage of their disease, it is very important for their self-esteem and sense of mastery over a deteriorating situation to continue to attend school when they wish to, if only for a few hours a day.

An explanation to the class about the child's illness will have been given by a member of the treatment team earlier in the course of the illness, usually soon after the diagnosis. At the outset, classmates are most frequently concerned about whether or not they can catch the disease from the patient.

In the event of the child becoming terminally ill, the child's teacher will have to confront and deal with the impending death of

Table 13.4.6 Books for children about death.

Alcott, L.M. (1968). *Little women*. Little, Brown, Boston.

Alex, M. and Alex, B. (1981). *Grandpa and me*. Lion Publishing, Hertford, UK

Bernstein, J.E. and Gullo, S.V. (1977). *When people die*. E. P. Dutton, New York

Fassler, J. (1971). *My grandpa died today*. Human Sciences Press, New York

Grollman, E.A. (1976). *Talking about death—A dialogue between parent and child*. Beacon Press, Boston, MA

White, E.B. (1952). *Charlotte's web*. Harper & Row, New York

Zim, H. and Bleeker, S. (1970). *Life and death*. William Morrow, New York the child and the resulting effects on the classmates, other teachers, and students at the school. Under these circumstances, it is wise to have made some preparation beforehand. Discussion at a staff meeting might take place involving other teachers and the principal to examine their attitudes to death and dying. This would assist staff to formulate an appropriate plan that the child's teacher could then implement with the class. The teacher should also confer with the child's parents, who need to be involved in these plans.

The child's treatment team, particularly the hospital school teacher, will liaise with the school and the child's school teachers to maximize his or her educational opportunities. Terminally ill children may wish to be included and need to be treated as normally as possible. A bean chair or similar comfortable support in the corner of the classroom close to the focus of interest may enable such children to enjoy many hours of satisfaction, even though they may not be able to participate actively in all lessons. Deterioration is usually gradual and death is not expected to occur suddenly or unexpectedly, for example, during class. If the terminally ill student deteriorated rapidly or collapsed unexpectedly, there still would be sufficient time to take him or her home or to hospital with the parents and family.

Saying goodbye: the child's preparation for death

Children who are seriously or terminally ill will usually take steps to put their affairs in order. During her preparation for a mismatched bone marrow transplant, one of the author's patients completed tapestries bearing personal notes of thanks for the author and another doctor. These were presented after her death by her parents, who reported that she had discussed her funeral with her friends, requesting that her two closest girlfriends sing a favoured hymn.

Another patient, a teenage boy dying of progressive non-Hodgkin's lymphoma, summoned all the ward staff to his room to say goodbye to each. Later, with many of his friends present, he bequeathed one of his possessions to each, including his most cherished possession, a CB radio.

The following example from the author's department provides even more striking evidence of preparation for and acceptance of imminent death.

Case history

Patient A had acute non-lymphoblastic leukaemia diagnosed at age 13. Following relapse 18 months later, she proceeded to a mismatched bone marrow transplant 3 months after relapse, with her mother as the donor. Patient A died 5 weeks after the transplant.

A's mother reported that during her last few months, A spoke more about the possibility of death and of the need to plan for the disposal of her material possessions. After her relapse she frequently spoke of not wanting to die, mainly confiding her thoughts to her mother. She attended three healing masses and was noted to have fewer periods of depression afterwards. One of the pages from her notebook on which she recorded her observations of what she thought death would be like, is reproduced with the family's permission in Fig. 13.4.2.

A's mother reported A's great self-control as she planned for the possibility of not surviving the transplant. She asked that the family have a holiday together before the transplant, she asked if she owned her bedroom furniture and her piano and about her right to make a will. Those attending her funeral were to wear bright colours. The service was to be held in her school chapel and the madrigal group of which she was a member was to sing a favourite hymn. A nominated a white coffin, named the clothing for her burial ('not a nightie, under any circumstances') and asked that a family photograph, a Bible, and her rosary beads be placed in her coffin. She purchased a remembrance gift for her parents and wrote them a personal letter. She recorded herself playing a special piece of music on the piano. She asked her parents not to remain sad, to be kind, and loving to each other and always to stay together.

These examples show that dying children may respond in a manner well beyond their years.

The dying child's premonition of imminent death

Terminally ill children often know when they are about to die and may even share this information with their parents.

One of the author's patients, a 9-year-old boy, died suddenly, shortly after the abrupt onset of severe interstitial pneumonitis, eight months after bone marrow transplant. His family owned one of a number of shops clustered in a marina and their son was well known to the other tenants. After he had died, the parents learnt that he had spent time chatting with each and every tenant in the marina, on the day before his death.

Another of the author's patients, a 5-year-old boy with terminal acute lymphoblastic leukaemia, died at home. On the night he died, he came into his parents' bedroom. He explained that he did not quite know what to say to them and, instead, sang a familiar children's song, *Sing a Rainbow*.

Needing permission to die

Young people who are dying may linger close to death for prolonged periods. They may simply need permission from their loved ones to die and will often die promptly when such permission is given. One of the author's patients, an 11-year-old boy with osteogenic sarcoma, was dying at home after a 5-year illness. Throughout his illness, he had demonstrated a notable tenacity to survive and willingness to endure continuing and painful treatment as long as it entailed some hope for further quality survival. After his death, his father reported that as the boy's death drew close, he lingered on in a coma for more than 7 days. An Aboriginal community nurse who was caring for the patient spoke with his father, informing him that the boy needed his parents' permission to die. The father and mother ushered the boy's grandmother and other relatives out of his room, sat down alone by the boy's bed, spoke to him of their love for him and gave him their permission to die. The boy died peacefully a few hours later.

Future prospects in paediatric palliative care

One can anticipate ongoing studies on psychological aspects of death and dying in both well and sick children. The challenge for the caregiver will be to keep abreast of current thought and to respond to new principles of care as they become validated.

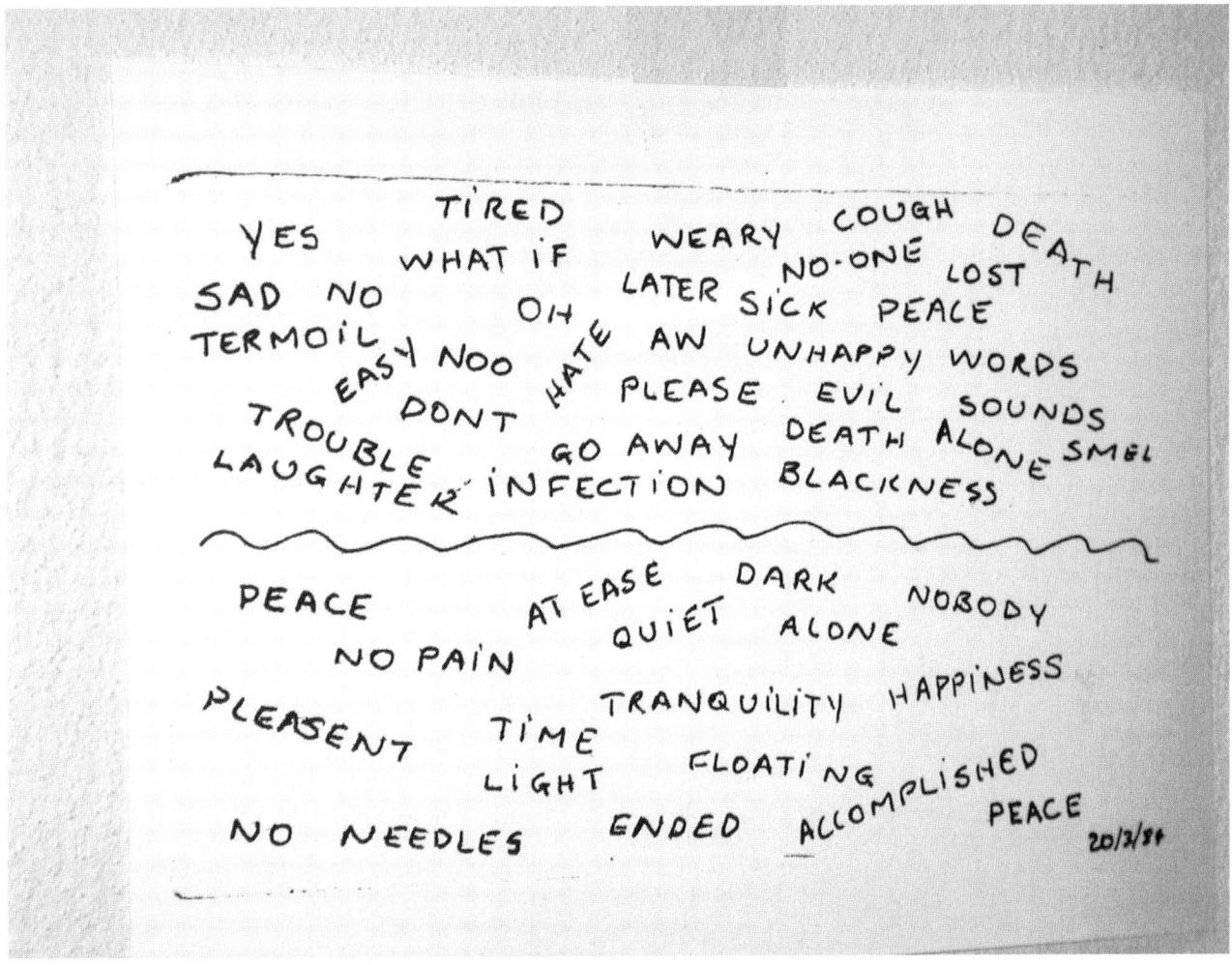

Figure 13.4.2 A page from A's notebook recording her own observations of what she thought death would be like (reproduced with her parents' permission).

Conclusion: implications for staff

Staff caring for terminally ill children face similar stresses to those confronted by the family. Because the family's outlook is greatly influenced by the personality and reactions of the staff, a special degree of maturity and caring is required. Staff should remember to recognize their own limitations and the importance of the support an inter-disciplinary team approach can offer. Staff should be realistic in the goals they set and use supports available to them. Regular periods of leave, and interests and commitments outside the work-place, will all help to ensure a continuing effective level of care to those in need.

It is often asked how one could work in such an emotionally charged field, to which the response (as most who work in this field will know) is that one enjoys the work and finds working with children such as these and their families rewarding, fascinating, frequently unpredictable, never boring, and always a privilege.

Further reading

Bearison, D.J. (2006). *When treatment fails: How medicine cares for dying children*. Oxford University Press, New York.

Corr, C.A. and Corr, D.M. (eds) (1985). *Hospice approaches to paediatric care*. Influential treatise on application of principles of palliative care to children, Springer, New York.

Foley, G.V. and Whittam, E.H. (1990). Care of the child dying of cancer: Part I. *CA—A Cancer Journal for Clinicians*, **40**, 327–54. Concise and valuable overview of paediatric palliative care.

Pettle, M.S.A. and Lansdown, R.G. (1986). Adjustment to the death of a sibling. *Archives of Disease in Childhood*, **61**, 278–83. Useful report of the experiences of siblings of a deceased child.

References

1. Piaget, J. and Inhelder, B. (1969). *The psychology of the child*. Translated from the French by Helen Weaver. Basic Books, New York.
2. Singer, D. and Revenson, T. (1978). *A Piaget primer: How a child thinks*. Universities Press, New York.
3. Rando, T.A. (1984). *Grief, dying and death: Clinical interventions for caregivers*, pp. 385–91. Research Press, Champaign, IL.
4. Wass, H. (1984). Concepts of death: A developmental perspective. In *Childhood and death* (eds. H. Wass and C.A. Corr). Hemisphere, Washington, DC.
5. Nagy, M. (1948). The child's theories concerning death. *Journal of Genetic Psychology*, **73**, 3–27.

6. Anthony, S. (1972). *The discovery of death in childhood and after.* Basic Books, New York.

7. Kane, B. (1979). Children's concepts of death. *Journal of Genetic Psychology,* **134,** 41–53.

8. Speece, M.W. and Brent, S.B. (1984). Children's understanding of death: A review of three components of a death concept. *Child Development,* **55,** 1671–86.

9. Lansdown, R. and Benjamin, G. (1985). The development of the concept of death in children aged 5–9 years. *Child: Care, Health and Development,* **11,** 13–20.

10. Schonfeld, D. (1989). Crisis intervention for bereavement support: A model of intervention in the children's school. *Clinical Pediatrics,* **28,** 29.

11. Schonfeld, D.J. and Kappelman, M. (1990). The impact of school-based education on the young child's understanding of death. *Developmental and Behavioural Pediatrics,* **11,** 247–52.

12. Wass, H. and Cason, L. (1984). Fears and anxieties about death. In *Childhood and death* (eds. H. Wass and C.A. Corr), pp. 25–45. Hemisphere, Washington, DC.

13. Anthony, S. (1972). *The discovery of death in childhood and after,* pp. 163–5. Basic Books, New York.

14. McNeil, J. (1983). Young mothers' communication about death with their children. *Death Education,* **6,** 323–39.

15. Knudson, A.G. and Natterson, J.M. (1960). Participation of parents in the hospital care of their fatally ill children. *Pediatrics,* **26,** 482–90.

16. Morrissey, J.R. (1965). Death anxiety in children with a fatal illness. In *Crisis intervention* (ed. H.J. Parad), pp. 324–38. Family Service Association of America, New York.

17. Natterson, J.M. and Knudson, A.G. (1960). Observations concerning fear of death in fatally ill children and their mothers. *Psychosomatic Medicine,* **22,** 456–65.

18. Richmond, J.B. and Waisman, H.A.(1955). Psychologic aspects of management of children with malignant diseases. *American Journal of Diseases in Childhood,* **89,** 42–7.

19. Vernick, J. and Karon, M. (1965). Who's afraid of death on a leukemia ward? *American Journal of Diseases of Children,* **109,** 393–7.

20. Karon, M. and Vernick, J. (1968). An approach to the emotional support of fatally ill children. *Clinical Pediatrics,* **7,** 274–80.

21. Waechter, E.H. (1971). Children's awareness of fatal illness. *American Journal of Nursing,* **71,** 1168–72.

22. Bluebond-Langner, M. (1978). *The private worlds of dying children.* Princeton University Press, Princeton, NJ.

23. Sarason, S.B. *et al.* (1960). *Anxiety in elementary school children.* Wiley, New York.

24. Murray, H.A. (1943). *Thermatic apperception test.* Harvard University Press, Cambridge, MA.

25. Glaser, B. and Strauss, A. (1965). *Awareness of dying: A study of social interaction.* Aldine, Chicago.

26. Spinetta, J.J., Rigler, D., and Karon, M. (1974). Personal space as a measure of a dying child's sense of isolation. *Journal of Consulting and Clinical Psychology,* **42,** 751–6.

27. Spinetta, J.J., Rigler, D., and Karon, M. (1973). Anxiety in the dying child. *Pediatrics,* **52,** 841–5.

28. Clunies-Ross, C. and Lansdown, R. (1988). Concepts of death, illness and isolation found in children with leukaemia. *Child: Care, Health and Development,* **14,** 373–86.

29. Adams-Greenly, M. (1984). Helping children communicate about serious illness and death. *Journal of Psychosocial Oncology,* **2**(2), 61–72.

30. Schmitt, B.B. and Guzzino, M.H. (1985). Expressive therapy with children in crisis: A new avenue of communication. In *Hospice approaches to paediatric care* (eds. C.A. Corr and D.M. Corr), pp. 155–77. Springer, New York.

31. Fagen, T.S. (1982). Music therapy in the treatment of anxiety and fear in terminal paediatric patients. *Music Therapy. Journal of the American Association for Music Therapy,* **2,** 13–23.

32. Corr, C.A. (1984). Books for adults. *In Childhood and death* (eds. H. Wass and C.A. Corr), pp. 367–71. Hemisphere Publishing Corporation, Washington, DC.

33. Wass, H. (1984). Books for children. In *Childhood and death,* (eds. H. Wass and C.A. Corr), pp. 373–6. Hemisphere Publishing Corporation, Washington, DC.

34. Lamers, E. (1986). Books for adolescents. In *Adolescence and death* (eds. C.A. Corr and J.N. McNeil), pp. 233–42. Springer, New York.

35. Aradire, C. (1976). Books for children about death. *Pediatrics,* **57,** 372.

13.5

Bereavement issues and staff support

Betty Davies and Stacy Orloff

Bereavement: significance of the concept

Most children in developing countries die of infectious diseases; those in the more developed countries, because of advances in medical technology and delivery of health care, most often die of trauma. For toddlers and older children, unintentional injuries are the leading causes of death accounting for 36 per cent of deaths in the 1–4 age group, 42 per cent in the 5–9 and 10–14 age groups and even higher among older adolescents. However, the leading cause of death varies according to age, with most children dying in the first year of life than in all other years combined and two-thirds of these occurring in the neonatal period from disorders related to congenital abnormalities and prematurity [1]. Despite such scientific progress, however, children continue to die of incurable disease such as cancer, congenital anomalies, and genetic defects. Though sometimes difficult to admit, the end result of the paediatric palliative care experience is the death of a child. A child's death is considered a greater loss because the child has not had the opportunity to live a full life as compared to the adult or aged individual; a child's death confounds our expectation that children will grow into adulthood and live a normal lifespan. A child's death confounds our hope that this child may be the one who recovers. All concerned—the parents, the child, siblings, grandparents, the physician, and the other professionals involved in the care—face difficulties in acknowledging the death of a child. A child's death evokes in each one of us the 'inner bereaved child'; it reawakens those painful and repressed effects of separation and loss from our earliest development and makes for a rapid withdrawal from the pain involved. The purpose of this chapter is to bridge the gap between theory and practice and to offer some practical suggestions to assist parents and siblings following the death of a child from a life limiting illness or condition, health-care professionals with this emotion-filled experience, and the greater community that is affected by the death of the child.

Death of a child: impact on the family

The family provides for its members the necessary relationships, both in quality and intensity, out of which normal growth and development occur. Because of these relationships, the system behaves, not as a simple composition of independent elements, but coherently and inseparably as a whole. Following this perspective, illness or death in any family member is a potential assault on the family system. The death of a child, therefore, affects not only individual family members, but also the family unit as a whole.

Empty space

The death of a child creates an empty space for surviving family members, a sense in the family that there is always something missing [2]. Interviews with 49 families, 7–9 years after a death from childhood cancer, suggested that three patterns of grieving characterized family members' responses to this sense of emptiness: getting over it, filling the emptiness, and keeping the connection. Those families who placed emphasis on getting over the grief tended to have a somewhat concrete plan for putting the death of the child behind them. They accepted the death matter of factly as either God's will or as something we all have to face. The second group of families filled the empty space by keeping busy (e.g. building a new house) or by substituting other problems or situations to take their mind off their grief. They acknowledged the emptiness, but made an effort to fill up the space with activities. The largest number of families accepted the empty space though they tried never to forget or become very busy. They acknowledged the empty space, allowed it to exist, treasured their remaining children more and valued life in general.

No pattern of grieving is suggested as superior to the others. The patterns only serve to emphasize that grief, for any family or family member, should not be expected to follow a specific path within specified time limits. Additional findings from this same study reported that the child's death requires individual reorganization and adjustments within the family system [3]. Changes in marital status and or the addition of other children required adjustments in the relationships of family members. Some changes were developmental in nature while others, according to the informants, were directly related to the death of the child. Regardless of the changes, however, a child's death is perceived as a significant event, a reference point to which all subsequent events can be related.

Levels of functioning

When a child dies, all aspects of family life are altered. How the family responds to and incorporates those changes are critical for all family members. Even before their child dies, families have characteristic ways of being in the world, responding to stress, sharing thoughts and feelings, and interacting with the external world.

When a child is ill and dies, these characteristic ways of coping come into play. These coping strategies are more or less functional and help health-care providers to understand the variability in family response[4,5].

Communicating openly

Some families communicate freely in discussing the child's illness, death, and family members' responses following the death. Such discussion occurs in the presence of other family members and all persons are allowed to express their own thoughts and feelings. Each member of the family offers a similar version of a story; there is an underlying sense of coherence among family members. Other families are more closed in that they do not have this freedom of expression. There may be considerable talk, but it is not focused on the questions being asked. Communication is limited or guarded; family members seem less connected to one another.

Dealing with feelings

Some families focus not only on events, but also on the thoughts and feelings associated with such events. As a result, they are more aware of the process; this awareness leads to action. The opposite is true for other families who are less able to focus on feelings and to anticipate potentially difficult occasions, such as special holidays, and consequently became stuck in their sadness.

Defining roles

Some families are more flexible in assuming new roles while acknowledging that no one could take the place of the child who died. Each family member is valued for himself and is perceived as an integral member of the group. In other families, roles are rigidly maintained; surviving siblings may be expected to fill the vacated role of 'older' child, or 'responsible' child, for example.

Utilizing resources

More functional families use a wide range of resources, accepting their vulnerabilities and their need for support. They seek out and request support from a variety of sources, and often express gratitude and satisfaction with the assistance they receive. Less functional families withdraw from sources of support, claiming that they are able to manage 'on their own' and sometimes denying the extent of their grief. They seem unable to communicate what their needs are, or what they want. Any assistance comes from formal sources rather than from informal networks of friends and family. They often feel angry and resentful due to their unfulfilled expectations.

Solving problems

Some families identify problems or difficulties as they occur, openly exchange information about the situation and develop strategies for dealing with the problem. Input is sought from all family members and others and creative solutions are developed. Other families approach problems by focusing on why the problem occurred and on who was at fault, rather than on generating solutions. There is little sense that change is occurring.

Incorporating change

All families struggle with incorporating the past into the present; it takes considerable effort to incorporate the changes associated with the loss of a loved one. Some families are able to reflect on this process, and identify ways in which they can be accommodating to the changes. Other families are resistant to reorganization; they seem static, lamenting that they will 'never be the same', and often feeling stuck at being sad, depressed, angry, or resentful.

Assessing a family for ways of coping provides some direction for assisting grieving families. For example, in families where communication is closed, health-care providers must make an effort to share information with all family members instead of relying on one member to convey the information to the others. In families where anger and sadness prevail, health-care providers must spend additional time listening to the distress and the perceived causes of the situation, while gently encouraging broader perspectives and insights. Most importantly, awareness of levels of family functioning helps care providers understand that different families cope in different ways. The goal is not to 'fix' families but to understand them and support them as much as possible.

Parental grief

The loss of a child through death is quite unlike any other loss known. In comparison with other individuals in different role relationships to the deceased (e.g. spouse, sibling, and child), the grief of parents is more intense, more complex, and longer lasting[6,7]. When a child dies, the parents feel each day as grey, hollow, empty; each day is a burden. Parents feel overwhelmed with feelings of anger, depression, uncontrollable tears, hopelessness, frustration, and fear for their remaining children. Parents can be reassured that the psychosomatic symptoms they experience are not congruent with mental illness. This reassurance is underscored by a study of parents two years after their child had died from cancer[8]. These parents presented a profile on a symptom checklist (Symptom Checklist 90—Revised) that was significantly different to the normal non-clinical and psychiatric outpatient group. This suggests that these bereaved mothers and fathers display a psychological pattern that is more symptomatic than normal, but less symptomatic than diagnosed outpatients. Despite the recognition of parental grief as an intensely difficult psychological experience, relatively few researchers have empirically addressed this issue. Study samples vary widely in composition and results have been contradictory. Four types of factors potentially related to bereavement outcome have been identified:

1 Demographic factors.

2 Factors related to parents' premorbid personalities or experiences.

3 Factors related to the child's hospitalization or death.

4 Post-death factors[9].

It is also very important to note that most of this research has traditionally focused on mothers' grief. However, research on fathers of severely ill children has not been the focus of many investigations. When fathers are included they are often grouped with mothers in studies where the majority of participants are mothers, or the number of fathers from which results are drawn is very low. Consequently, relatively little is known about fathers' unique experiences of having a child with life-limiting illness who dies. This significant knowledge gap limits our understanding of fathers, often resulting in stereotypical views about fathers. That is, fathers are commonly seen as less involved in their ill child's care, considered to be less emotional, grieve less intensely, and show less distress by the loss of their child when compared to mothers[10,11]. A pilot study of fathers' experiences of a child's life-limiting illness suggested that fathers are very involved in the care of their children, their grief is both profound and individually varied with some fathers showing strong emotions, while others are less expressively emotional, yet their suffering is immense[12]. Sadly, bereaved fathers reported feeling devalued by the health-care professionals who cared for their dying children. Moreover, cultural values, beliefs, and practices of all family members play a central role in how families respond to having a seriously ill child[13]. The influence of culture on families' experience of paediatric palliative care is an issue we can no longer afford to ignore, given our society's increasing ethnic and cultural diversity.

Duration and intensity of grief

It has often been assumed that the pain of grief decreases with the passing of time. However, some studies[9,14–16] report that parents who had been grieving for longer than 2 years reported similar patterns to parents who had experienced a loss within the past 2 years and that parental grief appears to remain fairly intense for at least four years. These findings concur with more recent conceptualizations of grief as an active process that occurs over time[17] rather than as an event from which individuals 'recover'. Additional research also highlights an optimal time frame for a child's terminal illness as it relates to the parents' grief experience. Parents whose children died between 6 and 18 months after diagnosis seemed to be the most prepared for the death and had a better adjustment in the bereavement process[18] than those whose child lived for more than 18 months after diagnosis.

Survival guilt

The unique difficulties inherent in the loss of a child stem from the view that the death of a child is not only inappropriate in the context of living, but its tragic and untimely nature is also a basic threat to the function of parenthood. Parents feel victimized by the loss of their child, by the loss of their hopes and dreams, and by their own loss of self-esteem because they feel they have failed as parents in protecting their child. This victimization is sometimes referred to as survival guilt[19]. This phenomenon lends evidence as to why coming to terms with their loss may be a difficult task and why bereaved parents face so many more difficulties than other bereaved individuals. Thoughts of suicide, self-accusations, inconsolable grief, and withdrawal from family and friends are common parental reactions to the loss.

Complicated grief

The experience of parental grief is profound, affected by a myriad of factors that predispose parents to be exceptionally vulnerable to complicated or unresolved grief. Complicated bereavement is characterized by an inability to adapt to the loss and bring grieving to a satisfactory conclusion[20]. Research into the elements of complicated parental bereavement has been limited. It is

inappropriate, therefore, to evaluate parental bereavement with traditional criteria. A new model of parental mourning must be developed. Until such a model is developed, the following behaviours remain the most useful for the clinician in assessing complicated bereavement. These behaviours, displayed years after the actual death, include, but are not limited to, maintaining the dead child's environment just as it was at the time of death, developing physical symptoms similar to those of the deceased, feeling unacceptable, and intense sadness at various anniversary times, being unable to talk about the deceased child without intense reactivation of the feelings experienced at the time of the death[21].

The marital dyad

Parents as individuals are affected by the death of their child; the marital dyad is also affected. Mothers and fathers may deal differently with expression of feelings, working, and doing daily activities, relating to things that trigger memories of the deceased child and searching for meaning in what has happened. One of the most difficult aspects of parental bereavement is that the death of a child strikes both partners in the marital dyad simultaneously and confronts them with the same overwhelming loss. Consequently, each partner's primary and most therapeutic source of support is taken away. The person to whom each would turn for support is confronting and working through his or her own grief.

Divorce

A common occurrence is that one spouse may misinterpret the behaviour of the other. The erroneous assumption that because partners suffer the same loss, they will experience the same grief, may set up unrealistic expectations that most likely will not be met. The expectation of going through the entire crisis together is often thwarted for bereaved parents. This in itself constitutes a loss for the couple as they may have been accustomed to pulling together through crises. When combined with other factors, this loss places additional burdens of grief, loss, and demands for adaptation on already over-burdened individuals. Such reactions have led to the assertion that there may be higher divorce rates in bereaved couples. However, the assumption that parental loss of a child invariably destroys the marital relationship is an erroneous interpretation of early research findings; these reports have failed to take into account normal divorce rates and longitudinal designs. Several studies[22–24] suggest that while stresses of childhood illness and subsequent death of the child are exceptionally high, and may exacerbate pre-existing marital discord, family relationships do not automatically have to be disrupted and end in divorce. In one study[3] of 56 families 7 to 9 years following a child's death from cancer, nine couples were divorced. Four of the nine divorced couples stated that the death of the child was a major factor contributing to their divorce. The other five couples did not attribute the divorce to the child's death but viewed it as a result of other problems that existed before the child was diagnosed with cancer.

Intimacy

The lack of synchronicity in grieving styles and grief experiences commonly results in dissimilar expectations and coping strategies. Husbands and wives may deal differently with expression of feelings, working, and doing daily activities, relating to things that trigger memories of the deceased and searching for the meaning of what has happened. One problem discussed frequently is the inhibition of sexual response and intimacy in bereaved parents. This area of difficulty may be the result of fear related to having and losing other children or guilt over experiencing pleasure. It may also be a symptom of grief or depression experienced by one partner or both partners[25]. Fathers, uncomfortable in communicating feelings verbally, may use sexual intimacy as a means of seeking comfort from their partners. It is not uncommon for the couple to sustain some sexual difficulties for up to 2 years following a child's death because of disinterest or grief-related symptomatology in one partner or both partners. In fact, in one cross-sectional study of 54 bereaved parents[26], the response pattern was characterized by a decrease in intensity of the grief experience in the second year following the child's death, followed by an increase in intensity in the third year. Mothers tended to exhibit more intense grief experiences and poorer subsequent adjustment than fathers. Parental bereavement may intensify rather than decline, over time.

Search for meaning

The death of a child is so profound that it ultimately sends bereaved parents into a deep and painful existential 'search for meaning' and this search may be a key factor in a positive 'growth' versus negative 'despair' resolution of the grief experience. Of the numerous comments made by 36 parents in one study[27], 40 responses indicated a positive outlook, whereas only 13 responses were negative. Positive growth responses included: learning to live each day to the fullest; being more understanding of others; having a stronger faith; being aware of the precariousness of life; and being a better person in general. Focusing on the potential for growth when a child has died is meant in no way to minimize the deep and long-lasting pain of grief; rather, it is meant to point out the importance of channelling the pain and rage into meaningful endeavours that can contribute to recovery.

Sibling grief

Paediatric palliative care is focused on families; this implies that health-care professionals must also pay attention to the needs of the siblings of children who die. The responses of children to the death of a sibling have not been extensively examined until recent years, yet to lose a brother or sister has potentially traumatic effects that last a lifetime. Davies[5] offers a comprehensive review of sibling bereavement research, with suggestions for interventions for children and the adults who care for them. She presents a model of sibling bereavement, which emphasizes that numerous variables must be taken into account when attempting to understand and assist grieving siblings. The model suggests that siblings exhibit four major responses to the death of a brother or sister: 'I hurt inside', 'I do not understand', 'I do not belong', and 'I am not enough'. The first two responses are similar to those most often described that focus on the behavioural/emotional reactions of children and the cognitive responses that result from children's developing understanding about death. Looking at the longer-term responses of siblings brought forth the additional two responses.

Sibling responses

'I hurt inside'

This response includes all the emotions typically associated with grief and the behavioural manifestations of such emotions in children. Siblings may exhibit a wide range of behavioural problems after the death of a brother or sister. Many studies, however, define the behavioural changes seen in bereaved children as problematic, if not even pathological, although positive responses also have been identified. Problems have included a range of behaviours, attitudes, emotions, symptoms, cognitions, and diagnoses (Table 13.5.1). Often ignored in children are psycho-physiological responses such as headaches, general aches and pains, stomach cramps, and disruptions in eating and sleeping patterns. These are common in grieving adults, so it is not surprising that grieving children experience them as well. Sleeping disturbances are common—children may not want to go to bed at night, especially if they shared a room with the deceased child; they may have bad dreams or nightmares, or walk in their sleep. Eating disturbances may include overeating or a loss of appetite. Anxiety may be evident and school performance may deteriorate. Children will frequently complain of loneliness. Some bereaved children also feel guilty for the death of their sibling even when they held no responsibility for the death.

Bereaved children's hurt derives from the vulnerability of being human, of feeling love for, and attachment to their brothers or sisters, so that when they are gone, siblings miss them. The other three responses derive from the vulnerability that children experience from being dependent on the adults in their lives. How adults interact with children determines the degree to which siblings feel that they do not understand, do not belong, or are not enough.

Table 13.5.1 Sibling responses to the death of a brother or sister from cancer[68].

Psychological
Fearful of own death and parents' death
Tearful
Anxiety (over people leaving, with new situations)
Loneliness
Angry outbursts or temper tantrums
Concerns about getting cancer
Attention-seeking from parents
Withdrawn (guarding feelings and thoughts)
Sadness
Daydreaming
Change in school performance (decreased concentration)
Physiological
Sleep disturbances (reluctant to go to bed, nightmares)
Eating disturbances (loss of appetite, lack of interest in food)
Bodily complaints (e.g. headaches, stomach aches, generalized aches)
Increased incidence of colds and influenza episodes
Frequent infections (urinary tract, respiratory tract)

'I do not understand'

This response is greatly influenced by a child's level of cognitive development. Younger children may not comprehend that their brother or sister is never coming back; they may not understand that death is forever. Children of all ages may be confused by the array of powerful feelings that surge within them; they may be mystified by the activity and reactions of others. They are confused and bewildered by all that is happening.

'I do not belong'

When children feel left out of what is happening, they feel as if they 'do not belong'. In the aftermath of a child's death, siblings often want to help, but do not know how; or, if they try to help, their efforts are not acknowledged or are even criticized. When children verbalize their natural curiosity in the form of questions and are ignored or told to be quiet, they get the message that they are inappropriate and they begin to feel as if they 'do not belong'. The reorganization of roles and responsibilities that accompany the death of any family member may leave the child feeling as if he has lost his place in the family. As well, bereaved children feel different from their non-bereaved peers and this too contributes to feelings of not belonging.

'I am not enough'

Siblings' feelings of 'I am not enough' arise from perceptions that they should have been the one to die since, in their view, the deceased child was the parents' favourite, or was the smartest, the prettiest, or the 'best' in some way[5,28]. Moreover, siblings see their parents' distress, and creatively attempt to lift their parents' spirits by behaving very well or by overachieving in school, for example. It is difficult for parents to manage their own grief; their personal resources are stretched to the limit, and their other children want their parents to 'get back to normal'. When parents continue to grieve, siblings may feel as if their efforts are in vain. They can feel they are not enough to make their parents happy ever again.

Influencing factors

The aforementioned responses do not occur in isolation but within a context of many interrelated variables. No one factor accounts for the total experience of any individual child. Three categories of factors come into play: individual, situational, and environmental. Individual factors include age, gender, temperament, and past experience with loss. For example, loss occurring at younger than 5 years of age or during early adolescence and the presence of pre-existing psychological difficulties are warning signs for children at risk.

Situational factors, such as the circumstances of the illness and death, affect sibling responses. For example, siblings who witness considerable pain and suffering in the ill child may be more troubled than siblings of children who die peacefully.

Environmental factors include the pre-death relationship between siblings. Siblings who shared close relationships with their brother or sister tend to demonstrate more internalizing behaviour after the death of the child. Emotional closeness between siblings exerts a stronger influence on bereavement outcome than closeness in age, length of illness, or number of surviving children in the family. Health-care professionals, therefore, need to be particularly sensitive to the needs of the children who shared a close relationship with their brother or sister. Environmental variables also include the social climate and functioning level of families and the social context of the family. For example, the greater the degree of commitment, help, and support family members provide for one another, the fewer withdrawing and acting out behaviour is reported for the bereaved children.[29] Furthermore, families with a greater emphasis on social, cultural, recreational, and religious involvement tended to have children with fewer behavioural problems following a sibling's death[5,29].

Intervening conditions and consequences

Davies' model emphasizes that intervening conditions either facilitate or constrain how siblings deal with their grief. The most significant conditions seem to be the ways in which adults interact with the siblings. When adults comfort those siblings who are hurting, teach those who do not understand, include siblings so they feel as if they belong and validate siblings' sense of worth, those children are more likely to have increased self-esteem and maturity, to be more sensitive and empathetic and better prepared to handle death. In contrast, when adults belittle children's expressions of hurt, disregard their questions and level of cognitive development, exclude them from day-to-day events and activities and shame them for not understanding, or for not responding as the adults expect, then the siblings are more likely to feel invisible, insecure, and insignificant. The impact of the death casts a dark shadow far into siblings' future[5].

Grandparent grief

Grandparent grief is often overlooked, both in the professional literature and in clinical practice. Grandparents frequently suffer a dual loss. Their hearts are filled with sadness while providing emotional support to their adult children and simultaneously mourning the loss of their grandchild. Bereaved grandparents often describe experiencing little familial support during this time. It may seem as though all the attention is on the bereaved parents and siblings. They feel as though their grief is disenfranchised; no one seems to acknowledge the loss they feel. Even when grandparents ask for emotional support many state they rarely feel they receive any from extended family members or the greater community. Bereaved grandparents often describe feeling a profound sense of helplessness. If possible, they would gladly 'change places' with their deceased grandchild. Providing clinical interventions, such as bereavement support groups, access to bibliotherapy, and individualized counselling is frequently helpful[30-34].

Summary

The death of a child has a potentially traumatic impact on the family. The death induces profound parental grief, which affects parents as individuals and as marital partners; the death alters the behaviour of siblings. From the literature reviewed, it can be concluded that the death of a child is not something to 'get over'. Instead, it is an event that surviving parents, siblings, and other family members must learn to integrate into the ongoing fabric of their lives. Only by understanding this to be the case, can health professionals offer the knowledgeable, sensitive, and long-term support that such families require.

Professional caregiver response

Helping a child die well, physically comfortable, psychologically and spiritually at peace; helping parents cope with the experience of their child's death as well as they possibly can; helping siblings and other children close to the dying child master the experience to the full potential of their developmental level—each of these is a challenge to health-care professionals, personally and professionally. Caregivers absorb much of the same stress experienced by the family members of a dying child and experience similar conflict. This stress, and the associated disruption, pressure, and depletion, requires significant personal and professional effort at adaptation and balance. Furthermore, the death of a child characteristically leads to a core conflict in persons caring for the child—a tendency to overprotect and become over-involved with the child and an opposing tendency to move away from the child to protect oneself from painful involvement.

Showing compassion

In order for those in caring professions to function effectively—to 'enjoy' being a good doctor, nurse, social worker/counsellor, clergyman or lawyer, professionals must allow themselves to approach, and to a degree share, the distress of those they are attempting to help[35,36]. They must show compassion. Yet, when confronted with a dying child, professionals are sometimes compelled to respond with analysis, clinical judgement, and 'doing' behaviours in an effort to maintain some sense of control and composure.

However, compassion and control seem incompatible. Professionals vary widely in the extent to which they can retain their compassion. Two things are crucial: the magnitude of the distress and the individual's own confidence in his or her ability to cope with it. As long as professionals feel that their participation is worthwhile, they will find themselves able to tolerate high levels of disturbance in others without disengaging. Confidence in one's ability to cope with the distress of others can be, and normally is, obtained by a process of attunement. By repeated, reflective exposure, professionals gradually discover what they can do to alleviate distress and how much of it is inevitable and insurmountable. Interdisciplinary teams can serve as a wonderful support for the health-care professional. Interdisciplinary teams provide health-care professionals a safe place in which to share their feelings and receive guidance—particularly when professional boundaries may be 'too close for comfort'.

Key attributes

Some health-care professionals are more suitable than others to the demanding role of working with dying children and adolescents[37,38]. Those who are best suited to this role have specific personal attributes, including a high tolerance for ambiguity, flexibility, and an appreciation for individual differences; good external support networks and a realistic awareness of personal limits; joie de vivre and sense of humour; an open communication style and tendency to value self-awareness as assets; and empathy and a willingness continually to learn[39,40]. Perhaps the most basic characteristic is one's comfort with death. Becoming a clinical practitioner who can move towards instead of away from children who are dying does not come easily. Only by coming to terms with one's own thoughts and feelings about death and about children, is it possible to adapt philosophically to working with children who might die. Self-awareness is integral to effective care of the dying; caregivers need to be conscious of their own agendas as they interface with patient, family, team, and institution directions and goals[41].

Health-care provider–family relationships

The duration of relationships with patients who have long-term, chronic illness provides health-care providers with both the opportunity and the obligation to establish relationships as persons as well as professionals. The nurse, counsellor, or physician may become a 'professional friend'. The relationship is a professional one—it is time limited, goal oriented, and patient centred with professional knowledge and skills employed on the patient's behalf[42]. However, the relationship may also assume some of the qualities usually described as part of a socially meaningful relationship. When the patient is a child, health-care providers often become professional friends, not only of the child, but also of the family. As the child enters the terminal phase, the closeness of the relationship may enhance personal and professional distress. Professional boundaries are almost always tested. One study[43] described the 'struggle' nurses experience while caring for children with chronic, life-limiting illness or condition who die. They struggled with grief but their expression of such distress was hampered by a code of conduct either self-imposed or imposed by their profession, their institution, or society in general. Nurses also struggled with moral distress when directives for painful, life-prolonging treatment for children in the dying process challenged their professional ethic to provide comfort for the patient.

Manifestations of stress: cost of caring

In a study of occupational stress in the care of the critically ill, the dying, and the bereaved, three major categories of stress—physical, psychological, and behavioural—were reported[41]. Of these, physical symptoms of stress were reported less often and psychological symptoms were reported more often than behavioural ones. Furthermore, younger caregivers reported more symptoms of stress and fewer coping strategies than older caregivers. By being aware of the manifestation of stress, professionals can monitor their own responses, taking appropriate action when they begin to experience such symptoms. Appropriate actions include approaches at both institutional and personal levels. Much of the literature cites the paediatric ward as a potential source of ultimate frustration, anguish, and personal and professional stress for caregivers; however, only a limited number of studies describe the stress experienced by staff working with such children[42,43]. In one of these published studies that describes staff stress in a paediatric hospice setting[42], a small but distinct subgroup of staff who manifested symptoms of psychological distress were characterized in two ways. First, they had experienced relatively recent bereavement in their personal lives. Second, they had failed to resolve their grief about a bereavement that had occurred some considerable time before. Deep distress can be rekindled when a trigger event echoes back to and resurrects a sense of personal loss. The very nature of the work serves as a constant reminder of their loss and may interfere with their own natural grieving.

Institutional actions

Within agencies, primary consideration must be given to staff selection. Individuals must want to work in paediatric palliative care and must come with a repertoire of coping abilities developed through previous work and personal experiences. They must be trained in the care of dying children. On the whole, physicians, nurses, counsellors, and chaplains are inadequately prepared to care for the dying; education has emphasized life-saving activities, maintenance of personal control, and the avoidance of failure. The lack of accountability for psychosocial care has also contributed to this lack of education for all health professionals; for example, issues of 'patient safety' have only referred to physical aspects of the situation.

The need for systematic education for nurses was identified more than 20 years ago[44]; however, in the interim, few such programmes have been described and even fewer programmes have been evaluated[45]. There are similar findings in medical literature pertaining to the education of physicians[46–48]. Other allied health-care professionals such as social workers/counsellors and chaplains are also infrequently provided with quality end-of-life care education. The need for appropriate training in the care of the dying remains strong[49,50].

The good news is that in the last several years new interdisciplinary end-of-life curricula have been developed and published. In the United States, for example, several key constituencies have developed training curricula for paediatric hospice and palliative care. The Initiative for Pediatric Palliative Care (IPPC) developed an interdisciplinary curriculum and training programme[51,52]. The National Hospice and Palliative Care Organization, through its paediatric special interest group, Children's Project on Palliative/Hospice Services (ChiPPS), has also published an interdisciplinary paediatric hospice/palliative care curriculum[53,54]. As well, the End-of-Life Nursing Education Consortium (ELNEC) was launched in 2000 by the American Colleges of Nursing and the City of Hope National Medical Center[55]. In the following year, the ELNEC-Pediatric Palliative Care Curriculum began. Other efforts are also underway throughout the world, including Canada, Great Britain, and Europe (to name only a few).

Recent findings suggest that the milieu of the ward when a child died affects the nurse's grief[44]. When it was acknowledged how difficult it might be for the nurse when her patient died, the nurse felt supported and felt better able to resolve her grief. When nursing care goals were clearly established as palliative, nurses experienced less distress since they were able to focus on making the patient comfortable and the family was satisfied with the care. The difficulty in an acute care setting, however, is that not all members of the team are able to acknowledge the child will not recover. As well, opportunities to brief, debrief, review, and analyse the situation in a safe, supportive environment with one another and with physician colleagues helped nurses cope with current and subsequent stresses in their practice settings.

Health-care providers who provide home-based care (particularly hospice care) to dying children may also struggle when the child dies. The very nature of hospice work requires the health-care professional to work in a very intimate environment with the ill child and family. Day in and day out, the home-care staff are providing care while sitting on the child's bed at home and seeing the family in their own environment. Families may be less guarded at home and home-care staff often witness feelings and behaviours that may not be as evident in the hospital. This experience may also allow the home-care staff to feel more at peace after the child's death as they have had the opportunity to see the child happy to be in his/her home. Given the greater opportunity for health-care providers to feel more a part of the family due to the intimate work environment, it is important to ensure that home-based health-care providers have an opportunity to de-brief with supervisors. Some health-care workers, finding it more difficult to manage professional boundaries when working in a child's home, will benefit from added support after experiencing a child's death.

The necessity of team building and support in interdisciplinary teamwork has been the focus of long-standing debate. There are three primary advantages to allowing staff as a group the time and means to understand and tackle the difficult issues that necessarily arise in any team[56]. First, understanding of interpersonal dynamics and pitfalls amongst the team will further the team's understanding of the families for whom they care. Second, while some may argue that teams are really too busy helping families to waste time on the unnecessary nicety of promoting understanding, the contrary is true in that time is saved. Prolonged and unresolved staff conflict saps and debilitates the individual and undermines his or her self-esteem, commitment, and efficiency. At its worst, it leads to high staff turnover with consequent fragmentation in care and delivery. Third, 'problems and difficulties encountered by those facing great distress have a way of echoing and reverberating in the service set up to help them, with the danger that a service inadvertently mirrors, and therefore remirrors, the very difficulties it aims to ease[56].' Any group claiming to work as a team should show their battle scars. 'If they don't have them, they haven't worked as a team!'[57]

Personal actions

The person best equipped to deal with the care of the dying child is that person who has developed a wide repertoire of coping skills through exposure to previous life stressors, both personally and professionally. Conversely, professionals who deal with feelings of helplessness and passivity by excessive intellectualization, flight into activity, denial, projection, rationalization, or withdrawal are going to experience personal distress as well as finding themselves in the middle of considerable staff conflict[36]. Effective coping requires a high degree of self-awareness and personal responsibility. Personal approaches, therefore, must include developing outlets for physical and emotional expression, creating periods of solitude for reflection and integration and finding meaning through one's personal philosophy.

Implications for practice

Helping the bereaved

According to the Committee for the Study of Health Consequences of the Stress of Bereavement[58], health-care providers and institutions are professionally and morally obligated to assist the bereaved by being sensitive to and knowledgeable about the impact of grief. To carry out this role responsibly, they should be able to communicate about sensitive issues, to understand the nature of normal and abnormal bereavement reactions and to be knowledgeable about community resources to which the bereaved can be referred for specialized help if needed. A recent review of models in the field of death, dying, and bereavement suggests the need to shift perspective from passive victimization to an opportunity for active processes whereby one can regain some measure of control and meaning in living with loss[17,59]. Limitations in the attention paid to the bereaved by health-care professionals appear to derive from three factors:

1   Their inadequate training about the nature of bereavement and their own personal feelings toward death

2   The failure of health-care institutions to acknowledge their responsibility for bereavement follow-up, the stress that caring for dying and bereaved persons puts on their staff, and the need for sufficient staff time for these activities

3   The financial constraints imposed by the current structure of third-party reimbursement arrangements, particularly in the United States.

Despite these constraints, it is necessary for health professionals to formulate some approach to the bereaved because, whether they are trained or untrained, those who interact with a bereaved person will have an impact—negative or positive—on that individual. It is clearly more beneficial to families for the health-care provider to be trained in bereavement. In recent years, there has been much more documentation in the literature addressing assessment and intervention strategies when working with bereaved individuals[60–62]. A limited number of studies examined the relationship between parental bereavement outcome and health-care professionals' interventions prior to, at the time of, and after the child's death[16,63]. Results revealed that, in many cases, actions that were considered helpful or not helpful varied according to each individual's personal perceptions and situations. Because of the uniqueness of every parent's grieving response, health-care professionals' interventions cannot simply be standardized but rather, must be individualized to meet the needs of each bereaved parent and each family. The most consistently helpful action was related to the attitude of the health-care providers—showing a caring, concerned attitude and demonstrating an ability to be involved with parents[63].

While one must always be weary of 'cookbook' approaches to grief counselling, consideration of some general principles for helping individuals may be beneficial. Any health-care professional providing support to bereaved families must, at a minimum, have a basic understanding of the theoretical perspectives, particularly with regard to families who have had a child die. The goal for health-care professionals is to help bereaved siblings (and parents) to integrate their losses in ways that are regenerative, rather than degenerative, in the continual unfolding of their lives.

Bereaved parents

Health-care professionals begin by making contact with the parents and letting them know that the health-care team is available to meet with them should they desire such contact. Parents often have many questions about the child's death and the team members who are willing to discuss these sensitive issues provide a meaningful service to the family. Parents especially value contact with those care providers who cared directly for their child and, in particular, with any health-care provider who was with the child at the moment of death.

In working with bereaved parents, it is critical to maintain a family systems perspective, recognizing the impact of the death on family members and on their interactions with one another. Health-care professionals are in a unique position to help families enhance their functioning following a death through offering insights that may provide them with different ways of being in the world. For example, the belongings of the deceased child have the potential of serving as memories and the meaning associated with a particular belonging determines whether or not it is kept[64]. Furthermore, memories may vary in meaning for individuals within the family. Memories may have a mutually held meaning for the family as a whole and private meaning for its individual members. Consequently, if asked, health-care professionals must avoid telling families what to do with their child's belongings. Rather, they can encourage families to be aware of the subtle meanings associated with various belongings that serve as memories. For example, when visible mementos of their child (e.g. photographs) are displayed within a grouping of photos of all children in the family, a different message is conveyed than if the photo is the only one displayed. In the first instance, the surviving children perceive that the deceased child was 'one of the family'; in the second instance, they may perceive that the deceased child is the 'most important' child in the family. Siblings in the first instance are likely to feel more special than siblings in the second family. Also, the greater the discrepancy between the family's mutually held meaning of the memory and the individual's private meanings of the memory, the less the integration of the loss by the family and its individual members. It is important, therefore, to encourage family members to share openly their private meanings and to help them realize that not having the same meanings and memories is acceptable. Often family members choose to maintain one of the deceased's favourite possessions. These linking objects help to bridge the transition from the immediacy of the child's death to a virtual presence with the surviving family members' present and future.

The importance of effective communication has been recognized as an essential element in facilitating individual and family coping with a childhood chronic, life-limiting illness, or condition. However, effective communication refers not just to the sharing of information but to the creation of a climate within the family that allows and encourages the expression of feelings. Several studies support the suggestion that parent–sibling communication differs before and after the death. Before the death, talking about the illness and death is related specifically to the events of day-to-day care. After the death, while open expression may pertain to many topics and areas of concern to family members, discussion about the feelings aroused by the death may be excluded. Similarly, the open expression of grief may not be supported, even in the most expressive families. This exclusion may not be, and is usually not, conscious. Often, it is communicated implicitly by the lack of willingness to experience and express openly the painful emotions associated with grief. Therefore, it seems that parents, including those who communicated openly with their children before the death, need encouragement in communicating openly with their surviving children after the death so that the sadness and sorrow is shared and expressed. It is also important to assess the communication style of the extended family. For many families, grandparents, aunts and uncles, other family members, and close friends may live close by and have participated in the child's care. They are grieving also and how information is shared with this extended family is important for health-care providers to know. All assessments must include a sensitivity and understanding of the family's cultural, religious, and spiritual background. It is not reasonable to use one standard as the measurement of effective communication with all families.

Almost all the evidence recommends professional intervention following the death of a child; the need for a trained professional in the area of bereavement seems evident. Follow-up by the care providers focuses on facilitating communication within the family, allowing parents to vent their anxieties and concerns, assessing the family's grief in order to promote the mental health of the family, and referring the parents and other family members to additional useful resources. One major resource may be books written for bereaved parents. A most potent resource available, however, is specific support groups for bereaved parents, which provide ongoing social support. Options include groups such as The Compassionate Friends, an international self-help group for all types of bereaved parents; Candlelighters, a group for parents of children with cancer, or other local groups or organizations (such as hospices) devoted to helping bereaved parents; CRUSE is a grief counselling service offered throughout the United Kingdom. Through mutual sharing, learning, modelling, and support, these groups support parents in their grief.

Probably the most critical realization for health-care providers who offer bereavement support to parents is that they cannot take away the parents' pain and suffering. Therefore, the follow-up offered must be supportive in nature and provided over time. Professionals providing bereavement support may feel helpless in such situations and want to do something more. Instead, they must value the 'gift of presence', of being there to share the pain. Table 13.5.2 provides a synthesis of principles and intervention strategies for working with bereaved parents[65,66].

Bereaved siblings

Two critical assumptions provide the foundation for interventions with bereaved siblings[5]. First, health-care providers must acknowledge the impact of a child's death on the surviving siblings. Until very recently, the focus of all attention has been the parents of the child who died; siblings have been relatively forgotten. Research into the long-term effects of sibling bereavement continues to validate the significance of this event for siblings.

Health-care professionals must be aware of the meaning of sibling responses. For example, children who demonstrate a pattern of behaviour that includes persistent sadness and withdrawal, decreased involvement in activities and hobbies, acting out, diminished self-esteem, and a loss of interest and achievement in school require individualized attention through referrals to the school counsellor or to a specialist in children's grief.

Many bereaved siblings have described their experience of participating in a specialized bereavement support group as an important part of their experience. Such bereavement groups may be helpful for any bereaved sibling not just those who show long-term psychological symptomatology. The number of grief groups for children has increased considerably during the past decade throughout North America, the United Kingdom, and Australia. Some groups are time-limited, offered for 6 or 8 weeks or over a weekend; others are open-ended and children may attend over many months. Most offer structured activities that form the basis for group discussion and individualized expression. The evaluation of one programme indicated that the children valued learning that they were 'not alone' in their thoughts and feelings; they were reassured by learning that they were 'not as different from other kids' as they had previously thought. The participants' parents perceived the group lessened their children's anxiety and acting-out behaviours[67].

Many hospices and grief centres also sponsor week-end bereavement retreats and camps for surviving siblings, bereaved parents, and the bereaved family as a whole. These camps and retreats offer opportunities for attendees to participate in a variety of specialized bereavement groups and activities intended to foster caring connections, support, and personal growth. Attendees describe these retreats and camps as very meaningful and often an important step in assisting them during their bereavement journey.

The second underlying assumption to helping siblings is that health-care providers must understand that a child's parents are often the best ones to help their own children. However, parents

Table 13.5.2 Principles and strategies for working with bereaved parents[20,66].

1	Make contact and assess the bereaved parents
2	Provide assurance that they can survive their loss, keeping in mind the parents' unique perspective
3	Provide times to grieve, remembering that grief has its own time
4	Facilitate the identification and expression of feelings, including anger, hostility, sadness, relief, and guilt
5	Encourage verbalization of thoughts and recollections of the deceased child; do not be afraid to mention the deceased child's name
6	Interpret 'normal' grieving behaviour and responses
7	Maintain a therapeutic and realistic perspective; do not rush to 'fix' the pain
8	Allow for individual differences relating to gender, age, personality, culture, ethnicity, religion, and characteristics of the death
9	Avoid analysing or interrupting parents' repeated stories and tears
10	Help to identify and resolve secondary losses, such as the hopes, dreams, and expectations the parents had for the deceased child
11	Examine defences and coping strategies; carefully examine resistance to the grief process
12	Assist in finding sources of continuing support
13	Identify and refer 'pathology'
14	Interpret 'recovery' for them; correct unrealistic expectations of themselves and of the grief process

Table 13.5.3 Helping children cope with grief: Remember the CHILD.

C—Consider
Consider the unique situation of the child, his/her developmental capacity to understand, his/her thoughts, his/her feelings, his/her relationship to their sibling
A child is a child: do not expect a child to be 'the man around the house' or the 'little mother'; it is unfair to the child's future development and often limiting to the grieving process to assign inappropriate role responsibilities to the child
H—Honesty
Use the 'd' word: death, die, dying
Realize that it is all right to not have all the answers
Avoid euphemisms—words which are confusing or have other meanings for the child
Avoid words such as gone away or went on a trip; expressions such as these can make everyday events—leaving on a vacation, going to work—very frightening for the child
Do not explain to a child that the dead person is sleeping; he/she will be afraid of sleeping
I—Involve
Let the child know what is happening; if possible, before the death occurs
Give the child factual knowledge about the cause of death—especially the school-age child
Involve the child in saying good-bye to the dying and deceased—allow the child the choice to participate in the funeral to the level at which he/she is comfortable
L—Listen
Concentrate on discussing the stumbling block of the moment—too often when the subject is sensitive, adults want to rush ahead to explain and reassure in order to finish the conversation; rather, let the child talk through what is on his/her mind
Let the child know that it is all right to not want to talk to anyone anymore about the death for a while
Give the child outlets for expressing his/her grief—art, drawing, play, writing letters, poetry, stories, hammering
Be aware of thoughts and fantasies children may have of being reunited with the person who has died; each child must be considered potentially at risk for suicide and any kind of communication that suggests this possibility should be promptly and fully evaluated; careful attention to any suggestion of suicidal risk, no matter what the age of the child, is essential
Clarify that death is not the result of the child's action or thoughts; be attuned to magical thinking involved in the child's explanation of the death and correct it to avoid guilt and inappropriate grief reactions
D—Do it over and over again
Appropriately share your grief: realize that children cannot do grief work without permission and role models; children need to see an honest expression of emotions from adults accompanied by explanations and reassurances
Keep in mind the developmental capacities of the child and his/her age-related concerns and needs

grieving over the loss of a child seldom have the personal energy to provide their grieving children as much support as the parents would like to give. Health-care professionals must support parents in supporting their children. This is not to say, however, that direct contact with siblings is unhelpful; indeed, direct interventions by caregivers can be particularly advantageous for children who need a less emotionally involved adult with whom to discuss their concerns. Such children often avoid discussing their own grief with their parents because they are trying to protect their parents from further distress.

There is considerable similarity between the techniques used to help children cope with a dying sibling and those used to help children adjust to the death of a sibling. In both cases, in order to guide parents in supporting their other children, health-care professionals must understand children's views of death and must be aware of the normal responses of children to death. This information then serves as the foundation upon which parents' questions and concerns about their surviving children can be discussed. Communication with siblings needs to be open, and must take into account each child's individual needs and developmental level. For all

children, however, parents and caregivers need to remember the CHILD when helping him or her to cope with grief (Table 13.5.3).

Conclusion

Facing the impending death of a child is an experience like no other. The unnaturalness of a child's death compounds the pain, the sorrow, and the sadness. Yet, children too must face life-limiting illnesses or conditions. It is crucial that we pay attention to this experience. The loss of a child triggers profound grief in all those who knew and cared for the child—the parents, siblings, grandparents, teachers, nurses, doctors, social workers, and chaplains, as well as other health providers who, on a daily basis, were witness to the plight of the child and his/her family. Health-care professionals can do much to facilitate optimal bereavement outcomes in the child's family. Such individuals must realize the child's need to be cared for in a style that promotes comfort and dignity. In addition, such individuals must remember that the experiences of the family during the dying process will affect significantly their future lives as survivors. Professionals must be aware of the various reactions that comprise 'normal' grief in parents and siblings, recognizing that such reactions may be influenced by a variety of mediating factors, some of which have been identified. Furthermore, health-care professionals must be aware that the intensity of the immediate impact does seem to diminish over time but the long-term effects, though not easily identified or measured, last a lifetime.

Health-care professionals who choose to care for dying children and their families do not engage in this work without needing support themselves. This is a challenging field, one which demands that professionals struggle with the difficult task of maintaining balance and perspective. In addition, however, working with such children and their families provides meaning to life. Working with these children helps to give a clear perspective on what is really valuable. Working with these children helps us to grow, to develop as both persons and professionals. It has been said that all of us need to learn about our own mortality, limitations, and vulnerabilities. These children and their families teach these lessons well.

References

1. NCHS (2001). Deaths: Final Data for 1999. *National Vital Statistics Report*, **49**(8), 1–15. [Online]. Available: http://www.cdc.gov/nchs/data/nvsr49/nvsr49_08.pdf

2. McClowry, S.G., Davies, E.B., May, K.A. *et al.* (1987). The empty space phenomenon: The process of grief in the bereaved family. *Death Studies*, **11**, 361–74.

3. Martinson, I.M., McClowry, S.G., Advies, B. *et al.* (1994). Changes over time: A study of family bereavement following childhood cancer. *Journal of Palliative Care*, **10**, 19–25.

4. Davies, B., Spinetta, J., Martinson, I. *et al.* (1986). Manifestations of levels of functioning in grieving families. *Journal of Family Issues*, **7**(3), 297–313.

5. Davies, B. (1999). *Shadows in the Sun: Experiences of sibling bereavement in childhood*. Bruner/Mazell, Philadelphia, PA.

6. Clayton, P., Desmarais, L., and Winokur, G. (1968). A study of normal bereavement. *American Journal of Psychiatry*, **125**, 168–787.

7. Sanders, C.M. (1979–80). A comparison of adult bereavement in the death of a spouse, child, and parent. *Omega*, **10**, 303–22.

8. Moore, I.M., Gilliss, C.L., and Martinson, I.M. (1988). Psychosomatic symptoms in parents 2 years after the death of a child with cancer. *Nursing Research*, **37**, 1046.

9. Hazzard, A., Weston, L., and Gutteres, C. (1992). After a child's death. Factors related to parental bereavement. *Developmental and Behavioral Pediatrics*, **13**, 24–30.

10. Lang, A. and Gottlieb, L. (1993). Parental grief reactions and marital intimacy following infant death. *Death Studies*, **17**, 233–55.

11. Yeh, C.H. (2002). Gender differences of parental distress in children with cancer. *Journal of Advanced Nursing*, **38**, 598–606.

12. Davies, B., Gudmundsdottir, M., Worden, W. *et al.* (2004). "Living in the dragon's shadow" –Fathers' experiences of a child's life-threatening illness. *Death Studies*, **28**, 1–25.

13. Rehm, R.S. (1999). Religious faith in Mexican-American families dealing with chronic childhood illness. *Journal of Nursing Scholarship*, **31**(1), 33–8.

14. Davies, B., Deveau, E., Papadatou, D. *et al.* (1998). Experiences of mothers of children who died from cancer—A cross cultural perspective. *Cancer Nursing*, **21**(5), 301–11.

15. Davies, B. (2001). Fathers' experiences in paediatric palliative care. Paper presented at International Conference on Death, Dying, and Bereavement, London, Ontario.

16. Neidig, I.R. and Dalgas-Pelish, P. (1991). Parental grieving and perceptions regarding health care professionals' interventions. *Issues in Comprehensive Nursing*, **14**, 179–91.

17. Attig, T.W. (1991). The importance of conceiving of grieving as an active process. *Death Studies*, **15**, 383–93.

18. Rando, T. (1993). *Readings in paediatric psychology*. Plenum Press, New York.

19. Miles, M.S. (1985). Helping adults mourn the death of a child. In *Issues in comprehensive paediatric nursing*, Vol. 1 (eds. H. Wass and C.A. Corr), pp. 219–41. Hemisphere Publishing, Washington, DC.

20. Worden, W. (1982).*Grief counseling and grief therapy: A handbook for the mental health practitioner*. Springer, New York.

21. Foley, G.V. and Whittham, E.H. (1991). Care of the child dying of cancer: Part II. *CA—A Cancer Journal for Clinicians*, **41**, 52–64.

22. Foster, D., O'Malley, E., and Koocher, G.P. (1981). The parent interviews. In *The Damocles syndrome: Psychosocial consequences of surviving childhood cancer* (eds. G.P. Koocher and E. O'Malley), pp. 86–100. McGraw-Hill, New York.

23. Lansky, S.B., Cairns, N.U., Hassanem, R. *et al.* (1978). Childhood cancer: Parental discord and divorce. *Pediatrics*, **62**, 184–8.

24. Spinetta, L., Swarner, L., and Sheoposh, L. (1981). Effective parental coping following death of a child from cancer. *Journal of Pediatric Psychology*, **6**, 251–63.

25. Rando, T.A. (1986). The unique issues and impact of the death of a child. In *Parental loss of a child* (ed. T.A. Rando), pp. 5–43. Research Press, Champaign, IL.

26. Rando, T.A. (1983). An investigation of grief and adaptation in parents whose children have died from cancer. *Journal of Pediatric Psychology*, **8**, 3–20.

27. Miles, M.S. and Crandall, E.K. (1983). The search for meaning and its potential for affecting growth in bereaved parents. *Health Values: Achieving High Level Wellness*, **7**, 19–23.

28. Martinson, I., Davies, B., and McClowry, S. (1987). The long-term effects of sibling death on self-concept. *Journal of Pediatric Nursing*, **2**, 227–35.

29. Davies, B. (1988). The family environment in bereaved families and its relationship to surviving sibling behaviour. *Children's Health Care*, **17**, 22–30.

30. Finkbeiner, A.K. (1996). *After the death of a grandchild: Living with loss through the years*. Free Press, NY.

31. Galinsky, N. (1999). *When a grandchild dies: What to do, what to say, how to cope*. Gal in the Sky Publ., Houston.

32. Gerner, M.H. (1990). *For bereaved grandparents*. Centering Corporation, Omaha.

33. Reed, M.L. (2000). *Grandparents cry twice*. Baywood, Amityville, NY.

34. Schweibert, P. (1996). *A grandparent's sorrow*. Perinatal Loss, Portland, OR.

35. Parkes, C.M. (1986). *Bereavement: Studies of grief in adult life*, 2nd edition. Tavistock Publications, New York.

36. Vachon, M.L.S. and Pakes, E. (1985). Staff stress in the care of the critically ill and dying child. *Issues in Comprehensive Pediatric Nursing*, **8**, 151–82.

37. Davies, B. and Eng, B. (1993). Factors influencing nursing care of children who are terminally ill: A selective review. *Pediatric Nursing*, **19**, 9–14.

38. Hilden, J.M., Emanuel, E.J., Fairclough, D.L. *et al.* (2001). Attitudes and practices among paediatric oncologists regarding end-of-life care: results of the American Society of Clinical Oncology Survey. *Journal of Clinical Oncology*, **19**(1), 205–12.

39. Benoliel, J.Q. (1986). The cancer patient's right to know and decide: An ethical perspective. In *Issues and topics in cancer nursing* (eds. R. McCorkle and G. Honglarom), pp. 5–17. Appleton-Century-Crofts, Norwalk, CN.

40. Zerwekh, J.Y. (1984). Professional stress and distress. In *Hospice and palliative nursing care* (eds. A.G. Blues and J.Y. Zerwekh), pp. 347–62. Grune and Stratton, New York.

41. Vachon, M.L.S. (1987). *Occupational stress in the care of the critically ill, the dying and the bereaved*. Hemisphere Publishing, New York.

42. Woolley, H., Stein, A., Forrest, G.C. *et al.* (1989). Staff stress and job satisfaction at a children's hospice. *Archives of Disease in Childhood*, **64**, 114–18.

43. Davies, B., Clark, D., Connaughty, S. *et al.* (1996). The experience of nursing care for chronically ill children who die. Final report. *Pediatric Nursing*, **22**, 500–7.

44. Quint, J.C. (1967). *The nurse and the dying patient*. Macmillan, New York.

45. Degner, L.F. and Gow, C.M. (1988). Evaluation of death education in nursing: A critical review. *Cancer Nursing*, **11**, 151–9.

46. Penney, J.C. (1987). The evolution of a medical school curriculum in death and dying. *Journal of Palliative Care*, **3**, 14–18.

47. Irwin, W.G. (1984). Teaching terminal care at Queen's University of Belfast. I-Course, sessional educational objectives and content. *British Medical Journal*, **289**, 1509–11.

48. Scofield, G.R. (1989). Terminal care and the continuing need for professional education. *Journal of Palliative Care*, **5**, 32–6.

49. Hilden, J.H., Emanuel, E.J., Fairclough, D.L. *et al.* (2001). Attitudes and practices among paediatric oncologists regarding end-of-life care: results of the 1998 American Society of Clinical Oncology Survey. *Journal of Clinical Oncology*, **19**(10), 205–12.

50. Papadatou, D. (1997). Training health professionals in caring for dying children and grieving families. *Death Studies*, **21**(6), 575–600.

51. Solomon, M.Z., Browning, D., Dokken, D. *et al.* (2003). The Initiative for Pediatric Palliative Care (IPPC) curriculum: Enhancing family-centered care for children with life-threatening conditions. (Modules 1-5). Education Development Center, Inc, Newton, MA. http://www.ippcweb.org.

52. Browing, D.M. and Solomon, M.Z. (2005). The initiative for paediatric palliative care: An interdisciplinary educational approach for healthcare professionals. *Journal of Pediatric Nursing*, **20**, 326–34.

53. National Hospice and Palliative Care Organization: Education and training curriculum in paediatric palliative care. (2003). http://www.nhpco.org.

54. Csikai, E. and Raymer, M. (2005). Social workers' educational needs in end-of-life care. *Social Work in Health Care*, **41**(1), 53–72.

55. American Association of Colleges of Nursing and City of Hope: End-of-Life Nursing Education Curriculum: Pediatric Palliative Care. (2006). http://www.aacn.nche.edu/elnec.

56. Stein, A. and Woolley, H. (1994). Care for the carers. In *Care of the dying child* (ed. A. Goldman), pp. 164–81. Oxford University Press, Oxford.

57. Mount, B.M. and Voyer, S. (1980). Staff stress in palliative hospice care. In *The Royal Victoria Hospital Manual on palliative hospice care* (eds. I. Ajemaian and B.M. Mount), p. 146. Arno Press.

58. Osterweiss, M., Solomon, F., and Green, M. (eds). (1984). Bereavement reactions, consequences, and care. Report by the Committee for the Study of Health Consequences of the Stress of Bereavement, Institute of Medicine, National Academy of Sciences. National Academy Press, Washington, DC.

59. Corr, C.A. and Doki, K.J. (1994). Current models of death, dying and bereavement. *Critical Care Nursing Clinics of North America*, **6**, 545–52.

60. McCollum, A. (1974). Counseling the grieving parent. In *Care of the child facing death* (ed. L. Burton), pp. 177–88. Routledge & Kegan Paul, London.

61. Pine, Y.R. and Brauer, C. (1986). Parental grief: A synthesis of theory research, and intervention. In *Parental loss of a child* (ed. T.A. Rando), pp. 59–96. Research Press, Champaign, IL.

62. Rando, T.A. (1984). *Grief, dying, and death: Interventions for caregivers*. Research Press, Champaign, IL.

63. Hasse, K.E. (1989). At the time of death: help for the child's parents. *Children's Health Care*, **18**, 146–52.

64. Davies, B. (1987). Family responses to the death of a child: The meaning of memories. *Journal of Palliative Care*, **3**, 9–15.

65. Rando, T.A. (1986). Individual and couples treatment following the death of a child. In *Parental loss of a child* (ed. T.A. Rando), pp. 341–414. Research Press, Champaign, IL.

66. Schmidt, L. (1987). Working with bereaved parents. In *The child and family facing life-threatening illness* (eds. T. Krulik, B. Holaday and I.M. Martinson), pp. 327–44. JB Lippincott, Philadelphia.

67. Collins, J.B., Davies, B., Steele, R. *et al.* (1999). Family voices: An evaluation of the impact of the Canuck Place Children's Hospice Program. Final Report to British Columbia Health Research Foundation. Community Grants Program, Vancouver, BC.

68. Davies, B. and Martinson, I.M. (1989). Care of the family: Special emphasis on siblings during and after the death of a child. In *Pediatric hospice care: What helps* (ed. B.B. Martin), pp. 186–99. Children's Hospital of Los Angeles, Los Angeles.

SECTION 14

Geriatric palliative medicine

14.1

Palliative medicine in dementia

Ladislav Volicer

Dementia is an acquired syndrome that causes progressive loss of intellectual abilities, such as memory, language (aphasia), the capacity to use tools (apraxia) or recognize objects (agnosia), and planning and thinking in abstract terms (executive function). Dementia is present if at least memory and one additional intellectual ability are impaired, and the impairment is severe enough to interfere with social or occupational functioning.

Dementia is the most common neurological disease in the elderly. Its incidence increases from 4.3 cases/1000 persons/year among 65–69 year olds to 85.6 cases/1000 persons/year among individuals 90 years old and older[1].

If a person exhibits symptoms of dementia, an evaluation should be performed to determine its cause. Many pathological disorders lead to dementia (Table 14.1.1). Although some disorders are reversible through medical or surgical treatment, the number of patients with remedial dementias is rather small. Most dementing conditions

Table 14.1.1 Some causes of dementia.

Potentially reversible dementias	Irreversible dementias
Tumors: both in brain and peripheral tissues	Neurodegenerative diseases:
	Alzheimer's disease
Metabolic disorders: thyroid disease, electrolyte imbalance, renal or hepatic failure	Dementia with Lewy bodies
	Fronto-temporal dementia
	Pick's disease
Head trauma	Huntington's disease
Poisoning: heavy metals, alcoholism, solvents, and insecticides	Parkinson's disease
	Progressive supranuclear palsy
Brain infections	Vascular dementias:
Autoimmune disorders: brain vasculitis, lupus erythematosus, multiple sclerosis	Multi-infarct dementia
	Binswanger's disease
Drug adverse effects	Occlusive cerebrovascular disease
Nutritional disorders: deficiency of vitamins B12, B6, B1, and folate	Cerebral embolism
	Anoxia secondary to cardiac arrest or carbon monoxide poisoning
Psychiatric disorders	
Normal pressure hydrocephalus	Infections:
AIDS encephalopathy	Creutzfeldt–Jakob disease
	Postencephalitic dementia

considered potentially reversible produce structural changes in the brain that do not respond to treatment[2].

The vast majority of dementias, especially in older individuals, is caused by degenerative changes in the brain that progress over time and lead to loss of independence. Despite recent advances in neuroscience and psychopharmacology, treatment of individuals suffering from progressive dementias cannot stop or reverse the course of these disorders. Although death is not a direct consequence of the dementing process, complications leading to death are inevitable consequences of the disease. Therefore, advanced dementia should be considered to be a terminal illness similar to untreatable cancer. The goals of care typically focus on palliative treatment for medical complications, striving for maximal comfort instead of maximal survival at any cost.

Progressive degenerative dementias

There are four main types of progressive degenerative dementias: Alzheimer's disease (AD), vascular dementia, dementia with Lewy bodies, and fronto-temporal dementia. It is sometimes difficult to distinguish different progressive dementias by clinical examination because their symptoms are similar, especially in the later stages of the disease. Also, it is not uncommon that an autopsy examination finds evidence for more than one cause of dementia and the relative contribution of these causes to the clinical syndrome is unclear.

Alzheimer's disease

Alzheimer's disease is the most common cause of progressive degenerative dementia. Autopsy studies have found that approximately 60 per cent of demented patients have pure AD and another 15 per cent have AD combined with other disorders. The diagnostic criteria for Alzheimer's disease include multiple cognitive deficits manifested by both memory impairment and at least one other cognitive disturbance (aphasia, apraxia, agnosia, or disturbance of executive functioning). This cognitive deficit must be severe enough to cause significant impairment in social or occupational functioning, and must represent a significant decline from a previous level of functioning. The course of the dementia must be characterized by gradual onset and continuing cognitive decline, and the cognitive impairment cannot be due to other brain disease, to systemic disturbances that can cause dementia, or to drug-induced effects. The possibility that the deficit is caused by other conditions, such as delirium or depression also has to be excluded.

The clinical diagnosis of AD is tentative and needs to be supported by neuropathological examination of the brain after the patient dies. Thus, the most definite clinical diagnosis of AD is 'probable Alzheimer's disease,' which is made when there are no other possible aetiological factors. Neuropathological criteria for AD include presence of senile or neuritic plaques and neurofibrillary tangles. The plaques and tangles each contain a specific protein that may play role in the pathogenesis of AD. Beta amyloid protein is present in the plaques and the tau protein is found in the tangles.

A small number of patients with AD have one of three mutations or trisomy of chromosome 21 that affect metabolism of β-amyloid. β-Amyloid is toxic for nerve cells and causes nerve cell dysfunction and ultimately cell death. There is also one gene that influences the age at which AD develops. Individuals who have apolipoprotein E4 develop AD earlier than individuals who have apolipoprotein E3 or E2. Environmental factors that increase the risk of development of AD are brain injury, low education, and stressful life.

Neuritic plaques and neurofibrillary tangles are present in small quantities even in brains of elderly individuals who were not demented before they died. This finding indicates that formation of plaques and tangles may be a part of normal aging process but that does not mean that everybody who develops plaques and tangles has to develop dementia. Only about one-half of individuals who on autopsy had enough plaques and tangles to be diagnosed as having AD but did not have any cerebrovascular changes were clinically demented before death[3]. This suggests the importance of vascular changes that can lead to development of dementia even in absence of Alzheimer changes.

Vascular dementia

Vascular dementia refers to impaired cognitive function caused by cerebral injury that is related to different forms of cerebral vascular disease. It is possible to distinguish five types of vascular dementia: multiple infarct dementia, strategic single infarct dementia, small vessel disease (Binswanger disease), hypoperfusion states, and haemorrhaghic lesions. The incidence and prevalence of vascular dementia varies widely. It is the leading cause of dementia in the elderly in Japan, China, and Russia, but appears to be declining in other regions, most likely related to improvements in the management of hypertension[4].

Vascular dementia is usually characterized by a sudden onset and stepwise progression of symptoms. However, there is a significant overlap between symptoms of Alzheimer's disease and vascular dementia. The diagnosis is also problematic because of frequent combination of Alzheimer and vascular changes found during autopsy. In the Honolulu Asia Aging Study, autopsy examination found that 31 per cent of individuals had only Alzheimer changes but 68 per cent had mixed pathology[5].

Dementia with Lewy bodies

Dementia with Lewy bodies (also sometimes called diffuse Lewy body disease) is characterized by a fluctuating course of cognitive impairment that includes episodic confusion and lucid intervals similar to delirium[6]. In addition there must be at least one of the following: (1) visual and/or auditory hallucinations resulting in paranoid delusions, (2) mild extrapyramidal symptoms (muscle rigidity, slow movements) or adverse extrapyramidal response to standard doses of neuroleptics, or (3) repeated unexplained falls. The clinical features of dementia with Lewy bodies persist over a long period of time, in contrast to the shorter time course of delirium, and dementia with Lewy bodies progresses to severe dementia. As with AD, other causes of the progressive cognitive decline have to be excluded.

Dementia with Lewy bodies is characterized during autopsy by the presence of round structures called Lewy bodies. These structures are found inside the nerve cells in the brain cortex. Lewy bodies are also present in Parkinson's disease, but in Parkinson's disease, they are limited to subcortical areas of the brain. Lewy bodies contain α-synuclein protein, a substance that plays role in apoptosis. Mutation of α-synuclein gene, which is present on chromosome 2, leads to development of severe dementia with Lewy bodies. α-Synuclein is also present in astrocytes in amyotrophic lateral sclerosis and in oligodendroglia in multiple system atrophy[7].

Frontotemporal dementia

There is no uniform terminology for frontotemporal dementia, which accounts for up to 10 per cent of the cases with progressive degenerative dementia[8]. Some investigators label all frontotemporal dementias as Pick's disease, while other consider Pick's disease to be a pathological subtype of frontotemporal dementia, which is characterized by specific neuropathological findings: Pick bodies inside nerve cells and balooned nerve cells. The diagnosis of frontotemporal dementia is based on personality changes and the presence of atrophy of the frontal brain areas in neuroimaging studies. The personality changes in frontotemporal dementia are similar to changes induced by damage of frontal lobes by other causes (injury, stroke) and include behavioural disinhibition, loss of social or personal awareness, or disengagement with apathy. Patients with frontotemporal dementia differ from Alzheimer patients because they maintain some abilities (e.g. elementary drawing and calculations) into the later stages of dementia.

Atrophy of frontal and temporal lobes of the brain and proliferation of non-neuronal glial cells in these areas characterize pathological findings in frontotemporal dementia. Frontotemporal dementia is one of the diseases that exhibit abnormality of the tau proteins. These diseases also are called hereditary tauopathies and include frontotemporal dementia and Pick's disease, progressive supranuclear palsy, corticobasal degeneration, dementia with parkinsonism and progressive subcortical gliosis. In some cases, the tau protein is missing and in some cases there is an imbalance between different isoforms of tau protein[9].

Characteristics of severe and terminal stages of progressive degenerative dementias

Pattern of decline in higher cortical functioning

Although there are some differences in symptomatology of different dementias in their early courses, the period with severe dementia, and the terminal stages, have very similar characteristics.

The course of these dementias can be characterized as a gradual loss of independence (Fig. 14.1.1). The course can be divided into four stages. During the mild stage, individuals develop memory problems and spatial disorientation, and they may have some personality changes. In the moderate stage, they start having language difficulties, become unable to use tools and utensils, and become confused. Confusion may lead to agitation and there also may be sleep disturbances.

The severe stage is characterized by further progression of cognitive deficits with impaired comprehension. In this stage, individuals often do not recognize the need for basic activities of daily living and resist when caregivers attempt to provide care. In the terminal stage, individuals become either mute or unable to have meaningful verbal communication, and they may not even be able to maintain eye contact.

This progressive course of cognitive deficits has been compared to reverse child development, with the most complex functions lost first. However, there is no exact relationship, and variation is great. For instance, some patients with severe dementia are still able to read and some individuals may be completely mute but still able to drive.

Functional decline

In the mild stage of dementia, the ability to perform instrumental activities of daily living may become gradually impaired. As dementia progresses and the individuals with dementia need assistance or reminders with basic activities of daily living, they enter the moderate stage of dementia. In this stage, individuals may not be able to use utensils, but may be still able to feed themselves if a finger food is provided. Progression into the severe stage is characterized by development of motor difficulties. Individuals may not be able to feed themselves at all, and start having difficulties walking. They develop either an unsteady or narrow-based gait (scissoring), and are at a high risk for falls. However, they may still be able to walk with assistance. Most individuals also develop incontinence. Once individuals are unable to walk even with assistance, they progress into the terminal phase of dementia. At that point, they often develop swallowing difficulties that causes choking on food and liquids, and may lead to aspiration of nasopharyngeal secretions.

Common chronic diseases and comorbidities

There is no known biological association between either AD or frontotemporal dementia and other physical illnesses. Individuals with dementia may develop the whole spectrum of diseases that accompany normal aging. However, some diseases are more common in individuals with AD, especially in the later stages. A case control study using 7195 death certificates found that patients who died with AD had a higher incidence of Parkinson's disease, epilepsy, sensory impairments, infections, malnutrition, hip fractures and other injuries, and pressure sores than did the control subjects[10]. These conditions fall into three main categories: neurological complications, intercurrent infections, and malnutrition. Hip fractures and other injuries are related to motor impairment that is a risk factor for development of infections, and pressure sores are related to both motor impairment and malnutrition.

Neurological complications

Neurological complications include parkinsonism, stroke, myoclonus, and seizures. Development of extrapyramidal symptoms in particular closely parallels psychotic symptoms and is associated with increased rate of progression of cognitive impairments, functional impairments, nursing home entry, or death[11].

Parkinsonism manifests mainly as bradykinesia and muscle rigidity, and may be induced by the use of neuroleptics. However, muscle rigidity often develops in patients who were not treated with neuroleptics and may be a consequence of dementia with Lewy bodies, which can either occur alone or in combination with AD. The association between Lewy bodies and extrapyramidal symptoms is not precise, however, and patients with a pathological diagnosis of dementia with Lewy bodies may not develop any extrapyramidal manifestations.

Extrapyramidal symptoms may occur in isolated AD and presumably would develop in all patients with this disorder if they

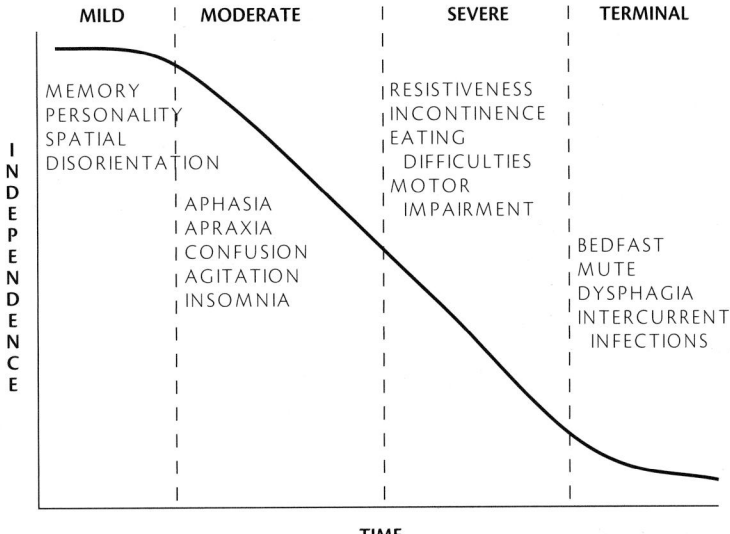

Figure 14.1.1 Course of progressive dementias. Reprinted from Mahoney, E.K. *et al.* (2000) *Management of Challenging Behaviors in Dementia* with permission from Health Professions Press, Baltimore.

survived long enough. The parkinsonism is probably caused by the atrophy of the substantia nigra, a common finding in autopsies of patients with AD. Dopaminergic deficits in the meso-cortical pathway also may contribute to these symptoms.

The incidence of stroke may be promoted by amyloid deposits in cerebral arteries. Such deposits are a common cause of death in hereditary cerebral haemorrhage, Dutch type. As mentioned above, brain infarctions increase the severity of dementia.

Myoclonus and seizures are other common neurological complications. The prevalence of myoclonus increases with progression of dementia and may be present in more than one-third of patients with AD. There is some evidence that myoclonus is associated with increased rate of dementia progression because patients with myoclonus have shorter durations of dementia and more cognitive impairments than patients without myoclonus. New onset seizures develop in one-quarter of patients with AD; they accelerate the progression of cognitive deficits and may lead to earlier institutionalization[12]. Seizures may be due to compensatory changes that occur in the brains of Alzheimer patients, such as increased kainic acid binding sites or axon sprouting.

Intercurrent infections

The most common infections in individuals with dementia affect the urinary tract, upper and lower respiratory tracts, skin and subcutaneous tissues, gastrointestinal tract, and eyes[13]. Generalized infections are the most common cause of death, with bronchopneumonia causing death in about 60 per cent of patients with AD. Patients with advanced dementia have increased susceptibility to these infections because of several factors: changes in immune function, incontinence, decreased mobility, and aspiration. Therefore, these infections are almost inevitable consequences of advanced dementia.

Patients with AD have impairment of cell-mediated immunity and changes in cytokine secretion and acute-phase proteins[14]. These changes may decrease immunological defenses. Incontinence is unavoidable once patients become unable to communicate and sit on a toilet, and the incidence of urinary tract infections is increased by the use of urinary catheters and by bowel incontinence. Incontinence also leads to impairment of skin integrity and development of pressure sores.

Decreased mobility is a consequence of both gait problems and perceptual impairments. An unsteady gait and gait abnormality (narrow-based gait) are secondary to increased muscle tone and rigidity. Patients also lose the ability to recognize obstacles in their path and may not be able to sit down safely in a chair. Inability to walk increases the risk for development of urinary tract infection by 3.4 times and risk of pneumonia by 6.6 times. Decreased mobility also is a risk factor for incidence of pressure sores, which may result in sepsis.

Aspiration of upper respiratory secretions occurs even in some healthy subjects during sleep. It is more common in those with depressed consciousness. The risk of aspiration increases in patients who have a hyperextended neck, myoclonus, and contractures, all of which are common consequences of advanced dementia.

Strategies to prevent aspiration pneumonia include oral hygiene, avoidance of smoking, potentiation of the cough reflex, and endotracheal intubation. Periodontal disease and dental plaques are risk factors for development of pneumonia. In dentate individuals, risk factors for development of aspiration pneumonia included requiring help with feeding, chronic obstructive pulmonary disease, diabetes mellitus, number of decayed teeth, number of functional teeth, and presence of specific microbes in the saliva. Oral care was shown to decrease the incidence of pneumonia, number of febrile days, and death from pneumonia[15]. Aspiration may also be prevented by medications that potentiate the cough reflex, such as angiotensin-converting enzyme inhibitors and amantadine[16].

Malnutrition

Patients with AD and other progressive dementias often lose weight. Weight loss may start several years before diagnosis of dementia[17]. The weight loss is probably not due to a hypermetabolic state because only minor differences were observed between demented patients and cognitively intact individuals who had similar food intake and physical activity, and resting energy expenditure was similar in institutionalized patients with AD and controls[18]. Weight loss may be due to decreased food intake or increased energy expenditure. Individuals with dementia living alone may forget to prepare food and eat. Visual spatial problems also may decrease food intake because the patient may not be able to recognize food. Decreased appetite with food refusal occurs commonly in patients with AD and may be a symptom of depression. When apraxia develops, patients become unable to feed themselves and require feeding by caregivers. As the disease progresses, swallowing difficulties develop, leading to choking on food and liquids. This may further compromise their food intake.

Increased energy expenditure may be caused by wandering and restlessness. Rapid pacing may increase energy expenditure by 1600 kcal/day. Even patients who no longer can ambulate may exhibit increased activity in bed; as result, bedfast patients may require up to 2800 kcal/day to maintain their body weights[19]. In patients with Parkinson's disease, muscle rigidity, which is common in late stage dementia, also is a source of increased energy expenditure.

Weight loss may not always be an indication of compromised nutritional status and is not associated with increased incidence of comorbid physical illness. In advanced dementia, when patients become unable to walk even with assistance, weight loss may be due to largely to muscle atrophy. In this setting, the use of ideal weight tables would be misleading[19].

Prognostication in advanced dementia

Dementia significantly decreases life expectancy. A population survey in Shanghai, China that investigated predictors of mortality found that the mortality risk ratio was 5.4 for AD and 7.2 for vascular dementia in patients aged 65–74 years,. The risk ratio for AD was similar to the mortality risk ratio for cancer. Among patients aged 75 years and older, the mortality risk ratios were 2.8 for AD, 3.5 for vascular dementia, and 3.6 for 'other dementias'. Because dementing disorders were common in subjects aged 75 years and older, 23.7 per cent of the risk of death could be attributed to these disorders[20]. Similar results have been obtained in Swedish, Italian, and French studies.

Several risk factors have been found to increase mortality risk in individuals with AD and other dementias. These include older age, male gender, low education, comorbidity, and functional disability[21]. Additional risk factors include language impairment at the earliest stages of AD, extrapyramidal symptoms, and more severe behavioural symptoms. Although these factors may be important in terms of health-care planning, they do not substantially increase the accuracy of prognostication in the individual case. It remains very difficult to estimate prognosis in an individual with advanced dementia because of the unpredictability of intercurrent diseases that are the most common cause of death.

Notwithstanding the challenges inherent in the estimation of individual prognosis, physicians often must prognosticate in order to access health-care services. In the United States, the Medicare hospice benefit, which provides comprehensive home care services, requires that two physicians attest that the patient's survival will be 6 months or less if the disease runs its expected course. This guideline is difficult to apply in the population with dementia.

Most recently, estimation of prognosis based on the clinical findings included in a standardized data collection instrument known as the Minimum Data Set was developed[22]. A risk score in this approach is directly proportional to the percent of individuals who die within six months, ranging from 2.7 per cent at a score of 0 to 75 per cent at a score of 12 or more. This may be clinically useful but does not provide a clear cut-off for a prognosis of 6 months, which would be needed to apply the model to the legal prognostication required to access hospice services in the United States. For instance, if the cut-off score is 9 or larger, 63 per cent of individuals will die within 6 months but 26 per cent or individuals with lower scores will also die within 6 months. Thus, significant number of individuals would be deprived of hospice services even though they die within the 6-month period. The difficulty in accessing comprehensive hospice services for demented patients in the United States reinforces the importance of targeting palliative care to patient and family need, rather than to an estimate of survival. There is a need for palliative care that cannot be based on prognostication.

Assessment and treatment of medical problems

Issues in treatment planning and decision-making for patients with advanced dementia

When there is a need for decisions regarding medical interventions, the first concern is determination of decision-making capacity of the individual requiring medical care. Health-care providers may err by overestimation or underestimation of capacity to make decisions regarding health care. Overestimation may occur because individuals are often not tested for their cognitive functioning and may be proficient in covering up their cognitive impairment. Overestimation of decision-making capacity is more common if the patient agrees with the health-care provider. Underestimation of decision-making capacity may occur if an individual carries diagnosis of AD or another progressive dementia and a health practitioner erroneously assumes that the diagnosis itself makes the person unable to make decisions[23]. Underestimation of decision-making capacity is especially common in residents of long-term care facilities who are often considered too impaired to make any decisions.

Individuals who can demonstrate understanding, appreciation, reasoning and expression of a choice regarding a medical intervention, and an understanding of the risks involved in foregoing the intervention are likely to have decision-making capacity. Decision-making capacity should be documented in the medical record, particularly if it has been questioned and a more detailed assessment has been undertaken to evaluate it. Depending on the context—both clinical and regulatory/legal—evaluation by a consultant (usually a neurologist or psychiatrist) may be required to establish a basis for concluding that capacity exists or not.

For individuals who lack decision-making capacity, the decisions have to be made by a proxy. The proxy may decide on the basis of previous patient's wishes if they are known (substituted judgement) or on the basis of the patient's best interest. The clinical and regulatory/legal issues surrounding proxy judgements vary greatly and require that clinicians understand these issues, or obtain consultative help to do so.

Decisions made on the basis of substituted judgement rely on patient's previous wishes that are known to the proxy. The proxy is supposed to act as if being in the 'patient's shoes'. Previous wishes of the patient could be expressed either formally as advance directives or a living will made before the patient became demented, or informally by oral communication between the patient and the proxy during which the patient clarifies his or her philosophy regarding medical interventions should dementia occur. The problem with living wills is that they are very often quite general and do not cover advanced dementia. It has been reported that choices for other conditions poorly predict what the individual would want if he or she developed dementia[24]. An opportunity for formulation of advance directives is mandated at the time of admission into a nursing home. However, this discussion is often focused primarily on preferences concerning cardiopulmonary resuscitation (CPR) and is reviewed only after the crisis of acute illness and hospitalization. Advance directive forms often contain inconsistent language and vague conditions for implementation. Therefore, the advance directives have to be often interpreted by the proxy.

Very often, an appointed proxy or a family member does not have any evidence of the patient's desires or values concerning the present situation. In that case, they have to decide on the basis of the best interest of the patient, as perceived by them. These decisions are very difficult and the proxies need guidance from the treatment team in this process. Otherwise, they may feel overwhelmed and guilty if they decide to forgo some treatment modalities. The caregivers of individuals with dementia, who are most often their proxies, more often select life-sustaining interventions than healthy older adults would want for themselves. It has been reported that family members are not well prepared for their decision-making roles and experience substantial burden, have limited understanding of dementia progression, are uncomfortable in setting the goals of care, have little experience with death, and are ambivalent about the anticipated death of their relative (considering it both a tragedy and a blessing)[25].

Treatment decisions should be made before the time of crisis at a meeting between the treatment team and the proxy and other family members or friends. The treatment team should include the physician or other medical provider, nursing staff representative, and a social worker. The social worker often acts as the meeting's moderator. The presence of a chaplain also is useful for answering concerns regarding religious or ethical matters.

The family conference is a good opportunity to answer all concerns expressed by the proxy and others close to the patient regarding patient's condition and treatment[26]. During the conference, the treatment team should clarify the patient's prognosis and describe options for management of complications and intercurrent diseases. Risk and benefits of all the management strategies should be clearly explained. The presence or absence of evidence concerning the patient's previous wishes should be determined at the beginning of the discussion. The discussion itself should be framed as an opportunity for decisions regarding the goals of care—survival at all costs, maintenance of function, or comfort care[27]. According to these goals, decisions are made to accept or forgo CPR, transfer to acute care setting should medical problems develop, treatment with antibiotics, and tube feeding. These decisions (advance proxy plan) are not permanent and may be changed by the proxy any time. Therefore, it is necessary to maintain good communication between the treatment team and the proxy, notifying the proxy of any significant change in patient's condition. The decisions should be reviewed periodically, and if the proxy dies or become incapacitated, a new proxy should update the advance proxy plan[28].

Informed decisions require knowledge of the benefits and burdens of proposed medical interventions. The relevant details are described below.

Cardiopulmonary resuscitation

The immediate survival of resuscitated nursing home residents is 18.5 per cent; only 3.4 per cent are discharged from the hospital alive[29]. Because the presence of dementia decreases the probability of successful CPR by three times, only 1 per cent of demented residents suffering cardiac arrest can be expected to be discharged alive from the hospital. Even this potential benefit may not be desirable in individuals with severe dementia because CPR is a stressful experience for those who survive. They may experience CPR-related injuries such as broken ribs, and often have to be on a respirator. The intensive care unit environment is not conducive to appropriate care for demented individuals, who may experience worsening confusion and often develop delirium. In addition, patients who are discharged alive from the hospital after CPR are much more impaired than they were before the arrest.

DNR orders in nursing home populations are associated with advanced age, cognitive dysfunction, physical dependency, presence of advance directives or durable power of attorney for health care, absence of Medicaid, and daily visitors. The presence of a DNR order also is influenced by nursing home characteristics and ethnicity of nursing home residents. DNR decisions are affected by the language used to describe CPR procedure and the probability of success presented to the resident. In a study of desire for CPR in a retirement village, 41 per cent of residents opted for CPR if they had an acute illness before learning about survival statistics. When a 10-17 per cent success rate was presented, only 22 per cent desired CPR. The preference decreased to 5 per cent when they were told that with a chronic illness present, the success rate of CPR is only 0–5 per cent[30].

Transfer to acute care setting

Transfer of demented individuals to an emergency room or hospital exposes them to serious risks. Even cognitively intact hospitalized elderly individuals develop depressed psychophysiological functioning that includes confusion, falling, not eating, and incontinence. These symptoms are often managed by medical interventions, such as psychotropic medications, restraints, nasogastric tubes, and urinary catheters, which expose the patient to possible complications, including thrombophlebitis, pulmonary embolus, aspiration pneumonia, urinary tract infection, and septic shock.

Transfer of long-term care facility residents to an emergency room or hospital for treatment of infections and other conditions may not be optimal for management of these problems. Immediate survival after an episode of pneumonia is similar in residents receiving treatment in a long-term care facility and in a hospital. Longer-term outcomes are actually better in residents treated in a nursing home. In one study, the 6-week mortality rate was 18.7 per cent in non-hospitalized residents and 39.5 per cent in hospitalized residents despite no significant differences between the hospitalized and non-hospitalized groups before diagnosis[31]. Similarly, a larger proportion of hospitalized individuals had worsening of their functional status or died at 2 months after the episode of pneumonia. Thus, the available data indicate that transfer to an emergency room or hospital has significant degree of risks and relatively few benefits for individuals with severe dementia. Therefore, this management strategy should be used only when it is consistent with overall goals of care, and not as a default option.

Artificial nutrition and hydration

Patients with severe dementia are unable to feed themselves and often develop swallowing difficulties that provoke choking on food and liquids. They may also start refusing food by not opening their mouth when they are fed. Choking and food refusal are often exhibited simultaneously. Swallowing difficulties and choking may be minimized by adjustment of diet texture and by replacing thin liquids with thick ones (e.g. yogurt instead of milk), and food refusal often responds to antidepressant treatment or to administration of appetite stimulants[32].

There is no evidence that the long-term feeding tubes are beneficial in individuals with advanced dementia. Tube feeding does not prevent aspiration pneumonia and actually might increase its incidence because it does not prevent aspiration of nasopharyngeal secretions and of regurgitated gastric contents. Tube feeding also does not prevent occurrence of other infections. Nasogastric tubes may cause infections of sinuses and middle ear, and gastrostomy tubes may cause cellulitis, abscesses, and even necrotizing fasciitis and myositis. Contaminated feeding solutions may cause gastrointestinal symptoms and bacteriuria.

Tube feeding also does not prevent malnutrition or increase survival in individuals with progressive degenerative dementia. Life-threatening arrhythmia can occur during insertion of a nasogastric tube and perioperative complications, including mortality, are possible following percutaneous endoscopic gastrostomy tube placement. The occurrence of pressure ulcers is not decreased by tube feeding and there is also no evidence that tube feeding promotes healing of pressure ulcers or improves functional status of individuals with severe dementia[33]. The risk of pressure ulcers actually may be increased when tube feeding is initiated because of the use of restraints and increased production of urine and stool.

Tube feeding may increase discomfort of the patients by the presence of the tube itself and by the use of restraints that are often necessary to prevent tube removal. Tube feeding also deprives the patient of taste of food and contact with the caregivers during the feeding process.

The many local, pleuropulmonary, abdominal, and other complications associated with tube feeding must be considered by clinicians and proxies. The imbalance between burdens and benefits justifies a recommendation that tube feeding generally should not be used in individuals with advanced dementia.

Antibiotic treatment of generalized infections

Antibiotic therapy is quite effective in the treatment of an isolated episode of pneumonia or other systemic infection. In most patients, it is possible to limit antibiotic therapy to oral preparations that are equally, if not more, effective as parenteral. It is preferable to limit the use of intravenous therapy in individuals with severe dementia, who do not understand the need for intravenous catheters, try to remove them, and may be restrained or given psychotropic drugs to allow the treatment to continue. In patients who have poor oral intake, intramuscular administration of cephalosporins can be used for treatment of infections.

However, the effectiveness of antibiotic therapy is limited by the recurrent nature of infections in advanced dementia. Antibiotic therapy does not prolong survival in cognitively impaired patients who are unable to ambulate even with assistance and who are mute[34]. Antibiotics also are not necessary for maintenance of comfort in demented individuals because their comfort can be maintained equally well with analgesics and antipyretics, and oxygen if necessary[35].

In addition, antibiotic use is not without adverse effects. Patients may develop gastrointestinal upset, diarrhoea, allergic reactions, hyperkalaemia, agranulocytosis, and *Clostridium difficile* infection. Diagnostic procedures, such as blood drawing and sputum suctioning, which are necessary for rational use of antibiotics, cause discomfort and confusion in demented individuals who do not understand the need for them. The decision to use antibiotics in patients with advanced dementia should, therefore, take into consideration the recurrent nature of infections, which is caused by persistent swallowing difficulties with aspiration and by other factors predisposing for development of infections[36], and the factors that significantly reduce the benefits of antibiotic treatment.

Strategies for maintaining quality of life in advanced dementia

Quality of life in severe dementia is a difficult concept because individuals with severe dementia are unable to report subjective perceptions. Therefore, caregivers must rely on non-verbal communication and observations, which are interpreted in terms of life satisfaction. Nonetheless, it is possible to postulate three important factors that determine quality of life in patients with severe dementia: management of physical symptoms, management of psychiatric symptoms, and provision of meaningful activities. It is also important to promote quality of life of family caregivers and to involve the whole treatment team in assessment of both the patient and the family[37].

Assessment and management of pain and selected other symptoms

Although pain may be a result of an acute condition (faecal impaction, urinary retention, unrecognized fracture), the most common causes are chronic conditions, such as arthritis, old fractures, neuropathy, and malignancy. Pain assessment is difficult in individuals who cannot provide verbal reports. It is necessary to observe these patients for non-verbal signs of discomfort that may indicate the presence of pain. It may be helpful to use a formal observational pain assessment scale that can evaluate pain severity and treatment response (Table 14.1.2)[38,39]. Pain should be treated aggressively, with an opioid if necessary.

Constipation is very common in individuals with advanced dementia and faecal impaction may even cause death. The usual treatment for constipation includes a high fibre diet and osmotic laxatives. Stimulating laxatives should be used only occasionally and stool softeners should be avoided because they often are not effective[40].

Presssure ulcers should be prevented if possible by frequent turning. This also may reduce the incidence of pneumonia. During the dying process, it is important to prevent discomfort due to dryness of the mouth by the use of artificial saliva spray or ice chips.

Assessment and management of behavioural symptoms

Management of psychiatric symptoms in severe dementia is as important for quality of life as management of pain in individuals with terminal cancer. Some behaviours are caused by environmental or physical causes, some by interaction between individuals with dementia and their caregivers, and some are due to dementing process itself. It is important to first eliminate the possibility that behaviours are due to environmental or physical causes, e.g. cold or hot temperature, noise, and hunger or thirst. The most common physical symptom that causes discomfort is unrecognized or undertreated pain[41]. The two most common and most important behavioural syndromes are resistiveness to care and agitation/apathy.

Resistiveness to care

Behavioural problems that occur during interaction between an individual with severe dementia and a caregiver are often erroneously labelled 'aggression'. They are actually caused by the lack of effective communication between the individual with dementia and the caregiver. The individual with dementia does not understand the need for caregiver activity and may resist undressing, bathing, dressing, being put to bed, etc. If the caregiver insists on providing the care, the individual with dementia defends him/herself and may even strike out because the individual with dementia considers the caregiver to be an aggressor. Therefore, this behaviour should be called resistiveness to care[42], which may escalate into combative behaviour.

It is important to prevent escalation of resistiveness to care into combative behaviour that may result in injury of the caregiver or patient. The appropriate non-pharmacological intervention for such a behaviour is improvement in communication, delaying the caregiving activity, or modifying caregiving strategy. Another approach is distraction during care that can be provided by informal discussion or by a planned reminiscence that utilizes remaining long-term memories. Reminiscence during bathing can decrease the stress of bathing, as measured by an increase in heart rate. Resistiveness to care also can be decreased by providing a relaxing environment before the intended procedure. A relaxation period

Table 14.1.2 Pain assessment in advanced dementia (PAINAD).

	0	1	2	Score
Breathing Independent of vocalization	Normal	Occasional laboured breathing. Short period of hyperventilation	Noisy laboured breathing. Long period of hyperventilation. Cheyne–Stokes respirations	
Negative vocalization	None	Occasional moan or groan. Low level speech with a negative or disapproving quality	Repeated troubled calling out. Loud moaning or groaning. Crying	
Facial expression	Smiling, or inexpressive	Sad. Frightened. Frown	Facial grimacing	
Body language	Relaxed	Tense. Distressed pacing. Fidgeting	Rigid. Fists clenched, Knees pulled up. Pulling or pushing away. Striking out	
Consolability	No need to console	Distracted or reassured by voice or touch	Unable to console, distract or reassure	
				TOTAL

provided by exposure to Snoezelen (colourful moving images and soothing music) decreased resistiveness during a teeth cleaning by dental hygienist.

The most effective strategy for management of resistiveness is modification of caregiver approaches. This may include changes in an environment, making bathrooms more homelike and comfortable, or changes in caregiving strategies. Substitution of bed bath for a shower or tub bath greatly decreases resistiveness to bathing without adverse hygienic consequences.

Agitation and apathy

Agitation and apathy may be caused by the dementing process itself. Agitation is a term that is sometimes used to label all behavioural symptoms in dementia but it is better to reserve it for behaviours that communicate to others that the patient is experiencing unpleasant state of excitement and which remain after interventions to reduce internal or external stimuli have been carried out[43]. Apathy is a condition different from depression and results in different pattern of blood flow changes in the brain. Agitation and apathy often occur in the same individual and are difficult to treat pharmacologically because sedatives used to decrease agitation often increase apathy and stimulants used to decrease apathy often increase agitation. The best treatment approach for agitation and apathy is provision of meaningful activities that will be described in the next section.

Meaningful activities and therapeutic environment

Individuals with dementia are unable to initiate meaningful activities themselves because of impairment of the executive function, aphasia resulting in inability to communicate and comprehend, and apraxia resulting in inability to continue their hobbies and activities. It is important to provide meaningful activities even for individuals with severe dementia because they rarely, if ever, progress into a persistent vegetative state. There are four different types of meaningful activities: activities of daily living (ADLs), physical activities, cognitive activities, and creative activities.

Activities of daily living

Activities of daily living include eating, dressing, bathing, toileting, continence, and transferring, and individuals with severe dementia require help in all these activities. The level of help should be appropriate for the level of cognitive impairment; too much help will eliminate patient's involvement, too little help will lead to frustration and agitated behaviour. The caregiver has to realize that he has to partner with a patient and provide care in as much cooperative way as possible. It would be useful to change our terminology and use 'care partner' instead of caregiver. Individuals with dementia benefit from having a stable routine for their activities. Activities of daily living can be made more meaningful even for individuals with severe dementia by using familiar procedures (e.g. shaving with a shaving cream).

Physical activities

Physical activities include adapted sports, exercises, walking programmes, and any other activity the person may be able to perform. Physical activities improve mood, muscle strength and tone, and sleep. They also improve balance and may help to maintain independent ambulation. With progression of dementia, the ability to ambulate independently becomes impaired. Individuals with severe dementia become unable to walk independently because of unsteady or narrow-based gait and inability to avoid obstacles. It is important to help them maintain ambulation for as long as possible and adaptive devices, such as Merry Walker, may help in that respect. When individuals can no longer ambulate even with assistance, physical activity can be provided by doing range of motion and by gentle massage.

Cognitive activities

Significant cognitive impairment prevents individuals with severe dementia from participating in many cognitive activities, such as reading, playing games or musical instruments, solving puzzles, and watching television. However, it is possible to involve them in activities utilizing long-term memories that they may still have. Reminiscence of pleasant memories can be evoked using individualized audiotapes that leave pauses for the patient to respond to the tape (Simulated Presence). This reminiscence therapy delivered by earphones and portable tape player resulted in happier facial expression and increased involvement, but did not change the degree of agitation when compared to placebo tapes and usual care[44].

Reminiscence therapy can be also used to stimulate all senses. A programme 'Bright Eyes' is organized around a theme, e.g. baseball.

With this theme in mind, sense of smell is stimulated by freshly cut grass and tactile sense is stimulated by touching a baseball cap and glove; psychomotor activity is stimulated by tossing a baseball, visual sense by a picture of well known ball park, hearing by singing 'Take me out to the ball game', and gustatory sense by serving non-alcoholic beer. In very severe dementia, reminiscence may be initiated by a familiar scent, artificial bird sounds, and familiar objects.

Creative activities

Creative activities include music, dance, drawing, painting, and craft activities. Even individuals who cannot participate in any cognitive activities may be able to use simple instrument in a group music session and do some drawing with finger prints. Music is an important component of the Snoezelen therapeutic environment and can be used even in severe dementia. Relaxing music together with coloured images may decrease resistiveness to care, as described above. Snoezelen experience also produced positive mood/behaviour change in women with dementia but the effect was not long-lasting. An art programme that uses paints to allow individuals with dementia to express themselves by creating colourful visual images on paper or fabric can result in pleasurable sustained activity and may improve an individual's sense of well-being.

There are also other modalities of meaningful activities that can be employed, such as massage, aromatherapy and pet therapy. Massage may be combined with aromatherapy and may decrease agitation. Aromatherapy using essential oils may assist in the treatment of agitation and neuropsychiatric symptoms, but carries a danger of an allergic reaction to the oils. Use of home-like scents, e.g. baking or cooking, might be also effective and safer. Animal-assisted therapy results in increased social interaction and decreased agitated behaviour and can be used even in severe dementia.

Ideally, the activities described above should be presented as an integrated programme that is available not only during workdays but also during evenings and weekends—continuous activity programming. The programme should be individualized as much as possible, taking into account personal preferences for the type of activity, type of music and like or dislike of pets. Continuous activity programming that involves an interdisciplinary team of care partners can double the hours of activity programming without increase in manpower, and was shown to decrease social isolation and use of psychotropic medications, to improve nutritional state, and to increase staff and family satisfaction[45]. A special activity programme for individuals with end-of life dementia was recently developed and described[46].

Assessment and management of family burden and distress

Functional dependence, together with unsafe behaviour and behavioural symptoms of dementia, create a need for constant supervision that poses a great burden for the caregivers. Since Alzheimer's disease and other progressive dementias last on the average 8 years, caregivers often have to cope with functional impairment and behavioural symptoms for many years. Caregiving in dementia is more stressful than caregiving for physically impaired older adults. Caregivers of individuals with dementia give up their vacation or hobbies more often, have less time for other family members, and report more work-related difficulties than caregivers of individuals with physical impairment. The burden of caregiving results in decreased health-related quality of life.

The degree of burden depends on several factors (Fig. 14.1.2). The primary stressors are caused by the dementia itself, which results in loss of ability to perform basic activities of daily living, presents problems related to psychiatric symptoms and conditions, and forces the caregiver to make decisions regarding the patient's care. Psychiatric symptoms and conditions are the most important factors for caregiver stress. Unfortunately, many caregivers attribute behavioural and psychological symptoms of dementia to causes other than the dementia itself and believe that the individual with dementia has control over his or her behaviour. Having to make decisions about care recipient's care can lead to a significant level of stress for the caregiver, which could be reduced considerably if the health care professionals discuss and support the caregiver's decision.

The secondary caregiver stressors are related to the consequences of caregiving that directly affect the caregiver. Since a spouse is very often the primary caregiver, caregiving may affect the quality of marital relationship. Dementia may cause changes in the patterns of sexual behaviour or loss of intimacy. Increased sexual demands may be difficult to handle for a wife who has to care for her husband like for a child. Another source of stress may be conflict between the primary caregiver and other family members. This conflict is especially serious if children from a previous marriage do not get along well with the caregiving spouse. Caregivers who report poor family functioning in the area of affective responsiveness, problem solving, and communication have higher ratings of strain and burden than caregivers who report good family functioning[47].

Job-related difficulties may also cause significant stress for the caregiver. Many caregivers have to quit their jobs to provide full-time care resulting in lost earnings. Caregivers who continue working may have to decrease their working hours and may miss new job opportunities or promotions.

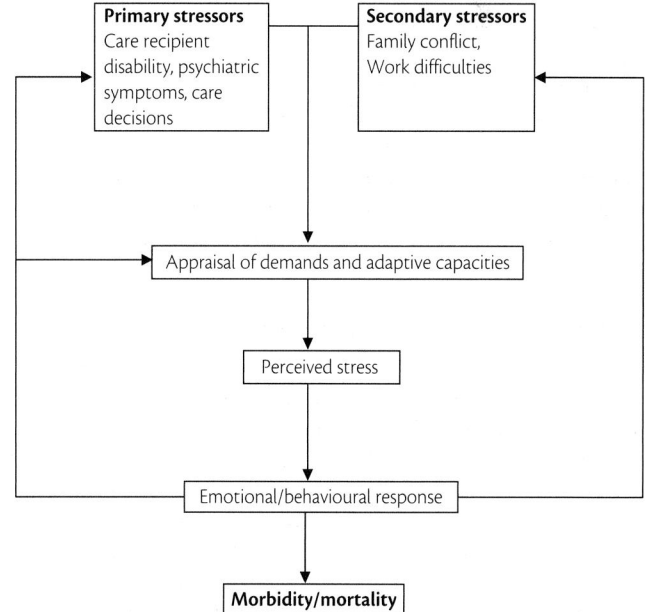

Figure 14.1.2 Caregiving burden according to the Stress/Health Model. Reprinted with permission from Volicer, L. (2005). Caregiver burden in dementia care: prevalence and health effects. *Current Psychosis & Therapeutics Reports*, **3**, 20–5.

Both primary and secondary stressors should be continually evaluated by the caregiver, who must decide whether the demands posed by the patient's illness can be met. The caregiver becomes stressed if she/he perceives a mismatch between the demand and her/his ability to meet them. The stress then affects emotional and behavioural responses of the caregiver. The responses could be maladaptive and result in increased primary and secondary stressors, or in decreased capacity to appraise the ability to cope with the demands, thus increasing the stress level further. Examples of such a maladaptive response could be physical altercation with the care recipient that would result in more severe behavioural symptoms, or a verbal fight with another family member. Chronic level of perceived stress results in psychiatric and physical consequences. The most significant psychiatric consequence of dementia caregiving is high incidence of depression and anxiety.

Physical consequences of caregiving include increased morbidity and mortality of the caregivers. Caregivers are less likely to engage in preventive health behaviours and experience consequences of chronic stress that include increased blood pressure and impaired immune function. The risk of experiencing physical illness or disability is increased in spousal caregivers and the greatest risk is associated with providing more daily living assistance. Spouses who provide care and experience caregiving stress have higher mortality risk than non-caregiving controls.

Although caregiver stress is related to the direct provision of care for the demented individual, the stress does not cease after the individual is institutionalized. Caregivers often feel guilty that they 'failed' their loved ones by placing them in an institution and the caregiver burden remains high. Bereavement support is very important for caregivers of individuals with dementia because almost half of them develop depression after patient's death and significant degree of depression was also found almost two years after the death of the care recipient[48]. Therefore, it is very important to monitor physical and mental status of caregivers not only during patients' life but also after his/her death.

Conclusion

Palliative treatment is very appropriate for individuals with severe dementia and their families. The treatment should address not only medical problems but also behavioural symptoms of dementia and should strive for highest quality of life possible. Support of family caregivers during severe dementia and after death is crucial for preserving their physical and mental health.

References

1. Ganguli, M., Dodge, H.H., Chen, P. *et al.* (2000). Ten-year incidence of dementia in a rural elderly US community population: The MoVIES Project. *Neurology*, **54**, 1109–16.
2. Alzheimer's Disease and Related Dementia Guideline Panel. (1996). *Recognition and initial assessment of Alzheimer's disease and related dementias.* Agency for Health Care Policy and Research, Rockville, MD.
3. Snowdon, D.A., Greiner, L.H., Mortimer, J.A. *et al.* (1997). Brain infarction and the clinical expression of Alzheimer disease—The nun study. *JAMA*, **277**, 813–17.
4. (1998). *Neuropathology of dementing disorders*, 1st edition. Oxford University Press, New York, NY.
5. White, L., Petrovitch, H., Ross, W. *et al.* (1996). Prevalence of dementia in older Japanese-American men in Hawaii— The Honolulu-Asia Aging Study. *JAMA*, **276**, 955–60.
6. McKeith, I.G., Ballard, C.G., Perry, R.H. *et al.* (2000). Prospective validation of Consensus criteria for the diagnosis of dementia with Lewy bodies. *Neurology*, **54**, 1050–8.
7. Duda, J.E., Lee, V.M.Y., and Trojanowski, J.Q. (2000). Neuropathology of synuclein aggregates: New insights into mechanisms of neurodegenerative diseases. *J Neurosci Res*, **61**, 121–7.
8. Mendez, M.F., Cherrier, M., Perryman, K.M. *et al.* (1996). Frontotemporal dementia versus Alzheimer's disease: Differential cognitive features. *Neurology*, **47**, 1189–94.
9. Spillantini, M.G., Murrell, J.R., Goedert, M. *et al.* (1998). Mutation in the tau gene in familial multiple system tauopathy with presenile dementia. *Proc Natl Acad Sci USA*, **95**, 7737–41.
10. Chandra, V., Bharucha, N.E., and Schoenberg, B.S. (1986). Conditions associated with Alzheimer's disease at death: Case-control study. *Neurology*, **36**, 209–11.
11. Volicer, L. and Hurley, A.C. (1997). Physical status and complications in patients with Alzheimer disease: Implications for outcome studies. *Alzheimer Dis Assoc Disord*, **11**, 60–5.
12. Volicer, L., Smith, S., and Volicer, B.J. (1995). Effect of seizures on progression of dementia of the Alzheimer type. *Dementia*, **6**, 258–63.
13. Perls, T.T. and Herget, M. (1995). Higher respiratory infection rates on an Alzheimer's special care unit and successful intervention. *JAGS*, **43**, 1341–4.
14. Chiappelli, M., Tumini, E., Porcellini, E. *et al.* (2006). Impaired regulation of immune responses in cognitive decline and Alzheimer's disease: Lessons from genetic association studies. *Expert Rev Neurother*, **6**, 1327–36.
15. Yoneyama, T., Yoshida, M., Ohrui, T. *et al.* (2002). Oral care reduces pneumonia in older patients in nursing homes. *J Am Geriatr Soc*, **50**, 430–33.
16. Volicer, L. (2007). Terminal stage. In *Clinical diagnosis and management of Alzheimer's disease* (ed. S. Gauthier), pp. 247–55. Informa Healthcare, Oxon, England.
17. Johnson, D.K., Wilkins, C.H., and Morris, J.C. (2006). Accelerated weight loss may precede diagnosis in Alzheimer disease. *Arch Neurol*, **63**, 1312–17.
18. Poehlman, E.T. and Dvorak, R.V. (2000). Energy expenditure, energy intake, and weight loss in Alzheimer disease. *Am J Clin Nutr*, **71**, 650S–5S.
19. Khodeir, M., Conte, E.E., Morris, J.J. *et al.* (2000). Effect of decreased mobility on body composition in patients with Alzheimer's disease. *Journal of Nutrition, Health & Aging*, **4**, 19–24.
20. Katzman, R., Hill, L.R., Yu, E.S.H. *et al.* (1994). The malignancy of dementia: Predictors of mortality in clinically diagnosed dementia in a population survey of Shanghai, China. *Arch Neurol*, **51**, 1220–5.
21. Aguero-Torres, H., Fratiglioni, L., Guo, Z. *et al.* (1999). Mortality from dementia in advanced age: A 5-year follow-up study of incident dementia cases. *J Clin Epidemiol*, **52**, 737–43.
22. Mitchell, S.L., Kiely, D.K., Hamel, M.B. *et al.* (2004). Estimating prognosis for nursing home residents with advanced dementia. *JAMA*, **291**, 2734–40.
23. Ganzini, L., Volicer, L., Nelson, W. *et al.* (2003). Pitfalls in assessment of decision-making capacity. *Psychosomatics*, **44**, 237–43.
24. Reilly, R.B., Teasdale, T.A., and McCullough, L.B. (1994). Projecting patients' preferences from living wills: An invalid strategy for management of dementia with life-threatening illness. *JAGS*, **42**, 997–1003.
25. Forbes, S., Bern-Klug, M., and Gessert, C. (2000). End-of-life decision-making for nursing home residents with dementia. *Journal of Nursing Scholarship*, **32**, 251–8.
26. Mahoney, M.A., Hurley, A.C., and Volicer, L. (1998). Advance proxy planning. In *Hospice care for patients with advanced progressive dementia* (eds. L. Volicer and A. Hurley), pp. 169–88. Springer Publishing Company, New York.
27. Gillick, M., Berkman, S., and Cullen, L. (1999). A patient-centered approach to advance medical planning in the nursing home. *JAGS*, **47**, 227–30.

28. Volicer, L., Cantor, M.D., Derse, A.R. *et al.* (2002). Advance care planning by proxy for residents of long-term care facilities who lack decision-making capacity. *J Am Geriatr Soc,* **50**, 761–7.

29. Finucane, T.E. and Harper, G.M. (1999). Attempting resuscitation in nursing homes: Policy considerations. *JAGS,* **47**, 1261–4.

30. Murphy, D.J., Burrows, D., Santili, S. *et al.* (1994). The influence of the probability of survival on patients' preference regarding cardiopulmonary resuscitation. *N Engl J Med,* **330**, 545–9.

31. Thompson, R.S., Hall, N.K., Szpiech, M. *et al.* (1997). Treatments and outcomes of nursing-home-acquired pneumonia. *J Am Board Fam Pract,* **10**, 82–7.

32. Morris, J. and Volicer, L. (2001). Nutritional management of individuals with Alzheimer's disease and other progressive dementias. *Nutrition in Clinical Care,* **4**, 148–55.

33. Gillick, M.R. (2000). Sounding board—Rethinking the role of tube feeding in patients with advanced dementia. *N Engl J Med,* **342**, 206–10.

34. Luchins, D.J., Hanrahan, P., and Murphy, K. (1997). Criteria for enrolling dementia patients in hospice. *J Am Geriatr Soc,* **45**, 1054–9.

35. Van der Steen, J.T., Ooms, M.E., Van der Wal, G. *et al.* (2002). Pneumonia: The demented patient's best friend? Discomfort after starting or withholding antibiotic treatment. *J Am Geriatr Soc,* **50**, 1681–8.

36. Volicer, L., Brandeis, G., and Hurley, A.C. (1998). Infections in advanced dementia. In *Hospice care for patient with advanced progressive dementia* (eds. L. Volicer and A. Hurley), pp. 29–47. Springer Publishing Company, New York.

37. Lane, P., Trudeau, S.A., Hewitt, S. *et al.* (2000). Interdisciplinary assessment of persons with Alzheimer's disease and other progressive dementias. *Alzheimer's Disease Quarterly,* **1**, 16–43.

38. Hutchison, R.W., Tucker, W.F., Jr, Kim, S. *et al.* (2006). Evaluation of a behavioral assessment tool for the individual unable to self-report pain. *American Journal of Hospice and Palliative Care,* **23**, 328–31.

39. Warden, V., Hurley, A.C., and Volicer, L. (2003). Development and psychometric evaluation of the PAINAD (Pain Assessment in Advanced Dementia) Scale. *JAMDA,* **4**, 9–15.

40. Volicer, L., Lane, P., Panke, J.A. *et al.* (2004). Management of constipation in residents with dementia: Sorbitol effectiveness and cost. *Journal of the American Medical Directors Association,* **5**, 239–41.

41. Cohen-Mansfield, J. and Creedon, M. (2002). Nursing staff members' perceptions of pain indicators in persons with severe dementia. *Clinical Journal of Pain,* **18**, 64–73.

42. Mahoney, E.K., Hurley, A.C., Volicer, L. *et al.* (1999). Development and testing of the resistiveness to care scale. *Res Nurs Health,* **22**, 27–38.

43. Hurley, A.C., Volicer, L., Camberg, L. *et al.* (1999). Measurement of observed agitation in patients with Alzheimer's disease. *J Mental Health Aging,* **5**, 117–33.

44. Camberg, L., Woods, P., Ooi, W.L. *et al.* (1999). Evaluation of Simulated Presence: A personalized approach to enhance well-being in persons with Alzheimer's disease. *JAGS,* **47**, 446–52.

45. Volicer, L., Simard, J., Pupa, J.H. *et al.* (2006). Effects of continuous activity programming on behavioral symptoms of dementia. *Journal of the American Medical Directors Association,* **7**, 42f6–31.

46. Simard, J. (2005). Namaste, giving life to the end of life. *Alzheimer's Care Quarterly,* **6**, 14–19.

47. Heru, A.M., Ryan, C.E., and Iqbal, A. (2004). Family functioning in the caregivers of patients with dementia. *Int J Ger Psychiat,* **19**, 533–7.

48. Bodnar, J.C. and Kiecolt-Glaser, J.K. (1994). Caregiver depression after bereavement: Chronic stress isn't over when it's over. *Psychol Aging,* **9**, 372–80.

49. Volicer, L. and Hurley, A. (1998). *Hospice Care for Patients with Advanced Progressive Dementia*, p. xii. Springer Publishing Company, New York, NY.

50. Schulz, R. and Martire, L.M. (2004). Family caregiving of persons with dementia: Prevalence, health effects, and support strategies. *American Journal of Geriatric Psychiatry,* **12**, 240–9.

14.2

Palliative medicine in older adults

Nathan E. Goldstein and Diane E. Meier

Palliative care differs for geriatric patients from what is usually appropriate in a younger patient because of the nature and duration of chronic illness during old age. Despite the fact that most deaths occur in older adults in the setting of chronic illness, clinical guidelines for palliative care have predominately focused on younger adults. Considerations such as maintaining functional status, the presence of discrete syndromes effecting older adults (e.g. dementia, delirium, frailty, falls), and physiologic changes that occur with aging necessitate an approach to the geriatric patient, which integrates the fundamental principles of geriatrics into the model of palliative care. In addition, older patients are cared for in a variety of settings, some of which (e.g. nursing homes) may be unfamiliar to clinicians. This chapter will outline the key principles fundamental to the care of older patients and explore how to employ these concepts when caring for geriatric patients in need of palliative care for symptoms, goal setting, or coordination of care across settings.

Demographics

Improvements in sanitation and nutrition combined with advances in medicine have produced a dramatic increase in life expectancy[1]. While a child born in the United States in 1900 could expect to live fewer than 50 years, life expectancy for a child born in 2025 is expected to increase to 84 years for a girl and 78 years for a boy[2]. By the year 2030, the percentage of the US population over 65 is projected to be near 20 percent as compared with 5 percent in 1900[3]. While modern medicine can save a patient from a potentially fatal heart attack, early stage cancer, and most bacterial diseases, these survivors will eventually go on to develop advanced, end-stage disease such as heart failure, dementia, debilitating arthritis, or Parkinson's disease—to name just a few. Indeed, today most adults die while old and sick and after a substantial period of disability[4].

Despite the fact death typically occurs in older adults in the setting of chronic illness, research in and clinical guidelines for palliative care have predominantly focused on younger adults—specifically those with cancer[5]. The prototypical example of a palliative care patient is that of a 45-year-old mother of three with advanced breast cancer. Care for this patient would include chemotherapy until it no longer meets the patient's goals of care, treating her symptoms (e.g. pain, anorexia), addressing her psychological and spiritual concerns, supporting her partner, and helping to arrange for care of her children after her death. The majority of this patient's

care occurs at home (with or without hospice) or in the hospital, and the period of functional debility is relatively brief (months). The care of this patient is markedly different from that of an 88-year-old widowed woman with advanced emphysema, osteoarthritis, hypertension, moderate cognitive impairment, and frailty. Palliative care for this patient involves treating the primary disease process (her lung disease); managing her multiple chronic medical conditions and co-morbidities (osteoarthritis, hypertension) and geriatric syndromes (cognitive impairment, frailty); assessing and treating the physical and psychological symptom distress associated with all of these medical issues; and establishing goals of care and treatment plans in the setting of an unpredictable prognosis. The needs of her caregiver(s) are also different from that of the younger patient. Individuals caring for geriatric patients are often adult children with their own family, work responsibilities, and medical conditions; and these roles must be balanced with the months to years of personal care that they must provide to their aging parent[5].

Data on the treatment of pain in old age suggests that elderly patients also receive less pain medication than younger persons for chronic and acute pain. In one study, nearly 30 per cent of elderly cancer patients living in long-term care facilities did not receive pain medication despite daily complaints of pain, and another 16 per cent received only acetaminophen; these percentages increased with age and minority ethnicity[6]. Age and female gender were predictors of under-treatment of pain in a study of ambulatory patients with cancer[7]. Geriatric patients with hip fracture also receive inadequate pain control, particularly if suffering from cognitive impairment[8,9]. Chronic pain syndromes such as arthritis, low-back pain, and other musculoskeletal problems affect 25–50 per cent of the community dwelling elderly and are also typically under-treated[10]. Given the prevalence of cognitive impairment, musculoskeletal disorders, and malignant disease in the elderly, these studies indicate that pain is inadequately identified and treated in the geriatric population.

Factors to consider in the approach to geriatric patients

Because of the functional, psychological, and physiologic changes that occur with aging, the basic approach to the geriatric patient differs from that of a younger patient. These differences include aspects of history taking and physical exam, a shift from the acute illness model to encompass multiple chronic diseases, and goals of care that maximize function and reduce burdens of treatment.

Functional assessment

While the basic elements of approach to the history taking in younger patients apply to older individuals (e.g. chief complaint, history of present illness), there are distinct aspects of the history applicable primarily to the elderly. A portion of the history must focus on the older patient's pre-morbid level of function. Traditionally functional status is assessed by using two separate categories—Activities of Daily Living (ADL)[11] and Instrumental Activities of Daily Living (IADL)[12]. The six ADLs include patients' self ability to use the toilet, eat (i.e. feed themselves), dress, groom (i.e. neatness of hair, nails, hands), ambulate, and bathe. The eight IADLs include patients' ability to carry out the following tasks on their own: use the telephone, shop, prepare food, clean house, clean their laundry, use transportation, take their medications, and manage finances. While both scales have formal rating systems that are useful within a research context, in a clinical setting patients are often rated as being independent, needing some assistance, or being totally dependent in their ADLs or IADLs. Knowledge of a patient's premorbid functional assessment is essential in the context of palliative care because this information can assist in setting realistic goals of treatment as well as aid in discharge planning. Older patients often have a relatively smaller functional reserve than younger patients, and so a previously independent 85-year-old woman may quickly become completely dependent within the context of a hospitalization for an acute illness. Clinicians encountering this patient for the first time during her hospitalization may wrongly assume she was always this infirm, unless baseline functional status is clarified in order to assure that goal-setting and treatment decisions do not underestimate a patient's potential for recovery

Social assessment

In addition to focusing on older patients' functional status, the palliative care clinician must take a detailed social history in assessing patients with advanced illness. It is important to get a sense of patients' caregivers, as older patients are often cared for by either an aged spouse (who may have some degree of debility and chronic illness as well) or children (who have to split their time caring for their aged parent with concerns about their own family or work). Each of these situations may increase caregiver burden and may pose a significant impediment for safe discharge planning. It is not uncommon to find older patients whose aged partner at home can no longer care for them—either physically or emotionally. Nor is it uncommon to find that children can no longer balance caring for an aged parent with their other responsibilities. In addition to caring for the patient and planning appropriate care transitions, the palliative care clinician will need to be aware of feelings of guilt or failure that this may evoke from these family caregivers and provide appropriate counselling and referral to supportive services. In addition to caregivers of older patients, with changes in family structure, palliative care clinicians are encountering an increasing number of younger patients whose primary care giver may be an older parent, a situation which encompasses many of the complexities mentioned above. Regardless of the demographics of the caregiver, older patients almost uniformly need assistance at home after a hospitalization or nursing home stay, and an interdisciplinary team of palliative care specialists can not only assist in

this organizing, but also refer family to community resources for emotional and psychological support to reduce caregiver strain. Research has shown that caregiver burden is a significant factor for both morbidity and mortality—even when controlling for other factors[13,14]. Caregiver burden has been linked to a wide array of ill effects on both caregivers and the patients for whom they care[15,16], and so assessing the needs of caregivers and assisting them is a key element of caring for older patients with advanced illness.

In addition to assessing the family caregiver for palliative care patients, clinicians must pay special attention to the social network of older patients. Older patients may be physically isolated for a multitude of reasons: difficulties with ambulation, inability to drive, lack of funds to participate in day programmes—to name just a few. Physical isolation may quickly lead to social isolation for an older adult. Many older patients have lost life-partners, friends, and family members, and thus may suffer from protracted grief and bereavement compounded by social isolation. This isolation may be particularly difficult for patients with serious illness as these individuals may not have anyone to assist them with their most basic needs or may be afraid to ask for help from friends, relatives, and neighbors due to a fear of becoming a burden. These patients should be referred to volunteer agencies aimed at assisting older patients, and may particularly benefit from referral to a hospice organization with a large volunteer base. For these patients, the process of 'life review' may be particularly important. This process involves patients recounting (either orally to a clinician, or recording on paper or audio/videotape) major events in their lives and what they believe are their most important accomplishments. This allows the patient to realize the legacy that they are leaving to their family or society and helps patients cope with the loss of self and existential suffering often encountered when confronting the possibility of death.

Rethinking goal-setting in the context of chronic illness in older adults

In younger patients, the focus of the palliative care clinician is usually on one acute, life-threatening illness. In older individuals, however, the focus is typically on multiple competing co-morbidities, any one of which could ultimately result in the patient's death. For example, a palliative care physician may be consulted on a 89-year-old man with moderate dementia, diabetes, peripheral vascular disease, and coronary artery disease who is admitted to the hospital with gangrene of the left foot resulting in sepsis. He then suffers a small myocardial infarction induced by rate-related ischaemia from his systemic infection. In this case, the palliative medicine clinician must focus on more than the basic decision as to whether the patient should undergo amputation. The approach to this patient and his family in the context of setting goals of care must relate to balancing the various chronic illnesses. Which plan is better—to have the patient undergo peripheral re-vascularization with the risk of a significant myocardial event or return to his previous location of care and combine antibiotic treatment and local wound management with palliative care? Care for a patient like this is no longer the exception, but has become the rule for many palliative medicine providers who must learn to balance the multiple competing co-morbid conditions of patients with chronic, eventually fatal illness. This re-framing of illness as the summed consequences of multiple chronic diseases is difficult for clinicians as the majority of medical training focuses on cure of discrete illness, and in older patients cure is rarely an option. Instead, the goal is to maximize function and quality of life. Patients and families must be educated on this as well. Popular culture considers growing old as being synonymous with decay and debility, an image in stark contrast to the fundamental geriatric principle, which aims to have patients 'age in place' (i.e. in their home and community), remaining as functionally and socially connected as possible. To assure the best quality of care for an aging population, this concept must become a cornerstone of palliative medicine as well.

The rethinking of palliative care in the context of older patients leads to another key concept of geriatrics—the primary goal is to keep the chronic disease as stable as possible. This assures that clinicians work to maximize patients' quality of life while maintaining their functional status and assuring that the benefits of disease-modifying treatments outweigh the burdens—where both benefit and burden are defined by the patient's overall goals of care. Physicians can help weigh the risks and benefits of procedures in light of the individual patient's current health status and previously stated goals of care. Some surgeries are clearly palliative. For example, cataract surgery can lead to tremendous improvement in a patient's quality of life; however, preventive repair of an asymptomatic abdominal aortic aneurysm may not be indicated in a patient with severe disability due to chronic illness. In addition, as a patient's underlying medical illness and functional status change, so too may their goals of care[17]. That is, some patients may opt for a focus on life-sustaining treatments as illness progresses, whilst others may prefer a largely palliative approach. Goals of care must be reassessed over time in patients with chronic illness[4], and at each juncture options for palliative and supportive services must be reconsidered in the context of a patient's changing goals.

The need to revisit goals of care over time has become more pressing in the last decade due to advances in medical technology. The advent of new therapies, particularly those designed for patients with end-stage lung or heart disease, have led to increases in longevity some for patients, but at a price. While 20 years ago, treatment of severe cardiac disease consisted of medications alone[18], high-tech devices such as implantable cardioverter defibrillators (ICDs) and left-ventricular assist devices (LVADs)[19] are now available to alter the natural course of the disease. Patients with severe primary pulmonary hypertension (increased resistance to lung blood flow) now may receive a constant infusion of the medication epoprostenol to maintain cardiac and lung function[20].

While there is no doubt that these interventions often improve quality and extend quantity of life, none are without complications. For example, LVAD patients require anti-coagulation to reduce risk of stroke or blood clots, with associated high risk of bleeding complications[21,22]. Currently available LVADs require patients to be permanently attached to an extracorporeal device[23], and clinicians must help patients decide if this machine dependency is acceptable to them. Patients with pulmonary hypertension on epoprostenol must carry an external pump with them at all times, and can die within hours if the pump fails or if the medication supply is exhausted. The current standard of care in the United States is to offer any device or procedure that might prolong life, with little attention to the long-term costs or other consequences of these choices.

The ICD is a particularly interesting example of a device with a dramatic shift in the benefit–burden ratio as patients near the end of life. An ICD is a device implanted in a patient's chest to monitor the heart rhythm and deliver shocks to terminate potentially lethal arrhythmias when necessary. While ICDs reduce sudden cardiac death[24–27], patients with these devices do eventually die of something, whether heart failure or other diseases. As a patient's clinical status worsens, physiologic changes (intrinsic and extrinsic to the heart) may affect the cardiac conduction system, leading to more arrhythmias and increasing the frequency of shocks. Since ICD shocks can cause pain and anxiety and may not prolong a life of acceptable quality[28–30], it is appropriate to consider ICD deactivation as a patient's clinical status worsens and death is near[31,32]. When an ICD is implanted, physicians believe the device is appropriate at *that particular* time given the patient's clinical status. But a device that is indicated at one point may not continue to be appropriate later, when a new benefit vs. burden calculation becomes necessary. When a patient's cardiac disease—or a new illness—worsens to a point where death is likely soon, the burdens of the ICD will exceed its benefits, and clinicians must address the issue of ICD deactivation at that time[33].

Palliative care for geriatric syndromes

The geriatric syndromes are clusters of illnesses, often multifactorial in aetiology, that are prevalent among older adults[34,35]. While numerous conditions have been defined as geriatric syndromes, the ones most likely to be encountered by palliative medicine clinicians are dementia, delirium, constipation, falls, frailty, and depression.

Dementia

Dementia is defined as an acquired decline in memory and in at least one other cognitive function (e.g. language, visual-spatial, executive) sufficient to interfere with daily life in an otherwise alert individual[36]. Dementia is usually, though not always, irreversible and is characterized by a slow decline in cognitive and other functioning overtime[37]. While the majority of patients diagnosed with dementia will have Alzheimer's disease, other forms include Lewy body dementia, vascular dementia, and Parkinson's disease with dementia. Understanding the differences between these forms is key to palliative medicine clinicians, because their symptoms vary. For example, Lewy body dementia is characterized by behavioural changes and visual hallucinations early in the disease, whereas patients with Alzheimer's often have personality and behavioural changes when they are in the middle to late stages[37]. These behavioural changes become more frequent as dementia progresses[38], and patients may suffer from paranoia, delusions, hallucinations, sleep disorders, agitation, and combativeness. Such symptoms are associated with rapid cognitive and functional decline[38,39]. These behavioural changes place an incredible burden on caregivers, not only because it becomes more difficult to provide daily care to these individuals but also because caregivers are simultaneously mourning the loss of the person they knew. Because behavioural changes in patients with dementia place such a large strain on caregivers, they are linked to an increased likelihood of nursing home placement[39,40].

Dementia is the prototype of chronic illness in the geriatric population. Providing palliative care to geriatric (and non-geriatric) patients with chronic illness means that at different stages of illness, patients will require preventive, life-prolonging, rehabilitative, and palliative measures based on individual needs. For examples of

Table 14.2.1 How palliative care and treatments change throughout the course of chronic illness.

Early	Middle	Late
Discuss diagnosis, prognosis, and course of disease	Assess efficacy of disease modifying therapy	Discuss/re-evaluate goals of care with patient and caregivers
Discuss disease-modifying therapies	Review course of disease	Re-evaluate and change advance directives as necessary
Discuss goals of care, hopes, and expectations	Confirm advance directives and ensure a health-care proxy is appointed	Actively manage symptoms
Discuss advance care planning	Recommend physical/occupational therapy to preserve function and promote socialization	Review financial resources and needs
Manage comorbidities	Behavioural and pharmacologic symptom control	Consider hospice referral/planning to ensure peaceful death
Advise financial planning/consultation with a social worker for future needs including long-term care	Treat mood disorders	Assess spiritual needs
Inform patients and family about support groups	Suggest support groups for patients and caregivers	Offer respite care
Offer social and emotional support to caregivers	Offer social and emotional support to caregivers	Inform patient and family that death is expected
Inquire about desire for spiritual support	Review long-term care options and resource needs	Support financial (assure affairs are in order) and emotional closure (five things to suggest families and patients to say to each other include: 'Thank you', 'I love you', 'Forgive me', 'I forgive you', 'Goodbye')[128]
Behavioural and pharmacologic symptom control		
Treat mood disorders		Provide social and emotional support to family and other caregivers

how palliative care may differ throughout the course of a patient's illness, see Table 14.2.1.

Delirium

Delirium is a medical illness characterized by a disturbance of level of consciousness, which develops rapidly, tends to fluctuate over the course of the day, and is caused by the physiologic consequences of an underlying medical condition, medication, or other substance[41]. It is distinguished from dementia by its effect on level of consciousness, fluctuation over time, and its rapid onset. While patients in the last days of life may suffer from delirium (also known as terminal delirium), older patients are particularly at risk for this condition. While delirium has been shown to have a prevalence of anywhere from 5–50 per cent of hospitalized older patients[42–45], depending on their underlying medical condition, it is often under-recognized[46–48]. This is due in part to the fact that delirium comes in two forms: hyperactive, hyperalert and hypoactive, hypoalert[49]. The hyperactive delirium is recognized quickly, as patients may be shouting, agitated, restless, aggressive, and even violent at times. Patients with hypoalert delirium, on the other hand, are often not diagnosed because they may be sleeping or unresponsive, and this type of delirium may be inaccurately attributed to fatigue or depression. Both hypo- and hyperalert delirium are often misdiagnosed as dementia in older patients if the patient's baseline pre-morbid function is not properly determined by clinicians.

To assist clinicians with diagnosing delirium, the Confusion Assessment Method can be used[50]. This screening tool, which has been shown to be 94 per cent sensitive and 90 per cent specific for diagnosing delirium when compared to Diagnostic and Statistical Manual of Mental Disorders (DSM) criteria[41] consists of four elements: (1) acute onset and fluctuating course; (2) inattention; (3) disorganized thinking; and (4) altered level of consciousness[50].

A positive screen includes both elements 1 and 2 and either 3 or 4. Diagnosing delirium is particularly important given that patients with delirium may have mortality rates as high as 35–40 per cent at one year[51]. Data also indicate that delirium in older patients may take several months to clear after they leave the hospital, and it is associated with increased rates of nursing home placement amongst elderly patients[52]. In some patients, delirium may never clear, and even if it does, patients may be so debilitated by it that they will never return to their baseline functional status. The persistent nature of delirium can thus influence patients' care needs after discharge as well as lead to increased caregiver strain.

Multiple factors place older patients at risk for delirium. Underlying (and possibly undiagnosed) dementia in an older hospitalized patient is one of the strongest and most consistent risk factors for delirium[48,53]. Many medications increase risk for delirium, especially in older patients. These include anticholinergics and anti-histamines (e.g. diphenhydramine), tricyclic antidepressants, anti-inflammatory medications (e.g. prednisone), benzodiazepines, gastrointestinal agents (e.g. ranitidine, cimetidine), opioid analgesics (especially meperidine), and some cardiovascular agents (e.g. digitalis)[54,55]. It is important for the palliative medicine clinician to recognize the potential of these agents to induce delirium because they are commonly prescribed for older adults and should be discontinued if they no longer contribute to meeting the patient's goals of care (e.g. cimetidine, ranitidine). Other precipitants of delirium in older patients include hypoxia, infection, constipation/faecal impaction, sensory impairment, withdrawal syndromes (from alcohol or benzodizepenes), electrolyte imbalance, renal/hepatic dysfunction, stroke, and urinary retention[48,54].

The cornerstone for treating delirium is to attempt to reverse/treat the underlying cause. In some cases this can result in a rather dramatic improvement; for example, treating a urinary tract infection in an older patient with metastatic bladder cancer incorrectly labeled as 'actively dying' may cause a dramatic improvement in mental status. However, many causes of delirium are not reversible, and older patients often have multiple aetiologies for their delirium—especially if they have advanced illness[49]. For patients whose delirium can not be reversed, a combination of medications and environmental/social support can be used. Antipsychotics (both typical and atypical) are the medications most often used in the treatment of delirium. Benzodiazepines should not be used as first line treatment (except in patients thought to be having delirium due to withdrawal of alcohol or benzodiazepines) because one randomized clinical trial[56] showed that while antipsychotics were helpful, benzodiazepines actually worsened delirium in patients with advanced HIV disease[57]. This trial showed that anti-psychotic medications helped patients with both hyperactive, hyperalert delirium as well as patients with hypoactive, hypoalert delirium[57]. The hypoactive delirium patients are often overlooked despite the fact that hypoactive delirium is associated with the same poor outcomes as is the more active forms of delirium. Patients with agitated delirium may benefit from environmental interventions such as frequent re-orientation (provided by objects such as dateboards, clocks with large faces); reducing ambient noise levels; putting familiar objects in the room; and encouraging family members to be near the bedside offering reassurance and calming words. In conjunction with other non-pharmacologic interventions, these environmental techniques have been shown to decrease delirium in hospitalized patients and subsequently improve both morbidity and mortality[52,58]. Not all older patients will experience delirium, but given both the physical and emotional toll it can take on patients and their caregivers in addition to the association of delirium with increased morbidity, mortality, increased likelihood of nursing home placement, and increased hospital length of stay[52,59–62], it is particularly important for clinicians to recognize this condition and attempt to reverse it.

Constipation

Constipation is a nearly universal complaint of elderly patients. Over half of the community dwelling elderly report constipation[63]. Risk factors include female gender, medications, depression, and immobility[64–66]. Many chronic diseases with high prevalence in older adults also predispose patients to constipation—Parkinson's disease, hypothyroidism, diabetes mellitus, diverticular disease, irritable bowel syndrome, and hemorrhoids to name only a few. It is also one of the few side effects of opioids that do not decrease with time. Other common medications that many elderly patients take that may dispose to constipation include iron and calcium supplements, calcium channel blockers, anti-histamines, and tricyclic antidepressants.

Because of its prevalence and complications in older patients, it is important that clinicians ask about this symptom when caring for elderly patients. Complications resulting from constipation include functional bowel obstruction, nausea and vomiting, anorexia, delirium, colonic perforation, and death. When taking a history of constipation, the clinician should ask about baseline bowel habits as well as current frequency of stools to ascertain changes in the patient's pattern. Prevention of constipation is particularly important in older patients, who may become more immobile as their underlying illness progresses. Older patients receiving opioid medications should simultaneously be started on a multi-component

(stool softener + laxative) prophylactic bowel regimen. A rectal exam or radiographic obstructive series should be performed in older patients to assure that fecal impaction is not present, as using an increasingly stronger regimen of oral laxatives in an impacted older adult is not only unlikely to improve constipation but may lead to bowel perforation. Diarrhoea in an older patient who has a history of constipation may be a sign of bowel inflammation and liquid stool leaking around an area of impaction. For a further discussion on laxatives and a guideline for prescribing these medications, please refer to Chapter 10.2.3.

Falls

Falling is a common geriatric syndrome that may lead to decreased mobility and is linked with serious injury and increased risk of nursing home placement[67,68]. It is often part of a vicious cycle in older individuals, which leads to fear of falling and change of gait and behaviour patterns leading to diminished mobility and subsequent increased frequency of falls. Falls are particularly important in palliative care patients because they may be a sign of worsening disease (e.g. pain from breast cancer which has metastasized to the femur may result in pain and fracture, either of which can result in a fall in an older adult) and may also result in increased caregiver strain and make formerly possible discharge plans unsafe.

Falls in older adults are often multi-factorial in nature and may result from medications, arthritis, impaired gait and balance, environmental factors, decreased strength, sensory impairment (e.g. vision, proprioception), and from underlying medical disease[68–70]. Many of the medications prescribed in palliative care (e.g. opioids, benzodiazepines, anti-psychotics)[71,72] may increase falls, and so the benefit must be weighed against the risk of falling. Impaired gait and balance may be due to general deconditioning, pain, or physiologic processes related to aging. Similarly, decreased strength and sensory impairment (including problems with vision, proprioception, or vibration sense) may be due to aging but may also be related to the patient's underlying terminal illness. Environmental factors may pose fall risks whether it be in the hospital—such as when an older patient is attached to several tubes or poles—or in the home due to factors such as cluttered walking paths, loose rugs, improper lighting, or a lack of grab-bars and railings[73]. An older patient who entered the hospital with relatively good muscle strength and tone may become debilitated in the setting of an acute worsening of their underlying disease and subsequent confinement to bed, and thus a previously safe home environment may no longer be a suitable discharge plan. Medical conditions can predispose patients to falls either as a direct result of the disease (e.g. Parkinson's disease) or due to a physical symptom of the underlying condition (e.g. heart failure resulting in hypotension). Delirious patients may be at increased risk for falls[74]. Multiple interventions have been shown to reduce the risk of falls in older patients, including reducing psychoactive and hypotensive medications, home safety assessment by health professionals and modification of environmental risks (e.g. securing rugs, removing cords, addition of grab-bars), gait-retraining, and use of assistive devices and appropriate footware[68,75–78].

Frailty

Frailty is a unique syndrome in older adults characterized as a progressive, physiologic process marked by declines in function and physiologic reserves as well as increased vulnerability to morbidity and mortality[79]. It is separate from (though often related to) disability, a condition marked by difficulty carrying out activities of daily living[80]. It is of particular importance in palliative care because frailty is often seen but not recognized in this population, which can cause a great deal of confusion and unnecessary diagnostic testing for both clinicians and families. Clinically, it is defined by generalized weakness, weight loss, fatigue, slowed performance, and a generalized state of low activity[81]. While it may coexist and be related to other comorbidities, it also exists as a separate clinical syndrome and has been shown to carry an increased risk of death when controlling for all other factors[81,82]. In practice it may be seen as a gradual progressive downward spiral in function and activity, and this decline in reserve and function leads to inability to recover from what may have been a trivial illness[79]. This syndrome is particularly confusing for families who may not understand that frailty is associated with risk of death similar to that of metastatic cancer or heart failure.

Researchers have shown that the frailty syndrome is related to a series of biological changes present in older patients[83]. Central to the model of frailty is sarcopenia—the loss of skeletal mass[79]. Several hormonal changes have also been associated with the frailty syndrome, and these include growth hormone, insulin-like growth factor-1, and changes in the hypothalamic-pituitary-adrenal axis[79]. Inflammation, characterized by chronically elevated levels of iterleukin-6 and chronic immune system activation appears to be present in large subpopulations of older adults who are frail[84]. For each of these systems, there is evidence that these age-related changes lead to vulnerability and poor outcomes in older adults, and that the aggregate alterations may have synergistic effects[79].

Palliative care is paramount for older patients who suffer from frailty[85]. This includes controlling pain and other symptoms, preventing hospital and nursing home admission, maintaining and improving functional status through rehabilitation and exercise, and improving overall sense of well-being through medical, psychological, and social interventions[79]. On an individual level, physical and occupational therapy, hormonal interventions, and anti-inflammatory medications may help to improve patients' symptoms[79]. For example, increased use of resistance exercise and Tai Chi have separately been associated with benefits in function and quality of life as well as a reduction in falls[86–88]. When added to resistance exercise, nutritional supplements have been shown to counteract frailty to some extent[86]. Uncontrolled pain has been associated with increasing frailty and debility in older adults[10,79,89], and as such it is of paramount importance to control pain in frail elders. Systematic interventions in the United States such as instituting inpatient (ACE—Acute Care for the Elderly, or GEM—Geriatric Evaluation and Management) or outpatient (PACE—Program of All-Inclusive Care for the Elderly) programmes have been shown to improve outcomes in frail, older patients[79]. Finally, using a team based approach to provide targeted geriatric assessment by pulling expertise from physicians, nurses, and social workers may improve outcomes for older patients with frailty[90,91].

Depression

While depression may be an issue in any patient near the end of life, depressive symptoms in older adults occur so frequently that it is recognized as a geriatric syndrome. While there is some controversy as to whether older adults suffer from higher rates of major depressive disorders as defined by DSM criteria, the prevalence of depressive symptoms is high in most research examining older adults[92]. The aetiology of prevalent depressive symptoms in older patients is likely multifactorial, but includes a combination of physical illness, neurologic disease, and changes in social support and economic resources as they relate to patient's baseline coping skills and behaviours[93]. Because of the multi-factorial aetiology of depression in older adults traditional screening tools relying on symptoms (such as anorexia, insomnia, fatigue, and weight loss) as markers may be non-specific for depression and instead reflect the consequences of co-morbid chronic medical illness[94]. It is more helpful to screen for psychological symptoms such as hopelessness, worthlessness, guilt, and suicidal ideation[95].

Easy-to-use screens for depression include the single item 'Are you depressed?[96]' and the two-item depression case finding instrument, which involves asking patients: (1) 'During the past month, have you often been bothered by feeling down, depressed, or hopeless?' and (2) 'During the past month, have you often been bothered by little interest or pleasure in doing things?[97]' Both tools have been shown to be excellent screens, and if patients answer 'no' to these questions then depression is unlikely[96,97]. Instruments, such as the Geriatric Depression Scale[98] have been developed for use and tested specifically in older populations, but regardless of which scale one uses, it is important to evaluate how the patient's mood interferes with his daily activities.

While sadness or difficulty coping may be 'normal' occurrences for older patients with chronic disease, depression, even in the face of terminal illness, is never 'normal' and must be addressed[94]. Prevalence rates of depression in patients with terminal illness are difficult to obtain, as studies report varying ranges[99]. It is clear, however, that patients with a history of depression, substance abuse, or uncontrolled pain are at higher risk for depression[96,100]. Treatment of depression in patients with serious illness is often multi-factorial, combining psychotherapy, cognitive–behavioural techniques, and medications. Appropriate antidepressants may include a selective serotonin reuptake inhibitor (SSRIs), a serotonin-in-noradrenaline reuptake inhibitor (SNRI), tricyclic antidepressants, or trazodone[95]. These agents may take several weeks to take effect, however, so for patients whose death is near psychostimulants (e.g. methylphenidate 2.5–5 mg at 8 am and 1 pm daily) may be of benefit. Medications used for depression in an older person may increase the frequency of delirium and falls[72], and so it is important to balance the benefits of a medication with its potential side-effects in an older frail patient near the end of life.

Physiologic changes associated with aging

While it appears that pain perception does not change with normal aging[101] there are changes in physiology that make evaluation and treatment more complex and difficult. Physical changes related to aging may complicate differential diagnosis of symptoms. For example, hip pain in an older woman with metastatic breast cancer may relate to spread of the disease to the femur, a stress fracture, osteoarthritis, or some combination of these. These conditions require different treatments, and a combination of diagnostic studies and treatments may be required.

Impact of hearing and vision changes on providing palliative care

Age-related changes in hearing and vision are particularly prevalent in older individuals and pose special challenges for the clinician.

Hearing loss is the most common sensory impairment in old age. Presbycusis is a term used to denote progressive bilaterally symmetric decrease in hearing primarily affecting high tones and associated with the aging process. It has been linked to physiologic changes in the cochlea, the organ of Corti, and the temporal bone[102]. Another common cause of hearing reduction in older adults relates to cerumen impaction, a correctable process that results from both age-related changes to the cerumen glands themselves (decrease in number and activity) as well as attempts to manually disimpact the cerumen with either fingers or swabs that may ultimately worsen the impaction[102]. Other age-related causes of hearing loss in older adults include vascular events, acoustic neuomas, and otosclerosis. Visual changes are also common in older patients, and sources include cataracts, glaucoma, age-related macular degeneration, and diabetic retinopathy.

These changes in sensation often complicate and slow the history and physical exam. In addition, they may result in social isolation as well as mistakes in both understanding and adhering to treatment plans. Older adults may be embarrassed about these changes as they are a stereotypical sign of aging, and they may not readily admit to their families and clinicians that they exist. Palliative medicine practitioners must be aware of the prevalence of these disorders and ask about them. Referral to audiologists and ophthalmologists for both diagnosis and treatment are warranted regardless of the stage of patient's illness, as either maintenance or improvement of function are possible with current treatments, and this can greatly improve patients' quality of life. In addition to referral to specialists, clinicians can assist patients by writing out clear, simple directions for medications in large print (which will assist patients with either visual or hearing difficulties) as well as use of large fonts on both patient handout materials and prescription bottles.

Dry mouth and tooth loss

Age-related changes in dentition and production of saliva can result in discomfort, weight loss, and exacerbation of the frailty syndrome. While dentures are often employed for patients with poor dentition, these prostheses are not without complications. Ill-fitting dentures can cause pain and difficulty with chewing and speaking, resulting in a worsening of the original problems as well as social isolation and embarrassment. Removal of teeth may result in loss of the gum structure making it more difficult for dentures to fit well, as well as restriction to softer foods. Since these foods are not as satisfactory in terms of taste and texture and interfere with social engagement, this may lead to both weight loss and a general decline in quality of life. It must be remembered that food is not only used for sustenance but is a central aspect of social identity and belonging—at home and in important religious and cultural groups. A loss of the ability to share in these traditions may result in social isolation, withdrawal, and depression.

Xerostomia is the subjective feeling of dry mouth and may be a particular problem in older adults. It is often multi-factorial in origin and may result from conditions relating to aging as well as a side effect of treatments. Medication use is the most common cause of dry mouth in older individuals, and may result from antidepressants, anticholinergics, antipsychotics, chemotherapy, antispasmodics, and opioid medications. Age-related conditions that may contribute to dry mouth include diabetes mellitus, Sjögren's syndrome, and bacterial infections of the salivary glands. In addition, older patients are particularly at risk of dehydration

not only because of underlying medical conditions such as dementia or decreased functional status making it difficult to feed themselves, but they also have a blunted thirst response as compared to younger patients. Because the functions of saliva include beginning digestion, protecting from dental caries, and lubricating and repairing oral tissues[103], conditions resulting in decreased saliva have multiple consequences and must be considered when evaluating patients with weight loss, anorexia, or dysphagia—all conditions that are encountered with some frequency in the older palliative care population.

Dysphagia and artificial hydration and nutrition

Dysphagia is any difficulty in swallowing food or transferring food from the mouth to the stomach. It may be related to physiologic changes such as poor dentition or xerostomia, or to other disease processes such as cancer, esophageal abnormalities, or neurological conditions (including Parkinson's disease and dementia). Dysphagia may be a result of medications used to treat these conditions or surgery/radiation to the mouth, pharynx, oesophagus, or stomach related to malignant disease. Environmental conditions such as improper diets, lack of assistance with feeding, and bland or uninteresting food may also contribute to dysphagia.

A common medical response to dysphagia is to provide artificial hydration or nutrition through either an enteral or parenteral route. Artificial hydration and nutrition is an emotionally charged issue for many caregivers, both familial and professional. Many believe that the patient would suffer hunger and thirst without artificial hydration and nutrition. While many older patients receive these treatments in the last months of life, there is no evidence that it prolongs life or relives suffering in patients with terminal dementia or other illnesses[104–107]. Family members should understand that loss of appetite is a normal part of the dying process and is associated with nearly all terminal conditions including dementia and frailty. Studies of terminally ill cognitively intact patients with anorexia have shown that they do not suffer hunger and that symptoms of dry mouth can be relieved with good oral hygiene, artificial saliva, and sips of water[108]. Tube feeding has not been shown to decrease the risk of aspiration pneumonia in older adults, and may actually increase this risk[109]. While artificial hydration and nutrition may seem like an attractive treatment for older patients with dysphagia, its benefits and burdens must be carefully analysed in the context of the patient's overall goals of care. Support and education for caregivers of patients who have to make decisions about providing these treatments is imperative and is often best provided with an interdisciplinary team approach and family meetings.

Changes in renal and hepatic function and their impact on prescribing

Age-related changes in renal and hepatic function are important in the older palliative care patient because of their implications for the prescribing of all medications—particularly with respect to opioids. Age-related declines in kidney function may make it more difficult for older patients to eliminate opioids as well as their metabolites. Similarly, decreases in glomerular filtration rates, increased susceptibility to volume depletion secondary to decreases in hypothalamic vasopressin, and decreased thirst all place older adults at higher risk of side effects. Changes in the liver also occur with aging and may result in a decreased ability to induce enzymes such as cytochrome p450, a key component in the metabolism of medications. Interactions between medications may further alter hepatic metabolism. Knowledge of changes in hepatic and renal function and their impact on drug metabolism are important for opioids as well as other pain medications such as acetaminophen and non-steroidal anti-inflammatory drugs (NSAIDs). Preferred opioids in renal insufficiency are hydromorphone and fentanyl because these agents are metabolized in the liver[110]. Acetaminophen should not be used in patients with liver disease. NSAIDs are contraindicated in patients with renal disease, and should be used with caution in the older patient because of their gastrointestinal side-effects and propensity to cause bleeding through platelet inhibition[10].

In general, it can be assumed that the elderly are more sensitive to medications, especially those with actions in the central nervous system, and thus have a greater potential for toxicity. These changes have important implications for prescribing—in terms of both medication strength and dosing intervals. The adage 'start low—go slow' holds for all prescribing in this patient population, but it is especially true in the context of symptom management.

Relationship of dermatologic changes to pressure ulcers and poor wound healing

Changes in both skin and subcutaneous adipose tissue that occur with aging have implications for providing palliative care to older adults. Epidermal thickness decreases with age and keratinocytes are smaller and have a lower proliferation rate in older individuals; both of these changes cause skin to be more sensitive to minor trauma and to heal more slowly[111]. Changes in the dermis relate to decreases in collagen, elastic fibres, and vascular structures, thus resulting in thinner skin, which heals slower, has a decreased inflammatory response, and appears more transparent[111]. Loss of subcutaneous fat, which can occur with any progressive chronic illness, also occurs independently as a natural part of the aging process. This makes older individuals more prone to pressure ulcers, but also has implications for rates of absorption of transdermal preparations of medications—as a loss of fat may result in both more rapid and more erratic absorption of medications. Because changes in the skin are visible and, from a societal perspective, may be one of the clearest markers of old age, these changes may result in social isolation, depression, and poor quality of life. While proper skin care through the use of lotions, lubricants, and sunscreens along with the prevention and treatment of pressure ulcers must be meticulously applied in older adults, the social and psychological implications of dermatologic changes that occur with older patients near the end of life should be considered as well.

Models of geriatric care

Unlike palliative care for younger patients, which is delivered in either the inpatient or outpatient setting, geriatric patients often require care across a more complex continuum including a hospice facility, the hospital, a rehabilitation facility, a nursing home, and their own home. Clinicians must understand and communicate with providers in each of these settings in order to assure safe and quality care for older palliative care patients and their family.

Palliative care in hospitals

More than 50 per cent of adults die in the hospital, and nearly 100 per cent of older adults spend some time in the hospital in the year before death[1,112]. Given these statistics, most older adults first encounter palliative medicine in the inpatient hospital setting. These services provide a multifaceted approach that integrates control of pain and other symptoms, improving communication between providers and patients/families, and creating effective discharge plans that will meet the older patients' needs and transition to a new setting of care[113]. Palliative medicine programmes may be housed within internal medicine, geriatrics, anesthesia, oncology, case management, and other programmes, depending on the locus of leadership and administrative support[114]. Because of the predominance of older adults in hospitals and on palliative care services, these teams must have expertise in the care of older frail patients to both understand their clinical needs but also to prevent functional decline. Hospitalization in older patients is associated with functional decline and a number of other complications (e.g. skin breakdown, deconditioning, falls, delirium, weight loss), which can leave an older patient in worse condition upon discharge than when they arrived in the hospital for the treatment of their admitting diagnosis[115,116]. Hospital palliative care clinicians must utilize services necessary to reduce the hazards of hospitalization, which often lead to increased morbidity and mortality[117].

Palliative care in nursing homes

Given the demography of old age with prolonged functional impairment in the context of multi-morbidity, some have argued that the new frontier of palliative care will be in the nursing home, which is likely to become the most common location of death by 2040[118]. Integration of palliative care principles in the nursing home is fraught with challenges. Staff in US nursing homes, under pressure of well intended but often counter productive regulations, often implement all life-sustaining treatments regardless of projected outcome and patients' goals of care. This results in hospital transfer at the first sign of illness without prior discussion about a plan of care. Recent interventions related to advanced care planning have shown promise[119,120]. Reimbursement patterns are also a disincentive to providing good palliative care, particularly in terms of the use of hospice services in nursing homes. In the United States, for example, hospice reimbursement may be below the standard Medicaid reimbursement for a nursing home bed or for provision of rehabilitation services, making it economically impossible for nursing homes to offer hospice to patients. Other barriers to palliative care in nursing homes include the near 100 per cent annual turnover of poorly paid and poorly trained 'hands on' staff and a nearly equivalent turnover of nursing and administrative directors, for similar reasons[121].

Because of the challenges of providing palliative care in nursing homes, clinicians must pay special attention in the transfer of care of patients to these settings. Regardless of destination, older patients who leave the inpatient setting are particularly vulnerable to poor hand-offs as they transition from one facility to another[122–124]. Especially in cases where patients have either complex care plans based on their goals or particularly difficult to treat symptoms, conversations upon transfer from one facility should occur directly from one physician to another to assure that the patient's history and plan are understood by all individuals who will be caring for the patient at the new facility. All too often, communication about plans of care are relegated to illegible and inadequate standardized forms completed by administrative staff who are not directly responsible for or familiar with patient care, and as a result the nuances and complexities of a plan of care—especially in terms of the treatment of vulnerable frail elders—is lost upon transition from one set to another. In addition to a legible and brief summary of the patient's medical conditions and hospital course, key elements of a transition document include names and contact information for surrogate/proxy; wishes for resuscitation/ventilation (DNR/DNI) and re-hospitalization; medication dosages, frequency of administration, and purpose; contact information for the physicians who took care of the patient in the hospital who can be reached if further information is necessary; contact information for agencies who will be providing care in the home; and follow-up appointments. It is not enough to simply create and complete documents—both the discharging and receiving facilities have a responsibility to communicate before, during, and after the patient's discharge. The core components of these responsibilities are outlined in Table 14.2.2. Patients and families are often confused about the nature, purpose, and goals of the transition. To assure that they understand the transfer and have the information that they need to assure a smooth transition, Table 14.2.3 provides a checklist of prompts that can be provided to help families ask appropriate questions of the health care team.

Palliative care in the home setting

Many older persons in need of palliative care prefer to be at home. Complexities of symptom management, caregiver burden and anxiety, need for medical equipment and procedures, and reimbursement for services and home visits can often make this difficult, however. Particularly among older frail individuals who have difficulty managing the health-care system and organizing complex discharge plans, it is the role of the palliative care physician to know and carefully organize the options for home-care support and services and to advocate for patients returning to their home.

A complete home-care team consists of a physician, social worker, and visiting nurse. Additional services that may be vital to the care of patients at home include physical or occupational therapists, speech pathologists, wound care specialists, and clergy. In the United States, many of these services are offered to individuals on the hospice benefit, but due to regulations requiring patients to forego life-sustaining treatments and be certified as within 6 months of death in order to access hospice, this benefit may not be available to all patients. The palliative care physician must remain in contact with patients and caregivers (both paid and unpaid) to assure a safe home-care plan. The role of the physician is to create the plan of care with respect to the patient's medical condition and to oversee the delivery of care for patients, though the administrative role of the physician in this team varies by country and reimbursement practices. Social workers provide emotional support and counselling to patients and their caregivers, both before and after the patient dies. They are also the coordinators of care in terms of assuring insurance eligibility, completing the appropriate paperwork, and acting as a liaison with home care and durable medical equipment agencies to assure that the necessary equipment and services are provided. Finally, the visiting nurse is often the principal professional in the care of homebound older patients, serving as the bridge between patient/family and physician, social worker, and other health-care professionals, and assuring that symptom and goal setting needs are addressed.

Palliative care at home often involves medical equipment in the patient's home. Care planning involves determining adequacy of

Table 14.2.2 Core elements of communication that must be provided before, during, and after transition of frail older patients from one health care setting to another.

Both the sending and receiving care teams are expected to:

◆ Shift their perspective from the concept of a patient discharge to that of a patient transfer with continuous management

◆ Begin planning for a transfer to the next care setting upon or before a patient's admission

◆ Elicit the preferences of patients and caregivers and incorporate these preferences into the care plan, where appropriate

◆ Identify a patient's system of social support and baseline level of function (i.e. how will this patient care for him- or herself after discharge?)

◆ Communicate and collaborate with practitioners across settings to formulate and execute a common care plan

◆ Use the preferred mode of communication (i.e. telephone, fax, e-mail) of collaborators in other settings

The sending health-care team is expected to ensure that:

◆ The patient is stable enough to be transferred to the next care setting

◆ The patient and caregiver understand the purpose of the transfer

◆ The receiving institution is capable of and prepared to meet the patient's needs

◆ All relevant sections of the transfer information form are complete

◆ The care plan, orders, and a clinical summary precede the patient's arrival to the next care setting. The discharge summary should include the patient's baseline functional status (both physical and cognitive) and recommendations from other professionals involved with the patient's care, including social workers, occupational therapists, and physical therapists

◆ The patient has a timely follow-up appointment with an appropriate health care professional

◆ A member of the sending health-care team is available to the patient, caregiver, and receiving health-care team for 72 h after the transfer to discuss any concerns regarding the care plan

◆ The patient and family understand their health-care benefits and coverage as they pertain to the transfer

The receiving health-care team is expected to ensure that:

◆ The transfer forms, clinical summary, discharge summary, and physician's orders are reviewed prior to or upon the patient's arrival

◆ The patient's goals and preferences are incorporated into the care plan

◆ Discrepancies or confusion regarding the care plan, the patient's status, or the patient's medications are clarified with the sending health-care team

Used with permission from Eric A. Coleman, MD, Care Transitions Program. www.caretransitions.org.

space for these elements as well as the means to deliver them (Is there an elevator? Will the hospital bed fit in it?) and support their use (Is there appropriate electrical power to supply the needed equipment?). Home safety must be considered in terms of both the use of specialized medical equipment (Are there smokers in the house that would prohibit the use of oxygen?) and to assure that patients can have 24-h access to emergency help. This may require that a caregiver is in the home at all times or the use of electronic devices that can summon help from either emergency support services or a nursing agency. There should also be a health-care

Table 14.2.3 Guidelines to assist patients and families ask appropriate questions before transition between health care settings.

Before I leave the care facility, the following tasks should be completed:

◆ I have been involved in decisions about what will take place after I leave the facility

◆ I understand where I am going after I leave this facility and what will happen to me once I arrive

◆ I have the name and phone number of a person I should contact if a problem arises during my transfer

◆ I understand what my medications are, how to obtain them, and how to take them. The critical medications I may need immediately (e.g. pain medications) are already in my home or at the pharmacy of my next location of care

◆ I understand the potential side effects of my medications and whom I should call if I experience any of them

◆ I understand what symptoms I need to watch out for and whom to call should I notice them

◆ I understand how to keep my health problems from becoming worse

◆ My doctor or nurse has answered my most important questions prior to my leaving the facility

◆ My family or someone close to me knows that I am coming home and what I will need once I leave the facility

◆ If I am going directly home, I have scheduled a follow-up appointment with my doctor, and I have transportation to this appointment

Adapted with permission from Eric A. Coleman, MD, Care Transitions Program. www.caretransitions.org

professional available at all times to answer patient/caregiver questions, make appropriate changes to treatment plans as necessary—regardless of time or day, and to perform home visits on an emergency basis if care needs can not be managed over the telephone. Recent trials show that this model of 'hospital at home' is associated with improved outcomes, greater patient satisfaction, and may be cost saving[125,126].

Depending on the patients' illness, functional status, and care needs, there are appropriate options for providing care for patients at home. Patients who are functionally independent may need no help on an ongoing basis but only a visiting nurse to periodically check on them. For those patients who need more assistance at home, a certified home health agency may be able to provide an aide who can assist with basic functions such as bathing and dressing as well as housekeeping and shopping. To a limited extent, these individuals are paid for by insurers (in the United States, Medicare and Medicaid). For those individuals needing more services who can afford it, a private pay aide can be hired to provide more hours and assist with more complex needs. Nursing home placement is often the option of last resort if the patient and family do not have resources to private pay for help at home. Finally, hospice provides an interdisciplinary team approach to care, and will provide a wide array of services but only for patients meeting eligibility criteria for hospice.

Advance care planning across transitions of care

Advance directives address two issues: who should speak for the patient if he or she cannot (health care proxy or durable power of attorney for health care) and the kinds of treatments that should or should not be undertaken (living will or health-care directive)[4]. An advance care plan anticipates these contingencies, in that it creates contingencies for worsening of disease and outlines not only what is to be done, but what is *not* to be done and who is to be contacted in the event of an emergency[4]. These documents often address the larger goals of care such as desired functional outcomes and acceptable vs. unacceptable states. In particular, these documents should describe the scenario the patient considers a 'fate worse than death' and so all clinicians caring for a patient will have a clear understanding of what outcomes are—and most importantly are *not*—acceptable to a patient. These larger goals of care then can help determine which therapies are appropriate and which

should be withheld. For example, a clinician might frame the question as follows: 'Some of my patients say that if they are permanently unconscious or unable to recognize and interact with their loved ones, that at that point they would want medical care focused on their comfort. Others of my patients say they would want all life-prolonging technologies used, regardless of their mental condition. Which kind of person are you?'

Advance care planning often beings with a conversation between the clinician and the patient/family. The next step is to operationalize this in a formal document, many of which are publicly available. One example, the Physicians Orders for Life-Sustaining Treatment (POLST), which was created in Oregon, is a document now adopted by many states in the US, which covers a wide range of medical treatments and options for patients with advanced illness. Data has shown that the POLST is effective in influencing the care plan—it is followed by health care providers in the outpatient setting and has been taken up with increasing frequency in nursing home settings[119,127]. An electronic copy of the POLST is available at www.polst.org.

These plans are only effective, however, if they are transferred from one location of care to another. Unfortunately, this does not always occur[124], either because the form is not transferred or because its instructions are not followed. It is of paramount importance that advance care plans are transferred from one location of care to another and that all parties involved in the care of a patient understand and agree to carry out a plan of care directed by the patient or surrogate as expressed in these documents. In addition to traditional documentation, out of hospital do not resuscitate forms should be given to all palliative care patients in the home when this is in line with their goals of care. Likewise, the use of an order not to re-hospitalize a patient should be considered in the care of patients at home. (Both of these orders are part of the standardized POLST form.) While these concepts apply to all patients with advanced illness, it is particularly important for older patients who might not be able to express their wishes due to dementia or delirium. Because frail older adults may suffer from multiple exacerbations of chronic disease, the care plan must be readdressed over time with patients, to assure that it reflects their current wishes and medical condition. Finally, palliative care clinicians should be comfortable with time-limited trials of therapies and express this concept to patients and their families. If a particular treatment does not yield the hoped-for improvement in a patients' quality of life or is no longer in line with the overall goals, then it should be discontinued. In the case of caregivers who insist on taking loved ones home, as may be encountered in the case of adult children caring for aging parents, palliative care clinicians should explain that even the best laid discharge plans often fail. This pre-emptive counselling can reduce feelings of guilt and inadequacy of caregivers who take loved ones home only to find that their care needs are too complex for them to meet in the home setting.

Conclusion

To provide the highest quality palliative care to older patients, clinicians must understand their unique needs as well as how the aging process affects the delivery of health care to the elderly. Older patients are afflicted by chronic, progressive illnesses that may persist for decades, and lead to increasing functional dependency and caregiver burden. Physicians are challenged to ameliorate symptoms, maintain patients' physical and social function, delay progression of disease, relive caregiver stress, and assist patients with planning for the future. The benefits and burdens of treatments in older patients with multiple diseases may be quite different than that in younger patients with only one life-threatening illness, and as a result clinicians must assess the older patient's goals of care and tailor treatments to those goals. Improvement in symptoms must be balanced with maintaining functional status and maximizing quality of life—a challenge that makes care of the frail older adult sometimes difficult but always rewarding.

References

1. Field, M.J. and Cassel, C.K. (eds.) (1997). *Approaching death: Improving care at the end of life*. National Academy Press, Washington, D.C.
2. United States Census Bureau. Projected Life Expectancy at Birth by Race and Hispanic Origin, 1999 to 2100. Available at: http://www.census.gov/population/www/projections/files/nation/summary/np2008-t10.xls Accessed on November 12, 2008.
3. United States Census Bureau. U.S. Interim Projections by Age, Sex, Race, and Hispanic Origin. Available at: http://www.census.gov/population/www/projections/files/nation/summary/np2008-t2.xls Accessed on November 12, 2008.
4. Lynn, J. and Goldstein, N.E. (2003). Advance care planning for fatal chronic illness: Avoiding commonplace errors and unwarranted suffering. *Ann Intern Med*, **138**(10), 812–18.
5. Goldstein, N.E. and Morrison, R.S. (2005). The intersection between geriatrics and palliative care: A call for a new research agenda. *J Am Geriatr Soc*, **53**(9), 1593–8.
6. Bernabei, R., Gambassi, G., Lapane, K. et al. (1998). Management of pain in elderly patients with cancer. Sage Study Group. Systematic assessment of geriatric drug use via epidemiology. *JAMA*, **279**(23), 1877–82.
7. Cleeland, C.S., Gonin, R., Hatfield, A.K. et al. (1994). Pain and its treatment in outpatients with metastatic cancer. *New England Journal of Medicine*, **330**(9), 592–6.
8. Feldt, K.S., Ryden, M.B., and Miles, S. (1998). Treatment of pain in cognitively impaired compared with cognitively intact older patients with hip-fracture. *J Am Geriatr Soc*, **46**(9), 1079–85.
9. Morrison, R.S. and Siu, A.L. (2000). A comparison of pain and its treatment in advanced dementia and cognitively intact patients with hip fracture. *J Pain Symptom Manage*, **19**(4), 240–8.
10. (2002). The Management of Persistent Pain in Older Persons. *J Am Geriatr Soc*, **50**(6 Suppl), S205–24.
11. Katz, S., Downs, T., Cash, H. et al. (1970). Progress in development of the index of ADL. *Gerontologist*, **10**(1), 20–30.
12. Lawton, M. and Brody, E. (1969). Assessment of older people: Self-maintaining and instrumental activities of daily living. *Gerontologist*, **9**(3), 179–86.
13. Schulz, R., Newsom, J., Mittelmark, M. et al. (1997). Health effects of caregiving: The caregiver health effects study: An ancillary study of the cardiovascular health study. *Annals of Behavioral Medicine*, **19**(2), 110–16.
14. Schulz, R. and Beach, S.R. (1999). Caregiving as a risk factor for mortality: The caregiver health effects study. *JAMA*, **282**(23), 2215–19.
15. Covinsky, K.E., Goldman, L., Cook, E.F. et al. (1994). The impact of serious illness on patients' families. Support Investigators. Study to understand prognoses and preferences for outcomes and risks of treatment. *JAMA*, **272**(23), 1839–44.
16. Beach, S.R., Schulz, R., Yee, J.L. et al. (2000). Negative and positive health effects of caring for a disabled spouse: Longitudinal findings from the caregiver health effects study. *Psychology & Aging*, **15**(2), 259–71.
17. Fried, T.R., Byers, A.L., Gallo, W.T. et al. (2006). Prospective study of health status preferences and changes in preferences over time in older adults. *Arch Intern Med*, **166**(8), 890–5.
18. Boxer, R., Yang, S.X., and Hager, W.D. (2003). Congestive heart failure and the elderly. *Conn Med*, **67**(8), 497–503.
19. Rose, E.A., Moskowitz, A.J., Heitjan, D.F. et al; Randomized Evaluation of Mechanical Assistance for the Treatment of Congestive Heart Failure (REMATCH) Study Group. (2001). Long-term mechanical left ventricular assistance for end-stage heart failure. *N Engl J Med*, **345**(20), 1435–43.
20. Humbert, M., Sitbon, O., and Simonneau, G. (2004). Treatment of pulmonary arterial hypertension. *N Engl J Med*, **351**(14), 1425–36.
21. Goldstein, D.J. and Beauford, R.B. (2003). Left ventricular assist devices and bleeding: Adding insult to injury. *Ann Thorac Surg*, **75**(6 Suppl), S42–7.
22. Kohmoto, T., Oz, M.C., and Naka, Y. (2004). Late bleeding from right internal mammary artery after heartmate left ventricular assist device implantation. *Ann Thorac Surg*, **78**(2), 689–91.
23. Copeland, J.G., Smith, R.G., Arabia, F.A. et al. (2004). Cardiac replacement with a total artificial heart as a bridge to transplantation. *N Engl J Med*, **351**(9), 859–67.
24. Buxton, A.E., Lee, K.L., Fisher, J.D. et al. (1993). A randomized study of the prevention of sudden death in patients with coronary artery disease. *New England Journal of Medicine*, **341**(25), 1882–90.
25. Bardy, G.H., Lee, K.L., Mark, D.B. et al. (2005). Amiodarone or an implantable cardioverter-defibrillator for congestive heart failure. *N Engl J Med*, **352**(3), 225–37.
26. Moss, A.J., Zareba, W., Hall, W.J. et al. (2002). Prophylactic implantation of a defibrillator in patients with myocardial infarction and reduced ejection fraction. *New England Journal of Medicine*, **346**(12), 877–83.
27. Moss, A.J., Hall, W.J., Cannom, D.S. et al. (1996). Improved survival with an implanted defibrillator in patients with coronary disease at high risk for ventricular arrhythmia. *New England Journal of Medicine*, **335**(26), 1933–40.
28. Glikson, M. and Friedman, P.A. (2001). The implantable cardioverter defibrillator. *Lancet*, **357**, 1107–17.
29. Eckert, M. and Jones, T. (2002). How does an implantable cardioverter defibrillator (ICD) affect the lives of patients and their families? *International Journal of Nursing Practice*, **8**, 152–7.
30. Sears, S.F. and Conti, J. (2002). Quality of life and psychological functioning of ICD patients. *Heart*, **87**, 488–93.
31. Solomon, M.Z., O'Donnell, L., Jennings, B. et al. (1993). Decisions near the end of life: Professional views on life-sustaining treatments. *Am J Public Health*, **83**(1), 14–23.

32. Faber-Langendoen, K. and Bartels, D.M. (1992). Process of forgoing life-sustaining treatment in a university hospital: An empirical study. *Crit Care Med*, **20**(5), 570–7.

33. Goldstein, N.E., Lampert, R., Bradley, E.H. *et al.* (2004). Management of implantable cardioverter defibrillators in end-of-life care. *Annals of Internal Medicine*, **141**, 835–8.

34. Olde Rikkert, M.G., Rigaud, A.S., van Hoeyweghen, R.J. *et al.* (2003). Geriatric syndromes: Medical misnomer or progress in geriatrics? *Neth J Med*, **61**(3), 83–7.

35. Rao, A.V., Seo, P.H., and Cohen, H.J. (2004). Geriatric assessment and comorbidity. *Semin Oncol*, **31**(2), 149–59.

36. Reuben, D.B, Herr, K.A., Pacala, J.T. *et al* (eds.) (2005). *Geriatrics at your fingertips*, 7th edition. The American Geriatrics Society, New York.

37. Cummings, J.L., Arslan, D., and Jarvik, L. (1997). Dementia. In *Geriatric Medicine*, 3rd edition, (eds. C.K. Cassel, H.J. Cohen, E.B. Larson *et al.*), pp. 897–916. Springer, New York.

38. Reisberg, B., Borenstein, J., Salob, S.P. *et al.* (1987). Behavioral symptoms in Alzheimer's Disease: Phenomenology and treatment. *J Clin Psychiatry*, **48** (Suppl), 9–15.

39. Chung, J.A. and Cummings, J.L. (2000). Neurobehavioral and neuropsychiatric symptoms in Alzheimer's Disease: Characteristics and treatment. *Neurol Clin*, **18**(4), 829–46.

40. Donaldson, C., Tarrier, N., and Burns, A. (1997). The impact of the symptoms of dementia on caregivers. *Br J Psychiatry*, **170**, 62–8.

41. (1994). *Diagnostic and statistical manual of mental disorders*, 4th edition. American Psychiatric Association, Washington, DC.

42. Marcantonio, E.R., Goldman, L., Mangione, C.M. *et al.* (1994). A clinical prediction rule for delirium after elective noncardiac surgery. *JAMA*, **271**(2), 134–9.

43. Levkoff, S.E., Evans, D.A., Liptzin, B. *et al.* (1992). Delirium. The occurrence and persistence of symptoms among elderly hospitalized patients. *Arch Intern Med*, **152**(2), 334–40.

44. Francis, J., Martin, D., and Kapoor, W.N. (1990). A prospective study of delirium in hospitalized elderly. *JAMA*, **263**(8), 1097–101.

45. Inouye, S.K., Viscoli, C.M., Horwitz, R.I. *et al.* (1993). A predictive model for delirium in hospitalized elderly medical patients based on admission characteristics. *Ann Intern Med*, **119**(6), 474–81.

46. Rincon, H.G., Granados, M., Unutzer, J. *et al.* (2001). Prevalence, detection and treatment of anxiety, depression, and delirium in the adult critical care unit. *Psychosomatics*, **42**(5), 391–6.

47. Pisani, M.A., Araujo, K.L., Van Ness, P.H. *et al.* (2006). A research algorithm to improve detection of delirium in the intensive care unit. *Crit Care*, **10**(4), R121.

48. Inouye, S.K. (2006). Delirium in older persons. *N Engl J Med*, **354**(11), 1157–65.

49. Gleason, O.C. (2003). Delirium. *Am Fam Physician*, **67**(5), 1027–34.

50. Inouye, S.K., van Dyck, C.H., Alessi, C.A. *et al.* (1990). Clarifying confusion: The confusion assessment method. A new method for detection of delirium. *Ann Intern Med*, **113**(12), 941–8.

51. Doran, J. and Mi, D. (2001). Delirium in the hospitalized elderly. *Aust J Hosp Pharm*, **31**, 35–40.

52. McAvay, G.J., Van Ness, P.H., Bogardus, S.T., Jr. *et al.* (2006). Older adults discharged from the hospital with delirium: 1-Year outcomes. *J Am Geriatr Soc*, **54**(8), 1245–50.

53. Cole, M.G. (2004). Delirium in elderly patients. *Am J Geriatr Psychiatry*, **12**(1), 7–21.

54. Francis, J. (1997). Delirium. In *Geriatric Medicine*, 3rd edition (eds. C.K. Cassel, H.J. Cohen, E.B. Larson *et al.*), pp. 917–22. Springer-Verlag, New York.

55. Agostini, J.V., Leo-Summers, L.S., and Inouye, S.K. (2001). Cognitive and other adverse effects of diphenhydramine use in hospitalized older patients. *Arch Intern Med*, **161**(17), 2091–7.

56. Casarett, D.J., Karlawish, J.H.T., and Byock, I. (2002). Advocacy and activism: Missing pieces in the quest to improve end-of-life care. *Journal of Palliative Medicine*, **5**(1), 3–12.

57. Breitbart, W., Marotta, R., Platt, M.M. *et al.* (1996). A double-blind trial of haloperidol, chlorpromazine, and lorazepam in the treatment of delirium in hospitalized aids patients. *Am J Psychiatry*, **153**(2), 231–7.

58. Inouye, S.K., Bogardus, S.T., Jr., Charpentier, P.A. *et al.* (1999). A multicomponent intervention to prevent delirium in hospitalized older patients. *N Engl J Med*, **340**(9), 669–76.

59. Ely, E.W., Shintani, A., Truman, B. *et al.* (2004). Delirium as a predictor of mortality in mechanically ventilated patients in the intensive care unit. *JAMA*, **291**(14), 1753–62.

60. Bogardus, S.T., Jr., Desai, M.M., Williams, C.S. *et al.* (2003). The effects of a targeted multicomponent delirium intervention on postdischarge outcomes for hospitalized older adults. *Am J Med*, **114**(5), 383–90.

61. Ely, E.W., Gautam, S., Margolin, R. *et al.* (2001). The impact of delirium in the intensive care unit on hospital length of stay. *Intensive Care Med*, **27**(12), 1892–900.

62. Inouye, S.K., Bogardus, S.T., Jr., Baker, D.I. *et al.* (2000). The hospital elder life program: A model of care to prevent cognitive and functional decline in older hospitalized patients. Hospital Elder Life Program. *J Am Geriatr Soc*, **48**(12), 1697–706.

63. Harari, D., Gurwitz, J.H., Avorn, J. *et al.* (1997). How do older persons define constipation? Implications for therapeutic management. *J Gen Intern Med*, **12**(1), 63–6.

64. Campbell, A.J., Busby, W.J., and Horwath, C.C. (1993). Factors associated with constipation in a community based sample of people aged 70 years and over. *J Epidemiol Community Health*, **47**(1), 23–6.

65. Harari, D., Gurwitz, J.H., and Minaker, K.L. (1993). Constipation in the elderly. *J Am Geriatr Soc*, **41**(10), 1130–40.

66. Whitehead, W.E., Drinkwater, D., Cheskin, L.J. *et al.* (1989). Constipation in the elderly living at home. Definition, prevalence, and relationship to lifestyle and health status. *J Am Geriatr Soc*, **37**(5), 423–9.

67. Tinetti, M.E. and Williams, C.S. (1997). Falls, injuries due to falls, and the risk of admission to a nursing home. *N Engl J Med*, **337**(18), 1279–84.

68. Tinetti, M.E. (2003). Clinical practice. Preventing falls in elderly persons. *N Engl J Med*, **348**(1), 42–9.

69. Agostini, J.V. and Tinetti, M.E. (2002). Drugs and falls: Rethinking the approach to medication risk in older adults. *J Am Geriatr Soc*, **50**(10), 1744–5.

70. Tinetti, M.E., Speechley, M., and Ginter, S.F. (1988). Risk factors for falls among elderly persons living in the community. *N Engl J Med*, **319**(26), 1701–7.

71. Leipzig, R.M., Cumming, R.G., and Tinetti, M.E. (1999). Drugs and falls in older people: A systematic review and meta-analysis: II. Cardiac and analgesic drugs. *J Am Geriatr Soc*, **47**(1), 40–50.

72. Leipzig, R.M., Cumming, R.G., and Tinetti, M.E. (1999). Drugs and falls in older people: A systematic review and meta-analysis: I. Psychotropic drugs. *J Am Geriatr Soc*, **47**(1), 30–9.

73. Tinetti, M.E. (1997). Falls. In *Geriatric Medicine*, (eds. C.K. Cassel, H.J. Cohen, E.B. Larson *et al.*), 3rd edition, pp. 787–99. Springer-Verlag, New York.

74. Marcantonio, E.R., Kiely, D.K., Simon, S.E. *et al.* (2005). Outcomes of older people admitted to postacute facilities with delirium. *J Am Geriatr Soc*, **53**(6), 963–9.

75. Gillespie, L.D., Gillespie, W.J., Robertson, M.C. *et al.* (2003). Interventions for preventing falls in elderly people. *Cochrane Database Syst Rev*, **4**, CD000340.

76. Campbell, A.J., Robertson, M.C., Gardner, M.M. *et al.* (1999). Psychotropic medication withdrawal and a home-based exercise program to prevent falls: A randomized, controlled trial. *J Am Geriatr Soc*, **47**(7), 850–3.

77. Cumming, R.G., Thomas, M., and Szonyi, G. *et al.* (1999). Home visits by an occupational therapist for assessment and modification of environmental hazards: A randomized trial of falls prevention. *J Am Geriatr Soc*, **47**(12), 1397–402.

78. Tinetti, M.E., Baker, D.I., McAvay, G. *et al.* (1994). A multifactorial intervention to reduce the risk of falling among elderly people living in the community. *N Engl J Med*, **331**(13), 821–7.

79. Walston, J.D. and Fried, L.P. (2003). Frailty and its implications for care. In *Geriatric Palliative Care* (eds. R.S. Morrison and D.E. Meier), pp. 93–109. Oxford University Press, New York.

80. Fried, L.P., Ferrucci, L., Darer, J. *et al.* (2004). Untangling the concepts of disability, frailty, and comorbidity: Implications for improved targeting and care. *J Gerontol A Biol Sci Med Sci*, **59**(3), 255–63.

81. Fried, L.P., Tangen, C.M., and Walston, J. *et al.* (2001). Frailty in older adults: Evidence for a phenotype. *J Gerontol A Biol Sci Med Sci*, **56**(3), M146–56.

82. Chin, A.P.M.J., Dekker, J.M., Feskens, E.J. *et al.* (1999). How to select a frail elderly population? A comparison of three working definitions. *J Clin Epidemiol*, **52**(11), 1015–21.

83. Walston, J., Hadley, E.C., Ferrucci, L. *et al.* (2006). Research agenda for frailty in older adults: Toward a better understanding of physiology and aetiology: Summary from the American Geriatrics Society/National Institute on Aging Research Conference on Frailty in Older Adults. *J Am Geriatr Soc*, **54**(6), 991–1001.

84. Leng, S., Chaves, P., Koenig, K. *et al.* (2002). Serum interleukin-6 and hemoglobin as physiological correlates in the geriatric syndrome of frailty: A pilot study. *J Am Geriatr Soc*, **50**(7), 1268–71.

85. Boockvar, K.S. and Meier, D.E. (2006). Palliative care for frail older adults: 'There are things I can't do anymore that i wish i could … '*JAMA*, **296**(18), 2245–53.

86. Fiatarone, M.A., O'Neill, E.F., Ryan, N.D. *et al.* (1994). Exercise training and nutritional supplementation for physical frailty in very elderly people. *N Engl J Med*, **330**(25), 1769–75.

87. Yarasheski, K.E., Pak-Loduca, J., Hasten, D.L. *et al.* (1999). Resistance exercise training increases mixed muscle protein synthesis rate in frail women and men ≥76 yr old. *Am J Physiol*, **277**(1 Pt 1), E118–25.

88. Province, M.A., Hadley, E.C., Hornbrook, M.C. *et al.* (1995). The effects of exercise on falls in elderly patients. A preplanned meta-analysis of the ficsit trials. Frailty and injuries: Cooperative studies of intervention techniques. *JAMA*, **273**(17), 1341–7.

89. Root, J. (2003). Pain and debility associated with spinal compression fractures. *J Okla State Med Assoc*, **96**(3), 147–9.

90. Dyer, C.B., Hyer, K., Feldt, K.S. *et al.* (2003). Frail older patient care by interdisciplinary teams: A primer for generalists. *Gerontol Geriatr Educ*, **24**(2), 51–62.

91. Wieland, D. (2003). The effectiveness and costs of comprehensive geriatric evaluation and management. *Crit Rev Oncol Hematol*, **48**(2), 227–37.

92. Koenig, H.G. and Blazer, D.G. (1992). Epidemiology of geriatric affective disorders. *Clin Geriatr Med*, **8**(2), 235–51.

93. Koenig, H.G., Blazer, D., and Hocking, L.B. (1997). Depression, anxiety, and other affective disorders. In *Geriatric Medicine*, 3rd edition (eds. C.K. Cassel, H.J. Cohen, E.B. Larson *et al.*), pp. 949–65. Springer-Verlag, New York.

94. Goldstein, N.E. and Morrison, R.S. (2005). Treatment of pain in older patients. *Crit Rev Oncol Hematol*, **54**(2), 157–64.

95. Breitbart, W., Rosenfeld, B., Pessin, H. *et al.* (2000). Depression, hopelessness, and desire for hastened death in terminally ill patients with cancer. *JAMA*, **284**(22), 2907–11.

96. Chochinov, H.M., Wilson, K.G., Enns, M. *et al.* (1997). 'Are you depressed?' Screening for depression in the terminally ill. *Am J Psychiatry*, **154**(5), 674–6.

97. Whooley, M.A., Avins, A.L., Miranda, J. *et al.* (1997). Case-finding instruments for depression. Two questions are as good as many. *J Gen Intern Med*, **12**(7), 439–45.

98. Yesavage, J.A., Brink, T.L., and Rose, T.L. *et al.* (1982). Development and validation of a geriatric depression screening scale: A preliminary report. *J Psychiatr Res*, **17**(1), 37–49.

99. Block, S.D. (2000). Assessing and managing depression in the terminally ill patient. ACP-ASIM end-of-life care consensus panel. American College of Physicians—American Society of Internal Medicine. *Ann Intern Med*, **132**(3), 209–18.

100. Chochinov, H.M. (2001). Depression in cancer patients. *Lancet Oncol*, **2**(8), 499–505.

101. Ferrell, B.A. (2003). Acute and chronic pain. In *Geriatric medicine: An evidence based approach*, (ed. C.K. Cassell) 4th Edition, pp. 323–42. Springer-Verlag, New York.

102. Mhoon, E.E. (1997). Otologic changes and disorders. In *Geriatric Medicine*, (eds. C.K. Cassel, H.J. Cohen, E.B. Larson *et al.*) 3rd edition. Springer, New York.

103. Gibson, G. and Niessen, L.C. (1997). Aging and the oral cavity. In *Geriatric Medicine*, (eds. C.K. Cassel, H.J. Cohen, E.B. Larson *et al.*) 3rd edition. Springer, New York.

104. Mitchell, S.L., Tetroe, J.M. (2000). Survival after percutaneous endoscopic gastrostomy placement in older persons. *J Gerontol A Biol Sci Med Sci*, **55**(12), M735–9.

105. Sanders, D.S., Carter, M.J., D'Silva, J. *et al.* (2000). Survival analysis in percutaneous endoscopic gastrostomy feeding: A worse outcome in patients with dementia. *Am J Gastroenterol*, **95**(6), 1472–5.

106. Abuksis, G., Mor, M., Segal, N. *et al.* (2000). Percutaneous endoscopic gastrostomy: High mortality rates in hospitalized patients. *Am J Gastroenterol*, **95**(1), 128–32.

107. Grant, M.D., Rudberg, M.A., and Brody, J.A. (1998). Gastrostomy placement and mortality among hospitalized medicare beneficiaries. *JAMA*, **279**(24), 1973–6.

108. Ganzini, L., Goy, E.R., Miller, L.L. *et al.* (2003). Nurses' experiences with hospice patients who refuse food and fluids to hasten death. *N Engl J Med*, **349**(4), 359–65.

109. Finucane, T.E. and Bynum, J.P. (1996). Use of tube feeding to prevent aspiration pneumonia. *Lancet*, **348**(9039), 1421–4.

110. Dean, M. (2004). Opioids in renal failure and dialysis patients. *J Pain Symptom Manage*, **28**(5), 497–504.

111. Goldfarb, M.T., Ellis, C.N., and Voorhees, J.J. (1997). Dermatologic disease and problems. In *Geriatric Medicine*, (eds. C.K. Cassel, H.J. Cohen, E.B. Larson *et al.*) 3rd edition. Springer, New York.

112. Teno, J. Brown atlas. Available at: www.chcr.brown.edu. Accessed on August 14, 2007.

113. National Consensus Project for Quality Palliative Care. *Clinical practice guidelines for quality palliative care.* Brooklyn, NY, May, 2004.

114. Meier, D.E. (2006). Palliative care in hospitals. *J Hosp Med*, **1**(1), 21–8.

115. Boyd, C.M., Xue, Q.L., Simpson, C.F. *et al.* (2005). Frailty, hospitalization, and progression of disability in a cohort of disabled older women. *Am J Med*, **118**(11), 1225–31.

116. Gill, T.M., Allore, H.G., Holford, T.R. *et al.* (2004). Hospitalization, restricted activity, and the development of disability among older persons. *JAMA*, **292**(17), 2115–24.

117. Creditor, M.C. (1993). Hazards of hospitalization of the elderly. *Ann Intern Med*, **118**(3), 219–23.

118. Teno, J.M. (2003). Now is the time to embrace nursing homes as a place of care for dying persons. *J Palliat Med*, **6**(2), 293–6.

119. Meyers, J.L., Moore, C., McGrory, A. *et al.* (2004). Physician orders for life-sustaining treatment form: Honouring end-of-life directives for nursing home residents. *J Gerontol Nurs*, **30**(9), 37–46.

120. Casarett, D., Karlawish, J., Morales, K. *et al.* (2005). Improving the use of hospice services in nursing homes: A randomized controlled trial. *JAMA*, **294**(2), 211–17.

121. Scalzi, C.C., Evans, L.K., Barstow, A. *et al.* (2006). Barriers and enablers to changing organizational culture in nursing homes. *Nurs Adm Q*, **30**(4), 368–72.

122. Boockvar, K., Fishman, E., Kyriacou, C.K. *et al.* (2004). Adverse events due to discontinuations in drug use and dose changes in patients transferred between acute and long-term care facilities. *Arch Intern Med*, **164**(5), 545–50.

123. Boockvar, K.S., Fridman, B., and Marturano, C. (2005). Ineffective communication of mental status information during care transfer of older adults. *J Gen Intern Med*, **20**(12), 1146–50.

124. Morrison, R.S., Olson, E., Meier, D.E. (1995). The inaccessibility of advance directives on transfer from ambulatory to acute care settings. *JAMA*, **274**(6), 478–82.

125. Leff, B., Burton, L., and Mader, S.L. *et al.* (2005). Hospital at home: Feasibility and outcomes of a program to provide hospital-level care at home for acutely ill older patients. *Ann Intern Med*, **143**(11), 798–808.

126. Harris, R., Ashton, T., Broad, J. *et al.* (2005). The effectiveness, acceptability and costs of a hospital-at-home service compared with acute hospital care: A randomized controlled trial. *J Health Serv Res Policy*, **10**(3), 158–66.

127. Hickman, S.E., Tolle, S.W., Brummel-Smith, K. *et al.* (2004). Use of the physician orders for life-sustaining treatment program in oregon nursing facilities: Beyond resuscitation status. *J Am Geriatr Soc*, **52**(9), 1424–9.

128. Byock, I. (1997). *Dying well*. Riverhead Books, New York.

SECTION 15

Psychiatric, psychosocial, and spiritual issues in palliative medicine

Spiritual issues in palliative medicine

Susan E. McClement and Harvey Max Chochinov

Introduction

'The spiritual dimension cannot be ignored, for it is what makes us human[1]' Viktor E. Frankl

Palliative care has as its focus care of the whole person, including biopsychosoical, cultural, and *spiritual* needs[2]. That end-of-life care should incorporate some consideration of spiritual care is consistent with the vision of Dame Cicely Saunders, champion of the hospice movement[3]. People confronted by serious illness often draw on religious or spiritual beliefs[4–6]. Ferrell and Coyle[7] posit that, 'if left un-addressed spiritual distress may stifle the opportunity for growth at the end of life, lead to poorly controlled symptoms, and result in an "unquiet death"'. Clearly, such outcomes are incommensurate with the aims and goals of palliative medicine.

The burgeoning literature examining the topic of spirituality within health care in general, and within palliative care in particular, underscores the notion that attending to patients' spiritual care needs is a vital part of providing optimal palliative care[8–10]. Competencies for spiritual care have been developed[11], guidance on how to discuss religious and spiritual concerns with dying patients has been published; courses on spirituality are becoming more common in medical schools in the United States, and chapters devoted to spirituality are readily apparent in authoritative palliative medicine and nursing textbooks[7,12,13]. Yet health-care providers frequently report that they feel ill equipped to provide spiritual care at the end of life and wrestle with many questions about it. What is spiritual care? What is spiritual suffering? Who should provide spiritual care? How is a spiritual assessment conducted? What are some spiritual interventions for end-of-life care? What are some future research directions in the area of spiritual care? Answers to these questions form the basis of this chapter.

What is spirituality?

An ancient Chinese proverb reminds us that, 'the beginning of wisdom is to call things by their right name'[14]. Such wisdom presupposes conceptual clarity. To date, such clarity concerning spirituality remains elusive. Despite the growing literature on spirituality, there is no consensus on a definition of this concept[15]. Increased secularization of society has resulted in a shift from the traditional explicitly religious meaning given to spirituality[12,13]. Numerous definitions of spirituality exist in the literature, such that the concept of spirituality in relation to health research is plagued by definitional ambiguity[9].

Amidst the myriad of definitions of spirituality found in the literature, however, are some common themes to inform our understanding of this concept. Unruh and colleagues[16]' critical review of definitions of spirituality found in diverse professional health literature identified seven thematic categories: (1) relationship to God, a spiritual being, a Higher Power, or reality greater than the self; (2) not of the self; (3) transcendence or connectedness unrelated to a belief in a higher being; (4) existential, not of the material world; (5) meaning and purpose in life; (6) life force of the person, integrating aspect o the person; and (7) summative definitions that combined multiple themes[16].

A helpful working definition offered by Mauk and colleagues[17] defines spirituality as 'the core of a person's being' ... usually conceptualized as a 'higher' experience or transcendence of oneself. Often, such an experience involves a perception of a personal relationship with a supreme being (such as God). However, many who consider themselves spiritual deny such identification with a higher power. Spirituality, then, also encompasses feelings and thoughts that bring meaning and purpose to human existence or to one's life journey.

In addition to the theoretical definitions of spirituality found in the literature, our understanding of the concept of spirituality should ideally also be informed by the insights of dying patients. How do these individuals define spirituality? The empirical work in this area, though limited, is instructive. A qualitative study conducted by Chao and colleagues[18] examining the essence of spirituality in a sample of terminally ill Buddhist and Christian patients ($n = 6$) identified four broad thematic areas: (1) communion with self (self-identity, wholeness, inner peace); (2) communion with others (love, reconciliation); (3) communion with nature (inspiration, creativity); and (4) communion with a higher being (faithfulness, hope, gratitude). These findings are consistent with Burkhardt and Jacobson's[19] observation that, 'spirituality is known and experienced in relationships'. The notions of communion and connectedness underscore the importance of 'relationship' in the spiritual well-being of patients, and the salience of spiritual care interventions that promote such connectedness.

Spirituality and religion (see also Chapter 4.4)

The term spirituality is sometimes used synonymously (and mistakenly) in place of the term religion[20]. Religion is typically equated with an organized system of beliefs, rituals, and practices an individual identifies and associates with that includes a relationship with a divine being. Religion may or may not be part of a person's spirituality[21]. A comparison of the characteristics associated with religion and spirituality identified by Robinson and colleagues[22] is detailed in Table 15.1.1.

Some authors object that that describing religion in term so of what it does is functionalist, reductionist, and implies negative attitudes towards religious belief[23]. Our purpose in seeking to distinguish between these two terms has no such nefarious purpose. Clinicians need to be aware of these related concepts because of the relative importance each may play in the lives of their patients. For example, research reviewed by Marler and Hadaway[24] indicates that some patients see themselves as both spiritual and religious. Other patients who are religious may express their spirituality through identification and involvement within a particular religion. Still yet other patients may claim to be highly spiritual, yet not religious. For these individuals, an important common denominator appears to be the notion of 'transcending the commonplace and searching their soul for deeper meaning'[20].

The concepts of spirituality and religion are also important because of their impact on health outcomes. Research has been conducted suggesting that religion and spirituality play a positive role in individuals coping with cancer and human immunodeficiency virus (HIV)[25,26]. Studies among advanced cancer patients suggest that spiritual well-being and meaning are important buffers against hopelessness, depression, and desire for hastened death[26–28]. These findings point to the need for interventions that address spiritual suffering.

Spirituality and patient perspectives

Do terminally ill patients and those with life-threatening illnesses want health-care providers to be attuned to spiritual needs? Public opinion and empirical literature suggest that such attention would be welcomed by at least some patients. A Gallup survey[29] conducted in 1977 examining spiritual beliefs and the dying process (n = 1200) indicated that in addition to turning to family (81 per cent), close friends (61 per cent), and clergy (36 per cent) for companionship and support at the end of life, 30 per cent of respondents would look to doctors for such support. Forty per cent of respondents indicated that it would be very important to have a physician who was spiritually attuned to them if they were dying.

King and Bushwick[30] conducted a cross-sectional survey of family practice adult inpatients at two hospitals in the United States (n = 203). Though limitations of the study include patient

homogeneity and variations in regional religiosity, the findings revealed that 77 per cent of patients felt that physicians should consider patients' spiritual needs, and 37 per cent of patients wanted their physicians to discussion religious beliefs with them more frequently. Of note is the finding that 68 per cent of the patients in the study reported that their physician never discussed religious beliefs with them.

Questionnaires completed by a convenience sample of ambulatory pulmonary outpatients (n = 177) examining patient acceptance of physicians asking them if they have spiritual or religious beliefs would influence their medical decisions if they became gravely ill revealed that 45 per cent of respondents felt that religious beliefs would influence their medical decisions if they were gravely ill[4]. Of those individuals, 94 per cent agreed or strongly agreed that the physician ask them whether they have such beliefs if they developed a grave illness. Respondents who denied having such beliefs also agreed that physicians should ask about them. It is important to note in this same study that while two-thirds of the patients welcomed the idea of discussing religion or spirituality with their doctor, nearly one-quarter of respondents found this prospect objectionable with just less than 10 per cent reporting strong reservations. Neither the nature of these objections nor demographic characteristics of patients offering them were articulated in the study.

Not all research regarding patients' attitudes towards spiritual dimensions is quite so definitive. A comparative qualitative study conducted by Murray and colleagues[31] that explored the spiritual needs of people dying of lung cancer (n = 20) and heart failure (n = 20) found the extent to which patients wish to have spiritual care incorporated into their health care was unclear. Some patients, though in need of spiritual support, either did not see the provision of such support as the purview of the health professional or worried about burdening 'busy' professionals with this issue. That spiritual needs may not be readily expressed speaks to the importance of health-care providers creating a climate wherein patients feel comfortable to engage in discussion about spiritual care issues should they wish to do so[31].

Spiritual pain and existential suffering

The Tibetan Book of the Living and Dying[32] notes that

> Often we forget that the dying are losing their whole world: their house, their job, their relationships, their body, and their mind – they're losing everything. All the losses we could possibly experience in life are joined together in one overwhelming loss when we die ....

Clearly, a multiplicity of spiritual issues arise in the wake of being diagnosed with a life-threatening illness. Patients, confronted with mortality, limitations, and loss wrestle with questions about their life's purpose and meaning amidst suffering. But what is suffering? Cassell[33] defined suffering as the state of distress brought about by an actual or perceived threat to the integrity or continued existence of the whole person. Suffering is 'an anguish that is experienced, not only as a pressure to change, but as a threat to our composure, our integrity, and the fulfillment of our intentions' (p.231).

The Concise Oxford Dictionary[34] defines suffering as 'to undergo, experience, be subjected to (pain loss, grief, defeat, change, punishment, wrong, etc.)'. A central notion in this definition is that those

Table 15.1.1 Concepts of religion and spirituality[22].

Religion	Spirituality
◆ Focused in institutions	◆ Not institutionally bound
◆ Concerned with defining orthodoxy and orthopraxy	
◆ Meaning transmitted through doctrine and stories of the community	◆ Concerned with discovery of meaning in the context of the level individual
◆ May provide a motivational and disciplined framework for spiritual growth	◆ Concerned with self-directed spiritual growth

who suffer submit (or are forced to submit) to a particular set of circumstances outside of their control. Such a situation has the potential to seriously erode one's autonomy[35], and foster hopelessness and loss of control. Strang and colleagues[36]' study of hospital chaplains, palliative care physicians, and pain specialists' definitions of the term existential pain suggests that the term is used as a metaphor for suffering. This acknowledges that suffering can include physical pain and the reciprocal interaction between somatic pain and existential suffering. Suffering based on a perception of lost autonomy and control may express itself in patient requests for death hastening measures. McClain and colleagues[28] demonstrated significant correlations between spiritual well-being and desire for hastened death ($r = -0.51$), hopelessness ($r = -0.68$), and suicidal ideation ($r = -0.41$). These findings suggest that spiritual well-being may confer some protection against end-of-life despair based on the additional findings that depression was significantly correlated with desire for hastened death in patients will low spiritual well-being ($r = 0.40$) but not in those high in spiritual well-being ($r = 0.20$)[27].

Research conducted by Chochinov and colleagues[37] also demonstrates the salience of existential issues as they affect the wish to go on living in the face of a progressing terminal illness. Examination of the concurrent influences on the will to live in a sample of 189 end-stage cancer patients revealed that physical variables played a secondary role to existential, psychiatric, and social variables; all of which were highly correlated with the will to live. Stepwise regression modeling was conducted to examine the relationship between the will to live and patient characteristics. Hopelessness, burden to others, and dignity entered into the final model, demonstrating that influential role existential variables play in this patient population. Given their prominent influence on will to live amongst patients nearing death, health-care providers are well advised to more fully appreciate their importance.

Providing spiritual care: who, me?

Glass and colleagues[38] note that, 'responding to the spiritual needs of patients and families is not solely the domain of the chaplain, clergy, or other officially designated professionals. All members of the health-care team share the responsibility of identifying and being sensitive to spiritual concerns'. Numerous barriers to the provisions of spiritual care at the end of life have been identified in the literature; however. Chibnall and colleagues[39] in their qualitative study with physicians ($n = 17$) at a university based hospital identified (1) the marginalization and devaluing of psychosocial and spiritual care during medical training; (2) lack of safe and supportive environment in which to discuss issues of loss and death; (3) time demands and busy clinical schedules; and (4) lack of training and skill regarding communication with patients regarding existential issues as significant barriers. Lack of training in spiritual assessment and care has also been identified by nurses as barriers to providing spiritual care to patients[40].

Health-care providers may assume that issues of spiritual care are best left to clergy or other types of spiritual leaders. Clearly, if the results of a spiritual assessment indicate the need for further specialized care, or specific information related to religion referrals to chaplains and clergy are warranted[41]. Research suggests, however, that health-care providers should be able to respond to most of the questions posed to chaplains. In a Swedish national survey of hospital chaplains, religious questions accounted for only 8 per cent of the questions regularly posed to them. Other questions concerned questions of meaning; death and dying; pain and illness; and relationships[43].

McSherry and Ross[42] caution that health-care providers cannot assume either that all patients have spiritual needs that require attention all of the time, or that they will look to health-care professionals to help meet these needs. This requires that the health-care team make some determination regarding the extent to which the patient is desirous of their involvement regarding spiritual care issues. Inevitably, it is the clinician's own comfort level with providing spiritual care that dictates involvement in it. Palliative care clinicians may have palliative care expertise, but are not necessarily specialists in spiritual assessment and care giving. It has been suggested that the provision of good spiritual care is dependent on the clinician's awareness of a spiritual dimension in his or her own life; honed communication skills[43], and the ability to establish a trusting relationship with patients, and drawing on one' own life experience and maturity[44]. Owing to differing spiritual or religious needs of both patient and caregiver, there will be individuals for whom we cannot provide spiritual care, but other members of the interdisciplinary team can. Thus an important part of spiritual care involves each member of the team recognizing their own limitations and that the needs of terminally ill person require multiple sets of skill and knowledge that may not be present in any one individual[45,46].

Spiritual assessment

Naming and acknowledging spiritual distress allows for a greater awareness of what the patient is experiencing and thus increases possibilities for resolution. Such acknowledgment presupposes that clinicians be able to evaluate spiritual well-being in the patients for whom they are caring. Owing to the sensitive and personal nature of spirituality, prefacing the spiritual assessment with an acknowledgment of the sensitivity of the questions as well as the need for the assessment are important in setting the tone for the conversation to follow. Suggestions regarding how clinicians might preface the spiritual assessment with patients have been published[47].

To the extent that a patient's physiological status will permit it, base-line spiritual assessment data is typically collected from patients at the time of admission to hospital or hospice. Far from being a one-off type of assessment, continuous evaluation of spiritual care needs should occur.

A variety of models for spiritual assessment exist in the literature. Many of these involve the use of direct open-ended questioning. Maugens[47] recommends the mnemonic SPIRIT as a way of structuring spiritual inquiry. The S in SPIRIT stands for *Spiritual belief system* that is the person's religious affiliation. *P* stands for personal spirituality and includes the person's spiritual views shaped by a person's unique life experiences. *I* stands for Integration and involvement with a spiritual community and speaks to the importance of assessing the patients' involvement in spiritual communities and other supportive spiritual groups. *R* relates to ritualized practices and restrictions that individuals embrace as part of their lifestyle that may influence health. *I* refers to implications for medical care and is concerned with how spiritual beliefs and practices may shape the patient's participation in health care.

T stands for terminal events planning and reminds the clinician about the importance of assessing patients' end-of-life concerns.

Puchalski and Romer[48] offer the mnemonic 'FICA' for remembering four components to cover during a spiritual assessment. 'FICA' stands for *F*aith or beliefs (e.g. What is your faith or belief?), *I*mportance and influence (e.g. What role do your beliefs play in regaining your health), *C*ommunity (e.g. are you part of a spiritual or religious community?), and *A*ddress (e.g. How should this issues be addressed by health-care providers?)

Ferszt *et al.*[49] developed an approach to spiritual assessment that examines the areas of connection, meaning and joy, and strength and comfort. Questions asked within each of these areas of life are designed to serve as a springboard to conversation with the patient and uses language that is accessible and comfortable for clinicians and patients. These questions are summarized in Table 15.1.2.

Many of the approaches to conducting a spiritual assessment described in the literature use a qualitative approach to gathering information from the patient. Paper and pencil questionnaires to elicit information about spirituality also exist that may serve as a means of identifying and codifying patients' spiritual status, needs, and resources[41]. Such tools are not designed to replace interaction between patient and health-care provider, but rather to facilitate ongoing assessment and communication regarding spiritual care issues.

No single assessment approach, whether qualitative or quantitative, is likely to be ideal in all situations. An assessment method that works well with one client may be inappropriate with another. The ideal assessment tool for use in practice will be, 'easy to use, flexible and take little time to assess the spiritual state of patients at different times and in different situations[50].

Spiritual care interventions for end-of-life care

Both general and specific spiritual care interventions are identified in the literature. Arguably, palliative care in and of itself is a general intervention aimed at improving patients' quality of life, enhancing well-being, and reducing suffering. This finding was demonstrated in a study conducted by Cohen and colleagues[51] of 88 patients admitted to five palliative care units in two distinct regions of Canada from whom scores on the McGill Quality of Life Scale were collected on admission and one week later. Qualitative data concerning patient changes in quality of life since admission to palliative care were also collected. The findings from this study indicated improved patient physical, psychological, and existential well-being following admission to the palliative care unit, as well as a sense of deeper spiritual awareness.

Kissane and associates[52] assert that demoralization syndrome, with its attendant hopelessness and loss of meaning represents an important expression of existential distress in palliative care patients. They advocate a broad range of approaches for the hopelessness, loss of meaning, and existential distress palliative patients may experience. These include (1) providing continuity of care and active symptom management; (2) exploring patients' attitudes toward hope and meaning in life; (3) balancing support for grief with promotion of hope; (4) fostering the search for a renewed purpose and role in life; (5) using cognitive therapy to reframe negative beliefs; (6) involving pastoral care for spiritual support; (7) promoting supportive relationships and use of volunteers; (8) enhancing family functioning by conducting family meetings; and (9) reviewing the goals of care in multi-disciplinary team settings. Preliminary reports regarding the validation of The Demoralization Scale have been published[53]; however, future research is needed to examine the feasibility and efficacy of the various interventions to manage demoralization syndrome.

Cole and Pargament[54] developed a pilot psychotherapy program of individuals with cancer that explored important existential issues identified to be important in those facing a life-threatening illness: control, identify, relationships, and meaning. Preliminary findings suggest that the majority of participants (*n* = 10) indicated they preferred to participate in this type of program over others that did not contain a spiritual focus.

Breitbart and associates[55] have utilized meaning-based psychotherapy in ambulatory advanced cancer patients. Using a combination of instruction, discussion, and experiential exercises, this eight session group intervention aims to help patients sustain or enhance their sense of meaning and purpose in their lives and to optimize each group member's remaining life span. Prior to the intervention, 40 per cent of group participants Preliminary evaluation of this approach found that none of the participants perceived as meaningless, compared to 40 per cent of participants who did not report a sense of meaning or purpose in their life prior to taking part in the meaning-centred group psychotherapy session.

Chochinov and colleagues' programmatic work examining dignity in the terminally ill has resulted in an empirically derived model of dignity towards the end of life, and the development of a therapeutic intervention called Dignity Therapy that targets depression and suffering along with enhancing palliative patients' sense of purpose, meaning, and will to live[56–59]. Patients are asked questions that provide them with the opportunity to address aspects of life they feel were most important or meaningful to them; to detail aspects of their personal history that they want remembered, and convey messages and sentiments they wish to impart. Questions that are asked during Dignity Therapy are outlined in Table 15.1.3.

Table 15.1.2 Spiritual assessment tool[42].

Area of assessment	Related questions
Connection	◆ Who are the persons or communities you look to for support? What role do they have in your care?
	◆ Do you have an image of a power greater than yourself?
	◆ Has your life situation now affected your feelings about yourself, your faith, or your relationships?
Meaning and joy	◆ What has been most important in your life?
	◆ What are you most thankful for?
	◆ What makes or has made you happy?
	◆ What do you feel the proudest of in your life?
Strength and comfort	◆ Is there anything that is comforting to you now?
	◆ What helped you get through difficult times in the past?
	◆ Who or what is your source of strength now?
Hope and concerns	◆ Is there anything that you hope for?
	◆ Is there anything that feels unfinished?

Table 15.1.3 Dignity therapy question protocol[55–58].

◆ Please tell me a little about your life history, particularly the parts that you either remember most or think are the most important. When did you feel most alive?

◆ Are there specific things that you would want your family to know about you, and are their particular things you would want them to remember?

◆ What are the most important roles you have played in life [family roles, vocational roles, community service roles, etc.]? Why were they so important to you and what do you think you accomplished in those roles?

◆ What are your most important accomplishments and what do you feel most proud of?

◆ Are there particular things that you feel still need to be said to your loved ones, or things that you would want to take the time to say once again?

◆ What are your hopes and dreams for your loved ones?

◆ What have you learned about life that you would want to pass along to others? What advice of words of guidance would you wish to pass along to your [son, daughter, husband, wife, parents, other(s)]?

◆ Are their words or perhaps even instructions you would like to offer your family, to help prepare them for the future?

◆ In creating this permanent record, are their other things that you would like included?

Engaging in the process of Dignity Therapy allows patients' to address grief-related issues, and impart wishes and instructions to loved ones. Patients' responses to the questions are tape-recorded transcribed, edited, and returned to the patient who then shares the document with friends and family members as desired. The transcribed document acts as a type of legacy that transcends the patient's death and offers comfort to bereft loved ones.

Dignity Therapy shows promise as a novel therapeutic intervention for suffering and distress at the end of life. Ninety-one per cent of the terminally ill patients who have participated in this intervention ($n = 100$) report being satisfied with it. A heightened sense of dignity was found in 76 per cent of patients; 68 per cent reported a heightened sense of meaning; 47 per cent had an increased will to life and 81 per cent reported that it had been (or would be) of help to family members with whom they had shared the transcribed document. Post-dignity therapy intervention measures of suffering were significantly improved ($P = 0.023$), and depressive symptoms were reduced ($P = 0.05$). Patients who reported that Dignity Therapy helped their loved ones reported a heightened sense of purpose ($r = 0.562$; $P < 0.0001$) and will to live ($r = 0.387$; $P < 0.0001$); and felt that life was more meaningful ($r = 0.480$; $P < 0.0001$)[58].

Directions for future research

Although research from a variety of disciplines has enhanced our understanding about the connections between spirituality and health, many questions remain unanswered[60]. Owing to its subjective, experiential, contextualized nature, some would argue that spirituality is not amenable to definition or measurement. This does not mean, however, that spirituality cannot be examined empirically. A methodological approach that honours the subjective meaning and experience of the individual within given historical, social, and cultural contexts can be realized through the use of qualitative research methods[61]. For researchers wishing to

operationalize and measure spirituality, however, conceptual ambiguity is highly problematic, because approaches to measurement of a given construct follow conceptual decisions[62]. Incongruencies in conceptual and operational definitions threaten the validity of the research and pose significant challenges in the development of appropriate spiritual outcomes measures[51].

A recent survey of spiritual care needs of hospitalized children and their families found that quality of spiritual care provided to be wanting, underscoring the need for ongoing research with this patient population[63]. Future work in this area might include an explication of the spiritual care needs and preferences of hospitalized paediatric and adolescent patients and their parents.

Research points to health-care providers feeling inadequately prepared to address the spiritual concerns of patients, and in need of ongoing education in matters of spiritual care[42]. The optimal timing, nature, duration, and outcomes of such educational intervention need further examination.

Walter[46] asserts that the language or discourse of spirituality and spiritual care is largely restricted to the English speaking world. Accordingly, the search for spirituality in health care has been cast in terms of primarily an Anglo-American debate[44]. Such an approach fails to encompass different notions of spirituality such as understood in many world religions[64]. Given that we live and provide palliative care in a multicultural context, research is needed with diverse populations that will broaden our understanding of the relationships between spirituality and culture and the spiritual care concepts and issues that are salient to different constituencies[8].

The provision of spiritual care is a multi-disciplinary endeavor[45]. This requires that clinicians and researchers come together to share their perspectives regarding spiritual care and jointly identify fruitful areas of collaborative investigation.

There is increasing awareness of the need for palliation of individuals living with illnesses other than cancer[65]. Expanding the focus of spiritual care research to include individuals with life-threatening illness apart from cancer is thus indicated.

Finally, a basic tenet of palliative care is that the patient and family constitute the unit of care[7]. Yet, little is known regarding the role that spirituality plays in affecting bereavement outcomes for family members. Retrospective research and prospective cohort studies indicate that the outcome of bereavement is affected by religious belief[66–68], suggesting that the absence of such belief may be a risk factor for delayed or complicated grief. Ongoing research is needed to examine the extent to which strong beliefs may be a proxy for better adjustment and less psychological distress in the bereavement period. Such work may help to identify those family members who may have difficulty in adjusting following the patient's death.

Conclusion

In defining palliative care, the World Health Organization emphasizes that the control pain, of other symptoms, and of psychological social and spiritual problems is paramount[69]. Patients experiencing life-threatening illnesses want and need meaning, perhaps more that at any other time in their lives. Thus, spiritual care is an aspect of palliative care that must not be undervalued. Attending to the spiritual needs of palliative care patients may provide them with the opportunity 'to find meaning in the midst of suffering and to have the opportunity for love, compassion, and partnership in their final journey'[70].

References

1. Frankl, V. (1955). *The doctor and the soul: An introduction to logotherapy*. Alfred A. Knopf, New York.

2. Poor, B. and Poirrier, G.P. (eds.) *End of life nursing care*, pp. 175–87. Jones & Bartlett Publishers Inc. and National League for Nursing, London.

3. Saunders, C. (2001). The evolution of palliative care. *J R Soc Med*, **94**, 430–2.

4. Ehman, J.W., Ott, B.B., Short, T.H. *et al.* (1999). Do patients want physicians to inquire about their spiritual or religious beliefs if they become gravely ill? *Arch Intern Med*, **159**, 1803–6.

5. Matthew, D., McCullough, M., Larson, D. *et al.* (1998). Religious commitment and health status: A review of the research and implications for family medicine. *Arch Intern Med*, **7**, 118–24.

6. Hamel, R. and Lysaught, M. (1994). Choosing palliative care: Do religious beliefs make a difference? *J Palliat Care*, **10**, 61–6.

7. Ferrell, B.R. and Coyle, N. (eds.) (2001). *Textbook of palliative nursing*. Oxford University Press, Oxford.

8. Chochinov, H.M. and Cann, B.J. (2005). Interventions to enhance the spiritual aspects of dying. *Journal Palliat Med*, **8**(1), S103–15.

9. Sinclair, S., Pereira, J. and Raffin, S. (2006). A thematic review of the spirituality literature within palliative care. *J Palliat Med*, **9**, 464–78.

10. Chiu, L. (2004). An integrative review of the concepts of spirituality in the health sciences. *West J Nurs Res*, **26**, 405–28.

11. Baldacchino, D.R. (2006). Nursing competencies for spiritual care. *J Clin Nurs*, **15**, 885–96.

12. Strang, S. and Strang, P. (2006). Spiritual care. In *Textbook of palliative medicine* (eds. E. Bruera, I. Higginson, C. Ripamonti, and C. von Gunten), pp. 1019–28. Hodder Arnold, London.

13. Cassidy, J.P. and Davies, D.J. (2003).Cultural and spiritual aspects of palliative medicine. In *Oxford textbook of palliative medicine*, (eds. D. Doyle, G. Hanks, N. Cherny, and K. Calman) 3rd edition, pp. 951–7. Oxford University Press, Oxford.

14. http://oneproverb.net/bwfolder/chinesebw.html (accessed on November 15, 2006).

15. Tanyi, R (2002). Towards clarification of the meaning of spirituality. *J Adv Nurs*, **39**, 500–9.

16. Unruh, A.M., Versnel, J., and Kerr, N. (2002). Spirituality unplugged: A review of commonalities and contentions, and a resolution. *Canad J Occup Ther*, **69**, 15–19.

17. Mauk, K.L. and Schmidt, N.K. (2004). *Spiritual care in nursing practice*. Lippincott Williams & Wilkins, Philadelphia.

18. Chao, C.C., Chen, C., and Yen, M. (2002). The essence of spirituality of terminally ill patients. *J Nurs Res*, **10**, 237–44.

19. Burkhardt, M.A. and Jacobson, M.G.N. (2000). Spirituality and health. In *Holistic nursing: A handbook for practice*, (eds. B.M. Dossey, L. Keegan, and C.E. Guzetaa) 3rd edition, pp. 91–121. Gaithersburg, MD: Aspen.

20. Schmidt, N.A. and Mauk, K.L. (2004). Spirituality as a life journey. In *Spiritual care in nursing practice*, (K.L. Mauk and N.K. Schmidt), pp. 2–19. Lippincott Williams Wilkins, Philadelphia.

21. Smith, A.R. (2006). Using the synergy model to provide spiritual nursing care in critical care settings. *Crit Care Nurs*, **26**, 41–7.

22. Robinson, S., Kendrick, K., and Brown, A. (2003). *Spirituality and the practice of healthcare*. Palgrave McMillan: Basingstoke.

23. Clarke, J. (2006). Religion and spirituality: A discussion paper about negativity, reductionism and differentiation in nursing texts. *International J Nurs Stud*, **43**, 775–85.

24. Marler, P.L. and Hadaway, C.K. (2002). 'Being religious' or 'being spiritual' in America: A zero-sum proposition? *J for the Scientific Study of Religion*, **41**, 289–300.

25. Baider, L., Russak, S.M., Perry, S. *et al.* (1999). The role of religious and spiritual beliefs in coping with malignant melanoma: An Israeli sample. *Psychooncology*, **8**, 27–35.

26. Nelson, C.J., Rosenfeld, B., Breitbart, W. *et al.* (2002). Spirituality, religion and depression in the terminally ill. *Psychosomatics*, **43**, 213–20.

27. Breitbart, W., Rosnefeld, B., Pressin, H. *et al.* (2000). Depression, hopelessness, and desire for death in terminally ill patients with cancer. *JAMA*, **284**, 2907–11.

28. McClain, C.S., Rosenfeld, B., and Breitbart, W. (2003). Effect of spiritual well-being on end-of-life despair in terminally ill cancer patients. *Lancet*, **361**, 1603–7.

29. The George, H. Gallup International Institute (1997). *Spiritual beliefs and the dying process*. The George, Princeton.

30. King, D.E. and Bushwick, B. (1994). Beliefs and attitudes of hospital inpatients about faith, healing and prayer. *J Fam Pract*, **39**, 349–52.

31. Murray, S.A., Kendall, M., Boyd, K. *et al.* (2004). Exploring the spiritual needs of people dying of lung cancer or heart failure: A prospective qualitative interview study of patients and their carers. *Palliat Med*, **18**, 39–45.

32. Rinpoche, S. (2002). *The Tibetan book of living and dying*, p. 176. Harper, San Francisco.

33. Cassell, E.J. (1991). *The nature of suffering and the goals of medicine*. Oxford University Press, New York.

34. Sykes, J.B. (1982).*The Oxford concise dictionary*. Clarendon Press, Oxford.

35. Younger, J.B. (1995). The alienation of the sufferer. *Adv Nurs Sci*, **17**, 53–72.

36. Strang, S. and Strang, P. (2002). Questions posed to hospital chaplains by palliative care patients. *J Palliat Med*, **5**, 857–64.

37. Chochinov, H.M., Hack, T., Hassard, T. *et al.* (2005). Understanding the will to live in patients nearing death. *Psychosomatics*, **46**, 7–10.

38. Glass, E., Cluxton, D., and Rancour, P. (2001). Principles of patient and family assessment. In *Textbook of palliative nursing* (eds. B.R. Ferrell and N. Coyle), pp. 37–50. Oxford University Press, Oxford.

39. Chibnall, J.T., Bennett, M.L., Videen, S.D. *et al.* (2004). Identifying barriers to psychosocial spiritual care at the end of life: A physician group study. *American Journal of Hospice & Palliative Medicine*, **21**, 419–26.

40. Oldnall, A. (1996). A critical analysis of nursing: Meeting spiritual needs of patients. *J Adv Nurs*, **23**, 138–44.

41. Taylor, E.J. (2001). Spiritual assessment. In *Textbook of palliative nursing* (eds. B.R. Ferrell and N. Coyle), pp. 397–406. Oxford University Press, Oxford.

42. McSherry, W. and Ross, L. (2002). Dilemmas of spiritual assessment: Considerations for nursing practice. *J Adv Nurs*, **38**, 479–88.

43. Tulsky, J.A. (2005). Interventions to enhance communication among patients, providers, and families. *J Palliat Med*, **8**(Suppl), S95–102.

44. Pronk, K. (2005). Role of the doctor in relieving spiritual distress at the end of life. *Am J Hosp Palliat Care*, **22**, 419–25.

45. Victoria Hospice Society (1998). Spiritual care. In *Medical care of the dying*, 3rd edition, pp.534–7, Author, Victoria, B.C.

46. Walter, T. (2002). Spirituality in palliative care: Opportunity of burden? *Palliat Med*, **16**, 133–9.

47. Maugens, T.A. (1996). The Spiritual history. *Arch Fam Med*, **5**,11–16.

48. Pulchaski, C.M. and Romer, A.L. (2000). Taking a spiritual history allows clinicians to understand patients more fully. *J Palliat Med*, **3**, 129–37.

49. Ferszt, G.G., Teegan-Case, S., and Taylor, P.B. (2001). Spiritual assessment tool. *End of life nursing care* (eds. B. Poor and G.P. Poirrier). Jones and Bartlett, Boston.

50. Catterall, R.A., Cox, M., Greer, B. *et al.* (1998). The assessment and audit of spiritual care. *Int J of Pall Nurs*, **4**, 162–8.

51. Cohen, S.R., Boston, P., Mount, B.M. *et al.* (2001). Changes in quality of life following admission to palliative care units. *Palliat Med*, **15**, 363–71.

52. Kissane, D., Clarke, D.M., and Street, A.F. (2001). Demoralization syndrome—A relevant psychiatric dianosis for palliative care. *J Palliat Care*, **17**,12–21.

53. Kissane, D.W. (2004). The demoralization scale: a report of its development and preliminary validation. *J Palliat Care*, **20**, 269–76.

54. Cole, B. and Pargament, K. (1999). Re-creating your life: A spiritual/psychotherapeutic intervention for people diagnosed with cancer. *Psychooncology*, **8**, 395–407.

55. Breitbart, W., Gibson, C., Poppito, S.R. *et al.* (2004). Psychotherapeutic interventions at the end of life: A focus on meaning and spirituality. *Can J Psychiatry*, **49**, 366–72.

56. Chochinov, H.M., Hack, T., McClement, S. *et al.* (2002). Dignity in the terminally ill: An empirical model. *Soc Sci Med*, **54**, 433–43.

57. Chochinov, H.M. (2002). Dignity conserving care: A new model for palliative care. *JAMA*, **287**, 2253–60.

58. Chochinov, H.M., Hack, T., Hassard, T. *et al.* (2005). Dignity therapy: A novel psychotherapeutic intervention for patients near the end of life. *J Clin Oncol*, **23**, 5520–5.

59. McClement, S.E., Chochinov, H.M., Hack, T.F. *et al.* (2004). Dignity conserving care: Application of research findings to practice. *Int J Palliat Nurs*, **10**,173–9.

60. Schmidt, N.A. (2004). Nursing research about spirituality and health. In *Spiritual care in nursing practice* (eds. K.L. Mauk and N.K. Schmidt), pp. 303–26. Lippincott Williams Wilkins, Philadelphia.

61. Streubert, H.J. and Carpenter, D.R. (1999). *Qualitative research in nursing: Advancing the humanistic imperative*. Lippincott, Philadelphia.

62. Kristjanson, L.J. (1992). Conceptual issues related to measurement in family research. *Can J Nurs Res*, **24**, 37–52.

63. Feudtner, C., Haney, J., and Dimmers, M.A. (2003). Spiritual care needs of hospitalized children and their families: A national survey of pastoral care providers' perceptions. *Paediatrics*, **111**, e67–72

64. Markham, I. (1998). Spirituality and the world faiths. In *The spiritual challenge of health care* (eds. M. Cobb and V. Robshaw), pp. 73–87. Churchill Livingstone, Edinburgh.

65. Addington-Hall, J.M. and Higginson, I.J. (eds.) (2001). *Palliative care for non-cancer patients*. Oxford University Press, Oxford.

66. Lauer, M.E., Muilhern, R.E., Schell, M.J. *et al.* (1989). Long term follow-up of parental adjustment following a child's death at home or hospital. *Cancer*, **63**, 988–94.

67. McIntosh, D.N., Silver, R.C., and Wortman, C.B. (1993). Religion's role in adjustment to a negative life event: coping with the loss of a child. *J Per Soc Psychol*, **65**, 812–21.

68. Rosik, C.H. (1989). The impact of religious orientation in conjugal bereavement among older adults. *Int J Ageing Hum Dev*, **28,** 251–60.

69. World Health Organization (2002). *National cancer control programmes: Policies and managerial guidelines*, 2nd edition, p. 1. Author: Geneva.

70. Pulchaski, C.M., Dorff, E., and Hendi, I.Y. (2004). Spirituality, religion, and healing in palliative care. *Clin Geriatr Med*, **20**, 689–714.

The emotional problems of the patient in palliative medicine

Mary L.S. Vachon

Emotional problems and psychosocial distress are common as individuals confront the palliative phase of illness and their impending death[1]. That palliative care goes beyond the management of physical symptoms is well known but can be illustrated by the fact that 57 per cent of 814 new referrals to the Macmillan Nurses in the UK were for emotional support[2].

As patients and families deal with these issues and distress, caregivers may become deeply involved with them in their distress, remain neutral, or may detach themselves from the patient/family experience. The approach of the caregiver to the patient/family unit may assist patients and family members to come to terms with their distress, may increase the distress or may not have any impact on the distress. The manner in which the professional caregiver deals with patients and their family members may also impact the amount of distress the professional caregiver feels[3,4]. Appropriate intervention at this critical point may decrease the immediate emotional suffering for all concerned. In addition, intervention can also ease the family bereavement period[5].

The assessment and treatment of the psychosocial distress associated with palliative illness involves the ability to distinguish between the normal symptoms of a person's adjustment to advanced illness, distress that requires intervention and the symptoms of a major psychiatric disorder. The skilled practitioner must be able to identify, assess, and, when possible, treat the physical symptoms of the disease together with the increasing debility and changes in social roles and social isolation associated with the disease and the dying process. At the same time she must be able to distinguish when the social isolation or change in social roles are signs of a major depression, when the pain and symptoms of the disease have a strong psychological overlay requiring psychiatric or psychological referral, or when such symptoms are reflective of suffering, requiring a different intervention and when apparent hallucinations and confusion may be reflections of a spiritual or existential end of life crisis. In addition, the caregiver requires self knowledge and understanding of the concept of countertransference in order to effectively help the patient with his or her process, using the self as an instrument, or at the very least not interfering with the process the dying person may be experiencing, or needing to experience at this point in his or her life[6].

Overview of chapter

Focus of the chapter

This chapter will outline some underlying assumptions of palliative care. There will then be a review of the epidemiological data on the psychosocial distress associated with palliative illness, identifying some of the factors associated with increased risk, and reviewing current approaches to intervention in psychosocial distress. This will be followed by a clinical discussion of the emotional and psychosocial/spiritual issues confronting dying persons and suggestions for interventions. Clinical examples as well as art and reflections from persons who have died of their illness will be used to give the reader better insight into the experience of the palliative care patient and family.

This chapter will not discuss the psychiatric problems of depression and anxiety and related concerns as these topics are covered in Chapter 15.5.

Palliative care is whole-person care

In *Crossing Over: Narratives of Palliative Care*, which describes the experience of palliative care in two settings in the United States and Canada[7], Barnard *et al.* state, 'palliative care is whole-person care not only in the sense that the whole person of the patient (body, mind, spirit) is the object of care, but also in that the whole person of the caregiver is involved. Palliative care is, par excellence, care that is given through the medium of a human relationship'[7].

More recently, Katz[6] has applied the psychiatric concept of countertransference to end-of-life care. Countertransference is defined as '... an "abbreviation" for the totality of our responses to our work—emotional, cognitive and behavioural—whether prompted by our patients, by the dynamics incumbent to our helping relationships, or by our own inevitable life experiences'[6]. End of life care professionals of all disciplines and levels of experience, not just therapists, are subject to powerful reactions to their work. These reactions are seen as being far more diverse than 'compassion fatigue' or 'vicarious traumatization'[6].

Drawing on the quantum physics concepts that the whole is greater than the sum of its parts, similarly to Kearney's

A Place of Healing: Working with Suffering in Living and Dying[8], Katz speaks the alchemical reaction that occurs when two individuals engage together at the most vulnerable time in human existence—the end of life. Alchemy is 'that space' that takes its own place in the poignant relationship between helper and patient. Through the experience both can be transformed.

Dr. Roger Cole, a palliative care physician[9], writes of this alchemy that occurred early in his career in a relationship with a young man dying of AIDS. 'In writing this book I am indebted to John. He made me wonder. He made me wonder why some people have to suffer. He made me wonder why we become "spiritually blind" and separated from our souls. He made me wonder what freedom from fear would be like; how it would be to experience the peace that was evident when he knew he was dying, and whether I would put it off until my own death to find out. By making me wonder, he made me seek understanding'[9].

Perhaps an explanation for the alchemy that occurs within relationships can be explained by findings contained in Daniel Goleman's recent book, *Social Intelligence: The New Science of Human Relationships*[4]. Goleman says that our brains have evolved to push us to act to ease the pain of others. Science is now telling us there is a net of neurons in the brain with the sole task of attuning us to the inner state of the person we're with. When we are with someone in distress our motor neurons make us want to act. The social brain prepares us to act appropriately—and the appropriate reaction to someone in dire distress is to help. We are wired to be compassionate and to help—but that help can go both ways, which might be part of the alchemy.

Neimeyer[10] addresses psychologists involved in end-of-life care, noting 'it can be understandably tempting to translate a patient's poignant anxieties about dying into simple medical symptoms to be managed or mitigated. Arguably, however, a psychologist's preoccupation with symptoms rather than their significance constitutes a form of professional abandonment of vulnerable and potentially needy patients at the end of their lives'[10].

Illness does not occur in a vacuum

Sir William Osler has been quoted as saying, 'Ask not what disease the person has, but rather what person the disease has'[11]. The underlying premise of the chapter is that illness does not occur in a vacuum. The individual has a personal history, personality characteristics, and coping mechanisms that may prove to be helpful or unhelpful in dealing with the present situation. In addition, most individuals are members of a social network. The manner in which an individual's significant others respond to the person and his or her illness may, in part, determine the individual's response to the disease. A diagnosis of AIDS in a young nurse with dependent children living in rural Africa, and needing to continue to work as long as she can to support her family will obviously have a different disease experience requiring a different response from that of a woman of the same age living in a western society who is diagnosed with inflammatory breast cancer, carefully assesses her options, chooses to have aggressive treatment, and then relapses.

An individual's process of adaptation to the disease will also be determined in part by a number of other variables including:

- Age and stage of family development.
- The nature of the disease.

- The trajectory or pattern of the illness.
- The individual and family's previous experience with illness and death.
- Socioeconomic status.
- Cultural variables[12].

The illness trajectory may affect adaptation

Both the person with life-threatening illness and the support network will respond differently depending on whether the illness was initially perceived as having been 'cured' and has now relapsed; whether the disease was perceived to be a chronic disease, which was expected to go on 'forever' and is now at the point where treatment aimed at prolonging survival is no longer appropriate; whether there were hopes to cure the disease with a procedure such as a stem-cell transplant, which then leads to, or potentially precipitates death; or whether the disease has had a fairly rapid trajectory to death[12].

Kafetz[13] notes that in elderly people, the process of dying tends to be less clear-cut than in younger people with malignancy. The 'dying trajectory' may last longer, and awareness may be clouded by cognitive dysfunction. He quotes Nuland[14] who says that death in old age is often a protracted affair. An elderly patient said to Nuland, 'Death keeps taking little bits of me'. Her physician commented: 'She saw that with each attack of dizziness or fainting or confusion she became a little older, a little weaker and a little more tired. She knew that for ten years or more, she had been moving step by step towards the grave'[13].

Lynn[15] noted that function and symptoms at the end of life generally follow one of three trajectories: (1) a short period of obvious decline at the end, typical of cancer; (2) long-term disability with periodic exacerbations and unpredictable timing of death that characterize dying with chronic organ or system failures (some cancers that respond to treatment and then relapse come into this category); and (3) self-care deficits and a slowly dwindling course to death from dementia. Only the first of these forms of death allows for an 'aware' death[13]. Relatives who expect aware deaths may become angry and turn their anger onto doctors and nurses when death takes other forms. It is noted that dying people need psychosocial support but this can only be given when it is clear that the dying phase is identified and that is not always possible in trajectories 2 and 3.

Early intervention may decrease later distress

The assumption is made that if the needs of the person with a life-threatening illness and the significant others are handled reasonably well from the time of diagnosis, then even if the final outcome is death, the problems associated with this outcome will be fewer and less complicated than would be the case if there were numerous unresolved problems during the early stages of the illness[12]. One of the major issues in palliative care involves when it is appropriate to refer a patient to a palliative care program or team.

A 76-year-old woman was diagnosed with metastatic breast cancer 9 years before her final illness trajectory. During these years she had an excellent quality of life, teaching skiing and sailing. When her disease recurred, she was referred for psychotherapy in which she explored the meaning of her illness in her life and was referred for home palliative care, while being given chemotherapy. She looked forward to the discussions with the psychotherapist, developed a good relationship with her palliative care physician, and the nurses who visited. At times she took a break from palliative care to travel, then resumed palliative care visits. The day before she died she was visited at home where she was dying overlooking her garden and a river. She said, 'Time has changed now. The flowers look totally different. I close my eyes and I think to myself, "oh, so that is what it is going to be like". I think to myself, "it is just what Mary said it would be."' The night before this woman died she said 'I want to go to my own bed'. Her family helped her to move from the hospital bed, which had been placed in the living room, up the stair glide into her bed where she died peacefully the next day.

This is in contrast to a young man who was referred for palliative care while still ambulatory, and planning a family holiday. The assumption was that if the palliative care physician met the man at this point then the physician would have a better idea of who he was when he was closer to dying. The palliative care physician visited and said that he was not usually asked to see patients who were still able to walk. The patient was discharged from the palliative care program causing problems to be discussed later. The problems with referral are not always with others in the system not referring soon enough.

The preface to the Canadian document, A Consensus-based Model to Guide Hospice Palliative Care[16], notes that people are living with illnesses for much longer. Faced with longer illness people must deal with many issues:

♦ How to get relief of symptoms?

♦ How can they carry on with life, as they have known it?

♦ How will the illness affect roles and relationships?

♦ What can be done to change the illness experience?

♦ How can people restore or maintain their capacity for meaningful and valuable experiences that give quality to their lives?

Each of these issues creates expectations, needs, hopes, and fears, which must be addressed in order for the ill person to carry on with life and find opportunities for growth within the illness experience. For many years, the approach used in hospice palliative care has helped patients and their families address these issues during the last stage of the illness experience: the process of dying. The same approach can now be used to enhance health-care delivery throughout the entire illness experience. All the skills developed in hospice palliative care can be applied early to help patients improve their quality of life, increase their ability to participate in therapy to fight their disease, and, potentially, prolong their lives[16].

Intervention should meet patient and family needs

It is not appropriate simply to intervene. Intervention must be done carefully and at a pace best matched to patient–family needs as opposed to caregiver expectations and agendas about what 'should' be done.

A 40-year-old man was diagnosed with amyloidosis and eventually experienced kidney failure and was put on dialysis. He had considerable difficulty in dealing with the diagnosis and preferred to stay in the city near medical treatment, rather than returning to the farming community in which he lived with his wife and 14-year-old son. Although others felt that he should be closer to his family during his final months, he avoided them until such time as he was ready to begin to face the possibility of his death at which time he returned home and in his own way prepared his wife and son for his death.

While caregivers sometimes inappropriately make the decision not to tell patients and their family members what is likely to happen, at other times caregivers may inappropriately err on the side of giving too much negative information too soon and too often, allowing for no possibility of hope.

Good palliative care involves options

People should have some choice with regard to how they choose to spend their final illness and where they choose to spend these days. To have this choice, people will need to be aware of the extent of their disease and its expected prognosis. Given this knowledge and the available resources, people should be able to choose to continue active treatment, albeit possibly within some limits; choose palliative treatment; choose to be removed from technological support; or choose to be at home with or without a support programme or choose to be in a hospital or hospice setting. Zimmerman and Rodin[17] review the literature on denial of death and palliative care and say that whereas the emphasis on a death denying society may have been appropriate in the early days of hospice, palliative care must now be open to serving 'all patients with life-threatening illness rather than only those who acknowledge that they are dying, we must develop novel ways of delivering palliative care … Many terminally ill patients are not ready to be labelled as "dying", but all wish to stop suffering'[17].

Obviously, not everyone has the ideal options and choices available to them due to a variety of social beliefs, economic constraints, and other issues. These variables range from cultural beliefs that people should not be told that they have cancer or that they are going to die; to settings that strongly encourage terminally ill patients to transfer to hospice settings because of the economic problems associated with expensive 'active treatment', which will not cure the patient; to problems in Africa where health-care workers are being infected at the same rate as the general population[18] and are continuing to work, both because of financial issues as well as the fact that there are not other professionals to take their place when they have to stop working. At the recent International Nurses' Forum, Nurses at the Forefront of HIV/AIDS, Sr. Christa Mary Jones, reported that at her hospital five student nurses and six staff nurses died in the past year. 'To access testing and treatment they must stand in the same queues as their clients, undermining the relationship of trust and authority that is fundamental to their effectiveness'[18]. In some setting, special Wellness Centers are being set up for these staff members and so they do not have to attend clinic with patients for whom they will be caring. In some cultures, there is not enough money for even the very basic necessities of health care. Here, people die at home or even on the streets, not because they choose to do so, but because there are no other options available.

In first-world countries, scientific advances in some areas such as advanced colorectal cancer have significantly prolonged life for those with advanced disease, but at considerable cost. More than

50 per cent of new colorectal cancer patients present with stage III or metastatic disease and half of all people with colorectal cancer are diagnosed with recurrent or metastatic disease[19,20]. The new drug therapies for metastatic colorectal cancer have almost doubled the life expectancy for patients. The median survival with new drugs has gone from 8 to more than 21 months[19,21]. The near-doubling of the median survival achieved over the past decade has been accompanied by a staggering 340-fold increase in drug costs—just for the initial 8 weeks of treatment. Costs have gone from $63 to $21 000. In 2004, 32 000 people in the United States received a diagnosis of stage IV colorectal cancer, and recurrent metastatic disease developed in an additional 24 000. The drug costs for an eight-week course of initial treatment for these 56 000 patients was estimated to be approximately $666 million—or $1.2 billion with the addition of monoclonal-antibody therapy. Societies will need to struggle with decision-making in this area[21].

While there are obviously benefits of prolonged survival, not all patients and their families are able to derive the same benefit from this time. Some family members feel torn as they know that, while the person with cancer feels that life should be prolonged at all costs, the financial cost the family is incurring for the extra time will cause the family long-term difficulty and they are not sure the extra time is worth the later financial burden they will have to assume. One young husband said, 'If she is going to die anyway, she might just as well do it sooner, rather than later. If I am going to be widowed, then I would just like to get on with my life.' Sometimes, the extra time allows couples to work through these issues and deal effectively with the impact of the person's dying on their relationship, as happened in this situation. Other patients and families are able to use much of the time they receive for increased closeness and planning for the future, but as patients continue to feel reasonably well it is easy to imagine that one has beaten the disease and hard when relapse occurs. As one palliative patient said, 'being palliative is to live in the meadow of "I don't know"'.

Von Gruenigen and Daly[22] reviewed the literature to determine the factors associated with the continuation of futile treatment in women with advanced ovarian cancer. Summarizing the number of women in the United States who would die of gynaecologic malignancies in 2004, they calculated that gynaecologic oncologists would have the discussion about medical futility 28 000 times that year.

In their review they concluded that there was 'little research investigating the reasoning of oncologists in decision-making regarding continued provision of high-burden treatment such as chemotherapy, in the face of no meaningful probability of physiologic benefit'[22]. Reviewing the literature involving physician's use of antibiotics, artificial nutrition and hydration, and mechanical ventilation, they found such decisions were influenced by personal and background factors such as gender, experience, and postgraduate education. African American physicians were six times more likely to prescribe aggressive treatments than were Caucasians. Younger physicians, who spent more time in clinical practice, were more willing to withdraw therapy. Physicians who denied medical futility were influenced by religion, the practice of legal defensiveness, aggressive practice style, and emotional detachment. Patient characteristics associated with futile treatments included recent treatment initiation, age of the patient and diagnosis. In a study comparing African American and white, terminally ill patients and their designated family caregivers[23] given a near death condition,

African American patients were more likely than white patients to desire each of the life-sustaining measures (all $P < 0.004$).

Von Gruenigen and Daly[22] quoted a study by Ramondetta et al.[24] who surveyed members of the Society of Gynecologic Oncologists in 2000 on end-of-life issues. Although only 35 per cent responded, 44 per cent of these believed that gynaecologic oncologists paternalistically influenced end-of-life decisions. When gynaecologic oncology patients were surveyed on end-of-life decisions, 96 per cent emphasized 'straight talk' and 64 per cent expected compassion. Donovan et al.[25] found that 25 per cent of recently diagnosed woman with ovarian cancer stated they would never switch to palliative care but would choose salvage therapy even if the expected survival was only one week.

Titrate information to patient needs (see also Chapters 5.5 and 6.2)

Given, that under ideal circumstances, people should have the choice of where and how to spend their final time, and so too should they have the option of choosing how much information they want about their illness including the option of choosing not to know their prognosis if this is their preference. The medical practitioner must be aware that, much as there is a 'right to know', there is also a corresponding 'right not to know' provided that the patient has given the health-care provider the clear message that this is his/her choice. Problems arise in this situation, however, if the patient chooses 'not-to-know' that the treatment she/he is demanding has almost no likelihood of success and the person refuses to acknowledge the possibility that death may result from this disease episode.

Haggerty et al.[26] studied 126 patients with metastatic cancer seeing 30 oncologists in 12 outpatient clinics in New South Wales, 95 per cent wanted information about side effects and treatment options, 85 per cent wanted to know the longest survival time with treatment, 80 per cent wanted 5 year survival rates, and 81 per cent wanted to know average survival. Fifty-nine per cent wanted to discuss expected survival when first diagnosed with metastatic disease. Thirty-eight and 44 per cent respectively wanted to negotiate when expected survival and dying, respectively, were discussed—they wanted information about life expectancy, dying, and palliative care only if they asked for it or after negotiation. Patients with an expected survival of years were more likely to want to discuss life expectancy when first diagnosed with metastasis. Sixty-five per cent wanted to know their shortest survival time without treatment and one year survival rates in order to allow themselves to prepare themselves and their families for the future and assist with decision-making and life planning. Many indicated that such information might best be given over several consultations, given that it takes time to understand and adjust to this information—especially if there is a shorter expected survival. However, the problem that may result then is that the time to have the conversation disappears.

A Japanese study of 529 patients[27] found that when receiving bad news, patients desired detailed information and a supportive environment. The Measure for Patient Preferences (MPP-J) demonstrated a 5-factor structure: support, facilitation, medical information, clear explanation, and encouraging question-asking. Regression analysis indicated that a female gender, the fighting spirit, and anxious preoccupation dimensions of the Mental Adjustment to Cancer (MAC) scale were positively associated with all 5 MPP-J factors. The US and Japanese populations were similar in that both placed importance on receiving information about their cancer and its treatment, the physician speaking in a manner that is honest and easy to understand, and the physician offering support. However, there were differences in the way that Japanese and American patients preferred to have information delivered. The highest rated item in Japan was being told in person, rather than over the phone, whereas that item was ranked 24th in the US. The lowest ranked item in both Japan and the US was 'the doctor holding my hand or touching my arm while telling me the news'. The study concluded that, contrary to the traditional paternalistic and hierarchical culture that does not encourage questioning, Japanese physicians should encourage patients to ask questions and should consider the gender, disease state, and psychological characteristics (fighting spirit and anxious preoccupation) of the patient when delivering bad news. Physicians were encouraged to provide emotional support and to understand the patients' communication style preferences regarding what information to receive and how to receive it, since patients might expect the information to automatically be provided by their physicians.

Haggerty et al.[26] concluded from their review of the literature that patients frequently misunderstood much of what they were told, incorrectly stated the extent of their disease and the goal of treatment and overestimated their prognosis. They suggested that such misunderstanding may lead patients to make decisions contrary to their best interests—for example choosing futile life-sustaining therapy at the expense of quality of life. They quote another Australian study by Gattelleri et al.[28] of initial consultations between oncologists and incurable cancer patients. Eighty-five per cent were informed of the aim of anticancer treatment and that the disease was incurable (75 per cent). Slightly more than half (58 per cent) were told about life expectancy, only one-third (35 per cent) received a quantitative estimate, and fewer than 10 per cent were given a time frame of life expectancy. Physicians in such situations experience tension between providing hope and realism[29], particularly because less than half of patients in that study wanted a quantitative estimate of their prognosis. Those with a poorer prognosis were less likely to want the information, however, a large majority wanted to know whether they would die from their disease[29].

Epidemiology of psychosocial distress

Psychosocial distress

The National Comprehensive Cancer Network[30] addressed the stigma attached to psychological problems and chose to use the word 'distress' because it is more readily accepted and less embarrassing than a psychological or psychiatric term. In the context of cancer, distress has been defined as 'a multifactorial unpleasant emotional experience of a psychological (cognitive, behavioural, emotional), social, or spiritual nature that may interfere with the ability to cope effectively with cancer, its physical symptoms, and its treatment'[30,31]. Feelings of distress range along a continuum, from sadness and vulnerability to disabling depression. Distress can be described in terms of suffering, hopelessness, and existential or spiritual crisis, can undermine the capacity for pleasure, take away a sense of meaning, diminish the ability to connect with others, and overall have a negative effect on quality of life[32,33].

Ambulatory cancer patients reported a range of distress, including depression, anxiety, and adjustment disorders from 18 to 50 per cent[33–36]. In a Jordanian sample of cancer inpatients the prevalence of distress was 70 per cent[37]. From 61 to 79 per cent of the palliative care subgroup ($N = 69$) in a stratified, randomized, Registry-based, Canadian community cancer sample of 1319 people living with cancer[34] currently had high distress on the General Health Questionnaire (GHQ) compared with 18–34 per cent of the general cancer population. In a replication of the original study at Toronto-Sunnybrook Regional Cancer Centre (T-SRCC)[38] 79 per cent of both terminally ill inpatients ($N = 31$) and terminally ill outpatients ($N = 14$) had high distress compared with 66 per cent of the total inpatient population ($N = 97$) and 30 per cent of the outpatient population ($N = 346$). Thirty-eight per cent of the total population ($N = 443$) had high distress[39].

Using the ICD-10 Diagnostic Criteria for Research, Durkin et al.[40] found 139 (62 per cent) of patients on a palliative care unit met criteria for psychiatric disorder. Thirty-three (24 per cent) of patients had dual diagnoses. The commonest diagnoses were organic disorders followed by neurotic and stress-related disorders (27, 16, and 16 per cent respectively). One hundred and twenty-six (91 per cent) of the patients with a psychiatric disorder had been symptomatic on admission. Of these, 35 per cent were receiving incorrect or inadequate treatment. They concluded that future research needs to identify effective methods of detecting and diagnosing these disorders to enable early and effective treatment programs be initiated.

Kafetz[13] noted that when Hinton looked at deaths in general wards in 1963, he found widespread distress. Thirty-four years later the SUPPORT study in the USA yielded very similar findings[41]. Despite great advances in palliative care in the intervening period, many dying patients were still troubled by pain and other symptoms. Despite the ubiquitous nature of psychological distress in palliative patients, their distress tends to be under-diagnosed and under-treated, with up to 50 per cent of psychiatric disorders going unrecognized by medical and nursing personnel[33,40].

Factors associated with psychosocial distress

In Zabora et al.'s study[35] of ambulatory cancer patients ($n = 4$, 496), diagnoses with a poorer prognosis and greater patient burden produced similar rates of distress. Pancreatic cancer patients had the highest mean scores for symptoms such as anxiety and depression, while Hodgkin's patients exhibited the highest mean scores for hostility. Those with a history of emotional difficulties are more apt to be distressed[42,43].

In the Canadian Needs study[44], pain, other symptoms, and treatment side-effects, as well as cancer-related fears, had direct and indirect effects on psychological symptoms of distress. Impaired role performance was a central mediator for the indirect effects. The model explained 34 per cent of the variance in GHQ scores and was equally applicable to all three provinces, both male and female subjects, rural and urban settings, and to all stages of illness. Pain was the single most important explaining variable, but other symptoms, including fatigue, had an impact on impaired role performance. However, impaired role performance also had a negative effect on distress over and above the effect of pain. Kaasa et al.[45] also found that patients who had impaired role performance in addition to pain were most distressed and that distress varied with severity of the pain and role impairment.

The variables associated with high distress in the Canadian study[34,38,39,44] included problems with physical functioning, physical integrity, emotional well-being, social relationships, illness adaptation, economic/occupational roles, and cognitive ability. A previous comparison of a number of studies of patients with advanced disease[39] showed that the most commonly reported problems associated with distress were pain, decreased energy or weakness, fatigue, appetite disturbances, psychological disturbance, breathing problems, sleep disturbances, nausea, and constipation. Problems with walking and climbing stairs, and confusion were more common in the Canadian studies[34,38,39,44].

Turner *et al.*[46] studied 83 elderly patients (aged 75 and above) being treated with palliative radiotherapy for lung cancer. Psychological distress and concerns were measured using the HADS and a Concerns Checklist. Fifty-five per cent of the group was described as being anxious pre-treatment and 63 per cent post-radiotherapy. Fifty-three per cent were depressed pre-treatment and 47 per cent post-treatment. Comparable figures for 49 patients 65 and younger were 54 per cent anxious pre-treatment and 52 per cent anxious post-treatment; 53 per cent depressed pre-treatment and 55 per cent depressed post-treatment. The median number of concerns identified by the elderly patients was 10 (range 1–18) before treatment, rising slightly to 10.5 at follow-up. The younger group reported somewhat more concerns (median 12), (range 0–18 before and after treatment). None of the concerns had a rating above 2, moderately concerned. There were non-significant shifts in problems over the course of treatment. Initially, the younger group rated the illness, the future relating to the illness and family highest concerns and energy as a moderate concern, but energy levels became a minor concern by the end of treatment. The elderly also ranked family as one of their most serious concerns before treatment but this improved at follow-up. Breathlessness was consistently rated as a moderate concern by the elderly patients, and their median scores for energy level and future relating to their illness increased from mild to moderate after radiotherapy. Patients said staff addressed their physical concerns such as breathlessness and pain, as well as concerns about the illness and its treatment. Staffs were less likely to have addressed concerns about psychosocial issues such as family and the future.

In the T-SRCC study[38], terminally ill inpatients reported a mean of 17.6 problems in the past month (median = 15) and terminally ill outpatients had a mean of 20.92 problems (median = 19.5). Ninety-four per cent of the terminally ill group reported a current biggest problem compared with 73 per cent of the total sample. The most commonly reported biggest problems were

- Physical side-effects of disease and treatment, 23 per cent.

- Changes in lifestyle, 14 per cent.

- Pain, 10 per cent.

- Dealing with recurrent disease/death, 8 per cent.

Pain was the current biggest problem most likely to be associated with high distress (88 per cent) for the total sample. This was followed by dealing with recurrent disease/death (70 per cent), physical side-effects of the disease and illness (54 per cent), and changes in lifestyle (38 per cent). In an Italian study by Morasso *et al.*,[47] the most frequent unmet needs were symptom control (62.1 per cent)

and emotional support (51.7 per cent). Low functional state was significantly associated with a high proportion of patients with unmet needs of personal care, information, communication, occupational functioning, and emotional closeness. Patients with unmet needs showed significantly higher psychological and symptom distress for most needs.

More recently, in a study of 209 terminally ill Japanese cancer patients[1], younger age, longer education, lower performance status, more severe pain, more severe constipation, more severe fatigue, greater concern about financial issues, pain, being a burden to others, loss of independence and dignity, less satisfaction with confidantes, and presence of past history of major depression were significant factors associated with the presence of psychological distress. Logistic regression analysis showed that lower performance status, greater concern about being a burden to others, and less satisfaction with confidantes were the final significant factors associated with psychological distress at baseline, when patients were registered for the program, before admission to the palliative care unit. The authors suggested that in looking at factors associated with adjustment disorders and major depression, multidimensional factors such as physical functioning, social support factors, and existential issues may underlie the psychological distress experienced by terminally ill cancer patients.

In a Greek study[48], significant associations were found between the desire for hastened death and pain, fatigue, loss of appetite, and feeling sad. Statistically significant associations were also found between Schedule of Attitudes toward Hastened Death (SAHD) scores, age, and ECOG. Twenty-six per cent of the patients reported high Desire for Hastened Death, while 41 per cent reported moderate desire. The contribution of pain, lack of appetite, and sadness accounted for 42 per cent of the variance in SAHD scores. The authors suggest that the desire for hastened death is significantly related to feeling sad, lack of appetite, pain and fatigue, after controlling for age, gender, and performance status according to ECOG in terminally ill cancer patients. Despite all the efforts being made in palliative care, these symptoms do not seem to be decreasing in the distress they cause.

Distress can also be a familial phenomenon[49]. A meta analysis of 21 studies comparing patient and caregiver distress found a positive association between patient and caregiver distress. Patients and carers did not experience either more or less distress than one another. There was a relationship between time since diagnosis and distress and it was suggested that early intervention with both patients and caregivers could decrease distress. Kissane *et al.*[50] studied palliative care families at risk of a morbid psychological outcome. The family types were identified as: Intermediate (51 per cent); Sullen (26 per cent); and Hostile (23 per cent). These were significantly associated with steadily increasing levels of distress.

Annabelle Cooper was an artist who was 53 when she was diagnosed with endometrial cancer. Four years later she was diagnosed with breast cancer. She died less than 2 years later. Annabelle used her art to help her to cope with the distress she experienced during her treatment for cancer.

During her chemotherapy in the middle of winter Annabelle became extremely distressed; having visions of going and sleeping with the poppies in the garden in $-32°C$ weather. In Picture 15.2.1, she shows herself as she experienced chemotherapy. She was a cork bobbing in the ocean. Nearby the HMS Chemotherapy sailed with a message for God to bless all who sailed on her. Picture 15.2.2

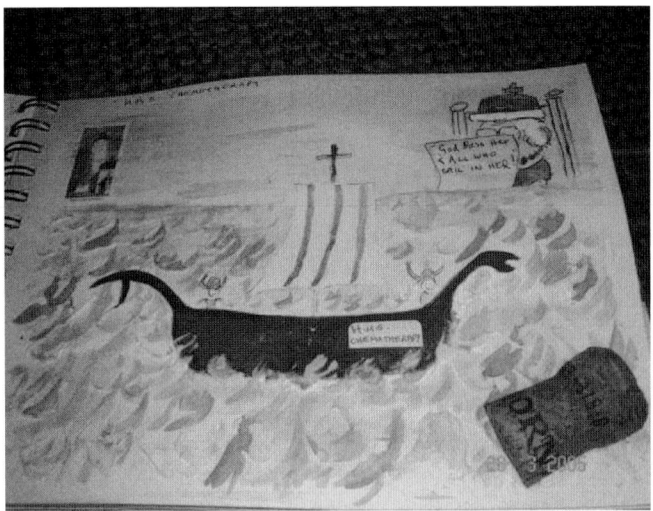

Picture 15.2.1 HMS Chemo.

shows her image of herself as Sisyphus, needing to push the rock of cancer up the hill, only to have it come down again and have to keep pushing it up the hill.

Assessment and intervention

Recent work with a new diagnostic tool, the Distress Thermometer (DT) has shown that a score of 4 or more on this single-item measure compares favourably with longer measures, such as the Hospital Anxiety and Depression Scale, an 18-item Brief Symptom Inventory[51], and the Center for Epidemiological Studies-Depression Scale (CES-D)[52]. A score of 4 or greater on the DT and accompanying Problem List (Fig. 15.2.1) can make it easier to screen patients in the clinic to identify distress stemming from emotional, spiritual or religious concerns, practical or family issues, or physical problems. Consensus-based guidelines developed by the Distress Management Panel of NCCN recommend screening all patients regularly for psychosocial distress as a part of routine cancer care[30]. These guidelines are based on evidence that oncologists and oncology nurses do not recognize psychological distress, despite its prevalence in the cancer population and its association with greater non-adherence to treatment recommendations, poorer satisfaction with care, and poorer quality of life across many domains[51]. When health-care

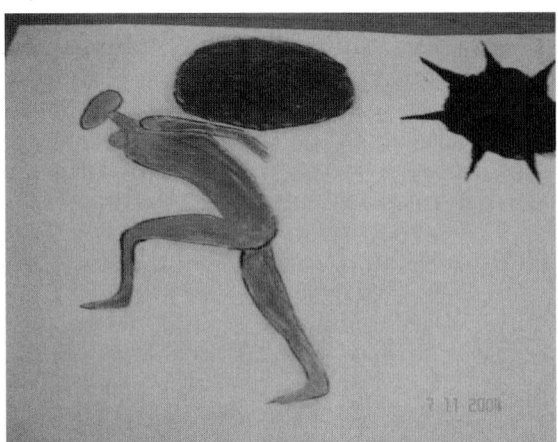

Picture 15.2.2 Sisyphus.

professionals fail to recognize distress, cancer patients do not receive effective pharmacologic and non-pharmacologic interventions for relieving it[51]. Bultz and Carlson[53] noted that the Canadian Strategy for Cancer Control (CSCC) recently suggested that distress be added as the sixth vital sign to the other five key indicators—temperature, respiration, heart rate, blood pressure, and more recently pain. They do not, however, suggest a particular instrument to be used.

The Distress Thermometer and guidelines to address each facet of distress are available at http://www.nccn.org. Murillo and Holland[54] provide guidelines for distress management in advanced illness. They suggest the primary oncology team use the distress thermometer to assess the patient for excessive worries, fear, sadness, unclear thinking, despair, severe family problems, and spiritual crisis. A score of 5 or more should result in referral to mental health, social work, or pastoral services. Mild distress or a score less than 5 can usually be dealt with by the oncology team. An algorithm of the management of distress identifying the professional group responsible for dealing with various aspects of distress is provided. They suggest that

> Standards for psychosocial care and clinical practice guidelines for supportive services should be endorsed by major organizations involved in end-of-life care. They should be promulgated in a manner similar to that used with pain management.
>
> Educational standards for end-of-life care must include training in the recognition of distress and its management by the primary care team. Such standards should also be included in the curricula of both mental health professionals (psychologists, psychiatrists, psychiatric social workers, and nurses) and the clergy qualifying as pastoral counsellors. Pastoral counselling should be included in psychosocial services, because they should not be fragmented and distanced from other aspects of care during the end of life.
>
> Patients and families must be educated to understand that the psychosocial/spiritual domains are an integral part of their end-of-life care and should not be viewed as disconnected and unrelated[54].

Neimeyer[10] has reviewed the role of the psychologist in assessing and dealing with those at the end of life and suggests the use of tools to assess and document different facets of death concerns. 'The best of these offer a refined view of different facets of death concerns, such as fears concentrating on the pain involved in dying, on spiritual issues, on existential questions regarding the confrontation with the unknown, on concerns for bodily integrity after death, on the inability to accomplish important life goals or purposes, and on the impact of one's death on others'[10]. He suggests that appropriate selection of instruments could help to target interviews and interventions to domains of concern to individual patients and to document the effects of treatment programs in ameliorating them.

Attachment theory and cancer

Previously, the author has written of personality and psychoneuroimmunological factors that may or may not be associated with cancer, its development, and progression[39]. Because of space limitations, this chapter will focus only on one aspect of this literature, attachment behaviour and possible psychoneuroimmunological links.

Tacón[55] reviewed the literature on attachment theory and the psychosocial literature in cancer to develop an integrative model of attachment theory and type C behaviour pattern possibly associated

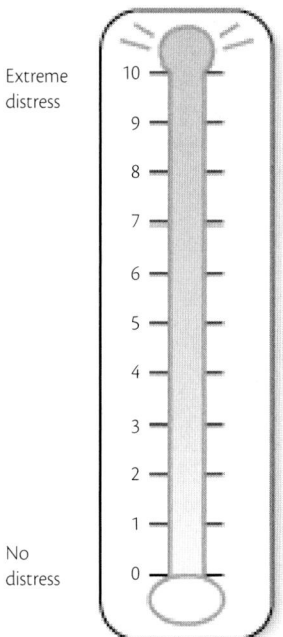

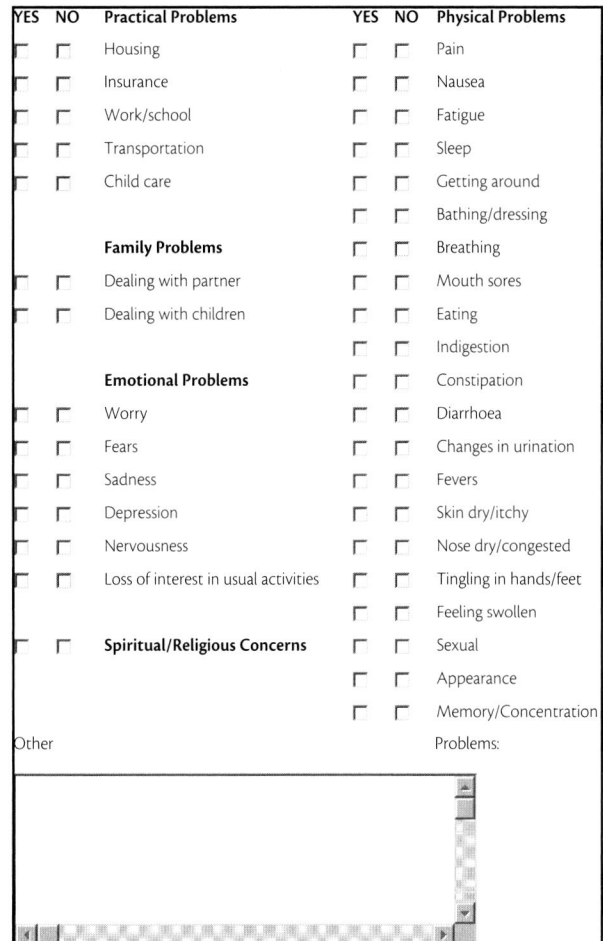

Please indicate if any of the following has been a cause of distress in the past week, including today. Be sure to check NO or YES for each.

YES	NO	Practical Problems	YES	NO	Physical Problems
☐	☐	Housing	☐	☐	Pain
☐	☐	Insurance	☐	☐	Nausea
☐	☐	Work/school	☐	☐	Fatigue
☐	☐	Transportation	☐	☐	Sleep
☐	☐	Child care	☐	☐	Getting around
			☐	☐	Bathing/dressing
		Family Problems	☐	☐	Breathing
☐	☐	Dealing with partner	☐	☐	Mouth sores
☐	☐	Dealing with children	☐	☐	Eating
			☐	☐	Indigestion
		Emotional Problems	☐	☐	Constipation
☐	☐	Worry	☐	☐	Diarrhoea
☐	☐	Fears	☐	☐	Changes in urination
☐	☐	Sadness	☐	☐	Fevers
☐	☐	Depression	☐	☐	Skin dry/itchy
☐	☐	Nervousness	☐	☐	Nose dry/congested
☐	☐	Loss of interest in usual activities	☐	☐	Tingling in hands/feet
			☐	☐	Feeling swollen
☐	☐	**Spiritual/Religious Concerns**	☐	☐	Sexual
			☐	☐	Appearance
			☐	☐	Memory/Concentration
		Other			Problems:

Figure 15.2.1 Screening tools for measuring distress.
Instructions: Please circle the number (0–10) that best describes how much distress you have been experiencing in the past week, including today.

with cancer[56]. The Typc C personality is characterized by being cooperative; overly patient; unassertive and appeasing; nonexpressive of emotions, especially anger; inattentive to or unaware of one's needs and signals, and compliant with authority. 'Attachment, a biobehavioural theory of development, provides an explanation for lifelong patterns acquired in childhood. It describes how early parent–child interactions establish patterns of social relations, stress response, and emotional regulation in offspring. Attachment may play a role in physical illness and in specific diseases such as cancer … Attachment is conceptualized as a behavioural control system rooted in neurophysiological processes within the central nervous system … Attachment figures appear to be the original regulators of the child's affective and physiological reactivity to stress as well as a model for using social support when needed'[55]. The traditional classification system is (1) secure and (2) insecure patterns—avoidant and ambivalent. Children of sensitive or responsive caregivers have been shown to develop a secure style, and as adults have a positive image of themselves and of others. They are comfortable with intimacy, are not restricted in affect, and have high self esteem. When a child receives inconsistent parenting he or she develops an ambivalent style, characterized by intense affect and emotional neediness, fear of abandonment, and low self-esteem. As adults, children whose caregivers were emotionally cold and rejecting develop the avoidant style characterized by compulsive self-reliance, high distrust with fear of intimacy, and hyperregulation of affect. The person with this style also has an inhibited display of negative emotions, masking negative affect, especially anger. Such persons also tend to restrict acknowledging distress, appearing unperturbed, while displaying physiological arousal during exploration of threatening issues. Tacón notes that the literature shows that security moderates stress reactivity, insecurely attached, inhibited children had the highest levels of cortisol post session in contrast to secure children. Attachment plays a contributory role in stress activation. Tacón et al.[57] studied 104 women with and without breast cancer and found the women in the breast cancer group scored significantly higher on avoidant attachment and emotional control than women in the control group. Tacón notes that further research needs to be done to differentiate between avoidance as a premorbid pattern or a coping response to cancer.

Integrating attachment theory with Temoshok's[56] research on the Type C personality, Tacón proposes a connection. She suggests that parent–child relations and emotional patterning involving the non expression of emotion are connected. She quotes the Johns Hopkins longitudinal study of 1337 white male medical students, followed for 40 years. The physicians who went on to develop cancer held less close relations, especially with their parents in the early years[58].

Tacón proposes an epigenetic model consisting of 5 levels: 'The developmental context (level I) consists of the family of origin and family variables. The socioemotional context (level II) involves precursors to attachment. The biobehavioural prototype (level III) represents the individual attachment style that emerges from experience. Next the psychophysiological and behavioural (level IV) refers to both internal psychophysiological activity such as cognitive perception, physiological stress, and immune reactivity and external behavioural manifestations (coping strategies and emotional regulation). Finally, there is a convergence of the individual (level V) with challenging life events that test the degree of accord between internal and external realities'[55].

Temoshok[59] commented on the article by Tacón[55] elaborating on the biological connections by which coping patterns developed in early life and based on genetic predisposition can affect the development and progression of disease in later life. Temoshok's work[56] focused on how the type C personality might influence the progression, rather than the development of disease. She has theorized that the goal of coping is to maintain psychological–physiological homeostasis and that the more closely a coping process resembles the inverted U-shaped function that characterizes homeostasis for most biological processes; the more likely it is to be adaptive and associated with positive health outcomes. 'Maladaptive learned coping patterns, such as type C coping represent deviations from homeostasis in that they fail to recognize, respond appropriately to, or resolve stressors, thus keeping the physiological stress response chronically engaged, with subsequent long-term damage to implicated biological systems'[59], Earlier work of hers showed that type C copers engaged in an inappropriate physiological stress response. 'Considerable psychoneuro–immunologic research has shown that the hormonal alterations induced by stress alter the synthesis and release of cytokines (small, soluble proteins that are secreted by all effector T cells, stimulated by specific recognition of antigen, and that are the principal mediators of CD4 T-cell effector actions). Cytokines have a generally immunosuppressive effect on natural killer cells activity, which has a key role in controlling metastases'[59]. Costanzo et al.[60] studied the relationship between interleukin-6 (IL-6), a proinflammatory cytokine, which has been shown to be related to psychosocial stress, depression and social support, and progression of disease in 61 advanced ovarian cancer patients. IL-6 is also associated with poorer prognosis among ovarian cancer patients and has been implicated in the metastasis of ovarian cancer. The patients completed assessments of social support, distressed mood, and quality of life before surgery. Peripheral blood was drawn preoperatively, and the plasma was assayed for IL-6, ascites samples were assayed for IL-6 for a subset of the sample. 'Both IL-6 levels and distressed mood were elevated among patients. After statistically adjusting effects of age and disease stage, social attachment was associated with lower levels of IL-6 in peripheral blood ($P = 0.03$), whereas poorer health-related quality of life was associated with higher IL-6 (P values ranged from 0.01 to 0.03 on different measures). This pattern of relations was also found in the ascites. Moreover, IL-6 levels in peripheral blood plasma correlated significantly with IL-6 in the ascites ($P < 0.001$), suggesting that peripheral IL-6 reflects IL-6 levels at the site of the tumour'[60]. Depressive and anxious symptoms were not related to IL-6 in either blood or ascetic fluid, but those women who reported a prior history of depression had higher ascites IL-6 levels. Poorer physical and functional well-being and greater fatigue were associated with higher IL-6 in peripheral blood over and above the effects of age and disease severity. The authors suggested that social support might play a protective role with respect to IL-6 elevations, and IL-6 may be an independent marker of health-related quality of life among ovarian cancer patients.

The authors note that to their knowledge theirs is the first study to find an association between psychosocial factors and a cytokine related to tumour production not only in peripheral blood but also in the vicinity of the tumour. Their finding of high scores on social attachment, reflecting a sense of intimacy and closeness with someone else, and lower levels of IL-6 are similar to other findings of women with heterogeneous gynecological cancers who more frequently seek social support having lower levels of IL-6 presurgery. The authors suggest that '(p)hysiologic mechanisms underlying behavioural-IL-6 relations may involve the interdependent relation between IL-6 and the hypothalamic pituitary adrenocortical (HPA) system. IL-6 is secreted during HPA activation and is closely involved in feedback loops with stress hormones, including adrenocorticotropic hormone (ACTH), corticotrophin-releasing hormone (CRH), and glucocorticoids. Social support has been associated with attenuated HPA activity and glucocorticoid levels … Thus, social support or depression may influence IL-6 levels through HPA activity'[60]. The authors suggest that given that social attachment and a history of depression, but not mood states were associated with IL-6, personality traits, or longstanding psychological characteristics may influence IL-6 secretion in the area of the tumour. Their laboratory has shown that stress hormones, including norepinephrine and epinephrine, as well as isoproterenol (a nonspecific β-adrenergic agonist), stimulate *in vitro* production of vascular endothelial growth factor (VEGF) by ovarian tumour cells, and these effects are blocked by propranolol (a β-adrenergic receptor antagonist). VEGF is a cytokine responsible for tumour angiogenesis. Its expression and secretion is induced by IL-6, and VEGF also stimulates IL-6 secretion. Given that stress hormones can stimulate VEGF through β-adrenergic receptors, then it is possible, but only speculative at present, that elevated stress hormones among chronically depressed individuals or among individuals with chronically poor or aversive social relationships may induce tumour production of IL-6 in a similar manner[60]. They suggest an alternative hypothesis as well, that high levels of IL-6 around the tumour and the periphery may trigger distress and malaise.

There has been recent interest in attachment behaviour in the end-of-life or palliative care setting[61,62]. Tan et al.[61] note that Western medicine patients at the end of their lives value strong relationships with their health-care providers and care that addresses the whole person and issues beyond their disease. Collaborative therapeutic relationships of this type provide the foundation for patients to explore and address biopsychosocial and spiritual aspects of dying, yet research shows that patients are often not satisfied with their communication with clinicians providing end-of-life care. Hunter et al.[62] draw on the work of Bowlby[63] who defined attachment across the lifespan as being 'any form of behaviour that results in a person attaining or retaining proximity to some other differentiated or preferred individual, who is usually conceived as stronger and/or wiser'[63].

Attachment behaviours are said to be activated at times of stress or ambiguity when there is a real or perceived threat. Differences in attachment styles affect both health seeking behaviour and the ability to be soothed by or accept help from others. '(T)he term attachment refers only to a propensity of an individual within relationships. This propensity may be shaped by the responsiveness of the provider and by the system of 'mutual regulation' that develops. From this perspective, the relationship that patients develop with clinicians depends not only on their attachment style but also depends upon the contributions from clinicians and caregivers … the empathic responsiveness of clinicians to specific attachment needs and fears may influence the success of the therapeutic relationship that develops'[61]. Hunter et al.[62] note that there are two models for viewing adult attachment behaviour—the three-group typology: secure, anxious–ambivalent, and avoidant, or the four–group typology: secure, preoccupied, dismissing–avoidant, and fearful–avoidant styles. 'Measures of adult attachment have also evolved into multi-item measures that load onto the two dimensions reflecting working models of attachment. As the names of these two dimensions suggest, attachment anxiety involves a habitual preoccupation with close relationships and a fear of separation and abandonment, whereas attachment avoidance involves a defensive tendency to over-value independence and dismiss the importance of close relationships'[62]. Hunter *et al.* suggest that working models of attachment should contribute to understanding why an individual's distress and experience of emotional support vary in the context of end-stage cancer. They also suggest that coping and support in the context of end stage cancer will be influenced by a fear of death. Previous research has shown that 'Secure people report less fear of death than insecure people, anxious-ambivalent people display greater fear both consciously and unconsciously, whereas avoidant people exhibited an unconscious fear of death'[62]. The authors studied 67 end-stage cancer patients who were either married or living with a partner, measuring the impact of attachment style as evidenced within the relationship, and emotional support on negative effect. There are limitations with the sample in that 71 per cent of eligible patients either refused to participate or were too unwell to participate. A further 8 per cent were unable to participate because of a decline in health between referral to the homecare service and the interview.

Path analysis showed that high levels of both attachment anxiety and attachment avoidance were associated with lower levels of emotional support, which in turn had a major adverse influence on patients' negative affect. In addition, attachment anxiety was also directly associated with distress. Patients who reported an emotionally supportive relationship with their spouse reported lower levels of negative affect. The authors state 'Put simply, the ability of dying cancer patients to benefit from discussions with their spouse is critical to how they feel in the final weeks of life'[62]. They suggest that emotional support in end-stage cancer is important for several reasons including the ability to make practical decisions, plan for the future, and expectant roles and reduce fear and anxiety; the expression of love and respect and a general valuing of the person, influencing self-worth at a time when self-worth is being tested for both patients and spouses; and perhaps most importantly emotional support facilitates the exploration of existential issues. 'Through this process a sense of purpose in the past and present is maintained and a sense of isolation and meaninglessness is attenuated'[62].

Tan *et al.*[61] apply the concept of attachment behaviour to relationships with palliative care professionals. They suggest that patients with a dismissing attachment style may be more open to a supportive relationship when a clinician not only communicates interest and availability but also pays respect to the person's need to retain autonomy. 'For those who have a preoccupied attachment style, feedback that provides assurance about the predictability of support may be important for them to feel secure and to maintain emotional equilibrium. The help-seeking of patients with a fearful attachment style may be concealed beneath a posture of avoidance or self-sufficiency. However, such individuals may come to trust clinicians who are reliable and not distracted by the contradictory signals from such patients about their need for support'[61]. The authors quote the work of Ciechanowski and colleagues[64,65]

who studied patients with diabetes. On the basis of glycosylated haemoglobin levels, they found that patients with diabetes mellitus who had a secure attachment demonstrated significantly better treatment adherence than those with a fearful, preoccupied, or dismissing attachment styles. However, if patients with a dismissing attachment style reported better communication with their health-care providers, they tended to achieve better metabolic control. 'This result suggests that although individuals with an insecure attachment style may have difficulty forming collaborative therapeutic relationships, the responsiveness of health-care providers may significantly influence the ultimate success of the relationship'[61].

The physical deterioration of advanced or terminal illness with its heightened dependency may trigger a crisis of attachment in many individuals. In palliative care, any attempt to define a patient as having an attachment disorder must also look at the 'attachment issues' of the health-care provider. In an important book, *When Professionals Weep*[6] dealing with countertransference in end-of-life issues, referred to above, Katz notes that end-of-life care professionals are subject to powerful reactions to their work. Some of these responses originate in the helper. Some 'belong' to the patient (but are knowingly or unknowingly incorporated by the empathic helping professional) and some belong to that 'alchemy', that 'space' that takes its own place in the poignant relationship between helper and patient. Professional caregivers may also have attachment issues. They may have a detached style, leading patients and family members to feel they don't care, or they may have anxious attachment, feeling they are the only one who can take care of patients, or they may have a secure attachment, allowing them to connect with patients, become appropriately involved, yet not be destroyed when patients die.

Attachment patterns are not only relevant to patients with cancer; they are also relevant to the care they receive. Kim and Carver[66] studied 400 spousal caregivers of patients with cancer. They found that how often spousal caregivers engaged in various types of care was a joint function of attachment and orientation. However, the difficulty that caregivers experienced in providing care was directly related to attachment orientation, without moderation by gender. Among husbands, insecure attachment qualities interfered with caregiving, and the secure quality did not foster more caregiving. Among wives, secure attachment was associated with more frequent emotional care, and anxious attachment was related to more frequent tangible care. It was hypothesized that husband's less frequent involvement in providing care for their wives' medical needs as a function of attachment anxiety might be due to their tending to be emotional upset, or their fear of abandonment, as they faced medical threats associated with their wife's cancer. Securely attached caregivers had less difficulty in providing care, while those with avoidant attachment had difficulty providing emotional care.

The patient's experience with terminal cancer

Living with terminal illness

For the purposes of this section, terminal illness is defined as advanced disease that is expected to end in death within the not too distant future. Patients with terminal disease might be receiving palliative treatment, including chemotherapy and radiotherapy, as well as other palliative treatment for symptom relief. Hutchinson[67] speaks of the 'migrations of identity' that patients with end-stage renal disease undergo. Three major constructs were identified: redefinition of self, quality of supports, and meanings of illness and treatment. The image of 'low self worth was captured in descriptors such as 'helplessness, dependence, humiliation and inadequacy'[67]. The redefinition of self concerns a change in identity. Gillies and Johnston[68] write of a similar concept of identity loss and maintenance in cancer and dementia. They note that both present a fundamental challenge to maintaining a sense of self over time. 'Both can affect the individual's memory, thinking, judgement, orientation, language, behaviour, personality and physical well-being. The effects are thus thought to be global, are progressive and are often irreversible'[68].

Theorists use a variety of terms to describe the completion of adaptation to major psychosocial transitions[67], using the terms 'integration', 'gaining a new identity', 'reincorporation', and 'return of the hero'. Hutchinson suggests that caregivers have the opportunity to help patients to re-establish a sense of integrity and wholeness at a time when their identity is being threatened by change, over which they have no control. The key element is providing a sense of safety, making it safe to suffer. He draws on the work of Michael Kearney[8], suggesting that providing a safe space where patients can regain a sense of integrity and wholeness in the face of illness and suffering is an ancient part of the health-care mandate.

This section will focus on the process of coping and adaptation in terminal illness and will discuss issues such as the meaning of the illness, accepting or denying the disease, trust and attachment, what do dying people want, hope, maintaining control and dignity, healing, anger, forgiveness, suffering, spirituality, and the respectful death model of care. The section will close with a clinical example that illustrates many of the concepts in the chapter.

Lynn[69] has said that excellence in caring for a person at the end of life requires that the clinician understand four critical elements:

- The patient's story including the patient's family and the ways the family make sense of life and its vicissitudes.

- The body and the limits and possibilities determined by its ailments over time.

- The care system and what can be done routinely and in exceptional circumstances.

- One only then can the practitioner be an effective instrument of healing in the context of fatal illness.

The meaning of the illness

The nature and extent of psychosocial vulnerability to life-threatening illness is specific to individuals and depends on the personal meaning of the disease. Meaning is defined as an 'individual's perception of the potential significance of an event, such as the occurrence of serious illness, for the self and one's plan of action'[70]. Meaning encompasses the individual's perception of the ability she/he has to accomplish future goals and to maintain the viability of interpersonal actions. The meaning of life-threatening illness comprises the set of physical, social, and intrapsychic changes that are associated with the illness. The changes associated with cancer include: (1) loss of personal control; (2) loss of self-esteem and self-worth; (3) changes in body image; (4) reduced social status; and (5) disruption of interpersonal relationships.

Singh,[71] a transpersonal psychologist who has worked in hospice for many years, developed a Psychospiritual Journey of the Dying Process that draws on many spiritual traditions. Her model includes phases of *Chaos, Surrender,* and *Transcendence. Chaos* involves the

five psychological phases enunciated by Kübler-Ross: denial, anger, bargaining, depression, and acceptance[72]. In addition, it involves the deeper experiences dying persons may pass through in the course of transformation: the experience of alienation, anxiety, the despair that leads to 'letting go', and the dread of engulfment.

'The movement into the present brings changes in identity, changes in levels of consciousness known and experienced. Arising at the same time come changes in meaning. Meaning is a powerful psychodynamic in the transformation from tragedy to grace. Meaning is the attribution of a purposeful construct to the suffering experienced. It is an important aspect of personhood and, as Viktor Frankl reveals[73], each of us struggles for meaning in the chaos of suffering. *Our ability to intuit meaning that has value, depth, and reality is related to the ease of our transformation*'[73].

More recently Zoellner and Maercker[74] reviewed the field of post-traumatic growth (PTG) from the perspective of psychology. They see both PTG as one construal of meaning and PTG within a meaning-making coping process as two of four possible personal growth coping strategies. PTG as one construal of meaning aims to answer the question, 'why did it happen?', but it may also answer the question 'what for'. According to this conceptualization, the subjective perception of personal growth would signify a benefit attribution. In PTG within a meaning-making coping process, a distinction is made between global and situational meaning. 'Global meaning encompasses a person's enduring beliefs and valued goals. Situational meaning, in contrast, is the meaning that is formed in the interaction between a person's global meaning and the circumstances of a particular person–environment interaction. A traumatic event threatens global meaning, thereby initiating the meaning-making process. It is the challenge of the coping process to integrate situational meaning (appraisal of trauma) with global meaning. Within this framework, different areas of post-traumatic growth would fall into different categories of meaning making: Finding benefits from the traumatic event (such as personal strength) would fall into the category of assimilation, i.e. changing the situational meaning to accommodate the global meaning. In contrast, a modified philosophy of life would address enduring changes in global meaning'[74]. The authors suggest that post-traumatic growth is still not clearly understood, nor is it reliably linked to measures of adjustment. In a longitudinal study of college students before and after September 11, 2001, 'positive emotions in the aftermath of crisis fully accounted for the relation between the pre-crisis resilience (personality trait) and post-crisis growth, conceptualized as increases in life satisfaction, optimism and tranquility. Without assessing positive emotions simultaneously, post crisis growth would have been predicted by pre-crisis resilience. However, it was not the personality factor of resilience that played the crucial role, but the existence of positive emotions'[74]. The authors suggest that traumatic events are more or less linked to life threat. 'These experiences may make individuals more aware of their own mortality and the fragility of life in general. This acknowledgement may lead to a heightened appreciation for life as one dimension of PTG'[74]. Psychotherapy constitutes a good context to explore positive changes in the aftermath of trauma.

John was a young, very successful businessman who entered into a spiritual transformation as a result of his experience with Stage 2 lymphoma, which was unresponsive to chemotherapy. He had been hoping for a cure with chemotherapy, then to be eligible for a stem-cell transplant, then to be able to have his disease kept under control for an extended time with chemotherapy. When it became clear that his disease was not responding to treatment, a physician covering for his oncologist with whom he had a very good relationship met with him and his wife. The author happened to be present for the conversation. The physician explained that his recent tests showed that his disease was progressing. John had already realized this and we had been discussing palliative care options when the physician entered the room. John pushed the physician to get information about his life expectancy. The physician reluctantly said his life would be only a very few weeks. John and his wife dealt with this information and then he said to the physician, 'there is a plan that my wife and I have had to establish a fund for others who might not have the resources to obtain some of the drugs and other things that we have been able to obtain, people who might need help with expenses such as babysitting and parking. We would like to establish a fund for such people. We would have done this if I lived, the fact that I am dying means that we should do this quickly.' The Hibiscus Fund was named for the flower the couple enjoyed on their trips to Bermuda. It is now being used to help other people dealing with lymphoma.

Accepting the disease and prognosis

Patients in the Canadian Needs Studies[34,38,39] were asked to identify the three biggest problems they had confronted since their diagnosis. Difficulty in accepting the illness was the first or second most commonly mentioned 'biggest problem', but by the time of the interview about two-thirds of those in the CCS study and three-quarters of those in the T-SRCC study, who described it as having been one of their three biggest problems, said they had managed to resolve the problem. People said they relied upon themselves, their spouse, physicians, and family members for help in learning to accept their illness. Their primary coping methods in helping them to accept their illness were to share their concern about the problem and to confront the situation in a practical way, for example, making plans for their family in the event of their death, making a will, and taking treatment.

Terminally ill patients did not feel they were having difficulty in accepting the thought of their illness but they did acknowledge having difficulty in coming to terms with the different stages of their disease, dealing with the physical symptoms of their disease, and with thoughts of their illness coming back or getting worse.

In an essay about her breast cancer experience, Dr Jane Poulson[75] writes of her feelings when confronted with a life-threatening illness.

'*Shockwaves*

There was anger. Even though I had exceeded recommended screening guidelines, this tumour presented out of the blue. I'd had regular radiologic and physical exams throughout the preceding 10 years. Everything had been fine, even at a routine visit 5 months earlier. then, despite my diligence, a nasty inflammatory carcinoma suddenly appeared and dramatically put an end to all normal activities … It appeared at the worst possible time in my career. I had just joined the Department of Medicine at the University of Toronto Hospital and the University of Toronto. This was not a good way to begin new professional relationships, but when I think about it now I ask myself, "Is there any good time to get cancer?"

There was fear. As a general internist I had cared for many patients with cancer. I was fascinated by the disease itself and really liked my patients. However, I could not imagine being able to cope

with having cancer myself. Eight years of experience in palliative care only served to heighten my fears. The Toronto Hospital had hired me to establish an academic program in palliative medicine and I had set up a clinic for symptom management only 6 months before my own diagnosis. My mind was flooded not with images of people dying peacefully with good symptom management but rather of patients with intolerable pain and global distress …

None of the diseases I have lived with—not juvenile diabetes, not blindness, not heart disease—has had the emotional impact of cancer. Although other diseases have potentially life-threatening consequences, cancer carries with it a unique terror'[75].

Dr Robert Cramb, an anaesthesiologist, journalled, 'I am sitting alone in mom's hospital with her … It is night time and this morning I got a call from her nurse saying that she had gone unconscious. Not thinking too clearly, I had one of my colleagues cover for me and then came to see mom. I feel like I am really stretching the good will of my department these last few weeks but I just wanted to be with my mom. She was indeed unconscious and not responding but I could still sense great strength in her and I was afraid this journey was not going to be over soon.

I called Susan and Sandra on the way to the hospital …When I came into the room her good friend of 41 years was with her. Ruth was a welcome sight and a great comfort. We chatted for some time and then I saw tears coming down her face but we kept on talking about mom. The Dr X came in and said the obvious that she had changed for the worse. He described her as courageous, very strong, and forward thinking through all this misery (my word). He looked at me directly but tears had started to fill my eyes. He said I must be strong as well for her. I honestly don't know what that means at this point. I think that I just feel love, sadness, and yes, glad the end is coming to send her along from this misery to a better place. There is no going back, no cure to be had. The words from the song Jewel sings comes to mind "Only kindness matters anymore".

What kindness can I offer at this stage? Only last night I had visited her and although she was very, very weak I could hear her speak in whispers from time to time. I asked if there was anything I could do and she roused and shook her head and said "Rob, I really don't know"….before I left I spent a couple of hours with her and listened to music and just held her hand.

I had made a CD compilation with Ronan Tyler's 'Going Home/ Amazing Grace' and Charlotte Church singing a prayer with Josh Groban. I put this one on first and she smiled that beautiful smile and said in a whisper "she has such a beautiful voice." I could see true joy in her face. How is that possible in such adverse situations I sat there for a long while pondering.

But I digress. Tonight, she is likely dying and I am sitting here watching her breath shallow breaths with some music in the background. Her mouth is open and eyes closed. She does not rouse to verbal or light stimuli. I am quite beside myself as I don't know what to do next. Is there something to do? I feel there is but wonder if that is just my nature and the kind of work I do.

I think back to when my friend Bill's mom died at St. Mike's Hospital. I was working out and lightly meditating when I saw in my mind's eye Bill standing at her bedside in the ICU in anguish. I then brought his hand over to his mother's and watched as the white light passed back and forth between them and hers went. I don't know where. He called me a little while later to tell me that she had passed on.

I am so agitated though I am not sure I can get into that mind space if that is what is required. Is anything required? I keep turning her to the light. I had them turn her today to the window where the sun was pouring into the room and felt better.

What am I going to do without her … but I don't want her to keep going through this horrible end of cancer experience. Wasting away molecule by molecule. Mind still intact. When the nurses turned her today her body stiffened and she grimaced like in pain. We all decide we will keep pressing her PCA button to ensure that she remains comfortable.

The only thing I want to do now is make sure that she is not alone at this time. We have been her advocates for so long. It is now 10 months (Dec. 15) since she was diagnosed with ovarian cancer. I can still remember being woken up at 9 am by her family doctor after having spent all night at St Mike's Hospital with my dad on the evening of his rescue surgery which was a fruitless effort. I think that I will read for a bit the book Mary gave me[76]. How am I going to heal from this loss? I am not sure …

Healing at a Distance

Sir William Osler, one of the fathers of modern medicine, is widely quoted as having said that objectivity is the essential quality of the true physician. What he actually said is different and far more profound than that. The original quote was in Latin and it is the Latin word aequanimatas which is usually translated as "objectivity". But aequanimatas means "calmness of mind", or "inner peace". Inner peace is certainly the ultimate resource for those dealing with suffering on a daily basis. But this isn't something achieved from distancing yourself from the suffering around you. Inner peace is more of a question of cultivating perspective, meaning and wisdom even as life touches you with its pain. It is more a spiritual quality than a mental quality'[76].

Denial and minimization in advanced disease

Patients who do not accept the prognosis of the treating physician or who are not making appropriate life plans based on a negative prognosis are often said to be denying their illness or its negative impact. 'Denial is how one simplifies the complexity of life … While downright denial can be harmful, denying itself is a phase of the coping process. It revises or reinterprets a portion of a painful reality avoiding what it threatens to be, and holding fast to the image of what has been'[77]. More than thirty years ago, Dr. Avery Weisman wrote in *On Death and Dying*[78] of three orders of denial. In first-order denial, the individual denies the main facts of the illness. Second-order denial may appear after the diagnosis is accepted; the individual denies the significance or implications of the illness. In third-order denial, there is an inability to believe that the illness will result in death—the person believes he or she will remain in this incapacitated state forever. More recently, Dr Fawzy Fawzy, a psycho-oncologist has contrasted denial with minimization. In contrast to denial, minimization involves acknowledging that one has the problem, but recognizing that one can still do things[79].

Some patients maintain control by minimizing or refusing to accept that a prognosis may be a bad as caregivers may be trying to help them to realize it is.

Melissa was a single mother of a 13-year-old son, Rory, and a 7-year-old daughter, Amanda. She had been diagnosed with low grade non-Hodgkin's lymphoma when Amanda was an infant, shortly after she had separated from her husband. She had a poor relationship with her ex husband who was verbally abusive and did not contribute to the maintenance of the family. Amanda had a fairly good relationship with her father, but Rory refused to see his father. Melissa realized that after her death Amanda would probably go to live with her father, but felt that Rory would probably live with her brother, Dan, although she realized that in the long run Rory might go to be with his father in order to maintain a relationship with his sister. Melissa did a videotape for her children in which she was able to comment to Rory that she understood his need to distance from her, as she had done the same with her parents. She was able to speak to Amanda about the fact that it had been hard for her to have a mother who had health problems from the time that she was an infant. With some encouragement, she had been able in this legacy to discuss the good things in her relationship with her ex-husband, the primary one being that he had given her the gift of her wonderful children.

Despite being strongly encouraged, and even pushed to discuss the situation of her impending death with Amanda, Melissa had refused to do so; saying that she was sure that her daughter could see that she was getting sicker and was going to die. She had a discussion with Rory about the fact that she would die. After considerable pushing, Melissa finally agreed to have a meeting with Amanda's social worker and the author the next week to discuss her impending death. Two days before the scheduled appointment, Dan called to say that Melissa was very sick. I went to do a home visit. Dan picked me up at the subway station and drove me to Melissa's home. As we arrived, Rory was sitting with Amanda in his lap on the front steps. He said, 'I told her'. The social worker had arrived at the same time. Amanda ran away from the adults and shut herself in her room. I went to speak with Melissa who said, 'it's hard to believe that this is happening.' I agreed that it was hard to believe, but she was indeed dying and she had to let the children know that she loved them. After a while Rory brought Amanda into Melissa's room. He asked Amanda to tell Melissa a funny story that had happened at school that day. Amanda did, then Melissa invited the children into her king size bed. She hugged them, they all cried as she told them that she loved them; she would miss them and would be with them always. The children now live together with their father, their relationship no doubt strengthened by this important bonding experience.

'The diagnosis of a devastating or terminal illness can precipitate a loss of control over virtually every aspect of a person's existence. If the loss of control is perceived as unacceptable, a patient can take on a denial response subconsciously. By denying the precipitating event, control is restored and integrity is maintained … Denial may have adaptive value by protecting an individual from devastating, life-threatening information, or it can be maladaptive by preventing an individual from participating in informed consent, closing important relationships, and reconciling final affairs'[80]. Denial is a fluid, interpersonal process that fluctuates over time, leaving 'windows of opportunity' when the resilience of denial may be temporarily weakened. Clinicians who recognize this 'will recognize the need to reassess denial frequently and eliminate the need to see it as either good or bad'[80].

Given that clinical prediction is as yet an inexact science and that minimization may be associated with prolonged survival, how should the physician and or other health-care team members respond when patients and their family members appear to be denying their prognosis? When possible, it is best to support the client's need for hope while gradually helping him/her to face the reality of current losses and the likelihood of impending death[81].

> Maguire[81] states that 'Patients use denial as a defense when the truth is too painful to bear. So, it should not be challenged unless it has created serious problems for the patient or relative. In challenging denial, it is important to be gentle so that the fragile defenses are not disrupted, but to be firm enough, that any awareness can be explored and developed'.

Ask the patient to give an account of what has happened since the illness was first discovered. Explore how the person felt at each key point—with the first symptom, seeing a specialist, being tested, being informed about the results.

Explore perceptions about what is wrong. This may provide glimpses of doubt … Patients maybe ambivalent about whether they want to face reality. It is useful to confront this by saying, 'It looks as though part of you prefers to believe that it is not serious, but another part of you is willing to consider your cancer is back and not responding to treatment. Which part of you should I relate to?'

If that strategy fails, gently challenge inconsistencies. If that does not work check whether there is a 'window' in it, 'I can understand that you think that it is an infection. Is there any time, even a moment, when you consider it might not be so simple?' If the person says no, accept that he or she finds it too painful to accept what is happening. If yes, explore what makes the individual think there might be something more serious.

Patients who are single parents with dependent children, or others whose failure to acknowledge their prognosis may jeopardise their family's future may require a somewhat more directive approach. Generally, if caregivers can be respectful of patient's difficulties in facing their illness, and be willing to stick by them, gradually introducing new information as it becomes available, acceptance will come. When denial still persists it is usually reflective of a lifetime coping pattern.

Issues of trust and attachment

Carol was a successful middle-aged professional woman with metastatic breast cancer. She was somewhat overweight with some issues of body image. In one therapy session, as we were discussing the impact of her deteriorating condition, she said, 'do you mean that I might become so infirm that I might not be able to wipe my own butt?' The thought was clearly quite difficult to comprehend. Soon after this discussion, Carol became quite ill and almost died. During this time she was found to have a large blackened ulcer in her sacral area. This needed to be dressed regularly. Initially Carol was quite ill and didn't care who did what to her, but as she recovered and returned home she said, 'you remember that I said no way I could cope with someone wiping my butt, now I know that is OK. I can trust people to take care of me and I have become very close to some of these nurses who clean my butt—the male nurse as well as the females'.

The earliest stage of development in the stages of Erik Erikson[82] is the stage of trust versus mistrust. Mathew Fox[83] writes that 'We begin to trust at the earliest stages of our lives and if, by bad parenting, we have been so deprived as to have missed this lesson of trust, then we must be healed elsewhere along the line many times to regain trust[83]' '… through trust one learns about love, life and

ecstasy and the pain that accompanies every layer of ecstatic living carries through in the death experience as well. Death too can be trusted. And in a real sense we are entrusted with death so that we ought to be reverencing that aspect of living as much as any other aspect ….The very awesomeness of death experiences unveils for us-and for some people for the very first time-the cosmic depth of our lives, the cosmic connection of our lives'[83].

About a year and a half before she died, thinking that she might be dying, Carol asked me to speak at her funeral. I said that I would be honoured, but what did she wish me to say. 'Teach them how not to be afraid of death as you have taught me not to be afraid.' I was unaware that I had taught her how not to be afraid of death.

Dr Roger Cole[9], a palliative care physician says that '(p)alliative care workers make a difference by knowing how to relieve suffering, by meeting information and communication needs, and by extending emotional, social and spiritual support. Through human interest and compassion, palliative care can help a patients move towards the deepest peace, love and understanding accessible to a human being. I am sure of this because of the times I have seen serenity emerge when someone reaches acceptance in the face of imminent death'[9].

Annabelle had an anxious, early attachment with her parents who had trouble being available to meet her needs. As a child she would often feel inadequately parented, but had the experience of being parented by The Light. The Light would tell her what good parents would do in the situations in which she found herself. She derived comfort from this. She married and received psychotherapy from a male and a female psychiatrist for many years, which allowed her to parent her own two children effectively. Periodically, throughout her adult life, Annabelle would check herself into the hospital when she felt anxious. Her psychiatrists were available to help her through her initial diagnosis of uterine cancer in her early fifties, but by the time she was diagnosed with breast cancer 5 years later both of her therapists had died. Through a loved and respected friend she was referred to the author when she developed her second malignancy. Perhaps because of her earlier experiences with her psychiatrist, she was able to form a very solid psychotherapeutic alliance. She was able to establish good relationships with her physicians who saw her as an individual. Her oncologist took the time to look at her art and to try to understand her. Her radiation oncologist, admired her collection of pearl neckties, and her surgeon recognized her as the

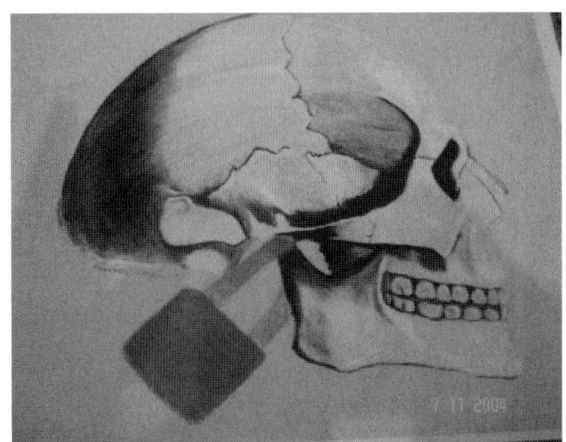

Picture 15.2.3 The Skull.

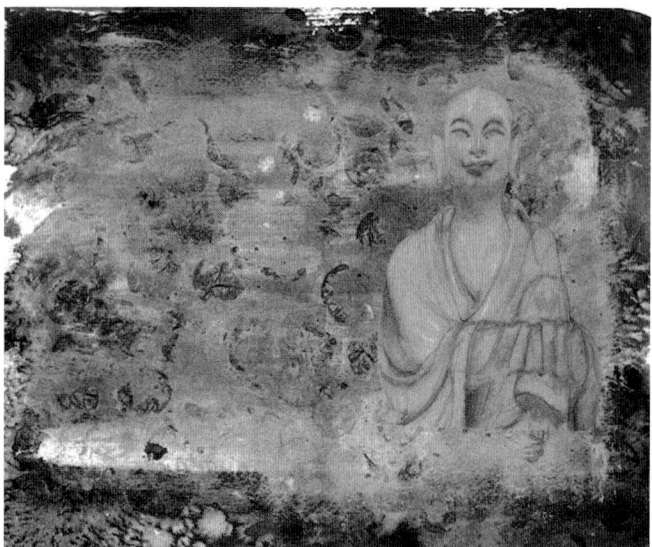

Picture 15.2.4 The Buddha.

author of numerous letters to the editor in the Globe and Mail, a Canadian newspaper. Annabelle used her art to communicate her feelings about her cancer and gave the author permission to share her art and her story with professional audiences, feeling that they needed to learn what patients went through during the experience of cancer.

Perhaps because of her attachment issues, Annabelle was very anxious that her family would not be able to care for her during her cancer treatment and went to Emergency often, as she had done throughout her life before cancer. A few weeks before being diagnosed with metastatic breast cancer, she related that she had a dream in which four angels came to her in a hovercraft. They told her they were the June angels and had come to take her to a safe place. During her radiotherapy for metastatic disease to her lungs she was admitted to the palliative care unit. When she arrived in her room on the PCU she said 'this is the room the angels used for their launching pad in my dream'. She felt fairly, but not completely secure there. However, after a couple of weeks, she screamed and cried out, despite heavy medications. She was unable to verbalize what she was screaming about. When her therapist visited she was able to relax and talk about the angels, and issues that concerned her, then she would resume screaming when the therapist was not there. Her daughters asked the staff what they usually did about patients who screamed this much and were told the staff had never had this experience.

On Wednesday evening I visited Annabelle. Her head was warm and her limbs were cold. Her mouth and throat were quite dry. I asked the nurse if she felt that she was dying soon and she said, no she had quite a bit of time left. The next day she was screaming so much that her daughters called to ask if I could visit, but I was with other clients. Annabelle died peacefully alone on Saturday morning. When I reviewed her chart to tell her daughters what she wanted done for her funeral, I saw that on 2 February, the Feast of St Blaise in the Catholic Church, when the blessings of the throats are carried out, Annabelle had said, 'I will not be silenced the way my father was'. Picture 15.2.3 shows her feeling of how her family of origin was unable to communicate. In the eastern tradition, the throat chakra is about speaking one's truth and being in touch with one's

creativity. Annabelle felt that in the time before she received her diagnosis of metastatic cancer her art had reached a new level. Picture 15.2.4 shows an image of the Buddha of which she was quite proud.

In the Buddhist tradition there is the dissolution of the elements of earth, water, fire and air in the process of dying[84]. The dissolution of the earth element involves the body losing all of its strength, we are drained of all energy, and we become weak and frail. 'Our mind is agitated and delirious, but then sinks into drowsiness'[84]. As the earth element withdraws into the water element, we begin to lose control of our bodily fluids, there may be incontinence and dryness of the tongue, eyes, and throat. 'Our mind becomes hazy, frustrated, irritable, and nervous. Some sources say we feel as if we were drowning in an ocean or being swept away by a huge river'[84]. With the fire element our mouth and nose dry up completely, all the warmth of the body begins to seep away, usually from the feet and hands toward the heart. Perhaps a steamy heat arises from the crown of our head. Our breath is cold as it passes through our mouth and nose. No longer can we eat or drink anything. The aggregate of perception is dissolving and our mind swings alternately between clarity and confusion[84]. As the air element is dissolving it becomes harder and harder to breathe. 'We begin to hallucinate and have visions: If there has been a lot of negativity in our lives, we may see terrifying forms. Haunting and dreadful moments of our lives are replayed, and we may even cry out in terror. If we have led lives of kindness and compassion, we may experience blissful, heavenly visions, and 'meet' loving friends or enlightened beings. For those who have led good lives, there is peace in death instead of fear'[84]. Before Annabelle was diagnosed with her recurrence she related a dream in which both of her parents were building a house in heaven, initially there was no room for her, then there was a room. If one analyses her experience using the Buddhist perspective, she was visited and prepared by the June angels, she then went through difficult times in which she screamed and told the angels that she was ready to die. She died in peace in April, after going through her agitated screaming experience, having already said in February that she would not be silenced.

What do dying people want?

Steinhauser *et al.*[85] surveyed patients, bereaved relatives, healthcare professionals, and hospice volunteers about what constituted a good death from their perspective. The participants identified six major components of a good death: pain and symptom management, clear decision-making, preparation for death, completion, contributing to others, and affirmation of the whole person.

Lynn[41] writes that medical texts attribute dying to severe physiological dysfunction. However, beyond pain and dysfunction, the dying are absorbed with the annihilation of the self, the impact on loved ones, the terror of the unknown, and the opportunity for transcendence beyond the mortal. To die peacefully—to die with the knowledge that life has had meaning and that one is connected through time and space to others, to God, and to the Universe—is to die well. Helping people to die well requires knowledge and skill, as well as a willingness to be intensely involved in the most intimate phases of another's life. Physical, spiritual, psychological, and social distress must be addressed with concern and compassion. In being with dying persons and their family members caregivers must confront their own mortality[86].

Dr David Kuhl[87], a palliative care physician, interviewed dying patients, using an existential phenomenological perspective in an attempt to come to understand, what is it like everyday to get up knowing that the disease within you will likely cause your death? He said that as a researcher 'I had to learn to listen, not only with my ears but with my heart as well. I had to learn to set aside biases, to stop seeking to predict, explain, or control the disease's progression. I had to suspend judgement and hear the testimony, to bear witness to the experience of living and dying with a terminal illness'[87]. The patients he interviewed spoke of:

- Changing perspectives of time, what it means, how to spend it.

- The suffering that resulted from hearing their terminal diagnosis for the first time and the need to communicate effectively with health-care professionals.

- Physical pain, its reality, and its effect on who they were.

- The importance of being touched, being in touch.

The major themes and concerns of those he interviewed were:

- The natural process of reviewing one's life (looking back) once one understands that dying is a reality.

- Speaking and hearing truth.

- Longing to belong, that is, to understand who they were in the past with regard to their original families, as well as in the present with regard to their chosen (adult) family.

- Asking the question Who am I? in the search to know who they were in the present, free of the expectation of others.

- Experiencing transcendence-meaning, value, God, spirituality, a higher being greater than oneself.

In his second book *Facing Death Embracing Life*[88], he states that in doing his first book he came to the realization 'that what dying people want is the same as what living people want, primarily a sense of connection to themselves, to those they love and who love them, and to a sense or essence of something greater than themselves. Physical pain, poor communication, and anxiety are some of the features that impede the process of connection. For many people knowing that they have a terminal illness serves as a catalyst for them to search for meaning, to make sense of their lives, to appreciate and to be honest with themselves and with those they love'[88].

I first met Mary Pocock, whose reflections and art were in the third edition of the *Oxford Textbook of Palliative Medicine*[39], when she was diagnosed with breast cancer in her early forties. She died in September 2004, shortly after turning 52. For many years Mary lived with metastatic disease. She dealt with her disease through meditation practices, yoga, art, journalling, spending time with others with cancer and those without the disease, humour, filming her experience, and growing deeper into her oneness with the universe, and her connection with others.

Mary came to speak with me about palliative care options a couple of years before her death. I suggested that, since she was a patient at Princess Margaret Hospital, she visit the new unit that was being planned. Instead of signing up on a palliative care waiting list, she signed up to do the art on the unit and produced large transparencies of nature scenes for each of the windows on the unit.

On her first admission to the PMH PCU Mary was frightened, and thought she was going to die. She awakened that first night and was able to enter into the scene on the window of her room. She saw the angels there and felt she was being cared for and watched over. Realizing how much comfort this image gave her she was able to realize how much comfort it would give to others—indeed she received feedback about the importance of her windows to other patients as well as to staff. She died in this same room with the angels on the window.

Mary had a website on which she shared her reflections. She wrote in The Pocock Diaries 'Since my hospital stay, my palliative status has been jimmied up a notch. My lungs have many tumours and I am on oxygen about five hours a day now. I call my oxygen generator O_2/D_2. It looks like a robot—too bad it can't vacuum. My mind states fluctuate, between worrying that I am dying to feeling fine and thinking I am on the mend. Then I come back to the present moment, accept what is and live my day. This is a difficult task; not getting caught up in mind states and emotion'.

As Mary's illness progressed she dealt with the issues that she needed to address. Drawing on the Buddhist image of the lotus we explored the fact that sometimes we thought the issues were resolved, only to have another layer of petals begin to open, drawing us deeper and deeper into the resolution of issues of concern. We spoke of Kathleen Dowling Singh's book The Grace of Dying[71], which Mary liked— and of how the process from Surrender to Transcendence was not an easy one. Mary reminded me of the fact that the lotus has its roots in the 'muck' in order to develop in the presence of the sun. She listened to Ann Mortife's songs on the CD This Is a Healing Journey and spoke of the poignancy of Ann's song 'I Always Thought I'd Have Tomorrow'.

The day before she died, Mary spoke of a dream she had the night before, after we had been discussing what the process of dying might be like. In her dream she had received permission from the City of Toronto to put up a Cirque de Soleil tent in Trinity Bellwoods Park across the street from her apartment. She would live there until she died. People could come and go. There was a clown with a dog, there were places for Centering prayers for the Christians, and meditation for the Buddhists. Mary was teaching her dharma and had a spot to meditate in the corner. The film she had been doing with Michael Mitchell was playing in the background and she was being filmed by CBC for a documentary, You Can Have Fun While You Are Dying.

On the night of her death Mary was awakened by a Code Red in her hospital room. This allowed her to have a conscious death with her husband Marcus[89]. She could no longer speak, but wrote to him, 'at last I feel safe, secure and loved'. Mary had attachment issues from her early years. Trusting that her needs would be met had been a major issue during her illness. At last she could feel safe, secure and loved.

She then wrote, 'I only want to have half the medication that is ordered to dry up my secretions. I want to be able to see if I can cough them up.' Her oncologist had said that he would know when Mary was dying when she stopped dictating what medications she wanted. She then wrote, 'I don't know what is happening'. It became obvious that she was dying and her husband called in Drolma, a Buddhist nun friend of Mary's and her sister.

Drolma was reading and chanting to her as she died and said that her rapid breathing became normal and she breathed her last just as the most sacred passage was being read. She died in the lotus position.

Mary wrote this poem to be read at her funeral

Live for me.
Laugh for me.
Do good and give to the world for me.
Grow for me
Share for me
Mourn for me,
But let your own spirit fill again
With friends, family and new laughter.
Or I'll come down and kick your ass.
As a gopher or horned owl—ha ha.

(some people at the funeral saw a baby skunk parade across the window outside the funeral home just as the gopher was mentioned)[89].

Mary spent a lot of time planning her funeral, drawing on The Dead Good Funerals Book[90]. *At her funeral people were encouraged to visit for a few hours before the service and to draw or write on the simple pine box which held her body. Her body was cremated after the service. I wrote to Mary's husband to request permission to write of Mary in this chapter. He responded that Mary's artistic efforts continue. Her ashes are to be part of an exhibit by Spring Hurlbut, a gifted artist who is doing a photographic exhibit using the ashes of her deceased father, a child, and a young artist. Mary's ashes are part of that exhibit. Spring felt that she was guided by Mary in her photographic use of Mary's ashes.*

I used the story of the lotus with many of my clients, discussing the need sometimes to go into more depth into their psyche than they might have thought necessary. After hearing the story, Melissa, referred to above, brought me a purple crystal lotus, which sits in my office. The day Melissa was dying, another client inadvertently brushed up against the lotus and a petal fell off. I gave this petal to Melissa's twin when we met.

Hope

Singh[71] speaks of the time when hope evaporates during the process of transformation in terminal illness—the process of realizing that hope is a clinging to something other than *what is*. 'During the transformative process, there are profound changes in the quality of hope. Hope in its previously known form (i.e. hope for the continuation of one's existence) is washed away like the dissolving letters of a prayer written on a beach. During the ups and downs of the ordeal of terminal illness, it is hard to say whether hope is taken away or hope is given up. Hope itself becomes difficult. The person is torn between the desire to live and the fear that allowing hope to emerge one more time would only create more misery if the treatment fails again'[71]. 'In the head-on collision between terminal illness and the personal consciousness of the ego, hope is almost always the first powerful dynamic to come to the forefront. It arises with the first intimation of tragedy. Hope is a powerful constellation of human emotions, beliefs, and ideas, but it is a painful playground.

For the mental ego faced with a terminal prognosis, hope typically signifies one thing, the continuance of self. This is the thought 'I know that all things are impermanent, that everything must pass, and yet … and yet'[91].

I visited Sean on the palliative care unit, where he had been admitted for symptom relief, in late January, soon after he had

returned from a trip to celebrate his 45th birthday with his family. During much of this time he needed to be pushed in a wheel chair, by his wife or one of his young children. He had already had what was thought to be a 'final' family trip, a few months earlier. He said, 'I managed OK with the trip last week. I think that it is reasonable to think that I could take my wife away for a cruise to celebrate her 40th in March. Don't you agree?' He had already taken her away for her 39th assuming he would not be around to take her for her 40th. Sean died 13 February.

In the opening page of his book, *The Anatomy of Hope: How People Prevail in the Face of Illness*[92], Jerome Groopman, a medical oncologist and chief of experimental medicine at Beth Israel Deaconess, who holds a chair in medicine at Harvard Medical School, writes, 'Pandora, the first mortal woman, received from Zeus a box that she was forbidden to open. The box contained all human blessings and all human curses. Temptation overcame restraint, and Pandora opened it. In a moment, all the curses were released into the world, and all of the blessings escaped and were lost-except one: hope. Without hope, mortals could not exist'[92].

Groopman describes hope as the elevating feeling we experience when we see in the mind's eye-a path to a better future. Hope acknowledges the significant obstacles and deep pitfalls along that path. True hope has no room for delusion. He reviews the physiology of hope noting that researchers have found that a change in mind-set has the power to alter neurochemistry. Belief and expectation—the key elements of hope—can block pain by releasing endorphins and enkephalins, mimicking the effects of morphine. In some cases, hope can effect physiological processes such as respiration, circulation, and motor functions.

'Hope can arrive only when you recognize that there are real options and you have genuine choices. Hope can flourish only when you believe that what you do can make a difference, that your actions can bring a future different from the present. To have hope, then is to acquire a belief in your ability to have some control over your circumstances. You are no longer entirely at the mercy of forces outside yourself'[92].

Groopman shares the story of a colleague, the chair of the Department of Pathology, whose specialty was stomach cancer. He was diagnosed with an 'untreatable' stomach cancer, for which he decided to seek aggressive treatment with high-dose chemotherapy and intensive radiotherapy. His colleagues felt 'It's madness, pure madness, what George is doing.' Groopman himself wondered '… whether George's intimate knowledge of death had triggered an extreme form of denial—so extreme that he was subjecting himself to iatrogenic torture. He risked hastening his demise, or at least robbing himself of the last tranquil days at home with his wife, his children, his friends. What Eric Paulsen termed 'madness' seemed rather a sad, self-defeating loss of judgement'[92]. George survived and thirteen years later Groopman interviewed him for this book. George was aware that all his colleagues disagreed with his decision.

'Once I decided to go for it, I thought of my forebears. They were pioneers who embarked on a journey west that was perilous and uncertain. Most knew they would perish on the way. But they persisted …'

And his faith, I asked how did that influence him?

'I recited the Twenty-third psalm—before, during, and after each treatment. It spoke so directly, so beautifully, to my plight…'

George also said that he had derived a great deal of comfort from knowing how many people were praying for him. The distances he had travelled in his career, and the diversity of the department he led, had brought him into contact with physicians and scientists of many faiths. Christians, Jews, Hindus, Buddhists, Muslims all had him in their prayers …

'Eunha (his wife) … had this sixth sense that I would be cured. I didn't. My survival has made her more devout, almost mystical. She was always convinced that I'd live. But scientifically, that was so remote. Like you, I didn't see the end that way'[92,93].

Maintaining control and dignity

Volker et al.[94] surveyed advanced practice nurses ($n = 9$ and patients $n = 7$) in Texas regarding their respective perspectives about the control and comfort patients with advanced disease want at the end of life. The nurses felt the patients want:

'Engagement with living: maintaining professional and personal role functions in the context of ongoing treatment.

Turning the corner: decisions, choices, circumstances, and struggles that influence the timing of or transition toward the dying process.

Comfort and dignity: desires for comfort in the end-of-life experience that are respectful of a person's sense of dignity and personal values.

Control over the dying process: patient and family concerns, desires and manifestations of control over the place, process and logistics of end-of-life care'[94].

The patients wanted:

1 'Protection of dignity: the desire to have personal dignity protected and respected.

2 Control of pain and other symptoms associated with disease: concern about past and present experiences with physical discomfort. Some expressed worry or an assumption that pain and symptoms would not be well controlled as disease progressed.

3 Management of treatment: desire to be involved actively in decisions regarding cancer treatment.

4 Management of how remaining time is spent: reflections regarding changing priorities on control over time.

5 Management of impact on family: actions to prepare family for both financial and emotional consequences.

6 Control over the dying process: concerns about the process of how death will occur'[94].

Chochinov and colleagues[95,96] studied dignity in palliative care patients and found 7.5 per cent of 213 patients felt they were not able to maintain their dignity. His dignity therapy intervention had a patient satisfaction rate of 91 per cent in the 100 patients (50 in Canada and 50 in Australia) with whom the intervention was used. Seventy-six per cent reported a heightened sense of dignity, 68 per cent an increased sense of purpose, 67 per cent a heightened sense of meaning, 47 per cent an increased will to live, and 81 per cent reported that it would be of help to their family. Chochinov's study is reported in more depth in Chapter 15.1. His intervention consisted of a series of questions, which patients with advanced illness were asked. Their responses were then transcribed and reshaped into a narrative, which ended with a statement or passage from the interview that provided an appropriate ending, given that

this was a generativity, legacy-making exercise, the ending needed to be appropriate to the patient's overall message. Once the edited transcript was completed, it was read to patients who could make changes as appropriate.

The author used Chochinov's questions with 7 parents who were dying and leaving young children. The children whose parent was dying ranged in age from 3 to 21, with most being pre-teen. Initially the interviews were tape recorded. In one, done in the patient's home, his children aged 5 and 7 could be heard playing outside. At the patients' suggestions, later interviews were videotaped, and then some couples asked to be videotaped together. The patient would speak about his or her early life and hopes and dreams, the parents would then discuss their relationship, the birth of their children, special memories and hopes and dreams for the children's future. Parents spoke of the special characteristics of their children, their hopes for the people they would turn out to be, and in one situation the father told his children he never wanted them to have credit cards—to pay cash for everything the way he did! The bereaved parents are pleased they have this legacy, although the tapes are too painful for them to watch at this point. The sister of one deceased single parent did watch the video around the anniversary of her sister's death. She was quite touched by it, liked to see how much healthier her sister looked when she did the video, was surprised at some of the feelings her sister expressed and felt it would be of great value to her children.

Healing

'Healing has been defined as a relational process involving movement towards an experience of integrity and wholeness, which may be facilitated by a caregiver's interventions but is dependent upon an innate potential within the patient. It is not dependent upon the presence of, or the capacity for, physical well-being. Indeed it is possible to die healed'[97]. Given the right support psycho/social/spiritual transitions can be a time of opportunity as well as spiralling loss.

Healing can occur within suffering. Healing is the process of becoming psychologically and spiritually more integrated and whole: a phenomenon that enables persons to become more completely themselves and more fully alive. Such healing can only come from the depths of the individual's psyche[8].

Caregivers can help to create the environment that might foster inner healing within the palliative patient. 'In practice this happens when a combination of effective care and human companionship helps to establish a secure, inner space for that person to be in. The process is further facilitated if the carers themselves have found ways of staying with and being in their own experience of suffering'[8].

Hutchinson[67], who has collaborated with Mount and Kearney, writes of patients with end-stage renal disease (ESRD): a cause of suffering or an opportunity for healing. He notes that patients with ESRD need to negotiate important transitions along their illness trajectory, as indeed do patients with other diseases. Drawing on the literature from family therapy, psychiatry, narrative therapy, and mythology, he notes that there is a remarkable similarity in all of these fields and with key authors. The adaptation processes described are remarkably similar. 'For example, they all agree that in the middle of this process there is a very difficult period before the person can experience a successful resolution. This period has been described as 'chaos' (Satir); 'the phase of disorganization and despair' (Parkes); 'the liminal or betwixt and between space when confusion and disorientation reigns' (White); and 'the Belly of the Whale' (Campbell)'[67].

Speaking of caregivers working with those with ESRD, Hutchinson offers suggestions to make dialysis and transplant units more healing. This would include an acknowledgement of the issue and an intention to provide help—dealing with issues such as pain and other symptoms, while recognizing that psychosocial and spiritual factors may be even more important. He suggests open supportive discussions with patients with ESRD about the difficulties and high mortality associated with the treatment. Appropriate patient-specific support should be organized at times of major transition. Caregivers of all disciplines must be provided with training in order to provide these discussions and this support. He suggests an approach that instead of asking whether dialysis will significantly prolong life, the question should be asked, will the prolongation of life achieved by dialysis be an extension of suffering or is there a reasonable possibility of healing and an acceptable quality of life? 'It is not simply a question of whether a given decision is likely to prolong life, but whether it is likely to be associated with effective adaptation to the anticipated life transitions. Of course such decisions must depend on the individual values of the patient and should be based on in-depth discussions involving the clinical triad (patient, family, and health-care worker). Patients need to know that they have realistic choices other than pursuing therapy aimed at prolonging life'[67].

Singh[71] writes of the process of transformation that may occur with serious illness—the turning point in the evolution of consciousness. 'Transformation occurs through subtraction. We begin, as we heal successive dualities, as we approach deeper and deeper levels of integration, to eliminate the nonessential. As we participate in the process, we find paradoxically, that the subtraction adds, that through the exclusion of the nonessential from our attention, we create movement and we become more inclusively essential'[71].

Kathy, a middle-aged lawyer, who lived alone, with good support from her friend and former husband, had intended to die at home, yet as the time to die approached she decided to move into a palliative care unit. She said, 'My possessions that were so important to me before are no longer important. I do not need to have them around me. I no longer need to be in control the way I used to need to be in control'.

In our final conversation as Kathy told me of her decision to move into the palliative care unit. I reminded her of a conversation we had 15 months previously when it looked like she was going to die. She had said, 'When I was in emergency waiting for a bed I had the experience of being in a boat, it was a beautiful boat with highly polished teak wood. There were oarsmen on the boat and I couldn't decide if the boat should go forward or backward. Then the boat turned into a beautiful garden; then the flowers in the garden turned into the faces of animals, like you see in those beautiful pictures'. I asked when we had the original conversation, whether she was alone in the boat. Her face lit with a beatific smile and she responded, 'No'. She then said, 'I guess, even though I didn't go to spirituality, spirituality came to me'. In our final conversation I reminded her of the previous conversation and said that originally I hadn't asked who had been in the boat with her. I asked if she remembered who had been there. She smiled and said, 'The Spirit of Love, and Light and Peace.'

I asked if that Spirit was still with her. She smiled another beatific smile and said, 'Yes'.

When I asked Kathy's brother's permission to use this anecdote he responded 'When Kathy finally did leave for the palliative care unit, she got on the gurney and when the attendants wheeled her down the hall she never once looked back or tried to have one last touch to her life's surroundings—they had obviously become irrelevant to her. That tough gal from Integra and I looked at each other and burst into tears'. Of note is that after I spoke at Kathy's funeral, giving the eulogy she had asked me to give, her brother handed me a gift from Kathy. He said that as Kathy was about to go to the palliative care unit she looked for a pin of a butterfly made from the bones of a woolly mammoth, which he had given her for Christmas. She said, this must go to Mary—my business card has a butterfly formed from my initials, a logo created from by a client who felt the image reflected the transformation I had undergone with my cancer experience, which I now attempt to bring to others.

Anger

'When denial cannot be maintained it is replaced in rapid succession by feelings of anger, rage, envy, and resentment ... When denial no longer has any blocking power, the scream of "NO!" turns quickly to the shout, "Why me?"[71]' Anger may arise from fear or feelings of impotence and is a reflection of one's response to a loss of control. A woman dying of colon cancer refused to allow her 10-year-old daughter to go to summer camp saying, 'if I have to stay in the hospital and die, there is no way you should be able to go to camp and have a good time.'

Anger can temporarily give a dying person the sense of being in control and can temporarily block off the emotion of fear. Anger can be healing and is closer to the truth than the repression of anger. Anger 'eventually, although usually painfully, works toward the experience of more and fuller life'[71].

Philip *et al.*[98] recently reviewed the literature on anger in palliative care. Reported rates of anger in cancer patients ranged from 9–18 per cent. There is some indication that anger is becoming more common in the clinical situation. Sixty-two per cent of Australian physicians reported being subjected to verbal abuse by patients in the previous year, while patients and their families were responsible for verbal abuse directed at nursing staff in 17 per cent and 25 per cent of instances. The authors suggest the possible increase in anger may be reflective of 'a variety of social factors, including a greater confidence to question doctors fallibility, a more acceptable emotional response to threat that does not admit vulnerability, a normalization of aggression and a recognition that the 'squeaky gate gets attention'. Perhaps there are wider social phenomena at play, such as an increasing culture of expectation of health that suggests there is fault in the event of poor physical outcome'[98].

In cancer care, anger can be seen as being an emotion that may later lead to a more constructive response. However, through making oneself available to deal with anger, professionals may be at some personal cost. The authors conducted 9 focus groups with 45 palliative care workers in a variety of settings including those in acute hospital palliative care, community, and inpatient palliative care services/hospice. 'Following a diagnosis of cancer or a terminal illness, a person is forced to deal with a series of losses: the loss of their role in life, or functional capacities, of livelihood, of independence, and ultimately of relationships. The anger associated with this may be named directly or may be expressed as other complaints such as their doctors' perceived or real neglect and sometimes abandonment'[99]. Doctors may also be criticized because of a delay in diagnosis, the way information is presented, or because breaking through a hopeful stance. Anger may also be associated with pain, both as a manifestation of pain, or as the awareness of dying complicating the experience of pain for several patients. Some patients may have persistent anger as a part of their response to life. Family members may also become angry at caregivers because of perceived inadequacies of care, personal frustration at not being able to provide care at home, or for the same reasons that patients experience.

Philip et al.[98] suggest a 7-step approach to anger:

Preparation—it is helpful to be prepared for the fact that the person is angry. This allows some personal preparation time for the clinician. It is helpful to conduct the meting in a quiet room, where everyone is seated so as to confer the message that there is time to discuss the issue and there are no power differentials caused by height differences.

Listen—engage the person in respectful communication, seeking to avoid personalization of the anger, considering the other person's worldview, review the usefulness of anger as a coping strategy, and ultimately invite the person to redirect their emotions into other psychological responses. Invite the person to tell their story, acknowledging the anger. 'Perhaps you could take me back to … This often involves returning to the beginning of the illness or diagnosis and the narrative should be allowed to unfold without interruption'[98].

Involve experienced clinicians—the capacity to interact with angry patients and families increases with experience, but is eroded by tiredness or burnout.

If anger persists, reconsider approach— 'If anger remains, despite a conscientious attempt by experienced staff to address patient or family concerns, then the approach should be reconsidered. The aims should move from attempting to resolve the anger, to support of the team of health-care professionals'[98].

Consider limits—it may be useful to put some limits on behaviour, interactions and responses. Staff must feel safe and not physically or verbally threatened when providing care.

Support the team—support of the team is essential when dealing with persistently angry patients or family members.

Involve and independent broker—another medical opinion or Clinical Ethics Service may help to defuse the situation.

It must also, of course, be recognized that as Lynn[15] reflected effective care of the dying needs to recognize what the health-care system can and cannot do and as caregivers we need to recognize that our personal issues, whether recognized or unrecognized may interfere in our work with dying people. Kuhl[88] writes that as he finished his first book *What Dying People Want*[87], he was simultaneously dealing with his grief for his sister who had died during the writing of the book. He experienced many emotions, one of which was anger. 'I was angry and frustrated with a system that seemed to allow her to slip through the cracks. In fact, at one point I was filled with rage. I understand the system, and I understand that things happen unintentionally. These same things have happened to people under my care over the years. But I understand it differently now. The system will never be perfect, but because it was my sister, I wanted perfection for her'. People at the end of life can benefit from the company of others who share that time with them, people who work hard to know and understand the needs and desires of the person at the end of life in the context of a complex health-care system, people who are willing and prepared to act as advocates on behalf of the person with the terminal illness'[88].

Forgiveness

A diagnosis of cancer often involves a reprioritizing of values that involve forgiveness issues. Tension often results between harbouring anger or bitterness and wanting to achieve reprioritized goals. Patients may use forgiveness to help them to resolve these issues[100].

Dr Ira Byock[101] suggests that there are five things that must be done in order to complete the relationships we will be leaving behind. These are

1 Forgive me.

2 I forgive you.

3 Thank you.

4 I love you.

5 Goodbye.

Forgiveness is not an easy task. Often there are family members, friends, and others whom we have hurt and who have hurt us. The general benefits of forgiveness include 'psychological and spiritual growth; reduction of negative emotions such as sadness, anger, or anxiety; ability to let go of the past and get on with life; cessation of hurtful behaviours; increase in ability to re establish or build new relationships; and transcendence … In addition forgiveness also may lead to a more accepting and peaceful death, help solidify a sense of meaning in life, help restore healthy relationships, and promote serenity in the dying process'[100].

Twenty patients receiving palliative or terminal care and five in remission were interviewed regarding their definition of forgiveness[100]. Participants were asked to describe an incident in their life that reflected forgiveness including misdiagnosis, rejection by a parent, and murder of a child. Many had eventually come to realize that their negativity was unhealthy and perhaps, even harmful. Their cancer diagnosis often compounded their growing tension between harbouring their emotions and being slowly consumed by them. Cancer led to rethinking their priorities and gaining focus on what was really important in their lives as the reality of the finiteness of life became obvious. As participants contemplated the meaning of their cancer diagnosis and focused on their enduring personal values, the tension between their negative emotions and trying to live out their personal values escalated, and for some became intolerable. This intolerability led to considering forgiveness as one possible means of alleviating the tension. Participants attempted to gain perspective, tried to analyse the situation—reflecting on the role of the other as well as themselves. They drew on their underlying beliefs, personal identities, moral principles, and religious beliefs to make sense of the situation. They used interpersonal, intrapersonal, and transpersonal means to understand and clarify their situation. Most participants achieved some degree of resolution and forgiveness. The degree of resolution varied considerably, but most were able to report that their anger and bitterness were gone and they were able to define more clearly and live more consistently with their personal values.

Suffering in the face of terminal illness (see also Chapter 3.1)

Singh[71] notes that as the pretence about prognosis ends, acceptance arises and opens the way to the naked experience of our alienation. 'We have cut ourselves off from our self, from others, and from Spirit. With mortality breathing down our necks, we begin to become aware of our myopic focus. Our attention shifts. This state of alienation becomes, in the dying process, painfully uncovered and revealed'[71]. This is an essential component of the experience of suffering in terminal illness.

Suffering has its source in challenges that threaten the intactness of the person as a complex social and psychological entity[102]. Cassel states that the relief of suffering as well as the care of disease must be seen as twin obligations of a medical profession that is truly dedicated to the care of the sick. The failure to understand the nature of suffering can result in intervention, which though technically adequate not only fails to relieve suffering but becomes a source of suffering itself.

Terry and Olson[103] surveyed 100 patients admitted to a hospice and asked them 'In what way are you suffering?' Twenty-four patients were unable to state the reason for hospice admission but none had any uncertainty in identifying the nature of their own suffering. Thirty-five patients identified their suffering as physical pain, although pain as a source of suffering was only weakly correlated with pain scores. Some patients with pain scores of 8–10/10 did not mention pain as a cause of suffering, while others with a score of 0/10 did identify pain as a source of suffering. Thirty patients identified their suffering with physical symptoms other than pain. Twenty-eight patients identified their suffering as entirely emotional in origin and seven patients identified their suffering as mixed somatic and emotional in origin.

Dr Yvonne Yi-Wood Mak is a palliative care physician in Hong Kong. She began to keep a diary in 2000 when she was researching the meaning of suffering and desire for early death in advanced cancer patients. She recorded her patients' subjective experiences and also her own reflections. In September 2003 she fractured her lower spine while preparing a barbeque for hospice colleagues. During her experience of being housebound she became impatient with her pain, and began to question what were her priorities in life and what were simply trivial pursuits. What was the importance of her role as a mother, was her role as a mother a greater or lesser mission than her role as a hospice physician? Then while having acupuncture for her back she became aware of a lump in her breast leading to a diagnosis of breast cancer. She continued with her journaling, which was published as a weekly column in the South China Morning Post and has now been published as *A Mother's Diary*[104]. Her father and other family elders had been struck with life-threatening illnesses and then she became ill. 'I wanted to keep a diary especially for my young children because I did not want them to live in the shadow of traumatic life events. Rather, I wanted to share with them the lessons I had learned, hoping that one day they would understand life constructively by reflecting on my journey'[104].

The value of a spiritual or religious belief system (see also Chapter 15.1)

'In the terminal phase of illness the self becomes increasingly conscious of its own disconnection from Spirit which it is beginning to intuit and encounter. Whether or not people have been religious or spiritual at other points in their lives, an experience with life-threatening illness will often lead to their exploring these issues'[71].

McClain *et al.*[105] studied spirituality in 160 patients with a life expectancy of less than 3 months. Spirituality was measured in two ways: Meaning the extent to which patients felt inner peace and Faith, the comfort and strength they got from religious beliefs. Patients who expressed a strong sense of either type of spirituality were less likely that those with low spiritual well-being to show symptoms of end-of-life despair. Among those with less than 3 months to live, those with a strong sense of spiritual well-being were less likely than others to feel hopeless, want to die, or consider suicide. Patients who were depressed only tended to want to die if they also had a low sense of spiritual well-being. In contrast, those with a strong sense of spirituality did not wish for hastened death, regardless of whether they were also depressed. Many terminally ill patients feel despair during their final days of life, which can manifest itself in a number of ways, such as hopelessness, wish for death, or suicidal thoughts. The current findings suggest that providing patients with a strong sense of spiritual well-being may enable them to avoid spending their last days in despair. The authors concluded that meaning-centred therapy may be more important as you get older and closer to death and have a more reflective perspective on life.

Lin and Bauer-Wu[106] did an integrative review of the literature on the psychospiritual well-being of people with advanced cancer. Their review covered the literature from 14 countries and researchers in nursing, medicine, psychology, and theology. Six major themes emerged as central components of psycho-spiritual well-being: self-awareness, coping and adjusting effectively with stress, relationships and connectedness with others, sense of faith, sense of empowerment and confidence, and living with meaning and hope. They concluded that patients with an enhanced sense of psycho-spiritual well-being are able to cope more effectively with the process of terminal illness and find meaning in the experience. Contributors to positive psycho-spiritual well-being included prognostic awareness, family and social support, autonomy, hope, and meaning in life. Factors that detract from psycho-spiritual well-being are emotional distress, anxiety, helplessness, hopelessness, and fear of death.

Singh[71] speaks of the period of Surrender into Transcendence as being a stage in which the individual can rest in the 'natural great peace'. In this phase, people frequently report seeing visions of spiritual figures, family members, or friends who have died. These visions may or may not be congruent with their previous belief systems. On the day before he died, a Jewish atheist with no belief in an afterlife found himself going back and forth between his hospital room and an incredibly beautiful garden. He said 'I don't believe in anything beyond this life, but it looks like I am going there.'

Singh says this period of transcendence is '*what occurs as consciousness coincides with the Ground of Being*'[71]. It is a time when 'dread dissipates in a profound healing and infusion'[71].

The respectful death model of care

Farber and Farber[107] suggest an approach for dealing with dying persons, which they call A Respectful Death Model of Care. Their model recognizes that many caregivers are committed to the concept of a 'good death', which is an acknowledgement of the inevitability of death. They suggest, however, that there is an inherently value-laden aspect to the term 'good' that implies a right and wrong way.

'It begs a judgement, but who is the right party to be that judge? Is it the helping professional with extensive clinical experience who may be watching a patient and family make decisions that are certain to add to their combined suffering? Is it the patient exercising his or her autonomy? Is it the family caregiver who has taken the courageous and compassionate act of caring for the loved one?'[107]. They propose a model of Respectful Death in which there is a non-judgemental relationship between parties 'an opportunity to weave expertise, values, and differences into a whole cloth that supports the common values of all parties'[107]. The model implies the patient, family members, and care professionals beginning to share knowledge, work towards a common goal, and create a shared story. Research shows that patients, family members and healthcare providers all recognize that the presence of a therapeutic relationship is very important to effective outcomes. The authors propose that integrating the Respectful Death model into clinical practice requires developing a relationship of discovery with patients *and* families. 'Patients, families and care professionals report that the components for achieving this level of care are as follows:

1 *Commitment.* Stressing that the helping professional will care for the patient and family through and beyond death.

2 *Connection.* Creating a special relationship that allows any topic of importance to the patient and family to be discussed regardless of whether it is medical or not. This aspect of relationship is related to Carl Roger's concept of unconditional positive regard.

3 *Consciousness.* Understanding the patient's and family's personal experience, as well as the helping professional's personal and professional meaning, within the ever-changing context of illness'[107].

This model creates a space for the patient, family, and healthcare professional to enter into a caring relationship and explore optimal outcomes congruent with the patient's values, experiences, and goals.

Conclusion

This chapter will conclude with the story of Roy whose story illustrates many of the concepts discussed above, including distress, attachment, countertransference and alchemy, dissolution of the elements, the appearance of religious figures, hope, suffering, spirituality, transcendence, intervention, the role of the therapist, and respectful death, while raising many other questions. It also brings to the chapter the concept of nearing death awareness. The story is used with the permission of his wife, son-in-law who wrote much of the story and the reiki practitioner who was with Roy shortly before his death.

Roy was a 72-year-old exceptionally intelligent, well read, and successful international business man who had been referred to the author many years ago after a traumatic life event. Over the years I came to know him and family members through a variety of professional and non-professional encounters.

Thirty-five years prior to Roy's death from non-Hodgkin's lymphoma, he had been diagnosed with Hodgkin's disease which had recurred several months prior to his death. While on treatment for Hodgkin's disease, he developed non-Hodgkin's lymphoma. During his hospitalization Roy appeared to become very disoriented and at night

time seemed to be revisiting many of the very traumatic experiences that he had undergone in his international work, much of which was very difficult.

I did a home visit. Roy started the conversation by saying, 'You're Catholic, aren't you? I need you to know that while I was very sick in the hospital I was told that I was going to need to review every scene of my life, and to examine my culpability in scene after scene. In these scenes it was not as though I was in a field with John. I was in the field forty paces from John, who was wearing his blue plaid shirt. I was actually there in the field with him, feeling the feelings that I felt at the time of the initial encounter. I needed to review my culpability in scene after scene, but during these scenes, which happened night after night I was being held by the Virgin Mary. I am not Catholic, although I suppose if I had to choose a religion that it the one I would choose. But I wasn't brought up in that religion'. Roy then proceeded to relate what happened in scene after scene around the world. Some of the scenes were very difficult for him to re-experience, involving as they did the deaths of other people.

Roy was unlike his normal polite self as he related these scenes. If I interjected at all he just patiently 'heard me out' and then resumed his monologue. At the end of the two hour visit I made arrangements to return in a couple of weeks.

A couple of days later, Virginia, his wife said that she had mentioned my visit to Roy and he did not remember that I had visited. His wife asked if I thought that his subconscious was speaking to me.

When I returned for the second visit I said that I understood that he did not recall our previous visit. He said that indeed that was the case and he was very upset about it, 'I had no right to tell you those stories. They were confidential, and other people were involved in the incidents.' I told him that in his conversation he had very much remained the man of great integrity that I had always known him to be. He had mentioned no names, had spoken so quickly that I did not remember much of what he said, and that totally unlike my normal self I had taken no notes. He was relieved with this reassurance. He spoke about some of his concerns as he was obviously deteriorating, his awareness of the challenges presented to his wife, and their respective children. He then told me that when he was hospitalized for his treatment for his Hodgkin's disease, 35 years ago he had a 'visitor' who came to see him quite regularly. At the time Roy was having this visitor, Roy was in California receiving his treatment and the visitor was a socially active priest on the East Coast. Roy said that the priest would come to see him every afternoon at the same time and they would have long conversations. The staff became quite interested in these visits and they were sorrier than Roy when the visits stopped.

At the end of the interview Roy asked, 'Are you learning anything from me?' I relied that I was indeed. I walked away from the conversation thinking that with Roy and a number of then other clients with whom I was then working, many of whom are mentioned in this chapter, I was indeed continuing to learn despite having been doing this work for over 35 years. These visits occurred about 9 months from when Roy died. Below are excerpts from his son-in-law, edited by his wife describing his last days. The reiki practitioner who was called in to help with Roy's passing then offers her version of what happened.

A week before he passed away, Roy and I had a wild experience. Roy was fading from the cancer, and had been in and out for a few days. There were times where he was confused, and other times, where he was sharp as ever.

It was dinner- time, and I was sitting with him, and was being called to come to the table. Something was keeping me with him, as I felt he was slipping away. Several times I was called, and yet couldn't tear myself away. I had spent many months with him, and had developed a pretty keen sense of what he was feeling. After about 20 min sitting quietly with him, I felt him relax, and thought it was safe to leave the room. Even as I left the room, I could not help but feel that he had been close to passing. There were a few last things that Roy had wanted to do, but it would seem that we would not get them done.

Each night as I would say goodnight to Roy, I always wondered if this would be the last time. He had struggled for so long with so many things, I only wanted for him to find peace. This night, I headed to bed fairly early, looking to get some sleep. We were taking turns helping the nurse to flip him, and I had the early shift. Out of a pretty deep sleep, Virginia woke me. My guess at the time would be about 2:30AM. She was pretty wired, and asked that I come up right away. Roy had woken up, and we needed to talk with him, and he was spot on. We chatted briefly about the things that still had to get done, and when I suggested that we take care of it in the morning, he insisted that we get it done right away. So here we were, in his room, with the oxygen going, in the middle of the night, taking care of details! When all was finished, I sent Virginia back to bed. I went out to the living room, and sat with the nurse.

We chatted about Roy. Roy was a pretty good patient, and the nurses were so kind to him and us. They are involved everyday caring for palliative patients, and they not only take care of the patient, but the family too. We had chatted for perhaps half and hour or so, when we heard what sounded like an alarm coming from Roy's room. We raced across the house to his room, and I came blasting in like there was a fire. The alarm sound was gone. Roy lay in his bed—not moving. The sound alone would have woken anyone—it was like a screech. We heard it from 80 feet away from his room. Roy didn't move. I came right up to the foot of the bed, and called his name loudly. No reaction. I came right next to him at his bedside—and placed my hand on his chest. There was no movement, and he was completely still. I looked at his eyes, and there was no movement—I had bumped the bed several times to get close to him, and there was nothing. I stayed there with my hand on him for maybe 20 sec. Nothing in that time gave me any reason to think he was still there. Twice in my life, I have had people take their last breath in my arms. I was positive that Roy was gone. The nurse was saying, 'Its OK, he has found peace.' 'Yeah', I said, 'it's good.' I stepped back from beside the bed, and just made the sign of the cross and said a Hail Mary. No sooner had I finished, than Roy opened his eyes. Without a beat the nurse said: 'It's OK Roy—we are just checking on you—everything is fine—go back to sleep. He closed his eyes pretty quickly, and we escaped from the room. I was very shaken—I was positive that he was gone.

We went back out to the living room, and sat and chatted. We could not figure out what had made the screeching sound … I said to Ingrid, the nurse, 'I am not sure what just happened there—I have been with people that passed, and I am sure Roy was gone.' We spoke about what had just happened, and about Roy and about patients that Ingrid had taken care of. We talked for perhaps an hour.

Suddenly again we were startled by another sound—the sound of Roy yelling. Only it was coming directly from his room—the monitor was not even on. We raced into his room to find him

trying to sit up. He was very excited. He grabbed onto me right away, and said: Don't leave me—hold onto me—don't let me go. You can't leave me—stay with me—promise you will stay right here beside me. There was real fear in him. He grabbed on to Ingrid as well and just kept repeating 'promise you will stay right here'. It took probably 15 min or more to get him calmed down. Roy was not an excitable patient, and this was so far out of the ordinary.

I had seen Roy in many situations, but never like this. I had seen him having his clothes cut off as they were going to look for bullet wounds—he was cool—he even apologized for calling me Mike. I sat with him while we watched them hose down his house from a fire—he was cool. I had sat in court watching him get roasted, while he tried to lead the lawyer to where he wanted him to go. I had stood beside him as they told him that his cancer was untreatable—he was a rock. He was entirely lucid. He did not mumble or stumble, he was very direct as to what he wanted. When he finally calmed down to the point that I felt he was OK, I said to him—'what happened Roy?—Something happened a while ago while you were sleeping—what happened to you Roy?'

He said, 'People—People came to get me'. 'Who were they Roy, who were these people?' 'I am not sure—I thought they might be bad people, so I ran away.' 'I don't think they were bad people Roy, I think they were just people you don't know yet—I think they are OK Roy'. 'They were looking for me and I just wanted to get away' 'It's OK Roy they are probably good people—I think they are OK'. We chatted on about how we would stay with him and that everything was OK—we are all safe here.

Dawn was starting to come, and you could see the outlines of the early sky around the window blinds …, I was sitting next to Roy's bed holding his hand, when he said, 'Well, we have a busy day to day'. I said 'we got everything done last night Roy—what do we have to get done today?' He said, 'We have a cremation today'. 'Who are we cremating Roy?'

Roy looked at me like I was an idiot. 'We have to cremate me'. 'We can't cremate you Roy—you aren't dead!!!!!!!' I was completely blown away. Roy was totally lucid. We had just spoken about the income trust situation not a minute before. I said, 'Roy you are still alive, we can't cremate you'. Roy was convinced that he was dead. He was convinced that he had died. He went through the motions of proving to himself that I was real. He pinched the skin on my arms, and then began to poke me in the forehead. He took on a look of wonderment—this did not compute for him. Roy was perhaps the most rational thinker that I have ever come across. If this blew his mind, it certainly did mine. He asked me if I could prove I was real. I said I knew something that only he and I could know—he had given my daughter a book and a figurine—I knew who the figurine had come from—his mother. This seemed to put him on the road to calming further. We just watched and chatted as the sunrise kicked in to full glory. Finally, at almost 7 AM, I was so worn out, I said to Roy that the house was waking up, and that lots of people would be around. I was beat and I was going to head off to bed now. My last comment to him was 'You know what this day is Roy?' 'I think this day is a gift Roy—I don't think you are supposed to be here—make sure you have a great day'—He just nodded and smiled.

Roy had quite a day. He made it out of bed and went to his chair in the living room, and had chats with Virginia's girls. He gave the girls gifts that had to be given before he died. He had a great day for being on the ball, and it wasn't till later in the afternoon that he began to wind down. That was the last day that he left his room. He had one last supper, and then stopped eating, drinking, and pretty much communicating—it was like he was trying to get back to where he had been—and it was on purpose.

On the last afternoon, we had a visit from the 'Reiki ladies'. These are two ladies that are Reiki Masters. When they arrived at 3, I headed down for a nap. I had a Reiki treatment once, and had gotten nothing out of it. To say I was sceptical of its benefits would be an apt description. When I came back upstairs at 6, they were still there. They collared me right away, and asked if I was Mark? Yes. They needed to talk to me. Sure what's up? No, they needed to talk to me in private. We went into a bedroom across from Roy's, and they shut the door. They said Roy was ready to go, and that he needed me to help him to go. I said we had been thru this about a week ago, and that he knew I wanted him to go. They said that I needed to help him—that he needed me to help get him there. They offered no ideas as to what to do. They packed up and disappeared shortly. I grabbed a glass of wine, and started to slug it back …. I realized that I couldn't stall just because I didn't know what to do. One of my great friends was in trouble, and needed help. I headed into his room, to find Ann the housekeeper sitting at the end of the bed. I slid down next to him beside the bed, held onto his arm, and began to stroke his head. I said: Roy—its all over—the game has ended. Its time for us to go and find those people that scared you—it's OK, its time to go and find them again. They are OK Roy—let's go find them. Come with me Roy—let's go and find the light together, we can find them Roy. I told him that it was safe, that everyone was safe … now its time for us to find your peace—let's go to the light Roy—lets go! I kept repeating these things to him for a minute or two—I told him that we loved him and that we would be happy for him to find peace. I felt Roy start to relax; I had the nurse go get the family. All the while I just kept repeating that it was time and that all would be OK—it was time for him now—that we needed to find the peace for him—he didn't need to keep on—it was his time now. Virginia came in and gave him a beautiful gentle kiss and sat on the other side of the bed. All the family had come in, and were standing at the end of the bed. I just kept on stroking his head and telling him that we all loved him and that it was OK. He took only a few deep breaths more, and then he became still. I felt great relief for him because I know where he is. He is back to where he should have been.

His reiki therapist wrote

Roy first came into my life in February of 2006. I had been hired to do nursing foot care for him. Little did I know the impact he and his family would have on me over the next 10 months.

On the first visit I am required to complete a medical history. When I explained this I was handed a three-page history beginning with his birth date. I was also provided with a list of medications and their purposes. The thoroughness was a little surprising but not unusual for someone who has been dealing with the medical profession for some time …

Roy's condition continued to deteriorate and we added Reiki near the beginning of September … One Reiki session that really stands out in my mind is one he had while in hospital. I didn't feel the usual warmth in my hands and gave only a half hour treatment. At the end Roy held my hand, looked straight at me and said 'Thank you, you have been so kind to me.' I felt he was looking deeply into my soul and felt a connection I had never experienced with a client before. I can still see his face and feel the intensity of that connection. It was an amazing moment.

In November Roy's condition had deteriorated so that some days he was alert and others he was confused. I felt he was between two realities, slipping in and out of each … At about this time Virginia wondered if continuing the Reiki was worthwhile and we decided to give it a break for a few weeks to see if there was any difference.

In the mean time Virginia was also receiving Reiki or reflexology treatments. After one of these she asked me if Reiki might help Roy let go and cross over. If there was ever a man who could hang onto life by sheer willpower Roy was that man. I told Virginia that I felt Reiki could help but I wanted the advice and help of my Reiki master and friend Gayle Moynes …

(W)e met at my home and I drove asking for help and guidance all the way to Roy and Virginia's home. When we got there the house was full of family but the main activity was in the bedroom with other family members cloistered around Roy's bed. He seemed quite agitated and uncomfortable. He had phlegm in his throat and couldn't cough it up. His son-in-law Mark kept asking if he could help him by attempting to suction the phlegm. Gayle quietly said to me 'We need to clear this room. Give Roy space and help him settle down.'

We asked everyone to leave and using Reiki we cleared the room of any negative energy.

With just the three of us in the room I then introduced Gayle to Roy …

We held Roy's hands, upper arms, shoulders, chest, solar plexus, and head. I asked Gayle about working the feet but she advised me that the feet keep us connected to the earth so we kept working the upper body. Gayle kept contact with two spots behind Roy's head.

Roy became quiet and less restless. We spoke to him quietly, reassuring him that it was okay for him to leave this world, that his guardian angels were here to protect him, any of his Indian guides who had crossed over would help guide him to where he had to go. That he was going to a safe place filled with complete unconditional love. Gayle told him there were others waiting for him on the other side. He seemed very calm then opened his eyes and said 'Bills, there's bills to pay I better not go.' I immediately said 'No, your work here is complete, it is time for you to go.' Again he became calm.

Gayle asked me to go and get Virginia and only Virginia to come in. While Gayle and I gave Roy Reiki from our side of the bed Virginia told Roy she loved him and always would and that someday they would be together again. She told him it was time for him to join his friends who had crossed over. She also assured him he was going to a safe place that there were no bad people and he would be safe …

Eventually our conversation got around to the fact that Gayle and I felt Roy needed assurance from one more person before he could go. That person was his son-in-law, Mark. Virginia asked if we would talk to him. Not sure it was our place to do so we agreed to take him aside.

… We told him that we felt he had a very special relationship with Roy and that although not aware of it somehow he was the reason Roy was holding on. We suggested Roy needed Mark's reassurance that it was okay for him to go, that Virginia would be looked after and that it was time for Roy to go to a better place, that his purpose here had been fulfilled. We both gave Mark a hug and felt it was time for us to go.

I told Virginia I felt sure Roy would pass that night. We said our goodbyes with hugs all around and left...

Sometime later that evening Virginia called to say Roy had passed with his family around him. I immediately called Gayle to let her know, I thought I heard a little sob, and we both agreed it was quite an experience, that Roy had an amazing family and that he must have been an incredible man.

References

1. Akechi, T., Toru, O., Sugawara, Y. et al. (2004). Major depression, adjustment disorders, and post traumatic stress disorder in terminally ill cancer patients: Associated and predictive factors. *Journal of Clinical Oncology*, **22**, 1957–65.

2. Skilbeck, J., Connor, J., Bath, P. et al. (2002). Part 1. A description of the Macmillan Nurse caseload. Clinical nurse specialists in palliative care. *Palliative Medicine*, **16**, 285–96.

3. Strazdins, L. (2002). Emotional work and emotional contagion. In *Managing feelings in the workplace* (eds. N. Ashkanasy, W J. Zerbe, and C. E. J. Hartel), pp. 232–50. M.E. Sharpe, Armonk, NY.

4. Goleman, D. (2006). *Social intelligence: The new science of human relationships*. Bantam Dell, New York.

5. Fakhoury, W.K.H., McCarthy, M., and Addington-Hall, J. (1997). Carers' health status: Is it associated with their evaluation of the quality of palliative care? *Scandinavian Journal of Social Medicine*, **25**, 296–301.

6. Katz, R. (2006). When our personal selves influence our professional work: An introduction to emotions and countertransference in end-of-life care. In *When professionals weep* (eds. R.S. Katz and T.A. Johnson), pp. 3–12. Routledge, Taylor Francis Group, New York.

7. Barnard, D., Towers, A., Boston, P. et al. (2000). *Crossing over: Narratives of palliative care*. Oxford, New York.

8. Kearney, M. (2000). *A place of healing: Working with suffering in living and dying*. Oxford University Press, Oxford.

9. Cole, R. (2005). *Mission of love: A spiritual guide to living and dying peacefully*. Rev. ed. Lothian Books, South Melbourne, Australia.

10. Neimeyer, R. (2005). From death anxiety to meaning-making at the end of life: Recommendations for psychological assessment. *Clinical Psychology: Science and Practice*, **12**, 354–7.

11. Sachs, O. (1995). *An anthropologist on Mars*. Alfred A. Knopf, New York.

12. Vachon, M.L.S. (1994). Psychosocial variables: Cancer morbidity and mortality. In *A challenge for living: Death, dying and bereavement* (eds. I. Corless, B. Germino, and M. Pittman-Lindeman), pp. 135–55. Jones and Bartlett Publishers, Boston.

13. Kafetz, K. (2002). What happens when elderly people die? *Journal of the Royal Society of Medicine*, **95**, 536–8.

14. Nuland, S.B. (1994). *How We Die*. Chatto and Windus, London.

15. Lynn, J. (2001). Perspectives on care at the close of life. *Journal of the American Medical Association*, **285**, 925–32.

16. Ferris, F.D., Balfour, H.M., Bowen, K. et al. A Consensus-based Model to Guide Hospice Palliative Care. Ottawa: Canadian Hospice Palliative Care Association, March 2002.

17. Zimmerman, C. and Rodin, G. (2004). The denial of death thesis: Sociological critique and implications for palliative care. *Palliative Medicine*, **18**, 121–8.

18. Canadian Nurses Association. (2006). *Nurses at the forefront of HIV/AIDS: Report of the international nurses' forum*. Canadian Nurses Association, Ottawa, Ontario.

19. Viale, P.H., Fung, A., and Zitella, L. (2005). Advanced colorectal cancer: Current treatment and nursing management with economic constraints. *Clinical Journal of Oncology Nursing*, **9**, 541–52.

20. Xiong, H.O. and Jaffer, J.A. (2004). Treatment of colorectal cancer metastasis: The role of chemotherapy. *Cancer and Metastasis Reviews*, **23**, 145–63.

21. Schrag, D. (2004). The price tag on progress-chemotherapy for colorectal cancer. *The New England Journal of Medicine*, **351**, 317–19.

22. Von Gruenigen, V.E. and Daly, B.J. (2005). Futility: Clinical decisions at the end-of-life in women with ovarian cancer. *Gynecologic Oncology*, **97**, 638–44. (And references in the original.)

23. Phipps, E., True, G., Harris, D. et al. (2003). Approaching the end of life: Attitudes, preferences, and behaviors of African-American and white patients and their family caregivers. *Journal of Clinical Oncology*, **21**, 549–54.

24. Ramondetta, L.M., Tortolero-Luna G., Bodurka D.C. et al. (2004). Approaches for end-of-life care in the field of gynecologic oncology: An exploratory study. *International Journal of Gynecologic Cancer*, **14**, 580–8.

25. Donovan, K.A., Greene, P.G., Shuster, J.L. et al. (2002). Treatment preferences in recurrent ovarian cancer. *Gynecologic Oncology*, **86**, 200–11.

26. Haggerty, R.G., Butow, P.N., Ellis P.A. et al. (2004). Cancer patients preferences for communication of prognosis in the metastatic setting. *Journal of Clinical Oncology*, 22, 1721–30.

27. Fujimori, M., Parker, P.A., Akechi T. et al. (2007). Japanese patients' communication style preference when receiving bad news. *Psycho-Oncology*, **16**, 617–25.

28. Gattellari, M., Voigt, K.J., Butow, P.N. et al. (2002). When the treatment goal is not cure: Are patients equipped to make informed decisions? *Journal of Clinical Oncology*, **20**, 503–13.

29. Kaplowitz, S.A., Osuch, J.R., Safron, D. et al. (1999). Physician communication with seriously ill cancer patients: Results of a survey of physicians. In *End of life issues: Interdisciplinary and multidimensional perspectives*. (ed. B de Vries). Springer Publishing, New York.

30. National Comprehensive Cancer Network. (2003). Distress management clinical practice guidelines. *J Natl Comp Cancer Network*, **1**, 344–74.

31. Barsevick, A. (2003). Depression. *CancerSourceRN.com*. 08/05/2003 accessed on 14/11/2003.

32. Breitbart, W., Bruera, E., Chochinov, M.H. et al. (1995). Neuropsychiatric syndromes and psychological symptoms in patients with advanced cancer. *Journal of Pain and Symptom Management*, **10**, 131–41.

33. Kelly, B., McClement, S., and Chochinov, H.M. (2006). Measurement of psychological distress in palliative care. *Palliative Medicine*, **20**, 779–89.

34. Vachon, M.L.S., Lancee, W.J., Conway, B. et al. (1990). *The needs of persons living with cancer in Manitoba*. Canadian Cancer Society, Toronto.

35. Zabora, J., BrintzenhofeSzoc, K., Curbow, B. et al. (2001). The prevalence of psychological distress by cancer site. *Psycho-Oncology*, **10**, 19–28.

36. Carlson, L.E. and Bultz, B.D. (2004). Efficacy and medical cost offset of psychosocial interventions in cancer care: Making the case for economic analysis, *Psychosocial-Oncology*, **13**, 837–49.

37. Khatib, J., Salhi, R., and Awad, G. (2004). Distress in cancer inpatients in King Hussein Cancer Center (KHCC): A study using the Arabic-modified version of the distress thermometer. *Psycho-Oncology*, **12**(1 Suppl), S42.

38. Vachon, M.L.S., Fitch, M., Greenberg, M. et al. (1995). The needs of cancer patients and their families attending Toronto–Sunnybrook Regional Cancer Centre, unpublished data.

39. Vachon, M.L.S. (2004). The emotional problems of the patient in palliative medicine. In *Oxford Textbook of Palliative Medicine*, 3rd edition (eds. D. Doyle, G. Hanks, N. Cherny, K. Calman). pp. 961–85. Oxford University Press, Oxford.

40. Durkin, I., Kearney, M., and O'Siorain, L. (2003). Psychiatric disorder in a palliative care unit. *Palliative Medicine*, **17**, 212–18.

41. Lynn, J., Teno, J.M., Phillips, R.J. et al. (1997). Perception by family members of the dying experience of older and seriously ill patients. *Annals of Internal Medicine*, **126**, 97–106.

42. Aass, N., Fosså, S.D., Dahl, A.A. et al. (1997). Prevalence of anxiety and depression in cancer patients seen at the Norwegian Radium Hospital. *European Journal of Cancer*, **33**, 1597–604.

43. Stommel, M., Kurtz, M.E., Kurtz, J.C. *et al.* (2004). A longitudinal analysis of the course of depressive symptomatology in Geriatric patients with cancer of the breast, colon, lung, or prostate. *Health Psychology*, **23**, 564–73.

44. Lancee, W.J., Vachon, M.L.S., Ghadirian, P. *et al.* (1994). The impact of pain and impaired role performance on distress in persons with cancer. *Canadian Psychiatric Association Journal*, **39**, 617–22.

45. Kaasa, S., Malt, U., Hagen, S. *et al.* (1993). Psychological distress in cancer patients with advanced disease. *Radiotherapy and Oncology*, **27**, 193–7.

46. Turner, N.J., Muers, M.F., Haward, R.A. *et al.* (2007). Psychological distress and concerns of elderly patients treated with palliative radiotherapy for lung cancer. *Psycho-Oncology*, **16**, 707–713.

47. Morasso, G., DiLeo, S., Fiore, M. *et al.* (1999). Psychosocial and symptom distress in terminal cancer patients with met and unmet needs. *Journal of Pain and Symptom Management*, **17**, 402–9.

48. Mystakidou, K., Parpa, E., Katsouda, E. *et al.* (2006). The role of physical and psychological symptoms in desire for death: A study of terminally ill cancer patients. *Psycho-Oncology*, **15**, 355–60.

49. Hodges, L.J., Humphris, G.M, and Macfarlane, G. (2005). A meta-analytic investigation of the relationship between the psychological distress of cancer patients and carers. *Social Science and Medicine*, **60l**, 1–12.

50. Kissane, D.W., McKenzie, M., McKenzie, D.P. *et al.* (2003). Psychosocial morbidity associated with patterns of family functioning in palliative care: Baseline data from the Family Focused Grief Therapy controlled trial. *Palliative Medicine*, **17**(6), 527–37.

51. Jacobsen, P.B., Donovan, K.A., Trask, P.C. *et al.* (2005). Screening for psychologic distress in ambulatory cancer patients. *Cancer*, **103**, 1494–502.

52. Ransom, S., Jacobsen, P.B., and Booth-Jones, M. (2006). Validation of the Distress Thermometer with bone marrow transplant patients. *Psycho-Oncology*, **15**, 604–12.

53. Bultz, B.D. and Carlson, L.E. (2006). Emotional distress: The sixth vital sign-future directions in cancer care. *Psycho-Oncology*, **15**, 93–5.

54. Murillo, M. and Holland, J.C. (2004). Clinical practice guidelines for the management of psychosocial distress at the end of life. *Palliative and Supportive Care*, **2**, 65–77.

55. Tacón, A.M. (2002). Attachment and cancer: A conceptual integration. *Integrative Cancer Therapies*, **1**, 371–81. (And references in the original.)

56. Temoshok, L. (1987). Personality, coping style, emotion and cancer: Towards an integrative model. *Imperial Cancer Research Fund*, **6**, 545–67.

57. Tacón, A.M., Caldera Y., and Bell. N. (2001). Attachment, emotional control and breast cancer. *Family Systems and Health*, **19**, 319–26.

58. Thomas, C. (1988). Cancer and the youthful mind: A forty year perspective. *Advances in Body Mind Medicine*, **5**, 42–58.

59. Temoshok, L.R. (2002). Connecting the dots linking mind, behavior, and disease: The biological concomitants of coping patterns: Commentary on "Attachment and cancer: a conceptual integration. *Integrative Cancer Therapies*, **1**,387–91. (And references in the original.)

60. Costanzo, E.S, Lutgendorf, S.K., Sood, A.K. *et al.* (2005). Psychosocial factors and interleukin-6 among women with advanced ovarian cancer. *Cancer*, **104**, 305–13. (And references in the original.)

61. Tan, A., Zimmerman, C., and Rodin, G. (2005). Interpersonal processes in palliative care: An attachment perspective on the patient-clinician relationship. *Palliative Medicine*, **19**, 143–50. (And references in the original.)

62. Hunter, M.J., Davis, P.J., and Tunstall, J.R. (2006). The influence of attachment and emotional support in end-stage cancer. *Psycho-Oncology*, **15**, 431–44. (And references in the original.)

63. Bowlby, J. (1977). The making and breaking of affectional bonds. Aetiology and psychopathology in the light of attachment theory. *British Journal of Psychiatry*, **130**, 201–10.

64. Ciechanowski, P.S., Katon, W.J., Russo, J.E. *et al.* (2001). The patient-provider relationship: attachment theory and adherence to treatment in diabetes. *American Journal of Psychiatry*, **158**, 29–35.

65. Ciechanowski, P.S., Hirsh, I.B., and Katon, W.J. (2002). Interpersonal predictors of HbAlc in patients with Type 1 diabetes. *Diabetes Care*, **25**, 731–6.

66. Kim, Y. and Carver, C.S. (in press). Frequency and difficulty in caregiving among spouses of individuals with cancer: Effects of adult attachment and gender. *Psycho-Oncology*, DOI: 10.1002/pon.1110.

67. Hutchinson, T.A. (2005). Transitions in the lives of patients with End Stage Renal Disease: A cause of suffering and an opportunity for healing. *Palliative Medicine*, 19, 270–7. (And references in the original.)

68. Gillies, B. and Johnston, G. (2004). Identity loss and maintenance: Commonality of experience in cancer and dementia. *European Journal of Cancer Care*, **13**, 436–42.

69. Lynn, J. (1997). An 88-year-old woman facing the end of life. *Journal of the American Medical Association*, **277**, 1633–40.

70. Fife, B.L. (1994). The conceptualization of meaning in illness. *Social Science and Medicine*, **38**, 309–16.

71. Singh, K.D. (1998). *The grace in dying: How we are transformed spiritually as we die*. Harper, San Francisco.

72. Kübler-Ross, E. (1969). *On Death and Dying*. Macmillan, New York.

73. Frankl, V. (1984). *Man's Search for meaning*. Washington Square Press, New York.

74. Zoellner, T., Maercker, A. (2006). Post-traumatic growth in clinical psychology-a clinical review and introduction of a two component model. *Clinical Psychology*, **26**, 626–53. (And references in the original.)

75. Poulson, J. (2002). *The doctor will not see you now*. Novalis, St. Paul University, Ottawa.

76. Remen, N. (1996). *Kitchen table wisdom*. Riverhead Books, New York.

77. Weisman, A. (1979).*Coping with cancer*. McGraw-Hill Book Co., New York.

78. Weisman, A. (1972). *On dying and denying*. Behavioral Publications, New York.

79. Vachon, M.L.S. (2002). Denial and minimization in advanced cancer. *Hot Spot*, **4**(1), 2. http://www.sunnybrook.ca/programs/tsrcc/treatmentprevention/rapidresponse.

80. Stephenson, P.S. (2004). Understanding denial. *Palliative Medicine*, **31**, 985–8.

81. Maguire, P. (2000). Communication with terminally ill patients and their relatives. In: *Handbook of psychiatry in palliative medicine* (eds. H.M. Chochinov and W. Breitbart), pp. 291–01. Oxford University Press, New York.

82. Erikson, E.H. (1959, reissued 1980). *Identity and the life cycle: Selected papers*. Norton, New York.

83. Fox, M. (1983). *Original blessing*. Jeremy P. Tarcher/Putnam, New York.

84. Rinpoche, S. (1992). *The Tibetan book of living and dying*. HarperSanFrancisco, San Francisco.

85. Steinhauser, K.E., Clipp, E.C., McNeilly, M. *et al.* (2000). In search of a good death: Observations of patients, families, and providers. *Annals of Internal Medicine*, **132**, 825–32.

86. Olson, M. and Dossey, B.M. (2005). Dying in peace. In *Holistic nursing: A handbook for practice* (eds. B.M. Dossey, L. Keegan, and C.E. Guzzetta), pp. 691–718. Jones and Bartlett Publishers, Sudbury, MA.

87. Kuhl, D. (2002). *What do dying people want?* Doubleday, Toronto.

88. Kuhl, D. (2006). *Facing death embracing life*. Doubleday, Toronto.

89. Vachon, M.L.S. (2004). Reflections on the life and death of Mary Pocock. *Hot Spot*, **6**, (2). http://www.sunnybrook.ca/programs/tsrcc/treatmentprevention/rapidresponse.

90. Gill, S. and Fox, J. (1996). *The dead good funerals book*. Engineers of the Imagination, Welfare State International, Ulverstone, Cumbria.

91. Kapleau, P. (1989). *The wheel of life and death: A practical and spiritual guide*. Anchor Books, New York.

92. Groopman, J. (2004). *The anatomy of hope: How people prevail in the face of illness*. Random House, New York.

93. Vachon, M.L.S. (2006). Hope in advanced disease. *Hot Spot*, **8**, 2–3 (February). http://www.sunnybrook.ca/programs/tsrcc/treatmentprevention/rapidresponse.

94. Volker, D.L, Kahn, D., and Penticuff, J.H. (2004). Patient control and end-of-life care. Part 1: The advanced nurse perspective. *Oncology Nursing Forum*, **31**, 945–53.

95. Chochinov, H.M. (2002). Dignity-conserving care-a new model for palliative care. *Journal of the American Medical Association*, **287**, 2253–60.

96. Chochinov, H.M., Hack, T., McClement, S. *et al.* (2002). Dignity in the terminally ill: A developing empirical model. *Social Science and Medicine*, **54**, 433–43.

97. Mount, B.M. and Kearney, M. (2003). Healing and palliative care: Charting our way forward. *Palliative Medicine*, **17**, 657–8.

98. Philip, J., Gold, M., Schwartz, M. *et al.* (2007). Anger in palliative care: A clinical approach. *Internal Medicine Journal*, **37**, 49–55. (And references in the original.)

99. Kissane D. (1994). Managing anger in palliative care. Aust Fam Physician, **23**, 1257–9

100. Mickley, J.R and Cowles, K. (2001). Ameliorating the tension: Use of forgiveness for healing. *Oncology Nursing Forum*, **28**, 31–7.

101. Byock, I. (1997). *Dying well: The prospect for growth at the end of life*. Riverhead Books, New York.

102. Cassel, E. (1982). The nature of suffering and the goals of medicine. *New England Journal of Medicine*, **306**, 639–45.

103. Terry, W. and Olson, L.G. (2004). Unobvious wounds: The suffering of hospice patients. *Internal Medicine Journal*, **34**, 604–7.

104. Dr. Hanna. (2006). *A mother's diary*. Yvonne Yi Wood Mak, Hong Kong.

105. McClain, C., Rosenfeld, B., and Breitbart, W. (2003). The effect of spiritual well-being on end of life despair in terminally ill cancer patients. *Lancet*, **361**, 1603–7.

106. Lin, H. and Bauer-Wu, S. (2003). Psycho-Spiritual well-being in patients with advanced cancer: An integrative review of the literature. *Journal of Advanced Nursing*, **44**, 1:69–80.

107. Farber, A. and Farber, S. (2006). The respectful death model: difficult conversations at the end-of-life. In *When professionals weep*. (eds. R.S. Katz and T.A. Johnson), pp. 221–36. Routledge, Taylor Francis Group, New York.

The family perspective

Joan T. Panke and Betty R. Ferrell

Introduction

Definition of the family

Advanced disease from any chronic illness impacts all of the family members surrounding the one with the diagnosis. Changing demographics of our society and an aggressive shift of health care into the living room makes the role of family caregivers in chronic and terminal illness even more significant. While the family was traditionally defined as an individual of blood relationship, a broad definition of family is most appropriate and best defined as those individuals considered as a family by the patient. Studies in oncology related to the family have generally found that approximately 70 per cent of primary family caregivers are spouses, approximately 20 per cent are children (of which daughters or daughters-in-law are most predominant), and approximately 10 per cent are friends or more distant relatives[1,2]. Family then includes biologic relatives as well as persons identified by the patient as significant in their lives, intimately involved with the patient, who love the patient, and have frequent contact with the patient[3,4]. A review of the literature on the topic of family and palliative care reveals that most of the research has focused on family care-giving demands, emotional responses to illness, and family bereavement.

It is important to note that opportunities for growth, healing, and support for both patient and family are tremendous even while they are coping with countless difficulties and sorrows as the patient's disease progresses. We may not be able to change the course of a disease or eventual death, yet professional caregivers can support and aggressively advocate for the needs of the patient and family by attending simultaneously to their physical, psychological, social, and spiritual needs and concerns. Patients and their loved ones can be given the opportunity to attend to what is important to them, ultimately bringing about a more peaceful death.

Dying is recognized as a uniquely individual experience. An interdisciplinary team approach to care is necessary in order to address and respond to the many needs of the patient and family. Palliative care is appropriate at every stage of the disease regardless of whether or not the patient is seeking curative treatment. By introducing palliative care earlier in the disease trajectory, it is possible to recognize subtle shifts that take place, reassess and adapt goals as necessary, and open the way for patients and families to begin to reframe hope, to find meaning, and to adapt as a disease progresses.

Fig. 15.3.1 presents a model of quality of life (QOL) for family caregivers that has evolved through research in this area at the City of Hope Medical Center since 1987. Family caregivers' QOL, similar to the patient, encompasses dimensions of physical, psychological, social, and spiritual well-being.

Appreciation for the caregivers' perspective is critical to the care of the patient. Decades of work in hospice and palliative care have demonstrated that support of family caregivers is an essential feature of quality care for patients with chronic advanced illness. Because family members are assuming a greater role with the shift of care to the home, quality care is dependent upon addressing family caregivers' needs[5,6].

Attention to family needs and concerns should occur throughout the trajectory of any potentially life-threatening illness. Family caregiving takes on distinct meaning in situations such as AIDS in which care is shifted to non-blood relatives and often to other individuals experiencing the same illness. Future trends in health care will also shift care from professionals to unlicensed caregivers as our society becomes increasingly dependent upon significant others such as an elderly spouse, whose ability to provide the intensive care of advanced disease is limited[7,8]. Distance caregiving is also an increasing social issue as middle aged children attempt to direct the care of parents who are hundreds or thousands of miles away and who have serious chronic illness or are at the end of life.

Terminal illness as a family experience

Families are profoundly influenced by acute and chronic illness. Day-to-day family activities, roles and relationships, and the meaning of life itself becomes altered, once life shifts from health to illness. Terminal illness adds an entire dimension, even for those who have faced years or decades of chronic illness. During terminal illness, patients and families struggle not only with the present and all that is included with terminal illness care but also with the overwhelming issues associated with death and transcendence beyond death[9–12].

Early work in palliative care focused attention on patients with advanced cancer. Patients with other chronic, progressive illnesses may have a less predictable and prolonged decline toward death. Family members of patients dying from heart disease and other chronic illnesses other than cancer may experience added burden due to repeated exacerbations and remissions over a longer trajectory of the illness[13,14]. While much of what has been learned

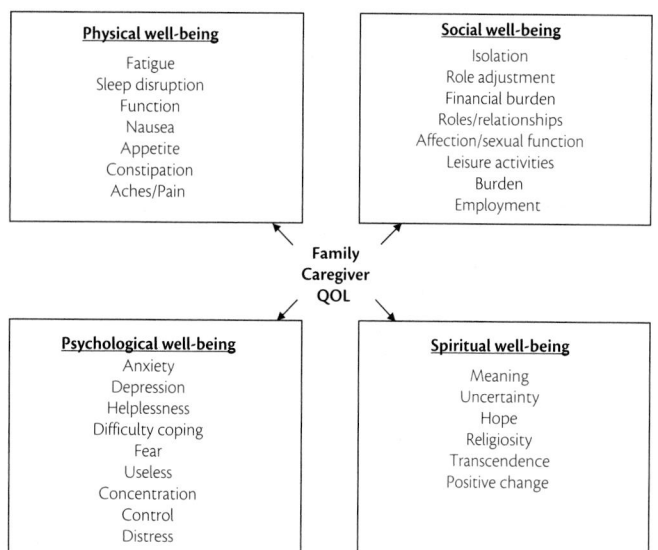

Figure 15.3.1 Family caregiver quality of life.

regarding the needs and concerns of patients and families with advanced cancer can be applied to patients with other illnesses, it is important to appreciate individual differences.

Palliative care has the ability to prevent family crisis and create cohesion in the light of even a life-threatening illness. In a study of parents of children with cancer, a mother described having a child diagnosed with cancer as an experience in which the family actually came closer together. Grandparents became supportive in the care of the child. Both parents worked together to provide comfort to the child, and siblings also became cooperative and concerned about their brother with cancer. However, the mother described the experience of having the child suffering pain by saying, 'It was as if someone threw a hand grenade in our living room'[15]. Having a child with uncontrolled symptoms created an opposite environment in which the grandparents became critical of the parents' care and the parents became critical of each other. The siblings were frightened of their brother's pain and thus isolated themselves from him.

As family caregivers observe physical and emotional suffering of a loved one who is dying, they also struggle with their own losses and changing roles while dealing with their concerns about their caregiving abilities[16]. Family intervention is needed to confront the many physical and emotional issues associated with palliative care. Intervention is dependent upon assessment of family functioning and use of an interdisciplinary team to meet the diverse needs of the family.

Coping with a terminal illness can challenge both the patient and the family in terms of their spiritual beliefs. When someone is dying, hope may seem diminished, but despair is not necessarily inevitable. Spiritual concerns may become more intense as death approaches and spirituality is a significant contributor to quality of life at the end of life. Through assessment and intervention, family caregivers have the opportunity to find comfort and strength from their spirituality that assists in their coping[17]. The dying person may search for deeper spiritual meaning of life's work or relationship to others or God. Family members may search for the meaning in a loved one's death. Assessing what hope or living with

uncertainty means to an individual assists the patient and family to set realistic goals for the time that they do have remaining (see Section 15 for further discussion on spirituality).

Role of the family caregivers in palliative care

Whether patients are receiving aggressive treatments aimed at curing a life-threatening illness or comfort, they are likely to have multiple physical, psychological, social, and spiritual needs. Family members often have to allocate more time to caring for the patient[18]. Furthermore, family caregivers may have to manage work outside the home along with caregiving roles. Many family caregivers assuming the demanding job of caring for someone they love are performing this care after completing 8 hours employment outside the home each day[19].

The role of the family caregiver involves both direct and indirect care needs. Direct care includes those aspects of care carried out directly with the patient, such as symptom management, emotional support, monitoring for changes in patient status, medication administration, and assistance with activities of daily living. Indirect care involves activities carried out on behalf of the patient, such as obtaining prescriptions and medications, transportation, scheduling and coordination of appointments, and dealing with financial issues[18]. In our research in the area of family caregivers' involvement in pain management, we have also found that family caregivers are commonly involved in 'night duty,' assuming total care; making decisions at night for patients who perhaps are more independent during the day hours[5].

Barriers to effective symptom management by family caregivers

It is notable given the extent of their involvement that there has been little attention given to family caregivers. In a study in 1998 to 1999, we analysed all end-of-life content in nursing textbooks as a part of our Robert Wood Johnson-funded work on end-of-life care[19]. We reviewed 50 textbooks used in schools of nursing comprising 45 683 pages to analyse nine end-of-life topics (i.e. pain, symptom management, bereavement, quality of life, legal issues, and ethical issues). Overall, only 2 per cent of content in textbooks had any relationship to any end of life topic, and the area most neglected was the needs and roles of family caregivers. Of the 45 683 pages, only 42 pages (or 0.1 per cent of content) were related to family. Seventy-one percent of the texts reviewed had no content at all related to family caregivers (see Table 15.3.1). Efforts to address knowledge deficits of professionals related to care of the family are underway through initiatives such as the End of Life Nursing Education Consortium (ELNEC), which includes care of the family as a common thread throughout the curriculum (see http://www.aacn.nche/ELNEC)[20].

Family caregivers frequently lack information regarding what to expect as a disease progresses, how to manage symptoms, and when to report symptoms or failure of treatments to control symptoms. Similarly, lack of adequate support has been identified as a barrier to care that negatively impacts symptom management.

Frequently cited barriers to effective pain management by family caregivers of patients with cancer include fear of respiratory depression, fear of drug tolerance, fear of drug addiction, and lack of knowledge regarding chronic pain. Investigators have documented that family members play an important role in pain management[2,21–23]. As family members assume the role of caregivers for patients, they are often required to manage complex

Table 15.3.1 Nursing textbook analysis of family caregiver content at the end of life (per cent of textbooks including content related to the topic of family).

Roles and needs of family caregivers	0	+	++
Importance of recognizing needs of family and caregivers at EOL	57	37	6
Assessment of family needs	57	26	17
Family dynamics	83	13	4
Recognition of ethnic or cultural influences on EOL care	91	2	7
Coping strategies and support systems	70	26	4
Average of all family content	71	21	8

Note: 0 = absent; + = present; ++ = commendable; EOL = end of life.

medication regimens, parenteral infusion devices, and other complex treatments in the home[24–27]. Thus, family members are assuming the responsibility for pain relief despite the need to understand basic pain-management principles. Family members often deny that the patient is in pain to avoid the realization that the disease is progressing[28], The family's decisions in pain management seem to range from giving pain medications aggressively (while often being quite concerned about their decisions in medicating) to restricting and withholding medications because of concern that they would be criticized for over-medicating the patient or using too much of the medications.

Caregiver burden

Caregiver burden can be described as the emotional and physical demands and responsibilities of an illness that are placed on family members, friends, or other individuals involved with the patient outside of the health-care system. Families often do not know how to provide physical care, adjust to role changes, and cope with the many losses faced during the dying process and after the death. Many caregivers have physical illnesses that may impact their ability to care for the patient and themselves. Patients worry about the emotional and financial burdens placed on family members. Some families have had to drain life savings to cover costs of care.

A study by Grobe, Ilstrup, and Ahmann[29] revealed that family members of terminally ill patients with cancer needed to learn new skills such as assisting with ambulation, comfort care, and pain management in order to provide effective care in the home. These family members reported that specific care-giving skills were not taught by their health-care providers, and they were left with a 'trial and error' method of skill acquisition.

Tringali[30] reinforced this conclusion by observing family members of patients with cancer at three different phases of illness including initial treatment, recurrent disease, and follow-up treatment. Family caregivers were evaluated regarding their cognitive, emotional, and physical needs. Regardless of the phase of illness, informational needs were identified as most important. The results suggest that the provision of information prepares family members to support the patient, reinforces the treatment goals, and assists in managing the side effects of therapy and disease. It is apparent from the reports of these investigators[29,30], and others[7,8,31,32], that the needs of family members are not being

met, and that understanding needs and assisting families in meeting those needs will contribute to improved care.

Caregivers may experience severe mood disruption in the areas of depression, anxiety, and fatigue. Providing adequate pain relief is of great comfort to caregivers, who express feelings of helplessness, frustration, and sadness when unable to provide comfort. Unfortunately, caregivers often receive limited instruction in the use of pharmacologic and non-pharmacologic pain management techniques and principles, and may tend to undermedicate the patient in response to their concerns about addiction, respiratory depression, and drug tolerance.

We have consistently seen a low correlation between patient and family caregivers regarding pain intensity levels and distress regarding pain. The level of concern, stress, and knowledge of the caregiver are different from the patient. Family caregiver's perception of pain may be influenced by the nature of the pain, its duration, and the patient's prognosis. An interesting finding from our recent studies is that the family caregivers' fear of addiction and tolerance was worse than the fear experienced by the patients themselves[1].

General fears and concerns of family members

Family caregivers expect that quality care will be provided to the patient. Families also look to health-care professionals to provide information regarding the disease and dying process, physical care, symptom management needs, emotional support, and for practical guidance[32,33].

A review of the research on the impact of cancer on the family[34] identified 11 separate issues of concern for family members. These included:

1 Emotional strain.

2 Physical demands.

3 Uncertainty.

4 Fear of the patient dying.

5 Altered roles and lifestyles.

6 Finances.

7 Ways to comfort the patient.

8 Perceived inadequacies of services.

9 Existential concern.

10 Sexuality.

11 Non-convergent needs among household members.

Studies of family members caring for persons with advanced cancer have shown that most experience stress in the caregiver role and significant stress in observing patient suffering. Family caregivers report distress from uncertainty about the course of the disease as well as feelings about their inability to provide care (such as effective symptom relief) or to manage the patient's psychological symptoms such as depression and anxiety.

Given, Given, and Kozachik[18] identified needs of family members of dying persons as including:

1 Need for information regarding the disease:

- Information about physical care and comfort measures.

- What symptoms to expect and how to manage them.

- Treatment regimens.

- Expectations for future care.
- Patient's emotional response.
- Household management procedures.
- Finances.
- Community resources.

2 Need for assistance with how to structure care activities:

- Monitoring and reporting symptoms.
- Monitoring disease status.
- Transportation.
- Nutritional considerations.
- Coordination of care (scheduling).
- Financial concerns.

3 Continued guidance to alleviate stressors, overall burden and associated depression:

- Escalation of care demands as patient's disease and functional status declines.
- Strategies to assist with coping with disease progression and patient decline.
- Detailed, specific information regarding unique psychological and social needs.

The needs of family caregivers are multiple and complex. A study by Borneman, Chu, Wagman, *et al.*[35], demonstrated that family caregivers of patients with cancer undergoing palliative surgery have important quality-of-life concerns and needs for support, both before and after surgery for advanced disease. In addition to common concerns including uncertainty, fears regarding the future, and loss, these caregivers had concerns regarding surgical risks and care after surgery. As an important component of palliative care, surgery profoundly impacts the family caregivers of patients with cancer, and it is important to assess their needs and provide interventions to help them cope. Examples of comments from these caregivers are depicted in Table 15.3.2.

Family communication

Issues of communication frequently influence family caregiving in palliative care. Understanding family information needs is central to providing the care necessary to maintain patients in any setting. It is important to assess the need for information and how information is best shared in a given family. The emotional and psychosocial needs of both patient and family reinforce the importance of interdisciplinary care in advanced illness. As our society becomes more diverse, it is also essential to consider the many cultural considerations in family communication and decision-making.

Vachon described many issues related to family communication during advanced illness. Family members, like patients, experience significant distress during the patient's illness. Three major problematic issues can be summarized from the research literature related to family communication and cancer:

1 Concealing feelings.
2 Acquiring information.
3 Coping with helplessness.

Table 15.3.2 Comments of family caregivers of patients with cancer undergoing palliative surgery[35].

'She lives separate from me, but I'm . . . always calling her every day, at least three to four times a day. I'm always just making sure she's feeling okay. I'm there for her a lot. I'm very there for her in her life'

'Especially because he went in thinking he might have an ulcer or a hiatal hernia. And one minute you're going in with that thought, and, a few hours later, the doctor came in . . . He knew it was cancer. Your life changes . . . It just seems like a death sentence as soon as you hear the word "cancer."'

'But he trusts [the doctor]. We both think he's wonderful. And he has just been, he's he's given us the hope that we need. Because even though he gave us those terrible statistics, he, he let us realize that there are 15 per cent of people who do make it. And he has done these kinds of surgeries before . . . He just made us feel like he was skilled, competent, knew what he was doing, and was going to give [my husband] the best chance that he could possibly. And you have to have that faith in the surgeon, otherwise you don't want to go on. You just say forget it.'

'I have to spend time with [my husband]. I have to spend time with my mother 'cause they're both at that point where . . . yeah. And one of them can go at any time. Who knows. And then you're working the other days so it's just sometimes I feel overwhelmed. It's, sometimes it's fine and other days I just feel like falling apart. But I can't 'cause I'm strong and I have to take care of everybody.'

'I'm scared. I worry about just him getting through it . . . For the first few days, I'll still be worried, and I'll just be glad when he comes home. I'll be glad to do anything, you know, just to have him come home again. I know it's good to know the truth, and I'm glad that [the doctor] was so up front with us. But it's just so hard to deal with. Surgery's very scary. The chemotherapy and radiation were not scary. I knew he would get sick, but I knew that there was no chance of him dying from it. This is a whole different animal.'

'We talk every once in a while, and I'm reading my book and he's watching TV and taking naps and going to the bathroom. But we're here together today. So, I just told my boss that I, I'm not going to be at work today.'

'It was more of a quality of life thing. They'd like to get her eating, like to get her home. Like to get her spending her time in a way that she finds, you know, enjoyable. But, um, they're not planning on curing her or anything like that. I think she is aware of the prognosis. But, you know, like she said, she wants to still be in the treatment category more than, she doesn't want hospice at this point. So, although she knows that, she's not ready to just say that's it and prepare to die. She's wanting to do whatever she can to keep going.'

Family communication can become restricted as family members withhold information to protect one another from difficult issues[36–38]. Patients often under-report symptoms to avoid distressing family caregivers. Three patterns of restricted communication among couples coping with the terminal phase of cancer were identified by Hinton[38]:

1 Consciously avoiding any discussion of the illness as a self-protective way of preventing one's distress level from rising.

2 Avoiding discussion of the illness in order to maintain the positive attitude felt to be essential to coping with the disease, thereby avoiding discussing any pessimistic feelings.

3 Those who had rarely spoken openly about emotional events in the past and maintained this pattern during the terminal illness.

An important intervention by health-care providers is to validate the family caregiver's contributions to the patient's comfort and reinforce their commitment. Health-care providers play a central role in enhancing communication between various family members, with the patient, and with other health-care professionals. In the terminal phase of illness, families often require greater support to overcome barriers to communication, which greatly affect patient care. Psychosocial services, such as the care provided by a clinical psychologist or psychiatrist, are important, but all team members can assist in improved family communication. Encouraging expression of concerns, facilitating discussions, active listening, and providing information are all important components of this care (see Section 4).

Clinical issues in supporting family caregivers

What family caregivers need most is information and support. Family caregivers increasingly assume 24-h care that in recent years was provided in acute, inpatient settings, perhaps having received little or no education and even more importantly, little emotional support. In many instances, family caregivers are now assuming procedures and treatments that have previously been confined to intensive care units. Health-care professionals provide this care with the support of colleagues and with the assurance that the 'next shift' will relieve them soon. Family caregivers seldom have such assurance. Much can be provided in the way of home care and hospice services and yet even for those individuals with access to such services, the majority of the responsibility rests on the family members themselves.

In recent research conducted at the City of Hope National Medical Center, we evaluated a structured pain education programme in both elderly patients and family caregivers. The educational programme was successful in improving knowledge and attitudes about pain, as well as direct outcomes such as improved pain intensity and overall quality of life. However, the study also revealed the unmet emotional needs of family caregivers arising from the perceived burden of responsibility for the relief of a loved one's suffering[39]. This study, and other literature, demonstrates that providing information alone is not sufficient, but that family caregivers desperately need support for the intense roles they assume and the burdens they shoulder associated with assuming responsibility for patient comfort.

Family members often feel helpless, despite their best attempts, if symptoms persist. Family caregivers also may deny the presence of symptoms as a means of coping with the situation. Our previous decade of research has revealed the ever-present metaphor of pain as a symbol of death. In this sense, pain is unlike treatment of other symptoms, such as nausea or constipation, in that it carries with it the existential issues of suffering and death.

Realistically, professionals cannot always be present as a team to address family needs. The one-to-one encounter is significant in that it may serve to uncover important issues or concerns of both the patient and the family, which can then be shared with other team members. The value of a team meeting cannot be stressed enough as an opportunity to explore important issues and to create and re-evaluate a realistic plan of care that is patient and family oriented.

Alternative therapies

Family caregivers often seek alternative therapies either as curative treatments or as palliative treatments for symptom management. Montbriand[40] reviewed alternative therapies in cancer care and categorized these as spiritual, psychological, or physical modalities.

Spiritual methods include faith healing, psychic surgery, and similar modalities. Psychological therapies include visualization or other cognitive therapies. The most common alternative treatment is the use of physical methods such as herbs, vitamins, health foods, and healers.

These methods may be a valuable component of the patient's care, enhancing the effects of traditional methods. However, health providers should assess the use of these modalities to determine the potential for misuse or to identify areas of fraud or financial burden too often associated with their use. Work by Montbriand[40] and others[41] serves as a useful guide to direct health-care providers in this important aspect of care.

Educating family caregivers to utilize alternative, non-pharmacologic approaches can enhance patient comfort. Use of gentle massage, incorporating music into daily activities, or cognitive behavioural techniques such as distraction, relaxation and imagery may benefit family caregivers by enhancing their sense of helpfulness and control (see Section 16).

Bereavement issues

Care provided to families during the course of a terminal illness has a profound influence on bereavement following death of the patient. All of the earlier cited suggestions for family support during illness will also influence subsequent bereavement. Positive bereavement outcomes result from a sense by family caregivers of having provided optimum care and relieved symptoms. The physical and psychological burdens of care giving may be relieved in part when family members feel that they were able to minimize the patient's distress and that the patient received appropriate professional care[9,12]. It is important that assessment of the family continue into the bereavement period, when physical symptoms can become apparent (see Section 19).

Ethical dilemmas encountered by family caregivers

An additional area of study is the ethical dilemmas associated with palliative care (see Section 5). The many ethical decisions and conflicts encountered by families may be in relation to the management of pain and other symptoms; initiation or withdrawing/withholding of treatments; medication management; physician relations; patient assessment; personal decisions; religious issues; balancing career and personal life; professional limitations; and nutrition and hydration[28].

Studies to date have identified the important role of family caregivers and their educational needs in assuming care for the person with cancer. Research has also begun to describe conflicts and burdens faced by caregivers. The impact of cancer care on caregivers, their ethical dilemmas and resultant distress, and their knowledge of pain management principles and techniques are areas for additional study[32,34].

Implications for future research

As care shifts into the home and family caregivers provide a greater extent of palliative care, research should also expand to understudied areas. It is important to evaluate outcomes of palliative care to include both patient and family caregivers. Outcomes should incorporate all aspects of quality of life including physical, psychological, social, and spiritual well-being (Fig. 15.3.1).

Opportunities exist to advance research collectively as a discipline and to strengthen clinical interventions for family caregivers in order to provide optimum support for these individuals and for families[19]. An example of family caregiver outcomes is the Quality of Life Questionnaire, Family Version and the Family Pain Questionnaire (questionnaires available on-line: http://prc.coh.org). The Quality of Life Questionnaire is a tool developed specifically for family caregivers, and is analogous to a questionnaire used to assess patients' quality of life[42]. This is an example of methodology that assesses the family caregiver's needs as distinct from those of the patient.

There is a need to extend family research beyond a single caregiver or beyond spouses alone. Clinical experience documents the impact of terminal care on all family members, yet the entire family unit, and particular individuals such as children, is seldom studied[43]. An effort to include family educational and supportive needs with chronic, progressive illnesses other than cancer is needed.

Future research should incorporate cost–benefit outcomes and include direct as well as indirect costs and the costs assumed by patients and families[44]. Cost measures are essential in the future restructuring of health care to establish the benefits of palliative care.

We have found important methodologic issues associated with conducting family research in pain management. Selection of instruments proves to be a constant challenge. A review of family literature revealed instruments frequently used in family caregiving research, including[45]:

1 Family APGAR (adaptation, partnership, growth, affection, resolved).

2 Family Pain Questionnaire.

3 Quality of Life - Caregiver.

4 Family communication tools.

5 Social support tools.

6 Family-functioning tools.

7 Care-giving demand assessments.

8 Caregiver burden instruments.

9 Barriers Questionnaire.

10 Instruments applied from patient outcomes (Coping, Anxiety).

11 Family Finances Survey.

12 Interview tools.

There is a need for rigorous work to develop or adapt instruments specific to the issues of family care giving and pain. Moreover, methodologic challenges exist when including family caregivers in pain research:

◆ Definition of family to determine who would be identified as a caregiver.

◆ Assessing individual versus family systems outcomes to ensure individual differences are measured.

◆ Distinguishing family caregiver response to illness versus pain since emotional responses often overlap.

◆ Distinguishing family versus patient outcomes to identify individual needs for education, management, and support.

◆ Assessing physical versus psychological or emotional burden and suffering.

◆ Use of qualitative methods to identify themes/concerns to help in gaining greater understanding of the caregiver role, and identification of issues in need of further investigation.

◆ Need for instruments that reflect the current reality of health care and responsibility of family caregivers.

◆ Determining the unit of analysis.

◆ Gaining access to family subjects when they are already experiencing time constraints due to increased patient care needs.

◆ Subject burden may complicate the measurement of needs, concerns, or physical symptoms.

◆ Assessing cultural meanings of family, religion, traditions, and ethnicity.

Sexuality and terminal illness

Sexuality is a critical issue to patients and their partners and yet it is often ignored within the context of palliative care. Sexuality encompasses not only sexual intercourse but also dimensions of intimacy, self-concept, and the expression of love, which is critical at this phase of life transition. Previous research has documented sexuality as a priority need of patients and family caregivers and that this need is often ignored[46]. Acts of intimacy and/or sexual intercourse have significant meaning during terminal illness, and are often important forms of communication during terminal illness. A failure to intervene with this equally important aspect of holistic care creates great distress for patients and their loved ones.

Sexuality can be addressed by first exploring with the patients their needs and assessment of physical or psychological issues associated with sexuality. Issues of sexuality are often examples of divergent needs between patients and family caregivers. Patients may have a continued or even stronger desire for sexual activity yet partners may be reluctant to reciprocate due to either fear of physical harm or avoidance of the intimacy with their loved one given the prognosis. Tension is best addressed by allowing both partners to express their feelings or concerns associated with illness or intimacy. There are also basic considerations such as a lack of privacy within institutional settings or physical changes such as altering the hospital bed so that both patient and partner can sleep together.

The first challenge is to facilitate communication with patient or partner regarding issues of sexuality and intimacy. We have found it useful within our Quality of Life Questionnaire, Family Version (available on-line: http://prc.coh.org) to ask questions regarding distress from illness and interference with relationships as ways to begin communication and lead on to more specific aspects of intimacy. This important need is also an example of where co-ordination of the palliative care team is important, to ensure that sexuality is assessed and services are routinely offered by a member of the team and that additional services by a sexual counsellor are available as needed.

Responding to the needs of the family

While the emotional problems facing patients and families are significant, there is much to be done to minimize the suffering of terminal illness. Palliative care programmes have demonstrated successful interventions to reduce the physical and emotional burdens of patients and families. Table 15.3.3 is a list of suggested interventions derived from the literature that serve as a guide to evaluate the adequacy of support in existing programmes as well as to guide interventions for individual families.

In order to meet the needs of the family, we must gain greater understanding and expertise in all aspects of both patient and family

Table 15.3.3 Suggested interventions to facilitate family coping with advanced illness.

1 **Communication:** Assess family communication patterns prior to and over the course of an illness

2 **Family relationships:** Acknowledge the relationship of the family member to the patient. Caregiving is significantly influenced by the distinct relationship (i.e. spouse, parent, child)

3 **Family developmental level:** Recognize the family's developmental level and its relationship to their coping with the illness. Family developmental crises (recent retirement, births, marriages, etc.), influence coping with illness. Assess whether multiple developmental crises are occurring

4 **Family conferences:** Establish mechanisms for conducting family conferences to facilitate shared communication between patient, family, and health care providers and to clarify changing goals of care

5 **Concurrent stressors:** Recognize areas of concurrent stress which may be unrelated to the patient or illness (i.e. job loss, stress in the extended family, coping with children)

6 **Financial concerns:** Provide counseling for the direct and indirect financial burdens associated with chronic illness

7 **Education:** Diminish caregiver's sense of helplessness by empowering them with knowledge and skills to enhance patient comfort (i.e. use of drug and non-drug modalities)

8 **Pain education:** Provide structured pain education to diffuse anxiety regarding issues such as addiction and tolerance

9 **Physical aspects of care:** Develop family education regarding the basic physical aspects of care giving (i.e. lifting, bathing, toileting)

10 **Encourage expression of fears and concerns:** Provide opportunities for family caregivers to express their emotions through individual or group support away from the patient

11 **Emotional strain:** Provide opportunities to verbalize the emotional strain inherent in care giving during terminal illness

12 **Risk for dysfunctional coping:** Identify families at risk for dysfunctional coping with terminal illness. Risk factors include families with poor communication patterns, prior history of family stress, and those with prior issues on non-compliance

13 **Issues of uncertainty:** Provide information regarding anticipated symptoms and discuss the distress associated with uncertainty

14 **The actual death:** Provide information regarding what to expect with the actual death event

15 **Sources of family support:** Evaluate and co-ordinate available sources of family support, i.e. social workers, spiritual support persons, clinical psychologists, psychiatrists, family counselling, peer support groups

care covered in the other sections of this text. Enhancing clinical skills in care of the patient automatically improves assessment of family issues since attention to the physical, psychological, social, and spiritual issues related to the patient can be translated to the assessment of the family. The interdisciplinary team approach is the key to assessing and responding to both patient and family needs. The reader is referred to Table 15.3.3 to for specific recommendations.

Summary

In summary, attention to family needs and concerns are an integral aspect of palliative care. Family care has been a cornerstone of the hospice philosophy and will remain so but such care demands professional support. A mother in our family research recently described having a child with cancer as 'being forced to watch your child dangled over a river'. She went on to say that having a child in pain, however, is like 'watching the child dropped into the river and drown'. Again, while experiencing terminal illness is a terrible event, and observing it perhaps even more so, the important lessons of palliative care demonstrate that much can be done to alleviate the suffering of both the patient and their family.

References

1. Ferrell, B.R., Ferrell, B.A., Rhiner, M. et al. (1991). Family factors influencing cancer pain management. *Post Graduate Medical Journal*, **67**(Suppl. 2), S64–9.

2. Glajchen, M. (2004). The emerging role and needs of family caregivers in cancer care. *The Journal of Supportive Oncology*, **2**, 145–55.

3. Egan, K.A. and Labyak, M.J. (2006). Hospice care. In *Textbook of Palliative Nursing* (eds. B.R. Ferrell and N. Coyle), pp. 13–46. Oxford University Press, New York.

4. Family caregiver alliance. Fact sheet: selected caregiver statistics. Available URL: http://www.caregiver.org/caregiver/jsp/content_node.jsp?nodeid=439. [Accessed September 18, 2006.]

5. Ferrell, B.R., Cohen, M.Z., Rhiner, M. et al. (1991). Pain as a metaphor for illness Part II: Family caregivers' management of pain. *Oncology Nursing Forum*, **18**, 1315–21.

6. Ferrell, B.R., Rhiner, M., Cohen, M.Z. et al. (1991). Pain as a metaphor for illness Part I: Impact of cancer pain on family caregivers. *Oncology Nursing Forum*, **18**, 1303–9.

7. Spillman, B.C. and Pezzin, L.E. (2000). Potential and active caregivers: changing networks and the "sandwich generation." *Milbank Quarterly*, **78**, 347–74.

8. Phipps, E. et al. (2003). Family care giving for patients at life's end: report from the cultural variations study (CVAS). *Palliative and Supportive Care*, **1**, 165–70.

9. Schulz, R. and Beach, S.R. (1999). Caregiving as a risk factor for mortality: the Caregiver Health Effects Study. *The Journal of the American Medical Association*, **282**, 2215–9.

10. Navaie-Waliser, M. et al. (2002). When the caregiver needs care: the plight of vulnerable caregivers. *American Journal of Public Health*, **92**, 409–13.

11. Northouse, L.L., Walker, J., Schafenacker, A. et al. (2002). A family-based program of care for women with recurrent breast cancer and their family members. *Oncology Nursing Forum*, **29**, 1411–9.

12. Haley, W.E., LaMonde, L.A., Han, B. et al. (2001). Family caregiving in hospice: effects on psychological and health functioning among spousal caregivers of hospice patients with lung cancer or dementia. *The Hospice Journal*, **15**, 1–18.

13. Emanuel, E.J., Fairclough, D.L., Slutsman, J. et al. (1999). Assistance from family members, friends, paid care givers, and volunteers in the care of terminally ill patients. *The New England Journal of Medicine*, **341**, 956–63.

14. Field, M.J. and Cassel, C.K. (1997). *Approaching Death: Improving Care at the End of Life* (Report of the Institute of Medicine Task Force). National Academy Press, Washington, DC.

15. Ferrell, B.R., Rhiner, M., Shapiro, B. et al. (1994). The experience of paediatric cancer pain, Part I: impact of pain on the family. *Journal of Paediatric Nursing*, **9**, 368–79.

16. Goetschius, S.K. (2001). Caring for families: the other patient in palliative care. In *Palliative Care Nursing: Quality Care to the End of Life* (eds. M.L. Matzo and D.W. Sherman), pp. 245–74. Springer Publishing Company, Inc., New York.

17. Johnson Taylor, E. (2006). Spiritual assessment. In *Textbook of Palliative Nursing* (eds. B.R. Ferrell and N. Coyle), pp. 581–94. Oxford University Press, New York.

18. Given, B.A., Given, C.W., and Kozachik, S. (2001). Family support in advanced cancer. *CA: A Cancer Journal for Clinicians*, **51**, 213–31.

19. Ferrell, B., Virani, R., and Grant, M. (1999). Analysis of end-of-life content in nursing textbooks. *Oncology Nursing Forum*, **26**, 869–76.

20. American Association of Colleges of Nursing and City of Hope National Medical Center (2000). *End of life nursing education consortium (ELNEC)*. http://www.aacn.nche.edu/ELNEC (20 August, 2006).

21. Glajchen, M. (2003). Caregiver burden and pain control. In *Cancer Pain* (eds. R. Portenoy and E. Bruera), Cambridge University Press, New York.

22. McMillan, S.C., Small, B.J., Weitzner, M. *et al.* (2006). Impact of coping skills intervention with family caregivers of hospice patients with cancer. *Cancer*, **106**, 214–22.

23. Cameron, J.I., Franche, R.L., Cheung, A.M. *et al.* (2002). Lifestyle interference and emotional distress in family caregivers of advanced cancer patients. *Cancer*, **94**, 521–7.

24. Wong, R.K.S., Franssen, E., Szumacher, E. *et al.* (2002). What do patients living with advanced cancer and their carers want to know? A needs assessment. *Supportive Care in Cancer*, **10**, 408–15.

25. Spross, J., McGuire, D., Schmitt, R. (1991). Oncology Nursing Society position paper on cancer pain. *Oncology Nursing Forum*, **17**, 595–614, 751–60, 943–4.

26. Scott, L.D. (2001). Technological caregiving: a qualitative perspective. *Home Health Care Management and Practice*, **13**, 227–35.

27. Schumacher, K.L. *et al.* (2000). Family caregiving skill: development of the concept. *Research in Nursing and Health*, **23**, 191–203d.

28. Ferrell, B.R., Johnson Taylor, E., Grant, M. *et al.* (1993). Pain management at home: struggle, comfort and mission. *Cancer Nursing*, **16**, 169–78.

29. Grobe, M.E., Ilstrup, E.M., and Ahmann, D.L. (1990). Skills needed by family members to maintain the care of an advanced cancer patient. *Cancer Nursing*, **4**, 371–5.

30. Tringali, C.A. (1986). The needs of family members of cancer patients. *Oncology Nursing Forum*, **13**, 65–9.

31. Flor, H., Turk, D.C., Scholz, O.B. (1987). Impact of chronic pain on the spouse: marital, emotional and physical consequences. *Journal of Psychosomatic Research*, **31**, 63–71.

32. Davies, B. (2006). Supporting families in palliative care. In *Textbook of Palliative Nursing* (eds. B.R. Ferrell and N. Coyle), pp. 545–60. Oxford University Press, New York.

33. Kristjanson, L.J., Leis, A., Koop, P. *et al.* (1997). Family members' care expectations, care perceptions, and satisfaction with advanced cancer care: results of a multi-site pilot study. *Journal of Palliative Care*, **13**, 5–13.

34. Lewis, F.M. (1986). The impact of cancer on the family: a critical analysis of the research literature. *Patient Education and Counselling*, **8**, 269–89.

35. Borneman, T., Chu, D.Z., Wagman, L. *et al.* (2003). Concerns of family caregivers of patients with cancer facing palliative surgery for advanced malignancies. *Oncology Nursing Forum*, **30**, 997–1005.

36. Chao, S.Y. and Roth, P. (2000). The experiences of Taiwanese women caring for parents-in-law. *Journal of Advanced Nursing*, **31**, 631–8.

37. Kinsella, G., Cooper, B., Picton, C. *et al.* (2000). Factors influencing outcomes for family caregivers of persons receiving palliative care. *Journal of Palliative Care*, **16**, 46–54.

38. Hinton, J. (1981). Sharing or withholding awareness of dying between husband and wife. *Journal of Psychosomatic Research*, **25**, 337–43.

39. Ferrell, B.R., Ferrell, B.A., Ahn, C. *et al.* (1994). Pain management for elderly patients with cancer at home. *Cancer*, **74**, 2139–46.

40. Montbriand, M.J. (1994). An overview of alternate therapies chosen by patients with cancer. *Oncology Nursing Forum*, **21**, 1547–54.

41. Berenson, S. (2006). Complementary and alternative therapies chosen by patients with cancer. In *Textbook of Palliative Nursing* (eds. B.R.Ferrell and N. Coyle), pp. 491–509. Oxford University Press, New York.

42. Ferrell, B.R., Grant, M., Chan, J. *et al.* (1995). The impact of cancer pain education on family caregivers of elderly patients. *Oncology Nursing Forum*, **22**, 1211–8.

43. Rhiner, M., Ferrell, B.R., Shapiro, B. *et al.* (1994). The experience of paediatric cancer pain, Part II: management of pain. *Journal of Paediatric Nursing*, **9**, 380–7.

44. Ferrell, B.R. (1995). How patients and families pay the price. *Proceedings of the Bristol Pain Symposium* — Johns Hopkins University, IASP Press.

45. Ferrell, B.R. (2001). Pain observed: the experience of pain from the family caregiver's perspective. *Clinics in Geriatric Medicine*, **17**, 595–609.

46. Lamb, M.A. (2006). Sexuality. In *Textbook of Palliative Nursing* (eds. B.R. Ferrell and N. Coyle), pp. 421–28. Oxford University Press, New York.

15.4

The stress of professional caregivers

Liz Jamieson, Emma Teasdale,
Alison Richardson, and Amanda Ramirez

Many different health professionals care for patients in the last years of their life—in the community, in hospitals, in hospices, care homes, and other institutions. Some health professionals devote the whole of their working time to palliative care, while for many it forms only a small part of their formal workload. Working with patients who have incurable disease and those who are dying exposes professionals to the physical, psychological, and spiritual suffering of patients, as well as the grief of carers and relatives. The deterioration and death of particular patients, such as those who are young or those with whom the professional identifies, can be particularly distressing. Working with people who are dying may also force professionals to face their own mortality[1]. Whilst caring for those with incurable disease and who are dying can be very demanding, it can equally be a source of great professional satisfaction. Because providing palliative care involves often intense experiences of caring, it is important to examine how this work might impact on the mental health of professional caregivers.

Further challenges for palliative care professionals include the broadening remit of their services to include end-of-life care for people with various life threatening conditions beyond cancer including dementia, AIDS, cardiac, respiratory and renal failure[2]. Palliative care services as a whole face the challenge of an increasing population of those living with cancer as survival from cancer continues to improve. Alongside this, there are rising patient expectations of access to palliative care services at the end of life.

The widening remit for palliative care services to non-cancer patients, and to greater numbers of patients in general, has contributed to palliative care now increasingly being delivered in a diverse range of settings, including home care, hospices, and hospitals. These different settings are likely to affect a palliative care professional's job-related stress or satisfaction. Many hospices are partly or entirely charitably funded and hospice-based palliative care professionals may therefore experience different levels of stress arising from the managerial and financial aspects of their work compared with those working in hospitals. Acute palliative care units focus to a greater extent on symptom management than on care of the dying. In these units, the nature of the patient relationship with staff may be more transient as length of stay is shorter and patients who are not immediately dying may be transferred to nursing homes or be sent home[3].

Understanding and eliciting patient preferences for place of care and death presents another challenge for palliative care staff. In the UK, well over 50 per cent of patients would choose to die at home[4] yet in many countries, including the UK, hospitals are the places where most people come to the end of life. In the UK, the proportion of home deaths for patients with cancer fell from 27 per cent in 1994 to 22 per cent in 2001[5].

The motivation and personal qualities of people providing palliative care may influence their mental health. Many of those who choose to work in palliative care do so because of a deep compassion for the suffering of the dying, coupled with an altruistic desire to help others[6]. Being open to pain and suffering may nevertheless increase their vulnerability to experiencing poor mental health. For some palliative care professionals, a strong spiritual element underpins their work. Less altruistic motives may also draw people to work with the dying. People may be attracted to palliative care in order to heal their own wounds sustained in childhood or adulthood by supporting others through their pain and are thus considered to be 'wounded healers'[7].

This chapter describes the levels of poor mental health experienced by palliative care professionals, as well as the risk factors and consequences of that poor mental health. Approaches and strategies for optimizing the well-being of palliative care professionals are also outlined.

Levels of mental health in palliative care professionals

The study of poor mental health among palliative care professionals has focused on both psychiatric morbidity, defined as a severe pervasive psychological distress, including clinically important anxiety and depression likely to benefit from a psychological intervention, and burnout defined as more specific work-related distress. Psychiatric morbidity is conventionally estimated by the General Health Questionnaire (GHQ)[8], a self-administered screening tool that detects common non-psychotic potential psychiatric morbidity and has been validated against a clinical psychiatric interview. Different versions of the GHQ are available with different cut-off points (representing 'caseness') where individuals are said to be suffering a level of psychiatric morbidity for which professional intervention is usually warranted.

Burnout is a less well-validated syndrome described as comprising emotional exhaustion (feeling emotionally overextended by work), depersonalization (an unfeeling and impersonal response towards people), and reduced personal accomplishment (feelings of competence and achievement at work) that can occur among individuals who work with people in some capacity[9]. The Maslach Burnout Inventory (MBI)[10] is the gold-standard measure for burnout and consists of emotional exhaustion, depersonalization, and personal accomplishment subscales. High scores in the emotional exhaustion or depersonalization scales, or low scores in the personal accomplishment scale, indicate high levels of burnout.

The mental health of palliative physicians has been examined in a number of robust studies. A UK questionnaire-based study of the mental health of over 1000 consultants found that about a quarter of consultant palliative physicians reported psychiatric morbidity using the GHQ, a level similar to that found among hospital consultants including cancer consultants (medical, surgical and clinical oncologists) as well as gastroenterologists and radiologists[11,12]. The levels of psychiatric morbidity among palliative medicine doctors in training in the UK are also estimated at a quarter using the GHQ and again similar to those found among trainee clinical and medical oncologists[13]. UK palliative physicians do however report lower levels of burnout compared with hospital consultants including emotional exhaustion, depersonalization, and personal accomplishment[11]. Palliative care consultants in Australia experience similar levels of psychiatric morbidity and burnout compared to UK colleagues[14], whilst a small study with a low response rate suggests that palliative physicians in Japan experience lower levels of both psychiatric morbidity and burnout compared with clinical oncologists[15].

There has been less robust work examining the psychiatric morbidity of nurses. However, findings from studies that do exist indicate that levels of psychiatric morbidity in palliative care and hospice nurses are similar to those of nurses working in other specialities, including home care nurses, health visitors, nurses working with patients with learning disabilities, and those working in hospitals[16–18].

Studies examining the mental health of nurses have focused more on burnout and suggest that hospice nurses experience lower levels of burnout compared with hospital nurses. Specifically, levels of emotional exhaustion and depersonalization appear to be consistently lower among hospice nurses compared with medical, surgical, and intensive care nurses[19]. However, levels of personal accomplishment tend to be fairly similar across all those nursing groups.

Interestingly, the levels of poor mental health of chaplains working within hospices in the United Kingdom appears similar to that of palliative care physicians, with approximately one quarter found to have identifiable psychiatric morbidity using the GHQ[20].

Overall, palliative care professionals appear to experience similar or somewhat better mental health when compared to other health professionals. Specifically, palliative care professionals experience similar levels of psychiatric morbidity and less burnout than other health professionals according to recent, robust studies[11,13,19]. These findings are supported in earlier, smaller studies[22].

Consequences of poor mental health among palliative care professionals

Whilst the levels of estimated psychiatric morbidity and burnout among palliative care professionals is not high compared with other health professionals; one quarter of palliative physicians, for example, report symptoms indicating psychiatric morbidity. This poor mental health among palliative care professionals is of concern because it involves the personal suffering of individual members of staff and their families, and also because it may compromise the quality of care they are able to deliver to patients and carers.

Doctors with poor mental health are more likely to lack empathy and to have poor communication skills[12,23]. They are also more likely to report being irritable with patients and colleagues as well as to report impaired clinical performance, including medical errors and adverse events[24,25]. Consultants with psychiatric morbidity are twice as likely to report drinking hazardous levels of alcohol and to report their intention to retire early[25]. They are also more likely to take long-term sick leave[26] and to be at greater risk of suicide than the general population, with female physicians having more elevated suicide rates than male physicians according to a meta-analysis based on the world literature[27].

There is less robust evidence for the consequences of poor mental health among nurses. A review by Lu *et al*[28]. found that research from various countries suggests that job satisfaction is a significant predictor of nursing absenteeism, burnout, turnover, and intention to quit. Sickness rates among nurses are two to three times higher than those among doctors. Other studies examining the consequences of poor mental health in nurses have focused on the importance of the nursing role on patient experience. One large hospital survey based on the report of patients and nurses found that patients cared for on units where nursing staff felt burnt out or frequently expressed an intention to quit were less satisfied with the various components of their care. Patients on units where nurses found their work meaningful were more satisfied with all aspects of their hospital stay[29].

A framework for understanding poor mental health among palliative care professionals

Understanding the factors that influence the mental health of palliative care professionals may help to explain why they experience lower levels of burnout compared with their hospital colleagues. It may be that health professionals with better mental health choose to work in palliative care. It is also possible that the approach or culture of palliative care protects those working in the specialty from the work-related distress experienced by doctors and nurses working in other specialties. Fig. 15.4.1 shows an evidence-based framework for understanding poor mental health among health-care professionals. Much of the evidence for the framework derives from studies of senior doctors[12,30]. The framework is based on an interactional model of stress[22], according to which the stresses inherent in providing health care precipitate burnout and psychiatric morbidity in those who are psychologically vulnerable. Previous psychiatric history, family psychiatric history, childhood experience of illness, death, and

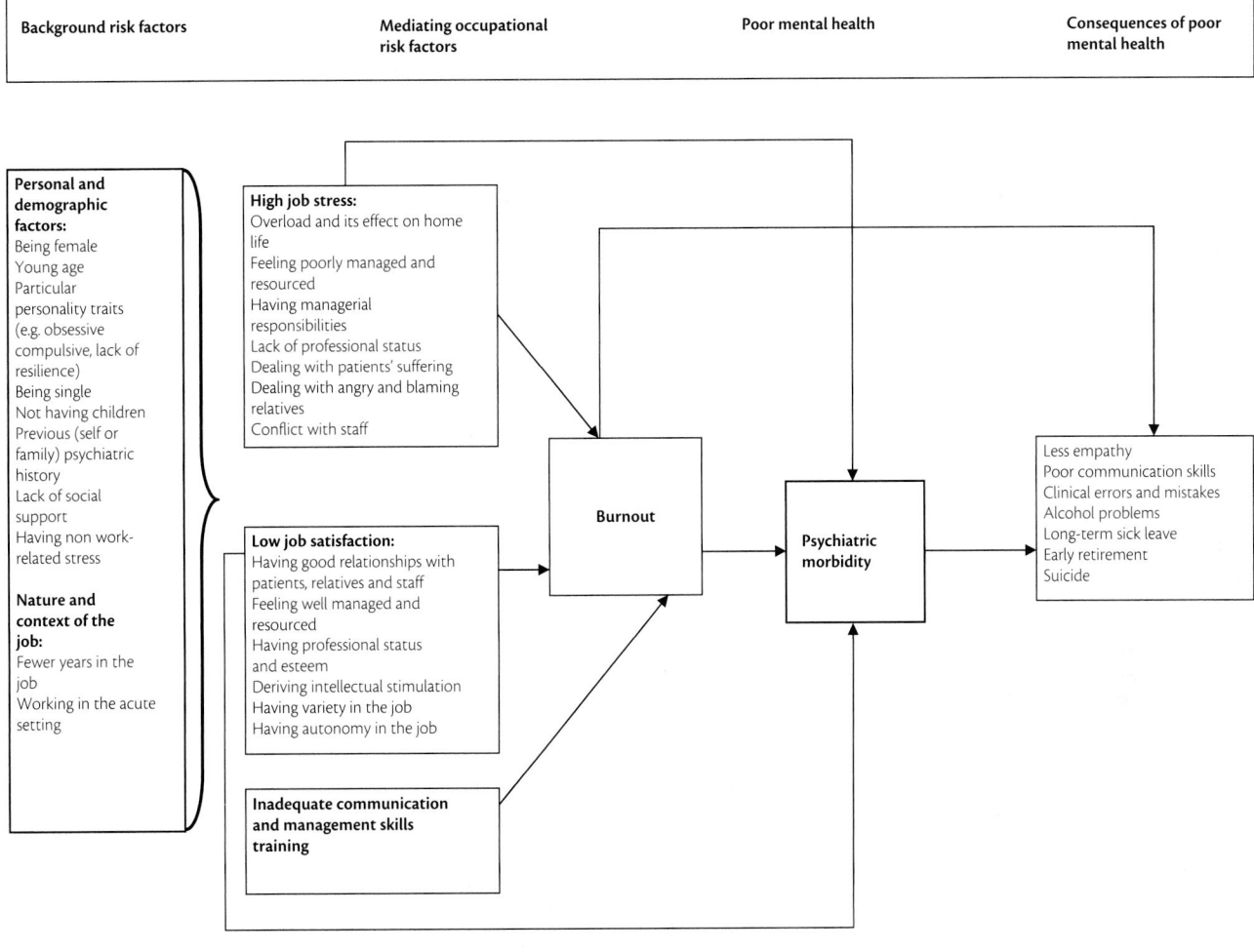

| Background risk factors | Mediating occupational risk factors | Poor mental health | Consequences of poor mental health |

Personal and demographic factors:
Being female
Young age
Particular personality traits (e.g. obsessive compulsive, lack of resilience)
Being single
Not having children
Previous (self or family) psychiatric history
Lack of social support
Having non work-related stress

Nature and context of the job:
Fewer years in the job
Working in the acute setting

High job stress:
Overload and its effect on home life
Feeling poorly managed and resourced
Having managerial responsibilities
Lack of professional status
Dealing with patients' suffering
Dealing with angry and blaming relatives
Conflict with staff

Low job satisfaction:
Having good relationships with patients, relatives and staff
Feeling well managed and resourced
Having professional status and esteem
Deriving intellectual stimulation
Having variety in the job
Having autonomy in the job

Inadequate communication and management skills training

Burnout

Psychiatric morbidity

Less empathy
Poor communication skills
Clinical errors and mistakes
Alcohol problems
Long-term sick leave
Early retirement
Suicide

Figure 15.4.1 Framework for understanding poor mental health among health professionals.

emotional neglect, lack of social support, and personality traits have all been described as vulnerability factors for poor mental health among doctors and nurses.

Precipitating occupational risk factors for poor mental health among health professionals include high levels of stress at work. High levels of job stress increase the risk of burnout and psychiatric morbidity. Conversely, job satisfaction has been shown to protect the mental health of consultants against the adverse effects of job stress[12,30]. So for any reported level of job stress, those consultants with low job satisfaction experience worse mental health than those with high job satisfaction. Adequacy of training appears to influence the mental health of consultants. In particular, feeling insufficiently trained in communication skills and management skills increases the risk of burnout[12]. These precipitating risk factors need to be understood in the wider context of the individual's demographic characteristics and the nature of the job they are doing and the context in which they are working.

Sources of job stress

Typically, lower levels of job stress have been reported among palliative care professionals compared to other health professionals[16,21,31]. The main sources of job stress reported by palliative care professionals include organizational stressors (e.g. overload, management, resources); patient-related stressors

(e.g. dealing with illness and dying), and work relationships (e.g. conflict with staff).

Organizational stressors
Overload

Feeling overloaded at work and the effect this has on home life was found to be a predominant source of job stress for UK palliative physicians[21]. Similarly, 'being over stretched at times', and 'the effect of hours of work on personal life' were shown to be frequently reported stressors by palliative physicians in training[13]. Nevertheless, compared to other hospital consultants, palliative physicians tend to experience significantly less stress from feeling overloaded at work[21].

Workload and the discordance between work and family obligations have also been found to be significant sources of stress for palliative care nurses[18,32,33]. As was evident in palliative physicians, palliative care nurses tend to experience less stress related to work overload than other nurse specialities such as medical-surgical nurses[31], nurses caring for people with learning disabilities[17], and district nurses, ward nurses, health visitors, and midwives[16].

Feeling poorly managed and resourced

Feeling that they are poorly managed and resourced has also been reported as a source of job stress for palliative physicians.

However, when compared to other hospital consultants, these issues are less stressful for palliative physicians[12,21].

Similarly, palliative care nurses were found to report higher levels of management support compared to home care nurses, ward nurses, and midwives[16], and higher satisfaction with their supervision compared to nurses caring for people with learning disabilities[18].

Having managerial responsibilities

Both palliative care physicians and other hospital consultants have reported similar levels of job stress from having managerial responsibilities[12, 21].

Low prestige

Feelings of low prestige regarding their specialty or feeling under-utilized were rated more highly as a source of stress by palliative care physicians in training than by clinical or medical oncologists in training. Similarly, a lack of recognition of their role by other members of staff was found as a major source of stress in chaplains working in palliative care[20].

Patient stressors

Dealing with patients' suffering, death, and dying

Perhaps surprisingly, dealing with patients' suffering, death and dying have not been identified as predominant sources of job stress among doctors working in palliative care. Indeed, both palliative physicians and other hospital consultants have reported similar levels of stress in relation to dealing with patients' suffering. However, palliative physicians report significantly less stress than hospital consultants specifically from working with patients who have incurable disease[12,21]. Similarly, palliative physicians in training report less stress in dealing with death and dying than trainees in medical or clinical oncology[13].

It is probable that caring for patients with incurable disease presents palliative physicians with the opportunity to fulfil their role in regard to pain management and symptom control. This differs from the role of consultants in acute hospitals, whose primary aim is to cure patients, and so may therefore experience a greater sense of failure if they can no longer offer any treatment to a patient.

Conversely, palliative care nurses have reported that their stress is primarily associated with dealing with death and dying[17,19]. Furthermore there is evidence to suggest that nurses from other specialties such as medicine, surgery, cardiovascular surgery and oncology also find dealing with patient death and dying stressful[32]. However, it is not clear whether palliative care nurses feel less stress than other nurses from dealing with death and dying. In the US palliative care nurses and intensive care nurses were found to report significantly more stress in relation to dealing with death and dying than medical/surgical nurses[31]. However, further research from the UK and US has indicated that palliative care nurses tend to report lower stress in relation to dealing with death and dying than oncology, coronary and critical care nurses[18,34].

Dealing with death and dying becomes particularly stressful for palliative care nurse specialists when the patient is young, when the nurse has formed a close relationship with the patient, or when several deaths occur in a short space of time[3,16]. Problems of attachment to dying patients and the inherently different nature of the nurse–patient relationship may explain why palliative care nurses find this more stressful than palliative physicians.

Communicating with patients and their families

Palliative physicians reported significantly less stress than hospital consultants from aspects of work involving communicating with patients and relatives in difficult situations, including 'having to deal with distressed, angry or blaming relatives' and 'having to break bad news to patients and their relatives'[21]. However, this difference was not found among trainee doctors in palliative medicine and clinical and medical oncology, who reported that the second most common stressful event was 'communicating with patients and families' and 'breaking bad news' when asked to describe a recent stressful event[13].

Work relationships
Conflict with other staff

Conflict with other staff appears to be a significant stressor for palliative care professionals. In particular, for UK palliative physicians 'encountering difficulties in relationships with nurses' was the only aspect of work which they rated more highly as a source of stress than other hospital consultants[21]. Also palliative doctors in training were found to have higher stress levels in regard to 'difficult relations with nursing staff' when compared to clinical and medical oncologist trainees[13].

In relation to nursing staff from various specialties, 'conflict with other staff' has been shown to be a significant stressor[32]. In a study of hospice palliative care nurses, conflict with other staff made the greatest overall contribution to the levels of burnout they experienced[19].

The higher level of stress from conflict with other staff experienced by palliative physicians compared to consultants from other specialties may result from a lack of clarity in the roles of consultants and senior nurses in hospice palliative care, since historically some (charitably-funded) hospices were run by nurse-matrons. Finlay[35] found that hospice medical directors reported their most stressful relationship was with 'matrons'. Hospice matrons described that their most stressful relationships were with home care nurses and other nurses generally. Role ambiguity, when an individual experiences a lack of clarity about the scope and responsibilities of his/her role and about colleagues' expectations of the role, has been reported as a major source of stress among staff working in a variety of occupations. Addressing this difficulty in palliative care may protect against burnout.

Sources of job satisfaction

Typically, research has focused on sources of job stress for palliative care professionals rather than sources of job satisfaction. Nevertheless, there is some evidence that palliative physicians and nurses have significantly higher levels of job satisfaction compared to consultants or nurses working in other specialities[16,18,21,32]. The main sources of job satisfaction reported by palliative care professionals relate to relationships with patients and relatives, management, resources and autonomy.

Having good relationships with patients, relatives and staff

Having good relationships with patients, relatives and staff is a predominant source of job satisfaction for UK palliative physicians. Furthermore, in comparison to other physicians, palliative physicians report higher levels of satisfaction from having good relationships[12,21]. Similarly, in the US, focus groups of palliative care staff reported that contact with dying patients and their families was a major source of job satisfaction[36].

Having personal relationships with patients and their families and experiencing positive feedback from the family regarding care were the greatest sources of job satisfaction among palliative care nurses[16,37].

Well managed and resourced

Being managed well and having good resources has been found to contribute more to palliative physicians' job satisfaction compared with other hospital consultants[21].

Having professional status and esteem and deriving intellectual stimulation

Palliative physicians and other hospital consultants report that they derive similar levels of job satisfaction from their professional status and esteem and opportunities for intellectual stimulation[21].

Having autonomy and variety in the job

The most highly rated sources of job satisfaction among consultants generally are having high levels of autonomy and variety in the job[12,21]. Interestingly, UK palliative physicians report more satisfaction than hospital consultants from having a high level of autonomy.

Managing symptoms and dying

Palliative care doctors reported more satisfaction than other consultants from helping patients through controlling their symptoms and managing death and dying well[21]. Not surprisingly, the one aspect of work that was rated more highly by the other consultants was 'helping patients through curing disease'[21].

Training and support

Eighty-one per cent of UK palliative physicians have reported that they feel insufficiently trained in management skills and over a third felt that they had received inadequate training in communication skills. Burnout was more prevalent among consultants who felt insufficiently trained in communication and management skills than among those who felt sufficiently trained[21]. Similarly, management training was highlighted by one quarter of UK Macmillan nurses as a necessary requirement to improve training on dealing with work stress[16]. Lack of staff support and lack of involvement in decision-making has also been associated with poor mental health in nurses[18].

Individual risk factors

Demographics

Gender

Female palliative physicians have been shown to experience a significantly higher prevalence of psychiatric morbidity (38 per cent) than male palliative physicians (16 per cent). However, no gender difference in levels of burnout or sources of job stress and satisfaction were found[21]. The lack of any gender differences in levels of burnout and sources of job stress and satisfaction provides no evidence that the difference arises directly from work.

This gender difference in psychiatric morbidity has also been found among hospital consultants and NHS managers but not other staff such as nurses, radiographers, technical/laboratory staff, and administrative staff[38]. It seems, therefore, that it is not being female per se, which is a risk factor, but being female in particular jobs, namely medicine and management, where NHS culture and hierarchies may have a more adverse impact on women than men[39].

Age

Younger palliative physicians and hospice staff (including nurses, social workers, and administrative staff) in the US have been found to report higher degrees of burnout[40,41].

Similarly, in Australia, younger age has been associated with higher depersonalization and an increased risk of emotional exhaustion in palliative doctors[14]. In UK consultants, young age (being under 55 years) or fewer years in post as a consultant have also been shown to be risk factors for burnout[12,42].

Marital status and dependants

Being single was an independent risk factor for burnout among UK hospital consultants including palliative physicians[11].

Personality and resilience

Some individuals possess personal characteristics, which make them resilient to the effects of stress. Among the personal characteristics that have been suggested as having this function are a *hardy personality*[43] and an ability to perceive one's world as meaningful and manageable, or *sense of coherence*[44].

Individuals who have a hardy personality exhibit tendencies believed to be very useful in coping with stressful events. These tendencies include a commitment to oneself and the areas in one's life, including work, so that there is meaning and purpose; a sense of control, a belief that one has the power to influence the course of events; and a sense of challenge in the face of change, regarding change as an opportunity for growth and development. Similarly, individuals with a sense of coherence feel they have the external and internal resources to meet any demands and see such demands as worthy challenges.

Nevertheless, whilst such personality attributes are likely to influence mental health, personality is a difficult construct to measure. Consequently, few robust studies have examined the relationship between personality and poor mental health in health-care professionals in general or specifically in palliative care professionals.

Culture of niceness

Being nice or good is seen as a central value in palliative care[3]. Palliative care professionals work extremely hard to provide high quality care for their patients and patients' relatives so that the dying patient can achieve a 'good' or 'nice' death. Being nice is a joint activity between caregivers and patients, which involves a friendly and informal approach. This may include polite greetings, exchanging pleasantries, talking about mundane things like the weather, cracking a joke, or sharing a sense of humour[45]. Such reciprocal relationships can be rewarding and therapeutic as they serve to distance and ameliorate any problems occurring in the worlds of the palliative care nurses and their patients.

Nevertheless, whilst there is no doubt that palliative caregivers are caring and dedicated people, this drive towards being nice has the potential to encourage an unhealthy culture of 'chronic niceness'[46]. Within such a culture, the negative aspects of caring daily for the dying tend to be ignored. This is disadvantageous as staff may feel unable to criticise the team or the support they receive in any way. As such, issues are not dealt with appropriately and stress can arise as palliative care professionals may feel unable to provide the high standard of care they desire[3].

Stress from outside of work

Stress arising from aspects of life outside of work has been found to be associated with poor mental health in health-care professionals.

In particular, NHS staff (including nurses, doctors, and ancillary staff) who had experienced a severe life event outside of work (e.g. death of a loved one, bankruptcy) in the previous year were more likely to experience poor mental health[47].

Different settings and patient groups

Palliative care is increasingly being delivered in a diverse range of settings, including home care, hospices, and hospitals. It is likely that these differing work environments may impact upon palliative care professionals' job stress or satisfaction in different ways.

Few studies have examined the sources of stress and poor mental health of palliative care professionals working in different settings. In the UK, hospice-based palliative physicians typically reported feeling better managed and resourced than hospital-based palliative physicians[21].

The nature of the patient group with which palliative care professionals are working may have also impact on their mental health. There is evidence to suggest that health-care professionals, in general, working with AIDS/HIV patients experience similar levels of poor mental health as health-care professionals working with cancer patients[48]. Nevertheless, this not been replicated with palliative care professionals.

Summary of risk factors for poor mental health

Being female and being younger have been highlighted as particular risk factors for poor mental health among senior doctors generally. The relative youth and high proportion of females among palliative physicians compared with consultants in other specialties should increase their risk of burnout, yet this does not appear to be the case. These demographic characteristics, therefore, do not adequately explain why palliative care professionals experience similar levels of psychiatric morbidity and less burnout compared with other health professionals.

Overall, palliative care professionals tend to experience lower job stress and higher job satisfaction than other health-care professionals. Typically, palliative care professionals tend to experience significantly less stress from feeling overloaded at work (the most predominant source of job stress for health-care professionals). Palliative care professionals also report less stress from dealing with fatal illness and death than other health-care professionals. Patients with incurable disease present opportunities to palliative care professionals to fulfil their role through pain management and symptom control, and through addressing psychosocial problems. In contrast, health-care professionals working in acute hospital-based specialties, in which the aims of treatment are to cure disease and prolong life, may experience a sense of failure with such patients through having nothing more to offer them.

Job satisfaction is important to mental health and has been shown to have a moderating impact on the relationship between job stress and both burnout and psychiatric morbidity in hospital consultants[12]. In particular, palliative care professionals report higher satisfaction than other health-care professionals from having good relationships with patients and relatives (the most predominant source of job satisfaction for health-care professionals). In addition, palliative care professionals report less stress and more satisfaction in relation to the way they are managed and resourced, as well as more satisfaction from having a high level of autonomy. Karasek[49] has shown that the amount of control an individual has over his/her work can influence mental health. For individuals working in jobs with high demands, such as health-care professionals, high levels of control and autonomy over work are particularly important in protecting against the harmful effects of stress. It is therefore likely that higher job satisfaction, particularly in relation to having good relationships with patients and having autonomy at work, explains why palliative care professionals typically experience less burnout.

There is some suggestion that job stress increases and job satisfaction decreases as palliative care moves into acute hospital settings[21]. Hospices are typically well resourced in comparison to acute hospital settings, and hospice-based palliative care professionals generally feel better managed.

Approaches to improving the mental health of palliative care professionals

Maintaining and improving professional caregivers' mental health is essential for their own well-being and for the quality of care they provide to patients and carers. This suggests the need to find ways to reduce the stress and maintain or improve the satisfaction that palliative care professionals experience from their work.

Strategies to reduce the risk of poor mental health among professional caregivers

Management and resources

Work overload and its disruptive effect on home life is the predominant aspect of job stress for palliative care professionals, and having good relationships with patients and relatives is the greatest source of job satisfaction. Palliative care professionals also derive great satisfaction from working autonomously and feeling well managed and resourced. Clearly, it is necessary to maintain existing levels of resources within palliative medicine, particularly with regard to human resources (workforce), so that high quality patient care can be delivered.

Training

The large proportion of palliative physicians who considered that they had received insufficient training in communication and management skills, have been shown to be at increased risk of burnout[11]. This underlies the need for more effective training in communication and management skills as an integral part of the undergraduate and postgraduate curricula for palliative medicine. This will ensure optimal patient care, as well as reduce the likelihood of poor mental health among professional caregivers.

Training in effective team working is also likely to be important in protecting the mental health of professional carers. The sense of belonging to an effective team has been shown to be an important coping mechanism in palliative care workers[50]. Training in effective team work has also been shown to be related to improved mental health in hospital-based health-care teams[51], reduced sickness absence in physicians[26] and increased job satisfaction in nurses[52].

Supervision and support

Effective clinical supervision is likely to promote the maintenance of core clinical skills among professional caregivers and thereby enhance clinical practice. In turn, such supervision is likely to benefit not only patients, but also professional caregivers. Such supervision should address the physical, psychological, social, spiritual, and communication dimensions of patient care. Such effective clinical supervision should be made available and individuals should be encouraged to regularly attend[3].

Typically, palliative physicians in training who were satisfied with the level of support they received experienced less job stress[13]. Similarly, lack of staff support was associated with poor mental health in hospice nurses[18]. Most UK hospices offer some means of formal support to staff, usually a combination of group and individual support, but only infrequently did hospices involve a psychologist, psychiatrist, or counselling service[53].

Managing poor mental health of professional caregivers

It is important to provide a confidential mental health service to which palliative care professionals can be referred to in order to manage any significant mental health problems. For independent hospices it may be important to have assessments carried out at another institution in order to preserve confidentiality, as concern over confidentiality is likely to be a barrier to palliative care professionals accessing such services[19,54]. Indeed, one large cancer treatment centre has developed a model known as the 3 Cs: complementary therapies, clinical supervision, and provision of confidential counselling separate from the organization[55].

Summary

Providing effective training in communication skills, management skills, and team-working alongside effective clinical supervision is likely to reduce the risk of poor mental health among palliative care professionals. In addition, existing levels of resourcing and management practices within palliative medicine should be, at the very least, maintained if not improved to ensure that palliative care professionals are able to provide care to patients without jeopardizing their own mental health.

The provision of a confidential mental health service for all staff that is independent of management and that offers support in managing both personal and work-related problems is another key component in improving the mental health of those working in palliative care.

References

1. Nash, A. (1989). A terminal case? Burnout in palliative care. *Professional Nurse*, 4(9), 443–4.
2. Addington-Hall, J.M. and Higginson, I. (2001). *Palliative care for non-cancer patients*. Oxford University Press, Oxford.
3. Aranda, S. (2004). Cost of caring. In *Palliative care nursing: Principles and evidence for practice* (edited. S. Payne, J. Seymour, and C. Ingleton), Chapter 32, pp. 620–35. Open University Press.
4. Higginson, I. and Sen-Gupta, G. (2000). Place of care in advanced cancer: A qualitative systematic review of patient preferences. *J Pall Med*, 3, 287–300.
5. Gomes, B. and Higginson, I. (2004). Home or hospital? Choices at the end of life. *J Royal Soc Med*, 97, 413–4.
6. Rokach, A. (2005). Caring for those who care for the dying: Coping with the demands on palliative care workers. *Palliative and Supportive Care*, 3, 325–32.
7. Mason, C. (2002). Basic themes. In *Journeys into palliative care: Roots and reflections* (ed. C. Mascon), pp. 15–31. Jessica Kingsley Publishers, London, UK.
8. Goldberg, D.P. and Williams, P. (1988). *A user's guide to the General Health Questionnaire*. NFER-Nelson Publishing Co, Windsor, Berkshire.
9. Maslach, C. and Jackson, S.E. (1986). *Maslach burnout inventory manual*, 2nd edition. Consulting Psychologists Press, Palo Alto, California.
10. Maslach, C. and Jackson, S.E. (1981). The measurement of experienced burnout. *Journal of Occupational Behaviour*, 2, 99–113.
11. Ramirez, A.J., Graham, J., Richards, M.A. *et al.* (1995). Burnout and psychiatric disorder among cancer clinicians. *Br J Cancer*, 71, 1263–69.
12. Ramirez, A.J., Graham, J., Richards, M.A. *et al.* (1996). Mental health of hospital consultants: The effects of stress and satisfaction at work. *Lancet*, 347(9003), 724–8.
13. Berman, R., Campbell, M., Makin, W. *et al.* (2007). Occupational Stress in palliative medicine, medical oncology and clinical oncology specialist registrars. *Clinical Medicine*, 7(3), 235–42.
14. Dunwoodie, D.A. and Auret, K. (2007). Psychological morbidity and burnout in palliative care doctors in Western Australia. *Internal Medicine Journal*, 21, 1–6.
15. Asai, M., Morita, T., Akechi, T. *et al.* (2007). Burnout and psychiatric morbidity among physicians engaged in end-of-life care for cancer patients: A cross-sectional nationwide survey in Japan. *Psycho-Oncology*, 16(5), 421–8.
16. Dunne, J.J. and Jenkins, L. (1991). Stress and coping in Macmillan nurses: A study in comparative context. Cancer Relief Macmillan Fund, London.
17. Power, K.G. and Sharp, G.R. (1988). A comparison of sources of nursing stress and job satisfaction among mental handicap and hospice nursing staff. *J Adv Nurs*, 13, 726–32.
18. Cooper, C.L. and Mitchell, S. (1990). Nursing the critically ill and dying. Human relations, 43(4), 297–311.
19. Payne, N. (2001). Occupational stressors and coping as determinants of burnout in female hospice nurses. *J Adv Nurs*, 33(3), 396–405.
20. Williams, M.L., Wright, M., Cobb, M. *et al.* (2004). A prospective study of the roles, responsibilities and stresses of chaplains working within a hospice. *Palliat Med*, 18, 638–45.
21. Graham, J., Ramirez, A.J., Cull, A. *et al.* (1996). Job stress and satisfaction among palliative physicians. *Palliat Med*, 10, 185–94.
22. Vachon, M.L.S. (2005). The stress of professional caregivers. In *Oxford textbook of palliative medicine*, 3rd edition (ed. Doyle), pp. 992–1004. Oxford University Press.
23. Heaven, C., Maguire, P, and Clegg, J. (1998). Impact of communication skills training on self-efficacy, outcome expectancy, and burnout. *Psycho-Oncology*, 7, 61.
24. Firth-Cozens, J. and Greenhalgh, J. (1997). Doctors' perceptions of the links between stress and lowered clinical care. *Soc Sci Med*, 44(7), 1017–22.
25. Taylor, C., Graham, J., Potts, H.W.W. *et al.* (2007). The impact of hospital consultants' poor mental health on patient care. *Br J Psychiatry*, 190, 268–9.
26. Kivimaki, M., Sutinen, R., Elovainio, M. *et al.* (2001). Sickness absence in hospital physicians: 2 Year follow up study on determinants. *Occup Environ Med*, 58, 361–6.
27. Schernhammer, E.S. and Colditz, G.A. (2004). Suicide rates among physicians: A quantitative and gender assessment (meta-analysis). *Am J Psychiatry*, 161, 2295–302.
28. Lu, H., While, A.E., and Barriball, L. (2005). Job satisfaction among nurses: A literature review. *Int J Nurs Stud*, 42, 211–27.
29. Leiter, M.P., Harvie, P, and Frizzell, C. (1998). The correspondence of patient satisfaction and nurse burnout. *Soc Sci Med*, 47(10), 1611–17.
30. Taylor, C., Graham, J., Potts, H.W.W. *et al.* (2005). Changes in mental health of U.K. hospital consultants since the mid 1990s. *Lancet*, 366, 742–44.
31. Foxall, M.J., Zimmermanm, L., Standley, R. *et al.* (1990). A comparison of frequency and sources of nursing job stress perceived by intensive care, hospice and medical-surgical nurses. *J Adv Nurs*, 15, 577–84.
32. Gray-Toft, P.A. and Anderson, J.G. (1981). Stress among hospital staff: its causes and effects. *Soc Sci Med*, 159, 639–47.
33. Alexander, D.A. and Ritchie, E. (1990). Stressors and difficulties in dealing with the terminal patient. *J Palliat Care*, 6(3), 28–33.

34. Mallett, K., Price, J.H., Jurs, S.G. *et al.* (1991). Relationships among burnout, death anxiety and social support in hospice and critical care nurses. *Psychological Reports*, **68**, 1347–59.

35. Finlay, I.G. (1990). Sources of stress in hospice medical directors and matrons. *Palliat Med*, **4**, 5–9.

36. Grunfeld, E., Zitzelsberger, L., Coristine, M. *et al.* (2005). Job stress and job satisfaction of cancer care workers. *Psycho-oncology*, b, 61–9.

37. Krikorian, D.A. and Moser, D.H. (1985). Satisfactions and stresses experienced by professional nurses in hospice programs. *American Journal of Hospice Care*, **2**(1), 25–33.

38. Wall, T.D., Bolden, R.I., Borrill, C.S. *et al.* (1997). Minor psychiatric disorder in NHS trust staff: occupational and gender differences. *Br J Psychiatry*, **171**, 519–23.

39. Graham J. and Ramirez, A.J. (1997). Mental health of hospital consultants. *J Psychosom Res*, **43**(3), 227–31.

40. Deckard, G., Meterko, M., and Field, D. (1994). Physician burnout: an examination of personal, professional and organisational relationships. *Med Care*, **32**, 745–54.

41. Masterson-Allen, S., Mor, V., Laliberte, L. *et al.* (1985). Staff burnout in a hospice setting. *Hospital Journal*, **1**, 1–15.

42. Agius, R., Blenkin, H., Deary, I. *et al.* (1996). Survey of perceived stress and work demands of consultant doctors. *Occup Environ Med*, **53**, 217–24.

43. Kobasa, S.C. (1979). Stressful live events, personality and health: an inquiry into hardiness. *J Pers Soc Psychol*, **37**, 1–11.

44. Antonovsky, A. (1987). *Unraveling the mystery of health—How people manage stress and stay well*. Jossey-Bass Publishers, San Francisco.

45. Li, S. (2004). 'Symbiotic niceness': Constructing a therapeutic relationship in psychosocial palliative care. *Soc Sci Med*, **58**(12), 2571–83.

46. Speck, P. (1994). Working with dying people: On being good enough. In *The unconscious at work: individual and organizational stress in human services* (eds. A. Obholtzer and V. Roberts), Chapter 10. Routledge, London.

47. Weinberg, A. and Creed, A. (1999). Stress and psychiatric disorder in healthcare professionals and hospital staff. *Lancet*, **355**, 533–37.

48. Catalan, J., Burgess, A., Pergami, A. *et al.* (1996). The psychological impact on staff of caring for people with serious diseases: The case of HIV infection and oncology. *J Psychosom Res*, **40**(4), 425–35.

49. Karasek, R.A. (1979). Job-demands, job-decision latitude and mental strain: Implications for job redesign. *Administrative Science Quarterly*, **24**, 285–308.

50. Vachon, M.L. (1995). Staff stress in hospice/palliative care: A review. *Palliat Med*, **9**(2), 91–122.

51. Borrill, C., West, M., Shapiro, D. *et al.* (2000). Team working and effectiveness in health care. *British Journal of Health Care Management*, **6**(8), 364–71.

52. Rafferty, A.M., Ball, J., and Aiken, L.H. (2001). Are teamwork and professional autonomy compatible, and do they result in improved hospital care? *Quality in Health Care*, **10**(Suppl II), ii32–7.

53. McKee, E. (1995). Staff support in hospices. *International Journal of Palliative Nursing*, **1**, 200–5.

54. Addington Hall, J. and Ramirez, A. (2006). The Carers. ABC Palliative Care. In *ABC of palliative care*, 2nd edition (M. Fallon and G. Hanks). BMJ books. Blackwell Publishing.

55. Mackereth, P.A., White, K., Cawthorn, A. *et al.* (2005). Improving stressful working lives: Complementary therapies, counselling and clinical supervision for staff. *European Journal of Oncology Nursing*, **9**, 147–54.

Psychiatric symptoms in palliative medicine

William Breitbart, Harvey Max Chochinov, and Steven D. Passik

Introduction

Often, it is not death that is feared, but rather the process that leads to death. Images of suffering, or dying in isolation, can be foremost on the minds of those with terminal illness. Unaddressed physical and psychiatric symptoms often interact and impact negatively on quality of life. Therefore, the prompt recognition and effective treatment of both psychiatric and physical symptoms becomes critically important to the well-being of the patient with advanced disease. In general, palliative care specialists are quite expert at managing a broad spectrum of difficult and complex physical symptoms. Managing psychiatric complications (such as anxiety, delirium, depression, suicide, and desire for hastened death) and difficult psychosocial issues (such as bereavement, loss, family dysfunction) facing patients with terminal illness and their families, however, can test the limits of even the most skilled and experienced palliative medicine practitioner. It is for this reason that a multi-disciplinary approach to the management of the patient with advanced disease has gained broad acceptance. A psychiatrist or psychologist can play a vital role as a member of such a treatment team. This role includes the assessment and treatment of the psychiatric complications of terminal illness and the application of psychological and psychiatric techniques to the management of physical symptoms. This chapter is designed to both provide psychiatric consultants with a knowledge base specific to terminal illness, and to give the palliative medicine practitioner a framework for approaching psychiatric issues in palliative care. The interested reader is referred to another Oxford University Press textbook, edited by two of the authors of this chapter, entitled the *Handbook of Psychiatry in Palliative Medicine*[1] for a more extensive review.

Prevalence of psychiatric disorders in the terminally ill

The patient with advanced disease faces many stressors during the course of illness, including fears of a painful death, disability, disfigurement, and dependency. While such concerns are universal, the level of psychological distress is quite variable depending on personality, coping ability, social support, and medical factors.

The Psychosocial Collaborative Oncology Group determined the prevalence of psychiatric disorders seen in 215 cancer patients (ambulatory or hospitalized, with a wide range of cancer diagnoses and stages of disease) in three cancer centres utilizing the criteria from the Diagnostic and Statistical Manual III classification of disorders[2]. About half (53 per cent) of the patients evaluated were adjusting normally to the stresses of cancer with no diagnosable psychiatric disorder; however, 47 per cent had clinically apparent psychiatric disorders. Of the 47 per cent who had psychiatric disorders, 68 per cent had reactive anxiety and depression (adjustment disorders with depressed or anxious mood), 13 per cent had major depression, 8 per cent had an organic mental disorder (delirium).

Cancer patients with advanced disease are a particularly vulnerable group in terms of the development of psychiatric complications[1–4]. The incidence of pain, depression, and delirium all increase with higher levels of physical debilitation and advanced illness[5–10]. Approximately 25 per cent of all cancer patients experience severe depressive symptoms, with the prevalence increasing to 77 per cent in those with advanced illness[7]. The prevalence of organic mental disorders (delirium) among cancer patients requiring psychiatric consultation has been found to range from 25 to 40 per cent and as high as 85–88 per cent during the terminal stages of illness[3,9,10]. Still, contrary to a common clinical assumption, the prevalence of depressive and anxiety disorders do not increase as death approaches[11]. Opioid analgesics such as meperidine, levorphanol, and morphine sulfate, commonly cause acute confusional states, particularly in the elderly and terminally ill[9,10]. Cancer patients with pain are twice as likely to develop a psychiatric disorder than patients without pain. Of the patients who received a psychiatric diagnosis, 39 per cent reported significant pain. In contrast, only 19 per cent of patients without a psychiatric diagnosis had significant pain[2]. The psychiatric diagnoses of these patients with pain were predominantly adjustment disorder with depressed or mixed mood (69 per cent) and major depression in 15 per cent. This finding of increased frequency of psychiatric disturbance in cancer patients with pain has been reported by others[12].

In a study by Minagawa *et al.*[4] using the Structured Clinical Interview for DSM-III-R (SCID) to evaluate the incidence of psychiatric disorders in a sample of 109 terminally ill cancer patients admitted to a palliative care unit, found that 53.7 per cent of patients met criteria for a specific psychiatric disorder (this finding is similar to the rate of 47 per cent found in earlier studies of general cancer patient populations). The most common psychiatric disorders among the terminally ill cancer patients were: delirium (28 per cent), dementia (10.7 per cent), adjustment disorders (7.5 per cent), amnestic disorder (3.2 per cent), major depression (3.2 per cent), and generalized anxiety disorder (1.1 per cent). This study dramatically under-represents the prevalence of depression in patients with advanced disease. The sample studied consisted of patients in the last week or two of life. Delirium and organic mental disorders were thus developing rapidly in this sample, masking pre-existing depression and other disorders that were likely present up to the stage of disease where delirium overwhelmed the clinical picture. While the palliative care literature has data on the prevalence of psychiatric disorders in cancer and AIDS patients (see below), data regarding the prevalence of psychiatric disorders in patients with end-stage heart, lung, liver, or neurodegenerative disorders is almost completely lacking.

Early descriptions of the prevalence of psychiatric disorders in patients with human immunodeficiency virus (HIV) disease and/or AIDS suggested rather significant rates of anxiety, depression, cognitive impairment disorders, and risk for suicide[13–16]. Tross and Hirsh[13], in 1988, reported the prevalence of psychiatric disorders in an ambulatory sample of 279 patients with AIDS spectrum disorders. The study included asymptomatic gay men, gay men with AIDS-related complex (ARC), and gay men with AIDS. All patients with organic mental disorders or obvious neurologic impairment were excluded. Men with ARC showed the greatest distress and frequency of psychiatric disorder. Three-quarters of the men with ARC, one-half of the AIDS patients, and two-fifths of the asymptomatic gay men were diagnosed as having a psychiatric disorder. The most common psychiatric diagnosis was adjustment disorder, seen in two-thirds of AIDS patients and more than half of patients with ARC. Depression was present in one-quarter of the entire study population. Patients with AIDS thus have quite comparable, if not higher, levels of psychiatric distress than cancer patients. There is a higher prevalence of psychiatric disorders seen in homosexual men (with or without HIV infection) as compared to the heterosexual men or the general population[14]. Atkinson et al.[14] found that homosexual men had higher lifetime rates of substance abuse, affective disorders, and anxiety disorders than the general population that may have predated their HIV infection.

There have been several reports of psychiatric diagnoses seen in AIDS patients who were hospitalized and more seriously ill. Karina et al. reported that of 357 patients hospitalized with AIDS, 49 (14 per cent) had at least one psychiatric diagnosis[15]. These patients were hospitalized an average 60 days longer than AIDS patients without such psychiatric illnesses. Differences in medical morbidity could not account for longer length of stay. Barbuto et al.[16] reviewed the psychiatric consultation data collected on 65 hospitalized patients with AIDS. Psychiatric consultations were most frequently requested to evaluate depressive symptoms, suicidal risk, and behaviour related to CNS impairment by delirium or dementia. In this study organic mental disorders, adjustment disorders, anxiety disorders, and affective disorders ranked in order of decreasing prevalence. Eighty per cent of AIDS patients, given a functional psychiatric diagnosis, had the diagnosis changed to an organic mental disorder as illness progressed and cognitive impairment became more obvious. Perry and Tross[17] reported on the prevalence of psychiatric disorders seen in medically hospitalized AIDS patients at New York Hospital. Sixty-five per cent of patients were diagnosed with an organic mental disorder, and 17 per cent were diagnosed with major depression. The organic mental disorders seen were predominantly AIDS dementia complex (ADC) and delirium, often in combination. Perry[18] later reported in 1999 that between 65 and 80 per cent of AIDS patients develop some type of organic mental disorder during the course of illness.

Over the last decade, the epidemiology of the AIDS epidemic, particularly in developed countries has changed from a disease of homosexual men to a disease of injection drug users and their sexual partners. In addition the introduction of protease inhibitors in the late mid-1990s began to change the medical course of HIV disease. With the widespread introduction of highly active antiretroviral therapies, mortality rates among patients with advanced HIV disease have declined dramatically, and this has had an impact on the prevalence of psychiatric disorders, primarily cognitive impairment disorders such as AIDS-related dementia. Despite these advances in AIDS therapies, substantially elevated rates of major depression and substance abuse were consistently observed. Rabkin et al.[19] reported rates of major depression of about 10 per cent, rates of anxiety disorders in the 8–13 per cent range, and current drug use disorders in the 14–17 per cent range. In addition, surveys indicate that psychological and physical symptom burden in ambulatory AIDS patients is rather significant. Vogl et al.[20] reported that ambulatory AIDS patients have an average of 17 symptoms on the Memorial Symptom Assessment Scale, with the most prevalent symptoms including: worrying (86 per cent), fatigue (85 per cent), sadness (82 per cent), and pain (76 per cent). Like cancer patients, patients with AIDS were more likely to have symptoms of psychological distress as disease advanced and when pain was a co-morbid symptom.

Controlling psychiatric symptoms

Anxiety in the patient with advanced illness

The terminally ill patient presents with a complex mixture of physical and psychological symptoms in a context of a frightening reality. Thus the recognition of anxious symptoms requiring treatment can be challenging. Patients with anxiety complain of tension or restlessness, or they exhibit jitteriness, autonomic hyperactivity, vigilance, insomnia, distractibility, shortness of breath, numbness, apprehension, worry, or rumination. Often the physical or somatic manifestations of anxiety overshadow the psychological or cognitive ones, and are the symptoms that the patient most often presents[21]. The consultant must use these symptoms as a cue to inquire about the patient's psychological state, which is commonly one of fear, worry, or apprehension. The assumption that a high level of anxiety is inevitably encountered during the terminal phase of illness is neither correct nor helpful or accurate for diagnostic and treatment purposes[11]. In deciding whether to treat anxiety during the terminal phase of illness, the patient's subjective level of distress is the primary impetus for the initiation of treatment. Other considerations include problematic patient behaviour such as non-compliance due to anxiety, family and staff reactions to the patient's distress, and the balancing of the risks and benefits of treatment[22].

Prevalence studies of anxiety, primarily in cancer populations, report a higher prevalence of mixed anxiety and depressive symptoms rather than anxiety alone[22]. Prevalence of anxiety increases with advancing disease and decline in the patient's physical status[19]. Brandenberg et al.[23] reported that 28 per cent of advanced melanoma patients were anxious compared to 15 per cent of controls. Anxiety, like fever, is a symptom in this population that can have many aetiologies. Anxiety may be encountered as a component of an adjustment disorder, panic disorder, generalized anxiety disorder, phobia, or agitated depression. Additionally, in the terminally ill cancer patient, symptoms of anxiety are most likely to arise from some medical complication of the illness or treatment such as organic anxiety disorder, delirium, or other organic mental disorders[3,7,21,22]. Hypoxia, sepsis, poorly controlled pain, and adverse drug reactions such as akathisia or withdrawal states are specific entities which often present as anxiety. Patients who had been managed for long periods of time with relatively high doses of benzodiazepines or opioid analgesics for the control of anxiety or pain, often become tolerant or physically dependent upon these drugs. During the terminal phase of illness, when patients become less alert, there is a tendency to minimize the use of sedating medications. It is important to consider the need to slowly taper benzodiazepines and opioid analgesics in order to prevent acute withdrawal states. Withdrawal states in terminally ill patients often present first as agitation or anxiety and become clinically evident days later than might be expected in younger, healthier patients due to impaired metabolism. Benzodiazepine withdrawal, for example, can present first as agitation or anxiety, though the diagnosis is often missed in terminally ill patients, and especially the elderly, where physiologic dependence on these medications is often unrecognized[24]. In the dying patient, anxiety can represent impending cardiac or respiratory arrest, pulmonary embolism, electrolyte imbalance, or dehydration.

Given the complexity of causative factors, the scarcity of studies on anxiety and its treatment in the palliative setting is unfortunate[25]. Apart from treating the causative factors, anxiety can be treated by psychotherapy, behavioural therapy, and pharmacotherapy[25]. Despite the fact that anxiety in terminal illness commonly results from medical complications, it is therefore important not to forget that psychological factors related to death and dying or existential issues, play a role in anxiety, particularly in patients who are alert and not confused[21,22]. Patients frequently fear the isolation and separation of death. Claustrophobic patients may be afraid of the idea of being confined and buried in a coffin. These issues can be disconcerting to consultants who may find themselves at a loss for words that are consoling to the patient. Nonetheless, one should not avoid eliciting these concerns, listening empathically to them, and enlisting pastoral involvement where appropriate.

The specific treatment of anxiety in the terminally ill often depends on aetiology, presentation, and setting. An example of how the specific aetiology of the anxious symptom is important is the case of hypoxia. Anxiety associated with hypoxia and dyspnoea in a patient with diffuse lung metastases is most responsive to treatment with oxygen and opioid analgesics. If the same patient's presentation included hallucinations and agitation, a neuroleptic would be added to the regimen. In the hospital setting, an arterial blood gas (ABG) can confirm the diagnosis of hypoxia. However, the good clinician caring for the terminally ill patient at home may

conclude on clinical grounds that hypoxia is present and therefore would treat anxiety associated with it in an identical fashion to that in the hospital. An ABG provides confirmatory information but is not essential to considering and treating hypoxia and so may be unnecessary when attempting to maximize the patient's comfort.

Pharmacologic treatment of anxiety in the terminally ill

The pharmacotherapy of anxiety in terminal illness (see Table 15.5.1) involves the judicious use of the following classes of medications: benzodiazepines, neuroleptics (typical and atypical), antihistamines,

Table 15.5.1 Anxiolytic medications used in patients with advanced disease.

Generic name	Approximate daily dosage range (mg)	Route[a]
Benzodiazepines		
Very short acting		
Midazolam	10–60 per 24 h	IV, SC
Short acting		
Alprazolam	0.25–2.0 TID–QID	PO,SL
Oxazepam	10–15 TID–QID	PO
Lorazepam	0.5–2.0 TID–QID	PO, SL IV, IM
Intermediate acting		
Chlordiazepoxide	10–50 TID–QID	PO, IM
Long acting		
Diazepam	5–10 BID–QID	PO, IM, IV, PR
Clorazepate	7.5–15 BID–QID	PO
Clonazepam	0.5–2.0 BID–QID	PO
Non-benzodiazepines		
Buspirone	5.0–20 TID	PO
Neuroleptics		
Haloperidol	0.5–5.0 Q 2–12 h	PO, IV, SC, IM
Methotrimeprazine	10–20 Q 4–8 h	IV, SC, PO
Thioridazine	10–75 TID–QID	PO
Chlorpromazine	12.5–50 Q 4–12 h	PO, IM, IV
Atypical neuroleptics		
Olanzapine	2.5–20 Q 12–24 h	PO
Risperidone	1.0–3.0 Q 12–24 h	PO
Quetiapine fumarate	25–200 Q 12–24 h	PO
Antihistamine		
Hydroxyzine	25–50 Q 4–6 h	PO, IV, SC
Tricyclic antidepressants		
Imipramine	12.5–150 h	PO, IM
Clomipramine	10–150 h	PO

[a] PO, per oral; IM, intramuscular; PR, *per rectum*; IV, intravenous; SC, sub-cutaneous; SL, sub-lingual; BID, two times a day; TID, three times a day; QID, four times a day. Parenteral doses are generally twice as potent as oral doses, intravenous bolus injections, or infusions should be administered slowly.

antidepressants, and opioid analgesics[3,7,21,22,26]. Still, the choice of anxiolytic drug is principally based upon studies in other populations, and the specific knowledge base on pharmacological treatment of anxiety in the palliative setting is limited[27].

Benzodiazepines

Benzodiazepines are the mainstay of the pharmacologic treatment of anxiety in the terminally ill patient. The shorter-acting benzodiazepines, such as lorazepam, alprazolam, and oxazepam, are safest in this population. The selection of these drugs avoids toxic accumulation due to impaired metabolism in debilitated individuals. Lorazepam, oxazepam, and temazepam are metabolized by conjugation in the liver and are therefore safest in patients with hepatic disease. This is in contrast to alprazolam and other benzodiazepines which are metabolized through oxidative pathways in the liver that are more vulnerable to interference with hepatic damage. The disadvantage of using short-acting benzodiazepines is that patients often experience breakthrough anxiety or end of dose failure. Such patients benefit from switching to longer-acting benzodiazepines such as diazepam or clonazepam. Dying patients often benefit from parenteral administration of these drugs. Common dosage regimens include: lorazepam 0.5–2.0 mg, PO, IV, or IM, 3–6 h; alprazolam 0.25–1.0 mg, PO, TID–QID; diazepam 2.5–10 mg, PO, PR, IM, or IV q3–6 h; clonazepam 1–2 mg, PO, BID–TID. Dying patients can be administered diazepam rectally when no other route is available, with dosages equivalent to oral regimens. Rectal diazepam[28] has been used widely in the palliative care field to control anxiety, restlessness, and agitation associated with the final days of life.

Midazolam, a very short-acting, water-soluble benzodiazepine, is usually administered as an intravenous infusion in critical care settings where sedation is the goal in an agitated or anxious patient on a respirator. Midazolam may also prove useful in controlling anxiety and agitation in terminal phases of illness[28–30]. Unlike diazepam, midazolam has a short duration of action and seems to be less irritating to subcutaneous tissues when given by subcutaneous infusion. Since it is several times as potent as diazepam, starting doses should be low and careful monitoring of effects should be initiated. Doses ranging from 2 to 10 mg/day have been found to be safe and effective for most patients. However, doses as high as 30–60 mg/day have been reported[31]. Clonazepam, a longer-acting benzodiazepine, has been found to be extremely useful in the palliative care setting for the treatment of anxiety, depersonalization, or derealization in patients with seizure disorders, brain tumours, and mild organic mental disorders. Patients who experience end of dose failure with recurrence of anxiety on shorter-acting drugs also find clonazepam helpful. It is not uncommon to switch patients from alprazolam to clonazepam when attempting to taper off alprazolam. Clonazepam is also useful in patients with organic mood disorders who have symptoms of mania, and as an adjuvant analgesic in patients with neuropathic pain[32–34].

Fears of causing respiratory depression should not prevent the clinician from using adequate dosages of benzodiazepines to control anxiety. The likelihood of respiratory depression is minimized when one utilizes shorter-acting drugs, increases the dosages in small increments in a carefully monitored setting, and ultimately switches to longer acting drugs.

Non-benzodiazepine anxiolytics

Typical neuroleptics, such as thioridazine and haloperidol, and some of the newer atypical neuroleptics, such as olanzapine, are useful in the treatment of anxiety when benzodiazepines are not sufficient for symptom control[19]. They are also indicated when an organic aetiology is suspected or when psychotic symptoms such as delusions or hallucinations accompany the anxiety. Neuroleptics are perhaps the safest class of anxiolytics in patients where there is legitimate concern regarding respiratory depression or compromise. Typically haloperidol 0.5–5 mg, PO, IV, or SC, q2–12 h, is sufficient to control anxious symptoms and avoid excessive sedation. Lower potency neuroleptics such as thioridazine (10–25 mg, PO, TID) are effective anxiolytics and can help with insomnia and agitation. Methotrimeprazine (10–20 mg, every 4–8 h, IM, IV, or SC) is a phenothiazine with unique analgesic and anxiolytic properties that is often used for the treatment of pain and anxiety in the dying patient[35,36]. Its side effects include sedation, anticholinergic symptoms and hypotension. Intravenous administration by slow infusion is preferable to avoid problems with hypotension. Chlorpromazine (12.5–50 mg, PO, IM, or IV, q4–12 h) has similar side effects that limit its application in this setting. However, it can be useful in patients where sedation is desirable. With typical neuroleptic drugs, such as those listed above, one must be aware of the potential for extrapyramidal side effects (particularly when patients are taking additional neuroleptics for antiemetic purposes) and the remote possibility of neuroleptic malignant syndrome. Tardive dyskinesia is rarely a concern given the generally short-term usage and low dosages of these medications in this population[37]. Typical neuroleptics all share the same properties of non-specific and potent CNS dopamine blocking activity. Atypical neuroleptics such as risperidone, olanzapine, and quetiapine may have the same anxiolytic properties as typical neuroleptics, but with significantly lower frequency of extrapyramidal side effects or tardive dyskinesia.

Hydroxyzine is an antihistamine with mild anxiolytic, sedative, and analgesic properties. It is particularly useful when treating anxious, terminally ill cancer patients with pain. One hundred milligrams of hydroxyzine given parenterally has analgesic potency equivalent to 8 mg of morphine and potentiates the analgesic effects of morphine[38]. As an anxiolytic, 25–50 mg of hydroxyzine q4–6 h PO, IV, or SC is effective.

Tricyclic, heterocyclic, and second generation antidepressants are the most effective treatment for anxiety accompanying depression and are helpful in treating panic disorder[39–41]. Guidelines for their use are discussed in the section 'Depression'. Their usefulness is often limited in the dying patient due to anticholinergic and sedative side effects. Very often the consultant is faced with the task of relieving symptoms in a short period of time and so drugs that require a period of weeks to achieve therapeutic effect are unsatisfactory.

Opioid drugs such as the narcotic analgesics are primarily indicated for the control of pain. However, these drugs are also effective in the relief of dyspnoea due to cardiopulmonary processes and the anxiety associated with them[42]. Opioid drugs are particularly useful in the treatment of dying patients who are in respiratory distress. Continuous intravenous infusions of morphine or other narcotic analgesics allow for careful titration and control of respiratory distress, anxiety, pain, and agitation[43]. Occasionally one must maintain the patient in a state of unresponsiveness in order to maximize comfort. When respiratory distress is not a major problem, it is preferable to use the opioid drugs solely for analgesic purposes and to add more specific anxiolytics (such as the benzodiazepines) to control concomitant anxiety.

Buspirone, is a non-benzodiazepine anxiolytic that is useful along with psychotherapy in patients with chronic anxiety or anxiety related to adjustment disorders. The onset of anxiolytic action is delayed in comparison to the benzodiazepines, taking 5–10 days for relief of anxiety to begin. Since buspirone is not a benzodiazepine, it will not block benzodiazepine withdrawal, and so one must be cautious when switching from a benzodiazepine to buspirone. The effective dose of buspirone is 10 mg orally three times a day[44]. Because of its delayed onset of action and indication for use in chronic anxiety states, buspirone may be of limited usefulness to the clinician treating anxiety and agitation in the terminally ill.

Non-pharmacologic treatment of anxiety in terminally ill patients

Non-pharmacologic interventions for anxiety and distress include supportive psychotherapy and behavioural interventions that are used alone or in combination. Brief supportive psychotherapy is often useful in dealing with both crisis-related issues as well as existential issues confronted by the terminally ill[45]. Psychotherapeutic interventions should include both the patient and family, particularly as the patient with advanced illness becomes increasingly debilitated and less able to interact. Mental-health professionals can assist in seeing that the emotional needs of patients and families are met during the terminal phase of illness. Such needs include continuous, updated information regarding the disease status and treatment options available. This information must be delivered repeatedly and with sensitivity as to what they are currently prepared and able to hear and absorb. Families, especially, require a great deal of reassurance that they and the medical staff have done everything possible for the patient. The goals of psychotherapy with the patient are to establish a bond that decreases the sense of isolation experienced with terminal illness, to help the patient face death with a sense of self worth, to correct misconceptions about the past and present, to integrate the present illness into a continuum of life experiences, and to explore issues of separation, loss, and the unknown that lies ahead. The therapist should emphasize past strengths and support previously successful ways of coping. This helps the patient mobilize inner resources, modify plans for the future, and perhaps even accept the inevitability of death.

It is during the terminal phase of illness that we have the greatest opportunity to affect the process of adaptation to loss. Mental health professionals must extend their supportive stance to include both the patient and family. Anticipatory bereavement is a common experience which allows patients, loved ones, and health care providers the opportunity to mentally prepare for the impending death. Patients and family members should be encouraged to use this period to reconcile differences, extend important final communications, and re-affirm feelings and wishes. It is a time is of vital importance that can often set the tone for the subsequent bereavement course[46].

Relaxation, guided imagery, and hypnosis may help reduce anxiety and thereby increase the patient's sense of control. Most patients with advanced illness are still appropriate candidates for useful application of behavioural techniques despite physical debilitation. In assessing the utility of such interventions for a terminally ill patient, the clinician should, however, take into account the mental clarity of the patient. Confusional states interfere dramatically with a patient's ability to focus attention and thus limit the usefulness of these techniques[3]. Occasionally these techniques

can be modified so as to include even mildly cognitive impaired patients. This often involves the therapist taking a more active role by orienting the patient, creating a safe and secure environment, and evoking a conditioned response to the therapist's voice or presence. A typical behavioural intervention for anxiety in a terminally ill patient would include a relaxation exercise combined with some distraction or imagery technique. Typically the patient is first taught to relax with passive breathing accompanied by either passive or active muscle relaxation. Once in such a relaxed state, the patient is taught a pleasant, distracting imagery exercise. In a randomized study comparing a relaxation technique with alprazolam in the treatment of anxiety and distress in non-terminally ill cancer patients, both treatments were demonstrated to be quite effective for mild to moderate degrees of anxiety or distress. The drug intervention (alprazolam) was more effective for greater levels of distress or anxiety and had more rapid onset of beneficial effect[47]. Relaxation techniques can be prescribed concurrently with anxiolytic medications in highly anxious cancer patients.

Depression in patients with advanced illness

The prevalence of depression in cancer patients ranges from 10 to 25 per cent and increases with higher levels of disability, advanced illness, and pain[3,8,48,49]. Closeness to death does not seem to increase the prevalence rate[11]. The prevalence of major depression in terminally ill cancer patients receiving care in palliative care units suggest that the prevalence of depression in patients during the last weeks to months of life ranges from 9 to 18 per cent[48,50] supported by the findings of a systematic review which demonstrated a median prevalence rate of 15 per cent[51]. Risk factors associated with depression have been identified for the general population and patients with advanced disease. Certain types of cancer, such as pancreatic cancer, are associated with an increased incidence of depression. Family history of depression and history of previous depressive episodes further increase the risk of developing a depressive episode in the context of advanced cancer. Many studies have also found a correlation between depression, pain, and functional status[52]. Tumours by their origin or metastases to the CNS can cause depressive symptoms[53]. In addition, any evaluation of depression must also include an examination of medications and physical conditions that may be the cause of depression. Corticosteroids[54], chemotherapeutic agents[55–58], (vincristine, vinblastine, asparaginase, intrathecal methotrexate, interferon, interleukin) amphotericin[59], whole brain radiation[60], CNS metabolic-endocrine complications[61], and paraneoplastic syndromes[62], can present as depression, and addressing these factors must precede initiation of treatment. Major depression also commonly co-occurs with other psychiatric disorders (called comorbidity)[63]. Loss of meaning and low scores on measures of spiritual well-being are also associated with higher levels of depressive symptoms, suggesting that the relationship between existential distress and depression in terminal illness warrants further investigation[64].

Assessment of depression in the terminally ill

Depressed mood and sadness can be appropriate responses as the terminally ill patient faces death. These emotions can be manifestations of anticipatory grief over the impending loss of one's life, health, loved ones, and autonomy. Despite this, major depressive syndrome is a common mental health problem arising in the palliative care setting. Depression is under-diagnosed and under-treated. Depression significantly diminishes quality of life and complicates symptom control, resulting in more frequent admission to inpatient care setting. The under-diagnosis of depression in the palliative care setting relates to the minimization of these symptoms by clinicians, the concern that severely medically ill patients will not be able to tolerate the side effects or drug interactions associated with the initiation of antidepressant therapy, and the difficulties of accurately diagnosing depression in the terminally ill[65].

The DSM-IV criteria for major depressive disorder, the most severe and well-documented diagnosis within the depression spectrum, are shown in Table 15.5.2. They include two core criterion symptoms, depressed mood and anhedonia, a marked loss of interest or pleasure in activities. In order to qualify for the diagnosis, a patient must exhibit one of these core symptoms, along with at least four other symptoms from the criterion list. A critical problem associated with diagnosing depression in medically ill patients' lies with the issue of how best to interpret the physical/somatic symptoms of depression. Five different approaches to the diagnosis of major depression have been proposed: an inclusive approach—includes all symptoms whether or not they may be secondary to advanced illness or treatment; an exclusive approach—deletes and disregards all physical symptoms from consideration, not allowing them to contribute to the diagnosis; an aetiologic approach—the clinician attempts to determine if the physical symptom is due to illness or treatment or due to a depressive disorder; a substitutive approach—where physical symptoms of uncertain aetiology are replaced by other non-somatic symptoms[66]. This approach is best exemplified by the Endicott Substitution Criteria also listed in Table 15.5.2. Finally, a fifth approach involves requiring a higher threshold number of diagnostic criteria symptoms to make a diagnosis (seven rather than five). This approach is best exemplified by Chochinov et al.[49] who studied the prevalence of depression in a cohort of 130 terminally ill patients in a palliative care facility. They reported that 9.2 per cent met Research Diagnostic Criteria (RDC) for major depression when using high-severity thresholds for RDC criteria A symptoms (equivalent to the symptom threshold judgements specified in DSM-IV). This approach yielded the identical prevalence of major depression whether or not one included somatic symptoms in the diagnostic criteria or used Endicott revised criteria[66] (involving replacement of somatic symptoms with non-somatic alternatives). While concern has been raised about the non-specificity of somatic symptoms in the medically ill, these results—along with those of other investigations[67,68]—indicate that their inclusion may not overly influence the diagnostic classification of major depression.

The diagnostic interview remains the most commonly used clinical tool and should directly assess commonly accepted criteria in addition to relying more on the psychological or cognitive symptoms of major depression (H). The diagnosis of a major depressive syndrome in a terminally ill patient often relies more on the psychological or cognitive symptoms of major depression (worthlessness, hopelessness, excessive guilt, and suicidal ideation), rather than the neuro-vegetative or somatic signs and symptoms of major depression. The strategy of relying on the psychological or cognitive signs and symptoms of depression for diagnostic specificity is itself not without problems. How is the clinician to interpret feelings of hopelessness in the dying patient when there is no hope for cure or recovery? Feelings of hopelessness, worthlessness, or suicidal ideation must be explored in detail. While many dying patients lose hope of a cure, they are able to maintain hope for better symptom control. For many patients hope is contingent on the ability to find continued meaning in their day to day existence. Hopelessness that is pervasive and accompanied by a sense of despair or despondency is more likely to represent a symptom of a depressive disorder. Similarly patients often state that they feel they are burdening their families unfairly, causing them great pain and inconvenience. Those beliefs are less likely to represent a symptom of depression than if the patient feels that their life has never had any worth, or that they are being punished for evil things they have done. Suicidal ideation, even rather mild and passive forms, is very likely associated with significant degrees of depression in terminally ill cancer patients[69,70].

Numerous assessment methods for depression including diagnostic classification systems, structured interview, and screening instruments have been used in research, as enumerated in Table 15.5.3. Unfortunately, few studies of depression in terminally ill or advanced cancer patients have used such research assessment methods to date. Chochinov et al.[71] studied brief screening instruments to measure depression in the terminally ill. His group compared the performance of four brief screening measures for depression in a group of terminally ill patients. The methods compared included: (1) a single-item interview assessing depressed mood—', Have you been depressed most of the time for the past two weeks?'; (2) a two-item interview assessing depressed mood and loss of interest in activities; (3) a visual analogue scale for depressed mood; and (4) the 13-item Beck depression inventory. Semi-structured diagnostic interviews were administered to 197 patients receiving palliative care for advanced cancer. The interview diagnoses served as the standard against which the screening performance of the four brief screening methods was assessed. As reported in other depression screening studies, the self-report instruments (i.e. the Beck and the mood visual analogue scale) demonstrated a low positive predictive value (0.27 and 0.17, respectively) and a high negative predictive value (0.96 and 0.92, respectively).

Table 15.5.2 DSM-IV symptoms of major depression and substitute symptoms suggested by Endicott.

DSM-IV criteria	Substitute symptoms
Depressed mood most of the day	
Markedly diminished interest or pleasure in all or almost all activities most of the day	
Weight loss or gain, or decreased or increased appetite	Depressed appearance, tearfulness
Insomnia or hypersomnia decreased	Social withdrawal, talkativeness
Psychomotor agitation or retardation	
Fatigue or loss of energy	Brooding, self-pity, or pessimism
Feeling of worthlessness or excessive or inappropriate guilt	
Diminished ability to think or concentrate, or indecisiveness	Lack of reactivity, cannot be cheered up

Recurrent thoughts of death, or suicidal ideation or planning or a suicide attempt

Table 15.5.3 Assessment methods for depression in patients with advanced disease.

Diagnostic classification systems
Diagnostic and Statistical Manual DSM-III, III-R, IV
Endicott Substitution Criteria
Research Diagnostic Criteria (RDC)
Structures diagnostic interviews
Schedule for Affective and Schizophrenia (SADS)
Diagnostic Interview Schedule (DIS)
Structured Clinical interview for DSM-IIIR (SCID)
Screening instruments—self-report
General Health Questionnaire-30 (GHQ)
Hospital Anxiety and Depression Scale (HADS)
Beck Depression Inventory—13 items (BDI)
Visual Analogue Scale for Depressed Mood

Most noteworthy, the single-item interview question, 'Have you been depressed most of the time for the past two weeks?', correctly identified the diagnosis of every patient, while not misidentifying any patient, substantially outperforming the questionnaire and visual analogue measures. Brief screening measures for depression are thus important clinical tools for terminally ill patients. The performance of the single-item interview, which essentially asks patients if they are depressed, speaks to the importance of mood inquiry in this particularly vulnerable patient population.

Passik and colleagues demonstrated that clinical depression is under-recognized in cancer patients, but that the Zung Depression Rating Scale could be utilized effectively by oncologists and nurses as a rapid screening tool for depression in advanced cancer patients, and that oncologists could be easily trained to diagnose and initiate further evaluation and treatment of clinical depression in advanced cancer patients[72–75]. More recently, the Hamilton Depression Rating Scale has shown good properties as an assessment tool[76].

Management of depression in the terminally ill

Depression in cancer patients with advanced disease is optimally managed utilizing a combination of supportive psychotherapy, cognitive behavioural techniques, and antidepressant medications[48]. Psychotherapy and cognitive behavioural techniques are useful in the management of psychological distress in cancer patients, and have been applied to the treatment of depressive and anxious symptoms related to cancer and cancer pain. Psychotherapeutic interventions, either in the form of individual or group counselling, have been shown to effectively reduce psychological distress and depressive symptoms in cancer patients[45,77,78]. Cognitive behavioural interventions, such as relaxation and distraction with pleasant imagery, have also been shown to decrease depressive symptoms in patients with mild to moderate levels of depression[47]. Psychopharmacological interventions (i.e. antidepressant medications) (see Table 15.5.4), however, are the mainstay of management in the treatment of cancer patients with severe depressive symptoms who meet criteria for a major depressive episode[48]. The efficacy of antidepressants

Table 15.5.4 Antidepressant medications used in patients with advanced disease.

Generic name	Approximate daily dosage range (mg)	Route[a]
Tricyclic antidepressants		
Amitriptyline	10–150	PO, IM, PR
Doxepin	12.5–150	PO, IM
Imipramine	12.5–150	PO, IM
Desipramine	12.5–150	PO, IM
Nortriptyline	10–125	PO
Clomipramine	10–150	PO
Serotonin-specific reuptake inhibitors		
Fluoxetine	20–160	PO
Sertraline	50–200	PO
Paroxetine	10–60	PO
Citalopram	10–60	PO
Escitalopram	10–40	PO
Fluvoxamine	50–300	PO
Serotonin–norepinephrine reuptake inhibitor		
Venlafaxine	75–225	PO
Serotonin 2 antagonists/serotonin reuptake inhibitors		
Trazodone	25–300	PO
Nefazodone	100–600	PO
Norepinephrine and dopamine reuptake blockers		
Buproprion	200–450	PO
Buproprion—SR[b]	150–300	PO
Mirtazapine	15–60	PO
Heterocyclic antidepressants		
Maprotiline	50–75	PO
Amoxapine	100–150	PO
Psychostimulants		
Dextroamphetamine	2.5–20 BID	PO
Methylphenidate	2.5–20 BID	PO
Modafinil	50–400	PO
Monoamine oxidase inhibitors		
Isocarboxazid	20–40	PO
Phenelzine	30–60	PO
Tranylcypromine	20–40	PO
Moclobemide	100–600	PO
Benzodiazepines		
Alprazolam	0.25–2.0 TID	PO
Lithium carbonate	600–1200	PO

[a] PO, per oral; IM, intramuscular; PR, *per rectum*; BID, two times a day; TID, three times a day; intravenous infusions of a number of tricyclic antidepressants are utilized outside of the United States. This route is, however, not FDA approved.

[b] SR, sustained release.

[c] Comes in chewable tablet form that can be absorbed without swallowing.

in the treatment of depression in cancer patients has been well established[40,48,79–81].

Pharmacologic treatment of depression in the terminally ill

Any treatment for major depression in the terminally ill will be less effective if given in a context devoid of psychotherapeutic support. Although both psychotherapy and cognitive behavioural therapy have proven effective in reducing psychological distress and mild to moderate depressive symptomatology in the cancer setting, pharmacotherapy is the mainstay for treating terminally ill patients meeting diagnostic criteria for major depression[44,65]. Factors such as prognosis and the timeframe for treatment may play an important role in determining the type of pharmacotherapy for depression. A depressed patient with several months of life expectancy can afford to wait the 2–4 weeks it may take to respond to a serotonin reuptake inhibitor or a tricyclic antidepressant. The depressed dying patient with less than 3 weeks to live may do best with a rapid-acting psychostimulant[65,82,83]. Patients who are within hours to days of death and in distress are likely to benefit most from the use of sedatives or opioid infusions.

Tricyclic antidepressants

Tricyclic antidepressants (TCAs) have been the cornerstone for treating depression in the general cancer setting since the early 1960s. Their application specifically to the terminally ill, however, requires a careful risk–benefit ratio analysis. Although nearly 70 per cent of patients treated with a tricyclic for non-psychotic depression can anticipate a positive response, these medications are associated with a side effect profile which can be particularly troublesome for terminally ill patients[65,84]. They have multiple pharmacodynamic actions accounting for these side effects, including blockade of muscarinic cholinergic receptors, alpha-adrenoceptor blockade, and H_1 histamine receptor blockade. The tertiary amines (amitriptyline, doxepin, imipramine) have a greater propensity to cause side effects than do secondary amines (nortriptyline, desipramine)[85]. The secondary amines are thus often a preferable choice for the terminally ill.

The anticholinergic side effects can include constipation, dry mouth, and urinary retention. To avoid exacerbating symptoms associated with genitourinary outlet obstruction, decreased gastric motility, or stomatitis, a relatively non-anticholinergic tricyclic, such as desipramine or nortriptyline, is a reasonable choice. Those patients who are receiving medication with anticholinergic properties (such as pethidine, atropine, diphenhydramine, phenothiazines) are at risk for developing an anticholinergic delirium, and thus antidepressants which are potently anticholinergic should be avoided[86]. The anticholinergic actions of TCAs can also cause serious tachycardia which can be problematic for terminally ill patients with cardiac insufficiency. The quinidine-like effects of TCAs can also lead to arrhythmias by virtue of their ability to delay conduction via the His–Purkinje system[87] (associated with nonspecific ST–T changes and T waves on the electrocardiograph). These effects are particularly concerning for those terminally ill patients with pre-existing conduction defects, especially second or third degree heart block.

Alpha1-blockade is associated with postural hypotension and dizziness. This can be of particular concern for the frail volume depleted patient who, because of these side effects, is at risk for falls and possible fractures. Nortriptyline and protriptyline are the TCAs least associated with alpha1-blockade. H_1 histamine receptor blockage is associated with sedation and drowsiness. For dying patients already exposed to a variety of sedating agents (e.g. narcotic analgesics, antiemetics, anxiolytics, neuroleptics) TCAs such as amitriptyline and doxepin are the most likely to accentuate the overall cumulative sedating effects of these medications.

TCAs should be started at low doses (10–25 mg qhs) and increased in 10–25 mg increments every 2–4 days, until a therapeutic dose is attained or side effects become a dose limiting factor. Depressed cancer patients often achieve a therapeutic response at significantly lower doses of TCAs (25–125 mg) than are necessary in the physically well (150–300 g)[44]. There is also evidence to suggest that patients with advanced cancer achieve higher serum tricyclic levels at modest doses[88]. In order to minimize drug toxicity and more carefully guide the process of drug titration, prescribing tricyclics (desipramine, nortriptyline, amitriptyline, imipramine) with well-established therapeutic plasma levels may be advantageous[89]. Desipramine and nortriptyline are generally better tolerated in this population than is amitriptyline or imipramine.

The choice of which specific TCA to use depends on a variety of factors, including the nature of the underlying terminal medical condition, the characteristics of the depressive episode, past responses to antidepressant therapy, and the specific drug side effect profile. Those patients who present with agitation and insomnia may respond favourably to more sedating tricyclics (amitriptyline, doxepin). For the terminally ill depressed patient, the choice of TCA is made on the basis of a side effect profile which will be least incompatible with the patient's overall medical condition. Most tricyclics are available as rectal suppositories for patients who are no longer able to take medication orally. Outside of the United States, certain tricyclics are given as intravenous infusion[90]. Although not very practical, amitriptyline, imipramine, and doxepin can also be given intramuscularly[48,65].

It must be borne in mind that a therapeutic response to TCAs (as with all antidepressants) has a latency time of 3–6 weeks. For the terminally ill depressed patient whose life expectancy is anticipated to be less than this, psychostimulants may offer a more viable, rapid response alternative.

Serotonin-specific reuptake inhibitors

The selective serotonin reuptake inhibitors (SSRIs) now have an important role in the pharmacotherapy of depression in the medically ill and those with advanced cancer and AIDS[48,65,82,91]. They have been found to be as effective in the treatment of depression as the tricyclics[92,93] and have a number of features which may be particularly advantageous for the terminally ill. The SSRIs have a very low affinity for adrenergic, cholinergic, and histamine receptors, thus accounting for negligible orthostatic hypotension, urinary retention, memory impairment, sedation, or reduced awareness[94]. They have not been found to cause clinically significant alterations in cardiac conduction and are generally favourably tolerated along with a wider margin of safety than the TCAs in the event of an overdose. They do not therefore require therapeutic drug level monitoring.

Most of the side effects of SSRIs result from their selective central and peripheral serotonin reuptake inhibition. These include increased intestinal motility (loose stools, nausea, vomiting, insomnia, headaches, and sexual dysfunction). Some patients may experience anxiety, tremor, restlessness, and akathisia (the latter is relatively rare but it can be problematic for the terminally ill patient with Parkinson's disease)[95]. These side effects tend to be dose related and may be problematic for patients with advanced disease.

There are different SSRIs being marketed, including fluoxetine, sertraline, paroxetine, citalopram, and fluvoxamine. With the exception of fluoxetine, whose elimination half-life is 2–4 days, the SSRIs have an elimination half-life of about 24 h. Fluoxetine is the only SSRI with a potent active metabolite, norfluoxetine, whose elimination half-life is 7–14 days. Fluoxetine can cause mild nausea and a brief period of increased anxiety as well as appetite suppression that usually lasts for a period of several weeks. Some patients can experience transient weight loss, but weight usually returns to baseline level. The anorectic properties of fluoxetine have not been a limiting factor in the use of this drug in cancer patients. Fluoxetine and norfluoxetine do not reach a steady state for 5–6 weeks, compared with 4–14 days for paroxetine, citalopram, fluvoxamine, and sertraline. These difference are important, especially for the terminally patient in whom a switch from an SSRI to another antidepressant is being considered. If a switch to a monamine oxidase inhibitor is required, the washout period for fluoxetine will be at least 5 weeks, given the potential drug interactions between these two agents. Since fluoxetine has entered the market, there have been several reports of significant drug–drug interactions[96,97]. Until it has been studied further in the medically ill, it should be used cautiously in the debilitated dying patient. Paroxetine, citalopram, fluvoxamine, and sertraline on the other hand require considerably shorter washout periods (10–14 days) under similar circumstances.

All the SSRIs have the ability to inhibit the hepatic isoenzyme P450 11D6, with sertraline and citalopram being least potent in this regard. Citalopram appears to be the SSRI with the least potential for serious drug–drug interactions. This is important with respect to dose/plasma level ratios and drug interactions, since the SSRIs are dependent upon hepatic metabolism. For the elderly patient with advanced disease, the dose response curve for sertraline appears to be relatively linear. On the other hand, particularly for paroxetine (which appears to most potently inhibit cytochrome P450 11D6), small dosage increases can result in dramatic elevations in plasma levels. Paroxetine, and to a somewhat lesser extent fluoxetine, appear to inhibit the hepatic enzymes responsible for their own clearance[98]. The co-administration of these medications with other drugs that are dependent on this enzyme system for their catabolism (e.g. tricyclics, phenothiazines, type IC antiarrhythmics, and quinidine) should be done cautiously. Fluvoxamine has been shown in some instances to elevate the blood levels of propranolol and warfarin by as much as twofold, and should thus not be prescribed together with these agents.

SSRIs can generally be started at their minimally effective doses. For the terminally ill, this usually means initiating therapy at approximately half the usual starting dose used in an otherwise healthy patient. For fluoxetine, patients can begin on 5 mg (available in liquid form) given once daily (preferably in the morning) with a range of 10–40 mg/day; given its long half-life, some patients may only require this drug every second day. Paroxetine can be started at 10 mg once daily (either morning or evening) for the patient with advanced disease, and has a therapeutic range of 10–40/day. Fluvoxamine, which tends to be somewhat more

sedating, can be started at 25 mg (in the evenings) and has a therapeutic range of 50–300 mg. Sertraline can be initiated at 50 mg, morning or evening, and titrated within a range of 50–200 mg/day. Citalopram can be initiated at 10 mg per day and titrated up to a dose of 40–60 mg/day. If patients experience activating effects on SSRIs, they should not be given at bedtime but rather moved earlier into the day. Gastrointestinal upset can be reduced by ensuring the patient does not take medication on an empty stomach[48,65].

Serotonin–norepinephrine reuptake inhibitor

Venlaflaxine (Effexor®), is the only antidepressant in this class. It is a potent inhibitor of neuronal serotonin and norepinephrine reuptake and appears to have no significant affinity for muscarinic, histamine, or alpha1-adrenergic receptors. Some patients may experience a modest sustained increase in blood pressure, especially at doses above the recommended initiating dose. Compared with the SSRIs, its protein binding (<35 per cent) is very low. Few protein binding induced drug interactions are thus expected. Like other antidepressants, Venlaflaxine should not be used in patients receiving monamine oxidase inhibitors. Its side-effect profile tends to generally be well tolerated with few discontinuations. While there is currently no data addressing at its use in the terminally ill depressed patient, its pharmacokinetic properties and side effect profile suggest it may have a role to play[48,65,82].

Serotonin 2 antagonists/serotonin reuptake inhibitors

Nefazodone and trazodone are chemically related antidepressants that block post-synaptic 5-HT$_2$ receptors. Nefazodone is much less sedating than trazodone, but more likely to cause gastrointestinal activation. Nefazodone can be started at a dose of 50 mg at bedtime and titrated up to a range of 100–500 mg/day. Nefazodone does not have significant sexual side effects. If given in sufficient doses (100–300 mg/day), Trazodone can be an effective antidepressant. Although its anticholinergic profile is almost negligible it has considerable affinity for alpha1-adrenoceptors and may thus predispose patients to orthostatic hypotension and its problematic sequelae (i.e. falls, fractures, head injuries). Trazedone is very sedating and in low doses (100 mg qhs) is helpful in the treatment of the depressed cancer patient with insomnia. It is highly serotonergic and its use should be considered when the patient requires adjunct analgesics effect in addition to antidepressant effects. Trazodone has little effect on cardiac conduction but can cause arrhythmias in patients with premorbid cardiac disease[99]. Trazodone has also been associated with priapism and should thus be used with caution in male patients[100]. It is highly sedating with drowsiness being its most common adverse side effect. In smaller doses it can thus be used as an effective sedative hypnotic.

Norepinephrine and dopamine reuptake blockers

Buproprion has not been studied extensively in patients with advanced disease. However, one might consider prescribing buproprion if patients have a poor response to a reasonable trial of other antidepressants. Buproprion may have a role in the treatment of the psychomotor retarded depressed terminally ill patient as it has energizing effects similar to the stimulant drugs[101,102]. However, because of the increased incidence of seizures, in patients with CNS disorders, bupropion has a limited role in the oncology population. Buproprion and its sustained release form buproprion SR have also been used as an adjunct to smoking cessation interventions, but this experience has generally limited to patients with earlier stages of cancer or in healthy populations[48,65,82].

Mirtazapine is the 6-aza analogue of the tetracyclic antidepressant mianserin. Mirtazapine enhances central noradrenergic and serotonergic activities with blockade of central presynaptic alpha2 inhibitory receptors and post-synaptic serotonin 5-HT$_2$ and 5-HT$_3$ receptors. It compares favourably with amitriptyline and trazodone, with further studies needed to compare the clinical efficacy of mirtazapine to serotonin reuptake inhibitors. Mirtazapine improves appetite resulting in weight gain, which is desirable in cancer patients. In addition, the marked sedative effect of this medication proves quite useful in patients with sleeping difficulties[48,65,82].

Heterocyclic antidepressants

The heterocyclic antidepressants have side-effect profiles that are similar to the TCAs. Maprotiline should be avoided in patients with brain tumours and in those who are at risk for seizures since the incidence of seizures is increased with this medication[103]. Amoxapine has mild dopamine blocking activity. Hence, patients who are taking other dopamine blockers (e.g. antiemetics) have an increased risk of developing extrapyramidal symptoms and dyskinesias[104]. Mianserin (not available in the United States) is a serotonergic antidepressant with adjuvant analgesic properties that is used widely in Europe and Latin America. Costa et al.[81] showed mianserin to be a safe and effective drug for the treatment of depression in cancer.

Psychostimulants

The psychostimulants (dextroamphetamine, methylphenidate, pemoline, and modafinil) offer an alternative and effective pharmacologic approach to the treatment of depression in the terminally ill[83,105–117]. These drugs have a more rapid onset of action than the SSRIs and are often energizing. They are most helpful in the treatment of depression in cancer patients with advanced disease and those where dysphoric mood is associated with severe psychomotor slowing and even mild cognitive impairment. Ocassionally treatment with an SSRI and a psychostimulant may be initiated concurrently so that patients with depression may receive the immediate benefits of the psychostimulant drug until the 1–2 weeks necessary for an SSRI to begin to work pass. At that point the psychostimulant may be withdrawn as symptoms of depression are monitored. A decision at that point can be made to either continue without the psychostimulant (if the SSRI has begun to take effect) or the psychostimulant drug can be restarted and continued. Psychostimulants have been shown to improve attention, concentration, and overall performance on neuropsychological testing in the medically ill[118]. In relatively low dose, psychostimulants stimulate appetite, promote a sense of well-being, and improve feelings of weakness and fatigue in cancer patients. Treatment with dextroamphetamine or methylphenidate usually begins with a dose of 2.5 mg at 8:00 am and at noon. The dosage is slowly increased over several days until a desired effect is achieved or side effects (overstimulation, anxiety, insomnia, paranoia, confusion) intervene. Typically a dose greater than 30 mg/day is not necessary although occasionally patients require up to 60 mg/day. Patients usually are maintained on methylphenidate for 1–2 months, and approximately two-thirds will be able to be withdrawn from methylphenidate without a recurrence of depressive symptoms. Those who do recur can be maintained on a psychostimulant for up to 1 year without significant abuse

problems. Tolerance will develop and adjustment of dose may be necessary. An additional benefit of such stimulants as methylphenidate and dextroamphetamine are that they have been shown to reduce sedation secondary to opioid analgesics and provide adjuvant analgesics in cancer patients[119]. Common side effects of stimulants include nervousness, overstimulation, mild increase in blood pressure and pulse rate, and tremor. More rare side effects include dyskinesias or motor tics as well as a paranoid psychosis or exacerbation of an underlying and unrecognized confusional state.

Pemoline was a unique psychostimulant chemically unrelated to amphetamine, which has recently been removed from the market by its manufacturer because of several deaths due to irreversible liver damage. It was a less potent stimulant with little abuse potential[109]. Advantages of pemoline as a psychostimulant in cancer patients included the lack of abuse potential, the lack of wfederal regulation through special triplicate prescriptions, the mild sympathomimetic effects, and the fact that it comes in a chewable tablet form that can be absorbed through the buccal mucosa and be used by cancer patients who have difficulty swallowing or have intestinal obstruction. Pemoline appeared to be as effective as methylphenidate or dextroamphetamine in the treatment of depressive symptoms in terminally ill cancer patients[120]. Pemoline can be started at a dose of 18.75 mg in the morning and at noon, and increased gradually over days. Typically patients require 75 mg a day or less. Pemoline should be used with caution in patients with liver impairment, and liver function tests should be monitored periodically with longer-term treatment[121].

Modafinil, a novel psychostimulant or 'wakefulness agent', has been approved for use in the United States for the treatment of excessive daytime sleepiness due to narcolepsy and other medical conditions. Although more controlled studies need to be completed, early case series reports suggest its efficacy as an adjuvant antidepressant[114–117]. Modafinil is a novel psychostimulant, whose mechanism of action is unclear, that does not have a similar pharmacological profile to the other sympathomimetic amines. Although modafinil may produce euphoric effects and has been shown to be reinforcing at high doses in monkeys during clinical trials, the subjective effects of modafinil are markedly different from those of amphetamine and methylphenidate. This suggests that modafinil may not have the same abuse liability as those drugs. Because of this lower abuse potential, modafinil is a Schedule IV prescription[114–117]. A case series by Menza et al.[114] showed modafinil to be a useful augmenting agent in treatment resistant depression, particularly when patients complain of fatigue as one of their symptoms. In this series, modafinil was used in combination with a number of different antidepressants and anticonvulsants, including SSRIs, buproprion, venlafaxine, and divalproex. The addition of modafinil was well tolerated and led to a marked reduction in depressive symptoms in all seven patients. Modafinil should be given in the morning and can be started at a dose of 100 mg for most patients. Starting at 50 mg is advisable for elderly or frail patients. The dose can then be titrated upwards. In his case series, Menza's modal dose was 200 mg. However, modafinil can be used in doses up to 400 mg/day. Modafinil may be a useful alternative to other psychostimulants for patients who are unable to tolerate or for whom the usual psychostimulants are contraindicated (e.g. in that modafinil is less sympathomimetic, has less potential for adverse cardiovascular effects, for example, tachycardia, lowers seizure threshold very minimally if at all, and has very low abuse potential).

Monamine oxidase inhibitors

In general monoamine oxidase inhibitors (MAOIs) have been considered a less desirable alternative for treating depression in the terminally ill. Patients who receive MAOIs must avoid foods rich in tyramine, sympathomimetic drugs (amphetamines, methylphenidate), and medications containing phenylpropranolamine and pseudoephedrine[95]. The combination of these agents with MAOIs may cause hypertensive crisis, leading to strokes and fatalities. MAOIs in combination with opioid analgesics have also been reported to be associated with myoclonus and delirium, and must therefore be used together cautiously[65]. The use of meperidine while on MAOIs is absolutely contraindicated and can lead to hyperpyrexia, cardiovascular collapses, and death. MAOIs can also cause considerable orthostatic hypotension. Avoiding this minefield of adverse interactions can be particularly problematic for the terminally ill. It is not surprising that MAOIs tend to be reserved in this patient population for those who have shown past preferential responses to them for treatment of their depression.

The new reversible inhibitors of monoamine oxidase-A (RIMAs) may reduce some of the problems associated with the older MAOIs (tranylcypromine, isocarboxazide). There are no studies on the role of RIMAs in the depressed terminally ill but there are interesting theoretical reasons to suggest they may eventually have a larger role to play than the non-selective MAOIs. RIMAs selectively inhibit MAO-A enzyme, therefore leaving MAO-B enzyme available to deal with any tyramine challenge. Moclobemide, a relatively novel RIMA, appears to be loosely bound to the MAO-A receptor and is thus relatively easily displaced by tyramine from its binding sight. It has a very short half-life which further reduces the possibility of any prolonged adverse effects, for example, hypertensive crisis. Dietary restrictions avoidant of tyramine-containing foods are thus not required. The side-effect profile of moclobemide is far more favourable than non-selective MAOIs and tends to be well tolerated. Although the risk of hypertensive crisis is significantly reduced, it is not, however, entirely eliminated. Agents such as meperidine, procarbazine, dextromethorphan, or other ephedrine-containing agents are still best avoided. Its short half-life requires that moclobemide be administered two times daily, with a total dosage range of 150–600 mg daily. Co-administration with cimetidine will increase its plasma concentration thus requiring appropriate dosage adjustments. While RIMAs may offer some advantages in the terminally ill depressed patient over tranylcypromine and isocarboxazid, they will likely remain a second line choice to other available non-MAOI antidepressants.

Lithium carbonate

Patients who have been receiving lithium carbonate, prior to a cancer illness, should be maintained on it throughout their cancer treatment, although close monitoring is necessary in the preoperative and postoperative periods when fluids and salt may be restricted[100]. Maintenance doses of lithium may need reduction in seriously ill patients. Lithium should be prescribed with caution for patients receiving cis-platinum because of the potential nephrotoxicity of both drugs. Several authors have reported possible beneficial effects from the use of lithium in neutropenic cancer patients. However, the functional capabilities of these leukocytes have not been determined. The stimulation effect appears to be transient; no mood changes have been noted in these patients[122,123].

Benzodiazepines

The triazolobenzodiazepine alprazolam has been shown to be a mildly effective antidepressant as well as an anxiolytic. Alprazolam is particularly useful in cancer patients who have mixed symptoms of anxiety and depression. Starting dose is 0.25 mg three times a day, effective doses are usually in the range of 4–6 mg daily[47].

Electroconvulsive therapy

Occasionally, it is necessary to consider electroconvulsive therapy (ECT) for depressed cancer patients who have depression with psychotic features or in whom treatment with antidepressants pose unacceptable side effects. The safe effective use of ECT in the medically ill has been reviewed by others[44].

Non-pharmacologic treatment of depression in terminally ill patients

Supportive psychotherapy is a useful treatment approach to depression in the terminally ill patient. Psychotherapy with the dying patient consists of active listening with supportive verbal interventions and the occasional interpretation[102]. Despite the seriousness of the patient's plight, it is not necessary for the psychiatrist or psychologist to appear overly solemn or emotionally restrained. Often it is only the psychotherapist, of all the patient's care givers, who is comfortable enough to converse lightheartedly and allow the patient to talk about their life and experiences, rather than focus solely on impending death. The dying patient who wishes to talk or ask questions about death should be allowed to do so freely, with the therapist maintaining an interested, interactive stance. It is not uncommon for the dying patient to benefit from pastoral counselling. If a chaplaincy service is available, it should be offered to the patient and family.

A number of psychotherapies, other than supportive psychotherapy, have been described as potentially useful in the treatment of depressive symptoms and distress in a palliative care population. A review of the applications of interpersonal, existential, life narrative, and group psychotherapy intervention in the palliative care population is available to the reader[1,124]. Recently, several novel psychotherapies have been developed and are being tested in the treatment of depression, hopelessness, loss of meaning, and demoralization. Two examples of such developing psychotherapies include: Meaning-Centered psychotherapy[125] and Dignity-Conserving care[126].

Suicide, assisted suicide, and desire for hastened death in the terminally ill

Suicide, suicidal ideation, and desire for hastened death are all important and serious consequences of unrecognized and inadequately treated clinical depression. While clinical depression has been demonstrated to be a critically important factor in desire for hastened death (through suicide or other means), understanding more fully why some patients with a terminal illness wish or seek to hasten their death remains an important element in the practice of palliative care. Despite the continued legal prohibitions against assisted suicide, a substantial number of patients think about and discuss those alternatives with their physicians, family, and friends[127].

Suicide

Cancer patients are at increased risk of suicide relative to the general population, particularly in the terminal stage of illness.

Table 15.5.5 Suicide vulnerability factors in patients with advanced disease.

Pain, suffering aspects
Advanced illness, poor prognosis
Depression, hopelessness
Delirium, disinhibition
Control, helplessness
Pre-existing psychopathology
Substance/alcohol abuse
Suicide history, family history
Fatigue, exhaustion
Lack of social support, social isolation

Factors associated with increased risk of suicide in patients with advanced disease[69,70] are listed in Table 15.5.5. Patients with advanced illness are at highest risk, perhaps because they are most likely to have such cancer complications as pain, depression, delirium, and deficit symptoms. Psychiatric disorders are frequently present in hospitalized cancer patients who are suicidal. A review of the psychiatric consultation data from Memorial Sloan-Kettering Cancer Center showed that one-third of suicidal cancer patients had a major depression, about 20 per cent suffered from a delirium, and 50 per cent were diagnosed with an adjustment disorder with both anxious and depressed features at the time of evaluation[69,70].

Suicide in cancer patients occurs most frequently among the newly diagnosed and among patients with advanced disease[128–131]. The suicide rate in cancer patients has steadily decreased during the last 30–40 years[131]. Eighty-six per cent of suicides studied by Farberow et al.[132] occurred in the preterminal or terminal stages of illness, despite greatly reduced physical capacity. Poor prognosis and advanced illness usually go hand-in-hand. It is thus not surprising that in Sweden, those who were expected to die within a matter of months were the most likely to commit suicide. Of 88 cancer suicides, 14 had an uncertain prognosis, and 45 had a poor prognosis[128]. With advancing disease, the incidence of significant cancer pain increases. Uncontrolled pain in cancer patients is a dramatically important risk factor for suicide. The vast majority of cancer suicides in several studies showed that these patients had severe pain which was often inadequately controlled and poorly tolerated[128,132].

Depression is a factor in 50 per cent of all suicides. Those suffering from depression are at 25 times greater risk of suicide than the general population[133,134]. The role depression plays in cancer suicide is equally significant. Approximately 25 per cent of all cancer patients experience severe depressive symptoms, with about 6 per cent fulfilling DSM-III criteria for the diagnosis of major depression[45,49]. Among those with advanced illness and progressively impaired physical function, symptoms of severe depression rise to 77 per cent[7]. Depression also appears to be important in terms of patient preferences for life-sustaining medical therapy. Ganzini et al. reported that among elderly depressed patients, an increase in desire for life-sustaining medical therapies followed treatment of depression in those subjects who had been initially more severely depressed, more hopeless, and

more likely to overestimate the risks and to underestimate the benefits of treatment[135]. They concluded that while patients with mild to moderate depression are unlikely to alter their decisions regarding life-sustaining medical treatment in spite of treatment for their depression, severely depressed patients—particularly those who are hopeless—should be encouraged to defer advance treatment directives. In these patients, decisions about life-sustaining therapy should be discouraged until after treatment of their depression.

Hopelessness is the key variable that links depression and suicide in the general population. Further, hopelessness is a significantly better predictor of completed suicide than is depression alone[136]. Chochinov et al. demonstrated that hopelessness was correlated more highly with suicidal ideation in terminally ill cancer patients than was the level of depression[137]. With the typical cancer suicide being characterized by advanced illness and poor prognosis, hopelessness is commonly experienced. In Scandinavia, the highest incidence of suicide was found in cancer patients who were offered no further treatment, and no further contact with the health-care system[128,131]. Being left to face illness alone creates a sense of isolation and abandonment that is critical to the development of hopelessness. The prevalence of organic mental disorders among cancer patients requiring psychiatric consultation has been found to range from 25 to 40 per cent[2,138], reaching as high as 85 per cent during the terminal stages of illness[9]. While earlier work suggested that delirium was a protective factor in regard to cancer suicide[129], clinical experience has found these confusional states to be a major contributing factor in impulsive suicide attempts, especially in the hospital setting.

Loss of control and a sense of helplessness in the face of cancer are important factors in suicide vulnerability. Control refers to both the helplessness induced by symptoms or deficits due to cancer or its treatments, as well as the excessive need on the part of some patients to be in control of all aspects of living or dying. Farberow et al. noted that patients who were accepting and adaptable were much less likely to commit suicide than cancer patients who exhibited a need to be in control of even the most minute details of their care[132]. This need to control may be prominent in some patients and cause distress with little provocation. However, it is not uncommon for cancer-related events to induce a great sense of helplessness even in those who are not typically controlling individuals. Impairments or deficits induced by cancer or cancer treatments include loss of mobility, paraplegia, loss of bowel and bladder functions, amputation, aphonia, sensory loss, and inability to eat or swallow. Most distressing to patients is the sense that they are losing control of their minds, especially when they are confused or sedated by medications. The risk of suicide is increased in cancer patients with such physical impairments, especially when accompanied by psychological distress and disturbed interpersonal relationships due to these deficit factors[132].

Fatigue, in the form of emotional, spiritual, financial, familial, communal and other resource exhaustion increases risk of suicide in the cancer patient[70]. Cancer is now often a chronic illness. Increased survival is accompanied by increased numbers of hospitalizations, complications, and expenses. Symptom control thus becomes a prolonged process with frequent advances and setbacks. The dying process also can become extremely long and arduous for all concerned. It is not uncommon for both family members and health care providers to withdraw prematurely from the cancer patient under these circumstances. A suicidal patient can thus feel even more isolated and abandoned. The presence of a strong support system for the patient that may act as an external control of suicidal behaviour reduces risk of cancer suicide significantly.

Holland[139] advises that it is extremely rare for a cancer patient to commit suicide without some degree of premorbid psychopathology that places them at increased risk. Farberow et al.[129] described a large group of cancer suicides as the 'Dependent Dissatisfied'. These patients were immature, demanding, complaining, irritable, hostile, and difficult ward management problems. Staff often felt manipulated by these patients and became irritable due to what they saw as excessive demands for attention. Suicide attempts or threats were often seen as 'hysterical' or manipulative. Consultation data from Memorial Sloan-Kettering on suicidal cancer patients showed that half had a diagnosable personality disorder[170].

The frequency of suicide attempts in cancer patients has not been well studied. While the frequency of suicidal thinking in the cancer setting may be in question, its relationship to suicide attempts or completions is clearer. Bolund[128] reports that half of all Swedish cancer suicides had previously conveyed suicidal thoughts or plans to their relatives. In addition, many of the completed cancer suicides had been preceded by an attempted suicide. This is consistent with the statistics of suicide in general, which show that a previous suicide attempt greatly increases the risk of completed suicide[140–142]. A family history of suicide is of increasing relevance in assessing suicide risk.

Suicidal ideation

Thoughts of suicide probably occur quite frequently, particularly in the setting of advanced cancer, and seem to act as a steam valve for feelings often expressed by patients as 'if it gets too bad, I always have a way out'. Once they develop a trusting and safe relationship, patients almost universally reveal occasional persistent thoughts of suicide as a means of escaping the threat of being overwhelmed by cancer. More recent published reports, however, suggest that suicidal ideation is relatively infrequent in cancer and is limited to those who are significantly depressed. Silberfarb et al.[143] found that only three of 146 breast cancer patients had suicidal thoughts, while none of the 100 cancer patients interviewed in a Finnish study expressed suicidal thoughts[144]. A study conducted at St Boniface Hospice in Winnipeg, Canada, demonstrated that only 10 of 44 terminally ill cancer patients were suicidal or desired an early death, and all 10 were suffering from clinical depression[145].

At Memorial Hospital, suicide risk evaluation accounted for 8.6 per cent of psychiatric consultations, usually requested by staff in response to a patient verbalizing suicidal wishes[70]. Among 185 cancer patients with pain studied at Memorial Hospital, suicidal ideation was found in 17 per cent of the study population[70]. The actual prevalence of suicidal ideation may be considerably higher in that patients often disclose these thoughts only after a stable, ongoing physician–patient relationship has been established.

Assessment and management of the suicidal terminally ill patient

Assessment of suicide risk and appropriate intervention are critical. Early and comprehensive psychiatric involvement with high-risk individuals can often avert suicide in the cancer setting[116]. A careful evaluation includes a search for the meaning of suicidal thoughts as well as an exploration of the seriousness of the risk. The clinician's ability to establish rapport and elicit a patient's thoughts are essential as he or she assesses history, degree of intent, and quality of internal and external controls. One must listen sympathetically, not appearing critical or stating that such thoughts are inappropriate. Allowing the patient to discuss suicidal thoughts often decreases the risk of suicide. The myth that asking about suicidal thoughts 'puts the idea in their head', is one that should be dispelled, especially in cancer[127]. Patients often reconsider and reject the idea of suicide when the physician acknowledges the legitimacy of their option and the need to retain a sense of control over aspects of their death.

The suicide vulnerability factors (Table 15.5.5) should be utilized as a guide to evaluation and management. Once the setting has been made secure, assessment of the relevant mental status and adequacy of pain control can begin. Analgesics, neuroleptics, or antidepressant drugs should be utilized when appropriate to treat agitation, psychosis, major depression, or pain. Underlying causes of delirium or pain should be addressed specifically when possible. Initiation of a crisis-intervention-oriented psychotherapeutic approach, mobilizing as much of the patient's support system as possible is important. A close family member or friend should be involved in order to support the patient, provide information, and assist in treatment planning. Psychiatric hospitalization can sometimes be helpful but is usually not desirable in the terminally ill patient. Thus, the medical hospital or home is the setting in which management most often takes place. While it is appropriate to intervene when medical or psychiatric factors are clearly the driving force in a cancer suicide, there are circumstances when usurping control from the patient and family with overly aggressive intervention may be less helpful. This is most evident in those with advanced illness where comfort and symptom control are the primary concerns.

Ultimately the palliative care clinician may not be able to prevent all suicides in all terminally ill patients that he or she cares for. The emphasis of intervention should be to aggressively attempt to prevent suicide that is driven by the desperation of uncontrolled physical and psychological symptoms such as uncontrolled pain, unrecognized delirium, and unrecognized and untreated depression. Prolonged suffering caused by poorly controlled symptoms can lead to such desperation, and it is the appropriate role of the palliative care team to provide effective management of physical and psychological symptoms as an alternative to desire for death, suicide, or request for assisted suicide by patients.

Requests for assisted suicide

A growing body of literature has emerged on the type of physical and psychological concerns that may give rise to a desire for hastened death and request for assisted suicide. Even if relatively little empirical research has addressed this issue, especially with medically ill patients, some authors found rates of support for legalization of assisted-suicide that were roughly comparable to those published in studies on the general population. In a survey study done by Breitbart et al., 64 per cent of AIDS patients supported assisted-suicide legalization[146]. In another study 55 per cent of terminally ill AIDS patients indicated a possible interest in assisted suicide. In a 1996 study of oncology patients, 25 per cent of cancer patients reported that they had thought seriously about euthanasia and 12 per cent had discussed this option with their physicians[147]. A number of social variables, such as fear of becoming a burden to family and friends and experience with the death of a friend or family, have been significant predictors of interest in assisted suicide among ambulatory patients with AIDS[146]. This joins a growing evidence of research demonstrating an important relationship between social support and desire for death, when no relationship was found with pain, physical symptoms, or stage of disease[127].

Desire for hastened death

Desire for hastened death may be thought of as a unifying construct underlying requests for assisted suicide or euthanasia, as well as suicidal thoughts in general. Literature has emerged on the type of physical and psychological concerns that may give rise to a desire for hastened death. Several studies have demonstrated that depression plays a significant role in the terminally ill patient's desire for hastened death. The precise intensity of this association between depression and desire for hastened death is still being investigated. Chochinov et al. found that of 200 terminally ill patients in a palliative care facility, 44.5 per cent acknowledged at least a fleeting desire to die—these episodes were brief and did not reflect a sustained or committed desire to die[148]. However, 17 patients (8.5 per cent) reported an unequivocal desire for death to come soon and indicated that they held this desire consistently over time. Among this group, 10 (58.8 per cent) received a diagnosis of depression, compared to a prevalence of 7.7 per cent in patients who did not endorse a genuine, consistent desire for death. Patients with depression were approximately six to seven times more likely to have a desire for hastened death than patients without depression. Patients with a desire for death were also found to have significantly more pain and less social support than those patients without a desire for death. Breitbart et al.[50] studied the relationships between depression, hopelessness, and desire for death in a sample of 92 terminally ill cancer patients. Sixteen patients (17 per cent) were classified as having a high desire for death, based on their scores on a validated self report measure of desire for hastened death called the Schedule of Attitudes Toward Hastened Death[149,150], and 16 per cent met criteria for a current major depressive episode. Of the patients who met criteria for major depressive episode, seven (47 per cent) were classified as having a high desire for hastened death while only 12 per cent without a desire for death met criteria for depression. Thus, patients with a major depression were four times more likely to have a high desire for hastened death. In addition, Breitbart and his colleagues found that both depression and hopelessness, characterized as a pessimistic cognitive style rather than an assessment of one's poor prognosis, appear to be unique and synergistic determinants of desire for hastened death[46]. No significant association with the presence or the intensity of pain was found. Desire for hastened death also appears to be primarily a function of psychological distress and social factors such as social support, spiritual well-being, quality of life and perception of oneself as a burden to others. Among dying patients, 'will to live', as measured with a visual analogue scale, tends to fluctuate rapidly over time and is correlated with anxiety, depression, and shortness of breath as death approaches[151].

Interventions for desire for hastened death and despair at the end of life

The response of a clinician to despair at the end of life as manifest by a patient's expression of desire for death or request for assisted suicide has important and obvious implications on all aspects of care which impact on patients, family, and staff[152]. These issues must be addressed both rapidly and thoughtfully, offering the patient a non-judgemental willingness to engage in a discussion of the factors that contribute to the suffering and despondency that leads patients to express such a desire for death. Some investigators speak of this suffering in using such terms as 'spiritual' suffering, 'demoralization', loss of 'dignity', 'loss of meaning'[125,153–156] and have developed interventions based on these concepts/themes.

Palliative care practitioners have begun to deal with the issue of spirituality in the dying and interventions for spiritual suffering. Rousseau[153] outlines an approach for the treatment of spiritual suffering which is composed of the following steps: (1) controlling physical symptoms; (2) providing a supportive presence; (3) encouraging life review to assist in recognizing purpose value and meaning; (4) exploring guilt, remorse, forgiveness, reconciliation; (5) facilitating religious expression; (6) reframing goals; and (7) encourage meditative practices, focus on healing rather than cure. Rousseau has presented an approach to spiritual suffering that is an interesting blend of basic psychotherapeutic principles.

Psychotherapeutic techniques that are particularly adaptive to psychotherapy with the dying, such as life narrative and life review, are also included. There is an emphasis on facilitating religious expression and confession that in fact may be extremely useful to many patients, but is not applicable to all patients and not necessarily an intervention that many clinicians feel comfortable providing. What Rousseau's work suggests is that novel psychotherapeutic interventions aimed at improving spiritual well-being, sense of meaning, and diminishing hopelessness, demoralization, and distress are critically necessary to develop at this stage in the development of palliative medicine.

Kissane et al.[154] have described a syndrome of 'demoralization' in the terminally ill which they propose is distinct from depression, and consists of a triad of hopelessness, loss of meaning, and existential distress expressed as a desire for death. It is associated with life-threatening medical illness, disability, bodily disfigurement, fear, loss of dignity, social isolation, and feelings of being a burden. Because of the sense of impotence and hopelessness, those with the syndrome predictably progress to a desire to die or commit suicide. Kissane et al. describe a treatment approach for demoralization syndrome[154]. This approach emphasizes a multi-disciplinary, multimodal approach consisting of: (1) ensuring continuity of care and active symptom management; (2) ensuring dignity in the dying process; (3) utilizing various types of psychotherapy to help sustain a sense of meaning, limit cognitive distortions, and maintain family relationships (i.e. meaning-based, cognitive behavioural, interpersonal, and family psychotherapy interventions); (4) use of life review and narrative, and attention to spiritual issues; and (5) pharmacotherapy for co-morbid anxiety, depression, and delirium.

Ensuring 'dignity' in the dying process is a critical goal of palliative care. Despite use of the term 'dignity' in arguments for and against a patient's self-governance in matters pertaining to death, there is little empirical research on how this term has been used by patients who are nearing death. Chochinov et al.[155] examined how dying patients understand and define the term 'dignity', in order to develop a model of dignity in the terminally ill (see Fig. 15.5.1). A semi-structured interview was designed to

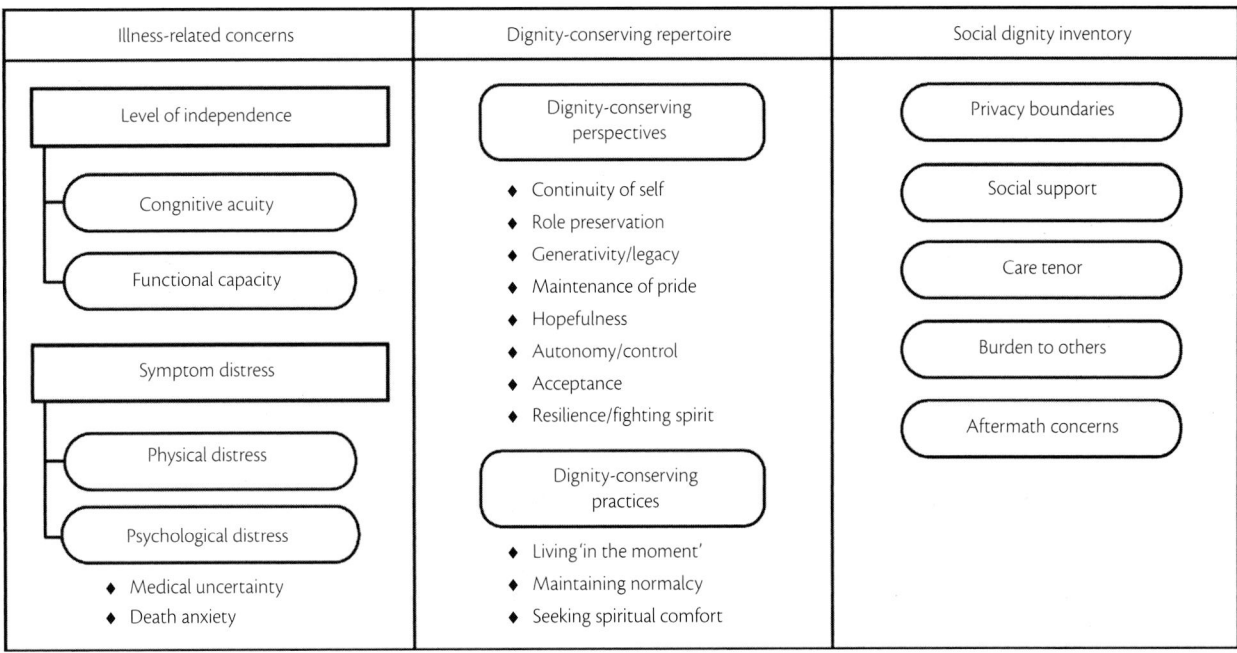

Figure 15.5.1 Major dignity categories, themes, and sub-themes.

explore how patients cope with their advanced cancer and to detail their perceptions of dignity. Three major categories emerged from a detailed qualitative analysis, including illness-related concerns (concerns that derive from or are related to the illness itself, and threaten to or actually do impinge on the patient's sense of dignity); dignity-conserving repertoire (internally held qualities or personal approaches or techniques that patients use to bolster or maintain their sense of dignity); and social dignity inventory (social concerns or relationship dynamics that enhance or detract from a patient's sense of dignity). These broad categories and their carefully defined themes and sub-themes form the foundation for an emerging model of dignity amongst the dying. The concept of dignity and the notion of dignity-conserving care offer a way of understanding how patients face advancing terminal illness, and presents an approach that clinicians can use to explicitly target the maintenance of dignity as a therapeutic objective, and principle of bedside care for patients nearing death. Chochinov, in fact, describes his technique of 'dignity conserving care' in a review[126] which interested readers can read for further details.

Interventions for hopelessness, loss of meaning and purpose in the terminally ill are of particular importance when addressing the issues of desire for death and despair at the end of life. Breitbart and colleagues[125,156] have developed an intervention they term 'meaning-centred' group psychotherapy for advanced cancer patients; an intervention based on the concepts and principles of Viktor Frankl's writings and logotherapy. The intervention is designed to help patients with advanced cancer sustain or enhance a sense of meaning, peace, and purpose in their lives even as they approach the end of life. Meaning-centred group psychotherapy is a manualized, 8-week (1.5 h weekly sessions) intervention which utilizes a mixture of didactics, discussion, and experiential exercises that focus around particular themes related to meaning and advanced cancer. The session themes include: Session 1—Concepts of Meaning and Sources of Meaning; Session 2—Cancer and Meaning; Session 3—Meaning and Historical Context of Life; Session 4—Storytelling, Life Project; Session 5—Limitations and Finiteness of Life; Session 6—Responsibility, Creativity, Deeds; Session 7—Experience, Nature, Art, Humor; Session 8—Termination, Goodbyes, Hopes for the Future. Patients are assigned readings and homework that are specific to each session's theme and which are utilized in each session. While the focus of each session is on issues of meaning/peace and purpose in life in the face of advanced cancer and a limited prognosis, elements of support and expression of emotion are inevitable in the context of each group session (but limited by the focus on experiential exercises, didactics and discussions related to themes focusing on meaning).

Most palliative care clinicians believe that aggressive management of physical and psychological symptoms and syndromes that have been demonstrated to contribute to desire for death will naturally prevent such expressions of distress or requests for assisted suicide. For instance, there is a general consensus that individuals with a major depression can be effectively treated in the context of terminal illness. No research has yet addressed if such treatment for depression directly influences desire for hastened death. Because depression and hopelessness are not identical constructs (although highly correlated) clinical interventions, such as those described above, developed to more specifically address hopelessness and related constructs such as dignity, loss of meaning, demoralization, and spiritual suffering or distress will be important to empirically test and utilize in general palliative care practice if they prove effective.

Cognitive disorders in the terminally ill

Cognitive failure is unfortunately all too common in patients with advanced illness. The Diagnostic and Statistical Manual of Mental Disorders, Fourth Edition (DSM-IV)[157] divides cognitive disorders into the sub-categories of: (1) delirium, dementia, amnesic, and other cognitive disorders; (2) mental disorders due to a general medical condition (including mood disorder, anxiety disorder, and personality change due to a general medical condition); and (3) substance-related disorders. While virtually all of these mental syndromes can be seen in the patient with advanced cancer, the most common include delirium, dementia, and mood and anxiety disorders due to a general medical condition. Lipowski[158] categorized organic mental disorders into those that were characterized by general cognitive impairment (i.e. delirium and dementia) and those where cognitive impairment was rather selective or limited (i.e. amnesic disorder, organic hallucinosis, and organic mood disorder). With organic mental disorders where cognitive impairment is selective, limited, or relatively intact, the more prominent symptoms tend to consist of either anxiety, mood disturbance, delusions, hallucinations, or personality change. For instance, the patient with mood disturbance meeting criteria for major depression, who is severely hypothyroid or on high-dose corticosteroids is most accurately diagnosed as having a mood disorder due to a general medical condition or substance-induced mood disorder, respectively (particularly if organic factors are judged to be the primary aetiology related to the mood disturbance). Similarly, the patient with hyponatremia, or the patient on acyclovir for CNS herpes who is experiencing visual hallucinations but has an intact sensorium with minimal cognitive deficits, is more accurately diagnosed as having a psychotic disorder due to a general medical condition or a substance-induced psychotic disorder, respectively.

In spite of very little being known about the neuropathogenesis of delirium, its symptoms suggest that it is a dysfunction of multiple regions of the brain[159]. Delirium has been characterized as an aetiologically non-specific, global, cerebral dysfunction characterized by concurrent disturbances of level of consciousness, attention, thinking, perception, memory, psychomotor behaviour, emotion, and the sleep–wake cycle. Disorientation, fluctuation, or waxing and waning of these symptoms, as well as acute or abrupt onset of such disturbances are other critical features of delirium. Delirium, in contrast with dementia, is conceptualized as a reversible process. Reversibility of the process of delirium (Fig. 15.5.2) is often possible even in the patient with advanced illness; however, it may not be reversible in the last 24–48 h of life. This is most likely due to the fact that irreversible processes such as multiple organ

failure are occurring in the final hours of life. Delirium occurring in these last days of life is often referred to as terminal restlessness or terminal agitation in the palliative care literature.

At times it is difficult to differentiate delirium from dementia since they frequently share such common clinical features as impaired memory, thinking, judgement, and disorientation. Dementia appears in relatively alert individuals with little or no clouding of consciousness. The temporal onset of symptoms in dementia is more sub-acute or chronically progressive, and one's sleep–wake cycle seems less impaired. Most prominent in dementia are difficulties in short- and long-term memory, impaired judgement, and abstract thinking as well as disturbed higher cortical functions (such as aphasia and apraxia). Occasionally one will encounter delirium superimposed on an underlying dementia, such as in the case of an elderly patient, an AIDS patient, or a patient with a paraneoplastic syndrome. Clinically, we often utilize a number of scales or instruments that aid us in the diagnosis of delirium, dementia, or cognitive failure.

Delirium in the terminally ill: prevalence, diagnosis, assessment, and management

Prevalence of delirium

Delirium is the most common and serious neuropsychiatric complication in the patient with advanced illness. Cognitive disorders, and delirium in particular, have enormous relevance to symptom control and palliative care. Delirium is highly prevalent in cancer and in AIDS patients with advanced disease, particularly in the last weeks of life, with prevalence rates ranging from 25 to 85 per cent[9,160–166]. Delirium is one of the most common mental disorders encountered in general hospital practice. Knight and Folstein[167] estimated that 33 per cent of hospitalized medically ill patients have serious cognitive impairments. Massie et al. found delirium in 25 per cent of 334 hospitalized cancer patients seen in psychiatric consultation and in 85 per cent (11 of 13) of terminal cancer patients[9]. Pereira et al. found the prevalence of cognitive impairment in cancer inpatients to be 44 per cent, and just prior to death, the prevalence rose to 62.1 per cent[168]. Delirium also occurs in up to 51 per cent of postoperative patients[158,169]. The incidence of delirium is currently increasing, which reflects the growing numbers of elderly, who are particularly susceptible[158]. Studies of elderly patients admitted to medical wards estimate that between 30 and 50 per cent of patients 70 years or older showed symptoms of delirium at some point during hospitalization[170–174]. Elderly patients who develop delirium during a hospitalization have been estimated to have a 22–76 per cent chance of dying during that hospitalization[175].

Delirium is associated with increased morbidity in the terminally ill, causing distress in patients, family members, and staff[161,176,177]. In a study of the 'delirium experience' of terminally ill cancer patients, Breitbart et al.[176] found that 54 per cent of patients recalled their delirium experience after recovery from delirium. Factors predicting delirium recall included the degree of short-term memory impairment, delirium severity, and the presence of perceptual disturbances (the more severe the less likely recall). Distress related to the episode of delirium was rated by patients, spouses/care givers, and nurses on a 0–4 numerical rating scale (with 4 being most severe). Patients averaged a rating of 3.2, spouses 3.75, and nurses a 3.2. The most significant factor predicting distress for

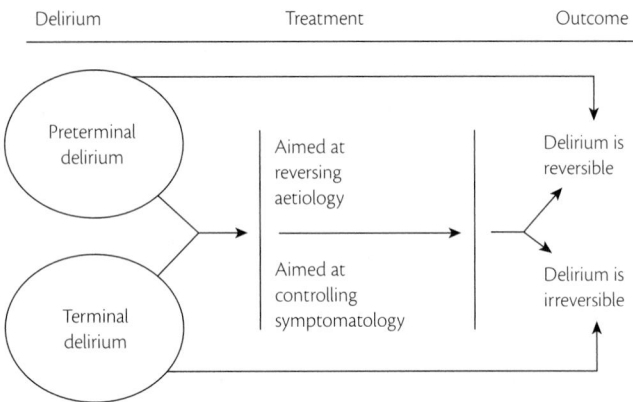

Figure 15.5.2 Overview of delirium management.

patients was the presence of delusions. Patients with hypoactive delirium were just as distressed as patients with hyperactive delirium. Predictors of spouse distress included the patients' Karnofsky Performance Status (the lower the Karnofsky, the worse the spouse distress), and nurse distress included delirium severity and perceptual disturbances. Delirium can interfere dramatically with the recognition and control of other physical and psychological symptoms such as pain[178–180] in later stages of illness. Often a preterminal event, delirium is a sign of significant physiologic disturbance, usually involving multiple medical aetiologies, including infection, organ failure, medication side effects (including opioids), as well as extremely rare paraneoplastic syndromes[54,166,181–183]. In spite of the prevalence of delirium in patients receiving palliative care, and the burden delirium represents for patients, relatives and staff, there is still a dearth of rigorous studies on delirium in the palliative care setting[166].

Lawlor *et al.*[184] reported on their experience in the management of delirium in advanced cancer patients in a palliative care unit. While 42 per cent of patients had delirium upon admission to their palliative care unit, terminal delirium occurred in 88 per cent of the deaths. Unfortunately delirium is often under-recognized or misdiagnosed, and inappropriately treated or untreated in terminally ill patients. Impediments to progress in the recognition and treatment delirium have included confusion regarding terminology and lack of consistency in utilizing diagnostic classification systems. In addition, the signs and symptoms of delirium can be diverse and are sometimes mistaken for other psychiatric disorders such as mood or anxiety disorders. Practitioners caring for patients with life-threatening illnesses must be able to diagnose delirium accurately, undertake appropriate assessment of aetiologies, and be knowledgeable about the benefits and risks of the pharmacologic and non-pharmacologic interventions currently available in managing delirium among the terminally ill.

Diagnosing delirium

The clinical features of delirium are quite numerous and include a variety of neuropsychiatric symptoms that are also common to other psychiatric disorders such as depression, dementia, and psychosis[185]. Clinical features of delirium include prodromal symptoms (restlessness, anxiety, sleep disturbance, and irritability), rapidly fluctuating course, reduced attention (easily distractible), altered arousal, increased or decreased psychomotor activity, disturbance of sleep–wake cycle, affective symptoms (emotional lability, sadness, anger, and euphoria), altered perceptions (misperceptions, illusions, delusions—poorly formed—and hallucinations), disorganized thinking and incoherent speech, disorientation to time, place, or person, and memory impairment (cannot register new material). Neurologic abnormalities can also be present during delirium, including cortical abnormalities (dysgraphia, constructional apraxia, dysnomic aphasia), motor abnormalities (tremor, asterixis, myoclonus, and reflex and tone changes), and electroencephalogram abnormalities (usually global slowing). It is this protean nature of delirious symptoms, the variability and fluctuation of clinical findings, and the unclear and often contradictory definitions of the syndrome that have made delirium so difficult to diagnose and treat.

Table 15.5.6 lists the DSM-IV[157] criteria for delirium. The essential defining features of delirium, based on DSM-IV criteria, have shifted, from the extensive list of typical symptoms and abnormalities

Table 15.5.6 DSM-IV criteria for delirium.

Delirium due to a general medical condition
1. Disturbance of consciousness (i.e. reduced clarity of awareness of the environment) with reduced ability to focus, sustain, or shift attention
2. Change in cognition (such as memory deficit, disorientation, language disturbance, or perceptual disturbance) that is not better accounted for by a pre-existing, established, or evolving dementia
3. The disturbance develops over a short period of time (usually hours to days) and tends to fluctuate during the course of the day
4. There is evidence from the history, physical examination, or laboratory findings of a general medical condition judged to be aetiologically related to the disturbance

described above, to a focus on the two essential concepts of disordered attention (arousal) and cognition (while continuing to recognize the importance of acute onset and organic aetiology). Associated phenomena such as psychomotor behavioural changes, perceptual disturbances, hallucinations, or delusions are no longer viewed as essential to the diagnosis of delirium. Delirium is now conceptualized primarily as 'a disorder of arousal and cognition'[186] in contrast to dementia, which is a disorder of cognition (with no arousal disturbance). It is this disorder of the arousal system, with consequent disturbances in level of consciousness and attention, that is pathognomonic of delirium and is, in part, the basis for classifying delirium into several subtypes.

Sub-types of delirium

Three clinical sub-types of delirium, based on arousal disturbance and psychomotor behaviour, have been described. These sub-types included the 'hyperactive' (hyperarousal, hyperalert, or agitated) sub-type, the 'hypoactive' (hypoarousal, hypoalert, or lethargic) sub-type, and a 'mixed' sub-type with alternating features of hyperactive and hypoactive delirium[186,187]. Researchers[188] suggest that the hyperactive form is most often characterized by hallucinations, delusions, agitation, and disorientation, while the hypoactive form is characterized by confusion and sedation, but is rarely accompanied by hallucinations, delusions, or illusions. In addition, there is evidence suggesting that specific delirium sub-types may be related to specific aetiologies of delirium, may have unique pathophysiologies, and may have differential responses to treatment[34,35]. It is estimated that approximately two-thirds of deliria are either of the hypoactive or mixed sub-type, hence, the prototypically agitated delirious patient most familiar to clinicians is actually a minority of the deliria which occur[187–189]. Additionally, irrespective of delirium sub-type, delusions and perceptual disturbances occur more commonly than previously anticipated[189].

Differential diagnosis

Many of the clinical features and symptoms of delirium can be also be associated with other psychiatric disorders such as depression, mania, psychosis, and dementia. For instance, delirious patients, not uncommonly, may exhibit emotional (mood) disturbances such as anxiety, fear, depression, irritability, anger, euphoria, apathy, and mood lability. Delirium, particularly the 'hypoactive' sub-type, is often initially misdiagnosed as depression. Symptoms of major depression, including altered level of activity (hypoactivity), insomnia, reduced ability to concentrate, depressed mood, and even suicidal ideation, can overlap with symptoms of delirium making accurate diagnosis more difficult. In distinguishing delirium from depression, particularly in the context of advanced disease, an evaluation of the onset and temporal sequencing of depressive and cognitive symptoms is particularly helpful. Importantly, the degree of cognitive impairment in delirium is much more severe and pervasive than in depression, with a more abrupt temporal onset. Also, in delirium the characteristic disturbance in arousal or consciousness is present, while it is usually not a feature of depression. Similarly, a manic episode may share some features of delirium, particularly a 'hyperactive' or 'mixed' subtype of delirium. Again, the temporal onset and course of symptoms, the presence of a disturbance of consciousness (arousal) as well as of cognition, and the identification of a presumed medical aetiology for delirium are helpful in differentiating these disorders. Delirium that is characterized by vivid hallucinations and delusions must be distinguished from a variety of psychotic disorders. In delirium, such psychotic symptoms occur in the context of a disturbance in consciousness or arousal, as well as memory impairment and disorientation, which is not the case in other psychotic disorders. Delusions in delirium tend to be poorly organized and of abrupt onset, and hallucinations are predominantly visual or tactile rather than auditory as is typical of schizophrenia. Finally, the development of these psychotic symptoms in the context of advanced medical illness makes delirium a more likely diagnosis.

The most common differential diagnostic issue is whether the patient has delirium, or dementia, or a delirium superimposed upon a pre-existing dementia. Both delirium and dementia are cognitive impairment disorders and so share such common clinical features as impaired memory, thinking, judgement, and disorientation. The patient with dementia is alert and does not have the disturbance of consciousness or arousal that is characteristic of delirium. The temporal onset of symptoms in dementia is more sub-acute and chronically progressive, and one's sleep–wake cycle seems less impaired. Most prominent in dementia are difficulties in short- and long-term memory, impaired judgement, and abstract thinking as well as disturbed higher cortical functions (such as aphasia and apraxia). Occasionally one will encounter delirium superimposed on an underlying dementia such as in the case of an elderly patient, an AIDS patient, or a patient with a paraneoplastic syndrome. Delirium, in contrast with dementia, is conceptualized as a reversible process. Reversibility of the process of delirium is often possible even in the patient with advanced illness; however, it may not be reversible in the last 24–48 h of life. This is most likely due to the fact that irreversible processes such as multiple organ failure are occurring in the final hours of life. Delirium occurring in these last days of life is sometimes referred to as 'terminal delirium' in the palliative care literature.

Delirium screening/diagnostic scales

A number of scales or instruments have been developed which can aid the clinician in rapidly screening for cognitive impairment disorders (dementia or delirium) or in establishing a diagnosis of delirium[190–198] (see Table 15.5.7). Such scales have been described and their relative strengths and weaknesses reviewed elsewhere[195,199]. Perhaps most helpful to clinicians are the Mini-Mental State Examination (a cognitive impairment screening tool)

Table 15.5.7 Assessment methods for delirium in cancer patients.

Diagnostic classification systems:
DSM-IV
ICD-9, ICD-10
Diagnostic interviews/instruments:
Delirium Symptom Interview[190](DSI)
Confusion Assessment Method[201](CAM)
Delirium rating scales:
Delirium Rating Scale[196](DRS)
Delirium Rating Scale—Revised 98[200](DRS-R-98)
Confusion Rating Scale[197](CRS)
Saskatoon Delirium Checklist[195](SDC)
Memorial Delirium Assessment Scale[191](MDAS)
Abbreviated Cognitive Test for Delirium[202](CTD)
Cognitive impairment screening instruments:
Mini-Mental State Exam[192](MMSE)
Short Portable Mental Status Questionnaire[198](SPMSQ)
Cognitive Capacity Screening Examination[202](CCSE)
Blessed Orientation Memory Concentration Test[194](BOMC)

and several delirium diagnostic/rating scales, including the Delirium Rating Scale, the Delirium Rating Scale—Revised 98, the Confusion Assessment Method, the Abbreviated Cognitive Test for Delirium, and the Memorial Delirium Assessment Scale. These tools are described briefly below.

Mini-mental state examination

The Mini-Mental State Examination (MMSE)[197] is useful in screening for cognitive failure, but does not distinguish between delirium or dementia. The MMSE provides a quantitative assessment of the cognitive performance and capacity of a patient, and is a measure of severity of cognitive impairment. It is also most sensitive to cortical dementias such as Alzheimer's disease, and less sensitive in detecting sub-cortical deficits such as those found in AIDS dementia. The MMSE assesses five general cognitive areas, including orientation, registration, attention and calculation, recall and language. Although a score of 23 or less has generally been considered the cutoff score for cognitive impairment, a three-tiered system is now often utilized suggesting that a score of 24–30 indicates no impairment, 18–23: mild impairment, and 0–17: severe impairment.

Delirium rating scale

The Delirium Rating Scale (DRS), developed by Trzepacz et al.[196] is a 10-item clinicianrated symptom rating scale for diagnosing delirium. The scale is based on DSM-III-R diagnostic criteria for delirium and is designed to be used by the clinician to identify delirium, and distinguish it reliably from dementia, or other neuropsychiatric disorders. Each item is scored by choosing one best rating and carries a numerical weight chosen to distinguish the phenomenological characteristic of delirium. A score of 12 or greater is diagnostic of delirium.

Delirium Rating Scale—Revised 98

The Delirium Rating Scale—Revised 98 (DRS-R-98) is a revision of the DRS. The DRS-R-98 has 13 severity and three diagnostic items with descriptive anchors for each rating level. It includes more items than the DRS and was designed for phenomenological and treatment research, though it can be used clinically. The DRS-R-98 is a valid, sensitive, and reliable instrument for rating delirium severity. It has advantages over the original DRS for repeated measures and phenomenological studies due to its enhanced breadth of symptoms and separation into severity and diagnostic sub-scales[200].

Confusion Assessment Method

The Confusion Assessment Method (CAM)[201] is a nine-item delirium diagnostic scale utilizing the DSM-III-R criteria for delirium, which can be administered rather quickly by a trained clinician. A unique and helpful feature of the CAM is that the CAM also can be given using a simplified diagnostic algorithm that includes only four items of the CAM, that is designed for rapid identification of delirium by non-psychiatrists. The four-item algorithm requires the presence of: acute onset and fluctuating course, inattention, and either disorganized thinking or altered level of consciousness.

Abbreviated Cognitive Test for Delirium

The Abbreviated Cognitive Test for Delirium[202] was developed as a tool to help identify delirium in patients in the intensive care unit setting who have limited ability to communicate verbally. This brief tool utilizes visualization span and recognition memory for pictures as two of nine content scores that produces a total score that reliably identifies delirium and can discriminate delirium from dementia, depression, and schizophrenia.

Memorial Delirium Assessment Scale

The Memorial Delirium Assessment Scale (MDAS) is a 10-item delirium assessment tool (see Table 15.5.8) validated among hospitalized inpatients with advanced cancer and AIDS[191]. The MDAS is both a good delirium diagnostic screening tool as well as a reliable tool for assessing delirium severity among patients with advanced disease. A cutoff score of 13 is diagnostic of delirium.

Table 15.5.8 Items from the Memorial Delirium Assessment Scale (MDAS).

1. Reduced level of consciousness (awareness)
2. Disorientation
3. Short-term memory impairment
4. Impaired digit span
5. Reduced ability to maintain and shift attention
6. Disorganized thinking
7. Perceptual disturbance
8. Delusions
9. Decreased or increased psychomotor
10. Sleep–wake cycle disturbance (disorder of arousal)

The MDAS has advantages over other delirium tools in that it is both a diagnostic as well as a severity measure that is ideal for repeated assessments and for use in treatment intervention trials. Lawlor et al.[203] further examined the clinical utility and validation of the MDAS in a population of advanced cancer patients in a palliative care unit. These investigators found the MDAS to be useful in this population, and found that a cutoff score of 7 out of 30 yielded the highest sensitivity (98 per cent) and specificity (76 per cent) for a delirium diagnosis in this palliative care population.

Management of delirium in the terminally ill

The standard approach to the managing delirium in the medically ill, and even in those with advanced disease, includes a search for underlying causes, correction of those factors, and management of the symptoms of delirium[37,50,51]. The desired and often achievable outcome is a patient who is awake, alert, calm, cognitively intact, not psychotic, and communicating coherently with family and staff. In the terminally ill patient who develops delirium in the last days of life ('terminal' delirium), the management of delirium is in fact unique, presenting a number of dilemmas, and the desired clinical outcome may be significantly altered by the dying process.

Assessment of aetiologies of delirium

When confronted with a delirium in the terminally ill or dying patient, a differential diagnosis should always be formulated as to the likely aetiology(ies). There is an ongoing debate as to the appropriate extent of diagnostic evaluation that should be pursued in a dying patient with a terminal delirium[204,207]. Most palliative care clinicians would undertake diagnostic studies only when a clinically suspected aetiology can be identified easily, with minimal use of invasive procedures, and treated effectively with simple, interventions that carry minimal burden or risk of causing further distress. Diagnostic work-up in pursuit of an aetiology for delirium may be limited by either practical constraints such as the setting (home, hospice) or the focus on patient comfort, so that unpleasant or painful diagnostics may be avoided. Most often, however, the aetiology of terminal delirium is multifactorial or may not be determined. Bruera et al.[161] report that an aetiology is discovered in less than 50 per cent of terminally ill patients with delirium. When a distinct cause is found for delirium in the terminally ill, it is often irreversible or difficult to treat. Studies, however, in patients with earlier stages of advanced cancer have demonstrated the potential utility of a thorough diagnostic assessment[161,179]. When such diagnostic information is available, specific therapy may be able to reverse delirium. One study found that 68 per cent of delirious cancer patients could be improved, despite a 30-day mortality of 31 per cent[162]. Another found that one-third of the episodes of cognitive failure improved following evaluation that yielded a cause for these episodes in 43 per cent[161].

In a prospective study of delirium in patients on a palliative care unit[184], investigators reported that the aetiology of delirium was multifactorial in the great majority of cases. Even though delirium occurred in 88 per cent of dying patients in the last week of life, delirium was reversible in approximately 50 per cent of episodes. Causes of delirium that were most associated with reversibility included dehydration and psychoactive/opioid medications. Hypoxic and metabolic encephalopathy were less likely to be reversed in terminal delirium. The diagnostic work-up should

Table 15.5.9 Causes of delirium in patients with advanced disease.

Direct central nervous system (CNS) causes
Primary brain tumour
Metastatic spread to CNS
Seizures
Indirect causes
Metabolic encephalopathy due to organ failure
Electrolyte imbalance
Treatment side effects from chemotherapeutic agents:
Steroids
Radiation
Narcotics
Anticholinergics
Antiemetics
Antivirals
Infection
Haematologic abnormalities
Nutritional deficiencies
Paraneoplastic syndromes

include an assessment of potentially reversible causes of delirium. A full physical examination should assess for evidence of sepsis, dehydration, or major organic failure. Medications that could contribute to delirium should be reviewed. A screen of laboratory parameters will allow assessment of the possible role of metabolic abnormalities, such as hypercalcemia, and other problems, such as hypoxia or disseminated intravascular coagulation. Imaging studies of the brain and assessment of the cerebrospinal fluid may be appropriate in some instances.

Delirium can have multiple potential aetiologies (see Table 15.5.9). In patients with advanced cancer, for instance, delirium can be due either to the direct effects of cancer on the central nervous system (CNS), or to indirect CNS effects of the disease or treatments (medications, electrolyte imbalance, failure of a vital organ or system, infection, vascular complications, and preexisting cognitive impairment or dementia)[161,184]. Given the large numbers of drugs cancer patients require, and the fragile state of their physiologic functioning, even routinely ordered hypnotics are enough to tip patients over into a delirium. Narcotic analgesics such as levorphanol, morphine sulfate, and meperidine, are common causes of confusional states, particularly in the elderly and terminally ill. Chemotherapeutic agents known to cause delirium include methotrexate, fluorouracil, vincristine, vinblastine, bleomycin, BCNU, *cis*-platinum, asparaginase, procarbazine, and the glucocorticosteroids[54–60,180]. Except for steroids, most patients receiving these agents will not develop prominent CNS effects. The spectrum of mental disturbances related to steroids includes minor mood lability, affective disorders (mania or depression), cognitive impairment (reversible dementia), and delirium (steroid psychosis). The incidence of these disorders range from 3 to 57 per cent in non-cancer populations, and they occur most commonly on higher doses. Symptoms usually develop within the first

2 weeks on steroids, but in fact can occur at any time, on any dose, even during the tapering phase[179]. These disorders are often rapidly reversible upon dose reduction or discontinuation[179].

Non-pharmacologic interventions

In addition to seeking out and potentially correcting underlying causes for delirium, symptomatic and supportive therapies are important[162,163,177,206]. In fact, in the dying patient they may be the only steps taken. Fluid and electrolyte balance, nutrition, vitamins, measures to help reduce anxiety and disorientation, interactions with and education of family members may be useful. Measures to help reduce anxiety and disorientation (i.e. structure and familiarity) may include a quiet, well-lit room with familiar objects, a visible clock or calendar, and the presence of family. Judicious use of physical restraints, along with one-to-one nursing observation may also be necessary and useful.

Inouye *et al.*[208] reported on a successful multicomponent intervention program to prevent delirium in hospitalized older patients. They focused on a set of risk factors that were highly predictive of delirium in the elderly which included: pre-existing cognitive impairment, visual impairment, hearing impairment, sleep deprivation, immobility, dehydration, and severe illness. Interventions directed at constant reorientation, correction of hearing and visual impairment, reversal of dehydration, and early mobilization appeared to significantly reduce the number and duration of episodes of delirium in hospitalized older patients. The applicability of these interventions and the likelihood that they would prevent delirium in the terminally ill, particularly in the last days of life, is likely minimal.

Pharmacologic interventions in delirium

Supportive techniques alone are often not effective in controlling the symptoms of delirium, and symptomatic treatment with neuroleptics or sedative medications are necessary (Table 15.5.10). Neuroleptic drugs (dopamine blocking drugs) such as haloperidol, are utilized frequently as antiemetics in the medical setting; however, only 0.5–2 per cent of hospitalized cancer patients, for instance, receive haloperidol for the management of the symptoms of delirium[209,210]. In terminally ill populations, as many as 17 per cent receive an antipsychotic for agitation or psychological distress, despite an estimated prevalence of delirium ranging from 25 per cent in the hospitalized cancer patient to 85 per cent in the terminally ill[211,212].

Neuroleptics

Haloperidol, a neuroleptic drug that is a potent dopamine blocker, is often the drug of choice in the treatment of delirium in patients with advanced disease[1,212–219]. Haloperidol in low doses, 1–3 mg/day, is usually effective in targeting agitation, paranoia, and fear. Typically 0.5–1.0 mg haloperidol (PO, IV, IM, SC) is administered, with repeat doses every 45–60 min titrated against target symptoms[204,220,221]. An intravenous route can facilitate rapid onset of medication effects. If intravenous access is unavailable, one can start with intramuscular or sub-cutaneous administration and switch to the oral route when possible. The majority of delirious patients can be managed with oral haloperidol. Parenteral doses are approximately twice as potent as oral doses. Delivery of haloperidol by the sub-cutaneous route is utilized by many palliative care practitioners[161,222]. Low doses of neuroleptic medication is usually sufficient in treating delirium in elderly terminally ill patients.

Table 15.5.10 Medications in managing delirium in patients with advanced disease.

Generic name	Approximate daily dosage range[a]	Route
Neuroleptics		
Haloperidol	0.5–5 mg every 2–12 h	PO, IV, SC, IM
Thioridazine	10–75 mg every 4–8 h	PO
Chlorpromazine	12.5–50 mg every 4–12 h	PO, IV, IM
Methotrimeprazine	12.5–50 mg every 4–8 h	IV, SC, PO
Molindone	10–50 mg every 8–12 h	PO
Droperidol	0.625 mg–2.5 mg every 4–8 h	IV, IM
Atypical neuroleptics		
Olanzapine	2.5–20 mg every 12–24 h	PO
Risperidone	1–3 mg every 12–24 h	PO
Quetiapine	25–200 mg every 12–24 h	PO
Benzodiazepines		
Lorazepam	0.5–2.0 mg every 1–4 h	PO, IV, IM
Midazolam	30–100 mg every 24 h	IV, SC
Anaesthetics		
Propofol	10–70 mg every hour	IV
	Upto 200–400 mg/h	

[a] Parenteral doses are generally twice as potent as oral doses; IV, intravenous infusions or bolus injections should be administered slowly; IM, intramuscular injections should be avoided if repeated use becomes necessary; PO, oral forms of medication are preferred; or SC, subcutaneous infusions are generally accepted modes of drug administration in the terminally ill.

In general, doses need not exceed 20 mg of haloperidol in a 24-h period; however, there are those that advocate high doses (upto 250 mg/24 h of haloperidol usually intravenously) in selected cases[215].

A common strategy in the management of symptoms related to delirium is to add parenteral lorazepam to a regimen of haloperidol[223,224]. Lorazepam (0.5–1.0 mg q1–2 h PO or IV), along with haloperidol may be more effective in rapidly sedating the agitated delirious patient, and may help minimize extrapyramidal side effects associated with haloperidol[224]. An alternative strategy is to switch from haloperidol to a more sedating neuroleptic such as chlorpromazine (see Fig. 15.5.3). In a double-blind, randomized comparison trial of haloperidol, chlorpromazine, and lorazepam, Breitbart et al. demonstrated that lorazepam alone, in doses up to 8 mg in a 12-h period, was ineffective in the treatment of delirium and in fact contributed to worsening delirium and cognitive impairment[160]. Both neuroleptic drugs, however, in low doses (approximately 2 mg of haloperidol equivalent/24 h), were highly effective in controlling the symptoms of delirium (dramatic improvement in DRS scores) and improving cognitive function (dramatic improvement in MMSE scores). In addition, both haloperidol and chlorpromazine were demonstrated to significantly improve the symptoms of delirium in both the 'hypoactive' as well as the 'hyperactive' sub-types of delirium[160]. Methotrimeprazine, a phenothiazine neuroleptic with properties similar to chlorpromazine, is often utilized parenterally (intravenously or by subcutaneous infusion) to control confusion and agitation in terminal delirium[225]. Dosages range from 12.5 to 50 mg every 4–8 h up to 300 mg/24 h for most patients, including the elderly where doses at the lower end of the range are preferable. Hypotension and excessive sedation are potential limitations of this drug; however, methotrimeprazine has the advantage of also being an analgesic, equipment to morphine, through non-opioid mechanisms[225].

Several new, atypical, antipsychotic agents with less or more specific dopamine blocking effects (less risk of extrapyramidal side effects or tardive dyskinesia) are now available and include such agents as clozaril, risperidone, and olanzapine[226–230]. Risperidone has been useful in the treatment of dementia and psychosis in AIDS patients at doses of 1–6 mg/day, suggesting safe use in patients with delirium[229]. There are a limited number of published studies of the use of these agents in the treatment of delirium[227–230]. Breitbart et al.[230] published a large (n = 82) open trial of olanzapine for the treatment of delirium in hospitalized patients with advanced cancer. Olanzapine was highly effective in the treatment of delirium, resolving delirium in 76 per cent of patients, with no incidence of extrapyramidal side effects. Several factors were found to be significantly associated with poorer response to olanzapine treatment for delirium, including age over 70, history of dementia, and hypoactive delirium. The average starting dose was in the 2.5–5 mg range and patients were given up to 20 mg/day of olanzapine. Sedation was the most common side effect. Many palliative care clinicians are using risperidone in low doses (e.g. 0.5–1.0 mg twice a day, orally) as well as olanzipine (2.5–20 mg/day in divided doses) in the management of delirium in terminally ill patients, particularly in those who have a demonstrated intolerance to the extrapyramidal side effects of the classic neuroleptics. A limitation on the use of these agents is the lack of availability in parenteral formulations. Still, the need for combined efforts in the assessment and treatment of delirium has recently been pointed to[231]. Fig. 15.5.3 illustrates an algorithm that has been developed for use by the Memorial Sloan-Kettering Cancer Center Psychiatry Service, for the management of delirium in hospitalized cancer patients.

While neuroleptic drugs such as haloperidol are most effective in diminishing agitation, clearing the sensorium, and improving cognition in the delirious patient, this is not always possible in delirium which complicates the last days of life. Processes causing delirium may be ongoing and irreversible during the active dying phase. Ventafridda et al.[232] and Fainsinger et al.[180] have reported that a significant group (10–20 per cent) of terminally ill patients experience delirium that can only be controlled by sedation to the point of a significantly decreased level of consciousness. Lawlor et al.[184] report that at least 50 per cent of terminal delirium is reversible. The goal of treatment with such agents as midazolam, propofol, and to some extent methotrimeprazine, is quiet sedation only. Midazolam, given by subcutaneous or intravenous infusion in doses ranging from 30 to 100 mg/24 h can be used to control agitation related to delirium in the terminal stages[29,30]. Propofol, a short-acting anaesthetic agent, has also begun to be utilized primarily as a sedating agent for the control of agitated patients with 'terminal' delirium. In several case reports of propofol's use in terminal care, an intravenous loading dose of 20 mg of propofol was followed by a continuous infusion of propofol with initial doses ranging from 10 to 70 mg/h, and with titration of doses up to as high as 400 mg/h over a period of hours to days in severely

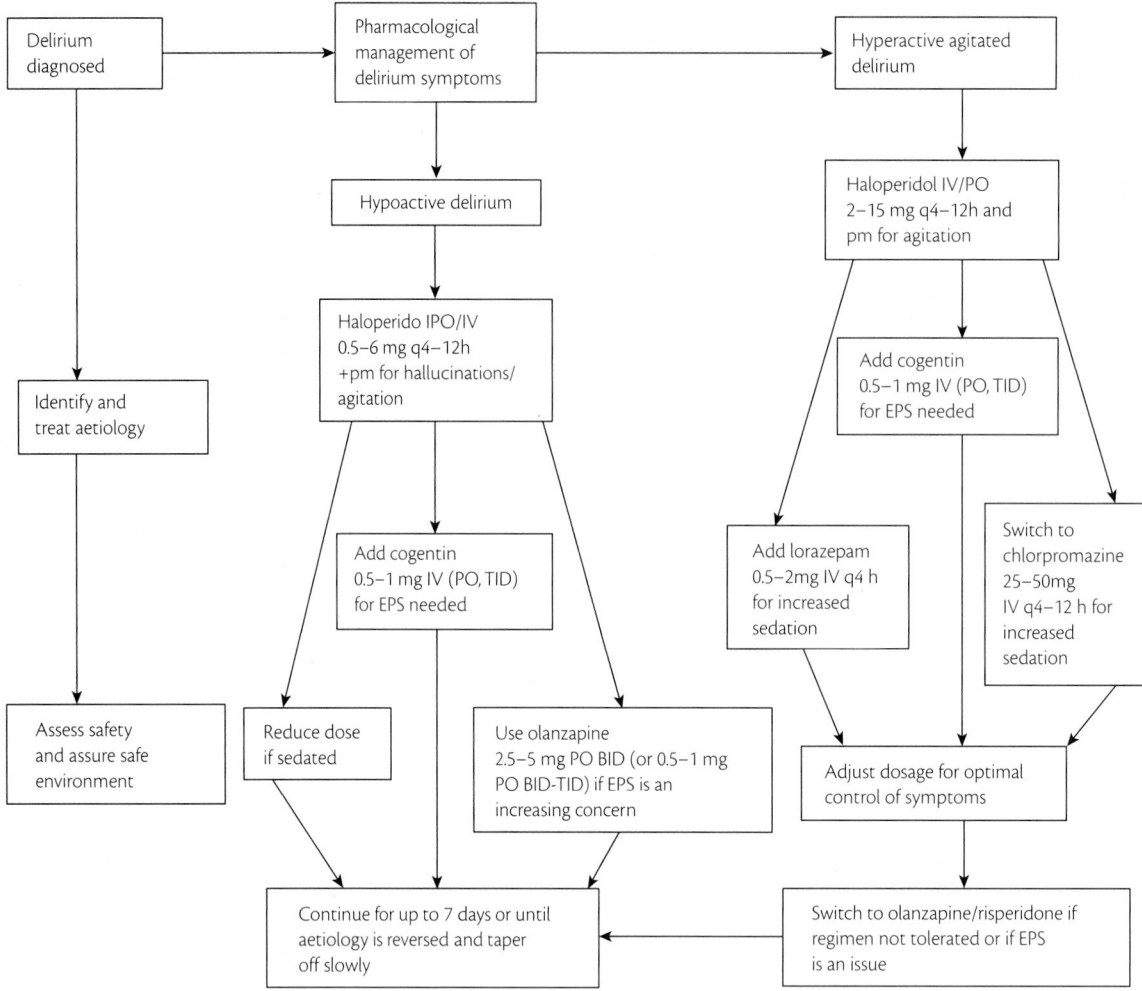

Figure 15.5.3 The delirium algorithm. Atypical neuroleptics.

agitated patients[233,234]. Propofol has an advantage over midazolam in that the level of sedation is more easily controlled and
recovery is rapid upon decreasing the rate of infusion[233].

Controversies in the management of terminal delirium

Several aspects of the use of neuroleptics and other pharmacologic
agents in the management of delirium in the dying patient remain
controversial in some circles. Some have argued that pharmacologic interventions with neuroleptics or benzodiazepines are inappropriate in the dying patient. Delirium is viewed by some as a
natural part of the dying process that should not be altered. In particular, there are clinicians who care for the dying who view hallucinations and delusions which involve dead relatives communicating
with or in fact welcoming dying patients to heaven, as an important
element in the transition from life to death. Clearly, there are many
patients who experience hallucinations and delusions during delirium that are pleasant and in fact comforting, and many clinicians
question the appropriateness of intervening pharmacologically in
such instances. Another concern that is often raised is that these
patients are so close to death that aggressive treatment is unnecessary. Parenteral neuroleptics or sedatives may be mistakenly
avoided because of exaggerated fears that they might hasten death

through hypotension or respiratory depression. Many are unnecessarily pessimistic about the possible results of neuroleptic treatment
for delirium. They argue that since the underlying pathophysiologic
process often continues unabated (such as hepatic or renal failure),
no improvement can be expected in the patient's mental status.
There is concern that neuroleptics or sedatives may worsen a delirium by making the patient more confused or sedated.

Clinical experience in managing delirium in dying patients suggests that the use of neuroleptics in the management of agitation,
paranoia, hallucinations, and altered sensorium is safe, effective,
and often quite appropriate[223]. Management of delirium on a case
by case basis seems wisest. The agitated, delirious dying patient
should probably be given neuroleptics to help restore calm. A 'wait
and see' approach, prior to using neuroleptics, may be appropriate
with some patients who have a lethargic or somnolent presentation
of delirium, or those who are having frankly pleasant or comforting
hallucinations. Such a 'wait and see' approach must however be
tempered by the knowledge that a lethargic or hypoactive delirium
may very quickly and unexpectedly become an agitated or hyperactive delirium that can threaten the serenity and safety of the
patient, family, and staff. An additional rationale for intervening
pharmacologically with patients who have a lethargic or hypoactive

delirium is more recent evidence that neuroleptics (i.e. haloperidol and chlorpromazine) are effective in controlling the symptoms of delirium in both hyperactive as well as hypoactive sub-types of delirium[160]. In fact neuroleptics improved both the arousal disturbance, as well as cognitive functioning in patients with hypoactive delirium. Also, some clinicians suggest that hypoactive delirium may respond to psychostimulants or combinations of neuroleptics and stimulants[235,236]. Similarly, hallucinations and delusions during a delirium that are pleasant and comforting can quickly become menacing and terrifying. It is important to remember that by nature, the symptoms of delirium are unstable, and fluctuate over time.

Finally, perhaps the most challenging of clinical problems is management of the dying patient with a 'terminal' delirium that is unresponsive to standard neuroleptic interventions, whose symptoms can only be controlled by sedation to the point of a significantly decreased level of consciousness. Before undertaking interventions such as midazolam or propofol infusions, where the best achievable goal is a calm, comfortable, but sedated and unresponsive patient, the clinician must first take several steps. The clinician must have a discussion with the family (and the patient if there are lucid moments when the patient appears to have capacity) eliciting their concerns and wishes for the type of care that can best honour their desire to provide comfort and symptom control during the dying process. The clinician should describe the optimal achievable goals of therapy as they currently exist. Family members should be informed that the goal of sedation is to provide comfort and symptom control, and not to hasten death. They should also be told to anticipate that sedation may result in a premature sense of loss, and that they may feel their loved one is in some sort of limbo state, not yet dead, but yet no longer alive in the vital sense. The distress and confusion that family members can experience during such a period can be ameliorated by including the family in the decision-making and emphasizing the shared goals of care. Sedation in such patients is not always complete or irreversible; some patients have periods of wakefulness despite sedation, and many clinicians will periodically lighten sedation to reassess the patient's condition. Ultimately, the clinician must always keep in mind the goals of care and communicate these goals to the staff, patients, and family members. The clinician must weigh each of the issues outlined above in making decisions, on how to best manage the dying patient who presents with delirium, that preserves and respects the dignity and values of that individual and family.

Behavioural interventions for the control of selected physical symptoms

While the diagnosis and treatment of psychiatric disorders in the patient with advanced illness is of importance, pain and other troublesome physical symptoms must also be aggressively treated in efforts aimed at the enhancement of the patient's quality of life[237]. The deleterious influence of uncontrolled pain on a patient's psychological state is often intuitively understood and recognized. However, physical symptoms other than pain can go undetected and cause significant emotional distress. This distress often dissipates when effective management is instituted. Coyle et al.[238] reported that 70 per cent of terminally ill patients have three or more physical symptoms other than pain. This finding replicates those of earlier papers that elucidate the multiple problems facing the terminally ill patient[239]. These symptoms must be assessed by the psychologist or psychiatrist concerned with the assessment and treatment of affective and other syndromes in the terminally ill population. In other chapters of this text, the management of a variety of physical symptoms experienced in terminal illness, including pain, dyspnoea, nausea, vomiting, asthenia, cachexia, and anorexia are discussed. In the following section, we will briefly review psychological interventions that may be useful in the management of some selected distressing symptoms.

Pain

The reader is directed to Chapter 10.1.13 for a detailed discussion of the use of behavioural, psychotherapeutic, and psychopharmacologic interventions in pain control. In brief, behavioural interventions are effective in the management of acute procedures-related cancer pain, and as an adjunct in the management of chronic cancer pain[240,241]. Hypnosis, biofeedback, and multicomponent cognitive behavioural interventions have been used to provide comfort and minimize pain in adults, children, and adolescents undergoing bone marrow aspirations, spinal taps, and other painful procedures[242–244]. Typically, behavioural interventions utilized in the management of acute procedure-related pain employ the basic elements of relaxation and distraction or diversion of attention. In chronic cancer pain, cognitive behavioural techniques are most effective when they are employed as part of a multimodal, multidisciplinary approach[221]. Adequate medical assessment and management of cancer pain is essential. Mild to moderate levels of residual pain can be effectively managed with behavioural techniques that are quite similar to those used for anxiety, phobias, and anticipatory nausea and vomiting. Relaxation techniques are utilized to help the patient achieve a relaxed state. Once in a relaxed state, the cancer patient with pain can use a variety of imagery techniques, including pleasant distracting imagery, transformational imagery, and dissociative imagery[221]. Transformational imagery involves the imaginative transformation of either the painful sensation itself, or the context of pain, or both. Patients can imaginatively transform a sensation of pain in their arm, for instance, into a sensation of warmth or cold. They can use such imagery as 'dipping their arm into a bucket of cold spring water', or 'into a vat of warm honey'. Such techniques can also be used to alter the context of the pain. Dissociative imagery or dissociated somatization refers to the use of one's imagination to disconnect or dissociate from the pain experience. Specifically, patients can sometimes imagine that they leave their pain racked body in bed and walk about for 5–10 min pain free. Patients can also imagine that a particularly painful part of their body becomes disconnected or dissociated from the rest of them, resulting in a period of freedom from pain. These techniques can provide much needed respite from pain. Even short periods of relief from pain can break the vicious pain cycle that entraps many cancer patients.

Anorexia and weight loss (see Chapter 10.3)

Cancer patients and their families find weight loss demoralizing, perplexing, and distressing. Weight loss and anorexia in the terminally ill patient are complex problems that can arise from a number of sources. While most often a variety of medical factors account for the anorexia and cachexia associated with terminal illness, psychological and psychiatric factors may also play a role in the aetiology of anorexia and weight loss. Among the most frequent of such causes are anxiety, depression, and conditioned food aversions[245].

The treatment of anorexia and weight loss begins with the identification and correction of its reversible causes. For example, when uncontrolled opioid-induced nausea is identified as a key factor in a patient's inability to eat, adding an antiemetic may completely control the subsequent anorexia. Once specific causes have been ruled out or corrected, subsequent treatment relies upon environmental manipulations[239]. Frequent administration of favourite foods, nutritional supplements, and fluids can reverse weight loss.

When poor appetite is a symptom of underlying major depression or significant anxiety, psychopharmacologic interventions with antidepressants and anxiolytics are indicated. Conditioned nausea and vomiting is often quite responsive to relaxation training and other behavioural techniques[246]. These interventions can be employed even by patients with advanced disease if their sensorium is clear and they are capable of concentrating.

Behavioural interventions are commonly used to treat a variety of eating disorders in cancer patients, including conditioned anorexia, swallowing difficulties, and nausea and vomiting. Dixon[247] reported on a study of 55 nutritionally at-risk cancer patients who were randomized to four intervention groups. One group received nutritional support alone, the other received relaxation training only, a third group received both supplementation and relaxation, and the fourth group was a no intervention control. Weight gain was greatest for the relaxation groups who were taught deep abdominal breathing, autosuggestion, progressive relaxation, and imagery. Campbell et al.[248] showed that a relaxation and imagery exercise program was associated with weight gain and improvement in performance status. Conditioned difficulties with eating, swallowing, and nausea have been managed successfully with systematic desensitization[249,250]. Hypnosis has been utilized in children with cancer[251] resulting in improved appetite and weight gain.

Asthenia/fatigue

Asthenia or fatigue is defined as generalized weakness, and physical or mental fatigue. Studies suggest that as many as two-thirds of advanced cancer patients complain of fatigue. Unfortunately, a treatable cause of asthenia will be identified and corrected in only a minority of cases. The role of psychiatric factors in the presentation of asthenia in the dying cancer patient is small in comparison to that of physical factors. However, psychiatric factors are probably enlisted too often by frustrated house staff who have seen a number of treatments fail, and then view the patient's continuing malaise as a sign of depression. More likely the cause of asthenia arises from some of the following aetiologies: malnutrition, infection, profound anaemia, metabolic abnormalities, and reactions to medication. Chemotherapeutic agents and radiotherapy are frequently employed as palliative therapies in patients with advanced cancer. Both can cause significant weakness that may resolve after treatment is completed.

The psychological and psychiatric treatment of patients with fatigue includes patient and family education (especially to address the non-psychological nature of the problem in many cases). An ongoing supportive relationship which permits the patient to express fears and concerns about the meaning of continued weakness and to address distorted ideas that they may have about its prognostic significance is important. Fatigue is generally recognized as a multidimensional construct, with a physical and cognitive dimension, and assessment and treatment of fatigue should reflect this[252]. Some patients who suffer with temporary fatigue from chemotherapy or radiotherapy feel that their weakness is a sign of imminent death. The literature in support of the pharmacotherapy of fatigue in cancer patients is relatively limited. Some patients respond to steroids (methylprednisone, 15–30 mg daily) with improvement in mood, appetite, and physical well-being. Unfortunately, this response tends to be fleeting. Also problematic is the fact that prolonged use of steroids can exacerbate weakness by causing proximal myopathy. Steroids have several other potentially distressing adverse effects including severe psychiatric syndromes such as organic mood syndromes and delirium. Psychostimulants have been used in the treatment of asthenia with good results[253]. In a randomized, double-blind, placebo-controlled trial, Breitbart et al.[235] demonstrated that the psychostimulants methylphenidate and pemoline were superior to placebo and provided clinically significant improvement in fatigue amongst a sample of ambulatory AIDS patients. The average dose of methylphenidate was approximately 50 mg/day and 100 mg/day for pemoline; minimal side effects and weight gain was noted with the stimulant drugs. Selected patients do respond well to amphetamine, methylphenidate, or pemoline, and it is thus appropriate to use stimulants not only for depressive syndromes but also for the asthenia/weakness syndrome. Despite the appetite suppressing effects of amphetamine-like drugs, stimulants often improve energy and appetite in fatigued terminally ill patients.

Nausea and vomiting

Approximately 50 per cent of patients with advanced cancer experience nausea and vomiting during the course of their illness[239,254]. Common causes of nausea and vomiting in cancer patients include radiation, medications, toxins, metabolic derangements, obstruction of the gastrointestinal tract, and chemotherapy. During the course of chemotherapy, many patients become sensitized to the treatment, develop phobic-like reactions, and even develop conditioned responses to stimuli in the hospital setting. As a result of being conditioned by the experience of profound nausea and vomiting secondary to highly emetic chemotherapy agents, patients report being nauseated in anticipation of treatment. A conservative estimate of the prevalence of anticipatory nausea and vomiting (ANV) is at least 33 per cent[255]. The factors that increase the likelihood of developing ANV are as follows: (1) severity of post-treatment nausea and vomiting (high density, duration, and frequency); (2) a pattern of increasing nausea and vomiting; and (3) receiving highly emetic drugs (cis-platinum) or combinations of chemotherapies[256].

Given the relationship between intensity of post-chemotherapy nausea and vomiting and the development of ANV, the efficacy of antiemetic regimens in the management of these symptoms becomes increasingly important. Antiemetic drugs are the mainstay of managing chemotherapy-induced nausea and vomiting in patients with advanced disease. Several antiemetic drugs have dopamine blocking properties and so can cause a variety of extrapyramidal side effects. Akathisia is a common extrapyramidal symptom experienced by the patient as an intense inner sense of restlessness, often accompanied by outward manifestations of agitation. This is often confused with anxiety related to illness by physicians and nurses. Patients can often differentiate feelings of anxiety and nervousness from a sense of motor restlessness. Additionally, akathisia is often accompanied by other extrapyramidal symptoms such as mild tremor or cogwheel rigidity. Treatment of akathisia secondary to antiemetics may involve lowering the dose of the antiemetic, switching to a non-dopamine blocking agent such as ondansetron, or the addition of a benzodiazepine or an anticholinergic agent.

Rapid onset, short-acting benzodiazepines are helpful in controlling ANV once it has developed. Alprazolam has been shown to be clinically effective in reducing ANV in doses of 0.25–0.5 mg TID to QID, given for 1–2 days prior to chemotherapy[257]. Behavioural control of anticipatory nausea and vomiting has proven to be highly effective[254]. The techniques that have been studied include relaxation training with guided imagery, video game distraction (in children), and systematic desensitization. It is unclear whether muscular relaxation or cognitive-attentional distraction is the key element in the efficacy of some of these techniques. Chemotherapy nurses trained in these techniques can remarkably improve the quality of life in chemotherapy patients.

Insomnia (see Chapter 10.12)

Behavioural interventions have been successfully applied to the treatment of insomnia in cancer patients. Cannici et al.[258] studied 15 patients suffering from secondary insomnia due to cancer, and showed a marked reduction in mean sleep onset latency after progressive muscle relaxation training. Stam and Bultz[259] showed an increase in duration of sleep utilizing relaxation and imagery techniques. Such techniques are useful non-pharmacologic interventions that help keep medication use to a minimum. Occasionally sleep disturbance in cancer patients may be due to a concomitant psychiatric disorder such as depression or delirium. Obviously in these cases specific treatment for the underlying disorder is a preferred approach. Pharmacotherapy utilizing benzodiazepines, neuroleptics, or antidepressants may also be indicated when sleep disturbance is due to medication side effects or some other organic aetiology. Sleep disturbances are common in palliative medicine, but many patients do not seek medical attention for sleep disturbances, and under-diagnosis and under-treatment are probably common[260].

Conclusion

As the possibility of cure or prolongation of life becomes remote in the care of the patient with advanced cancer or AIDS, the focus of treatment shifts to symptom control and enhancement of quality of life. Such patients are uniquely vulnerable to both physical and psychiatric complications. The high prevalence of distressing physical symptoms, such as pain, make the assessment of psychiatric symptoms difficult. It is critical that physicians and nurses working in the palliative care setting recognize the unique knowledge and skills of psychiatrists and psychologists and the contributions they can make to the care of the terminally ill patient. The role of the psychiatrist, or other mental health professional, in the care of the terminally ill or dying patient is critical to both adequate symptom control and integration of the physical, psychological, and spiritual dimensions of human experience in the last weeks of life. To be most effective in this role, the psychiatrist must not only have specialized knowledge of the psychiatric complications of terminal illness and the existential issues confronted those at the end of life,

but also must be familiar with the common physical symptoms that plague the patient with advanced disease and contribute so dramatically to suffering.

References

1. Chochinov, H.M.C. and Breitbart, W., ed. *Handbook of Psychiatry in Palliative Medicine*. New York: Oxford University Press, 2009.
2. Derogatis, L.R. *et al.* (1983). The prevalence of psychiatric disorders among cancer patients. *Journal of the American Medical Association,* **249**, 751–7.
3. Breitbart, W. *et al.* (1995). Neuropsychiatric syndromes and psychological symptoms in patients with advanced cancer. *Journal of Pain and Symptom Management,* **10**, 131–41.
4. Minagawa, H. *et al.* (1996). Psychiatric morbidity in terminally ill cancer patients. *Cancer,* **78**, 1131–7.
5. Foley, K.M. (1985). The treatment of cancer pain. *New England Journal of Medicine,* **313**, 84–95.
6. Chochinov, H.M.C. (2000). Psychiatry and the terminally ill. *Canadian Journal of Psychiatry,* **45**, 143–50.
7. Breitbart, W., Jaramillo, J.R., and Chochinov, H.M.C. (1998). Palliative and terminal care. In *Psycho-Oncology* (ed. J.C. Holland *et al.*), pp. 437–49. New York: Oxford University Press.
8. Bukberg, J., Penman, D., and Holland, J. (1984). Depression in hospitalized cancer patients. *Psychosomatic Medicine,* **43**, 199–212.
9. Massie, M.J., Holland, J.C., and Glass, E. (1983). Delirium in terminally ill cancer patients. *American Journal of Psychiatry,* **140**, 1048–50.
10. Lawlor, P.G. *et al.* (2000). Occurrence, causes and outcomes of delirium in patients with advanced cancer. *Archives of Internal Medicine,* **160**, 786–94.
11. Lichtental, W.G. *et al.* (2009). Do rates of mental disorders and existential distress among advanced stage cancer patients increase as death approaches? *Psycho-Oncology,* **18**, 50–61.
12. Ahles, T.A., Blanchard, E.B., and Ruckdeschel, J.C. (1983). The multidimensional nature of cancer related pain. *Pain,* **17**, 277–88.
13. Tross, S. and Hirsch, D.A. (1988). Psychological distress and neuropsychological complications of HIV infection and AIDS. *American Psychologist,* **43**, 929–34.
14. Atkinson, J.H., Grant, I., and Kennedy, C.J. (1988). Prevalence of psychiatric disorders among men infected with human immunodeficiency virus. *Archives of General Psychiatry,* **45**, 859–64.
15. Karina, K. *et al.* (1994). Psychiatric comorbidity and length of stay in hospitalized AIDS patients. *American Journal of Psychiatry,* **151**, 1475–8.
16. Barbuto, J., Fleishman, S., and Holland, J. (1987). *Prevalence of Psychiatric Disorders in AIDS Patients. Current Concepts in Psycho-Oncology and AIDS.* Memorial Sloan-Kettering Cancer Center, 17–19 September.
17. Perry, J.S.W. and Tross, S. (1984). Psychiatric problems of AIDS inpatients at the New York Hospital: a preliminary report. *Public Health Reports,* **99**, 200–5.
18. Perry, S.W. (1990). Organic mental disorders caused by HIV: update on early diagnosis and treatment. *American Journal of Psychiatry,* **147**, 696–710.
19. Rabkin, J. *et al.* (1997). Prevalence of axis I disorders in an AIDS cohort: a cross-sectional, controlled study. *Comprehensive Psychiatry,* **38**, 146–54.
20. Vogl, D. *et al.* (1999). Symptom prevalence, characteristics, and distress in AIDS outpatients. *Journal of Pain and Symptom Management,* **18**, 253–62.
21. Holland, J.C. (1989). Anxiety and cancer: the patient and family. *Journal of Clinical Psychiatry,* **50**, 20–5.
22. Massie, M.J. and Payne, D.K. (2000). Anxiety in palliative care. In *Handbook of Psychiatry in Palliative Medicine* (ed. H.M.C. Chochinov and W. Breitbart), pp. 63–74. New York: Oxford University Press.
23. Brandenberg, Y., Bolund, C., and Sigurdardotti, V. (1992). Anxiety and depressive symptoms at different stages of malignant melanoma. *Psycho-oncology,* **1**, 71–8.

24. Whitcup, S.M. and Miller, F. (1987). Unrecognized drug dependence in psychiatrically hospitalized elderly patients. *Journal of American Geriatric Society*, **35**, 297–301.

25. Roth, A.J. and Massie, M.J. (2007). Anxiety and its management in advanced cancer. *Current Opinion in Supportive and Palliative Care*, **1**, 50–6.

26. Wald, T. *et al. Rapid Relief of Anxiety in Cancer Patients with Both Alprazolam and Placebo* Vol. 34.4. Washington DC: American Psychiatric Press, 1994–1995.

27. Jackson, K.C. and Lipman, A.G. (2007). Drug therapy for anxiety in palliative care. *Cochrane Database of Systematic Reviews* 1,CD004596.

28. Twycross, R.G. and Lack, S.A. (1984). *Therapeutics in Terminal Disease*. London: Pitman, pp. 99–103.

29. Bottomley, D.M. and Hanks, G.W. (1990). Subcutaneous midazolam infusion in palliative care. *Journal of Pain and Symptom Management*, **5**, 259–61.

30. Mendoza, R. *et al.* (1987). Midazolam in acute psychotic patients with hyperarousal. *Journal of Clinical Psychiatry*, **48**, 291–3.

31. De Sousa, E. and Jepson, A. (1988). Midazolam in terminal care. *Lancet*, **1**, 67–8.

32. Chouinard, G., Young, S.N., and Annable, L. (1983). Antimanic effect of clonazepam. *Biological Psychiatry*, **18**, 451–66.

33. Keck, P., McElroy, S., and Nemeroff, C. (1992). Anticonvulsants in the treatment of bipolar disorder. *The Journal of Neuropsychiatry and Clinical Neurosciences*, **4**, 395–405.

34. Walsh, T.D. (1990). Adjuvant analgesic therapy in cancer pain. In *Advances in Pain Research and Therapy* Vol. 16 (ed. K.M. Foley, J.J. Bonica, and V. Ventafridda), pp. 155–66. Second International Congress on Cancer Pain. New York: Raven Press.

35. Beaver, W.T. *et al.* (1966). A comparison of the analgesic effect of methotrimeprazine and morphine in patients with cancer. *Clinical and Pharmacological Therapy*, **7**, 436–46.

36. Oliver, D.J. (1985). The use of methotrimeprazine in terminal care. *British Journal of Clinical Practice*, **39**, 339–40.

37. Breitbart, W. (1986). Tardive dyskinesia associated with high dose intravenous metaclopramide. *New England Journal of Medicine*, **315**, 518.

38. Beaver, W.T. and Feise, G. (1976). Comparison of the analgesic effects of morphine, hydroxyzine and their combination in patients with postoperative pain. In *Advances in Pain Research and Therapy* (ed. J.J. Bonica and Albe-Fessard), pp. 553–7. New York: Raven Press.

39. Liebowitz, M.R. (1985). Imipramine in the treatment of panic disorder and its complications. *Psychiatry Clinics of North America*, **8**, 37–47.

40. Massie, M.J. and Popkin, M.K. (1998). Depression. In *Psycho-oncology* (ed. J.C. Holland *et al.*), pp. 518–41. New York: Oxford University Press.

41. Mavissakalian, M. (1993). Combined behavioral and pharmacological treatment of anxiety disorders. In *American Psychiatric Press Review of Psychiatry* Vol. 12. Washington DC: American Psychiatric Press.

42. Bruera, E. *et al.* (1990). Effects of morphine on the dyspnoea of terminal cancer patients. *Journal of Pain and Symptom Management*, **5**, 341–4.

43. Portenoy, R.K. *et al.* (1986). Intravenous infusions of opioids in cancer pain: clinical review and guidelines for use. *Cancer Treatment Reports*, **70**, 575–81.

44. Robinson, D., Napoliello, M.J., and Schenk, J. (1988). The safety and usefulness of buspirone as an anxiolytic drug in elderly versus young patients. *Clinical Therapy*, **10**, 740–6.

45. Massie, M.J., Holland, J.C., and Straker, N. (1989). Psychotherapeutic interventions. In *Handbook of Psycho-oncology: Psychological care of the Patient with Cancer* (ed. J.C. Holland and J.H. Rowland), pp. 455–69. New York: Oxford University Press.

46. Chochinov, H.M.C. and Holland, J.C. (1989). Bereavement. In *Handbook of Psycho-oncology: Psychological Care of the Patient with Cancer* (ed. J.C. Holland and J.H. Rowland), pp. 612–27. New York: Oxford University Press.

47. Holland, J.C. *et al.* (1991). A randomized clinical trial of alprazolam versus progressive muscle relaxation in cancer patients with anxiety and depressive symptoms. *Journal of Clinical Oncology*, **9**, 1004–11.

48. Wilson, K.G. *et al.* (2000). Diagnosis and Management of Depression in Palliative Care. In *Handbook of Psychiatry in Palliative Medicine* (ed. H.M.C. Chochinov and W. Breitbart), pp. 25–44. New York: Oxford University Press.

49. Chochinov, H.M.C. *et al.* (1994). Prevalence of depression in the terminally ill: effects of diagnostic criteria and symptom threshold judgements. *American Journal of Psychiatry*, **151** (April), 4.

50. Breitbart, W. *et al.* (2000). Depression, hopelessness, and desire for hastened death in terminally ill patients with cancer. *Journal of the American Medical Association*, **284**, 2907–11.

51. Hotopf, M. *et al.* (2002). Depression in advanced disease: a systematic review Part 1. Prevalence and case finding. *Palliative Medicine*, **16**, 81–97.

52. Spiegel, D., Sands, S., and Koopman, C. (1994). Pain and depression in patients with cancer. *Cancer*, **74**, 2570–8.

53. Lynch, M.E. (1995). The assessment and prevalence of affective disorders in advanced cancer. *Journal of Palliative Care*, **11**, 10–18.

54. Stiefel, F.C., Breitbart, W., and Holland, J.C. (1989). Corticosteroids in cancer: neuropsychiatric complications. *Cancer Investigation*, **7**, 479–91.

55. Young, D.F. (1982). Neurological complications of cancer chemotherapy. In *Neurological Complications of Therapy: Selected topics* (ed. A. Silverstein), pp. 57–113. New York: Futura Publishing.

56. Holland, J.C., Fassanellos, and Ohnuma, T. (1974). Psychiatric symptoms associated with L-asparaginase administration. *Journal of Psychiatric Research*, **10**, 165.

57. Adams, F., Quesada, J.R., and Gutterman, J.U. (1984). Neuropsychiatric manifestations of human leukocyte interferon therapy in patients with cancer. *Journal of the American Medical Association*, **252**, 938–41.

58. Denicoff, K.D. *et al.* (1987). The neuropsychiatric effects of treatment with interleukin-w and lymphokine-activated killer cells. *Annals of Internal Medicine*, **107** (3), 293–300.

59. Weddington, W.W. (1982). Delirium and depression associated with amphotericin B. *Psychosomatics*, **23**, 1076–8.

60. DeAngelis, L.M., Delattre, J., and Posner, J.B. (1989). Radiation-induced dementia in patients cured of brain metastases. *Neurology*, **39**, 789–96.

61. Breitbart, W.B. (1989). Endocrine-related psychiatric disorders. In *The Handbook of Psycho-oncology: The Psychological Care of the Cancer Patient* (ed. J. Holland and J. Rowland), pp. 356–66. New York: Oxford University Press.

62. Posner, J.B. (1988). Nonmetastatic effects of cancer on the nervous system. In *Cecil's Textbook of Medicine* (ed. J.B. Wyngaarden and L.H. Smith), pp. 1104–7. Philadelphia PA: WB Saunders.

63. Wilson, K.G. *et al* (2007). Depression and anxiety disorders in palliative care. *Journal of Pain and Symptom Management*, **33**, 118–29.

64. Nelson, C.J. *et al.* (2002). Spirituality, religion, and depression in the terminally ill. *Psychosomatics*, **43**, 213–20.

65. Block S. (2000). Assessing and managing depression in the terminally ill patient. *Annals of Internal Medicine*, **132**, 209–18.

66. Endicott, J. (1983). Measurement of depression patients with cancer. *Cancer*, **53**, 2243–8.

67. Kathol, R.G. *et al.* (1990). Diagnosis of major depression in cancer patients according to four sets of criteria. *American Journal of Psychiatry*, **147**, 1021–4.

68. Zimmerman, M., Coryell, W.H., and Black, D.W. (1990). Variability in the application of contemporary diagnstic criteria: endogenous depression as an example. *American Journal of Psychiatry*, **147**, 1173–9.

69. Breitbart, W. (1990). Cancer pain and suicide. In *Advances in Pain Research and Therapy* Vol. 16 (ed. K. Foley *et al.*), pp. 399–412. New York: Raven Press.

70. Breitbart, W. (1987). Sucide in cancer patients. *Oncology* **1**, 49–53.

71. Chochinov, H.M.C. *et al.* (1997). Are you depressed? Screening for depression in the terminally ill. *American Journal of Psychiatry, 154,* 674–6.

72. Passik, S. *et al.* (1998). Oncologists' recognition of depression in their patients with cancer. *Journal of Clinical Oncology, 16,* 1594–600.

73. McDonald, M. *et al.* (1999). Nurses' recognition of depression in patients with cancer. *Oncology Nursing Forum, 10,* 185–93.

74. Passik, S. *et al.* (2000). Oncology staff recognition of depressive symptoms on videotaped interviews of depressed cancer patients: implications for designing a training program. *Journal of Pain and Symptom Management, 19,* 329–38.

75. Passik, S. *et al.* (2001). An attempt to employ the zung self-rating depression scale as a lab test to trigger follow-up in ambulatory oncology clinics: criterion validation and detection. *Journal of Pain and Symptom Management, 21,* 273–81.

76. Olden, S. *et al.* (2009). Measuring depression at the end of life: is the Hamilton Depression rating Scale a valid instrument? *Assessment, 16,* 43–54.

77. Spiegel, D., Bloom, J.R., and Yalom, I.D. (1981). Group support for patients with metastatic cancer: a randomized prospective outcome study. *Archives of General Psychiatry, 38,* 527–33.

78. Spiegel, D. and Bloom, J.R. (1983). Group therapy and hypnosis reduce metastatic breast carcinoma pain. *Psychosomatic Medicine, 4,* 333–9.

79. Rifkin, A. *et al.* (1985). Trimipramine in physical illness with depression. *Journal of Clinical Psychiatry, 46,* 4–8.

80. Purohit, D.R. *et al.* (1978). The role of antidepressants in hospitalized cancer patients. *Journal of the Association of Physicians in India, 26,* 245–8.

81. Costa, D., Mogos, I., and Toma, T. (1985). Efficacy and safety of mianserin in the treatment of depression of women with cancer. *Acta Psychiatric Scand, 72,* 85–92.

82. Tremblay, A. and Breitbart, W. (2001). Psychiatric dimensions of palliative care. *Neurology Clinics, 19,* 949–67.

83. Homsi, J. *et al.* (2001). A phase II study of methylphenidate for depression in advanced cancer. *American Journal of Hospice and Palliative Care, 18,* 403–7.

84. Davis, J.M. and Glassman, A.H. (1989). Antidepressant drugs. In *Comprehensive Textbook of Psychiatry,* 5th edn. (ed. H.I. Kaplan and B.J. Sadock), Baltimore MD: Williams and Wilkins.

85. Preskorn, S.H. (1993). Recent pharmacologic advances in antidepressant therapy for the elderly. *American Journal of Medicine, 94* (Suppl. 5A).

86. Breitbart, W. and Passik, S.D. (1993). Psychiatric aspects of palliative care. In *Oxford Texbook of Palliative Medicine* (ed. D. Doyle, G.W. Hanks, and MacDonald), Oxford: Oxford University Press.

87. Le Melledo, J.M. and Bradwejn, J. (1993). Psychopharmacology of depression. In *Pharmacotherapy of Depression; Pharmanual* Vol. 20 (ed. Yvon D. Lapiere), pp. 25–46. Montreal: Chicago; Pharmalibri.

88. Stoudemire, A. and Fogel, B.S. (1987). Psychopharmacology in the medically ill. In *Principles of Medical Psychiatry* (ed. A. Stoudemire, B.S. Fogel, and F.L. Orlando), pp. 79–112. Grune and Stratton, Inc.

89. Preskorn, S.H. and Jerkovich, G.S. (1990). Central nervous system toxicity of tricyclic antidepressants: phenomenology, course, risk factors, and role of therapeutic drug monitoring. *Journal of Clinical Psychopharmacology, 10,* 88–95.

90. Massie, M.J. and Holland, J.C. (1984). Diagnosis and treatment of depression in the cancer patient. *Journal of Clinical Psychiatry, 42,* 25–8.

91. Fisch, M.J. *et al.* (2002). Fluoxetine versus placebo in advanced cancer outpatients: a placebo controlled, double-masked trial of the Hoosier Oncology Group. In *Proceedings of the 37th Annual Meeting of ASCO,* May 12–15, San Francisco, CA, abstract # 383A.

92. Glassman, A.H. (1984). The newer antidepressant drugs and their cardiovascular effects. *Psychopharmacological Bulletin 20,* 272–9.

93. Mendels, J. (1987). Clinical experience with serotonin reuptake inhibiting antidepressants. *Journal of Clinical Psychiatry, 48* (Suppl.), 26–30.

94. Cooper, G.L. (1988). The safety of fluoxetine—an update. *British Journal of Psychiatry, 153,* 77–86.

95. Preskorn, S. and Burke, M. (1992). Somatic therapy for major depressive disorder: selection of an antidepressant. *Journal of Clinical Psychiatry, 53* (Suppl.), 1–14.

96. Ciraulo, D.A. and Shader, R.I. (1990). Fluoxetine drug–drug interactions. I. Antidepressants and antipsychotics. *Journal of Clinical Psychopharmacology, 10,* 48–50.

97. Pearson, H.J. (1990). Interaction of fluoxetine with carbamazepine. *Journal of Clinical Psychiatry, 51,* 126.

98. Armstrong, S.C. and Cozza, K.L. (2001). Consultation-liaison psychiatry drug–drug intractions update. *Psychosomatics, 42,* 269–72.

99. Rudorfer, M.V. and Potter, W.Z. (1989). Anti-depressants. A comparative review of the clinical pharmacology and therapeutic use of the 'newer' versus the 'older' drugs. *Drugs, 37,* 713–38.

100. Sher, M., Krieger, J.N., and Juergen, S. (1983). Trazodone and priapism. *American Journal of Psychiatry, 140,* 1362–4.

101. Shopsin, B. (1983). Buproprion: a new clinical profile in the psychobiology of depression. *Journal of Clinical Psychiatry, 44,* 140–2.

102. Peck, A.W., Stern, W.C., and Watkinson, C. (1983). Incidence of seizures during treatment with tricyclic antidepressant drugs and buproprion. *Journal of Clinical Psychiatry, 44,* 197–201.

103. Lloyd, A.H. (1977). Practical consideration in the use of maprotiline (ludiomil) in general practice. *Journal of Internal Medical Research 5,* 122–5.

104. Ayd, F. (1979). Amoxapine: a new tricyclic antidepressant. *International Drug Therapy Newsletter, 14,* 33–40.

105. Fernandez, F. *et al.* (1987). Methylphenidate for depressive disorders in cancer patients. *Psychosomatics, 28,* 455–61.

106. Katon, W. and Raskind, M. (1980). Treatment of depression in the medically ill elderly with methylphenidate. *American Journal of Psychiatry, 137,* 963–5.

107. Kaufmann, M.W., Muarray, G.B., and Cassem, N.H. (1982). Use of psycho-stimulants in medically ill depressed patients. *Psychosomatics, 23,* 0817–19.

108. Fisch, R. (1985–1986). Metylphenidate for medical inpatients. *International Journal of Psychiatry in Medicine, 15,* 75–9.

109. Chiarillo, R.J. and Cole, J.O. (1987). The use of psychostimulants in general psychiatry. A reconsideration. *Archives of General Psychiatry, 44,* 286–95.

110. Satel, S.L. and Nelson, C.J. (1989). Stimulants in the treatment of depression: a critical overview. *Journal of Clinical Psychiatry, 50,* 241–9.

111. Woods, S.W. *et al.* (1986). Psychostimulant treatment of depressive disorders secondary to medical illness. *Journal of Clinical Psychiatry, 47,* 12–15.

112. Burns, M.M. and Eisendrath, S.J. (1994). Dextroamphetamine treatment for depression in terminally ill patients. *Psychosomatics, 35* (11), 80–2.

113. Olin, J. and Masand, P. (1996). Psychostimulants for depression in hospitalized cancer patients. *Psychosomatics, 37*(1), 57–61.

114. Menza, M.A., Kaufman, K.R., and Castellanos, A.M. (2000). Modafinil augmentation of antidepressant treatment in depression. *Journal of Clinical Psychiatry, 61,* 378–81.

115. Gold, L.H. and Balster, R.L. (1996). Evaluation of the cocaine-like discriminative stimulus effects and reinforcing effects of modafinil. *Psychopharmacology (Berlin), 126,* 286–92.

116. Warot, D. *et al.* (1993). Subjective effects of modafinil, a new central adrenergic stimulant in healthy volunteers: a comparison with amphetamine, caffeine, and placebo. *European Psychiatry, 8,* 201–8.

117. Cox, J.M. and Pappagallo, M. (2001). Modafinil: a gift to portmanteau. *American Journal of Hospice and Palliative Medicine, 18,* 408–10.

118. Fernandez, F. *et al.* (1988). Cognitive impairment due to AIDS related complex and its response to psychostimulants. *Psychosomatics, 29,* 38–46.

119. Bruera, E. *et al.* (1987). Methylphenidate associated with narcotics for the treatment of cancer pain. *Cancer Treatment Reports, 71,* 67–70.

120. Breitbart, W. and Mermelstein, H. (1992). Pemoline: an alternative psychostimulant for the management of depressive disorders in cancer patients. *Psychosomatics*, **33**, 352–6.

121. Nehra, A. *et al.* (1990). Pemoline associated hepatic injury. *Gastroenterology*, **99**, 1517–19.

122. Greenberg, D.B., Younger, J., and Kaufman, S.D. (1993). Management of lithium in patients with cancer. *Psychosomatics*, **34**, 388–94.

123. Stein, R.S., Flexner, J.H., and Graber, S.E. (1980). Lithium and granulocytopenia during induction therapy of acute myelogenous leukemia: update of an ongoing trial. *Advances in Experimental Medical Biology*, **127**, 187–98.

124. Cassem, N.H. (1987). The dying patient. In *Massachusetts General Hospital Handbook of General Hospital Psychiatry*, 2nd edn. (ed. T.P. Hackett and N.H. Cassem), pp. 332–52. Littleton MA: PSG Publishing Co. Inc.

125. W. Breitbart, W. (2002). Spirituality and meaning in supportive care: spirituality and meaning-centered group psychotherapy interventions in advanced cancer. *Supportive Care in Cancer*, **10**, 272–80.

126. Chochinov, H.M.C. (2002). Dignity-conserving care—a new model for palliative care. *Journal of the American Medical Association*, **287**, 2253–60.

127. Rosenfeld, B. *et al.* (2002). Suicide, assisted suicide, and euthanasia in the terminally ill. In *Handbook of Psychiatry in Palliative Medicine* (ed. H.M.C. Chochinov and W. Breitbart), pp. 51–62. New York: Oxford University Press.

128. Bolund, C. (1973–1976). Suicide and cancer: II. Medical and care factors in suicide by cancer patients in Sweden. *Journal of Psychosocial Oncology*, **3**, 17–30.

129. Farberow, N.L., Schneidman, E.S., and Leonard, C.V. Suicide among general medical and surgical hospital patients with malignant neoplasms. *Medical Bulletin 9*, Washington DC: US Veterans Administration, 1963.

130. Fox, B.H. *et al.* (1982). Suicide rates among cancer patients in Connecticut. *Journal of Chronic Diseases*, **35**, 85–100.

131. Hem, E. *et al.* (2004). Suicide risk in cancer patients from 1960 to 1999. *Journal of Clinical Oncology*, **22**, 4209–16.

132. Farberow, N.L. *et al.* (1971). An eight year survey of hospital suicides. *Suicide and Life-Threatening Behavior*, **1**, 20.

133. Robins, E. *et al.* (1950). Some clinical considerations in the prevention of suicide based on 134 successful suicides. *American Journal of Public Health*, **49**, 888–9.

134. Guze, S. and Robins, E. (1970). Suicide and primary affective disorders. *British Journal of Psychiatry*, **117**, 437–8.

135. Ganzini, L. *et al.* (1994). The effect of depression treatment on elderly patients' preferences for life-sustaining medical therapy. *American Journal of Psychiatry*, **151**, 1613–16.

136. Beck, A.T., Kovacs, M., and Weissman, A. (1975). Hopelessness and suicidal behavior: an overview. *Journal of the American Medical Association*, **234**, 1146–9.

137. Chochinov, H.M.C. *et al.* (1998). Depression, hopelessness, and suicidal ideation in the terminally ill. *Psychosomatics* **39**, 366–70.

138. Levine, P.M., Silberfarb, P.M., and Lipowski, Z.J. (1978). Mental disorders in cancer patients. *Cancer*, **42**, 1385–90.

139. Holland, J.C. (2003). Psychological aspects of cancer. In *Cancer Medicine*, 6th edn. (ed. J.F. Holland and E. Frei), pp. 1039–54. Philadelphia PA: Lea and Febiger.

140. Zweig, R. and Hinrichsen, G. (1993). Factors associated with suicide attempts by depressed older adults: a prospective study. *American Journal of Psychiatry*, **150**, 1687–92.

141. Dubovsky, S.L. (1978). Averting suicide in terminally ill patients. *Psychosomatics*, **19**, 113–15.

142. Murphy, G.E. (1977). Suicide and attempted suicide. *Hospital Practice*, **12**, 78–81.

143. Silberfarb, P.M., Maurer, L.H., and Cronthamel, C.S. (1980). Psychosocial aspects of breast cancer patients during different treatment regimens. *American Journal of Psychiatry*, **137**, 450–5.

144. Achte, K.A. and Vanhkouen, M.L. (1971). Cancer and the psyche. *Omega*, **2**, 46–56.

145. Brown, J.H. *et al.* (1986). Is it normal for terminally ill patients to desire death? *American Journal of Psychiatry*, **143**, 208–11.

146. Breitbart, W., Rosenfeld, B., and Passik, S.D. (1996). Interest in physician-assisted suicide among ambulatory HIV-infected patients. *American Journal of Psychiatry*, **153**, 238–42.

147. Emmanuel, E.J. *et al.* (1996). Euthanasia and physician-assisted suicide: Attitudes and experiences of oncology patients, oncologists and the public. *Lancet*, **347**, 1805–10.

148. Chochinov, H.M.C. *et al.* (1995). Desire for death in the terminally ill. *American Journal of Psychiatry*, **152**, 1185–91.

149. Rosenfeld, B. *et al.* (1999). Measuring desire for death among patients with HIV/AIDS: the schedule of attitudes toward hastened death. *American Journal of Psychiatry*, **156**, 94–100.

150. Rosenfeld, B. *et al.* (2000). The schedule of attitudes toward hastened death: measuring desire for hastened death in terminally ill cancer patients. *Cancer*, **88**, 2868–75.

151. Chochinov, H.M.C. *et al.* (1999). Will to live in the terminally ill. *Lancet*, **354**, 816–19.

152. Breitbart, W., Chochinov, H.M.C., and Passik, S. (1998). Psychiatric aspects of palliative care. In *Oxford Textbook of Palliative Medicine* (ed. D. Doyle, G.E.C Hanks, and N. McDonald), pp. 933–54. Oxford: Oxford University Press.

153. Rousseau, P. (2000). Spirituality and the dying patient. *Journal of Clinical Oncology*, **18**, 2000–2.

154. Kissane, D., Clarke, D.M., and Street, A.F. (2001). Demoralization syndrome—a relevant psychiatric diagnosis for palliative care. *Journal of Palliative Care*, **17**, 12–21.

155. Chochinov, H.M.C. *et al.* (2002). Dignity in the terminally ill: an empirical model. *Social Science and Medicine*, **54**, 433–43.

156. Greenstein, M. and Breitbart, W. (2000). Cancer and the experience of meaning: a group psychotherapy program for people with cancer. *American Journal of Psychotherapy*, **54**, 486–500.

157. American Psychiatric Association. *Diagnostic and Statistical Manual of Mental Disorders* 4th edn. Washington DC: American Psychiatric Association, 1994.

158. Lipowski, Z.J. (1990). *Delirium: Acute Confusional States*. New York: Oxford University Press.

159. Lipowski, Z.J. (1983). Transient cognitive disorders (delirium, acute confusional states) in the elderly. *American Journal of Psychiatry*, **140**, 1426–36.

160. Breitbart, W. *et al.* (1996). A double-blind trial of haloperidol, chlorpromazine, and lorazepam in the treatment of delirium in hospitalized AIDS patients. *American Journal of Psychiatry*, **153**, 231–7.

161. Bruera, E. *et al.* (1992). Cognitive failure in patients with terminal cancer: a prospective study. *Journal of Pain and Symptom Management*, **7**, 192–5.

162. Fainsinger, R. and Young, C. (1991). Cognitive failure in a terminally ill patient. *Journal of Pain and Symptom Management*, **6**, 492–4.

163. Leipzig, R. *et al.* (1987). Reversible narcotic associated mental status impairment in patients with metastatic cancer. *Pharmacology*, **35**, 47–54.

164. Levine, P.M., Silberfarb, P., and Lipowski, Z.J. (1978). Mental disorders in cancer patients. *Cancer*, **42**, 1385–91.

165. Murray, G.B. (1987). Confusion, delirium, and dementia. In *Massachusetts General Hospital Handbook of General Hospital Psychiatry* 2nd edn. (ed. T.P. Hackett and N.H. Cassem), pp. 84–115. Littleton MA: PSG Publishing.

166. Leonard, M. *et al.* (2008). Delirium issues in palliative care settings. *Journal of Psychosomatic Research*, **65**, 289–98.

167. Knight, E.B. and Folstein, M.F. (1977). Unsuspected emotional and cognitive disturbance in medical patients. *Annals of Internal Medicine*, **87**, 723–4.

168. Pereira, J., Hanson, J., and Bruera, E. (1997). The frequency and clinical course of cognitive impairment in patients with terminal cancer. *Cancer*, **79**, 835–41.

169. Tune, L.E. (1991). Postoperative delirium. *International Psychogeriatrics*, **3**, 325–32.

170. Gillick, M.R., Serrel, N.A., and Gillick, L.S. (1982). Adverse consequences of hospitalization in the elderly. *Social Science in Medicine*, **16**, 1033–8.

171. Warsaw, G.A. *et al.* (1982). Functional disability in the hospitalized elderly. *Journal of the American Medical Association*, **248**, 847–50.

172. Berman, K. and Eastham, E.J. (1974). Psychogeriatric ascertainment and assessment for treatment in an acute medical ward setting. *Aging*, **3**, 174–88.

173. Seymour, D.J. *et al.* (1980). Acute confusional states and dementia in the elderly: the role of dehydration/volume depletion, physical illness and age. *Aging*, **9**, 137–46.

174. Hodkinson, H.M. (1973). Mental impairment in the elderly. *Journal of the Royal College of Physicians London*, **7**, 305–17.

175. Varsamis, J., Zuchowski, T., and Maini, K.K. (1972). Survival rates and causes of death in geriatric psychiatric patients: a six year follow-up study. *Canadian Psychiatry Association Journal*, **17**, 17–22.

176. Breitbart, W., Gibson, C., and Tremblay, A. (2002). The delirium experience: Delirium recall and delirium related distress in hospitalized patients with cancer, their spouses/caregivers, and their nurses. *Psychosomatics*, **43**, 183–9.

177. Trzepacz, P.T., Teague, G.B., and Lipowski, Z.J. (1985). Delirium and other organic mental disorders in a general hospital. *General Hospital Psychiatry*, **7**, 101–6.

178. Bruera, E. *et al.* (1992) The assessment of pain intensity in patients with cognitive failure: a preliminary report. *Journal of Pain and Symptom Management*, **7(5)**, 267–70.

179. Coyle, N. *et al.* (1994). Delirium as a contributing factor to 'Crescendo' pain: three case reports. *Journal of Pain and Symptom Management*, **9**, 44–7.

180. Fainsinger, R. *et al.* (1991). Symptom control during the last week of life in a palliative care unit. *Journal of Palliative Care*, **7**, 5–11.

181. Bruera, E. *et al.* (1989). The cognitive effects of the administration of narcotic analgesics in patients with cancer pain. *Pain*, **39**, 13–16.

182. Silberfarb, P.M. (1983). Chemotherapy and cognitive defects in cancer patients. *Annual Review of Medicine*, **34**, 35–46.

183. Stiefel, F., Fainsinger, R., and Bruera, E. (1992). Acute confusional states in patients with advanced cancer. *Journal of Pain and Symptom Management*, **7**, 94–8.

184. Lawlor, P.G. *et al.* (2002). The occurrence, causes and outcomes of delirium in advanced cancer patients: a prospective study. *Archives of Internal Medicine*, **160**, 786–94.

185. Wise, M.G. and Brandt, G.T. (1992). Delirium. In *Textbook of Neuropsychiatry* 2nd edn (ed. S.C. Yudofsky and R.E. Hales), pp. 89–107. Washington DC: American Psychiatric Press.

186. Ross, C.A. (1991). CNS arousal systems: possible role in delirium. *International Psychogeriatrics*, **3**, 353–71.

187. Lipowski, Z.J. (1980). Delirium: acute brain failure in man. Springfield IL: Charles C Thomas, 1980.

188. Breitbart, W. *et al.* (1995). Neuropsychiatric syndromes and psychological symptoms in patients with advanced cancer. *Journal of Pain and Symptom Management*, **10**, 131–41.

189. Stagno, D., Gibson, C., and Breitbart, W. (2004). The delirium subtypes: a review of prevalence, phenomenology, pathophysiology, and treatment response. *Palliative and Supportive Care*, **2**, 171–9.

190. Albert, M.S. *et al.* (1991). The delirium symptom interview: an interview for the detection of delirium symptoms in hospitalized patients. *Journal of Geriatric Psychiatry and Neurology*, **5**, 14–21.

191. Breitbart, W. *et al.* (1997). The Memorial Delirium Assessment Scale. *Journal of Pain and Symptom Management*, **13**, 128–37.

192. Folstein, M.F., Folstein, S.E., and McHugh, P.R. (1975). 'Mini-mental status': a practical method for grading the cognitive state of patients for clinicians. *Journal of Psychiatric Research*, **12**, 189–98.

193. Jacobs, J.C. *et al.* (1977). Screening for organic mental syndromes in the medically ill. *Annals of Internal Medicine*, **86**, 40–6.

194. Katzman, R. *et al.* (1983). Validation of a short orientation-memory-concentration test of cognitive impairment. *American Journal of Psychiatry*, **140**, 734–9.

195. Hjermstad, M.J., Loge, J.H., and Kaasa, S. (2004). Methods for assessment of cognitive failure and delirium in palliative care patients: implications for practice and research. *Palliative Medicine*, **3**, 494–506.

196. Trzepacz, P.T., Baker, R.W., and Greenhouse, J. (1988). A symptom rating scale for delirium. *Psychiatric Research*, **1**, 89–97.

197. Williams, M.A. (1991). Delirium/acute confusional states: evaluation devices in nursing. *International Psychogeriatrics*, **3**, 301–8.

198. Wolber, G. *et al.* (1984). Validity of the short Portable Mental Status Questionnaire with elderly psychiatric patients. *Journal of Consultational and Clinical Psychology*, **52**, 712–13.

199. Smith, M.J., Breitbart, W.S., and Platt, M.M. (1995). A critique of instruments and methods to detect, diagnose, and rate delirium. *Journal of Pain and Symptom Management*, **10**, 35–77.

200. Trzepacz, P.T. *et al.* (1999). *Validity of the Delirium Rating Scale—Revised-98 (DRS-R-98)*. Abstract #41. In *Proceedings of the 46th Annual Meeting of the Academy of Psychosomatic Medicine*, 18–21 November, New Orleans, LA.

201. Inouye, B.K. *et al.* (1990). Clarifying confusion: the confusion assessment method, a new method for detection of delirium. *Annals of Internal Medicine*, **113**, 941–8.

202. Hart, R.P. *et al.* (1997). Abbreviated cognitive test for delirium. *Journal of Psychosomatic Research*, **43**, 417–23.

203. Lawlor, P.G. *et al.* (2000). Clinical utility, factor analysis and further validation of the Memorial Delirium Assessment Scale (MDAS). *Cancer*, **88**, 2859–67.

204. American Psychiatric Association (1999). Practice Guidelines for the Treatment of Patients with Delirium. *American Journal of Psychiatry*, **156**, S1–20.

205. Bruera, E. (1991). Case report. Severe organic brain syndrome. *Journal of Palliative Care*, **7**, 36–8.

206. Lichter, I. and Hunt, E. (1990). The last 48 hours of life. *Journal of Palliative Care*, **6(4)**, 7–15.

207. Tuma, R. and DeAngelis, L. (1992). Acute encephalopathy in patients with systemic cancer. *Annals of Neurology*, **32**, 288–9.

208. Inouye, B.K. *et al.* (1999). A multicomponent intervention to prevent delirium in hospitalized older patients. *New England Journal of Medicine*, **340**, 669–76.

209. Derogatis, L.R. *et al.* (1979). A survey of psychotropic drug prescriptions in an oncology population. *Cancer*, **44**, 1919–29.

210. Steifel, F., Kornblith, A., and Holland, J. (1990). Changes in prescription patterns of psychotropic drugs for cancer patients during a 10-year period. *Cancer*, **65**, 1048–53.

211. Goldberg, G. and Mor, V. (1985). A survey of psychotropic use in terminal cancer patients. *Psychosomatics*, **26**, 745–51.

212. Jaeger, H., Morrow, G., and Brescia, F. (1985). A survey of psychotropic drug utilization by patients with advanced neoplastic disease. *General Hospice Psychiatry*, **7**, 353–60.

213. Akechi, T. *et al.* (1996). Usage of haloperidol for delirium in cancer patients. *Support Care in Cancer*, **4**, 390–2.

214. Fernandez, F. *et al.* (1988). Treatment of severe, refractory agitation with a haloperidol drip. *Journal of Clinical Psychiatry*, **49**, 239–41.

215. Fernandez, F, Levy, J.F., and Mansell, P.W.A. (1989). Management of delirium in terminally ill AIDS patients. *International Journal of Psychiatry in Medicine*, **19**, 165–72.

216. Rosen, J.H. (1979). Double-blind comparison of haloperidol and thioridazine in geriatric outpatients. *Journal of Clinical Psychiatry*, **40**, 17–20.

217. Smith, G.R., Taylor, C.W., and Linkons, P. (1974). Haloperidol versus thioridazine for the treatment of psychogeriatric patients: a double-blind clinical trial. *Psychosomatics,* **15,** 134–8.

218. Thomas, H., Schwartz, E., and Petrilli, R. (1992). Droperidol versus haloperidol for chemical restraint of agitated and combative patients. *Annals of Emergency Medicine,* **21,** 407–13.

219. Gagnon, P.R. (2008). Treatment of delirium in supportive and palliative care. *Current Opinion in Supportive and Palliative Care,* **2,** 60–6.

220. Breitbart, W. (1988). Psychiatric complications of cancer. In *Current Therapy in Hematology Oncology-3* (ed. M.C. Brain and P.P. Carbone), pp. 268–74. Toronto: BC Decker.

221. Breitbart, W. (1989). Psychiatric management of cancer pain. *Cancer,* **63,** 2336–42.

222. Twycross, R.G. and Lack, S.A. Symptom Control in Far Advanced Cancer: Pain Relief. London: Pitman Books, 1983.

223. Breitbart, W. (2001), Diagnoisis and management of delirium in the terminally ill. In *Topics in Palliative Care* Vol. 5 (ed. R. Portenoy and E. Bruera), pp. 303–21. New York: Oxford University Press

224. Menza, M., Murray, G., and Holmes, V. (1988). Controlled study of extrapyramidal reactions in the management of delirious medically ill patients: intravenous haloperidol versus intravenous haloperidol plus benzodiazepines. *Heart and Lung,* **17,** 238–241.

225. Oliver, D.J. (1985). The use of methotrimeprazine in terminal care. *British Journal of Clinical Practice,* **39,** 339–40.

226. Alici-Evciman, Y. Breitbart, W. (2008). An update on the use of antipsychotics in the treatment of delirium. *Palliative and Supportive Care,* **6,** 177–82.

227. Passik, S.D. and Cooper, M. (1999). Complicated delirium in a cancer patient successfully treated with olanzipine. *Journal of Pain and Symptom Management,* **17,** 219–23.

228. Sipahimalani, A. and Massand, P.S. (1998). Olanzipine in the treatment of delirium. *Psychosomatics,* **39,** 422–30.

229. Sipahimalani, A., Sime, R.M., and Masand, P.S. (1997). Treatment of delirium with risperidone. *International Journal of Geriatric Psychopharmacology,* **1,** 24–6.

230. Breitbart, W., Tremblay, A., and Gibson, C. (2002). An open trial of olanzapine for the treatment of delirium in hospitalized cancer patients. *Psychosomatics,* **43,** 175–6.

231. Caraceni, A. and Simonetti, F. (2009). Palliating delirium in patients with cancer. *Lancet Oncology,* **10,** 164–72.

232. Ventafridda, V. *et al.* (1990). Symptom prevalence and control during cancer patients' last days of life. *Journal of Palliative Care,* **6,** 7–11.

233. Mercadante, S., De Conno, F., and Ripamonti, C. (1995). Propofol in terminal care. *Journal of Pain and Symptom Management,* **10,** 639–42.

234. Moyle, J. (1995). The use of propofol in palliative medicine. *Journal of Pain and Symptom Management,* **10,** 643–6.

235. Fainsinger, R. and Bruera, E. (1992). Treatment of delirium in a terminally ill patient. *Journal of Pain and Symptom Management,* **7,** 54–6.

236. Stiefel, F. and Bruera, E. (1991). Psychostimulants for hypoactive-hypoalert delirium? *Journal of Palliative Care,* **3,** 25–6.

237. Bruera, E. (1990). Symptom control in patients with cancer. *Journal of Psychosocial Oncology,* **8,** 47–73.

238. Coyle, N. *et al.* (1990). Character of terminal illness in the advanced cancer patient: pain and other symptoms during the last four weeks of life. *Journal of Pain and Symptom Management,* **5,** 83–93.

239. Levy, M. and Catalano, R. (1985). Control of common physical symptoms other than pain in patients with terminal disease. *Seminars in Oncology,* **12,** 411–30.

240. Fotopoulos, S.S., Graham, C., and Cook, M.R. (1979). *Psychophysiologic control of cancer pain.* In Advances in Pain Research and Therapy Vol. 2. (ed. J.J. Bonica and V. Ventafridda), pp. 231–44. New York: Raven Press.

241. Turk, D. and Rennert, K. (1981). *Pain and the terminally ill cancer patient: a cognitive-social learning perspective.* In Behavior Therapy in Terminal Care (ed. H.J. Sobel), pp. 137–54. Cambridge: Ballinger.

242. Hilgard, E. and LeBaron, S. (1982). Relief of anxiety and pain in children and adolescents with cancer: quantitative measures and clinical observations. *International Journal of Clinical Experimental Hypnosis,* **30,** 417–42.

243. Jay, S., Elliott, C., and Varni, J. (1986). Acute and chronic pain in adults and children with cancer:*Journal of Consulting and Clinical Psychology,* **54,** 601–7.

244. Kellerman, J. *et al.* (1983). Adolescents with cancer: hypnosis for the reduction of acute pain and anxiety associated with medical procedures. *Journal of Adolescent Health Care,* **4,** 85–90.

245. Lesko, L. (1989). *Anorexia.* In Handbook of Psycho-oncology: Psychological Care of the Patient with Cancer (ed. J.C. Holland and J. Rowland), pp. 434–43. New York: Oxford University Press.

246. Redd, W.H., Andresen, G.V., and Minagawa, R.Y. (1982). Hypnotic control of anticipatory emesis in patients receiving cancer chemotherapy. *Journal of Consulting and Clinical Psychology,* **50,** 14–19.

247. Dixon, J. (1984). Effect of nursing interventions on nutritional and performance status in cancer patients. *Nursing Research,* **33,** 330–5.

248. Campbell, D. *et al.* (1984). Relaxation: its effect on the nutritional status and performance status of clients with cancer. *Journal of the American Dietary Association,* **84,** 201–4.

249. Redd, W.H. (1980). In vivodesensitization in the treatment of chronic emesis following gastrorintestinal surgery. *Behavior Therapy,* **11,** 421–7.

250. West, B. and Piccionne, C. (1982). Cognitive behavioral techniques in treating anorexia and depression in a cancer patient. *The Behavioral Therapist,* **5,** 115–17.

251. LeBaw, W. *et al.* (1975). The use of self hypnosis by children with cancer. *American Journal of Clinical Hypnosis,* **17,** 233–8.

252. Radbruch, L. *et al.* (2008). Fatigue in palliative care patients – an EAPC approach. *Palliative Medicine,* **22,** 13–32.

253. Breitbart, W. *et al.* (2001). A randomized, double-blind, placebo-controlled trial of psychostimulants for the treatment of fatigue in ambulatory patients with human immunodeficiency virus disease. *Archives of Internal Medicine,* **161,** 411–20.

254. Barnes, M. (1988). Nausea and vomiting in the patient with advanced cancer. *Journal of Pain and Symptom Management,* **3,** 81–5.

255. Morrow, G.R. and Morrell, B.S. (1982). Behavioral treatment for the anticipatory nausea and vomiting induced by cancer chemotherapy. *New England Journal of Medicine,* **307,** 1476–80.

256. Jacobsen, P.B. *et al.* (1988). Non pharmacologic factors in the development of post treatment nausea with adjuvant chemotherapy for breast cancer. *Cancer,* **61,** 379–85.

257. Greenberg, D.B. *et al.* (1987). Alprazolam for phobic nausea and vomiting related to cancer chemotherapy. *Cancer Treatment Reports,* **71,** 549–50.

258. Cannici, J., Malcolm, R., and Peck, L.A. (1983). Treatment of insomnia in cancer patients using muscle relaxant training. *Journal of Behavior Therapy and Experimental Psychiatry,* **14,** 251–6.

259. Stamm, H., Bultz, B., and Pittman, C. (1986). Psychosocial problems and interventions in a referred sample of cancer patients. *Psychosomatic Medicine,* **48,** 539–48.

260. Hajjar, R.R. (2008). Sleep disturbance in palliative care. *Clinics in Geriatric Medicine,* **24,** 83–91.

15.6

Bereavement

David W. Kissane and Talia Zaider

Introduction

Mourning is an essential adaptive response to the inevitable experience of loss. In many ways it is the debt that has to be repaid for investment in the joys of life. Familiarity with and confidence in responding to grief is a *sine qua non* for all clinicians working in palliative medicine, including the capacity to differentiate healthy from maladaptive adjustment. Many losses are experienced as patients and their families move through the phases of progressive illness towards death. Related grief is thus current as well as anticipatory of future loss. Support for the grieving process in both the patients and their carers clearly begins during palliative care and places the clinician in an ideal position to sustain continuity of this care into bereavement.

Family-centred care is integral to this supportive process as the family's understanding of the illness and its treatment influences their later adjustment. Every word uttered by the treating team, the related tone, and sensitivity shown contributes to the experience for the bereaved, who generally need to understand the process of death and discuss any features of concern. Palliative care teams are ideally placed to recognize those at greater risk of poor outcome and provide care prophylactically to prevent bereavement morbidity.

Although words such as grief, mourning, and bereavement are commonly used interchangeably, the following definitions indicate their use in this chapter:

- *Bereavement* is the state of loss resulting from death[1].
- *Grief* is the emotional response associated with loss[2].
- *Mourning* is the process of adaptation, including the cultural and social rituals prescribed as accompaniments[3].
- *Anticipatory grief* precedes the death and results from the expectation of that event[3].
- *Pathological grief* represents an abnormal outcome involving psychological, social, or physical morbidity[4].
- *Disenfranchised grief* represents the hidden sorrow of the marginalized where there is less social permission to express many dimensions of loss[5].

In this chapter, the theoretical models that have been developed to explain bereavement phenomena and the process of mourning are considered with a view to generating an understanding of the clinical features of grief. Recognition of those at risk of complicated outcome is mandatory to offer preventative interventions. Models of follow-up and management of complicated grief are fully explored, as is variation across the lifecycle and the impact of stigmatized deaths. Spiritual aspects of bereavement highlight the contributions of the world's major religions in supporting the bereaved. Bereavement research in the future will be aided by use of validated measures, which are summarized towards the chapter's end as a handy resource. Finally, to conclude, the recognition that personal growth is a common outcome despite the sadness of loss reminds us that creativity often emerges as a result of resolution of the mourning process.

Theoretical models of bereavement phenomena

Dating from Darwin's observation of monkeys 'weeping' from grief, ethology has pointed out that social birds and mammals do grieve[6]. Indeed, mourning appears to be the price paid for the evolutionary adaptiveness of social relationships. This universality of grief suggests it is imprinted into the biological processes of the species, consistent with the experience that death seems to be difficult for people everywhere. Yet, social constructionists remind us that the shape and content of grief is culturally determined. It varies markedly across places, times, and social groups, with noteworthy differences in the expression of anger, emotionality, self-mutilation, rituals, and public versus private grief[7].

A conceptual framework that illuminates what underpins the phenomena of bereavement aids our clinical understanding of the experience of the bereaved (see Table 15.6.1). Explanatory models favoured by bereavement researchers were ranked in the following order of importance: attachment, psychodynamic, sociological, cognitive behavioural, and ethology[8]. Although limited by the available list of potential theories (for instance, continuing bonds, interpersonal, systemic, and traumatic were not offered), these models help practitioners work flexibly with pertinent issues.

Attachment theory posits that the development of close affectionate bonds to particular others generates security and survival potential[9]. From a secure base, the capacity for curiosity emerges to generate creativity in autonomous adult life. Parents, especially the mother, constitute the usual subject of primary attachments, but these behaviours become enduring throughout adult life and the spouse eventually replaces the parents as the recipient of the strongest bonds. The family thus forms the setting for the major constellation of bonds. Through studying parent–child relationships, Mary Ainsworth differentiated secure from insecure attachments, the latter appearing as either anxious, avoidant, or disorganized/hostile[10]. A transgenerational influence is evident between the parental style of attachment and that found in children,

Table 15.6.1 Theoretical models explaining bereavement phenomena.

Name of model	Key contributors	Main features
Attachment theory	Bowlby, Ainsworth, Parkes, Weiss	The bonds of close relationships are severed by loss
Psychodynamic theory	Freud, Klein, Horowitz, Kohut	Early relationships lay down a template that guide future relationships
Interpersonal model	Sullivan, Bonnano, Horowitz, Benjamin	Relational influences are dominant in grief outcome
Psychosocial transition	Parkes, Janoff-Bulman	Changed assumptive world view
Sociological model	Rosenblatt, Klass, Walter	Cultural influences shape the form and content of grief
Family systems theory	Walsh, McGoldrick, Kissane, Shapiro	Family are the main source of support; family functioning determines outcome
Cognitive stress coping theory	Stroebe, Kavanagh	Conditioned or learnt patterns become entrenched
Traumatic model	Horowitz, Pynoos, Prigerson, Jacobs	Intrusive aspects of trauma dominate
Ethology	Darwin, Lorenz	Biological and physiological processes underpin the phenomena across species

such that families can transmit insecure patterns of relating through the generations. The nature of attachments in a person's life influences the impact of loss when these bonds are changed, determining the work of mourning as this separation is dealt with[11,12].

While related to attachment theory, the psychodynamic model places greater emphasis on the development of the person, with all of their childhood and earlier life influences, including their sense of self, confidence, and resilience that comes with a robust self-esteem, and their learnt capacity to mourn. Schematic representations of early relationships construct a template (technically termed object relations) that lays down the operating principles guiding the emotional experience of relationships. Once the infant has developed feelings of concern for its mother, Klein described the early pining evident when the mother was absent[13]. Mourning was thus recognized as a life-long mechanism of adaptation to cope with the inevitable traumas of life.

Interpersonal theories have emerged recently to throw further light on bereavement[14] and complement the psychodynamic model. Cyclical relational patterns are understood to result from current relational selections based on their resonance with the past, often confirming previous expectations. Schemas of the 'who the self is' are constructed through relational interactions to establish a role for the person pertaining to these relationships. Horowitz has made particular use of these schemas using a stress-response model for grief[15]. For instance, ambivalence towards the deceased is associated with greater distress, but restructuring the 'ambivalent' schema is possible through its observation in current relational patterns and the introduction of strategic variations to alter this habitually dysfunctional pattern. Horowitz and colleagues have tested a model of therapy based on these premises[16].

Transition theorists highlight the adaptation to change that is inherent in any resolution of grief. Parkes suggested that alteration to an individual's set of ideas and beliefs about their environment—their assumptive world—was central to adaptation[17]. Development of acceptance of change is implicit in such a view.

In their contribution to a sociological model of bereavement, post-modern writers emphasize the various discourses that indicate a multiplicity of perspectives. The notion of the 'breaking of the bonds' of relationship, first hinted at by Freud in 1912[18], is thus socially determined. Klass and colleagues highlighted the process of continuing bonds through reverence for the dead as both ancestors and moral guides[19]. Walter noted that conversations about and with the deceased served as one means of sustaining

a relationship[20]. It becomes a personal choice whether the bereaved moves on to a new relationship or sustains the attitude of a 'broken heart'.

The sociological view also recognizes the loneliness of the bereaved and the value of groups or networks, including the family, to counter the social isolation that otherwise might prevail. Patterns of socialization of the bereaved vary with cultures, but networks of support have a vital influence on adjustment. The manner in which a family grieves and how its members continue to relate to each other is crucial to outcome. Families wreaked by conflict, reduced cohesion, and poor communication struggle to support each other—high rates of psychosocial morbidity are found in dysfunctional families[21]. Family systems theory makes particular use of intergenerational and family lifecycle perspectives[22].

Mourning can be triggered by unexpected life events, natural disasters, and traumas that violate the person and introduce an unwelcome element to the experience that is described as 'shocking'. Traumatic grief captures something that is unique to the trauma and challenges the bereaved with the intrusion of any resultant distressing memories. Prigerson and Jacobs have argued for recognition of the specifically traumatic nature of some deaths and their impact on grief[23].

Finally, behavioural models offer their contribution to bereavement theory through the challenge of chronic grief, in which the bereaved become stuck in an entrenched state of distress[24]. Patterns such as social withdrawal, 'memorialization' of the deceased through preserving their bedroom, clothes, and possessions intact as if a shrine, or chronic weeping upon mention of the deceased's name illustrate these behaviours. Cognitive behavioural approaches such as activity scheduling generate clinical improvement and point to an element of conditioned response in chronic grief.

The number of overlapping dimensions to these conceptual models is noteworthy, yet none by itself is a sufficient and complete explanation of bereavement phenomena. However, the intrapsychic, interpersonal, systemic, and sociological features of these models deliver an intersecting and overall coherence, which aids our eventual understanding of the complex phenomena observed in grief.

Stroebe and Schut have pointed out that while these general theories of grief explain the broad range of phenomena observed, they do not inform fully about the specific coping pathways that grieving individuals go down[25]. They have suggested a dual process model of bereavement-specific coping, in which oscillation occurs between loss-orientation, in which there is a focus on the loss itself, and restoration-orientation, in which the focus shifts to attending to ongoing life. Active 'grief work' occurs when the bereaved are loss-oriented, but excessive negative emotion could lead to a deterioration in coping, and so active confrontation of grief sits in a dynamic equilibrium with some degree of avoidance of grief. The individual needs at times to pull back and take 'time out' from the distress of the loss. They may do so through use of the restorative track in which the negative emotions are countered by some degree of positive reappraisal and of construction of meaning about the event. This promotes positive affects and eventually opens up new goals and plans for the future. Complex regulation exists in getting this balance right between grieving and restoring, with both interpersonal and cultural influences guiding this balance. Dissonance between bereaved members of a family, for instance, will challenge the balance and lead systemically to some readjustment by some or more members.

The bereaved cope therefore through adjusting the balance between expression of negative and positive emotions in emotion-based coping, and incorporating appropriate degrees of problem-solving and meaning-generation to guide their sense of purpose and control. They need to sustain the normal operation and functioning in their lives while also grieving the loss that has occurred irrevocably.

The nature of normal grief

The expression of normal grief is evident through its emotional, cognitive, physical, and behavioural features[1]. Eric Lindemann provided the first systematic study of these through his observations of people who lost a relative in Boston's *Cocoanut Grove Nightclub* fire[26]. Somatic distress with numbness, preoccupation with sad memories of the deceased, guilt, anger, loss of the regular patterns of conduct, and identification with symptoms of the deceased formed the key dimensions that Lindemann observed.

Emotional distress occurs in waves that last for minutes at a time and involves unavoidable crying, loss of concentration and purpose while preoccupied with thoughts about the deceased, and a range of associated affects including sadness, anger, despair, anxiety, and guilt. Cognitive processes become dominated by memories, reflected in story telling, reminiscences, and conversations about the deceased. Physical responses include numbness, restlessness, tension, tremors, sleep disturbance, anorexia, weight loss, fatigue, and a variety of aches and pains. Finally, behavioural aspects are variously reflected in social withdrawal, wandering, searching, and seeking company and consolation.

A number of physiological changes have been identified in neuroendocrine functioning[27] (for instance, challenge studies like the dexamethasone suppression test), immune indices[28] (e.g. natural killer cell functioning), and sleep efficiency[29]. Exploration of these physiological changes not only suggests that grief and depression lie on a biological continuum but also provides understanding for the morbidity, both somatic and psychosocial, that is associated with bereavement.

The clinical presentations of grief

As the family journey through palliative care, the clinical phases progress from anticipatory grief through to the immediate news of the death, to the stages of acute grief and, potentially for some, the complications of bereavement.

Anticipatory grief

When news of cancer recurrence or disease progression reaches the patient and family, grief is initiated as they anticipate eventual death. However, not all of this grief is about the final loss, as many changes unfold with the illness and its treatment. Loss of health can be accompanied by loss of work, leisure activities, financial security, independence, sense of certainty about life and further physical impairments, body image change, and altered perception of well-being. The clinician is challenged to understand the meaning of the loss to each person and evaluate therein their grief response.

Anticipatory grief generally draws the supportive family into a configuration of mutual comfort and greater closeness as the news of the illness and its proposed management is grappled with. For a time this perturbation advantages the care of the sick, until the pressures of daily life draw the family back towards their prior constellation. Movement back and forth is evident thereafter as news of illness progression unfolds. Periods of grief become interspersed with phases of contentment and happiness. When the family is engaged in the domiciliary care of their ill member, their cohesion potentially increases as they share their fears, hopes, joy, and distress.

In contrast, difficulties emerge for some families as they express their anticipatory grief. Impaired coping is exhibited through protective avoidance, denial of the seriousness of the threat, anger, or withdrawal from involvement. Sometimes family dysfunction is so glaring that clinicians are rapidly drawn into its snares. More commonly, however, subthreshold or mild depressive or anxiety disorders develop gradually as individuals struggle to adapt to unwelcome changes. While anticipatory grief was historically suggested to reduce post-mortem grief[30], intense distress is now well recognized as a marker of risk for complicated grief.

During this phase of anticipatory grief, clinicians can usefully help the family that is capable of effective communication by encouraging them to openly share their feelings as they pay attention to the material needs of their dying family member or friend. Saying goodbye needs to be recognized as a process that evolves over time, with opportunities for reminiscence, celebration of the life and contribution of the dying person, expressions of gratitude, and completion of any unfinished business[31]. These tasks have the potential to generate creative and positive emotional aspects of what is otherwise a sad time for all.

Grief of family and friends gathered around the death bed

When relatives or close friends gather to keep watch by the bed of a dying person, not only do they support the sick, but they also help their own subsequent adjustment. The solidarity shared through this experience cements these carers into mutually supportive relationships. As staff go about nursing the ill patient, they need to comfortably relate to the family, whether in the home, hospice, or hospital. For years to come, these poignant moments will be recalled in immense detail—the sensitivity and courteous respect of health professionals is crucial[32]. Clinicians can helpfully comment on the process of dying, explaining the breathing patterns, and commenting on any noises, secretions, patient reactions, and comfort. The experience needs to be normalized empathically and the family reassured whenever concern develops. Discussion about pain, reasons for medications, and skilled prediction of events will assuage worry and build a collaborative approach to the care of the dying.

Religious rituals warrant active facilitation, including appropriate notification of a religious minister or pastoral care worker. Respect for the body remains paramount once death has occurred and the expression of sympathy from clinicians is greatly appreciated. The family will be invariably grateful for time spent alone with the deceased, while regard for cultural approaches to the laying out of the body is essential[33] (discussed later in the section on cross-cultural bereavement practices). The bereaved are commonly bewildered and benefit from guidance about what to do next—making contact with the undertaker is an obvious example.

When relatives have not been present at the moment of death, informing them by telephone of the fact is generally undesirable. The invitation for them to attend in person is often based on a stated deterioration in the patient's condition. On arrival, the news can be sensitively shared in an appropriate setting before accompanying them to see the deceased. To help the family to integrate an understanding of all that has occurred, clinicians should explain the sequence of medical events culminating in the death. Questions need to be sensitively answered and time taken to comfort the bereaved in their distress.

From time to time, the cause of death will remain uncertain and an autopsy may be indicated. A senior clinician should outline the pertinent issues, emphasizing the positive aspects of the information that will be gleaned and indicating that it will be subsequently shared with the family in a follow-up meeting. Unless there is a legal requirement for a coroner's post-mortem, the family's views on autopsy need to be fully respected.

Sometimes staff will have concerns about the emotional response of the bereaved. If there is uncertainty about its cultural appropriateness, consultation with an informed cultural intermediary may prove helpful. The prescription of short-acting benzodiazepines will help some, while others will prefer to manage without medication. A follow-up telephone call on the next day is worthwhile to check on coping and identify the need for continued support.

Caution is needed in settings where grief could be marginalized, well exemplified by ageism[5]. If a death is normalized because it appears in step with the lifecycle, family members can be given less support and reduced permission to express many aspects of their loss. In the process, the disenfranchised can be ignored in their sorrow.

Acute grief and time course of bereavement

The sequence or phases through which the bereaved move over time are never rigidly demarcated but merge gradually one into the other[1,3]. They assist the clinician to recognize aberration from the normal evolution. From the (1) initial numbness and sense of unreality, (2) waves of distress begin to occur as the bereaved suffer intense pining and yearning for their lost one. Memories of the deceased trigger these acute pangs of grief. Then as the pain of separation grows, (3) a phase of disorganization emerges as loneliness resulting from the loss sets in. Hofer described this phase aptly as a constant background disturbance of restlessness, inattention, sadness, and despair with social withdrawal that can last for several months[34]. Eventually (4) a

phase of reorganization and recovery develops as nostalgia replaces sadness, morale improves, and an altered world view is constructed. Personal growth can be recognized at this stage and new creativity is expressed[35].

The time course of mourning is proportional to the strength of attachment to the lost person and also varies with cultural expression, there being no sharply defined end point to grief. Just as a mother's grief following sudden infant death syndrome lasts longer than grief following a neonatal death, so to with adult loss, the mourning that follows many years of marriage is generally longer than brief relationships. Older widows and widowers may continue to display their grief for several years[36]. This can correspond with a continuing relationship with the deceased, which for some is their choice and leads to chronic grief. The clinical task is then to differentiate those who remain within the spectrum of normality from those who cross the threshold of complicated grief.

Pathological grief

Normal and abnormal responses to bereavement span a spectrum in which intensity of reaction, presence of a range of related grief behaviours, and time course determine the differentiation. Psychiatric conditions that commonly accompany grief include clinical depression, anxiety disorders, alcohol abuse or other substance abuse and dependence, psychotic disorders, and post-traumatic stress disorder (PTSD). When frank psychiatric disorders complicate bereavement, their recognition and management is straightforward; subthreshold states present the greater clinical challenge as studies of the bereaved indicate groups in which clusters of intense grief symptoms are distinct from the normal trajectory of grief[37–39]. Their recognition calls for an experienced clinical judgement that does not normalize the distress as necessarily understandable (see Table 15.6.2). In practice, a set of criteria by which these patients can be identified as high-risk and the application of preventive models of bereavement care eliminate some of the academic debate about their characteristics.

Inhibited or delayed grief

While use of avoidance may serve some as a temporary coping mechanism, its persistence is sometimes associated with relationship

Table 15.6.2 Clinical presentations of pathological grief.

Category	Features
Inhibited or delayed grief	Avoidance postpones expression
Complicated grief	Perpetuation of mourning chronically
Traumatic grief	Unexpected and shocking form of death
Depressive disorders	Both major and minor depressions
Anxiety disorders	Insecurity and relational problems
Alcohol and substance abuse/dependence	Excessive use of substances impairs adaptive coping
Post-traumatic stress disorder	Persistent, intrusive images with cues
Psychotic disorders	Manic, severe depressive states, and schizophrenia

difficulties or the emergence of a hypomanic state in individuals with bipolar disorder. There are scenarios, however, in which the absence of significant distress and impairment immediately following loss may be understandable, perhaps indicative of resilience. Bonanno cogently argues that the prevailing model of grief that has become popularized in our culture (e.g. the need for 'grief work') is based on poorly supported assumptions, and does not allow for the full range of grief responses that may prove adaptive among the bereaved[40]. In keeping with this view, Bonnano identifies a subgroup of individuals who show little distress or disruption to normal functioning following a loss, with relatively stable, healthy functioning up to 2 years following the event. Rather than consider them delayed or avoidant in their grief, Bonnano instead refers to this group as resilient, noting that research to date has failed to find any evidence for the phenomenon of delayed grief. On this basis, he challenges the assumption that the absence of grief is necessarily pathological, that it indicates a superficial bond with the deceased or that it necessarily warrants clinical intervention. Still, it is important to highlight that cultural variation influences grief expression. Additionally, among those who present with symptoms of complicated grief (see below), avoidance of activities or situations reminiscent of the loss is common and may indeed require targeted intervention.

Complicated grief

An impressive body of empirical work supports the validity of complicated grief as a clinical entity, distinct from normal grief responses and related pathological states (e.g., major depression). Although there continues to be some debate about whether complicated grief constitutes a bona fide psychiatric disorder[41], mounting evidence argues for its inclusion in the fifth edition of the *Diagnostic and Statistical Manual of Mental Disorders (DSM)*[42]. Despite apparent overlap between symptoms of complicated grief and other *DSM-IV* disorders (e.g. major depression, post-traumatic stress disorder)[43], its central features (e.g. disbelief regarding the death, yearning and longing for the deceased, loss of meaning, and distrust of others) are not accounted for by existing diagnostic categories[44,45]. As a result, patients with complicated grief may go unrecognized if we rely solely on our current diagnostic system to characterize this subgroup of bereaved individuals. Of particular concern is the unique morbidity and functional impairment shown to be associated with this syndrome. Even after accounting for the confounding influence of concurrent disorders such as major depression, the presence of complicated grief was independently associated with risk for a range of health problems, including cardiac distress, hypertension, increased alcohol and cigarette consumption, and suicidal ideation.

Prigerson and her colleagues derived a diagnostic algorithm for assessing complicated grief, based initially on the consensus of an expert panel, and then refined with further empirical testing[46]. Using the Inventory of Complicated Grief[44], cases of complicated grief were identified with high sensitivity and specificity[46]. Moreover, a substantial and growing number of cross-validation studies have successfully replicated the unique clustering of the proposed criteria as a coherent and distinct syndrome[47]. The essential feature of complicated grief is intense separation distress, exemplified by strong feelings of yearning and longing for the deceased and persistent protest against the death. In addition, four of eight possible symptoms must be endorsed, as experienced daily or to a marked degree. These include having great difficulty accepting the death, feeling life is meaningless, feeling unable to trust others, experiencing excessive irritability or anger, feeling the future is bleak and feeling unable to carry on with one's usual activities. Results from a *DSM-V* field trial conducted with a community sample of 317 bereaved persons indicated that the presence of complicated grief at 6–12 months post-loss predicted much higher risk for morbidity than its presence within the first 6 months following loss[42]. In keeping with these results, and to avoid the premature diagnosis of a normal grief response, criteria were established that complicated grief symptoms must persist for at least 6 months, with evidence of significant impairment accompanying the diagnosis.

Who is most likely to develop complicated grief in response to the death of a loved one? Attachment processes are believed to play a central role in predicting the grief response, with separation distress most strongly activated following the loss of a 'security-enhancing attachment bond'[48]. The loss of a close and stabilizing attachment figure may be especially harrowing to those with a history of childhood neglect or abuse. Indeed, evidence suggests that these subgroups are especially prone to develop complicated grief[49]. Bereaved individuals who suffered a traumatic or unexpected loss had an intimate relationship with the deceased, and experienced little support following the death are also at heightened risk for complicated grief (for review, see refs. 42 and 49).

Chronic grief, the prior term used for complicated grief, is particularly associated with overly dependent relationships in which a sense of abandonment is avoided by perpetuation of the relationship through memorialization of the deceased and maintenance of continuing bonds. A stuck situation emerges in which the tearfulness is induced by any reminder of the deceased without any cognitive transition being achieved in the world view of the bereaved. Social withdrawal and depression are common. A fantasy of re-union with the deceased can cause suicide to be an increasingly attractive option. Active treatment using pharmacology for depression and cognitive behavioural therapy to reality test the loss and promote socialization (via activity scheduling) is appropriate for chronic grief.

Traumatic grief

When death has been unexpected or its nature in some way shocking—traumatic, violent, stigmatized, or perceived as undignified—its integration and acceptance may be interfered with by the arousal and increased distress that memories can trigger. Intensive recollections including flashbacks, nightmares, and recurrent intrusive memories cause hyperarousal, disbelief, insomnia, irritability, and disturbed concentration, which distorts normal grieving[23]. The shock of the death can precipitate mistrust, anger, detachment, and an unwillingness to accept its reality. These reactions at a subthreshold level merge with the full features of PTSD, but the subthreshold state has been observed to persist for years and contribute substantial morbidity.

Depressive disorders

Rates of major depression in the bereaved have varied between 16 and 50 per cent, peaking over the first 2 months[40,41], and gradually decreasing to 15 per cent across the next 2 years[42,43]. The features of any major depressive episode post-bereavement resemble major depression at other points of the lifecycle[44].

There is a tendency to chronicity, considerable social morbidity, and risk of inadequate treatment.

Anxiety disorders

These take the form of adjustment disorders, generalized anxiety disorder, and phobic states and occur in up to 30 per cent of the bereaved[45]. Patients present commonly to general practitioners with a range of somatic concerns. Separation anxiety of a heightened nature can be distinguished from anxiety symptoms of a general kind.

Alcohol and substance abuse/dependence

Typically an exacerbation of pre-existing psychiatric states, individuals predisposed to alcohol abuse or dependence on other substances such as benzodiazepines relapse during bereavement[45]. Other family members often raise the alarm.

Post-traumatic stress disorder

While clearly related to unnatural deaths, deaths involving profound breakdown of bodily surfaces, gross disfigurement due to head and neck cancers, or other causes of relatives perceiving the illness to cause loss of dignity may generate traumatic memories in the bereaved. Schut and colleagues found that PTSD was often correlated with the perceived inadequacy of the goodbye, and suggested that rituals to complete this be incorporated into related grief therapies[46].

Psychotic disorders

Bereavement is a common precipitant of relapse of psychotic illnesses such as bipolar disorder or schizophrenia in individuals so predisposed; occasionally, mania presents for the first time in such a setting.

Family grief

Family therapists have long recognized the salience of family processes to mourning and their systemic influence on outcome[47]. Exploration of the association between family functioning and bereavement morbidity highlighted the manner in which family dysfunction predicts increased rates of psychosocial morbidity in the bereaved[21]. Family-centred care that focuses on the well-being of the family during palliative care is uniquely placed to reduce rates of morbidity in those subsequently bereaved.

A typology of family functioning during both palliative care and bereavement was created using cluster analysis in the Melbourne-based family grief studies[21,48]. Dimensions of cohesiveness, expressiveness, and conflict from the Family Environment Scale[49] determined five classes of families illustrated in Table 15.6.3. While over half the families met in a palliative care setting demonstrate resilience through their family functioning, and do not need particular psychological assistance to achieve an adaptive outcome from bereavement, the remainder have identifiable characteristics predictive of a higher risk of morbid outcome and can be specifically targeted through a preventive model of family care[51].

During early bereavement, families at risk have been shown to decompensate through deterioration in their functioning with loss of cohesiveness, communication breakdown, and increased conflict. A proportion of families with *Intermediate* characteristics of functioning changes to become *Sullen* or *Hostile* in type. Importantly, these dysfunctional families carry the bulk of the psychosocial morbidity observed to occur during bereavement, thus highlighting the potential benefits of a family form of intervention. Screening of families on their admission to palliative care through the use of a well-validated measure such as the Family Relationships Index[49] provides an ideal means to recognize those families at greater risk of morbid outcome during bereavement. Rules to interpret family functioning and thus recognize those at risk when screening (on admission to the palliative care service) are summarized in Table 15.6.4.

Recognizing those at risk of complicated bereavement outcome

Palliative care teams are ideally placed to recognize those at increased risk of complicated grief and plan preventive interventions in an endeavour to circumvent morbidity. To accomplish this, bereavement care planning does not begin post-death but at the point of entry into the palliative care service. The continuity of supportive care that flows from this builds a strong therapeutic alliance, which will be more likely to survive ambivalence about the death than if a bereavement counsellor attempts to begin post-death. Avoidance hinders many attempts to engage the bereaved after the death.

In times of resource scarceness and economic rationalism, services are under pressure to direct their clinical staff to appropriate areas of need. When relatives appear resilient and well-supported, clinicians can wisely respect their capacity to cope with loss adaptively. Indeed, empirical evidence confirms that when preventive interventions are targeted to those at risk, benefits ensue[53], whereas when they are broadly offered to a bereaved population regardless of risk, no such benefit is discernible[54]. In the latter type of study, the well functioning dilute any evidence of benefit to those at risk. In contrast with a broadly supportive bereavement follow-up programme that utilizes condolence cards and invitations to memorial services, seriously intended preventive interventions should be directed towards those at increased risk.

Risk factors to aid recognition of those at greater risk of complicated grief are summarized in Table 15.6.5. These should be assessed at entry to the service and upgraded during the phase of palliative care, including revision shortly after the death. Completion of the family genogram presents an ideal time for such assessment as relationships, prior losses, and coping are considered. Some palliative care services have developed checklists based on such risk factors to generate a numerical measure of risk. There has been insufficient validation of such scales at this stage, but the presence of any single factor in Table 15.6.5 signifies greater risk. Continued observation of the pattern of grief evolution over time is appropriate whenever such concern exists.

Health consequences of bereavement

Over 15 studies of mortality following bereavement provide evidence for an increased rate of deaths in the 45–75 age range, with these occurring over the first year post-loss, particularly the first 6 months from acute cardiovascular causes[55]. While some

Table 15.6.3 Typology of palliative care and bereaved families[21,50].

Category	Family type	Rate of occurrence (%)	Features
Well functioning types	Supportive	32	Strongly cohesive families who grieve adaptively
	Conflict resolving	20	Cohesion and effective communication empowers tolerance of difference of opinions
Dysfunctional types	Hostile	6–12	Poorly cohesive with high conflict, ineffective communication, and fractured relationships;families resist help
	Sullen	9–18	Muted anger generates highest levels of depression; families seek help
	Intermediate	20–33	Mid-range levels of communication, cohesion, and conflict place these families at risk of deterioration when stressed by life events

studies have only identified increased mortality in men, a well-controlled study of 12, 522 spouse pairs in a prepaid health care plan showed increased mortality for both women and men, |adjusting for age, education, and other mortality predictors[56]. Other noteworthy causes of death in addition to cardiovascular events include accidents, suicide, alcohol and substance abuse, and cirrhosis, while the association evident in large epidemiological studies of increased mortality with social isolation and alienation is also relevant[57].

Early studies by Saunders[58] and Parkes[59] identified the increased use of health services—both greater consultations and hospitalizations—by the recently bereaved, with increased psychological distress, somatic health complaints, more days of disability, and greater reliance on medications. Some 20–25 per cent were noted to develop depressive disorders,[40] but increased rates of anxiety disorders, including PTSD in settings of traumatic loss, also occur[45]. Some of the explanations for these health consequences lie in the development of complicated grief, others in altered behaviours and life-style including diet, smoking, and alcohol consumption. Studies have also highlighted effects on the cardiovascular, neuroendocrine, and immunological systems: several studies have shown increased rates of myocardial infarction post-bereavement[53]; altered cortisol levels were seen in parents following death of their children from leukaemia[50]; altered

lymphocyte response to mitogens and lowered natural killer cell activity were also seen in bereaved spouses[60–62]. Immunosuppressed patients, either chemically induced or as a result of AIDS, develop specific malignancies such as lymphomas or Kaposi's sarcomas. However, the clinical relevance of the immunological changes described in bereavement is uncertain in the light of a series of large epidemiological studies that fail to show increased rates of cancer in the bereaved[63–65].

Table 15.6.5 Risk factors for complicated grief.

Category	Range of circumstances
Nature of the death	Untimely within the lifecycle (e.g. death of child)
	Sudden and unexpected (e.g. death from septic neutropaenia during chemotherapy)
	Traumatic (e.g. gross cachexia and debility)
	Stigmatized (e.g. AIDS or suicide)
Strengths and vulnerabilities of the carer/bereaved	Past history of psychiatric disorder (e.g. depression)
	Personality and coping style (e.g. intense worrier, low self-esteem)
	Cumulative experience of losses
Nature of the relationship with the deceased	Overly dependent (e.g. clinging, symbiotic)
	Ambivalent (e.g. angry and insecure with alcohol abuse, infidelity, gambling)
Family and support network	Dysfunctional family (e.g. poor cohesiveness and communication, high conflict)
	Isolated (e.g. new migrant, new residential move)
	Alienated (e.g. perception of poor support)

Table 15.6.4 Screening rules to recognize families at greater risk of dysfunction and complicated grief through use of the Family Relationships Index (FRI).[a][52]

FES[a] subscales	Typical range of scores for family types		
	Intermediate	Sullen	Hostile
Expressiveness	1–3	1–2	0–2
Cohesiveness	3–4	2–3	0–2
Conflict	0–1	1–2	1–4
FRI total	8–9	5–7	0–4

[a] FRI (Family Relationships Index) is derived from the FES (Family Environment Scale).[49] FRI is the sum of the cohesiveness, expressiveness, and reversed (out of 4)conflict score; its maximum sum is 12.

Bereavement follow-up by the treatment team

Once the patient has died, the palliative care team should routinely review the death and the bereavement-related risk factors in the next available multi-disciplinary team meeting. Was the death perceived to impact significantly on key family members? What level of bereavement follow-up should be adopted?

Two broad levels of follow-up are possible. The first involves the expression of condolences via the telephone, sympathy card, visit by the nurse or general practitioner, staff attendance at the funeral, and subsequent family invitation to a periodic commemorative service arranged by the palliative care team. This model provides both encouragement and support while normalizing the grief that relatives express and respecting their mourning process without undue intrusion. Where greater concern does emerge, an opportunity presents to intervene appropriately. The staff who have developed the closest relationships with the family are wisely selected by the team to take up this observing model of follow-up as it provides them with a means of gradual farewell. Their formal identification and documentation is nonetheless important to ensure completion of the process over time. Final contact is often shortly after the first anniversary.

The second model of follow-up is for those individuals or families judged to be at greater risk and thought likely to benefit from a preventive intervention. Studies have shown that such prevention effectively reduces morbidity when delivered to those 20 per cent likely otherwise to develop complicated grief[53]. Teams vary in their pursuit of this depending on staff availability; in other instances, general practitioners provide active individual support. Individual, group, or family approaches are valid and selected on the basis of personal needs. Where continuity of involvement of the counsellor from palliative care into bereavement is possible, direct knowledge of the deceased is advantageous, as is the continuing relationship with the bereaved. Attempts to establish bereavement counselling only after the death meet high rates of defensive avoidance blocking this form of support. Where social isolation is noteworthy, the additional support derived from a group approach maximizes connectedness[66,67]. Others will seek the personal support of individual therapy. For many, a family approach is cost-effective in reaching several at risk when the nature of the family's functioning has been shown by screening to be dysfunctional. *Family Focused Grief Therapy* (FFGT) offers continuity from palliative care through to bereavement and, in promoting family functioning, it fosters the role of the family as a prime source of support[52]. Asian cultures including the Chinese and Japanese are especially suited to family models of care[68].

The diverse range of clinicians in palliative care teams, including chaplains or pastoral care workers, nurses, social workers, psychologists or psychiatrists, general practitioners, volunteers, and generic bereavement counsellors ensure that there is no shortage of staff to support the bereaved. Nevertheless, staff caught up with the business of acute patient care will neglect the bereaved despite their best of intentions. Team leadership needs to actively monitor programmes of bereavement follow-up to ensure its adherence to an intended protocol and to initiate appropriate cross-referral of those at greater risk.

Grief therapies

As loss is so ubiquitous within palliative care, all clinicians need skill in the application of grief therapies. The most basic model is a supportive–expressive intervention in which the person is invited to share their feelings about the loss to a health professional who will listen and seek to understand the other's distress in a comforting manner. The key therapeutic aspects of this encounter are the sharing of distress and, through the relational understanding that is acknowledged, some shift in cognitive appraisal of the reality that has been forever altered. There are hundreds of small losses involving aspects of health and well-being as well as hopes and dreams that are experienced by the patient during their terminal illness. Support is needed from all members of the treatment team in response to these before the major loss of the patient is ultimately experienced through death.

Formal interventions that are possible for bereaved people are multiple, but the very first question is whether 'an intervention' is actually warranted. For the majority, although bereavement is painful, their personal resilience will ensure their normal adaptation. There can, therefore, be no justification for routine intervention as grief is not a disease. Those considered at risk of maladaptive outcome are the ones that should be treated preventatively and those who later develop complicated bereavement need active treatments.

The spectrum of interventions spans individual, group, and family oriented therapies, and encompasses all schools of psychotherapy as well as appropriately indicated pharmacotherapies. Adoption of any model (or parts thereof) is predicated on the clinical issues and associated predicaments that arise. Thus, variation will be influenced by age, perception of support, the nature of the death, the personal health of the bereaved, and the presence of co-morbid states. Clinicians generally plan for an intervention to proceed as six to eight sessions over several months and do well to map this out at the beginning. In this sense, grief therapy is focused and time-limited, but multi-modal therapies are commonplace. Thus, group as well as individual therapies better support the lonely so that socialization complements interpersonally any intrapersonal change.

Guided mourning

Guided mourning as an approach to 'grief work' promotes narrative review with repetitive recollections of the deceased being actively encouraged to relive and eventually revise the relationship experienced, ultimately redefining the reality of self and situation[69,70]. In the process, Worden emphasized the accomplishment of four basic tasks of mourning: accepting the reality of loss, working through the pain of grief, adjusting to a new environment without the loved person, and establishing a collection of positive and useful memories of the deceased for future reference[71]. Reality testing and adaptation to the separation leads to what Parkes termed an altered assumptive world in which the ideas, attitudes, and beliefs about the self and the world are fundamentally altered[17,72,73]. The inherent cognitive change is vital to future equanimity. Even when culture prescribes some level of continuing bonds with one's ancestors, creativity and generativity emerge from resolution of the mourning process[35]. Raphael has tended to understand much of this guided grief therapy within the rubric of 'crisis' intervention, placing additional emphasis on the mobilization of support to assist and comfort the bereaved[53] (Table 15.6.6).

Interpersonal psychotherapy

As well as the supportive–expressive model described above, interpersonal psychotherapy (IPT) places emphasis on the nature

Table 15.6.6 Models of grief therapy.

Name of model of therapy	Potential focus for the model's application	Clinical issues when indicated
Supportive–expressive therapy (guided grief work, crisis intervention)	Individual or group	Avoidance of emotional expression
		Inhibited or delayed grief
		Isolated and needing support
		Established psychiatric disorders including depression
Interpersonal or psychodynamic therapy	Individual or group	Relational issues dominate
		Role transition difficulties
Cognitive behavioural therapy	Individual or group	Chronic grief with stuckness of behaviours
		Traumatic grief
		Post-traumatic stress disorder
Family focused grief therapy	Family	Family either at risk or clearly dysfunctional in its relating
		Adolescents or children at risk
Combined pharmacotherapies with any of the psychotherapeutic models	Individual	Depressive disorders
		Anxiety disorders
		Sleep disorders
Complicated grief treatment	Individual	Complicated grief

Group interventions can be given in parallel with individual approaches to intervention.

of relationships and how the bereaved functions within these[74]. The psychodynamic model overlaps considerably with these interpersonal approaches[75]. The mixed feelings underpinning ambivalent relationships warrant expression and understanding, while the past influences on insecure and overly dependent patterns of relating help to consider future needs. The nature of the continuing relationship with the deceased is explored alongside any desire to replace the lost person. The urge for reunion with the deceased merits active discussion as suicidal desire easily grows out of persistence of such ideas. Gersie highlighted the dangerous pull that reunion fantasies can have when the dependent bereaved lament their loss and search to re-establish connection[76]. Increased suicide risk also occurs among socially isolated, elderly widowers, those who abuse alcohol, and those with a current or past history of depressive disorder.

Cognitive behavioural therapy

Cognitive behavioural therapy offers a special contribution to chronic grief[24]. Here, continued connectivity with the deceased may be valued and bring benefits to the bereaved that are cherished, promoting some memorialization as 'stuckness' that prevents other progress in life. Furthermore, repeated exposure to cues that induce sadness may deepen depressive illness in these circumstances. Behavioural approaches regulate exposure to these cues, optimize socialization through activity scheduling, moderate inappropriate drug and alcohol use, and promote graduated involvement in new roles and experiences. Related cognitive reframing of negative ideas such as unfairness and hopelessness steers towards a constructive adaptation.

Complicated grief treatment

Complicated grief treatment (CGT), a form of therapy recently developed and evaluated by Shear and colleagues[87], integrates techniques from interpersonal- and cognitive behavioural therapies in order to specifically target symptoms of complicated grief. CGT draws from the dual-process model of adaptive coping[25], thus focusing simultaneously on discussion of the loss and restoration of adaptive functioning. Attention to the loss and associated affect is alternated with pragmatic facilitation of identified life goals. To address the trauma-like symptoms presented in complicated grief (e.g. intrusive thoughts of death, avoidance of reminders of death), exposure-based exercises are adapted from cognitive behavioural therapies for PTSD. To address loss-related symptoms (e.g. yearning and longing for deceased) and encourage a revised connection to the deceased, the bereaved is invited to engage in an imaginal conversation with the deceased and to generate a list of positive memories. A randomized controlled trial compared standard interpersonal psychotherapy (IPT) with CGT among 95 men and women who met criteria for complicated grief[87]. Treatment response was evident in 51 per cent of participants who received CGT, compared to only 28 per cent of those treated with IPT. Furthermore, CGT was associated with significantly better outcome than IPT on self-report measures of complicated grief symptoms, depression, work, and social functioning. Interestingly, among participants who had experienced a violent or traumatic loss, response rates were higher for CGT than for IPT. Furthermore, response to CGT varied by type of loss, with loss of a spouse, friend, or relative associated with higher response to CGT than loss of a child.

Addressing the bereaved's self-image

When an overly dependent relationship has formed the basis of a complicated grief reaction, the bereaved's self-image changes from 'being valued and cared for' to being now 'alone and useless'. Patterns of perceived abandonment may re-emerge from earlier relationships. Therapy needs to target boosting self-esteem, confidence, and sense of security. The combination of both group and individual therapy has special merit since the group process promotes socialization in an individual otherwise at risk of isolation[88]. Brief group psychotherapy[76] can be offered as a complementary programme of support for the more needy, and both variety and creativity can enhance such programmes, exemplified by one programme that combined group behaviour therapy with art therapy[89].

Family focused grief therapy (FFGT)

A family approach to grief intervention is exemplified by FFGT[61]. Such a model aims to improve family functioning while also supporting the expression of grief and, as mentioned, can be applied preventatively to those families judged through screening to be at high risk of such morbid outcome[61]. Commencing thus during palliative care and including the ill member in the family work, FFGT continues through the early phases of bereavement until there is confidence that morbidity has been prevented or appropriately treated. This approach invites the family to identify and agree to work on aspects of family life that they recognize as a cause of concern. Through enhancing cohesion, promoting open communication of thoughts and feelings, and teaching effective problem-solving to reduce conflict and optimize tolerance of different opinions, the improved functioning of the family as a unit becomes the means to accomplish adaptive mourning. The continuity of care and the personal knowledge that the therapist achieves of the dying family member empowers considerable maturation in the family unit not only as carers but also as comforters of the bereaved.

Basic aids in grief counselling

Basic aids to any form of grief counselling include the use of evocative rather than sensitive language to assist the expression of feelings, the sharing of photo albums and special letters from the loved person, writing about any unfinished business to draw it to a close, and optimizing attendance at cultural or religious rituals to support the process of mourning. Children can be encouraged to make up a 'scrap' or memory book about a deceased parent as an aide to their adaptive mourning. Complementary forms of therapy such as art[90] and music[91] therapy can also make a valuable contribution to any programme for the bereaved. Any individual differences in the intensity and progress of mourning need to be normalized as appropriate. For instance, research has repeatedly confirmed that mothers express grief more intensely than fathers do[59]. Time must be allowed to permit the process to unfold naturally and the length of mourning is helpfully appraised as proportional to the strength of attachment to the deceased.

Pharmacotherapy

Where the experience of death has been in some manner 'shocking', incomplete assimilation of the event can develop, leading to intrusive recollections and numbing. Here, the bereaved need to make clear sense of the loss, understanding the mechanisms involved in the death, and attributing responsibility to appropriate factors[92]. Benzodiazepines have a particular role in reducing autonomic arousal, lessening intrusive symptoms, and allaying anxiety so that avoidant responses are minimized[57]. The treatment team helps further by bringing the bereaved back in the weeks after the death to review overall understanding of events and report on findings from any autopsy. Whenever a coroner's inquiry follows a death, the bereaved are to be encouraged to attend to increase their integration of understanding of such events.

Pharmacotherapies are widely used to support the bereaved—judicious prescribing is nonetheless important. Benzodiazepines allay anxiety and assist sleep, but words of caution should be offered about intermittent use to avoid tachyphylaxis and dependence. Antidepressants are indicated whenever bereavement is complicated by the development of depressive disorder, panic attacks, and moderate to severe adjustment disorders[93,94]. If insomnia is prominent, tricyclics (e.g. dothiepin, nortriptyline, desipramine) or tetracyclics (e.g. mianserin) are beneficial; otherwise, selective serotonergic reuptake inhibitors (e.g. sertraline, paroxetine, citalopram, fluvoxamine, fluoxetine) or combined noradrenergic and serotonergic reuptake inhibitors (e.g. venlafaxine, mirtazapineduloxetine) are indicated. Occasionally, antipsychotics are needed for hypomania or other forms of psychosis.

Predictors of outcome from grief interventions

The best predictors of an adaptive outcome include a gradually resolving trajectory of emotional distress that began from a moderate rather than excessive initial level, open communication with others, good supports, robust self-esteem, and evidence of personal competency in the daily tasks that are ordinarily pursued[95]. In contrast, pathological grief can be considered dimensionally through greater degrees of separation distress, emotional numbing and dissociation, mood symptoms, impaired social functioning, and maladaptive coping styles. Categorical approaches to pathological grief incorporate elements of avoidance or denial, distortion through excessive anger, despair, guilt, idealization or somatization, and prolongation that culminates in chronicity of distress. An integrated approach to the treatment of complicated grief incorporates balanced combinations of pharmacology (e.g. antidepressants or antianxiety agents), individual psychotherapy, and socialization through family or group work[57].

The notion of recovery is important and recognized by the return of equanimity in discussion of the deceased. A process of social transition has been accomplished[96]. New interests or roles are adopted, with new friendships emerging. Eventually, the bereaved see their future with reprioritized and altered world views. As ultimate evidence of completed mourning, new generativity and creativity emerges in the activities and lives of the bereaved[35].

Special types of loss

Particular needs arise for bereaved children, the very elderly, and when loss is especially stigmatized, for instance death from AIDS. The timing of such deaths within the lifecycle explains some of the special considerations that arise.

Children and bereavement

The general principle of open communication with children about cancer or serious illness, its nature and meaning, treatment, and prospect of death is important[97,98]. Concepts need to be presented in an age-appropriate manner, recognizing that the finality of death only becomes more completely understood around the age of 9–10 years[99]. Younger children believe that death is reversible; after age 5, the understanding is more in terms of separation with a gradual recognition of its irreversibility. Families can teach children a healthy understanding of the lifecycle and support the child through identification of and reassurance by available, surviving adults who commit to remaining involved with the child in the future. Such processes may help a child to mature more rapidly and grow in their appreciation of death as cessation of life. Children display a variety of bereavement symptoms including sadness, fear, guilt, insecurity, and behavioural problems[100]. A programme that guides parents in what to say and do to assist their children was found to be helpful[101].

The death of either a parent or sibling is a significant and distressing occurrence that prompts many children to ask questions such as: 'Why? Did I cause it? Who will care for me?' Careful discussion of death causation is worthwhile to avoid prophylactically any misinterpretation by the child. In the setting of advanced cancer, when death can be anticipated, preparation of the child through involvement in care activities and open discussion of realities facilitates acceptance and adjustment. Subsequent involvement of children in funeral and anniversary rituals[102] normalizes the experience of loss and promotes the family as the continuing, supportive environment[103].

The long-term effects of childhood bereavement are not completely clear, as studies have been hampered by being retrospective, but they have suggested that the loss of a mother prior to age 12 predicts an increased risk of adult depression. However, the quality of the relationship to subsequent careproviders may be more significant in determining outcome than the parental loss[104]. Nonetheless, should such children develop cancer themselves in adult life, their memories of their dying parent and related identifications are powerful influences on their overall adjustment.

After accidents, cancer is the second leading cause of death in childhood. The family typically focuses on the dying child with the risk of relative neglect of other children. They in turn may try to replace the dead child and experience survivor guilt. Openness of family communication about all aspects of the illness and death is the best formula to promote normal grieving and family meetings can especially model this. The grief of the parents needs support alongside the grief of the children, empowering the parents to attend to their children's grief, rather than the children being parentified as a support for their parents. Parents may become hypervigilant about their surviving children's health, unwittingly promoting hypochondriasis in later life if too much attention is placed on somatic symptoms and fear of cancer. Attention to the functioning of the family provides the most useful model for recognition of those at greater risk of poorer outcome[105]. Families that block discussion, suppress sharing of feelings, and concentrate rigidly on concrete events fare more poorly than families that comfort one another with empathy and teamwork.

The elderly and bereavement

When couples have been married for many years, the length and depth of their attachment may predispose them to profound grief, further complicated by the acute loneliness they can experience if many of their friends and sources of support have already died. Elderly bereaved men can have particular needs in these circumstances[106]. Moreover, despite apparent support from within the family, the bereaved spouse may carry an especially painful level of loneliness[107]. The social support of the elderly bereaved warrants special consideration, including use of volunteer programmes[108].

Bereavement during adulthood

Although the loss of a spouse has received most attention in research, loss of a parent or sibling during adult life is a common event and will generate distress proportional to the degree of emotional closeness to the deceased. Increased maturity is one potential outcome of such losses[109]. Where there is a high familial incidence of cancer raising questions of genetic risk, as in familial polyposis, breast, or colon cancer, the death of a sibling increases the sense of vulnerability of family members and highlights the importance of genetic testing and counselling when relevant.

When comparisons have been made between the death of a spouse, parent, or child, the most intense bereavement reactions are found following the death of a child, an event clearly out of step with lifecycle expectations[110,111]. Parents have a strong and powerful investment in their children such that their premature death shakes the adult personality to its very roots[112]. Its impact is life-long—although the distress slowly declines with the passage of time, it plateaus eventually to a steady state of continued influence, although the meaning of this continues to change throughout the lifecycle[113]. For many it is a disruptive and life-shattering experience, necessitating a continuing life-long accommodation, but this is affected to some degree by the quality of the relationship before the child's death and the relationship that exists with other surviving children.

Aware of such inherent challenges, palliative care teams do well to involve parents in the care of terminally ill children (including adult offspring), foster open communication of feelings about the death, and seek views on their philosophy of life. Where parents can find some meaning and sense of purpose in their child's life, their acceptance of the death, despite its inherent unfairness, is likely to be greater[114]. The incorporation of parents into the model of family-centred care remains important when a middle-aged adult is dying and predeceasing elderly parents; often the focus of the palliative care team is on the nuclear family, supporting the spouse and children to the neglect of parental grief.

Hospices for dying children allow particular care to be taken of the family, including continuity of this care into bereavement. Active discussion of the choice between death at home or in the hospice is important and a family-centred model of care will consider the potential impact on usually three generations of family membership. Well-functioning families are perceived to cope better with death in the home, while respite admissions can bring relief to those families more stressed by the emotional demands of caring for the dying child. Irrespective of whether death is affecting a young child, an adolescent, or young adult, grief is intense and potentially protracted; sustained support of family members is especially important when the functioning of the family has been stressed or is clearly dysfunctional.

Bereavement and AIDS

The stigma associated with human immunodeficiency virus (HIV) infection handicaps the adjustment of both patients and their families and adds a risk factor for complicated grief. Caregiving partners of men with AIDS experience several stressors that induce role conflict and burden[115]. Mean scores for depressive symptoms were found in one longitudinal study to remain at one standard deviation above the general community norm 3 years after the death[116]. The families also display complex dynamics related to their degree of acceptance of a homosexual relationship, any ambivalence about which potentially complicates the mourning process[117].

Spirituality and bereavement

The existential quest to understand the meaning of life creates an endeavour to understand the uniqueness and special contribution of each and every person. This spiritual orientation influences adaptation both to dying and to bereavement. Clinicians do well to inquire about the spiritual dimensions and philosophy of life of both their patients and families[118]. For some, this will be expressed in the language of their religious beliefs; for others, cultural custom and traditions will inform their set of values and the philosophy by which they have lived. Using these values to understand the life of the deceased helps in appraising their accomplishments, the sort of person they were, and the meaning their life had. When consensus about this can be achieved with the bereaved, it assists their acceptance of the death. Moreover, when the latter has been peaceful, this will console the bereaved, but when the death was difficult, disappointing, or in some manner horrifying, there is considerable work to do in helping the bereaved to understand and come to terms with this final outcome. A spiritual understanding of the person's life may help in accepting the limitations of palliative care or coming to terms with any unfinished business that remained in the deceased's life. Philosophically this may be akin to letting go of the ideal and accepting a life lived with a goodness that is sufficient.

Ritual is an important component of religious and cultural tradition as it creates a proven pathway down which the bereaved tread[119]. The wisdom of centuries is often woven into such rituals as a means of assisting the bereaved to mourn. Respect for such ritual is important and clinicians help the bereaved by endorsing its value. Familiarity with different ethnic traditions is worthwhile in palliative care. Nonetheless, should a clinician meet an unfamiliar ethnic group, they should seek from the relatives an understanding of their tradition and strive to co-operate with them in a culturally sensitive manner.

Bereavement practices across cultures

Palliative care practitioners need at least some rudimentary knowledge of cross-cultural bereavement customs to inform sensitive clinical practice. Most cultures do sanction the expression of emotions such as crying, fear, and anger, while each of the world's major religions have developed comprehensible practices to guide

their bereaved. Eastern religions sustain greater belief in a spirit world, reflecting an animism underlying Asian religious traditions. Western religions in contrast are theistic in nature. An overview of the contribution of the world's major religions to bereavement practices follows, but further information about other ethnic and religious practices can be found in the references listed in the further reading section.

Hindu bereavement practices

Hindus believe in rebirth with transmigration of the *jeevatma* or subtle personality of the person into another life until eventually the *atma* (soul) merges with God[120]. The theory of *karma* and its reciprocal reactions explains suffering that can be endured through detachment. Fear of death is reduced through belief in rebirth. It is the sacred duty (*dharma*) of the family to follow the teachings of the *shastras*, the sacred religious texts, and to perform the rituals and acts of piety and charity to ensure the peaceful repose of the departed soul, although variation occurs according to caste, regions, and finances.

Death is preferred at home and with the patient on the floor. A drop or two of water from the Ganges is sprinkled from a basil leaf onto the lips or mouth of the person just before or soon after death[121]. Loud shrieks of emotion are able to be expressed when death has happened. Then a ritual washing of the body occurs, and the widow removes her wedding mark from her forehead, while the heads of the men can be shaved and all dress in white. Condolences are shared freely. Priests read from sacred texts, recite verses from the *Bhagavad Gita*, and sing devotional songs. In India, after the body is anointed and garlanded, it would be cremated at the burning ghat, where the eldest son would ignite the pyre. Mourners chant or wail. The spirit is said to depart the body when the skull cracks. The funeral rites last for a traditional 12 days, during which all sleep on the floor and eat vegetarian food. After ablutions, the recital of prayers occurs twice daily and special gatherings of the mourners—termed *markha* or *utthama* ceremonies— ensure the open sharing of grief by all involved. The empty handed display of the palms of the hands symbolizes their sense of devastation. After 12 days, the ashes would be traditionally scattered into the waters of the Ganges and charitable acts performed to aid beggars.

Hindu death outside of India can still respect traditional customs such as ritualistic washing, preparation of the body, pall-bearing to gain virtue, and the prayer ceremonies as described. Hindu traditions are indeed the most ancient of the world religions.

Buddhist bereavement practices

Buddhist tradition also began in India during the sixth century BC and believed in repeated rebirth. Through attaining the state of a clear and calm mind undisturbed by worldly events and full of compassion, the diligent person can escape the continuous cycle of rebirth to attain enlightenment (*nirvana*). Theravada Buddhism, which concentrates on teachings found in the Four Noble Truths and the Eightfold Path, is found in Sri Lanka, Myanmar, Thailand, Cambodia, and Laos. Mahayana Buddhism in its various faith and devotional forms is practised widely in China, Japan, Korea, Taiwan, and Vietnam. Vajrayana Buddhism places emphasis on rituals and initiation rites and is found in Tibet, Nepal, Mongolia, and parts of India[122]. While the Vietnamese prefer death at home, for instance, the vast majority of Chinese families seek admission to hospital to directly avoid death in the home.

As the Buddhist person approaches death, chanting certain *sutras* has a calming effect on the mind and helps concentrate on the Buddha or Pure Land. Ceremonial instructions can be quietly read to the dead to guide it through the *bardo* (transitional state) between life forms. The ceremony can be repeated for 49 days until rebirth is assured. The body is wrapped in a white silk cloth; incense and votive papers are burned; both cremation and below-ground burial are practiced; and a series of prayer ceremonies are conducted. Mourners wear white clothes and head bands and can walk with sticks, symbolizing that their grief has left them in need of support. An altar of commemoration for the dead is usually erected in the home; daily offerings are made and prayers recited. Family dinners are held on the 49th, 100th, and 365th days after the death; temple ceremonies are observed on the first and 15th days of each lunar month, the lunar new year, and the first anniversary. Filial duty is particularly laid down for the first son to commemorate his family's ancestors; custom requires the open display of grief as a mark of loyalty.

Confucianism and death

Confucius taught the right way of relating to others to achieve peace, harmony, and happiness[123]. Social rituals optimized the expression of mutual respect. The attitude of the living towards the dead is similarly respectful and one of continuous remembrance and affection. Family-centred rituals are at the core of such expressions of gratitude and grief, consistent with strong traditions of filial duty, and they guide members to follow the middle way, always avoiding extremes[124]. These rituals model the ultimate dignity of human relationships and bring grace and beauty to human behaviour through continuity with the past and tradition.

Confucian philosophy views the human person as part of an infinite biological chain, the value of each person lying in their part of one's family and society. Accepting one's fate and bearing sorrow in silence is part of the maintenance of human dignity[125]. Public prescribed rituals are the place to express grief. For the Chinese to be buried in China or have their ashes returned to China means reunion with their ancestors in the town their family originated from—understanding the significance of such wishes can help to reassure and comfort the dying.

Taoism and death

The second great spiritual tradition that originated in China focuses more on nature than man in providing a means of transcending the limits of one's world[125]. Everything is in a state of continuous change, necessitating acceptance of the spontaneity of things. Spiritual tranquillity is achieved by freeing oneself from worldly pursuits, even by adopting an element of playful fun.

The circle of the yin and yang is the symbol of the Supreme Reality and the cosmic forces underpinning natural change[123]. Yin is the feminine, passive, dark, cold, wet, and soft aspects of life while yang represents the masculine, active, bright, hot, dry, and hard elements. Their complementary and interactional relationship leads to ceaseless transformations in the forms of life and death. Positive admiration of such beauty in nature promotes acceptance and counters any anxiety about death.

Grief is recognized as part of the normal emotions of life, but it is moderated in intensity by acceptance of the unending change of nature and the transformation of the spirit within the cosmic world. Taoist philosophy clearly posits that the dominant perspective on death is one of acceptance[124].

Jewish bereavement practices

Judaism splits into several denominations ranging from the Orthodox to the Reform, with further variations being culturally based on Ashkenazic (Central-Eastern European) or Sephardic (Spanish-African) origins. Basic beliefs include the concept of one God, the sanctity of the person created in the image of God, the immortality of the soul and an afterlife following judgement, and a period of purification. The Talmud states that one should not hasten death. Visitation of the sick and accompaniment of the dying are ancient traditions. The rabbi should be called at the approach of death to say a confessional prayer (the *Vidui*) and recite the fundamental affirmation of faith, the *Shema*.

The process of life review prior to death has generated one interesting tradition taking the form of writing an ethical will. In this document, the dying person records his/her legacy to his/her family. It states the hopes and dreams held for the family, the values considered important, and any thoughts or messages that the family should remember. Such ethical wills are usually warmly and lovingly written and thus are a source of great comfort to the bereaved.

After death, the body should be cleansed and prepared by the burial society (*Chevrah Kadisha*) through a religious ritual (*Taharah*). Dressed in white and robed in a prayer shawl (*tallit*), burial of the body in the ground is desirable within 24 h and fulfils the notion of 'returning to dust'. Post-mortem examinations, embalming, and cremation are prohibited. A simple funeral service honours the dead with an eulogy, psalms, and a reading of the Memorial Prayer. The family, whose garments may be torn as a symbol of grief, then accompany the coffin to the cemetery to conclude the burial.

While the period between death and burial is termed the *Aninut*, the time of intense shock, the first 3 days following the funeral are seen as the time for weeping and lamentation at home in private mourning. The period of 7 days following the burial corresponds with the tradition of *shiva*, in which the primary mourners sit on low stools and allow others to prepare their food. Their energy is focused on grief, knowing that their friends will take care of them. The community gathers at the home to make up a *minyan* (quorum of 10) so that the mourner's prayer, The *Kaddish*, may be recited. The *Kaddish* affirms faith in God and hope in an everlasting resurrection. The burning of a memorial candle is also a common tradition during this time.

The period of 30 days following the burial is termed the *sheloshim*, a time when business can be resumed but grief continues and due allowance is made for the distress of the mourners. In the 10 months after the *sheloshim*, lives are expected to gradually return to normal, but the *Kaddish* is recited at Sabbath services each week, thus supporting the bereaved's grief within their community. At the first anniversary, the commemorative tombstone is unveiled at the cemetery and the formal period of mourning is concluded. The dead are, however, remembered each year during the *Yizkor* memorial service and at the *Yahrzeit* (the family meeting on the anniversary of the day of death).

Christian bereavement practices

Many of the rituals of Christianity are derived from their Jewish origins. The basic tenets are that *Jesus* of Nazareth was the *Messiah*, the Son of God, who was crucified to redeem the sins of mankind, and rose from the dead on the third day as evidence of his divinity. Reconciliation with monotheism is achieved through the doctrine of the *Trinity* (God the Father, Son, and Holy Spirit), three persons in one God. Christ's teachings were laid down in the *Gospels* and *Acts of the Apostles* as the *New Testament*, which was then added to the Jewish Bible. There is belief in the soul, forgiveness of wrong-doing, resurrection of the body, and everlasting life in the place commonly termed heaven. The *Eastern Orthodox Churches* split from the *Roman Catholic Church* in the 11th century, while the *Protestant Reformation* occurred during the 16th century[126].

Priesthood is followed in the tradition of the rabbis, with study in preparation and ordination bringing responsibility for the conduct of the major rituals. These are perceived as a source of spiritual grace and connectedness with God and are known as the *sacraments*. *Baptism* with water is an initial cleansing ritual celebrating entry into the community, while the *Mass* is the major sacrament celebrating the life of Jesus in the form of a Jewish Passover meal with communion, the sharing of the sacred bread and wine. Christian tradition recognizes *Mary* as the mother of Jesus, introducing a female element missing from other major world religions.

For the sick, in the Roman Catholic rite both the sacrament of *Confession or Reconciliation*, in which sins are repented before a priest and forgiven, and the sacrament of *Anointing the sick*, formerly called *Extreme Unction* in keeping with the blessed oils that are used, are a means of spiritual uplifting and prayerful connectedness with God. In the Eastern rites, the priest will chant the *Office for the Sick* and the *Office for the Parting of the Soul*, while in the Anglican rite, *Prayers for the Sick* are said. Contact with a priest or minister of the appropriate church is important for Christians to access these rituals before death. The family would traditionally gather around the bed of the dying keeping prayerful watch, including recital of the *Rosary* prayer to invoke the support of Mary in the Roman Catholic tradition.

Once death has occurred, funeral directors play a dominant role in arranging services with the priest and plans for burial or cremation. Viewing of the body is common and may be accompanied by prayers. The funeral occurs when practical within a few days of the death, usually occurring in a church or chapel. Traditionally, a *Vigil* service on the night preceding the funeral involves prayers, psalms, or recitation of the *Rosary*. In Roman Catholicism, the *Requiem Mass* incorporates the regular sacrament with a commemorative service, while in Orthodox services, mourners prostrate themselves and kiss the cross. If there is a burial, a *Service of Internment* takes place at the graveside; if cremated, the ashes are placed in an urn for later internment or scattering by the family.

Within the Eastern rites, memorial services (*Panikhidi*) are held 3, 8, and 40 days after the funeral with chanting of traditional psalms and anthems (*Contakion & Trepanion*). Catholic rites include the offering of *Votive Masses* to commemorate the dead, especially at times of the anniversary and at the calendar *Feasts of All Saints and All Souls*. Considerable variation occurs across the range of Protestant and Free Churches of Christian tradition, incorporating differing emphasis on beliefs about communion, Bible interpretation, and church rules. Members of African communities converted to Christianity retain some beliefs in Voodoo, spirit healing, and witchcraft, while fundamentalist practice has emerged in many churches to counter the drift away from religious practice. *Mormons* (*Church of the Latter-Day Saints*) wear a sacred undergarment, which should not be removed after death.

Thus, within Christian tradition, the prayers for the sick before death play a potentially spiritual healing role, while the bereavement practices orientate around church services but provide continuing support for the bereaved from their church communities.

Islamic bereavement practices

Muhammad saw himself around 610 AD as one of a succession of Semitic prophets following in the tradition of Moses, Abraham, and Jesus who preached God's judgement on each person according to their works, culminating in the resurrection of the dead. The Islamic religion has been based on the *Quran* and teachings of its prophet and quickly spread across the Arabic nations from Morocco to Egypt to Pakistan to Indonesia[127].

As death approaches, the Imam should be called to attend the dying. They may be helped to sit up or turn their face towards Mecca and their confession of faith is prayed as their relatives gather around and provide support. Following death, ritual washing occurs to prepare the body. As a rule, only men wash a man's body and only women a woman's. A *Quran* reader chants from the holy book during this cleansing ablution. Washing proceeds in a fixed pattern and with great respect for the body, which is then wrapped in three pieces of white cloth and thus prepared for burial. Cremation is forbidden through belief in resurrection of the body. Cultural variation exists within Islamic sects with regard to the expression of grief: it ranges from extreme wailing to restrained composure. Burial is encouraged within 24 h. News of the death and invitation to pray for the deceased is announced by loudspeaker from the village minaret.

During the final ceremony, the face of the deceased is made visible for the mourners to look at and bid farewell. Recitation from the *Quran* or construction of a personal dirge is common. The Imam invites the community to forgive the deceased any wrong deeds and the *Prayer for the Dead* is recited. The body is then ready for burial. The body lying on a bier is carried in procession to the graveside and lowered into the grave, positioning the face and eyes towards Mecca and laying a board across the face to permit a little room. The *Quran* is read while the grave is filled with soil and the Imam gives a final blessing. Then, while the mourners leave in silence, Islamic belief states that two angels visit the deceased to ask the final five questions as an expression of their faith. The Imam, standing at the head of the grave acts for the angels and calls the deceased to answer these questions: Who is your God? Prophet? Book? Iman? Qibla (prayer direction)? The Imam listens for the head of the dead to bump against the wooden board in reply and continues to call the name of the deceased until the response is heard.

In North Africa, bereaved women wear white, while in the Middle East, they wear black—young women for 3 months; older women for 1 year. Special sweet food is eaten on the third, seventh, and 40th days and prayers are offered. The story of the prophet's birth is read on the 40th day as a source of consolation and a special stone is laid at the tomb on the anniversary of the burial. Traditionally, children have been excluded from Islamic burial ceremonies although these practices appear to be changing. The rituals

Table 15.6.7 Psychometric properties of grief and bereavement self-report measures.

Instrument name	Item number and response style	Subscale or factor structure	Reliability	Validity	Comments on utility
Texas Revised Inventory of Grief (TRIG)[128]	21-item, 5-point response	Past behaviour at time of death; Present feelings	Cronbach's α 0.77–0.87	Satisfactory predictive validity	Comparison between past and present responses invalidated by memory; subscale 2 useful as a change measure
Grief Experience Inventory (GEI)[129]	135-item, true–false response	Validity scales of denial, atypical response, and social desirability; Clinical scales of despair anger, guilt, isolation, control, rumination, despersonalization, somatization and death, anxiety	Cronbach's α 0.34–0.84; test–retest 0.53–0.87 over 9 weeks	Satisfactory concurrent and predictive validity	Long measure, some items using past tense wording in a fixed manner; true–false response style less useful as a change measure
Core Bereavement Items (CBI)[130] and Bereavement Phenomenology Questionnaire (BPQ)[106, 131]	17-item, CBI and 22-item BPQ; 4-point response	CBI—1 scale BPQ—1 factor[132]	Cronbach's α 0.91 (CBI); 0.93 (BPQ)	Satisfactory concurrent and predictive validity	Sensible focus on core bereavement phenomena. CBI best measure of normal responses; BPQ better as measure to include symptoms of non-resolution. CBI derived in part from BPQ
Inventory of Complicated Grief (ICG)[38]	19-item, 5-point response	Separation distress Traumatic grief	Cronbach's α 0.94; test-retest 0.80 over 6 months	Satisfactory concurrent and predictive validity	Derived from research on bereaved elderly spouses whose loss resulted from cancer
Inventory of Traumatic Grief (ITG)[23]	30-item, 5-point response	Separation distress Traumatic grief	Cronbach's α 0.95	Concurrent validity with SF-36	Permits application of proposed diagnostic criteria for traumatic grief
Sibling Inventory of Bereavement (SIB)[133]	46-item, 5-point response	Grief factor; Personal growth	Cronbach's α 0.88–0.95	Satisfactory predictive validity	Instrument only used with adolescents (13–18 years) although developed from qualitative data from children
Grief Experience Questionnaire (GEQ)[134]	55-item, 5-point response	Eight factors from principal components analysis: abandonment, stigma, searching, guilt, somatic, personal responsibility, self-destructive, and shame	Cronbach's α 0.68–0.89	Differentiates suicidally bereaved from other losses	Useful for stigmatized deaths from suicide, AIDS

clearly draw in community support for the bereaved as they foster hope in the belief of resurrection.

Secular bereavement practices

Many in society are non-religious, whether agnostic or atheistic, and see death as a natural process, albeit considerably medicalized. There is grief at the closure of life and mourning for those left behind. The funeral industry provides support for the bereaved and helps them celebrate the life of the deceased person with appropriate eulogy, poetry, and story, conducting a secular service in the funeral parlour, while other self-help groups are available to support the bereaved. For the non-religious, such processes continue to nurture the expression of grief and affirm the normality of mourning.

Research and measurement in bereavement

Although generic measures of psychiatric symptomatology (see Chapter 5.5) are commonly used in bereavement research, a number of self-report measures of bereavement phenomena make it now possible to specifically evaluate the process and outcome of both the grief over the loss and the supportive therapies used by palliative care services to intervene. The psychometric properties and key references of these bereavement measures are summarized in Table 15.6.7 as a resource for researchers.

Qualitative studies of bereavement are ideally suited to reveal the unique meanings that inform the reactions of individuals or cultural groups to death and loss[135]. They are derived from constructivist philosophy that recognizes the socially and personally constructed realities of human experience and are helpful in generating theory, but limited in providing causal explanations for grief phenomena or demonstrating the efficacy of particular interventions. Yet mixed qualitative–quantitative methodologies continue to provide valuable insights, well exemplified by the work of Folkman's group in studying the bereavement experience of carer's of gay men dying from AIDS[136]. Here, they recognized the value of positive emotion and spirituality, leading to an enriched understanding of the contribution of meaning-based coping to the adaptive responses of the bereaved. There is a substantial need for qualitatively based observational and interventional studies in bereavement.

Positive outcome and personal growth

The adaptation that follows the wrenching loss of bereavement is associated with personal growth for a sizeable proportion. Although this personal growth manifests itself most clearly after the acute pain of grief, it is actually identifiable across all phases of the bereavement process[137]. Renewed sense of meaning, self-awareness, increased empathy, appreciation of family and relationships, independence, reprioritized goals and values, deepened spirituality, and increased altruism can all result from positive reappraisal, seeking for help and enhanced social resources.

Clinicians can helpfully reassure bereaved people about these beneficial outcomes, especially at times when the going is hard. Providing information about the longitudinal course of the mourning process including the prospect of such personal growth creates a feedback loop that nurtures adaptive recovery through cognitive appraisal and active coping.

Conclusion

Bereavement care is an integral dimension of palliative medicine as clinicians sustain continuity of care in assisting the family or carers of their deceased patient. Knowledge of and competence in assessing grief is essential to enable recognition of the 20 per cent of the bereaved who get into difficulties and need additional assistance. Routine assessment of the bereaved for risk factors for complicated grief provides a responsible method through which treatment teams can intervene preventatively or early to reduce unnecessary morbidity. Effective therapies are available to assist in the management of complicated grief and palliative care practitioners should be skilled in their application or understand the circumstances when referral for further specialist help is appropriately made. Grief is an inevitable dimension of our humanity, an adaptive adjustment process, and one that with support can be approached with courage. Grief that is shared is grief that is healed.

Further reading

Irish, D.P., Lundquist, K.F., and Nelsen, V.J. (ed.) (1993). *Ethnic variations in dying, death and grief: Diversity in universality.* Taylor & Francis, Washington, DC. A useful resource to cross-cultural bereavement.

Jacobs, S. (1993). *Pathologic grief. Maladaptation to loss.* American Psychiatric Press, Washington, DC. A concise account of complicated mourning.

Kissane, D.W. and Bloch, S. (2002). *Family focused grief therapy. A model of family-centered care during palliative care and bereavement.* Open University Press, Buckingham. An innovative, integrated and preventive approach to family care.

Parkes, C.M. (1998). *Bereavement. Studies of grief in adult life,* 3rd edition. International Universities Press, Madison. A classic and worthwhile introduction.

Parkes, C.M., Laungani, P., and Young, B. (ed.) (1997). *Death and bereavement across cultures.* Routledge, London. Useful reference to cross-cultural bereavement practices.

Raphael, B. (1983). *Anatomy of bereavement.* Basic Books, New York. A classic work with excellent discussion of grief across the life cycle.

Stroebe, M.S., Hansson, R.O., Stroebe, W. *et al.* (ed.) (2001). *Handbook of bereavement research. Consequences, coping, and care.* American Psychological Association, Washington, DC. An excellent, up-to-date review of recent research that comprehensively explores theory, culture, coping and intervention.

Stroebe, M.S., Stroebe, W., and Hansson, R.O. (ed.) (1993). *Handbook of bereavement. Theory, research and intervention.* Cambridge University Press, Cambridge. Excellent compilation of phenomenology, bereavement studies and approaches.

References

1. Parkes, C. (1998). *Bereavement: Studies of grief in adult life,* 3rd edition. International Universities Press, Madison.
2. Stroebe, M., Stroebe, W., and Hansson, R. (eds.) (1993). *Handbook of bereavement.* Cambridge University Press, Cambridge.
3. Raphael, B. (1983). *The anatomy of bereavement.* Hutchinson, London.
4. Rando, T. (1993). *Treatment of complicated mourning.* Research Press, Illinois.
5. Doka, K. (1989). Disenfranchised grief. In *Disenfranchised grief: Recognizing hidden sorrow* (ed. K. Doka), pp. 3–11. Lexington Books, Lexington, MA.
6. Darwin, C. (1872). *The expression of the emotions in man and animals.* Murray, London.
7. Rosenblatt, P. (2001). A social constructionist perspective on cultural differences in grief. In *Handbook of bereavement research. Consequences, coping, and care* (eds. M. Stroebe, R. Hansson, W. Stroebe, and H. Schut), pp. 285–300. American Psychological Association, Washington, DC.
8. Middleton, W., Moylan, A., Raphael, B. *et al.* (1993). An international perspective on bereavement related concepts. *Australian and New Zealand Journal of Psychiatry,* **27,** 457–63.
9. Bowlby, J. (1977). The making and breaking of affectional bonds I & II. *British Journal of Psychiatry,* **130,** 201–10 and 421–31.
10. Ainsworth, M., Blehar, M., Waters, E. *et al.* (1978). *Patterns of attachment: A psychological study of the strange situation.* Erlbaum, Hillsdale, NJ.
11. Parkes, C. (1985). Bereavement. *British Journal of Psychiatry,* **146,** 11–17.
12. Jacobs, S., Kosten, T., Kasl, S. *et al.* (1987/88). Attachment theory and multiple dimensions of grief. *Omega,* **18,** 41–52.
13. Klein, M. (1940). Mourning and its relation to manic-depressive states. *International Journal of Psycho-analysis,* **21,** 125–53.
14. Shapiro, E. (2001). Grief in interpersonal perspective: Theories and their implications. In *Handbook of bereavement research. Consequences, coping, and care* (eds. M. Stroebe, R. Hansson, W. Stroebe, and H. Schut), pp. 301–27. American Psychological Association, Washington, DC.
15. Horowitz, M. (1989). A model of mourning: Change in schemas of self and other. *Journal of the American Psychoanalytic Association,* **38,** 297–324.
16. Horowitz, M., Bonanno, G., and Holen, A. (1993). Pathological grief: Diagnosis and explanations. *Psychosomatic Medicine,* **55,** 260–73.

17. Parkes, C. (1975). What becomes of redundant world models? A contribution to the study of adaptation to change. *British Journal of Medical Psychology*, **48**, 131–7.

18. Freud, S. (1912). *Totem and taboo*. Hogarth Press, London.

19. Klass, D., Silverman, P., and Nickman, S. (eds.) (1996). *Continuing bonds: New understandings of grief*. Taylor & Francis, Washington, DC.

20. Walter, T. (1996). A new model of grief: Bereavement and biography. *Mortality*, **1**, 7–25.

21. Kissane, D., Bloch, S., Dowe, D. *et al.* (1996). The Melbourne family grief study I & II. *American Journal of Psychiatry*, **153**, 650–8 and 659–66.

22. Walsh, F. and McGoldrick, M. (eds.) (1991). *Living Beyond Loss*. Norton, New York.

23. Prigerson, H. and Jacobs, S. (2001). Traumatic grief as a distinct disorder: A rationale, consensus criteria, and a preliminary empirical test. In *Handbook of bereavement research. Consequences, coping, and care* (eds. M. Stroebe, R. Hansson, W. Stroebe, and H. Schut), pp. 613–37. American Psychological Association, Washington DC.

24. Kavanagh, D. (1990). Towards a cognitive behavioural intervention for adult grief reactions. *British Journal of Psychiatry*, **157**, 373–83.

25. Stroebe, M. and Schut, H. (2001). Models of coping with bereavement: A review. In *Handbook of bereavement research. Consequences, coping, and care* (eds. M. Stroebe, R. Hansson, W. Stroebe, and H. Schut), pp. 375–403. American Psychological Association, Washington, DC.

26. Lindemann, E. (1944). Symptomatology and management of acute grief. *American Journal of Psychiatry*, **101**, 141–8.

27. Jacobs, S., Bruce, M., and Kim, K. (1997). Adrenal function predicts demoralisation after losses. *Psychosomatics*, **38**, 529–34.

28. Esterling, B., Kiecolt-Glaser, J., and Glaser, R. (1996). Psychosocial modulation of cytokine-induced natural killer cell activity in older adults. *Psychosomatic Medicine*, **58**, 264–72.

29. Hall, M., Baum, A., Buysse, D. *et al.* (1998). Sleep as a mediator of the stress–immune relationship. *Psychosomatic Medicine*, **60**, 48–51.

30. Parkes, C. (1975). Determinants of outcome following bereavement. *Omega*, **6**, 303–23.

31. Meares, R. (1981). On saying goodbye before death. *Journal of the American Medical Association*, **246**, 1227–9.

32. Maguire, P. (1985). Barriers to psychological care of the dying. *British Medical Journal*, **291**, 1711–13.

33. Parkes, C., Laungani, P., and Young, B. (eds.) (1997). *Death and bereavement across cultures*. Routledge, London.

34. Hofer, M. (1984). Relationships as regulators: A psychobiologic perspective on bereavement. *Psychosomatic Medicine*, **46**, 183–97.

35. Polloch, G. (1989). *The mourning-liberation process*. International University Press, New Haven, CT.

36. Zisook, S. and Schuchter, S. (1985). The first four years of widowhood. *Psychiatric Annals*, **16**, 288–94.

37. Parkes, C. and Weiss, R. (1983). *Recovery from bereavement*. Basic Books, New York.

38. Prigerson, H., Maciejewski, P., Newson, J. *et al.* (1995). Inventory of complicated grief. *Psychiatry Research*, **59**, 65–79.

39. Prigerson, H., Frand, E., and Kasl, S. (1995). Complicated grief and bereavement-related depression as distinct disorders: Preliminary empirical validation in elderly bereaved spouses. *American Journal of Psychiatry*, **152**, 22–30.

40. Bonanno, G.A. (2004). Loss, trauma and human resilience: Have we underestimated the human capacity to thrive after extremely aversive events? *American Psychologist*, **59**(1), 20–8.

41. Stroebe, M., van Son, M., Stroebe, W. *et al.* (2000). On the classification and diagnosis of pathological grief. *Clinical Psychology Review*, **20**, 57–75.

42. Prigerson, H.G., Vanderwerker, L.C., and Maciejewski, P.K. (2007). Complicated grief as a mental disorder: Inclusion in DSM (Chapter 8). In *Handbook of bereavement research and practice: 21st century perspectives* (eds. M. Stroebe, R. Hansson, H. Schut, and W. Stroebe). American Psychological Association Press, Washington, D.C.

43. Hogan, N.S., Worden, J.W., and Schmidt, L.A. (2003–2004). An empirical study of the proposed Complicated Grief Disorder Criteria. *Omega: The Journal of Death and Dying*, **48**, 263–77.

44. Prigerson, H.G., Maciejewski, P.K., Reynolds, C.F. *et al.* (1995). Inventory of complicated grief: A scale to measure maladaptive symptoms of loss. *Psychiatry Research*, **59**(1), 65–79.

45. Prigerson, H.G., Bierhals, A.J., Kasl, S.V. *et al.* (1996). Complicated grief as a disorder distinct from bereavement-related depression and anxiety: A replication study. *American Journal of Psychiatry*, **153**, 1484–6.

46. Prigerson, H.G., Bridge, J., Maciejewski, P.K. *et al.* (1999). Influence of traumatic grief on suicidal ideation among young adults. *American Journal of Psychiatry*, **156**, 1994–5.

47. Prigerson, H.G. and Maciejewski, P.K. (2005–2006). A call for sound empirical testing and evaluation of criteria for complicated grief proposed for DSM-V. *Omega: The Journal of Death and Dying*, **52**(1), 1541–3764.

48. Neimeyer, R.A. (2005–2006). Complicated grief and the quest for meaning: A constructivist contribution. *Omega: The Journal of Death and Dying*, **52**(1), 37–52.

49. Silverman, G.K., Johnson, J.G., and Prigerson, H.G. (2001). Preliminary explorations of the effects of prior trauma and loss on risk of psychiatric disorders in recently widowed people. *Israel Journal of Psychiatry and Related Science*, **38**, 202–15.

50. Kissane, D., Bloch, S., Burns, W. *et al.* (1994). Perceptions of family functioning and cancer. *Psycho-oncology*, **3**, 259–69.

51. Clayton, P. (1990). Bereavement and depression. *Journal of Clinical Psychiatry*, **51**, 34–8.

52. Parkes, C. (1984). The effects of bereavement on physical and mental health: A study of the case records of widows. *British Medical Journal*, **2**, 274–80.

53. Zisook, S. and Schuchter, S. (1991). Depression through the first year after the death of a spouse. *American Journal of Psychiatry*, **148**, 1346–52.

54. Harlow, S., Goldberg, E., and Comstock, G. (1991). A longitudinal study of the prevalence of depressive symptomatology in elderly widowed and married women. *Archives of General Psychiatry*, **48**, 1065–8.

55. Zisook, S., Schuchter, S., and Sledge, P. (1994). The spectrum of depressive phenomena after spousal bereavement. *Journal of Clinical Psychiatry*, **55**(Suppl. 4), 29–36.

56. Karam, E. (1994). The nosological status of bereavement-related depressions. *British Journal of Psychiatry*, **165**, 48–52.

57. Jacobs, S. (1993). *Pathological grief*. American Psychiatric Association Press, Washington, DC.

58. Schut, H., Stroebe, M., de Keijser, J. *et al.* (1997). Intervention for the bereaved: Gender differences in the efficacy of two counselling programmes. *British Journal of Clinical Psychology*, **36**, 63–72.

59. Kissane, D. and Bloch, S. (1994). Family grief. *British Journal of Psychiatry*, **164**, 728–40.

60. Moos, R. and Moos, B. (1981). *Family environment scale manual*. Consulting Psychologists' Press, Palo Alto, CA.

61. Kissane, D. and Bloch, S. (2002). *Family focused grief therapy: A model of family-centered care during palliative care and bereavement*. Open University Press, Buckingham.

62. Raphael, B. (1977). Preventive intervention with the recently bereaved. *Archives of General Psychiatry*, **34**, 1450–4.

63. Parkes, C. (1981). Evaluation of a bereavement service. *Journal of Preventive Psychiatry*, **1**, 179–88.

64. Stroebe, M. and Stroebe, W. (1993). The mortality of bereavement: A review. In *Handbook of bereavement. theory, research, and intervention* (eds. M. Stroebe, W. Stroebe, and R. Hansson), pp. 175–95. Cambridge University Press, Cambridge.

65. Schaefer, C., Quesenberry, C., and Wi, S. (1995). Mortality following conjugal bereavement and the effects of a shared environment. *American Journal of Epidemiology*, **141**, 1142–52.

66. House, J., Landi, K., and Umberson, D. (1988). Social relationship and health. *Science*, **241**, 540–5.

67. Saunders, C. (1999). *Grief: The mourning after: Dealing with adult bereavement*, 2nd edition. Wiley, New York.

68. Hofer, M., Wolff, C., Freedman, S. *et al.* (1972). A psycho-endocrine study of bereavement: parts I & II. *Psychosomatic Medicine*, **34**, 481–507.

69. Bartrop, R., Lazarus, L., Luckhurst, E. *et al.* (1977). Depressed lymphocyte function after bereavement. *Lancet*, **1**, 834–6.

70. Schleifer, S., Keller, M., Camerino, J. *et al.* (1983). Suppression of lymphocyte stimulation following bereavement. *Journal of the American Medical Association*, **250**, 374–7.

71. Irwin, M., Daniels, M., and Weiner, H. (1987). Immune and neuro-endocrine changes after bereavement. *Psychiatric Clinics of North America*, **10**, 449–65.

72. Jones, D. and Goldblatt, P. (1986). Cancer mortality following widow(er)hood: Some further results from the Office of Population Censuses and Surveys Longitudinal Study. *Stress Medicine*, **2**, 129–40.

73. Kaprio, J., Koskenvuo, M., and Rita, H. (1987). Mortality after bereavement: A prospective study of 95,647 widowed persons. *American Journal of Public Health*, **77**, 283–7.

74. Helsing, K., Comstock, G., and Szklo, M. (1982). Causes of death in a widowed population. *American Journal of Epidemiology*, **116**, 524–32.

75. Yalom, I. and Vinogradov, S. (1988). Bereavement groups: Techniques and themes. *International Journal of Group Psychotherapy*, **38**, 419–46.

76. Lieberman, M. and Yalom, I. (1992). Brief group therapy for the spousally bereaved: A controlled study. *International Journal of Group Psychotherapy*, **42**, 117–32.

77. Kissane, D. (2000). Family grief therapy: A new model of family-centered care during palliative care and bereavement. In *Cancer and the family*, 2nd edition (eds. L. Baider, G. Cooper, and Kaplan De Nour). Wiley, Chichester.

78. Kissane, D. (1999). Importance of family-centred care to palliative medicine. *Japanese Journal of Clinical Oncology*, **29**, 1–3.

79. Melges, F. and Demaso, D. (1980). Grief-resolution therapy: reliving, revising and revisiting. *American Journal of Psychotherapy*, **34**, 51–61.

80. Mawson, D., Marks, I., Ramm, L. *et al.* (1981). Guided mourning for morbid giref: A controlled study. *British Journal of Psychiatry*, **138**, 185–93.

81. Worden, J. (1991). *Grief counseling and grief therapy: A handbook for the mental health practitioner*, 2nd edition. Springer, New York.

82. Janoff-Bulman, R. (1989). Assumptive worlds and the stresss of traumatic events: Application of the schema concept. *Social Cognition*, **7**, 113–36.

83. Janoff-Bulman, R. (1992). *Shattered assumptions. Towards a new psychology of trauma*. Free Press, New York.

84. Klerman, G., Weissman, M., and Rounsaville, B. (1984). *Interpersonal psychotherapy of depression*. Basic Books, New York.

85. Horowitz, M., Marmar, C., Weiss, D. *et al.* (1984). Brief psychotherapy of bereavement reactions. *Archives of General Psychiatry*, **41**, 438–48.

86. Gersie, A. (1991). *Storymaking in bereavement. Dragons fight in the meadow*. Jessica Kingsley Publishers, London.

87. Shear, K., Frank, E., Houck, P.R. *et al.* (2005). Treatment of complicated grief: A randomized controlled trial. *JAMA*, **293**, 2601–8.

88. Vachon, M., Sheldon, A., Lancee, W. *et al.* (1980). A controlled study of self-help intervention for widows. *American Journal of Psychiatry*, **137**, 1380–4.

89. Schut, H., de Keijser, J., van den Bout, J. *et al.* (1996). Cross modality grief therapy: Description and assessment of a new program. *Journal of Clinical Psychology*, **52**, 357–65.

90. Simon, R. (1982). Bereavement art. *American Journal of Art Therapy*, **20**, 135–43.

91. Bright, R. (1986). *Grieving: A handbook for those who care*. MMB Music Inc, St Louis, MO.

92. Rynearson, E. (1987). Psychotherapy of pathologic grief. *Psychiatric Clinics of North America*, **10**, 487–99.

93. Jacobs, S., Nelson, J., and Zisook, S. (1987). Treating depressions of bereavement with antidepressants: A pilot study. *Psychiatric Clinics of North America*, **10**, 501–10.

94. Pasternak, R., Reynolds, C., and Schlernitzauer, M. (1991). Acute open-trial nortriptyline therapy of bereavement-related depression in late life. *Journal of Clinical Psychiatry*, **52**, 307–10.

95. Lund, D., Caserta, M., and Dimond, M. (1993). The course of spousal bereavement. In *Handbook of bereavement: theory, research and intervention* (eds. M. Stroebe, W. Stroebe, and R. Hansson), pp. 240–54. Cambridge University Press, Cambridge.

96. Silverman, P. (1986). *Widow to widow*. Springer, New York.

97. Adams-Greenly, M. (1984). Helping children communicate about serious illness and death. *Journal of Psychosocial Oncology*, **2**, 62–72.

98. Eiser, C. and Havermans, T. (1992). Children's understanding of cancer. *Psycho-oncology*, **1**, 169–81.

99. Rowland, J. (1989). Developmental stage and adaptation: Child and adolescent model. In *Handbook of psycho-oncology* (eds. J. Holland and J. Rowland), pp. 519–43. Oxford University Press, Oxford.

100. Webb, N. (ed.) (1993). *Helping bereaved children*. Guilford, London.

101. Adams-Greenly, M. and Moynihan, R. (1983). Helping the children of fatally ill parents. *American Journal of Orthopsychiatry*, **53**, 219–29.

102. Silverman, P. and Worden, J. (1992). Children's understanding of the funeral ritual. *Omega*, **25**, 319–31.

103. Wells, R. (1988). *Helping children cope with grief*. Sheldon, London.

104. Tennant, C., Bebbington, P., and Hurry, J. (1980). Parental death in childhood and risk of adult depressive disorders: A review. *Psychological Medicine*, **10**, 289–99.

105. Davies, B., Spinetta, J., Martinson, I. *et al.* (1986). Manifestations of levels of functioning in grieving families. *Journal of Family Issues*, **7**, 297–313.

106. Byrne, G. and Raphael, B. (1994). A longitudinal study of bereavement phenomena in recently widowed elderly men. *Psychological Medicine*, **24**, 411–21.

107. Large, T. (1989). Some aspects of loneliness in families. *Family Process*, **28**, 25–35.

108. Lopata, H. (1986). Becoming and being a widow: Reconstruction of the self and support systems. *Geriatric Psychiatry*, **19**, 203–14.

109. Malinak, D., Hoyt, M., and Patterson, V. (1979). Adults' reactions to the death of a parent: A preliminary study. *American Journal of Psychiatry*, **136**, 1152–6.

110. Saunders, C. (1979). A comparison of adult bereavement in the death of spouse, child, and parent. *Omega*, **10**, 303–22.

111. Middleton, W., Raphael, B., Burnett, P. *et al.* (1998). A longitudinal study comparing bereavement phenomena in recently bereaved spouses, adult children and parents. *Australian and New Zealand Journal of Psychiatry*, **32**, 235–41.

112. Rubin, S. (1993). The death of a child is forever: The life course impact of child loss. In *Handbook of bereavement* (eds. M. Stroebe, W. Stroebe, and R. Hansson), pp. 285–99. Cambridge University Press, Cambridge.

113. Neimeyer, R., Keese, B., and Fortner, M. (2000). Loss and meaning reconstruction: Propositions and procedures. In *Traumatic and non-traumatic loss and bereavement: Clinical theory and practice* (eds. R. Malkinson, S. Rubin, and E. Witztum), pp. 197–230. Psychosocial Press/International Universities Press, Madison CT.

114. Spinetta, J., Swarner, J., and Shepost, J. (1981). Effective parental coping following death of a child from cancer. *Journal of Paediatric Psychology*, **6**, 251–63.

115. Folkman, S., Chesney, M., and Christopher-Richards, A. (1994). Stress and coping in caregiving partners of men with AIDS. *Psychiatric Clinics of North America*, **17**, 35–53.

116. Moskowitz, J., Acree, M., and Folkman, S. (1998). Depression and AIDS-related bereavement: A 3-year follow-up. New perspectives on

depression in AIDS-related caregiving and bereavement. In *Annual Meeting of the American Psychological Association*, San Francisco, CA. Cited by Folkman, S. Revised coping theory and the process of bereavement, In *Handbook of bereavement research* (eds. M.S. Stroebe, R.O. Hansson, W. Stroebe, and H. Schut), pp. 563–84. American Psychological Association, Washington, DC.

117. Wolfe, B. (1993). AIDS and bereavement. In *Death and spirituality* (eds. K. Doka and J. Morgan), pp. 257–78. Baywood, New York.

118. Doka, K. (1993). The spiritual crisis of bereavement. In *Death and spirituality* (eds. K. Doka and J. Morgan), pp. 185–93. Baywood, New York.

119. Imber-Black, E. (1991). Rituals and the healing process. In *Living beyond loss: Death in the family* (eds. F. Walsh and M. McGoldrick). Norton, New York.

120. Sharma, D. (1990). Hindu attitude toward suffering, dying and death. *Palliative Medicine*, **4**, 235–8.

121. Laungani, P. (1997). Death in a Hindu family. In *Death and bereavement across cultures* (eds. C. Parkes, P. Laungani, and B. Young), pp. 52–72. Routledge, London.

122. Truitner, K. and Truitner, N. (1993). Death and dying in Buddhism. In *Ethnic variations in dying, death, and grief: Diversity in universality* (eds. D. Irish, K. Lundquist, and V. Nelsen), pp. 125–36. Taylor & Francis, Washington, DC.

123. Ryan, D. (1993). Death: eastern perspectives. In *Death and spirituality* (eds. K. Doka and J. Morgan), pp. 76–92. Baywood, Amityville.

124. Joachim, C. (1986). *Chinese Religions*. Prentice-Hall, Englewood Cliffs, NJ.

125. Overmyer, D. (1987). *Religions of China*. Harper & Row, New York.

126. Ter Blanche, H. and Parkes, C. (1997). Christianity. In *Death and bereavement across cultures* (eds. C. Parkes, P. Laungani, and B. Young), pp. 131–46. Routledge, London.

127. Jonker, G. (1997). The many facets of Islam. Death, dying and disposal between orthodox rule and historical convention. In *Death and bereavement across cultures* (eds. C. Parkes, P. Laungani, and B. Young), pp. 147–65. Routledge, London.

128. Faschingbauer, T. (1981). *Texas revised inventory of grief manual*. Honeycomb, Houston, TX.

129. Saunders, C., Mauger, P., and Strong, P. (1985). *A manual for the grief experience inventory*. Center for the Study of Separation and Loss, Blowing Rock, NC.

130. Burnett, P., Middleton, W., Raphael, B. *et al.* (1997). Measuring core bereavement phenomenon. *Psychological Medicine*, **27**, 49–57.

131. Burnett, P., Middleton, W., Raphael, B. *et al.* (1993). Concepts of normal bereavement. Journal of Traumatic Stress, **24**, 8–30.

132. Kissane, D., Bloch, S., and McKenzie, D.P. (1997). The bereavement phenomenology questionnaire. *Australian and New Zealand Journal of Psychiatry*, **31**, 370–4.

133. Hogan, N. and Greenfield, D. (1991). Adolescent sibling bereavement symptomatology in a large community sample. *Journal of Adolescent Research*, **6**, 97–112.

134. Barrett, T. and Scott, T. (1989). Development of the Grief Experience Questionnaire. *Suicide and Life-Threatening Behaviour*, **19**, 201–15.

135. Neimeyer, R. and Hogan, N. (2001). Quantitative or qualitative? Measurement issues in the study of grief. In *Handbook of bereavement research* (eds. M. Stroebe, R. Hansson, W. Stroebe, and H. Schut), pp. 89–118. American Psychological Association, Washington, DC.

136. Folkman, S. (2001). Revised coping theory and the process of bereavement. In *Handbook of bereavement research. Consequences, coping, and care* (eds. M. Stroebe, R. Hansson, W. Stroebe, and H. Schut), pp. 563–84. American Psychological Association, Washington, DC.

137. Hogan, N., Morse, J., and Tason, M. (1996). Toward an experiential theory of bereavement. *Omega*, **33**, 43–65.

SECTION 16

Medical rehabilitation and the palliative care patient

Deborah Franklin and Andrea Cheville

Introduction

The integration of rehabilitation and palliation may sound unlikely to those who do not regularly participate in the care of patients with palliative or hospice needs. Experienced care providers, however, have long recognized the power of incorporating key elements of rehabilitation medicine into the delivery of comprehensive palliative or hospice care. In some countries, such as the UK, the integration has existed since the inception of modern hospice care and is part of palliative care. In other countries, the integration involves distinct services as well as integrated services. This chapter concentrates largely on the non-UK hospice models, especially those existing in the USA. The integration of rehabilitation medicine and palliative care is, however, of global relevance.

This integration is facilitated by a fundamental alignment between rehabilitation medicine and palliative care, which both emphasize the importance of all elements of the biopsychosocial model. Both employ interdisciplinary teams to develop care plans that respond not just to the physiological but also the psychological and social needs of patients and their caregivers. Both rehabilitation medicine and palliative care medicine seek multi-dimensional outcomes that are not related specifically to disease state, such as the functional independence measures (FIM) or, quality of life (QOL) parameters.

Rehabilitation strategies contribute to palliative care by maintaining and, if possible, promoting functional independence during a period of expected physiological decline. In addition to maximizing function through patient and caregiver training, rehabilitation strategies can prevent deleterious complications such as skin breakdown, joint contractures, pneumonia, and generalized deconditioning. The judicious selection of durable medical equipment (DME) is best done in collaboration with Physical Medicine and Rehabilitation (PM&R) specialists who can combine extensive knowledge of available componentry with an understanding of the salient medical and prognostic characteristics of a given patient.

This chapter highlights aspects of rehabilitation medicine that are of greatest value for patients requiring palliative care in hospital or hospice. Section I describes where and how such rehabilitation services can be obtained. Section II reviews the timing of rehabilitation interventions and the associated concept of functional patient goal-setting. Section III provides in-depth examples of specific rehabilitation interventions available to patients with advanced disease processes, including the important areas of caregiver training and support. Section IV examines current barriers to the effective use of rehabilitation strategies in palliative care medicine and outlines some emerging approaches for improving outcomes.

Section I: delivery of rehabilitation services in palliative care

The delivery of rehabilitation services as part of palliative care varies between health-care systems. Many regional and international rehabilitation organizations have special interest groups that address the distinct needs of palliative care populations. Among physicians these include oncological rehabilitation groups, geriatric-focused groups and pain management specialists. Rehabilitation medicine specialists as well as exercise physiologists involved in the care of palliative care populations have begun producing evidence-based care guidelines for treating patients with advanced disease[1]. Others have participated in clinical trials demonstrating the efficacy of their techniques in patients with advanced disease[2]. Health-care professionals who specialize in lymphoedema management or myofascial techniques may already have considerable experience with medically complex, terminally ill patients, as may givers who have worked in acute and sub-acute inpatient facilities.

Physical Medicine & Rehabilitation (PM&R), also called Physiatry or Rehabilitation Medicine is the primary medical specialty responsible for the provision of rehabilitation services in the USA. Board certification has been available since 1948 for physicians who complete 4 years of post-graduate specialty training and pass both written and oral competency examinations[3]. In the USA, Rehabiliation Medicine specialists who can document at least 2 years or 100 h of participation in a palliative care team and involvement in the care of at least 50 palliative care patients will be eligible for subspecialty certification in palliative care (until 2012) without completion of a formal palliative care fellowship. After 2012 completion of a palliative care fellowship will be necessary to achieve dual board certification.

Some, but not all, of the traditional members of the interdisciplinary rehabilitation team continue to provide services as patients transfer from active treatment to palliative care (Table 16.1.1).

Table 16.1 The rehabilitation team by discipline.

Rehabilitation Medicine Specialist	Rehabilitation psychologist
Rehabilitation Nurse	Prosthetist/Orthotist
Physiotherapist (PT)	Recreational therapist
Occupational Therapist (OT)	Adaptive driving specialist
Speech and swallowing Therapist (ST)	Music therapist
Speech/communication	Art therapist
Language/cognition	Horticultural therapist
Swallowing	Pastoral carer/Chaplain
Respiratory therapist	Vocational rehabilitator counsellors
Social worker	DME Vendor

The level of training and competency-based certification required for the delivery of rehabilitation team services varies between countries. In the USA, physiotherapists (PTs) complete a 2-year master's level degree programme or 3-year doctorate but can delegate some of their active treatment to physiotherapy assistants (PTAs) or restorative aides. Physiotherapists are asked to attend to issues of strength, endurance and mobility. This includes wheelchair skills and other adaptive mobility as well as gait training on increasingly challenging surfaces for ambulatory patients. Programmes should be tailored to reflect the environmental challenges of the home, such as stairs to enter, size of home, location of bed, bathroom modifications, etc. Transfers from wheelchair to car, van, or adapted vehicle should be reviewed. For patients with gradual but inexorably progressive disability from diseases such as muscular dystrophy (MD) or progressive multiple sclerosis (MS), purchase or lease of a vehicle with full wheelchair carrying capacity may be a sound and meaningful investment. Easy transportation helps patients to continue working with their medical team for symptom management or treatment of reversible complications but also makes it possible for patients to participate in a much wider variety of family and community activities.

Occupational therapists (OTs) may treat isolated upper extremity impairments or focus on essential functional activities such as dressing, bathing, toileting, and self feeding. Many use validated cognitive assessment tools regularly, such as the Boston Diagnostic Aphasia Examination, a modified Token Test, the Wisconsin Card Sorting Test or parts of the Wechsler Adult Intelligence Scale, during their initial patient assessment and, if indicated, at subsequent times[4]. OT assessment of cognitive function and the impact of any impairment on patient function becomes especially vital when the treating team does not have easy access to speech and language therapists (SLPTs) or quantitative neuropsychologists. The longer battery of testing offered by neuropsychologists may exceed the endurance of terminally ill patients and offers more nuanced, detailed information than might be needed for patients who are not, for the most part, anticipating returning to work or school. Often tools with fewer items, administered by occupational or speech language therapists can provide the rehabilitation team with adequate information about patient cognition. Accurate cognitive assessment enables the selection and tailoring of realistic rehabilitation goals and interventions. It may be necessary for explaining to caregivers that 24-h supervision will be necessary to care for a specific patient. Earlier in gradually progressing diseases, the input of quantitative neuropsychologists may be used by patients who

want to learn strategies for limiting the effect of emerging cognitive deficits. In other situations, neuropsychologists may be asked to help differentiate the memory and attention deficits stemming from untreated depression or anxiety, from symptoms of progressive dementia or other reversible and irreversible causes of cognitive decline. Physicians on the patient's team may want to use this information to initiate pharmacological management of anxiety, attentional, and arousal deficits as well as mood disorders. Neuropsychometric data may be needed to persuade patients to handover financial or legal affairs to designated executors, or conversely, to persuade family members that the patient is still able to manage for themselves. Supportive psychotherapists and counsellors are too well appreciated within palliative care to warrant discussion here but are also core members of all but the sparsest rehabilitation teams. Rehabilitation psychologists have extensive experience in discussing loss of function, acceptance of disability and illness experience with patients but may need to adjust to the impact of treating terminally ill and actively dying patients.

During the 1970s the field of OT expanded its toolbox for promoting function by introducing dance, music, horticulture, and comparable therapy programmes. Graduates from these programmes are frequently employed by palliative caregivers along with other allied health professionals, such as massage therapists and meditation teachers. Integration of patients' spiritual beliefs are central to both palliative and rehabilitation medicine. Pastoral care representatives are often active on general rehabilitation units as well as in palliative care programmes and can use these tandem roles to improve collaboration between specialists. Other members of the traditional rehabilitation team can help maximize QOL and minimize burden of care for patients with advanced disease. Physiatrists, PTs, and OTs will also often work closely with DME suppliers to select optimal adaptive equipment for patients developing progressive dependence at home. These can include automatic lifts, bathing, and toileting aides and wheelchairs as well as smaller items that facilitate autonomy with self care (e.g. reachers, buttonhole assists, sock donners).

Funding in the USA for all level of rehabilitation services is achieved through a mixture of reimbursable services, philanthropically supported care and private payment. Social workers and case managers promote access to care by facilitating communication among payers, patients, and prescribers. They often assist families in applying for small financial grants from the American Cancer Society to pay for home-care equipment need or transportation benefits to and from a rehabilitation centre. Some local health-care system both in the USA and other countries, may make certain rehabilitation services more readily available to palliative care patients than others.

Despite the enormous overlap between members of the palliative care team and the general rehabilitation team, certain distinctions need to be respected when asking rehabilitation specialists to treat palliative care patients. Rehabilitation has traditionally been associated with the restoration of function, which may not be possible in the palliative population. Rehabilitation resources are allocated preferentially to those for whom they will provide the greatest and most enduring benefits and less to persons with progressive disabilities and starkly limited life expectancy. Nonetheless, PM&R has a strong history of contributing to the maintenance of dignity and autonomy at the end of life. During the 1960s, John Dietz, MD created one of the first cancer rehabilitation programmes through a collaboration between Memorial Sloan-Kettering Hospital and the Rusk Institute of New York University. Dietz is best remembered for introducing a widely used, four-track model for the rehabilitation of patients with cancer:

1 preventive;

2 restorative;

3 supportive; and

4 palliative[5].

Dietz's fourth track, palliative, produced a mandate to provide rehabilitation services tailored to patients with advanced disease. The efficacy of rehabilitation services at the end of life has been studied mostly among cancer patients, but Rehabiliation Medicine Specialists and therapists have also garnered experience with the application of rehabilitation interventions for patients with end-stage cardiac, neuro-degenerative, pulmonary, or renal disease, frailty syndromes or other progressive disability.

Palliative care patients can obtain comprehensive rehabilitation evaluations through several avenues. In well-served areas, patients may already have productive, working relationships with rehabilitation specialists from earlier phases in their disease processes. If not, direct consultations can be requested for patients hospitalized prior to or following transition to a palliative care plan. The primary treating team may request a Rehabilitation Medicine consultation for a comprehensive approach, addressing all associated impairments and resulting disability, or they may choose to prescribe therapeutic interventions administered by PTs, OTs, speech language and respiratory therapists, music therapists, and psychologists. While many of these treatments can be initiated directly by patients and their families in the community, they usually require medical staff to drive requests in a hospital setting. Rehabilitation Medicine specialists will focus on functional goals for patients and will advocate for more aggressive treatment of symptoms that limit functional participation. Patient haemoglobin levels below 9 g/dl, for instance, may be acceptable to palliative care team members if they do not produce symptomatic breathlessness, tachycardia, or hypotension. However, Rehabilitation Medicine Specialists may find themselves advocating for palliative transfusions of blood products or judicious use of erythropoietin for what they see as a reversible cause of suboptimal patient function and endurance.

Integration of PM&R specialists, therapists, and other rehabilitation service givers in palliative care programmes occurs more easily in the centralized setting of an inpatient hospital. Rehabilitation Medicine Specialists can serve as standing members of palliative care teams and therapists can be asked to develop particular expertise in the treatment of a greater volume of patients with advanced disease. Several large, well-organized cancer centres in the USA and Europe have established successful in-house rehabilitation programmes to meet the needs of their patients throughout the disease continuum. These centres have produced clinical research on the efficacy and safety of rehabilitation treatments in advanced disease and have served as training programmes for more than two generations of rehabilitation specialists interested in end-of-life care[6] Smaller cancer centres have sought to follow suit by funding part-time positions for Rehabilitation Medicine Specialists, or paying for specialized training for therapy staff. The presence of

rehabilitation specialists on palliative care teams is often reassuring to patients and their families at a time when they feel restorative services may be withdrawn prematurely.

In some cases, palliative care patients may require separate admission to an inpatient rehabilitation programme. In the USA, such admissions are funded with the expectation that they will enable a terminally ill patient to return to home and not proceed to another type of institutional care. If further residential care is anticipated, rehabilitation services should be pursued at that location. Short, targeted rehabilitation stays for palliative care patients may be entirely for family or care-giver training, with little expectation of independent functional gains by the patient. In other cases, a combination of functional gains and caregiver training are used to ensure safety, decrease burden of care and maximize independence for patients returning home. Maximal functional restoration enhances independence and psychological stability for palliative care patients, while reducing the risk of medical co-morbidities associated with falls, deconditioning and compromised self care. Rehabilitation units associated with cancer centres have often accumulated decades of expertise in designing realistic and effective treatment plans for patients towards the end of life. In some countries, free-standing inpatient rehabilitation facilities (IRF) that wish to begin treating palliative care patients may need to reinforce programme development with educational opportunities for staff who may not have as much experience in treating patients with advanced disease. The psychological demands of working with patients and their families towards the end-of-life need to be addressed as well, particularly for staff who may have chosen rehabilitation because it was a part of health care that focuses on survivorship and recovery. Some rehabilitation facilities may want to enhance around-the-clock medical and nursing services to provide an appropriate level of care for those patients who may have increasing symptom control requirements. Lack of around-the-clock services may result in acute rehospitalization for patients who have already expressed the wish to complete their care at home.

Inpatient rehabilitation programmes can be offered at various levels of intensity. In the USA, IRF stays may only be reimbursed if they provide a minimum of 3 h of specific rehabilitation services a day with documented need for daily medical supervision. IRFs are designed to offer patients access to concentrated services that would otherwise be difficult to obtain and coordinate. Neuropsychologists, speech language therapists, rehabilitation certified nurses and, in some cases, orthotists, prosthetists and equipment vendors work with the treating Rehabiliation Medicine Specialist to return patients to the community. Sub-acute programmes and skilled nursing facilities (SNF) offer access to some rehabilitation services but for 1–2 h a day in a sub-acute rehabilitation programme and as needed, but for rarely more than one hour daily in a SNF setting. Some SNFs are able to provide longer term care if a patient is ultimately unable to return to a community setting for medical or social reasons.

Rehabilitation services are provided routinely as part of home care for patients with many diagnoses and should not be denied to patients due to disease stage. Home services have the advantage of tailoring functional solutions and home programmes for the environment where the patient spends most of their time. The goals of treatment in the home setting focus on the essentials of self care, transfers, household ambulation, ascending and descending stairs and perhaps some early community re-entry. If higher level goals, including vocational reintegration, remain realistic, patients should be reassessed by the prescribing physician for possible referral to an outpatient therapy centre. For patients, with reduced function, PTs and OTs can provide home assessments and direction for effective management.

Strength, endurance and functional performance gains can be achieved or maintained through supervised home programmes. Therapists should encourage patients and caregivers to become independent, with home exercise programmes reserving skilled therapy benefits for episodes in the disease trajectory when further declines in function warrant reassessment and the introduction of new or different rehabilitation interventions. For patients able to leave their homes, Rehabilitation Medicine outpatient visits every 4–8 weeks serve as opportunities for readjusting the overall rehabilitation treatment plan during disease progression. Symptom management including neurolytic procedures for excess spasticity, trigger point injections, advanced wound care and pharmacological pain management are available through most outpatient Rehabilitation Medicine practices. Patients with metastatic bone lesions, hemi- or paraparesis may require customized wheelchairs. Improperly selected seating systems can, for instance, result in skin breakdown as well as reduced performance. Most rehabilitation centres offer skilled medical equipment selection with medical justification for requested components. The introduction of new equipment often requires a period of supervised training for patients and caregivers. Rehabilitation centres should be able to coordinate delivery of these services through outpatient as well as home visits.

Patients who are, at least initially, able to seek rehabilitation services at an outpatient facility should be encouraged to do so. In many cases the intensity and complexity of PT and OT treatment available in an outpatient practice far exceeds what can be delivered in the home. Symptom-focused treatments such as complex decongestive therapy (CDT) for lymphoedema are usually offered in outpatient clinics, although home visits can be arranged. Palliative care patients may draw inspiration from their own functional gains and those of other patients at an outpatient centre. They may also find that the more intense programme and the energy expended in travel becomes too difficult as disability accrues. At such times of transition, outpatient therapists and treating Rehabilitation Medicine Specialists should ensure that patients and their caregivers are equipped with a realistic, home-based maintenance programme.

In the final stages of end-of-life care, the role of rehabilitation services evolves. Goals shift towards preventing injury and the safe delivery of dependent care rather than emphasizing functional independence. Positioning, maintenance of skin integrity, pain control, continence, and safe alimentation become priorities. Therapists may return briefly to teach a previously ambulatory patient and their caregivers wheelchair skills or proper use of mechanical lifts (Fig. 16.1). The impact of rehabilitation services for patients at inpatient hospices has not been widely evaluated, however. Yoshioka's 1994 study showed functional gains and improved patient and family satisfaction associated with PT services in an inpatient hospice[7].

Integrative medicine practitioners can also address some of the rehabilitation needs of patients with advanced disease. Today's

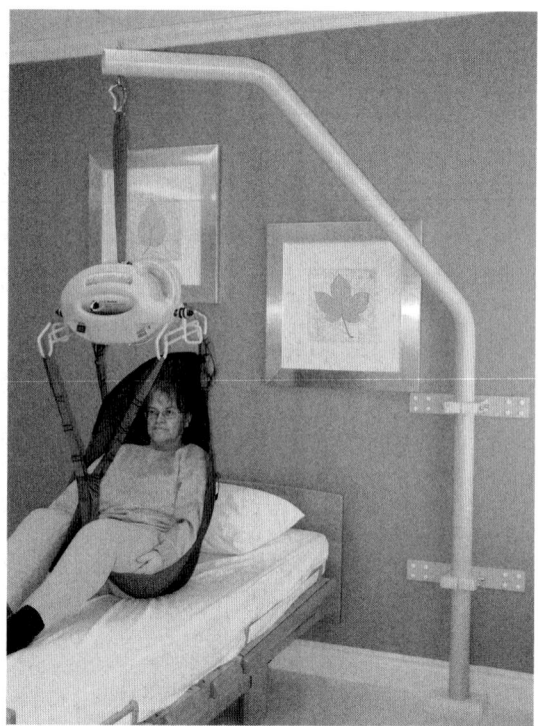

Figure 16.1 Mechanical lift 562724 (with courtesy: Sammons Preston: A Paterson Medical Co).

patients benefit from several decades-worth of collaborative practice between rehabilitation medicine specialists and integrative, complementary or alternative medicine departments. The holistic model embraced by integrative practitioners is shared by rehabilitation specialists, as are specific interventions including acupuncture, many manual or myofascial treatments, movement therapies, and relaxation techniques. Rehabiliation Medicine Specialists and therapists who have experience with complementary modalities can explain the risks and benefits of available treatments. They should also be familiar with certification requirements for various givers and, if possible, be able to provide the names and addresses of local practitioners who have the training and experience needed for the treatment of patients with advanced disease. Receiving treatment for pain management or musculoskeletal symptoms in the less medical environment of an integrative care centre, spa, or private clinic is often a welcome relief for patients who may have completed challenging months or years of aggressive medical treatment.

Bodywork is offered internationally under many rubrics. Some approaches require greater patient participation such as therapeutic yoga or Feldenkrais training, while others, such as massage, permit a more passive role. At a minimum, massage refers to the manipulation of superficial muscle groups and tissue. Certain techniques achieve deeper effects through specialized strokes or manoeuvres. Massage contributes to rehabilitation goals by direct mechanical effects as well as reflexive and psychological effects. The mechanical effects include the mobilization of oedema within soft tissue and improvements in vascular perfusion. The term *reflexive effect* is used to describe the influence of cutaneous stimulation on the autonomic nervous system and the spinal cord. The psychological benefits of massage therapy are reflected in the subjective sense of relaxation and well-being experienced during and after treatment. The rediscovery of the body as a source of pleasurable and positive input is particularly important for patients who may have come to see their physical bodies as burdensome and disappointing. Revival of a more positive mind–body connection is essential for encouraging ongoing efforts at compassionate self care and self efficacy in patients requiring palliative care services.

More participatory forms of bodywork, such as Feldenkrais, Trager psychophysical integration, or the application of Alexander Technique, address pain and functional deficits by treating underlying systemic dysfunction. Some mechanical low back pain, for instance, can be understood as the result of musculoskeletal malalignment during gait and at rest. The Feldenkrais method achieves its goals by increasing conscious awareness of bodily positioning and movement habits. This may be extremely important for patients seeking to limit painful and functional side effects of new hemiparesis or increased tone. Other techniques seek to relieve physical symptoms through a combination of bodily, emotional, and cognitive interventions. Trager psychophysical integration uses gentle mobilization via rhythmic oscillations and rocking with the intention of affecting the subconscious mind as well as the body. Bodyworkers in any tradition should be able to supply patients and their physicians with literature outlining the nature of the treatment they are proposing.

While many types of bodywork require one-to-one giver–patient sessions several movement therapies can be delivered in a group or class setting. Qigong and Tai Chi can offer low impact, minimal resistance programmes that improve balance, strength, and endurance[8]. Modified yoga positions can make the benefits of this several thousand-year-old movement therapy available to even the most medically compromised patients[9].

Relaxation-orientated therapies act synergistically with rehabilitation interventions. Anxiety causes many palliative care patients to limit their activities leading to a cycle of deconditoning and decreased capacity that precipitates further anxiety. Diminished anxiety and depression improves patients' ability to retain and apply rehabilitative strategies during functional tasks and has been shown to correlate with improved function and QOL markers[10]. Cancer and other palliative care centres often subsidize formal relaxation programmes for patients who may lack the resources to pay privately. In other cases, friends and family members can be encouraged to obtain massage treatment or other gift vouchers for palliative care patients during the final stages of illness. Lay and professional treatment givers must be familiar with and comfortable with weight-bearing, spinal, cardiac, and other precautions that may be indicated for a given patient. Many rehabilitation interventions that are used safely in other patient populations, carry increased risk of injury for patients with advanced disease. However, many of these complications can also occur spontaneously. Pathological fractures, for instance, can occur when a patient reaches in bed or repositions. Armed with this information patients and givers may choose to proceed with interventions that will improve function and QOL, even if there is accompanying risk. Risks, such as the ones inherent in the remobilization of patients with known bony metastases should be discussed prior to the initiation of treatment. Physicians caring for the patient should be able to provide guidelines and precautions for weight-bearing status, range of motion, cardiovascular parameters, and other limitations if indicated.

Throughout the disease trajectory, direct and indirect constraints influence the delivery of rehabilitation services for palliative care patients. Transportation is often a problem for patients who could benefit from outpatient services. In some health-care systems, the cost of an eight session course of treatment may be unmanageable for patients whose income may have been reduced by progressive disability. In the USA, patients who elect to have hospice care are often allocated a relatively finite amount of funding, only a small portion of which can be responsibly spent on rehabilitation services or even more sophisticated DME.

Section II: assessment of needs, timing and integration of interventions and goal setting

Assessment

A strong association between functional status and health-related quality of life (HRQOL) has been established for many disease states. This association is particularly well-documented for cancer patients. As a result, almost all QOL metrics used for cancer patients (e.g. EORTC-QLQ-C30, Functional Assessment of Cancer Treatment (FACT), Functional Living Index Cancer (FLIC) and Cancer Rehabilitation Evaluation System (CARES) specifically measure function[11–14]. Studies have shown that in some cultural settings, functional decline undermines cancer patients' QOL to the point that they may engage in passive suicidal ideation and ultimately express interest in physician-assisted suicide[15–17]. In fact, functional status was among the strongest predictors of desire for hastened death and pursuit of euthanasia in several studies[17,18]. Cancer patients wish to remain functionally autonomous. Eighty-eight per cent of 301 hospice inpatients expressed a strong desire to recover independent mobility[19]. An equally robust study showed that, 'loss of ability to do what one wants', was rated highest among end-of-life concerns[20].

Cancer patients with advanced disease express interest in receiving rehabilitation services and generally find them useful. For example, over 80 per cent of patients with advanced breast cancer and Karnofsky Performance Scores (KPS) between 40 and 50, expressed interest in receiving therapy to improve their mobility[21]. Similarly, 70 per cent of hospice patients found conventional physiotherapy to be 'useful' with almost two-thirds describing it as 'highly effective'[22]. Empirical evidence indicates that substantial improvement can be achieved in multiple domains including mobility, self-care, vocational capacity, and communication[23]. Reports describe improved outcomes in both inpatient and outpatient settings with patients with central nervous system involvement making functional gains comparable to those of patients with similar impairments of ischaemic and traumatic origin[24,25,26]. Hospice inpatients can improve their mobility indices through standard rehabilitation therapies[27]. Prevention and mitigation of functional decline through the proactive use of rehabilitation has been demonstrated in patients with inexorably progressive conditions, such as AIDS prior to the availability of effective treatment, progressive MS, and other advanced disease states[28,29,30]. Similar functional and QOL improvement should be achievable for a proportion of cancer patients as well as those with less well-studied disease processes.

Timing

Joann Lynn and her colleagues have identified trajectories of functional decline in cancer and other illnesses[31]. Trajectories are generally characterized by an extended period during which functional capacity remains almost at baseline, with several episodes of transient decline in response to disease progression, recurrence or major disease-modifying therapies. The final phase in advanced disease is often characterized by a dramatic drop in function in the final year or months of life, with marked physical dependency. A significant proportion of patients with terminal disease are elderly, which means that their functional reserve is more likely already to have been reduced by medical co-morbidities. Many patients arrive at the terminal phase of their disease trajectory having already acquired associated or independent neuropathies, cognitive deficits, and degenerative arthropathies that place them at risk of abrupt decline. Although many patients are poised for severe functional problems, determining when to intervene is not always self evident.

The timing of rehabilitation within the complex management of advanced disease is a particularly challenging and under-researched issue. Ideally, rehabilitation integrates restorative, supportive, preventative, and palliative strategies in a concerted fashion that allows patients to retain maximum autonomy for as long as possible. In order to achieve this, effective treatments must be delivered expeditiously to patients when they are able to derive the greatest benefits. Several barriers prevent the realization of this seemingly straightforward mandate. (1) Clinicians caring for patients with advanced disease are not necessarily familiar with either the substance or potential benefits of rehabilitation interventions. Consequently, reliable local referral patterns are not always established[32]. (2) Non-rehabilitation clinicians are less likely to screen patients routinely for functional decline. When functional evaluation is not a component of routine care, disability generally receives clinical attention only late in its course, when interventions tend to be less effective. (3) Clinicians may believe that at the stage of illness when disease modifying therapies are of no further benefit, rehabilitation has similarly little to offer. Ultimately, many non-rehabilitation clinicians have difficulty determining accurately who, when, and why to refer for rehabilitation evaluation and services.

Patient-related barriers also impede the timely involvement of rehabilitation services. Function is a broad and multi-dimensional concept that most patients are not accustomed to discussing with their medical caregivers. Until mobility or activity of daily living (ADL) performance is in imminent danger, patients may not bring their difficulties to clinicians' attention[33]. Patients may consider functional decline an inevitable and irremediable consequence of their conditions and therefore not worth mentioning. Because most rehabilitation interventions require active and ongoing patient participation, patient and support system 'buy in' is essential. Patients must appreciate the need for rehabilitation, recognize future benefit in the process and perceive meaning in its goals. This level of patient endorsement may occur only after significant functional decline when patients confront dependency. Unfortunately, data from non-terminal populations suggest that once patients become significantly debilitated, rehabilitation is more demanding and the gains from treatment may be fewer.

The situation is exacerbated by the fact that little time during outpatient visits is devoted to the discussion of emerging disability.

Inpatient hospitalizations appear to provide a better opportunity for overcoming this obstacle with a 559 (95 per cent CI, 187–1670) odds ratio favouring detection of physical impairments in an inpatient as opposed to an outpatient setting[34]. As delivery of care shifts increasingly to the outpatient setting, the need for effective communication both between patients and caregivers, as well as patients and their physician will be essential if disability is to be addressed effectively. Failure to address cumulative disability results in patients living at lower levels of function and experiencing more difficulty and distress than is necessary.

Factors inherent in functional decline and its measurement also aggravate the problem. Often functional decline in terminal conditions, such as cancer, cardiac disease, and COPD is insidiously progressive without the abrupt changes that herald the need for intervention[35]. We do not have definitive data that indicate at what points along the trajectory of functional decline rehabilitation involvement will do the most good. At present, characterizing the magnitude and rate of patients' decline is a challenge. Current functional metrics lack sensitivity across the broad range of performance seen among patients with advanced disease. Patients' baseline function, from which they subsequently decline, is also highly variable. Difficulty with an ADL such as dressing or bathing may reflect a drastic and precipitous decline for some patients and virtually no change for others.

It is usually neither fiscally nor logistically possible to have all palliative care patients evaluated by a rehabilitation physician. Even if it were, functional status changes constantly in patients with advanced disease, often creating an entirely new collection of problems within months, if not weeks, after evaluation. Nonetheless, early intervention allows physical impairments to be treated in an efficient manner without excessive cost. For this reason, elderly patients, or those with multiple co-morbidities and/or a disability at baseline, should be referred for more extensive assessment of their rehabilitation needs. At the very least, such referrals establish a relationship between patients and a rehabilitation team that can be developed in the future. The timing for referral of patients without these risk factors can be based on the following guidelines:

- any ADL difficulty;

- any new or significant instrumental activity of daily living (IADL) difficulty;

- any difficulty with household or conservative community mobility;

- any new or significant deterioration in mobility;

- frail, ill, or disabled caregiver;

- significant change in medical status (e.g. diagnosis with brain metastases, episode of ventilator dependency, pathological fracture); and

- symptom (e.g. pain, dyspnoea) interference with function.

Goal setting: foundation, components, and barriers
Foundation

The link between physical impairment and disability has been studied in different populations with advanced disease. In stage IV breast cancer, for example, leading physical impairments include paraplegia, steroid myopathy, and joint pains[36]. These impairments are generally related to disease progression and changes in treatment and may be associated with abrupt functional decline in the absence of rehabilitation interventions. Pleural or pulmonary compromise can undermine acutely aerobic reserve leading to severe exertional intolerance. Malignant lesions, particularly bone metastases, can undermine the essential supporting structures of the musculoskeletal system. Non-surgical, anti-cancer treatments, including radiotherapy and chemotherapy, can produce disability by injuring muscles and nerves. Additional sources of functional decline have been identified. Cross-sectional studies in cohorts with advanced lung cancer have demonstrated correlations between fatigue, pain, and functional status[37]. Pain also correlates strongly with function in other cancer cohorts[38,39]. Breakthrough pain (BTP), defined as transient increases above baseline that warrant analgesic use, has been identified as an important cause of compromised functional status[40,41]. Unfortunately, the available cross-sectional studies did not isolate aetiological factors so it remains unclear whether a confounding factor such as unstable bone or dural metastases could be responsible for both pain and poor function. To date, longitudinal studies which may allow more precise characterization of the genesis of disability in advanced disease are still lacking.

The degree to which pain and fatigue create disability in advanced disease has immediate and practical implications. It has been shown that 75–95 per cent of cancer pain can be controlled through non-invasive means but that these interventions continue to be under-utilized in the home care setting[42–46] Targeting pain not only addresses an important symptom and source of distress but has the additional documented benefit of limiting functional decline. Similar dual efficacy for symptom mitigation and functional preservation or restoration can be achieved by targeting fatigue in patients with advanced disease[47].

Enhancing caregiver–patient communication is essential for the integration of effective rehabilitation approaches into palliative care. Several studies have documented significant barriers to this type of communication[48–51]. One study of the caregivers of cancer patients followed by a palliative care service characterized family communication as 'difficult'. However, this study also found that the challenges of caregiving and illness can enhance family solidarity[52]. Other studies have determined that patients and their families strive to minimize discussion about caregiving preferences and other disability-related issues, partly because of reluctance to confront the patient's impending decline and partly in a perhaps misguided effort to protect one another from psychological stress[53–55]. Studies that have examined communication patterns between patients and physicians and between caregiver and physicians have shown that the needs and desires of patients and caregivers may conflict. In an effort to deny the consequences of their illnesses, patients may attempt to limit discussion with their physicians[56] Studies of caregivers, after patients' deaths, reveal a strikingly different pattern, suggesting that caregivers would prefer more physician communication regarding the patient's illness[57]. These studies indicate that communication preferences cannot be summarized easily. Moreover, they reveal that patients and caregivers may, at times, have diametrically opposed communication needs which in turn can interfere with the selection and implementation of optimal rehabilitation strategies.

In an effort to understand communication challenges at the end of life better, Fried et al. assessed levels of patient and caregiver agreement with statements regarding illness-related communication[58]. Almost 40 per cent of the study cohort (n = 193)

had advanced cancer while the remainder included patients with congestive heart failure and chronic obstructive pulmonary disease. Virtually all patients (88.6 per cent) and caregivers (93.8 per cent) felt that it was important to talk about the patients' illness. Approximately 40 per cent of caregivers desired more communication with patients and found communication difficult. In 33.2 per cent of pairs, the caregiver desired more communication when the patient did not, compared with 13.5 per cent of pairs in which the patient desired more communication when the caregiver did not. Caregivers' desire for increased communication was associated independently with increased caregiver burden, which was measured in terms of emotional distress. Fried's study, the most comprehensive to date regarding patient–caregiver communication, suggests the presence of barriers that stem partially from patients' reluctance to discuss their illness. No studies have extended this examination of communication patterns to focus specifically on discussion of disability in the palliative care setting. As previously stated, this gap is problematic for several reasons: (1) many patients with advanced disease experience significant disability; (2) disability extracts a heavy psychological and fiscal toll on patients and caregivers; (3) when properly addressed, disability can often be mitigated with conventional interventions; (4) successful intervention requires active patient and caregiver participation; (5) this participation requires effective communication for goal setting and for mutual effort. Additional qualitative and quantitative research is needed to facilitate the optimal selection and integration of proven rehabilitation strategies into the delivery of palliative care.

Goal setting: components

Rehabilitation goals should reflect patient age, disease type and stage, medical co-morbidities, baseline fitness level and psychological, social, educational, and financial resources. Dietz's four-part approach to rehabilitation goal setting for cancer patients remains broadly applicable for other patients with progressive disease processes[59]. Deitz described rehabilitation strategies that could achieve four complementary yet distinct function-oriented goals: *preventive, restorative, supportive,* and *palliative.*

Preventive rehabilitation goals seek to avoid the expected impairments that accompany disease progression. Sitting protocols, for example, limit the physiological impact of prolonged bed rest. The positioning of paralysed limbs and pressure relief techniques are other examples of common preventive interventions. Caregiver education is often a highly effective preventative approach. Empowering and informing caregivers can help reduce predictable complications, such as skin breakdown, that result from immobility or unmanaged urinary incontinence.

Restorative rehabilitation has as its goal the return of the patient to his or her premorbid level of functioning when no lasting impairment need occur. Such approaches are often utilized following intensive oncological or other treatment. Pulmonary rehabilitation can be helpful after thoracotomy. Other restorative approaches are used to regain upper extremity strength and range of motion after mastectomy or radiation. Structured progressive aerobic conditioning represents a very effective restorative technique for patients undergoing bone marrow transplantation. It can be used judiciously to allow even patients with progressive disease to recover some portion of their premorbid fitness levels.

Supportive rehabilitation attempts to optimize functioning in patients with irreversible impairments. Supportive programmes include the multi-modal techniques used to rehabilitate patients after limb salvage procedures such as internal hemi-pelvectomy. Combined interventions focusing on strength, endurance, proprioception and balance can create functional ambulatory patterns that compensate for impaired limb and pelvic biomechanics.

Palliative rehabilitation includes supportive approaches designed to reduce patients' dependence in mobility and self-care activities. Emotional reinforcement and comfort should be provided concurrently. There are many opportunities for effective intervention. Preservation of bowel and bladder continence, for example, is an important goal for patients with advanced disease. Incontinence often precipitates profound psychological distress. Simple rehabilitation interventions can often extend patients' ability to toilet independently until the very terminal stages of cancer. Anasarca and progressive lymphoedema are common among end-stage cancer patients. Palliative rehabilitation approaches such as lymphatic drainage techniques and multi-layer compression bandaging can minimize oedema, thereby enhancing patient comfort and mobility. These measures also function preventatively to reduce the likelihood of local skin breakdown and associated infections.

Goal setting: barriers

Uncontrolled pain remains one of the best understood components of functional decline in advanced disease. A sturdy evidence basis for the relationship between pain control and function exists for cancer patients. It is likely that pain plays an important role in the production of disability associated with other terminal conditions but no research initiatives have confirmed this association to date. Integration of rehabilitation specialists in palliative care makes it more likely that movement-related escalation in pain intensity will be identified and managed with pharmacological as well as non-pharmacological interventions. Management of movement-related pain is essential for maintaining functional independence. Movement-related pain is also referred to as incident pain or break through pain. When poorly controlled it contributes to a cycle of decreased activity and decreased functional autonomy. Effective control of activity-associated or incident pain should be incorporated into patients' overall pain management plan and is best accomplished through one prescribing giver with other team members providing recommendations as appropriate to their expertise.

Inadequate pain control will undermine even the most expert rehabilitation efforts. Disease processes that destroy bone, joint, or nerve structures frequently cause pain when the affected structures are recruited for mobility and self-care tasks. When pain increases with weight-bearing or on movement, many patients will respond by limiting activities, including those needed for autonomous mobility and self-care. The resulting deconditioning can and should be avoided through the proactive elimination of incident or activity-associated pain. Lost functional capacity is much harder to restore, particularly in patients with significant disease burden. A proactive approach to baseline and incident pain management thus preserves function as well as contributing to overall HRQOL in patients with advanced disease.

Palliative caregivers and rehabilitation specialists share an interest in achieving pain control in the home setting. Inpatient pain management teams often achieve excellent control of baseline pain but have inadequate opportunity to address movement-related, incident pain. Most patients' situations change dramatically upon discharge. Few can or wish to remain indefinitely in bed with 24-h support. Their activity profiles must change, generally becoming more arduous. If no effort has been expended during the hospitalization to manage pain induced by typical, at-home activities, then a valuable opportunity has been lost. Rehabilitation services can play a vital role is assuring that such opportunities are recognized and exploited in order to provide comprehensive pain management that promotes increased activity. Pharmacological approaches alone may not suffice. For this reason, an iterative process is required whereby interventional and pharmacological analgesic approaches coordinate with rehabilitative efforts, all of which must remain exquisitely responsive to ongoing patient feedback. Patients are active participants in this process. It becomes clear in the chapter's description of rehabilitation interventions that far more than ubjective pain rating is required. Patients and their caregivers must be engaged fully in order to learn and to practise compensatory strategies and perform therapeutic exercises. Sources of poor patient participation must actively be sought and definitely addressed whenever possible.

Rehabilitation's role in controlling incident pain can generally be fulfilled by using the following steps:

1 Ensure that all sources of pain potentially amenable to specific treatments (e.g. spinal cord compression, bone metastases) are addressed.

2 Ensure that baseline or 'at rest' pain is adequately controlled.

3 Ensure that patients have recourse to 'as needed' or 'rescue' analgesic dosing for incident or movement-related pain.

4 Collect a realistic profile of the patient's activities following discharge.

5 Educate patients regarding the general approach and the need to attend carefully to incident or movement-related pain.

6 Trial the full spectrum of activities with current analgesics, soliciting pain ratings for each activity. (Only if no clear history of incident or movement-related pain is available.)

7 If incident or movement-related pain intensity is unacceptable, retrial with proactive use of 'as needed' or 'rescue' analgesics. Depending on the agent's pharmacokinetics, a full hour may be required after ingestion before maximal serum levels are achieved.

8 Retrial painful activities, soliciting pain ratings for each activity.

9 If incident or movement-related pain intensity remains unacceptable, deconstruct painful activities to identify evocative motions and positions.

10 Implement compensatory strategies and determine whether assistive devices and/or orthoses reduce incident pain.

11 Retrial painful activities, particularly when patients are fatigued, and solicit pain ratings for each activity.

12 If pain intensity remains unacceptable, determine which activities provoke pain as well as the intensity, frequency, duration, quality, and location of the pain.

13 If the pain occurs with high frequency, adjustment of patients' baseline regimen may be indicated.

14 If incident or movement-related pain is severe and focal, interventional analgesic approaches may be indicated.

15 Increase 'as needed' medication dosing, change medication and/or add additional medications specifically targeting incident or movement-related pain.

16 Retrial painful activities, soliciting pain ratings for each activity.

17 If incident or movement-related pain intensity remains unacceptable, continue to iteratively refine the 'as needed' analgesic regimen.

The analgesic principles governing management of incident pain have been detailed by several authors elsewhere and in Chapter 10.1[60–62]. The main challenge is in achieving an adequate balance between analgesia and unwanted side effects, especially drowsiness when the patient is at rest. Patients and their caregivers should be educated to assess pain needs throughout the day and time breakthrough medication use appropriately. The negative impact of decreased activity that accompanies overmedication should be explained. All patients started on opioid analgesia should be educated about the need for a concomitant bowel programme and should be instructed in several pharmacological and non-pharmacological management strategies. Efficacy of the accompanying bowel programme should be assessed at each outpatient visit and frequently for patients receiving homecare. Patients and their caregivers should be encouraged to bring inadequate pain control or troublesome side effects to their care team's attention so that adjustments can be made.

Symptoms other than pain routinely undermine patients' function in terminal disease. Dyspnoea, anxiety, nausea, and orthostatic hypotension and other symptoms threaten patients' autonomy. Using an iterative approach similar to that outlined above for pain management, the rehabilitation team can work with patients and their palliative caregivers to ensure that symptoms are controlled during activity. Rehabilitation techniques, compensatory strategies, assistive devices, and orthotics can be used in, for example chronic obstructive pulmonary disease (COPD) in conjunction with supplemental oxygen and inhalers to minimize the effect on the functional performance. Activity-associated anxiety similarly can be managed with behavioural techniques and titration of anxiolytics coupled with rehabilitative strategies. Limiting the functional impact of symptoms requires ongoing assessment by therapists during treatment sessions, effective interdisciplinary communication when control is inadequate and the coordinated efforts of palliative and rehabilitative clinicians.

When multi-disciplinary rehabilitation teams communicate openly and effectively they are marvellous vehicles for realizing patients' potential in an expeditious and humane fashion. However, there are many challenges and actual interactions too often fall short of the ideal usually as a result of lack of time and isolation of specialities. All disciplines struggle with limited time and resources but the latter challenge is more specific to rehabilitation. Each specialty; e.g. rehabilitation physicians and nurses, physical and occupational therapy, is charged with specific tasks. In physicians' cases this includes mediating between the particulars of patients' medical conditions and the rehabilitation process. When physicians fail to keep the team appraised of changes in patients' medical status or when the team fails to alert physicians to changes in patients' performance status the rehabilitation process suffers. Sedation, poorly controlled pain, lack of initiative due to depression, unrecognized instability of a bone and dyspnoea will undermine rehabilitation efforts but can often be mediated with

medical and rehabilitation interventions[63,64]. Physical and occupational therapists cannot promote or preserve function in the absence of comprehensive pharmacological and non-pharmacological symptom control. At the same time, physicians must monitor their patients' functional progress, or lack thereof, in order to determine when additional interventions may be needed. The importance of ongoing and effective communication between all team members cannot be overemphasized. Infrastructure and practice patterns that support effective communication should be cultivated constantly. For all palliative care in addition to hospice patients, this requires strong representation of rehabilitation services in home-care networks, as well as throughout a range of inpatient facilities.

Medical team leaders for palliative care patients are expected to coordinate with other medical specialties and to share changes in treatment plan or prognoses with givers of rehabilitation services, as these clearly impact on rehabilitation goals, the discharge and future equipment needs. The rehabilitation team can deploy its resources most effectively when equipped with current and accurate medical information concerning individual patient status.

Section IV: rehabilitation strategies for specific palliative care populations

Ideally, rehabilitation interventions in palliative care constitute a new stage in an ongoing integration of rehabilitation services that may have begun with the initial diagnosis or treatment of the patient's underlying disease. Patients who arrive at a palliation-only phase in their disease process, without previous access to rehabilitation services, are no less able to benefit from carefully selected rehabilitation interventions designed to maintain or, in some cases even restore, key elements of independent function. Preservation of function is central to a sense of autonomy for many patients. Lost ability to 'do what one wants' has been identified as a leading concern of patients and caregivers at the end of life[65]. At times, fear of progressive disability and dependence on others exceeds fear of impending death[66]. It is equally notable that loss of function contributes to painful and costly medical complications such as pressure ulcers, falls, and accompanying fractures. Many of the rehabilitation strategies used to reduce the impairments and disability produced by acute and chronic illness offer significant benefit for patients with advanced disease. In the USA, inpatient rehabilitation units develop treatment plans based on the six functional domains for FIM scores. These are mobility, self care, sphincter control (bowel and bladder), communication, and social cognition including social interaction, problem solving, and memory. Goals in these areas can be assigned by any member of the treatment team and discrepancies should be resolved in interdisciplinary team meetings and with input from the patient and their caregivers. Rehabilitation specialists working with patients who are still able to attend outpatient clinics may find themselves operating more independently, but should make every effort to share their treatment plans with all members of the extended treatment team. Although rehabilitation services can be obtained on an ad hoc basis, patient needs are best served when specific rehabilitation specialists are consistently part of a palliative care team. Medically-trained rehabilitation specialists assist in the selection of appropriate goals for patients by combining knowledge of rehabilitation potential with an understanding of the underlying disease processes. In many cases they may be able to diagnose and treat disease-related impairments that result in disability.

Rehabilitation of palliative care patients with motor deficits

Specific myopathies as well as neurologically mediated motor weakness occur in many patients with advanced disease. Progressive dystrophies, such as Duchenne's muscular dystrophy or fascio-scapular-humeral dystrophy, create an increasing reliance on compensatory strategies and adaptive devices for many years prior to a final or more complete phase of dependence. Patients with these diagnoses and their families have experienced a gradual loss of function over time and may have a wealth of knowledge and equipment that can be built on, as needs progress. Other patients experience more abrupt onset of motor deficits when vertebral metastases result in paraparesis or a metastatic brain lesion causes dense haemiplegia. Almost all patients also experience a more generalized loss of motor function due to the complex interaction of cardiovascular, nutritional and musculoskeletal changes associated with prolonged bedrest or other precipitents of deconditioning. Understanding the aetiology and physiology of impairments that contribute to motor deficits is essential to optimizing rehabilitation interventions.

Certain impairment groups have been the subject of more extensive clinical research. Paraparesis and, to a lesser extent, tetraparesis from malignant spinal cord compression (SCC) occur relatively commonly in patients with advanced cancers. In the USA, extensive experience with traumatic spinal cord injury (SCI) through the federally-funded model systems programme enables many rehabilitation teams to effectively address the functional needs of comparably impaired palliative care patients with a minimum of retraining or programme development. Palliative care populations with SCC require careful modification of SCI protocols as they have different life expectancies and co-morbidities. Shared goals include strengthening the paralysed patient's ability to direct care, integration of compensatory strategies and adaptive equipment and acceptance of realistic goals based on physiological as well as social and environmental constraints. Unlike complete traumatic SCI, the restoration of motor function in cancer-related SCC is thought to occur in proportion to the duration of deficits prior to treatment usually with radiation or surgery[67]. In many cases, surgical intervention for very new onset SCC, even in older patients with advanced cancer, preserves lower extremity function for as much as 6 months to a year, whereas comparable interventions in younger traumatic SCI may offer little chance of benefit. The higher incidence of co-morbidities including irradiated skin and simultaneous disease progression, however, may limit the functional restoration of systemically ill patients, even if the cause of their myelopathy can be addressed effectively.

Patients with intracranial processes resulting in motor weakness benefit greatly from the vast experience rehabilitation specialists have with stroke and brain injury patients. Studies comparing specifically the outcomes of terminally ill patients with intracranial lesions who receive rehabilitation services with the outcomes achieved for stroke patients have consistently shown comparable performance in multiple domains but with cancer patients having a higher rate of interruption of services due to medical complications[68].

Patients with pure upper motor neuron or mixed upper and lower motor neuron involvement often have increased tone or spasticity that may benefit from neurolytic or pharmacological interventions. Local injections of phenol or botulinum toxin can be used to prevent contractures and joint deformities for patients with advanced disease states as can passive range of motion and splinting programmes.

Lower motor neuron impairments result in more focal motor deficits producing a flaccid paralysis, although leptomeningeal disease and certain non-oncological diagnoses can produce more diffuse patterns of lower motor neuron weakness. Lower motor neuron lesions require greater attention to bracing and positioning, to limit pain or further injury to the affected body parts. Understanding the aetiology and pathophysiology of the motor weakness again directs the selection of rehabilitation interventions. The functional benefits of increased tone that can be used to assist with transfers for patients with upper motor lesions is absent in lower motor injury. Earlier introduction of assistive devices rather than pure compensatory strategies may be required. A universal cuff (Fig. 16.2) for holding utensils, grooming, and hygiene aids can improve significantly autonomy for patients with hand weakness from a tumour-related compression of the C8 and T1 nerve roots. A balanced forearm orthosis (Fig. 16.3) enhances upper extremity function for patients with compromised proximal strength but preserved dexterity. Orthotics may be introduced to stabilize vulnerable joints, although their added weight can be counterproductive in the setting of significant weakness. Isolated 'foot drop' or anterior tibialis weakness can be treated with dynamic or static ankle–foot orthoses (AFO) depending on clinical presentation. In some cases enhanced knee control can be achieved, despite quadriceps, or hamstring weakness, by altering the degree of dorsiflexion or plantarflexion specified in the orthotic prescription. Orthoses can be extended to encompass the knee (KAFO) but the added weight and cumbersome profile limits their utility. The probable co-presence of more proximal hip flexor or gluteal weakness in these cases further diminishes the likelihood of effective bracing for purposes of ambulation. Nonetheless, distal stabilization with a solid and supportive AFO may facilitate transfers, even in a patient with flaccid hemiplegia, while also providing some degree of joint protection.

Instruction in compensatory strategies enables patients with motor deficits to remain mobile and accomplish self-care activities. Patients are taught to capitalize on the strength of preserved muscle groups and to modify posture and body mechanics to minimize the secondary complications that result from focal weakness. Appropriately selected assistive devices also facilitate mobility and self care for patients with motor deficits. Reachers, for instance, permit partially paralysed patients to retrieve objects while other devices reduce the amount of energy expended on specific tasks.

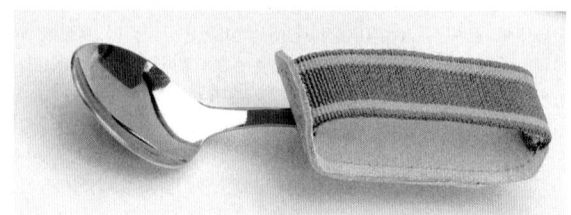

Figure 16.2 Universal cuff 1485 (with courtesy: Sammons Preston: A Patterson Medical Co.).

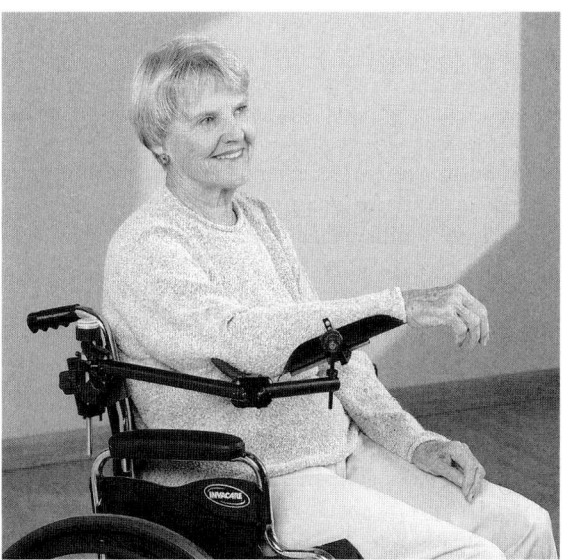

Figure 16.3 Balanced forearm orthosis 71330101 (with courtesy: Sammons Preston: A Patterson Medical Co.).

Investment in more expensive DME, particularly power wheelchairs, presents a challenging dilemma for rehabilitation specialists treating patients with advanced disease. Many practices circumvent some of the payment issues by collaborating with patient advocacy groups to pool devices that can be given to patients, requiring perhaps only the purchase of some customized componentry. The risks of providing imprecisely prescribed DME should not be ignored as improper seat cushioning or positioning, for example, can result in pressure ulcers, contractures, or other complications that may lead to an earlier or more painful death. Early, proactive identification of developing deficits results in the prescription of equipment for more meaningful periods. In these cases, prescribing physicians and suppliers should incorporate the expectation of further functional decline into the selection of components. Many amyotrophic lateral sclerosis (ALS)/motor neuron disease clinics, for instance, begin by providing power wheelchairs with patient-controlled toggle-steering initially, but with the ability to convert to a companion control, as many patients will lose the ability to operate the device safely.

Rehabilitation strategies for sensory deficits

Sensory deficits may be the result of progressive disease such as diabetes, peripheral nerve impingement by tumour, or neurotoxic effects of previous treatments with radiation or specific chemotherapies. Simultaneous damage to proprioceptive nerve fibres can have enormous functional impact on standing balance, ambulation as well as the dexterity needed for many self-care activities. In some cases, sensory deficits can be expected to subside even in advanced disease, if neurotoxic treatments are stopped or there is tumour response to palliative radiotherapy. The devastating sensory and proprioceptive deficits accompanying advanced diabetes, however, are not reversible.

Protection becomes the primary principle in selection of rehabilitation goals and interventions for patients with sensory deficits. Injury to insensate skin must be avoided at all costs, particularly as healing is often impaired due to a number of factors including nutritional status and overall decreased mobility. All patients with insensate skin and their caregivers should be taught a thorough approach to skin inspection and pressure relief through weight shifts and positioning. Less cosmetically appealing braces such as a double metal upright AFO (Fig. 16.4) may be necessary as in-shoe orthoses easily lead to non-healing wounds. Impaired hand or upper extremity sensation can also lead to non-healing wounds but the relative visibility of these body parts often results in better protection and more prompt treatment. Patients with impaired upper extremity sensation can benefit from consultation with an OT for an introduction to devices that restore some degree of fine motor function in the absence of sensory input. Enlarged utensil handles, buttoners and even sock donners allow independent performance of ADLs despite impaired sensation, especially if visual function is spared.

Increased reliance on visual cues enables patients with proprioceptive deficits to achieve some degree of compensation. In addition, indirect positional information or proprioceptive feedback can be transmitted through assistive devices such as canes and walkers or rollators for patients with primarily lower extremity proprioceptive losses. In addition to proprioceptive feedback, broad-based devices such as walkers/rollators and Zimmer frames provide mechanical stabilization for persons with impaired balance. The risk of injury from a fall requires careful assessment of when to limit ambulation or at least unsupervised ambulation altogether. Many patients achieve greater autonomy and even levels of aerobic activity safely propelling a manual wheelchair rather than walking shorter distances precariously. Nonetheless the goal of 'walking again' often drives patients to select less safe and efficient forms of mobility. Assistive devices, particularly walkers/rollators/ Zimmer frames and wheelchairs can be viewed as publicly embarrassing emblems of disease and declining function. As with the rehabilitation of acute and chronic conditions, rehabilitation in palliative care requires skilful introduction of solutions that may be unpalatable initially. Interdisciplinary rehabilitation teams including rehabilitation psychologists have experience helping patients move from wishing for a cure to making the most of remaining abilities. Frequently, underlying depression needs to be addressed pharmacologically as well as psychotherapeutically

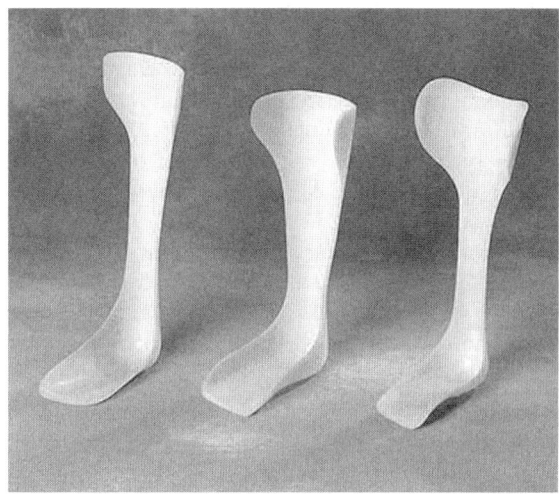

Figure 16.4 Ankle foot orthosis (AFO) A368LSL or 554721012 (with courtesy: Sammons Preston: A Patterson Medical Co.).

before rehabilitation strategies can be integrated effectively. The importance of patient and family being united with professional management is central and is explored more extensively in our concluding remarks.

Rehabilitation for patients with cerebellar dysfunction or movement disorders

Profound mobility and self-care deficits are associated with the cerebellar injuries and movement disorders that occur in several malignancies, including primary brain tumours and paraneoplastic syndromes, specifically ovarian and lung[69,70]. Patients with movement disorders such as parkinsonism or other causes of dysmetria, with or without tremor, may benefit from weighted utensils and assistive devices, particularly as motor strength is often preserved in these conditions. Safety awareness and fall prevention must be emphasized repeatedly as denial and other causes of diminished insight often cause patients with ataxia to underestimate the impact of their deficits. Therapists can build on patients' instinctive protective mechanisms, such as adoption of a widened base of support to establish safe movement patterns. Home and environmental modification can improve safety vastly and prevent falls for all patients with movement disorders, including the more diffuse bradykinesia and loss of protective reflexes seen in advanced dementias. Advanced alcohol-related encephalopathies, hereditary, and non-hereditary spinal cerebellar ataxias, or Huntington's chorea require a sophisticated approach to DME prescription. Wheelchair seating systems, for instance, must be selected to provide maximal postural support without compromising freedom of movement more than necessary. Patient ability to self-propel manually, as well as power mobility may need to be reassessed at intervals. Power mobility settings including speed and responsiveness often can be adjusted to prolong the period of independent mobility in the face of decreasing motor coordination.

Rehabilitation for patients with cranial nerve and mechanical oral motor deficits

Cranial nerve involvement from neoplastic disease, ALS or MS or other diagnoses can have severe medical and social consequences due to disruption of vision, speech, swallowing and management of oral secretions. Collaboration with speech therapists, head and neck surgeons and respiratory therapists may be needed to prevent aspiration pneumonia and insure adequate oxygenation. Dysphagia and odynophagia can easily compromise nutrition, leading to the various functional and medical problems. Compensatory strategies are available for cognitively intact patients with focal swallowing deficits to help avoid tube feedings or restrictive food consistencies.

Dysarthria can be a devastating symptom for patients who experience a decreasing ability to make their needs known during a period of increasing dependence. In certain cases intelligibility can be enhanced through compensatory strategies that increase respiratory support for vocalization, by introducing energy conservation techniques and the use of rest breaks. In other cases, augmentive communication devices from simple picture boards to computer interfaces that permit word or letter selection are more helpful. Family and caregiver education and training is also essential for diffusing some of the inevitable frustration of patients who lose the ability to communicate as part of a terminal illness.

Many, but not all, rehabilitation interventions for visual loss, field cuts, or oculomotor compromise remain effective in the palliative care setting. Few patients are going to learn to read Braille during the terminal phases of a disease but many of the other resources developed for the visually impaired in general, such as recorded books, textured organizational tools, and other adaptive equipment, can be used by persons with diabetic retinopathy, optic chiasm tumours or other diagnoses that impair visual function.

Rehabilitation opportunities for patients with cognitive dysfunction

Cognitive dysfunction complicates many progressive and terminal conditions. These deficits increase caregiver burden, create safety concerns and degrade interpersonal relations. Brain metastases can create focal deficits such as apraxia, alexia, and aphasia that have wide-reaching impact on numerous areas of independent function. Neurodegenerative processes often impair higher level cognitive function, short-term memory, and attention, while also creating disturbances in executive function and emotional control. Treating clinicians need to be very familiar with algorithms for distinguishing reversible from irreversible causes of cognitive dysfunction among palliative care patients. Urinary tract infections, medication effects and other reversible causes of delirium are especially prevalent in medically compromised populations. Non-reversible deficits may resemble the more discrete aphasias associated with specific central nervous system (CNS) lesions or present as more diffuse cognitive slowing and near-somonolence which can occur as a delayed effect of cranial irradiation.

Speech language therapy and cognitive interventions used for stroke and brain injury patients can result in modest but helpful functional gains for terminally ill patients. Memory books and computerized prosthetics as well as pharmacological management of agitation or disrupted sleep–wake cycles can improve overall cognitive performance. Training of family, friends, and caregivers is often necessary to ensure continuity and incorporation of compensatory strategies and other tools. Although time-consuming and only partially effective, these efforts engage patients and their support networks, often creating a sense of helping to make things better at a time that may otherwise be characterized by an overwhelming sense of helplessness and futility.

Rehabilitation strategies for patients with deconditioning

Deconditioning is probably one of the most widespread and, sometimes at least partially, reversible deficits to occur during end-of-life care. Many factors including anaemia, dyspnoea, pain, disrupted sleep, nausea, fatigue, orthostasic hypotension, and malnutrition along with cachexia result in decreased activity tolerance and an accelerating downward spiral of further deconditioning. Rehabilitation interventions for patients with deconditioning in the setting of advanced disease can be divided into approaches that restore or preserve function and those that mitigate the effects of decreased endurance through compensatory strategies and environmental modification.

Therapeutic exercise, particularly for patients with advanced disease, should always be prescribed with careful attention to intensity, modality and duration as well as the clear articulation of necessary precautions. Safe intensities are best understood for patients with advanced cardiac conditions but guidelines are emerging for other diagnoses as well[71]. Realistic goal selection will determine the choice of modalities although optimal programmes generally mix some proportion of flexibility, aerobic, and resistance or strengthening exercises tailored to the patient's current potential. Active and passive range of motion programmes are important for maintaining the ability to achieve comfortable positioning while also preventing pressure ulcers and limiting joint contractures that may impede hygiene, dressing, and other aspects of self care. Therapeutic aerobic programmes in patients with advanced cancer have demonstrated the possibility of physiological as well as functional improvement provided that disease progression does not outstrip training effect. A graded conditioning programme can be prescribed for motivated patients. Studies of the efficacy of resistance training and strengthening programmes in androgen-deprived men with prostate cancer have proven the possibility of maintaining or even improving strength in the context of malignancy[72]. Improved peripheral muscle efficiency often allows patients with pulmonary and cardiac compromise to accomplish more, despite fixed or worsening respiratory and cardiovascular function. Combining strength training with functional activities, such as sit to stand transfers is often an efficient way to design exercise programmes for compromised patients with little time or endurance for multi-modal protocols.

Patient safety and, at times, medical liability require careful delineation of exercise precautions. These should include limitations for patients with thrombocytopenia, weight bearing restrictions for patients with bone metastases or bracing requirements for patients with spinal instability.

Caregiver support

Palliative care has long recognized that effective interventions require attention to the larger context of patient, family and social support networks. As disability accumulates these family and social networks may begin providing an increasing proportion of daily care, particularly when funding for paid care workers is not available or such care is not desired. In their recent analysis of the needs of family caregivers, Rabow, Hauser, and Adams identified five burdens that can overwhelm giver resources: (1) time and logistics; (2) physical tasks; (3) financial costs; (4) emotional and mental health risks; and (5) other health risks[73]. Rehabilitation Medicine and rehabilitation services can reduce if not eliminate several of these burdens through organized caregiver training programmes. Short, focused inpatient rehabilitation stays or intensive teaching prior to discharge from an acute medical service can improve markedly patient safety and decrease caregiver burden. Caregivers should understand the biomechanics of patient transfers that protect both their own and the patient's body. Review of bowel and bladder programmes limits symptomatic and medical complications after discharge and is central to theprotection of sacral skin, the prevention of sacral wounds and minimization of the psychological distress accompanying adult incontinence. Rehabilitation nurses have experience of teaching complex wound care techniques as well as skin protection through pressure relief and positioning. They also teach patients and caregivers proper medication management in the home, including the use of 'as needed' dosing for symptom management. All members of the interdisciplinary team contribute to important goals, such as fall prevention, while select disciplines may focus more on sleep–wake cycle regularization, pain control, or functional endurance. The therapy suite or inpatient rehabilitation unit becomes a practice setting where family and other caregivers can

develop competence and confidence in caring for the patient on their own. On occasions, it will become evident that the identified support system is not adequate for meeting the patient's needs and alternative disposition will need to be arranged. Reasoned modification of care plans at this level, however, is preferable to unrealistic discharges home and crisis-based readmissions. Caregiver training by rehabilitation specialists reduces the risk of injury to patients or their assistants and can conserve time and energy for both by introducing labour-saving devices such as mechanical lifts, stair glides, ramps, wheelchairs, transfer boards, and bathing aides (Fig. 16.5). Follow up training can be provided by home therapists as needs change. Caregiver training also alleviates some of the emotional and psychological stressors that burden patients and those around them. Preservation of functional autonomy or even the ability to be out doors or attend a community event, may offer tremendous psychological and emotional return for the patient. Involving caregivers in the resolution of speech language and communication deficits can diffuse some of the anger and frustration that would otherwise develop for patients who lose the ability to communicate effectively. Effective caregiver training includes the patient as much as possible given their current functional capacity. At a minimum, efforts must be made to explain techniques carefully to patients and to maximize their ability to direct their own self care. Caregivers and, to some extent, patients should be trained to instruct additional givers in the future to allow for respite intervals of different durations. Although the goals of rehabilitation services at this time may be primarily caregiver training, inclusion of strengthening and endurance activities for the patients may continue, as improved functional performance on the part of the patient markedly reduces caregiver burden and may prolong a patient's ability to remain comfortably in their home.

Section IV: barriers

Patients wish to remain in control of their bodies for as along as possible despite the ravages of disease. Dame Cicely Saunders acknowledged this unassailable truth in describing the hospice mission as enabling the 'dying person to live . . . at his own maximum potential performing to the limit of his physical . . . capacity with control and independence whenever possible'[74]. Dame Cicely recognized the now well-established association

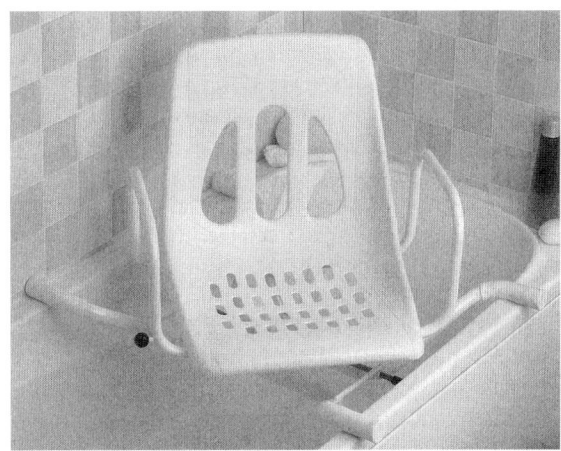

Figure 16.5 Bathing aide: 554959 or AA1104 (with courtesy: Sammons Preston: A Patterson Medical Co.).

between functional decline and reduced HRQOL, depression, passive suicidal ideation, and interest in euthanasia. Despite patients' distress at the prospect of dependency, rehabilitation medicine has often remained marginal in the spectrum of palliative care in some cultures. Careful examination of rehabilitation's role in ameliorating the advanced stages of terminal disease is overdue. The price of failing to do so may be a tremendous loss of potential.

An important barrier to the integration of rehabilitation services is widespread lack of familiarity with the field on the part of clinicians' caring for patients with advanced disease. The breadth of rehabilitation medicine, both in the spectrum of its treatments, as well as the range of conditions treated, makes it challenging to encapsulate with a pithy sound bite. However, a general rule of thumb not only summarizes rehabilitation's *raison d'etre* but also emphasizes its close kinship with palliative care. Rehabilitation medicine, like palliative care, does not seek to halt or eliminate disease processes. Just as palliation focuses on symptom control, rehabilitation focuses on function. All rehabilitation medicine's diagnostic and therapeutic effort is expended on enhancing or preserving patients' capacity for independent mobility, self-care, communication, and cognition. Diseases, their treatments, and their symptoms are only relevant to the rehabilitation paradigm in the manner in which they threaten or potentiate function.

Palliative care and rehabilitation medicine have not produced comparable empirical evidence-bases for practice. Palliative care has enjoyed continued expansion of a now growing supportive literature. Very few publications guide rehabilitation specialists in the care of dying patients. Many of these are anecdotal or involve small convenience samples. As a result, current clinical practices are largely based on the consensus statements for specific disease types (e.g. NCCN), evidence derived from the early or acute stages of disease (e.g. aerobic conditioning during adjuvant chemotherapy), isolated case reports and common sense. In areas where literature exists, e.g. acute rehabilitation of cancer patients, study cohorts are generally defined by diagnoses rather than disease stage. Therefore uncertainty remains as to subjects' prospects for disease modification or cure and the proportion of their care delivered with palliative intent. As a result, limited inferences can be made as to the efficacy of rehabilitative interventions in far advanced disease. The absence of high quality, empirical data is a decided shortcoming at a time when evidence-based medicine is increasingly expected to address some of the more pressing inadequacies of modern medical systems, including resource allocation. At present, honest recognition of rehabilitation's incomplete evidence-base in the palliative setting is the best means of preventing inappropriate adherence to therapies of equivocal benefit. The clinician must continuously ground him- or herself by asking, 'Will this improve my patient's function?'

References

1. Sliwa, J.A., and Marciniak, C. (1998). Physical rehabilitation of the cancer patient. In *Palliative care and rehabilitation of cancer patients* (Ed. von Gunten, C.F.). pp. 76–90, Kluwer Academic Publishers, Boston; Headley, J.A., Ownby, K.K., and John, L.D. (2004). The effect of seated exercise on fatigue and quality of life in women with advanced breast cancer. *Oncology Nursing Forum*, **31**, 977–83 or National Comprehensive Cancer Network Practice Guidelines in Oncology: Cancer Related Fatigue (2007) Version 2: FT-1. Available at www.nccn.org.

2. Dimeo, F., Fetsher, S., Lange, W. *et al.* (1998). Effects of aerobic exercise on the physical performance and incidence of treatment-related complications after high-dose chemotherapy. *Blood*, **90**, 3390–94.

3. Stevens, R. (1998). *American medicine and the public interest.* University of California Press, Los Angeles, 330.

4. Zorowitz, R.D., and Adamovich, B.B. (2000). Assessment of communication. In *Physical medicine and rehabilitation: the complete approach* (eds. Grabois, M. *et al.*), pp. 263–76. Blackwell Science, Malden, MA.

5. Dietz, J.H.(1969). Rehabilitation of the cancer patient. *Medical Clinics in North America*, **53**, 607–24.

6. Recognized examples in the United States include M. D. Anderson Cancer in Texas, Memorial Sloan Kettering Cancer in New York and the Mayo Clinic in Minesotta.

7. Yoshioka, H. (1994). Rehabilitation for the terminal cancer patient. *American Journal of Physical Medicine & Rehabilitation*, **73**, 199–206

8. Lee, M.S., Chen, K.W., Sancier, K.M. (2007). Qigong for cancer treatment: a systematic review of controlled clinical trials. *Acta Oncologica* **46**, 171–722. Vlukelatos, A., Cumming, R.G., Lord, S.R. *et al.* (2007) A randomized, controlled trial of tai chi for the prevention of falls: the central Sydney tai chi trial. *Journal of the American Geriatrics Society*, **55**, 1185–91.

9. Farrel, S.J., Ross, A.D.M., and Sehgal, K.V. (1999). Eastern movement therapies. *Physical Medicine and Rehabilitation Clinics of North America*, **10**, 617–29 and Chen, K.M., Tseng, W.S., Ting, L.F., *et al.* (2007), Development and evaluation of a yoga exercise program for older adults. *Journal of Advanced Nursing*, **57**, 432–41.

10. Dimeo, F.C., Stieglitz, R.D., Novelli-Fischer, U. *et al.* (1999). Effects of physical activity on the fatigue and psychologic status of cancer patients during chemotherapy, *Cancer*, **85**, 2273–7.

11. Osoba, D., Zee, B., Pater, J. *et al.* (1994). Psychometric properties and responsiveness of the EORTC quality of Life Questionnaire (QLQ-C30) in patients with breast, ovarian and lung cancer. s*Quality of Life Research*, **3**(5), 353–64.

12. Cella, D.F., Tulsky, D.S., Gray, G., *et al.* (1993). The Functional Assessment of Cancer Therapy scale: development and validation of the general measure. *Journal of Clinical Oncology*, **11**(3), 570–9.

13. Schipper, H., Clinch, J., McMurray, A. *et al.* (1984). Measuring the quality of life of cancer patients: the Functional Living Index-Cancer: development and validation. *Journal of Clinical Oncology*, **2**(5), 472–83.

14. Heinrich, R.L., Schag, C.C., and Ganz, P.A. (1984). Living with cancer: the Cancer Inventory of Problem Situations. *Journal of Clinical Oncology*, **40**(4), 972–80.

15. Mystakidou, K., Parpa, E., Katsouda, E. *et al.* (2006). The role of physical and psychological symptoms in desire for death: a study of terminally ill cancer patients. *Psychooncology*, **15**(4), 355–60.

16. Fairclough, D.L.(1998). Quality of life, cancer investigation, and clinical practice. *Cancer Investigation,* **16**(7), 478–84.

17. O'Mahony, S., Goulet, J., Kornblith, A. *et al.* (2005). Desire for hastened death, cancer pain and depression: report of a longitudinal observational study. *Journal of Pain and Symptom Management*, **29**(5), 446–57.

18. van der Maas, P.J., van der Wal, G., Haverkate, I. *et al.* (1996). Euthanasia, physician-assisted suicide, and other medical practices involving the end of life in the Netherlands, 1990–1995. *New England Journal of Medicine*, **335**(22), 1699–705.

19. Yoshioka, H. (1994). Rehabilitation for the terminal cancer patient. *American Journal of Physical Medicine and Rehabilitation*, **73**(3), 199–206.

20. Axelsson, B., and Sjoden, P.O. (1998). Quality of life of cancer patients and their spouses in palliative home care. *Palliative Medicine*, **12**(1), 29–39.

21. Cheville, A.L.T., Basford, J.R., and Kornblith, A.B. Physical impairments in patients with metastatic breast cancer: prevalence and treatment pattern. *Journal of Clinical Oncology*. In press.

22. Yoshioka, H. (1994). Rehabilitation for the terminal cancer patient. *American Journal of Physical Medicine and Rehabilitation*, **73**(3), 199–206.

23. Harvey, R.F., Jellinek, H.M., and Habeck, R.V. (1982). Cancer rehabilitation. An analysis of 36 program approaches. *JAMA*, **247**(15), 2127–31.

24. McKinley, W.O., Huang, M.E., and Brunsvold, K.T. (1999). Neoplastic versus traumatic spinal cord injury: an outcome comparison after inpatient rehabilitation. *Archieves of Physical Medicine and Rehabilitation*, **80**(10):1253–1257.

25. McKinley WO, Huang ME, Tewksbury MA. (2000). Neoplastic vs. traumatic spinal cord injury: an inpatient rehabilitation comparison. *American Journal of Physical Medicine and Rehabilitation*, **79**(2), 138–44.

26. O'Dell, M.W., Barr, K., Spanier, D. (1998). Functional outcome of inpatient rehabilitation in persons with brain tumours. *Archieves of Physical Medicine and Rehabilitation*, **79**(12), 1530–4.

27. Yoshioka H. (1994). Rehabilitation for the terminal cancer patient. *American Journal of Physical Medicine and Rehabilitation*, **73**(3), 199–206.

28. Yarasheske, K.R., and Roubenoff, R. (2001). Exercise treatment for HIV-associated metabolic and anthropomorphic complications. *Exercise and Sport Sciences Reviews*, 29, 170–4.

29. Kraft, G., and Alquist, A. (1996). Effect of resistive exercise on physical function in multiple sclerosis. *Veterans Aff Rehabil Res Dev Prog Rep*, **33**, 328–9.

30. Hicks, J.E. (1999). Exercise in patients with inflammatory arthritis and connective tissue disease. *Rheumatic Diseases Clinics of North America* **16**(4), 845–70.

31. Lunney, J.R., Lynn, J., Foley, D.J. *et al.* (2003). Patterns of functional decline at the end of life. *JAMA*, **289**(18), 2387–92.

32. Beck, L.C., Cheville, A.L., Petersen, T. *et al.* (2006). Functional problems in cancer patients: medical record documentation and associated characteristics. *American Academy of Physical Medicine and Rehabilitation Annual Assembly*. Honolulu, HI

33. Detmar, S.B., Muller, M.J., Wever, L.D. *et al.* (2001). The patient–physician relationship. Patient-physician communication during outpatient palliative treatment visits: an observational study. *JAMA*, **285**(10), 1351–7.

34. Cheville, A.L., Troxel, A.B., Basford, J.R. *et al.* (2008). Prevalence and patterns of physical impairments in patients with metastatic breast cancer. *Journal of Clinical Oncology*, **26**(16), 2621–9.

35. Lunney, J.R., Lynn, J., Foley, D.J. *et al.* (2003). Patterns of functional decline at the end of life. *JAMA*. **289**(18), 2387–92.

36. Cheville, A.L., Troxel, A.B., Basford, J.R. *et al.* (2008). Prevalence and patterns of physical impairments in patients with metastatic breast cancer. *Journal of Clinical Oncology* **26**(16), 2621–9.

37. Fox, S.W., and Lyon, D.E. (2006). Symptom clusters and quality of life in survivors of lung cancer. *Oncology Nursing Forum*, **33**(5), 931–6.

38. Beck, L.C., Cheville, A.L., Petersen, T. *et al.* (2006). Functional problems in cancer patients: medical record documentation and associated characteristics. *American Academy of Physical Medicine and Rehabilitation Annual Assembly*. Honolulu, HI

39. Palmore, E., and Cleveland, W. (1976). Aging, terminal decline, and terminal drop. *Journals of Gerontology*,. **31**(1), 76–81.

40. Portenoy, R.K., Hagen, N.A. (1990). Breakthrough pain: definition, prevalence and characteristics. *Pain*, **41**(3), 273–81.

41. Portenoy, R.K., Payne, D., and Jacobsen, P.(1999). Breakthrough pain: characteristics and impact in patients with cancer pain. *Pain*, **81**(1–2), 129–34.

42. Foley, K.M. (1985). The treatment of cancer pain. *New England Journal of Medicine*, **313**(2), 84–95.

43. Levy, M.H. (1996). Pharmacologic treatment of cancer pain. *New England Journal of Medicine*, **335**(15), 1124–32.

44. McCarberg, B.H. (2007). The treatment of breakthrough pain. *Pain Medicine*, **8**(Suppl 1), S8–13.

45. Miaskowski, C. (2005). The next step to improving cancer pain management. *Pain Management Nursing*, **6**(1), 1–2.

46. Ferrell, B.R., Juarez, G., and Borneman, T. (1999). Use of routine and breakthrough analgesia in home care. *Oncology Nursing Forum*. **26**(10), 1655–61.

47. Hanna, A., Sledge, G., Mayer, M.L. *et al.* (2006). A phase II study of methylphenidate for the treatment of fatigue. *Supportive Care in Cancer*, **14**(3), 210–5.

48. Edwards, H., and Forster, E. (1999). Avoidance of issues in family caregiving. *Contemporary Nurse*. **8**(2), 5–13

49. Payne, S., Smith, P., and Dean, S. (1999). Identifying the concerns of informal carers in palliative care. *Palliative Medicine*, **13**(1), 37–44.

50. Pecchioni, L. (2001). Implicit decision-making in family caregiving. *Journal of Social and Personal Relationships*, **18**, 219–37.

51. Zhang, A.Y., and Siminoff, L.A. (2003). Silence and cancer: why do families and patients fail to communicate? *Health Communication*, **15**(4), 415–29.

52. Payne, S., Smith, P., and Dean, S. (1999). Identifying the concerns of informal carers in palliative care. *Palliative Medicine*, **13**(1), 37–44.

53. Edwards, H., and Forster, E. (1999). Avoidance of issues in family caregiving. *Contemporary Nurse*. **8**(2), 5–13

54. Pecchioni, L. (2001). Implicit decision-making in family caregiving. *Journal of Social and Personal Relationships*, **18**:219-237.

55. Zhang, A.Y., and Siminoff, L.A. (2003). Silence and cancer: why do families and patients fail to communicate? *Health Communication*, **15**(4), 415–29.

56. Leydon, G.M., Boulton, M., Moynihan, C., *et al.* (2000). Cancer patients' information needs and information seeking behaviour: in depth interview study. *BMJ*, **320**(7239), 909–13.

57. Hanson, L.C., Danis, M., and Garrett, J. (1997). What is wrong with end-of-life care? Opinions of bereaved family members. *Journal of American Geriatrics Society*, **45**(11), 1339–44.

58. Fried, T.R., Bradley, E.H., O'Leary, J.R. *et al.* (2005). Unmet desire for caregiver-patient communication and increased caregiver burden. *Journal of American Geriatrics Society*, **53**(1), 59–65.

59. Herbert Dietz, J. Jr. (1981). *Rehabilitation oncology*. John Wiley & Sons, New York, 25–31.

60. Portenoy, R.K., Payne, D., and Jacobsen, P. (1999). Breakthrough pain: characteristics and impact in patients with cancer pain. *Pain*, **81**(1–2):129–34.

61. Portenoy, R.K.H., and Hagen, N.A. (1990). Breakthrough pain: definition, prevalence and characteristics. *Pain*, **41**(3), 273–81.

62. McCarberg, B.H. (2007). The treatment of breakthrough pain. *Pain Medicine*, **8**(Suppl 1), S8-S13.

63. Hanna, A., Sledge, G., Mayer, M.L. *et al.* (2006). A phase II study of methylphenidate for the treatment of fatigue. *Supportive Care in Cancer*, **14**(3), 210–5.

64. Portenoy, R.K., Thaler, H.T., Kornblith, A.B. *et al.* (1994). Symptom prevalence, characteristics and distress in a cancer population. *Quality of Life Research*, **3**(3), 183–9.

65. Axelsson, B., and Sjoden, P.O. (1998). Quality of life of cancer patients and their spouses in palliative home care. *Palliative Medicine*, **12**, 29–39.

66. Breitbart, W., Chochinov, H., and Passik, S. (1998). Psychiatric aspects of palliative care. In *Oxford textbook of palliative medicine*. (eds. Doyle, D., Hanks, G., MacDonald, N.), pp. 993–54.

67. Guo, Y.B., Young, J.L., Palmer, Y. *et al.* (2003). Prognostic factors for survival in metastatic spinal cord compression: a retrospective study in a rehabilitation setting," *American Journal of Physical Medicine and Rehabilitation*, **82**, 665–8; Helwig-Larsen, S. (1996). Clinical outcome in metastatic spinal cord compression: a prospective study of 153 patients *Acta Neurologica Scandinavica*, 269–27.

68. Marciniak, C., Sliwa, J., Spill, G. *et al.* (1996). Functional outcome following rehabilitation of the cancer patient. *Archives of Physical Medicine and Rehabilitation*, **77**, 54–7.

69. Peterson, K., Rosenblum, M.K., Kotanides, H. *et al.* (1992). Paraneoplastic cerebellar degeneration. I. A clinical analysis of 55 anti-Yo antibody positive patients. *Neurology*, 42:1931–7.

70. Clouston, P.D., Sapre, C.B., Arbizu, T. *et al.* (1992). Paraneoplastic cerebellar degeneration. III Cerebellar degeneration, cancer and the Lambert–Eaton myasthenic syndrome. *Neurology*, **42**, 144–50.

71. Bartels, M.N. (2000). Cardiac rehabilitation. In *Physical medicine and rehabilitation: the complete approach* (eds. M. Grabois *et al.*), pp. 1436–56, Blackwell Science, Malden, MA.

72. Segal, R.J., Reid, R.D., Courneya, K.S. *et al.* (2003). Resistance exercise in men receiving androgen deprivation therapy for prostate cancer. *Journal of Clinical Oncology*, **21**, 1653–9.

73. Rabow, M.W., Hauser, J.M., Adams, J. (2004). Supporting family caregivers at the end-of-life: "they don't know what they don't know." *JAMA*, **291**, 483–91.

74. Saunders, C.M. (2006). *Cicely Saunders: Selected writings, 1958–2004.* Oxford University Press, Oxford.

Complementary therapies in palliative medicine

Gary Deng and Barrie Cassileth

Introduction

Patients with advanced illness who are receiving palliative care, facing a poor prognosis, and experiencing a heavy symptom burden, often seek health-care practices and agents outside the realm of mainstream medicine. Collectively these modalities often are termed 'Complementary and Alternative Medicine (CAM)'. CAM therapies are diverse, ranging from unproved alternative 'cures' that offer false hope to adjunctive complementary therapies that provide legitimate supportive care. Although complementary therapies and alternative approaches often are discussed under the umbrella of CAM, it is clinically and conceptually necessary to distinguish between the two categories because they comprise profoundly different modalities.

Alternative therapies generally are promoted for use instead of mainstream therapy. Purveyors cater to people who have lost confidence or grown antagonistic to mainstream medicine. These may be patients aware of their poor prognosis and limited therapeutic options, but unready to give up the hope of cure. Unfortunately, alternative therapies, by definition, are not supported by evidence. They are alternative, not accepted as viable treatments by mainstream medicine, because they lack solid data in support of efficacy and safety. Alternative regimens are usually very expensive and potentially harmful. They may harm directly through physiologic activity, or indirectly when patients forego receipt of mainstream care. Patients with advanced illness may be especially vulnerable to these approaches, as they often promise cure even in the setting of end-stage disease.

Complementary therapies, on the other hand, are used for symptom management and to enhance a sense of physical, mental and spiritual well-being. They serve as adjuncts to mainstream care. They are promoted not as cures, but as means to enhance patients' quality of life. They may be supported by evidence, although the strength of the evidence varies. They also generally have a favourable risk/benefit ratio. Complementary therapies can be considered a useful component in palliative care because they may offer the promise of salutary effects on body, mind and spirit, aiming to control pain and other symptoms and to optimize quality of life for patients and families. Although the origin of some complementary therapies predates the advent of modern biomedicine, they have not been incorporated into mainstream medical care until recently. The goal of complementary therapies is essentially the same as that proposed by the World Health Organization for palliative care[1].

The distinction between alternative and complementary therapies therefore has profound implications. Health professionals should steer patients away from harmful or useless alternative therapies while making helpful complementary therapies available. Whereas alternative therapies typically are sought by patients outside of mainstream medical care, complementary therapies are increasingly available not only directly to patients on a private basis, but also in hospitals, clinics, and homes as a component of symptom control and the effort to ease the physical, psychosocial, and spiritual distresses associated with advanced life-threatening illnesses such as cancer.

In this chapter, we will summarize the state of CAM in the current health-care system, review the alternative therapies that are so widely and temptingly proffered to patients and families, and discuss helpful complementary therapies applicable to palliative medicine.

Complementary and alternative medicine in the current health-care system

Long available, CAM therapies became increasingly visible in the USA during the 1990s. This phenomenon was driven by public fascination with unconventional therapies, a higher tolerance and acceptance of therapies from other cultures, legislative and regulatory changes propelled by strong political and economical interest groups, and publications documenting the impact of complementary modalities. The popularity of CAM has affected every component of the health-care system and all specialties of medicine, including palliative care. It has left its mark on the thinking and practice of physicians and other health professionals, and has broadened patients' involvement and influence in their own care.

Prevalence

A survey done in the early 1990s estimated that about one-third of adults in the USA reported using at least one unconventional therapy in the past year, and one-third of these visited providers for these therapies[2]. No longer a collection of covert practices[3], CAM today is highly visible. Thanks to the Internet, information about CAM is widely available to the general public. A Google search of 'alternative therapy' yielded 16 million hits in November 2006. It is a multi-billion dollar business in the USA, and of equivalent impact and importance throughout the developed world[2,4].

Surveys conducted in the USA and internationally have demonstrated that the prevalence of CAM therapy use in the general population varies from <10 per cent to more than 70 per cent. The wide range can be attributed primarily to variable understandings and definitions of CAM. Some surveys define CAM in a very broad sense, including lifestyle activities such as weight loss efforts, exercise, church attendance, and support activities such as group counselling. Others specify only the use of herbal products. Prevalence rates also vary among geographic regions and prevailing cultures.

A recent report presented the most comprehensive and reliable findings to date on the state CAM in the USA. The National Center for Health Statistics' 2002 National Health Interview Survey involved 31 044 adults from the general public. Seventy-five per cent of the respondents used some form of CAM[5]. Even when prayer for health was excluded, the percentage was still close to 50 per cent. Consistent with virtually all previous surveys, CAM use was most common among women, better educated people, those hospitalized in the previous year, and former smokers. Some of these groups presumably represent a more health conscious segment of the population.

The use of CAM among cancer patients is widespread. A systematic review[6] of 26 surveys of cancer patients in 13 countries showed that the average prevalence of CAM use across all studies was 31 per cent. Therapies most commonly adopted around the world included dietary treatments, herbs, homeopathy, hypnotherapy, imagery or visualization, meditation, megavitamins, relaxation, and spiritual healing. The prevalence of CAM use in the USA ranged from 7 per cent to 50 per cent. Recent large surveys from Europe showed that 36 per cent of cancer patients use some form of CAM (range among countries 15–73 per cent)[7]. Herbal remedies were most common. A nation-wide survey in Japan showed a prevalence of 45 per cent among cancer patients and 26 per cent among patients with benign tumours[8]. A strong association between being in a palliative care unit and the use of CAM modalities was found. The most popular CAM therapies are herbs or other dietary supplements. Another consistent finding in cancer patient surveys is that users typically are younger, more educated and more affluent—again likely indicators of a desire and ability to play an active role in their own care.

CAM use by cancer patients has grown in recent years[6]; a secondary analysis of approximately 3000 cancer patients estimates a 64 per cent increase after 1987[10]. This may reflect expanded variety of over-the-counter remedies, broader availability of complementary therapies in mainstream cancer programmes and centres, and greater ease in access to health-related information over the Internet.

US legislation, passed in 1994, allowed herbal medicines and other 'dietary supplements' to be sold without US Food and Drug Administration (FDA) review as long as no claims were made about the ability of these products to prevent or treat disease. An estimated doubling of dietary supplement sales resulted in the following 6 years. According to the National Nutritional Food Association, annual sales of dietary supplements reached $19.8 billion in 2003, an amount that included $4.2 billion in herbs.

Although the sale of most supplements has increased each year, the sale of herbs declined by 3 per cent in 2002 and 1.8 per cent in 2003[9]. This decline is presumed due to unrealistically high public expectations, media reports about safety concerns and questionable effectiveness, and public confusion about the vast array of products.

Public access to information

Patients get most of their CAM information not from their physicians, but rather, for better or worse, from sources more knowledgeable about these therapies. CAM is an open and public issue today, discussed in mass media and readily found on the Internet. Magazines articles and television specials provide the general public with details about new CAM therapies. CAM practitioners openly advertize on radio, television, Internet, and in telephone directories. CAM product marketers sponsor infomercials on television, send newsletters and product catalogues via mass mailing, and are engaged in multi-level marketing schemes. Information available to the public varies widely in accuracy, and misinformation about health issues is widespread. In 1999, the US Federal Trade Commission (FTC) announced that it had identified hundreds of websites promoting and selling phoney cures for cancer and other serious ailments among the estimated 15 000–17 000 health-related websites. Because today there are approximately 874 000 000 such sites, it is likely that those selling bogus treatments have increased accordingly.

Recognition by mainstream medicine

Health insurance programmes increasingly cover CAM services and providers[11]. More than 30 major insurers in the USA cover more than one method. Expanding insurance coverage of complementary therapies reflects consumer demand. It also represents efforts of managed care organizations to control costs despite the dearth of cost-effectiveness data. CAM users often have chronic conditions and use more health-care resources. If they are helped by complementary therapies or steered toward less expensive treatment regimens, overall health-care costs may be reduced.

In the USA, insurance coverage for CAM also varies by state. Some require prescription or supervision by a physician. Naturopathic care is covered by approximately 100 insurance companies in the USA; most are concentrated in Alaska, Connecticut, and Washington State.

Within the last decade, increasing numbers of research articles focused on CAM therapies have been published in mainstream medical journals. Articles about CAM in major journals shifted from commentaries expressing concerns about quackery through the 1970s, to surveys of patients' knowledge and use of unproved methods in the 1980s and 1990s, to reports of actual research results starting primarily in the mid-1990s. In 1996 and 1997, the National Library of Medicine added many new CAM search terms to its medical subject headings, and began to cover alternative medicine journals previously not reviewed for inclusion in Medline. Opposition by the scientific community is being replaced by emphasis on the importance of methodologically sound research, which now increasingly takes place in numerous respected institutions around the world.

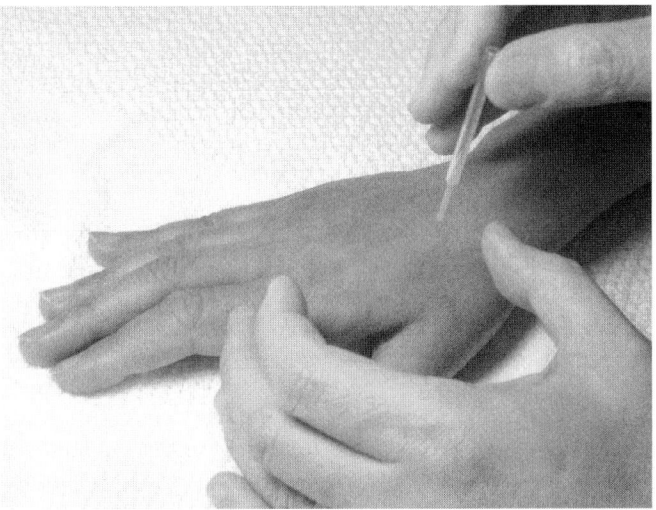

Figure 17.1 Acupuncture: removal of the guide tube after insertion of the acupuncture needle at LI-4 acupuncture point.

Table 17.1 Reputable sources of online information on complementary and alternative medicine.

Medline Plus:
http://www.nlm.nih.gov/medlineplus/druginformation.html
British Medical Journal:
http://www.biomedcentral.com/bmccomplementalternmed/
Memorial Sloan-Kettering Cancer Center:
http://www.mskcc.org/aboutherbs
National Center for Complementary and Alternative Medicine (NCCAM): http://nccam.nih.gov
American Cancer Society: http://www.cancer.org/docroot/ETO/ETO_5. asp?sitearea=ETO
NIH Office of Dietary Supplements: http://dietary-supplements.info.nih.gov
U.S. Pharmacopeia: http://www.usp.org/dietarySupplements

Theories and practices of complementary and alternative therapies

CAM therapies are a diverse group of modalities that may be grouped into four general categories: biologically based practices; mind–body medicine; manipulative and body-based practices, and energy medicine. These groups overlap. For example, yoga practice is body-based, but it also has mind–body and energy medicine components. In addition, there are whole medical systems that cut across all domains. Traditional Chinese Medicine, for example, includes biologically active botanicals, mind–body practices, manipulative techniques and acupuncture (Fig. 17.1).

Biologically-based practices

The biologically-based practices encompass therapies that involve ingestion, or rarely, injection of substances said to induce physiologic changes that prevent and treat disease. The regimens may be a specified dietary plan, herbs, vitamins, or other constituents extracted from natural sources. The rationale usually is based on laboratory findings, e.g. anti-tumour activity *in vitro* or in animal models, or traditional use, such as herbal preparations from Traditional Chinese Medicine, Naturopathy, or Homeopathy.

In palliative care, unproved biological therapies tend to be adopted for one of two reasons. First, patients may use them in a final effort to treat end-stage disease. Laboratory data may have suggested that value of a particular natural substance, and despite the absence of clinical data, patients want to try them in an effort to leave no stone unturned. Second, patients may use them as supportive measures to 'strengthen the body', to 'boost the immune system' or to 'improve nutrition'.

Unfortunately, many of these therapies are based on no research or on preliminary laboratory studies, and their clinical relevance has been untested. Some products are outright commercial operations with exaggerated claims based on pseudoscience. In addition, because many of these agents are biologically active, their side effects, and interaction with other drugs cannot be overlooked (Table 17.1)[12]. The public apparently is not aware that herbs are essentially dilute natural drugs that contain scores of different chemicals, most of which are not yet documented. Effects are not always predictable.

A prominent example in this group of unproved or disproved biological therapies is shark cartilage. Interest in shark cartilage as a cancer therapy was activated by a 1992 book, *Sharks Don't Get Cancer*, by William Lane, and by a television special that displayed apparent remissions in patients treated with shark cartilage in Cuba. The televised outcome was strongly disputed by oncologists in the USA. Advocates promote the therapy based on its putative anti-angiogenic properties. Shark cartilage was found to contain a substance with anti-angiogenic activity *in vitro*[13], but the active component appears to be a large molecule proteoglycan with a molecular weight of 10 000 daltons[14]. Whether such large molecules can be absorbed via the digestive tract and reach the target tumour tissue at a sufficiently high local concentration is questionable. Clinical studies have yet to show that ingestion of shark cartilage yields survival benefit or improved quality of life in advanced cancer patients[15,16]. The product was poorly tolerated due to its unpleasant taste.

Another example is caesium therapy. According to the theory, an alkaline environment discourages tumour growth. By taking caesium chloride, one can alkalinize the body and kill the cancer cells. Unfortunately, the activity of caesium chloride does not appear to be cancer tissue-specific. Excessive alkalization creates electrolyte and pH imbalance that disrupt the normal function of cells. Caesium therapy has resulted in life-threatening cardiac arrhythmia[17,18].

Metabolic therapies, offered primarily through clinics situated in Tijuana, Mexico, are another example of alternative therapies targeting advanced cancer patients desperate for anything that may offer the hope of cure. These therapies involve practitioner-specific combinations of diet plus vitamins, minerals, enzymes, and 'detoxification'. One of the best known sites for metabolic therapy is the Gerson clinic, where treatment is based on the belief that toxic products of cancer cells accumulate in the liver, leading to liver failure and death. The Gerson treatment aims to counteract liver damage with a low-salt, high-potassium diet, coffee enemas, and a gallon of fruit and vegetable juice daily[19]. The clinic's use of liquefied raw calf liver injections was suspended in 1997 following sepsis in a number of patients.

The potential for herb–drug interaction is problematic in patients who are receiving other medications. Some herbs interfere with coagulation and produce dangerous blood pressure swings and unwanted interactions with anaesthetics[12]. Herbs such as feverfew, garlic, ginger, and ginkgo have anticoagulant effects and should be avoided by patients receiving warfarin sodium, heparin sodium, aspirin, and related agents. The risk of herb–drug interactions appears to be greatest for patients with kidney or liver problems. Herbs can alter metabolism of prescription medicines via the cytochrome P450 system, possibly worsening side effects or compromising efficacy[12]. Similar cautions are necessary for patients receiving radiation, as some herbs photosensitize the skin and cause severe reactions.

This category of CAM therapies also has been sullied by unscrupulous business practices. For example, 'coral calcium'[20] became popular for a while thanks to blanket promotion that falsely claimed its ability to cure cancer; therapy became unavailable after a crackdown by government. Unscrupulous CAM providers may use a commercially successful sales approach known as multi-level marketing, in which an army of motivated sales 'associates' promote unsubstantiated claims while shielding the root provider from liability.

Palliative care health professionals may encounter elaborate dietary plans such as the macrobiotic diet, detoxification regimens, mega-dose vitamin therapy, laetrile, Essiac tea, Iscador, immuno-augmentive therapy, etc. The specific therapies are too numerous to be discussed here. Several online sources (Table 17.1) provide reliable information for patients and health-care professionals about such products and regimens (Table 17.2).

In contrast to these ineffective therapies, there are numerous, biologically active natural substances that have been formally evaluated and are now in use as therapeutic agents. Some of the most successful chemotherapeutic agents (paclitaxel, topotecan, irinotecan, vincristine, vinorelbine, etc.) were extracted from botanicals or their derivatives. Other natural substances have shown promise in supportive care, such as carnitine for the treatment of cancer-related fatigue[21,22] and glutamine to prevent taxane-induced neuropathy[23,24].

Biological CAM agents should be used, if at all, under the supervision of professionals who are familiar with the specific agents and their potential benefits and risks, taking into consideration a patient's particular medical conditions and concurrent medications.

Any questionable agents should be used in a clinical trial setting with close monitoring of adverse events.

Mind–body techniques

The very existence of the placebo effect, in which suggestion and expectancy can induce biological change, demonstrates the connection between mind and body. The potential to influence health with our minds is an appealing concept and an under-utilized opportunity. It affirms the power of the individual. Some mind–body interventions have moved from the category of alternative, unconventional therapies into mainstream complementary or supportive care. For example, the effectiveness of meditation, biofeedback, and yoga in stress reduction and the control of some physiologic reactions have been documented[25,26].

Mind–body therapies in palliative care are geared to decrease distress and promote relaxation in different ways. They can be an element among a variety of strategies that attend to patients' psychological health. Support groups, good doctor–patient relationships, and the emotional and instrumental help of family and friends are vital, and mind–body strategies can support these benefits as well. For some patients, mind–body interventions satisfy spiritual needs.

The benefits of the mind–body therapies should not be overstated, however. The idea that patients can influence the course of their disease through mental or emotional work is not substantiated and can evoke feelings of guilt and inadequacy when disease continues to advance despite patients' best spiritual or mental efforts[27–29].

Hypnotherapy has been shown to reduce chemotherapy-related nausea and vomiting in children, and possibly to control anxiety and nausea. Hypnosis for pain is well supported[30]. Hypnotherapy can be integrated into different stages (the Initial Crisis, Transition, Acceptance, and Preparation for Death) of a patient's reaction to the lack of curative options[31,32]. Other techniques, including visualization and progressive relaxation, also decrease pain and promote well-being[33].

Meditation can help in stress reduction. In a randomized study of 109 cancer patients that compared participation in a 7-week Mindfulness-Based Stress Reduction Programme with a wait-list control, the programme was associated with significant improvement in mood disturbance and symptoms of stress[34]. A single-arm study of another programme in a cohort of breast and prostate cancer patients showed significant improvement in overall quality of life, stress and sleep quality, but symptom improvement was not

Table 17.2 Herbal products with potentially serious adverse effects.

Product (responsible constituents if known)	Adverse effects
Aristolochia, *Bragantia*, or *Asarum* species (aristolochic acid)	Renal toxicity that can lead to renal failure
Common comfrey, prickley comfrey, and Russian comfrey (pyrrolizidine alkaloids)	Hepatotoxicity, veno-occlusive disease
Ephedra, Ma huang (ephedrine alkaloids)	Sympathomimetic activity, hypertension, tachycardia, increased risks for stroke, heart attack, and heart failure
Products containing androstenedione, or 'andro'	Androgenic and oestrogenic effects
Kava	Hepatotoxicity
St John's Wort	Potent cytochrome P450 3A4 inducer, altered metabolism of many drugs

Source: US Food and Drug Administration.

significantly correlated with programme attendance or minutes of home practice[35].

Yoga, which combines physical movement, breath control and meditation, improved sleep quality in a controlled trial of 39 lymphoma patients. Practising a form of yoga that incorporates controlled breathing and visualization significantly decreased sleep disturbance when compared with wait-list controls[36]. Mindfulness-Based Stress Reduction techniques must be practised regularly to produce beneficial effects[37].

Manipulative and body-based methods

This group of therapies aims to reduce tension and malfunction by manipulation of the musculoskeletal system with various techniques. Osteopathic and chiropractic doctors were among the earliest groups to use manual methods. The benefit of chiropractic treatment on low back pain was supported by a National Institutes of Health consensus conference[38], but its value is widely disputed by mainstream physicians and its potential to harm frail patients is a concern.

Numerous approaches involve touch and manipulation techniques, including hands-on massage, very light touch or no touch at all. No-touch therapies such as Reiki or therapeutic touch have been termed 'energy medicine', but more recently deemed to be mind–body interventions. A similar method is therapeutic touch (TT), which, despite its name, involves no direct contact. In TT, healers move their hands a few inches above a patient's body and sweep away 'blockages' to the patient's energy field. Although a study in the *Journal of the American Medical Association* showed that experienced TT practitioners were unable to detect the investigator's 'energy field'[39], and despite mainstream scientists' unwillingness to accept its fundamental premises, TT is taught in North American nursing schools and is practised by nurses in the USA and other countries. Reiki is defined as spiritually guided life force, the manipulation of energy surrounding the patient. This energy is called 'Ki' in Japanese lore or 'Qi or Chi' in Chinese tradition. It involves no touch. A small study reported better pain control in advanced cancer patients receiving Reiki when compared with usual care[40]. Reduction of heart rate and diastolic blood pressure was reported in a randomized controlled trial of 45 subjects[41]. However, the relationship between the clinical effect and the purported bioenergy field, as well as its subjection to a practitioner's manipulation, has never been convincingly demonstrated.

Massage therapists apply pressure to muscle and connective tissue to reduce tension and pain, improve circulation, and encourage relaxation. Swedish massage, the most common type in the USA, is gentle and comprised five basic strokes (stroking, kneading, friction, percussion, and vibration). The movement is rhythmic and free-flowing. Other variations include reflexology (foot massage), shiatsu and tui-na (acupressure). The practice of massage therapy requires State certification or licensure.

The benefits of massage therapy are documented in palliative care populations[42]. This intervention is well documented for pain reduction in cancer patients at various stages of illness[43]. In the largest study to date, 87 hospitalized cancer patients were randomized to reflexology or to control on a crossover basis. Pain and anxiety scores fell with massage, with differences between groups achieving substantial significance ($p = 0.001$)[44]. Pain scores fell by two-thirds immediately after the first massage of patients. The improvements appeared to be cumulative. No similar changes were seen in controls. Other studies found similar results for patients with postoperative pain. In an analysis of 1290 patient reports of symptom severity pre- and post-massage therapy, 0–10 ratings of pain, fatigue, stress/anxiety, nausea, depression, and 'other' were reduced by approximately 50 per cent, even for patients reporting high baseline scores. Benefits persisted with no return toward baseline scores throughout 48-h follow-up[45].

Tai-Chi is an exercise regimen derived from martial arts. A person practicing tai chi moves the body and limbs in a slow, relaxed, fluid, and graceful series of movements. Attention is also paid to breathing and meditation. Tai-Chi practice has been shown to improve agility and reduce risk of falls in frail and elderly patients[46,47]. In a randomized controlled study of 256 elderly patients, a Tai-Chi exercise programme resulted in significantly fewer falls, and fewer injurious falls when compared with the stretching control group. The risk for multiple falls in the Tai Chi group was 55 per cent lower than that of the stretching control group. The Tai Chi participants showed significant improvements in measures of functional balance, physical performance, and reduced fear of falling[48].

Music therapy

Music can evoke deep-seated emotion. A particular music may hold special meaning to an individual depending on his/her life experience. Music therapy, which can be receptive or participatory, is provided by professional musicians who are also trained music therapists. They often hold professional degrees in music therapy, and are adept in dealing with the psychosocial as well as clinical issues faced by patients and family members.

Music therapy is particularly effective in the palliative care setting. Music offers creative; lyrical and symbolic means to address existential and spiritual needs, is aesthetically beautiful and expressive; brings form, order, comfort and hope; transcends predicaments, space and time; and affirms or re-establishes relationship with self, others, and the universe. Formal music therapy programmes in palliative medicine exist in many major institutions. Although music therapy extends back to folklore and Greek mythology (Apollo was the god of both music and medicine), it has been studied scientifically only in recent years.

Controlled trials indicate that music therapy produces emotional and physiological benefits, reducing anxiety, stress, depression, and pain. Music interventions significantly reduce heart rate, respiratory rate, and anxiety scores among inpatients after myocardial infarction, during ventilatory assistance, and when undergoing flexible sigmoidoscopy[49]. Live music more effectively reduced anxiety than recorded music.

In the preoperative setting, randomized trials have found that music reduced anxiety and its physiologic correlates such as blood pressure and salivary cortisol, a biochemical marker of stress and anxiety. Music lowered blood pressure and anxiety scores during and after eye surgery[50] and among women undergoing hysterectomies in a randomized, controlled trial[51].

Music therapy was shown to be effective against laboratory-induced pain, among cancer patients[44] and among cancer patients with chronic pain[52]. Music reduced intraoperative analgesic requirements compared with controls, and patients randomized to a music intervention reported significantly less pain and required less pain medication. In what was possibly the largest trial of its type, 500 surgical patients were randomized to control, recorded music, jaw relaxation, or a music/jaw relaxation combination.

Music led to significant decreases in both pain intensity and related distress associated with pain[53]. Music also can help reduce depression[54]. A randomized controlled trial of cancer patients undergoing autologous stem-cell transplantation showed that anxiety, depression and total mood disturbance scores were significantly lower in the music therapy group than the standard care controls[55].

Energy medicine

Therapies in this category involve manipulation of a putative human energy field. This may be provided by a 'healer', an individual with a special gift for energy healing. Healing of this type, which has remained popular over the centuries in less developed areas of the world[56], has gained increasing public interest and acceptance in the USA. Healers in many areas of the USA claim the ability to cure people of cancer. Although they may cause only minor difficulties when patients also receive mainstream care, many patients are firmly convinced of healers' abilities and decline even to have tumours removed surgically in favour of healers' ministrations.

The purported manipulation of energy field may also be provided by devices that sell for hundreds of dollars. One such device is the 'BioResonance Therapy Device' which is claimed to detect 'electromagnetic emissions' from the patient's cancer cells, modify them and send them back to the patients to correct the defects in the cancer cells. Obviously, no one with a basic understanding of the pathogenesis and treatment of cancer would subscribe to such a theory[57], but that did not stop the manufacturer of these devices from propagating the myth and promoting the equipment in the international market.

Acupuncture

Acupuncture involves the insertion and stimulation of needles at selected body points to achieve a therapeutic effect (Fig. 17.1). Although it is based on the theory that needling regulates the flow of vital energy, recent neuroscience research suggests that acupuncture induces clinical responses through modulation of the nervous system[58,59].

Most acupuncture research was done in analgesia models. Acupuncture was shown to relieve both acute (e.g. postoperative dental pain) and chronic (e.g. headache) pain[60,61]. A recent randomized controlled trial of 570 patients with osteoarthritis of the knee found that a 26-week course of acupuncture significantly improved pain and dysfunction when compared with sham-acupuncture control. All patients received other usual care for osteoarthritis. Improvement in function but not in pain was observed at week 8, suggesting that long-term treatment maybe required to achieve full effect[62].

A randomized placebo-controlled trial tested auricular acupuncture for cancer patients with pain despite stable medication. Ninety patients were randomized to needles placed at correct acupuncture points (treatment group), versus acupuncture or pressure at non-acupuncture points. Pain intensity decreased by 36 per cent at 2 months from baseline in the treatment group, a statistically significant difference compared with the two control groups, for whom little pain reduction was seen[63]. Skin penetration per se showed no significant analgesic effect. The authors selected acupuncture points by measuring electrodermal signals. These results are especially important because most of the patients had neuropathic pain, which is generally considered to be more difficult to treat than pain related to tissue injury.

Acupuncture also helps lessen nausea and vomiting associated with chemotherapy, surgery, pregnancy, and motion sickness[64–67]. In one study, 104 breast cancer patients receiving highly emetogenic chemotherapy were randomized to receive electroacupuncture at the PC6 acupuncture point, minimal needling at non-acupuncture points, or pharmacotherapy alone. Electroacupuncture significantly reduced the number of episodes of total emesis when compared with pharmacotherapy only. Most patients did not know the group to which they had been assigned[68]. The effects of acupuncture do not appear entirely due to attention, clinician-patient interaction, or simple placebo effect.

Acupuncture has been reported to reduce xerostomia (dry mouth) caused by salivary gland injury from head and neck radiotherapy. Acupuncture improved Xerostomia Inventory scores in 18 patients with head and neck cancer and pilocarpine-resistant xerostomia in uncontrolled trials.

Patients with breast or prostate cancer may experience vasomotor symptoms (hot flashes) during oestrogen or androgen ablation therapy. A few uncontrolled studies investigated acupuncture to treat these symptoms and the results of these and subsequent trials remain inconclusive. Earlier studies showed that acupuncture may reduce vasomotor symptoms (hot flashes) in postmenopausal women[69]. Self-stimulation of implanted miniature acupuncture needles attenuated tamoxifen-related hot flashes in 8 of 12 patients with breast cancer[70], and similar results were found in a case series of patients with breast[71] and prostate cancer[72]. However, subsequent controlled trials demonstrated that such reduction can also be seen in patients receive sham acupuncture controls. The difference in reduction of hot flashes was not statistically significant between traditional acupuncture and sham acupuncture[73,74].

Post-chemotherapy fatigue has few reliable treatments in patients without a correctable cause, such as anaemia. It can be a major contributing factor in lowering the quality of life in cancer patients. In an uncontrolled trial of fatigue after chemotherapy, acupuncture reduced fatigue 31 per cent after 6 weeks of treatment. Among those with severe fatigue at baseline, 79 per cent had non-severe fatigue scores at follow-up[75], whereas fatigue was reduced only in 24 per cent of patients receiving usual care in another centre[76].

Other therapies

Other complementary therapies, such as spiritual care, counselling, exercise and fitness programme, and group support, have been part of supportive, rehabilitative and palliative care for decades. Many of these behavioural interventions fall in the grey area between mainstream treatment and CAM.

Pet therapy (the use of pet animals) is thought to help reduce loneliness and improve quality of life, especially for those who are elderly, alone or demented. Most pet therapy research has been conducted in psychiatric settings. A randomized clinical trial with pain and palliative care cancer patients, conducted at the NIH Clinical Centre, was launched in 2005. This study will examine how animal-assisted therapy affects pain in cancer patients receiving pain and palliative care at the NIH Clinical Center.

Art therapy is a behavioural modality that uses creative expression to help develop coping skills. Many cancer centres provide access to artistic expression on a recreational basis or guided by professional art therapists. A few reports showed an association between art therapy with better collaboration of children with leukaemia with painful procedures, and with reduced stress and lowered anxiety in family caregivers of patients with cancer. Although scientific study of art therapy is minimal, it is clear that many patients enjoy creative activity, and the enjoyment per se is an important end in and of itself.

Summary

The public in general and palliative care patients in particular are interested in complementary and alternative therapies. These therapies are diverse and have variable benefits and risks. Some are clearly fraudulent. Patients should be advised to avoid them.

Complementary therapies, on the other hand, can help reduce many symptoms experienced by patients with advanced illnesses. Although many of these therapies have been practised over time as components of traditional medical systems, efforts to subject complementary therapies to rigorous scientific research started only in the past decade or so. This research has resulted in an increasing body of evidence that supports the use of acupuncture, massage, music, mind–body therapies, and other complementary modalities to reduce physical and emotional symptoms.

Mainstream medical centres and practices have established Integrative Medicine services to incorporate complementary therapies into multi-disciplinary treatment plans. These therapies should be applied particularly when conventional treatments produce unwarranted side effects to bring satisfactory symptom relief. In some cases, complementary therapies also may reduce the level of opioids required for pain control, and thereby mitigate opioid-related side effects.

In providing patient-centred medical care, complementary therapies must be tailored to the needs and preferences of each patient. Economic concerns, patients' belief systems, and cultural backgrounds also influence selection of therapies. In light of product quality control issues and potential interactions with prescription medications, it is important to access or refer patients and families to sources of reliable information about common herbs and dietary supplements[12].

Professional societies have been established to raise awareness and encourage the use of evidence-based complementary therapies in palliative and supportive care (www.IntegrativeOnc.com). By properly integrating complementary therapies into palliative care, we can help reduce troubling symptoms, promote family involvement and patient self-care, improve the patient's sense of well-being, and enhance the physician–patient relationship.

References

1. WHO (1990). *Cancer pain and relief (Technical Report Series 804)*. World Health Organization, Geneva.
2. Eisenberg, D.M., Kessler, R.C, Foster, C. *et al.* (1993). Unconventional medicine in the United States. Prevalence, costs, and patterns of use. *New England Journal of Medicine*, **328**, 246–52.
3. Cassileth, B.R., Lusk, E.J., Strouse, T.B. *et al.*(1984). Contemporary unorthodox treatments in cancer medicine. A study of patients, treatments, and practitioners. *Annals of Internal Medicine*, **101**, 105–12.
4. Eisenberg, D.M., Davis, R.B., Ettner, S.L, *et al.* (1998). Trends in alternative medicine use in the United States, 1990–1997: results of a follow-up national survey. *JAMA*, **280**, 1569–75.
5. Barnes, P.M., Powell-Griner, E., McFann, K. *et al.* (2004). Complementary and alternative medicine use among adults: United States, 2002. *Advance Data*, 1–19.
6. Ernst, E., and Cassileth, B.R. (1998). The prevalence of complementary/alternative medicine in cancer: a systematic review. *Cancer*, **83**, 777–82.
7. Molassiotis, A., Fernadez-Ortega, P., Pud, D. *et al.* (2005). Use of complementary and alternative medicine in cancer patients: a European survey. *Annals of Oncology*, **16**, 655–63.
8. Hyodo, I., Amano, N., Eguchi, K. *et al.* (2005). Nationwide survey on complementary and alternative medicine in cancer patients in Japan. *Journal of Clinical Oncology*, **23**, 2645–54.
9. http://www.nnfa.org/facts/index.htm. Accessed 19 December 2006.
10. Abu-Realh, M.H., Magwood, G., Narayan, M.C. *et al.* (1996). The use of complementary therapies by cancer patients. *Nursingconnections*, **9**, 3–12.
11. Kilgore, C. (1998). Perspectives. Expanding coverage signals growing demand, acceptance for alternative care. *Medicine and Health*, **52**(suppl) 1–4.
12. AboutHerbs. http://www.mskcc.org/aboutherbs Accessed 19 December 2006.
13. Lee, A., and Langer, R. (1983). Shark cartilage contains inhibitors of tumour angiogenesis. *Science*, **221**, 1185–7.
14. Liang, J.H., and Wong, K.P. (2000). The characterization of angiogenesis inhibitor from shark cartilage. *Advances in Experimental Medicine and Biology*, **476**, 209–23.
15. Miller, D.R., Anderson, G.T., Stark, J.J. *et al.* (1998). Phase I/II trial of the safety and efficacy of shark cartilage in the treatment of advanced cancer. *Journal of Clinical Oncology*, **16**, 3649–55.
16. Loprinzi, C.L., Levitt, R., Barton, D.L. *et al.* (2005). Evaluation of shark cartilage in patients with advanced cancer. *Cancer*
17. Pinter, A., Dorian, P., and Newman, D. (2002). Cesium-induced torsades de pointes. *New England Journal of Medicine*, **346**, 383–4.
18. Satoh, T., Zipes, D.P. (1998). Cesium-induced atrial tachycardia degenerating into atrial fibrillation in dogs: atrial torsades de pointes? *Journal of Cardiovascular Electrophysiology*, **9**, 970–5.
19. Green S (1992). A critique of the rationale for cancer treatment with coffee enemas and diet. *JAMA*, **268**, 3224–7.
20. Marcason W (2003). What is the lowdown on Coral Calcium? *Journal of the American Dietetic Association* **103**, 1319.
21. Cruciani, R.A., Dvorkin, E., Homel, P. *et al.* (2004). L-carnitine supplementation for the treatment of fatigue and depressed mood in cancer patients with carnitine deficiency: a preliminary analysis. *Annals of the New York Academy of Sciences* **1033**, 168–76.
22. Graziano, F., Bisonni, R., Catalano, V. *et al.* (2002). Potential role of levocarnitine supplementation for the treatment of chemotherapy-induced fatigue in non-anaemic cancer patients. *British Journal of Cancer*, **86**, 1854–7.
23. Stubblefield, M.D., Vahdat, L.T., Balmaceda, C.M. *et al.* (2005). Glutamine as a neuroprotective agent in high-dose paclitaxel-induced peripheral neuropathy: a clinical and electrophysiologic study. *Clinical Oncology (Royal College of Radiologists)*, **17**, 271–6.
24. Savarese, D.M., Savy, G. *et al.* (2003). Prevention of chemotherapy and radiation toxicity with glutamine. *Cancer Treatment Reviews*, **29**, 501–13.
25. (1996). Integration of behavioral and relaxation approaches into the treatment of chronic pain and insomnia. NIH Technology Assessment Panel on Integration of Behavioral and Relaxation Approaches into the Treatment of Chronic Pain and Insomnia. *JAMA*, **276**, 313–8.
26. Deng, G., and Cassileth, B.R. (2005). Integrative oncology: complementary therapies for pain, anxiety, and mood disturbance. *CA: A Cancer Journal For Clinicians*, **55**, 109–16.
27. Cunningham, A.J., Edmonds, C.V., Jenkins, G.P. *et al.* (1998). A randomized controlled trial of the effects of group psychological therapy on survival in women with metastatic breast cancer. *Psychooncology*, **7**, 508–17.
28. Gellert, G.A., Maxwell, R.M., and Siegel, B.S. (1993). Survival of breast cancer patients receiving adjunctive psychosocial support therapy: a 10-year follow-up study. *Journal of Clinical Oncology*, **11**, 66–9.
29. Cassileth, B.R. (1989). The social implications of mind–body cancer research. *Cancer Investigation*, **7**, 361–4.
30. Sellick, S.M., and Zaza, C. (1998). Critical review of 5 nonpharmacologic strategies for managing cancer pain. *Cancer Prevention & Control*, **2**, 7–14.

31. Marcus, J., Elkins, G., Mott F (2003). A model of hypnotic intervention for palliative care. *Advances in Mind-Body Medicine*, **19**, 24–7.

32. Marcus, J., Elkins, G., Mott F (2003). The integration of hypnosis into a model of palliative care. *Integrative Cancer Therapies*, **2**, 365–70.

33. Walker, L.G., Walker, M.B., Ogston, K. *et al.* (1999). Psychological, clinical and pathological effects of relaxation training and guided imagery during primary chemotherapy. *British Journal of Cancer*, **80**, 262–8.

34. Speca, M., Carlson, L.E., Goodey, E. *et al.* (2000). A randomized, wait-list controlled clinical trial: the effect of a mindfulness meditation-based stress reduction program on mood and symptoms of stress in cancer outpatients. *Psychosomatic Medicine*, **62**, 613–22.

35. Carlson, L.E., Speca, M., Patel, K.D. *et al.* (2004). Mindfulness-based stress reduction in relation to quality of life, mood, symptoms of stress and levels of cortisol, dehydroepiandrosterone sulfate (DHEAS) and melatonin in breast and prostate cancer outpatients. *Psychoneuroendocrinology*, **29**, 448–74.

36. Cohen, L., Warneke, C., Fouladi, R.T. *et al.* (2004). Psychological adjustment and sleep quality in a randomized trial of the effects of a Tibetan yoga intervention in patients with lymphoma. *Cancer*, **100**, 2253–60.

37. Shapiro, S.L., Bootzin, R.R., Figueredo, A.J. *et al.* (2003). The efficacy of mindfulness-based stress reduction in the treatment of sleep disturbance in women with breast cancer: an exploratory study. *Journal of Psychosomatic Research*, **54**, 85–91.

38. Lawrence, D.J. (1990). Report from the Consensus Conference on the Validation of Chiropractic Methods. *Journal of Manipulative And Physiological Therapeutics*, **13**, 295–6.

39. Rosa, L., Rosa, E., Sarner, L. *et al.*(1998). A close look at therapeutic touch. *JAMA*, **279**, 1005–10.

40. Olson, K., Hanson, J., Michaud M (2003). A phase II trial of Reiki for the management of pain in advanced cancer patients. *Journal of Pain and Symptom Management*, **26**, 990–7.

41. Mackay, N., Hansen, S., McFarlane O (2004). Autonomic nervous system changes during Reiki treatment: a preliminary study. *Journal of Alternative and Complementary Medicine*, **10**, 1077–81.

42. Wilkinson, S., Aldridge, J., Salmon, I. *et al.* (1999). An evaluation of aromatherapy massage in palliative care. *Palliative Medicine*, **13**, 409–17.

43. Ferrell-Torry, A.T., and Glick, O.J. (1993). The use of therapeutic massage as a nursing intervention to modify anxiety and the perception of cancer pain. *Cancer Nursing*, **16**, 93–101.

44. Beck, S.L. (1991). The therapeutic use of music for cancer-related pain. *Oncology Nursing Forum*, **18**, 1327–37.

45. Cassileth, B.R., Vickers, A.J. (2004). Massage therapy for symptom control: outcome study at a major cancer center. *Journal of Pain and Symptom Management*, **28**, 244–9.

46. Lin, M.R., Hwang, H.F., Wang, Y.W. *et al.* (2006). Community-based tai chi and its effect on injurious falls, balance, gait, and fear of falling in older people. *Physical Therapy*, **86**, 1189–201.

47. Faber, M.J., Bosscher, R.J., Chin, A.P.M.J. *et al.* (2006). Effects of exercise programs on falls and mobility in frail and pre-frail older adults: A multicenter randomized controlled trial. *Archives of Physical Medicine and Rehabilitation*, **87**, 885–96.

48. Li, F., Harmer, P., Fisher, K.J., *et al.* (2005). Tai Chi and fall reductions in older adults: a randomized controlled trial. *Journals of Gerontology. Series A, Biological Sciences and Medical Sciences*, **60**, 187–94.

49. Chlan, L., Evans, D,., Greenleaf, M., Walker J (2000). Effects of a single music therapy intervention on anxiety, discomfort, satisfaction, and compliance with screening guidelines in outpatients undergoing flexible sigmoidoscopy. *Gastroenterology and Nursing*, **23**, 148–56.

50. Allen, K., Golden, L.H., Izzo, J.L., Jr. *et al.* (2001). Normalization of hypertensive responses during ambulatory surgical stress by perioperative music. *Psychosomatic Medicine*, **63**, 487–92.

51. Mullooly, V.M., Levin, R.F., Feldman, H.R. (1988). Music for postoperative pain and anxiety. *The Journal of the New York State Nurses' Association*, **19**, 4–7.

52. Zimmerman, L., Pozehl, B., Duncan, K. *et al.* (1989). Effects of music in patients who had chronic cancer pain. *Western Journal of Nursing Research*, **11**, 298–309.

53. Good, M., Stanton-Hicks, M., Grass, J.A., *et al.* (2001). Relaxation and music to reduce postsurgical pain. *J Adv Nurs*, **33**, 208–15.

54. Hanser, S.B., and Thompson, L.W. (1994). Effects of a music therapy strategy on depressed older adults. *Journal of Gerontology*, **49**, P265–P269.

55. Cassileth, B.R., Vickers, A.J., and Magill, L.A. (2003). Music therapy for mood disturbance during hospitalization for autologous stem cell transplantation: a randomized controlled trial. *Cancer*, **98**, 2723–9.

56. Cassileth, B.R., Vlassov, V.V., and Chapman, C.C. (1995). Health care, medical practice, and medical ethics in Russia today. *JAMA*, **273**, 1569–73.

57. Ernst E (2004). Bioresonance, a study of pseudo-scientific language. *Forsch Komplementarmed Klass Naturheilkd*, **11**, 171–3.

58. Kaptchuk, T.J. (2002). Acupuncture: theory, efficacy, and practice. *Annals of Internal Medicine*, **136**, 374–83.

59. Han, J.S. (2004). Acupuncture and endorphins. *Neuroscience Letter*, **361**, 258–61.

60. NIH Consensus Conference (1998). Acupuncture. *JAMA*, **280**, 1518–24.

61. Melchart, D., Linde, K,. Fischer, P. *et al.* (1999). Acupuncture for recurrent headaches: a systematic review of randomized controlled trials. *Cephalalgia* **19**, 779–86; discussion 65.

62. Berman, B.M., Lao, L., Langenberg, P. *et al.* (2004). Effectiveness of acupuncture as adjunctive therapy in osteoarthritis of the knee: a randomized, controlled trial. *Annals of Internal Medicine*, **141**, 901–10.

63. Alimi, D., Rubino, C., Pichard-Leandri, E. *et al.* (2003). Analgesic effect of auricular acupuncture for cancer pain: a randomized, blinded, controlled trial. *Journal of Clinical Oncology*, **21**, 4120–6.

64. Ezzo, J.M., Richardson, M.A., Vickers, A. *et al.* (2006). Acupuncture-point stimulation for chemotherapy-induced nausea or vomiting. *Cochrane Database of Systematic Reviews* CD002285.

65. Chernyak, G.V., and Sessler, D.I. (2005). Perioperative acupuncture and related techniques. *Anesthesiology*, **102**, 1031–49; quiz 77–8.

66. Lee, A., and Done, M.L. (2004). Stimulation of the wrist acupuncture point P6 for preventing postoperative nausea and vomiting. *Cochrane Database of Systematic Reviews*, CD003281.

67. Jewell, D., and Young, G. (2003). Interventions for nausea and vomiting in early pregnancy. *Cochrane Database of Systematic Reviews*, CD000145.

68. Shen, J., Wenger, N., Glaspy, J. *et al.* (2000). Electroacupuncture for control of myeloablative chemotherapy-induced emesis: A randomized controlled trial. *JAMA*, **284**, 2755–61.

69. (2004). Treatment of menopause-associated vasomotor symptoms: position statement of The North American Menopause Society. *Menopause*, **11**, 11–33.

70. Towlerton, G., Filshie, J., O'Brien, M. *et al.* (1999). Acupuncture in the control of vasomotor symptoms caused by tamoxifen. *Palliative Medicine*, **13**, 445.

71. Porzio, G., Trapasso, T., Martelli, S. *et al.* (2002). Acupuncture in the treatment of menopause-related symptoms in women taking tamoxifen. *Tumori*, **88**, 128–30.

72. Hammar, M., Frisk, J., Grimas, O. *et al.* (1999). Acupuncture treatment of vasomotor symptoms in men with prostatic carcinoma: a pilot study. *Journal of Urology*, **161**, 853–6.

73. Vincent, A., Barton, D.L., Mandrekar, J.N. *et al.* (2006). Acupuncture for hot flashes: a randomized, sham-controlled clinical study. *Menopause*.

74. Huang, M.I., Nir, Y., Chen, B., Schnyer, R., Manber R (2006). A randomized controlled pilot study of acupuncture for postmenopausal hot flashes: effect on nocturnal hot flashes and sleep quality. *Fertility and Sterility*, **86**, 700–10.

75. Vickers, A.J., Straus, D.J., Fearon, B. *et al.* (2004). Acupuncture for postchemotherapy fatigue: a phase II study. *Journal of Clinical Oncology*, **22**, 1731–5.

76. Escalante, C.P., Grover, T., Johnson, B.A. *et al.* (2001). A fatigue clinic in a comprehensive cancer center: design and experiences. *Cancer*, **92**, 1708–13.

SECTION 18

Palliative care in the home

18.1

Palliative care in the home: an overview

Derek Doyle

The principles of palliative care are the same whether it is provided in the home, in a hospital, or in a hospice. There are, however, several unique challenges when palliative care is offered in the home. They will be the focus of this section.

The confusing kaleidoscope of models of care and nomenclature

By 'care in the home' is meant that offered to patients living in their own home or that of a relative, in a nursing or care home, in a hostel for the homeless, or in a prison or similar institution. That is to say, all care *not* given in a hospital. Patients may still be attending a hospital for investigations, day care or specialist consultations. In what follows the term Primary Care will, where possible, be avoided because of different meanings in different countries. In some it refers to care by doctors and nurses working exclusively with patients living in one of the settings listed above. In others, it refers to the doctor or nurse of first contact, often one working in a hospital, who may never see a patient at home or speak to any relative except the one accompanying the patient.

The subject is unfortunately complicated by the fact that, worldwide, so many different words are used to describe the professionals involved in home care. Whereas in many European countries the doctor is a 'general practitioner' (GP), in North America he or she will be called either a 'family doctor' or 'family physician.' The attending nurse may be a 'community nurse', a 'district nurse', or a 'clinical nurse specialist' (e.g. cardiac, diabetic, COPD (chronic obstructive pulmonary disease), paediatric, psychiatric or dialysis nurse) The clinical nurse specialists who care for those with advanced cancer in Britain will include 'Macmillan nurses', 'Marie Curie nurses', and 'site specific clinical nurse specialists'—terms reflecting specialist training and expertise in palliative care nursing or the care of patients with site specific malignancy. Whereas in Britain the person employed to provide domestic assistance in the home is a 'Home Help', in North America such a person will be called a 'Home Maker'. Even the hospital departments have differing names. In Britain and countries in the same tradition, patients coming for consultations will be seen in a Health Centre staffed by GPs, or a hospital Out-Patient Department. In North America and countries following that tradition, they are seen in a hospital's Ambulatory Care Department. The Accident and Emergency Department (A&E) of Britain is the Emergency Room (ER) of North America.

The situation becomes more complicated when the patterns of care for those at home are described. Few countries have the same systems. In Britain and countries following its traditions, the GP is responsible for patients who have asked to be his/her responsibility. He or she is the professional who makes the initial assessment, orders investigations, decides whether or not specialist expertise is needed and, in many cases, selects the specialist colleague who he or she wants to see the patient. Working with the GP will be nurses employed by the GP or their practice, as well as community nurses (employed by the local health authority) each attending patients in their homes. Together they will decide whether bringing in the services of a Home Help would be useful, and what else needs to be done to enable the patients to have optimal care at home. The quality of their collaboration and communication is, as we shall see, crucially important when providing palliative care. Traditionally GPs made house calls to those too ill or frail for whatever reason to visit their health-centre consulting rooms (or 'surgery'). Home visits are now done less frequently than even a decade ago and out-of-hours home visits are done by doctors employed by a cooperative or agency, again of relevance in palliative care[1]. In a system such as the British National Health Service (NHS) just described, the doctor and nurses are paid by the state, the patient only having to pay for prescribed drugs (unless exempt because of age and certain chronic conditions).

In other parts of the world family doctors not only see patients who visit them in their offices but may have admitting rights in local hospitals and direct access to the most sophisticated investigations. Few home visits are done and most out-of-hours problems, even if not true emergencies, are dealt with in the ER of the nearest hospital. Fees are paid directly by the patient or through an insurance agency. Attending hospital can be a frustrating experience for terminally ill patients. They have to wait to be seen, may miss meals because of investigations being done, have to give the same personal details to several different staff members, and then find that there are poor transport arrangements to return home[2].

In a few countries, even where secondary and tertiary referral hospitals are highly developed, there may be no 'primary care' of the types described but clinics, staffed by doctor(s) and nurses serving a large, scattered population. Specialist advice and diagnostic services such as x-ray, bacteriology, and biochemistry may only be available in a distant hospital. Many of the medicines regarded as essential in a 'developed' country may not be available and, even when they are, may be too expensive for most patients to be able to afford. In such countries opioids, if available, can only be obtained from the pharmacies of tertiary referral specialist hospitals and then only for limited periods such as 30 days and with a legal ceiling on the dose permitted. In yet other places out-patient (ambulatory) palliative care services are available in major hospitals for patients under care at home[3].

The picture, therefore, is a mixed one ranging from the sophistication of the developed countries to the scanty services without basic medications and diagnostic services of the developing world. In the former most GPs and family doctors will have been taught something, albeit usually far from enough, about palliative care whilst in the poorer countries where it might be argued palliative care is even more needed than in the developed world because the means to cure such conditions as malignancy are non-existent, they will have been taught nothing about palliative care. It is clearly difficult if not impossible to discuss comprehensively how palliative care might be offered across this spectrum. This chapter has been written in the hope that readers will study how best to provide high quality palliative care in their country whatever its pattern of 'primary care', its economics, culture, sophistication and development. What is not intended is that anyone shall attempt to clone what appears to them a perfect service. There is no such thing.

What do we know about palliative care in the home today?

The least important thing we know is that palliative care at home may save money![4,13] Infinitely more important is that most patients do not achieve their wish to die at home[5]. It has long been claimed that everyone wants to die at home. In fact, in Britain, 61 per cent of 16–24-year olds do so, and 49 per cent of 65+ do so[6–9]. One study[6] found that 55 per cent of cancer patients hoped to die at home but only 23 per cent did so. Only 12 per cent of patients with malignant and non-malignant conditions wanted to die in hospital but 55 per cent did so. Less than 5 per cent wanted a nursing home death but 20 per cent died there. Patient choice was not evident. On the other hand Marie Curie researchers in the UK found that 90 per cent of patients under their care died at home as they had wished[10]. Is it more accurate to say that whilst many would like to die at home, most certainly want to spend as long at home as possible? The subject is clearly neither simple nor straight forward.

Whether or not there is a Community Palliative Care Service does not seem crucial in determining place of death[11]. Deaths at home are decreasing even when the provision of palliative care in the community is of a high standard, a community palliative care service is being used, and specialist palliative care advice is available around the clock[12]. Data show that in many places the level of poorly relieved suffering in both dying children and adults, is higher in hospitals than in patients' homes, but presumably that is something both public and patients are unaware of. The factors determining where they die seem to be as much societal as medical[11]. In this recent systematic review data from 58 studies involving 1.5 million patients were analysed. Those patients most likely to be cared for and to die at home are those who not only want to die there but have expressed this preference, those with low functional status, those aware of the imminence of dying, those who have lived with the caring relative for some time and, on

weaker evidence, those with solid tumours. Those with non-solid tumours and those with more than one illness are more likely to die in hospital. Bradshaw found that those referred for in-patient care were older, less likely to have a carer and in need of more nursing[13]. This would suggest that as our populations age more will die in institutions.

According to Higginson the factors determining where people die and why vary greatly from country to country[11]. In Italy, 75 per cent of patients under a community palliative care service died at home[14] whereas in Sweden 37 per cent died at home[15]. In the UK, USA, France, Germany, and Switzerland the percentage of people dying at home is steadily falling. In the UK in 1994, 27 per cent died at home. By 2003, the figure had fallen to 22 per cent. In some countries rooms are too small for satisfactory home nursing with its equipment, seats for attendants and streams of visitors. In yet others most of the care is given in hospital but patients ask to be taken home, often in the last 24 h, to die there. The problems of continuity of care, timing of medications and continuity of emotional support are obvious. According to one study place of death is more related to the role and influence of the GP than of any nurse[16–18]. Other factors are the relatives, the handling of emergencies, and the availability of medications and equipment. In Italy, on the other hand, whether or not a person died at home depended on whether a Community Palliative Care Service was involved and that itself depended on whether the patient was married and well educated[19,74]. De Conno working in Milan also reported on the effect of a community service[20] whilst Toscani in Cremona found that most wanted home deaths because hospital care was so poor for the dying[21]. A UK study found that those dying at home were usually married, had had less depression and anxiety, and were well supported[22]. In contrast to the Italian studies, Grande and colleagues (in the UK) found that a comprehensive community palliative service did not lead to more patients staying at home but to better care before eventual admission. The study (of 94 GPs, 225 community nurses and 144 carers) found night cover and support were better, the GPs finding that patients' anxiety and depression were less at home, the carers feeling that the patients had less pain and nausea[12,23].

What seems clear is that while good palliative care in the home is something to strive for, it may not result in more people dying there even if that is their wish. It follows that care in the home should be improved for its own sake and not solely to ensure that death takes place there.

Transferring a patient to hospital to die is often requested by a relative or done by a doctor because of perceived suffering and exhaustion of a relative, or because there are difficulties getting doctors to do house calls at night, a problem likely to increase in countries where GPs are opting out of all evening, night, and weekend work[1]. The need for on-call nurses has also been investigated[24]. Palliative care patients expect, and usually need, a fast response from their doctor. However, it seems that few GPs routinely hand over information to GP cooperatives. They and community nurses are not satisfied with current arrangements for 'out-of-hours' care and both groups agree that 24 h availability of palliative care nurses and medical specialists is essential, as are improved communication and collaboration[25].

Many relatives assume that caring for a person at home is beyond their physical, emotional, or intellectual ability (see below)[26]. There are reports of societal pressures brought to bear on a relative hoping to care for a patient at home, especially when the hospital to which they could be transferred has its own specialist hospital palliative care service.

Every patient under care at home has the right to have all treatment options explained, preferably in the presence of the caring relatives, and to select those they feel are best for them. Most important is that the professionals realize patients are seldom seeking life prolongation at any cost, but good quality of life if only for a short time. Their decisions, particularly about transfer to hospital or hospice, often reflect the patient's wish to ease the burden of care on relatives as much as achieving comfort for themselves. It has been said that the nearer a person is to death the more unselfish and considerate they are to others, especially carers in the home.

The commonest complaints about care in the home

Though few spontaneous complaints are received about the quality of home care both patients and carers are willing to express disappointments when invited to do so by researchers. These principally relate to bad communications and insufficient information[27–29]. One study found that 51 per cent of carers felt they did not get the clinical information they needed about the patient. In another study only 28 per cent found communication easy with their doctor whilst 30 per cent found him/her unsympathetic. Many carers have said that, so far as they can see, communication between doctors and nurses is poor, as is communication between hospital consultants and GPs/family doctors. One group never seems to know what the others have said[30]. Higginson reported on communication issues in three European countries[31].

Many studies have reported that carers did not get information about help and benefits that might have helped them—nursing equipment available on loan, financial help, Home Helps, night sitters, dietary advice. Others complain that they were not informed where the patient might be cared for—hospital, palliative care unit, nursing home, etc. This applied as much to cardiac and respiratory disease patients as to those with malignancy[32–34].

Several papers have highlighted the level of poorly relieved suffering experienced at home. GPs cannot be expected to be familiar with rare conditions or symptoms but the basics of pain and symptom control should be known. A study of 450 GPs in England found that they knew of the WHO analgesic ladder and the basics of pain management but little about uncommon conditions, converting from oral to subcutaneous (SC) medication and about drugs that can be used in a syringe driver[35]. A Canadian study found good commitment to palliative care but deep concerns about opioids, particularly in respiratory disease[36], whilst a German study found gross under-treatment of pain[37], Another UK study of newly qualified doctors found low confidence in their communication skills, and hands-on care in spite of considerable undergraduate teaching[38]. A British study, reports that 90 per cent of home-based patients had pain treated by their GP but the patients achieved adequate relief in only 52 per cent. In spite of that patient satisfaction with care was high. In the same study hospitals were rated but overall had poor ratings[39]. An Italian study of home care in the final weeks of life found that 76 per cent died at home, that pain was better controlled than other suffering, but 25 per cent were rendered unconscious for their final 12 h of life[14]. An Australian study found that GPs recognize the place and

importance of palliative care but felt they missed some of the suffering because they knew they did not have the skills to relieve it. Murray interviewed the GPs of 40 terminally ill patients[40]. They all recognized that there might be spiritual needs but either waited for a cue or felt they had insufficient time or the necessary skills to help. Mitchell found that patients and carers valued the time to talk with their doctors but, nevertheless, it was felt that palliative care in the home was less well provided than in palliative care units and hospitals[41]. Having said that, a Scottish survey found GPs aware that their palliative care skills could be improved[42], a finding borne out by the numbers attending training courses. Murray describes how palliative care in the community can be developed[43]. Oxenham demonstrated how it is possible to conduct a detailed and useful audit of pain management with the cooperation of GPs[44].

In Britain it is increasingly said by GPs that the principal reason they seek hospice admission is not for pain or symptom control, or because such patients take up much of their time which they are happy to give, but for the patient's need of nursing care, borne out by a 1996 study[45]. Paradoxically patients may come to appreciate how lacking in knowledge and skills their own doctor is when he/she calls in a palliative medicine specialist who changes all the medications and doses with immediate benefit. That doctor, however, knew that care could be improved and where to turn for help.

The challenge of pain management in children will be addressed in another section of this book but it is worth mentioning a Swedish study. It found a relationship between parental knowledge that death was imminent and unrelieved pain which in hospital was as high as 15.3 per cent and in the home 11.6 per cent[46].

It is not only doctors who have less-than-optimal knowledge and skills. A major US study of nurses showed only 56 per cent giving correct answers about pain management though 65 per cent were realistic about their knowledge levels, with 37 per cent thinking they were better or worse than the results showed[47]. It has also been found that palliative care nurses successfully diagnose only 25 per cent of patients with treatable depression and that the communication skills of specialist palliative care nurses are no better than other nurses, the most effective communicators being pharmacists.

Emergencies in the home

Studies have also shown that doctors are judged by how they cope with emergencies in the home. Such events can be crises for relatives when, in a hospital, they know they would easily be dealt with by the staff on duty. Carers rate home care in terms of how quickly a doctor responded to a house call, whether or not he seemed to know what to do; where, if it was necessary, the patient could be admitted and what specialist advice on the crisis was available in the home. It is difficult to exaggerate the anxiety and sense of helplessness felt by carers when something unexpected happens at home. Emergencies will be dealt with in detail later in this section.

The needs of the patient

Experience world-wide has shown that people receiving palliative care, whether in an institution or at home, need:

◆ To be cared for by health-care professionals who can recognize and diagnose their suffering and know how to deal with it-whether it is physical, emotional, social, or spiritual. Education and training in palliative care are therefore essential.

- To be assured that their autonomy and right to choose will be respected with regard to place of care (and place of death) and all treatments available and appropriate for them.

- Particularly in the home, they need to know that their relatives, especially those caring for them, are being supported, guided, and prepared for what lies ahead. *This is one feature that makes palliative care in the home different from such care in an institution.*

It is equally important to understand what is *not* essential for such patients, what they do not expect or ask for. Contrary to what most professionals believe, palliative care patients at home do not expect that the doctor will spend longer with them than he/she would with someone not near the end of life. The nearer patients are to death the more conscious are they of time and eager not to 'waste' it. Neither, in the later stages of their illnesses, do they want long, detailed explanations of the illness, treatment, and prognosis. Neither are they eager for more investigations, particularly invasive ones. Though they appreciate what all the professionals are doing to help them they do not want to have to develop relationships with more of them, something that needs to be remembered when different doctors and nurses (and students working with them) visit them. One British oncologist/palliative medicine physician found that the 'average' patient came into contact with 92 different professionals in the final months of life.

All these patients ask is to feel 'safe'—a word often used by them, unlikely and inappropriate as it seems. By this, so they tell us, they mean safe to suffer, safe to express their every emotion, safe to have faith, and safe to admit if it is weak or inadequate—safe to be themselves and not as relatives and friends may have seen them or want to see them. Lastly, they expect and value honesty at all times.

The part played by lay carers

It is impossible to exaggerate the role of lay carers. It is no wonder that so many researchers have come to the conclusion that the success or otherwise of care at home lies in the hands of the relatives as much as the professionals. They find themselves having to do a daunting range of things (see Table 18.1.1).

Many of these tasks they have not done before, nor have they been told in advance about them. Add to that the sense of isolation and loneliness at this time, the difficulty in explaining what they are going through, and the tempting option of having the patient admitted to a hospital where, they assume, care will be better and their own stamina not eroded[48].

Many studies have shown how stressful it can be caring for a patient at home, and how little health-care professionals recognize this. Feeling understood and supported *before* the loved one's death is a factor in reducing subsequent bereavement pain and morbidity[49]. They often report the patient having more pain and anxiety than is the case, possibly reflecting their own sense of helplessness[50].

The needs of lay carers

Lay carers in the home need as much time spent with them as with the patient. Studies continue to show that whether or not the patient stays at home or is admitted to an institution depends as much on the lay carers as anything else[3,39,51,52]. The help they need can often be anticipated and planned in advance, by the

Table 18.1.1 What lay carers find themselves having to learn.

- How to move, and especially lift, a helpless patient?
- How to cook for and often feed the patient?
- How to help with toileting, commode—emptying, washing and bathing?
- How to give medication (including liquid preparations of oral morphine, something that worries many)?
- How to listen to the patient's outpouring of fear, sadness, frustration, bewilderment, disappointment?
- How to respond to the patient's moods and answer the patient's questions?
- How to keep their own fears about what lies ahead from the patient?
- How to keep the family informed, and involved if they wish to be?
- How to deal with the hundreds of telephone or e-mail enquiries about the patient?
- How to maintain their own health and energy?
- How to keep the seriousness of the situation from the patient—what is often described as maintaining the conspiracy of silence. As is explained elsewhere in this book, even though the patient is known to be aware of the diagnosis and its outcome many relatives prefer to feel that they have succeeded in keeping them ignorant of what lies ahead?
- How to cope with different members of their extended family, some of whom they may not have seen for years, others with whom they have little in common, and yet others who increase tensions wherever they go?

professional care team. Their questions are 'What lies ahead and where do I fit into the picture, bearing in mind that I have never done this before and never been taught anything about this?' What they tell us they need to know is listed in Table 18.1.2

One problem in the home, but less so in hospitals, is that so many different relatives feel they should be told everything and be

Table 18.1.2 What lay carers say they want to know.

- Everything possible about the patient's illness and care plan
- About the nursing that will be involved and who will teach them
- About the reasons for, and methods of giving, medications

Research has shown that not only do patients and relatives, but also some nurses, have difficulty understanding treatments, medication regimens, and recognizing unusual pain[53]

- About any dietary needs or modifications
- About any emergencies/crises that *might* occur and how they as should deal with them (see later)
- About how to handle the never-ending stream, of visitors and enquirers
- About how to maintain their own health and stamina
- About the availability or otherwise of a Day Hospice/Palliative Day Care facility or the possibility of specialist palliative care advice when needed. (see later)
- About whom to contact in the event of a care problem even if it is not an emergency
- About any financial assistance they are eligible for
- About any domestic assistance they might get for the home
- About any equipment that they might borrow/buy to assist in the nursing (see later) and, crucially important, who is the lead clinician, coordinating the professional care team, how and when they will see him/her, and who will maintaining contact and communication with the hospital

able to speak to a doctor or nurse at any time convenient to them. Explanations or illustrations intended to help their understanding end up confusing them because they are different from those given by other members of the care team. 'The doctors and nurses all disagreed with each other'.

Addressing the needs of the carers

There are five ways of addressing most of the needs listed above

- The simplest is to advise carers to *use a small notebook* which they carry around with them, bringing it out when the doctor or nurses visit. At the front they write in advice, suggestions, instructions from the palliative care team members each time they visit. At the back they write in things about the patient and his/her care they want to ask the care team when next they see one of them.

- The doctor to set aside an hour (no more) with the main carers to *outline the palliative care principles and plans*, to tell them what help and resources are available whether or not they yet feel or recognize the need for such help, and to answer questions.

- Arranging for a member of the palliative care team (preferably a nurse) to spend about an hour with the key carers *demonstrating basic nursing procedures*—lifting, bathing, feeding, toileting, giving medications. If time permits it should be repeated after a week or two when they will have other questions. When patients attend Palliative Day Care units the opportunity is often taken to demonstrate basic nursing techniques to carers, whilst the patients are enjoying their own activities next door. People learn basic nursing quickly.

- Discuss whether having the patient attend a *Palliative Day Care Unit* will help both the patient and the carers. (See later in this section.)

- Particularly when there is rising tension and dysfunction in the family consider calling a *Family Conference*. All members of the family are warmly urged to come and told it will last less than an hour. It is led by the doctor and a nurse member of the team should be here too. The doctor explains that he will start with a brief update on the patient's illness, the stage it has reached, the likely prognosis and (more importantly) what care problems may lie ahead, what is being done (and what might need to be done) to relieve suffering. After that, he/she explains, each person present will be invited to ask questions and to say what most worries or upsets them. It is explained to them that other family members will not be allowed to interrupt them, or to speak at the same time. After each has spoken the doctor explains family dynamics, showing how each can and should understand and help each other but, at the same time, how even one person can make life hell for all the others. Finally they are asked to nominate one of the family to be the channel for all future communications, explaining that it is impracticable (and potentially confusing) for a doctor or nurse to keep meeting with different members of the family. Giving the family members responsibilities and, at the same time, demonstrating how they can and must strengthen each other, can be helpful.

Of course the best way to help such carers is not a technique or form of therapy but the reassurance that comes when they see that the doctor and nurses know what they are doing, are sensitive to need and are appropriately trained. We shall address that now.

The roles and needs of professional carers in the home

This is another area where home care differs from hospital care. The doctor will still have to be a diagnostician, watchful for complications, preventable emergencies and the need for changes in regimens. In addition he/she may need to be the leader of a large multi-professional team, knowing what each member of the team can contribute, what level of information each needs to contribute to the full—a conductor of an orchestra of skilled performers. On other occasions the best conductor may be someone else, perhaps the senior nurse, perhaps the local palliative medicine physician if one is available for consultation.

The nurse may find herself spending most of the time listening to the patient or relative rather than giving hands-on care; explaining what doctors and hospital staff have said and, on occasions having to decide whether or not to ask for medical help[54,55]. Different family members cope in their own way in their homes and all differently again when the patient is in hospital. Nurses have to learn to work with a spectrum of coping strategies in the lay carers[56]. Much of the nurse's time may be spent giving emotional care. Skilbeck, reviewing the work of clinical nurse specialists in palliative care found that 57 per cent was emotional care, 27 per cent was helping with pain, 33 per cent for non-pain symptoms. Thirteen per cent of patients died within a week of referral and 40 per cent within 6 weeks. On average they had two face-to-face meetings and made two phone calls in the 8-week period these patients were under their care[51,57,143]. Researchers in Hong Kong, found that pain and other physical symptoms were relatively easy to relieve but emotional, psychosocial, and spiritual ones were much more difficult[51].

Though members of a temporary team, created for one patient, they may not even be based in the same building. It is nevertheless vital that they meet on a regular basis, that they pass on important information to the others as efficiently as possible.

Barclay reminds us that we depend on computers but must not ignore the telephone[30]. Studies have been done on Patient Held Records small enough for the patient to take to clinics and hospital appointments, for each professional involved to insert salient facts of use to fellow professionals, as well as medications and the results of any investigations. They sound ideal for palliative care in the home but have not been shown to improve communications because some were not kept up to date, others were seen as unnecessary extra work by hospital doctors and some professionals were not sure how to record sensitive, confidential conversations with the patient, conversations that gave insight into how the patient was feeling and coping[58]. Some teams have found it helpful to make audio tapes of explanations and advice, as has for some time been used in oncology departments. The needs of team members are listed in Table 18.1.3.

Will we soon find ourselves using both telephones and computers in our cars, doing away with hardcopy records, preferring to send messages by e-mail, video conferencing team, meetings, and supplying each patient with electronic communication aids at our first meeting with them!?

Table 18.1.3 The needs of palliative care team members.

◆ Appropriate training in community palliative medicine

Thulesius stresses that any training must be tailored to the specific needs of community staff, not generic palliative care, so different are the demands on, and the health needs of workers in community palliative care[59]

◆ Training in how to deal with emergencies that might arise in the home

◆ An educated understanding of what each member of the care can contribute

◆ An understanding of how much information each needs to function properly and how best to convey that information

◆ Easy access to patient records

◆ A means of getting in touch with team members at short notice

◆ Detailed knowledge of local hospitals—where they are, how patients can be referred for consultation and/or admission

◆ Detailed knowledge of any specialist palliative care services or personnel in the locality—where they are based, how they may be contacted, how they might help in the home

◆ Knowledge of transport facilities for the seriously ill and their relatives—ambulance, voluntary services etc.

◆ Knowledge of what palliative care patients are entitled to and can apply for—financial assistance, discount holidays, reduced prescription charges, tax rebates, assistance in the house (Home Helps or Homemakers)

Pharmacy, diagnostic and emergency services

Palliative medicine in the home often involves frequent changes of drug regimens, many different medications (the mean is 4 but can be as high as 11), access to some medications at short notice, even

Table 18.1.4 Predictable complications.

Complications which can be anticipated in home-based palliative care

◆ Anaemia in myelomatosis

◆ Ascites in ovarian malignancy

◆ Bladder haemorrhage

◆ Blocked oesophagal stents

◆ Blocked urinary catheters

◆ Changed sleep pattern in cerebral malignancies

◆ Chest infections in COPD

◆ Confusional states with most infections

◆ Hiccup with renal impairment

◆ Hypercalcaemia Iatrogenic confusional states

◆ Increasing dyspnoea in cardiac failure

◆ Increasing dyspnoea in COPD

◆ Infection at dialysis site

◆ Leakage from paracentesis site

◆ Malodour from fungating lesion or colostomy

◆ Opiod-induced myoclonus

◆ Opioid-induced constipation

◆ Pain in bone metastases

◆ Pathological fractures

◆ Personality change in cerebral malignancies

◆ Spinal cord compression

◆ Superior vena caval obstruction

---

at night, with as little bureaucracy as possible[60]. Face-to-face negotiation with a pharmacist on how this can be achieved is useful. Also useful is the provision of a medicine box so that a relative or nurse can lay out all the regularly-taken pills at the time of the day they must be taken. Leaflets about pain control and the drugs used can be most helpful[142]. What is simple and obvious to a health care professional is unlikely to be seen as such by a distressed relative. Time spent explaining why each is being prescribed, when it should be taken, and what common adverse effects might be experienced, is never wasted time.

As an illness moves into the terminal phase diagnostic services are less needed (and can actually become an exhausting burden for many patients) but chest radiographs can be useful, films of bones if fractures are suspected. Rarely will MRI and CT scans be needed. Likewise haematological and biochemical tests are seldom useful except to confirm a suspicion of hypercalcaemia, or electrolyte upset explaining confusion. Too readily do we hide behind x-rays and sheets of laboratory tests when we should be listening and speaking to these patients.

What makes for successful palliative care in the home?

Skilled palliation of all suffering whatever its nature

The spectrum and intensity of pain and other symptoms are no different in the home from the hospital ward. Their pharmacological and psychological care is the same wherever the patient is cared for. Many problems occur so frequently that they can be anticipated and looked for whenever the doctor or nurses see the patient (Table 18.1.4).

What is different—and often very different—is that relatives feel nervous, untrained and inadequate about almost every aspect of patient care. They cannot differentiate between an annoying but not otherwise significant symptom and one that presages death (or so they suspect). Neither can they gauge intensity of pain with the result that they may regard the patient as having more pain than is the case[50]. A comprehensive systematic review of the literature identifies the interventions and strategies most likely to help carers[48].

Speedy, skilled handling of emergencies

A list of the commonest emergencies likely to be met in the home is shown in Table 18.1.5. Palliative care, wherever it is offered but especially in the home, should be an exercise in *pro-activity* rather than *reactivity*. Many of these emergencies cannot be prevented but the possibility of them happening can make the doctor's response speedier and better informed. They are also reminders that regular careful history-taking and examination are still needed even in advanced disease—learning of a patient's polydipsia leading to suspicions of diabetes or early hypercalcaemia, retention of urine or weakness when trying to walk to the toilet suggesting early (and possibly reversible) spinal cord compression, newly-developed confusion calling for urgent review of medication and biochemical profiling.

The doctor will need to ensure that all necessary drugs in high enough doses are in his/her emergency bag (see Table 18.1.6) and know exactly where he/she can transfer the patient if urgent investigation or consultation are needed. (Does a patient with spinal cord compression go to neuro-surgery or radiation oncology,

Table 18.1.5 Emergencies that might occur in the home.

Emergencies that can be encountered in home-based palliative care
◆ Acute confusional state
◆ Acute malignant hypercalcaemia
◆ Acute paranoia
◆ Blocked oesophageal stent
◆ Convulsions
◆ Intestinal obstruction
◆ Massive haemorrhage
◆ Panic attacks
◆ Pathological fracture
◆ Pericardial effusion
◆ Pleural effusion
◆ Spinal cord compression
◆ Superior vena caval obstuction
◆ Urinary retention

Table 18.1.7 Essential equipment for home care.

◆ Firm mattress (a bed is not essential)
◆ Anti-pressure sore mattresses / pads
◆ Feeding cup and spoons
◆ Medicine measuring cup/syringe
◆ Duvet or light blankets
◆ Air freshener
◆ Supply of ice cubes
◆ Commode
◆ Male urinal
◆ Back rest / triangular pillow
◆ Bedside table or equivalent
◆ Electric pad / hot water bottle
◆ Night lamp/ candle
◆ Chair for carer

Useful but not essential equipment

◆ TV set
◆ Radio
◆ Cordless telephone
◆ Bell to call carer
◆ Bed table/ laptop tray with non-slip mat
◆ Bedside fan
◆ Drinking straws
◆ Hoist
◆ Liquidizer
◆ Wheelchair

or a patient with superior vena caval obstruction go to radiation oncology or medical oncology?)

Knowing that emergencies might occur the doctor should always ensure the lay carers know where he/she (or a deputy) can be contacted. After the crisis has been dealt with it is important that he/she has a short meeting with the patient and carers to explain what has happened and, crucially important, to reassure that they are not to blame because often this is their first reaction—'What did I do wrong?'

Nursing equipment for care in the home

Table 18.1.7 lists equipment some of which can be regarded as essential, others useful but not essential. Without many of the items care in the home will not be easy and may prejudice patient care and comfort. It is the responsibility of the palliative care team to advise on each item and, if needs be, explain where they can be purchased or borrowed and at what cost. However, the carers must never be given the impression that without everything on these lists care in the home is not worth attempting.

Table 18.1.6 Essential drugs for the doctor's emergency bag.

◆ Morphine injection*
◆ Diamorphine injection (UK only)
◆ Dexamethasone injection **
◆ Hyoscine butylbromide injection
◆ Midazolam injection
◆ Methotrimeprazine injection
◆ Haloperidol injection
◆ Promethazine injection
◆ Cyclizine injection (UK only)
◆ Diazepam rectal solution***

* Important to have available sufficient for patients who may be on 300mg or more via a syringe driver

** May need to give up to 20 mg i.e. 5 ampoules of 4mg / ampoule

*** Useful as an anticonvulsant that can be used by lay carers

If space permits it is worth checking that the 'sick room' is laid out for maximum patient comfort and ease of nursing. The patient's bed should face the window which it should be possible to open. By the bed should be a small table on one side (for a lamp, water, medications, tissues, sputum mug if needed, a small hand bell and TV remote control) a chair on the other and space on each side of the bed, and behind the patient's head for attendants to move the patient. Every effort should be made to prevent kitchen and toilet smells reaching the sick room, and the noise of TV and telephone disturbing them.

Specialist palliative care services for home-bound patients

Community palliative care services are of two types.

Comprehensive ('Hospice at Home') with specialist palliative medicine physicians not only advising but taking charge of all medical care of the patient, his nursing colleagues doing all the professional nursing and, if needs be, staying with the patient round the clock. All essential equipment, even hospital beds and special mattresses is supplied by them. Such services make for better care at home but do not lead to more staying or dying at home [12,15,61]. A British study found that Hospice at Home was much more acceptable than care in a hospital—more personal, more 'therapeutic' and lay carers did not feel the service imposed any extra burden on them[52]. Whether such a service deskills GPs and community nurses has not been investigated. Might this become the preferred model of care now that GPs work shorter hours and do fewer home visits?

Advisory where specialist community trained palliative care nurses from the local palliative care unit, backed up by a specialist physician, visit the patient on the invitation of the GP or family physician. The nurses continue to visit and phone whilst the physician remains available to advise or visit when requested to. The GP retains clinical control at all times, writing prescriptions, ordering any investigations (in discussion with the palliative medicine physician)and supporting the relatives. Patients who regard the GP as their main prescriber have been found to be the best adherents to regimens[62].

What does the literature tell us about the effects and acceptance of community palliative care services that are now such major features of palliative care provision world-wide?

They are appropriate in non-malignant disease[63,135,139] including motor neuron disease (AML) patients on non-invasive ventilation at home,[64] and in those with Parkinson's disease[65]. The care of patients dying of cardiorespiratory failure[66] and cardiac failure have been examined[32,33] and comparisons made between patients with malignant and non-malignant diseases[67,68].

The use of community palliative care services has been reported in India[69], in Saudi Arabia[70], in Japan[71], in Germany[37] where a 3-year study found severe under-treatment of pain; in Spain where 22 638 people annually receive palliative care, 80 per cent of them for malignant disease, using 75 home-care programmes[72–74]; in Paris[54,75] and in Sicily where Mercadente has looked at the impact of symptoms on patients and the patterns of drug use in cancer patients receiving home care[76,77] in Italy[14,78]; and finally in Sweden[15].

The interface between GPs and such services is critically important[16]. GPs have a right to expect palliative medicine specialists to be available and accessible to advise them[30]. On the whole British GPs are happy with the role of advisory community palliative care services but want better 24-h cover and are prepared to assist with this[79] but a report on the care of the black population in London is challenging![80] Thirty years of home care of cancer and non-cancer patients have been reviewed[81], the key role of the family carers examined[3] as well as the barriers to cancer pain management[82], the taking of medication[62], and the value of explanatory leaflets[137]. Finally there is an interesting paper on why GPs use community palliative care services[83] and cancer patients' and carers' assessments of out-of-hours care[84].

Several studies, in addition to those already cited, have looked at whether or not community care services enable more to die at home[6–9,12,19,20,26,48,63,85].

There are a few patients who, in spite of the quality of care and emotional and social support provided at home, continue to feel a burden, or continue to lament loss of autonomy or independence or, to the end of life, still have some uncontrolled pain. Rarely, but it does happen, some might take their own lives[87]. For the vast majority of patients home care can maintain an acceptable quality of life[86].

Palliative day care/day hospice

In Britain such units are now common and popular with patients and their carers. For some reason they have not developed as much in other countries.

They are operated in whatever accommodation is available—a small hall/room attached to a hospital or palliative care unit, a church or community hall provided there is wheelchair access in the entrance, toilet, and a small room that might be used as an office/nursing procedures room. Cooking facilities are not essential provided prepared meals can be delivered and served hygienically. It is staffed by a nurse, physiotherapist, occupational therapist (all part time), selected and appropriately trained volunteers, all led by a coordinator with leadership skills and a background in palliative care.

Patients under care at home are brought in to the unit about twice weekly by volunteer transport arriving at about 10 a.m., enjoy a welcoming tea or coffee, and then seen by the coordinator or therapist who helps them with whatever creative work they want to do that day. It might be woodwork, pottery, indoor gardening, card making, baking, honing computer skills—the list is endless. Before a light lunch they are offered a little drink and after lunch (if not dozing) there is entertainment from visiting singers, actors, TV chefs and other celebrities, poets, interesting speakers, until their cars take them home at 3 p.m.

Opportunities are taken to review medication, change dressings, check that constipation has not recurred and that new clinical problems are not developing in which case a doctor sees them and immediately contacts the GP/family physician with advice.

Contrary to what some people think it is not 'divertional therapy—helping them to forget what lies ahead for them' but very creative, in the company of others in the same position as themselves. People ask to be allowed to do things or to learn skills that they have always wanted from computing to oil colour painting to calligraphy. They report that instead of feeling confined in their house and sensing they are a burden to carers they look forward to these days as the highlights of the week.

Day care should be considered as part and parcel of community palliative care, enabling people to stay at home longer with a reasonable quality of life. The cost implications have been studied[88] (as has the possibility of such care replacing in-patient care for cancer patients)[89]. The challenges of researching such a service has been addressed by Goodwin[90] and the literature on them thoroughly reviewed[91,92].

Community hospitals

In Britain and several other countries there are still a few hospitals staffed entirely by GPs/Family physicians to which they can admit their patients and, when needs be, invite consultants from nearby secondary and tertiary referral hospitals to advise. They can contribute to better palliative care in the community enabling pain and other symptoms to be brought under control and reducing the number dying in specialist units but not in the home. On the other hand, as already explained, community palliative care services do not affect the percentage of patients dying in specialist units or in the home[93].

Doctors and nurses working in them must have as much palliative care training as they would if they worked in a major city hospital.

Whether such hospitals are going to be the generic palliative care units of the future is too early to say. Before then, better 24-h medical cover by local doctors trained and experienced in palliative care will have to be restored and guaranteed.

Nursing homes/residential care homes

In this section these two terms are used interchangeably. They refer to institutions run commercially for the medium and long term residence and care of elderly people. There are many models. Some are primarily homes for those unable, for whatever reason, to remain in their own homes. Some are primarily for nursing care for those who, whilst not needing hospital care need more than simple residential care because of their level of disability and dependency. Yet others accept residents with minimal dependency and have the facilities and the staff to care for them through the period of palliative care to death. They range in size from those caring for very small numbers of residents to those with a hundred or more, often with their own fulltime doctor and nurses qualified in palliative care[94]. Whether or not nursing homes and their residents make greater demands on GPs has been studied in Britain. The question in important for any country where GPs and family physicians are making fewer 'house' calls (and that would include nursing homes) and few, if any, consultations between 6 p.m.–8 a.m. the following day[95]. Already most developed countries are seeing increasing numbers of old people spending their final years in nursing/care homes[55]. It has been suggested, such homes may become the generic palliative care units for the elderly of the future[96]. The implications for that to be successful are that consultants need to be available and nurses appropriately trained and managed. At present they are often poorly paid, and both inadequately trained and experienced in palliative care nursing[96,97] though the experience and commitment of such nurses needs to be recognized especially when devising a focused training programme for them[98–100]. It has been shown that good educational courses for the nursing staff do not always ensure organizational change[100]. Excellent studies of nursing home care of the elderly, including palliative care for them, have been published and can be commended[101–105].

Interesting and important differences have been noted in how pain and other symptoms are assessed in nursing homes and specialist palliative care centres[144]. Horton looked at how patients and nurses in the two viewed suffering. Both agreed about pain and physical symptom control but differed about patient's thoughts, emotional suffering, and practical matters[106]. Jordhoy and colleagues found that nursing home patients with advanced cancer had more severe anorexia, fatigue, and functional and cognitive impairment than other dying patients[107]. The recognition and assessment of pain was much improved in nursing homes when pain assessment scales were introduced[108]. Closs and co-workers developed and tested five pain assessment scales for nursing home residents with varying degrees of cognitive impairment[109]. Wu and colleagues studied the records of 9613 nursing home residents who had died, some receiving 'hospice care'/palliative care and some not. Those receiving palliative care had more and higher doses of opioids for severe pain than the others. They also had better reported and diagnosed pain[110]. The situation in Taiwanese nursing homes has been reported[111], as has such care in the USA[112,136], where Sloan and co-workers found that most of those dying in residential care/nursing home died where they had lived for some time (that is to say they were not transferred to a hospital/hospice). More than half of them died alone though their deaths were seen as imminent by staff and relatives in nursing homes but not in residential care homes. Overall suffering was minimal and, perhaps surprisingly, the highest approvals ratings were for

residential home care, and not nursing home palliative care[113]. Weiner, researching in the USA found attitudinal barriers to effective management of persistent pain in American nursing homes—fears related to addiction, increasing dependence with nurses feeling that they might have been able to help the residents if they had been given the time to do so[143]. According to Miller and colleagues 6 per cent of people dying in US nursing homes have received palliative care funded by Medicare for an average of 90 days[139].

If, as is being suggested, increasing numbers of elderly palliative care patients will be transferred to nursing homes, possibly from specialist palliative care units, can it be assumed that the quality of care will be maintained in the nursing home? One study found a definite falling off in quality of care and support for both patient and relatives[114]. In view of its prevalence it must be asked whether nursing homes where many, if not all, of the nursing staff have had no additional training in the care of demented patients, and the ambience has not been structured for dementia care, are the best place for such patients[115,116].

If much of this gives a disappointing picture of palliative care in nursing homes, much more positive and hopeful views and proposals have recently been advanced in Britain, Australia and the USA. The Scottish Partnership for Palliative Care (SPPC)—an umbrella organization representing all palliative care providers in the country—has published its discussion document 'Making Good Care Better' pointing to the need for, and means of achieving better palliative care in Scotland's nursing homes[117]. Excellent research and fieldwork in nursing homes in Edinburgh formed the basis of a PhD thesis by Hockley[118]. A multi-disciplinary working party with representatives of the Royal College of Physicians of London, the Royal College of Nursing of the UK and the British Geriatric Society published its report—'The health and care of older people in care homes: a comprehensive interdisciplinary approach. (2000)[119]. From Australia has come The National Palliative Care Program: Guidelines for a Palliative Approach in Residential Aged Care, prepared by Edith Cowan University, Australia (2004)[120]. Buchanan has demonstrated the usefulness of Minimum Data Sets in studying patients in nursing homes and how they are cared for[121], research supported by a paper looking at the usefulness of such tools in the UK 1997–1998[122].

Three groups have received little or no mention in this chapter. The first are those in custody, usually in jail or in police custody after arrest. Though little research has been done on this group palliative medicine consultants are occasionally asked to see and advise on a prisoner in need of palliative care. Few if any of the nurses staffing prison hospital wards have been trained in palliative care and many of the inmates have histories of drug misuse. In the UK representation has been made at the highest level to the prison service authorities to ensure that staff get some training, that consultants are called in as would happen outside prisons, and that should it be advised that the prisoner be admitted to a specialist palliative care unit (usually for terminal care) he/she be treated with as much consideration and dignity as any other patient. This was seen as a necessary request after reports of 'dangerous' prisoners being chained to hospital beds in their final days of life, still accompanied at all times by prison officers.

Another group are those living in hostels/shelters for the homeless, usually with no GP, accessible clinical records or means of contacting relatives. Their care has been studied by Podymow[123].

Table 18.1.8 Essential knowledge for home-based palliative care providers.

Specialist palliative care

- Where is the nearest unit?
- What are its policies for admitting patients?
- How are admissions arranged ? By phone, e-mail, letter, or form sent on request?
- Who can make the request for admission? Doctor, nurse, social worker, lawyer, patient, or relative?
- Are payments necessary and, if so, for what?
- Does the unit have a telephone advice service?
- Does the palliative medicine specialist do home visits?
- Do specialist palliative care nurses do home visits?
- Is there a designated community palliative care service? How is it accessed?
- Is advice available from a clinical pharmacist?
- Is advice available from a physiotherapist?
- Is advice available from an occupational therapist?
- Is advice available from a pastoral care worker / priest / minister/ religious teacher?

Tertiary (Specialist) hospital

- Does it accept patients specifically for palliative care rather than 'curative' care?
- Does it have its own Hospital Palliative Care Team / Service?
- What does it offer that the Palliative Care Unit does not?
- Does the medical specialist in the Palliative Care Unit also work there?

Resources available in the community where the patient lives

- Is there a community nursing service?
- Are these nurses trained in modern palliative care?
- Does this service operate 24 hours?
- Where can essential nursing equipment be accessed?
- Is there a laundry service for soiled bed linen?
- What does it cost and how does it operate?
- Can essential nursing equipment be accessed on loan, at what charge?
- Who delivers it and takes it back?
- Are Home Helps / Homemakers available and are they accessed?
- Are precooked meals available for housebound patients and carers?
- Is there a pharmacy service which collects prescriptions and delivers medications to patients' homes?
- Is there a transport service to take patients to clinics, hospital, day unit, and other services?
- How is it accessed, booked, and paid for?

Financial matters

- Where can patients, relatives, and professionals find out about grants, pensions, financial matters?
- Where can a patient or relative get legal advice on wills, benefits, advanced directives etc?

Planning a funeral

- Where can sensitive advice be obtained and how is it accessed?

Religious and spiritual matters

- Where can such people, relevant to each patient's religious affiliation, be accessed?
- Do local church or religious communities provide special services for the old, frail or dying in the community?

The third group, a very large and important one, are the ethnic minorities in our cities[70]. Readers are advised to read discussion documents published by the National Council for Palliative Care: *Opening Doors*[124], Council's 2006 document *Ethnicity, Older people and Palliative Care*[125], and *Wider Horizons: Care of the Dying in Multicultural Society*[126].

Accounts of first generation black Caribbean carers' satisfaction with end-of-life care comparing it with that received by Caucasians make salutary reading[127]. A problem faced by Afro-Americans in New York City is that of obtaining opioids for severe pain, because pharmacies in some areas of the city do not stock sufficient quantities of such analgesics[60].

In the USA Kagawa-Singer and Blackhall studied the complex cultural issues involved in palliative care provision, issues and differences that cannot be avoided or denied. When health-care professionals themselves increasingly come from many different backgrounds the possibilities of misunderstanding and hampering good care are legion[128], something further studied in Chinese patients in Taiwan, where the need for respect for different cultures and patient dignity are eloquently addressed[129].

Respite care

The main focus of this chapter has been on the carers. To a large extent whether or not the terminally ill patient will be able to stay, and possibly even die at home, depends on the physical and emotional health and stamina of the lay carers. For this reason it is often asked whether respite care, more for the sake of the carers than for the patient, might be of some use. Sadly little research has been done on this. We shall have to depend on anecdotes of which there are many.

It is assumed that respite care will be provided within a palliative care unit but how often can such units book a bed weeks in advance for such a patient? Do they have sufficient beds to use them in this way? Might it upset a patient to be admitted for a week or two to a unit where most of the other patients are frailer than him, and act as a painful reminder that he/she too will be in that state in the near future or, as some suggest, might it be reassuring to find what it is like there?

What many units report is that many 'respite care' patients have such far advanced disease by the time they are admitted to give their carers a rest that they go downhill rapidly and never return home. This *might* be explained by the GP and nurses not realizing how ill the patient was, but far more likely that the GP had repeatedly suggested a respite admission and the family carers had declined, feeling that for the patient to go to hospital primarily for their health and strength, and not that of the patient, was selfish of them. They kept going until at last they were at breaking point and agreed to the admission but by then the patient was near to death. The patient did not get his/her wish to die at home and the relatives are filled with guilt and a lasting sense of having failed their loved one at the end.

If there is any lesson in this it is that palliative care in the home should be started as early as possible, long before urgent admissions, for whatever reason, are needed. The GP can discuss how the relatives will be supported and, at this early stage, one of the options that can be discussed and described can be respite care. Pro-activity is the secret of effective palliative care in the home (Table 18.1.9).

Table 18.1.9 Home to hospital transfer list.

(Use before a patient is moved from home to a hospital/palliative care unit)

	Yes/No
Has the transfer been discussed with the patient?	Y/N
Have all the patient's questions been answered?	Y/N
Has the transfer been discussed with the relatives?	Y/N
Have they all had a chance to air anxieties?	Y/N
Has the receiving doctor been told:	
◆ The primary diagnosis	Y/N
◆ The secondary diagnoses	Y/N
◆ The previous treatment	Y/N
◆ The present treatment	Y/N
◆ How much the patient understands	Y/N
◆ What anxieties he/she has expressed	Y/N
◆ What anxieties the relatives have expressed	Y/N
Has the community nurse been told of the transfer?	Y/N
Have Social Services been told of the transfer?	Y/N
Has the community palliative care team been told?	Y/N

Table 18.1.10 Hospital/hospice to home transfer check-list.

(Use before sending a patient home from a hospital or palliative care unit)

	Yes/No
Has transfer been discussed with the patient?	Y/N
Has the patient had a chance to discuss any anxieties?	Y/N
Have the immediate relatives been informed?	Y/N
Have all their anxieties been addressed?	Y/N
Has it been discussed with the GP/FP?	Y/N
Has a home assessment been done by occupational therapist or community nurse?	Y/N
Has the patient been assessed for Activities of Daily Living?	Y/N
Have any necessary aids been provided/ordered?	Y/N
Has a medication chart been provided?	Y/N
Have follow-up arrangements been made?	Y/N
Has a detailed report been prepared for the GP/FP?	Y/N
Has transport been arranged for the patient?	Y/N

Transferring patients between home and hospital or palliative care unit

All professionals, and indeed many patients and lay carers, are aware that there can be breaks in the continuity of care and the conveying of essential information when patients area moved to or from their home to a hospital or palliative care unit. The results can include recurrence of pain, changes in regimens, the stress of forming relationships with doctors, nurses, and even domestic and clerical staff.

When life is changing fast and it is proving difficult to make sense of what is happening, changing the place of care—no matter how justified it was—can be extremely stressful. How may this be reduced?

The secret lies in the way essential information is passed from one carer to another, whether they are nurses, doctors, professions allied to medicine or clerical staff. Sample information charts can be found in Tables 18.1.9 and 18.1.10.

The benefits of such modest paperwork can be supplemented by such simple things as having the patient met and warmly welcomed as soon as they arrive in their new 'home' whether it is hospital or hospice, staff demonstrating that they have already read the communication sheets, relatives being invited to stay with the patient much longer than they might otherwise do and enjoying a meal with them, being introduced to carers and the routine of the unit.

Beyond question the biggest advance in this respect in the UK in recent years has been the introduction of the Integrated Palliative Care Pathways[130,131]. making the provision of palliative care as near seamless as it is possible to be, and the introduction of the Macmillan Gold Standards Framework slowly being introduced countrywide[132].

Research

This chapter is evidence that considerable research is being done but more is urgently needed. Collaboration should be possible now that so many GPs/family physicians are espousing the principles of palliative care and so many specialist services are operating.

Lip service is being paid to palliative care for non-malignant conditions but each of the life-threatening conditions needs to be studied—cardiac, respiratory, neurological, infections etc.

Little is known about the most appropriate educational methods and techniques for the different professional groups at different stages of learning and practising.

Though excellent work has started in training nursing home staff far more is needed and will continue to be needed as more people are admitted there primarily for palliative care.

Why are patients transferred from one care unit (including their home) to another? Is it essential? Is it dignified and in the patient's best interest and what factors influence such a momentous step? Is it evidence of patient autonomy or professional paternalism or pragmatism? Casarrret looked at differences between patients admitted to a palliative care service from academic versus non-academic units. Those from academic units were young, had higher incomes, were less likely to have DNR orders (Living Wills) and had higher medical and nursing needs that those from non-academic units[133].

Lastly, if palliative care—whoever practises it, whatever their professional role—is truly holistic embodying hope, then we must research how to recognize spiritual need, how and when to offer spiritual care without embarrassment or fear of being seen as proselytizing; research how/when to share our own humanity with our patients so that palliative care never degenerates into an exercise in prescribing or a test of our therapeutic skills or a reflection of our secularized, materialistic society[134].

If, as has been calculated, all whose lives end with chronic illness and frailty (that is to say 50 per cent of all deaths in the western world) in a few years time all palliative care will start in the home and continue there for longer than is usually spent in hospital. Are we ready for this?

References

1. Borgsteede, S.D. *et al.* (2006). Good end-of-life care according to patients and their general practitioners. *British Journal of General Practice*, **56**, 20–6.

2. Raynes, N.V. *et al.* (2000). Palliative care services: view of terminally ill patients. *Palliative Medicine*, **14**, 159–60.

3. Rabow, M.W. *et al.* (2003). Patient perception of an out patient palliative care intervention. *Journal of Pain and Symptom Management*, **26**(5), 1010–5.

4. Burke, K. (2004). Palliative care at home to get further funds if it saves money. *BMJ*, **328**, 544.

5. Thomas, C. *et al.* (2004). Place of death: preferences among cancer patients and their carers. *Social Science & Medicine*, **58**, 2431–44.

6. Higginson, I.J., and Gupta, S. (2000). Place of care in advanced cancer: a qualitative literature review of patient preferences. *Journal of Palliative Medicine*, **3**, 287–300.

7. Higginson, I.J. *et al.* (1998). Where do cancer patients die? Ten-year trends in the place of cancer deaths in England. *Palliative Medicine*, **12**, 353–63.

8. Higginson, I. *et al.* (2003). *Priorities and preferences for end of life care in England, Wales and Scotland*. National Council for Palliative Care, London.

9. Karlsen, S., and Addington-Hall, J. (1998). How do cancer patients who die at home differ from those who die elsewhere? *Palliative Medicine*, **12**, 279–86.

10. Wilkinson, S. (2000). Fulfiling patients' wishes: palliative care at home. *Journal of Palliative Nursing*, **6**(5), 212.

11. Gomes, B., and Higginson, I. (2006). Factors influencing death at home in terminally ill patients with cancer: systematic review. *BMJ*, **332**, 515–21.

12. Grande, G.E. *et al.* (2000). A randomised controlled trail of a hospital at home service for the terminally ill. *Palliative Medicine*, **14**, 375–85.

13. Bradshaw, P. (1993). Characteristics of clients referred to home, hospice and palliative care services in Western Australia. *Palliative Medicine*, **7**, 101–7.

14. Peruselli, C. (1999). Home palliative care for terminal cancer patients: a survey on the final week of life. *Palliative Medicine*, **13**, 233–41.

15. Rosenquist, A., Bergman, K., and Strang, P. (1999). Optimizing hospital-based home care for dying cancer patients: a population based study. *Palliative Medicine*, **13**, 393–7.

16. Aabom, B. *et al.* (2005). Population-based study of the place of death of patients with cancer: Implications for GPs. *British Journal of General Practice*, **55**(518), 684–9.

17. Bradley, E.H. *et al.* (2000). Referral of terminally ill patients for hospice: frequency and correlates. *Journal of Palliative Care*, **16**(4), 20–6.

18. Deschepper, R. *et al.* (2006). Communications on end-of-life decisions with patients wishing to die at home *British Journal of General Practice*, **56**, 14–9.

19. Costantini, M. (1993). Palliative home care. *Palliative Medicine*, **7**, 323–31.

20. De Conno, F. *et al.* (1996). Effect of home care on the place of death of advanced cancer patients. *European Journal of Cancer*, **32A**, 1142–7.

21. Toscani, F. and Mancini, C. (1990). Inadequacies of care in far advanced cancer patients: a comparison between home and hospital in Italy. *Palliative Medicine*, **4**, 31–6.

22. Dunphy, K., and Amesbury, B. (1990). A comparison of hospice and home care patients: patterns of referral, patient characteristics and predictors of place of death. *Palliative Medicine*, **4**, 105–11.

23. Dale, J. *et al.* (1996). Creating a shared vision of out-of-hours care using rapid appraisal methods to create an interagency, community-oriented approach to service development. *BMJ*, **312**, 1206–10.

24. Thomas, K. (2000). Out-of-hours palliative care: bridging the gap. *European Journal of Palliative Care*, **7**(1), 22–5.

25. Shipman, C. *et al.* (2000). Providing palliative care in primary care: how satisfied are GPs and district nurses with current out-of-hours arrangements? *British Journal of General Practice*, **50**(455), 477–8.

26. Hinton, J. (1994). Which patients with terminal cancer are admitted from home care? *Palliative Medicine*, **8**, 197–210.

27. Sykes, N., Pearson, S.E., and Chell, S. (1992). Quality of care of the terminally ill: the care's perception. *Palliative Medicine*, **6**, 227–36.

28. Seabrook, D. *et al.* (1998). Dying from cancer in community hospitals or a hospice: closest lay carers' perceptions. *British Journal of General Practice*, **48**, 1317–21.

29. Hockey, L. (1991). St Columba's hospice home care service: an evaluation study. *Palliative Medicine*, **5**, 315–22.

30. Barclay, S. (2000). Interprofessional communications. *Palliative Care Today*, **9**(1), 6.

31. Higginson, J., and Costantini, M. (2002). Communication in end-of-life cancer care. A comparison of team assessments in three European countries. *Journal of Clinical Oncology*, **20**, 3674–82.

32. McCarthy, M. *et al.* (1996). Dying from heart disease. *Journal of he Royal College of Physicians*, **30**(4), 325–8.

33. McCarthy, M. *et al.* (1997). Communication and choice in dying from heart disease. *J of the Royal Society of Medicine*, **90**, 128–31.

34. Halliwell, J. *et al.* (2004). GP discussion of prognosis with patients with severe COPD: a qualitative study *British Journal of General Practice*, **54**(509), 904–8.

35. Barclay, S. *et al.* (2002). Controlling cancer pain in primary care: the prescribing habits and knowledge base of general practitioners. *Journal of Pain and Symptom Management*, **23**(5), 383–92.

36. Burge, F. *et al.* (2000). Family medicine residents knowledge and attitudes about end-of-life care. *Journal of Palliative Care*, **16**(3), 5–12.

37. Zenz, M. *et al.* (1995). Severe under treatment of cancer pain: a 3-year survey of the German situation. *Journal of Pain and Symptom Management*, **10**, 3, 187–91.

38. Charlton, R. (2000). Perceived skills in palliative medicine in newly-qualified doctors in the UK. *Journal of Palliative Care*, **16**(4), 27–32.

39. Hanratty, B. (2000). Palliative care provided by GP' the carer's viewpoint. *British Journal of General Practice*, **50**, 653–4.

40. Murray, S.A. *et al.* (2003). GPs and their possible role in providing spiritual care: a qualitative study. *British Journal of General Practice*, **53**(497), 957–60.

41. Mitchell, G.K. (2002). How well do general practitioners deliver palliative care? A systematic review. *Palliative Medicine*, **16**, 457.

42. Millar, D.G. *et al.* (1998). Palliative care at home: an audit of cancer deaths in Grampian Region, Scotland. *British Journal of General Practice*, **48**, 1299–302.

43. Murray, S.A. *et al.* (2004). Developing primary palliative care. *BMJ*, **329**, 1056–7.

44. Oxenham, D. *et al.* (2003). Cancer pain management in Lanarkshire: a community-based audit. *Palliative Medicine*, **17**, 708–13.

45. Pugh, E.M.G. (1996). An investigation of general practitioner referrals to palliative care services. *Palliative Medicine*, **10**, 251–7.

46. Surkan, P.J. *et al.* (2006). Home care of a child dying of a malignancy and parental awareness of a child's impending death. *Palliative Medicine*, **20**, 161–9.

47. Glajchen, M., and Bookbinder M. (2001). Knowledge and perceived competence of home care nurses in pain management: USA National Study. *Journal of Pain and Symptom Management*, **21**(4), 307–16.

48. Harding, R., and Higginson, I.J. (2003). What is the best way to help caregivers in cancer and palliative care? A systematic literature review of interventions and their effectiveness. *Palliative Medicine*, **17**, 63–74.

49. Main, J. *et al.* (2000). Improving management of bereavement in GP based on a survey of recently bereaved subjects in a single general practice. *British Journal of General Practice*, **50**(460), 863–6.

50. Spiller, J., and Alexander, D. (1993). Domiciliary care: a comparison of the views of terminally ill patients and their family caregivers. *Palliative Medicine*, **7**, 109–115.

51. Mok, E. *et al.* (2003). Family experience caring for terminally ill patients with cancer in Hong Kong. *Hong Kong Cancer Nursing*, **26**(4), 267–75.

52. Wilson, A. *et al.* (2002). Patient and carer satisfaction with 'Hospital at Home' a quantitative and qualitative study from a randomised clinical trial. *British Journal of General Practice,* **52**(474), 9–13.

53. Schumacher, K. *et al.* (2002). Putting cancer pain management regimens into practice at home. *Journal of Pain and Symptom Management,* **23**(5), 369–82.

54. Douay, B. (1993). Morning and evening nursing in the home: urgent treatment *Palliative Medicine,* **7**(Suppl. 1), 61–63d.

55. Li, I.C., and Yin, T.J. (2005). Care needs of residents in community-based long-term care facilities in Taiwan. *Journal of Clinical Nursing,* **14**, 711–8.

56. Copp, G., and Dunn, V. (1993). Frequent and difficult problems perceived by nurses caring for the dying in community, hospice and acute care settings. *Palliative Medicine,* **7**, 19–25.

57. Skilbeck, J. *et al.* (2002). Clinical nurse specialists in palliative care. Part 1. A description of the Macmillan Nurse workload. *Palliative Medicine,* **16**, 285–96.

58. Cornbleet, M.A. *et al.* (2002). Patient-held records in cancer and palliative care: a randomised prospective trial. *Palliative Medicine,* **16**, 205–12.

59. Thulesius, H. *et al.* (2002). Learner-centred education in end-of life care improved well-being in home care staff: a prospective controlled study. *Palliative Medicine,* **16**, 347–54.

60. Morrison, R.S. *et al.* (2000). 'We don't carry that' Failure of pharmacies I predominantly non-white neighbourhoods to stock opioid analgesics. *NEJM,* **342**(14), 1023–6.

61. Zeppettella, G. (1999). How do terminally ill patients at home take their medication. *Palliative Medicine,* **13**, 469–75.

62. Addington-Hall, J., Fakhoury, W., and McCarthy, M. (1998). Specialist palliative care in non-malignant disease. *Palliative Medicine,* **12**, 417–27.

63. Eng, D. (2006). Management guidelines for motor neuron disease patients on non-invasive ventilation at home. *Palliative Medicine,* **20**, 69–79.

64. Hudson, P.L. *et al.* (2006). Would people with Parkinson's disease benefit from palliative care? *Palliative Medicine,* **20**, 87–94.

65. Lehman, R. (2004). Editorial: How long can I go on like this? Dying from cardio-respiratory disease. *British Journal of General Practice,* **54**(509), 892–3.

66. McKinlay, R.K. *et al.* (2004). Care of people dying with malignant and cardio-respiratory disease in general practice. British Journal of General Practice, **54** (509), 909–13.

67. Edmonds, P. *et al.* (2001). A comparison of the palliative care needs of patients dying from chronic respiratory diseases and lung cancer. *Palliative Medicine,* **15**, 287–95.

68. Ajithakumari, K. *et al.* (1997). Palliative home care – the Calicut experience (S India). *Palliative Medicine,* **11**, 451–4.

69. Ahmed, N. *et al.* (2004). Systemic review of the problems and issues of accessing specialist palliative care by patients, carers and health and social work professionals. *Palliative Medicine,* **18**, 525–42.

70. Ida, E. *et al.* (2002). Current status of hospice cancer deaths both in-patient and at home (1995–2000) and prospects of home care services in Japan. *Palliative Medicine,* **16**, 179–84.

71. Centeno, C. *et al.* (2000). The reality of palliative care in Spain. *Palliative Medicine,* **14**, 387–94.

72. Centeno, C. *et al.* Spain (2002). Palliative care progress in Spain: a national survey. *Journal of Pain and Symptom Management,* **24**(2), 245–51.

73. Gomez-Batiste, X. *et al.* (2002). The WHO Demonstration Project of Palliative care Implementation in Catalonia: Results 10 Years (1991–2001). *Journal of Pain and Symptom Management,* **24**(2), 239–44.

74. Gomas, J.-M. (1993). Palliative care at home: reality or mission impossible? *Palliative Medicine,* **7**(Suppl. 1), 45–59.

75. Mercadente, S. *et al.* (2000). The impact of home palliative care on symptoms in advanced cancer patients. *Supportive Care in Cancer,* **8**, 307–10.

76. Mercadente, S. (2001). Pattern of drug use by advanced cancer patients followed at home. *Journal of Palliative Care,* **17**(1), 37–40.

77. Ventafridda, V. *et al.* (1985). Palliative care in the home. *Tumori,* **71**, 449–54.

78. Boyd, K. (1995). The role of specialist home care teams: views of general practitioners in south London. *Palliative Medicine,* **9**, 138–44.

79. Koffman, J., and Higginson, I. (2001). Accounts of carers' satisfaction with health care at the end of life: a comparison of first generation black Caribbeans and white patients with advanced disease. *Palliative Medicine,* **15**, 337–45.

80. Morch, M.M. (1999). Thirty years experience with cancer and non-cancer patients in palliative home care. *Journal of Palliative Care,* **15**, 43–8.

81. Randall-David, E. *et al.* (2003). Barriers to cancer pain management: home-health and hospice nurses and patients. *Support Care Cancer,* **11**, 660–5.

82. Shipman, C. *et al.* (2002). How and why do GPs use specialist palliative care services? *Palliative Medicine,* **16**, 241–6.

83. Worth, A. *et al.* (2006). Out-of-hours palliative care: a qualitative study of cancer patients, carers and professionals. *British Journal of General Practice,* **56**, 6–13.

84. Hammes, B.J. (1998). Death and end-of life planning in one Midwestern Community. *Archive of Internal Medicine,* **158**, 383–90.

85. Hinton, J. (1994). Can home care maintain an acceptable quality of life for patients with terminal cancer and their relatives? *Palliative Medicine,* **8**, 1183–96.

86. Filiberti, A. *et al.* (2001). Characteristics of terminal cancer patients who committed suicide during a home palliative care programme. *Journal of Pain and Symptom Management,* **22**(1), 544–53.

87. Douglas, H.-R. *et al.* (2003). Palliative Day Care: what does it cost to run a service and does attendance affect use of other services? *Palliative Medicine,* **17**, 628–37.

88. Mor, V., Stalkewr, M.Z., and Gralla, R.R. (1998). Day hospital as an alternative to in-patient care for cancer patients: a random assignment trial. *Journal of Clinical Epidemiology,* **41**, 771–85.

89. Goodwin, D.M. *et al.* (2000). Methodological issues in evaluating palliative day care: a multicentre study. *Palliative Medicine,* **14**, 232.

90. Spencer, D.J., and Daniels, I.E. (1998). Day hospice care – a review of the literature. *Palliative Medicine,* **12**, 219–29.

91. Higginson, I.J. *et al.* (2000). Palliative day care. What do services do? *Palliative Medicine,* **14**, 277–86.

92. Thorne, C.P. *et al.* (1994). The influence of general practitioner community hospitals on the place of death of cancer patients. *Palliative Medicine,* **8**, 122–8.

93. Baar, F. (1999). Palliative care for the terminally ill in the Netherlands: the unique role of nursing homes. *European Journal of Palliative Care,* **6**, 169–72.

94. Pell, J., and Williams, S. (1999). Do nursing home residents make greater demands on GPs? A prospective, comparative study. *British Journal of General Practice,* **49**(44), 527–30.

95. Coady, D.A., and Wynne, H.A. (2001). Are continuing care beds in private nursing homes the answer to providing care for the longer term dying? *Palliative Medicine,* **15**, 155–6.

96. Komaromy, C., Sidell, M., and Katz, J.T. (2000). The quality of terminal care in residential and nursing homes. *International Journal of Palliative Nursing,* **6**, 192–200.

97. Froggatt, K.A. (2001). Palliative care in nursing homes: where next? *Palliative Medicine,* **15**, 42–8.

98. Froggatt, K.A. (2001). Evaluating a palliative care education project in nursing homes. *International Journal Palliative Care Nursing,* **6**, 140.

99. Froggatt, K. (2001). Life and death in English nursing homes: sequestration or transition? *Ageing & Society,* **21**, 319–32.

100. Froggatt, K. (2004). *Palliative care in care homes for older people.* National Council for Palliative Care, London.

101. Froggatt, K., Hasnip, J., and Smith, P. (2000). The challenges of end of life care. *Elderly Care,* **12**(2), 11–3.

102. Froggatt, K., and Hoult, L. (2002). Developing palliative care practice in nursing and residential care homes: the role of the clinical nurse specialist. *Journal of Clinical Nursing,* **11**(6), 802–8.

103. Hockley, J., and Clark, D. (eds.) (2002). *Palliative care for older people in care homes.* Open University Press, Buckingham

104. Horton, R. (2002). Differences in assessment of symptoms and quality of life between patients with advanced cancer and their specialist palliative care nurses in a home care setting. *Palliative Medicine,* **16**, 488–94.

105. Jordhoy, M.S. *et al.* (2003). Which cancer patients die in nursing homes? Quality of life, medical and socio-demographic characteristics. *Palliative Medicine,* **17**, 433–44.

106. Kamel, H.K. *et al.* (2001). Utilising pain assessment scales increased the of diagnosing pain among elderly nursing home residents. *Journal of Pain and Symptom Management,* **21**, 450–5.

107. Closs, S.J. *et al.* (2004). A comparison of 5 Pain Assessment Scales for Nursing Home residents with varying degrees of cognitive impairment. *Journal of Pain and Symptom Management,* **27**(3), 196–205.

108. Wu, N. *et al.* (2003). The problem of assessment bias when measuring the hospice effect using a nursing Home residents' pain tool. *Journal of Pain and Symptom Management,* **25**(5), 998–1009.

109. Tsai, Y.F. *et al.* (2004). Pain prevalence, experiences and management strategies among the elderly in Taiwanese nursing homes *Journal of Pain and Symptom Management,* **28**, 579–84.

110. Oliver, D.P., Porock, D., and Zweig, S. (2004). End of life care in, U.S. nursing homes: a review of the evidence. *Journal of the American Medical Directors Association,* **5**(3), 147–55.

111. Sloan, P.D. *et al.* (2003) End of life care in assisted living and related residential care settings: Comparison with Nursing Homes *Journal of the American geriatrics Society,* **51**, 1587–94.

112. Maccabee, J. (1994). The effect of transfer from a palliative care unit to nursing homes – are patients' and relatives' needs met? *Palliative Medicine,* **8**, 211–4.

113. Mitchell, S.L. *et al.* (2004). Terminal care for persons with advanced dementia in the nursing home and home care setting. *Journal of Palliative Medicine,* **7**, 6, 808–16.

114. Mitchell S.L., Kiely, D.K., and Hamel, M.B. (2004). Dying with advanced dementia in the nursing home. *Archives of Internal Medicine,* **164**(3), 321–6.

115. *Making good care better: National practice statements for general palliative care in adult care homes in Scotland.* 2006 Scottish Partnership for Palliative Care and the Scottish Executive, www.palliativecarescotland.org.uk

116. Hockley, J. (2006). PhD thesis [Refer to Librarian, University of Edinburgh].

117. RCP, RCN, BGS (2000). *The health and care of older people in care homes: a comprehensive interdisciplinary approach.* A report of a joint working party. Royal College of Physicians of London, London.

118. The National Palliative Care Program (2004). *Guidelines for a Palliative Approach in Residential Aged Care.* Prepared by: Edith Cowan University. (Australia) Download from Buckingham: http://www.health.gov.au/internet/wcms/publishing.nsf/Content/palliativecare-pubs-workf-guide.htm

119. Buchanan, J. *et al.* (2002). Analyses of nursing home residents in hospice care using the Minimum Data Sets USA. *Palliative Medicine,* **16**, 465–80.

120. Eve, A., and Higginson, I.J. (2000). Minimum dataset activity for hospice and hospital palliative care services in the UK 1997/1998. *Palliative Medicine,* **14**, 395–404.

121. Podymow, T. *et al.* (2006). Shelter-based palliative care for the homeless terminally ill. *Palliative Medicine,* **20**, 81–6.

122. *Opening doors: Improving access to Hospice and Specialist Palliative Care Services by members of the Black and Ethnic Minority Communities.* Occasional Paper No. 7, 1995 National Council for Palliative Care, London www.ncpc.org.uk.

123. Ethnicity, Older People and Palliative Care: a joint publication from the Policy Research Institute on ageing and ethnicity and the National Council for Palliative Care. 2006 www.ncpc.org.uk.

124. Firth, S. (2001). *Wider horizons: care of the dying in a multicultural society.* National Council for Palliative Care, London. <www.ncps.org.uk>.

125. Koffman, J. *et al.* (1999). Care in the last year of life: satisfaction with health services in the Black Caribbean population in an Inner London Health Authority. *Palliative Medicine,* **13**, 522.

126. Kagawa-Singer, M., and Blackhall, L.J. (2001). Negotiating cross-cultural issues at the end of life. *JAMA,* **286**, 2993–3001.

127. Tang, S.T. (2000). Meaning of death at home for Chinese patients in Taiwan with terminal cancer. *Cancer Nursing,* **23**(5), 367–70.

128. Ellershaw, J., and Wilkinson, S. (2003). *Care of the dying, a pathway to excellence.* Oxford University Press, Oxford.

129. Campbell, H., Hotchkiss, R., Bradshaw, N., and Porteous, M. (1998). Integrated care pathways. *British Medical Journal,* **316**, 133–7.

130. Thomas, K. (2003). *Care for the dying at home: companions on the journey.* Radcliffe Medical Press, Oxford.

131. Casarett, D.J. (2001). Differences between patients referred to hospice from academic versus non-academic settings. *Journal of Pain and Symptom Management,* **21**(3), 197.

132. Benzein, E. *et al.* (2001). The meaning of the lived experience of hope in patients with cancer in palliative home care. *Palliative Medicine,* **15**, 117–26.

133. Hayman, J.A. *et al.* (2001). Estimating the cost of informal care-giving for elderly patients with cancer. *Journal of Clinical Oncology,* **19**, 3219–25.

134. Kite, S. *et al.* (1999). Specialist palliative care and patients with non-cancer diagnoses: the experiences of a service. *Palliative Medicine,* **13**, 477–84.

135. Miller, S.C., and Mor, V. (2001). The emergence of Medicare hospice care in US nursing homes. *Palliative Medicine,* **15**, 471–80.

136. Rabow, M.W. *et al.* (2004). Supporting family carers. *JAMA,* **291**(4), 483–91.

137. Walker, J. (1992). Leaflet about pain control on MST. *Palliative Medicine,* **6**, 65.

138. Weiner, D.K. *et al.* (2002). Attitudinal barriers to effective treatment of persistent pain in nursing home residents. *Journal of American Geriatric Society,* **50**(12) 2035–40.

139. *Wong, F.K.Y. et al.* (2004). Health problems encountered by dying patients receiving palliative home care. *Cancer Nursing,* **27**(3), 244–51.

140. Gibbs, G. (1995). Nurses in private nursing homes: a study of their knowledge and attitudes to pain management in palliative care. *Palliative Medicine,* **9**, 245–53.

Palliative care in the home: North America

S. Lawrence Librach

The United States of America and Canada, two large democratic North American countries, share the longest undefended border in the world. These two countries have complex and comprehensive health-care systems, although both have developed different approaches to health-care and therefore to hospice/palliative care. Both countries have developed fairly sophisticated home-care systems. The quantity and complexity of these home-care services has increased and will continue to increase in the future.

Generally, in both countries, the purpose of home-care programmes is to provide:

◆ a substitution function for services provided by hospitals and long-term care facilities;

◆ a maintenance function that allows patients to remain independent in their current environment rather than moving to a new and more costly venue; and

◆ a preventative function, which invests in patient service and monitoring at additional short-term but lower long-term costs[1].

Similarities and differences between the USA and Canada which impact on the provision of hospice/palliative home care

Both countries physically are quite large in size. Although most of the population of both countries is based in urban areas, provision of health-care, particularly in Canada's more isolated northern areas, remains a major challenge. Over 80 per cent of the Canadian population lives within 100 km of the American border, the largest provinces being Ontario and Quebec. The densest populations in the USA are in the eastern seaboard area and in the west coast state of California.

The estimated population of the USA in 2006 (300 million) was almost 10 times the population of Canada (32 million). Both countries are built on waves of immigrant populations. The USA has had more of a 'melting pot' philosophy where immigrants maintain a little of their cultural identity but are expected to melt their traditions into American culture. The black (35 million) and Hispanic (33 million) population groups in the USA are the largest minority groups with the Hispanic group growing rapidly. Canada, a bilingual country (English and French), has a policy of multiculturalism and so the cultural identity of continuous waves of immigrants has been reasonably maintained. In both countries, the provision of hospice/palliative care is often challenged by different cultural traditions especially in large urban areas. Both countries also have native populations not only with different spiritual and cultural traditions but also with significant social and economic problems. Serving these mostly rural and often remote populations with appropriate palliative care is an issue.

In any country, inner city poor populations have always provided a challenge to serve with home palliative care. This is a much more significant problem in the USA where the inner city population is most often black or Hispanic and poor, lacking medical coverage and socio-economic resources. The per cent of blacks, especially those in the inner city areas, served by hospice programmes in the USA is still a concern. Both countries have social assistance providing somewhat of a safety net for these populations with the Canadian safety net being more comprehensive. Violence and drugs have been a much more prevalent problem in inner city US populations than in similar large cities in Canada.

The basic political systems differ. The USA is a republic with 50 states and several offshore territories. There is no national universal health-care scheme. Much of health care in the USA is legislated centrally, particularly institutional accreditation and the home hospice benefit from US Medicare. Canada with 10 provinces and three territories has developed in the British system of parliamentary government. The federal government has responsibility for the overall direction of health care and exercises this control through the Canada Health Act and transfer of federal tax income. Recently, the Canadian Federal Government moved to create a federal Secretariat for Palliative and End of Life Care although in 2006 the funding for this enterprise has been severely cut back. The actual provision of health care is the responsibility of each province and territory, supplementing federal funds with provincial and territorial tax revenues. The relationship of both US and Canadian federal governments with provinces or states and territories over the issue of health care is a source of continuing conflict and concern.

Canada has a universal national health-care scheme financed through taxes. All Canadians are guaranteed basic but comprehensive health-care services including home care without cost within the principles of the Canada Health Act: accessibility, universality, comprehensiveness, portability, and public administration. In only 3 of 10 provinces is palliative care considered a core health service.

All Canadian provinces and territories provide home-care services and thus serve dying patients in the home. Co-payments for drugs and services exist in some provinces. About 30 per cent of health-care costs are the responsibility of individuals and families in Canada, these costs including medication, semi-private hospital rooms and some equipment. About one-third of Canadians are covered by private insurance that provides extended health benefits that cover some of these costs as well as dental coverage, equipment, and some private duty nursing. All Canadians over age 65, those who are disabled, those on provincial home-care programmes and most persons on social assistance can access provincial drug formularies with minimal co-payments providing ready access to most drugs used in hospice palliative care.

The USA provides for health care through a combination of Medicare, national health-care coverage for citizens over age 65 and for those who are disabled, and private insurance schemes. Part of Medicare is a hospice benefit. About 42 million people in the USA have no health-care coverage[2]. Recently a national drug coverage scheme for the elderly was instituted in the USA but there still is considerable co-payment and the programmes are funded through individual contracts with private insurance companies. Most of the hospice programmes in the USA derive income from multiple sources: Medicare, private insurance, private funds, and donations. The percentage of gross domestic product spent on health care in the USA is considerably greater and unit costs for service are also generally much more expensive than in Canada. Recently a drug plan for patients over age 65 was introduced in the USA.

Both countries are challenged by similar demographics in planning hospice/palliative home-care services: an aging population, an increasing prevalence of cancer, preference of people for care at home, the transfer of care from hospitals to community settings, and a need to control health-care costs. The prevalence of HIV disease in the USA is greater than in Canada although death rates from HIV disease have dropped dramatically in both countries in the last 5 years.

In both countries, public polls have shown an overwhelming preference (>70 per cent in Canada and >90 per cent in the USA) for dying in the home. This has been a major stimulus for the development of home hospice/palliative care programmes.

In both countries, professional education in palliative care and in home care is limited. National continuing education programmes in palliative care for physicians have developed in both countries: the Educating Physicians in End of Life Care Project (the EPEC Project) and End-of-Life Nursing Education Consortium in the USA and the Ian Anderson Education Program in End-of-Life Care and the Pallium Project in Canada. In both countries, there are also numerous other palliative care continuing education programmes for health-care professionals.

Canada has a strong presence of general or family practitioners (50 per cent of all physicians) whereas the USA physician population is mostly specialist based. The ability of family physicians to participate in home palliative care should be much greater in Canada but currently there is a shortage of family physicians in many areas and significant changes in family physician practice patterns that have decreased the home-care role of family physicians, particularly in large urban areas. Most physicians in Canada work on a fee-for-service basis although alternate salary-type arrangements are increasing. Physician fees for home care in many Canadian provinces are quite low compared to office fees

and the number of physicians providing home care is decreasing. In Canada, the Education of Future Physicians in Palliative and End of Life Care (EFPPEC) Project has succeeded in introducing undergraduate medical competencies in the 17 medical schools as well as developing the expected competencies in postgraduate training. Both countries have developed postgraduate physician programmes in palliative medicine. Graduate nursing programmes producing nurse specialists in home care or in palliative care are limited in both countries.

Standards for accreditation of hospice/palliative care services exist in the USA. Hospices who wish to receive home hospice benefits through Medicare need to be accredited. Recently the national accrediting body in Canada has added a section on palliative care to its accreditation standards. Both countries have national hospice or palliative care organizations that are involved in these standards processes.

Home hospice care in the USA (Table 18.2.1)

Hospice care and programmes have increased rapidly in America. Hospice care including home care is funded mostly by the federal Medicare Hospice Benefit with further funding coming from Medicaid benefits provided by 43 of 50 states, private insurance, and other sources. To be a Medicare programme, a hospice must undergo regular accreditation and regular financial scrutiny. The Medicare Hospice Benefit was established in 1983, covering 82.4 per cent of hospice patients and stimulating the rapid growth of hospice care including home hospice care.

Those persons eligible for hospice Medicare benefits have to meet the following criteria:

◆ They are over 65 years of age, a citizen or permanent resident in the USA, or less than 65 if they have a disability or end-stage renal disease.

◆ They are certified by their doctor and the hospice medical director as having a prognosis less than 6 months.

◆ Patients must sign a statement choosing hospice care rather than curative treatment and standard Medicare benefits.

◆ They must enrol in a Medicare-approved programme.

The 6-month prognosis in the Medicare benefit has been a source of controversy as it expects an ability to prognosticate accurately, impedes access to patients who may require hospice care earlier in their illness, and trapped some patients without funding if they survived beyond 6 months although recently a renewal programme has been instituted. However, hospice programmes in the USA commit to providing care beyond 6 months as necessary and hospital palliative care consult teams are able to provide care at earlier phases of a patient's illness.

The hospice benefits covered by Medicare include both home and inpatient treatment by interdisciplinary teams, medical equipment and supplies, drugs, and volunteer support services. Hospice benefits do not cover expenses of care unrelated to the terminal illness. Regular home care is provided by experienced registered nurses and licensed practical nurses, home health aides and homemakers, and by visiting physicians. Counselling and spiritual support is also provided under the framework of hospice care in the home. Respite care, to give families a break in caring for a patient at home, can be provided in an appropriate facility. Co-payments may be required

Table 18.2.1 Home hospice care in the USA, 2006[3].

1.3 million patients received services from hospice in 2006
55.9 per cent non cancer illnesses and 44.1 per cent cancer
Three out of every four hospice patients (74.1 per cent) died in a private residence, nursing home, or other residential facility versus acute care hospital settings. Only 8.8 per cent died in acute care settings
4500 operating or planned hospice programmes:
Most of these facilities are either freestanding or located within a hospital and provide a mix of acute and residential care. Growth in small freestanding hospices
18.4 per cent of hospices reported they operate an inpatient facility
17 per cent home health-based
4 per cent nursing home or others
49 per cent of hospice programmes non-profit with continuing growth in the for profit sector
One in three people who died in the USA were looked after by a hospice
Average length of enrolment in hospice care was 56 days with a median of 20 days
81.7 per cent of hospice patients were over 65 years of age

to pay for outpatient drugs and for respite care but the expenses are set at only 5 per cent of the costs of such services.

Hospice care and its home-care component continue to grow rapidly in the USA under the expanding influence of well-organized and comprehensive hospice/palliative care programmes.

Home hospice/palliative care in Canada

All Canadians are covered by comprehensive, universal health care that includes home care as a part of the system. Home care in Canada has been defined as[4]: an array of services which enables clients, incapacitated in whole or in part, to live at home, often with the effect of preventing, delaying, or substituting for long-term care or acute care alternatives.

Home care may be delivered under numerous organizational structures, and similarly numerous funding and client payment mechanisms. It may address needs specifically associated with a medical diagnosis (e.g. diabetes therapy), and/or may compensate for functional deficits in the activities of daily living (e.g. bathing, cleaning, food preparation). Home care is a health programme, with health broadly defined; to be effective it may have to provide services which in other contexts might be defined as social or educational services (e.g. home maintenance, volunteer visits).

Home care may be appropriate for people with minor health problems and disabilities, and for those who are acutely ill requiring intensive and sophisticated services and equipment. There are no upper or lower limits on the age at which home care may be required, although as in other segments of the health system, utilization tends to increase with age.

In all 13 jurisdictions (10 provinces and 3 territories) in Canada, ministries or departments of health are responsible for the implementation of home-care policy and services. Most provinces have delegated responsibility for funding allocation and service delivery to regional or local health authorities. However, in most cases the provincial and territorial departments set overall policy guidelines and standards for regional service delivery, reporting

requirements, and monitoring outcomes. All provinces and territories have single points of access for home-care services.

There is considerable variation from province to province in the way home care is delivered and the services provided. In some provinces, public employees deliver all services. In others, there is combination of public and home-care agency funded employees or a contracting out of all services to for-profit and not-for-profit agencies. The patient assessment and the consequent care plan determine services to be delivered and the extent of public funding in full or in part. The assessment process itself and nursing services are typically provided free of charge, while fees may apply in some provinces for personal care and homemaking services. In some provinces, payment in part for certain equipment, supplies, and drugs may be the responsibility of the patient and family. Income or means-testing is done in some provinces to determine what the patient can contribute. In all provinces, persons over age 65 receive drugs with minimum charge or without any charge. Patients on home care under age 65 in some provinces are eligible for these drug benefits. There may also be direct charges or income tested co-payments to the patient for prescription drugs, medical supplies, and/or adaptive equipment[5]. There may be some restrictions on the amount of service that can be provided monthly but service may be provided for many months. In a number of areas, home palliative care patients may receive enhanced services over the usual services provided. All provinces through their home-care agencies can provide special equipment such as continuous subcutaneous infusion pumps, oxygen tanks or concentrators, hospital beds, intravenous supplies, and other equipment. However, recent budget cuts and policy changes have forced some increase in co-payments for some of these supplies and equipment after a certain amount of time with some means-testing in some areas. If the patient wants services or equipment beyond those assessed for public coverage, the patient and family may pay for them privately out-of-pocket or with private third-party insurance.

There is no specific benefit for hospice/palliative care within the Canadian health-care system. Palliative care units, nursing homes, and acute hospital beds are all part of the universal coverage. However, the lack of such a hospice benefit as exists in the USA has resulted in less comprehensive development of specific hospice/palliative care programmes in Canada. Only three provinces have made palliative care a core service and therefore the flow of government funding for palliative care programmes has been inconsistent across the country. Almost all acute care hospitals in Canada have palliative care programmes with variable interdisciplinary resources depending on the flow of funding from each individual institution. Full service interdisciplinary formal home palliative care programmes are becoming more common with the development of regional home palliative care programmes. Family physicians may provide physician services for palliative care patients at home. In other areas, specialist palliative medicine physicians provide consult back-up for family physicians or may provide direct primary care in the home. There are a number of regions with home palliative care programmes integrated into the overall health system. Most areas of Canada also have community volunteer hospice services providing volunteer support but they may not be part of formal interdisciplinary palliative care programmes. Cancer centres in Canada are often regional in nature and recently there has been much more presence of palliative care within those centres.

Canada has limited data on hospice/palliative care services. It is estimated that there are over 1000 palliative care programmes but the cumulative service data from those programmes are not known on a national basis. The percentage of home palliative care patients dying at home ranges from 20 to 70 per cent. Factors influencing this figure include presence or absence of specific home palliative care programmes, the availability of physicians to make home visits, the availability of inpatient palliative care unit beds, the presence of sufficient family support, and socioeconomic status. Efforts are now underway to begin to collect national data on palliative care.

Although Canada has a universal health-care system, the application of home-care services appropriate for palliative care patients varies across the country. A recent agreement between the federal government and provinces and territories has brought funding specifically designated for home palliative care. To support provincial and territorial government efforts to fulfil their commitment, the Canadian Hospice Palliative Care Association in partnership with the Canadian Home Care Association has defined the 'gold standard' for each of the four home-care services to be funded by government: case management, nursing, palliative-specific pharmaceuticals and personal care at the end of life. The gold standards establish the ideal level of care and support that all jurisdictions should strive to provide for people receiving hospice palliative care at home. They are designed to encourage and support a consistent approach across the country to palliative care services at home. The recommendations from this initiative and the standards statements include:

◆ Adopting strategies that will give their citizens timely access (i.e. 24 hours a day, 7 days a week) to hospice palliative care at home—including appropriate pharmaceuticals and equipment—so they feel confident that they can choose to die at home.

◆ Establishing interdisciplinary hospice palliative care teams that make effective use of the skills of each member to support clients/patients and families/caregivers.

◆ Supporting ongoing hospice palliative care education for members of the health-care team and family caregivers.

◆ Investing in home-care case management and information systems that support the interdisciplinary teams and provide information that can be used to evaluate home-care services at end of life.

◆ Supporting ongoing research into good practices for hospice palliative care at home, including the cultural, ethical, and spiritual aspects of care.

The lack of specific funding for formal interdisciplinary home palliative care programmes in some provinces will continue to limit the number of Canadians who can access expert palliative care. The identification of palliative care and home palliative care as core services within the health-care system in Canada in the future hopefully will change this situation in the future.

References

1. Health Canada. (1990). *Report on home care* (prepared by the Federal/Provincial/Territorial Working Group on Home Care, a Working Group of the Federal/Provincial/Territorial Subcommittee on Long Term Care), p. 2.
2. Data from the United States National Centre for Health Statistics. (2001).
3. Excerpted from National Hospice and Palliative Care Organization document. *NHPCO Facts and Figures 2006*.
4. Federal/Provincial/Territorial Working Group on Home Care, a Working Group of the Federal/Provincial/Territorial Subcommittee on Long Term Care. (1990). *Report on home care*, Health Canada, p. 2.
5. Federal-Provincial-Territorial Advisory Committee on Health Services Working Group on Continuing Care. (1999). *Provincial and Territorial Home Care Programs: A Synthesis for Canada*, Health Canada, May, p. 22.

SECTION 19

The terminal phase

The terminal phase

Mike Harlos

The terminal phase of illness can be one of the most challenging aspects of palliative care, with many of the factors that have impacted on quality of life throughout the illness demanding increasing clinical vigilance towards the end of life. Issues of symptom management, psychosocial and spiritual distress, functional decline, communication, and decision-making may come increasingly into focus through the lens of proximate death. While these challenges may present as sudden changes in status requiring urgent attention, they are often nonetheless predictable, comprising patterns of change that reflect a final common pathway of many progressive illnesses.

An anticipatory approach to foreseeable challenges is fundamental to ensuring the best possible quality of life for patient and family during the terminal phase of illness. Rather than be regarded as planning for what 'might go wrong', many issues are sufficiently common and predictable that they can hardly be considered as having 'gone wrong'… they are simply going as they are inclined to.

The clinical challenges commonly encountered in the final weeks, days, and hours of progressive illness are generally not unique to the terminal phase, however their progression and the limited time to address them imparts an urgency to their management. The preferred location of care may influence options for investigations and interventions, as supporting a hoped-for home death may not allow for rapid access to laboratory or imaging services, and complex routes of medication administration such as continuous infusions by central venous lines or intrathecal catheters may not be possible with local resources.

In this chapter, an overview of the terminal phase will be presented, with consideration of the challenges in symptom management, communication, ethical issues, and practical planning for care as influenced by care setting and goals/expectations.

Definition of the terminal phase

At what point does one define a terminal illness as having reached its 'terminal phase'? This is more than simply an exercise in semantics, as its definition enables the recognition and thus the appropriate management of needs, including pre-emptive planning for clinical challenges that might arise, addressing matters of end-of-life closure for patient and family, and facilitating communication around topics including hopes, goals, expectations, and fears.

The terminal phase can be considered as the period of inexorable and irreversible decline in functional status prior to death. This may unfold gradually over days or weeks with a fluctuating but nonetheless ongoing decline in a progressive illness, or precipitously

following an unexpected and devastating neurological event such as a stroke, or following a planned withdrawal of life-sustaining interventions such as haemodialysis or ventilatory support.

Overarching approach to care in the terminal phase

'Thank you for giving me aliveness.'[1]

This poignant statement by Jonathan, a terminally ill 6-year-old boy, captures the essence of palliative care with the succinct simplicity so characteristic of children. Even as death approaches, palliative care is focused on living as best as possible, an imperative which may require increasing vigilance and expertise to fulfil near the end of illness.

Much as the clinical challenges in the final days to weeks of terminal illness are similar to those presenting throughout the illness, the approach to care should be grounded in the same fundamental principles. Both the patient and family are the focus of comprehensive palliative care, and the health-care team should strive towards:

1 Ensuring the best possible quality of life for the patient—the cornerstone of care goals in palliative care, to which others are secondary. This goal is equally relevant in the final days of life as throughout the course of illness; the concept of quality of life may be reframed with time, but the need to maximize it remains.

2 Supporting families during the course of illness and after the patient's death; helping navigate the 'path of least regret' when considering care options, being mindful of how families may look back on care decisions month or years later.

Each family has unique dynamics of interaction, decision-making, and communication that are based on patterns of behaviour that have evolved over a lifetime. Much as if visiting an unfamiliar part of the world, the newcomer to this family microculture is well served by an approach including respect, naïveté, observation, and curiosity. Issues around death and dying are particularly intense and complex, taking families into unfamiliar areas of consideration and discussion.

Approaching decisions when choices are limited

In the final phase of terminal illness there will be health-care decisions which may become increasingly challenging, with little evidence to specifically guide choices in such advanced disease.

may prolong a very natural dying process, can aggravate oedema in severe hypoproteinemia, requires technology that may not be available in the chosen care setting, and maintains urine output with resultant toileting or catheterization needs and risk of skin excoriation if incontinent.

There is not a clear correlation between hydration status and the severity of terminal respiratory secretions ('death rattle')[19], although this is a common argument presented against hydration when speaking to families.

In view of an inconclusive body of evidence and the widely disparate approaches within the community of experienced palliative care clinicians, one can hardly justify a dogmatic stance on issues of hydration at the end of life. As with other potential interventions, each circumstance should be considered in its unique context, reviewing the hoped-for goals and the likelihood of their achievement.

A family wishing for artificial hydration to prevent thirst in a patient who is deeply comatose and near death following a massive cerebral haemorrhage can be reassured that thirst will not be experienced, in view of decreased level of consciousness. For the patient presenting with dehydration and hypercalcaemia, or opioid-induced neurotoxicity, or potentially reversible small bowel obstruction complicating metastatic ovarian cancer, there may be reasonable confidence that hydration will be beneficial.

Families may indicate cultural or religious beliefs, or strong personal convictions that it would be an abandonment of their loved one to not provide hydration, which they may consider a minimum obligation of care. In the absence of clear harm to the patient it would be difficult to justify a stance against hydration if technically feasible. Without risking compromise of the primary goal of patient comfort and quality of life, the support of family by helping navigate the 'path of least regret' is an important task in the terminal phase.

Parenteral hydration—subcutaneous vs. intravenous routes

If hydration is decided upon and the enteral route is not available, the most commonly used routes are subcutaneous (hypodermoclysis) or intravenous. Potential advantages of hypodermoclysis include:

◆ ease of administration when venous access is no longer possible due to limited choice of peripheral veins, or the care setting not having policy on intravenous hydration;

◆ comparable effectiveness and adverse effects to intravenous hydration in frail patient populations[20,21], with potentially less risk of volume overload;

◆ broader variety of potential sites of administration, including abdomen, thigh, scapula, axillary, sub-clavicular chest wall; in confused patients who may try to remove the subcutaneous cannula, the interscapular region may minimize this risk;

◆ infusions can be interrupted without concern of cannula thrombosis;

◆ has not been shown to cause septicaemia.

Solutions commonly used subcutaneously are normal saline, isotonic dextrose saline solutions, and 5 per cent dextrose solutions, in volumes of 1–2 l/day in adults[22].

The intravenous route should be chosen when aggressive rehydration is indicated for haemodynamic compromise and to correct significant electrolyte disturbances.

Arguably, in the dehydrated patient with excellent venous access and no technical barriers of administration, the intravenous route provides a means of rehydration that may have more acceptance by patient and families[23] and also allows for parenteral medications to be coadministered. The choice of route should be dictated by consideration of clinical factors and informed discussion with patients/families.

Route of medication administration

Ensuring timely access to needed medications is a fundamental component of effective palliative care throughout the course of illness, often assuming an added urgency as death nears. The loss of the oral route is a predictable eventuality which may occur suddenly, and the need for medications may be urgent due to the proximity of death and rapid clinical changes such as dyspnoea due to a terminal pneumonia or agitation with end-of-life delirium. It may not be possible to obtain medications such as parenteral opioids and sedatives after hours, particularly for the patient at home. Potentially needed medications should be stocked preemptively, using routes of administration that are practical under the circumstances. Consider pre-drawing individual doses for families if this may help simplify care.

There should be an ongoing review of all medications, with a view to discontinuing those which may no longer be needed, and exploring non-oral routes for others. Some medications, such as lipid-lowering agents, should be discontinued long before the final weeks of life-limiting illness. Antihypertensives can usually be tapered off in the terminal phase, as hypertension is not usually an issue with ongoing weight loss and diminishing fluid intake. Continuation of medications for diabetes mellitus, angina, or congestive heart failure should be guided by clinical assessment of need; poor control of such conditions can adversely affect quality of life even in the final weeks, although not likely so in the final days. Anticonvulsants are generally maintained, however the need for their initial prescription should be scrutinized—at times they have been initiated for neuropathic pain or seizure prophylaxis, which may not need ongoing treatment.

Carefully consider the pharmacotherapeutic implications of the removal of central venous access devices and feeding tubes prior to doing so. These are sometimes removed in pursuit of a 'palliative' aesthetic, taking away a very effective means of administering medications. Even when their use for maintaining hydration or continuing nutritional support has been decided against, they may remain helpful in administering medications such as anticonvulsants for which subcutaneous administration options are limited.

Choosing between non-oral routes

There are a wide variety of non-oral routes of medication administration, which differ in their availability across care settings (generally influenced by technical complexity and cost), acceptance by patient and family, and degree of sound clinical evidence supporting their use. By the time the oral route of medication administration is lost, some non-oral routes will likewise not be feasible, such as inhalational (due to general weakness) or spinal (due to care setting limitations, or overall frailty). The following are potential non-oral routes:

Feeding tube

If already in place, a feeding tube may be a convenient and well-tolerated means of medication administration. Some medications are available in liquid preparations, particularly if there are paediatric formulations available. Some tablets may be crushed, while others such as long-acting formulations and some enteric-coated medications such as omeprazole must not be. Even a liquid preparation may block a feeding tube, as with the antibiotic clarithromycin.

Rectal

With the increasing number of medications which can be given by subcutaneous injection, transmucosally (buccal, sublingual, or nasal), and transdermally, the rectal route is used less often. There may be physical discomfort from turning the patient and inserting the medication, and the patient/family may find rectal medications difficult or socially unacceptable. Nonetheless, for some medications such as acetaminophen (paracetamol) this may be the most readily available route.

Most opioids are either available commercially as suppositories (morphine, hydromorphone), or can be formulated as such by a compounding pharmacist.

Antinauseants available rectally include metoclopramide, domperidone (UK), prochlorperazine, chlorpromazine, and dimenhydrinate. A compounding pharmacist can be consulted regarding producing suppository formulations of other antinauseants.

The non-steroidal anti-inflammatory drugs diclofenac and ketoprofen are available in UK as suppositories.

Cautions regarding rectal administration of medications include ensuring the rectum is not blocked by stool or tumour, avoiding rectal administration of drugs in situations of severe thrombocytopenia or coagulopathy, and avoiding the rectal route in severe neutropenia if risk of infection remains a concern.

Nasal and oral (buccal, sublingual) transmucosal

Some medications are specifically formulated for buccal or sublingual use, including opioids such as Actiq® (fentanyl) and buprenorphine; benzodiazepines (lorazepam sublingual tablets), the phenothiazine prochlorperazine (a useful antinauseant), and the atypical antipsychotic olanzapine (can be used for nausea[24,25], and delirium).

Sublingual[26] and nasal[27] absorption of the intravenous preparations of several opioids has been demonstrated (in the range of 35–70 per cent), with an increasing body of literature regarding the lipid-soluble anilinopiperidine opioids fentanyl, sufentanil, and alfentanil. These medications generally have onset of action within 15 minutes by nasal or sublingual administration, and their effectiveness has been clearly demonstrated[28-31]. Their use in managing pain or dyspnoea crisis in the absence of a parenteral route of administration should be strongly considered.

Other medications whose injectable formulations have been shown to be absorbed by this route include the benzodiazepines midazolam[32,33] and lorazepam[34], and the NMDA antagonist ketamine[35]. A general guideline for sublingual or nasal dosing of an intravenous preparation is to start with the recommended intravenous dose and titrate to response; bioavailability will not exceed the intravenous route of administration, providing an inherent safety factor.

Atropine 1 per cent ophthalmic drops, 1–2 drops sublingually every 6 hours as needed, may help in reducing oral secretions[36,37], although literature support is inconsistent[38].

Many medications have commercially available liquid formulations intended for oral use, or can be compounded as such using an original powder form. For example, morphine oral elixir is available in concentrations as high as 50 mg/ml, hydromorphone is available as a 1 mg/ml elixir in North America, and methadone can be compounded in oral preparations up to 50 mg/ml approximately. Small buccal or sublingual doses (1 ml or less) in an unresponsive patient tend to be swallowed reflexively, and the effectiveness of this route is judged empirically. Doses requiring more than 1 ml can be administered in aliquots at 10–15-min intervals if necessary. This approach may enable symptom management in the absence of other options.

Transdermal

The transdermal patch formulation of fentanyl has been available for many years, with an established effectiveness as an opioid analgesic. It should not be used in opioid-naïve patients, and vigilance for drug accumulation is required as doses are incremented. Increased absorption occurs with elevated temperature, as with fever or local heating pad application. The long duration of action and the lag between dose change and observed effect preclude the use of transdermal fentanyl for responding to rapidly changing symptoms in the final days.

Buprenorphine is available in UK in transdermal patch form.

The transdermal scopolamine patch can be used for nausea that may have a vestibular component, and to diminish respiratory secretions.

Diclofenac is a nonsteroidal anti-inflammatory drugs which is commercially available in gel formulation.

There is an increasing trend for topical compounding of a variety of analgesics, analgesic adjuvants, antiemetics, and other medications. There is a paucity of randomized placebo-controlled trials in this burgeoning area of palliative pharmacotherapeutics, although some literature for topical ketamine is mounting, albeit conflicting[39,40].

Subcutaneous (intermittent injection, continuous infusion)

A wide variety of medications can be administered subcutaneously using the parenteral formulation. This is an ever-changing area, with new evidence frequently becoming available. Table 19.1.1 lists some medications often used in the terminal phase that can be administered by this route, either through either intermittently or continuous infusions using a syringe driver. In general, up to 3 ml/hour is tolerated and effective for medication administration by continuous subcutaneous infusion[41].

Oral-to-subcutaneous equivalences for opioids is variably reported, however it is generally safe and reasonable to assume that parenteral (subcutaneous, intravenous) opioids are approximately twice as potent as by oral route, due to bypassing first pass hepatic metabolism.

Intravenous (peripheral or central line)

The intravenous route for medications is not always available in the palliative setting, due limitations of the care setting, poor venous access, or a chosen approach by patient/family. If available, it provides a ready and reliable means of administration of a wide variety of medications, with minimal patient burden for pre-existing lines. Consideration should be given to leaving central venous access devices in place if the chosen care setting can support them, particularly in patients with unstable seizure disorders or for whom a symptom crisis such as pain, dyspnoea, or acute haemorrhage may require rapid administration of medications.

Table 19.1.1 Medications via subcutaneous route.

Drug class	Common indications	Drug	Beginning intermittent subcutaneous dose (adults)*	Beginning continuous infusion dose over 24 h (adults)*	Comments
Opioids	Pain, dyspnoea	Morphine	2.5–5 mg q4 h**	15–30 mg	
		Diamorphine (UK)	2.5 mg q4 h	15 mg(49)	
		Hydromorphone	0.5–1 mg q4 h	3–6 mg	
		Fentanyl	Use by continuous Infusion	150–300 mcg	
		Sufentanil	Use by continuous infusion	Must be individualized	Approx. 10 times the potency of fentanyl; useful when volume limits fentanyl administration
		Methadone (UK, USA; not available in Canada)	Individualized as per existing opioid tolerance	Individualized as per existing opioid tolerance	May be irritating; caution with dose titration
Benzodiazepines	Agitation, anxiety, seizure disorder	Midazolam	2.5 mg q4–6 h	20–40 mg for seizures(49)	
Neuroleptics	Agitation, anxiety, nausea and vomiting	Haloperidol	0.5–2.5 mg q6–8 h	2.5–10 mg(49)	The lower dose ranges are often effective for nausea
		Levomepromazine (methotrimeprazine)	Nausea may be improved with doses as low as 2.5 mg q8 h; restlessness and agitation: 2.5–5 mg q6 h	5–25 mg(49)	May be irritating; for severe agitation, doses as high as 300 mg/day may be needed; watch for paradoxical delirium due to anticholinergic effects
Barbiturates	Seizures, agitated delirium	Phenobarbital	60 mg q6–8 h¥	240 mg and higher; dose ranges of 200–2400 mg/24 h has been reported(50,51)	
Prokinetics	Nausea and vomiting	Metoclopramide	10 mg q6 h	30–100 mg(49)	
Anticholinergics	Secretions	Hyoscine hydrobromide (scopolamine)	0.3–0.6 mg q2–4 h	0.6–2.4 mg(49)	Likely to cause sedation and delirium in an alert patient
		Glycopyrrolate	0.2–0.4 mg q4–6 h	0.6–1.2 mg(49)	Less sedating than scopolamine
Corticosteroids	Anti-inflammatory; numerous and varied indications	Dexamethasone	Wide variation; depends on clinical indication	Wide variation; depends on clinical indication	Incompatible when mixed with midazolam or haloperidol(52); general vigilance advised for evidence of incompatibility in combinations (precipitation)
Antihistamines	Nausea and vomiting	Cyclizine (UK)	50 mg q8 h	150 mg(49)	May be irritating; caution regarding precipitation with diamorphine or other drugs
Diuretics	Fluid overload	Furosemide(53)	10–40 mg	No Information	
Somatostatin analogue	Bowel obstruction	Octreotide	100–200 mcg q8 h	300–600 mcg(49)	

* Consider lower doses in patients with impaired renal or liver function, compromised respiratory status, or body weight <50 kg.

** qXh indicates the dosing interval, where *X* is the # hours between doses.

¥ Conservative starting dose, based on the author's experience.

Notes: the following medications are irritating when administered subcutaneously and are not recommended by this route: chlorpromazine, prochlorperazine, diazepam;(49) dimenhydrinate(54).

Management of specific symptoms in the final days of life

Symptoms present in the terminal phase of illness are likely to reflect those experienced earlier for that patient; there will generally be a need for continued management of pre-existing pain, dyspnoea, nausea, pruritus, anxiety, and other symptoms.

There are also specific symptoms which the clinician must be prepared to address without delay in the final days, regardless of their existence previously, namely:

1 Pain.

2 Dyspnoea.

3 Agitation (usually associated with delirium).

4 Respiratory secretions.

Some basic principles of anticipatory preparation for their development apply to the management of these and other clinical issues:

◆ There should be proactive communication with patient/family about anticipated symptoms, exploring expectations around their investigation and management and to what degree these expectations are achievable. In the final days, reversing underlying conditions will generally not be possible. Investigations seeking to identify problems which cannot be addressed should not be pursued.

◆ Anticipated medications should be available by appropriate routes of administration, taking into consideration the implications of the care setting and the capabilities of the caregivers.

◆ There must be ongoing evaluation of patient comfort and family support needs.

◆ The health-care team must be available, accessible, and ready to respond in a timely manner to concerns that arise.

Pain

The prevalence of pain in advanced terminal illness is generally reported in the range of 70–80 per cent, regardless of the underlying diagnosis. The SUPPORT study found that 40 per cent of patients 'had severe pain most of the time' in the last 3 days of life[42].

Pain management in palliative care is comprehensively addressed elsewhere in this text (see Section 10.1), and the key components of assessment and management are unchanged in the final days. If decreased level of consciousness and/or confusion affects the patient's ability to report pain, the family and health-care team work together in assessing comfort. Disease-related pain that was present a few days earlier is likely to remain present, and its treatment should continue.

Investigations should only be pursued if pain management treatment will be influenced; in the final days it is unlikely that radiation therapy, surgery, or interventional analgesia will be considered.

Long-acting opioid preparations should be changed to their short-acting equivalents, in order to facilitate titration. For example, 120 mg twice a day of long-acting morphine can be changed to 20 mg orally every 4 hours, or 10 mg subcutaneously every 4 hours, or a continuous subcutaneous or intravenous infusion of 2.5 mg/h.

When a patient with transdermal fentanyl patch is in the last few days of life with escalating opioid needs, one could consider removal of the patch and initiating an estimated replacement equivalent of morphine or other opioid. However, this approach unnecessarily introduces new variables (diminishing serum fentanyl levels and imprecise opioid equivalence estimates) into an already unstable pain management situation, with limited time left. Consideration should be given to leaving the transdermal fentanyl unchanged as a stable foundation on which to titrate an additional short-acting opioid.

Alternatively, the fentanyl patch may be directly switched to a subcutaneous fentanyl infusion at the same dose, and adjusted to response.

Pain experienced specifically in relation to planned activity such as turning the patient or dressing changes (incident pain) can be managed using sublingual fentanyl or sufentanil preemptively[31], or oral transmucosal fentanyl citrate (Actiq®).

Dyspnoea

The prevalence of dyspnoea commonly increases with illness progression[43]; a study of children dying from cancer found a prevalence dyspnoea exceeding 80 per cent in the last month of life, with only 16 per cent receiving successful treatment.

Causes of dyspnoea in advanced cancer include directly tumour-related (parenchymal involvement, lymphangitic spread), indirect tumour causes (airway obstruction, pleural or pericardial effusions, ascites, superior vena cava obstruction, asthenia), illness complications (pneumonia, pulmonary embolism, haemoptysis, anaemia), and treatment-related (radiation or chemotherapy-induced pulmonary fibrosis, cardiomyopathy). Reversal of underlying causes as death nears becomes increasingly implausible, however consideration might be given to relatively straightforward interventions such as:

◆ treating an underlying infection;

◆ transfusing for low haemoglobin;

◆ corticosteroids (dexamethasone) for airway or superior vena cava obstruction;

◆ thoracentesis for large pleural effusions.

Non-pharmacological approaches to dyspnoea include elevating the head of the bed to a comfortable height and having a fan blowing cool air towards the patient.

If available, oxygen may be helpful in relieving dyspnoea; generally nasal prongs at 3–5 l/min will suffice, titrated to empirical effect rather than pulse oximetry.

Opioids are the main pharmacological intervention for relieving shortness of breath in the dying patient. Dosing is titrated to comfort, which is usually achieved without significant changes in respiratory rate or blood gases[44]. The respiratory rate may in fact remain high (tachypnoea) without distress, which does not require treatment. Generally, when opioids are being used to treat both pain and dyspnoea near the end of life, it will be dyspnoea that drives the opioid titration.

When anxiety is present, benzodiazepines such as midazolam[45] or lorazepam[46] may help, or the neuroleptic levomepromazine (methotrimeprazine)[46].

Dyspnoea in the final days of life is a very potent stimulus for distress, whose effective management may not be achievable without the patient becoming sedated. When death is near, it may not be possible to strike the balance between alertness and comfort, a fact which may be concerning for family and which requires open dialogue.

Withdrawing oxygen

In the unresponsive patient who is nearing death and appears comfortable to family and staff, continued administration of oxygen is not likely to be achieving a goal of improving comfort, and may well be prolonging the dying process. Consideration can be given to removing the oxygen, following discussion with family in the context of what the patient would want. The oxygen may perhaps be tapered over 1–2 h while observing for signs of distress.

Agitated delirium at the end of life

Delirium reaches a prevalence of 80 per cent or more in the final days[47,48], and may be associated with restlessness, agitation, paranoia, and combativeness. This constellation of symptoms is extremely upsetting for family, leaving a lasting image after the patient's death that is far from the gentle passing that is so much hoped for. Such a situation would be equally devastating for patients if they were aware of their behaviour and its impact on family.

Potential causes of delirium are legion, and efforts towards their diagnosis and reversal must not delay immediate and effective management of agitation with sedation. Factors ranging from infection, medication effects, brain or leptomeningeal involvement by tumour, hypoxia, metabolic disturbances such hypercalcaemia or hyponatremia, and hypo- or hyperglycaemia are but a few possible causes. Not uncommonly, more than one possible aetiology is implicated.

If it is felt that death may be hours or perhaps a day or two away, there is no purpose served in attempting to define and reverse possible causes of delirium. A possible exception to this is hypoglycaemia, which can be both diagnosed and treated immediately. With a prognosis of days to a week or more, there is more potential to either investigate possible causes, or empirically try interventions such as treating an infection, reviewing and changing medications, or starting dexamethasone if cerebral oedema complicating a known brain tumour is suspected.

Sedation for agitation will usually require combinations of neuroleptics such as levomepromazine (methotrimeprazine) or haloperidol with a benzodiazepine, most commonly midazolam. The subcutaneous route is preferred, as it does not require patient compliance and is easily administered.

Levomepromazine (methotrimeprazine) may be administered by intermittent subcutaneous injection, with doses ranging from 2.5 mg q6–8 h to as high as 50 mg q4h. Continuous infusion doses are described as ranging from 12.5–200 mg/24 h[49]. There is a potential for its inherent anticholinergic effects to aggravate a delirium with ongoing use.

Haloperidol doses for agitated delirium generally range from 0.5 mg q12 h to as high as 5 mg q4 h subcutaneously. It is not as sedating as levomepromazine (methotrimeprazine). Continuous infusions of haloperidol for agitation are described as ranging from 5–15 mg/24 h[49].

Midazolam can be added to a neuroleptic for added sedating effect. Used alone in the management of agitated delirium, benzodiazepines may result in disinhibition and increased restlessness. Typical intermittent subcutaneous doses range from 2.5 mg q6–8 h up to 5–10 mg q4 h. Continuous infusions of midazolam for agitation are described as ranging from 20–100 mg/24 h[49]. If the sublingual route is tolerated, lorazepam is a reasonable alternative to midazolam. Sublingual doses for adults generally range from 0.5 mg q6–8 h to as high as 1–2 mg q4 h in more severe agitation.

Occasionally, phenobarbital may need to be added to the above medications in order to achieve adequate sedation. Intermittent subcutaneous doses may begin with 50–100 mg q8h, adjusted empirically to effect. Continuous infusions have been described in doses ranging widely from 200–2400 mg/24 h[50,51].

It is important to have 'as needed' doses of sedatives available at doses that reflect those currently administered; this may be equal to the regularly scheduled intermittent dose, or equivalent to 2 h of a continuous infusion. The interval between allowed 'as needed' doses should generally not exceed 1 h; the results of the medication will be evident by that time, and if ineffective a repeat dose will allow some cumulative effect. It does not make sense to condemn the patient, family, and staff to wait several hours simply to repeat an ineffective dose.

Supporting the family

Family will be understandably distraught at the restlessness and confusion they are observing, and eager for its resolution. It is important that they understand the probable irreversibility of the need for sedation, given the short time expected until death. Otherwise, they may expect that the situation is one of temporary sedation followed by alertness and communication. Once the patient is more calm, family should be encouraged to visit, hold the patient's hand if they wish, play favourite music, and talk to the patient. None of this would be possible if the agitation were not aggressively managed.

If changes had occurred quickly, some family members may arrive having missed the opportunity for meaningful interaction. They should be supported in having private time alone with the patient should they wish, without other family members present. This might not be an intuitive step for families, and encouragement from staff may be needed.

Respiratory secretions—the 'death rattle'

Excessive respiratory tract secretions at the end of life, typically in the unresponsive patient within hours to days of dying (the 'death rattle') has a reported prevalence as high as 92 per cent[19]. The patient is not usually responsive at this time, and it is not always clear whether treatment is aimed at improving potential patient distress, or improving the visiting environment for family and friends. Both are important objectives, and the distinction is perhaps irrelevant.

For management of pulmonary secretions in the terminal phase, an anticholinergic such as scopolamine (hyoscine hydrobromide), or glycopyrrolate is commonly used. Intermittent subcutaneous dosing is generally preferred initially rather than a continuous infusion, since sometimes only one or two doses are required to achieve improvement.

Glycopyrrolate does not cross the blood-brain barrier as readily as scopolamine, and thus is less likely to cause sedation and delirium. However, it does not seem as effective as scopolamine in clinical practice. If the patient is still having periods of interactive and clear wakefulness, then glycopyrrolate is a reasonable first choice antisecretory. Intermittent subcutaneous doses range from 0.2–0.4 mg q4h as needed. Consideration of a continuous infusion would usually indicate a poor response intermittent dosing, in which case changing to scopolamine is warranted.

Commonly the patient with the 'death rattle' is not responsive; the sedating effects of scopolamine are generally moot at this time. Typical doses for intermittent subcutaneous administration are 0.3–0.6 mg q2 h as needed, and in situations of ongoing symptoms a continuous subcutaneous infusion of 0.6–2.4 mg/24 h[(49)] or higher may be needed.

For the patient in a care setting where the subcutaneous route is not available, the transdermal scopolamine patch may be tried. Its indicated use is for motion sickness, and it delivers about 1 mg scopolamine over 72 h. This is much less than the usual dose given subcutaneously for secretions. On occasion, the author has applied 2 to 3 transdermal scopolamine patches at once in order to try to achieve a similar dose to the usual subcutaneous dosing, which was anecdotally effective.

Suctioning in order to relieve terminal secretions is generally not recommended unless they are easily accessible in the oropharynx. Deeper suctioning is traumatic, and likely to cause further secretions.

Symptom crisis at the end of life

The sudden development of severe symptom distress may occur during the final phase of illness, and in fact may represent a fatal event. Although not common overall, such situations are traumatic for everyone and may leave unforgettable images for family. When possible, preemptive planning can facilitate rapid symptom management, and in the absence of such preparation the patient may die before effective treatment is administered.

Potential crises include:

♦ Respiratory—airway obstruction, pulmonary embolism, haemoptysis, fulminant pneumonia, pericardial tamponade. (Note—superior vena cava obstruction tends to be subacute in palliative patients).

♦ Pain—pathological fracture, perforated viscus, occasionally acute spinal cord compression.

♦ Haemorrhage—haematemesis, massive epistaxis, head and neck vessel erosion, haemoptysis, lower GI haemorrhage.

♦ Seizures.

Many of the above complications occur in individuals with a known vulnerability for them, and planning for their possible development involves:

♦ Preparing involved health-care staff, through information, education, formulating clear care plans for crisis management.

♦ Discussions with patient and family as guided by the judgement of the involved health-care professionals. Family caregivers supporting a home death will need clear and open discussions about the management of potential circumstances that may arise. Their information needs are generally broader and more comprehensive than the patient's in such circumstances, in order to ensure a rapid and effective response to a variety of potential symptoms challenges.

♦ Having potentially needed medications pre-drawn and available on hand.

♦ Practical measures such as having green rather than white towels available in case of an acute haemorrhage.

Management of crisis generally involves aggressive use of opioids and sedatives in order to achieve rapid comfort, most commonly with the aim of addressing pain and dyspnoea and to have the patient sedated and therefore not aware of the circumstances. Short-acting medications should be used; routes of administration include:

♦ Intravenous—rapid and reliable onset.

♦ Subcutaneous—readily available, however may have an unacceptably delayed onset of effect, particularly if the subcutaneous tissues are poorly perfused due to the physiologic effects of the crisis.

♦ Nasal or buccal/sublingual—for midazolam, fentanyl, sufentanil, and alfentanil; may have a more rapid and reliable onset of action that subcutaneous administration, particularly if poor subcutaneous perfusion as noted above.

♦ Intramuscular—although this route has lost favour in the palliative care community due to injection discomfort, in haemodynamic compromise the deep muscles will be more reliably perfused than the subcutaneous tissues. One might consider the use of lorazepam 2–4 mg intramuscularly for an acute seizure rather than subcutaneous midazolam; injection pain is not a compelling concern in this circumstance.

Specific doses will depend on existing tolerance to medications; typically an opioid dose for crisis will be at least double the current breakthrough dose, and sedative doses would be at minimum 5 mg midazolam subcutaneously or 2–4 mg lorazepam intramuscularly or intravenously. Methotrimeprazine 25–50 mg subcutaneously can also be considered for severe distress.

A common barrier to the effective use of opioids in managing symptom crisis at the end of life is the misconception that they will compromise the patient and potentially hasten death. There is no evidence that opioids compromise palliative patients when given in doses proportionate to the degree of distress.

The clinical context of a symptom crisis almost always involves agitation and a rapid respiratory rate. In the final moments, irregularly spaced apneic episodes interject, resulting in an erratic breathing pattern with clusters of rapid breaths and increasingly frequent and prolonged apneic episodes. This typically unfolds quickly - over a few seconds to several minutes - following which breathing ceases.

In contrast, excessive opioid doses cause a progressive slowing of breathing which tends to unfold more gradually (unless following a large intravenous bolus), with the respiratory pattern remaining regular. Level of consciousness progressively decreases, and pupils are generally pinpoint. This is an important distinction to recognize, as staff and family may be concerned that repeated opioid doses may contribute to the decline or in fact may have hastened death. When administering medications to a patient who is dying, there will invariably be a point at which the patient dies after (but not due to) receiving a medication dose. Caregivers should be reassured that the medications administered do not compromise the patient.

Sedation for anguish

The complex topic of palliative sedation is more thoroughly addressed elsewhere in this text (see Chapter 19.2). In aggressively managing severe pain and dyspnoea at the end of life as described above, sedation is often an inescapable outcome due to the doses required and the patient's overall condition. In terminal delirium, sedation is the primary intent of the medication administration, although it remains the only available intervention under the circumstances and if alternative effective measures existed they would selected.

On occasion, a patient nearing death who is not experiencing refractory physical symptoms or suffering from delirium indicates that wakefulness is unbearable, and in view of the proximity to dying he or she would rather remain asleep for the remainder of time left.

These are very challenging situations for all involved, including patient, family, and health-care team. If one does not feel conflicted in consideration of circumstances such as this, then perhaps not all of its implications are being appreciated.

As with any refractory suffering, reasonable efforts to address emotional and spiritual anguish should be pursued. However, in the patient with hours or days to live one must be mindful that such distress is not going to be subject to a 'quick fix', if any type of fix at all. Support by pastoral care and psychosocial clinicians should be offered, as well as skilled exploration of potentially addressable issues (such as fear of dying in poorly controlled pain).

In the absence of remediable factors and with the informed consent of the competent patient, sedation can be accomplished using medications as described above for delirium, although generally the lower dose range is effective as there is not stimulus of an agitated delirium.

There must be ongoing review of sedation effectiveness, and open dialogue with family and with the health-care team in order to provide a welcoming forum for discussing concerns.

The signs of dying

The final changes seen in the hours preceding death generally include:

- Decreasing level of consciousness.
- Decreasing interaction.
- Minimal intake, progressing to no oral intake.
- Decreasing urine output.
- Haemodynamic decline, with tachycardia, weak/thready pulse, cool extremities, and mottling (purplish reticular discolouration of the skin) beginning from distal extremities.
- Respiratory changes including tachypnoea, accessory muscle utilization, and shallow breathing.
- In the final minutes or hours, the breathing pattern often becomes irregular, with clusters of breathing such as the Cheyne–Stokes pattern or agonal clusters of breaths separated by apneic periods of several seconds to 1–3 min (on rare occasions longer).
- The breathing will ultimately stop, followed several minutes later by cessation of the heart beat.

These physical changes of dying can be upsetting to those at the bedside. Changes in skin colour and breathing patterns reflect inescapable physiological changes occurring in the dying process. It may be comforting for families to distinguish between who their loved one is—the person to whom they are so connected in thought and spirit—versus the physical changes that are happening to their loved one's body.

The family may wish to be left alone during the final moments of the patient's life, and should be allowed such privacy and time. Following the death, they may wish to have other family members and friends visit.

There may be family members who were not able to be present at the time of death, and perhaps feel guilty because of this. It may be helpful to talk about the meaningfulness of their connection in thought and spirit as distinguished from the purely physical proximity that they are regretting having missed. Whether they were at the bedside, or had stepped out of the room for a much needed break, or were in fact in a different country, their connection in spirit was not diminished by physical distance.

References

1. Sourkes, B. (1995). *Armfuls of time.* University of Pittsburgh Press, Pittsburgh, p. 167.
2. British Medical Association. (2001). *Withholding and withdrawing life-prolonging medical treatment*, 2nd edition. BMJ Publishing Group, London, p. 69.
3. The SUPPORT Principal Investigators. (1995). A controlled trial to improve care for seriously ill hospitalized patients. The study to understand prognoses and preferences for outcomes and risks of treatments (SUPPORT). *JAMA*, **274**, 1591–98.
4. Chochinov, H.M., Tataryn, D.J., Wilson, K.G. *et al.* (2000). Prognostic awareness and the terminally ill. *Psychosomatics*, **41**, 500–4.
5. Barnett, M.M. (2006). Does it hurt to know the worst?–psychological morbidity, information preferences and understanding of prognosis in patients with advanced cancer. *Psychooncology*, **15**, 44–55.
6. Jenkins, V., Fallowfield, L., and Saul, J. (2001). Information needs of patients with cancer: results from a large study in UK cancer centres. *British Journal of Cancer*, **84**, 48–51.
7. Fallowfield, L.J., Jenkins, V.A., and Beveridge, H.A. (2002). Truth may hurt but deceit hurts more: communication in palliative care. *Palliative Medicine*, **16**, 297–303.
8. Reisfield, G.M., Wallace, S.K., Munsell, M.F. *et al.* (2006). Survival in cancer patients undergoing in-hospital cardiopulmonary resuscitation: a meta-analysis. *Resuscitation*, **71**, 152–60.
9. Torelli, G.F., Campos, A.C., and Meguid, M.M. (1999). Use of TPN in terminally ill cancer patients. *Nutrition*, **15**, 665–7.
10. Rabeneck, L., McCullough, L.B., and Wray, N.P. (1997). Ethically justified, clinically comprehensive guidelines for percutaneous endoscopic gastrostomy tube placement. *Lancet*, **349**, 496–8.
11. Cervo, F.A., Bryan, L., and Farber, S. (2006). To PEG or not to PEG: a review of evidence for placing feeding tubes in advanced dementia and the decision-making process. *Geriatrics*, **61**, 30–5.
12. Galicia-Castillo, M. (2006). The PEG dilemma: feeding tubes are not the answer in advanced dementia. *Geriatrics*, **61**, 12–3.
13. McClement, S.E., Degner, L.F., and Harlos, M. (2004). Family responses to declining intake and weight loss in a terminally ill relative. Part 1: fighting back. *Journal of Palliative Care*, **20**, 93–100.
14. McClement, S.E., Degner, L.F., and Harlos, M.S. (2003). Family beliefs regarding the nutritional care of a terminally ill relative: a qualitative study. *Journal of Palliative Medicine*, **6**, 737–48.

15. Burge, F.I. (1993). Dehydration symptoms of palliative care cancer patients. *Journal of Pain and Symptom Management*, 8, 454–464.

16. McCann, R.M., Hall, W.J., and Groth Juncker, A. (1994). Comfort care for terminally ill patients. The appropriate use of nutrition and hydration [see comments]. *JAMA*, 272, 1263–6.

17. Morita, T., Tei, Y., Tsunoda, J., Inoue, S., and Chihara, S. (2001). Determinants of the sensation of thirst in terminally ill cancer patients. *Supportive Care in Cancer*, 9, 177–86.

18. Bliss, M.R. (1998). Pressure injuries: causes and prevention. *Hospital Medicine*, 59, 841–4.

19. Ellershaw, J.E., Sutcliffe, J., and Saunders, C.M. (1995). Dehydration and the dying patient. *Journal of Pain and Symptom Management*, 10, 192–7.

20. Turner, T., and Cassano, A.M. (2004). Subcutaneous dextrose for rehydration of elderly patients—an evidence-based review. *BMC Geriatrics*, 4, 2.

21. Slesak, G., Schnurle, J.W., Kinzel, E. *et al.* (2003). Comparison of subcutaneous and intravenous rehydration in geriatric patients: a randomized trial. *Journal of American Geriatrics Society*, 51, 155–60.

22. Farrand, S., and Campbell, A.J. (1996). Safe, simple subcutaneous fluid administration. *British Journal of Hospital Medicine*, 55, 690–2.

23. Mercadante, S., Ferrera, P., Girelli, D., and Casuccio, A. (2005). Patients' and relatives' perceptions about intravenous and subcutaneous hydration. *Journal of Pain and Symptom Management*, 30, 354–8.

24. Navari, R.M., Einhorn, L.H., Passik, S.D. *et al.* (2005). A phase II trial of olanzapine for the prevention of chemotherapy-induced nausea and vomiting: a Hoosier Oncology Group study. *Supportive Care in Cancer*, 13, 529–34.

25. Jackson, W.C., and Tavernier, L. (2003). Olanzapine for intractable nausea in palliative care patients. *Journal of Palliative Medicine*, 6, 251–5.

26. Weinberg, D.S., Inturrisi, C.E., Reidenberg, B. *et al.* (1988). Sublingual absorption of selected opioid analgesics. *Clinical Pharmacology and Therapeutics*, 44, 335–42.

27. Dale, O., Hjortkjaer, R., and Kharasch, E.D. (2002). Nasal administration of opioids for pain management in adults. *Acta anaesthesiologica Scandinavica*, 46, 759–70.

28. Borland, M., Jacobs, I., King, B., and O'brien, D. (2006). A randomized controlled trial comparing intranasal fentanyl to intravenous morphine for managing acute pain in children in the emergency department. *Annals of Emergency Medicine*.

29. Brenchley, J., and Ramlakhan, S. (2006). Intranasal alfentanil for acute pain in children. *Emergency Medicine Journal*, 23, 488.

30. Mathieu, N., Cnudde, N., Engelman, E., and Barvais, L. (2006). Intranasal sufentanil is effective for postoperative analgesia in adults. *Canadian Journal of Anaesthesia*, 53, 60–6.

31. Gardner-Nix, J.S. (2001). Oral transmucosal fentanyl and sufentanil for incident pain [Letter]. *Journal of Pain and Symptom Management*, 22, 627–30.

32. Wolfe, T.R., and Macfarlane, T.C. (2006). Intranasal midazolam therapy for paediatric status epilepticus. *American Journal of Emergency Medicine*, 24, 343–6.

33. Dale, O., Nilsen, T., Loftsson, T. *et al.* (2006). Intranasal midazolam: a comparison of two delivery devices in human volunteers. *Journal of Pharmacy and Pharmacology*, 58, 1311–8.

34. Wermeling, D.P., Miller, J.L., Archer, S.M. *et al.* (2001). Bioavailability and pharmacokinetics of lorazepam after intranasal, intravenous, and intramuscular administration. *Journal of Clinical Pharmacology*, 41, 1225–31.

35. Carr, D.B., Goudas, L.C., Denman, W.T. *et al.* (2004). Safety and efficacy of intranasal ketamine for the treatment of breakthrough pain in patients with chronic pain: a randomized, double-blind, placebo-controlled, crossover study. *Pain*, 108, 17–27.

36. Comley, C., Galletly, C., and Ash, D. (2000). Use of atropine eye drops for clozapine induced hypersalivation. *The Australian and New Zealand Journal of Psychiatry*, 34, 1033–4.

37. Hyson, H.C., Johnson, A.M., and Jog, M.S. (2002). Sublingual atropine for sialorrhea secondary to parkinsonism: a pilot study. *Movement Disorders*, 17, 1318–20.

38. De Simone, G.G., Eisenchlas, J.H., Junin, M. *et al.* (2006). Atropine drops for drooling: a randomized controlled trial. *Palliative Medicine*, 20, 665–71.

39. Lockhart, E. (2004). Topical combination of amitriptyline and ketamine for post herpetic neuralgia (abstract). *Journal of Pain*, 5, 82.

40. Lynch, M.E., Clark, A.J., Sawynok, J., and Sullivan, M.J. (2005). Topical 2% amitriptyline and 1% ketamine in neuropathic pain syndromes: a randomized, double-blind, placebo-controlled trial. *Anesthesiology*, 103, 140–6.

41. Anderson, S.L., and Shreve, S.T. (2004). Continuous subcutaneous infusion of opiates at end-of-life. *The Annals of Pharmacotherapy*, 38, 1015–23.

42. Lynn, J., Teno, J.M., Phillips, R.S. *et al.* (1997). Perceptions by family members of the dying experience of older and seriously ill patients. SUPPORT Investigators. Study to Understand Prognoses and Preferences for Outcomes and Risks of Treatments. *Annals of Internal Medicine*, 126, 97–106.

43. Reuben, D.B., and Mor, V. (1986). Dyspnoea in terminally ill cancer patients. *Chest*, 89, 234–6.

44. Bruera, E., Macmillan, K., Pither, J., and MacDonald, R.N. (1990). Effects of morphine on the dyspnoea of terminal cancer patients. *Journal of Pain and Symptom Management*, 5, 341–4.

45. Navigante, A.H., Cerchietti, L.C., Castro, M.A. *et al.* (2006). Midazolam as adjunct therapy to morphine in the alleviation of severe dyspnoea perception in patients with advanced cancer. *Journal of Pain and Symptom Management*, 31, 38–47.

46. Davis, C.L. (1997). ABC of palliative care. Breathlessness, cough, and other respiratory problems. *BMJ*, 315, 931–6.

47. Fainsinger, R.L., De Moissac, D., Mancini, I., and Oneschuk, D. (2000). Sedation for delirium and other symptoms in terminally ill patients in Edmonton. *Journal of Palliative Care*, 16, 5–10.

48. Bruera, E., Miller, L., McCallion, J. *et al.* (1992). Cognitive failure in patients with terminal cancer: a prospective study. *Journal of Pain and Symptom Management*, 7, 192–5.

49. Joint Formulary Committee. (2006). *British National Formulary London*, 52nd edition. London.

50. Stirling, L.C., Kurowska, A., and Tookman, A. (1999). The use of phenobarbitone in the management of agitation and seizures at the end of life. *Journal of Pain and Symptom Management*, 17, 363–8.

51. Sykes, N., and Thorns, A. (2003). Sedative use in the last week of life and the implications for end-of-life decision-making. *Archives of Internal Medicine*, 163, 341–4.

52. Negro, S., Azuara, M.L., Sanchez, Y. *et al.* (2002). Physical compatibility and in vivo evaluation of drug mixtures for subcutaneous infusion to cancer patients in palliative care. *Supportive Care in Cancer*, 10, 65–70.

53. Verma, A.K., da Silva, J.H., and Kuhl, D.R. (2004). Diuretic effects of subcutaneous furosemide in human volunteers: a randomized pilot study. *Annals of Pharmacothery*, 38, 544–9.

54. Brent, N.J. (1986). Right drug, wrong route. *Nursing Life*, 6, 72.

19.2

Sedation in palliative medicine

Eric L. Krakauer and Thomas E. Quinn

Introduction

The need for palliative sedation

The most fundamental task of palliative medicine, and indeed of medicine in general, is to relieve suffering[1,2]. Among terminally ill patients whose primary goal is comfort, severe suffering occurs occasionally that is refractory to standard palliative interventions. Controlled sedation, sometimes to unconsciousness, may be the only effective means of relieving suffering in these unusual situations.

Patients and their families fearful of severe, refractory terminal suffering may feel quite relieved when informed that palliative sedation is available as an option should all standard interventions fail. Thus, clinicians who are fully prepared to provide sedation for refractory terminal suffering often will be able to comfort fearful patients simply by discussing it with them[3]. Few patients will actually require palliative sedation to unconsciousness.

While there is consensus in the literature about the need for and permissibility of sedation for refractory suffering of a terminally ill patient, there remains debate about nomenclature, about the definition of palliative sedation, and about the ethics of specific practices. Rather than offering a thorough review of the literature, this chapter will provide guidance for palliative sedation based upon a synthesis of current debates.

Definitions

Palliative sedation may be defined as controlled induction of sedation, sometimes to the point of unconsciousness, to relieve severe refractory suffering of a terminally ill patient.

Severe, refractory suffering may be a result of severe, refractory physical symptoms such as pain, dyspnoea, or vomiting or severe, refractory neuro-psychiatric problems such as seizure, agitated delirium, anxiety, or depression. While severe psychosocial problems such as extreme complicated grief, shame, discrimination, rejection or guilt also may cause severe suffering in a terminally ill patient, they are unlikely to be refractory to intensive interventions including non-sedating medication, psychological counselling, spiritual guidance, and social interventions such as emotional, legal, and financial support[4]. Thus, palliative sedation should be considered as a response to psychosocial problems only in the most extraordinary circumstances.

Suffering is refractory when it cannot be adequately relieved despite aggressive and concerted efforts both to determine its causes and to treat them using standard palliative interventions without inducing sedation. Adequate relief is reduction of the patient's suffering to a tolerable level. Because pain, many other physical and neuro-psychiatric symptoms, and psycho-social suffering are subjective and not amenable to easy measurement, both 'tolerability' and 'adequate relief' can be defined only by each individual patient. Aggressive and concerted efforts are those that make use of the best available diagnostic techniques, palliative medications and other interventions and have enlisted the help of the best available experts (see below 'Practical guidelines for palliative sedation,' item A3).

The determination of refractoriness should be made only after all available diagnostic, therapeutic, and consultative possibilities have been exhausted that might bring adequate relief within a reasonable timeframe without intolerable adverse effects and without inducing sedation (Table 19.2.1). If possible, the determination of refractoriness should be made by a physician who knows the patient well and who has obtained the consensus of the team caring for the patient.

Nomenclature

Various names have been used for sedation for refractory suffering of dying patients. It is important to distinguish between ordinary sedation and palliative sedation to unconsciousness. Ordinary sedation is sedation that occurs commonly in the standard practice of palliative care for a variety of reasons. First, it may be an unintended side effect of medications—opioids or anticholinergics

Table 19.2.1 Criteria for determination of refractoriness of a severe symptom.

1 **Diagnosis**: aggressive efforts to diagnose the severe symptom are either successful or are exhaustive but unsuccessful within a reasonable time frame
2 **Treatment**: aggressive efforts to relieve the severe symptom using all available resources are unsuccessful within a reasonable time frame
3 **Consultation**: all available colleagues who might assist in diagnosing or treating the symptom or in providing psychosocial support to the patient or family within a reasonable time frame have been consulted
4 **Transfer**: transfer to another location where more potentially helpful resources are available is either not feasible or has been refused by the patient
5 **Persistent suffering**: the patient continues to report intolerable suffering despite all above interventions, or a patient lacking the ability to communicate verbally appears to the surrogate decision maker, the responsible physician, and at least one other clinician to be in severe distress despite all above interventions

for example—used to treat symptoms such as pain, dyspnoea, or troublesome respiratory secretions. Second, it may be an intended effect of ordinary sedating medications such as benzodiazepines or neuroleptics used to treat problems for which a sedative is ordinarily indicated such as anxiety, agitation, insomnia, or for an invasive procedure such as endoscopy. Ordinary sedation also includes sedation of a terminally ill patient to reduce the patient's awareness of a distressing symptom or condition without intending to induce unconsciousness. Underlying medical conditions including severe brain injury, metabolic derangements such as hypercalcaemia or hyperammonaemia, or severe sepsis may cause sedation themselves or may predispose the patient to an exaggerated response to potentially sedating medications. Finally, it may be due to a combination of causes. Palliative sedation to unconsciousness designates sedation for severe suffering that is refractory to all reasonable and aggressive interventions including ordinary sedation[5].

The term 'terminal sedation' is irreducibly ambiguous and should not be used in palliative care. By definition, death is never intended by palliative sedation. Because 'terminal sedation' inevitably connotes sedation intended to terminate or euthanasia, the term may be upsetting to many patients and their families, may undermine patients' trust in their clinicians, and may confuse clinicians and dissuade them from considering palliative sedation when it offers the only chance to relieve a terminally ill patient's severe refractory suffering[6].

Experience with palliative sedation to unconsciousness

The frequency and success of palliative sedation to unconsciousness is impossible to determine accurately because of lack of consensus and clarity in the literature about the definition of palliative sedation and about indications, goals, and appropriate medication regimens. Reports of the frequency of palliative sedation in palliative care programmes range from 1 to 88 per cent[7]. Practice patterns vary widely in part due to differing cultural beliefs and values[8–10]. In some studies, it is unclear whether patients received partial or deep sedation or were sedated to varying degrees. The frequency of palliative sedation also may be changing in settings where palliative care is becoming better and more available and where medical, ethical, and legal debates about end-of-life care are defining acceptable practice[11–13].

There is some consistency in the literature about some aspects of palliative sedation. Multiple studies list some or all of the same refractory symptoms as the most common indications for palliative sedation: pain, dyspnoea, agitated delirium, or vomiting[10,14,15]. Studies of physicians from multiple countries and cultures reveal a widespread opinion that palliative sedation for refractory suffering is sometimes needed and is ethically acceptable[9,10,16,17]. In addition, there is some concurring evidence that survival of patients in palliative care settings requiring palliative sedation for refractory suffering does not differ from non-sedated patients in the same settings and thus that palliative sedation may not hasten death[7,18].

Ethical issues

Moral imperative

There is broad agreement that physicians have a moral imperative to respond to the suffering of terminally ill patients, particularly when the suffering is extreme[19,20]. While severe refractory suffering is uncommon, it demands that physicians be prepared to provide palliative sedation as 'the end of the continuum of symptom management'[21].

Informed consent

There is broad agreement that patients have the right to decide on their own medical care free from limitations including undue interference from others and inadequate information (see chapter on 'Truth-Telling and Consent')[22]. When patients lack decision-making capacity, their autonomy is respected when a legitimate surrogate makes substituted judgements on behalf of the patient.

The physician should determine the goal or goals of care for any patient with a terminal illness in consultation with the patient or surrogate. When a terminally ill patient is experiencing severe, refractory suffering, palliative sedation should be considered only if the overriding goal of care is comfort[23]. In addition, the patient or surrogate must have decided to forego cardio-pulmonary resuscitation and to forego or have withdrawn invasive and non-invasive mechanical ventilation for respiratory failure[23].

Even when these conditions obtain and palliative sedation is being considered, it may not be initiated without informed consent[24]. The patient or surrogate should be informed of and capable of understanding both the clinical predicament that makes palliative sedation a legitimate treatment option and any alternative options. Religious or ethical concerns of the patient should be explored and religious counselling from a chaplain should be offered if appropriate. Because a decision about palliative sedation may have a lasting emotional impact on the patient's family and loved ones, efforts should be made to achieve consensus[3]. However, the clear request of a competent patient or a legal surrogate decision maker should be honoured even over objections of other family members or friends.

In the rarest of cases, there may be a terminally ill patient with severe, refractory suffering who lacks both decision-making capacity and any surrogate decision maker. If palliative sedation is being considered in such a case, consensus should be sought from at least one other senior physician—a palliative care specialist if possible—and from the hospital ethics committee.

Principle of double effect

The principle of double effect provides guidance for decisions when all possible actions risk bad consequences[25]. Its applicability to decisions about treatments to relieve suffering in dying patients is widely accepted. The principle states that an action with two or more possible effects, including at least one possible good and one possible bad effect, is morally permissible if four provisos are met[26,27]:

◆ The action must not be immoral in itself.

◆ The action must be undertaken with the *intention* of achieving only the good effect or effects. Possible bad effects may be *foreseen* but must not be *intended*.

◆ The action must not achieve the good effect by means of a bad effect.

◆ The action must be undertaken for a proportionally grave reason (the rule of proportionality).

When applied to standard palliative care, the principle directs that an intervention intended to relieve the severe suffering of a terminally ill patient is acceptable even at the risk of causing foreseen but unintended side effects. For example, opioids may be given to relieve the pain or dyspnoea of a terminally ill patient even at the risk of sedation, respiratory depression, hypotension, and hastening death. In cases of severe *refractory* suffering when palliative sedation is considered, sedation as a means to relieve suffering would be the intended good effect. Possible side effects of the sedative such as respiratory depression, hypotension, and hastening death may be foreseen but not intended. The act of giving medication to relieve suffering is not immoral as long as the patient or surrogate requests relief and accepts the risk of side effects and there are no safer means to achieve an acceptable degree of relief. Such serious side effects must be risked only for a proportionally grave reason such as the relief of severe refractory suffering of a terminally ill patient who does not wish to suffer[28].

Because clinical intentions may be complex and ambiguous, physicians working to relieve the suffering of frail terminally ill patients should think through their intentions carefully, document them in the medical record, and demonstrate them with their actions[29]. The least toxic medications should be used at the minimum doses that achieve the desired effect. The patient's response to the medication and level of comfort should be assessed frequently and changes in the dose or type of medication should be made based on these assessments. In this way, clinical intentions are made as clear as possible, the benefits of the intervention maximized, and the risk of bad effects minimized[30].

Distinction from voluntary active euthanasia and physician-assisted suicide

Palliative sedation can and should be clearly distinguished in theory and in practice from both voluntary active euthanasia and physician-assisted suicide (see Chapter 5.5)[31]. In palliative sedation, the physician intends only to relieve severe refractory suffering using sedation as a last resort. There is no intention to end the patient's life as in euthanasia and physician-assisted suicide[3].

In practice, palliative sedation entails titration of medications to comfort. The physician administers just enough medication to induce sedation and thereby assure comfort. Once comfort is achieved, the lowest doses that maintain comfort are used. Euthanasia and physician-assisted suicide entail no titration: no calculation or maintenance of minimum doses needed for comfort[29].

Even in the Netherlands, the only country where euthanasia is legal and more than a marginal practice[32], the Royal Dutch Medical Association's guidelines for palliative sedation clearly distinguish it from euthanasia[33]. Palliative sedation is deemed by the Association to be a means of relieving suffering that does not accelerate death[34].

Withholding and withdrawal of artificial nutrition and hydration

When palliative sedation is being considered, informed consent should be sought to withhold or withdraw artificial nutrition and hydration. It is neither euthanasia nor physician-assisted suicide to withhold or withdraw artificial nutrition and hydration from a terminally ill patient who declines them and whose severe refractory suffering is being treated with palliative sedation. The decision whether or not to use any medical intervention, including artificial nutrition and hydration, should be based on the patients goals, values, and

medical condition. Frequently, patients who have a terminal illness and are unable to eat frequently decline artificial nutrition and hydration. To provide these interventions against patients' wishes would not only infringe on their right to autonomy. Because these interventions also may cause harm by, for example, prolonging the dying process or exacerbating pulmonary oedema or ascites, providing them also risks violating the principle of non-maleficence.

The situation is morally no different when a patient is receiving palliative sedation for severe refractory suffering. For patients still able to eat prior to sedation, it is the patient's terminal illness that makes the sedation necessary and thereby precludes further eating. When the overriding goal is comfort and the patient or surrogate does not request artificial nutrition or hydration for religious reasons, there should be no presumption that an unwanted and potentially noxious intervention should be provided. When artificial nutrition and hydration are withheld or withdrawn in this situation, the patient dies of the terminal illness, not at the hand of the physician[35].

There may be patients whose religious or cultural beliefs require that artificial hydration and/or nutrition not be withheld or withdrawn during palliative sedation as long as the harms of these medical interventions do not grossly outweigh the potential benefits by the patient's own criteria[3]. Thus, there should be no absolute prohibition of artificial nutrition and hydration in patients receiving palliative sedation. Religious and cultural beliefs should be explored as carefully as possible and every effort made to assure that palliative sedation or any proposed treatment is compatible with cherished beliefs and values of the patient.

Misuse of palliative sedation

Studies from several countries have revealed that physicians occasionally provide interventions intended to hasten death even where euthanasia and physician-assisted suicide are illegal[36-40]. These data raise the concern that palliative sedation may be used to intentionally hasten death and that physicians may try to hide their intention by invoking the principle of double effect. Therefore, it is extremely important for physicians who provide palliative sedation to demonstrate their intentions as clearly as possible by documenting carefully in the medical record the regimen used and the patient's response.

An additional concern is raised by studies showing that use of palliative sedation decreased at some centres as pain control and palliative care became more available[11,12]. This suggests that suffering in terminally ill patient may sometimes be deemed refractory and palliative sedation provided simply for lack of standard palliative care. Patients in resource-constrained settings and other areas where palliative care is not available may be particularly vulnerable to premature consideration of palliative sedation. This is one of many reasons compelling reasons for development of palliative care services in poor countries and wherever they are not yet available[41,42].

Informing other clinicians

It is often helpful to involve key members of the patient's care team such as the primary nurse and social worker in the process of decision-making about palliative sedation. Before initiating palliative sedation, the physician always should inform all members of the patient's care team of the plan, the indication for palliative sedation, and the receipt of informed consent[3]. No clinicians should be required to participate in non-emergent palliative sedation—or in withdrawal of life-sustaining treatment—if they conscientiously object[21].

Legal issues

Laws in most rich western countries recognize the right of a competent patient to refuse any medical treatment including life-sustaining treatment. In the same countries, interventions to relieve the severe, refractory suffering of terminally ill patients generally are tolerated even if they might unintentionally hasten death.[32] In United States criminal law, for example, actions that might put another's life at risk are justifiable if the potential benefits of the action are likely and important enough. This precept reflects the rule of proportionality that is part of the principle of double effect[26].

In 1997, the United States Supreme Court found unanimously that there is no constitutional right to physician-assisted suicide. But it simultaneously found that permissible interventions to relieve suffering that may hastened death can be distinguished from impermissible hastening of death based on the physician's intentions[43,44]. Three justices wrote concurring opinions that support use of medications to relieve terminal suffering even to the point of causing unconsciousness[21,43]. Thus, while the Court did not support intentional hastening of death by physicians, it did support palliative sedation as a last resort to relieve severe, refractory suffering of terminally ill patients.

Practical guidelines for palliative sedation

A. Indications and prerequisites

Palliative sedation should be considered only under the following circumstances:

1   The patient must have a *severe, chronic, life-threatening illness* such as, but not limited to:

   a) Advanced incurable cancer.

   b) End-stage major organ failure, organ transplantation or organ replacement therapy not feasible or declined by the patient.

   c) Advanced AIDS, antiretroviral therapy no longer effective, causes intolerable side effects, or declined by the patient.

   d) Advanced neuromuscular disease.

   e) Advanced dementia, unable to take adequate oral nutrition.

2   The patient must be suffering from one or more *severe physical or neuro-psychiatric symptoms* such as, but not limited to pain, dyspnoea, vomiting, seizures, agitated delirium, anxiety, or depression.

3   The distressing symptom or symptoms must be *refractory to standard palliative interventions* such as, but not limited to:

   a) Medications such as opioids, neuroleptics, anticonvulsants, anxiolytics, and antidepressants.

   b) Neuromodulatory procedures for pain such as nerve block and intrathecal analgesia.

   c) Palliative radiation therapy.

   d) Palliative endoscopic or surgical procedures.

   e) Consultation by the best available medical specialists from disciplines relevant to the patient's disease or symptoms

such as palliative care, pain medicine, or psychiatry and by those who can provide psycho-social support such as social workers and chaplains.

4   *Comfort must be the overriding goal* of the patient's care according to the patient or, if the patient does not have capacity to make medical decisions, according to the legal surrogate decision maker.

   a) If there is doubt about a patient's capacity to make a specific medical decision, psychiatric consultation is recommended.

   b) If a patient does not have capacity and there is no legal surrogate decision maker, the goals of care should be determined by a non-legal surrogate who is the most knowledgeable person available about the patient's values, goals and preferences for care.

   c) If no surrogate decision maker is available, consensus on the goals of care should be sought from at least one other senior physician—a palliative care specialist if possible—and from the hospital ethics committee if one exists.

   d) In any case, both the goal of comfort and the discussion in which this goal was decided upon must be documented in the medical record.

5   Where possible, *an active order must exist to withhold life-sustaining treatments* including at least the following:

   a) Chest compressions.

   b) Defibrillation.

   c) Endotracheal intubation.

   d) Mechanical ventilation.

   e) Non-invasive ventilatory support.

6   *Informed consent* for palliative sedation that may unintentionally hasten death must be obtained in advance from the patient or from an appropriate surrogate decision maker identified following the procedure outlined in item 4 a–d above. The informed consent or decision-making process must be documented in the medical record.

7   If possible, all *staff members involved in caring for the patient should be informed* in advance of the plan to initiate palliative sedation. In particular, the patient's nurse and pharmacist should be informed.

   a) Once palliative sedation has been initiated, clinical staff who will be assigned to the case should be informed in advance of the plan of care.

   b) In non-emergent situations, staff members who conscientiously object to the care plan should be given the opportunity to excuse themselves from participation in the patient's care once a replacement is found. Every effort should be made in keeping with any institutional policies on conscientious objection to find a replacement for any essential staff member.

B. Special circumstances

1. Severe, refractory psycho-social suffering

Very rarely, a patient's severe psychosocial problems such as extreme complicated grief, shame, or guilt may cause severe suffering that is refractory to intensive and sustained intervention by the best available clinicians and supporters. In these very rare cases, respite sedation to unconsciousness may be considered (see below). Only after respite sedation has been tried at least once in addition to all other intensive palliative interventions without an acceptable reduction in the patient's suffering should permanent palliative sedation be considered[45,46].

2. Respite sedation

Time-limited sedation to unconsciousness or respite sedation may be used in terminally ill patients with severe refractory suffering in a variety of situations:

1 *Incident pain*: Some patients may experience particularly severe pain or other symptoms due to therapeutic or diagnostic procedures or to necessary movement for cleaning or other clinical care[47].

2 *Severe refractory psycho-social suffering*: One or more trials of respite sedation may 'break a cycle of anxiety and distress' that has evoked a request for palliative sedation[45,46].

3 *Patient requests trial of temporary sedation to unconsciousness*: Some patients with severe refractory physical or neuro-psychiatric symptoms who are not imminently dying may benefit from a temporary respite from their discomfort. The respite may relieve severe fatigue that could influence the patient's perception that the symptoms or the attempts to alleviate them are intolerable[3]. The patient may then decline further palliative sedation.

The mandatory informed consent discussion for respite sedation to unconsciousness should include the possibility that the patient may not reawaken and that death may be unintentionally hastened. Respite sedation may be provided for as little as a few minutes or as long as a few days. In general, artificial hydration should be provided if respite sedation is expected to last longer than a few hours. A decision on monitoring of heart rate and rhythm, blood pressure, and oxygen saturation should be based on the patient's specific goals and values and the clinical situation.

3. Terminal discontinuation of mechanical ventilation

In terminally ill patients receiving mechanical ventilation for respiratory failure, terminal extubation of the trachea or discontinuation of mechanical ventilation without extubation is likely to cause dyspnoea unless the patient is well pre-medicated, unconscious, or in a persistent vegetative state. Some patients may wish to receive only enough medication to reduce to a tolerable level the feeling of air hunger in the hope that they can remain awake during the process. However, it is reasonable to offer palliative sedation to unconsciousness when a patient or the surrogate of a patient not in a persistent vegetative state decides to terminally discontinue mechanical ventilation and identifies comfort as the overriding goal of care.

Palliative sedation to unconsciousness for terminal discontinuation of mechanical ventilation is medically and ethically slightly different from palliative sedation for severe refractory symptoms.

1 Sedation to unconsciousness may be intended not to relieve existing severe refractory symptoms but rather to assure that the patient does not experience severe dyspnoea in the time between removal of the ventilator and death.

a) The other prerequisites for palliative sedation apply in this situation as well: terminal illness, a decision that the overriding goal of care is comfort, an order to withhold or withdraw life-sustaining treatment, informed consent, an informed and prepared staff.

2 If the patient already is receiving sedation to treat or prevent discomfort from mechanical ventilation, this sedation should continue and adjustments should be made to assure comfort during and after the removal of the ventilator.

3 Because most agents used for palliative sedation have no analgesic effect and do not specifically relieve dyspnoea, opioid therapy usually should be continued or added to the sedative regimen.

a) In the absence of pain or other indications for opioid therapy, the opioid dose should be titrated to a normal respiratory rate and the absence of laboured breathing while the sedative is titrated to unconsciousness.

4 Sedation and opioid therapy should be initiated before the ventilator is removed. The adequacy of the treatment should be checked by setting the fraction of inspired oxygen at room air and changing the ventilation mode to pressure support at a setting adequate only to overcome the resistant of the endotracheal tube (approximately 5 cm H_2O for a tube 7.5 mm in internal diameter). Patients should be observed for 10–15 min on this ventilator setting (to allow their arterial partial pressure of oxygen to decrease and the partial pressure of carbon dioxide to increase).

a) If the patient develops tachypnoea, agitation, grimacing, or other evidence of discomfort, the patient's previous, more comfortable ventilator settings should be re-instituted, the doses of sedative and/or opioid should be increased, and the assessment repeated.

b) If the patient is apnoeic and is not thought to have pain, the opioid dose and/or sedative dose should be reduced and the trial repeated once the effects of the higher opioid and/or sedative doses have worn off. However, the sedative should not be reduced to the point of allowing the patient to wake up.

c) If the minimum opioid and/or sedative doses necessary to control the patient's pain and/or maintain an unconscious state also cause apnoea, and there are no other reversible causes of apnoea, the removal of the ventilator may proceed.

5 Any neuromuscular blocking agents should be stopped and the effects allowed to wear off before initiating palliative sedation so that the patient's respirations are not unnecessarily depressed and the effects of the sedation can be assessed.

a) If the effects of a neuromuscular blocking agent persist longer than 24 h after the last dose and there is a compelling reason to withdraw the ventilator quickly, the withdrawal may proceed but care must be taken to assure that the patient is well sedated since the patient will be paralysed and unable to show any signs of discomfort[48,49].

C. Medications

Ideal medications for palliative sedation have a rapid onset of action and a short duration of action that facilitate titration to the desired effect. They should reliably induce unconsciousness and

Table 19.2.2 Protocol for palliative sedation to unconsciousness using continuous intravenous infusion of midazolam, pentobarbital, or propofol.

Physician responsibilities

1 Confirm that:

   a) The patient's overriding goal of care is comfort

   b) The patient has an advanced terminal illness

   c) The patient is suffering from severe refractory physical or neuropsychiatric symptoms or psychosocial problems

   d) There is an order to withhold life-sustaining treatment

   e) Informed consent for palliative sedation to unconsciousness has been obtained

2 Document all of the above in the medical record

3 Inform the patient's clinical team of the plan

4 Specify in the orders:

   a) The loading dose, if any

   b) The initial infusion rate

   c) The amount of drug in mg/h and time interval for infusion rate increases

   d) The dose and time interval for any bolus doses

5 Ensure that the medication is titrated optimally by frequent assessment of the patient and/or by reading the documentation by nurses of all dose adjustments and of comfort levels before and after dose adjustments

6 Document in the medical record the efficacy of this therapy at least daily

Nurse responsibilities

1 Administer the medication as a continuous infusion by an infusion pump that is clearly labelled with the name of the medication

2 Once the desired level of sedation is achieved, reduce the infusion to the lowest rate that maintains the desired level

3 Should the patient exhibit any evidence of pain or other distress, increase the infusion rate as ordered

4 Once an initial steady dose rate is found that maintains the desired level of sedation, document the reason (intention) for any dose adjustment and the level of comfort before and after the adjustment

5 Do not reduce the infusion rate for low blood pressure, low respiratory rate, or other abnormal vital signs if the patient exhibits any evidence of pain or other distressing symptoms

6 When the medication is running out, call for additional medication well in advance so that there is no interruption in the infusion

Midazolam administration	Pentobarbital administration	Propofol administration
1 Inspect midazolam solution prior to administration. If precipitation is present, do not use	1 Inspect pentobarbital solution prior to administration. If precipitation is present, do not use	1 Use strict aseptic technique when administering propofol. Change infusion tubing every 12 h. Discard vial and any unused drug if not fully infused after 12 h
2 Loading dose for benzodiazepine-naïve patient: 0.03–0.05 mg/kg slow intravenous push (over 2–5 min)	2 Loading dose: 2–3 mg/kg slow intravenous push (no faster than 50 mg/min)	2 Infuse only through central venous catheter
3 Loading dose may be repeated every 5 min to achieve desired effect	3 A physician should give loading dose and remain at bedside for 15 min to observe the effect	3 Start infusion at 2.5–5 mcg/kg/min (for adults approximately 10–20 mg/h) and titrate to desired level of sedation every 10 min by increments of 10–20 mg/h
4 A physician should give each loading dose and remain at bedside for 10 min to observe the effect	4 At time of loading dose, start infusion at 1–2 mg/kg. Titrate to desired level of sedation	4 Use bolus doses of 10–20 mg every 10 min only for rapid control of extreme symptoms
5 At time of loading dose, start infusion at 0.02–0.1 mg/kg/h depending on patient's prior exposure to and tolerance for benzodiazepines. Titrate to desired level of sedation	5 Because tolerance may develop rapidly, assess the patient's comfort level frequently and adjust infusion rate as needed	5 During initiation of therapy, a physician should be present and remain at the bedside for 5 min to observe the effects. Any initial bolus doses should be given by a physician
6 Additional bolus doses equal to the hourly infusion dose may be given as often as every 15 min. A physician or nurse should remain at the bedside for 10 min to observe the effects of each bolus dose		6 During subsequent dose titration and bolus dosing, a physician or nurse should remain at the beside for 5 min to observe the effects
		7 The infusion should not be interrupted longer than 60 s when changing vials or tubing

cause minimal side effects. Agents mentioned in the literature include opioids, benzodiazepines, neuroleptics, barbiturates, and other general anesthetic induction agents[28]. In general, medications for palliative sedation to unconsciousness should be given via continuous and/or intermittent intravenous or subcutaneous infusion. Intramuscular injections generally should be avoided as the injections themselves may be painful. Administration of sedatives transdermally, rectally, or via tube gastrostomy or jejunostomy generally is not suitable for palliative sedation to unconsciousness because of the delayed onset of action and the greater difficulty in titrating the dose to the desired effect.

1. Opioids

Opioids such as morphine, hydromorphone, or fentanyl are the best available agents to relieve dyspnoea and many types of pain, but they are not reliable sleep-inducing agents by themselves. While opioids often cause drowsiness and may occasionally induce unconsciousness, especially in patients obtunded by other medications or by their medical conditions, increasing the opioid dose beyond that needed for relief of pain or dyspnoea puts the patient at increased risk of counter-productive and uncomfortable side effects such as myoclonus, hyperalgesia, and agitated delirium. Thus, opioids should not be used alone for palliative sedation. When pain or dyspnoea are present or expected, opioid therapy should be continued or added in combination with the sedative.

2. Benzodiazepines

Several benzodiazepines are cited in the literature on palliative sedation, lorazepam and midazolam most frequently[20,50]. Midazolam has the most rapid onset of action and is the easiest to titrate. However, benzodiazepines sometimes fail to provide adequate sedation[28,51]. In addition, they may cause paradoxical agitation and psychotic reactions particularly in elderly patients and those with impaired liver function[52–54]. Therefore, benzodiazepines should be used with caution for palliative sedation and are not ideal agents for palliative sedation to unconsciousness.

3. Neuroleptics

Antipsychotic drugs available in parenteral forms such as haloperidol, chlorpromazine and levomeprazine (formerly called methotrimeprazine) are cited in the literature on palliative sedation. Levomeprazine also has analgesic properties while haloperidol and chlorpromazine are good treatments for agitated delirium. However, none of these drugs alone reliably induce unconsciousness.

4. Barbiturates

Barbiturates including pentobarbital, thiopental, and phenobarbital reliably induce unconsciousness. All are available in parenteral form. Pentobarbital and especially thiopental have rapid onset and short duration of action for ease of titration. Pentobarbital also has beneficial antiemetic and anticonvulsant properties. Either thiopental or pentobarbital are excellent agents for palliative sedation to any degree including unconsciousness[55,56]. Pentobarbital may be easier to obtain outside of an intensive care unit.

5. Aesthetic induction agents

Anesthetic induction agents proposed for palliative sedation include propofol and ketamine. While ketamine has both sedative and analgesic properties and does not cause hypotension and respiratory depression like propofol and barbiturates, it commonly causes unpleasant dissociative or dysphoric reactions. It is not recommended as a single agent for palliative sedation. Propofol has an onset of action, duration of action, and half-life shorter than midazolam and any of the barbiturates. This greatly facilitates titration to the desired effect. Liver and renal disease do not appear to significantly affect its pharmacokinetics[57]. It also has anxiolytic, antiemetic, antipruritic, anticonvulsant, antimyoclonic, and muscle relaxant effects. Propofol therefore appears to be an excellent agent for palliative sedation to any degree including unconsciousness[28,58].

6. Combinations of sedatives

Many patients who require palliative sedation already will be receiving standard palliative medications such as an opioid and/or a benzodiazepine and/or a neuroleptic. Opioid therapy for pain should be continued despite the risk of hypotension and respiratory depression when a barbiturate or propofol is added because these latter agents have no analgesic effect. A benzodiazepine generally may be tapered once adequate sedation is achieved with another agent. However, if the sedative does not have strong anticonvulsant properties, the taper should proceed slowly to minimize the risk of seizure. Neuroleptic therapy may be reduced or discontinued provided adequate sedation can be maintained easily without it. Ketamine should be used only in combination with a benzodiazepine[59].

D. Recommended protocols

Recommended protocols for palliative sedation with midazolam, pentobarbital and propofol are provided in Table 19.2.2.

Conclusions

Palliative sedation is a well-accepted therapy that should be considered in the rare situations when a terminally ill patient whose overriding goal is comfort experiences severe suffering that is refractory to all available standard palliative interventions. Its availability alone may be very comforting to patients fearful of terminal suffering. Informed consent must be obtained and strict medical and ethical guidelines for providing, monitoring, and documenting palliative sedation should be followed.

Further reading

Cherny, N.I., and Portenoy, R.K. (1994). Sedation in the management of refractory symptoms: guidelines for evaluation and treatment. *Journal of Palliative Care*, **10**, 31–8.

Krakauer, E.L., Penson, R.T., Truog, R.D., King, L.A., Chabner, B.A., and Lynch, T.J. (2000). Sedation for intractable distress of a dying patient: acute palliative care and the principle of double effect. *The Oncologist*, **5**, 53–62.

Quill, T.E., and Byock, I.R. (2000). Responding to intractable terminal suffering: the role of terminal sedation and voluntary refusal of food and fluids. *Annals of Internal Medicine*, **132**, 408–14.

Tännsjö, T. (ed.) (2004). *Terminal sedation: euthanasia in disguise?* Kluwer, Dordrecht.

References

1. World Health Organization (2006). WHO Definition of Palliative Care. http://www.who.int/cancer/palliative/definition/en/ (accessed Nov. 19, 2006).
2. Cassell, E.J. (1982). The nature of suffering and the goals of medicine. *The New England Journal of Medicine*, **306**, 639–45.

3. Cherny, N.I. (2006). Sedation for the care of patients with advanced cancer. *Nature Clinical Practice. Oncology*, **3**, 492–500.

4. Jansen, L.A., and Sulmasy, D.P. (2002). Sedation, alimentation, hydration, and equivocation: careful conversation about care at the end of life. *Annals of Internal Medicine*, **136**, 845–9.

5. American Academy of Hospice and Palliative Care (2006). Statement on Palliative Sedation. http://www.aahpm.org/positions/sedation.html (accessed Nov. 19, 2006)

6. Krakauer, E.L. (2000). Responding to intractable terminal suffering. *Annals of Internal Medicine*, **133**, 560.

7. Sykes, N., and Thorns, A. (2003). The use of opioids and sedatives at the end of life. *Lancet Oncology*, **4**, 312–8.

8. Willems, D.L., Daniels, E.R., van der Wal, G. *et al.* (2000). Attitudes and practices concerning the end of life: a comparison between physicians from the United States and from the Netherlands. *Archives of Internal Medicine*, **160**, 63–8.

9. Chiu, T.Y., Hu, W.Y., Lue, B.H. *et al.* (2001). Sedation for refractory symptoms of terminal cancer patients in Taiwan. *Journal of Pain and Symptom Management*, **21**, 467–72.

10. Fainsinger, R.L., Waller, A., and Bercovici, M. *et al.* (2000). A multicentre international study of sedation for uncontrolled symptoms in terminally in patients. *Palliative Medicine*, **14**, 257–65.

11. Fainsinger, R.L., de Moissac, D., Mancini, I., and Oneschuk, D. (2000). Sedation for delirium and other symptoms in terminally ill patients in Edmonton. *Journal of Palliative Care*, **16**, 5–10.

12. Meunier-Cartal, J., Souberbielle, J.C., and Boureau, F. (1995). Morphine and the "lytic cocktail" for terminally ill patients in a French general hospital: evidence for an inverse relationship. *Journal of Pain and Symptom Management*, **10**, 267–73.

13. Muller-Busch, H.C., Andres, I., and Jehser, T. (2003). Sedation in palliative care – a critical analysis of, **7** years experience. *BMC Palliative Care*, **2**, 2. http://www.biomedcentral.com/1472-684X/2/2 (accessed Nov. 19, 2006)

14. Rousseau, P. (2000). The ethical validity and clinical experience of palliative sedation. *Mayo Clinic Proceedings*, **75**, 1064–9.

15. Cowan, J.D., and Walsh, D. (2001). Terminal sedation in palliative medicine – definition and review of the literature. *Supportive Care in Cancer*, **9**, 403–7.

16. Chater, S., Viola, R., Paterson, J., and Jarvis, V. (1998). Sedation for intractable distress in the dying – a survey of experts. *Palliative Medicine*, **12**, 255–69.

17. Morita, T., Akechi, T., Sugawara, Y. *et al.* (2002). Practices and attitudes of Japanese oncologists and palliative care physicians concerning terminal sedation: a nationwide survey. *Journal of Clinical Oncology*, **20**, 758–64.

18. Sykes, N., and Thorns, A. (2003). Sedative use in the last week of life and the implications for end-of-life decision-making. *Archives of Internal Medicine*, **163**, 341–4.

19. Wanzer, S.H., Federman, D.D., and Adelstein, J. *et al.* (1989). The physician's responsibility toward hopelessly ill patients: a second look. *The New England Journal of Medicine*, **320**, 844–9.

20. Levy, M.H., and Cohen, S.D. (2005). Sedation for the relief of refractory symptoms in the imminently dying: a fine intentional line. *Seminars in Oncology*, **32**, 237–46.

21. Quill, T.E., and Byock, I.R. (2000). Responding to intractable terminal suffering: the role of terminal sedation and voluntary refusal of food and fluids. *Annals of Internal Medicine*, **132**, 408–414.

22. Beauchamp, T.L., and Childress, J.F. (2001). *Principles of biomedical ethics*, fifth edition. Oxford University Press, New York, pp. 57–112.

23. Cherny, N.I., and Portenoy, R.K. (1994). Sedation in the management of refractory symptoms: guidelines for evaluation and treatment. *Journal of Palliative Care*, **10**, 31–8.

24. Quill, T.E., Lo, B., and Brock, D.W. (1997). Palliative options of last resort: a comparison of voluntary stopping of eating and drinking, terminal sedation, physician-assisted suicide, and voluntary active euthanasia. *JAMA*, **278**, 2099–104.

25. Boyle, J. (2004). Medical ethics and double effect: the case of terminal sedation. *Theoretical Medicine*, **25**, 51–60.

26. Quill, T.E., Dresser, R., and Brock, D.W. (1997). The rule of double effect – a critique of its role in end-of-life decision-making. *The New England Journal of Medicine*, **337**, 1768–71.

27. Sulmasy, D.P., and Pellegrino, E.D. (1999). The rule of double effect: clearing up the double talk. *Archives of Internal Medicine*, **159**, 545–50.

28. Krakauer, E.L., Penson, R.T., Truog, R.D. *et al.* (2000). Sedation for intractable distress of a dying patient: acute palliative care and the principle of double effect. *The Oncologist*, **5**, 53–62.

29. Hallenbeck, J.L. (2000). Terminal sedation: ethical implications in different situations. *Journal of Palliative Medicine*, **3**, 313–20.

30. Twycross, R. (1999). Palliative care physicians always have their patients' best interests in mind. *BMJ*, **319**, 639.

31. Wein, S. (2000). Sedation in the imminently dying patient. Oncology, **14**, 585-592.

32. Van der Heide, A., van Delden, J.J.M., and van der Wal, G. (2004). Doctor-assisted dying: what difference does legalization make? *Lancet*, **364**, 24–5.

33. Committee on National Guidelines for Palliative Sedation (2005). Royal Dutch Medical Association (KNMG) guidelines for palliative sedation. http://knmg.artsennet.nl/uri/?uri=AMGATE_6059_100_TICH_R171322439726668 (accessed Dec. 12, 2006).

34. Sheldon, T. (2005). Dutch doctors are given guidance on sedation. *BMJ*, **331**, 1422.

35. Callahan, D. (2004). Terminal sedation and artefactual fallacy. In *Terminal sedation: euthanasia in disguise?* (ed. T. Tännsjö), pp. 93–102. Kluwer, Dordrecht.

36. Van der Heide, A., Deliens, L., and Faisst, K. *et al.* (2003). End-of-life decision-making in six European countries: descriptive study. *Lancet*, **362**, 345–50.

37. Ward, B.J., and Tate, P.A. (1994). Attitudes among NHS doctors to requests for euthanasia. *BMJ*, **308**, 1332–4.

38. Førde, R., Aasland, O.G., and Falkum, E. (1997). The ethics of euthanasia – attutides and practice among Norwegian physicians. *Social Science & Medicine*, **45**, 887–92.

39. Wilson, W.C., Smedira, N.G., Fink, C. *et al.* (1992). Ordering and administration of sedatives and analgesics during the withholding and withdrawal of life support from critically ill patients. *JAMA*, **267**, 949–53.

40. Meier, D.E., Emmons, C.A., Wallenstein, S. *et al.* (1998). A national survey of physician-assisted suicide and euthanasia in the United States. *The New England Journal of Medicine*, **338**, 1193–201.

41. Harding, R., and Higginson, I.J. (2005). Palliative care in sub-Saharan Africa. *Lancet*, **365**, 1971–7.

42. Krakauer, E.L. Just palliative care: responding responsibly to the suffering of the poor. Journal of Pain and Symptom Management, **36**, 505 – 512.

43. Alpers, A., and Lo, B. (1999). The Supreme Court addresses physician-assisted suicide. Archives of Family Medicine, **8**, 200–5.

44. Burt, R.A. (1997). The Supreme Court speaks: not assisted suicide but a constitutional right to palliative care. *The New England Journal of Medicine*, **337**, 1234–6.

45. Cherny, N.I. (1998). Sedation in response to refractory existential distress: walking the fine line. *Journal of Pain and Symptom Management*, **16**, 404–6.

46. Rousseau, P. (2001). Existential suffering and palliative sedation: a brief commentary with a proposal for clinical guidelines. *Am J Hos Palliat Care*, **18**, 151–3.

47. Del Rosario, M.A.B., Martín, A.S., Ortega, J.J.M., and Feria, M. (2001). Temporary sedation with midazolem for control of severe incident pain. *Journal of Pain and Symptom Management*, **21**, 439–42.

48. Brody, H., Campbell, M.L., Faber-Langendoen, K., and Ogle, K.S. (1997). Withdrawing intensive life-sustaining treatment – recommendations

for compassionate clinical management. *The New England Journal of Medicine*, **336**, 652–7.

49. Truog, R.D., Burns, J.P., Mitchell, C. *et al.* (2000). Pharmacologic paralysis and withdrawal of mechanical ventilation at the end of life. *The New England Journal of Medicine*, **342**, 508–11.

50. Cowan, J.D., and Palmer, T.W. (2002). Practical guide to palliative sedation. *Current Oncology Reports*, **4**, 242–9.

51. Cheng, C., Roemer-Becuwe, C., and Pereira, J. (2002). When midazolam fails. *Journal of Pain and Symptom Management*, **23**, 256–65.

52. Breitbart, W., Marotta, R., and Platt, M.M. *et al.* (1996). A double-blind trial of haloperidol, chlorpromazine, and lorazepam in the treatment of delirium in hospitalized AIDS patients. *The American Journal of Psychiatry*, **153**, 231–7.

53. Twycross, R., Wilcock, A., Charlesworth, S., and Dickman, A. (2002). *Palliative care formulary*, 2nd edition. Radcliffe Medical Press, Oxon, pp. 64–74.

54. Shafer, A. (1998). Complications of sedation with midazolam in the intensive care unti and a comparison with other sedative regimens. *Critical Care Medicine*, **26**, 947–56.

55. Truog, R.D., Berda, C.B., Mitchell, C., and Grier, H.E. (1992). Barbiturates in the care of the terminally ill. *The New England Journal of Medicine*, **327**, 1678–82.

56. Greene, W.R., and Davis, W.H. (1991). Titrated intravenous barbiturates in the control of symptoms in patients with terminal cancer. *Southern Medical Journal*, **84**, 332–7.

57. Mirenda, J., and Broyles, G. (1995). Propofol as used for sedation in the ICU. *Chest*, **108**, 539–48.

58. Lundström, S., Zachrisson, U., and Fürst, C.J. (2005). When nothing helps: propofol as sedative and antiemetic in palliative cancer care. *Journal of Pain and Symptom Management*, **30**, 570–7.

59. Berger, J.M., Ryan, A., Vadivelu, N. *et al.* (2000). Ketamine-fentanyl-midazolam infusion for the control of symptoms in terminal life care. *American Journal of Hospice and Palliative Care*, **17**, 127–32.

SECTION 20

Education and training in palliative medicine

Introduction

Kenneth Calman

We are all now part of a learning society and medicine and medical education must be part of that process. Medical education itself is a continuum, beginning at the undergraduate level, progressing to specialist training and then entering the phase of continuing education. This continuum is critical for those involved in palliative medicine in that at each stage there are different levels of knowledge, skills and attitudes required. These three factors need emphasizing, as all are important. The clinician in palliative care needs an effective and growing knowledge base, together with a widening range of skills. In addition, the attitudes adopted will be the component with which patients are likely to identify and are the focus of much of the dissatisfaction with the care provided. However, all three are essential. There is not much point in a caring and communicative doctor if the knowledge base is not up to date and technical skills are limited. Here lies the ethical justification for continuing education. Patients expect their doctors to be fully aware of advances in diagnosis and treatment. Anything less would be doing patients a disservice.

Much of the debate on this subject relates to the purpose of medicine and of medical education. It is concerned with the attributes of the doctor and the relationship between these attributes to the curriculum and the educational process. It is also concerned about the concept of a profession and what it means to be a professional. These are very important issues that should be considered before entering into the more detailed aspects of education and training in palliative care[1].

The profession of medicine

It is suggested that the purpose of medicine is to serve the community by continually improving health, health care and quality of life, for the individual and the population by health promotion, prevention of illness, treatment and care and the effective use of resources, all within the context of a team approach. In terms of palliative medicine, this emphasizes the issues of quality of life, care and the team approach. It also highlights the importance of service to patients and this leads to a discussion of the concept of a profession.

It is not easy to define a profession but it has some, or all of the following characteristics. It is a vocation or calling and implies service to others. It has a distinctive knowledge base that is kept up to date and determines its own standards and sets its own examinations. It has a special relationship with those whom it serves—patients, clients. It has particular ethical principles, the ethical base, and is self-regulating and accountable to patients and to the profession itself[2–6].

Following from this it is possible to list a series of attributes that might be expected of the doctor, or other health professional. These include:

1 A high standard of ethical practice. This is a key part of the role of the doctor and in a medical world that is changing and developing constantly and within which the principles are challenged regularly. There is greater scrutiny of medical practice and this is to be welcomed.

2 Continuing professional development is an issue that is broader than continuing education. It is concerned with personal growth and satisfaction with performance. Its main feature is that it emphasizes the need to keep up to date.

3 Ability to work as part of a team. As medicine and palliative care increase in complexity, it is necessary to ensure that all the skills of team members are used to the full.

4 Patient focused. This should be an explicit part of the role of the doctor and of the palliative care service.

5 A concern with standards, outcomes effectiveness and audit. This must be part of the practice of palliative medicine. There are considerable variations in standards across the world and it is our patients who suffer when these standards are low.

6 An interest in change, improvement, research, and development. Medicine cannot and should not stand still. It is evolving and changing continually. All professionals need to be involved in that quest for improvement.

7 Ability to communicate. This is a key attribute of the doctor. Arrogance and discourtesy reflect badly on a profession whose primary purpose is to care for patients.

Some of these attributes will be discussed in more detail later in this chapter and in other sections of the book. They are set out here because the purpose of medical education is to pursue these attributes and, in addition to factual knowledge, provide a basis for the wider range of skills and attitudes to be developed. The concept of personal growth alluded to above is an interesting one. It includes how we spend our time, our outside interests and everything that makes us a broader person. It is about being a whole person with connections beyond medicine into hobbies, art, literature and all aspects of recreation in the original sense of the word. In practical terms, the process of education should assist the doctor to answer the following questions, posed by the patient and by the professional:

1 What is wrong with me? What is the diagnosis, and while this may be difficult, patients are often seeking an explanation for their symptoms.

2 What does this mean for me? The prognosis. This may be the most difficult issue of all. In spite of considerable experience in palliative care it is easy to get this aspect wrong.

3 What can be done for me? This is the caring and management component and can and should be explained to the patient and the family.

4 What can I learn from this patient? The research dimension. How will an understanding of this patient's problems help others in the future?

5 What can I teach others from this experience? This identifies the educational opportunities for both patients and professionals.

Education and learning

This therefore is the justification for a section in this textbook on the subject of education. It is a complex process about which we still have much to learn and before looking at the subject in more detail a few definitions will be set out. Teaching is the process by which learning is facilitated by another person who guides, directs and assesses progress. Learning is the outcome of a process that results in a change in knowledge, skills, attitudes and/or behaviour. It is usually assessed in a variety of different ways to reflect acquisition of the knowledge, skills, or attitudes that have been learned. A wide variety of methods have been used for this purpose. In this chapter, the use of the term 'student' covers all levels of the continuum and not just the undergraduate level.

The process of learning in a formal sense is brought together in a curriculum that has three components. The objectives (what will the student be expected to know or do at the end of the module or course). This includes the content of the course; the methods used (small group, lecture, computer-based, problem based, etc.) and the methods of assessment [essay, multiple choice, clinical or practical, oral, dissertation, Objective Structured Clinical Examination (OSCE), etc.]. The assessment may be formative in which the process takes place throughout the course, or summative, which takes place at the end. Both have advantages and disadvantages.

Two further definitions are important. The first is that of training. This implies the learning of specific knowledge, skills, or attitudes to tackle a particular clinical problem. For example, the doctor might be trained to manage pain, or understand pain mechanisms. Education, on the other hand, is not concerned only with task-based problems, but is broader and deeper. Education always has a value base while training does not have to have one. You can be trained to steal, pick pockets, or break into cars. You could not be educated to do these activities. Perhaps the best way of illustrating this difference is to note that 'to be trained is to have arrived, to be educated is to continue to travel'. Not surprisingly, both are necessary in the field of palliative medicine.

For those interested in further reading on the general aspects of education a short reading list is appended. Several journals are published specifically on medical education and are a most useful source of reference. It should be emphasized again that there is a strong moral imperative for the clinician in palliative care to keep up-to-date and for those involved in the education of professionals to be aware of the range of methods of teaching and assessment now available. The remainder of this chapter will deal with more specific topics and which are developed further in subsequent chapters.

The process of learning

There are many different theories of how learning occurs and its molecular and psychological basis. In general, it must involve memory and the ability to solve problems using existing knowledge or by thinking out new solutions. Learning can be superficial (some facts are recalled) or deep (when the mechanism behind the facts is understood); in general deep learning is preferable. Learning may be active (the student is positively involved in searching for information or developing skills) or passive (they sit in a lecture class being 'taught'). Again there are advantages and disadvantages to both. Increasingly, medical schools are using problem-based learning where the process is student-centred and its purpose is to engage the student in the topic and to encourage critical thinking and analysis, as well as the acquisition of factual knowledge. This method of learning is self-directed and sometimes called 'learning from experience'. For the student beyond the undergraduate phase, the learning can be even more self-directed and be related specifically to deficiencies in practice or in the development of new skills.

The learning cycle is a useful way of summarizing the above discussion (Fig. 20.1.1). It begins with the assessment of the learning needs of the group, class, or individual student. This is then translated into a curriculum. The next stage is the planning of the learning experience and the choice of method and setting to be used. This is then implemented and the process, including the student learning, is evaluated. The cycle is completed by a review of the learning requirements and the progression to the next stage of the learning experience.

A phrase that occurs frequently in other chapters is that of the 'reflective practitioner', or 'reflective learning'. This refers to the process by which the student takes time to think through a particular problem or patient issue, or to think about the process of care through an audit of a particular group of patients or type of problem. In some instances, a diary of work can be helpful for this purpose and the use of creative writing[7] may be particularly useful. The process of audit is a particularly powerful one. It involves the critical analysis of outcome and compares these to those in the literature or by other colleagues. It is an educational process that should lead to changes or modifications in practice.

Increasingly therefore, learning is student centred, relevant to their needs and the outcome of the defined learning process. A key part of the process is feedback on performance, and letting the student know how they are progressing. This can be both formal and informal but is an important role of the supervisor or mentor. There is no point in allowing a young clinician from any professional background to progress up the career ladder if the competencies that he or she demonstrates are inadequate. There is room for remedial work, but this should occur during the process of education when deficiencies can be remedied, not at the end. This is unfair to the student.

Learning palliative medicine

Students require support during their time in a palliative care service. It is not an easy area to work in, particularly if the placement is part

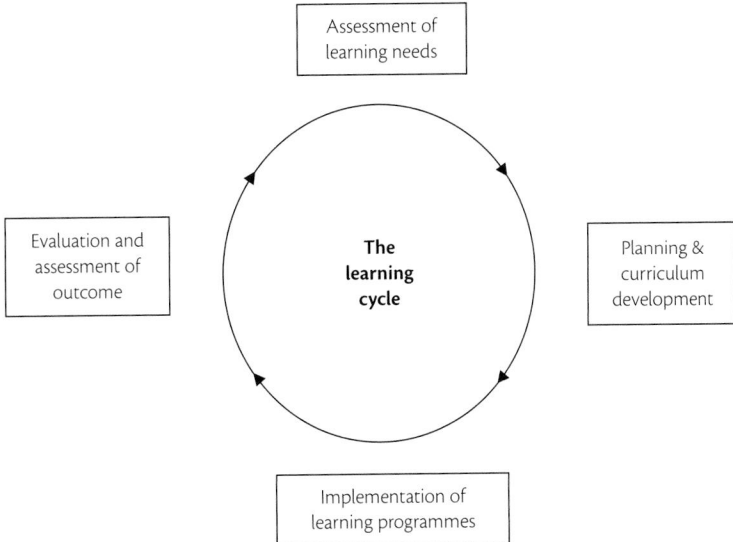

Figure 20.1.1 The learning cycle.

of a rotational programme and the student intends practising in a different branch of medicine. They may not have been exposed to the problems in the same way before, nor been as closely involved with patients who are dying. They will need help and the team as a whole needs to be alert to potential problems and to identifying those who are vulnerable. This is relevant at all levels of the continuum of medical education. Of particular interest is the development of a trusting environment in which it is easy for the student to seek help or support or to talk through their own feelings and concerns.

In many medical schools the student is encouraged to consider special study modules. These allow the student to spend time in a specialist area and increase their understanding of the subject. This is an ideal way to gain experience in palliative care and directors of services should be alert to the opportunities available.

In all of this role models are of particular importance. If a student attends a seminar on communication skills, practises their skills and reflects on them, only to be confronted in clinical practice with a clinician, from any professional background who demonstrates exactly the opposite attributes, then confusion will arise. The student picks up attitudes and approaches to patients by such mechanisms. This is sometimes called the 'hidden curriculum'. The apprenticeship model is a very powerful one and where it works well it can enthuse and enlighten the student. Habits learned by osmosis, by watching the senior person in action, are copied and personalized. The formal curriculum may be powerless to interfere with this and it needs to be recognized by those who teach. The process of 'socialization' into a profession is part of the ritual of becoming a professional and to change attitudes in clinical practice in those working in other specialties may be an important part of the work of the palliative care unit.

Facilitating learning

A wide variety of methods may be used to facilitate learning and each has advantages and disadvantages which are discussed in more detail in subsequent chapters. This is well illustrated by the process of learning communication skills, at the heart of palliative care practice. In educational terms there are several implications for the methods employed, which are also relevant to many other aspects of professional practice. First, should this be a short course, or should it be seen as a continuing thread throughout the curriculum? Second, should it be seen as a topic that is taught outside the clinical setting or at the bedside? Third, how can it be evaluated and what is the role of the patient in that process? Finally, what happens when the young professional meets resistance to new thinking on communication skills in a clinical setting when his or her superior does not agree with the approach? These questions are not specific to communication skills but reflect the kinds of difficulties in converting good practice into real life situations. Similar issues are raised in the teaching of ethical issues.

In the development of the curriculum, a balance will need to be struck between the scientific basis of medicine and those aspects of clinical practice that use the social sciences or the arts. This is of particular relevance in palliative medicine where both are required. The second dichotomy is between research and practice. How much learning needs a research focus? There is certainly an agreement that practice needs to be evidence based and the role of case conferences, literature searches, the use of the Internet are all relevant to this. Patients now expect their professional carers to be up to date and aware of recent developments in their own and related fields.

Advances in clinical management come about in several ways, one of which is the curiosity of the doctor; a wish to find out more and do things better. This curiosity leads to new methods of thinking, to observations that are built on and repeated and the hypothesis developed is then tested against the best available therapy. The methodology for such developments is part of the work of the doctor and should be a component of the curriculum. Palliative medicine needs research and an attitude of questioning should be part of the practice of the doctor or other professional.

The assessment of learning

Part of the educational process is the assessment of the outcome of the learning. This can be done in a wide variety of ways[8]. The most common ways include written essays, short questions, multiple choice questions and OSCEs. Such methods are particularly good at determining the knowledge base and, in some instances, clinical skills. Clinical examination of patients by students provides an additional way of assessing skills. However, attitudes are more difficult to assess and increasingly patients are used for this purpose.

It is also useful to consider the role of assessment in education and why it is needed. It has a clear role in the motivation of students, and in the facilitation of learning. It helps facilitate choices and options and gives feedback on the learning outcome. It is also used to satisfy accrediting bodies and determine student progression. It is a fundamental part of learning. Outside bodies use such assessments to compare the clinical unit or institution against known benchmark standards. Such processes are increasingly widespread and the clinician of the future will need to be sure that the standards that are in place meet the external quality requirements. The assessment procedures also serve to inform and assure patients and the public.

Increasingly, the end point of education is the assessment of the competence of the professional to perform tasks or to solve problems. This is more than just the assessment of factual knowledge and the ability to recall certain packets of information, important as that is. It is also about putting this information into practice. It is the component of medical education that the patient sees and experiences.

Relevant to this is the question as to who should assess the student? The most obvious answer is the relevant professional body, but it should be more than this. The role of the nurse or the dietician in the assessment of medical competence also has a place, as would the role of the patient. Increasingly, input from patients is informing the way in which professionals are assessed. The use of actors, professional patients, or simulated patients is a good way of finding out how students will cope with difficult situations and how they will communicate with patients. Communication remains the major cause of concern for many patients and the object of most complaints. Anything that will improve this position should be welcome.

In recent years, the role of the humanities in the teaching of palliative care has increased, hence the chapter on this topic in this section of the textbook. The use of the arts, such as literature and music, can help to encourage students to think in different ways about patients and their feelings and emotions. There is now considerable experience worldwide on this topic[9–11]. The use of narrative and stories to help understand the patient perspective are also relevant. Doctors and other health professionals are privileged to listen to patient's stories (histories, narratives) and help interpret them and in doing so facilitate the healing of the patient. Writing down what has happened, sharing it with others can be a powerful therapeutic and educational experience.

In this context, Howard Brody uses an interesting phrase. He recalls a patient who said 'My story is broken, can you help me fix it'. A comment that encapsulates so many of the issues in palliative care and uses the language of narrative to describe the problem.

Traditionally, learning takes place in classes and adopts several forms including lectures, seminars and tutorials. Nowadays learning is much more problem based and involves the student in finding out for himself or herself what the answers are to the problems set. In addition, especially for more experienced staff, learning sets provide an effective method of sharing and improving practice. Such sets, usually of five to seven people, meet on a regular basis and draw up an agenda for their own learning and find the people or the resource to help. They also share their own problems and experiences. Groups, for example, of newly appointed palliative care physicians would be ideal for this as a supportive and cohesive group facing many similar problems.

Increasingly, the use of electronic media will be used to assist in learning both for patients and professionals. Increasingly e-learning is forming an important place in the learning cycle for many purposes including assessment. Newer methods such as 'podcasts' are becoming available to undergraduates and postgraduates. The chapter in this section (Chapter 20.5) devoted to this topic highlights the major issues. The availability of large databases on the World Wide Web, and the access to journals and literature make the acquirement of the knowledge base much easier. However, this needs to be placed in the context of the clinical practice of the individual doctor and the facilities available. It can lead to the development of special interest groups and bulletin boards on the web facilitating discussion and problem-solving.

Mentoring is another useful (and growing) innovation. In this process a colleague, often not in the particular clinical field, acts as a sounding board and reflects back to the person views and experience. He or she can guide or be simply a person to listen. For those working in palliative care where there are difficult clinical issues to deal with, where the stress and strain of every day work can become overwhelming, such mentors can not only be of educational value but can assist in the performance of the clinical work.

Competencies of the specialist in palliative medicine

Increasingly, there is discussion about the competencies required of the clinician and how such competencies are generally defined by the specialist body[12,13]. Competence should cover the three aspects of learning and reflect not only the level of knowledge, skills and attitudes but the ability to solve problems, think critically, work as part of a team and show an appetite for continued learning. For most specialties such competencies against which individuals can be assessed are now published.

Multi-disciplinary learning: learning in teams

A further theme that is developed throughout the volume is that of teamwork. This applies equally to inter-disciplinary learning. How this is carried out will vary from setting to setting but in each instance requires that the team members learn from each other and respect the skills of other professionals. Again this may best be done with specific problems and involve the use of different experience and expertise to manage the problem. The use of the humanities is another vehicle that can assist in this process.

Teaching the teachers

So far it has been assumed that all professionals are natural teachers, able to inspire and motivate students. This is clearly not always the case. Teaching requires a special series of skills, many of which can be learned and improved with practice. In professional terms, most people who are involved in educational programmes will be asked to produce a portfolio of teaching activity along with evidence of student feedback as the end point of the process. External accrediting organizations will also wish to see evidence that teaching is being taken seriously and that those involved are aware of new developments in methods, curricular design and assessment of learning. The reading list develops these themes further. The teacher is also an academic leader whose function as a role model is critical. In education as in other areas of clinical practice, the early experiences are vital in sending messages of enthusiasm for the subject, of its excitement, its place in medicine as a whole and its value to patients and the public. Palliative care needs such teachers and leaders if it is to continue to grow and develop as a specialty. As public scrutiny of professional practice increases, so will the need for such professional leadership in setting out professional standards and values.

Further reading

Carlisle, C., Donovan, T., and Mercer, D. (eds.) (2005). *Interprofessional education. An agenda for health care professionals.* Quay Books, Dinton.

Cox, K.R., and Ewan, E. (1988). *The medical teacher*, 2nd edition. Churchill Livingstone, Edinburgh.

David, T., Patel, L., Burdett, K., and Rangachari, P. (1999). *Problem based learning in medicine.* Royal Society of Medicine Press, London.

Dent, J.A., and Harden, R.M. (eds) (2005). *A practical guide for medical teachers.* Churchill Livingstone, Edinburgh.

Miller, G.E. (1980). *Educating medical teachers.* Harvard University Press.

Newble, D., and Cannon, R. (1987). *A Handbook for medical teachers*, 2nd edition. MTP Press Ltd, Kluwer Academic Publishing Group, Lancaster.

Peyton, J.W.R. (1998). *Teaching and learning in medical practice.* Manticore Europe Ltd, Rickmansworth.

Sweet, J., Huttly, S., and Taylor, I. (2003). *Effective learning and teaching in medical, dental and veterinary education.* Kogan Page Ltd., London.

Wear, D., and Bickel, J. (ed.) (2000). *Educating for professionalism. Creating a culture of humanism in medical education.* University of Iowa Press, Iowa City.

Journals

The list below does not include specialist journals in palliative care, nor other medical and professional journals which include regular articles on education.

Academic Medicine. Journal of the Association of Medical Colleges. Washington. Previously the *Journal of Medical Education.*

Education for Primary Care. Radcliffe Medical Press, Abingdon, Oxford.

Journal of Medical Ethics. British Medical Journal Publishing Group, UK. Medical Humanities, special edition of the *Journal of Medical Ethics.*

Medical Education. Published for the Association for the study of Medical Education. Blackwell Science, Oxford, UK.

Medical Teacher. An International Journal of Education in the Health Sciences. In collaboration with the Association for Medical Education in Europe. Taylor and Francis Ltd, Basingstoke, Hants, UK.

References

1. Calman, K.C. (2006). *Medical education: past, present and future.* Elsevier, Edinburgh.
2. Freidson, E. (1975). *Profession of medicine. a study of the sociology of applied knowledge.* Dodd, Mead and Co., New York.
3. Calman, K.C. (1994). The profession of medicine. *British Medical Journal,* **309,** 1140–3.
4. Irvine, D. (2003). *The Doctor's Tale. Professionalism and public trust.* Radcliffe Medical Press, Oxford.
5. Alberti, G. (2003). Professionalism—time for a new look. *Clinical Medicine,* **3,** 91.
6. Medical Professionalism Project. (2002). Medical professionalism in the new millennium: a physician's charter. *Lancet,* **359,** 520–2.
7. Bolton, G. (2005). *Reflective Practice . Writing and professional development*, 2nd edition, Sage Publication.
8. Grant, J. (2002). Learning needs assessment: assessing the need. *British Medical Journal,* **324,** 156–9.
9. Greenhalgh T. and Hurwitz, B. (1998). *Narrative based medicine. Dialogue and discourse in clinical practice.* British Medical Journal Publishing Group, London.
10. Greenhalgh, T. (2006). *What seems to be the trouble? Stories in illness and healthcare.* Nuffield Trust, London.
11. Calman, K.C. (2000). *Storytelling, humour and learning in medicine.* The Stationery Office, London.
12. Calman, K.C. (2000). Postgraduate specialist training and continuing professional development. *Medical Teacher,* **22,** 448–51.
13. Gilmore, I. (2006). The future for specialists and the Medical Royal Colleges. *Lancet,* **368,** 1559–60.

Postgraduate education in palliative medicine

Meg Hegarty and David Currow

Introduction

For my initial two years of medical school, I had sat in lecture halls absorbing a wealth of information about anatomy, physiology, pharmacology and pathology. During the last two years, I had stood rapt at the bedside, taking in the words of master clinicians who revealed the subtleties of physical examination and the fine points of medical treatment. Brimming with new knowledge, I thought I was fully ready to assume the care of people. **I mistook information for insight**. While I was well prepared for the science, I was pitifully prepared for the soul[1].

Knowledge is knowing that a tomato is a fruit, not a vegetable. Wisdom is *not putting it into a fruit salad*[2].

Writers in palliative care education have long stressed the complex and holistic nature of palliative care practice and the need for education programmes which develop clinicians with superb, evidence-based clinical skills as well as capacities to engage therapeutically with patients and families, using a whole person approach and a well-developed 'therapeutic imagination'[3].

Undergraduate training in medicine, nursing and allied health disciplines continues to be reported as providing graduates with a less than adequate preparation for the appropriate management of issues of life-limiting illness, along with death and dying, despite some advances in this area[4]. Clinicians, either newly graduated or more experienced, therefore need to continue to recognize their learning needs and to access the most appropriate form(s) of postgraduate education for their situation. The mentoring and support of more experienced members of the local palliative care team may be important in this discerning process.

For the purposes of this chapter 'postgraduate education' is defined broadly, to include formal university-based postgraduate studies and other methods of facilitating the further learning of clinicians following the completion of their basic training, such as short courses and mentoring programmes. The scope of postgraduate education in palliative medicine includes education for clinicians whose practice will be within both specialist palliative care and generalist areas. This chapter does not provide a discussion of specialist, vocational training in palliative care, as this will be covered elsewhere in this section. We have used the term 'clinician' to refer to all palliative care workers, whether their clinical work is medical, social work, nursing, pastoral care, administration or any other role in palliative care.

This chapter aims to describe, in part, the changing and challenging landscape of palliative care education. Firstly, the underlying aim of postgraduate palliative care education is explored. Secondly, we outline what capabilities are required of a palliative care practitioner in current practice and the role education can play in developing these capabilities. Thirdly, the assessment of and feedback to students.

Fourthly, evaluating effective teaching approaches and, lastly, current developments and innovations.

However, before moving onto a detailed look at the above, a discussion of the context in which these changes and challenges are occurring needs to take place.

Context of postgraduate education in palliative care: trends and challenges

Palliative care postgraduate education occurs in the context of several trends: the magnitude of new work in palliative care, the emergence of new research areas, the explosion of professional and lay literature, the drive to develop an evidence-based practice and finally, changing clinician-patient relationships, with increasingly informed patients who have a desire to be involved in decision-making about their health care.

These evolving trends each present challenges for clinicians to develop continually their knowledge, practice, therapeutic skills and awareness of changing patient needs and expectations. These challenges fall into three main areas. Firstly, for any practitioner, there is a challenge of maintaining currency of practice as new evidence emerges. This challenge is typified by the large number of publications that become available on a weekly basis from all around the world. For example, across the spectrum of peer-reviewed articles typified by Medline, more than 20 000 listings are added weekly. Clearly, no practitioner is able to keep up with even a small fraction of this new work.

Secondly, clinicians have the added challenge of needing not only to keep up-to-date in areas related to symptom control, psychosocial support, pharmacology, family dynamics and bereavement, but also to be aware of current practice in the many fields of clinical care covering life-limiting illnesses. Any change in therapies that:

♦ prolong life;

♦ improve function;

- affect directly the course of disease in order to lessen symptomsis crucial for palliative care practitioners to know about and understand.

Thirdly, there is the challenge of basing clinical decisions on the best evidence rather than long established practice. Practitioners who originally established palliative care services in many parts of the world, did so in response to social and clinical imperatives. These 'pioneers' in the field were required to set up and maintain services, often with very few resources. The knowledge base for the evolving discipline of palliative care was necessarily small and based more in clinical experience than in research. Day-to-day practice that developed in such an environment needs to move from 'best experience' to 'best evidence', given the burgeoning evidence base available to inform practice. The transition from experience to evidence-based practice is a difficult one in any emerging area of clinical practice, a difficulty reflected in recent decades in other growing practice areas such as rehabilitation, sexual health, and sports medicine. As these 'first generation' practitioners become mentors of the second generation, this transition is important in introducing and fostering balanced approaches to evidence-based practice in new clinicians, so that their role is one of life-long learning and not simply a one-off training in established dogma.

The challenges inherent in the emerging trends are not insurmountable. Addressing them requires postgraduate education which evolves content and methodology continually to meet the new needs of changing practice milieux, while maintaining strong education in fundamental areas, such as the principles of clinical assessment and management.

The aim of postgraduate education in palliative care

The ultimate aim of postgraduate palliative care education is wise practice. Education facilitates a growth in students from acquiring knowledge to developing understanding (the move from information to insight alluded to in the opening quote) and then to applying this understanding wisely in practice. This development in many ways parallels the movement from novice to expert clinician.

A move from knowledge, to understanding, to wisdom in practice

For postgraduate education to facilitate the move from knowledge to wisdom successfully, educators need to understand each of these steps and the interplay of the many components of clinical thinking and judgement in practice.

Knowledge

Knowledge is a broad term, encompassing both received *information* (data) and the different *ways of knowing*[5,6], the processes by which the data is accepted.

Received information includes:

- *Stocks of knowledge*[7], which includes information gained through research findings, theory and concepts, clinical experience, and personal knowledge. The latter includes a person's cultural and emotional knowledge.

- *Situational knowledge*[7] that knowledge which provides information about a particular person's context, for example the person's age, living conditions, support system and personal resources.

Ways of knowing include analytical reasoning, emotional knowing, tacit (intuitive) knowing, practical/technical knowing, aesthetic knowing, and moral knowing[5,6,8]. Each of these ways or patterns of knowing produces part of the total knowledge about a situation. They are separate, but interrelated, each adding perspective to the others.

However, the acquisition of knowledge alone does not guarantee that it will be used wisely in practice. Coming to an understanding of the situation plays an important role in the transition of knowledge to wise practice.

Understanding

It is important for educators and students to recognize how understanding (or insight) differs from knowledge. From a competency-based approach to education, the difference is often not recognized[7]. However, understanding is a more complex phenomenon than knowledge involving 'an inner grasp of what is at issue', which can be developed and refined over time[9]. Understanding involves the use of a range of ways of knowing, including tacit knowledge, the ability to imagine possibilities[5], and emotional knowing, which may perceive what cannot be articulated, but can be expressed, for example a patient's unnamed fears. In the clinical setting, understanding can include an ability to perceive both the meaning and the significance of the situation—for the patient, for carers and for the clinical service. Self-knowledge is also a type of understanding.

While situational knowledge contextualizes stocks of knowledge cognitively, understanding takes this a step further, by synthesizing knowledge from different domains, resulting in insight and a fuller perception of what is happening. This then provides the raw material for more comprehensive clinical judgement and an appropriate empathetic response, both important aspects of exercising wisdom in practice.

Wisdom in practice

Wisdom in practice incorporates a critical and creative use of knowledge and evidence to inform an *ability to make sound judgements in difficult, complex and uncertain situations*[7]. Making these judgements involves the processes of clinical thinking and decision-making. It is often believed that clinical thinking and judgement are purely rational processes. However, as we have seen, both rational and non-rational ways of knowing and understanding are necessary. In fact, clinical intuition increases with practice experience[8,10]. Other factors also operate (mostly unconsciously) and inform the process of clinical thinking and judgement— values, beliefs, assumptions, attitudes, expectations, feelings and past experiences[11].

Developing wisdom in practice takes time. It is an iterative and ongoing process. Teaching clinicians, through all forms of postgraduate education, to become conscious of the unconscious aspects of their decision-making, through reflective practice, leads to understanding of the basis and potential biases of judgements. It develops in students a level of *metacognition*, an understanding of the processes of clinical thinking and the dangers of faulty clinical thinking. This provides clinicians with a *framework for incorporating both new evidence and the values of our patients into our clinical decisions*[12]. They also learn of the *elaborated learning*[13] by which they develop continually their own knowledge and understanding through integrating professional and life experiences, theory and research evidence.

Capabilities of a palliative care practitioner

What is expected of practitioners as they seek to maintain currency of practice? How does postgraduate education best enable this?

As well as the capability to understand their processes of clinical thinking and practice discussed above, today's practitioners need excellence in clinical assessment and ethical decision-making, management of symptoms, disease processes and treatment; communication skills; understanding of the impact of life-long illness on the human psyche and spirit and the skills and attitudes required in engaging therapeutically with people undergoing this process; and the capacity for interdisciplinary teamwork. Lifelong learning capacities include the capacity for both professional and personal development; reflective practice; and facility with tools for knowledge retrieval and use. Leadership skills include the ability to bring new knowledge to the field through research and collaboration and the ability to disseminate new knowledge through teaching and publication.

Postgraduate education develops these capacities through learning opportunities which build on existing skills and knowledge, challenging and mentoring clinicians through a range of adult learning models.

While ongoing development of all of these capabilities is important, several, with particular significance to current practice of palliative care, will be discussed more fully below.

Clinical assessment and management

Having learnt the basics of general clinical assessment and symptom management in undergraduate courses, postgraduate palliative care education deepens clinicians' understanding of why and how people die; of likely illness trajectories and pathophysiology; of contextualizing assessment and consideration of management options (including the significance and meaning of the symptom for the patient); and of effective interdisciplinary clinical practice. Advanced assessment and decision-making skills include recognizing when interventions would be futile; recognizing the difference between futility and clinical futility and making this clear in team decision-making processes; and clinical decision-making in complex or refractory suffering. Teaching methodologies found to be effective in clinical teaching include the use of multiple teaching approaches, both didactic and experiential, clinical placement in palliative care services, multi-media approaches and clinical supervision[14,15].

Communication

There is widespread evidence that effective communication skills improve disclosure of patient concerns[16]; increase patient satisfaction[17]; increase patient understanding and recall[18]; improve symptom management[19]; decrease emotional distress[20]; and improve physiological outcomes[21]. Clinician burnout is related to a lack of training in communication skills. There remains the perception that good communication skills will be developed through practice experience, despite evidence to the contrary[22]. Poor communication skills remain in evidence in palliative care settings. While many clinicians are unsure of ways to identify what patients want to know[23], up to 60 per cent of patient concerns remain undisclosed in hospice settings[24]. Patient cues are often missed, blocked, or distanced by palliative care staff[25].

Particular communication skills in which clinicians need to learn excellence include: assessing pain, breaking bad news, facilitating a goal-setting family meeting, discussing the use of artificial hydration or nutrition and discussing transitions, such as referral to hospice or a palliative care service. *Experiential learning methods*, such as *role plays and simulated situations*, *video- and audio-taping*, combined with reflective opportunities, allow students practice in using different communication techniques for these situations. While *face-to-face teaching* is the most common form of this education, *videoconferencing* has been used effectively with students in rural and remote areas[26] and *online comparison of transcripts, audio- and video-tapes of simulated patient/clinician encounters* teach graphically the role of non-verbal language and silence in communication. *Theory and research evidence* are more effective in facilitating learning and skill development when incorporated into experiential sessions to illustrate points of practice[27]. *Cultural nuances* in expectations of roles in communication styles, decision-making, 'truth-telling' etc., should be woven through case studies and discussions.

While *self-awareness* is noted as a skill within most approaches to communication skills training, Katz and associates have developed a programme which takes this further, encouraging *clinician mindfulness* and *bodily awareness* as integral approaches and tools in understanding what is happening within therapeutic interactions[28].

Feedback from the 'patient' and observers, both peers and tutor, is an important learning tool in both one-on-one and small group learning situations. The agenda-led outcome-based analysis (ALOBA) feedback and analysis model improves on the traditional rules of feedback. ALOBA is more focused, beginning with the learner identifying his or her agenda and the problems encountered in the role play or clinical experience[29]. The principles of this model are outlined in Box 20.2.1.

General principles of constructive feedback are summarized in Box 20.2.2. Although they have been acknowledged since the 1960s, they are still not widely used in medical education[22].

Sensitive topics

Communication about sensitive issues such as sexuality and intimacy remains difficult for many clinicians, with little overt discussion of them within palliative care teams as clinical issues. These are issues of which patients hesitate to speak with health professionals, yet are significant aspects of life for people when facing a life-limiting illness and death[30]. Teaching clinicians ways of communicating about such issues in sensitive ways involves not only knowledge of theory, understanding of their own attitudes and beliefs and blocks to communication, but opportunities actively to practice communication skills in these areas, using role play. Obviously, a safe learning environment is important. Where culturally appropriate, the sensitive use of shared humour can relieve some of the common awkwardness students may feel initially.

Teaching spiritual and existential care

Spiritual and existential concerns are significant for people with a life-limiting illness[31]. The human spirit and a person's spirituality, expressed in individual ways, are rich and often under-estimated resources for patients, at a time when many other resources are diminishing. Existential and spiritual suffering must always be considered as potential components of patient suffering or unrelieved pain[32]. Yet training in assessment and care in this area is widely lacking, leaving clinicians often with a sense of discomfort

Box 20.2.1 Principles of agenda-led outcome-based analysis.

Organizing the feedback process

◆ Start with the learner's agenda
  • Ask what problems the learner experienced and what help he would like from the rest of the group

◆ Look at the outcomes that the learner and the patient are trying to achieve
  • Discuss where the learner is aiming for and how to get there—effectiveness in communication is always dependent on what the interviewer and the patient are trying to achieve

◆ Encourage self-assessment and self-problem solving first
  • Allow the learner space to make suggestions before the group shares its ideas

◆ Involve the whole group in problem solving
  • Encourage the group to work together to generate solutions not only to help the learner but also to help themselves in similar situations

Giving useful feedback to each other

◆ Use descriptive feedback to encourage a non-judgemental approach
  • Descriptive feedback ensures that non-judgemental and specific comments are made and prevents vague generalization

◆ Provide balanced feedback
  • Encourage all group members to provide a balance in feedback of what worked well and what didn't work so well, thus supporting each other and maximizing learning. We learn as much by analysing why something works as why it doesn't

◆ Make offers and suggestions; generate alternatives
  • Make suggestions rather than prescriptive comments and reflect them back to the learner for consideration; think in terms of alternative approaches

◆ Be well intentioned, valuing and supportive
  • It is the group's responsibility to be respectful and sensitive to each other

Ensuring that analysis and feedback actually lead to deeper understanding and development of specific skills

◆ Rehearse suggestions
  • Try out alternative phrasing and practice suggestions—when learning any skill, observation, feedback and rehearsal are required to effect change

◆ Value the interview as a gift of raw material for the group
  • Use the interview as a gift of raw material around which the whole group can explore communication problems, issues and skills—group members can learn as much as the learner being observed who should not be the constant centre of attention. All group members have a responsibility to make and rehearse suggestions

◆ Opportunistically introduce theory, research evidence and wider discussion
  • Offer to introduce concepts, principles, research evidence and wider discussion at opportune moments to illuminate learning for the group as a whole

◆ Structure and summarize learning so that a constructive end-point is reached
  • Structure and summarize learning throughout the session using the Calgary-Cambridge Guides to ensure that learners piece together the individual skills that arise into an overall conceptual framework[22]

Source: Kurtz, *et al.* (2005)[22].

or ineptitude and patients with unaddressed suffering. Learning to take a simple spiritual history and being able to discuss existential concerns provides clinicians with a fuller understanding of patients, their resources and needs[33]. Learning skills and the qualities of presence required will involve clinicians' reflection on their own spirituality, philosophy and ways of nurturing their own spirits. This awareness is the highest predictor of ability to provide spiritual care[34]. Spiritual care training itself has been shown to produce a statistically significant improvement in participant spiritual well-being and attitudes, including compassion and attitude towards colleagues[35].

Developing the ethical imagination

Palliative care practitioners are practising in increasingly pluralistic societies, which hold a range of (sometimes competing) ethical views. *Teaching clinical decision-making* therefore needs to include

explicitly the role of patient and clinician values and include opportunities for developing the clinician's *skills of ethical imagination and interpretation*[36]. This entails developing an understanding of different ethical perspectives and approaches, including the traditional principles-, rights- and duties-based approaches; the newer ethical frameworks which suggest a relational basis for ethical decision-making; and the growing awareness of indigenous ethical frameworks. Knowledge and understanding of a range of frameworks allows clinicians to arrive at their own ethical positions better and to understand the thinking behind other perspectives, a crucial skill in negotiating complex clinical decision-making in pluralistic societies.

Learning applied ethics begins with recognizing that ethics reflect societal mores and evolve with changing attitudes and values. Education in the evolving nature of ethics puts into context ethical practice for clinicians and raises challenges for clinical and societal

Box 20.2.2 Principles of constructive feedback.

Feedback should be descriptive rather than judgemental or evaluative

◆ Make feedback specific rather than general

◆ Focus feedback on behaviour rather than on personality

◆ Feedback should be for the learner's benefit

◆ Focus feedback on sharing information rather than giving advice

◆ Check out interpretations of feedback

◆ Limit feedback to the amount of information that the recipient can use rather than the amount we would like to give

◆ Feedback should be solicited rather than imposed

◆ Give feedback only about something that can be changed

Source: adapted from Kurtz *et al.* (2005)[22].

leadership and change agency. Autonomy as an ethical principle provides a rich example. In most of the developed world, individual autonomy now ranks as the first ethical principle. This is the case both in societal attitudes generally and in health-care ethics. A quick glance at the contents pages of ethics textbooks printed in the last few decades reveals a reversal of the previous list of ethical principles—non-malfeasance, beneficence, justice and autonomy. Autonomy now usually ranks first, a reflection of the rise of individualism over the last few decades in much of the developed world. Yet acceptance of autonomy as the ultimate adjudicator needs to be seen within the broader ethical, clinical, cultural and social contexts. Justice or non-maleficence, for example, may have a greater ethical claim in some cases.

Curricula need to provide students with appropriate theory and skills practice in nuanced application of ethics, as well as, importantly, critical reflection on the attitudes and assumptions underpinning their own ethical thinking.

Cultural values and nuanced differences in understanding and expression of ethics in areas such as 'truth-telling' provide *teaching points* which can open discussions about the complexities of practice in this area.

Experiential learning has much to offer in putting flesh on dry ethical principles and theoretical frameworks. *Case studies and simulated situations* can involve students taking or being assigned a role other than their usual clinical role and arguing an ethical position from this perspective. This technique is a powerful tool for allowing students to consider professional, cultural and social factors which impinge on decision-making and which may form an ethical stance diametrically opposed to their usual position. It challenges clinicians to appraise their own positions and the factors leading to these. Skills in negotiating an ethical clinical decision with stakeholders who hold a range of differing ethical positions are also considered, practised, and then evaluated in peer discussions. This teaching technique has been used effectively within a formal postgraduate programme[37].

Another approach is to discuss students' current cases; clinician responses including emotional reactions, the impact of these responses on outcomes for patients and clinicians; and strategies for improving outcomes. Individual, institutional, societal and political influences on palliative care practice are also discussed[38].

Challenging the mantras

Within any field of practice, mantras evolve over time. Originally encapsulating a core belief of practice in a pithy manner, mantras can become sacrosanct, reiterated, and passed on in unreflective and unchallenged ways to each new generation of practitioners as part of their admission and socialization into the field. Palliative care certainly has its fair share of such mantras—*No-one should die alone; the unit of care is the patient and family; we're always here for you . . .*

However, some people choose to die alone; the specialist palliative care team may not be the most appropriate ones to be available 24 h a day. This does not necessarily mean relinquishing the mantra altogether, but interpreting its application differently and more thoughtfully in changing contexts. Mantras contain seeds of truth and may well apply to many, or even most, situations, yet an uncritical application of them as rules in every situation is poor practice. As with all aphorisms, they are generalizations, which hold immense power unless critiqued and applied wisely.

Postgraduate education offers opportunities to train clinicians in a reflective awareness of the ways mantras operate within their own practice and within the structures and policies which impinge on it. This creates questioning, creative clinicians, capable of articulating and owning the necessary, and often subtle, changes in focus as palliative care continues to evolve in response to changing demographic and clinical needs.

Attitudinal change

Educational objectives include not only the development of knowledge and skills, but also the development of attitudes or *professional dispositions*[39]. This is the most difficult area in which to effect change. It is relatively easy to increase levels of knowledge or skills, but attitudes are often longer-standing, embedded, unconscious, unrecognized, and unchallenged and are linked with (often unquestioned) beliefs, values, and assumptions.

In planning educational programmes, one learning objective in each module should be an attitudinal objective[40]. Teaching strategies for developing attitudes can include *mentoring* and *face-to-face or online small group discussion* of the different assumptions that clinicians bring to a clinical situation. *Group rules* of confidentiality and respectful listening and feedback should be articulated at the outset and agreed to by the group. *Reflective writing exercises* in which students reflect on their own attitudes and beliefs about, for example, pain and pain relief, what 'health' means, whose role is it to provide care etc. may provide the clinician's first experience of exploring consciously their own attitudes and the sources of these. *Clinical experience and reflections on narratives* can also effect attitudinal change[41] while didactic teaching alone does not[42].

While the acquisition of new knowledge and skills has effects on people's professional and personal lives, attitudinal change has a more profound effect in that it creates a shift, not just in a person's thinking, but in their way of seeing and operating in the world. This mirrors the shifts which often occur in their patients as they live with a life-limiting illness. Dying is so very often a process of *'transformative education';* when well facilitated, postgraduate palliative care education can also be transformative for clinicians (and educators!).

Learning to use the evidence: critical appraisal and applying evidence

Accessing and using the data sources that can inform best practice as new evidence becomes available are essential skills to be developed in clinicians. Newly published medical literature is proliferating and is of uneven quality. Within the peer-reviewed literature that relates to palliative care, the vast majority of papers are case series or randomized trials assessing efficacy. This means that the findings apply to the discreet population researched, but may not be effective if applied to palliative care populations more broadly. Few studies are available that establish effectiveness, or indeed are powered by the adverse outcomes (safety studies) rather than by efficacy.

Teaching clinicians to assess critically and use newly published data means ensuring their awareness of both the advantages and disadvantages of different types of evidence.

Systematic reviews

There has been a recent important trend to systematize the process of identifying, evaluating, and presenting high level summaries of data. Such systematic reviews (including Cochrane reviews) are an important step forward in helping current practitioners to understand current best evidence. They include literature from a wide range of difficult-to-find sources within a format that allows for easy digestion of the synthesized material. However, systematic reviews still rely on defining inclusion and exclusion criteria which may allow bias. The reviewers may also be the authors of significant papers in the area of the review. To date, the list of questions for systematic reviews that are relevant to palliative care are themselves a fairly eclectic collection of investigator-driven interests that do not reflect a systematic approach to improving clinical care and health service policy.

Consensus guidelines/clinical pathways/clinical practice guidelines

These are used widely in palliative care. As with all new tools, it is imperative to train clinicians to consider:

1   Who was part of the consensus group and, specifically, did it include practitioners whose practice is *not* in palliative care but from other disciplines and backgrounds?

2   What process of consultation took place in order to define the question?

3   How has the guideline or pathway been prospectively evaluated?

4   What is the ongoing evaluation of the effectiveness of the pathway in daily clinical practice?

Many guidelines from either systematic reviews or from consensus are also limited by the data that may be extrapolated from other areas of clinical practice. Generalization of data from non-palliative populations needs to be made, but is no substitute for the subsequent rigorous evaluation in a palliative population which has differing underlying mechanisms and contexts. Postgraduate education should alert clinicians to these limitations and their implications for practice.

Qualitative research

To complement guidelines written using quantitative methods, there have been initiatives to include qualitative data more systematically[43]. Deriving evidence from qualitative sources is likely to lead to a richness of data not currently reflected in systematic reviews that rely only on a hierarchy of evidence from (mostly) interventional studies. Yet, with its focus on individual, subjective human experiences and the contexts in which meaning is made, qualitative research often defies broad generalization and must be assessed using other criteria as well. In areas such as social policy with overlap that includes health, initiatives such as the Campbell Collaboration are creating a framework into which qualitative research can be assimilated for systematic reviews[44]. Learning to use and critique such frameworks and reviews, using criteria specific to qualitative data, is a skill needing to be developed by clinicians.

Critical appraisal skills

Whatever the source of data that practitioners access in order to inform evolving practice, there is the need to evaluate the evidence in a framework that is systematic and reproducible. Such skills are variably taught at under-and postgraduate level. For effective life-long learners, these skills are a key tool to sifting through the clinical literature for data that can truly improve clinical practice. This includes being able to define the question that needs to be posed in order to improve practice and to define the best methodology for answering a particular question. Frameworks and tools for appraising the literature are now more widely available via online resources such as www.caresearch.com.au

Learning to appraise critically and apply research evidence is best learnt by doing research. This will be discussed in the next session.

Learning for research quality

Training clinicians in research to improve the quality of palliative care is an ethical imperative for care of future patients. Close links between postgraduate programmes and research units provide opportunities to work with experienced research teams. Formal research training is offered by some universities, for example the *Strategic Training Program in Palliative Care Research* at McGill University, University Laval and University of Ottawa, funded by The Institute of Cancer Research & National Cancer Institute of Canada. A Masters by Research in Health Research with a focus on end-of-life care and a summer school research programme are offered by Lancaster University. Where programmes do not have specific research training, Masters programmes can easily incorporate the learning of publication and presentation skills by setting publishable papers rather than essays as assessment tasks and by mentoring learners through the processes of preparing a manuscript for publication.

Evaluating learning

Formal education programmes use a range of assessment tools and types of feedback. Assessment and assessment feedback perform two roles: (1) *to assess learning* and (2) *as learning processes in themselves.* Written or oral feedback, rather than simply a numerical mark, provides teaching at the most valuable learning points for the learner, as it is a targeted response, addressing the aspects of knowledge or skills wherein lie problems for this learner. The principles of constructive feedback in Box 20.2.2 apply to both written and oral feedback.

Evaluating learners assesses:

◆ *Knowledge—do you know it?*

◆ *Competence—can you show it?*

- *Performance—do you (choose to) do it?*
- *Outcomes—what results do you obtain from using it?*[22]

Designing assessment depends on which of the above are being assessed. Written and oral examinations or assessment tasks demonstrate *knowledge*; *competence* can effectively be assessed in the objective structured clinical examination (OSCE) or via observation of videotaped or live clinical interactions. (Competence includes the ability to demonstrate appropriate professional dispositions or attitudes.) More difficult to assess, apart from self-rating tools, are *confidence* (in knowledge, skills and ability to effect change), *development in ways of thinking or approaching a topic, self awareness* and *attitudinal change* itself. Portfolios and reflective journals can be effective tools for recording and contributing to these and the assessment of student awareness of development in these areas.

Clinical outcomes of professional postgraduate education are rarely assessed, with good reason. Translating knowledge into practice involves factors beyond the scope and control of educators alone, including organizational support and the use of key opinion leaders[45].

Evaluating postgraduate education: what works and why?

Understanding the ways adult learners learn provides the rationale for the effectiveness of certain educational approaches. Following are a few approaches which recognize and use this well.

Case-based and narrative approaches

Current studies demonstrate that clinical knowledge is largely held in the memory in the form of stories and templates, not as a series of facts[46]. Clinicians' experiences put into context the theory they were taught as undergraduates, building a repertoire of clinical memories. Learning, therefore, is more likely to happen and to be retained when case studies, simulation of clinical situations and narrative in its many forms are used as teaching tools. These methods go beyond *illustrating* theory to providing an *experience* of its application, either in reality or vicariously. The use and impact of literature and the arts ('the Medical Humanities') in palliative care education is discussed more fully elsewhere in this section.

Teaching from the 'tension points'[40]

Adult learners learn best when they see the content and learning as relevant to their practice[47]. Many clinicians seek postgraduate education to help them address clinical dilemmas. Identifying the 'tension points' and using these as starting points for teaching connects the teaching directly with students' most significant concerns[40].

Small group work teaching skills

Small group work is a technique with particular benefits for complex skill development, used in a range of teaching approaches including problem-based or case-based learning, the practising of clinical and professional skills, and reflective discussions[48]. Goal setting and eliciting and providing feedback are long, established teaching practices in small groups[49]. A new framework for development of skills with both cognitive and affective components adds

the skills of *identifying a* (participant's) *learning edge, proposing and testing hypotheses, and calibrating learners' self-assessments*[50].

Changing practice: academic detailing and clinical supervision

The evidence of clinical practice change as a result of new information from informal education through conference attendance, journal clubs, and team clinical meetings is, sadly, largely lacking[45]. However, sustainable practice change has been achieved using academic detailing, a technique long used by pharmaceutical company representatives. Sustained changes have occurred in practitioners' prescribing, screening and the ordering of pathology tests[45]. Such detailing entails:

- use of evidence based material to generate key messages;
- key objectives for change in behaviour;
- a specifically trained detailer who can quickly establish credibility;
- an understanding of the practitioners' current understanding and practice;
- a focused intervention that allows for new evidence to be presented in a succinct and practitioner friendly way with a positive feedback loop for changed behaviour[51].

Adapting this approach in postgraduate education may have benefits in producing targeted, quantifiable changes in clinical practice. However, sustained change in more complex skills, knowledge, and attitudes, such as the development of communication skills, is best achieved with clinical supervision following teaching sessions.

Research outcomes for different methods in teaching communication skills

Research into different methodologies for teaching communication skills has yielded useful findings. An intensive short course teaching communication skills, followed by a series of educational sessions has been shown to improve sustainability of learned *knowledge, competence, and confidence*. Training in communication skills increases *competence in simulated situations*[52], but not necessarily performance in real patient encounters[23,24]. It is clinical supervision following training which has been shown to improve *skill transfer to practice settings*[34].

Moving beyond 'what works?' in educational research

Research in postgraduate education in palliative care needs not only to provide evidence of effective practices, but also an increased understanding of why they work. This allows the various factors operating within the 'blackbox' of a particular educational programme to be teased out, individually assessed and their effects known. Teaching and learning methodologies and techniques can then be combined appropriately in designing curricula which will facilitate desired outcomes most effectively. Rather than simply asking '*What works and what doesn't?*', palliative care educational research needs to ask '*What's happening here?*'[53] and '*Why?*'.

Currently, evaluation of palliative care postgraduate education is largely ad hoc and is still in its early stages. Educational research most often asks '*What works?*', rather than '*Why?*' Most published evaluations of individual short courses rely on student self-assessment and report self-rated increases in confidence, knowledge, and skill competence in the short term, with some reporting sustained improvement over slightly longer periods. Self-reporting of changes in practice and learner instigation of practice innovations, either individually or at an organizational level, have been reported as direct outcomes of attending postgraduate education[54]. Formal, objective evaluation of university postgraduate programmes, teaching and student knowledge and skill levels are frequently conducted, but results rarely published.

Further effectiveness studies of teaching methodologies for palliative care are needed, as is further enquiry into why these are or are not effective.

Developments and innovations in postgraduate education

In 2006, a survey of postgraduate education in palliative care worldwide was conducted by the authors and the International Association for Hospice and Palliative Care. Much of the information on innovations below is derived from the questionnaire responses. Development and innovations fall broadly into the areas of new specialty areas of practice, collaborations in providing education, and the development of widely available resources. With a mix of interdisciplinary and discipline-specific courses represented, new courses specifically for palliative care practitioners in allied health fields seem still in their infancy and largely focused in social work.

Evolving specialty areas in palliative care

Emerging topics and courses within formal postgraduate programmes both reflect and contribute to the evolving of specialty areas with palliative care, such as palliative aged care and indigenous palliative care. Development of such new education programmes involves innovative, collaborative partnerships across formerly unconnected fields. Recent developments in postgraduate programmes include:

- *Interagency Collaboration for Palliative Care and Mental Health Nurses* (The National University of Ireland).

- *Health Promoting Palliative Care* (La Trobe University, Australia).

- *Pharmaco-economics and rehabilitation in palliative care* (Trivandrum Institute of Palliative Sciences, India).

- *Art and spirituality in palliative care* (UNITRE, Argentina).

- *Master of Medical Psychology* (Universidad Andres Bello, Latin America).

- *Palliative Care for Indigenous Populations topic* (Flinders University, Australia).

- *MSc in palliative care specifically for generalist care contexts* (University of Luton; Canterbury Christ Church University, UK).

Development of educational resources

In recent years, electronic resources, available in the public domain or as shared professional resources, have been developed as train-the-trainer programmes or educational resources for use by individual clinicians.

Significant among these are:

- *EPERC, End-of-Life Physician Education Resource Center* (www. eperc.mcw.edu).—*EPEC Education of Physicians in End-of-life Care train-the-trainer curriculum* (www.epec.net).

- *The Pallium Project* (www.pallium.ca).

- *ELNEC End-of-Life Nursing Education Consortium* (www.aacn. nche.edu/elnec).

- *Knowledge Network, incorporating Caresearch* (www.caresearch. com.au).

Collaborations

Local, national, and international collaborations among universities, clinical services, non-governmental organizations, and governmental agencies provide creative and productive education opportunities.

For example, the LEIFartsen and LEIFnurses forums are postgraduate short courses in ethics at the end of life, financially supported by the Belgian government, with mentorship provided by interdisciplinary faculty members of all universities in Flanders (physicians, philosophers, registered nurses, psychologists, psychiatrists, chaplains, moral consultants, medical ethicists). Similarly, all universities in the French Rhone area have collaborated to produce a Graduate Diploma in palliative care with a common curriculum. Programmes from Kent and Canterbury Christ Church University share modules, with complementary courses, focusing on different palliative care settings.

Other collaborations include: national approaches to palliative medicine training, as in UK and Canada; and international collaborative partnerships among universities, sharing resources and expertise.

Communities of learners have been set up to provide mutual learning opportunities and 'lateral mentoring' for clinicians in rural and remote areas. An example is the Alberta Rural Telelearning Project. Videoconferencing and online audioconferencing are other means of communication for such communities[55].

Conclusion

Practice experience alone is unlikely to be enough to develop wisdom in practice. Postgraduate education, in its many forms, facilitates clinician development and learning for clinical practice and leadership in palliative care. In doing this, postgraduate education is evolving to meet changing needs as palliative care itself evolves. Yet not all learning leads to wise practice. Further research is needed to understand better the effectiveness of educational approaches and methodologies and how best to construct models of developing wise practice in palliative care, responsive to evolving practice settings and demographic demands.

References

1. Groopman, J. (2004). *The anatomy of hope: how people prevail in the face of illness*. Random House, New York.
2. Anonymous.
3. Barnard, D. (2000). *Developing the therapeutic imagination*. (Abstract) Bas Solais ('Death with Illumination') International Palliative Care Conference, Dublin.
4. Block, S. (2002). Medical education in end-of-life care: the status of reform. *Journal of Palliative Medicine*, **5**(2), 243–8.

5. Heron, J. (1992). *Feeling and personhood: psychology in other key*. Sage Publications, London.

6. Carper, B.A. (1978). Fundamental patterns of knowing in nursing. In *Philosophical and theoretical perspectives for advanced nursing practice* (ed. Janet W. Kenney), pp. 5–13. Jones & Bartlett Publishers, Boston.

7. O'Sullivan, T. (2005). Some theoretical propositions on the nature of practice wisdom. *Journal of Social Work*, **5**(2), 221–42.

8. Greenhalgh, T. (2002). Uneasy bedfellows? Reconciling intuition and evidence based practice. *Youngminds Magazine*, **59**, 23–7.

9. Barnett, R. (1994). The limits of competence: knowledge, higher education and society. Open University Press, Buckingham, pp. 99–101.

10. Dreyfus, H.L., and Dreyfus, S.E. (1986). *Mind over machine: The power of human intuition and expertise in the era of the computer*. Blackwell, Oxford.

11. Hillier, R., and Wee, B. (2001). From cradle to grave: palliative medicine education in the UK. *Journal of the Royal Society of Medicine*, **94**, 468–71.

12. Del Mar, C., Doust, J., and Glasziou, P. (2006). Clinical thinking. evidence, communication and decision-making. Blackwell Publishing Ltd, Carlton, p. 2.

13. Coles, C. (1991). Is Problem-based learning the only way? In *The challenge of problem-based learning* (eds. D. Boud and G. Feletti), pp. 295–307. Kogan Page, London.

14. von Gunten, C.F., Twaddle, M., Preodor, M. *et al.* (2005). Evidence of improved knowledge and skills after an elective rotation in a hospice and palliative care program for internal medicine residents. *American Journal of Hospice and Palliative Care*, **22**(3), 195–203.

15. Thompson, A.R., Savidge, M.A., Fulper-Smith, M. *et al.* (1999). Testing a multimedia module in cancer pain management. *Journal of Cancer Education*, **14**(3), 161–3.

16. Maguire, P., Faulkner, A., Booth, K. *et al.* (1996). Helping cancer patients disclose their concerns. *European Journal of Cancer*, **32A**, 78–81.

17. Griffith, C.H. III, Wilson, J.F., Langer, S., and Haist, S.A. (2003). House staff non-verbal communication skills and standardized patient satisfaction. *Journal of General Internal Medicine*, **18**, 170–4.

18. Ley, P. (1988). *Communication with patients: improving satisfaction and compliance*. Croon Helm, London.

19. Stewart, M., Brown, J., Donner, A. *et al.* (2000). The impact patient-centred care on outcomes. *Journal of Family Practice*, **49**, 796–804.

20. Fallowfield, L.J., Hall, A., Maguire, G., and Baum, M. (1990). Psychological outcomes of different treatment policies in women with early breast cancer outside a clinical trial. *British Medical Journal*, **301**, 575–80.

21. Rost, K.M., Flavin, K.S., Cole, K., and McGill, J.B. (1991). Change in metabolic control and functional status after hospitalization. *Diabetes care*, **14**, 881–9.

22. Kurtz, S., Silverman, J., and Draper, J. (2005). Teaching and learning communication skills in medicine. Radcliffe Publishing, Oxford.

23. Fallowfield, L.J., Jenkins, V., Farewell, V. *et al.* (2002). Efficacy of a Cancer research UK communication skills training model for oncologists: a randomized controlled trial. *Lancet*, **359**, 650–6.

24. Heaven, C.M., and Maguire, P. (1997). Disclosure of concerns by hospice patients and their identification by nurses. *Palliative Medicine*, **11**, 283–90.

25. Heaven, C., Clegg, J., and Maguire, P. (2006). Transfer of communication skills training from workshop to workplace: the impact of clinical supervision. *Patient Education and Counseling*, March, **60**(3), 313–25.

26. Girgis, A., Cockburn, J., Butow, P. *et al.* (2006). *Training in communication skills from a distance: an oxymoron or reality?* (Abstract) 8th World Congress of Psycho-oncology, Venice.

27. Rollnick, S., Kinnersley, P., and Butler, C. (2002). Context-bound communication skills training: development of a new method. *Medical Education*, **36**, 377–83.

28. Katz, M., Cestelli, C., and Miccinesi, G. (2006). To communicate with the patient: putting the subjective experience of the doctors in the spotlight. *Psycho-oncology*, **15**(2) (Suppl.), S97–8.

29. Silverman, J., Kurtz, S.M., and Draper, J. (1996). The Calgary–Cambridge approach to communication skills teaching. 1. Agenda led outcome-based analysis of the consultation. *Education General Practice*, **7**, 288–99.

30. Lemieux, L., Kaiser, S., Pereira, J., and Meadows, L. (2004). Sexuality in palliative care: patient perspective. *Palliative Medicine*, **18**, 630–7.

31. Williams, A. (2006). Perspectives on spirituality at the end of life: a meta-summary. *Palliative and Supportive Care*, **4**, 407–17.

32. Mako, C., Galek, K., and Poppito, S. (2006). Spiritual pain among patients with advanced cancer in palliative care. *Journal of Palliative Medicine*, **9**(5), 1106–13.

33. Puchalski, C., and Romer, A.L. (2000). Taking a spiritual history allows clinicians to understand patients more fully. *Journal of Palliative Medicine*, **3**(1), 129.

34. Meyer, C.L. (2003). How effectively are nurse educators preparing students to provide spiritual care? *Nurse Educator*, **28**, 185–90.

35. Wasner, M., Longaker, C., Fegg, M.J., and Borasio, G.D. (2005). Effects of spiritual care training for palliative care professionals. *Palliative Medicine*, **19**(2), 99.

36. Hall, K. (2002). Medical decision-making: an argument for narrative and metaphor. [Journal Article. Research Support, Non-U.S. Gov't]. *Theoretical Medicine & Bioethics*, **23**(1), 55–73.

37. Formal Student Feedback, Advanced Palliative Care Topic, Master of Palliative Care Course, Department of Palliative and Supportive Services, Flinders University, Adelaide, 2005.

38. Fins, J., and Nilson, E. (2000). An approach to educating residents about palliative care and clinical ethics. *Academic Medicine*, **75**(6), 662–5.

39. Markakis, K.M., Beckman, H.B., Suchman, A.L., and Frankel, R.M. (2000). The path to professionalism: cultivating humanistic values and attitudes in residency training. *Academic Medicine*, **75**(2), 141–50.

40. Weissman, W.E. (2006). Palliative care education. What works, what doesn't. (Presentation) EFPPEC Interprofessional Symposium on Palliative and End-of-life care Education, Ontario.

41. Olthuis, G., and Dekkers, W. (2003). Medical education, palliative care and moral attitude: some objectives and future perspectives. *Medical Education*, **37**, 928–33.

42. Fischer, S.M., Gozansky, W.S., Kutner, J.S. *et al.* (2003). Palliative care education: an intervention to improve medical residents' knowledge and attitudes. *Journal of Palliative Medicine*, **6**(3), 391–9.

43. Dixon-Woods, M., and Fitzpatrick, R. (2001). Qualitative research in systematic reviews. *British Medical Journal*, **323**, 765–6.

44. Davies, P., and Boruch, R. (2001). The Campbell Collaboration. *British Medical Journal*, **323**, 294–5.

45. Davis, D.A., O'Brien, M.A., Freemantle, N. *et al.* (1999). Impact of formal continuing medical education: do conferences, workshops, rounds, and other traditional continuing education activities change physician behaviour or health-care outcomes? *JAMA*, **282**(9), 867–74.

46. Norman, G. (2005). Research in clinical reasoning: past history and current trends. *Medical Education*, **39**, 418–27.

47. Knowles, M. (1988). *Self-directed learning*. Association Press, New York.

48. Jacques, D. (2003). Teaching small groups. *BMJ*, **326**, 492–4.

49. Branch, W.T., and Paranjape, A. (2002). Feedback and reflection: teaching methods for clinical settings. *Academic Medicine*, **77**, 1185–8.

50. Fryer-Edwards, K., Arnold, R.M., Baile, W. *et al.* (2006). Reflective teaching practices: an approach to teaching communication skills in a small-group setting. *Academic Medicine*, **81**(7), 638–44.

51. Soumerai, S.B. (1990). Principles of education outreach ('academic detailing') to improve clinical decision-making. *JAMA*, **263**(4), 549–56.

52. Razavi, D., Delvaux, N., Marchal, S. *et al.* (2000). Testing health-care professionals' communication skills: the usefulness of highly emotional standardized role-playing sessions with simulators. *Psycho-Oncology*, July–August, **9(4)**, 293–302. Maguire Press.

53. Regehr, G. (2006). *The research and evaluation imperative in education.* (Presentation) EFPPEC Interprofessional Symposium on Palliative and End-of-life Education, London.

54. Kelly, L.J. (2001). Education in palliative care: making a difference to practice? *International Journal of Palliative Nursing*, **7(8)**, 401–7.

55. Hebert, M. (2006). Coming full circle in hospice palliative care telelearning: a case study approach. Final Evaluation Report, Telehealth/e-Health Research and Training Program, University of Calgary, Alberta.

Education and training in palliative medicine: training specialists in palliative medicine

Charles F. von Gunten, Gary Buckholz, and Frank D. Ferris

Palliative medicine is the physician discipline within the broad therapeutic model known as palliative care. Education and training in this discipline and model of care are devoted to producing an expert physician who participates in achieving the best possible quality of life for patients facing a life-threatening illness and for their families. The goals of the palliative medicine specialist are realized through the relief of suffering and the control of symptoms throughout the course of illness, including the time of death and the period of bereavement.

The practice of palliative medicine requires comprehensive age-appropriate assessment of the patient and family and participation in interdisciplinary, inter-professional care that can address physical, psychological, social, and spiritual needs. Palliative care helps the patient and family manage advanced illness and the prospect of death, assured that comfort will be a priority, values and decisions will be respected, spiritual and psychosocial needs will be addressed, practical support will be available, and opportunities for emotional growth and closure will exist.

Training in palliative medicine extends beyond competency in clinical care. A specialist in palliative medicine will want to acquire competency in education, programme-building, research, administration, and process (quality) improvement. In addition, because the specialist serves as a consultant to other physicians, a mastery of consultation etiquette is required.

The structure of a training programme in a particular country or setting will need to relate to the structure of the larger 'house' of medicine for which all physicians are trained. This chapter presumes that some readers want to make the case for specialist training in palliative medicine as well as advocate the development of new programmes to train specialist physicians in their own centres or countries. We imagine that this chapter, which has a US focus, adapted for a specific country, could serve as the document that could be submitted to a Minister of Health or Minister of Education in support of the development of palliative medicine training. Therefore, we start broadly with a rationale for specialist palliative medicine training as part of the professionalism of medicine and its social contract. Then we describe how training programmes are

structured as they relate to the prevailing scheme for training of doctors. Finally, we give some specifics about structuring a training programme, including evaluation of specialist competencies.

Rationale

The training of a physician requires the acquisition of knowledge and skill that exceeds that of others in society. In return for the benefit of that special knowledge and skill, society grants the medical profession semi-autonomous control over regulating its affairs and determining the standards for the admission and training of new members of the profession.

Formal training and recognition of a specialty must relate to formal training of physicians in general. Specialty training enhances professionalism in medicine by creating practice standards and well-defined competencies within a field of medical practice. The major clinical skills central to palliative medicine are the assessment and management of physical, psychological, and spiritual suffering faced by patients, with life-limiting illnesses, and their families. Communication and teamwork are critically important to achieving desired patient and family outcomes. Domains of knowledge and skill in palliative medicine can be subdivided further as shown in Table 20.3.1.

While these knowledge domains and skills overlap with the knowledge, attitudes, and skills that characterize other disciplines that care for patients with advanced illnesses, the specialty practice of palliative medicine is distinguished from other specialties by: (1) a higher level of clinical expertise in addressing the multidimensional needs of patients with life-threatening illnesses, including a practical skill set in symptom control interventions; (2) a high level of expertise in both clinical and non-clinical issues related to death and dying; (3) a commitment to working within an interdisciplinary team approach; and (4) the strong focus on the patient and family as the unit of care. Specialist level palliative medicine complements the core competency that should be maintained by other physician disciplines, particularly as it addresses the quality-of-life concerns of patients and families during the

Table 20.3.1 Domains of training in palliative medicine.

- Communication
- Ethical and legal decision-making
- Pain in cancer and non-cancer patients
- Management of non-pain symptoms
- Medical co-morbidities and complications in populations with life-threatening diseases
- Neuropsychiatric co-morbidities in populations with life-threatening diseases
- Psychosocial and spiritual support
- Death and dying
- Bereavement support for the family
- Quality improvement and research methodology in populations with advanced illnesses
- Interdisciplinary team work
- Legal and regulatory requirements
- Education
- Leadership and administration

period of advanced illness and the needs that arise specifically in the period surrounding the patient's death. Specialist level palliative medicine also seeks to improve the field through advocacy, teaching, research, and building new programmes.

The application of these specialist competencies improves the health and health care of the public. Formal recognition of these competencies by the larger 'house' of medicine lays the foundation for sustained, long-term excellence in the relief of suffering and compassionate care of the seriously ill and dying, by the medical profession.

The medical knowledge needed to relieve suffering and improve quality of life is greater now than in it has ever been in the history of medicine. Yet consistent application of this knowledge is not yet routine[1]. Specialization, and specialist training, can be seen as responses to the growth in medical knowledge and the need to make that knowledge available practically to patients and their families[2].

Palliative medicine needs to be integrated throughout the care system in a manner that mirrors other specialties. Generalist (sometimes called primary) palliative medicine is the responsibility of all physicians[3]. These generalist skills ensure that basic approaches to the relief of suffering and improving quality of life for the whole person and his or her family are made broadly available. As an analogy, every physician needs to be able to recognize angina pectoris. Specialist (sometimes called secondary) palliative medicine is the responsibility of trained professionals and hospital or community-based palliative care or hospice programmes. As an analogy, cardiologists and cardiology programmes only provide advice or care for some patients with heart disease. The role of the secondary specialist or programme is to provide consultation and assist the managing service with challenging cases. Tertiary palliative medicine is the province of academic centres where new knowledge is discovered through research, and new knowledge is disseminated through education. In addition, tertiary palliative care centres are likely to care for the most challenging cases.

Specialists in palliative medicine are needed to provide advanced care for patients and families whose needs exceed the capabilities of generalist or other specialist physicians. Palliative medicine specialists also have larger responsibilities to the field. They provide training and education to physicians and other health professionals, spearhead quality improvement initiatives, and undertake the research that will ultimately yield the evidence on which general medical practice should be based. Since the field is new, specialist physicians are called upon to advocate for the specialty as well as to participate in building programmes and administering them.

How does formal training lead to improved care?

Formal training sets standards on which the public can rely. Formal recognition of that training also represents the judgement of knowledgeable peers that a field is worthy of pursuit. Thus a formally recognized field can attract the 'best and the brightest' to commit their careers to developing the field further. This means that researchers will pursue efforts to extend and refine the knowledge base of the field, teachers will train the next generation of specialists, and administrators will devote resources to the clinical, research, and teaching needs of the specialty. Highly skilled specialists will be available to help with the most difficult patients and support their colleagues in improving care for all patients.

Are there risks associated with formal training of palliative medicine specialists?

Creation of another specialty does carry risks. Specialization can fragment health care further and drive up costs by adding yet another round of specialist consultations. Additionally, some are concerned that other physicians will 'dump' responsibility for palliative medicine exclusively into the lap of the specialist, when what patients desire and need is continuity. Alternatively, there may be a risk of alienating physicians already doing good palliative care, but not identifying themselves or practising as palliative medicine specialists. Proponents of palliative medicine specialty training address these concerns through careful delineation of the appropriate collaborative relationship between the consulting specialist and the primary attending physician.

An additional concern is that the development of a specialty will lead to physician domination of a field that values interdisciplinary-team-care using a bio-psycho-socio-spiritual model. Some also worry that widespread dissemination of palliative care throughout the health-care system will lead to a dilution or co-option of some essential essence of good palliative care. For instance, skeptics fear that hospital-based palliative care services—because of the culture inherent in hospitals—will be less likely to help patients return to their own homes and will be more likely to overuse diagnostic tests and procedures than in separate hospice programmes. Finally, some predict that the emergence of a cadre of academic palliative medicine specialists will engender a rift between teaching centres and the much larger world of community medicine.

These concerns are neither unique to palliative medicine nor inevitable. Specialist training in itself neither increases nor decreases the likelihood of these outcomes occurring. The root causes for these potential problems must be sought and prevented or redressed. They do not mitigate the driving rationale for professionalization of a field of new knowledge and practice of importance to the health of the public.

What are the criteria for recognition of a specialty?

In every country, the development of specialist training and its recognition by the medical profession rests on three criteria. First, the establishment of a specialist training programme signifies the differentiation of a new specialty, based on major new concepts in medical science. Second, the new specialty must represent a distinct and well-defined field of medical practice. Finally, the needed training must be sufficiently complex or extended that it is not feasible to include it in established training programmes.

Palliative medicine fulfils all of these criteria. The emergence of specialized journals, well-regarded textbooks, and formal curricula are all indicators of the development of a new and distinct body of knowledge. Research in the area of palliative medicine appears in general medical journals (like *The Lancet*, *The New England Journal of Medicine*) and at least seven specialized peer-reviewed journals: *Journal of Palliative Care* (Canada), *Journal of Pain and Symptom Management* (including supportive and palliative care, United States), *Journal of Palliative Medicine* (United States), *American Journal of Hospice and Palliative Care* (United States), *Palliative Medicine* (United Kingdom), *Progress in Palliative Care* (United Kingdom), and *European Journal of Palliative Care* (United Kingdom).

Models of physician practice in the field have been widely disseminated in the world. Physicians' work in hospice programmes, hospital-based palliative care consultation services and outpatient-based and home-based practices.

Formal training of specialists exists in each of the countries that have recognized the specialty. Curricula and training standards for each have been published[4–19].

Structure of training programmes

Conceptualizing a training scheme for palliative medicine requires relating it to the structure of training for all physicians in the country. Understanding how various countries organize medical training,

rationalizes some of the differences between the variability in required years of training for recognition as a specialist in palliative medicine. Entry into the profession is variable among countries. Table 20.3.2 shows a few examples that illustrate this variation. As a general rule, public education means the provision of 'grade school' to all its citizens without differentiation into a specialized track. In some countries, entry into the medical training occurs immediately after public school or 'grade' school. In others, the differentiation toward training in a profession happens earlier in the grade school curriculum. In only one country, the United States of America, a baccalaureate degree is required before entry into medical school. In others, the elements of a baccalaureate education are included in the medical school curriculum. Not all countries consider graduation from medical school to constitute a university doctorate; such countries require additional training for that distinction. Another way of conceptualizing a specialist training scheme is to answer the question, 'what knowledge and skills are expected of the physician before entering the palliative medicine training programme?'

What clinical resources are required?

All medical education is based on the observation that doctors learn their art through practice. A programme that trains specialists in palliative medicine relies on a well-functioning clinical programme that delivers palliative care to patients and their families. Since physician-training requires a graduated increase in responsibility for patient care in order to progress in skill, the trainee must be able to exercise supervised decision-making capacity in the provision of palliative care as part of the training experience.

The palliative medicine specialist provides care in two roles: consultant, and managing physician. Those roles are exercised in a variety of settings: hospitals, specialist units, specialty hospitals, long-term care including nursing homes, day hospitals, outpatient clinics, and home care. The clinical programme in which palliative medicine training is based needs to have enough breadth and depth

Table 20.3.2 Variation in training schemes for physician among example countries.

	Undergraduate medical education			Graduate medical education		
	Baccalaureate degree	Pre-clinical medical sciences	Clinical clerkships	Rotating internship or generalist training	Specialist	Subspecialty
Australia	2–3 years		2–3 years	1 year	2+ years	1+ year
Great Britain	5–6 years			2 years	2 years	4 years	
Germany	2 years		4 years		5–8 years	
Italy	3 years		3 years		3+ years	
Poland	2 years		4 years	1 year	3 years	1+ year
Portugal	4 years		2 years		3+ years	
Russia	2 years		4 years		1 year	
S. Africa	3 years		2 years	2 years	3+ years Registrar	
Sweden	2 years		4 years		3–5 years	1+ year
Switzerland	4 years		2 years		3+ years	
USA	4 years	2 years	2 years		3+ years residency	1+ year fellowship

of clinical experiences so that the trainee can demonstrate routinely the skills of a specialist before graduating from the programme.

At a minimum, training in three clinical sites is encouraged: (1) inpatient; (2) community; and (3) outpatient settings. Trainees should be exposed to patients with a wide variety of disease conditions and socioeconomic and cultural backgrounds. Trainees will want to have the opportunity to see patients in inpatient and community settings. Training programmes will demonstrate that clinical care and clinical teaching in all settings is provided in a collaborative manner among physicians and other health-care professionals. This collaborative practice model will use interdisciplinary team meetings for review and clinical decision-making. A consultation model, longitudinal care, and exposure to bereavement support need to be part of the training experience.

A programme in palliative medicine will allow trainees to acquire the knowledge and skills of consultative and managing palliative medicine as well as prepare them for a career in academic or community-based practice, focusing on the needs of patients with advanced chronic and terminal illnesses. Training is organized to provide a well-supervised experience at a level that allows trainees to acquire the competence of a specialist physician in the field.

What is needed institutionally?

One sponsoring institution takes responsibility for each training programme, even if training occurs among many institutions or clinical programmes. This sponsoring institution is responsible to ensure the existence and availability of those basic educational and patient care resources necessary to provide the palliative medicine trainee with meaningful involvement and responsibility in all aspects of the training programme. If training occurs across institutions and programmes, then a formal written affiliation agreement best acknowledges mutual responsibilities to provide high-quality care, adequate resources, and administrative support for the educational mission. In addition, the director at each site needs appropriate authority at that setting to carry out that portion of the training programme. Trainees need adequate supervision when present at participating institutions.

Modern facilities, to the same standard as elsewhere in the country, are needed to accomplish the overall educational programme. These facilities/resources will include a patient population adequate to meet the needs of the training programme in which the educational experiences take place. A diverse population of patients and their families representing a broad range of diagnoses and of palliative care needs, including patients with terminal illness, must be available for the trainees to provide meaningful care in a supervised environment. Exposure to special populations including children, the frail elderly, and cognitively impaired, patients with HIV disease, and patients with a history of chemical dependency is encouraged.

For each programme, the following clinical settings are needed: (1) inpatient acute care; (2) community (such as long-term care or specialist home care); and (3) outpatient care. It is necessary to have the support of nursing, social services, pastoral care, and allied therapies (including physical, occupational, and speech therapies), so that the trainee may collaborate in an interdisciplinary manner in the total care of the patient and family.

Access to a library with appropriate journals and texts in palliative medicine needs to be available. Library services should include electronic retrieval of information from medical databases.

Trainees need to learn the importance of life-long self-directed learning.

What faculty or training committee are needed?

A physician programme director will need considerable experience and expertise in palliative medicine and be committed strongly to the programme, in order to devote sufficient time to achieve the educational goals and objectives. This commitment is demonstrated by a level of institutional support that facilitates the management of the training programme by the programme director without other excessive responsibilities. The programme director will be experienced and qualified as a teacher, clinician, and administrator. The director will also demonstrate a career commitment to academic palliative medicine with participation in education and scholarly activity, including relevant research activities. The director will also demonstrate significant achievement in medical education, such as serving as a clinical supervisor in an inpatient or outpatient setting, performing curriculum development, or participating in didactic activities. It is strongly recommended in the United States that the programme director devotes an average of at least 20 h per week throughout the year to the training programme. In other countries the time devoted is usually less.

In addition to the programme director, each programme will need at least one other physician faculty member who devotes a substantial portion of professional time to the training programme. For programmes with more than two physician trainees, there should be at least 0.5 full-time equivalent additional physician faculty members for each additional trainee. Trainees need access to faculty engaged in administration and education as well as in clinical practice.

Potential physician faculty or training committee members will be designated as training faculty by the programme director. Criteria for being such a faculty member are included in Table 20.3.3. Some of the faculty may be drawn from collaborating programmes.

Because of the interdisciplinary nature of palliative medicine, the programme will maintain meaningful relationships with other medical specialty disciplines. Additional training faculty may include representatives from at least oncology, geriatric medicine, neurology, psychiatry, paediatrics, and anaesthesiology.

Given the importance of the team in specialist-level palliative medicine, the following health-care professional staff are identified in the United States as core members of the faculty, with major

Table 20.3.3 Criteria for physician faculty.

1	Extensive clinical experience in palliative medicine, typically amounting to at least 3 years during which at least 50 per cent of professional activities were related to palliative medicine or completion of an approved residency in palliative medicine
2	Evidence of substantial knowledge and skills in the discipline, based on interviews or letters of support, as well as evidence of attendance at courses, training programmes, visiting programmes in palliative medicine, etc.
3	Evidence of significant achievement in medical education, such as serving as a clinical supervisor in an inpatient or outpatient setting, designing and giving courses, etc.
4	Evidence of substantial achievement in academic palliative medicine in the form of publications or presentations at local or national meetings

responsibilities for the teaching of trainees: nurse, psychosocial clinician (such as a social worker or psychologist), and chaplain. In other countries, such as the United Kingdom, it is implicit that such professionals participate in training but are not usually members of the training committee.

What kind of interdisciplinary team (IDT) is needed?

An interdisciplinary team is an essential and fundamental aspect of palliative care. Palliative medicine trainees need access on an ongoing basis to an interdisciplinary team and need experience managing patient care in an interdisciplinary manner in all settings. Essential members of the interdisciplinary team are a physician, a nurse, a psychosocial clinician (such as a social worker or psychologist), and a chaplain. Additional desirable members of the team include a variety of individuals representing disciplines such as psychology, psychiatry, social work, dietetics, volunteers, nursing assistants, pharmacy, physiotherapy, occupational therapy, and music therapy.

How should the education programme be organized?

Traditionally, specialist training programmes are designed primarily with the criterion of time. A series of sites is selected, and a corresponding amount of time required in each setting is stipulated. The components are based on the local health-care system and the prevailing way that patients with advanced life-threatening illnesses are cared for.

Unfortunately, time alone does not ensure that a trainee will acquire the required attitudes, knowledge, and skills. Therefore, contemporary training schemes are moving to organizational structure based on the acquisition of competencies. A new programme will look at the competencies that are needed, and the average amount of time a well-selected trainee will need both to acquire and develop confidence in the practice of his or her new skills.

One way to organize the competencies needed in palliative medicine is to relate them to the six core competencies of all physicians described by the Accreditation Council for Graduate Medical Education (Table 20.3.4). Using this scheme, the palliative medicine training programme will require its trainees to broadly demonstrate competencies to the level expected of a new specialist practitioner. Individual training programmes provide the educational and clinical experiences for their trainees to be able to acquire the desired competency.

Clinical experiences will include opportunities to consult on and manage patients in a variety of settings. Trainees need the opportunity to provide ongoing care with responsibility for decision-making and management as well as consultative care for patients in all settings. This fosters the acquisition of assessment and management skills necessary for a specialist's evaluation and care of patients with complex palliative care needs.

A unique feature of the specialist role is that of clinical consultant. The trainee needs to develop skill in working collaboratively with referring physicians. Prior to specialist education, trainees with a general practice background assume that the patient and family is the primary object of professional attention; the 'customer' is always the patient. In contrast, when the specialist is a consultant to the managing service, the 'customer' is the managing service. The managing service may or may not implement the consultant's suggestions. New trainees to palliative medicine should

Table 20.3.4 Core physician competencies.

1	**Patient Care** that is compassionate appropriate, and effective for the treatment of health problems and the promotion of health
2	**Medical Knowledge** about established and evolving biomedical, clinical, and cognate (e.g. epidemiological and social–behavioural) sciences and the application of this knowledge to patient care
3	**Practice-Based Learning and Improvement** that involves investigation and evaluation of their own patient care, appraisal, and assimilation of scientific evidence and improvements in patient care
4	**Interpersonal and Communication Skills** that result in effective and age-appropriate information exchange and collaboration with patients, their families, and other health professionals
5	**Professionalism,** as manifested through a commitment to carrying out professional responsibilities, adherence to ethical principles, and sensitivity to a diverse patient population
6	**Systems-Based Practice,** as manifested by actions that demonstrate an awareness of and responsiveness to the larger context and system of health-care and the ability to effectively call on system resources to provide care that is of optimal value

not be expected to know the, frequently unwritten, rules of consultation etiquette (Table 20.3.5). Development of consultant skills facilitates both better patient care and education of the referring service. It also prevents conflict over who has power and control. Secondarily, skillful consultants help the palliative care programme grow and develop. They also model how to develop and nurture a clinical programme. Communication with all health-care team members, including the referring physician, prior to initiating new approaches to patient care is emphasized.

The programme should include a component that permits the trainee to acquire knowledge about the epidemiology and

Table 20.3.5 Consultation etiquette.

1	Respond to the request in a timely way
2	Determine the question to be answered by contacting the managing service.
3	Triage urgency
4	See the patient and family and review medical records
5	Contact the managing service BEFORE you write anything in the medical record to preliminarily communicate your initial clinical impression and suggestions and negotiate mutual roles and strategies
	a) Be brief and address the question asked
	b) Be specific about what you suggest (e.g. specific drugs, doses, and routes and titration schedules)
	c) Anticipate the future with contingency plans
6	Honour the managing service's authority; do not initiate communication and/or therapy with which they do not agree or know about
7	Teach with tact
8	Personal contact facilitates communication; Do not argue in the medical record
9	Follow-up; Be involved; Don't just disappear

pathophysiology of progressive chronic illnesses in persons of all ages, the management of these diseases in all settings, and the multiple issues associated with death and dying.

Attention will be directed not only to the physical but also to the behavioural, psychological, social, and spiritual aspects of illness. Communication skills and team-building are emphasized. All issues considered routinely by an interdisciplinary team, such as socioeconomic factors, cultural and ethnic diversity, religious background, and ethical and legal implications of practice decisions are addressed. Issues of regulatory compliance and quality improvement as applied to each setting will also be covered. An awareness of the potential for personal and family growth at the time of terminal illness is part of the educational programme. The programme encourages and facilitates professional self-care. Basic administrative concepts of programme management, financing for different care settings and public policy/advocacy are addressed.

Appropriate supervision and evaluation of the trainees is provided during all of the educational experiences.

Inpatient care

The inpatient setting may only take the form of a consultative team, but principal care management is highly desirable for at least a portion of training in the inpatient setting. Longitudinal follow-up is important so that the trainee participates in and experiences the outcomes of the care. An interdisciplinary team management approach to patients with acute medical and/or psychosocial problems will involve a full range of services usually ascribed to an acute-care general hospital, including the participation of nursing, social work, chaplaincy, diagnostic laboratory and imaging services, as well as personnel trained in state-of-the-art interventional palliation of pain and other symptoms. It is desirable that trainees have patient care experiences in both acute-care general hospitals and dedicated palliative care/hospice units as part of the training scheme. Learning objectives for this experience may include:

◆ Demonstrate expertise in acute physical symptom management and establish appropriate treatment plans by working closely with the pharmacist and other interdisciplinary team members:

• Choose appropriate medications and therapies.

• Recognize and respond to medication side effects.

• Titrate doses of medications using standard prescribing guidelines.

• Manage opioid infusions and patient-controlled analgesia (PCAs).

◆ Recognize the signs and likelihood of non-physical suffering by working closely with the interdisciplinary team:

• Demonstrate effective counselling skills and integrate other team members appropriately.

• Demonstrate an understanding of the concept of total pain.

◆ Determine goals of care collaboratively with patient and family by facilitating family meetings with other team members.

◆ Demonstrate effective teaching and teamwork and leadership skills:

• Choose appropriate times and methods to teach medical students, physician trainees, and others in an inpatient setting.

• Counsel and teach family members and staff around patients' last hours of living.

• Lead patient care rounds effectively and efficiently.

• Communicate effectively with other physicians important to the patient's care.

Specialist home care

This experience is designed to deliver care, with a team approach, to patients living in their homes who may require the services of multiple disciplines (including but not limited to nursing, social work, pastoral care, and bereavement counselling). The opportunity to deliver continuing care and to coordinate the implementation of recommendations from the interdisciplinary team is essential. Trainees will be involved in interdisciplinary team meetings while in this setting. The trainee will also be exposed to the organizational and administrative aspects of specialist community palliative care. Learning objectives for this experience may include:

◆ Demonstrate administrative and leadership skills with a home-care team.

◆ Demonstrate clinical skills such as assessment, communication, decision-making, and care-planning in the home environment.

◆ Demonstrate skills specific to the home-care environment such as adapting to limitations of the home as a setting for care and facilitating continuity of care.

◆ Care for a panel of home-care patients longitudinally to gain experience of continuity of care.

◆ Describe the roles, responsibilities, and potential contributions of all members of the team and demonstrate skills at working together as a team on a level playing field.

• Demonstrate family meeting skills in the home.

◆ Describe regulatory requirements unique to the home-care setting, such as safety around opioids.

◆ Demonstrate techniques to develop improved care within the community.

• Communicate with the patient's primary-care physician.

Long-term care

One or more long-term care institutions, such as a skilled nursing facility or chronic-care hospital, are a suggested component of the palliative medicine training programme. Trainees will be able to contribute to the care of the institution's patients through the provision of principal care or involvement in a consultative team, specialty clinic, or dedicated unit. Emphasis during this longitudinal experience will focus on: (1) the approach to diagnosis and treatment of the chronically ill patient (including acute-care needs) in a less technologically sophisticated environment than the acute-care hospital and/or specialist palliative care or hospice unit; (2) working within the limits of a decreased staff-to-patient ratio compared with acute-care hospitals; (3) the challenge of the clinical and ethical dilemmas that occur when caring for the terminally ill and the very old who are living in an institution designed for long-term care. Learning objectives for this experience may include:

◆ Perform geriatric assessments relevant to end-of-life care such as the Mini-Mental Status Examination, CAM clock, and three-item recall, Activities of Daily Living, Instrumental Activities of Daily Living, Braden pressure sore risk, fall risk, FAST dementia assessment, Karnofsky Performance Status Scale, World Health Organization Performance Status Scale, and New York Heart Association classification of congestive heart failure.

- Manage common geriatric syndromes and diseases such as frailty, dementia, depression, delirium, falls, pressure ulcers, incontinence, pain, urinary tract infections, urinary retention, constipation, Parkinson's disease, and stroke.

- Practice effective and meaningful primary and consultative hospice and palliative care in the long-term setting.

- Demonstrate the necessary knowledge of skilled nursing facility regulations that affect physician practice.

- Participate in interdisciplinary team work focusing on older adults.

- Develop prescribing patterns appropriate for older adults; address polypharmacy.

- Evaluate elderly patients for hospice services.

- Assess and manage elder abuse.

Outpatient care

An outpatient care setting, such as an outpatient palliative care, day hospital, hospice care clinic, or other clinic providing relevant palliative intervention is a desirable component of the training programme. The availability of multiple health-care professionals, capable of providing input to the patient's care is needed. Learning objectives for this experience may include:

- Demonstrate expertise in management of chronic physical symptoms and establish appropriate treatment plans:

  - Choose appropriate medications and therapies.

  - When chronic opioids are a viable option, learn proper use of partnership agreements and medication contracts/process of prescribing.

- Establish suitable therapies for patients with a high level of psychological distress associated with chronic illness, collaboratively with team members.

- Facilitate the progression referral for hospice care when appropriate.

- Demonstrate techniques to develop the specialist practice within the community:

  - Communicate with the patient's primary-care physician.

Continuity of care

Each trainee will participate meaningfully in the care of a panel of patients throughout the training period, following these patients where possible across multiple care settings. This fosters an understanding of the continuum of care for the palliative patient. In one of the community settings, the trainee will assume responsibility for a panel of patients, providing ongoing care. A log of patients and primary diseases will document this component.

Electives

No programme, no matter how well designed, meets all of the needs of its trainees. Therefore, it is highly desirable that at least some elective time be made available. Elective time in a clinically relevant field is recommended and may include:

- Interventional pain service.

- Paediatrics.

- Clinical Psychology.

- Psychiatry.

- Clinical/radiation oncology.

- Medical oncology.

- HIV/AIDS Care.

- General Practice.

- Additional geriatric medicine.

- International palliative medicine.

- Integrative/complementary medicine.

- Business development.

- Wound care.

- Respiratory, cardiology, or neurology clinics, etc.

Conferences

Didactic as well as clinical learning opportunities will be provided to the trainee. Conferences or seminars/workshops in palliative medicine should be designed specifically for the trainee to augment the clinical experiences. Specific consideration of articles published in the medical literature or other activities that foster interaction and development of skills in interpreting the medical literature are necessary. Trainees will participate both as learners and teachers in supplemental, educational opportunities such as the conferences listed earlier, communication-skills workshops, lecture series, and in both medical undergraduate education. It is also important that trainees participate in multi-disciplinary teaching and in teaching to multi-disciplinary groups.

Appropriate experiences designed to refine educational and teaching skills of the trainees need to be part of the programme.

Research and quality improvement programme

Palliative care research spans a very broad spectrum, and it is unlikely that the training faculty will have all the research knowledge and skills to meet the needs of all trainees. Therefore, working relationships with faculty from other relevant disciplines will be important, and some may be selected as research mentors for trainees. However, the primary responsibility for the trainee resides with the palliative medicine programme director. The completion of a scholarly project or quality improvement project by each trainee during the training programme is strongly encouraged in some programmes. Any trainee who desires an academic career in palliative medicine will want to complete training beyond that required for clinical competency, which will probably include the development and completion of a research project and, in some settings, a higher degree by research.

Mentorship

Mentorship results from the direct and personal relationship that develops between a trainee and someone more senior in the field. A trainee needs guidance through extensive and repeated contact with someone who has 'been there and done that' during their palliative medicine education. Mentorship includes teaching awareness of the professional stages of development. One model describes the emotional responses to training in palliative care as proceeding from intellectualization to emotional distancing for emotional survival to aspects of depression, to the development of emotional coping strategies, to the development of deep and sustainable compassion. Without mentorship, these predictable emotional responses to specialist training may cause the trainee prematurely to leave the field or develop maladaptive coping strategies. Mentors encourage self-reflection and help acknowledge counter-transference, secondary traumatic stress or vicarious traumatization through case review. Inevitable conflict within the training environment requires an experienced ear to learn the needed coping skills. The trainee will need help choosing the right career path and negotiating job opportunities. After the palliative medicine education is complete, the graduate continues to need a colleague/mentor for challenging cases or situations in the months and years that follow.

While the role of mentorship is essential, it is difficult to determine the best way to assure mentorship for trainees. Mentors can be assigned by the programme or chosen by the trainee. When assigned, it may not be the ideal match. When the trainee has been handed the task of finding a mentor, it can be intimidating to establish the relationship. Early in the months of training, the programme director will want to encourage trainees to choose or name a mentor among the faculty. The mentor could be a physician or another professional from the interdisciplinary team. Trainees can be told that faculty members are expecting the possible question 'Will you be my mentor?' It is helpful to label the relationship.

What should the curriculum be?

A curriculum, strictly defined, is a series of educational experiences designed to achieve defined learning objectives. In the case of specialist palliative medicine training, the curriculum is the sum of all experiences, clinical and didactic, which produce the new specialist physician. These experiences occur not just during 'regular business hours' but when the trainee is 'on call' or involved in conferences. The curriculum needs to ensure the opportunity for trainees to achieve the knowledge, skills, attitudes, and behaviours, as well as the reservoir of practical experience that engenders confidence. The specialist palliative medicine curriculum will contain the content and skill areas listed in Table 20.3.6.

The question that is most often asked is, 'how long' should a trainee rotate in each of the areas described in the section on structure? This is a challenging question to answer.

From an ideal point of view, each component of the programme is long enough to achieve the competencies expected of a specialist. As an appendix to this chapter, a list of competencies developed in the United States represents an attempt to help a prospective programme director answer this question.

Who is a good candidate for training?

A programme will decide the pre-requisites for consideration of a candidate for training. Criteria will vary depending on the country and programme. Some criteria will be contingent on the laws and regulations. The admission policy needs to ensure that all trainees have demonstrable competence in assessment and treatment of the range of medical conditions likely to be encountered in a palliative medicine population. Alternatively, the training programme needs

Table 20.3.6 Content and skills covered in the palliative medicine curriculum.

Epidemiology, natural history, and treatment options for patients with common chronic diseases and life-threatening medical conditions including paediatrics
History of the development of the discipline of palliative medicine
Age-appropriate comprehensive assessment including physical, cognitive, functional, social, psychological, and spiritual domains using history, examination, and appropriate laboratory evaluation; assessment of suffering and quality of life should be included
The role, function, and development of the inter-disciplinary team and its component disciplines in the practice of palliative care
Management of common co-morbidities and complications in patients with life-threatening illness
Management of neuropsychiatric co-morbidities in patients with life-threatening illnesses
Management of symptoms in palliative care patients, including various pharmacologic and non-pharmacologic modalities, and pharmacodynamics of commonly used agents; symptom management shall also include patient and family education, psychosocial and spiritual support, and appropriate referrals for other modalities such as invasive procedures
Management of palliative-care emergencies, e.g. spinal cord compression, suicidal ideation
Management of psychological, social, and spiritual issues of palliative care patients and their families
The natural history, phenomenology, and management of grief and bereavement, and the role of the interdisciplinary team in providing support to bereaved family members
Assessment and management of patients in community settings, such as home, long-term care
Care of the dying patient including managing terminal symptoms, patient/family education, bereavement, and organ donation
Economic and regulatory aspects of palliative care including national health policy issues and national financing mechanisms
Ethical and legal aspects of palliative care including but not limited to those pertinent to infants, children, adults, and geriatric populations
Cultural aspects of palliative care including issues relating to geographic location (urban vs. rural) ethnicity and socioeconomic status
Communication skills with patients, families, professional colleagues, and community groups
Ability to function as a consultant
Scholarship including research methodologies enabling interpretation of the medical literature and research methodologies appropriate to end-of-life-care settings and populations
Skills in quality improvement methodologies applicable in end-of-life-care settings
Teaching skills relevant to the practice of palliative care
Leadership and teamwork skills
Administrative and regulatory requirements for the practice of palliative medicine.
Professional self-care, e.g. self-reflection, lifelong learning, balancing work and personal interests

Table 20.3.7 Characteristics of a potential palliative medicine trainee.

Characteristic	Rationale
Positive perspective on life	Able to identify 'hope' in challenging situations
Spirit of inquiry, curiosity, learning	Palliative care is about accompanying the patient/family on a journey. Work is suited to an 'explorer' not a 'hero' or 'rescuer'
Altruistic	Oriented to the 'other' rather than the 'self'
Professional orientation	Able to be energized, nourished, and sustained by professional accomplishment rather than by patient/family praise
Committed to own discipline	Avoids boundary issues with other team members
Patient-focused, family-centred	This model supports palliative care goals
History of positive functioning within teams, groups, community organizations	Not a place to escape due to previous frustrations in these settings; avoid the 'lone ranger' that wants to do everything/be everything to the patient/family; avoid the 'angry' person who has an axe to grind with the health-care system
Maturity	Look for seasoning in life and a breadth of experience; (now unlikely in some countries due to changes in postgraduate training)
Recent losses	History of recent losses may indicate need to 'work out' personal needs rather than focus on patient/family needs

to ensure that these competencies are acquired before completion of the training programme.

Additional criteria are more challenging to identify. The training programme will want to identify the kind of specialist physician it wants to produce. Table 20.3.9 lists some general guidelines for choosing someone who will work well in the team environment of palliative care.

The interview is the most important part of the recruitment process. It is best to combine enthusiasm about your programme with honesty about shortcomings. Do not describe the programme as you wish it to be. Focus on getting information that is not in the written materials the candidate has already read. Try to get a personal 'gut' sense of the candidate. Encourage the candidate to describe specific instances in some detail rather than talk in generalities. For example, instead of asking, 'Why do you want a career in palliative medicine?' ask the question, 'Describe a patient that really captured why you want to go into this field'. While you will want to find out about the person's interests, experience, and accomplishments, include the following areas in your interview. Is this someone you could imagine working with for a year or more? Do you like this person? Does this person seem to have good judgement? Maturity? Is this person open to feedback from non-physician team members? Do you trust this person independently to take care of your patients and their families? Do you share similar enthusiasm for the work? Is this someone that works well in an interdisciplinary team model? Will the candidate fit in with the culture at your institution or programme? Is this person a cheerful problem-solver or an inveterate complainer? Is this person interested in working hard or in coming to your city or programme for reasons unrelated to the work? Is the person working toward something or looking to escape? The composite answers to these questions will help lead you to the candidates you seek. In the United Kingdom, 'Modernising Medieval Careers' has led to a number of problems with appointing trainees, including, for now, an undermining of the 'traditional interview'.

A particular challenge lies with the programme that has a number of 'slots' for trainees that need to be filled in order to meet the needs of the patients it serves. If you are interviewing to 'fill a slot' rather than selecting candidates who will do the best in your training environment, you are less likely to choose candidates that are ideal for your setting.

How should palliative medicine trainees be evaluated?

Programme faculty will want to provide regular evaluation of trainees' knowledge, skills, and attitudes in relation to the practice of medicine in general, and the competencies of palliative medicine in particular. Components of an evaluation will include, at a minimum, assessment of competence in patient care, clinical knowledge, interpersonal skills and communication, professionalism, knowledge of clinical systems, and commitment to continuous learning and quality improvement. Written criteria and standards will be developed to assess each of these domains.

In collaboration with members of the programme, teaching staff, and the interdisciplinary team, the programme director will want to provide a formal evaluation of the knowledge, attitudes, skills,

Table 20.3.8 Domains of programme evaluation by trainees.

- Quality of the curriculum
- Required and elective clinical experiences
- Trainees' needs
- Quality of one-on-one supervision and mentoring
- Faculty teaching responsibilities
- Feedback procedures
- Availability of financial and administrative resources and support
- Contribution of different clinical services to teaching
- Volume and variety of patients available for educational purposes
- Performance of members of the teaching staff
- Research experiences (if offered)

and professional growth of the trainees, at least semi-annually. The formal evaluation will include the development of a process for progressive improvement of assessment measures to evaluate competencies. The programme will want to implement the use of assessment tools that measure the trainee's actual attainment of competency rather than resting solely on faculty opinions about the general nature of the trainee's progress. The programme will also want to provide feedback to the trainee about his/her performance at the completion of each clinical rotation, not less than quarterly. Many programmes ask the trainee to develop an activity log and monitor trainee progress in completing appropriate clinical activities and procedures; (an 'activity log' is documentation with countersignature by supervising faculty of successful completion of the determined minimum number of activities and procedures). There should be an increase in the responsibilities of the trainee, commensurate with evidence of his/her ability to meet expected standards of practice. The programme will also want to maintain a permanent record of evaluation for each trainee and make it accessible to the trainees, site visitors, and other authorized personnel as required. Finally, at the conclusion of the programme, the programme director will provide a final written evaluation for each trainee who completes the programme, including documentation that the trainee has demonstrated a minimal level of competency in the core domains of palliative medicine, to practice independently and competently, and retain this evaluation as part of the trainee's permanent record. In cases of problematic performance, the programme will want to provide verbal and written feedback to trainees about strengths and weaknesses in performance, and a written plan of remediation with delineation of consequences of performance below the minimum standards set by the programme. Finally, the programme will want to establish fair procedures, as established by the sponsoring institution, regarding academic discipline and trainee complaints or grievances. It is also helpful to decide prospectively when, and how, a trainee will be asked to leave the programme.

How should palliative medicine faculty be evaluated?

A formal mechanism for regular written evaluation of the teaching staff by the programme director needs to exist, including provisions for confidential participation by trainees. Faculty evaluations should address: teaching ability, clinical knowledge, communication skills, professional attitudes, and role-modelling competencies. The results of such evaluations can be used for faculty counselling and for selecting faculty members for specific teaching assignments.

How should the training programme as a whole be evaluated?

The training programme should use trainee feedback and performance for the purpose of continuous quality improvement. The teaching staff will want to meet regularly with at least one trainee representative to review programme goals, objectives, structure and resources, and overall educational effectiveness. The balance between clinical service, teaching, and research should be assessed. The domains in Table 20.3.6 should be reviewed and documented. Pertinent accreditation standards will provide another approach to evaluating the programme as a whole.

Provision will be made for trainees to evaluate the training programme in writing at least annually. The results of such evaluations should be used to improve individual trainee and overall programme performance.

How should graduates of the programme be evaluated?

Each programme will want to maintain a system of evaluation of its graduates. The training programme will want to obtain feedback on demographic and practice profiles, licensure, and specialist advisory committee/board certification, and suggestions for programme development from the graduates after they have entered into practice. The performance of trainees on any certification examinations will be reviewed as data about attainment of educational goals.

Summary

The content and processes of Palliative Medicine Training described earlier will not be appropriate for every setting; however, the idea is to provide a template, which can be adapted for different countries/settings.

References

1. Sepulveda, C., Marlin, A., Yoshida, T., Ullrich, A. (2002). Palliative Care: The World health Organization's global Perspective. *Journal of Pain and Symptom Management*, **24**, 91–6.
2. Field, M.J. and Cassel, C.K. (eds.) (1997) *Approaching death: improving care at the end of life*. Washington, DC: National Academy Press.
3. von Gunten, C.F. (2002). Secondary and Tertiary Palliative Care in US Hospitals. *Journal of the American Medical Association*, **287**, 875–81.
4. Billings, J.A. and Block, S. (1997). Palliative care in undergraduate medical education. *Journal of the American Medical Association*, **278**, 733–43.
5. Block, S.D., Bernier, G.M., Crawley, L.M. *et al.* (1998). Incorporating palliative care into primary care education. *Journal of General Internal Medicine*, **13**, 768–73.
6. Barnard, D., Quill, T., Hafferty, F., Arnold, R., Plumb, J. *et al.* (1999). Preparing the ground: contributions of the pre-clinical years to medical education for care near the end-of-life. *Academic Medicine*, **74**, 499–505.
7. Meier, D.E., Morrison, R.S. and Cassel, C.K. (1997). Improving Palliative Care. *Annals of Internal Medicine*, **127**, 225–30.
8. Arnold, R. (2003). The challenges of integrating palliative care into postgraduate training. *Journal of Palliative Medicine*, **5**, 801–7.
9. Association for Palliative Medicine of Great Britain and Ireland (http://www.palliative-medicine.org).
10. Canadian Society of Palliative Care Physicians (http://www.cspcp.ca).
11. Australia & New Zealand Society of Palliative Medicine (http://www.anzspm.org.au).
12. Von Gunten, C.F., Sloan, P., Portenoy, R., Schonwetter, R. (2000). Physician board certification in hospice and palliative medicine. *Journal of Palliative Medicine*, **3**, 441–7.
13. Emanuel, L.L., von Gunten, C.F., Ferris, F.D. (eds.) (1999) *The Education for Physicians on End-of-life Care (EPEC) Curriculum*, www.epec.net.
14. Schonwetter, R.S., Hawke, W., Knight, C.F., (eds.) (1999). *Hospice and Palliative Medicine Core Curriculum and Review Syllabus*. American Academy of Hospice and Palliative Medicine. Dubuque, Iowa: Kendall/Hunt Publishing Company.
15. Ferris, F., Balfour, H., Bowen, K. *et al.* (2002). A model to guide patient and family care. Based on nationally accepted principles and norms of practice. *Journal of Pain and Symptom Management*, **24**(2), 106–23.

16. Billings, J.A. (2000). Palliative medicine fellowship programs in the United States: Year 2000 survey. *Journal of Palliative Medicine*, **3**, 391–6.
17. Billings, J.A., Block, S.D., Finn, J.W. *et al.* (2002) Initial Voluntary Program Standards for Fellowship Training in Palliative Medicine. *Journal of Palliative Medicine*, **5**, 23–33.

Appendix 20.3.1
Hospice and palliative medicine core competencies version 2.1

Patient and family care

The specialist trainee in palliative medicine should demonstrate compassionate, appropriate, and effective care, based on the existing evidence base in palliative medicine, aimed at maximizing well-being and quality of life for patients with advanced, progressive, life-threatening illnesses, and their families, and provide care in collaboration with an interdisciplinary team.

Gathers comprehensive and accurate information from all pertinent sources, including patient, family members, health-care proxies, other health-care providers, interdisciplinary team members, and medical records

Obtains a comprehensive medical history and physical exam, including:

- Patient understanding of illness and prognosis.
- Goals of care/advance care planning/proxy decision-making.
- Spirituality.
- Detailed symptom history (including use of validated scales).
- Psychosocial and coping history including loss history.
- Functional assessment.
- Quality-of-life assessment.
- Depression evaluation (including stressors and areas of major concern).
- Pharmacologic history including substance dependency or abuse.
- Detailed neurological exam, including mental status exam.

Correctly interprets existing diagnostic tests/procedures

Performs appropriate diagnostic workup; reviews primary source information and evaluation; determines prognosis and appropriate palliative course

Utilizes information technology; accesses on-line evidence-based medicine resources; uses electronic repositories of information, and medical records

Synthesizes and applies information in the clinical setting

Develops a prioritized differential diagnosis and problem list

Develops recommendations based on patient and family values

Routinely obtains additional clinical information (from other physicians, nurses, pharmacists, social workers, case managers, chaplains, respiratory therapists) when appropriate

Bases care on patient and family preferences and goals of care, evidence, clinical experience and judgement, and input from the interdisciplinary team (IDT)

Demonstrates a patient-family-centred approach to care

Makes recommendations to consulting physicians as appropriate

Makes recommendations to patient and family based on patient's past history, current clinical status, prognostic information, and patient and family and goals

Provides patient and family education

Educates families in maintaining and improving level of function to maximize quality of life

Explains palliative care services, recommendations, and latest developments to patients and families

Educates patient and family about disease trajectory and how and when to access palliation in future

Demonstrates care that shows respectful attention to age, gender, sexual orientation, culture, religion/spirituality, as well as family interactions and disability

Demonstrates use of the interdisciplinary approach in regard to their influence on the clinical situation as well as the individual's disability

Managing physical symptoms, psychosocial, and spiritual distress of the patient and family

Adjusts care plan according to the patient's care setting, values, and goals of care

Recognizes/reassesses physical and seeks to preserve opportunities within psychosocial and spiritual dimensions of individual and family life in the context of life-threatening illness and injury

Recognizes the potential value of completing personal affairs/unfinished business and relationships may have to patients and members of their families

Reassesses psycho-spiritual symptoms frequently, and makes therapeutic adjustments as needed

Seeks to maximize the patient's level of function and quality of life for patients and families

Evaluates level of function and functional decline

Evaluates quality of life over time

Provides expertise in maximizing patient's level of function and quality of life

Coordinates and facilitates with other members of the interdisciplinary team family meetings, consultation on goals of care, advance directive completion, and conflict resolution, continued but more moderate life-extending care and forgoing interventions

Recognizes signs and symptoms of impending death and appropriately cares for the imminently dying patient and family members

Effectively prepares family, other health-care professionals, and caregivers for the patient's death

Provides appropriate information about all settings of the palliative care continuum: acute and palliative care unit hospital, home and inpatient hospice, nursing home, and other community resources, to ensure smooth transitions across settings

Initiates care-setting planning early in course of care

Provides timely information to patients and families, and facilitates decision-making, about palliative care treatment settings

Works effectively as part of an interdisciplinary team to formulate optimal care-setting planning from health-care institutions

Provides support to the bereaved

Involves interdisciplinary team members in supporting the bereaved

Interprets and communicates eligibility for the Medicare/Medicaid hospice benefit and explains the integration of hospice services into the existing care plan

Provides treatment to the bereaved

Involves interdisciplinary team members in treating the bereaved

Appropriately refers family members to bereavement programmes

Recognizes the developmental stages in bereavement

Recognizes and differentiates complicated from non-complicated bereavement among family members of the deceased patients with life-threatening illnesses

Identifies individuals at high risk of complicated grief

Recognizes concept of suicidal risk in the dying and in the bereaved

Refers patients and family members to other health-care professionals to assess, treat, and manage patient- and family-care issues outside the scope of palliative care practice

Recognizes the need for collaborative disease-directed and palliation referral in order to deliver good medical care

Effectively collaborates with and makes referrals to paediatricians with expertise relevant to the care of children with advanced, progressive, and life-threatening illness

Accesses specialized paediatric and geriatric palliative care resources appropriately

Medical knowledge

The specialist trainee in palliative medicine should demonstrate knowledge about established and evolving biomedical, clinical, population science, and social–behavioural sciences relevant to the care of patients with life-threatening illnesses and to their families, and relate this knowledge to hospice and palliative care practice.

Explains the scope and practice of hospice and palliative medicine, including:

Domains of hospice and palliative care

History of hospice and palliative medicine

Settings where hospice and palliative care are provided

Elements of patient assessment and management across different hospice and palliative care settings, including home visit, nursing home visit, inpatient hospice unit visit, outpatient clinic visit, and in hospital patient visit

The Medicare/Medicaid Hospice Benefit, including essential elements of the programme, eligibility, and key regulations for all levels of hospice care

Barriers for patients and families to access hospice and palliative care

Recognizes the role of the interdisciplinary team in hospice and palliative care

Describes the role of the palliative physician in the interdisciplinary team

Identifies the various members of the interdisciplinary team and their roles and responsibilities

Recognizes how and when to collaborate with other allied health professionals, such as nutritionists, physical therapists, respiratory therapists, occupational therapists, speech therapists, and case managers

Describes concepts of team process and recognizes psychosocial and organizational elements that promote or hinder successful interdisciplinary team function

Explains how to assess and communicate prognosis

Identifies what elements of history and physical are critical to formulating prognosis for a given patient

Describes common chronic illness diagnoses with prognostic factors, expected natural course and trajectories, common treatments, complications, and the range of usual course

Describes effective strategies to communicate prognostic information to patients, families, and health-care providers

Recognizes the presentation and management of common cancers, including their evaluation, prognosis, treatment, patterns of advanced or metastatic disease, emergencies, complications, associated symptoms, and symptomatic treatments

Identifies common diagnostic and treatment methods in the initial evaluation and ongoing management of cancer

Identifies common elements in prognostication for solid tumours and hematological malignancies at various stages, including the natural history of untreated cancers

Describes patterns of advanced disease, associated symptoms, and symptomatic treatments for common cancers

Describes the presentation and management of common complications of malignancy, i.e. hypercalcaemia and brain metastases, and emergencies, i.e. seizures and haemorrhage

Describes the presentation and management of common non-cancer life-threatening conditions, including their evaluation, prognosis, treatment, patterns of disease progression, complications, emergencies, associated symptoms, and symptomatic treatments

Identifies markers of advanced disease in common non-cancer life-threatening conditions, such as congestive heart failure, chronic obstructive pulmonary disease, and dementia

Recognizes patterns of advanced disease, associated symptoms, i.e. dyspnoea for congestive heart failure and dysphagia for dementia, and symptomatic treatments for common non-cancer life-threatening conditions

Recognizes the presentation and management of common complications of non-cancer life-threatening conditions, i.e. pulmonary oedema and psychosis, and emergencies, i.e. myocardial infarction for coronary artery disease and stroke for cerebrovascular disease

Describes palliative management of common life-threatening conditions in such special settings as the intensive care unit and emergency department

Explains principles of assessing pain and other common non-pain symptoms

Describes the concept of 'total pain'

Explains the relevant basic science, pathophysiology, associated symptoms and signs, and diagnostic options useful in differentiating among different aetiologies of pain and non-pain symptoms

Describes a thorough assessment of pain and other symptoms, including the use of appropriate diagnostic methods and symptom-measurement tools

Describes how to complete a functional assessment of pain and non-pain symptoms

Names common patient, family, health-care professional, and health-care system barriers to the effective treatment of symptoms

Describes the use of opioids in pain and non-pain symptom management

Lists the indications, clinical pharmacology, alternate routes, equianalgesic conversions, appropriate titration, toxicities, and management of common side effects for opioids

Describes appropriate opioid prescribing, monitoring of treatment outcomes, and toxicity management in chronic, urgent, and emergency pain conditions

Describes appropriate opioid prescribing in different clinical care settings: home, specialist trainee in palliative medicinal hospice, hospital, long-term care facility

Describes the concepts of addiction, pseudo-addiction, dependence, and tolerance, and describes their significance in pain management, as well as approaches to managing pain in patients with current or prior substance abuse

Explains the legal and regulatory issues surrounding opioid prescribing

Describes the use of non-opioid analgesics, adjuvant analgesics, and other pharmacologic approaches to the management of both pain and non-pain symptoms

Identifies the indications, clinical pharmacology, alternate routes, appropriate titration, toxicities, and management of common side effects for: acetaminophen, aspirin, NSAIDs, corticosteroids, anticonvulsants, anti-depressants, and local anaesthetics used in the treatment of pain and non-pain symptoms

Identifies the collaborative role of pharmacists in safe and effective pain management

Describes the use of non-pharmacologic approaches to the management of pain and non-pain symptoms

Identifies indications, toxicities, and appropriate referral for interventional pain management procedures

Identifies indications, toxicities, management of common side effects, and appropriate referral for radiation therapy

Identifies indications, toxicities, and appropriate referral for surgical procedures commonly used for pain and non-pain symptom management, i.e. venting gastrostomy

Identifies indications, toxicities, and appropriate referral for commonly used complementary and alternative therapies, i.e. acupuncture, aromatherapy, guided imagery

Explains the role of allied health professions in pain and non-pain symptom management, such as speech, physical, respiratory, and occupational therapy

Describes the aetiology, pathophysiology, diagnosis, and management of common neuropsychiatric disorders encountered in palliative care practice, such as depression, delirium, seizures, and brain injury

Recognizes how to evaluate and treat common neuropsychiatric disorders

Describes how to refer appropriately to neurological and mental health professionals

Describes knowledge of the indications, contraindications, pharmacology, appropriate prescribing practice, and side effects of common psychiatric medications

Recognizes the diagnostic criteria and management issues of brain death, persistent vegetative state, and minimally conscious state

Recognizes common psychological stressors and disorders experienced by patients and families facing life-threatening conditions, and describes appropriate clinical assessment and management.

Recognize psychological distress

Describes concepts of coping styles, psychological defenses, and developmental stages relevant to the evaluation and management of psychological distress

Describes how to provide basic supportive counselling and to strengthen coping skills

Recognizes the needs of minor children when an adult parent or close relative is seriously ill or dying, and provides appropriate basic counselling or referral

Recognizes the needs of parents and siblings of children who are seriously ill or dying and to provides appropriate basic counselling or referral

Explains appropriate utilization of consultation with specialists in psychosocial assessment and management

Recognizes common social problems experienced by patients and families facing life-threatening conditions and describes appropriate clinical assessment and management

Able to assess, counsel, support, and make appropriate referrals to alleviate the burden of caregiving

Able to assess, provide support, and make appropriate referral around fiscal issues, insurance coverage, and legal concerns

Recognizes common experiences of distress around spiritual, religious, and existential issues for patients and families facing life-threatening conditions, and describes elements of appropriate clinical assessment and management

Describes the role of hope, despair, meaning, and transcendence in the context of severe and chronic illness

Describes how to perform a basic spiritual/existential/religious evaluation

Describes how to provide basic spiritual counselling

Identifies the indications for referral to chaplaincy or other spiritual counsellors and resources

Knows the developmental processes, tasks, and variations of life completion and life closure

Able to recognize, evaluate, and support diverse cultural values and customs with regard to information-sharing, decision-making, expression and treatment of physical and emotional distress, and preferences for sites of care and death

Recognizes major contributions from non-medical disciplines, such as sociology, anthropology, and health psychology in understanding and managing the patient's and family's experience of serious and life-threatening illness

Able to manage the syndrome of imminent death

Identifies common symptoms, signs, complications, and variations in the normal dying process and their management

Describes strategies to communicate with patient and family about the dying process and to provide support

Recognizes the elements of appropriate care of the patient and family at the time of death and immediately thereafter

Describes appropriate and sensitive pronouncement of death

Identifies the standard procedural components and psychosocial elements of post-death care

Recognizes the potential importance and existence of post-death rituals and how to facilitate them

Describes the basic science, epidemiology, clinical features, natural course, and management options for normal and pathologic grief

Demonstrates knowledge of elements of bereavement follow-up, including assessment, treatment, and referral options for bereaved family members

Recognizes the risk factors, diagnostic features, epidemiology, and management of depression, and complicated grief, and how they differ from normal grief

Describes common issues in the palliative care management of paediatric and geriatric patients and their families that differ from caring for adult patients, in regard to physiology, vulnerabilities, and developmental stages

Describes ethical and legal issues in palliative and end-of-life care and their clinical management

Discusses ethical principles and frameworks for addressing clinical issues

Describes federal, state, and local laws and practices that impact on palliative care practice

Consults clinical ethicist appropriately

Describes professional and institutional ethical policies relevant to palliative care practice

Practice-based learning and improvement

The specialist trainee in palliative medicine should be able to investigate, evaluate, and improve their practices in caring for patients and families and appraise and assimilate scientific evidence relevant to palliative care.

Maintains safe and competent practice, including self-evaluation and continuous learning

Demonstrates an ability to self-reflect on personal learning deficiencies and develop a plan for improvement

Demonstrates knowledge of and commitment to continuing professional development and life-long learning

Demonstrates knowledge of the roles and responsibilities of the trainee/mentor

Demonstrates the ability to reflect on his/her personal learning style and use different opportunities for learning

Demonstrates the ability to actively seek and utilize feedback

Demonstrates the ability to develop an effective learning relationship with members of the medical community faculty

Accesses, analyses, and applies the evidence base to clinical practice in palliative care

Demonstrates knowledge of, and recognizes limitations of evidence-based medicine in palliative care

Actively seeks to apply the best available evidence to patient care and encourages others to do so

Shows ability to apply evidence-based medicine to facilitate safe, up-to-date palliative clinical practice

Develops competencies as an educator

Recognizes the importance of assessing learning needs in initiating a teaching encounter

Reflects on benefits and drawbacks of alternative approaches to teaching, and the role of different teaching techniques to address knowledge, attitudes, and skills

Shows respect towards other learners

Describes the importance of defining learning goals and objectives as a basis for developing educational sessions

Demonstrates the ability to supervise clinical trainees and give constructive feedback

Demonstrates knowledge of the process and opportunities for research in palliative medicine

Recognizes and values the importance of addressing ethical issues in palliative care research

Is realistic about the benefits and challenges of palliative care research and supports research as appropriate to the setting

Recognizes and values the uses of data to demonstrate clinical, utilization, and financial outcomes of palliative care

Describes common approaches to quality and safety assurance

Demonstrates an openness and willingness to evaluate and participate in practice and service improvement

Demonstrates knowledge of palliative care's clinical, financial, and quality-of-care outcome measures

Demonstrates awareness of and adherence to patient safety standards

Interpersonal and communication skills

The specialist trainee in palliative medicine should be able to demonstrate interpersonal and communication skills that result in effective relationship-building, information exchange, emotional support, shared decision-making and teaming with patients, their patients' families, and professional associates.

Initiates informed relationship-centred dialogues about care

Assesses patient/family wishes regarding the amount of information they wish to receive and the extent of their participation in clinical decision-making

Determines, in collaboration with patient/family, the appropriate participants in discussions concerning a patient's care

Assesses patient's and family members' decision-making capacity, and other strengths and limitations on understanding and communication

Enlists legal surrogates to speak on behalf of a patient when making decisions for a patient without decision-making capacity

Recognizes differences between relationship-centred dialogues in adult and paediatric palliative based on physiology, vulnerabilities, and developmental stages

Demonstrates empathy

Uses empathic and facilitating verbal behaviours such as: naming, affirmation, normalization, reflection, silence, listening, self-disclosure, and humor in an effective and appropriate manner

Employs empathic and facilitating non-verbal behaviours such as: touch, eye contact, open posture, and eye-level approach in an effective and appropriate manner

Demonstrates ability to effectively recognize and respond to own emotions

Expresses awareness of own emotional state before, during, and after patient and family encounters

Reflects on own emotions after patient and family encounter or related event

Effectively processes own emotions in clinical setting in order to focus on the needs of the patient and family

Responds to requests to participate in spiritual or religious activities and rituals, in a manner that preserves respect for both the patient and family, as well as one's own integrity and personal and professional boundaries

Self-corrects communication miscues

Demonstrates the ability to educate patients/families about the medical, social, and psychological issues associated with life-limiting illness

Demonstrates self-awareness and ability to recognize differences between the clinician's own and the patient and family's values, attitudes, assumptions, hopes, and fears related to illness, dying, and grief

Recognizes the importance of serving as an educator for patient/family

Identifies gaps in knowledge for patients/families

Communicates new knowledge to patients/families adjusting language and complexity of concepts based on the patient/family's level of sophistication, understanding, and values, as well as on developmental stage of patient

Educates patients/families about normal developmental processes for life review, completion of practical affairs and relationships, and achievement of a satisfactory sense of life completion and closure

Identifies patients/families who may benefit from a language-translation service or interpreter

Refers patients/families with special needs to appropriate resources

Educates legal surrogates in preparation for role as medical decision-makers

Uses age, gender, and culturally-appropriate concepts and language when communicating with families and patients

Routinely assesses patients/families to identify individuals who might benefit from age, gender, and culturally-appropriate interventions or support

Shows sensitivity to developmental stages and processes in approaching patients/families

Appreciates the need to adjust communication strategies to honour different cultural beliefs

Demonstrates the above skills in the following paradigmatic situations with patients or families and documents an informative, sensitive note in the medical record:

◆ Giving bad news.

◆ Discussing transitions in goals of care from a curative and/or life prolonging focus to palliative care.

◆ Introducing option of palliative care consultation.

◆ Discussing goals of care including advance care planning and resuscitation status.

◆ Discussing appropriate care settings.

◆ Discussing the end-of-life care needs of a dying child with parents.

◆ Discussing the needs of minor children of dying adults.

◆ Withholding and withdrawing of any life-sustaining therapy.

◆ Continuing life-sustaining therapy with focus on palliation.

◆ Discussing enrollment into hospice.

◆ Dealing with requests for physician aid in dying.

◆ Discussing palliative sedation.

◆ Discussing artificial hydration and nutrition.

- Discussing severe spiritual or existential suffering.
- Referring to tasks-of-life review, completion of personal affairs, including relationships and sexuality, and social and spiritual aspects of life completion and closure.
- Saying good-bye to patients or families.
- Pronouncing death in presence of patient's family.
- Writing condolence notes and making bereavement calls.

Organizes and leads or co-facilitates a family meeting

Identifies when a family meeting is needed

Identifies appropriate goals for a family meeting

Demonstrates a step-wise approach in leading a family meeting

Demonstrates techniques for mediating intra-family or family–health-care team conflict

Documents the course and outcome of a family meeting in the medical record

Collaborates effectively with others as member or leader of Interdisciplinary Team (IDT)

Facilitates efficient team meetings

Accepts and solicits insights from IDT members regarding patient and family needs in evolving the patient's plan of care

Manages and recognizes the need for conflict resolution in IDT meetings

Provides constructive feedback to IDT members

Accepts feedback from IDT members

Develops effective relationships with referring physicians, consultant physicians, and other health-care providers

Provides a concise verbal history and physical exam presentation for a new palliative care patient

Summarizes the active palliative care issues and treatment recommendations for a known patient in signing out to or updating a colleague

Communicates with referring and consultant clinicians about the care plan/recommendations for the patient and family

Communicates with health-care providers when there is disagreement about treatment plans

Works toward consensus building about treatment plans and goals of care

Supports and empowers colleagues to lead and participate in family meetings

Elicits concerns from and provides emotional support and education to staff around difficult decisions and care scenarios

Maintains comprehensive, timely, and legible medical records

Documents legible notes in the medical record in a timeframe consistent with individual programme and institutional requirements

Adapts documentation to different medical record formats available or required in different settings

Follows documentation guidelines pertinent to local settings and regulatory agencies

Completes the major domains of palliative care (as per the National Consensus Project) in the initial history and physical exam

Consistently includes all relevant domains of palliative care (as per the National Consensus Project) in progress notes and follow-up documentation

Appropriately documents death pronouncement in the medical record and completes death certificate in a correct and timely manner

Professionalism

The specialist trainee in palliative medicine should be able to demonstrate a commitment to carrying out professional responsibilities, possess an awareness of their role in reducing suffering and enhancing quality of life, adherence to ethical principles, and sensitivity to a diverse patient population.

Achieves appropriate balance between needs of patients/family/team, while balancing one's own need for self-care

Describes effective strategies for self-care, including balance, emotional support, and dealing with burn-out and personal loss

Contributes to team wellness

Explains how to set appropriate boundaries with colleagues and with patients and families

Recognizes own role and the role of the system in disclosure and prevention of medical error

Assesses personal behaviour and accepts responsibility for errors when appropriate

Discloses medical errors in accord with institutional policies and professional ethics

Demonstrates accountability to patients, society, and the profession; and a commitment to excellence

Describes role of hospice medical director in terms of quality of care, compliance, and communication with other professionals

Fulfils professional commitments

Responds in a timely manner to requests from patients and families for medical information

Responds appropriately to requests for help from colleagues

Demonstrates accountability for personal actions and plans

Fulfils professional responsibilities and works effectively as a team member

Appropriately addresses concerns about quality of care and impaired performance among colleagues

Treats co-workers with respect, dignity, and compassion

Demonstrates knowledge of ethics and law that should guide care of patients, including special considerations around these issues in paediatric and adult palliative care, including:

- Foregoing life-sustaining treatment.
- Confidentiality.
- Truth-telling.
- Decision-making for children, and adolescents, and older patients with dementia.

- Limits of surrogate decision-making.
- Decision-making capacity.
- Conflicts of interest.
- Use of artificial hydration and nutrition.
- Requests for aid in dying.
- Research ethics.
- Nurse–physician collaboration.
- Principle of double effect.
- Organ donation.

Demonstrates respect and compassion towards all patients and their families, as well as towards other clinicians

Demonstrates willingness and ability to identify own assumptions, individual and cultural values, hopes, and fears related to life-limiting illness and injury, disability, dying, death, and grief

Displays sensitivity to issues surrounding age, ethnicity, sexual orientation, culture, spirituality and religion, and disability

Effectively communicates the mission of palliative medicine to hospital administrators, clinicians, and community at large

Systems-based practice

The specialist trainee in palliative medicine should be able to demonstrate an awareness of and responsiveness to the larger context and system of health-care, including hospice and other community-based services for patients, including children, and families, and the ability to effectively call on system resources to provide high-quality care.

Demonstrates care that is cost-effective and represents best practices

Recognizes relative costs of medications and other therapeutics/interventions

Implements best evidence-based practices for common palliative medicine clinical scenarios across settings

Explains the rationale for the use of medication formularies

Identifies similarities and differences between reimbursements for palliative medicine vs. hospice vs. hospital, vs. home health vs. long-term care

Describes basic concepts and patterns of physician billing, coding, and reimbursement across settings

Evaluates and implements systems improvement based on clinical practice or patient and family satisfaction data, in either personal practice, team practice, or within institutional settings

Reviews pertinent clinical or patient/family satisfaction data about personal, team, or institutional practice patterns

Integrates knowledge of health-care system in developing plan of care

Describes policies and procedures of pertinent health-care systems

Describes philosophy, admissions criteria, range of services, and structure of hospice care

Recognizes resources and barriers relevant to the care of specialized populations in palliative medicine, and has basic knowledge of how to mobilize appropriate support for these populations (e.g. paediatric patients, HIV patients, etc.)

Describes differences in admission criteria for various settings such as hospitals, palliative care units, skilled-nursing and assisted-living facilities, acute/sub-acute rehab facilities, and long-term acute-care settings as well as traditional home hospice

Collaborates effectively with all elements of the palliative care continuum, including hospitals, palliative care units, nursing homes, home and inpatient hospice, and other community resources

Effectively utilizes members of interdisciplinary team to create smooth and efficient transitions across health-care settings for patients and families

Communicates with care managers/appropriate staff across sites to enable seamless transitions between settings

Communicates with clinicians at time of care transitions to clarify and coordinate care plan across settings

Advocates for quality patient and family care and assists patients and families in dealing with system complexities

Communicates and supports patient and family decision-making about discharge planning—including settings of care, service options, and reimbursement/payer systems

Coordinates and facilitates dialogue between patients/families and service provider representatives (e.g. hospice liaison nurses, nursing home administrators; and inter-hospital departments including but not limited to ICU, intermediate care, emergency department)

Partners with health-care managers and providers to assess, coordinate, and improve patient safety and health care, and understands how these activities can affect system performance

Describes hospital and palliative medicine programme continuous quality improvement programmes and their goals and processes

Demonstrates ability to work with managers of varying disciplines to improve patient safety and system-based factors that affect care delivery

20.4

The role of the humanities in palliative medicine

Deborah Kirklin

My journey has two intertwined threads, elements which mirror each other as exactly as the two chains of the double helix. One is the medical history: the physical injury, the illness, the happening, the happened, the inevitable, and the unavoidable. The parallel thread is my emotional response: the disbelief, the grief, the doubt, the flung out, the banter, the bargaining, the accepting, the clenching of teeth, the sick to the teeth, the pain, the no-gain. Why me? Why me now?

(From The healing touch: the necessity for humanity in medicine and the humanities in medical education.
Michele Petrone)[1]

All journeys have highs and lows. Palliative medicine has come a long way in its own physical and spiritual journey. The care of those whose condition is not amenable to cure has, for many, been transformed by Cicely Saunders' determination to allow patients to chart their own courses. By including the humanities in the education section of this volume, the editors are encouraging practitioners and educators to draw on the wealth of human experience and wisdom embodied in the arts and humanities in their important work. This chapter will examine the potential role of the humanities in the education and training of all those looking after other human beings in the final part of their life journey. Firstly, the power of words, to reflect our conception of palliative medicine and to shape its nature, will be examined. Secondly, an overview of the framework whereby educational initiatives are and could be delivered, will be provided. Thirdly, the educational objectives that can be addressed specifically in this way will be illustrated with extracts from poetry and prose. Finally, the special area of caring for dying children will be highlighted. Educational resources which may be of interest to practitioners and educators will be suggested.

Background

A biomedical education cannot equip someone in their late teens or early 20s to understand the reactions of a bereaved person, the reactions of someone terrified to learn they have a life-threatening condition or the devastation of long-term disability.
(From Portfolio learning: the humanities in medical education.
Ilora Finlay)[2]

(What I'm looking for is a doctor) who is a close reader of illness and a good critic of medicine . . . someone who can treat body and soul . . . I'd like my doctor to scan me, to grope for my spirit as well as my prostate.
(From The patient examines the doctor Anatole)[3]

The last decade has seen an increasing enthusiasm amongst health-care professionals and educators to establish a role for the arts and humanities in both undergraduate and postgraduate medical education, and in continuing professional development. The humanities place expressing, exploring and interpreting the human condition as central to human philosophical and artistic endeavour. It is the deceptively simple imperative to make these pursuits integral to daily clinical practice that is fundamental to the humane practice of medicine. There is, however, no consensus about precisely which disciplines constitute the inter-disciplinary field of medical humanities. Literature, art, medical history, anthropology, theology and philosophy are integral to many courses. Creative writing, music, medical journalism and drama are also widely used.

Learning how to address the complex and important needs of those requiring palliative care poses as many emotional as it does intellectual challenges[4,5]. Willingness to think about and be open to new and sometimes uncomfortable ideas, an ability to use metaphors of life and death to help explain feelings there are no other words for, and a capacity to engage with the person at the centre of the medical drama are all vital. Later in this chapter three educational objectives, that among them aim to facilitate this ideal of learning, will be detailed. First, however, the importance of the words used to describe the subjects of those doctors' concern will be examined.

The power of words
Definitions and their consequences

Palliative medicine is 'the study and management of patients with active, progressive, far-advanced disease for whom the prognosis is limited and the focus of care is the quality of life'.

. . . the active total care of patients whose disease is not responsive to curative treatment. Control of pain, of other symptoms, of

psychological, social and spiritual problems is paramount. The goal of palliative care is achievement of the best quality of life for the patients and their families.

WHO definition[6]

In attempting to mark out the area of medical practice that falls within the province of palliative care, the importance of an ability to evaluate critically and select the language used in medicine, and more specifically in this field, will be illustrated. These terms have practical implications for patients and their families that are increasingly apparent as palliative medicine develops as a speciality with its own guiding principles, clinical goals and established practices. The words used to categorize the condition of patients help decide who does and does not fall under the care of palliative physicians. This, in turn, affects the resources that can be made available to the patient and family both in terms of medical and nursing care and social support. Use of the language of palliative care for a particular person implies changed expectations, for patients, carers and professionals, about the quality and length of life of the patient and the nature of the medical interventions they will be offered. Thinking about the words used in this field and examining what these terms imply is a practical way to initiate the learning process, discussed above, whereby learners must be willing to think about and be open to new and sometimes uncomfortable ideas.

Cure, care, and compassion

Above all else, those with distressing chronic or terminal illnesses need continuity of care—that is, the attention and friendship of one doctor whom they can come to trust and with whom they can share their hopes and fears.

(From *The Inhumanity of Medicine* David Weatherall)[7].

He was so pathetically reduced that Pelagia felt no shame in remaining with him even when he was naked, and she did not have to resort to delivering instructions from the far side of the door. His muscle was gone, and the skin hung about his bones in flaccid sheets.

She did not feel very much like a healer when she saw those feet, however; they were unrecognisable as such. They were a necrotic, multi-hued pulp . . . The stench was inconceivably stupefying, and at last Pelagia felt herself flood with the sacred compassion whose absence had so previously appalled her.

(From *Captain Corelli's Mandolin* Louis de Bernieres)[8]

'The surgeons
Are not going
To operate.
They've had a look
At your scan,'
He said,
'And it's too near
All the lymph glands
And all like that,
The arteries.'
He said.
It was too dangerous.
I was
Disappointed.
I think that

Was more disappointing
Than being told
I had cancer,
Because that
Was my cure.
To cut it out
And then it was
Away.

(From *I knew . . .* Presented by S. Murray *et al.*)[9]

Palliative medicine has of course already been defined on numerous occasions throughout this book. One part of those definitions inevitably focuses on the incurable nature of the conditions being addressed. Pellegrino and Thomasma equate cure with 'the eradication of the cause of an illness or disease, to the radical interruption and reversal of the natural history of the disorder'[10]. One danger of the cure-orientated model of health care is that, when cure is no longer possible, words and phrases such as 'untreatable' and 'beyond help' become all too easy to employ[11]. In contrast to the bleak, defeatist and demoralizing assumptions implied by these terms, the palliative care model requires strident and proactive efforts to be directed towards the alleviation of distressing symptoms and the maximization of quality of life. Words do matter and the words used in palliative care can and should provide hope, dignity, control and choice at a time when they are sorely needed.

The use of the word care in this context is also worthy of attention. Care is emphasized in palliative medicine and yet surely caring for patients is something that all physicians should do. Care is juxtaposed to treatment and treatment is somehow associated with cure. Caring is a positive goal and one which all patients would surely wish their doctors to aspire to. The implicit trade-off between care and treatment is not only erroneous given that the ongoing treatment of distressing symptoms is central to good palliative medicine and the care inherent in curative treatment, but potentially distressing to patients and their families who fear that the initiation of palliative care means the ending of the treatment of any conditions. The fostering of the inherent ability of all human beings to care for others is to be encouraged in all doctors. Caring should be integral to all medical care whether curative or palliative.

Finally, if care involves compassion, then the response of Louis de Bernières', Pelagia to the diseased and pitiful form of her ex-lover, Mandras, provides an interesting paradox. Only when Pelagia gains some psychological detachment from Mandras does she finally feel a sense of compassion for him. Before then her private anxieties and physical revulsion left this emotion disturbingly absent. This apparent contradiction, that only through emotional distance was compassion made possible, in some sense underlies the friendship that David Weatherall says a good doctor–patient relationship entails[7]. Whilst we will not always like our patients and would not perhaps choose them as friends in our private lives, nevertheless our compassion for them can enable us to value them and we would hope thereby to earn their trust and friendship.

Terminal

Of course, if incurability were the only element characterizing those conditions where care was deemed palliative, then much of medical practice would fall within the remit of palliative medicine. In chronic conditions such as arthritis and asthma, despite the clear intention to prevent premature death, we currently have no cure.

A significant emphasis is placed on the alleviation of distressing symptoms. These conditions are kept under control rather than cured and often contribute to the person's death.

In order to define more precisely those areas for which palliative care physicians might be responsible, the terminal nature of the condition is usually emphasized, as in the WHO definition. This emphasis, however, raises its own questions. Brief consideration of just two of those questions will serve to exemplify the sort of conundrum that might keep philosophers, linguists and physicians engaged for a considerable time. Firstly, precisely how long need the remaining (predicted) life span be to qualify as terminal, and secondly, is old age terminal? Few in this field would argue with the assertion that the answer to the first question is inevitably arbitrary depending as much on matching workload to available resources as on logic and consistency, although this statement might come as more of a surprise to the lay public. Whilst the mere posing of the second question is contentious, it is not easily dismissed[12]. Ironically, if we choose not to designate old age as incurable and terminal, then the need to develop and deliver properly resourced and co-ordinated care, now considered core in palliative care, might not be acknowledged adequately. Given the physical, social, and psychological vulnerability of very old and frail people this is precisely the sort of care from which they would benefit. The answers given by a society, a health-care system or by individual practitioners to questions like these can, and daily does, have profound effects on the patient's experience of the last part of their life. The irony inherent in this apparently sharp demarcation between curative medicine and palliative medicine has not of course escaped the attention of the latter's practitioners, and indeed the proper areas of concern of the palliative care team constitute an ongoing debate.

The emphasis on the terminal nature of conditions, although of value in helping define educational and training objectives, has the potential to distract the gaze of caregivers from the life being lived as attention is paid to the act of dying. Palliative care physicians are, therefore, often at pains to point out that palliative care is concerned with the life lived as well as the death of the individual concerned. For individuals, there is no sharp demarcation between the life they are living before and after the designation of incurable and terminal is made and so the emphasis on caring in palliative medicine is one that we would do well to re-embrace in curative medicine. Moreover, with the growing debate in recent years about the provision of palliative care and training in the context of both critical care and long-term care, the relevance of palliative care training to all physicians is once more underlined.

An appreciation of the tendency of patients, their families and their professional carers to focus on the impending death of the patient is important in understanding a number of important educational needs that the humanities can help address. Nevertheless it behoves us all to remember that the emotional and spiritual needs of those who are ill and those who care for them do not magically appear when the patient becomes eligible for the services of the palliative care team. Thus, any lessons the humanities can offer to the palliative care physician must surely be of value to all those living through the experience of illness. Carefully facilitated discussions involving health-care practitioners, patient representatives, managers, economists and policy makers about these and other issues would be beneficial, not only for palliative care, but also for areas of patient care outside the palliative physicians' remit.

Unbearable words

'You know perfectly well you can do nothing to help me, so leave me alone.'
'We can ease your suffering,' said the doctor.
'You can't even do that; leave me alone.'
. . . The doctor said [to the patient's wife] his physical suffering was dreadful, and that was true; but even more dreadful was his moral agony, and it was this that tormented him most.
. . . What had induced his moral agony was that during the night . . . It occurred to him that what had seemed utterly inconceivable before—that he had not lived the kind of life he should have— might be true.

(From *The Death of Ivan Ilyich* Leo Tolstoy)[13]

The physical, moral and spiritual agony of Ivan Ilyich stands in sharp contrast to Cicely Saunders' vision. A good education in palliative care should equip physicians with the knowledge, skills and attitudes to do much to minimize all of these agonies. Unfortunately, not all of the causes of such suffering, particularly the moral and spiritual ones, will be either apparent or amenable to physician directed intervention. Seeing this anguish at first hand can be unbearable for all concerned and can result in a protective distance being placed between the patient and carer. Leo Tolstoy feared a death like Ivan Ilyich's for himself and chose to confront his own fears in his writing. Palliative care physicians, although not perceiving their patient's death as a failure, may interpret suffering like Ivan Ilyich's as just that. Meeting him on paper and trying to understand the origin of his difficulties may provide some preparation for patients they meet who are struggling to find peace.

Unspeakable words

Other words have the potential to be so unbearable that they can become unspeakable. These include the words of patients who are thinking about ending their own lives or seeking help to do so. In many ways, this appears to be a taboo subject within palliative medicine and Cicely Saunders' sincerely felt opinion, that a call for euthanasia is an indictment of the care being given, is often quoted in response. Undoubtedly, there will be cases in which more can be done to ease the many types of suffering already alluded to and as a consequence people may well change their minds and want to live out what remains of their natural life span. However, there will remain cases where, despite optimal symptom control and psychosocial support, the patient remains steadfast in their wish to control the manner and time of their death. A recent UK legal case, involving a woman in the terminal phase of motor neuron disease wanting her right to assisted suicide to be recognized as a human right, provides an example of this.

Whilst death is clearly not viewed as a sign of failure in palliative care, it would seem that a call from the patient for help in dying often is. It is not my intention to discuss the case either for or against euthanasia and for a more detailed discussion of this important issue readers are encouraged to read Randall and Downie's excellent book about palliative care ethics. It is, however, important to consider the potential consequences that could flow from the over-simplistic equation that calls for euthanasia equal failure of palliative care. There is a danger that the wishes of the individual concerned would then be de-emphasized in the efforts of the team to 'get it right' and 'sort things out'. Some things cannot be sorted out and no matter how disturbing and distressing and contrary to the values of the attending physician, the wishes of the patient deserve to be listened to and acknowledged. One can only assume that the public support given by her GP to the lady with motor neuron disease mentioned above was very important to her. I do not know what that GP's personal moral views were in this case but his support of his patient's right to have her views listened to are an example to us all.

Spiritual words

When the priest came and heard his confession, he relented, seemed to feel relieved of his doubts and therefore of his agony, and experienced a brief moment of hope.

(From *The Death of Ivan Ilyich* Leo Tolstoy)[14]

The dying man was still screaming desperately and flailing his arms. One hand fell on the boy's head. The boy grasped it, pressed it to his lips, and began to cry. At that very moment Ivan Ilyich fell through and saw a light, and it was revealed to him that his life had not been what it should have been but that he could still rectify the situation.

(He then feels overwhelming compassion for his daughter and wife, who, he now realises, are suffering enormously. The focus of his concern is to ease their pain, not his own. Finally his life is what it should be.)

He searched for his accustomed fear of death and could not find it. Where was death? What death? There was no fear because there was no death. Instead of death there was light.

…

'It is all over,' said someone standing beside him.
He heard these words and repeated them to his soul.
'Death is over,' he said to himself. 'There is no more death.'
He drew in a breath, broke off in the middle of it, stretched himself out, and died.

(From *The Death of Ivan Ilyich* Leo Tolstoy)[15]

Happy the man, and happy he alone,
He who can call today his own; he who, secure within, can say,
Tomorrow, do thy worst, for I have lived today.

(John Dryden (1631–1700))[16]

Whilst it is clearly beyond the scope of this chapter to give even a cursory overview of the many sources of spiritual comfort and distress, I offer this prose and poetry to encourage quiet contemplation about the spiritual journeys that patients make a short time before the rest of us. For some, the journey is eased by religious belief, for others the love of close friends and family allows peace. Sadly, the journey is often lonely and demanding. The palliative care practitioner has both the honour and the duty to be a true and steadfast travelling companion.

Delivering education and training

… too many patients are unprepared for death, too many have symptoms left untreated and too many families are left to face this time feeling isolated and alone.

(From Emmanuel 1997 quoted in MacLeod)[17]

There is and always will be more to do in the education and training of physicians and the humanities can only hope to contribute to that important work. By describing work currently taking place in this field, this chapter is intended to offer the reader

insight into some of the approaches which the humanities can offer. By providing suggestions for further reading as well as highlighting available educational resources, it is hoped that those interested in this work will feel encouraged to include the humanities in their educational programmes. Like all areas of education, clear learning objectives need to be identified and appropriate assessment of students and evaluation of teaching effectiveness undertaken.

The General Medical Council (GMC)

When, in 1993, the GMC document *Tomorrow's doctors*[18] suggested that the humanities could be gainfully employed in undergraduate medical education, the media suggested were already familiar to those working with patients in palliative care. Art therapy and poetry therapy are just two examples of widely used approaches to enable patients to contemplate their own responses to their illness. *Tomorrow's Doctors* required medical schools to develop and deliver optional undergraduate courses called special study modules (SSMs) to allow students to pursue areas of particular interest to them in further depth. Specifically, those planning SSMs were encouraged to provide humanities modules such as literature and medicine[19]. A number of medical schools in the United Kingdom have responded by doing just that.

Moreover, the GMC's plans for revalidation will require all physicians to provide evidence of reflective practice, good communication skills, sensitivity to ethical concerns and a demonstration of both appropriate attitudes and patient-centred practice. The humanities can offer palliative care physicians practical and enjoyable ways to meet those expectations.

Undergraduate medical education

The development of humanities courses in this field has been patchy but encouraging. Many of these courses remain unreported and those developing them often work in relative isolation, unaware of similar efforts elsewhere. In the United States and Canada, work began several years ago to collate all available information about medical humanities courses on one universally accessible on-line database. This initiative has proven both popular and practical, with a large number of courses now listed of which many are directly or indirectly relevant to palliative care. Many of these courses in North America remain optional but in an increasing number of centres this work is now core and compulsory. In the United Kingdom details of a growing number of courses have been published and a database of UK medical humanities courses is now available on-line. Details of how to access both of these databases are provided under Further reading.

Postgraduate training

Postgraduate training in palliative care should address not only the clinical and psychosocial needs of patients and relatives but also those of the practitioner. There are encouraging signs in medicine as a whole that issues beyond the clinical management of a patient are being given more weight. Beginning in 2001 and for the first time since the Royal College of Physicians (RCP) began to examine doctors for membership, communication skills and appreciation of ethical and legal concerns are now systematically assessed. As a result, postgraduate training will now need to address these issues. In the same year the RCP published the first UK textbook in Medical Humanities thus endorsing the educational value that such courses can offer. Despite these promising signs, a lack of familiarity with the techniques and learning opportunities afforded by the humanities, as well as variable access to expert support in this area, will remain a problem for the foreseeable future. One of the important tasks facing academics in this field is, therefore, the development of educational resources to support those wishing to incorporate medical humanities into local training programmes; details of existing resources will be provided at this end of this chapter. In addition, training courses need to be available to interested clinicians and educators to enhance their confidence and skills base as well as guiding them to local expertise and support. Again details will be given below.

Continuing professional development

The concept of continuing professional development (CPD) represents a learning ideal where the educational and support needs of the maturing practitioner are addressed from the perspective of all those involved in the therapeutic context of his or her work. Thus, the needs of patients, their families, the community, the health-care team and those of the practitioner all determine the ongoing programme of education and support that should be CPD. Implicit in this definition of CPD are three elements that medical humanities purport to address. The first requires the doctor to appreciate the varied and often conflicting perspectives of patients, families and professionals. The second involves reflection on the strengths and weaknesses of the individual's practice—an ability to build on the former and address the reasons behind the latter. The third focuses on the support required by a practitioner engaged in caring for the sick, both as a professional and as a person. These three educational objectives will be considered below with examples from existing educational initiatives.

An integrated approach

Films, music, poetry, artworks, other visual stimuli may all be potent sources of learning and directly relevant to the problems of the patient being studied.

(From *Medical Humanities* Ilora Finlay)[20]

Although optional courses such as SSMs are extremely valuable in allowing students to consider important areas in greater depth, there is a compelling argument for the incorporation of training in palliative care into the core curriculum. If the humanities are to contribute to this training then this too will need to be within the core curriculum possibly either as part of the standard clinical training described earlier in this volume, or as a complementary but independent component of the courses. The value of this is attested below in the section 'Painting a roomful of bad news', which also provides a practical example of how this can be done.

Educational objectives

Reflecting

A key objective for medical humanities educators is to enable practitioners to reflect on their own thoughts, feelings, inclinations, practice and experience. Importantly, the process of reflection offers individuals an opportunity to gain new insights into the strengths and weaknesses of their own practice and into the nature of their own spiritual journey. This objective acknowledges both the participation of practitioners in the lived experience of illness,

and the fact that illness affects not only patients and their families but also those caring for them. The response of physicians to illness is far more than a scientific answer to biomedical challenges. Recognition of the individual needs, fears and values of physicians is, therefore, essential if they are to move beyond their own feelings and concerns and be able to place those of the patient central to their endeavours. To illustrate how the humanities might enable this reflection, I will describe the use of practical art in enabling both students and established practitioners to understand how fears for their own mortality can be evoked by the illness of patients. Recognizing this is an important step if practitioners are to be prepared psychologically to help another individual face their own death.

The wounded healer

The ailing physician remains a paradox to the average mind, a questionable phenomenon. May not his scientific knowledge tend to be clouded and confused by his own participation, rather than enriched and morally reinforced? He cannot face disease in clear-eyed hostility to her; he is a prejudiced party, his position is equivocal. With all due reserve it must be asked whether a man who himself belongs among the ailing can give himself to the cure or care of others as can a man who is himself entirely sound.

(From *Magic Mountain*, Thomas Mann)[21]

While (the doctor) inevitably feels superior to me because he is the doctor and I am the patient, I'd like him to know that I feel superior to him, too, that he is my patient, and I have my diagnosis of him.

(From 'The patient examines the doctor' Anatole Broyard)[3]

*O body swayed to music, O brightening glance,
How can we know the dancer from the dance?*

(From *Among school children* W.B. Yeats)[22]

How can we know the physician from the care he gives, the doctor from the therapy? In medicine, the practitioner not only diagnoses and administers treatment he is part of the diagnosis and part of the treatment. In the curative model of medicine, being a patient is about being sick and maybe dying and being a doctor is about making the patient better and sending death packing. But as Anatole Broyard points out, diagnosing is also the domain of the patient. This may involve a conscious act as in Broyard's case. More often perhaps an unconscious recognition of the healer's own wounds, psychological and spiritual, acts as an empathic bridge to the shared humanity which underpins a close doctor–patient relationship. This recognition of the wounds of the healer has led some to wonder who it is in fact that is the greatest beneficiary in the therapeutic relationship between doctor and patient.

The concept of the wounded healer underlies a psychological interpretation of the nature of the doctor–patient relationship that has resonance for many experienced practitioners. At the same time as the healer within the doctor reaches out to the wounded within the patient, so the wounded within the doctor reaches out to the patient for healing. Moreover, the participation of the wounded part of the healer in the relationship is essential for its success. Without this part of his or herself, the doctor cannot connect fully with the patient. The wounds of the healer may be overt and apparent or the doctor may not even be conscious of their existence. These wounds, which evidence the mortality of both patient and healer, represent the shared vulnerability that enable human beings to relate with one another at an emotional and psychological level. If these wounds remain unacknowledged, even at the subconscious level, then the result may be an inability to forge a fully therapeutic relationship between doctor and patient. Put simply, it will be difficult to establish rapport and trust.

Mortality

Now if, as Thomas Mann asserts, the ailing physician is a paradox to the average mind then, presumably, the mortal physician is a paradox too. And, in the cartoon world of doctors doing battle with death, there is indeed a paradox if the doctor's own mortality, his personal identity with death, is acknowledged. Yet, the palliative care physician, like all other practitioners, has at least one very important thing in common with his or her patient—they will both die. Uncertainty is something humans deal with poorly but this particular certainty, that we will all die, is one we seem psychologically adept at ignoring. The diagnosing of a 'terminal' condition is an unwelcome and public affirmation of this certainty for the individual concerned. The shunning experienced by dying patients or those diagnosed with conditions such as cancer (often equated in the lay mind with death), reflects in part the unwelcome reminder this gives to us all of our own mortality. The psychological sleight of hand by which we maintain our illusion of immortality is found wanting. The trick is exposed as cheap and flawed. Yet, unlike the lay public, doctors cannot shun the bearers of this uncomfortable reminder of their own mortality. In bringing himself or herself, the wounded healer, to the therapeutic relationship, doctors must face not only their patient's mortality but also their own. They must face their own fears as well as those of the patient. What follows is a description of how practical art can be used with both students and practitioners to help them do just that.

Painting a roomful of bad news

Clinical communication skills, now formally taught as part of all undergraduate medical courses, are also beginning to be introduced into the postgraduate training of various specialities. Breaking bad news is one of the topics frequently included. Understandably, students are often daunted by the enormity of the task involved when conveying bad news. Moreover, they find it difficult to believe that anyone can be taught how to break bad news and phrases such as 'you'll only know when you actually try it' and 'each time must be different' are familiar to communications skills tutors. There is of course some truth in these assertions although there are doubtless many approaches and ideas that can be usefully worked through before the student or young doctor is faced with a real patient in genuine distress. Nevertheless, the objections raised draw our attention to the importance of responding to the individual needs of the patient or carer with whom the conversation is taking place. Implicit in this apparently obvious statement is the requirement for a good doctor–patient relationship. This in turn, as I have argued above, hinges on a recognition by the practitioner, at some level, of his or her own vulnerability and, when the news is of impending death, of his or her own mortality.

The exercise described below has been used with numerous students and experienced practitioners. The following description relates to a group of students scheduled for a communications skills class about 'breaking bad news'. They were not self-selected, had minimal warning of what the class would involve and had not been primed with any theoretical information about the psychology discussed above. Instead they had been told that we

would use, amongst other things, painting to think about what would constitute bad news.

Twenty students took part in the class. The students were asked to close their eyes and using guided visual meditation they were taken to a room with 'bad news' written on the door. In their mind's eye they were asked to walk down a long corridor to this door, to look at and decide whether to go in. Once inside, they were instructed to look around the room and were given time to do so. They were then instructed to leave the room and walk back up the corridor. The students were then told to open their eyes and, without talking, to spend 10 minutes drawing or painting the room they had visited. Whilst initially quite nervous about the proposed painting ('I can't paint', 'help', 'I'm no artist'), all 20 set about their tasks with focus and care. Once the work was complete, the students were asked to describe what they had drawn with one other person in the group. The discussions were lively and good humoured with anxiety broken by smiles and encouraging words between peers. Students were invited, if they wished, to tell the larger group about their painting. The process became infectious as it became apparent that between them they had only painted two rooms.

The first room was grey, bare, dusty and depressing, It seemed that hope, joy and pleasure were not to be found in this room. Any small signs of life, indistinct and remote, were only to be glimpsed through a grimy window. The second room was, by contrast, bright and pleasant. A neat bed with colourful cover, beautiful flowers in a vase, a painting hanging on the wall and a carefully curtained window onto a world filled with sunshine. As the students described their pictures it became clear to them what these pictures were about. The first was what life would be like after bad news. The second represented the future life, on which they had previously counted, which would now be very different.

Using practical art, these students, and many others in similar groups, have used their own creativity to gain greater insight into hopes and fears of which they were often not conscious. This recognition of one's own feelings is a powerful preparation for the development of empathy.

Connecting

Fortunately, most doctors, qualifying in their mid-twenties, have little personal experience of death, although it is important to realize that a significant number will. This may be the death or terminal illness of an elderly relative such as a grandparent, a closer relative such as a parent or sibling, or of a friend or fellow pupil at school. As a young doctor, they often experience death as the end result of a failed resuscitation attempt. When the death is anticipated then they may well be called after the event and required to make legal confirmation of this event and to talk to the recently bereaved relatives. By the time the doctor has completed postgraduate training and is responsible for training others then, depending on the speciality chosen, that doctor will be expected to guide the healthcare team as they care for those with incurable conditions in the final part of their lives. MacLeod[19] talks of the 'turning points' described by experienced practitioners in palliative care: the moment when they first began to understand what their work was all about. This invariably occurred when they found themselves in an intimate and caring situation with a patient. Like Cicely Saunders caring for a relative stranger and suddenly understanding what was needed, so these doctors learnt from these close and moving experiences.

MacLeod's turning points play a key role in enabling the practitioner to appreciate how illness impacts on patients and their families. These important insights are, in turn, essential prerequisites for any meaningful attempt to empathize with those affected by illness. One view of empathy, as vicarious introspection, comes close to describing the way in which the arts can be used to connect health-care professionals and patients. Creative outlets, such as practical art, writing, and drama require practitioners to step outside of their professional role and to think, feel and listen person-to-person, and not professional to patient. I will now illustrate the use of literature to facilitate this process and thereby to improve understanding of the perspective of patients, carers and professionals in palliative care with reference to specific poetry and prose.

The patient's perspective

As soon as you're diagnosed the medical profession sees you as being the illness with the patient attached. Actually you are an ordinary person, with something dreadful that has happened to you, absolutely dreadful. That doesn't mean that all the rest of your life isn't carrying on. Maybe you're going to have to withdraw from some of it because of the physical limits, but things like relationships will still be there.

(Tracey quoted in *The healing touch* Michele Petrone)[23]

I opened this chapter with a quote from Michele Petrone, a professional artist who has painted and written about his experience of Hodgkin's lymphoma. When Michele was in isolation following a stem cell transplant he painted square pictures to fill the glass pane on his door. These paintings reveal his emotional journey of illness in ways of which even he was initially unaware. This collection of pictures has toured widely and been used in formal and informal settings to allow all of those caring for patients with serious illness to explore the feelings that are so often generated.

Fortunately, there are many generous individuals willing to share their emotional journeys with us through their writing, art, music, drama and dance. This growing body of work constitutes a rich and varied teaching resource. The authenticity of such work is appreciated by students of all ages and can provide convincing and useful guides to the agendas and priorities of patients. In his writing and through his subsequent work with patients, Michele Petrone has chosen to give a voice to others, like Tracey, struggling to cope in a world that has been turned upside down by illness. He reinforces Tracey's plea to all doctors to not let the person be hidden by their illness, not to view patients as illnesses with people attached. Through reading and discussing what patients write and say we can all help ensure that those voices are heard.

The carer's perspective

Why is a scar on a man a mark of distinction,
on a woman a mark of disfigurement?
I don't know.
Why is it funny when a man loses his hair,
And tragic when a woman loses hers?
I don't know.
What will you tell her
when the X-Rays turn the scar
on her breast raw-
hamburger red?
I don't know.

When she's bald, lost the hair
From her eyebrows,
And lies with closed eyes,
With a skeletal look,
Will you kiss her
and tell her
she's beautiful?
I don't know.
What do you do
In the bedroom,
When she is thinking
of death,
and she cries?
I hold her hand, and I breathe.

(From *I don't know* Joe Milosch)[24]

… I am relieved to leave you, relieved to be in the bus. New York is beautiful as we come in, at dusk. There is a patch of green under the flyover, and a man lives there, alone, in a shack he has made himself ….
It is not until tomorrow, in Manhattan, as I am crossing the street to post a letter, that a sense of your unhappiness will come crashing down on me, it will be as though you are with me, and in the road, in the traffic, a desolation will overwhelm me, which is both yours and mine. I will hurry back to your loft and as I close the door behind me the telephone will be ringing and it will be you: you unhappy, alone and lost.

(From *Flight* James Loader)[25]

I don't know, is a moving poem written by a husband trying to come to terms with his wife's breast cancer and the physical and psychological anguish that followed. Aware of the many issues this man would have to deal with, the medical team asked him lots of questions, to see how he was going to cope. These questions made him angry and this poem began as an angry poem. Subsequently, it also became a love poem—a poem full of pain, uncertainty, anger, love. Through writing the poem, he came to accept the fact that not knowing is OK, acceptable, appropriate. All this wisdom and more can be accessed and understood by reading this poem.

Flight by James Loader is a wonderful description of the lonely and claustrophobic experience that caring for the sick and dying can be. Students reading this piece feel themselves intuitively disapprove of the narrator and his desire to run away, not to be responsible. As they read on, as he runs only to know he must return, they begin to see the fuller picture, the man behind the carer with needs, fears and hopes of his own. This story has many analogies in the world they are more familiar with. The late night admission of a dying woman who'd be better off at home but whose partner says he can't cope anymore can all too easily be interpreted by the young admitting house officer as the consequence of a selfish and heartless carer. The snap-shot of the human tragedy seen in casualty almost certainly is just that—a two-dimensional representation of a moment in time—and gives only a limited idea of what has brought patient, carer and doctor to this place at this time. And yet, the admission history will purport to do just that, to sum up the situation, when instead it can only offer a fragment of the emerging narrative of illness. Analysis of the feelings pieces such as *Flight* evokes in the reader, can provide unanticipated insights into the carer's perspective and this in turn can have direct relevance to subsequent clinical work.

The professional's perspective

The frisson you get from a fine line of poetry comes chiefly, I think, from the sheer pleasure that someone has recorded something you thought only you had felt before. More that that, it comes from the realisation that many others have shared and will share with you this moment that you had thought was unique and inexpressible. The loneliness of the individual life is dissolved briefly in the flicker of that same sensation, of coherence.

(From *Odd Man Out* Martyn Harris)[26]

Most students have little idea of what being a doctor is really like. They will have been exposed to many and varied representations and interpretations of doctors. Examining how doctors are portrayed in popular culture provides insights into the expectations that society and patients have of doctors and doctors have of themselves. For a detailed description of how this can work the reader is referred to Glasser's paper[27]. In palliative medicine, the doctor's perspective can be ignored all too easily and the problems this can cause are discussed in the next section.

Support

The third objective is to enable those working in this field to draw on the arts and humanities for their own personal development and support. Given the demanding nature of the work and the well-documented stress felt by numerous professionals in this area, this last objective addresses a pressing need.

Crying in stairwells

I mumbled condolences to the parents and hurried from the room. Walking rapidly down the hall, looking neither right nor left, finally I reached the stairwell . . . A soft wail emanated from some place deep within me. Warm tears began to flow down my cheeks as I wept quietly for Joshua. Soon, however, angry sobs racked my body as all the frustration and impotence overwhelmed me.

(From *Joshua knew* Liana Roxanne Clark)[28]

When this piece was published it provoked a flurry of impassioned correspondence. Why, the letters asked, was the only support available to most doctors in this position still so inadequate and why do doctors still feel a need to hide their own feelings by crying in stairwells? Fortunately, for an increasing number of health professionals writing allows creative expression of the emotions elicited by their work and there is a growing body of publicly available doctor-generated literature in this field. However, for many doctors, nurses and others working in, for example, palliative care, the burdens are great and the sources of support few. MacLeod[19] has written about the types of stress encountered by young doctors. For many the experience of becoming close emotionally to a dying patient is formative and yet this experience is seldom acknowledged or considered from the viewpoint of the professionals concerned. As Copp and Dunn have reported[29], nurses also suffer from emotional stress when looking after dying patients. Not surprisingly, they report that patients who have not accepted their prognosis are particularly upsetting to look after. They also report that poor inter-professional communication and support can be frustrating and demoralizing. The opportunity exists, therefore, not only to use the humanities to support individuals but also to support teamwork and the mutual respect and understanding that are its prerequisites.

In some centres, there have been welcome attempts to address these issues either by using existing resources or by inviting in outside facilitators. This is, however, far from universally available. Support of this sort could be a valuable resource for doctors in palliative care and a proactive approach to the provision of these continuing educational needs throughout the speciality, would benefit not only doctors but also the patients they would feel more equipped to help.

Mutual support through listening

Another source of support, familiar to those working in medical humanities, is that which comes from listening to each other's stories. Work involving patients, carers and professionals listening to each other can be particularly powerful. Turner describes the support received by both carers and professionals when, as part of an educational exercise, carers were asked to tell their story to a student[30]. The carers were very pleased to be able to tell someone their story and felt that they were in some sense heard for the first time. The students felt that they gained far more from the storytelling than information. They felt a closeness to the teller which they found supportive and accepting. Sharing of stories, as opposed to eliciting histories, can facilitate mutual respect, greater understanding of alternative perspectives and can reduce the sense of isolation and loneliness sometimes felt by those involved in palliative care either as patient, carer or professional.

The care of dying children

He straightens, looks up, and our eyes lock. 'What happened?' he repeats softly, but more clearly.
I only have to look into those eyes for a second to know what he is asking . . . what happened to the baby he already loved more than he thought it was possible to love.
. . .
I stand in the centre of the room. I don't know what to say, and very quickly I am unable to say anything. It is all I can do to suppress the ball of grief that is growing in my chest. Images of my own son fill my mind: the toothless grins and sweet breast-milk breath as a baby, the squeals of laughter of a mischievous toddler, the warmth of his sleeping body nestled in my protecting arms, the innocent questions that challenge me, make me pause, make me smile.

(From *A father's eyes* Stephen Schultz)[31]

As I leaned over to listen to his chest with my stethoscope, Joshua awakened. His teal blue eyes fixed on my face.
'I don't need this anymore,' he said, and pulled off the oxygen mask. 'I'm ready to die now.'
I looked at his mother trying to hide my shock. For three weeks I had struggled to make this child well enough to go home for what would inevitably be his last Christmas. Now, on December 17, Joshua was telling me that the fight was over.
. . . as I left the room, I struggled with my emotions. I had felt so helpless, standing by, watching Joshua die, unable to heal him.

(From *Joshua knew* Liana Roxanne Clark)[28]

The care of dying children is one that many of us find particularly difficult[32]. Few of us feel emotionally prepared to deal with the death of a child and yet, faced with parental grief the professionals involved often view their own feelings as intrusive and relatively insignificant. In addition, the circumstances in which the child will die can be very different to those in which adults die. Parents, often capable of providing most if not all of the personal care, may not need or want outside help. Reading, writing and discussing literature like *A father's eyes* and *Joshua knew* enables the practitioner, not only to reflect on his or her one own practice and feelings, but also to share these with their peers. As in all other areas of life it can be a deep source of comfort to find out that someone else has felt just as you now feel.

Conclusion

'I will not profess bravery,' said Lydgate, smiling, 'but I acknowledge a good deal of pleasure in fighting, and I should not care for my profession, if I did not believe that better methods were to be found and enforced there as well as everywhere else.'
(From *Middlemarch* George Eliot)[33]

Palliative medicine has a history of setting standards by which other specialities are subsequently measured, of continually looking for better methods. Expertise in symptom control including pain relief is, to a great extent, now concentrated in the palliative care team and indeed team members often provide advice in these areas to those in other specialities. One of the reasons for this success may be the rather introspective nature of the speciality. Every intervention is questioned, the patient's wishes are paramount and every effort is made to ensure that the emotional, spiritual, and physical needs of the patient and family are met. Nevertheless, addressing the complex and diverse educational needs of those who will be involved in the care of individuals with incurable conditions has not proved easy. It remains a challenge to ensure that doctors in training have direct experience of caring for the dying and where training is provided to young doctors the retention of skills and knowledge can be poor. Thanks to concerted efforts, both in the United Kingdom and in numerous other countries, an increasing number of both undergraduate and post-graduate medical programmes do now incorporate some element of training in palliative care.

By emphasizing the powerful role that the humanities could play in the education, training, and support of doctors and other health-care professionals, who care for patients who cannot be cured, the editors of this volume have shown foresight and courage. It is now up to educators and clinicians in palliative medicine to embrace this opportunity to draw on the wealth of human wisdom and understanding embodied in the arts. In doing so they will, once more, be at the forefront of constructive change in medicine.

Acknowledgements

I would like to thank all the writers—patients, carers and professionals—who have so generously shared their deepest feelings with us all. I would also like to commend the editors of this volume for their vision in including the humanities in this important and influential clinical textbook.

Further reading

The arts and medicine: general works

Cassell, E.J. (1991). *The nature of suffering and the goals of medicine.* Oxford University Press, Oxford.

Downie, R.S. (ed.) (1994). *The healing arts: an anthology.* Oxford University Press, Oxford.

Evans, M., and Finlay, I. (ed.) (2001). *Medical humanities.* BMJ Publishing, London.

Fox, J. (1997). *Poetic medicine: the healing art of poem-making.* Tarcher/Putnam, New York.

Kirklin, D., and Richardson, R. (ed.) (2001). *Medical humanities: a practical introduction.* Royal College of Physicians, London.

Philipp, R., Baum, M., Mawson, A., and Calman, K. (2000). *Humanities in medicine: beyond the millennium.* Nuffield Trust, London.

The role of narrative in medicine

Campo, R. (1997). *The desire to heal—a doctor's education in empathy, identity and poetry.* WW Norton, London.

Greenhalgh, T., and Hurwitz, B. (ed.) (1998). *Narrative-based medicine.* BMJ Publishing, London.

Montgomery Hunter, K. (1991). *Doctors' stories: the narrative structure of medical knowledge.* Princeton University Press, Princeton.

Patient perspectives

Brighton, J., and Savage, A. (ed.) (1997). *The patient knows.* Marches Cancer Care, Cardiff.

Diamond, J.C. (1998). *. . . because cowards get cancer too.* Vermillion, London.

Harris, M. (1996). *Odd man out.* Pavilion Books Ltd.

Picardie, R. (1998). *Before I say goodbye.* Penguin Books, Middlesex.

Zola, I. (1982). *Ordinary lives: voices of disability and disease.* Applewood Books, Cambridge.

The doctor as patient

Vaughan, C. (1996). Teach me to hear mermaids singing. *British Medical Journal,* **313,** 565.

Wyoka, J. (1995). Hospice at home. *British Medical Journal,* **311,** 1687–8.

The carer's perspective

Herriot, B. (1996). The need to protect colleagues. *British Medical Journal,* **313,** 369.

Jayes, A. (1996). Open letter from a carer. *British Medical Journal.* **313,** 370.

Loader, J. (ed.) (1996). *Cold comfort.* Serpents Tail, London.

Martz, S. (ed.) (1992). *If I had my life over I would pick more daisies.* Papier Mache Press, Watsonville.

Spark, D. (1994). *Last things.* Ploughshares, Boston.

The doctor's perspective

Clark, L. (1993). Joshua knew. *Journal of the American Medical Association,* **270,** 2902.

Schultz, S. (1994). A father's eyes. *Journal of the American Medical Association,* **271,** 1146.

Seigel, B. (1994). Crying in stairwells: how should we grieve for dying patients? *Journal of the American Medical Association,* **272,** 659.

Singh, S. (1996). Around every tumour there's a person. *British Medical Journal,* **316,** 560.

Illness, patients, and doctors in fiction

De Bernières, L. (1995). *Captain Corelli's Mandolin.* Minerva, London.

Solzenitsyn, A. (1979). *Cancer ward.* Penguin, Middlesex.

Welsh, I. (1993). *Trainspotting.* Secker & Warburg, London.

Informative texts in humanities subjects relevant to this field

Randall, F., and Downie, R. (1999). *Palliative care ethics. a companion for all specialties.* Oxford University Press.

Porter, R. (1997). *The greatest benefit to mankind: a medical history of humanity from antiquity to the present.* Fontana Press, London.

Educational resources

http://www.mhrd.ucl.ac.uk, Database of UK medical humanities courses including reviews of the texts, images and films used in the courses.

http://endeavor.med.nyu.edu, Database of literature and medicine including details of courses available throughout North America.

Kirklin, D., Meakin, R., Lloyd, M., and Singh, S. (2001). *Living with and dying from cancer: an educational pack incorporating teaching materials for tutors and students.* Centre for Medical Humanities, London.

References

1. Petrone, M. (2001). The healing touch: the necessity for humanity in medicine and the humanities in medical education In *Medical humanities: a practical introduction* (eds. D. Kirklin and R. Richardson), p. 33. RCP, London.

2. Finlay, I. (2001). Portfolio learning: the humanities in medical education In *Medical humanities* (eds. M. Evans and I. Finlay), p. 156. BMJ Books, London.

3. Shapiro, J. (2000). Literature and the arts in medical education. *Family Medicine,* **32**(3), 157–8.

4. Field, D. (1995). Education for palliative care: formal education about death, dying and bereavement in UK medical schools in 1983 and 1994. *Medical Education,* **29,** 414–9.

5. Oliver, D. (1998). Training and knowledge of palliative care of junior doctors. *Palliative Medicine,* **12,** 297–9.

6. World Health Organization. http://www.who.int/cancer/palliative/definition/en/ accessed 17 April 2008.

7. Weatherall, D. (1994). The inhumanity of medicine. *British Medical Journal,* **309,** 24–31.

8. De Bernières, L. (1995). *Captain Corelli's Mandolin,* pp. 135–6. Minerva, London.

9. Murray, S., Kendall, M., Boyd, K. Volume 51. I knew … *BJGP,* (**51**) (470), 777.

10. Pellegrino, E., and Thomasma, D. (1993). *The virtues in medical practice.* Oxford University Press, New York.

11. Fox, E. (1997). Predominance of the curative model of medical care. *Journal of the American Medical Association,* **278**(9), 761–3.

12. Steel, K., Ribble, M., Ahronheim, J. (1999). Incorporating education on palliative care into the long-term care setting. *Journal of the American Geriatrics Society,* **47,** 904–7.

13. Tolstoy, L. (1981). *The Death of Ivan Ilyich,* p. 126. Bantam Classics, New York.

14. Tolstoy, L. (1981). *The Death of Ivan Ilyich,* p. 128. Bantam Classics, New York.

15. Tolstoy, L. (1981). *The Death of Ivan Ilyich,* pp. 132–3. Bantam Classics, New York.

16. Dryden, J. (1958). *Horat. Ode 29. Book 3. Paraphras'd in Pindarique Verse,* pt vii (1685). In *The Poems of John Dryden,* vol. **1,** (ed. J. Kinsley), p. 436. Clarendon Press, Oxford.

17. MacLeod, R. (2001). On reflection: doctors learning to care for people who are dying. *Social Science and Medicine,* **52,** 1719–27.

18. General Medical Council. (1993). *Tomorrow's Doctors— Recommendations on Undergraduate Medical Education.* General Medical Council, London.

19. Calman, K. (1999). Literature in the education of the doctor. *Lancet,* **29,** 1622–5.

20. Finlay, I. (2001). Portfolio learning: the humanities in medical education In *Medical humanities* (eds. M. Evans, and I. Finlay), p. 159. BMJ Books, London.

21. Mann, T. (1999). *Magic mountain,* p. 133. Vintage, London.

22. Yeats, WB. (2000) Among school children. In *The Collected Poems of W.B. Yeats* Wordsworth Editions, London, pp. 183–4.

23. Petrone, M. (2001). The healing touch: the necessity for humanity in medicine and the humanities in medical education. In *Medical humanities: A practical introduction* (eds. D. Kirklin, and R. Richardson) p. 34. RCP, London.

24. Milosch, J. (1997). I don't know. In *Poetic medicine* (ed. J. Fox), pp. 26–7. Tarcher/Putnam, New York.

25. Loader, J. (1996). Flight. In *Cold comfort* (ed. J. Loader), pp. 172–80. Serpents Tail, London.

26. Harris, M. (1996). *Odd man out,* p. 302. Pavilion Books Ltd, London.

27. Glasser, B. (2001). From Kafka to casualty doctors and medicine in popular culture & the arts—a special studies module. *The Journal of Medical Ethics: Medical Humanities,* **27**(2), 99–101.

28. Clark, L. (1993). Joshua knew. *Journal of the American Medical Association,* **270,** 2902.

29. Copp, G., and Dunn, V. (1993). Frequent and difficult problems perceived by nurses caring for the dying. *Palliative Medicine,* **7,** 19–25.

30. Turner, P., Sheldon, F., Coles, C. (2000). Listening to and learning from the family carer's story: an innovative approach in interprofessional education. *Journal of Interprofessional Care,* **14**(4), 387–95.

31. Schultz, S. (1994). A father's eyes. *Journal of the American Medical Association,* **271,** 1146.

32. Charlton, R. (1996). Addressing the needs of the dying child. *Palliative Medicine,* **10,** 240–6.

33. Eliot, G. (Edition pub 1981). *Middlemarch,* p. 152. Penguin Books, London.

Informatics in palliative medicine

Jose Pereira

Introduction

Information is at the core of much that is done in health care. Information on patients' presenting problems, past medical history, treatments, and wishes is used to make decisions about care provision. Health-care services are planned on the basis of information related to resources utilization and needs. Health professionals acquire new information through formal educational programmes or by informal learning opportunities. Patients and their families go in search of information in order to be better informed about their care options. Research is driven by the collection and analysis of information or data. Information has been described as the data and knowledge that intelligent systems, either human or artificial, use to support their decisions[1]. Information is the result of processing, manipulating and organizing data in a way that adds to the knowledge of the user and the receiver.

The last two decades have witnessed an unprecedented explosion of information and access to it. This has been driven largely by computer-based systems and digital technologies. With some noticeable exceptions, particularly in developing countries or countries in which access to information is controlled by state systems, health professionals, administrators, patients and families now have relatively easy access to what is the Internet (Net) and its subsidiary the World Wide Web (Web), the largest repository and conduit of information in history. It is not surprising therefore that the age we now live in is being referred to as the *Information Age* where information- and communication-related technologies are ubiquitous.

Palliative care is not immune to these profound influences and is already harnessing many of the technologies to improve the care of terminally ill patients and their families. This section explores some of these influences and opportunities as they may relate to palliative care, focusing largely on the role of informatics in supporting education of health professionals, patients and their families.

Defining informatics, health informatics and e-health

It is difficult to arrive at a single all-encompassing definition of *informatics*. As a concept it bears a diversity of meanings and dimensions. Informatics, according to the University of Edinburgh's School of Informatics, 'studies the representation, processing and communication of information in natural and engineered systems' and has 'computational, cognitive and social aspects'. It can be viewed as the collection, classification, storage, retrieval, dissemination and application of information. Others have looked at it more narrowly as the study of the application of computer-based technologies to the management of information, including the design and implementation of the hardware and software systems in support of this.

As an extension of *informatics, medical* or *health informatics* is the field that deals with the storage, retrieval, sharing and optimal use of biomedical information, data and knowledge for problem solving and decision-making. More broadly, the University of Iowa defines it as the 'study of information processing as it is used in healthcare'. This includes how medical knowledge is created, shaped, shared and applied. It involves the way we think about patients, and their information and decision-making needs, the way that treatments are defined, selected and developed, and how we organize ourselves to create and run health-care organizations[1]. Health informatics, as Coiera proposes, helps health professionals with their decisions and actions and improves patient outcomes by making better use of information[2]. It is closely associated with modern information technologies, notably in the areas of computing and communications.

Informatics in support of medical education

Information skills required by health professionals

Health professionals are inundated with information. It arrives through journals, pamphlets, letters, e-mail, the Web and the press. Some of it is highly relevant to their scopes of practice, and some irrelevant or even inaccurate. Keeping pace with new information, including triaging, storing and retrieving it rapidly when the need arises, has become a daunting task. Coeira has proposed some essential skills for health professionals to manage information[2]. They include:

- Understand the dynamic nature of medical knowledge.

- Know how to search for and assess knowledge according to the principals of evidence-based medicine.

- Understand models that explain the diagnostic process.

- Interpret uncertain clinical data and deal with artefact and error.

- Apply and adapt clinical knowledge to the individual circumstances of patients.

- Access, assess, select and apply a treatment guideline, adapt it to local circumstances, communicate it and record variations in treatment plan and outcome.

- Structure and record clinical data in a form appropriate for the immediate clinical task, for communication with colleagues, or for epidemiological purposes.

- Select and operate the most appropriate communication method for a given task (eg. face-to-face conversation, telephone, e-mail, video, voice mail, letter).

- Structure and communicate messages in a manner most suited to the recipient, task and chosen communication medium.

E-learning and telemedicine

Defining e-health and e-learning

E-health is a broad term that refers to health care that is delivered, supported or enhanced by electronic-, digital- or computer-based technologies. These include the Internet and the Web and their many associated technologies. It embraces technologies such as handheld computers including personal digital assistants (PDAs), MP3 players and multimedia CD- or DVD-ROMs. The notion of information and knowledge management is embedded in the term. However, a single clear definition remains elusive[3]. *E-learning*, a component of e-health, refers to the use of the same technologies in pursuit of supporting or enhancing education and learning. It also encompasses application of learning theories and the cognitive and social aspects of the learning process. Numerous other terms are used to refer to subdivisions of e-learning. These include *Web-based learning or Web learning*, when the delivery medium is the Web and its related technologies, and *computer-assisted learning* (CAL), when the learning is supported by computer-based technologies. Despite the overlaps between web-learning and CAL, the latter increasingly refers to learning opportunities supported by a laptop or desktop computer where the materials are stored on that computer. This includes case simulations, educational CD- or DVD-ROMS and intranet materials.

E-learning has revolutionized distance learning. One of the most challenging aspects of distance learning in the past, when it relied on regular mail, was the lack of immediacy which often resulted in the learner feeling isolated. Strategies to address this such as long-distance telephone and video conferencing were often prohibitively expensive. New communication and instructional technologies, many of them web-based, are bridging the immediacy barrier and making voice and video conferencing more accessible. It is also changing the way educational institutions view students. The term 'distributed' is now preferred over 'distance' to emphasize the increasing focus on the learner and the ability to support learning at a place, time and method of the learner's choosing[4]. It is therefore not only a medium for delivering distance learning, it also supports learner-centred education and can enhance traditional classroom-based learning.

Increasingly, medical and nursing faculties are adopting elements of e-learning in their undergraduate and postgraduate curricula[5]. In some cases the entire curriculum, including the goals and objectives of each course, the class and clinical rotation schedules and learning materials (print-based and digitalized), is available online while in other cases it is limited to specific content areas[6,7].

E-learning and its many associated technologies and methods appear to be well suited to support workplace, life-long and 'just-in-time' learning. The ability to pack a whole text book on a personal PDA or handheld computer and the capability of going online at short notice to find a site with the answers to a specific question generated while examining a patient, are two examples of how it can support these. Access to resources such as PubMed and a variety of online journals enhances continuing professional development, life-long learning and evidence-based practice.

Defining telehealth, telemedicine, and telelearning

The distinctions between *e-health* and *telemedicine*, and *e-learning* and *telelearning*, are increasingly blurred. Historically, *telemedicine* and *telelearning* preceded *e-health* and *e-learning* and referred to the use of communication media, specifically telephone-, cable- and satellite-based communication, for the delivery or enhancement of clinical care and education at a distance. This included audio- and videoconferencing and the transfer of data and images.

Telemedicine covers a broad spectrum of activities and can include two professionals discussing a case over the telephone, e-mail or videoconferencing[8–10], videoconferencing or videophones to support care directly[11–15] or telephone help lines[16,17]. It can also be as complex as biomedical robots and devices being used to perform surgery at a distance. A number of terms using the 'tele' prefix now describe various aspects of telemedicine. Examples include *teleconsulting, telenursing, teleradiology, telemonitoring* and *telesurgery*. Some suggest that although the terms *telemedicine and telehealth* are often used interchangeably, *telemedicine* is more appropriately used to refer only to the provision of clinical services while *telehealth* includes clinical and non-clinical services such as medical education, administration and research conducted at a distance.

The increased use of computer, digitalized and Internet-based technologies to support these activities underlies the increased use of the term *e-health* as an umbrella term that includes telemedicine, telehealth, telelearning, e-learning and health informatics, including electronic health records.

Concepts, tools, and methods supporting e-learning

E-learning and Web-learning encompass many different technologies and learning activities. They range from the simple posting of information to a web site, such as resources or clinical practice guidelines, to sophisticated learning management systems that support several functions, including course administration and content, interactive modules for independent self-learning and synchronous or asynchronous learning. Synchronous communication involves real-time interaction among two or more persons, using text, audio or video, while asynchronous communication is independent of time. Participants receive, read and post messages at times of their own choosing. Applications that support online conferencing are referred to as 'web-conferencing' tools and the process as 'computer mediated conferencing (CMC)'. Technologies that support asynchronous CMC include e-mailing, Listservs, bulletin boards, electronic discussion forums, 'blogs' and 'podcasts'. Electronic discussion forums hold an advantage over e-mailing in that postings can be organized as *threads*. Synchronous and asynchronous CMC (aCMC) have their respective advantages and limitations. Synchronous CMC provides real time contact between learners and instructors and builds a sense of community and belonging more rapidly than asynchronous methods. However, the logistics of organizing a time that is convenient for all participants, across time zones in the case of international courses, is a limiting factor. Asynchronous communication provides more independence with respect to time and place and may nurture reflection more than with synchronous learning [18]. With the appropriate design, asynchronous learning is a powerful tool to support reflective and constructive learning[19]. Learners have noted that the exercise of writing their online responses prompts them to reflect more deeply and articulate their thoughts more clearly. A combination of synchronous CMC and aCMC capitalizes on the advantages of both[20].

Learning management systems (LMSs) are software systems that enable the management and delivery of learning content and resources. At a minimum, LMSs usually allow for a common space to provide course information and content, student registration, communication tools, organization of user group, and tracking of learner and instructor activity. They may also support testing and online surveys. Word documents, digital slides, audio and video files, images and graphics can be stored and organized in them. Most systems allow for log-in security through password protection. There are many 'off the shelf' LMSs available. *Moodle* is open sourced and available for free downloading and use while most of the others require the purchase of licences. Developing new custom-built LMS programs de novo is costly and time-intensive.

Online instructors are not restricted to using an LMS if they wish to deliver e-learning. Depending on the needs of the courses and the competencies to be achieved, they may use a program that supports only synchronous conferencing or the creation and delivery of independent self-learning modules. Alternatively, they may opt to develop their own website using off-the-shelf software programs. Audio and video files can be made available through streaming. Large files containing video, audio and graphic material may be saved onto CD-or DVD-ROM discs, copied and distributed to learners, once copyright issues have been addressed.

E-learning and Web-learning can be integrated into education in different ways. These range from using the Web simply as a medium in which to store and distribute learning materials in a traditional classroom-based course, to delivering courses entirely online. Hybrid programmes that combine e-learning and traditional classroom-based-learning and take advantage of the strengths of both media are increasingly popular[20]. E-learning elements may constitute a minor or a major part of learning programmes. In blended e-learning, various technologies and methods are combined. These may include asynchronous and synchronous CMC and digitalized audio or videos files. E-learning may support independent self-learning (such as free-standing online modules), group-based learning with extensive interaction between learners and instructors, or combinations of both in a course. E-learning methods can provide open learning opportunities where learners register and complete the programme in their own time, or paced programmes which begin and end at pre-specified times and learners have to complete assignments or exercises within a pre-defined period of time.

Formal and informal learning through e-learning

Education is often perceived as formal events that are organized and delivered by instructors and for which learners register. However, some of the most effective learning occurs informally. Examples include corridor conversations between clinicians and consultants about a medical problem, online searches by clinicians for information on treatment options, or the use of a handheld computer to look up a clinical practice guideline. E-learning is particularly well suited to support informal learning particularly as it relates to life-long learning, just-in-time learning and learning at the workplace. The boundary between formal and informal learning is rapidly becoming blurred as interest in capturing or codifying these learning moments for purposes of obtaining continuing education credits increases.

Successful implementation of e-learning

Successful implementation of e-learning requires consideration of some important principles and guidelines. The reason for implementing e-learning should not be to replace traditional learning methods but rather to address barriers to accessing learning and enhancing learning. The basic principles of adult learning should be honoured[21]. The same processes involved in curriculum development with traditional courses, including conducting a needs assessment, establishing learning objectives, identifying instructional methods and evaluation, apply[22]. Special attention is required to choosing the appropriate designs, media and the technologies for a particular e-learning programme. The individual characteristics of the various technologies may influence learning outcomes[23].

The degree of interaction required by learners is an important instructional design consideration. Some online resources simply require that learners either read what is posted or download files. Others require extensive interaction, either with the software program or with other learners and instructors. Some software programs allow instructors to develop online learning events that prompt learners to interact with the software by, for example, responding to questions around cases. Immediate feedback can be programmed so that learners know immediately whether or not their responses were correct. Multimedia may be integrated to enhance the course, including graphics, audio and video files. Access to the internet, including the presence of firewalls, preparedness for the technology and costs are all important instructional design considerations[24]. A 'common denominator' approach which incorporates a technology base that is appropriate for the widest range of students is advised. Costs for implementing e-learning may be relatively high up front, but diminish with subsequent iterations[25].

At times, older technologies such as telephone conferencing may work better than newer more complex technologies. Some older technologies are being enhanced by newer adaptations. In the Canadian Pallium Project, for example, Aherne, Pereira, and colleagues used a telephone conferencing system to reach out to learners across Canada through monthly seminars and saved these to MP4 audio files that are made available for downloading (http://www.pallium.ca/index.php?s=events&e=15).

Familiarizing learners and instructors with the technology and the learning methods is critical. Garrison and colleagues have proposed a framework called the 'community of inquiry' with which to implement e-learning in a way that supports active cognitive processes such as creating, problem-solving, reasoning, decision-making and evaluation[26]. It also assists instructors in providing social, cognitive and instructional presences, all important elements of asynchronous CMC. Salmon has described a five-stage model to implement CMC[27]. Stage 1 involves activities to facilitate access and motivation of the learners. This is followed by techniques to increase socialization of the learners and enhancement of a sense of community (Stage 2). Stage 3 involves active information exchange, which includes strategies to increase feedback and learner participation. This stage precedes the actual construction of knowledge (Stage 4) in which most of the exchange of knowledge and attitudes occur. Included are strategies to deal with 'lurking' where some learners read the online messages and postings but do not actively contribute by posting themselves; a phenomenon which can be frustrating for learners and instructors alike. Stage 5 involves reflections on the learning process.

Effectiveness of e-learning

The broad question 'How effective is e-learning?' is difficult to answer because of the many different combinations of models, technologies and approaches in e-learning. How effective a particular e-learning programme is in achieving the learning objectives is dependent on many different factors, including the design, the technology used, the motivation of the learners and the enthusiasm of the instructors, amongst others. Nonetheless, with the appropriate attention to pedagogical and instructional design, e-learning is at least as effective as conventional classroom-based courses[28,29]. Clearly, it is not able to provide experiential learning opportunities, such as those required for learning communication skills.

Models of e-learning in medical education and palliative care

Despite initial doubts[30]. e-learning is increasingly being used in medical education, from undergraduate and postgraduate education to continuing professional development. It includes use of e-mailing, and asynchronous conferencing[31–34]. E-learning should not be seen as replacing traditional instructor-led learning, particularly at the bed-side, but as a complement to it[35]. E-learning within medical education can include digital curricula with learning materials, images and digital libraries, to manage learning and interaction between learners and instructors[36]. It can host and support modules that enhance problem-based learning. Importantly, the integration of e-learning into medical education can catalyse the shift toward applying adult learning theory, where educators will no longer serve mainly as the distributors of content, but will become more involved as facilitators of learning and assessors of competency.

E-learning is increasingly being used in palliative care education. Some diploma- and masters-level degree programmes, for example, now use multimedia and web-based learning to support their courses. Several groups have reported hybrid models. Between 1999 and 2001, Pereira and Murzyn used a hybrid approach, with online learning (asynchronous CMC), classroom-based learning and patient visits in hospices, to introduce a Canadian undergraduate pharmacy class to palliative care[37]. Since 2002, Pereira and colleagues have also used a hybrid approach with online learning (asynchronous CMC) and face-to-face learning, including the use of standardized patients, to provide palliative care education for rural family medicine residents in Alberta, Canada; a mean of 18 students per year have participated[20]. The course has evolved over the last 6 years and currently uses a blend of technologies to support synchronous (Elluminate®) and asynchronous (BlackBoard®) learning online as well self-standing modules (Adobe Breeze®). More recently the group has evaluated the impact of the course knowledge, attitudes and skills using validated instruments by assessing these pre- versus post-course. Significant improvements in knowledge, attitudes, and skills, with moderate to high effect sizes, were demonstrated[38]. The same group previously developed an entirely online interdisciplinary course for mainly rural and remote-based family physicians, nurses and pharmacists (PallCare EdNet) which relied on asynchronous CMC[39]. This course now includes self-standing modules and synchronous CMC in addition to asynchronous CMC (BlackBoard®).

Others have also reported courses that are delivered entirely online. Kinghorn delivered a 16-week interdisciplinary module online on psychosocial care of patients with advanced cancer using asynchronous CMC and e-mailing[40]. Twenty-nine students participated and low attrition rates were reported. Hinkka et al. used asynchronous CMC in a 12-month long course for general physicians in Finland[41]. They compared the 79 participants in the course with a control group of 100 general physicians who had not participated in the course. Doctors who had received the education chose CPR less often, were more likely to discontinue antibiotic treatment in a dying patient, and significantly more often agreed with the statement 'Terminal care is satisfying' than the control group doctors. The Open University in the United Kingdom has described an interdisciplinary distance learning course that uses multimedia, print-based materials and asynchronous CMC[42]. Weissman and team at the Medical College of Wisconsin, United States have been presenting a 1-year multi-disciplinary online continuing professional development programme relying largely on e-mail. Kim et al. evaluated an online course that used asynchronous CMC to introduce 42 undergraduate medical students to palliative care[43]. Most comments by students lacked critical thinking skills in linking evidence from the literature with ongoing discussions. Although the faculty prompted student discussions and posed questions, they unfortunately rarely highlighted learning points, corrected student errors, or summarized discussions, key strategies to ensure success of the online learning experience. This highlights the importance of educating the faculty on how to facilitate online learning. Palacios, Pereira, and Lyndon have developed an 8-week online course that prepares palliative care educators for online instruction[44]. The course, called 'Online Guide', has prepared palliative care educators in Canada, Argentina, Wales, Portugal and South Africa and spawned online courses for physicians and nurses in Argentina under the leadership of Dr. Roberto Wenk [personal communication].

A number of self-standing modules for independent learning online have been developed. Some of the noteworthy ones are listed in Table 20.5.1. This table also lists some innovative online resources that are not courses but complement education of health professionals.

E-learning in palliative care has not been limited to Web-based education. Wilkie and colleagues have described a multimedia toolkit for palliative care nurse educators called TNEEL that is available in CD-ROM format[45]. It includes engaging strategies for teaching and learning about end-of-life care. It can be downloaded from the Internet. Distance education using synchronous video-conferencing and telephone conferencing has been described. Regnard has described the use of videoconferencing in a programme called Interactive Multimedia Palliative Care Training Project (IMPACT)[46]. Although based in England, the programme linked 22 sites worldwide on a regular basis, reaching 136 professionals without the costs or time needed to travel. It supported presentations, discussions, and journal clubs and links rarely failed. Van Boxell et al. randomized 20 nurses to alternating videoconferencing and face-to-face modes of presentation[47]. Although the learners

Table 20.5.1 Examples of some Internet-based education resources for palliative care clinicians.

	Web site	Developer	Comments	URL (Web address)
Online modules	CLIPS	Help the Hospices, United Kingdom	Short, interactive online modules. Largely text-based. Problem-based learning. Free of charge	http://www.helpthehospices.org.uk/elearning/intro.htm
	Online E-learning modules	Department of Pain Medicine and Palliative Care at the Beth Israel Medical Centre in New York	Use audio-visual materials. Require registration fee	http://www.stoppain.org/for_professionals/content/education/elearning.asp
Online evidence-based references	PC-FACS online	The American Academy of Hospice and Palliative Medicine	Clinician editors systematically review and filter the most important and pertinent articles from more than 60 medical and scientific journals and make summaries of these available to its subscribers[105]	www.aahpm.org/membership/PC-FACS.HTML
	Shaare Zedek Cancer Pain and Palliative Medicine Reference Database	Dr. Nathan I. Cherny, Shaare Zedek Cancer Centre, Jerusalem, Israel	Free online bibliographic database of over 20 000 palliative care-related references (Bibliography system EndNotes is required)	http://www.chernydatabase.org/
Online communities of learning	Palliative Drugs Online	Oxford and Nottingham Palliative Care Programmes, United Kingdom	International web site dedicated to information on the use of drugs, both for licenced and unlicenced uses. Attached to it is an international listserv allowing professionals to communicate with one another	http://www.palliativedrugs.com/
Web sites with clinical information for palliative care providers	Palliative Info	Palliative Care Programme, Winnipeg, Canada. Dr. Mike Harlos	Contains comprehensive list of links to palliative care web sites	http://palliative.info/and http://palliative.info/pages/Tools.htm
	FastFacts and other education resources	EPERC College of Medicine, Wisconsin. Dr. David Weissman		http://www.eperc.mcw.edu/
	IAHPC Manual of Palliative Care	International Association for Hospice and Palliative Care		http://www.hospicecare.com/manual/IAHPCmanual.htm
	IAHPC Getting started series	International Association for Hospice and Palliative Care		http://www.hospicecare.com/gs/
	BMJ ABC in palliative care	*British Medical Journal* Fallon M, Hanks G.		http://www.hospice-spc-council.org.uk/informat.ion/abcofpc.htm
	Innovations in end of life care		An international peer-reviewed journal for leaders in end-of-life care published online from 1999–2003	http://www.edc.org/lastacts
	EPEC Project		Standardized modules to support palliative care education available for free online	http://www.epec.net/EPEC/webpages/index.cfm
	HACPM: Hypermedia Cancer Pain Managemnt Resource	Pain Research Center, University of Utah, Salt Lake City, USA	These tools include a calculator for converting drug dosages, and an interactive dermatome map These include video clips of pain experts and cancer patients addressing issues regarding pain management in patients with cancer. Also included are animated tutorials on the neurological processes involved in pain	http://www.painresearch.utah.edu/cancerpain/
	Palliative Care TIPS	Edmonton Palliative Care Programme, Canada	Short information sheets	http://www.palliative.org/PC/ClinicalInfo/PCareTips/PCareTipsIDX.html
	PDQ Supportive Care in Cancer, National Cancer Institutes, USA	National Institutes of Health, Bethesda, United States		http://www.nci.nih.gov/cancerinfo/pdq/supportivecare

(continued)

Table 20.5.1 (Continued) Examples of some Internet-based education resources for palliative care clinicians.

	Web site	Developer	Comments	URL (Web address)
Guidelines to assess web sites	DISCERN		http://www.discern.org.uk/	Guidelines to assess web sites
	QUICK	UK Centre for Health Information Quality	http://www.quick.org.uk/index2.htm	

preferred face-to-face workshops, they learnt as much from videoconferenced workshops. Videoconferencing was less suitable for psychological or emotional discussions, but this may have been due to the time constraints on the workshops. Lynch and colleagues used videoconferencing successfully to provide interdisciplinary continuing education to primary health-care physicians and nurses across Ontario, Canada[48]. The Canadian Pallium Project describes, on its web site (www.pallium.ca), a monthly audioconferencing professional development programme that was delivered over 14 months from February 2005 to March 2006. Each session linked a mean of 71 sites per session (range 32–117) across Canada, many in rural and remote regions, and a mean of 238 registered professionals from a variety of disciplines (range 147–430 per session). The first 40 min of each 1-h session is a semi-structured interview between a guest expert and a palliative care advanced practice nurse convener, based on questions submitted by those registered. The following 20 min was a question and answer period. The sessions were saved digitally and have been made available as MP3 podcasts on the web site to support asynchronous independent learning. The same project has also captured live-event grand rounds and deployed these via broadband web and PDA computing (in MPEG2 format) to support asynchronous learning.

Informatics in support of health care

The growing blurriness between formal and informal learning has been alluded to previously. Although much of this phenomenon may be attributed to the Internet, other emerging technologies may also be contributing to it. They include electronic health records and computer-based clinical decision support systems.

Electronic health records

Generally electronic health records refer to the field of informatics that is responsible for digitalizing patient-related information and making it available across settings. They do this by collating all or part of the information on a patient into one package that is accessible at the different locations a patient is cared for and by various caregivers.

Multiple terms have been used to define electronic records, often with overlapping definitions. The terms electronic health record (EHR) and electronic medical record (EMR) are in widespread use and are frequently used interchangeably. However, in health informatics, an EMR is considered to be one of several types of EHR. At the most basic level some digital records may be incorporated into what is largely a paper-based record. At an intermediate level is the EMR which contains a large amount of electronic data locally. At the highest level is the EHR which combines information from different institutions and sources and adds other health-related information that is not necessarily related to disease.

A wide spectrum of information may be contained in an EHR, depending on the needs, resources and wishes of the service provider and its clients[49]. This includes information relating to current and historical health, including demographic and other administrative information, medical progress notes and treatments, diagnoses, care plan recommendations, medications, prescription writing, investigation ordering systems, making referrals, and preparing consultation notes and results of investigations (including images). They can also be linked to practice management systems that support medical office functions such as scheduling, billing, appointment reminders and preventative health reminders. Copies of advance directives and health-care proxy forms may be added.

Electronic records may either be generated de novo or created from already existing hardcopy formats. In the latter, sometimes referred to as 'digital format records', records originally produced in a paper or other hardcopy form (including radiological images and photographs) are scanned or imaged and converted to a digital form. The process involved in converting these records to EHRs is expensive and time-consuming and must be done with accuracy. The accuracy and utility of the scanned images or documents should be verified before any consideration is given to disposing of the physical records.

Those responsible for the management of EHRs should ensure that the hardware, software and media used to manage the information remain safe, viable and do not degrade or become obsolete. The regular generation of backup copies of the data and protection is essential. Considerable planning and budgeting is therefore required prior to making decisions to convert physical medical records to digital formats. National and international standards and norms to ensure quality and achieve compatibility and interoperability between independent systems, as well as to enable modularity, are being developed.

In palliative care, a growing number of services are using computer-based technologies, specifically portable and handheld computers, including personal data assistants (PDAs), to assist in collecting clinical data in daily clinical use. Some pain and symptom assessment instruments have been transformed into PDA- and laptop-based interfaces and are being used on a daily basis to collect patient symptom profiles. The advantage of these symptoms is that the data can be easily saved into a database. Chung et al. have advocated for the use of portable information technologies, including PDAs and handheld computers, to support care at the bed-side, including the use of reference resources and assistance in collecting patient data and filling out electronic forms for clinical measurements by providing real-time prompts, clues, alerts, or other types of feedback, along with features such as pre-defined values in specific fields[51]. Another innovation has been the use of digital pens to assess patient symptoms at home[52].

Despite their potential benefits, a slow rate of adoption has been documented in some parts of the world[49]. In addition to the costs of the hardware systems, the expensive and time-consuming digitalizing process of converting from hardcopy formats, and the expertise and infrastructure required, there are other factors at play. These include interoperability issues where different health-care providers and vendors have different standards and protocols and privacy concerns where patient confidentiality has to be ensured. Multiple access points increase possible patient data interception. In the European Union for example, several Directives of the European Parliament and of the Council protect the processing and free movement of personal data, including for purposes of health care. The organizations and individuals charged with the management of this information and systems are required to ensure compliance with legal requirements and adequate protection of confidential data.

Computer-based clinical decision support systems (CDSSs)

CDSSs are interactive computer programs which are designed to assist clinicians with decision-making tasks[53]. They form a significant part of the field of health informatics in their role of supporting the clinical process and use of knowledge, from diagnosis to investigation and treatment. They also have the potential, whether specifically designed to do so or indirectly, of triggering and supporting just-in-time learning and workplace learning. While most are attached to the internal informatics systems of hospital and clinics, some can be used on handheld computers and PDAs[54,55].

A systematic review of controlled studies evaluating the effects of computer-based clinical decision supports on physician performance and patient outcomes found that CDSSs can enhance clinical performance for drug dosing, preventive care and other aspects of medical care, but not convincingly for diagnosis[56]. CDSSs have been shown in one study to decrease the rate of non-intercepted serious medication errors by more than half[57]. Stand-alone PDA-based CDSSs have been shown favourably to alter physicians prescribing of medications and reduce unsafe treatment decisions[54,55].

Four features have been found to be independent predictors of improved clinical practice with CDSSs[58]. These include: (1) automatic provision of decision support as part of clinician work flow; (2) provision of recommendations rather than just assessments; (3) provision of decision support at the time and location of decision-making; and (4) computer-based decision support. The ability to share recommendations with patients was also found to be important. However, not all studies report success; highlighting the complexity of using CDSSs in the decision-making process[59]. They may even introduce their own sources of errors[60].

Handheld computers at the point of care

The use of handheld computers is rising[61]. As a data entry tool, handheld computers have a number of advantages over paper-based data collection including reduced paperwork, transcription errors, time and cost[62]. Handheld computers may save nurses a considerable amount of time in daily administrative tasks. Lau and colleagues surveyed Canadian palliative care physicians and found that 58 per cent of them used PDAs on a daily basis, mostly to organize their practice and to look up medical references[50]. Some used PDAs to store patient information and to access electronic patient records (electronic patient record keeping). The physicians used a number of PDA-based reference resources, including C-Tools, Hopkins Opioid Programme, Lexi-Com, and EPERC Fast Facts. The authors suggest that, in addition to the above, PDAs can be used in palliative care for workflow analysis and collecting clinical data at the point of care (e.g. collecting symptom profiles). In support of research, some caution has been advised. In an Australian palliative care study that used PDAs to collect data at the point of care, high error rates occurred with the data collection[64]. Training and ongoing monitoring are clearly needed to reduce error rates.

Informatics in support of patient and family education

Patients and families on the Internet

Whether or not directed by their caregivers, an increasing number of patients and their families are accessing the Web to address their needs[65,66]. In North America, for example, up to 40 per cent of patients with cancer access the Web for more information on their illnesses and to find resources and support[67]. This number appears to be increasing[68,69]. The reasons why patients with life-threatening and terminal illnesses go on-line are diverse and include desire for more information, second opinions, search for cures and purchase of alternative and complementary therapies[70–72]. Internet-based online support groups have been used to provide support to patients with cancer and their families[73,74]. Patients with breast cancer found that the Internet improved their ability to communicate with their physicians and ask the right questions about their treatment options[71].

Guidelines to assist patients in identifying reputable web sites have been published. Although the usefulness of these has been challenged[75], some provide a useful framework with which to begin to evaluate the quality of a web site. These include DISCERN and QUICK (See Table 20.5.1 for their web addresses). It appears, however, that the quality of information available to patients on the Internet is improving, including palliative care related sites[76]. Although negative outcomes have been reported[77] the net outcome of patients' and families' internet activity seems positive[72]. Patients should be encouraged to discuss information that they obtain from the Internet with their clinicians[78] and professionals may direct their patients and families to web sites with accurate and detailed information that is specially tailored for the public[79,80].

Computers and multi-media in patient education

Computer-based patient education is gaining increasing recognition in health care[81–83]. Given that a significant part of a traditional patient-physician encounter is dedicated to providing patients with information, it is anticipated that computer-based patient education may enhance this process[84]. A number of technology-supported strategies have been proposed to enhance the exchange of information, including audiotapes of the patient-physician encounter, audio-visual aids such as audiotapes and videotapes, multimedia resources such as CD-ROM and DVD-ROM-based products and the Internet, telephone help-lines, and touch-screen computer programs[85].

Structured computer-delivered patient education, where clinicians print off information pamphlets that address specific patient needs at the point of care, improves patient satisfaction without adding to the consultation time[86]. In one review of the use of computer-based approaches to patient education, 13 studies were identified that described improvements in knowledge scores and clinical outcomes when computer-based patient education was compared with traditional education[87]. In addition, computer-based patient education programmes may enhance the communication that occurs between patient and health provider[71,88].

Audiocassette recordings of the consultations, given to patients, have been shown to increase their overall recall of the specific advice given during the consultation[89,90]. In one study, patients preferred audiotapes of the consultation over summary letters[90]. A systematic review of the effect of giving tape recordings or written summaries of consultations to patients with cancer showed that most people (between 83 and 96 per cent) who received summaries or audiotapes consistently found them helpful[91]. Although audiotapes improve recall and satisfaction appears to improve, they do not necessarily increase quality of life[92].

CD-ROM based products have been used in palliative care to educate patients and their families and assist in decision-making. An educational CD-ROM entitled *Completing a Life* covers a wide range of information for the user to choose from, spanning physical, emotional, family and spiritual issues[93]. The CD contains video narratives of individuals who tell their own stories of living with terminal illness. The goal is to assist patients and families in decision-making and in providing the user with a form of virtual support group.

Computer-based decision-aids for patients, usually in the form of online or CD-ROM-based resources, appear to result in higher knowledge scores, lower decision conflict scores and more active participation of patients[94,95]. The impact on satisfaction with the decision-making process has been mixed.

Computer touch-screen technology shows promise. Laptops with tablet-type screens or free-standing computer stations facilitate the collection and provision of information. Patients are able to pick the specific information they want and complete questionnaires with real time saving and collation of the data into databases. A role for this technology in clinical research is clear.

Preparatory education prior to undergoing radiotherapy or chemotherapy using video-based programmes appears beneficial. In one study, 30 patients received standard information and an information booklet while another 30 patients were shown a 12-min slide-tape programme describing practical information about treatment, correcting common misconceptions and encouraging questions[96]. Compared with the standard cohort, patients shown the slide-tape programme had better treatment-related knowledge at the beginning of treatment and showed less emotional distress at the end of treatment. Thomas and colleagues randomly assigned patients who were to receive radiotherapy or chemotherapy to receive standard written-information booklets with or without a video cassette[97]. Patients who viewed the videotape were substantially more satisfied than those who received only the written information and had lower degrees of anxiety during treatment than at the initial pre-treatment assessment. However, another study did not find differences in anxiety levels[98].

Patients prefer information that is as individualized as possible for their specific needs[86,99]. Compared with individual tapes of consultations, general information tapes may inhibit recall of information from the consultation[100]. As electronic medical records become more widespread, personalized computer-based information will be increasingly available.

Jefford and Tattersall have developed a checklist for producing patient information resources[101]. Patient involvement and the use of best-evidence is encouraged throughout the process. Deciding on the most appropriate medium for distribution is essential. Other items include using patient questions as the starting point, ensuring that common concerns and misconceptions are addressed, referring to relevant treatment or management options, including quantitative information, where possible, and questions to ask the doctor, stating references to sources of information and providing information on authorship, sponsorship and publication date.

Informatics and their influence on the patient-physician relationship

The wide availability of online health information is impacting on the practitioner-patient relationship[102]. Health professionals are no longer the 'keepers' of medical knowledge, but increasingly need to take the role of knowledge arbitrators and guides. Some are even beginning to use e-mail to communicate with patients and families[103]. Clearly, physicians and patients now have unique technological resources available and these can be harnessed to improve the patient–physician relationship. How they both utilize online medical information will influence the course of their relationship and possibly influence health outcomes. The decision-making process may improve if efforts are made to share the burden of responsibility for knowledge and further benefits are likely to arise when physicians assist patients in the information-gathering process[104].

Conclusions

Clearly, new information and communication technologies are complementing and enhancing health care across a number of domains, from service delivery to research and education. Many of these technologies are already being used in palliative care, while adoption of others should be considered. Although the hospice movement and palliative care promotes avoiding the inappropriate use of technology to prolong life where death is inevitable and imminent, newer technologies are now able to improve palliative care in a way that remains true to and consistent with its mission of improving the care and quality of life of patients with progressive incurable illnesses and their families. Palliative care administrators, clinicians, educators, and researchers should become acquainted with the myriad informatics-related technologies and methods in order to to adopt and adapt them in ways that improve patient care.

For a more comprehensive list, readers are referred to publications on the topic[106–110].

References

1. Wyatt, J.C., and Sullivan, F. (2005). What is health information? *BMJ*, **331**(7516), 566–8.
2. Coiera. E. (1998). Medical Informatics meets medical education. *Medical Journal of Australia*, **168**, 319–20.
3. Oh, H., Rizo, C., Enkin, M., and Jadad, A. (2005). What is eHealth (3): a systematic review of published definitions. *Journal of Medical Internet Research*, **7**(1), e1.

4. Holmberg, B. (1995). *Theory and practice of distance education*. Routledge Press, London.

5. William, J. Montelpare, W.J., and Williams, A. (2000). Web-based learning: Challenges in using the Internet in the undergraduate curriculum. *Education and Information Technologies*, **5**(2), 85–101.

6. Ross, N. (1999). AMEE Guide No. 14: Outcome-based education: Part 4-Outcome-based learning and the electronic curriculum at Birmingham Medical School. *Medical Teacher*, **21**(1), 26–31.

7. Dornan, T., Maredia, N., Hosie, L., Lee, C., and Stopford, A. (2003). Web-based presentation of an undergraduate clinical skills curriculum. *Medical Education*, **37**(6), 500–8.

8. Saysell, E., and Routley, C. (2003). Telemedicine in community-based palliative care: evaluation of a videolink teleconference project. *International Journal of Palliative Nursing*, **9**(11), 489–95.

9. Norum, J., and Jordhoy, M.S. (2006). A university oncology department and a remote palliative care unit linked together by email and videoconferencing. *Journal of Telemedicine & Telecare*, **12**(2), 92–6.

10. Kuebler, K.K., and Bruera, E. (2000). Interactive collaborative consultation model in end-of-life care. *Journal of Pain & Symptom Management*, **20**(3), 202–9.

11. De Conno, F., and Martini, C. (1997). Video communication and palliative care at home. *European Journal of Palliative Care*, **4**, 172–4.

12. Hebert, M.A., Jansen, J.J., Brant, R. *et al.* (2004). Successes and challenges in a field-based, multi-method study of home telehealth. *Journal of Telemedicine & Telecare*, **10**(Suppl. 1), 41–4.

13. Bensink, M., Armfield, N., Russell, T. *et al.* (2004). Paediatric palliative home care with Internet-based video-phones: lessons learnt. *Journal of Telemedicine and Telecare*, **10**(Suppl. 1), 47–9.

14. Miyazaki, M., Stuart, M., Liu, L. *et al.* (2003). Use of ISDN video-phones for clients receiving palliative and antenatal home care. *Journal of Telemedicine & Telecare*, **9**(2), 72–7.

15. Oyama, H., Wakao, F., and Okamura, H. (1997). Virtual reality support system in palliative medicine. *Studies in Health Technology & Informatics*, **39**, 60–3.

16. Lloyd-Williams, M. (2001). Out-of-hours palliative care advice line. *British Journal of General Practice*, **51**(469), 677.

17. Wilkes, L., Mohan, S., White, K., and Smith, H. (2004). Evaluation of an after hours telephone support service for rural palliative care patients and their families: a pilot study. *Australian Journal of Rural Health*, **12**(3), 95–8.

18. Garrison, D.R., Anderson, T., and Archer, W. (2000). Critical inquiry in a text-based environment: Computer conferencing in higher education. *The Internet and Higher Education*, **2**(2–3), 87–105.

19. Jonassen, D., Davidson, M., Collins, M. *et al.* (1995). Constructivism and computer-mediated communication in distance education. *The American Journal of Distance Education*, **9**(2), 7–26.

20. Pereira, J., Wedel, R., Murray, A. *et al.* (2005). Rural family care education: results of a hybrid distance course for rural family medicine residents. [Abstract]. *Journal of Palliative Care*, **21**(3), 225.

21. Norman, G.R. (1999). The adult learner: a mythical species. *Acad Med*, **74**, 886–9.

22. Clarke, D. (1999). Getting results with distance education. *The American Journal of Distance Education*, **12**(1), 38–51.

23. Kozma, R. (1994). Will media influence learning? Reframing the debate. *Educational Technology Research and Development*, **42**(2), 7–19.

24. Shearer, R. (2003). Instructional design in distance education: an overview. In *Handbook of distance education* (eds. M.G. Moore, and W.G. Anderson), pp. 275–86. Lawrence Erlbaum Associates Publishers, Mahwah.

25. Hulsmann, T. (1999). The costs of distance education. In *Higher education through open and distance learning* (ed. K. Harry), pp. 72–84. Routledge Press, New York.

26. Garrison, D.R., Anderson, T., and Archer, W. (2001). Critical thinking, cognitive presence and computer conferencing in distance education. *American Journal of Distance Education*, **15**(1), 7–23.

27. Salmon, G. (2000). *E-moderating the key to teaching and learning online*. Kogan Page, London.

28. Johnson, S.D., Aragon, S.R., Shaik, N., and Palma-Rivas, N. (2000). Comparative analysis of learner satisfaction and learning outcomes in online and face-to-face learning environments. *Journal of Interactive Learning Research*, **11**(1), 29–49.

29. Chumley-Jones, H.S., Dobbie, A., and Alford, C.L. (2002). Web-based learning: sound educational method or hype? A review of the evaluation literature. *Academic Medicine*, **77**(10), S86–S93.

30. Friedman, R.B. (1996). Top ten reasons the world wide web may fail to change medical education. *Academic Medicine*, **71**(9), 979–81.

31. Curran, V., Kirby, F., Parsons, E., and Lockyer, J. (2003). Discourse analysis of computer-mediated conferencing in World Wide Web-based continuing medical education. *Journal of Continuing Education in the Health Professions*, **23**, 229–38.

32. Chan, D.H., Leclair, K., and Kaczorowski, J. (1999). Problem-based small-group learning via the Internet among community family physicians: a randomised controlled trial. *MD Computing*, **16**(3), 54–8.

33. Sargeant, J.M., Purdy, R.A., Allen, M.J., and Shailesh, N. (2000). Evaluation of a CME problem-based learning Internet discussion. *Academic Medicine*, **76**, S50–S52.

34. Atack, L. (2003). Becoming a web-based learner: registered nurses' experiences. *Journal of Advanced Nursing*, **44**(3), 289–97.

35. Ruiz, J.G., Mintzer, M.J., and Leipzig, R. (2006). The impact of e-learning in medical education. *Academic Medicine*, **81**, 207–212.

36. Ellaway, R., Dewhurst, D., and Cumming, A. (2003). Managing and supporting medical education with a virtual learning environment: the Edinburgh Electronic Medical Curriculum. *Medical Teacher*, **25**(4), 372–80.

37. Pereira, J., and Murzyn, T. (2001). Integrating the 'new' with the 'traditional': an innovative education model. *Journal of Palliative Medicine*, **4**(1), 31–7.

38. Pereira Jose, L. (2007). The development and psychometric assessment of an instrument to assess palliative care competencies [microform]. Ottawa: Library and Archives Canada = Bibliothèque et Archives Canada. AMICUS No. 33360867.

39. Pereira, J. (2002). *Web-based learning: comparing two online palliative care courses*. Abstracts of the 2nd Congress of the EAPC Research Network, Lyon, France, May 23–25.

40. Kinghorn, S. (2005). Delivering multiprofessional web-based psychosocial education: the lessons learnt. *International Journal of Palliative Nursing*, **11**(8), 432–7.

41. Hinkka, H., Kosunen, E., Metsanoja, R. *et al.* (2002). General practitioners' attitudes and ethical decisions in end-of-life care after a year of interactive Internet-based training. *Journal of Cancer Education*, **17**(1), 12–8.

42. Silverdale, N., and Katz, J. (2005). The impact of a distance learning death and dying course: an analysis of student self-reported changes. *Nurse Education Today*, **25**(7), 509–18.

43. Kim, S., Farber, S., Kolko, B.E. *et al.* (2006). Faculty and student participation in online discussions of palliative care scenarios. *Family Medicine*, **38**(7), 494–9.

44. Palacios, M., Pereira, J., and Lyndon, J. (2005). Preparing palliative care educators for online facilitation: results of an international course. *Journal of Palliative Care*, **21**(3), 226 [abstract].

45. Wilkie, D.J., Kay, M., Judge, M., Wells, M.J., and Berkley, I.M. (2001). Excellence in teaching end-of-life care: a new multimedia toolkit for nurse educators. *Nursing and Health Care Perspectives*, **22**(5), 226–230.

46. Regnard, C. (2000). Using videoconferencing in palliative care. *Palliative Medicine*, **14**(6), 519–28.

47. van Boxell, P., Anderson, K., and Regnard, C. (2003). The effectiveness of palliative care education delivered by videoconferencing compared with face-to-face delivery. *Palliative Medicine*, **17**(4), 344–58.

48. Lynch, J., Weaver, L., Hall, P. *et al.* (2004). Using telehealth technology to support CME in end-of-life care for community physicians in Ontario. *Telemedicine Journal & E-Health*, **10**(1), 103–7.

49. Burt, C.W., and Hing, E. (2005). Use of computerized clinical support systems in medical settings: United States, 2001–2003. *Advanced Data*, **2**(353), 1–8.

50. Lau, F., Yang, J., Pereira, J., Daeninck, P., and Aherne, M. (2006). A survey of PDA use by palliative medicine practitioners. *Journal of Palliative Care*, **22**(4), 267–74.

51. Chung, K., Bell, R., and Lee, D. (2006). A point of care clinical documentation system for hospice care providers. *Journal of Medical Systems*, **30**(1), 33–7.

52. Lind, L., and Karlsson, D. (2004). A system for symptom assessment in advanced palliative home healthcare using digital pens. *Medical Informatics & the Internet in Medicine*, **29**(3–4), 199–210.

53. Purcell, G.P. (2005). What makes a good clinical decision support system. *BMJ*, **330**, 740–741.

54. Rubin, M.A., Bateman, K., Donnelly S. *et al.* (2006). Use of a personal digital assistant for managing antibiotic prescribing for outpatient respiratory tract infections in rural communities. *Journal of the American Medical Informatics Association*, **13**, 627–34.

55. Berner, E.S., Houston, T.K., Ray, M.N. *et al.* (2006). Improving ambulatory prescribing safety with a handheld decision support system: a randomized controlled trial. *Journal of the American Medical Informatics Association*, **13**(2), 171–9.

56. Hunt, D.L., Haynes, R.B., Hanna, S.E., and Smith, K. (1998). Effects of computer-based clinical decision support systems (CDSSs) on physician performance and patient outcomes. *JAMA*, **280**, 1339–46.

57. Bates, D.W., Leape, L.L., Cullen, D.J. *et al.* (1998). Effect of computerized physician order entry and a team intervention on prevention of serious medication errors. *JAMA*, **280**, 1311–6.

58. Kawamoto, K., Houlihan, C.A., Balas, E.A., and Lobach, D.F. (2005). Improving clinical practice using clinical decision support systems: a systematic review of trials to identify features critical to success. *BMJ*, **330**(7494), 765.

59. Wears, R.L., and Berg, M. (2005). Computer technology and clinical work: still waiting for Godot. *JAMA*, **293**, 1261–3.

60. Koppel, R., Metlay, J.P., Cohen, A. *et al.* (2005). Role of computerized physician order entry systems in facilitating medication errors. *JAMA*, **293**, 1197–203.

61. Kuziemsky, C.E., Lau, F., and Leung, R.C. (2005). A review on diffusion of personal digital assistants in healthcare. *Journal of Medical Systems*, **29**(4), 334–52.

62. Shaw, S., and May, V. (2004). An Australian agency revolutionizes home care with the palm pilot. *Caring*, **23**, 30–2.

63. Shaohui, M. (2005). Workflow analysis to identify opportunities for improving information management and nurses' work efficiency in palliative care. (Thesis). School of Information Technology and Computer Science. (available at www.library.uow.edu.au/adt-NWU/uploads/approved/adt-NWU20060522.115855/public/02Whole.pdf).

64. Shelby-James, T.M., Abernethy, A.P., McAlindon, A., and Currow, D. (2007). Handheld computers for data entry: High tech has its problems too. *Trials*, **8**, 5.

65. Eysenbach, G., Sa, E., and Diepgen, T.L. (1999). Shopping around the internet today and tomorrow: towards the millennium of cybermedicine. *British Medical Journal*, **319**, 1294.

66. Eng, T.R., Maxfield, A., Patrick, K., Deering, M.J., Ratzan, S.C., and Gustafson, D.H. (1998). Access to Health Information and Support. A Public Highway or a Private Road? *JAMA*, **280**, 1371–5.

67. Eysenbach, G. (2003). The impact of the Internet on Cancer outcomes. *CA Cancer J Clin*, **53**, 356–71.

68. Potts, H., and Wyatt, J.C. (2002). Online survey of doctors' experience of patients using the Internet. *Journal of Medical Internet Research*, **4**(1), e5.

69. Helft, P.R., Hlubocky, F., and Daugherty, C.K. (2003). American oncologists' views of internet use by cancer patients: a mail survey of American Society of Clinical Oncology members. *Journal of Clinical Oncology*, **21**, 942–7.

70. Jadad, A.R., Rizo, C.A., and Enkin, M.W. (2003). I am a good patient, believe it or not. *BMJ*, **326**, 1293–5.

71. Pereira, J., Koski, S., Hanson, J., and Bruera, E.D. (2000). Internet usage among women with breast cancer: an exploratory study. *Clinical Breast Cancer*, **1**(2), 148–53.

72. Pereira, J., Bruera, E., Macmillan, K., and Kavanagh, S. (2000). Patients with advanced cancer and their families on the Internet: motivation and impact. *Journal of Palliative Care*, **16**(4), 13–9.

73. Klemm, P., Reppert, K., and Visich, L. (1998). A nontraditional cancer support group. The Internet. *Computers in Nursing*, **16**, 31–6.

74. Winzelberg, A.J., Classen, C., Aplers, G.W. *et al.* (2003). Evaluation of an Internet support group for women with primary breast cancer. *Cancer*, **97**, 1164–73.

75. Jadad, A.R., and Gagliardi, A. (1998). Rating health information on the Internet: navigating to knowledge or to Babel? *JAMA*, **279**, 611–14.

76. Eysenbach, G., Powell, J., Kuss, O., and Sa, E. (2002). Empirical studies assessing the quality of health information for consumers on the World Wide Web. *JAMA*, **287**, 2691–700.

77. Stephenson, J. (1998). Patient pretenders weave tangled 'Web' of deceit. *JAMA*, **280**, 1297.

78. Pereira, J., and Jadad, A. (2005). 'I found this on the Internet': palliative care in the information age. In *The Oxford Case-Based Book on Palliative Care* (eds. N. Macdonald, N. Hagen, and D. Onsechuk), 2nd edition. Oxford Universtiy Press, New York.

79. Wilkes, L., White, K., and O'Riordan, L. (2000). Empowerment through information: supporting rural families of oncology patients in palliative care. *Australian Journal of Rural Health*, **8**, 41–6.

80. Back, I. (2001). Syringe driver drug compatibility database and patient information leaflets on the Internet. *Palliative Medicine*, **15**(1), 77.

81. Lovell, N.H., and Celler, B.G. (1999). Information technology in primary health care. *International Journal of Medical informatics*, **55**, 9–22.

82. Lewis, D. (1999). Computer-based approaches to patient education: A review of the literature. *JAMIA*, **6**, 272–82.

83. McPherson, C.J., Higginson, I.J., and Hearn, J. (2001). Effective methods of giving information in cancer: a systematic literature review of randomized controlled trials. *Journal of Public Health Medicine*, **23**, 227–34.

84. Calkins, D.R., Davis, R.B., Reiley, P. *et al.* (1997). Patient-physician communication at hospital discharge and patients' understanding of the postdischarge treatment plan. *Archives of Internal Medicine*, **157**, 1026–30.

85. Jefford, M., and Tattersall, M.N.H. (2002). Informing and involving patients in their own care. *Lancet Oncology*, **3**, 629–37.

86. Panasetis, P., Harris, M., Lovell, N.H., Celler, B.G., Sloggett, S., Dumlao, V.J., and Knowlden, S. (1998). EDUCATE Computer access to education: the computerised patient education leaflets project. *Informatics in Health Care Australia*, **7**(4), 154–8.

87. Lewis, D. (1999). Computer-based approaches to patient education: A review of the literature. *JAMIA*, **6**, 272–82.

88. Juge, C.F., and Assal, J.P. (1992). Designing computer-assisted instruction programmes for diabetic patients: how can we make them really useful? *Proceedings / the … Annual Symposium on Computer Application [sic] in Medical Care*, 215–9.

89. Bruera, E., Pituskin, E., Calder, K., Neumann, C.M., and Hanson, J. (1999). The addition of an audiocassette recording of a consultation to written recommendations for patients with advanced cancer: A randomized, controlled trial. *Cancer*, **86**, 2420–5.

90. Tattersall, M.H., Butow, P.N., Griffin, A.M., and Dunn, S.M. (1994). The take-home message: patients prefer consultation audiotapes to summary letters. *Journal of Clinical Oncology*, **12**, 1305–11.

91. Scott, J.T., Entwistle, V.A., Sowden, A.J., and Watt, I. (2001). Giving tape recordings or written summaries of consultations to people with cancer: a systematic review. *Health Expect*, **4**, 162–69.

92. Ong, L.M., Visser, M.R., Lammes, F.B. *et al.* (2000). Effect of providing cancer patients with the audiotaped initial consultation on satisfaction, recall, and quality of life: a randomized, double-blind study. *Journal of Clinical Oncology*, **18**, 3052–60.

93. Ogle, K., Greene, D.D., Winn, B. *et al.* (2003). Completing a Life: Development of an interactive multimedia CD-ROM for patient and family education in end-of-life care. *Journal of Palliative Medicine*, **6**(5), 841–50.

94. Molenaar, S., Sprangers, M.A., Postma-Schuit, F.C. *et al.* (2000). Feasibility and effects of decision aids. *Medical Decision Making*, **20**, 112–27.

95. Molenaar, S., Sprangers, M.A., Rutgers, E.J. *et al.* (2001). Decision support for patients with early stage breast cancer: effects of an interactive breast cancer CDROM on treatment decision, satisfaction, and quality of life. *Journal of Clinical Oncology*, **19**, 1676–87.

96. Rainey, L.C. (1985). Effects of preparatory patient education for radiation oncology patients. *Cancer*, **56**, 1056–61.

97. Thomas, R., Daly, M., Perryman, B., and Stockton, D. (2000). Forewarned is forearmed—benefits of preparatory information on video cassette for patients receiving chemotherapy or radiotherapy: a randomised controlled trial. *European Journal of Cancer*, **36**, 1536–43.

98. Harrison, R., Dey, P., Slevin, N.J. *et al.* (2001). Randomized controlled trial to assess the effectiveness of a videotape about radiotherapy. *British Journal of Cancer*, **84**, 8–10.

99. Jones, R., Pearson, J., McGregor, S. *et al.* (1999). Randomised trial of personalised computer based information for cancer patients. *BMJ*, **319**, 1241–47.

100. Dunn, S.M., Butow, P.N., Tattersall, M.H. *et al.* (1993). General information tapes inhibit recall of the cancer consultation. *Journal of Clinical Oncology*, **11**, 2279–85.

101. Jefford, M., and Tattersall, M.N.H. (2002). Informing and involving patients in their own care. *Lancet Oncology*, **3**, 629–37.

102. Murray, E., Lo, B., Pollack, L. *et al.* (2003). The impact of health information on the physician-patient relationship. Patient Perceptions. *Archives of Internal Medicine*, **163**, 1727–34.

103. Baker, L., Wagner, T.H., Singer, S., and Bundorf, M.K. (2003). Use of the Internet and e-mail for health care information: results from a national survey. *JAMA*, **289**, 2400–6.

104. Gerber, B.S., and Eiser, A.R. (2001). The patient–physician relationship in the internet age: future prospects and the research agenda. *Journal of Medical Internet Research*, **3**(2), e15.

105. Abernethy, A.P., and Arnold, R.M. (2006). PC-FACS: a real-time evidence resource for busy palliative care clinicians. *Journal of Palliative Medicine*, **9**(1), 24–8.

106. Deitrick, G.E., Timlin, A., Gardner, B., and Polomano, R.C. (2006). Palliative care and end-of-life care World Wide Web resources for geriatrics. *Journal of Pain & Palliative Care Pharmacotherapy*, **20**(3), 47–56.

107. Eisenberg, E. (2006). European pain and palliative care perspectives: new online resource for physicians and other health professionals. *Journal of Pain & Palliative Care Pharmacotherapy*, **20**(3), 29–30.

108. Williams, M. (2005). Palliative care web sites. *Home Healthcare Nurse*, **23**(11), 736–7.

109. Chambers, L., McDowall, J., and Gelb, B. (2005). A global children's hospice and palliative care website. *International Journal of Palliative Nursing*, **11**(6), 292–3.

110. Smith-Stoner, M., and Oliver, M. (2003). Ten palliative home care resources. *Home Healthcare Nurse*, **21**(11), 731–3.

Index